PRINCIPLES OF NEURAL SCIENCE

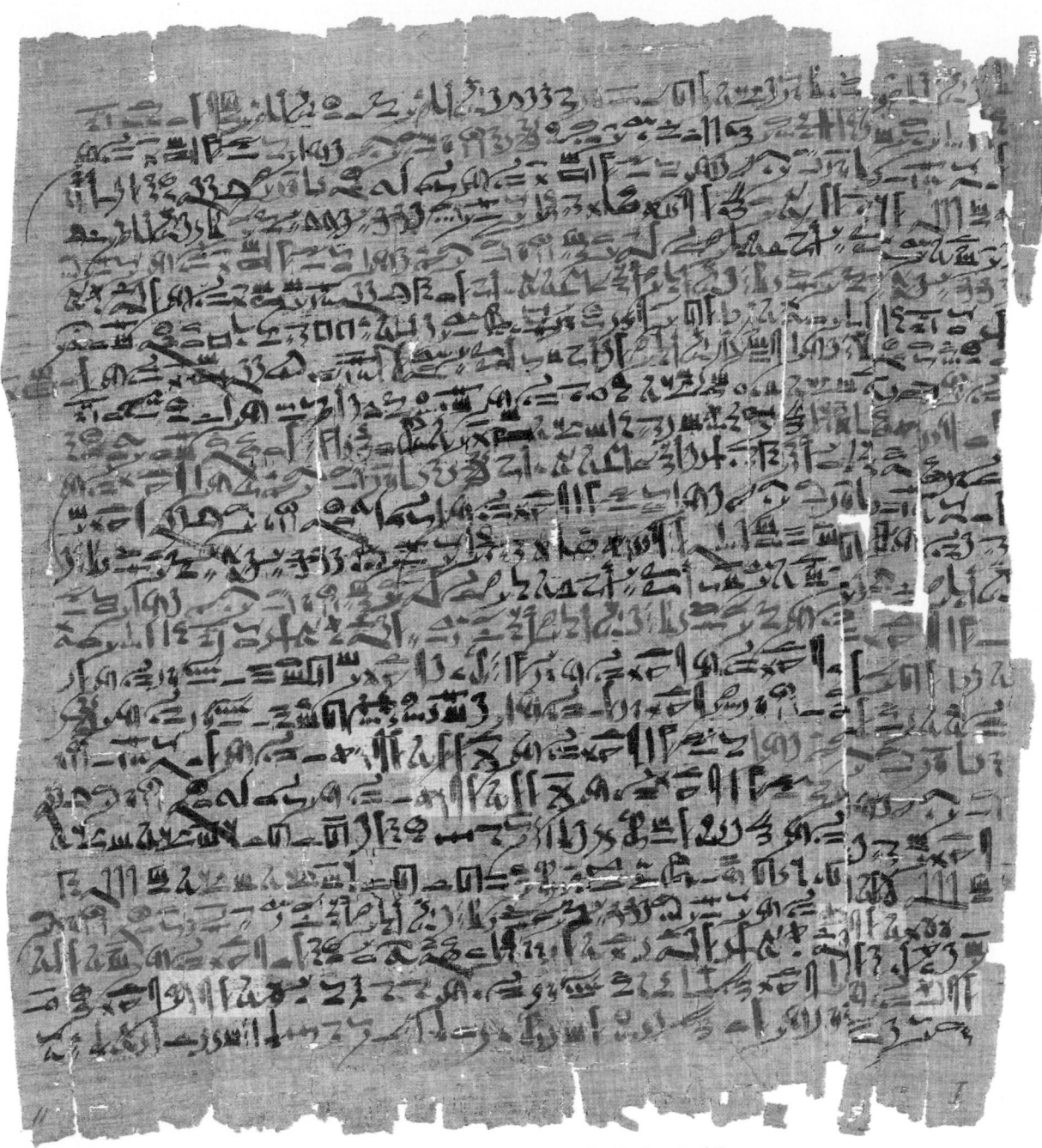

Columns II (left) and IV (right) of the Edwin Smith Surgical Papyrus

This papyrus, transcribed in the Seventeenth Century B.C., is a medical treatise that contains the earliest reference to the brain anywhere in human records. According to James Breasted, who translated and published the document in 1930, the word brain 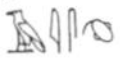 occurs only 8 times in ancient Egyptian, 6 of them on these pages. The papyrus describes here the symptoms, diagnosis, and prognosis of two patients with compound fractures of the skull, and compares the surface of the brain to "those ripples that happen in copper through smelting, with a thing in it that throbs and flutters under your fingers like the weak spot of the crown of a boy before it becomes whole for him." The red ink highlights the patients' ailments and their prognoses. (Reproduced, with permission, from the New York Academy of Medicine Library.)

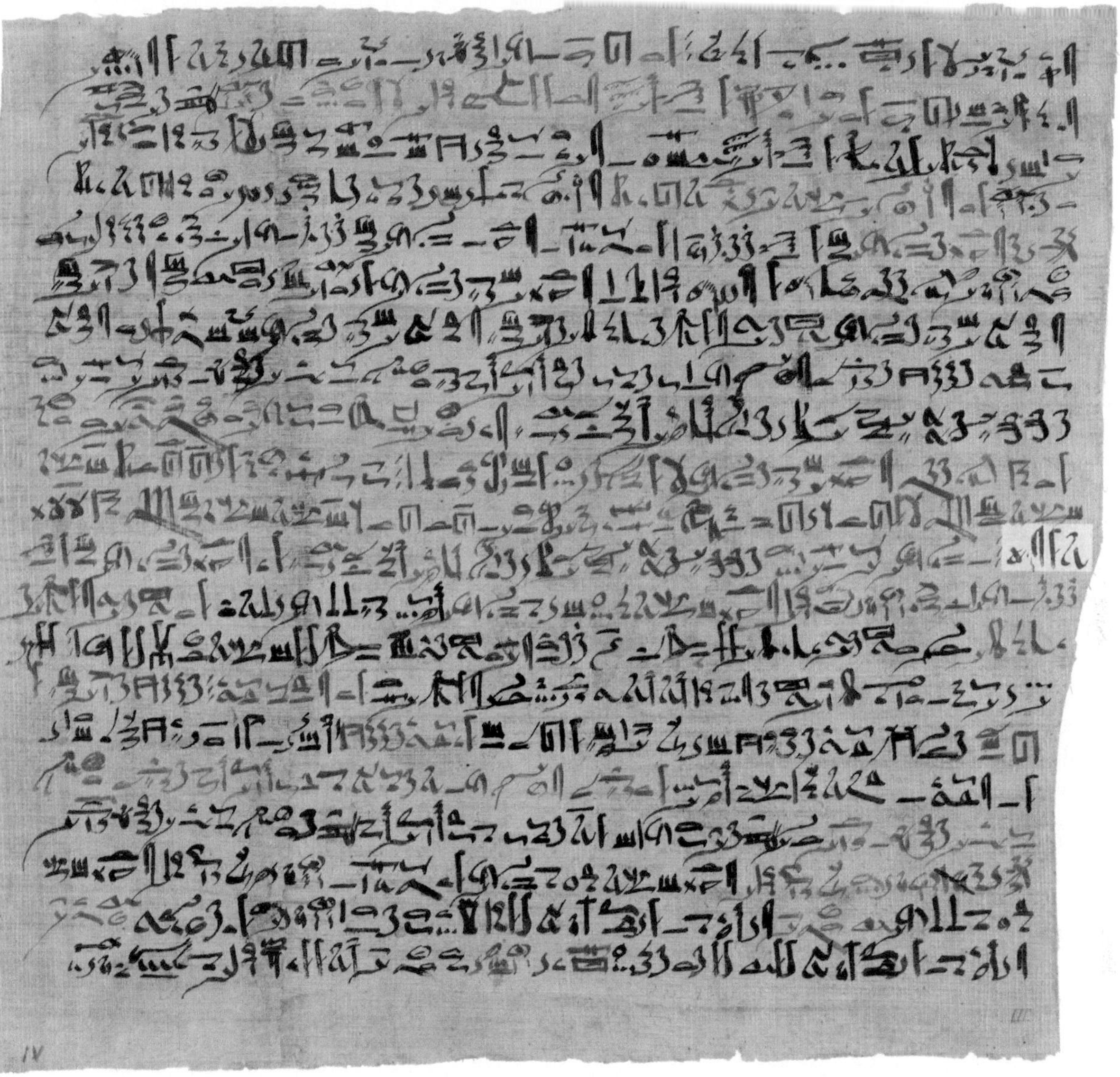

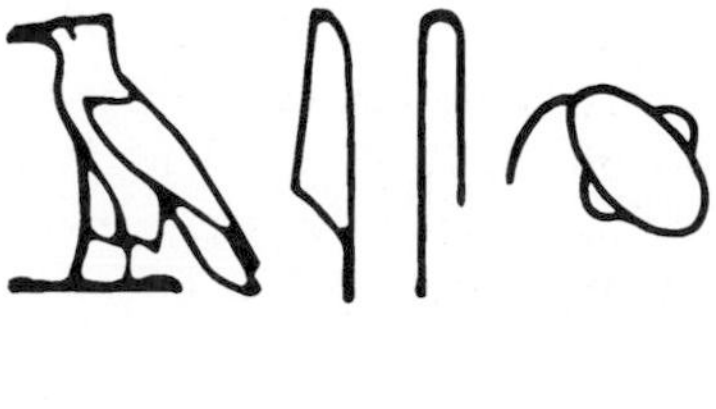

Men ought to know that from the brain, and from the brain only, arise our pleasures, joys, laughter and jests, as well as our sorrows, pains, griefs and tears. Through it, in particular, we think, see, hear, and distinguish the ugly from the beautiful, the bad from the good, the pleasant from the unpleasant. . . . It is the same thing which makes us mad or delirious, inspires us with dread and fear, whether by night or by day, brings sleeplessness, inopportune mistakes, aimless anxieties, absent-mindedness, and acts that are contrary to habit. These things that we suffer all come from the brain, when it is not healthy, but becomes abnormally hot, cold, moist, or dry, or suffers any other unnatural affection to which it was not accustomed. Madness comes from its moistness. When the brain is abnormally moist, of necessity it moves, and when it moves neither sight nor hearing are still, but we see or hear now one thing and now another, and the tongue speaks in accordance with the things seen and heard on any occasion. But when the brain is still, a man can think properly.

attributed to Hippocrates
Fifth Century, B.C.

PRINCIPLES OF NEURAL SCIENCE

Fifth Edition

Edited by

ERIC R. KANDEL

JAMES H. SCHWARTZ

THOMAS M. JESSELL

STEVEN A. SIEGELBAUM

A. J. HUDSPETH

Art Editor
Sarah Mack

McGraw Hill Medical

New York Chicago San Francisco Lisbon London Madrid Mexico City
Milan New Delhi San Juan Seoul Singapore Sydney Toronto

The McGraw-Hill Companies

Principles of Neural Science, Fifth Edition

1 2 3 4 5 6 7 8 9 0 DOW/DOW 17 16 15 14 13 12

ISBN 978-0-07-139011-8
MHID 0-07-139011-1

This book was set in Palatino by Cenveo Publisher Services.
The editors were Anne Sydor and Harriet Lebowitz.
The production supervisor was John Williams.
The art manager was Armen Ovsepyan.
The illustrators were Precision Graphics.
The editorial manager was Clayton Eccard.
The art consultant was Eve Siegel.
Project management was provided by Rajni Pisharody, Cenveo Publisher Services.
RR Donnelley was printer and binder.

This book is printed on acid-free paper.

Library of Congress Cataloging-in-Publication Data

Principles of neural science / edited by Eric R. Kandel ... [et al.] ; art editor, Sarah Mack. — 5th ed.
p. 1760; cm.
Includes bibliographical references and index.
ISBN 978-0-07-139011-8 (hard cover : alk. paper)
I. Kandel, Eric R.
[DNLM: 1. Central Nervous System—physiology. 2. Mental Processes—physiology.
3. Nervous System Diseases. 4. Neuropsychology. WL 300]
LC classification not assigned
612.8—dc23

2012023071

Cover image: This image is a lithograph by F. Schima from a drawing by Sigmund Freud of the spinal ganglion of the lamprey *Petromyzon*. Before he discovered the unconscious, Freud had a promising career as a neural scientist. The cover thus recognizes that, a century after Freud's discovery, progress in the study of cognition has reemphasized the importance of unconscious mental processes for perception and action. (Reproduced, with permission, from Sigmund Freud, "Über Spinalganglien und Rückenmark der Petromyzon," *Sitzungsberichte der Mathematisch-Naturwissenschaftlichen Classe der Kaiserlichen Akademie der Wissenschaften*, LXXVIII. Band I. Abtheilung, 1878, copyright New York Academy of Medicine.)

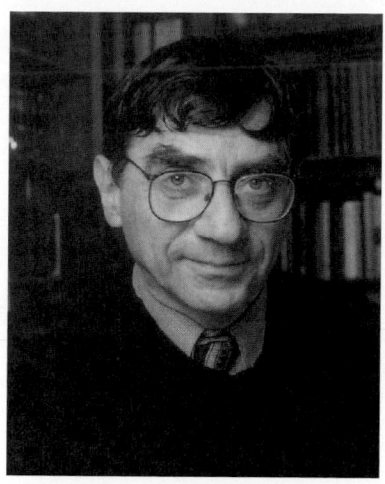

James H. Schwartz
1933–2006

WE WISH TO DEDICATE THIS FIFTH EDITION of *Principles of Neural Science* to our friend and colleague, James H. Schwartz, one of the founding editors who died on March 13, 2006. Jimmy was an outstanding neuroscientist and scholar. His talent for science and his extraordinary erudition were evident from his days as a medical student at New York University. While at NYU he worked with Werner Maas in the microbiology department and carried out an important set of studies on feedback inhibition in bacterial metabolism. This work was so impressive that upon completing medical school, Jimmy was nominated for the highly selective graduate program in biology that had just been established at The Rockefeller University by Detlev Bronk. By the time Jimmy obtained his Ph.D. in Fritz Lippman's laboratory and graduated from Rockefeller in 1964, he had established himself as an outstanding biochemist. He was therefore eagerly recruited back to NYU in 1965 as an Assistant Professor in the Department of Microbiology.

There Jimmy turned to studying the nerve cells of the snail *Aplysia*, which were so large and uniquely identifiable that they seemed likely candidates for a study of neuronal biochemical identity. The immediate success of his initial studies encouraged him to devote himself completely to the nervous system. He rapidly became one of the leading biochemists on the nervous system and one of the leading thinkers regarding the relationship of brain to behavior.

The idea of going from molecules to behavior was the organizing theme of the first edition of *Principles of Neural Science,* which Jimmy co-edited. He simply loved working on *Principles*. A superb writer, he demanded precision in language both in himself and in others. This made him an exceptional editor. He read and avidly edited every chapter. In addition, Jimmy contributed his sense of historical scholarship. It was his idea to open *Principles* with the images of hieroglyphics from the Egyptian papyrus, the earliest reference to the brain in human record, which we include as the opening images in this edition as well. But perhaps most importantly, Jimmy championed the idea that this book should delineate fundamental principles rather than serve as an encyclopedia of facts. Thus, Jimmy's vision and editorial skill greatly enriched each of the five editions. In his absence we have striven to make the final product an edition that will continue to meet the high standards of readability and scholarship he set for all of us.

Contents in Brief

Appendices

Contents

Part V
Perception

Preface

The ultimate goal of neural science is to understand how the flow of electrical signals through neural circuits gives rise to mind—to how we perceive, act, think, learn, and remember. Although we are still many decades away from achieving this level of understanding, neuroscientists have made significant progress in gaining insight into the neural mechanisms underlying behavior, the observable output of the nervous systems of humans and other organisms. We are also beginning to understand the disorders of behavior associated with neurological and psychiatric disease. As in the earlier editions of this book, we emphasize in this edition that behavior can be examined in terms of the electrical activity of both individual neurons and systems of nerve cells by seeking answers to five basic questions. How does the brain develop? How do nerve cells in the brain communicate with one another? How do different patterns of interconnections give rise to different perceptions and motor acts? How is the communication between neurons modified by experience? How is that communication altered by disease?

When we published the first edition of this book in 1981, these questions could be addressed only in terms of cellular biology. By the fourth edition in 2000 the same problems were being studied at the molecular level. In the decade intervening between the fourth and the present edition, molecular biology has continued to enlighten the analysis of neurobiological problems. Molecular biology has made it possible to probe the pathogenesis of many neurological diseases, including several devastating genetic disorders: muscular dystrophy, retinoblastoma, neurofibromatosis, Huntington disease, and certain forms of Alzheimer disease. Molecular biology also has greatly expanded our understanding of how the brain develops. Genetically modified worms, flies, and mice have allowed us to relate single genes, including the mutant genes underlying neurological disease, to signaling in nerve cells and to an organism's behavior. At the same time new molecular and optical tools have made it possible to image the activity of individual neurons in the intact brain and to manipulate the electrical activity of neurons and neural circuits to alter behavior. Such experiments have made it possible to examine the molecular dynamics of nerve cells in the circuits responsible for cognitive processes.

Every disease that affects the nervous system has some inherited component. Now that the 20,000 genes of the human genome have been sequenced, it is possible to identify which genes make us susceptible to certain disorders and thus to predict an individual's predisposition to a particular illness. This knowledge of the human genome is beginning to transform the practice of medicine. An individual genome scan can quantify the personal risk for neurological and psychiatric disorders at levels of increasing detail and complexity. We therefore again stress vigorously our view—advocated since the first edition—that the future of clinical neurology and psychiatry depends on the progress of neural science.

Despite the power of molecular biology to elucidate molecular mechanisms of neural function and disease, any detailed understanding of how neurons act to generate complex behaviors requires an analysis of the circuitry in which the neurons participate. Thus, key questions in neuroscience include: How are neuronal assemblies formed during development? What are the computations performed by those neural circuits and how does this activity generate behavior? How are circuits modified during learning and memory? What are the changes in neural circuits that give rise to neurological and psychiatric disease? Although the cellular and molecular biological approaches emphasized in the previous editions will certainly continue to yield important information, knowledge of the function of assemblies of neurons in defined circuits must be attained to arrive at a comprehensive cognitive neuroscience.

To study how we perceive, act, think, learn, and remember, we must develop new approaches and conceptual schemes for understanding the behavior of systems that range from single nerve cells to the substrate of cognition. As a result, in this edition we discuss more fully how the cognitive and behavioral functions of the sensory and motor systems expand our treatment of cognitive processes, and incorporate into our discussion the increasing power and importance of computational neural science. Our ability to record the electrical activity and visualize functional changes in the brain during normal and abnormal mental activity permits even complex cognitive processes to be studied directly. No longer are we constrained simply to infer mental functions from observable behavior. Indeed, a new appreciation of Freud's original insight about the importance of unconscious processes—one of the major new themes to emerge in cognitive neural science—re-emphasizes the great limitation of restricting our analysis of mind to observable behaviors. As a result of its progress in describing unconscious mental processes, neural science may soon develop the tools needed to probe the deepest of biological mysteries—the biological basis of consciousness and free will.

The intuitive insights that guided thinking about the mind at the time of our first edition in 1981 are proving inadequate in the 21st century. To give but one example, we intuitively sense that we perceive an object before interacting with it and we therefore fully expect that the brain acts in this sequential way. But recent studies indicate that at the highest levels the motor and sensory systems act in parallel, not in series, and that the motor system has considerable cognitive capability.

As a result of this progress, it has become easier to write a coherent introduction to the nervous system for students of behavior, biology, and medicine. Indeed, we think such a coherent summary is even more necessary now than it was with the first edition. Today neurobiology is central to the biological sciences—and indeed to science as a whole. Students of biology increasingly want to become familiar with neural science, and most students of psychology consider themselves to be studying the biological basis of behavior. At the same time progress in neural science is providing clearer guidance to clinicians, particularly in the treatment of psychiatric disorders. In fact, perhaps the most significant change in the clinical landscape since the first edition is the realization that psychiatry can be a clinical neural science, that the progress of psychotherapy can be assessed quantitively using brain imaging. We therefore believe it is particularly important to clarify the major principles and mechanisms governing the functions of the nervous system in health and disease without becoming lost in details.

This book provides the detail necessary to meet the interests and requirements of students in particular fields but is organized in such a way that excursions into special topics are not necessary for grasping the major principles of neural science. Toward that end we have continued to refine the illustrations in the book to allow students to understand the fundamental concepts of neural science.

Throughout this book we document the central principle that all behavior is an expression of neural activity and illustrate the insights into behavior that neural science provides. With this fifth edition we again hope to encourage the next generation of undergraduate, graduate, and medical students to approach the study of behavior in a way that unites its biological and social dimensions. From ancient times, understanding human behavior has been central to civilized cultures. Engraved at the entrance to the Temple of Apollo at Delphi was the famous maxim "Know thyself." For us, the study of mind and consciousness defines the frontier of biology.

Eric R. Kandel
Thomas M. Jessell
Steven A. Siegelbaum
A. J. Hudspeth

Acknowledgments

We were fortunate to have had the creative editorial assistance of Howard Beckman once again, who worked on the ongoing revisions of the fifth edition of *Principles of Neural Science* with the same characteristic demand for clarity of style and logic of argument that he has brought to previous editions. Without his assistance this edition would be a pale reflection of its previous editions.

Working on the other side of Manhattan at The Rockefeller University, away from the other editors at Columbia, Jim Hudspeth was responsible for the sections on Perception and Movement. In this lonely task Amy Miller, who cheerfully and accurately corrected the preliminary drafts of the relevant chapters, assisted him.

We owe a special debt to Sarah Mack who once again reinvented the entire art program. With her remarkable insight into science and detail, she produced remarkably clear, didactic, and artistically pleasing diagrams and images. We would like to thank our colleague Jane Dodd as well as Charles Lam, Becky Oles, and Terri Hamer for their help with the art program, and particularly Ann Canapary for her artistic contribution to the illustrations. We appreciate the generous help that Neil McMillan, Jackie Stewart, and Mariah Widman provided with the figures.

A great debt is also owed to Clayton Eccard who managed the editorial project with intelligence and diligence, allowing us to bring the book to fruition.

We thank Millie Pellan, Kathy MacArthur, and especially Maria Palileo at Columbia University, who typed the many versions of the manuscript through the various editorial stages.

We are indebted to our colleagues at McGraw-Hill, Harriet Lebowitz, Eve Siegel, and Ann Sydor, for their invaluable help in the production of this edition and grateful for the assistance of Rajni Pisharody in the composition of the book.

Many other colleagues have helped the editors by critically reading many chapters of the book. We are especially indebted to John Krakauer and John Koester for their efforts, which proved to be invaluable. Most importantly we owe the greatest debt to the contributing authors of this edition.

We finally thank our spouses and families for their support and forbearance during the editorial process.

Contributors

Laurence F. Abbott, PhD
William Bloor Professor of Theoretical Neuroscience
Co-Director, Center for Theoretical Neuroscience
Department of Neuroscience, and Department of Physiology and Cellular Biophysics
Columbia University College of Physicians and Surgeons

Thomas D. Albright, PhD
Conrad T. Prebys Professor and Chair,
Systems Neurobiology Laboratories
Salk Institute for Biological Studies, La Jolla, CA

David G. Amaral, PhD
Professor and Research Director,
The M.I.N.D. Institute
University of California, Davis

Gary Aston-Jones, PhD
William E. Murray SmartState Endowed Chair in Neuroscience
Director, Center for Cognitive Neuroscience
Director, Neuroscience Institute
Professor, Department of Neurosciences
Medical University of South Carolina

Cornelia I. Bargmann, PhD
Professor and Head of Laboratory
Investigator, Howard Hughes Medical Institute
The Rockefeller University

Ben A. Barres, MD, PhD
Professor and Chair, Department of Neurobiology
Stanford University School of Medicine

Allan I. Basbaum, PhD
Professor and Chair, Department of Anatomy
University of California, San Francisco

Robert H. Brown, Jr., MD
Professor and Chair, Department of Neurology
University of Massachusetts Medical School

John C. M. Brust, MD
Professor of Clinical Neurology,
Department of Neurology
Columbia University College of Physicians and Surgeons
Neurological Institute of New York at Columbia University Medical Center

Linda B. Buck, PhD
Investigator, Howard Hughes Medical Institute
Member, Division of Basic Sciences
Fred Hutchinson Cancer Research Center
Affiliate Professor of Physiology and Biophysics
University of Washington

Stephen C. Cannon, MD, PhD
Professor, Neurology and Neurotherapeutics
Associate Dean for Undergraduate Medical Education, Basic Sciences
University of Texas Southwestern Medical Center

David E. Clapham, MD, PhD
Investigator, Howard Hughes Medical Institute
Aldo R. Castañeda Professor of Cardiovascular Research
Department of Cardiology, Boston Children's Hospital
Professor of Neurobiology, Harvard Medical School

Jonathan D. Cohen, MD, PhD
Eugene Higgins Professor of Psychology
Co-Director, Princeton Neuroscience Institute
Princeton University
Professor of Psychiatry
University of Pittsburgh

Carol L. Colby, PhD
Professor,
Department of Neuroscience
University of Pittsburgh

Antonio R. Damasio, MD, PhD
University Professor
David Dornsife Professor of Neuroscience
Director, Brain and Creativity Institute
University of Southern California

Mahlon R. DeLong, MD
Professor, Department of Neurology
Emory University School of Medicine

Allison J. Doupe, MD, PhD
Professor, Departments of Physiology and Psychiatry
Center for Integrative Neuroscience
University of California, San Francisco

Roger M. Enoka, PhD
Professor, Department of Integrative Physiology
University of Colorado, Boulder

Christopher D. Frith, PhD, FMedSci, FRS, FBA
Emeritus Professor of Neuropsychology,
Wellcome Trust Centre for Neuroimaging
University College London
Visiting Professor, Interacting Minds Centre
Aarhus University, Denmark
Fellow, All Souls College, Oxford, UK

Uta Frith, PhD, FMedSci, FBA, FRS
Emeritus Professor of Cognitive Development,
Institute of Cognitive Neuroscience, University College London
Aarhus University Research Foundation Professor
CFIN, University of Aarhus, Denmark

Stefano Fusi, PhD
Associate Professor,
Center for Theoretical Neuroscience, Department of Neuroscience
Columbia University College of Physicians & Surgeons

Esther P. Gardner, PhD
Professor of Physiology and Neuroscience,
Department of Physiology and Neuroscience
New York University School of Medicine

Claude P. J. Ghez, MD
Professor of Neuroscience, Neurology, Physiology and Cellular Biophysics
Columbia University College of Physicians and Surgeons
Research Scientist, New York State Psychiatric Institute

Charles D. Gilbert, MD, PhD
Arthur and Janet Ross Professor
The Rockefeller University

T. Conrad Gilliam, PhD
Dean for Research and Graduate Education,
Biological Sciences Division
Marjorie I. and Bernard A. Mitchell Professor,
Department of Human Genetics
University of Chicago

Michael E. Goldberg, MD
David Mahoney Professor of Brain and Behavior in the Department of Neuroscience,
Departments of Neurology, Psychiatry, and Ophthalmology
Columbia University College of Physicians and Surgeons
Chief, Division of Neurobiology and Behavior
The New York State Psychiatric Institute

James E. Goldman, MD, PhD
Professor, Department of Pathology and Cell Biology
Columbia University College of Physicians and Surgeons

Gary W. Goldstein, MD
President and CEO, Kennedy Krieger Institute
Professor of Neurology and Pediatrics,
Professor of Environmental Health Sciences,
Johns Hopkins University School of Medicine

James E. Gordon, EdD
Professor and Associate Dean,
Division of Biokinesiology and Physical Therapy
University of Southern California

Francesca G. Happé, PhD
Professor of Cognitive Neuroscience,
MRC Social, Genetic and Developmental Psychiatry Centre
Institute of Psychiatry, King's College London

David J. Heeger, PhD
Professor of Psychology and Neural Science,
Department of Psychology and Center for Neural Science
New York University

Fay B. Horak, PhD
Professor of Neurology,
Neurological Sciences Institute
Oregon Health Sciences University

John Paul Horn, PhD
Professor, Department of Neurobiology and Center for Neuroscience
Associate Dean of Graduate Studies
University of Pittsburgh

A. J. Hudspeth, MD, PhD
Investigator, Howard Hughes Medical Institute
F. M. Kirby Professor and Head of Laboratory
The Rockefeller University

Steven E. Hyman, MD
Harvard University Distinguished Service Professor
Director, Stanley Center for Psychiatric Research
Broad Institute of Massachusetts Institute of Technology and Harvard University

Jonathan A. Javitch, MD, PhD
Lieber Professor of Experimental Therapeutics in Psychiatry, and Professor of Pharmacology
Columbia University College of Physicians and Surgeons
Chief, Division of Molecular Therapeutics
The New York State Psychiatric Institute

Thomas M. Jessell, PhD
Claire Tow Professor,
Department of Neuroscience
Departments of Biochemistry & Molecular Biophysics
Co-Director, Kavli Institute for Brain Science
Investigator, Howard Hughes Medical Institute
Columbia University

Kenneth O. Johnson, PhD*
Professor, Department of Neuroscience and Biomedical Engineering
Director, Zanvyl Krieger Mind/Brain Institute
Johns Hopkins University

John F. Kalaska, PhD
Professeur titulaire,
Département de physiologie
Université de Montréal

Eric R. Kandel, MD
University Professor, Department of Neuroscience
Professor and Director, Kavli Institute for Brain Science
Senior Investigator, Howard Hughes Medical Institute
Columbia University

John Koester, PhD
Professor Emeritus of Clinical Neuroscience
College of Physicians and Surgeons
Columbia University

Arnold R. Kriegstein, MD, PhD
John G. Bowes Distinguished Professor in Stem Cell and Tissue Biology
Director, The Eli and Edythe Broad Center of Regeneration Medicine and Stem Cell Research
Professor, Department of Neurology
University of California, San Francisco

*Deceased

Patricia K. Kuhl, PhD
Bezos Family Foundation Endowed Chair in Early Childhood Learning
Co-Director, Institute for Learning and Brain Sciences
Professor, Department of Speech & Hearing Sciences
University of Washington

John L. Laterra, MD, PhD
Professor of Neurology, Oncology, and Neuroscience
The Kennedy Krieger Institute
Johns Hopkins School of Medicine

Joseph E. LeDoux, PhD
University Professor,
Henry and Lucy Moses Professor of Science,
Professor of Neuroscience and Psychology,
Center for Neural Science, New York University
Director, Emotional Brain Institute
New York University, Nathan Kline Institute

Stephen G. Lisberger, PhD
George Barth Geller Professor and Chair,
Department of Neurobiology
Investigator, Howard Hughes Medical Institute
Duke University

Andrew G. S. Lumsden, PhD, FRS, FMedSci
Director, MRC Centre for Developmental Neurobiology
King's College London

Jane M. Macpherson, PhD
Professor Emeritus
Neurological Sciences Institute
Oregon Health & Science University

David A. McCormick, PhD
Professor, Department of Neurobiology
Yale University School of Medicine

Markus Meister, PhD
Professor of Biology,
Division of Biology
California Institute of Technology

Kenneth D. Miller, PhD
Professor, Neuroscience, Physiology & Cellular Biophysics
Co-Director, Center for Theoretical Neuroscience,
Department of Neuroscience
Columbia University College of Physicians and Surgeons

Donata Oertel, PhD
Professor of Neurophysiology,
Department of Neuroscience
University of Wisconsin

Carl R. Olson, PhD
Professor, Center for the Neural Basis of Cognition
Mellon Institute, Carnegie Mellon University

Keir G. Pearson, PhD
Professor, Department of Physiology
University of Alberta

George B. Richerson, MD, PhD
Professor and Head, Department of Neurology
The Roy J. Carver Chair in Neuroscience
Professor, Department of Molecular Physiology & Biophysics
University of Iowa, Carver College of Medicine
Attending Neurologist, Iowa City VA Hospital

Giacomo Rizzolatti, MD
Professor of Human Physiology,
Department of Neurosciences
University of Parma, Italy

Joshua R. Sanes, PhD
Paul J. Finnegan Family Director,
Center for Brain Science
Professor, Department of Molecular and Cellular Biology
Harvard University

Clifford B. Saper, MD, PhD
James Jackson Putnam Professor of Neurology and Neuroscience
Professor and Head, Department of Neurology
Beth Israel Deaconess Medical Center
Harvard Medical School

Daniel L. Schacter, PhD
William R. Kenan, Jr. Professor of Psychology,
Department of Psychology
Harvard University

James H. Schwartz, MD, PhD*
Professor of Physiology & Cellular Biophysics,
Psychiatry, and Neurology,
Center for Neurobiology and Behavior
Columbia University College of Physicians &
Surgeons

Sebastian Seung, PhD
Professor of Physics,
Professor of Computational Neuroscience,
Department of Brain and Cognitive Sciences
Massachusetts Institute of Technology

Nirao M. Shah, MD, PhD
Associate Professor,
Department of Anatomy
University of California, San Francisco

Peter B. Shizgal, PhD
Professor and Concordia University Research Chair,
Department of Psychology
FRQ-S Groupe de recherche en neurobiologie
comportementale
Concordia University

Steven A. Siegelbaum, PhD
Chair of Neuroscience, and Professor of Pharmacology
Investigator, Howard Hughes Medical Institute
Department of Neuroscience, Columbia University
College of Physicians & Surgeons

Scott A. Small, MD
Herbert Irving Professor of Neurology,
Taub Institute, Department of Neurology
Columbia University College of Physicians &
Surgeons

Peter L. Strick, PhD
VA Senior Research Career Scientist,
Director, Systems Neuroscience Institute
Co-Director, Center for the Neural Basis of Cognition
Distinguished Professor of Neurobiology
University of Pittsburgh

Thomas C. Südhof, MD
Avram Goldstein Professor,
Department of Molecular and Cellular Physiology
Stanford University School of Medicine

Larry W. Swanson, PhD
University Professor,
Appleman Professor of Biological Sciences,
Neurology, and Psychiatry
University of Southern California

Marc Tessier-Lavigne, PhD
Professor, Laboratory of Brain Development and
Repair
President, The Rockefeller University

W. Thomas Thach, Jr., MD
Professor of Neurobiology,
Departments of Anatomy and Neurobiology,
Neurology, and Physical Therapy
Washington University School of Medicine

Anthony D. Wagner, PhD
Professor, Department of Psychology and
Neuroscience Program
Stanford University

Mark F. Walker, MD
Associate Professor of Neurology,
Case Western Reserve University
Staff Neurologist, Cleveland VA Medical Center
Staff Neurologist, University Hospital Case
Medical Center

*Deceased

Stephen T. Warren, PhD
William Patterson Timmie Professor,
Charles Howard Candler Chair,
Department of Human Genetics
Emory University School of Medicine

Gary L. Westbrook, MD
Senior Scientist and Co-Director, Vollum Institute
Julie and Rocky Dixon Professor of Neurology
Oregon Health and Science University

Thomas Wichmann, MD
Associate Professor of Neurology,
Department of Neurology
Emory University School of Medicine

Daniel M. Wolpert, PhD, FMedSci, FRS
Department of Engineering,
University of Cambridge

Robert H. Wurtz, PhD
NIH Distinguished Investigator,
Laboratory of Sensorimotor Research
Chief, Section on Visual Motor Integration
National Eye Institute, National Institutes of Health

Rafael Yuste, MD, PhD
University Professor,
Department of Biological Sciences
Department of Neuroscience
Investigator, Howard Hughes Medical Institute
Columbia University

Huda Y. Zoghbi, MD
Professor, Baylor College of Medicine
Investigator, Howard Hughes Medical Institute
Director, Jan and Dan Duncan Neurological Research Institute
Texas Children's Hospital

Part I

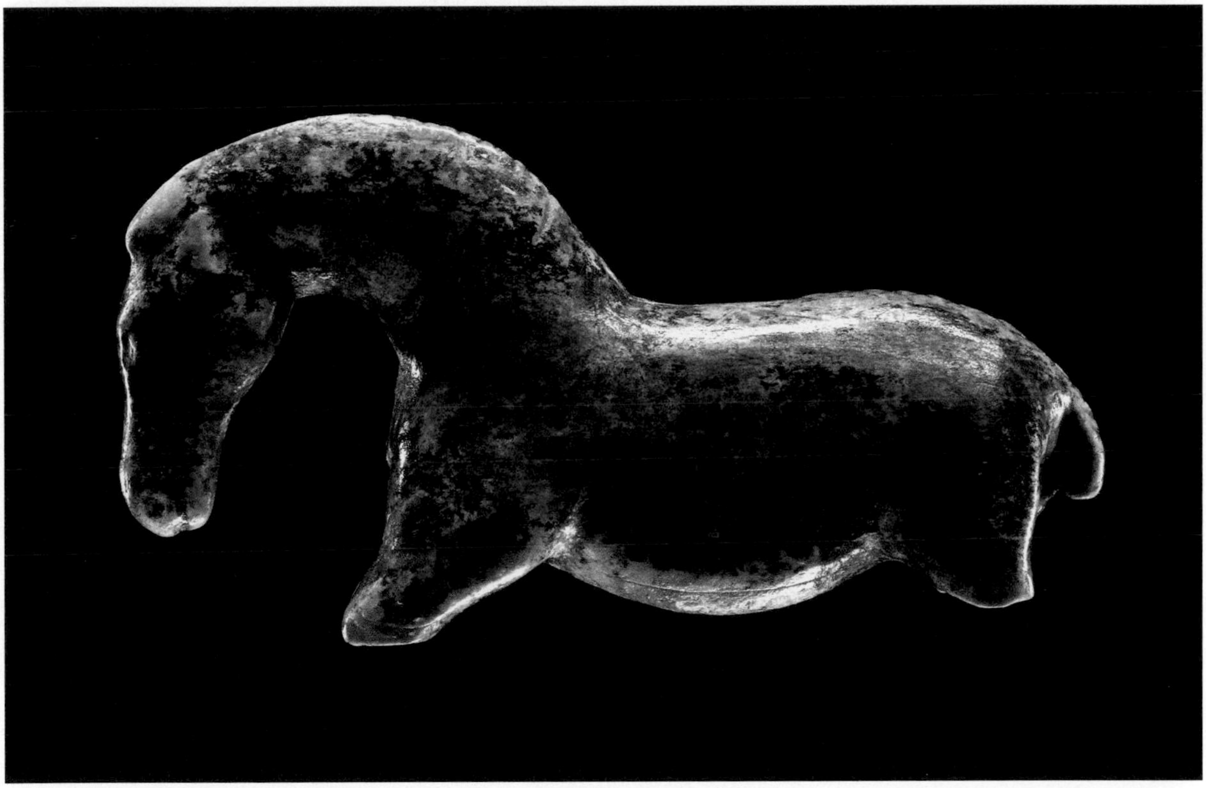

Preceding Page

Over 30,000 years old, this paleolithic sculpture of a horse was discovered in the Vogelherd caves of southern Germany. Measuring only 5 cm and carved from mammoth ivory, this elegant sculpture is evidence of early human's capacity for remarkable perceptiveness and creativity. (Reproduced, with permission, from the University of Tübingen, copyright for Vogelherd, Horse. Photo: Hilde Jensen.)

I Overall Perspective

DURING THE SECOND HALF OF THE 20TH CENTURY, the central focus of biology was on the gene. Now in the first half of the 21st century, the central focus of biology has shifted to neural science and specifically to the biology of the mind. We need to understand the processes by which we perceive, act, learn, and remember. How does the brain—an organ weighing only three pounds—conceive of the infinite, discover new knowledge, and produce the remarkable individuality of human thoughts, feelings, and actions? How are these extraordinary mental capabilities distributed within the organ? How are different mental processes localized to specific combinations of regions in the brain? What rules relate the anatomical organization and the cellular physiology of a region to its specific role in mentation? To what extent are mental processes hardwired into the neural architecture of the brain? What do genes contribute to behavior, and how is gene expression in nerve cells regulated by developmental and learning processes? How does experience alter the way the brain processes subsequent events, and to what degree is that processing unconscious? Finally, what is the neural basis underlying neurological and psychiatric disease? In this introductory section of *Principles of Neural Science*, we attempt to address these questions. In so doing, we describe how neural science is attempting to link the logic of neural circuitry to the mind—how the activities of nerve cells within defined, neural circuits are related to the complexity of mental processes.

In the last several decades, technological advances have opened new horizons for the scientific study of the brain. Today, it is possible to link the molecular dynamics of interconnected circuits of cells to the internal representations of perceptual and motor acts in the brain and to relate these internal mechanisms to observable behavior. New imaging techniques permit us to visualize the human brain in action—to identify specific regions of the brain associated with particular modes of thinking and feeling and their patterns of interconnections.

In the first part of this book, we consider the degree to which mental functions can be located in specific regions of the brain. We also examine the extent to which the behavior so localized can be understood in terms of the properties of individual nerve cells and their interconnections in their specific region of the brain. In the later parts of the book, we examine in detail the cognitive and affective functions of the brain: perception, action, motivation, emotion, development, learning, and memory.

The human brain is a network of more than 100 billion individual nerve cells interconnected in systems—neural circuits—that construct our perceptions of the external world, fix our attention, and control the machinery of our actions. A first step toward understanding the mind, therefore, is to learn how neurons are organized into signaling pathways and how they communicate by means of synaptic transmission. One of the chief ideas we shall develop in this book is that the specificity of the synaptic connections established during development underlie perception, action, emotion, and learning. We must also understand both the innate (genetic) and environmental determinants of behavior. Specifically, we want to know how genes contribute to behavior. Behavior itself, of course, is not inherited—what is inherited is DNA. Genes encode proteins that are important for the development and regulation of the neural circuits that underlie behavior. The environment, which begins to exert its influence in utero, becomes of prime importance after birth, and environmental contingencies can in turn influence behavior by altering gene expression.

By means of the merger of molecular biology, neurophysiology, anatomy, developmental biology, and cell biology with the study of cognition, emotion, and behavior in animals and people, modern neural science has given rise to a new science of mind. Along with astute clinical observation, modern neural science has reinforced the idea first proposed by Hippocrates more than two millennia ago that the proper study of mind begins with study of the brain. Cognitive psychology and psychoanalytic theory in turn have emphasized the diversity and complexity of human mental experience. By emphasizing functional mental structure and internal representation, cognitive psychology has stressed the logic of mental operations and of internal representations. Experimental cognitive psychology and clinical psychotherapy can now be strengthened by insights into the neural science of behavior and by imaging mental processes in action in real time. The task for the years ahead is to produce a study of mental processes, grounded firmly in empirical neural science, yet still fully concerned with problems of how internal representations and states of mind are generated.

Part I

1

The Brain and Behavior

THE LAST FRONTIER OF THE BIOLOGICAL SCIENCES—the ultimate challenge—is to understand the biological basis of consciousness and the brain processes by which we feel, act, learn, and remember. During the past few decades, a remarkable unification within the biological sciences has set the stage for addressing this great challenge. The ability to sequence genes and infer the amino acid sequences of the proteins they encode has revealed unanticipated similarities between proteins in the nervous system and those encountered elsewhere in the body. As a result, it has become possible to establish a general plan for the function of cells, a plan that provides a common conceptual framework for all of cell biology, including cellular neural science. The current challenge in the unification within biology, which we outline in this book, is the unification of the study of behavior—the science of the mind—and neural science—the science of the brain.

Such a unified approach, in which mind and body are not viewed as separate entities, rests on the view that all behavior is the result of brain function. What we commonly call the mind is a set of operations carried out by the brain. Brain processes underlie not only simple motor behaviors such as walking and eating but also all the complex cognitive acts and behavior that we regard as quintessentially human—thinking, speaking, and creating works of art. As a corollary, all the behavioral disorders that characterize psychiatric illness—disorders of affect (feeling) and cognition (thought)—result from disturbances of brain function.

How do the billions of individual nerve cells in the brain produce behavior and cognitive states, and how are those cells influenced by the environment, which includes social experience? Explaining behavior in terms of the brain's activities is the task of neural science, and the progress of neural science in explaining human behavior is a major theme of this book.

Neural science must continually confront certain fundamental questions. Is a particular mental process carried out in specific regions of the brain, or does it involve the brain as a whole? If a mental process can be localized to discrete brain regions, what is the relationship between the functions of those regions in perception, movement, or thought and the anatomy and physiology of those regions? Are these relationships more likely to be understood by examining each region as a whole or by studying individual nerve cells?

To answer these questions we shall examine how modern neural science describes language, one of the most human of cognitive behaviors. In so doing we shall focus on the cerebral cortex, the part of the brain that is most highly developed in humans. We shall see how the cortex is organized into functionally distinct regions, each made up of large groups of neurons, and how the neural apparatus of a highly complex behavior can be analyzed in terms of the activity of specific sets of interconnected neurons within specific regions. In Chapter 2 we describe how neural circuits function at the cellular level, using a simple reflex behavior to show how the interplay of sensory signals and motor signals culminate in a motor act.

Two Opposing Views Have Been Advanced on the Relationship Between Brain and Behavior

Our views about nerve cells, the brain, and behavior emerged during the 20th century from a synthesis of five experimental traditions: anatomy, embryology, physiology, pharmacology, and psychology.

The 2nd century Greek physician Galen proposed that nerves convey fluid secreted by the brain and spinal cord to the body's periphery. His views dominated Western medicine until the microscope revealed the true structure of the cells in nervous tissue. Even so, nervous tissue did not become the subject of a special science until the late 1800s, when the Italian Camillo Golgi and the Spaniard Santiago Ramón y Cajal produced detailed, accurate descriptions of nerve cells.

Golgi developed a method of staining neurons with silver salts that revealed their entire cell structure under the microscope. He could see clearly that each neuron typically has a cell body and two types of processes: branching dendrites at one end and a long, cable-like axon at the other. Using Golgi's technique, Ramón y Cajal discovered that nervous tissue is not a syncytium, a continuous web of elements, but a network of discrete cells. In the course of this work Ramón y Cajal developed some of the key concepts and much of the early evidence for the *neuron doctrine*—the principle that individual neurons are the elementary building blocks and signaling elements of the nervous system.

In the 1920s support for the neuron doctrine was provided by the American embryologist Ross Harrison, who showed that dendrites and the axon grow from the cell body and that they do so even when each neuron is isolated from others in tissue culture. Harrison also confirmed Ramón y Cajal's suggestion that the tip of the axon gives rise to an expansion, the *growth cone,* which leads the developing axon to its target, either to other nerve cells or muscles. The final and definite proof of the neuron doctrine came in the mid-950s with the introduction of electron microscopy. A landmark study by Sanford Palay unambiguously demonstrated the existence of synapses, specialized regions that permit chemical or electrical signaling between neurons.

Physiological investigation of the nervous system began in the late 1700s when the Italian physician and physicist Luigi Galvani discovered that muscle and nerve cells produce electricity. Modern electrophysiology grew out of work in the 19th century by three German physiologists—Johannes Müller, Emil du Bois-Reymond, and Hermann von Helmholtz—who succeeded in measuring the speed of conduction of electrical activity along the axon of the nerve cell and further showed that the electrical activity of one nerve cell affects the activity of an adjacent cell in predictable ways.

Pharmacology made its first impact on our understanding of the nervous system and behavior at the end of the 19th century when Claude Bernard in France, Paul Ehrlich in Germany, and John Langley in England demonstrated that drugs do not act just anywhere on a cell, but rather bind discrete receptors typically located in the surface membrane of the cell. This insight led to the discovery that nerve cells can communicate with each other by chemical means.

Psychological thinking about behavior dates back to the beginnings of Western science when the ancient Greek philosophers speculated about the causes of behavior and the relation of the mind to the brain. In the 17th century René Descartes distinguished body and mind. In Descartes' dualistic view the brain mediates perception, motor acts, memory, appetites, and passions—everything that can be found in the lower animals. But the *mind*—the higher mental functions, the conscious experience characteristic of human behavior—is not represented in the brain or any other part of the body but in the soul, a spiritual entity that communicates with the machinery of the brain by means of the pineal gland, a tiny structure in the midline of the brain. Later in the 17th century Baruch Spinoza began to develop a unified view of mind and body.

In the 18th century Western ideas about the mind split along new lines. Empiricists believed that the brain is initially a blank slate (*tabula rasa*) that is later filled by sensory experience, whereas idealists, notably Immanuel Kant, believed that our perception of the world is determined by inherent features of our mind or brain. In the mid-19th century Charles Darwin set the stage for the modern understanding of the brain as the seat of all behavior. He also advanced the even more radical idea that animals could serve as models of human behavior. Thus the study of evolution gave rise to ethology, the investigation of the behavior of animals in their natural setting, and later to experimental psychology, the study of human and animal behavior under controlled conditions. At the beginning of the 20th century Sigmund Freud introduced psychoanalysis. As the first systematic cognitive psychology, psychoanalysis framed the enormous problems that confront us in understanding the human mind.

Attempts to join biological and psychological concepts in the study of behavior began as early as 1800, when Franz Joseph Gall, a Viennese physician and neuroanatomist, proposed two radically new ideas. First, he advocated that the brain is the organ of the mind and that all mental functions emanate from the brain. In so doing, he rejected the idea that mind and body are separate entities. Second, he argued that the cerebral cortex did not function as a single organ but contained within it many organs, and that particular regions of the cerebral cortex control specific functions. Gall enumerated at least 27 distinct regions or organs of the cerebral cortex; later many more were added, each corresponding to a specific mental faculty. Gall assigned intellectual processes, such as the ability to evaluate causality, to calculate, and to sense order, to the front of the brain. Instinctive characteristics such as romantic love (*amativeness*) and combativeness were assigned to the back of the brain. Even the most abstract of human behaviors—generosity, secretiveness, and religiosity—were assigned a spot in the brain (Figure 1–1).

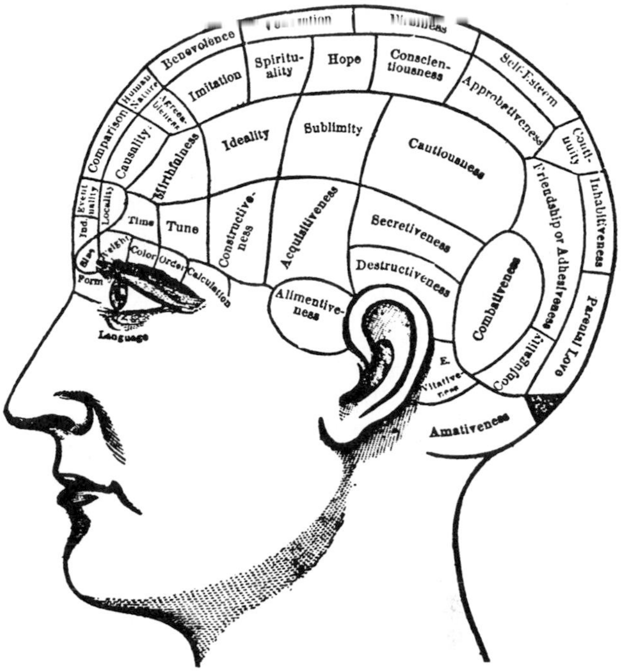

Figure 1–1 An early map of functional localization in the brain. According to the 19th century doctrine of phrenology, complex traits such as combativeness, spirituality, hope, and conscientiousness are controlled by specific areas in the brain, which expand as the traits develop. This enlargement of local areas of the brain was thought to produce characteristic bumps and ridges on the overlying skull, from which an individual's character could be determined. This map, taken from a drawing of the early 1800s, purports to show 42 intellectual and emotional faculties in distinct areas of the skull and the cerebral cortex underneath.

Although Gall's theory of localization was prescient, his experimental approach to localization was extremely naive. Rather than localize functions empirically, by looking into the brain and correlating defects in mental attributes with lesions in specific regions following tumor or stroke, Gall spurned all evidence derived from examination of brain lesions, discovered clinically or produced surgically in experimental animals. Influenced by physiognomy, the popular science based on the idea that facial features reveal character, Gall believed that the bumps and ridges on the skulls of people well endowed with specific faculties identified the centers for those faculties in the brain. He assumed that the size of an area of brain was related to the mental faculty represented in that area. Accordingly, exercise of a given mental faculty would cause the corresponding brain region to grow and this growth in turn would cause the overlying skull to protrude.

Gall first had this idea as a young boy when he noticed that those of his classmates who excelled at memorizing school assignments had prominent eyes. He concluded that this was the result of an overdevelopment of regions in the front of the brain involved in verbal memory. He developed this idea further when, as a young physician, he was placed in charge of an asylum for the insane in Vienna. There he began to study patients suffering from monomania, a disorder characterized by an exaggerated interest in some key idea or a deep urge to engage in some specific behavior—theft, murder, eroticism, extreme religiosity. He reasoned that, because the patient functioned well in all other behaviors, the brain defect must be discrete and in principle could be localized by examining the skulls of these patients. Based on these findings Gall drew cortical maps such as those of Figure 1–1. Gall's studies of localized brain functions led to *phrenology*, a discipline concerned with determining personality and character based on the detailed shape of the skull.

In the late 1820s Gall's ideas were subjected to experimental analysis by the French physiologist Pierre Flourens. By systematically destroying Gall's functional centers in the brains of experimental animals, Flourens attempted to isolate the contribution of each "cerebral organ" to behavior. From these experiments Flourens concluded that specific brain regions are not responsible for specific behaviors, but that all brain regions, especially the cerebral hemispheres of the forebrain, participate in every mental operation. Any part of a cerebral hemisphere, Flourens proposed, is able to perform all the hemisphere's functions. Injury to any one area of the cerebral hemisphere should therefore affect all higher functions equally. Thus in 1823 Flourens wrote: "All perceptions, all volitions occupy the same seat in these (cerebral) organs; the faculty of perceiving, of conceiving, of willing merely constitutes therefore a faculty which is essentially one."

The rapid acceptance of this belief, later called the *holistic* view of the brain, was based only partly on Flourens's experimental work. It also represented a cultural reaction against the materialistic view that the human mind is a biological organ. It represented a rejection of the notion that there is no soul, that all mental processes can be reduced to activity within the brain, and that the mind can be improved by exercising it, ideas that were unacceptable to the religious establishment and landed aristocracy of Europe.

The holistic view was seriously challenged, however, in the mid-19th century by the French neurologist Paul Pierre Broca, the German neurologist Carl Wernicke, and the British neurologist Hughlings Jackson. For example, in his studies of focal epilepsy, a disease characterized by convulsions that begin in a particular part of the body, Jackson showed that different motor and sensory functions could be traced to specific parts of the cerebral cortex. The regional studies of Broca, Wernicke, and Jackson were extended to the cellular level by Charles Sherrington and by

Box 1–1 The Central Nervous System

The Central Nervous System Has Seven Main Parts.

The **spinal cord,** the most caudal part of the central nervous system, receives and processes sensory information from the skin, joints, and muscles of the limbs and trunk and controls movement of the limbs and the trunk. It is subdivided into cervical, thoracic, lumbar, and sacral regions (Figure 1–2A).

The spinal cord continues rostrally as the **brain stem**, which consists of the medulla oblongata, pons, and midbrain. The brain stem receives sensory information from the skin and muscles of the head and provides the motor control for the head's musculature. It also conveys information from the spinal cord to the brain and from the brain to the spinal cord, and regulates levels of arousal and awareness through the reticular formation.

The brain stem contains several collections of cell bodies, the cranial nerve nuclei. Some of these nuclei receive information from the skin and muscles of the head; others control motor output to muscles of the face, neck, and eyes. Still others are specialized to process information from three of the special senses: hearing, balance, and taste.

The **medulla oblongata,** directly rostral to the spinal cord, includes several centers responsible for vital autonomic functions, such as digestion, breathing, and the control of heart rate.

The **pons,** rostral to the medulla, conveys information about movement from the cerebral hemispheres to the cerebellum.

The **cerebellum** lies behind the pons and is connected to the brain stem by several major fiber tracts called *peduncles.* The cerebellum modulates the force and range of movement and is involved in the learning of motor skills.

The **midbrain,** rostral to the pons, controls many sensory and motor functions, including eye movement and the coordination of visual and auditory reflexes.

The **diencephalon** lies rostral to the midbrain and contains two structures. The *thalamus* processes most of the information reaching the cerebral cortex from the rest of the central nervous system. The *hypothalamus* regulates autonomic, endocrine, and visceral functions.

The **cerebrum** comprises two cerebral hemispheres, each consisting of a heavily wrinkled outer layer (the *cerebral cortex*) and three deep-lying structures (the *basal ganglia,* the *hippocampus,* and the *amygdaloid nuclei*). The cerebral cortex is divided into four distinct lobes: frontal, parietal, occipital, and temporal (Figure 1–2B).

The basal ganglia participate in regulating motor performance; the hippocampus is involved with aspects of memory storage; and the amygdaloid nuclei coordinate the autonomic and endocrine responses of emotional states.

The brain is also commonly divided into three broader regions: the *hindbrain* (medulla oblongata, pons, and cerebellum), *midbrain,* and *forebrain* (diencephalon and cerebrum). The hindbrain (excluding the cerebellum) and midbrain together include the same structures as the brain stem.

Ramón y Cajal, who championed the view of brain function called *cellular connectionism.* According to this view individual neurons are the signaling units of the brain; they are arranged in functional groups and connect to one another in a precise fashion. Wernicke's work and that of the French neurologist Jules Dejerine in particular revealed that different behaviors are produced by different interconnected brain regions.

The first important evidence for localization emerged from studies of how the brain produces language. Before we consider the relevant clinical and anatomical studies, we shall first review the overall structure of the brain. (The anatomical organization of the nervous system is described in some detail in Chapter 17.)

The Brain Has Distinct Functional Regions

The central nervous system is a bilateral and essentially symmetrical structure with two main parts, the spinal cord and the brain. The brain comprises seven major structures: the medulla oblongata, pons, cerebellum, midbrain, diencephalon, and cerebrum (Box 1–1 and Figure 1–3).

Radiographic imaging techniques have made it possible to see these structures in living people. Brain imaging is now commonly used to evaluate the metabolic activity of discrete regions of the brain while people are engaged in specific tasks under controlled conditions. Such studies provide direct evidence that specific types of behavior involve particular regions of the brain. As a result, Gall's original idea that discrete

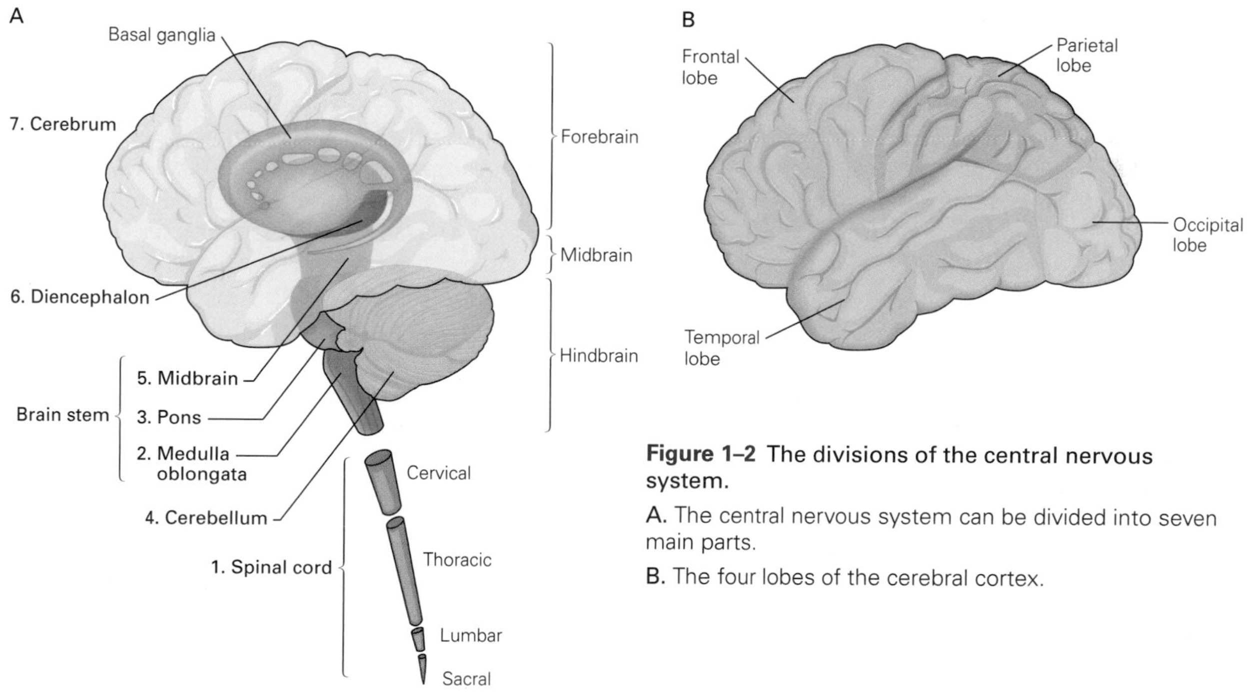

Figure 1–2 The divisions of the central nervous system.

A. The central nervous system can be divided into seven main parts.

B. The four lobes of the cerebral cortex.

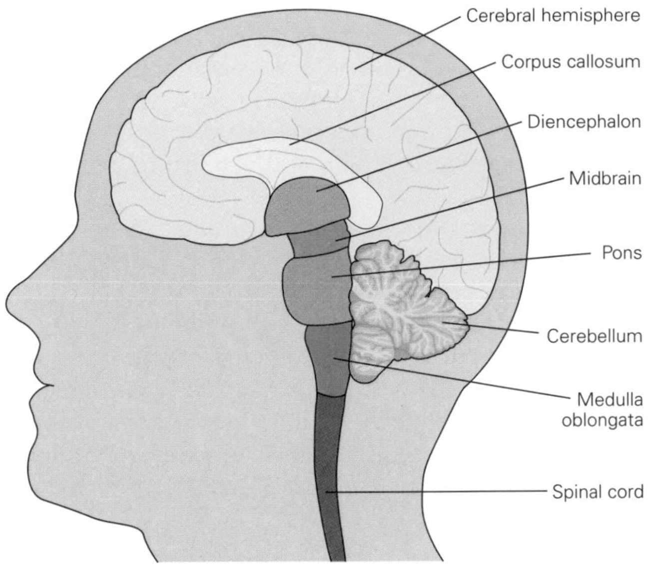

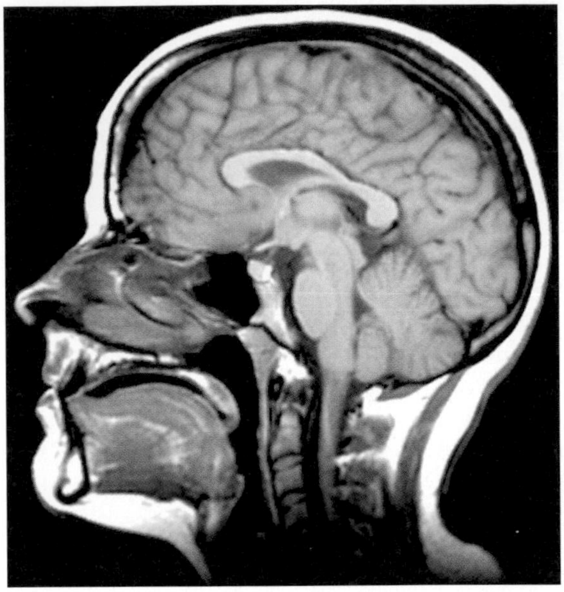

Figure 1–3 The main divisions are clearly visible when the brain is cut down the midline between the two cerebral hemispheres.

A. This schematic drawing shows the position of major structures of the brain in relation to external landmarks. Students of brain anatomy quickly learn to discern the major internal landmarks, such as the corpus callosum, a large bundle of nerve fibers that connects the left and right hemispheres.

B. The major brain divisions drawn in **A** are also evident in a magnetic resonance image of a living human brain.

regions are specialized for different functions is now one of the cornerstones of modern brain science.

Students of the brain taking a cellular connectionist approach have found that the operations responsible for our cognitive abilities occur primarily in the *cerebral cortex,* the furrowed gray matter covering the two cerebral hemispheres. In each of the hemispheres the overlying cortex is divided into *frontal, parietal, occipital,* and *temporal* lobes (see Figure 1–2B), named for the skull bones that overlie them. Each lobe has several characteristic deep infoldings, an evolutionary strategy for packing more nerve cells into a limited space. The crests of these convolutions are called *gyri,* whereas the intervening grooves are called *sulci* or *fissures.* The more prominent gyri and sulci, which are quite similar from person to person, bear specific names. For example, the *central sulcus* separates the *precentral gyrus,* an area concerned with motor function, from the *postcentral gyrus,* an area that deals with sensory function (Figure 1–4A).

Each lobe has a specialized set of functions. The frontal lobe is largely concerned with short-term memory and planning future actions and with control of movement; the parietal lobe with somatic sensation, with forming a body image and relating it to extrapersonal space; the occipital lobe with vision; and the temporal lobe with hearing and—through its deep structures, the hippocampus and amygdaloid nuclei—with learning, memory, and emotion.

Two important features characterize the organization of the cerebral cortex. First, each hemisphere is concerned primarily with sensory and motor processes on the contralateral (opposite) side of the body. Thus sensory information that reaches the spinal cord from the left side of the body crosses to the right side of the nervous system on its way to the cerebral cortex. Similarly, the motor areas in the right hemisphere exert control over the movements of the left half of the body. The second feature is that the hemispheres, although similar in appearance, are neither completely symmetrical in structure nor equivalent in function.

The First Strong Evidence for Localization of Cognitive Abilities Came from Studies of Language Disorders

The areas of the cortex that were first pinpointed to be important for cognition were concerned with language. These come from studies of *aphasia,* a language disorder that most often occurs when certain areas of brain tissue are destroyed by a stroke, the occlusion or rupture of a blood vessel to a portion of a cerebral hemisphere. Many of the important discoveries in the study of aphasia occurred in rapid succession during the last half of the 19th century. Taken together, these advances form one of the most exciting and important chapters in the neural science of human behavior.

Pierre Paul Broca, a French neurologist, was the first to identify specific areas of the brain concerned with language. Broca was influenced by Gall's efforts to map higher functions in the brain, but instead of correlating behavior with bumps on the skull he correlated clinical evidence of aphasia with brain lesions discovered post mortem. In 1861 he wrote, "I had thought that if there were ever a phrenological science, it would be the phrenology of convolutions (*in the cortex*), and not the phrenology of bumps (*on the head*)." Based on this insight Broca founded *neuropsychology*, a science of mental processes that he distinguished from the phrenology of Gall.

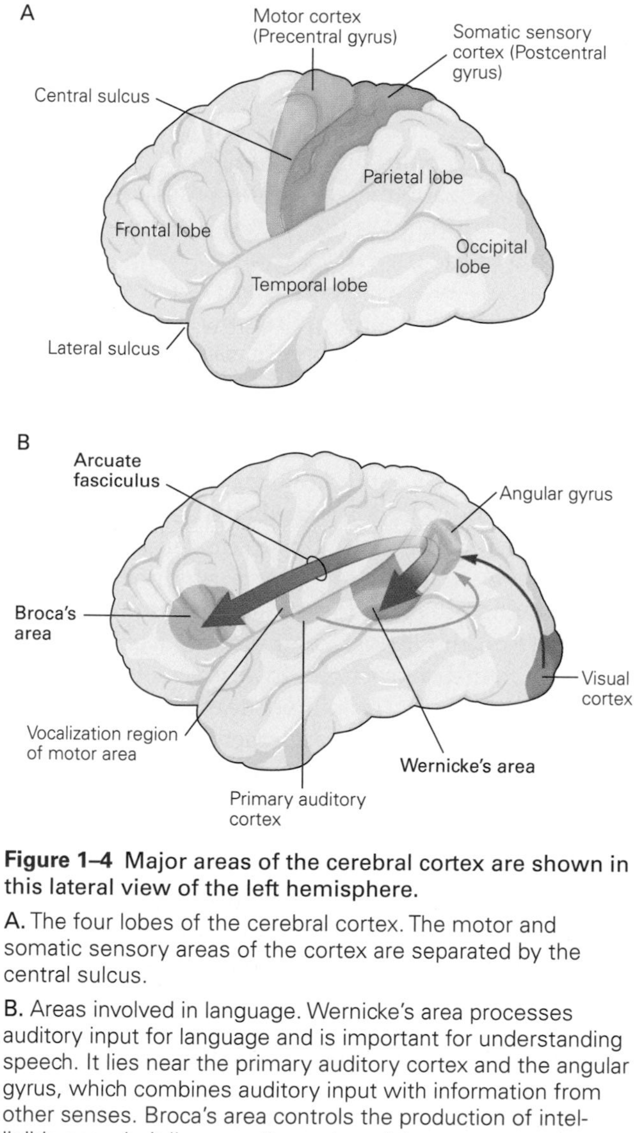

Figure 1–4 **Major areas of the cerebral cortex are shown in this lateral view of the left hemisphere.**

A. The four lobes of the cerebral cortex. The motor and somatic sensory areas of the cortex are separated by the central sulcus.

B. Areas involved in language. Wernicke's area processes auditory input for language and is important for understanding speech. It lies near the primary auditory cortex and the angular gyrus, which combines auditory input with information from other senses. Broca's area controls the production of intelligible speech. It lies near the region of the motor area that controls the mouth and tongue movements that form words. Wernicke's area communicates with Broca's area by a bidirectional pathway, part of which is made up of the arcuate fasciculus. (Adapted, with permission, from Geschwind 1979.)

In 1861 Broca described a patient, Leborgne, who as a result of a stroke could not speak, although he could understand language perfectly well. This patient had no motor deficits of the tongue, mouth, or vocal cords that would affect his ability to speak. In fact, he could utter isolated words, whistle, and sing a melody without difficulty. But he could not speak grammatically or create complete sentences, nor could he express ideas in writing. Postmortem examination of this patient's brain showed a lesion in the posterior region of the frontal lobe, now called *Broca's area* (Figure 1–4B). Broca studied eight similar patients, all with lesions in this region, and in each case the lesion was located in the left cerebral hemisphere. This discovery led Broca to announce in 1864: "*Nous parlons avec l'hémisphère gauche!*" (We speak with the left hemisphere!)

Broca's work stimulated a search for cortical sites associated with other specific behaviors—a search soon rewarded. In 1870 Gustav Fritsch and Eduard Hitzig galvanized the scientific community when they showed that characteristic limb movements of dogs, such as extending a paw, could be produced by electrically stimulating discrete regions of the precentral gyrus. These regions were invariably located in the contralateral motor cortex. Thus the right hand, the one most used for writing and skilled movements, is controlled by the left hemisphere, the same hemisphere that controls speech. In most people, therefore, the left hemisphere is regarded as *dominant*.

The next step was taken in 1876 by Karl Wernicke, who at age 26 published a now-classic paper, "The Symptom-Complex of Aphasia: A Psychological Study on an Anatomical Basis." In it he described another type of aphasia, a failure of comprehension rather than speech: a *receptive* as opposed to an *expressive* malfunction. Whereas Broca's patients could understand language but not speak, Wernicke's patient could form words but could not understand language. Moreover, the locus of this new type of aphasia was different from that described by Broca: The lesion occurred in the posterior part of the cortex where the temporal lobe meets the parietal and occipital lobes (Figure 1–4B).

On the basis of this discovery, and the work of Broca, Fritsch, and Hitzig, Wernicke formulated a neural model of language that attempted to reconcile and extend the two predominant theories of brain function at that time. Phrenologists and cellular connectionists argued that the cortex was a mosaic of functionally specific areas, whereas the holistic aggregate-field school claimed that every mental function involved the entire cerebral cortex. Wernicke proposed that only the most basic mental functions, those concerned with simple perceptual and motor activities, are mediated by neurons in discrete local areas of the cortex. More complex cognitive functions, he argued, result from interconnections between several functional sites. In placing the principle of localized function within a connectionist framework, Wernicke realized that different components of a single behavior are likely to be processed in several regions of the brain. He was thus the first to advance the idea of *distributed processing,* now a central tenet of neural science.

Wernicke postulated that language involves separate motor and sensory programs, each governed by distinct regions of cortex. He proposed that the motor program that governs the mouth movements for speech is located in Broca's area, suitably situated in front of that region of the motor area that controls the mouth, tongue, palate, and vocal cords (Figure 1–4B). He next assigned the sensory program that governs word perception to the temporal-lobe area that he had discovered, which is now called *Wernicke's area.* This region is conveniently surrounded by the auditory cortex and by areas now known collectively as *association cortex,* a region of cortex that integrates auditory, visual, and somatic sensations.

Thus Wernicke formulated the first coherent neural model for language that—with important modifications and elaborations we shall encounter in Chapter 60—is still useful today. According to this model, the initial steps in neural processing of spoken or written words occur in separate sensory areas of the cortex specialized for auditory or visual information. This information is then conveyed to a cortical association area, the angular gyrus, specialized for processing both auditory and visual information. Here, according to Wernicke, spoken or written words are transformed into a neural sensory code shared by both speech and writing. This representation is conveyed to Wernicke's area, where it is recognized as language and associated with meaning. It is also relayed to Broca's area, which contains the rules, or grammar, for transforming the sensory representation into a motor representation that can be realized as spoken or written language. When this transformation from sensory to motor representation cannot take place, the patient loses the ability to speak and write.

The power of Wernicke's model was not only its completeness but also its predictive utility. This model correctly predicted a third type of aphasia, one that results from disconnection. Here the receptive and expressive zones for speech are intact, but the neuronal fibers that connect them are destroyed. This *conduction aphasia,* as it is now called, is characterized by an incorrect use of words (*paraphasia*). Patients with conduction aphasia understand words that they hear and read and have no motor difficulties when they speak. Yet they cannot speak coherently; they omit parts of words or substitute incorrect sounds and in particular they have difficulties repeating phrases. Although painfully aware of their own errors, they are unable to put them right.

Inspired in part by Wernicke's advances and led by the anatomist Korbinian Brodmann, a new school of cortical localization arose in Germany at the beginning of the 20th century, one that distinguished functional areas of the cortex based on the shapes of cells and variations in their layered arrangement. Using this *cytoarchitectonic* method, Brodmann distinguished 52 anatomically and functionally distinct areas in the human cerebral cortex (Figure 1–5).

Even though the biological evidence for functionally discrete areas in the cortex was compelling, the aggregate-field view of the brain, not cellular connectionism, continued to dominate experimental thinking and clinical practice until 1950. This surprising state of affairs owed much to several prominent neural scientists who advocated for the aggregate-field view, among them the British neurologist Henry Head, the German neuropsychologist Kurt Goldstein, the Russian behavioral physiologist Ivan Pavlov, and the American psychologist Karl Lashley.

Most influential was Lashley, who was deeply skeptical of the cytoarchitectonic approach to functional mapping of the cortex. "The 'ideal' architectonic map is nearly worthless," Lashley wrote. "The area subdivisions are in large part anatomically meaningless, and misleading as to the presumptive functional divisions of the cortex." His skepticism was reinforced by his studies of the effects of various brain lesions on the ability of rats to learn to run a maze. From these studies Lashley concluded that the severity of a learning defect depended on the size of the lesion, not on its precise location. Disillusioned, Lashley—and after him many other psychologists—concluded that learning and other higher mental functions have no special locus in the brain and consequently cannot be attributed to specific collections of neurons.

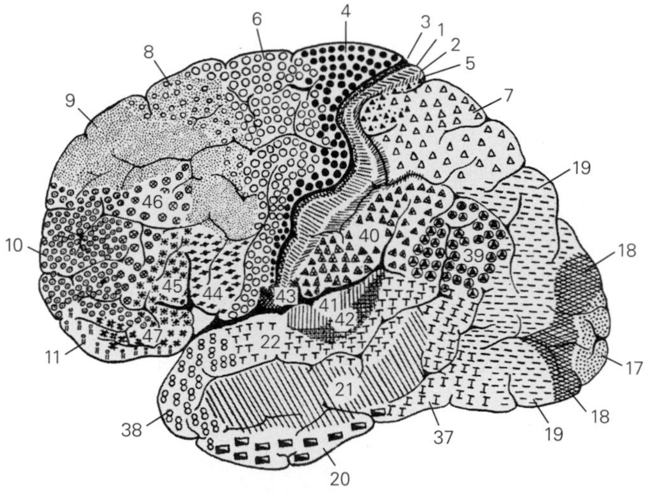

Figure 1–5 **Brodmann's division of the human cerebral cortex into 52 discrete functional areas. Brodmann identified these areas on the basis of distinctive nerve cell structures and characteristic arrangements of cell layers.** This scheme is still widely used today and is continually updated. Several areas defined by Brodmann have been found to control specific brain functions. For instance, area 4 is the motor cortex, responsible for voluntary movement. Areas 1, 2, and 3 constitute the primary somatosensory cortex, which receives sensory information primarily from the skin and joints. Area 17 is the primary visual cortex, which receives sensory signals from the eyes and relays them to other areas for further processing. Areas 41 and 42 constitute the primary auditory cortex. The drawing shows only areas visible on the outer surface of the cortex.

On the basis of his observations Lashley reformulated the aggregate-field view by further minimizing the role of individual neurons, specific neuronal connections, and even specific brain regions in the production of specific behavior. According to Lashley's theory of *mass action,* it is the full mass of the brain, not its regional components, that is crucial to function. Applying this idea to aphasia, Head and Goldstein asserted based on their clinical studies that language disorders can result from injury to almost any cortical area.

Lashley's experiments with rats and Head's clinical observations have now been reinterpreted. A variety of studies have shown that the maze-learning used by Lashley is unsuited to the search for local cortical functions because it involves so many motor and sensory capabilities. Deprived of one sensory capability, say vision, a rat can still learn to run a maze using touch or smell. Besides, as we shall see later in the book, many mental functions are mediated by more than one region or neuronal pathway. Thus a given function may show anatomical redundancy and not be eliminated by a single lesion.

Soon the evidence for localization of function became overwhelming. Beginning in the late 1930s, Edgar Adrian in England and Wade Marshall and Philip Bard in the United States discovered that touching different parts of a cat's body elicits electrical activity in distinct regions of the cerebral cortex. By systematically probing the body surface they established a precise map of the body surface in specific areas of the cerebral cortex described by Brodmann. This result showed that functionally distinct areas of cortex *can* be defined unambiguously according to anatomical criteria such as cell type and cell layering, connections of cells, and—most importantly—behavioral function. As we shall see in later chapters, functional specialization is a key organizing principle in the cerebral cortex, extending even to individual columns of cells within a functional area. Indeed, the brain is divided into many more functional regions than Brodmann envisaged.

More refined methods have now made it possible to learn even more about the function of different brain regions involved in language. In the late 1950s Wilder Penfield, and later George Ojemann, reinvestigated the cortical areas that produce language. While locally anesthetized during brain surgery for epilepsy, awake patients were asked to name objects (or use language in other ways) while different areas of the exposed cortex were stimulated with small electrodes. If an area of the cortex was critical for language, application of the electrical stimulus blocked the patient's ability to name objects. In this way Penfield and Ojemann were able to confirm—in the living, awake, and conscious brain—the language areas of the cortex described by Broca and Wernicke. In addition, Ojemann discovered other sites essential for language, in particular the insula, a region that lies deep to Broca's area. As we shall learn in Chapter 60 the neural networks for language are far more extensive and complex than those described by Broca and Wernicke.

Initially almost everything known about the anatomical organization of language came from studies of patients with brain lesions. Today positron emission tomography (PET) and functional magnetic resonance imaging (fMRI) allow anatomical analysis to be conducted on healthy people engaged in reading, speaking, and thinking (Chapter 20). Functional MRI, a noninvasive imaging technique for visualizing activity in the brain, has not only confirmed that reading and speaking activate different brain areas but has also revealed that the act of *thinking* about a word's meaning in the absence of sensory inputs activates a still different area in the left frontal cortex (Figure 1–6).

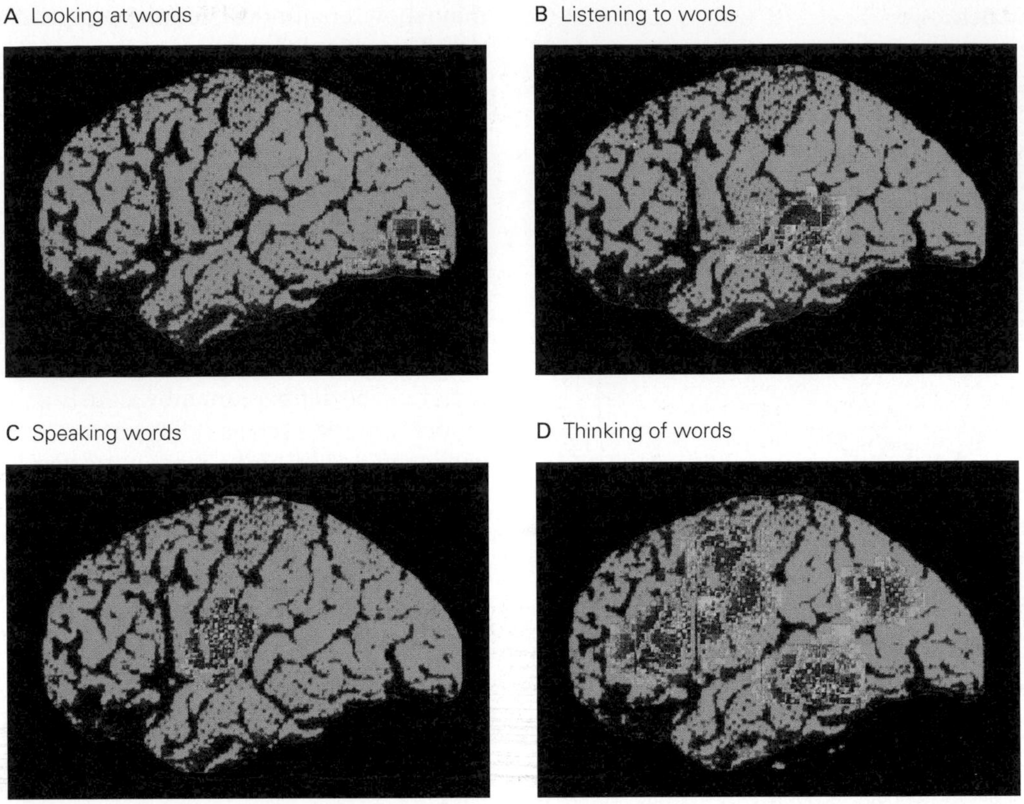

Figure 1–6 Specific regions of the cortex involved in the recognition of a spoken or written word can be identified with positron emission tomography (PET). Each of the four images of the human brain shown here (from the left side of the cerebrum) actually represents the averaged brain activity of several normal subjects. In these PET images **white** indicates areas of highest activity, **red** and **yellow** quite high activity, and **blue** and **gray** the areas of minimal activity. The "input" component of language (reading or hearing a word) activates the regions of the brain shown in **A** and **B**. The "output" component of language (speech or thought) activates the regions shown in **C** and **D**. (Reproduced, with permission, from Cathy Price.)

A. The reading of a single word produces a response both in the primary visual cortex and in the visual association cortex (see Figure 1–5).

B. Hearing a word activates the temporal cortex and the junction of the temporal-parietal cortex (see Figure 1–2). The same list of words used in the reading test (A) was used in the listening test. The results of the reading and listening tests show that the brain does not use the auditory pathway to convey a transformed visual signal.

C. Subjects were asked to repeat a word presented through earphones or on a screen. The spoken word activates the supplementary motor area of the medial frontal cortex. Broca's area is activated whether the word is heard or read. Thus both visual and auditory pathways converge on Broca's area, the common site for the motor articulation of speech.

D. Subjects were asked to respond to the word "brain" with an appropriate verb, for example, "to think." This type of task activates the frontal cortex as well as Broca's and Wernicke's areas. These areas play a role in all cognition and abstract representation.

In separate studies, Joy Hirsch and her colleagues, and Mariacristina Musso, Andrea Moro, and their colleagues used fMRI to explore more deeply Wernicke's idea that Broca's area contains the grammatical rules of language. Hirsch and her colleagues made the interesting discovery that processing of one's native language and processing of a second language occur in distinct regions within Broca's area. If the second language is acquired in adulthood, it is represented in a region separate from that which represents the native language. If the second language is acquired early, however, both the native language and the second language are represented in a common region in Broca's area. These studies indicate that the age at which a language is acquired is a significant factor in determining the functional organization of Broca's area. In contrast, there is no evidence of such separate processing of different languages in Wernicke's area (Figure 1–7).

Further evidence for the fundamental role of Broca's area in processing grammatical rules emerges from the fMRI studies of Musso and Morro on the *language instinct.* Because language is a uniquely human capability, Charles Darwin suggested that the acquisition of language is an inborn instinct comparable to that for upright posture. Children acquire the grammar of their native language simply by listening to their parents speak. They do not have to be taught the specific rules of grammar. In 1960 the linguist Noam Chomsky elaborated on Darwin's notion. He proposed that children acquire a language so easily and naturally because humans, unlike other primates, have the innate capability of generalizing to a complete and coherent language from a limited sample of sentences. Based on an analysis of the structure of sentences in various languages, Chomsky argued that all natural languages share a common design, which he called *universal grammar*. The existence of universal grammar, he argued, implies that there is an innate system in the human brain that evolved to mediate this grammatical design of language.

This, of course, raised the question: Where in the brain does such a system reside? Is it in Broca's area, as Wernicke's model would suggest? Musso, Moro, and their colleagues asked this question and found that the region of Broca's area concerned with second language becomes established and increases in activity only when an individual learns a second language that is "natural," that is, one that shares the universal grammar. If the second language is an *artificial language,* a language that violates the rules of universal grammar, activity in Broca's area does not increase. Thus Broca's area must contain some kind of constraints that determine the structure of all natural languages.

Studies of patients with brain damage continue to afford important insight into how the brain is organized for language. One of the most impressive results comes from a study of deaf people who have lost their ability to communicate through American Sign Language (ASL) after suffering cerebral damage. ASL uses hand gestures rather than sound and is perceived by sight rather than sound but has the same structural

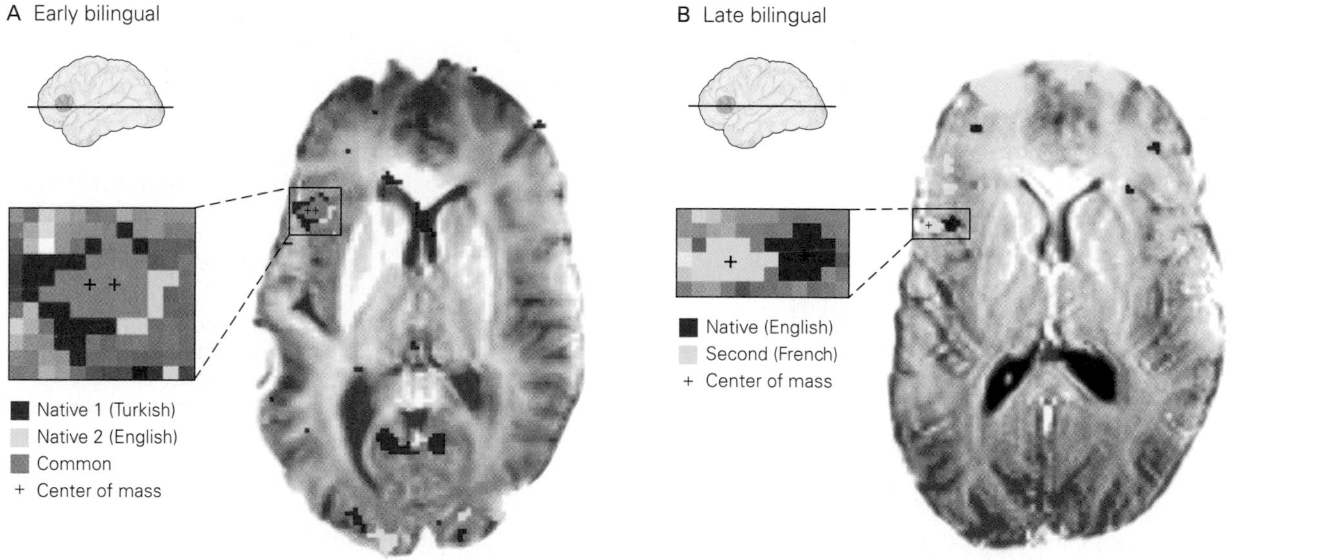

Figure 1–7 Functional magnetic resonance images of the brains of bilingual subjects during generation of narratives in two languages. These bilingual subjects were either "early" or "late" bilingual speakers; "early" bilinguals had learned two languages together prior to the age of 7 years, whereas "late" bilinguals acquired a second language after age 11 years. Axial slices of brain that intersect Broca's area are shown for one representative "early" bilingual subject and one representative "late" bilingual subject. Regions of the brain that responded during the narrative tasks are shown in **red** (native language) and **yellow** (native and second languages). In high-resolution views of these areas centroids of activity associated with each language are indicated by (+) and areas of overlap between the two areas are shown in **orange**. (Reproduced, with permission, from Kim et al. 1997.)

A. In the early bilingual subject the locations of the centers and spread of activity for both languages are indistinguishable at the resolution of functional magnetic resonance imaging (fMRI) (1.5 × 1.5 mm) as indicated by the close proximity of the two (+) and the orange region indicating sensitivity to both languages.

B. In the late bilingual subject both the locations of the centers (+) and the spread of the native and second language are distinguishable at the same resolution.

complexity as spoken languages. Signing is also localized to the left hemisphere; deaf people can become aphasic for sign language as a result of lesions in the left hemisphere, but not as a result of lesions in the right hemisphere. Damage to the left hemisphere can have quite specific consequences for signing just as for spoken language, affecting sign comprehension (following damage in Wernicke's area), grammar (following damage in Broca's area), or fluency.

These observations illustrate three points. First, the cognitive processing for language occurs in the left hemisphere and is independent of pathways that process the sensory and motor modalities used in language. Second, fully functional auditory and motor systems are not necessary conditions for the emergence and operation of language capabilities in the left hemisphere. Third, spoken language represents only one of a family of language skills mediated by the left hemisphere.

Similar conclusions that the brain has distinct cognitive systems have been reached from investigations of behaviors other than language. These studies demonstrate that complex information processing requires many distinct but interconnected cortical and sub-cortical areas, each concerned with processing some particular aspects of sensory stimuli or motor movement and not others. For example, in the visual system, a dorsal cortical pathway is concerned with *where* an object is located in the external world while a ventral pathway is concerned with *what* that object is.

Affective States Are Also Mediated by Local, Specialized Systems in the Brain

Despite the persuasive evidence for localized systems in the cortex dedicated to language, the idea nevertheless persisted that affective (emotional) functions could not be mediated by discrete specialized systems. Emotion, it was believed, must be an expression of whole-brain activity. Only recently has this view been modified. Although the neural systems governing emotion have not been mapped as precisely as the sensory, motor, and cognitive systems, distinct emotions can be elicited by stimulating specific parts of the brain in humans or experimental animals. The localization of neural systems regulating emotion has been dramatically demonstrated in patients with certain language disorders and in patients with a particular type of epilepsy that affects the regulation of affective states.

Some aphasic patients not only manifest cognitive defects in language but also have trouble with the affective aspects of language, such as intonation (prosody). These affective aspects are represented in the right hemisphere and, rather strikingly, the neural organization of the affective elements of language mirrors the organization of the logical content of language in the left hemisphere. Damage to the right temporal area corresponding to Wernicke's area in the left temporal region leads to disturbances in comprehending emotional aspects of speech, for example the ability to appreciate from a person's tone of voice whether he is describing a sad or happy event. In contrast, damage to the right frontal area corresponding to Broca's area leads to difficulty in expressing emotional aspects of speech.

Thus some neurons needed for language also exist in the right hemisphere. Indeed, there is now considerable evidence that an intact right hemisphere is necessary to appreciate semantic subtleties of language, such as irony, metaphor, and wit, as well as the emotional content of speech. There is also preliminary evidence that the ability to enjoy and perform music involves systems in the right hemisphere.

Aprosodias, disorders of affective aspects of language that are localized to the right hemisphere, are classified as sensory, motor, or conductive, following the classification used for aphasias.

Although the localization of language appears to be inborn, it is by no means completely determined until the age of seven or eight. Young children in whom the left cerebral hemisphere is severely damaged early in life can still develop an essentially normal grasp of language, but they do so at a cost, for the ability of these children to locate objects in space or to reason spatially is much reduced compared to that of normal children.

Studies of patients with chronic temporal lobe epilepsy provide further clues to the areas in the brain that regulate affective states. These patients manifest characteristic emotional changes, some of which occur only fleetingly during the seizure itself (the so-called *ictal phenomena*). Common ictal phenomena include feelings of unreality; déjà vu, the sensation of having been in a place before or of having had a particular experience before; transient visual or auditory hallucinations; feelings of depersonalization, fear, or anger; delusions; inappropriate sexual feelings; and paranoia.

More enduring emotional changes, however, are evident when patients are not having seizures. These *interictal phenomena* are interesting because they resemble a coherent psychiatric syndrome. Such patients lose all interest in sex, and the decline in sexual interest is often paralleled by an increase in social aggressiveness. Most have one or more distinctive personality traits; they can be intensely emotional, ardently religious, extremely moralistic, or totally lacking in humor. In striking contrast, patients with epileptic foci outside the temporal lobe typically show no abnormal emotion and behavior.

Recent studies have found that high-frequency electrical stimulation of the subthalamic nucleus, part of the motor system, can markedly improve the tremor characteristic of Parkinson disease, a movement disorder we consider in Chapter 41. Alim-Louis Benabid and his colleagues have found that stimulation of this region also induces unusual emotional states including euphoria, increased libido, feelings of merriment, infectious laughter, and hilarity—aspects of emotional expression that are depressed in Parkinson disease. One patient who previously was depressed and had suicidal thoughts began to enjoy himself again and abandoned his thoughts about suicide. He became creative once again, began a number of different projects, bought himself a new sports car, and began flirting with women.

Finally, one other important structure involved in the regulation of emotion is the amygdala, which lies deep within the cerebral hemispheres. Its role in emotion was discovered through studies of the effects of the lesions within the temporal lobe that produce epilepsy. The consequences of irritative lesions are exactly the opposite of those of destructive lesions resulting from a stroke or injury. Whereas destructive lesions bring about loss of function, often through the disconnection of related functional systems, the electrical activity brought about by epilepsy can increase activity in the regions in which the epileptic seizure occurs. In the case of amygdala seizures the increased activity leads to excessive expression of emotion. We consider the neurobiology of emotion in Part VII of this book.

Mental Processes Are the End Product of the Interactions Between Elementary Processing Units in the Brain

There are several reasons why the evidence for the localization of brain functions, which seems so obvious and compelling in retrospect, had been rejected so often in the past. Phrenologists introduced the idea of localization in an exaggerated form and without adequate evidence. They imagined each region of the cerebral cortex as an independent mental organ dedicated to a complete and distinct aspect of personality, much as the pancreas and the liver are independent digestive organs. Flourens's rejection of phrenology and the ensuing dialectic between proponents of the aggregate-field view (against localization) and the cellular connectionists (for localization) were responses to a theory that was simplistic and without adequate experimental evidence.

In the aftermath of Wernicke's discovery of the modular organization of language in the brain—interconnected serial and parallel processing centers with more-or-less independent functions—we now think that all cognitive abilities result from the interaction of many processing mechanisms distributed in several regions of the brain. Specific brain regions are not responsible for specific mental faculties but instead are *elementary processing units*. Perception, movement, language, thought, and memory are all made possible by the interlinkage of serial and parallel processing in discrete brain regions, each with specific functions. As a result, damage to a single area need not result in the complete loss of a cognitive function (or faculty) as many earlier neurologists believed. Even if a behavior initially disappears, it may partially return as undamaged parts of the brain reorganize their linkages.

Thus it is not accurate to think of a mental process as being mediated by a chain of nerve cells connected in series—one cell connected directly to the next—for in such an arrangement the entire process breaks down when a single connection is disrupted. A more realistic metaphor is that of a process consisting of several parallel pathways in a communications network that can interact and ultimately converge upon a common set of target cells. The malfunction of a single pathway affects the information carried by it but need not disrupt the entire system. The remaining parts of the system can modify their performance to accommodate the breakdown of one pathway.

Modular processing in the brain was slow to be accepted because, until recently, it was difficult to demonstrate which components of a mental operation a particular pathway or brain region represented. Nor is it easy to define mental operations in a manner that leads to testable hypotheses. Only during the last several decades, with the convergence of modern cognitive psychology and the brain sciences, have we begun to appreciate that all mental functions can be broken down into subfunctions.

To illustrate this point, consider how we learn, store, and recall information about objects, people, and events. Simple introspection suggests that we store each piece of our knowledge as a single representation that can be recalled by memory-jogging stimuli or even by the imagination alone. Everything you know about your grandmother, for example, seems to be stored in one complete representation that is equally accessible whether you see her in person, hear her voice, or simply think about her. Our experience, however, is not a faithful guide to how knowledge is stored in memory. Knowledge about grandmother is not stored as a single representation but rather is subdivided into distinct categories and stored separately. One region of the brain stores information about the invariant physical features that trigger your visual recognition of her.

Information about changeable aspects of her face—her expression and lip movements that relate to social communication—is stored in another region. The ability to recognize her voice is mediated in yet another region.

The most astonishing example of the modular organization of mental processes is the finding that our very sense of self—a self-aware coherent being, the sum of what we mean when we say "I"—is achieved through the connection of independent circuits in our two cerebral hemispheres, each mediating its own sense of awareness. The remarkable discovery that even consciousness is not a unitary process was made by Roger Sperry, Michael Gazzaniga, and Joseph Bogen in the course of studying patients in whom the corpus callosum—the major tract connecting the two cerebral hemispheres—was severed as a treatment for epilepsy. They found that each hemisphere had a consciousness that was able to function independently of the other.

Thus while one patient was reading a favorite book held in his left hand, the right hemisphere, which controls the left hand but cannot read, found that simply looking at the book was boring. The right hemisphere commanded the left hand to put the book down! Another patient would put on his clothes with the left hand while taking them off with the other. Each hemisphere has a mind of its own! In addition, the dominant hemisphere sometimes commented on the performance of the nondominant hemisphere, frequently manifesting a false sense of confidence regarding problems to which it could not know the solution, as the information was provided exclusively to the nondominant hemisphere.

Such studies have brought the study of consciousness to center stage in neural science. As we shall learn in Chapters 19, 20, and 61, consciousness, including self-consciousness, once the domain of philosophy, has been studied by neurobiologists such as Francis Crick, Christof Koch, Gerald Edelman, and Stanislas Dehaene. Neurobiologists do not concern themselves with the issue of subjectivity in conscious experience. Rather, they concentrate on understanding the neural correlates of consciousness—the pattern of neuronal activity associated with a specific conscious experience. Crick and Koch have focused on what they considered to be the simplest manifestation of consciousness: selective attention in visual perception. They believe a special and restricted population of neurons—perhaps only a few thousand cells—are responsible for this component. By contrast, Dehaene and Edelman believe that consciousness is a global property of the brain that involves vast numbers of nerve cells and a complex system of feed-forward broadcasting and feedback reentrant circuits.

As these examples illustrate, the main reason it has taken so long to appreciate which higher mental activities are mediated by particular regions of the brain is that we are dealing with biology's deepest riddle: the neural representation of consciousness and self-awareness. To be able to study the relationship between a mental process and specific brain regions, we must first identify the components of the mental process that we are attempting to explain. Of all behaviors, however, the higher mental processes are the most difficult to describe, to measure objectively, and to break down into elementary components. In addition, the brain's anatomy is immensely complex, and the structure and interconnections of its many parts are still not fully understood.

To analyze how a specific mental activity is processed in the brain, we must determine not only which aspects of the activity occur in which regions of the brain, but also how the mental activity is represented. Only in the last decade has this become possible. By combining the conceptual tools of cognitive psychology with new physiological techniques and brain-imaging methods, we are beginning to visualize the regions of the brain involved in particular behaviors. And we are beginning to discern how these behaviors can be described by a set of simpler mental operations and mapped to interconnected areas of the brain. Indeed, the excitement evident in neural science today stems from the conviction that at last we have the proper tools to explore empirically the organ of mental function and eventually to fathom the biological principles that underlie human behavior.

Eric R. Kandel
A. J. Hudspeth

Selected Readings

Bear DM. 1979. The temporal lobes: an approach to the study of organic behavioral changes. In: MS Gazzaniga (ed). *Handbook of Behavioral Neurobiology.* Vol. 2, *Neuropsychology,* pp. 75–95. New York: Plenum.

Caramazza A. 1995. The representation of lexical knowledge in the brain. In: RD Broadwell (ed). *Neuroscience, Memory, and Language.* Vol. 1, *Decade of the Brain,* pp. 133–147. Washington, DC: Library of Congress.

Churchland PS. 1986. *Neurophilosophy: Toward a Unified Science of the Mind-Brain.* Cambridge, MA: MIT Press.

Cooter R. 1984. *The Cultural Meaning of Popular Science: Phrenology and the Organization of Consent in Nineteenth-Century Britain.* Cambridge: Cambridge Univ. Press.

Cowan WM. 1981. Keynote. In: FO Schmitt, FG Worden, G Adelman, SG Dennis (eds). *The Organization of the Cerebral Cortex: Proceedings of a Neurosciences Research Program Colloquium*, pp. xi–xxi. Cambridge, MA: MIT Press.

Crick F, Koch C. 2003. A framework for consciousness. Nat Neurosci 6:119–126.

Edelman G. 2004. *Wider than the Sky: The Phenomenal Gift of Consciousness.* New Haven: Yale Univ. Press.

Ferrier D. 1890. *The Croonian Lectures on Cerebral Localisation.* London: Smith, Elder.

Geschwind N. 1974. *Selected Papers on Language and the Brain.* Dordrecht, Holland: Reidel.

Gregory RL. (ed). 1987. *The Oxford Companion to the Mind.* Oxford: Oxford Univ. Press.

Harrington A. 1987. *Medicine, Mind, and the Double Brain: A Study in Nineteenth-Century Thought.* Princeton, NJ: Princeton Univ. Press.

Harrison RG. 1935. On the origin and development of the nervous system studied by the methods of experimental embryology. Proc R Soc Lond B Biol Sci 118:155–196.

Jackson JH. 1884. The Croonian lectures on evolution and dissolution of the nervous system. Br Med J 1:591–593; 660–663; 703–707.

Kandel ER. 1976. The study of behavior: the interface between psychology and biology. In: *Cellular Basis of Behavior: An Introduction to Behavioral Neurobiology*, pp. 3–27. San Francisco: Freeman.

Kosslyn SM. 1988. Aspects of a cognitive neuroscience of mental imagery. Science 240:1621–1626.

Marshall JC. 1988. Cognitive neurophysiology: the lifeblood of language. Nature 331:560–561.

Marshall JC. 1988. Cognitive neuropsychology: sensation and semantics. Nature 334:378.

Ojemann GA. 1995. Investigating language during awake neurosurgery. In: RD Broadwell (ed). *Neuroscience, Memory, and Language.* Vol. 1, *Decade of the Brain*, pp. 117–131. Washington, DC: Library of Congress.

Petersen SE. 1995. Functional neuroimaging in brain areas involved in language. In: RD Broadwell (ed). *Neuroscience, Memory, and Language.* Vol. 1, *Decade of the Brain*, pp. 109–116. Washington DC: Library of Congress.

Posner MI, Petersen SE, Fox PT, Raichle ME. 1988. Localization of cognitive operations in the human brain. Science 240:1627–1631.

Ross ED. 1984. Right hemisphere's role in language, affective behavior and emotion. Trends Neurosci 7:342–346.

Shepherd GM. 1991. *Foundations of the Neuron Doctrine.* New York: Oxford Univ. Press.

Sperry RW. 1968. Mental unity following surgical disconnection of the cerebral hemispheres. Harvey Lect 62:293–323.

Young RM. 1990. *Mind, Brain and Adaptation in the Nineteenth Century.* New York: Oxford Univ. Press.

References

Adrian ED. 1941. Afferent discharges to the cerebral cortex from peripheral sense organs. J Physiol (Lond) 100: 159–191.

Bernard C. 1878–1879. *Leçons sur les Phénomènes de la vie Communs aux Animaux et aux Végétaux.* Vols. 1, 2. Paris: Baillière.

Boakes R. 1984. *From Darwin to Behaviourism: Psychology and the Minds of Animals.* Cambridge: Cambridge Univ. Press.

Broca P. 1865. Sur le siége de la faculté du langage articulé. Bull Soc Anthropol 6:377–393.

Brodmann K. 1909. *Vergleichende Lokalisationslehre der Grosshirnrinde in ihren Prinzipien dargestellt auf Grund des Zeelenbaues.* Leipzig: Barth.

Damasio H, Tranel D, Grabowski TJ, Adolphs R, Damasio AR. 2004. Neural systems behind word and concept retrieval. Cognition 92:179–229.

Darwin C. 1872. *The Expression of the Emotions in Man and Animals.* London: Murray.

Descartes R. [1649] 1984. *The Philosophical Writings of Descartes.* Cambridge: Cambridge Univ. Press.

DuBois-Reymond E. 1848–1849. *Untersuchungen über thierische Elektrizität.* Vols. 1, 2. Berlin: Reimer.

Ehrlich P. 1913. Chemotherapeutics: scientific principles, methods, and results. Lancet 2:445–451.

Flourens P. 1824. Recherches expérimentales. Archiv Méd 2:321–370; Cited and translated by P Flourens, JMD Olmsted. In: EA Underwood (ed). 1953. *Science, Medicine and History*, 2:290–302. London: Oxford Univ. Press.

Flourens P. 1824. *Recherches Expérimentales sur les Propriétés et les Fonctions du Système Nerveux, dans les Animaux Vertébrés.* Paris: Chez Crevot.

Fritsch G, Hitzig E. 1870. Über die elektrische Erregbarkeit des Grosshirns. Arch Anat Physiol Wiss Med, pp. 300–332; 1960. Reprinted in: G. von Bonin (transl). *Some Papers on the Cerebral Cortex*, pp. 73–96. Springfield, IL: Thomas.

Gall FJ, Spurzheim G. 1810. *Anatomie et Physiologie du Système Nerveux en Général, et du Cerveau en Particulier, avec des Observations sur la Possibilité de Reconnoître Plusieurs Dispositions Intellectuelles et Morales de l'Homme et des Animaux, par la Configuration de leurs Têtes.* Paris: Schoell.

Galvani L. [1791] 1953. *Commentary on the Effect of Electricity on Muscular Motion.* RM Green (transl). Cambridge, MA: Licht.

Gazzaniga MS, LeDoux JE. 1978. *The Integrated Mind.* New York: Plenum.

Geschwind N. 1979. Specializations of the human brain. Sci Am 241(3):180–199.

Goldstein K. 1948. *Language and Language Disturbances: Aphasic Symptom Complexes and Their Significance for Medicine and Theory of Language.* New York: Grune & Stratton.

Golgi C. [1906] 1967. The neuron doctrine: theory and facts. In: *Nobel Lectures: Physiology or Medicine, 1901–1921*, pp. 189–217. Amsterdam: Elsevier.

Head H. 1921. Release of function in the nervous system. Proc R Soc Lond B Biol Sci 92:184–209.

Head H. 1926. *Aphasia and Kindred Disorders of Speech.* Vols. 1, 2. Cambridge: Cambridge Univ. Press; 1963. Reprint. New York: Hafner.

Heilman KM, Scholes R, Watson RT. 1975. Auditory affective agnosia. Disturbed comprehension of affective speech. J Neurol Neurosurg Psychiatry 38:69–72.

Kim KSH, Relkin NR, Lee KM, Hirsch J. 1997. Distinct cortical areas associated with native and second languages. Nature 388: 171–174.

Krack P, Kumar R, Ardouin C, Dowsey PL, McVicker JM, Benabid A-L, Pollak P. 2001. Mirthful laughter induced by subthalamic nucleus stimulation. Mov Disord 16: 867–75.

Langley JN. 1906. On nerve endings and on special excitable substances in cells. Proc R Soc Lond B Biol Sci 78:170–194.

Lashley KS. 1929. *Brain Mechanisms and Intelligence: A Quantitative Study of Injuries to the Brain.* Chicago: Univ. Chicago Press.

Lashley KS, Clark G. 1946. The cytoarchitecture of the cerebral cortex of *Ateles:* a critical examination of architectonic studies. J Comp Neurol 85:223–305.

Locke J. 1690. *An Essay Concerning Human Understanding. In Four Books.* London: printed for T. Bassett.

Loeb J. 1918. *Forced Movements, Tropisms and Animal Conduct.* Philadelphia: Lippincott.

Marshall WH, Woolsey CN, Bard P. 1941. Observations on cortical somatic sensory mechanisms of cat and monkey. J Neurophysiol 4:1–24.

McCarthy RA, Warrington EK. 1988. Evidence for modality-specific meaning systems in the brain. Nature 334: 428–430.

Müller J. 1834–1840. *Handbuch der Physiologie des Menschen für Vorlesungen.* Vols. 1, 2. Coblenz: Hölscher.

Musso M, Moro A, Glanche V, Rijntes M, Reichenbach J, Büchel C, Weiler C. 2003. Broca's area and the language instinct. Nat Neurosci 6:774–781.

Nieuwenhuys R, Voogd J, van Huijzen, Chr. 1988. *The Human Central Nervous System: A Synopsis and Atlas,* 3rd rev. ed. Berlin: Springer.

Pavlov IP. 1927. *Conditioned Reflexes: An Investigation of the Physiological Activity of the Cerebral Cortex.* GV Anrep (transl). London: Oxford Univ. Press.

Penfield W. 1954. Mechanisms of voluntary movement. Brain 77:1–17.

Penfield W, Rasmussen T. 1950. *The Cerebral Cortex of Man: A Clinical Study of Localization of Function.* New York: Macmillan.

Penfield W, Roberts L. 1959. *Speech and Brain-Mechanisms.* Princeton, NJ: Princeton Univ. Press.

Petersen SE, Fox PT, Posner MI, Mintun M, Raichle ME. 1989. Positron emission tomographic studies of the processing of single words. J Cogn Neurosci 1:153–170.

Posner MI, Carr TH. 1992. Lexical access and the brain: anatomical constraints on cognitive models of word recognition. Am J Psychol 105:1–26.

Ramón y Cajal S. [1892] 1977. A new concept of the histology of the central nervous system. DA Rottenberg (transl). (See also historical essay by SL Palay, preceding Ramón y Cajal's paper.) In: DA Rottenberg, FH Hochberg (eds). *Neurological Classics in Modern Translation,* pp. 7–29. New York: Hafner.

Ramón y Cajal S. [1906] 1967. The structure and connexions of neurons. In: *Nobel Lectures: Physiology or Medicine, 1901–1921,* pp. 220–253. Amsterdam: Elsevier.

Ramón y Cajal S. [1908] 1954. *Neuron Theory or Reticular Theory? Objective Evidence of the Anatomical Unity of Nerve Cells.* MU Purkiss, CA Fox (transl). Madrid: Consejo Superior de Investigaciones Científicas Instituto Ramón y Cajal.

Ramón y Cajal S. 1937. *1852–1934. Recollections of My Life.* EH Craigie (transl). Philadelphia: American Philosophical Society; 1989. Reprint. Cambridge, MA: MIT Press.

Rose JE, Woolsey CN. 1948. Structure and relations of limbic cortex and anterior thalamic nuclei in rabbit and cat. J Comp Neurol 89:279–347.

Ross ED. 1981. The aprosodias: functional-anatomic organization of the affective components of language in the right hemisphere. Arch Neurol 38:561–569.

Sherrington C. 1947. *The Integrative Action of the Nervous System,* 2nd ed. Cambridge: Cambridge Univ. Press.

Spurzheim JG. 1825. *Phrenology, or the Doctrine of the Mind,* 3rd ed. London: Knight.

Swazey JP. 1970. Action proper and action commune: the localization of cerebral function. J Hist Biol 3:213–234.

von Helmholtz H. 1850. On the rate of transmission of the nerve impulse. Monatsber Preuss Akad Wiss Berlin, pp. 14–15. Translated in: W Dennis (ed). 1948. *Readings in the History of Psychology,* pp. 197–198. New York: Appleton-Century-Crofts.

Wernicke C. 1908. The symptom-complex of aphasia. In: A Church (ed). *Diseases of the Nervous System,* pp. 265–324. New York: Appleton.

Zurif E. 1974. Auditory lateralization, prosodic and syntactic factors. Brain Lang 1:391–401.

2

Nerve Cells, Neural Circuitry, and Behavior

THE REMARKABLE RANGE OF HUMAN behavior depends on a sophisticated array of sensory receptors connected to a highly flexible neural organ—the brain—that selects from among the stream of sensory signals those events in the environment that are important to the individual. In other words, the brain actively organizes perception, some of which is stored in memory for future reference, and some of which is transformed into immediate behavioral responses. All this is accomplished by interconnected nerve cells.

Individual nerve cells or neurons are the basic units of the brain. The human brain contains a huge number of these cells, on the order of 10^{11} neurons, that can be classified into at least a thousand different types. Yet the complexity of human behavior depends less on the variety of neurons than on their organization into anatomical circuits with precise functions. One key organizational principle of the brain, therefore, is that nerve cells with similar properties can produce different actions because of the way they are interconnected.

Because relatively few principles of organization give rise to considerable complexity, it is possible to learn a great deal about how the nervous system produces behavior by focusing on five basic features of the nervous system:

1. The structural components of individual nerve cells;
2. The mechanisms by which neurons produce signals within and between nerve cells;
3. The patterns of connections between nerve cells and between nerve cells and their targets: muscles and gland effectors;
4. The relationship of different patterns of interconnection to different types of behavior; and
5. How neurons and their connections are modified by experience

The various parts of this book are organized around these five major topics. In this chapter we provide an overview of the neural control of behavior by introducing these topics together. We first consider the structure and function of neurons and the glial cells that surround and support them. We then examine how individual cells organize and transmit signals and how signaling between a few interconnected nerve cells produces a simple behavior, the knee-jerk reflex. Finally, we consider how changes in signaling by specific cells can modify behavior.

The Nervous System Has Two Classes of Cells

There are two main classes of cells in the nervous system: nerve cells, or neurons, and glial cells, or glia.

Nerve Cells Are the Signaling Units of the Nervous System

A typical neuron has four morphologically defined regions: (1) the cell body, (2) dendrites, (3) axon, and (4) presynaptic terminals (Figure 2–1). As we shall see later, each region has a distinct role in generating signals and communicating with other nerve cells.

The cell body or *soma* is the metabolic center of the cell. It contains the nucleus, which contains the genes of the cell, and the endoplasmic reticulum, an extension of the nucleus where the cell's proteins are synthesized. The cell body usually gives rise to two kinds of processes: several short *dendrites* and one long, tubular *axon*. Dendrites branch out in tree-like fashion and are the main apparatus for receiving incoming signals from other nerve cells. The axon typically extends some distance from the cell body and carries signals to other neurons. An axon can convey electrical signals over distances ranging from 0.1 mm to 2 m. These electrical signals, called *action potentials,* are initiated at a specialized trigger region near the origin of the axon

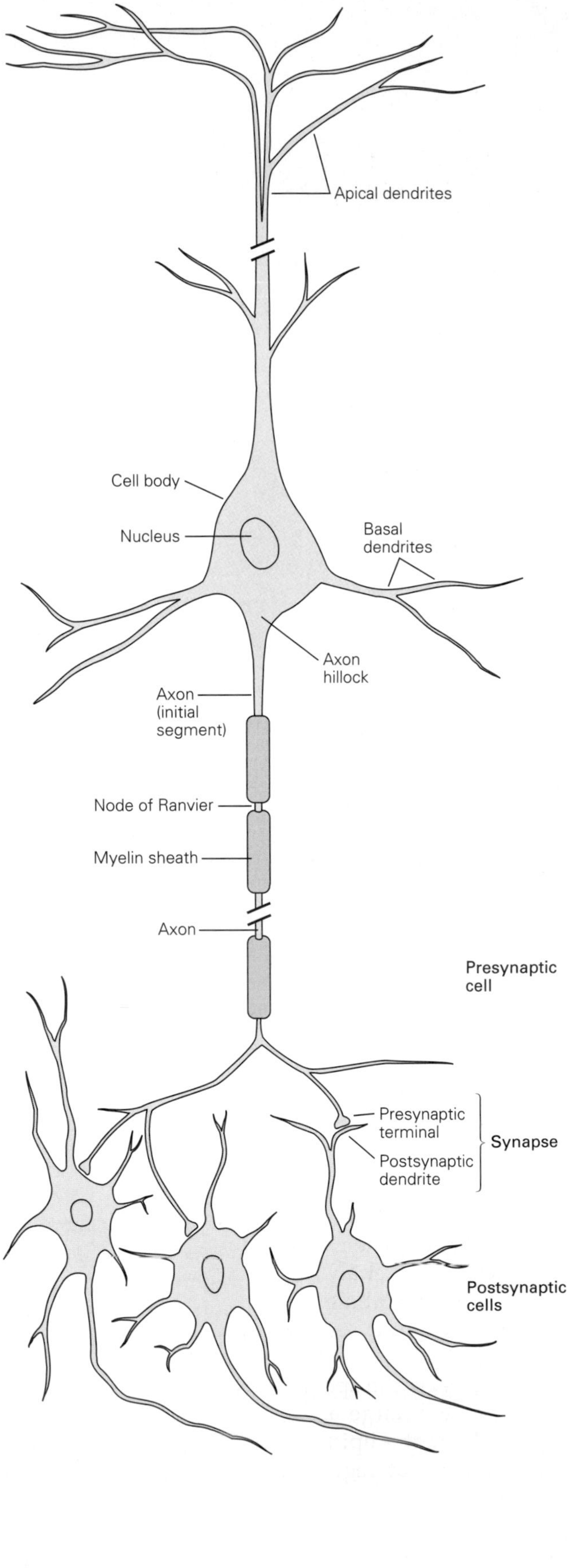

Figure 2–1 The structure of a neuron. Most neurons in the vertebrate nervous system have several main features in common. The cell body contains the nucleus, the storehouse of genetic information, and gives rise to two types of cell processes: axons and dendrites. Axons are the transmitting element of neurons; they vary greatly in length, some extending more than 2 m within the body. Most axons in the central nervous system are very thin (between 0.2 μm and 20 μm in diameter) compared with the diameter of the cell body (50 μm or more). Many axons are insulated by a sheath of fatty myelin that is regularly interrupted at gaps called the nodes of Ranvier. The action potential, the cell's conducting signal, is initiated at the initial segment of the axon and propagates to the synapse, the site at which signals flow from one neuron to another. Branches of the axon of the presynaptic neuron transmit signals to the postsynaptic cell. The branches of a single axon may form synapses with as many as 1,000 postsynaptic neurons. The apical and basal dendrites together with the cell body are the input elements of the neuron, receiving signals from other neurons.

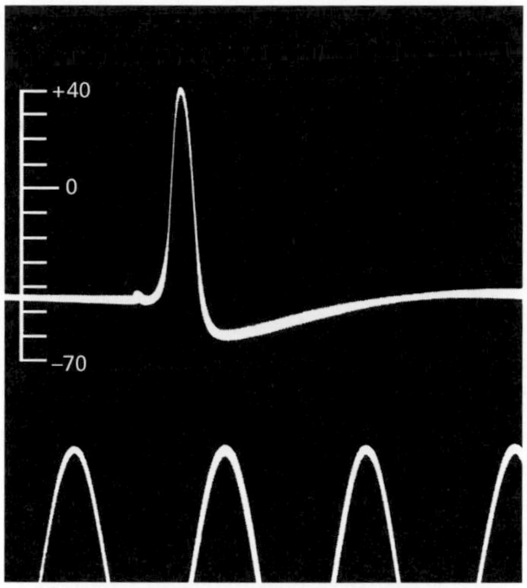

Figure 2–2 This historic tracing is the first published intracellular recording of an action potential. It was recorded in 1939 by Hodgkin and Huxley from a squid giant axon, using glass capillary electrodes filled with sea water. The timing pulses are separated by 2 ms. The vertical scale indicates the potential of the internal electrode in millivolts, the sea water outside being taken as zero potential. (Reproduced, with permission, from Hodgkin and Huxley 1939.)

called the *initial segment* from which they propagate down the axon without failure or distortion at speeds of 1 to 100 m/s. The amplitude of an action potential traveling down the axon remains constant at 100 mV because the action potential is an all-or-none impulse that is regenerated at regular intervals along the axon (Figure 2–2).

Action potentials are the signals by which the brain receives, analyzes, and conveys information. These signals are highly stereotyped throughout the nervous system, even though they are initiated by a great variety of events in the environment that impinge on our bodies—from light to mechanical contact, from odorants to pressure waves. The signals that convey information about vision are identical to those that carry information about odors. Here we see a key principle of brain function: the information conveyed by an action potential is determined not by the form of the signal but by the pathway the signal travels in the brain. The brain analyzes and interprets patterns of incoming electrical signals and their pathways, and in turn creates our sensations of sight, touch, smell, and sound.

To increase the speed by which action potentials are conducted, large axons are wrapped in an insulating sheath of a lipid substance, *myelin*. The sheath is interrupted at regular intervals by the nodes of Ranvier, uninsulated spots on the axon where the action potential is regenerated. We shall learn more about myelination in Chapter 4 and about action potentials in Chapter 7.

Near its end the axon divides into fine branches that contact other neurons at specialized zones of communication known as *synapses*. The nerve cell transmitting a signal is called the *presynaptic cell*; the cell receiving the signal is the *postsynaptic cell*. The presynaptic cell transmits signals from specialized enlarged regions of its axon's branches, called *presynaptic terminals* or *nerve terminals*. The presynaptic and postsynaptic cells are separated by a very narrow space, the *synaptic cleft*. Most presynaptic terminals end on the postsynaptic neuron's dendrites; but the terminals may also terminate on the cell body or, less often, at the beginning or end of the axon of the receiving cell (see Figure 2–1).

As we saw in Chapter 1, Ramón y Cajal provided much of the early evidence for the neuron doctrine, the principle that each neuron is a discrete cell with distinctive processes arising from its cell body and that neurons are the signaling units of the nervous system. In retrospect it is hard to appreciate how difficult it was to persuade scientists of this elementary idea. Unlike other tissues, whose cells have simple shapes and fit into a single field of the light microscope, nerve cells have complex shapes. The elaborate patterns of dendrites and the seemingly endless course of some axons initially made it extremely difficult to establish a relationship between these elements. Even after the anatomists Jacob Schleiden and Theodor Schwann put forward the cell theory in the early 1830s—and the idea that cells are the structural units of all living matter became a central dogma of biology—most anatomists did not accept that the cell theory applied to the brain, which they thought of as a continuous, web-like reticulum of very thin processes.

The coherent structure of the neuron did not become clear until late in the 19th century, when Ramón y Cajal began to use the silver-staining method introduced by Golgi. Still used today, this method has two advantages. First, in a random manner that is not understood, the silver solution stains only about 1% of the cells in any particular brain region, making it possible to examine a single neuron in isolation from its neighbors. Second, the neurons that do take up the stain are delineated in their entirety, including the cell body, axon, and full dendritic tree. The stain reveals that there is no cytoplasmic continuity between neurons, even at synapses between two cells.

Ramón y Cajal applied Golgi's method to the embryonic nervous systems of many animals as well as humans.

By examining the structure of neurons in almost every region of the nervous system, he could describe classes of nerve cells and map the precise connections between many of them. In this way Ramón y Cajal adduced, in addition to the neuron doctrine, two other principles of neural organization that would prove particularly valuable in studying communication in the nervous system.

The first of these has come to be known as the *principle of dynamic polarization.* It states that electrical signals within a nerve cell flow only in one direction: from the receiving sites of the neuron, usually the dendrites and cell body, to the trigger region at the axon. From there the action potential is propagated along the entire length of the axon to its terminals. In most neurons studied to date electrical signals in fact travel in one direction. Later in this chapter we describe the physiological basis of this principle.

The other principle advanced by Ramón y Cajal is that of *connectional specificity,* which states that nerve cells do not connect randomly with one another in the formation of networks. Rather each cell makes specific connections—at particular contact points—with certain postsynaptic target cells but not with others. The principles of dynamic polarization and connectional specificity are the basis of the modern connectionist approach to studying the brain.

Ramón y Cajal was also among the first to realize that the feature that most distinguishes one type of neuron from another is form, specifically the number of the processes arising from the cell body. Neurons are thus classified into three large groups: unipolar, bipolar, and multipolar.

Unipolar neurons are the simplest because they have a single primary process, which usually gives rise to many branches. One branch serves as the axon; other branches function as receiving structures (Figure 2–3A). These cells predominate in the nervous systems of invertebrates; in vertebrates they occur in the autonomic nervous system.

Bipolar neurons have an oval soma that gives rise to two distinct processes: a dendritic structure that receives signals from the periphery of the body and an axon that carries information toward the central nervous system (Figure 2–3B). Many sensory cells are bipolar, including those in the retina and in the olfactory epithelium of the nose. The receptor neurons that convey touch, pressure, and pain signals to the spinal cord, are variants of bipolar cells called *pseudo-unipolar* cells. These cells develop initially as bipolar cells but the two cell processes fuse into a single continuous structure that emerges from a single point in the cell body. The axon splits into two branches, one running to the periphery (to sensory receptors in the skin, joints, and muscle) and another to the spinal cord (Figure 2–3C).

Multipolar neurons predominate in the nervous system of vertebrates. They typically have a single axon and many dendritic structures emerging from various points around the cell body (Figure 2–3D). Multipolar cells vary greatly in shape, especially in the length of their axons and in the extent, dimensions, and intricacy of their dendritic branching. Usually the extent of branching correlates with the number of synaptic contacts that other neurons make onto them. A spinal motor neuron with a relatively modest number of dendrites receives about 10,000 contacts—1,000 on the cell body and 9,000 on dendrites. The dendritic tree of a Purkinje cell in the cerebellum is much larger and bushier, receiving as many as a million contacts!

Nerve cells are also classified into three major functional categories: sensory neurons, motor neurons, and interneurons. Sensory neurons carry information from the body's peripheral sensors into the nervous system for the purpose of both perception and motor coordination. Some primary sensory neurons are called afferent neurons, and the two terms are used interchangeably. The term *afferent* (carried toward the central nervous system) applies to all information reaching the central nervous system from the periphery, whether or not this information leads to sensation. The term *sensory* should, strictly speaking, be applied only to afferent inputs that lead to perception. Motor neurons carry commands from the brain or spinal cord to muscles and glands (efferent information). Interneurons are the most numerous and are subdivided into two classes: relay and local. Relay or projection interneurons have long axons and convey signals over considerable distances, from one brain region to another. Local interneurons have short axons because they form connections with nearby neurons in local circuits.

Each functional classification can be subdivided further. Sensory system interneurons can be classified according to the type of sensory stimuli to which they respond; these initial classifications can be broken down still further, into many subgroups according to location, density, and size. For example, the retinal ganglion cell interneurons, which respond to light, are classified into 13 types based on the size of the dendritic tree, the branching density, and the depth of its location in specific layers of the retina (Figure 2–4).

Glial Cells Support Nerve Cells

Glial cells greatly outnumber neurons—there are 2 to 10 times more glia than neurons in the vertebrate central nervous system. The name for these cells derives

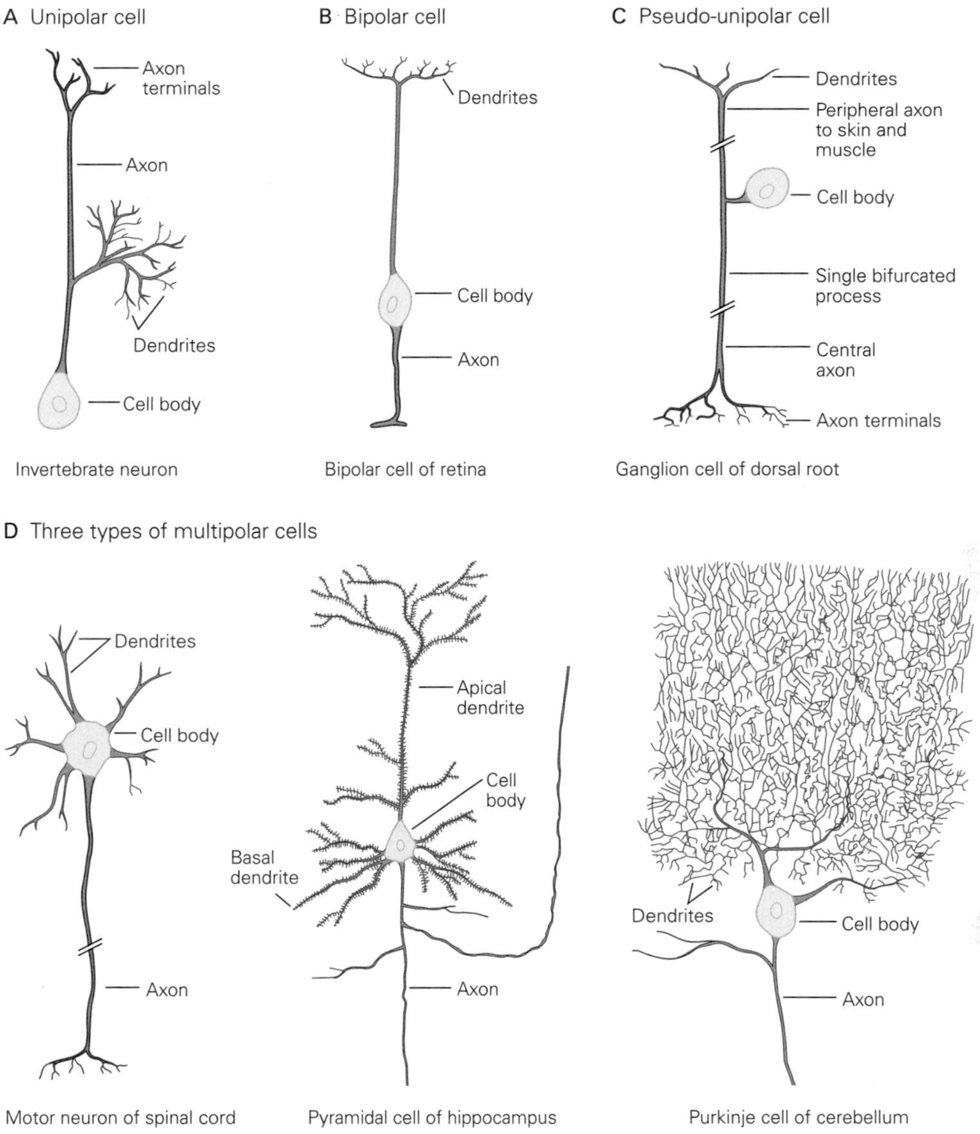

Figure 2–3 Neurons are classified as unipolar, bipolar, or multipolar according to the number of processes that originate from the cell body.

A. Unipolar cells have a single process emanating from the cell. Different segments serve as receptive surfaces or releasing terminals. Unipolar cells are characteristic of the invertebrate nervous system.

B. Bipolar cells have two types of processes that are functionally specialized. The dendrite receives electrical signals and the axon transmits signals to other cells.

C. Pseudo-unipolar cells are variants of bipolar cells that carry somatosensory information to the spinal cord. During development the two processes of the embryonic bipolar cell fuse and emerge from the cell body as a single process that has two functionally distinct segments. Both segments function as axons; one extends to peripheral skin or muscle, the other to the central spinal cord. (Adapted, with permission, from Ramón y Cajal 1933.)

D. Multipolar cells have a single axon and many dendrites. They are the most common type of neuron in the mammalian nervous system. Three examples illustrate the large diversity of these cells. Spinal motor neurons innervate skeletal muscle fibers. Pyramidal cells have a roughly triangular cell body; dendrites emerge from both the apex (the apical dendrite) and the base (the basal dendrites). Pyramidal cells are found in the hippocampus and throughout the cerebral cortex. Purkinje cells of the cerebellum are characterized by a rich and extensive dendritic tree that accommodates an enormous synaptic input. (Adapted, with permission, from Ramón y Cajal 1933.)

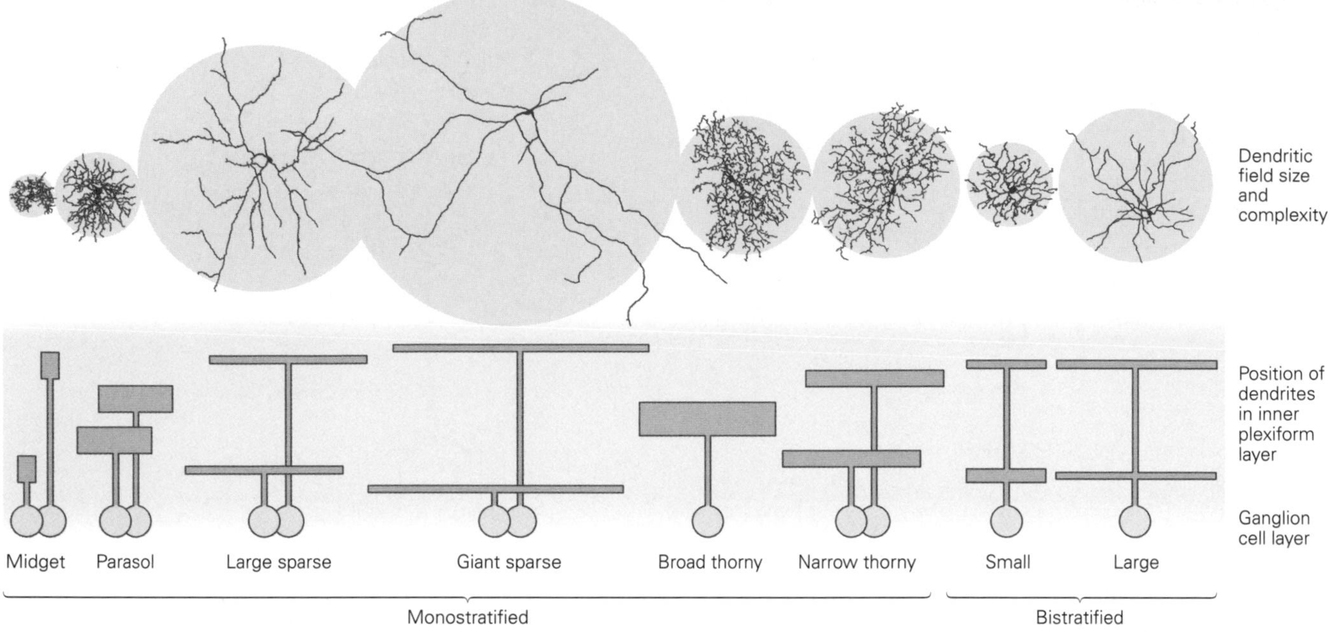

Figure 2–4 Sensory neurons can be subdivided into functionally distinct groups. Photodynamic staining distinguishes 13 types of retinal ganglion cells on the basis of their dendritic shape and depth of position in the retina. (Reproduced, with permission, from Dacey et al. 2003.)

from the Greek for glue, but glia do not commonly hold nerve cells together. Rather, they surround the cell bodies, axons, and dendrites of neurons. Glia differ from neurons morphologically; they do not form dendrites and axons. Glia also differ functionally. Although they arise from the same embryonic precursor cells, they do not have the same membrane properties as neurons; are not electrically excitable; and are not directly involved in electrical signaling, which is the function of nerve cells.

There are many kinds of glial cells. As we will discuss in Chapter 4, the diversity in morphology of glial cells suggests that glia are probably as heterogeneous as neurons. Nonetheless, glia in the vertebrate nervous system can be divided into two major classes: microglia and macroglia. Microglia are immune system cells that are mobilized to present antigens and become phagocytes during injury, infection, or degenerative diseases. There are three main types of macroglia: oligodendrocytes, Schwann cells, and astrocytes. In the human brain about 80% of all the cells are macroglia. Of these, approximately half are oligodendrocytes and half are astrocytes.

Oligodendrocytes and Schwann cells are small cells with relatively few processes. Both cells form the myelin sheath that insulates an axon by tightly winding their membranous processes around the axon in a spiral. Oligodendrocytes are found in the central nervous system; each cell envelops from one to 30 axonal segments (called internodes), depending on axon diameter (Figure 2–5A). Schwann cells occur in the peripheral nervous system, where each envelops a single segment of one axon (Figure 2–5B). Upon myelination, oligodendrocytes and Schwann cells influence axons by enhancing signal conduction and by segregating voltage-sensitive ion channels into distinct axonal domains (called node of Ranvier).

Astrocytes, the third main class of glial cells, owe their name to their irregular, roughly star-shaped cell bodies and large numbers of processes (Figure 2–5C). They comprise two major types. Protoplasmic astrocytes are found in the gray matter; their many processes end in sheet-like appendages. Fibrous astrocytes are found in the white matter and have long, fine processes that contain large bundles of tightly packed intermediate filaments. Both types of astrocytes have end-feet, dilatations that contact and surround capillaries and arterioles throughout the brain (Figure 2–5C). The sheet-like processes of protoplasmic astrocytes envelop nerve cell bodies and synapses, whereas the end-feet of fibrous astrocytes contact axons at the nodes of Ranvier.

The functions of astrocytes are still mysterious. It is generally thought that astrocytes are not essential

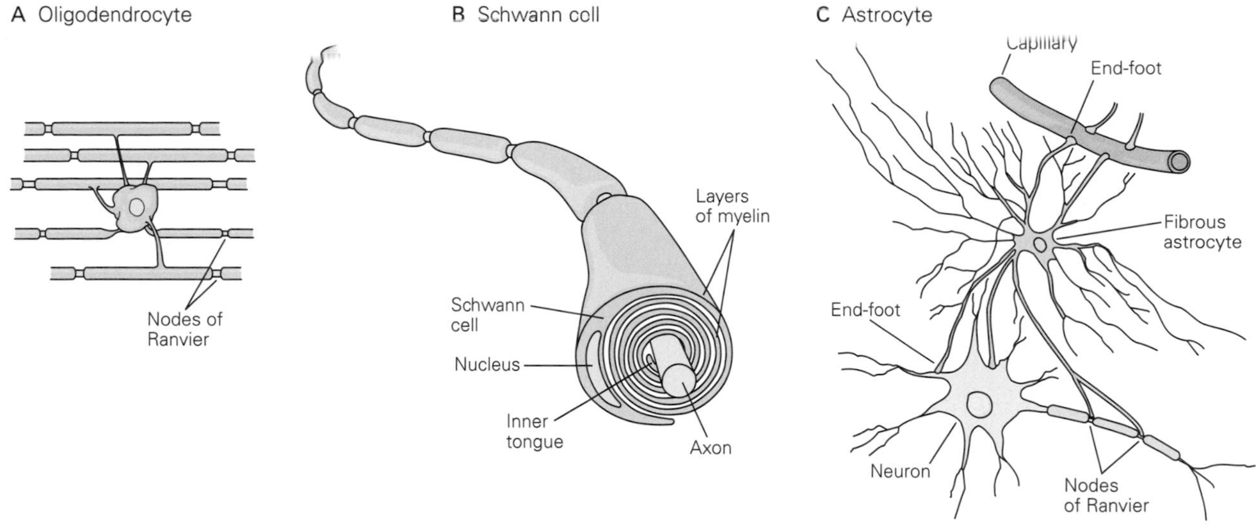

Figure 2–5 The principal types of glial cells are oligodendrocytes and astrocytes in the central nervous system and Schwann cells in the peripheral nervous system.

A. Oligodendrocytes are small cells with relatively few processes. In the white matter of the brain, as shown here, they provide the myelin sheaths that insulate axons. A single oligodendrocyte can wrap its membranous processes around many axons. In the gray matter perineural oligodendrocytes surround and support the cell bodies of neurons.

B. Schwann cells furnish the myelin sheaths for axons in the peripheral nervous system. During development several Schwann cells are positioned along the length of a single axon. Each cell forms a myelin sheath approximately 1 mm long between two nodes of Ranvier. The sheath is formed as the inner tongue of the Schwann cell turns around the axon several times, wrapping the axon in layers of membrane. In actuality the layers of myelin are more compact than what is shown here. (Adapted, with permission, from Alberts et al. 2002.)

C. Astrocytes, a major class of glial cells in the central nervous system, are characterized by their star-like shape and the broad end-feet on their processes. Because these end-feet put the astrocyte into contact with both capillaries and neurons, astrocytes are thought to have a nutritive function. Astrocytes also play an important role in maintaining the blood-brain barrier (See Appendix D).

for information processing but support neurons in four ways:

1. Astrocytes separate cells, thereby insulating neuronal groups and synaptic connections from each other.
2. Because astrocytes are highly permeable to K^+, they help regulate the K^+ concentration in the space between neurons. As we shall learn below, K^+ flows out of neurons when they fire. Repetitive firing may create excess extracellular K^+ that could interfere with signaling between cells in the vicinity. Astrocytes can take up the excess K^+ and thus maintain the efficiency of signaling between neurons.
3. Astrocytes perform other important housekeeping chores that promote efficient signaling between neurons. For example, as we shall learn later, they take up neurotransmitters from synaptic zones after release.
4. Astrocytes help nourish surrounding neurons by releasing growth factors.

Although glial cells do not generate action potentials, they have recently been found to participate in neuron-glial signaling processes. The significance of this signaling is still poorly understood, but it may actively help regulate synapse development and function (Chapter 4).

Each Nerve Cell Is Part of a Circuit That Has One or More Specific Behavioral Functions

Every behavior is mediated by specific sets of interconnected neurons, and every neuron's behavioral function is determined by its connections with other neurons. We can illustrate this with a simple behavior, the knee-jerk reflex. The reflex is initiated when a transient imbalance of the body stretches the quadriceps extensor muscles of the leg. This stretching elicits sensory information that is conveyed to motor neurons, which in turn sends commands to the extensor muscles to contract so that balance is restored. This reflex is useful for clinically, but the underlying mechanism is important because it continuously maintains normal tone in the quadriceps and prevents our knees from buckling when we stand or walk.

The tendon of the quadriceps femoris, an extensor muscle that moves the lower leg, is attached to the tibia through the tendon of the kneecap. Tapping this tendon just below the patella stretches the quadriceps femoris. This stretch initiates reflex contraction of the quadriceps muscle to produce the familiar knee jerk. By increasing the tension of a select group of muscles, the stretch reflex changes the position of the leg, suddenly extending it outward (Figure 2–6).

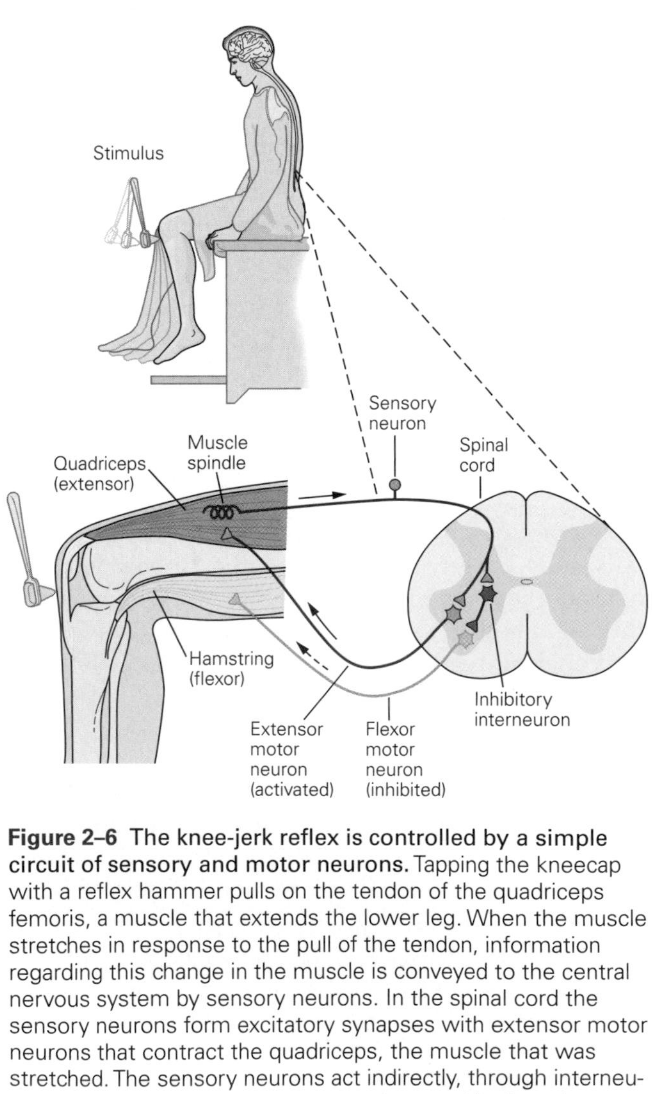

Figure 2–6 The knee-jerk reflex is controlled by a simple circuit of sensory and motor neurons. Tapping the kneecap with a reflex hammer pulls on the tendon of the quadriceps femoris, a muscle that extends the lower leg. When the muscle stretches in response to the pull of the tendon, information regarding this change in the muscle is conveyed to the central nervous system by sensory neurons. In the spinal cord the sensory neurons form excitatory synapses with extensor motor neurons that contract the quadriceps, the muscle that was stretched. The sensory neurons act indirectly, through interneurons, to inhibit flexor motor neurons that would otherwise contract the opposing muscle, the hamstring. These actions combine to produce the reflex behavior. In the drawing each extensor and flexor motor neuron represents a population of many cells.

The cell bodies of the sensory neurons involved in the knee-jerk reflex are clustered near the spinal cord in the dorsal root ganglia. They are pseudo-unipolar cells; one branch of each cell's axon runs to the quadriceps muscle at the periphery, whereas the other runs centrally into the spinal cord. The branch that innervates the quadriceps makes contact with stretch-sensitive receptors (muscle spindles) and is excited when the muscle is stretched. The branch reaching the spinal cord forms excitatory connections with the motor neurons that innervate the quadriceps and control its contraction. This branch also contacts local interneurons that *inhibit* the motor neurons controlling the opposing flexor muscles (Figure 2–6). These local interneurons are not involved in producing the stretch reflex itself, but by coordinating motor action they increase the stability of the reflex. Thus the electrical signals that produce the stretch reflex carry four kinds of information:

1. Sensory information is conveyed to the central nervous system (the spinal cord) from muscle.
2. Motor commands from the central nervous system are issued to the muscles that carry out the knee jerk.
3. Inhibitory commands are issued to motor neurons that innervate opposing muscles, providing coordination of muscle action.
4. Information about local neuronal activity related to the knee jerk is sent to higher centers of the central nervous system, permitting the brain to coordinate different behaviors either simultaneously or in series.

The stretching of just one muscle, the quadriceps, activates several hundred sensory neurons, each of which makes direct contact with 45 to 50 motor neurons. This pattern of connection, in which one neuron activates many target cells, is called *divergence* (Figure 2–7A). It is especially common in the input stages of the nervous system; by distributing its signals to many target cells, a single neuron can exert wide and diverse influence. Conversely, a single motor cell in the knee jerk circuit receives 200 to 450 input contacts from approximately 130 sensory cells. This pattern of connection is called *convergence* (Figure 2–7B). It is common at the output stages of the nervous system; a target motor cell that receives information from many sensory neurons is able to integrate information from many sources. Convergence also ensures that a motor neuron is activated only if a sufficient number of sensory neurons become activated together.

A stretch reflex such as the knee-jerk reflex is a simple behavior produced by two classes of neurons

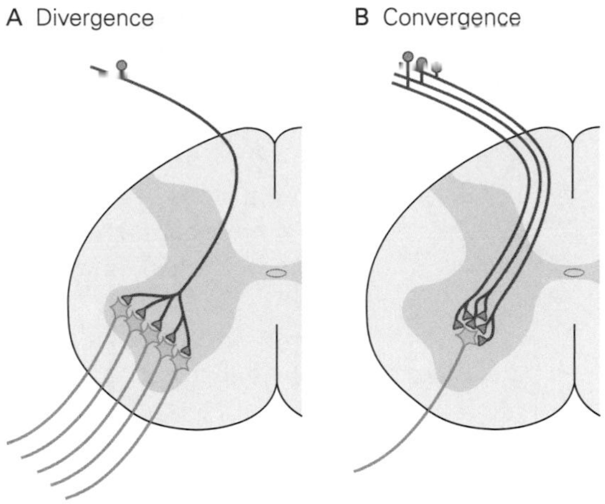

Figure 2–7 **Diverging and converging neuronal connections are a key organizational feature of the brain.**

A. In the sensory systems each receptor neuron usually contacts several neurons that represent the second stage of processing. At subsequent processing stages the incoming connections diverge even more. This allows sensory information from a single site to be distributed more widely in the spinal cord and brain.

B. By contrast, motor neurons are the targets of progressively converging connections. With this arrangement input from many presynaptic cells is required to activate the motor neuron.

Signaling Is Organized in the Same Way in All Nerve Cells

To produce a behavior, a stretch reflex for example, each participating sensory and motor nerve cell must generate four different signals in sequence, each at different site within the cell: an input signal, a trigger signal, a conducting signal, and an output signal. Regardless of cell size and shape, transmitter biochemistry, or behavioral function, almost all neurons can be described by a model neuron that has four functional

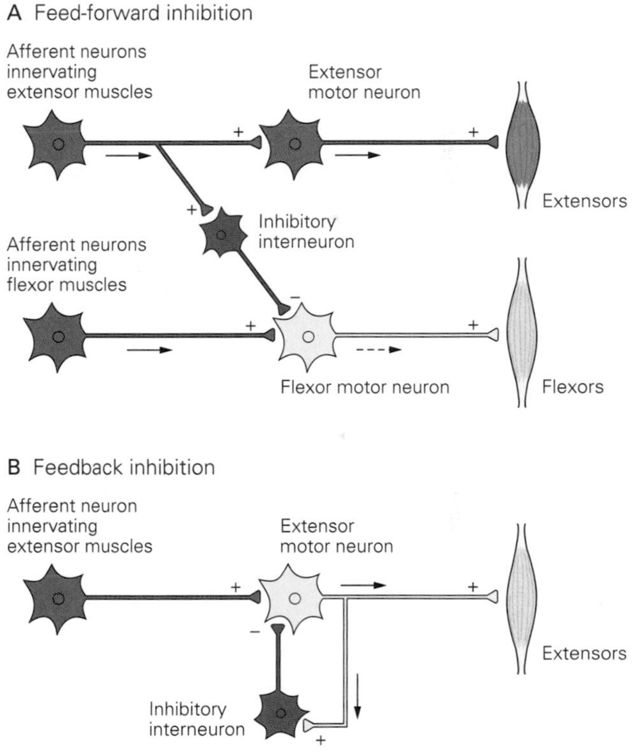

Figure 2–8 **Inhibitory interneurons can produce either feed-forward or feedback inhibition.**

A. Feed-forward inhibition enhances the effect of the active pathway by suppressing the activity of pathways mediating opposing actions. Feed-forward inhibition is common in monosynaptic reflex systems. For example, in the knee-jerk reflex circuit (Figure 2–6) afferent neurons from extensor muscles excite not only the extensor motor neurons but also inhibitory interneurons that prevent the firing of the motor cells innervating the opposing flexor muscles.

B. Feedback inhibition is a self-regulating mechanism. Here extensor motor neurons act on inhibitory interneurons that in turn act on the extensor motor neurons themselves and thus reduce their probability of firing. The effect is to dampen activity within the stimulated pathway and prevent it from exceeding a certain critical level.

connecting at excitatory synapses. But not all important signals in the brain are excitatory. Many neurons produce inhibitory signals that reduce the likelihood of firing. Even in the simple knee-jerk reflex the sensory neurons make both excitatory and inhibitory connections. Excitatory connections in the leg's extensor muscles cause these muscles to contract, whereas connections with inhibitory interneurons prevent the antagonist flexor muscles from contracting. This feature of the circuit is an example of *feed-forward inhibition* (Figure 2–8A). In the knee-jerk reflex, feed-forward inhibition is *reciprocal*, ensuring that the flexor and extensor pathways always inhibit each other so that only muscles appropriate for the movement and not those opposed to it are recruited.

Neurons can also have connections that provide *feedback inhibition*. For example, a motor neuron may have excitatory connections with both a muscle and an inhibitory interneuron that in turn inhibits the motor neuron. The inhibitory interneuron is thus able to limit the ability of the motor neuron to excite the muscle (Figure 2–8B). We will encounter many examples of feed-forward and feedback inhibition when we examine more complex behaviors in later chapters.

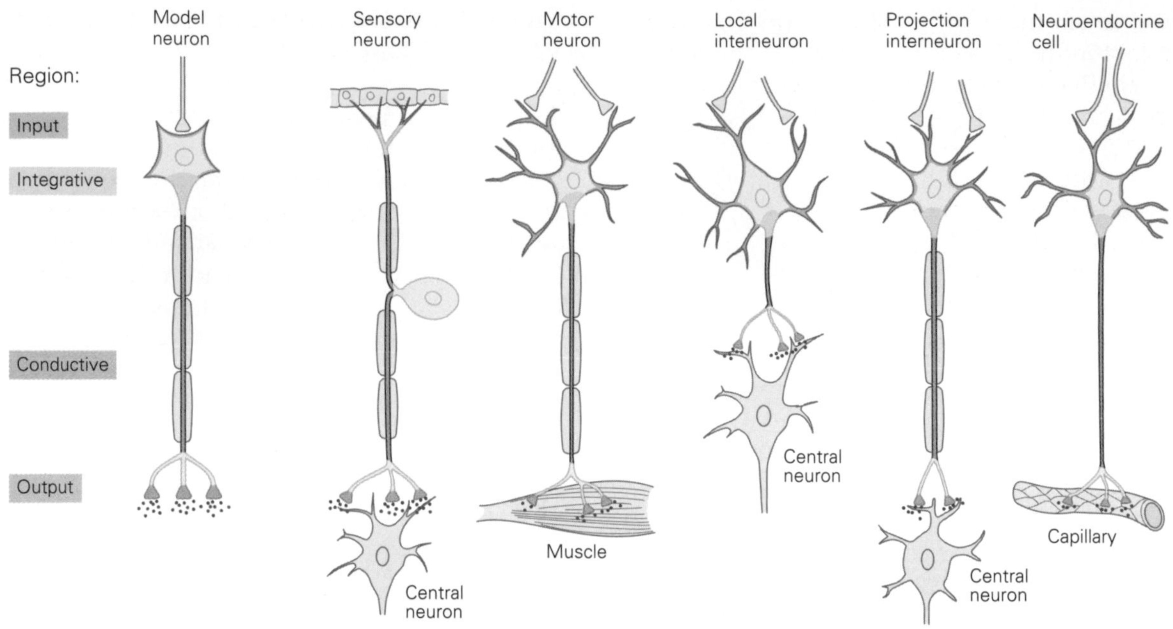

Figure 2–9 Most neurons, regardless of type, have four functional regions in which different types of signals are generated. Thus the functional organization of most neurons can be represented schematically by a model neuron. The input, integrative, and conductive signals are all electrical and integral to the cell, whereas the output signal is a chemical substance ejected by the cell into the synaptic cleft. Not all neurons share all these features; for example, local interneurons often lack a conductive component.

components that generate the four types of signals: a receptive component, a summing or integrative component, a long-range signaling component, and a secretory component (Figure 2–9). This model neuron is the physiological expression of Ramón y Cajal's principle of dynamic polarization.

The different types of signals generated in a neuron are determined in part by the electrical properties of the cell membrane. Every cell, including a neuron, maintains a certain difference in the electrical potential on either side of the plasma membrane when the cell is at rest. This is called the *resting membrane potential*. In a typical resting neuron the voltage of the inside of the cell is about 65 mV more negative than the voltage outside the cell. Because the voltage outside the membrane is defined as zero, we say the resting membrane potential is –65 mV. The resting potential in different nerve cells ranges from –40 to –80 mV; in muscle cells it is greater still, about –90 mV. As we shall see in Chapter 6, the resting membrane potential results from two factors: the unequal distribution of electrically charged ions, in particular the positively charged Na^+ and K^+ ions, and the selective permeability of the membrane.

The unequal distribution of positively charged ions on either side of the cell membrane is maintained by two main mechanisms. Intracellular Na^+ and K^+ concentrations are largely controlled by a membrane protein that actively pumps Na^+ out of the cell and K^+ back into it. This *Na^+-K^+ pump,* about which we shall learn more in Chapter 6, keeps the Na^+ concentration in the cell low (about one-tenth the concentration outside the cell) and the K^+ concentration high (about 20 times the concentration outside). The extracellular concentrations of Na^+ and K^+ are maintained by the kidneys.

The cell membrane is selectively permeable to K^+ because the otherwise impermeable membrane contains proteins that form pores called *ion channels.* The channels that are active when the cell is at rest are highly permeable to K^+ but considerably less permeable to Na^+. The K^+ ions tend to leak out of these open channels, down the ion's concentration gradient. As K^+ ions exit the cell, they leave behind a cloud of unneutralized negative charge on the inner surface of the membrane, so that the net charge inside the membrane is more negative than that outside.

A cell, such as nerve and muscle, is said to be excitable when its membrane potential can be quickly and significantly altered. This change serves as a signaling mechanism. In some neurons reducing the membrane potential by 10 mV (from –65 to –55 mV) makes the membrane much more permeable to Na^+ than to K^+. The resultant influx of positively charged Na^+ neutralizes the negative charge inside the cell and causes a brief and explosive change in membrane potential to +40 mV. This *action potential* is conducted down the cell's axon to the axon's terminal, where it initiates an elaborate chemical communication with other neurons or muscle cells. The action potential is actively propagated along the axon so that its amplitude does not diminish by the time it reaches the axon terminal. An action potential typically lasts approximately 1 ms, after which the membrane returns to its resting state, with its normal separation of charges and higher permeability to K^+ than to Na^+.

We shall learn more about the mechanisms underlying the resting potential and action potential in Chapters 6 to 7. In addition to the long distance signals represented by the action potential, nerve cells also produce local signals—receptor potentials and synaptic potentials—that are not actively propagated and that typically decay within just a few millimeters.

The change in membrane potential that generates long-range and local signals can be either a decrease or an increase from the resting potential. The resting membrane potential therefore provides the baseline on which all signaling occurs. A reduction in membrane potential is called *depolarization*. Because depolarization enhances a cell's ability to generate an action potential, it is excitatory. In contrast, an increase in membrane potential is called *hyperpolarization*. Hyperpolarization makes a cell less likely to generate an action potential and is therefore inhibitory.

The Input Component Produces Graded Local Signals

In most neurons at rest no current flows from one part of the cell to another, so the resting potential is the same throughout. In sensory neurons current flow is typically initiated by a physical stimulus, which activates specialized receptor proteins at the neuron's receptive surface. In our example of the knee-jerk reflex, stretching of the muscle activates specific ion channels that open in response to stretch of the sensory neuron membrane, as we shall learn in Chapter 5. The opening of these channels when the cell is stretched permits the rapid influx of Na^+ ions into the sensory cell. This ionic current changes the membrane potential, producing a local signal called the *receptor potential*.

The amplitude and duration of a receptor potential depend on the intensity of the muscle stretch: The larger or longer-lasting the stretch, the larger or longer-lasting the resulting receptor potential (Figure 2–10A). Thus, unlike the action potential, which is all or none, receptor potentials are graded. Most receptor potentials are depolarizing (excitatory). However, hyperpolarizing (inhibitory) receptor potentials are found in the retina.

The receptor potential is the first representation of stretch to be coded in the nervous system. This signal spreads passively, however, and therefore does not travel much farther than 1 to 2 mm. In fact, 1 mm down the axon the amplitude of the signal is only about one-third what it was at the site of generation. To be carried successfully to the central nervous system, the local signal must be amplified—it must generate an action potential. In the knee-jerk reflex the receptor potential in the sensory neuron must reach the first node of Ranvier in the axon. If it is large enough, the signal triggers an action potential that then propagates without failure to the axon terminals in the spinal cord (Figure 2–10C). At the synapse between the sensory neuron and a motor neuron, the action potential produces a chain of events that results in an input signal to the motor neuron.

In the knee-jerk reflex the action potential in the presynaptic terminal of the sensory neuron initiates the release of a chemical substance, or neurotransmitter, into the synaptic cleft (Figure 2–10D). After diffusing across the cleft, the transmitter binds to receptor proteins in the postsynaptic membrane of the motor neuron, thereby directly or indirectly opening ion channels. The ensuing flow of current alters the membrane potential of the motor cell, a change called the *synaptic potential*.

Like the receptor potential, the synaptic potential is graded; its amplitude depends on how much transmitter is released. In the same cell the synaptic potential can be either depolarizing or hyperpolarizing depending on the type of receptor molecule that is activated. Synaptic potentials, like receptor potentials, spread passively and thus are local changes in potential unless the signal reaches beyond the axon's initial segment and thus can give rise to an action potential. The features of receptor and synaptic potentials are summarized in Table 2–1.

The Trigger Zone Makes the Decision to Generate an Action Potential

Sherrington first pointed out that the function of the nervous system is to weigh the consequences of different types of information and then decide on appropriate responses. This *integrative* function of the nervous system is clearly seen in the actions of the trigger zone of the neuron, the initial segment of the axon.

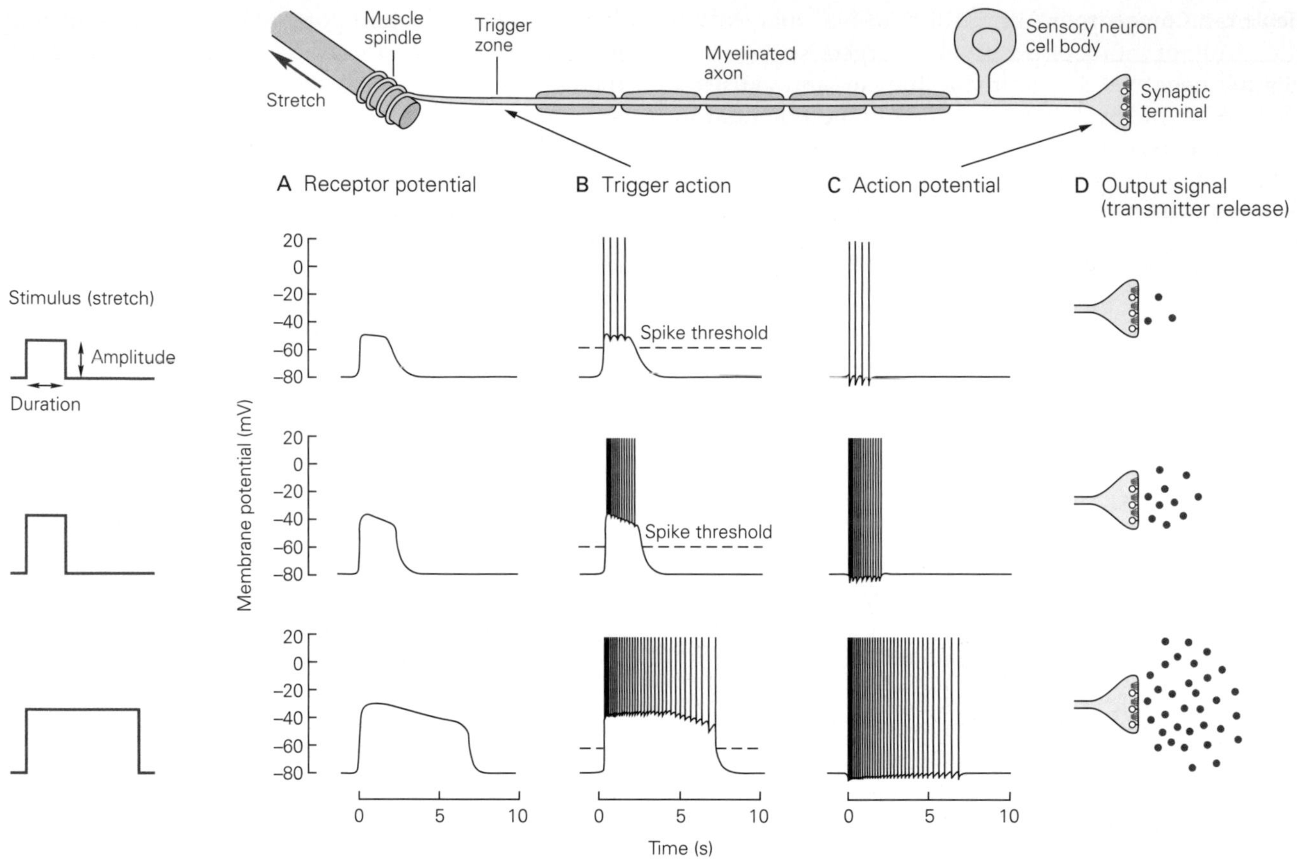

Figure 2–10 Each of the neuron's four signaling components produces a characteristic signal. The figure shows a sensory neuron activated by stretching of a muscle, which the neuron senses through a specialized receptor, the muscle spindle.

A. The input signal, called a receptor potential, is graded in amplitude and duration, proportional to the amplitude and duration of the stimulus.

B. The trigger zone sums the depolarization generated by the receptor potential. An action potential is generated only if the receptor potential exceeds a certain voltage threshold. Once this threshold is surpassed, any further increase in amplitude of the receptor potential can only increase the frequency with which the action potentials are generated, because action potentials have a constant amplitude. The duration of the receptor potential determines the duration of the train of action potentials. Thus the graded amplitude and duration of the receptor potential is translated into a frequency code in the action potentials generated at the trigger zone. All action potentials produced are propagated faithfully along the axon.

C. Action potentials are all-or-none. Because all action potentials have a similar amplitude and duration, the frequency and duration of firing represents the information carried by the signal.

D. When the action potential reaches the synaptic terminal, it initiates the release of a neurotransmitter, the chemical substance that serves as the output signal. The frequency of action potentials determines exactly how much neurotransmitter is released by the cell.

Action potentials are generated by a sudden influx of Na^+ through channels in the cell membrane that open and close in response to changes in membrane potential. When an input signal (a receptor potential or synaptic potential) depolarizes an area of membrane, the local change in membrane potential opens local Na^+ channels that allow Na^+ to flow down its concentration gradient, from outside the cell where the Na^+ concentration is high to inside where it is low.

Because the initial segment of the axon has the highest density of voltage-sensitive Na^+ channels and therefore the lowest threshold for generating an action potential, an input signal spreading passively along the cell membrane is more likely to give rise to an action potential at the initial segment than at other sites in the cell. This part of the axon is therefore known as the *trigger zone*. It is here that the activity of all receptor (or synaptic) potentials is summed and where, if the

Table 2–1 Comparison of Local (Passive) and Propagated Signals

Signal type	Amplitude (mV)	Duration	Summation	Effect of signal	Type of propagation
Local (passive) signals					
Receptor potentials	Small (0.1–10)	Brief (5–100 ms)	Graded	Hyperpolarizing or depolarizing	Passive
Synaptic potentials	Small (0.1–10)	Brief to long (5 ms–20 min)	Graded	Hyperpolarizing or depolarizing	Passive
Propagated (active) signals					
Action potentials	Large (70–110)	Brief (1–10 ms)	All-or-none	Depolarizing	Active

sum of the input signals reaches threshold, the neuron generates an action potential.

The Conductive Component Propagates an All-or-None Action Potential

The action potential is all-or-none: Stimuli below the threshold do not produce a signal, but stimuli above the threshold all produce the signals of the same amplitude. However much the stimuli vary in intensity or duration, the amplitude and duration of each action potential are pretty much the same. In addition, unlike receptor and synaptic potentials, which spread passively and decrease in amplitude, the action potential does not decay as it travels along the axon to its target—a distance that can be as great as 2 m—because it is periodically regenerated. This conducting signal can travel at rates as fast as 100 m/s.

The remarkable feature of action potentials is that they are highly stereotyped, varying only subtly (but in some cases importantly) from one nerve cell to another. This feature was demonstrated in the 1920s by Edgar Adrian, one of the first to study the nervous system at the cellular level. Adrian found that all action potentials have a similar shape or wave-form (see Figure 2–2). Indeed, the action potentials carried into the nervous system by a sensory axon often are indistinguishable from those carried out of the nervous system to the muscles by a motor axon.

Only two features of the conducting signal convey information: the number of action potentials and the time intervals between them (Figure 2–10C). As Adrian put it in 1928, summarizing his work on sensory fibers: "all impulses are very much alike, whether the message is destined to arouse the sensation of light, of touch, or of pain; if they are crowded together the sensation is intense, if they are separated by long intervals the sensation is correspondingly feeble." Thus, what determines the intensity of sensation or speed of movement is the frequency of the action potentials. Likewise, the duration of a sensation or movement is determined by the period over which action potentials are generated.

In addition to the frequency of the action potentials, the pattern of action potentials also conveys important information. For example, some neurons are not silent in the absence of stimulation but are spontaneously active. Some spontaneously active nerve cells (beating neurons) fire action potentials regularly; other neurons (bursting neurons) fire in brief bursts of action potentials. These diverse cells respond differently to the same excitatory synaptic input. An excitatory synaptic potential may initiate one or more action potentials in a cell that does not have a spontaneous activity, but in spontaneously active cells that same input will modulate the rhythm by increasing the rate of firing of action potentials.

An even more dramatic difference is seen when the input signal is inhibitory. Inhibitory inputs have little information value in a silent cell. By contrast, in spontaneously active cells inhibition can have a powerful *sculpting* role. By establishing periods of silence in otherwise ongoing activity, inhibition can produce a complex pattern of alternating firing and silence where none existed. These subtle differences in firing patterns may have important functional consequences for the information transfer between neurons. This has led mathematical modelers of neuronal networks to attempt to delineate neural codes in which information is also carried by the fine-grained pattern of firing—the exact timing of action potentials (Figure 2–11).

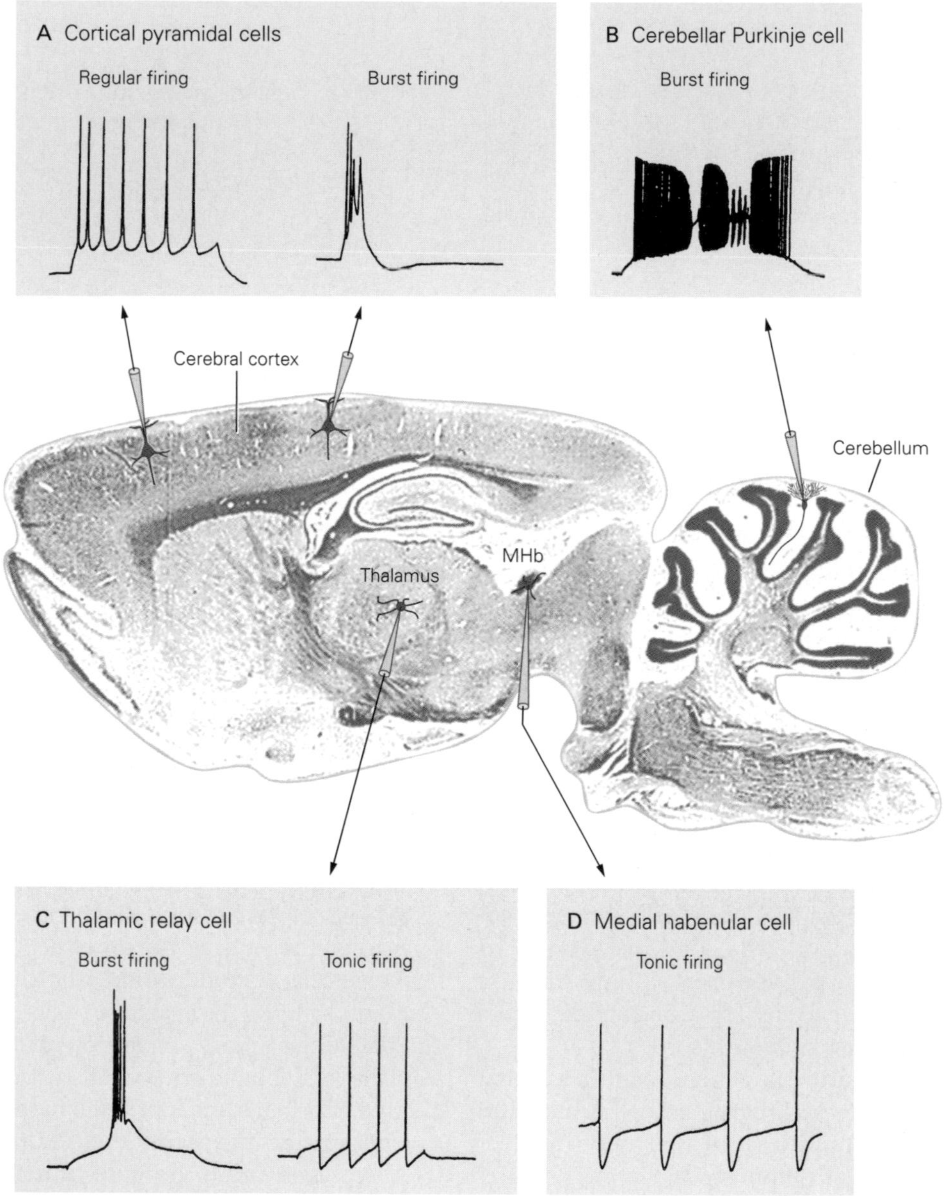

Figure 2–11 Neurons in the mammalian brain exhibit widely varying electrophysiological properties. (Reproduced, with permission, from McCormick, 2004.)

A. Intracellular injection of a depolarizing current pulse in a cortical pyramidal cell results in a train of action potentials that decline in frequency. This pattern of activity is known as regular firing. Some cortical cells generated bursts of three or more action potentials, even when depolarized only for a short period.

B. Cerebellar Purkinje cells generate high-frequency trains of action potentials in their cell bodies that are disrupted by the generation of Ca^{2+} action potentials in their dendrites. These cells can also generate plateau potentials from the persistent activation of Na^{+} conductances.

C. Thalamic relay cells may generate action potentials either as bursts or tonic trains of action potentials owing to the presence of a large low-threshold Ca^{2+} current.

D. Medial habenular cells generate action potentials at a steady and slow rate, in a pacemaker fashion.

If signals are stereotyped and reflect only the most elementary properties of the stimulus, how can they carry the rich variety of information needed for complex behavior? How is a message that carries visual information about a bee distinguished from one that carries pain information about the bee's sting, and how are these sensory signals distinguished from motor signals for voluntary movement? The answer is simple and yet is one of the most important organizational principles of the nervous system: Pathways of connected neurons, not individual neurons, convey information. Interconnected neurons form anatomically and functionally distinct pathways. The neural pathways activated by receptor cells in the retina that respond to light are completely distinct from the pathways activated by sensory cells in the skin that respond to touch.

The Output Component Releases Neurotransmitter

When an action potential reaches a neuron's terminal it stimulates the release of chemical substances from the cell. These substances, called *neurotransmitters,* can be small organic molecules, such as L-glutamate and acetylcholine, or peptides like substance P or LHRH (luteinizing hormone releasing hormone).

Neurotransmitter molecules are held in subcellular organelles called *synaptic vesicles,* which accumulate at specialized release sites in the terminals of the axon called *active zones.* To eject their transmitter substance into the synaptic cleft, the vesicles move up to and fuse with the neuron's plasma membrane, then burst open, a process known as *exocytosis.* The molecular machinery of neurotransmitter release is described in Chapters 11 and 12.

Once released, the neurotransmitter is the neuron's output signal. Like the input signal, it is graded. The amount of transmitter released is determined by the number and frequency of the action potentials that reach the presynaptic terminals (Figure 2–10C,D). After release the transmitter diffuses across the synaptic cleft and binds to receptors on the postsynaptic neuron. This binding causes the postsynaptic cell to generate a synaptic potential. Whether the synaptic potential has an excitatory or inhibitory effect depends on the type of receptor in the postsynaptic cell, not on the particular chemical neurotransmitter. The same transmitter substance can have different effects at different receptors.

The Transformation of the Neural Signal from Sensory to Motor Is Illustrated by the Stretch-Reflex Pathway

We have seen that the properties of a signal are transformed as the signal moves from one component of a neuron to another or between neurons. This transformative chain of events can be seen in the relay of signals for the stretch reflex.

When a muscle is stretched, the amplitude and duration of the stimulus are reflected in the amplitude and duration of the receptor potential generated in the sensory neuron (Figure 2–12A). If the receptor potential exceeds the threshold for an action potential in that cell, the graded signal is transformed at the trigger zone into an action potential, an all-or-none signal. The more the receptor potential exceeds threshold, the greater the depolarization and consequently the greater the frequency of action potentials in the axon. The duration of the input signal also determines the duration of the train of action potentials.

The information encoded by the frequency and duration of firing is faithfully conveyed along the axon to its terminals, where the firing of action potentials determines the amount of transmitter released. These stages of signaling have their counterparts in the motor neuron (Figure 2–12B) and in the muscle (Figure 2–12C).

Nerve Cells Differ Most at the Molecular Level

The model of neuronal signaling we have outlined is a simplification that applies to most neurons but there are some important variations. For example, some neurons do not generate action potentials. These are typically local interneurons without a conductive component; they have no axon or such a short one that regeneration of the signal is not required. In these neurons the input signals are summed and spread passively to the presynaptic terminal region nearby where transmitter is released. Neurons that are spontaneously active do not require sensory or synaptic inputs to fire action potentials because they have a special class of ion channels that permit Na^+ current flow even in the absence of excitatory synaptic input.

Even cells that are similar morphologically can differ importantly in molecular details. For example, they can have different combinations of ion channels. As we shall learn in Chapter 7, different ion channels provide neurons with various thresholds, excitability properties, and firing patterns (Figure 2–11). Neurons with different ion channels can therefore encode synaptic potentials into different firing patterns and thereby convey different information.

Neurons also differ in the chemical substances they use as transmitters and in the receptors that receive transmitter substances from other neurons. Indeed, many drugs that act on the brain do so by modifying the actions of specific chemical transmitters or receptors.

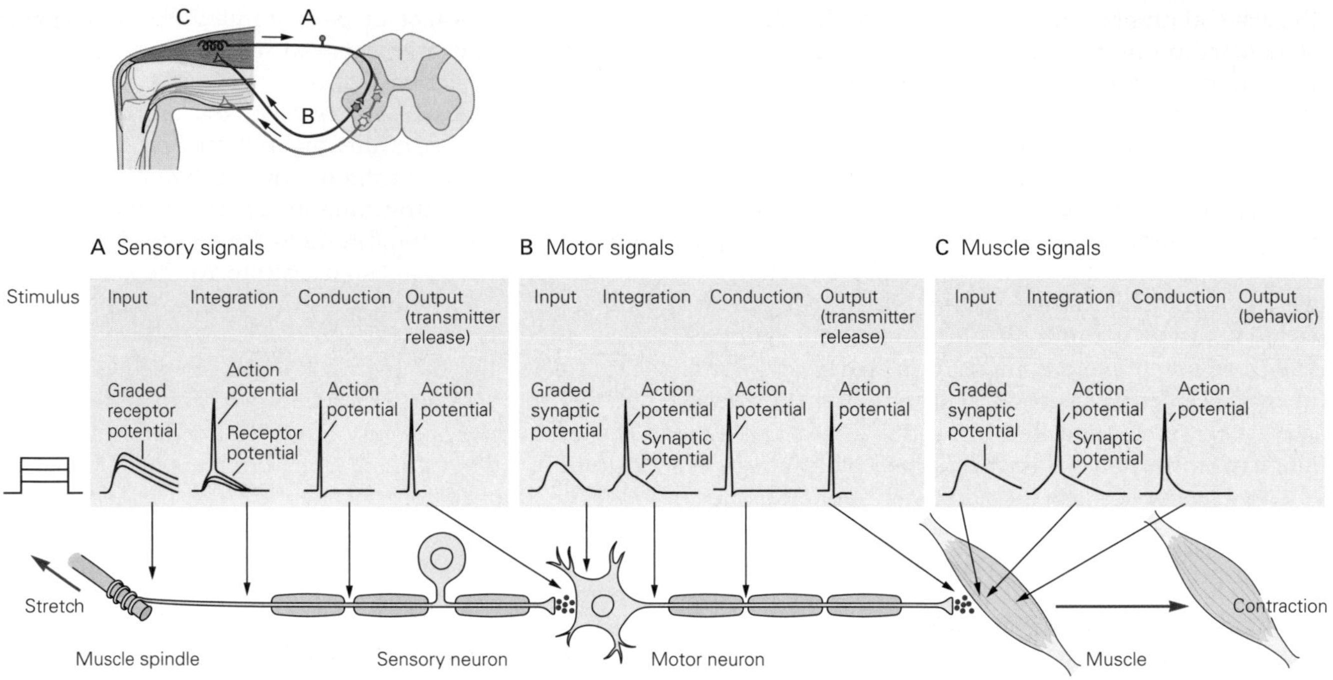

Figure 2–12. The sequence of signals that produces a reflex action.

A. The stretching of a muscle produces a receptor potential in the specialized receptor (the muscle spindle). The amplitude of the receptor potential is proportional to the intensity of the stretch. This potential spreads passively to the integrative or trigger zone at the first node of Ranvier. If the receptor potential is sufficiently large, it triggers an action potential that then propagates actively and without change along the axon to the axon terminal. At specialized sites in the terminal the action potential leads to an output signal, the release of a chemical neurotransmitter. The transmitter diffuses across the synaptic cleft between the axon terminal and a target motor neuron that innervates the stretched muscle; it then binds to receptor molecules on the external membrane of the motor neuron.

B. This interaction initiates a synaptic potential that spreads passively to the trigger zone of the motor neuron's axon, where it initiates an action potential that propagates actively to the terminal of the motor neuron's axon. The action potential releases a neuro transmitter where the axon terminal meets a muscle fiber.

C. The neurotransmitter binds receptors on the muscle fiber, triggering a synaptic potential in the muscle. If sufficiently large, or if combined with signals from other motor neurons, the synaptic potential will generate an action potential in the muscle, causing contraction of the muscle fiber.

Because of physiological differences among neurons, a disease may affect one class of neurons but not others. Certain diseases strike only motor neurons (amyotrophic lateral sclerosis and poliomyelitis), whereas others affect primarily sensory neurons (tabes dorsalis, a late stage of syphilis). Parkinson disease, a disorder of voluntary movement, damages a small population of interneurons that use dopamine as a neurotransmitter. Some diseases are selective even within the neuron, affecting only the receptive elements, the cell body, or the axon. In Chapter 14 we describe how research into myasthenia gravis, a disease caused by a faulty transmitter receptor in the muscle membrane, has provided important insights into synaptic transmission. Indeed, because the nervous system has so many cell types and variations at the molecular level, it is susceptible to more diseases (psychiatric as well as neurological) than any other organ system of the body.

Despite the differences among nerve cells, the basic mechanisms of electrical signaling are surprisingly similar. This simplicity is fortunate, for understanding the molecular mechanisms of signaling in one kind of nerve cell aids the understanding of these mechanisms in many other nerve cells.

Neural Network Models Simulate the Brain's Parallel Processing of Information

The stretch reflex illustrates how interactions between just a few types of nerve cells can constitute a functional circuit that produces a simple behavior, even though the number of neurons involved is large (the stretch reflex circuit has perhaps a few hundred sensory neurons and a hundred motor neurons). Can the individual neurons implicated in a complex behavior be identified with the same precision?

In invertebrate animals, and in some lower-order vertebrates, a single cell (a so-called command cell) can initiate a complex behavioral sequence. But as far as we know no complex human behavior is initiated by a single neuron. Rather, each behavior is generated by the actions of many cells. Broadly speaking, as we have seen, there are three components of the neural control of behavior: sensory input, intermediate processing, and motor output. In vertebrates each component is likely to be mediated by a single group or several distinct groups of neurons.

Moreover, each component may have multiple neural pathways that simultaneously provide the same or similar information. The deployment of several neuronal groups or pathways to convey similar information is called *parallel processing*. Parallel processing also occurs in a single pathway when different neurons in the pathway perform similar computations simultaneously. Parallel processing makes enormous sense as an evolutionary strategy for building a more powerful brain, for it increases both the speed and reliability of function within the central nervous system.

The importance of abundant, highly specific parallel connections has long been recognized by scientists attempting to construct theoretical models of the brain. The branch of computer science known as artificial intelligence originally used serial processing to simulate the brain's cognitive processes—pattern recognition, learning, memory, and motor performance. These serial models performed many tasks rather well, including playing chess. However, they performed poorly with other computations that the brain does almost instantaneously, such as recognizing faces or comprehending speech.

Many theoretical neurobiologists have turned to different types of models that include parallel processing, which they call *neural networks*. In these models, elements of the system process information simultaneously using both feed-forward and feedback connections. Interestingly, in systems with feedback circuits it is the dynamic activity of the system that determines the outcome of computation, not inputs or initial conditions.

Neural network models capture well the highly recurrent architecture of most actual neural circuits and also the ability of the brain to function in the absence of specific sensory input from outside the body such as during thinking, sleep, and the generation of endogenous rhythms, something with which traditional deterministic models have difficulty. Neural network models also show that analysis of individual elements of a system may not be enough to decode the *action potential code*. According to this neural network view, what makes the brain a remarkable information processing organ is not the complexity of its neurons but the fact that it has many elements interconnected in a variety of complex ways. Neural network modeling is discussed in Appendices E and F.

Neural Connections Can Be Modified by Experience

Most learning results in behavioral changes that endure for years, but even simple reflexes can be modified briefly. The fact that behavior is learned raises an interesting question: How is behavior modified if the nervous system is wired so precisely? How can changes in the neural control of behavior occur when connections between the signaling units, the neurons, are set during early development?

Several solutions for this dilemma have been proposed. The proposal that has proven most farsighted is the *plasticity hypothesis*, first put forward at the turn of the 20th century by Ramón y Cajal. A modern form of this hypothesis was advanced by the Polish psychologist Jerzy Konorski in 1948:

> The application of a stimulus leads to changes of a twofold kind in the nervous system . . . [T]he first property, by virtue of which the nerve cells *react* to the incoming impulse . . . we call *excitability*, and . . . changes arising . . . because of this property we shall call *changes due to excitability*. The second property, by virtue of which certain permanent functional transformations arise in particular systems of neurons as a result of appropriate stimuli or their combination, we shall call *plasticity* and the corresponding changes *plastic changes*.

There is now considerable evidence for functional plasticity at chemical synapses. These synapses often have a remarkable capacity for short-term physiological changes (lasting seconds to hours) that increase or decrease synaptic effectiveness. Long-term changes (lasting days) can give rise to further physiological changes that lead to anatomical alterations, including pruning of preexisting synapses and even growth of new ones.

As we shall see in later chapters, chemical synapses are functionally and anatomically modified through experience and learning as much as during early development. Functional alterations, physiological changes, are typically short-term and result in changes in the effectiveness of existing synaptic connections.

Anatomical alterations are typically long-term and consist of the growth of new synaptic connections between neurons. It is this functional plasticity of neurons that endows each of us with our individuality.

Eric R. Kandel
Ben A. Barres
A. J. Hudspeth

Selected Readings

Adrian ED. 1928. *The Basis of Sensation: The Action of the Sense Organs.* London: Christophers.

Gazzaniga MS (ed). 1995. *The Cognitive Neurosciences.* Cambridge, MA: MIT Press.

Jones EG. 1988. The nervous tissue. In: L Weiss (ed). *Cell and Tissue Biology: A Textbook of Histology,* 6th ed., pp. 277–351. Baltimore: Urban and Schwarzenberg.

Newan EA. 1993. Inward-rectifying potassium channels in retinal glial (Muller) cells. J Neurosci 13:3333–3345.

Perry VH. 1996. Microglia in the developing and mature central nervous system. In: KR Jessen, WD Richardson (eds). *Glial Cell Development: Basic Principles & Clinical Relevance,* pp. 123–140. Oxford: Bios.

Ramón y Cajal S. 1937. *1852–1937. Recollections of My Life.* EH Craigie (transl). Philadelphia: American Philosophical Society; 1989. Reprint. Cambridge, MA: MIT Press.

References

Adrian ED. 1932. *The Mechanism of Nervous Action: Electrical Studies of the Neurone.* Philadelphia: Univ. Pennsylvania Press.

Alberts B, Johnson A, Lewis J, Raff M, Roberts K, Walter JD. 2002. *Molecular Biology of the Cell,* 4th ed. New York: Garland.

Dacey DM, Peterson BB, Robinson FR, Gamlin PD. 2003. Fireworks in the primate retina: in vitro photodynamics reveals diverse LGN-projecting ganglion cell types. Neuron 37:15–27.

Erlanger J, Gasser HS. 1937. *Electrical Signs of Nervous Activity.* Philadelphia: Univ. Pennsylvania Press.

Hodgkin AL, Huxley AF. 1939. Action potentials recorded from inside a nerve fiber. Nature 144:710–711.

Hopfield JJ, Tank DW. 1986. Computing with neural circuits: a model. Science 233:625–633.

Kandel ER. 1976. The study of behavior: the interface between psychology and biology. In: *Cellular Basis of Behavior: An Introduction to Behavioral Neurobiology,* pp. 3–27. San Francisco: WH Freeman.

Konorski J. 1948. *Conditioned Reflexes and Neuron Organization.* Cambridge, MA: Cambridge Univ. Press.

Martinez PFA. 1982. *Neuroanatomy: Development and Structure of the Central Nervous System.* Philadelphia: Saunders.

McCormick DA. 2004. Membrane potential and action potential. In: JH Byrne and JL Roberts (eds.) *From Molecules to Networks: An Introduction to Cellular Neuroscience,* 2nd ed., p. 130. San Diego, CA: Elsevier.

Newman EA. 1986. High potassium conductance in astrocyte endfeet. Science 233:453–454.

Nicholls JG, Wallace BG, Fuchs PA, Martin AR. 2001. *From Neuron to Brain,* 4th ed. Sunderland, MA: Sinauer.

Penfield W (ed). 1932. *Cytology & Cellular Pathology of the Nervous System,* Vol. 2. New York: Hoeber.

Ramón y Cajal S. 1933. *Histology,* 10th ed. Baltimore: Wood.

Sears ES, Franklin GM. 1980. Diseases of the cranial nerves. In: RN Rosenberg (ed). *The Science and Practice of Clinical Medicine.* Vol. 5, *Neurology,* pp. 471–494. New York: Grune & Stratton.

Sherrington C. 1947. *The Integrative Action of the Nervous System,* 2nd ed. Cambridge, MA: Cambridge Univ. Press.

3

Genes and Behavior

All behaviors are shaped by the interplay of genes and the environment. The most stereotypic behaviors of simple animals are influenced by the environment, and the highly evolved behaviors of humans are constrained by innate properties specified by genes. Genes do not control behavior directly, but the RNAs and proteins encoded by genes act at different times and at many levels to affect the brain. Genes specify the developmental programs that assemble the brain and are essential to the properties of neurons and synapses that allow neuronal circuits to function. Genes that are stably inherited over generations create the machinery that allows new experiences to change the brain during learning.

In this chapter we ask how genes contribute to behavior. We begin with an overview of the evidence that genes do influence behavior, and then review basic principles of molecular biology and genetic transmission. We then provide a few examples of the way that genetic influences on behavior have been documented. Many persuasive links between genes and human behavior have emerged from the analysis of human brain development and function. However, a deep understanding of the ways that genes regulate behavior has emerged primarily from studies of worms, flies, and mice, animals whose genomes are accessible to experimental manipulation. Despite formidable challenges in studying complex genetic traits in humans, recent progress has revealed the genetic basis of some developmental and psychiatric disorders, and holds the promise of future understanding.

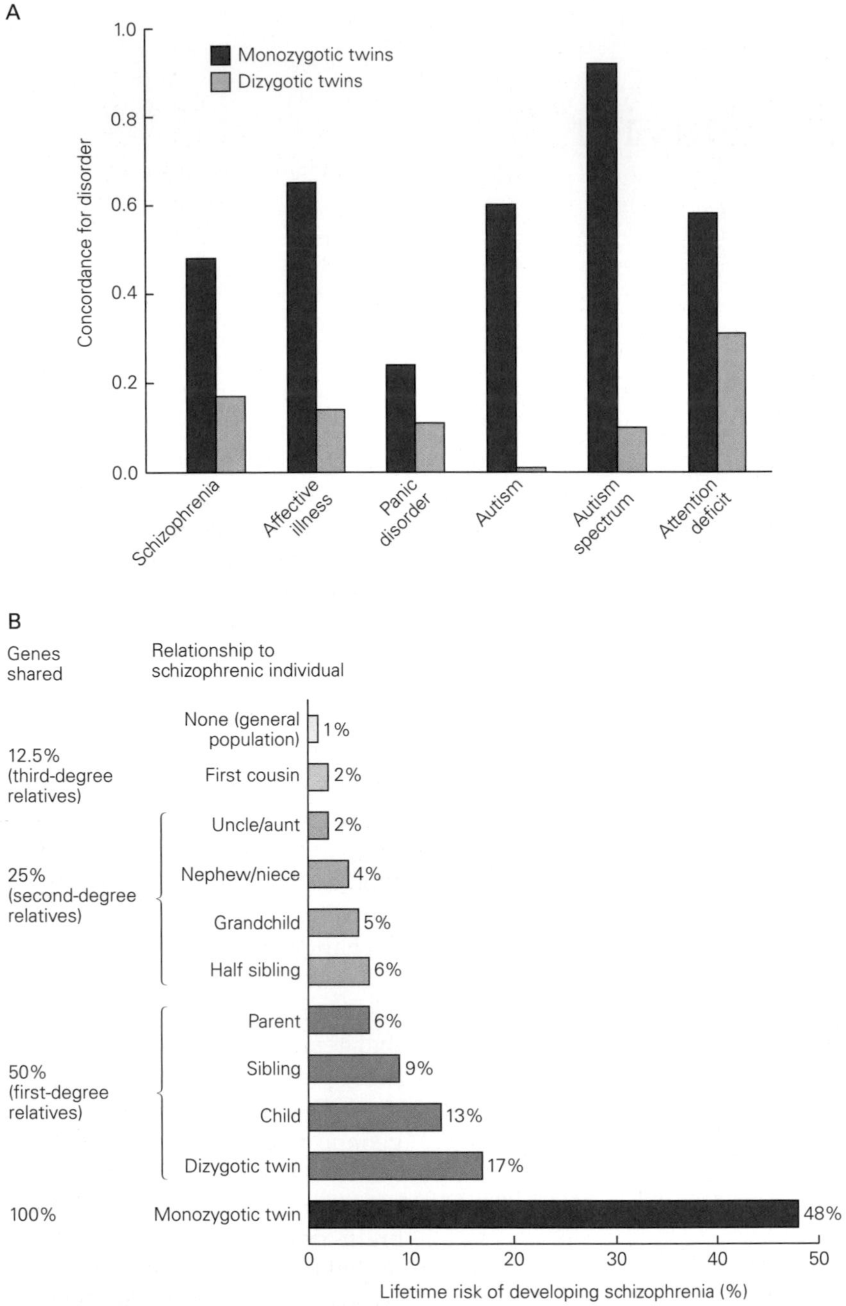

Figure 3–1 Familial risk of psychiatric disorders provides evidence of heritability.

A. Correlations between monozygotic twins for psychiatric disorders are considerably greater than those between dizygotic twins. Monozygotic twins share nearly all genes and have a high (but not 100%) risk of sharing the disease state. Dizygotic twins share 50% of their genetic material. A score of zero represents no correlation (the average result for two random people), whereas a score of 1.0 represents a perfect correlation. (Adapted, with permission, from McGue and Bouchard 1998.)

B. The risk of developing schizophrenia is greater in close relatives of a schizophrenic patient. Like dizygotic twins, parents and children, as well as brothers and sisters, share 50% of their genetic material. If only a single gene accounted for schizophrenia, the risk should be the same for parents, siblings, children, and dizygotic twins of patients. The variation between family members shows that more complex genetic and environmental factors are in play. (Modified, with permission, from Gottesman 1991.)

Genes, Genetic Analysis, and Heritability in Behavior

Many human psychiatric disorders and neurological diseases have a genetic component. The relatives of a patient are more likely than the general population to have the disease. The extent to which genetic factors account for traits in a population is called *heritability*. The strongest case for heritability is based on twin studies, first used by Francis Galton in 1883. Identical twins develop from a single fertilized egg that splits into two soon after fertilization; such monozygotic twins share all genes. In contrast, fraternal twins develop from two different fertilized eggs; these dizygotic twins, like normal siblings, share on average half their genetic information. Systematic comparisons over many years have shown that identical twins tend to be more similar (concordant) for neurological and psychiatric traits than fraternal twins, providing evidence of a heritable component of these traits (Figure 3–1A).

In an extension of the twin study model, Thomas Bouchard and colleagues in the Minnesota Twin Study examined identical twins that were separated early in life and raised in different households. Despite sometimes great differences in their environment, twins shared predispositions for the same psychiatric disorders and even tended to share personality traits, like extraversion. Thus genetic variation contributes to normal human differences, not just to disease states.

Heritability for human diseases and behavioral traits is usually substantially less than 100%, demonstrating that the environment is an important factor in acquiring diseases or traits. Estimates of heritability for many neurological, psychiatric, and behavioral traits from twin studies range around 50%, but heritability can be higher or lower for particular traits (Figure 3–1B). Although studies of identical twins and other kinships provide support for the idea that human behavior has a hereditary component, they do not tell us which genes are important, let alone how specific genes affect behavior. These questions can be addressed more easily by genetic studies in experimental animals in which both the gene and the environment are strictly controlled.

The Nature of the Gene

The related scientific areas of molecular biology and transmission genetics are central to our modern understanding of genes. The following primer introduces these ideas; a glossary at the end of the chapter defines commonly used terms.

Genes are made of DNA, and it is DNA that is passed on from one generation to the next. Through DNA replication exact copies of each gene are provided to all cells in an organism as well as to succeeding generations. DNA is made of two strands, each of which has a deoxyribose-phosphate backbone attached to a series of four subunits: the nucleotides adenine (A), guanine (G), thymine (T), and cytosine (C). The two strands are paired so that an A on one strand is always paired with a T on the complementary strand, and a G with a C (Figure 3–2). This complementarity ensures accurate copying of DNA during DNA replication and drives *transcription* of DNA into RNA. RNA differs from DNA in that it is single-stranded, has a ribose rather than a deoxyribose backbone, and uses the nucleoside base uridine (U) in the place of thymine.

Most genes encode protein products, which are generated by *translation* of the linear messenger RNA (mRNA) sequence into a linear polypeptide (protein) sequence composed of 20 different amino acids. A typical gene consists of a coding region, which is translated into a protein, and noncoding regions (Figure 3–3). The coding region is usually broken into small segments called *exons* that are separated by noncoding stretches called *introns*. The introns are deleted from the mRNA before its translation into protein.

Some functional RNAs do not encode protein. These include ribosomal RNAs (rRNAs) and transfer RNAs (tRNAs), essential components of the machinery for mRNA translation; small nuclear RNAs (snRNAs), which guide mRNA splicing; and microRNAs (miRNAs), small RNAs that pair with complementary sequences in specific mRNAs to inhibit their translation.

Each cell in the body contains the DNA for every gene but only expresses a specific subset of the genes as RNAs. The part of the gene that is transcribed into RNA is flanked by noncoding DNA regions, called *promoters* and *enhancers*, that allow accurate expression of the RNA in the right cells at the right time. Promoters and enhancers are typically found close to the beginning of the region to be transcribed, but can also act at a distance. A unique complement of DNA-binding proteins within each cell interacts with promoters and enhancers to regulate gene expression and resulting cellular properties.

The brain expresses a greater number of genes than any other organ in the body, and within the brain diverse populations of neurons express different groups of genes. The selective gene expression controlled by promoters, enhancers, and the DNA-binding proteins that interact with them permits a fixed number of genes to generate a vastly larger number of neuronal cell types and connections in the brain.

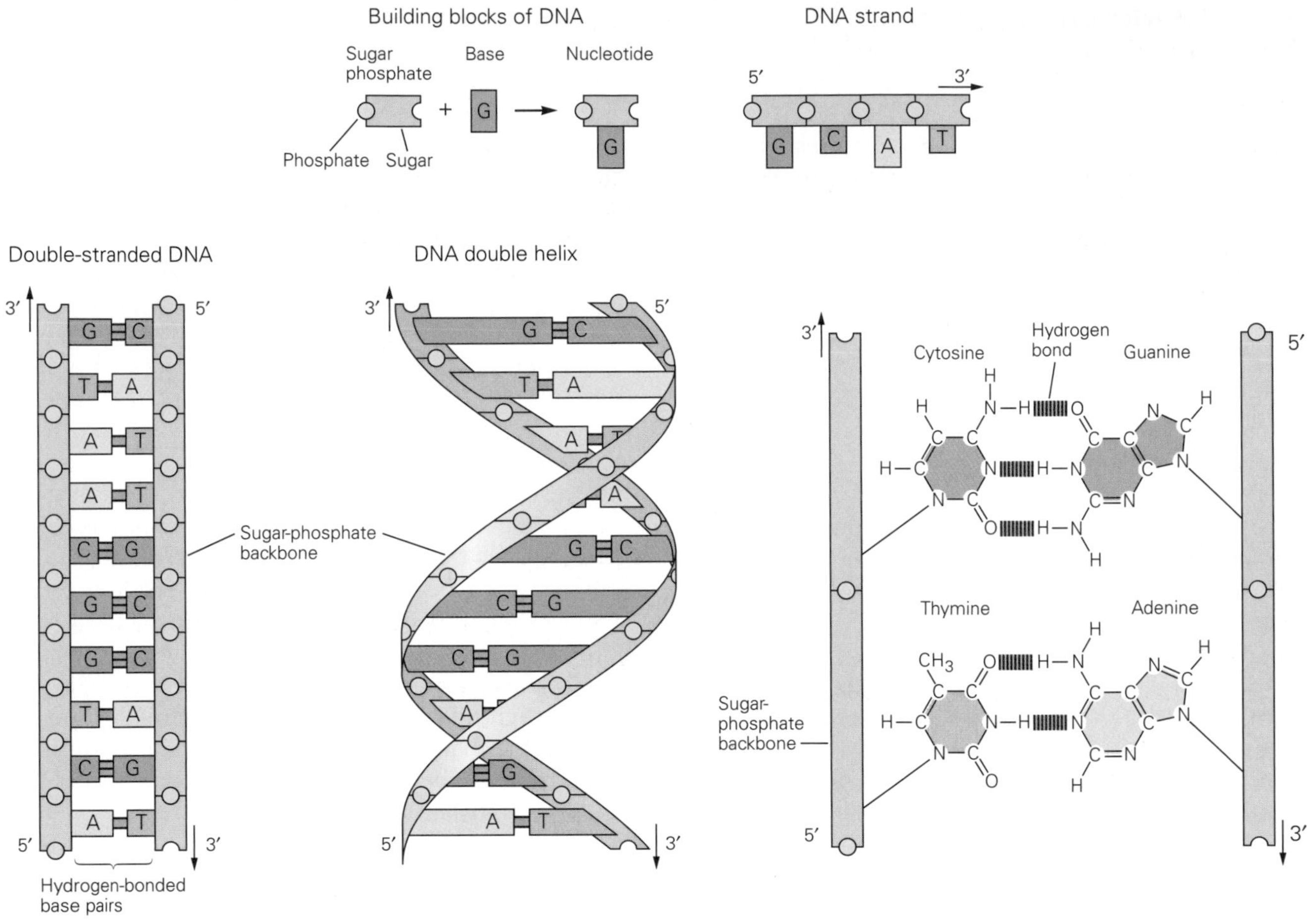

Figure 3–2 Structure of DNA. Four different nucleotide bases, adenine (**A**), thymine (**T**), cytosine (**C**), and guanine (**G**), are assembled on a sugar phosphate backbone in the double-stranded DNA helix.

Although genes specify the initial development and properties of the nervous system, the experience of an individual and the resulting activity in specific neural circuits can itself alter the expression of genes. In this way environmental influences are incorporated into the structure and function of neural circuits. The goal of genetics is to unravel the ways that individual genes affect a biological process, the ways that networks of genes affect each other's activity, and the ways that genes interact with the environment.

Genes Are Arranged on Chromosomes

The genes in a cell are arranged in an orderly fashion on long, linear stretches of DNA called *chromosomes.* Each gene in the human genome is reproducibly located at a characteristic position (locus) on a specific chromosome, and this genetic "address" can be used to associate biological traits with a gene's effects. Most multicellular animals (including worms, fruit flies, mice, and humans) are *diploid;* every somatic cell carries two complete sets of chromosomes, one from the mother and the other from the father.

Humans have about 25,000 genes but only 46 chromosomes: 22 pairs of autosomes (chromosomes that are present in both males and females) and 2 sex chromosomes (2 X chromosomes in females, 1 X and 1 Y chromosome in males) (Figure 3–4). Each parent supplies one copy of each autosome to the diploid offspring. Each parent also supplies one X chromosome to female (XX) offspring, but XY males inherit their single X chromosome from their mothers and their single Y chromosome from their fathers. Sex-linked inheritance was discovered in fruit flies by Thomas Hunt Morgan in 1910. This pattern of sex-linked inheritance associated with the single X chromosome has been highly significant in human genetic studies, where certain X-linked genetic diseases are commonly observed only in males but are genetically transmitted from mothers to their sons.

In addition to the genes on chromosomes, a very small number of an organism's genes are transmitted through cytoplasmic organelles called *mitochondria*, which carry out metabolic processes. Mitochondria in all children come from the ovum and therefore are transmitted from the mother to the child. Certain human disorders, including some neuromuscular degenerative diseases, mental retardation, and some forms of deafness, are caused by mutations in the mitochondrial DNA.

The Relationship Between Genotype and Phenotype

Because an individual has two copies of each autosomal gene, it is important to distinguish the *genotype* of an organism (its genetic makeup) and the *phenotype* (its appearance). The two copies of a particular autosomal gene in an individual are called *alleles*. If the two alleles are identical, the individual is said to be *homozygous* at that locus. If the alleles vary because of mutations, the individual is *heterozygous* at that locus. Males are *hemizygous* for genes on the X chromosome. A population can have a large number of alleles of a gene; for example, a single gene that affects human eye color called OCA2 can have alleles that encode shades of blue, green, hazel, or brown. In the broad sense a genotype is the entire set of alleles forming the genome of an individual; in the narrow sense it is the specific alleles of one gene. By contrast, a phenotype is a description of a whole organism, and is a result of the expression of the organism's genotype in a particular environment.

The difference between genotype and phenotype is evident when considering the consequences of having one normal (wild-type) allele and one mutant allele of the same gene. Most proteins are able to function even if only half their wild-type levels are present, so inactivating one copy of most genes does not lead to a change in phenotype. Thus, two organisms with different genotypes (two wild-type alleles, or one wild-type and one mutant allele) can have the same phenotype. The organism with two mutant alleles has a different phenotype. The phenotype of an animal can change over its lifetime,

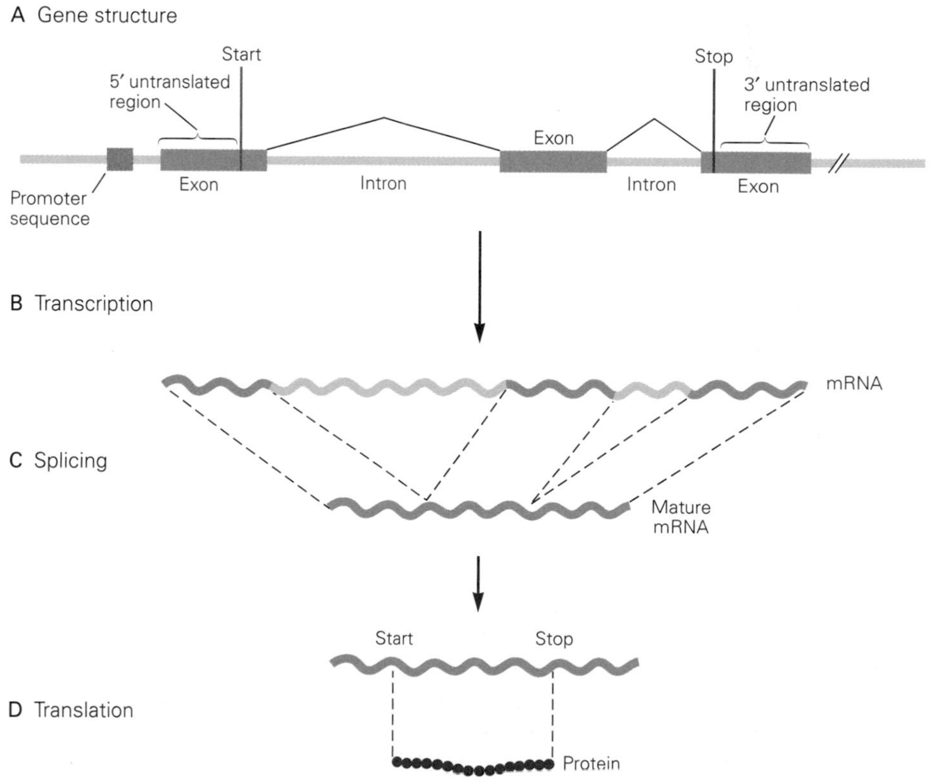

Figure 3–3 Gene structure and expression.

A. A gene consists of coding regions (exons) separated by noncoding regions (introns). Its transcription is regulated by noncoding regions such as promoters and enhancers that are frequently found near the beginning of the gene.

B. Transcription leads to production of a primary single-stranded RNA transcript that includes both exons and introns.

C. Splicing removes introns from the immature transcript and ligates the exons into a mature messenger RNA (mRNA), which is exported from the nucleus of the cell.

D. The mature mRNA is translated into a protein product.

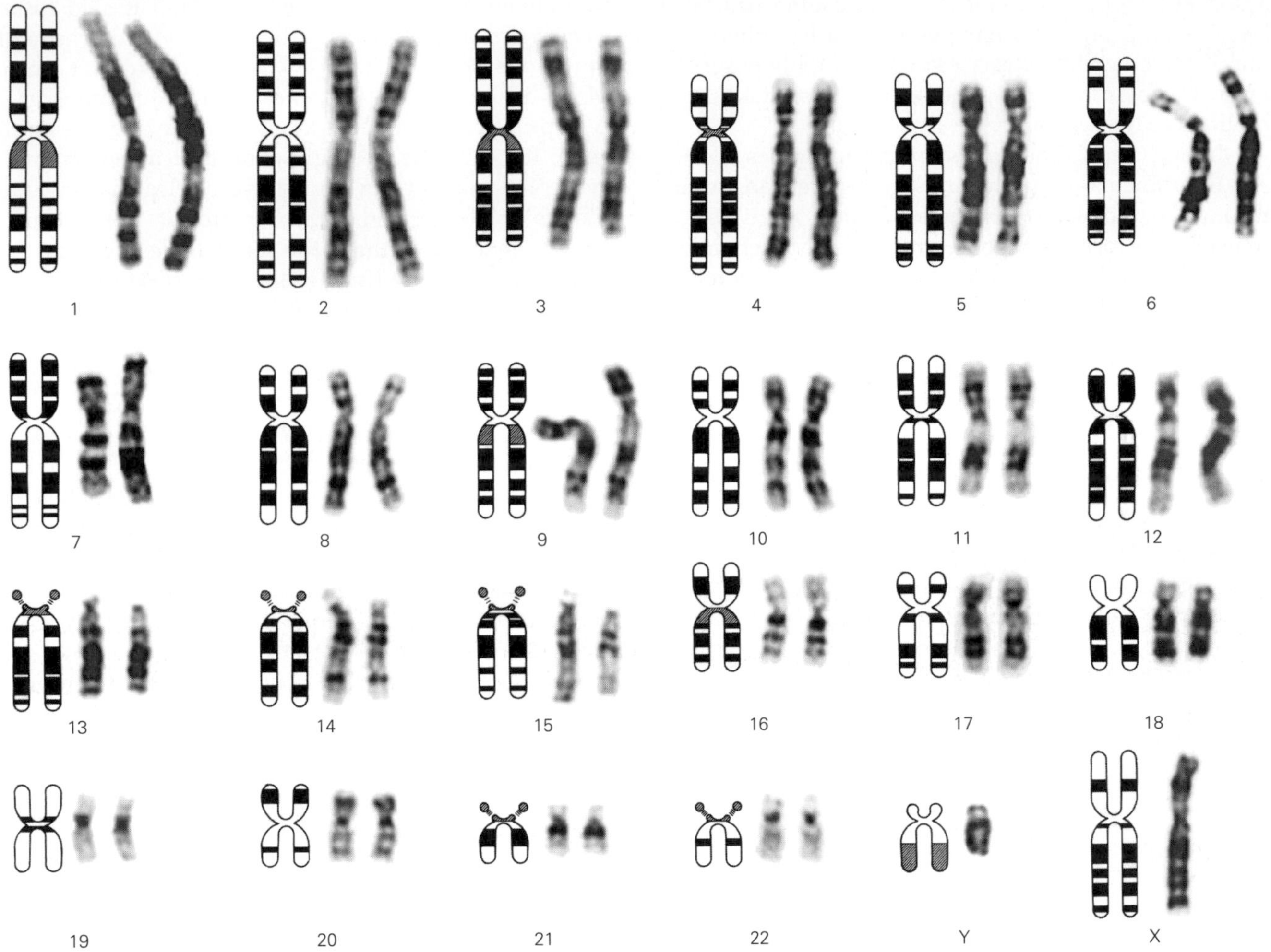

Figure 3–4 Map of normal human chromosomes at metaphase illustrating the distinctive morphology of each chromosome. Characteristic sizes and characteristic light and dark regions allow chromosomes to be distinguished from one another. (Adapted, with permission, from Watson et al. 1983.)

whereas the genotype remains constant (except for sporadic mutations in cancer cells and DNA rearrangements in the immune system).

If a mutant phenotype is expressed only when both alleles of a gene are mutated (that is, only individuals homozygous for the mutant allele exhibit the phenotype) the phenotypic trait as well as the mutant allele are said to be *recessive.* Recessive mutations usually result from loss or reduction of a functional protein. Recessive inheritance of mutant traits is commonly observed in humans and experimental animals.

If a mutant phenotype results from a combination of one mutant and one wild-type allele, the phenotypic trait and mutant allele are said to be *dominant.* In general, dominant mutations are more rare than recessive mutations. Some mutations are dominant because 50% of the gene product is not enough for a normal phenotype. Other dominant mutations lead to the production of an abnormal protein by the mutant gene or to expression of the wild-type gene product at an inappropriate time or place.

Genes and proteins are resilient in the face of small changes, so not every sequence change in a gene is deleterious. Most mutations are simply allelic polymorphisms that are silent; that is, they do not have any effect on the phenotype. Some are not silent but are expressed in ways that are benign, for example in eye color. Only rare mutations cause disturbance in

Box 3–1 Mutation: The Origin of Genetic Diversity

Although DNA replication generally is carried out with high fidelity, spontaneous errors called *mutations* do occur. Mutations can result from damage to the purine and pyrimidine bases in DNA, mistakes during the DNA replication process, and recombinations that occur during meiosis. It is these mutations that give rise to genetic polymorphisms.

The rate of spontaneously occurring mutations is low but measurable; spontaneous mutations make a significant contribution to human genetic disease. The frequency of mutations greatly increases when the organism is exposed to chemical mutagens or ionizing radiation during experimental genetic studies.

Chemical mutagens tend to induce *point mutations* involving changes in a single DNA base pair or the deletion of a few base pairs. By contrast, ionizing radiation can induce large insertions, deletions, or translocations. Both spontaneous and induced mutations can lead to changes in the structure of the protein encoded by the gene or to a partial decrease or absence of gene expression.

Functional changes in a single base pair within a coding region can be of three kinds: (1) a *missense mutation*, where the point mutation results in one amino acid in a protein being substituted for another; (2) a *nonsense mutation*, where a codon (a triplet of nucleotides) within the coding region is replaced by a stop codon, resulting in a shortened (truncated) protein product; or (3) a *frameshift mutation*, in which small insertions or deletions of nucleotides change the reading frame, leading to the production of a truncated or abnormal protein.

Large-scale mutations involve changes in chromosome structure that can affect the function of one gene or many contiguous genes. Such mutations include rearrangement of genes without the addition or deletion of material (*inversion*), or deletion or duplication of genes in a chromosome (*copy number variation*).

Although most single-gene traits are recessive, rearrangements that lead to duplication or deletion of multiple genes often have dominant effects. For example, individuals with three copies of chromosome 21 have Down syndrome due to the increased expression of multiple genes; no single gene when present in three copies is known to cause the cognitive and physical manifestations of Down syndrome.

development, cell function, or overt behavior. Some mutations are pathogenic, however, and these lead to disease (Box 3–1).

Genes Are Conserved Through Evolution

The nearly complete nucleotide sequence of the human genome was reported in 2000, and the complete nucleotide sequences of many animal genomes have also been decoded. Comparisons between these genomes leads to a surprising conclusion: the unique human species did not result from the invention of unique new human genes.

Humans and chimpanzees are profoundly different in their biology and behavior, yet they share 99% of their protein-coding genes. Moreover, most of the approximately 25,000 genes in humans are also present in other mammals like mice, and over half of all human genes are very similar to genes in invertebrates such as worms and flies (Figure 3–5). The conclusion from this surprising discovery is that ancient genes that humans

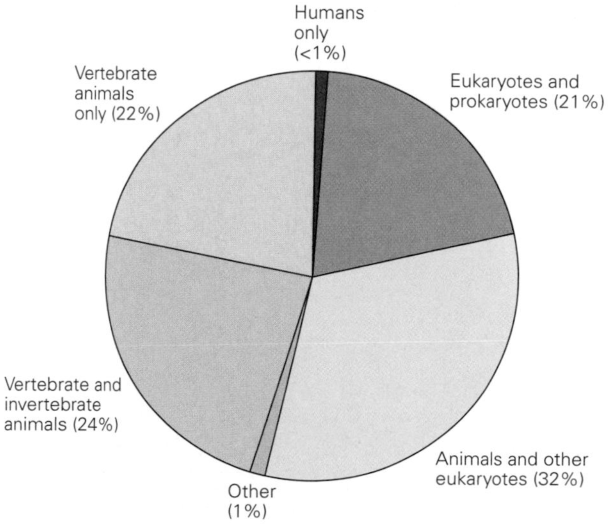

Figure 3–5 Most human genes are related to genes in other species. Less than 1% of genes are specific to humans; other genes may be shared by all living things, by all eukaryotes, by animals only, or by vertebrate animals only. (Modified, with permission, from Lander et al. 2001.)

share with other animals are regulated in new ways to produce novel human properties, like the capacity to generate complex thoughts and language.

Because of this conservation of genes throughout evolution, insights from studies of one animal can often be applied to other animals with related genes, an important fact as animal experiments are often possible when experiments on humans are not. For example, a gene from a mouse that encodes an amino acid sequence similar to a human gene usually has a similar function to the *orthologous* human gene.

Approximately one-half of the human genes have functions that have been demonstrated or inferred from orthologous genes in other organisms (Figure 3–6). A set of genes shared by humans, flies, and even unicellular yeasts encodes the proteins for intermediary metabolism, synthesis of DNA, RNA, and protein, cell division, and for cytoskeletal structures, protein transport, and secretion.

The evolution from single-celled organism to multicellular animals was accompanied by an expansion of genes concerned with intercellular signaling and gene regulation. The genomes of multicellular animals, such as worms, flies, mice, and humans, typically encode thousands of transmembrane receptors, many more than are present in unicellular organisms. These transmembrane receptors are used in cell-to-cell communication in development, in signaling between neurons, and as sensors of environmental stimuli. The genome of a multicellular animal also encodes 1,000 or more different DNA-binding proteins that regulate the expression of other genes. Many of the transmembrane receptors and DNA-binding proteins in humans are related to specific orthologous genes in other vertebrates and invertebrates. By enumerating the shared genetic heritage of the animals, we can infer that the basic molecular pathways for neuronal development, neurotransmission, electrical excitability, and gene expression were present in the common ancestor of worms, flies, mice, and humans. Moreover, studies of animal and human genes have demonstrated that the most important genes in the human brain are those that are most conserved throughout animal phylogeny. Differences between mammalian genes and their invertebrate counterparts most often result from gene duplication in mammals or subtle changes in gene expression and function, rather than the creation of entirely new genes.

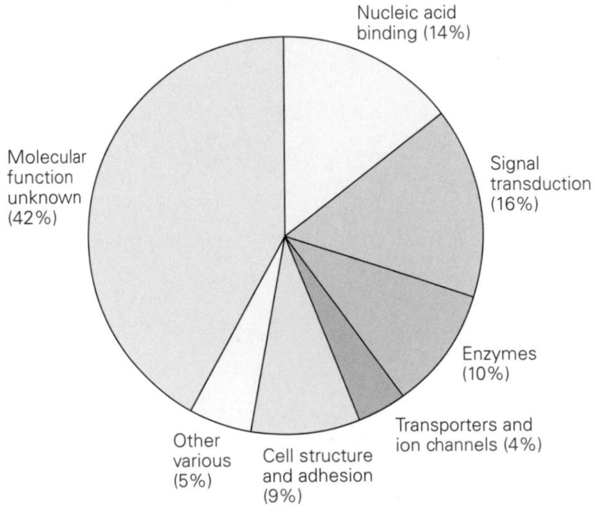

Figure 3–6 The predicted molecular functions of 26,383 human genes. (Modified, with permission, from Venter et al. 2001.)

The Role of Genes in Behavior Can Be Studied in Animal Models

Because of the conservation between human and animal genes, the relationships between the genes, proteins, and neural circuits that underlie behavior can be studied in animal models that are experimentally tractable. Two important strategies have been applied with great success in the study of gene function.

In *classical genetic analysis* organisms are first subjected to mutagenesis with a chemical or irradiation that induces random mutations, and then screened for heritable changes that affect the behavior of interest, say, sleep. This approach does not impose a bias as to the kind of gene involved; it is a random search of all possible mutations that cause detectable changes. Genetic tracing of heritable changes allows the identification of the individual genes that are altered in the mutant organism. Thus the pathway of discovery in classical genetics moves from phenotype to genotype, from organism to gene. In *reverse genetics* a specific gene of interest is targeted for alteration, a genetically modified animal is produced, and the animals with these altered genes are studied. This strategy is both focused and biased—one begins with a candidate gene—and the pathway of discovery moves from genotype to phenotype, from gene to organism.

These two experimental strategies and their more subtle variations form the basis of experimental genetics. Gene manipulation by classical and reverse genetics is conducted in experimental animals, not in humans.

Circadian Rhythm Is Generated by a Transcriptional Oscillator in Flies, Mice, and Humans

The first large-scale studies of the influence of genes on behavior were initiated by Seymour Benzer and his colleagues around 1970. They used random mutagenesis and classical genetic analysis to identify mutations that affected learned and innate behaviors in the fruit fly *Drosophila melanogaster*: circadian (daily) rhythms, courtship behavior, movement, visual perception, and memory (Boxes 3–2 and 3–3). These induced mutations have had an immense influence on our understanding of the role of genes in behavior.

We have a particularly complete picture of the genetic basis of the circadian control of behavior. An animal's circadian rhythm couples certain behaviors to a 24-hour cycle linked to the rising and setting of the sun. The core of circadian regulation is an intrinsic biological clock that oscillates over a 24-hour cycle. Because of the intrinsic periodicity of the clock, circadian behavior persists even in the absence of light or other environmental influences.

The clock can be reset, so that changes in the day-night cycle eventually result in a matching shift in the intrinsic oscillator, a phenomenon that is familiar to any traveler recovering from jet lag. Light-driven signals are transmitted by the eye to the brain to reset the clock. Finally, the clock drives output pathways for specific behaviors, such as sleep and locomotion.

Benzer's group searched through thousands of mutant flies to look for rare flies that failed to follow circadian rhythms because of mutations in the genes that direct circadian oscillation. From this work emerged the first insight into the molecular machinery of the circadian clock. Mutations in the *period,* or *per,* gene affected all circadian behaviors generated by the fly's internal clock.

Interestingly, *per* mutations could change the circadian clock in several ways (Figure 3–9). Arrhythmic *per* mutant flies, which exhibited no discernible intrinsic rhythms in any behavior, lacked all function of the *per* gene, so *per* is essential for rhythmic behavior. *Per* mutations that maintained some function of the gene resulted in abnormal rhythms. Long-day alleles produced 28-hour behavioral cycles, whereas short-day alleles produced a 19-hour cycle. Thus *per* is not just an essential piece of the clock, it is actually a timekeeper whose activity can change the rate at which the clock runs.

The *per* mutant has no major adverse effects other than the change in circadian behavior. This observation is important because, prior to the discovery of *per,* many had questioned whether there could be true "behavior genes" that were not required for the other physiological needs of an animal. *Per* does seem to be such a "behavior gene."

How does *per* keep time? The protein product PER is a transcriptional regulator that affects the expression of other genes. Levels of PER are regulated throughout the day. Early in the morning PER and its mRNA are low. Over the course of the day the PER mRNA and protein accumulate, reaching peak levels after dusk and during the night. The levels then decrease, falling before the next dawn. These observations provide an answer to the circadian rhythm puzzle—a central regulator appears and disappears throughout the day. But they are also unsatisfying because they only push the question back one step—what makes PER cycle? The answer to this question required the discovery of additional clock genes, which were discovered in flies and also in mice.

Emboldened by the success of the fly circadian rhythm screens, Joseph Takahashi began similar but far more labor-intensive genetic screens in mice in the 1990s. He screened hundreds of mutant mice for the rare mice with alterations in their circadian locomotion period, and found a single gene mutation that he called *clock* (Figure 3–10). When mice homozygous for the *clock* mutation are transferred to darkness, they initially experience extremely long circadian periods and later a complete loss of circadian rhythmicity. The *clock* gene therefore appears to regulate two fundamental properties of the circadian rhythm: the length of the circadian period and the persistence of rhythmicity in the absence of sensory input. These properties are conceptually identical to the properties of the *per* gene in flies.

The mouse *clock* gene, like the *per* gene in flies, encodes a transcriptional regulator whose activity oscillates through the day. The mouse CLOCK and fly PER proteins also shared a domain called a *PAS domain,* characteristic of a subset of transcriptional regulators. This observation suggests that the same molecular mechanism—oscillation of PAS-domain transcriptional regulation—controls circadian rhythm in flies and mice.

More significantly, parallel studies of flies and mice showed that similar groups of transcriptional regulators affected the circadian clock in both animals. After the mouse *clock* gene was cloned, a fly circadian rhythm gene was cloned and found to be closely related to mouse *clock,* even more so than *per.* In a different study a mouse gene similar to fly *per* was identified and inactivated by reverse genetics. The mutant mouse had a circadian rhythm defect, like fly *per* mutants. In other words, both flies and mice use both *clock* and *per* genes to control their circadian rhythms. A group of genes, not one gene, are conserved regulators of the circadian clock.

Box 3–2 Generating Mutations in Experimental Animals

Random Mutagenesis in Flies

Genetic analysis of behavior in the fruit fly (*Drosophila*) is carried out on flies in which individual genes have been mutated. Mutations can be made by chemical mutagenesis or by insertional mutagenesis. Chemical mutagenesis, for example with ethyl methanesulfonate (EMS), typically creates random point mutations in genes. Insertional mutagenesis occurs when mobile DNA sequences called *transposable elements* randomly insert themselves into other genes.

The most widely used transposable elements in *Drosophila* are the P elements. P elements may be modified to carry genetic markers for eye color, which makes them easy to track in genetic crosses, and they may also be modified to alter expression of the gene into which they are inserted.

To cause P element transposition, *Drosophila* strains that carry P elements are crossed to those that do not. This genetic cross leads to destabilization and transposition of the P elements in the resulting offspring. The mobilization of the P element causes its transposition into a new location in a random gene.

Chemical mutagenesis and transposable element mutagenesis are *random mutagenesis* strategies that can affect any gene in the genome. Similar random mutagenesis strategies are used to create mutations in the nematode worm *Caenorhabditis elegans*, the zebra fish, and mice.

Targeted Mutagenesis in Mice

Advances in molecular manipulation of mammalian genes have permitted precise replacement of a known normal gene with a mutant version. The process of generating a strain of mutant mice involves two separate manipulations. A gene on a chromosome is replaced by homologous recombination in a special cell line known as embryonic stem cells, and the modified cell line is incorporated into the germ cell population of the embryo.

The gene of interest must first be cloned. The gene is mutated and a selectable marker, usually a drug-resistance gene, is then introduced into the mutated fragment. The altered gene is then introduced into embryonic stem cells, and clones of cells that incorporate the altered gene are isolated. DNA samples of each clone are tested to identify a clone in which the mutated gene has been integrated into the homologous (normal) site, rather than some other random site.

When a suitable clone has been identified, the cells are injected into a mouse embryo at the blastocyst stage (3 to 4 days after fertilization), when the embryo consists of approximately 100 cells. These embryos are then reintroduced into a female that has been hormonally prepared for implantation and allowed to come to term. The resulting embryos are chimeric mixtures between the stem cell line and the host embryo.

Embryonic stem cells in the mouse have the capability of participating in all aspects of development, including the germline. Thus injected cells can become germ cells and pass on the altered gene to future generations of mice. This technique has been used to generate mutations in various genes crucial to development or function in the nervous system.

Altering Gene Function by RNA Interference

RNA interference takes advantage of the fact that most double-stranded RNAs in eukaryotic cells are targeted for destruction; the whole RNA is destroyed even if only part of it is double-stranded. By artificially causing a selected mRNA to become double-stranded, researchers can activate this process to reduce the mRNA levels for specific genes.

To reduce the function of a gene by RNA interference, small-sequence RNA is introduced that will pair with the endogenous mRNA because of complementarity between the small RNA sequence and the desired mRNA. Small RNA is usually 21 or 22 bases in length, and is known as *small interfering RNA* (siRNA) or *small hairpin RNA* (shRNA).

Pairing of siRNA or shRNA with mRNA leads to destruction of the endogenous mRNA by ribonucleases within the cell. The siRNA can be introduced by direct transfection of RNA into cells, or transgenes can be introduced into cells that drive expression of siRNA or shRNA.

If the complementarity between the siRNA and mRNA is perfect, the mRNA is usually destroyed. If the complementarity is close but not perfect, the translation of the mRNA is arrested. Although siRNAs and shRNAs are experimental tools, endogenous small miRNAs with imperfect matches to mRNAs are emerging as an important regulator of translation in many contexts.

RNA interference has great potential to increase the power of genetic analysis because it can be used on any species where transgenes or double-stranded RNA can be delivered to cells. It should allow researchers to change the activity of genes in animals that are not now used in classical genetic analysis such as long-lived birds and fish, and even primates.

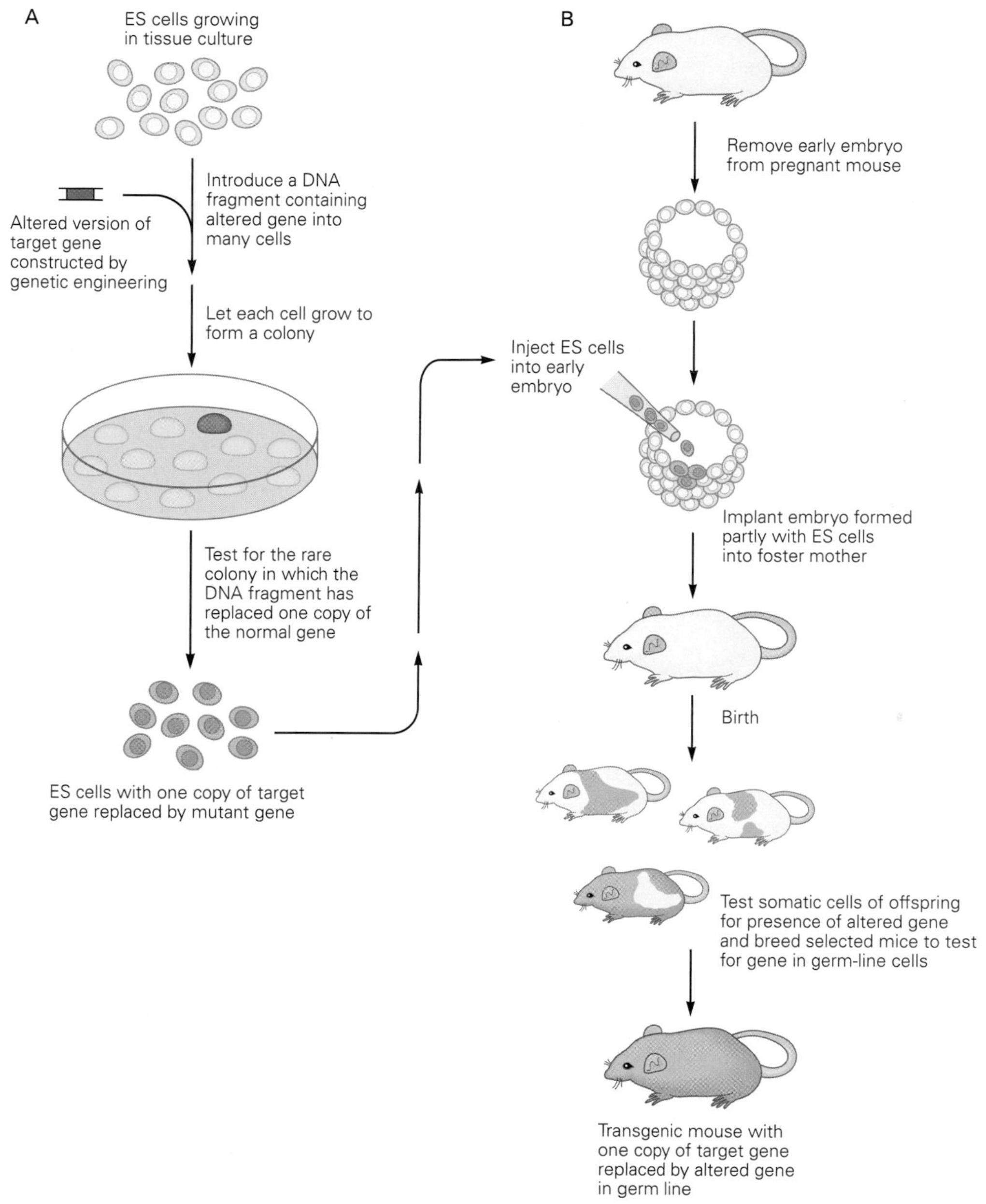
A
ES cells growing in tissue culture
Altered version of target gene constructed by genetic engineering
Introduce a DNA fragment containing altered gene into many cells
Let each cell grow to form a colony
Test for the rare colony in which the DNA fragment has replaced one copy of the normal gene
ES cells with one copy of target gene replaced by mutant gene
B
Remove early embryo from pregnant mouse
Inject ES cells into early embryo
Implant embryo formed partly with ES cells into foster mother
Birth
Test somatic cells of offspring for presence of altered gene and breed selected mice to test for gene in germ-line cells
Transgenic mouse with one copy of target gene replaced by altered gene in germ line

Figure 3–7 Creating mutant mice strains.

A. Creating mouse stem cells with specific targeted mutations.

B. Using altered embryonic stem (ES) cells to create genetically modified mice. (Reproduced, with permission, from Alberts et al. 2002.)

Box 3–3 Introducing Transgenes in Flies and Mice

Genes can be manipulated in mice by injecting DNA into the nucleus of newly fertilized eggs (Figure 3–8). In some of the injected eggs the new gene, or transgene, is incorporated into a random site on one of the chromosomes. Because the embryo is at the one-cell stage, the incorporated gene is replicated and ends up in all (or nearly all) of the animal's cells, including the germline.

Gene incorporation is illustrated with a coat color marker gene rescued by injecting a gene for pigment production into an egg obtained from an albino strain. Mice with patches of pigmented fur indicate successful expression of DNA. The transgene's presence is confirmed by testing a sample of DNA from the injected animals.

A similar approach is used in flies. The DNA to be injected is cloned into a transposable element (P element). When injected into the embryo, the DNA becomes inserted into the DNA of germ cell nuclei. P elements can be engineered to express genes at specific times and in specific cells. Transgenes may be wild-type genes that restore function to a mutant, or *designer genes* that activate other genes in new locations or code for a specifically altered protein.

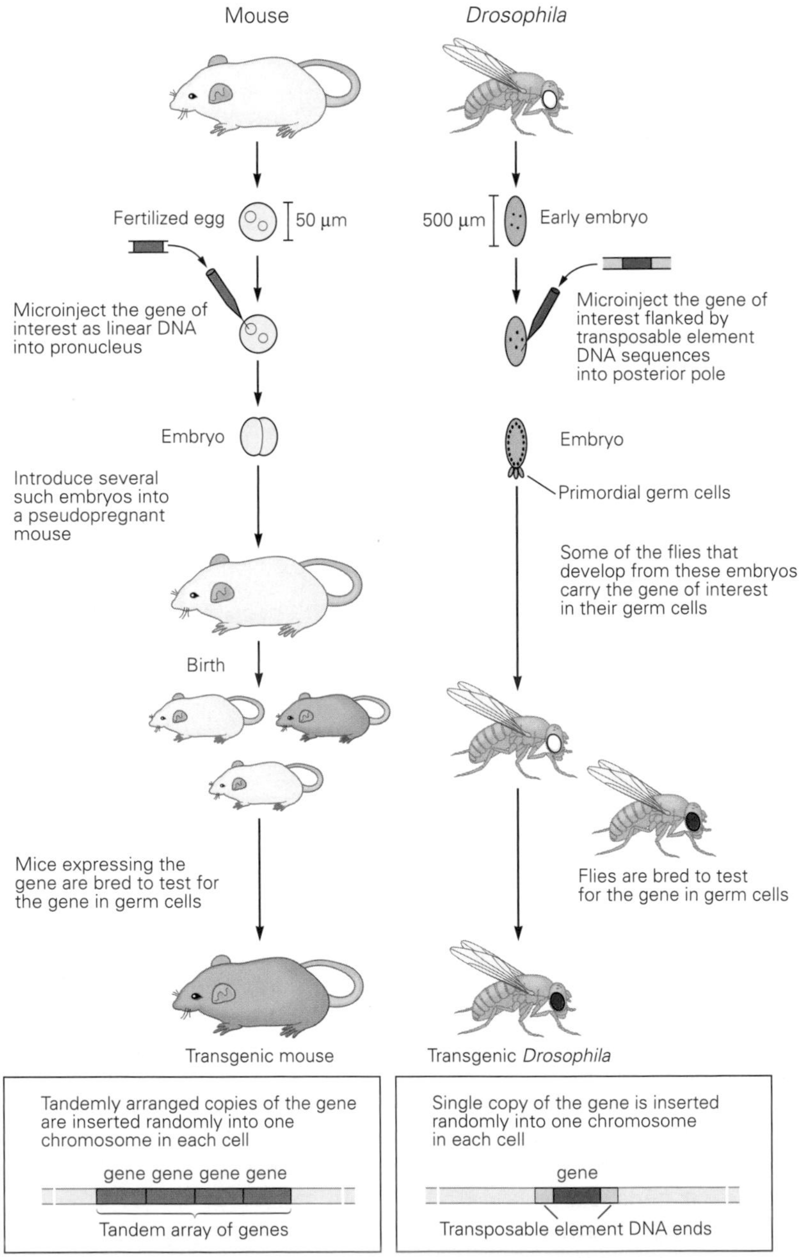

Figure 3–8 Generating transgenic mice and flies. Here the gene injected into the mouse causes a change in coat color, while the gene injected into the fly causes a change in eye color. In some transgenic animals of both species the DNA is inserted at different chromosomal sites in different cells (see illustration at bottom). (Reproduced, with permission, from Alberts et al. 2002.)

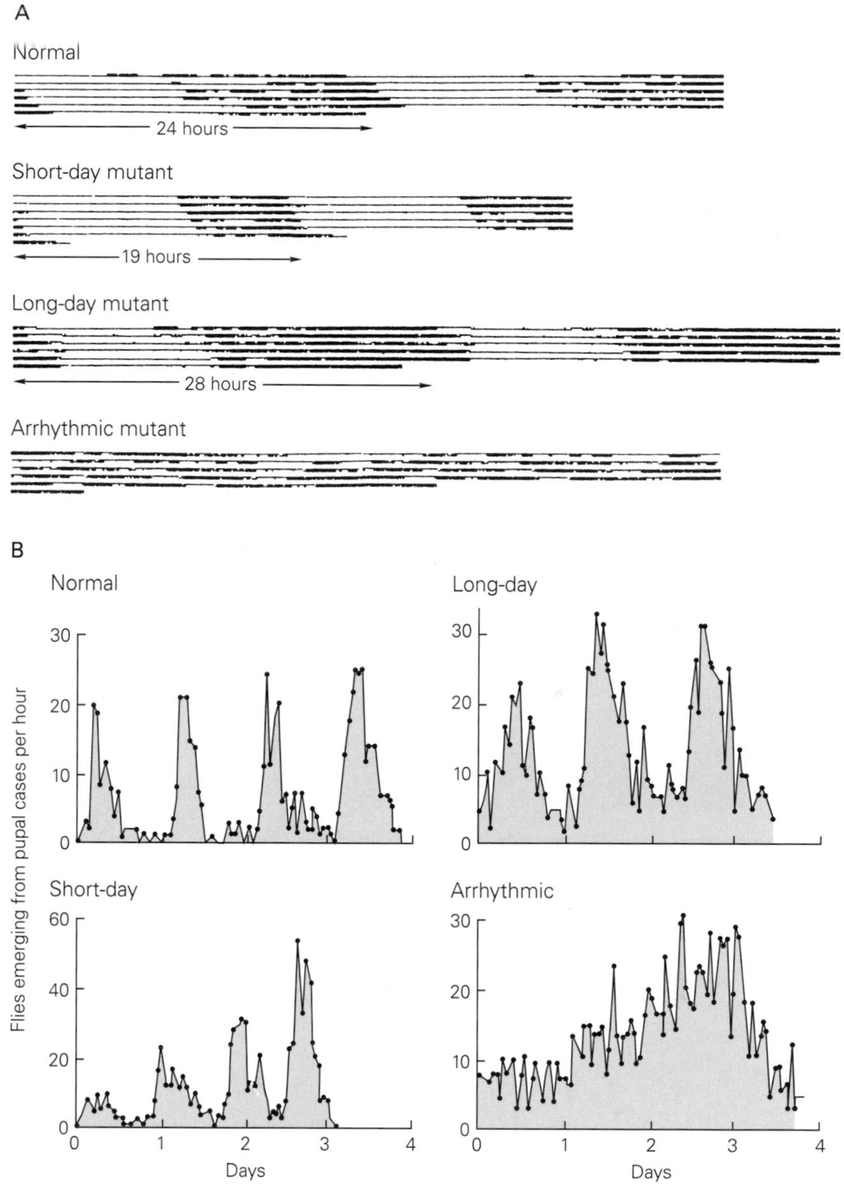

Figure 3–9 A single gene governs the circadian rhythms of behaviors in *Drosophila*. Mutations in the *period*, or *per*, gene affect all circadian behaviors regulated by the fly's internal clock. (Reproduced, with permission, from Konopka and Benzer 1971).

A. Locomotor rhythms in normal *Drosophila* and three strains of *per* mutants: short-day, long-day, and arrhythmic. Files were shifted from a cycle of 12 hours of light and 12 hours of dark into continuous darkness, and activity was then monitored under infrared light. Heavy lines indicate activity.

B. Normal adult fly populations emerge from their pupal cases in cyclic fashion, even in constant darkness. The plots show the number of flies (in each of four populations) emerging per hour over a 4-day period of constant darkness. The arrhythmic mutant population emerges without any discernible rhythm.

Characterization of these genes has led to an understanding of the molecular mechanisms of circadian rhythm, and a dramatic demonstration of the similarity of these mechanisms in flies and mice. In both flies and mice the CLOCK protein is a transcriptional activator. Together with a partner protein, it controls the transcription of genes that determine output behaviors such as locomotor activity levels. CLOCK and its partner also stimulate the transcription of the *per* gene. However, PER protein represses CLOCK's ability to stimulate *per* expression, so as PER protein accumulates, *per* transcription falls (Figure 3–11). The 24-hour cycle comes about because the accumulation and activation of PER protein is delayed by many hours after the transcription of *per*, a result of PER phosphorylation, PER instability, and interactions with other cycling proteins.

The molecular properties of *per*, *clock*, and related genes generate all properties essential for circadian rhythm. The key elements of the regulatory process are:

1. The transcription of circadian rhythm genes varies with the 24-hour cycle: PER activity is high at night, CLOCK activity is high during the day.
2. The circadian rhythm genes are transcription factors that affect each other's mRNA level,

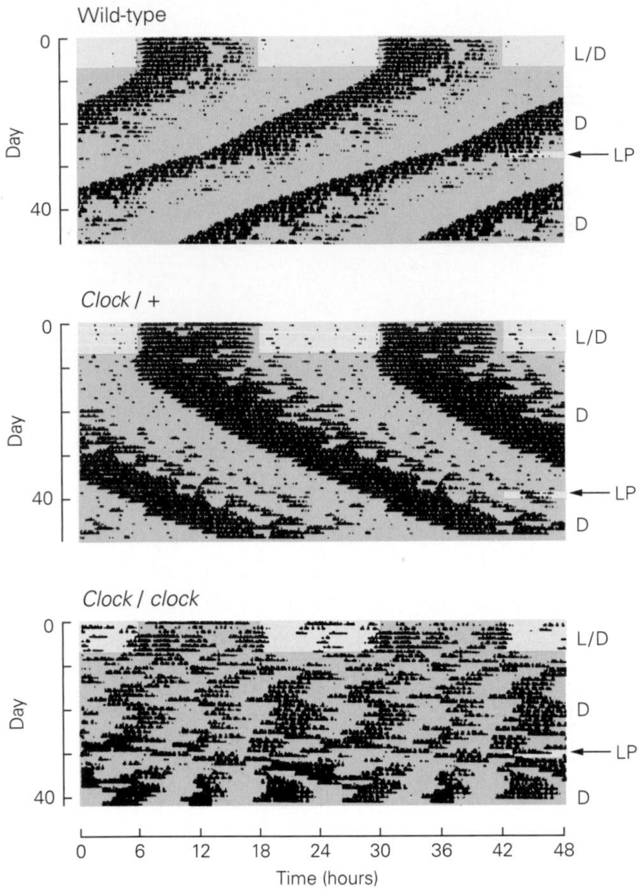

Figure 3–10 Rhythmicity in *clock* mutant mice. The records show periods of locomotor activity by three animals: wild-type, heterozygous, and homozygous. All animals were kept on a light-dark (**L/D**) cycle of 12 hours for the first 7 days, then transferred to constant darkness (**D**). They later were exposed to a 6-hour light period (**LP**) to reset the rhythm. The circadian rhythm for the wild-type mouse has a period of 23.1 hours. The period for the heterozygous *clock/+* mouse is 24.9 hours. The homozygous *clock/clock* mice experience a complete loss of circadian rhythmicity on transfer to constant darkness and transiently express a rhythm of 28.4 hours after the light period. (Reproduced, with permission, from Takahashi et al. 1994.)

generating the oscillations. CLOCK activates *per* transcription and PER represses CLOCK function.

3. The circadian rhythm genes also control the transcription of output genes that affect many downstream responses. For example, in flies the neuropeptide gene *pdf* controls locomotor activity levels.
4. The oscillation of these genes can be reset by light.

Recent work has shown that the same genetic network controls circadian rhythm in humans. People with advanced sleep-phase syndrome have short 20-day cycles and an extreme early-to-bed, early-to-rise "morning lark" phenotype. Louis Ptáček and Ying-hui Fu found that these individuals have mutations in a human *per* gene. These results demonstrate that genes for behavior are conserved from insects to humans. Advance sleep-phase syndrome is discussed in detail in the chapter on sleep (see Chapter 51).

Natural Variation in a Protein Kinase Regulates Activity in Flies and Honeybees

In the genetic studies of circadian rhythm described above, random mutagenesis was used to identify genes of interest in a biological process. All normal individuals have functional copies of *per, clock,* and the related genes; only after mutagenesis were different alleles generated. Another, more subtle question about the role of genes in behavior is to ask which genetic changes make normal individuals behave differently from each other. Work by Marla Sokolowski and her colleagues led to the identification of the first gene associated with variation in behavior among normal individuals in a species.

Larvae of *Drosophila* vary in activity level and locomotion. Some larvae, called rovers, move over long distances (Figure 3–12). Others, called sitters, are relatively stationary. *Drosophila* larvae isolated from the wild can be either rovers or sitters, indicating that these are natural variations and not laboratory-induced mutations. These traits are heritable; rover parents have rover offspring and sitter parents have sitter offspring.

Sokolowski used crosses between different wild flies to investigate the genetic differences between rover and sitter larvae. These crosses showed that the difference between rover and sitter larvae lies in a single major gene, the *for* (forager) locus. The *for* gene encodes a signal transduction enzyme, a protein kinase activated by the cellular metabolite cyclic guanosine 3′-5′monophosphate (cGMP). Thus this natural variation in behavior arises from altered regulation of signal transduction pathways. Many neuronal functions are regulated by protein kinases such as the cGMP-dependent kinase encoded by the *for* gene. Molecules such as protein kinases are particularly significant at transforming short-term neural signals into long-term changes in the property of a neuron or circuit.

Why would variability in signaling enzymes be preserved in wild populations of *Drosophila*, which typically include both rovers and sitters? The answer is that variations in the environment favor alternative genetic

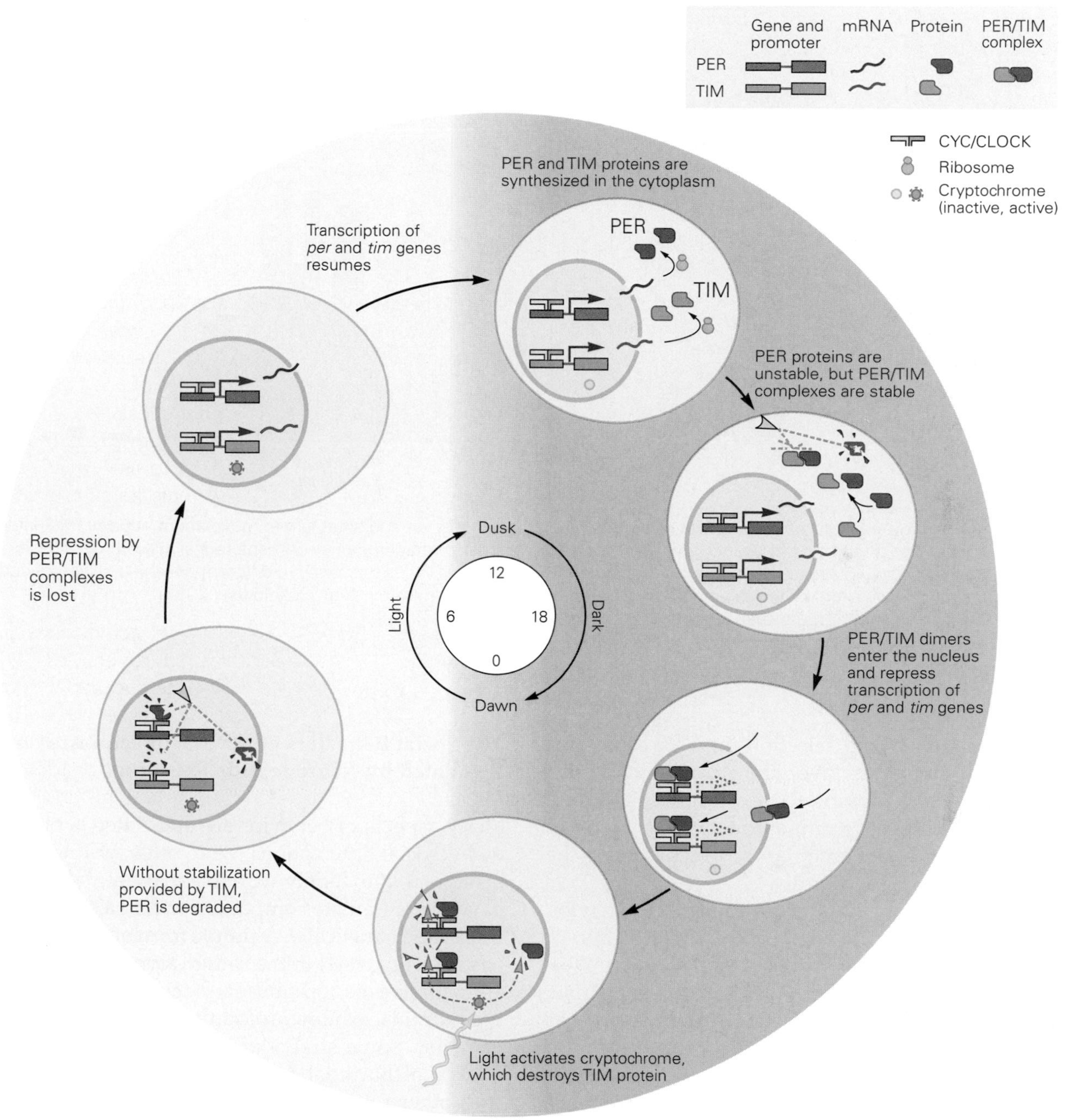

Figure 3–11 Molecular events that drive circadian rhythm. The genes that control the circadian clock are regulated by two nuclear proteins, PER and TIM, that slowly accumulate and then bind to one another to form dimers. When PER and TIM accumulate enough to dimerize, they enter the nucleus and shut off the expression of circadian genes including themselves. They do so by inhibiting CLOCK and CYCLE, which stimulate the transcription of *per* and *tim* genes. PER is highly unstable; most of the protein is degraded so quickly that it never has a chance to repress CLOCK-dependent *per* transcription. The degradation of PER is regulated by at least two different phosphorylation events by different protein kinases. When PER binds to TIM, PER is protected from degradation. As CLOCK drives more and more *per* and *tim* expression, enough PER and TIM eventually accumulate that the two can bind and stabilize each other, at which point they enter the nucleus to repress their own transcription. As a result, *per* and *tim* mRNA levels fall; thereafter, PER and TIM protein levels fall and CLOCK can (once again) drive expression of *per* and *tim* mRNA. During daylight TIM protein is degraded by signaling pathways that are regulated by light (including cryptochrome), so PER/TIM complexes form only at night. The CLOCK protein induces PER and TIM expression but is inhibited by PER and TIM proteins.

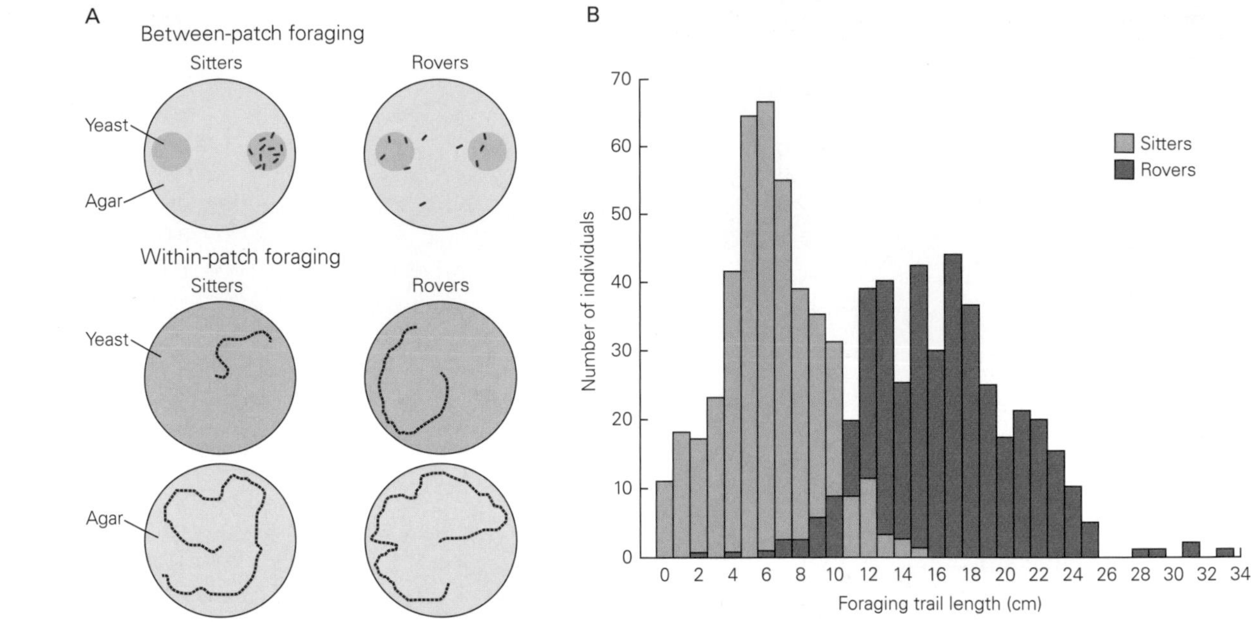

Figure 3–12 Foraging behavior of *Drosophila melanogaster* larvae. The larvae feast on patches of yeast. Rover-type larvae move from patch to patch, whereas sitter-type larvae stay put on a single patch for a long time. When foraging within a single patch, rover larvae move about more than sitter larvae. On agar alone, rover and sitter larvae move about equally. This difference in foraging behavior maps to a single protein kinase gene, *for*, that varies in activity in different fly larvae. (Reproduced, with permission, from Sokolowski 2001.)

forms: There is balanced selection for both behaviors. Crowded environments favor the rover larva, which is more effective at moving to new, unexploited food sources in advance of competitors, whereas sparse environments favor the sitter larva, which exploits the current source more thoroughly.

The *for* gene also affects honeybee behavior. Honeybees exhibit different behaviors at different stages of their life; in general, young bees are nurses, while older bees become foragers that leave the hive. The *for* gene is expressed at high levels in the brains of active foraging honeybees, and at low levels in the younger and more stationary nurse bees. Activation of cGMP signaling in young bees can cause them to enter the forager stage prematurely. Presumably, this change is normally programmed by an environmental stimulus or the bee's advancing age. Thus the same gene controls variation in a behavior in two different insects, the fruit fly and the bee. However, in the fruit fly the variation is expressed in different individuals, whereas in the honeybee it is expressed in one individual at different ages. The difference illustrates how an important regulatory gene can be recruited to different behavioral strategies in different species.

The Social Behaviors of Several Species Are Regulated by Neuropeptide Receptors

Many aspects of behavior are associated with an animal's social interactions with other animals. Social behaviors are highly variable between species, yet have a large innate component within a species that is controlled genetically. A simple form of social behavior has been analyzed in the roundworm *C. elegans.* These animals live in soil and eat bacteria. Different wild-type strains exhibit profound differences in feeding behavior. Some strains are solitary, dispersing across a lawn of bacterial food and failing to interact with each other. Other strains have a social feeding pattern, joining large feeding groups of dozens or hundreds of animals (Figure 3–13). The difference between these strains is genetic, as both feeding patterns are stably inherited.

The difference between social and solitary worms is caused by a single amino acid substitution in a single gene, a member of a large family of genes involved in signaling between neurons. This gene, *npr-1*, encodes a neuropeptide receptor. Neuropeptides have long been appreciated for their roles in coordinating behaviors across networks of neurons. For example, a neuropeptide hormone of the marine snail *Aplysia* stimulates a complex set of movements and behavior patterns associated with a single behavior, egg laying. Mammalian neuropeptides have been implicated in feeding behavior, sleep, pain, and many other behaviors and physiological processes. The existence of a mutation in the neuropeptide receptor that alters social behavior suggests that this kind of signaling molecule is important both for generating the behavior and for generating the variation between individuals.

Neuropeptide receptors have also been implicated in the regulation of mammalian social behavior. The neuropeptides oxytocin and vasopressin stimulate mammalian affiliative behaviors such as pair bonding and parental bonding with offspring. Oxytocin is required in mice for social recognition, the ability to identify a familiar individual. Oxytocin and vasopressin have been studied in depth in prairie voles, rodents that form lasting pairs to raise their young. Oxytocin released in the brain of female prairie voles during mating stimulates pair-bond formation. Likewise, vasopressin released in the brain of male prairie voles during mating stimulates pair-bond formation and paternal behavior.

The extent of pair-bonding varies substantially between mammalian species. Male prairie voles form pair-bonds with females and help them raise their offspring, but the closely related male montane voles breed widely and do not engage in paternal behavior. The difference between the behaviors of males in these species correlates with differences in the expression of the V1a class of vasopressin receptors in the brain. In prairie voles V1a vasopressin receptors are expressed at high levels in a specific brain region, the ventral pallidum (Figure 3–14). In montane voles the levels are much lower in this region, although high in other brain regions.

The importance of oxytocin and vasopressin and their receptors has been confirmed and extended by reverse genetic studies in mice, which are genetically easier to manipulate than voles. For example, introducing the V1a vasopressin receptor gene from prairie voles into male mice, which behave more like montane voles, increases the expression of the V1a vasopressin receptor in the ventral pallidum and increases the affiliative behavior of the male mice toward females. Thus differences between species in the pattern of expression of the vasopressin receptor can contribute to differences in social behaviors.

The analysis of vasopressin receptors in different rodents provides insight into the mechanisms by which genes and behaviors can change during evolution. Genetic changes in evolution alter the pattern of expression of the V1a vasopressin receptor in the ventral forebrain. These changes in turn alter the activity of a neural circuit, so that the function of the ventral forebrain is linked to the function of the vasopressin-secreting neurons that are activated by mating. As a result, social behaviors are altered.

The importance of oxytocin and vasopressin in human social behavior is not known, but the central role of pair-bonding and pup rearing in mammalian species suggests that these molecules might play a role in our species as well.

Genetic Studies of Human Behavior and Its Abnormalities

Human genetics is studied by observing traits that vary between individuals, analyzing pedigrees to trace the transmission of genetic traits across generations, and identifying functional variants using molecular

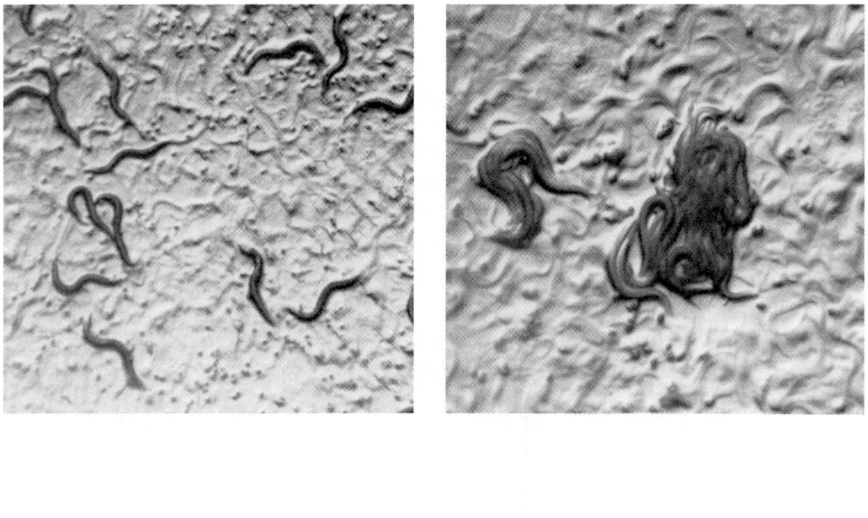

Figure 3–13 Feeding behavior of the roundworm *Caenorhabditis elegans* **depends on the level of activity of a neuropeptide receptor gene.** In one strain individual worms graze in isolation (**left**), whereas in another strain individuals mass together to feed. The difference is explained by a single amino acid substitution in the neuropeptide receptor gene. (Reproduced, with permission, from Mario de Bono and Cell Press.)

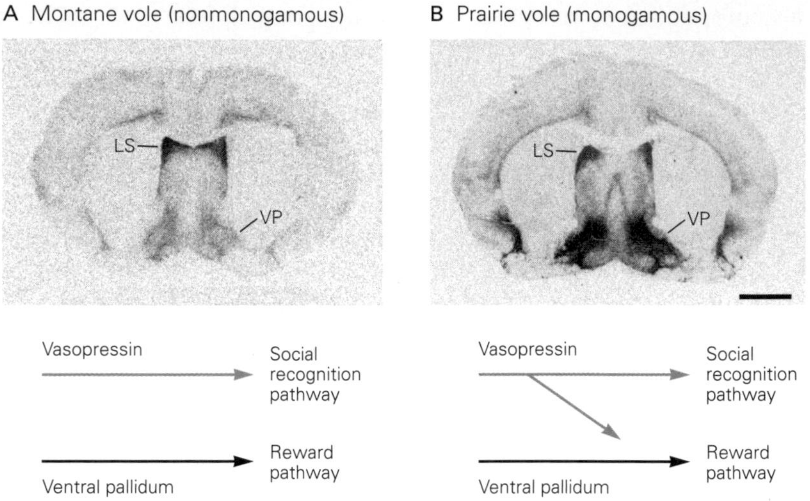

Figure 3–14 **Distribution of vasopressin (V1a) receptor binding in the ventral pallidum of montane voles (nonmonogamous) and prairie voles (monogamous).** (Adapted, with permission, from Young et al. 2001.)

A. V1a receptor expression is high in the lateral septum (LS) but low in the ventral pallidum (VP) in the nonmonogamous montane vole.

B. Expression is high in the ventral pallidum of the monogamous prairie vole. Expression of the receptor in the ventral pallidum allows vasopressin to link the social recognition pathway to the reward pathway.

biology. Human genetics is more challenging than experimental genetics because one cannot do inbreeding or crossbreeding experiments in people as one can in worms, flies, or mice.

Nonetheless, careful pedigree tracing has identified a variety of mutations that affect the human brain and behavior, including mutations that lead to neurodegenerative diseases, neurological disorders, and developmental disorders. In some cases mutations in a single gene have large effects on a neurological or behavioral trait. However, most neurological or psychiatric diseases are believed to reflect interactions between multiple genes and the environment, and our ability to tease apart these influences is still limited.

The first gene discovered to be important for a neurological disease in humans was the gene responsible for phenylketonuria (PKU), described by Asbørn Følling in Norway in 1934. This rare disease affects 1 in 15,000 children and results in severe impairment of cognitive function. Children with this disease have two abnormal copies of the gene that codes for phenylalanine hydroxylase, the enzyme that converts the amino acid phenylalanine to tyrosine. The mutation is recessive; heterozygous carrier individuals have no symptoms. Children who lack normal function in both copies of the gene accumulate high blood concentrations of phenylalanine from dietary proteins, which in turn leads to the production of toxic metabolites that interfere with neuronal function. The specific biochemical processes by which phenylalanine adversely affects the brain are still not understood.

The PKU phenotype (mental retardation) results from the interaction of the genotype (the homozygous *pku* mutation) and the environment (the diet). The treatment for PKU is thus simple and effective: Mental retardation can be prevented by a low-protein diet. The molecular and genetic analysis of gene function in PKU has led to dramatic improvements in the life of PKU patients. Since the early 1960s the United States has instated mandatory testing for PKU in newborns. By identifying children with the genetic disorder and modifying their diet before the disease appears many aspects of the disorder can be prevented.

Later chapters of this book describe many examples of single-gene traits that, like PKU, have led to insights into brain function and dysfunction. Certain themes have emerged from these studies. A number of rare neurodegenerative disorders such as Huntington disease and spinocerebellar ataxia result from the pathological, dominant expansion of glutamate residues within proteins. The discovery of these polyglutamine repeat disorders highlighted the danger to the brain of unfolded and aggregated proteins. The discovery that epileptic seizures can be caused by a variety of mutations in ion channels led to the realization that these disorders are primarily disorders of neuronal excitability.

The single-gene disorders mentioned earlier are rare compared to the total burden of neurodegenerative and psychiatric disease. One might wonder why we study rare single-gene variants if they represent a tiny fraction of the total disease burden. The reason is that rare, relatively simple disorders can provide insight into the biological processes affected in more common, complex forms of the disease. For example, among the prominent successes of human genetics has been the discovery of rare genetic variants that lead to early-onset Alzheimer disease or Parkinson disease.

Individuals with these severe rare variants represent a tiny subset of all individuals with Alzheimer disease or Parkinson disease, but the rare variants uncovered cellular processes that are also disrupted in the larger patient pool, pointing the way to general therapeutic avenues.

In the remainder of this chapter we discuss the genetics of autism and schizophrenia, two psychiatric disorders that manifest themselves in childhood or adolescence, respectively. Compared to the polyglutamine repeat diseases or ion channel-related seizure disorders, the biological causes of autism and schizophrenia are still largely unknown. Nonetheless, in some cases we can begin to see how certain genes, and the associated biological processes, affect complex brain functions such as language, learning, and emotion.

Neurological Disorders in Humans Suggest That Distinct Genes Affect Different Brain Functions

Autism is a common, devastating developmental disorder characterized by deficiencies in language acquisition, difficulties in social interactions, and stereotyped interests. About 1 in 200 children are diagnosed with autism (the exact frequency varies with diagnostic criteria), with about three times as many boys affected as girls. The clinical symptoms of autism typically emerge in the first 3 years of life and often include a regression phase in which children lose the language skills they mastered when younger.

There is considerable variability between autistic individuals. Children affected with autism have a higher frequency of seizures and cognitive problems than the general population, and some are severely disabled. However, many autistic individuals have normal or above-normal intelligence, and can, with appropriate care, goes on to lead highly successful lives.

Autism has a very strong heritable component (see Figure 3–1A), which should increase the chances of identifying the underlying genes. Autism is also a disorder of broader significance because it provides insight into behaviors that are unique to humans: language, complex intelligence, and interpersonal interactions. The fact that autistic defects in social communication can coexist with normal intelligence in other domains suggests that the brain is modular, with distinct cognitive functions that can vary independently.

The idea that distinct genes affect different cognitive domains is supported by the contrasting effects of a rare genetic syndrome called Williams syndrome. Children with Williams syndrome acquire language late, but they ultimately overcome their early deficits to develop strong language skills and normal social behavior. Indeed, these children exhibit extreme sociability; for example, they lack the shyness children typically have in the presence of strangers. However, Williams children are profoundly defective in spatial processing, and they score as poorly as, or even worse than, autistic children on IQ tests. The different patterns of impairments in autism and Williams syndrome suggest that language and social skills can be separated from some other brain functions. Brain areas concerned with language are impaired in autistic children but active or accented in Williams syndrome children. By contrast, general and spatial intelligence is more impaired in Williams syndrome than in many autistic children.

Williams syndrome is genetically simple; it is caused by a heterozygous deletion of chromosome region 7q11.23. The simplest interpretation of this defect is that the level of expression of one or more genes within this interval is reduced because there is only one copy instead of two of each gene in the region. The precise genes in this region that affect sociability and spatial processing are not yet known, but they are of great interest because of their potential to provide insight into the genetic regulation of human behaviors.

Another rare syndrome has shed light on genetic requirements for human language. A study of a human family with defects in speech articulation, as well as grammatical and linguistic impairment, led to the identification of a specific mutation in the transcriptional regulator *FOXP2*. This gene is not uniquely human—it is present in all mammals and birds—but several changes in the gene have appeared since the divergence of humans and other primates. A human-specific pattern of development of the brain, larynx, or mouth under the control of *FOXP2* might be one of the genetic adaptations that made human speech possible.

Autism-Related Disorders Exemplify the Complex Genetic Basis of Behavioral Traits

Autism is a common disorder, yet there is no single genetic location for autism as there is for the much rarer Williams syndrome. At least part of the explanation for this difference is that autism is not really one disorder caused by a single kind of genetic lesion, but rather a cluster of related disorders caused by a variety of different genetic changes. The recognition of this genetic complexity is providing inroads into autism and related syndromes that affect social communication and language.

The symptoms of classical autism partly overlap with those of a number of genetic disorders whose genetic basis is understood. For example like autism, fragile X syndrome affects mostly boys, and patients have poor social cognition, high social anxiety, and repetitive behavior. However, fragile X syndrome is associated with broader cognitive defects, along with certain physical characteristics, like an elongated face and protruding ears. Fragile X syndrome has been genetically associated with a mutation that reduces expression of a single gene on the X chromosome. This gene regulates the translation of mRNAs into proteins in neurons, a process that is regulated during synaptic plasticity and learning. The male preponderance of fragile X syndrome is explained because males have only a single X chromosome, and therefore lose all expression of the relevant gene when it is mutated. Since females have two X chromosomes, they can be carriers of the disease without being strongly affected.

Another autism-like syndrome whose genetic basis is understood is Rett syndrome, which we consider in detail in Chapter 64. Rett syndrome is an X-linked, progressive neurodevelopmental disorder and one of the most common causes of mental retardation in females. The disease is confined to females because Rett syndrome is lethal in the developing male embryo, which has a single X chromosome. Affected girls seem to develop normally until they are 6 to 18 months of age, when they fail to acquire speech and purposeful hand use is replaced by compulsive, uncontrolled hand-wringing.

Huda Zoghbi and her colleagues found that the major cause of this disease is a mutation in the methyl CpG binding protein 2 (*MeCP2*) gene. Methylation of specific CpG sequences in DNA alters expression of nearby genes, and it is thought that *MeCP2* binds methylated DNA as part of a process that regulates mRNA transcription. This discovery shows that acquisition of complex developmental properties such as language is associated with specific patterns of gene expression, most likely in the brain. Current research on Rett syndrome focuses on identifying the affected brain regions and the inappropriately transcribed genes in these children.

Psychiatric Disorders and the Challenge of Understanding Multigenic Traits

The observation that common diseases such as autism are less well understood than rare diseases such as Rett syndrome applies broadly to psychiatric disorders. Schizophrenia affects about 1% of all young adults, causing a pattern of thought disorders and emotional withdrawal that profoundly impairs life. It is strongly heritable (see Figure 3–1B), but its genetic basis is poorly understood. Despite evidence of heritability, and despite progress in research on individual diseases using experimental animal models, it has been difficult to identify the genes associated with many common human psychiatric diseases like chronic depression and anxiety disorders, which affect a substantial fraction of people. In this final section of the chapter we survey the approaches that are being developed to address these shortfalls.

Complex Inheritance and Genetic Imprinting in Human Genetics

Understanding Mendelian inheritance is not always sufficient for understanding human genetic disorders. For example, studies of human developmental disorders have shown important effects of an unusual form of gene regulation called *parental imprinting*. Although humans have two copies of all autosomes, they sometimes express mRNA from only one of the two copies of a gene, either the copy from the mother or the copy from the father. Angelman syndrome and Prader-Willi syndrome are examples of genetic diseases with a complex heritability caused by parental imprinting. To understand these diseases, one must not only know the DNA lesion associated with the disease but also understand whether the DNA lesion was inherited from the father or the mother (Figure 3–15).

Angelman syndrome is an inherited disorder that can include severe mental retardation, epilepsy, absence of speech, hyperactivity, and inappropriate laughter. The syndrome results from deletion of multiple genes on one copy of the chromosome region 15q11-q13. In this region some genes are expressed only from the maternally derived chromosome, and a different set of genes are expressed only from the paternally derived chromosome. The genes implicated in Angelman syndrome are expressed only from the maternally derived chromosome. Therefore, if a child receives a normal chromosome from her mother and an abnormal chromosome with a deletion from her father, she will not have Angelman syndrome. However, if she receives a normal chromosome from her father and an abnormal chromosome from her mother, she will have Angelman syndrome.

For Angelman syndrome the most important gene in this region appears to be the gene that encodes UBE3A, a ubiquitin-protein ligase that is expressed only from the maternally derived chromosome. Ubiquitin ligases stimulate the degradation and turnover of other proteins. The important targets of UBE3A are thought to regulate general brain plasticity, perhaps by regulating the activity of neurotransmitter receptors.

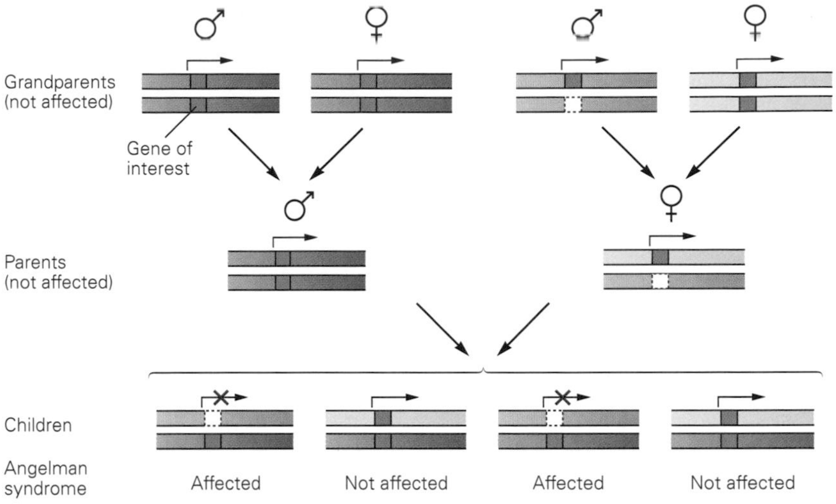

Figure 3–15 Expression of an imprinted gene. Imprinted genes are expressed from only one of two chromosomes, either the chromosome derived from the father or the one derived from the mother. In this example the gene responsible for Angelman syndrome is expressed only from the maternally derived chromosome. If this chromosome has a deletion (dashed region), the child has symptoms of the disease.

A different neurodevelopmental behavioral disorder, Prader-Willi syndrome, is also caused by a deletion of multiple genes on chromosome 15q11-q13, but the genes implicated in Prader-Willi syndrome are expressed only from the paternally derived chromosome. Therefore, Prader-Willi syndrome results from the reciprocal of the pattern of inheritance in Angelman syndrome: A child must receive the abnormal chromosome from his father to develop Prader-Willi syndrome. Prader-Willi syndrome is associated with obesity, and psychiatric symptoms include obsessive-compulsive behavior, bipolar disorder, and pervasive developmental disorders.

Parental imprinting is an example of the complexity that can confound expectations in human gene mapping. Recent studies in mice by Catherine Dulac's group suggest that parental imprinting is more common in the brain than it is in other tissues in the body. If this observation holds true in humans, it could help explain why mapping human behavioral traits is difficult.

Multigenic Traits: Many Rare Diseases or a Few Common Variants?

Genetic mapping methods that follow linkage across generations are highly effective in identifying single-gene traits (Box 3–4). However, most common genetic disorders in humans cannot be followed through pedigrees as single-gene traits, and they are suspected or known to involve multiple genes as well as genetic interactions with the environment. Schizophrenia, autism, and depression fall into this category, as do diabetes, coronary artery disease, and asthma.

In contrast to single-locus Mendelian traits, multigenic traits do not have a simple recognizable pattern of inheritance (autosomal dominant, recessive, or X-linked), and thus the relative contributions of several genes to one trait are difficult to analyze. Nevertheless, determining which genes contribute to complex human traits has profound implications for the care and treatment of human disease and therefore is an area of intense study.

To understand complex psychiatric disorders it will be important to distinguish between various models of transmission. According to one (monogenic) model, many genes in the population can contribute to a disorder, but each gene mutation is individually rare and has a strong effect. Taking the examples described earlier in the chapter, it is known that *MeCP2* mutations (Rett syndrome) and fragile X mutations each account for 1–2% of children with autism-related disorders. In a rare monogenic model there might be 100 other mutations, each individually rare, that can result in autism.

A second (polygenic) model assumes that a small number of relatively common mutations, each of which has only a small effect on risk, interact together to cause a disorder. The latter model is sometimes called the "common variant – common disease" hypothesis. Common human variants are known to increase the risk of some common diseases such as macular degeneration, which leads to adult-onset blindness. Thus, there are well-understood examples of both the monogenic and polygenic models in human genetics. An important question is the extent to which each model contributes to the burden of psychiatric diseases.

Box 3–4 Genetic Polymorphisms and Linkage Mapping

The most common strategy for finding genes that affect humans has been *linkage analysis,* which takes advantage of the fact that two random individuals differ in their DNA sequences at many positions in the genome. The sequence variants, which are usually functionally neutral, are called *DNA polymorphisms,* and the most restricted changes are called *single nucleotide polymorphisms.*

DNA polymorphisms are tracked by a variety of methods, usually by amplifying specific regions from an individual's DNA and examining the sequence of those regions. In linkage mapping the segregation of many different DNA polymorphisms is correlated with the segregation of the genetic trait of interest in the same families. Coinheritance of a DNA marker and mutant phenotype (or disease state) suggests that the marker and the mutant gene lie close together on the chromosome (Figure 3–16).

A DNA marker that is linked to a mutant gene is almost always coinherited with the mutant gene, whereas DNA marker and mutant gene that are not linked are coinherited only by chance. The chance that any two unlinked loci—for example, loci from different chromosomes—will be inherited together is 1/2, and the chance that they will be coinherited in n siblings is $(1/2)^n$. Thus, if two loci are coinherited in all eight affected siblings from a single family, the odds against this being a random event would be $(1/2)^8 = 256{:}1$.

A statistically rigorous linkage value based on family trait mapping and specific models of inheritance is called the *lod* (logarithm of odds) score. For practical purposes a lod score equal to or greater than 3 indicates that a DNA marker is significantly linked to a genetic trait. The discovery of a high lod score is the first step in finding the right gene.

Typically, the region is narrowed down by seeking many additional polymorphic DNA markers that are on chromosome regions near the first linked DNA marker. A careful analysis is then conducted to ask which polymorphic DNA markers are coinherited with the genetic trait most frequently. Genes involved in many human neurological diseases have been pinpointed using this approach.

Despite its power, classical linkage analysis failed to reveal genes for schizophrenia and bipolar disorder, and this failure inspired the development of alternative strategies for mapping human genetic traits. One strategy continues to rely on tracking transmission through families but uses models that are less rigid than those of classical linkage analysis. This method does not make assumptions about whether a mutation is dominant or recessive but assumes only that linked DNA will tend to be coinherited in two affected siblings. Another strategy uses quantitative models to assist the identification of genes that contribute some genetic variance to a multigenic trait (*quantitative trait loci*).

Finally, the completion of the human genome sequence is being followed by identification of many DNA polymorphisms in the human genome and resequencing of many regions of the genome from hundreds of individuals. A fuller understanding of the genetic variance in our human heritage may provide clues about how to identify the DNA polymorphisms that lead to psychiatric illness.

In both the "rare monogenic" model and the "common variant – common disease" model, it is challenging to identify the effects of individual mutations. Therefore, current psychiatric genetic studies usually involve international consortia cooperating in the diagnosis of very large clinical groups of patients. These studies can be analyzed using both monogenic and polygenic models of inheritance, and an increasingly sophisticated array of genotyping methods to assess correlations between regions of the genome and traits of interest (Box 3–4). Promising results have emerged from a variety of studies. Verification of these results will require independent replication of results and very large numbers of patients. With that caveat, some of the first fruits of these studies are described below.

A successful single-gene mapping study of a large Scottish family with a high rate of schizophrenia led to the identification of the risk gene *Disc1* (for Disrupted in Schizophrenia). In mice *Disc1* has effects on neuronal development, neuronal signaling, and the incorporation of newborn neurons into neural circuits. In humans a *Disc1* mutation greatly increases the risk of schizophrenia, but it is mutated only in a small fraction of schizophrenic patients. Other candidate genes for

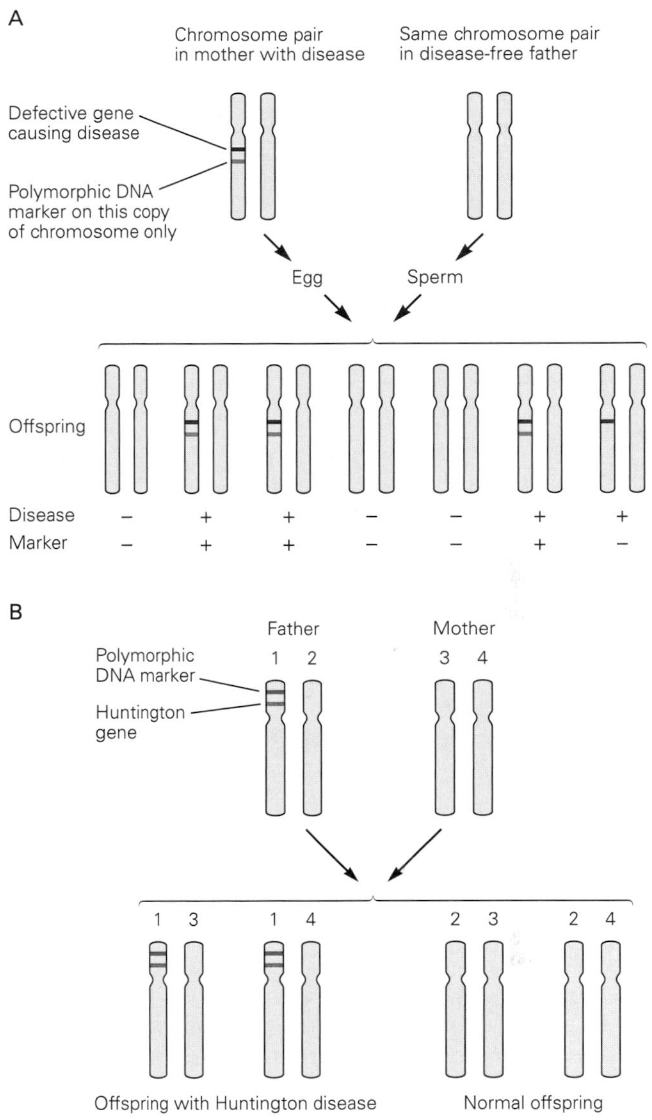

Figure 3–16 Methods for mapping human genes.

A. Genetic linkage analysis detects the coinheritance of a mutated gene responsible for a human disease and a nearby polymorphic DNA marker. In this example the gene responsible for the disease is inherited in four offspring, three of which coinherit the marker. Thus the gene responsible for the disease is located close to the polymorphic DNA marker on this chromosome. The presence of the polymorphic marker is scored by direct sequencing of the human DNAs or by physical techniques that detect nucleotide mismatches between a reference sequence and the sequence being tested.

B. Inheritance of the gene responsible for Huntington disease can be traced by following the inheritance of a particular polymorphic DNA marker on chromosome 4.

schizophrenia have been identified from the alternative approach of looking for statistical associations between the disorder and specific loci in the genome in a sample of thousands of schizophrenic patients from different families. One risk gene identified in this way is *neuregulin*, a developmental signaling gene that affects cell migration and synapse formation. Together the studies of *Disc1* and *neuregulin* begin to suggest that a developmental defect in the brain can underlie schizophrenia.

Similar large-scale studies of thousands of autistic children and their families have led to the repeated identification of mutations in certain autism risk genes. Several mutations in autistic patients affect transmembrane signaling proteins called neurexins and neuroligins, which affect the strength of synapses. These results and other genetic results suggest that subtle alterations in synaptic transmission play a role in autism. Sophisticated genetic analysis suggests that an increased risk for autism exists at many locations in the genome (Figure 3–17). Some of these loci may be rare monogenic high-risk variants and others may be more common, low-risk variants.

One remarkable discovery made by Michael Wigler's group while trying to understand the genetic basis of

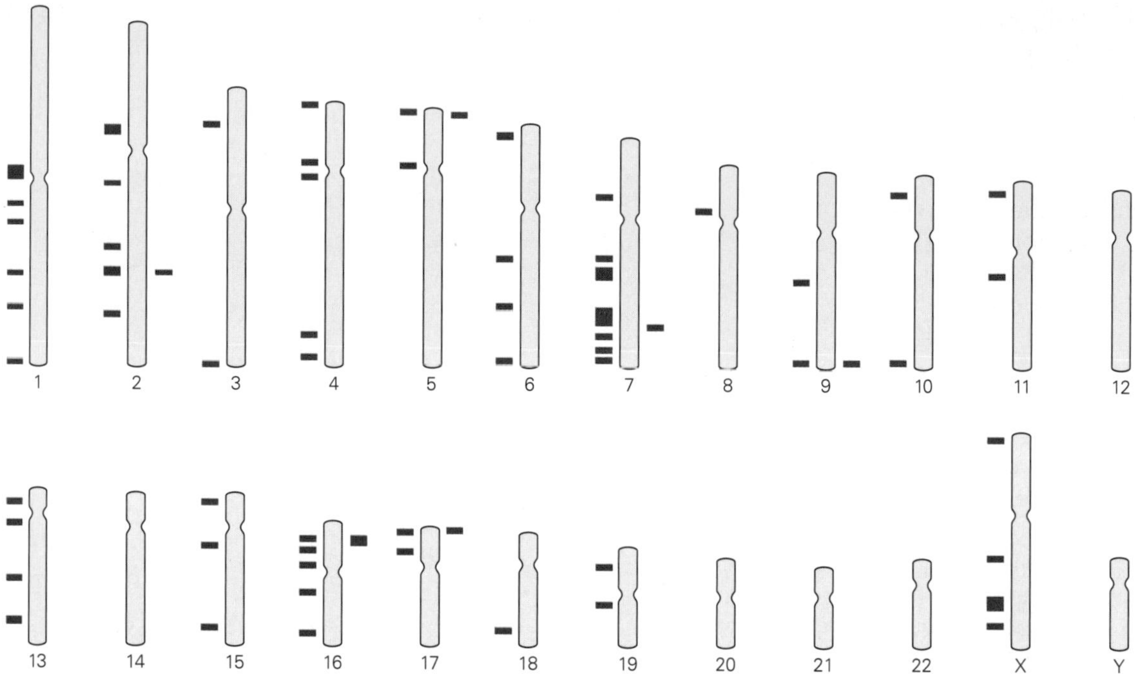

Figure 3–17 Candidate loci that contribute to autism spectrum disorders. The loci were identified in several published genome screens. Many different loci may increase the risk of autism. The most consistent signal reported in multiple studies is on the long arm of chromosome 7, but there is also overlap of different studies on chromosomes 2 and 16. No one locus appears in all studies. (Reproduced, with permission, from Folstein et al. 2001.)

autism is that a fraction of the mutations associated with autism are not actually inherited from either parent. They are new mutations in the autistic child that arose in the sperm or the oocyte prior to fertilization. Identical monozygotic twins that separate after fertilization will both have the trait, the classical definition of heritability. Moreover, once the mutation arises, the affected child has a trait that can be passed on to his or her children, so it is indeed a heritable trait. However, classical genetic linkage studies rely on the assumption that virtually all disease-causing mutations are preexisting mutations inherited across many generations, and the finding of new mutations in autism violate that expectation. Human biology is a constant source of surprises.

New tools are being developed to help address the complexities of multigenic traits. For example, brain imaging techniques are being used to pinpoint anatomical loci underlying clinical syndromes that might be caused by specific mutations. At this writing, it will soon be possible to sequence the complete genomes of individual psychiatric patients to discover genetic variants. Even when these sequences are available, however, we will still need sophisticated approaches to ask which of the many variations that distinguish one human being from every other human being represent the risk factors for disease.

An Overall View

Genes affect many aspects of behavior. There are remarkable similarities in personality traits and psychiatric illnesses in human twins, even those raised separately; domestic and laboratory animals can be bred for particular, stable behavioral traits; a few specific genes are associated with human behaviors.

In recent years we have seen great success in identifying the genes associated with neurological diseases such as Alzheimer disease, Parkinson disease, Huntington disease, and spinocerebellar ataxias, as well as those associated with developmental disorders such as Rett syndrome and Angelman syndrome. What we have learned about the genetic basis of these diseases may help us fashion approaches to researching the more difficult psychiatric diseases such as schizophrenia, depression, and autism.

Human behavioral traits are multigenic in origin. Although alterations in a single gene account for individual differences in social behavior in nematodes and activity levels in *Drosophila*, only rarely will genetic alteration at a single gene fully explain a psychiatric disease or a behavior in humans. More frequently, several different genes will each act independently to affect a trait, or have effects only in combination with each other. Model organisms such as the fly, the worm, and the mouse are important for genetics because they are experimentally tractable. By studying genes in these simple animals, where the genome and environment can be rigorously controlled, it is possible to identify the conserved biological pathways that mediate behavior in humans. Several successes have emerged from this approach. The *per* gene in the fruit fly led to an understanding of human advanced sleep phase syndrome, and the gene for narcolepsy in dogs has led to an understanding of the underlying biology of sleep in humans (see Chapter 51).

There is still much to learn about the ways that genes affect the brain. Biologists are becoming more skilled at delineating the role of individual genes within particular neurons and circuits. There are important insights to be gained about the genetics of psychiatric disease and the genetic influences on normal psychological, physiological, and cognitive traits. Yet it is the interplay of genetics, environment, chance, and individual choice that ultimately determines the behavioral differences between individuals. The challenge of genetics is to understand the undeniable effects of genes, while acknowledging that many factors influence human mental processes and behavior.

Glossary[1]

Allele. Humans carry two sets of chromosomes, one from each parent. Equivalent genes in the two sets might be different, for example, because of single nucleotide polymorphisms. An allele is one of the two (or more) forms of a particular gene.

Centromere. Chromosomes contain a compact region known as a centromere, where sister chromatids (the two exact copies of each chromosome that are formed after replication) are joined.

Cloning. The process of generating sufficient copies of a particular piece of DNA to allow it to be sequenced or studied in some other way.

Complementary DNA (cDNA). A DNA sequence made from a messenger RNA molecule, using an enzyme called *reverse transcriptase*. cDNAs can be used experimentally to determine the sequence of messenger RNAs after their introns (nonprotein-coding sections) have been spliced out.

Conservation of genes. Genes that are present in two distinct species are said to be conserved, and the two genes from the different species are called *orthologous genes*. Conservation can be detected by measuring the similarity of the two sequences at the base (RNA or DNA) or amino acid (protein) level. The more similarities there are, the more highly conserved the two sequences.

Copy number variation (CNV). A deletion or duplication of a limited genetic region that results in an individual having more or fewer than the usual two copies of some genes. Copy number variations are observed in some neurological and psychiatric disorders.

Euchromatin. The gene-rich regions of a genome (see also heterochromatin).

Eukaryote. An organism with cells that have a complex internal structure, including a nucleus. Animals, plants, and fungi are all eukaryotes.

Genome. The complete DNA sequence of an organism.

Genotype. The set of genes that an individual carries; usually refers to the particular pair of alleles (alternative forms of a gene) that a person has at a given region of the genome.

Haplotype. A particular combination of alleles (alternative forms of genes) or sequence variations that are closely linked—that is, are likely to be inherited together—on the same chromosome.

Heterochromatin. Compact, gene-poor regions of a genome, which are enriched in simple sequence repeats.

Introns and exons. Genes are transcribed as continuous sequences, but only some segments of the resulting messenger RNA molecules contain information that encodes a protein product. These segments are called *exons*. The regions between exons are known as *introns* and are spliced from the RNA before the product is made.

Long and short arms. The regions on either side of the centromere are known as arms. As the centromere is not in the center of the chromosome, one arm is longer than the other.

Messenger RNA (mRNA). Proteins are not synthesized directly from genomic DNA. Instead, an RNA template (a precursor mRNA) is constructed from the sequence of the gene. This RNA is then processed in various ways, including splicing. Spliced RNAs destined to become templates for protein synthesis are known as mRNAs.

Mutation. An alteration in a genome compared to some reference state. Mutations do not always have harmful effects.

Phenotype. The observable properties and physical characteristics of an organism.

Polymorphism. A region of the genome that varies between individual members of a population. To be called a polymorphism, a variant should be present in a significant number of people in the population.

[1] From P. Bork and R. Copley. 2001. Genome speak. *Nature* 409:815.

Prokaryote. A single-celled organism with a simple internal structure and no nucleus. Bacteria and Archaebacteria are prokaryotes.
Proteome. The complete set of proteins encoded by the genome.
Recombination. The process by which DNA is exchanged between pairs of equivalent chromosomes during egg and sperm formation. Recombination has the effect of making the chromosomes of the offspring distinct from those of the parents.
Restriction endonuclease. An enzyme that cleaves DNA at a particular short sequence. Different types of restriction endonuclease cleave at different sequences.
RNA interference (RNAi). A method for reducing the function of a specific gene by introducing into a cell small RNAs with complementarity to the targeted mRNA. Pairing of the mRNA with the small RNA leads to destruction of the endogenous mRNA.
Single nucleotide polymorphism (SNP). A polymorphism caused by the change of a single nucleotide. SNPs are often used in genetic mapping studies.
Splicing. The process that removes introns (noncoding portions) from transcribed RNAs. Exons (protein-coding portions) can also be removed. Depending on which exons are removed, different proteins can be made from the same initial RNA or gene. Different proteins created in this way are *splice variants* or *alternatively spliced*.
Transcription. The process of copying a gene into RNA. This is the first step in turning a gene into a protein, although not all transcripts lead to proteins.
Transcriptome. The complete set of RNAs transcribed from a genome.
Translation. The process of using a messenger RNA sequence to build a protein. The messenger RNA serves as a template on which transfer RNA molecules, carrying amino acids, are lined up. The amino acids are then linked together to form a protein chain.

Cornelia I. Bargmann
T. Conrad Gilliam

Selected Readings

Alberts B, Johnson A, Lewis J, Raff M, Roberts K, Walter P. 2002. *Molecular Biology of the Cell*, 4th ed. New York: Garland Publishing. Also searchable at http://www.ncbi.nlm.nih.gov/entrez/query.fcgi?db=Books.

Allada R, Emery P, Takahashi JS, Rosbash M. 2001. Stopping time: the genetics of fly and mouse circadian clocks. Annu Rev Neurosci 24:1091–119.

Botstein D, Risch N. 2003. Discovering genotypes underlying human phenotypes: past successes for mendelian disease, future approaches for complex disease. Nat Genet 33:228–337. Suppl.

Bouchard TJ Jr, Lykken DT, McGue M, Segal NL, Tellegen A. 1990. Sources of human psychological differences: the Minnesota Study of Twins Reared Apart. Science 250: 223–228.

Griffiths AJF, Gelbart WM, Miller JH, Lewontin RC. 1999. *Modern Genetic Analysis*. New York: Freeman. Also searchable at http://www.ncbi.nlm.nih.gov/entrez/query.fcgi?db=Books.

Insel TR, Young LJ. 2001. The neurobiology of attachment. Nat Rev Neurosci 2:129–136.

International Human Genome Sequencing Consortium. 2001. Initial sequencing and analysis of the human genome. Nature 409:860–921.

Online Mendelian Inheritance in Man, OMIM™. McKusick-Nathans Institute of Genetic Medicine, Johns Hopkins University (Baltimore, MD) and National Center for Biotechnology Information, National Library of Medicine (Bethesda, MD), World Wide Web URL: http://www.ncbi.nlm.nih.gov/omim/

Novina CD, Sharp PA. 2004. The RNAi revolution. Nature 430:161–164.

Shahbazian MD, Zoghbi HY. 2002. Rett syndrome and MeCP2: linking epigenetics and neuronal function. Am J Hum Genet 71:1259–1272.

Venter JG, Adams MD, Myers EW, Li PW, Mural RJ, Sutton GG, Smith HO, et al. 2001. The sequence of the human genome. Science 291:1304–1351.

References

Amir RE, Van den Veyver IB, Wan M, Tran CQ, Francke U, Zoghbi HY. 1999. Rett syndrome is caused by mutations in X-linked MECP2, encoding methyl-CpG-binding protein 2. Nat Genet 23:185–188.

Antoch MP, Song EJ, Chang AM, Vitaterna MH, Zhao Y, Wilsbacher LD, Sangoram AM, King DP, Pinto LH, Takahashi JS. 1997. Functional identification of the mouse circadian Clock gene by transgenic BAC rescue. Cell 89:655–667.

Arnold SE, Talbot K, Hahn CG. 2004. Neurodevelopment, neuroplasticity, and new genes for schizophrenia. Prog Brain Res 147:319–345.

Bellugi U, Lichtenberger L, Jones W, Lai Z, St George M. 2000. I. The neurocognitive profile of Williams Syndrome: a complex pattern of strengths and weaknesses. J Cogn Neurosci 12:7–29. Suppl.

Ben-Shahar Y, Robichon A, Sokolowski MB, Robinson GE. 2002. Influence of gene action across different time scales on behavior. Science 296:741–744.

Brunner HG, Nelen M, Breakefield XO, Ropers HH, van Oost BA. 1993. Abnormal behavior associated with a point mutation in the structural gene for monoamine oxidase A. Science 262:578–580.

Caron H, van Schaik B, van der Mee M, Baas F, Riggins G, van Sluis P, Hermus MC, et al. 2001. The human transcriptome map: clustering of highly expressed genes in chromosomal domains. Science 291:1289–1292.

De Bono M, Bargmann CI. 1998. Natural variation in a neuropeptide Y receptor homolog modifies social behavior and food responses in *C. elegans*. Cell 94:679–689.

Folstein SE, Rosen-Sheidley B. 2001. Genetics of autism: complex aetiology for a heterogeneous disorder. Nat Rev Genet 2:943–955.

Gottesman II. 1991. *Schizophrenia Genesis. The Origins of Madness*. New York: Freeman.

Gross C, Hen R. 2004. The developmental origins of anxiety. Nat Rev Neurosci 5:545–552.

Holmes A, Lit Q, Murphy DL, Gold E, Crawley JN. 2003. Abnormal anxiety-related behavior in serotonin transporter null mutant mice: the influence of genetic background. Genes Brain Behav 2:365–380.

Kahler SG, Fahey MC. 2003. Metabolic disorders and mental retardation. Am J Med Genet C Semin Med Genet 117:31–41.

Khaitovich P, Muetzel B, She X, Lachmann M, Hellmann I, Dietzsch J, Steigele S, et al. 2004. Regional patterns of gene expression in human and chimpanzee brains. Genome Res 14:1462–1473.

Konopka RJ, Benzer S. 1971. Clock mutations of Drosophila melanogaster. Proc Natl Acad Sci U S A 68:2112–2116.

Lai CS, Fisher SE, Hurst JA, Vargha-Khadem F, Monaco AP. 2001. A forkhead-domain gene is mutated in a severe speech and language disorder. Nature 413:519–523.

Lander, ES, Linton, LM, Birren, B, Nusbaum, C, Zody, MC, Baldwin J, Devon K, et al. 2001. Initial sequencing and analysis of the human genome. Nature 409:860-921.

Lim MM, Wang Z, Olazabal DE, Ren X, Terwilliger EF, Young LJ. 2004. Enhanced partner preference in a promiscuous species by manipulating the expression of a single gene. Nature 429:754–757.

McGue, M, Bouchard, TH Jr. 1998. Genetic and environmental influences on human behavioral differences. Ann Rev Neurosci 21:1–24.

Mendel G. 1866. Versuche über Pflanzen-hybriden. Verh Naturforsch 4:3–47;1966. Translated in: C Stern, ER Sherwood (eds). *The Origin of Genetics: A Mendel Source Book*. San Francisco: Freeman.

Sokolowski MB. 1980. Foraging strategies of *Drosophila melanogaster*: a chromosomal analysis. Behav Genet 10: 291–302.

Sokolowski MB. 2001. Drosophila: genetics meets behavior. Nat Rev Genet 2:879–890.

Stefansson H, Sigurdsson E, Steinthorsdottir V, Bjornsbottir S, Sigmundsson T, Ghosh S, Brynjolfsson J, et al. 2002. Neuregulin 1 and susceptibility to schizophrenia. Am J Hum Genet 71:877–892.

Takahashi JS, Pinto LH, Vitaterna MH. 1994. Forward and reverse genetic approaches to behavior in the mouse. Science 264:1724–1733.

Toh KL, Jones CR, He Y, Eide EJ, Hinz WA, Virshup DM, Ptacek LJ, Fu YH. 2001. An hPer2 phosphorylation site mutation in familial advanced sleep phase syndrome. Science 291:1040–1043.

Walter J, Paulsen M. 2003. Imprinting and disease. Semin Cell Dev Biol 14:101–110.

Watson JD, Tooze J, Kurtz DT (eds). 1983. *Recombinant DNA: A Short Course*. New York: Scientific American; distr. by W.H. Freeman.

Whitfield CW, Cziko AM, Robinson GE. 2003. Gene expression profiles in the brain predict behavior in individual honey bees. Science 302:296–299.

Young LJ, Lim MM, Gingrich B, Insel TR. 2001. Cellular mechanisms of social attachment. Horm Behav 40: 133–138.

Zondervan KT, Cardon LR. 2004. The complex interplay among factors that influence allelic association. Nat Rev Genet 5:89–100.

Part II

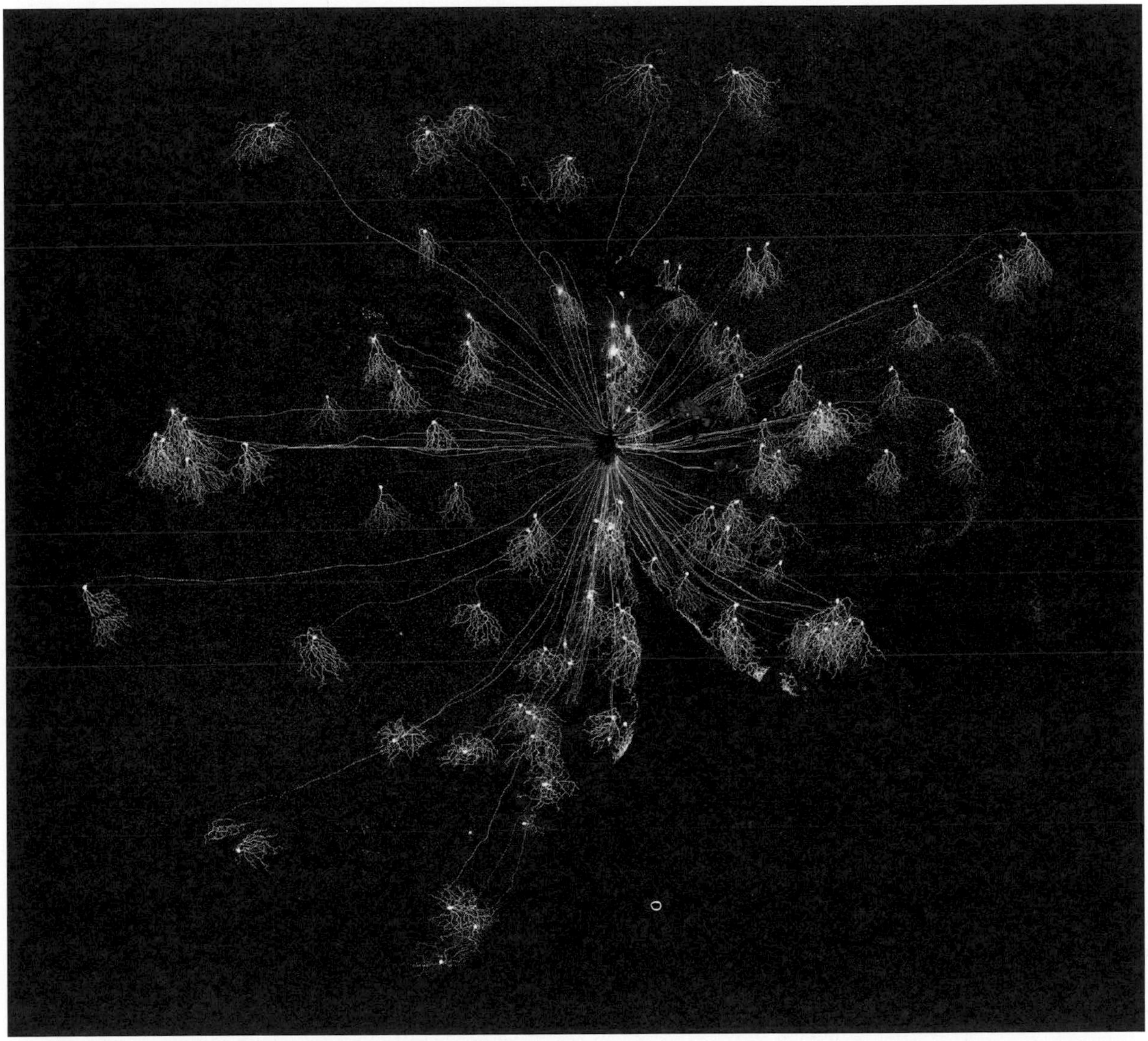

Preceding Page

Retinal ganglion cells arrayed across the retina are illuminated by a transgenic marker (junctional adhesion molecule B [JAM-B]). Whereas the axons of all ganglion cells converge at the back of the eye and exit the retina as the optic nerve en route to the brain, the dendrites of this particular set of neurons also share the same orientation, branching downward from the cell bodies. Their common form reflects a common function: detection of upward motion in the visual field. (Reproduced, with permission, from In-Jung Kim and Joshua Sanes.)

II

Cell and Molecular Biology of the Neuron

IN ALL BIOLOGICAL SYSTEMS, from the most primitive to the most advanced, the basic building block is the cell. Cells are often organized into functional modules that are repeated in complex biological systems. The vertebrate brain is the most complex example of a modular system. Complex biological systems have another structural feature: They are architectonic—that is, their anatomy, fine structure, and biochemistry all reflect a specific physiological function. Thus, the construction of the brain and the cell biology, biophysics, and biochemistry of its component neurons reflect its fundamental function, which is to mediate behavior.

The great diversity of nerve cells—the fundamental units from which the modules of the nervous systems are assembled—is derived from one basic cell plan. Three features of this plan give nerve cells the unique ability to communicate with one another precisely and rapidly over long distances. First, the neuron is polarized, possessing receptive dendrites on one end and communicating axons with synaptic terminals at the other. This polarization of functional properties is commonly used to restrict the flow of impulses to one direction. Second, the neuron is electrically and chemically excitable. Its cell membrane contains specialized proteins—ion channels and receptors—that permit the influx and efflux of specific inorganic ions, thus creating electrical currents that alter the voltage across the membrane. Third, the neuron contains proteins and organelles that endow it with specialized secretory properties that allow it to release neurotransmitters at synapses.

In this part of the book, we shall be concerned with the properties of the neuron that give it the ability to generate electrical signals in the form of synaptic and action potentials (see Chapter 4). The initiation of a signal depends on ion channels in the cell membrane that open in response to changes in membrane voltage and to neurotransmitters released by other nerve cells. In Chapter 5, we consider general properties of ion channels. Neurons use three major classes of channels for signaling: (1) resting channels generate the resting potential and underlie the passive properties of neurons that determine the time course of synaptic potentials, their spread along dendrites, and the threshold for firing an action potential, as discussed in Chapter 6; (2) voltage-gated channels are responsible for the active currents that generate the action potential, which is discussed in Chapter 7; and (3) ligand-gated channels open in response to neurotransmitters to generate synaptic potentials. In this section, we focus mainly on resting and voltage-gated channels. In the next section, we consider in more detail ligand-gated channels.

Part II

4

The Cells of the Nervous System

NEURONS AND GLIA—the cells from which the nervous system is assembled—share many characteristics with cells in general. However, neurons are specially endowed with the ability to communicate precisely and rapidly with other cells at distant sites in the body. Two features give neurons this ability.

First, they have a high degree of morphological and functional asymmetry: Neurons have receptive dendrites at one end and a transmitting axon at the other. This arrangement is the structural basis for unidirectional neuronal signaling.

Second, neurons are both electrically and chemically excitable. The cell membrane of neurons contains specialized proteins—ion channels and receptors—that facilitate the flow of specific inorganic ions, thereby redistributing charge and creating electrical currents that alter the voltage across the membrane. These changes in charge can produce a wave of depolarization in the form of action potentials along the axon, the usual way a signal travels within the neuron. Glia are less excitable, but their membranes contain transporter proteins that facilitate the uptake of ions as well as proteins that remove neurotransmitter molecules from the extracellular space, thus regulating neuronal function.

There are about 100 distinct types of neurons. This cytological diversity is also apparent at the molecular level. Although neurons all inherit the same complement of genes, each expresses a restricted set and thus produces only certain molecules—enzymes, structural proteins, membrane constituents, and secretory products—and not others. In large part this expression depends on the cell's developmental history. In essence each cell *is* the set of molecules that it makes.

Neurons and Glia Share Many Structural and Molecular Characteristics

Neurons and glia develop from common neuroepithelial cells of the embryonic nervous system and thus

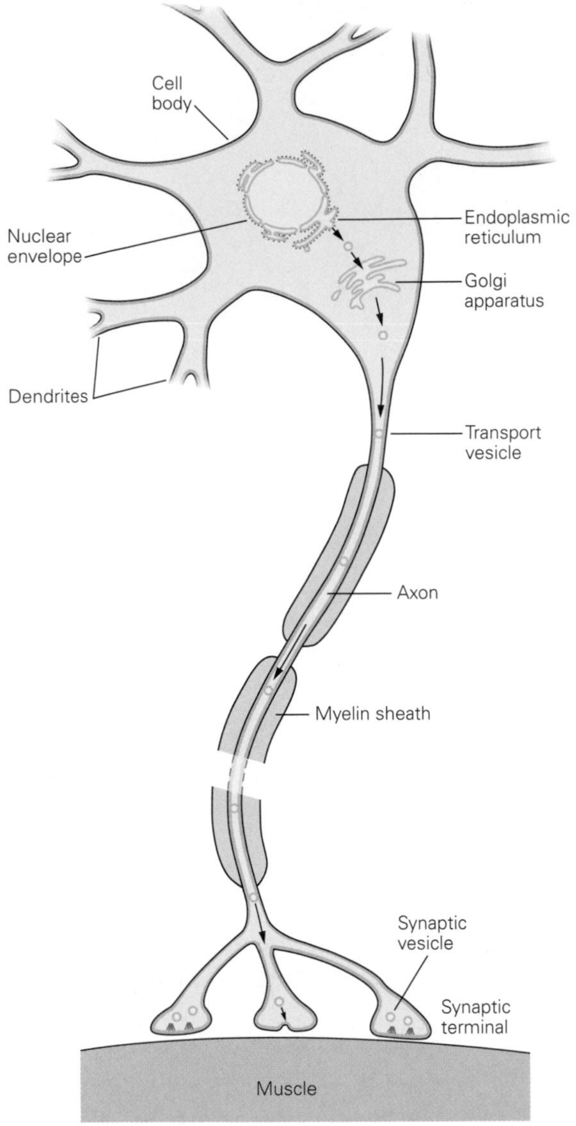

Figure 4–1 The structure of a neuron. The cell body and nucleus of a spinal motor neuron are surrounded by a double-layered membrane, the nuclear envelope, which is continuous with the endoplasmic reticulum. The space between the two membrane layers that constitutes the nuclear envelope is continuous with the lumen of the endoplasmic reticulum. Dendrites emerge from the basal aspect of the neuron, the axon from the apical aspect. (Adapted, with permission, from Williams et al. 1989.)

share many structural and molecular characteristics (Figure 4–1). The boundaries of these cells are defined by the cell membrane or *plasmalemma*, which has the asymmetric bilayer structure of all biological membranes and provides a hydrophobic barrier impermeable to most water-soluble substances. Cytoplasm has two main components: cytosol and membranous organelles.

Cytosol is the aqueous phase of cytoplasm. In this phase only a few proteins are actually free in solution. With the exception of some enzymes that catalyze metabolic reactions, most proteins are organized into functional complexes. A recent subdiscipline called *proteomics* has determined that these complexes can consist of many distinct proteins, none of which are covalently linked to another. For example, the cytoplasmic tail of the *N*-methyl-D-aspartate (NMDA)-type glutamate receptor, a membrane-associated protein that mediates excitatory synaptic transmission in the central nervous system, is anchored in a large complex of more than 100 scaffold proteins and protein-modifying enzymes. (Many cytosolic proteins involved in second-messenger signaling, discussed in later chapters, are embedded in the cytoskeletal matrix immediately underneath the plasmalemma.) Ribosomes, the organelle on which messenger RNA (mRNA) molecules are translated, are made up of several protein subunits. Proteasomes, large multienzyme organelles that degrade ubiquitinated proteins (a process described later in this chapter), are also present throughout the cytosol of neurons and glia.

Membranous organelles, the second main component of cytoplasm, include mitochondria and peroxisomes as well as a complex system of tubules, vesicles, and cisternae called the *vacuolar apparatus.* Mitochondria and peroxisomes process molecular oxygen. Mitochondria generate adenosine triphosphate (ATP), the major molecule by which cellular energy is transferred or spent, whereas peroxisomes prevent accumulation of the strong oxidizing agent hydrogen peroxide. Thought to be derived from symbiotic organisms that invaded eukaryotic cells early in evolution, these two organelles are not functionally continuous with the vacuolar apparatus.

The vacuolar apparatus includes the rough endoplasmic reticulum, the smooth endoplasmic reticulum, the Golgi complex, secretory vesicles, endosomes, lysosomes, and a multiplicity of transport vesicles that interconnect these various compartments (Figure 4–2). Their lumen corresponds topologically to the outside of the cell; consequently, the inner leaflet of their lipid bilayer corresponds to the outer leaflet of the plasmalemma.

The major subcompartments of this system are anatomically discontinuous, but they remain functionally connected because membranous and lumenal material is moved from one compartment to another by means of transport vesicles. For example, proteins and phospholipids synthesized in the rough endoplasmic reticulum (the portion of the reticulum nearest the nucleus and studded with ribosomes) and the smooth endoplasmic reticulum are transported to the Golgi complex and then to secretory vesicles, which empty their contents when the vesicle membrane fuses with the

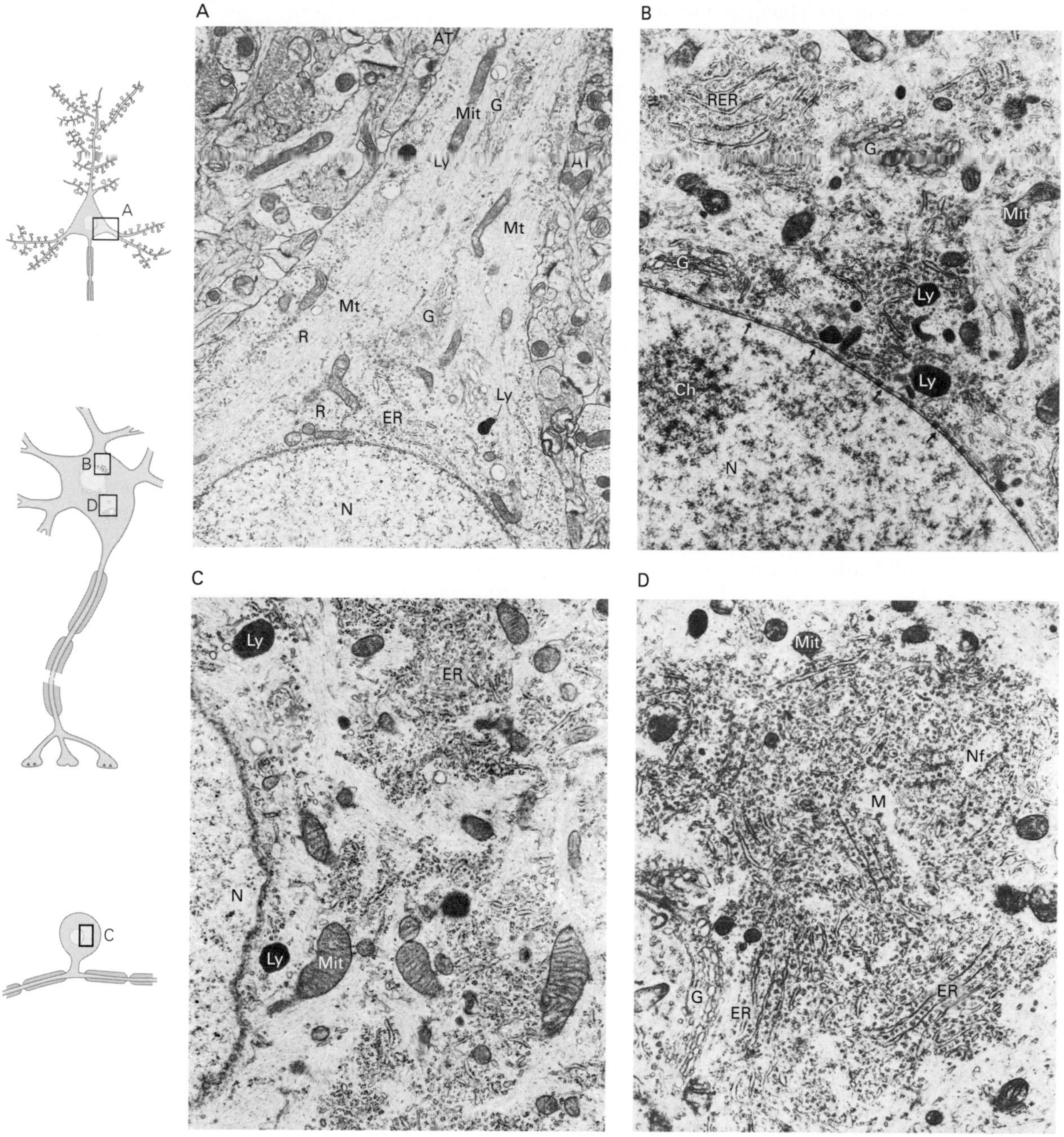

Figure 4–2 Organelles of the neuron. Electron micrographs show cytoplasm in four different regions of the neuron. (Adapted, with permission, from Peters et al. 1991.)

A. A dendrite emerges from a pyramidal neuron's cell body, which includes the endoplasmic reticulum (**ER**) above the nucleus (**N**) and a portion of the Golgi complex (**G**) nearby. Some Golgi cisternae have entered the dendrite, as have mitochondria (**Mit**), lysosomes (**Ly**), and ribosomes (**R**). Microtubules (**Mt**) are prominent cytoskeletal filaments in the cytosol. Axon terminals (**AT**) making contact with the dendrite are seen at the top and right.

B. Some components of a spinal motor neuron that participate in the synthesis of macromolecules. The nucleus (**N**), containing masses of chromatin (**Ch**), is bounded by the nuclear envelope, which contains many nuclear pores (**arrows**). The mRNA leaves the nucleus through these pores and attaches to ribosomes that either remain free in the cytoplasm or attach to the membranes of the endoplasmic reticulum to form the rough endoplasmic reticulum (**RER**). Regulatory proteins synthesized in the cytoplasm are imported into the nucleus through the pores. Several parts of the Golgi apparatus (**G**) are seen, as are lysosomes (**Ly**) and mitochondria (**Mit**).

C–D. Micrographs of a dorsal root ganglion cell (**C**) and a motor neuron (**D**) show the organelles in the cell body that are chiefly responsible for synthesis and processing of proteins. The mRNA enters the cytoplasm through the nuclear envelope and is translated into proteins. Free polysomes, strings of ribosomes attached to a single mRNA, generate cytosolic proteins and proteins to be imported into mitochondria (**Mit**) and peroxisomes. Proteins destined for the endoplasmic reticulum are formed after the polysomes attach to the membrane of the endoplasmic reticulum (**ER**). The particular region of the motor neuron shown here also includes membranes of the Golgi apparatus (**G**), in which membrane and secretory proteins are further processed. Some of the newly synthesized proteins leave the Golgi apparatus in vesicles that move down the axon to synapses; other membrane proteins are incorporated into lysosomes (**Ly**) and other membranous organelles. The microtubules (**M**) and neurofilaments (**Nf**) are components of the cytoskeleton.

plasmalemma (a process called *exocytosis*). This secretory pathway serves to add membranous components to the plasmalemma and also to discharge any contents of the secretory vesicles into the extracellular space.

Conversely, plasmalemmal membrane is taken into the cell in the form of endocytic vesicles (*endocytosis*). These are incorporated into early endosomes, sorting compartments that are concentrated at the cell's periphery. The incorporated membrane, which typically contains specific proteins such as receptors, is then either shuttled back to the plasmalemma by vesicles for recycling or directed to late endosomes and eventually to mature lysosomes for degradation. (Exocytosis and endocytosis are discussed in detail later in this chapter and in Chapter 12.) The smooth endoplasmic reticulum also acts as a regulated internal Ca^{2+} store throughout the neuronal cytoplasm (see Chapter 11 on Ca^{2+} release).

A specialized portion of the rough endoplasmic reticulum forms the nuclear envelope, a spherical flattened cisterna that surrounds chromosomal DNA and its associated proteins (histones, transcription factors, polymerases, and isomerases) and defines the nucleus (Figure 4–1). Because the nuclear envelope is continuous with other portions of the endoplasmic reticulum and to the other membranes of the vacuolar apparatus, it is presumed to have evolved as an invagination of the plasmalemma to ensheathe eukaryotic chromosomes. The nuclear envelope is interrupted by nuclear pores, where fusion of the inner and outer membranes of the envelope results in the formation of hydrophilic channels through which proteins and RNA are exchanged between the cytoplasm proper and the nuclear cytoplasm.

Even though nucleoplasm and cytoplasm are continuous domains of cytosol, only molecules with molecular weights less than 5,000 can pass through the nuclear pores freely by diffusion. Larger molecules need help. Some proteins have special nuclear localization signals, domains that are composed of a sequence of basic amino acids (arginine and lysine) that are recognized by soluble proteins called *nuclear import receptors* (importins). At a nuclear pore this complex is guided into the nucleus by another group of proteins called *nucleoporins*.

The cytoplasm of the nerve cell body extends into the dendritic tree without functional differentiation. Generally, all organelles in the cytoplasm of the cell body are also present in dendrites, although the densities of the rough endoplasmic reticulum, Golgi complex, and lysosomes rapidly diminish with distance from the cell body. In dendrites the smooth endoplasmic reticulum is prominent at the base of thin processes called *spines* (Figures 4–3 and 4–4), the receptive portion of excitatory synapses. Concentrations of polyribosomes in dendritic spines are presumed to serve local protein synthesis (see below and Figure 4–4).

In contrast to the continuity of the cell body and dendrites, a sharp functional boundary exists between the cell body at the axon hillock, where the axon emerges. Ribosomes, rough endoplasmic reticulum, and the Golgi complex—the organelles that comprise the main biosynthetic machinery for proteins in the neuron—are generally excluded from axons (see Figure 4–3). Lysosomes and certain proteins are also excluded. However, axons are rich in synaptic vesicles and their precursor membranes.

The Cytoskeleton Determines Cell Shape

The cytoskeleton determines the shape of a cell and is responsible for the asymmetric distribution of organelles within the cytoplasm. It includes three filamentous structures: microtubules, neurofilaments, and microfilaments. These filaments and associated proteins account for approximately a quarter of the total protein in the cell.

Microtubules form long scaffolds that extend from one end of a neuron to the other and play a key role in developing and maintaining cell shape. A single microtubule can be as long as 0.1 mm. Microtubules are constructed of protofilaments, each of which consists of multiple pairs of α- and β-tubulin subunits arranged longitudinally along the microtubule (Figure 4–5A). Tubulin subunits bind to neighboring subunits along the protofilament and also laterally between adjacent protofilaments. The tubulin dimer has a polar structure: The negative end is oriented to the center of the cell while the positive end extends out to the periphery, to the dendrites and axon.

Microtubules grow by addition of guanosine triphosphate (GTP)-bound tubulin dimers at their positive end, the end that points to the periphery. Shortly after polymerization the GTP is hydrolyzed to guanosine diphosphate (GDP). When a microtubule stops growing, its positive end is capped by a GDP-bound tubulin monomer. Given the low affinity of the GDP-bound tubulin for the polymer, this would lead to catastrophic depolymerization unless the microtubules were stabilized by interaction with other proteins.

In fact, while microtubules undergo rapid cycles of polymerization and depolymerization in dividing cells, in mature dendrites and axons they are much more stable. This stability is caused by microtubule-associated proteins (MAPs) that promote the oriented polymerization and assembly of the tubulin polymers. MAPs in axons differ from those in dendrites. For example, MAP2

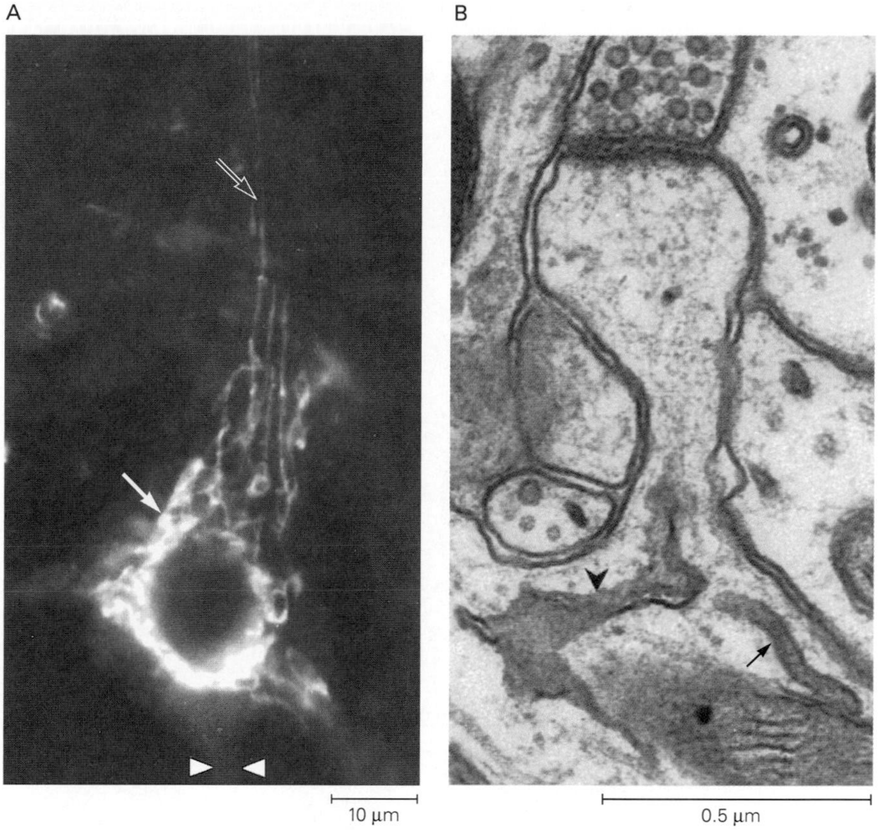

Figure 4–3 Golgi and endoplasmic reticulum membranes extend from the cell body into dendrites.

A. The Golgi complex (**solid arrow**) appears under the light microscope as several filaments that extend into the dendrites (**open arrow**) but not into the axon. The **arrowheads** at the bottom indicate the axon hillock. For this micrograph a large neuron of the brain stem was immunostained with antibodies specifically directed against the Golgi complex. (Reproduced, with permission, from De Camilli et al. 1986.)

B. Smooth endoplasmic reticulum (**arrowhead**) extends into the neck of a dendritic spine, while another membrane compartment sits at the origin of the spine (**arrow**). (Reproduced, with permission, from Cooney et al. 2002.)

is present in dendrites but not in axons, whereas tau and MAP3 are present. In Alzheimer disease and some other degenerative disorders tau proteins are modified and abnormally polymerized, forming a characteristic lesion called the *neurofibrillary tangle* (Box 4–1).

Tubulins are encoded by a multigene family. At least six genes code the α- and β-subunits. Because of the expression of the different genes or post transcriptional modifications more than 20 isoforms of tubulin are present in the brain.

Neurofilaments, 10 nm in diameter, are the bones of the cytoskeleton (see Figure 4–5B). They are the most abundant fibrillar component in axons; on average there are 3 to 10 times more neurofilaments than microtubules in an axon. Neurofilaments are related to intermediate filaments of other cell types, including the cytokeratins of epithelial cells (hair and nails), glial fibrillary acidic protein in astrocytes, and desmin in muscle. Unlike microtubules, neurofilaments are stable and almost totally polymerized in the cell.

At 3–7 nm in diameter microfilaments are the thinnest of the three main types of fibers that make up the cytoskeleton (Figure 4–5C). Like thin filaments of muscle, microfilaments are made up of two strands of polymerized globular actin monomers, each bearing an ATP or adenosine diphosphate (ADP), wound into a double-stranded helix. Actin is a major constituent of all cells, perhaps the most abundant animal protein in nature. There are several closely related molecular forms: the α actin of skeletal muscle and at least two other molecular forms, β and γ. Each is encoded by a different gene. Neural actin in higher vertebrates is a mixture of the β and γ species, which differ from muscle actin by a few amino acid residues. Most actin molecules are highly conserved, not only in different cell types of a species but also in organisms as distantly related as humans and protozoa.

Unlike microtubules and neurofilaments, actin filaments are short. They are concentrated at the cell's periphery in the cortical cytoplasm just underneath the plasmalemma, where they form a dense network with many actin-binding proteins (eg, spectrin-fodrin, ankyrin, talin, and actinin). This matrix plays a key role in the dynamic function of the cell's periphery, such as the motility of growth cones (the growing tips of axons) during development, generation of specialized microdomains at the cell surface, and the formation of pre- and postsynaptic morphological specializations.

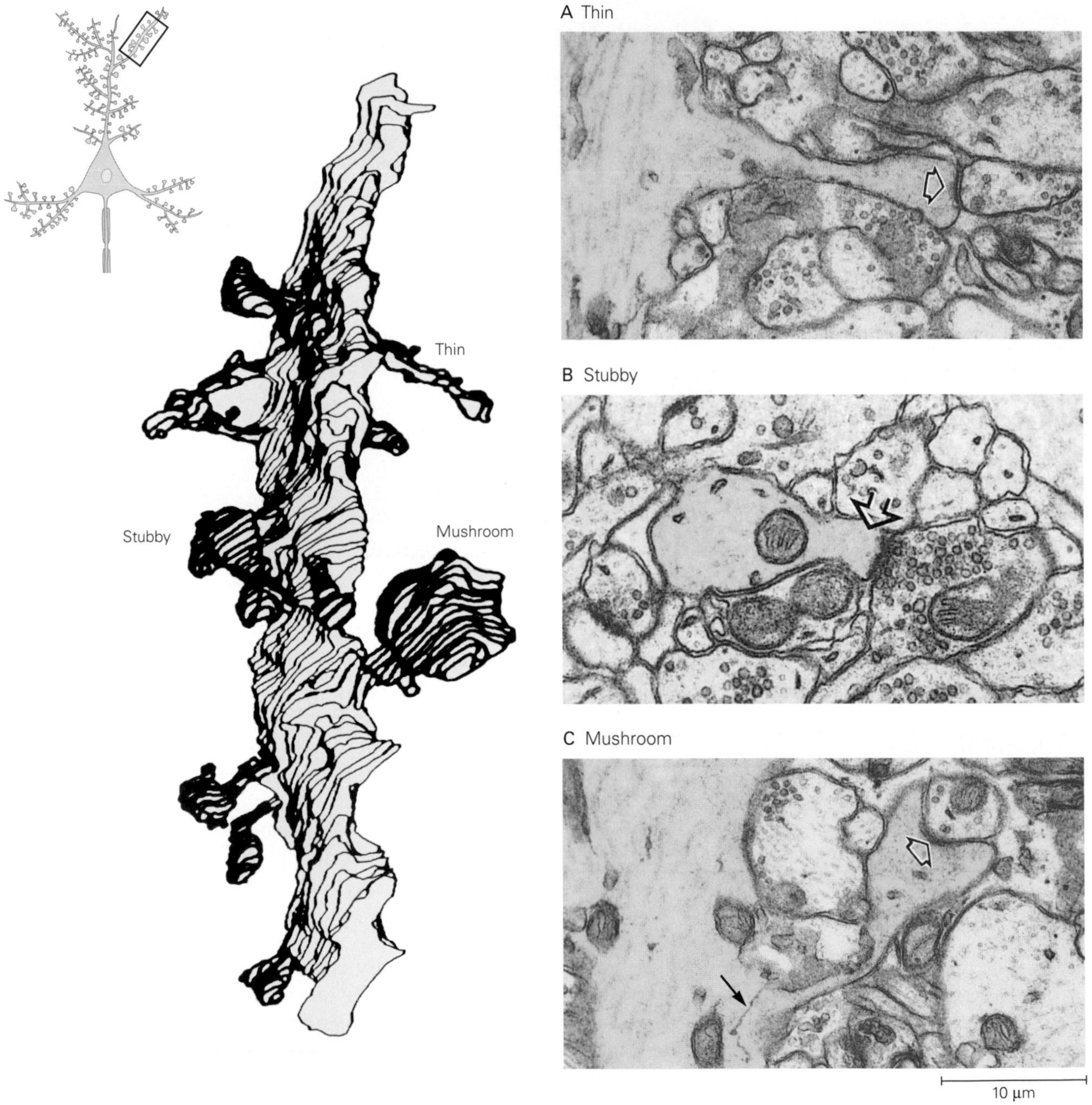

Figure 4–4 Types of dendritic spines. Three types of dendritic spine shapes are shown in a mature dendrite in a pyramidal cell in the CA1 region of the hippocampus. The drawing is based on a series of electron micrographs. (Reproduced, with permission, from Harris and Stevens 1989.)

A. In this thin dendritic spine the thickened receptive surface (**open arrow**), located across from the presynaptic axon, contains synaptic receptors. The tissue shown here and in B and C is from the hippocampus of a postnatal day-15 rat brain.

B. Stubby spines containing postsynaptic densities (**arrow**) are both small and rare in the mature hippocampus. Their larger counterparts (not shown) predominate in the immature brain.

C. Mushroom-shaped spines have a larger head. The immature spine shown here contains flat cisternae of smooth endoplasmic reticulum, some with a beaded appearance (**solid arrow**). The postsynaptic density is indicated by the **open arrow**. (A, B, and C are reproduced, with permission, from Sorra and Harris 1993.)

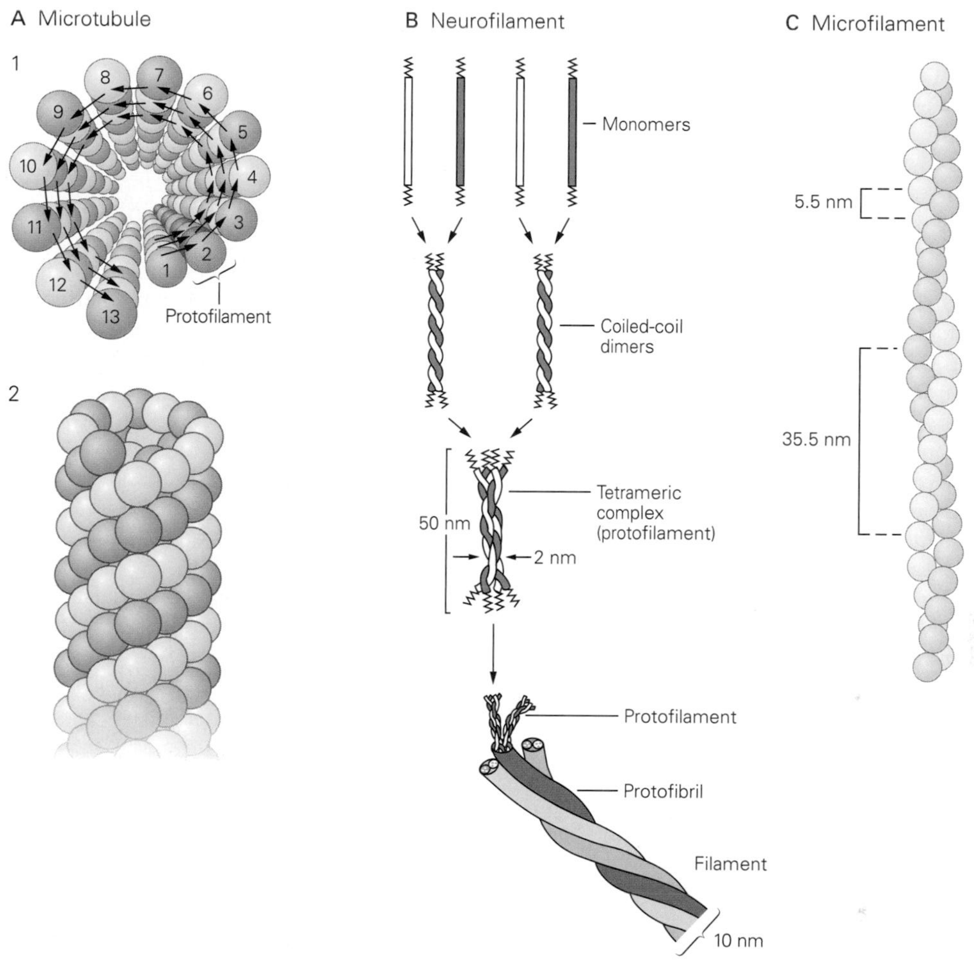

Figure 4–5 Atlas of fibrillary structures.

A. Microtubules, the largest-diameter fibers (25 nm), are helical cylinders composed of 13 protofilaments, each 5 nm in width. Each protofilament is made up of a column of alternating α- and β-tubulin subunits (each subunit has a molecular weight of approximately 50,000). Adjacent subunits bind to each along the longitudinal protofilaments and laterally between subunits of adjacent protofilaments.

A tubulin molecule is a heterodimer consisting of one α- and one β-tubulin subunit. **1.** View of a microtubule. The arrows indicate the direction of the right-handed helix. **2.** A side-view of a microtubule shows the alternating α- and β-subunits.

B. Neurofilaments are built with fibers that twist around each other to produce coils of increasing thickness. The thinnest units are monomers that form coiled-coil heterodimers. These dimers form a tetrameric complex that becomes the protofilament. Two protofilaments become a protofibril, and three protofibrils are helically twisted to form the 10 nm diameter neurofilament. (Adapted, with permission, from Bershadsky and Vasiliev 1988.)

C. Microfilaments, the smallest diameter fibers (approximately 7 nm), are composed of two strands of polymerized globular actin (G-actin) monomers arranged in a helix. At least six different (but closely related) actins are found in mammals. Each variant is encoded by a separate gene. Microfilaments are polar structures because the globular monomers are asymmetric.

Like microtubules, microfilaments undergo cycles of polymerization and depolymerization. At any one time approximately half the total actin in a cell can exist as unpolymerized monomers. The state of actin is controlled by binding proteins, which facilitate assembly and limit polymer length by capping the rapidly growing end of the filament or by severing it. Other binding proteins crosslink or bundle microfilaments. The dynamic state of microtubules and microfilaments permits a mature neuron to retract old axons and dendrites and extend new ones. This structural plasticity is thought to be a major factor in changes of synaptic connections and efficacy, and therefore cellular mechanisms of long-term memory and learning.

Box 4–1 Abnormal Accumulations of Proteins Are Hallmarks of Many Neurological Disorders

Tau is a microtubule-binding protein normally present in nerve cells. In Alzheimer disease abnormal aggregates of tau are visible in the light microscope in neurons and glia as well as in the extracellular space. Highly phosphorylated tau molecules arranged in long, thin polymers wind around one another to form paired helical filaments (Figure 4–6A and see Chapter 59). Bundles of the polymers, known as *neurofibrillary tangles*, accumulate in neuronal cell bodies, dendrites, and axons (Figure 4–6A).

In normal neurons tau is either bound to microtubules or free in the cytosol. In the tangles it is not bound to microtubules but is highly insoluble. The tangles form at least in part because tau is not proteolytically degraded. The accumulations disturb the polymerization of tubulin and therefore interfere with axonal transport. Consequently, the shape of the neuron is not maintained.

Tau accumulations are also found in neurons of patients with progressive supranuclear palsy, a movement disorder, and in patients with frontotemporal dementias, a group of neurodegenerative disorders that affect the frontal and temporal lobes (see Chapter 59). The familial forms of fronto temporal dementias are caused by mutations in the *tau* gene. Abnormal aggregates are also found in glial cells, both astrocytes and oligodendrocytes, in progressive supranuclear palsy, cortico-basoganglionic degeneration, and fronto temporal dementias.

The peptide β-amyloid also accumulates in the extracellular space in Alzheimer disease (Figure 4–6B and see Chapter 57). It is a small proteolytic product of a much larger integral membrane protein, amyloid precursor protein, which is normally processed by several proteolytic enzymes associated with intracellular membranes. The proteolytic pathway that generates β-amyloid requires the enzyme β-secretase.

For unknown reasons, in Alzheimer disease abnormal amounts of the amyloid precursor are processed by β-secretase. Some patients with early-onset familial Alzheimer disease either have mutations in the amyloid precursor gene or in the genes coding for the membrane proteins presenilin 1 and 2, which are closely associated with β-secretase activity.

In Parkinson disease abnormal aggregates of α-synuclein accumulate in cell bodies of neurons. Like tau, α-synuclein is a normal soluble constituent of the cell. But in Parkinson disease it becomes insoluble, forming spherical inclusions called *Lewy bodies* (Figure 4–6C and see Chapter 44).

These abnormal inclusions also contain ubiquitin. Because ubiquitin is required for proteasomal degradation of proteins, its presence suggests that affected neurons have attempted to target α-synuclein or other molecular constituents for proteolysis. Apparently, degradation does not occur, possibly because of misfolding or the abnormal aggregation of the proteins or because of faulty proteolytic processing in the cell.

Do these abnormal protein accumulations affect the physiology of the neurons and glia? On the one hand, the accumulations may form in response to altered post-translational processing of the proteins and serve to isolate the abnormal proteins, permitting normal cell activities. On the other hand, the accumulations may disrupt cellular activities such as membrane trafficking and axonal and dendritic transport. In addition, the altered proteins themselves, aside from the aggregations, may have deleterious effects. With β-amyloid there is evidence that the peptide itself is toxic.

In addition to serving as cytoskeleton, microtubules and actin filaments act as tracks along which organelles and proteins are rapidly driven by molecular motors. The motors used by the actin filaments, the *myosins*, also mediate other types of cell motility, including extension of the cell's processes, and the translocation of membranous organelles from the bulk cytoplasm to the region adjacent to the plasma membrane. (Actomyosin is responsible for muscle contraction.) Because the microtubules and actin filaments are polar, each motor drives its organelle cargo in only one direction.

As already mentioned, microtubules are arranged in parallel in the axon with positive ends pointing away from the cell body and negative ends facing the cell body. This regular orientation permits some organelles to move toward nerve endings and others to move away from nerve endings, the direction being determined by the specific type of molecule motor, thus maintaining the distinctive distribution of axonal organelles (Figure 4–7). In dendrites, however, microtubules with opposite polarities are mixed together, explaining why the organelles of the cell body and dendrites are similar.

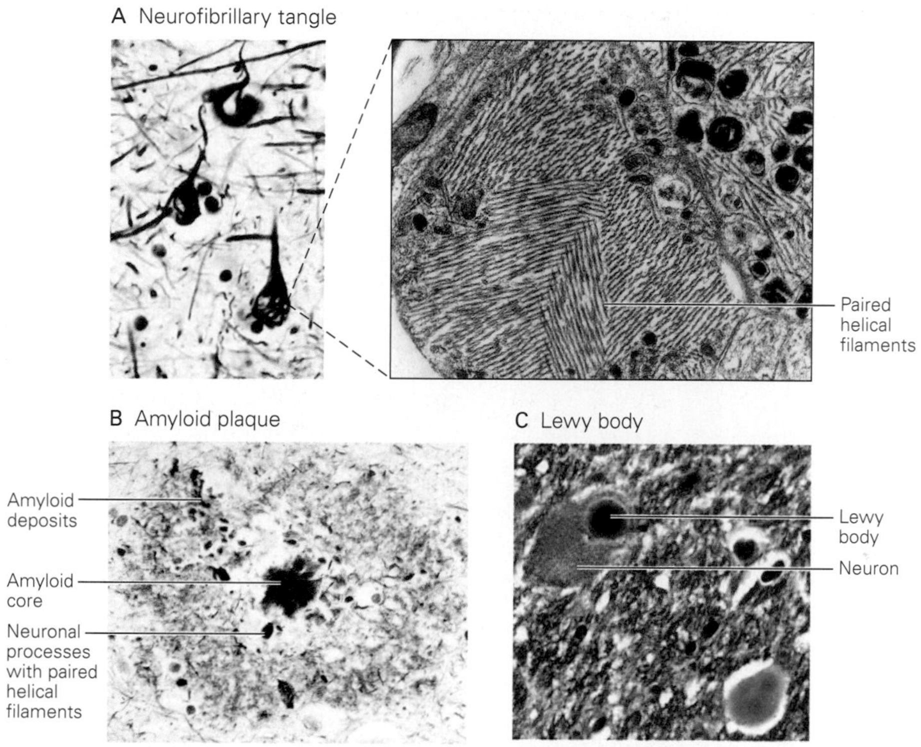

Figure 4–6 Abnormal aggregates of proteins inside neurons in Alzheimer and Parkinson diseases.

A. Intracellular neurofibrillary tangles of Alzheimer disease, labeled here with a dark silver stain (left). (Reproduced, with permission, from J.P. Vonsattel.) The electron micrograph of a tangle (right) shows the bundles of abnormal filaments, here filling a dendrite. The filaments are composed of altered tau protein. (Reproduced, with permission, from Esiri et al. 2002.)

B. Extracellular deposits of polymerized β-amyloid peptides in Alzheimer disease create an amyloid plaque. This plaque has a dense core of amyloid as well as a surrounding halo of deposits. Note the neuronal processes in the plaque with tangle pathology. (Reproduced, with permission, from J.P. Vonsattel.)

C. A Lewy body in the substantia nigra of a patient with Parkinson disease contains accumulations of abnormal filaments made up of α-synuclein, among other proteins. (Reproduced, with permission, from J.P. Vonsattel.)

Protein Particles and Organelles Are Actively Transported Along the Axon and Dendrites

In neurons most proteins are made in the cell body from mRNAs in the cell body. Important examples are synthesis of neurotransmitter biosynthetic enzymes, synaptic vesicle membrane components, and neurosecretory peptides. Because axons and terminals often lie at great distances from the cell body, transport mechanisms are crucial for sustaining the function of these remote regions.

The axon terminal, the site of secretion most important for neuronal signaling, is considerably distant from the cell body. For example, in a motor neuron that innervates a muscle of the leg in humans, the distance of the nerve terminal from the cell body can exceed 10,000 times the cell-body diameter. Passive diffusion is far too slow to deliver vesicles, particles, or even single macromolecules over this great distance. Membrane and secretory products formed in the cell body must be actively transported to the end of the axon (Figure 4–8).

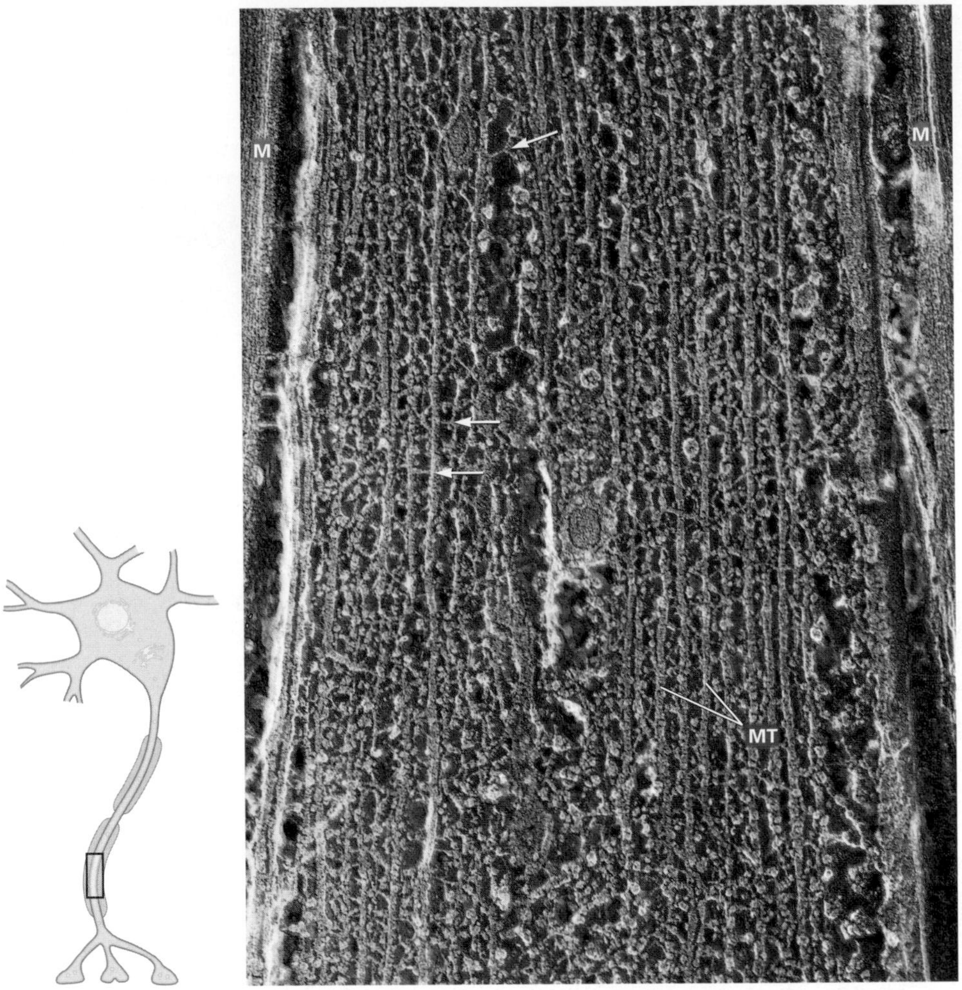

Figure 4–7 The cytoskeletal structure of an axon. The micrograph shows the dense packing of microtubules and neurofilaments linked by cross bridges (**arrows**). Organelles are transported in both the anterograde and retrograde directions in the microtubule-rich domains. Visualization in the micrograph was achieved by quick freezing and deep etching. **M**, myelin sheath; **MT**, microtubules × 105,000. (Adapted, with permission, from Schnapp and Reese 1982.)

In 1948 Paul Weiss first demonstrated axonal transport when he tied off a sciatic nerve and observed that axoplasm in the nerve accumulated with time on the proximal side of the ligature. He concluded that axoplasm moves at a slow, constant rate from the cell body toward terminals in a process he called *axoplasmic flow*. Today we know that the flow Weiss observed consists of two discrete mechanisms, one fast and the other slow.

Membranous organelles move toward terminals (anterograde direction) and back toward the cell body (retrograde direction) by *fast axonal transport*, a form of transport that is faster than 400 mm per day in warm-blooded animals. In contrast, cytosolic and cytoskeletal proteins move only in the anterograde direction by a much slower form of transport, *slow axonal transport*. These transport mechanisms in neurons are adaptations of processes that facilitate intracellular movement of organelles in all secretory cells. Because these mechanisms all operate along axons, they have been used by neuroanatomists to trace the axon distribution of neurons (Box 4–2).

Fast Axonal Transport Carries Membranous Organelles

Large membranous organelles are carried to and from the axon terminals by fast transport (Figure 4–10). These organelles include synaptic vesicle precursors, large dense-core vesicles, mitochondria, elements of the smooth endoplasmic reticulum, as well as protein

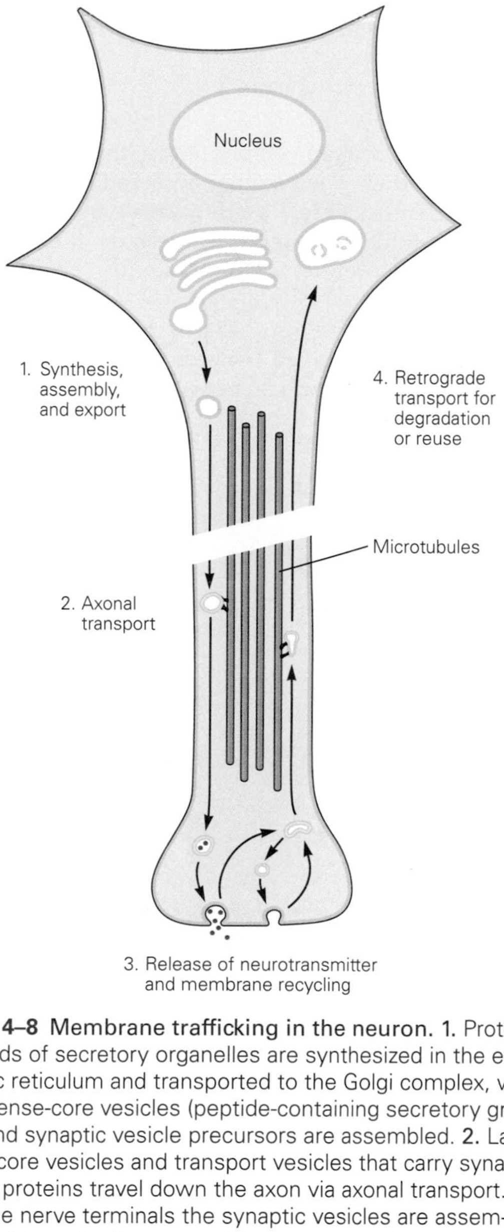

Figure 4–8 Membrane trafficking in the neuron. 1. Proteins and lipids of secretory organelles are synthesized in the endoplasmic reticulum and transported to the Golgi complex, where large dense-core vesicles (peptide-containing secretory granules) and synaptic vesicle precursors are assembled. **2.** Large dense-core vesicles and transport vesicles that carry synaptic vesicle proteins travel down the axon via axonal transport. **3.** At the nerve terminals the synaptic vesicles are assembled and loaded with nonpeptide neurotransmitters. Synaptic vesicles and large dense-core vesicles release their contents by exocytosis. **4.** Following exocytosis, large dense-core vesicle membranes are returned to the cell body for reuse or degradation. Synaptic vesicle membranes undergo many cycles of local exocytosis and endocytosis in the presynaptic terminal.

particles carrying RNAs. Direct microscopic analysis reveals that fast transport occurs in a stop-and-start (saltatory) fashion along linear tracks of microtubules aligned with the main axis of the axon. The saltatory nature of the movement results from the periodic dissociation of an organelle from the track or from collisions with other particles.

Early experiments on dorsal root ganglion cells showed that anterograde fast transport depends critically on ATP, is not affected by inhibitors of protein synthesis (once the labeled amino acid injected is incorporated), and does not depend on the cell body, because it occurs in axons severed from their cell bodies. In fact, active transport can occur in reconstituted cell-free axoplasm.

Microtubules provide an essentially stationary track on which specific organelles can be moved by molecular motors. The idea that microtubules are involved in fast transport emerged from the finding that certain alkaloids that disrupt microtubules and block mitosis, which depends on microtubules, also interfere with fast transport.

Molecular motors were first visualized in electron micrographs as cross bridges between microtubules and moving particles (Figure 4–7). The motor molecules for anterograde transport (toward the positive end of microtubules) are *kinesin* and a variety of kinesin-related proteins. The kinesins represent a large family of adenosine triphosphatases (ATPase), each of which transports different cargoes. Kinesin is a heterotetramer composed of two heavy chains and two light chains. Each heavy chain has three domains: (1) a globular head (the ATPase domain) that acts as the motor when attached to microtubules, (2) a coiled-coil helical stalk responsible for dimerization with the other heavy chain, and (3) a fan-like carboxyl-terminus that interacts with the light chains.

The organelles moved by retrograde fast transport are primarily endosomes generated by endocytic activity at nerve endings, mitochondria, and elements of the endoplasmic reticulum. Many of these components degrade in lysosomes. Retrograde fast transport also delivers signals that regulate gene expression in the neuron's nucleus. For example, activated growth factor receptors are taken up into vesicles at nerve endings and carried back along the axon to their site of action in the nucleus. Transport of transcription factors informs the gene transcription apparatus in the nucleus of conditions in the periphery. Retrograde transport of these molecules is especially important during nerve regeneration and axon regrowth (see Chapter 54). Certain toxins (tetanus toxin) as well as pathogens (herpes simplex, rabies, and polio viruses) are also transported toward the cell body along the axon.

The rate of retrograde fast transport is approximately one-half to two-thirds that of anterograde fast transport. As in anterograde transport, particles move along microtubules. The motor molecule for retrograde transport is a microtubule-associated ATPase called MAP-1C. This molecule is similar to the dyneins

Box 4–2 Neuroanatomical Tracing Makes Use of Axonal Transport

Neuroanatomists typically locate axons and terminals of specific nerve cell bodies by microinjection of dyes; expression of fluorescent proteins; or autoradiographically tracing specific proteins soon after administering radioactively labeled amino acids, certain labeled sugars (fucose or amino sugars, precursors of glycoprotein), or specific transmitter substances.

Similarly, particles, proteins, or dyes that are readily taken up at nerve terminals by endocytosis and transported back to cell bodies are used to identify the cell bodies. The enzyme horseradish peroxidase has been most widely used for this type of study because it readily undergoes retrograde transport and its reaction product is conveniently visualized histochemically.

Axonal transport is also used by neuroanatomists to label material exchanged between neurons, making it possible to identify neuronal networks (Figure 4–9).

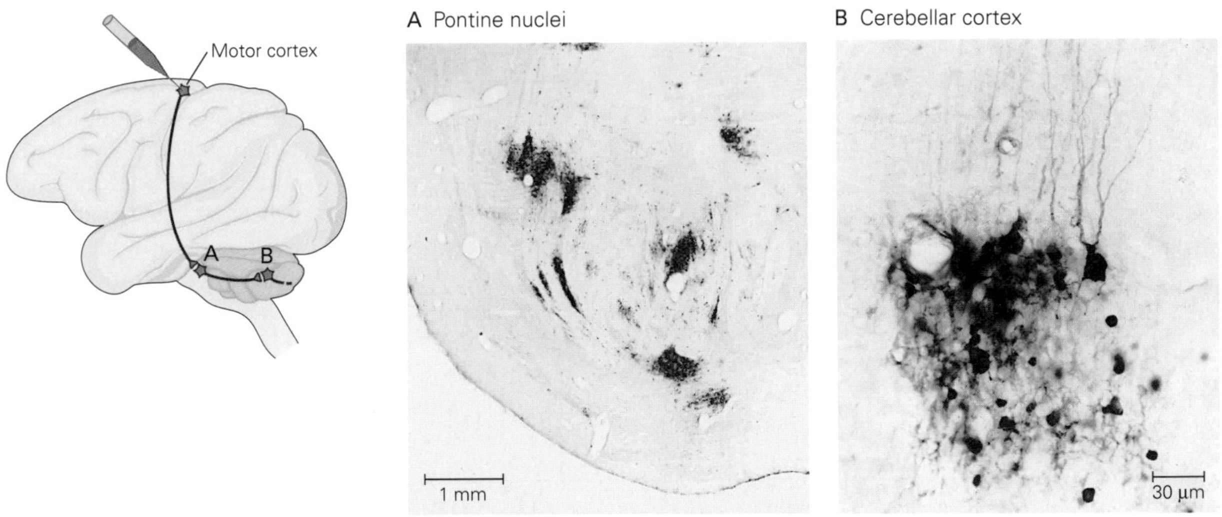

Figure 4–9 Axonal transport of the herpes simplex virus (HSV) is used to trace cortical pathways in monkeys. Depending on the strain, the virus moves in the anterograde or retrograde direction by axonal transport. In either direction it enters a neuron with which the infected cell makes synaptic contact. Here the projections of cells in the primary motor cortex to the cerebellum in monkeys were traced using an anterograde-moving strain (HSV-1 [H129]). Monkeys were injected in the region of the primary motor cortex that controls the arm. After 4 days the brain was sectioned and immunostained for viral antigen. Micrographs show the virus was transported from the primary motor cortex to second-order neurons in pontine nuclei (**A**) and then to third-order neurons in the cerebellar cortex (**B**). (Reproduced, with permission, from P. L. Strick.)

in cilia and flagella of other cells and consists of a multimeric protein complex with two globular heads on two stalks connected to a basal structure. The globular heads attach to microtubules and act as motors, moving toward the negative end of the polymer. As with kinesin, the other end of the complex attaches to the organelle being moved.

Microtubules also transport mRNAs and ribosomal RNA carried in particles formed with RNA-binding proteins. These proteins have been characterized in both vertebrate and invertebrate nervous systems and include the cytoplasmic polyadenylation element binding protein (CPEB), the fragile X protein, Hu proteins, NOVA, and Staufen. The activities of these proteins are critical. Humans with mutations in the fragile X gene are mentally retarded and have spinal defects. For example, CPEB keeps select mRNAs dormant during transport from the cell body to nerve endings;

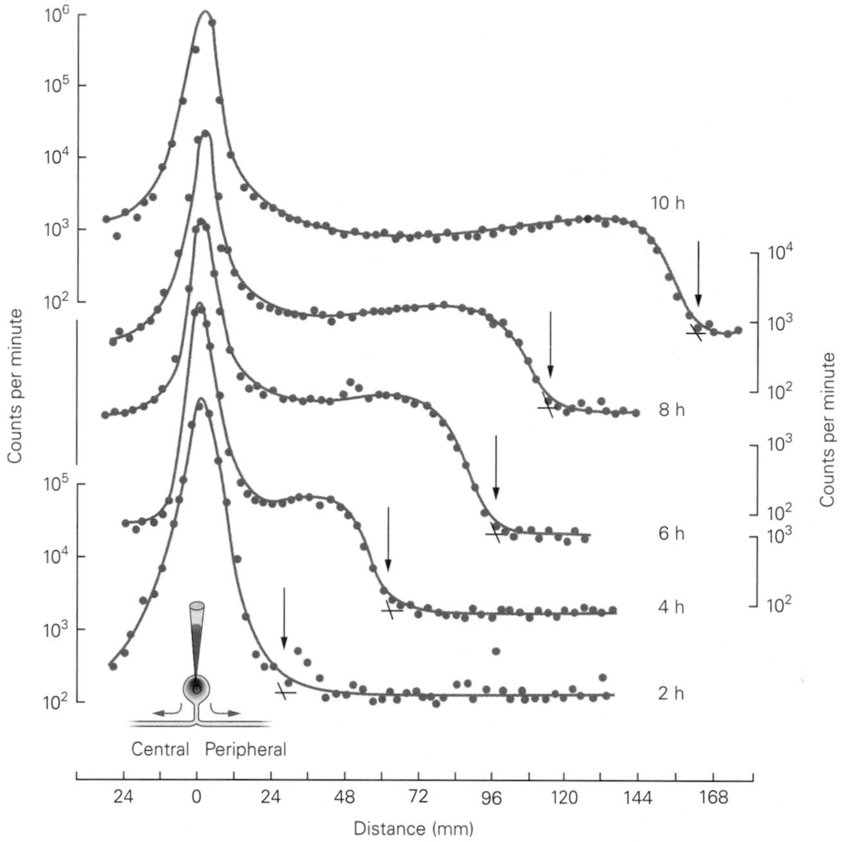

Figure 4–10 Early experiments on anterograde axonal transport used radioactive labeling of proteins. In the experiment illustrated here the distribution of radioactive proteins along the sciatic nerve of the cat was measured at various times after injection of [^{3}H]-leucine into dorsal root ganglia in the lumbar region of the spinal cord. To show transport curves from various times (2, 4, 6, 8, and 10 hours after the injection) in one figure, several ordinate scales (in logarithmic units) are used. Large amounts of labeled protein stay in the ganglion cell bodies but, with time, move out along axons in the sciatic nerve, so the advancing front of the labeled protein is progressively farther from the cell body (**black arrows**). The velocity of transport can be calculated from the distances of the front displayed at the various times. From experiments of this kind Sidney Ochs found that the rate of fast axonal transport is constant at 410 mm per day at body temperature. (Adapted, with permission, from Ochs 1972.)

once there (upon stimulation), the binding protein can facilitate the local translation of the RNA by mediating polyadenylation and activation of the messenger. Both CPEB and Staufen were discovered in *Drosophila* where they maintain maternal mRNAs dormant in unfertilized eggs and, upon fertilization, distribute and localize mRNA to various regions of the dividing embryo.

Proteins, ribosomes, and mRNA are concentrated at the base of dendritic spines (Figure 4–11). Only a select group of mRNA are transported to the nerve terminals. These include mRNA for actin- and cytoskeletal-associated proteins MAP2 and the α-subunit of the Ca^{2+}/calmodulin-dependent protein kinase. They are translated in the dendrites in response to activity in a presynaptic neuron. This local protein synthesis is thought to be important in sustaining the molecular changes at the synapse that underlie long-term memory and learning. Likewise, the mRNA for myelin basic protein is transported to the distant ends of the oligodendrocytes, where it is translated as the myelin sheath grows, as discussed later in this chapter.

Slow Axonal Transport Carries Cytosolic Proteins and Elements of the Cytoskeleton

Cytosolic proteins and cytoskeletal proteins are moved from the cell body by slow axonal transport. Slow transport occurs only in the anterograde direction and consists of at least two kinetic components that carry different proteins at different rates.

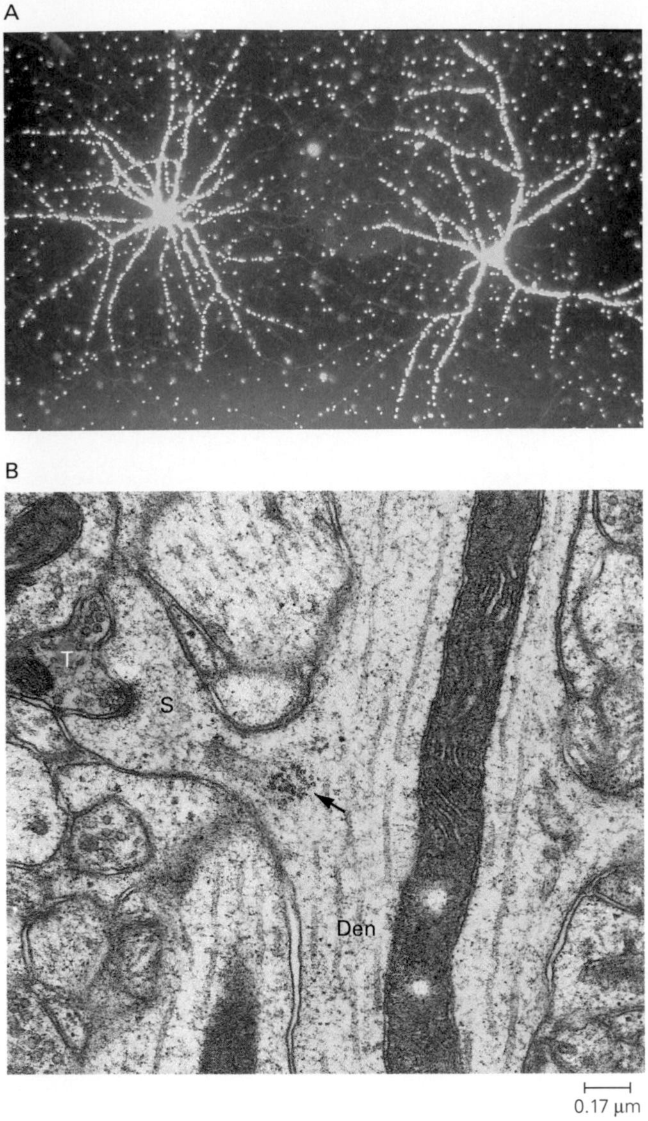

Figure 4–11 Ribosomes in the dendritic arbor. (Images reproduced, with permission, from Oswald Steward.)

A. Some ribosomes are dispatched from the cell body to dendrites where they are used in local protein synthesis. This autoradiograph shows the distribution of ribosomal RNA (rRNA) in hippocampal neurons in low-density cultures using in situ hybridization. The photomicrograph was taken with dark field illumination, in which silver grains reflect light and thus appear as bright spots. Silver grains, denoting the rRNA, are heavily concentrated over cell bodies and dendrites but are not detectable over the axons that crisscross among the dendrites.

B. Ribosomes in dendrites are selectively concentrated at the junction of the spine and main dendritic shaft (**arrow**), where the spine contacts the axon terminal of a presynaptic neuron. This electron micrograph shows a mushroom-shaped spine of a neuron in the hippocampal dentate gyrus. Note the absence of ribosomes in the dendritic shaft. **S**, spine head; **T**, presynaptic terminal; **Den**, main shaft of the dendrite containing a long mitochondrion. × 60,000.

The slower component travels at 0.2 to 2.5 mm per day and carries the proteins that make up the fibrillar elements of the cytoskeleton: the subunits of neurofilaments and α- and β-tubulin subunits of microtubules. These fibrous proteins constitute approximately 75% of the total protein moved in the slower component. Microtubules are transported in polymerized form by a mechanism involving microtubule sliding in which relatively short preassembled microtubules move along existing microtubules. Neurofilament monomers or short polymers move passively together with the microtubules because they are cross-linked by protein bridges.

The other component of slow axonal transport is approximately twice as fast as the slower. It carries clathrin, actin, and actin-binding proteins as well as a variety of enzymes and other proteins.

Proteins Are Made in Neurons as in Other Secretory Cells

Secretory and Membrane Proteins Are Synthesized and Modified in the Endoplasmic Reticulum

The mRNAs for secretory and membrane proteins are translated in conjunction with the membrane of the rough endoplasmic reticulum, and their polypeptide products are processed extensively within the lumen of the endoplasmic reticulum. Most polypeptides destined to become proteins are translocated across the membrane of the rough endoplasmic reticulum during synthesis, a process called *cotranslational transfer.*

Transfer is possible because ribosomes, the site where proteins are synthesized, attach to the cytosolic surface of the reticulum (Figure 4–12). Complete transfer of the polypeptide chain into the lumen of the reticulum produces a secretory protein (recall that the inside of the reticulum is related to the outside of the cell). Important examples are the neuroactive peptides. If the transfer is incomplete, an integral membrane protein results. Because a polypeptide chain can thread its way through the membrane many times during synthesis, several membrane-spanning configurations are possible depending on the primary amino acid sequence of the protein. Important examples are neurotransmitter receptors and ion channels (see Chapter 5).

Some proteins transported into the endoplasmic reticulum remain there. Others are moved to other compartments of the vacuolar apparatus or to the plasmalemma, or are secreted into the extracellular space. Proteins that are processed in the endoplasmic reticulum are extensively modified. One important modification is the formation of intramolecular disulfide

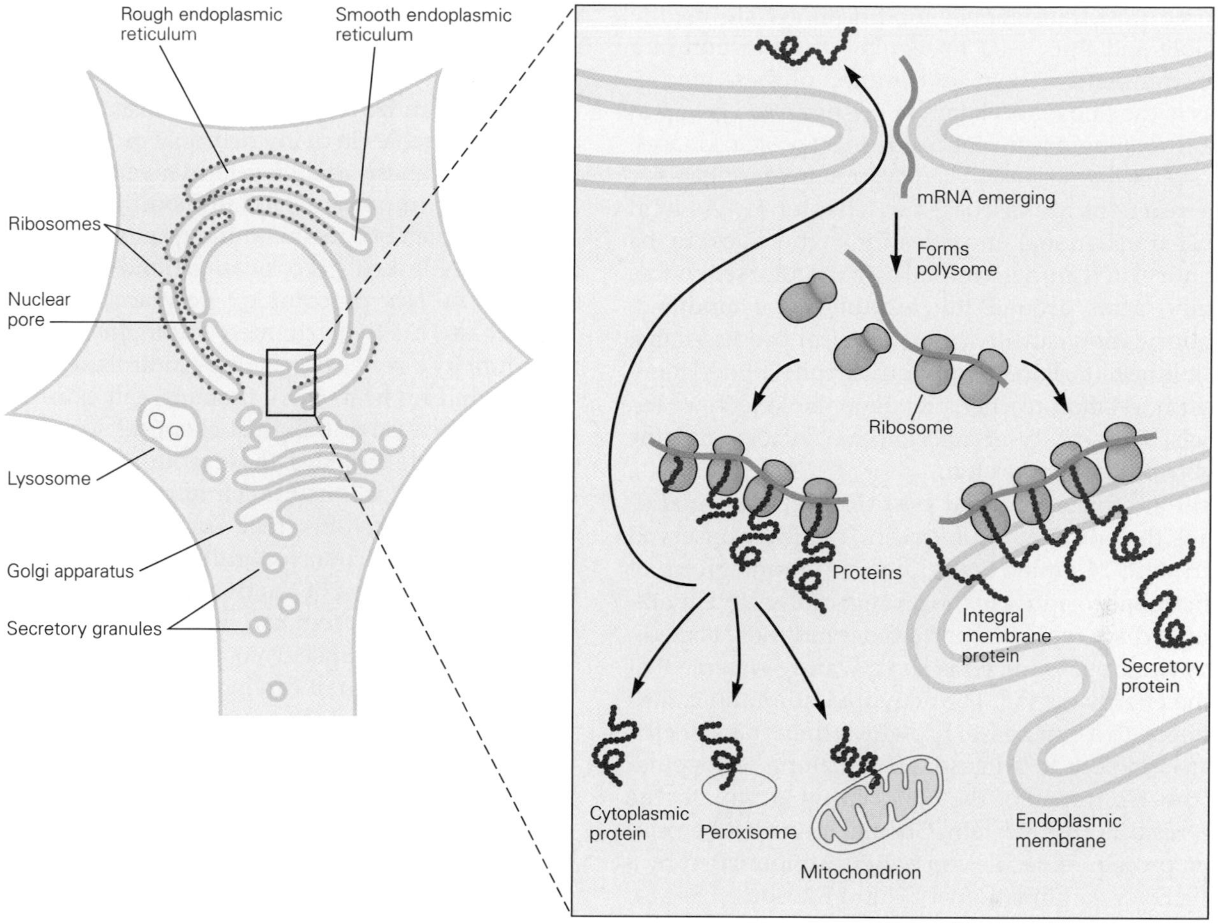

Figure 4–12 Protein synthesis in the endoplasmic reticulum. Free and membrane-bound polysomes translate mRNA that encodes proteins with a variety of destinations. Messenger RNA, transcribed from genomic DNA in the neuron's nucleus, emerges into the cytoplasm through nuclear pores (enlargement) to form polyribosomes. The polypeptides that become secretory and membrane proteins are translocated across the membrane of the rough endoplasmic reticulum.

linkages (Cys-S-S-Cys) caused by oxidation of pairs of free sulfhydryl side chains, a process that cannot occur in the reducing environment of the cytosol. Disulfide linkages are crucial to the tertiary structure of these proteins.

Proteins may be modified by cytosolic enzymes either during synthesis (cotranslational modification) or afterward (post-translational modification). One example is N-acylation, the transfer of an acyl group to the N-terminus of the growing polypeptide chain. Acylation by a 14-carbon fatty acid myristoyl group permits the protein to anchor in membranes through the lipid chain.

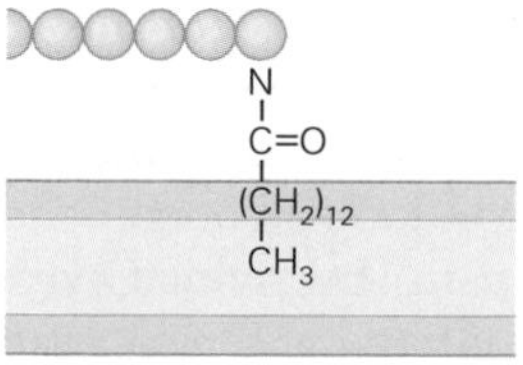

Other fatty acids can be conjugated to the sulfhydryl group of cysteine, producing a thioacylation:

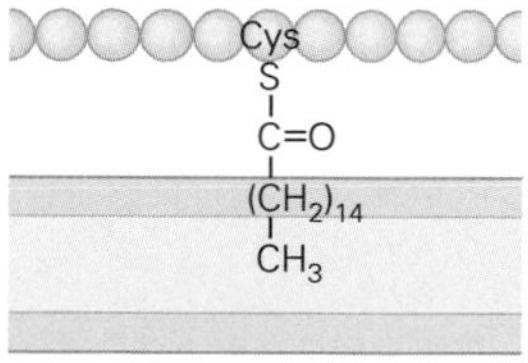

Isoprenylation is another post-translational modification important for anchoring proteins to the cytosolic side of membranes. It occurs shortly after synthesis of the protein is completed and involves a series of enzymatic steps that result in thioacylation by one of two long-chain hydrophobic polyisoprenyl moieties (farnesyl, with 15 carbons, or geranyl-geranyl, with 20) of the sulfhydryl group of a cysteine at the C-terminus of proteins.

Some post-translational modifications are readily reversible and thus used to regulate the function of a protein transiently. The most common of these modifications is the phosphorylation at the hydroxyl group in serine, threonine, or tyrosine residues by protein kinases. Dephosphorylation is catalyzed by protein phosphatases. (These reactions are discussed in Chapter 11.) As with all post-translational modifications, the sites to be phosphorylated are determined by particular sequences of amino acids around the residue to be modified. Phosphorylation can alter physiological processes in a reversible fashion. For example, protein phosphorylation-dephosphorylation reactions regulate the kinetics of ion channels, the activity of transcription factors, and the assembly of the cytoskeleton.

Still another important post-translational modification is the addition of ubiquitin, a highly conserved protein with 76 amino acids, to the ∊-amino group of specific lysine residues in the protein molecule. Ubiquitination, which regulates protein degradation, is mediated by three enzymes. E1 is an activating enzyme that uses the energy of ATP. The activated ubiquitin is next transferred to a conjugase, E2, which then transfers the activated moiety to a ligase, E3. E3 alone or together with the E2 transfers the ubiquitinyl group to the lysine residue in a protein. Specificity arises because a given protein molecule can only be ubiquinated by a specific E3 or combination of E3 and E2. Some E3s also require special cofactors—ubiquitination occurs only in the presence of E3 and a cofactor protein.

Monoubiquitination tags a protein for degradation in the endosomal-lysosomal system. This is especially important in endocytosis and recycling of surface receptors. Ubiquitinyl monomers are successively linked to the ∊-amino group of a lysine residue in the previously added ubiquitin moiety. Addition of more than five ubiquitins to the multiubiquitin chain tags the protein for degradation by the proteasome, a large complex containing multifunctional protease subunits that cleave proteins into short peptides.

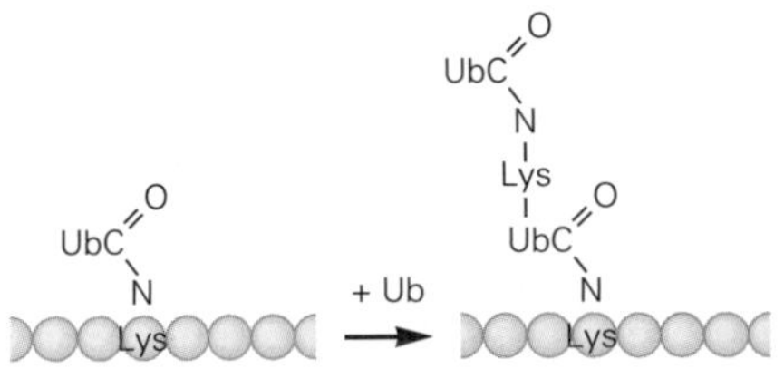

The ATP-ubiquitin-proteasome pathway is a mechanism for the selective and regulated proteolysis of proteins that operates in the cytosol of all regions of the neuron—dendrites, cell body, axon, and terminals. Until recently this process was thought to be primarily directed to poorly folded, denatured, or aged and damaged proteins. We now know that ubiquitin-mediated proteolysis can be regulated by neuronal activity and plays specific roles in many neuronal processes, including synaptogenesis and long-term memory storage.

Another important protein modification is glycosylation, which occurs on amino groups of asparagine residues (N-linked glycosylation) and results in the addition *en bloc* of complex polysaccharide chains. These chains are then trimmed within the endoplasmic reticulum by a series of reactions controlled by chaperones, including heat shock proteins, calnexin, and calreticulin. Because of the great chemical specificities of oligosaccharide moieties, these modifications can have important implications for cell function. For example, cell-to-cell interactions that occur during development rely on molecular recognition between glycoproteins on the surfaces of the two interacting cells. Also, because a given protein can have somewhat different oligosaccharide chains, glycosylation can diversify the function of a protein. It can increase the hydrophilicity of the protein (useful for secretory proteins), fine-tune its ability to bind macromolecular partners, and delay its degradation.

An interesting post-translational modification of mRNA is RNA interference (RNAi), the targeted destruction of double-stranded RNAs. This mechanism, which is believed to have arisen to protect cells against viruses and other rogue fragments of nucleic acids, shuts down the synthesis of any targeted protein. Double-stranded RNAs are taken up by an enzyme complex that cleaves the molecule into oligomers. The RNA sequences are retained by the complex. As a result, any homologous hybridizing RNA strands, either double- or single-stranded, will be destroyed. The process is regenerative: The complex retains a hybridizing fragment and goes on to destroy another RNA molecule until none remain in the cell. Although the physiological role of RNA interference (RNAi) in normal cells is unclear, transfection or injection of RNAi into cells is of great research and clinical importance (see Chapter 3).

Secretory Proteins Are Modified in the Golgi Complex

Proteins from the endoplasmic reticulum are carried in transport vesicles to the Golgi complex where they are modified and then moved to synaptic terminals and other parts of the plasmalemma. The Golgi complex appears as a grouping of membranous sacks aligned with one another in long ribbons.

The mechanism by which vesicles are transported between stations of the secretory and endocytic pathways is remarkably conserved from simple unicellular prokaryotes (yeast) to neurons and glia of multicellular organisms. Transport vesicles develop from membrane, beginning with the assembly of proteins that form *coats*, or coat proteins, at selected patches of the cytosolic surface of the membrane. A coat has two functions. It forms rigid cage-like structures that produce evagination of the membrane into a bud shape and it selects the protein cargo to be incorporated into the vesicles.

There are several types of coats. Clathrin coats assist in evaginating Golgi complex membrane and plasmalemma during endocytosis. Two other coats, COPI and COPII, cover transport vesicles that shuttle between the endoplasmic reticulum and the Golgi complex. Coats usually are rapidly dissolved once free vesicles have formed. The fusion of vesicles with the target membrane is mediated by a cascade of molecular interactions, the most important of which is the reciprocal recognition of small proteins on the cytosolic surfaces of the two interacting membranes: vesicular soluble *N*-ethylmaleimide-sensitive factor attachment protein receptors (v-SNAREs) and t-SNAREs (target-membrane SNAREs). The actions of these small proteins are discussed in Chapter 12 in connection with how synaptic vesicles release neurotransmitters at synapses.

Vesicles from the endoplasmic reticulum arrive at the *cis* side of the Golgi complex (the aspect facing the nucleus) and fuse with its membranes to deliver their contents into the Golgi complex. These proteins travel from one Golgi compartment (cisterna) to the next, from the *cis* to the *trans* side, undergoing a series of enzymatic reactions. Each Golgi cisterna or set of cisternae is specialized for a particular type of reaction. Several types of protein modifications, some of which begin in the endoplasmic reticulum, occur within the Golgi complex proper or within the transport station adjacent to its *trans* side, the *trans-Golgi network* (the aspect of the complex typically facing away from the nucleus toward the axon hillock). These modifications include the addition of N-linked oligosaccharides, O-linked (on the hydroxyl groups of serine and threonine) glycosylation, phosphorylation, and sulfation.

Both soluble and membrane-bound proteins that travel through the Golgi complex emerge from the trans-Golgi network in a variety of vesicles that have different molecular compositions and destinations. Proteins transported from the trans-Golgi network include secretory products as well as newly synthesized components for the plasmalemma, endosomes, and other membranous organelles (see Figure 4–1). One class of vesicles carries newly synthesized plasmalemmal proteins and proteins that are continuously secreted (*constitutive secretion*). These vesicles fuse with the plasmalemma in an unregulated fashion. An important type of these vesicles delivers lysosomal enzymes to late endosomes.

Still other classes of vesicles carry secretory proteins that are released by an extracellular stimulus (*regulated secretion*). One type stores secretory products, primarily neuroactive peptides in high concentrations. Called *large dense-core vesicles* because of their electron-dense (osmophilic) appearance in the electron microscope, these vesicles are similar in function and biogenesis to peptide-containing granules of endocrine cells. Large dense-core vesicles are targeted primarily to axons but can be seen in all regions of the neuron. They accumulate in the cytoplasm just beneath the plasma membrane and are highly concentrated at axon terminals, where they undergo Ca^{2+}-regulated exocytosis (see Figure 4–8). The optimal stimulus for their secretion is a train of action potentials.

An important, but as yet unanswered, question is how synaptic vesicles—the small lucent vesicles responsible for the rapid release of neurotransmitter at axon terminals—reach the terminals. It is thought that proteins that make up synaptic vesicles are carried to endosomes and the plasmalemma of axon terminals in large precursor vesicles from the trans-Golgi network. Once at the terminals the proteins are processed into synaptic vesicles as they pass through endosomes during the exocytosis/recycling process described in Chapter 12. The neurotransmitter molecules stored in synaptic vesicles are released by exocytosis regulated by Ca^{2+} influx through channels close to the release site.

Surface Membrane and Extracellular Substances Are Recycled in the Cell

Vesicular traffic toward the cell surface is continuously balanced by *endocytic traffic* from the plasmalemma to internal organelles. This traffic is essential for maintaining the area of the plasmalemma in a steady state. It can alter the activity of many important regulatory molecules on the cell surface (eg, by removing receptors and adhesion molecules). It also removes nutrients and molecules, such as expendable receptor ligands and damaged membrane proteins, to the degradative compartments of the cells. Finally, it serves to recycle synaptic vesicles at nerve terminals (see Chapter 12).

A significant fraction of endocytic traffic is carried in clathrin-coated vesicles. The clathrin coat interacts selectively through transmembrane receptors with extracellular molecules that are to be taken up into the cell. For this reason clathrin-mediated uptake is often referred to as *receptor-mediated endocytosis*. The vesicles eventually shed their clathrin coats and fuse with the early endosomes, in which proteins to be recycled to the cell surface are separated from those destined for other intracellular organelles. Patches of the plasmalemma can also be recycled through larger, uncoated vacuoles that also fuse with early endosomes (*bulk endocytosis*).

Glial Cells Play Diverse Roles in Neural Function

Glia Form the Insulating Sheaths for Axons

A major function of oligodendrocytes and Schwann cells is to provide the insulating material that allows rapid conduction of electrical signals along the axon. These cells produce thin sheets of myelin that wrap concentrically, many times, around the axon. Central nervous system myelin, produced by oligodendrocytes, is similar, but not identical to peripheral nervous system myelin, produced by Schwann cells.

Both types of glia produce myelin only for segments of axons. This is because the axon is not continuously wrapped in myelin, a feature that facilitates propagation of action potentials (see Chapter 6). One Schwann cell produces a single myelin sheath for one segment of one axon, whereas one oligodendrocyte produces myelin sheaths for segments of as many as 30 axons (Figure 4–13).

The number of layers of myelin on an axon is proportional to the diameter of the axon—larger axons have thicker sheaths. Axons with very small diameters are not myelinated; nonmyelinated axons conduct action potentials much more slowly than do myelinated axons because of their smaller diameter and lack of myelin insulation (see Chapter 6).

The regular lamellar structure and biochemical composition of the sheath are consequences of how myelin is formed from the glial plasma membrane. In the development of the peripheral nervous system, before myelination takes place, the axon lies within a trough formed by Schwann cells. Schwann cells line up along the axon at regular intervals that become the myelinated segments of axon. The external membrane of each Schwann cell surrounds the axon to form a double membrane structure called the *mesaxon,* which elongates and spirals around the axon in concentric layers (Figure 4–13C). As the axon is ensheathed, the cytoplasm of the Schwann cell is squeezed out to form a compact lamellar structure.

The regularly spaced segments of myelin sheath are separated by unmyelinated gaps, called *nodes of Ranvier,* where the plasma membrane of the axon is exposed to the extracellular space for approximately 1 μm (Figure 4–14). This arrangement greatly increases the speed at which nerve impulses are conducted (up to 100 m/s in humans) because the signal jumps from one node to the next, a mechanism called *saltatory conduction* (see Chapter 6). Nodes are easily excited because they have a low threshold. In the axon membrane at the nodes the density of Na^+ channels, which generate the action potential, is approximately 50 times greater than in myelin-sheathed regions of membrane. Several cell adhesion molecules in the paranodal regions keep the myelin boundaries stable.

In the human femoral nerve the primary sensory axon is approximately 0.5 m long and the internodal distance is 1 to 1.5 mm; thus approximately 300 to 500 nodes of Ranvier occur along a primary afferent fiber between the thigh muscle and the cell body in the dorsal root ganglion. Because each internodal segment is formed by a single Schwann cell, as many as 500 Schwann cells participate in the myelination of each peripheral sensory axon.

Myelin has bimolecular layers of lipid interspersed between protein layers. Its composition is similar to that of the plasmalemma, consisting of 70% lipid and 30% protein with high concentrations of cholesterol and phospholipid. In the central nervous system myelin has two major proteins: myelin basic protein, a small, positively charged protein that is situated on the cytoplasmic surface of compact myelin, and proteolipid protein, a hydrophobic integral membrane protein. Presumably, both provide structural stability for the sheath. Both have also been implicated as important autoantigens against which the immune system can react to produce the demyelinating disease, multiple sclerosis. In the peripheral nervous system myelin contains a major protein, P_0, as well as the hydrophobic protein PMP22. Autoimmune reactions to these proteins produce a demyelinating peripheral neuropathy, the Guillain-Barré syndrome. Mutations in myelin protein genes also cause a variety of demyelinating diseases in both peripheral and central axons (Box 4–3). Demyelination slows down, or even stops, conduction of the action potential in an affected axon, because it allows electrical current to leak out of the axonal membrane. Thus, demyelinating diseases have devastating effects on neuronal circuits in the brain, spinal cord, and peripheral nervous system.

Astrocytes Support Synaptic Signaling

Astrocytes are star-shaped glia found in all areas of the brain; indeed, they constitute nearly half the number of brain cells. They play important roles in nourishing

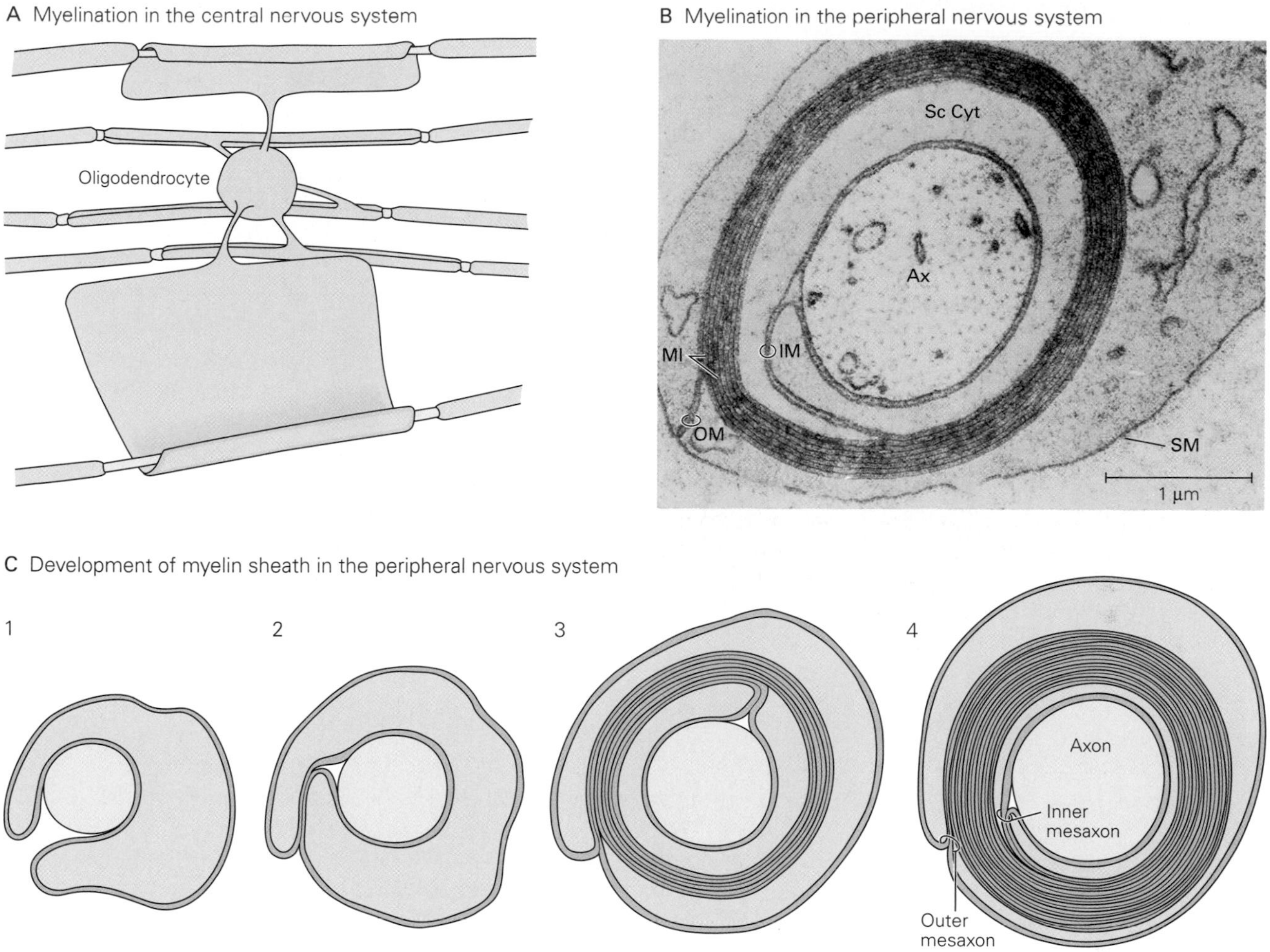

Figure 4–13 Myelin insulates the axons of both central and peripheral neurons.

A. Axons in the central nervous system are wrapped in several layers of myelin produced by oligodendrocytes. Each oligodendrocyte can myelinate many axons. (Reproduced, with permission, from Raine 1984.)

B. This electron micrograph of a transverse section through an axon (**Ax**) in the sciatic nerve of a mouse shows the origin of a sheet of myelin (**MI**) at a structure called the inner mesaxon (**IM**). The sheet arises from the surface membrane (**SM**) of a Schwann cell, which is continuous with the outer mesaxon (**OM**). The Schwann cell cytoplasm (**Sc Cyt**) still surrounds the axon; eventually, it is squeezed out and the myelin layers become compact. (Reproduced, with permission, from Dyck et al. 1984.)

C. A peripheral nerve fiber is myelinated by a Schwann cell in several stages. In stage 1 the Schwann cell surrounds the axon. In stage 2 the outer aspects of the plasma membrane have become tightly apposed in one area. This membrane fusion reflects early myelin membrane formation. In stage 3 several layers of myelin have formed because of continued rotation of the Schwann cell cytoplasm around the axon. In stage 4 a mature myelin sheath has formed; much of the Schwann cell cytoplasm has been squeezed out of the innermost loop. (Adapted, with permission, from Williams et al. 1989.)

neurons and in regulating the concentrations of ions and neurotransmitters in the extracellular space. But astrocytes and neurons also communicate with each other to modulate synaptic signaling in ways that are still poorly understood.

Astrocytes have large numbers of thin processes that enfold all the blood vessels of the brain, and ensheath synapses or groups of synapses. By their intimate physical association with synapses, often closer than 1 μm, astrocytes are positioned to regulate extracellular concentrations of ions, neurotransmitters, and other molecules (Figure 4–17).

How do astrocytes regulate axonal conduction and synaptic activity? The first recognized physiological

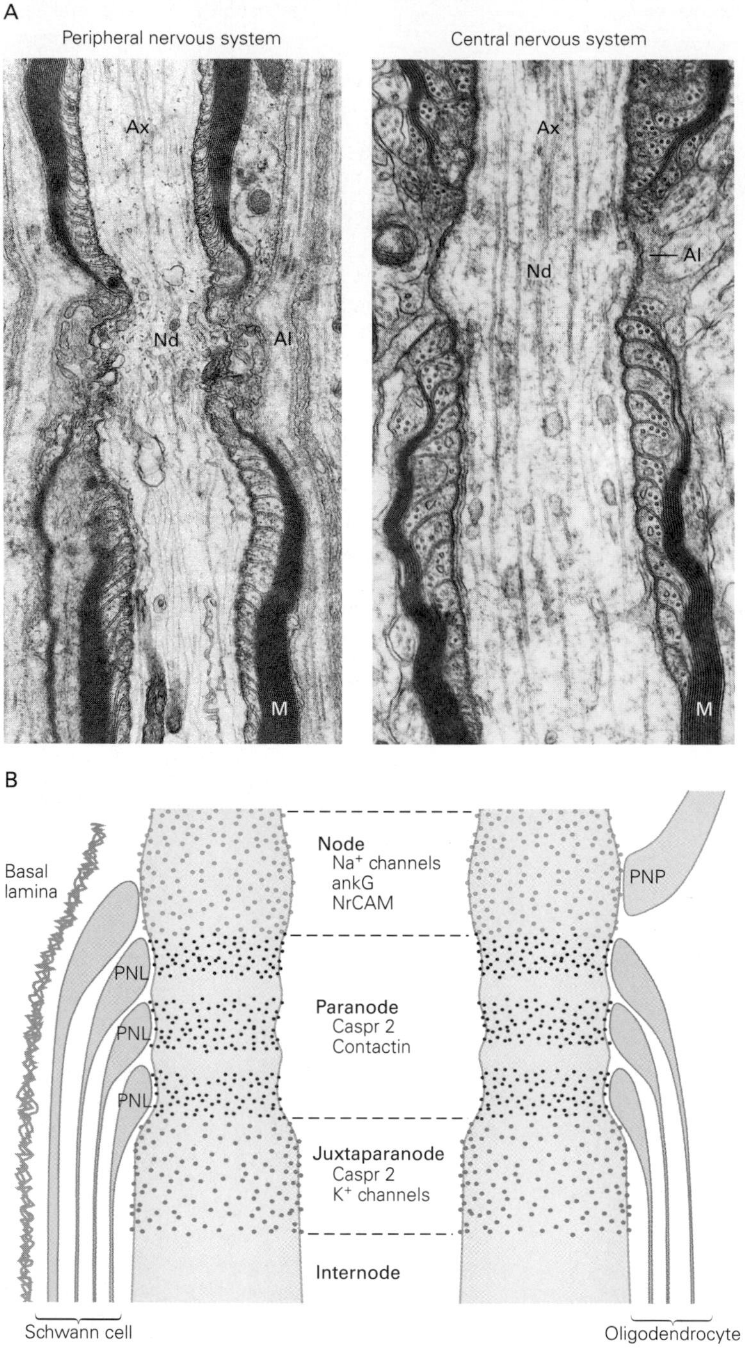

Figure 4–14 The myelin sheath of axons has regular gaps called the *nodes of Ranvier.*

A. Electron micrographs show the region of nodes in axons from the peripheral nervous system and spinal cord. The axon **(Ax)** runs vertically in both micrographs. The layers of myelin **(M)** are absent at the nodes **(Nd)**, where the axon's membrane (axolemma, **Al**) is exposed. (Reproduced, with permission, from Peters et al. 1991.)

B. Regions on both sides of a node of Ranvier are rich in stable contacts between myelinating cells and the axon, to ensure that the nodes do not move or change in size and to restrict the localization of K^+ and Na^+ channels in the axon. Potassium permeable channels and the adhesion protein Caspr2 are concentrated in the juxtaparanode. Paranodal loops **(PNL)** of Schwann cell or oligodendrocyte cytoplasm form a series of stable junctions with the axon. The paranode region is rich with adhesion proteins such as Caspr2, contactin, and neurofascin (NF155). At the nodes in central axons, perinodal astroglial processes **(PNP)** contact the axonal membrane, which is enormously rich with Na^+ channels. This localization of Na^+ permeability is a major basis for the saltatory conduction in myelinated axons. The membrane-cytoskeletal linker ankyrin G **(ankG)** and the cell adhesion molecules NrCAM and NF186 are also concentrated at the nodes. (Reproduced, with permission, from Peles and Salzer 2000.)

Box 4–3 Defects in Myelin Proteins Disrupt Conduction of Nerve Signals

Because in myelinated axons normal conduction of the nerve impulse depends on the insulating properties of the myelin sheath defective myelin can result in severe disturbances of motor and sensory function.

Many diseases that affect myelin, including some animal models of demyelinating disease, have a genetic basis. The *shiverer* (or *shi*) mutant mice have tremors and frequent convulsions and tend to die young. In these mice the myelination of axons in the central nervous system is greatly deficient and the myelination that does occur is abnormal.

The mutation that causes this disease is a deletion of five of the six exons of the gene for myelin basic protein, which in the mouse is located on chromosome 18. The mutation is recessive; a mouse develops the disease only if it has inherited the defective gene from both parents. *Shiverer* mice that inherit both defective genes have only approximately 10% of the myelin basic protein found in normal mice.

When the wild-type gene is injected into fertilized eggs of the *shiverer* mutant with the aim of rescuing the mutant, the resulting transgenic mice express the wild-type gene but produce only 20% of the normal amounts of MBPs. Nevertheless, myelination of central neurons in the transgenic mice is much improved. Although they still have occasional tremors, the transgenic mice do not have convulsions and have a normal life span (Figure 4–15).

In both the central and peripheral nervous systems myelin contains a protein termed myelin-associated glycoprotein (MAG). MAG belongs to the immunoglobulin superfamily that includes several important cell surface proteins thought to be involved in cell-to-cell recognition, eg, the major histocompatibility complex of antigens, T-cell surface antigens, and the neural cell adhesion molecule (NCAM).

MAG is expressed by Schwann cells early during production of myelin and eventually becomes a component

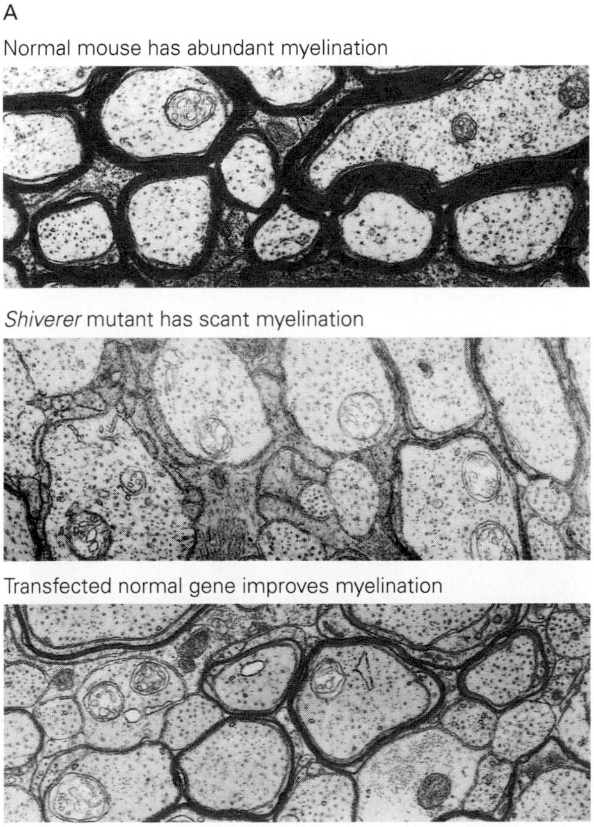
A
Normal mouse has abundant myelination
Shiverer mutant has scant myelination
Transfected normal gene improves myelination

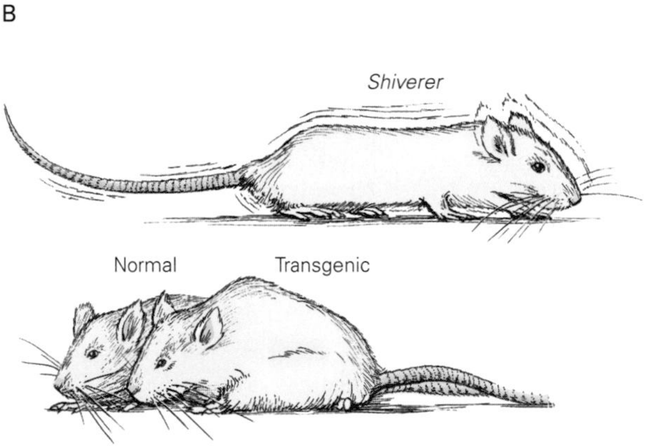
B
Shiverer
Normal
Transgenic

Figures 4–15 A genetic disorder of myelination in mice can be partially cured by transfection of the normal gene that encodes myelin basic protein.

A. Electron micrographs show the state of myelination in the optic nerve of a normal mouse, a *shiverer* mutant, and a mutant transfected with the gene for myelin basic protein.

B. The *shiverer* mutant exhibits poor posture and weakness. Injection of the wild-type gene into the fertilized egg of the mutant improves myelination; the treated mutant looks as perky as a normal mouse. (Reproduced, with permission, from Readhead et al. 1987.)

(continued)

Box 4–3 Defects in Myelin Proteins Disrupt Conduction of Nerve Signals (continued)

of mature (compact) myelin. Its early expression, subcellular location, and structural similarity to other surface recognition proteins suggest that it is an adhesion molecule important for the initiation of the myelination process. Two isoforms of MAG are produced from a single gene through alternative RNA splicing.

More than half of the protein in myelin in central axons is the proteolipid protein (PLP), which has five membrane-spanning domains. Proteolipids differ from lipoproteins in that they are insoluble in water. Proteolipids are soluble only in organic solvents because they contain long chains of fatty acids that are covalently linked to amino acid residues throughout the proteolipid molecule. In contrast, lipoproteins are noncovalent complexes of proteins with lipids and often serve as soluble carriers of the lipid moiety in the blood.

Many mutations of PLP are known in humans as well as in other mammals, eg, the *jimpy* mouse. One example is Pelizaeus-Merzbacher disease, a heterogeneous X-linked disease in humans. Almost all PLP mutations occur in a membrane-spanning domain of the molecule. Mutant animals have reduced amounts of (mutated) PLP, hypomyelination, and degeneration and death of oligodendrocytes. These observations suggest that PLP is involved in the compaction of myelin.

The major protein in mature peripheral myelin, myelin protein zero (MPZ or P_0), spans the plasmalemma of the Schwann cell. It has a basic intracellular domain and, like MAG, is a member of the immunoglobulin superfamily. The glycosylated extracellular part of the protein, which contains the immunoglobulin domain, functions as a homophilic adhesion protein during myelin ensheathing by interacting with identical domains on the surface of the apposed membrane. Genetically engineered mice in which the function of P_0 has been eliminated have poor motor coordination, tremors, and occasional convulsions.

Observation of *trembler* mouse mutants led to the identification of peripheral myelin protein 22 (PMP22). This Schwann cell protein spans the membrane four times and is normally present in compact myelin. PMP22 is altered by a single amino acid in the mutants. A similar protein is found in humans, encoded by a gene on chromosome 17.

Mutations of the PMP22 gene on chromosome 17 produce several hereditary peripheral neuropathies, while a duplication of this gene causes one form of Charcot-Marie-Tooth disease (Figure 4–16). Charcot-Marie-Tooth disease, the most common inherited peripheral neuropathy, and is characterized by progressive muscle weakness, greatly decreased conduction in peripheral nerves, and cycles of demyelination and remyelination. Because both duplicated genes are active, the disease results from *increased* production of PMP22 (a two- to three-fold increase in gene dosage). Mutations in a number of genes expressed by Schwann cells can produce inherited peripheral neuropathies.

A

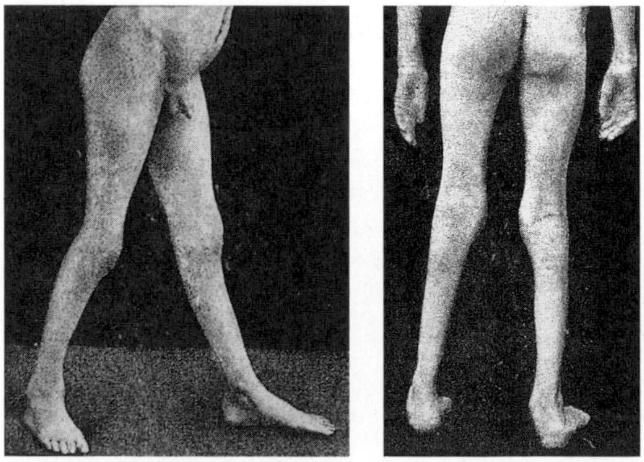

Figure 4–16 Charcot-Marie-Tooth disease (type 1A) results from increased production of peripheral myelin protein 22.

A. A patient with Charcot-Marie-Tooth disease shows impaired gait and deformities. (Reproduced, with permission, from Charcot's original description of the disease, Charcot and Marie 1886.)

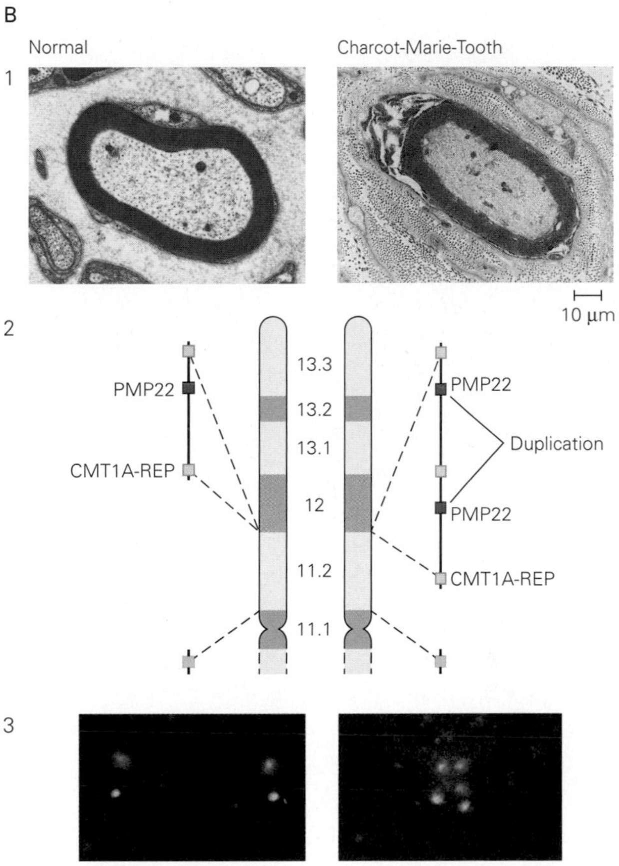

B. The disordered myelination in Charcot-Marie-Tooth disease (type 1A) results from increased production of peripheral myelin protein 22 (PMP22).

1. Sural nerve biopsies from a normal individual (Reproduced, with permission, from A. P. Hays) and from a patient with Charcot-Marie-Tooth disease. (Reproduced, with permission, from Lupski and Garcia 1992.) In the patient's biopsy the myelin sheath is slightly thinner than normal and is surrounded by concentric rings of Schwann cell processes. These changes are typical of the recurrent demyelination and remyelination seen in this disorder.

2. The increase in PMP22 is caused by a duplication of a normal 1.5 megabase region of the DNA on the short arm of chromosome 17 at 17p11.2-p12. The PMP22 gene is flanked by two similar repeat sequences (CMT1A-REP), as shown in the normal chromosome 17 on the left. Normal individuals have two normal chromosomes. In patients with the disease (right) the duplication results in two functioning PMP22 genes, each flanked by a repeat sequence. The normal and duplicated regions are shown in the expanded diagrams indicated by the **dashed lines**. (The repeats are thought to have given rise to the original duplication, which was then inherited. The presence of two similar flanking sequences with homology to a transposable element is believed to increase the frequency of unequal crossing-over in this region of chromosome 17 because the repeats enhance the probability of mispairing of the two parental chromosomes in a fertilized egg.)

3. Although a large duplication (3 megabases) cannot be detected in routine examination of chromosomes in the light microscope, evidence for the duplication can be obtained using fluorescence in situ hybridization. The PMP22 gene is detected with an oligonucleotide probe tagged with the dye Texas Red. An oligonucleotide probe that hybridizes with DNA from region 11.2 (indicated by the green segment close to the centromere), is used for in situ hybridization on the same sample. A nucleus from a normal individual **(left)** shows a pair of chromosomes, each with one red site (PMP22 gene) for each green site. A nucleus from a patient with the disease **(right)** has one extra red site, indicating that one chromosome has one PMP22 gene and the other has two PMP22 genes. (Adapted, with permission, from Garcia et al. 1991.)

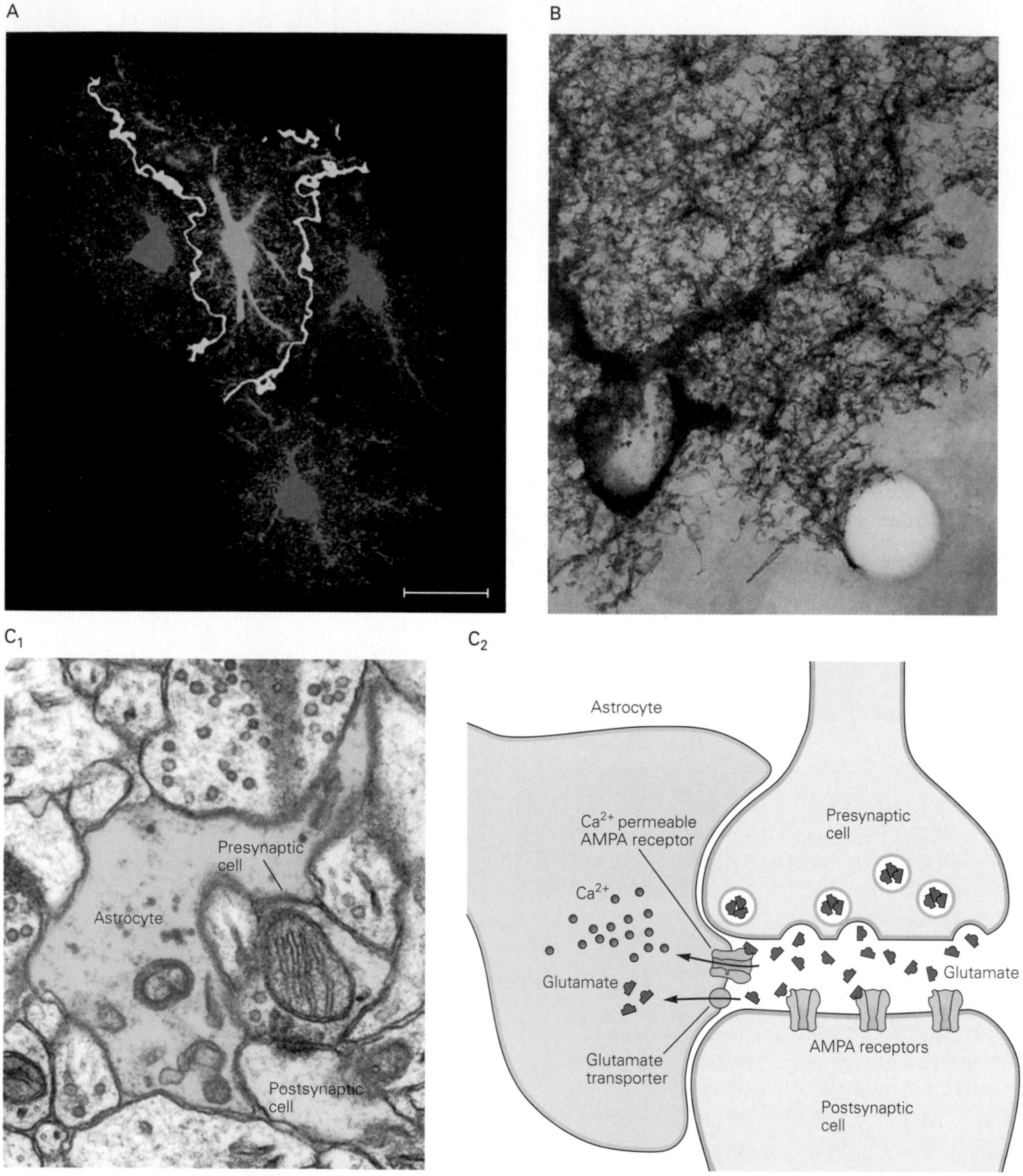

Figure 4–17 Astrocyte processes are intimately associated with synapses.

A. Each of four adjacent astrocytes appears to occupy a distinct volume, with only a small overlap at the ends of their processes. In this overlap area astrocytes are connected to each other by gap junctions. Bar = 20 μm. (Reproduced, with permission, from Bushong et al. 2002.)

B. This high-voltage electron micrograph shows several thick processes emanating from the cell body of an astrocyte and branching into extraordinarily fine processes. The typical astrocyte envelopment of a blood vessel is shown at lower right. (Reproduced, with permission, from Hama, Ari, and Kosaka 1994.)

C. The processes of astrocytes are intimately associated with both presynaptic and postsynaptic elements. **1.** The close association between astrocyte processes and synapses is seen in this electron micrograph of hippocampal cells. (Reproduced, with permission, from Ventura and Harris 1999.) **2.** Glutamate released from the presynaptic neuron activates not only receptors on the postsynaptic neuron but also α-amino-3-hydroxy-5-methylisoxazole-4-propionate (**AMPA**) receptors on astrocytes. Astrocytes remove glutamate from the synaptic cleft by uptake through high-affinity transporters. (Reproduced, with permission, from Gallo and Chittajallu 2001.)

role was that of K^+ buffering. When neurons fire action potentials they release K^+ ions into the extracellular space. Because astrocytes have high concentrations of K^+ channels in their membranes, they can act as *spatial buffers*: They take up K^+ at sites of neuronal activity, mainly synapses, and release it at distant contacts with blood vessels. Astrocytes can also accumulate K^+ locally within their cytoplasmic processes along with Cl^- ions and water. Unfortunately, accumulation of ions and water in astrocytes can contribute to severe brain swelling after head injury.

Astrocytes also regulate neurotransmitter concentrations in the brain. For example, high-affinity transporters located in the astrocyte's plasma membrane rapidly clear the neurotransmitter glutamate from the synaptic cleft (Figure 4–17C). Once within the glial cell, glutamate is converted to glutamine by the enzyme glutamine synthetase. Glutamine is then transferred to neurons, where it serves as an immediate precursor of glutamate (see Chapter 13). Interference with these uptake mechanisms results in high concentrations of extracellular glutamate that can lead to the death of neurons, a process termed excitotoxicity. Astrocytes also degrade dopamine, norepinephrine, epinephrine, and serotonin.

Astrocytes sense when neurons are active because they are depolarized by the K^+ released by neurons and have neurotransmitter receptors similar to those of neurons. For example, Bergmann glia in the cerebellum express glutamate receptors. Thus, the glutamate released at cerebellar synapses affects not only postsynaptic neurons but also astrocytes near the synapse. The binding of these ligands to glial receptors increases the intracellular free Ca^{2+} concentration, which has several important consequences. The processes of one astrocyte connect to those of neighboring astrocytes through gap junctions, allowing transfer of ions and small molecules between many cells. An increase in free Ca^{2+} within one astrocyte increases Ca^{2+} concentrations in adjacent astrocytes. This spread of Ca^{2+} through the astrocyte network occurs over hundreds of micrometers. It is likely that this Ca^{2+} wave modulates nearby neuronal activity by triggering the release of nutrients and regulating blood flow. An increase in Ca^{2+} in astrocytes leads to the secretion of signals that enhance synaptic function, but the specific molecular components of these signals are not understood.

Astrocytes also are important for the development of synapses. They prepare the surface of the neuron for synapse formation and stabilize newly formed synapses. For example, astrocytes secrete substances called thrombospondins that promote the formation of new synapses. In pathological states, such as chromatolysis produced by axonal damage, astrocytes and presynaptic terminals temporarily retract from the damaged postsynaptic cell bodies. Astrocytes release neurotrophic and gliotrophic factors that promote the development and survival of neurons and oligodendrocytes. Astrocytes also protect other cells from the effects of oxidative stress. For example, the glutathione peroxidase in astrocytes detoxifies toxic oxygen free radicals released during hypoxia, inflammation, and neuronal degeneration.

Finally, astrocytes ensheath small arterioles and capillaries throughout the brain, forming contacts between the ends of astrocyte processes and the basal lamina around endothelial cells. The central nervous system is sequestered from the general circulation so that macromolecules in the blood do not passively enter the brain and spinal cord (the "blood-brain barrier"). The barrier is largely the result of tight junctions between endothelial cells and cerebral capillaries, a feature not shared by capillaries in other parts of the body (see Appendix D). Nevertheless, endothelial cells have a number of transport properties that allow some molecules to pass through them into the nervous system. Because of the intimate astrocyte–blood vessel contacts, the transported molecules, such as glucose, come into contact with and can be taken up by astrocyte end-feet.

Choroid Plexus and Ependymal Cells Produce Cerebrospinal Fluid

Cells of the ependyma and choroid plexus are derived from immature neuroepithelium. The ependyma, a single layer of ciliated cuboidal cells, lines all the ventricles of the brain, helping to move cerebrospinal fluid through the ventricular system (Figure 4–18A). At several places in the lateral and fourth ventricles the ependyma is continuous with cells of the choroid plexus, which covers thin blood vessels that project into the ventricles (Figure 4–18B). These choroid plexus epithelial cells filter plasma from the blood and secrete this ultrafiltrate as cerebrospinal fluid. Cerebrospinal fluid production and the properties of choroid plexus cells are considered in detail in Appendix D.

Microglia in the Brain Are Derived from Bone Marrow

Unlike neurons, astrocytes, and oligodendrocytes, microglia do not belong to the neuroectodermal lineage. Instead they derive from bone marrow. Entering the central nervous system early in development,

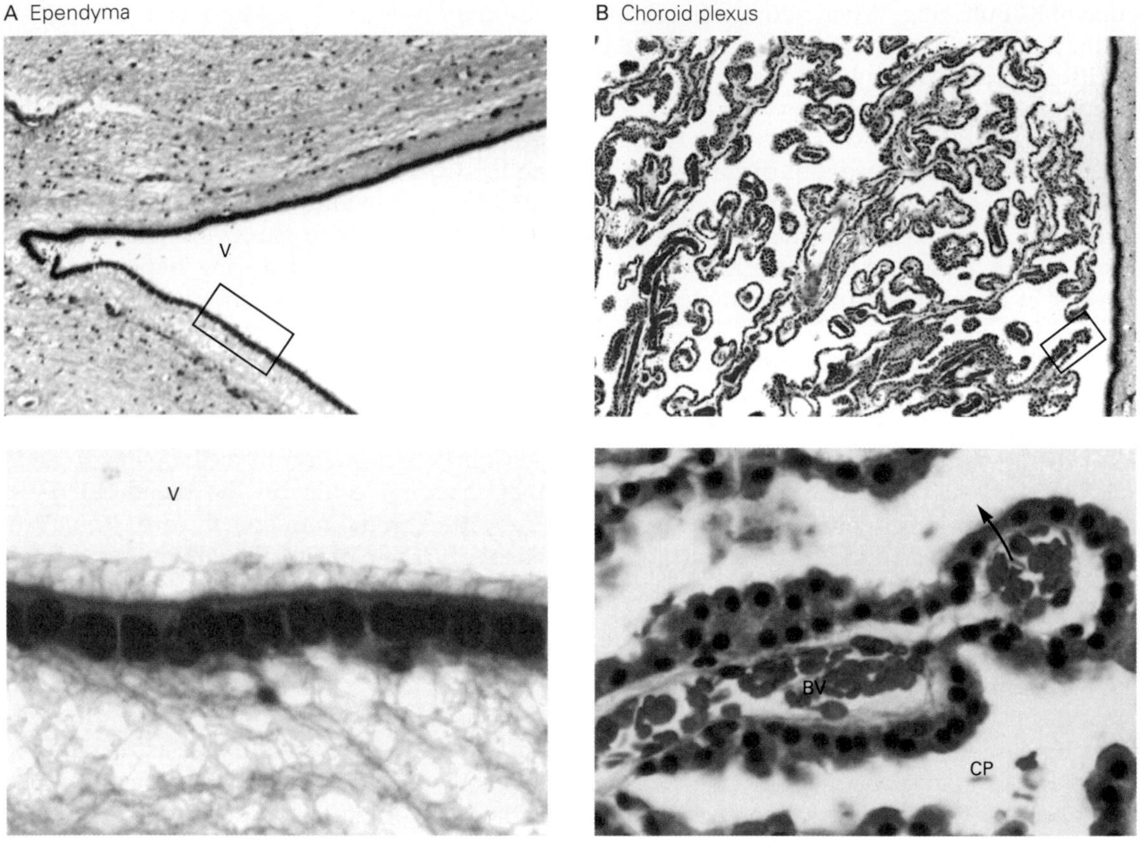

Figure 4–18 Ependyma and choroid plexus.

A. The ependyma is a single layer of ciliated, cuboidal cells lining the cerebral ventricles (V). High magnification of the ependymal lining (rectangle in upper image) shows the cilia on the ventricular side of the ependymal cells.

B. The choroid plexus is continuous with the ependyma but projects into the ventricles, where it covers thin blood vessels and forms a highly-branched, papillary structure. This is the site of cerebrospinal fluid formation. High magnification shows the blood vessel core (**BV**) and overlying choroid plexus (**CP**). The **arrow** denotes the direction of fluid flow from capillary into ventricle during the formation of cerebrospinal fluid.

they reside in all regions of the brain throughout life (Figure 4–19). Their functions are not well understood, although they probably play an important role in immunological surveillance in the CNS, poised to react to foreign invaders.

Of all of the cells in the central nervous system, microglia are the best at processing and presenting antigens to lymphocytes and secreting cytokines and chemokines during inflammation. Thus they serve to bring lymphocytes, neutrophils, and monocytes into the central nervous system and expand the lymphocyte population, important immunological activities in infection, stroke, and immune-mediated demyelinating disease. Microglia can also become macrophages, clearing debris after infarcts (strokes) or other degenerative neurological disorders.

An Overall View

The morphology of neurons is elegantly suited to receive, conduct, and transmit signals. Dendrites provide a highly branched, elongated surface for receiving signals. Axons conduct electrical impulses rapidly over long distances to their synaptic terminals, which release neurotransmitters onto target cells. Although all neurons conform to the same basic cell plan, different types of neurons vary widely in their specific morphological features.

Neurons in different locations differ in the complexity of their dendritic trees, extent of axon branching, as well as in the number of synaptic terminals that they form and receive. The functional significance of these morphological differences is plainly evident. For example,

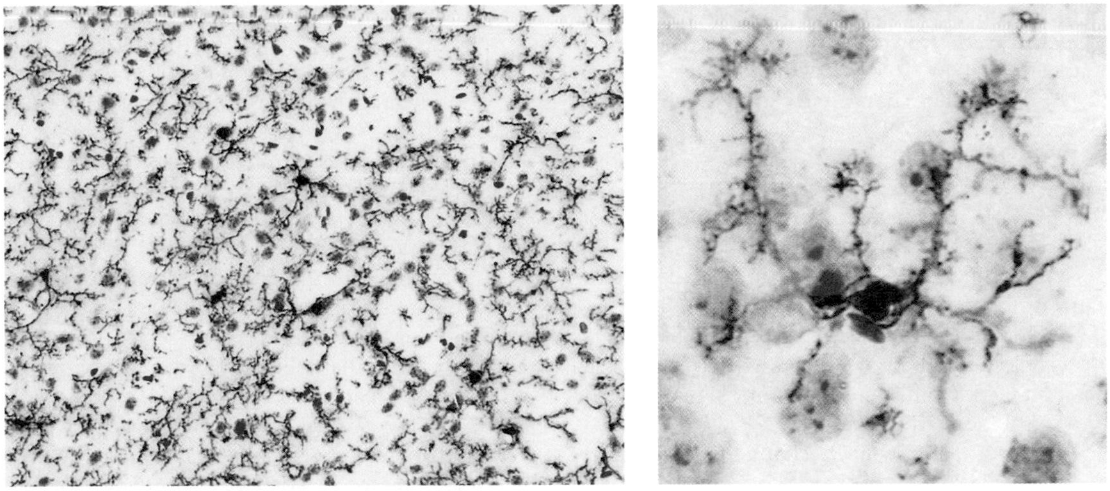

Figure 4–19 Large numbers of microglia reside in the mammalian central nervous system. The micrograph on the left shows microglia in the cerebral cortex of an adult mouse (in **brown**, immunocytochemistry). The **blue** spots are the nuclei of nonmicroglial cells. The microglial cells have fine, lacy processes, as shown in the higher magnification micrograph on the right. (Reproduced, with permission, from Berry et al. 2002.)

motor neurons must have a more complex dendritic tree than sensory neurons, as even simple reflex activity requires integration of many excitatory and inhibitory inputs. As we shall see in subsequent chapters, different types of neurons have different neurotransmitters, ion channels, and neurotransmitter receptors. Together, these biochemical, morphological, and electrophysiological differences contribute to the great complexity of information processing in the brain.

Most neuronal proteins are synthesized in the cell body, but some synthesis occurs in dendrites and axons. The newly synthesized proteins are folded with the assistance of chaperones, and their final structure is often modified by permanent or reversible post-translational modifications. The final destination of a protein in the neuron depends on signals encoded in its amino acid sequence. Transport of proteins and RNA occurs with great specificity and results in the vectorial transport of selected membrane components. The cytoskeleton provides an important framework for the transport of organelles to different intracellular locations in addition to controlling neuronal shape.

As we shall see in later chapters, all these fundamental cell-biological processes are profoundly controlled by electrical activity, which produces the dramatic changes in cell structure and function by which neural circuits adapt to experience (learning).

Finally, the nervous system also contains several types of glial cells. Oligodendrocytes and Schwann cells produce the myelin insulation that enables axons to conduct electrical signals rapidly. Astrocytes ensheath other parts of the neuron, particularly synapses. Glia control extracellular ion and neurotransmitter concentrations, and actively participate in the formation and function of synapses.

James H. Schwartz
Ben A. Barres
James E. Goldman

Selected Readings

Alberts B, Johnson A, Lewis J, Raff M, Roberts K, Walter P (eds). 2002. *Molecular Biology of the Cell,* 4th ed. New York: Garland.

Brown A. 2003. Axonal transport of membranous and nonmembranous cargoes: a unified perspective. J Cell Biol 160:817–821.

Dyck PJ, Thomas PK, Griffin JW, Low PA, Poduslo JF (eds). 1993. *Peripheral Neuropathy,* 3rd ed. Philadelphia: Saunders.

Dyck PJ, Thomas PK, Lambert EH, Bunge R (eds). 1984. *Peripheral Neuropathy,* 2nd ed., Vols. 1, 2. Philadelphia: Saunders.

Giraudo CG, Hu C, You D, Slovic AM, Mosharov EV, Sulzer D, Melia TJ, Rothman JE. 2005. SNAREs can promote complete fusion and hemifusion as alternative outcomes. J Cell Biol 170:249–260.

Glickman MH, Ciechanover A. 2002. The ubiquitin-proteasome proteolytic pathway: destruction for the sake of construction. Physiol Rev 82:373–428.

Hartl FU. 1996. Molecular chaperones in cellular protein folding. Nature 381:571–579.

Holtzman E. 1989. *Lysosomes. (Cellular Organelles).* New York: Plenum.

Kelly RB. 1993. Storage and release of neurotransmitters. Cell 72:43–53.

Kimelberg HK. 2010. Functions of mature mammalian astrocytes: a current view. The Neuroscientist 16:79–106.

Kreis T, Vale R (eds). 1999. *Guidebook to the Cytoskeletal and Motor Proteins,* 2nd ed. Oxford: Oxford Univ. Press.

Nigg EA. 1997. Nucleocytoplasmic transport: signals, mechanisms and regulation. Nature 386:779–787.

Pemberton LF, Paschal BM. 2005. Mechanisms of receptor-mediated nuclear import and nuclear export. Traffic 6:187–198.

Rothman JE. 2002. Lasker Basic Medical Research Award: the machinery and principles of vesicle transport in the cell. Nat Med 8:1059–1062.

Schatz G, Dobberstein B. 1996. Common principles of protein translocation across membranes. Science 271:1519–1526.

Schwartz JH. 2003. Ubiquitination, protein turnover, and long-term synaptic plasticity. Sci STKE 190:26.

Siegel GJ, Albers RW, Brady S, Price DL (eds). 2005. *Basic Neurochemistry: Molecular, Cellular, and Medical Aspects,* 7th ed. Amsterdam: Elsevier.

Signor D, Scholey JM. 2000. Microtubule-based transport along axons, dendrites and axonemes. Essays Biochem 35:89–102.

St Johnston D. 2005. Moving messages: the intracellular localization of mRNAs. Nat Rev Mol Cell Biol 6:363–375.

Stryer L. 1995. *Biochemistry,* 4th ed. New York: Freeman.

Tahirovic S, Bradke F. 2009. Neuronal polarity. Cold Spring Harb Perspect Biol 1:a001644.

Zhou L, Griffin JW. 2003. Demyelinating neuropathies. Curr Opin Neurol 16:307–313.

References

Berry M, Butt AM, Wilkin G, Perry VH. 2002. Structure and function of glia in the central nervous system, in *Greenfield's Neuropathology*. Graham DI and Lantos PL eds., 7th ed., pp. 104–105. London: Arnold.

Bershadsky AD, Vasiliev JM. 1988. *Cytoskeleton.* New York: Plenum.

Bushong EA, Martone ME, Jones YZ, Ellisman MH. 2002. Protoplasmic astrocytes in CA1 stratum radiatum occupy separate anatomical domains. J Neurosci 22:183–192.

Charcot J-M, Marie P. 1886. Sur une forme particulière d'atrophie musculaire progressive, souvent familiale, dábutant par les pieds et les jambes et atteignant plus tard les mains. Rev Med 6:97–138.

Ciechanover A, Brundin P. 2003. The ubiquitin proteasome system in neurodegenerative diseases: sometimes the chicken, sometimes the egg. Neuron 40:427–446.

Cooney JR, Hurlburt JL, Selig DK, Harris KM, Fiala JC. 2002. Endosomal compartments serve multiple hippocampal dendritic spines from a widespread rather than a local store of recycling membrane. J Neurosci 22:2215–2224.

De Camilli P, Moretti M, Donini SD, Walter U, Lohmann SM. 1986. Heterogeneous distribution of the cAMP receptor protein RII in the nervous system: evidence for its intracellular accumulation on microtubules, microtubule-organizing centers, and in the area of the Golgi complex. J Cell Biol 103:189–203.

Divac I, LaVail JH, Rakic P, Winston KR. 1977. Heterogeneous afferents to the inferior parietal lobule of the rhesus monkey revealed by the retrograde transport method. Brain Res 123:197–207.

Duxbury MS, Whang EE. 2004. RNA interference: a practical approach. J Surg Res 117:339–344.

Esiri MM, Hyman BT, Beyreuther K, Masters C. 1997. Ageing and dementia, in *Greenfield's Neuropathology*. 6th ed. Graham DI and Lantos PL eds.,Vol II. London: Arnold.

Gallo V, Chittajallu R. 2001. Neuroscience. Unwrapping glial cells from the synapse: what lies inside? Science 292:872– 873.

Goldberg AL. 2003. Protein degradation and protection against misfolded or damaged proteins. Nature 426:895–899.

Görlich D, Mattaj IW. 1996. Nucleocytoplasmic transport. Science 271:1513–1518.

Hama K, Arii T, Kosaka T. 1994.Three-dimensional organization of neuronal and glial processes: high voltage electron microscopy. Microsc Res Tech 29:357–367.

Harris KM, Jensen FE, Tsao B. 1992. Three-dimensional structure of dendritic spines and synapses in rat hippocampus (CA1) at postnatal day 15 and adult ages: implications for the maturation of synaptic physiology and long-term potentiation. J Neurosci 12:2685–2705.

Harris KM, Stevens JK. 1989. Dendritic spines of CA1 pyramidal cells in the rat hippocampus: serial electron microscopy with reference to their biophysical characteristics. J Neurosci 9:2982–2997.

Hirokawa N. 1997. The mechanisms of fast and slow transport in neurons: identification and characterization of the new Kinesin superfamily motors. Curr Opin Neurobiol 7:605–614.

Hirokawa N, Pfister KK, Yorifuji H, Wagner MC, Brady ST, Bloom GS. 1989. Submolecular domains of bovine brain kinesin identified by electron microscopy and monoclonal antibody decoration. Cell 56:867–878.

Hoffman PN, Lasek RJ. 1975. The slow component of axonal transport: identification of major structural polypeptides of the axon and their generality among mammalian neurons. J Cell Biol 66:351–366.

Lemke G. 2001. Glial control of neuronal development. Annu Rev Neurosci 24:87–105.

Lupski JR, Garcia CA. 1992. Molecular genetics and neuropathology of Charcot-Marie-Tooth disease type 1A. Brain Pathol 2:337–349.

Lupski JR, de Oca-Luna RM, Slaugenhaupt S, Pentao L, Guzzetta V, Trask BJ, Saucedo-Cardenas O, Barker DF, et al. 1991. DNA duplication associated with Charcot-Marie-Tooth disease type 1A. Cell 66:219–232.

McNew JA, Goodman JM. 1996. The targeting and assembly of peroxisomal proteins: some old rules do not apply. Trends Biochem Sci 21:54–58.

Mirra SS, Hyman BT. 2002. Aging and dementia. In: DI Graham, PL Lantos (eds). *Greenfield's Neuropathology,* 7th ed., Vol. 2, p. 212. London: Arnold.

Ochs S. 1972. Fast transport of materials in mammalian nerve fibers. Science 176:252–260.

Peles E, Salzer JL. 2000. Molecular domains of myelinated axons. Curr Opin Neurobiol 10:558–565.

Peters A, Palay SL, Webster H deF. 1991. *The Fine Structure of the Nervous System,* 3rd ed. New York: Oxford University Press.

Raine CS. 1984. Morphology of myelin and myelination. In *Myelin,* Morell P ed. New York: Plenum Press.

Ramón y Cajal S. [1901] 1988. Studies on the human cerebral cortex. IV. Structure of the olfactory cerebral cortex of man and mammals. In: J DeFelipe, EG Jones (eds, transl). *Cajál on the Cerebral Cortex,* pp. 289–362. New York: Oxford Univ. Press.

Ramón y Cajal S. [1909] 1995. *Histology of the Nervous System of Man and Vertebrates.* N Swanson, LW Swanson (transl). Vols. 1, 2. New York: Oxford Univ. Press.

Readhead C, Popko B, Takahashi N, Shine HD, Saavedra RA, Sidman RL, Hood L. 1987. Expression of a myelin basic protein gene in transgenic Shiverer mice: correction of the dysmyelinating phenotype. Cell 48:703–712.

Roa BB, Lupski JR. 1994. Molecular genetics of Charcot-Marie-Tooth neuropathy. Adv Human Genet 22:117–152.

Schnapp BJ, Reese TS. 1982. Cytoplasmic structure in rapid-frozen axons. J Cell Biol 94:667–679.

Sorra KE, Harris KM. 1993. Occurrence and three-dimensional structure of multiple synapses between individual radiatum axons and their target pyramidal cells in hippocampal area CA1. J Neurosci 13:3736–3748.

Sossin W. 1996. Mechanisms for the generation of synapse specificity long-term memory: the implications of a requirement for transcription. Trends Neurosci 19:215–218.

Takei K, Mundigl O, Daniell L, De Camilli P. 1996. The synaptic vesicle cycle: a single vesicle budding step involving clathrin and dynamin. J Cell Biol 1335:1237–1250.

Ventura R, Harris KM. 1999. Three-dimensional relationships between hippocampal synapses and astrocytes. J Neurosci 19:6897–6906.

Weiss P, Hiscoe HB. 1948. Experiments on the mechanism of nerve growth. J Exp Zool 107:315–395.

Wells DG, Richter JD, Fallon JR. 2000. Molecular mechanisms for activity-regulated protein synthesis in the synapto-dendritic compartment. Curr Opin Neurobiol 10:132–137.

Williams PL, Warwick R, Dyson M, Bannister LH (eds). 1989. *Gray's Anatomy,* 37th ed., pp 859–919. Edinburgh: Churchill Livingstone.

Zemanick MC, Strick PL, Dix RD. 1991. Direction of transneuronal transport of herpes simplex virus 1 in the primate motor system is strain-dependent. Proc Natl Acad Sci U S A 88:8048–8051.

5

Ion Channels

Signaling in the brain depends on the ability of nerve cells to respond to very small stimuli with rapid and large changes in the electrical potential difference across the cell membrane. In sensory cells, the membrane potential changes in response to minute physical stimuli: Receptors in the eye respond to a single photon of light; olfactory neurons detect a single molecule of odorant; and hair cells in the inner ear respond to tiny movements of atomic dimensions. These sensory responses ultimately lead to the firing of an action potential during which the membrane potential changes up to 500 volts per second.

The rapid changes in membrane potential that underlie signaling throughout the nervous system are mediated by ion channels, a class of integral membrane proteins found in all cells of the body. The ion channels of nerve cells are optimally tuned to respond to specific physical and chemical signals. They are also heterogeneous—in different parts of the nervous system different types of channels carry out specific signaling tasks.

Because of their key roles in electrical signaling, malfunctioning of ion channels can cause a wide variety of neurological diseases (see Chapter 14). Diseases caused by ion channel malfunction are not limited to the brain; cystic fibrosis, skeletal muscle disease, and certain types of cardiac arrhythmia, for example, are also caused by ion channel malfunction. Moreover, ion channels are often the site of action of drugs, poisons, or toxins. Thus ion channels have crucial roles in both the normal physiology and pathophysiology of the nervous system.

In addition to ion channels, nerve cells contain a second important class of proteins specialized for moving ions across cell membranes, the ion transporters or pumps. These proteins do not participate in rapid neuronal signaling but rather are important for establishing and maintaining the concentration gradients of physiologically important ions between the inside and outside of the cell. As we will see in this chapter and Chapter 6, ion transporters differ in important aspects from ion channels, but also share certain common features.

Rapid Signaling in the Nervous System Depends on Ion Channels

Ion channels have three important properties: (1) They recognize and select specific ions, (2) they open and close in response to specific electrical, mechanical, or chemical signals, and (3) they conduct ions across the membrane. The channels in nerve and muscle conduct ions across the cell membrane at extremely rapid rates, thereby providing a large flow of electric charge. Up to 100 million ions can pass through a single channel each second. This current causes the rapid changes in membrane potential required for signaling, as will be discussed in Chapter 7. The fast flow of ions through channels is comparable to the turnover rate of the fastest enzymes, catalase and carbonic anhydrase, which are limited by diffusion of substrate. (The turnover rates of most other enzymes are considerably slower, ranging from 10 to 1,000 per second.)

In light of such an extraordinary rate of ion flow, channels are surprisingly selective for the ions they allow to permeate. Each type of channel allows only one or a few types of ions to pass. For example, the negative resting potential of nerve cells is largely determined by a class of K^+ channels that are 100-fold more permeable to K^+ than to Na^+. In contrast, during the action potential a class of Na^+ channels is activated that are 10- to 20-fold more permeable to Na^+ than to K^+. Thus a key to the great versatility of neuronal signaling is the regulated activation of different classes of ion channels, each of which is selective for specific ions.

Many channels open and close in response to a specific event: Voltage-gated channels are regulated by changes in membrane potential, ligand-gated channels by chemical transmitters, and mechanically gated channels by pressure or stretch. However, some channels are normally open in the cell at rest. The ion flux through these "resting" channels contributes significantly to the resting potential.

Ion channels are limited to catalyzing the passive movement of ions down their thermodynamic concentration and electrical gradients. For example, Na^+ ions enter a cell through voltage-gated Na^+ channels during an action potential because the external Na^+ concentration is much greater than the internal concentration; the open channels allow Na^+ to diffuse into the cell down its concentration gradient. With such passive ion movement the Na^+ concentration gradient would eventually dissipate were it not for ion pumps. Different types of ion pumps maintain the concentration gradients for Na^+, K^+, Ca^{2+}, Cl^-, and other ions.

These pumps differ from ion channels in two important details. First, whereas open ion channels have a continuous water-filled pathway through which ions flow unimpeded from one side of the membrane to the other, each time a pump moves an ion, or a group of a few ions, across the membrane, it must undergo a series of conformational changes. As a result, the rate of ion flow through pumps is 100 to 100,000 times slower than through channels. Second, pumps that maintain ion gradients use energy, often in the form of adenosine triphosphate (ATP), to transport ions against their electrical and chemical gradients. Such ion movements are termed *active transport*. The function and structure of ion pumps is considered in detail at the end of this chapter and in Chapter 6.

In this chapter we examine four questions: Why do nerve cells have channels? How can channels conduct ions at such high rates and still be selective? How are channels gated? How are the properties of these channels modified by various intrinsic and extrinsic conditions? In addition, we compare the molecular structure of various channels and consider how channel structure explains function. Finally, we compare ion movements through channels and transporters. In succeeding chapters we consider how resting channels and pumps generate the resting potential (Chapter 6), how voltage-gated channels generate the action potential (Chapter 7), and how ligand-gated channels produce synaptic potentials (Chapters 8, 9, and 10).

Ion Channels Are Proteins That Span the Cell Membrane

To appreciate why nerve cells use channels, we need to understand the nature of the plasma membrane and the physical chemistry of ions in solution. The plasma membrane of all cells, including nerve cells, is approximately 6 to 8 nm thick and consists of a mosaic of lipids and proteins. The core of the membrane is formed by a double layer of phospholipids. Embedded within this continuous lipid sheet are integral membrane proteins, including ion channels.

The lipids of the membrane do not mix with water—they are hydrophobic. In contrast, the ions within the cell and those outside strongly attract water molecules—they are hydrophilic (Figure 5–1). Ions attract water because water molecules are dipolar: Although the net charge on a water molecule is zero, charge is separated within the molecule. The oxygen atom in a water molecule tends to attract electrons and so bears a small net negative charge, whereas the

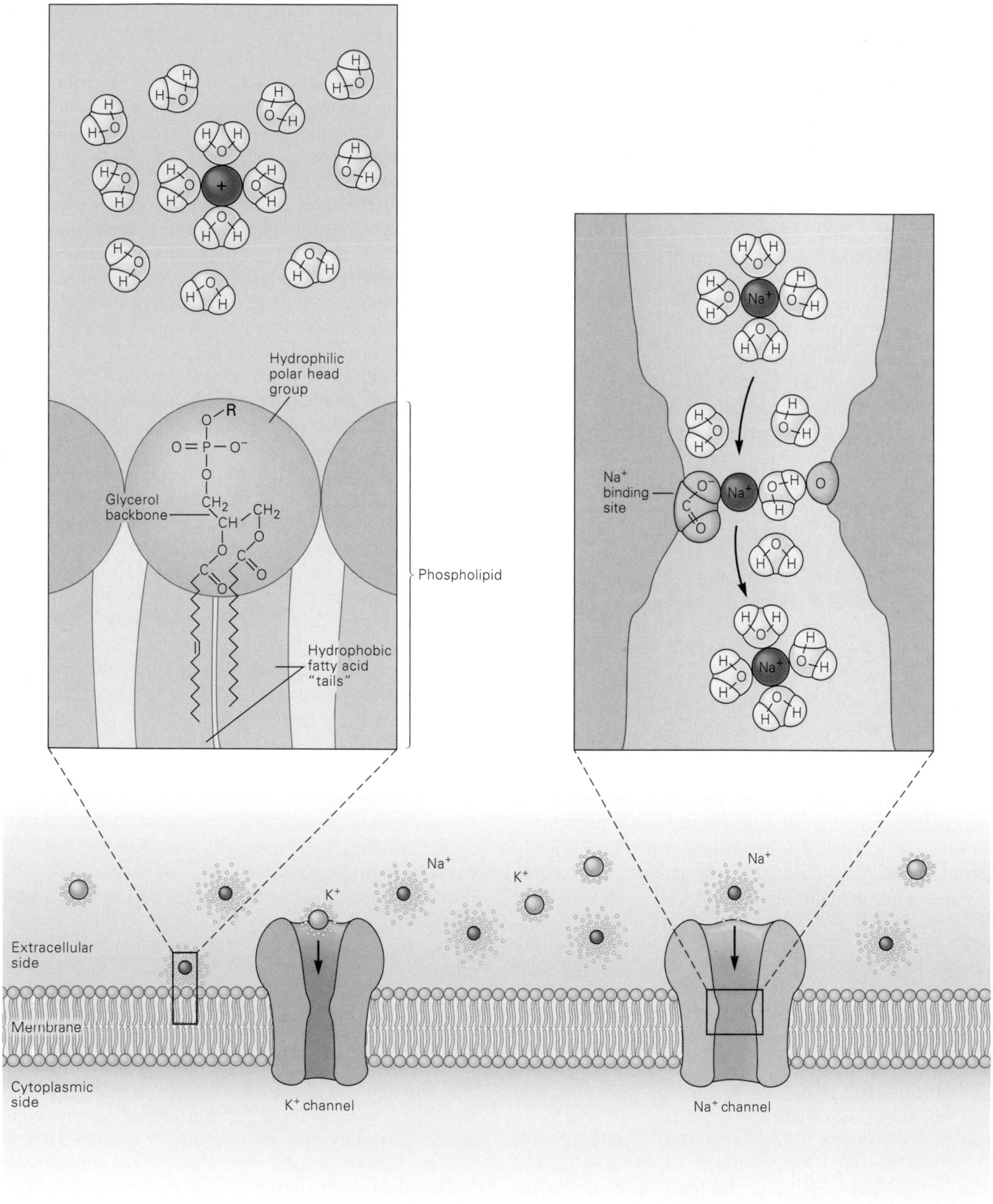

Hydrophilic polar head group
Glycerol backbone
Hydrophobic fatty acid "tails"
Phospholipid
Na+ binding site
Extracellular side
Membrane
Cytoplasmic side
K+
Na+
K+ channel
Na+ channel

hydrogen atoms tend to lose electrons and therefore carry a small net positive charge. As a result of this unequal distribution of charge, positively charged ions (cations) are strongly attracted electrostatically to the oxygen atom of water, and negatively charged ions (anions) are attracted to the hydrogen atoms. Similarly, ions attract water; in fact they become surrounded by electrostatically bound *waters of hydration* (see Figure 5–1).

An ion cannot move away from water into the noncharged hydrocarbon tails of the lipid bilayer in the membrane unless a large amount of energy is expended to overcome the attraction between the ion and the surrounding water molecules. For this reason it is extremely unlikely that an ion will move from solution into the lipid bilayer, and therefore the bilayer itself is almost completely impermeable to ions. Rather, ions cross the membrane through ion channels, specialized pores or openings in the membrane where, as we shall see, the energetics favor ion movement.

Ion channels are not simply holes in the lipid membrane but are distinct protein structures that span the lipid bilayer. Although their molecular nature has been known with certainty for only approximately 25 years, the idea of ion channels dates to the work of Ernst Brücke at the end of the 19th century. Physiologists had long known that, despite the fact that the cell membrane acts as a barrier, cell membranes are nevertheless permeable to water and many small solutes, including some ions. To explain osmosis, the flow of water across biological membranes, Brücke proposed that membranes contained channels or pores that allow water but not larger solutes to flow. Over 100 years later Peter Agre found that a family of proteins termed aquaporins form channels with a high selective permeability to water. At the beginning of the 20th century William Bayliss suggested that water-filled channels would permit ions to cross the cell membrane easily, as the ions would not need to be stripped of their waters of hydration.

The idea that ions move through channels leads to a question: How can a water-filled channel conduct ions at high rates and yet be selective? How, for instance, does a channel allow K^+ ions to pass while excluding Na^+ ions? Selectivity cannot be based solely on the diameter of the ion because K^+, with a crystal radius of 0.133 nm, is larger than Na^+ (crystal radius of 0.095 nm). Because ions in solution are surrounded by waters of hydration, the ease with which an ion moves in solution (its mobility or diffusion constant) depends on the size of the ion together with the shell of water surrounding it.

The smaller an ion, the more highly localized is its charge and the stronger its electric field. As a result, smaller ions attract water more strongly. Thus, as Na^+ moves through solution its stronger electrostatic attraction for water causes it to have a larger water shell, which tends to slow it down relative to K^+. Because of its larger water shell, Na^+ behaves as if it is larger than K^+. In fact, there is a precise relationship between the size of an ion and its mobility in solution: the smaller the ion, the lower its mobility. We therefore can construct a model of a channel that selects K^+ rather than Na^+ simply on the basis of the interaction of the two ions with water in a water-filled channel (Figure 5–1).

Although this model explains how a channel can select K^+ and exclude Na^+, it does not explain how a

Figure 5–1 **(Opposite) The permeability of the cell membrane to ions is determined by the interaction of ions with water, the membrane lipid bilayer, and ion channels.** Ions in solution are surrounded by a cloud of water molecules (waters of hydration) that are attracted by the net charge of the ion. This cloud is carried along by the ion as it diffuses through solution, increasing the effective size of the ion. It is energetically unfavorable, and therefore improbable, for the ion to leave this polar environment to enter the nonpolar environment of the lipid bilayer formed from phospholipids. Phospholipids have a hydrophilic head and a hydrophobic tail. The hydrophobic tails join to exclude water and ions, whereas the polar hydrophilic heads face the aqueous environments of the extracellular fluid and cytoplasm. The phospholipid is composed of a backbone of glycerol in which two –OH groups are linked by ester bonds to fatty acid molecules. The third –OH group of glycerol is linked to phosphoric acid. The phosphate group is further linked to one of a variety of small, polar alcohol head groups (**R**).

Ion channels are integral membrane proteins that span the lipid bilayer, providing a pathway for ions to cross the membrane. The channels are selective for specific ions.

Potassium channels have a narrow pore that excludes Na^+. Although a Na^+ ion is smaller than a K^+ ion, in solution the effective diameter of Na^+ is larger because its local field strength is more intense, causing it to attract a larger cloud of water molecules. The K^+ channel pore is too narrow for the hydrated Na^+ ion to permeate.

Sodium channels have a selectivity filter that weakly binds Na^+ ions. According to the hypothesis developed by Bertil Hille and colleagues, a Na^+ ion binds transiently at an active site as it moves through the filter. At the binding site the positive charge of the ion is stabilized by a negatively charged amino acid residue on the channel wall and also by a water molecule that is attracted to a second polar amino acid residue on the other side of the channel wall. It is thought that a K^+ ion, because of its larger diameter, cannot be stabilized as effectively by the negative charge and therefore will be excluded from the filter. (Modified, with permission, from Hille 1984.)

channel could select Na^+ and exclude K^+. Moreover, the model cannot account quantitatively for the very high ionic selectivity exhibited by biological K^+ channels. This problem led many physiologists in the 1930s and 1940s to abandon the channel theory in favor of the idea that ions cross cell membranes by first binding to a specific carrier protein, which then shuttles the ion through the membrane. In this carrier model selectivity is based on the chemical binding between the ion and the carrier protein, not on the mobility of the ion in solution.

Even though we now know that ions can cross membranes by means of a variety of transport macromolecules, the Na^+-K^+ pump being a well-characterized example (Chapter 6), many properties of membrane ion conductances do not fit the carrier model. Most important is the rapid rate of ion transfer across membranes. This transfer rate was first examined in the early 1970s by measuring the transmembrane current initiated when the neurotransmitter acetylcholine (ACh) binds its receptor in the cell membrane of skeletal muscle fibers at the synapse between nerve and muscle. Using measurements of membrane current noise, small statistical fluctuations in the mean ionic current induced by ACh, Bernard Katz and Ricardo Miledi concluded that the current conducted by a single ACh receptor is 10 million ions per second. In contrast, the Na^+-K^+ pump transports at most 100 ions per second.

If the ACh receptor acted as a carrier, it would have to shuttle an ion across the membrane in 0.1 μs (one ten-millionth of a second), an implausibly fast rate. The 100,000-fold difference in rates strongly suggests that the ACh receptor (and other ligand-gated receptors) must conduct ions through a channel. Later measurements in many voltage-gated pathways selective for K^+, Na^+, and Ca^{2+} also demonstrated large currents carried by single macromolecules, indicating that they too are channels.

But we are still left with the problem of what makes a channel selective. To explain selectivity, Bertil Hille extended the pore theory by proposing that channels have narrow regions that act as molecular sieves. At this *selectivity filter* an ion must shed most of its waters of hydration to traverse the channel; in their place weak chemical bonds (electrostatic interactions) form with polar (charged) amino acid residues that line the walls of the channel (Figure 5–1). Because shedding its waters of hydration is energetically unfavorable, the ion will traverse a channel only if its energy of interaction with the selectivity filter compensates for the loss of the energy of interaction with its waters of hydration. Ions traversing the channel are normally bound to the selectivity filter for only a short time (less than 1 μs), after which electrostatic and diffusional forces propel the ion through the channel. In channels where the pore diameter is large enough to accommodate several water molecules, an ion need not be stripped completely of its water shell.

How is this chemical recognition and specificity established? One theory was developed in the early 1960s by George Eisenman to explain the properties of ion-selective glass electrodes (which are similar to pH electrodes but select among the alkali metal cations). According to this theory, a binding site with a high negative field strength—for example, one formed by negatively charged carboxylic acid groups of glutamate or aspartate—will bind Na^+ more tightly than K^+. This selectivity results because the electrostatic interaction between two charged groups, as governed by Coulomb's law, depends inversely on the distance between the two groups.

Because Na^+ has a smaller crystal radius than K^+, it will approach a negative site more closely than K^+ and thus will derive a more favorable free-energy change on binding. This compensates for the requirement that Na^+ lose some of its waters of hydration to traverse the narrow selectivity filter. In contrast, a binding site with a low negative strength—one that is composed, for example, of polar carbonyl or hydroxyl oxygen atoms—would select K^+ over Na^+. At such a site the binding of Na^+ would not provide a sufficient free-energy change to compensate for the loss of the ion's waters of hydration, which Na^+ holds strongly. However, such a site would be able to compensate for the loss of a K^+ ion's associated water molecules as the larger K^+ ions interact more weakly with water. It is currently thought that ion channels are selective both because of specific chemical interactions and because of molecular sieving based on pore diameter.

Currents Through Single Ion Channels Can Be Recorded

A complete understanding of how channels work requires three-dimensional structural information. X-ray crystallographic and other structural analyses have been informative in the study of enzymes and other soluble proteins but have only recently been applied to integral membrane proteins, such as ion channels, because their transmembrane hydrophobic regions make them difficult to crystallize. Nevertheless, for the past 35 years single-channel recording has provided important functional information that has yielded significant insights into channel structure.

Before it became possible to resolve the small amount of current that flows through a single ion channel in biological membranes, channel function was studied in artificial lipid bilayers. In the early 1960s Paul Mueller and Donald Rudin developed a technique for forming functional lipid bilayers by painting a thin drop of phospholipid over a hole in a nonconducting barrier that separates two salt solutions. Although lipid membranes are highly impermeable to ions, ionic permeability of the membrane increases dramatically when certain peptide antibiotics are added to the salt solution. Early studies with gramicidin A, a 15-amino acid cyclic peptide, were especially informative. Application of low concentrations of gramicidin A brings about small step-like changes in current across the membrane. These brief pulses of current reflect the all-or-none opening and closing of the single ion channel formed by the peptide.

The current through a single gramicidin channel varies with membrane potential in a linear manner; that is, the channel behaves as a simple resistor (Figure 5–2). The amplitude of the single-channel current can thus be obtained from Ohm's law, $i = V/R$, where i is the current through the single channel, V is the voltage across the membrane, and R is the resistance of the open channel. The resistance of a single open channel is approximately 8×10^{10} ohms (Figure 5–2C). In dealing with ion channels it is more useful to speak of the reciprocal of resistance or conductance ($\gamma = 1/R$), as this provides an electrical measure related to ion permeability. Thus, Ohm's law can be expressed as $i = \gamma \times V$. The conductance of the gramicidin A channel is approximately 12×10^{-12} siemens (S), or 12 picosiemens (pS), where 1 S equals 1/ohm.

The insights into basic channel properties obtained from artificial membranes were later confirmed in biological membranes by the patch-clamp technique, developed by Erwin Neher and Bert Sakmann in 1976 (Box 5–1). A glass micropipette containing ACh—the

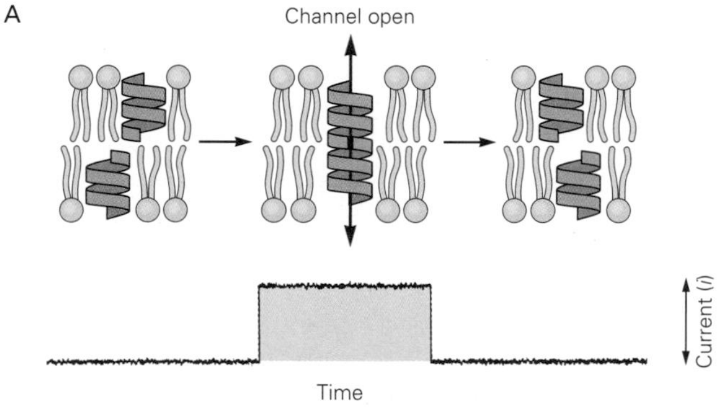

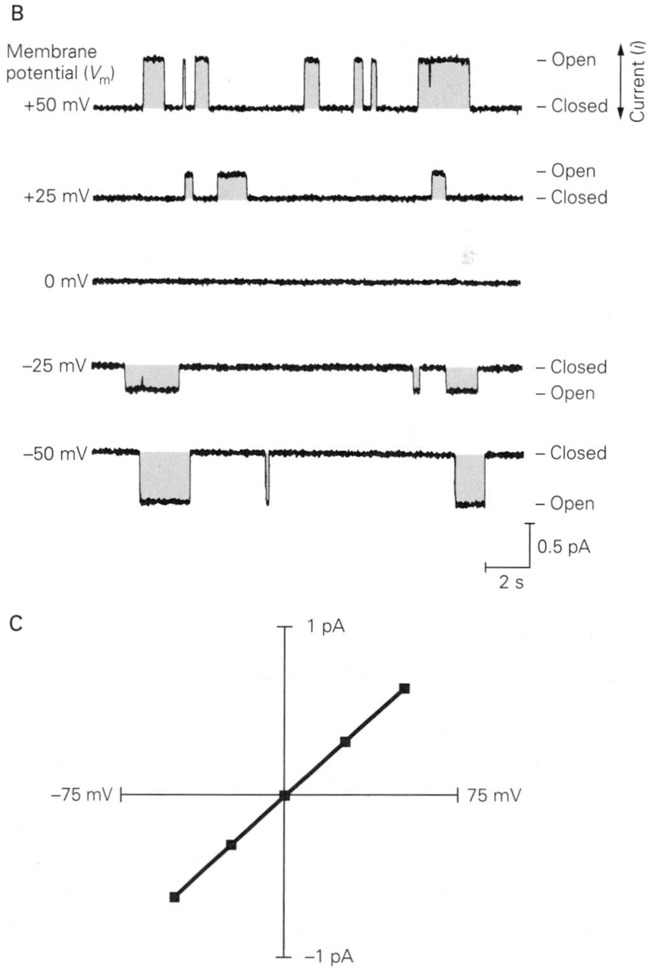

Figure 5–2 Characteristics of the current in a single ion channel. The data presented here were obtained from a channel formed by the addition of gramicidin A molecules to the solution bathing an artificial lipid bilayer.

A. A functional gramicidin A channel is thought to form by end-to-end dimerization of two gramicidin peptides. (Reproduced, with permission, from Sawyer, Koeppe, and Andersen 1989.)

B. The channel opens and closes in an all-or-none fashion, resulting in brief current pulses through the membrane. If the electrical potential across the membrane (V_m) is varied, the current through the channel (i) changes proportionally. V_m is measured in millivolts (mV); i is measured in picoamperes (pA).

C. A plot of the current through the channel versus the potential difference across the membrane reveals that the current is linearly related to the voltage; in other words, the channel behaves as an electrical resistor that follows Ohm's law ($i = V/R$ or $i = \gamma \times V$). (Data reproduced, with permission, from Olaf Andersen and Lyndon Providence.)

Box 5–1 Recording Current in Single Ion Channels: The Patch Clamp

The patch-clamp technique was developed in 1976 by Erwin Neher and Bert Sakmann to record current from single ion channels. It is a refinement of the original voltage clamp technique (see Box 7–1).

A small fire-polished glass micropipette with a tip diameter of approximately 1 μm is pressed against the membrane of a skeletal muscle fiber that has been treated with proteolytic enzymes to remove connective tissue from the muscle surface. The pipette is filled with a salt solution resembling that normally found in the extracellular fluid.

A metal electrode in contact with the electrolyte in the micropipette connects the pipette to a special electrical circuit that measures the current through channels in the membrane under the pipette tip (Figure 5–3A).

In 1980 Neher discovered that applying a small amount of suction to the patch pipette greatly increased the tightness of the seal between the pipette and the membrane. The result was a seal with extremely high resistance between the inside and the outside of the pipette. The seal lowered the electronic noise and extended the usefulness of the patch-clamp technique to the whole range of channels involved in electrical excitability, including those with small conductances.

Since this discovery Neher and Sakmann, and many others, have used the patch-clamp technique to study all three major classes of ion channels—voltage-gated, ligand-gated, and mechanically gated—in a variety of neurons and other cells (Figure 5–3B).

Christopher Miller independently developed a method for incorporating channels from biological membranes into artificial lipid bilayers. Biological membranes are first homogenized in a laboratory blender; centrifugation of the homogenate then separates out a portion composed only of membrane vesicles. Under appropriate ionic conditions these membrane vesicles will fuse with a planar lipid membrane, incorporating any ion channel in the vesicle into the planar membrane.

This technique has two experimental advantages. First, it allows recording from ion channels in regions of cells that are inaccessible to patch clamp; for example, Miller has successfully studied a K^+ channel isolated from the internal membrane of skeletal muscle (the sarcoplasmic reticulum). Second, it allows researchers to study how the composition of the membrane lipids influences channel function.

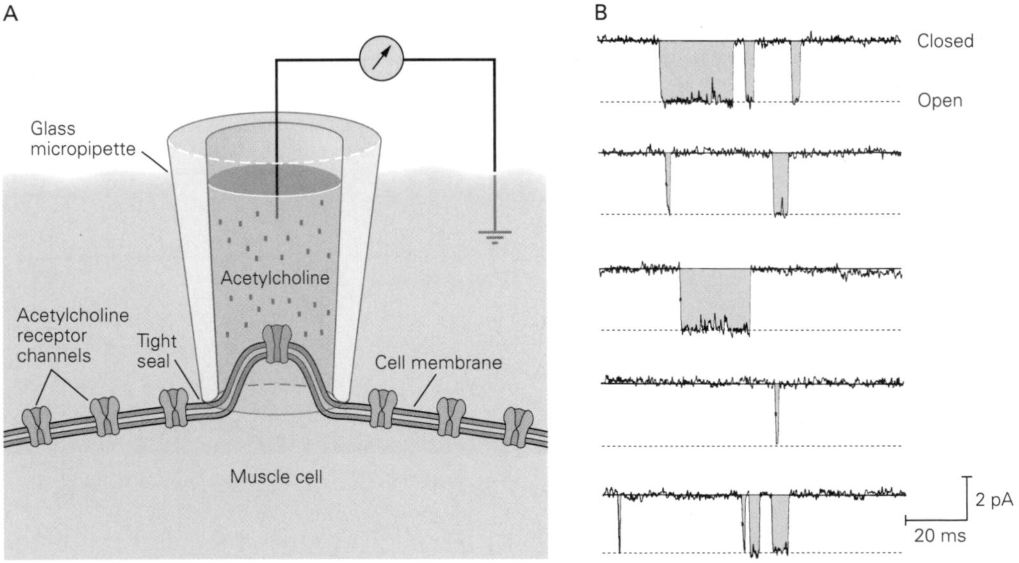

Figure 5–3 Patch-clamp setup and recording.

A. A pipette containing a low concentration of acetylcholine (ACh) in saline solution is used to record current through ACh receptor channels in skeletal muscle. (Adapted, with permission, from Alberts et al. 1994.)

B. Patch-clamp recording of the current through a single ACh receptor channel as the channel switches between closed and open states. (Reproduced, with permission, from B. Sakmann.)

neurotransmitter that activates the ACh receptors in the membrane of skeletal muscle—was pressed tightly against a frog muscle membrane. Small unitary current pulses representing the opening and closing of a single ACh receptor channel were recorded from the area of the membrane under the pipette tip. As with gramicidin A channels, the relation between current and voltage in the ACh receptor channel is linear (Figure 5–2), with a single-channel conductance of approximately 25 pS. This generates a unitary current of 2 pA (picoamperes) at a membrane potential of –80 mV (millivolts), which corresponds to a flux of around 12.5 million ions per second.

Ion Channels in All Cells Share Several Characteristics

Most cells are capable of local signaling, but only nerve and muscle cells are specialized for rapid signaling over long distances. Although nerve and muscle cells have a particularly rich variety and high density of membrane ion channels, their channels do not differ fundamentally from those of other cells in the body. In this section we describe the general properties of ion channels found in a wide variety of cells.

The Flux of Ions Through a Channel Is Passive

The flux of ions through ion channels is passive, requiring no expenditure of metabolic energy by the channels. The direction and eventual equilibrium for this flux are determined not by the channel itself, but rather by the electrostatic and diffusional driving forces across the membrane.

Ion channels allow particular types of ions to cross the membrane, selecting either cations or anions to permeate. Some types of cation-selective channels allow the cations that are usually present in extracellular fluid—Na^+, K^+, Ca^{2+}, and Mg^{2+}—to pass almost indiscriminately. However, many other cation-selective channels are permeable primarily to a single type of ion, whether it is Na^+, K^+, or Ca^{2+}. Most types of anion-selective channels are also highly discriminating; they conduct only one physiological ion, chloride (Cl^-).

The kinetic properties of ion permeation are best described by the channel's conductance, which is determined by measuring the current (ion flux) through the open channel in response to an electrochemical driving force. The net electrochemical driving force is determined by two factors: the electrical potential difference across the membrane and the concentration gradients of the permeant ions across the membrane. Changing either one can change the net driving force (see Chapter 6).

As we have seen, in some open channels the current varies linearly with driving force—that is, the channels behave as simple resistors. In others the current is a nonlinear function of driving force. This type of channel behaves as a rectifier—it conducts ions more readily in one direction than in the other because of asymmetry in the channel's structure or environment. Whereas the conductance of a resistor-like channel is constant—it is the same at all voltages—the conductance of a rectifying channel is variable and must be determined by plotting current versus voltage over the entire physiological range of membrane potential (Figure 5–4).

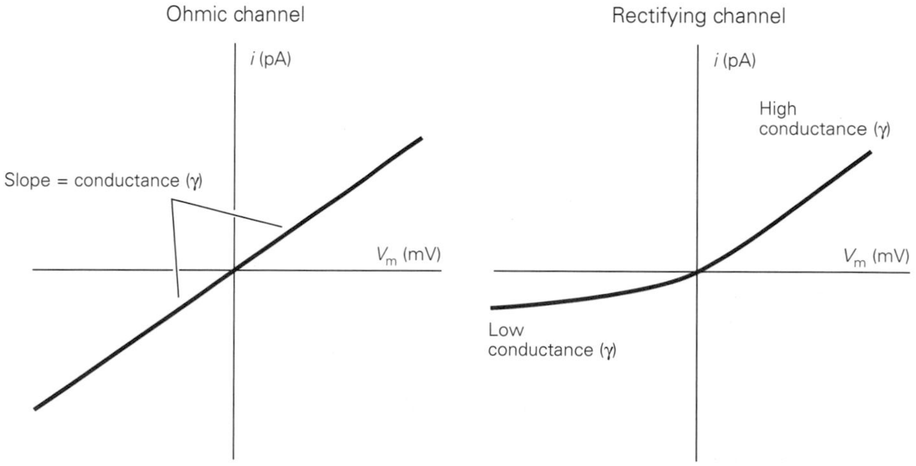

Figure 5–4 Current–voltage relations. In many ion channels the relation between current through the open channel and membrane voltage is linear (left plot). Such channels are said to be "ohmic" because they follow Ohm's law, $i = V_m/R$ or $V_m \times \gamma$, where γ is conductance. In other channels the relation between current and membrane potential is nonlinear. This kind of channel is said to "rectify," in the sense that it conducts current more readily in one direction than the other. The right plot shows an outwardly rectifying channel where positive current is larger than the negative current for a given absolute value of voltage.

The rate of net ion flux (current) through a channel depends on the concentration of the permeant ions in the surrounding solution. At low concentrations the current increases almost linearly with concentration. At higher concentrations the current tends to reach a point at which it no longer increases. At this point the current is said to *saturate*.

This saturation effect is consistent with the idea that ion flux across the cell membrane is not strictly a function of laws of electrochemical diffusion in free solution but also involves the binding of ions to specific polar sites within the pore of the channel. A simple electrodiffusion model would predict that the ionic current should continue to increase as long as the ionic concentration also increases; that is, the more charge carriers in solution, the greater the current.

The relation between current and ionic concentration for a wide range of ion channels is well described by a simple chemical binding equation, identical to the Michaelis-Menten equation for enzymes, suggesting that a single ion binds within the channel during permeation. The ionic concentration at which current reaches half its maximum defines the *dissociation constant*, the concentration at which half of the channels will be occupied by a bound ion. The dissociation constant in plots of current versus concentration is typically quite high, approximately 100 mM, indicating weak binding. (In typical interactions between enzymes and substrates the dissociation constant is below 1 μM.) This weak interaction indicates that the bonds between the ion and the channel are rapidly formed and broken. In fact, an ion typically stays bound in the channel for less than 1 μs. The rapid rate at which an ion unbinds is necessary for the channel to achieve the very high conduction rates responsible for the rapid changes in membrane potential during signaling.

Some ion channels are susceptible to occlusion by certain free ions or molecules in the cytoplasm or extracellular fluid. Passage through the channel can be blocked by particles that bind either to the mouth of the aqueous pore or somewhere within the pore. If the blocker is an ionized molecule that binds to a site within the pore, it will be influenced by the membrane electric field as it enters the channel. For example, if a positively charged blocker enters the channel from outside the membrane, then making the cytoplasmic side of the membrane more negative—which, according to convention, corresponds to a more negative membrane potential (see Chapter 6)—will drive the blocker into the channel through an electrostatic attraction, increasing the block. Although blockers are often toxins or drugs that originate outside the body, some are common ions that are normally present in the cell or its environment. Physiological blockers of certain classes of channels include Mg^{2+}, Ca^{2+}, Na^{+}, and polyamines such as spermine.

The Opening and Closing of a Channel Involve Conformational Changes

In all ion channels so far studied the channel protein has two or more conformational states that are relatively stable. Each of these stable conformations represents a different functional state. For example, each ion channel has at least one open state and one or two closed states. The transition of a channel between these different states is called *gating*.

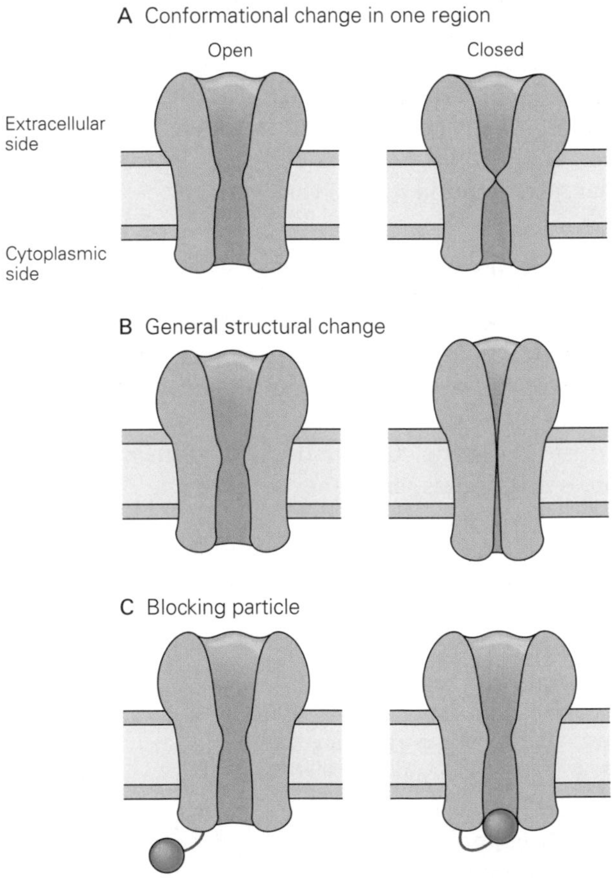

Figure 5–5 Three physical models for the opening and closing of ion channels.

A. A localized conformational change occurs in one region of the channel.

B. A generalized structural change occurs along the length of the channel.

C. A blocking particle swings into and out of the channel mouth.

Relatively little is known about the molecular mechanisms of gating. Although the picture of a gate swinging open and shut is a convenient image, it probably is accurate only for certain cases (for example the inactivation of Na^+ and K^+ channels, which we describe in Chapter 7). More commonly, channel gating involves widespread changes in the channel's conformation. For example, evidence from high-resolution electron microscopy and image analysis suggests that the opening and closing of gap junction channels (which we consider in Chapter 8) involve a concerted twisting and tilting of the six subunits that make up the channel. Similar evidence indicates that ACh receptor channels open through a coordinated twisting and bending of the α-helixes of each of the five subunits that form the channel pore. In K^+ channels movement of a ring of α-helixes that forms the internal mouth of the pore is thought to act as a gate. The molecular rearrangements that occur during the transition from closed to open states appear to enhance ion conduction through the channel not only by creating a wider lumen, but also by positioning relatively more polar amino acid constituents at the surface that lines the aqueous pore.

The primary function of ion channels in neurons is to generate transient electrical signals, and three major gating mechanisms have evolved to control channel opening (Figure 5–5). Certain channels are opened by the binding of chemical ligands, known as agonists. Some ligands bind directly to the channel either at an extracellular or intracellular site; transmitters bind at extracellular sites whereas certain cytoplasmic constituents, such as Ca^{2+}, cyclic nucleotides and GTP-binding proteins, bind at intracellular sites. Other ligands activate cellular signaling cascades, which can covalently modify a channel through protein phosphorylation. Other ion channels are regulated by changes in membrane potential. Some voltage-gated channels act as temperature sensors; changes in temperature shift their voltage gating to higher or lower membrane potentials, giving rise to heat- or cold-sensitive channels. Finally, some channels are regulated by mechanical stretch of the membrane (Figure 5–6).

The rapid gating actions necessary for moment-to-moment signaling may also be influenced by certain long-term changes in the metabolic state of the cell. For example, the gating of some K^+ channels is sensitive to intracellular levels of ATP. Some channel proteins contain a subunit with an integral oxidoreductase catalytic domain that is thought to alter channel gating in response to the redox state of the cell.

These regulators control the entry of a channel into one of three functional states: closed and activatable

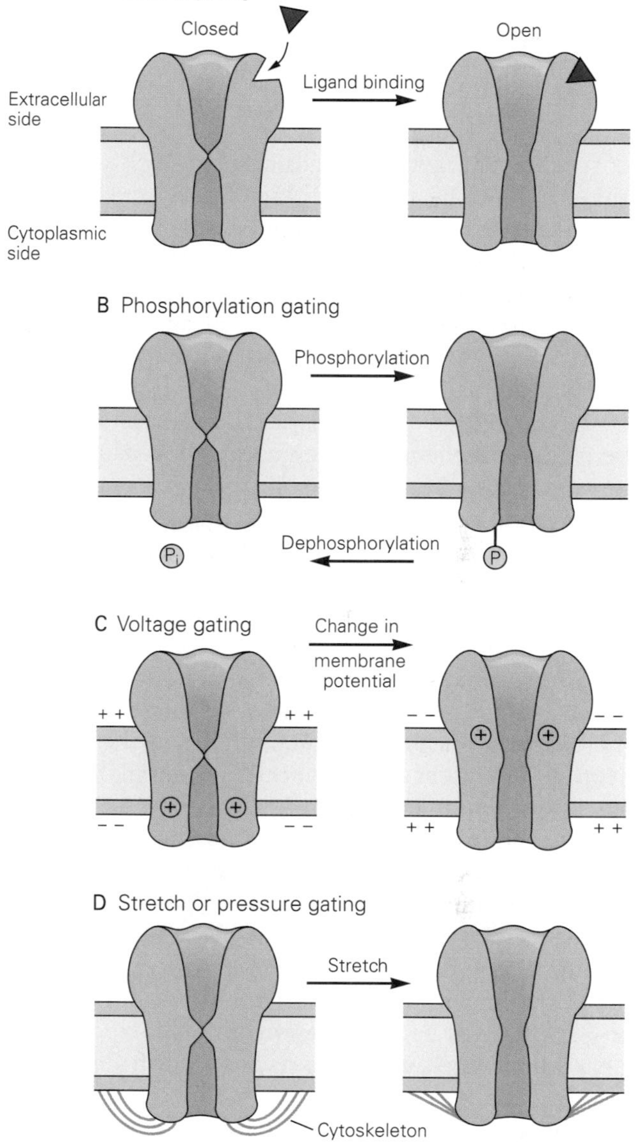

Figure 5–6 Several types of stimuli control the opening and closing of ion channels.

A. A ligand-gated channel opens when a ligand binds a receptor site on the external surface of the channel protein. The energy from ligand binding drives the channel toward an open state.

B. Some channels are regulated by protein phosphorylation and dephosphorylation. The energy for channel opening comes from the transfer of the high-energy phosphate, P_i.

C. Voltage-gated channels open and close with changes in the electrical potential difference across the membrane. The change in membrane potential causes a local conformational change by acting on a region of the channel that has a net charge.

D. Some channels open and close through stretch or pressure. The energy for gating may come from mechanical forces that are passed to the channel through the cytoskeleton.

(resting), open (active), or closed and nonactivatable (refractory). A change in the functional state of a channel requires energy. In voltage-gated channels the energy is provided by the movement of a charged region of the channel protein through the membrane's electric field. This region, the *voltage sensor*, contains a net electric charge because of the presence of basic (positively charged) or acidic (negatively charged) amino acids. The movement of the charged voltage sensor through the electric field imparts a change in free energy to the channel that alters the equilibrium between the closed and open states of the channel. For most voltage-gated channels, channel opening is favored by making the inside of the membrane more positive (depolarization).

In transmitter-gated channels gating is driven by the change in chemical-free energy that results when the transmitter binds to a receptor site on the channel protein. For mechanically activated channels the energy associated with membrane stretch is thought to be transferred to the channel either through the cytoskeleton or more directly by changes in tension of the lipid bilayer.

The stimuli that gate the channel also control the rates of transition between the open and closed states of a channel. For voltage-gated channels the rates are steeply dependent on membrane potential. Although the time scale can vary from several microseconds to a minute, the transition tends to require a few milliseconds on average. Thus, once a channel opens it stays open for a few milliseconds before closing, and after closing it stays closed for a few milliseconds before reopening. Once the transition between open and closed states begins, it proceeds virtually instantaneously (in less than 10 μs, the present limit of experimental measurements), thus giving rise to abrupt, all-or-none, step-like changes in current through the channel.

Ligand-gated and voltage-gated channels enter refractory states through different processes. Ligand-gated channels can enter the refractory state when their exposure to the agonist is prolonged. This process, called *desensitization,* is discussed in Chapter 11. The mechanisms underlying desensitization of ion channels are not yet completely understood. In some channels desensitization appears to be an intrinsic property of the interaction between ligand and channel, although in others it is a result of phosphorylation of the channel molecule by a protein kinase.

Many, but not all, voltage-gated channels enter a refractory state after opening, a process termed *inactivation*. In the inactive state the channel is closed and can no longer be opened by positive voltages. Rather, the membrane potential must be returned to its initial negative resting level before the channel can recover from inactivation so that it can again open in response to depolarization. In voltage-gated Na^+ and K^+ channels inactivation is thought to result from a conformational change, controlled by a subunit or region of the channel separate from that which controls activation. In contrast, the inactivation of certain voltage-gated Ca^{2+} channels is thought to require Ca^{2+} influx. An increase in internal Ca^{2+} concentration inactivates the Ca^{2+} channel by binding to the regulatory molecule calmodulin, which is permanently associated with the Ca^{2+} channel protein (Figure 5–7).

Exogenous factors, such as drugs and toxins, can also affect the gating control sites of an ion channel. Most of these agents tend to close the channel but a few open it. Some bind to the same site at which the endogenous agonist normally binds and thereby interfere with normal gating. The binding can be weak and reversible, as in the blockade of the nicotinic ACh-gated channel in skeletal muscle by curare, a South American arrow poison (see Chapter 9). Or it can be strong and irreversible, as in the blockade of the same channel by the snake venom α-bungarotoxin.

Some exogenous substances act in a noncompetitive manner and affect the normal gating mechanism without directly interacting with the transmitter-binding site. For example, binding of the drug diazepam (Valium) to a regulatory site on Cl^- channels that are gated by γ-aminobutyric acid (GABA), an inhibitory neurotransmitter, prolongs the opening of the channels in response to GABA (Figure 5–8). This type of indirect, allosteric effect is found in voltage- or stretch-gated channels as well.

The Structure of Ion Channels Is Inferred from Biophysical, Biochemical, and Molecular Biological Studies

What do ion channels look like? How does the channel protein span the membrane? What happens to the structure of the channel when it opens and closes? Where along the length of the channel protein do drugs and transmitters bind?

Biochemical and molecular biological studies have provided a basic understanding of channel structure and function. All ion channels are large integral-membrane proteins with a core transmembrane domain that contains a central aqueous pore spanning the entire width of the membrane. The channel protein often contains carbohydrate groups attached to its external surface. The pore-forming region of many channels is made up of two or more subunits, which may be identical or different.

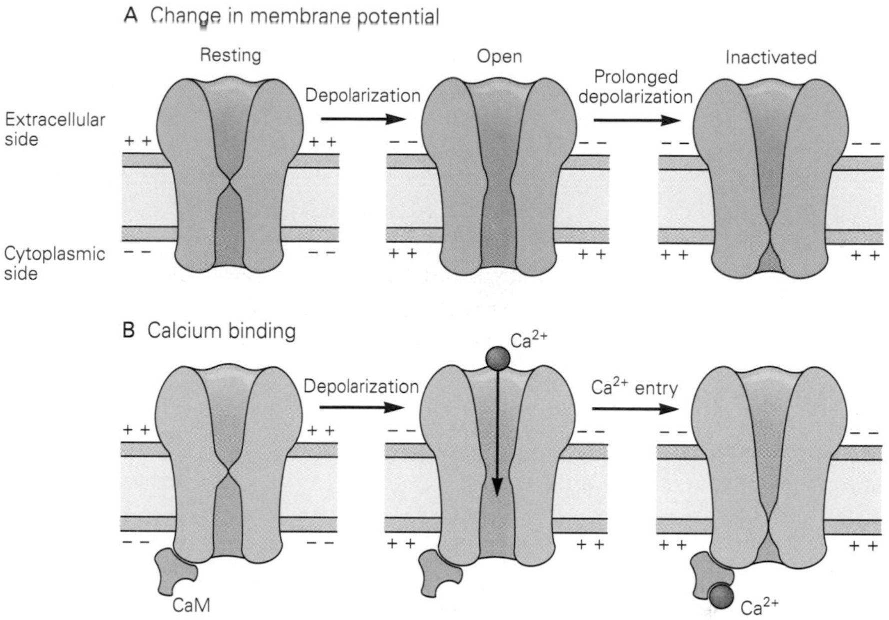

Figure 5–7 Voltage-gated channels are inactivated by two mechanisms.

A. Many voltage-gated channels enter a refractory (inactivated) state after briefly opening when the membrane is depolarized. They recover from the refractory state and return to the resting state only after the membrane potential is restored to its resting value.

B. Some voltage-dependent Ca^{2+} channels inactivate when the internal Ca^{2+} level increases following channel opening. The internal Ca^{2+} binds to calmodulin (CaM), a specific regulatory protein associated with the channel.

In addition, some channels have auxiliary subunits that modify their functional properties. These subunits may be cytoplasmic or embedded in the membrane (Figure 5–9).

The genes for all the major classes of ion channels have been cloned and sequenced. The amino acid sequence of a channel, inferred from its DNA sequence, can be used to create a structural model of the channel protein. Regions of secondary structure—the arrangement of the amino acid residues into α-helixes and β-sheets—as well as regions that are likely to correspond to membrane-spanning domains

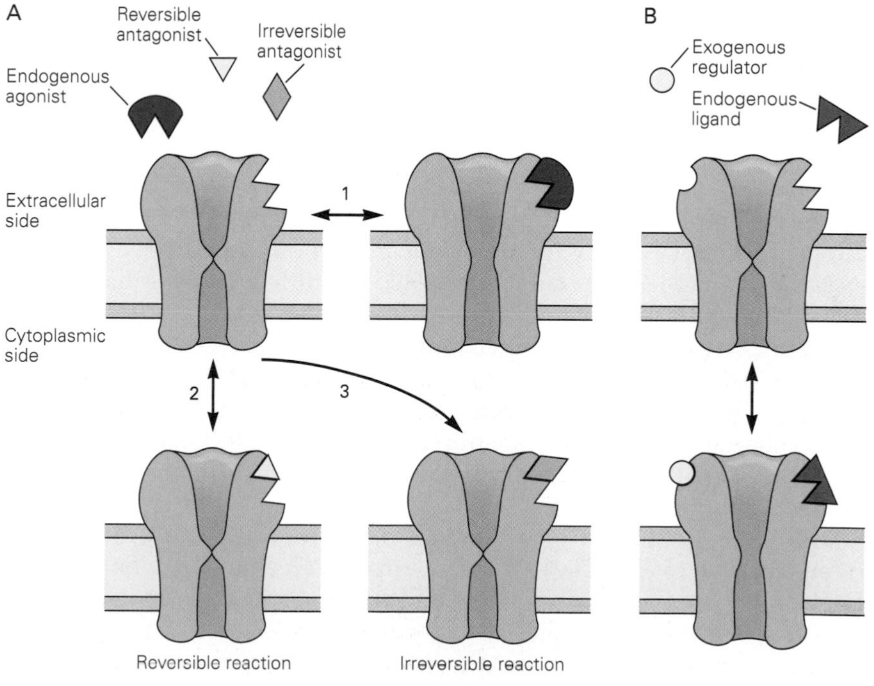

Figure 5–8 Exogenous ligands, such as drugs, can bias an ion channel toward an open or closed state.

A. In channels that are normally opened by the binding of an endogenous ligand (**1**), a drug or toxin may block the binding of the agonist by means of a reversible (**2**) or irreversible (**3**) reaction.

B. Some exogenous agents can bias a channel toward the open state by binding to a regulatory site, distinct from the ligand-binding site that normally opens the channel.

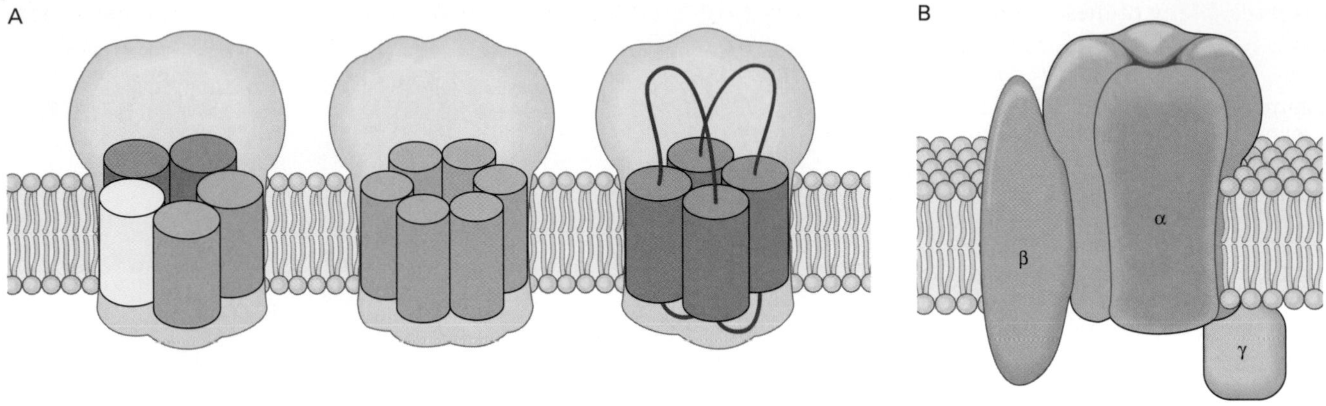

Figure 5–9 Ion channels are integral membrane proteins composed of several subunits.

A. Ion channels can be constructed as hetero-oligomers from distinct subunits (**left**), as homo-oligomers from a single type of subunit (**middle**), or from a single polypeptide chain organized into repeating motifs, where each motif functions as the equivalent of one subunit (**right**).

B. In addition to one or more α-subunits that form a central pore, some channels contain auxiliary subunits (β or γ) that modulate the gating of the pore.

of the channel are predicted based on the structures of related proteins that have been experimentally determined using electron and X-ray diffraction analysis. This type of analysis identified the presence of four hydrophobic regions, each around 20 amino acids in length, in the amino acid sequence of a subunit of the ACh receptor channel. Each of these regions is thought to form an α-helix that spans the membrane (Figure 5–10).

Additional insights into channel structure and function have been obtained by comparing the amino acid sequences of the same type of channel from different species. Regions that show a high degree of similarity (that is, have been highly conserved through evolution) are likely to be important in maintaining the structure and function of the channel. Likewise, conserved regions in different but related channels are likely to serve a common biophysical function. For example, voltage-gated channels selective for different cations have a specific membrane-spanning segment that contains positively charged amino acids (lysine or arginine) spaced at every third position along an α-helix. This motif is observed in all voltage-gated cation channels, but not in transmitter-gated channels, suggesting that this charged region is important for voltage gating (see Chapter 7).

Once a structure for a channel has been proposed, it can be tested in several ways. For example, antibodies can be raised against synthetic peptides that correspond to different hydrophilic regions in the protein sequence. Immunocytochemistry can then be used to determine whether the antibody binds to the extracellular or cytoplasmic surface of the membrane, thus defining whether a particular region of the channel is extracellular or intracellular.

The functional consequences of changes in a channel's primary amino acid sequence can be explored through a variety of techniques. One particularly versatile approach is to use genetic engineering to construct channels with parts that are derived from the genes of different species—so-called *chimeric channels*. This technique takes advantage of the fact that the same type of channel can have somewhat different properties in different species. For example, the bovine ACh receptor channel has a slightly greater single-channel conductance than the ACh receptor channel in electric fish. By comparing the properties of a chimeric channel to those of the two original channels, one can assess the functions of specific regions of the channel. This technique has been used to identify the membrane-spanning segment that forms the lining of the pore of the ACh receptor channel (see Chapter 9).

The roles of different amino acid residues or stretches of residues can be tested using site-directed mutagenesis, a type of genetic engineering in which specific amino acid residues are substituted or deleted. Finally, one can exploit the naturally occurring mutations in channel genes. A number of inherited and spontaneous mutations in the genes that encode ion channels in nerve or muscle produce changes in channel function that can underlie certain neurological diseases. Many of these mutations are caused by localized changes in single amino acids within channel proteins, demonstrating the importance of that region for channel function.

Ion Channels Can Be Grouped into Gene Families

The great diversity of ion channels in a multicellular organism is underscored by the recent sequencing of the human genome. Our genome contains nine genes encoding variants of voltage-gated Na^+ channels, 10 genes for different Ca^+ channels, over 75 genes for K^+ channels, 70 genes for ligand-gated channels, and more than a dozen genes for Cl^- channels. Fortunately, the evolutionary relationships between the genes that encode ion channels provide a relatively simple framework with which to categorize them.

Most of the ion channels that have been described in nerve and muscle cells fall into a few gene superfamilies. Members of each gene superfamily have similar amino acid sequences and transmembrane topology and, importantly, related functions. Each superfamily is thought to have evolved from a common ancestral gene by gene duplication and divergence. Several superfamilies can be further classified into families of genes with more closely related structure and function.

One superfamily encodes ligand-gated ion channels that are receptors for the neurotransmitters ACh, GABA, glycine, or serotonin. All of these receptors are composed of five subunits, each of which has four

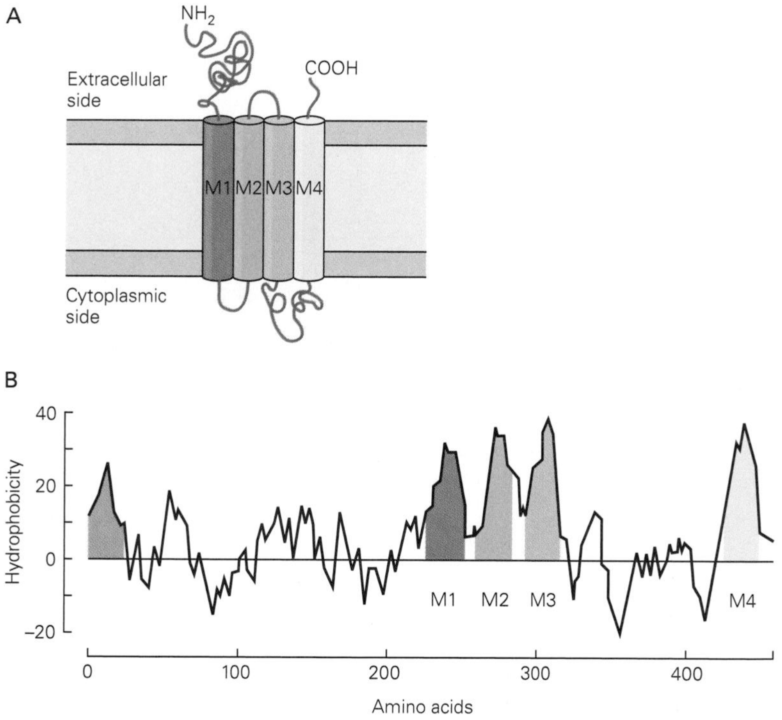

Figure 5–10 The secondary structure of membrane-spanning proteins.

A. A proposed secondary structure for a subunit of the nicotinic acetylcholine (ACh) receptor channel present in skeletal muscle. Each cylinder (**M1–M4**) represents a putative membrane-spanning α-helix comprised of approximately 20 hydrophobic amino acid residues. The membrane segments are connected by cytoplasmic or extracellular segments (**loops**) of hydrophilic residues. The amino terminus (**NH_2**) and carboxy terminus (**COOH**) of the protein lie on the extracellular side of the membrane.

B. The membrane-spanning regions of an ion channel protein can be identified using a hydrophobicity plot. Here a running average of hydrophobicity is plotted for the entire amino acid sequence of the α-subunit of the nicotinic ACh receptor. Each point in the plot represents an average hydrophobic index of a sequence of 19 amino acids and corresponds to the midpoint of the sequence. The amino acid sequence of the subunit is inferred from the nucleotide sequence of the cloned receptor subunit gene. Four of the hydrophobic regions (M1–M4) correspond to the membrane-spanning segments. The hydrophobic region at the far left in the plot is the signal sequence that positions the hydrophilic amino terminus of the protein on the extracellular surface of the cell during protein synthesis. The signal sequence is cleaved from the mature protein. (Reproduced, with permission, from Schofield et al. 1987.)

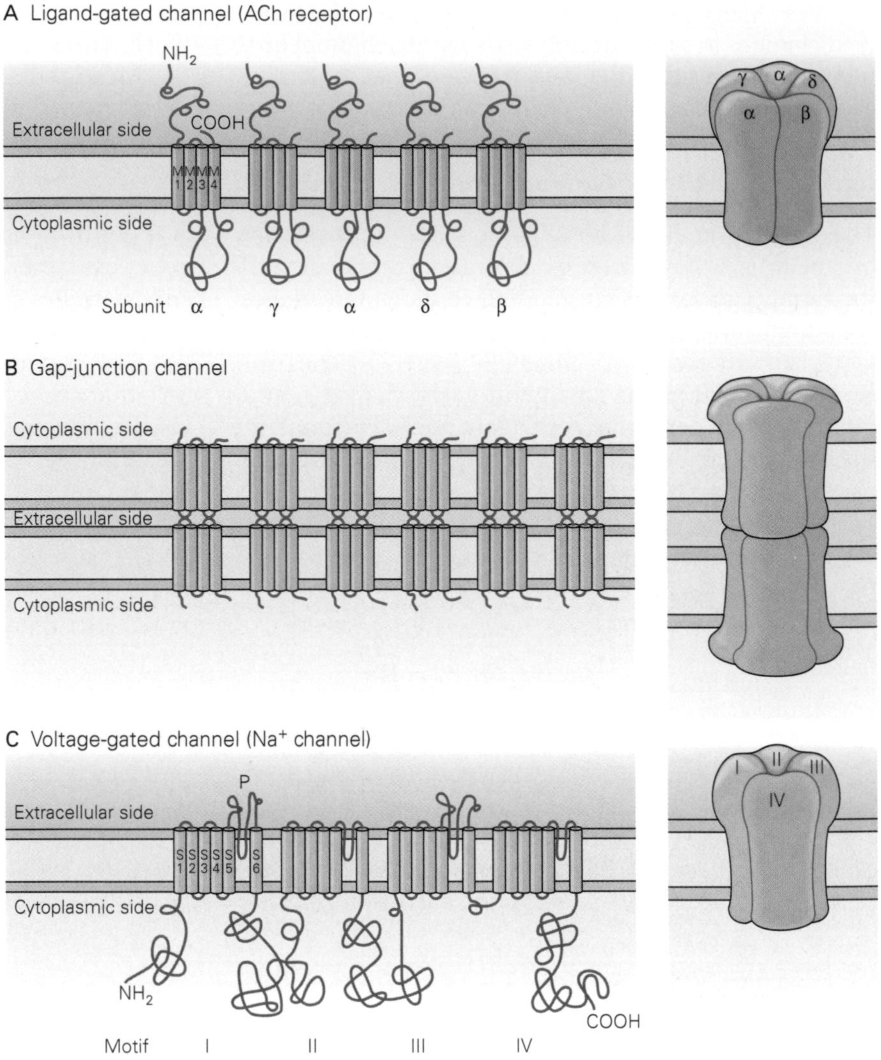

Figure 5–11 Three superfamilies of ion channels.

A. Members of a large family of ligand-gated channels, such as the acetylcholine receptor channel, have five closely related subunits, each of which contains four transmembrane α-helixes (**M1–M4**). Each cylinder in the figure represents a single transmembrane α-helix.

B. The gap-junction channel is formed from a pair of hemichannels, one each in the pre- and postsynaptic cell membranes that join in the space between two cells. Each hemichannel is made of six identical subunits, each containing four transmembrane α-helixes. Gap-junction channels serve as conduits between the cytoplasm of the pre- and postsynaptic cells at electrical synapses (see Chapter 8).

C. The voltage-gated Na^+ channel is formed from a single polypeptide chain that contains four homologous domains or repeats (**motifs I–IV**), each with six membrane-spanning α-helixes (**S1–S6**). The S5 and S6 segments are connected by an extended strand of amino acids, the P-region, which dips into and out of the external surface of the membrane to form the selectivity filter of the pore.

transmembrane α-helixes (Figure 5–11A). In addition, the extracellular domain that forms the receptor for the ligand contains a conserved loop of 13 amino acids flanked by pair of cysteine residues that form a disulfide bond. As a result, this receptor superfamily is referred to as the cys-loop receptors. Ligand-gated channels can be classified by their ion selectivity in addition to their agonist. The genes that encode glutamate receptor channels belong to a separate gene family.

Gap-junction channels, which bridge the cytoplasm of two cells at electrical synapses (see Chapter 8), are encoded by a separate gene superfamily. A gap-junction channel is composed of 12 identical subunits, each of which has four membrane-spanning segments (Figure 5–11B).

The genes that encode the voltage-gated ion channels responsible for generating the action potential belong to another family. These channels are usually activated by membrane depolarization and are selective for Ca^{2+}, Na^+, or K^+. All voltage-gated channels have a similar architecture, with a core motif composed of six transmembrane segments termed S1–S6 (Figure 5–11C). The S5 and S6 segments are connected by a highly conserved P-region, which loops into and out of the extracellular face of the membrane and forms the selectivity filter of the channel. Voltage-gated Na^+ and Ca^{2+} channels are composed of a large subunit that contains four repeats of this basic motif. Voltage-gated K^+ channels are composed of four separate subunits, each containing one motif. This structure is shared by other, more distantly related channel families (see Chapter 7).

The major gene family encoding the voltage-gated K^+ channels is distantly related to two families of K^+ channels, each with distinctive properties and structure (Figure 5–12). One family consists of the genes encoding inward-rectifying K^+ channels, which are open at the resting potential and close rapidly during depolarization. Each channel subunit has only two transmembrane segments connected by a pore-forming P-region. A second family is composed of subunits with two repeated pore-forming segments. These channels may also contribute to the resting K^+ conductance.

The sequencing of the genomes of a variety of species has led to the identification of additional ion channel gene families, found in organisms from bacteria to humans. Channels with related P-regions have been identified that are only very distantly related to the family of voltage-gated channels. These channels include the glutamate-gated channels, in which the P-region is inverted: It enters and leaves the internal surface of the membrane (see Figure 5–12D). Finally, the transient receptor potential (TRP) family of nonselective cation channels (named after a mutant *Drosophila* strain in which light evokes an abnormal transient receptor potential in photoreceptors) comprises a very large group of channels that contain a P-region. Like the voltage-gated K^+ channels, TRP channels also contain six transmembrane segments but are usually gated by intracellular ligands. TRP channels are important for Ca^{2+} metabolism in all cells, visual signaling in insects, and pain, heat, and cold sensation in the nervous system of higher animals. Recent evidence implicates TRP channels in mechanosensation and hearing in insects and fish and in certain taste sensations in mammals.

A number of other families of channels have been identified, distinct from those considered above. These include Cl^- channels that help set the resting potential of certain nerve and skeletal muscle cells, and a class of ligand-gated cation channels activated by ATP, which functions as a neurotransmitter at certain synapses.

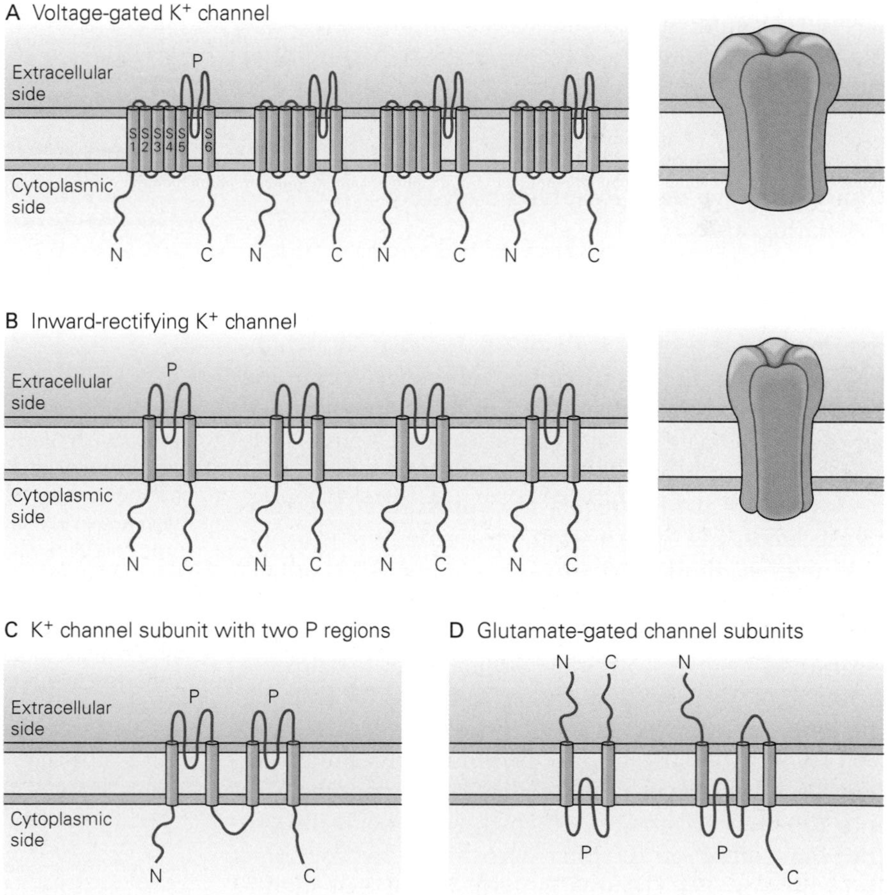

Figure 5–12 Four related families of ion channels with P-regions

A. Voltage-gated K^+ channels are composed of four subunits. Each K^+ channel subunit corresponds to one repeated domain of a voltage-gated Na^+ channel, with six transmembrane segments and a pore-forming P-region.

B. Inward-rectifying K^+ channels are composed of four subunits, each of which has only two transmembrane segments connected by a P-region.

C. A third type of K^+ channel is composed of subunits that contain two repeats of the inward-rectifying K^+ channel subunit, with each repeat containing a P-region. Two of these subunits are presumed to form a channel with four P-regions.

D. Glutamate receptor channels form a distinct P-region channel family. In these receptors the amino terminus is extracellular and the P-region enters and exits the cytoplasmic side of the membrane. The bacterial GluR0 subunit contains two transmembrane segments (**left**). In higher organisms the subunits contain a third transmembrane segment (**right**).

With the completion of the human genome project, it is likely that nearly all of the major classes of ion channel genes have now been identified.

However, the diversity of ion channels is even greater than the large number of ion channel genes. Because most channels in a given subfamily are composed of multiple subunits, each of which may be encoded by a family of closely related genes, combinatorial permutations of these subunits can generate a diverse array of heteromultimeric channels with different functional properties. Further diversity can be produced by alternative splicing of precursor mRNA transcribed from a single gene. Finally, the sequence of a transcript can be altered by a process termed RNA editing. As with enzyme isoforms, variants of a channel with slightly different properties may be expressed at distinct stages of development (Figure 5–13), in different cell types throughout the brain (Figure 5–14), and even in different regions within a cell. These subtle variations in structure and function presumably allow channels to perform highly specific functions.

The rich variety of ion channels in different types of neurons may make it possible to develop drugs that can activate or block channels in selected regions of the nervous system. Such drugs would, in principle, have maximum therapeutic effectiveness with minimum side effects.

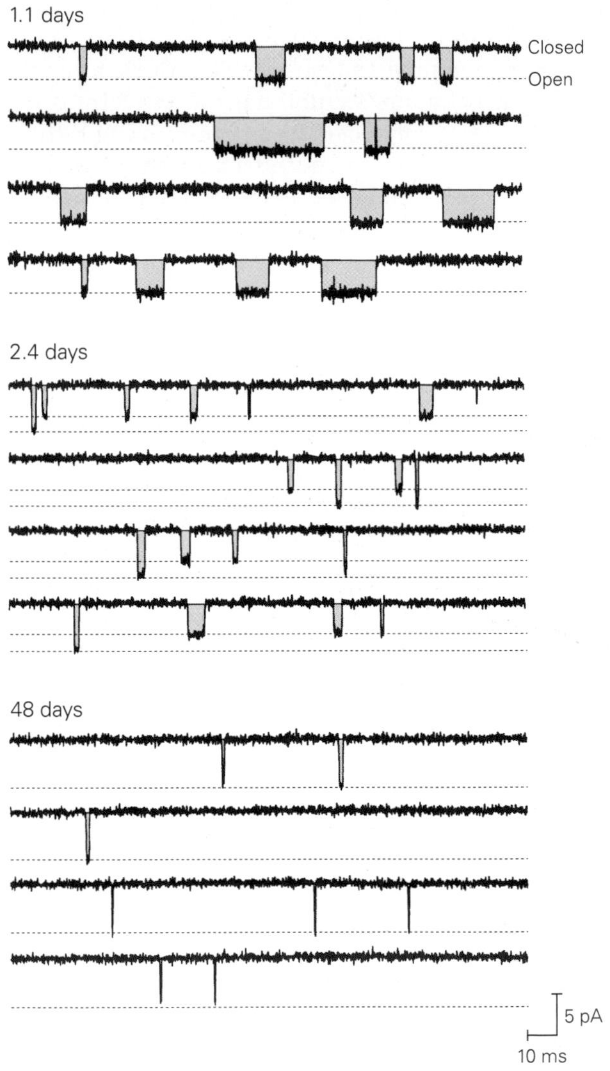

Figure 5–13 Variants of an ion channel gene can be expressed at different points in development to fine tune channel properties. These examples of currents through individual acetylcholine receptor channels were recorded from frog skeletal muscle at three stages of development: early (1.1 days), intermediate (2.4 days), and late (48 days). In immature muscle the single channels have a relatively small conductance and a relatively long open time. In mature muscle the channel conductance is larger and the average open time is shorter. At intermediate stages of development the population of channel variants is mixed; both brief, large-conductance channel openings and longer-lasting, small-conductance channel openings are evident. This functional difference results from a developmental switch in subunit composition caused by a change in gene expression. Both immature and mature forms of the receptor have α-, β-, and δ-subunits. However, the γ-subunit expressed early in development is replaced by the ε-subunit as the animal matures. (Reproduced, with permission, from Owens and Kullberg 1989.)

The Closed and Open Structures of Potassium Channels Have Been Resolved by X-Ray Crystallography

Rod MacKinnon and his colleagues provided the first high-resolution X-ray crystallographic analysis of the molecular architecture of an ion-selective channel. To overcome the difficulties inherent in obtaining crystals of integral membrane proteins, they initially focused on a bacterial K^+ channel, termed KcsA. These channels were useful for crystallography as they can be expressed at high levels for purification, are relatively small, and have a simple transmembrane topology that is similar to inward-rectifier K^+ channels present in higher organisms, including mammals (see Figure 5–12B). The structure of the channel was further simplified using molecular engineering to truncate cytoplasmic regions that are not essential for forming the ion-selective pore.

The crystal structure determined from the modified KcsA protein provides several important insights into the mechanisms by which the channel facilitates the movement of K^+ ions across the hydrophobic lipid bilayer. The channel is made up of four identical subunits arranged symmetrically around a central

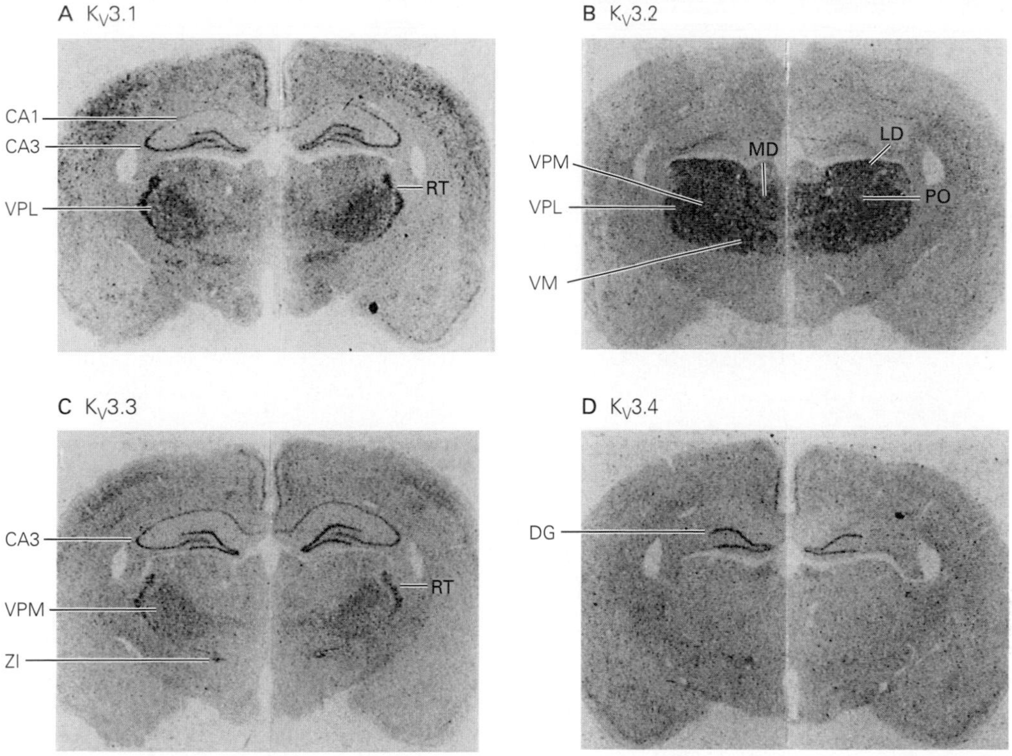

Figure 5–14 Variants of a potassium channel are expressed in different regions of the brain. Autoradiograms show the expression patterns of mRNA transcripts of the four genes comprising the K_V3 subfamily of voltage-gated K^+ channel subunits (determined by in situ hybridization). In each autoradiogram the dark areas represent high densities of expression. The brain was sectioned at the level of the posterior thalamus. The thalamic nuclei shown are **VPL**, ventral posterior lateral; **VPM**, ventral posterior medial; **MD**, medial dorsal; **LD**, lateral dorsal; **VM**, ventromedial; **PO**, posterior; and **RT**, reticular. Hippocampal regions **CA1 and CA3; DG**, dentate gyrus; and **ZI**, zona incerta. (Reproduced, with permission, from Weiser et al. 1994.)

pore (Figure 5–15A). Each subunit has two membrane-spanning α-helixes, an inner and outer helix, that are connected by the P-loop, which forms the selectivity filter of the channel. At the extracellular end of the channel the two α-helixes tilt away from the central axis of the pore so that the structure resembles an inverted teepee.

The four inner α-helixes from each of the subunits line the cytoplasmic end of the pore. At the intracellular mouth of the channel these four helixes cross, forming a very narrow opening—the "smoke hole" of the teepee. The inner helixes are homologous to the S6 membrane-spanning segment of voltage-gated K^+ channels. At the extracellular end of the channel the pair of transmembrane helixes from each subunit are connected by a region consisting of three elements: (1) a chain of amino acids that surrounds the mouth of the channel (the turret region); (2) an abbreviated α-helix (the pore helix) approximately 10 amino acids in length that projects toward the central axis of the pore; and (3) a stretch of 5 amino acids near the C-terminal end of the P-region that forms the selectivity filter (Figure 5–15B).

The shape and structure of the pore determine its ion-conducting properties. Both the inner and outer mouths of the pore are lined by acidic amino acids with negative charges that help attract cations from the bulk solution. Going from inside to outside, the pore consists of a medium wide tunnel 18 Å in length that leads into a wider (10 Å diameter) spherical inner chamber (Figure 5–15D). This chamber is lined predominantly by the side chains of hydrophobic amino acids. These relatively wide regions are followed by the very narrow selectivity filter, only 12 Å in length, which is rate-limiting for the passage of ions. A high ion throughput rate is ensured by the fact that the inner 28 Å of the pore, from the cytoplasmic entrance to the selectivity filter, lacks polar groups that could delay ion passage by binding and unbinding the ion.

An ion passing from the polar solution through the nonpolar lipid bilayer encounters the least energetically

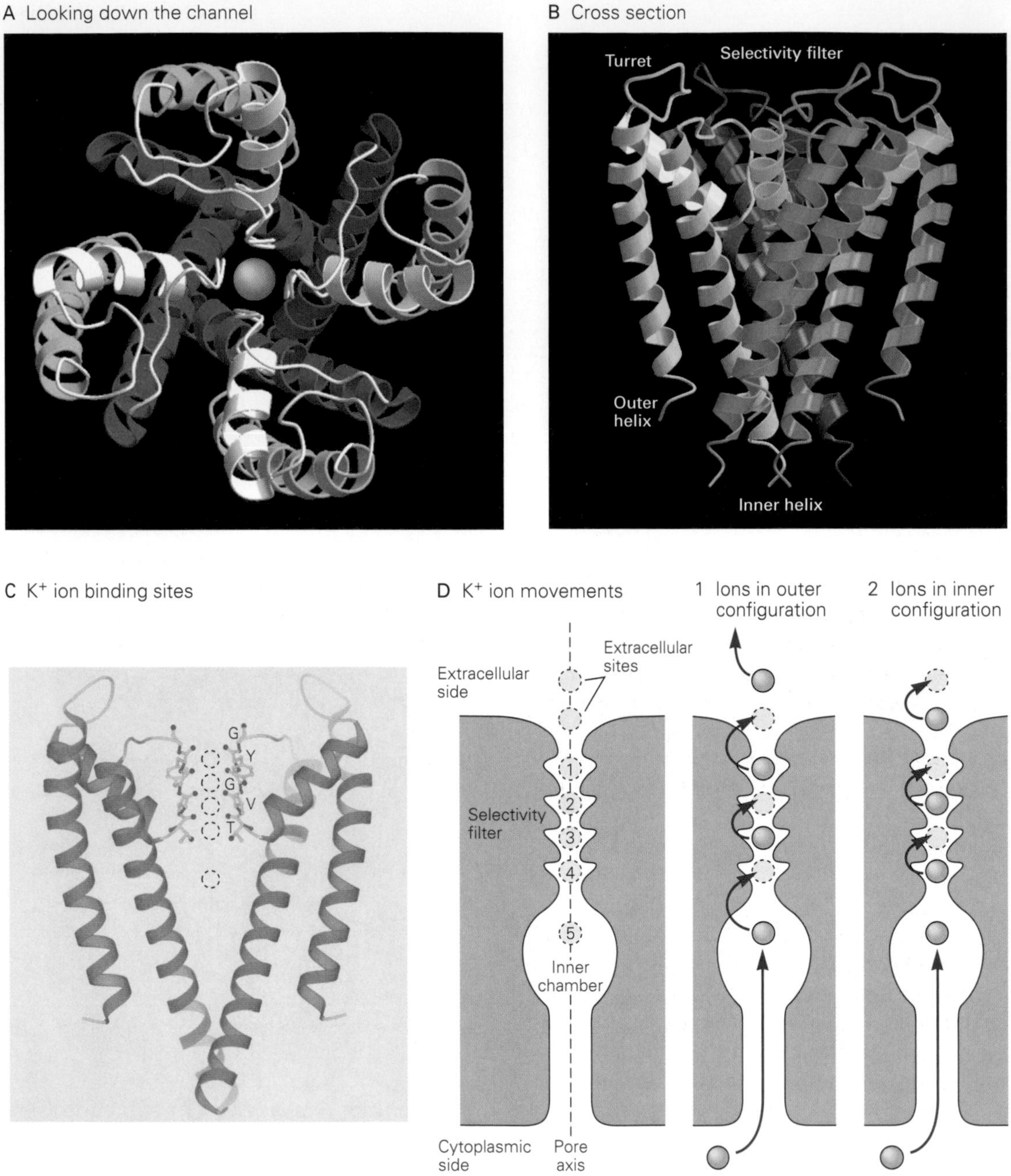

Figure 5–15 The X-ray crystal structure of a bacterial potassium channel. (Reproduced, with permission, from Doyle et al. 1998.)

A. Each of the four subunits of the K^+ channel KcsA contributes two membrane-spanning helixes, the outer helix (**blue**) and the inner helix (**red**). The P-region (**white**) lies near the extracellular surface of the channel pore and consists of a short α-helix (pore helix) and a loop that forms the selectivity filter of the channel. A K^+ ion is in the center of the pore. The view is looking down the channel from outside the cell.

B. The channel is seen in a cross section in the plane of the membrane. The four subunits are shown in different colors.

C. Another view in the same orientation as in part B shows only two of the four subunits. The channel contains five K^+ binding sites (**dashed**). Four of the sites lie in the selectivity filter (**yellow**) and the fifth site lies in an inner chamber near the center of the channel. The four K^+ binding sites of the selectivity filter are formed by successive rings of oxygen atoms (**red**) from five amino acid residues per subunit. Four of the rings are formed by carbonyl oxygen atoms from the main chain backbone of four consecutive amino acid residues—glycine (**G**), tyrosine (**Y**), glycine (**G**), and valine (**V**). A fifth ring of oxygen near the internal end of the selectivity filter is formed by the side-chain hydroxyl oxygen of threonine (**T**). Each ring contains four oxygen atoms, one from each subunit. Only the oxygen atoms from two of the four subunits are shown in this view. (Reproduced, with permission, from Zhou et al. 2001.)

D. A view of ion permeation through the channel illustrates the changes in occupancy of the various K^+ binding sites. A pair of ions hops in concert between a pair of binding sites in the selectivity filter. In the initial state, the "outer configuration," a pair of ions is bound to sites 1 and 3. As an ion enters the inner mouth of the channel, the ion in the inner chamber jumps to occupy the innermost binding site of the selectivity filter (site 4). This causes the pair of ions in the outer configuration to hop outward, expelling an ion from the channel. The two ions now in the inner configuration (sites 2 and 4) can hop to binding sites 1 and 3, returning the channel to its initial state (the outer configuration), from which it can conduct a second K^+ ion. (Adapted, with permission, from Miller 2001.)

favorable region in the middle of the bilayer. The high energetic cost for a K^+ ion to enter this region is minimized by two details of channel structure. The inner chamber is filled with water, which provides a highly polar environment, and the pore helixes provide a dipole whose electronegative carboxyl ends point toward this inner chamber (Figures 5–15C and 5–18A).

The high energetic cost incurred as a K^+ ion sheds its waters of hydration is partially compensated by the presence of 20 oxygen atoms that line the walls of the selectivity filter and form favorable electrostatic interactions with the permeant ion. Each of the four subunits contributes four main-chain carbonyl oxygen atoms from the protein backbone and one side-chain hydroxyl oxygen atom to form a total of four binding sites for K^+ ions. Each bound K^+ ion is thus stabilized by interactions with a total of eight oxygen atoms, which lie in two planes above and below the bound cation. In this way the channel is able to compensate for the loss of the K^+ ion's waters of hydration. The amino acid side chains of the selectivity filter, which are directed away from the central axis of the channel, help to stabilize the filter at a critical width, such that it provides optimal electrostatic interactions with K^+ ions as they pass but is too wide for smaller Na^+ ions to interact effectively with all eight carbonyl oxygens atoms at any point along the length of the filter (Figure 5–15C).

In light of the extensive interactions between a K^+ ion and the channel, how does the KcsA channel manage its high rate of conduction? Although the channel contains a total of five potential binding sites for K^+ ions—four in the selectivity filter and one in the inner chamber—X-ray analysis shows that the channel can be occupied by at most three K^+ ions at any instant. One ion is normally present in the wide inner chamber, and two ions occupy two of the four binding sites within the selectivity filter (Figure 5–15D). Because of electrostatic repulsion, two K^+ ions never simultaneously occupy adjacent binding sites within the selectivity filter; rather, a water molecule is always interspersed between K^+ ions.

During conduction a pair of K^+ ions within the selectivity filter hop in tandem between pairs of binding sites. If only one ion were in the selectivity filter it would be bound rather tightly, and the throughput rate for ion permeation would be compromised. But the mutual electrostatic repulsion between two K^+ ions occupying nearby sites ensures that the ions will linger only briefly, thus resulting in a high overall rate of K^+ conduction.

X-ray crystallographic analysis has also begun to provide insight into the conformational changes that underlie the opening and closing of K^+ channels. Studies by Clay Armstrong in the 1960s suggested that a gate exists at the intracellular mouth of voltage-gated K^+ channels of higher organisms. Small organic compounds such as tetraethylammonium can enter and block the channel only when this internal gate is opened by depolarization. We now know that this internal gate is the narrow opening formed by the crossing of the four α-helixes at the intracellular mouth of the channel. The small opening at the helix bundle crossing in KcsA revealed by X-ray crystallography turns out to be too narrow to allow ions to pass. Thus the X-ray crystal structure is that of a closed channel.

What do K^+ channels look like when they are open? Although we do not know the answer for KcsA, MacKinnon and his colleagues determined the open structure for a related bacterial K^+ channel, MthK. Each subunit of this channel has two transmembrane segments, similar to KcsA. Unlike KcsA, MthK has a cytoplasmic binding domain for Ca^{2+} and can be opened by high concentrations of internal Ca^{2+}. MacKinnon and colleagues determined the structure of the open state by growing crystals of MthK in the presence of Ca^{2+}. Remarkably, the inner helixes that form the tight bundle crossing in KcsA are bent in MthK at a flexible glycine residue that causes them to splay outward, forming an internal orifice that is dilated to 20 Å in diameter, wide enough to pass K^+ as well as larger compounds such as tetraethylammonium (Figure 5–16). This mechanism is likely to be a general one because the inner helixes of many K^+ channels of bacteria and higher organisms have a conserved glycine residue at this position. The presence of a bend at this glycine gating hinge was recently confirmed in the X-ray crystal structure of a mammalian voltage-gated K^+ channel.

The Structural Basis of Chloride Selectivity Reveals a Close Relation Between Ion Channels and Ion Transporters

Ions move across cell membranes by active transport by ion transporters (or pumps) as well as diffusion through ion channels. Ion transporters are distinguished from ion channels because (1) they require a source of energy to actively transport ions against their electrochemical gradients and (2) they transport ions at rates much lower than those of ion channels, too low to support fast neuronal signaling. Nevertheless, some types of transporters and certain ion channels may have a similar structure according to studies of a bacterial membrane protein that transports protons and Cl^-. These studies also yield insights into the structural basis for Cl^- channel selectivity.

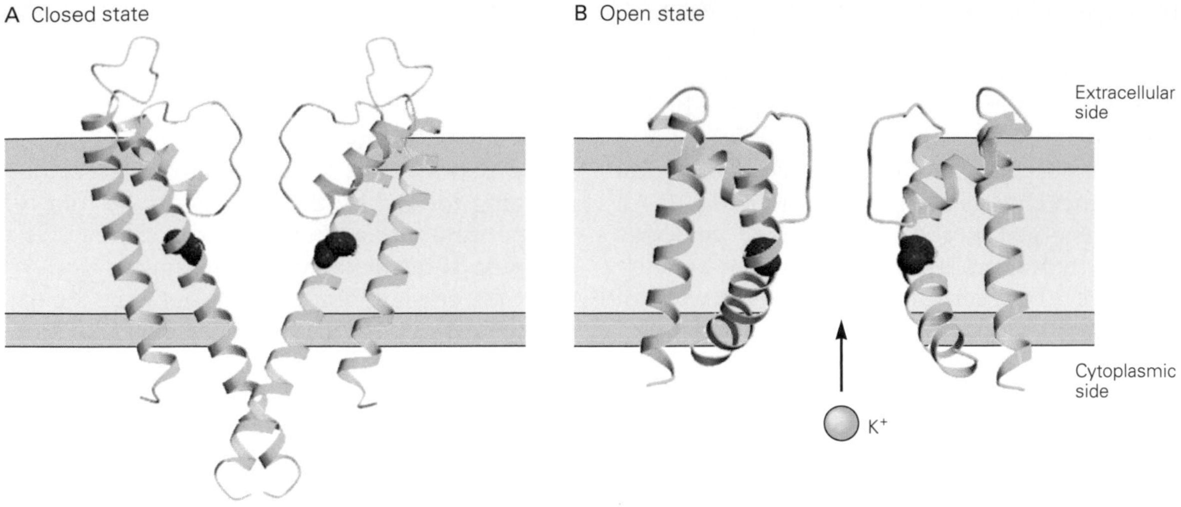

Figure 5–16 **Gating of bacterial potassium channels.** Only two of four subunits are shown.

A. In the closed state the internal mouth of the pore formed by the inner helixes is too narrow to allow K^+ to pass (based on the X-ray crystal structure of the KcsA channel).

B. In the open state the inner helixes are bent at a conserved glycine residue (**red**), widening the internal mouth of the pore (based on the X-ray crystal structure of the MthK channel). (Reproduced, with permission, from Yu et al. 2005; after Jiang et al. 2002.)

A large family of Cl^- channels, the ClC channels, is widely expressed in neurons and other cells of vertebrates. In vertebrate skeletal muscle the ClC-1 channels are important in maintaining the resting potential. Mutations in the genes for these channels underlie certain inherited forms of myotonia; the loss of Cl^- channel activity leads to a depolarizing after-potential following an action potential, resulting in repetitive firing of action potentials that produces abnormally prolonged muscle contraction. MacKinnon and his colleagues obtained a high-resolution X-ray crystal structure for a ClC protein from the bacterium *Escherichia coli*. Based on the close similarity of their amino acid sequences, it seems likely that the three-dimensional structures of the *E. coli* protein and vertebrate ClC channels would be very similar. Indeed, the *E. coli* ClC structure is consistent with the findings of a large number of previous studies of the effects of mutagenesis of vertebrate ClC channels.

It therefore came as a surprise when Chris Miller and colleagues found that the *E. coli* ClC is a transporter, not a channel. The *E. coli* ClC transporter uses the energy stored in a H^+ gradient across the cell membrane to move Cl^- against its electrochemical gradient from the inside of the cell to the outside in exchange for the transport of H^+ from the outside of the cell to the inside, down its electrochemical gradient. This type of transporter is termed an ion exchanger. In the *E. coli* ClC two Cl^- ions are transported in exchange for one proton. The rate of Cl^- transport through the *E. coli* ClC by this exchange mechanism is 100- to 1,000-fold slower than that of vertebrate ClC channels.

The *E. coli* ClC protein, similar to vertebrate ClC channels, is a homodimer composed of two identical subunits. Each vertebrate ClC channel subunit forms a separate Cl^--conducting pore that gates independently from the other half (Figure 5–17A,B). The structure of the *E. coli* ClC transporter is much more complex than that of a K^+ channel. Each subunit contains 18 α-helixes divided into related N-terminal and C-terminal halves, each containing nine helixes (Figure 5–17C,D). Surprisingly, the two halves are found in a head-to-head arrangement so that the helixes in each half have an opposite orientation in the membrane (helix 1 is related to helix 18, not helix 10). Unlike the pore of a K^+ channel, which is widest in the central region, each pore of the *E. coli* ClC has an hourglass profile (Figure 5–18B). The neck of the hourglass, a tunnel 12 Å in length that forms the selectivity filter, is just wide enough to contain fully dehydrated Cl^- ions.

Although the structures of the *E. coli* ClC transporter and K^+ channel differ in significant respects, the two structures have evolved in four similar ways to achieve a high degree of ion selectivity. First, both can be occupied by multiple ions. The *E. coli* ClC contains three binding sites for Cl^- ions within each selectivity filter. It appears that they can all be occupied

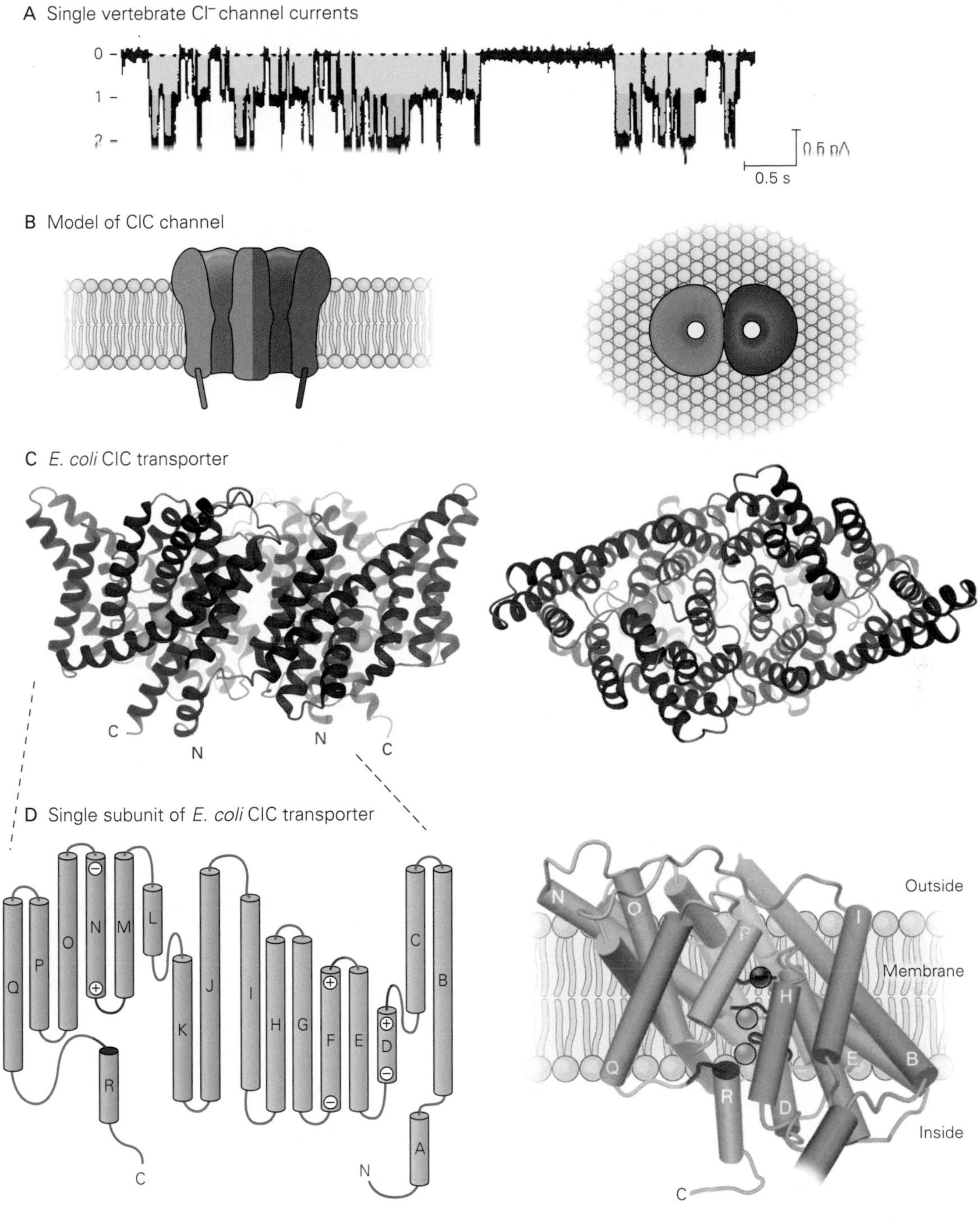

Figure 5–17 The vertebrate ClC family of chloride channels and transporters are double-barrel channels with two identical pores.

A. Recordings of current through a single vertebrate Cl^- channel show three levels of current: both pores closed (**0**), one pore open (**1**), and both pores open (**2**). (Reproduced, with permission, from Miller 1982.)

B. The ClC channels are dimers composed of two identical subunits, each forming a Cl^--selective pore. The channel is shown from the side (**left**) and looking down on the membrane from outside the cell (**right**). Each subunit contains its own ion transport pathway and gate. In addition, the dimer has a gate shared by both subunits (not shown). The drawing illustrates the functional properties of the channel.

C. The X-ray crystal structure of the *Escherichia coli* ClC Cl^-/H^+ exchanger in a side view (left) and top-down view (right). The ribbon diagram shows that each subunit is composed of a large number of α-helixes. Two Cl^- ions (**green spheres**) are shown bound to each subunit: one ion is bound to the selectivity filter and a second is bound to an internal site closer to the cytoplasmic side of the membrane. (Reproduced, with permission, from Dutzler et al. 2002; Dutzler 2004.)

D. Left: The linear arrangement of the two cytoplasmic helixes (A and R) and 16-membrane helixes (B–Q) in a single subunit of the *E. coli* ClC transporter. The helixes from the N-terminal half of a subunit are shown in **green**, while the helixes from the C-terminal half are shown in **cyan**. (Reproduced, with permission, from Dutzler et al. 2002.) **Right:** The three-dimensional arrangement of the helixes in a single *E. coli* ClC subunit. The regions in **red** help form the Cl^- permeation path. The Cl^- ions at the selectivity filter (**top**) and an internal site (**bottom**) are illustrated as **green spheres**. A negative charge on the channel wall that may serve as the channel's gate is illustrated as a **red sphere**. (Reproduced, with permission, from Jentsch 2002.)

simultaneously, thus creating a metastable state that ensures that the ions pass through the pore quickly. Second, in both cases the ion binding sites are formed by polar, partially charged atoms, not by fully ionized atoms. Thus the Cl^- binding sites are formed by main chain amide nitrogen atoms, which bear a partial positive charge, and by side-chain hydroxyl groups. The binding energy provided by these polar groups is relatively weak, ensuring that the Cl^- ions do not become too tightly bound. Third, in both structures permeant ions are stabilized in the center of the membrane by the partial charges of α helixes (Figure 5–18). In *E. coli* ClC the positively polarized (N-terminal) ends of two α-helixes dip partway into the membrane to lower the energetic barrier for Cl^- ions within the nonpolar environment of the membrane. Fourth, in both cases wide water-filled vestibules at either end of the selectivity filter allow ions to approach the filter in a partially hydrated state (see Figure 5–18).

Thus we see that, although the K^+ channel and *E. coli* ClC pores differ fundamentally in amino acid sequence and in secondary, tertiary, and quaternary structures, strikingly similar functional features have evolved in these two classes of membrane proteins to ensure both a high degree of ion selectivity and efficient throughput. These features have been conserved with surprising fidelity from prokaryotes through humans.

Why does the *E. coli* ClC function as a H^+/Cl^- exchanger, whereas the vertebrate ClC proteins function as conventional channels? A likely explanation is that, unlike ion channels, the *E. coli* ClC does not have a continuous open pathway for ion movement from the outside of the membrane to the inside. Rather, like other pumps it is thought to have two gates, one external and one internal. Importantly, the two gates would never open simultaneously. Rather, ion movements and gate movements are presumed to be highly coupled in a tight cycle of reactions (Figure 5–19).

The relatively slow opening and closing of two gates in each cycle of ion transport, which takes place on a scale of milliseconds, explains why the rate of ion transfer through a transporter is several orders of magnitude slower than that of an ion channel. In the crystal structure of the *E. coli* ClC transporter the Cl^- ion in the selectivity filter is trapped by a negatively charged side chain of a nearby glutamate residue on one side and an electronegative hydroxyl group from a serine residue on the other side. Protonation of this glutamate is likely to cause its side chain to rotate out of the way, permitting Cl^- movement.

One or both of the *E. coli* ClC gates is thought to be missing in vertebrate ClC channels, providing an unobstructed pathway for the rapid diffusion of Cl^- down its electrochemical gradient. Thus, despite the

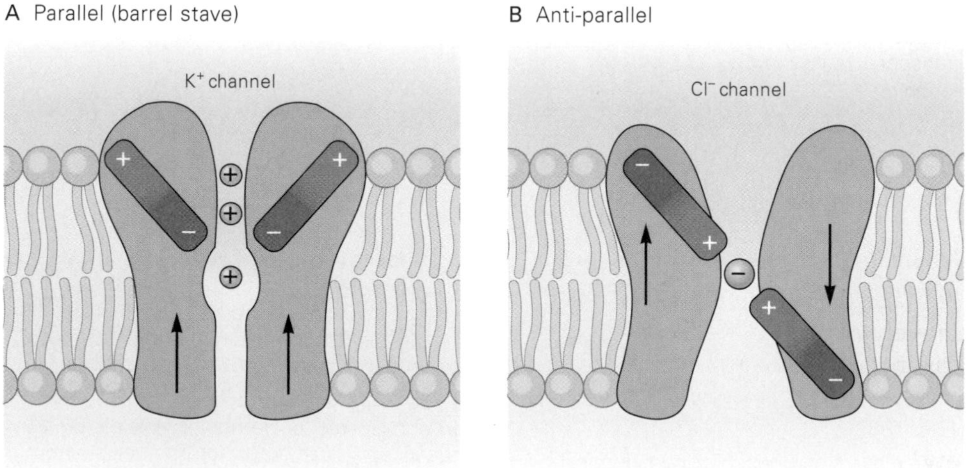

Figure 5–18 Comparison of general architectures of potassium and chloride channels. (Reproduced, with permission, from Dutzler et al. 2002.)

A. In K^+ channels the pore helixes (only two of four are shown here) are in a more or less parallel orientation, like the staves of a barrel. Their negatively charged dipoles point in the same direction to stabilize a K^+ ion in the internal vestibule of the channel.

B. In Cl^- channels the two pore helixes are in an antiparallel arrangement. Their positive dipole ends point toward the center of the channel to stabilize a Cl^- ion in the middle of the channel. Only one subunit of the dimeric Cl^- channel is shown.

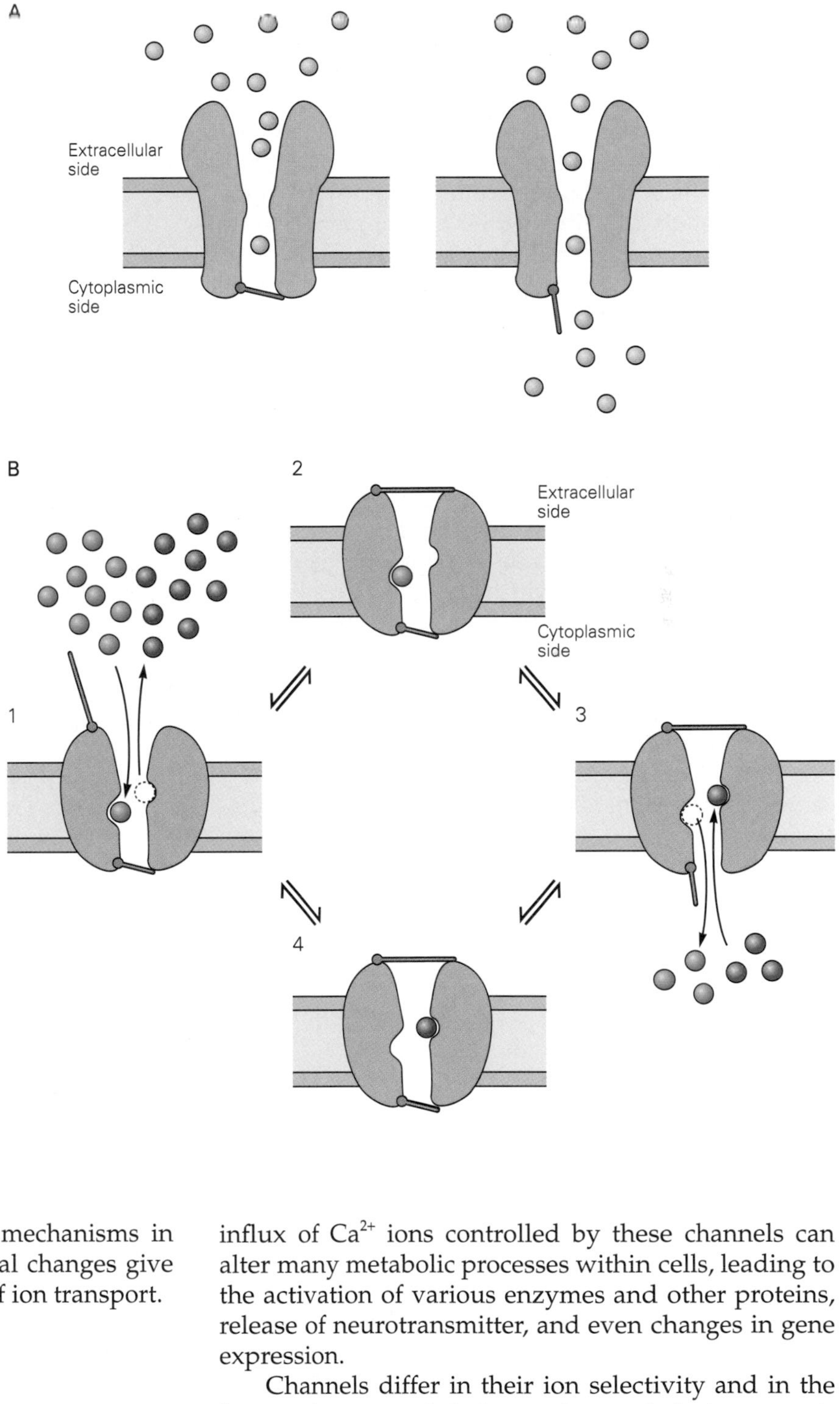

Figure 5–19 The functional difference between ion channels and pumps. (Adapted, with permission, from Gadsby 2004.)

A. Channels have a continuous aqueous pathway for ion conduction across the membrane. This pathway can be occluded by the closing of a gate.

B. Pumps have two gates in series that control ion flux. The gates are never open simultaneously, but both can close to trap one or more ions in the pore. The type of pump illustrated here moves two different types of ions in opposite directions and is termed an *exchanger* or *antiporter*. Ion movement is tightly linked to a cycle of opening and closing of the two gates. When the external gate is open, one type of ion (**red**) leaves while the other type (**blue**) enters the channel (**1**). This triggers a conformational change, causing the external gate to shut, thereby trapping the incoming ion (**2**). A second conformational change then causes the internal gate to open, allowing the trapped ion to leave and a new ion to enter (**3**). A further conformational change opens the external gate, allowing the cycle to continue (**4**). With each cycle, one type of ion is transported from the outside to the inside of the cell, whereas the other type is transported from the inside to the outside of the cell. By coupling the movements of two or more ions, an exchanger can use the energy stored in the concentration gradient of one ion to actively transport another ion against its concentration gradient.

conservation of certain fundamental mechanisms in ClC proteins, relatively small structural changes give rise to two very distinct mechanisms of ion transport.

An Overall View

In all cells ion channels permit the flow of ions across an otherwise impermeable membrane. In nerve and muscle cells ion channels are important for controlling the rapid changes in membrane potential associated with the action potential, receptor potentials and postsynaptic potentials of target cells. In addition, the influx of Ca^{2+} ions controlled by these channels can alter many metabolic processes within cells, leading to the activation of various enzymes and other proteins, release of neurotransmitter, and even changes in gene expression.

Channels differ in their ion selectivity and in the factors that control their opening and closing, or gating. Ion selectivity is achieved through physical–chemical interactions between the ion and various amino acid residues that line the walls of the channel pore. Gating involves a change of the channel's conformation in response to an extrinsic stimulus, such as voltage, a ligand, or stretch or pressure.

Three methodological advances have greatly increased our understanding of channel function. First, the patch-clamp technique has made it possible to record the current through single channels. Second, genome-wide sequencing has determined the primary amino acid sequences of nearly all genes that encode ion channels. From these results many of the channels described so far can be grouped into three major gene families: voltage-gated channels and related subfamilies, a large family of ligand-gated channels, and gap-junction channels. Finally, X-ray crystallography has provided a detailed view of the three-dimensional structure of two types of channels.

The activity of channels can be modified by cellular metabolic reactions, including protein phosphorylation; by various ions that act as blockers; and by toxins, poisons, and drugs. Channels are also important targets in various diseases. Certain autoimmune neurological disorders, such as myasthenia gravis, result from the actions of specific antibodies that interfere with channel function. Other diseases, such as hyperkalemic periodic paralysis, result from ion channel defects because of genetic mutations. Detailed knowledge of the genetic basis of channel structure and function may one day make it possible to devise more specifically targeted pharmacological therapies for various neurological and psychiatric disorders.

Steven A. Siegelbaum
John Koester

Selected Readings

Armstrong CM, Hille B. 1998. Voltage-gated ion channels and electrical excitability. Neuron 20:371–380.

Ashcroft FM. 2000. *Ion Channels and Disease: Channelopathies.* New York: Academic Press.

Bezanilla F. 2008. Ion channels: from conductance to structure. Neuron 60:456–468.

Hille B. 2001. *Ion Channels of Excitable Membranes,* 3rd ed. Sunderland, MA: Sinauer.

Jentsch TJ. 2008. CLC chloride channels and transporters: from genes to protein structure, pathology and physiology. Crit Rev Biochem Mol Biol 43:3–36.

Miller C. 1987. How ion channel proteins work. In: LK Kaczmarek, IB Levitan (eds). *Neuromodulation: The Biological Control of Neuronal Excitability,* pp. 39–63. New York: Oxford Univ. Press.

Yu FH, Yarov-Yarovoy V, Gutman GA, Catterall WA. 2005. Overview of molecular relationships in the voltage-gated ion channel superfamily. Pharmacol Rev 57:387–395.

References

Accardi A, Miller C. 2004. Secondary active transport mediated by a prokaryotic homologue of ClC Cl^- channels. Nature 427:803–807.

Alberts B, Bray D, Lewis J, Raff M, Roberts K, Watson JD. 1994. *Molecular Biology of the Cell,* 3rd ed. New York: Garland.

Andersen OS, Koeppe RE II. 1992. Molecular determinants of channel function. Physiol Rev 72:S89–S158.

Bayliss WM. 1918. *Principles of General Physiology,* 2nd ed., rev. New York: Longmans, Greene.

Brücke E. 1843. Beiträge zur Lehre von der Diffusion tropfbarflüssiger Korper durch poröse Scheidenwände. Ann Phys Chem 58:77–94.

Doyle DA, Cabral JM, Pfuetzner RA, Kuo A, Gulbis JM, Cohen SL, Chait BT, MacKinnon R. 1998. The structure of the potassium channel: molecular basis of K^+ conduction and selectivity. Science 280:69–77.

Dutzler R. 2004. Structural basis for ion conduction and gating in ClC chloride channels. FEBS Lett 564:229–233.

Dutzler R, Campbell EB, Cadene M, Chait BT, MacKinnon R. 2002. X-ray structure of a ClC chloride channel at 3.0 Å reveals the molecular basis of anion selectivity. Nature 415:287–294.

Eisenman G. 1962. Cation selective glass electrodes and their mode of operation. Biophys J 2:259–323. Suppl 2.

Frech GC, VanDongen AM, Schuster G, Brown AM, Joho RH. 1989. A novel potassium channel with delayed rectifier properties isolated from rat brain by expression cloning. Nature 340:642–645.

Gadsby DC. 2004. Ion transport: spot the difference. Nature 427:795–797.

Guharay F, Sachs F. 1984. Stretch-activated single ion channel currents in tissue-cultured embryonic chick skeletal muscle. J Physiol (Lond) 352:685–701.

Hamill OP, Marty A, Neher E, Sakmann B, Sigworth FJ. 1981. Improved patch-clamp techniques for high-resolution current recording from cells and cell-free membrane patches. Pflugers Arch 391:85–100.

Henderson R, Unwin PNT. 1975. Three-dimensional model of purple membrane obtained by electron microscopy. Nature 257:28–32.

Hille B. 1984. *Ionic Channels of Excitable Membranes.* Sunderland, MA: Sinauer.

Hladky SB, Haydon DA. 1970. Discreteness of conductance change in bimolecular lipid membranes in the presence of certain antibiotics. Nature 225:451–453.

Horn R, Patlak J. 1980. Single channel currents from excised patches of muscle membrane. Proc Natl Acad Sci U S A 77:6930–6934.

Jentsch TJ. 2002. Chloride channels are different. Nature 415:276-277.

Jiang Y, Lee A, Chen J, Cadene M, Chait BT, MacKinnon R. 2002. The open pore conformation of potassium channels. Nature 417:523–526.

Katz B, Miledi R. 1970. Membrane noise produced by acetylcholine. Nature 226:962–963.

Katz B, Thesleff S. 1957. A study of the "desensitization" produced by acetylcholine at the motor end-plate. J Physiol (Lond) 138:63–80.

Kyte J, Doolittle RF. 1982. A simple method for displaying the hydropathic character of a protein. J Mol Biol 157:105–132.

Miller C. 1982. Open-state substructure of single chloride channels from *Torpedo electroplax*. Philos Trans R Soc Lond B Biol Sci 299:401–411.

Miller C (ed). 1986. *Ion Channel Reconstitution*. New York: Plenum.

Miller C. 2001. See potassium run. Nature 414:23–24.

Miller C. 2006. ClC chloride channels viewed through a transporter lens. Nature 440:484–489.

Morais-Cabral JH, Zhou Y, MacKinnon R. 2001. Energetic optimization of ion conduction rate by the K^+ selectivity filter. Nature 414:37–42.

Mueller P, Rudin DO, Tien HT, Wescott WC. 1962. Reconstitution of cell membrane structure *in vitro* and its transformation into an excitable system. Nature 194:979–980.

Mullins LJ. 1961. The macromolecular properties of excitable membrane. Ann N Y Acad Sci 94:390–404.

Neher E, Sakmann B. 1976. Single-channel currents recorded from membrane of denervated frog muscle fibres. Nature 260:799–802.

Noda M, Takahashi H, Tanabe T, Toyosato M, Kikyotani S, Furutani Y, Hirose T, et al. 1983. Structural homology of *Torpedo californica* acetylcholine receptor subunits. Nature 302:528–532.

Owens JL, Kullberg R. 1989. *In vivo* development of nicotinic acetylcholine receptor channels in *Xenopus* myotomal muscle. J Neurosci 9:1018–1028.

Sawyer DB, Koeppe RE II, Andersen OS. 1989. Induction of conductance heterogeneity in gramicidin channels. Biochemistry 28:6571–6583.

Schofield PR, Darlison MG, Fujita N, Burt DR, Stephenson FA, Rodriguez H, Rhee LM, Ramachandran J, Reale V, Glencorse TA, Seeburg PH, Barnard EA. 1987. Sequence and functional expression of the $GABA_A$ receptor shows a ligand-gated receptor super-family. Nature 328: 221–227.

Tempel BL, Papazian DM, Schwarz TL, Jan YN, Jan LY. 1987. Sequence of a probable potassium channel component encoded at *Shaker* locus of *Drosophila*. Science 237: 770–775.

Urry DW. 1971. The gramicidin A transmembrane channel: a proposed $\Pi_{(L,D)}$ helix. Proc Natl Acad Sci U S A 68: 672–676.

Venkatachalam K, Montell C. 2007. TRP channels. Annu Rev Biochem 76:387–417.

Weiser M, Vega-Saenz de Miera E, Kentros C, Moreno H, Franzen L, Hillman D, Baker H, Rudy B. 1994. Differential expression of Shaw-related K^+ channels in the rat central nervous system. J Neurosci 14:949–972.

Zhou Y, Morais-Cabral JH, Kaufman A, MacKinnon R. 2001. Chemistry of ion coordination and hydration revealed by a K^+ channel-Fab complex at 2.0 Å resolution. Nature 414:43–48.

6

Membrane Potential and the Passive Electrical Properties of the Neuron

INFORMATION IS CARRIED WITHIN neurons and from neurons to their target cells by electrical and chemical signals. Transient electrical signals are particularly important for carrying time-sensitive information rapidly and over long distances. These transient electrical signals—receptor potentials, synaptic potentials, and action potentials—are all produced by temporary changes in the electric current into and out of the cell, changes that drive the electrical potential across the cell membrane away from its resting value. This current represents the flow of negative and positive ions through ion channels in the cell membrane.

Two types of ion channels—resting and gated—have distinctive roles in neuronal signaling. Resting channels are primarily important in maintaining the resting membrane potential, the electrical potential across the membrane in the absence of signaling. Some types of resting channels are constitutively open and are not gated by changes in membrane voltage; other types are gated by voltage but can open at the negative resting potential of neurons. Most voltage-gated channels, in contrast, are closed when the membrane is at rest and require membrane depolarization to open.

In this and the next several chapters we consider how transient electrical signals are generated in the neuron. We begin by discussing how resting ion channels establish and maintain the resting potential and briefly describe the mechanism by which the resting potential can be perturbed, giving rise to transient electrical signals such as the action potential. We then consider how the passive electrical properties of neurons—their resistive and capacitive characteristics—contribute to the integration and local propagation of synaptic and receptor potentials within the neuron. In Chapter 7 we shall examine the detailed mechanisms by which voltage-gated Na^+, K^+, and Ca^{2+} channels generate the action potential, the electrical signal conveyed along the axon. Synaptic and receptor potentials are considered in Chapters 8 to 11 in the contexts of synaptic signaling between neurons and sensory reception.

The Resting Membrane Potential Results from the Separation of Charge Across the Cell Membrane

The neuron's cell membrane has thin clouds of positive and negative ions spread over its inner and outer surfaces. At rest the extracellular surface of the membrane has an excess of positive charge and the cytoplasmic surface an excess of negative charge (Figure 6–1). This separation of charge is maintained because the lipid bilayer of the membrane is a barrier to the diffusion of ions, as explained in Chapter 5. The charge separation gives rise to a difference of electrical potential, or

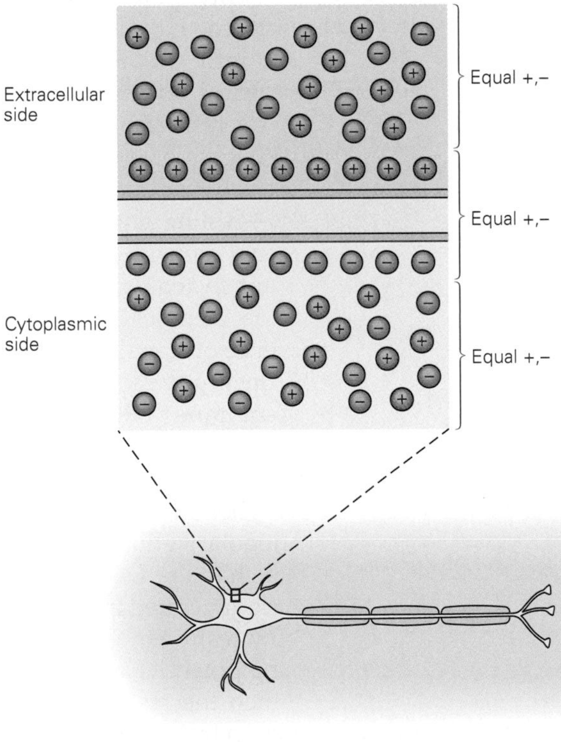

Figure 6–1 The cell membrane potential results from the separation of net positive and net negative charges on either side of the membrane. The excess of positive ions outside the membrane and negative ions inside the membrane represents a small fraction of the total number of ions inside and outside the cell at rest.

voltage, across the membrane called the *membrane potential* (V_m), defined as

$$V_m = V_{in} - V_{out},$$

where V_{in} is the potential on the inside of the cell and V_{out} the potential on the outside.

The membrane potential of a cell at rest is called the *resting membrane potential* (V_r). Since by convention the potential outside the cell is defined as zero, the resting potential is equal to V_{in}. Its usual range is –60 mV to –70 mV. All electrical signaling involves brief changes in the resting membrane potential that are caused by electrical currents across the cell membrane.

The electric current is carried by ions, both positive (cations) and negative (anions). The direction of current is conventionally defined as the direction of *net movement of positive charge.* Thus, in an ionic solution cations move in the direction of the electric current and anions move in the opposite direction. In the nerve cell at rest there is no net charge movement across the membrane. When there is a net flow of cations or anions into or out of the cell, the charge separation across the resting membrane is disturbed, altering the electrical potential of the membrane. A reduction or reversal of charge separation, leading to a less negative membrane potential, is called *depolarization.* An increase in charge separation, leading to a more negative membrane potential, is called *hyperpolarization.*

Changes in membrane potential that do not lead to the opening of gated ion channels are passive responses of the membrane and are called *electrotonic potentials.* Hyperpolarizing responses are almost always passive, as are small depolarizations. However, when depolarization approaches a critical level, or threshold, the cell responds actively with the opening of voltage-gated ion channels, which produces an all-or-none *action potential* (Box 6–1).

The Resting Membrane Potential Is Determined by Nongated and Gated Ion Channels

The resting membrane potential is the result of the passive flux of individual ion species through several classes of resting channels. Understanding how this passive ionic flux gives rise to the resting potential enables us to understand how the gating of different types of ion channels generates the action potential, as well as the receptor and synaptic potentials.

Box 6–1 Recording the Membrane Potential

Reliable techniques for recording the electrical potential across cell membranes were developed in the late 1940s. These techniques allow accurate recordings of both the resting membrane potential and action potentials.

Glass micropipettes filled with a concentrated salt solution serve as electrodes and are placed on either side of the cell membrane. Wires inserted into the back ends of the pipettes are connected via an amplifier to an oscilloscope, which displays the amplitude of the membrane potential in volts. Because the diameter of a microelectrode tip is small (< 1 μm), it can be inserted into a cell with relatively little damage to the cell membrane.

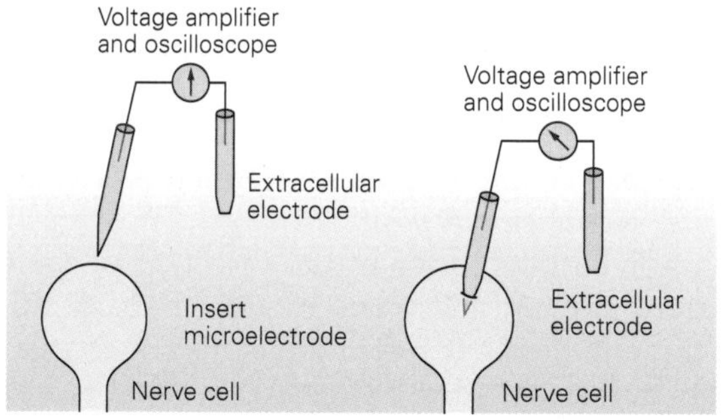

Figure 6–2A The recording setup.

When both electrodes are outside the cell, no electrical potential difference is recorded. But as soon as one microelectrode is inserted into the cell, the oscilloscope shows a steady voltage, the resting membrane potential. In most nerve cells at rest the membrane potential is approximately –65 mV.

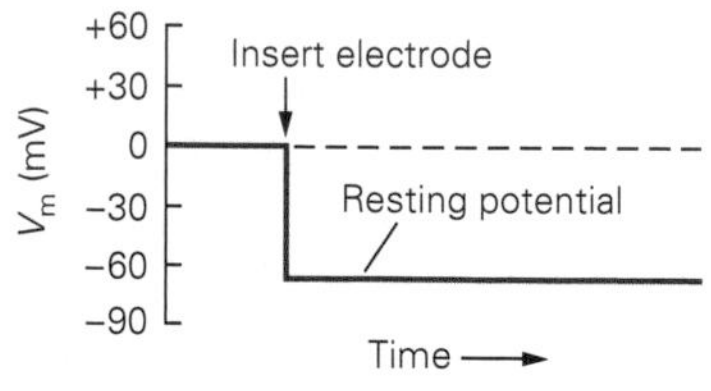

Figure 6–2B Oscilloscope display.

The membrane potential can be experimentally changed using a current generator connected to a second pair of electrodes—one intracellular and one extracellular. When the intracellular electrode is made positive with respect to the extracellular one, a pulse of positive current from the current generator causes positive charge to flow into the neuron from the intracellular electrode. This current returns to the extracellular electrode by flowing outward across the membrane.

As a result, the inside of the membrane becomes more positive while the outside of the membrane becomes more negative. This progressive *decrease* in the normal separation of charge is called *depolarization.*

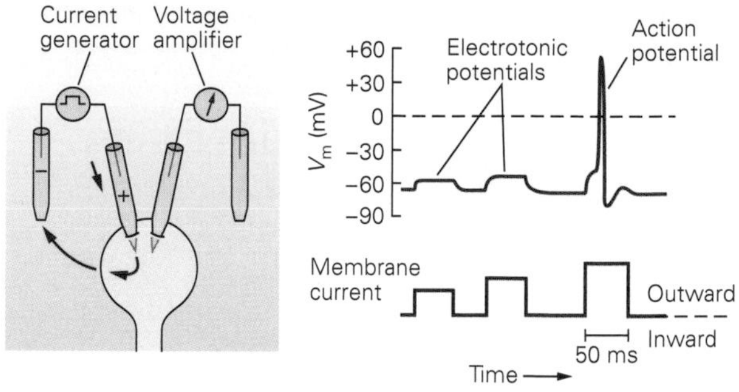

Figure 6–2C Depolarization.

Small depolarizing current pulses evoke purely electrotonic (passive) potentials in the cell—the size of the change in potential is proportional to the size of the current pulses. However, a sufficiently large depolarizing current triggers the opening of voltage-gated ion channels. The opening of these channels leads to the action potential, which differs from electrotonic potentials in the way in which it is generated as well as in magnitude and duration.

Reversing the direction of current—making the intracellular electrode negative with respect to the extracellular electrode—makes the membrane potential more negative. This *increase* in charge separation is called *hyperpolarization.*

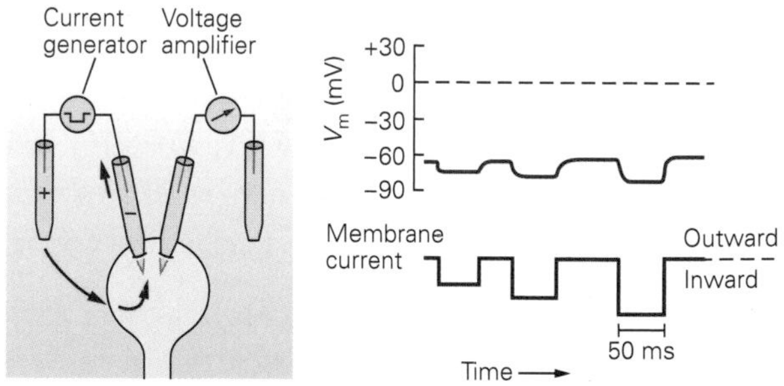

Figure 6–2D Hyperpolarization.

The responses of the cell to hyperpolarization are usually purely electrotonic—as the size of the current pulse increases, the hyperpolarization increases proportionately. Hyperpolarization does not trigger an active response in the cell.

Table 6–1 Distribution of the Major Ions Across a Neuronal Membrane at Rest: The Giant Axon of the Squid

Species of ion	Concentration in cytoplasm (mM)	Concentration in extracellular fluid (mM)	Equilibrium potential[1] (mV)
K^+	400	20	−75
Na^+	50	440	+55
Cl^-	52	560	−60
A^- (organic anions)	385	none	none

[1]The membrane potential at which there is no net flux of the ion species across the cell membrane.

No single ion species is distributed equally on the two sides of a nerve cell membrane. Of the four most abundant ions found on either side of the cell membrane, Na^+ and Cl^- are concentrated outside the cell and K^+ and organic anions (A^-, primarily amino acids and proteins) inside. Table 6–1 shows the distribution of these ions inside and outside of one particularly well-studied nerve cell process, the giant axon of the squid, whose extracellular fluid has a salt concentration similar to that of seawater. Although the absolute values of the ionic concentrations for vertebrate nerve cells are two- to threefold lower than those for the squid giant axon, the *concentration gradients* (the ratio of the external to internal ion concentration) are similar.

The unequal distribution of ions raises several important questions. How do ionic gradients contribute to the resting membrane potential? What prevents the ionic gradients from dissipating by diffusion of ions across the membrane through the resting channels? These questions are interrelated, and we shall answer them by considering two examples of membrane permeability: the resting membranes of glial cells, which are permeable to only one species of ion, and the resting membranes of nerve cells, which are permeable to three. For the purposes of this discussion, we shall only consider the resting channels that are not gated by voltage and thus are always open.

Open Channels in Glial Cells Are Permeable to Potassium Only

The permeability of a cell membrane to particular ion species is determined by the relative proportions of the various types of ion channels that are open. The simplest case is that of the glial cell, which has a resting potential of approximately −75 mV. Like most cells, a glial cell has high concentrations of K^+ and negatively charged organic anions on the inside and high concentrations of Na^+ and Cl^- on the outside. However, most resting channels in the membrane are permeable only to K^+.

Because K^+ ions are present at a high concentration inside the cell, they tend to diffuse across the membrane from the inside to the outside of the cell down their chemical concentration gradient. As a result, the outside of the membrane accumulates a net positive charge (caused by the slight excess of K^+) and the inside a net negative charge (because of the deficit of K^+ and the resulting slight excess of anions). Because opposite charges attract each other, the excess positive charges on the outside and the excess negative charges on the inside collect locally on either surface of the membrane (see Figure 6–1).

The flux of K^+ out of the cell is self-limiting. The efflux of K^+ gives rise to an electrical potential difference—positive outside, negative inside. The greater the flow of K^+, the more charge is separated and the greater is the potential difference. Because K^+ is positive, the negative potential inside the cell tends to oppose the further efflux of K^+. Thus ions are subject to two forces driving them across the membrane: (1) a *chemical driving force,* a function of the concentration gradient across the membrane, and (2) an *electrical driving force,* a function of the electrical potential difference across the membrane.

Once K^+ diffusion has proceeded to a certain point, the electrical driving force on K^+ exactly balances the chemical driving force. That is, the outward movement of K^+ (driven by its concentration gradient) is equal to the inward movement of K^+ (driven by the electrical potential difference across the membrane). This potential is called the K^+ *equilibrium potential,* E_K (Figure 6–3). In a cell permeable only to K^+ ions, E_K determines the resting membrane potential, which in most glial cells is approximately −75 mV.

The equilibrium potential for any ion X can be calculated from an equation derived in 1888 from basic

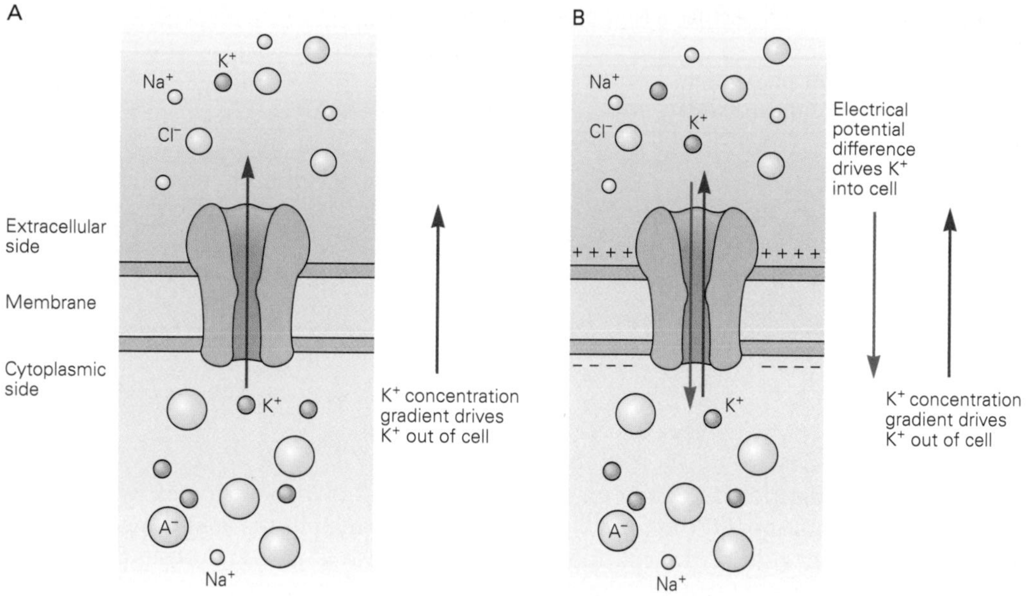

Figure 6–3 The flux of K^+ across a cell membrane is determined by both the K^+ concentration gradient and the membrane potential.

A. In a cell permeable only to K^+, the resting potential is generated by the efflux of K^+ down its concentration gradient.

B. The continued efflux of K^+ builds up an excess of positive charge on the outside of the cell and leaves behind an excess of negative charge inside the cell. This buildup of charge leads to a potential difference across the membrane that impedes the further efflux of K^+, so eventually an equilibrium is reached: The electrical and chemical driving forces are equal and opposite, and as many K^+ ions move in as move out.

thermodynamic principles by the German physical chemist Walter Nernst:

$$E_X = \frac{RT}{zF} \ln \frac{[X]_o}{[X]_i}, \qquad \textbf{Nernst Equation}$$

where R is the gas constant, T the temperature (in degrees Kelvin), z the valence of the ion, F the Faraday constant, and $[X]_o$ and $[X]_i$ the concentrations of the ion outside and inside the cell. (To be precise, chemical activities rather than concentrations should be used.)

Since RT/F is 25 mV at 25°C (77°F, room temperature), and the constant for converting from natural logarithms to base 10 logarithms is 2.3, the Nernst equation can also be written as follows:

$$E_X = \frac{58\,\text{mV}}{z} \log \frac{[X]_o}{[X]_i}.$$

Thus, for K^+, since $z = +1$ and given the concentrations inside and outside the squid axon in Table 6–1:

$$E_K = \frac{58\,\text{mV}}{1} \log \frac{[20]}{[400]} = -75\,\text{mV}.$$

The Nernst equation can be used to find the equilibrium potential of any ion that is present on both sides of a membrane permeable to that ion (the potential is sometimes called the *Nernst potential*). The Na^+, K^+, and Cl^- equilibrium potentials for the distributions of ions across the squid axon are given in Table 6–1.

In our discussion so far we have treated the generation of the resting potential as a passive mechanism—the diffusion of ions down their chemical gradients—one that does not require the expenditure of energy by the cell, for example through hydrolysis of adenosine triphosphate (ATP). However, energy (from ATP hydrolysis) is required to set up the initial concentration gradients and to maintain them in neurons, as we shall see below.

Open Channels in Resting Nerve Cells Are Permeable to Several Ion Species

Unlike glial cells, nerve cells at rest are permeable to Na^+ and Cl^- ions in addition to K^+ ions. Of the abundant ion species in nerve cells, only the large organic anions (A^-) are unable to permeate the cell membrane. How are the concentration gradients for the three permeant ions (Na^+, K^+, and Cl^-) maintained across the membrane of a single cell, and how do these three gradients interact to determine the cell's resting membrane potential?

To answer these questions, it is easiest to examine first only the diffusion of K^+ and Na^+. Let us return to the simple example of a cell having only K^+ channels, with concentration gradients for K^+, Na^+, Cl^-, and A^- as shown in Table 6–1. Under these conditions the resting membrane potential, V_r, is determined solely by the K^+ concentration gradient and is equal to E_K (–75 mV) (Figure 6–4A).

Now consider what happens if a few resting Na^+ channels are added to the membrane, making it slightly permeable to Na^+. Two forces drive Na^+ into the cell: Na^+ tends to flow into the cell down its chemical concentration gradient, and it is driven into the cell by the negative electrical potential difference across the membrane (Figure 6–4B). The influx of Na^+ depolarizes the cell, but only slightly from the K^+ equilibrium potential (–75 mV). The new membrane potential does not come close to the Na^+ equilibrium potential of +55 mV because there are many more resting K^+ channels than Na^+ channels in the membrane.

As soon as the membrane potential begins to depolarize from the value of the K^+ equilibrium potential, K^+ flux is no longer in equilibrium across the membrane. The reduction in the negative electrical force driving K^+ into the cell means that there is now a net flow of K^+ out of the cell, tending to counteract the Na^+ influx. The more the membrane potential is depolarized and driven away from the K^+ equilibrium potential, the greater is the net electrochemical force driving K^+ out of the cell and consequently the greater the net K^+ efflux. Eventually, the membrane potential reaches a new resting level at which the increased outward movement of K^+ just balances the inward movement of Na^+ (Figure 6–4C). This balance point (usually approximately –65 mV) is far from the Na^+ equilibrium potential (+55 mV) and is only slightly more positive than the K^+ equilibrium potential (–75 mV).

To understand how this balance point is determined, bear in mind that the magnitude of the flux of an ion across a cell membrane is the product of its *electrochemical driving force* (the sum of the electrical and chemical driving forces) and the conductance of the membrane to the ion:

$$\text{ion flux} = (\text{electrical driving force} + \text{chemical driving force}) \times \text{membrane conductance}.$$

In a resting nerve cell relatively few Na^+ channels are open, so the membrane conductance of Na^+ is quite low. Thus, despite the large chemical and electrical forces driving Na^+ into the cell, the influx of Na^+ is small. In contrast, many K^+ channels are open in the membrane of a resting cell so that the membrane conductance of K^+ is relatively large. Because of the high relative conductance of Na^+ to K^+ in the cell at rest, the small net outward force acting on K^+ is enough to produce a K^+ efflux equal to the Na^+ influx.

The Electrochemical Gradients of Sodium, Potassium, and Calcium Are Established by Active Transport of the Ions

For a cell to have a steady resting membrane potential, the charge separation across the membrane must be constant over time. That is, at every instant the influx of positive charge must be balanced by the efflux of positive charge. If these fluxes were not equal, the charge separation across the membrane, and thus the membrane potential, would vary continually.

As we have seen, the passive movement of K^+ out of the resting cell through open channels balances the passive movement of Na^+ into the cell. However, this steady leakage of ions cannot be allowed to continue unopposed for any appreciable length of time because the Na^+ and K^+ gradients would eventually run down, reducing the resting membrane potential.

Dissipation of ionic gradients is prevented by the sodium-potassium pump (Na^+-K^+ pump), which moves Na^+ and K^+ *against* their electrochemical gradients: It extrudes Na^+ from the cell while taking in K^+. The pump therefore requires energy, and the energy comes from hydrolysis of ATP (Figure 6–5A). Thus at the resting membrane potential the cell is not in equilibrium but rather in a *steady state*: There is a continuous passive influx of Na^+ and efflux of K^+ through resting channels that is exactly counterbalanced by the Na^+-K^+ pump. As we saw in the previous chapter, pumps are similar to ion channels in that they catalyze the movement of ions across cell membranes. However they differ in two important respects. First, whereas ion channels are passive conduits that allow ions to move down their electrochemical gradient, pumps transport ions against their electrochemical gradient by expending chemical energy. Second, ion transport is much faster in channels: Ions typically flow through channels at a rate of 10^7 to 10^8 per second, whereas pumps operate at speeds more than 10,000 times slower.

The Na^+-K^+ pump is a large membrane-spanning protein with catalytic binding sites for Na^+ and ATP on its intracellular surface and for K^+ on its extracellular surface. With each cycle the pump hydrolyzes one molecule of ATP. (Because the Na^+-K^+ pump hydrolyzes ATP, it is also referred to as the *Na^+-K^+ ATPase*.)

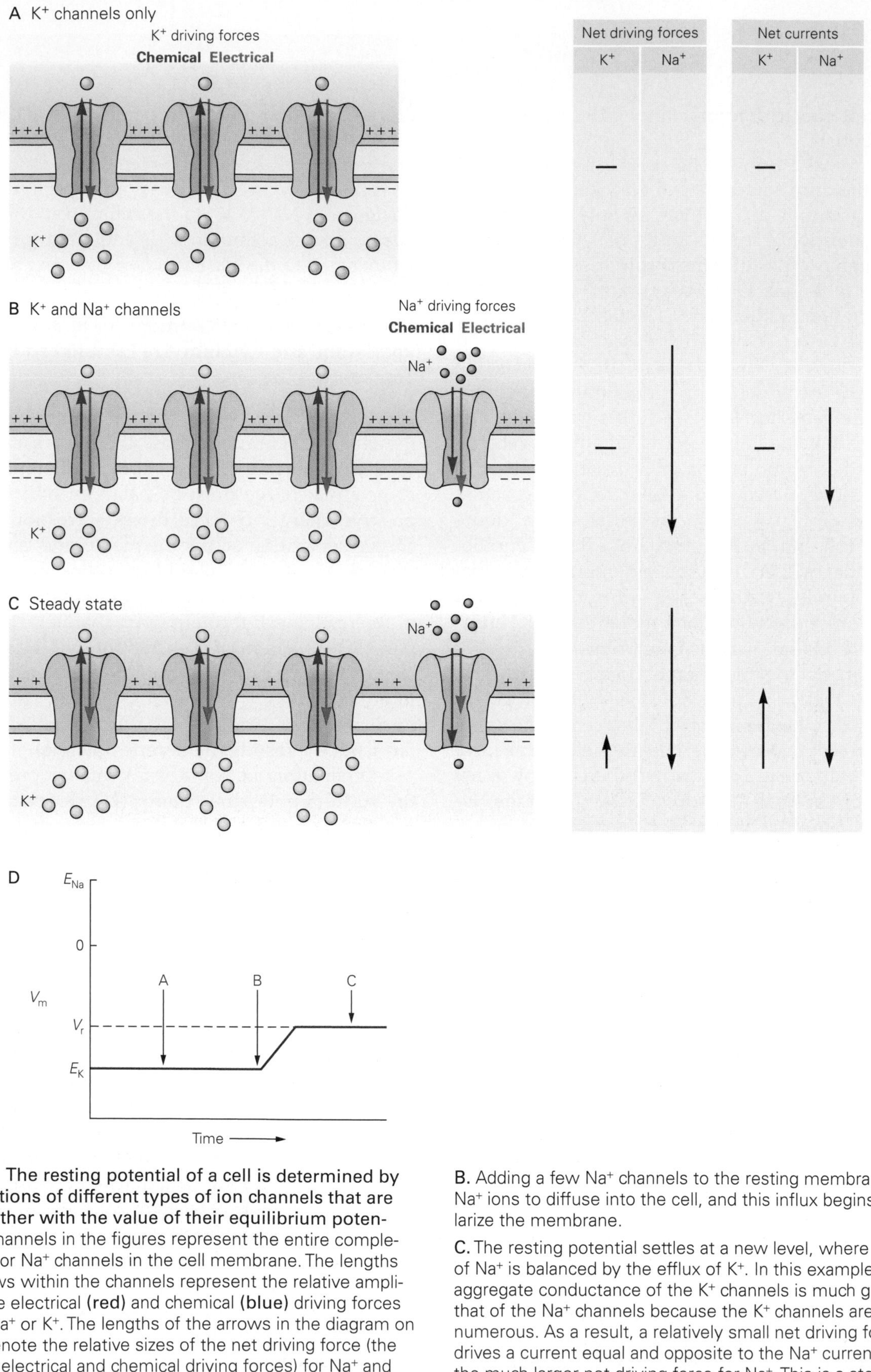

Figure 6–4 The resting potential of a cell is determined by the proportions of different types of ion channels that are open, together with the value of their equilibrium potentials. The channels in the figures represent the entire complement of K^+ or Na^+ channels in the cell membrane. The lengths of the arrows within the channels represent the relative amplitudes of the electrical **(red)** and chemical **(blue)** driving forces acting on Na^+ or K^+. The lengths of the arrows in the diagram on the right denote the relative sizes of the net driving force (the sum of the electrical and chemical driving forces) for Na^+ and K^+ and the net ion currents. Three hypothetical situations are illustrated.

A. In a resting cell in which only K^+ channels are present, K^+ ions are in equilibrium and $V_m = E_K$.

B. Adding a few Na^+ channels to the resting membrane allows Na^+ ions to diffuse into the cell, and this influx begins to depolarize the membrane.

C. The resting potential settles at a new level, where the influx of Na^+ is balanced by the efflux of K^+. In this example the aggregate conductance of the K^+ channels is much greater than that of the Na^+ channels because the K^+ channels are more numerous. As a result, a relatively small net driving force for K^+ drives a current equal and opposite to the Na^+ current driven by the much larger net driving force for Na^+. This is a steady-state condition, in which neither Na^+ nor K^+ is in equilibrium but the net flux of charge is null.

D. Membrane voltage changes during the hypothetical situations illustrated in **A**, **B**, and **C**.

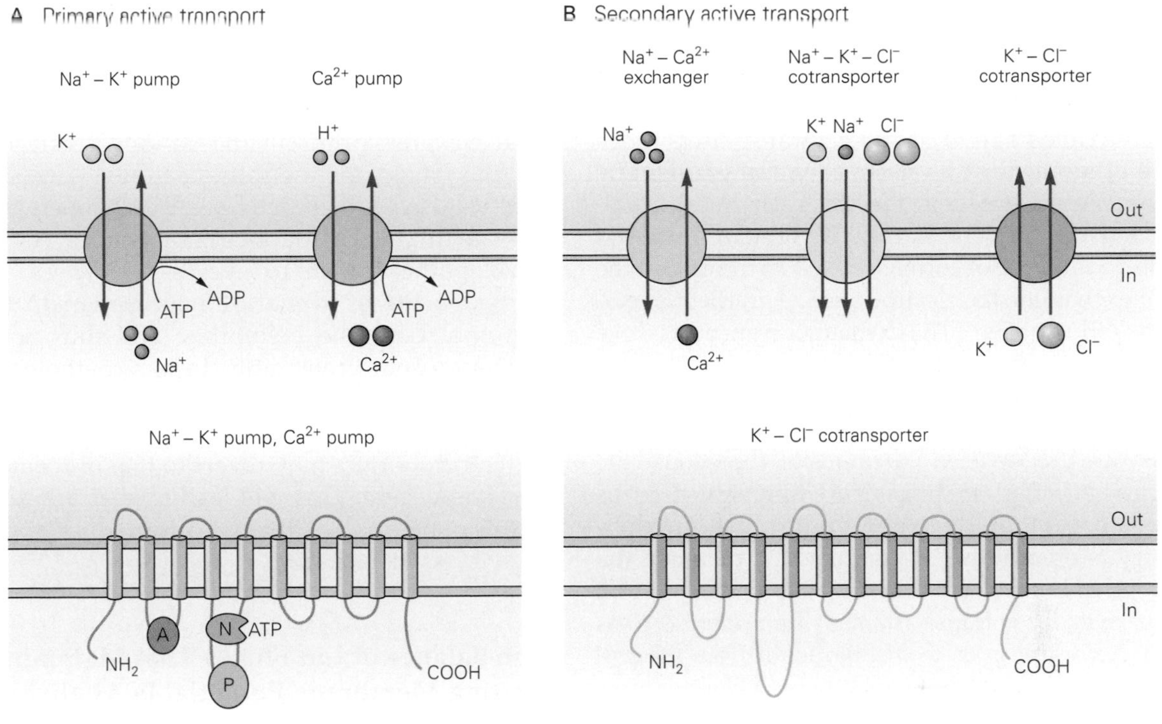

Figure 6–5 Pumps and transporters regulate the chemical concentration gradients of Na^+, K^+, Ca^{2+}, and Cl^- ions.

A. The Na^+-K^+ pump and Ca^{2+} pump are two examples of active transporters that use the energy of adenosine triphosphate (ATP) hydrolysis to transport ions against their concentration gradient. The α-subunit of a Na^+-K^+ pump or homologous Ca^{2+} pump (**below**) has 10 transmembrane segments, a cytoplasmic amino terminus, and a cytoplasmic carboxyl terminus. There are also cytoplasmic loops important for binding ATP (**N**), ATP hydrolysis and phosphorylation of the pump (**P**), and transducing phosphorylation to transport (**A**). The Na^+-K^+ pump also contains a smaller β-subunit with a single transmembrane domain (not shown).

B. The Na^+-Ca^{2+} exchanger uses the potential energy of the electrochemical gradient of Na^+ to transport Ca^{2+} out of a cell. The Na^+-Ca^{2+} exchanger contains nine transmembrane segments, two reentrant membrane loops important for ion transport, and a large cytoplasmic regulatory loop. Chloride ions are transported into the cell by the Na^+-K^+- Cl^- cotransporter and out of the cell by the K^+-Cl^- cotransporter. These transporters are members of a family of Cl^- transport proteins with 12 transmembrane segments.

It uses this energy of hydrolysis to extrude three Na^+ ions from the cell and bring in two K^+ ions. The unequal flux of Na^+ and K^+ ions causes the pump to generate a net outward ionic current. Thus, the pump is said to be *electrogenic.* This pump-driven efflux of positive charge tends to set the resting potential a few millivolts more negative than would be achieved by the passive diffusion mechanisms discussed above. During periods of intense neuronal activity the increased influx of Na^+ leads to an increase in Na^+-K^+ pump activity that generates a prolonged outward current, leading to a prolonged hyperpolarizing after-potential that can last for several minutes, until the normal Na^+ concentration is restored. The Na^+-K^+ pump is inhibited by ouabain or digitalis plant alkaloids, an action that is important in the treatment of heart failure.

The Na^+-K^+ pump is a member of a large family of pumps known as P-type ATPases (because the phosphoryl group of ATP is temporarily transferred to the pump). P-type ATPases include a Ca^{2+} pump that transports Ca^{2+} across cell membranes (see Figure 6–5A). All cells normally maintain a very low cytoplasmic Ca^{2+} concentration, between 50 and 100 nM. This concentration is more than four orders of magnitude lower than the external concentration, which is approximately 2 mM. Calcium pumps in the plasma membrane transport Ca^{2+} out of the cell; other Ca^{2+} pumps located in internal membranes, such as the smooth endoplasmic reticulum, transport Ca^{2+} from the cytoplasm into these intracellular Ca^{2+} stores. Calcium pumps are thought to transport two Ca^{2+} ions for each ATP molecule that is hydrolyzed, with two protons transported in the opposite direction. The Na^+-K^+ pump and Ca^{2+} pump have similar structures. They are formed from 110 kD α-subunits, whose large transmembrane domain contains 10 membrane-spanning α-helixes (see Figure 6–5A).

Most neurons have relatively few Ca^{2+} pumps in the plasma membrane. Instead, Ca^{2+} is transported out of the cell by the Na^+-Ca^{2+} exchanger (Figure 6–5B). This membrane protein is not an ATPase but a different type of molecule called a *cotransporter*. Cotransporters move one type of ion against its electrochemical gradient by using the energy stored in the electrochemical gradient of a second ion. (The *E. coli* ClC protein discussed in Chapter 5 is a type of cotransporter.) In the case of the Na^+-Ca^{2+} exchanger, the electrochemical gradient of Na^+ drives the efflux of Ca^{2+}. The exchanger transports three or four Na^+ ions into the cell (down the electrochemical gradient for Na^+) for each Ca^{2+} ion it removes (against the electrochemical gradient of Ca^{2+}). Because Na^+ and Ca^{2+} are transported in opposite directions, the exchanger is termed an *antiporter.* Ultimately, it is the hydrolysis of ATP by the Na^+-K^+ pump that provides the energy (stored in the Na^+ gradient) to maintain the function of the Na^+-Ca^{2+} exchanger. For this reason, ion flux driven by cotransporters is often referred to as *secondary active transport,* to distinguish it from the primary active transport driven directly by ATPases.

Chloride Ions Are Also Actively Transported

So far, for simplicity, we have ignored the contribution of chloride (Cl^-) to the resting potential. However, in most nerve cells the Cl^- gradient is controlled by one or more active transport mechanisms so that E_{Cl} will differ from V_r. As a result, the opening of Cl^- channels will bias the membrane potential toward its Nernst potential. Chloride transporters typically use the energy stored in the gradients of other ions—they are cotransporters.

Cell membranes contain a number of different types of Cl^- cotransporters (Figure 6–5B). Some transporters increase intracellular Cl^- to levels greater than those that would be passively reached if the Cl^- Nernst potential was equal to the resting potential. In such cells E_{Cl} is positive to V_r so that the opening of Cl^- channels depolarizes the membrane. An example of this type of transporter is the Na^+-K^+-Cl^- cotransporter. This protein transports two Cl^- ions into the cell together with one Na^+ and one K^+ ion. As a result, the transporter is electroneutral. The Na^+-K^+-Cl^- cotransporter differs from the Na^+-Ca^{2+} exchanger in that the former transports all three ions in the same direction—it is a *symporter.*

However, in most neurons the Cl^- gradient is determined by cotransporters that move Cl^- out of the cell. This action lowers the intracellular concentration of Cl^- so that E_{Cl} is typically more negative than the resting potential. As a result, the opening of Cl^- channels leads to an influx of Cl^- that hyperpolarizes the membrane. The K^+-Cl^- cotransporter is an example of such a transport mechanism; it moves one K^+ ion out of the cell for each Cl^- ion it exports.

Interestingly, in early neuronal development cells tend to express primarily the Na^+-K^+-Cl^- cotransporter. At this stage the neurotransmitter γ-aminobutyric acid (GABA), which activates Cl^- channels, typically has an excitatory (depolarizing) effect. As neurons develop they begin to express the K^+-Cl^- cotransporter, such that in mature neurons GABA typically hyperpolarizes the membrane and thus acts as an inhibitory neurotransmitter. In some pathological conditions in adults, such as certain types of epilepsy or chronic pain syndromes, the expression pattern of the Cl^- cotransporters may revert to that of the immature nervous system. This will lead to aberrant depolarizing responses to GABA that can produce abnormally high levels of excitation.

The Balance of Ion Fluxes That Maintains the Resting Membrane Potential Is Abolished During the Action Potential

In the nerve cell at rest the steady Na^+ influx is balanced by a steady K^+ efflux, so that the membrane potential is constant. However, this balance changes when the membrane is depolarized toward the threshold for an action potential. As the membrane potential approaches this threshold, voltage-gated Na^+ channels open rapidly. The resultant increase in membrane conductance to Na^+ causes the Na^+ influx to exceed the K^+ efflux once threshold is exceeded, creating a net influx of positive charge that causes further depolarization. The increase in depolarization causes still more voltage-gated Na^+ channels to open, resulting in a greater influx of Na^+, which accelerates the depolarization even further.

This regenerative, positive feedback cycle develops explosively, driving the membrane potential toward the Na^+ equilibrium potential of +55 mV:

$$E_{Na} = \frac{RT}{F}\ln\frac{[Na]_o}{[Na]_i} = 58 \text{ mV} \log\frac{[440]}{[50]} = +55 \text{ mV}.$$

However, the membrane potential never quite reaches E_{Na} because K^+ efflux continues throughout the depolarization. A slight influx of Cl^- into the cell also counteracts the depolarizing effect of the Na^+ influx. Nevertheless, so many voltage-gated Na^+ channels open during the rising phase of the action potential that the cell membrane's Na^+ conductance is much greater than the conductance of either Cl^- or K^+. Thus, at the peak of the action potential the membrane potential approaches the Na^+ equilibrium potential, just as at rest (when permeability to K^+ is predominant) the membrane potential tends to approach the K^+ equilibrium potential.

The membrane potential would remain at this large positive value near the Na^+ equilibrium potential indefinitely but for two processes that repolarize the membrane, thus terminating the action potential. First, following the peak of the action potential the voltage-gated Na^+ channels gradually close by the process of inactivation (see Chapters 5 and 7). Second, opening of the voltage-gated K^+ channels causes the K^+ efflux to gradually increase. The increase in K^+ conductance is slower than the increase in Na^+ conductance because of the slower rate of opening of the voltage-gated K^+ channels. The slow increase in K^+ efflux together with the decrease in Na^+ influx produces a net efflux of positive charge from the cell, which continues until the cell has repolarized to its resting membrane potential.

The Contributions of Different Ions to the Resting Membrane Potential Can Be Quantified by the Goldman Equation

Although K^+, Na^+, and Cl^- fluxes set the value of the resting potential, V_m is not equal to E_K, E_{Na}, or E_{Cl} but lies at some intermediate value. As a general rule, when V_m is determined by two or more species of ions, the contribution of one species is determined not only by the concentrations of the ion inside and outside the cell but also by the ease with which the ion crosses the membrane. One convenient measure of how readily the ion crosses the membrane is the permeability (P) of the membrane to that ion, which has units of velocity (cm/s). This measure is similar to that of a diffusion constant, which determines the rate of solute movement in solution driven by a local concentration gradient. The dependence of membrane potential on ionic permeability and concentration is given by the Goldman equation:

$$V_m = \frac{RT}{F} \ln \frac{P_K[K^+]_o + P_{Na}[Na^+]_o + P_{Cl}[Cl^-]_i}{P_K[K^+]_i + P_{Na}[Na^+]_i + P_{Cl}[Cl^-]_o}.$$

Goldman Equation

This equation applies only when V_m is not changing. It states that the greater the concentration of an ion species and the greater its membrane permeability, the greater its contribution to determining the membrane potential. In the limit, when permeability to one ion is exceptionally high, the Goldman equation reduces to the Nernst equation for that ion. For example, if $P_K >> P_{Cl}$ or P_{Na}, as in glial cells, the equation becomes as follows:

$$V_m \cong \frac{RT}{F} \ln \frac{[K^+]_o}{[K^+]_i}.$$

Alan Hodgkin and Bernard Katz used the Goldman equation to analyze changes in membrane potential in the squid giant axon. They measured the variations in membrane potential in response to systematic changes in the extracellular concentrations of Na^+, Cl^-, and K^+. They found that if V_m is measured shortly after the extracellular concentration is changed (before the internal ionic concentrations are altered), $[K^+]_o$ has a strong effect on the resting potential, $[Cl^-]_o$ has a moderate effect, and $[Na^+]_o$ has little effect. The data for the membrane at rest could be fit accurately by the Goldman equation using the following permeability ratios:

$$P_K : P_{Na} : P_{Cl} = 1.0 : 0.04 : 0.45.$$

At the peak of the action potential there is an instant in time when V_m is not changing and the Goldman equation is applicable. At that point the variation of V_m with external ionic concentrations is fit best if a quite different set of permeability ratios is assumed:

$$P_K : P_{Na} : P_{Cl} = 1.0 : 20 : 0.45.$$

For these values of permeability the Goldman equation approaches the Nernst equation for Na^+:

$$V_m \cong \frac{RT}{F} \ln \frac{[Na^+]_o}{[Na^+]_i} = +55 \text{ mV}.$$

Thus at the peak of the action potential, when the membrane is much more permeable to Na^+ than to any other ion, V_m approaches E_{Na}. However, the finite permeability of the membrane to K^+ and Cl^- results in K^+ efflux and Cl^- influx that partially counterbalance Na^+ influx, thereby preventing V_m from quite reaching E_{Na}.

The Functional Properties of the Neuron Can Be Represented as an Electrical Equivalent Circuit

The usefulness of the Goldman equation is limited because it cannot be used to determine how rapidly the membrane potential changes in response to a change in permeability. It is also inconvenient for determining the magnitude of the individual Na^+, K^+, and Cl^- currents.

This information can be obtained using a simple mathematical model derived from electrical circuits. The model, called an *equivalent circuit*, represents all of the important electrical properties of the neuron by a circuit consisting of conductors or resistors, batteries, and capacitors.[1]

Equivalent circuits provide us with an intuitive understanding as well as a quantitative description of how current caused by the movement of ions generates signals in nerve cells.

The first step in developing an equivalent circuit is to relate the membrane's discrete physical properties to its electrical properties. We start by considering the lipid bilayer, which endows the membrane with electrical *capacitance*, the ability of an electrical nonconductor (insulator) to separate electrical charges on either side of it. The nonconducting phospholipid bilayer of the membrane separates the cytoplasm and extracellular fluid, both of which are highly conductive environments. The presence of a thin layer of opposing charges on the inside and outside surfaces of the cell membrane, acting as a capacitor, gives rise to the electrical potential difference across the membrane. The electrical potential difference or voltage across a capacitor is

$$V = Q/C,$$

where Q is the net excess positive or negative charge on each side of the capacitor and C is the capacitance. Capacitance is measured in units of farads (F), and charge is measured in coulombs (where 96,500 coulombs of a univalent ion is equivalent to 1 mole of that ion). A charge separation of 1 coulomb across a capacitor of 1 F produces a potential difference of 1 volt. A typical value of membrane capacitance for a nerve cell is approximately 1 μF per cm^2 of membrane area. Very few charges are required to produce a large potential difference across such a capacitance. For example, the excess of positive and negative charges separated by the membrane of a spherical cell body with a diameter of 50 μm and a resting potential of –60 mV is 29×10^6 ions. Although this number may seem large, it represents only a tiny fraction (1/200,000) of the total number of positive or negative charges in solution within the cytoplasm. The bulk of the cytoplasm and the bulk of the extracellular fluid are electroneutral.

The membrane is a *leaky capacitor* because it is studded with ion channels that can conduct charge. Ion channels endow the membrane with conductance and with the ability to generate electromotive force (emf). The lipid bilayer itself has effectively zero conductance or infinite resistance. However, because ion channels are highly conductive, they provide pathways of finite electrical resistance for ions to cross the membrane. Because neurons contain many types of channels selective for different ions, we must consider each class of ion channel separately.

In an equivalent circuit we can represent each K^+ channel as a resistor or conductor of ionic current with a single-channel conductance γ_K (remember, conductance = 1/resistance) (Figure 6–6). If there were no K^+ concentration gradient, the current through a single K^+ channel would be given by Ohm's law: $i_K = \gamma_K \times V_m$. However, since there is normally a K^+ concentration gradient, there is also a chemical force driving K^+ across the membrane, represented in the equivalent circuit by a battery. (A source of electrical potential is called an *electromotive force* and an electromotive force generated by a difference in chemical potentials is called a battery.) The electromotive force of this battery is given by E_K, the Nernst potential for K^+ (Figure 6–7).

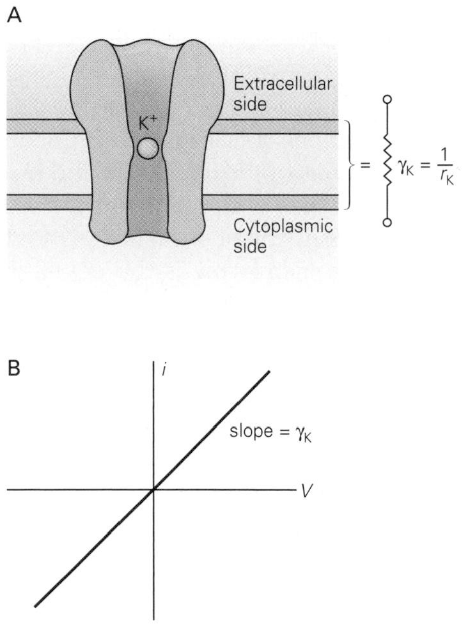

Figure 6–6 Electrical properties of a single K^+ channel.

A. A single K^+ channel can be represented as a conductor or resistor (conductance, γ, is the inverse of resistance, r).

B. The relationship of current (i) and voltage (V) for a single K^+ channel in the absence of a concentration gradient. The slope of the line is equal to γ_K.

[1]The electrical concepts underlying the equivalent circuit are described in detail in Appendix A.

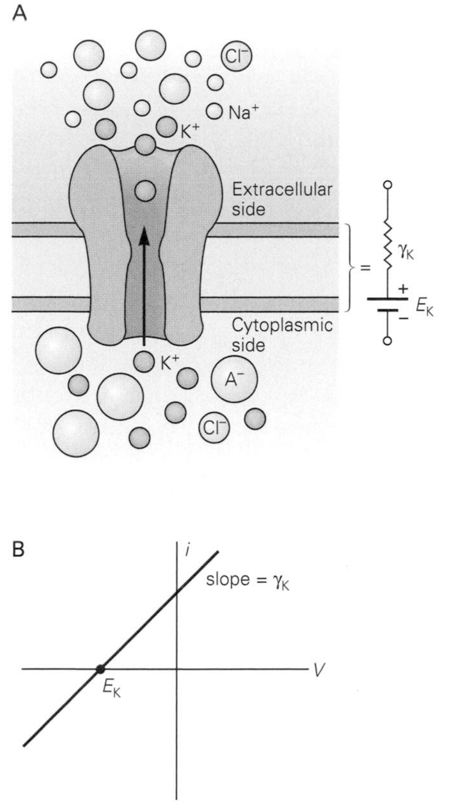

Figure 6–7 Chemical and electrical forces contribute to current through an ion channel.

A. A concentration gradient for K^+ gives rise to an electromotive force, which has a value equal to E_K, the Nernst potential for K^+. This can be represented by a battery. In this circuit the battery E_K is in series with the conductor γ_K, representing the conductance of the K^+ channel.

B. The current-voltage relation for a K^+ channel in the presence of both electrical and chemical driving forces. The potential at which the current is zero is equal to the K^+ Nernst potential.

In the absence of voltage across the membrane, the normal K^+ concentration gradient causes an outward K^+ current. According to our convention for current, an outward movement of positive charge across the membrane corresponds to a positive current. According to the Nernst equation, when the concentration gradient for a positively charged ion, such as K^+, is directed outward (ie, the K^+ concentration inside the cell is higher than outside), the equilibrium potential for that ion is negative. Thus the K^+ current that flows solely because of its concentration gradient is given by $i_K = -\gamma_K \times E_K$ (the negative sign is required because a negative equilibrium potential produces a positive current at 0 mV).

Finally, for a real neuron that has both a membrane voltage and a K^+ concentration gradient, the net K^+ current is given by the sum of the currents caused by the electrical and chemical driving forces:

$$i_K = (\gamma_K \times V_m) - (\gamma_K \times E_K) = \gamma_K \times (V_m - E_K).$$

The term $(V_m - E_K)$ is called the *electrochemical driving force*. It determines the direction of ionic current and (along with the conductance) its magnitude. This equation is a modified form of Ohm's law that takes into account the fact that ionic current through a membrane is determined not only by the voltage across the membrane but also by the ionic concentration gradients.

A cell membrane has many resting K^+ channels, all of which can be combined into a single equivalent circuit consisting of a conductor in series with a battery (Figure 6–8). In this equivalent circuit the total conductance of all the K^+ channels (g_K), ie, the K^+ conductance of the cell membrane in its resting state, is equal to the number of resting K^+ channels (N_K) multiplied by the conductance of an individual K^+ channel (γ_K):

$$g_K = N_K \times \gamma_K.$$

Because the battery in this equivalent circuit depends solely on the concentration gradient for K^+ and is independent of the number of K^+ channels, its value is the equilibrium potential for K^+, E_K.

Like the population of resting K^+ channels, all the resting Na^+ channels can be represented by a single conductor in series with a single battery, as can the resting Cl^- channels (Figure 6–9). Because the K^+, Na^+, and Cl^- channels account for the bulk of the passive ionic current through the membrane in the cell at rest, we can calculate the resting potential by incorporating these three pathways into a simple equivalent circuit of a neuron.

To construct this circuit we need only connect the elements representing each type of channel at their two ends with elements representing the extracellular fluid and cytoplasm. The extracellular fluid and cytoplasm are both good conductors (compared with the membrane) because they have relatively large cross sectional areas and many ions available to carry charge. In a small region of a neuron, the extracellular and cytoplasmic resistances can be approximated by a *short circuit*—a conductor with zero resistance (Figure 6–10). The membrane capacitance (C_m) is determined by the insulating properties of the lipid bilayer, which separates the extracellular and cytoplasmic conductors.

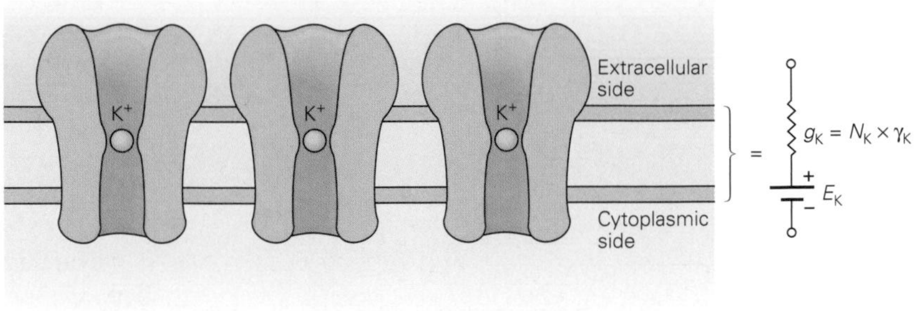

Figure 6–8 All the resting K^+ channels in a nerve cell membrane can be lumped into a single equivalent circuit comprised of a battery in series with a conductor. The K^+ conductance of the membrane at rest is $g_K = N_K \times \gamma_K$, where N_K is the number of passive K^+ channels and γ_K is the conductance of a single K^+ channel.

The equivalent circuit can be made more realistic by incorporating the active ion fluxes driven by the Na^+-K^+ pump, which extrudes three Na^+ ions from the cell for every two K^+ ions it pumps in. This electrogenic ATP-dependent pump, which keeps the ionic batteries charged, can be added to the equivalent circuit in the form of a current generator (Figure 6–11).

The use of the equivalent circuit to analyze neuronal properties quantitatively is illustrated in Box 6–2. There we see how the equivalent circuit can be used to calculate the resting potential, V_m. We also see how the equivalent circuit can be simplified by combining all of the resting Na^+, K^+, and Cl^- channels into a single resting current pathway, with a conductance g_r and a battery E_r, which is equal to the resting potential.

The Passive Electrical Properties of the Neuron Affect Electrical Signaling

Once an electrical signal is generated in part of a neuron, for example in response to a synaptic input on a branch of a dendrite, it is integrated with the other inputs to the neuron and then propagated to the axon initial segment, the site of action potential generation. During signaling, when a stimulus generates action potentials or local (synaptic or sensory generator) potentials in a neuron, the membrane potential changes frequently.

What determines the rate of change in potential with time or distance? What determines whether a stimulus will or will not produce an action potential? Here we consider the neuron's passive electrical properties and geometry and how these relatively constant properties affect the cell's electrical signaling. In the next five chapters we shall consider the properties of the gated channels and how the active ionic currents they control change the membrane potential.

Neurons have three passive electrical properties that are important for electrical signaling. We have already considered the resting membrane conductance or resistance ($g_r = 1/R_r$) and the membrane capacitance, C_m. A third important property that determines signal propagation along dendrites or axons is their intracellular axial resistance (r_a). Although, as mentioned above, the resistivity of cytoplasm is much lower than that of the membrane, the axial resistance along the entire length of an extended thin neuronal process can

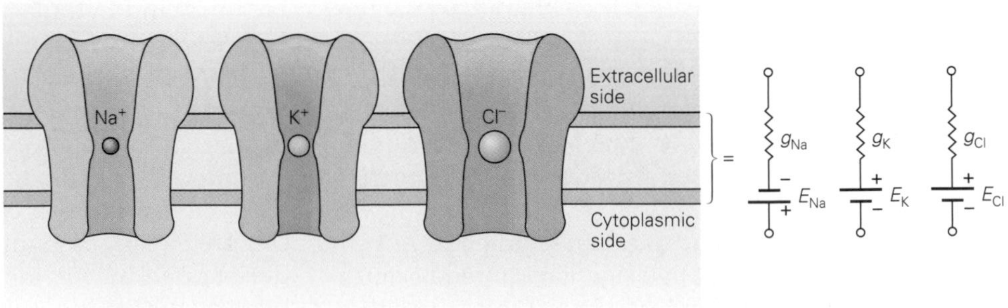

Figure 6–9 The populations of Na^+, K^+, and Cl^- ion channels can each be represented by a battery in series with a conductor. The directions of the battery poles reflect the electromotive force generated by each ionic flux, inside negative for K^+ and Cl^- and positive for Na^+.

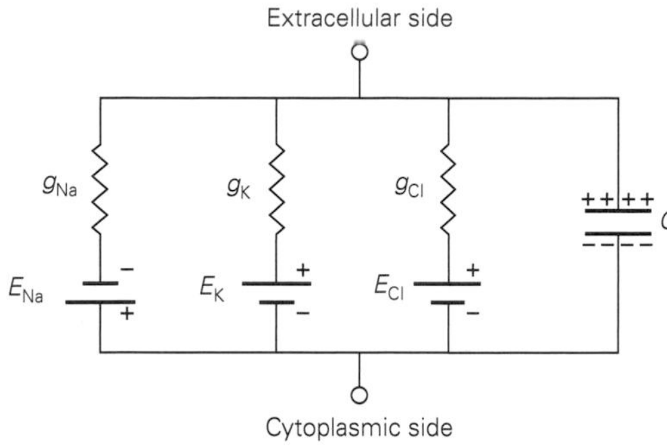

Figure 6–10 An equivalent circuit of the neuronal membrane. The elements of the circuit include pathways representing the Na^+, K^+, and Cl^- ion channels and short-circuit pathways provided by the cytoplasm and extracellular fluid. The lipid bilayer and the conducting solutions on its intracellular and extracellular surfaces endow the membrane with electrical capacitance (C_m).

be considerable. Because these three elements provide the return pathway to complete the electrical circuit when active ionic currents flow into or out of the cell, they determine the time course of the change in synaptic potential generated by the synaptic current. They also determine whether a synaptic potential generated in a dendrite will depolarize the trigger zone on the axon initial segment enough to fire an action potential. Finally, the passive properties influence the speed at which an action potential is conducted.

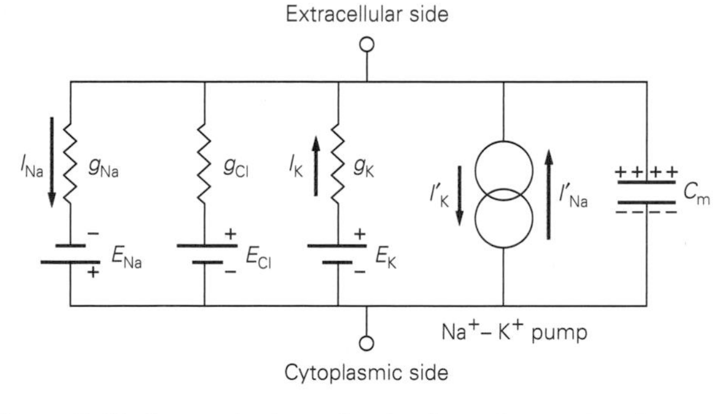

Figure 6–11 An equivalent circuit of passive and active current in a neuron. Under steady-state conditions the passive Na^+ and K^+ currents are balanced by active Na^+ and K^+ fluxes (I'_{Na} and I'_K) driven by the Na^+-K^+ pump. The active Na^+ flux (I'_{Na}) is 50% greater than the active K^+ flux (I'_K), and therefore I_{Na} is 50% greater than I_K, because the Na^+-K^+ pump transports three Na^+ ions out for every two K^+ ions it transports into the cell.

Membrane Capacitance Slows the Time Course of Electrical Signals

The steady-state change in a neuron's voltage in response to subthreshold current resembles the behavior of a simple resistor, but the initial *time course* of the change does not. A true resistor responds to a step change in current with a similar step change in voltage, but the neuron's membrane potential rises and decays more slowly than the step change in current (Figure 6–15). This property of the membrane is caused by its *capacitance.*

To understand how the capacitance slows down the voltage response, recall that the voltage across a capacitor is proportional to the charge stored on the capacitor. To alter the voltage, charge (Q) must be added to or removed from the capacitor (C):

$$\Delta V = \Delta Q/C.$$

To change the charge across the capacitor (the neuron's lipid bilayer), current must flow across the capacitor (I_c). Since current is the flow of charge per unit time ($I_c = \Delta Q/\Delta t$), the change in voltage across a capacitor is a function of the magnitude of the current and the time that the current flows:

$$\Delta V = I_c \cdot \Delta t/C.$$

Thus the magnitude of the change in voltage across a capacitor in response to a current pulse depends on the duration of the current, because time is required to deposit and remove charge across the capacitor.

If the membrane had only resistive properties, a step pulse of outward current would change the membrane potential instantaneously. Conversely, if the membrane had only capacitive properties, the membrane potential would change linearly with time in response to the same step of current. Because the membrane has both capacitive and resistive properties in parallel, the actual change in membrane potential combines features of the two pure responses. The initial slope of the relation between V_m and time reflects a purely capacitive element, whereas the final slope and amplitude reflect a purely resistive element (Figure 6–15, upper plot).

In the simple case of the spherical cell body of a neuron, the time course of the potential change is described by the following equation:

$$\Delta V_m(t) = I_m R_m (1 - e^{-t/\tau}),$$

where e is the base of the system of natural logarithms and has a value of approximately 2.72, and τ is the *membrane time constant,* given by the product of the

Box 6–2 Using the Equivalent Circuit Model to Calculate Resting Membrane Potential

An equivalent circuit model of the resting membrane can be used to calculate the resting potential. To simplify the calculation we shall initially ignore Cl^- channels and begin with just two types of resting channels, K^+ and Na^+, as illustrated in Figure 6–12. Moreover, we ignore the electrogenic influence of the Na^+-K^+ pump because it is small.

Because we consider only steady-state conditions, where the membrane potential, V_m, is not changing, we can also ignore membrane capacitance. (Membrane capacitance and its delaying effect on changes in V_m are discussed below.)

Because there are more resting channels for K^+ than for Na^+, the membrane conductance for K^+ is much greater than that for Na^+. In the equivalent circuit in Figure 6–12, g_K (10×10^{-6} S) is 20 times higher than g_{Na} (0.5×10^{-6} S). Given these values and the values of E_K and E_{Na}, V_m is calculated as follows.

Under the above conditions where the membrane potential is constant, there is no net current across the membrane. Therefore I_{Na} is equal and opposite to I_K:

$$-I_{Na} = I_K$$

or

$$I_{Na} + I_K = 0. \quad \textbf{(6–1)}$$

We can easily calculate I_{Na} and I_K in two steps. First, we add up the separate potential differences across the Na^+ and K^+ branches of the circuit. Going from the inside to the outside across the Na^+ branch, the total potential difference is the sum of the potential differences across E_{Na} and across g_{Na}:*

$$V_m = E_{Na} + I_{Na}/g_{Na}.$$

Similarly, for the K^+ conductance branch

$$V_m = E_K + I_K/g_K.$$

Next, we rearrange and solve for I:

$$I_{Na} = g_{Na} \times (V_m - E_{Na}) \quad \textbf{(6–2a)}$$

*Because we have defined V_m as $V_{in} - V_{out}$, the following convention must be used for these equations. Outward current (in this case I_K) is positive and inward current is negative. Batteries whose positive pole is directed toward the inside of the membrane (eg, E_{Na}) are given positive values in the equations. The reverse is true for batteries whose negative pole is directed toward the inside, such as the K^+ battery.

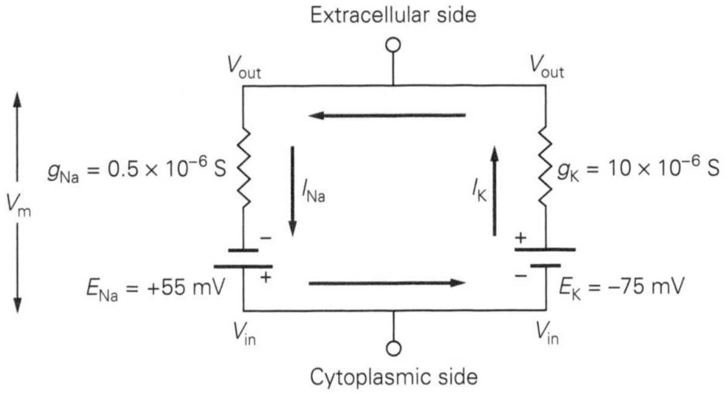

Figure 6–12 In this simple electrical equivalent circuit the resting membrane potential depends on the resting K^+ and Na^+ channels only.

$$I_K = g_K \times (V_m - E_K). \quad \textbf{(6–2b)}$$

As these equations illustrate, the ionic current through each conductance branch is equal to the conductance of that branch multiplied by the net electrical driving force. For example, with the K^+ current the conductance is proportional to the number of open K^+ channels, and the driving force is equal to the difference between V_m and E_K. If V_m is more positive than E_K (–75 mV), the driving force is positive and the current is outward; if V_m is more negative than E_K, the driving force is negative and the current is inward.

Similar equations are used in a variety of contexts in this book to relate the magnitude of a particular ionic current to its membrane conductance and driving force.

As we saw in Equation 6–1, $I_{Na} + I_K = 0$. If we now substitute Equations 6–2a and 6–2b for I_{Na} and I_K in Equation 6–1, multiply through, and rearrange, we obtain the following expression:

$$V_m \times (g_{Na} + g_K) = (E_{Na} \times g_{Na}) + (E_K \times g_K).$$

Solving for V_m we obtain an equation for the resting membrane potential that is expressed in terms of membrane conductances and batteries:

$$V_m = \frac{(E_{Na} \times g_{Na}) + (E_K \times g_K)}{g_{Na} + g_K} \quad \textbf{(6–3)}$$

From this equation, using the values in our equivalent circuit (Figure 6–12), we calculate $V_m = -69$ mV.

Equation 6–3 states that V_m approaches the value of the ionic battery that has the greater conductance. This principle can be illustrated by considering what happens during the action potential. At the peak of the

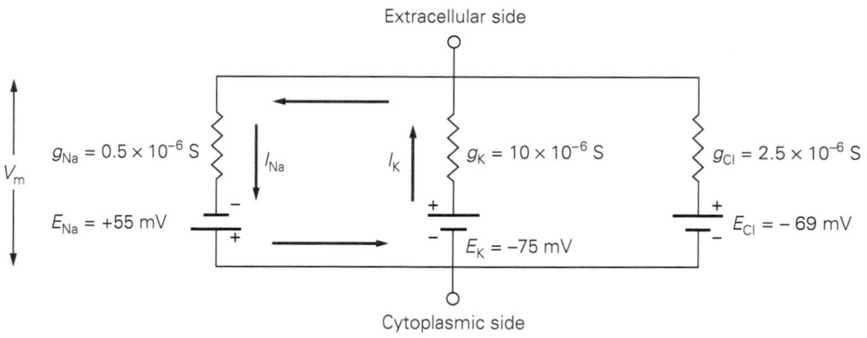

Figure 6–13 This electrical equivalent circuit includes the Cl^- pathway. There is no current through the Cl^- channels because V_m is at E_{Cl}.

action potential g_K is essentially unchanged from its resting value, but g_{Na} increases as much as 500-fold. This increase in g_{Na} is caused by the opening of voltage-gated Na^+ channels. In the equivalent circuit in Figure 6–12, a 500-fold increase would change g_{Na} from 0.5×10^{-6} S to 250×10^{-6} S.

If we substitute this new value of g_{Na} into Equation 6–3 and solve for V_m, we obtain +50 mV. V_m is closer to E_{Na} than to E_K at the peak of the action potential because g_{Na} is now 25-fold greater than g_K, so that the Na^+ battery becomes much more important than the K^+ battery in determining V_m.

The real resting membrane has open channels for Cl^- as well as for Na^+ and K^+. One can derive a more general equation for V_m, following the steps outlined above, from an equivalent circuit that includes a conductance pathway for Cl^- with its associated Nernst battery (Figure 6–13):

$$V_m = \frac{(E_{Na} \times g_{Na}) + (E_K \times g_K) + (E_{Cl} \times g_{Cl})}{g_{Na} + g_K + g_{Cl}}. \qquad \textbf{(6–4)}$$

This equation is similar to the Goldman equation in that the contribution to V_m of each ionic battery is weighted in proportion to the conductance of the membrane for that particular ion. In the limit, if the conductance for one ion is much greater than that for the other ions, V_m approaches the value of that ion's Nernst potential.

The contribution of Cl^- ions to the resting potential can now be determined by comparing V_m calculated for the Na^+ and K^+ circuits only (Figure 6–12) and for all three ions (Figure 6–13). For most nerve cells the value of g_{Cl} ranges from one-fourth to one-half of g_K. In the simplified example in Figure 6–13 Cl^- ions flow passively across the membrane, so that E_{Cl} is equal to the value of V_m, which is determined by Na^+ and K^+.

Because $E_{Cl} = V_m$ (−69 mV in this case), there is no current through the Cl^- channels. As a result when we include g_{Cl} and E_{Cl} in the circuit (Figure 6–13), the calculated value of V_m does not differ from that when the Cl^- conductance is absent (Figure 6–12). However, in most neurons Cl^- is actively transported out of the cell so that E_{Cl} is more negative than the resting potential. Adding the Cl^- pathway to the calculation would shift V_m to a slightly more negative value.

The equivalent circuit can be further simplified by lumping the conductance of all the resting channels that contribute to the resting potential into a single conductance, g_r, and replacing the battery for each conductance channel with a single battery whose value, E_r, is given by Equation 6–4 (Figure 6–14). Here the subscript r stands for the resting channel pathway. Because the resting channels provide a pathway for the steady leakage of ions across the membrane, they are sometimes referred to as *leakage channels* (see Chapter 7). This consolidation of resting pathways will prove useful when we consider the effects on membrane voltage of current through voltage-gated and ligand-gated channels in later chapters.

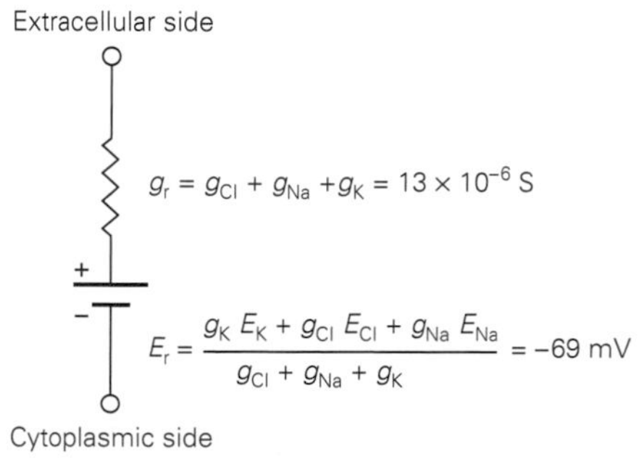

Figure 6–14 The Na^+, K^+, and Cl^- resting channels can be represented together by a single conductance and battery. The total resting membrane conductance (g_r) and the electromotive force or battery (E_r) give the resting potential determined by Equation 6–4.

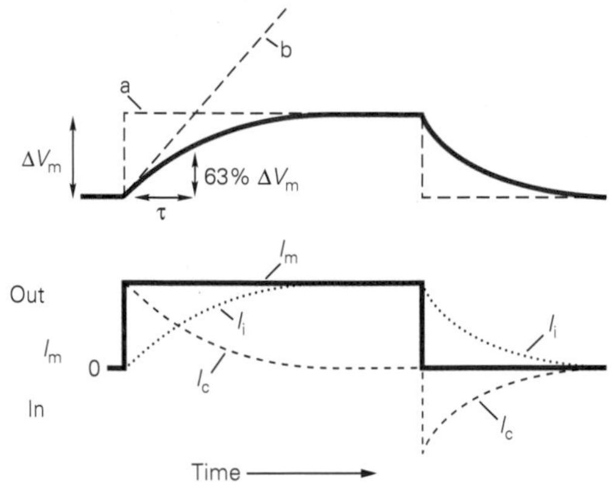

Figure 6–15 The rate of change in the membrane potential is slowed by the membrane capacitance. The upper plot shows the response of the membrane potential (ΔV_m) to a step current pulse (I_m). The shape of the actual voltage response (**red line**) combines the properties of a purely resistive element (**dashed line a**) and a purely capacitive element (**dashed line b**). The time taken to reach 63% of the final voltage defines the membrane time constant, τ. The lower plot shows the two elements of the total membrane current (I_m) during the current pulse: the ionic current (I_i) across the resistive elements of the membrane (ion channels) and the capacitive current (I_c).

membrane resistance and capacitance (R_mC_m). The time constant can be measured experimentally as the time it takes the membrane potential to rise to $1 - 1/e$, or approximately 63% of its steady-state value (Figure 6–15, upper plot). Typical values of τ for neurons range from 20 to 50 ms. We shall return to the time constant in Chapter 10 where we consider the temporal summation of synaptic inputs in a cell.

Membrane and Axoplasmic Resistance Affect the Efficiency of Signal Conduction

So far we have considered the effects of the passive properties of neurons on signaling only within the cell body. Distance is not a factor in the propagation of a signal in the neuron's soma because the cell body can be approximated as a tiny sphere whose membrane voltage is uniform. However, a subthreshold voltage signal traveling along extended structures such as dendrites, axons, and muscle fibers decreases in amplitude with distance from the site of initiation. To understand how this attenuation occurs, we will consider how the geometry of a neuron influences the distribution of current.

If current is injected into a dendrite at one point, how will the membrane potential change along the length of the dendrite? For simplicity, consider how membrane potential varies with distance after a constant-amplitude current pulse has been on for some time ($t \gg \tau$). Under these conditions the membrane capacitance is fully charged, so membrane potential reaches a steady value. The variation of the potential with distance thus depends solely on the relative values of the *membrane resistance* in a unit length of dendrite, r_m (units of $\Omega \cdot$ cm), and the *axial resistance* per unit length of dendrite, r_a (units of Ω/cm). The change in membrane potential becomes smaller with distance along the dendrite away from the current electrode (Figure 6–16A). This decay with distance is exponential and expressed by

$$\Delta V(x) = \Delta V_0 e^{-x/\lambda},$$

where λ is the membrane *length constant*, x is the distance from the site of current injection, and ΔV_0 is the change in membrane potential produced by the current at the site of injection ($x = 0$). The length

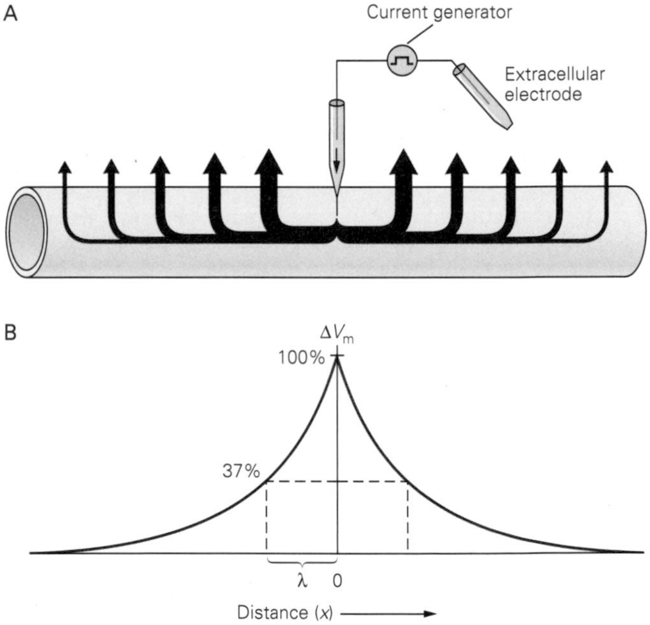

Figure 6–16 The change in membrane potential along a neuronal process during electrotonic conduction decreases with distance.

A. Current injected into a neuronal process by a microelectrode follows the path of least resistance to the return electrode in the extracellular fluid. (The thickness of the arrows represents the magnitude of membrane current.)

B. The change in V_m decays exponentially with distance from the site of current injection. The distance at which ΔV_m has decayed to 37% of its value at the point of current injection defines the length constant, λ.

constant is the distance along the dendrite to the site where ΔV_m has decayed to $1/e$, or 37% of its initial value (Figure 6–16B). It is a measure of the efficiency of electrotonic conduction, the passive spread of voltage changes along the neuron, and is determined by the values of membrane and axial resistance as follows:

$$\lambda = \sqrt{(r_m / r_a)}.$$

The better the insulation of the membrane (that is, the greater r_m) and the better the conducting properties of the inner core (the lower r_a), the greater the length constant of the dendrite. That is because current is able to spread farther along the inner conductive core of the dendrite before leaking across the membrane at some point x to alter the local membrane potential:

$$\Delta V(x) = i(x) \cdot r_m.$$

The length constant is also a function of the diameter of the neuronal process. Neuronal processes vary greatly in diameter, from as much as 1 mm for the squid giant axon to 1 μm for fine dendritic branches in the mammalian brain. For neuronal processes with similar ion channel densities (number of channels per unit membrane area) and cytoplasmic composition, the larger the diameter, the longer the length constant. Thus thicker axons and dendrites have longer length constants than do narrower processes and hence can transmit passive electrical signals for greater distances. Typical values for neuronal length constants range from 0.1 to 1.0 mm.

To understand how the diameter affects the length constant, we must consider how the diameter (or radius) of a process affects r_m and r_a. Both r_m and r_a are measures of resistance for a unit length of a neuronal process of a given radius. The axial resistance r_a of the process depends inversely on the number of charge carriers (ions) in a cross section of the process. Therefore, given a fixed cytoplasmic ion concentration, r_a depends inversely on the cross sectional area of the process, $1/(\pi \cdot \text{radius}^2)$. The resistance of a unit length of membrane r_m depends inversely on the total number of channels in a unit length of the neuronal process. Channel density, the number of channels per μm^2 of membrane, is often similar among different-sized processes. As a result, the number of channels per unit length of a neuronal process increases in direct proportion to increases in membrane area, which depends on the circumference of the process times its length; therefore, r_m varies as $1/(2 \cdot \pi \cdot \text{radius})$. Because r_m/r_a varies in direct proportion to the radius of the process, the length constant is proportional to the square root of the radius.

The efficiency of electrotonic conduction has two important effects on neuronal function. First, it influences spatial summation, the process by which synaptic potentials generated in different regions of the neuron are added together at the trigger zone at the axon hillock (see Chapter 10). Second, electrotonic conduction is a factor in the propagation of the action potential. Once the membrane at any point along an axon has been depolarized beyond threshold, an action potential is generated in that region. This local depolarization spreads passively down the axon, causing successive adjacent regions of the membrane to reach the threshold for generating an action potential (Figure 6–17). Thus the depolarization spreads along the length of the axon by local current driven by the difference in potential between the active and resting regions of the axon membrane. In axons with longer length constants local current spreads a greater distance down the axon, and therefore the action potential propagates more rapidly.

Large Axons Are More Easily Excited Than Small Axons

The influence of axonal geometry on action potential conduction plays an important role in a common neurological exam. In the examination of a patient for diseases of peripheral nerves, the nerve often is stimulated by passing current between a pair of external cutaneous electrodes placed over the nerve, and the population of resulting action potentials (the *compound action potential*) is recorded farther along the nerve by a second pair of cutaneous voltage-recording electrodes. In this situation the total number of axons that generate action potentials varies with the amplitude of the current pulse.

To drive a cell to threshold, a stimulating current from the positive electrode must pass through the cell membrane into the axon. There it travels along the axoplasmic core, eventually exiting the axon into the extracellular fluid through the membrane to reach the second (negative) electrode. However, most of the stimulating current does not even enter the axon, moving instead through neighboring axons or through the low-resistance pathway of the extracellular fluid. Thus, the axons into which current enters most easily are the most excitable.

In general, axons with the largest diameter have the lowest threshold for excitation. The greater the diameter of the axon, the lower the axial resistance to the flow of current down the axon because the number of charge carriers (ions) per unit length of the axon is greater. Because more current enters the larger axon, the axon is depolarized more efficiently than a smaller

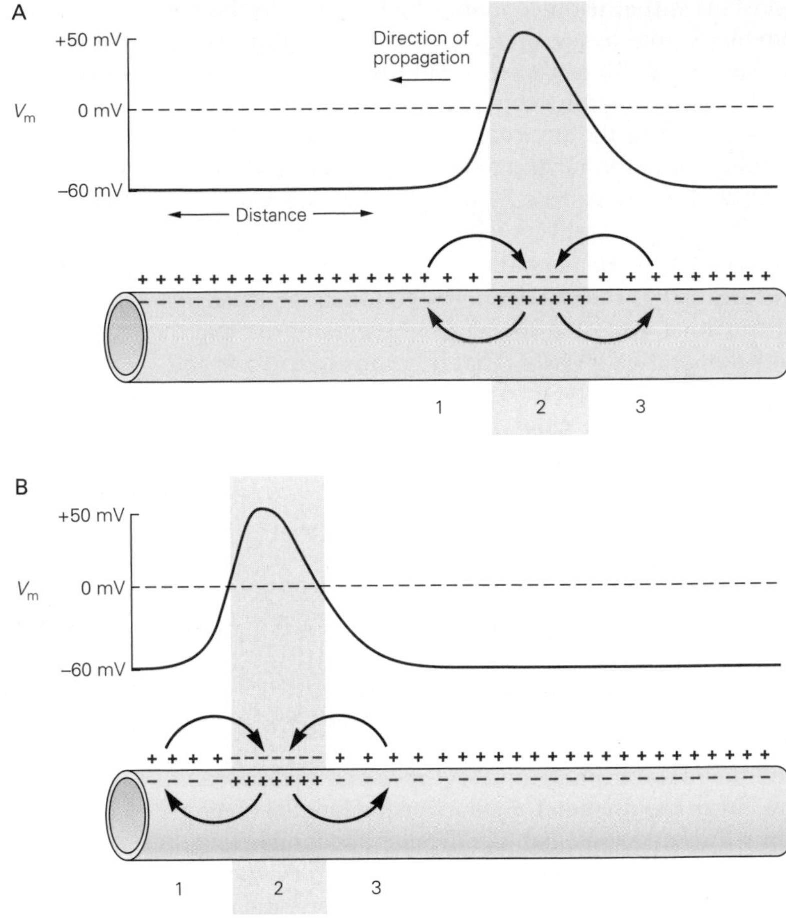

Figure 6–17 Electrotonic conduction contributes to propagation of the action potential.

A. An action potential propagating from right to left causes a difference in membrane potential in two adjacent regions of the axon. The difference creates a local-circuit current that causes the depolarization to spread passively. Current spreads from the more positive active region (**2**) to the less positive resting region *ahead* of the action potential (**1**), as well as to the less positive area *behind* the action potential (**3**). However, because there is also an increase in membrane K^+ conductance in the wake of the action potential (see Chapter 7), the buildup of positive charge along the inner side of the membrane in area 3 is more than balanced by the local efflux of K^+, allowing this region of membrane to repolarize.

B. A short time later, the action potential has traveled down the axon and the process can be repeated.

axon. For these reasons, larger axons are recruited at low values of current; axons with smaller diameter are recruited only at relatively greater current strengths.

The fact that larger axons conduct more rapidly and have a lower current threshold for excitation aids in the interpretation of clinical nerve-stimulation tests. Neurons that convey different types of information (eg, motor versus sensory) often differ in axon diameter and thus conduction velocity (see Table 22–1). In addition, a specific disease process may preferentially affect a subset of the functional classes of axons. Thus, using conduction velocity as a criterion to determine which classes of axons have defective conduction properties can help one infer the neuronal basis for the neurological deficit.

Passive Membrane Properties and Axon Diameter Affect the Velocity of Action Potential Propagation

The passive spread of depolarization during conduction of the action potential is not instantaneous. In fact, electrotonic conduction is a rate-limiting factor in the propagation of the action potential. We can understand this limitation by considering a simplified equivalent circuit of two adjacent segments of axon membrane connected by a segment of axoplasm.

An action potential generated in one segment of membrane supplies depolarizing current to the adjacent membrane, causing it to depolarize gradually toward threshold (see Figure 6–17). According to Ohm's law, the larger the axoplasmic resistance, the smaller the current between adjacent membrane segments ($I = V/R$) and thus the longer it takes to change the charge on the membrane of the adjacent segment.

Recall that, since $\Delta V = \Delta Q/C$, the membrane potential changes slowly if the current is small because ΔQ, equal to current multiplied by time, changes slowly. Similarly, the larger the membrane capacitance, the more charge must be deposited on the membrane to change the potential across the membrane, so the current must flow for a longer time to produce a given depolarization. Therefore, the time it takes for depolarization to spread along the axon is determined by both the axial resistance r_a and the capacitance per unit length of the axon c_m (units F/cm). The rate of passive spread varies inversely with the product $r_a c_m$. If this product is reduced, the rate of passive spread increases and the action potential propagates faster.

Rapid propagation of the action potential is functionally important, and two adaptive strategies have evolved to increase it. One is an increase in the diameter of the axon core. Because r_a decreases in proportion to the square of axon diameter, whereas c_m increases in direct proportion to diameter, the net effect of an increase in diameter is a decrease in $r_a c_m$. This adaptation has been carried to an extreme in the giant axon of the squid, which can reach a diameter of 1 mm. No larger axons have evolved, presumably because of the competing need to keep neuronal size small so that many cells can be packed into a limited space.

The second strategy to increase conduction velocity is the wrapping of a myelin sheath around an axon (see Chapter 4). This process is functionally equivalent to increasing the thickness of the axonal membrane by as much as 100 times. Because the capacitance of a parallel-plate capacitor such as the membrane is inversely proportional to the thickness of the insulation material (see Appendix A), myelination decreases c_m and thus $r_a c_m$. Myelination results in a proportionately much greater decrease in $r_a c_m$ than does the same increase in the diameter of the axon core because the many layers of membrane wrapped in the myelin sheath produce a very large decrease in c_m. For this reason, conduction in myelinated axons is faster than in nonmyelinated axons of the same diameter.

In a neuron with a myelinated axon the action potential is triggered at the nonmyelinated initial segment of membrane just distal to the axon hillock. The inward current that flows through this region of membrane is available to discharge the capacitance of the myelinated axon ahead of it. Even though the capacitance of the axon is quite small (because of the myelin insulation), the amount of current down the core of the axon from the trigger zone is not enough to discharge the capacitance along the *entire* length of the myelinated axon.

To prevent the action potential from dying out, the myelin sheath is interrupted every 1 to 2 mm by bare patches of axon membrane approximately 1 μm in length, the nodes of Ranvier (see Chapter 4). Although the area of membrane at each node is quite small, the nodal membrane is rich in voltage-gated Na^+ channels and thus can generate an intense depolarizing inward Na^+ current in response to the passive spread of depolarization down the axon. These regularly distributed nodes thus boost the amplitude of the action potential periodically, preventing it from decaying with distance.

The action potential, which spreads quite rapidly along the internode because of the low capacitance of the myelin sheath, slows down as it crosses the high-capacitance region of each bare node. Consequently, as the action potential moves down the axon it jumps quickly from node to node (Figure 6–18A). For this reason, the action potential in a myelinated axon is said to move by *saltatory conduction* (from the Latin *saltare,* to jump). Because ionic membrane current flows only at the nodes in myelinated fibers, saltatory conduction is also favorable from a metabolic standpoint. Less energy must be expended by the Na^+-K^+ pump in restoring the Na^+ and K^+ concentration gradients, which tend to run down as the action potential is propagated.

Various diseases of the nervous system are caused by demyelination, such as multiple sclerosis and Guillain-Barré syndrome. As an action potential goes from a myelinated region to a bare stretch of demyelinated axon, it encounters a region of relatively high c_m and low r_m. The inward current generated at the node just before the demyelinated segment may be too small to provide the capacitive current required to depolarize the segment of demyelinated membrane to threshold. In addition, this local-circuit current does not spread as far as it normally would because it is flowing into a segment of axon that has a short length constant because of its low r_m (Figure 6–18B). These two factors can combine to slow, and in some cases actually block, the conduction of action potentials, causing devastating effects on behavior (see Chapter 7).

An Overall View

The lipid bilayer, which is virtually impermeant to ions, is an insulator separating two conducting solutions, the cytoplasm and the extracellular fluid. Ions can cross the lipid bilayer only by passing through ion channels in the cell membrane. When the cell is at rest, passive ionic fluxes into and out of the cell are balanced, so the charge separation across the membrane remains constant and the membrane potential is maintained at its resting value.

The value of the resting membrane potential in nerve cells is determined primarily by resting channels that conduct K^+, Cl^-, and Na^+. In general, the membrane potential is closest to the equilibrium (Nernst) potential of the ion (or ions) with the greatest membrane

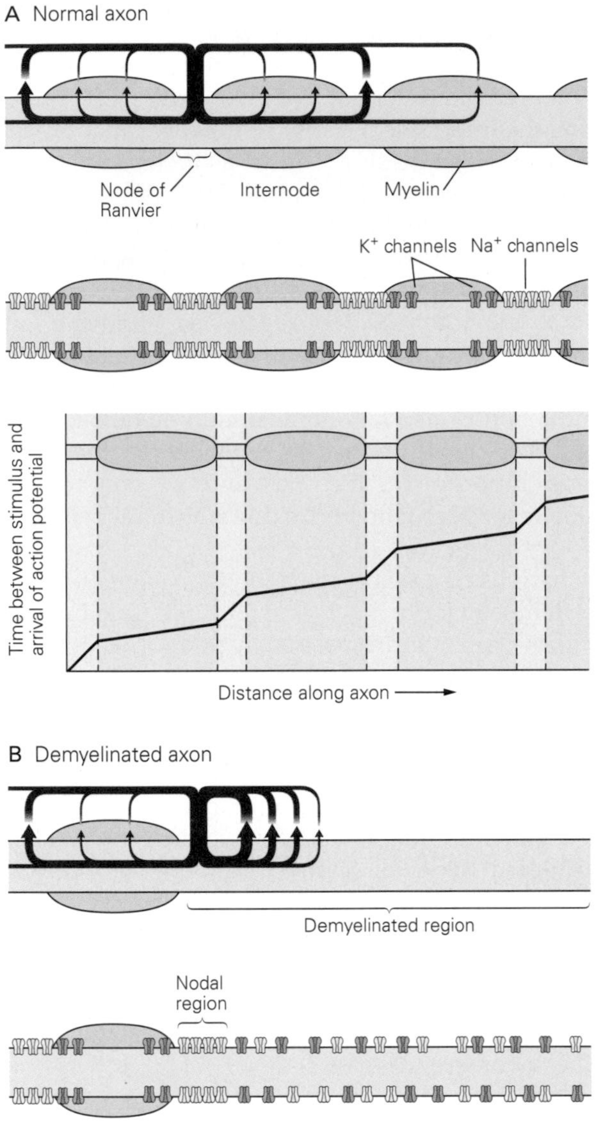

Figure 6–18 Action potentials in myelinated nerves are regenerated at the nodes of Ranvier.

A. The densities of capacitive and ionic membrane currents (membrane current per unit area of membrane) are much higher at the nodes of Ranvier than in the internodal regions. (In the figure the density of membrane current at any point along the axon is represented by the thickness of the arrows.) Because of the higher capacitance of the axon membrane at the nodes, the action potential slows down as it approaches each node and thus appears to skip rapidly from node to node as it propagates from left to right.

B. In regions of the axon that have lost their myelin, the spread of the action potential is slowed down or blocked. The local-circuit currents must discharge a larger membrane capacitance and, because of the shorter length constant (caused by the low membrane resistance in demyelinated stretches of axon), they do not spread well down the axon.

permeability. The permeability of a cell membrane for an ion species is proportional to the number of open channels that allow passage of that ion.

The resting membrane potential is close to the Nernst potential for K^+, the ion to which the membrane is most permeable. The membrane is also somewhat permeable to Na^+, however, and therefore an influx of Na^+ shifts the membrane potential slightly positive to the K^+ Nernst potential. At this potential the electrical and chemical driving forces acting on K^+ are no longer in balance, so K^+ diffuses out of the cell. The passive fluxes of K^+ and Na^+ are each counterbalanced by active fluxes driven by the Na^+-K^+ pump.

Chloride is actively transported out of most but not all neurons in the adult nervous system. When it is not, it is passively distributed so as to be at equilibrium inside and outside the cell. Under most physiological conditions the bulk concentrations of Na^+, K^+, and Cl^- inside and outside the cell are constant. Changes in membrane potential that generate neuronal signals (action potentials, synaptic potentials, and receptor potentials) are caused by substantial changes in the membrane's relative permeabilities to these three ions. These changes in permeability, caused by the opening of gated ion channels, change the net charge separation across the membrane, but produce only negligible changes in the bulk concentrations of ions.

Two competing requirements determine the functional design of neurons. First, to maximize the computing power of the nervous system, neurons must be small so that large numbers of them can fit into the brain and spinal cord. Second, to maximize the ability of the animal to respond to changes in its environment, neurons must conduct signals rapidly. These two adaptive features are constrained by the materials from which neurons are made.

Because the nerve cell membrane is thin and surrounded by two conducting media, it has a high capacitance. In addition, the currents that change the charge on the membrane capacitance along the length of an axon or dendrite flow through a relatively poor conductor—a thin column of cytoplasm. These two factors combine to slow down the conduction of voltage signals. Moreover, the various ion channels that are open at rest and that give rise to the resting potential also degrade the signaling function of the neuron, as they make the cell leaky and limit how far a signal can travel passively.

To compensate for these physical constraints neurons use voltage-gated channels to generate action potentials. The action potential is continually regenerated along the axon and thus conducted without attenuation. For pathways in which rapid signaling is particularly important, conduction of the action potential is enhanced by either myelination of the axon or an increase in axon diameter, or by both.

John Koester
Steven A. Siegelbaum

Selected Readings

Finkelstein A, Mauro A. 1977. Physical principles and formalisms of electrical excitability. In: ER Kandel (ed). *Handbook of Physiology: A Critical, Comprehensive Presentation of Physiological Knowledge and Concepts.* Sect. 1, *The Nervous System.* Vol. 1, *Cellular Biology of Neurons,* Part 1, pp. 161–213. Bethesda, MD: American Physiological Society.

Hille B. 2001. *Ionic Channels of Excitable Membranes,* 3rd ed. Sunderland, MA: Sinauer.

Hodgkin AL. 1992. *Chance and Design.* Cambridge: Cambridge Univ. Press.

Hodgkin AL. 1964. Saltatory conduction in myelinated nerve. In: *The Conduction of the Nervous Impulse. The Sherrington Lecture, VII,* pp. 47–55. Liverpool: Liverpool University Press.

Jack JB, Noble D, Tsien RW. 1975. Chapters 1, 5, 7, and 9. In: *Electric Current Flow in Excitable Cells,* pp. 1–4, 83–97, 131–224, 276–277. Oxford: Clarendon.

Johnston D, Wu M-S. 1995. Functional properties of dendrites. In: *Foundations of Cellular Neurophysiology,* pp. 55–120. Cambridge, MA: MIT Press.

Koch C. 1999. *Biophysics of Computation,* pp. 25–48. New York: Oxford Univ. Press.

Moore JW, Joyner RW, Brill MH, Waxman SD, Najar-Joa M. 1978. Simulations of conduction in uniform myelinated fibers: relative sensitivity to changes in nodal and internodal parameters. Biophys J 21:147–160.

Rall W. 1977. Core conductor theory and cable properties of neurons. In: ER Kandel (ed). *Handbook of Physiology: A Critical, Comprehensive Presentation of Physiological Knowledge and Concepts,* Sect. 1. *The Nervous System,* Vol. 1, *Cellular Biology of Neurons,* Part 1, pp. 39–97. Bethesda, MD: American Physiological Society.

References

Bernstein J. [1902] 1979. Investigations on the thermodynamics of bioelectric currents. Pflügers Arch 92:521–562. Translated in: GR Kepner (ed). *Cell Membrane Permeability and Transport,* pp. 184–210. Stroudsburg, PA: Dowden, Hutchinson & Ross.

De Koninck Y. 2007. Altered chloride homeostasis in neurological disorders: a new target. Curr Opin Pharmacol 7:93-99.

Gadsby DC. 2009. Ion channels versus ion pumps: the principal difference, in principle. Nat Rev Mol Cell Biol 10:344–352.

Goldman DE. 1943. Potential, impedance, and rectification in membranes. J Gen Physiol 27:37–60.

Hodgkin AL, Katz B. 1949. The effect of sodium ions on the electrical activity of the giant axon of the squid. J Physiol 108:37–77.

Hodgkin AL, Rushton WAH. 1946. The electrical constants of a crustacean nerve fibre. Proc R Soc Lond Ser B 133:444–479.

Huxley AF, Stämpfli R. 1949. Evidence for saltatory conduction in peripheral myelinated nerve fibres. J Physiol 108:315–339.

Jorgensen PL, Hakansson KO, Karlish SJ. 2003. Structure and mechanism of Na,K-ATPase: functional sites and their interactions. Annu Rev Physiol 65:817–849.

Lytton J. 2007. Na^+/Ca^{2+} exchangers: three mammalian gene families control Ca^{2+} transport. Biochem J 406:365–382.

Nernst W. [1888] 1979. Zur Kinetik der in Lösung befindlichen Körper. [On the kinetics of substances in solution.] Z Physik Chem 2:613–622, 634–637. Translated in: GR Kepner (ed). *Cell Membrane Permeability and Transport,* pp. 174–183. Stroudsburg, PA: Dowden, Hutchinson & Ross.

Orkand RK. 1977. Glial cells. In: ER Kandel (ed). *Handbook of Physiology: A Critical, Comprehensive Presentation of Physiological Knowledge and Concepts,* Sect. 1, *The Nervous System,* Vol. 1, *Cellular Biology of Neurons,* Part 2 pp. 855–875. Bethesda, MD: American Physiological Society.

Siegel GJ, Agranoff BW, Albers RW (eds). 1999. *Basic Neurochemistry: Molecular, Cellular, and Medical Aspects,* 6th ed. Philadelphia: Lippincott-Raven.

Stokes DL, Green NM. 2003. Structure and function of the calcium pump. Annu Rev Biophys Biomol Struct 32: 445–468.

7

Propagated Signaling: The Action Potential

NERVE CELLS ARE ABLE TO CARRY electrical signals over long distances because the long-distance signal, the action potential, is continually regenerated and thus does not attenuate as it moves down the axon. In Chapter 6 we saw how an action potential arises from sequential changes in the membrane's permeability to Na^+ and K^+ ions. We also considered how the membrane's passive properties influence the speed at which action potentials are conducted. In this chapter we focus on the voltage-gated ion channels that are critical for generating and propagating action potentials and consider how these channels are responsible for many important features of a neuron's electrical excitability.

Action potentials have four properties important for neuronal signaling. First, they have a threshold for initiation. As we saw in Chapter 6, in many nerve cells the membrane behaves as a simple resistor in response to small hyperpolarizing or depolarizing current steps. The membrane voltage changes in a graded manner as a function of the size of the current step according to Ohm's law, $\Delta V = \Delta I \cdot R$ (in terms of conductance, $\Delta V = \Delta I / G$). However, as the size of the depolarizing current increases, eventually a threshold voltage is reached, typically at around –50 mV, at which point an action potential is generated (see Figure 6–2C). Second, the action potential is an all-or-none event. The size and shape of an action potential initiated by a large depolarizing current is the same as that of an action potential evoked by a current that just surpasses the threshold.[1] Third, the action potential is conducted without decrement. It has a self-regenerative feature that keeps the amplitude constant, even when it is conducted over great distances. Fourth, the action potential is followed by a refractory period. For a brief time after an action potential is generated, the neuron's ability to fire a second action potential is suppressed. The refractory period limits the frequency at which a nerve can fire action potentials, and thus limits the information-carrying capacity of the axon.

These four properties of the action potential—initiation threshold, all-or-none nature, conduction without decrement, and refractory period—are unusual for biological processes, which typically respond in a graded fashion to changes in the environment. Biologists were puzzled by these properties for almost 100 years after the action potential was first measured in the mid 1800s. Finally, in the late 1940s and early 1950s studies of the membrane properties of the giant axon of the squid by Alan Hodgkin, Andrew Huxley, and Bernard Katz provided the first quantitative insight into the mechanisms underlying the action potential.

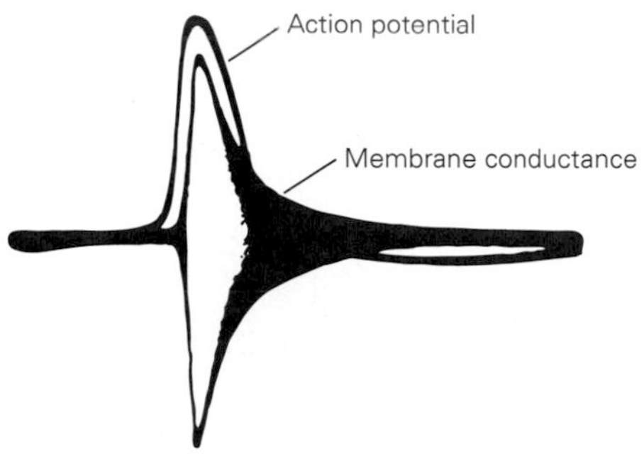

Figure 7–1 The action potential results from an increase in ionic conductance of the axon membrane. This historic recording from an experiment conducted in 1939 by Kenneth Cole and Howard Curtis shows the oscilloscope record of an action potential superimposed on a simultaneous record of membrane conductance.

The Action Potential Is Generated by the Flow of Ions Through Voltage-Gated Channels

An important early insight into how action potentials are generated came from an experiment performed by Kenneth Cole and Howard Curtis. While recording from the giant axon of the squid they found that ion conductance across the membrane increases dramatically during the action potential (Figure 7–1). This discovery provided the first evidence that the action potential results from changes in the flux of ions through channels in the membrane. It also raised two central questions: Which ions are responsible for the action potential, and how is the conductance of the membrane regulated?

A key insight into this problem was provided by Alan Hodgkin and Bernard Katz, who found that the amplitude of the action potential is reduced when the external Na^+ concentration is lowered, indicating that Na^+ influx is responsible for the rising phase of the action potential. They proposed that depolarization of the cell above threshold causes a brief increase in the cell membrane's permeability to Na^+, during which Na^+ permeability overwhelms the dominant K^+ permeability of the resting cell membrane, thereby driving the membrane potential towards E_{Na}. Their data also suggested that the falling phase of the action potential was caused by a later increase in K^+ permeability.

Sodium and Potassium Currents Through Voltage-Gated Channels Are Recorded with the Voltage Clamp

This insight of Hodgkin and Katz raised a further question. What mechanism is responsible for regulating the changes in the Na^+ and K^+ permeabilities of the membrane? Hodgkin and Andrew Huxley reasoned that the Na^+ and K^+ permeabilities were regulated directly by the membrane voltage. To test this hypothesis they systematically varied the membrane potential in the squid giant axon and measured the resulting changes in the conductance of voltage-gated Na^+ and K^+ channels. To do this they made use of a new apparatus, the voltage clamp, developed by Kenneth Cole.

Prior to the availability of the voltage-clamp technique, attempts to measure Na^+ and K^+ conductance as a function of membrane potential had been limited by the strong interdependence of the membrane potential and the gating of Na^+ and K^+ channels. For example, if the membrane is depolarized sufficiently to open some of the voltage-gated Na^+ channels, the influx of Na^+ through these channels causes further depolarization. The additional depolarization causes still more

[1]The all-or-none property describes an action potential that is generated under a specific set of conditions. The size and shape of the action potential *can* be affected by changes in membrane properties, ion concentrations, temperature, and other variables, as discussed later in the chapter.

Na^+ channels to open and consequently induces more inward Na^+ current:

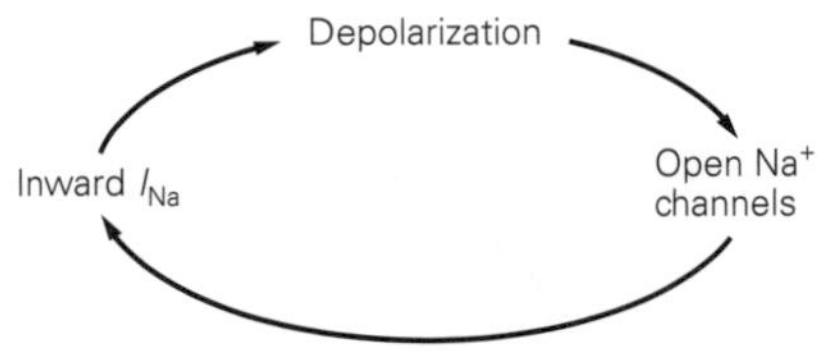

This positive feedback cycle, which eventually drives the membrane potential to the peak of the action potential, makes it impossible to achieve a stable membrane potential. A similar coupling between current and membrane potential complicates the study of the voltage-gated K^+ channels.

The voltage clamp interrupts the interaction between the membrane potential and the opening and closing of voltage-gated ion channels. It does so by adding or withdrawing a current from the axon that is equal to the current flowing through the voltage-gated membrane channels. In this way the voltage clamp prevents the membrane potential from changing. The amount of current that must be generated by the voltage clamp to keep the membrane potential constant provides a direct measure of the current flowing across the membrane (Box 7–1). Using the voltage-clamp

Box 7–1 Voltage-Clamp Technique

The voltage-clamp technique was developed by Kenneth Cole in 1949 to stabilize the membrane potential of neurons for experimental purposes. It was used by Alan Hodgkin and Andrew Huxley in the early 1950s in a series of experiments that revealed the ionic mechanisms underlying the action potential.

The voltage clamp permits the experimenter to "clamp" the membrane potential at predetermined levels, preventing changes in membrane current from influencing the membrane potential. By controlling the membrane potential one can measure the effect of changes in membrane potential on the membrane's conductance of individual ion species.

The voltage clamp consists of one intracellular and extracellular pair of electrodes used to measure the membrane potential and one intracellular and extracellular pair of electrodes used to pass current across the membrane (Figure 7–2). Through the use of a negative feedback amplifier, the voltage clamp is able to pass the correct amount of current across the cell membrane to rapidly step the membrane to a constant predetermined potential.

Depolarization opens voltage-gated Na^+ and K^+ channels, initiating movement of Na^+ and K^+ across the membrane. This change in membrane current ordinarily would change the membrane potential, but the voltage clamp maintains the membrane potential at a predetermined (commanded) level.

When Na^+ channels open in response to a moderate depolarizing voltage step, an inward ionic current develops because Na^+ ions are driven through these channels by their electrochemical driving force. This Na^+ influx would normally depolarize the membrane by increasing the positive charge on the inside of the membrane and reducing the positive charge on the outside.

The voltage clamp intervenes in this process by simultaneously withdrawing positive charges from the cell and depositing them in the external solution. By generating a current that is equal and opposite to the ionic current through the membrane, the voltage-clamp circuit automatically prevents the ionic current from changing the membrane potential from the commanded value. As a result, the *net* amount of charge separated by the membrane does not change and therefore no significant change in V_m can occur.

The voltage clamp is a negative feedback system. A negative feedback system is one in which the value of the output of the system (V_m in this case) is fed back as the input to a system and compared to a reference value (the command signal). Any difference between the command signal and the output signal activates a "controller" (the feedback amplifier in this case) that automatically reduces the difference. Thus the actual membrane potential automatically and precisely follows the command potential.

For example, assume that an inward Na^+ current through the voltage-gated Na^+ channels ordinarily causes the membrane potential to become more positive than the command potential. The input to the feedback amplifier is equal to ($V_{command} - V_m$). The amplifier generates an output voltage equal to this error signal multiplied by the gain of the amplifier. Thus, both the input and the resulting output voltage at the feedback amplifier will be negative.

This negative output voltage will make the internal current electrode negative, withdrawing net positive charge from the cell through the voltage-clamp circuit. As the current flows around the circuit, an equal amount of net positive charge will be deposited into the external solution through the other current electrode.

A refinement of the voltage clamp, the patch-clamp technique, allows the functional properties of single ion channels to be analyzed (see Box 5–1).

technique, Hodgkin and Huxley provided the first complete description of the ionic mechanisms underlying the action potential.

One advantage of the voltage clamp is that it readily allows the ionic and capacitive components of membrane current to be analyzed separately. As described in Chapter 6, the membrane potential V_m is proportional to the charge Q_m on the membrane capacitance C_m. When V_m is not changing, Q_m is constant, and no capacitive current ($\Delta Q_m/\Delta t$) flows. Capacitive current flows *only* when V_m is changing. Therefore when the membrane potential changes in response to a very rapid step of command potential, capacitive current flows only at the beginning and end of the step. Because the capacitive current is essentially instantaneous, the ionic currents that subsequently flow through the voltage-gated channels can be analyzed separately.

Measurements of these ionic currents can be used to calculate the voltage and time dependence of changes in membrane conductance caused by the opening and closing of Na^+ and K^+ channels. This information provides insights into the properties of these two types of channels.

A typical voltage-clamp experiment starts with the membrane potential clamped at its resting value. When a 10 mV depolarizing step is applied, a very brief outward current instantaneously discharges the

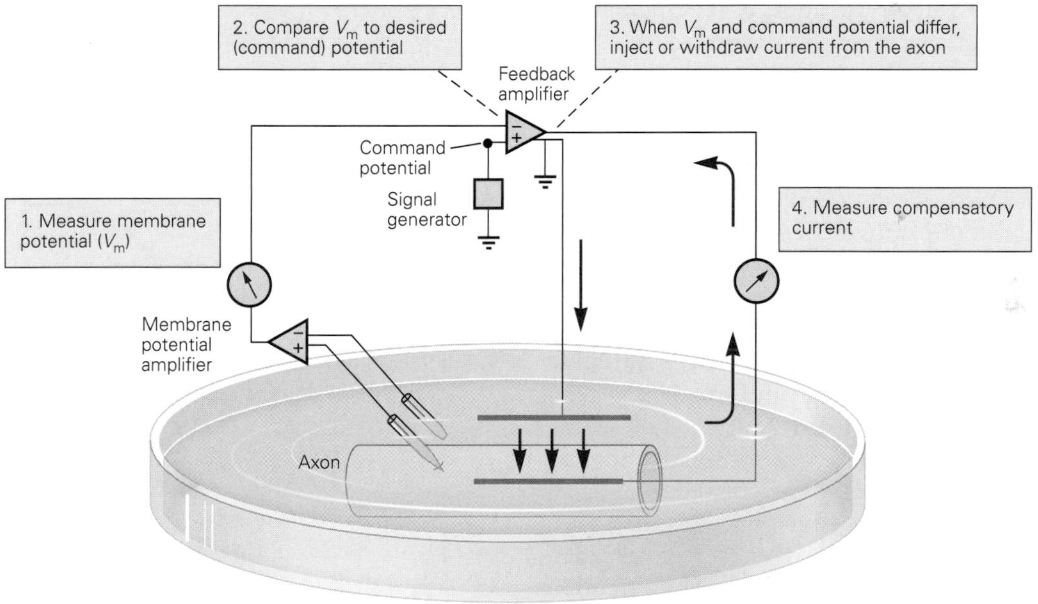

Figure 7–2 The negative feedback mechanism of the voltage clamp. Membrane potential (V_m) is measured by one amplifier connected to an intracellular electrode and an extracellular electrode in the bath. The membrane potential signal is displayed on an oscilloscope and is also fed into the negative terminal of the voltage-clamp feedback amplifier. The command potential, which is selected by the experimenter and can be of any desired amplitude and waveform, is fed into the positive terminal of the feedback amplifier. The feedback amplifier then subtracts the membrane potential from the command potential and amplifies any difference between these two signals. The voltage output of the amplifier is connected to the internal current electrode, a thin wire that runs the length of the axon core. The negative feedback ensures that the voltage output of the amplifier drives a current across the resistance of the current electrode that alters the membrane voltage to minimize any difference between V_m and the command potential. To accurately measure the current-voltage relationship of the cell membrane, the membrane potential must be uniform along the entire surface of the axon. This is made possible by the highly conductive internal current electrode, which short-circuits the axoplasmic resistance, reducing axial resistance to zero (see Chapter 6). This low-resistance pathway eliminates all variations in electrical potential along the axon core.

membrane capacitance by the amount required for a 10 mV depolarization. This capacitive current (I_c) is followed by a smaller outward current that persists for the duration of the voltage step. This steady ionic current flows through the nongated resting ion channels of the membrane, which we refer to here as *leakage channels* (see Box 6–2). The current through these channels is called the *leakage current*, I_l. The total conductance of this population of channels is called the *leakage conductance* (g_l). At the end of the step a brief inward capacitive current repolarizes the membrane to its initial voltage and the total membrane current returns to zero (Figure 7–3A).

If a large depolarizing step is commanded, the current record is more complicated. The capacitive and leakage currents both increase in amplitude. In addition, shortly after the end of the capacitive current and the start of the leakage current, an inward (negative) current develops; it reaches a peak within a few milliseconds, declines, and gives way to an outward current. This outward current reaches a plateau that is maintained for the duration of the voltage step (Figure 7–3B).

A simple interpretation of these results is that the depolarizing voltage step sequentially turns on two types of voltage-gated channels that select for two distinct ions. One type of channel conducts ions that generate an inward current, while the other conducts ions that generate an outward current. Because these two oppositely directed currents partially overlap in time, the most difficult task in analyzing voltage-clamp experiments is to determine their separate time courses.

Hodgkin and Huxley achieved this separation by changing ions in the bathing solution. By replacing Na^+ with a larger, impermeant cation (choline·H^+), they eliminated the inward Na^+ current. Later, the task of separating inward and outward currents was made easier by the discovery of drugs or toxins that selectively block the different classes of voltage-gated channels (Figure 7–4). Tetrodotoxin, a poison from a certain Pacific puffer fish, blocks the voltage-gated Na^+ channel with a very high potency in the nanomolar range of concentration. (Ingestion of only a few milligrams of tetrodotoxin from improperly prepared puffer fish, consumed as the Japanese sushi delicacy *fugu*, can be fatal.) The cation tetraethylammonium specifically blocks the squid axon voltage-gated K^+ channel.

When tetraethylammonium is applied to the axon to block the K^+ channels, the total membrane current (I_m) consists of I_c, I_l, and I_{Na}. The leakage conductance, g_l, is constant; it does not vary with V_m or with time. Therefore the leakage current I_l can be readily calculated and subtracted from I_m, leaving I_{Na} and I_c. Because

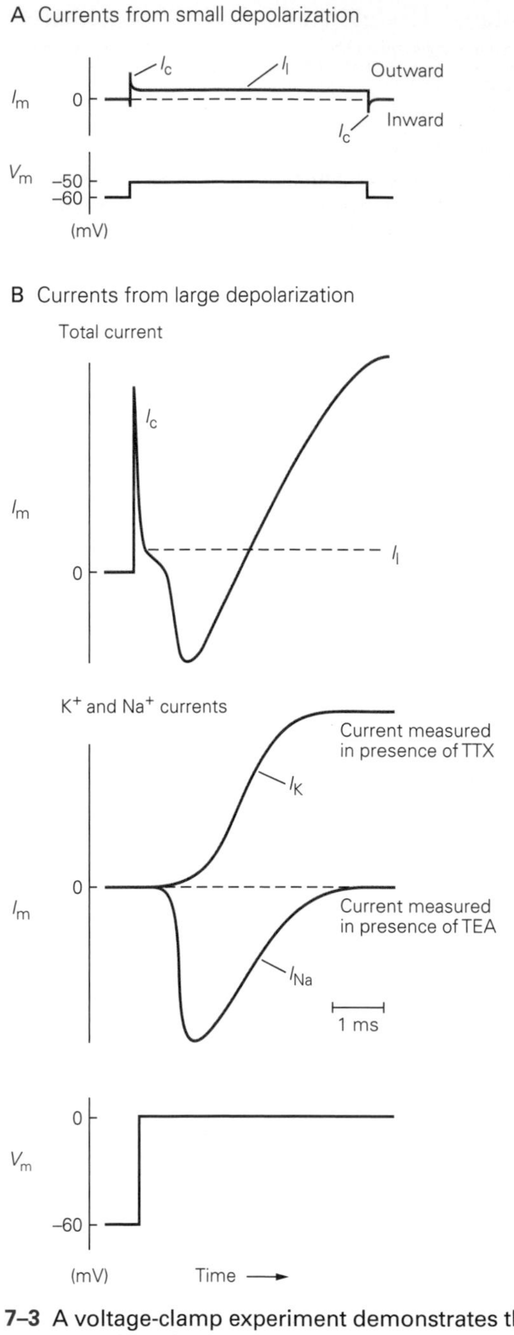

Figure 7–3 A voltage-clamp experiment demonstrates the sequential activation of two types of voltage-gated channels.

A. A small depolarization (10 mV) elicits capacitive and leakage currents (I_c and I_l, respectively), the components of the total membrane current (I_m).

B. A larger depolarization (60 mV) results in larger capacitive and leakage currents, plus a time-dependent inward ionic current followed by a time-dependent outward ionic current.

Top: Total (net) current in response to the depolarization. **Middle**: Individual Na^+ and K^+ currents. Depolarizing the cell in the presence of tetrodotoxin (TTX), which blocks the Na^+ current, or in the presence of tetraethylammonium (TEA), which blocks the K^+ current, reveals the pure K^+ and Na^+ currents (I_K and I_{Na}, respectively) after subtracting I_c and I_l. **Bottom**: Voltage step.

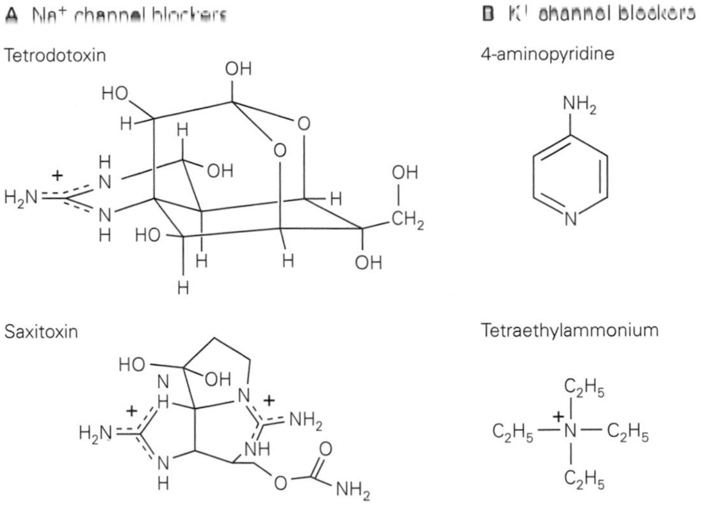

Figure 7–4 Drugs that block voltage-gated Na$^+$ and K$^+$ channels.

A. Tetrodotoxin and saxitoxin both bind to Na$^+$ channels with a very high affinity. Tetrodotoxin is produced by certain puffer fish, newts, and frogs. Saxitoxin is synthesized by the dinoflagellates *Gonyaulax*, which are responsible for red tides. Consumption of clams or other shellfish that have fed on the dinoflagellates during a red tide causes paralytic shellfish poisoning.

B. Tetraethylammonium is a cation that blocks certain voltage-gated K$^+$ channels with a relatively low affinity. The plus signs represent positive charge. 4-Aminopyridine is another blocker of K$^+$ channels. It is used to improve conduction of nerve impulses in patients with multiple sclerosis.

I_c occurs only briefly at the beginning and end of the pulse, it is easily isolated by visual inspection, revealing the pure I_{Na}. Similarly, I_K can be measured when the Na$^+$ channels are blocked by tetrodotoxin (Figure 7–3B).

By stepping the membrane to a wide range of potentials, Hodgkin and Huxley were able to measure the Na$^+$ and K$^+$ currents over the entire voltage extent of the action potential (Figure 7–5). They found that the Na$^+$ and K$^+$ currents vary as a graded function of the membrane potential. As the membrane voltage is made more positive, the outward K$^+$ current becomes larger. The inward Na$^+$ current also becomes larger with increases in depolarization, up to a certain extent. However, as the voltage becomes more and more positive, the Na$^+$ current eventually declines in amplitude. When the membrane potential is +55 mV, the Na$^+$ current is zero. Positive to +55 mV, the Na$^+$ current reverses direction and becomes outward.

Hodgkin and Huxley explained this behavior by a very simple model in which the size of the Na$^+$ and K$^+$ currents is determined by two factors. The first is the magnitude of the Na$^+$ or K$^+$ conductance, g_{Na} or g_K, which reflects the number of Na$^+$ or K$^+$ channels open at any instant (see Chapter 6). The second factor is the electrochemical driving force on Na$^+$ ions ($V_m - E_{Na}$) or K$^+$ ions ($V_m - E_K$). The model is thus expressed as:

$$I_{Na} = g_{Na} \times (V_m - E_{Na})$$

$$I_K = g_K \times (V_m - E_K).$$

According to this model the amplitudes of I_{Na} and I_K change as the voltage is made more positive because there is an increase in g_{Na} and g_K. The Na$^+$ and K$^+$ conductances increase because the opening of the Na$^+$ and K$^+$ channels is voltage-dependent. The currents also change in response to changes in the electrochemical driving forces.

Both I_{Na} and I_K initially increase in amplitude as the membrane is made more positive because g_{Na} and g_K increase steeply with voltage. However, as the membrane potential approaches E_{Na} (+55 mV), I_{Na} declines because of the decrease in inward driving force, even though g_{Na} is large. That is, the positive membrane voltage now opposes the influx of Na$^+$ down its chemical concentration gradient. At +55 mV the chemical and electrical driving forces are in balance so there is no net I_{Na}, even though g_{Na} is quite large. As the membrane is made positive to E_{Na}, the driving force on Na$^+$ becomes positive. That is, the electrical driving force pushing Na$^+$ out is now greater than the chemical driving force pulling Na$^+$ in, and hence I_{Na} becomes outward. The behavior of I_K is simpler; because E_K is quite negative (–75 mV), both g_K and the outward driving force on K$^+$ become larger as the membrane is made more positive, thereby increasing the outward K$^+$ current.

Voltage-Gated Sodium and Potassium Conductances Are Calculated from Their Currents

From the two preceding equations Hodgkin and Huxley were able to calculate g_{Na} and g_K by dividing measured Na$^+$ and K$^+$ currents by the known Na$^+$ and K$^+$ electrochemical driving forces. Their results provide direct insight into how membrane voltage controls channel opening because the values of g_{Na} and g_K reflect the number of open Na$^+$ and K$^+$ channels (Box 7–2).

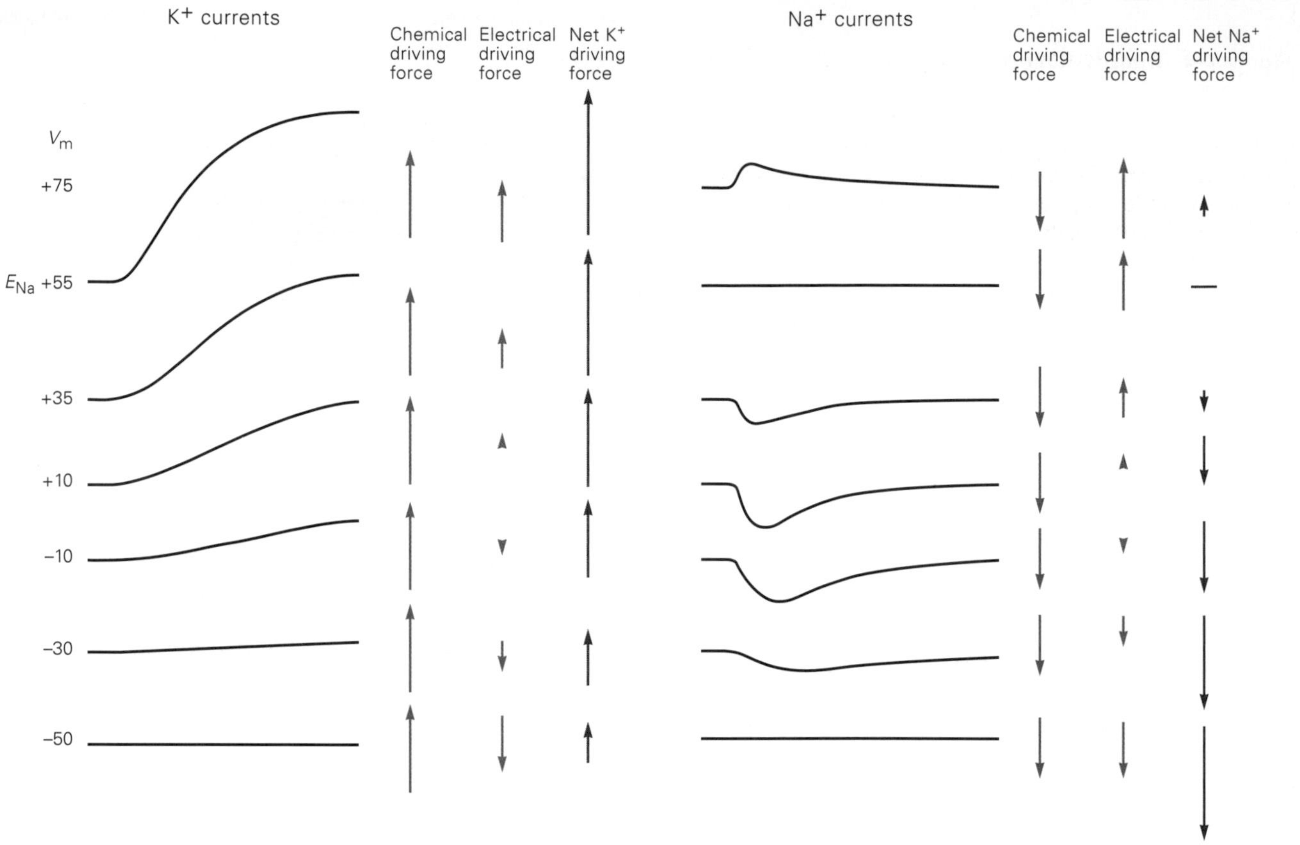

Figure 7–5 The magnitude and polarity of the Na^+ and K^+ membrane currents vary with the amplitude of membrane depolarization. Left: With progressive depolarization the voltage-clamped membrane K^+ current increases monotonically, because both g_K and $(V_m - E_K)$, the driving force for K^+, increase with increasing depolarization. The voltage during the depolarization is indicated at left. The direction and magnitude of the chemical (E_K) and electrical driving force on K^+, as well as the net driving force, is given by arrows at the right of each trace. (Up arrows = outward force; down arrows = inward force.)

Right: At first the Na^+ current becomes increasingly inward with increasing depolarization due to the increase in g_{Na}. However, as the membrane potential approaches E_{Na} (+55 mV) the magnitude of the inward Na^+ current begins to decrease due to the decrease in inward driving force $(V_m - E_{Na})$. Eventually, I_{Na} goes to zero when the membrane potential reaches E_{Na}. At depolarizations positive to E_{Na}, the sign of $(V_m - E_{Na})$ reverses, and I_{Na} becomes outward. Arrows at the right of each trace show chemical (E_{Na}) and electrical driving forces and net Na^+ driving force.

Measurements of g_{Na} and g_K at various levels of membrane potential reveal two functional similarities and two differences between the Na^+ and K^+ channels. Both types of channels open in response to depolarization. Also, as the size of the depolarization increases, the probability and rate of opening increase for both types of channels. The Na^+ and K^+ channels differ, however, in the rate at which they open and in their responses to prolonged depolarization. At all levels of depolarization the Na^+ channels open more rapidly than K^+ channels (Figure 7–7). When the depolarization is maintained for some time, the Na^+ channels begin to close, leading to a decrease of inward current. The process by which Na^+ channels close during a prolonged depolarization is termed *inactivation*.

Thus depolarization causes Na^+ channels to switch between three different states—resting, activated, or inactivated—which represent three different conformations of the Na^+ channel protein (see Figure 5–7). In contrast, squid axon K^+ channels do not inactivate; they remain open as long as the membrane is depolarized, at least for voltage-clamp depolarizations lasting up to tens of milliseconds (Figure 7–7).

In the inactivated state the Na^+ channel cannot be opened by further membrane depolarization. The inactivation can be reversed only by repolarizing the membrane to its negative resting potential, whereupon the channel switches to the resting state. This switch takes some time because channels leave the inactivated state relatively slowly (Figure 7–8).

Box 7–2 Calculation of Membrane Conductances from Voltage-Clamp Data

Membrane conductances can be calculated from voltage-clamp currents using equations derived from an equivalent circuit (Figure 7–6) that includes the membrane capacitance (C_m); the leakage conductance (g_l), representing the conductance of all of the resting (nongated) K^+, Na^+, and Cl^- channels (see Chapter 6); and g_{Na} and g_K, the conductances of the voltage-gated Na^+ and K^+ channels.

In the equivalent circuit the ionic battery of the leakage channels, E_l, is equal to the resting membrane potential, and g_{Na} and g_K are in series with their appropriate ionic batteries.

The current through each class of voltage-gated channel may be calculated from a modified version of Ohm's law that takes into account both the electrical (V_m) and chemical (E_{Na} or E_K) driving forces on Na^+ and K^+:

$$I_K = g_K(V_m - E_K)$$

and

$$I_{Na} = g_{Na}(V_m - E_{Na}).$$

Rearranging and solving for g gives two equations that can be used to compute the conductances of the active Na^+ and K^+ channel populations:

$$g_K = \frac{I_K}{(V_m - E_K)}$$

and

$$g_{Na} = \frac{I_{Na}}{(V_m - E_{Na})}.$$

In these equations the independent variable V_m is set by the experimenter. The dependent variables I_K and I_{Na} can be calculated from the records of voltage-clamp experiments (see Figure 7–5). The parameters E_K and E_{Na} can be determined empirically by finding the values of V_m at which I_K and I_{Na} reverse their polarities, that is, their *reversal potentials*.

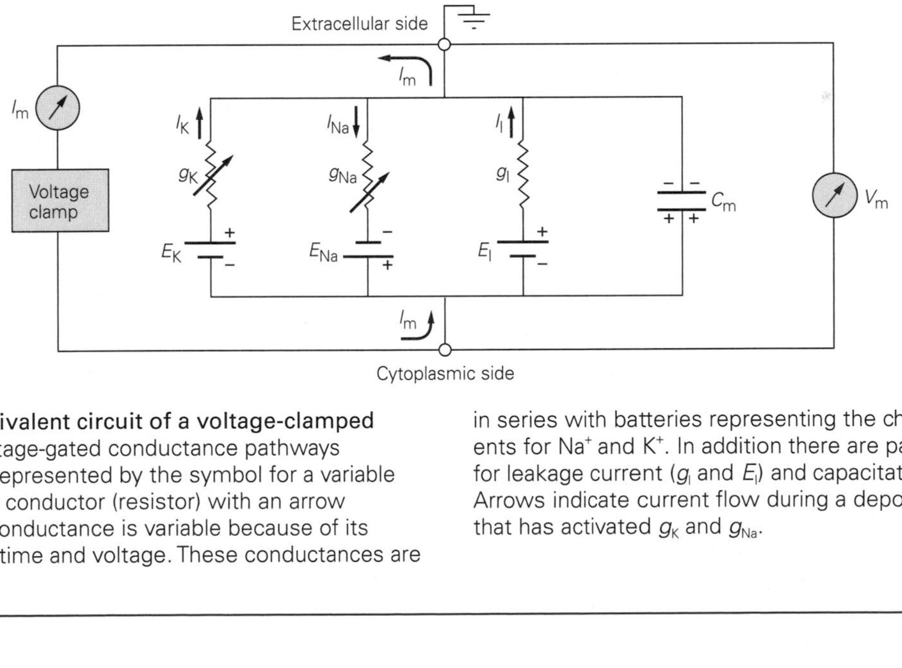

Figure 7–6 Equivalent circuit of a voltage-clamped neuron. The voltage-gated conductance pathways (g_K and g_{Na}) are represented by the symbol for a variable conductance—a conductor (resistor) with an arrow through it. The conductance is variable because of its dependence on time and voltage. These conductances are in series with batteries representing the chemical gradients for Na^+ and K^+. In addition there are parallel pathways for leakage current (g_l and E_l) and capacitative current (C_m). Arrows indicate current flow during a depolarizing step that has activated g_K and g_{Na}.

These variable, time-dependent effects of depolarization on g_{Na} are determined by the kinetics of two gating mechanisms in Na^+ channels. Each Na^+ channel has an *activation gate* that is closed while the membrane is at the resting potential and opened by depolarization. An *inactivation gate* is open at the resting potential and closes after the channel opens in response to depolarization. The channel conducts Na^+ only for the brief period during depolarization when *both* gates are open (Figure 7–9). Repolarization reverses the two processes, closing the activation gate and then opening the inactivation gate.

The Action Potential Can Be Reconstructed from the Properties of Sodium and Potassium Channels

Hodgkin and Huxley were able to fit their measurements of membrane conductance to a set of empirical equations that completely describe the Na^+ and K^+ conductances as a function of membrane potential and time. Using these equations and measured values for the passive properties of the axon, they computed the shape and conduction velocity of the action potential.

The calculated waveform of the action potential matched the waveform recorded in the unclamped axon almost perfectly. This close agreement indicates that the mathematical model developed by Hodgkin and Huxley accurately describes the properties of the channels that are essential for generating and propagating the action potential. More than a half-century later the Hodgkin-Huxley model stands as the most successful quantitative model in neural science if not in all of biology.

According to the Hodgkin-Huxley model an action potential involves the following sequence of events. Depolarization of the membrane causes Na^+ channels to open rapidly (an increase in g_{Na}), resulting in an inward Na^+ current. This current, by discharging the membrane capacitance, causes further depolarization, thereby opening more Na^+ channels, resulting in a further increase in inward current. This regenerative process drives the membrane potential toward E_{Na}, causing the rising phase of the action potential.[2]

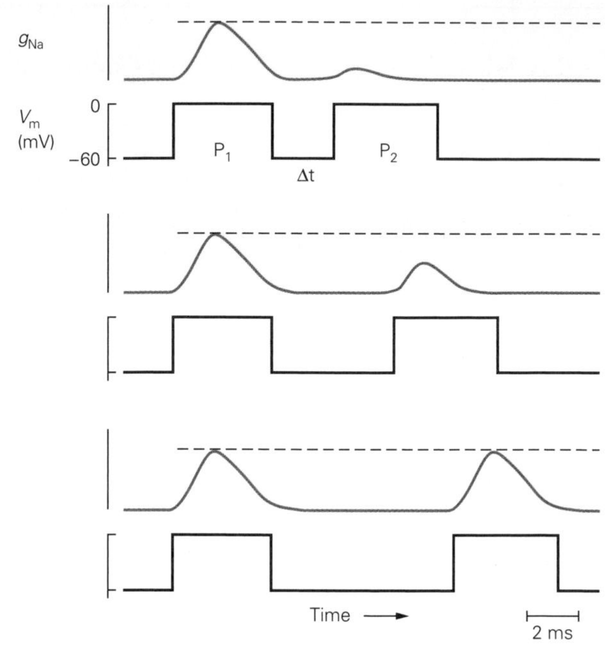

Figure 7–8 Sodium channels remain inactivated for a few milliseconds after a depolarizing current. If the interval (Δt) between two depolarizing pulses (P_1 and P_2) is brief, the second pulse produces a smaller increase in g_{Na} because many of the Na^+ channels remain inactivated after the first pulse. The longer the interval between pulses, the greater the increase in g_{Na} during the second pulse, because a greater fraction of channels will have recovered from inactivation during the period of repolarization and returned to the resting state when the second pulse begins. The time course of recovery from inactivation following repolarization contributes to determining the time course of the refractory period of an action potential.

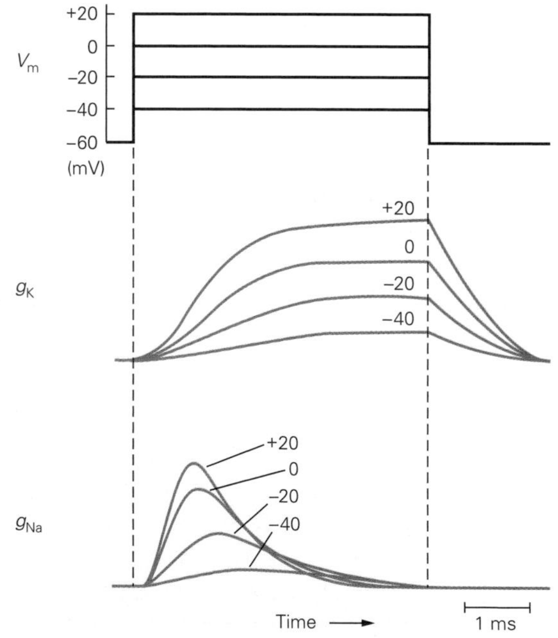

Figure 7–7 The responses of K^+ and Na^+ channels to prolonged depolarization. Increasing depolarizations elicit graded increases in K^+ and Na^+ conductance (g_{Na} and g_K), which reflect the proportional opening of thousands of voltage-gated K^+ and Na^+ channels. The Na^+ channels open more rapidly than the K^+ channels. During a maintained depolarization the Na^+ channels close after opening because of the closure of an inactivation gate. The K^+ channels remain open because they lack a fast inactivation process.

[2]It may at first seem inconsistent to say that current flows *outward* across the membrane when a cell is depolarized experimentally (see Figure 6–2C), while attributing the depolarization during the upstroke of the action potential to an *inward* Na^+ current. However, in both cases the current across the capacitance of the membrane (C_m) is actually outward. It is simply as a matter of convention that we describe the direction of current injected through a microelectrode as the direction in which the injected current leaves the cell across the membrane capacitance, whereas we describe the direction of the ionic membrane current as the direction of charge movement through the channels.

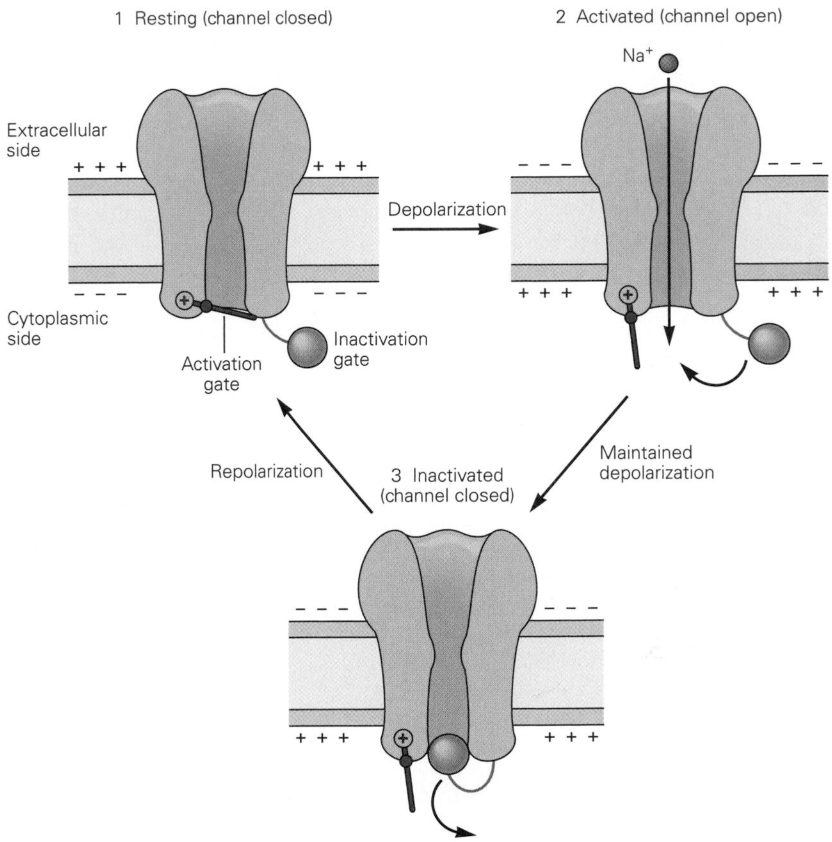

Figure 7–9 Voltage-gated Na^+ channels have two gates that respond in opposite ways to depolarization. In the resting state the activation gate is closed and the inactivation gate is open (**1**). A depolarizing stimulus results in opening of the activation gate, allowing Na^+ to flow through the channel, followed by closing of the inactivation gate (**2**). Once the inactivation gate has closed, the channel enters the inactivated state (**3**). On repolarization the inactivation gate opens and the activation gate closes as the channel returns to the resting state (**1**). The channel is only open during the brief period when both the activation and inactivation gates are open (**2**).

The depolarization limits the duration of the action potential in two ways: (1) It gradually inactivates the voltage-gated Na^+ channels, thus reducing g_{Na}, and (2) it opens, with some delay, the voltage-gated K^+ channels, thereby increasing g_K. Consequently, the inward Na^+ current is followed by an outward K^+ current that tends to repolarize the membrane (Figure 7–10).

In most nerve cells the action potential is followed by a hyperpolarizing *after-potential*, a transient shift of the membrane potential to values more negative than the resting potential. This brief negative change in V_m occurs because the K^+ channels that open during the repolarizing phase of the action potential remain open for some time after V_m has returned to its resting value. It takes a few milliseconds for all of the K^+ channels to return to the closed state. During this time, when the permeability of the membrane to K^+ is greater than during the resting state, V_m is slightly greater (more negative) than its normal resting value, resulting in a V_m closer to E_K (Figure 7–10).

The combined effect of this transient increase in K^+ conductance and the residual inactivation of the Na^+ channels (see Figure 7–10) underlies the *absolute refractory period*, the brief period of time following an action potential when it is impossible to elicit another action potential. As some K^+ channels begin to close and some Na^+ channels recover from inactivation, the membrane enters the *relative refractory period*, during which it is possible to trigger an action potential, but only by applying stimuli that are stronger than those normally required to reach threshold. Together, these refractory periods typically last just 5–10 ms.

Two features of the action potential predicted by the Hodgkin-Huxley model are its threshold and all-or-none behavior. A fraction of a millivolt can be the difference between a subthreshold stimulus and a stimulus that generates a full-sized action potential. This all-or-none phenomenon may seem surprising when one considers that g_{Na} increases in a strictly *graded* manner as depolarization increases (see Figure 7–7). Each increment of depolarization increases the number of voltage-gated Na^+ channels that open, thereby gradually increasing I_{Na}. How then can there be a discrete threshold for generating an action potential?

Although a small subthreshold depolarization increases the inward I_{Na}, it also increases two *outward*

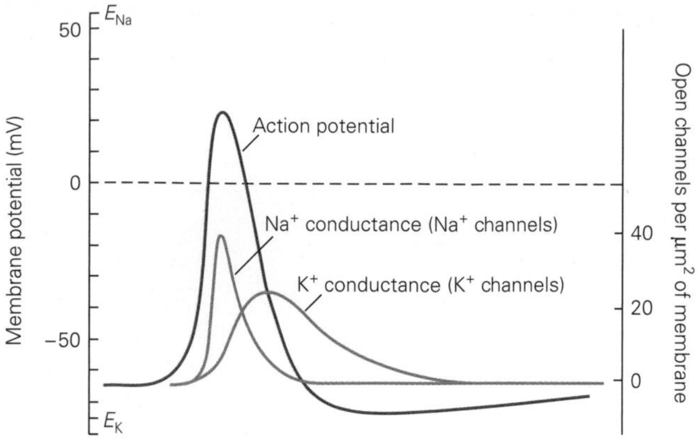

Figure 7–10 The sequential opening of voltage-gated Na^+ and K^+ channels generates the action potential. One of Hodgkin and Huxley's great achievements was to dissect the change in conductance during an action potential into separate components attributable to the opening of Na^+ and K^+ channels. The shape of the action potential and the underlying conductance changes can be calculated from the properties of the voltage-gated Na^+ and K^+ channels. (Adapted, with permission, from Hodgkin and Huxley 1952.)

currents, I_K and I_l, by increasing the electrochemical driving forces acting on K^+ and Cl^-. In addition, the depolarization augments g_K by gradually opening more voltage-gated K^+ channels (Figure 7–7). As the outward I_K and I_l increase with depolarization they repolarize the membrane and resist the depolarizing action of the Na^+ influx. However, because of the high voltage sensitivity and more rapid kinetics of activation of the Na^+ channels, the depolarization eventually reaches a point where the increase in inward I_{Na} exceeds the increase in outward I_K and I_l. At this point there is a net inward ionic current. This produces a further depolarization, opening even more Na^+ channels, so that the depolarization becomes regenerative, driving the membrane potential all the way to the peak of the action potential. The specific value of V_m at which the net ionic current ($I_{Na} + I_K + I_l$) just changes from outward to inward, depositing a net positive charge on the inside of the membrane capacitance, is the threshold.

Variations in the Properties of Voltage-Gated Ion Channels Expand the Signaling Capabilities of Neurons

The basic mechanism of electrical excitability identified by Hodgkin and Huxley in the squid giant axon appears to be universal in all excitable cells: Voltage-gated channels conduct an inward Na^+ current followed by an outward K^+ current. However, we now know that there are many types of voltage-gated Na^+ and K^+ channels encoded by families of related genes that are expressed in different nerve and muscle cells.

The biophysical properties of the various Na^+ and K^+ channels can differ both quantitatively and qualitatively from the channels characterized by Hodgkin and Huxley. Other gene families encode voltage-gated channels that select for Ca^{2+} ions or have mixed permeability to Na^+ and K^+. Moreover, the distribution of these channels can vary between different types of neurons, and can even vary as a function of locale within a single neuron. These differences in the pattern of ion channel expression have important consequences for membrane excitability, as we shall now explore.

The Nervous System Expresses a Rich Variety of Voltage-Gated Ion Channels

Voltage-gated Na^+ and K^+ channels similar to those described by Hodgkin and Huxley have been found in almost every type of neuron examined. In addition, most neurons contain voltage-gated Ca^{2+} channels that open in response to membrane depolarization. A strong electrochemical gradient drives Ca^{2+} into the cell, so these channels give rise to an inward I_{Ca} that helps depolarize the cell.

Some neurons and muscle cells have voltage-gated Cl^- channels that contribute to membrane repolarization. Many neurons have cation channels that are slowly activated by hyperpolarization (instead of the usual depolarization). These hyperpolarization-activated cation (or HCN) channels are permeable to both K^+ and Na^+ and have a reversal potential around −40 to −30 mV. As a result, they give rise to an inward depolarizing current, referred to as I_h, when the membrane repolarizes to negative resting potentials or becomes hyperpolarized during synaptic inhibition.

Each basic type of ion channel has many variants. For example, several types of voltage-activated K^+ channels differ in their kinetics of activation, voltage-activation range, and sensitivity to various ligands. Four of these variants are particularly important in the nervous system. (1) The slowly activating K^+ channel described by Hodgkin and Huxley is called the *delayed rectifier*. (2) The *calcium-activated K^+ channel* is activated by an increase in intracellular Ca^{2+} when nearby voltage-gated Ca^{2+} channels open in response to depolarization. One subclass of calcium-activated K^+ channels is voltage-dependent. However, in the absence of Ca^{2+} the channel requires very large, nonphysiological depolarization to open. The binding of Ca^{2+} to a site on the cytoplasmic surface of the channel shifts its voltage-gating to allow the channel to open at more negative potentials. (3) The *A-type K^+ channel* is activated rapidly by depolarization, almost as rapidly as the Na^+ channel; like the Na^+ channel, it also inactivates rapidly if the depolarization is prolonged. (4) The *M-type K^+ channel* requires only small depolarizations from the resting potential to open; however, it activates very slowly, requiring tens of milliseconds to open. One distinctive feature of the M-type channel is that it is *closed* by a neurotransmitter, acetylcholine.

Similarly, at least five major types of voltage-gated Ca^{2+} channels and eight types of voltage-gated Na^+ channels are expressed in the nervous system. Each of these major subtypes is encoded by a different gene and has several structural and functional variants that are generated through alternative splicing or by combining the pore-forming α-subunit with different types of auxiliary subunits.

The squid axon can generate an action potential with just two types of voltage-gated channels. Why then are so many types of voltage-gated ion channels found in the nervous system? The answer is that neurons with a greater variety of voltage-gated channels have much more complex information-processing abilities than those with only two types of channels. Some ways in which various voltage-gated channels influence neuronal function are described below.

Gating of Voltage-Sensitive Ion Channels Can Be Influenced by Various Cytoplasmic Factors

In a typical neuron the opening and closing of certain voltage-gated ion channels can be modulated by various cytoplasmic factors, thus affording the neuron's excitability properties greater flexibility. Changes in the levels of such cytoplasmic factors may result from the activity of the neuron itself or from the influences of other neurons.

Calcium concentration is one important cytoplasmic factor that modulates ion channel activity. The ionic current through membrane channels during an action potential generally does not result in appreciable changes in the intracellular concentrations of most ion species. Calcium is a notable exception to this rule. The concentration of free Ca^{2+} in the cytoplasm of a resting cell is extremely low, about 10^{-7} M, several orders of magnitude below the external Ca^{2+} concentration, which is approximately 2 mM. For this reason the intracellular Ca^{2+} concentration may increase many fold above its resting value as a result of the influx of Ca^{2+} through voltage-gated Ca^{2+} channels. The transient increase in Ca^{2+} concentration near the inside of the membrane enhances the probability that calcium-activated, voltage-sensitive K^+ channels will open. Some Ca^{2+} channels are themselves sensitive to levels of intracellular Ca^{2+}, becoming inactivated when incoming Ca^{2+} binds to their intracellular surface. Changes in the intracellular concentration of Ca^{2+} can also influence a variety of cellular metabolic processes, including neurotransmitter release and gene expression.

The activity of voltage-gated channels can also be regulated by the action of neurotransmitters through the recruitment of second-messenger pathways (see Chapter 11). These pathways can alter channel activity through a number of mechanisms, including direct phosphorylation of the intracellular domains of a channel or direct binding of cyclic nucleotides or membrane phosphoinositides to specialized binding domains in certain types of channels. As is true for the effects of Ca^{2+} binding, these pathways typically affect the kinetics or voltage sensitivity of channel gating rather than ion permeability of the open channel. The importance of cytoplasmic Ca^{2+} and other second messengers in the control of neuronal activity will become evident in many contexts throughout this book.

Excitability Properties Vary Between Regions of the Neuron

Different regions of a neuron have different types of ion channels that support the specialized functions of each region. The axon, for example, specializes in carrying signals faithfully over long distances; as such it functions as a relatively simple relay line. In contrast, the input, integrative, and output regions of a neuron (see Figure 2–9) typically perform more complex processing of the information they receive before passing it along.

Dendrites in many types of neurons have voltage-gated ion channels, including Ca^{2+}, K^+, HCN, and Na^+ channels. When activated, these channels help shape the amplitude, time course, and propagation of the synaptic potentials to the cell body. In some neurons action potentials may be propagated from the trigger zone at the initial segment of the axon back into the dendrites, thereby influencing synaptic integration in the dendrites. In other neurons the density of voltage-gated channels in the dendrites is sufficient to support the generation of a local action potential, which may then be conducted through the cell soma to the axon initial segment.

The trigger zone at the axon initial segment has the lowest threshold for action potential generation in part because it has an exceptionally high density of voltage-gated Na^+ channels. In addition, it typically has voltage-gated ion channels that are sensitive to relatively small deviations from the resting potential.

These channels thus play a critical role in the transformation of graded synaptic or receptor potentials into a train of all-or-none action potentials. Examples include the M-type and certain A-type K^+ channels, and a class of low voltage-activated Ca^{2+} channels (see below).

Conduction of the action potential down the axon is mediated primarily by voltage-gated Na^+ and K^+ channels that function much like those in the squid axon. In peripheral myelinated axons the mechanism of action potential repolarization at the nodes of Ranvier is particularly simple—the spike is terminated by fast inactivation of Na^+ channels combined with a large outward K^+ leakage current. Voltage-gated K^+ channels play a relatively minor role in action potential repolarization in these peripheral axons. In contrast, some central myelinated axons have significant numbers of voltage-gated K^+ channels at their nodes important for repolarization. Moreover, both central and peripheral myelinated axons have fairly high densities of K^+ channels under the myelin sheath near the two ends of each internodal segment. The normal function of these K^+ channels is to suppress any action potential that may be generated by axon membrane under the myelin sheath. In demyelinating diseases these channels become exposed and thus inhibit the ability of the bare axon to conduct action potentials (see Chapter 6).

Presynaptic nerve terminals at chemical synapses commonly have a high density of voltage-gated Ca^{2+} channels. Arrival of an action potential in the terminal opens these channels, causing an influx of Ca^{2+} that triggers transmitter release (Chapter 12).

Excitability Properties Vary Between Types of Neurons

Through the expression of a distinct complement of ion channels, the electrical properties of a neuron can be fine-tuned to match the dynamic demands of the information that it processes. Thus, although the function of a neuron is defined to a great extent by its synaptic inputs and outputs to other neurons, the excitability properties of the cell are also a critical factor in cell function.

Two aspects of excitability are important: (1) control of the shape of the action potential and (2) spike encoding, the process by which receptor potentials or synaptic potentials are converted into a temporal pattern of action potentials. Both of these features vary widely between different types of neurons. Of the voltage-gated channels, the K^+ channels exhibit the greatest functional diversity. Differences in K^+ channel expression are a key factor in determining the distinctive excitability properties of different classes of neurons.

How a neuron responds to synaptic input is determined by the proportions of different types of voltage-gated channels in the cell's input and integrative regions. For example, cells with different combinations of channels respond differently to a constant excitatory input. Some cells respond with only a single action potential, others with a train of action potentials at a constant rate of firing, and still others with either an accelerating or decelerating train of action potentials. The combined presence of certain voltage-gated Ca^{2+} channels and HCN channels generates pacemaker currents that allow some neurons to fire spontaneously in the absence of any external input (Figure 7–11D).

The firing rate of most neurons saturates as the strength of synaptic input increases, with a maximal rate that is not particularly high. However, certain classes of neurons have an unusually wide dynamic range and are able to fire at very high frequencies because of an unusually brief refractory period. This high firing rate is of particular importance in the auditory system, where neurons must respond to sound waves of very high frequencies. The short refractory period is caused, in part, by the expression in the auditory neurons of the voltage-gated K^+ channel Kv3, whose activation gates close extremely rapidly following repolarization, resulting in a very short hyperpolarizing after-potential.

Some types of synaptic inputs to a neuron modulate the function of voltage-gated channels and thereby modulate the cell's response to other inputs. For example, in some neurons a steady hyperpolarizing synaptic input makes the cell less excitable by reducing the extent of inactivation of the A-type K^+ channels that occurs at the normal resting potential of the cell. In other neurons such a steady hyperpolarization makes the cell *more* excitable because it reduces the inactivation of a particular class of voltage-gated Ca^{2+} channels. The firing properties of neurons can also be modulated by changing the function of certain voltage-gated ion channels, such as the M-type K^+ channels, through synaptic activation of second messengers (Figure 7–11A–C).

Although the action potentials in a neuron under constant conditions are constant in shape, action potential duration and amplitude can vary depending on intrinsic neuronal activity and extrinsic synaptic inputs. Such changes can be particularly prominent in the input and output regions of the neuron. The longer the duration of the action potential, the longer the voltage-gated ion channels stay open and thus the greater the Ca^{2+} influx through voltage-gated Ca^{2+} channels. Changes in duration of the action potential therefore can play an important role in influencing events that are sensitive to cytoplasmic Ca^{2+} levels, such as ion channel

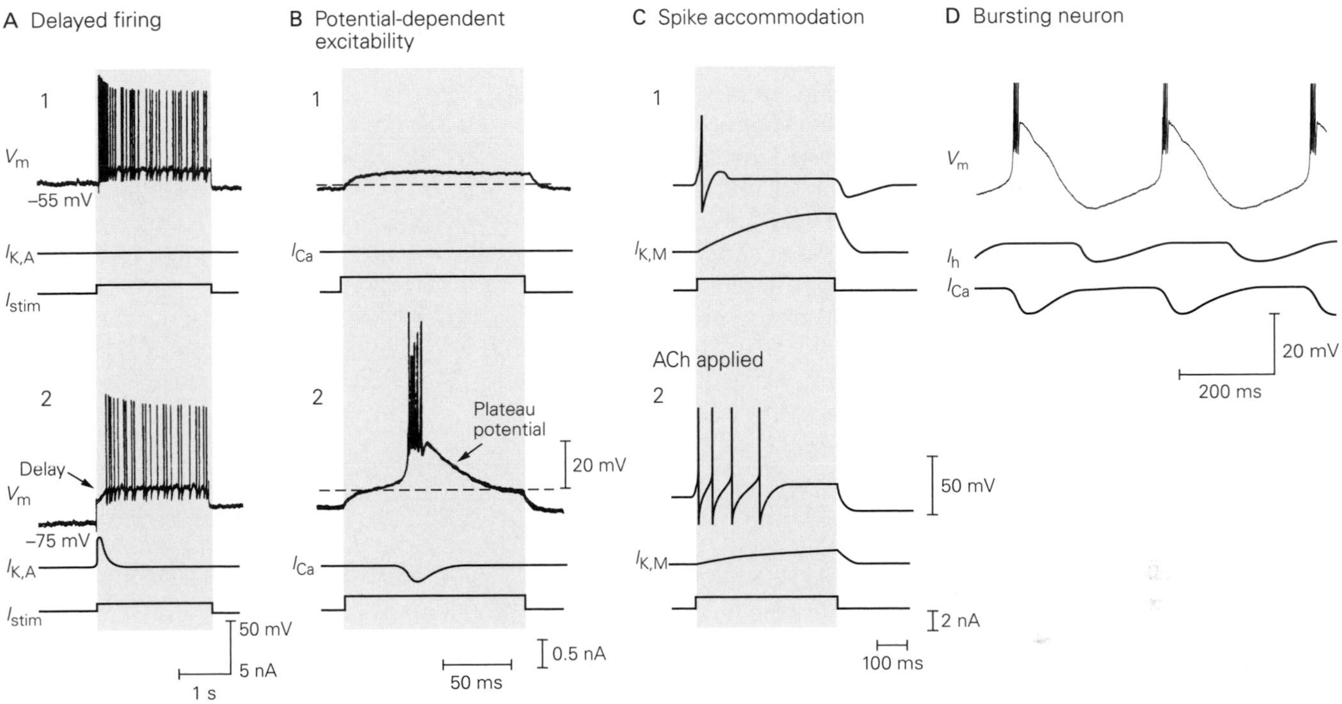

Figure 7–11 The response of a neuron to synaptic input is determined by its complement of voltage-gated ion channels. The waveform of the ionic current traces in the figure is drawn to reflect the activation and inactivation of the underlying conductances during the slow subthreshold changes in membrane potential. In reality, the currents will also show rapid changes during any triggered action potentials because of large, rapid changes in driving force.

A. Injection of a depolarizing current pulse (I_{stim}) into a neuron in the nucleus tractus solitarius normally triggers an immediate train of action potentials (**1**). If the cell is first held at a hyperpolarized membrane potential, the spike train is delayed (**2**). The delay is caused by A-type K^+ channels, which are activated by depolarizing synaptic input. The opening of these channels generates a transient outward K^+ current, $I_{K,A}$, that briefly drives V_m away from threshold. These channels typically are inactivated at the resting potential (–55 mV), but steady hyperpolarization removes the inactivation. (Reproduced, with permission, from Dekin and Getting 1987.)

B. A small depolarizing current pulse injected into a thalamic neuron at rest generates a subthreshold depolarization (**1**). If the membrane potential is held at a hyperpolarized level, the same current pulse triggers a burst of action potentials (**2**). The effectiveness of the current pulse is enhanced because the hyperpolarization causes a type of voltage-gated Ca^{2+} channel to recover from inactivation. Depolarizing inward current through the Ca^{2+} channels (I_{Ca}) generates a plateau potential of about 20 mV that triggers a burst of action potentials. The dashed line indicates the level of the normal resting potential. (Reproduced, with permission, from Llinás and Jahnsen 1982.)

The data in parts A and B demonstrate that steady hyperpolarization, such as might be produced by inhibitory synaptic input to a neuron, can profoundly affect the spike train pattern of a neuron. This effect varies greatly among cell types and depends on the presence or absence of particular types of voltage-gated Ca^{2+} and K^+ channels.

C. The firing properties of sympathetic neurons in autonomic ganglia are regulated by a neurotransmitter. (**1**) A prolonged depolarizing current normally results in a single action potential. The depolarization turns on a slowly activated K^+ current, the M current ($I_{K,M}$). The slow activation kinetics of the M-type channels allow the cell to fire one action potential before the efflux of K^+ through the M-type channels becomes sufficient to shift the membrane to more negative voltages and prevent the cell from firing more action potentials (a process termed *accommodation*). (**2**) Synaptic release of the neurotransmitter acetylcholine (ACh) onto this neuron activates a second-messenger pathway that closes the M-type channels, allowing the cell to fire many action potentials in response to the same stimulus. (See also Figure 11–11.) (Reproduced, with permission, from Jones and Adams 1987.)

D. In the absence of synaptic input, thalamocortical relay neurons can fire spontaneously in brief bursts of action potentials. These bursts are produced by current through two types of voltage-gated ion channels. The gradual depolarization that leads to a burst is driven by inward current through HCN channels (I_h), which have the unusual property of opening in response to hyperpolarizing voltage steps. The firing burst is triggered by an inward Ca^{2+} current through voltage-gated Ca^{2+} channels that are activated at relatively low levels of depolarization. This Ca^{2+} influx generates sufficient depolarization to reach threshold and drive a brief burst of Na^+-dependent action potentials. The strong depolarization during the burst causes the HCN channels to close and inactivates the Ca^{2+} channels, allowing hyperpolarization to develop between bursts of firing. This hyperpolarization then opens the HCN channels, initiating the next cycle in the rhythm. (Reproduced, with permission, from McCormick and Huguenard 1992.)

gating, transmitter release, long-term changes in synaptic strength, and gene expression.

Extrinsic synaptic inputs can modulate action potential shape by activating second-messenger pathways that modulate the activity of certain voltage-gated ion channels (see Chapter 11). The most common intrinsic modulation occurs during high-frequency firing, when there is a progressive buildup of inactivation of voltage-gated K^+ channels that leads to a progressive increase in the duration of the later action potentials in a train. Some of the functional implications of these changes in action potential shape are considered in later chapters.

The Mechanisms of Voltage-Gating and Ion Permeation Have Been Inferred from Electrophysiological Measurements

The empirical equations derived by Hodgkin and Huxley are quite successful in describing how the flow of ions through the Na^+ and K^+ channels generates the action potential. However, these equations describe the process of excitation primarily in terms of changes in membrane conductance and current. They tell little about the mechanisms that activate or inactivate channels in response to changes in membrane potential or selectivity for specific ions.

Our understanding of the properties of ion channel molecules was greatly enhanced by patch-clamp studies of current through single channels (see Box 5–1). Patch-clamp experiments demonstrate that voltage-gated channels generally have only two conductance states, open and closed. Recordings of single voltage-gated Na^+ channels show that, in response to a depolarization, a channel opens in an all-or-none fashion, conducting brief current pulses of constant amplitude but variable duration (Figure 7–12). During a maintained depolarization the open state of a channel is rapidly terminated by inactivation. Typical conductances of single voltage-gated Na^+, K^+, and Ca^{2+} channels range from 1 to 20 pS, depending on channel type. One class of calcium-activated K^+ channel has an unusually large conductance of approximately 200 pS.

Voltage-Gated Sodium Channels Open and Close in Response to Redistribution of Charges Within the Channel

In their original study of the squid axon, Hodgkin and Huxley suggested that a voltage-gated channel has a net charge, the *gating charge,* somewhere within the membrane. They postulated that a change in membrane

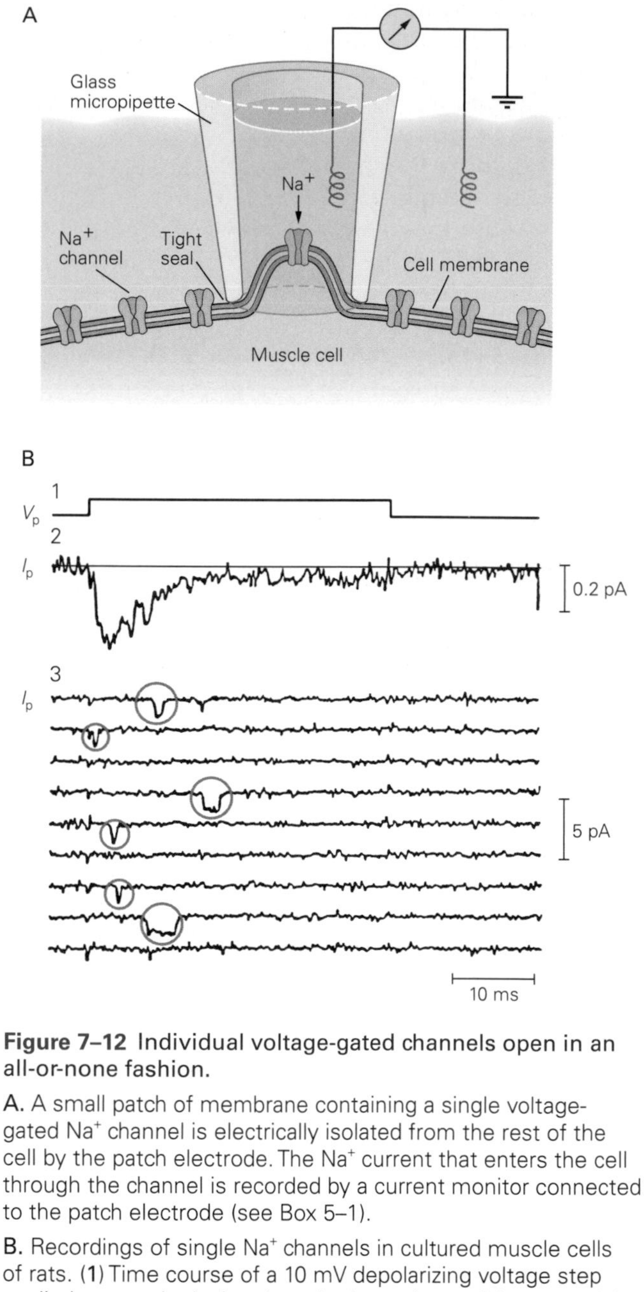

Figure 7–12 Individual voltage-gated channels open in an all-or-none fashion.

A. A small patch of membrane containing a single voltage-gated Na^+ channel is electrically isolated from the rest of the cell by the patch electrode. The Na^+ current that enters the cell through the channel is recorded by a current monitor connected to the patch electrode (see Box 5–1).

B. Recordings of single Na^+ channels in cultured muscle cells of rats. **(1)** Time course of a 10 mV depolarizing voltage step applied across the isolated patch of membrane (V_p = potential difference across the patch). **(2)** The sum of the inward current through the Na^+ channel in the patch during 300 trials (I_p = current through the patch). The trace was obtained by blocking the K^+ channels with tetraethylammonium and subtracting the leakage and capacitive currents electronically. **(3)** Nine individual trials from the set of 300, showing six openings of the channel **(circles).** These data demonstrate that the total Na^+ current recorded in a conventional voltage-clamp record (see Figure 7–3B) can be accounted for by the all-or-none opening and closing of a large number of Na^+ channels. (Reproduced, with permission, from Sigworth and Neher 1980.)

potential causes this charge to move across the electric field of the membrane, resulting in conformational changes that open or close the channel.

They further predicted that the movement of charge would be measurable. For example, they postulated that depolarization would move a positive gating charge from near the inner surface toward the outer surface of the membrane, owing to the interaction of the charge with the membrane electric field. This displacement would reduce the net separation of charge across the membrane and hence tend to hyperpolarize the membrane. To keep the membrane potential constant in a voltage-clamp experiment, a small extra component of outward capacitive current, called *gating current,* would have to be generated by the voltage clamp to counteract this rearrangement of charge within the membrane.

These predictions of Hodgkin and Huxley were later confirmed when the membrane current was examined by means of very sensitive techniques. The gating current was found to flow at the beginning and end of a depolarizing voltage-clamp step prior to the opening or closing of the Na^+ channels (Figure 7–13).

Analysis of the gating current has provided additional insights into the mechanisms of voltage-gating. For example, it has revealed that activation and inactivation of Na^+ channels are coupled processes. During a short depolarizing pulse the net outward movement of gating charge within the membrane at the beginning of the pulse is balanced by an equal and opposite movement of gating charge at the end of the pulse. However, if the pulse lasts long enough for Na^+ channel inactivation to take place, the movement of gating charge back across the membrane at the end of the pulse is delayed. Some of the gating charge is thus temporarily immobilized; only as the Na^+ channels recover from inactivation is that charge free to move back across the membrane. This charge immobilization indicates that some of the gating charges cannot move while the inactivation gate is closed.

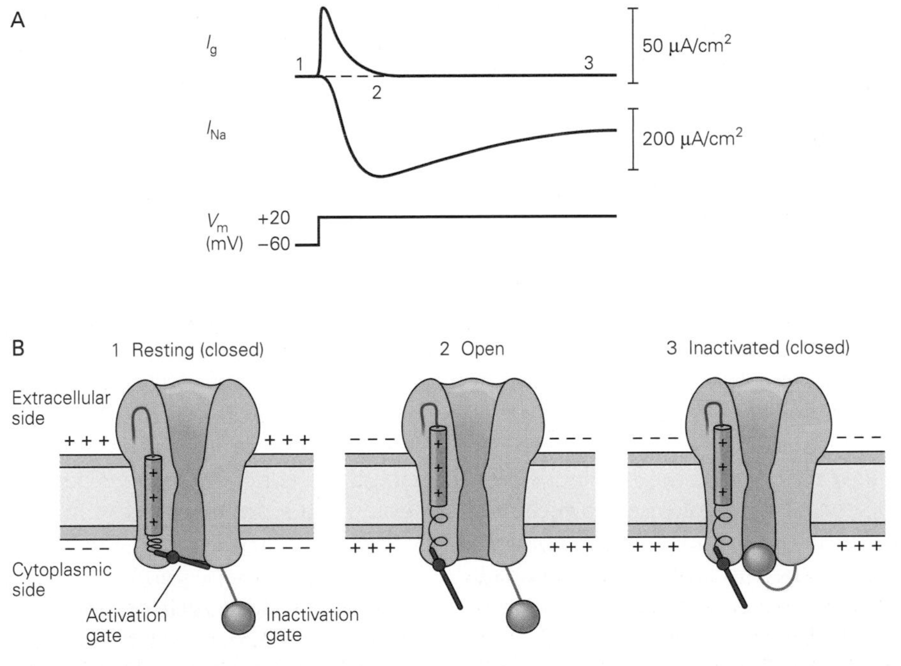

Figure 7–13 Changes in charge distribution within the Na^+ channel are associated with opening and closing of the channel.

A. When the membrane is depolarized, the Na^+ current (I_{Na}) is activated and then inactivated. The activation of the Na^+ current is preceded by a brief outward current (I_g), reflecting the outward movement of positive charges within the Na^+ channels associated with the opening of their activation gates. To detect this small gating current it is necessary to block the flow of ionic current through the Na^+ and K^+ channels and mathematically subtract the capacitive current due to charging of the lipid bilayer. (Adapted, with permission, from Armstrong and Gilly 1979).

B. The redistribution of gating charge and positions of the activation and inactivation gates when the channel is at rest, open, and inactivated. The **red cylinder** represents a positively charged region containing the gating charge that is thought to move through the membrane electric field in response to voltage changes. Depolarization from the resting state causes the gating charge to move outward, opening the activation gate. Inactivation closes the channel, immobilizing the gating charge.

To explain this immobilization phenomenon, Clay Armstrong and Francisco Bezanilla proposed that Na^+ channel inactivation occurs when the open (activated) channel is blocked by a tethered plug (a ball and chain mechanism), thereby preventing the closure of the activation gate (Figure 7–13B). In support of this idea, exposing the inside of the axon to proteolytic enzymes selectively eliminates inactivation and its effect on gating charge. The Na^+ channels remain open during a depolarization, and gating charge immobilization at the end of the pulse is eliminated—presumably because the enzymes clip off the inactivation "ball."

Voltage-Gated Sodium Channels Select for Sodium on the Basis of Size, Charge, and Energy of Hydration of the Ion

In Chapter 5 we saw how the structure of the K^+ channel pore could explain how such channels are able to select for K^+ over Na^+ ions. The narrow diameter of the K^+ channel selectivity filter (around 0.3 nm) requires that a K^+ or Na^+ ion must shed nearly all of its waters of hydration to enter the channel, an energetically unfavorable event.

The energetic cost of dehydration of a K^+ ion is well compensated by its close interaction with a cage of electronegative carbonyl oxygen atoms contributed by the peptide backbones of the four subunits of the K^+ channel selectivity filter. Because of its smaller radius, a Na^+ ion has a higher local electric field than does a K^+ ion and therefore interacts more strongly with its waters of hydration than does K^+. On the other hand, the small diameter of the Na^+ ion precludes close interaction with the cage of carbonyl oxygen atoms in the selectivity filter; the resultant high energetic cost of dehydrating the Na^+ ion excludes it from entering the channel.

How then does the selectivity filter of the Na^+ channel select for Na^+ over K^+ ions? Bertil Hille was able to deduce a model for the Na^+ channel's selectivity mechanism from measurements of the channel's relative permeability to several types of organic and inorganic cations that differ in size and hydrogen-bonding characteristics. As we learned in Chapter 5, the channel behaves as if it contains a filter or recognition site that selects partly on the basis of size, thus acting as a molecular sieve (see Figure 5–1). Based on the size of the largest organic cation that could readily permeate the channel, Hille deduced that the selectivity filter had rectangular dimensions of 0.3×0.5 nm. This cross section is just large enough to accommodate one Na^+ ion contacting one water molecule. Cations that are larger in diameter cannot pass through the pore. Cations smaller than this critical size pass through the pore, but only after losing most of the waters of hydration they normally carry in free solution.

The ease with which organic cations with good hydrogen-bonding characteristics pass through the channel suggests that part of the inner wall of the channel is made up of negatively polarized or charged amino acid residues that can substitute for the ion's waters of hydration. Lowering the pH of the fluid surrounding the cell reduces the conductance of the open channel, consistent with the titration of an important negatively charged carboxylic acid residue.

Based on these findings, Hille proposed that Na^+ channels select for ions by the following mechanism. Negatively charged carboxylic acid groups of glutamate or aspartate residues at the outer mouth of the pore perform the first step in the selection process by attracting cations and repelling anions. The negative carboxylic acid groups, as well as other oxygen atoms that line the pore, can substitute for waters of hydration, but the degree of effectiveness of this substitution varies among ion species. For example, the negative charge of a carboxylic acid is able to form a stronger coulombic interaction with the smaller Na^+ ion compared to the larger K^+ ion. Because the Na^+ channel is large enough to accommodate a cation in contact with several water molecules, the energetic cost of dehydration is not as great as it is in a K^+ channel. As a result of these two features, the Na^+ channel is able to select for Na^+ over K^+. A recent X-ray crystal structure of a bacterial voltage-gated Na^+ channel has confirmed many of the key features of Hille's model.

Voltage-Gated Potassium, Sodium, and Calcium Channels Stem from a Common Ancestor and Have Similar Structures

Detailed molecular studies have revealed that all voltage-gated cation channels—those permeant to K^+, Na^+, or Ca^{2+}—have a similar underlying architecture. In fact, there is now strong evidence from studies of bacteria, plants, invertebrates, and vertebrates that most voltage-sensitive cation channels stem from a common ancestral channel—perhaps a K^+ channel—that can be traced to a single-cell organism living more than 1.4 billion years ago, before the evolution of separate plant and animal kingdoms. The amino acid sequences that are highly conserved through evolution help identify the domains within contemporary voltage-gated cation channels that are critical for function.

Voltage-gated cation channels are composed of pore-forming α-subunits that each contain a motif consisting of six transmembrane segments (S1–S6). A seventh hydrophobic region, the "P-region," connects the S5 and S6 segments. It forms a loop that dips into and out of the extracellular side of the membrane and forms the channel's selectivity filter. All voltage-gated K^+ channels consist of four pore-forming subunits, each of which contributes one P-region to the pore of the fully assembled channel. Voltage-gated Na^+ and Ca^{2+} channels consist of one large pore-forming subunit containing four internal repeats of this basic motif (Figure 7–14). The amino acid sequence of the S5-P-S6 region of voltage-gated K^+ channels is homologous to that of bacterial K^+ channels with two transmembrane segments.

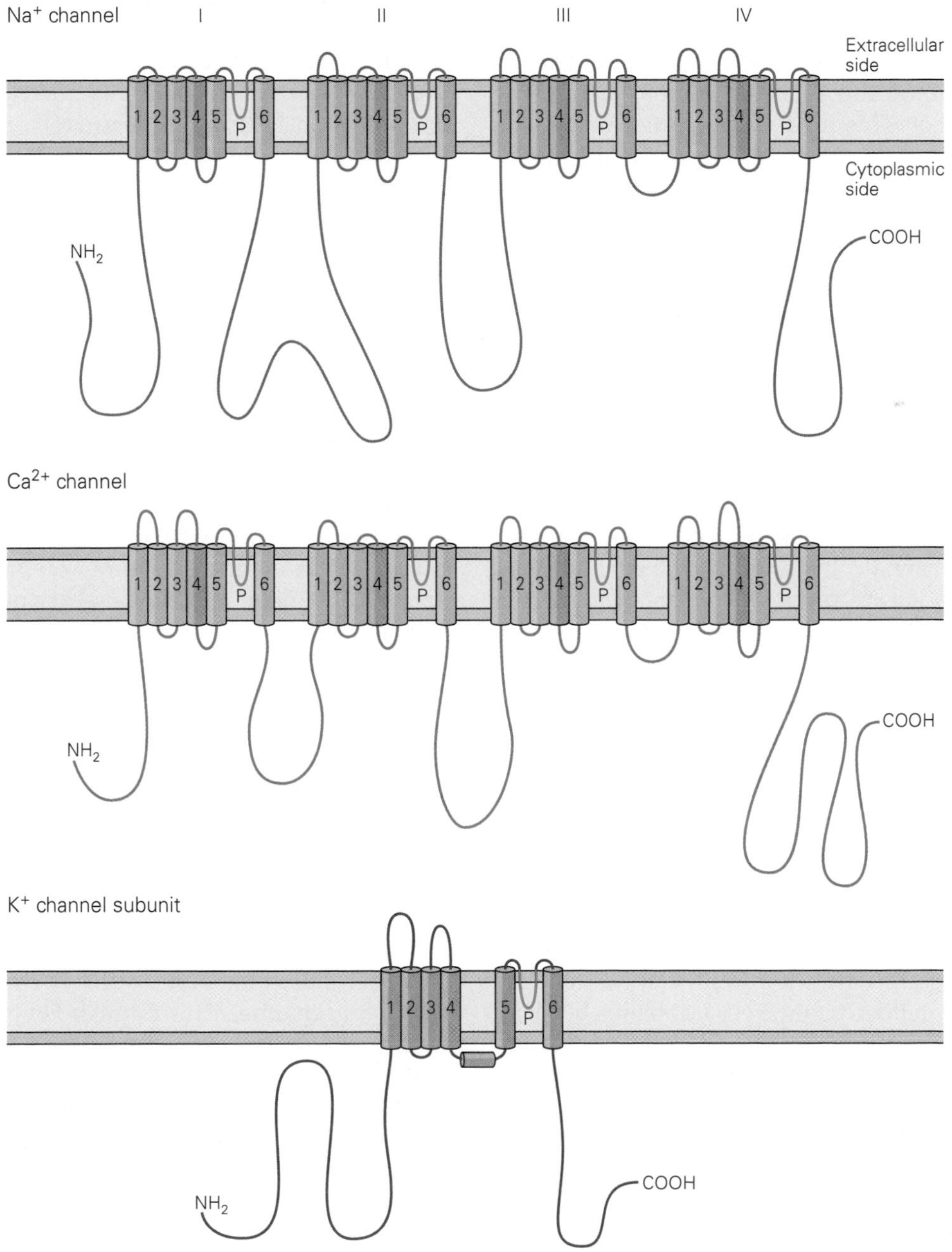

Figure 7–14 The voltage-gated cation channels have homologous α-subunit domains. The α-subunit of the Na^+ and Ca^{2+} channels consists of a single polypeptide chain with four homologous repeats (I–IV) of a basic motif that contains six membrane-spanning α-helixes (S1–S6). The P-region between α-helixes 5 and 6 that dips into and out of the membrane forms the selectivity filter. The S4 segment has a net positive charge. The α-subunit of the K^+ channel, in contrast, has only one domain with six α-helixes and a P-region; four K^+ channel α-subunits are assembled to form a complete channel (see Figure 5–12A). (Adapted, with permission, from Catterall 1988; Stevens 1991.)

The S4 segment is thought to play a particularly important role in voltage-gating. This transmembrane segment contains a distinctive pattern of amino acids in which every third position contains a positively charged arginine or lysine residue. The presence of so many positive charges within a single transmembrane segment is highly unusual. Because this pattern of positive charges is present in all voltage-gated channels but is absent in channels that are not voltage-gated, it is thought that this region might be the voltage sensor—that part of the protein that transduces depolarization of the cell membrane into a conformational change that opens the channel. This idea is supported by experiments using site-directed mutagenesis, which show that neutralization of positive charges in S4 decreases the gating current and voltage sensitivity of channel activation.

X-Ray Crystallographic Analysis of Voltage-Gated Channel Structures Provides Insight into Voltage-Gating

How do the positive charges in S4 move through the membrane electric field during channel gating? How is S4 movement coupled to gating? What is the relationship of the voltage-sensing region to the pore-forming region of the channel? Insights into such questions have been provided by recent X-ray crystallographic structures of mammalian delayed rectifier voltage-gated K^+ channels performed by Rod MacKinnon and his colleagues, as well as by a number of studies using mutagenesis and other biophysical approaches.

The X-ray crystal structures of the Kv1.2 channel and a Kv1.2-2.1 chimera show that a K^+ channel subunit is composed of two domains. The S1–S4 segments form a voltage-sensing domain at the periphery of the channel while the S5-P-S6 region forms the pore domain at the central axis of the channel (Figure 7–15). The idea that the S1–S4 voltage sensor is a separate domain is consistent with the recent finding that certain bacterial proteins contain S1–S4 domains but lack a pore domain. One such protein is a voltage-sensitive phosphatase and a second protein forms a voltage-gated proton channel.

In the two-transmembrane segment bacterial K^+ channels the four inner transmembrane helixes, which correspond to the S6 helixes in voltage-gated K^+ channels, form a tight bundle crossing at their cytoplasmic ends to form the gate of the channel (see Figure 5–16). In the open state the inner ends of these helixes were seen to splay out to open the gate by bending at flexible glycine hinges. The structure of the Kv1.2-2.1 chimera indicates that the S6 helix is also bent at this conserved glycine hinge so that the channel adopts an open conformation. It is not surprising that the Kv channel is in the open state as there is no voltage gradient across the channel in the crystals. This is similar to the situation in a membrane that has been depolarized to 0 mV, a voltage at which the channels are normally open.

One long-standing question in studies of voltage-gating is how the charges on the voltage-sensor overcome the unfavorable energy change associated with their positioning within the nonpolar membrane where they must sense the electric field. The crystal structure provides some answers to this question. Mutagenesis studies indicate that four positively charged arginine residues in the external half of the S4 segment are likely to carry most of the gating charge. In the open state the four positive charges face outward toward the extracellular side of the membrane, where they may undergo energetically favorable interactions with water or the negatively charged head groups of the phospholipid bilayer. Positive charges on other S4 residues that lie more deeply within the lipid bilayer are stabilized by interactions with negatively charged acidic residues on the S1–S3 transmembrane helixes.

At present a crystal structure for the closed state of the channel is lacking. However, MacKinnon and colleagues have proposed a plausible model for voltage-gating based on the structures of the open voltage-gated K^+ channel and the closed two-transmembrane segment bacterial K^+ channel (Figure 7–16). According to this model, a negative voltage inside the cell exerts a force on the positively charged S4 helix that causes it to move inward by about 1.0 to 1.5 nm. As a result, the four positively charged S4 residues that in the depolarized state face the external environment and sense the extracellular potential now face the intracellular side of the membrane and sense the intracellular potential. In this manner movement of each S4 segment will translocate 3–4 electronic charges across the membrane electric field as the channel transitions between the closed and open states, for a total of 12–16 charges moved per tetrameric channel. This number is very similar to the total charge movement determined from gating current measurements.

How are S4 movements coupled to the gate of the channel? According to the model, the inward movement of the S4 segment when the membrane voltage becomes negative exerts a downward force on an α-helix that couples the S4 and S5 transmembrane segments. This S4-S5 coupling helix lies roughly parallel to the membrane at its cytoplasmic surface. In the open state the S4-S5 helix rests on the inner end of the S6 helix gate. As a result, downward movement of the helix applies force to S6, closing the gate. Thus voltage gating is thought to rely on the electromechanical coupling between the voltage-sensing domain and the pore domain of the channel. Although this electromechanical coupling model provides a very satisfying picture for how changes in membrane voltage lead to channel gating, a definitive answer to this key problem will require resolution of the structure of the closed state of a voltage-gated channel.

The Diversity of Voltage-Gated Channel Types Is Generated by Several Genetic Mechanisms

The conservative mechanism by which evolution proceeds—creating new structural or functional entities by duplicating, modifying, shuffling, and recombining existing gene-coding sequences—is illustrated by the modular design of the members of the extended gene family that encodes the voltage-gated Na^+, K^+, and Ca^{2+} channels. This family also includes genes that encode calcium-activated K^+ channels, the hyperpolarization-activated HCN channels, and a voltage-independent cyclic nucleotide-gated cation channel important for phototransduction and olfaction.

The functional differences between these channels are caused by differences in amino acid sequence in their core transmembrane domains as well as by the addition of regulatory domains to the C-terminal cytoplasmic end of the proteins. Some of these cytoplasmic domains bind either Ca^{2+} or cyclic nucleotides, enabling these agents to regulate channel gating (Figure 7–17).

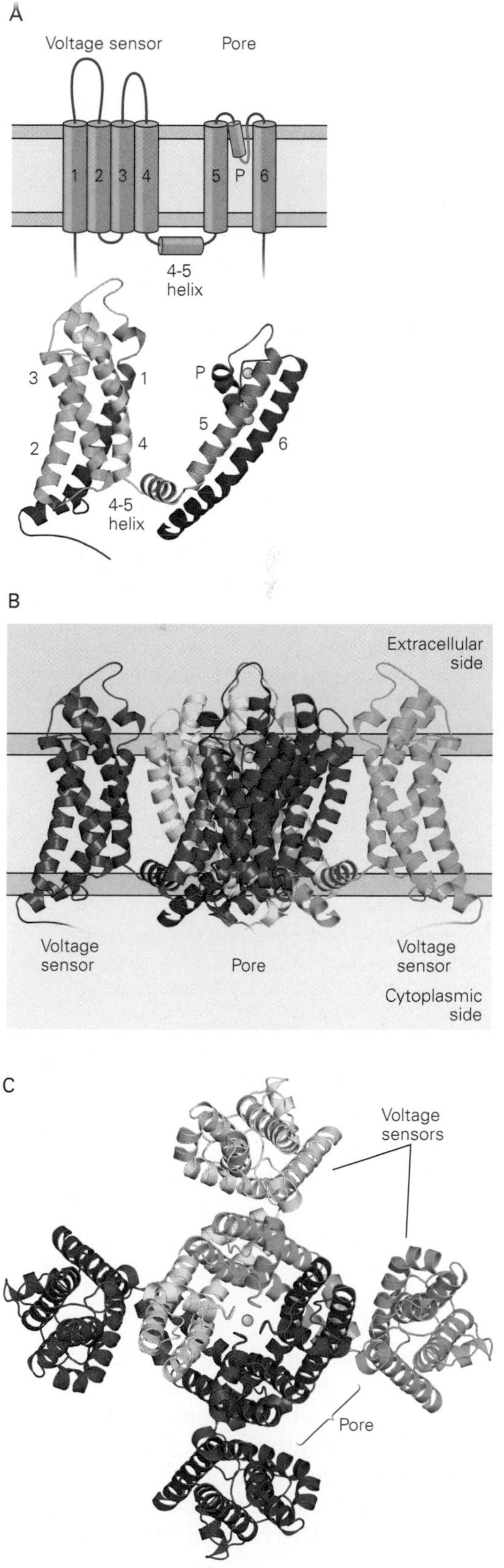

Figure 7–15 X-ray crystal structure of a voltage-gated K^+ channel. (Adapted, with permission, from Long et al. 2007.)

A. **Top**: In addition to its six transmembrane α-helixes (S1–S6), a voltage-gated K^+ channel subunit contains a short α-helix (the P helix) that is part of the P-region selectivity filter, as well as an α-helix on the cytoplasmic side of the membrane that connects transmembrane helixes S4 and S5 (4-5). **Bottom**: An X-ray structural model of a single subunit shows the positions of the six membrane-spanning helixes, the P helix, and the 4-5 linker helix. Note how the S1–S4 voltage-sensing region and S5-P-S6 pore-forming region are localized in separate domains. Two potassium ions bound in the pore are shown in **pink**.

B. Side view of the tetrameric voltage-gated K^+ channel. Each individual subunit is highlighted in a different color. The red subunit is in the same orientation as the subunit shown above in panel part A. The approximate position of the lipid bilayer is indicated (**tan colors**).

C. A view looking down on the tetrameric channel from outside the cell. The four voltage-sensors (S1–S4) are located on the periphery and the S5-P-S6 pore-forming region of the channel is in the center. A potassium ion is shown in the center of the pore (**pink**). (Adapted, with permission, from Long et al. 2007.)

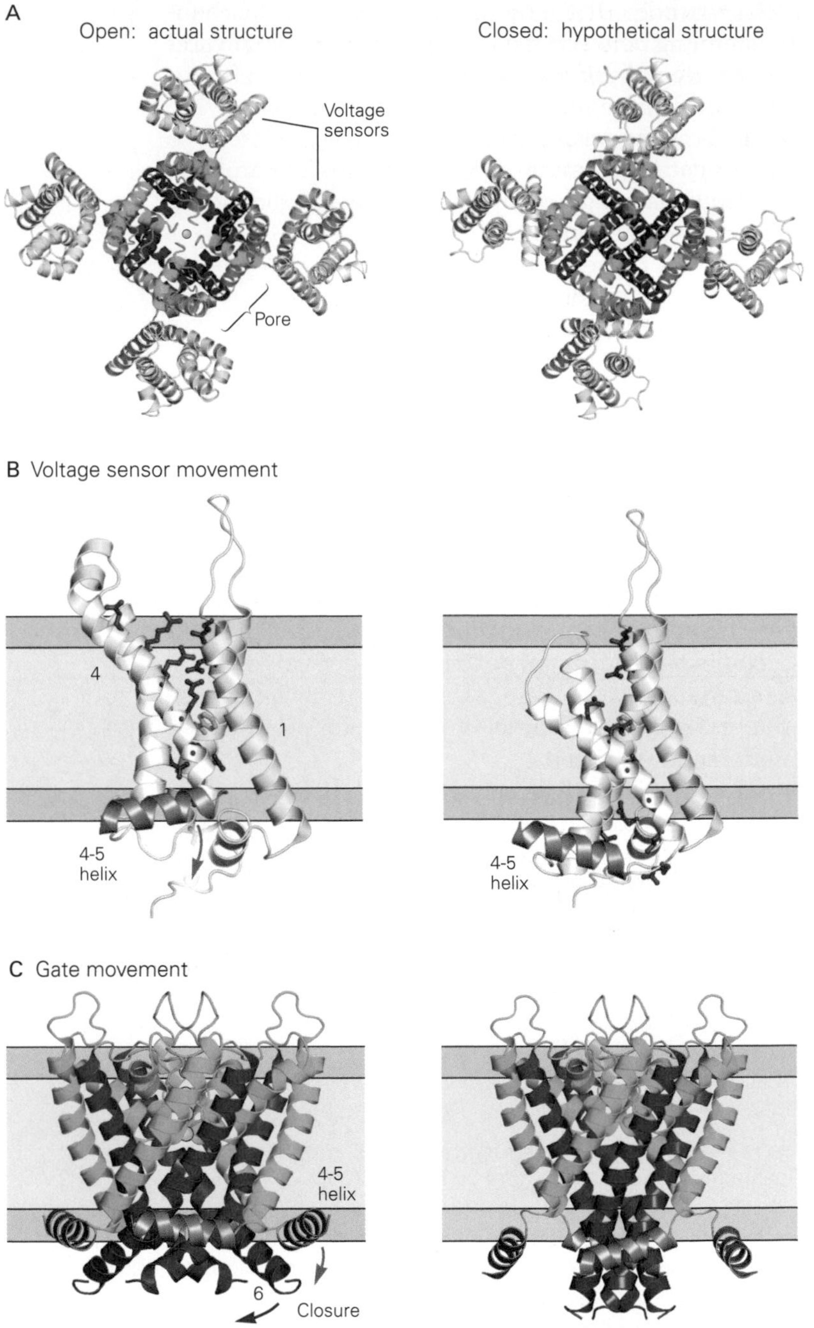

Figure 7–16 Model for voltage-gating based on X-ray crystal structures of two K⁺ channels. The drawings on the left show the actual structure of an open voltage-gated K^+ channel (from the crystal structure shown in Figure 7–15). The drawings on the right show the hypothetical structure of a closed voltage-gated K^+ channel, based in part on the structure of the pore region of the two-transmembrane segment bacterial K^+ channel KcsA in the closed state. (Adapted, with permission, by Yu-hang Chen from Long et al. 2007.)

A. A view looking down on the open and closed channel from outside the cell. Note how the central pore is constricted in the closed state. This constriction prevents K^+ flow through the channel.

B. A view of the S1–S4 voltage-sensing domain from the side, parallel to the plane of the membrane. Positively charged residues in S4 are shown as **blue sticks**. In the open state, when the membrane is depolarized, four positive charges on the S4 helix are located in the external half of the membrane, facing the external solution. The positive charges in the interior of the membrane are stabilized by interactions with negatively charged residues in S1 and S2 (**red sticks**). In the closed state, when the membrane potential is negative, the S4 region moves inward so that its positive charges now lie in the inner half of the membrane. The inward movement of S4 causes the cytoplasmic S4-S5 coupling helix to move downward.

C. The putative conformational change in the channel pore upon voltage-gating. A side view of the tetrameric S5-P-S6 pore region of the channel shows the S4-S5 coupling helix. Membrane repolarization causes the downward movement of the S4-S5 helix, applying force to the S6 inner helix of the pore. This causes the S6 helix to bend at its glycine hinge, thereby closing the gate of the channel.

As we saw in Chapter 5, the four subunits that comprise the inward-rectifying K^+ channels are truncated versions of the fundamental structural motif; they consist of only the P region and its two flanking membrane-spanning regions. Evolution has provided many of these channels with an extrinsic mechanism of voltage sensitivity through the addition of an internal cationic binding site. When the cell is depolarized, cytoplasmic Mg^{2+} or positively charged polyamines (small organic molecules that are normal constituents of the cytoplasm) are electrostatically driven to this binding site from the cytoplasm, plugging the channel.

Inactivation of voltage-gated ion channels is also mediated by different molecular modules. For example, the rapid inactivation of both the A-type K^+ channel and the voltage-gated Na^+ channel is mediated by a tethered plug that binds to the inner mouth of the channel when the activation gate opens. In the A-type K^+ channel the plug is formed by the cytoplasmic N-terminus of the channel protein, whereas in voltage-gated Na^+ channels it is formed by the cytoplasmic loop connecting domains III and IV of the α-subunit.

The wide range of firing properties of different neurons and the ability of a single neuron to adapt its firing to a range of synaptic inputs depends on the large diversity of ion channels expressed throughout the nervous system. Even a single ion species, such as K^+, can cross the membrane through several distinct types of channels, each with its own characteristic kinetics, voltage dependence, and sensitivity to different modulators. For voltage-gated channels five different mechanisms are responsible for this diversity. (1) More than one gene may encode related α-subunits within one class of channel. For example, eight different genes that encode voltage-gated Na^+ channel α-subunits are expressed in the mammalian nervous system. (2) The four α-subunits that form a K^+ channel may be encoded by different genes. After translation the α-subunits are in some cases mixed and matched in various combinations, thus forming different subclasses of heteromultimeric channels. (3) A single gene product may be alternatively spliced, resulting in

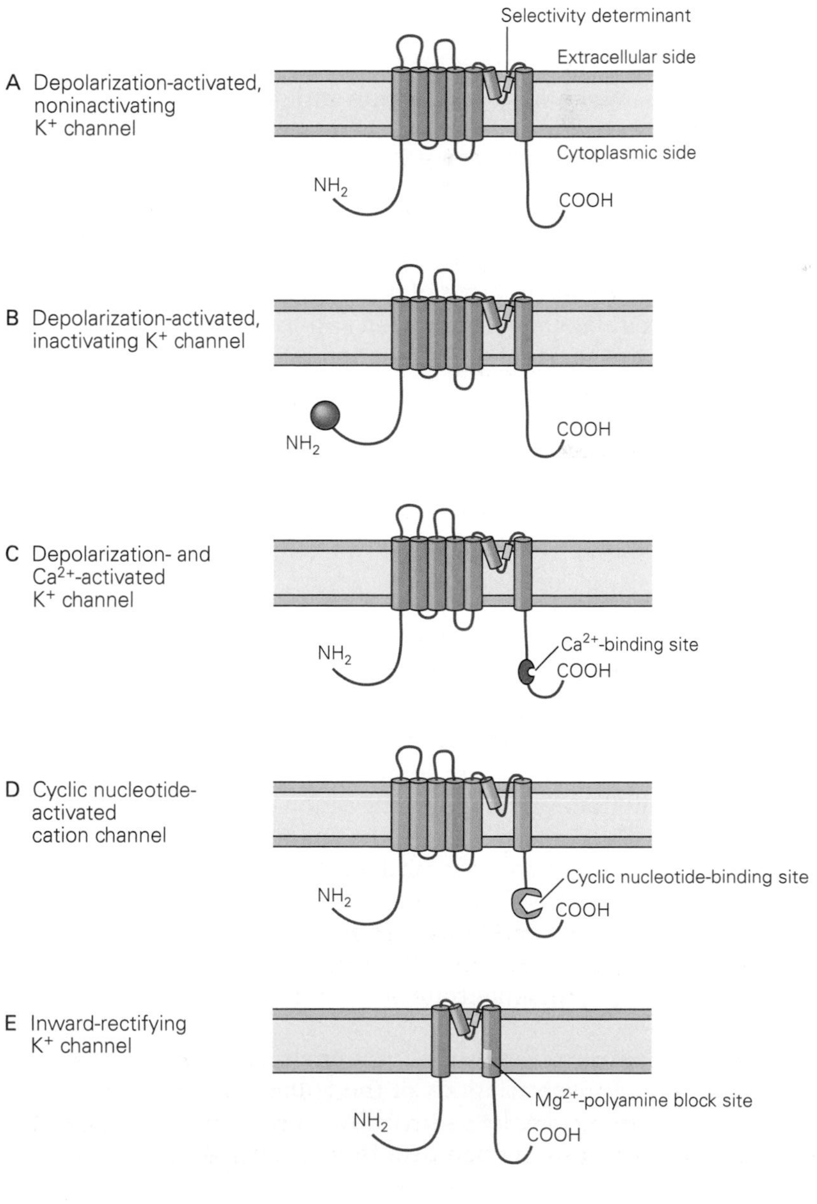

Figure 7–17 The extended gene family of voltage-gated channels produces variants of a common molecular design.

A. The basic transmembrane topology of an α-subunit of a voltage-gated K^+ channel.

B. Many K^+ channels that are first activated and then inactivated by prolonged depolarization have a ball-and-chain segment at their N-terminal end that inactivates the channel by plugging its inner mouth.

C. Some K^+ channels that require both depolarization and an increase in intracellular Ca^{2+} to activate have a Ca^{2+}-binding sequence attached to the C-terminal end of the channel.

D. Cation channels gated by cyclic nucleotides have a cyclic nucleotide-binding domain attached to the C-terminal end. One class of such channels includes the voltage-independent, cyclic nucleotide-gated channels important in the transduction of olfactory and visual sensory signals. Another subclass consists of the hyperpolarization-activated (HCN) channels important for pacemaker activity (see Figure 7–11D). The P loops in these channels lack key amino acid residues required for K^+ selectivity. As a result, these channels do not show a high degree of discrimination between Na^+ and K^+.

E. Inward-rectifying K^+ channels, which are gated by blocking particles available in the cytoplasm, are formed from a truncated version of the basic building block, with only two membrane-spanning regions and a P-region.

variations in the messenger RNA (mRNA) molecules that encode the α-subunit. (4) The RNA that encodes an α-subunit may be edited by chemical modification of a single nucleotide, thereby changing the composition of a single amino acid in the channel subunit. (5) One type of α-subunit may be combined with different accessory subunits to form functionally different channel types.

These accessory subunits (often termed β-, γ-, or δ-subunits) may be either cytoplasmic or membrane-spanning and can produce a wide range of effects on channel function. For example, some β-subunits enhance the efficiency with which the channel is trafficked to the membrane. Other subunits regulate channel gating, either enhancing or inhibiting the coupling of depolarization to channel opening. In some K^+ channels the α-subunit lacks a tethered inactivation plug; the association of such α-subunits with β-subunits that contain their own N-terminal tethered plugs can endow the channel with the ability to rapidly inactivate. In contrast to the α-subunits, there is no known homology among the β-, γ-, and δ-subunits from the three major subfamilies of voltage-gated channels.

These various sources of channel diversity also vary widely between different areas of the nervous system, between different types of neurons, and within different subcellular compartments of a given neuron. A corollary of this regional differentiation is that mutations or epigenetic mechanisms that alter voltage-gated channel function can have very selective effects on neuronal or muscular function. The result is a large array of neurological diseases called channelopathies (see Chapter 14).

An Overall View

An action potential is produced when ions move across the cell membrane through voltage-gated channels and thereby change the charge separation across the membrane. An influx of Na^+, and in some cases Ca^{2+}, depolarizes the membrane and initiates the action potential. An efflux of K^+ then repolarizes the membrane by restoring the initial charge separation. A particularly important subset of voltage-gated channels opens primarily when the membrane potential nears the threshold for an action potential; these channels have a profound effect on the spike-train encoding properties of a neuron.

We know much about how channels function from studies that use variations of the voltage-clamp technique—these studies let us eavesdrop on a channel at work. And we know a good deal from biochemical, molecular biological, and X-ray crystallographic studies about the channel's structure—about the primary amino acid sequence of the proteins that form them and how these proteins adopt their detailed secondary, tertiary, and quaternary structures in the membrane.

Now these two approaches are being combined in a concerted effort to understand the relationship between structure and function in these channels: how the detailed three-dimensional structure of the molecule and the chemical and physical properties of its individual residues gives rise to the remarkable gating and ion permeation properties of the voltage-gated channels. Thus, we may soon be able to understand the molecular mechanism for the remarkable ability of voltage-gated channels to generate the action potential. These insights into channel function have two important practical implications. They will allow us to understand better the molecular bases of certain genetic diseases that involve mutations in ion channel genes, and they will enable us to design safer and more effective drugs to treat a variety of diseases that involve disturbances in electrical signaling (such as epilepsy, multiple sclerosis, myotonia, and ataxia).

John Koester
Steven A. Siegelbaum

Selected Readings

Armstrong CM, Hille B. 1998. Voltage-gated ion channels and electrical excitability. Neuron 20:371–380.

Bezanilla F. 2008. How membrane proteins sense voltage. Nat Rev Mol Cell Biol 9:323–332.

Hille B. 2001. *Ion Channels of Excitable Membranes,* 3rd ed. Sunderland, MA: Sinauer.

Hodgkin AL. 1992. *Chance & Design: Reminiscences of Science in Peace and War.* Cambridge: Cambridge Univ. Press.

Jan LY, Jan YN. 1997. Cloned potassium channels from eukaryotes and prokaryotes. Annu Rev Neurosci 20: 91–123.

Llinás RR. 1988. The intrinsic electrophysiological properties of mammalian neurons: insights into central nervous system function. Science 242:1654–1664.

MacKinnon R. 2003. Potassium channels. FEBS Lett 555:62–65.

Rudy B, McBain C. 2001. Kv3 channels: voltage-gated K^+ channels designed for high-frequency repetitive firing. Trends Neurosci 24:517–526.

Smart T. 2004. The state of ion channel research in 2004. Nat Rev Drug Discov 3:239–278.

Yu FH, Catterall WA. 2003. Overview of the voltage-gated sodium channel family. Genome Biol 4(3):207.

References

Armstrong CM, Bezanilla F. 1977. Inactivation of the sodium channel. II. Gating current experiments. J Gen Physiol 70:567–590.

Armstrong CM, Gilly WF. 1979. Fast and slow steps in the activation of sodium channels. J Gen Physiol 59:388–400.

Catterall WA. 1988. Structure and function of voltage-sensitive ion channels. Science 242:50–61.

Cole KS, Curtis HJ. 1939. Electric impedance of the squid giant axon during activity. J Gen Physiol 22:649–670.

Dekin MS, Getting PA. 1987. In vitro characterization of neurons in the vertical part of the nucleus tractus solitarius. II. Ionic basis for repetitive firing patterns. J Neurophysiol 58:215–229.

Heinemann SH, Terlau H, Stühmer W, Imoto K, Numa S. 1992. Calcium channel characteristics conferred on the sodium channel by single mutations. Nature 356:441–443.

Hodgkin AL, Huxley AF. 1952. A quantitative description of membrane current and its application to conduction and excitation in nerve. J Physiol 117:500–544.

Hodgkin AL, Katz B. 1949. The effect of sodium ions on the electrical activity of the giant axon of the squid. J Physiol 108:37–77.

Isom LL, DeJongh KS, Catterall WA. 1994. Auxiliary subunits of voltage-gated ion channels. Neuron 12:1183–1194.

Jiang Y, Lee A, Chen J, Ruta V, Cadene M, Chait BT, MacKinnon R. 2003. X-ray structure of a voltage-dependent K^+ channel. Nature 423:33–41.

Jones SW. 1985. Muscarinic and peptidergic excitation of bull-frog sympathetic neurones. J Physiol 366:63–87.

Jones SW, Adams PR. 1987. The M current and other potassium currents of vertebrate neurons. In: LK Kaczmarek, IB Levitan (eds). *Neuromodulation: The Biological Control of Neuronal Excitability*, pp. 159–178. New York: Oxford Univ. Press.

Llinás R, Jahnsen H. 1982. Electrophysiology of mammalian thalamic neurones *in vitro*. Nature 297:406–408.

Long SB, Tao X, Campbell EB, MacKinnon R. 2007. Atomic structure of a voltage-dependent K^+ channel in a lipid membrane-like environment. Nature 450:376–382.

McCormick DA, Huguenard JR. 1992. A model of electrophysiological properties of thalamocortical relay neurons. J Neurophysiol 68:1384–1400.

Noda M, Shimizu S, Tanabe T, Takai T, Kayano T, Ikeda T, Takahashi H, et al. 1984. Primary structure of *Electrophorus electricus* sodium channel deduced from cDNA sequence. Nature 312:121–127.

Papazian DM, Schwarz TL, Tempel BL, Jan YN, Jan LY. 1987. Cloning of genomic and complementary DNA from *Shaker*, a putative potassium channel gene from *Drosophila*. Science 237:749–753.

Payandeh J, Scheuer T, Zheng N, Catterall WA. 2011. The crystal structure of a voltage-gated sodium channel. Nature 475:353–59.

Sigworth FJ, Neher E. 1980. Single Na^+ channel currents observed in cultured rat muscle cells. Nature 287:447–449.

Stevens CF. 1991. Making a submicroscopic hole in one. Nature 349:657–658.

Vassilev PM, Scheuer T, Catterall WA. 1988. Identification of an intracellular peptide segment involved in sodium channel inactivation. Science 241:1658–1661.

Yang N, George AL Jr, Horn R. 1996. Molecular basis of charge movement in voltage-gated sodium channels. Neuron 16:113–122.

Part III

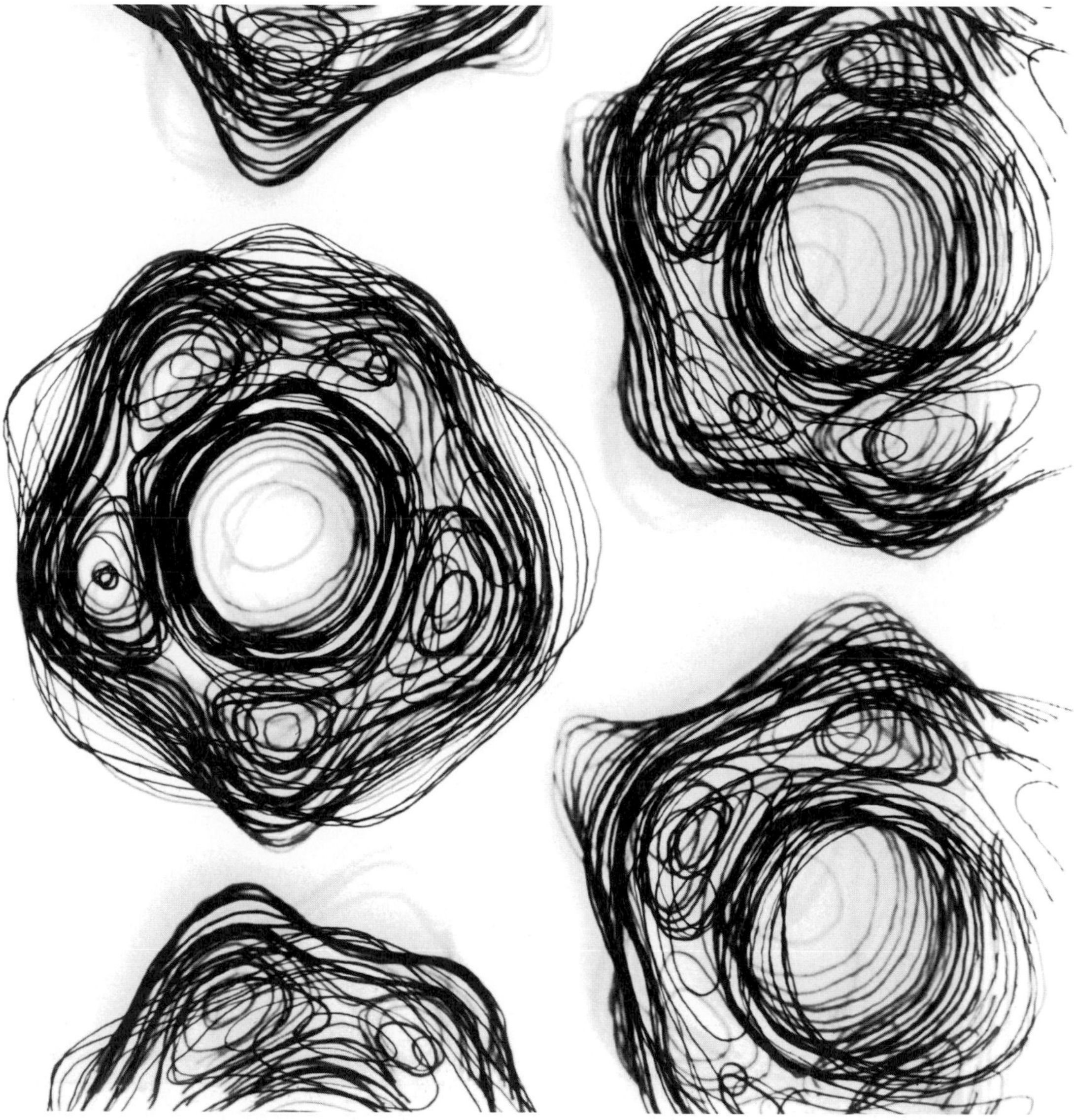

Preceding Page

The structure of nicotinic acetylcholine receptor channels is revealed through electron microscope images. This reconstruction shows the receptor-channel pore and the contours of its surrounding five subunits as they would be seen from the perspective of the synaptic cleft. (Reproduced, with permission, from Nigel Unwin.)

III Synaptic Transmission

In Part II, we examined how electrical signals are initiated and propagated within an individual neuron. We now turn to synaptic transmission, the process by which one nerve cell communicates with another. An average neuron forms and receives 1,000 to 10,000 synaptic connections, and the human brain contains at least 10^{11} neurons. Thus 10^{14} to 10^{15} synaptic connections are formed in the brain. There are 1,000-fold more synapses in one brain than the 100 billion stars in our galaxy! Fortunately, only a few basic mechanisms underlie synaptic transmission at these many connections.

With some exceptions, the synapse consists of three components: (1) the terminals of the presynaptic axon, (2) a target on the postsynaptic cell, and (3) a zone of apposition. Based on the structure of the apposition, synapses are categorized into two major groups: electrical and chemical. At electrical synapses, the presynaptic terminal and the postsynaptic cell are in very close apposition at regions termed *gap junctions*. The current generated by an action potential in the presynaptic neuron directly enters the postsynaptic cell through specialized bridging channels called *gap junction channels*, which physically connect the cytoplasm of the presynaptic and postsynaptic cells. At chemical synapses, a cleft separates the two cells, and the cells do not communicate through bridging channels. Rather, an action potential in the presynaptic cell leads to the release of a chemical transmitter from the nerve terminal. The transmitter diffuses across the synaptic cleft and binds to receptor molecules on the postsynaptic membrane, which regulates the opening and closing of ion channels in the postsynaptic cell. This leads to changes in the membrane potential of the postsynaptic neuron that can either excite or inhibit the firing of an action potential.

Receptors for transmitters can be classified into two major groups depending on how they control ion channels in the postsynaptic cell. One type, the ionotropic receptor, is an ion channel that opens when the transmitter binds. The second type, the metabotropic receptor, acts indirectly on ion channels by activating a biochemical second-messenger cascade within the postsynaptic cell. Both types of receptors can result in excitation or inhibition. The sign of the signal depends not on the identity of the transmitter but on the properties of the receptor with which the transmitter interacts. A single transmitter can produce several distinct effects by activating different types of receptors. Thus, receptor diversity permits a relatively small number of transmitters to produce a wide variety of synaptic actions. Most transmitters are low-molecular-weight molecules, but certain peptides also can act as messengers at synapses. The methods of electrophysiology, biochemistry, and molecular biology have been used to characterize the receptors in postsynaptic cells that respond to these various chemical messengers. These methods have also clarified how second-messenger pathways transduce signals within cells.

In this part of the book, we consider synaptic transmission in its most elementary forms. We first compare and contrast the two major classes of synapses, chemical and electrical (see Chapter 8). We then focus on a model chemical synapse in the peripheral nervous system, the neuromuscular junction between a presynaptic motor neuron and postsynaptic skeletal muscle fiber (see Chapter 9). Next we examine the principles of chemical synapses between neurons in the central nervous system, focusing on the postsynaptic cell and its integration of thousands of synaptic signals from multiple presynaptic inputs, which involve both ionotropic receptor-mediated signals (see Chapter 10) as well as metabotropic receptor-mediated signals (see Chapter 11). We then turn to the presynaptic terminal and consider the mechanisms by which neurons release transmitter from their presynaptic terminals, how transmitter release can be regulated by neural activity (see Chapter 12), and the chemical nature of the neurotransmitters (see Chapter 13). Because the molecular architecture of chemical synapses is complex, many diseases can affect chemical synaptic transmission (see Chapter 14). One disorder that we consider in detail in this section is myasthenia gravis, a disease that disrupts transmission at synapses between spinal motor neurons and skeletal muscle. Analysis of abnormalities in synaptic transmission associated with human disease is important clinically. At the same time clinical studies have provided critical insight into mechanisms that underlie normal synaptic function.

Part III

8

Overview of Synaptic Transmission

WHAT GIVES NERVE CELLS THEIR SPECIAL ABILITY to communicate with one another rapidly and with such great precision? We have already seen how signals are propagated *within* a neuron, from its dendrites and cell body to its axonal terminals. With this chapter we begin to consider the signaling *between* neurons through the process of synaptic transmission.

The specialized site at which one neuron communicates with another is called a *synapse*, and synaptic transmission is fundamental to the neural functions we consider later in the book, such as perception, voluntary movement, and learning.

The average neuron forms several thousand synaptic connections and receives a similar number. The Purkinje cell of the cerebellum receives up to 100,000 synaptic inputs. Although many of these connections are highly specialized, all neurons make use of one of the two basic forms of synaptic transmission: electrical or chemical. Moreover, the strength of both forms of synaptic transmission can be enhanced or diminished by cellular activity. This *plasticity* of synapses is crucial to memory and other higher brain functions.

Electrical synapses are employed primarily to send rapid and stereotyped depolarizing signals. In contrast, chemical synapses are capable of more variable signaling and thus can produce more complex behaviors. They can mediate either excitatory or inhibitory actions in postsynaptic cells and produce electrical changes in the postsynaptic cell that last from milliseconds to many minutes. Chemical synapses also serve to amplify neuronal signals, so even a small presynaptic nerve terminal can alter the response of large postsynaptic cells. Not surprisingly, most synapses in the brain are chemical. Because chemical synaptic transmission is so central to understanding brain and behavior, it is examined in detail in the next four chapters.

Synapses Are Either Electrical or Chemical

The term *synapse* was introduced at the beginning of the twentieth century by Charles Sherrington to describe the specialized zone of contact at which one neuron communicates with another. This site had first been described histologically at the level of light microscopy by Ramón y Cajal in the late 19th century.

All synapses were initially thought to operate by means of electrical transmission. In the 1920s, however, Otto Loewi discovered that the chemical compound acetylcholine (ACh) conveys signals from the vagus nerve to the heart. Loewi's discovery provoked considerable debate in the 1930s over whether chemical signaling existed at other synapses, including synapses between motor nerve and skeletal muscle as well as synapses in the brain.

Two schools of thought emerged, one physiological and the other pharmacological. Each championed a single mechanism for all synaptic transmission. Led by John Eccles (Sherrington's student), the physiologists argued that synaptic transmission is electrical, that the action potential in the presynaptic neuron generates a current that flows passively into the postsynaptic cell. The pharmacologists, led by Henry Dale, argued that transmission is chemical, that the action potential in the presynaptic neuron leads to the release of a chemical substance that in turn initiates current in the postsynaptic cell. When physiological and ultrastructural techniques improved in the 1950s and 1960s, it became clear that both forms of transmission exist. Although a chemical transmitter is used at most synapses, some operate purely by electrical means.

Once the fine structure of synapses was made visible with the electron microscope, chemical and electrical synapses were found to have different structures. At chemical synapses the presynaptic and postsynaptic neurons are completely separated by a small space, called the synaptic cleft; there is no continuity between the cytoplasm of one cell and the next. In contrast, at electrical synapses the pre- and postsynaptic cells communicate through special channels, the *gap-junction channels,* that directly connect the cytoplasm of the two cells.

The main functional properties of the two types of synapses are summarized in Table 8–1. The most important difference can be observed by injecting a positive current into the presynaptic cell to elicit a depolarization. At both types of synapses outward current across the presynaptic cell membrane deposits positive charge on the inside of the presynaptic cell membrane, thereby depolarizing the cell (see Chapter 6). At electrical synapses some of the current will enter the postsynaptic cell through the gap-junction channels, depositing a positive charge on the inside of the membrane and depolarizing it. The current leaves the postsynaptic cell across the membrane capacitance and through resting channels (Figure 8–1A). If the depolarization exceeds threshold, voltage-gated ion channels in the postsynaptic cell open and generate an action potential. By contrast, at chemical synapses there is no direct low-resistance pathway between the pre- and postsynaptic cells. Instead, the action potential in the presynaptic neuron initiates the release of a chemical transmitter, which diffuses across the synaptic cleft to interact with receptors on the membrane of the postsynaptic cell (Figure 8–1B).

Electrical Synapses Provide Instantaneous Signal Transmission

During excitatory synaptic transmission at an electrical synapse, voltage-gated ion channels in the presynaptic cell generate the current that depolarizes the postsynaptic cell. Thus these channels not only depolarize the presynaptic cell above the threshold for an action potential but also generate sufficient ionic current to produce a change in potential in the postsynaptic cell.

To generate such a large current, the presynaptic terminal must be big enough for its membrane to contain many ion channels. At the same time, the postsynaptic

Table 8–1 Distinguishing Properties of Electrical and Chemical Synapses

Type of synapse	Distance between pre- and postsynaptic cell membranes	Cytoplasmic continuity between pre- and postsynaptic cells	Ultrastructural components	Agent of transmission	Synaptic delay	Direction of transmission
Electrical	4 nm	Yes	Gap-junction channels	Ion current	Virtually absent	Usually bidirectional
Chemical	20–40 nm	No	Presynaptic vesicles and active zones; postsynaptic receptors	Chemical transmitter	Significant: at least 0.3 ms, usually 1–5 ms or longer	Unidirectional

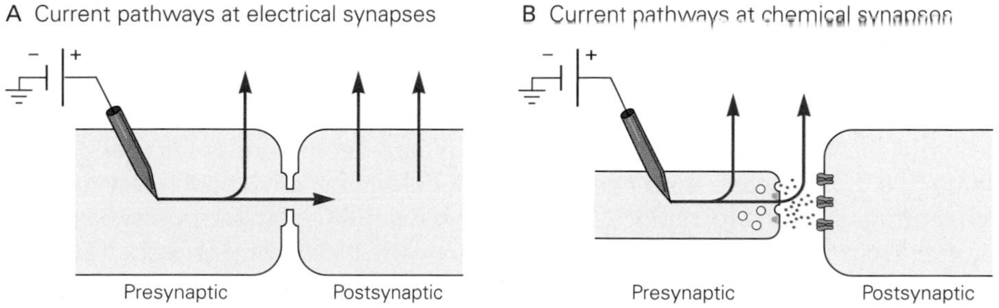

Figure 8–1 Functional properties of electrical and chemical synapses.

A. At an electrical synapse some current injected into the presynaptic cell escapes through resting (nongated) ion channels in the cell membrane. However, some current also enters the postsynaptic cell through gap-junction channels that connect the cytoplasm of the pre- and postsynaptic cells and that provide a low-resistance (high-conductance) pathway for electrical current.

B. At chemical synapses all current injected into the presynaptic cell escapes into the extracellular fluid. However, the resulting depolarization of the presynaptic cell membrane can produce an action potential that causes the release of neurotransmitter molecules that bind receptors on the postsynaptic cell. This binding opens ion channels that initiate a change in membrane potential in the postsynaptic cell.

cell must be relatively small. This is because a small cell has a higher input resistance (R_{in}) than a large cell and, according to Ohm's law ($\Delta V = I \times R_{in}$), undergoes a greater voltage change (ΔV) in response to a given presynaptic current (I).

Electrical synaptic transmission was first described by Edwin Furshpan and David Potter in the giant motor synapse of the crayfish, where the presynaptic fiber is much larger than the postsynaptic fiber (Figure 8–2A). An action potential generated in the presynaptic fiber

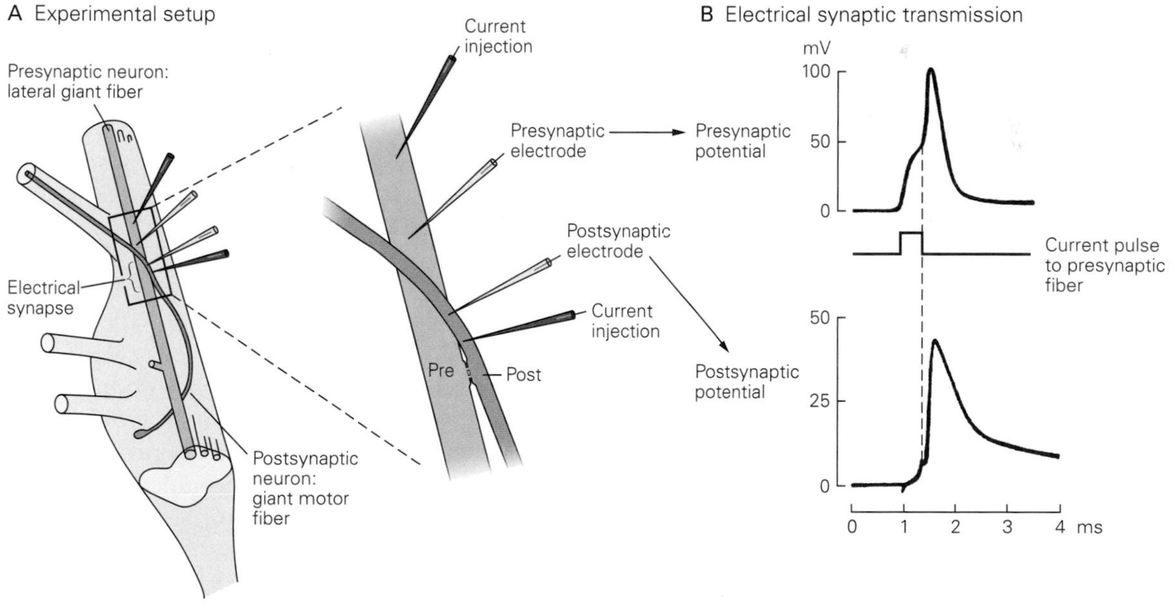

Figure 8–2 Electrical synaptic transmission was first demonstrated at the giant motor synapse in the crayfish. (Adapted, with permission, from Furshpan and Potter 1957 and 1959.)

A. The lateral giant fiber running down the nerve cord is the presynaptic neuron. The giant motor fiber, which projects from the cell body in the ganglion to the periphery, is the postsynaptic neuron. Electrodes for passing current and for recording voltage are placed within the pre- and postsynaptic cells.

B. Transmission at an electrical synapse is virtually instantaneous—the postsynaptic response follows presynaptic stimulation in a fraction of a millisecond. The **dashed line** shows how the responses of the two cells correspond in time. At chemical synapses there is a delay (the synaptic delay) between the pre- and postsynaptic potentials (see Figure 8–8).

produces a depolarizing postsynaptic potential that often exceeds the threshold to fire an action potential. At electrical synapses, the synaptic delay—the time between the presynaptic spike and the postsynaptic potential—is remarkably short (Figure 8–2B).

Such a short latency is not possible with chemical transmission, which requires several biochemical steps: release of a transmitter from the presynaptic neuron, diffusion of transmitter molecules to the postsynaptic cell, binding of transmitter to a specific receptor, and subsequent gating of ion channels (all described later in this chapter). Only current passing directly from one cell to another can produce the near-instantaneous transmission observed at the giant motor synapse.

Another feature of electrical transmission is that the change in potential of the postsynaptic cell is directly related to the size and shape of the change in potential of the presynaptic cell. Even when a weak subthreshold depolarizing current is injected into the presynaptic neuron, some current enters the postsynaptic cell and depolarizes it (Figure 8–3). In contrast, at a chemical synapse the current in the presynaptic cell must reach the threshold for an action potential before it can release transmitter and elicit a response in the postsynaptic cell.

Most electrical synapses can transmit both depolarizing and hyperpolarizing currents. A presynaptic action potential with a large hyperpolarizing afterpotential produces a biphasic (depolarizing-hyperpolarizing) change in potential in the postsynaptic cell. Signal transmission at electrical synapses is similar to the passive propagation of subthreshold electrical signals along axons (see Chapter 6) and therefore is also referred to as *electrotonic transmission.* At some specialized gap junctions the channels have voltage-dependent gates that permit them to conduct depolarizing current in only one direction, from the presynaptic cell to the postsynaptic cell. These junctions are called *rectifying synapses.* (The crayfish giant motor synapse is an example.)

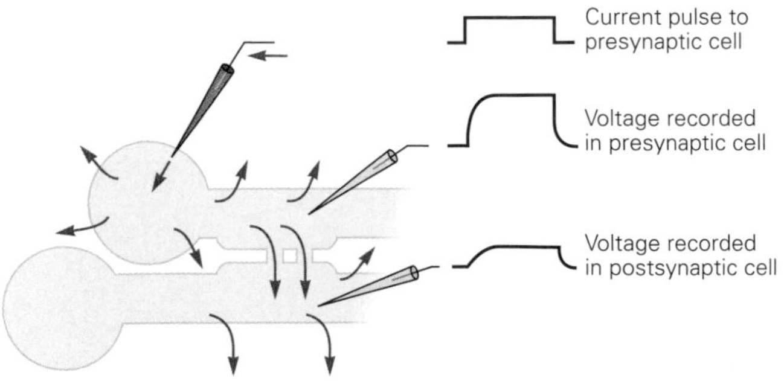

Figure 8–3 Electrical transmission is graded and occurs even when the current in the presynaptic cell is below the threshold for an action potential. This can be demonstrated by depolarizing the presynaptic cell with a small current pulse through one electrode while the membrane potential is recorded with a second electrode. A subthreshold depolarizing stimulus causes a passive depolarization in the presynaptic and postsynaptic cells. (Depolarizing or outward current is indicated by an upward deflection.)

Cells at an Electrical Synapse Are Connected by Gap-Junction Channels

The specialized region of contact between two neurons at an electrical synapse is termed the *gap junction.* Here the separation between the two neurons (4 nm) is much less than the normal nonsynaptic space between neurons (20 nm). This narrow gap is bridged by the gap-junction channels, specialized protein structures that conduct ionic current from the presynaptic to the postsynaptic cell.

A gap-junction channel consists of a pair of *hemichannels,* or connexons, one in the presynaptic and the other in the postsynaptic cell membrane. These hemichannels thus form a continuous bridge that provides a direct communication path between the two cells (Figure 8–4). The pore of the channel has a large diameter of approximately 1.5 nm, which permits inorganic ions and small organic molecules and experimental markers such as fluorescent dyes to pass between the two cells.

Each hemichannel or connexon is composed of six identical subunits, called *connexins.* Connexins in different tissues are encoded by a large gene family containing more than 20 members. All connexin subunits have an intracellular N- and C-terminus with four interposed α-helixes that span the cell membrane (Figure 8–4C). Many gap-junction channels in different cell types are formed by the products of different connexin genes and thus respond differently to modulatory factors that control their opening and closing. For example, although most gap-junction channels close in response to lowered cytoplasmic pH or elevated cytoplasmic Ca^{2+}, the sensitivity of different channel isoforms to these factors varies widely. This pH and Ca^{2+}-dependent closing of gap-junction channels plays an important role in the decoupling of damaged cells from healthy cells, because damaged cells contain elevated Ca^{2+} levels and a high concentration of protons. Finally, neurotransmitters released from nearby chemical synapses can modulate the opening of gap-junction channels through intracellular metabolic reactions (see Chapter 11).

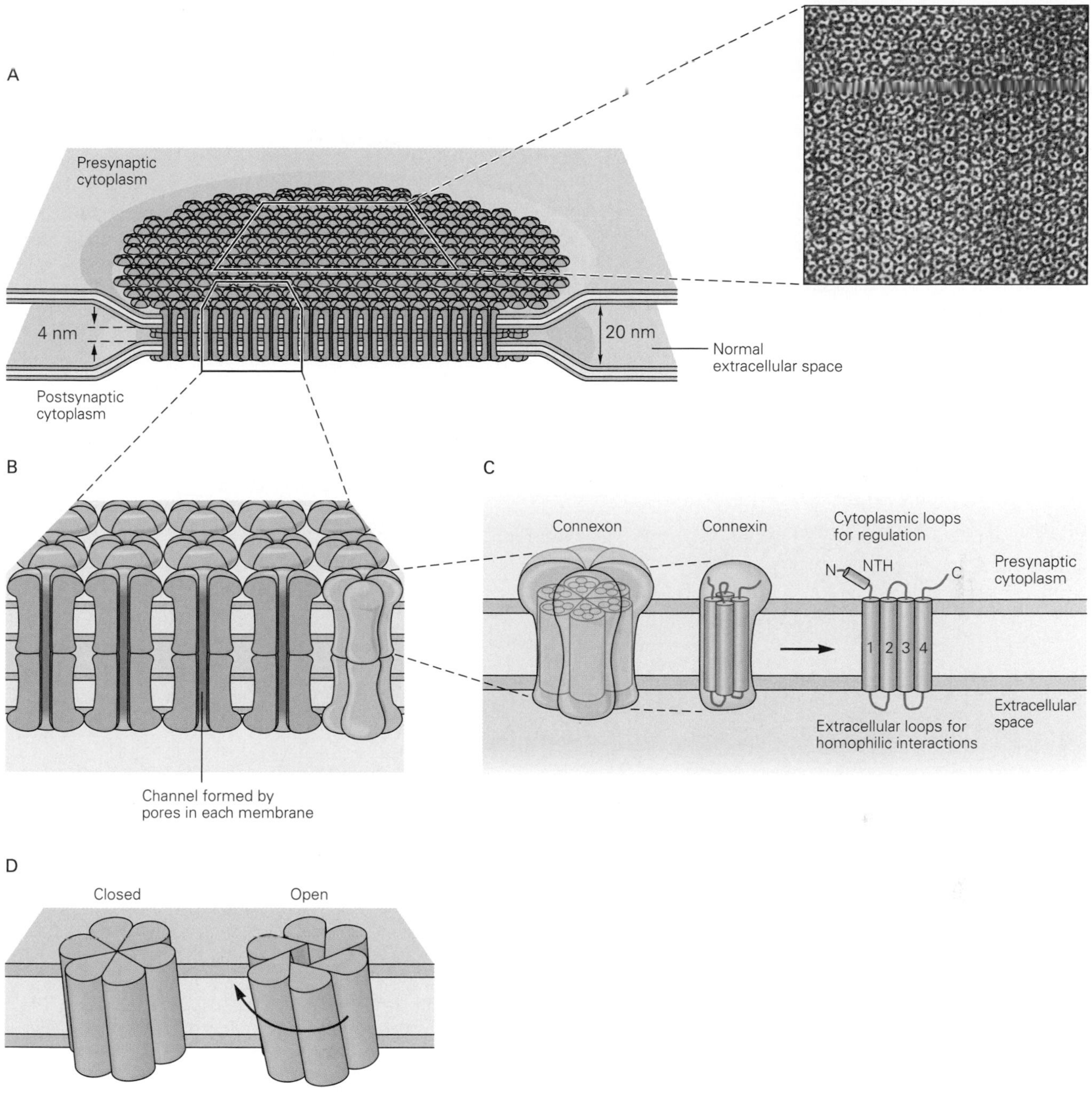

Figure 8–4 A three-dimensional model of the gap-junction channel, based on X-ray and electron diffraction studies.

A. The electrical synapse, or gap junction, is composed of numerous specialized channels that span the membranes of two neurons. These gap-junction channels allow current to pass directly from one cell to the other. The array of channels shown in the electron micrograph was isolated from the membrane of a rat liver. The tissue has been negatively stained, a technique that darkens the area around the channels and in the pores. Each channel appears hexagonal in outline. Magnification ×307,800. (Reproduced, with permission, from N. Gilula.)

B. A gap-junction channel is actually a pair of hemichannels, one in each apposite cell that connects the cytoplasm of the two cells. (Adapted, with permission, from Makowski et al. 1977.)

C. Each hemichannel, or connexon, is made up of six identical subunits called connexins. Each connexin is approximately 7.5 nm long and spans the cell membrane. A single connexin has intracellular N- and C-termini, including a short intracellular N-terminal α-helix (NTH), and four membrane-spanning α-helixes (1–4). There are regions of similarity in the amino acid sequences of gap-junction proteins from many different kinds of tissue. These include the transmembrane helixes and the extracellular regions, which are involved in the homophilic matching of apposite hemichannels.

D. The connexins are arranged in such a way that a pore is formed in the center of the structure. The resulting connexon, with a pore diameter of approximately 1.5 to 2 nm, has a characteristic hexagonal outline, as shown in part A. In some gap-junction channels the pore is opened when the subunits rotate approximately 0.9 nm at the cytoplasmic base in a clockwise direction. (Reproduced, with permission, from Unwin and Zampighi 1980.)

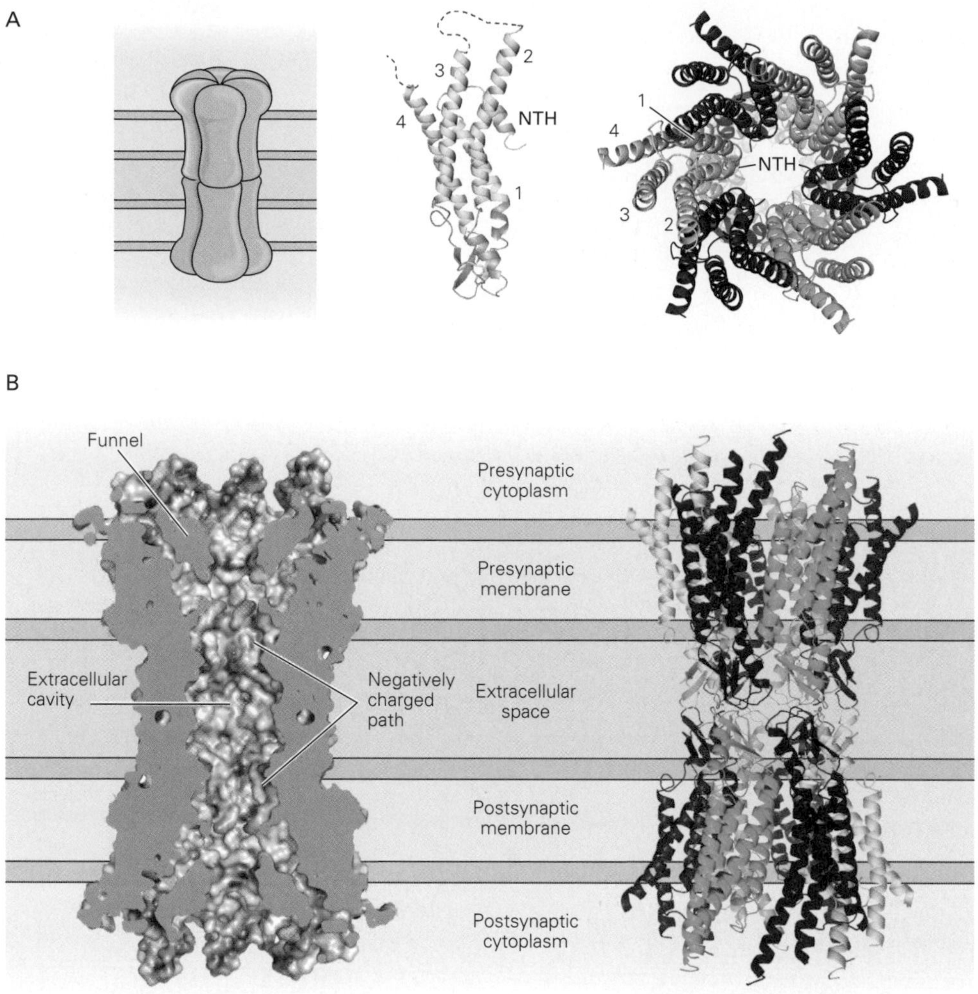

Figure 8–5 High-resolution three-dimensional structure of a gap-junction channel. All structures were determined by X-ray crystallography of gap-junction channels formed by the human connexon 26 subunit. (Reproduced, with permission, from Maeda et al., 2009.)

A. Left: Diagram of an intact gap-junction channel showing the pair of apposed hemichannels in the pre- and postsynaptic cells. **Middle:** High-resolution structure of a single connexin subunit showing the presence of four transmembrane α-helixes (1–4) and a short N-terminal helix (NTH). The orientation of the subunit corresponds to that of the yellow subunit in the diagram to the left. **Right:** Bottom-up view looking into a hemichannel from the cytoplasm. Each of the six subunits has a different color. The helixes of the yellow subunit are numbered. The orientation corresponds to that of the yellow hemichannel in the diagram at left, following a 90° rotation toward the viewer.

B. Two side views of the gap-junction channel in the plane of the membrane show the two apposed hemichannels. The orientation is the same as in the panel of part A. **Left:** Cross-section through the channel shows the internal surface of the channel pore. **Blue** indicates positively charged surfaces, and **red** indicates negatively charged surfaces. The **green mass** inside the pore at the cytoplasmic entrance (funnel) is thought to represent the channel gate formed by the N-terminal helix. **Right:** A side view of the channel shows each of the six connexin subunits in the same color scheme as in part A. The entire gap-junction channel is approximately 9 nm wide by 15 nm tall.

The three-dimensional structure of a gap-junction channel formed by the human connexin 26 subunit has recently been determined by X-ray crystallography. This structure shows in detail how the membrane-spanning α-helixes assemble to form the central pore of the channel and how the extracellular loops connecting the transmembrane helixes interdigitate to connect the two hemichannels (Figure 8–5). The pore is lined with polar residues that facilitate the movement of ions. An N-terminal α-helix may serve as the voltage gate of the connexin 26 channel, plugging the cytoplasmic mouth of the pore in the closed state. A separate gate at the extracellular side of the channel, formed by the extracellular loop connecting the first two membrane helixes, has been inferred from functional studies. This loop gate is thought to close isolated hemichannels that are not docked to a hemichannel partner in the apposing cell.

Electrical Transmission Allows the Rapid and Synchronous Firing of Interconnected Cells

How are electrical synapses useful? As we have seen, transmission across electrical synapses is extremely rapid because it results from the direct passage of current between cells. Speed is important for escape responses. For example, the tail-flip response of goldfish is mediated by a giant neuron in the brain stem (known as the Mauthner cell), which receives sensory input at electrical synapses. These electrical synapses rapidly depolarize the Mauthner cell, which in turn activates the motor neurons of the tail, allowing rapid escape from danger.

Electrical transmission is also useful for orchestrating the actions of large groups of neurons. Because current crosses the membranes of all electrically coupled cells at the same time, several small cells can act coordinately as one large cell. Moreover, because of the electrical coupling between the cells, the effective resistance of the coupled network of neurons is smaller than the resistance of an individual cell. Thus, from Ohm's law, the synaptic current required to fire electrically coupled cells is larger than that necessary to fire an individual cell. That is, electrically coupled cells have a higher firing threshold. Once this high threshold is surpassed, however, electrically coupled cells fire synchronously because voltage-activated Na^+ currents generated in one cell are very rapidly conducted to other cells.

Thus a behavior controlled by a group of electrically coupled cells has an important adaptive advantage: It is triggered explosively. For example, when seriously perturbed, the marine snail *Aplysia* releases massive clouds of purple ink that provide a protective screen. This stereotypic behavior is mediated by three electrically coupled motor cells that innervate the ink gland. Once the action potential threshold is exceeded in these cells, they fire synchronously (Figure 8–6). In certain fish, rapid eye movements (called saccades) are also mediated by electrically coupled motor neurons

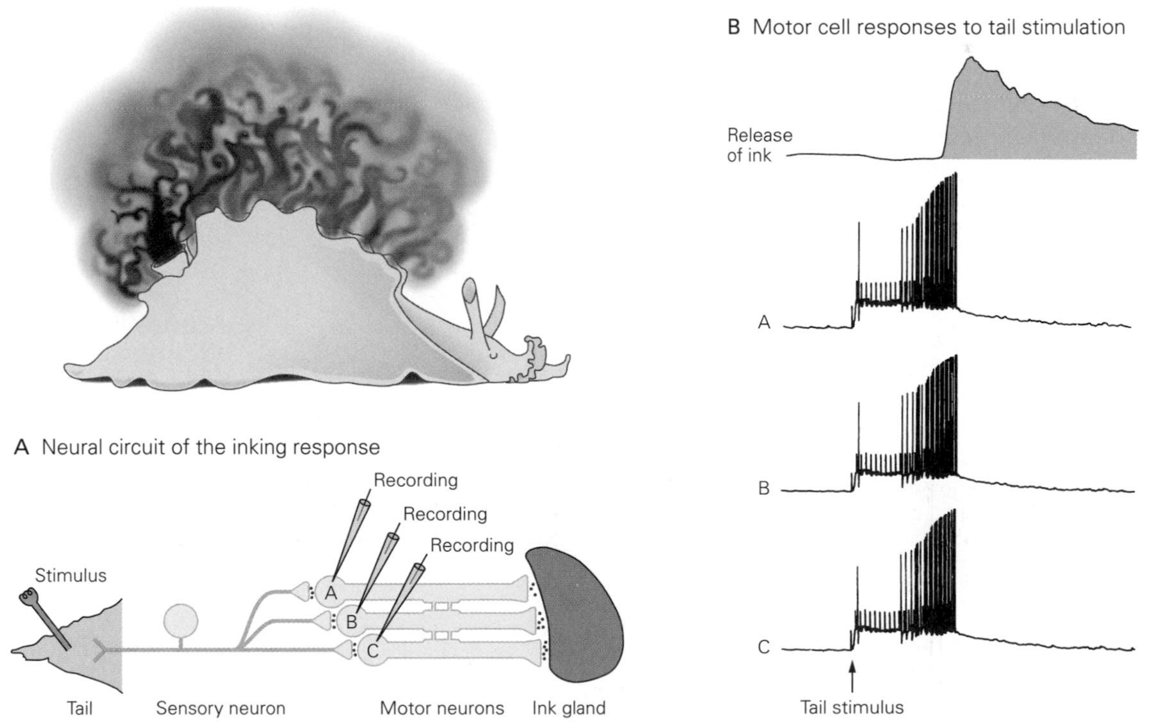

Figure 8–6 Electrically coupled motor neurons firing together can produce synchronous behaviors. (Adapted, with permission, from Carew and Kandel 1976.)

A. In the marine snail *Aplysia* sensory neurons from the tail ganglion form synapses with three motor neurons that innervate the ink gland. The motor neurons are interconnected by electrical synapses.

B. A train of stimuli applied to the tail produces a synchronized discharge in all three motor neurons that results in the release of ink.

firing together. Gap junctions are also important in the mammalian brain, where the synchronous firing of electrically coupled inhibitory interneurons generates synchronous, high-frequency oscillations.

In addition to providing speed or synchrony in neuronal signaling, electrical synapses also can transmit metabolic signals between cells. Because gap-junction channels are relatively large and nonselective, they conduct a variety of inorganic cations and anions, including the second messenger Ca^{2+}, and even allow moderate-sized organic compounds (less than 1,000 Da molecular weight)—such as the second messengers inositol 1,4,5-trisphosphate (IP_3), cyclic adenosine monophosphate (cAMP), and even small peptides—to pass from one cell to the next.

Gap Junctions Have a Role in Glial Function and Disease

Gap junctions are formed between glial cells as well as between neurons. In glia the gap junctions mediate both intercellular and intracellular communication. In the brain individual astrocytes are connected to each other through gap junctions, which mediate communication between them, forming a glial cell network. Electrical stimulation of neuronal pathways in brain slices can release neurotransmitters that trigger a rise in intracellular Ca^{2+} in certain astrocytes. This produces a wave of Ca^{2+} that propagates at a rate of approximately 1 μm/s, traveling from astrocyte to astrocyte by diffusion through gap-junction channels. Although the precise function of the waves is unknown, their existence suggests that glia may play an active role in signaling in the brain.

Gap-junction channels also enhance communication *within* certain glial cells, the Schwann cells that produce the myelin sheath of axons in the peripheral nervous system. Successive layers of myelin formed by a single Schwann cell are connected by gap junctions. These gap junctions may help to hold the layers of myelin together and promote the passage of small metabolites and ions across the many layers of myelin. The importance of the Schwann cell gap-junction channels is underscored by certain genetic diseases. For example, the X chromosome-linked form of Charcot-Marie-Tooth disease, a demyelinating disorder, is caused by single mutations in a connexin gene (*connexin 32*) expressed in the Schwann cell that blocks gap-junction channel function. Inherited mutations that prevent the function of a connexin expressed in the cochlea (connexin 26) underlie up to half of all instances of congenital deafness. This connexin normally forms gap-junction channels that are important for fluid secretion in the inner ear.

Chemical Synapses Can Amplify Signals

In contrast to electrical synapses, at chemical synapses there is no structural continuity between pre- and postsynaptic neurons. In fact, the separation between the two cells at a chemical synapse, the synaptic cleft, is usually wider (20–40 nm) than the nonsynaptic intercellular space (20 nm). Chemical synaptic transmission depends on the diffusion of a neurotransmitter across the synaptic cleft. A neurotransmitter is a chemical substance that binds receptors in the postsynaptic membrane of the target cell. At most chemical synapses transmitter is released from specialized swellings of the axon, the presynaptic terminals, which typically contain 100 to 200 synaptic vesicles, each of which is filled with several thousand molecules of the neurotransmitter (Figure 8–7).

The synaptic vesicles are clustered at specialized regions of the presynaptic membrane called *active zones*, which are the sites of neurotransmitter release. During a presynaptic action potential, voltage-gated Ca^{2+} channels at the active zone open, allowing Ca^{2+} to enter the presynaptic terminal. The rise in intracellular Ca^{2+} concentration triggers a biochemical reaction that causes the vesicles to fuse with the presynaptic membrane and release neurotransmitter into the synaptic cleft, a process termed *exocytosis*. The transmitter

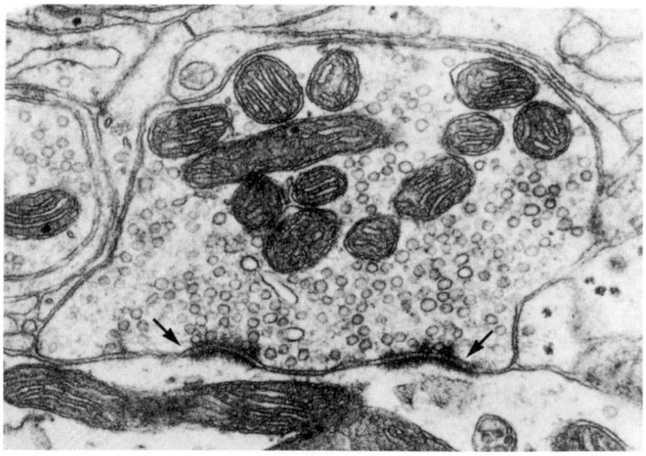

Figure 8–7 The fine structure of a presynaptic terminal. This electron micrograph shows a synapse in the cerebellum. The large dark structures are mitochondria. The many small round bodies are vesicles that contain neurotransmitter. The fuzzy dark thickenings along the presynaptic membrane (**arrows**) are the active zones, specialized areas that are thought to be docking and release sites for synaptic vesicles. The synaptic cleft is the space just outside the presynaptic terminal separating the pre- and postsynaptic cell membranes. (Reproduced, with permission, from J. E. Heuser and T. S. Reese.)

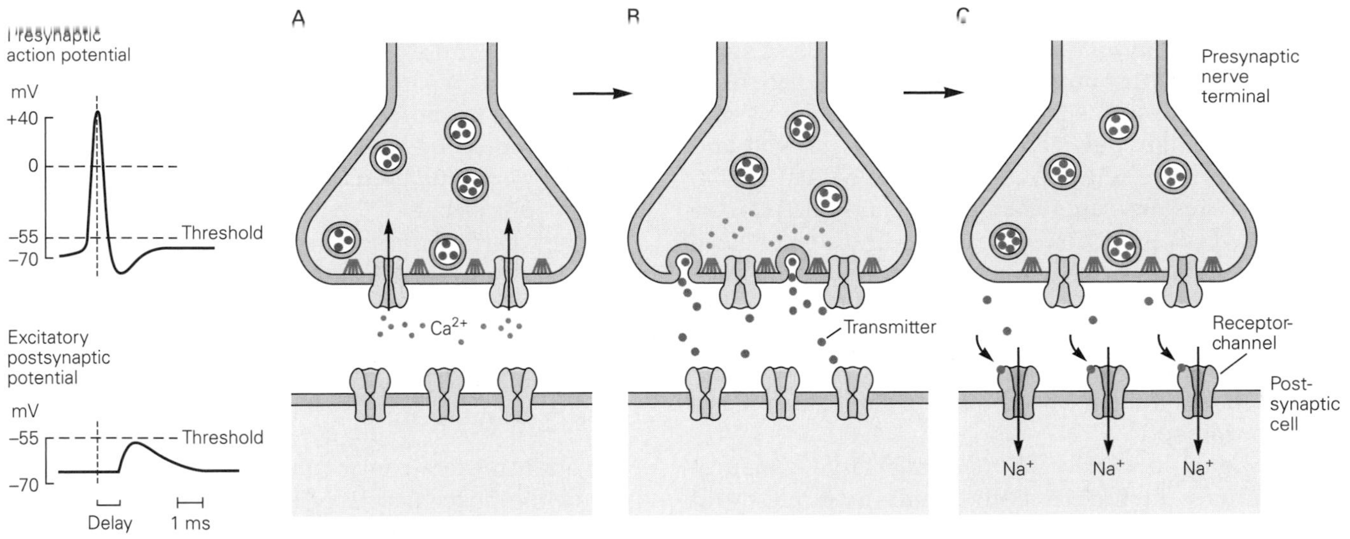

Figure 8–8 Synaptic transmission at chemical synapses involves several steps. The complex process of chemical synaptic transmission accounts for the delay between an action potential in the presynaptic cell and the synaptic potential in the postsynaptic cell compared with the virtually instantaneous transmission of signals at electrical synapses (see Figure 8–2B).

A. An action potential arriving at the terminal of a presynaptic axon causes voltage-gated Ca^{2+} channels at the active zone to open. The **gray filaments** represent the docking and release sites of the active zone.

B. The Ca^{2+} channel opening produces a high concentration of intracellular Ca^{2+} near the active zone, causing vesicles containing neurotransmitter to fuse with the presynaptic cell membrane and release their contents into the synaptic cleft (a process termed *exocytosis*).

C. The released neurotransmitter molecules then diffuse across the synaptic cleft and bind specific receptors on the postsynaptic membrane. These receptors cause ion channels to open (or close), thereby changing the membrane conductance and membrane potential of the postsynaptic cell.

molecules then diffuse across the synaptic cleft and bind to their receptors on the postsynaptic cell membrane. This in turn activates the receptors, leading to the opening or closing of ion channels. The resulting flux of ions alters the membrane conductance and potential of the postsynaptic cell (Figure 8–8).

These several steps account for the synaptic delay at chemical synapses, a delay that can be as short as 0.3 ms but often lasts several milliseconds. Although chemical transmission lacks the speed of electrical synapses, it has the important property of *amplification*. Just one synaptic vesicle releases several thousand molecules of transmitter that together can open thousands of ion channels in the target cell. In this way a small presynaptic nerve terminal, which generates only a weak electrical current, can depolarize a large postsynaptic cell.

Neurotransmitters Bind to Postsynaptic Receptors

Chemical synaptic transmission can be divided into two steps: a transmitting step, in which the presynaptic cell releases a chemical messenger, and a receptive step, in which the transmitter binds to and activates the receptor molecules in the postsynaptic cell. The transmitting process resembles endocrine hormone release. Indeed, chemical synaptic transmission can be seen as a modified form of hormone secretion. Both endocrine glands and presynaptic terminals release a chemical agent with a signaling function, and both are examples of regulated secretion (Chapter 4). Similarly, both endocrine glands and neurons are usually some distance from their target cells. There is one important difference, however, between endocrine and synaptic signaling. Whereas the hormone released by a gland travels through the blood stream until it interacts with all cells that contain an appropriate receptor, a neuron usually communicates only with the cells with which it forms synapses. Because the presynaptic action potential triggers the release of a chemical transmitter onto a target cell across a distance of only 20 nm, the chemical signal travels only a small distance to its target. Therefore, neuronal signaling has two special features: It is fast and precisely directed.

To accomplish this directed or focused release, most neurons have specialized secretory machinery, the active zones, which are directly apposed to the transmitter receptors in the postsynaptic cell. In neurons without active zones, the distinction between neuronal and hormonal transmission becomes blurred.

For example, the neurons in the autonomic nervous system that innervate smooth muscle reside at some distance from their postsynaptic cells and do not have specialized release sites in their terminals. Synaptic transmission between these cells is slower and relies on a more widespread diffusion of transmitter. Furthermore, the same transmitter substance can be released differently from different cells. From one cell a substance can be released as a conventional transmitter acting directly on neighboring cells. From other cells it can be released in a less focused way as a modulator, producing a more diffuse action; and from still other cells it can be released into the blood stream as a neurohormone.

Although a variety of chemicals serve as neurotransmitters, including both small molecules and peptides (see Chapter 13), the action of a transmitter depends on the properties of the postsynaptic receptors that recognize and bind the transmitter, not the chemical properties of the transmitter. For example, ACh can excite some postsynaptic cells and inhibit others, and at still other cells it can produce both excitation and inhibition. It is the receptor that determines the action of ACh, including whether a cholinergic synapse is excitatory or inhibitory.

Within a group of closely related animals, a transmitter substance binds conserved families of receptors and can be often associated with specific physiological functions. In vertebrates ACh acts on excitatory ACh receptors at all neuromuscular junctions to trigger contraction and it acts on inhibitory ACh receptors to slow the heart.

The notion of a receptor was introduced in the late 19th century by the German bacteriologist Paul Ehrlich to explain the selective action of toxins and other pharmacological agents and the great specificity of immunological reactions. In 1900 Ehrlich wrote: "Chemical substances are only able to exercise an action on the tissue elements with which they are able to establish an intimate chemical relationship . . . [This relationship] must be specific. The [chemical] groups must be adapted to one another . . . as lock and key."

In 1906 the English pharmacologist John Langley postulated that the sensitivity of skeletal muscle to curare and nicotine was caused by a "receptive molecule." A theory of receptor function was later developed by Langley's students (in particular, A.V. Hill and Henry Dale), a development that was based on concurrent studies of enzyme kinetics and cooperative interactions between small molecules and proteins. As we shall see in the next chapter, Langley's "receptive molecule" has been isolated and characterized as the ACh receptor of the neuromuscular junction.

All receptors for chemical transmitters have two biochemical features in common:

1. They are membrane-spanning proteins. The region exposed to the external environment of the cell recognizes and binds the transmitter from the presynaptic cell.
2. They carry out an effector function within the target cell. The receptors typically influence the opening or closing of ion channels.

Postsynaptic Receptors Gate Ion Channels Either Directly or Indirectly

Neurotransmitters control the opening of ion channels in the postsynaptic cell either directly or indirectly. These two classes of transmitter actions are mediated by receptor proteins derived from different gene families.

Receptors that gate ion channels directly, such as the ACh receptor at the neuromuscular junction, are composed of four or five subunits that form a single macromolecule. Such receptors contain both an extracellular domain that forms the binding site for the transmitter and a membrane-spanning domain that forms an ion-conducting pore (Figure 8–9A). This kind of receptor is often referred to as *ionotropic*. Upon binding neurotransmitter, the receptor undergoes a conformational change that opens the channel. The actions of ionotropic receptors, also called *receptor-channels* or *ligand-gated channels*, are discussed in detail in Chapters 9 and 10.

Receptors that gate ion channels indirectly, like the several types of receptors for norepinephrine or dopamine in neurons of the cerebral cortex, are normally composed of one or at most two subunits that are distinct from the ion channels they regulate. These receptors, which commonly have seven membrane-spanning α-helixes, act by altering intracellular metabolic reactions and are often referred to as *metabotropic receptors*. Activation of these receptors often stimulates the production of second messengers, small freely diffusible intracellular metabolites such as cAMP or diacylglycerol. Many of these second messengers activate protein kinases, enzymes that phosphorylate different substrate proteins. In many instances the protein kinases directly phosphorylate ion channels, leading to their opening or closing (Figure 8–9B). The actions of metabotropic receptors are examined in detail in Chapter 11.

Ionotropic and metabotropic receptors have different functions. The ionotropic receptors produce relatively fast synaptic actions lasting only milliseconds. These are commonly found at synapses in neural circuits that mediate rapid behaviors, such as the stretch

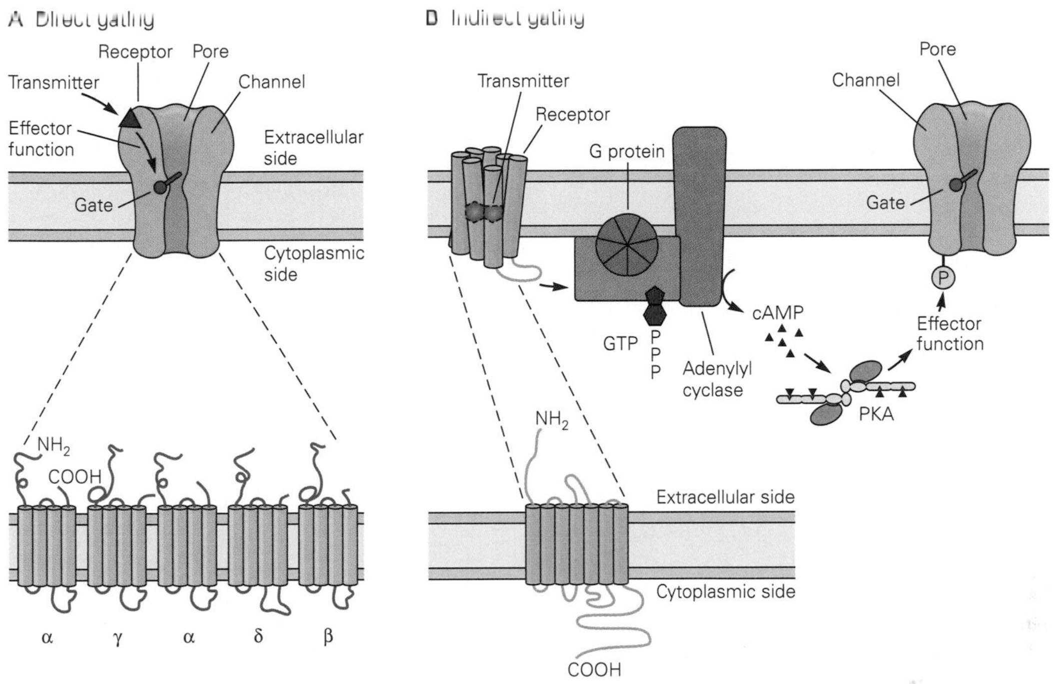

Figure 8–9 Neurotransmitters open postsynaptic ion channels either directly or indirectly.

A. A receptor that directly opens ion channels is an integral part of the macromolecule that also forms the channel. Many such ligand-gated channels are composed of five subunits, each of which is thought to contain four membrane-spanning α-helical regions.

B. A receptor that indirectly opens an ion channel is a distinct macromolecule separate from the channel it regulates. In one large family of such receptors, the receptors are composed of a single subunit with seven membrane-spanning α-helical regions that bind the ligand within the plane of the membrane. These receptors activate a guanosine triphosphate (GTP)–binding protein (G protein), which in turn activates a second-messenger cascade that modulates channel activity. In the cascade illustrated here the G protein stimulates adenylyl cyclase, which converts adenosine triphosphate (ATP) to cAMP. The cAMP activates the cAMP-dependent protein kinase (PKA), which phosphorylates the channel (P), leading to a change in function.

receptor reflex. The metabotropic receptors produce slower synaptic actions lasting seconds to minutes. These slower actions can modulate behavior by altering the excitability of neurons and the strength of the synaptic connections of the neural circuitry mediating behavior. Such modulatory synaptic actions often act as crucial reinforcing pathways in the process of learning.

Steven A. Siegelbaum
Eric R. Kandel

Selected Readings

Bennett MV, Zukin RS. 2004. Electrical coupling and neuronal synchronization in the mammalian brain. Neuron 19:495–511.

Colquhoun D, Sakmann B. 1998. From muscle endplate to brain synapses: a short history of synapses and agonist-activated ion channels. Neuron 20:381–387.

Cowan WM, Kandel ER. 2000. A brief history of synapses and synaptic transmission. In: MW Cowan, TC Südhof, CF Stevens (eds). *Synapses,* pp. 1–87. Baltimore and London: The Johns Hopkins Univ. Press.

Eccles JC. 1976. From electrical to chemical transmission in the central nervous system. The closing address of the Sir Henry Dale Centennial Symposium. Notes Rec R Soc Lond 30:219–230.

Furshpan EJ, Potter DD. 1959. Transmission at the giant motor synapses of the crayfish. J Physiol 145:289–325.

Goodenough DA, Paul DL. 2009. Gap junctions. Cold Spring Harb Perspect Biol 1:a002576.

Jessell TM, Kandel ER. 1993. Synaptic transmission: a bidirectional and a self-modifiable form of cell-cell communication. Cell 72:1–30.

Nakagawa S, Maeda S, Tsukihara T. 2010. Structural and functional studies of gap junction channels. Curr Opin Struct Biol 20:423–430

References

Beyer EC, Paul DL, Goodenough DA. 1987. Connexin 43: a protein from rat heart homologous to a gap junction protein from liver. J Cell Biol 105:2621–2629.

Bruzzone R, White TW, Scherer SS, Fischbeck KH, Paul DL. 1994. Null mutations of connexin 32 in patients with x-linked Charcot-Marie-Tooth disease. Neuron 13: 1253–1260.

Carew TJ, Kandel ER. 1976. Two functional effects of decreased conductance EPSP's: synaptic augmentation and increased electrotonic coupling. Science 192:150–153.

Cornell-Bell AH, Finkbeiner SM, Cooper MS, Smith SJ. 1990. Glutamate induces calcium waves in cultured astrocytes: long-range glial signaling. Science 247:470–473.

Dale H. 1935. Pharmacology and nerve-endings. Proc R Soc Lond 28:319–332.

Eckert R. 1988. Propagation and transmission of signals. In: *Animal Physiology: Mechanisms and Adaptations*, 3rd ed., pp. 134–176. New York: Freeman.

Ehrlich P. 1900. On immunity with special reference to cell life. Croonian Lect Proc R Soc Lond 66:424–448.

Furshpan EJ, Potter DD. 1957. Mechanism of nerve-impulse transmission at a crayfish synapse. Nature 180:342–343.

Harris AL. 2009. Gating on the outside. J Gen Physiol 133:549–553.

Heuser JE, Reese TS. 1977. Structure of the synapse. In: ER Kandel (ed). *Handbook of Physiology: A Critical, Comprehensive Presentation of Physiological Knowledge and Concepts*, Sect. 1. *The Nervous System*, Vol. 1 *Cellular Biology of Neurons*, Part 1, pp. 261–294. Bethesda, MD: American Physiological Society.

Jaslove SW, Brink PR. 1986. The mechanism of rectification at the electrotonic motor giant synapse of the crayfish. Nature 323:63–65.

Langley JN. 1906. On nerve endings and on special excitable substances in cells. Proc R Soc Lond B Biol Sci 78:170–194.

Loewi O, Navratil E. 1926. Über humorale Übertragbarkeit der Herznervenwirkung. X. Mitteilung: über das Schicksal des Vagusstoffs. Pflügers Arch 214:678–688; 1972. Translated in: On the humoral propagation of cardiac nerve action. Communication X. The fate of the vagus substance. In: I Cooke, M Lipkin Jr (eds). *Cellular Neurophysiology: A Source Book*, pp. 478–485. New York: Holt, Rinehart and Winston.

Maeda S, Nakagawa S, Suga M, Yamashita E, Oshima A, Fujiyoshi Y, Tsukihara T. 2009. Structure of the connexin 26 gap junction channel at 3.5 Å resolution. Nature 458:597–602.

Makowski L, Caspar DL, Phillips WC, Goodenough DA. 1977. Gap junction structures. II. Analysis of the X-ray diffraction data. J Cell Biol 74:629–645.

Pappas GD, Waxman SG. 1972. Synaptic fine structure: morphological correlates of chemical and electronic transmission. In: GD Pappas, DP Purpura (eds). *Structure and Function of Synapses*, pp. 1–43. New York: Raven.

Ramón y Cajal S. 1894. La fine structure des centres nerveux. Proc R Soc Lond 55:444–468.

Ramón y Cajal S. 1911. *Histologie du Système Nerveux de l'Homme & des Vertébrés*, Vol. 2. L Azoulay (transl). Paris: Maloine, 1955. Reprint. Madrid: Instituto Ramón y Cajal.

Sherrington C. 1947. *The Integrative Action of the Nervous System*, 2nd ed. New Haven: Yale Univ. Press.

Unwin PNT, Zampighi G. 1980. Structure of the junction between communicating cells. Nature 283:545–549.

Whittington MA, Traub RD. 2003. Interneuron diversity series: inhibitory interneurons and network oscillations in vitro. Trends Neurosci 26:676–682.

9

Signaling at the Nerve-Muscle Synapse: Directly Gated Transmission

Communication between neurons in the brain relies mainly on chemical synapses. Much of our present understanding of the function of these synapses is based on studies of synaptic transmission at the nerve-muscle synapse, the junction between a motor neuron and a skeletal muscle fiber. This is the site where synaptic transmission was first studied and remains best understood. Moreover, the nerve-muscle synapse is the site of a number of inherited and acquired neurological diseases. Therefore, before we examine the complexities of synapses in the central nervous system, we will examine the basic features of chemical synaptic transmission at the nerve-muscle synapse.

The nerve-muscle synapse is an ideal site for studying chemical signaling because it is relatively simple and accessible to experimentation. The muscle cell is large enough to accommodate the two or more microelectrodes needed to make electrical measurements. Also the muscle cell normally receives signals from just one presynaptic axon, in contrast to the convergent connections on central nerve cells. Most importantly, chemical signaling at the nerve-muscle synapse involves a relatively simple mechanism: Release of neurotransmitter from the presynaptic nerve directly opens a single type of ion channel in the postsynaptic membrane.

The Neuromuscular Junction Is a Well-Studied Example of Directly Gated Synaptic Transmission

The motor neuron innervates the muscle at a specialized region of the muscle membrane called the *end-plate,* where the motor axon loses its myelin sheath and splits into several fine branches. The ends of the fine branches form multiple expansions or varicosities, called *synaptic boutons,* from which the motor neuron releases its transmitter. Each bouton is positioned over a specialized region of the muscle membrane containing deep depressions, or *junctional folds,* which contain the transmitter receptors (Figure 9–1). The transmitter released by the motor axon terminal is acetylcholine

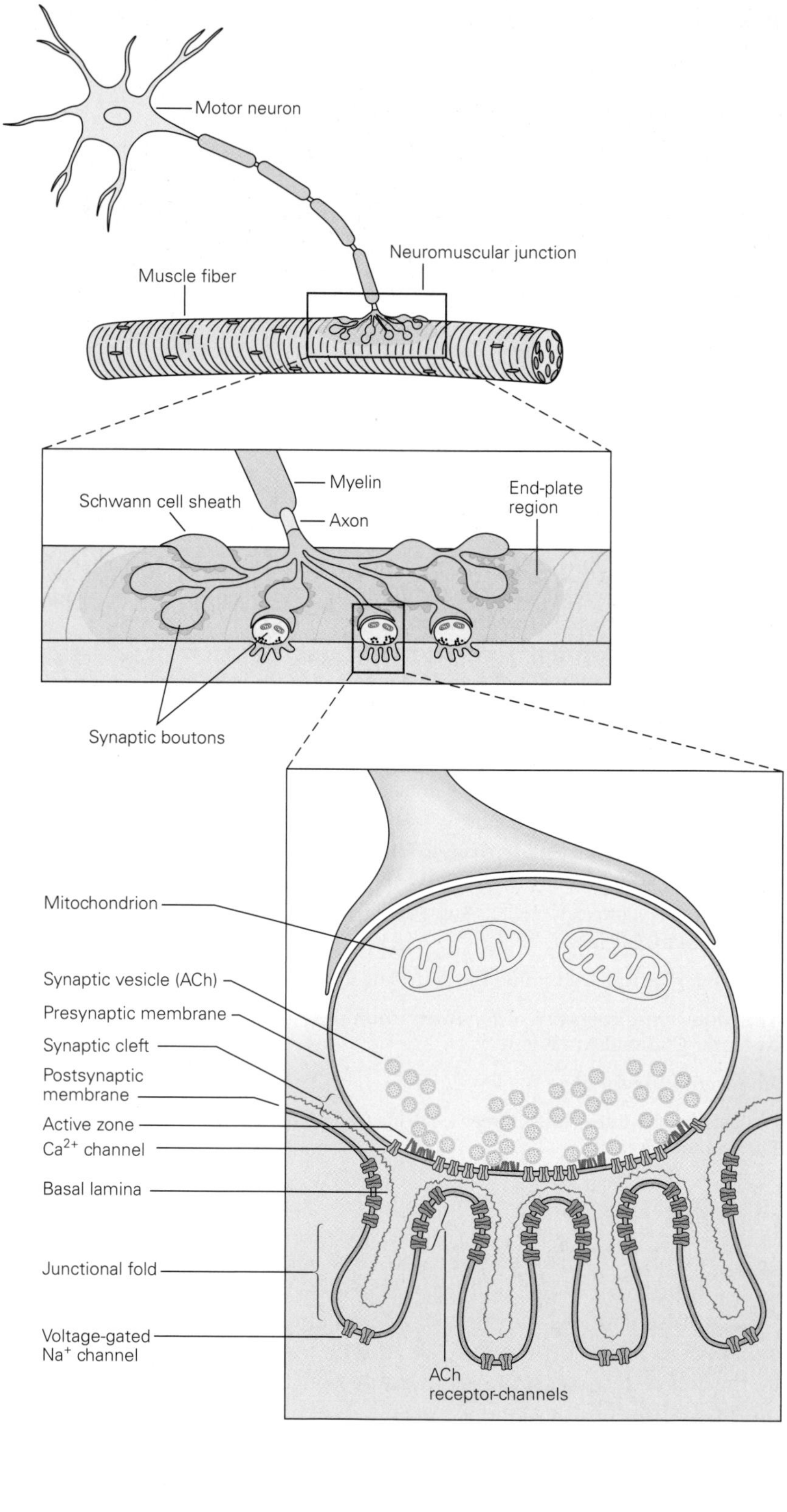

Figure 9–1 The neuromuscular junction is an ideal site for studying chemical synaptic signaling. At the muscle the motor axon ramifies into several fine branches approximately 2 μm thick. Each branch forms multiple swellings called *synaptic boutons*, which are covered by a thin layer of Schwann cells. The boutons lie over a specialized region of the muscle fiber membrane, the *end-plate*, and are separated from the muscle membrane by a 100-nm synaptic cleft. Each bouton contains mitochondria and synaptic vesicles clustered around *active zones*, where the neurotransmitter acetylcholine (ACh) is released. Immediately under each bouton in the end-plate are several junctional folds, the crests of which contain a high density of ACh receptors.

The muscle fiber and nerve terminal are covered by a layer of connective tissue, the basal lamina, consisting of collagen and glycoproteins. Unlike the cell membrane, the basal lamina is freely permeable to ions and small organic compounds, including the transmitter. Both the presynaptic terminal and the muscle fiber secrete proteins into the basal lamina, including the enzyme acetylcholinesterase, which inactivates the ACh released from the presynaptic terminal by breaking it down into acetate and choline. The basal lamina also organizes the synapse by aligning the presynaptic boutons with the postsynaptic junctional folds. (Adapted, with permission, from McMahan and Kuffler 1971.)

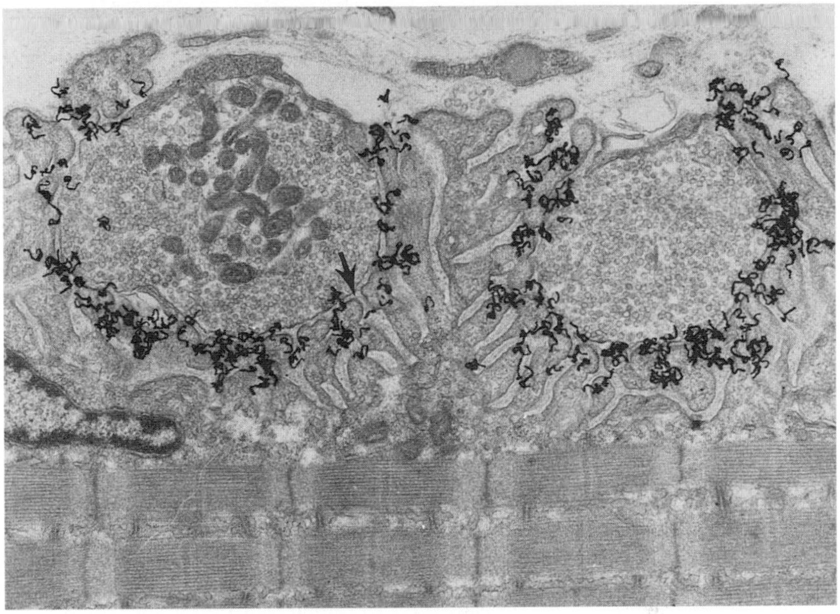

Figure 9–2 Acetylcholine receptors in the vertebrate neuromuscular junction are concentrated at the top one-third of the junctional folds. This receptor-rich region is characterized by an increased density of the postjunctional membrane (**arrow**). The autoradiograph shown here was made by first incubating the membrane with radiolabeled α-bungarotoxin, which binds to the ACh receptor (**black grains**). Radioactive decay results in the emittance of a particle that causes overlaid silver grains to become fixed along its trajectory (**black grains**). Magnification ×18,000. (Reproduced, with permission, from Salpeter 1987.)

(ACh) and the receptor on the muscle membrane is the nicotinic type of ACh receptor.[1]

The presynaptic and postsynaptic membranes are separated by a synaptic cleft approximately 100 nm wide. Within the cleft is a basal lamina (or basement membrane) composed of collagen and other extracellular matrix proteins. The enzyme acetylcholinesterase, which rapidly hydrolyzes ACh, is anchored to the collagen fibrils of the basal laminae. In the muscle cell, in the region below the crest of the junctional fold and extending into the fold, the membrane is rich in voltage-gated Na^+ channels (Figure 9–1).

Each synaptic bouton contains all the machinery required to release neurotransmitter. This includes the synaptic vesicles, which contain the transmitter ACh, and the active zones, regions of the membrane specialized for release of transmitter, where the synaptic vesicles are clustered (Figure 9–1). In addition, each active zone contains voltage-gated Ca^{2+} channels that permit Ca^{2+} to enter the terminal with each action potential (see Figure 9–1). This influx of Ca^{2+} triggers the fusion of the synaptic vesicles with the plasma membrane at the active zones, releasing the contents of the synaptic vesicle into the synaptic cleft by the process of exocytosis (see Chapter 12). Every active zone in the presynaptic membrane is positioned opposite a junctional fold in the postsynaptic cell. At the crest of each fold the receptors for ACh are clustered in a lattice, with a density of approximately 10,000 receptors per μm^2 (Figure 9–2). The nicotinic ACh receptor is a ligand-gated channel: It is an integral membrane protein that both binds ACh and forms an ion channel (Figure 9–3).

The Motor Neuron Excites the Muscle by Opening Ligand-Gated Ion Channels at the End-Plate

The release of transmitter from the motor nerve terminal opens ACh receptor-channels in the muscle membrane at the end-plate, and this action rapidly depolarizes the membrane. The resulting excitatory postsynaptic potential (EPSP), also called the *end-plate potential* at the nerve-muscle synapse, is very large; stimulation of a single motor cell produces a synaptic potential of approximately 70 mV.

This change in membrane potential usually is large enough to rapidly activate the voltage-gated Na^+ channels in the junctional folds, converting the end-plate potential into an action potential, which then propagates along the muscle fiber. In contrast, in the central nervous system most presynaptic neurons produce postsynaptic potentials less than 1 mV in amplitude. As a result, input from many presynaptic neurons is needed to generate an action potential in most neurons.

[1] There are two basic types of receptors for ACh: nicotinic and muscarinic, so called because the alkaloids nicotine and muscarine bind exclusively to and activate one or the other type of ACh receptor. The nicotinic receptor is an ionotropic receptor, whereas the muscarinic receptor is a metabotropic receptor (see Chapter 8). We shall learn more about muscarinic ACh receptors in Chapter 11.

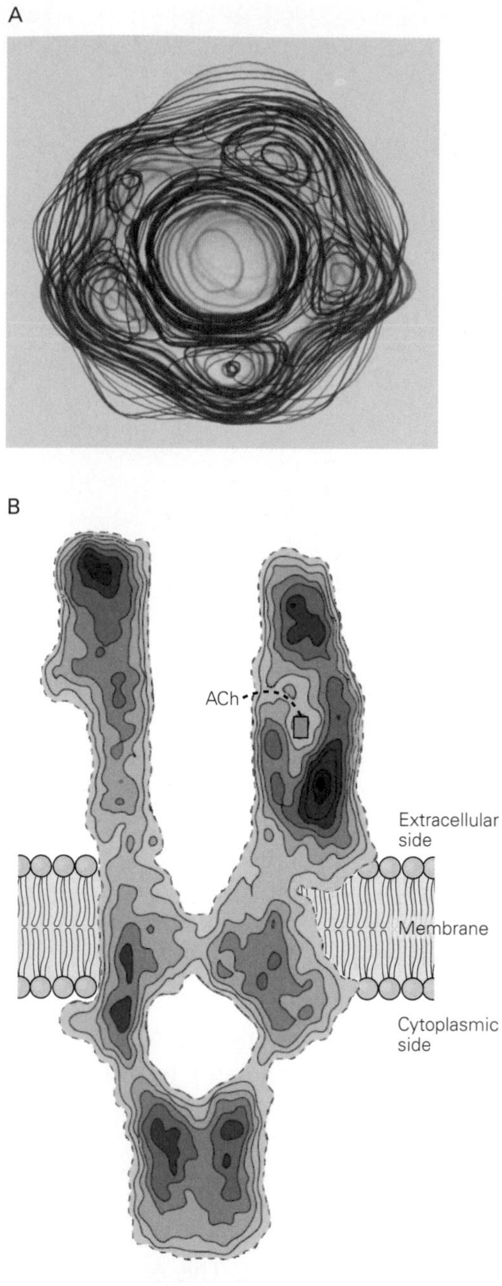

Figure 9–3 Low-resolution structure of the acetylcholine (ACh) receptor-channel. These reconstructed electron microscope images were obtained by computer processing of negatively stained images of ACh receptors in the fish *Torpedo californica*. The resolution is fine enough to see overall structures but too coarse to resolve individual atoms.

A. View looking down on the receptor from the extracellular space. The overall diameter of the receptor and its channel is approximately 8.5 nm. (Reproduced, with permission, from Brisson and Unwin 1985.)

B. Side view of the receptor in the lipid bilayer. The pore is wide at the external and internal surfaces of the membrane but narrows considerably within the lipid bilayer. The channel extends some distance into the extracellular space. A molecule of ACh enters a crevice in the wall of the receptor. (Adapted, with permission, from Karlin 2002; Miyazawa et al. 1999.)

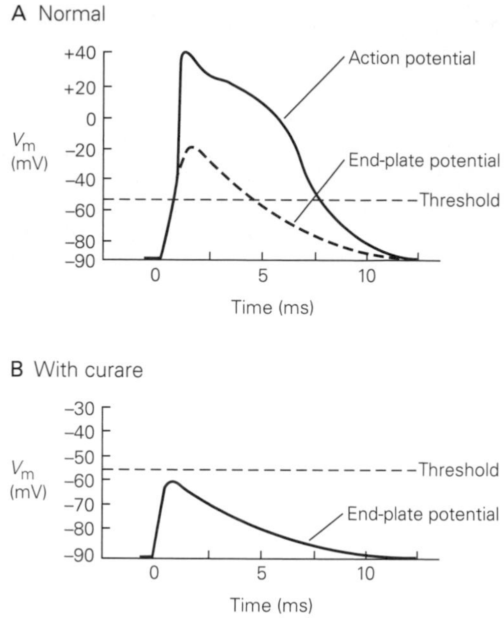

Figure 9–4 The end-plate potential can be isolated pharmacologically for study.

A. Under normal circumstances stimulation of the motor axon produces an action potential in a skeletal muscle cell. The **dashed line** shows the inferred time course of the end-plate potential that triggers the action potential.

B. Curare blocks the binding of acetylcholine (ACh) to its receptor and so prevents the end-plate potential from reaching the threshold for an action potential (**dashed line**). In this way the currents and channels that contribute to the end-plate potential, which are different from those producing an action potential, can be studied. The end-plate potential shown here was recorded in the presence of a low concentration of curare, which blocks only a fraction of the ACh receptors. The values for the resting potential (–90 mV), end-plate potential, and action potential in these intracellular recordings are typical of a vertebrate skeletal muscle.

The End-Plate Potential Is Produced by Ionic Current Through Acetylcholine Receptor-Channels

The end-plate potential was first studied in detail in the 1950s by Paul Fatt and Bernard Katz using intracellular voltage recordings. Fatt and Katz were able to isolate the end-plate potential by applying the drug curare[2] to reduce the amplitude of the postsynaptic potential below the threshold for the action potential (Figure 9–4). They found that the EPSP in muscle cells

[2]Curare is a mixture of plant toxins used by South American Indians, who apply it to arrowheads to paralyze their quarry. Tubocurarine, the purified active agent, blocks neuromuscular transmission by binding to the nicotinic ACh receptor, preventing its activation by ACh.

was largest at the end-plate and decreased progressively with distance (Figure 9–5).

From this, Fatt and Katz concluded that the end-plate potential is generated by an inward ionic current that is confined to the end-plate and then spreads passively away. (Remember, an inward current corresponds to an influx of positive charge, which depolarizes the inside of the membrane.) Inward current is confined to the end-plate because the ACh receptor-channels are concentrated there, opposite the presynaptic terminal from which transmitter is released.

The end-plate potential rises rapidly but decays more slowly. The rapid rise is caused by the sudden release into the synaptic cleft of ACh, which diffuses rapidly to the receptors at the end-plate. (Not all the ACh reaches receptors, however, because ACh is quickly removed from the synaptic cleft by hydrolysis by acetylcholinesterase and diffusion.)

The current that generates the end-plate potential was first studied in voltage-clamp experiments (see Box 7–1). These studies revealed that the end-plate current rises and decays more rapidly than the resultant end-plate potential (Figure 9–6). The time course of the end-plate current is directly determined by the rapid opening and closing of the ACh receptor-channels. Because it takes time for an ionic current to charge or discharge the muscle membrane capacitance, and thus alter the membrane voltage, the EPSP lags behind the synaptic current (see Figure 6–15 and the Postscript at the end of this chapter).

The Ion Channel at the End-Plate Is Permeable to Both Sodium and Potassium

Why does the opening of the ACh receptor-channels lead to an inward current that produces the depolarizing end-plate potential? And which ions move through the ACh-gated channels to produce this inward current? One important means of identifying the ion (or ions) responsible for the synaptic current is to measure the value of the chemical driving force (the chemical battery) propelling ions through the channel. Remember, the current through a set of membrane channels is given by the product of the membrane conductance and the electrochemical driving force on the ions conducted through the channels (see Chapter 6). The end-plate current that underlies the EPSP is determined by:

$$I_{\text{EPSP}} = g_{\text{EPSP}} \times (V_{\text{m}} - E_{\text{EPSP}}), \qquad \textbf{(9–1)}$$

where I_{EPSP} is the end-plate current, g_{EPSP} is the conductance of the ACh receptor-channels, V_{m} is the membrane potential, and E_{EPSP} is the chemical driving force or battery generated by the transmembrane concentration gradients of the ions conducted through the channels.

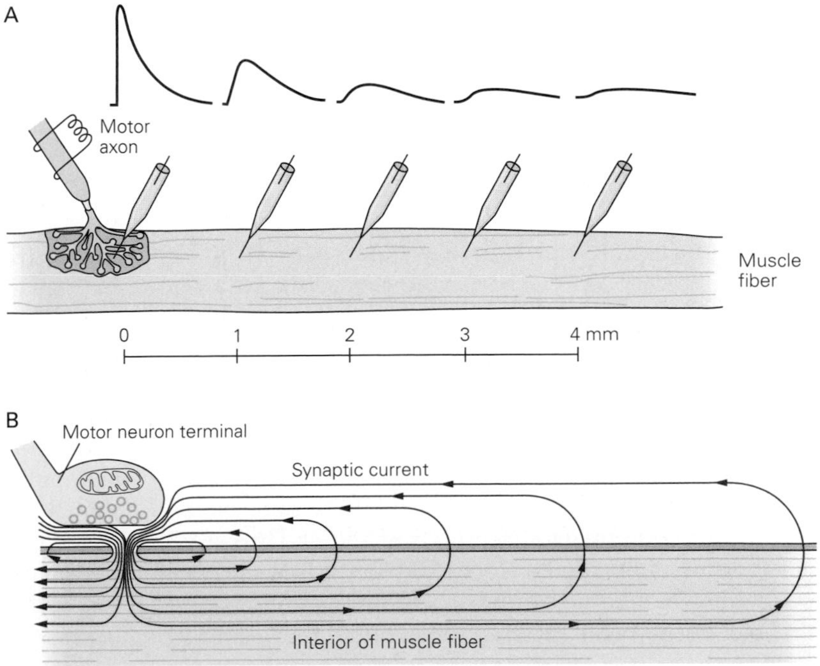

Figure 9–5 The end-plate potential decreases with distance as it passively propagates away from the end-plate. (Adapted, with permission, from Miles 1969.)

A. The amplitude of the postsynaptic potential decreases and the time course of the potential slows with distance from the site of initiation in the end-plate.

B. The decay results from leakiness of the muscle fiber membrane. Because charge must flow in a complete circuit, the inward synaptic current at the end-plate gives rise to a return outward current through resting channels and across the membrane (the capacitor). This return outward flow of positive charge depolarizes the membrane. Because current leaks out all along the membrane, the outward current decreases with distance from the end-plate.

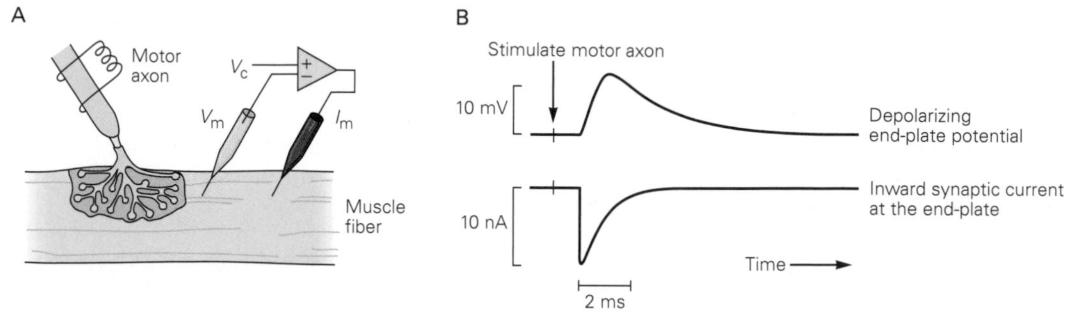

Figure 9–6 The end-plate current increases and decays more rapidly than the end-plate potential.

A. The membrane at the end-plate is voltage-clamped by inserting two microelectrodes into the muscle at the end-plate. One electrode measures membrane potential (V_m) and the second passes current (I_m). Both electrodes are connected to a negative feedback amplifier, which ensures that sufficient current (I_m) is delivered so that V_m will remain clamped at the command potential V_c. The synaptic current evoked by stimulating the motor nerve can then be measured at constant V_m, for example −90 mV (see Box 7–1).

B. The end-plate potential (measured when V_m is not clamped) changes relatively slowly and lags behind the more rapid inward synaptic current (measured under voltage-clamp conditions). This is because synaptic current must first alter the charge on the membrane capacitance of the muscle before the muscle membrane is depolarized.

The fact that current through the end-plate is inward at the normal resting potential of a muscle cell (−90 mV) indicates that there is an inward (negative) electrochemical driving force on the ions that carry current through the ACh receptor-channels at this potential. Thus, E_{EPSP} must be positive to −90 mV.

The value of E_{EPSP} in Equation 9–1 can be determined by altering V_m in a voltage-clamp experiment and determining its effect on I_{EPSP}. Depolarizing the membrane reduces the net inward electrochemical driving force, thus decreasing the magnitude of the inward end-plate current. If V_m is set equal to E_{EPSP}, there will be no net current through the end-plate channels because the electrical driving force (V_m) will exactly balance the chemical driving force (E_{EPSP}). The potential at which the net ionic current is zero is the *reversal potential* for current through the synaptic channels; by determining the reversal potential we can experimentally measure the value of E_{EPSP}. If V_m is made more positive than E_{EPSP}, there will be a net outward driving force. In that case stimulation of the motor nerve leads to an outward ionic current (by opening the ACh receptor-channels) that hyperpolarizes the membrane.

If an influx of Na^+ were solely responsible for the end-plate potential, the reversal potential for the excitatory postsynaptic potential would be the same as the equilibrium potential for Na^+ (E_{Na} = +55 mV). Thus, if V_m is experimentally altered from −100 to +55 mV, the end-plate current should diminish progressively because the electrochemical driving force on Na^+ ($V_m - E_{Na}$) is reduced. At +55 mV the inward current should be abolished, and at potentials more positive than +55 mV the end-plate current should reverse in direction and become outward.

Instead, experiments at the end-plate showed that as V_m is reduced, the inward current rapidly becomes smaller and is abolished at 0 mV. At values more positive than 0 mV the end-plate current reverses direction and becomes outward (Figure 9–7). This reversal potential is not equal to the equilibrium potential for Na^+ or any of the other major cations or anions. In fact, this chemical potential is produced not by a single ion species but by a combination of ions: The ligand-gated channels at the end-plate are almost equally permeable to both major cations, Na^+ and K^+. Thus, during the end-plate potential Na^+ flows into the cell and K^+ flows out. The reversal potential is at 0 mV because this is a weighted average of the equilibrium potentials for Na^+ and K^+ (Box 9–1). At the reversal potential the influx of Na^+ is balanced by an equal efflux of K^+ (Figure 9–7).

Why are the ACh receptor-channels at the end-plate not selective for a single ion species like the voltage-gated Na^+ or K^+ channels? This is because the diameter of the pore of the ACh receptor-channel is substantially larger than that of the voltage-gated channels. Electrophysiological measurements suggest that it may be up to 0.8 nm in diameter, an estimate based on the size of the largest organic cation that can permeate the channel. For example, the permeant cation tetramethylammonium (TMA) is approximately 0.6 nm in diameter. In contrast, the voltage-gated Na^+

channel is only permeant to organic cations that are smaller than 0.5 × 0.3 nm in cross section, and voltage-gated K^+ channels will only conduct ions less than 0.3 nm in diameter.

The relatively large diameter of the ACh receptor pore is thought to provide a water-filled environment that allows cations to diffuse through the channel relatively unimpeded, much as they would in free solution. This explains why the pore does not discriminate between Na^+ and K^+. It also explains why even divalent cations, such as Ca^{2+}, can permeate the channel. Anions are excluded, however, by the presence of fixed negative charges in the channel, as described later in this chapter.

The Current Through Single Acetylcholine Receptor-Channels Can Be Measured Using the Patch Clamp

The synaptic current at the end-plate is generated by a couple of hundred thousand channels. Recordings of the current through single ACh receptor channels, using the patch-clamp technique (see Box 5–1), have provided us with insight into the molecular events underlying the end-plate potential.

Individual Receptor-Channels Conduct All-or-None Unitary Currents

The first successful recordings of single ACh receptor-channel currents from skeletal muscle cells, by Erwin Neher and Bert Sakmann in 1976, showed that the opening of an individual channel generates a very small rectangular step of ionic current (Figure 9–8). At a given resting potential a channel will always generate the same-size current pulse. At −90 mV the current steps are approximately −2.7 pA in amplitude. Although this is a very small current, it corresponds to a flow of approximately 17 million ions per second!

The current steps change in size with changes in membrane potential because the current depends on

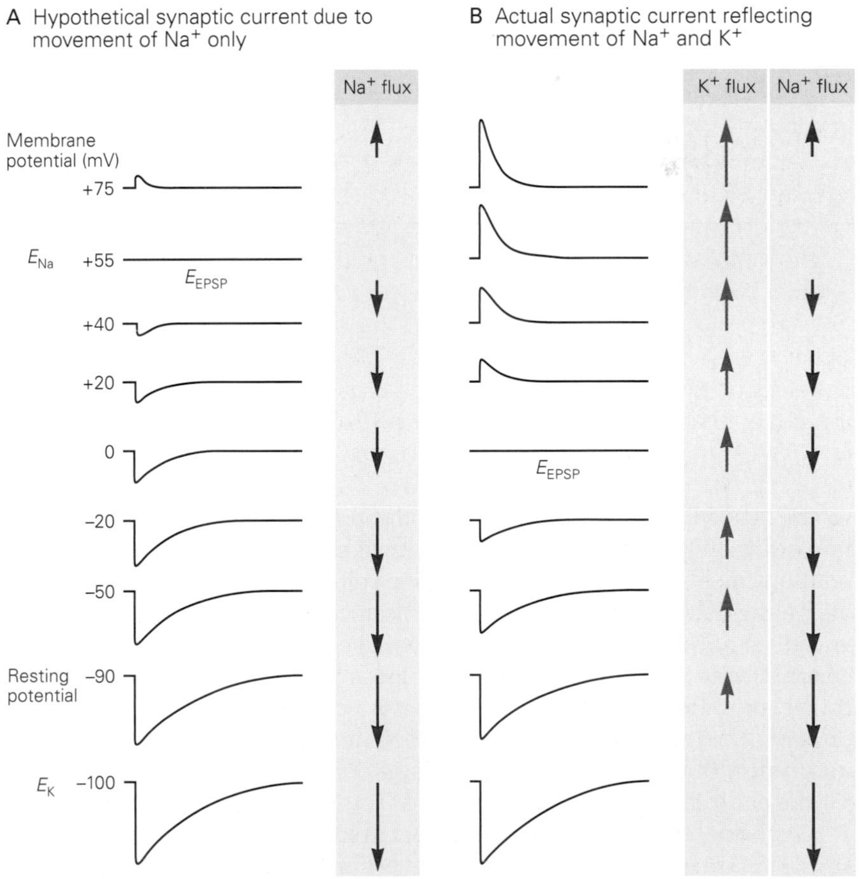

Figure 9–7 The end-plate potential is produced by the simultaneous flow of Na^+ and K^+ through the same receptor-channels. The ionic currents responsible for the end-plate potential can be determined by measuring the reversal potential of the end-plate current using a voltage clamp.

A. In the hypothetical case in which Na^+ flux alone is responsible for the end-plate current, the reversal potential would occur at +55 mV, the equilibrium potential for Na^+ (E_{Na}). The arrow at the right of each current record reflects the magnitude of the net Na^+ flux at that membrane potential. (Down arrows = inward; up arrows = outward).

B. In the actual case in which the ACh receptor-channel is permeable to both Na^+ and K^+, experimental results show that the end-plate current reverses at 0 mV because the ion channel allows Na^+ and K^+ to move into and out of the cell simultaneously (see Box 9–1). The net current is the sum of the Na^+ and K^+ fluxes through the end-plate channels. At the reversal potential (E_{EPSP}) the inward Na^+ flux is balanced by an outward K^+ flux so that no net charge flows.

Box 9–1 Reversal Potential of the End-Plate Potential

The reversal potential of a membrane current carried by more than one ion species, such as the end-plate current through the ACh receptor-channel, is determined by two factors: (1) the relative conductance for the permeant ions (g_{Na} and g_K in the case of the end-plate current) and (2) the equilibrium potentials of the ions (E_{Na} and E_K).

At the reversal potential for the ACh-gated current, inward current carried by Na^+ is balanced by outward current carried by K^+:

$$I_{Na} + I_K = 0. \quad \textbf{(9–2)}$$

The individual Na^+ and K^+ currents can be obtained from

$$I_{Na} = g_{Na} \times (V_m - E_{Na}) \quad \textbf{(9–3a)}$$

and

$$I_K = g_K \times (V_m - E_K). \quad \textbf{(9–3b)}$$

Remember that these currents do not result from Na^+ and K^+ flowing through separate channels (as occurs during the action potential) but through the same ACh receptor-channel. We can substitute Equations 9–3a and 9–3b for I_{Na} and I_K in Equation 9–2, replacing V_m with E_{EPSP} (because at the reversal potential $V_m = E_{EPSP}$):

$$g_{Na} \times (E_{EPSP} - E_{Na}) + g_K \times (E_{EPSP} - E_K) = 0. \quad \textbf{(9–4)}$$

Solving this equation for E_{EPSP} yields

$$E_{EPSP} = \frac{(g_{Na} \times E_{Na}) + (g_K \times E_K)}{g_{Na} + g_K}. \quad \textbf{(9–5)}$$

If we divide the top and bottom of the right side of this equation by g_K, we obtain

$$E_{EPSP} = \frac{E_{Na}\,(g_{Na}/g_K) + E_K}{(g_{Na}/g_K) + 1}. \quad \textbf{(9–6)}$$

If $g_{Na} = g_K$, then $E_{EPSP} = (E_{Na} + E_K)/2$.

These equations can also be used to solve for the ratio g_{Na}/g_K if one knows E_{EPSP}, E_K, and E_{Na}. Thus, rearranging Equation 9–6 yields

$$\frac{g_{Na}}{g_K} = \frac{E_{EPSP} - E_K}{E_{Na} - E_{EPSP}}. \quad \textbf{(9–7)}$$

At the neuromuscular junction, $E_{EPSP} = 0$ mV, $E_K = -100$ mV, and $E_{Na} = +55$ mV. Thus, from Equation 9–7, g_{Na}/g_K has a value of approximately 1.8, indicating that the conductance of the ACh receptor-channel for Na^+ is slightly higher than for K^+. A comparable approach can be used to analyze the reversal potential and the movement of ions during excitatory and inhibitory synaptic potentials in central neurons (see Chapter 10).

---

the electrochemical driving force ($V_m - E_{EPSP}$). For single ion channels the equivalent of Equation 9–1 is

$$i_{EPSP} = \gamma_{EPSP} \times (V_m - E_{EPSP}),$$

where i_{EPSP} is the amplitude of current through one channel and γ_{EPSP} is the conductance of a single channel. The relationship between i_{EPSP} and membrane voltage is linear, indicating that the single-channel conductance is constant and does not depend on membrane voltage; that is, the channel behaves as a simple resistor. From the slope of this relation the channel is found to have a conductance of 30 pS. The reversal potential of 0 mV, obtained from the intercept of the membrane voltage axis, is identical to that for the end-plate current (Figure 9–9B).

Although the amplitude of the current through a single ACh channel is constant for every opening, the duration of each opening and the time between openings vary considerably. These variations occur because channel openings and closings are stochastic; they obey the same statistical law that describes radioactive decay. Because of the random thermal motions and fluctuations that a channel experiences, it is impossible to predict exactly how long it will take any one channel to bind ACh or how long that channel will stay open before the ACh dissociates and the channel closes. However, the average length of time a particular type of channel stays open is a well-defined property of that channel, just as the half-life of radioactive decay is an invariant property of a particular isotope. The mean open time for ACh receptor-channels is approximately 1 ms. Thus each channel opening permits the movement of approximately 17,000 ions.

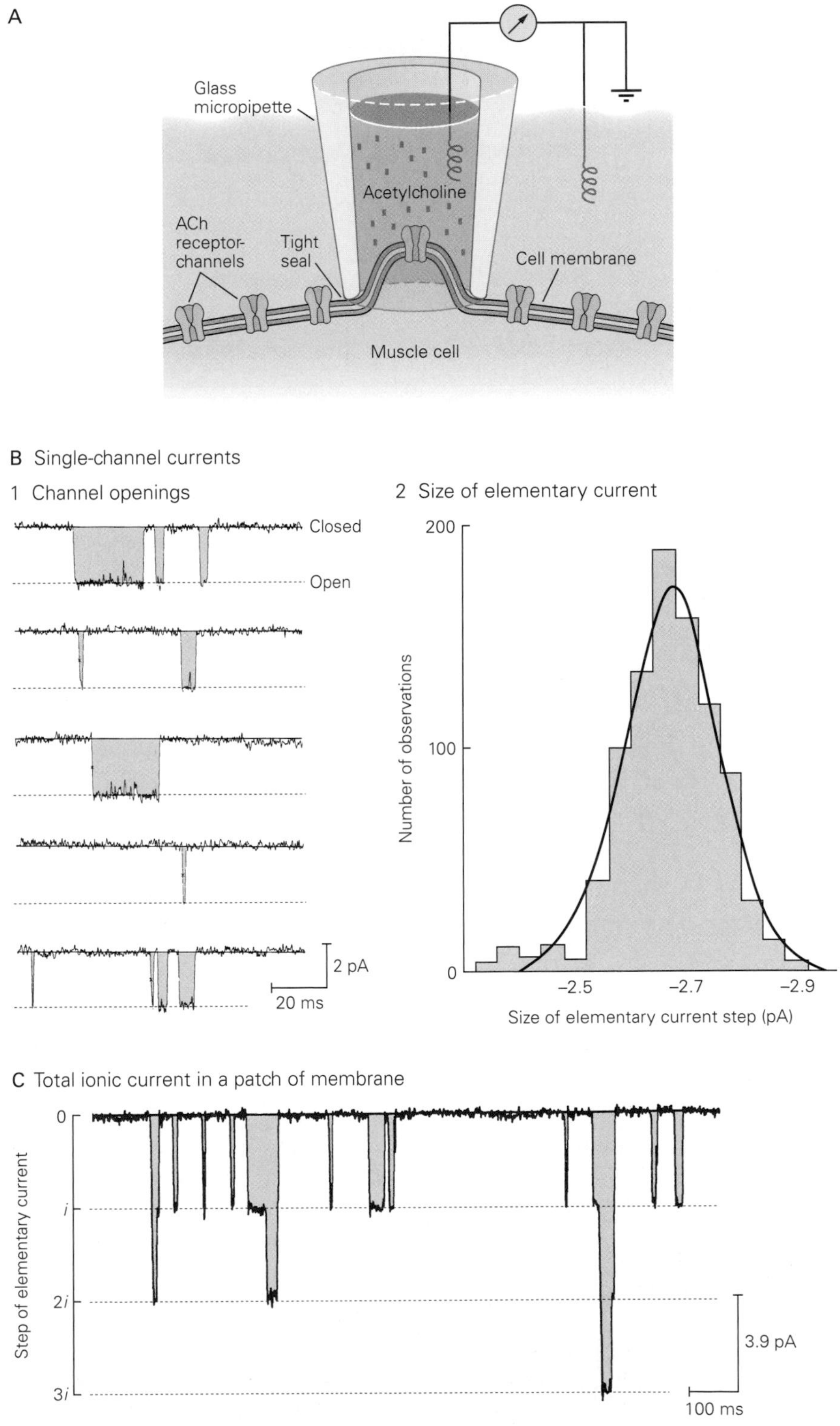

Figure 9–8 Individual ACh receptor-channels conduct an all-or-none elementary current.

A. The patch-clamp technique is used to record currents from single ACh receptor-channels. The patch electrode is filled with salt solution that contains a low concentration of ACh and is then brought into close contact with the surface of the muscle membrane (see Box 5–1). The patch may contain one or many receptor-channels.

B. Single-channel currents from a patch of frog muscle membrane with a resting potential of –90 mV were recorded in the presence of 100 nM ACh. (**1**) The opening of a channel results in an influx of positive charge (recorded as a downward current step). The patch contained a large number of ACh receptor-channels so that successive openings in the record probably arise from different channels. (**2**) A histogram plotting the amplitudes of these rectangular pulses (in pA) versus the number of observed pulses with the given amplitude. The histogram has a single peak, indicating that the patch of membrane contains only a single type of active channel with an elementary current that varies randomly around a mean of –2.7 pA (1 pA = 10^{-12} A). This mean, the *elementary current,* represents an elementary conductance of 30 pS. (Reproduced, with permission, from B. Sakmann.)

C. When the membrane potential is increased to –130 mV, the individual channel currents increase to –3.9 pA because of the increase in electrical driving force. The elementary conductance remains equal to 30 pS. When several channels open simultaneously, the individual current pulses add linearly. The record shows one, two, or three channels open at different times in response to application of ACh. (Reproduced, with permission, from B. Sakmann.)

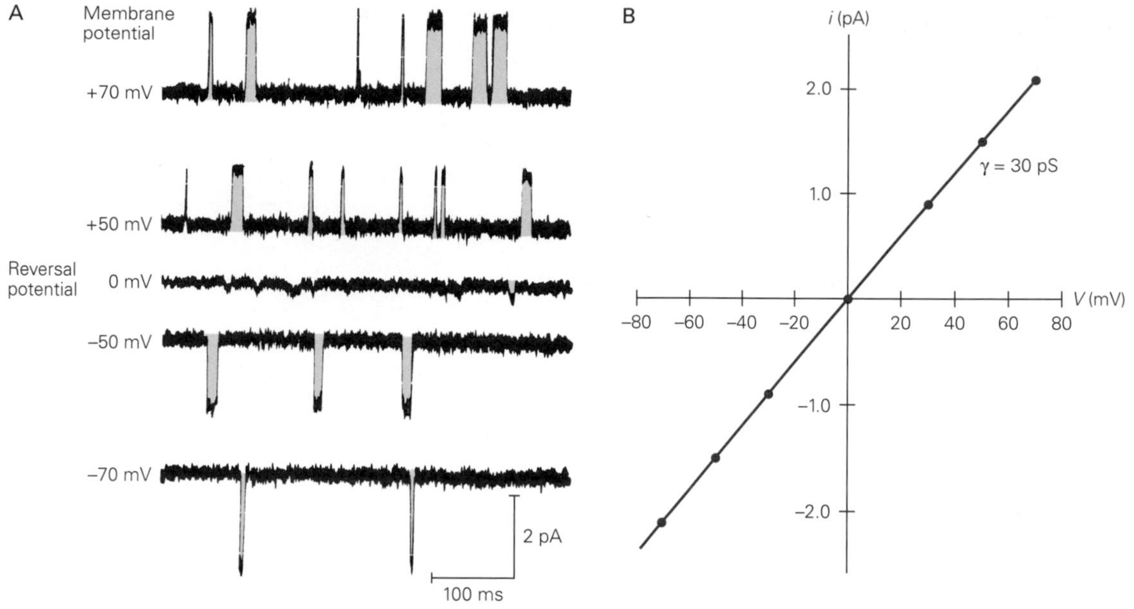

Figure 9–9 The ACh receptor-channel behaves as a simple resistor.

A. The voltage across a patch of membrane was systematically varied during exposure to 2 μM ACh. The current recorded at the patch is inward at voltages negative to 0 mV and outward at voltages positive to 0 mV, thus defining 0 mV as the reversal potential.

B. The linear relation between current through a single ACh receptor-channel and membrane voltage shows that the channel behaves as a simple resistor with a single-channel conductance (γ) of about 30 pS.

Each ACh receptor-channel has two binding sites for ACh; both sites must be occupied by transmitter for the channel to open efficiently. Once a channel closes, the ACh molecules dissociate and the channel remains closed until it binds ACh again.

Four Factors Determine the End-Plate Current

Stimulation of a motor nerve releases a large quantity of ACh into the synaptic cleft. The ACh rapidly diffuses across the cleft and binds to the ACh receptors, causing more than 200,000 receptor-channels to open almost simultaneously. (This number is obtained by comparing the total end-plate current, approximately –500 nA, with the current through a single channel, approximately –2.7 pA.) How do small step-like changes in current through 200,000 individual ACh receptor-channels produce the smooth waveform of the end-plate current?

The rapid opening of so many channels causes a large increase in the total conductance of the end-plate membrane, g_{EPSP}, and produces the rapid increase in end-plate current. The ACh in the cleft decreases rapidly to zero (in less than 1 ms) because of enzymatic hydrolysis and diffusion, after which the channels begin to close in the random manner described above. Each closure produces a small step-like decrease in end-plate current because of the all-or-none nature of single-channel currents. However, because each unitary current step is tiny relative to the large current carried by many thousands of channels, the random closing of a large number of small unitary currents causes the total end-plate current to appear to decay smoothly (Figure 9–10).

The summed conductance of all open channels in a large population of ACh receptor-channels is the total synaptic conductance, $g_{EPSP} = n \times \gamma$, where n is the average number of channels opened and γ is the conductance of a single channel. The number of open channels is the product of the total number of channels in the end-plate membrane (N) and the probability that any given channel is open, $n = N \times p_{open}$. The probability that a channel is open depends largely on the concentration of the transmitter at the receptor, not on the value of the membrane potential, because the channels are opened by the binding of ACh, not by voltage. The total end-plate current is therefore given by

$$I_{EPSP} = N \times p_{open} \times \gamma \times (V_m - E_{EPSP}),$$
$$= n \times \gamma \times (V_m - E_{EPSP}).$$

This equation shows that the total end-plate current depends on four factors: (1) the total number of end-plate channels (N); (2) the probability that a channel is open (p_{open}); (3) the conductance of each open channel (γ); and (4) the driving force on the ions ($V_m - E_{EPSP}$).

The relationships between total end-plate current, end-plate potential, and single-channel current are shown in Figure 9–11 for a wide range of membrane potentials.

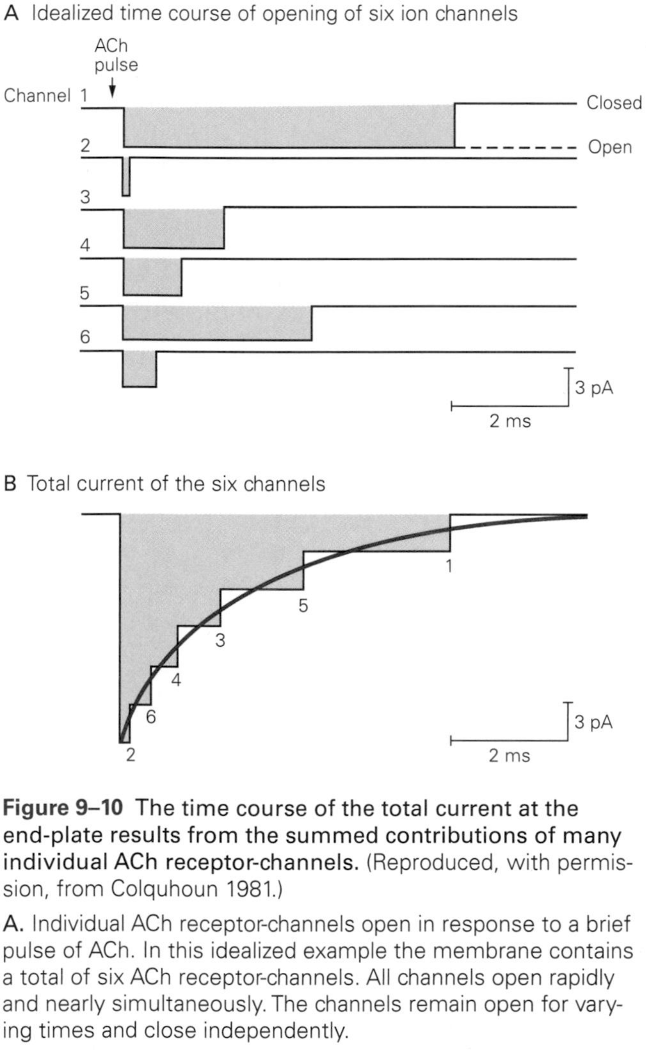

Figure 9–10 The time course of the total current at the end-plate results from the summed contributions of many individual ACh receptor-channels. (Reproduced, with permission, from Colquhoun 1981.)

A. Individual ACh receptor-channels open in response to a brief pulse of ACh. In this idealized example the membrane contains a total of six ACh receptor-channels. All channels open rapidly and nearly simultaneously. The channels remain open for varying times and close independently.

B. The stepped trace shows the sum of the six single-channel current records in part A. It represents the current during the sequential closing of each channel (the number indicates which channel has closed) in a hypothetical end-plate containing only six channels. In the final period of current only channel 1 is open. In a current record from a whole muscle fiber, with thousands of channels, the individual channel closings are not visible because the current scale needed to display the total end-plate current (hundreds of nanoamperes) is so large that the contributions of individual channels cannot be resolved. As a result, the total end-plate current appears to decay smoothly.

The Molecular Properties of the Acetylcholine Receptor-Channel Are Known

The ACh receptors that produce the end-plate potential differ in two important ways from the voltage-gated channels that generate the action potential in muscle. First, the action potential is generated by two distinct classes of voltage-gated channels that are activated sequentially, one selective for Na^+ and the other for K^+. In contrast, the ACh receptor-channel alone generates the end-plate potential by allowing both Na^+ and K^+ to pass with nearly equal permeability.

Second, the Na^+ flux through voltage-gated channels is regenerative: By increasing the depolarization of the cell, the Na^+ influx opens more voltage-gated Na^+ channels. This regenerative feature is responsible for the all-or-none property of the action potential. In contrast, the number of ACh receptor-channels opened during the synaptic potential is fixed by the amount of ACh available. The depolarization produced by Na^+ influx through these ligand-gated channels does not lead to the opening of more ACh-gated channels and cannot produce an action potential. To trigger an action potential, a synaptic potential must recruit neighboring voltage-gated channels (Figure 9–12).

As might be expected from these two differences in physiological properties, the ACh-gated and voltage-gated channels are formed by different macromolecules that exhibit different sensitivities to drugs and toxins. Tetrodotoxin, which blocks the voltage-gated Na^+ channel, does not block the influx of Na^+ through the nicotinic ACh receptor-channels. Similarly, α-bungarotoxin, a snake venom protein that binds tightly to the nicotinic receptors and blocks the action of ACh, does not interfere with voltage-gated Na^+ or K^+ channels (α-bungarotoxin has proved useful in the biochemical characterization of the ACh receptor).

The nicotinic ACh receptor at the nerve-muscle synapse is an ionotropic receptor: It is part of a single macromolecule that includes the pore in the membrane through which ions flow. Where in the molecule is the binding site located? How is the pore of the channel formed? What are its properties? Insights into these questions have been obtained from molecular studies of the ACh receptor proteins and their genes.

Biochemical studies by Arthur Karlin and Jean-Pierre Changeux indicate that the mature nicotinic ACh receptor is a membrane glycoprotein formed from five subunits: two α-subunits and one β-, one γ-,

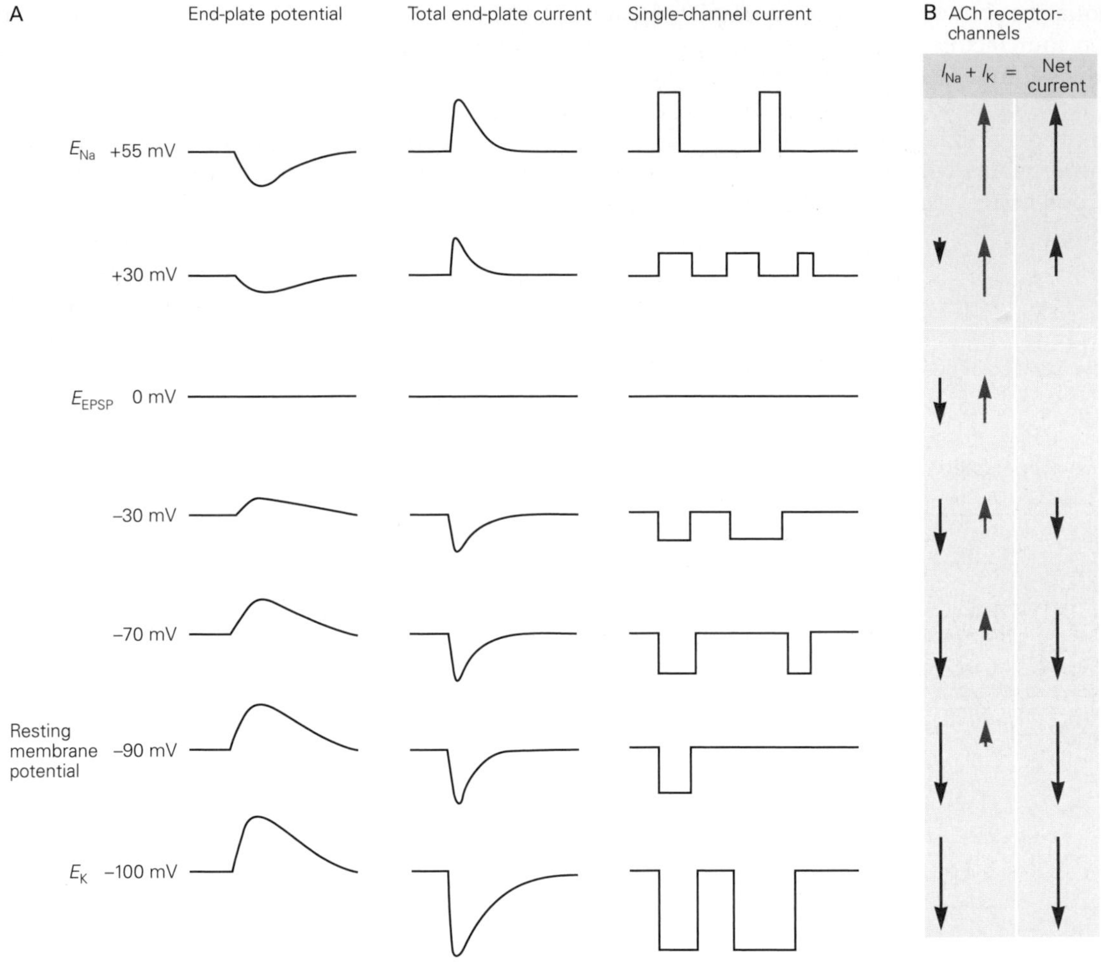

Figure 9–11 Membrane potential has a similar effect on the end-plate potential, total end-plate current, and ACh-gated single-channel current.

A. At the normal resting potential of the muscle membrane (–90 mV) the current through single ACh receptor-channels is large and inward because of the large inward driving force on Na^+ and small outward driving force on K^+. The resulting total end-plate current (made up of currents from more than 200,0000 channels) produces a large depolarizing end-plate potential. At more positive levels of membrane potential (increased depolarization), the inward driving force on Na^+ is less and the outward driving force on K^+ is greater. This results in a decrease in the size of the single-channel and total end-plate current, thus reducing the size of the end-plate potential. At the reversal potential (0 mV) the inward Na^+ flux is balanced by the outward K^+ flux, so there is no net current at the end-plate and no change in V_m. Further depolarization to +30 mV inverts the direction of the end-plate current, as there is now a much larger outward driving force on K^+ and a small inward driving force on Na^+. As a result, the outward flow of K^+ hyperpolarizes the membrane. Note that on either side of the reversal potential the end-plate current drives the membrane potential toward the reversal potential.

B. The direction of Na^+ and K^+ fluxes in individual channels changes with V_m. The algebraic sum of the Na^+ and K^+ currents, I_{Na} and I_K, gives the *net current* through the ACh receptor-channels. (Arrow length represents the relative magnitude of a current. Up = out, down = in.)

and one δ-subunit. The amino terminus of each of the subunits is exposed on the extracellular surface of the membrane and contains the ACh-binding site. Karlin and his colleagues have identified two extracellular binding sites for ACh on each receptor-channel in the clefts between each α-subunit and its neighboring γ- or δ-subunit. One molecule of ACh must bind at each of the two sites for the channel to open efficiently (Figure 9–13). The inhibitory snake venom α-bungarotoxin also binds to the ACh-binding sites on the α-subunit.

Insight into the structure of the channel has come from analysis of the primary amino acid sequences of the receptor's subunits as well as from biophysical studies. The work of Shosaku Numa and his colleagues demonstrated that the four subunit types are encoded by distinct but related genes. Sequence comparison of the subunits shows a high degree of similarity among them: One-half of the amino acid residues are identical or conservatively substituted. This similarity suggests that all subunits have a similar structure. Furthermore, all four of the genes for the subunits are homologous; that is, they are derived from a common ancestral gene.

The distribution of the polar and nonpolar amino acids of the subunits provides important clues as to how the subunits are threaded through the membrane bilayer. Each subunit contains four hydrophobic regions of approximately 20 amino acids called M1 to M4, each of which is thought to form an α-helix that spans the membrane. The amino acid sequences of the subunits suggest that the subunits are symmetrically arranged like the staves of a barrel, creating a central pore through the membrane (Figure 9–14).

The walls of the channel pore are formed by the M2 membrane-spanning segment and by the loop connecting M2 to M3. Three rings of negative charges that flank the external and internal boundaries of the M2 segment play an important role in the channel's selectivity for cations. Certain local anesthetic drugs block the channel by interacting with one ring of polar serine residues and two rings of hydrophobic residues in the central region of the M2 helix, midway through the membrane (Figure 9–14D).

A three-dimensional model of the entire receptor-channel complex has been proposed by Arthur Karlin and Nigel Unwin based on neutron scattering and electron diffraction images respectively (see Figure 9–3). The complex is divided into three regions: a large extracellular portion that contains the ACh binding site, a narrow transmembrane pore selective for cations, and a large exit region at the internal membrane surface (Figure 9–14C). The extracellular region is surprisingly large, approximately 6 nm in length. In addition, the extracellular end of the pore has a wide mouth approximately 2.5 nm in diameter. Within the bilayer of the membrane the pore gradually narrows.

More detailed insight into the structure of the extracellular domain of the ACh receptor has come

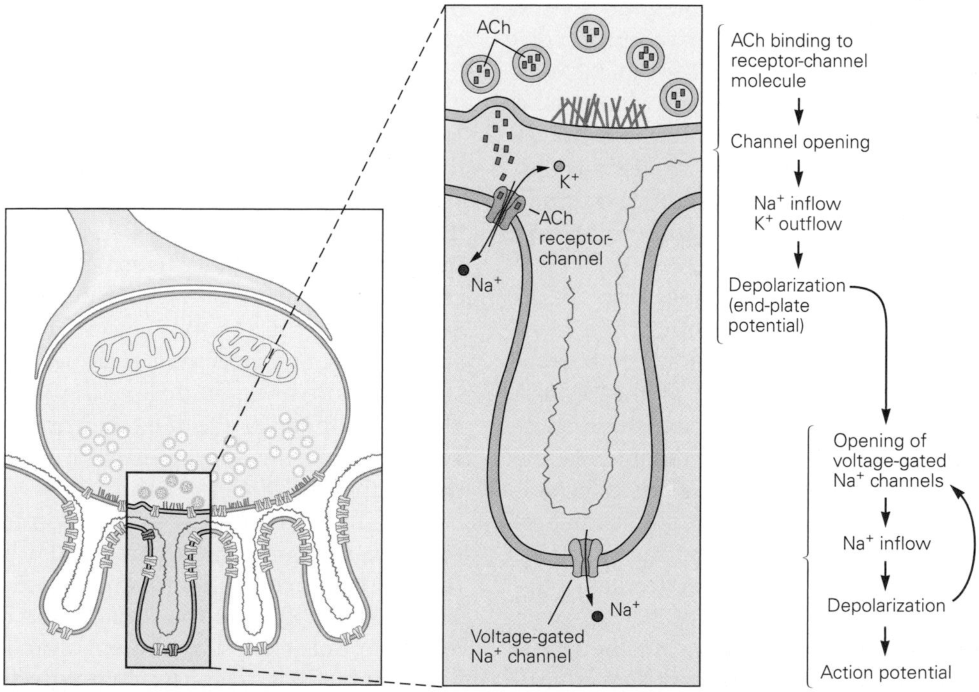

Figure 9–12 The depolarization resulting from the opening of ACh receptor-channels at the end-plate opens voltage-gated Na^+ channels. The depolarization of the muscle membrane during the end-plate potential opens neighboring voltage-gated Na^+ channels in the muscle membrane. The depolarization is normally large enough to open a sufficient number of Na^+ channels to exceed the threshold for an action potential. (Reproduced, with permission, from Alberts et al. 1989.)

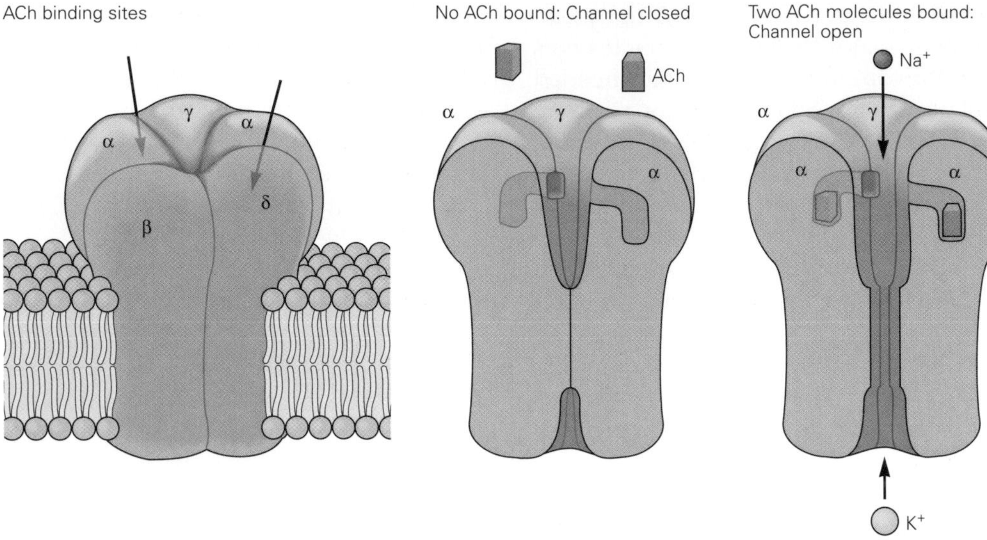

Figure 9–13 The nicotinic ACh receptor-channel is a pentameric macromolecule. The receptor-channel is a single macromolecule consisting of five subunits, which form a pore through the cell membrane (see Figure 9–14). The channel is composed of two identical α-subunits, and one each of the β-, γ-, and δ-subunits. When two molecules of **ACh** bind to the extracellular binding sites—formed at the interfaces of the two α-subunits and their neighboring γ- and δ-**subunits**—the receptor-channel molecule changes conformation. This change opens the pore through which both K^+ and Na^+ flow down their electrochemical gradients.

from X-ray crystallographic studies of a molluscan ACh-binding protein, which is homologous to the amino terminus of the nicotinic ACh receptor subunit at the end-plate. Remarkably, unlike typical ACh receptors, the molluscan ACh-binding protein is a soluble protein secreted by glial cells into the extracellular space. At cholinergic synapses in snails it acts to reduce the size of the excitatory postsynaptic potential, perhaps by buffering the free concentration of ACh in the synaptic cleft.

In a crystal structure of the molluscan ACh-binding protein in the presence of nicotine, five identical subunits are assembled into a symmetric pentameric ring (Figure 9–15A). The walls of the protein are seen to surround a large vestibule, which presumably funnels ions toward the narrow transmembrane domain of the receptor. Each subunit binds one molecule of nicotine at the ACh binding site, which is located at the interface between neighboring subunits; thus, the pentamer binds a total of five molecules of ligand. Although nicotinic ACh receptors at the end-plate have only two binding sites for ligand, some neuronal nicotinic ACh receptors are composed of five identical subunits and are thought to bind five molecules of ACh. Although the overall similarity of the amino acid sequences of the molluscan protein and nicotinic ACh receptors is fairly low (25%), the residues that form the ACh binding site are highly conserved, suggesting that the structure of the site is similar to that of the molluscan protein.

Our picture of the transmembrane region of the nicotinic ACh receptor is still incomplete. However, recent electron diffraction data from Unwin suggest that the four transmembrane segments of each subunit are indeed α-helixes that traverse the 3 nm length of the lipid bilayer (Figure 9–15B). The pore-lining M2 segments are inclined toward the central axis of the channel, so that the pore narrows continuously from the outside of the membrane to the inside. In the closed state a ring of hydrophobic residues is thought to constrict the pore in the middle of the M2 helix to a diameter of less than 0.6 nm. This hydrophobic ring may act as the channel's gate, providing a steric and energetic barrier that prevents ion conduction.

The binding of ACh to the receptor is thought to trigger a rotation of the extracellular binding domain that is somehow coupled to an opposite rotation in the M2 helixes, widening the constriction in the middle of M2 to around 0.8 to 0.9 nm, enabling ion permeation. This diameter is in reasonable agreement with electrophysiological estimates based on the pore's permeability to organic cations. The work of Karlin, however, suggests that the gate lies near the cytoplasmic mouth of the channel.

An Overall View

The terminals of motor neurons form synapses with muscle fibers at specialized regions in the muscle membrane called end-plates. When an action potential reaches the terminals of a presynaptic motor neuron it causes release of ACh. The transmitter diffuses across the synaptic cleft and binds to nicotinic ACh receptors in the end-plate, thus opening channels that allow Na^+, K^+, and Ca^{2+} to flow across the postsynaptic muscle. A net influx of Na^+ ions produces a depolarizing synaptic potential called the end-plate potential.

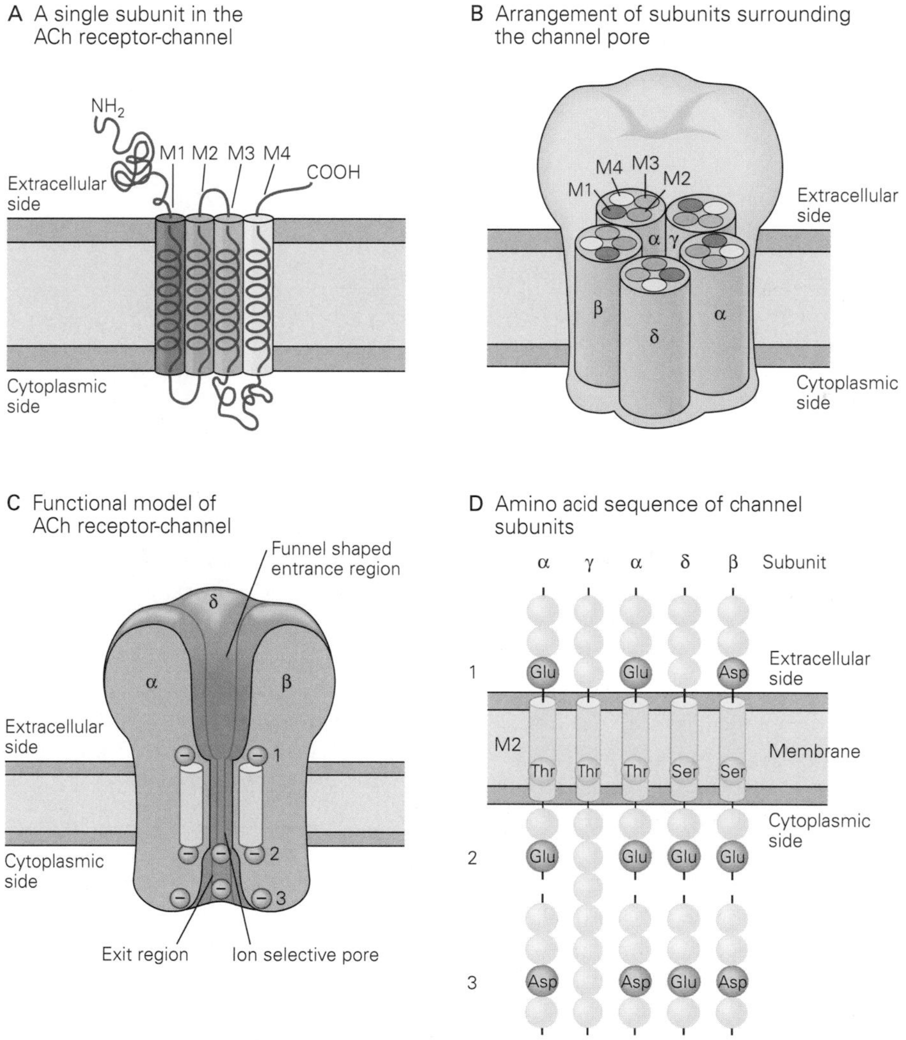

Figure 9–14 The ACh receptor subunits are homologous membrane-spanning proteins.

A. Each subunit contains a large extracellular N-terminus, four membrane-spanning α-helixes (**M1–M4**), and a short extracellular C-terminus. The N-terminus contains the ACh-binding site, and the membrane helixes form the pore.

B. The five subunits are arranged such that they form a central aqueous channel, with the M2 segment of each subunit forming the lining of the pore. Note that the γ-subunit lies between the two α-subunits. (Dimensions are not to scale.)

C. According to one model, negatively charged amino acids on each subunit form three rings of negative charge around the pore. As an ion traverses the channel it encounters these rings of charge. The rings at the external (**1**) and internal (**3**) surfaces of the cell membrane may serve as prefilters that help repel anions and form divalent cation blocking sites. The central ring near the cytoplasmic side of the membrane bilayer (**2**) may contribute more importantly to establishing the specific cation selectivity of the selectivity filter, which is the narrowest region of the pore.

D. The amino acid sequences of the M2 and flanking regions of each of the five subunits. The horizontal series of amino acids numbered **1, 2,** and **3** constitute the three rings of negative charge (part C). The aligned serine and threonine residues within M2 help form the selectivity filter.

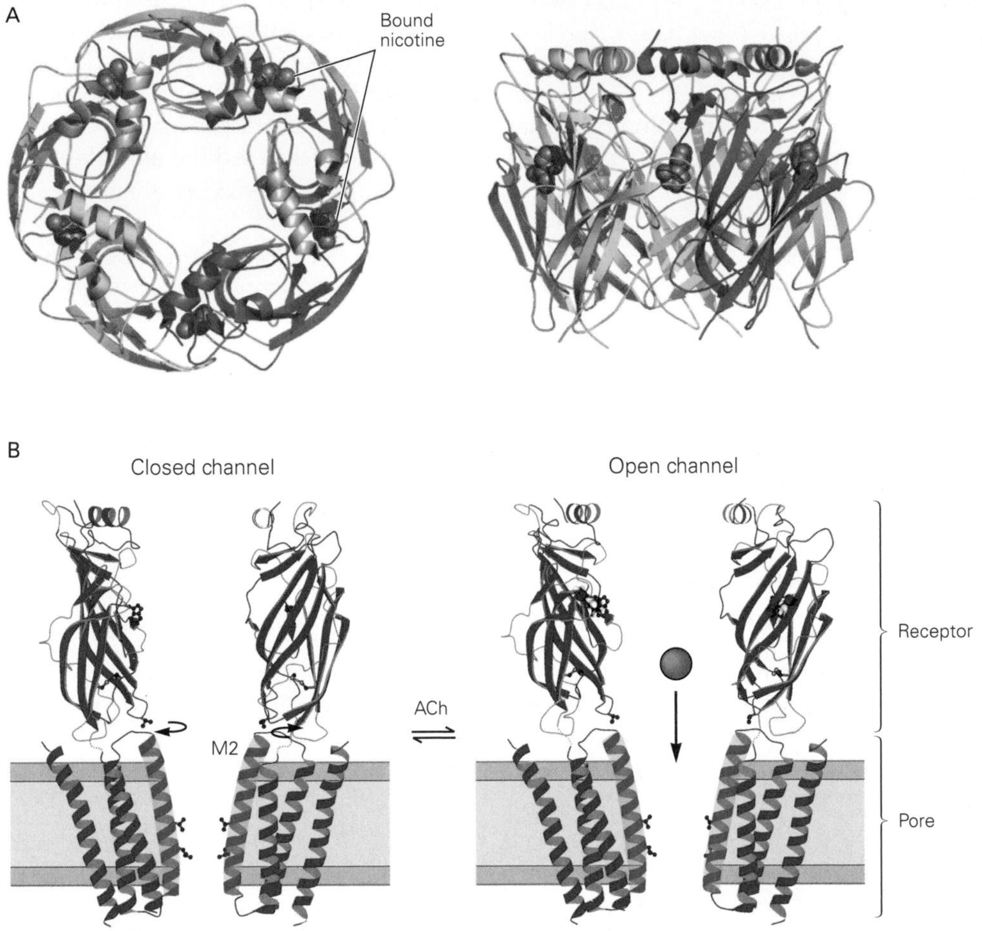

Figure 9–15 A high-resolution three-dimensional structural model of the nicotinic ACh receptor-channel.

A. A structural model of the ACh-binding protein, secreted by glial cells in mollusks, in the presence of nicotine. Five identical subunits assemble into a pentameric macromolecule that contains a large central cavity. The ACh-binding protein is homologous to the extracellular ligand-binding domain of the ACh receptor-channel, which is thus thought to resemble this structure. The view on the left shows the ACh-binding protein in an orientation that corresponds to looking down at the ACh receptor-channel from the extracellular side of the membrane. The view on the right shows the ACh-binding protein in an orientation that corresponds to looking at the side of the extracellular portion of the ACh receptor-channel with the membrane below. (Reproduced, with permission, from Celie et al. 2004.)

B. A model for the ACh-receptor channel in the open and closed states. View looking at the side of the channel, showing two of five subunits. The structure of the extracellular region is based on the structure of the ACh-binding protein. The structure of the membrane helixes is based on electron diffraction analysis of two-dimensional crystals of the ACh receptor-channel from electric fish. The M2 helixes line the pore (see Figure 9–14B). In the closed channel (left) a hydrophobic girdle of leucine and valine residues constricts the pore, preventing ion permeation. The channel opens (right) when ACh binding induces a rotation in the extracellular binding domain that leads to a corresponding rotation in the M2 helix, widening the pore and permitting ion permeation. (Reproduced, with permission, from Unwin 2003.)

Because the ACh-activated channels are concentrated at the end-plate, the opening of these channels produces only a local depolarization that spreads passively along the muscle fibers. However, this local depolarization is very large. In a healthy individual it is always suprathreshold. Thus the local depolarization activates a sufficient number of voltage-gated Na^+ channels in the end-plate to generate an action potential that actively propagates along the length of the muscle.

The protein that forms the nicotinic ACh receptor-channel has been purified, its genes cloned, and its amino acids sequenced. It is composed of five subunits, two of which—the α-subunits that recognize and bind ACh—are identical. Each subunit has four hydrophobic regions that are thought to form membrane-spanning α-helixes. The protein also contains two sites for recognizing and binding ACh. This channel is thus gated directly by a chemical transmitter. The functional molecular domains of the ACh receptor have been identified, and the steps that link ACh-binding to the opening of the channel are now being investigated. Although the atomic-level structure of the ACh receptor-channel has not been resolved, the structures of bacterial ligand-gated channels that are closely related to the ACh receptor have been resolved. Thus we may soon be able to see in atomic detail the molecular dynamics of the ACh receptor-channel's physiological functions.

The large number of ACh receptor-channels at the end-plate ensures that synaptic transmission will proceed with a high safety factor. In the autoimmune disease myasthenia gravis, antibodies to the ACh receptor decrease the number of ACh receptors, thus seriously compromising transmission at the neuromuscular junction (see Chapter 14). Certain congenital mutations in the ACh receptor subunits also contribute to a family of diseases of the neuromuscular junction termed congenital myasthenic syndrome. In some instances these mutations shorten the duration of channel opening, decreasing current during an excitatory postsynaptic potential. Other mutations prolong the opening of the ACh receptor-channels (slow channel syndrome). This leads to excessive Ca^{2+} influx, which is thought to promote degeneration of the end-plate.

Acetylcholine is only one of many neurotransmitters in the nervous system, and the end-plate potential is just one example of chemical signaling. Do transmitters in the central nervous system act in the same fashion, or are other mechanisms involved? In the past such questions were virtually unanswerable because of the small size and great variety of nerve cells in the central nervous system. However, advances in experimental technique—in particular, the patch clamp—have made synaptic transmission at central synapses easier to study. Already it is clear that many neurotransmitters operate in the central nervous system much as ACh operates at the end-plate, although other transmitters produce their effects in quite different ways. Some of the many variations of synaptic transmission that characterize the central and peripheral nervous systems are discussed in the next two chapters.

Postscript: The End-Plate Current Can Be Calculated from an Equivalent Circuit

The current through a population of ACh receptor-channels can be described by Ohm's law. However, to fully describe how the electrical current generates the end-plate potential, all the resting channels in the surrounding membrane must be considered. Because channels are proteins that span the bilayer of the membrane, we must also take into consideration the capacitive properties of the membrane and the ionic batteries determined by the distribution of Na^+ and K^+ inside and outside the cell.

The dynamic relationship of these various components can be explained using the same rules we used in Chapter 6 to analyze the current in passive electrical devices that consist only of resistors, capacitors, and batteries. We can represent the end-plate region with an equivalent circuit that has three parallel branches: (1) one representing the synaptic current through the transmitter-gated channels; (2) one representing the return current through resting channels (the nonsynaptic membrane); and (3) one representing current across the lipid bilayer, which acts as a capacitor (Figure 9–16).

Because the end-plate current is carried by both Na^+ and K^+, we could represent the synaptic branch of the equivalent circuit as two parallel branches, each representing the flow of a different ion species. At the end-plate, however, Na^+ and K^+ flow through the same ion channel. It is therefore more convenient (and correct) to combine the Na^+ and K^+ current pathways into a single conductance (g_{EPSP}), representing the ACh-gated channels.

The conductance of this pathway depends on the number of channels opened, which in turn depends on the concentration of transmitter. In the absence of transmitter no channels are open, and the conductance is zero. When a presynaptic action potential causes the release of transmitter, the conductance of this pathway increases to a value of approximately 5×10^{-6} S (or a resistance of 2×10^5 Ω). This is about five times the conductance of the parallel branch representing the resting or leakage channels (g_l).

The end-plate conductance is in series with a battery (E_{EPSP}), with a value given by the reversal potential for synaptic current (0 mV) (Figure 9–16). This value is the weighted algebraic sum of the Na^+ and K^+ equilibrium potentials (see Box 9–1).

The current during the excitatory postsynaptic potential (I_{EPSP}) is given by

$$I_{EPSP} = g_{EPSP} \times (V_m - E_{EPSP}).$$

Using this equation and the equivalent circuit of Figure 9–16 we can now analyze the end-plate potential in terms of ionic currents (Figure 9–17).

At the onset of the excitatory synaptic action (the dynamic phase), an inward current (I_{EPSP}) is generated

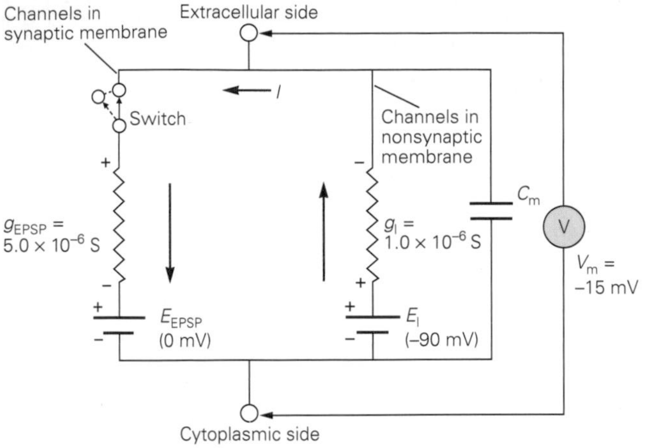

Figure 9–16 The equivalent circuit of the end-plate. The circuit has three parallel current pathways. One conductance pathway represents the end-plate current and consists of a battery, E_{EPSP}, in series with the conductance of the ACh receptor-channels, g_{EPSP}. Another conductance pathway represents current through the nonsynaptic membrane and consists of a battery representing the resting potential (E_l) in series with the conductance of the resting channels (g_l). In parallel with both of these conductance pathways is the membrane capacitance (C_m). The voltmeter (V) measures the potential difference between the inside and the outside of the cell.

When no ACh is present, the end-plate channels are closed and carry no current. This state is depicted as an open electrical circuit in which the synaptic conductance is not connected to the rest of the circuit. The binding of ACh opens the synaptic channel. This event is electrically equivalent to throwing the switch that connects the gated conductance pathway (g_{EPSP}) with the resting pathway (g_l). In the steady state there is an inward current through the ACh-gated channels and an outward current through the resting channels. With the indicated values of conductances and batteries, the membrane will depolarize from –90 mV (its resting potential) to –15 mV (the peak of the end-plate potential).

by the ACh-gated channels because of the increased conductance to Na^+ and K^+ and the large inward driving force on Na^+ at the resting potential of –90 mV (Figure 19-17B, time 2). Because charge must flow in a closed loop, the inward synaptic current must leave the cell as outward current. The equivalent circuit includes two parallel pathways for outward current: a conductance pathway (I_l) representing current through the resting (or leakage) channels and a capacitive pathway (I_c) representing current across the membrane capacitance. Thus,

$$I_{EPSP} = -(I_l + I_c).$$

During the earliest phase of the end-plate potential the membrane potential, V_m , is still close to its resting value, E_l. As a result, the outward driving force on current through the resting channels ($V_m - E_l$) is small. Therefore most of the current leaves the cell as capacitive current and the membrane depolarizes rapidly (Figure 9–17B, time 2). As the cell depolarizes, the outward driving force on current through the resting channels increases, while the inward driving force on synaptic current through the ACh receptor-channels decreases. Concomitantly, as the concentration of ACh in the synapse decreases, the ACh receptor-channels begin to close, and eventually the inward current through the gated channels is exactly balanced by outward current through the resting channels ($I_{EPSP} = -I_l$). At this point there is no current into or out of the capacitor, ($I_c = 0$). Because the rate of change of membrane potential is directly proportional to I_c,

$$I_c / C_m = \Delta V / \Delta t,$$

the membrane potential will have reached a peak or new steady-state value, $\Delta V/\Delta t = 0$ (Figure 9–17B, time 3).

As the ACh-gated channels close, I_{EPSP} decreases further. Now I_{EPSP} and I_l are no longer in balance and the membrane potential starts to repolarize, because the outward current through leak channels (I_l) becomes larger than the inward synaptic current. During most of the declining phase of the synaptic action there is no current through the ACh receptor-channels because all these channels are closed. Instead, current passes through the membrane only as outward current carried by resting channels balanced by inward current across the membrane capacitor (Figure 9–17B, time 4).

When the end-plate potential is at its peak or steady-state value, $I_c = 0$ and therefore the value of V_m can be easily calculated. The inward current through the ACh-gated channels (I_{EPSP}) must be exactly balanced by outward current through the resting channels (I_l):

$$I_{EPSP} + I_l = 0. \qquad \textbf{(9–8)}$$

The current through the ACh receptor-channels (I_{EPSP}) and resting channels (I_l) is given by Ohm's law:

$$I_{EPSP} = g_{EPSP} \times (V_m - E_{EPSP}),$$

and

$$I_l = g_l \times (V_m - E_l).$$

By substituting these two expressions into Equation 9–8, we obtain

$$g_{EPSP} \times (V_m - E_{EPSP}) + g_l \times (V_m - E_l) = 0.$$

To solve for V_m we need only expand the two products in the equation and rearrange them so that

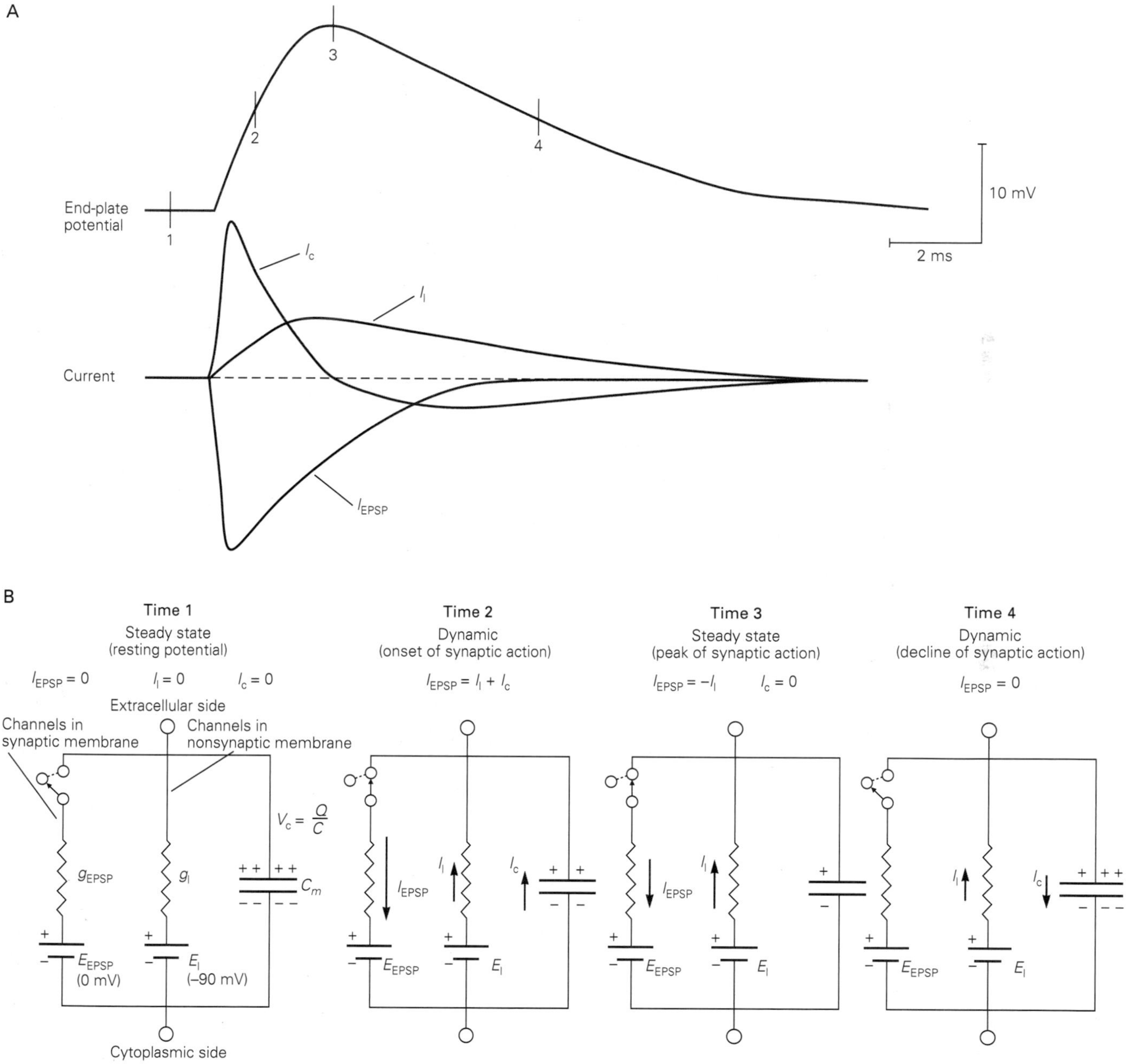

Figure 9–17 Both the ACh-gated synaptic conductance and the passive membrane properties of the muscle cell determine the time course of the end-plate potential.

A. The time course of the end-plate potential and the component currents through the ACh receptor-channels (I_{EPSP}), the resting (or leakage) channels (I_l), and the capacitor (I_c). There is a capacitive current only when the membrane potential is changing. In the steady state, such as at the peak of the end-plate potential, the inward flow of positive charge through the ACh receptor-channels is exactly balanced by the outward ionic current across the resting channels, and there is no capacitive current.

B. Equivalent circuits for the current at times 1, 2, 3, and 4 shown in part A. (The relative magnitude of a current is represented by the arrow length.)

all terms in voltage appear on the left side:

$$(g_{EPSP} \times V_m) + (g_l \times V_m) = (g_{EPSP} \times E_{EPSP}) + (g_l \times E_l).$$

By factoring out V_m on the left side, we finally obtain

$$V_m = \frac{(g_{EPSP} \times E_{EPSP}) + (g_l \times E_l)}{g_{EPSP} + g_l}. \qquad \textbf{(9–9)}$$

This equation is similar to that used to calculate the resting and action potentials (see Chapter 6). According to Equation 9–9, the peak voltage of the end-plate potential is a weighted average of the electromotive forces of the two batteries for ACh-gated and resting currents. The weighting factors are given by the relative magnitude of the two conductances. If the ACh-gated conductance is much smaller than the resting conductance ($g_{EPSP} \ll g_l$), $g_{EPSP} \times E_{EPSP}$ will be negligible compared with $g_l \times E_l$. Under these conditions V_m will remain close to E_l. This situation occurs when only a few ACh receptor-channels are opened, because the ACh concentration is low. Conversely, if g_{EPSP} is much larger than g_l, Equation 9–9 states that V_m approaches E_{EPSP}, the synaptic reversal potential. This situation occurs when a large number of ACh-activated channels are open, because the concentration of ACh is high. At intermediate ACh concentrations, with a moderate number of ACh-activated channels open, the peak end-plate potential lies somewhere between E_l and E_{EPSP}.

We can now calculate the peak end-plate potential for the specific case shown in Figure 9–16, where $g_{EPSP} = 5 \times 10^{-6}$ S, $g_l = 1 \times 10^{-6}$ S, $E_{EPSP} = 0$ mV, and $E_l = -90$ mV. Substituting these values into Equation 9–9 yields

$$V_m = \frac{[(5 \times 10^{-6}\ \text{S}) \times (0\ \text{mV})] + [(1 \times 10^{-6}\ \text{S}) \times (-90\ \text{mV})]}{(5 \times 10^{-6}\ \text{S}) + (1 \times 10^{-6}\ \text{S})}.$$

or

$$V_m = \frac{(1 \times 10^{-6}\ \text{S}) \times (-90\ \text{mV})}{(6 \times 10^{-6}\ \text{S})}$$

$$= -15\ \text{mV}.$$

The peak amplitude of the end-plate potential is then

$$\Delta V_{EPSP} = V_m - E_l = -15\ \text{mV} - (-90\ \text{mV}) = 75\ \text{mV}.$$

As a check for consistency we can see whether, at the peak of the end-plate potential, the synaptic current is equal and opposite to the nonsynaptic current so that the net membrane current is indeed equal to zero:

$$I_{EPSP} = (5 \times 10^{-6}\ \text{S}) \times (-15\ \text{mV} - 0\ \text{mV}) = -75 \times 10^{-9}\ \text{A}$$

and

$$I_l = (1 \times 10^{-6}\ \text{S}) \times [-15\ \text{mV} - (-90\ \text{mV})] = 75 \times 10^{-9}\ \text{A}.$$

Here we see that Equation 9–9 ensures that $I_{EPSP} + I_l = 0$.

Eric R. Kandel
Steven A. Siegelbaum

Selected Readings

Changeux JP. 2010. Allosteric receptors: from electric organ to cognition. Annu Rev Pharmacol Toxicol 50:1–38.

Fatt P, Katz B. 1951. An analysis of the end-plate potential recorded with an intra-cellular electrode. J Physiol 115:320–370.

Heuser JE, Reese TS. 1977. Structure of the synapse. In: ER Kandel (ed). *Handbook of Physiology: A Critical, Comprehensive Presentation of Physiological Knowledge and Concepts*, Sect. 1 *The Nervous System*, Vol. 1 *Cellular Biology of Neurons*, Part 1, pp. 261–294. Bethesda, MD: American Physiological Society.

Hille B. 2001. *Ion Channels of Excitable Membranes*, 3rd ed., pp. 169–199. Sunderland, MA: Sinauer.

Imoto K, Busch C, Sakmann B, Mishina M, Konno T, Nakai J, Bujo H, Mori Y, Fukuda K, Numa S. 1988. Rings of negatively charged amino acids determine the acetylcholine receptor-channel conductance. Nature 335:645–648.

Karlin A. 2002. Emerging structure of the nicotinic acetylcholine receptors. Nat Rev Neurosci 3:102–114.

Neher E, Sakmann B. 1976. Single-channel currents recorded from membrane of denervated frog muscle fibres. Nature 260:799–802.

Unwin N. 2005. Refined structure of the nicotinic acetylcholine receptor at 4 Å resolution. J Mol Biol 346:967–989.

References

Akabas MH, Kaufmann C, Archdeacon P, Karlin A. 1994. Identification of acetylcholine receptor-channel lining residues in the entire M2 segment of the α-subunit. Neuron 13:919–927.

Alberts B, Bray D, Lewis J, Raff M, Roberts K, Watson JD. 1989. *Molecular Biology of the Cell*, 2nd ed. New York: Garland.

Brejc K, van Dijk WJ, Klaassen RV, Schuurmans M, van der Oost J, Smit AB, Sixma TK. 2001. Crystal structure of an ACh-binding protein reveals the ligand-binding domain of nicotinic receptors. Nature 411:269–276.

Brisson A, Unwin PN. 1985. Quaternary structure of the acetylcholine receptor. Nature 315:474–477.

Celie PH, van Rossum-Fikkert SE, van Dijk WJ, Brejc K, Smit AB, Sixma TK. 2004. Nicotine and carbamylcholine binding to nicotinic acetylcholine receptors as studied in AChBP crystal structures. Neuron 41:907–914.

Charnet P, Labarca C, Leonard RJ, Vogelaar NJ, Czyzyk L, Gouin A, Davidson N, Lester HA. 1990. An open channel blocker interacts with adjacent turns of α-helices in the nicotinic acetylcholine receptor. Neuron 4:87–95.

Claudio T, Ballivet M, Patrick J, Heinemann S. 1983. Nucleotide and deduced amino acid sequences of Torpedo californica acetylcholine receptor γ-subunit. Proc Natl Acad Sci U S A 80:1111–1115.

Colquhoun D. 1981. How fast do drugs work? Trends Pharmacol Sci 2:212–217.

Dwyer TM, Adams DJ, Hille B. 1980. The permeability of the endplate channel to organic cations in frog muscle. J Gen Physiol 75:469–492.

Fertuck HC, Salpeter MM. 1974. Localization of acetylcholine receptor by 125I-labeled α-bungarotoxin binding at mouse motor endplates. Proc Natl Acad Sci U S A 71:1376–1378.

Heuser JE, Salpeter SR. 1979. Organization of acetylcholine receptors in quick-frozen, deep-etched, and rotary-replicated Torpedo postsynaptic membrane. J Cell Biol 82: 150–173.

Ko C-P. 1984. Regeneration of the active zone at the frog neuromuscular junction. J Cell Biol 98:1685–1695.

Kuffler SW, Nicholls JG, Martin AR. 1984. *From Neuron to Brain: A Cellular Approach to the Function of the Nervous System*, 2nd ed. Sunderland, MA: Sinauer.

McMahan UJ, Kuffler SW. 1971. Visual identification of synaptic boutons on living ganglion cells and of varicosities in postganglionic axons in the heart of the frog. Proc R Soc Lond B Biol Sci 177:485–508.

Miles FA. 1969. *Excitable Cells*. London: Heinemann.

Miyazawa A, Fujiyoshi Y, Stowell M, Unwin N. 1999. Nicotinic acetylcholine receptor at 4.6 Å resolution: transverse tunnels in the channel wall. J Mol Biol 288:765–786.

Miyazawa A, Fujiyoshi Y, Unwin N. 2003. Structure and gating mechanism of the acetylcholine receptor pore. Nature 424:949–955.

Noda M, Furutani Y, Takahashi H, Toyosato M, Tanabe T, Shimizu S, Kikyotani S, et al. 1983. Cloning and sequence analysis of calf cDNA and human genomic DNA encoding α-subunit precursor of muscle acetylcholine receptor. Nature 305:818–823.

Noda M, Takahashi H, Tanabe T, Toyosato M, Kikyotani S, Furutani Y, Hirose T, et al. 1983. Structural homology of Torpedo californica acetylcholine receptor subunits. Nature 302:528–532.

Palay SL. 1958. The morphology of synapses in the central nervous system. Exp Cell Res 5:275–293. Suppl.

Raftery MA, Hunkapiller MW, Strader CD, Hood LE. 1980. Acetylcholine receptor: complex of homologous subunits. Science 208:1454–1457.

Revah F, Galzi J-L, Giraudat J, Haumont PY, Lederer F, Changeux J-P. 1990. The noncompetitive blocker [3H] chlorpromazine labels three amino acids of the acetylcholine receptor gamma subunit: implications for the alpha-helical organization of regions MII and for the structure of the ion channel. Proc Natl Acad Sci U S A 87:4675–4679.

Salpeter MM (ed). 1987. *The Vertebrate Neuromuscular Junction*, pp. 1–54. New York: Liss.

Takeuchi A. 1977. Junctional transmission. I. Postsynaptic mechanisms. In: ER Kandel (ed). *Handbook of Physiology: A Critical, Comprehensive Presentation of Physiological Knowledge and Concepts*, Sect. 1 *The Nervous System*, Vol. 1 *Cellular Biology of Neurons*, Part 1, pp. 295–327. Bethesda, MD: American Physiological Society.

Toyoshima C, Unwin N. 1988. Ion channel of acetylcholine receptor reconstructed from images of postsynaptic membranes. Nature 336:247–250.

Verrall S, Hall ZW. 1992. The N-terminal domains of acetylcholine receptor subunits contain recognition signals for the initial steps of receptor assembly. Cell 68:23–31.

Villarroel A, Herlitze S, Koenen M, Sakmann B. 1991. Location of a threonine residue in the alpha-subunit M2 transmembrane segment that determines the ion flow through the acetylcholine receptor-channel. Proc R Soc Lond B Biol Sci 243:69–74.

Unwin N. 1995. Acetylcholine receptor-channel imaged in the open state. Nature 373:37–43.

Unwin N. 2003. Structure and action of the nicotinic acetylcholine receptor explored by electron microscopy. FEBS Lett 555:91–95.

10

Synaptic Integration in the Central Nervous System

LIKE SYNAPTIC TRANSMISSION at the neuromuscular junction, most rapid signaling between neurons in the central nervous system involves ionotropic receptors in the postsynaptic membrane. Thus, many principles that apply to the synaptic connection between the motor neuron and skeletal muscle fiber at the neuromuscular junction also apply in the central nervous system. Synaptic transmission between central neurons is more complex, however, for several reasons. First, although most muscle fibers are innervated by only one motor neuron, a central nerve cell (such as the motor neuron in the spinal cord) receives connections from hundreds or even thousands of neurons. Second, muscle fibers receive only excitatory inputs, whereas central neurons receive both excitatory and inhibitory inputs. Third, all synaptic actions on muscle fibers are mediated by one neurotransmitter, acetylcholine (ACh), which activates only one type of receptor (the ionotropic nicotinic ACh receptor); however, a single central neuron can respond to different types of inputs, each mediated by a distinct transmitter that alters the activity of specific types of receptor. These receptors include both ionotropic receptors, where binding of transmitter directly opens an ion channel, and metabotropic receptors, where transmitter binding indirectly regulates a channel by activating second messengers. As a result, unlike muscle fibers, central neurons must integrate diverse inputs into a single coordinated action. Finally, the nerve–muscle synapse is a model of efficiency—every action potential in the motor neuron produces an action potential in the muscle fiber. In comparison, connections made by a presynaptic neuron onto the motor neuron are only modestly effective—often 50 to 100 excitatory neurons must fire together to produce a synaptic potential large enough to trigger an action potential in a motor cell.

The first insights into synaptic transmission in the central nervous system came from experiments by John Eccles and his colleagues in the 1950s on the synaptic inputs onto spinal motor neurons that control the stretch reflex, the simple behavior we considered in Chapter 2. The spinal motor neurons remain particularly useful for examining central synaptic mechanisms because they have large, accessible cell bodies and, most important, they receive both excitatory and inhibitory connections and therefore allow us to study the integrative action of the nervous system on the cellular level.

Central Neurons Receive Excitatory and Inhibitory Inputs

To analyze the synapses that mediate the stretch reflex, Eccles activated a large population of axons of the sensory cells that innervate the stretch receptor organs in the quadriceps (extensor) muscle (Figure 10–1A,B). Nowadays the same experiments can be done by stimulating a single sensory neuron. For example, passing sufficient current through a microelectrode into the cell body of a stretch-receptor neuron that innervates the extensor muscle generates an action potential in the sensory cell. This in turn produces a small excitatory postsynaptic potential (EPSP) in the motor neuron that innervates precisely the same muscle (in this case the quadriceps) monitored by the sensory neuron (Figure 10–1B upper panel). The EPSP produced by the one sensory cell, the unitary EPSP, depolarizes the extensor motor neuron by less than 1 mV, often only 0.2 to 0.4 mV, far below the threshold for generating an action potential (typically, a depolarization of 10 mV or more is required to reach threshold).

The generation of an action potential requires the near-synchronous firing of a number of sensory neurons. This can be observed in an experiment in which a population of sensory neurons is stimulated by passing current through an extracellular electrode. As the strength of the extracellular stimulus is increased, more sensory afferent fibers are excited, and the depolarization produced by the EPSP becomes larger. The depolarization eventually becomes large enough to bring the membrane potential of the axon initial segment (the integrative component of the motor neuron) to the threshold for an action potential.

In contrast to the EPSP produced in the extensor motor neuron, stimulation of the extensor stretch-receptor neuron produces a small inhibitory postsynaptic potential (IPSP) in the motor neuron that innervates the flexor muscle, which is antagonistic to the extensor muscle (Figure 10–1B lower panels). This hyperpolarizing action is mediated by an inhibitory interneuron, which receives excitatory input from the sensory neurons of the extensor muscle and in turn makes synapses with the motor neurons that innervate the flexor muscle. In the laboratory a single interneuron can be stimulated intracellularly to directly elicit a small unitary IPSP in the motor neuron. Extracellular activation of an entire population of interneurons elicits a larger IPSP.

Although a single EPSP in the extensor motor neuron is not nearly large enough to elicit an action potential, the neuron integrates many EPSPs from a large number of afferent sensory fibers to initiate an action potential. At the same time, IPSPs, if strong enough, can counteract the sum of the excitatory actions and prevent the membrane potential from reaching threshold. In addition to counteracting synaptic excitation, synaptic inhibition can exert powerful control over action potential firing in neurons that are spontaneously active because of the presence of intrinsic pacemaker channels. This function, called the *sculpting* role of inhibition, shapes the pattern of firing in such cells (Figure 10–2).

Excitatory and Inhibitory Synapses Have Distinctive Ultrastructures

As we learned in Chapter 8, the effect of a synaptic potential—whether it is excitatory or inhibitory—is determined not by the type of transmitter released from the presynaptic neuron but by the type of ion channels in the postsynaptic cell activated by the transmitter. Although some transmitters can produce both excitatory and inhibitory postsynaptic potentials, by acting on distinct classes of ionotropic receptors at different synapses, most transmitters produce a single predominant type of synaptic response; that is, a transmitter is usually inhibitory or excitatory. For example, in the vertebrate brain neurons that release glutamate typically act on receptors that produce excitation; neurons that release γ-aminobutyric acid (GABA) or glycine act on receptors that produce inhibition.

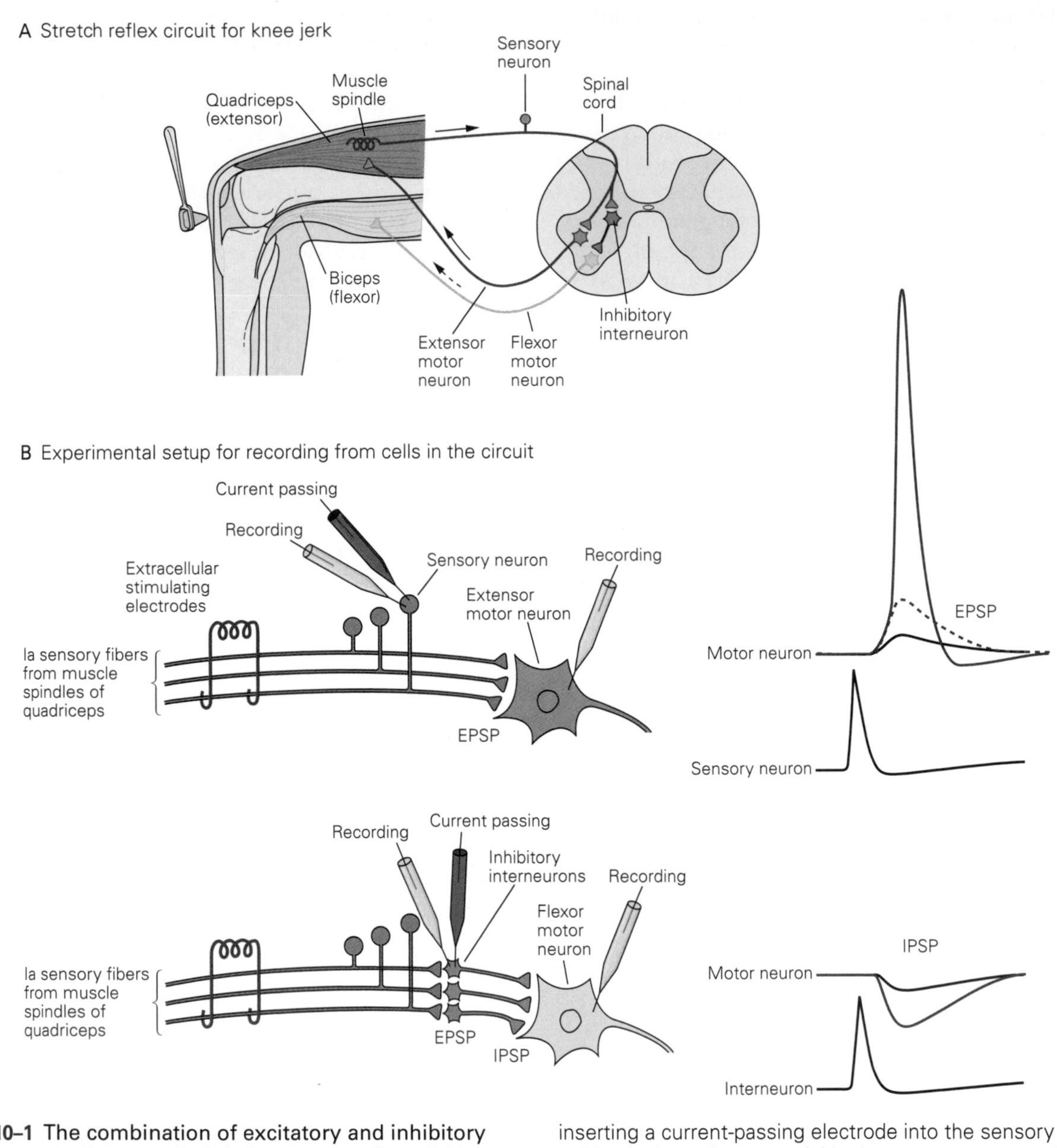

Figure 10–1 The combination of excitatory and inhibitory synaptic connections mediating the stretch reflex of the quadriceps muscle is typical of circuits in the central nervous system.

A. The stretch-receptor sensory neuron at the extensor (quadriceps) muscle makes an excitatory connection with an extensor motor neuron that innervates this same muscle group. It also makes an excitatory connection with an interneuron, which in turn makes an inhibitory connection with a flexor motor neuron that innervates the antagonist biceps femoris muscle group. Conversely, an afferent fiber from the biceps (not shown) excites an interneuron that makes an inhibitory synapse on the extensor motor neuron.

B. This idealized experimental setup shows the approaches to studying the inhibition and excitation of motor neurons in the pathway illustrated in part A. **Above:** Two alternatives for eliciting excitatory postsynaptic potentials (EPSPs) in the extensor motor neuron. A single presynaptic axon can be stimulated by inserting a current-passing electrode into the sensory neuron cell body. An action potential in the sensory neuron stimulated in this way triggers a small EPSP in the extensor motor neuron **(black trace).** Alternatively, the whole afferent nerve from the quadriceps can be stimulated electrically with extracellular electrodes. The excitation of many afferent neurons through the extracellular electrode generates a synaptic potential **(dashed trace)** large enough to initiate an action potential **(red trace).** **Below:** The setup for eliciting and measuring inhibitory potentials in the flexor motor neuron. Intracellular stimulation of a single inhibitory interneuron receiving input from the quadriceps pathway produces a small inhibitory (hyperpolarizing) postsynaptic potential (IPSP) in the flexor motor neuron **(black trace).** Extracellular stimulation recruits numerous inhibitory neurons and generates a larger postsynaptic IPSP **(red trace).** (Action potentials from the sensory neuron and interneuron appear smaller because they were recorded at lower amplification than the motor neuron action potentials).

The synaptic terminals of excitatory and inhibitory neurons can be distinguished by their morphology. Two morphological types are common in the brain: Gray type I and type II (named after E. G. Gray, who described them). Most type I (asymmetric) synapses are glutamatergic and therefore excitatory, whereas most type II synapses (symmetric) are GABAergic and therefore inhibitory. Type I synapses have round synaptic vesicles, an electron-dense region at the active zone of the presynaptic membrane, and an even larger dense region in the postsynaptic membrane apposed to the active zone, known as the *postsynaptic density* (PSD). Type II synapses have oval or flattened synaptic vesicles with less obvious presynaptic membrane specializations and PSD (Figure 10–3). Although type I synapses are mostly excitatory and type II inhibitory, the two morphological types have proved to be only a first approximation to transmitter biochemistry. As we shall learn in Chapter 13, immunocytochemistry affords much more reliable distinctions between transmitter types based on the biochemical nature of the transmitters or the enzymes involved in their synthesis.

Excitatory Synaptic Transmission Is Mediated by Ionotropic Glutamate Receptor-Channels That Are Permeable to Sodium and Potassium

The excitatory transmitter released from the presynaptic terminals of stretch-receptor neurons is the amino acid L-glutamate, the major excitatory transmitter in the brain and spinal cord. Eccles and his colleagues discovered that the EPSP in spinal motor cells results from the opening of glutamate-gated channels permeable to both Na^+ and K^+. This ionic mechanism is similar to that produced by ACh at the neuromuscular junction described in Chapter 9. Like the ACh-gated channels, the glutamate-gated channels conduct both Na^+ and K^+ with nearly equal permeability. As a result, the reversal potential for current flow through these channels is 0 mV (see Figure 9–7).

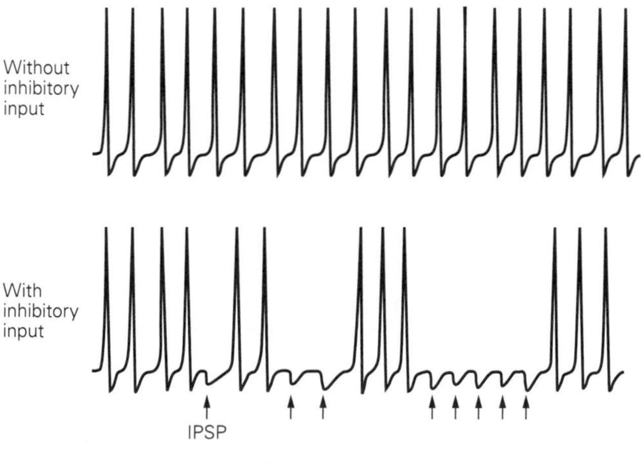

Figure 10–2 Inhibition can shape the firing pattern of a spontaneously active neuron. Without inhibitory input the neuron fires continuously at a fixed interval. With inhibitory input **(arrows)** some action potentials are inhibited, resulting in a distinctive pattern of impulses.

Glutamate receptors can be divided into two broad categories: the ionotropic receptors, which are ligand-gated channels where glutamate binding directly opens the channel, and metabotropic receptors, which are G protein-coupled receptors that indirectly gate channels through the production of second messengers (Figure 10–4). There are three major subtypes of ionotropic glutamate receptors: AMPA, kainate, and NMDA, named according to the types of synthetic agonists that activate them (α-amino-3-hydroxy-5-methylisoxazole-4-propionic acid, kainate, and *N*-methyl-D-aspartate, respectively). The NMDA receptor is selectively blocked by the drug APV (2-amino-5-phosphonovaleric acid). The AMPA and kainate receptors are not affected by APV but both are blocked by the drug CNQX (6-cyano-7-nitroquinoxaline-2,3-dione), and thus they are sometimes called the *non-NMDA receptors*. The metabotropic glutamate receptors can be selectively activated by *trans*-(1S,3R)-1-amino-1,3-cyclopentanedicarboxylic acid (ACPD). The action of ionotropic glutamate receptors is always excitatory or depolarizing, as the reversal potential of their ionic current is near zero, whereas the metabotropic receptors can produce either excitation or inhibition, depending on the reversal potential of the ionic currents that they regulate.

The NMDA receptor has several interesting properties. First, this ligand-gated channel is permeable to Ca^{2+} as well as to Na^+ and K^+ (Figure 10–4A). Second, opening the channel requires extracellular glycine as a cofactor. Under normal conditions the concentration of extracellular glycine is sufficient to allow the NMDA receptor-channel to be activated efficiently by glutamate. Third, the NMDA receptor is unique among ligand-gated channels thus far characterized because its opening depends on membrane voltage as well as transmitter. The voltage-dependence is caused by a mechanism that is quite different from that employed by the voltage-gated channels that generate the action potential. In the latter, changes in membrane potential are translated into conformational changes in the channel by an intrinsic voltage-sensor. In the NMDA receptors,

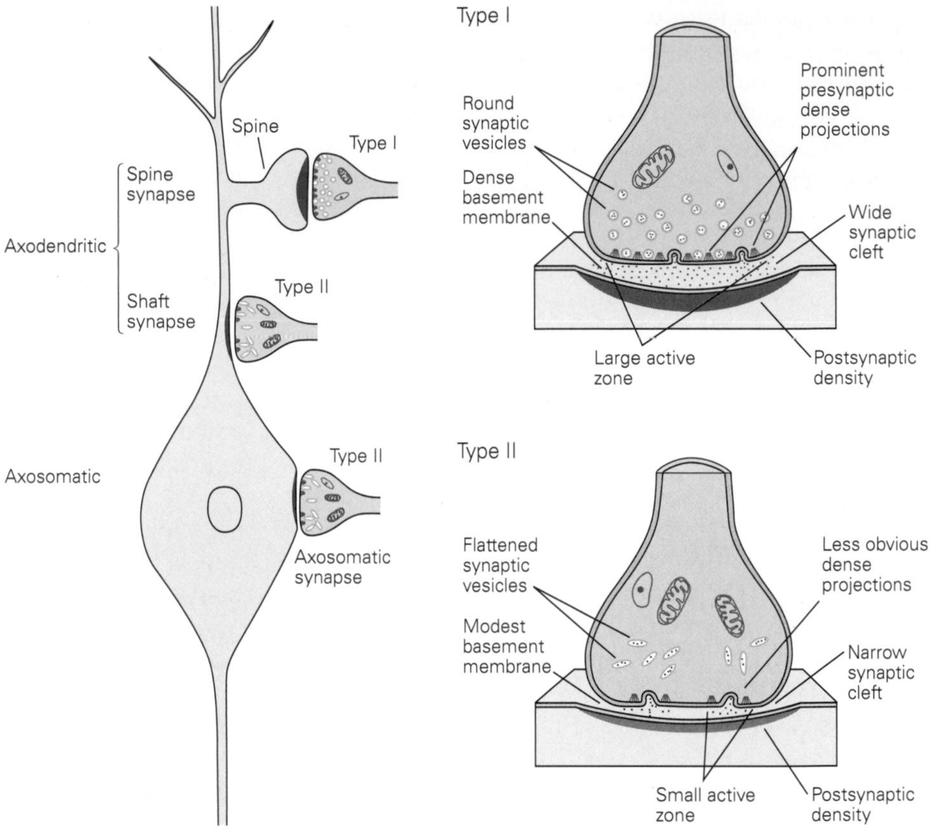

Figure 10–3 The two most common morphological types of synapses in the central nervous system are Gray type I and type II. Type I is usually excitatory, exemplified by glutamatergic synapses; type II is usually inhibitory, exemplified by GABAergic synapses. Differences include the shape of vesicles, prominence of presynaptic densities, total area of the active zone, width of the synaptic cleft, and presence of a dense basement membrane. Type I synapses typically contact specialized projections on the dendrites, called spines, and less commonly contact the shafts of dendrites. Type II synapses often contact the cell body and dendritic shaft.

however, depolarization removes an extrinsic plug from the channel. At the resting membrane potential (–65 mV) extracellular Mg^{2+} binds tightly to a site in the pore of the channel, blocking ionic current. But when the membrane is depolarized (for example, by the opening of AMPA receptor-channels), Mg^{2+} is expelled from the channel by electrostatic repulsion, allowing Na^+ and Ca^{2+} to enter (Figure 10–5).

The NMDA receptor has the further interesting property that it is inhibited by the hallucinogenic drug phencyclidine (PCP, also known as angel dust) and by MK801, both of which bind to a site in the pore of the channel that is distinct from the Mg^{2+} binding site (Figure 10–4A). Indeed, blockade of NMDA receptors produces symptoms that resemble the hallucinations associated with schizophrenia, whereas certain antipsychotic drugs enhance current flow through the NMDA receptor-channels. This has led to the hypothesis that schizophrenia may involve a defect in NMDA receptor function.

At most central synapses that use glutamate as the transmitter, the postsynaptic membrane contains both NMDA and AMPA receptors. The contributions of current through NMDA and AMPA receptors to the total excitatory postsynaptic current (EPSC) can be dissected using pharmacological antagonists in a voltage-clamp experiment (Figure 10–6). At the normal resting potential of most neurons, the NMDA receptor-channels are largely inhibited by Mg^{2+}. As a result, the EPSC is predominantly determined by charge flow through the AMPA receptors, which generate a current with a very rapid rising phase and very rapid decay phase. However, as a neuron becomes depolarized, Mg^{2+} is driven out of the mouth of the NMDA receptors and more charge flows through these channels. Thus, the NMDA receptor conducts current maximally when two conditions are met: Glutamate is present, and the cell is depolarized (Figure 10–6). That is, the NMDA receptor acts as a "coincidence detector," detecting a timing relationship between activation of the presynaptic and postsynaptic cells. In addition, because of the intrinsic kinetics of ligand gating, the current through the NMDA receptor rises and decays with a much slower time course than the AMPA receptor current. As a result, the NMDA receptors contribute to a late, slow phase of the EPSC and EPSP.

As most glutamatergic synapses contain AMPA receptors that are capable of triggering an action potential, what is the function of the NMDA receptor? At first glance the function of these receptors is even more puzzling because they are normally blocked by Mg^{2+} at the resting potential. However, when glutamate is paired with depolarization, the NMDA receptors uniquely conduct Ca^{2+} into the postsynaptic cell. This leads to a rise in intracellular [Ca^{2+}] that can activate various calcium-dependent signaling cascades, including calcium-calmodulin-dependent protein kinase II (CaMKII) (see Chapter 11). Thus NMDA receptor activation can translate electrical signals into biochemical ones. Some of these biochemical reactions lead to long-lasting changes in synaptic strength, a set of processes called long-term synaptic plasticity that are thought to be important during synapse development and for regulating neural circuits in the adult brain. In particular, an NMDA receptor-dependent long-term potentiation (LTP) of excitatory synaptic transmission has been implicated in certain forms of memory storage (see Chapters 66 and 67).

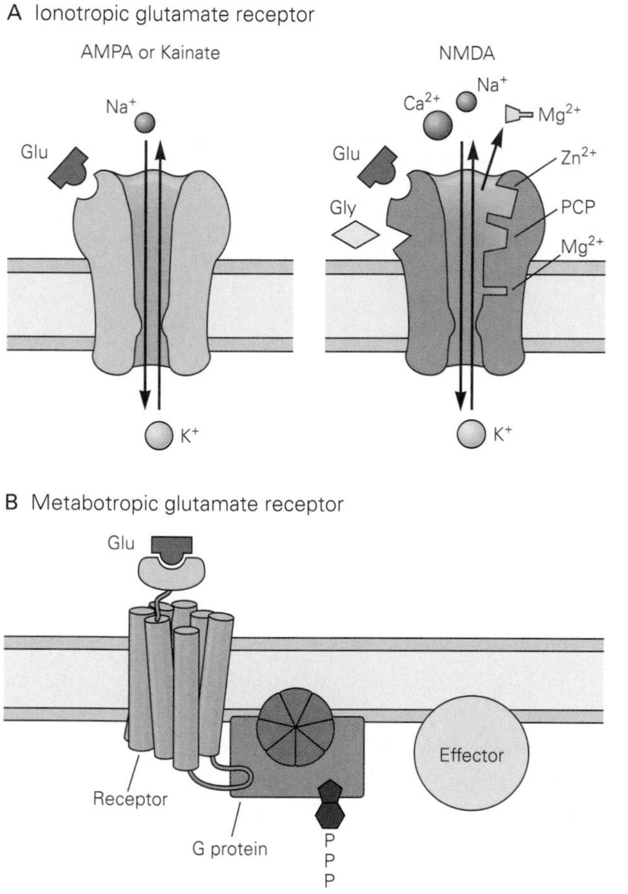

Figure 10–4 Different classes of glutamate receptors regulate excitatory synaptic actions in neurons in the spinal cord and brain.

A. Three classes of ionotropic glutamate receptors directly gate ion channels permeable to cations. The AMPA and kainate type of receptors bind the glutamate agonists AMPA or kainate, respectively. These receptors contain a channel that is permeable to Na^+ and K^+. The NMDA receptor, which binds the glutamate agonist NMDA, contains a channel permeable to Ca^{2+}, K^+, and Na^+. It has binding sites for glutamate, glycine, Zn^{2+}, phencyclidine (PCP, or *angel dust*), MK801 (an experimental drug), and Mg^{2+}, each of which regulates the functioning of the channel differently.

B. The metabotropic glutamate receptors indirectly gate ion channels by activating a GTP-binding protein, which in turn interacts with effector molecules that alter metabolic and ion channel activity (see Chapter 11).

However, there is also a potential downside to the entry of Ca^{2+} through the NMDA receptors. Excessively high concentrations of glutamate are thought to result in an overload of Ca^{2+} in the postsynaptic neurons. Such high levels of Ca^{2+} can be toxic to neurons. In tissue culture even a brief exposure to high concentrations of glutamate can kill many neurons, an action called *glutamate excitotoxicity*. The high concentrations of intracellular Ca^{2+} are thought to activate calcium-dependent proteases and phospholipases and lead to the production of free radicals that are toxic to the cell. Glutamate toxicity may contribute to cell damage after stroke, to the cell death that occurs with episodes of rapidly repeated seizures experienced by patients who have status epilepticus, and to degenerative diseases such as Huntington disease. Agents that selectively block the NMDA receptor may protect against the toxic effects of glutamate and have been tested clinically. Unfortunately, the hallucinations that accompany NMDA receptor blockade have so far limited the usefulness of such compounds. A further complication of attempts to control excitotoxicity by blocking NMDA receptor function is that physiological levels of NMDA receptor activation can actually protect neurons from damage and cell death.

The Excitatory Ionotropic Glutamate Receptors Are Encoded by a Distinct Gene Family

What are the molecular bases for the biophysical function of glutamate receptors and how are these receptors related to other ligand-gated ion channels? Over the past 20 years the genes coding for the subunits of all the major neurotransmitter receptors have been identified. This molecular analysis demonstrates evolutionary linkages among the structure of receptors that enable us to classify them into three distinct

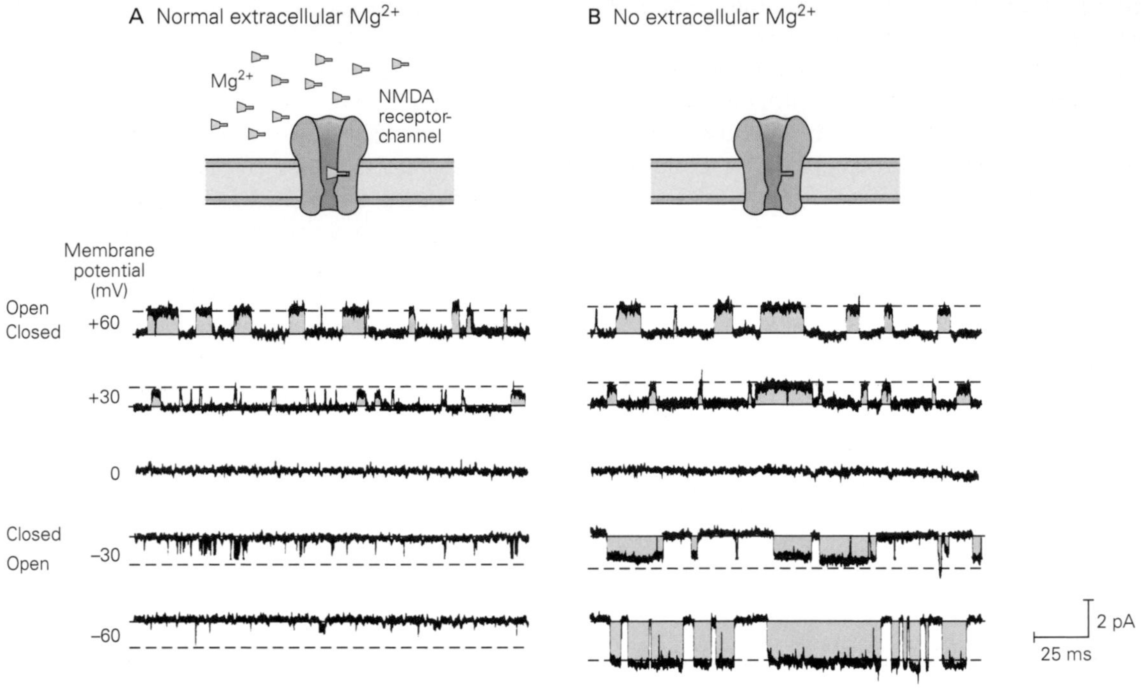

Figure 10–5 Opening of single NMDA receptor-channels depends on voltage in addition to glutamate. These recordings are from individual NMDA receptor-channels (from rat hippocampal cells in culture). Downward deflections indicate pulses of inward (negative) current; upward deflections indicate outward (positive) current. (Reproduced, with permission, from J. Jen and C. F. Stevens.)

A. When Mg^{2+} is present in normal concentration in the extracellular solution (1.2 mM), the channel is largely blocked at the resting potential (–60 mV). At negative membrane potentials only brief, flickery, inward currents are seen upon channel opening because of the Mg^{2+} block. Substantial depolarization (to +30 mV or +60 mV) relieves the Mg^{2+} block, permitting longer-lasting pulses of outward current through the channel.

B. When Mg^{2+} is removed from the extracellular solution, the opening and closing of the channel do not depend on voltage. The channel is open at the resting potential of –60 mV, and the synaptic current reverses near 0 mV, like the total synaptic current (see Figure 10–6B).

families (Figure 10–7). One family includes the genes encoding the kainate, AMPA, and NMDA receptors; the genes encoding the AMPA and kainate receptors are more closely related to one another than are the genes encoding the NMDA receptors. Surprisingly this gene family bears little resemblance to the two other gene families that encode ionotropic receptors (one that encodes the ACh, GABA, and glycine receptors, and one that encodes ATP receptors, as described below).

Unlike the pentameric nicotinic ACh receptor family, the AMPA, kainate, and NMDA receptors are tetrameric proteins with four subunits arranged around a central pore. The AMPA receptor subunits are encoded by four separate genes (*GluA1-GluA4*), and there are five different kainate receptor subunit genes (*GluK1-GluK5*). Most of the AMPA and kainate receptors are heteromers composed of two different types of *GluA* and *GluK* subunits, respectively. The NMDA receptors are encoded by a family consisting of five genes that fall into two groups, the single *GluN1* gene and the four *GluN2A-D* genes. Each NMDA receptor contains two GluN1 subunits and two of the different types of GluN2 subunits.[1] In addition, many of these subunit genes are alternatively spliced, generating further diversity. Autoantibodies to the AMPA receptor GluA3 subunit are thought to play an important role in some forms of epilepsy. These antibodies actually mimic glutamate by activating

[1]This nomenclature used for the glutamate receptor subunits conforms to recent naming conventions. In previous nomenclature used in the literature, the four AMPA receptor subunit genes were referred to as *GluR1-4* or *GluRA-D*, the kainate receptor subunit genes were referred to as *GluR5-6*, *KA1* and *KA1*, and the NMDA receptor subunit genes as *NR1* and *NR2A-D*.

GluA3-containing receptors, resulting in excessive excitation and seizures.

The amino acid sequence of the ionotropic glutamate receptor subunits and subsequent functional and biochemical studies provided the initial compelling evidence that the transmembrane topology of these subunits is very different from that of the nicotinic ACh receptor (Figure 10–7). Our understanding of the ionotropic glutamate receptors was then greatly expanded by Eric Gouaux and colleagues' determination of the high-resolution X-ray crystal structures of the isolated AMPA receptor ligand binding domain and of an intact AMPA receptor-channel formed by GluA2 subunits (Figure 10–8).

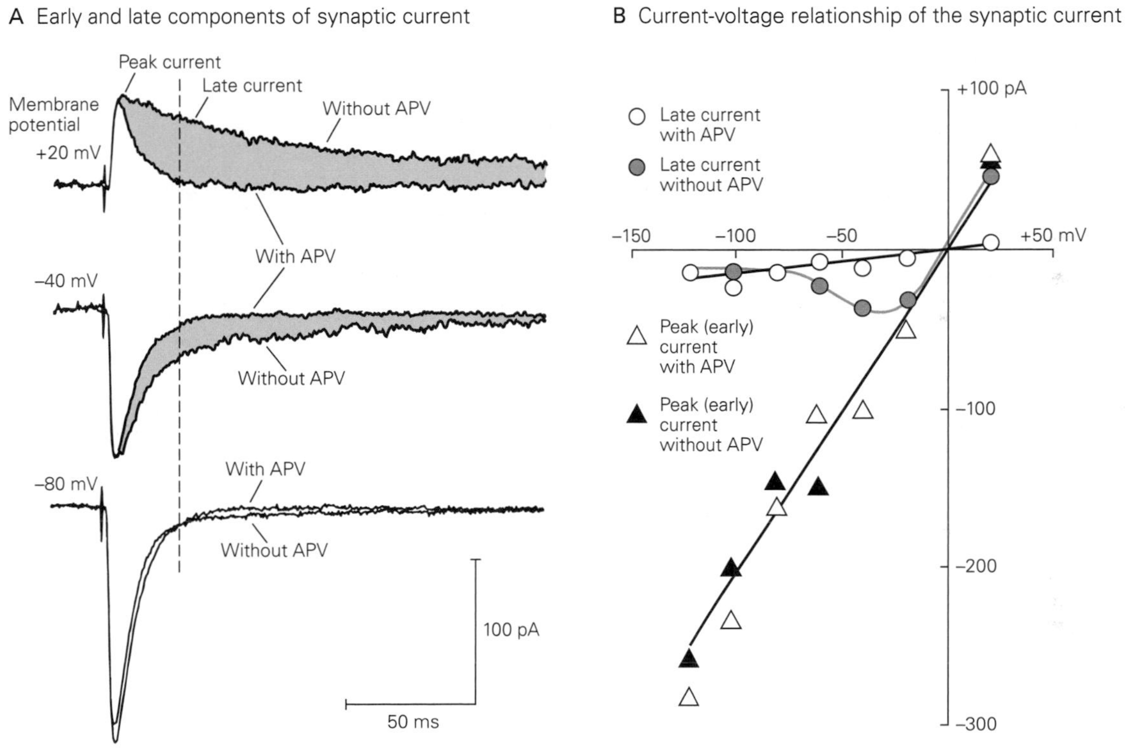

Figure 10–6 The contributions of the AMPA and NMDA glutamate receptor-channels to the excitatory postsynaptic current. These voltage-clamp current records are from a cell in the hippocampus. Similar receptor-channels are present in motor neurons and throughout the brain. (Adapted, with permission, from Hestrin et al. 1990.)

A. The drug APV selectively binds to and blocks the NMDA receptor. Shown here is the excitatory postsynaptic current (EPSC) before and during application of 50 μM APV at three different membrane potentials. The difference between the traces **(blue region)** represents the contribution of the NMDA receptor-channel to the EPSC. The current that remains in the presence of APV is the contribution of the AMPA receptor-channels. At –80 mV there is no current through the NMDA receptor-channels because of pronounced Mg^{2+} block (see Figure 10–5). At –40 mV a small late inward current through NMDA receptor-channels is evident. At +20 mV the late component is more prominent and has reversed to become an outward current. The vertical dotted line indicates the time 25 ms after the peak of the synaptic current, which is used for the calculations of late current in part B.

B. The postsynaptic currents through the NMDA and AMPA receptor-channels differ in their dependence on the membrane potential. The current through the AMPA receptor-channels contributes to the early phase of the synaptic current **(filled triangles).** The early phase is measured at the peak of the synaptic current and plotted here as a function of membrane potential. The current through the NMDA receptor-channels contributes to the late phase of the synaptic current **(filled circles).** The late phase is measured 25 ms after the peak of the synaptic current **(dotted line** in part A), a time at which the AMPA receptor component has decayed almost to zero. Note that the AMPA receptor-channels behave as simple resistors; current and voltage have a linear relationship. In contrast, current through the NMDA receptor-channels is nonlinear and increases as the membrane is depolarized from –80 to –40 mV, owing to progressive relief of Mg^{2+} block. The reversal potential of both receptor-channel types is at 0 mV. The components of the synaptic current in the presence of 50 μm APV are indicated by the unfilled circles and triangles. Note how APV blocks the late (NMDA receptor) component but not the early (AMPA receptor) component of the EPSC.

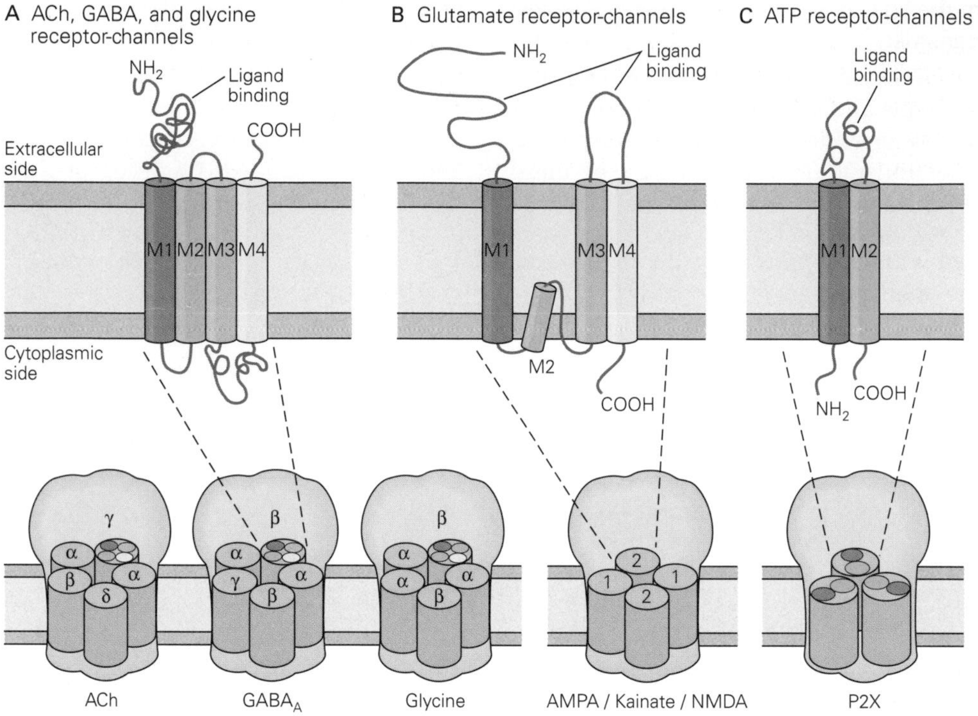

Figure 10–7 The three families of ligand-gated channels.

A. The nicotinic ACh, $GABA_A$, and glycine receptor-channels are all pentamers composed of several types of related subunits. As shown here, the ligand-binding domain is formed by the extracellular amino-terminal region of the protein. Each subunit has a membrane domain with four membrane-spanning α-helixes (M1–M4) and a short extracellular carboxyl terminus. The M2 helix lines the channel pore.

B. The glutamate receptor-channels are tetramers, often composed of two different types of closely related subunits (here denoted 1 and 2). The subunits have a large extracellular amino terminus, a membrane domain with three membrane-spanning α-helixes (M1, M3, and M4), a large extracellular loop connecting the M3 and M4 helixes, and an intracellular carboxyl terminus. The M2 segment forms a loop that dips into and out of the cytoplasmic side of the membrane, contributing to the selectivity filter of the channel. The glutamate binding site is formed by residues in the extracellular amino terminus and in the M3-M4 extracellular loop.

C. The ATP receptor-channels (or purinergic P2X receptors) are trimers. Each subunit possesses two membrane-spanning α-helixes (M1 and M2) and a large extracellular loop that binds ATP. The M2 helix lines the pore.

Glutamate Receptors Are Constructed from a Set of Modules

AMPA receptors are composed of three distinct modules: an extracellular amino-terminal domain, an extracellular ligand-binding domain, and a transmembrane domain (Figure 10–8A,B). The transmembrane domain contains three transmembrane α-helixes (M1, M3, and M4) and a loop (M2) between the M1 and M3 helixes that dips into and out of the cytoplasmic side of the membrane. This M2 loop is thought to form the selectivity filter of the channel. It adopts a structure similar to the pore-lining P loop of K^+ channels, except that in K^+ channels the P loop dips into and out of the extracellular surface of the membrane (see Figure 5–15).

Both the extracellular amino-terminal domain and the extracellular ligand binding domain are homologous to bacterial amino acid binding proteins. Each domain forms a bi-lobed clamshell-like structure similar to the structure of the bacterial proteins, in which the amino acid is bound within the clamshell. The amino-terminal domain does not bind glutamate but is homologous to the glutamate binding domain of metabotropic glutamate receptors. In the ionotropic glutamate receptors this domain is involved in subunit assembly, the modulation of receptor function by ligands other than glutamate, and the interaction with other synaptic proteins to regulate synapse development.

The ligand-binding domain is formed by two distinct regions in the linear sequence of the protein. One region is located in the extracellular amino terminus of the protein from the end of the amino terminal domain up to the M1 transmembrane helix; the second region is formed by the large extracellular loop connecting the M3 and M4 helixes. In the ionotropic receptors, the binding of a molecule of glutamate within the clamshell triggers the closure of the lobes of the clamshell; competitive antagonists also bind to the clamshell but fail to trigger clamshell closure. Thus the conformational change associated with clamshell closure is thought to be coupled to the opening of the ion channel.

Given the homology among the various subtypes of glutamate receptors, it is likely that the kainate and NMDA receptors adopt an overall structure similar to that of the homomeric GluA2 receptor. However, there are also likely to be some important differences that give rise to the distinct physiological functions of the different receptors. As we saw previously, the NMDA receptor-channels are permeable to Ca^{2+}, whereas most AMPA receptors are not. These differences have been localized to a single amino acid residue in the pore-forming M2 loop (Figure 10–9A). All NMDA receptor subunits contain the neutral residue asparagine at this position in the pore. In most types of AMPA receptor subunits this residue is the uncharged amino acid glutamine. However,

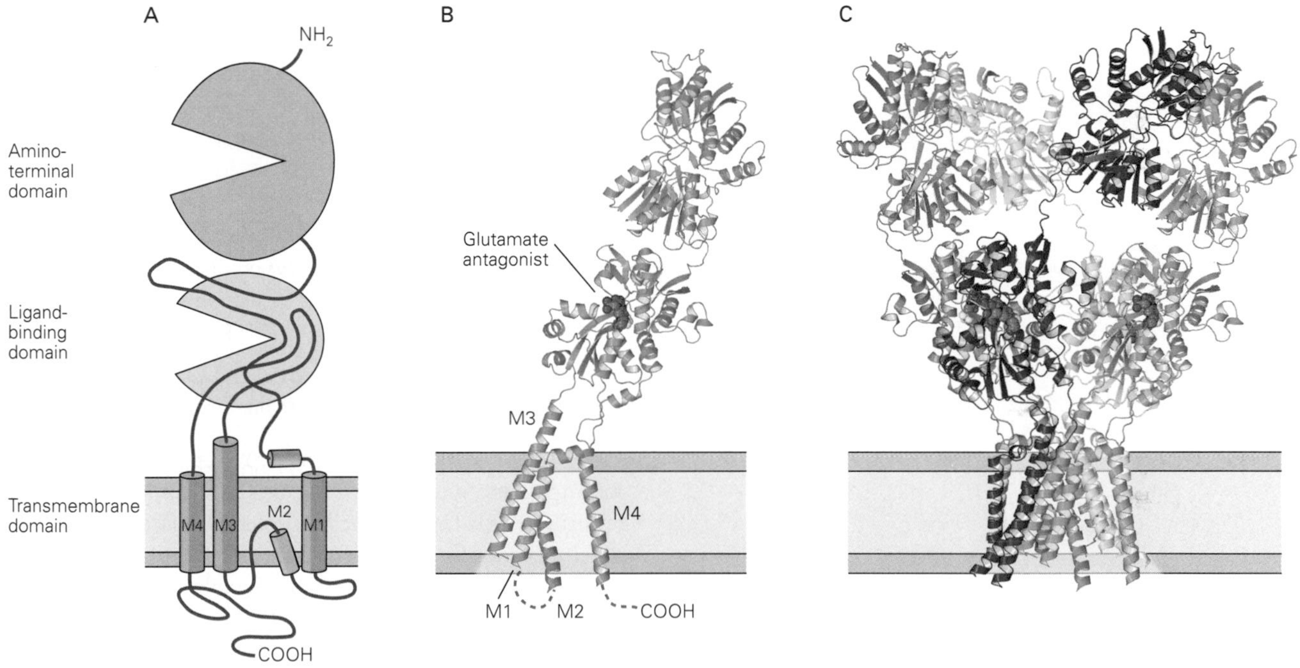

Figure 10–8 Structure of an ionotropic glutamate receptor.

A. Schematic organization of the ionotropic glutamate receptors. The receptors contain a large extracellular amino terminus, followed by a transmembrane domain containing three membrane-spanning α-helixes (M1, M3, and M4) and a loop that dips into the cytoplasmic side of the membrane (M2). The ligand-binding domain is formed by the extracellular region of the receptor on the amino-terminal side of the M1 segment and by the extracellular loop connecting M3 and M4. These two regions intertwine to form a clamshell structure that binds glutamate and various pharmacological agonists and competitive antagonists. A second clamshell structure is formed at the extreme amino terminus of the receptor. This amino-terminal domain is thought to modulate receptor function and synapse development. It does not bind glutamate in the ionotropic receptors. (Reproduced, with permission, from Armstrong et al. 1998.)

B. Three-dimensional X-ray crystal structure of an AMPA receptor composed solely of GluA2 subunits. A side view of the structure of a single GluA2 subunit showing the amino-terminal domain, ligand-binding domain, and transmembrane domain. The M1, M3, and M4 transmembrane α-helixes are indicated, as is the short α-helix in the M2 loop. A molecule of a competitive antagonist of glutamate bound to the ligand-binding domain is shown in a space-filling representation. The cytoplasmic loops connecting the membrane α-helixes were not resolved in the structure and have been drawn as dashed lines. (Reproduced, with permission, from Sobolevsky, Rosconi and Gouaux, 2009.)

C. A side view of the structure of the tetrameric receptor. The four GluA2 subunits associate through the extracellular domains as a pair of dimers (two-fold symmetry). In the amino-terminal domain, one dimer is formed by the blue and yellow subunits, and the other dimer is formed by the red and green subunits. In the ligand-binding domain, the subunits change partners. In one dimer the blue subunit associates with the red subunit, whereas in the other dimer the yellow subunit associates with the green subunit. In the transmembrane region the subunits associate as a four-fold symmetric tetramer. This is a highly unusual subunit arrangement whose significance is not fully understood. (Reproduced, with permission, from Sobolevsky, Rosconi and Gouaux, 2009.)

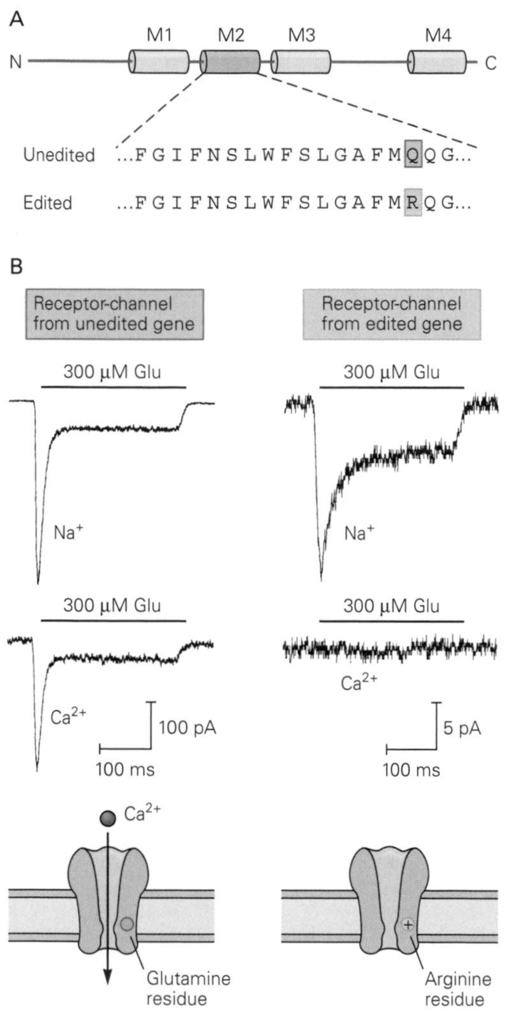

Figure 10–9 Determinants of Ca^{2+} permeability of the AMPA receptor.

A. Comparison of amino acid sequences in the M2 region of the AMPA receptor-channel coded by unedited and edited transcripts of the *GluA2* gene. The unedited transcript codes for the polar residue glutamine (**Q**, using the single-letter amino acid notation), whereas the edited transcript codes for the positively charged residue arginine (**R**). In the adult the GluA2 protein exists almost exclusively in the edited form.

B. AMPA receptor-channels expressed from unedited transcripts conduct Ca^{2+} (left traces), whereas those expressed from edited transcripts do not (right traces). The top and bottom traces show currents elicited by glutamate with either extracellular Na^+ (top traces) or Ca^{2+} (bottom traces) as the predominant permeant cation. (Reproduced, with permission, from Sakmann 1992.)

in the GluA2 subunit the corresponding M2 residue is arginine, a positively charged basic amino acid. Inclusion of even a single GluA2 subunit causes the AMPA receptor-channels to have a very low permeability to Ca^{2+}, most likely as a result of strong electrostatic repulsion by the arginine. Some cells form AMPA receptors that lack the GluA2 subunit. Such AMPA receptor-channels generate a significant Ca^{2+} influx, because their pores lack the positively charged arginine residue.

Peter Seeburg and his colleagues made the remarkable discovery that the DNA of the *GluA2* gene does not actually encode an arginine residue at this position in the M2 loop but rather codes for a glutamine residue. After transcription the codon for glutamine in the *GluA2* mRNA is replaced with one for arginine because of a chemical modification of a single nucleotide base through an enzymatic process termed RNA editing (Figure 10–9A). The importance of this RNA editing is underscored by a genetically engineered mouse that Seeburg and colleagues designed to express a *GluA2* gene in which the glutamine residue could no longer be edited to an arginine. Such mice develope seizures and die within a few weeks after birth, presumably caused by excess intracellular Ca^{2+} as all the AMPA receptors in these mice have a high Ca^{2+} permeability.

NMDA and AMPA Receptors Are Organized by a Network of Proteins at the Postsynaptic Density

How are the different glutamate receptors localized and arranged at excitatory synapses? Like most ionotropic receptors, glutamate receptors are normally clustered at postsynaptic sites in the membrane, opposed to glutamatergic presynaptic terminals. The vast majority of excitatory synapses in the mature nervous system contain both NMDA and AMPA, whereas in early development synapses containing only NMDA receptors are common. How are synaptic receptors clustered and targeted to appropriate sites? We are now beginning to appreciate that a large number of regulatory proteins that constitute the postsynaptic density help organize the three-dimensional structure of the postsynaptic cell membrane, including the localization of postsynaptic receptors (Figure 10–10).

The postsynaptic density is a remarkably stable structure, permitting its biochemical isolation, purification and characterization. Electron microscopic studies of intact and isolated postsynaptic densities provide a strikingly detailed view of their structure. By using gold-labeled antibodies it is possible to identify specific protein components of the postsynaptic membrane, including the location and number of glutamate receptors. A typical PSD of around 350 nm in diameter contains about

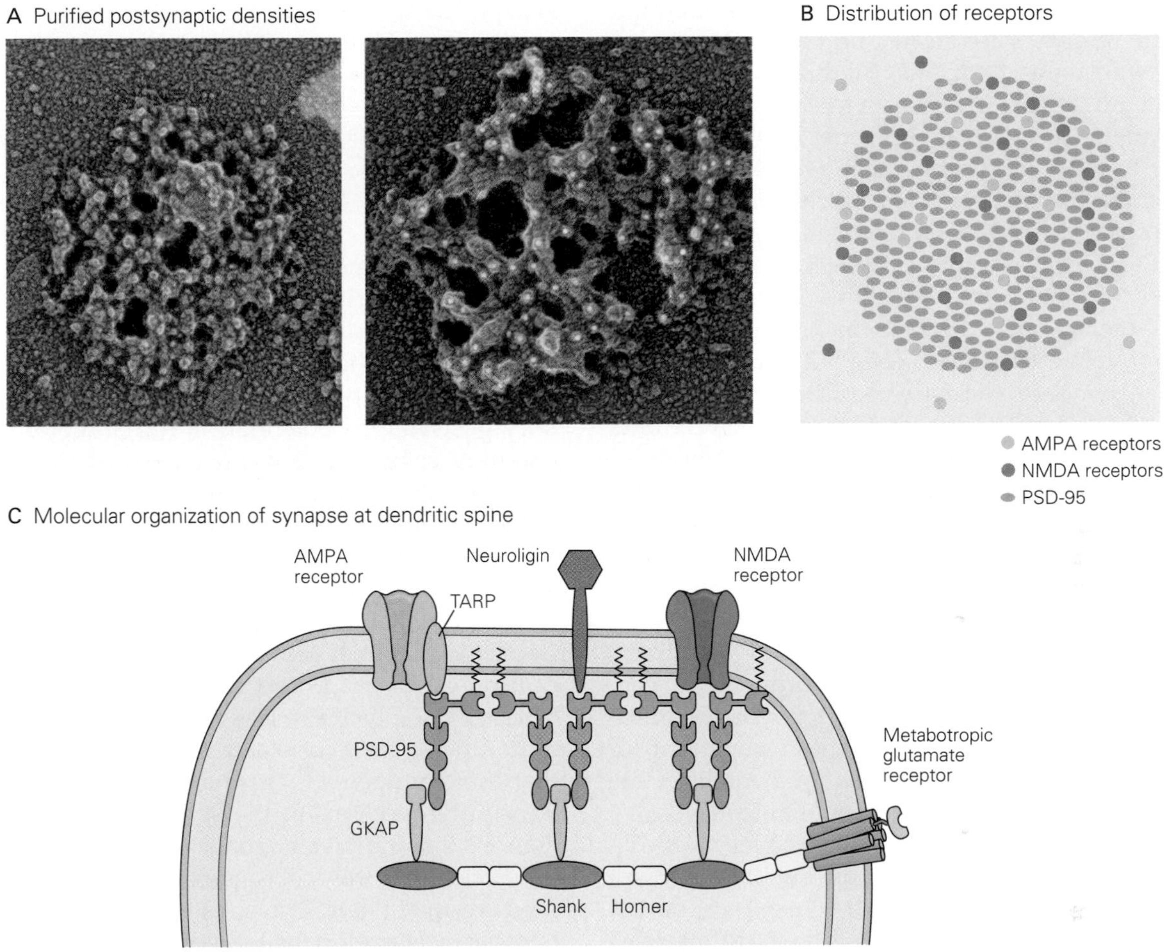

Figure 10–10 The postsynaptic cell membrane is organized into a macromolecular complex at excitatory synapses.

Proteins containing PDZ domains help organize the distribution of AMPA and NDMA receptors of the postsynaptic membrane at the postsynaptic density. (Reproduced, with permission, from Sheng and Hoogenrad 2007. Micrographs originally provided by Thomas S. Reese and Xiaobing Chen, National Institutes of Health, USA.)

A. Electron microscope images of biochemically purified postsynaptic densities, showing organization of protein network. The membrane lipid bilayer is no longer present. **Left**: View of postsynaptic density from what would normally be the outside of the cell. This image consists of the extracellular domains of various receptors and membrane proteins. **Right**: View of a postsynaptic density from what would normally be the cytoplasmic side of the membrane. White dots show immunolabeled guanylate kinase anchoring protein, an important component of the PSD.

B. Schematic view of localization and typical number of NMDA receptors, AMPA receptors, and PSD-95, a prominent postsynaptic density protein, at a synapse.

C. Schematic view of the network of receptors and their interacting proteins in the postsynaptic density. PSD-95 contains three PDZ domains at its amino terminus and two other protein interacting motifs at its carboxyl terminus, an SH3 domain and guanylate kinase (GK) domain. Certain PDZ domains of PSD-95 bind to the carboxyl terminus of the GluN2 subunit of the NMDA receptor. PSD-95 does not directly interact with AMPA receptors but binds to the carboxyl terminus of the TARP family of membrane proteins, which interact with the AMPA receptors as auxiliary subunits. PSD-95 also acts as a scaffold for various cytoplasmic proteins by binding to the guanylate-kinase-associated protein (GKAP), which interacts with Shank, a large protein that associates into a meshwork linking the various components of the postsynaptic density. PSD-95 also interacts with the cytoplasmic region of neuroligin. The metabotropic glutamate receptor is localized on the periphery of the synapse. It interacts with the protein Homer, which in turn binds to Shank.

20 NMDA receptors, which tend to be localized near the center of the PSD, and 10 to 50 AMPA receptors, which are less centrally localized. The metabotropic glutamate receptors are located on the periphery, outside the main area of the PSD. All three receptor types interact with a wide array of cytoplasmic and membrane proteins to ensure their proper localization.

One of the most prominent proteins in the postsynaptic density important for the clustering of glutamate receptors is PSD-95 (postsynaptic density protein of 95 kD molecular weight). PSD-95 is a membrane-associated protein that contains three repeated regions—the so-called PDZ domains—important for protein-protein interactions. The PDZ domains bind to specific sequences at the extreme carboxy terminus of a number of cellular proteins. They are named PDZ after the three proteins in which they were first identified: PSD-95, the DLG tumor suppressor protein in *Drosophila*, and a protein termed ZO-1. The PDZ domains of PSD-95 bind the NMDA receptor and the Shaker-type voltage-gated K^+ channel, thereby localizing and concentrating these channels at postsynaptic sites. PSD-95 also interacts with the postsynaptic membrane protein neuroligin, which forms an extracellular contact in the synaptic cleft with the presynaptic membrane protein neurexin, an interaction important for synapse development. Mutations in neuroligin are thought to contribute to some cases of autism.

Although PSD-95 does not directly bind to AMPA receptors, it does interact with an auxiliary subunit of these receptors termed the *transmembrane AMPA receptor regulatory protein* (TARP). The TARP proteins contain four transmembrane segments with a cytoplasmic C-terminus. These proteins strongly regulate the trafficking, synaptic localization, and gating of the AMPA receptors. The first TARP family member to be identified was stargazin, which was isolated through a genetic screen in the *stargazer* mutant mouse, so named because these animals have a tendency to tip their heads backward and stare upward. Loss of stargazin leads to a complete loss of AMPA receptors from cerebellar granule cells, which results in cerebellar ataxia and frequent seizures. Other members of the TARP family are similarly required for AMPA receptor trafficking to the surface membrane of other types of neurons.

The proper localization of AMPA receptors by stargazin depends on the interaction between its C-terminus and PSD-95. AMPA receptors also bind to a distinct PDZ domain protein called GRIP, and metabotropic glutamate receptors interact with yet another PDZ domain protein called Homer. In addition to interacting with receptors, proteins with PDZ domains interact with many other cellular proteins, including proteins that bind to the actin cytoskeleton, providing a scaffold around which a complex of postsynaptic proteins is constructed. Indeed, a biochemical analysis of the postsynaptic density has identified dozens of proteins that participate in NMDA or AMPA receptor complexes.

Inhibitory Synaptic Action Is Usually Mediated by Ionotropic GABA and Glycine Receptor-Channels That Are Permeable to Chloride

Although glutamatergic excitatory synapses account for the vast majority of synapses in the brain, inhibitory synapses play an essential role in the nervous system both by preventing too much excitation and by helping coordinate activity among networks of neurons. Inhibitory postsynaptic potentials in spinal motor neurons and most central neurons are generated by the amino acid neurotransmitters GABA and glycine. GABA is a major inhibitory transmitter in the brain and spinal cord. It acts on two receptors, $GABA_A$ and $GABA_B$. The $GABA_A$ receptor is an ionotropic receptor that directly opens a Cl^- channel. The $GABA_B$ receptor is a metabotropic receptor that activates a second-messenger cascade, which often indirectly activates a K^+ channel (see Chapter 11). Glycine, a less common inhibitory transmitter in the brain, also activates ionotropic receptors that directly open Cl^- channels. Glycine is the major transmitter released in the spinal cord by the interneurons that inhibit antagonist muscles.

Eccles and his colleagues determined the ionic mechanism of the IPSP in spinal motor neurons by systematically changing the level of the resting membrane potential in a motor neuron and stimulating a presynaptic inhibitory interneuron (Figure 10–11). When the motor neuron membrane is held at the normal resting potential (–65 mV), a small hyperpolarizing potential is generated when the interneuron is stimulated. When the motor neuron membrane is held at –70 mV, no change in potential is recorded when the interneuron is stimulated. But at potentials more negative than –70 mV the motor neuron generates a *depolarizing* response following stimulation of the inhibitory interneuron. This reversal potential of –70 mV corresponds to the Cl^- equilibrium potential in spinal motor neurons (the extracellular concentration of Cl^- is much greater than the intracellular concentration). Thus, at –70 mV the tendency of Cl^- to diffuse into the cell down its chemical concentration gradient is balanced by the electrical force (the negative membrane potential) that opposes Cl^- influx. Replacement of extracellular Cl^- with an impermeant anion reduces the size of the IPSP and shifts the reversal potential to more positive values in accord with the predictions of the Nernst equation. Thus, the IPSP results from an increase in Cl^- conductance.

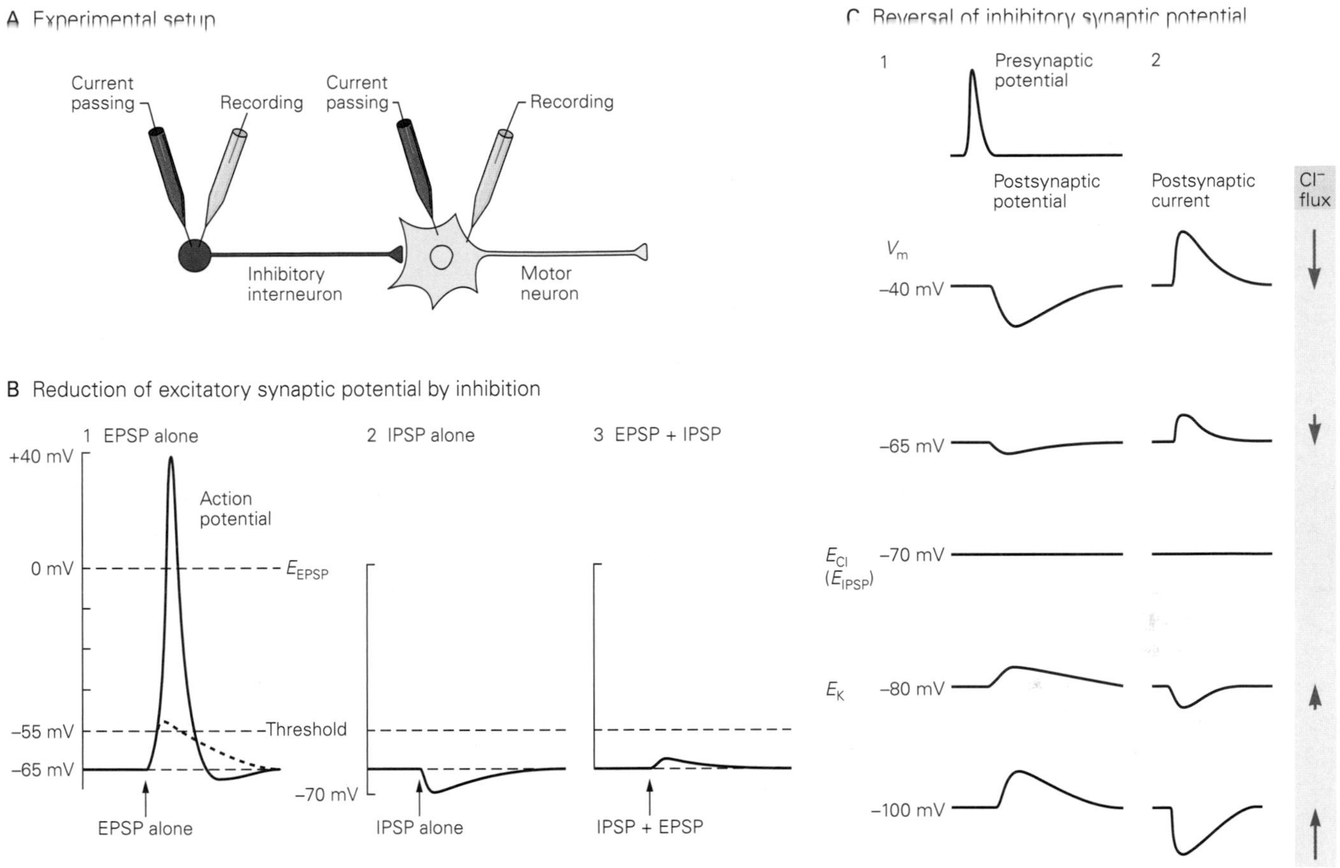

Figure 10–11 Inhibitory actions at chemical synapses result from the opening of ion channels selective for Cl^-.

A. In this hypothetical experiment two electrodes are placed in the presynaptic interneuron and two in the postsynaptic motor neuron. The current-passing electrode in the presynaptic cell is used to produce an action potential; in the postsynaptic cell it is used to alter the membrane potential systematically prior to the presynaptic input.

B. Inhibitory actions counteract excitatory actions. **1.** A large EPSP occurring alone depolarizes the membrane toward E_{EPSP} and exceeds the threshold for generating an action potential. **2.** An IPSP alone moves the membrane potential away from the threshold toward E_{Cl}, the Nernst potential for Cl^- (–70 mV). **3.** When inhibitory and excitatory synaptic potentials occur together, the effectiveness of the EPSP is reduced, preventing it from reaching the threshold for an action potential.

C. The IPSP and inhibitory synaptic current reverse at the equilibrium potential for Cl^-. **1.** A presynaptic spike produces a hyperpolarizing IPSP at the resting membrane potential (–65 mV). The IPSP is larger when the membrane potential is set at –40 mV due to the increased driving force on Cl^-. When the membrane potential is set at –70 mV the IPSP is nullified. This reversal potential for the IPSP occurs at E_{Cl}. With further hyperpolarization of the membrane the IPSP is inverted to a depolarizing postsynaptic potential (at –80 and –100 mV) because the membrane potential is negative to E_{Cl}. **2.** The reversal potential of the inhibitory postsynaptic current measured under voltage clamp. An inward (negative) current flows at membrane potentials negative to the reversal potential (corresponding to an efflux of Cl^-) and an outward (positive) current flows at membrane potentials positive to the reversal potential (corresponding to an influx of Cl^-). (Up arrows = efflux, down arrows = influx.)

Currents Through Single GABA and Glycine Receptor-Channels Can Be Recorded

The currents through single GABA and glycine receptor-channels, the unitary currents, have been measured using the patch-clamp technique. Both transmitters activate Cl^- channels that open in an all-or-none manner, similar to the opening of ACh and glutamate-gated channels. The conductance of a glycine receptor-channel (46 pS) is larger than that of a $GABA_A$ receptor-channel (30 pS). As a result, the unitary current through glycine-gated channels is somewhat larger than that of $GABA_A$ receptor-channels (Figure 10–12). This difference results because the diameter of the glycine receptor-channel pore is slightly larger than that of the $GABA_A$ receptor-channel pore.

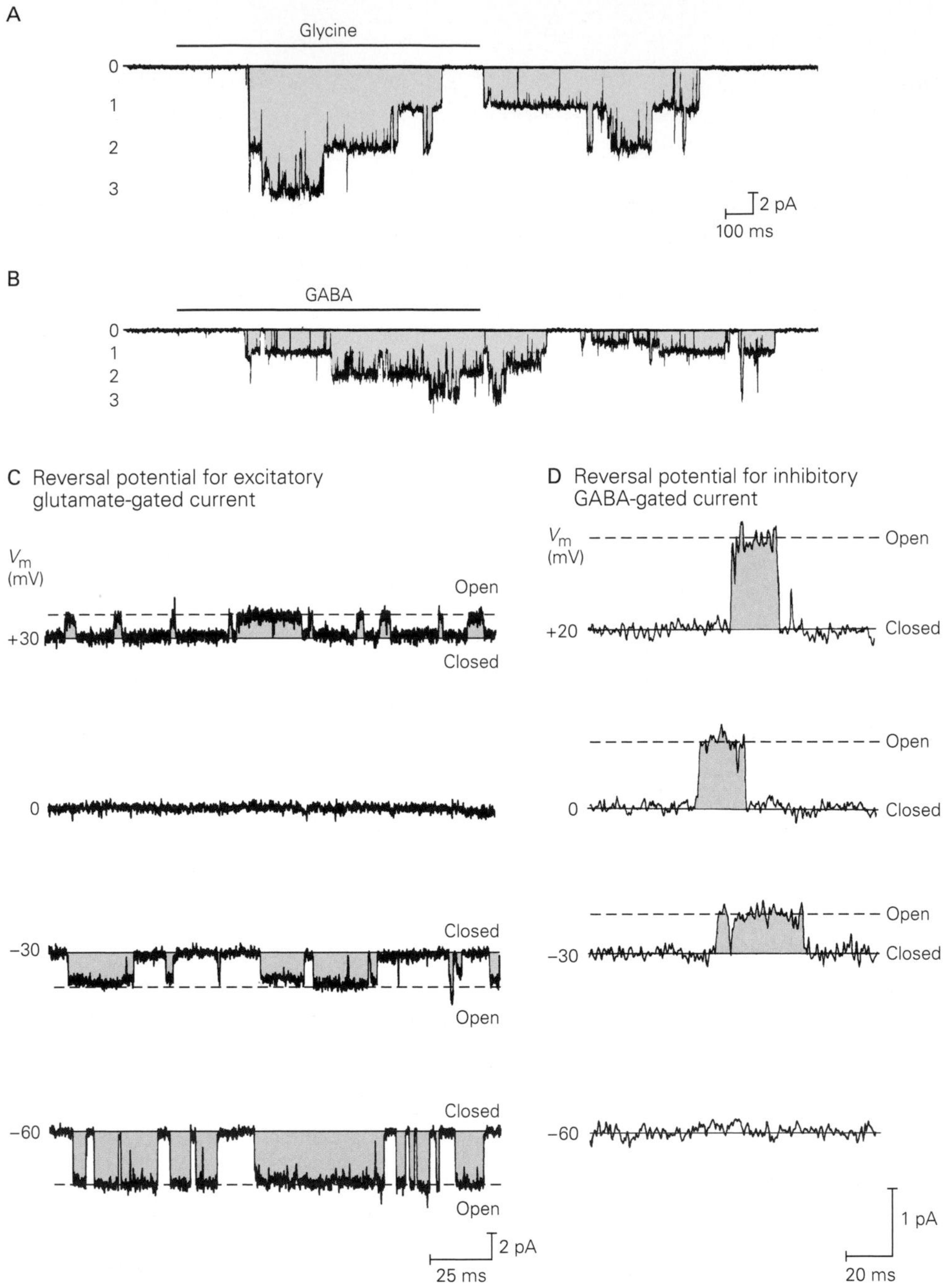

Figure 10–12 Comparison of single-channel excitatory currents activated by glutamate and inhibitory currents activated by GABA and glycine.

A. Single-channel currents through three glycine receptor-channels in a patch from a mouse spinal neuron. (Reproduced, with permission, from Bormann et al. 2007.)

B. Single-channel currents through GABA receptor-channels in the same patch. In A and B the membrane was held at a voltage negative to the Cl^- equilibrium potential, so channel openings generate an inward current owing to an efflux of Cl^-. (Reproduced, with permission, from Bormann et al. 2007.)

C. Excitatory current through a single NMDA receptor-channel in a rat hippocampal neuron. As the membrane potential is moved in a depolarizing direction (from –60 to –30 mV), the current pulses become smaller. At 0 mV (the reversal potential for the EPSP) the current pulses are nullified, and at +30 mV they invert and are outward. The reversal potential at 0 mV is the weighted average of equilibrium potentials for Na^+, Ca^{2+}, and K^+, the three ions responsible for generating this current. Note: In this recording there was no Mg^{2+} in the external solution so the NMDA receptor-channel openings are voltage-independent. (Reproduced, with permission, from J. Jen and C. F. Stevens.)

D. Inhibitory current through a single GABA-activated channel in a rat hippocampal neuron. The current is nullified at approximately –60 mV (the reversal potential for the IPSP in this cell). At more depolarized levels the current pulses are outward (corresponding to the influx of Cl^-). This reversal potential lies near the equilibrium potential for Cl^-, the only ion contributing to this current. (Reproduced, with permission, from B. Sakmann.)

The inhibitory action of these Cl^- channels can be demonstrated by comparing the reversal potentials of current through a $GABA_A$ receptor-channel and a glutamate receptor-channel. The excitatory current reverses at 0 mV (Figure 10–12C). Therefore, opening of glutamate receptor-channels at the normal resting potential generates an inward current (influx of positive charge), driving the membrane past threshold. In contrast, the inhibitory current becomes nullified and begins to reverse at values more negative than –60 mV (Figure 10–12D). Thus, the opening of $GABA_A$ receptor-channels at typical resting potentials normally generates an outward current (influx of negative charge), preventing the membrane from reaching threshold.

Chloride Currents Through Inhibitory $GABA_A$ and Glycine Receptor-Channels Normally Inhibit the Postsynaptic Cell

In a typical neuron the resting potential of –65 mV is slightly more positive than E_{Cl} (–70 mV). At this resting potential the chemical force driving Cl^- into the cell is slightly greater than the electrical force opposing Cl^- influx—that is, the electrochemical driving force on Cl^- ($V_m - E_{Cl}$) is positive. As a result, the opening of Cl^- channels leads to a positive current, based on the relation $I_{Cl} = g_{Cl}(V_m - E_{Cl})$. Because the charge carrier is the negatively charged Cl^- ion, the positive current corresponds to an influx of Cl^- into the neuron, down its electrochemical gradient. This causes a net increase in the negative charge on the inside of the membrane—the membrane becomes hyperpolarized.

Some central neurons have a resting potential that is approximately equal to E_{Cl}. In such cells an increase in Cl^- conductance does not change the membrane potential—the cell does not become hyperpolarized—because the electrochemical driving force on Cl^- is nearly zero. However, the opening of Cl^- channels in such a cell still inhibits the cell from firing an action potential in response to a near-simultaneous EPSP. This is because the depolarization produced by an excitatory input depends on a weighted average of the batteries for all types of open channels—that is, the batteries for the excitatory and inhibitory synaptic conductances and the resting conductances—with the weighting factor equal to the total conductance for a particular type of channel (see Chapter 9, Postscript). Because the battery for Cl^- channels lies near the resting potential, opening these channels helps hold the membrane near its resting potential during the EPSP by increasing the weighting factor for the Cl^- battery.

The effect that the opening of Cl^- channels has on the magnitude of an EPSP can also be described in terms of Ohm's law. Accordingly, the amplitude of the depolarization during an EPSP, ΔV_{EPSP}, is given by:

$$\Delta V_{EPSP} = I_{EPSP}/g_1$$

where I_{EPSP} is the excitatory synaptic current and g_1 is the total conductance of all other channels open in the membrane, including resting channels and any contributions from the transmitter-gated Cl^- channels. Because the opening of the Cl^- channels increases the resting conductance, the depolarization during the EPSP decreases. This consequence of synaptic inhibition is called the *short-circuiting* or *shunting* effect.

The different biophysical properties of synaptic conductances can be also understood as distinct mathematical operations carried out by the postsynaptic neuron. Thus, inhibitory inputs that hyperpolarize the cell perform a *subtraction* on the excitatory inputs, whereas those that shunt the excitation perform a *division*. Adding excitatory inputs (or removing nonshunting inhibitory inputs) results in a *summation*. Finally, the combination of an excitatory input with the removal of an inhibitory shunt produces a *multiplication*.

In some cells, such as those with metabotropic $GABA_B$ receptors, inhibition is caused by the opening of K^+ channels. Because the K^+ equilibrium potential of neurons (E_K = –80 mV) is always negative to the resting potential, opening K^+ channels inhibits the cell even more profoundly than opening Cl^- channels (assuming a similar-size synaptic conductance). $GABA_B$ responses turn on more slowly and persist for a longer time compared with $GABA_A$ responses.

Paradoxically, under some conditions the activation of $GABA_A$ receptors in brain cells can cause excitation. This is because the influx of Cl^- after intense periods of stimulation can be so great that the intracellular Cl^- concentration increases substantially. It may even double. As a result, the Cl^- equilibrium potential may become more positive than the resting potential. Under these conditions the opening of Cl^- channels leads to Cl^- efflux and depolarization of the neuron. Such depolarizing Cl^- responses occur normally in some neurons in newborn animals, where the intracellular Cl^- concentration tends to be high even at rest. This is because the K^+-Cl^- cotransporter is expressed at low levels during early development, as discussed in Chapter 6. Depolarizing Cl^- responses may also occur in the distal dendrites of more mature neurons and perhaps also at their axon initial segment. Such excitatory $GABA_A$ receptor actions in adults may contribute to epileptic discharges in which large, synchronized, and depolarizing GABA responses are observed.

Ionotropic Glutamate, GABA, and Glycine Receptors Are Transmembrane Proteins Encoded by Two Distinct Gene Families

The genes coding for the $GABA_A$ and glycine receptors are closely related to each other. More surprisingly, the $GABA_A$ and glycine receptors are structurally related to the nicotinic ACh receptors, even though the latter select for cations. Thus, these receptors are members of one large gene family (Figure 10–7A). In contrast, the glutamate receptors have evolved from a different class of proteins and thus represent a second gene family of ligand-gated channels (Figure 10–7B).

Ionotropic $GABA_A$ and Glycine Receptors Are Homologous to Nicotinic ACh Receptors

Like nicotinic ACh receptor-channels, the $GABA_A$ and glycine receptor-channels are each composed of five subunits that are encoded by related gene families (Figure 10–7A). The $GABA_A$ receptors are usually composed of two α-, two β-, and one γ- or δ-subunit. The receptors are activated by the binding of two molecules of GABA in clefts formed between the two α- and β-subunits. The glycine receptors are composed of three α- and two β-subunits and require the binding of up to three molecules of ligand to open. The transmembrane topology of each $GABA_A$ and glycine receptor subunit is similar to that of a nicotinic ACh receptor subunit, consisting of a large extracellular ligand-binding domain followed by four hydrophobic transmembrane α-helices (labeled M1, M2, M3, and M4), with the M2 helix forming the lining of the channel pore. However, the amino acids flanking the M2 domain are strikingly different from those of the nicotinic ACh receptor. As discussed in Chapter 9, the pore of the ACh receptor contains rings of negatively charged acidic residues that help the channel select for cations over anions. In contrast, the GABA and glycine receptor-channels contain either neutral or positively charged basic residues at the homologous positions, which contributes to the selectivity of these channels for anions.

Most of the classes of receptor subunits are encoded by multiple related genes. Thus, there are six subtypes of $GABA_A$ α-subunits (α1-α6), three β-subunits (β1-β3), three γ-subunits (γ1-γ3) and one δ-subunit. The genes for these different subtypes are often differentially expressed in different types of neurons, endowing their inhibitory synapses with distinct properties. The possible combinatorial arrangements of these subunits in a fully assembled pentameric receptor provides an enormous potential diversity of receptor subtypes.

The $GABA_A$ and glycine receptors play important roles in disease and in the actions of drugs. $GABA_A$ receptors are the target for several types of drugs that are clinically important and socially abused, including general anesthetics, benzodiazepines, barbiturates, and alcohol. General anesthetics can be either gases or injectable compounds that induce a loss of consciousness and are therefore widely used during surgery. Benzodiazepines are antianxiety agents and muscle relaxants that include diazepam (Valium), lorazepam (Ativan), and clonazepam (Klonopin). Zolpidem (Ambien) is a non-benzodiazepine compound that promotes sleep. The barbiturates comprise a distinct group of hypnotics that includes phenobarbital and secobarbital. The different classes of compounds—GABA, general anesthetics, benzodiazepines, barbiturates, and alcohol—bind to different sites on the receptor but act similarly to increase the opening of the GABA receptor-channel. For example, whereas GABA binds to a cleft between the α- and β-subunits, benzodiazepines bind to a cleft between the α- and γ-subunits. In addition, the binding of any one of these classes of drug influences the binding of the others. For example, a benzodiazepine (or a barbiturate) binds more strongly to the receptor-channel when GABA also is bound, and this tight binding helps stabilize the channel in the open state. In this manner, the various compounds all enhance inhibitory synaptic transmission.

How do these various compounds that all act on $GABA_A$ receptors to promote channel opening produce such diverse behavioral and psychological effects, for example, reducing anxiety versus promoting sleep? It turns out that many of these compounds interact selectively with specific subunit subtypes, which can be localized to different regions of the brain. For example, zolpidem binds selectively to $GABA_A$ receptors containing the α1-subtype of subunit. In contrast, the anxiolytic effect of benzodiazepines requires binding to the α2- and γ-subunits.

In addition to being important pharmacological targets, the $GABA_A$ and glycine receptors are targets of disease and poisons. Missense mutations in the α subunit of the glycine receptor underlie an inherited neurological disorder called *familial startle disease* (or *hyperekplexia*), characterized by abnormally high muscle tone and exaggerated responses to noise. These mutations decrease the opening of the glycine receptor and so reduce the normal levels of inhibitory transmission in the spinal cord. The poison strychnine, a plant alkaloid compound, causes convulsions by blocking the glycine receptor and decreasing inhibition. Nonsense mutations that result in truncations of $GABA_A$ receptor α- and γ-subunits have been implicated in congenital forms of epilepsy.

Some Synaptic Actions Depend on Other Types of Ionotropic Receptors in the Central Nervous System

Certain fast excitatory synaptic actions are mediated by the neurotransmitter serotonin (5-HT) acting at the 5-HT_3 class of ionotropic receptor-channels. These ionotropic receptors have four transmembrane segments and are structurally similar to the nicotinic ACh receptors. Like the ACh receptor-channels, 5-HT_3 receptor-channels are permeable to monovalent cations and have a reversal potential near 0 mV.

Finally, ionotropic receptors for adenosine triphosphate (ATP), which serves as an excitatory transmitter at selected synapses, constitute a third major family of transmitter-gated ion channels. These so-called purinergic receptors (named for the purine ring in adenosine) occur on smooth muscle cells innervated by sympathetic neurons of the autonomic ganglia as well as on certain central and peripheral neurons. At these synapses ATP activates an ion channel that is permeable to both monovalent cations and Ca^{2+}, with a reversal potential near 0 mV. Several genes coding for this family of ionotropic ATP receptors (termed the P2X receptors) have been identified. The amino acid sequence and subunit structure of these ATP receptors is different from the other two ligand-gated channel families. An X-ray crystal structure of the P2X receptor reveals that it has an exceedingly simple organization in which three subunits, each containing only two transmembrane segments, surround a central pore (Figure 10–7C).

Excitatory and Inhibitory Synaptic Actions Are Integrated by the Cell into a Single Output

Up to now we have mostly focused on the physiological and molecular properties of excitatory or inhibitory synapses in isolation. However, each neuron in the central nervous system is constantly bombarded by an array of synaptic inputs from many other neurons. A single motor neuron, for example, may be innervated by as many as 10,000 different presynaptic endings. Some are excitatory, others inhibitory; some are strong, others weak. Some inputs contact the motor cell on the tips of its apical dendrites, others on proximal dendrites, some on the dendritic shaft, others on the soma. The different inputs can reinforce or cancel one another. How does a given neuron integrate these signals into a coherent output?

As we saw earlier, the synaptic potentials produced by a single presynaptic neuron typically are not large enough to depolarize a postsynaptic cell to the threshold for an action potential. The EPSPs produced in a motor neuron by most stretch-sensitive afferent neurons are only 0.2 to 0.4 mV in amplitude. If the EPSPs generated in a single motor neuron were to sum linearly, at least 25 afferent neurons would have to fire together and release transmitter to depolarize the trigger zone by the 10 mV required to reach threshold. But at the same time the postsynaptic cell is receiving excitatory inputs, it may also be receiving inhibitory inputs that prevent the firing of action potentials by either a subtractive or shunting effect. The net effect of the inputs at any individual excitatory or inhibitory synapse will therefore depend on several factors: the location, size, and shape of the synapse, the proximity and relative strength of other synergistic or antagonistic synapses, and the resting potential of the cell.

Inputs are coordinated in the postsynaptic neuron by a process called *neuronal integration.* This cellular process reflects the task that confronts the nervous system as a whole: decision making. A cell at any given moment has two options: to fire or not to fire an action potential. Charles Sherrington described the brain's ability to choose between competing alternatives as the *integrative action of the nervous system.* He regarded this decision making as the brain's most fundamental operation.

Synaptic Inputs Are Integrated to Fire an Action Potential at the Axon Initial Segment

In most neurons the decision to initiate an action potential is made at one site: the initial segment of the axon (see Chapter 2). Here the cell membrane has a lower threshold for action potential generation than at the cell body or dendrites because it has a higher density of voltage-dependent Na^+ channels (Figure 10–13). With each increment of membrane depolarization, more Na^+ channels open, thus generating a higher density of inward current (per unit area of membrane) at the axon initial segment than elsewhere in the cell. At the initial segment the depolarization increment required to reach the threshold for an action potential (–55 mV) is only 10 mV from the resting level of –65 mV. In contrast, the membrane of the cell body must be depolarized by 30 mV before reaching its threshold (–35 mV). Therefore, synaptic excitation first discharges the region of membrane at the initial segment, also called the *trigger zone.* The action potential generated at this site then depolarizes the membrane of the cell body to threshold and at the same time is propagated along the axon.

Because neuronal integration involves the summation of synaptic potentials that spread to the trigger zone, it is critically affected by two passive membrane properties of the neuron (see Chapter 6). First, the

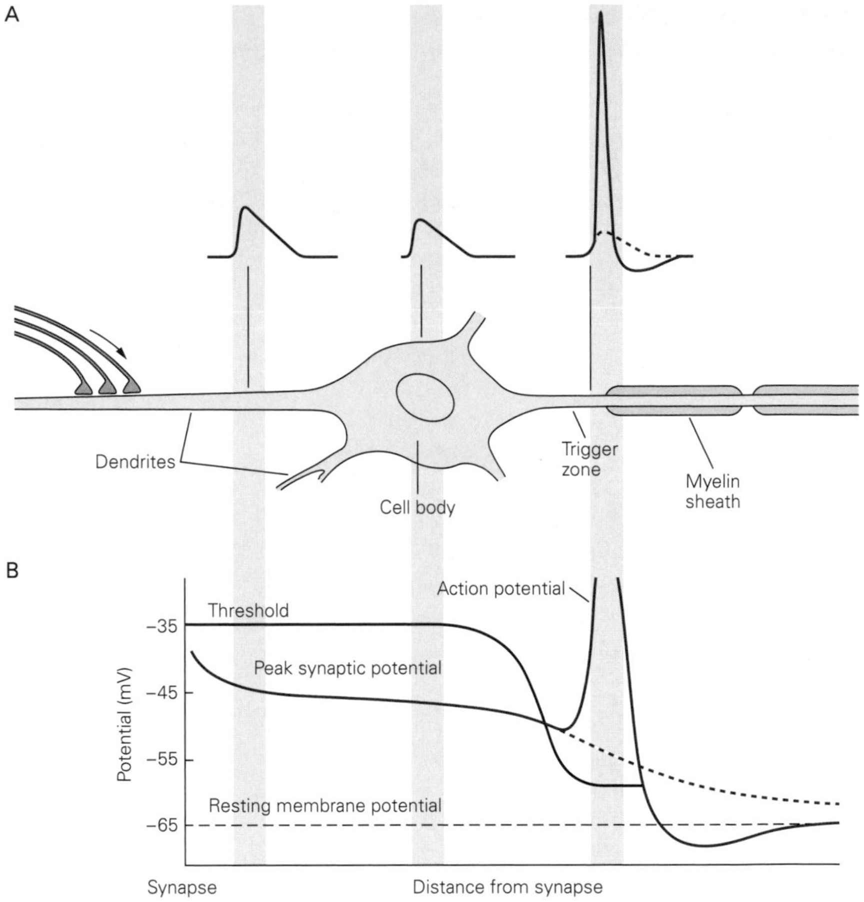

Figure 10–13 A synaptic potential arising in a dendrite can generate an action potential at the axon initial segment. (Adapted, with permission, from Eckert et al. 1988.)

A. An excitatory synaptic potential originating in the dendrites decreases with distance as it propagates passively to the soma. Nevertheless, an action potential can be initiated at the trigger zone (the axon initial segment) because the density of the Na^+ channels in this region is high, and thus the threshold is low.

B. Comparison of the threshold for initiation of the action potential at different sites in the neuron (corresponding to drawing A). An action potential is generated when the amplitude of the synaptic potential exceeds the threshold. The **dashed line** shows the decay of the synaptic potential if no action potential is generated at the axon initial segment.

membrane time constant helps determine the time course of the synaptic potential and thereby controls *temporal summation,* the process by which consecutive synaptic potentials at the same site are added together in the postsynaptic cell. Neurons with a large membrane time constant have a greater capacity for temporal summation than do neurons with a shorter time constant (Figure 10–14A). As a result, the longer the time constant, the greater the likelihood that two consecutive inputs from an excitatory presynaptic neuron will summate to bring the cell membrane to its threshold for an action potential.

Second, the *length* constant of the cell determines the degree to which a local depolarization decreases as it spreads passively from a synapse along the length of the dendrite. In cells with a longer length constant, signals spread to the trigger zone with minimal decrement; in cells with a short length constant, the signals decay rapidly with distance. Because the depolarization produced at one synapse is almost never sufficient to trigger an action potential at the trigger zone, the inputs from many presynaptic neurons acting at different sites on the postsynaptic neuron must be added together. This process is called *spatial summation.* Neurons with a large length constant are more likely to be brought to threshold by inputs arising from different sites than are neurons with a short length constant (Figure 10–14B).

Dendrites Are Electrically Excitable Structures That Can Fire Action Potentials

Propagation of signals in dendrites was originally thought to be purely passive. However, intracellular recordings from the cell body of neurons in the 1950s and from dendrites beginning in the 1970s demonstrated that dendrites could produce action potentials. Indeed, we now know that the dendrites of most neurons contain voltage-gated Na^+, K^+, and Ca^{2+} channels in addition to ligand-gated channels and leakage channels. In fact, the rich diversity of dendritic conductances suggests that central neurons rely on a sophisticated repertory of electrophysiological properties to integrate synaptic inputs.

One function of the voltage-gated Na^+ and Ca^{2+} channels in dendrites may be to amplify the EPSP. In some neurons there are sufficient concentrations of voltage-gated channels in the dendrites to serve as a local trigger zone. This can further amplify weak excitatory input that arrives at remote parts of the dendrite. When a cell has several dendritic trigger zones, each one sums the local excitation and inhibition produced by nearby synaptic inputs; if the net input is above threshold, a dendritic action potential may be generated, usually by voltage-dependent Na^+ or Ca^{2+} channels (Figure 10–15). Nevertheless, the number of voltage-gated Na^+ or Ca^{2+} channels in the dendrites is usually not sufficient to support the all-or-none regenerative propagation of these action potentials to the cell body. Rather, action potentials generated in the dendrites are local events that propagate electrotonically to the cell body and axon initial segment, where they are integrated with all other input signals in the cell.

Do active conductances influence dendritic integration? There is currently a vigorous debate as to what arithmetic rules dendrites use to summate inputs. While some results indicate that dendrites are highly nonlinear devices that work by firing local spikes in individual dendritic branches, others argue that dendrites behave essentially as linear integrators (ie, they sum inputs arithmetically). In this linear scenario, dendritic conductances would balance each other to achieve a stable integration regime.

The dendritic voltage-gated channels also permit action potentials generated at the axon initial segment to propagate backward into the dendritic tree. These *back-propagating* action potentials are found in most

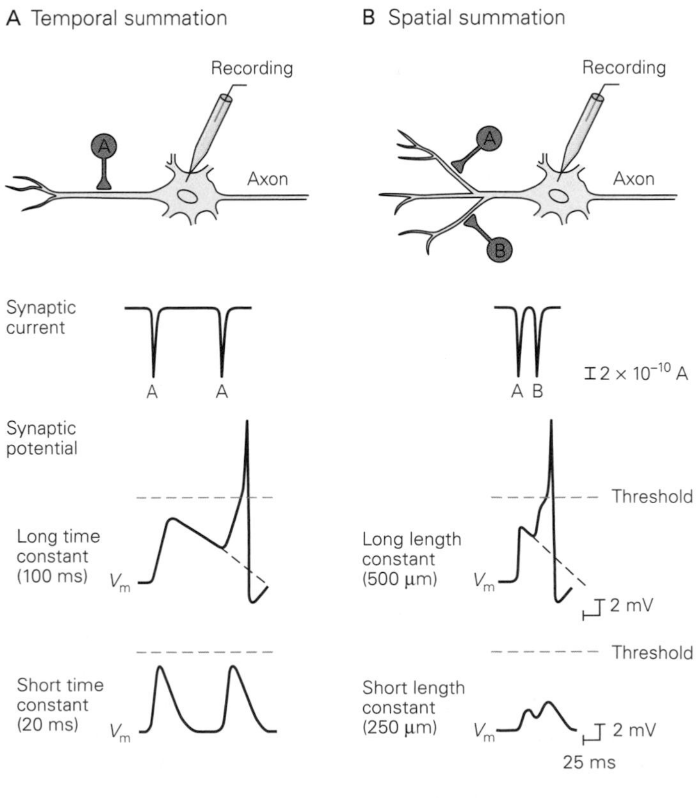

Figure 10–14 Central neurons are able to integrate a variety of synaptic inputs through temporal and spatial summation of synaptic potentials.

A. The time constant of a postsynaptic cell (see Figure 6–15) affects the amplitude of the depolarization caused by consecutive EPSPs produced by a single presynaptic neuron (**A**). Here the synaptic current generated by the presynaptic neuron is nearly the same for both EPSPs. In a cell with a *long* time constant the first EPSP does not fully decay by the time the second EPSP is triggered. Therefore, the depolarizing effects of both potentials are additive, bringing the membrane potential above the threshold and triggering an action potential. In a cell with a *short* time constant the first EPSP decays to the resting potential before the second EPSP is triggered. The second EPSP alone does not cause enough depolarization to trigger an action potential.

B. The length constant of a postsynaptic cell (see Figure 6–16) affects the amplitudes of two excitatory postsynaptic potentials produced by two presynaptic neurons (A and B). For illustrative purposes, both synapses are the same (500 µm) distance from the postsynaptic cell's trigger zone at the axon initial segment, and the current produced by each synaptic contact is the same. If the distance between the site of synaptic input and the trigger zone in the postsynaptic cell is only one length constant (that is, the postsynaptic cell has a length constant of 500 µm), the synaptic potentials produced by each of the two presynaptic neurons will decrease to 37% of their original amplitude by the time they reach the trigger zone. Summation of the two potentials results in enough depolarization to exceed threshold, triggering an action potential. If the distance between the synapse and the trigger zone is equal to two length constants (ie, the postsynaptic cell has a length constant of 250 µm), each synaptic potential will be less than 15% of its initial amplitude, and summation will not be sufficient to trigger an action potential.

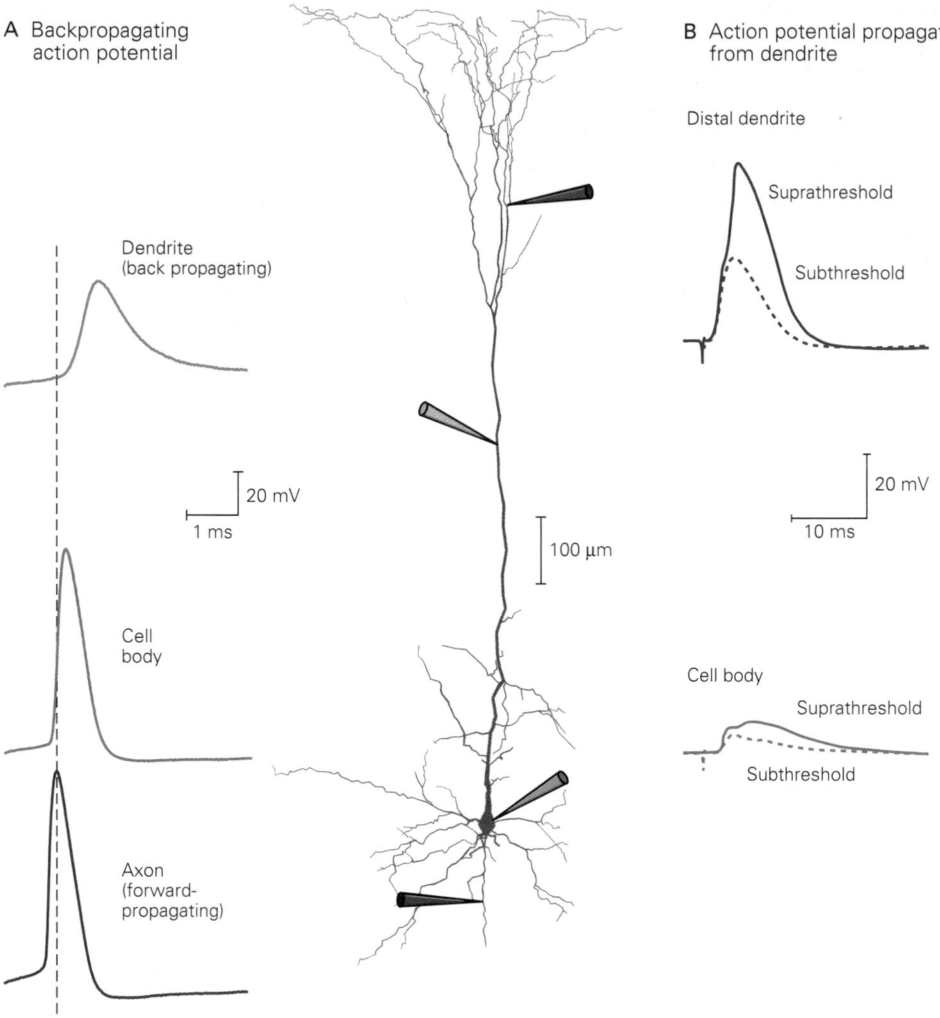

Figure 10–15 Dendrites support propagation of action potentials to and from the axon initial segment. The figure illustrates an experiment in which several electrodes are used to record membrane voltage and pass stimulating currents in the axon, the soma, and at several locations along the dendritic tree. The recording electrode and corresponding voltage trace are matched according to color. (Adapted, with permission, from Stuart et al. 2000.)

A. An action potential can be propagated from the axon initial segment to the dendrites. Such backpropagation depends on activation of voltage-gated Na^+ channels in the dendrites. Unlike the action potential that is continually regenerated along an axon, the amplitude of a backpropagating action potential decreases as it travels along a dendrite due to the relatively low density of voltage-gated Na^+ channels in dendrites.

B. A strong depolarizing EPSP at a dendrite can generate an action potential that travels to the cell body. Such forward-propagating action potentials are often generated by dendritic voltage-gated Ca^{2+} channels and have a high threshold. They propagate relatively slowly and decrement with distance, often failing to reach the cell body. The **solid line** shows a suprathreshold response generated in the dendrite, and the **dotted line** shows a subthreshold response.

neurons and are largely generated by dendritic voltage-gated Na^+ channels. Although the precise role of backpropagating action potentials is unclear, they may provide a temporally precise mechanism for regulating current through the NMDA receptor by providing the depolarization necessary to remove the Mg^{2+} block (see Figure 10–5).

Synapses on a Central Neuron Are Grouped According to Physiological Function

All four regions of the nerve cell—axon, terminals, cell body, and dendrites—can in principle be presynaptic or postsynaptic sites. The most common types of contact, illustrated in Figure 10–16, are axodendritic, axosomatic, and axo-axonic (by convention, the presynaptic element is identified first). Axodendritic synapses can occur on the dendritic shaft or on spines. Dendrodendritic and somasomatic contacts are also found, but they are rare.

The proximity of a synapse to the trigger zone is traditionally thought to be important to its effectiveness. A postsynaptic current generated at an axosomatic site should produce a greater change in membrane potential at the trigger zone, and therefore a greater influence on action potential output, than does an equal current at more remote axodendritic contacts, because of the passive cable properties of a dendrite (Figure 10–17). Nevertheless, it seems that some neurons compensate for this effect by placing more glutamate receptors at distal synapses than at proximal synapses, ensuring that inputs along the dendritic tree have a more equivalent strength at the initial segment, thereby minimizing spatial effects in dendritic integration.

In contrast to axodendritic and axosomatic input, most axo-axonic synapses have no direct effect on the trigger zone of the postsynaptic cell. Instead, they affect the activity of the postsynaptic neuron by controlling the amount of transmitter released from the presynaptic terminals (see Chapter 12).

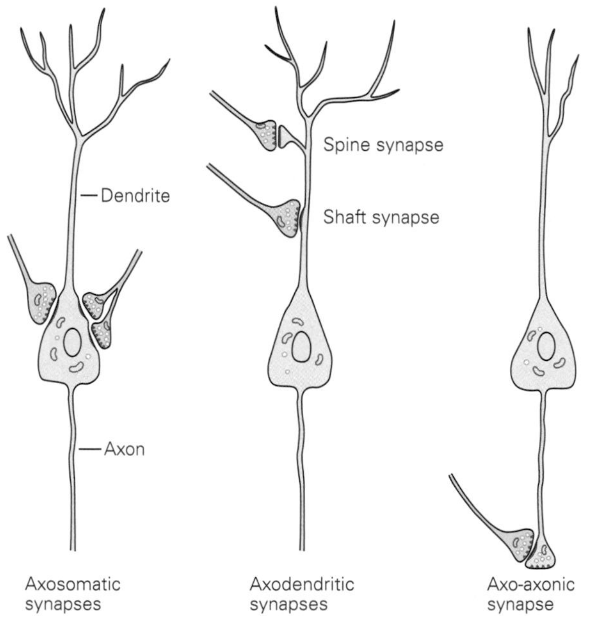

Figure 10–16 Synaptic contact can occur on the cell body, the dendrites, or the axon of the postsynaptic cell. The names of various kinds of synapses—axosomatic, axodendritic, and axo-axonic—identify the contacting regions of both the presynaptic and postsynaptic neurons (the presynaptic element is identified first). Axodendritic synapses can occur on either the shaft of a dendrite or on a specialized input zone, the spine.

The location of inhibitory inputs in relation to excitatory ones is critical for the effectiveness of the inhibitory stimuli. Inhibitory shunting is more significant when initiated at the cell body near the axon hillock. The depolarization produced by an excitatory current from a dendrite must pass through the cell body as it moves toward the axon initial segment. Inhibitory actions at the cell body open Cl^- channels, thus increasing Cl^- conductance and reducing by shunting much of the depolarization produced by the spreading excitatory current. As a result, the influence of the excitatory current on the membrane potential at the trigger zone is strongly curtailed (Figure 10–17). In contrast, inhibitory actions at a remote part of a dendrite are much less effective in shunting excitatory actions or in affecting the more distant trigger zone. Thus, it is not surprising that in the brain significant inhibitory input frequently occurs on the cell body of neurons.

Even though some excitatory inputs occur on dendritic shafts, close to 95% of all excitatory inputs in the brain terminate on dendritic spines, surprisingly avoiding dendritic shafts (see Figure 10–3). Although the function of spines is not completely understood, their thin necks provide a barrier to diffusion of various signaling molecules from the spine head to the dendritic shaft. As a result a relatively small Ca^{2+} current through the NMDA receptors can lead to a relatively large increase in [Ca^{2+}] that is localized to the head of the individual spine that is synaptically activated (Figure 10–18A). Moreover, because action potentials can backpropagate from the cell body to the dendrites (see below), spines also serve as sites at which information about presynaptic and postsynaptic activity is integrated. Indeed, when a backpropagating action potential is paired with presynaptic stimulation, the spine Ca^{2+} signal is greater than the linear sum of the individual Ca^{2+} signals from synaptic stimulation alone or action potential stimulation alone. This "supralinearity" is specific to the activated spine and occurs because depolarization during the action potential causes Mg^{2+} to be expelled from the NMDA receptor, allowing it to conduct Ca^{2+} into the spine (see Figure 10–5). The resultant Ca^{2+} accumulation thus provides, at an individual synapse, a biochemical detector of the near simultaneity of the input (EPSP) and output (backpropagating action potential), which is thought to be a key requirement of memory storage.

As the thin spine neck, at least partly, restricts the rise in Ca^{2+}, and thus long-term plasticity, to the spine that receives the synaptic input, spines also ensure that activity-dependent changes in synaptic function, and

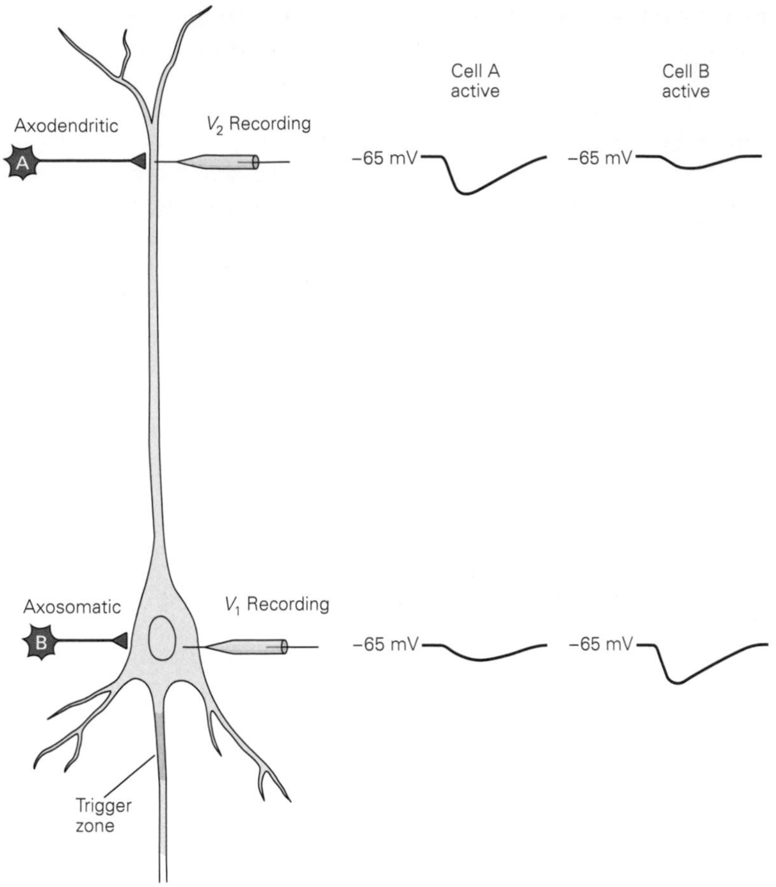

Figure 10–17 The effect of an inhibitory current in the postsynaptic neuron depends on the distance the current travels from the synapse to the cell's trigger zone. In this hypothetical experiment the inputs from inhibitory axosomatic and axodendritic synapses are compared by recording from both the cell body (V_1) and the dendrite (V_2) of the postsynaptic cell. Stimulating the axosomatic synapse from presynaptic cell B produces a large IPSP in the cell body. Because the synaptic potential is initiated in the cell body it will undergo little decrement before arriving at the trigger zone in the initial segment of the axon. The IPSP decays as it propagates up the dendrite, producing only a small hyperpolarization at the site of dendritic recording. Stimulating the axodendritic synapse from presynaptic cell **A** produces a large local IPSP in the dendrite but only a small IPSP in the cell body because the synaptic potential decays as it propagates down the dendrite to the cell body. Thus the axosomatic IPSP is more effective than the axodendritic IPSP in inhibiting action potential firing in the postsynaptic cell.

thus memory storage, are restricted to the synapses that are activated. The ability of spines to implement such synapse-specific local learning rules may be of fundamental importance for the ability of neural networks to store meaningful information (see Appendix E). Finally, the local synaptic potentials in some spines are filtered as they propagate through the spine neck and enter the dendrite, reducing the size of the EPSP at the soma. The regulation of this electrical filtering could control the efficacy with which local EPSPs are conducted to the soma.

An Overall View

The past several years have seen a remarkable growth in our understanding of the diversity of molecules and mechanisms underlying the postsynaptic responses of neurons in the central nervous system to transmitter released from their presynaptic inputs. Nonetheless, nearly all fast synaptic actions in the brain are mediated by only three main amino acid neurotransmitters: the excitatory transmitter glutamate and the inhibitory transmitters GABA and glycine. These produce rapid changes in the postsynaptic membrane potential by acting on specific classes of ligand-gated channels, known as ionotropic receptors. Glutamate depolarizes a postsynaptic cell by acting on three types of ionotropic receptors: the kainate, AMPA, and NMDA receptors. In addition, glutamate acts on metabotropic receptors to produce slower modulatory synaptic actions that can be either excitatory or inhibitory. The fast inhibitory transmitters hyperpolarize cells by acting on $GABA_A$ receptors or glycine receptors. GABA also binds to inhibitory metabotropic $GABA_B$ receptors,

The inhibitory $GABA_A$ and glycine receptors belong to the same superfamily of receptors as do the excitatory nicotinic ACh receptors present at the neuromuscular junction. They are composed of five homologous subunits, with each subunit containing four membrane-spanning α-helixes. The three types of glutamate receptors belong to a separate receptor gene family. They are composed of four homologous subunits, with each subunit containing two extracellular ligand binding regions and a transmembrane domain containing three membrane-spanning α-helixes and a reentrant P-loop that forms the selectivity filter of the channel.

Despite the fact that fast synaptic transmission in the brain depends on only three major neurotransmitters acting on five main classes of ionotropic receptors, there is an enormous diversity in the postsynaptic properties of synapses in the brain. This is due, in part, to the presence of a large number of subtypes of the different receptors, resulting from the presence of multiple isoforms of receptor subunits encoded by distinct but related genes. Further diversity is generated through posttranscriptional processing, including differential RNA splicing and RNA editing. For $GABA_A$ receptors alone it has been estimated that there is a potential for the existence of up to 800 different receptor subtypes due to combinatorial arrangements of the different subunit isoforms, although it is likely that far fewer are actually generated in the brain.

Clearly, a major challenge is the identification of which receptor subunit combinations actually exist in the brain and where those subunits are located. Although this is a daunting task, the potential payoff is great, offering the possibility of subtype-specific drugs

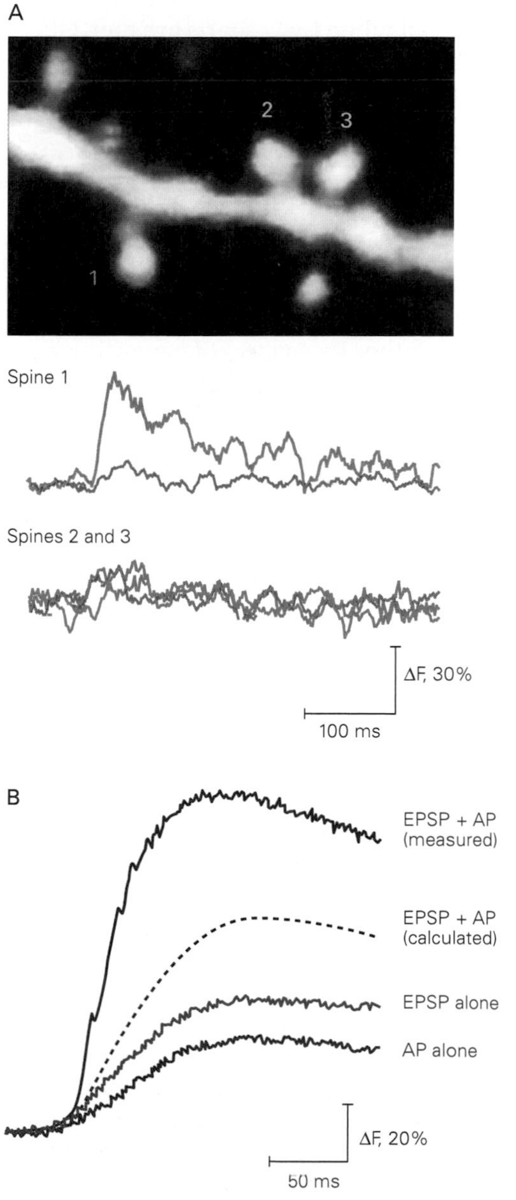

Figure 10–18 Dendritic spines compartmentalize calcium influx through NMDA receptors.

A. This fluorescence image of a hippocampal CA1 pyramidal neuron filled with a calcium-sensitive dye shows the outline of a dendritic shaft with several spines. When the dye binds Ca^{2+} its fluorescence intensity increases. The traces plot fluorescence intensity as a function of time following the extracellular stimulation of the presynaptic axon. Spine 1 shows a large, rapid fluorescence increase (ΔF) in response to synaptic stimulation (**red trace**), reflecting Ca^{2+} influx through the NMDA receptors. In contrast, there is little change in the fluorescence intensity in the neighboring dendrite shaft (**grey trace**), showing that Ca^{2+} accumulation is restricted to the head of the spine. Spines 2 and 3 show little increase in fluorescence in response to synaptic stimulation because their presynaptic axons were not activated by the external stimulus. (Reproduced, with permission, from Lang et al. 2004.)

B. Calcium accumulation is greatest in spines when synaptic stimulation is paired with postsynaptic action potentials. The vertical axis is proportional to the intracellular Ca^{2+} concentration in a dendritic spine. The Ca^{2+} signal generated when an EPSP and a backpropagating action potential are evoked at the same time (EPSP + AP [measured]) is greater than the expected sum of the individual Ca^{2+} signals (EPSP + AP [calculated]) when either an EPSP or a backpropagating action potential (AP) is evoked alone. (Adapted, with permission, from Yuste and Denk, 1995.)

that produce highly specific actions. For example, whereas compounds that produce a nonspecific blockade of all types of $GABA_A$ receptors lead to excess excitation and seizures, a drug that selectively blocks the subtype of $GABA_A$ receptor containing the α5-subunit has a beneficial effect on memory storage. A different drug that activates the $GABA_A$ α2/α3-subtype of receptors alleviates neuropathic pain.

As we have seen in this chapter and will return to throughout the book, one of the key properties of neuronal synapses is that their function can be modulated by experience. Some forms of synaptic plasticity involve long-term changes in receptor expression. One of the best characterized examples of activity-dependent synaptic plasticity depends on the properties of the NMDA receptors, which conduct Ca^{2+} into a postsynaptic cell when two criteria are met: Glutamate must be released from the presynaptic terminal and the postsynaptic neuron must be sufficiently depolarized to expel Mg^{2+} from the pore of the receptor through electrostatic repulsion. In normal amounts, Ca^{2+} triggers signaling pathways that enhance excitatory synaptic transmission, a process essential for certain types of memory (see Chapters 66 and 67). In excess, as occurs during stroke and certain neurodegenerative diseases, Ca^{2+} leads to neuronal death and brain damage.

Another key aspect of synaptic transmission in the CNS is the fact that individual excitatory or inhibitory inputs normally produce relatively small changes in a neuron's membrane potential. A neuron must therefore integrate information from thousands of excitatory and inhibitory inputs before deciding whether the threshold for an action potential (–55 mV) has been reached. The summation of these inputs within a single cell depends critically on the cell's passive properties, namely on its time and length constants. Moreover, a synapse's location is critically important to its efficacy. Excitatory synapses tend to be located on spines on neuronal dendrites, whereas inhibitory synapses predominate on the cell body, where they can effectively interrupt and override the excitatory inputs traveling down the cell's dendrites to the soma. The final summing of inputs to the cell is made at the axon initial segment, which contains the highest density of Na^+ channels in the cell and thus has the lowest threshold for spike initiation. The consequences of mixed excitatory and inhibitory inputs in neural networks is discussed in Appendix E.

Much of the discussion in this chapter has been based on the schematic model of the neuron outlined in Chapter 2. According to this model, the dendritic tree is specialized as the receptive pole of the neuron, the axon is the signal-conducting portion, and the axon terminal is the transmitting pole. This model implies that the neuron, the signaling unit of the nervous system, merely sends and receives information. In reality, neurons in most brain regions are more complex. As we have seen in this chapter, active conductances allow dendrites to propagate action potentials, which interact with synaptic events to produce long-lasting changes in synaptic transmission. Moreover, dendritic spines appear ideally suited to implement input-specific learning rules. Thus, our current view is that dendrites are complex, integrative compartments in neurons that can powerfully affect the propagation of synaptic potentials to the cell body and the relay of activity-dependent information from the cell body and initial segment back to synapses on the dendrites. Although crucial to neuronal integration, the electrical properties of dendrites and spines remain rather poorly understood and are an area of active investigation. In fact, as we shall see when considering the sensory and motor systems, the integrative properties of neurons in many brain regions allow the neurons to perform essential transformations on their inputs, rather than serve as simple relay stations.

Steven A. Siegelbaum
Eric R. Kandel
Rafael Yuste

Selected Readings

Arundine M, Tymianski M. 2004. Molecular mechanisms of glutamate-dependent neurodegeneration in ischemia and traumatic brain injury. Cell Mol Life Sci 61:657–668.

Bredt DS, Nicoll RA. 2003. AMPA receptor trafficking at excitatory synapses. Neuron 40:361–379.

Colquhoun D, Sakmann B. 1998. From muscle endplate to brain synapses: a short history of synapses and agonist-activated ion channels. Neuron 20:381–387.

Hausser M, Spruston N, Stuart GJ. 2000. Diversity and dynamics of dendritic signaling. Science 290:739–744.

Kash TL, Trudell JR, Harrison NL. 2004. Structural elements involved in activation of the gamma-aminobutyric acid type A ($GABA_A$) receptor. Biochem Soc Trans 32:540–546.

Mayer ML, Armstrong N. 2004. Structure and function of glutamate receptor ion channels. Annu Rev Physiol 66:161–181.

Olsen RW, Sieghart W. 2009. $GABA_A$ receptors: subtypes provide diversity of function and pharmaocology. Neuropharmacology 56:141–148.

Peters A, Palay SL, Webster HD. 1991. *The Fine Structure of the Nervous System.* New York: Oxford Univ. Press.

Sheng M, Hoogenraad CC. 2007. The postsynaptic architecture of excitatory synapses: a more quantitative view. Ann Rev Biochem 76:823–847.

References

Armstrong N, Sun Y, Chen GQ, Gouaux E. 1998. Structure of a glutamate-receptor ligand-binding core in complex with kainate. Nature 395:913–917.

Bormann J, Hamill O, Sakmann B. 1987. Mechanism of anion permeation through channels gated by glycine and γ-aminobutyric acid in mouse cultured spinal neurones. J. Physiol. 385:243-286.

Cash S, Yuste R. 1999. Linear summation of excitatory inputs by CA1 pyramidal neurons. Neuron 22:383–394.

Coombs JS, Eccles JC, Fatt P. 1955. The specific ionic conductances and the ionic movements across the motoneuronal membrane that produce the inhibitory post-synaptic potential. J Physiol 130:326–373.

Eccles JC. 1964. *The Physiology of Synapses.* New York: Academic.

Eckert R, Randall D, Augustine G. 1988. Propagation and transmission of signals. In: *Animal Physiology: Mechanisms and Adaptations,* 3rd ed., pp. 134–176. New York: Freeman.

Finkel AS, Redman SJ. 1983. The synaptic current evoked in cat spinal motoneurones by impulses in single group Ia axons. J Physiol 342:615–632.

Gray EG. 1963. Electron microscopy of presynaptic organelles of the spinal cord. J Anat 97:101–106.

Grenningloh G, Rienitz A, Schmitt B, Methsfessel C, Zensen M, Beyreuther K, Gundelfinger ED, Betz H. 1987. The strychnine-binding subunit of the glycine receptor shows homology with nicotinic acetylcholine receptors. Nature 328:215–220.

Hamill OP, Bormann J, Sakmann B. 1983. Activation of multiple-conductance state chloride channels in spinal neurones by glycine and GABA. Nature 305:805–808.

Hestrin S, Nicoll RA, Perkel DJ, Sah P. 1990. Analysis of excitatory synaptic action in pyramidal cells using whole-cell recording from rat hippocampal slices. J Physiol 422: 203–225.

Heuser JE, Reese TS. 1977. Structure of the synapse. In: ER Kandel (ed), *Handbook of Physiology: A Critical, Comprehensive Presentation of Physiological Knowledge and Concepts,* Sect. 1 *The Nervous System.* Vol. 1, *Cellular Biology of Neurons,* Part 1 pp. 261–294. Bethesda, MD: American Physiological Society.

Hollmann M, O'Shea-Greenfield A, Rogers SW, Heinemann S. 1989. Cloning by functional expression of a member of the glutamate receptor family. Nature 342:643–648.

Jia H, Rochefort NL, Chen X, Konnerth A. 2010. Dendritic organization of sensory input to cortical neurons in vivo. Nature 464:1307–1312.

Lang C, Barco A, Zablow L, Kandel ER, Siegelbaum SA, Zakharenko SS. 2004. Transient expansion of synaptically connected dendritic spines upon induction of hippocampal long-term potentiation. Proc Natl Acad Sci U S A 101:16665–16670.

Llinas R. 1988. The intrinsic electrophysiological properties of mammalian neurons: insights into central nervous system function. Science 23:242:1654–1664.

Llinas R, Sugimori M. 1980. Electrophysiological properties of in vitro Purkinje cell dendrites in mammalian cerebellar slices. J Physiol 305:197–213.

Magee JC, Cook EP. 2000. Somatic EPSP amplitude is independent of synapse location in hippocampal pyramidal neurons. Nat Neurosci 3:895–903.

Markram H, Lubke J, Frotscher M, Sakmann B. 1997 Regulation of synaptic efficacy by coincidence of postsynaptic APs and EPSPs. Science 275:213–215.

Masu M, Tanabe Y, Tsuchida K, Shigemoto R, Nakanishi S. 1991. Sequence and expression of a metabotropic glutamate receptor. Nature 349:760–765.

Moriyoshi K, Masu M, Ishii T, Shigemoto R, Mizuno N, Nakanishi S. 1991. Molecular cloning and characterization of the rat NMDA receptor. Nature 354:31–37.

Palay SL. 1958. The morphology of synapses in the central nervous system. Exp Cell Res Suppl 5:275–293.

Pritchett DB, Sontheimer H, Shivers BD, Ymer S, Kettenmann H, Schofield PR, Seeburg PH. 1989. Importance of a novel $GABA_A$ receptor subunit for benzodiazepine pharmacology. Nature 338:582–585.

Redman S. 1979. Junctional mechanisms at group Ia synapses. Prog Neurobiol 12:33–83.

Sakmann B. 1992. Elementary steps in synaptic transmission revealed by currents through single ion channels. Neuron 8:613–629.

Sommer B, Köhler M, Sprengel R and Seeburg, PH. 1991. RNA editing in brain controls a determinant of ion flow in glutamate-gated channels. Cell 67:11–19.

Sheng M, Hoogenraad C. 2007. The postsynaptic architecture of excitatory synapses: a more quantitative view. Ann Rev Biochem 76:823–847.

Sherrington CS. 1897. The central nervous system. In: M Foster. *A Text Book of Physiology,* 7th ed. London: Macmillan.

Sobolevsky AI, Rosconi MP, Gouaux E. 2009. X-ray structure, symmetry and mechanism of an AMPA-subtype glutamate receptor. Nature 462:745–56.

Stuart G, Spruston N, Häuser M (eds). 1999. *Dendrites.* Oxford, England, and New York: Oxford Univ. Press.

Surprenant A, Buell G, North RA. 1995. P_{2x} receptors bring new structure to ligand-gated ion channels. Trends Neurosci 18:224–229.

Yuste R. 2010. *Dendritic Spines.* Cambridge, MA and London, England: MIT Press.

Yuste R, Denk W. 1995. Dendritic spines as basic functional units of neuronal integration. Nature 375:682–684.

11

Modulation of Synaptic Transmission: Second Messengers

THE BINDING OF NEUROTRANSMITTER to postsynaptic receptors produces a postsynaptic potential either directly, by opening ion channels, or indirectly, by altering ion channel activity through changes in the postsynaptic cell's biochemical state. As we saw in Chapter 8, the type of action depends on the type of receptor. Activation of *ionotropic receptors* directly opens ion channels that are part of the receptor macromolecule itself. In contrast, activation of *metabotropic receptors* regulates the opening of ion channels indirectly through biochemical signaling pathways. The receptor and ion channels that are affected are distinct macromolecules (Figure 11–1).

Whereas the action of ionotropic receptors is fast and brief, metabotropic receptors produce effects that begin slowly and persist for long periods, ranging from hundreds of milliseconds to many minutes. The two types of receptors also differ in their functions. Ionotropic receptors *mediate* behaviors, from simple reflexes to complex cognitive processes. Metabotropic receptors *modulate* behaviors; they modify reflex strength, help focus attention, set emotional states, and contribute to long-lasting changes in neural circuits that underlie learning and memory. Metabotropic receptors are responsible for many of the actions of transmitters, hormones, and growth factors.

Ionotropic receptors change the balance of charge across the neuron's membrane quickly. As we have seen, this change is local at first but is propagated as an action potential along the axon if the change in membrane potential is suprathreshold. Activation of metabotropic receptors also begins as a local action that can spread to a wider region of the cell. A neurotransmitter reacting with a metabotropic receptor activates proteins that in

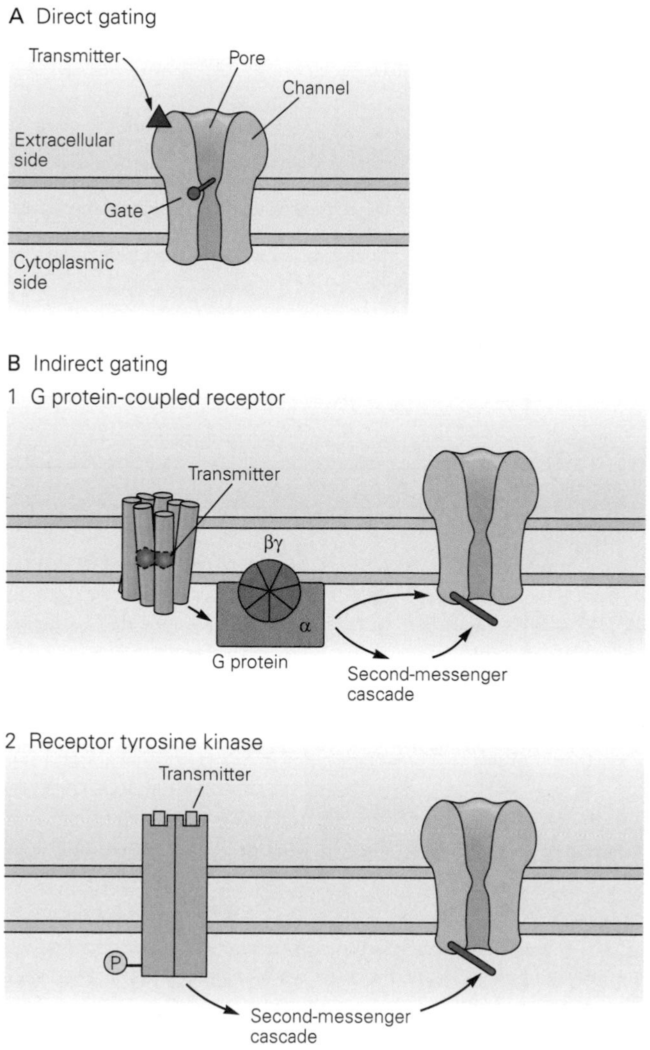

Figure 11–1 Neurotransmitter actions can be divided into two groups according to the way in which receptor and effector functions are coupled.

A. Direct transmitter actions are produced by ionotropic receptors, ligand-gated channels in which the receptor and ion channel are domains formed by a single macromolecule. The binding of transmitter to the receptor on the extracellular aspect of the protein directly opens the ion channel embedded in the cell membrane.

B. Indirect transmitter actions are caused by binding of transmitter to metabotropic receptors that are separate macromolecules from the ion channels that they regulate. There are two families of these receptors. **1.** G protein-coupled receptors activate guanosine triphosphate (GTP)-binding proteins that engage a second-messenger cascade or act directly on ion channels. **2.** Receptor tyrosine kinases initiate a cascade of protein phosphorylation reactions, beginning with autophosphorylation of the kinase itself on tyrosine residues.

turn activate effector enzymes. The effector enzymes then often produce second-messenger molecules that can diffuse within a cell to activate still other enzymes that catalyze modifications of a variety of target proteins, greatly changing their activities.

There are two major families of metabotropic receptors: G protein-coupled receptors and receptor tyrosine kinases. We first describe the G protein-coupled receptor family and later discuss the receptor tyrosine kinase family.

The G protein-coupled receptors are coupled to an effector by a trimeric guanine nucleotide-binding protein, or G protein (Figure 11–1B). This receptor family contains α- and β-adrenergic receptors for norepinephrine, muscarinic acetylcholine (ACh) receptors, γ-aminobutyric acid B ($GABA_B$) receptors, certain glutamate and serotonin receptors, all receptors for dopamine, receptors for neuropeptides, odorant receptors, rhodopsin (the protein that reacts to light, initiating visual signals, see Chapter 26), and many others. Many of these receptors are thought to be involved in neurological and psychiatric disease and are key targets for the actions of important classes of therapeutic drugs.

G protein-coupled receptors activate a variety of effectors. Typically the effector is an enzyme that produces a diffusible second messenger. These second messengers in turn trigger a biochemical cascade, either by activating specific protein kinases that phosphorylate the hydroxyl group of specific serine or threonine residues in various proteins or by mobilizing Ca^{2+} ions from intracellular stores, thus initiating reactions that change the cell's biochemical state. In some instances the G protein or the second messenger act directly on an ion channel.

The Cyclic AMP Pathway Is the Best Understood Second-Messenger Signaling Cascade Initiated by G Protein-Coupled Receptors

The adenosine 3′,5′-cyclic monophosphate (cyclic AMP or cAMP) pathway is a prototypic example of a second-messenger cascade. It was the first second-messenger pathway to be discovered, and our conception of other second-messenger pathways is based on it.

The binding of transmitter to receptors linked to the cAMP cascade first activates a specific G protein, G_s (named for its action to *stimulate* cAMP synthesis). In its resting state G_s, like all G proteins, binds a molecule of guanosine diphosphate (GDP). The interaction of G_s with a ligand-bound receptor promotes the exchange

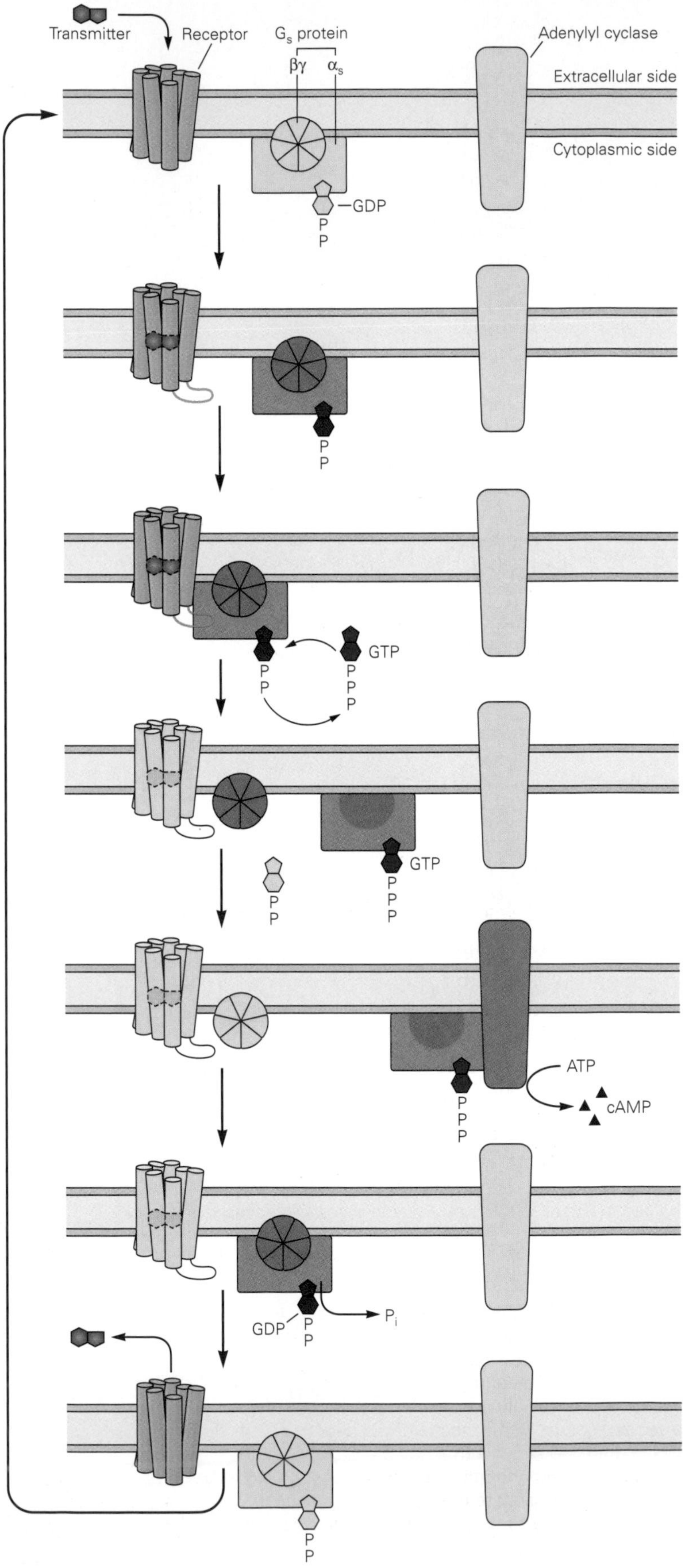

Transmitter binding alters conformation of receptor, exposing binding site for G_s protein.

Diffusion in the bilayer leads to association of transmitter receptor complex with G_s protein, thereby activating it for GTP-GDP exchange.

Displacement of GDP by GTP causes the α-subunit to dissociate from the G_s complex, exposing a binding site for adenylyl cyclase on the α-subunit.

The α-subunit binds to and activates the cyclase to produce many molecules of cAMP.

Hydrolysis of the GTP by the α-subunit returns the subunit to its original conformation, causing it to dissociate from the cyclase (which becomes inactive) and reassociate with the βγ complex.

The activation of the cyclase is repeated until the dissociation of transmitter returns the receptor to its original conformation.

of the bound GDP for guanosine triphosphate (GTP), leading to a conformational change that activates the G protein. In its activated state G_s stimulates the integral membrane protein adenylyl cyclase to catalyze the conversion of adenosine triphosphate (ATP) to cAMP. When associated with the cyclase, G_s also acts as a GTPase, hydrolyzing its bound GTP to GDP. When GTP is hydrolyzed, the G protein becomes inactive and dissociates from the cyclase, thereby stopping the synthesis of cAMP (Figure 11–2). Typically, a G_s protein remains active for a few seconds before its bound GTP is hydrolyzed.

Once a G protein-coupled receptor binds a ligand, it can interact sequentially with more than one G protein macromolecule. As a result, the sequential binding of relatively few molecules of transmitter to a small number of receptors can activate a large number of cyclase complexes. The signal is further amplified in the next step in the cAMP cascade, the activation of the protein kinase.

The major target of cAMP in most cells is the cAMP-dependent protein kinase (also called protein kinase A or PKA). This kinase, identified and characterized by Edward Krebs and colleagues, is a heterotetrameric enzyme consisting of a dimer of two regulatory (R) subunits and two catalytic (C) subunits. In the absence of cAMP the R subunits bind to and inhibit the C subunits. In the presence of cAMP each R subunit binds two molecules of cAMP, leading to a conformational change that causes the R and C subunits to dissociate (Figure 11–3). Dissociation frees the C subunits to transfer the γ-phosphoryl group of ATP to the hydroxyl groups of specific serine and threonine residues in substrate proteins.

Protein kinase A is distantly related through evolution to other serine and threonine protein kinases that we shall consider: the Ca^{2+}/calmodulin-dependent protein kinases and protein kinase C. These kinases also have regulatory and catalytic domains, but both domains are within the same polypeptide molecule (see Figure 11–6).

In addition to blocking enzymatic activity, the R subunits of PKA also target the C subunits to distinct sites within cells. Human PKA has two types of R subunits, each with two subtypes: $R_{I\alpha}$, $R_{I\beta}$, $R_{II\alpha}$, and $R_{II\beta}$. The genes for each are distinct but derive from a common ancestor. The two R subunits in a molecule of PKA are present as a dimer, formed when the R subunits are synthesized. Because the dimer never separates, hybrid types of the kinase do not exist in the cell. This is functionally important because the types have different properties. For example, type II PKA (containing R_{II}-type subunits) is targeted to the membrane by A kinase attachment proteins (AKAPs). One AKAP targets PKA to the *N*-methyl-D-aspartate (NMDA)-type glutamate receptor by binding both PKA and the postsynaptic density protein PSD-95, which binds to the cytoplasmic tail of the NMDA receptor (see Chapter 10). In addition, this AKAP also binds a protein phosphatase, which removes the phosphate group from substrate proteins (see Figure 11–14). By localizing PKA and other signaling components near their substrate, AKAPs form local signaling complexes that increase the specificity, speed, and efficiency of second-messenger cascades. Because AKAPs have only a weak affinity for R_I subunits, most type I PKA is free in the cytoplasm.

Kinases can only phosphorylate proteins on serine and threonine residues that are embedded within a context of specific *phosphorylation consensus sequences* of amino acids. For example, phosphorylation by PKA usually requires a sequence of two contiguous basic amino acids—either lysine or arginine—followed by any amino acid, and then by the serine or threonine residue that is phosphorylated (for example, Arg-Arg-Ala-Thr).

Several important protein substrates for PKA have been identified in neurons. These include voltage-gated and ligand-gated ion channels, synaptic vesicle proteins, enzymes involved in transmitter biosynthesis, and proteins that regulate gene transcription. As a result, the cAMP pathway has widespread effects on the electrophysiological and biochemical properties of neurons. We shall consider some of these actions later in this chapter.

Figure 11–2 The cAMP cycle. (Opposite) The binding of a transmitter to certain metabotropic receptors activates the stimulatory G protein (G_s). The G protein is a heterotrimer consisting of α-, β-, and γ-subunits. The β- and γ-subunits form a unit that binds tightly to the membrane. In its resting state the α-subunit of G_s, termed α_s, binds a molecule of guanosine diphosphate (GDP). When activated by its interaction with a ligand-bound receptor, the GDP bound to α_s is exchanged for guanosine triphosphate (GTP), causing α_s to functionally dissociate from the βγ complex. Next α_s associates with an intracellular domain of adenylyl cyclase, thereby activating the enzyme to produce cAMP from adenosine triphosphate (ATP). When bound to the cyclase, α_s is a GTPase. The hydrolysis of GTP to GDP and inorganic phosphate (P_i) leads to the dissociation of α_s from the cyclase and its reassociation with the βγ complex. The cyclase then stops producing the second messenger. At some point during this cycle the transmitter dissociates from the receptor. The system returns to an inactive state when the transmitter-binding site on the receptor is empty, the three subunits of the G protein reassociate, and the guanine nucleotide-binding site on the α-subunit is occupied by GDP. (Adapted, with permission, from Alberts et al. 1994.)

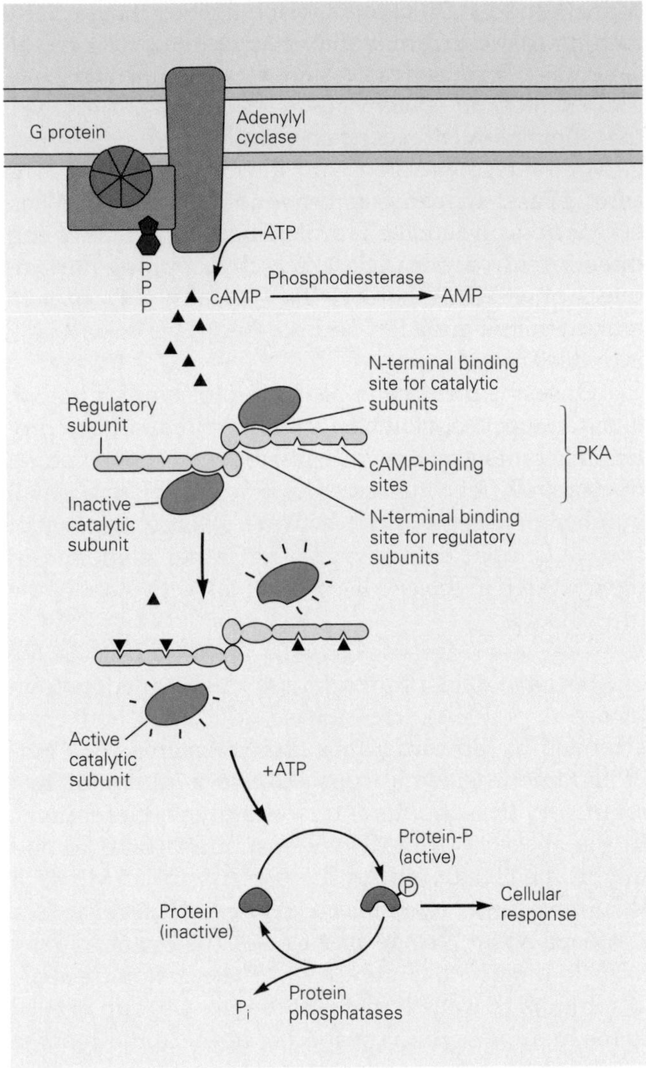

Figure 11–3 **The cAMP pathway activates protein kinase A.** Adenylyl cyclase converts adenosine triphosphate (ATP) into cAMP. Four cAMP molecules bind to the two regulatory subunits of the protein kinase A (PKA), liberating the two catalytic subunits, which are then free to phosphorylate specific substrate proteins on certain serine or threonine residues, thereby producing a cellular response. Two kinds of enzymes regulate this pathway. Phosphodiesterases convert cAMP to adenosine monophosphate (which is inactive), and protein phosphatases remove phosphate groups (P) from the substrate proteins, releasing inorganic phosphate, P_i (see also Figure 11–14).

The Second-Messenger Pathways Initiated by G Protein-Coupled Receptors Share a Common Molecular Logic

Approximately 800 of the roughly 23,000 genes thought to comprise the human genome code for G protein-coupled receptors. Although many of these are odorant receptors in olfactory neurons (see Chapter 32), many others are receptors for well-characterized neurotransmitters used throughout the nervous system. Despite their enormous diversity, all G protein-coupled receptors consist of a single polypeptide with seven characteristic membrane-spanning regions (serpentine receptors) (Figure 11–4).

The number of substances that act as second messengers in synaptic transmission is much fewer than the number of transmitters. Approximately 100 substances serve as transmitters; each can activate several types of receptors on the cell surface. The few second messengers that have been well characterized fall into two categories, intracellular and transcellular. Intracellular messengers are molecules whose actions are confined to the cell in which they are produced. Transcellular messengers are molecules that can readily cross the cell membrane and thus can leave the cell in which they are produced to act as intercellular signals, or first messengers, on neighboring cells.

A Family of G Proteins Activates Distinct Second-Messenger Pathways

The first G protein, G_s (where "s" stands for stimulatory), was identified more than 30 years ago by

Martin Rodbell, Al Gilman, and their colleagues. Since that time a large family of G proteins has been identified. The G proteins are associated with the inner leaflet of the plasma membrane, where they interact with G protein-coupled receptors.

The G proteins that couple receptor activation to intracellular effectors are trimers that consist of three subunits: α, β, and γ (Figure 11–2). The α-subunit is only loosely associated with the membrane and is usually the agent that couples the receptor to its primary effector enzyme. The β- and γ-subunits form a strongly bound complex that is more tightly associated with the membrane. As we shall learn later in this chapter, the βγ complex of G proteins can also regulate the activity of certain ion channels directly.

Approximately 20 types of α-subunits have been identified, 5 types of β-subunits, and 12 types of γ-subunits. G proteins with different α-subunits couple different classes of receptors and effectors, and therefore have different physiological actions. The β-adrenergic receptor activates adenylyl cyclase by acting on G_s proteins; these contain the α_s type of α-subunit. Some muscarinic ACh receptors inhibit the cyclase by acting on G_i proteins (where "i" stands for inhibitory); these contain the α_i type subunit. Still other G proteins ($G_{q/11}$ proteins, which contain α_q- or α_{11}-subunits) activate phospholipase C and probably other signal transduction mechanisms not yet identified. The G_o protein, which contains the α_o-subunit, is expressed at particularly high levels in the brain. Compared with other organs

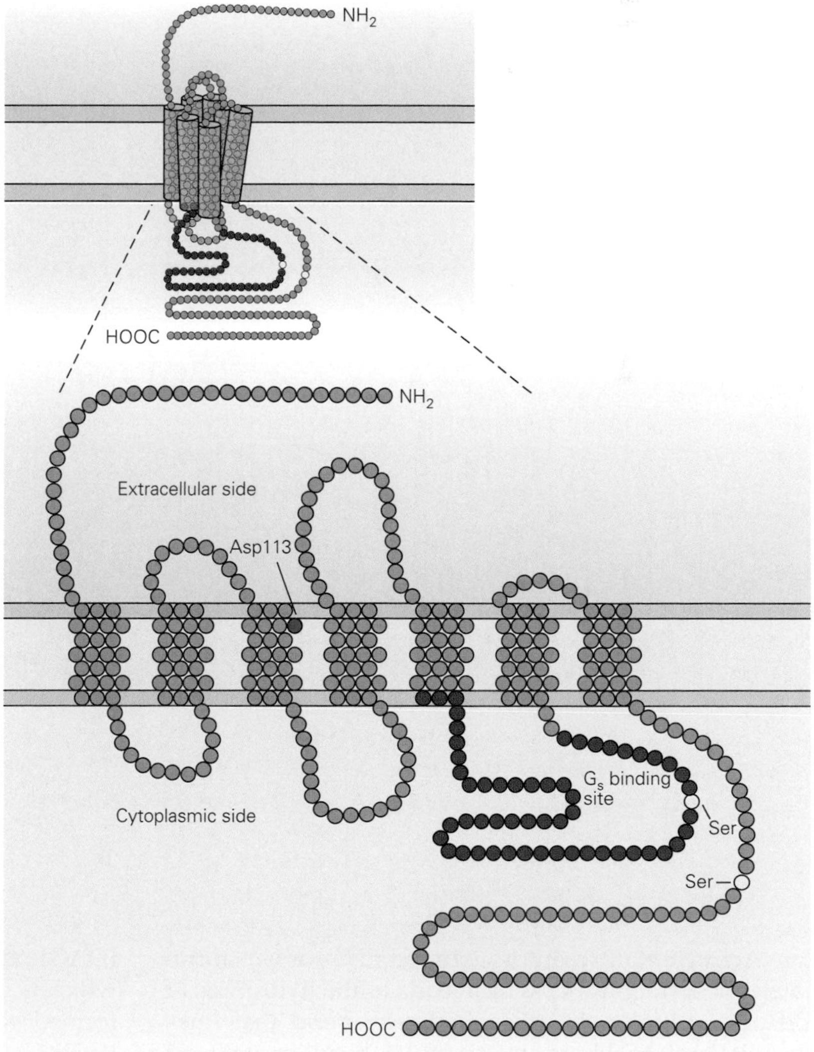

Figure 11–4 G protein-coupled receptors contain seven membrane-spanning domains. The β_2-adrenergic receptor shown here is representative of G protein-coupled receptors, including the β_1-adrenergic and muscarinic acetylcholine (ACh) receptors and rhodopsin. It consists of a single subunit with an extracellular amino terminus, intracellular carboxy terminus, and seven membrane-spanning α-helixes. The binding site for the neurotransmitter lies in a cleft in the receptor formed by the transmembrane helixes. The amino acid residue aspartic acid (Asp)-113 participates in binding. The part of the receptor indicated in **brown** associates with G protein α-subunits. Two serine (Ser) residues in the intracellular carboxy-terminal tail are sites for phosphorylation by specific receptor kinases, which helps inactivate the receptor. (Adapted, with permission, from Frielle et al. 1989.)

of the body, the brain contains an exceptionally large variety of G proteins. Even so, because of the limited number of classes of G proteins, one type of G protein can often be activated by different classes of receptors.

The known effector targets for G proteins are more limited than the types of G proteins. Important effectors include certain ion channels that are activated by the βγ complex, adenylyl cyclase in the cAMP pathway, phospholipase C in the diacylglycerol-inositol polyphosphate pathway, and phospholipase A_2 in the arachidonic acid pathway. Each of these effectors (except for the ion channels) initiates changes in specific target proteins within the cell, either by generating second messengers that bind to the target protein or by activating a protein kinase that phosphorylates it. Despite their differences, second-messenger pathways activated by G protein signaling share a common design (Figure 11–5).

Hydrolysis of Phospholipids by Phospholipase C Produces Two Important Second Messengers, IP_3 and Diacylglycerol

Many important second messengers are generated through the hydrolysis of phospholipids in the inner leaflet of the plasma membrane. This hydrolysis is catalyzed by three enzymes—phospholipase C, phospholipase D, and phospholipase A_2—named for the ester bonds they hydrolyze in the phospholipid. The phospholipases each can be activated by different G proteins coupled to different receptors.

The most commonly hydrolyzed phospholipid is phosphatidylinositol 4,5-bisphosphate (PIP_2), which typically contains the fatty acid stearate esterified to the glycerol backbone in the first position and the unsaturated fatty acid arachidonate in the second:

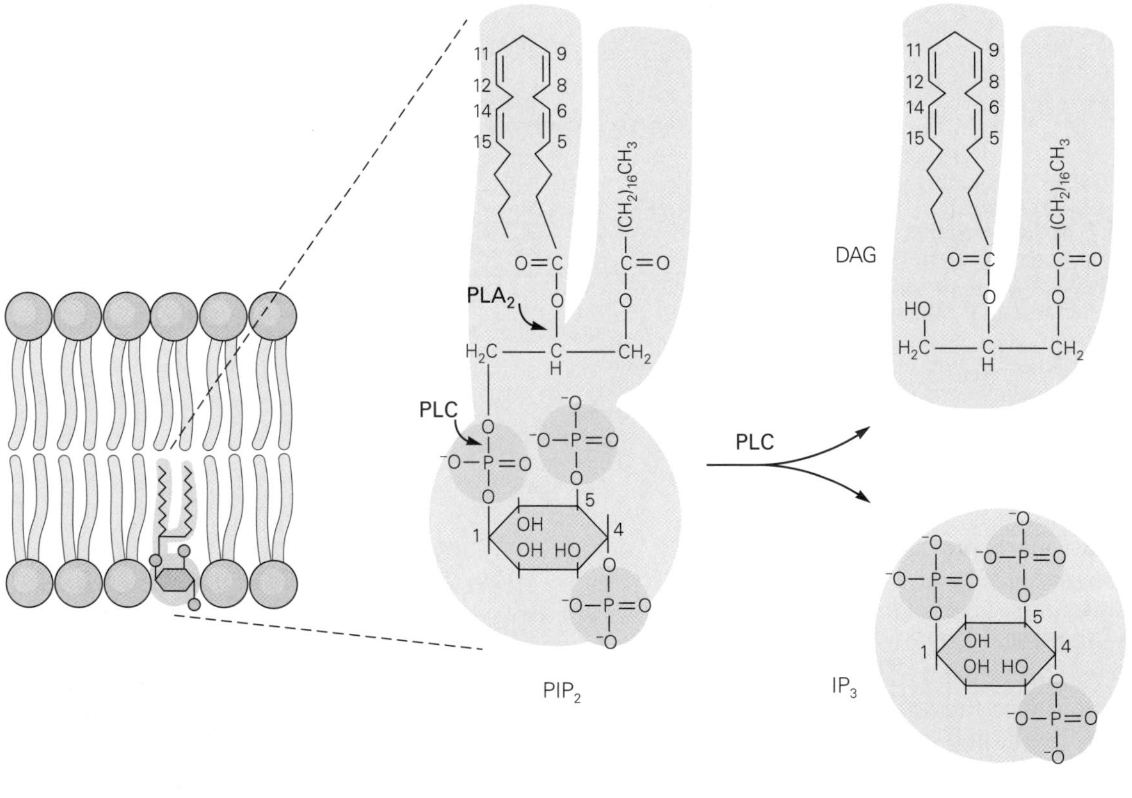

Activation of receptors coupled to G_q or G_{11} stimulates phospholipase C, which leads to the hydrolysis of PIP_2 (specifically the phosphodiester bond that links the glycerol backbone to the polar head group) and production of two second messengers, diacylglycerol (DAG) and inositol 1,4,5-trisphosphate (IP_3). DAG, which is hydrophobic, remains in the membrane when formed, where it recruits the cytoplasmic protein kinase C (PKC). PKC and DAG together with certain membrane phospholipids form an active complex that can

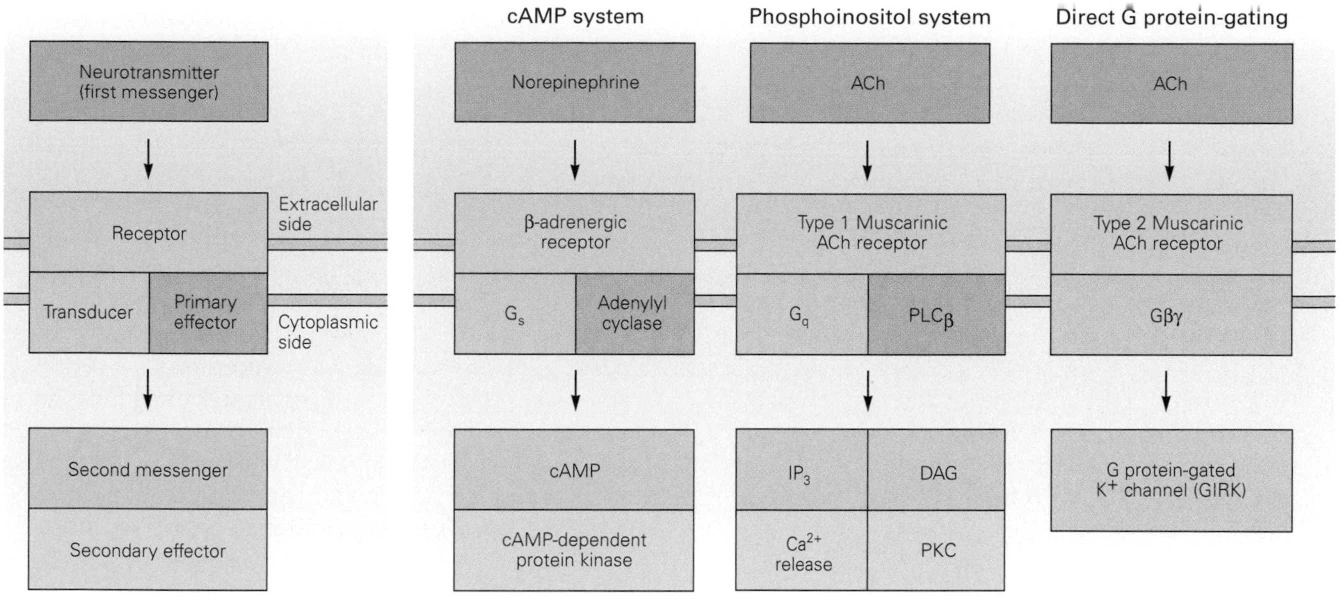

Figure 11–5 Synaptic second-messenger systems involving G protein coupling follow a common sequence. The signal transduction pathways illustrated here involve similar steps (**left**). Chemical transmitters arriving at receptor molecules in the plasma membrane activate a closely related family of G proteins (the transducers) that activate different enzymes or channels (the primary effectors). The activated enzymes produce a second messenger that activates a secondary effector or acts directly on a target (or regulatory) protein.

cAMP system. This pathway can be activated by a transmitter-bound β-adrenergic receptor, which acts through the G_s protein α_s-subunit to activate adenylyl cyclase. Adenylyl cyclase produces the second messenger cAMP, which activates PKA. The G protein here is termed G_s because it stimulates the cyclase. Some receptors activate a G_i protein that inhibits the cyclase.

Phosphoinositol system. This pathway, activated by a type 1 muscarinic acetylcholine (ACh) receptor, uses the G_q or G_{11} type of G protein (with α_q- or α_{11}-subunits, respectively) to activate a primary effector, phospholipase Cβ (PLC_β). This enzyme hydrolyzes the phospholipid, phosphatidylinositol 4,5-bisphosphate (PIP_2), yielding a pair of second messengers: diacylglycerol (DAG) and inositol 1,4,5-trisphosphate (IP_3). In turn, IP_3 releases Ca^{2+} from internal stores, whereas DAG activates protein kinase C (PKC). The drop in membrane PIP_2 levels can directly alter the activity of some ion channels.

Direct G protein-gating. This pathway represents the simplest synaptic mechanism for G protein-coupled receptor action. Acetylcholine (ACh) acting on type 2 muscarinic receptors activates the G_i protein, leading to functional dissociation of the α_i-subunit and βγ complex. The βγ complex interacts directly with a G protein-gated inward-rectifying K^+ channel (GIRK), leading to channel opening and membrane hyperpolarization.

phosphorylate many protein substrates in the cell, both membrane-associated and cytoplasmic (Figure 11–6A). Activation of some isoforms of PKC requires elevated levels of cytoplasmic Ca^{2+} in addition to DAG (Box 11–1).

The second product of the phospholipase C pathway, IP_3, stimulates the release of Ca^{2+} from intracellular membrane stores in the lumen of the smooth endoplasmic reticulum. The membrane of the reticulum contains a large integral membrane macromolecule, the IP_3 receptor, which forms both a receptor for IP_3 on its cytoplasmic surface and a Ca^{2+}-permeant channel that spans the membrane of the reticulum. When this macromolecule binds IP_3 the channel opens, releasing Ca^{2+} into the cytoplasm (Figure 11–6A).

The increase in intracellular Ca^{2+} triggers many biochemical reactions and opens calcium-gated channels in the plasma membrane. Calcium can also act as a second messenger to trigger the release of additional Ca^{2+} from internal stores by binding to another integral protein in the membrane of the smooth endoplasmic reticulum, the ryanodine receptor (so called because it binds the plant alkaloid ryanodine, which inhibits the receptor; in contrast, caffeine opens the ryanodine receptor). Like the IP_3 receptor to which it is distantly related, the ryanodine receptor forms a Ca^{2+}-permeant channel that spans the reticulum membrane; however, cytoplasmic Ca^{2+}, not IP_3, gates the ryanodine receptor-channel.

Calcium often acts by binding to the small cytoplasmic protein calmodulin. An important function of the calcium/calmodulin complex is to activate the Ca^{2+}/calmodulin-dependent protein kinase (CaM kinase). This enzyme is a complex of many similar subunits, each

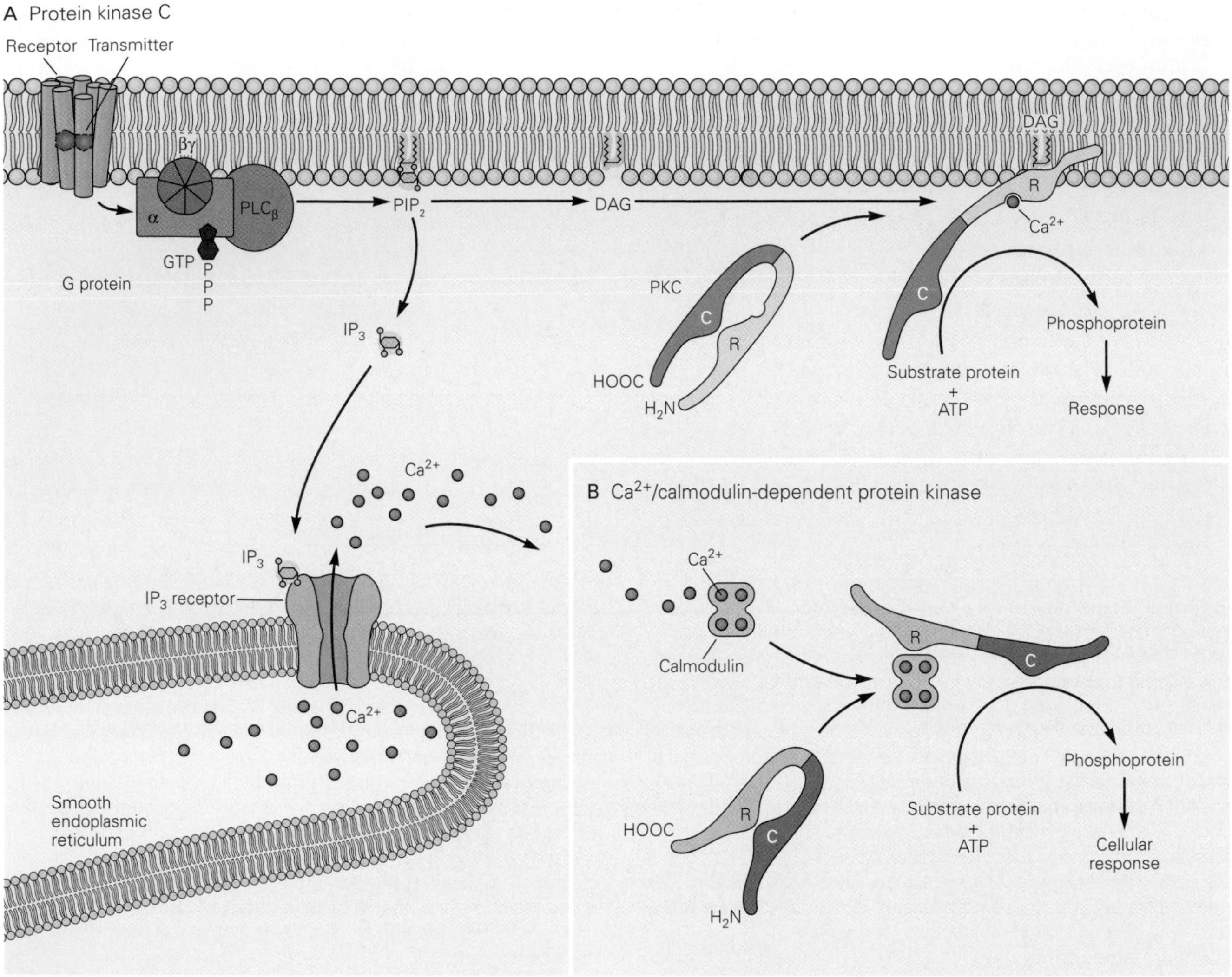

Figure 11–6 **Hydrolysis of phospholipids in the cell membrane activates three major second-messenger cascades.**

A. The binding of transmitter to a receptor activates a G protein that activates phospholipase Cβ (PLC_{β}). This enzyme cleaves phosphatidylinositol 4,5-bisphosphate (PIP_2) into the second messengers, inositol 1,4,5-trisphosphate (IP_3) and diacylglycerol (DAG). IP_3 is water-soluble and diffuses into the cytoplasm, where it binds to a receptor-channel on the smooth endoplasmic reticulum, the IP_3 receptor, to release Ca^{2+} from internal stores. DAG remains in the membrane, where it activates protein kinase C (PKC). Membrane phospholipid is also a necessary cofactor for PKC activation. Some isoforms of PKC also require Ca^{2+} for activation. PKC is composed of a single protein molecule that has both a regulatory domain that binds DAG and a catalytic domain that phosphorylates proteins on serine or threonine residues.

B. The Ca^{2+}/calmodulin-dependent protein kinase is activated when Ca^{2+} binds to calmodulin. The Ca^{2+}/calmodulin complex then binds to a regulatory domain of the kinase, causing its activation. The kinase is composed of many similar subunits (only one of which is shown here), each having both regulatory and catalytic functions. The catalytic domain phosphorylates proteins on serine or threonine residues. (**ATP**, adenosine triphosphate; **C**, catalytic subunit; **COOH**, carboxy terminus; **H_2N**, amino terminus; **R**, regulatory subunit.)

containing both regulatory and catalytic domains within the same polypeptide chain. When the Ca^{2+}/calmodulin complex is absent, the C-terminal regulatory domain of the kinase binds and inactivates the catalytic portion. Binding to the Ca^{2+}/calmodulin complex causes conformational changes of the kinase molecule that unfetter the catalytic domain for action (Figure 11–6B). Once activated, CaM kinase can phosphorylate itself through intramolecular reactions at many sites in the molecule. Autophosphorylation has an important functional effect:

It converts the enzyme into a form that is independent of Ca^{2+}/calmodulin and therefore persistently active even in the absence of Ca^{2+}.

Persistent activation of protein kinases is a general and important mechanism for maintaining biochemical processes underlying long-term changes in synaptic function associated with certain forms of memory. In addition to the persistent activation of Ca^{2+}/calmodulin-dependent protein kinase, PKA can also become persistently active following a transient increase in cAMP, because of the enzymatic degradation of its regulatory subunits through the ubiquitin pathway. The decline in regulatory subunit concentration results in the long-lasting presence of free catalytic subunits, even after cAMP levels have declined, leading to the continued phosphorylation of substrate proteins. PKC can also become persistently active through proteolytic cleavage of its regulatory and catalytic domains or expression of a PKC isoform that lacks a regulatory domain.

Hydrolysis of Phospholipids by Phospholipase A_2 Liberates Arachidonic Acid to Produce Other Second Messengers

Phospholipase A_2 hydrolyzes phospholipids distinct from PIP_2 by cleaving the fatty acyl bond between the 2′ position of the glycerol backbone and arachidonic acid. This releases arachidonic acid, which is then converted through enzymatic action to one of a family of active metabolites called *eicosanoids*, so called because of their 20 (Greek *eicosa*) carbon atoms.

Three types of enzymes metabolize arachidonic acid: (1) cyclooxygenases, which produce prostaglandins and thromboxanes; (2) several lipoxygenases, which produce a variety of metabolites to be discussed below; and (3) the cytochrome P450 complex, which oxidizes arachidonic acid itself as well as cyclooxygenase and lipoxygenase metabolites (Figure 11–7).

Arachidonic acid and its metabolites are soluble in lipids and thus readily diffuse through membranes. Therefore, in addition to acting within the cell in which they are produced, these substances can act on neighboring cells, including a presynaptic neuron. In this way they act as transcellular synaptic messengers (discussed in the next section).

Synthesis of prostaglandins and thromboxanes in the brain is dramatically increased by nonspecific stimulation such as electroconvulsive shock, trauma, or acute cerebral ischemia (localized absence of blood). Many of the actions of prostaglandins are mediated in the plasma membrane by a family of G protein-coupled receptors. The members of this receptor family can activate or inhibit adenylyl cyclase or activate phospholipase C.

Box 11–1 Isoforms of Protein Kinase C

At least nine isoforms of protein kinase C (PKC) have been found in nervous tissue. Rather than having regulatory and catalytic functions in different subunits, like PKA, most PKC isoforms contain regulatory and catalytic domains in a single continuous polypeptide chain (see Figure 11–6A).

Two functionally interesting differences have thus far been found among these isoforms. The so-called major forms (α, β_I, β_{II}, and γ) all have a calcium-binding site and are activated by Ca^{2+} ions together with diacylglycerol. The minor forms (eg, δ, ε, and ζ) lack the calcium-binding domain, and therefore their activity is independent of Ca^{2+}.

The second interesting difference is that, of the major forms, only PKCγ is activated by low concentrations of arachidonic acid, a membrane fatty acid, although all the isoforms respond to diacylglycerol or phorbol esters (plant toxins that bind to PKC and promote tumors).

With one exception, PKC isoforms also contain a site between the regulatory and catalytic domains that is sensitive to proteolysis. High levels of cytoplasmic Ca^{2+} can activate proteases that cleave PKC at this site, releasing a cytoplasmic form of PKC called protein kinase M (PKM). This protein fragment is constitutively active because it lacks the regulatory domain. As a result, elevations in Ca^{2+} can lead to prolonged activation of the kinase.

Long-lasting activation of PKC can also be produced through expression of the gene encoding PKCζ. This isoform is unique in that it lacks a regulatory domain and is therefore constitutively active. Expression of PKCζ produces persistent PKC activity in hippocampal neurons during the induction of long-term potentiation, which is thought to underlie certain forms of learning and memory in the hippocampus (see Chapter 67).

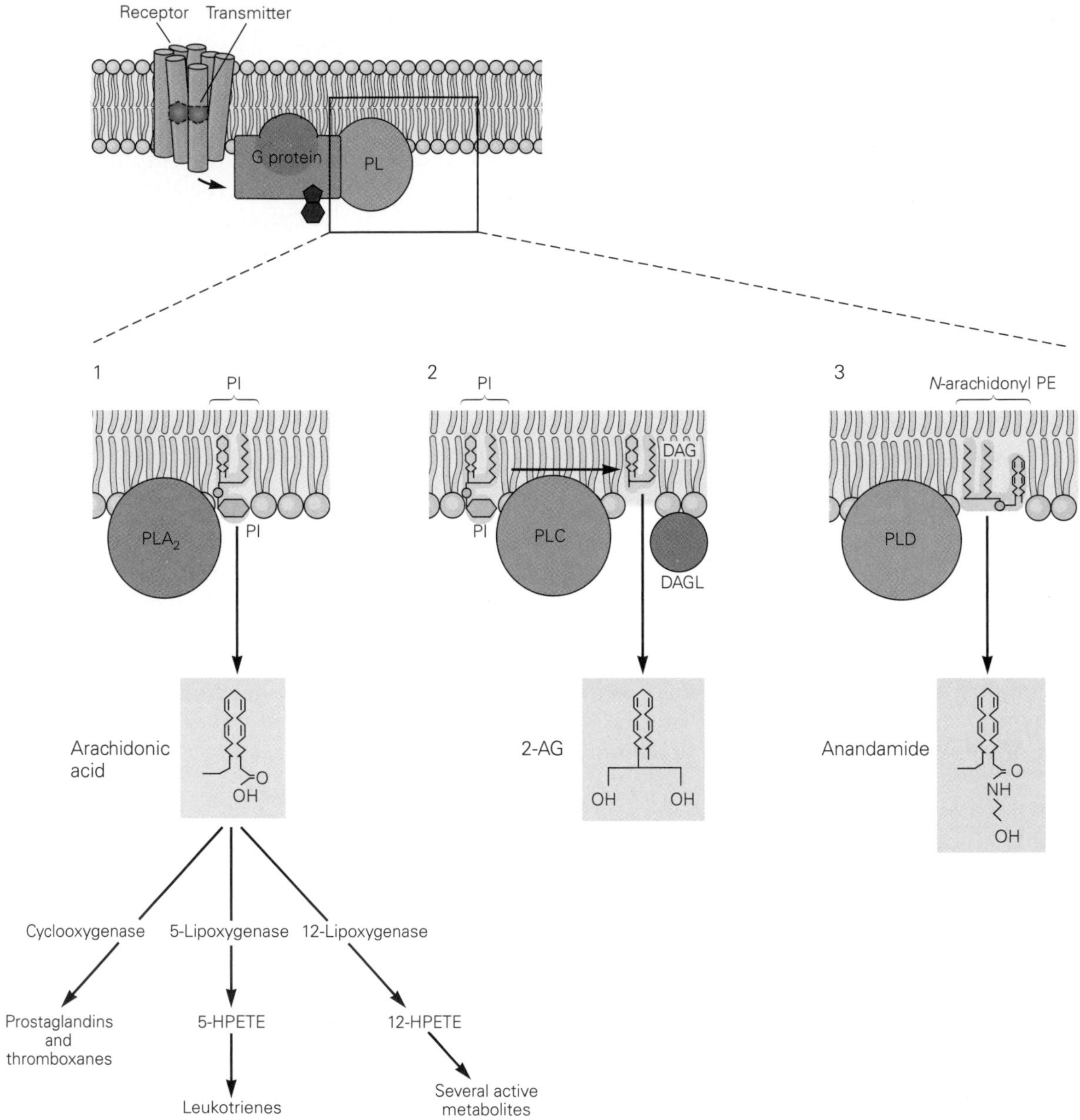

Figure 11–7 Three phospholipases generate distinct second messengers by hydrolysis of phospholipids containing arachidonic acid.

Pathway 1. Stimulation of G protein-coupled receptors leads to activation of phospholipase A_2 (PLA_2) by the free βγ subunit complex. Phospholipase A_2 hydrolyzes phosphatidylinositol (PI) in the plasma membrane, leading to the release of arachidonic acid, a 20-carbon fatty acid that is a component of many phospholipids. Once released, arachidonic acid is metabolized through several pathways, three of which are shown. The 12- and 5-lipoxygenase pathways both produce several active metabolites; the cyclooxygenase pathway produces prostaglandins and thromboxanes. Cyclooxygenase is inhibited by indomethacin, aspirin, and other nonsteroidal anti-inflammatory drugs. Arachidonic acid and many of its metabolites modulate the activity of certain ion channels.

Pathway 2. Other G proteins activate phospholipase C (PLC), which hydrolyzes PI in the membrane to generate DAG (see Figure 11–6). Hydrolysis of DAG by a second enzyme, diacylglycerol lipase (DAGL), leads to production of 2-arachidonylglycerol (2-AG), an endocannabinoid that is released from neuronal membranes and then activates G protein-coupled endocannabinoid receptors in the plasma membrane of other neighboring neurons.

Pathway 3. Elevation of intracellular Ca^{2+} activates phospholipase D (PLD), which hydrolyzes phospholipids that have an unusual polar head group containing arachidonic acid (*N*-arachidonylphosphatidylethanolamine [*N*-arachidonyl PE]). This action generates a second endocannabinoid termed anandamide (arachidonylethanolamide). (**HPETE**, hydroperoxyeicosatetraenoic acid.)

Lipoxygenases introduce an oxygen molecule into the arachidonic acid molecule, generating hydroperoxyeicosatetraenoic acids (HPETEs). These metabolites are synthesized in response to depolarization of brain slices with high concentrations of extracellular K^+, glutamate, or NMDA. The compounds 5-HPETE, 12-HPETE, and some of their downstream metabolites modulate certain ion channels. These metabolites may also be important in mediating pain sensation by activating transient receptor potential (TRP) ion channels in certain sensory neurons (see Chapter 5). They also can act as transcellular second messengers, a function that appears to be important for long-term synaptic changes in the hippocampus.

Transcellular Messengers Are Important for Regulating Presynaptic Function

Our understanding of the physiological importance of transcellular messengers is continuing to evolve. In addition to the lipoxygenase metabolites of arachidonic acid, two other important classes of transcellular messengers are the endocannabinoids and gases, both of which readily diffuse through the membrane into the extracellular space.

Endocannabinoids Are Derived from Arachidonic Acid

In the early 1990s researchers identified two types of G protein-coupled receptors, CB1 and CB2, which bind with high affinity the active compound in marijuana, Δ^9-tetrahydrocannabinol (THC). Both classes of receptors are coupled to G_i and G_o types of G proteins.

The CB1 receptors are the most abundant type of G protein-coupled receptor in the brain and are found predominantly on axons and presynaptic terminals in the central and peripheral nervous systems. Activation of these receptors inhibits release of several types of neurotransmitters, including the inhibitory neurotransmitter GABA and the excitatory transmitter glutamate. The CB2 receptors are found mainly on lymphocytes, where they modulate the immune response.

The identification of the cannabinoid receptors led to the purification of their endogenous ligands, the endocannabinoids. Two major endocannabinoids have been identified. Anandamide (Sanskrit *ananda*, bliss) consists of arachidonic acid coupled to ethanolamine (arachidonylethanolamide); 2-arachidonylglycerol (2-AG) consists of arachidonic acid esterified at the 2 position of glycerol. Both are produced by the enzymatic hydrolysis of phospholipids containing arachidonic acid, a process that is initiated either when certain G protein-coupled receptors are stimulated or the internal Ca^{2+} concentration is elevated (Figure 11–7). The two endocannabinoids bind to both CB1 and CB2 receptors.

Because the endocannabinoids are lipid metabolites that can diffuse through the membrane, they also can act as transcellular retrograde signals (Figure 11–8). Production of these metabolites is often stimulated in postsynaptic neurons by the increase in intracellular Ca^{2+} that results from postsynaptic excitation. Once produced, the endocannabinoids diffuse through the cell membrane to nearby presynaptic terminals, where they bind to CB1 receptors and inhibit transmitter release. In this manner the postsynaptic cell can control activity of the presynaptic neuron. There is now intense interest in understanding how the activation of these receptors in the brain leads to the various behavioral effects of marijuana.

The Gaseous Second Messengers, Nitric Oxide and Carbon Monoxide, Stimulate Cyclic GMP Synthesis

The two best studied gaseous transcellular messengers are nitric oxide (NO) and carbon monoxide (CO). Like other second messengers, NO and CO are not unique to neurons but operate in other cells of the body. For example, NO is a local hormone released from the endothelial cells of blood vessels, causing relaxation of the smooth muscle of vessel walls. Like the metabolites of arachidonic acid, NO and CO readily pass through cell membranes. They affect nearby cells without acting on a surface receptor, and they are extremely short-lived.

How do NO and CO produce their actions? Both gases stimulate the synthesis of guanosine 3′,5′-cyclic monophosphate (cyclic GMP or cGMP), which like cAMP is a cytoplasmic second messenger that activates a protein kinase. Specifically, NO and CO activate guanylyl cyclase, the enzyme that converts GTP to cGMP. There are two types of guanylyl cyclase. One is an integral membrane protein with an extracellular receptor domain and an intracellular catalytic domain that synthesizes cGMP. The other is cytoplasmic (soluble guanylyl cyclase) and is the isoform that is activated by NO.

Cyclic GMP has two major actions. It acts directly to open cyclic nucleotide-gated channels (important for phototransduction and olfactory signaling, as described in Chapters 26 and 32, respectively), and it activates the cGMP-dependent protein kinase (PKG). PKG differs from the cAMP-dependent protein kinase in that it is a single polypeptide with both regulatory (cGMP-binding) and catalytic domains, which are

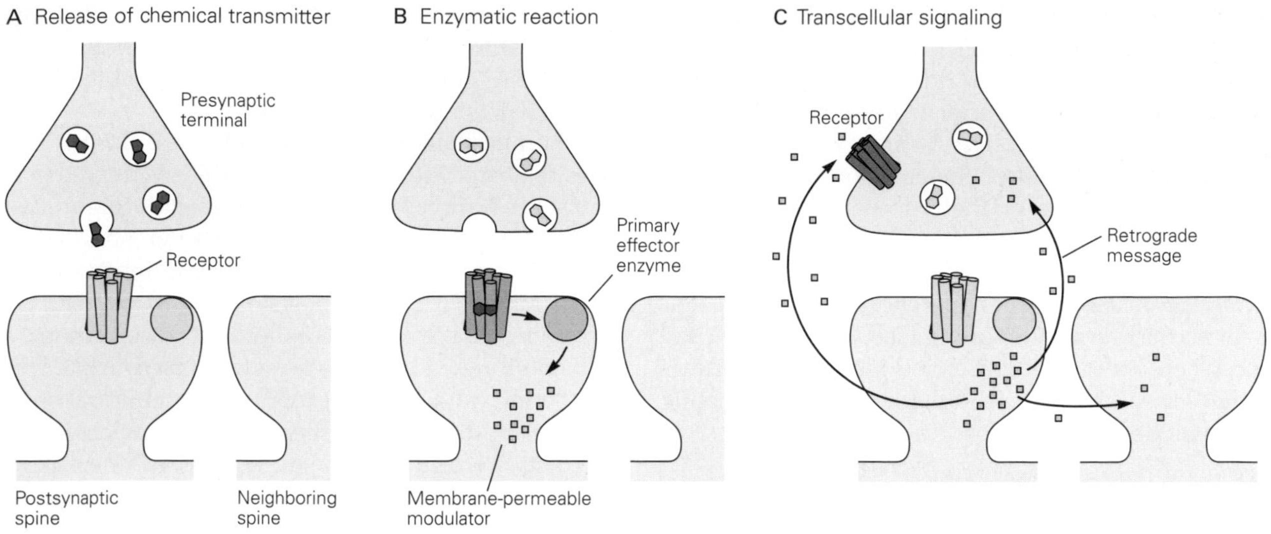

Figure 11–8 Transcellular signaling can occur from the postsynaptic neuron to the presynaptic neuron (retrograde transmission) and between postsynaptic cells. Until recently, synaptic signaling was thought to occur only from the presynaptic neuron to the postsynaptic cell. Transcellular signaling is initiated by a presynaptic signal. A presynaptic terminal releases a neurotransmitter at the synapse and that transmitter reacts with a G protein-coupled receptor in a postsynaptic dendritic spine (**A**). The receptor activates enzymes that produce a membrane-permeable modulator (**B**). The modulator is released from the postsynaptic spine and diffuses to neighboring postsynaptic spines as well as presynaptic terminals (**C**). There it can produce either first-messenger effects, by acting on G protein-coupled receptors in the surface membrane, or second-messenger-like effects, by entering the cell to act within. This kind of modulator of the presynaptic terminal is called a *retrograde messenger* rather than a second messenger, and its action is called *transcellular signaling*.

homologous to regulatory and catalytic domains in other protein kinases.

Cyclic GMP-dependent phosphorylation of proteins is prominent in Purkinje cells of the cerebellum, large neurons with copiously branching dendrites. There the cGMP cascade is activated by NO produced and released from the presynaptic terminals of granule cell axons (the parallel fibers) that make excitatory synapses onto the Purkinje cells. This increase in cGMP in the Purkinje neuron reduces the response of the AMPA receptors to glutamate, thereby depressing fast excitatory transmission at the parallel fiber synapse.

A Family of Receptor Tyrosine Kinases Mediates Some Metabotropic Receptor Effects

The receptor tyrosine kinases comprise the second major family of receptors that gate ion channels indirectly. These receptors are integral membrane proteins composed of a single subunit with an extracellular ligand-binding domain connected to a cytoplasmic region by a single transmembrane segment. The cytoplasmic region contains a protein kinase domain that phosphorylates both itself (autophosphorylation) and other proteins on tyrosine residues (Figure 11–9). This phosphorylation results in the activation of a large number of proteins, including other kinases that are capable of acting on ion channels.

The ligands for the receptor tyrosine kinases are peptide hormones, including epidermal growth factor (EGF), fibroblast growth factor (FGF), nerve growth factor (NGF), brain derived neurotrophic factor (BDNF), and insulin. Cells also contain important nonreceptor cytoplasmic tyrosine kinases, such as the protooncogene *src*. These nonreceptor tyrosine kinases are often activated by interactions with receptor tyrosine kinases and are important in regulating growth and development.

Many (but not all) of the receptor tyrosine kinases exist as monomers in the plasma membrane in the absence of ligand. Ligand binding causes one receptor subunit to associate with another to form a homodimer thereby activating the intracellular kinase. Each monomer phosphorylates its counterpart at a tyrosine residue, an action that enables the kinase to phosphorylate other proteins. Like the serine and threonine protein kinases, tyrosine kinases regulate the activity of neuronal proteins they phosphorylate, including the activity of certain ion channels. Tyrosine kinases also activate an isoform of phospholipase C, phospholipase Cγ, which like PLCβ, cleaves PIP_2 into IP_3 and diacylglycerol.

Receptor tyrosine kinases initiate cascades of reactions involving several adaptor proteins and other protein kinases that often lead to changes in gene transcription. The mitogen-activated protein kinases (MAPKs) are an important group of serine-threonine kinases that can be activated by a signaling cascade initiated by receptor tyrosine kinase stimulation. MAP kinases are activated by cascades of protein-kinase reactions (kinase kinases), each cascade specific to one of three types of MAP kinase: extracellular signal regulated kinase (ERK), p38 MAP kinase, and *c-Jun* N-terminal kinase (JNK).

MAP kinase signaling cascades are initiated when a specific adaptor protein binds to a phosphotyrosine residue on the cytoplasmic tail of an activated receptor tyrosine kinase. The binding is mediated by the SH2 domain of the adaptor protein, named for the domain's homology to a region of src. A second adaptor protein domain, SH3 (named for its homology to another region of src), binds to proline-rich regions of effector proteins, thereby coupling the activated receptor to the effector. The signaling complex ultimately binds to a small monomeric GTP-binding protein (MW 20,000–40,000), such as Ras or one of its relatives. Ras was first identified because it acts as a protooncogene. These small GTP-binding proteins are distantly related to the α-subunit of the heterotrimeric G proteins discussed earlier in this chapter.

Ras becomes active following the exchange of a bound molecule of GDP for GTP, similar to the activation

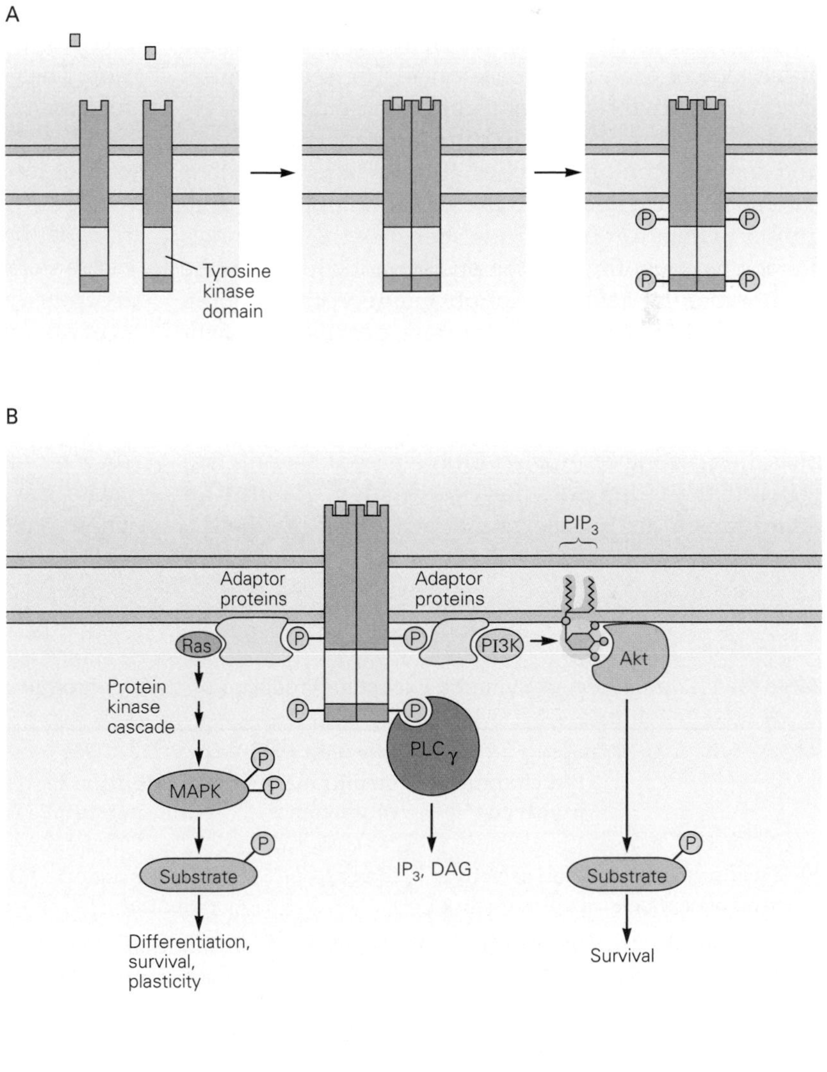

Figure 11–9 Receptor tyrosine kinases are a major class of metabotropic receptors.

A. Receptor tyrosine kinases are monomers in the absence of a ligand. The receptor contains a large extracellular binding domain that is connected by a single transmembrane segment to a large intracellular region that contains a catalytic tyrosine kinase domain. Ligand binding to the receptor often causes two receptor subunits to form dimers, enabling the enzyme to phosphorylate itself on various tyrosine residues on the cytoplasmic side of the membrane.

B. After the receptor is autophosphorylated, several downstream signaling cascades become activated through the binding of specific adaptor proteins to the receptor phosphotyrosine residues (P). The signaling cascade on the left illustrates the activation of mitogen-activated protein kinase (MAPK). A series of adaptor proteins recruits the small guanosine triphosphate (GTP)-binding protein Ras, which activates a protein kinase cascade, leading to the dual phosphorylation of MAP kinase on nearby threonine and tyrosine residues. The activated MAP kinase then phosphorylates substrate proteins on serine and threonine residues, including ion channels and transcription factors. Signaling pathways on the right illustrate the activation of the Akt protein kinase (also called PKB). Adaptor proteins first activate phosphoinositide 3-kinase (PI3K), which adds a phosphate group to PIP_2, yielding PIP_3, which then enables Akt activation. In yet another pathway, phospholipase Cγ becomes activated on binding to a different phosphotyrosine residue, providing a mechanism for producing inositol 1,4,5-trisphosphate (IP_3) and diacylglycerol (DAG) that does not rely on G proteins. (**PLCγ**, phospholipase Cγ.)

of trimeric G proteins. The activated Ras protein then initiates a cascade of reactions involving two upstream kinase kinases that lead to the phosphorylation and activation of MAP kinase. Activated MAP kinases have several important actions. They translocate to the nucleus where they turn on gene transcription by phosphorylating certain transcription factors. This action is thought to be important in stabilizing long-term memory formation. MAP kinases also phosphorylate cytoplasmic and membrane proteins to produce short-term modulatory actions (Figure 11–9).

The Physiological Actions of Ionotropic and Metabotropic Receptors Differ

Second-Messenger Cascades Can Increase or Decrease the Opening of Many Types of Ion Channels

The structural differences between metabotropic and ionotropic receptors are reflected in their functional effects (Table 11–1). Metabotropic receptor actions are much slower than ionotropic ones. The physiological action of the two classes of receptors also differs.

Ionotropic receptors regulate channels that function as simple on-off switches, those whose main job is either to excite a neuron to fire an action potential or to inhibit the neuron from firing. Because these channels are normally confined to the postsynaptic region of the membrane, the action of ionotropic receptors is local. Conversely, metabotropic receptors, because they activate diffusible second messengers, can act on channels some distance from the receptor. As a result, metabotropic receptors regulate a variety of channel types, including resting channels, voltage-gated channels that generate the action potential or provide Ca^{2+} influx for neurotransmitter release, and ligand-gated channels.

Finally, whereas transmitter binding always leads to an increase in the opening of ionotropic receptor-channels, the activation of metabotropic receptors can lead to either an increase or a decrease in channel opening. For example, MAP kinase phosphorylation of an inactivating (A-type) K^+ channel in the dendrites of hippocampal pyramidal neurons decreases the K^+ current magnitude, thereby enhancing dendritic action potential firing.

The slow synaptic actions of metabotropic receptors normally are insufficient to cause a cell to fire an action potential. But they can greatly influence electrophysiological properties of a neuron. By acting on resting and voltage-gated channels in the neuron's cell body and dendrites, metabotropic receptor actions can alter resting potential, input resistance, length and time constants, threshold potential, action potential duration, and repetitive firing characteristics. By acting on channels in axon terminals and the postsynaptic membrane, metabotropic receptors can also modulate, respectively, neurotransmitter release and the opening of ionotropic receptor-channels, thereby regulating synaptic transmission. These various actions of metabotropic receptors are referred to as *modulatory synaptic actions* (Figure 11–10).

The distinction between direct and indirect regulation of ion channels is nicely illustrated by cholinergic synaptic transmission in autonomic ganglia. Stimulation of the presynaptic nerve releases ACh from the nerve terminals. This directly opens nicotinic ACh receptor-channels, producing a fast EPSP in the postsynaptic neuron. The fast EPSP is followed by a slow EPSP that takes approximately 100 ms to develop but which then lasts for several seconds. The slow EPSP is produced by the activation of metabotropic muscarinic ACh receptors that close a delayed-rectifier K^+ channel called the muscarine-sensitive (or M-type) K^+ channel. These voltage-gated channels are partially activated

Table 11–1 Comparison of Synaptic Excitation Produced by the Opening and Closing of Ion Channels

	Ion channels involved	Effect on total membrane conductance	Contribution to action potential	Time course	Second messenger	Nature of synaptic action
EPSP caused by opening of channels	Non selective cation channel	Increase	Triggers action potential	Usually fast (milliseconds)	None	Mediating
EPSP caused by closing of channels	K^+ channel	Decrease	Modulates action potential	Slow (seconds or minutes)	Cyclic AMP (or other second messengers)	Modulating

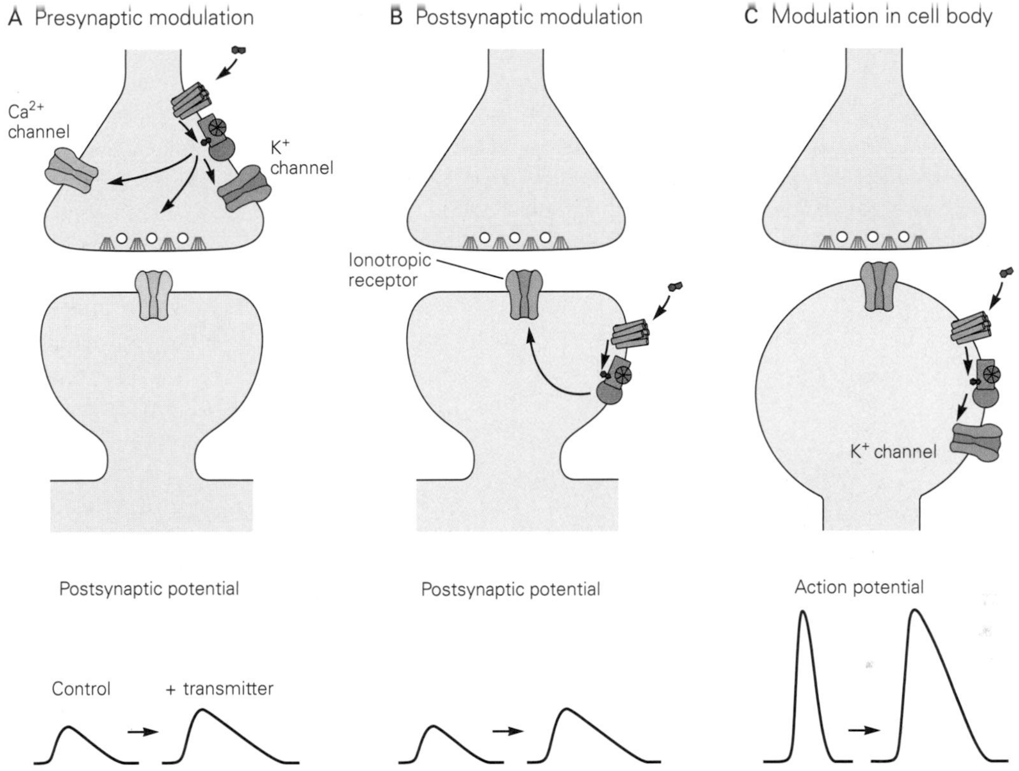

Figure 11–10 The modulatory actions of second messengers can occur at three cellular sites.

A. In the presynaptic neuron second messengers can modulate the activity of K^+ and Ca^{2+} channels, as well as the transmitter release machinery, to regulate the efficacy of transmitter release and thus the size of the fast postsynaptic potential mediated by ionotropic receptors.

B. In the postsynaptic neuron second messengers can alter directly the amplitude of postsynaptic potentials by modulating ionotropic receptors.

C. Second messengers can also affect the function of resting and voltage-gated channels in the soma and dendrites, thus altering a variety of electrical properties of the cell, including resting potential, input resistance, length and time constants, threshold, and action potential duration (as illustrated here).

when the cell is at rest, and the current through them helps determine the cell resting potential and input resistance (Figure 11–11).

The M-type K^+ channel is distinguished from other delayed-rectifier K^+ channels by its slow activation. It requires several hundred milliseconds to fully activate on depolarization. Closure of the M-type channels in response to muscarinic stimulation causes a decrease in K^+ efflux from the cell at the resting potential. As a result, K^+ efflux no longer balances the Na^+ influx through resting channels, and the net influx of Na^+ leads to membrane depolarization (Figure 11–11).

How far will the membrane depolarize? Membrane depolarization decreases the inward driving force on Na^+ and increases the outward driving force on K^+, such that the net inward current decreases. Thus the membrane will depolarize until the decrease in K^+ conductance (resulting from the closure of the M-type channels) is offset by the increase in the outward driving force on K^+ and the decrease in the inward driving force on Na^+ (as a result of the depolarization). At this new steady-state membrane potential the outward K^+ current and inward Na^+ current are again in balance.

Although the magnitude of the slow EPSP caused by closure of the M-type K^+ channels is relatively modest, the decrease in K^+ conductance profoundly increases action potential firing in response to a fast excitatory input. What are the special properties of the slow EPSP that produce this effect? First, the depolarization resulting from the reduction in resting K^+ conductance drives the membrane closer to threshold. Second, the increase in input resistance decreases the amount of excitatory current necessary to depolarize the cell by a given voltage. Third, the reduction in the

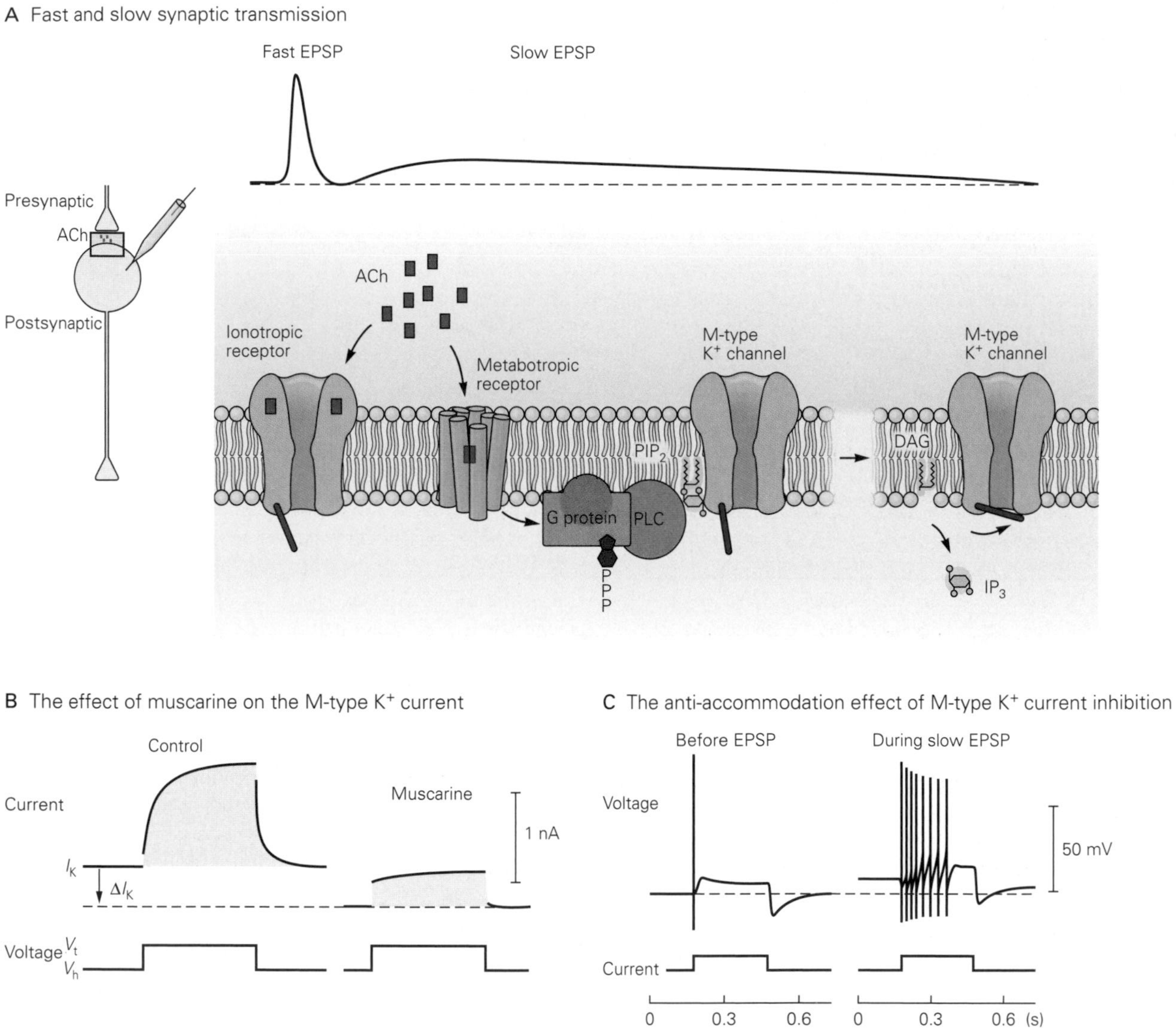

Figure 11–11 Fast ionotropic and slow metabotropic synaptic actions at autonomic ganglia.

A. The release of ACh onto a postsynaptic neuron in autonomic ganglia produces a fast excitatory postsynaptic potential (EPSP) followed by a slow EPSP. The fast EPSP is produced by activation of ionotropic nicotinic ACh receptors. The slow EPSP is produced by activation of metabotropic muscarinic ACh receptors. This receptor stimulates PLC to hydrolyze PIP_2, yielding IP_3 and DAG. The decrease in PIP_2 causes the closure of the M-type delayed-rectifier K^+ channel.

B. Voltage clamp recordings indicate that ACh decreases the magnitude of the current carried by the M-type K^+ channel. The depolarization of the membrane from a negative holding potential (V_h, typically –60 mV) to a more positive test potential (V_t, typically –30 mV) normally causes a slow increase in outward K^+ current (I_K) as the M-type K^+ channels activate (control). Application of muscarine, a plant alkaloid that selectively stimulates the muscarinic ACh receptor, decreases the outward K^+ current at the holding potential (note the shift in base line current, ΔI_K) by closing the M-type K^+ channels that are open at rest. The functional loss of M-type channels also decreases the magnitude of the slowly activated K^+ current in response to the step depolarization. (Adapted, with permission, from Adams et al. 1986.)

C. In the absence of muscarinic ACh receptor stimulation, the neuron fires only a single action potential in response to a prolonged depolarizing current stimulus, a process termed accommodation (**left**). This is because the slow activation of the M-type K^+ channel repolarizes the membrane below threshold. When the same current stimulus is applied during a slow EPSP, the neuron fires a more sustained train of action potentials (**right**) because the decrease in M-type current decreases the extent to which the membrane repolarizes during the stimulus. (Adapted, with permission, from Adams et al. 1986.)

delayed K^+ current enables the cell to produce a more sustained firing of action potentials in response to a prolonged depolarizing stimulus.

In the absence of ACh, a ganglionic neuron normally fires only one or two action potentials and then stops firing in response to prolonged excitatory stimulation that is just above threshold. This process, termed *accommodation*, results in part from the increase in M-type K^+ current in response to the prolonged depolarization, which helps repolarize the membrane below threshold. As a result, if the same prolonged stimulus is applied during a slow EPSP (when the M-type K^+ channels are closed), the neuron remains depolarized above threshold during the entire stimulus and thus fires a prolonged burst of impulses, a process termed *anti-accommodation* (Figure 11–11C). As this modulation by ACh illustrates, the M-type K^+ channels do more than help set the resting potential—they also control excitability.

A G protein mediates the modulation of the M-type channel by muscarinic receptor activation. However, until recently the target effector of the G protein remained a mystery. Although a number of lines of evidence implicated the PIP_2 hydrolysis pathway, neither PKC nor IP_3 seemed to play a role in regulating M-type channel opening. It is now known that PIP_2 is a necessary cofactor required for the proper function of many types of channels, including the M-type channels. As a result, stimulation of muscarinic ACh receptors that activate phospholipase C leads to closure of the M-type channels because of the decrease in PIP_2 levels in the membrane. Thus, M-type channels are regulated by the degradation of a substance rather than the synthesis of a chemical messenger. How PIP_2 binding enables proper functioning of the M-type channels remains unknown.

Although we do not know precisely the molecular mechanisms regulating M-type channels, we do have a more detailed understanding of how effectors in other types of modulatory actions regulate channel function. We shall first describe the simplest mechanism, the direct gating of ion channels by G proteins, and then consider a more complex mechanism dependent on protein phosphorylation by PKA.

G Proteins Can Modulate Ion Channels Directly

The simplest mechanism for activating an ion channel is direct gating of an ionotropic receptor-channel, as when ACh binds and opens the nicotinic ACh receptor-channel. The simplest mechanism for the indirect gating of a channel is when a metabotropic receptor releases a G protein subunit that directly interacts with the channel to modify its opening. This mechanism is used to gate two kinds of ion channels: the G protein-gated inward-rectifier K^+ channel (GIRK) and a voltage-dependent Ca^{2+} channel. With both kinds of channels, the G protein's βγ complex is the mediator (Figure 11–12A).

The GIRK channel, like other inward-rectifier channels, passes current more readily in the inward than the outward direction, although in physiological situations K^+ current is always outward. As we learned in Chapter 5, inward-rectifier channels resemble a truncated voltage-gated K^+ channel in having two transmembrane regions connected by a P-region loop that forms the selectivity filter in the channel (see Figure 5–12).

In the 1920s Otto Loewi described how the release of ACh in response to stimulation of the vagus nerve slows the heart rate (Figure 11–12B). We now know that the ACh activates muscarinic receptors to stimulate G protein activity, which directly opens the GIRK channel. For many years this transmitter action was puzzling because it has properties of both ionotropic and metabotropic receptor actions. The time course of activation of the K^+ current following release of ACh is slower (50 to 100 ms rise time) than that of ionotropic receptors (submillisecond rise time). However, the rate of K^+ channel activation is much faster than that of second-messenger-mediated actions that depend on protein phosphorylation (which can take many seconds to turn on). Although biochemical and electrophysiological studies clearly demonstrated that a G protein was required for this action, patch-clamp experiments showed that the G protein did not trigger production of a diffusible second messenger (Figure 11–12C). These findings were reconciled when it was found that activation of the muscarinic receptors releases the G protein's βγ-subunits, which directly open the K^+ channel.

Activation of GIRK channels hyperpolarizes the membrane in the direction of E_K (–80 mV). In certain classes of spontaneously active neurons the outward K^+ current through these channels acts predominantly to decrease the neuron's intrinsic firing rate, opposing the slow depolarization caused by excitatory pacemaker currents carried by the hyperpolarization-activated, cyclic nucleotide-regulated (HCN) channels (see Chapter 7). Because GIRK channels are activated by neurotransmitters, they provide a means for regulating the firing rate of excitable cells. These channels are regulated in a wide variety of neurons by a large number of transmitters and neuropeptides that act on different G protein-coupled receptors to activate either G_i or G_o, thereby releasing β_γ subunits.

Several G protein-coupled receptors also act to inhibit the opening of certain voltage-gated Ca^{2+} channels, again as a result of the direct binding to the channel of the βγ complex of G_i or G_o. Because Ca^{2+}

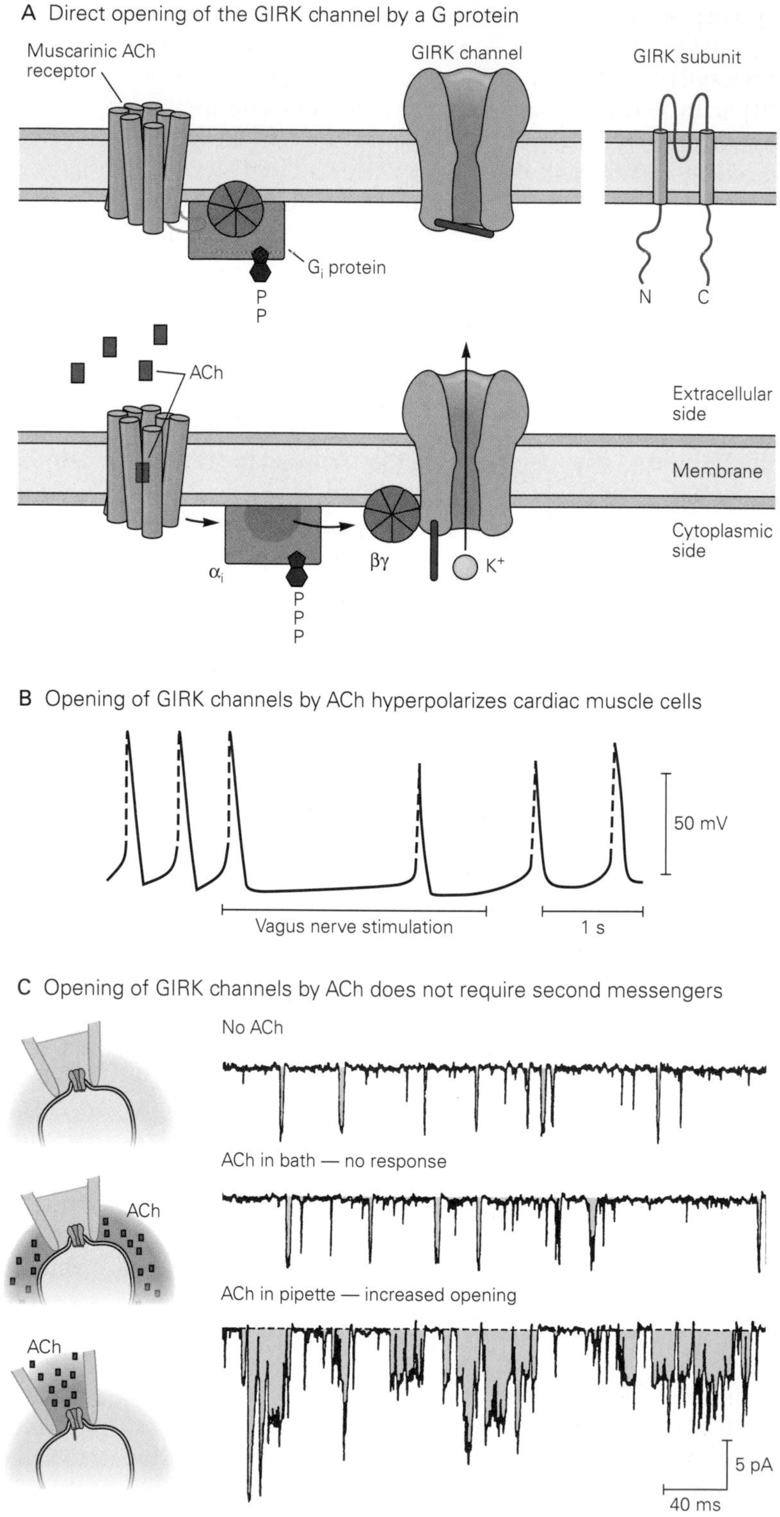

Figure 11–12 Some G proteins open ion channels directly without employing second messengers.

A. An inward-rectifying K$^+$ channel (GIRK) is opened directly by a G protein. Binding of ACh to a muscarinic receptor causes the dissociation of the G$_i$ protein $\alpha_i\beta\gamma$-complex; the free $\beta\gamma$-subunits bind to a cytoplasmic domain of the channel, causing the channel to open.

B. Stimulation of the parasympathetic vagus nerve releases ACh, which acts at muscarinic receptors to open GIRK channels in cardiac muscle cell membranes. The current through the GIRK channel hyperpolarizes the cells, thus helping to slow the heart rate. (Adapted, with permission, from Toda and West 1967.)

C. Three single-channel records show that opening of GIRK channels does not involve a freely diffusible second messenger. In this experiment the pipette contained a high concentration of K$^+$, which makes E_K less negative. As a result, when GIRK channels open, they generate brief pulses of inward (downward) current. In the absence of ACh, channels open briefly and infrequently (top record). Application of ACh in the bath (outside the pipette) does not increase channel opening in the patch of membrane under the pipette (middle record). The ACh must be in the pipette to activate the channel (bottom record). This is because the free $\beta\gamma$-subunits, released by the binding of ACh to its receptor, remain tethered to the membrane near the receptor and can only activate nearby channels. The subunits are not free to diffuse to the channels under the patch pipette. (Reproduced, with permission, from Soejima and Noma 1984.)

influx through voltage-gated Ca^{2+} channels normally has a depolarizing effect, the dual action of G protein βγ-subunits—Ca^{2+} channel inhibition and K^+ channel activation—strongly inhibits neuronal firing. As we will see in Chapter 12, inhibition of voltage-gated Ca^{2+} channels in presynaptic terminals through G protein βγ-subunits can suppress the release of neurotransmitter, a process termed *presynaptic inhibition*.

Cyclic AMP-Dependent Protein Phosphorylation Can Close Potassium Channels

In the marine mollusk *Aplysia*, stimulation of certain interneurons results in the release of the transmitter serotonin. This produces a slow EPSP in a group of mechanoreceptor sensory neurons. These sensory neurons initiate defensive withdrawal reflexes in response to tactile stimuli through fast, excitatory synapses with motor neurons. Serotonin sensitizes this reflex, enhancing the animal's response to a stimulus, resulting in a simple form of learning (see Chapter 66).

The modulatory action of serotonin depends on its binding to a G protein-coupled receptor that activates a G_s protein, which elevates cAMP and thus activates PKA. This leads to the direct phosphorylation and subsequent closure of the serotonin-sensitive (or S-type) K^+ channel that acts as a resting channel (Figure 11–13). Like the closing of the M-type K^+ channel with ACh, closure of the S-type K^+ channel decreases K^+ efflux from the cell, thereby depolarizing the cell and decreasing its resting membrane conductance.

The opening of the same S-type channels can be enhanced by the neuropeptide FMRFamide, acting through 12-lipoxygenase metabolites of arachidonic acid. This enhanced K^+ channel opening leads to a slow hyperpolarizing IPSP associated with an increase in resting membrane conductance. Thus a single channel can be regulated in opposing ways by distinct second-messenger pathways that produce opposing effects on neuronal excitability. A resting K^+ channel with two pore-forming domains in each subunit (TREK) in mammalian neurons is also dually regulated by PKA and arachidonic acid in a manner very similar to the dual regulation of the S-type channel in *Aplysia*.

Synaptic Actions Mediated by Phosphorylation Are Terminated by Phosphoprotein Phosphatases

Synaptic actions mediated by phosphorylation are terminated by phosphoprotein phosphatases, enzymes that remove phosphoryl groups from proteins, thereby generating inorganic phosphate. One class of phosphatases dephosphorylates proteins at serine or threonine residues and hence can reverse the actions of PKA, PKC, and Ca^{2+}/calmodulin kinase (Figure 11–14). A second class dephosphorylates proteins at tyrosine residues. Finally, a third group is specific for the pair of adjacent phosphorylated residues that mediate activation of MAP kinases.

Phosphatase activity can be regulated by different mechanisms. One of the major serine-threonine phosphatases in neurons, phosphatase-1, is under the control of a regulatory protein called inhibitor-1. Inhibitor-1 binds to and inhibits phosphatase-1 only after the inhibitor has itself been phosphorylated by PKA (Figure 11–14). An increase in cAMP therefore has two effects that enhance levels of protein phosphorylation: It increases the rate of phosphorylation by activating PKA and decreases the rate of dephosphorylation by inhibiting phosphatase-1.

Another serine-threonine phosphatase, calcineurin, is activated in response to an increase in the concentration of Ca^{2+} inside a cell. The Ca^{2+} binds to calmodulin and the Ca^{2+}/calmodulin complex then activates the phosphatase. One of the important functions of calcineurin is to dephosphorylate inhibitor-1. In neurons of the basal ganglia, Paul Greengard and colleagues showed that dopamine (acting through metabotropic D_1 receptors and cAMP production) activates PKA, which in turn phosphorylates inhibitor-1 (called DARPP-32 in these cells). The resulting inhibition of phosphatase-1 leads to an overall enhancement of phosphorylation in the neuron. However, if NMDA receptors are activated by release of glutamate, the resultant Ca^{2+} influx can stimulate calcineurin. This leads to the dephosphorylation of inhibitor-1, which relieves the inhibition of phosphatase-1, resulting in a decrease in overall levels of phosphorylation in the basal ganglion neurons. As we shall learn later in Chapter 67, a similar calcineurin cascade is thought to underlie a long-lasting depression of synaptic transmission in the hippocampus.

Second Messengers Can Endow Synaptic Transmission with Long-Lasting Consequences

So far we have described how synaptic second messengers alter the biochemistry of neurons for periods of time lasting seconds to minutes. Second messengers can also effect long-term changes lasting days to weeks as a result of alterations in a cell's expression of specific genes (Figure 11–15). Such changes in gene expression result from the ability of second-messenger cascades to control the activity of transcription factors, regulatory proteins that control mRNA synthesis.

The activity of some transcription factors can be directly regulated by phosphorylation. For example, a transcription factor termed the cAMP response element-binding protein (CREB) is activated when

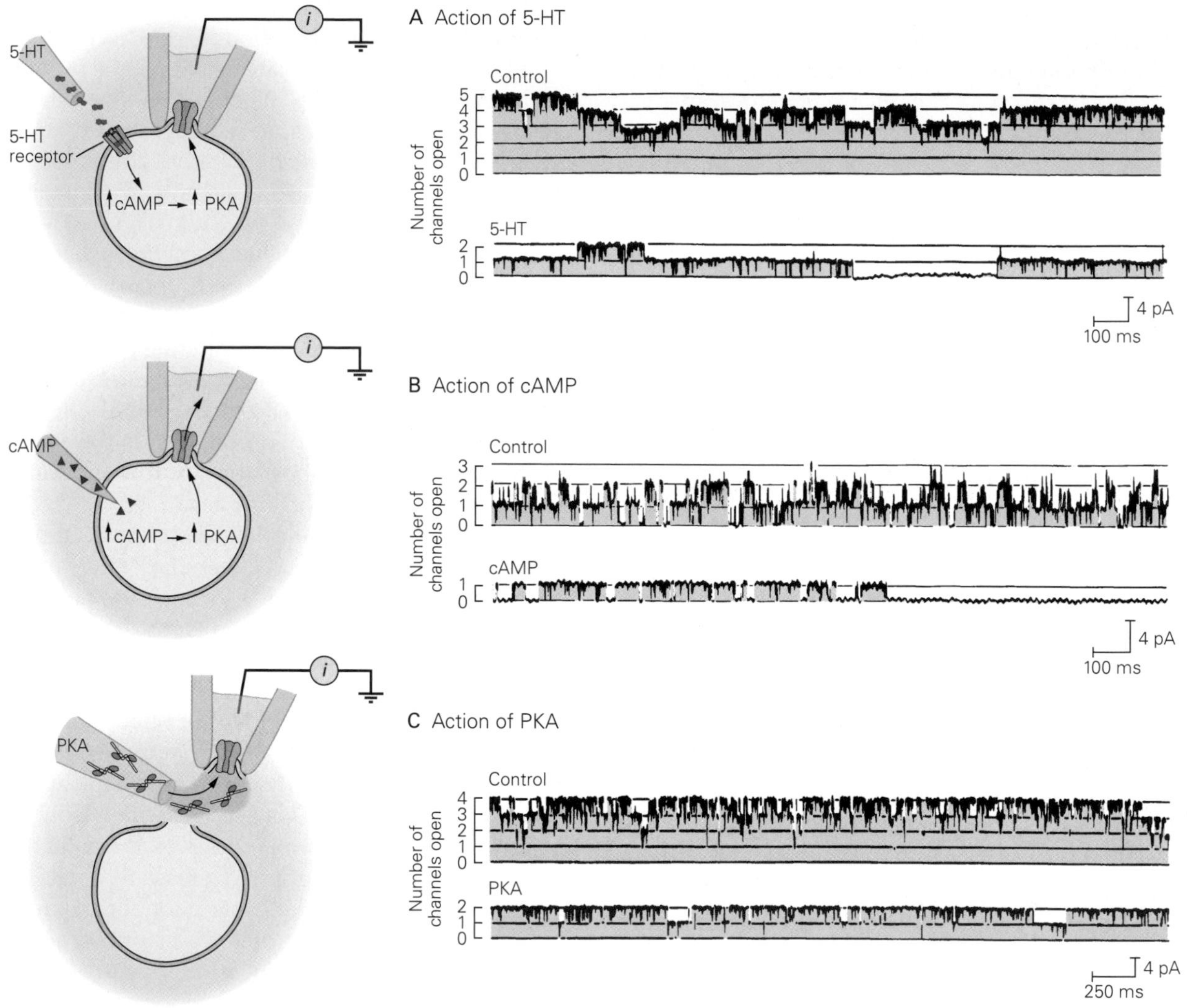

Figure 11–13 Serotonin closes a K$^+$ channel through the diffusible second-messenger cAMP. Serotonin (5-HT) produces a slow excitatory postsynaptic potential (EPSP) in *Aplysia* sensory neurons by closing the serotonin-sensitive or S-type K$^+$ channels. The 5-HT receptor is coupled to G_s, which stimulates adenylyl cyclase. The increase in cAMP activates cAMP-dependent protein kinase A (PKA), which phosphorylates the S-type channel, leading to its closure. Single-channel recordings illustrate the actions of 5-HT, cAMP, and PKA on the S-type channels.

A. Addition of 5-HT to the bath closes three of five S-type K$^+$ channels active in this cell-attached patch of membrane. The experiment implicates a diffusible messenger, as the 5-HT applied in the bath has no direct access to the S-type channels in the membrane under the pipette. Each channel opening contributes an outward (positive) current pulse. (Adapted, with permission, from Siegelbaum, Camardo, and Kandel 1982.)

B. Injection of cAMP into a sensory neuron through a microelectrode closes all three active S-type channels in this patch. The bottom trace shows the closure of the final active channel in the presence of cAMP. (Adapted, with permission, from Siegelbaum, Camardo, and Kandel 1982.)

C. Application of the purified catalytic subunit of PKA to the cytoplasmic surface of the membrane closes two out of four active S-type K$^+$ channels in this cell-free patch. ATP was added to the solution bathing the inside surface of the membrane to provide the source of phosphate for protein phosphorylation. (Adapted, with permission, from Shuster et al. 1985.)

phosphorylated by PKA, Ca^{2+}/calmodulin-dependent protein kinases, PKC, or MAP kinases. Once activated, CREB enhances transcription by binding a component of the transcription machinery, the CREB-binding protein (CBP). CBP activates transcription by recruiting RNA polymerase II and by functioning as a histone acetylase, adding acetyl groups to certain histone lysine residues. The acetylation weakens the binding between histones and DNA, which opens up the chromatin structure and enables specific genes to be transcribed. The changes in transcription and chromatin structure are important for regulating neuronal development, as well as for long-term learning and memory (see Chapters 66 and 67).

An Overall View

Signaling between neurons occurs when neurotransmitters bind to their postsynaptic receptors. Two distinct classes of receptors, ionotropic and metabotropic, differ widely in biochemical mechanism, duration of action, and physiological function.

Binding of transmitter to an ionotropic receptor directly opens an ion channel that is part of the receptor macromolecule. These ligand-gated receptor-channels produce the fastest and briefest type of synaptic action, lasting only a few milliseconds. This fast synaptic transmission mediates most motor actions and sensory processing.

Longer-lasting effects of transmitters are mediated by two major types of metabotropic receptors: G protein-coupled receptors and receptor tyrosine kinases. G protein-coupled receptors are proteins with seven transmembrane segments. They are members of a large gene superfamily and all act through G proteins, either to activate second-messenger cascades or directly alter ion channel activity. Prominent second messengers are cAMP and the products of hydrolysis of phospholipids: IP_3, diacylglycerol, and arachidonic acid.

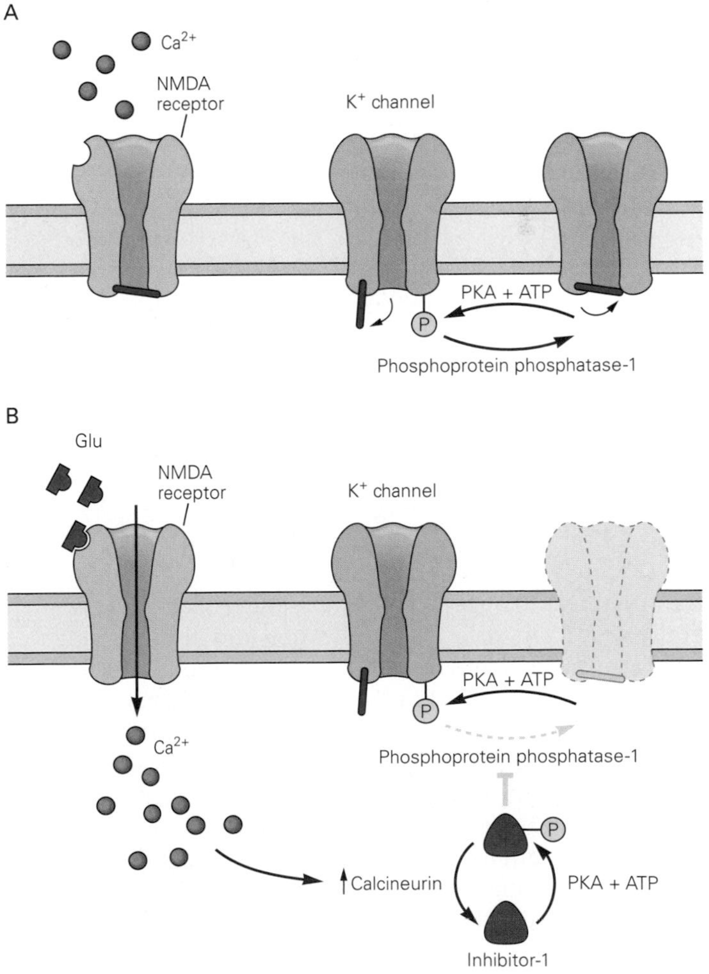

Figure 11–14 **Phosphoprotein phosphatases end the actions of protein kinases.**

A. The forward rate of phosphorylation of substrate proteins (here a K^+ channel) is controlled by protein kinases, the reverse rate by phosphoprotein phosphatases.

B. The extent and duration of phosphorylation can be controlled by regulation of phosphatase activity through a protein called inhibitor-1. When inhibitor-1 is phosphorylated by cAMP-dependent protein kinase (PKA), it binds to and blocks the activity of phosphoprotein phosphatase-1. The extent of phosphorylation of inhibitor-1 is controlled by another phosphatase, calcineurin, which is activated by the Ca^{2+}/calmodulin complex. In this manner Ca^{2+} entering the cell through the *N*-methyl-D-aspartate (NMDA)-type glutamate receptors activates calcineurin and triggers dephosphorylation of inhibitor-1. This in turn leads to the disinhibition of phosphoprotein phosphatase-1, which then dephosphorylates many substrates, including the K^+ channel. (**ATP**, adenosine triphosphate; **P**, phosphate; **Glu**, glutamate.) (Adapted, with permission, from Halpain, Girault, and Greengard 1990.)

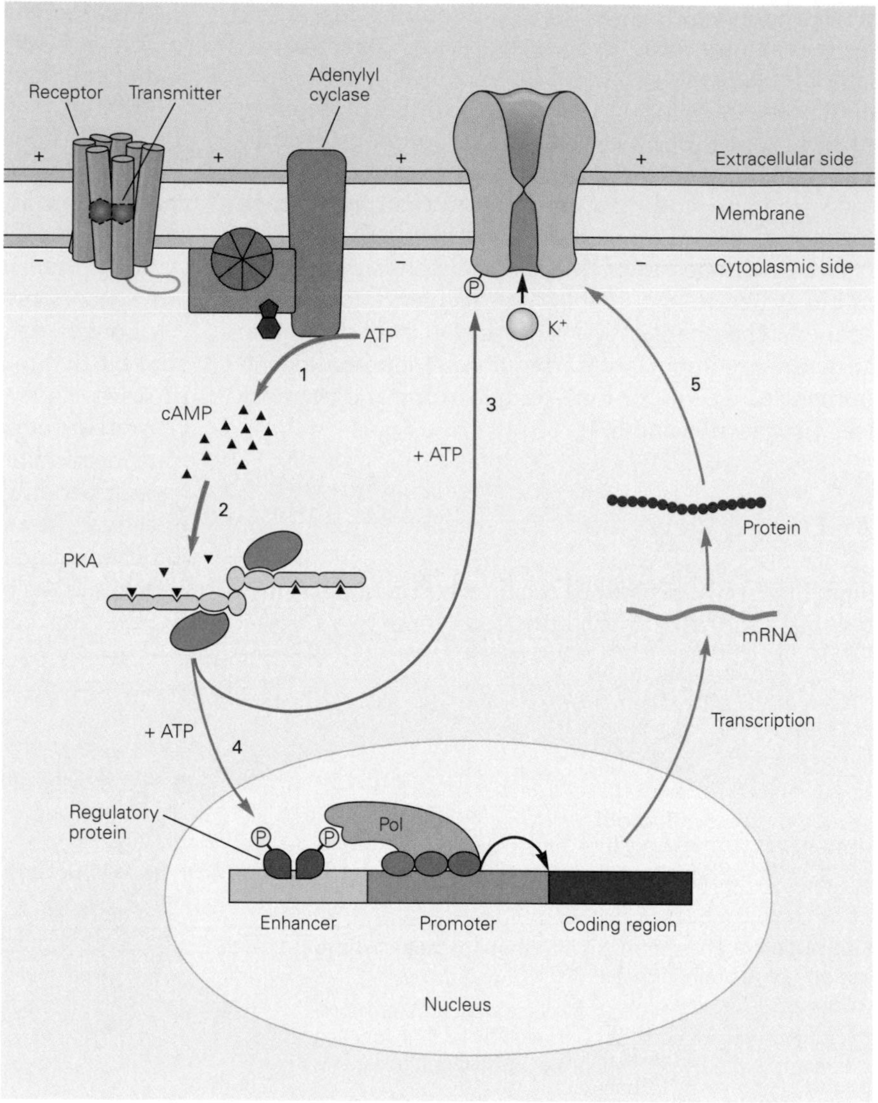

Figure 11–15 A single neurotransmitter can have either short-term or long-term effects on an ion channel. In this example a short exposure to transmitter activates the cAMP second-messenger system (**1**), which in turn activates PKA (**2**). The kinase phosphorylates a K^+ channel; this produces a synaptic potential that lasts for several minutes and modifies the excitability of the neuron (**3**). With sustained activation of the receptor, the kinase translocates to the nucleus, where it phosphorylates one or more transcription factors that turn on gene expression (**4**). As a result of the new protein synthesis, the synaptic actions are prolonged—closure of the channel and changes in neuronal excitability last days or longer (**5**). (**Pol**, polymerase.)

Many second-messenger actions involve phosphorylation of a variety of target proteins, including ion channels, thereby changing the functional state of the channels. These second-messenger actions generally last from seconds to minutes and thus do not mediate rapid behaviors. Rather they modulate the strength and efficacy of fast synaptic transmission—by modulating transmitter release or the responsiveness of ionotropic receptors to their ligand—or the electrical excitability of postsynaptic cells. Second-messenger actions not only open ion channels, as do the fast synaptic actions, but also close channels that are normally open in the absence of transmitter, thereby decreasing membrane conductance.

These modulatory actions are important in producing emotional states, mood, arousal, and simple forms of learning and memory. Many neurological and psychiatric disorders, including Parkinson disease, depression, anxiety, and schizophrenia, are thought to involve alterations in metabotropic receptor-dependent forms of synaptic transmission. Drugs that act to enhance or depress metabotropic receptor activation are important for treating these diseases.

The longest-lasting effects of neurotransmitters involve changes in gene expression, changes that can persist for days or longer. These more permanent actions are mediated by many of the same types of receptors and second-messenger pathways that operate in the shorter-term modulatory actions of transmitters. The long-term processes, however, may require repeated stimulation of the receptors and more prolonged action of the second messengers. As we shall see in Chapters 66 and 67, synaptically induced changes in gene expression are critical for long-term memory storage.

Steven A. Siegelbaum
David E. Clapham
James H. Schwartz

Selected Readings

Berridge MJ. 2009. Inositol trisphosphate and calcium signalling mechanisms. Biochim Biophys Acta 1793:933–940.

Brown DA, Passmore GM. 2009. Neural KCNQ (Kv7) channels. Br J Pharmacol 156:1185–1195.

Greengard P. 2001. The neurobiology of slow synaptic transmission. Science 294:1024–1030.

Hernandez CC, Zaika O, Tolstykh GP, Shapiro MS. 2008. Regulation of neural KCNQ channels: signalling pathways, structural motifs and functional implications. J Physiol 586:1811–1821.

Kano M, Ohno-Shosaku T, Hashimotodani Y, Uchigashima M, Watanabe M. 2009. Endocannabinoid-mediated control of synaptic transmission. Physiol Rev 89:309–380.

Levitan IB. 1999. Modulation of ion channels by protein phosphorylation. How the brain works. Adv Second Messenger Phosphoprotein Res 33:3–22.

Milligan G, Kostenis E. 2006. Heterotrimeric G-proteins: a short history. Br J Pharmacol 147 (Suppl 1):S46–55.

Nishizuka Y. 2003. Discovery and prospect of protein kinase C research: epilogue. J Biochem 133:155–158.

Schwartz JH. 2001. The many dimensions of cAMP signaling. Proc Natl Acad Sci U S A 98:13482–13484.

Suh BC, Hille B. 2008. PIP2 is a necessary cofactor for ion channel function: how and why? Annu Rev Biophys 37:175–195.

References

Adams PR, Jones SW, Pennefather P, Brown DA, Koch C, Lancaster B. 1986. Slow synaptic transmission in frog sympathetic ganglia. J Exp Biol 124:259–285.

Alberts B, Bray D, Lewis J, Raff M, Roberts K, Watson JD. 1994. *Molecular Biology of the Cell,* 3rd ed. New York: Garland.

Carnegie GK, Means CK, Scott JD. 2009. A-kinase anchoring proteins: from protein complexes to physiology and disease. IUBMB Life 61:394–406.

Chen Z, Gibson TB, Robinson F, Silvestro L, Pearson G, Xu B, Wright A, Vanderbilt C, Cobb MH. 2001 MAP kinases. Chem Rev 101:2449–2476.

Fantl WJ, Johnson DE, Williams LT. 1993. Signalling by receptor tyrosine kinases. Annu Rev Biochem 62:453–481.

Francis SH, Corbin JD. 1994. Structure and function of cyclic nucleotide-dependent protein kinases. Annu Rev Physiol 56:237–272.

Frielle T, Kobilka B, Dohlman H, Caron MG, Lefkowitz RJ. 1989. The β-adrenergic receptor and other receptors coupled to guanine nucleotide regulatory proteins. In: S Chien (ed). *Molecular Biology in Physiology,* pp. 79–91. New York: Raven.

Greenberg SM, Castellucci VF, Bayley H, Schwartz JH. 1987. A molecular mechanism for long-term sensitization in *Aplysia.* Nature 329:62–65.

Halpain S, Girault JA, Greengard P. 1990. Activation of NMDA receptors induces dephosphorylation of DARPP-32 in rat striatal slices. Nature 343:369–372.

Logothetis DE, Kurachi Y, Galper J, Neer EJ, Clapham DE. 1987. The βγ subunits of GTP-binding proteins activate the muscarinic K^+ channel in heart. Nature 325:321–326.

Murphy RC, Fitzpatrick FA (eds). 1990. Arachidonate related lipid mediators. Methods Enzymol 187:1–683.

Needleman P, Turk J, Jakschik BA, Morrison AR, Lefkowith JB. 1986. Arachidonic acid metabolism. Annu Rev Biochem 55:69–102.

Osten P, Valsamis L, Harris A, Sacktor TC. 1996. Protein synthesis-dependent formation of protein kinase Mzeta in long-term potentiation. J Neurosci 16:2444–2451.

Pfaffinger PJ, Martin JM, Hunter DD, Nathanson NM, Hille B. 1985. GTP-binding proteins couple cardiac muscarinic receptors to a K channel. Nature 317:536–538.

Piomelli D, Volterra A, Dale N, Siegelbaum SA, Kandel ER, Schwartz JH, Belardetti F. 1987. Lipoxygenase metabolites of arachidonic acid as second messengers for presynaptic inhibition of *Aplysia* sensory cells. Nature 328:38–43.

Shuster MJ, Camardo JS, Siegelbaum SA, Kandel ER. 1985. Cyclic AMP-dependent protein kinase closes the serotonin-sensitive K+ channels of Aplysia sensory neurones in cell-free membrane patches. Nature 313:392–395.

Siegel GJ, Agranoff BW, Albers RW, Molinoff PB (eds). 1994. *Basic Neurochemistry: Molecular, Cellular and Medical Aspects,* 7th ed. Amsterdam: Elsevier.

Siegelbaum SA, Camardo JS, Kandel ER. 1982. Serotonin and cyclic AMP close single K^+ channels in *Aplysia* sensory neurones. Nature 299:413–417.

Soejima M, Noma A. 1984. Mode of regulation of the ACh-sensitive K-channel by the muscarinic receptor in rabbit atrial cells. Pflugers Arch 400:424–431.

Takai Y, Sasaki T, Matozaki T. 2001. Small GTP-binding proteins. Physiol Rev 81:153–208.

Tedford HW, Zamponi GW. 2006. Direct G protein modulation of Cav2 calcium channels. Pharmacol Rev 58:837–862.

Toda N, West TC. 1967. Interactions of K, Na, and vagal stimulation in the S-A node of the rabbit. Am J Physiol 212:416–423.

Wayman GA, Lee YS, Tokumitsu H, Silva AJ, Soderling TR. 2008. Calmodulin-kinases: modulators of neuronal development and plasticity. Neuron 59:914–931.

12

Transmitter Release

Some of the brain's most remarkable abilities, such as learning and memory, are thought to emerge from the elementary properties of chemical synapses, where presynaptic terminals release chemical transmitters that activate receptors in the membrane of the postsynaptic cell. In the last three chapters we saw how postsynaptic receptors control ion channels that generate the postsynaptic potential. Here we consider how electrical and biochemical events in the presynaptic terminal lead to the secretion of neurotransmitters. In the next chapter we examine the chemistry of the neurotransmitters themselves.

Transmitter Release Is Regulated by Depolarization of the Presynaptic Terminal

What are the signals at the presynaptic terminal that lead to the release of transmitter? Bernard Katz and Ricardo Miledi first demonstrated the importance of depolarization of the presynaptic membrane through the firing of a presynaptic action potential. For this purpose they used the giant synapse of the squid, a synapse large enough to permit insertion of electrodes into both pre- and postsynaptic structures. Two electrodes are inserted into the presynaptic terminal—one for stimulating and one for recording—and one electrode is inserted into the postsynaptic cell for recording the excitatory postsynaptic potential (EPSP), which provides an index of transmitter release (Figure 12–1A).

When the presynaptic neuron is stimulated it fires an action potential, and after a brief delay an EPSP large enough to trigger an action potential is recorded in the

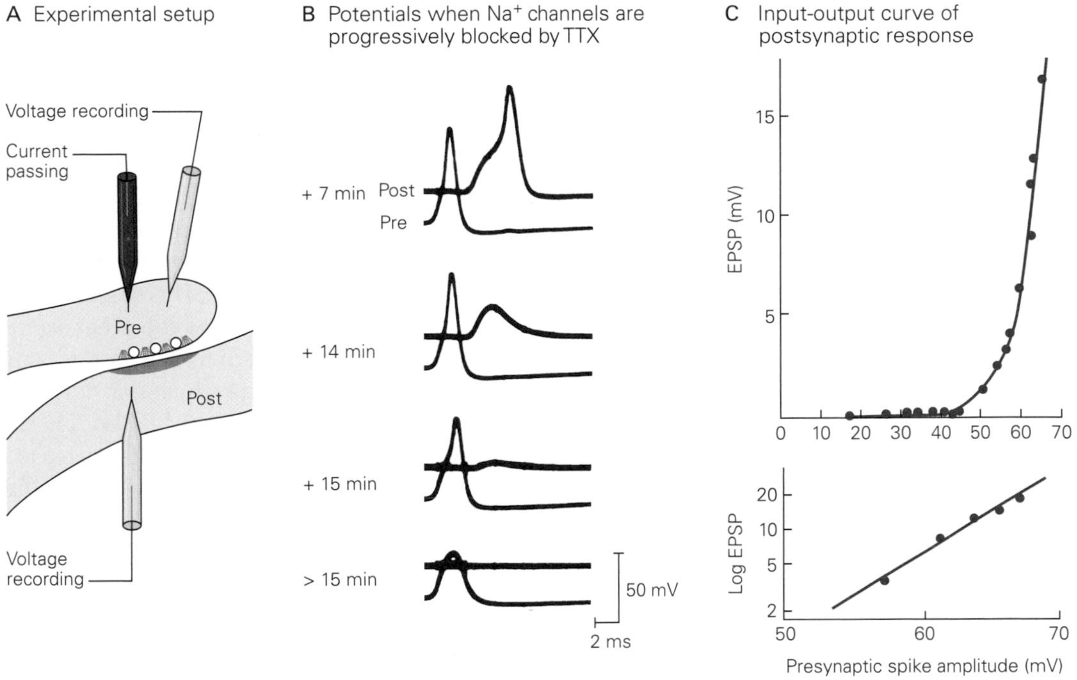

Figure 12–1 Transmitter release is triggered by changes in presynaptic membrane potential. (Adapted, with permission, from Katz and Miledi 1967a.)

A. Voltage recording electrodes are inserted in both the pre- and postsynaptic fibers of the giant synapse in the stellate ganglion of a squid. A current-passing electrode is also inserted presynaptically to elicit a presynaptic action potential.

B. Tetrodotoxin (TTX) is added to the solution bathing the cell to block the voltage-gated Na^+ channels that underlie the action potential. The amplitudes of both the presynaptic action potential and the excitatory postsynaptic potential (EPSP) gradually decrease as more and more Na^+ channels are blocked. After 7 min the presynaptic action potential can still produce a suprathreshold EPSP that triggers an action potential in the postsynaptic cell. After about 14 to 15 min the presynaptic spike gradually becomes smaller and produces smaller postsynaptic depolarizations. When the presynaptic spike is reduced to 40 mV or less, it fails to produce an EPSP. Thus the size of the presynaptic depolarization (here provided by the action potential) controls the magnitude of transmitter release.

C. An input–output curve for transmitter release is determined from the dependence of the amplitude of the EPSP on the amplitude of the presynaptic action potential. This relation is obtained by stimulating the presynaptic nerve during the onset of the blockade by TTX of the presynaptic Na^+ channels, when there is a progressive reduction in the amplitude of the presynaptic action potential and postsynaptic depolarization. The upper plot demonstrates that (1) a 40 mV presynaptic action potential is required to produce a postsynaptic potential. Beyond this threshold there is a steep increase in amplitude of the EPSP in response to small increases in the amplitude of the presynaptic potential and (2) the relationship between the presynaptic spike and the EPSP is logarithmic, as shown in the lower plot. A 10 mV increase in the presynaptic spike produces a 10-fold increase in the EPSP.

postsynaptic cell. Katz and Miledi then asked how the presynaptic action potential triggers transmitter release. They found that as voltage-gated Na^+ channels are blocked by application of tetrodotoxin, successive action potentials become progressively smaller. As the action potential is reduced in size, the EPSP decreases accordingly (Figure 12–1B). When the Na^+ channel blockade becomes so profound as to reduce the amplitude of the presynaptic spike below 40 mV (positive to the resting potential), the EPSP disappears altogether. Thus the amount of transmitter release (as measured by the size of the postsynaptic depolarization) is a steep function of the amount of presynaptic depolarization (Figure 12–1C).

Katz and Miledi next investigated how presynaptic depolarization triggers transmitter release. The action potential is produced by an influx of Na^+ and an efflux of K^+ through voltage-gated channels. To determine whether Na^+ influx or K^+ efflux is required to trigger transmitter release, Katz and Miledi first blocked the Na^+ channels with tetrodotoxin. They then asked whether direct depolarization of the presynaptic membrane, by current injection, would still trigger transmitter release. Indeed, depolarization of the presynaptic membrane beyond a threshold of about 40 mV positive to the resting potential elicits an EPSP in the postsynaptic cell. Beyond that threshold, progressively greater depolarization leads to progressively greater amounts of transmitter release. This result shows that during a normal action potential presynaptic Na^+ influx is not necessary for release. Rather Na^+ influx is important only insofar as it depolarizes the membrane enough for transmitter release to occur (Figure 12–2B).

To examine the contribution of K^+ efflux to transmitter release, Katz and Miledi blocked the voltage-gated K^+ channels with tetraethylammonium at the same time they blocked the voltage-sensitive Na^+ channels with tetrodotoxin. They then injected a depolarizing current into the presynaptic terminals and found that the EPSPs were of normal size, indicating that normal transmitter release occurred (Figure 12–2C). Thus neither Na^+ nor K^+ flux is required for transmitter release.

In the presence of tetraethylammonium the current pulse elicits a maintained presynaptic depolarization because the K^+ current that normally repolarizes the presynaptic membrane is blocked. As a result, transmitter release is sustained throughout the current pulse as reflected in the prolonged depolarization of the postsynaptic cell. The sustained depolarization increased the accuracy of the measurements and permitted Katz and Miledi to determine a complete input–output curve relating presynaptic depolarization to transmitter release (Figure 12–2D). They confirmed the steep dependence of transmitter release on presynaptic depolarization. In the range of depolarization over which transmitter release increases (40–70 mV positive

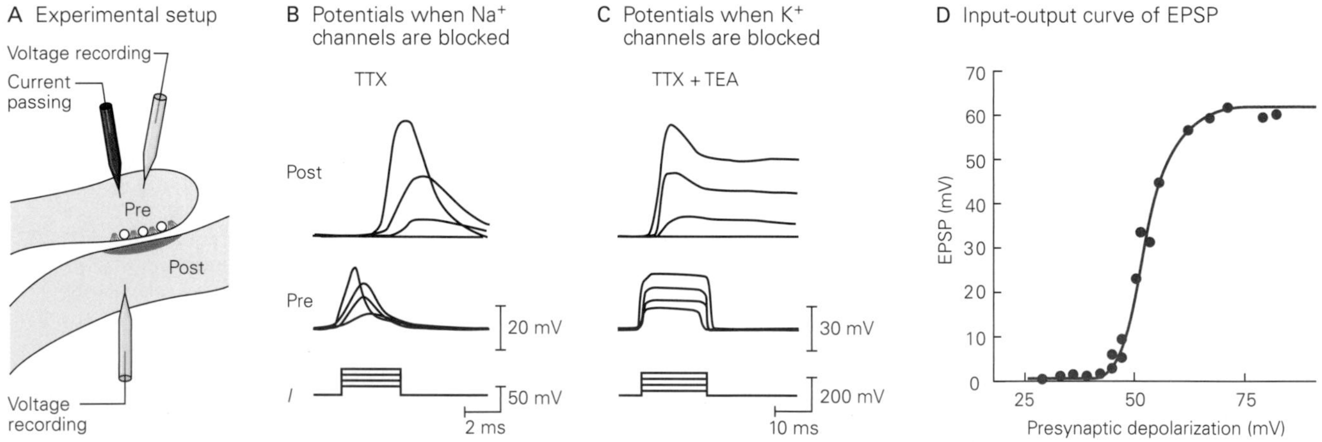

Figure 12–2 Transmitter release is not directly triggered by the opening of presynaptic voltage-gated Na^+ or K^+ channels. (Adapted, with permission, from Katz and Miledi 1967a.)

A. Voltage recording electrodes are inserted in both the pre- and postsynaptic fibers of the giant synapse in the stellate ganglion of a squid. A current-passing electrode has also been inserted into the presynaptic cell.

B. Depolarizing the presynaptic terminal with direct current injection through a microelectrode can trigger transmitter release even after the voltage-gated Na^+ channels are completely blocked by adding tetrodotoxin (TTX) to the cell-bathing solution. Three sets of traces represent (from bottom to top) the depolarizing current pulse injected into the presynaptic terminal (*I*), the resulting potential in the presynaptic terminal (**Pre**), and the EPSP generated by the release of transmitter onto the postsynaptic cell (**Post**). Progressively stronger current pulses in the presynaptic cell produce correspondingly greater depolarizations of the presynaptic terminal. The greater the presynaptic depolarization, the larger the EPSP. The presynaptic depolarizations are not maintained throughout the duration of the depolarizing current pulse because delayed activation of the voltage-gated K^+ channels causes repolarization.

C. Transmitter release occurs even after the voltage-gated Na^+ channels have been blocked with TTX *and* the voltage-gated K^+ channels have been blocked with tetraethylammonium (TEA). In this experiment TEA was injected into the presynaptic terminal. The three sets of traces represent the same measurements as in part B. Because the presynaptic K^+ channels are blocked, the presynaptic depolarization is maintained throughout the current pulse. The large sustained presynaptic depolarization produces large sustained EPSPs.

D. Blocking both the Na^+ and K^+ channels permits accurate control of presynaptic voltage and the determination of a complete input–output curve. Beyond a certain threshold (40 mV positive to the resting potential) there is a steep relationship between presynaptic depolarization and transmitter release, as measured from the size of the EPSP. Depolarizations greater than a certain level do not cause any additional release of transmitter. The initial presynaptic resting membrane potential was approximately –70 mV.

to the resting level) a 10 mV increase in depolarization produces a 10-fold increase in transmitter release. Depolarization of the presynaptic membrane above an upper limit produces no further increase in the postsynaptic potential.

Release Is Triggered by Calcium Influx

Katz and Miledi next turned their attention to Ca^{2+} ions. Earlier, Katz and José del Castillo had found that increasing the extracellular Ca^{2+} concentration enhanced transmitter release, whereas lowering the concentration reduced and ultimately blocked synaptic transmission. Because transmitter release is an intracellular process, these findings implied that Ca^{2+} must enter the cell to influence transmitter release.

Previous work on the squid giant axon membrane had identified a class of voltage-gated Ca^{2+} channels, the opening of which results in a large Ca^{2+} influx because of the large inward electrochemical driving force on Ca^{2+}. The extracellular Ca^{2+} concentration, approximately 2 mM in vertebrates, is normally four orders of magnitude greater than the intracellular concentration, approximately 10^{-7} M at rest. However, because these Ca^{2+} channels are sparsely distributed along the axon they cannot, by themselves, provide enough current to produce a regenerative action potential.

Katz and Miledi found that the Ca^{2+} channels were much more abundant at the presynaptic terminal. There, in the presence of tetraethylammonium and tetrodotoxin, a depolarizing current pulse was sometimes able to trigger a regenerative depolarization that required extracellular calcium, a *calcium spike*. Katz and Miledi therefore proposed that Ca^{2+} serves dual functions. It is a carrier of depolarizing charge during the action potential (like Na^+), and it is a special chemical signal—a second messenger—conveying information about changes in membrane potential to the intracellular machinery responsible for transmitter release. Calcium ions are able to serve as an efficient chemical signal because of their low resting concentration, approximately 10^5 fold lower than the resting concentration of Na^+. As a result, the small amounts of ions that enter or leave a cell during an action potential can lead to large percentage changes in intracellular Ca^{2+} that can trigger various biochemical reactions. Proof of the importance of Ca^{2+} channels in release has come from more recent experiments showing that specific toxins that block Ca^{2+} channels also block release.

The properties of the voltage-gated Ca^{2+} channels at the squid presynaptic terminal were measured by Rodolfo Llinás and his colleagues. Using a voltage clamp, Llinás depolarized the terminal while blocking the voltage-gated Na^+ channels with tetrodotoxin and the K^+ channels with tetraethylammonium. He found that graded depolarizations activated a graded inward Ca^{2+} current, which in turn resulted in graded release of transmitter (Figure 12–3). The Ca^{2+} current is graded because the Ca^{2+} channels are voltage-dependent like the voltage-gated Na^+ and K^+ channels. Calcium ion channels in squid terminals differ from Na^+ channels, however, in that they do not inactivate quickly but stay open as long as the presynaptic depolarization lasts.

Calcium ion channels are concentrated in presynaptic terminals at *active zones,* the sites where neurotransmitter is released, exactly opposite the postsynaptic receptors (Figure 12–4). Calcium ions do not diffuse long distances from their site of entry because free Ca^{2+} ions are rapidly buffered by calcium-binding proteins. As a result, Ca^{2+} influx creates a sharp local

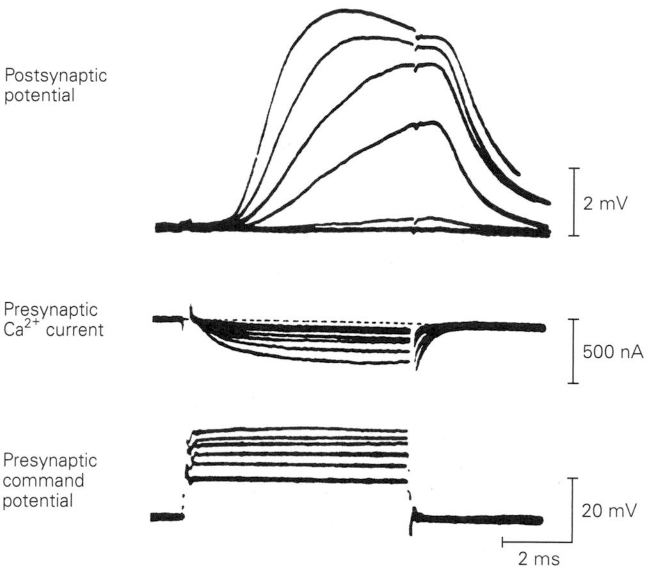

Figure 12–3 Transmitter release is regulated by Ca^{2+} influx into the presynaptic terminals through voltage-gated Ca^{2+} channels. The voltage-sensitive Na^+ and K^+ channels in a squid giant synapse were blocked by tetrodotoxin and tetraethylammonium. The membrane of the presynaptic terminal was voltage-clamped and membrane potential stepped to six different command levels of depolarization (**bottom**). The amplitude of the postsynaptic depolarization (**top**) varies with the size of the presynaptic inward Ca^{2+} current (**middle**) because the amount of transmitter release is a function of the concentration of Ca^{2+} in the presynaptic terminal. The notch in the postsynaptic potential trace is an artifact that results from turning off the presynaptic command potential. (Adapted, with permission, from Llinás and Heuser 1977.)

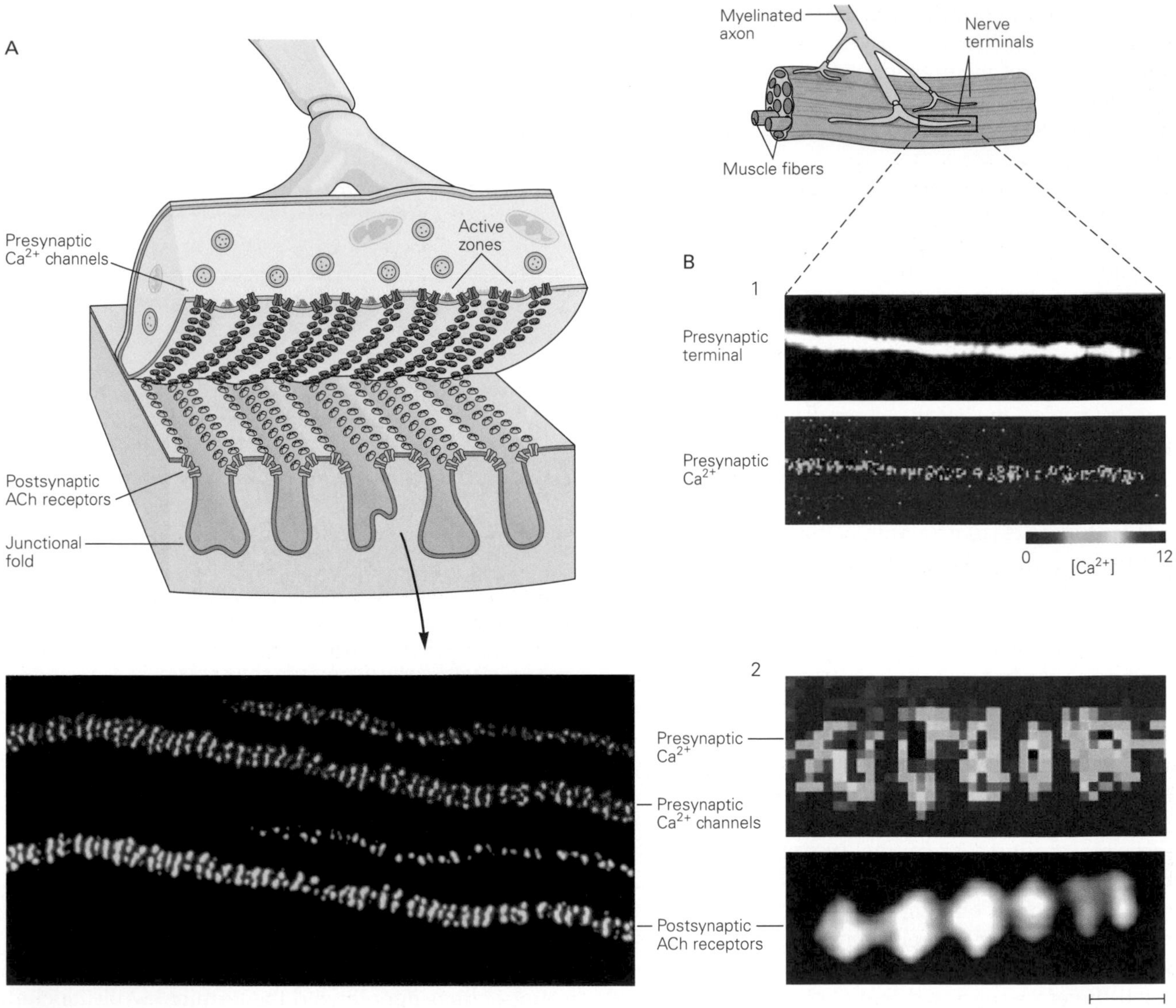

Figure 12–4 Calcium flowing into the presynaptic nerve terminal during synaptic transmission at the neuromuscular junction is concentrated at the active zone. Calcium channels in presynaptic terminals at the end-plate are concentrated opposite clusters of nicotinic acetylcholine (ACh) receptors on the postsynaptic muscle membrane. Two drawings show the frog neuromuscular junction.

A. The enlarged view shows the microanatomy of the neuromuscular junction with the presynaptic terminal peeled back. A fluorescent image shows the presynaptic Ca^{2+} channels (labeled with a Texas red-coupled marine snail toxin that binds to Ca^{2+} channels), and postsynaptic ACh receptors (labeled with fluorescently tagged α-bungarotoxin, which binds selectively to ACh receptors). The two images are normally superimposed but have been separated for clarity. The patterns of labeling with both probes are in almost precise register, indicating that the active zone of the presynaptic neuron is in almost perfect alignment with the postsynaptic membrane containing the high concentration of ACh receptors. (Reproduced, with permission, from Robitaille, Adler, and Charlton 1990.)

B. Calcium influx in presynaptic terminals is localized at active zones. Calcium can be visualized using calcium-sensitive fluorescent dyes. **1.** A presynaptic terminal at a neuromuscular junction filled with the dye fura-2 under resting conditions is shown in the black and white image. The fluorescence intensity of the dye changes as it binds Ca^{2+}. In the color image, color-coded fluorescence intensity changes show local hot-spots of intracellular Ca^{2+} in response to a single presynaptic action potential. **Red** indicates regions with a large increase in Ca^{2+}; **blue** indicates regions with little increase in Ca^{2+}. Regular peaks of Ca^{2+} are seen along the terminal, corresponding to the localization of Ca^{2+} channels at the active zones. **2.** The color image shows a high-magnification view of the peak increase in terminal Ca^{2+} levels. The corresponding black-and-white image shows fluorescence labeling of nicotinic ACh receptors in the postsynaptic membrane, illustrating the close spatial correspondence between areas of presynaptic Ca^{2+} influx and areas of postsynaptic receptors. The scale bar represents 2 μm. (Reproduced, with permission, from Wachman et al. 2004.)

rise in Ca^{2+} concentration at the active zones. This rise in Ca^{2+} in the presynaptic terminals can be visualized using Ca^{2+}-sensitive fluorescent dyes (Figure 12–4B). One striking feature of transmitter release at all synapses is its steep and nonlinear dependence on Ca^{2+} influx; a twofold increase in Ca^{2+} influx can increase the amount of transmitter released by 16-fold. This relationship indicates that at some site, the *calcium sensor,* the cooperative binding of several Ca^{2+} ions is required to trigger release.

The Relation Between Presynaptic Calcium Concentration and Release

How much Ca^{2+} is necessary to induce release of neurotransmitters? To address this question Bert Sakmann and Erwin Neher and their colleagues measured synaptic transmission in the calyx of Held, a large synapse in the mammalian brain stem that is part of the auditory pathway. This synapse is specialized for very rapid and reliable transmission to allow for precise localization of sound in the environment.

The calyx forms a cup-like presynaptic terminal that engulfs a postsynaptic cell body (Figure 12–5A). To ensure that every action potential results in reliable synaptic transmission, the calyx synapse includes almost a thousand active zones that function as independent synapses. In contrast, synaptic terminals of a typical neuron in the brain contain only a single active zone. Because the calyx terminal is large, it is possible to insert electrodes into both the pre- and postsynaptic structures, much as with the squid giant synapse, and directly measure the synaptic coupling between the two compartments. This paired recording allows a precise determination of the time course of activity in the presynaptic and postsynaptic cells (Figure 12–5B).

These recordings revealed a brief lag of 1 to 2 ms between the onset of the presynaptic action potential and the postsynaptic excitatory synaptic potential, which accounts for what Sherrington termed the *synaptic delay.* Because Ca^{2+} channels open more slowly than Na^{+} channels, Ca^{2+} does not begin to enter the presynaptic terminal until the membrane has begun to repolarize. Surprisingly, once Ca^{2+} enters the terminal, transmitter is rapidly released with a delay of only a few hundred microseconds. Thus the synaptic delay is largely attributable to the time required to open Ca^{2+} channels. The astonishing speed of Ca^{2+} action indicates that, prior to Ca^{2+} influx, the biochemical machinery underlying the release process must already exist in a primed and ready state.

A presynaptic action potential normally produces only a brief rise in presynaptic Ca^{2+} concentration because the Ca^{2+} channels open only for a short time. In addition, Ca^{2+} influx is localized at the active zone. These two properties contribute to a concentrated local pulse of Ca^{2+} that induces a burst of transmitter release (Figure 12–5B). As we shall see later in this chapter, the duration of the action potential regulates the amount of Ca^{2+} that flows into the terminal and thus the amount of transmitter release.

To determine how much Ca^{2+} is needed to trigger release, the Neher and Sakmann groups introduced into the presynaptic terminal an inactive form of Ca^{2+} that was complexed within a light-sensitive *chemical cage.* They also loaded the terminals with a fluorescent dye that alters its fluorescence upon binding Ca^{2+} and so can be used to assay the intracellular Ca^{2+} concentration. By uncaging the Ca^{2+} ions with a flash of light they could trigger transmitter release through a uniform, known increase in Ca^{2+} concentration. These experiments revealed that a rise in Ca^{2+} concentration of less than 1 μM is sufficient to induce release of some transmitter, but approximately 10 to 30 μM Ca^{2+} is required to release the amount normally observed during an action potential. Here again the relationship between Ca^{2+} concentration and transmitter release is highly nonlinear, consistent with a model in which four or five Ca^{2+} ions must bind to the Ca^{2+} sensor to trigger release (Figure 12– 5C,D).

Several Classes of Calcium Channels Mediate Transmitter Release

Calcium channels are found in all nerve cells and in many non-neuronal cells. In skeletal and cardiac muscle cells Ca^{2+} channels are important for excitation-contraction coupling; in endocrine cells they mediate release of hormones. Neurons contain five classes of voltage-gated Ca^{2+} channels: the L-type, P/Q-type, N-type, R-type, and T-type, each encoded by distinct genes or gene families. Each type has specific biophysical and pharmacological properties and physiological functions (Table 12–1).

Calcium channels are multimeric proteins whose distinct properties are determined by their pore-forming subunit, the α_1-subunit. The α_1-subunit is homologous to the α-subunit of the voltage-gated Na^{+} channel, comprised of four repeats of a domain with six membrane-spanning segments that includes the S4 voltage-sensor and pore-lining P region (see Figure 7–14). Calcium channels also have auxiliary subunits (termed α_2, β, γ, and δ) that modify the properties of the channel formed by the α_1-subunit.

Four of the voltage-gated Ca^{2+} channels—the L-type, P/Q-type, N-type, and R-type—require fairly strong

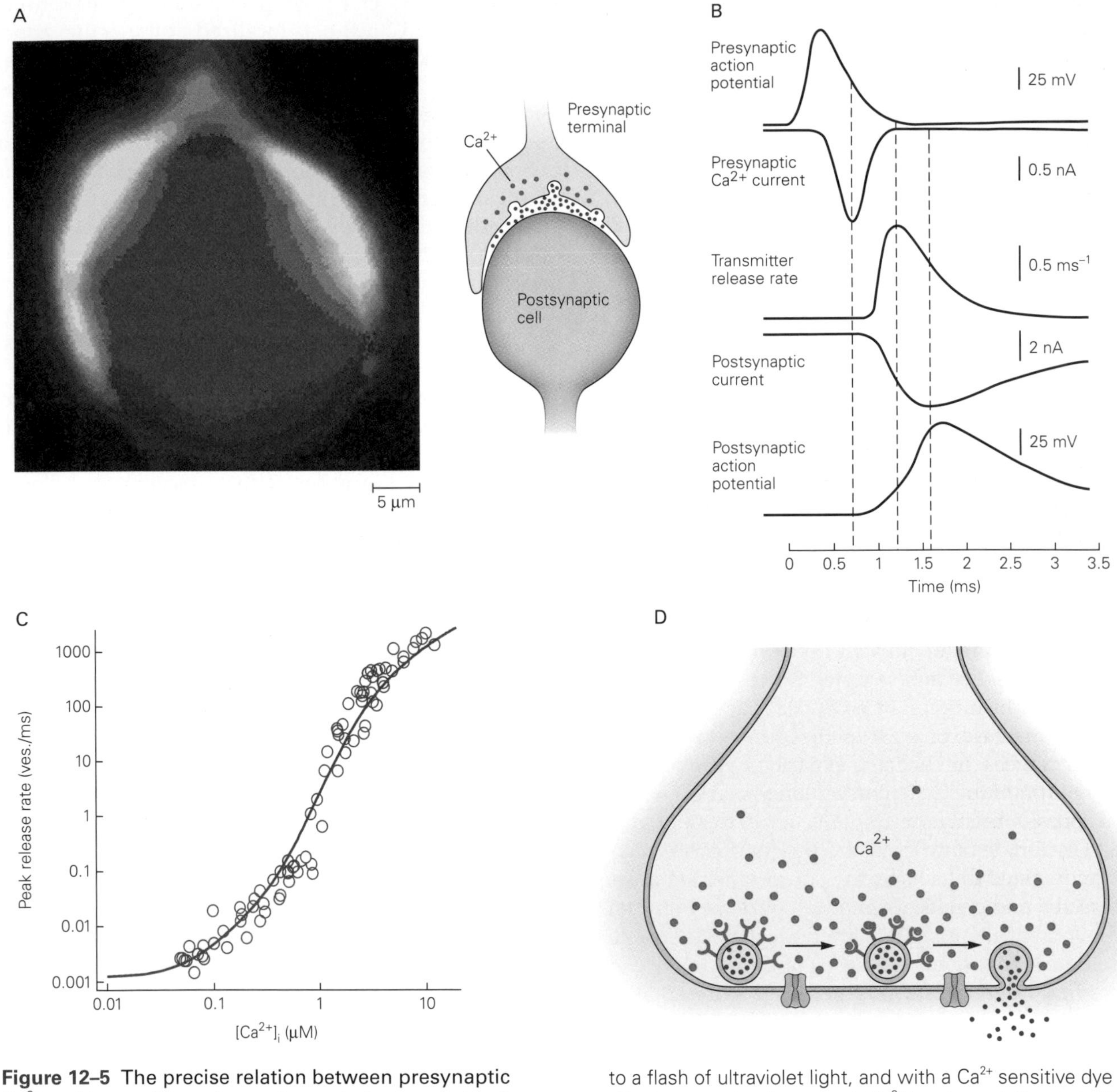

Figure 12–5 The precise relation between presynaptic Ca^{2+} and transmitter release at a central synapse has been measured. (Reproduced, with permission, from Meinrenken, Borst, and Sakmann 2003, and Sun et al. 2007.)

A. The large presynaptic terminal of the calyx of Held in the mammalian brain stem (**yellow**) engulfs a postsynaptic cell body (**blue**). Fluorescence image on left shows a calyx filled with a calcium-sensitive dye.

B. Time courses of the presynaptic action potential, presynaptic Ca^{2+} current, transmitter release rate, postsynaptic current through glutamate receptors, and the postsynaptic action potential. The **dashed lines** indicate the timing of the peak responses for the Ca^{2+} current, transmitter release, and postsynaptic action potential.

C. Transmitter release is steeply dependent on the Ca^{2+} concentration in the presynaptic terminal. The calyx was loaded with a caged Ca^{2+} compound that releases its bound Ca^{2+} in response to a flash of ultraviolet light, and with a Ca^{2+} sensitive dye that allows measuring how much Ca^{2+} is released. By controlling the intensity of light one can regulate the increase in Ca^{2+} in the presynaptic terminal. The plot, on a logarithmic scale, shows the relation between the rate of vesicle release and intracellular Ca^{2+} concentration. The circles depict measurements from individual experiments, and the blue line depicts a fit of the data by a model that assumes that release is triggered by a major Ca^{2+} sensor that binds five Ca^{2+} ions, resulting in a Ca^{2+} cooperativity of five. Due to the non-linear relationship between Ca^{2+} and release small increments in Ca^{2+} at concentrations of more than one μm cause massive increases in release.

D. The release of transmitter from a vesicle requires the binding of five Ca^{2+} ions to a calcium-sensing synaptic vesicle protein. In the figure Ca^{2+} binding is shown to trigger exocytosis by binding to five sensors present on a single vesicle. In reality, a single sensor binds several Ca^{2+} ions to trigger release.

depolarization to be activated (voltages positive to −40 to −20 mV are required) and thus are often referred to as *high-voltage-activated* Ca^{2+} channels. In contrast, T-type channels open in response to small depolarizations around the threshold for generating an action potential (−60 to −40 mV) and are therefore called *low-voltage-activated* Ca^{2+} channels. Because they are activated by small changes in membrane potential, the T-type channels help control excitability at the resting potential and are an important source of the excitatory current that drives the rhythmic pacemaker activity of certain cells in both brain and heart.

In neurons the rapid release of conventional transmitters associated with fast synaptic transmission is mediated mainly by the P/Q-type and N-type Ca^{2+} channels because these are the channel types concentrated at the active zone. The localization of N-type Ca^{2+} channels at the frog neuromuscular junction has been visualized using a fluorescence-labeled snail toxin that binds selectively to these channels (see Figure 12–4A). The L-type channels are not found in the active zone and thus do not normally contribute to the fast release of conventional transmitters such as ACh and glutamate. However, Ca^{2+} influx through L-type channels is important for slower forms of release that do not occur at specialized active zones, such as the release of neuropeptides from neurons and of hormones from endocrine cells. As we shall see below, regulation of Ca^{2+} influx into presynaptic terminals controls the amount of transmitter release and hence the strength of synaptic transmission.

Voltage-gated Ca^{2+} channels are responsible for certain acquired and genetic diseases. A point mutation in the α_1-subunit of P/Q-type channels underlies an inherited form of migraine. A mutation in the α_1-subunit of L-type channels inhibits the voltage-dependent inactivation of these channels, and underlies Timothy syndrome, a pervasive developmental disorder involving both impaired cognitive function and a severe form of autism. Patients with Lambert-Eaton syndrome, an autoimmune disease associated with muscle weakness, make antibodies to the L-type channel α_1-subunit that decrease total Ca^{2+} current.

Transmitter Is Released in Quantal Units

How does the influx of Ca^{2+} trigger release? Katz and his colleagues provided the key insight into this question by showing that transmitter is released in discrete amounts they called *quanta*. Each quantum of transmitter produces a postsynaptic potential of fixed size, called the *quantal synaptic potential*. The total postsynaptic potential is made up of a large number of quantal potentials. EPSPs seem smoothly graded in amplitude only because each quantal (or unit) potential is small relative to the total potential.

Katz and Fatt obtained the first clue as to the quantal nature of synaptic transmission in 1951 when they observed spontaneous postsynaptic potentials of approximately 0.5 mV in the nerve-muscle synapse of the frog. Like end-plate potentials evoked by nerve stimulation, these small depolarizing responses were largest at the site of nerve-muscle contact and decayed electrotonically with distance (see Figure 9–5). Small spontaneous potentials have since been observed in mammalian

Table 12–1 Voltage-Gated Ca^{2+} Channels of Neurons

Gene	Former name	Ca^{2+} channel type	Tissue	Blocker	Voltage-dependence[1]	Function
$Ca_V1.1-1.4$	$\alpha_{1C,D,F,S}$	L	Muscle, neurons	Dihydropyridines	HVA	Contraction, slow release
$Ca_V2.1$	α_{1A}	P/Q	Neurons	ω-Agatoxin (spider venom)	HVA	Fast release +++
$Ca_V2.2$	α_{1B}	N	Neurons	ω-Conotoxin (cone snail venom)	HVA	Fast release ++
$Ca_V2.3$	α_{1E}	R	Neurons	SNX-482 (tarantula venom)	HVA	Fast release +
$Ca_V3.1-3.3$	$\alpha_{1G,H,I}$	T	Muscle, neurons	Mibefradil (limited selectivity)	LVA	Pacemaker firing

[1]**HVA**, high voltage activated; **LVA**, low voltage activated.

muscle and in central neurons. Because the postsynaptic potentials at vertebrate nerve-muscle synapses are called *end-plate potentials,* Fatt and Katz called these spontaneous potentials *miniature end-plate potentials.*

Several results convinced Fatt and Katz that the miniature end-plate potentials represented responses to the release of small amounts of ACh, the neurotransmitter used at the nerve-muscle synapse. The time course of the miniature end-plate potentials and the effects of various drugs on them are indistinguishable from the properties of the end-plate potential. Like the end-plate potentials, the miniature end-plate potentials are enhanced and prolonged by prostigmine, a drug that blocks hydrolysis of ACh by acetylcholinesterase. Conversely, they are reduced and finally abolished by agents that block the ACh receptor. The miniature end-plate potentials represent responses to small packets of transmitter that are spontaneously released from the presynaptic nerve terminal in the absence of an action potential. Their frequency can be increased by a small depolarization of the presynaptic terminal. They disappear if the presynaptic motor nerve degenerates and reappear when a new motor synapse is formed.

What could account for the small, fixed size of the miniature end-plate potential (around 0.5–1 mV)? Del Castillo and Katz first tested the possibility that each event represents a response to the opening of a *single* ACh receptor-channel. Small amounts of ACh applied to the frog muscle end-plate elicited depolarizing postsynaptic responses that were much smaller than the 0.5 mV response of a miniature end-plate potential. This finding made it clear that the miniature end-plate potential represents the opening of more than one ACh receptor-channel. In fact, Katz and Miledi were later able to estimate the voltage response to the elementary current through a single ACh receptor-channel as being only approximately 0.3 μV (see Chapter 9). Based on this estimate a miniature end-plate potential of 0.5 mV would represent the summation of the elementary currents of approximately 2,000 channels. Later work showed that a miniature end-plate potential is the response to the synchronous release of approximately 5,000 molecules of ACh.

What is the relationship of the large end-plate potential evoked by nerve stimulation and the small, spontaneous miniature end-plate responses? This question was addressed by del Castillo and Katz in a study of synaptic signaling at the nerve-muscle synapse bathed in a solution low in Ca^{2+}. Under this condition the end-plate potential is reduced markedly, from the normal 70 mV to about 0.5 to 2.5 mV. Moreover, the amplitude of each successive end-plate potential now varies randomly from one stimulus to the next; often no response can be detected at all (termed *failures*). However, the minimum response above zero—the unit EPSP in response to a presynaptic action potential—is identical in amplitude (approximately 0.5 mV) and shape to the spontaneous miniature end-plate potentials. Importantly, the amplitude of each end-plate potential is an integral multiple of the unit potential (Figure 12–6).

Now del Castillo and Katz could ask: How does the rise of intracellular Ca^{2+} that accompanies each action potential affect the release of transmitter? They found that increasing the external Ca^{2+} concentration does not change the amplitude of the unit synaptic potential. However, the proportion of failures decreases and the incidence of higher-amplitude responses (composed of multiple quantal units) increases. These observations show that an increase in external Ca^{2+} concentration does not enhance the *size* of a quantum of transmitter (that is, the number of ACh molecules in each quantum) but rather acts to increase the average number of quanta that are released in response to a presynaptic action potential (Box 12–1). The greater the Ca^{2+} influx into the terminal, the larger the number of transmitter quanta released.

Thus three findings led del Castillo and Katz to conclude that transmitter is released in packets with a fixed amount of transmitter, a quantum: The amplitude of the end-plate potential varies in a stepwise manner at low levels of ACh release, the amplitude of each step increase is an integral multiple of the unit potential, and the unit potential has the same mean amplitude as that of the spontaneous miniature end-plate potentials.

In the absence of an action potential the rate of quantal release is low—only one quantum per second is released spontaneously at the end-plate. In the presence of a normal concentration of extracellular Ca^{2+} the firing of an action potential in the presynaptic terminal at the vertebrate nerve-muscle synapse releases approximately 150 quanta, each approximately 0.5 mV in amplitude, resulting in a large end-plate potential. Thus when Ca^{2+} enters the presynaptic terminal during an action potential, it dramatically increases the rate of quantal release by a factor of 150,000, triggering the synchronous release of about 150 quanta in about one millisecond.

Transmitter Is Stored and Released by Synaptic Vesicles

What anatomical features of the cell might account for the quantum of transmitter? The physiological observations indicating that transmitter is released in fixed quanta coincided with the discovery, through electron microscopy, of accumulations of small clear vesicles in

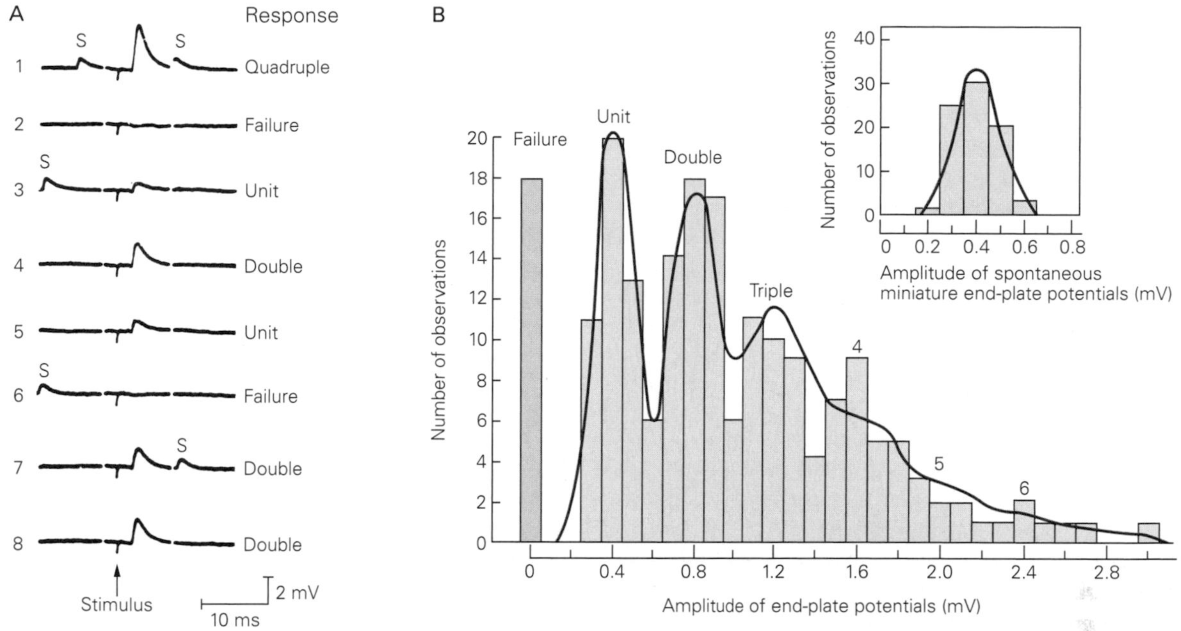

Figure 12–6 Neurotransmitter is released in fixed increments. Each increment or quantum of transmitter produces a unit excitatory postsynaptic potential (EPSP) of fixed amplitude. The amplitude of the EPSP evoked by nerve stimulation is thus equal to the amplitude of the unit EPSP multiplied by the number of quanta of transmitter released.

A. Intracellular recordings from a muscle fiber at the end-plate show the change in postsynaptic potential when eight consecutive stimuli of the same size are applied to the motor nerve. To reduce transmitter release and to keep the end-plate potentials small, the tissue is bathed in a calcium-deficient (and magnesium-rich) solution. The postsynaptic responses to the nerve stimulus vary. Two presynaptic impulses elicit no EPSP (failures), two produce unit potentials, and the others produce EPSPs that are approximately two to four times the amplitude of the unit potential. Note that the spontaneous miniature end-plate potentials (**S**), which occur at random intervals in the traces, are the same size as the unit potential. (Adapted, with permission, from Liley 1956.)

B. After many end-plate potentials are recorded, the number of EPSPs corresponding to a given amplitude is plotted as a function of this amplitude in the histogram shown here. The distribution of responses falls into a number of peaks. The first peak, at 0 mV, represents failures. The first peak of responses, at 0.4 mV, represents the unit potential, the smallest elicited response. The unit response has the same amplitude as the spontaneous miniature end-plate potentials (inset), indicating that the unit response is caused by the release of a single quantum of transmitter. The other peaks in the histogram are integral multiples of the amplitude of the unit potential; that is, responses are composed of two, three, four, or more quantal events.

The number of responses under each peak divided by the total number of events in the entire histogram is the probability that a single presynaptic action potential triggers the release of the number of quanta that corresponds to the peak. For example, if there are 30 events in the peak corresponding to the release of two quanta out of a total of 100 events recorded, the probability that a presynaptic action potential releases exactly two quanta is 30/100 or 0.3. This probability follows a Poisson distribution (**red curve**). This theoretical distribution is composed of the sum of several Gaussian functions. The spread of the unit peak (standard deviation of the Gaussian function) reflects the fact that the amount of transmitter in a quantum, and hence the amplitude of the quantal postsynaptic response, varies randomly about a mean value. The successive Gaussian peaks widen progressively because the variability associated with each quantal event sums linearly with the number of quanta. The distribution of amplitudes of the spontaneous miniature potentials (inset) is fit by a Gaussian curve whose width is identical to that of the Gaussian curve for the unit synaptic responses. (Adapted, with permission, from Boyd and Martin 1956.)

the presynaptic terminal. Del Castillo and Katz speculated that the vesicles are organelles for the storage of transmitter, each vesicle stores one quantum of transmitter (amounting to several thousand molecules), and each vesicle releases its entire contents into the synaptic cleft in an all-or-none manner at sites specialized for release.

The sites of release, the active zones, contain a cloud of synaptic vesicles that cluster above a fuzzy electron-dense material attached to the internal face of the presynaptic membrane (see Figure 12–4A). At all rapid synapses the vesicles are typically clear, small, and ovoid, with a diameter of approximately 40 nm. Although most synaptic vesicles do not contact the

Box 12–1 Calculating the Probability of Transmitter Release

The release of a quantum of transmitter is a random event. The fate of each quantum of transmitter in response to an action potential has only two possible outcomes—the quantum is or is not released. This event resembles a binomial or Bernoulli trial (similar to tossing a coin in the air to determine whether it comes up heads or tails).

The probability of a quantum being released by an action potential is independent of the probability of other quanta being released by that action potential. Therefore, for a population of releasable quanta, each action potential represents a series of independent binomial trials (comparable to tossing a handful of coins to see how many coins come up heads).

In a binomial distribution p stands for the average probability of success (ie, the probability that any given quantum will be released) and q (equal to $1 - p$) stands for the mean probability of failure. Both the average probability (p) that an individual quantum will be released and the store (n) of readily releasable quanta are assumed to be constant. (Any reduction in the store is assumed to be quickly replenished after each stimulus.) The product of n and p yields an estimate m of the mean number of quanta that are released to make up the end-plate potential. This mean is called the *quantal content* or *quantal output*.

Calculation of the probability of transmitter release can be illustrated with the following example. Consider a terminal that has a releasable store of five quanta ($n = 5$). If we assume that $p = 0.1$, then q (the probability that an individual quantum is not released from the terminals) is $1 - p$, or 0.9. We can now determine the probability that a stimulus will release no quanta (failure), a single quantum, two quanta, three quanta, or any number of quanta (up to n).

The probability that none of the five available quanta will be released by a given stimulus is the product of the individual probabilities that each quantum will not be released: $q^5 = (0.9)^5$, or 0.59. We would thus expect to see 59 failures in a hundred stimuli. The probabilities of observing zero, one, two, three, four, or five quanta are represented by the successive terms of the binomial expansion:

$$(q+p)^5 = q^5 \text{ (failures)} + 5\,q^4p \text{ (1 quantum)}$$
$$+ 10\,q^3p^2 \text{ (2 quanta)} + 10\,q^2p^3 \text{ (3 quanta)}$$
$$+ 5\,qp^4 \text{ (4 quanta)} + p^5 \text{ (5 quanta)}.$$

Thus, in 100 stimuli the binomial expansion would predict 33 unit responses, 7 double responses, 1 triple response, and 0 quadruple or quintuple responses.

Values for m vary from approximately 100 to 300 at the vertebrate nerve-muscle synapse, the squid giant synapse, and *Aplysia* central synapses, to as few as 1 to 4 in the synapses of the sympathetic ganglion and spinal cord of vertebrates. The probability of release p also varies, ranging from as high as 0.7 at the neuromuscular junction in the frog and 0.9 in the crab down to around 0.1 at some central synapses. Estimates for n range from 1,000 (at the vertebrate nerve-muscle synapse) to 1 (at single terminals of central neurons).

The parameters n and p are statistical terms; the physical processes represented by them are not yet completely understood. As discussed in this chapter, transmitter is packaged in synaptic vesicles and a quantum of transmitter corresponds to the all-or-none release of the contents of a vesicle. Although the parameter n was initially assumed to represent the number of readily releasable (or available) quanta of transmitter, it is now thought to reflect the number of release sites or active zones in the presynaptic terminals that are loaded with vesicles containing neurotransmitter.

Although an active zone has a number of docked vesicles, there is evidence that a presynaptic action potential can trigger the exocytosis of at most one vesicle per active zone. Although the number of release sites is thought to be fixed, the fraction that is loaded with vesicles is thought to be variable.

The parameter p probably represents a compound probability depending on at least two processes: the number of vesicles that have been loaded or docked onto a release site (a process referred to as vesicle mobilization) and the probability that an action potential will discharge a quantum of transmitter from a given vesicle docked at the active zone. This probability is thought to depend on Ca^{2+} influx during an action potential.

The quantal size a is the response of the postsynaptic membrane to the release of a single quantum of transmitter. Quantal size depends largely on the properties of the postsynaptic cell, such as the input resistance and capacitance (which can be independently estimated) and the responsiveness of the postsynaptic membrane to the transmitter substance. This can also be measured by the postsynaptic membrane's response to the application of a constant amount of transmitter.

The mean size of a synaptic response E evoked by an action potential thus depends on the product of the total number of quanta present, the probability that an individual quantum is released, and the size of the response to a quantum: $E = n \cdot p \cdot a$.

active zone, some are physically bound. These are called the *docked* vesicles and are thought to be the ones immediately available for release. At the neuromuscular junction the active zones are linear structures (see Figure 12–4), whereas in central synapses they are disc-shaped structures approximately 0.1 μm^2 in area with dense projections pointing into the cytoplasm. Active zones are always precisely apposed to the postsynaptic membrane patches that contain the neurotransmitter receptors. Thus presynaptic and postsynaptic specializations are functionally and morphologically attuned to each other. As we shall learn later, several key active zone proteins involved in transmitter release have now been identified and characterized.

Quantal transmission has been demonstrated at all chemical synapses so far examined with only one exception: at the synapse between photoreceptors and bipolar neurons in the retina (Chapter 26). Nevertheless, the efficacy of transmitter release from a single presynaptic cell onto a single postsynaptic cell varies widely in the nervous system and depends on several factors: (1) the number of synapses between a pair of presynaptic and postsynaptic cells (ie, the number of presynaptic boutons that contact the postsynaptic cell); (2) the number of active zones in an individual synaptic terminal; and (3) the probability that a presynaptic action potential will trigger release of one or more quanta of transmitter at an active zone (Box 12–1).

In the central nervous system most presynaptic terminals have only a single active zone where an action potential usually releases at most a single quantum of transmitter in an all-or-none manner. However at some central synapses, such as the calyx of Held, the presynaptic terminal may contain many active zones and thus can release a large number of quanta in response to a single presynaptic action potential. Central neurons also differ in the number of synapses that a typical presynaptic cell makes with a typical postsynaptic cell. Whereas most central neurons form only a few synapses with any one postsynaptic cell, a single climbing fiber forms up to 10,000 terminals on a single Purkinje neuron in the cerebellum! Finally, the mean probability of transmitter release from a single active zone also varies widely among different presynaptic terminals, from less than 0.1 (that is, a 10% chance that a presynaptic action potential will trigger release of a vesicle) to greater than 0.9. This wide range of probabilities can even be seen among the individual boutons at different synapses between one specific type of presynaptic cell and one specific type of postsynaptic cell.

Thus central neurons vary widely in the efficacy and reliability of synaptic transmission. Synaptic reliability is defined as the probability that an action potential in a presynaptic cell leads to some measurable response in the postsynaptic cell—that is, the probability that a presynaptic action potential releases one or more quanta of transmitter. Efficacy refers to the mean amplitude of the synaptic response, which depends on both the reliability of synaptic transmission and on the mean size of the response when synaptic transmission does occur.

Most central neurons communicate at synapses that have a low probability of transmitter release. The high failure rate of release at most central synapses (ie, their low release probability) is not a *design defect* but serves a purpose. As we discuss below, this feature allows transmitter release to be regulated over a wide dynamic range, which is important for learning and memory. In synaptic connections where a low probability of release is deleterious for function, this limitation is overcome by simply having many active zones in one synapse, as is the case at the calyx of Held and the nerve-muscle synapse. Both contain hundreds of independent active zones, so an action potential reliably releases 150 to 250 quanta, ensuring that a presynaptic signal is always followed by a postsynaptic action potential. Reliable transmission at the neuromuscular junction is essential for survival. An animal would not survive if its ability to move away from a predator was hampered by a low-probability response.

Not all chemical signaling between neurons depends on synapses. Some substances, such as certain lipid metabolites and the gas nitric oxide (see Chapter 11), can diffuse across the lipid bilayer of the membrane. Others can be moved out of nerve endings by carrier proteins if their intracellular concentration is sufficiently high. Plasma membrane transporters for glutamate or γ-aminobutyric acid (GABA) normally take up transmitter into a cell from the synaptic cleft following a presynaptic action potential (see Chapter 13). However, in certain glial cells of the retina, the direction of glutamate transport can be reversed under certain conditions, causing glutamate to leave the cell through the transporter into the synaptic cleft. Still other substances simply leak out of nerve terminals at a low rate. Surprisingly, approximately 90% of the ACh that leaves the presynaptic terminals at the neuromuscular junction does so through continuous leakage. This leakage is ineffective, because it is diffuse and not targeted to receptors at the end-plate region, and because it is continuous and low level rather than synchronous and concentrated.

Synaptic Vesicles Discharge Transmitter by Exocytosis and Are Recycled by Endocytosis

The quantal hypothesis of del Castillo and Katz has been amply confirmed by direct experimental evidence that synaptic vesicles do indeed package neurotransmitter and that they release their contents by directly fusing with the presynaptic membrane, a process termed *exocytosis.*

Forty years ago Victor Whittaker discovered that the synaptic vesicles in the motor nerve terminals of the electric organ of the fish *Torpedo* contain a high concentration of ACh. Later, Thomas Reese and John Heuser and their colleagues obtained electron micrographs that caught vesicles in the act of exocytosis. To observe the brief exocytotic event, they rapidly froze the nerve-muscle synapse by immersing it in liquid helium at precisely defined intervals after the presynaptic nerve was stimulated. In addition, they increased the number of quanta of transmitter discharged with each nerve impulse by applying the drug 4-aminopyridine, a compound that blocks certain voltage-gated K^+ channels, which increases the duration of the action potential, thereby enhancing Ca^{2+} influx.

These techniques provided clear images of synaptic vesicles at the active zone during exocytosis. Using a technique called *freeze-fracture electron microscopy,* Reese and Heuser noted deformations of the presynaptic membrane along the active zone immediately after synaptic activity, which they interpreted as invaginations of the cell membrane caused by fusion of synaptic vesicles. These deformations lay along one or two rows of unusually large intramembranous particles, visible along both margins of the presynaptic density and now thought to be the voltage-gated Ca^{2+} channels (Figure 12–7). The particle density (approximately 1,500 per μm^2) is approximately that of the Ca^{2+} channels essential for transmitter release. Moreover, the proximity of the particles to the release site is consistent with the short time interval between the onset of the Ca^{2+} current and the release of transmitter.

Finally, Heuser and Reese found that these deformations are transient; they occur only when vesicles are discharged and do not persist after transmitter has been released. Thin-section electron micrographs revealed a number of omega-shaped (Ω) structures that have the appearance of synaptic vesicles that have just fused with the membrane, prior to the complete collapse of the vesicle membrane into the plasma membrane (Figure 12–7B). Heuser and Reese confirmed this idea by showing that the number of Ω-shaped structures is directly correlated with the size of the EPSP when they varied the concentration of 4-aminopyridine to alter the amount of transmitter release. These morphological studies provide striking evidence that transmitter is released from synaptic vesicles by means of exocytosis.

Following exocytosis, the excess membrane added to the presynaptic terminal is retrieved. When Heuser and Reese obtained images of presynaptic terminals 10 to 20 seconds after stimulation, they observed new structures at the plasma membrane, the coated pits, which represent membrane retrieval through the process of endocytosis (Figure 12–7C). Several seconds later the coated pits are seen to pinch off from the membrane and appear as coated vesicles in the cytoplasm. As we will see below, endocytosis through coated pit formation represents one of several means of vesicle membrane retrieval.

Capacitance Measurements Provide Insight into the Kinetics of Exocytosis and Endocytosis

In certain neurons with large presynaptic terminals the increase in surface area of the plasma membrane during exocytosis can be detected in electrical measurements as increases in membrane capacitance. As we saw in Chapter 6, the capacitance of the membrane is proportional to its surface area. Neher discovered that one could use measurements of capacitance to monitor exocytosis in secretory cells.

In adrenal chromaffin cells (which release epinephrine and norepinephrine) and in mast cells of the rat peritoneum (which release histamine and serotonin) individual dense-core vesicles are large enough to permit measurement of the increase in capacitance associated with fusion of a single vesicle. Release of transmitter in these cells is accompanied by stepwise increases in capacitance, followed somewhat later by stepwise decreases, which reflect the retrieval and recycling of the excess membrane (Figure 12–8).

In neurons the changes in capacitance caused by fusion of single, small synaptic vesicles are usually too low to resolve. In certain favorable synaptic preparations that release large numbers of vesicles (such as the giant presynaptic terminals of bipolar neurons in the retina), membrane depolarization triggers a transient smooth rise in the total capacitance of the terminal as a result of the exocytosis and retrieval of the membrane from hundreds of individual synaptic vesicles (Figure 12–8C). These results provide direct measurements of the rates of membrane fusion and retrieval.

Exocytosis Involves the Formation of a Temporary Fusion Pore

Morphological studies of mast cells using rapid freezing suggest that exocytosis depends on the formation of a temporary fusion pore that spans the membranes of the vesicle and plasma membranes. In electrophysiological studies of capacitance increases in mast cells, a channel-like fusion pore was detected in

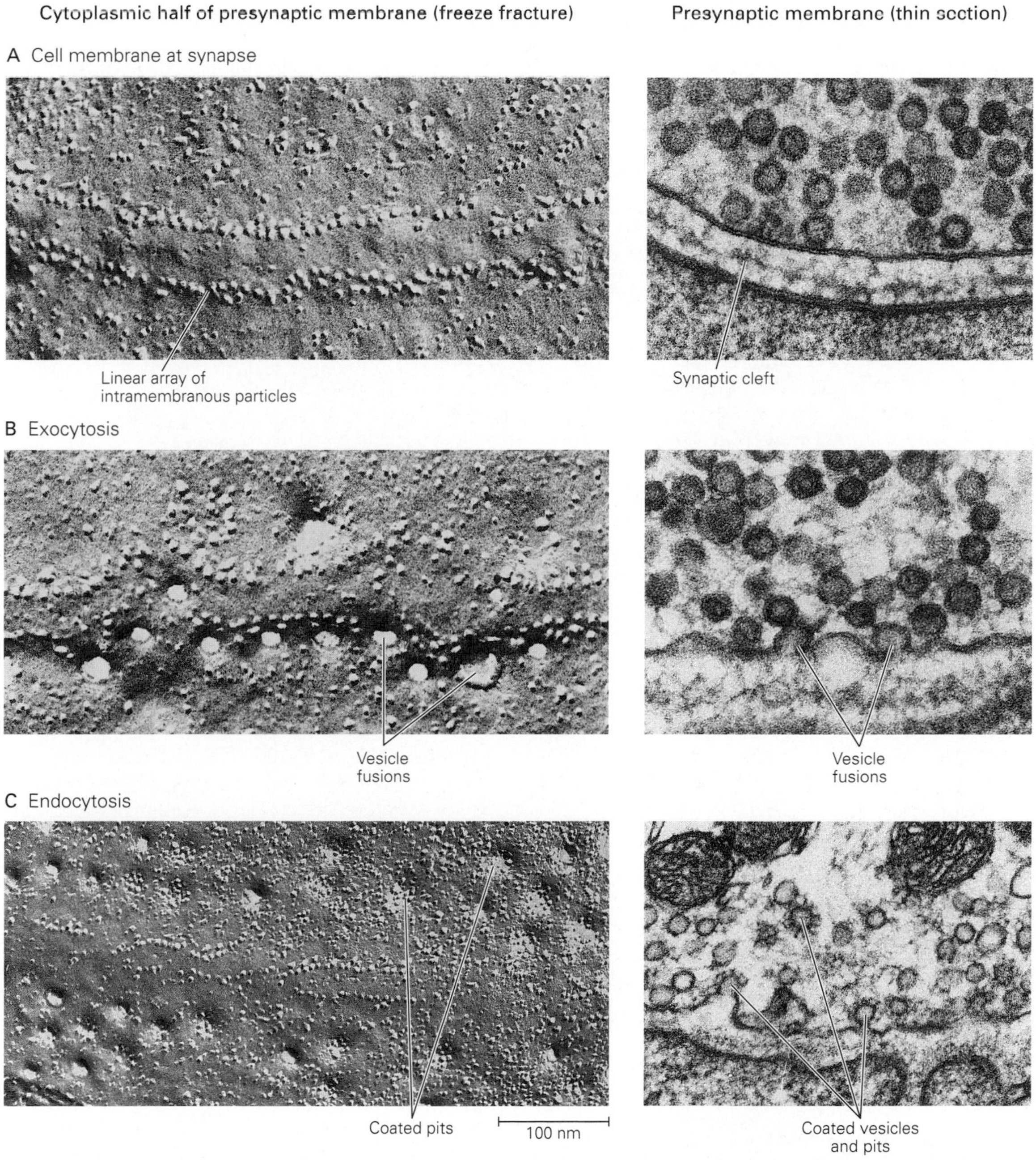

Figure 12–7 Synaptic vesicles release transmitter by exocytosis and are retrieved by endocytosis. The images on the left are freeze-fracture electron micrographs at a neuromuscular junction. The views shown are of the cytoplasmic leaflet of the presynaptic membrane looking up from the synaptic cleft. The images on the right are thin-section electron micrographs showing cross-section views of the presynaptic terminal, synaptic cleft, and postsynaptic muscle membrane. (Reproduced, with permission, from Heuser and Reese 1981.)

A. Parallel rows of intramembranous particles arrayed on either side of an active zone are thought to be the voltage-gated Ca^{2+} channels essential for transmitter release. The thin-section image at right shows the synaptic vesicles adjacent to the active zone.

B. Synaptic vesicles release transmitter by fusing with the plasma membrane (exocytosis). Here synaptic vesicles are caught in the act of fusing with the plasma membrane by rapid freezing of the tissue within 5 ms after a depolarizing stimulus. Each depression in the plasma membrane represents the fusion of one synaptic vesicle. In the micrograph at right vesicle fusion is observed as Ω-shaped structures.

C. After exocytosis, synaptic vesicle membrane is retrieved by endocytosis. Within approximately 10 seconds after fusion of the vesicles with the presynaptic membrane, coated pits form. After another 10 seconds the coated pits begin to pinch off by endocytosis to form coated vesicles. These vesicles include the membrane proteins of the original synaptic vesicle and also molecules captured from the external medium. The vesicles are recycled at the terminals or are transported to the cell body, where the membrane constituents are degraded or recycled (see Chapter 4).

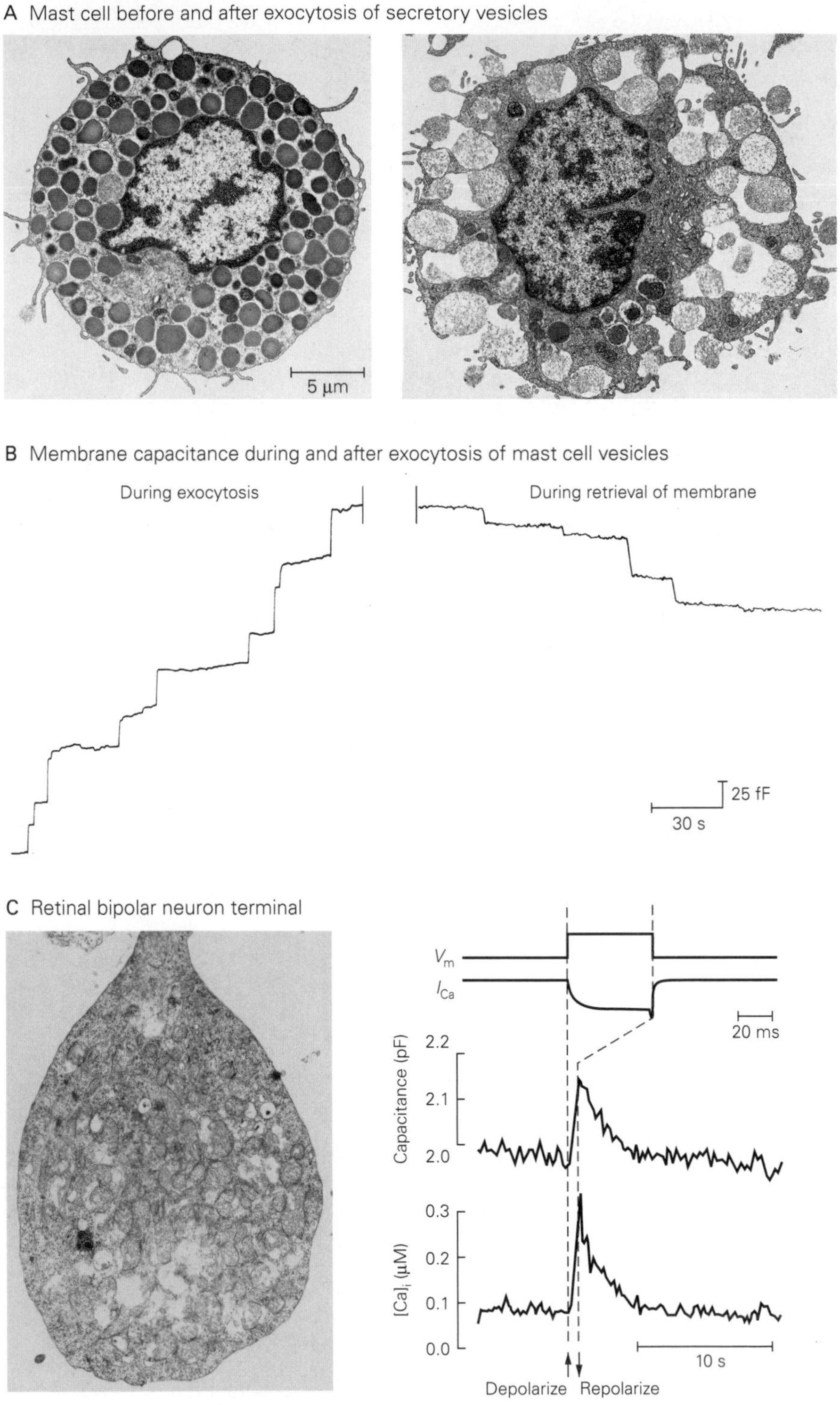
A Mast cell before and after exocytosis of secretory vesicles
5 µm
B Membrane capacitance during and after exocytosis of mast cell vesicles
During exocytosis
During retrieval of membrane
25 fF
30 s
C Retinal bipolar neuron terminal
Vm
ICa
20 ms
Capacitance (pF)
2.2
2.1
2.0
[Ca]i (µM)
0.3
0.2
0.1
0.0
10 s
Depolarize
Repolarize

the electrophysiological recordings prior to complete fusion of vesicles and cell membranes. This fusion pore starts out with a single-channel conductance of approximately 200 pS, similar to that of gap-junction channels, which also bridge two membranes. During exocytosis the pore rapidly dilates, probably from around 5 to 50 nm in diameter, and the conductance increases dramatically (Figure 12–9A).

The fusion pore is not just an intermediate structure leading to exocytosis of transmitter, as transmitter can be released through the pore prior to full fusion. This was first shown by amperometry, a method that uses an extracellular carbon-fiber electrode to detect certain amine neurotransmitters, such as serotonin, based on an electrochemical reaction between the transmitter and the electrode that generates an electrical current proportional to the local transmitter concentration. Firing of an action potential in serotonergic cells leads to a large transient increase in electrode current, corresponding to the exocytosis of the contents of a single dense-core vesicle. In some instances these large transient increases are preceded by smaller, longer-lasting current signals that reflect leakage of transmitter through a fusion pore that flickers open and closed several times prior to complete fusion (Figure 12–9B).

Transmitter can also be released solely through transient fusion pores, that is, without full collapse of the vesicle membrane into the plasma membrane. Capacitance measurements for exocytosis of both large dense-core vesicles and small clear vesicles in neuroendocrine cells show that the fusion pore can open and close rapidly and reversibly. The reversible opening and closing of a fusion pore represents a very rapid method of membrane retrieval. The circumstances under which the small clear vesicles at fast synapses discharge transmitter through a fusion pore, as opposed to full membrane collapse, are uncertain.

The Synaptic Vesicle Cycle Involves Several Steps

When firing at high frequency, a typical neuron is able to maintain a high rate of transmitter release. This can result in the exocytosis of a large number of vesicles, more than the number originally present within the presynaptic terminal. To prevent the supply of vesicles from being rapidly depleted, used vesicles are rapidly retrieved and recycled. Because nerve terminals are usually some distance from the cell body, replenishing vesicles by synthesis in the cell body and transport to the terminals would be too slow to be practical.

Synaptic vesicles are released and reused in a simple cycle (Figure 12–10A). Vesicles fill with neurotransmitter and cluster in the nerve terminal. They then dock at the active zone where they undergo a complex *priming* process that makes vesicles competent to respond to the Ca^{2+} signal that triggers the fusion process.

Three mechanisms exist for retrieving the synaptic vesicle membrane following exocytosis and each has a distinct time course. The first, most rapid mechanism involves the reversible opening and closing of the fusion pore, without the full collapse of the vesicle membrane into the plasma membrane (Figure 12–10B1). In the *kiss-and-stay* pathway the vesicle remains at the active zone after the fusion pore closes, ready for a second

Figure 12–8 (Opposite) **Changes in capacitance reveal the time course of exocytosis and endocytosis.**

A. Electron micrographs show a mast cell before (**left**) and after (**right**) inducing exocytosis. Mast cells are secretory cells of the immune system that contain large dense-core vesicles filled with the transmitter histamine. Exocytosis of the secretory vesicles is normally triggered by the binding of antigen complexed to an immunoglobulin (IgE). Under experimental conditions massive exocytosis can be triggered by the inclusion of a nonhydrolyzable analog of guanosine triphosphate (GTP) in an intracellular recording electrode. (Reproduced, with permission, from Lawson et al. 1977.)

B. Stepwise increases in capacitance reflect the successive fusion of individual secretory vesicles with the mast cell membrane. The step increases are unequal because of variability in the membrane area of the vesicles. After exocytosis the membrane added through fusion is retrieved through endocytosis. Endocytosis of individual vesicles gives rise to the stepwise decreases in membrane capacitance. In this way the cell maintains a constant size. (The units are in femtofarads, fF, where 1 fF = 0.1 μm^2 of membrane area.) (Adapted, with permission, from Fernandez, Neher, and Gomperts 1984.)

C. The giant presynaptic terminals of bipolar neurons in the retina are more than 5 μm in diameter, permitting direct patch-clamp recordings of membrane capacitance and Ca^{2+} current. A brief depolarizing voltage-clamp step in membrane potential (V_m) elicits a large sustained Ca^{2+} current (I_{Ca}) and a rise in the cytoplasmic Ca^{2+} concentration, $[Ca]_i$. This results in the fusion of several thousand small synaptic vesicles with the cell membrane, leading to an increase in total membrane capacitance. The increments in capacitance caused by fusion of individual vesicles are too small to resolve. As the internal Ca^{2+} concentration falls back to its resting level upon repolarization, the extra membrane area is retrieved and capacitance returns to its baseline value. The increases in capacitance and Ca^{2+} concentration outlast the brief depolarization and Ca^{2+} current (note different time scales) because of the relative slowness of endocytosis and Ca^{2+} metabolism. (Micrograph reproduced, with permission, from Zenisek et al. 2004; traces adapted, with permission, from von Gersdorff and Matthews 1994.)

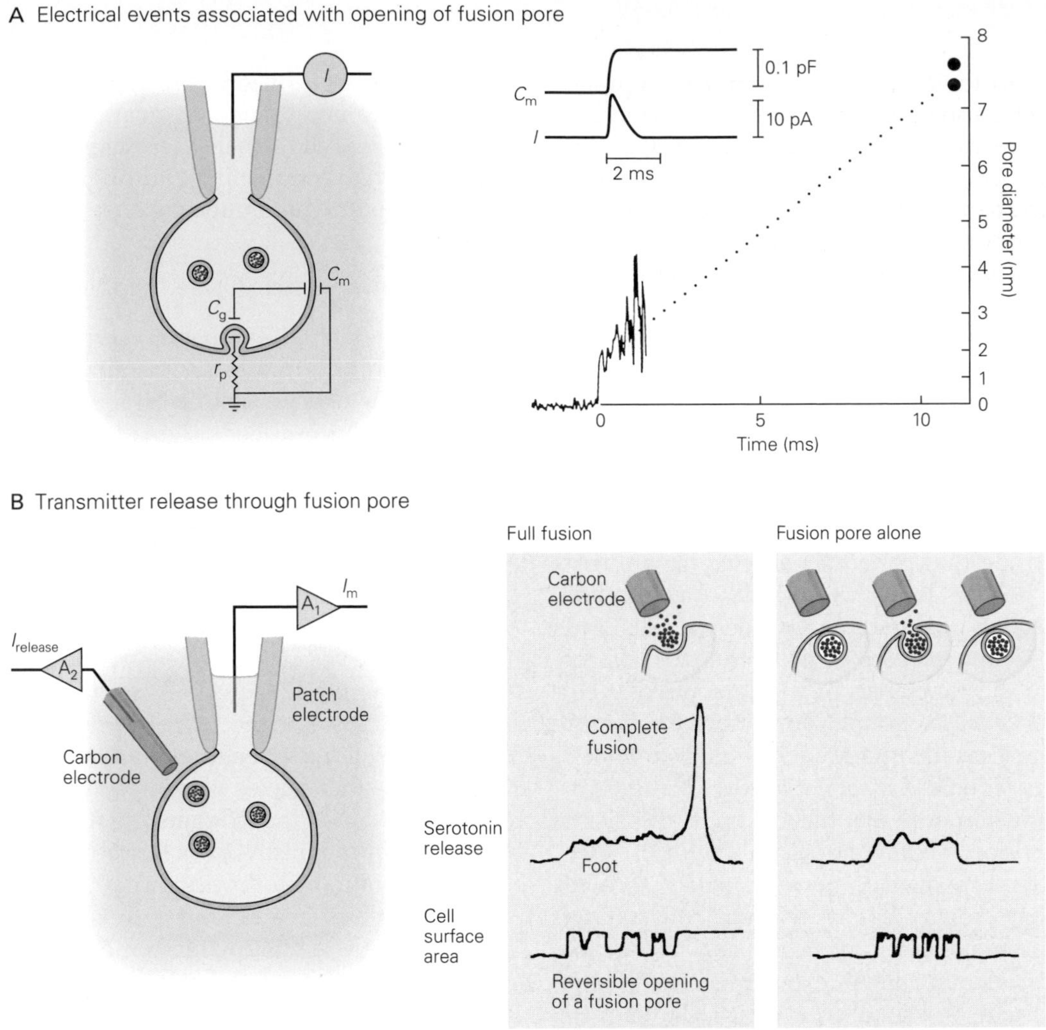

Figure 12–9 Some transmitter is released through temporary fusion pores.

A. A patch clamp is used to record membrane current associated with the opening of a fusion pore. As a vesicle fuses with the plasma membrane, the capacitance of the vesicle (C_g) is initially connected to the capacitance of the rest of the cell membrane (C_m) through the high resistance of the fusion pore (r_p). Because the membrane potential of the vesicle (lumenal side negative) is normally much more negative than the membrane potential of the cell, charge flows from the vesicle to the cell membrane during fusion. This transient current (I) is associated with the increase in membrane capacitance (C_m). The magnitude of the conductance of the fusion pore (g_p) can be calculated from the time constant of the transient current according to $\tau = C_g r_p = C_g / g_p$. The pore diameter can be calculated from the pore conductance, assuming that the pore spans two lipid bilayers and is filled with a solution whose resistivity is equal to that of the cytoplasm. In the plot on the right the pore shows an initial conductance of approximately 200 pS, similar to the conductance of a gap-junction channel, corresponding to a pore diameter of approximately 2 nm. The poor diameter and conductance rapidly increase as the pore dilates to approximately 7 to 8 nm in 10 ms (**filled circles**). (Adapted, with permission, from Monck and Fernandez 1992; Spruce et al. 1990.)

B. Transmitter release is measured by amperometry. A cell is voltage-clamped with an intracellular patch electrode while an extracellular carbon fiber is pressed against the cell surface. A large voltage applied to the tip of the carbon electrode oxidizes certain amine transmitters (such as serotonin or norepinephrine). This oxidation of one molecule generates one or more free electrons, which results in an electrical current that is proportional to the amount of transmitter release. The current can be recorded through an amplifier (A_2) connected to the carbon electrode. Membrane current and capacitance are recorded through the patch electrode amplifier (A_1). Recordings of transmitter release and capacitance measurements from mast cell secretory vesicles are shown at the right. These records indicate that serotonin may be released through the reversible opening and closing of the fusion pore prior to full fusion or by reversible fusion pore opening and closing through the fusion pore alone, that is without full fusion. During the brief fusion pore openings small amounts of transmitter escape through the pore, resulting in a low-level signal (a *foot*) that precedes a large spike of transmitter release upon full fusion (see inset for illustration). During the foot the cell membrane capacitance (proportional to cell surface area) undergoes reversible step-like changes as the fusion pore opens and closes. Sometimes the reversible opening and closing is not followed by full fusion, such that transmitter is released through the fusion pore alone. (Adapted, with permission, from Neher 1993.)

release event. In the *kiss-and-run* pathway the vesicle leaves the active zone after the fusion pore closes, but is competent for rapid rerelease. Vesicles are thought to be preferentially recycled through these pathways during stimulation at low frequencies.

Stimulation at higher frequencies recruits a second, slower recycling pathway that uses clathrin to retrieve the vesicle membrane after fusion with the plasma membrane (see Figure 12–10B2). (The clathrin-coated vesicle membranes are the coated pits observed by Heuser and Reese.) In this pathway the retrieved vesicular membrane must be recycled through an endosomal compartment before the vesicles can be reused. Clathrin-mediated recycling requires up to a

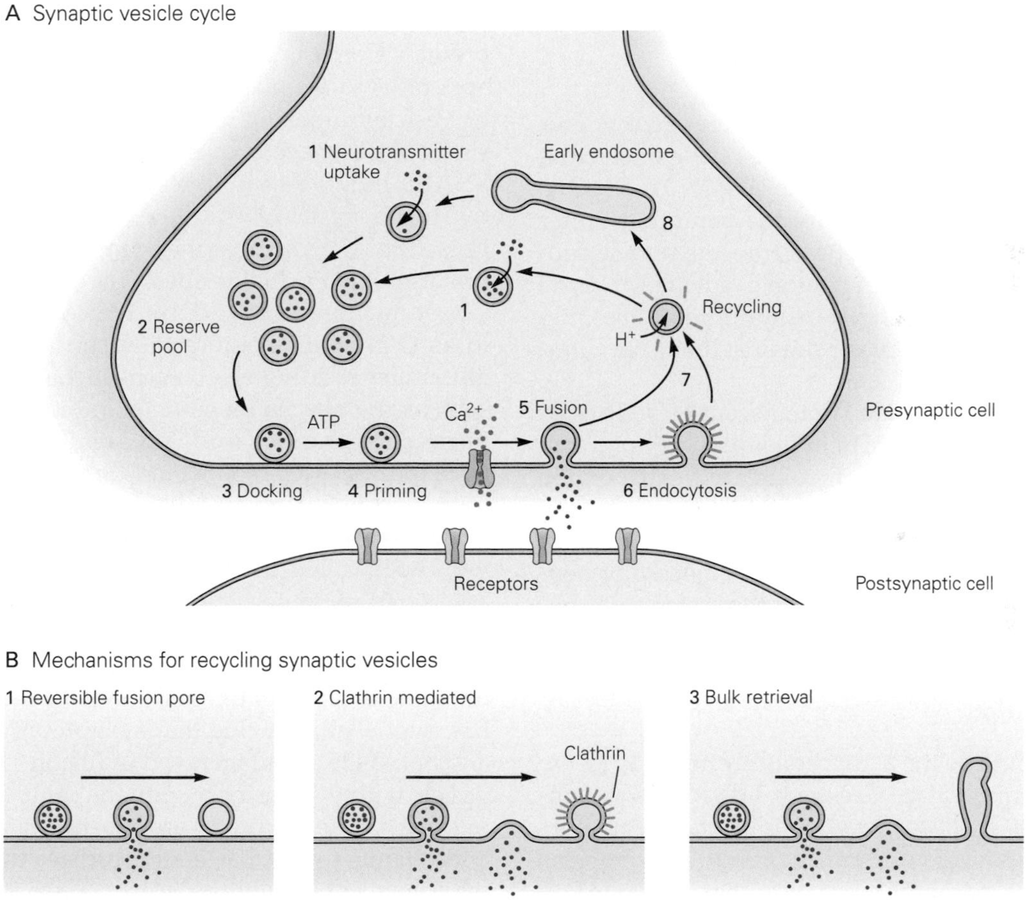

Figure 12–10 The synaptic vesicle cycle.

A. Synaptic vesicles are filled with neurotransmitters by active transport (**step 1**) and join the vesicle cluster that may represent a reserve pool (**step 2**). Filled vesicles dock at the active zone (**step 3**) where they undergo an ATP-dependent priming reaction (**step 4**) that makes them competent for calcium-triggered fusion (**step 5**). After discharging their contents, synaptic vesicles are recycled through one of several routes (see part B). In one common route, vesicle membrane is retrieved via clathrin-mediated endocytosis (**step 6**) and recycled directly (**step 7**) or by endosomes (**step 8**).

B. Retrieval of vesicles after transmitter discharge is thought to occur via three mechanisms, each with distinct kinetics. **1.** A reversible fusion pore is the most rapid mechanism for reusing vesicles. The vesicle membrane does not completely fuse with the plasma membrane and transmitter is released through the fusion pore. Vesicle retrieval requires only the closure of the fusion pore and thus can occur rapidly, in tens to hundreds of milliseconds. This pathway may predominate at lower to normal release rates. The spent vesicle may either remain at the membrane (kiss-and-stay) or relocate from the membrane to the reserve pool of vesicles (kiss-and-run). **2.** In the classical pathway excess membrane is retrieved through endocytosis by means of clathrin-coated pits. These pits are found throughout the axon terminal except at the active zones. This pathway may be important at normal to high rates of release. **3.** In the bulk retrieval pathway, excess membrane reenters the terminal by budding from uncoated pits. These uncoated cisternae are formed primarily at the active zones. This pathway may be used only after high rates of release and not during the usual functioning of the synapse. (Adapted, with permission, from Schweizer, Betz, and Augustine 1995; Südhof 2004.)

minute for completion, and appears to shift from the active zone to the membrane surrounding the active zone (see Figure 12–7).

A third mechanism operates after prolonged high-frequency stimulation. Under these conditions large membranous invaginations into the presynaptic terminal are visible, which are thought to reflect membrane recycling through a process called *bulk retrieval* (Figure 12–10B3).

Exocytosis of Synaptic Vesicles Relies on a Highly Conserved Protein Machinery

Biochemists have isolated and purified many key proteins of synaptic vesicles, as well as their interacting partners in the plasma membrane (Figure 12–11). One key class of vesicle proteins are the neurotransmitter transporters (Chapter 13). These transmembrane proteins use energy stored in a proton gradient across the vesicle membrane to pump transmitter molecules into the vesicle from the cytoplasm, against their concentration gradient.

Other synaptic vesicle proteins target vesicles to their release sites, participate in the discharge of transmitter by exocytosis, and mediate recycling of the vesicle membrane. The protein machinery involved in these three steps is conserved from worms to humans, and forms the basis for the regulated release of neurotransmitter. We consider each of these steps in turn.

The Synapsins Are Important for Vesicle Restraint and Mobilization

The vesicles outside the active zone represent a reserve pool of transmitter. Paul Greengard discovered a family of proteins, *synapsins*, that are important regulators of the reserve pool of vesicles (Figure 12–11). Synapsins are peripheral membrane proteins that are bound to the cytoplasmic surface of synaptic vesicles. They also bind adenosine triphosphate (ATP) and actin.

The synapsins are substrates for both protein kinase A and Ca^{2+}/calmodulin-dependent protein kinase I. When the nerve terminal is depolarized and Ca^{2+} enters, the synapsins become phosphorylated by the kinase and are thus released from the vesicles, a step that is thought to mobilize the reserve pool of vesicles for transmitter release. Indeed, genetic deletion of synapsins or application of a synapsin antibody leads to a decrease in the number of synaptic vesicles in the nerve terminal and a decrease in the ability of a terminal to maintain a high rate of transmitter release during repetitive stimulation.

SNARE Proteins Catalyze Fusion of Vesicles with the Plasma Membrane

Because a membrane bilayer is a stable structure, fusion of the synaptic vesicle and plasma membrane must overcome a large unfavorable activation energy. This is accomplished by a family of fusion proteins now referred to as SNAREs (soluble *N*-ethylmaleimide–sensitive factor attachment receptors) (Figure 12–12).

SNAREs are universally involved in membrane fusion, from yeast to humans. They mediate both constitutive membrane trafficking during the movement of proteins from the endoplasmic reticulum to the Golgi apparatus to the plasma membrane, as well as synaptic vesicle trafficking important for regulated exocytosis. SNAREs have a conserved protein sequence, the SNARE motif, that is 60 residues long. They come in two forms. Vesicle SNAREs or v-SNAREs (also referred to as R-SNAREs because they contain an important central arginine residue) reside in the vesicle membranes. Target-membrane SNAREs or t-SNAREs (also referred to as Q-SNAREs because they contain an important glutamine residue) are present in target membranes, such as the plasma membrane. In biochemical experiments using purified v-SNAREs and t-SNAREs in solution, four SNARE motifs bind tightly to each other to form an α-helical coiled-coil complex (Figure 12–12B).

Each synaptic vesicle contains a single type of v-SNARE called synaptobrevin (also called vesicle-associated membrane protein or VAMP). By contrast, the presynaptic active zone contains two types of t-SNARE proteins, syntaxin and SNAP-25. (Synaptobrevin and syntaxin have one SNARE motif; SNAP-25 has two.) The first clue that synaptobrevin, syntaxin, and SNAP-25 are all involved in fusion of the synaptic vesicle with the plasma membrane came from the finding that all three proteins are substrates for botulinum and tetanus toxins, bacterial proteases that are potent inhibitors of transmitter release. James Rothman then provided the crucial insight that these three proteins interact in a tight biochemical complex.

How does formation of the SNARE complex drive synaptic vesicle fusion? During exocytosis the SNARE motif of synaptobrevin, on the synaptic vesicle, forms a tight complex with the SNARE motifs of SNAP-25 and syntaxin, on the plasma membrane (Figure 12–12). The crystal structure of the SNARE complex suggests that this complex draws the membranes together. The ternary complex of synaptobrevin, syntaxin, and SNAP-25 is extraordinarily stable. The energy released in its assembly is thought to draw the negatively charged phospholipids of the vesicle and plasma membranes in close apposition, forcing them into a prefusion

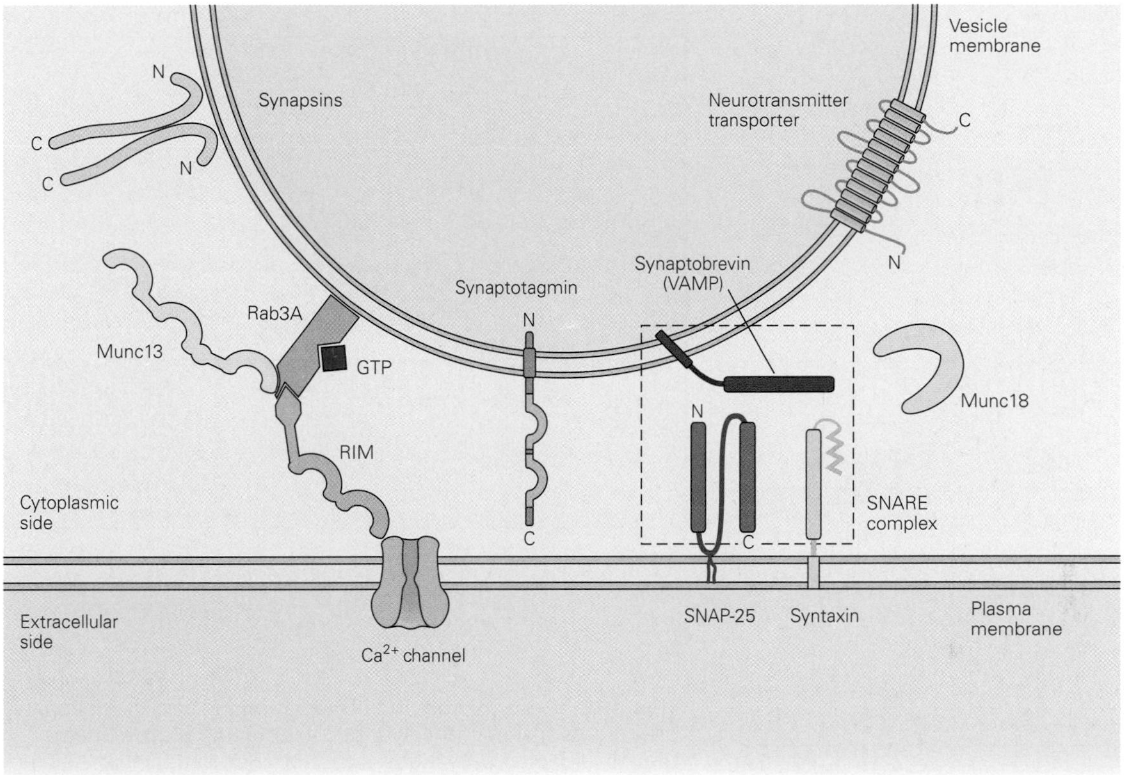

Figure 12–11 A protein network regulates synaptic vesicle exocytosis and membrane cycling. The drawing shows some of the key synaptic vesicle and plasma membrane proteins at the active zone and their interactions. Exocytosis is mediated by the formation of the SNARE complex (**dotted lines**), which results from the tight interaction between the protein synaptobrevin (or VAMP) in the vesicle membrane and the proteins syntaxin and SNAP-25 in the plasma membrane. Munc18 interacts with the SNARE complex and is essential for vesicle fusion. A second protein complex occurs when the vesicle protein Rab3 binds to the cytoplasmic proteins Munc13 and RIM. The SNARE and Rab3 complexes are functionally linked because of an interaction between syntaxin and Munc13. The syntaxin-Munc13 complex likely inhibits the formation of the SNARE complex. The vesicle protein synaptotagmin serves as the Ca^{2+} sensor for exocytosis and may also interact with RIM. Synaptic vesicles also contain membrane transporters necessary for neurotransmitter uptake. A peripheral vesicle protein, synapsin, is important in regulating the availability of vesicles from the reserve pool.

intermediate state (Figure 12–12). Such an unstable state may start the formation of the fusion pore and account for the rapid opening and closing (flickering) of the fusion pore observed in electrophysiological measurements. The SNARE proteins may form part of the fusion pore based upon studies that have shown that mutations in the transmembrane region of syntaxin alter the single-channel conductance of the fusion pore.

However, the SNAREs do not fully account for fusion of the synaptic vesicle and plasma membranes. Reconstitution experiments with purified proteins in lipid vesicles indicate that synaptobrevin, syntaxin, and SNAP-25 can catalyze fusion; but the in vitro reaction shows little regulation by Ca^{2+} and the reaction is much slower and less efficient than vesicle fusion in a real synapse. One important additional protein required for exocytosis of synaptic vesicles is Munc18 (mammalian unc18 homolog). Homologs of Munc18, referred to as SM proteins (sec1/Munc18-like proteins), are essential for intracellular fusion reactions in general. Munc18 binds to syntaxin before the SNARE complex assembles by an unknown mechanism. Deletion of Munc18 prevents all synaptic fusion in neurons. The core fusion machinery is thus composed of SNARE and SM proteins that are modulated by various accessory factors specific for particular fusion reactions.

After fusion, the SNARE complex must be disassembled for efficient vesicle recycling to occur. Rothman discovered that a cytoplasmic ATPase called NSF (*N*-ethylmaleimide-sensitive fusion protein) binds to SNARE complexes via an adaptor protein called

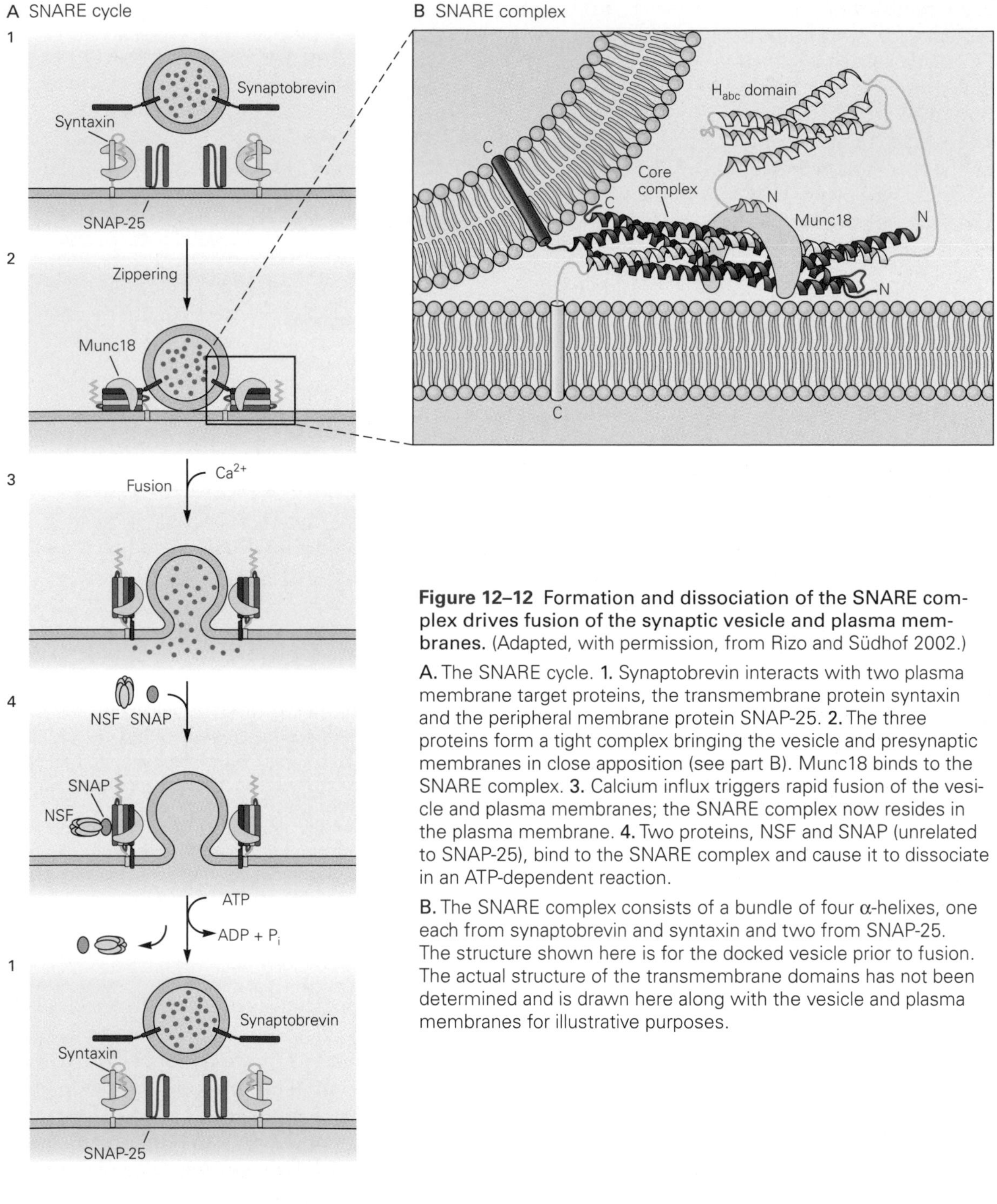

Figure 12–12 Formation and dissociation of the SNARE complex drives fusion of the synaptic vesicle and plasma membranes. (Adapted, with permission, from Rizo and Südhof 2002.)

A. The SNARE cycle. **1.** Synaptobrevin interacts with two plasma membrane target proteins, the transmembrane protein syntaxin and the peripheral membrane protein SNAP-25. **2.** The three proteins form a tight complex bringing the vesicle and presynaptic membranes in close apposition (see part B). Munc18 binds to the SNARE complex. **3.** Calcium influx triggers rapid fusion of the vesicle and plasma membranes; the SNARE complex now resides in the plasma membrane. **4.** Two proteins, NSF and SNAP (unrelated to SNAP-25), bind to the SNARE complex and cause it to dissociate in an ATP-dependent reaction.

B. The SNARE complex consists of a bundle of four α-helixes, one each from synaptobrevin and syntaxin and two from SNAP-25. The structure shown here is for the docked vesicle prior to fusion. The actual structure of the transmembrane domains has not been determined and is drawn here along with the vesicle and plasma membranes for illustrative purposes.

SNAP (soluble NSF-attachment protein, not related to the SNARE protein SNAP-25). NSF and SNAP use the energy of ATP hydrolysis to dissociate SNARE complexes, thereby regenerating free SNARE (Figure 12–12A). NSF also participates in the cycling of AMPA-type glutamate receptors in dendritic spines.

Calcium Binding to Synaptotagmin Triggers Transmitter Release

Because fusion of synaptic vesicles with the plasma membrane must occur within a fraction of a millisecond, it is thought that most proteins responsible for fusion are assembled prior to Ca^{2+} influx. According to this view, once Ca^{2+} enters the presynaptic terminal it binds a Ca^{2+} sensor on the vesicle, triggering immediate fusion of the membranes.

A family of closely related synaptic vesicle proteins, the synaptotagmins, has been identified as the major Ca^{2+} sensors that trigger fusion. The synaptotagmins are membrane proteins with a single N-terminal transmembrane region that anchors them to the synaptic vesicle (Figure 12–13A). The cytoplasmic region of each synaptotagmin protein is largely composed of two domains, the C2 domains, which are a common protein motif homologous to the Ca^{2+} and phospholipid-binding C2 domain of protein kinase C. That the C2 domains bind not only Ca^{2+} but also phospholipids is consistent with their importance in calcium-dependent exocytosis. Moreover, the synaptotagmins bind Ca^{2+} over a concentration range similar to the Ca^{2+} concentration required to trigger transmitter release.

The two C2 domains bind a total of five Ca^{2+} ions, the same number of Ca^{2+} ions that electrophysiological experiments reveal are required to trigger release of a quantum of transmitter (Figure 12–13B). The binding of the Ca^{2+} ions to synaptotagmin is thought to act as a switch, promoting the interaction of the C2 domains with phospholipids. The C2 domains of synaptotagmin also interact with SNARE proteins, through both calcium-independent and calcium-dependent reactions.

Studies with mutant mice in which synaptotagmin 1 is deleted or its Ca^{2+} affinity is altered provide further evidence that synaptotagmin is the physiological Ca^{2+} sensor. When the affinity of synaptotagmin for Ca^{2+} is decreased twofold, the Ca^{2+} required for transmitter release is changed by the same amount. When synaptotagmin 1 is deleted in mice, flies, or worms, an action potential is no longer able to trigger fast synchronous release. However, Ca^{2+} is still capable of stimulating a slow form of release referred to as asynchronous release (Figure 12–13C). Thus, although synaptotagmin 1 is not required for all forms of calcium-mediated transmitter release, it is essential for fast synaptic transmission.

The Fusion Machinery Is Embedded in a Conserved Protein Scaffold at the Active Zone

A defining feature of fast synaptic transmission is that neurotransmitter is released by exocytosis at the active zone. Other types of exocytosis, such as that which occurs in the adrenal medulla, do not require a specialized domain of the plasma membrane. The active zone is thought to coordinate and regulate the docking and priming of synaptic vesicles to ensure the speed and tight regulation of release. This is accomplished through a conserved set of proteins that form one large macromolecular structure.

An exceedingly detailed view of the structure of the active zone at the frog neuromuscular junction has been obtained by Jack MacMahan using a powerful ultrastructural technique called scanning electron microscopic tomography. This technique has shown how synaptic vesicles are tethered to the membrane by a series of electron-dense projections, termed *ribs* and *beams,* that attach to defined sites on the vesicles and to particles (*pegs*) in the presynaptic membrane that may correspond to voltage-gated Ca^{2+} channels (Figure 12–14).

A key goal in understanding how the various synaptic vesicle and active zone proteins are coordinated during exocytosis is to fit the various proteins that have been identified into this high-resolution electron micrograph. Several cytoplasmic proteins have been identified that are thought to be components of a cytoskeletal matrix at the active zone. These include two large cytoplasmic multidomain proteins, Munc13 (not related to the Munc18 protein discussed above) and RIM, which form a tight complex with each other and may well comprise part of the ribs and beams. The binding of RIM and Munc13 is an important component of the priming of synaptic vesicles for exocytosis. Phosphorylation of RIM by cAMP-dependent protein kinase is likely to be a key regulatory mechanism in the long-term enhancement of transmitter release implicated in certain forms of learning and memory. As we will see below, regulation of Munc13 by second messengers is involved in short-term forms of synaptic plasticity. RIM binds several other synaptic vesicle proteins, including the Rab3 family of low molecular weight guanosine triphosphatases (GTPases). There are four Rab3 isoforms (Rab3A, B, C, and D) that transiently associate with synaptic vesicles as the GTP–Rab3 complex (Figure 12–11). The binding of RIM and Rab3 is thought to regulate the interaction of synaptic vesicles with the active zone during the vesicle cycle.

Modulation of Transmitter Release Underlies Synaptic Plasticity

The effectiveness of chemical synapses can be modified for short and long periods, a property called *synaptic plasticity.* Such functional modification can be effected by intrinsic or extrinsic signals. An example of an intrinsic signal is rapid firing; extrinsic signals include direct synaptic input from other neurons and more diffuse actions of neuromodulators.

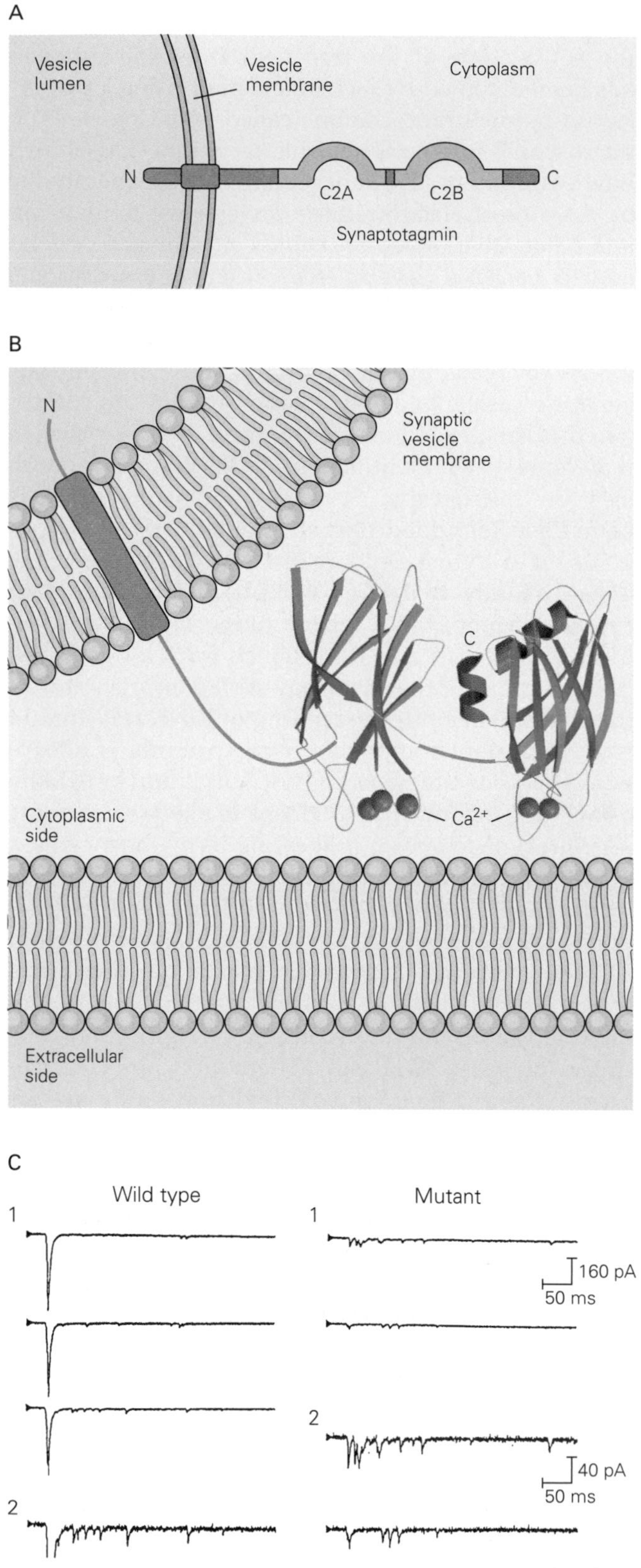

Figure 12–13 The structure of synaptotagmin and genetic evidence for its role in transmitter release.

A. Synaptotagmin is an integral membrane protein of synaptic vesicles. The short N-terminal tail, which resides in the vesicle lumen, is followed by a single hydrophobic domain that spans the vesicle membrane and a long cytoplasmic tail that contains two C2 domains (C2A and C2B) near the C terminus. The C2 domains are calcium- and phospholipid-binding motifs found in many other proteins, including PKC.

B. The X-ray crystal structure of the two C2 domains is shown here. The C2A domain binds three Ca^{2+} ions and the C2B domain two Ca^{2+} ions. The structures of the other regions of synaptotagmin have not yet been determined and are drawn here for illustrative purposes. The membrane and structures are drawn to scale.

C. Fast calcium-triggered transmitter release is absent in mutant mice lacking synaptotagmin. Recordings show excitatory postsynaptic currents evoked in vitro by stimulation of cultured hippocampal neurons from wild-type mice or mutant mice in which synaptotagmin has been deleted by homologous recombination (1). Neurons from wild-type mice show large, fast excitatory postsynaptic currents evoked by three successive presynaptic action potentials, reflecting the fact that synaptic transmission is dominated by the rapid synchronous release of transmitter from a large number of synaptic vesicles. In the bottom trace, where the synaptic current is shown at a highly expanded current scale (2), one can see that a small, prolonged phase of asynchronous release of transmitter follows the fast phase of synchronous release. During this slow phase there is a prolonged increase in frequency of individual quantal responses. In neurons from a mutant mouse a presynaptic action potential triggers only the slow asynchronous phase of release; the rapid synchronous phase has been abolished.

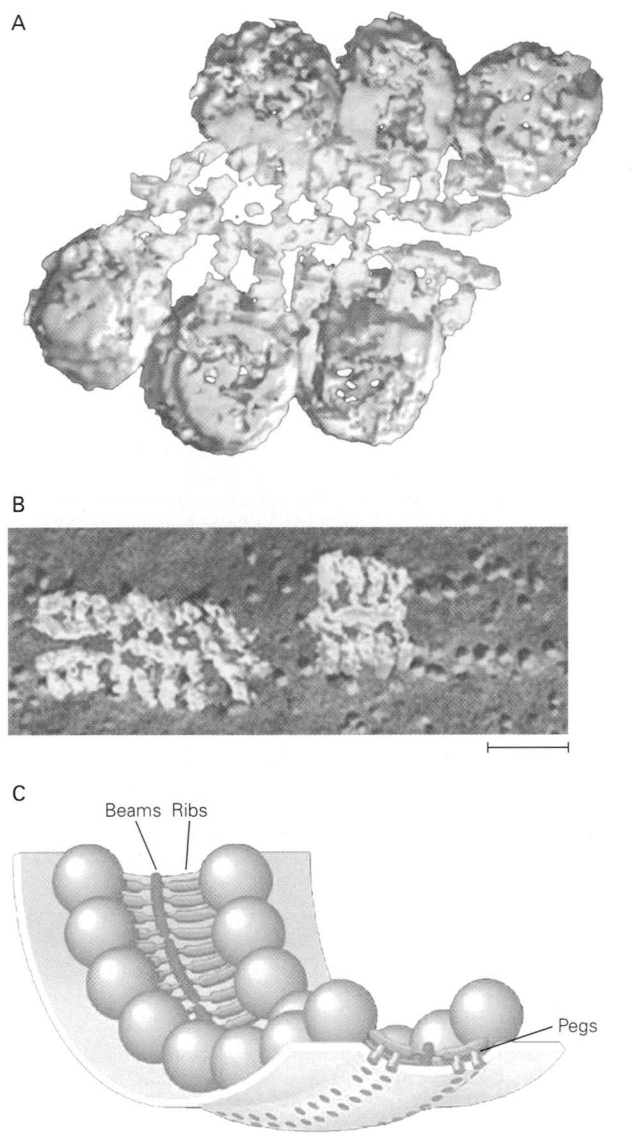

Figure 12–14 Synaptic vesicles at the active zone. The images are obtained from electron microscopic tomography. (Reproduced, with permission, from Harlow et al. 2001.)

A. Vesicles are tethered to filamentous proteins of the active zone. Three distinct filamentous structures are resolved: pegs, ribs, and beams. Ribs protruding from the vesicles are attached to long horizontal beams, which are anchored to the membrane by vertical pegs.

B. Ribs and beams superimposed on a freeze fracture view of intramembranous particles at the active zone show how the ribs are aligned with the particles, some of which are presumed to be voltage-gated Ca^{2+} channels. Scale bar = 100 nm.

C. A model for the structure of the active zone shows the relation between synaptic vesicles, pegs, ribs, and beams.

Synaptic strength can be modified presynaptically, by altering the release of neurotransmitter, or postsynaptically, by modulating the response to transmitter, or both. Long-term changes in presynaptic and postsynaptic mechanisms are crucial to development and learning (Chapters 66 and 67). Here we focus on how synaptic strength changes through modulation of the amount of transmitter released.

Transmitter release can be modulated dramatically and rapidly—by several-fold in a matter of seconds—and this change can be maintained for seconds, to hours, or even days. In principle, such changes can be mediated by two different mechanisms: changes in Ca^{2+} influx or changes in the amount of transmitter released in response to a given Ca^{2+} concentration.

Synaptic strength commonly is enhanced by intense activity. In many neurons a high-frequency train of action potentials is followed by a period during which a single action potential produces successively larger postsynaptic potentials (Figure 12–15A). High-frequency stimulation of the presynaptic neuron, which in some cells can generate 500 to 1,000 action potentials per second, is called *tetanic stimulation*. The increase in size of the EPSP during tetanic stimulation is called *potentiation*; the increase that persists after tetanic stimulation is called *post-tetanic potentiation* (Figure 12–15A). This enhancement usually lasts several minutes, but it can persist for an hour or more at some synapses. The opposite effect, a decrease in the size of postsynaptic potentials, occurs in response to more prolonged periods of high-frequency stimulation. This effect is referred to as synaptic *depression* (Figure 12–15B).

Activity-Dependent Changes in Intracellular Free Calcium Can Produce Long-Lasting Changes in Release

Because transmitter release depends strongly on the intracellular Ca^{2+} concentration, mechanisms that affect the concentration of free Ca^{2+} in the presynaptic terminal also affect the amount of transmitter released. Normally the rise in Ca^{2+} in the presynaptic terminal in response to an action potential is rapidly buffered by cytoplasmic calcium-binding proteins and mitochondria; Ca^{2+} is also actively transported out of the neuron by pumps and transporters.

However, during tetanic stimulation so much Ca^{2+} flows into the axon terminals that the Ca^{2+} buffering and clearance systems become saturated. This leads to a temporary excess of Ca^{2+}, called *residual* Ca^{2+}. The residual free Ca^{2+} enhances synaptic transmission for many minutes or longer by activating certain enzymes

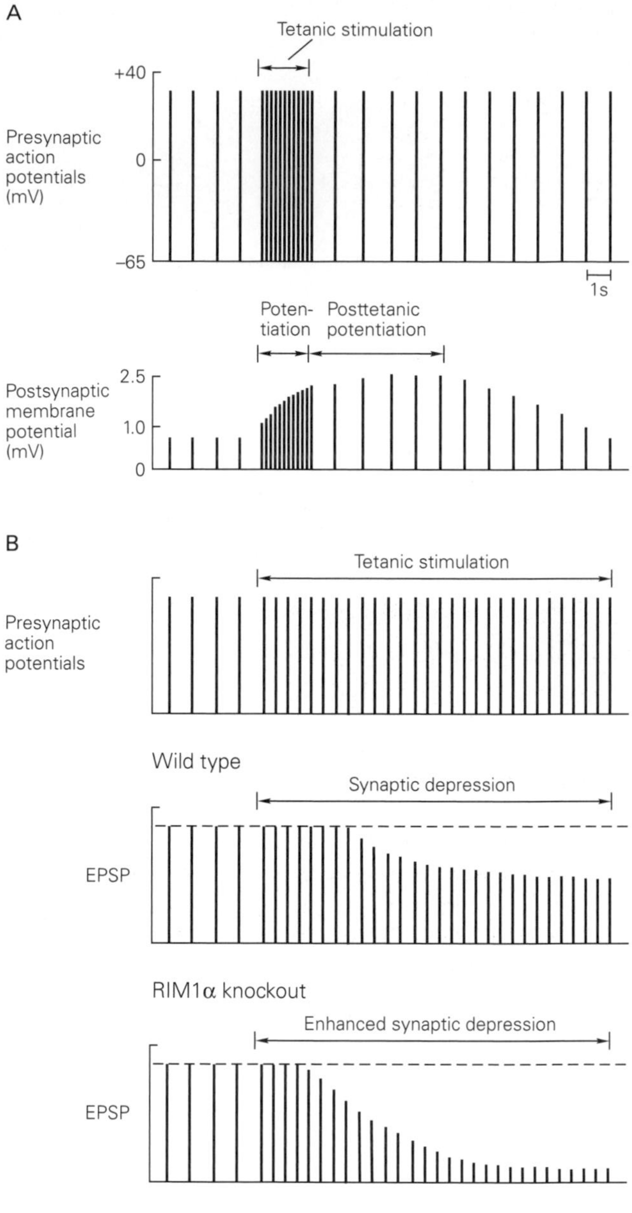

Figure 12–15 Repetitive presynaptic firing produces persistent changes in transmitter release.

A. A brief burst of high-frequency stimulation leads to a sustained enhancement in transmitter release. The time scale of the experimental records here has been compressed (each presynaptic and postsynaptic potential appears as a simple line indicating its amplitude). A stable excitatory postsynaptic potential (EPSP) of around one mV is produced when the presynaptic neuron is stimulated at a relatively low rate of one action potential per second. The presynaptic neuron is then stimulated for a few seconds at a higher rate of 50 action potentials per second. During this *tetanic stimulation* the EPSP increases in size because of enhanced release, a phenomenon known as *potentiation.* After several seconds of stimulation, the presynaptic neuron is returned to the initial rate of stimulation (1 per second). However, the EPSPs remain enhanced for minutes, and in some cells for several hours. This persistent increase is called *posttetanic potentiation.*

B. Prolonged tetanic stimulation can decrease the amplitude of the EPSP, a phenomenon called *synaptic depression.* In this example the presynaptic neuron produces a stable postsynaptic response of 1 mV when stimulated at a rate of 1 action potential per second. When the rate of stimulation is increased to 15 action potentials per second, the EPSP eventually declines in amplitude. This synaptic depression is thought to result from the temporary depletion of the store of releasable synaptic vesicles. Deletion of the active zone protein RIM1α enhances synaptic depression. (Adapted, with permission, from Schoch et al. 2002.)

that are sensitive to enhanced levels of resting Ca^{2+}, such as, the Ca^{2+}/calmodulin-dependent protein kinase. Activation of such calcium-dependent enzymatic pathways is thought to increase the priming of synaptic vesicles in the terminals.

Here then is the simplest kind of cellular memory! The presynaptic cell stores information about the history of its activity in the form of residual Ca^{2+} in its terminals. This Ca^{2+} acts by multiple pathways that have different halftimes of decay. In Chapters 66 and 67 we shall see how posttetanic potentiation at certain synapses is followed by an even longer-lasting process (also initiated by Ca^{2+} influx), called *long-term potentiation,* which can last for many hours or even days.

During prolonged tetanic stimulation synaptic vesicles become depleted at the active zone, resulting in synaptic depression. To counteract this depression, the synapse utilizes multiple mechanisms that often involve a complex of two of the active zone proteins discussed above, Munc13 and RIM. For example, prolonged tetanic stimulation activates phospholipase C, which produces inositol 1,4,5-trisphosphate (IP_3) and diacylglycerol. Diacylglycerol directly interacts with a protein domain on Munc13 called the C1 domain (no relation to the C2 domain) homologous to the diacylglycerol-binding domain in protein kinase C. Binding of diacylglycerol to Munc13 during prolonged repetitive stimulation helps maintain a high rate of transmitter release even in the face of depression by accelerating the rate of synaptic vesicle recycling. As a result, deletion of Munc13 or RIM results, among other actions, in an enhancement in depression (Figure 12–15B).

Axo-axonic Synapses on Presynaptic Terminals Regulate Transmitter Release

Synapses are formed on axon terminals as well as the cell body and dendrites of neurons (see Chapter 10). Although axosomatic synaptic actions affect all branches of the postsynaptic neuron's axon (because they affect the probability that the neuron will fire an action potential), axo-axonic actions selectively control individual terminals of the axon. One important action of axo-axonic synapses is to increase or decrease Ca^{2+} influx into the presynaptic terminals of the postsynaptic cell, thereby enhancing or depressing transmitter release, respectively.

As we saw in Chapter 10, when one neuron releases transmitter that hyperpolarizes the cell body (or dendrites) of another, it decreases the likelihood that the postsynaptic cell will fire; this action is called *postsynaptic inhibition.* In contrast, when a neuron makes synapses onto the axon terminal of another cell, it can reduce the amount of transmitter that will be released by the postsynaptic cell onto a third cell; this action is called *presynaptic inhibition* (Figure 12–16A). Other axo-axonic synaptic actions can increase the amount of transmitter released by the postsynaptic cell; this action is called *presynaptic facilitation* (Figure 12–16B). Both presynaptic inhibition and facilitation can occur in response to activation of ionotropic or metabotropic receptors in the membrane of the presynaptic terminals. For reasons that are not well understood, presynaptic modulation usually occurs early in sensory pathways.

The best-analyzed mechanisms of presynaptic inhibition and facilitation are in invertebrate neurons and vertebrate mechanoreceptor neurons (whose cell bodies lie in dorsal root ganglia). Three mechanisms for presynaptic inhibition have been identified in these cells. One mechanism depends on the activation of ionotropic GABA receptor-channels in the presynaptic terminal. The opening of these channels leads to an increased conductance to Cl^-, which decreases (or short-circuits) the amplitude of the action potential in the presynaptic terminal. The smaller depolarization activates fewer Ca^{2+} channels, thereby decreasing transmitter release.

The other two mechanisms both result from the activation of presynaptic G protein-coupled metabotropic receptors. One type of action results from the modulation of ion channels. As we saw in Chapter 11, the βγ-subunit complex of G proteins can simultaneously close voltage-gated Ca^{2+} channels and open K^+ channels. This decreases the influx of Ca^{2+} and enhances repolarization of the presynaptic terminal, thus diminishing transmitter release. The second type of G protein-dependent action depends on a direct action by the βγ-subunit complex on the release machinery itself, independent of any changes in ion channel activity or Ca^{2+} influx. This second action is thought to involve a decrease in the Ca^{2+} sensitivity of the release machinery.

In contrast, presynaptic facilitation can be caused by enhanced influx of Ca^{2+}. In certain molluscan neurons serotonin acts through cAMP-dependent protein phosphorylation to close K^+ channels in the presynaptic terminal (including the *Aplysia* S-type K^+ channel discussed in Chapter 11). This action increases the duration of the presynaptic action potential, thereby increasing Ca^{2+} influx by enabling the voltage-dependent Ca^{2+} channels to remain open for a longer period. In other cells activation of presynaptic ionotropic receptors increases transmitter release. This facilitation can be caused directly in the case of Ca^{2+}-permeable receptor-channels by directly enhancing Ca^{2+} influx, or indirectly in the case of voltage-gated Ca^{2+} channels through depolarization of the presynaptic terminal, which leads to increased Ca^{2+} influx.

Thus, presynaptic terminals are endowed with a variety of mechanisms that allow for the fine-tuning of the strength of synaptic transmission. Although we know a fair amount about short-term changes in synaptic strength—changes that last minutes and hours—we are only beginning to learn about mechanisms that support changes that persist for days, weeks, and longer. These long-term changes often require alterations in gene expression and growth of presynaptic and postsynaptic structures in addition to alterations in Ca^{2+} influx and enhancement of transmitter release from existing terminals.

An Overall View

In his book *Ionic Channels of Excitable Membranes,* Bertil Hille summarizes the importance of calcium in neuronal function as follows:

> Electricity is used to gate channels and channels are used to make electricity. However, the nervous system is not primarily an electrical device. Most excitable cells ultimately translate their electrical excitation into another form of activity. As a broad generalization, excitable cells translate their electricity into action by Ca^{2+} fluxes modulated by voltage-sensitive Ca^{2+} channels. Calcium ions are intracellular messengers capable of activating many cell functions. Calcium channels… serve as the only link to transduce depolarization into all the nonelectrical activities controlled by excitation. Without Ca^{2+} channels our nervous system would have no outputs.

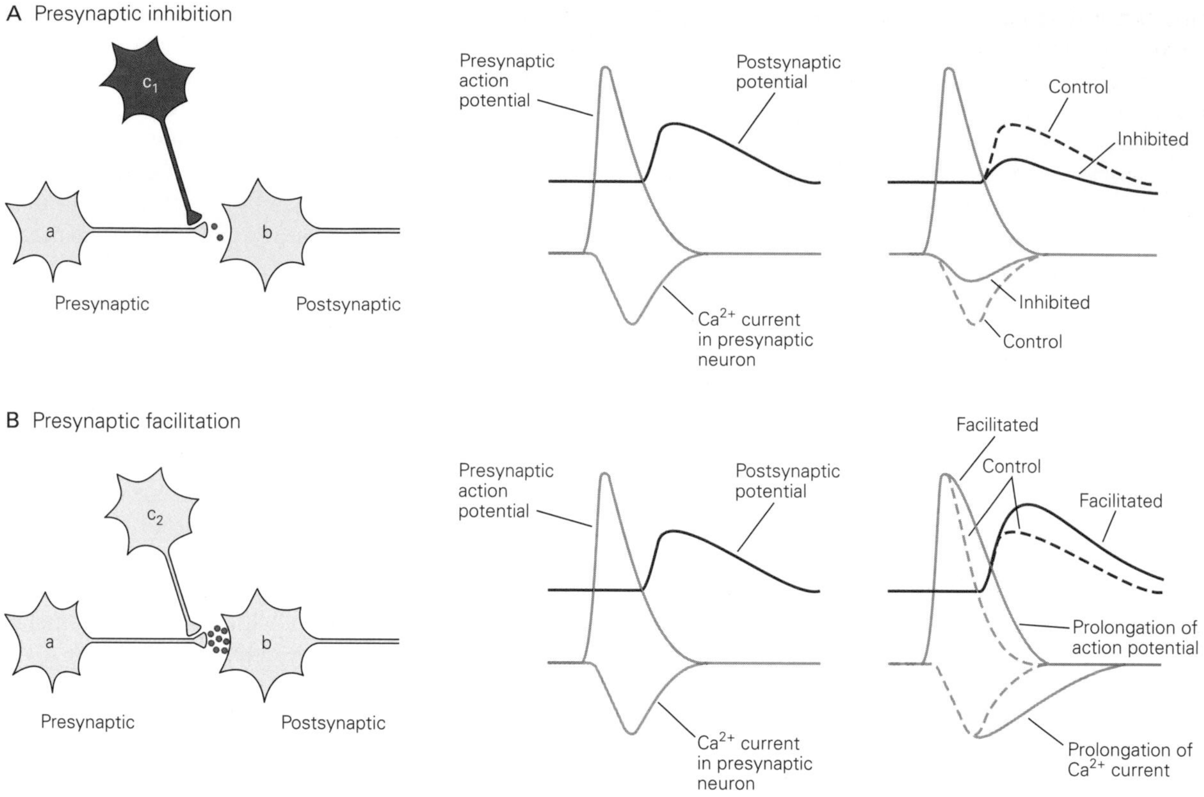

Figure 12–16 Axoaxonic synapses can inhibit or facilitate transmitter release by the presynaptic cell.

A. An inhibitory neuron (c_1) forms a synapse on the axon terminal of neuron a. Release of transmitter by cell c_1 activates a metabotropic receptor on the terminals of cell a, which inhibits the Ca^{2+} current in these terminals, thereby reducing the amount of transmitter released by cell a onto cell b. The reduction of transmitter release from cell a in turn reduces the amplitude of the excitatory postsynaptic potential in cell b, a process termed presynaptic inhibition.

B. A facilitating neuron (c_2) forms a synapse on the axon terminal of neuron a. Release of transmitter by cell c_2 activates a metabotropic receptor on the terminals of cell a, which decreases a K^+ current in the terminals, thereby prolonging the action potential and increasing Ca^{2+} influx into cell a. This increases transmitter release from cell a onto cell b, thereby increasing the size of the EPSP in cell b, a process termed presynaptic facilitation.

Neither Na^+ influx nor K^+ efflux is required to release neurotransmitter at a synapse. Only Ca^{2+}, which enters the cell through voltage-gated channels in the presynaptic terminal, is essential. Synaptic delay—the time between the onset of the action potential and the release of transmitter—largely reflects the time it takes for voltage-gated Ca^{2+} channels to open and for Ca^{2+} to trigger the discharge of transmitter from synaptic vesicles.

Transmitter is packaged in vesicles that each contain approximately 5,000 transmitter molecules. The all-or-none release of transmitter from a single vesicle results in a quantal synaptic potential. Synaptic potentials evoked by nerve stimulation are comprised of integral multiples of the quantal potential caused by the release of transmitter from multiple synaptic vesicles. Increasing the extracellular Ca^{2+} does not change the size of the quantal synaptic potential. Rather, it increases the probability that a vesicle will discharge its transmitter. As a result, the number of vesicles that release transmitter is increased, leading to a larger postsynaptic potential. In addition, transmitter is spontaneously released at low rates from synaptic vesicles, producing what are called *spontaneous miniature synaptic potentials.*

Electron microscopic images of presynaptic terminals that have been rapidly frozen following electrical stimulation reveal that synaptic vesicles release transmitter by exocytosis. The vesicle membrane fuses with the plasma membrane in the vicinity of the active zone, allowing the transmitter to flow out of the cell toward receptors on a postsynaptic cell. A conserved protein machinery mediates the exocytosis and rapid retrieval of synaptic vesicles that allows nerve terminals to maintain a high rate of transmitter release, even during prolonged trains of action potentials.

Vesicle fusion is thought to be catalyzed by the assembly of a synaptic vesicle SNARE protein (v-SNARE) with a pair of SNARE proteins in the presynaptic target membrane (t-SNARES) into a tight complex that forces the synaptic vesicle and plasma membrane into close proximity. Two other proteins, Munc13 and Munc18, are essential for synaptic vesicle fusion, probably because they enable SNARE complex assembly. Calcium triggers the opening of the vesicles during a late step in the synaptic vesicle cycle by binding to synaptotagmin, a synaptic vesicle protein that serves as the major Ca^{2+} sensor in exocytosis. The machinery that executes fusion and Ca^{2+} triggering is embedded in the active zone by a conserved protein scaffold that also regulates transmitter release. A critical component of this scaffold is a large multidomain protein called RIM that binds to Rab3, a GTP-binding protein on synaptic vesicles, and also interacts with Munc13.

The amount of transmitter released from a neuron is not fixed but can be modified by both intrinsic and extrinsic modulatory processes. High-frequency stimulation produces an increase in transmitter release called posttetanic potentiation. This potentiation, which lasts a few minutes, is caused by an action of the residual Ca^{2+} remaining in the terminal after the large Ca^{2+} signal that occurs during the train of action potentials has been largely dissipated by diffusion, buffering, and extrusion. Neurotransmitters acting at axo-axonic synapses can facilitate or inhibit release of transmitter by altering the steady-state level of resting Ca^{2+}, the Ca^{2+} influx during the action potential, or the functioning of the release machinery.

Steven A. Siegelbaum
Eric R. Kandel
Thomas C. Südhof

Selected Readings

Katz B. 1969. *The Release of Neural Transmitter Substances.* Springfield, IL: Thomas.

Lonart G. 2002. RIM1: an edge for presynaptic plasticity. Trends Neurosci 25:329–332.

Meinrenken CJ, Borst JG, Sakmann B. 2003. Local routes revisited: the space and time dependence of the Ca^{2+} signal for phasic transmitter release at the rat calyx of Held. J Physiol 547:665–689.

Reid CA, Bekkers JM, Clements JD. 2003. Presynaptic Ca^{2+} channels: a functional patchwork. Trends Neurosci 26:683–687.

Stevens CF. 2003. Neurotransmitter release at central synapses. Neuron 40:381–388.

Südhof TC. 2004. The synaptic vesicle cycle. Annu Rev Neurosci 27:509–547.

References

Akert K, Moor H, Pfenninger K. 1971. Synaptic fine structure. Adv Cytopharmacol 1:273–290.

Baker PF, Hodgkin AL, Ridgway EB. 1971. Depolarization and calcium entry in squid giant axons. J Physiol 218: 709–755.

Bollmann JH, Sakmann B, Gerard J, Borst G. 2000. Calcium sensitivity of glutamate release in a calyx-type terminal. Science 289:953–957.

Borst JG, Sakmann B. 1996. Calcium influx and transmitter release in a fast CNS synapse. Nature 383:431–434.

Boyd IA, Martin AR. 1956. The end-plate potential in mammalian muscle. J Physiol 132:74–91.

Couteaux R, Pecot-Dechavassine M. 1970. Vésicules synaptiques et poches au niveau des "zones actives" de la jonction neuromusculaire. C R Acad Sci Hebd Seances Acad Sci D 271:2346–2349.

Del Castillo J, Katz B. 1954. The effect of magnesium on the activity of motor nerve endings. J Physiol 124:553–559.

Enoki R, Hu YL, Hamilton D, Fine A. 2009. Expression of long-term plasticity at individual synapses in hippocampus is graded, bidirectional, and mainly presynaptic: optical quantal analysis. Neuron 62:242–53.

Fatt P, Katz B. 1952. Spontaneous subthreshold activity at motor nerve endings. J Physiol 117:109–128.

Fawcett DW. 1981. *The Cell,* 2nd ed. Philadelphia: Saunders.

Fernandez JM, Neher E, Gomperts BD. 1984. Capacitance measurements reveal stepwise fusion events in degranulating mast cells. Nature 312:453–455.

Fernandez-Chacon R, Konigstorfer A, Gerber SH, Garcia J, Matos MF, Stevens CF, Brose N, Rizo J, Rosenmund C, Südhof TC. 2001. Synaptotagmin I functions as a calcium regulator of release probability. Nature 410:41–49.

Geppert M, Goda Y, Hammer RE, Li C, Rosahl TW, Stevens CF, Südhof TC. 1994. Synaptotagmin I. A major Ca^{2+} sensor for transmitter release at a central synapse. Cell 79:717–727.

Harlow LH, Ress D, Stoschek A, Marshall RM, McMahan UJ. 2001. The architecture of active zone material at the frog's neuromuscular junction. Nature 409:479–484.

Heuser JE, Reese TS. 1981. Structural changes in transmitter release at the frog neuromuscular junction. J Cell Biol 88:564–580.

Hille B. 2001. *Ionic Channels of Excitable Membranes,* 3rd ed. Sunderland, MA: Sinauer.

Kandel ER. 1981. Calcium and the control of synaptic strength by learning. Nature 293:697–700.

Katz B, Miledi R. 1967a. The study of synaptic transmission in the absence of nerve impulses. J Physiol 192:407–436.

Katz B, Miledi R. 1967b. The timing of calcium action during neuromuscular transmission. J Physiol 189:535–544.

Klein M, Shapiro E, Kandel ER. 1980. Synaptic plasticity and the modulation of the Ca^{2+} current. J Exp Biol 89:117–157.

Kretz R, Shapiro E, Connor J, Kandel ER. 1984. Post-tetanic potentiation, presynaptic inhibition, and the modulation of the free Ca^{2+} level in the presynaptic terminals. Exp Brain Res Suppl 9:240–283.

Kuffler SW, Nicholls JG, Martin AR. 1984. *From Neuron to Brain: A Cellular Approach to the Function of the Nervous System,* 2nd ed. Sunderland, MA: Sinauer.

Lawson D, Raff MC, Gomperts B, Fewtrell C, Gilula NB. 1977. Molecular events during membrane fusion. A study of exocytosis in rat peritoneal mast cells. Cell Biol 72: 242–259.

Liley AW. 1956. The quantal components of the mammalian end-plate potential. J Physiol 133:571–587.

Llinás RR. 1982. Calcium in synaptic transmission. Sci Am 247:56–65.

Llinás RR, Heuser JE. 1977. Depolarization-release coupling systems in neurons. Neurosci Res Program Bull 15:555–687.

Llinás R, Steinberg IZ, Walton K. 1981. Relationship between presynaptic calcium current and postsynaptic potential in squid giant synapse. Biophys J 33:323–351.

Lynch G, Halpain S, Baudry M. 1982. Effects of high-frequency synaptic stimulation on glumate receptor binding studied with a modified in vitro hippocampal slice preparation. Brain Res 244:101–111.

Magee JC, Johnston D. 1997. A synaptically controlled, associative signal for Hebbian plasticity in hippocampal neurons. Science 275:209–213.

Magnus CJ, Lee PH, Atasoy D, Su HH, Looger LL, Sternson SM. 2011. Chemical and genetic engineering of selective ion channel-ligand interactions. Science 333:1292–1296.

Martin AR. 1977. Junctional transmission. II. Presynaptic mechanisms. In: ER Kandel (ed). *Handbook of Physiology: A Critical, Comprehensive Presentation of Physiological Knowledge and Concepts,* Sect. 1 *The Nervous System,* Vol. 1 *Cellular Biology of Neurons,* Part 1, pp. 329–355. Bethesda, MD: American Physiological Society.

Monck JR, Fernandez JM. 1992. The exocytotic fusion pore. J Cell Biol 119:1395–1404.

Neher E. 1993. Cell physiology. Secretion without full fusion. Nature 363:497–498.

Nicoll RA. 1982. Neurotransmitters can say more than just "yes" or "no." Trends Neurosci 5:369–374.

Park M, Penick EC, Edwards JG, Kauer JA, Ehlers MD. 2004. Recycling endosomes supply AMPA receptors for LTP. Science 305:1972–1975.

Peters A, Palay SL, Webster H deF. 1991. *The Fine Structure of the Nervous System: Neurons and Supporting Cells,* 3rd ed. Philadelphia: Saunders.

Redman S. 1990. Quantal analysis of synaptic potentials in neurons of the central nervous system. Physiol Rev 70:165–198.

Rhee JS, Betz A, Pyott S, Reim K, Varoqueaux F, Augustin I, Hesse D, et al. 2002. Beta phorbol ester- and diacylglycerol-induced augmentation of transmitter release is mediated by Munc13s and not by PKCs. Cell 108:121–133.

Rizo J, Südhof TC. 2002. Snares and Munc18 in synaptic vesicle fusion. Nat Rev Neurosci 3:641–653.

Robitaille R, Adler EM, Charlton MP. 1990. Strategic location of calcium channels at transmitter release sites of frog neuromuscular synapses. Neuron 5:773–779.

Schneggenburger R, Neher E. 2000. Intracellular calcium dependence of transmitter release rates at a fast central synapse. Nature 406:889–893.

Schoch S, Castillo PE, Jo T, Mukherjee K, Geppert M, Wang Y, Schmitz F, Malenka RC, Südhof TC. 2002. RIM1alpha forms a protein scaffold for regulating neurotransmitter release at the active zone. Nature 415:321–326.

Schoch S, Deak F, Konigstorfer A, Mozhayeva M, Sara Y, Südhof TC, Kavalali ET. 2001. SNARE function analyzed in synaptobrevin/VAMP knockout mice. Science 294:1117–1122.

Schweizer FE, Betz H, Augustine GJ. 1995. From vesicle docking to endocytosis: intermediate reactions of exocytosis. Neuron 14:689–696.

Smith SJ, Augustine GJ, Charlton MP. 1985. Transmission at voltage-clamped giant synapse of the squid: evidence for cooperativity of presynaptic calcium action. Proc Natl Acad Sci U S A 82:622–625.

Söllner T, Whiteheart SW, Brunner M, Erdjument-Bromage H, Geromanos S, Tempest P, Rothman JE. 1993. SNAP receptors implicated in vesicle targeting and fusion. Nature 362:318–324.

Spruce AE, Breckenridge LJ, Lee AK, Almers W. 1990. Properties of the fusion pore that forms during exocytosis of a mast cell secretory vesicle. Neuron 4:643–654.

Sun JY, Wu LG. 2001. Fast kinetics of exocytosis revealed by simultaneous measurements of presynaptic capacitance and postsynaptic currents at a central synapse. Neuron 30:171–182.

Sun JY, Wu XS, Wu LG. 2002. Single and multiple vesicle fusion induce different rates of endocytosis at a central synapse. Nature 417:555–559.

Sutton RB, Fasshauer D, Jahn R, Brunger AT. 1998. Crystal structure of a SNARE complex involved in synaptic exocytosis at 2.4 A resolution. Nature 395(6700):347–353.

von Gersdorff H, Matthews G. 1994. Dynamics of synaptic vesicle fusion and membrane retrieval in synaptic terminals. Nature 367:735–739.

Wachman ES, Poage RE, Stiles JR, Farkas DL, Meriney SD. 2004. Spatial distribution of calcium entry evoked by single action potentials within the presynaptic active zone. J Neurosci 24:2877–2885.

Wernig A. 1972. Changes in statistical parameters during facilitation at the crayfish neuromuscular junction. J Physiol 226:751–759.

Zenisek D, Horst NK, Merrifield C, Sterling P, Matthews G. 2004. Visualizing synaptic ribbons in the living cell. J Neurosci 24:9752–9759.

Zucker RS. 1973. Changes in the statistics of transmitter release during facilitation. J Physiol 229:787–810.

13

Neurotransmitters

CHEMICAL SYNAPTIC TRANSMISSION can be divided into four steps—(1) synthesis and storage of a transmitter substance, (2) release of the transmitter, (3) interaction of the transmitter with receptors at the postsynaptic membrane, and (4) removal of the transmitter from the synaptic cleft. In the previous chapter we considered steps 2 and 3: the release of transmitters and how they interact with postsynaptic receptors. We now turn to the initial and final steps of chemical synaptic transmission: the synthesis of transmitter molecules and their removal from the synaptic cleft after synaptic action.

A Chemical Messenger Must Meet Four Criteria to Be Considered a Neurotransmitter

Before considering the biochemical processes involved in synaptic transmission, it is important to make clear what is meant by a chemical transmitter. The concept is empirical rather than logical and has changed over the years with increased understanding of synaptic transmission.

The concept that nerve stimulation led to release of chemical signals was elaborated as early as 1905 by the physiologist John Newport Langley, who demonstrated that adrenomedullary extracts elicited tissue responses comparable to sympathetic nerve stimulation. However, Thomas Renton Elliott is generally credited with the first experimental evidence of chemical neurotransmission in his observations that the physiological effects of sympathetic nerve stimulation were due to release of adrenaline. In 1921 Otto Loewi demonstrated the release of acetylcholine (ACh) from vagus nerve terminals in frog hearts. Henry Dale extended Loewi's work on ACh, later sharing the Nobel Prize with Loewi. In 1946 Ulf von Euler reported further work on adrenergic transmission. The terms *cholinergic* and *adrenergic* were introduced to indicate that a neuron makes and releases ACh or norepinephrine (or epinephrine), the two substances first recognized as neurotransmitters.

Since that time many other substances have been identified as transmitters. Furthermore, because of the work of Bernard Katz in the 1950s on quantal release (see Chapter 12), it is usually taken for granted that substances acting as transmitters are stored in vesicles at synapses and released by exocytosis. Nevertheless some substances considered to be neurotransmitters are released into the synaptic cleft directly from the cytoplasm as well as by exocytosis. Thus ideas about neurotransmitters have had to be modified continually to accommodate new information about the cell biology of neurons and the pharmacology of receptors.

As a first approximation, a neurotransmitter can be defined as a substance that is released by a neuron and that affects a specific target in a specific manner. A target can be either another neuron or an effector organ, such as muscle or gland. As with many other operational concepts in biology, the concept of a transmitter is not precise. Neurotransmitters are protean, resembling other released agents in many regards yet also differing from them depending on the site of action and circumstances. Although the actions of hormones and neurotransmitters are quite similar, neurotransmitters usually act on targets that are close to the site of transmitter release, whereas hormones are released into the bloodstream to act on distant targets.

Neurotransmitters differ from autacoids in that a transmitter typically acts on a target other than the releasing neuron itself, whereas an autacoid acts only on the cell from which it was released. Nevertheless, at some synapses transmitters activate not only receptors in the postsynaptic cell but also autoreceptors on the presynaptic terminal. Autoreceptors usually modulate synaptic transmission that is in progress, for example, by limiting further release of transmitter or inhibiting subsequent transmitter synthesis. Receptors can also exist on presynaptic terminals at axo-axonic synapses, where the presynaptic terminal receives synaptic input from another neuron. These receptors function as heteroreceptors that regulate terminal excitability and transmitter release (see Chapter 12).

Importantly, the interaction of neurotransmitters with receptors is typically transient, lasting from milliseconds to minutes. Nevertheless, neurotransmitter action can result in long-term changes within target cells lasting hours or days. Lastly, increasing evidence suggests that a non-neural cell, the astrocyte, can also synthesize, store, and release neurotransmitters as well as express receptors that modulate astrocyte function.

Despite these difficulties in arriving at a strict definition, a limited number of substances of low molecular weight are generally accepted as neurotransmitters. Even so, it is often difficult to demonstrate that a specific transmitter operates at a particular synapse, particularly given the diffusibility and rapid reuptake or degradation of transmitters at the synaptic cleft. Because of this difficulty, many neurobiologists believe that a substance should not be accepted as a neurotransmitter unless the following four criteria are met:

1. It is synthesized in the presynaptic neuron.
2. It is present in the presynaptic terminal and is released in amounts sufficient to exert a defined action on the postsynaptic neuron or effector organ.
3. When administered exogenously in reasonable concentrations it mimics the action of the endogenous transmitter (for example, it activates the same ion channels or second-messenger pathway in the postsynaptic cell).
4. A specific mechanism usually exists for removing the substance from the synaptic cleft.

The nervous system makes use of two main classes of chemical substances for signaling: small-molecule transmitters and neuroactive peptides, which are short polymers of amino acids. Both classes of neurotransmitters are contained in vesicles, large and small. Neuropeptides are packaged in large dense-core vesicles (approximately 70–250 nm in diameter), which release their contents by exocytosis, similar to those seen in secretory glands and mast cells. Small-molecule transmitters are packaged in small electron-lucent vesicles (~40 nm in diameter), which release their contents through exocytosis at active zones closely associated with specific Ca^{2+} channels (see Chapter 12). Large dense-core vesicles can contain both small-molecule transmitters and neuropeptides.

Both types of vesicles are found in most neurons but in different proportions. Small synaptic vesicles are characteristic of neurons that use ACh, glutamate, γ-aminobutyric acid (GABA), and glycine as transmitters, whereas large dense-core vesicles are typical of neurons that use catecholamines and serotonin as transmitters. The adrenal medulla, once used as a model for studying exocytosis, contains only secretory granules that are similar to large dense-core vesicles. Because dense-core vesicles can contain both small-molecule transmitters and neuropeptides, they are important in co-transmission, which is discussed later in this chapter.

Only a Few Small-Molecule Substances Act as Transmitters

A relatively small number of low-molecular-weight substances are generally accepted as neurotransmitters, including ACh, amino acids or their amine-containing derivatives, adenosine triphosphate (ATP), and ATP

Table 13–1 Small-Molecule Transmitter Substances and Their Precursors

Transmitter	Precursor
Acetylcholine	Choline
Biogenic amines	
Dopamine	Tyrosine
Norepinephrine	Tyrosine
Epinephrine	Tyrosine
Serotonin	Tryptophan
Histamine	Histidine
Melatonin	Serotonin
Amino acids	
Aspartate	Oxaloacetate
γ-Aminobutyric acid	Glutamine
Glutamate	Glutamine
Glycine	Serine
ATP	ADP
Adenosine	ATP
Arachidonic acid	Phospholipids
Carbon monoxide	Heme
Nitric oxide	Arginine

metabolites (Table 13–1). The amine chemical messengers share many biochemical similarities. All are charged small molecules that are formed in relatively short biosynthetic pathways and synthesized either from essential amino acids or from precursors derived from the major carbohydrate substrates of intermediary metabolism. Like other pathways of intermediary metabolism, synthesis of these neurotransmitters is catalyzed by enzymes that, almost without exception, are cytosolic. ATP, which originates in mitochondria, is abundantly present throughout the cell.

As in any biosynthetic pathway, the overall synthesis of amine transmitters typically is regulated at one rate-limiting enzymatic reaction. The rate-limiting step often is characteristic of one type of neuron and usually is absent in other types of mature neurons.

Acetylcholine

Acetylcholine is the only low-molecular-weight amine transmitter substance that is not an amino acid or derived directly from one. The biosynthetic pathway for ACh has only one enzymatic reaction, catalyzed by choline acetyltransferase (step 1 in the reaction shown below). This transferase is the characteristic and limiting enzyme in ACh biosynthesis. Nervous tissue cannot synthesize choline, which is derived from the diet and delivered to neurons through the blood stream. The co-substrate, acetyl coenzyme A (acetyl CoA), participates in many general metabolic pathways and is not restricted to cholinergic neurons.

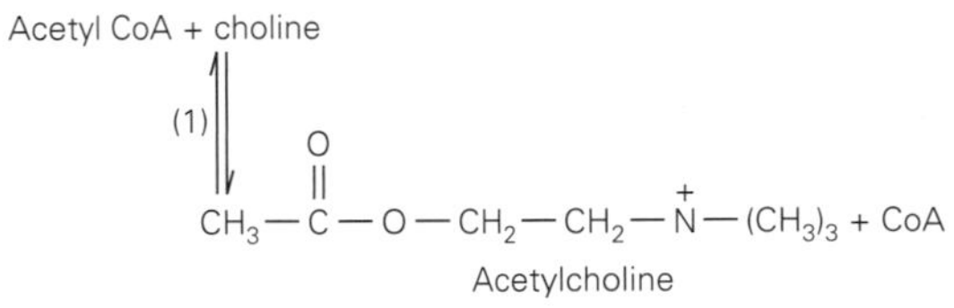

Acetylcholine is released at all vertebrate neuromuscular junctions by spinal motor neurons (see Chapter 9). In the autonomic nervous system it is the transmitter for all preganglionic neurons and for parasympathetic postganglionic neurons as well (see Chapter 47). Cholinergic neurons form synapses throughout the brain; those in the nucleus basalis have particularly widespread projections to the cerebral cortex. Acetylcholine (together with a noradrenergic component) is a principle neurotransmitter of the reticular activating system, which modulates arousal, sleep, wakefulness, and other critical aspects of human consciousness.

Biogenic Amine Transmitters

The term *biogenic amine,* although chemically imprecise, has been used for decades to designate certain neurotransmitters. This group includes the catecholamines and serotonin. Histamine, an imidazole, is also often referred to as a biogenic amine, although its biochemistry is remote from the catecholamines and the indolamines.

Catecholamine Transmitters

The catecholamine transmitters—dopamine, norepinephrine, and epinephrine—are all synthesized from the essential amino acid tyrosine in a common biosynthetic pathway containing five enzymes: tyrosine hydroxylase, pteridine reductase, aromatic amino acid decarboxylase, dopamine β-hydroxylase, and phenylethanolamine-*N*-methyl transferase. Catecholamines have the catechol nucleus, a 3,4-dihydroxylated benzene ring.

The first enzyme, tyrosine hydroxylase (step 1 below), is an oxidase that converts tyrosine to L-dihydroxyphenylalanine (L-DOPA). This enzyme is rate-limiting for the synthesis of both dopamine and norepinephrine. It is present in all cells producing catecholamines and requires a reduced pteridine cofactor, Pt-2H, which is regenerated from pteridine (Pt) by another enzyme, pteridine reductase, which uses nicotinamide adenine dinucleotide (NADH) (step 4 below). This reductase is not specific to neurons.

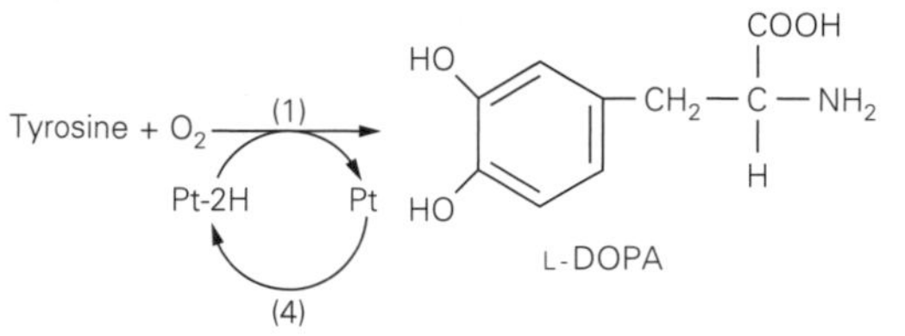

L-DOPA is next decarboxylated by aromatic amino acid decarboxylase, also called L-DOPA decarboxylase (step 2 below), to yield dopamine and CO_2:

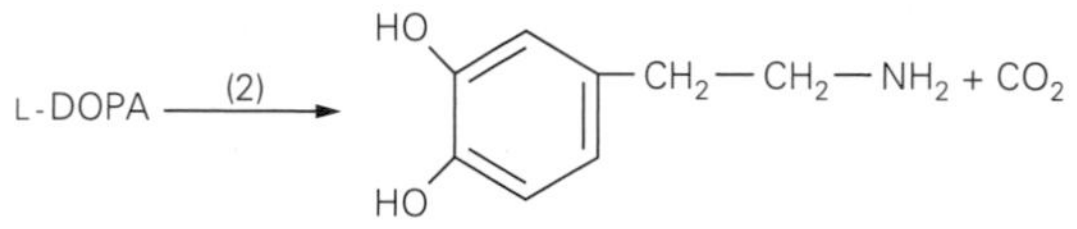

Dopamine

The third enzyme in the sequence, dopamine β-hydroxylase (step 3 below), converts dopamine to norepinephrine. Unlike all other enzymes in the biosynthetic pathways of small-molecule neurotransmitters, dopamine β-hydroxylase is membrane-associated. It is bound tightly to the inner surface of aminergic vesicles as a peripheral protein. Consequently, norepinephrine is the only transmitter synthesized within vesicles.

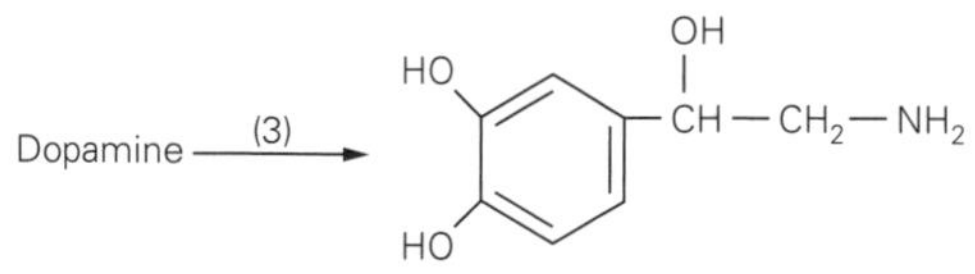

Norepinephrine

In the central nervous system norepinephrine is used as a transmitter by neurons with cell bodies in the locus ceruleus, a nucleus of the brain stem with many complex modulatory functions (see Chapter 46). Although these adrenergic neurons are relatively few in number, they project diffusely throughout the cortex, cerebellum, and spinal cord. In the peripheral nervous system norepinephrine is the transmitter of the postganglionic neurons in the sympathetic nervous system (see Chapter 47).

In addition to these four catecholaminergic biosynthetic enzymes, a fifth enzyme, phenylethanolamine-*N*-methyltransferase (step 5 below), methylates norepinephrine to form epinephrine (adrenaline) in the adrenal medulla. This reaction requires *S*-adenosylmethionine as a methyl donor. The transferase is a cytoplasmic enzyme. Thus, for epinephrine to be formed, its immediate precursor, norepinephrine, must exit from vesicles into the cytoplasm. For epinephrine to be released, it must then be taken up into vesicles. Only a small number of neurons in the brain use epinephrine as transmitter.

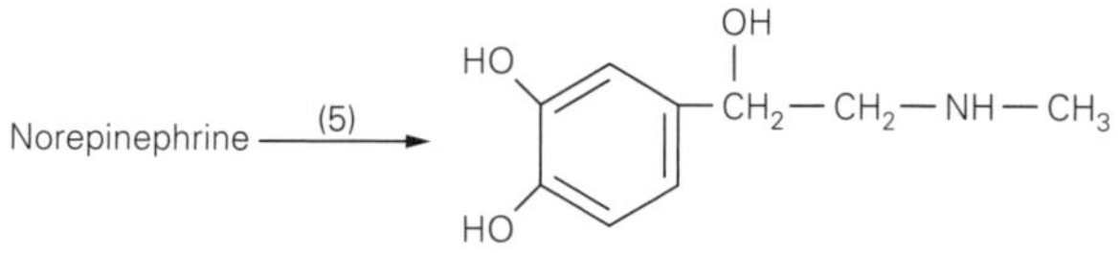

Epinephrine

The production of these catecholamine neurotransmitters is controlled by feedback regulation of the first enzyme in the pathway. Not all cells that release catecholamines express all five biosynthetic enzymes, although cells that release epinephrine do. During development the expression of the genes encoding these synthetic enzymes is independently regulated and the particular catecholamine produced by a cell is determined by which enzyme(s) in the step-wise pathway are not expressed. Thus, neurons that release norepinephrine do not express the methyltransferase, and neurons that release dopamine do not express the transferase or dopamine β-hydroxylase.

Of the four major dopaminergic nerve tracts, three arise in the midbrain (see Chapter 46). Dopaminergic neurons in the substantia nigra that project to the striatum are important for the control of movement and are affected in Parkinson disease and other disorders of movement. The mesolimbic and mesocortical tracts are critical for affect, emotion, attention, and motivation and are implicated in schizophrenia and drug addiction (see Chapters 48, 49, and 62). A fourth dopaminergic tract, the tuberoinfundibular pathway, originates in the arcuate nucleus of the hypothalamus and projects to the pituitary gland, where it regulates secretion of hormones (see Chapter 46).

The synthesis of biogenic amines is highly regulated and can be rapidly increased. As a result, the amounts of transmitter available for release can keep up with wide variations in neuronal activity. Opportunities for regulating both the synthesis of catecholamine transmitters and the production of enzymes in the step-wise catecholamine pathway are discussed in Box 13–1.

Trace amines, naturally occurring catecholamine derivatives, may also be transmitters. In invertebrates the tyrosine derivatives tyramine and octopamine play key roles in numerous physiological processes

Box 13–1 Catecholamine Production Varies with Neuronal Activity

The production of norepinephrine is able to keep up with wide variations in neuronal activity because it is highly regulated. In autonomic ganglia the amount of norepinephrine is regulated transsynaptically. Activity in the presynaptic neurons, which are both cholinergic and peptidergic, first induces short-term changes in second messengers in the postsynaptic adrenergic cells.

These changes increase the supply of norepinephrine through the cAMP-dependent phosphorylation of tyrosine hydroxylase, the first enzyme in the norepinephrine biosynthetic pathway. Phosphorylation enhances the affinity of the hydroxylase for the pteridine cofactor and diminishes feedback inhibition by end products such as norepinephrine. Phosphorylation of tyrosine hydroxylase lasts only as long as cAMP remains elevated, as the phosphorylated hydroxylase is quickly dephosphorylated by protein phosphatases.

If presynaptic activity is sufficiently prolonged, however, other changes in the production of norepinephrine will occur. Severe stress to an animal results in intense presynaptic activity and persistent firing of the postsynaptic adrenergic neuron, placing a greater demand on transmitter synthesis. To meet this challenge, the tyrosine hydroxylase gene is induced to increase production of the enzyme protein. Elevated amounts of tyrosine hydroxylase are observed in the cell body within hours after stimulation and at nerve endings days later.

This induction of increased levels of tyrosine hydroxylase begins with the persistent release of chemical transmitters from the presynaptic neurons and prolonged activation of the cAMP pathway in postsynaptic adrenergic cells, which activates the cAMP-dependent protein kinase (PKA). This kinase phosphorylates not only existing tyrosine hydroxylase molecules, but also a transcription factor, cAMP response element binding protein (CREB).

Once phosphorylated, CREB binds a specific DNA enhancer sequence called the cAMP-recognition element (CRE), which lies upstream (5′) of the gene for the hydroxylase. Binding of CREB to CRE facilitates the binding of RNA polymerase to the gene's promoter, increasing tyrosine hydroxylase transcription. Induction of tyrosine hydroxylase was the first known example of a neurotransmitter altering gene expression.

There is a high degree of similarity in amino acid and nucleic acid sequences encoding three of the biosynthetic enzymes: tyrosine hydroxylase, dopamine β-hydroxylase, and phenylethanolamine-*N*-methyltransferase. This similarity suggests that the three enzymes arose from a common ancestral protein.

Moreover, long-term changes in the synthesis of these enzymes are coordinately regulated in adrenergic neurons. At first, this discovery suggested that the genes encoding these enzymes might be located sequentially along the same chromosome and be controlled by the same promoter, like genes in a bacterial operon. But in humans the genes for the biosynthetic enzymes for norepinephrine are not located on the same chromosome. Therefore, coordinate regulation is likely achieved by parallel activation through similar but independent transcription activator systems.

including behavioral regulation. Trace amine receptors also have been identified in mammals, where their function is still a matter of some controversy.

Serotonin

Serotonin (5-hydroxytryptamine or 5-HT) and the essential amino acid tryptophan from which it is derived belong to a group of aromatic compounds called indoles, with a five-member ring containing nitrogen joined to a benzene ring. Two enzymes are needed to synthesize serotonin: tryptophan (Trp) hydroxylase (step 1 in the following reaction), an oxidase similar to tyrosine hydroxylase, and aromatic amino acid decarboxylase, also called 5-hydroxytryptophan (5-HTP) decarboxylase (step 2 in the following reaction).

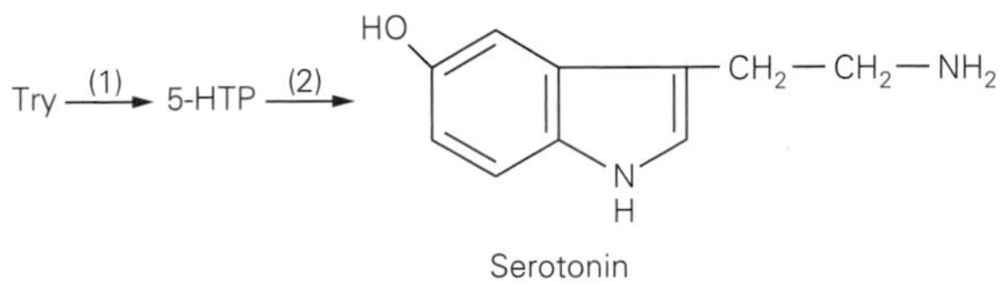

The limiting reaction is catalyzed by the first enzyme in the pathway, tryptophan hydroxylase. Tryptophan hydroxylase is similar to tyrosine hydroxylase not only in catalytic mechanism but also in amino acid sequence. The two enzymes are thought to stem from a common ancestral protein by gene duplication because the two hydroxylases are syntenic, that is, they are encoded by genes close together on the same chromosome (tryptophan hydroxylase, 11p15.3-p14;

tyrosine hydroxylase, 11p15.5). The second enzyme in the pathway, 5-hydroxytryptophan decarboxylase, is identical to L-DOPA decarboxylase. Enzymes with similar activity, L-aromatic amino acid decarboxylases, are present in non-nervous tissues as well.

The cell bodies of serotonergic neurons are found in and around the midline raphe nuclei of the brain stem and are involved in regulating attention and other complex cognitive functions (Chapter 46). The projections of these cells (like those of noradrenergic cells in the locus ceruleus) are widely distributed throughout the brain and spinal cord. Serotonin and the catecholamines norepinephrine and dopamine are implicated in depression, a major mood disorder. Antidepressant medications inhibit the uptake of serotonin, norepinephrine, and dopamine, thereby increasing the magnitude and duration of the action of these transmitters, which in turn leads to altered cell signaling and adaptations (see Chapter 63).

Histamine

Histamine, derived from the essential amino acid histidine by decarboxylation, contains a characteristic five-member ring with two nitrogen atoms. It has long been recognized as an autacoid, active when released from mast cells in the inflammatory reaction and in the control of vasculature, smooth muscle, and exocrine glands (eg, secretion of highly acidic gastric juice). Histamine is a transmitter in both invertebrates and vertebrates. It is concentrated in the hypothalamus, one of the centers for regulating the secretion of hormones (see Chapter 47). The decarboxylase catalyzing its synthesis (step 1 below), although not extensively analyzed, appears to be characteristic of histaminergic neurons.

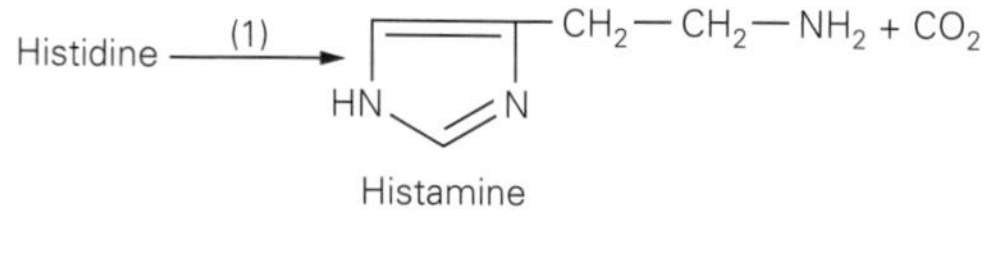

Amino Acid Transmitters

In contrast to acetylcholine and the biogenic amines, which are not intermediates in general metabolic pathways and are produced only in certain neurons, the amino acids glutamate and glycine are not only neurotransmitters but also universal cellular constituents. Because they can be synthesized in neurons, neither are essential amino acids.

Glutamate, the neurotransmitter most frequently used at excitatory synapses throughout the central nervous system, is produced from α-ketoglutarate, an intermediate in the tricarboxylic acid cycle of intermediary metabolism. After it is released, glutamate is taken up from the synaptic cleft by specific transporters in the membrane of both neurons and glia (see below). The glutamate taken up by astrocytes is converted to glutamine by the enzyme glutamine synthase. This glutamine then diffuses back into neurons that use glutamate as a transmitter, where it is hydrolyzed back to glutamate. Phosphate-activated glutaminase (PAG), which is present at high concentrations in these neurons, is responsible for salvaging the molecule for reuse as a transmitter.

Glycine is the major transmitter used by inhibitory interneurons of the spinal cord. It is also an allosteric modulator of the *N*-methyl-D-aspartate (NMDA) subtype of glutamate receptors (see Chapter 10). Glycine is synthesized from serine. Its specific biosynthesis in neurons is not well understood, but its biosynthetic pathway in other tissues is well known. The amino acid GABA is synthesized from glutamate in a reaction catalyzed by glutamic acid decarboxylase (step 1 below):

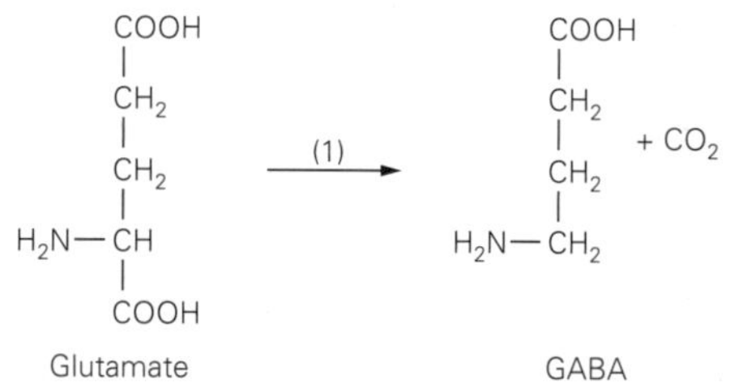

GABA is present at high concentrations throughout the central nervous system and is also detectable in other tissues. It is used as a transmitter by an important class of inhibitory interneurons in the spinal cord. In the brain GABA is the major transmitter of various inhibitory neurons and interneurons, such as the medium spiny neurons of the striatum, striatal interneurons, basket cells of both the cerebellum and the hippocampus, the Purkinje cells of the cerebellum, granule cells of the olfactory bulb, and amacrine cells of the retina.

ATP and Adenosine

ATP and its degradation products (eg, adenosine) act as transmitters at some synapses. Adenosine has an inhibitory effect through a number of adenosine receptors in the central nervous system and caffeine's stimulatory effects depend on inhibition of adenosine binding to its receptors. Adenine and guanine and their sugar-containing derivatives are called purines; the evidence for transmission at purinergic receptors is especially strong for autonomic neurons that innervate the vas deferens, bladder, and muscle fibers of the heart; for nerve plexuses on smooth muscle in the gut; and for some neurons in the brain. Purinergic transmission is particularly important for nerves mediating pain (see Chapter 22).

ATP released by tissue damage acts to transmit pain sensation through one type of ionotropic purine receptor present on the terminals of peripheral axons of nociceptor dorsal root ganglion cells. ATP released from terminals of the central axons of the dorsal root ganglion cells excites another type of ionotropic purine receptor on neurons in the dorsal horn of the spinal cord.

Small-Molecule Transmitters Are Actively Taken Up into Vesicles

Common amino acids act as transmitters in some neurons but not in others, indicating that the presence of a substance in a neuron, even in substantial amounts, is not in itself sufficient evidence that the substance is used as a transmitter. For example, at the neuromuscular junction of the lobster (and other arthropods) GABA is inhibitory and glutamate is excitatory. The concentration of GABA is approximately 20 times greater in inhibitory cells than in excitatory cells, supporting the idea that GABA is the inhibitory transmitter at the lobster neuromuscular junction. In contrast, the concentration of the excitatory transmitter, glutamate, is similar in both excitatory and inhibitory cells. Glutamate therefore must be compartmentalized within these neurons; that is, *transmitter* glutamate must be kept separate from *metabolic* glutamate. In fact, transmitter glutamate is compartmentalized in synaptic vesicles.

Although the presence of a specific set of biosynthetic enzymes can determine whether a small molecule can be used as a transmitter, it does not mean that the molecule will be used. Before a substance can be released as a transmitter it usually must first be concentrated in synaptic vesicles. Transmitter concentrations within vesicles are high, on the order of several hundred millimolar. Neurotransmitter substances are concentrated in vesicles by transporters that are specific to each type of neuron and energized by a vacuolar-type H^+-ATPase (V-ATPase) common to neurons of all types (and found also in glandular tissue, such as the adrenal medulla).

Using the energy generated by the hydrolysis of cytoplasmic ATP, the V-ATPase creates a H^+ electrochemical gradient by promoting the influx of protons into the vesicle. Transporters use this proton gradient to drive transmitter molecules into the vesicles against their concentration gradient. A number of different vesicular transporters have been identified in mammals that are responsible for concentrating different transmitter molecules in vesicles (Figure 13–1). These proteins span the vesicle membrane 12 times, and are distantly related to a class of bacterial transporters that mediate drug-resistance. (Although related in function, vesicular transporters differ structurally and mechanistically from the transporters in the plasma membrane, which are driven by the Na^+ electrochemical gradient rather than by H^+. See below.)

Transmitter molecules are taken up into a vesicle by vesicular transporters in exchange for the transport of two protons out of the vesicle. Because the maintenance of the pH gradient requires the hydrolysis of ATP, the uptake of transmitter into vesicles is energy-dependent. Vesicular transporters can concentrate neurotransmitters up to 100,000-fold relative to their concentration in the cytoplasm. Uptake of transmitters by the transporters is extremely rapid, enabling vesicles to be quickly refilled after they release their transmitter and are retrieved by endocytosis; this is important for maintaining the supply of releasable vesicles during periods of rapid nerve firing (see Chapter 12).

Although the specificity of transporters is quite marked—the ACh transporter does not transport choline or any other transmitter, and the glutamate transporter hardly carries any aspartate at all—the affinity for their transmitters can be quite low. For example, the Michaelis constant (K_m) for ACh or glutamate transport is approximately 0.3 mM, and for GABA 5 to 10 mM. This low affinity for transmitter presumably does not limit synaptic transmission, however, because the concentrations of these substances in the cytoplasm are normally very high. In contrast, amine transporters have a substantially higher affinity for monoamines (K_m of approximately 1–15 μM), appropriate for the lower cytoplasmic concentration of these substances.

Transporters and V-ATPases are present in the membranes of both small synaptic vesicles and large dense-core vesicles. Vesicular transporters are the targets of several important pharmacological agents. Reserpine and tetrabenazine both inhibit uptake of amine transmitters by binding to the vesicular monoamine transporter and have played a historic role in development of the biogenic amine hypothesis of depression (see Chapter 63). The psychostimulants amphetamine and 3,4-methylenedioxy-*N*-methylamphetamine (MDMA or ecstasy) deplete vesicles of amine transmitter

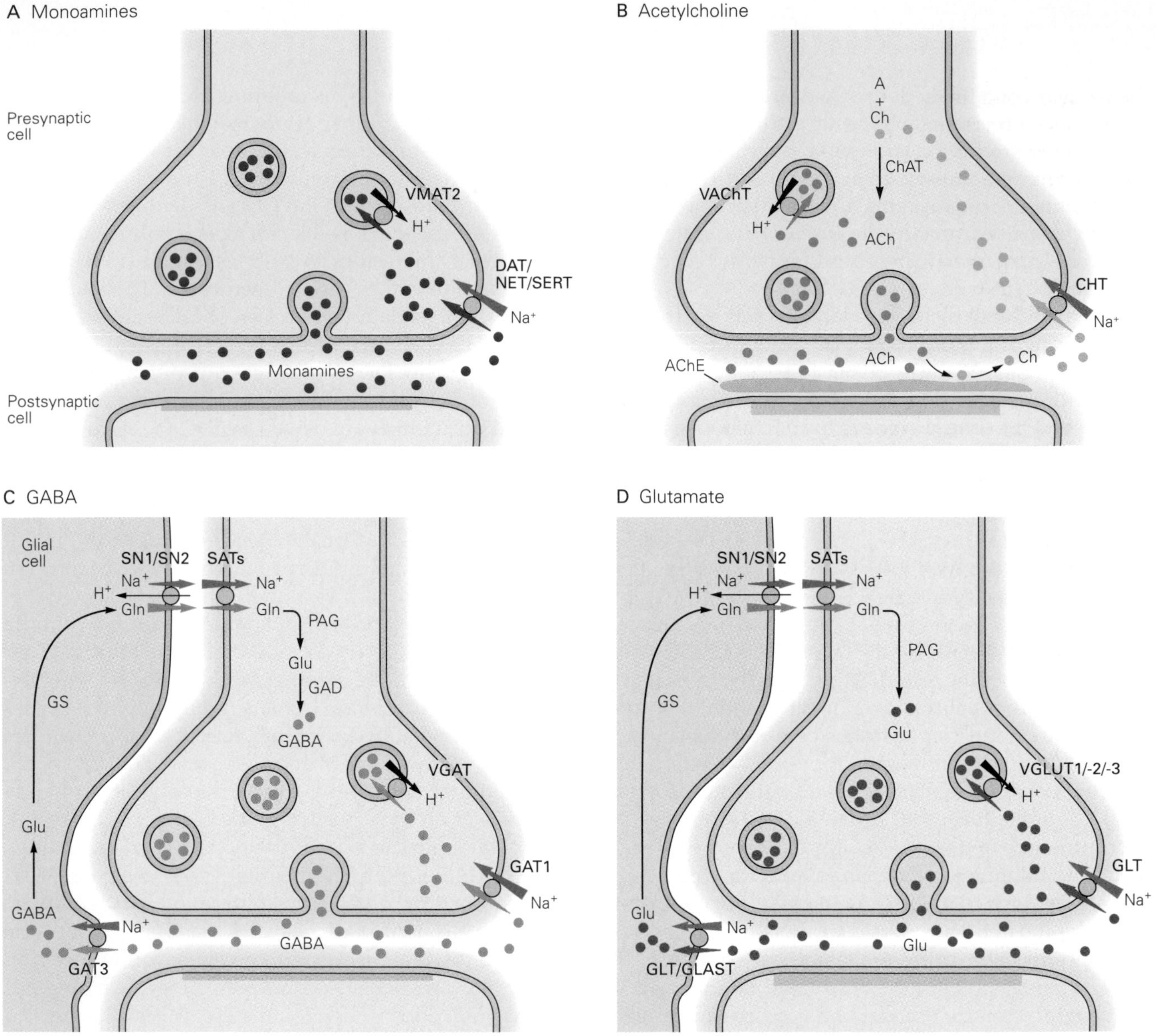

Figure 13–1 Small-molecule transmitters are transported from the cytosol into vesicles or from the synaptic cleft to the cytosol by transporters. Most small-molecule neurotransmitters are released by exocytosis from the nerve terminal and act on specific postsynaptic receptors. The signal is terminated and transmitter recycled by specific transporter proteins located at the nerve terminal or in surrounding glial cells. Transport by these proteins (**orange circles**) is driven by the H^+ (**black arrows**) or Na^+ (**red arrows**) electrochemical gradients. (Adapted, with permission, from Chaudhry et al. 2008.)

A. Three distinct transporters mediate reuptake of monoamines across the plasma membrane. The dopamine transporter (DAT), norepinephrine transporter (NET), and serotonin transporter (SERT) are responsible for the reuptake (**dark blue arrows**) of their cognate transmitters. The vesicular monoamine transporter VMAT2 transports all three monoamines into synaptic vesicles for subsequent exocytotic release.

B. Cholinergic signaling is terminated by metabolism of acetylcholine (ACh) to the inactive choline and acetate by acetylcholinesterase (AChE), which is located in the synaptic cleft. Choline (Ch) is transported back into the nerve terminal (**light blue arrow**) by the choline transporter (CHT), where choline acetyltransferase (ChAT) subsequently catalyzes acetylation of choline to reform ACh. The ACh is transported into the vesicle by the vesicular ACh transporter (VAChT).

C. At GABAergic and glycinergic nerve terminals the GABA transporter (GAT1) and glycine transporter (GLYT2, not shown) mediate reuptake of GABA and glycine (**gray arrow**), respectively. GABA may also be taken up by surrounding glial cells (eg, by GAT3). In the glial cells glutamate (Glu) is converted by glial glutamine synthetase to glutamine (Gln). Glutamine is transported back to the nerve terminal by the concerted action of the system N transporter (SN1/SN2) and system A transporter (SAT) (**brown arrows**). The glial transporter GLYT1 (not shown) also contributes to the clearance of glycine.

D. After release from excitatory neuronal terminals the majority of glutamate is taken up by surrounding glial cells (eg, by GLT and GLAST) for conversion to glutamine, which is subsequently transported back to the nerve terminals by SN1/SN2 and a type of SAT (SATx) (**brown arrows**). Reuptake of glutamate (**purple arrow**) at glutamatergic terminals also has been demonstrated for a GLT isoform.

molecules, most likely by dissipating the pH gradient. These compounds may also compete with the amine transmitters for uptake, and are presumed to interact directly with the transporters, though it is not yet clear whether these drugs and the actual transmitters bind to the same or different sites on the transporters.

Drugs that are sufficiently similar to the normal transmitter substance can act as *false transmitters.* These are packaged in vesicles and released by exocytosis as if they were true transmitters, but they often bind only weakly or not at all to the postsynaptic receptor for the natural transmitter. Therefore, their release decreases the efficacy of transmission. Several drugs that have been used to treat hypertension, such as phenylethylamines, are taken up into adrenergic terminals and replace norepinephrine in synaptic vesicles. When released, these drugs are not as potent as norepinephrine at postsynaptic adrenergic receptors. Some of these drugs must be actively taken up into neurons by transporters in the external membrane of the cell. These transporter molecules are discussed later in this chapter.

Many Neuroactive Peptides Serve as Transmitters

With the exception of dopamine β-hydroxylase, the enzymes that catalyze the synthesis of the low-molecular-weight neurotransmitters are found in the cytoplasm. These enzymes are synthesized on free polysomes in the cell body and are distributed throughout the neuron by axoplasmic flow. Thus small-molecule transmitter substances can be formed in all parts of the neuron; most importantly, they can be synthesized at nerve terminals where they are released.

In contrast, neuroactive peptides are derived from secretory proteins that are formed in the cell body. Like other secretory proteins, neuroactive peptides or their precursors are first processed in the endoplasmic reticulum and then move to the Golgi apparatus to be processed further. They then leave the Golgi apparatus in secretory granules that are destined to become large dense-core vesicles, which are moved to axon terminals by fast axonal transport.

More than 50 short peptides are pharmacologically active in nerve cells (Table 13–2). Some act as hormones on targets outside the brain (eg, angiotensin and gastrin) or are products of neuroendocrine secretion (eg, oxytocin, vasopressin, somatostatin, luteinizing hormone, and thyrotropin-releasing hormone). In addition to being hormones in some tissues, they also act as neurotransmitters when released close

Table 13–2 Neuroactive Mammalian Brain Peptides Categorized According to Tissue Localization

Category	Peptide
Hypothalamic releasing hormones	Thyrotropin-releasing hormone
	Gonadotropin-releasing hormone
	Somatostatin
	Corticotropin-releasing hormone
	Growth hormone-releasing hormone
Neurohypophyseal hormones	Vasopressin
	Oxytocin
Pituitary peptides	Adrenocorticotropic hormone
	β-Endorphin
	α-Melanocyte-stimulating hormone
	Prolactin
	Luteinizing hormone
	Growth hormone
	Thyrotropin
Pineal hormones	Melatonin
Invertebrate peptides	FMRFamide
	Hydra head activator
	Proctolin
	Small cardiac peptide
	Myomodulins
	Buccalins
	Egg-laying hormone
	Bag cell peptides
Gastrointestinal peptides	Vasoactive intestinal polypeptide
	Cholecystokinin
	Gastrin
	Substance P
	Neurotensin
	Methionine-enkephalin
	Leucine-enkephalin
	Insulin
	Glucagon
	Bombesin
	Secretin
	Somatostatin
	Thyrotropin-releasing hormone
	Motilin
Heart	Atrial natriuretic peptide
Other	Angiotensin II
	Bradykinin
	Sleep peptide(s)
	Calcitonin
	CGRP
	Neuropeptide Y
	Neuropeptide Yy
	Galanin
	Substance K (neurokinin A)

FMRFamide, Phe-Met-Arg-Phe-amide; CGRP, calcitonin gene-related peptide. (Adapted, with permission, from Krieger 1983.)

to a target neuron, where they can cause inhibition or excitation, or both.

Neuroactive peptides have been implicated in modulating sensory perception and emotions. Some peptides, including substance P and enkephalins, are preferentially located in regions of the central nervous system involved in the perception of pain. Other neuropeptides regulate complex responses to stress; these peptides include γ-melanocyte stimulating hormone, corticotropin-releasing hormone (CRH), adrenocorticotropin (ACTH), and β-endorphin.

Although the diversity of neuroactive peptides is enormous, as a class these chemical messengers share a common cell biology. The most direct way to determine relatedness between peptides is to compare either the amino acid sequences of the peptides or the nucleotide base sequences in the genes that encode them. A striking generality is that neuroactive peptides are grouped in families with members that have similar sequences of amino acid residues. At least 10 have been identified; the seven main families are listed in Table 13–3.

Several different neuroactive peptides can be encoded by a single continuous messenger RNA (mRNA), which is translated into one large polyprotein precursor (Figure 13–2). Polyproteins can serve as a mechanism for amplification by providing more than one copy of the same peptide from the one precursor. As an example, the precursor of glucagon contains two copies of the hormone. Polyproteins generate diversity by producing several distinct peptides cleaved from one precursor, as in the case of the opioid peptides.

The processing of more than one functional peptide from a single polyprotein is not unique to neuroactive peptides. The mechanism was first described for proteins encoded by small RNA viruses. Several viral polypeptides are produced from the same viral polyprotein, and all contribute to the generation of new virus particles. As with the virus, where the different proteins obviously serve a common biological purpose (formation of new viruses), a neuronal polypeptide will in many instances yield peptides that work together to serve a common physiological goal. Sometimes the biological functions appear to be more complex, as peptides with related or antagonistic activities can be generated from the same precursor.

A particularly striking example of this form of synergy is the group of peptides formed from the precursor of egg-laying hormone (ELH), a set of neuropeptides that govern diverse reproductive behaviors in the marine mollusk *Aplysia*. Egg-laying hormone can act as a hormone causing the contraction of duct muscles; it can also act as a neurotransmitter to alter the firing of several neurons involved in producing behaviors, as do the other peptides cut from the polyprotein.

The processing of polyproteins to neuroactive peptides takes place within the neuron's major intracellular membrane system and in vesicles. Several peptides are produced from a single polyprotein by limited and specific proteolytic cleavage catalyzed by proteases present within these internal membrane systems. Some of these enzymes are serine proteases, a class that also includes the pancreatic enzymes trypsin and chymotrypsin. As with trypsin, the site of the peptide bond cleaved is determined by the presence of one or two dibasic amino acid residues (lysine and arginine) in the substrate protein. Cleavage occurs between residue X and two dibasic residues (eg, X-Lys-Lys, -X-Lys-Arg,

Table 13–3 Some Families of Neuroactive Peptides

Family	Peptide members
Opioids	Opiocortin, enkephalins, dynorphin, FMRFamide
Neurohypophyseal hormones	Vasopressin, oxytocin, neurophysins
Tachykinins	Substance P, physalaemin, kassinin, uperolein, eledoisin, bombesin, substance K
Secretins	Secretin, glucagon, vasoactive intestinal peptide, gastric inhibitory peptide, growth hormone releasing factor, peptide histidine isoleucine amide
Insulins	Insulin, insulin-like growth factors I and II
Somatostatins	Somatostatins, pancreatic polypeptide
Gastrins	Gastrin, cholecystokinin

FMRFamide, Phe-Met-Arg-Phe-amide.

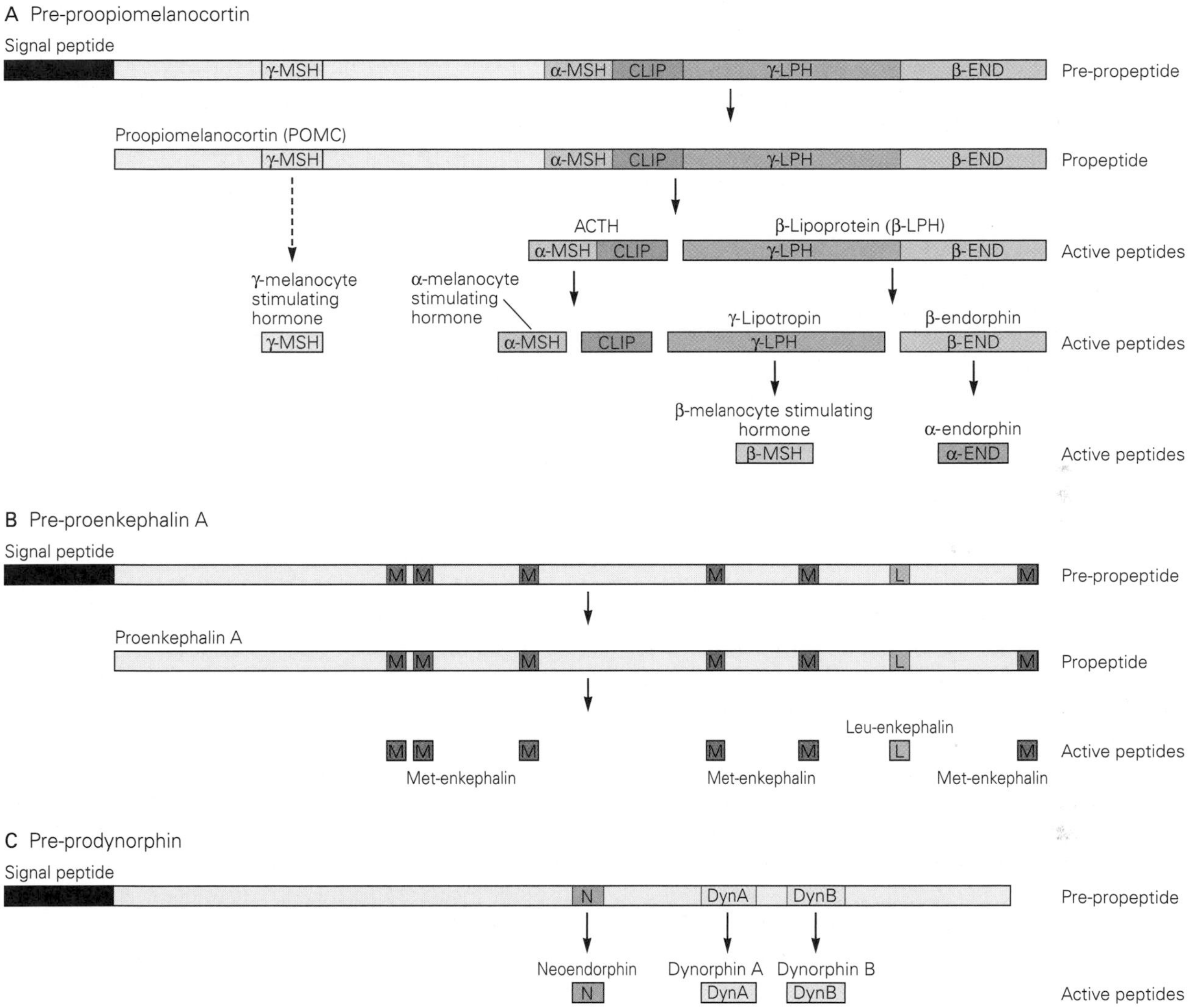

Figure 13–2 Hormone and neuropeptide precursors are processed differentially. In several instances neuropeptides and hormones arise from larger precursor molecules that require multiple rounds of proteinase-mediated cleavage. These precursors are processed differentially to yield their specific peptide products. Transport of these precursors through the membrane of the endoplasmic reticulum is initiated by a hydrophobic signal sequence. Internal cleavages often occur at basic residues within the polypeptide. Moreover, these precursors have key cysteine residues and sugar moieties that play roles in their processing and function. Generally, the first iteration of processing begins with the newly synthesized polyprotein precursor (known as the pre-propeptide form), which contains an amino-terminal signal sequence that is cleaved to generate a smaller molecule, the propeptide. Differential processing of the three families of peptides gives rise to the opioid peptides—POMC (proopiomelanocortin), enkephalin, and dynorphin.

A. The POMC precursor is processed differently in different lobes of the pituitary gland, resulting in α-melanocyte stimulating hormone (α-MSH) and γ-MSH, corticotropin-like intermediate lobe peptide (CLIP), and β-lipotropin (β-LPH). β-LPH is cleaved to yield γ-LPH and β-endorphin (β-END), which themselves yield β-melanocyte stimulating hormone (β-MSH) and α-endorphin (α-END), respectively. The endoproteolytic cleavages within ACTH (adrenocorticotropic hormone) and β-LPH take place in the intermediate lobe but not the anterior lobe.

B. Similar principles are evident in the processing of the enkephalin precursor, which gives rise to six Met-enkephalin peptides and one Leu-enkephalin peptide.

C. The dynorphin precursor is also cleaved into at least three peptides, including α-neoendorphin (N), dynorphin A (Dyn A), and dynorphin B (Dyn B), which are related to Leu-enkephalin since the amino-terminal sequences of all three peptides contain the sequence of Leu-enkephalin.

-X-Arg-Lys, or -X-Arg-Arg). Although cleavage is common at dibasic residues, it can also occur at single basic residues, and polyproteins sometimes are cleaved at other peptide bonds.

Other types of peptidases also catalyze the limited proteolysis required for processing polyproteins into neuroactive peptides. Among these are thiol endopeptidases (with catalytic mechanisms like that of pepsin), amino peptidases (which remove the N-terminal amino acid of the peptide), and carboxypeptidase B (an enzyme that removes an amino acid from the N-terminal end of the peptide if it is basic).

Neurons that produce the same polyprotein may release different neuropeptides as a consequence of differences in the way the polyprotein is processed. An example is proopiomelanocortin (POMC), one of the three branches of the opioid family. POMC is found in neurons of the anterior and intermediate lobes of the pituitary, in the hypothalamus and several other regions of the brain, as well as in the placenta and the gut. The same mRNA for POMC is found in all of these tissues, but different peptides are produced from POMC in different tissues in a regulated manner. One possibility is that two neurons that process the same polyprotein differently might contain proteases with different specificities within the lumina of the endoplasmic reticulum, Golgi apparatus, or vesicles. Alternatively, the two neurons might contain the same processing proteases, but each cell might glycosylate the common polyprotein at different sites, thereby protecting different regions of the polypeptide from cleavage.

Peptides and Small-Molecule Transmitters Differ in Several Ways

The metabolism of peptides differs from that of small-molecule transmitters in several important ways: their site of synthesis, the type of vesicle in which they are stored, and the mechanism of exocytotic release. Whereas small-molecule transmitters are chiefly synthesized at axon terminals, neuroactive peptides are made only in the cell body because their synthesis as secretory proteins requires the transfer of the nascent polypeptide chain into the lumen of the endoplasmic reticulum (see Chapter 4).

The large dense-core vesicles in which peptides are stored originate from the trans-Golgi network through a pathway different from that of the synaptic vesicles transporting small-molecule transmitters. Large dense-core vesicles are homologous to the secretory granules of non-neuronal cells and follow the *regulated* secretory pathway. Biogenesis of synaptic vesicles also begins in the trans-Golgi network in the form of precursor vesicles produced in the cell body. These vesicles are then transported down the axon to presynaptic terminals, where the precursor vesicle is thought to first fuse with the presynaptic membrane through the *constitutive* secretory pathway. The precursor vesicle membrane is then retrieved through endocytosis and processed through local endosomes to yield a mature synaptic vesicle capable of participating in the release of neurotransmitter through regulated exocytosis.

Although both types of vesicles contain many similar proteins, dense-core vesicles lack several proteins needed for release at the active zones. The membranes from dense-core vesicles are used only once; new dense-core vesicles must be synthesized in the cell body and transported to the axonal terminals by anterograde transport. Moreover no uptake mechanisms exist for neuropeptides. Thus once a peptide is released, a new supply must arrive from the cell body before release can take place again. There is increasing evidence for local protein synthesis in axons, and this might also be a source of new peptide for release.

The large dense-core vesicles release their contents by an exocytotic mechanism that is not specialized to nerve cells and that does not require active zones; release can thus take place anywhere along the membrane of the axon terminal. As in other examples of regulated secretion, exocytosis of the dense-core secretory vesicles depends on a general elevation of intracellular Ca^{2+} through voltage-gated Ca^{2+} channels that are not localized to the site of release. As a result, this form of exocytosis is slow and requires high stimulation frequencies to raise Ca^{2+} to levels sufficient to trigger release. This is in contrast to the rapid exocytosis of synaptic vesicles following a single action potential, which results from the large, rapid increase in Ca^{2+} through voltage-gated Ca^{2+} channels tightly clustered at the active zone.

Peptides and Small-Molecule Transmitters Coexist and Can Be Co-released

Neuroactive peptides, small-molecule transmitters, and other neuroactive molecules can coexist in the same dense-core vesicles of a neuron (see Chapter 4). In mature neurons the combination usually consists of one of the small-molecule transmitters and one or more peptides derived from a polyprotein. For example, ACh and vasoactive intestinal peptide (VIP) can be released together and work synergistically on the same target cells.

Another example is calcitonin gene–related peptide (CGRP), which in most spinal motor neurons is packaged together with ACh, the transmitter used at the neuromuscular synapse. CGRP activates adenylyl cyclase, raising cyclic adenosine monophosphate (cAMP) levels and cAMP-dependent protein phosphorylation in the target muscles (see Chapter 11). Increased protein phosphorylation results in an increase in the force of contraction. One other example is the co-release of glutamate and dynorphin in neurons of the hippocampus, where glutamate is excitatory and dynorphin inhibitory. Because postsynaptic target cells have receptors for both chemical messengers, all of these examples of co-release are also examples of cotransmission.

As already described, the dense-core vesicles that release peptides differ from the small clear vesicles that release only small-molecule transmitters. The peptide-containing vesicles may or may not contain small-molecule transmitter, but both types of vesicles contain ATP. As a result ATP is released by exocytosis of both large dense-core vesicles and synaptic vesicles. Moreover, it appears that ATP may be stored and released in a number of distinct ways: (1) ATP is co-stored and co-released with transmitters, (2) ATP release is simultaneous but independent of transmitter release, and (3) ATP is released alone. Co-release of ATP (which after release can be degraded to adenosine) may be an important illustration that coexistence and co-release do not necessarily signify cotransmission. ATP, like many other substances, can be released from neurons but still not be effective if there are no receptors nearby.

As mentioned above, one criterion for judging whether a particular substance is used as a transmitter is that the substance is present in high concentrations in a neuron. Identification of transmitters in specific neurons has been important in understanding synaptic transmission and a variety of histochemical methods are used to detect chemical messengers in neurons (Box 13–2).

An interesting example of co-release of two small-molecule transmitters is that of glutamate and dopamine by neurons projecting to the ventral striatum. This co-release may have important implications for modulation of motivated behaviors. It has been established that the vesicular transporter VGlut2 gathers glutamate into vesicles in these dopaminergic terminals, and glutamate is released together with dopamine in response to different patterns of dopaminergic neuron firing. In addition, glutamate uptake also enhances vesicular monoamine storage by increasing the pH gradient that drives vesicular monoamine transport, providing a novel presynaptic mechanism to regulate quantal size.

Removal of Transmitter from the Synaptic Cleft Terminates Synaptic Transmission

Timely removal of transmitters from the synaptic cleft is critical to synaptic transmission. If transmitter molecules released in one synaptic action were allowed to remain in the cleft after release, they would prevent new signals from getting through. The synapse would become refractory, mainly because of receptor desensitization resulting from continued exposure to transmitter. Transmitters are removed from the cleft by three mechanisms: diffusion, enzymatic degradation, and reuptake. Diffusion removes some fraction of all chemical messengers.

Enzymatic degradation of transmitter is used only by cholinergic synapses. At the neuromuscular junction the active zone of the presynaptic nerve terminal is situated just above the junctional folds of the muscle membrane. The ACh receptors are located at the surface of the muscle facing the release sites and do not extend deep into the folds (see Figure 9–1), whereas acetylcholinesterase is anchored to the basement membrane within the folds. This anatomical arrangement of transmitter, receptor, and degradative enzyme serves two functions.

First, on release ACh reacts with its receptor; after dissociation from the receptor the ACh diffuses into the cleft and is hydrolyzed to choline and acetate by acetylcholinesterase. As a result, the transmitter molecules are used only once. Thus one function of the esterase is to punctuate the synaptic message. The second function is to recapture the choline that otherwise might be lost by diffusion away from the synaptic cleft. Once hydrolyzed by the esterase, the choline lingers in the reservoir provided by the junctional folds and is later taken back up into cholinergic nerve endings by a high-affinity choline transporter. (There is no uptake mechanism for ACh itself.) In addition to acetylcholinesterase, ACh is also degraded by another esterase, butyrylcholinesterase, which can degrade other molecules including cocaine and the paralytic drug succinylcholine. However, the precise functions of butyrylcholinesterase remain to be more fully understood.

Many other enzymatic pathways that degrade released transmitters are not involved in terminating synaptic transmission but are important for controlling the concentration of the transmitter within the neuron or for inactivating transmitter molecules that have diffused away from the synaptic cleft. Many of these degradation enzymes are important clinically—they provide sites for drug action and serve as diagnostic indicators. For example, monoamine oxidase (MAO) inhibitors,

Box 13–2 Detection of Chemical Messengers and Their Processing Enzymes within Neurons

Powerful histochemical techniques are available for detecting both small-molecule transmitter substances and neuroactive peptides in histological sections of nervous tissue.

Catecholamines and serotonin, when reacted with formaldehyde vapor, form fluorescent derivatives. In an early example of transmitter histochemistry, the Swedish neuroanatomists Bengt Falck and Nils Hillarp found that the reaction can be used to locate transmitters with fluorescence microscopy under properly controlled conditions.

Because individual vesicles are too small to be resolved by the light microscope, the exact position of the vesicles containing the transmitter can be inferred by comparing the distribution of fluorescence under the light microscope with the position of vesicles under the electron microscope.

Histochemical analysis can be extended to the ultrastructure of neurons under special conditions. Fixation of nervous tissue in the presence of potassium permanganate, chromate, or silver salts intensifies the electron density of vesicles containing biogenic amines and thus brings out the large number of dense-core vesicles that are characteristic of aminergic neurons.

It is also possible to identify neurons that express the gene for a particular transmitter enzyme or peptide precursor. Many methods for detecting specific mRNAs depend on the nucleic acid hybridization. One such method is in situ hybridization.

Two single strands of a nucleic acid polymer will pair if their sequence of bases is complementary. With in situ hybridization the strand of noncoding DNA (the negative or antisense strand or its corresponding RNA) is applied to tissue sections under conditions suitable for hybridizing with endogenous (sense) mRNA. If the probes are radiolabeled, autoradiography reveals the locations of neurons that contain the complex formed by the labeled complementary nucleic acid strand and the mRNA.

Hybrid oligonucleotides synthesized with nucleotides containing base analogs tagged chemically, fluorescently, or immunoreactively can be localized cytochemically. Both labels can be used at the same time (Figure 13–3A). More recent modifications of these approaches involve viral or transgenic expression of proteins fused to variants of green fluorescent protein (Figure 13–3B).

Transmitter substances can also be localized by immunocytochemistry. Amino acid transmitters, biogenic

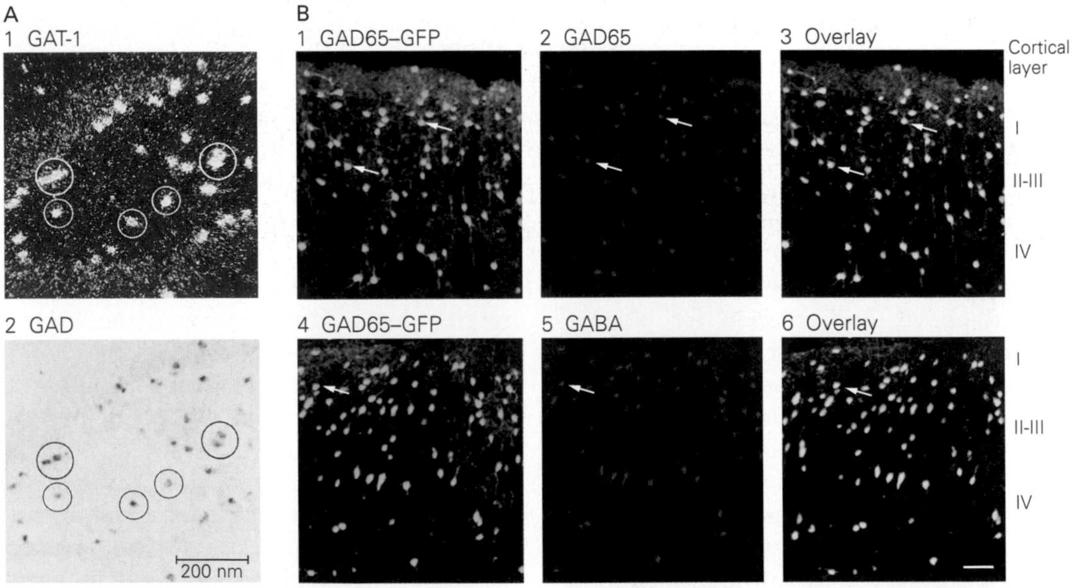

Figure 13–3 Histochemical techniques for visualizing chemical messengers.

A. A light-microscope section of the hippocampus of a rat. **1.** In situ hybridization using a probe for the mRNA encoding GAT-1, a GABA transporter. The probe was end-labeled with α-^{35}S-dATP and visualized by clusters of silver grains in the overlying autoradiographic photographic emulsion. Neurons expressing both transcripts were labeled by the phosphatase reaction product and by silver grains. **Circles** enclose nerve cell bodies that contain both labels. **2.** In situ hybridization of the mRNA for glutamic acid decarboxylase (GAD), the specific biosynthetic enzyme for GABA, was carried out with an oligonucleotide probe linked to the enzyme alkaline phosphatase. The GAD probe was visualized by accumulation of colored alkaline phosphatase reaction product in the cytoplasm. **Circles** enclose areas containing cells with the greatest reactivity. (Reproduced, with permission, from Sara Augood.)

B. Images of neocortex from a GAD65GFP transgenic mouse in which green fluorescent protein (GFP) is expressed under the control of the GAD65 promotor. GFP is co-localized with GAD65 (1-3) and GABA (4-6) (both detected by indirect immunofluorescence) in neurons in the supragranular layers. Most of the GFP-positive neurons are immunopositive for GAD65 and GABA (**arrows**). Scale bar = 100 μm. (Adapted, with permission, from López-Bendito et al. 2004.)

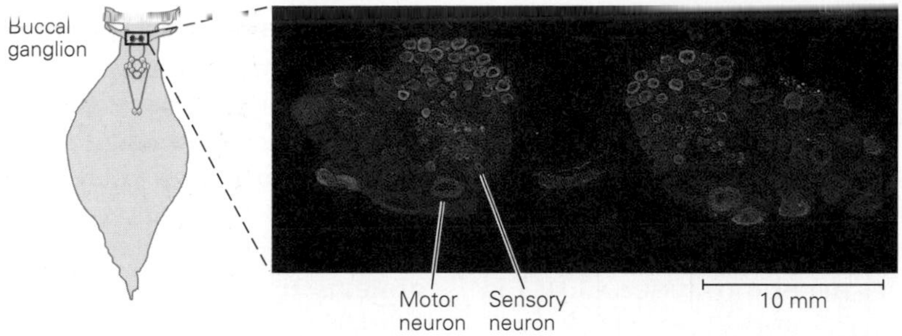

Figure 13–4 An immunochemical technique visualizes a neuropeptide. The buccal ganglion of the marine snail *Aplysia* contains the sensory, motor, and interneurons that control the rhythmic movements of the feeding apparatus of the animal. A cryostat section of the bilaterally symmetrical buccal ganglion is labeled with an antibody raised against FMRFamide. The staining shows immunoreactive FMRFamide in certain sensory neurons (most of the cells with the small cell bodies) as well as certain motor neurons (cells with larger cell bodies). Some of these cells contain one or more other peptides or conventional transmitters such as ACh. (Reproduced, with permission, from Lloyd et al. 1987.)

amines, and neuropeptides have a primary amino group that becomes covalently fixed within the neurons; this group becomes cross-linked to proteins by aldehydes, the usual fixatives used in microscopy.

For immunohistochemical localization, specific antibodies against the transmitter substances are necessary. Antibodies specific to serotonin, histamine, and many neuroactive peptides can be detected by a second antibody (in a technique called *indirect immunofluorescence*). As an example, if the first antibody is rabbit-derived, the second antibody can be goat antibody raised against rabbit immunoglobulin.

These commercially available secondary antibodies are tagged with fluorescent dyes and used under the fluorescence microscope to locate antigens in regions of individual neurons—cell bodies, axons, and sometimes terminals (Figures 13–3, 13–4).

Ultrastructure localization can be achieved by immunochemical techniques, usually involving a peroxidase-antiperoxidase system. Another method is to use antibodies linked to gold particles, which are electron-dense (Figure 13–5). Spheres of colloidal gold can be generated with precise diameters in the nanometer range, and because they are electron-dense they can be seen in the electron microscope. This technique has the additional useful feature that more than one specific antibody can be examined in the same tissue section if each antibody is linked to gold particles of different sizes.

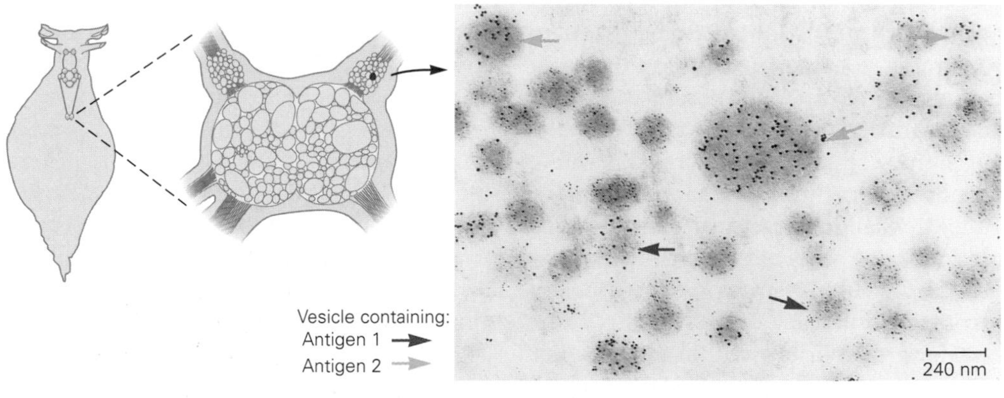

Figure 13–5 Electron-opaque gold particles linked to antibody are used to locate antigens in tissue at the ultrastructural level. The electron micrograph shows a section through the cell body of an *Aplysia* bag cell. Bag cells control reproductive behavior by releasing a group of neuropeptides cleaved from the egg-laying hormone (ELH) precursor. The cells contain several kinds of dense-core vesicles. The cell shown here was treated with two antibodies against different regions of the ELH precursor. One antibody was raised in rabbits and the other in rats. These antibodies were detected with anti-rabbit or anti-rat immunoglobulins (secondary antibodies) raised in goats. Each secondary antibody was coupled to colloidal gold particles of a distinct size. Vesicles identified by antigen 1 are smaller than vesicles identified by antigen 2, indicating that the specific fragments cleaved from the precursor are localized in different vesicles. (Reproduced, with permission, from Fisher et al. 1988.)

which block the degradation of amine transmitters, are used to treat depression and Parkinson disease. Determination of the concentrations of the metabolites of catechol-*O*-methyltransferase (COMT), which is important for degrading biogenic amines and found in the cytoplasm of most cells, provides an index of the efficacy of drugs that affect the synthesis or degradation of the biogenic amines in nervous tissue. COMT is thought to play a particularly important role in regulating cortical dopamine levels due to the low levels of the dopamine uptake transporter.

The mechanisms for removing neuropeptides from the synaptic cleft are slow diffusion and proteolysis by extracellular peptidases. In contrast, small-molecule transmitters are removed more quickly from the synaptic cleft.

The critical mechanism for inactivation of most neurotransmitters is reuptake at the plasma membrane. This mechanism serves the dual purposes of terminating the synaptic action of the transmitter as well as recapturing transmitter molecules for subsequent reuse. High-affinity uptake, with binding constants of 25 μM or less for the released transmitter, is mediated by transporter molecules in the membranes of nerve terminals and glial cells. Unlike vesicular transporters, which are powered by the H^+ electrochemical gradient in a countertransport mechanism, plasma membrane transporters are driven by the Na^+ electrochemical gradient through a symport mechanism in which Na^+ ions and transmitter move in the same direction.

Each type of neuron has its own characteristic uptake mechanism. For example, noncholinergic neurons do not take up choline with high affinity. Certain powerful psychotropic drugs can block uptake processes. For example, cocaine blocks the uptake of dopamine, norepinephrine, and serotonin; the tricyclic antidepressants and selective serotonin reuptake inhibitors, such as fluoxetine (Prozac), block uptake of serotonin or norepineprhine. The application of appropriate drugs that block transporter molecules can prolong and enhance synaptic signaling by the biogenic amines and GABA. In some instances drugs act both on transporter molecules on the neuron's surface and on vesicular transporters within the cell. For example, amphetamines must be actively taken up by the dopamine transporter on the external membrane of the neuron before they can operate on the vesicular transporter for amine transmitters.

Transporter molecules for neurotransmitters belong to two distinct groups that are different in both structure and mechanism. High-resolution structures of bacterial homologs from each of these families have been solved recently, which has greatly advanced our understanding of transporter mechanisms. One group, the neurotransmitter sodium symporters (NSS), is a superfamily of transmembrane proteins that thread through the plasmalemma 12 times and includes the transporters of GABA, glycine, norepinephrine, dopamine, serotonin, osmolytes, and amino acids. The other consists of transporters of glutamate; these proteins traverse the plasmalemma eight times and contain two helical hairpins that seem to serve a role in gating access of substrate from each side of the membrane. Each group includes several transporters for each transmitter substance; for example, there are multiple GABA, glycine, and glutamate transporters, each with somewhat different localization, function, and pharmacology.

The two groups can be distinguished functionally. Although both are driven by the electrochemical potential provided by the Na^+ gradient, transport of glutamate requires the countertransport of K^+, whereas transport by the NSS usually requires the cotransport of a Cl^- ion. During transport of glutamate one negatively charged molecule of the transmitter is imported with three Na^+ ions and one proton (symport) in exchange for the export of one K^+. This leads to a net influx of two positive charges for each transport cycle, generating an inward current. As a result of this charge transfer, the negative resting potential of the cell generates a large inward driving force that results in an enormous gradient of glutamate across the cell membrane. In contrast, the NSS proteins transport one to three Na^+ ions and one Cl^- ion together with their substrates. Under most conditions the electrochemical driving force is sufficient for transporters to transport transmitter into the cell, thereby concentrating it inside the cell.

An Overall View

Information carried by a neuron is encoded in electrical signals that travel along its axon to a synapse, where these signals are transformed and carried across the synaptic cleft by one or more chemical messengers.

The two major classes of chemical messengers, small-molecule transmitters and neuroactive peptides, are packaged in vesicles within the presynaptic neuron. After their synthesis in the cytoplasm, small-molecule transmitters are taken up and concentrated in vesicles, where they are protected from degradative enzymes that maintain a constant level of transmitter substance in the cytoplasm. Synaptic vesicles are highly concentrated in nerve endings. Because they are quickly replenished during synaptic activity, much of the small-molecule transmitter in the neuron must be synthesized locally at the terminals.

In contrast, the protein precursors of neuroactive peptides are synthesized only in the cell body; the neuropeptides become packaged in secretory granules and vesicles that are carried from the cell body to the terminals by axoplasmic transport. Unlike the vesicles that contain small-molecule transmitters, these vesicles are not refilled at the terminal.

Given their central importance in brain function, it is not surprising that the enzymes that regulate transmitter biosynthesis are under tight regulatory control. Changes in neuronal activity can produce homeostatic changes in the levels of these enzymes. This regulation can occur both post-translationally in the cytoplasm, as a result of phosphorylation and dephosphorylation reactions, and by transcriptional contol in the nucleus.

Precise mechanisms for terminating transmitter actions represent a key step in synaptic transmission that is nearly as important as transmitter synthesis and release. Some released transmitter is lost as a result of simple diffusion out of the synaptic cleft. However, for the most part, transmitter actions are terminated by specific molecular reactions. For example, acetylcholine is rapidly hydrolyzed by acetylcholinesterase to choline and acetate, whereas glutamate is taken up into presynaptic terminals and glia by specific transporters that are driven by ion gradients. Some of the most potent psychoactive compounds act by interfering with transmitter reuptake. The psychostimulatory effects of cocaine result from its action to prevent reuptake of catecholamines whereas the blockade of serotonin transporters are responsible for the antidepressant effects of the selective serotonin reuptake inhibitors (SSRIs).

Can we arrive at a comprehensive and precise definition of a neurotransmitter? Probably not, as the definition is empirical. The first step in understanding the molecular strategy of chemical transmission usually involves identifying the contents of synaptic vesicles. Except for those instances in which transmitter is released by transporter molecules or by diffusion through the membrane (in the case of gases and lipid metabolites, see Chapter 11), only molecules suitably packaged in vesicles can be released from a neuron's terminals. But not all molecules released by a neuron are chemical messengers—only those that bind to appropriate receptors and initiate functional changes in that target neuron can usefully be considered neurotransmitters.

Information is transmitted when transmitter molecules bind to receptor proteins in the membrane of another cell, causing them to change shape. Once the molecules of transmitter are bound, the receptor generates electrical or metabolic signals in the postsynaptic cell. The co-release of several neuroactive substances onto appropriate postsynaptic receptors permits great diversity of information to be transferred in a single synaptic action.

James H. Schwartz
Jonathan A. Javitch

Selected Readings

Alberts B, Johnson A, Lewis J, Raff M, Roberts K, Walter P. 2002. Membrane transport of small molecules and the electrical properties of membranes. In: *Molecular Biology of the Cell*, 4th ed. New York and Oxford: Garland Science.

Cooper JR, Bloom FE, Roth RH. 2003. *The Biochemical Basis of Neuropharmacology*, 8th ed. New York: Oxford Univ. Press.

Edwards RH. 2007. The neurotransmitter cycle and quantal size. Neuron 55:835-58.

Koob GF, Sandman CA, Strand FL (eds). 1990. A decade of neuropeptides: past, present and future. Ann N Y Acad Sci 579:1–281.

Mortensen OV, Amara SG. 2003. Dynamic regulation of the dopamine transporter. Eur J Pharmacol 479(1–3):159–170.

Siegel GJ, Agranoff BW, Albers RW, Molinoff PB (eds). 1998. *Basic Neurochemistry: Molecular, Cellular, and Medical Aspects*, 6th ed. Philadelphia: Lippincott.

Snyder SH, Ferris CD. 2000. Novel neurotransmitters and their neuropsychiatric relevance. Am J Psychiatry 157:1738–1751.

Toei M, Saum R, Forgac M. 2010. Regulation and isoform function of the V-ATPases. Biochemistry 49:4715-23.

Torres GE, Amara SG. 2007. Glutamate and monoamine transporters: new visions of form and function. Curr Opin Neurobiol 17:304-12.

Weihe E, Eiden LE. 2000. Chemical neuroanatomy of the vesicular amine transporters. FASEB J 15:2435–2449.

References

Augood SJ, Herbison AE, Emson PC. 1995. Localization of GAT-1 GABA transporter mRNA in rat striatum: cellular coexpression with GAD_{67} mRNA, GAD_{67} immunoreactivity, and paravalbumin mRNA. J Neurosci 15:865–874.

Burnstock G. 1986. Purines and cotransmitters in adrenergic and cholinergic neurones. Prog Brain Res 68:193–203.

Chaudhry FA, Boulland JL, Jenstad M, Bredahl MK, Edwards RH. 2008. Pharmacology of neurotransmitter transport into secretory vesicles. Handb Exp Pharmacol 184:77–106.

Dale H. 1935. Pharmacology and nerve endings. Proc R Soc Med (Lond) 28:319–332.

Danbolt NC, Chaudhry FA, Dehnes Y, Lehre KP, Levy LM, Ullensvang K, Storm-Mathisen J. 1998. Properties and localization of glutamate transporters. Prog Brain Res 116:23–43.

Falck B, Hillarp N Å, Thieme G, Torp A. 1982. Fluorescence of catecholamines and related compounds condensed with formaldehyde. Brain Res Bull 9(1–6):11–15.

Fisher JM, Sossin W, Newcomb R, Scheller RH. 1988. Multiple neuropeptides derived from a common precursor are differentially packaged and transported. Cell 54:813–822.

Gouaux E. 2009. The molecular logic of sodium-coupled neurotransmitter transporters. Philos Trans R Soc Lond B Biol Sci 364:149–54.

Henry LK, Meiler J, Blakely RD. 2007. Bound to be different: neurotransmitter transporters meet their bacterial cousins. Mol Interv 7:306–309.

Hnasko TS, Chuhma N, Zhang H, Goh GY, Sulzer D, Palmiter RD, Rayport S, Edwards RH. 2010. Vesicular glutamate transport promotes dopamine storage and glutamate corelease in vivo. Neuron 65:643–56.

Iversen LL. 1995. Neuropeptides: promise unfulfilled? Trends Neurosci 18(2):49–50.

Jiang J, Amara SG. 2011. New views of glutamate transporter structure and function: advances and challenges. Neuropharmacology 60:172–181.

Katz B. 1969. *The Release of Neural Transmitter Substances.* Springfield, IL: Thomas.

Krieger DT. 1983. Brain peptides: what, where, and why? Science 222:975–985.

Lloyd PE, Frankfurt M, Stevens P, Kupfermann I, Weiss KR. 1987. Biochemical and immunocytological localization of the neuropeptides FMRFamide SCPA, SCPB, to neurons involved in the regulation of feeding in Aplysia. J Neurosci 7:1123–1132.

Loewi O. 1960. An autobiographic sketch. Perspect Biol Med 4:3–25.

López-Bendito G, Sturgess K, Erdélyi F, Szabó G, Molnár Z, Paulsen O. 2004. Preferential origin and layer destination of GAD65-GFP cortical interneurons. Cereb Cortex 14:1122–1133.

Liu Y, Kranz DE, Waites C, Edwards RH. 1999. Membrane trafficking of neurotransmitter transporters in the regulation of synaptic transmission. Trends Cell Biol 9:356–363.

Okuda T, Haga T. 2003. High-affinity choline transporter. Neurochem Res 28:483–488.

Otsuka M, Kravitz EA, Potter DD. 1967. Physiological and chemical architecture of a lobster ganglion with particular reference to γ aminobutyrate and glutamate. J Neurophysiol 30:725–752.

Rubin RP. A brief history of great discoveries in pharmacology: in celebration of the centennial anniversary of the founding of the American Society of Pharmacology and Experimental Therapeutics. 2007. Pharmacol Rev 59: 289–359.

Scheller RH, Axel R. 1984. How genes control an innate behavior. Sci Am 250(3):54–62.

Singh SK. 2008. LeuT: a prokaryotic stepping stone on the way to a eukaryotic neurotransmitter transporter structure. Channels 2:380–389.

Sossin WS, Fisher JM, Scheller RH. 1989. Cellular and molecular biology of neuropeptide processing and packaging. Neuron 2:1407–1417.

Stuber GD, Hnasko TS, Britt JP, Edwards RH, Bonci A. 2010. Dopaminergic terminals in the nucleus accumbens but not the dorsal striatum corelease glutamate. J Neurosci 30:8229–8233.

Thoenen H. 1974. Trans synaptic enzyme induction. Life Sci 14:223–235.

Yamashita A, Singh SK, Kawate T, Jin Y, Gouaux E. 2005. Crystal structure of a bacterial homologue of Na^+/Cl^--dependent neurotransmitter transporters. Nature 437:205–223.

Yernool D, Boudker O, Jin Y, Gouaux E. 2004. Structure of a glutamate transporter homologue from Pyrococcus horikoshii. Nature 431:811–818.

14

Diseases of the Nerve and Motor Unit

... to move things is all that mankind can do, for such the sole executant is muscle, whether in whispering a syllable or in felling a forest.

Charles Sherrington, 1924

THE MAJOR CONSEQUENCE OF THE elaborate information processing that takes place in the brain is the contraction of skeletal muscles. Indeed, animals are distinguishable from plants by their ability to make precise, goal-directed movements of their body parts. As we shall see in Chapter 16, the problem of deciding when and how to move is, to a large degree, the driving force behind the evolution of the nervous system.

In all but the most primitive animals, specialized muscle cells generate movement. There are three general types of muscles: Smooth muscle is used primarily for internal actions such as peristalsis and control of blood flow; cardiac muscle is used exclusively for pumping blood; and skeletal muscle is used primarily for moving bones. In this chapter we examine a variety of neurological disorders in mammals that affect movement by altering action potential conduction in a motor nerve, synaptic transmission from nerve to muscle, or muscle contraction itself.

In 1925 Charles Sherrington introduced the term *motor unit* to designate the basic unit of motor function—a motor neuron and the group of muscle fibers it innervates (see Chapter 34). The number of muscle fibers innervated by a single motor neuron varies widely throughout the body, depending on the dexterity of the movements controlled and the mass of the body part to be moved. Thus motor units with fewer than 100 muscle fibers finely control eye movements, whereas in the leg a single motor unit contains up to 1,000 muscle fibers. In each case all the muscles innervated by a motor unit are of the same type. Moreover, motor units are recruited in a fixed order for both voluntary and reflex movements. The smallest motor units are the first to be recruited, joined later by larger units as muscle force increases.

The motor unit is a common target of disease. The distinguishing features of diseases of the motor unit vary depending on which functional component is primarily affected: (1) the cell body of the motor or sensory neuron, (2) the corresponding axons, (3) the neuromuscular junction (the synapse between the motor axon and muscle), or (4) the muscle fibers that are innervated by the motor neuron. Accordingly, disorders of the motor unit have traditionally been classified as motor neuron diseases, peripheral neuropathies, disorders of the neuromuscular junction, or primary muscle diseases (myopathies) (Figure 14–1).

Peripheral neuropathies arise from abnormal function of motor neurons or their axons, leading to weakness of movement. Most peripheral neuropathies also involve sensory neurons, leading to problems in sensation. In some rare motor neuron diseases the motor neurons and motor tracts in the spinal cord degenerate but sensory nerves are spared. In *myopathies* weakness is caused by degeneration of the muscles with little or no change in motor neurons. In neuromuscular junction diseases alterations in the synapse lead to weakness that may be intermittent. Clinical and laboratory studies usually allow one to distinguish disorders of peripheral nerves from those of the neuromuscular junction or muscle (see Postscript to this chapter).

Disorders of the Peripheral Nerve, Neuromuscular Junction, and Muscle Can Be Distinguished Clinically

When a peripheral nerve is cut, the muscles innervated by that nerve immediately become paralyzed and then waste progressively. Because the nerve carries sensory as well as motor fibers, sensation in the area innervated by the nerve is also lost and tendon reflexes are lost immediately. The term *atrophy* (literally, lack of nourishment) refers to the wasting away of a once-normal muscle. Because of historical usage *atrophy* appears in the names of several diseases that are now regarded as neurogenic.

The main symptoms of the myopathies often include difficulty in walking or lifting. Other, less common symptoms include inability of the muscle to relax (myotonia), cramps, pain (myalgia), or the appearance in the urine of the heme-containing protein that gives muscle its red color (myoglobinuria). The muscular dystrophies are myopathies with special characteristics: The diseases are inherited, all symptoms are caused by

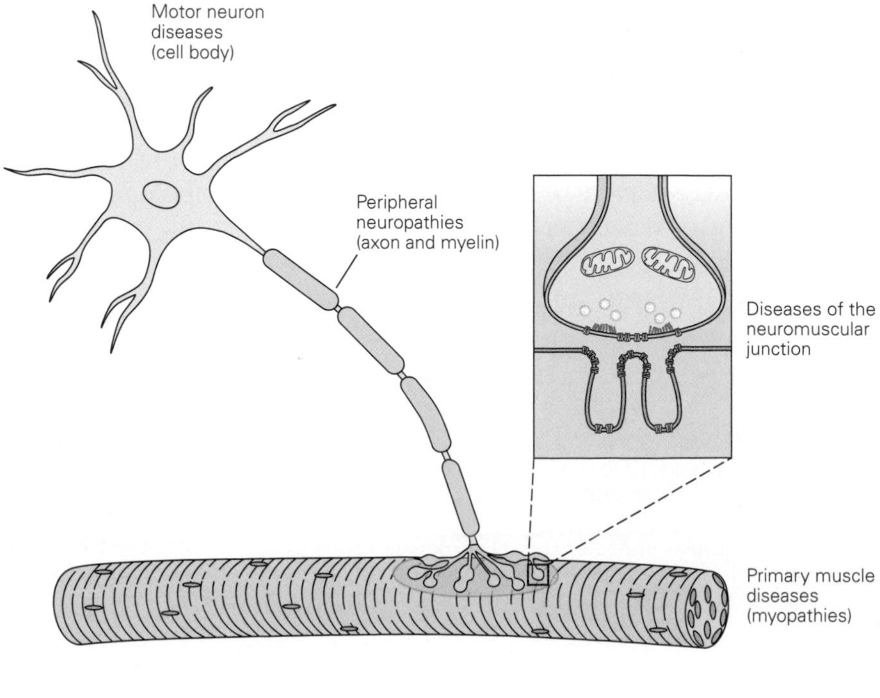

Figure 14–1 Classification of the four types of motor unit disorders is based on the part of the motor unit that is affected.

weakness, the weakness becomes progressively more severe, and signs of degeneration and regeneration are seen histologically.

Distinguishing neurogenic and myopathic diseases may be difficult because both produce weakness of muscle. Classification and differential diagnosis of these diseases involve both clinical and laboratory criteria. As a first approximation, weakness of the distal limbs most often indicates a neurogenic disorder, whereas proximal limb weakness signals a myopathy. *Fasciculations*—twitches of muscle that are visible through the skin—are often signs of neurogenic diseases. They result from involuntary but synchronous contractions of all muscle fibers in a motor unit. *Fibrillations*—spontaneous contractions of single muscle fibers—can also be signs of on going denervation of muscle. Fibrillations are not visible but can be recorded with an electromyogram (EMG). The electrical record of a fibrillation is a low-amplitude potential that reflects electrical activity in a single muscle cell. Electrophysiological studies suggest that fasciculations arise in the motor nerve terminal.

In diagnosing motor neuron disorders, clinical neurologists distinguish between lower and upper motor neurons. *Lower motor neurons* are motor neurons of the spinal cord and brain stem that directly innervate skeletal muscles. *Upper motor neurons* are neurons in the premotor cortex that issue commands for movements to the lower motor neurons through their axons in the corticospinal (pyramidal) tract. The distinction between upper and lower motor neurons is important clinically because diseases involving each class of neurons produce distinctive symptoms. Disorders of lower motor neurons cause atrophy, fasciculations, decreased muscle tone, and loss of tendon reflexes; disorders of upper motor neurons and their axons result in spasticity, overactive tendon reflexes, and an abnormal plantar extensor reflex (the Babinski sign).

The primary symptom of disorders of the neuromuscular junction is weakness; in some neuromuscular junction diseases this weakness is quite variable even during the course of a single day.

A Variety of Diseases Target Motor Neurons and Peripheral Nerves

Motor Neuron Diseases Do Not Affect Sensory Neurons

The best-known disorder of motor neurons is amyotrophic lateral sclerosis (Lou Gehrig disease). *Amyotrophy* is another word for neurogenic atrophy of muscle; *lateral sclerosis* refers to the hardness felt when the pathologist examines the spinal cord at autopsy. This hardness results from the proliferation of astrocytes and scarring of the lateral columns of the spinal cord caused by degeneration of the corticospinal tracts. Some motor neurons are spared, notably those supplying ocular muscles and those involved in voluntary control of bladder sphincters.

The symptoms of amyotrophic lateral sclerosis (ALS) usually start with painless weakness of the arms or legs. Typically the patient, often a man in his 40s or 50s, discovers that he has trouble in executing fine movements of the hands; typing, playing the piano, playing baseball, fingering coins, or working with tools all become awkward.

Most cases of ALS involve both upper and lower motor neurons. Thus the typical weakness of the hand is associated with wasting of the small muscles of the hands and feet and fasciculations of the muscles of the forearm and upper arm. These signs of lower motor neuron disease are often associated with hyperreflexia, an increase in tendon reflexes characteristic of corticospinal upper motor neuron disease.

The cause of most (95%) cases of ALS is unknown; the disease is progressive and ultimately affects muscles of respiration. There is no effective treatment for this fatal condition.

Approximately 10% of cases are inherited as dominant traits. Of these, approximately 25% arise from mutations in the gene encoding the protein copper/zinc cytosolic superoxide dismutase, or SOD1. The fact that this form of the disease is dominantly inherited suggests that the disorder arises from some acquired toxic property of the mutant SOD1 protein. This is underscored by the observation that nearly all mutations causing this form of ALS are missense changes that substitute one or more amino acids in the wild-type, normal protein. The exact neurotoxic property of the mutant enzyme remains unclear.

Strikingly, mice and rats that have high levels of the mutant SOD1 develop an adult-onset form of motor neuron disease that leads to death. By contrast, mice expressing equivalently high levels of normal SOD1 do not develop paralysis. These findings are consistent with the concept that the mutant molecule has acquired one or more forms of cytotoxicity. As with other aspects of normal and abnormal functions of the brain and spinal cord, mouse models of motor neuron disease have proven highly instructive for the study of potential treatments as well as the molecular pathogenesis of the disease.

There are other variants of motor neuron disease. The first symptoms may be restricted to muscles innervated by cranial nerves, with resulting dysarthria (difficulty speaking) and dysphagia (difficulty swallowing). When cranial symptoms occur alone, the syndrome is called progressive bulbar palsy. (The term *bulb* is used interchangeably with *pons,* the structure at the base of the brain where motor neurons that innervate the face and swallowing muscles reside, and *palsy* means weakness.) If only lower motor neurons are involved, the syndrome is called progressive spinal muscular atrophy.

Progressive spinal muscular atrophy is a developmental disorder of motor neurons and is characterized by weakness, wasting, loss of reflexes, and fasciculations. Most cases arise in infants and are caused by recessively inherited mutations in the gene encoding a protein called survival motor neuron or SMN. Some rare cases begin in late childhood or even early adulthood. The SMN protein is implicated in the trafficking of RNA in and out of the nucleus and in the formation of complexes that are important in RNA splicing. In humans the SMN locus on chromosome 5 has two almost identical copies of the SMN gene. One produces a full length SMN protein, whereas the second expresses a small amount of full-length SMN and a shortened SMN. The loss of full-length SMN from mutations at the main locus can be mitigated to some degree by the shortened SMN protein expressed at the second locus.

Amyotrophic lateral sclerosis and its variants are restricted to motor neurons; they do not affect sensory neurons or autonomic neurons. The acute viral disease poliomyelitis is also confined to motor neurons. These diseases illustrate dramatically the individuality of nerve cells and the principle of selective vulnerability. The basis of this selectivity is, in general, not understood.

Diseases of Peripheral Nerves Affect Conduction of the Action Potential

Diseases of peripheral nerves may affect either axons or myelin. Because motor and sensory axons are bundled together in the same peripheral nerves, disorders of peripheral nerves usually affect both motor and sensory functions. Some patients with peripheral neuropathy report abnormal, frequently unpleasant, sensory experiences similar to the sensations felt after local anesthesia for dental work. These sensations are variously called numbness, pins-and-needles, or tingling. When the sensations occur spontaneously without an external sensory stimulus they are called paresthesias.

Patients with paresthesias usually have impaired perception of cutaneous sensations (pain and temperature), often because the small myelinated fibers that carry these sensations are selectively affected. Proprioceptive sensations (position and vibration) may be lost without loss of cutaneous sensation. Lack of pain perception may lead to injuries. The sensory disorders are more prominent distally (called a glove-and-stocking pattern), possibly because the distal portions of the nerves are most remote from the cell body and therefore most susceptible to disorders that interfere with axonal transport of essential metabolites and proteins.

Peripheral neuropathy is first manifested by weakness that is usually distal. Tendon reflexes are usually depressed or lost, fasciculation is seen only rarely, and wasting does not ensue unless the weakness has been present for many weeks.

Neuropathies may be either acute or chronic. The best-known acute neuropathy is Guillain-Barré syndrome. Most cases follow respiratory infection or infectious diarrhea, but the syndrome may occur without preceding illness. The condition may be mild or so severe that mechanical ventilation is required. Cranial nerves may be affected, leading to paralysis of ocular, facial, and oropharyngeal muscles. The disorder is attributed to an autoimmune attack on peripheral nerves by circulating antibodies. It is treated by removing the offending antibodies by infusions of gamma globulin and plasmapheresis. The blood is removed from a patient, cells are separated from plasma which has the antibodies, and the cells alone are returned to the patient.

The chronic neuropathies vary from the mildest manifestations to incapacitating or even fatal conditions. There are many varieties, including genetic diseases (acute intermittent porphyria, Charcot-Marie-Tooth disease), metabolic disorders (diabetes, vitamin B_{12} deficiency), intoxication (lead), nutritional disorders (alcoholism, thiamine deficiency), carcinomas (especially carcinoma of the lung), and immunological disorders (plasma cell diseases, amyloidosis). Some chronic disorders, such as neuropathy caused by vitamin B_{12} deficiency in pernicious anemia, are amenable to therapy.

In addition to being acute or chronic, neuropathies may be categorized as demyelinating (in which the myelin sheath breaks down) or axonal (in which the axon is affected). In demyelinating neuropathies, as might be expected from the role of the myelin sheath in saltatory conduction, conduction velocity is slowed because the axons have lost myelin (discussed below). In axonal neuropathies the myelin sheath is not affected and conduction velocity is normal.

Axonal and demyelinating neuropathies may lead to positive or negative symptoms and signs. The negative signs consist of weakness or paralysis, loss of tendon reflexes, and impaired sensation resulting from loss of motor and sensory nerves. The positive symptoms of peripheral neuropathies consist of paresthesias that arise from abnormal impulse activity in sensory fibers, and either spontaneous activity of injured nerve fibers or electrical interaction (cross-talk) between abnormal axons, a process called *ephaptic transmission* to distinguish it from normal synaptic transmission. For unknown reasons damaged nerves also become hyperexcitable. Lightly tapping the site of injury can evoke a burst of unpleasant sensations in the region over which the nerve is distributed.

Negative symptoms, which have been studied more thoroughly than positive symptoms, can be attributed to three basic mechanisms: conduction block, slowed conduction, and impaired ability to conduct impulses at higher frequencies. Conduction block was first recognized in 1876 when the German neurologist Wilhelm Erb observed that stimulation of an injured peripheral nerve below the site of injury evoked a muscle response, whereas stimulation above the site of injury produced no response. He concluded that the lesion blocked conduction of impulses of central origin, even when the segment of the nerve distal to the lesion was still functional. Later studies confirmed this conclusion by showing that selective application of diphtheria and other toxins produces conduction block by causing demyelination only at the site of application.

Why does demyelination produce nerve block and how does it lead to slowing of conduction velocity? As discussed in Chapter 6, conduction velocity is much more rapid in myelinated fibers than in unmyelinated axons for two reasons. First, there is a direct relationship between conduction velocity and axon diameter, and myelinated axons tend to be larger in diameter. Second, membrane capacitance in the myelinated regions of the axon is less than at the unmyelinated nodes of Ranvier, greatly speeding up the rate of depolarization and thus conduction. In contrast, when an action potential propagates along long stretches of demyelinated axon it becomes severely attenuated.

When myelination is disrupted by disease, the action potentials in different axons of a nerve begin to conduct at slightly different velocities. As a result, the nerve loses its normal synchrony of conduction in response to a single stimulus (measurement of conduction velocities in peripheral nerves is described in Figure 14–2). This slowing and loss of synchrony are thought to account for some early clinical signs of demyelinating neuropathy. For example, functions that normally depend on the arrival of synchronous bursts of neural activity, such as tendon reflexes and vibratory sensation, are lost soon after the onset of a chronic neuropathy. As demyelination becomes more severe, conduction becomes blocked. Conduction failure may be intermittent, occurring only at high frequencies of neural firing, or complete.

The Molecular Bases of Some Inherited Peripheral Neuropathies Have Been Defined

Myelin proteins have been found to be affected in some demyelinating hereditary peripheral neuropathies, termed Charcot-Marie-Tooth disease. As in other peripheral neuropathies, muscle weakness and wasting, loss of reflexes, and loss of sensation in the distal parts of the limbs characterize the condition. These symptoms appear in childhood or adolescence and are slowly progressive.

One form (type 1) has the features of a demyelinating neuropathy. Conduction in peripheral nerves is slow, with histological evidence of demyelination followed by remyelination. Sometimes the remyelination leads to gross hypertrophy of the nerves. Type 1 disorders are inexorably progressive, without remissions or exacerbations. Another form (type 2) has normal nerve conduction velocity and is considered an axonal neuropathy without demyelination. Both types 1 and 2 are inherited as autosomal dominant diseases.

In the 1990s the genetic defects in these conditions began to be localized. The type 1 disease was attributed to mutations on two different chromosomes (locus heterogeneity). A more common form (type 1A) was linked to chromosome 17, whereas a less common form (1B) was localized to chromosome 1. To a remarkable degree the genes at these loci have been directly implicated in myelin physiology (Figure 14–3). Type 1A involves a defect in peripheral myelin protein 22, and type 1B the myelin protein P_0. Moreover, as discussed in Chapter 8, an X-linked form of demyelinating neuropathy occurs because of mutations in the gene expressing connexin-32, a subunit of the gap-junction channels that interconnect myelin folds near the nodes of Ranvier (Figure 14–3B). Still other genes have been implicated in inherited demyelination.

Some proteins implicated in axonal neuropathies are identified in Figure 14–4 and Table 14–1. Genes encoding the neurofilament light subunit and an axonal motor protein related to kinesin, which is important for transport along microtubules, are mutated in two types of axonal neuropathies. Defects in these genes are associated with peripheral neuropathies with prominent weakness. The mechanisms by which genes alter axonal function in other axonal neuropathies are less evident.

As noted earlier, a wide range of problems other than genetic mutations lead to peripheral neuropathies. Particularly striking are nerve defects associated with the presence of autoantibodies directed against ion channels in distal peripheral nerves. For example, some individuals with motor unit instability (cramps and fasciculations), as well as sustained or exaggerated muscle contractions caused by hyperexcitability of motor nerves, have serum antibodies directed against one or more axonal voltage-gated K^+ channels. The prevailing view is that binding the autoantibodies to the channels reduces K^+ conductance and thereby depolarizes the axon, leading to augmented and sustained firing of the distal motor nerve and associated muscle contractions. Alterations in ion channel function underlie a variety of neurological disorders, as in acquired disorders of channels in the neuromuscular junction and inherited defects in voltage-gated channels in muscle (discussed below).

Diseases of the Neuromuscular Junction Have Multiple Causes

Many diseases involve disruption of chemical transmission between neurons and their target cells. By analyzing such abnormalities researchers have learned a great deal about the mechanisms underlying normal synaptic transmission as well as disorders caused by dysfunction at the synapse.

Diseases that disrupt transmission at the neuromuscular junction fall into two broad categories:

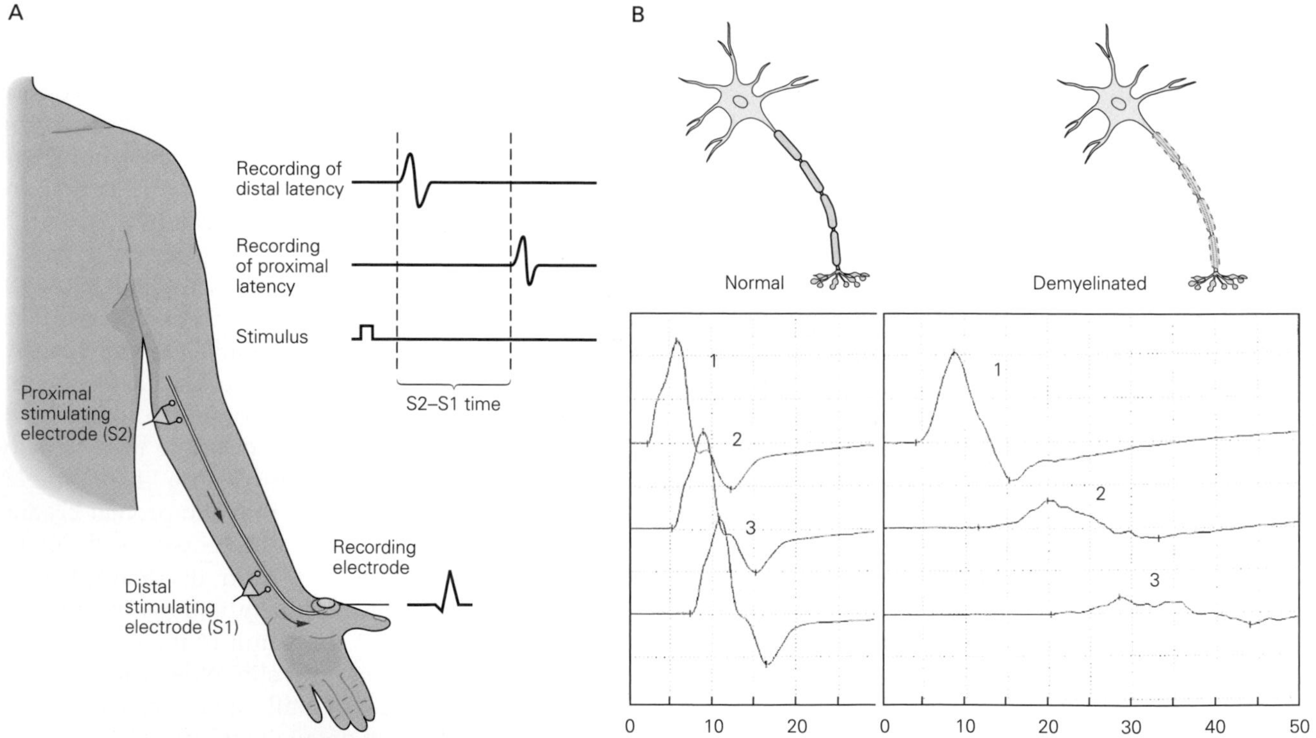

Figure 14–2 Measurement of motor nerve conduction velocity.

A. A shock is applied through a proximal (S2) or distal (S1) stimulating electrode, and the extracellular action potential is measured by the recording electrode. The time it takes the action potential to propagate from S2 to the muscle (t_{S2}) is the proximal latency; the time from S1 to the muscle (t_{S1}) is the distal latency. The distance between S1 and S2 divided by ($t_{S2} - t_{S1}$) gives the conduction velocity.

B. The waveforms of motor nerve action potentials are recorded in the thumb muscles after stimulation of the motor nerve at the wrist (**1**), just below the elbow (**2**), and just above the elbow (**3**). The action potentials from a normal nerve have the same waveforms regardless of the site of stimulation. They are distinguished only by the longer time period required for the waveform to develop as the site of the stimulus is moved up the arm (away from the recording site). When the motor nerve is demyelinated just distal to the elbow but above the wrist, the motor nerve action potential is normal when stimulation occurs at the wrist (**1**) but delayed and desynchronized when stimulation is proximal to the nerve lesion (**2, 3**). (Reproduced, with permission, from Bromberg 2002.)

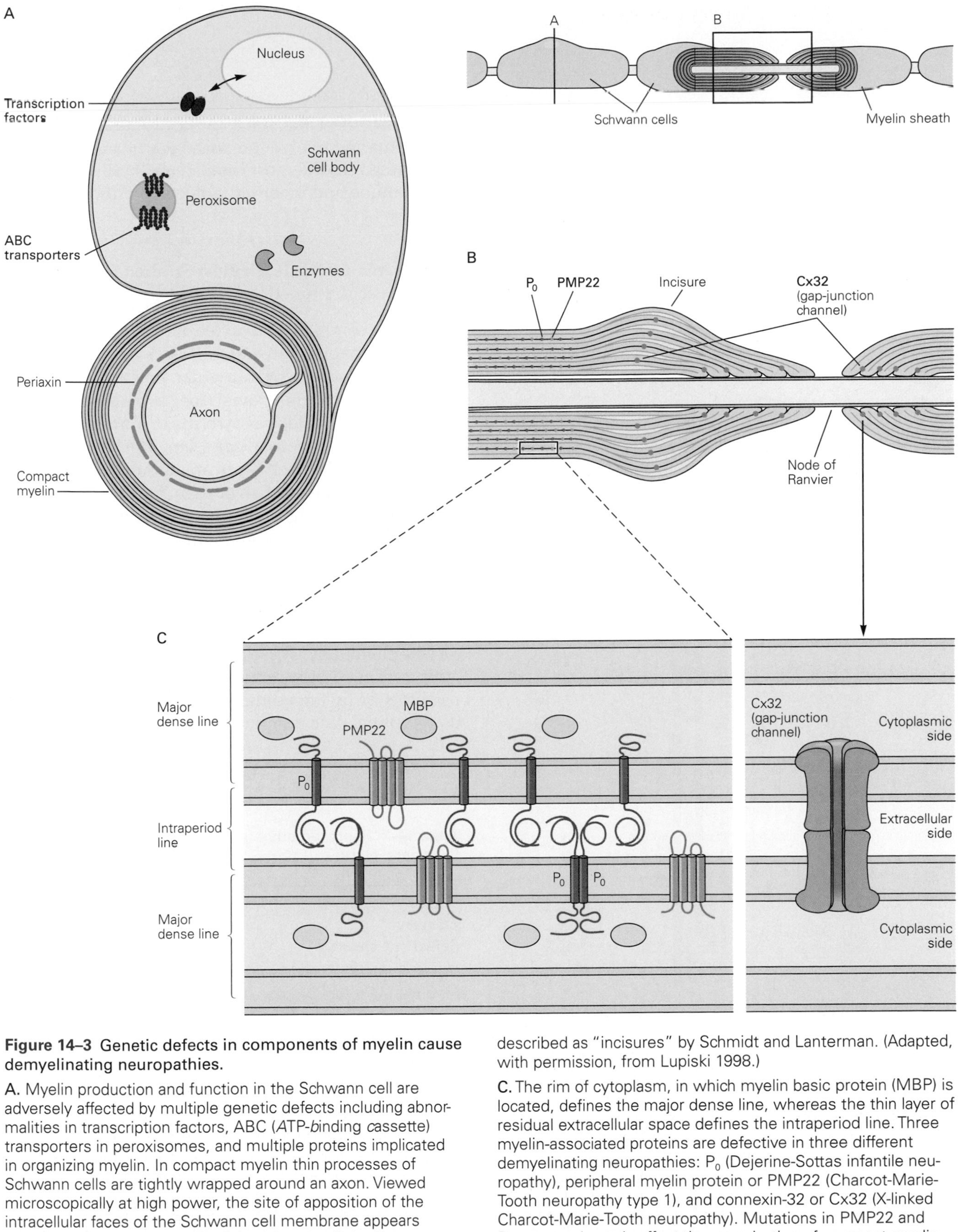

Figure 14–3 Genetic defects in components of myelin cause demyelinating neuropathies.

A. Myelin production and function in the Schwann cell are adversely affected by multiple genetic defects including abnormalities in transcription factors, ABC (*ATP-binding cassette*) transporters in peroxisomes, and multiple proteins implicated in organizing myelin. In compact myelin thin processes of Schwann cells are tightly wrapped around an axon. Viewed microscopically at high power, the site of apposition of the intracellular faces of the Schwann cell membrane appears as a dense line, whereas the apposed extracellular faces are described as the *intraperiod line* (see definition in part C). (Adapted, with permission, from Lupiski 1998.)

B. Peripheral axons are wrapped in myelin, which is compact and tight except near the nodes of Ranvier and at focal sites described as "incisures" by Schmidt and Lanterman. (Adapted, with permission, from Lupiski 1998.)

C. The rim of cytoplasm, in which myelin basic protein (MBP) is located, defines the major dense line, whereas the thin layer of residual extracellular space defines the intraperiod line. Three myelin-associated proteins are defective in three different demyelinating neuropathies: P_0 (Dejerine-Sottas infantile neuropathy), peripheral myelin protein or PMP22 (Charcot-Marie-Tooth neuropathy type 1), and connexin-32 or Cx32 (X-linked Charcot-Marie-Tooth neuropathy). Mutations in PMP22 and P_0 genes adversely affect the organization of compact myelin. (Adapted, with permission, from Brown and Amato 2002.)

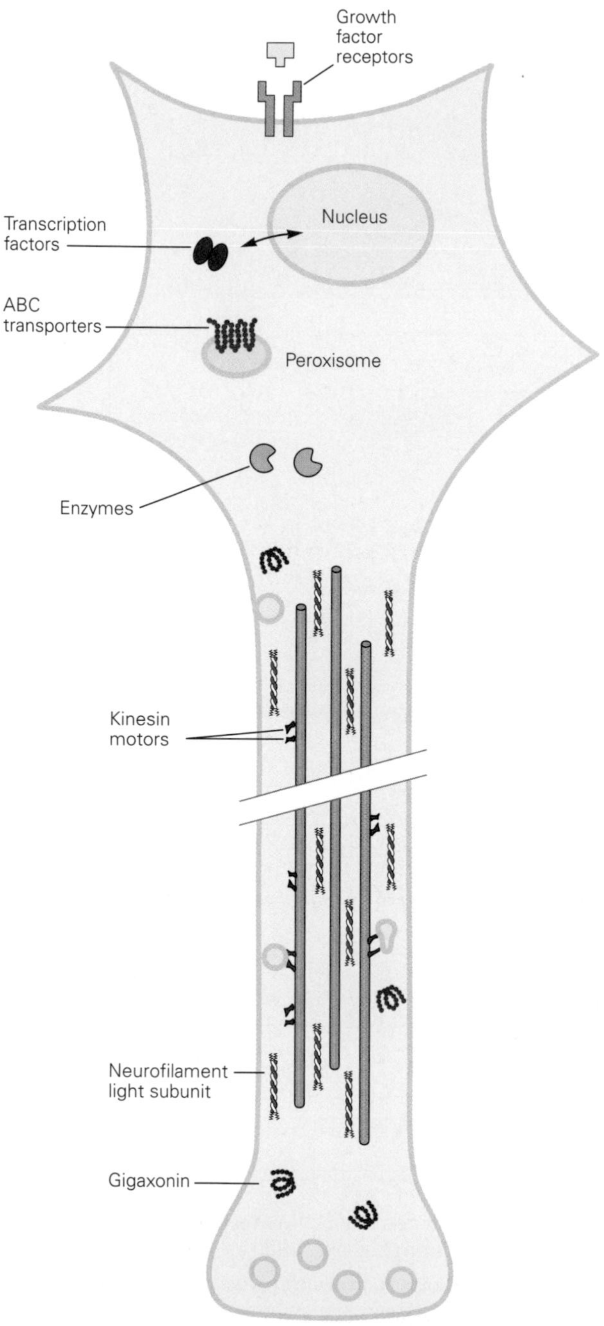

Figure 14–4 Genetic defects in a number of cell constituents cause axonal neuropathies. These include defects in receptors for growth factors, ABC (ATP-binding cassette) transporters in peroxisomes, cytosolic enzymes, microtubule motor proteins like the kinesins, neurofilament proteins, and other structural proteins such as gigaxonin. (Adapted, with permission, from Brown and Amato 2002.)

those that affect the presynaptic terminal and those that primarily involve the postsynaptic membrane. In both categories the most intensively studied cases are autoimmune and inherited defects in critical synaptic proteins.

Myasthenia Gravis Is the Best Studied Example of a Neuromuscular Junction Disease

The most common and extensively studied disease affecting synaptic transmission is myasthenia gravis, a disorder at the neuromuscular junction in skeletal muscle. Myasthenia gravis (the term means severe weakness of muscle) has two major forms. The most prevalent is the autoimmune form. The second is congenital and heritable; it is not an autoimmune disorder and is heterogeneous. Fewer than 500 cases have been identified, but analysis of the congenital syndromes has provided information about the organization and function of the human neuromuscular junction. This form is discussed later in the chapter.

In autoimmune myasthenia gravis antibodies are produced against the nicotinic acetylcholine (ACh) receptor in muscle. These antibodies interfere with synaptic transmission by reducing the number of functional receptors or by impeding the interaction of ACh with its receptors. As a result, communication between the

Table 14–1 Representative Inherited Disorders of Peripheral Nerves

Site of primary defect	Protein	Disease
Myelin	Proteolipid myelin protein 22	Charcot-Marie-Tooth disease (CMT)
	Proteolipid protein P_0	Infantile CMT (Dejerine-Sottas neuropathy)
	Connexin-32	X-linked CMT
Axon	Kinesin KIF1Bβ motor protein	Motor predominant neuropathy
	Heat shock protein 27	Motor predominant neuropathy
	Neurofilament light subunit	Motor predominant neuropathy
	Tyrosine kinase A receptor	Congenital sensory neuropathy
	ABC 1 transporter	Tangier disease
	Transthyretin	Amyloid neuropathy

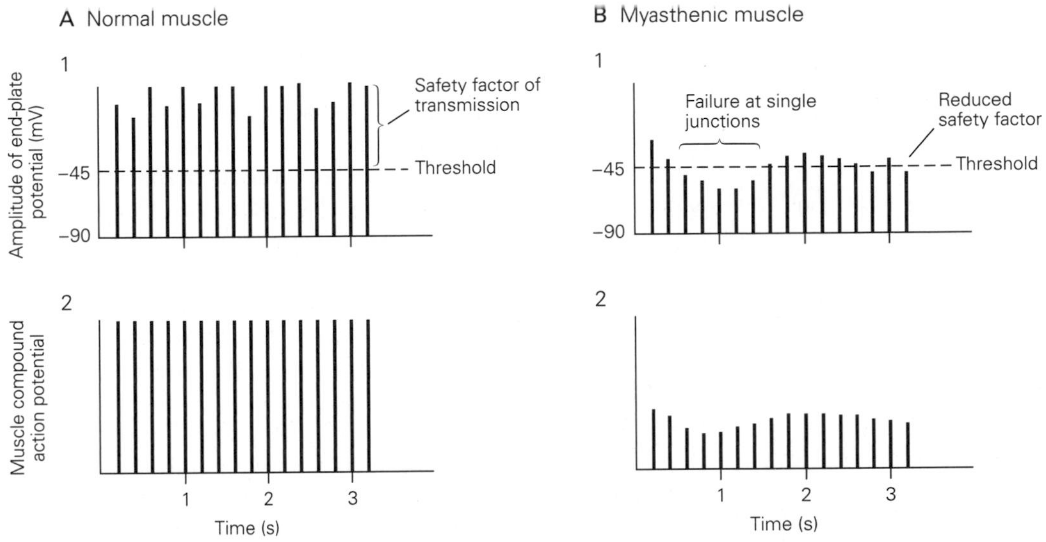

Figure 14–5 Synaptic transmission at the neuromuscular junction fails in myasthenia gravis. (Reproduced, with permission, from Lisak and Barchi 1982.)

A. In the normal neuromuscular junction the amplitude of the end-plate potential is so large that all fluctuations in the potential occur well above the threshold for an action potential. That is, there is a large safety factor in synaptic transmission (**1**). Therefore, during repetitive stimulation of the motor nerve the amplitude of the compound action potentials, representing the action potentials in all muscle fibers innervated by the nerve, is constant and invariant (**2**).

B. In the myasthenic neuromuscular junction postsynaptic changes reduce the amplitude of the end-plate potential so that under optimal circumstances the end-plate potential may be just sufficient to produce a muscle action potential. Fluctuations in transmitter release that normally accompany repeated stimulation now cause the end-plate potential to drop below this threshold, leading to conduction failure at that synapse (**1**). The amplitude of the compound action potentials in the muscle declines progressively and shows only a small and variable recovery (**2**).

motor neuron and the skeletal muscle becomes weakened. This weakness has four special characteristics:

1. It almost always affects cranial muscles—eyelids, eye muscles, and oropharyngeal muscles—as well as limb muscles.
2. The severity of symptoms varies in the course of a single day, from day to day, or over longer periods (giving rise to periods of remission or exacerbation), making myasthenia gravis unlike most other diseases of muscle or nerve.
3. There are no conventional clinical or electromyographic signs of denervation.
4. The weakness is reversed by drugs that inhibit acetylcholinesterase, the enzyme that degrades ACh.

Myasthenia gravis is a disorder of neuromuscular transmission. When a motor nerve is stimulated at rates of 2 to 5 per second, the amplitude of the compound action potential evoked in normal human muscle remains constant. In myasthenia gravis the amplitude decreases rapidly. This abnormality resembles the pattern induced in normal muscle by *d*-tubocurarine (the active compound in curare), which blocks nicotinic ACh receptors and inhibits the action of ACh at the neuromuscular junction. Neostigmine (Prostigmin), which inhibits acetylcholinesterase and thus prolongs the action of ACh at the neuromuscular junction, reverses the decrease in amplitude of evoked compound action potentials in myasthenic patients (Figure 14–5).

The decrease in the compound muscle action potential in response to repetitive stimulation of the motor nerve mirrors the clinical symptom of fatigability in myasthenia. For example, when patients are asked to look upward in a sustained gaze, the eyelids tire after several seconds and droop downward (ptosis). Like decremental responses on electromyography, this fatigability and drooping reverse after treatment with inhibitors of acetylcholinesterase (Figure 14–6).

Approximately 15% of adult patients with myasthenia have benign tumors of the thymus (thymomas). As the symptoms in myasthenic patients are often improved by removal of these tumors, some element of the thymoma may stimulate autoimmune

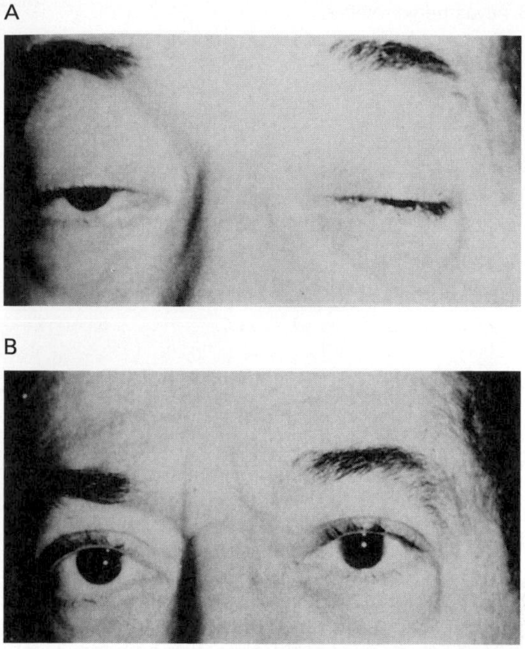

Figure 14–6 Myasthenia gravis often selectively affects the cranial muscles. (Reproduced, with permission, from Rowland, Hoefer, and Aranow 1960.)

A. Severe drooping of the eyelids, or ptosis, is characteristic of myasthenia gravis. This patient also could not move his eyes to look to either side.

B. One minute after an intravenous injection of 10 mg edrophonium, an inhibitor of acetylcholinesterase, both eyes are open and can be moved freely. The inhibition of acetylcholinesterase prolongs the action of ACh in the synaptic cleft, thus compensating for the reduced number of ACh receptors in the muscle (see Figure 14–7).

pathology. Indeed, myasthenia gravis often affects people who have other autoimmune diseases, such as rheumatoid arthritis, systemic lupus erythematosus, or Graves disease (hyperthyroidism).

The modern concept of myasthenia emerged with the isolation and characterization of the nicotinic ACh receptor. In 1973 Douglas Fambrough and Daniel Drachman, using radioactive α-bungarotoxin to label the receptor in human end-plates, found fewer binding sites in myasthenic muscle than in controls. In addition, morphological studies revealed a smoothing of the junctional folds, the site of receptor localization (Figure 14–7).

That same year James Patrick and Jon Lindstrom demonstrated in rabbits that the generation of antireceptor antibodies was accompanied by the onset of myasthenia-like symptoms when they injected animals with nicotinic ACh receptors purified from eel electroplax (which is related to the skeletal muscles of higher vertebrates). The weakness was reversed by the cholinesterase inhibitors neostigmine or edrophonium. As in humans with myasthenia gravis, the animals were abnormally sensitive to neuromuscular blocking agents such as curare, and the evoked compound action potentials in muscle decreased with repetitive stimulation. It was later found that a similar syndrome could be induced in mice and other mammals by immunization with nicotinic ACh receptor protein (Figure 14–8).

By 1975 all the essential characteristics of the human disease had been reproduced in experimental

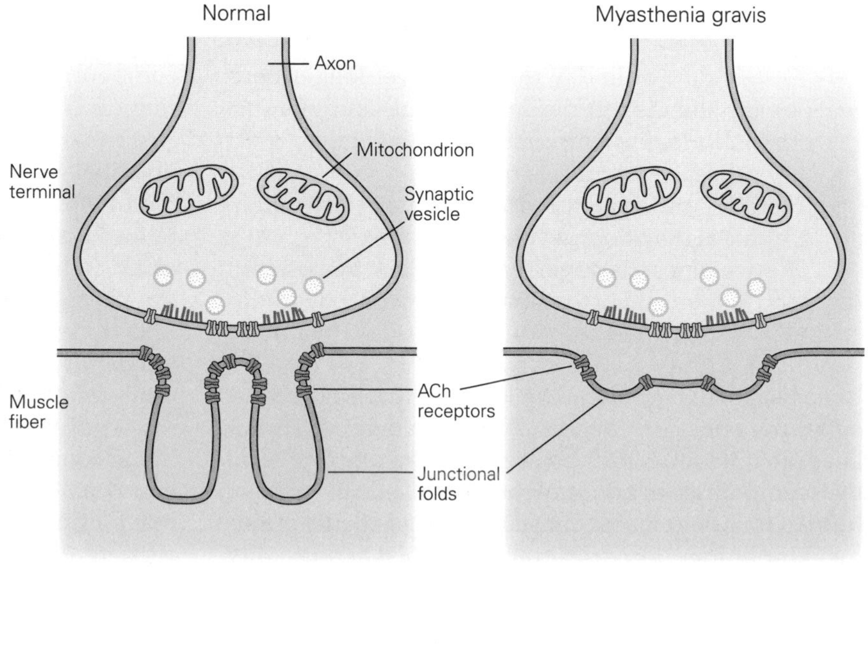

Figure 14–7 Morphological abnormalities of the neuromuscular junction in myasthenia gravis. At the neuromuscular junction ACh is released by exocytosis of synaptic vesicles at active zones in the nerve terminal. Acetylcholine flows across the synaptic cleft to reach receptors that are concentrated at the peaks of junctional folds. Acetylcholinesterase in the cleft rapidly terminates transmission by hydrolyzing ACh. The myasthenic neuromuscular junction has a reduced number of ACh receptors, simplified synaptic folds, and a widened synaptic space, but a normal nerve terminal.

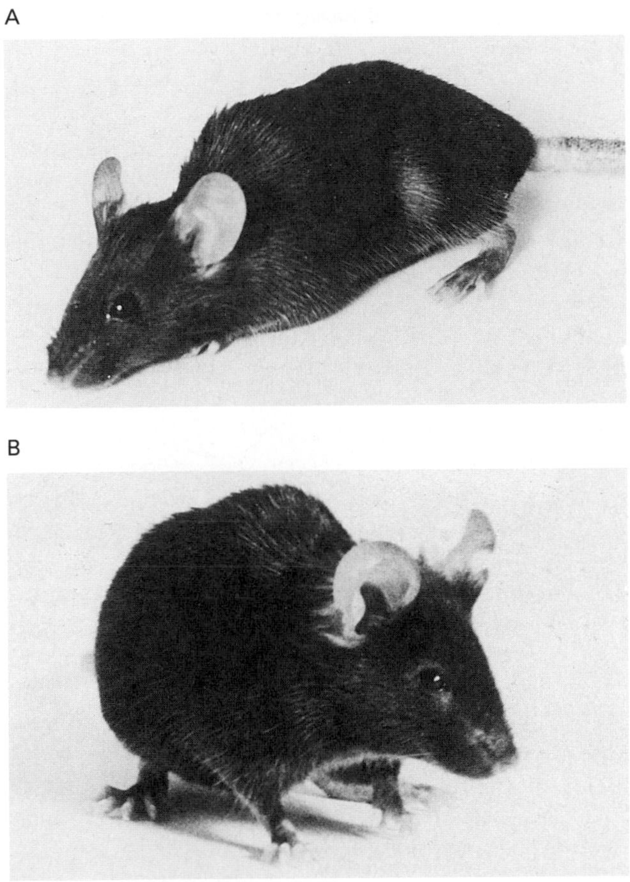

Figure 14–8 The posture of a myasthenic mouse improves after treatment with neostigmine. To produce the syndrome the mouse was immunized with 15 μg of purified nicotinic ACh receptor protein. (Reproduced, with permission, from Berman and Patrick 1980.)

A. Before treatment the mouse is inactive.

B. The mouse is standing 12 minutes after receiving an intraperitoneal injection of 37.5 μg/kg neostigmine bromide, which inhibits acetylcholinesterase and thus increases the availability of ACh in the synaptic cleft of the neuromuscular junction.

autoimmune myasthenia gravis in mice, rabbits, and monkeys. After experimental myasthenia gravis was characterized, antibodies directed against nicotinic ACh receptors were found in the serum of many patients with myasthenia. How do these immunological observations account for the characteristic decrease in the response of myasthenic muscle to repeated stimulation?

An action potential in a motor axon normally releases enough ACh to induce a large excitatory end-plate potential with an amplitude of approximately 70 to 80 mV relative to the resting potential of –90 mV (see Chapter 9). Thus the normal end-plate potential is greater than the threshold needed to initiate an action potential, approximately –45 mV. In normal muscle the difference between the threshold and the actual end-plate potential amplitude—the safety factor—is therefore quite large (Figure 14–5A). In fact, in many muscles the amount of ACh released during synaptic transmission can be reduced to as little as 25% of normal before it fails to initiate an action potential.

A reduction in the density of ACh receptors, as in myasthenia, reduces the probability that a molecule of ACh will find a receptor before it is hydrolyzed by the enzyme acetylcholinesterase. In addition, in myasthenia the geometry of the end-plate is also disturbed. The normal infolding at the junctional folds is reduced and the synaptic cleft is enlarged (Figure 14–7). These morphological changes promote diffusion of ACh away from the synaptic cleft and thus further reduce the probability of ACh interacting with the few remaining functional receptors. As a result, the amplitude of the end-plate potential is reduced to the point where it is barely above threshold (Figure 14–5B).

Thus in myasthenia synaptic transmission is readily blocked even though the vesicles in the presynaptic terminals contain normal amounts of ACh and the process of transmitter release is intact. Both the physiological abnormality (the decremental response) and the clinical symptoms (muscle weakness) are partially reversed by drugs that inhibit acetylcholinesterase (Figures 14–6 and 14–8).

How do antibodies cause the symptoms of myasthenia? The antibodies do not simply occupy the site of ACh binding. Rather, they appear to react with epitopes elsewhere on the receptor molecule. This increases the destruction of nicotinic ACh receptors, probably because myasthenic antibodies bind and cross-link the receptors, triggering their degradation (Figure 14–9). In addition, some myasthenic antibodies bind proteins of the complement cascade of the immune system, causing lysis of the postsynaptic membrane.

Despite the evidence documenting the primary role of antibodies against the nicotinic ACh receptor in myasthenia, approximately one-fifth of patients with myasthenia, including some who respond to anti-immune therapy like plasmapheresis, do not have these antibodies. Instead, most of these patients have antibodies against another postsynaptic protein, known as MuSK (*mu*scle-*s*pecific Trk-related receptor with a *k*ringle domain). MuSK is a receptor tyrosine kinase that interacts with agrin, a protein released from the motor nerve terminal that helps to organize the nicotinic ACh receptors into clusters at the neuromuscular junction.

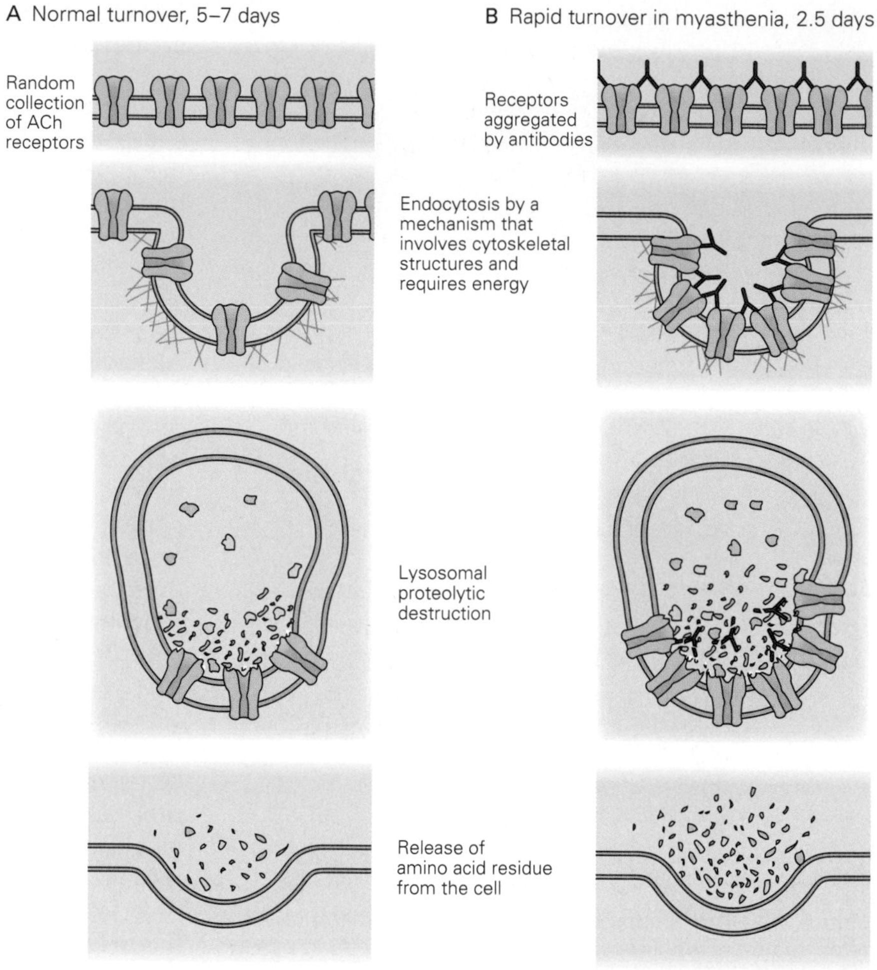

Figure 14–9 Turnover of ACh receptors increases in myasthenia. (Adapted, with permission, from Lindstrom 1983, and Drachman 1983.)

A. Normal turnover of randomly spaced ACh receptors takes places every 5 to 7 days.

B. In myasthenia gravis and experimental myasthenia gravis, the cross-linking of ACh receptors by antibodies facilitates endocytosis and the phagocytic destruction of the receptors, which leads to a two- to threefold increase in the rate of receptor turnover. Binding of antireceptor antibody activates the complement cascade, which is involved in focal lysis of the postsynaptic membrane. This focal lysis is probably primarily responsible for the characteristic morphological alterations of postsynaptic membranes in myasthenia (see Figure 14–7).

It appears to be functionally important both during development and in the adult. Although the adverse effects of the anti-MuSK antibodies have not yet been defined, the antibodies block some of the normal clustering of the nicotinic ACh receptors following the interaction of agrin with MuSK.

Treatment of Myasthenia Targets the Physiological Effects and Autoimmune Pathogenesis of the Disease

Anticholinesterases, especially pyridostigmine, provide symptomatic relief, but the treatment is rarely complete and does not alter the basic disease. Immunosuppressive therapies include corticosteroids and azathioprine or related drugs that suppress antibody synthesis.

Plasmapheresis—removing the plasma and the antibodies to the nicotinic ACh receptors or to MuSK—often ameliorates symptoms within days or a few weeks, as does infusion of immunoglobulin.

Although the benefit is transient, it may be sufficient to prepare a patient for thymectomy or to support the patient through more severe episodes. Intravenous administration of immunoglobulins also reduces the titer of antibodies to the nicotinic ACh receptor and to MuSK by mechanisms that are unclear.

There Are Two Distinct Congenital Forms of Myasthenia Gravis

There are two distinct types of myasthenia in which symptoms may be present from birth. In neonatal myasthenic syndrome the mother herself has autoimmune myasthenia that is transmitted passively to the newborn via the immune system. By contrast, in congenital myasthenia the infant has an inherited defect in some component of the neuromuscular junction, rather than an autoimmune disease, and thus does not have serum antibodies to the nicotinic ACh receptor or MuSK.

Congenital myasthenic syndromes fall into three broad groups based on the site of the defect in the neuromuscular synapse: presynaptic, synaptic cleft, and postsynaptic forms. Clinical features common to these disorders include a positive family history, weakness with easy fatigability (present since infancy), drooping of the eyelids (ptosis), a decremental response to repetitive stimulation on electromyography, and negative screening for anti-nicotinic ACh receptor antibodies. A striking feature of many of these diseases is the subnormal development of the skeletal muscles, reflecting the fact that normal function at the neuromuscular synapse is required to maintain normal muscle bulk.

In one presynaptic form of congenital myasthenia the enzyme choline acetyltransferase is absent or reduced in the distal motor terminal. This enzyme is essential for the synthesis of ACh from choline and acetyl coenzyme A (see Chapter 13). In its absence the synthesis of ACh is impaired. The result is weakness that usually begins in infancy or early childhood. In another presynaptic form of congenital myasthenia the number of quanta of ACh released after an action potential is less than normal. The molecular basis for this defect is unknown.

Congenital myasthenia may also result from the absence of acetylcholinesterase in the synaptic cleft. In this circumstance end-plate potentials and miniature end-plate potentials are not small, as in autoimmune myasthenia, but are rather markedly prolonged, which may explain the repetitive response of the evoked muscle potential in those patients. Cytochemical studies indicate that ACh-esterase is absent from the basement membranes. At the same time, nicotinic ACh receptors are preserved.

The physiological consequence of ACh-esterase deficiency is sustained action of ACh on the end-plate and ultimately the development of an end-plate myopathy. This myopathy indicates that skeletal muscle can react adversely to excessive electrical stimulation at the neuromuscular junction. In treating this disorder it is critical to avoid using agents like inhibitors of ACh-esterase that can increase firing in the end-plate and thereby exacerbate the muscle weakness.

Most congenital myasthenia cases are caused by primary mutations in the genes encoding different subunits of the nicotinic ACh receptor. The *slow channel syndrome* is characterized by prominent limb weakness but little weakness of cranial muscles (the reverse of the pattern usually seen in autoimmune myasthenia, where muscles of the eyes and oropharynx are almost always affected). End-plate currents are slow to decay and channel opening is abnormally long. The mutations probably act both by increasing the affinity of the nicotinic ACh receptor for ACh, thereby prolonging the effects of this transmitter, and by directly slowing the channel closing rate. In some instances quinidine is effective therapy for slow channel syndrome because it blocks the open receptor-channel. As in ACh-esterase mutations, the end-plate degenerates because of excessive postsynaptic stimulation, and thus anticholinesterase medications are potentially dangerous.

In the *fast channel syndrome* a different set of mutations in one or more subunits of the nicotinic ACh receptor leads to an accelerated rate of channel closing and end-plate current decay. The fast channel syndrome may respond either to acetylcholinesterase inhibitors or to 3,4-diaminopyridine, which increases presynaptic firing and ACh quantal release, probably by blocking a presynaptic K^+ conductance.

Lambert-Eaton Syndrome and Botulism Are Two Other Disorders of Neuromuscular Transmission

Some patients with cancer, especially small-cell cancer of the lung, have a syndrome of proximal limb weakness and a neuromuscular disorder with characteristics that are the opposite of those seen in myasthenia gravis. Instead of a decline in synaptic response to repetitive nerve stimulation, the amplitude of the evoked potential increases; that is, neuromuscular transmission is facilitated. The first postsynaptic potential is abnormally small, and subsequent responses increase in amplitude so that the final summated potential is two to four times the amplitude of the first potential.

This disorder, *Lambert-Eaton syndrome*, is attributed to the action of antibodies against voltage-gated Ca^{2+} channels in the presynaptic terminals. It is thought that these antibodies react with an antigen in the channels, degrading the channels as the antibody-antigen complex is internalized. Calcium channels similar to those in presynaptic terminals are found in cultured cells from the small-cell carcinoma of the lung; development of antibodies against these antigens in the tumor might be followed by pathogenic action against nerve terminals, another kind of molecular mimicry.

A facilitating neuromuscular block also occurs in human botulism, because the botulinum toxin also impairs release of ACh from nerve terminals. Both botulism and Lambert-Eaton syndrome are ameliorated by administration of calcium gluconate or guanidine, agents that promote the release of ACh. These drugs are less effective than immunosuppressive treatments for long-term control of Lambert-Eaton syndrome, which is chronic. However, botulism is transient, and if the patient is kept alive during the acute phase by treating symptoms, the disorder disappears in weeks as the infection is controlled and botulinum toxin is inactivated.

Diseases of Skeletal Muscle Can Be Inherited or Acquired

The weakness seen in any myopathy is usually attributed to degeneration of muscle fibers. At first the missing fibers are replaced by regeneration of new fibers. Ultimately, however, renewal cannot keep pace and fibers are lost progressively. This leads to compound potentials of brief duration and reduced amplitude in the motor unit. The decreased number of functioning muscle fibers accounts for the diminished strength. Skeletal muscle diseases are conveniently divided into those that are inherited and those that appear to be acquired.

Dermatomyositis Exemplifies Acquired Myopathy

The prototype of an acquired myopathy is dermatomyositis, defined by two clinical features: rash and myopathy. The rash has a predilection for the face, chest, and extensor surfaces of joints, including the fingers. The myopathic weakness primarily affects proximal limb muscles. Both rash and weakness usually appear simultaneously and become worse in a matter of weeks. The weakness may be mild or life-threatening.

This disorder affects children or adults. Approximately 10% of adult patients have malignant tumors. Although the pathogenesis is unknown, dermatomyositis is thought to be an autoimmune disorder of small intramuscular blood vessels.

Muscular Dystrophies Are the Most Common Inherited Myopathies

The best-known inherited muscle diseases are the muscular dystrophies; several major types are distinguished by clinical and genetic patterns. Some types are characterized by weakness alone (Duchenne, facioscapulohumeral and limb girdle dystrophies); others have additional clinical features (such as the myotonic muscular dystrophies). Most are recessively inherited and begin in early childhood (Duchenne, Becker, and limb girdle dystrophy); less frequently, the dystrophies are dominantly inherited (facioscapulohumeral or myotonic dystrophy). In the limb-girdle dystrophies progressive weakness of the proximal limbs is a cardinal trait. In the myotonic muscular dystrophies progressive weakness is accompanied by severe muscle stiffness.

Duchenne muscular dystrophy affects only males because it is transmitted as an X-linked recessive trait. It starts in early childhood and progresses relatively rapidly, so patients are in wheelchairs by age 12 years and usually die in their third decade. This dystrophy is caused by mutations that severely reduce levels of dystrophin, a skeletal muscle protein that apparently confers tensile strength to the muscle cell. In a related inherited muscle disorder known as *Becker muscular dystrophy,* dystrophin is present but is either abnormal in size or reduced in quantity (approximately 10%). Becker dystrophy is thus much milder; individuals with Becker dystrophy typically are able to walk well into adulthood, albeit with weakness of the proximal leg and arm muscles.

The dystrophin gene is the second largest human gene, spanning approximately 2.5 million base pairs, or 1% of the X chromosome and 0.1% of the total human genome. It contains at least 79 exons that encode a 14-kb mRNA. The inferred amino acid sequence of the dystrophin protein suggests a rod-like structure and a molecular weight of 427,000, with domains similar to those of two cytoskeletal proteins, alpha-actinin and spectrin. Dystrophin is localized to the inner surface of the plasma membrane. The amino terminus of dystrophin is linked to cytoskeletal actin, whereas the carboxy terminus is linked to the extracellular matrix by transmembrane proteins (Figure 14–10).

Most boys with Duchenne muscular dystrophy have a deletion in the dystrophin gene; approximately a third have point mutations. In both cases the mutations introduce premature stop codons in the mutant RNA transcripts that prevent synthesis of full-length dystrophin. Becker dystrophy is also caused by deletions and missense mutations, but the mutations do not introduce stop codons. The resulting dystrophin protein is nearly normal in length and can at least partially substitute for normal dystrophin (Figure 14–11).

The discovery of the affected gene product in Duchenne muscular dystrophy by Louis Kunkel in the mid-1980s was rapidly followed by the discovery of numerous other novel muscle proteins, some with an intimate relationship to dystrophin. As a result, the primary genetic and protein defects underlying most major muscular dystrophies have now been identified (Table 14–2). Thus it may be more constructive now to change the system of classifying the dystrophies to one based on the component of the muscle cell that is implicated. Most of the dystrophies, best represented

Table 14–2 Representative Muscular Dystrophies

Site of primary defect	Protein	Disease
Extracellular matrix	Collagen VI α1, α2, and α3	Bethlem myopathy
	Merosin laminin α2-subunit	Congenital myopathy
Transmembrane	α-sarcoglycan	LGMD-2D
	β-sarcoglycan	LGMD-2E
	χ-sarcoglycan	LGMD-2C
	σ-sarcoglycan	LGMD-2F
	Dysferlin	LGMD-2B, Miyoshi myopathy
	Caveolin-3	LGMD-1C, rippling muscle disease
	α7-integrin	Congenital myopathy
	Na^+ channel	Hyperkalemic paralysis
	Ca^{2+} channel	Hypokalemic paralysis
	Cl^- channel	Myotonia congenita
	XK protein	McLeod syndrome
Submembrane	Dystrophin	Duchenne, Becker dystrophies
Sarcomere/myofibrils	Tropomyosin B	Nemaline rod myopathy
	Calpain	LGMD-2A
	Titin	Distal (Udd) dystrophy
	Nebulin	Nemaline rod myopathy
	Telethonin	LGMD-2G
	Skeletal muscle actin	Nemaline rod myopathy
	Troponin	Nemaline rod myopathy
Cytoplasm	Desmin	Desmin storage myopathy
	αβ-crystallin	Distal myofibrillar myopathy
	Selenoprotein	Rigid spine syndrome
	Plectin	Epidermolysis bullosa simplex
Sarcoplasmic reticulum	Ryanodine receptor	Central core disease, malignant hyperthermia
	SERCA1	Brody myopathy
Nucleus	Emerin	Emery-Dreifuss dystrophy
	Lamin A/C	Emery-Dreifuss dystrophy
	Poly A binding protein, repeat	Oculopharyngeal dystrophy
Enzymes/miscellaneous	Myotonin kinase, CTG repeat	Myotonic dystrophy
	Zinc finger 9, CCTG repeat	Proximal myotonic dystrophy
	Epimerase	Inclusion body myositis
	Myotubularin	Myotubular myopathy
	Chorein	Chorea-acanthocytosis
Golgi apparatus	Fukutin	Fukuyama congenital dystrophy
	Fukutin-related peptide	Limb-girdle dystrophy
	POMT1	Congenital muscular dystrophy
	POMGnT1	Congenital muscular dystrophy

LGMD, limb-girdle muscular dystrophy.

by dystrophin deficiency, are believed to arise because of accelerated muscle injury and breakdown. A small group, associated with deficiency of the protein dysferlin, is a consequence of slower repair of muscle membrane after injury (Figure 14–10).

Many of these disorders are characterized by slowly progressive weakness of the proximal arms and legs and thus are limb-girdle dystrophies. Most are recessively inherited; mutations in both copies of a particular gene prevent expression of the normal protein product and thus lead to loss of function of that protein.

Primary genetic defects in a diverse group of skeletal muscle proteins lead to the limb-girdle phenotype (Table 14–2) in which weakness is prominent in the torso and in proximal muscles of the arms and legs. Why this pattern of degeneration is so common is unknown, especially because the affected proteins are expressed in both distal and proximal muscles. The pattern likely reflects muscle use. The proximal muscles are, on average, more subject to low-level but chronic contractile activity because they serve as antigravity muscles.

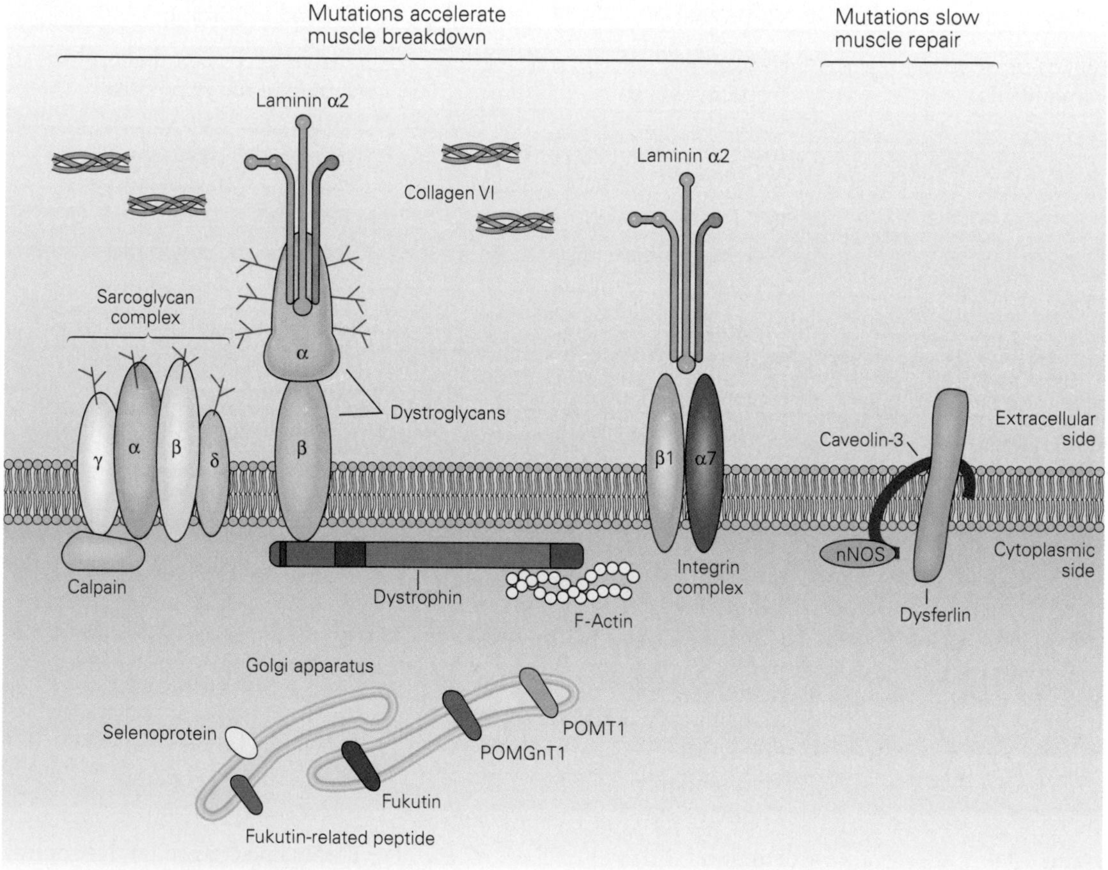

Figure 14–10 In muscular dystrophy mutant proteins either weaken the muscle cell membrane or slow its repair after injury. For example, a deficiency of dystrophin, a submembrane protein, causes Duchenne muscular dystrophy. Dystrophin interacts with complexes of other membrane proteins that are mutant in other dystrophies, including the dystroglycans and the sarcoglycans, which are closely associated with extracellular proteins such as laminin α2 and collagen. Several other proteins that are normally present in the Golgi apparatus and essential for adding sugar groups to membrane proteins are found to be mutant in different forms of muscular dystrophy. These include POMT1 (protein *O*-mannosyl transferase 1), POMGnT1 (protein *O*-mannosyl β1,2-*N*-acetylglucosaminyl transferase), fukutin, fukutin-related peptide, and a selenoprotein. Dysferlin, which is mutated in still other dystrophies, is involved in the repair of skeletal muscle membrane after injury. (Modified, with permission, from Brown and Mendell 2005.)

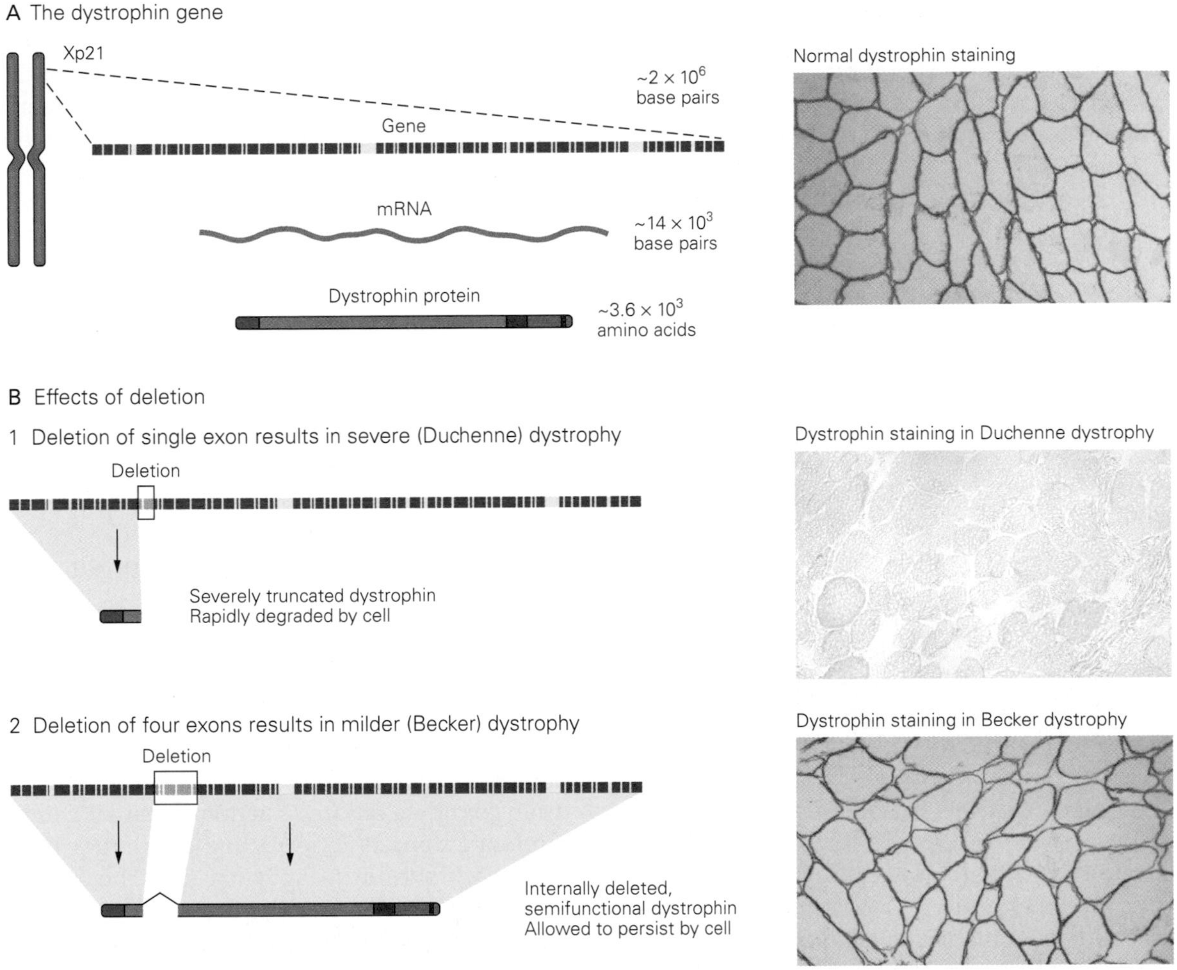

Figure 14–11 Two forms of muscular dystrophy are caused by deletion mutations in the dystrophin gene. (Adapted, with permission, from Hoffman and Kunkel 1989; photos, reproduced with permission, from Arthur P. Hays.)

A. The relative position of the dystrophin gene within the Xp21 region of the X chromosome. An enlargement of this locus shows the 65 exons (**light blue**) and introns (**dark blue**) defining the gene with approximately 2.0×10^6 base pairs. Transcription of the gene gives rise to mRNA (approximately 14×10^3 base pairs), and translation of this mRNA gives rise to the protein dystrophin (mol wt 427,000). Expression of dystrophin in a normal muscle is shown in an immunoperoxidase stain photo at right.

B. A deletion of genomic DNA encompassing only a single exon results in the clinically severe Duchenne muscular dystrophy. A larger deletion encompassing four exons results in the clinically milder Becker muscular dystrophy. In both cases the gene is transcribed into mRNA, and the exons flanking the deletion are spliced together. **1.** If a single exon is deleted and a nonintegral set of codons is missing, the borders of neighboring exons may not match, causing the translational reading frame to shift. As a result, incorrect amino acids are inserted into the growing polypeptide chain until an abnormal stop codon is reached, causing premature termination of the protein. The truncated protein may be unstable, may fail to be localized in the membrane, or may fail to bind to glycoproteins. Functional dystrophin is then almost totally absent. A muscle biopsy of Duchenne dystrophy (right) shows no detectable immunoreactive dystrophin. **2.** If the deletion is larger but an integral number of codons are deleted, the reading frame can be maintained in the mRNA. This produces a dystrophin molecule with an internal deletion but intact ends. Although the protein is smaller than normal and may be present in less than normal amounts, some muscle function is preserved. Immunoperoxidase staining of dystrophin is minimally reduced in a muscle biopsy of Becker dystrophy (right).

Myotonic dystrophy has several distinctive features, including an autosomal inheritance pattern, weakness that is predominantly distal, involvement of nonmuscle tissues, and striking muscle stiffness (myotonia). The stiffness is induced by excessive electrical discharges of the muscle membrane associated with voluntary muscle contractions or percussive or electrical stimulation of the muscle. It is most intense with the first few movements after a period of rest and improves with continued muscular activity (*warm-up* phenomenon). Typical features are difficulty relaxing the grip of a handshake for several seconds, difficulty opening the eyelids after forceful squinting, or stiffness in the legs with the first few steps after rising from a chair.

Electromyography demonstrates that the muscle cell membrane is electrically hyperexcitable; after a contraction, bursts of repetitive action potentials wax and wane in amplitude and frequency (20–100 Hz) over several seconds and thereby delay relaxation (Figure 14–12A). This sustained contraction is truly independent of nerve supply because it persists after blockade of either the incoming motor nerve impulse or neuromuscular transmission with agents such as curare.

The symptoms are not confined to muscles. Almost all patients have cataracts; affected men commonly have testicular atrophy and baldness and often develop cardiac conduction system defects that lead to irregularities in the heartbeat. The primary genetic defect is a dominantly transmitted expansion of a triplet of base pairs (CTG) in a noncoding region of a gene (myotonin kinase) on chromosome 19. RNA transcripts of the expanded CTG segments accumulate in the nucleus and alter splicing of several critical genes, including the gene for a Cl^- channel, ClC-1 (see Chapter 5). Loss of function of this channel leads to excessive electrical activity in skeletal muscle and, as a consequence, myotonia. As discussed below, direct mutations in the same Cl^- channel gene can lead to a similar abnormal pattern of muscle activity.

Some Inherited Diseases of Skeletal Muscle Arise from Genetic Defects in Voltage-Gated Ion Channels

The normal electrical excitability of skeletal muscle is essential to the rapid and nearly synchronous contraction of an entire muscle fiber. The depolarizing end-plate potential at the neuromuscular junction triggers an action potential that propagates longitudinally along the surface of the muscle fiber and radially inward along the transverse tubules, invaginations of the fiber membrane that come into close apposition with the sarcoplasmic reticulum (see Chapter 34).

Depolarization of the transverse tubules induces a conformational change in L-type voltage-gated Ca^{2+} channels. The conformational change is directly transmitted to a particular class of Ca^{2+} release channels (ryanodine receptors) in the sarcoplasmic reticulum, causing the channels to open. The release of Ca^{2+} from the sarcoplasmic reticulum raises myoplasmic Ca^{2+} and thus activates ATP-dependent movement of actin-myosin filaments.

Normally, one action potential is generated in a muscle fiber for each end-plate potential. Repolarization of the muscle action potential depends on inactivation of Na^+ channels and the opening of delayed-rectifier voltage-gated K^+ channels similar to those in axons. In addition, Cl^- influx through the ClC-1 channels is important in maintaining the normal negative resting potential. Mutations in any one of these channels contribute to inherited muscle disease.

Periodic Paralysis Is Associated with Altered Muscle Excitability and Abnormal Levels of Serum Potassium

The electrical coupling of the end-plate potential to depolarization of the transverse tubules is disrupted in several inherited diseases of muscle. These disorders reflect a variety of defects in excitability ranging from complete failure of action potential generation to prolonged bursts of repetitive discharges in response to a single stimulus (Figure 14–12). The derangements of muscle fiber excitability are transient and result in *periodic paralysis*. Between episodes muscle function is normal. These are rare diseases of skeletal muscle, with a prevalence of 1 per 100,000 or less. Inheritance is autosomal dominant, except for one form of myotonia.

Weakness may be so severe during an attack of periodic paralysis that a patient is bedridden for hours, unable to raise an arm or leg off the bed. Fortunately, during such attacks the muscles of respiration and swallowing are spared, so life-threatening respiratory arrest does not occur. Attack frequency is variable from almost daily to only a few episodes in a lifetime. Consciousness and sensation are not impaired.

During an attack the resting potential of affected muscles is depolarized from a normal value of –90 mV to approximately –60 mV. At this depolarized potential most Na^+ channels are inactivated, rendering the muscle fiber chronically refractory and thus unable to generate action potentials. Recovery of strength occurs spontaneously and is associated with repolarization to a resting potential within a few millivolts of normal and recovery of excitability.

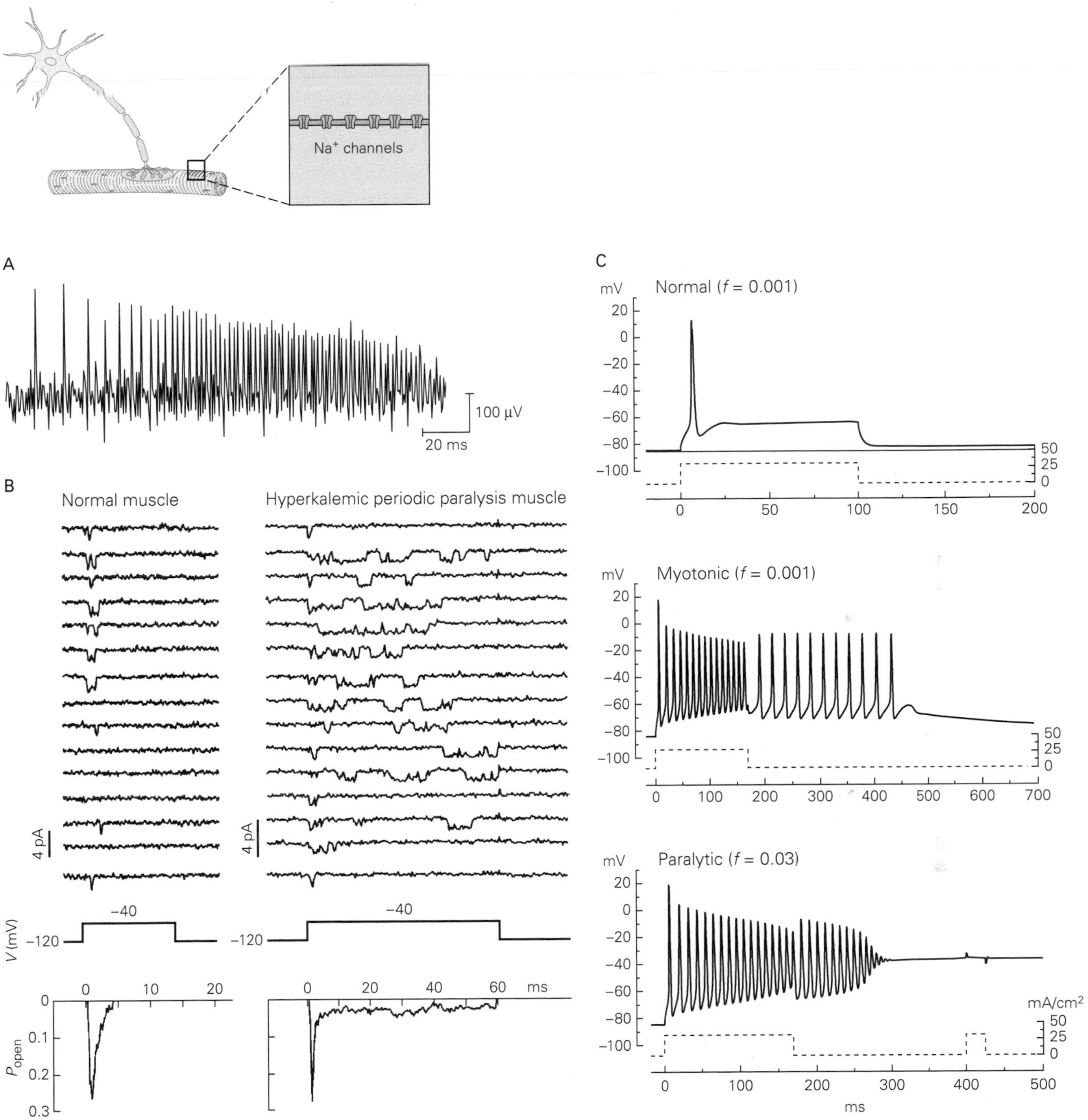

Figure 14–12 Myotonia or paralysis may result from impaired inactivation of Na⁺ channels in skeletal muscle.

A. The electrical signature of myotonia (muscle stiffness) is a rapid burst of action potentials in response to a single stimulus. The action potentials, shown here from extracellular recordings, vary in amplitude and wax and wane in frequency. Such a burst may be triggered by a voluntary muscle contraction or a mechanical stimulus such as percussion of the muscle.

B. Cell-attached patch recordings from cultured human muscle cells. In normal muscle the Na^+ channels open early and briefly in response to a voltage-clamp depolarization from –120 mV to –40 mV. In muscle from patients with hyperkalemic periodic paralysis (M1592V Na^+ channel mutation) the prolonged openings and reopenings indicate impaired inactivation. The probability of channel opening (obtained by averaging individual records) remains elevated in the hyperkalemic muscle following inactivation. (Reproduced, with permission, from Cannon, Brown, and Corey 1991.)

C. Even modest disruption of Na^+ channel inactivation is sufficient to produce bursts of myotonic discharges or depolarization-induced loss of excitability. These computer simulation records show muscle voltage in response to an injected depolarizing current (**dashed line**). The fraction of mutant channels that actually fails to inactivate normally (*f*) varies within a population over time. In these simulations *f* was varied from normal to values appropriate for myotonic or paralytic muscle. (Reproduced, with permission, from Cannon, Brown, and Corey 1993.)

Two variants of periodic paralysis have been delineated. Hyperkalemic periodic paralysis attacks occur during periods of high venous K^+ (6.0 mM or higher versus normal levels of 3.5–4.5 mM). Ingesting foods with high K^+ content such as bananas or fruit juice may trigger an attack. Conversely, hypokalemic periodic paralysis presents as episodic weakness in association with low blood K^+ (2.5 mM or lower). Affected muscle is paradoxically depolarized in the setting of reduced extracellular K^+, which shifts the reversal potential for K^+ to more negative values. Both forms are inherited as autosomal dominant traits.

Genetic analyses have demonstrated that hyperkalemic periodic paralysis is caused by missense mutations in a gene that encodes the pore-forming subunit of a voltage-gated Na^+ channel expressed in skeletal muscle. Inactivation of mutant Na^+ channels is disrupted. Subtle defects of inactivation produce myotonia; more pronounced changes result in chronic depolarization and loss of excitability with paralysis (Figure 14–12B, C). Hypokalemic paralysis is usually caused by mutations in a gene that encodes the main subunit of a voltage-sensitive Ca^{2+} channel in skeletal muscle. Andersen's syndrome, a rare form of periodic paralysis characterized by weakness, developmental defects, and cardiac irritability, is caused by primary mutations in the gene for an inward-rectifying K^+ channel important for establishing the resting potential (Figure 14–13).

In myotonia congenita muscle stiffness is present from birth and is not progressive. Unlike myotonic dystrophy there is no muscle wasting, permanent muscle weakness, or other organ involvement. Myotonia congenita is a consequence of mutations in the gene coding for the ClC-1 Cl^- channel in skeletal muscle membrane. The resultant decrease in Cl^- influx leads to membrane depolarization and repetitive firing. The disease is inherited as a dominant, semidominant, or recessive trait.

An Overall View

Studies of the diseases of the peripheral nervous system represent a powerful synergy between clinical and basic neuroscience and the fruitful interaction of both approaches with molecular genetics and molecular immunology. Progress in the last decade in defining the molecular basis for these disorders has been extraordinary. Molecular genetic analyses of most disorders inherited as Mendelian traits, beginning only with clinical data in affected families and DNA from family members, have led to the description of causative defects in muscle and nerve proteins.

In some diseases, such as primary muscular dystrophies and inherited neuropathies, little is known about the normal function of the newly discovered disease genes. Thus, the investigation of these diseases has generated new opportunities to learn about the basic molecular and cellular biology of nerve and muscle. In other diseases, such as familial amyotrophic lateral sclerosis and the ion channel diseases, the disease genes and proteins have previously been identified and studied extensively; there is already a large body of biological and biophysical information on which to base further studies.

Also remarkable is the convergence of the discovery of the primary gene defects in the inherited nerve and muscle disorders with new technologies for manipulating the DNA of mice. We now have mouse models of the human diseases with precisely defined genetic defects (using transgenes to over express specific mutant proteins or gene knock-out technology to disrupt the function of proteins). These are already proving invaluable for the analysis of the function of novel proteins, the mechanism of disease evolution, and studies of new treatment strategies.

In general, the development of new therapies for these disorders has lagged behind discovery of

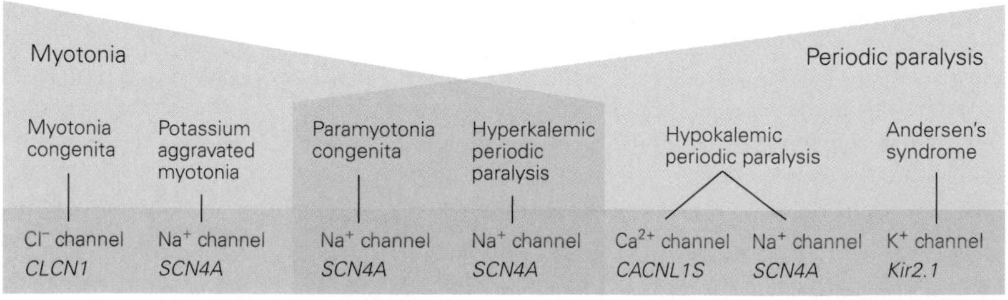

Figure 14–13 The myotonias and periodic paralyses are caused by mutations in genes for diverse voltage-gated ion channels in the skeletal muscle membrane. Some channel disorders are characterized only by myotonia, some only by periodic paralysis, and some by myotonia and paralysis. Some clinical disorders (eg, hypokalemic periodic paralysis) may arise from defects in different channels in different individuals.

the offending genetic or immune defects. The best exception to this generalization is myasthenia gravis; anti-immune therapies have dramatically reduced myasthenia mortality. Converting new molecular insights from other neuromuscular diseases into effective treatments will be a central challenge for clinical neuroscience in the next decade.

The primary therapy for recessively inherited, loss-of-function diseases will ultimately be some form of replacement of the missing protein; the use of viral-mediated gene therapy has already been explored in a pilot study of adults with a sarcoglycan deficiency. It is conceivable that newer methods to replace the missing proteins will not require viral delivery systems.

A major therapeutic challenge across all of human genetics is how to treat the dominantly inherited diseases in which the primary pathology involves cytotoxic effects of the gene mutations. Exciting strategies are evolving to inactivate the mutant allele. These include developing small molecules and proteins that inactivate the promoters for the genes and infusing either antisense oligonucleotides or inhibitory RNA molecules to inactivate the RNA templates made from the genes. Moreover, as the cellular pathways activated by the mutant genes and proteins become known, more downstream targets for the development of more conventional drug therapies will be identified.

For all these reasons we can be optimistic that the molecular analysis of these neuromuscular disorders will continue to illuminate important neurobiological principles in the neuromuscular system while at the same time opening new avenues for primary treatments of these often devastating diseases.

Postscript: Diagnosis of Motor Unit Disorders Is Aided by Laboratory Criteria

When the sole manifestation of a disease is limb weakness (with no fasciculation or upper motor neuron signs) clinical criteria may be insufficient to distinguish neurogenic and myopathic diseases. To assist in this differentiation, clinicians rely on several laboratory tests: measurement of muscle enzyme activity in serum, electromyography and nerve conduction studies, muscle biopsy, and DNA analysis.

One test that helps distinguish myopathic from neurogenic diseases is the measurement of serum enzyme activities. The sarcoplasm of muscle is rich in soluble enzymes that are normally found in low concentrations in the serum. In many muscle diseases the concentration of these sarcoplasmic enzymes in serum is elevated, presumably because the diseases affect the integrity of surface membranes of the muscle that ordinarily keep soluble enzymes within the sarcoplasm. The enzyme activity most commonly used for diagnosing myopathy is creatine kinase, an enzyme that phosphorylates creatine and is important in the energy metabolism of muscle.

Some abnormalities can be diagnosed by electromyography, a clinical procedure in which a small needle is inserted into a muscle to record extracellularly the electrical activity of several neighboring motor units. Three specific measurements are important: spontaneous activity at rest, the number of motor units under voluntary control, and the duration and amplitude of action potentials in each motor unit.

In normal muscle there is usually no activity outside the end-plate in the muscle at rest. During a weak voluntary contraction a series of motor unit potentials is recorded as different motor units become recruited. In fully active normal muscles these potentials overlap in an interference pattern so that it is impossible to identify single potentials (Figure 14–14A). Normal values have been established for the amplitude and duration of motor unit potentials. The amplitude of the motor unit potential is determined by the number of muscle fibers within the motor unit.

In neurogenic disease the partially denervated muscle is spontaneously active even at rest. The muscle may still contract in response to voluntary motor commands; but because some motor axons have been lost, the number of motor units under voluntary control is smaller than normal. During a maximal voluntary contraction the loss of motor units is evident in the EMG, which shows a discrete pattern of motor unit potentials instead of the profuse interference pattern for normal muscles (Figure 14–14B).

In recently denervated muscle the EMG may also show fibrillation potentials, low-amplitude electrical potentials that correspond to the firing of a single muscle fiber. As the neurogenic disease progresses, the amplitude and duration of individual motor unit potentials may increase, because the remaining axons give off small branches that innervate the muscle fibers denervated by the loss of other axons. Accordingly, surviving motor units contain more than the normal number of muscle fibers.

In myopathic diseases there is no activity in the muscle at rest and no change in the number of motor units firing during a contraction. But because there are fewer surviving muscle fibers in each motor unit, the motor unit potentials are of shorter duration and smaller in amplitude (Figure 14–14C).

The conduction velocities of peripheral motor axons can also be measured through electrical stimulation and recording (see Figure 14–2). The conduction velocity of motor axons is slowed in demyelinating neuropathies but is normal in neuropathies without demyelination (axonal neuropathies).

The histochemical appearance of muscle in a biopsy can provide a useful diagnostic tool. Human muscle fibers are identified by histochemical reactions as type I or type II, which respectively are either aerobic (enriched for oxidative enzymes) or anaerobic (abundant glycolytic enzymes) (see Chapter 34). All muscle fibers innervated by a single motor neuron are of the

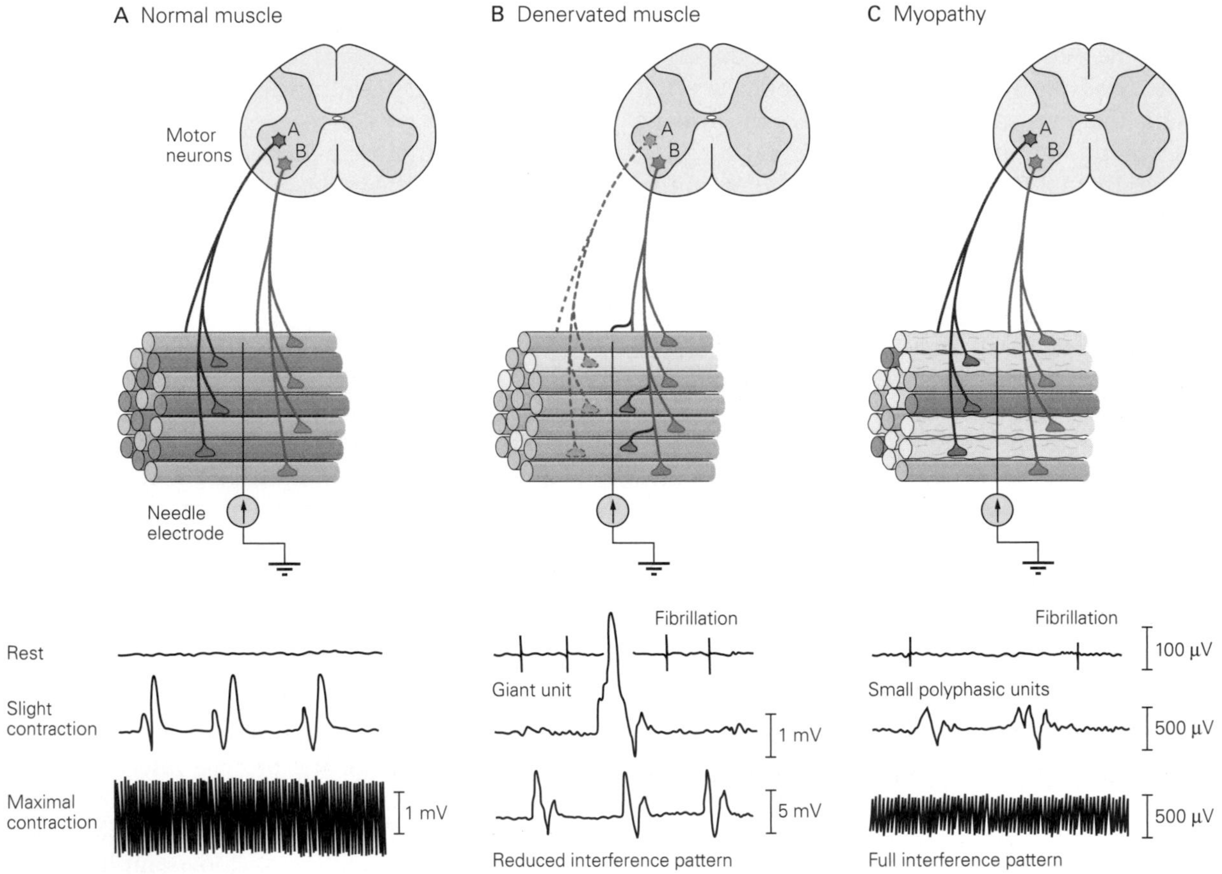

Figure 14–14 Neurogenic and myopathic diseases have different effects on the motor unit.

A. A motor unit potential is recorded by inserting a needle electrode into the muscle. The muscle fibers innervated by a single motor neuron are not usually adjacent to one another, yet the highly effective transmission at the neuromuscular junction ensures that each muscle fiber innervated by the same neuron will generate an action potential and contract in response to an action potential in the motor neuron. Activation of one or a few motor neurons produces a simple extracellular voltage signal and a small contraction (middle trace). A larger contraction activates a greater number of motor neurons and a larger number of muscle fibers, producing a strong contraction (lower trace). The extracellular voltage signal is more complex. Interference from the extracellular currents through the large number of muscle fibers, which are activated at slightly different times by the large number of motor neurons.

B. When motor neurons are diseased, the number of motor units under voluntary control is reduced. The muscle fibers supplied by the degenerating motor neuron (cell A) become denervated and atrophic. However, the surviving neuron (cell B) sprouts axonal branches that reinnervate some of the denervated muscle fibers. The electromyogram shows larger than normal motor unit potentials (middle trace) because the surviving motor neuron innervates more than the usual number of muscle fibers (it also innervates formerly denervated fibers). Axons of the surviving motor neuron fire spontaneously even at rest, giving rise to fasciculations, another characteristic of motor neuron disease. Single denervated fibers also fire spontaneously, producing fibrillations (top trace). Under conditions of maximal contraction the interference pattern is reduced (lower trace) because muscle fiber action potentials are more synchronized due to the reduced number of motor neuron inputs.

C. When muscle is diseased the number of muscle fibers in each motor unit is reduced. Some muscle fibers innervated by the two motor neurons shrink and become nonfunctional. In the electromyogram the motor unit potentials do not decrease in number but are smaller and of shorter duration than normal.

Table 14–3 Differential Diagnosis of Disorders of the Motor Unit

Finding	Nerve	Neuromuscular junction	Muscle
Clinical			
Weakness	++	+	++
Wasting	++	–	+
Fasciculations	+	–	–
Cramps	+	–	+/–
Sensory loss	+/–	–	–
Hyperreflexia, Babinski	+ (ALS)	–	–
Laboratory			
Elevated serum CPK	–	–	++
Elevated cerebrospinal fluid protein	+/–	–	–
Slowed nerve conduction	+	–	–
Response to repetitive stimulation	Normal	Decremental (MG) Incremental (LEMS)	Normal
Electromyography			
Fibrillation, fasciculation	++	–	+/–
Duration of potentials	Increased	Normal	Decreased
Amplitude of potentials	Increased	Normal	Decreased
Muscle Biopsy			
Isolated fiber atrophy	++	Normal	+/–
Grouped fiber atrophy	++	Normal	Normal
Muscle necrosis	Normal	Normal	++

ALS, amyotrophic lateral sclerosis; CPK, creatine phosphokinase; LEMS, Lambert-Eaton myasthenic syndrome; MG, myasthenia gravis.

same histochemical type. However, the muscle fibers of one motor unit are normally interspersed among the muscle fibers of other motor units. Enzyme stains of a cross section of healthy muscle show that oxidative or glycolytic fibers are intermixed in a *checkerboard* pattern.

In chronic neurogenic diseases the muscle innervated by a dying motor neuron becomes atrophic and some muscle fibers disappear. Axons of surviving neurons tend to sprout and reinnervate some of the nearby remaining muscle fibers. Because the motor neuron determines the biochemical properties of a muscle fiber, the reinnervated muscle fibers assume the histochemical properties of the innervating neuron. As a result, the fibers of a muscle in neurogenic disease become clustered by type (a pattern called *fiber-type grouping*).

If the disease is progressive and the neurons in the surviving motor units also become affected, atrophy occurs in groups of adjacent muscle fibers belonging to the same histochemical type, a process called *group atrophy*. In contrast, the muscle fibers in myopathic diseases are affected in a more or less random fashion. Sometimes an inflammatory cellular response is evident and sometimes there is prominent infiltration of the muscle by fat and connective tissue.

The main clinical and laboratory features used for the differential diagnosis of diseases of the motor unit are listed in Table 14–3.

Robert H. Brown
Stephen C. Cannon
Lewis P. Rowland

Selected Readings

Cannon SC. 2006. Pathomechanisms in channelopathies of skeletal muscle and brain. Annu Rev Neurosci 29:387–415.

Engel AG, Sine SM. 2005. Current understanding of congenital myasthenic syndromes. Curr Opin Pharmacol 3:308–321.

Irobi J, deJonghe P, Timmerman V. 2004. Molecular genetics of distal hereditary motor neuropathies. Hum Mol Genet 13 (Spec No 2):R195–R202.

Newsom-Davis J. 2005. Neuromuscular junction channelopathies: a brief overview. Acta Neurol Belg 105:181–186.

Ranum LP, Day JW. 2004. Pathogenic RNA repeats: an expanding role in genetic disease. Trends Genet 20:506–512.

References

Bansal D, Campbell KP. 2004. Dysferlin and the plasma membrane repair in muscular dystrophy. Trends Cell Biol 14:206–213.

Berman PW, Patrick J. 1980. Experimental myasthenia gravis: a murine system. J Exp Med 151:204–223.

Boillee S, Yamanaka K, Lobsiger CS, et al. 2006. Onset and progression in inherited ALS determined by motor neurons and microglia. Science 312:1389–1392.

Bonilla E, Samitt CE, Miranda AF, et al. 1988. Duchenne muscular dystrophy: deficiency of dystrophin at the muscle cell surface. Cell 54:447–452.

Bromberg MB. 2002. Acute and chronic dysimmune polyneuropathies. In: Brown WF, Bolton CF, Aminoff MJ (eds). *Neuromuscular Function and Disease*, p. 1048, Fig. 58–2. New York: Elsevier Science.

Brown RH Jr. Amato AA. 2002. Inherited peripheral neuropathies: classification, clinical features and review of molecular pathophysiology. In: Brown WF, Bolton CF, Aminoff MJ (eds). *Neuromuscular Function and Disease*, p. 624, Fig. 35–2. New York: Elsevier Science.

Brown RH Jr., Mendell J. 2005. The muscular dystrophies. In: Kasper DL, Fauci AS, Longo DL, Braunwald E, Hauser SL, Jameson JL (eds). *Harrison's Principles of Internal Medicine*, 16th ed, pp. 2527–2540. New York, NY: McGraw-Hill.

Cannon SC, Brown RH Jr, Corey DP. 1991. A sodium channel defect in hyperkalemic periodic paralysis: potassium-induced failure of inactivation. Neuron 6:619–626.

Cannon SC, Brown RH Jr, Corey DP. 1993. Theoretical reconstruction of myotonia and paralysis caused by incomplete inactivation of sodium channels. Biophys J 66:270–288.

Cossu G, Sampaolesi M. 2004. New therapies for muscular dystrophy: cautious optimism. Trends Mol Med 10: 516–520.

Cull-Candy SG, Miledi R, Trautmann A. 1979. End-plate currents and acetylcholine noise at normal and myasthenic human endplates. J Physiol 86:353–380.

Dalakas MC. 2004. Inflammatory disorders of muscle: progress in polymyositis, dermatomyositis and inclusion body myositis. Curr Opin Neurol 17:561–567.

Drachman DB. 1983. Myasthenia gravis: immunology of a receptor disorder. Trends Neurosci 6:446–451.

Drachman DB. 1994. Myasthenia gravis. N Engl J Med 330:1797–1810.

Famborough DM, Drachman DB, Satyamurti S. 1973. Neuromuscular junction in myasthenia gravis: decreased acetylcholine receptors. Science 182:293–295.

Fink JK. Hereditary spastic paraplegia. Curr Neurol Neurosci Rep 6:65–76.

Haliloglu G, Topaloglu H. 2004. Glycosylation defects in muscular dystrophies. Curr Opin Neurol 5:521–527.

Harper CM. 2004. Congenital myasthenic syndromes. Semin Neurol 24:111–123.

Hoffman EP, Brown RH, Kunkel LM. 1987. Dystrophin: the protein product of the Duchenne muscular dystrophy locus. Cell 51:919–928.

Hoffman EP, Kunkel LM. 1989. Dystrophin in Duchenne/Becker muscular dystrophy. Neuron 2:1019–1029.

Lindstrom J. 1983. Using monoclonal antibodies to study acetylcholine receptors and myasthenia gravis. Neurosci Comment 1:139–156.

Lisak RP, Barchi RL. 1982. *Myasthenia Gravis*. Philadelphia: Saunders.

Lupiski JR. 1998. Molecular genetics of peripheral neuropathies. In: JB Martin (ed). *Molecular Neurology*, pp. 239–256. New York: Scientific American.

Milone M, Fukuda T, Shen XM, et al. 2006. Novel congenital myasthenic syndromes associated with defects in quantal release. Neurology 66:1223–1229.

Newsom-Davis J, Buckley C, Clover L, et al. 2003. Autoimmune disorders of neuronal potassium channels. Ann N Y Acad Sci 998:202–210.

Nowak KJ, Davies KE. 2004. Duchenne muscular dystrophy and dystrophin: pathogenesis and opportunities for treatment. EMBO Rep 5:872–876.

Ozawa E, Mizuno Y, Hagiwara Y, et al. 2005. Molecular and cell biology of the sarcoglycan complex. Muscle Nerve 32:563–576.

Pasinelli P, Brown RH Jr. 2006. Molecular biology of amyotrophic lateral sclerosis: insights from genetics. Nat Rev Neurosci 7:710–723.

Ralph GS, Radcliffe PA, Day DM, et al. 2005. Silencing mutant SOD1 using RNAi protects against neurodegeneration and extends survival in an ALS model. Nat Med 11:429–433.

Rosen DR, Siddique T, Patterson D, Figelwicz DA, et al. 1993. Mutations in Cu/Zn superoxide dismutase gene are associated with familial amyotrophic lateral sclerosis. Nature 362:59–62.

Rowland LP, Hoefer PFA, Aranow H Jr. 1960. Myasthenic syndromes. Res Publ Assoc Res Nerv Ment Dis 38: 548–600.

Shy ME. 2004. Charcot-Marie-Tooth disease: an update. Curr Opin Neurol 17:579–585.

Verpoorten N, De Jonghe P, Timmerman V. 2006. Disease mechanisms in hereditary sensory and autonomic neuropathies. Neurobiol Dis 21:247–255.

Vincent A. 2006. Immunology of disorders of neuromuscular transmission. Acta Neurol Scand Suppl 183:1–7.

Zatz M, Starling A. 2005. Calpains and disease. N Engl J Med 352:2413–2423.

Zuchner S, Vance JM. 2005. Emerging pathways for hereditary axonopathies. J Mol Med 83:935–943.

Part IV

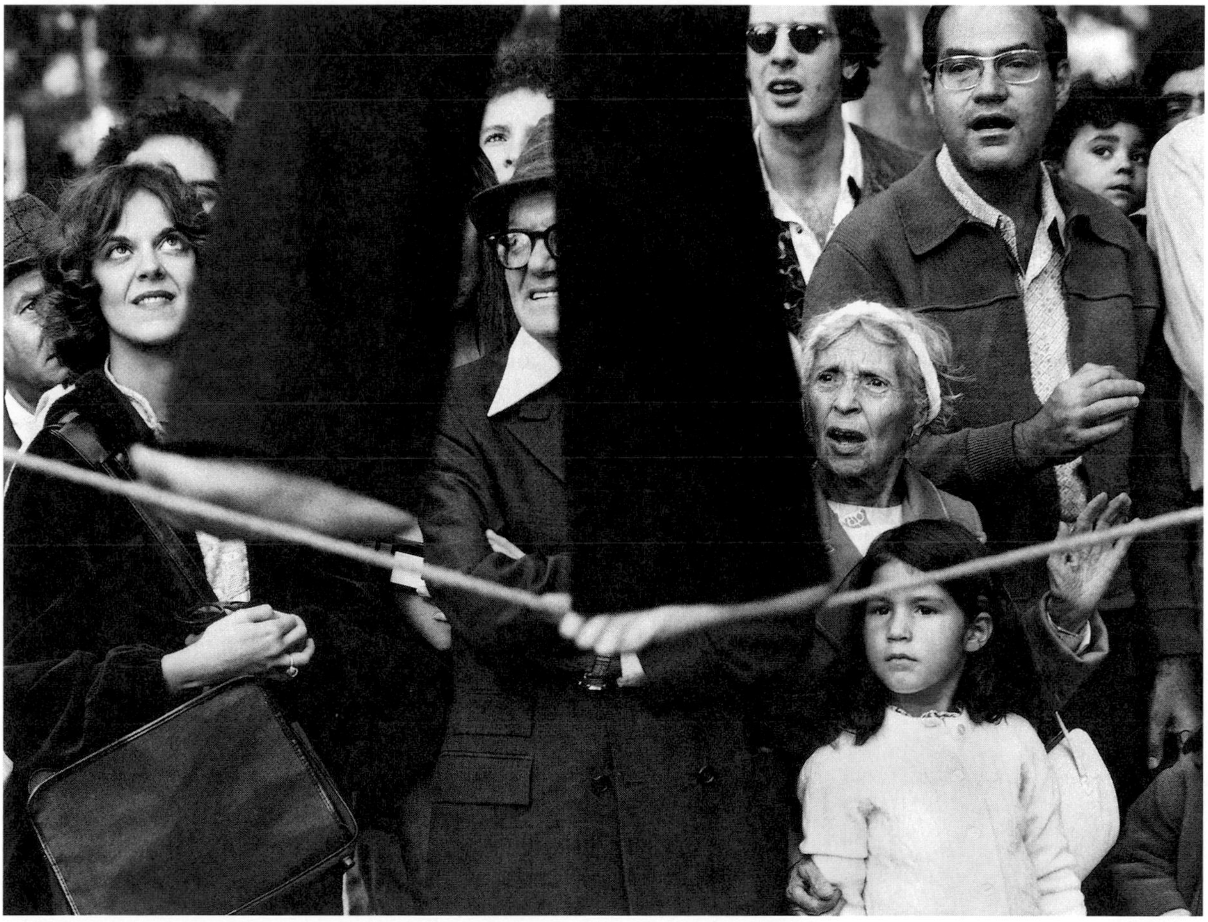

Preceding Page

A crowd watches a tightrope walker. The specific movements and perilous position of the acrobat are thought to resonate with viewers by engaging their system of mirror neurons. These neurons are activated both when an individual performs a set of movements, and when he or she observes those same movements performed by others. Similar neural systems may underlie social cognition as well, allowing us to perceive and comprehend the mental states of others. (Reproduced, with permission, from Arthur Paxton.)

IV The Neural Basis of Cognition

So far in this book we have examined the properties of individual nerve cells and how they communicate at synapses to produce simple reflex behaviors. We now begin to consider larger, interconnected networks of neurons, the complex circuits that give rise to mental activity: perception, planned action, and thought. The field of systems neuroscience aims to understand how these networks produce the cognitive functions of the brain, one of the ultimate challenges of science. We need to know how sensory information is perceived, and how perceptions are assembled into inner representations and recruited into plans for immediate behavior or concepts for future actions. It is still unclear how complex memories are made and how percepts, ideas, and feelings are transformed into language.

Neural science first emerged in the mid-1950s with the development of powerful techniques for exploring the cellular dynamics of the nervous system and with the convergence into a single discipline of several previously separate disciplines concerned with the brain and behavior: molecular biology, neuroanatomy, electrophysiology, and cell and developmental biology. The modern science of mind is the pragmatic result of the attempt to merge neural science with cognitive psychology. New techniques permit us to observe the system properties of the brain directly, not only in animal models, but in controlled behavioral experiments in alert, behaving people. As a result neural science is able to address testable hypotheses about how brain functions lead to mental processes such as perception, memory, decisions, and actions.

The aim of the new science of mind is to examine classical philosophical and psychological questions about mental functions in the light of modern cell and molecular biology. This is a bold undertaking. How do we begin to think about perception, ideas, action, and feelings in biological terms? So far, progress in understanding the major functional systems of the brain—the sensory, motor, motivational, memory, and attentional systems—has benefited from a reductionist approach to mental function. This approach is based on the assumption that these functions will emerge from the biological properties of nerve cells and of their pattern of interconnections. According to this view, which was introduced in Chapter 1, brain and mind are inseparable. Mind can be considered a set of operations carried out by the brain, an information-processing organ made powerful by the enormous number, variety, and interactions of its nerve cells and by the complexity of interconnection among these cells. In this section and later parts of this book, we describe the attempt to extend this cell biological approach beyond the neuron doctrine to the neuronal circuit doctrine, to the cognitive functions of the brain. We focus specifically on the major domains of cognitive neural science: perception, action, motivation, attention, learning, and memory.

An understanding of the biological basis of cognitive functions requires deep appreciation of the anatomy of the neural systems that subserve these functions in the brain. In the same way that the detailed structure of a protein reveals important principles of its action, knowledge of neuroanatomy and physiology can provide profound insight into how the nervous system functions. Just as many contemporary ideas about the dynamic mechanisms underlying the development of connectivity in the nervous system were anticipated a century ago by Ramón y Cajal on the basis of Golgi images of neurons in histological specimens, we predict that much of our understanding of higher brain function will depend on refined mapping of neuronal circuits and analysis of the signals that pass through those circuits.

Modern anatomical, physiological, and imaging techniques are revealing how neural circuits are organized. For example, the sensory pathways from one brain region to the next are organized in such a way that neighboring groups of neurons in the brain maintain the spatial relationship of sensory receptors in the periphery of the body. This topological organization is an important way of conveying spatial information about sensory events. In recent years, the study of connectivity in the brain has been advanced even further with new imaging techniques, such as diffusion-tensor imaging. These techniques have made visible the patterns of interconnectivity of different regions of the living human brain during specific behaviors. As a consequence, a much clearer idea of the brain regions involved in many complex cognitive functions is emerging.

In this part of the book, we first review in Chapters 15 and 16 the anatomical organization of the three major functional subdivisions of the nervous system: sensory, motor, and modulatory. We also take a closer look at the structural and functional organization of the central nervous system by following the flow of sensory information from the periphery into the spinal cord and brain, the transformation of that information into a motor command, and the effect of that command on muscle, the organ of behavior. We then examine in Chapters 17 and 18 the cognitive processes of the brain that are concerned with visual perception, planned action, memory, and selective conscious attention. Many of these activities are represented in higher-order-association regions of the cerebral cortex, areas that bring together information from various sensory systems to provide coordinated plans for action. A number of major insights in action and perception are now emerging. Perhaps most importantly, we examine in Chapter 19 why we no longer conceive of sensory and motor and cognitive processes as occurring sequentially. Rather perception and the planning for action occur simultaneously, and the higher motor systems have cognitive functions. One of the important questions that we shall examine in this section is how mental functions are represented in different regions of the brain. In doing so we shall explore what approaches can be used to render cognitive processes such as attention, motivation, and even consciousness accessible to rigorous physiological and anatomical analysis.

In later parts of the book we shall explore each functional system of the brain in detail, examining how the specific structure and cellular interconnections of a system determine its particular function.

Part IV

15

The Organization of the Central Nervous System

In the earlier chapters of this book we emphasized that modern neuroscience is based importantly on two tenets. First, the brain is organized into functionally specific areas, and second, neurons in different parts of the vertebrate nervous system, indeed in all nervous systems, are quite similar. What distinguishes one functionally distinct brain region from another, and one brain from the next, are the number and types of neurons in each and how they are interconnected through development. The specific patterns of interconnection and the resulting functional organization of neural circuits in distinct brain regions underlie the individuation of behavior.

All behavior, from simple reflex responses to complex mental acts, is the product of signaling between appropriately interconnected neurons. Consider the simple act of hitting a tennis ball (Figure 15–1). Visual information about the motion of the approaching ball is analyzed in the visual system. This information is combined with proprioceptive information about the position of the arms, legs, and trunk to calculate the movement necessary to intercept the ball. Once the swing is initiated, many minor adjustments of the motor program are made based on a steady stream of sensory information about the trajectory of the approaching ball. Finally, this entire act is accessible to consciousness, and thus may elicit memories and emotions. Of course, as the swing is being executed, the brain is also engaged in maintaining the player's heart rate, respiration, and other autonomic functions that are typically outside the awareness of the player.

Thus, to understand the neural control of any behavior it is necessary to break down that behavior into key components, to then identify the regions of the brain responsible for each component, and to analyze the neural connections between those regions. Although the anatomy of the brain and its interconnections appear complex, brain anatomy is easier to grasp if one understands the relatively simple set of principles that underlie the fundamental organization of the nervous system. In this and the next five

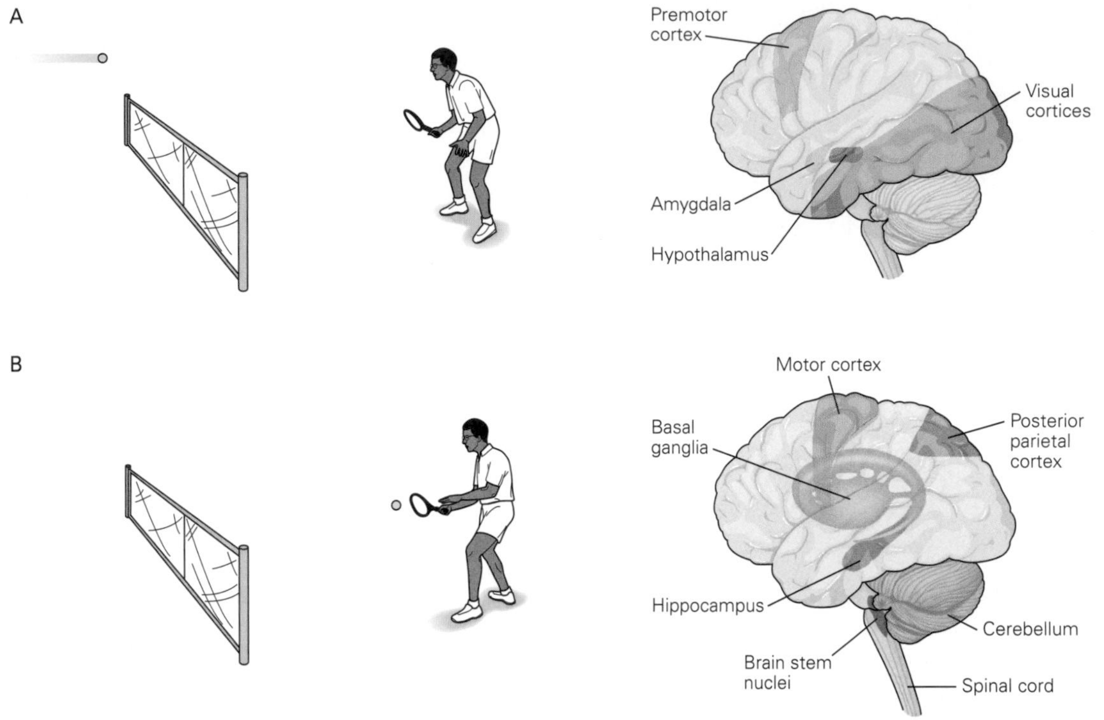

Figure 15–1 A simple behavior is mediated by many parts of the brain.

A. A tennis player watching an approaching ball uses the visual cortex to judge the size, direction, and velocity of the ball. The premotor cortex develops a motor program to return the ball. The amygdala acts in conjunction with other brain regions to adjust the heart rate, respiration, and other homeostatic mechanisms and also activates the hypothalamus to motivate the player to hit well.

B. To execute the shot the player must use all of the structures illustrated in part A as well as others. The motor cortex sends signals to the spinal cord that activate and inhibit many muscles in the arms and legs. The basal ganglia become involved in initiating motor patterns and perhaps recalling learned movements to hit the ball properly. The cerebellum adjusts movements based on proprioceptive information from peripheral sensory receptors. The posterior parietal cortex provides the player with a sense of where his body is located in space and where his racket arm is located with respect to his body. Throughout the movement, brain stem neurons regulate heart rate, respiration, and arousal. The hippocampus is not involved in hitting the ball but is involved in storing the memory of the return so that the player can brag about it later.

chapters we examine the relationship between anatomy and behavior in a series of progressively more complex examples.

In this chapter and the next we review the major anatomical components of the central nervous system by outlining the organization of the major functional systems that recruit these components. In Chapters 17 and 18 we examine how complex cognitive functions are constructed from the interaction of cortical association areas. In Chapter 19 we describe how in higher cortical association areas perception—the product of the sensory systems—and action—the product of the motor systems—work in parallel. Finally, in Chapter 20 we explore how complex cognitive functions of humans, including attention and consciousness, can be studied by means of brain imaging.

The Central Nervous System Consists of the Spinal Cord and the Brain

The location and orientation of components of the central nervous system within the body are described with reference to three axes: the rostral-caudal, dorsal-ventral, and medial-lateral axes (Figure 15–2).

The spinal cord is the most caudal part of the central nervous system and in many respects the simplest part. It extends from the base of the skull to the first lumbar vertebra. The spinal cord receives sensory information from the skin, joints, and muscles of the trunk and limbs, and contains the motor neurons responsible for both voluntary and reflex movements. Along its length the spinal cord varies in size and shape, depending on whether the emerging motor

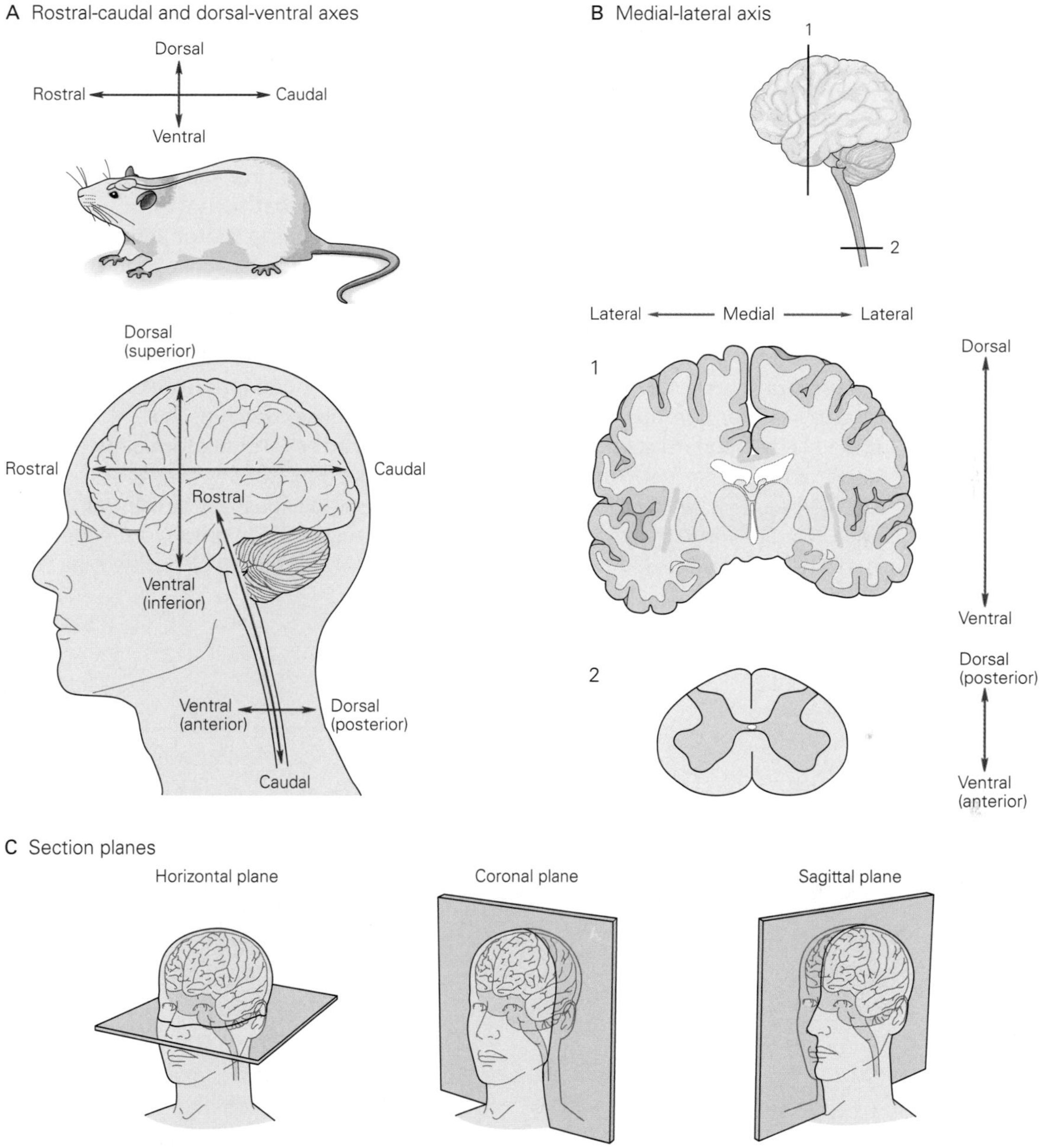

Figure 15–2 The central nervous system is described along three major axes. (Adapted, with permission, from Martin 2003.)

A. *Rostral* means toward the nose and *caudal* toward the tail. *Dorsal* means toward the back of the animal and *ventral* toward the belly. In lower mammals the orientations of these two axes are maintained through development into adult life. In humans and other higher primates the longitudinal axis flexes in the brain stem by approximately 110°. Because of this flexure the same positional terms have different meanings when referring to structures below and above the flexure. Below the flexure, in the spinal cord, rostral means toward the head, caudal means toward the coccyx (the lower end of the spinal column), ventral (anterior) means toward the belly, and dorsal (posterior) means toward the back. Above the flexure, rostral means toward the nose, caudal means toward the back of the head, ventral means toward the jaw, and dorsal means toward the top of the head. The term *superior* is often used synonymously with dorsal, and *inferior* means the same as ventral.

B. *Medial* means toward the middle of the brain and *lateral* toward the side.

C. When brains are sectioned for analysis, slices are typically made in one of three cardinal planes: horizontal, coronal, or sagittal.

nerves innervate the limbs or trunk; it is thicker at levels that innervate the arms and legs.

The spinal cord is divided into a core of central gray matter and surrounding white matter. The gray matter, which contains nerve cell bodies, is typically divided into dorsal and ventral horns (so-called because the gray matter appears H-shaped in transverse sections). The *dorsal horn* contains an orderly arrangement of sensory relay neurons that receive input from the periphery, whereas the *ventral horn* contains groups of motor neurons and interneurons that regulate motor neuronal firing patterns. The axons of motor neurons innervate specific muscles. The white matter is made up in part of rostral-caudal (longitudinal) ascending and descending tracts of myelinated axons. The ascending pathways carry sensory information to the brain, while the descending pathways carry motor commands and modulatory signals from the brain to the muscles.

The nerve fibers to and from the spinal cord are bundled in 31 spinal nerves, each of which has a sensory and a motor division. The sensory division (the *dorsal root*) carries information from muscles and skin into the spinal cord and terminates in the dorsal aspect of the cord. Different classes of axons within the dorsal roots convey pain, temperature, touch, and visceral sensory information. The motor division (the *ventral root*) emerges from the ventral aspect of the cord and comprises the axons of motor neurons that innervate muscles. Ventral roots from certain levels of the spinal cord also include sympathetic and parasympathetic axons. The motor neurons of the spinal cord comprise the "final common pathway" through which all higher brain levels controlling motor activity must act.

The brain, which lies rostral to the spinal cord, is composed of six regions: the medulla, pons, midbrain, cerebellum, diencephalon, and cerebral hemispheres or telencephalon (Figure 15–3). Each of these divisions is found in both hemispheres of the brain with slight bilateral differences. Each of the six divisions is further subdivided into several anatomically and functionally distinct areas.

The three divisions of the central nervous system immediately rostral to the spinal cord—the medulla, pons, and midbrain—are collectively termed the *brain stem*.

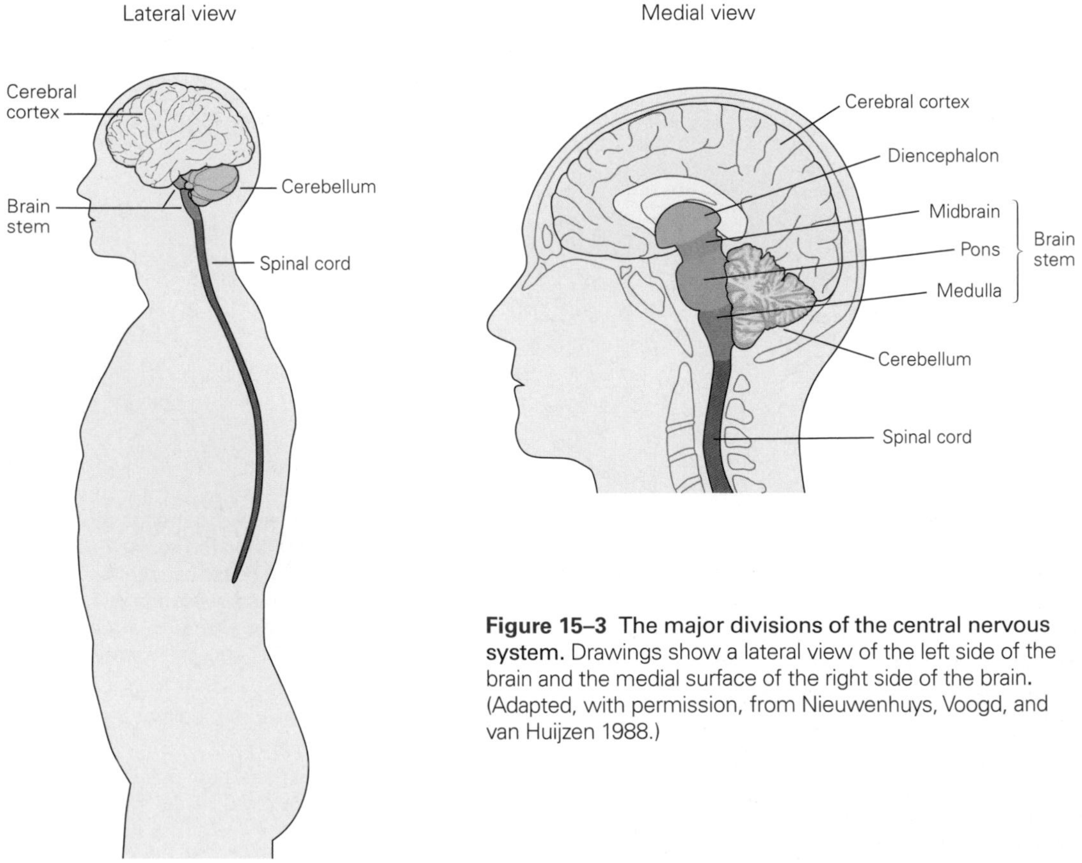

Figure 15–3 The major divisions of the central nervous system. Drawings show a lateral view of the left side of the brain and the medial surface of the right side of the brain. (Adapted, with permission, from Nieuwenhuys, Voogd, and van Huijzen 1988.)

The *medulla*, the most caudal portion of the brain stem, is a direct extension of the spinal cord and resembles the spinal cord both in organization and function. Neuronal groups in the medulla participate in regulating blood pressure and respiration. The medulla also contains neuronal groups that are early components of pathways that mediate taste, hearing, and maintenance of balance as well as the control of neck and facial muscles.

The *pons* lies rostral to the medulla and protrudes from the ventral surface of the brain stem. The ventral portion of the pons contains the pontine nuclei, groups of neurons that relay information about movement and sensation from the cerebral cortex to the cerebellum. The dorsal portion of the pons contains structures involved in respiration, taste, and sleep.

The *midbrain*, the smallest part of the brain stem, lies rostral to the pons. Nuclei in the midbrain provide important linkages between components of the motor system, particularly the cerebellum, basal ganglia, and cerebral hemispheres. For example, the substantia nigra provides important input to a portion of the basal ganglia that regulates voluntary movements. The substantia nigra is the focus of intense interest as damage to its dopaminergic neurons is responsible for the pronounced motor disturbances that are characteristic of Parkinson disease (see Chapter 43). The midbrain also contains components of the auditory and visual systems. Finally, several regions of the midbrain give rise to pathways that are connected to the extraocular muscles that control eye movements.

The brain stem has five distinct functions. First, just as the spinal cord mediates sensation and motor control of the trunk and limbs, the brain stem mediates sensation and motor control of the head, neck, and face. The sensory input and motor output of the brain stem is carried by 12 cranial nerves that are functionally analogous to the 31 spinal nerves. Second, the brain stem is the site of entry for information from several specialized senses, such as hearing, balance, and taste. Third, specialized neurons in the brain stem mediate parasympathetic reflexes, such as decreases in cardiac output and blood pressure, increased peristalsis of the gut, and constriction of the pupils. Fourth, the brain stem contains ascending and descending pathways that carry sensory and motor information to other divisions of the central nervous system. Fifth, a relatively diffuse network of neurons distributed throughout the core of the brain stem, known as the *reticular formation*, receives a summary of much of the incoming sensory information and is important in regulating alertness and arousal.

The *cerebellum* lies over the pons and is divided into several lobes by distinct fissures. The cerebellum is important for maintaining posture and coordinating head, eye, and arm movements, and is also involved in minute regulation of motor output and learning motor skills. Until recently, the cerebellum was considered a purely motor structure, but new anatomical information about its interconnections with the cerebral cortex and functional imaging studies have shown that it is also involved in language and other cognitive functions. The cerebellum contains far more neurons than any other single subdivision of the brain, including the cerebral hemispheres. Its internal circuitry, however, is well understood because relatively few types of neurons are involved. The cerebellum receives information about somatic sensation from the spinal cord, information about balance from the vestibular organs of the inner ear, and motor and sensory information from various areas of the cerebral cortex via the pontine nuclei.

The *diencephalon* contains two major subdivisions: the thalamus and hypothalamus. The thalamus is an essential link in the pathway of sensory information from the periphery (other than olfactory receptors in the nose) to sensory regions of the cerebral hemispheres. It once was thought to act only as a relay station for sensory information traveling to the neocortex, but now it is clear that it also determines which sensory information reaches the neocortex. The thalamus also interconnects the cerebellum and basal ganglia with regions of the cerebral cortex concerned with movement and cognition. Like the reticular formation, the diencephalon also has regions that are thought to influence levels of attention and consciousness.

The hypothalamus lies ventral to the thalamus and regulates homeostasis and several reproductive behaviors. For example, it plays an important role in somatic growth, eating, drinking, and maternal behavior by regulating the hormonal secretions of the pituitary gland. The hypothalamus also influences behavior through its extensive afferent and efferent connections with practically every region of the central nervous system. It is an essential component of the motivational systems of the brain, initiating and maintaining behaviors the organism finds aversive or rewarding. Finally, one group of neurons in the hypothalamus, the suprachiasmatic nucleus, regulates circadian rhythms, cyclical behaviors that are entrained to the daily light–dark cycle.

The *cerebral hemispheres* are the largest part of the human brain. They consist of the cerebral cortex, the underlying white matter, and three deep-lying structures: the basal ganglia, amygdala, and hippocampal formation. The cerebral hemispheres have perceptual, motor, and cognitive functions, including memory and emotion. The two hemispheres are interconnected by the corpus callosum, which is visible on the medial surface of the hemispheres. The corpus callosum is the largest of the commissures (large bundles of axons that mainly link similar regions of the left and right sides of the brain). The amygdala is concerned with the expression of emotion, the hippocampus with memory formation, and the basal ganglia with the control of movement and aspects of motor learning.

While the spinal cord, brain stem, and diencephalon mediate many life-sustaining functions, it is the cerebral cortex—the thin outer layer of the cerebral hemispheres—that is responsible for much of the planning and execution of actions in everyday life. The cerebral cortex is divided into four major lobes—frontal, parietal, temporal, and occipital—named after the overlying cranial bones (Figure 15–4). Each lobe includes many distinct functional subregions. The temporal lobe, for example, has distinct regions with auditory, visual, or memory functions.

Two additional regions of the cerebral cortex are the cingulate cortex, which surrounds the dorsal surface of the corpus callosum and is involved in the regulation of emotion and cognition, and the insular cortex (insula), which is not visible on the surface owing to the overgrowth of the frontal, parietal, and temporal lobes (Figure 15–5) and is concerned with emotion and the regulation of homeostasis. The overhanging portion of the cerebral cortex that buries the insula within the lateral sulcus is called the operculum.

Although the cerebral cortex on both sides of the brain is generally similar, some areas of cortex on the two sides are functionally distinct. In right-handed people, for example, portions of the left cerebral cortex are specialized for language, whereas the right side of the brain is more related to visuospatial information processing.

In the mid-19th century Pierre Paul Broca first called attention to portions of the frontal, parietal, and temporal lobes that encircle the fluid-filled ventricles of the brain, forming a continuous region at the border of the cerebral cortex. He named this region the limbic lobe (Latin *limbus*, border). The limbic lobe is no longer considered one of the major subdivisions of the cerebral cortex. However, the cingulate gyrus, which surrounds the corpus callosum and occupies much of Broca's limbic lobe (Figure 15–4), is a separate division of the neocortex, much like the insular cortex.

Distinct functional components of the neural system are connected to each other via discrete pathways, that is, tracts of bundled axons from one discrete population of neurons that terminate in another discrete population. Some of these pathways are very large and can be seen with the unaided eye in the gross brain. The pyramidal tracts, for example, project conspicuously from the cerebral cortex to the spinal cord. Most pathways are not nearly as prominent but can be demonstrated with neuroanatomical tracing techniques (see Box 4–2).

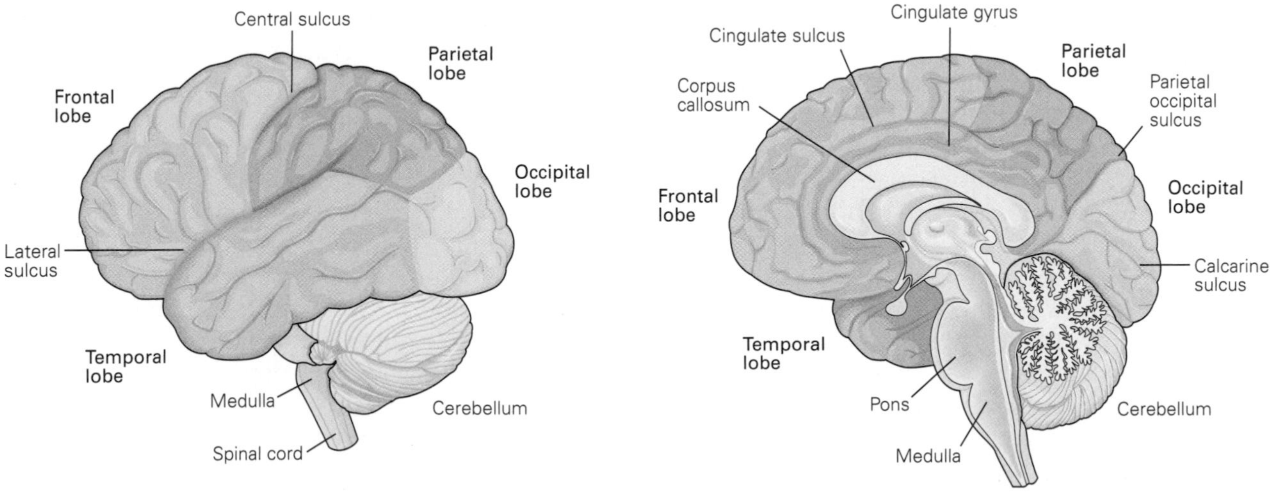

Figure 15–4 The major lobes and some prominent sulci of the human cerebral cortex. A lateral view of the left side of the brain is shown at left and a medial view of the right side of the brain at right. (Reproduced, with permission, from Martin 2003.)

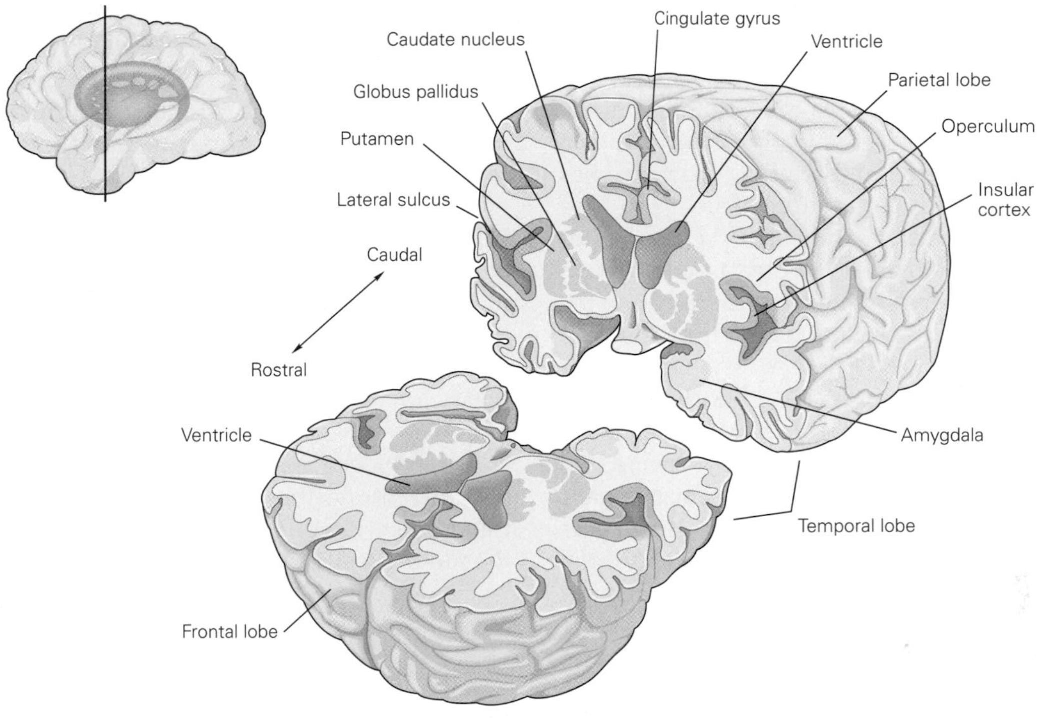

Figure 15–5 **Structures in the middle of the cerebral hemispheres.** These include the basal ganglia (caudate nucleus and globus pallidus) and insular cortex. Large cavities in the brain called ventricles are filled with cerebrospinal fluid. (Adapted, with permission, from England and Wakely 1991.)

The Major Functional Systems Are Similarly Organized

The central nervous system consists of several functional systems that are relatively autonomous. There are, for example, discrete systems for each of the five special senses (touch, vision, hearing, taste, smell), for different classes of movement (eye movements, arm movements, hand movements), and for language. Each functional system comprises numerous interconnected anatomical sites throughout the brain.

These several functional systems of the brain must act together cooperatively. In sensory systems, for example, sensory neurons in the periphery project, directly or indirectly, to one or more regions in the spinal cord, brain stem, and thalamus. The thalamus projects to the primary sensory areas of cerebral cortex, which in turn project to other regions of cortex.

Information Is Transformed at Each Synaptic Relay

The output of each synaptic relay in a functional pathway is rarely the same as its input. For example, information may be amplified or attenuated depending on the arousal level of the animal. A single neuron typically receives signals from thousands of presynaptic neurons, and the summation of all of these inputs determines the output of the neuron. The information encoded by each successive neuron in a functional pathway is typically more complex than the output of the preceding neuron.

Neurons at Each Synaptic Relay Are Organized into a Neural Map of the Body

One of the most striking features of the organization of most sensory systems is that the inputs from peripheral receptive surfaces—the retina of the eye, the cochlea of the inner ear, and the surface of the skin—are arranged *topographically* throughout successive stages of processing. Neighboring groups of cells in the retina, for example, project to neighboring groups of cells in nuclei of the thalamus, which, in turn, project to neighboring regions of the visual cortex. In this way the neurons at each successive relay of a sensory pathway form an orderly *neural map* of information from the receptive surface.

These neural maps reflect not only the spatial arrangement of receptors but also the variation in receptor density throughout the receptive surface. The density of innervation in an area of skin, for example, determines the degree of sensitivity of that area to tactile stimuli. The central region of the retina, the fovea, has the highest density of photoreceptors of any part of the retina and thus the greatest visual acuity. Correspondingly, the area of visual cortex devoted to information from the fovea is greater than the areas representing the peripheral portions of the retina, where the density of receptors (and visual acuity) is lower.

Similarly, in successive stages of cortical motor pathways the neurons that regulate particular body parts are clustered together to form a motor map; the most well-defined motor map is in the primary motor cortex. Motor maps, like sensory maps, do not represent every part of the body equally. The extent of the representation of a body part in a motor map reflects the density of innervation of that part, and thus the fineness of control required for movements in that part.

Each Functional System Is Hierarchically Organized

Information processing in sensory and motor systems is organized hierarchically. Within a system some areas of the cerebral cortex are designated as primary, secondary, or tertiary areas, depending on their functional sequence within the pathway. For example, the primary motor cortex mediates voluntary movements of the limbs and trunk; it is called primary because it contains neurons that directly activate somatic motor neurons in the spinal cord. The primary sensory areas receive most of their information from the thalamus, which receives signals from the peripheral receptors with only a few intervening synaptic relays. Whereas the primary sensory areas of cortex are the *initial* site of cortical processing of sensory information, the primary motor cortex is the *final* site in the cortex for processing motor commands.

The primary visual cortex is located caudally in the occipital lobe and is predominantly associated with the prominent calcarine sulcus (see Figure 15–4). The primary auditory cortex is located in the temporal lobe, where it is associated with a series of gyri (Heschl's gyri) on the lateral sulcus. The primary somatosensory cortex is located caudal to the central sulcus on the postcentral gyrus, in the parietal lobe.

Each primary sensory area conveys information to an adjacent, higher-order area, a unimodal association area where individual neurons selectively encode specific features of sensory stimuli and together represent complex information. At very advanced stages of the visual system, individual neurons are responsive to highly integrated information, such as the shape of a face.

Each higher-order sensory area sends its outputs to one or another of three major multimodal association areas that integrate information from two or more sensory modalities and coordinate this information with plans for action (see Chapter 18). Complex sensory information is also sent to higher-order motor areas, located rostral to the primary motor cortex in the frontal lobe, where programs for movement, or potential movements, are calculated and conveyed to the primary motor cortex for implementation. Some of the motor areas in the frontal lobe also send commands directly to the spinal cord. Cells in the primary motor cortex influence neurons in the ventral horn of the spinal cord responsible for muscle movements, and thus the primary motor cortex is intimately associated with the motor systems of the spinal cord.

Functional Systems on One Side of the Brain Control the Other Side of the Body

Most pathways in the central nervous system are bilaterally symmetrical and cross over to the opposite (contralateral) side of the brain or spinal cord. As a result, sensory and motor activities on one side of the body are mediated by the cerebral hemisphere on the opposite side. Thus, movement on the left side of the body is largely controlled by neurons in the right motor cortex.

The pathways of different systems cross at different anatomical levels within the brain. For example, the ascending pathways for pain cross in the spinal cord almost immediately upon entering the central nervous system. The sensory pathway for fine touch, however, ascends on the same side of the spinal cord that it enters. At the medulla, where it makes its first synapse, second-order fibers cross over to the thalamus on the contralateral side. Crossings of this kind within the brain stem and spinal cord are called *decussations*.

The Cerebral Cortex Is Concerned with Cognition

Phylogenetically, humans have the most elaborate cerebral cortex. The four lobes of the cerebral cortex have a highly convoluted shape, formed by indentations or grooves (*sulci*) that separate elevated regions (*gyri*), which occupy a relatively consistent position across individuals. One of the most prominent indentations, the lateral sulcus or sylvian fissure, separates the temporal lobe from the frontal and parietal lobes (see Figure 15–4). Another prominent indentation, the central sulcus, runs medially and laterally on the dorsal surface of the hemisphere and separates the frontal and parietal lobes.

It is likely that this convoluted shape arose during evolution as a strategy for packing ever-increasing numbers of neurons into the limited space of the skull, as the thickness of the cortex does not vary substantially in different species (always approximately 2 to 4 mm thick), although the surface area is dramatically larger in higher primates, particularly in humans. By allowing for a greater number of cortical neurons, an increase in the surface area of the cortex provides a greater capacity for processing information.

Neurons in the Cerebral Cortex Are Organized in Layers and Columns

The neocortex—the region of cerebral cortex nearest the surface of the brain—is organized into layers and columns, an arrangement that increases the computational efficiency of the cerebral cortex. As we shall see below, the subcortical regions have a nuclear organization.

The neocortex receives inputs from the thalamus, other cortical regions on both sides of the brain, and other structures. Its output is directed to other regions of the neocortex, basal ganglia, thalamus, pontine nuclei, and the spinal cord. These complex input–output relationships are efficiently organized in the orderly layering of cortical neurons; each layer contains different inputs and outputs. Most of the neocortex contains six layers, numbered from the outer surface (pia mater) of the cortex to the white matter (Figure 15–6).

Layer I, the *molecular layer*, is occupied by the dendrites of cells located in deeper layers and axons that travel through this layer to make connections in other areas of the cortex.

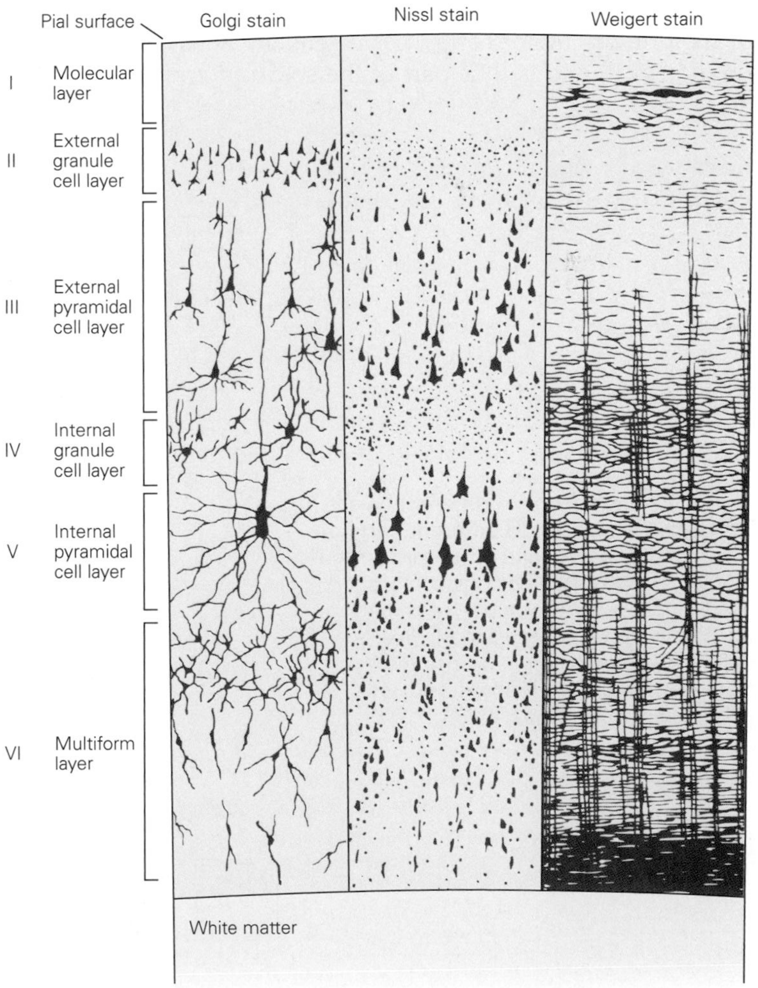

Figure 15–6 The neurons of the neocortex are arranged in distinctive layers. The appearance of the neocortex depends on what is used to stain it. The Golgi stain reveals a subset of neuronal cell bodies, axons, and dendritic trees. The Nissl method shows cell bodies and proximal dendrites. A Weigert stain reveals the pattern of myelinated fibers. (Reproduced, with permission, from Heimer 1994.)

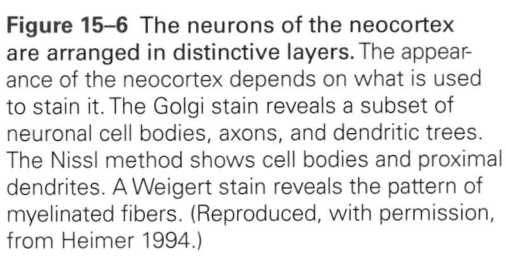

Layers II and III contain mainly small pyramidal shaped cells. Layer II, the *external granular cell layer*, is one of two layers that contain small spherical neurons. Layer III is called the *external pyramidal cell layer* (an internal pyramidal cell layer lies at a deeper level). The neurons located deeper in layer III are typically larger than those located more superficially. The axons of pyramidal neurons in layers II and III project locally to other neurons within the same cortical area as well as to other cortical areas, thereby mediating intracortical communication (Figure 15–7).

Layer IV contains a large number of small spherical neurons and thus is called the *internal granular cell layer*. It is the main recipient of sensory input from the thalamus and is most prominent in primary sensory areas. For example, the region of the occipital cortex that functions as the primary visual cortex has an extremely prominent layer IV (Figure 15–8). Layer IV in this region is so heavily populated by neurons and so complex that it is typically divided into three sublayers. Areas with a prominent layer IV are called *granular cortex*. In contrast the precentral gyrus, the site of the primary motor cortex, has essentially no layer IV (Figure 15–8) and is thus part of the so-called *agranular* frontal cortex. These two cortical areas are among the easiest to identify in histological sections.

Layer V, the *internal pyramidal cell layer*, contains mainly pyramidally shaped cells that are typically larger than those in layer III. Pyramidal neurons in this layer give rise to the major output pathways of the cortex, projecting to other cortical areas and to subcortical structures (Figure 15–7).

The neurons in layer VI are fairly heterogeneous and thus this layer is called the *polymorphic* or *multiform layer*. It blends into the white matter that forms the deep limit of the cortex and carries axons to and from areas of cortex.

Although each layer of the neocortex is defined primarily by the presence, absence, and packing density of distinctive cell types, each layer also contains the dendrites of specific cortical neurons. Layers I through III contain the apical dendrites of neurons that have their cell bodies in layers V and VI, as well as in layers II and III, whereas layers V and VI contain the basal dendrites of neurons with cell bodies in layers III and IV, as well as in layers V and VI (Figure 15–7). The inputs to a cortical neuron thus depend on the location of its dendrites and cell body.

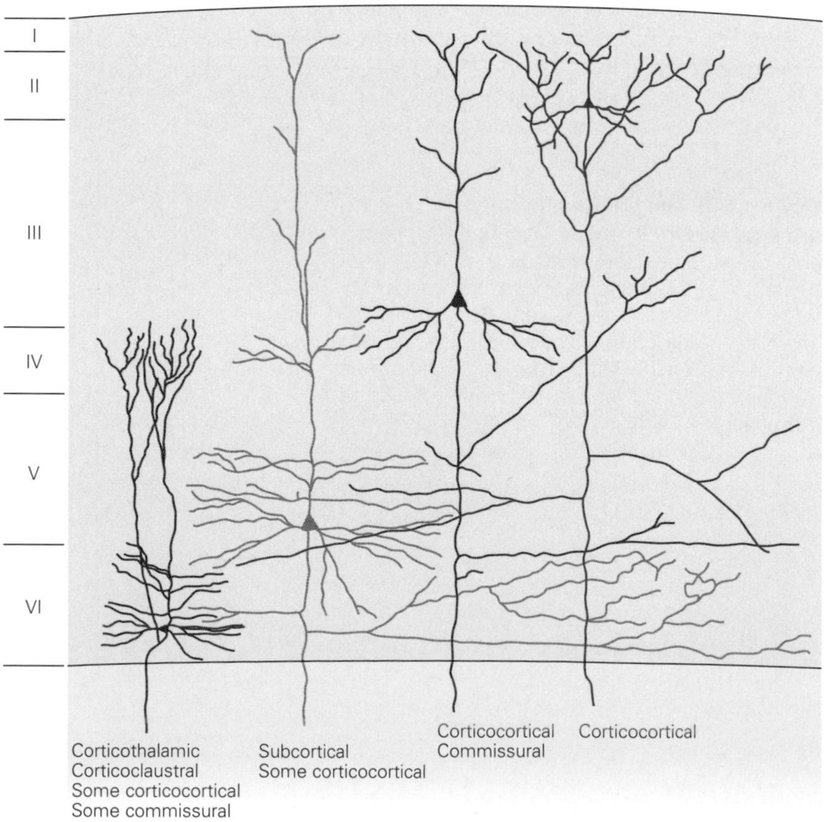

Figure 15–7 Neurons in different layers of neocortex project to different parts of the brain. Projections to other parts of the neocortex, the so-called corticocortical or associational connections, arise primarily from neurons in layers II and III. Projections to subcortical regions arise mainly from layers V and VI. (Reproduced, with permission, from Jones 1986.)

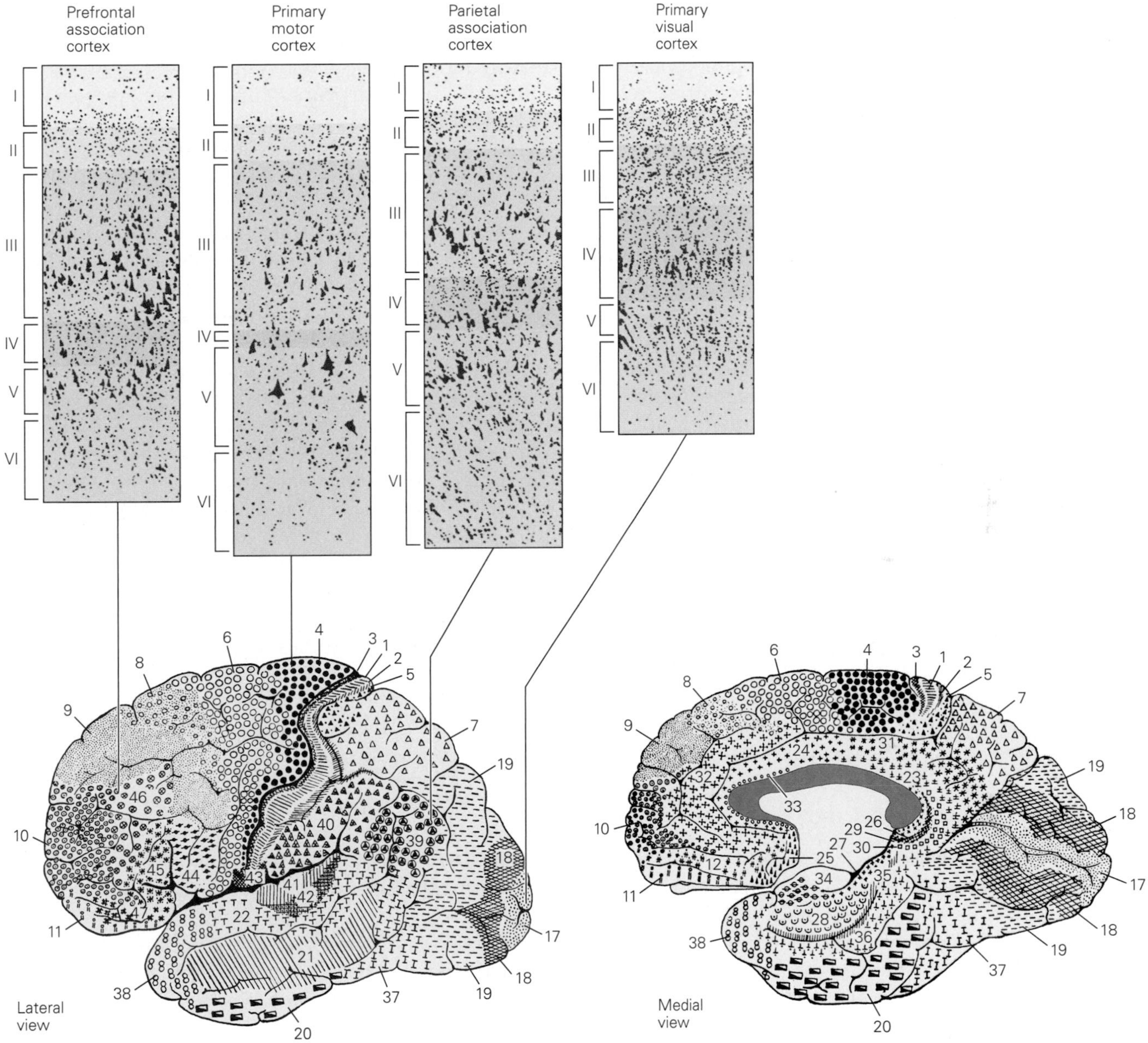

Figure 15–8 The extent of each cell layer of the neocortex varies throughout the cortex. Sensory areas of cortex, such as the primary visual cortex, tend to have a very prominent internal granular cell layer (layer IV), the site of sensory input. Motor areas of cortex, such as the primary motor cortex, have a very meager layer IV but prominent output layers, such as layer V. These differences led Korbinian Brodmann and others working at the turn of the 20th century to divide the cortex into various cytoarchitectonic regions. Brodmann's 1909 subdivision shown here is a classic analysis but was based on a single human brain. (Reproduced, with permission, from Martin 2003.)

The thickness of individual layers and the details of their functional organization vary throughout the cortex. An early student of the cerebral cortex, Korbinian Brodmann, used the relative prominence of the layers above and below layer IV, cell size, and packing characteristics to distinguish different areas of the neocortex. Based on such cytoarchitectonic differences, Brodmann in 1909 divided the cerebral cortex into 47 regions (Figure 15–8).

Although Brodmann's demarcation coincides, in part, with recent information on localized functions in the neocortex, the cytoarchitectonic method alone does not capture the subtlety or variety of function of all the distinct regions of the cortex. For example, Brodmann identified five regions (areas 17–21) as being concerned with visual function in the monkey. In contrast, modern connectional neuroanatomy and electrophysiology have identified more than 35 functionally distinct cortical regions within the five regions studied by Brodmann.

Within the neocortex information passes from one synaptic relay to another using feedforward and feedback connections. In the visual system, for example, feedforward projections from the primary visual cortex to secondary and tertiary visual areas originate mainly in layer III and terminate mainly in layer IV of the target cortical area. In contrast, feedback projections to earlier stages of processing originate from cells in layers V and VI and terminate in layers I, II, and VI (Figure 15–9).

Neurons in the neocortex are often organized into columns that run from the white matter to the pial surface, thus traversing the layers. (This columnar organization is not particularly evident in standard histological preparations.) Each column is a fraction of a millimeter in diameter. Neurons within a column tend to have very similar response properties, presumably because they form a local processing network. Columns are thought to be the fundamental computational modules of the neocortex (see Chapter 22).

The Cerebral Cortex Has a Large Variety of Neurons

The neurons of the cortex have a variety of shapes and sizes. Raphael Lorente de Nó, a student of Santiago Ramón y Cajal, used the Golgi stain to identify more than 40 different types of cortical neurons based only on the distribution of their dendrites and axons. The neurons of the cortex, as elsewhere, can be broadly defined as either principal (projection) neurons or local interneurons. Projection neurons typically have pyramid-shaped cell bodies (Figure 15–10). They are located mainly in layers III, V, and VI and use the amino acid glutamate as their primary transmitter at excitatory synapses. The axons of principal neurons convey information to the next synaptic relay in the system.

Local interneurons have axons that remain within the same area where their cell body is located and use the neurotransmitter γ-aminobutyric acid (GABA) at inhibitory synapses. These interneurons constitute 20% to 25% of the neurons in the neocortex and are located in all layers. Interneurons may receive inputs from the same sources as the principal cells.

Several types of GABAergic interneurons have been distinguished based on their pattern of connections and the cotransmitters they use with GABA (Figure 15–11). Basket cells form axosomatic synapses, that is, their axons terminate on the cell bodies of target neurons. Other interneurons form axo-axonic synapses, that is, their axons terminate exclusively on the axons of target neurons. The multiple arrays of synaptic terminals formed by these cells resemble a chandelier and thus these cells are typically called *chandelier cells*.

The neocortex also has a population of excitatory interneurons, located primarily in layer IV. These cells have star-shaped dendritic trees and use glutamate as a transmitter. These excitatory interneurons are the primary recipients of sensory information from the thalamus.

Subcortical Regions of the Brain Are Functionally Organized into Nuclei

Three major structures lie deep within the cerebral hemispheres: the basal ganglia, the hippocampal formation, and the amygdala. These three subcortical structures act to regulate cortical activity.

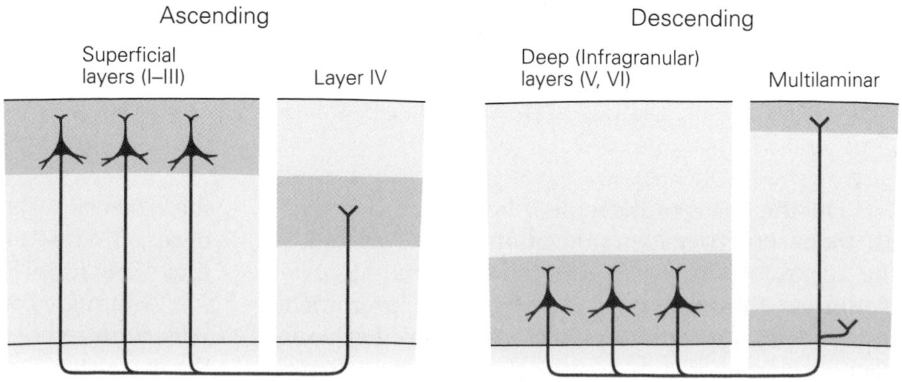

Figure 15–9 Ascending and descending cortical pathways are distinguished by the organization of their pre- and postsynaptic connections within the cortical layers. Ascending or feedforward pathways generally originate in superficial layers of the cortex and invariably terminate in layer IV. Descending or feedback pathways generally originate from deep layers and terminate in layers I and VI. (Adapted, with permission, from Felleman and Van Essen 1991.)

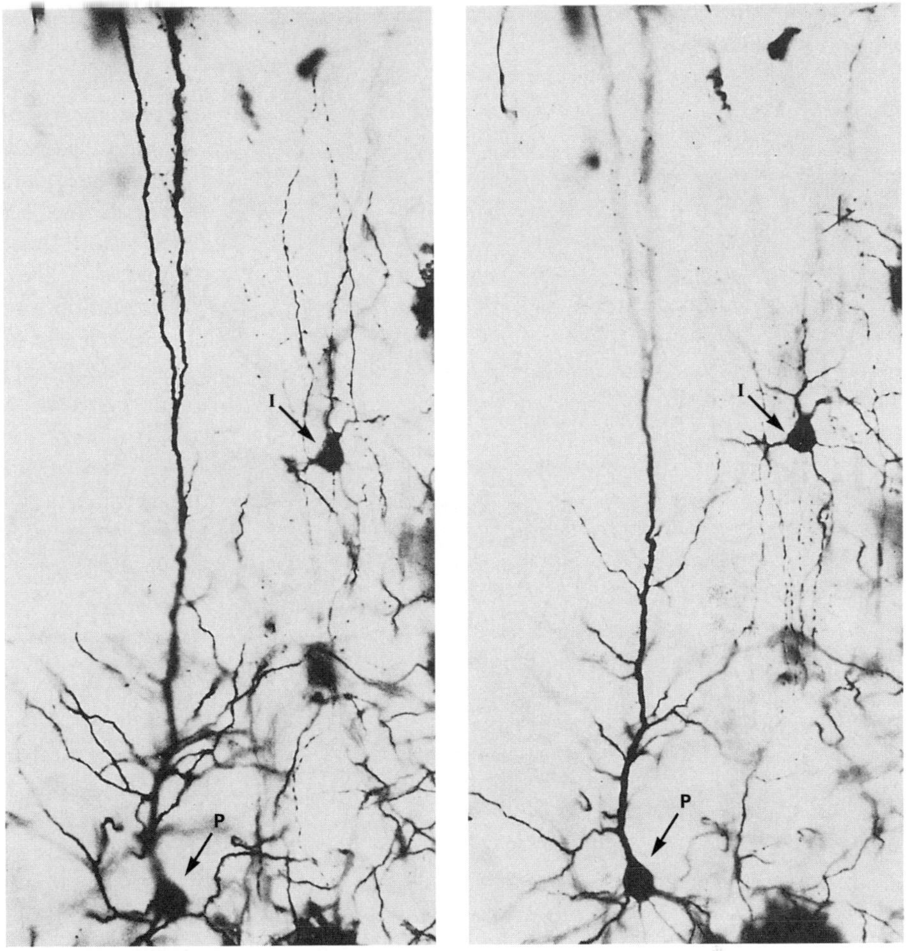

Figure 15–10 A projection neuron and interneuron in the somatic sensory cortex of a monkey. These photomicrographs were made at different depths of focus through the same Golgi-stained preparation. A Golgi type I pyramidal cell (**P**) in layer V is seen better on the left, whereas a Golgi type II interneuron (**I**) in layers II–III is seen better on the right. (Reproduced, with permission, from Jones 1986.)

Neurons in the basal ganglia regulate movement and contribute to certain cognitive functions such as the learning of motor skills. The basal ganglia receive input from all parts of the cerebral cortex but send their output largely through the thalamus to the frontal lobe. The basal ganglia have five major functional subcomponents: the caudate nucleus, putamen, globus pallidus, subthalamic nucleus, and substantia nigra (Figure 15–12).

The hippocampal formation includes the hippocampus, dentate gyrus, and subiculum. The hippocampus and associated cortical regions form the floor of the temporal horn of the lateral ventricle (Figure 15–12). Together these structures are responsible for the formation of long-term memories about our daily experiences, so-called episodic memories, but are not the permanent storage site of these memories (see Chapter 65). Damage to the hippocampus interferes with people's ability to form new memories but does not significantly impair the ability to retrieve old memories.

The amygdala, which lies just rostral to the hippocampus, is involved in analyzing the emotional or motivational significance of sensory stimuli. It receives input directly from the major sensory systems. Neurons in the amygdala project to the neocortex, basal ganglia, hippocampus, and a variety of subcortical structures including the hypothalamus. Projections to the brain stem can modulate somatic and visceral components of emotion. For example, the amygdala mediates the unconscious responses to danger—changes in heart rate, respiration, and pupillary dilation—as well as the conscious emotional perception of fear.

Thin histological sections through the diencephalon and brain stem reveal the structure of several nuclei. Most nuclei are not homogeneous populations of cells but instead comprise a variety of cells of different sizes and shapes organized into subnuclei, divisions, or layers. A nucleus that appears homogeneous when viewed with the nonspecific Nissl stain (Figure 15–13) may

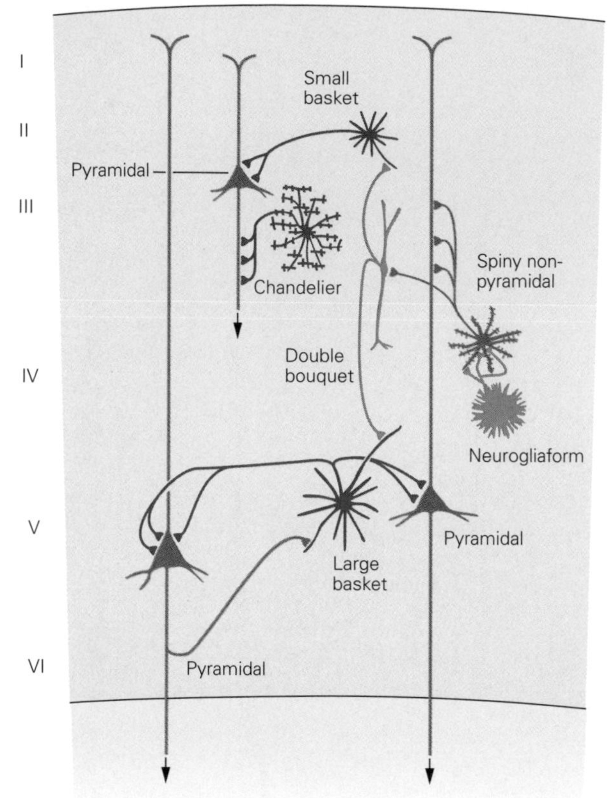

Figure 15–11 The cerebral cortex has several types of GABAergic interneurons. Known types of GABAergic neurons **(dark gray)** and putative types **(light gray)** have different connections with projection neurons in the neocortex. The known GABAergic cells include chandelier cells, which terminate exclusively on the axons of pyramidal neurons, and the large and small basket cells, whose axons terminate mainly on the cell bodies of pyramidal neurons. Double bouquet and neurogliaform cells may also be GABAergic. The neurogliaform cells form axosomatic synapses on spiny pyramidal neurons. (Adapted, with permission, from Houser et al. 1986.)

actually prove to be organizationally complex when viewed with other stains that highlight the structure of dendrites (such as the Golgi technique) or the chemical composition of the neurons (such as histochemistry or immunohistochemistry). Neurons in the lateral geniculate nucleus of the thalamus, for example, are grouped into alternating bands of neurons with different functions (Figure 15–14).

The characterization of a nucleus in the brain thus depends on the method by which the neurons are visualized. Indeed, modern neuroanatomy, based on the molecular characterization of different nerve cell types, has contributed greatly to the definition of brain regions. One particularly telling example occurred in the 1970s when Bengt Falck and Nils Hillarp developed a histofluorescence technique for staining monoamine neurotransmitters (see Box 13–2). This technique allowed researchers to deconstruct the reticular formation, a region of the brain stem so named because of its diffuse and seemingly chaotic appearance. We now understand that this region is finely organized into groups of cells characterized by transmitter phenotype (serotonergic, noradrenergic, or dopaminergic). Many other powerful techniques for defining the chemical or genetic composition of neuronal types have emerged in the last few decades. For example, in situ hybridization allows neurons to be visualized based on the genes they express (see Box 13–2). This has led to the tongue-in-cheek saying that "the gains in brain lie mainly in the stain."

Modulatory Systems in the Brain Influence Motivation, Emotion, and Memory

Some areas of the brain are neither purely sensory nor purely motor but instead modify specific sensory or motor functions. Modulatory systems are often involved in behaviors that respond to a primary need such as hunger, thirst, or sleep. For example, sensory and modulatory systems in the hypothalamus determine blood glucose levels. When blood sugar drops below a certain critical level, we feel hunger. To satisfy hunger, modulatory systems in the brain focus vision, hearing, and smell on stimuli that are relevant to feeding.

Distinct modulatory systems within the brain stem modulate attention and arousal. Small groups of adrenergic and serotonergic modulatory neurons in the brain stem set the general arousal level of an animal through their connections with forebrain structures. As we will discuss further in Chapter 46, a group of cholinergic modulatory neurons, the basal nucleus of Meynert, is also involved in arousal or attention. It is located beneath the basal ganglia in the basal forebrain portion of the telencephalon. The axons of the neurons in this nucleus project to essentially all portions of the neocortex.

If a predator finds potential prey, a variety of cortical and subcortical systems determine whether the prey is edible. Once food is recognized, other cortical and subcortical systems initiate a comprehensive voluntary motor program to bring the animal into contact with the prey, capture it and place it in the mouth, and chew and swallow.

Finally, the physiological satisfaction the animal experiences in eating reinforces the behaviors that

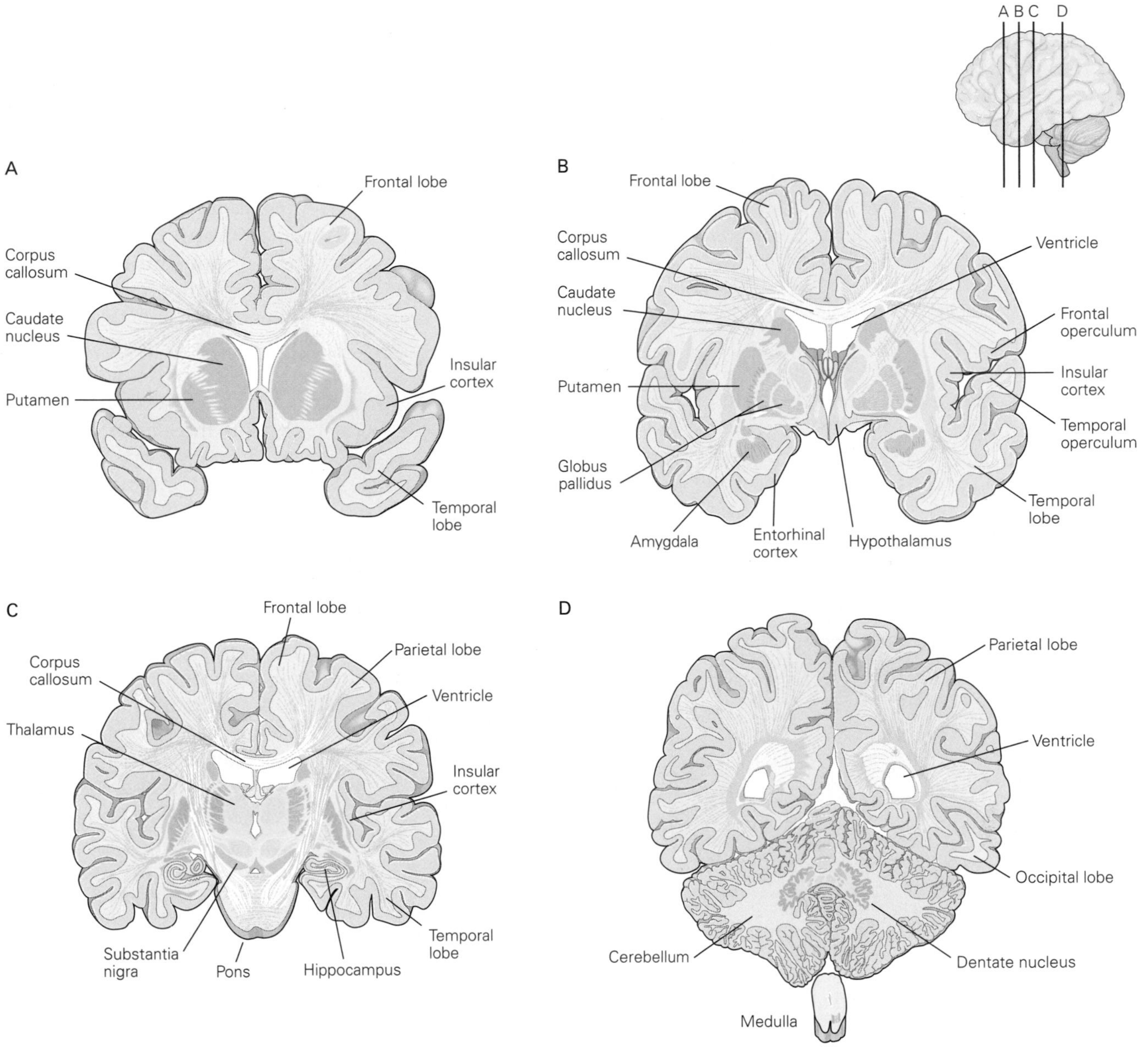

Figure 15–12 Subcortical regions. Four sequential coronal sections (A–D) were made in the rostral-caudal sequence indicated on the lateral view of the brain. (Reproduced, with permission, from Nieuwenhuys, Voogd, and van Huijzen 1988.)

led to the successful predation. A group of dopaminergic neurons in the midbrain are important for monitoring reinforcements and rewards. The power of the dopaminergic modulatory systems has been demonstrated by experiments in which electrodes were implanted into the reward regions of rats and the animals were freely allowed to press a lever to electrically stimulate their brains. They preferred this self-stimulation to obtaining food or water, engaging in sexual behavior, or any other naturally rewarding activity.

How the brain's modulatory systems concerned with reward, attention, and motivation interact with the sensory and motor systems is one of the most interesting questions in neuroscience, one that is also fundamental to our understanding of learning and memory storage. We take up this discussion in detail in Chapter 46

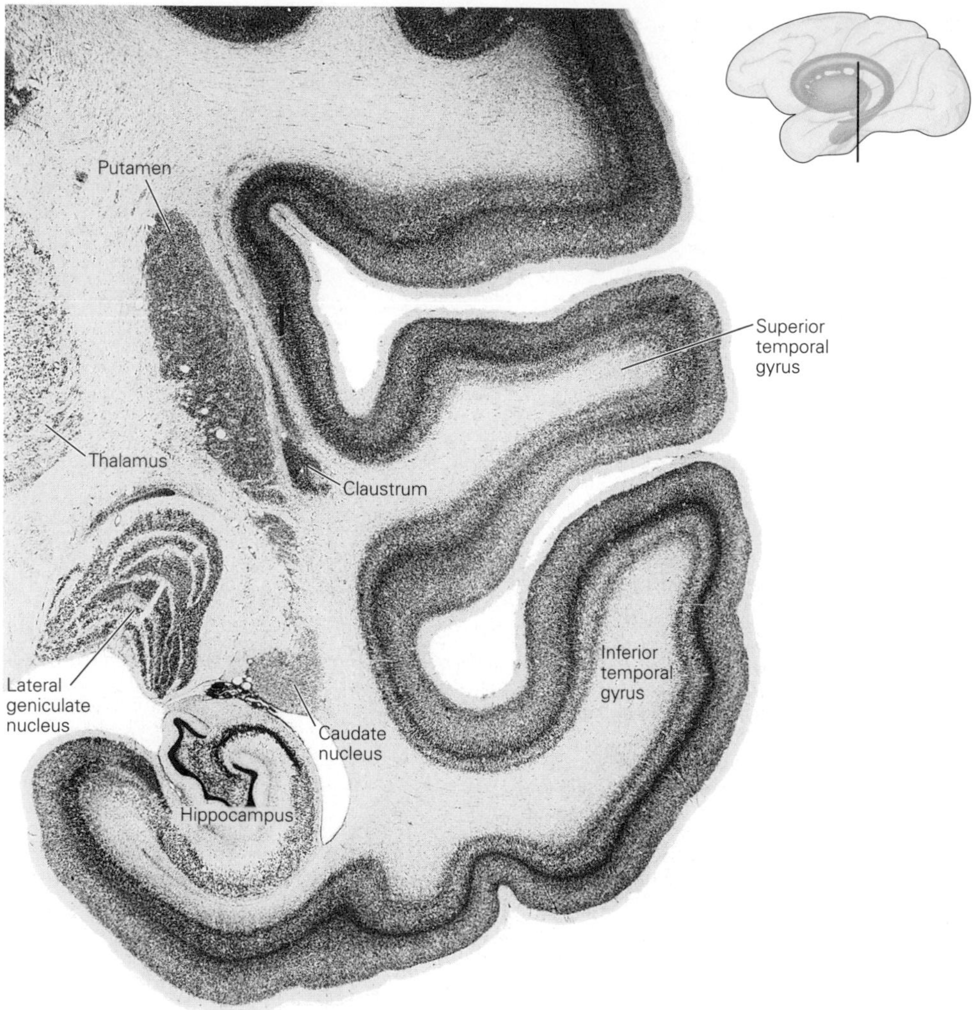

Figure 15–13 Several nuclei and cortical areas are visible in the right hemisphere of a Macaque monkey brain. Neuronal and glial cell bodies show up as the grainy dark portions of this low-magnification photograph of a Nissl-stained coronal section. The layering of the neurons of the lateral geniculate nucleus of the thalamus can be seen (see also Figure 15–14). Layering also occurs in the hippocampus and the neocortex of the temporal lobe. Other nuclei are more homogeneous, such as the caudate nucleus, putamen, and claustrum. The white regions between the clusters of neurons constitute the white matter where axons run from one brain region to one or more other regions.

The Peripheral Nervous System Is Anatomically Distinct from the Central Nervous System

The peripheral nervous system supplies the central nervous system with a continuous stream of information about both the external environment and the internal environment of the body. It has somatic and autonomic divisions (Figure 15–15).

The *somatic division* includes the sensory neurons that receive information from the skin, muscles, and joints. The cell bodies of these sensory neurons lie in the dorsal root ganglia and cranial ganglia. Receptors associated with these cells provide information about muscle and limb position and about touch and pressure at the body surface. In Part V (Perception) we shall see how remarkably specialized these receptors are in transducing one or another type of physical energy (such as deep pressure or heat) into the electrical signals used by the nervous system. In Part VI (Movement) we shall see that sensory receptors in the muscles and joints are crucial to shaping coherent movement of the body.

The *autonomic division* of the peripheral nervous system mediates visceral sensation as well as motor control of the viscera, vascular system, and exocrine glands. It consists of the sympathetic, parasympathetic, and enteric systems. The sympathetic system participates in the body's response to stress, whereas the parasympathetic system acts to conserve body resources and restore homeostasis. The enteric nervous system, with neuronal cell bodies located in or adjacent to the viscera, controls the function of smooth muscle of the gut. The functional organization of the autonomic nervous system is described in Chapter 47 and its role in emotion and motivation in Chapters 48 and 49.

An Overall View

The nervous system receives sensory information from the environment, evaluates the significance of the information, and generates appropriate behavioral responses. Accomplishing these tasks requires an anatomical plan of considerable complexity. The human nervous system is comprised of approximately 100 billion neurons, each of which receives and gives rise to thousands of connections. Some of these connections are formed nearly a meter from the cell body of the neuron.

Despite this complexity, the structure of the nervous system is similar in individuals of a species. Knowledge of neuronal structure and the pathways of information flow in the brain is important not only for understanding the normal function of the brain but also for identifying specific regions that are disturbed during neurological illness.

The nervous system has two anatomically distinct components. The central nervous system consists of the brain and spinal cord, while the peripheral nervous system is composed of specialized clusters of neurons (ganglia) and peripheral nerves. The peripheral nervous system relays information to the central nervous system and executes motor commands generated in the brain and spinal cord. Even the simplest behavior involves the integrated activity of several sensory, motor, and functional pathways are precisely arranged synaptic relays made up of clusters or layers of neurons called nuclei. Each functional pathway normally has the same anatomical arrangement in every individual.

Although neuroanatomy may seem to provide only a static picture of the nervous system, it can provide profound insight into how the nervous system functions, in the same way that the detailed structure of proteins reveals important principles of protein function. Understanding brain function therefore depends on an understanding of both structure and function, and crucially, of the relation between the two.

As we shall see in later chapters, modern neuroimaging has revolutionized the study of the cognitive

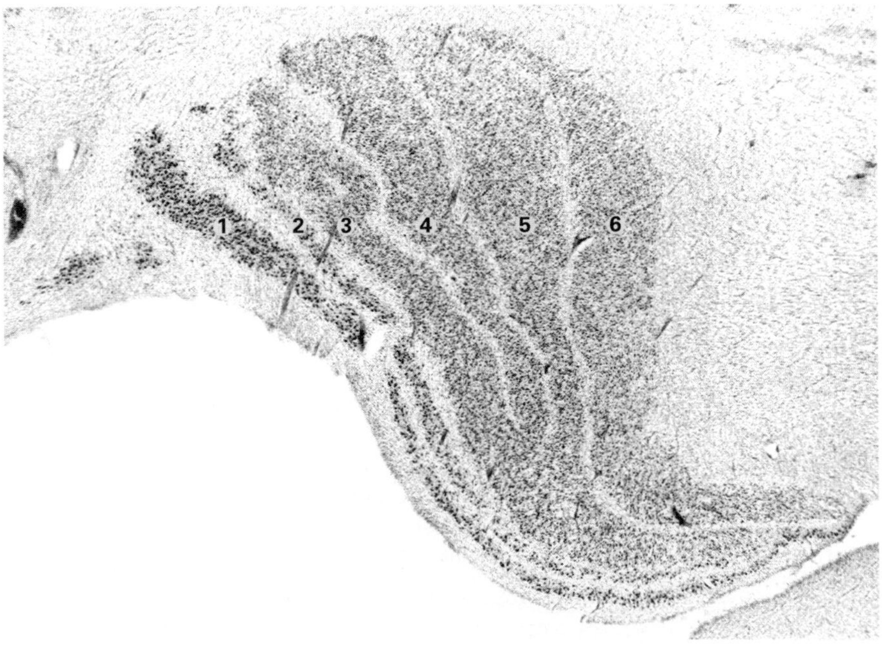

Figure 15–14 The lateral geniculate nucleus is an example of a complex nucleus. The nucleus is shown in a Nissl-stained coronal section of the right hemisphere of a human brain. Axons from different types of neurons in the retina terminate in different layers (1–6) of the nucleus. In addition, each layer receives input from only one eye. Each layer contains both projection neurons and interneurons. (The nucleus is described in detail in Chapter 26 in the discussion of visual perception.)

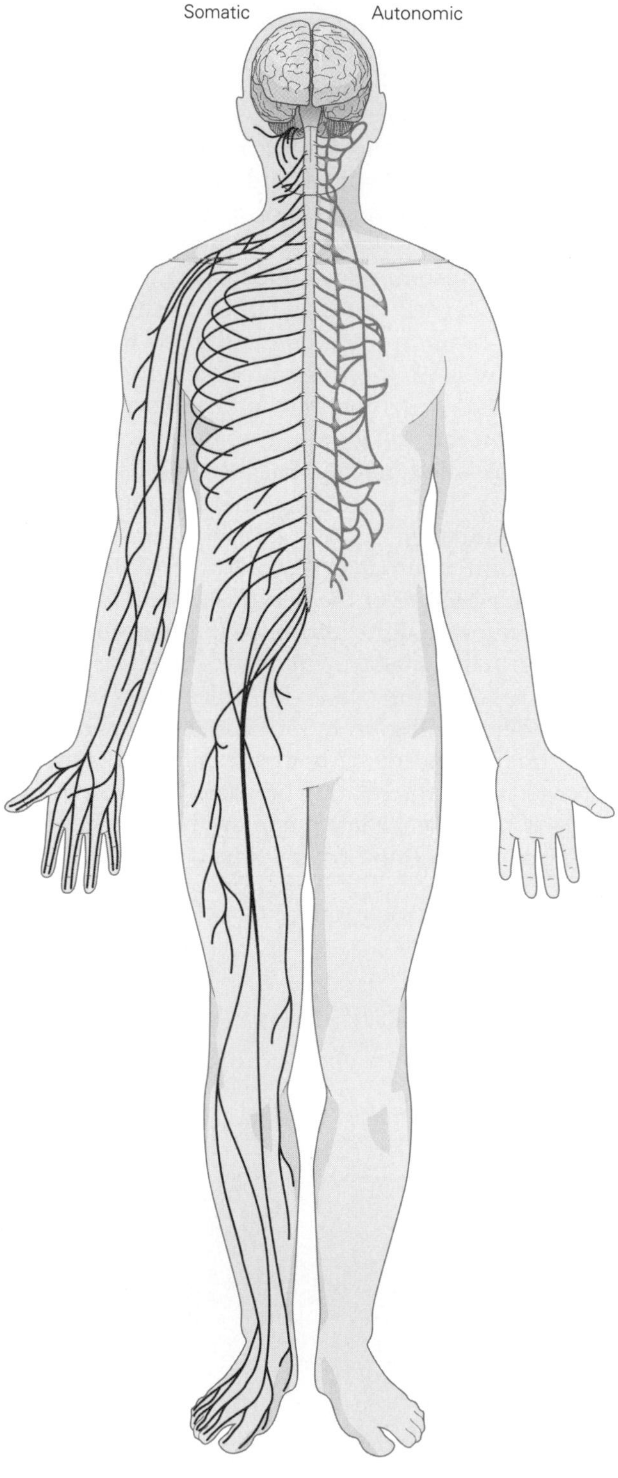

Figure 15–15 The peripheral nervous system has somatic and autonomic divisions. The somatic division carries information from the skin to the brain and from the brain to muscles. The autonomic division regulates involuntary functions, including activity of the heart and smooth muscles in the gut and glands.

operations of the brain. In particular, positron emission tomography (PET) and magnetic resonance imaging (MRI) have made the functional organization of the intact human brain visible during behavioral experiments. These techniques, in addition to being important tools for diagnosing diseases of the central nervous system, have given us a much clearer idea of the functional specialization of the nervous system. Importantly, they have placed neurology and psychiatry on a firmer empirical footing.

David G. Amaral
Peter L. Strick

Selected Readings

Brodal A. 1981. *Neurological Anatomy in Relation to Clinical Medicine*, 3rd ed. New York: Oxford Univ. Press.

England MA, Wakely J. 1991. *Color Atlas of the Brain and Spinal Cord: An Introduction to Normal Neuroanatomy*. St. Louis: Mosby Year Book.

Martin JH. 2003. *Neuroanatomy: Text and Atlas*, 3rd ed. New York: McGraw-Hill.

Nauta WJH, Feirtag M. 1986. *Fundamental Neuroanatomy*. New York: Freeman.

Nieuwenhuys R, Voogd J, van Huijzen Chr. 1988. *The Human Central Nervous System: A Synopsis and Atlas*, 3rd rev. ed. Berlin: Springer-Verlag.

Paxinos G, Mai K. 2003. *The Human Nervous System*. San Diego: Academic Press.

References

Amaral DG. 2003. The amygdala, social behavior, and danger detection. Ann N Y Acad Sci 1000:337–347.

Broca P. 1878. Anatomie comparée des circonvolutions cérébrales. Le grand lobe limbique et le scissure limbique dans le serie des mammitères. Rev Anthropol 12:646–657.

Brodmann K. 1909. *Vergleichende Lokalisationslehre der Grosshirnrinde in ihren Prinzipien dargestellt auf Grund des Zellenbaues*. Leipzig: Barth.

Dahlström A, Carlsson A. 1986. Making visible the invisible. In: MJ Parnam, J Bruinnvels (eds), *Discoveries in Pharmacology*. Vol. 3, *Pharmacological Methods, Receptors and Chemotherapy*, pp. 97–125. Amsterdam: Elsevier.

Falck B, Hillarp NA, Thieme G, Torp A. 1962. Fluorescence of catecholamines and related compounds condensed with formaldehyde. J Histochem Cytochem 10:348–354.

Felleman DJ, Van Essen DC. 1991. Distributed hierarchical processing in the primate cerebral cortex. Cereb Cortex 1:1–47.

Freund TF, Buzsaki G. 1996. Interneurons of the hippocampus. Hippocampus 6:347–470.

Heimer L. 1994. *The Human Brain and Spinal Cord: Functional Neuroanatomy and Dissection Guide*, 2nd ed. New York: Springer.

Houser CR, Vaughn JE, Hendry SHC, et al. 1986. GABA neurons in the cerebral cortex. In: EG Jones, A Peters (eds), *Cerebral Cortex,* Vol. 2, Chapter 3: Functional Properties of Cortical Cells, pp. 63–89. New York/London: Plenum.

Jones EG. 1986. Connectivity of the primate sensory-motor cortex. In: EG Jones, A Peters (eds), *Cerebral Cortex*, Vol. 5, Chapter 4: Sensory-Motor Areas and Aspects of Cortical Connectivity, pp. 113–183. New York/London: Plenum.

Lorente de Nó R. 1949. Cerebral cortex. Architecture, intracortical connections, motor projections. In: JF Fulton (ed), *Physiology of the Nervous System*, 3rd ed., pp. 288–330. New York: Oxford Univ. Press.

Ramón y Cajal S. 1995. *Histology of the Nervous System of Man and Vertebrates*, 2 vols. N Swanson, LW Swanson (transl). New York: Oxford Univ. Press.

West MJ. 1990. Stereological studies of the hippocampus: a comparison of the hippocampal subdivisions of diverse species including hedgehogs, laboratory rodents, wild mice and men. Prog Brain Res 83:13–36.

16

The Functional Organization of Perception and Movement

The human brain identifies objects and carries out actions in ways no current computer can even begin to approach. Merely to see—to look onto the world and recognize a face or facial expression—entails amazing computational achievements. Indeed, all our perceptual abilities—seeing, hearing, smelling, tasting, and touching—are analytical triumphs. Similarly, all of our voluntary actions are triumphs of engineering. The brain accomplishes these computational feats because its information processing units—its nerve cells—are wired together in very precise ways.

In this chapter we outline the neuroanatomical organization of perception and action. We focus on touch because the somatosensory system is particularly well understood and because touch clearly illustrates the interaction of sensory and motor systems—how information from the body surface ascends through the sensory relays of the nervous system to the cerebral cortex and is transformed into motor commands that descend to the spinal cord to produce movements.

We now have a fairly complete understanding of how the physical energy of a tactile stimulus is transduced by mechanoreceptors in the skin into electrical activity, and how this activity at different relays in the brain correlates with specific aspects of the experience of touch. Moreover, because the pathways from one relay to the next are well delineated, we can see how sensory information is coded at each relay.

Trying to comprehend the functional organization of the brain might at first seem daunting. But as we saw in the last chapter, the organization of the brain is simplified by three anatomical considerations. First, there are relatively few types of neurons. Each of the many thousands of spinal motor neurons or millions of neocortical pyramidal cells has a similar structure and serves a similar function. Second, neurons in the brain and spinal cord are clustered in discrete functional groups called nuclei, which are connected to form functional systems. Third, specific regions of the cerebral cortex are specialized for sensory, motor, or, as we shall learn in detail in Chapters 17 and 18, associational functions.

Sensory Information Processing Is Illustrated in the Somatosensory System

Complex behaviors, such as using touch alone to differentiate a ball from a book, require the integrated action of several nuclei and cortical regions. Information is processed in the brain in a hierarchical fashion. Thus information about a stimulus is conveyed through a succession of subcortical and then cortical regions and at each level of processing the information becomes increasingly complex. In addition, different types of information, even within a single sensory modality, are processed in several anatomically discrete pathways. In the somatosensory system a light touch and a painful pin prick to the same area of skin are mediated by different pathways in the brain.

Somatosensory Information from the Trunk and Limbs Is Conveyed to the Spinal Cord

Sensory information from the trunk and limbs enters the spinal cord, which has a core H-shape region of gray matter surrounded by white matter. The gray matter on each side of the cord is divided into dorsal (or posterior) and ventral (or anterior) horns (Figure 16–1). The dorsal horn contains groups of sensory neurons

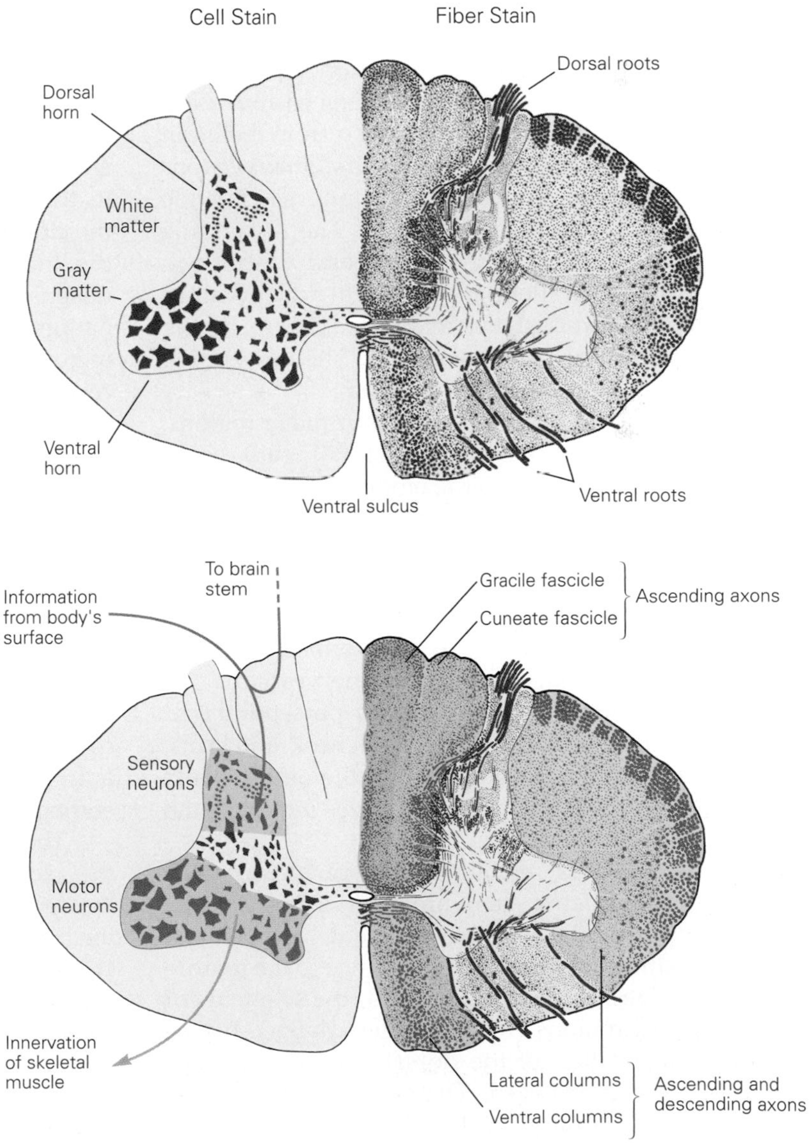

Figure 16–1 The major anatomical features of the spinal cord. **Top:** The left side depicts a cell stain of the gray matter and the right side a fiber-stained section. **Bottom:** The ventral horn (**green**) contains large motor neurons, whereas the dorsal horn (**orange**) contains smaller neurons. Fibers of the gracile fascicle carry somatosensory information from the lower limbs, whereas fibers of the cuneate fascicle carry somatosensory information from the upper body. Fiber bundles of the lateral and ventral columns include both ascending and descending fiber bundles.

(sensory nuclei) whose axons receive stimulus information from the body's surface. The ventral horn contains groups of motor neurons (motor nuclei) whose axons exit the spinal cord and innervate skeletal muscles.

Unlike the sensory nuclei, the motor nuclei form columns that run the length of the spinal cord. Interneurons of various types in the gray matter inhibit the output of the spinal cord neurons. These inhibitory interneurons thus modulate both sensory information flowing toward the brain and motor commands descending from the brain to the spinal motor neurons. Motor neurons can also adjust the output of other motor neurons via the interneurons.

The white matter surrounding the gray matter contains bundles of ascending and descending axons that are divided into dorsal, lateral, and ventral columns. The dorsal columns, which lie between the two dorsal horns of the gray matter, contain only ascending axons that carry somatic sensory information to the brain stem (Figure 16–1). The lateral columns include both ascending axons and axons descending from the brain stem and neocortex that innervate spinal interneurons and motor neurons. The ventral columns also include ascending and descending axons. The ascending somatic sensory axons in the lateral and ventral columns constitute parallel pathways that convey information about pain and thermal sensation to higher levels of the central nervous system. The descending axons control axial muscles and posture.

The spinal cord is divided into four major regions: cervical, thoracic, lumbar, and sacral (Figure 16–2). These regions are related to the embryological somites from which muscles, bones, and other components of the body develop (see Chapters 52 and 53). Axons projecting from the spinal cord to body structures that develop at the same segmental level join together in the intervertebral foramen with axons entering the spinal cord to form spinal nerves. Spinal nerves at the cervical level are involved with sensory perception and motor function of the back of the head, neck, and arms; nerves at the thoracic level innervate the upper trunk; whereas lumbar and sacral spinal nerves innervate the lower trunk, back, and legs.

Each of the four regions of the spinal cord contains several segments; there are 8 cervical segments, 12 thoracic segments, 5 lumbar segments, and 5 sacral segments. Although the actual substance of the mature spinal cord does not look segmented, the segments of the four spinal regions are nonetheless defined by the number and location of the dorsal and ventral roots that enter or exit the cord. The spinal cord varies in size and shape along its rostrocaudal axis because of two organizational features.

First, relatively few sensory axons enter the cord at the sacral level. At higher levels (lumbar, thoracic, and cervical) the number of sensory axons entering the cord increases progressively. Conversely, most descending axons from the brain terminate at cervical levels, with progressively fewer descending to lower levels of the spinal cord. Thus the number of fibers in the white matter is highest at cervical levels (where there are the highest numbers of both ascending and descending fibers) and lowest at sacral levels. As a result, sacral levels of the spinal cord have much less white matter than gray matter, whereas the cervical cord has more white matter than gray matter (Figure 16–2).

The second organizational feature is variation in the size of the ventral and dorsal horns. The ventral horn is larger at the levels where the motor nerves that innervate the arms and legs exit the spinal cord. The number of ventral motor neurons dedicated to a body region roughly parallels the dexterity of movements of that region. Thus a larger number of motor neurons is needed to innervate the greater number of muscles and to regulate the greater complexity of movement in the limbs as compared with the trunk. Likewise, the dorsal horn is larger where sensory nerves from the limbs enter the cord. Limbs have a greater density of sensory receptors to mediate finer tactile discrimination and thus send more fibers to the cord. These regions of the cord are known as the lumbosacral and cervical enlargements.

The Primary Sensory Neurons of the Trunk and Limbs Are Clustered in the Dorsal Root Ganglia

The sensory neurons that convey information from the skin, muscles, and joints of the limbs and trunk to the spinal cord are clustered together in dorsal root ganglia within the vertebral column immediately adjacent to the spinal cord (Figure 16–3). These neurons are pseudo-unipolar in shape; they have a bifurcated axon with central and peripheral branches. The peripheral branch terminates in skin, muscle, or other tissue as a free nerve ending or in association with specialized receptors.

The central process enters the spinal cord. On entry the axon forms branches that either terminate within the spinal gray matter or ascend to nuclei located near the junction of the spinal cord with the medulla (Figure 16–3). These local and ascending branches provide two functional pathways for somatosensory information entering the spinal cord from dorsal root ganglion cells. The local branches can activate local reflex circuits while the ascending branches carry information into the brain, where this information becomes the raw material for the perception of touch, position sense, or pain.

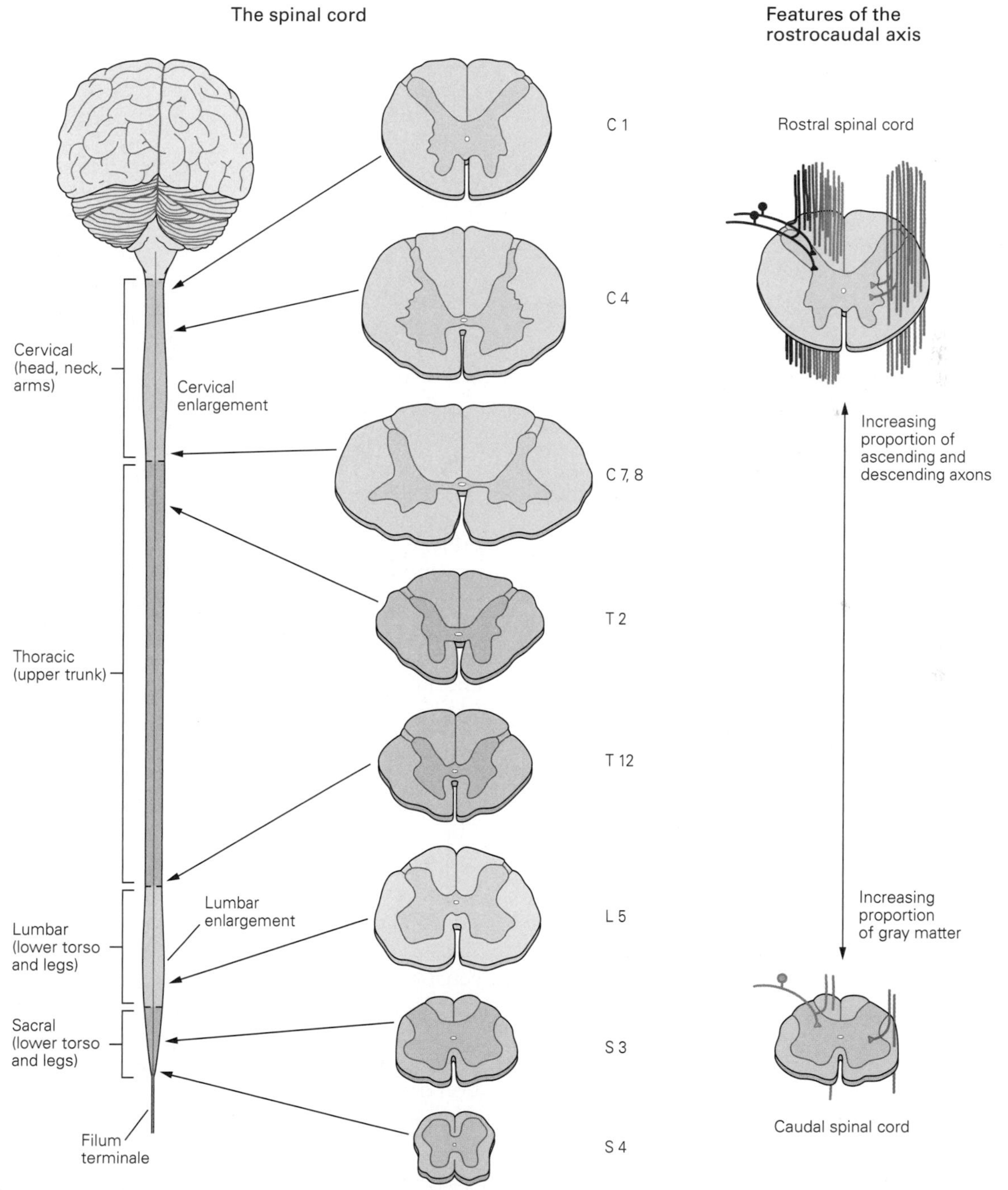

Figure 16–2 The internal and external appearances of the spinal cord vary at different levels. The proportion of gray matter (the H-shaped area within the spinal cord) to white matter is greater at sacral levels than at cervical levels. At sacral levels very few incoming sensory fibers have joined the spinal cord, whereas most of the motor fibers have already terminated at higher levels of the spinal cord. The cross-sectional enlargements at the lumbar and cervical levels are regions where the large number of fibers innervating the limbs enter or leave the spinal cord.

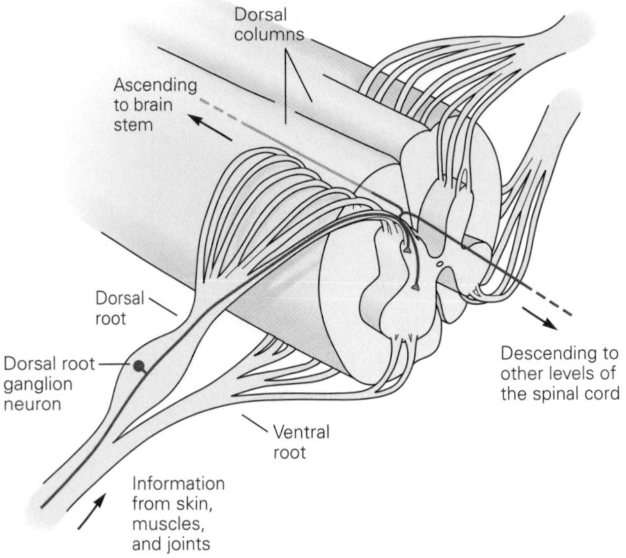

Figure 16–3 Dorsal root ganglia and spinal nerve roots. The cell bodies of neurons that bring sensory information from the skin, muscles, and joints lie in the dorsal root ganglia, clusters of cells that lie adjacent to the spinal cord. The axons of these neurons are bifurcated into peripheral and central branches. The central branch enters the dorsal portion of the spinal cord.

The Central Axons of Dorsal Root Ganglion Neurons Are Arranged to Produce a Map of the Body Surface

The central axons of the dorsal root ganglion cells form a neural map of the body surface when they terminate in the spinal cord. This orderly somatotopic distribution of inputs from different portions of the body surface is maintained throughout the entire ascending somatosensory pathway.

Axons that enter the cord in the sacral region ascend in the dorsal column near the midline, whereas those that enter at successively higher levels ascend at progressively more lateral positions within the dorsal columns. Thus, in the cervical cord, where axons from all portions of the body have already entered, sensory fibers from the lower body are located medially in the dorsal column, while fibers from the trunk, the arm and shoulder, and finally the neck occupy progressively more lateral areas. At cervical levels of the cord the axons forming the dorsal columns are divided into two bundles: a medially situated gracile fascicle and a more laterally situated cuneate fascicle (Figure 16–4).

Each Somatic Submodality Is Processed in a Distinct Subsystem from the Periphery to the Brain

The submodalities of somatic sensation—touch, pain, and position sense—are processed in the brain through different pathways that end in different brain regions. To illustrate the specificity of these parallel pathways, we will follow the path of information for the submodality of touch.

The primary afferent fibers that carry information about touch enter the ipsilateral dorsal column and, without crossing to the contralateral column, ascend to the medulla. Fibers from the lower body run in the gracile fascicle and terminate in the gracile nucleus, whereas fibers from the upper body run in the cuneate fascicle and terminate in the cuneate nucleus. Neurons in the gracile and cuneate nuclei give rise to axons that cross to the other side of the brain and ascend to the thalamus in a long fiber bundle called the medial lemniscus (Figure 16–4).

As in the dorsal columns of the spinal cord, the fibers of the medial lemniscus are arranged somatotopically. Because the sensory fibers cross the midline to the other side of the brain, the right side of the brain receives sensory information from the left side of the body, and vice versa. The fibers of the medial lemniscus end in a specific subdivision of the thalamus called the ventral posterior nucleus (Figure 16–4). There the fibers maintain their somatotopic organization such that those carrying information from the lower body end laterally and those carrying information from the upper body and face end medially.

The Thalamus Is an Essential Link Between Sensory Receptors and the Cerebral Cortex for All Modalities Except Olfaction

The thalamus is an egg-shaped structure that constitutes the dorsal portion of the diencephalon. It conveys sensory input to the primary sensory areas of the cerebral cortex but is more than simply a relay. It acts as a gatekeeper for information to the cerebral cortex, preventing or enhancing the passage of specific information depending on the behavioral state of the animal.

The thalamus is a good example of a brain region made up of several well-defined nuclei. As many as 50 thalamic nuclei have been identified. Some nuclei receive information specific to a sensory modality and project to a specific area of the neocortex. Cells in the ventral posterior lateral nucleus (where the medial lemniscus terminates) process somatosensory information,

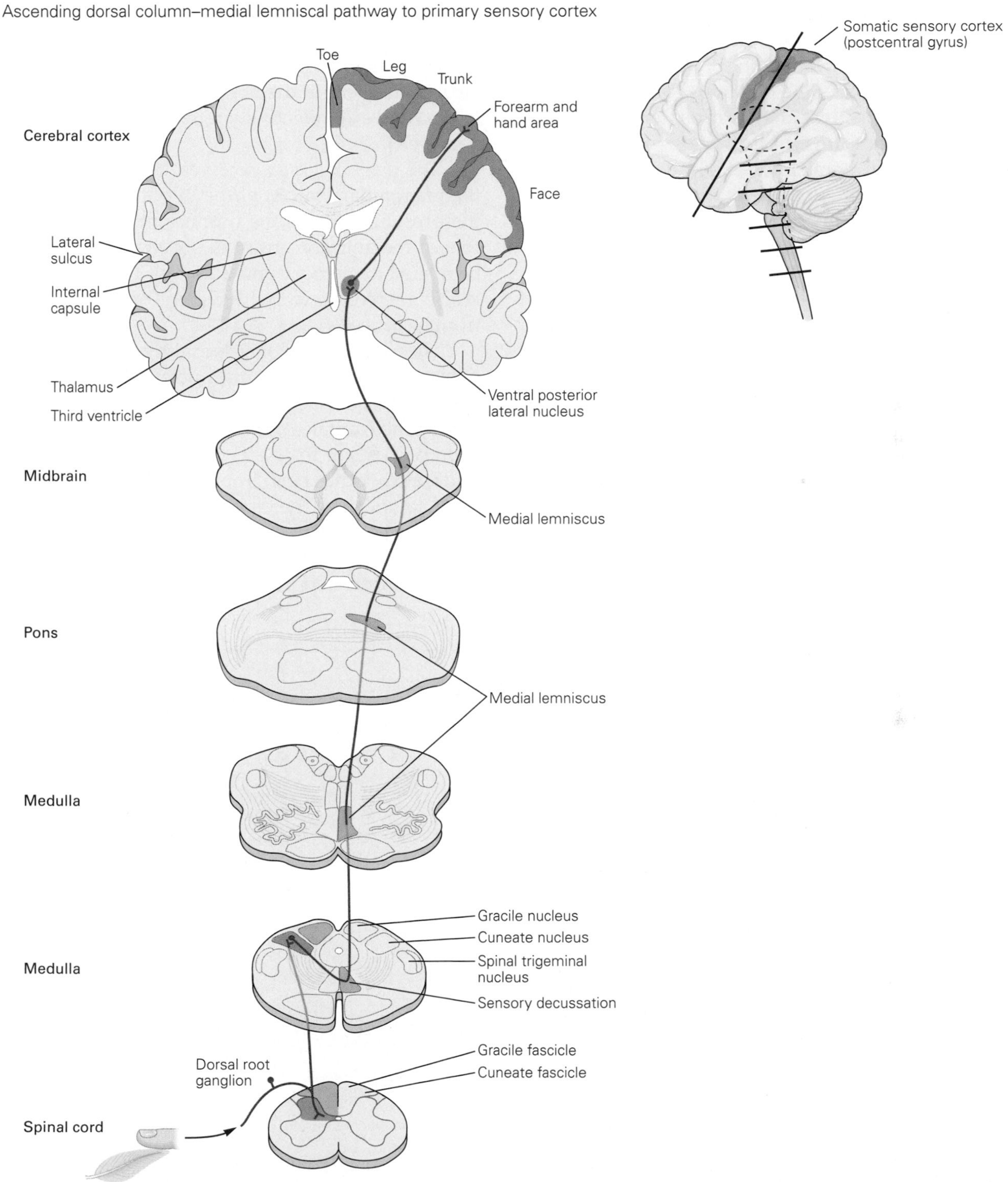

Figure 16–4 The medial lemniscus is a major afferent pathway for somatosensory information. Somatosensory information enters the central nervous system through the dorsal root ganglion cells. The flow of information ultimately leads to excitation of the somatosensory cortex. Fibers that relay information from different parts of the body maintain an orderly relationship to each other and form a neural map of the body surface in their pattern of termination at each synaptic relay.

and their axons project to the primary somatosensory cortex (Figure 16–4). Other portions of the thalamus participate in motor functions, transmitting information from the cerebellum and basal ganglia to the motor regions of the frontal lobe.

Axons from cells of the thalamus that project to the neocortex travel in the internal capsule, a large fiber bundle that carries most of the axons running to and from the cerebral hemispheres. Through its connections with the frontal lobe, the thalamus may also play a role in cognitive functions, such as memory. Some nuclei that may play a role in attention project diffusely to large but distinctly different regions of cortex. The reticular nucleus, which forms the outer shell of the thalamus, does not project to the neocortex at all. Its largely inhibitory neurons receive inputs from other fibers as they exit the thalamus en route to the neocortex and in turn to the other thalamic nuclei.

The nuclei of the thalamus are most commonly classified into four groups—anterior, medial, ventrolateral, and posterior—with respect to the internal medullary lamina, a sheet-like bundle of fibers that runs the rostrocaudal length of the thalamus (Figure 16–5). Thus the medial group of nuclei is located medial to the internal medullary lamina, whereas the ventral and posterior groups are located lateral to it. At the rostral pole of the thalamus the internal medullary lamina splits and surrounds the anterior group. The caudal pole of the thalamus is occupied by the posterior group, dominated by the pulvinar nucleus. Groups of neurons are also located within the fibers of the internal medullary lamina and are collectively referred to as the intralaminar nuclei.

The *anterior group* receives its major input from the mammillary nuclei of the hypothalamus and from the presubiculum of the hippocampal formation. The role of the anterior group is uncertain but thought to be related to memory and emotion. The anterior group is also interconnected with regions of the cingulate and frontal cortices.

The *medial group* consists mainly of the mediodorsal nucleus. This large thalamic nucleus has three subdivisions, each of which is connected to a particular portion of the frontal cortex. The nucleus receives inputs from portions of the basal ganglia, the amygdala, and midbrain and has been implicated in memory.

The nuclei of the *ventral group* are named according to their position within the thalamus. The ventral anterior and ventral lateral nuclei are important for motor control and carry information from the basal

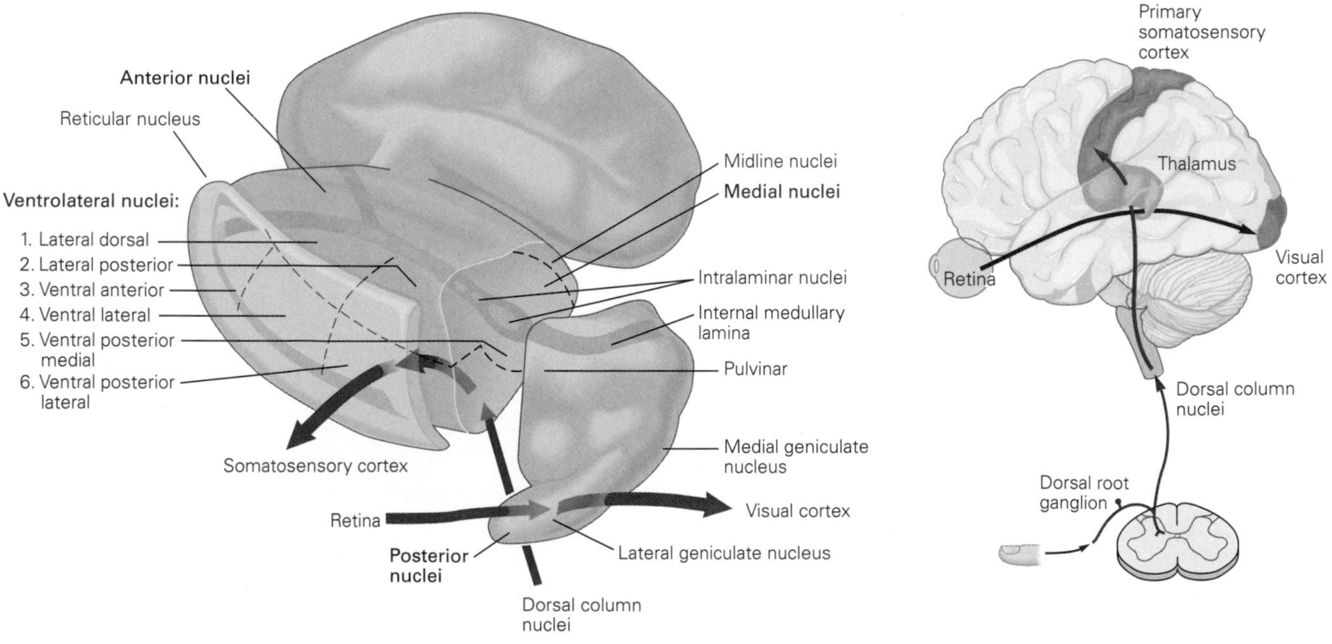

Figure 16–5 The major subdivisions of the thalamus. The thalamus is the critical relay for the flow of sensory information from peripheral receptors to the neocortex. Somatosensory information is conveyed from dorsal root ganglia to the ventral posterior lateral nucleus and from there to the primary somatosensory cortex. Likewise, visual information from the retina reaches the lateral geniculate nucleus, which conveys it to the primary visual cortex in the occipital lobe. Each of the sensory systems, except olfaction, has a similar processing step within a distinct region of the thalamus.

ganglia and cerebellum to the motor cortex. The ventral posterior lateral nucleus conveys somatosensory information to the neocortex.

The *posterior group* includes the medial and lateral geniculate nucleus, lateral posterior nucleus, and the pulvinar. The medial and lateral geniculate nuclei are located near the posterior part of the thalamus. The medial geniculate nucleus is a component of the auditory system; it is organized tonotopically, and conveys auditory information to the superior temporal gyrus of the temporal lobe. The lateral geniculate nucleus receives information from the retina and conveys it to the primary visual cortex in the occipital lobe. The pulvinar is most enlarged in the primate brain, especially in the human brain, and its development seems to parallel the enlargement of the association regions of the parietal-occipital-temporal cortex (see Chapter 18). It has been divided into at least three subdivisions and is extensively interconnected with widespread regions of the parietal, temporal, and occipital lobes, as well as with the superior colliculus and other nuclei of the brain stem related to vision.

The thalamus not only projects to the visual areas of the neocortex but also receives extensive return inputs back from the neocortex. In fact, in the lateral geniculate nucleus the number of synapses formed by axons from the return projection from the occipital cortex is greater than the number of synapses that the lateral geniculate nucleus receives from the retina. Most nuclei of the thalamus receive a similarly prominent return projection from the cerebral cortex, although the functional significance of these projections is unclear.

The thalamic nuclei described thus far are called the *relay* (or *specific*) *nuclei* because they have a specific and selective relationship with a particular portion of the neocortex. Other thalamic nuclei, called *nonspecific nuclei,* project to several cortical and subcortical regions. These nuclei are located either on the midline of the thalamus (the midline nuclei) or within the internal medullary lamina (the intralaminar nuclei). The largest of the midline nuclei are the paraventricular, parataenial, and reuniens nuclei; the largest of the intralaminar cell groups is the centromedian nucleus. The intralaminar nuclei project to medial temporal lobe structures, such as the amygdala and hippocampus, but also send projections to components of the basal ganglia. These nuclei receive inputs from a variety of sources in the spinal cord, brain stem, and cerebellum and are thought to mediate cortical arousal and perhaps to participate in the integration of sensory submodalities that we shall learn about in Chapters 21 and 22.

Finally, the outer covering of the thalamus is formed by a unique sheet-like structure, the *reticular nucleus*. The majority of its neurons use the inhibitory transmitter γ-aminobutyric acid (GABA), whereas most of the neurons in the other thalamic nuclei use the excitatory transmitter glutamate. Moreover, the neurons of the reticular nucleus are not interconnected with the neocortex. Rather, their axons terminate on the other nuclei of the thalamus. These other nuclei also provide the input to the reticular nucleus via collaterals of their axons that exit the thalamus through the reticular nucleus. Thus the reticular nucleus modulates activity in other thalamic nuclei based on its monitoring of the entirety of the thalamocortical stream of information. This portion of the thalamus thus acts like a filter that gates information flow to the neocortex.

We see, then, that the thalamus is not a passive relay station where information is simply passed on to the neocortex. Rather it is a complex brain region where substantial information processing is possible. To give but one example, the output of somatosensory information from the ventral posterior lateral nucleus is subject to four types of processing: (1) local processing within the nucleus; (2) modulation by brain stem inputs, such as the noradrenergic and serotonergic systems; (3) inhibitory feedback from the reticular nucleus; and (4) excitatory feedback from the neocortex.

Sensory Information Processing Culminates in the Cerebral Cortex

Somatosensory information from the ventral posterior lateral nucleus is conveyed mainly to the primary somatosensory cortex (Brodmann's area 3b). The neurons here are exquisitely sensitive to tactile stimulation of the skin surface. As in subcortical synaptic centers of the somatosensory system, the neurons in different parts of the cortex are somatotopically organized.

When the neurosurgeon Wilder Penfield stimulated the surface of the somatic sensory cortex in patients undergoing brain surgery, he found that sensation from the lower limbs is mediated by neurons located near the midline of the brain, whereas sensations from the upper body, hands and fingers, the face, lips, and tongue are mediated by neurons located laterally. As we shall learn in more detail in Chapter 17, Penfield found that although all parts of the body are represented in the cortex somatotopically, the area of cortex devoted to each body part is not proportional to its mass. Instead, it is proportional to the density of innervation, which translates to the fineness of discrimination in the body part. Thus the area of cortex devoted to the fingers is larger than that for the arms.

Likewise, the representation of the lips and tongue occupies more cortical surface than that of the remainder of the face (Figure 16–6).

The cerebral cortex is organized functionally into columns of cells extend from the white matter to the surface of the cortex. The cells in each column comprise a computational module with a highly specialized function. The larger the area of cortex dedicated to a function, the greater the number of computational columns that are dedicated to that function (see Chapter 19). The highly discriminative sense of touch in the fingers is a result of the large area of cortex dedicated to processing somatosensory information from the hand.

A second major insight from the early electrophysiological studies was that the somatosensory cortex contains not one but several somatotopic arrays of inputs from the skin and therefore several neural maps of the body surface. The primary somatosensory cortex (anterior parietal cortex) has four complete maps of the skin, one each in areas 3a, 3b, 1, and 2. Basic processing of tactile information takes place in area 3, whereas more complex or higher-order processing occurs in area 1. In area 2 tactile information is combined with information concerning limb position to mediate the tactile recognition of objects. Neurons in the primary somatosensory cortex project to neurons in adjacent areas, and these neurons in turn project to other adjacent cortical regions (Figure 16–7). At higher levels in the hierarchy of cortical connections somatosensory information is used in motor control, eye–hand coordination, and memory related to touch.

The cortical areas involved in the early stages of sensory processing are concerned only (or primarily) with a single modality. Such regions are called unimodal association areas. Information from the unimodal association areas converges on multimodal association areas of the cortex concerned with combining sensory modalities. As we shall learn in the next two chapters and again in Chapter 62, these multimodal associational areas, which are heavily interconnected with the hippocampus, appear to be particularly important for two tasks: (1) the production of a unified percept and (2) the representation of the percept in memory.

Thus, from the mechanical pressure on a receptor in the skin to the perception that a finger has been touched by a friend shaking your hand, somatosensory

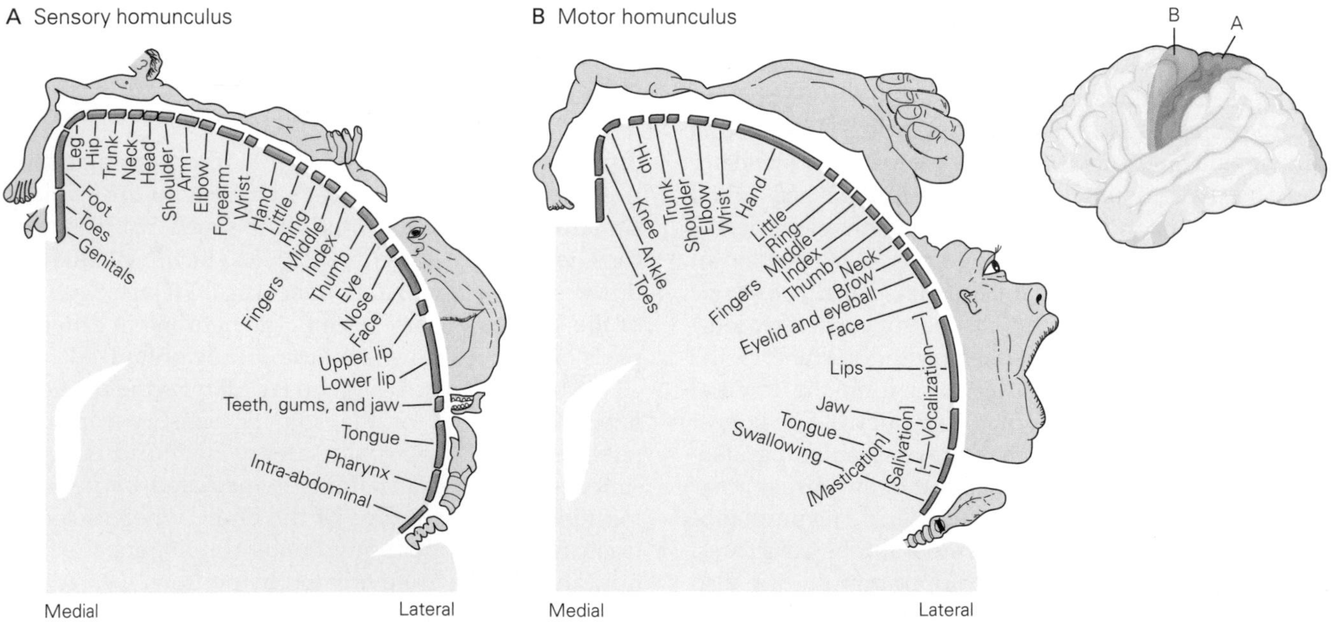

Figure 16–6 A homunculus illustrates the relative amounts of cortical area dedicated to individual parts of the body. (Adapted, with permission, from Penfield and Rasmussen 1950.)

A. The entire body surface is represented in an orderly array of somatosensory inputs in the cortex. The area of cortex dedicated to processing information from a particular part of the body is not proportional to the mass of the body part but instead reflects the density of sensory receptors in that part. Thus sensory input from the lips and hands occupies more area of cortex than, say, that from the elbow.

B. Output from the motor cortex is organized in similar fashion. The amount of cortical surface dedicated to a part of the body is related to the degree of motor control of that part. Thus in humans much of the motor cortex is dedicated to moving the muscles of the fingers and the muscles related to speech.

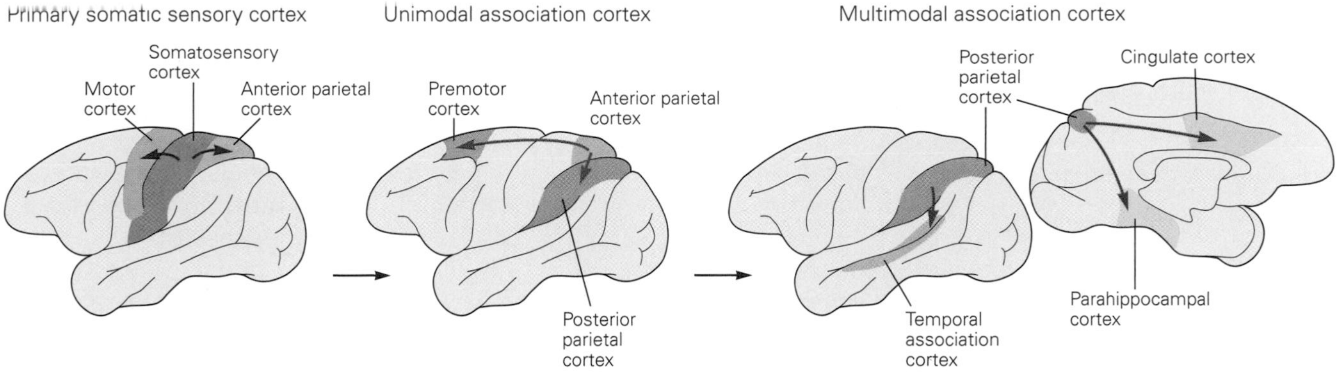

Figure 16–7 The processing of sensory information in the cerebral cortex begins with primary sensory areas, continues in unimodal association areas, and is completed in multimodal association areas. Sensory systems also communicate with portions of the motor cortex. For example, the primary somatosensory cortex projects to the motor area in the frontal lobe and to the somatosensory association area in the parietal cortex. The somatosensory association area, in turn, projects to higher-order somatosensory association areas and to the premotor cortex. Information from different sensory systems converges in the multimodal association areas, which include the parahippocampal, temporal association, and cingulate cortices.

information is processed in serial and parallel pathways from the dorsal root ganglia to the somatosensory cortex, to unimodal association areas, and finally to multimodal association areas. One of the primary purposes of somatosensory information is to guide directed movement. As one might imagine, there is a close linkage between the somatosensory and motor functions of the cortex.

Voluntary Movement Is Mediated by Direct Connections Between the Cortex and Spinal Cord

As we shall see in Chapter 18 a major function of the perceptual systems is to provide the sensory information necessary for the actions mediated by the motor systems. The primary motor cortex is organized somatotopically like the somatic sensory cortex (Figure 16–6B). Specific regions of the motor cortex influence the activity of specific muscle groups.

The axons of neurons in layer V of the primary motor cortex project through the corticospinal tract to the ventral horn of the spinal cord. The human corticospinal tract consists of approximately one million axons, of which approximately 40% originate in the motor cortex. These axons descend through the subcortical white matter, the internal capsule, and the cerebral peduncle in the midbrain (Figure 16–8). In the medulla the fibers form prominent protuberances on the ventral surface called the medullary pyramids, and thus the entire projection is sometimes called the pyramidal tract.

Like the ascending somatosensory system, the descending corticospinal tract crosses to the opposite side of the spinal cord. Most of the corticospinal fibers cross the midline in the medulla at a location known as the pyramidal decussation. However, approximately 10% of the fibers do not cross until they reach the level of the spinal cord at which they will terminate. The corticospinal fibers make monosynaptic connections with motor neurons, connections that are particularly important for individuated finger movements. They also form synapses with interneurons in the spinal cord. These indirect connections are important for coordinating larger groups of muscles in behaviors such as reaching and walking.

The motor information carried in the corticospinal tract is significantly modulated by both sensory information and information from other motor regions. A continuous stream of tactile, visual, and proprioceptive information is needed to make voluntary movement both accurate and properly sequenced. In addition, the output of the motor cortex is under the substantial influence of other motor regions of the brain, including the cerebellum and basal ganglia, structures that are essential for smoothly executed movements. These two subcortical centers provide feedback essential for the smooth execution of skilled movements and thus are also important for motor learning, the improvement in motor skills through practice (Figure 16–9, and see Chapter 65).

The cerebellum receives somatosensory information directly from primary afferents originating in the spinal cord as well as from corticospinal axons descending

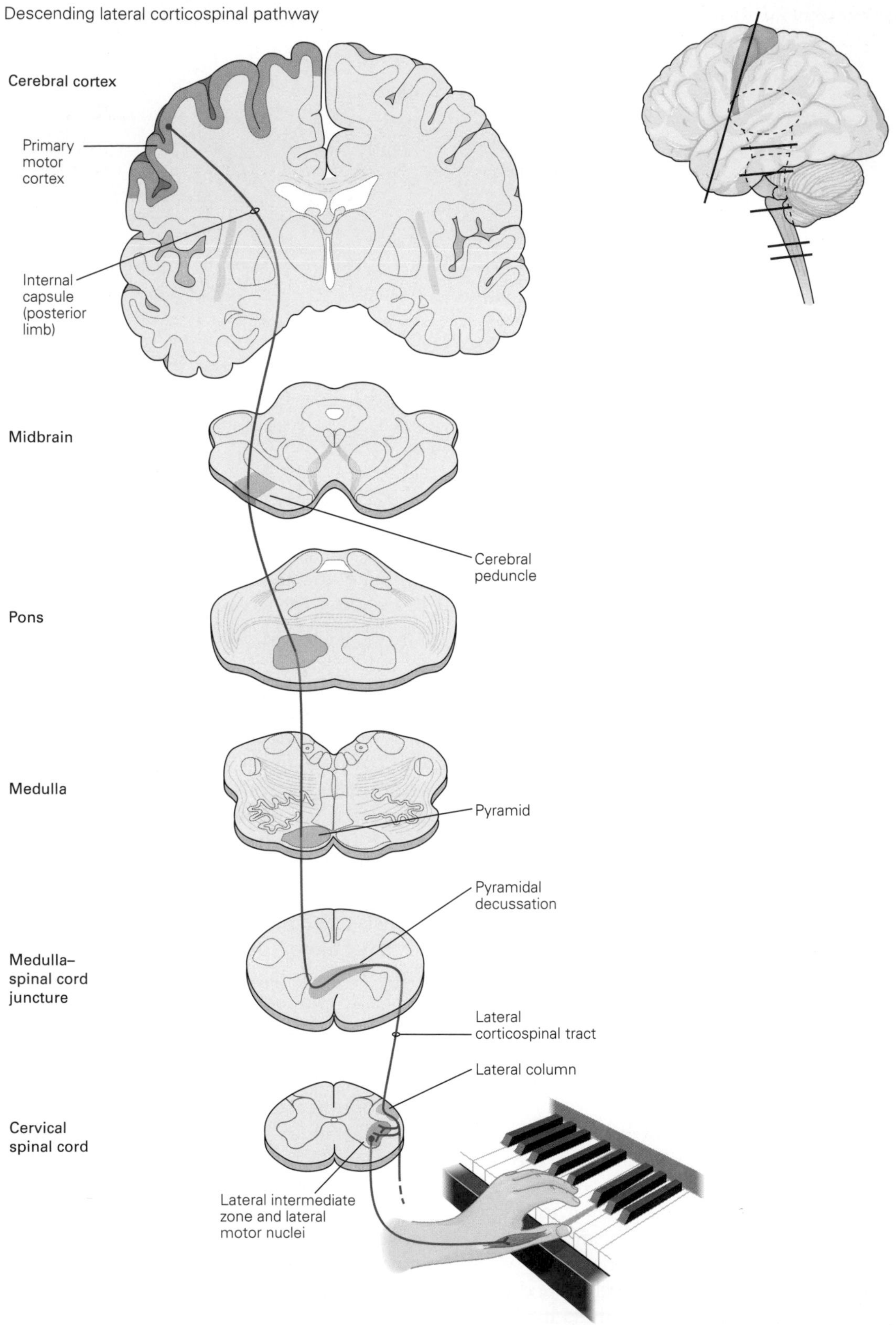

Figure 16–8 Fibers that originate in the primary motor cortex and terminate in the ventral horn of the spinal cord constitute a significant part of the corticospinal tract. The same axons are at various points in their projection part of the internal capsule, the cerebral peduncle, the medullary pyramid, and the lateral corticospinal tract.

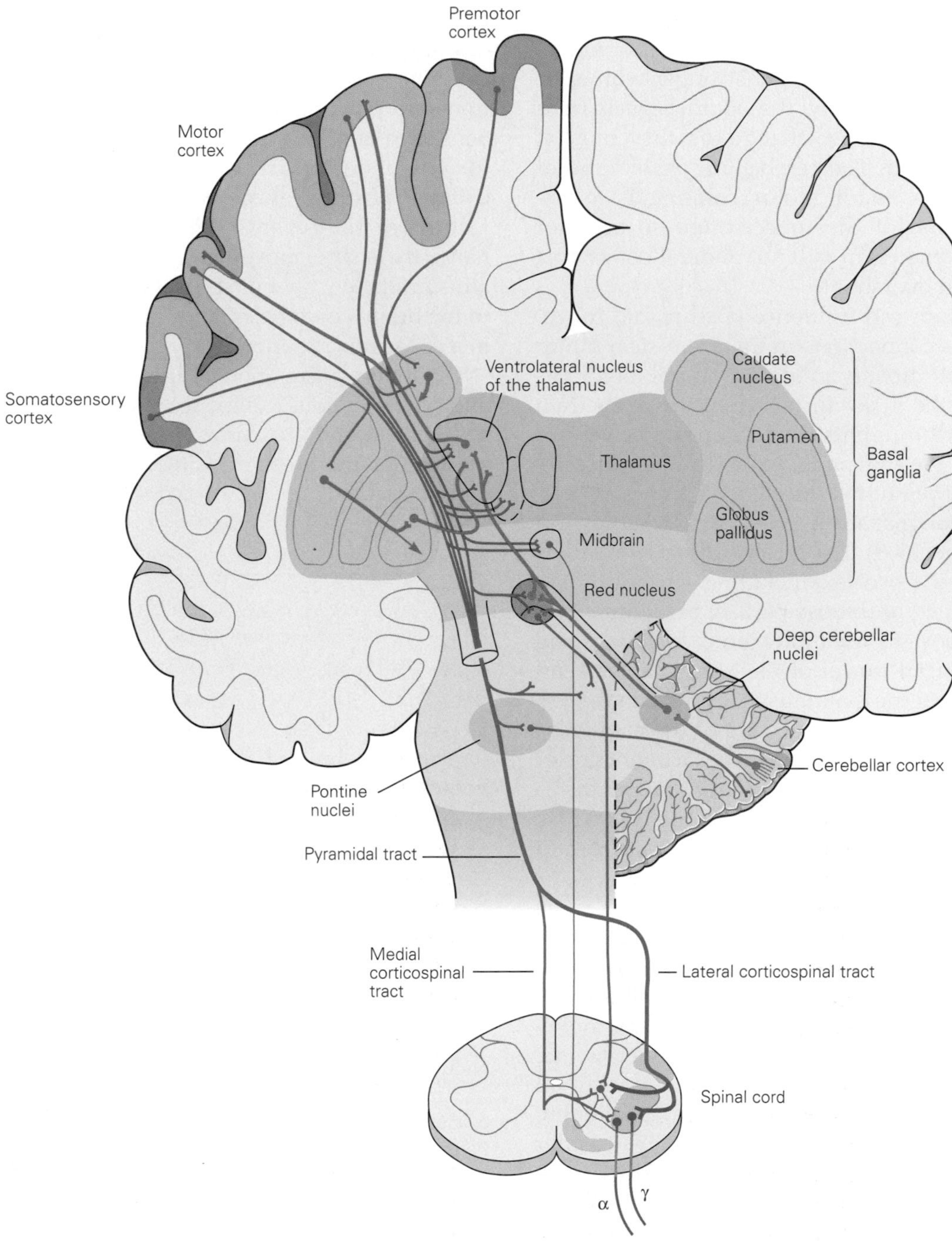

Figure 16–9 Voluntary movement requires coordination of all components of the motor system. The principal components are the motor cortex, basal ganglia, thalamus, midbrain, cerebellum, and spinal cord. The principal descending projections are shown in **green**; feedback projections and local connections are shown in **purple**. All of this processing is incorporated in the inputs to the motor neurons of the ventral horn of the spinal cord, the so-called "final common pathway" that innervates muscle and elicits movements. (This figure is a composite view made from sections of the brain taken at different angles.)

from the neocortex. The cerebellum is thought to be part of an error-correcting mechanism for movements because it can compare movement commands from the cortex with somatic sensory information about what actually happened. Thus the cerebellum is thought to be important in "predictive control" of movements, in which commands for movements are adjusted based on information about the effectiveness of prior movement. In addition, as muscles get stronger with exercise and as our bodies grow, the neural signals for a particular movement must change, as they must if muscles are damaged. The cerebellum enables motor control systems to adapt motor commands to the changing condition of the musculature so that, for example, a weakened arm will not undershoot its goal or a stronger arm overshoot.

The cerebellum can influence posture and movement through its connections in the brain stem motor nuclei, which can directly modulate spinal motor circuits. However, the major influence of the cerebellum on movement is through its connections in the ventrolateral nuclei of the thalamus, which connect directly to the motor and premotor cortex.

The basal ganglia are a collection of subcortical nuclei (see Figure 16–9) that receive direct projections from much of the neocortex, including sensory, motor, and premotor areas, and those parts of association cortex that are important for motivation, cognition, and emotion. The output nuclei of the basal ganglia send signals to regions of the thalamus that project to the cerebral cortex. Although the functions of the basal ganglia have remained surprisingly elusive, dysfunction of the basal ganglia results in particularly striking disorders of movement characteristic of Parkinson disease (tremor at rest, rigidity, and disinclination to move) and of Huntington disease (choreiform movements).

Thus an important consequence of basal ganglia dysfunction is that the abnormal signals sent to cortical motor areas have a major, negative, impact on motor output. Indeed, cortical lesions that limit voluntary movement also abolish the involuntary movements associated with disorders of the basal ganglia. This capacity of the basal ganglia to create marked disorders of movement when they are functioning abnormally must in some way be matched by a similar profound influence over normal motor function.

An Overall View

Sensory and motor information is processed in the brain in a variety of discrete pathways that are active simultaneously. A functional pathway is formed by the serial connection of identifiable groups of neurons, and each group processes more complex or specific information than the preceding group. Thus different pathways that run through the spinal cord, brain stem, and into the cortex mediate the sensations of touch and pain. All sensory and motor systems follow the pattern of hierarchical and parallel processing.

As we shall see in later chapters, contrary to an intuitive analysis of our personal experience, perceptions are not precise copies of the world around us. Sensation is an abstraction, not a replication, of reality. The brain constructs an internal representation of external physical events after first analyzing various features of those events. When we hold an object in the hand, the shape, movement, and texture of the object are simultaneously but separately analyzed according to the brain's own rules, and the results are integrated in a conscious experience.

How this integration occurs—the *binding problem*—and how conscious experience emerges from the brain's selective attention to incoming sensory information are two of the most pressing questions in cognitive neural science.

David G. Amaral

Selected Readings

Brodal A. 1981. *Neurological Anatomy in Relation to Clinical Medicine,* 3rd ed. New York: Oxford Univ. Press.

Carpenter MB. 1991. *Core Text of Neuroanatomy,* 4th ed. Baltimore: Williams and Wilkins.

England MA, Wakely J. 1991. *Color Atlas of the Brain and Spinal Cord: An Introduction to Normal Neuroanatomy.* St. Louis: Mosby Year Book.

Martin JH. 2003. *Neuroanatomy: Text and Atlas,* 3rd ed. Stamford, CT: Appleton & Lange.

Nieuwenhuys R, Voogd J, van Huijzen Chr. 1988. *The Human Central Nervous System: A Synopsis and Atlas,* 3rd rev. ed. Berlin: Springer-Verlag.

Peters A, Jones EG (eds). 1984. *Cerebral Cortex.* Vol. 1, *Cellular Components of the Cerebral Cortex.* New York: Plenum.

Peters A, Palay S, Webster H de F. 1991. *The Fine Structure of the Nervous System,* 3rd ed. New York: Oxford Univ. Press.

References

Brodmann K. 1909. *Vergleichende Lokalisationslehre der Grosshirnrinde in ihren Prinzipien dargestellt auf Grund des Zellenbaues.* Leipzig: Barth.

Felleman DJ, Van Essen DC. 1991. Distributed hierarchical processing in the primate cerebral cortex. Cereb Cortex 1:1–47.

Kaas JH. 2006. Evolution of the neocortex. Curr Biol 16: R910–914.

Kaas JH, Qi HX, Burish MJ, Gharbawie OA, Onifer SM, Massey JM. 2008. Cortical and subcortical plasticity in the brains of humans, primates, and rats after damage to sensory afferents in the dorsal columns of the spinal cord. Exp Neurol 209:407–16.

McKenzie AL, Nagarajan SS, Roberts TP, Merzenich MM, Byl NN. 2003. Somatosensory representation of the digits and clinical performance in patients with focal hand dystonia. Am J Phys Med Rehabil 82:737–749.

Penfield W, Boldrey E. 1937. Somatic motor and sensory representation in the cerebral cortex of man as studied by electrical stimulation. Brain 60:389–443.

Penfield W, Rasmussen T. 1950. *The Cerebral Cortex of Man: A Clinical Study of Localization of Function*. New York: Macmillan.

Ramón y Cajal S. 1995. *Histology of the Nervous System of Man and Vertebrates*. 2 vols. N Swanson, LW Swanson (transl). New York: Oxford Univ. Press.

Rockland KS, Ichinohe N. 2004. Some thoughts on cortical minicolumns. Exp Brain Res 158:265–277.

17

From Nerve Cells to Cognition: The Internal Representations of Space and Action

NEURAL SCIENTISTS BELIEVE THAT a cellular approach is necessary to understand how the brain works. Considering that the brain has a hundred billion nerve cells, it is remarkable how much can be learned about mental activity by examining one nerve cell at a time. Progress is particularly good when we understand the anatomy and connections of functionally important pathways.

Cellular studies of the sensory systems, for example, provide important insight into how stimuli at the body's surface are translated by the brain into sensations and planned action. In the visual system, the sensory system most thoroughly studied at the cellular level, information arrives in the brain from the retina in parallel pathways dedicated to analyzing different aspects of the visual image—form, movement, and color. These separate inputs are eventually integrated into coherent images according to the brain's own rules, rules that are embodied in the circuitry of the visual system.

Different modalities of perception—an object seen, a face touched, or a melody heard—are processed similarly by the different sensory systems. Receptors in each system first analyze and deconstruct stimulus information. Receptors at the periphery of the body for each system are sensitive to a particular kind of physical event—light, pressure, tone, or chemical odorants. When a receptor is stimulated—when, for example, a receptor cell in the retina is excited by light—it responds with a distinct pattern of firing that represents certain properties of the stimulus. Each sensory system obtains information about the stimulus in this way and this information is conveyed along a pathway of cells leading to a specific (unimodal) region of cerebral cortex. In the cortex different unimodal regions representing different sensory modalities communicate with multimodal association areas through specific intracortical pathways, and in this network signals are selected and combined into an apparently seamless perception.

The brain thus produces an integrated perception because nerve cells are wired together in precise and orderly ways according to a general plan that does not vary greatly among normal individuals. Nevertheless, the connections are not exactly the same in all individuals. As we shall learn in later chapters, connections between cells can be altered by activity and by learning. We remember specific events because the structure and function of the connections between nerve cells are modified by those events.

Despite its success, neural scientists believe that a cellular approach alone is not sufficient for understanding how the integrative action of the brain—the simultaneous activity of discrete sets of neurons—produces cognition. For this task the brain must be studied as an information processing organ. This is the approach of *cognitive neural science*, which uses a combination of methods from a variety of fields—cell biology, systems neural science, brain imaging, cognitive psychology, behavioral neurology, and computational neuroscience.

Ulric Neisser, one of the pioneers of cognitive psychology, defined the challenge of this field in the following terms:

> It has been said that beauty is in the eye of the beholder. As a hypothesis . . . it points clearly enough to the central problem of cognition—the world of experience is produced by the man who experiences it . . . . There certainly is a real world of trees and people and cars and even books, and it has a great deal to do with our experience of these objects. However, we have no direct immediate access to the world, nor to any of its properties. . . .
>
> Whatever we know about reality has been mediated not only by the organs of sense but by complex systems which interpret and reinterpret sensory information. . . . The term "cognition" refers to all the processes by which the sensory input is transformed, reduced, elaborated, stored, recovered and used. . . .

In this chapter we first discuss how cognitive neural science evolved from otherwise disparate disciplines. We illustrate the success of the approach by considering what has been learned about one complex mental state: the experience of personal and extrapersonal space, both real and imagined. We then discuss how the unconscious and conscious mental processes are modeled by cognitive neural science. A great deal of cognitive processing goes on unconsciously. Sigmund Freud likened the conscious perception of mental processes to the perception of the external world by sense organs. We also discuss the profound challenges to a scientific study of consciousness. The five major subjects of cognitive neural science—perception, action, emotion, language, and memory—are discussed in detail in the subsequent five parts of the book beginning with Chapter 21.

The Major Goal of Cognitive Neural Science Is to Understand Neural Representations of Mental Processes

Until the end of the 19th century the chief method for understanding the mind was introspection. In fact, the scholarly study of the mind was a branch of philosophy. By the middle of the 19th century, however, the philosophical approach was giving way to empirical analysis and eventually the formation of the independent discipline of experimental psychology. In its early years experimental psychology was concerned primarily with the sequence of events by which an external stimulus becomes an internal sensation. By the end of the 19th century the interests of psychologists turned to how behavior is generated, how it is modified by learning and attention, and how it is stored in memory.

The discovery of simple experimental ways of studying learning and memory—first in human beings by Hermann Ebbinghaus in 1885 and a few years later in experimental animals by Ivan Pavlov and Edgar Thorndike—led to a rigorous empirical school of psychology called *behaviorism*. Behaviorists, notably J. B. Watson and B. F. Skinner in the United States, argued that behavior could be studied with the precision of the physical sciences, but only if psychologists abandoned speculation about what occurs in the mind and focused exclusively on the observable aspects of behavior. For example, the behaviorists argued that one cannot base a psychology on the idea that people do certain things because they believe they are the right things to do or because they want to do them.

Behaviorists regarded these unobservable mental processes, especially anything as abstract as motivations, feeling, or conscious awareness, as inaccessible to scientific study. They concentrated instead on evaluating—objectively and precisely—the relationship between specific physical stimuli and observable responses in intact animals. Their early successes in studying simple forms of behavior and learning encouraged them to treat all cognitive processes that intervene between the stimulus (input) and behavior (output) as irrelevant.

During behaviorism's most influential period, in the 1950s, many psychologists accepted the most radical behaviorist position: that observable behavior is all there is to mental life. As a result, the scientific concept of behavior largely depended on the techniques used to study it. This emphasis reduced the domain of experimental psychology to a restricted set of problems and excluded some of the most fascinating features of mental life.

By the 1960s it was not difficult for the founders of cognitive psychology—notably Edwin Tolman, Frederick Bartlett, George Miller, Noam Chomsky, Ulric Neisser, and Herbert Simon—to convince the scientific community that behaviorism was too limiting Building on earlier evidence from Gestalt psychology, psychoanalysis, and neurology, these early cognitive psychologists sought to demonstrate that our knowledge of the world is based on our biological equipment for perceiving the world, that perception is a constructive process that depends not only on the stimulus but also on the mental apparatus of the perceiver—the organization of the sensory and motor systems in the brain. We now realize that this constructive process also involves emotion, motivation, and reward.

What ultimately distinguished the cognitivists from the behaviorists was not only their conceptual approach to behavior but also the complexity of the methods they used. Cognitivists realized that only relatively few input–output relationships are stereotyped, that these relationships vary significantly because of mental states, past history, and expectations, the very factors that the behaviorists tended to ignore. Thus these variables must also be observable in behavior (or *output*) but are just more difficult to identify than the behavior defined by behaviorists.

This new perspective relied on neural network modeling and fortunately it coincided with the emergence of large-scale computers in the period following World War II. Computers allowed the modeling and testing of ideas about large neural networks that in principle are capable of higher mental functions. However, once psychologists acknowledged that mental activity was equivalent to computational processes in the brain, they had to face the fact that most mental processes were still largely inaccessible in living subjects. Without direct access to the brain, it would be difficult if not impossible to choose between various rival theories.

Fortunately, new tools for the empirical study of mental processes quickly became available, and significant progress was soon made in cellular analyses of the neural mediation of vision, touch, and action in intact primates engaged in ordinary behavior. Single-neuron recording and noninvasive imaging and recording techniques have allowed researchers to describe how neural activity in different sensory and motor pathways encodes sensory stimuli and planned actions. Moreover, imaging methods permit direct visualization of the brain in human subjects engaged in mental activity, allowing insight into attention and aspects of consciousness under controlled conditions (Chapter 20). Thus we can now study directly neural representations of the environment and motor action by comparing cellular recordings in primates engaged in purposeful activity with imaging of the human brain at work.

Cognitive neural science, as now practiced, emerged from four major technical and conceptual developments. First, in the 1960s and 1970s techniques were developed by Robert Wurtz and Edward Evarts at the National Institutes of Health for studying the activity of single cells in the brains of animals, including primates, engaged in controlled behavior in the laboratory. This allowed investigators to correlate the activity of specific populations of neurons with specific perceptual and motor processes. From these microelectrode studies we have been able to see that the mechanisms of perception are much the same in humans, monkeys, and even simpler animals.

These cellular studies in monkeys also made it possible to identify the importance of different combinations of areas of the brain involved in specific cognitive functions, such as attention and decision-making. These approaches changed the way the biology of behavior is studied both in experimental animals and in humans.

Second, developments in neural science and cognitive psychology stimulated a renewed interest in the behavioral analysis of patients with brain lesions that interfere with mental functioning. This area, *neuropsychology,* had remained a strong subspecialty of neurology in Europe but was neglected for a time in the United States. Lesions of different regions of the brain can result in quite specific cognitive deficits. The behavioral consequences of brain lesions thus tell us much about the function of specific neural pathways. Lesion studies have shown that cognition is the product of several specialized systems, each with many components. For example, the visual system has specialized pathways for processing information about color and form on the one hand and movement on the other.

Third, the development of imaging techniques such as positron emission tomography (PET) and functional magnetic resonance imaging (MRI), as well as the development of magnetoencephalography, has made it possible to relate changes in the activity of large populations of neurons to specific mental acts in living humans (see Chapter 20). This advance has been paralleled by two further developments. The use of voltage and calcium-sensitive dyes has permitted the study of neuronal activity in large ensembles of neurons, both in vitro and in the brains of behaving animals. The more recent use of light-sensitive ion channels has permitted the activation or inactivation of the activity of specific neurons or groups of neurons in the neural circuits of intact behaving animals.

Finally, improvement in computers and the emergence of a powerful subdiscipline of computational neural science has made it possible to model the activity of large populations of neurons and to test ideas about the roles of specific components of neural circuits in the brain in particular behaviors. To understand the neural organization of a complex behavior like speech we must understand not only the properties of individual cells and pathways but also the network properties of circuits in the brain. Although network properties depend on the properties of individual neurons in the network, they are not identical or even similar to those properties but are an *emergent* property of the way those different cells are interconnected.

When computational approaches are combined with detailed behavioral studies, for example with the psychophysical study of a specific perceptual act, the combined analysis can help to characterize the properties of a system. Thus psychophysics can describe what the system is capable of doing whereas computational modeling can describe how the properties of constituent cells could account for system properties of the neural circuits involved (see Appendices E and F).

The work of cognitive and computational neuroscientists is providing enormous insight into the workings of the brain. However, it also raises a difficult set of questions about the relationship between observed neurophysiological and mental processes, and particularly between these cellular biological processes and consciousness. The answers to these questions are yet unknown, but the mere fact that scientists are addressing them is a major advance.

To illustrate how cognitive neural science describes a mental act, in the next few sections we summarize what neural science has learned about the brain's representation of personal space (one's body) and peripersonal space, the space within arm's length ("near space"). We shall see how the brain constructs mental representations of space from external sensory input; how this representation gives rise to imagined and remembered space; and how it is selected by action, modified by normal experience, and distorted by

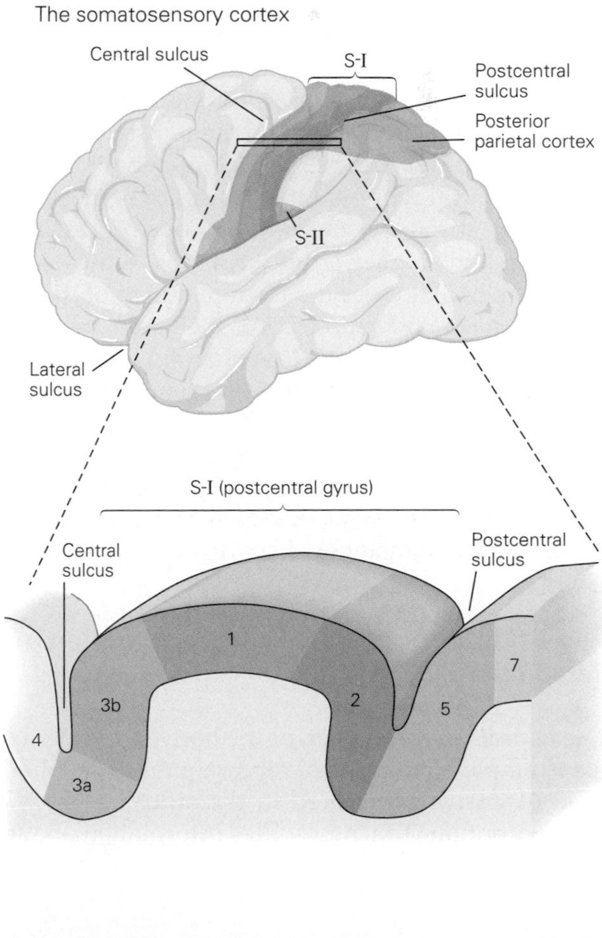

Figure 17–1 The somatosensory system in the cerebral cortex. A lateral view of a cerebral hemisphere illustrates the location of the primary somatic sensory cortex in the parietal lobe. The somatic sensory cortex has three major divisions: the primary (S-I) and secondary (S-II) somatosensory cortices and the posterior parietal cortex. A sagittal section shows the distinct cytoarchitectonic regions of S-I (Brodmann's areas 3a, 3b, 1, and 2) and the adjacent posterior parietal cortex (areas 5 and 7) and motor cortex (area 4).

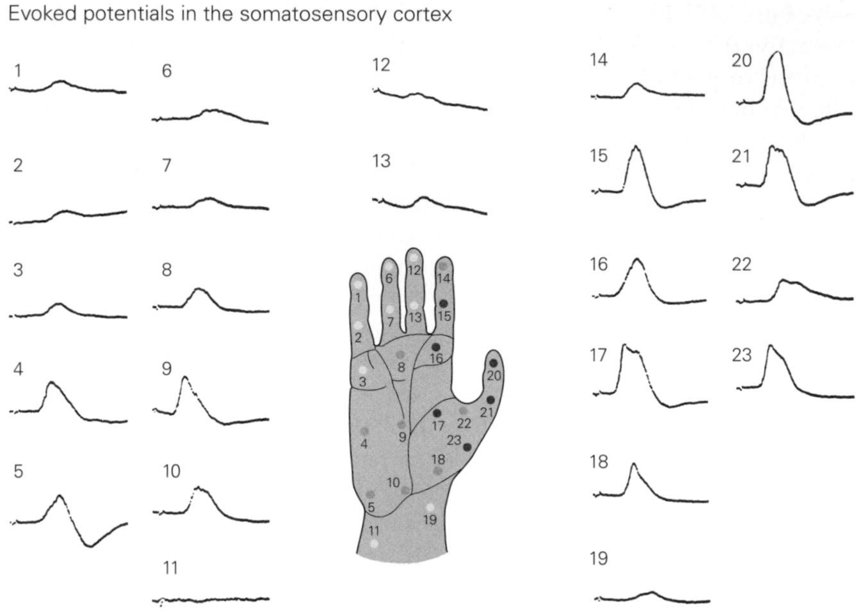

Figure 17–2 Evoked potentials in the somatosensory cortex elicited by stimulation of the hand. The evoked potentials shown here are the summed activity of one large group of neurons in the left postcentral gyrus of a monkey, elicited by a light touch at different points on the right palm. The evoked potentials were strongest when the thumb or forefinger was stimulated (points 15, 16, 17, 20, 21, and 23) and weakest when the middle or small finger was stimulated (points 1, 2, 3, 12, and 13). (Adapted, with permission, from Marshall, Woolsey, and Bard 1941.)

abnormal experience such as loss of a body part. This discussion illustrates a key principle that we will consider again in Chapter 19, that action has a key role in perception. The cognitive functions of the premotor areas provide for flexibility in behavior, preventing an otherwise stereotypic relationship between sensory input and behavioral output. By interpreting sensory input based on experience and mental state, these cognitive premotor processes shape our behavior.

The neural representation of space is most clearly evident in the early stages of sensory processing—in primary and higher-order areas of somatosensory cortex—where it takes the form of a map of the tactile sensors on the body surface. We shall see how this map can be modified after the loss of a body part and how those modifications can create a phantom representation. We shall also see how representations of personal and peripersonal space differ from extrapersonal space, the space beyond arm's length ("far space"), and how representations of extrapersonal space can give rise to imagined and remembered space.

The Brain Has an Orderly Representation of Personal Space

The neural representation of the body surface is a simple example of an internal representation, one that has been extensively explored in the study of touch and proprioception. Touch provides information about the properties of objects, such as their shape, texture, and solidity; proprioception provides information about the static position and movement of fingers and limbs.

An internal representation can be thought of as a certain pattern of neural activity that has at least two aspects: (1) the pattern of activation within a particular population of neurons (some cells are active and others not) and (2) the pattern of firing in individual cells.

Sensory neurons with receptors in the skin translate the mechanical energy of a stimulus into neural signals that are then conveyed along pathways that end in the somatosensory areas of the parietal lobe of the cerebral cortex (Figure 17–1). Each pathway includes one or more synaptic relays. At each relay, where thousands of afferent axons terminate on a cluster of similar neurons, the arrangement of the presynaptic fibers preserves the spatial relations of the receptors on the body surface. This somatotropic order thus creates a neural map of the body surface at each synaptic relay in the somatosensory system—information from neighboring receptors in the skin is conveyed to neighboring cells in each synaptic relay.

Neural maps of the body surface were first detected in laboratory animals using gross recording and stimulation techniques on the surface of the postcentral gyrus of the parietal cortex, the only portion of the cortex accessible with the experimental techniques available at that time. In the late 1930s Wade Marshall found that he could produce an evoked potential in the cortex by touching a specific part of the animal's body surface (Figure 17–2). Evoked potentials are electrical signals that represent the summed activity of thousands of cells and are recorded with external macroelectrodes on the brain surface. The evoked response method was used by Marshall, Clinton Woolsey, and Phillip Bard to map the neural representation of the body surface in the postcentral gyrus of monkeys (Figure 17–3).

The human somatosensory cortex was similarly mapped in the late 1940s by the Canadian neurosurgeon Wilder Penfield during operations for epilepsy and other brain disorders. Working with locally anesthetized conscious patients, Penfield stimulated various points on the surface of the postcentral gyrus

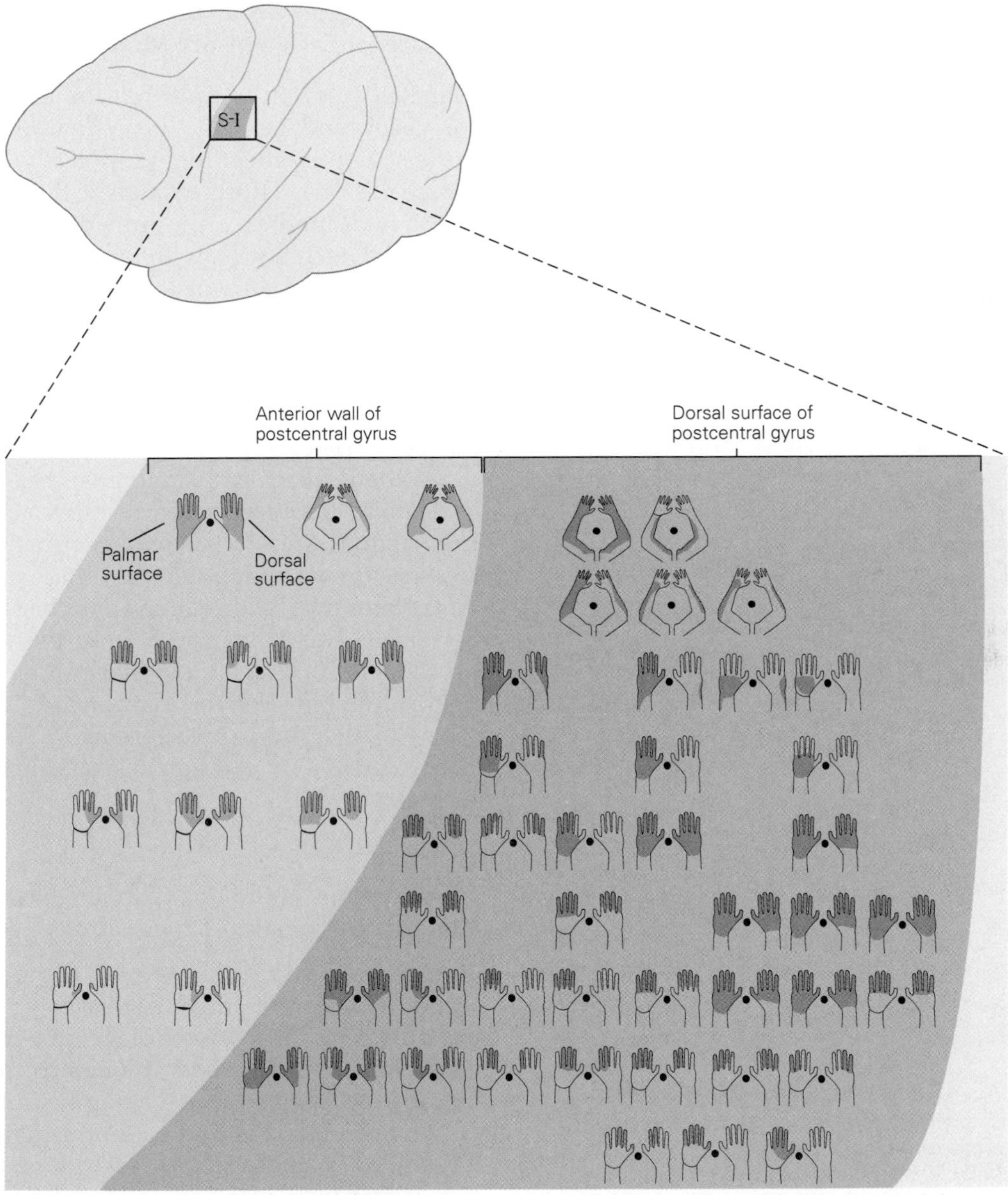

Figure 17–3 An early map of the representation of the hands in the monkey cortex. Recordings were made in the primary somatic sensory cortex (S-I) in the postcentral gyrus. The lateral view of the brain shows the recording site. Sites in Brodmann's areas 3b and 1 that responded to stimulation of the palmar and dorsal surfaces of the right hand are identified by **black dots** in a schematic map of these areas. The area of the hand that evoked a response at each site is indicated by the **colored portion** of the hand. The sites in the anterior wall of the postcentral gyrus are roughly in areas 3b and 3a (see Figure 17–1). The sites on the dorsal surface of the postcentral gyrus are roughly in area 1. (Adapted, with permission, from Marshall, Woolsey, and Bard 1941.)

and asked the patients to report what they felt. This procedure was necessary to ascertain where the epilepsy started and therefore to avoid damage to healthy brain tissue during surgery. Penfield found that activation of specific populations of cells in the postcentral gyrus reasonably simulated natural activation of these populations, producing sensations of touch and pressure in the contralateral hand or leg. From these studies Penfield constructed the neural map of the human body in the primary somatosensory cortex.

In this map the leg is represented in the most medial area of cortex followed by the trunk, arms, face, and finally, most laterally, the teeth, tongue, and esophagus. The area devoted to each part of the body reflects the relative importance of that part in sensory perception. Thus the area for the face is large compared with that of the back of the head, that of the index finger is gigantic compared with the big toe, and the torso is represented in the smallest area of all (Figure 17–4).

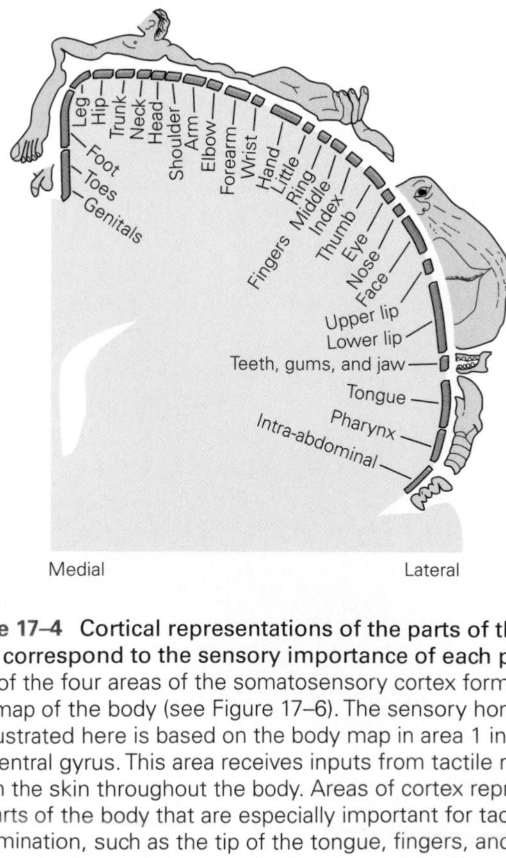

Figure 17–4 Cortical representations of the parts of the body correspond to the sensory importance of each part. Each of the four areas of the somatosensory cortex forms its own map of the body (see Figure 17–6). The sensory homunculus illustrated here is based on the body map in area 1 in the postcentral gyrus. This area receives inputs from tactile receptors in the skin throughout the body. Areas of cortex representing parts of the body that are especially important for tactile discrimination, such as the tip of the tongue, fingers, and hand, are disproportionately large, reflecting the greater degree of innervation in these parts. (Adapted, with permission, from Penfield and Rasmussen 1950.)

Such differences reflect differences in innervation density throughout the body. Similar relationships are observed in other animals. In rabbits, for example, the face and snout have the largest cortical representation because they are the most important sensory surfaces a rabbit uses to explore its environment (Figure 17–5).

The Cortex Has a Map of the Sensory Receptive Surface for Each Sensory Modality

Marshall went on to find that the receptive surfaces for vision and hearing, the retina and the cochlea, are also represented topographically in the cortex. Marshall's early efforts to analyze these sensory maps of the body probed only limited areas of the cortex and used techniques with poor spatial resolution. His work in the area of touch led to the conclusion that there is a single large representation of the body surface in the cerebral cortex. Later studies based on single-neuron recordings revealed four fairly complete maps in the four areas of the primary somatosensory cortex (Figure 17–6).

Although each of the four areas has essentially the same body map, each area processes a distinct type of information. Area 3a receives information from muscles and joints, important for limb proprioception. Area 3b receives information from the skin, important for touch. This information from the skin is further processed within area 1 and then combined with information from muscles and joints in area 2. This explains why a small lesion in area 1 impairs tactile discrimination, whereas a small lesion in area 2 impairs the ability to recognize the shape of a grasped object.

Cortical Maps of the Body Are the Basis of Accurate Clinical Neurological Examinations

The existence in the brain of maps of the sensory receptive surface and a similar motor map for movement explains why clinical neurology can be an accurate diagnostic discipline, even though for many decades before brain imaging came along neurology relied on only the simplest tools: a wad of cotton, a safety pin, a tuning fork, and a rubber reflex hammer. For example, disturbances in the somatic sensory system can be located with remarkable accuracy because there is a direct relationship between the anatomical organization of the functional pathways in the brain and specific perceptual and motor behaviors.

A dramatic example of this relationship is the Jacksonian march, a characteristic sensory seizure first

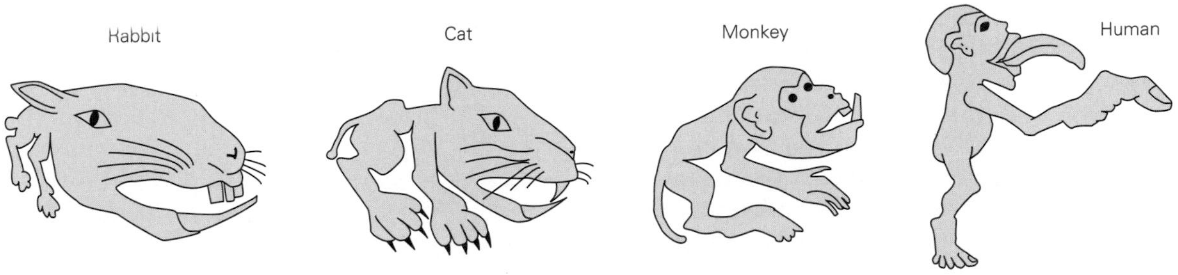

Figure 17–5 Cortical somatosensory maps in different species reflect different somatic sensibilities. These drawings show the relative importance of body regions in the somatosensory cortex of four species, based on evoked potentials in the thalamus and cortex.

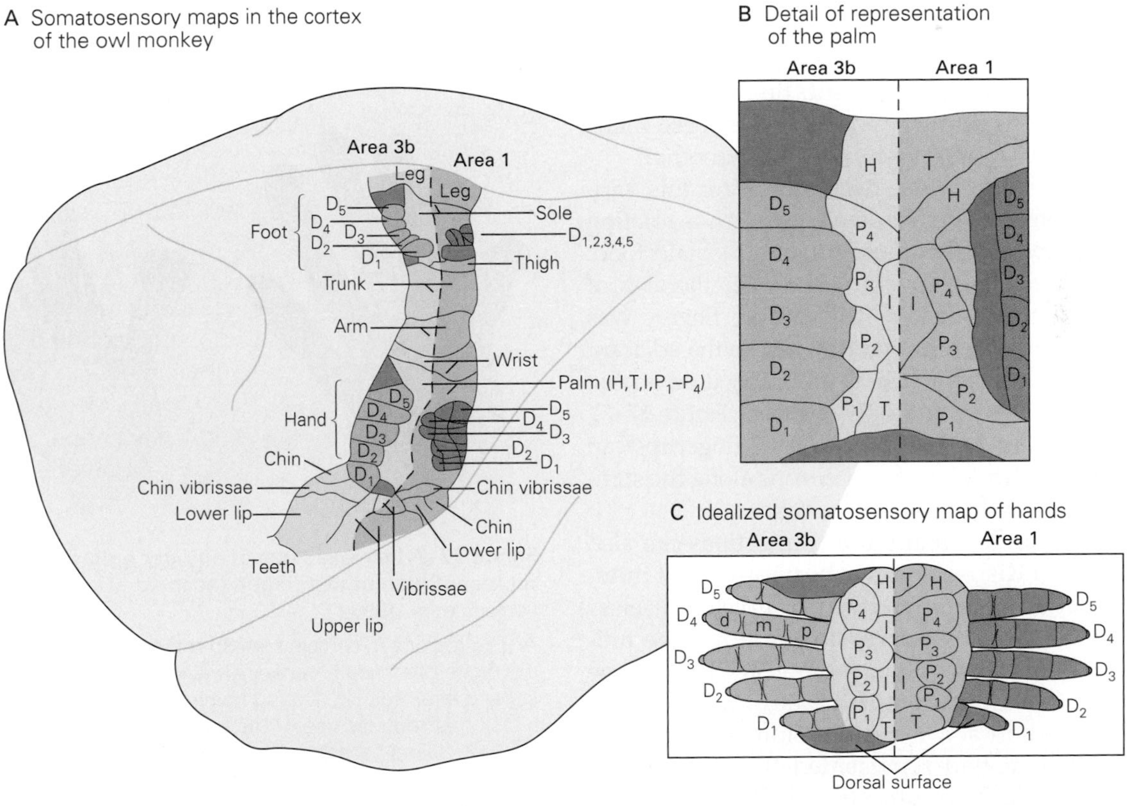

Figure 17–6 Each of the four areas of the primary somatic sensory cortex forms its own complete representation of the body surface. (Adapted with permission, from Kaas et al. 1981.)

A. Somatosensory maps of the body in Brodmann's areas 3b and 1 are shown in this dorsolateral view of the brain of an owl monkey. The two maps are roughly mirror images. Each digit of the hands and feet is individually represented (**D_1 to D_5**). Areas 2 and 3a (not shown) have a similar organization.

B. This more detailed illustration of the representation of the palm in areas 3b and 1 shows discrete areas of representation of the palmar pads (**P_4 to P_1**), two insular pads (**I**), two hypothenar pads (**H**), and two thenar pads (**T**).

C. This idealized representation of the hands in the somatosensory cortex is based on studies of a large number of monkeys. The areas of cortex devoted to the palm and digits reflect the extent of innervation of each part of the hand. The five digital pads (**D_1 to D_5**) include distal, middle, and proximal segments (**d, m, p**).

described by the British neurologist John Hughlings Jackson. In this type of seizure there is, in addition to a motor progression, a sensory progression. Numbness and paresthesia (inappropriate sensations such as burning or prickling) begin in one place and spread throughout the body. For example, numbness might start at the fingertips, spread to the hand, up the arm, across the shoulder into the back, and down the leg on the same side. This sequence is explained by the arrangement of inputs from the body in the somatosensory cortex (Figure 17–4); the seizure starts in the lateral region of the cortex, in the area where the hand is represented, and propagates across the cortex toward the midline.

The Internal Representation of Personal Space Can Be Modified by Experience

Until recently it was thought that the sensory maps of the body surface in the cortex were hard-wired, and the pathways from the receptors in the skin to the cortex are fixed early in development. But cortical maps do change, even in adults, and details of these maps vary considerably from one individual to another.

To show that experience can account for this variability, owl monkeys were trained to touch a rotating disk with the tips of the middle fingers to obtain food. After several months of touching the disk, the area of cortex devoted to the tips of the middle fingers was greatly expanded, whereas that devoted to the adjacent proximal phalanges, which had not been used in the experiment, was correspondingly reduced (Figure 17–7). These results demonstrate that use of the fingertips can strengthen connections between neurons along the somatosensory pathway from skin to cortex.

Dramatic changes in afferent connections can also occur because of disuse. In one study of several monkeys an upper limb was rendered completely useless by severing all sensory nerves to the arm. The animals were monitored for 10 or more years. In all these monkeys the representation of the face, where innervation remained intact, expanded into the adjacent area of cortex that had represented the hand before deafferentation. As a result, stimulation of the face evoked responses in the area of cortex that normally represented the hand. These changes occurred in a wide area of cortex: A third of the entire body map was taken over by new connections from the face.

How do these changes occur? Afferent connections to neurons in the somatic sensory cortex are thought to be fine-tuned during development when the firing of pre- and postsynaptic cells is correlated. Cells that

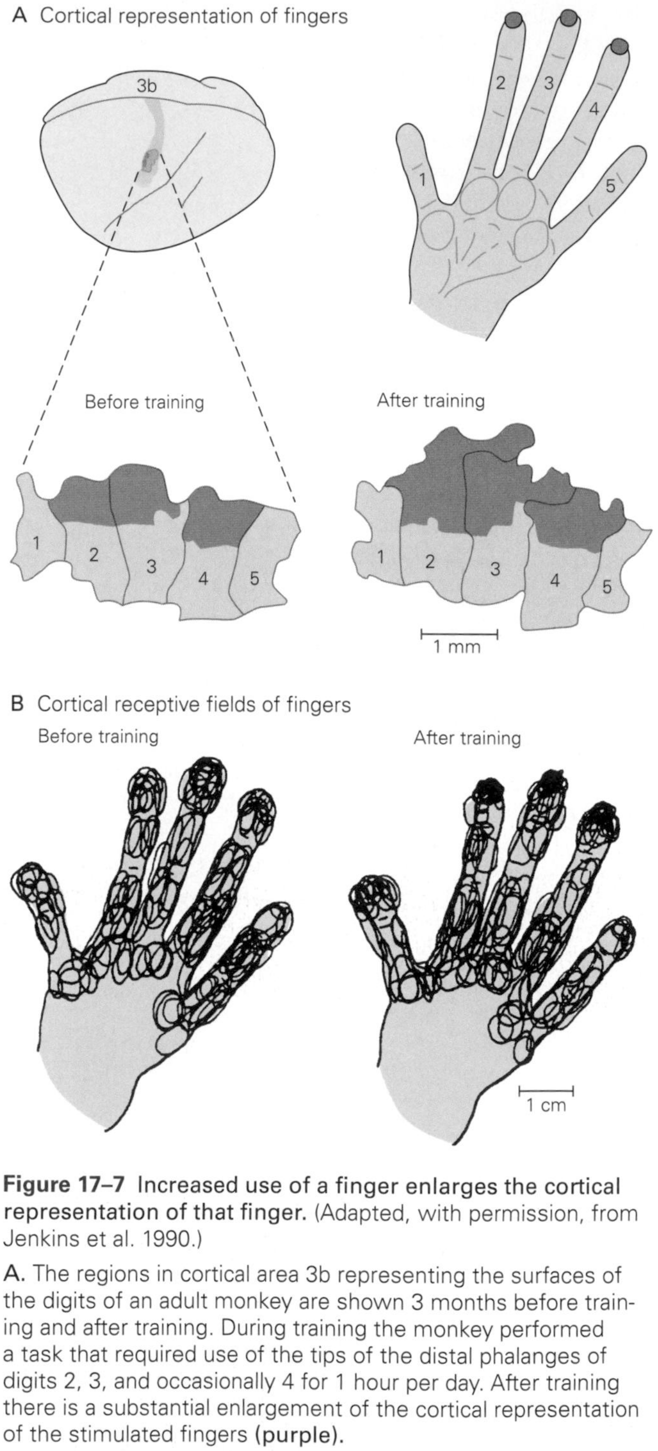

Figure 17–7 Increased use of a finger enlarges the cortical representation of that finger. (Adapted, with permission, from Jenkins et al. 1990.)

A. The regions in cortical area 3b representing the surfaces of the digits of an adult monkey are shown 3 months before training and after training. During training the monkey performed a task that required use of the tips of the distal phalanges of digits 2, 3, and occasionally 4 for 1 hour per day. After training there is a substantial enlargement of the cortical representation of the stimulated fingers **(purple)**.

B. All receptive fields on the surfaces of the digits were identified before and after training to determine recording sites within area 3b. The receptive field for a cortical neuron is the area on the skin where a tactile stimulation either excites or inhibits a cell. Training increased the number of receptive fields in the distal tips of the phalanges of digits 2, 3, and 4.

fire together are thought to strengthen their connection together. Michael Merzenich and his colleagues tested this idea by surgically connecting the skin of two adjacent fingers of a monkey. This procedure assures that the connected fingers are always used together and therefore increases the correlation of their inputs from the skin. Increasing the correlation of activity from adjacent fingers in this way abolishes the sharp discontinuity normally evident between the zones in the somatosensory cortex that receive inputs from these digits. Thus, although patterns of connections are genetically programmed, they are also modified by experience.

Magnetic encephalography, a method for recording the magnetic field produced by local electrical activity, has been used to construct cortical maps of the hand with a precision of millimeters (Figure 17–8). This technique has been used to compare the hand area in the cortex of normal adult humans with that of patients with a congenital fusion of the fingers (syndactyly). Patients with this syndrome do not have individual fingers—their hand is like a fist—so that neural activity in one part of the hand is always correlated with activity in all the other parts. The representation in the cortex of the syndactylic hand is considerably less than that of a normal person, and within this shrunken representation the neurons that receive signals from the fingers are not organized somatotopically (Figure 17–9A).

When the fingers of one syndactylic patient were surgically separated, however, each newly separate finger became individually represented in the cortex within weeks. The new neural organization occupied an area of cortex closely corresponding to that of normal individuals, with normal distances between each digit (Figure 17–9B).

These results raise an important question that is even more urgent in the study of phantom limbs. How are changes in cortical maps interpreted by the brain, and how do they shape perception? Many patients with amputated limbs continue to have a vivid sensory experience of the missing limb, a disorder known as the *phantom limb syndrome.* The patient senses the presence of the missing limb, feels it move around, and even feels it try to shake hands when greeting someone. Terrible pain is often felt in the phantom limb.

Phantom limb sensation and the pain associated with it have been attributed to impulses entering the spinal cord from the scar of nervous tissue in the stump. In fact, removing the scar or cutting the sensory nerves just above it may relieve pain in some cases. But imaging studies of the somatosensory cortex of patients who have lost a hand suggest that phantom limb sensations are caused by a rearrangement of cortical circuits. As the afferents from the lost hand wither, adjacent afferent fibers expand into their place, just as in the monkeys with deafferented limbs.

In several patients the area of cortex that represented a hand before amputation now receives afferents from at least one other site on the skin. This has been called *remapping of referred sensations.* Stimuli applied to the face and upper arm are selectively capable of eliciting referred sensations in the phantom hand; both areas are represented in the brain next to the hand area (Figure 17–10). Thus changes in the arrangement of sensory afferents force changes in the readout of the

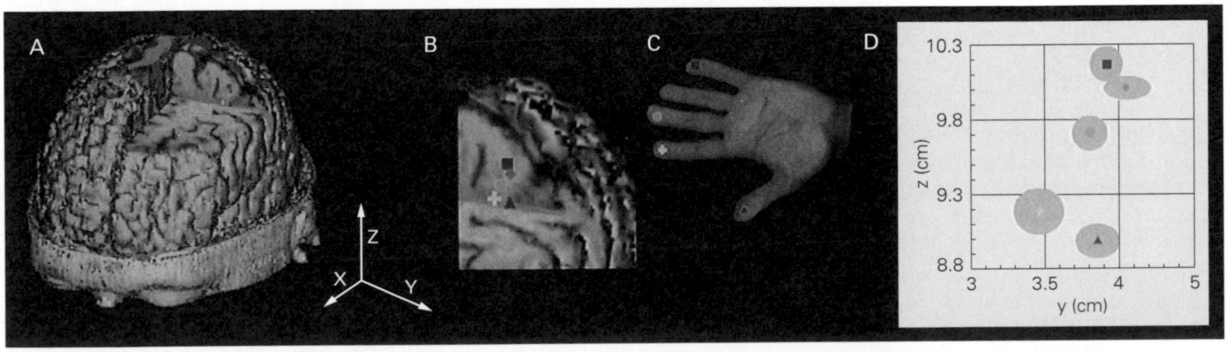

Figure 17–8 The representation of the hand in the somatosensory cortex can be visualized with magnetic encephalography. (Reproduced, with permission, from Mogilner et al. 1993.)

A–C. The areas of representation of the fingers are indicated on a three-dimensional reconstruction of a subject's brain (color key is shown in C).

D. A two-dimensional plot of the cortex in the coronal phase shows discrete areas of representation for each finger. The data points are averages, the **gray ovals** indicate standard errors.

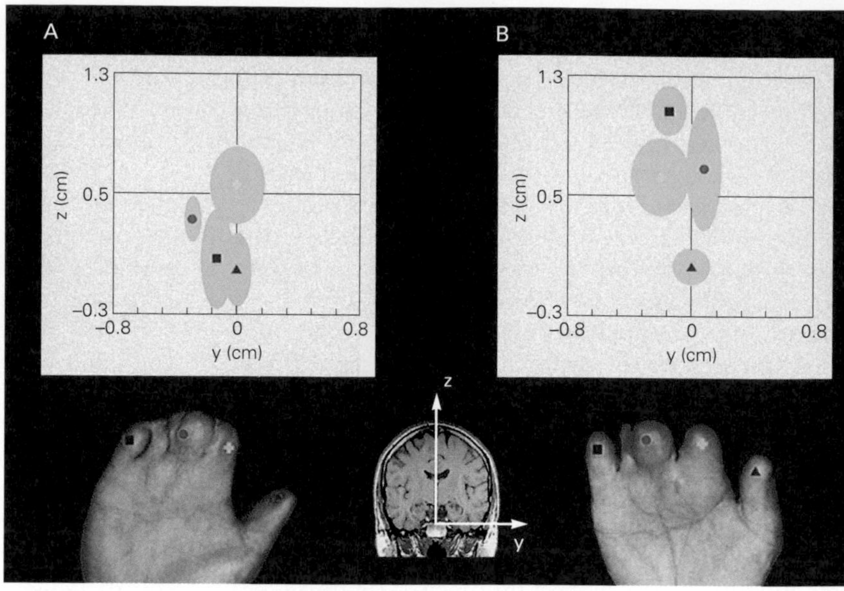

Figure 17–9 Cortical representation of the hand changes following surgical correction of syndactyly of digits 2 to 5. (Reproduced, with permission, from Mogilner et al. 1993.)

A. A preoperative map shows that the cortical representation of the thumb, index, middle, and little fingers is abnormal and lacks any somatotopic organization. For example, the distance between sites of representation of the thumb and little finger is significantly smaller than normal (see Figure 17–8D).

B. Twenty-six days after surgical separation of the digits, the organization of the inputs from the digits is somatotopic. The distance between the sites of representation of the thumb and little finger has increased to 1.06 cm.

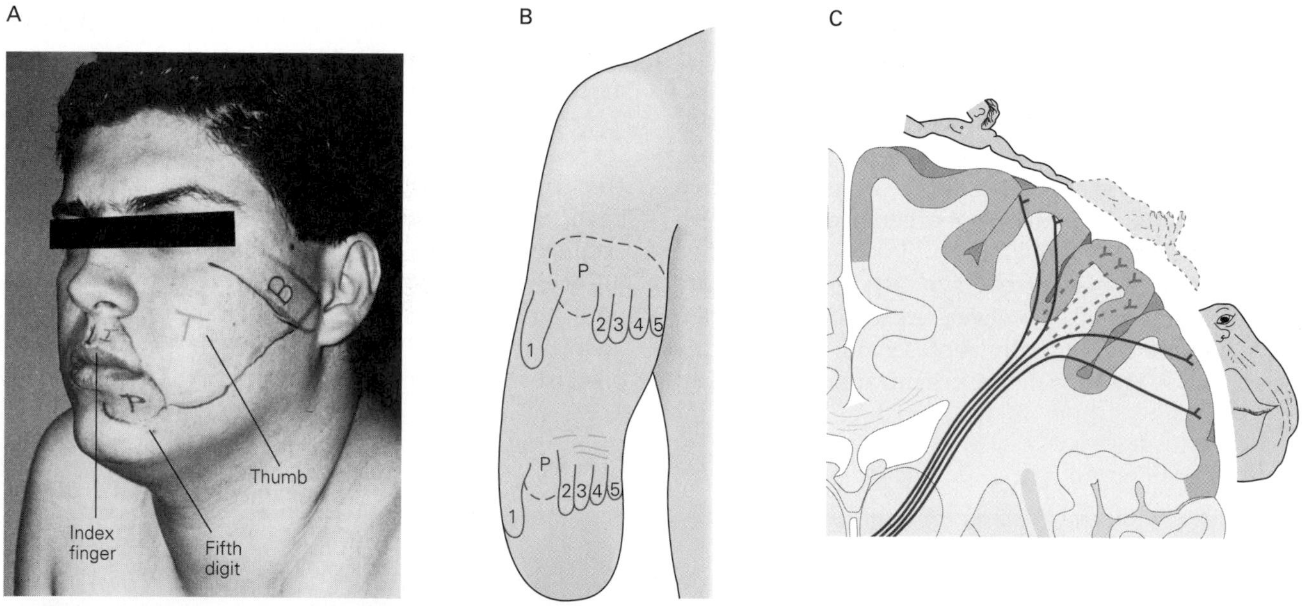

Figure 17–10 Phantom limb sensations can be evoked by stimulating particular areas of skin. Patients who have had an arm amputated experience sensation of the missing hand when their faces and upper arms are touched. (Reproduced, with permission, from Ramachandran 1993.)

A. The face of a patient whose arm was amputated above the left elbow is marked to show where stimulation (brushing the face with a cotton swab) elicits sensation referred to the phantom digits. Regions of the body that evoke referred sensations are called *reference fields*. Stimulation of the region labeled **T** always evokes sensations of the phantom thumb. Stimulation of facial areas marked **I**, **P**, and **B** evoke sensation of the phantom index finger, pinkie, and ball of the thumb, respectively. This patient was tested 4 weeks after amputation.

B. Another patient experienced referred sensation in two distinct areas on the arm—one area close to the line of amputation and a second area 6 cm above the elbow crease—in addition to sites on the face. Each area of referred sensation is a precise spatial map of the lost digits; the maps are almost identical except for the absence of fingertips in the upper map (P, palm). When the patient imagined pronating his phantom lower arm, the entire upper map shifted in the same direction by approximately 1.5 cm. Stimulating the skin region between these two maps did not elicit sensations of the phantom limb.

C. Portion of a sensory homunculus showing how the cortical area receiving inputs from the hand is flanked by the regions devoted to the face and the arm. Rearrangement of these cortical inputs is thought to be responsible for some types of phantom limb sensation.

sensory map—the brain learns to interpret activity on the patch of cortex receiving information from the face and upper arm as emanating from the amputated limb.

Extrapersonal Space Is Represented in the Posterior Parietal Association Cortex

Neurons in the primary somatosensory cortex areas 3a, 3b, and 1 project to higher-order unimodal areas of the anterior parietal lobe (Brodmann's area 2), and to multimodal association areas in the posterior parietal cortex (Brodmann's areas 5 and 7). The latter also receive input from the visual and auditory systems and from the hippocampus. The parietal association areas thus integrate somatic sensory information with other sensory modalities to form spatial percepts of objects in extrapersonal or far space.

Indeed, the connection between higher mental processes and specific nerve cells has been most dramatically demonstrated in these association areas in the posterior parietal cortex. Lesions here produce complex defects in personal or peripersonal spatial perception, visuomotor integration, and selective attention. Damage to the posterior parietal lobe produces object agnosia, a modality-specific inability to recognize certain kinds of objects even though afferent sensory pathways function normally. For example, some patients with posterior parietal damage are unable to recognize objects through touch (*astereognosis*). In fact, the most common agnosias result from lesions in the posterior parietal cortex.

Many patients with parietal lesions also show a striking deficit in awareness of one side of their body. For example, such patients may not dress, undress, or wash the affected side (*personal neglect syndrome*). They may even deny or disown their left arm or leg, going so far as to ask, "Who put this arm in bed with me?" Because the idea of having a left limb is foreign to them, patients may also deny the paralysis in this limb and attempt to leave the hospital prematurely because they feel nothing is wrong with them. Such denial about a disease or disability is referred to as *anosognosia.*

In some patients with right parietal lesions the sensory neglect extends from near space to far space. In these cases the ability to copy the left side of a drawing is severely disturbed. The patient may sketch the petals of a flower on the right side only. When asked to copy a clock, the patient may ignore the numbers on the left, try to cram all the numbers into the right half of the clock, or draw them on one side running off the clock face (Figure 17–11). A particularly dramatic example of spatial neglect is seen in self-portraits by

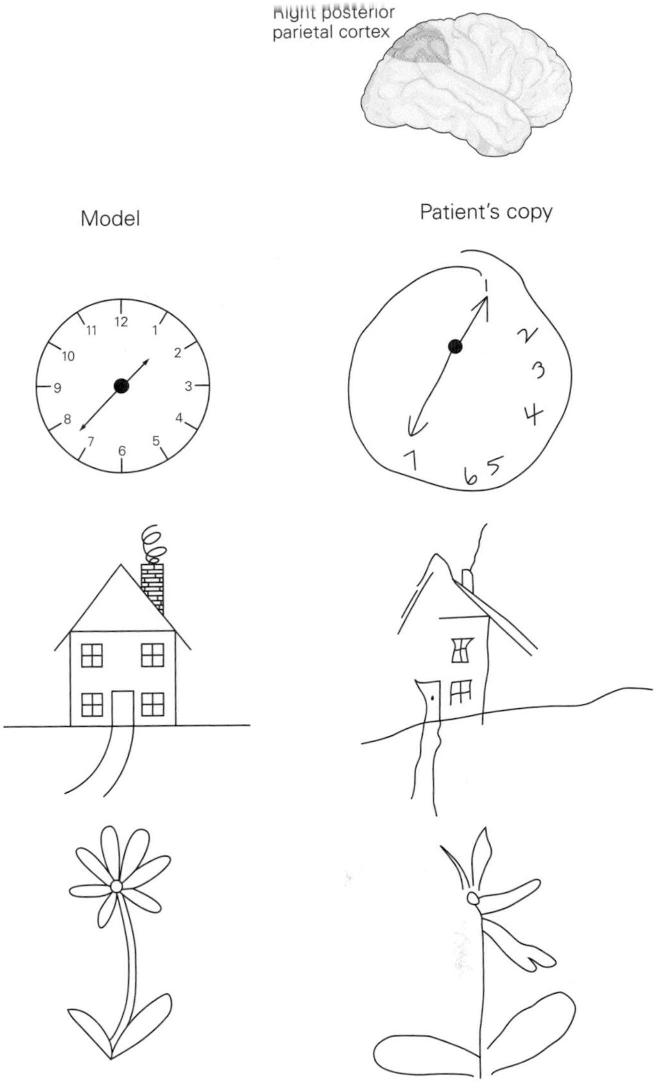

Figure 17–11 **The drawings on the right were made by patients with unilateral visual neglect following lesion of the right posterior parietal cortex.** (Reproduced, with permission, from Bloom and Lazerson 1988.)

a German artist who suffered a stroke that affected his right posterior parietal cortex. The portraits done in the two months after the stroke show a profound neglect of the left side of the face (Figure 17–12).

Spatial neglect can be quite selective. Some patients with neglect syndrome after injury to the right hemisphere have deficits in the perception of the form of objects. A patient may recognize an entire object but not all its parts, even though the visual pathways are intact (Figure 17–13).

Another form of spatial neglect is the neglect of one half of a remembered image, called *representational*

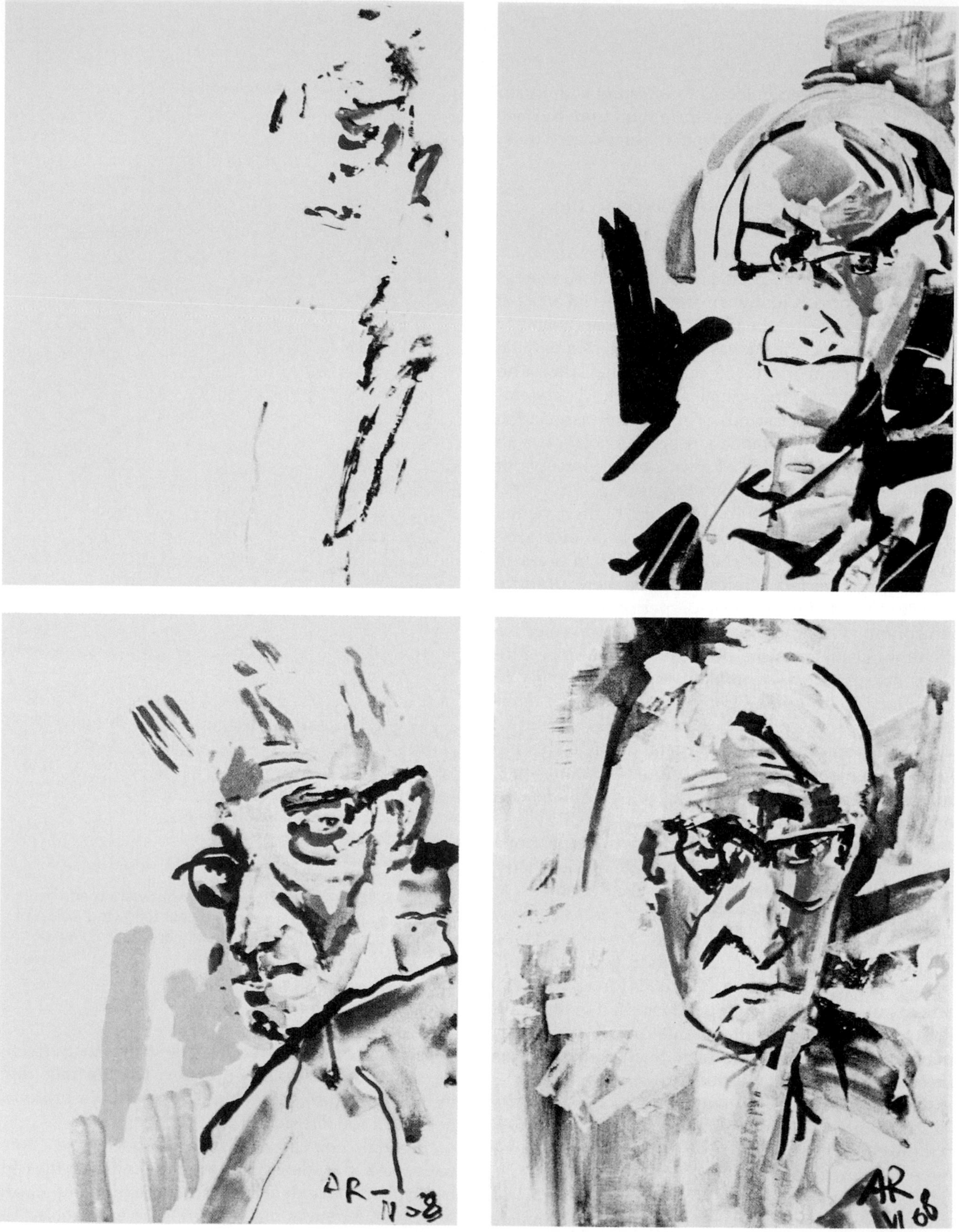

Figure 17–12 Self-portraits by an artist following damage to his right posterior parietal cortex. Each portrait was drawn at a different time after the stroke: at 2 months (upper left), at 3.5 months (upper right), at 6 months (lower left), and at 9 months (lower right), by which time the artist had largely recovered. The early portraits show severe neglect of the left side of face, the side opposite the lesion. (Reproduced, with permission, from Jung 1974.)

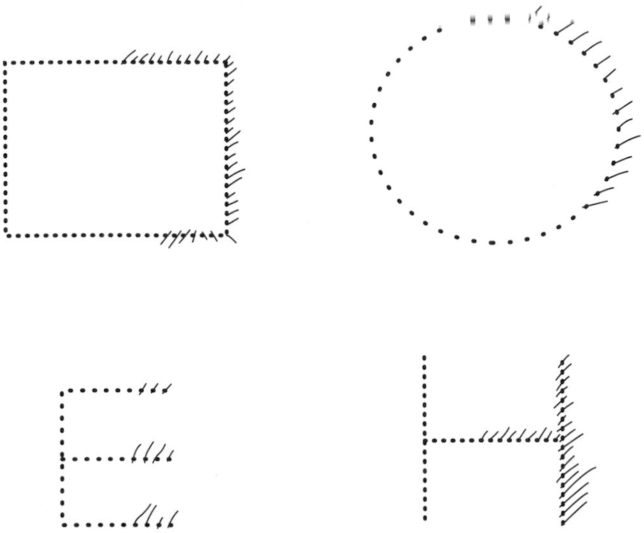

Figure 17–13 The neglect of space following injury to the right posterior parietal cortex is selective. Patients were shown drawings in which the shape of an object is drawn in dots (or other tiny forms) and then asked to mark with a pencil each dot. The figures here show the responses of one patient who neglected the left half of each object even though she was able to report accurately each shape (square, circle, letter E, letter H). (Adapted, with permission, from Marshall and Halligan 1995.)

neglect. This was first observed by the Italian neurologist Edoardo Bisiach in a group of patients in Milan, all of whom had injury to their right parietal lobe. Patients were asked to imagine that they were standing in the city's main public square, the Piazza del Duomo, facing the cathedral, and to describe from memory the buildings around the square (Figure 17–14). These subjects were able to identify all the buildings on the right side of the square (ipsilateral to the lesion) but could not recall the buildings on the left, even though these buildings were thoroughly familiar to them. The patients were then asked to imagine that they were standing on the steps of the cathedral, so that right and left were reversed. In this imagined position the patients were again asked to identify the buildings around the plaza. This time they identified only the buildings that they previously failed to name.

These results suggest that memory of external space is perceived in relation to the vantage point of the observer, not simply of that of objects in the environment. These Milanese patients clearly had stored a complete memory of the entire piazza and had complete access to that memory. But when they remembered the piazza they neglected the left half, depending on the vantage point of the remembered image, because they were unable to recall images associated with their left side, contralateral to the side of the lesion. Thus, Bisiach concluded, memories for each half of the visual field are accessed through the contralateral hemisphere.

Recent PET studies indicate that when normal subjects close their eyes and imagine an object such as the letter "a," the visualization recruits activity in the primary visual cortex, just as when an actual object is seen with the eyes. Patients with representational neglect presumably lack such an orienting mechanism. Thus damage to the posterior parietal cortex, which impairs real-time visual perception, can also impair remembered or imagined visual images.

Much of Mental Processing Is Unconscious

In 1860 Herman Helmholtz, one of the pioneers in applying physical methods to perception, succeeded in measuring the conduction velocity of the nerve impulse to be approximately 90 m/s. He then went on to study reaction time—the time it took a subject to react to a stimulus—and found it to be much slower than the time required for the information to reach the brain by means of conduction time alone. This caused Helmholtz to realize that the brain must require a considerable amount of time to process sensory information before that information reaches conscious perception. Helmholtz proposed that this was the time the brain needed to evaluate, transform, and reroute the neural signals prior to our being aware of the significance of these signals. This *unconscious inference*, he argued, was required for perception and voluntary movement.

In the beginning of the 20th-century Sigmund Freud elaborated on Helmholtz's idea that much of mental activity is unconscious, pointing out that our unconscious mental life is not a single process but has at least three components: implicit, dynamic, and preconscious unconscious. Implicit unconscious is Helmholtz's unconscious inference. It includes, as we shall learn in Chapters 65 and 66, implicit memory, the type of memory that underlies learning perceptual and motor skills and which we now attribute to the striatum, the cerebellum, and the amygdala. The dynamic unconscious is that part of unconscious mental activity that involves our conflicts, repressed thoughts, and sexual as well as aggressive urges. This component of unconscious mental processes was the major focus of Freud's work. Finally, the preconscious unconscious is that part of the unconscious that is most readily accessible to consciousness. This component is

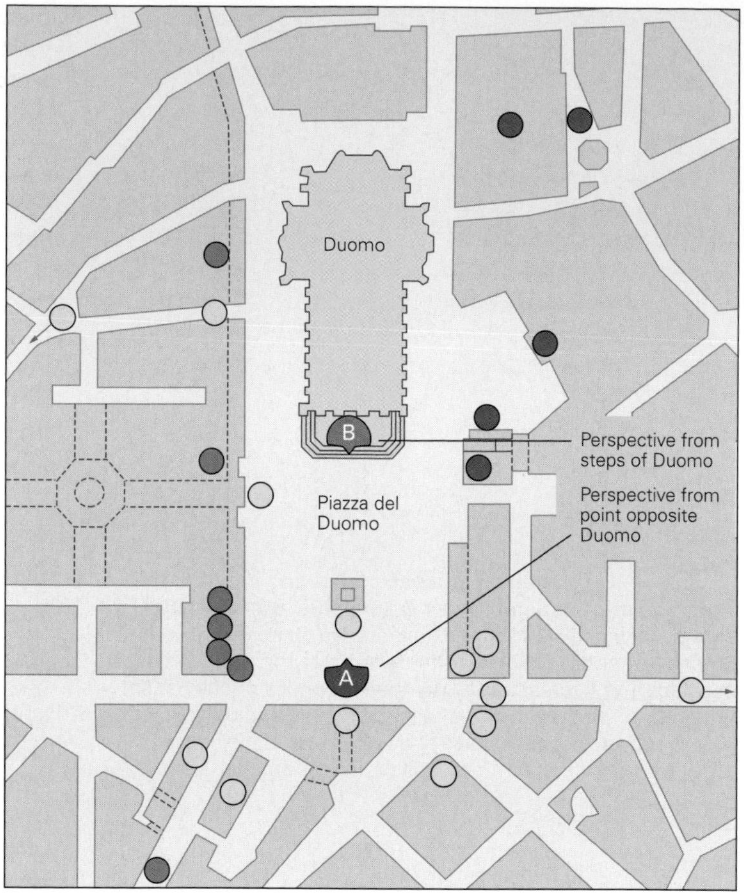

Figure 17–14 Milanese patients with lesions of the right posterior parietal cortex are able to recall only landmarks on their right in the Piazza del Duomo in Milan. Patients were asked to recall landmarks from memory from two points in the square. The **blue circles** in the map represent landmark buildings recalled from perspective A opposite the Duomo; the **green circles** represent landmark buildings recalled from perspective B on the steps of the Duomo. (Adapted, with permission, from Bisiach and Luzzatti 1978.)

concerned with organizing and planning for immediate actions, functions we now attribute to the prefrontal cortex.

The insight of Helmholtz and Freud that much of our mental life is unconscious raised the following related questions: What is left for freedom of action? What is the nature of free will? A major step in addressing this issue empirically was a study by Benjamin Libet. The study was based on an earlier finding that any voluntary movement is preceded by a *readiness potential,* a small electrical response recorded from the surface of the skull that occurs approximately one second before the movement. Libet asked subjects to will a movement and found to his surprise that a subject's awareness of his own willingness to move a finger followed, rather than preceded, the readiness potential and did so by as much as a full second. By recording neural activity we can predict a subject's desire to move a finger before the subject is aware of his own desire to move that finger! Thus what we consider acts of free will may have a significant unconscious step.

Is Consciousness Accessible to Neurobiological Analysis?

Consciousness Poses Fundamental Problems for a Biological Theory of Mind

Exploration of the nature of spatial neglect and free will touches on one of the great issues of cognitive neural science, and in fact of all science: the nature of consciousness. The unique character of consciousness has attracted fierce interest and debate among philosophers of mind because it is difficult to see how consciousness might be explained in reductionist physical terms.

At the beginning of this book we stated that what we commonly call *mind* is a set of operations carried out by the brain. Because consciousness is a fundamental property of mind, it too must be a function of the brain and in principle we should be able to identify neural circuits that give rise to it. However, before we can develop theories of consciousness that can be tested by empirical science, we must first define consciousness in operational terms.

Here we should emphasize that, in general, the concepts that neuroscientists initially use to describe mental processes—such as learning, memory, or consciousness—are those developed by philosophers. Such concepts were formed without knowledge of how mental processes are mediated by the brain. Once neuroscientists define a specific mental process in psychological terms—and we can now do so quite precisely—they then can attempt to localize and analyze the neuronal systems that mediate the process. This approach, as we shall see, can now even be applied to consciousness.

Consciousness is ordinarily thought of as a state of self-awareness. Philosophers of mind such as John Searle and Thomas Nagel have defined three essential features of self-awareness: subjectivity, unity, and intentionality.

The *subjectivity* of self-awareness is the characteristic that poses the greatest philosophical and scientific challenge. Each of us has an awareness of a self that is the center of experience. Each of us experiences a world of sensations that feel unique and private. Our own experience seems much more real to us than the experiences of others. Our own ideas, moods, and sensations—our successes and disappointments, joys and pains—are experienced directly, whereas we can only indirectly appreciate other people's ideas, moods, and sensations. Is the aroma of lavender that I smell identical to your experience of lavender? This is not simply a question of our sensory capability. Even when sensory capabilities are measurably identical, the aroma of lavender is not only determined by the lavender but also by our personal history—the experience we recall from memory—and since experiential history is highly individualized, lavender may not produce the same subjective sensation in each of us.

Once we know how the aroma of lavender is mediated by neural signals that announce the presence of chemical molecules, how does our sensation, the conscious awareness of an aroma, arise from other neural networks of the brain?

The fact that conscious experience is fundamentally subjective raises the question of whether it is even possible to determine objectively some characteristics of consciousness that transcend individual experience. If the senses produce only subjective experience, the argument goes, those same senses cannot be the means of arriving at an objective understanding of experience.

The *unity* of self-awareness refers to the fact that our experience of the world at any given moment is felt as a single unified experience. All of the various sensory modalities are blended into a single experience. When we sit down to dinner we experience the chair against our back, the sound of music, and the fruity flavor of the wine as connected and simultaneous. When we speak to our dinner partners we do so in whole sentences; we are aware that we are completing an idea but pay little if any attention to the process of constructing sentences.

Finally, self-awareness has *intentionality*. That is, our conscious experience connects successive moments and we have the sense that successive moments are directed to some goal.

In earlier times these features of consciousness led some philosophers to a dualistic view of mind, a view that the body and the mind are very different substances—the body being physical and the mind existing in some nonphysical, spiritual medium. Today almost all philosophers of mind agree that what we call consciousness derives from physical properties of the brain. Thinkers about consciousness fall into two groups. The first group, of which Daniel Dennett is the most prominent advocate, thinks there is no problem of consciousness. Consciousness emerges quite simply from an understanding of neuronal activity. Dennett argues, much as did the neurologist John Hughlings Jackson a century earlier, that consciousness is not a discrete operation of the brain but the outcome of the computational activity of the association areas of the brain. The second group, which includes Francis Crick, Christof Koch, John Searle, Thomas Nagel, Antonio Damasio, and Gerald Edelman, believes that consciousness is a discrete phenomenon and that the issues of subjectivity, unity, and intentionality must be confronted if we are to understand how our experience is constructed.

Because consciousness has properties that other mental functions do not, a biological explanation poses a formidable problem, a problem so inherently difficult that the philosopher Colin McGinn has argued that consciousness is simply inaccessible to empirical study because of limitations inherent in human intelligence. Just as monkeys cannot understand quantum theory, humans cannot understand consciousness, McGinn argues. Conversely, Searle and Nagel argue that consciousness *is* accessible to analysis but we have been unable to explain it because it is a highly subjective and complex property of the brain unlike any function of the brain we understand—indeed, unlike any other subject of scientific inquiry.

Of the three features of consciousness, subjectivity is the most difficult to analyze empirically. Nagel and Searle illustrate the precise difficulty in the following way. Assume we succeed in studying a person's consciousness by recording the electrical activity of neurons in a region known to be important for consciousness while that person carries out a particular task requiring conscious attention. How do we then analyze the results? Can we say that the firing of a group of neurons *causes* a private subjective experience? Does a burst of action potentials in the thalamus and somatic sensory cortex switch information into consciousness so that a person now perceives an object in his hand and perceives it as round or square, hard or malleable? What empirical grounds do we have for believing that when a mother looks at her infant child the firing of cells in the inferotemporal cortex concerned with face recognition causes conscious recognition of her child's face?

As yet we do not know even in the simplest case how the firing of specific neurons leads to conscious perception. In fact, Searle argues that we lack even an adequate theoretical model of how an ontologically objective phenomenon—electrical signals in another person's brain—can cause an ontologically subjective experience such as pain. Because consciousness is irreducibly subjective, it lies beyond the reach of science as we currently practice it.

Similarly, Nagel argues that because current science is essentially a reductionist approach to understanding phenomena it cannot address consciousness without a significant change in method, one in which the elements of subjective experience are defined. These elements are likely to be basic components of brain function much as atoms and molecules are basic components of matter. According to Nagel, object-to-object reductions are not problematic because we understand, at least in principle, how the properties of a given type of matter arise from the molecules of which it is made. What we lack are rules for extrapolating subjective experience from the physicochemical properties of interconnected nerve cells.

Nagel argues that our complete lack of insight into the elements of subjective experience should not prevent us from discovering rules that relate conscious phenomena to cellular processes in the brain. In fact, Nagel believes that the knowledge needed to think about a more fundamental type of analytical reduction—from something subjective (experience) to something objective (physical)—can be gained only through the accumulation of cell-biological information. Only after we have developed a theory of mind that supports this novel and fundamental reduction will the limitations of the current reductionism become apparent. The discovery of the elementary components of subjective consciousness, Nagel argues, may require a revolution in biology and most likely a complete transformation of scientific thought.

Neurobiological Research on Cognitive Processes Does Not Depend on a Specific Theory of Consciousness

Most neural scientists whose work touches on the question of consciousness are not necessarily working toward or anticipating a revolution in scientific thought. Although neural scientists working on issues such as sensory perception and cognition must struggle with the difficulties of defining consciousness experimentally, these difficulties do not appear to preclude productive research. The physicist Steven Weinberg perhaps best expressed this attitude:

> I don't see how anyone but George will ever know how it feels to be George. On the other hand, I can readily believe that at least in principle we will be able to explain all of George's behavior reductively, including what he says about what he feels, and that consciousness will be one of the emergent higher-level concepts appearing in this equation.

Indeed, neural science has made considerable progress in understanding the neurobiology of sensory perception without having to account for individual experience. Understanding the neural basis of perception of color and form, for example, does not depend on resolving the question of whether each of us sees the same blue. Despite the fact that perception of an object is constructed by the brain from piecemeal sensory information, and despite individual differences caused by experience, perception of an object is not arbitrary and appears to correspond to objective physical properties of the object. What we do not understand is the step from action potentials to awareness of an object.

Although the subjectivity of consciousness makes the neurobiological study of consciousness especially difficult, in principle such a study may not be insurmountable using current methods. The subjective nature of perception does not prevent one person from objectively studying what another person perceives. We have been able to correlate some regularities of perception with specific patterns of neuronal activity in different individuals under a variety of circumstances. The correlation between a neural event and a mental event, based on rigorous criteria, should be a sufficient first approximation of the neural process mediating a mental operation by any reasonable standards of scientific explanation. For this reason Crick and Koch emphasized that the first step in the analysis of consciousness is to find the neural correlates of consciousness, the minimal set of neural events that give rise to a conscious percept.

Finding the neural systems that mediate consciousness may not be simple. Gerald Edelman and

Stanislas Dehaene have argued that the neural correlates of consciousness are unlikely to be localized but rather widely distributed throughout the cerebral cortex and thalamus. There is extensive evidence of massive feedforward broadcasting as well as, feedback or recursive connections between cortical areas, which Dehaene believes may be essential for the conversion of unconscious to conscious perception.

By contrast, Crick and Koch believed that the most elementary neural correlates of consciousness are likely to involve only a small set of neurons, and therefore one should be able to determine the neural circuits to which they belong. Crick and Koch proposed a search for the neural activity that produces specific instances of consciousness, such as perception of the movement of an object, its shape, and its color. Having done that we may eventually be in a position to meet Searle's and Nagel's higher demands: to develop a theory of the correlations we discover empirically, to state the laws of correlation between neural phenomena and subjective experience.

Because at any moment we can be conscious of one of a large variety of sounds, smells, and objects as well as actions, consciousness must involve modulatory control over a variety of neural systems. Thus consciousness is required for many aspects of mental activity: visual perception, thinking, emotion, action, and the perception of self. Because we understand the visual system best, Crick and Koch argued that our efforts should be focused on visual perception and in particular on two phenomena: binocular rivalry and selective attention.

Studies of Binocular Rivalry Have Identified Circuits That May Switch Unconscious to Conscious Visual Perception

When two different images are presented simultaneously to the two eyes—horizontal bars to one eye, vertical bars to the other—the subject's perception alternates spontaneously from one monocular view to the other. Erik Lumer and his colleagues found in functional imaging experiments that whenever an individual switches from one eye to the next—from one conscious percept to the next—three sets of cortical areas are recruited. One is the ventral visual pathway of the temporal lobe, which is concerned with perceptions of objects and people. The others are the parietal and frontal regions, which are known to be involved in visual attention to space. Lumer and his colleagues suggest that the frontal and parietal areas are critical for conscious perception and that these areas focus awareness on specific internal representations of visual images.

Nikos Logothetis has carried out similar analyses at the level of individual neurons and confirmed that the competition between rivalrous stimuli in the two halves of the visual field is resolved late in the ventral pathway, in the inferior temporal cortex and the lower layers of the superior temporal sulcus. These regions in turn project to and receive connections from the prefrontal cortex. In light of these findings Crick and Koch argued that the pathways for conscious visual perception course through the inferior temporal cortex to the prefrontal and parietal cortices.

Selective Attention to Visual Stimuli Can Be Studied on the Cellular Level in Nonhuman Primates

Selective attention in vision is another useful starting point for a cell-biological approach to the study of consciousness. At any given moment we are aware of only a small fraction of the sensory stimuli that impinge on us. As we look out on the world, we focus on specific objects or scenes that have particular interest and exclude others.

If you raise your eyes from this book to look at a person entering the room, you are no longer attending to the words on this page. Nor are you attending to the decor of the room or other people in the room. This focusing of the sensory apparatus is an essential feature of all sensory processing, as Williams James first noted in his *Principles of Psychology* (1890):

> Millions of items . . . are present to my senses which never properly enter my experience. Why? Because they have no interest for me. My experience is what I agree to attend to. . . . Everyone knows what attention is. It is the taking possession by the mind, in clear and vivid form, of one out of what seem several simultaneously possible objects of trains of thought. Focalization, concentration of consciousness, are of its essence. It implies withdrawal from some things in order to deal effectively with others.

Cellular studies of the posterior parietal cortex in monkeys have provided important insight into the neural mechanisms of focusing attention on specific objects in the visual field. Like neurons in other visual processing centers, each parietal neuron fires when a visual stimulus enters its receptive field (see Chapter 25 for a description of the receptive fields of cortical neurons in the visual system). The strength of the neuron's response depends on whether the animal is paying attention to the stimulus. The response is moderate when the animal's gaze is directed away from the stimulus but vigorous when the monkey attends to the stimulus (Figure 17–15).

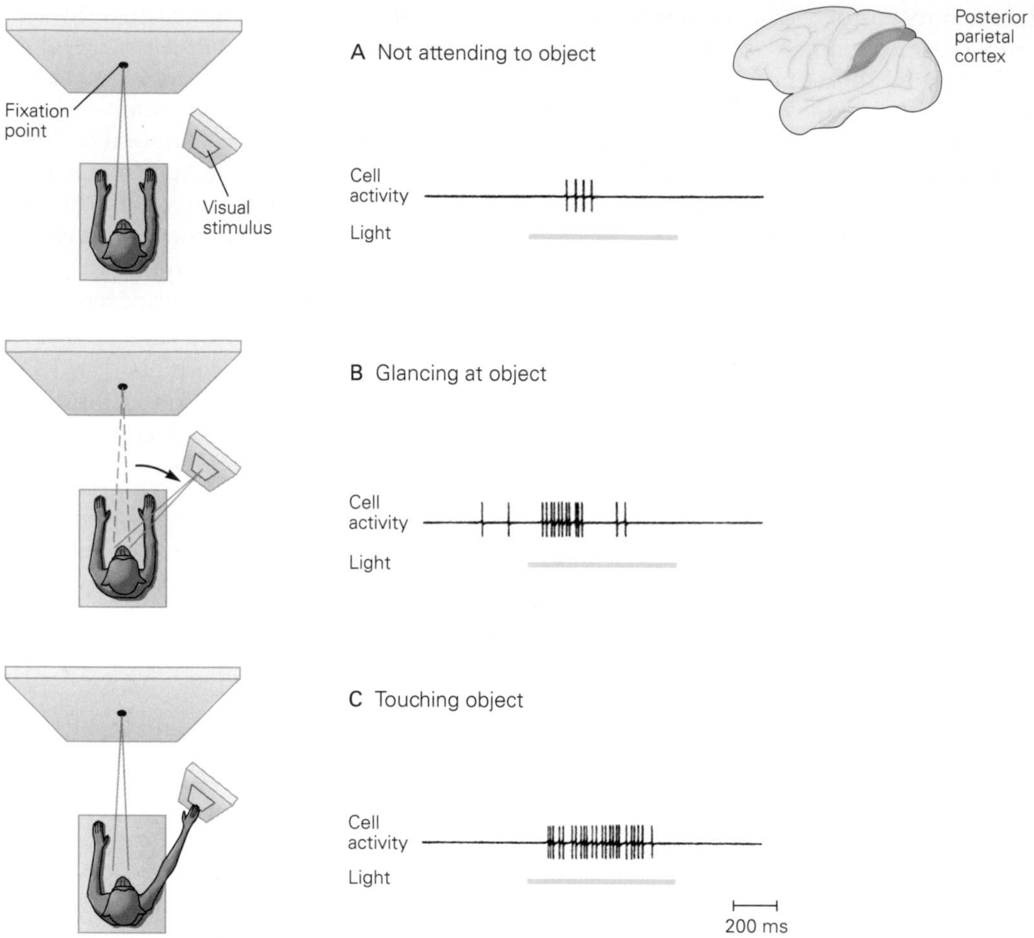

Figure 17–15 Neurons in the posterior parietal cortex of a monkey respond more vigorously to a stimulus when the animal is attentive to the stimulus. (Reproduced, with permission, from Wurtz, Goldberg, and Robinson 1982.)

A. A spot of light elicits only a few action potentials in a cell when the animal's gaze is directed away from the stimulus.

B. The same cell's firing increases when the animal's eyes move to the stimulus.

C. The cell's firing increases even more when the monkey touches the spot without moving his eyes.

These findings are consistent with the clinical observation that the parietal cortex is involved in focusing on objects in space. The response of the neuron is independent of how the animal attends to the stimulus. The firing rate of the neuron increases by about the same amount whether the animal merely looks at the stimulus or reaches for it while continuing to look elsewhere (Figure 17–15). This independence is significant because the posterior parietal cortex makes connections with structures in the prefrontal cortex that are involved in the planning and execution of movements of the eyes and hands.

When an object induces slightly disparate images in the two retinas, we do not see double images. Instead we perceive a single object in front of or behind the plane of fixation. Three-dimensional movies and Magic Eye books take advantage of this phenomenon, displaying slightly different images to each eye to induce a conscious perception of depth. Neurons in the primary visual cortex, the first synaptic relay of the visual system in the cerebral cortex, are sensitive to this retinal disparity and could therefore provide the basis for depth perception. However, these same neurons respond differently to black and white images that are anticorrelated and disparate—images in which each black pixel presented to one eye corresponds to a white pixel in the other, and vice versa. Although the neural synapse should give rise to a conscious perception of depth, in fact such images are not perceived as a single image having depth; instead they are treated as rivalrous alternating images. One sees either a white-on-black or black-on-white image, and the perceptual switch occurs spontaneously every few seconds, without any separation of depth.

Both retinal disparity and anticorrelated images produce an ocular reflex that adjusts the eyes to a depth of field equal to the plane of the image fixated, yet anticorrelated images are not perceived as one image with a single depth of field. The signal of depth triggers a cellular response in the primary visual cortex that is not consciously perceived and therefore does not have a direct role in conscious depth perception. It is thought that later stages of visual processing are responsible for depth perception and somehow reject the depth information computed for anticorrelated images in the primary visual cortex.

The study is important because it shows how neural activity can be dissociated from conscious perception. Disparate anticorrelated images are consciously perceived as rivalrous images—you see one input or the other but you do not see them fused into one object. However, neurons in the primary visual cortex do detect the anticorrelated images as fused and compute the depth of the fused image. In addition, the eyes make automatic vergence movements to the computed depth of the fused image that the brain does not consciously perceive.

These findings reinforce the idea that sensory input alone does not give rise to consciousness; higher-level interpretation of that input is needed.

How Is Self-Awareness Encoded in the Brain?

If visual attention is presently the most tractable example of consciousness, self-awareness is probably the deepest problem. Although aspects of self-awareness are evident in nonhuman primates, self-awareness is central to human identity and has evolved in parallel with language and other forms of symbolic communication.

A more promising approach to the study of consciousness may lie in the latest advances in neural prosthetics that give people the ability to voluntarily modulate neural signals to achieve a goal (move a cursor on the screen). Similarly, some individuals can achieve great control of their breathing and heart rate. These feats suggest that studies of how people can consciously control signals that are normally unconscious may shed light on the neural processes of self-awareness.

An Overall View

To come to grips with the biological processes of cognition, it is necessary to move beyond the individual neuron and consider how information is processed in neural networks. This requires not only the methods and approaches of cellular and systems neuroscience but also the insights of cognitive psychology.

The anterior regions of the parietal lobe contain elementary internal representations of the body surface and peripersonal space that can be modified by experience. Analysis of such modifications in the posterior parietal association cortex indicates that selective attention is a factor in integrating the internal representation of the body with perception of extrapersonal space. The representation of the body is integrated with the representation of actual, imagined, or remembered visual space, and self-consciousness functions within this integrated representation. Indeed, the Russian neuropsychologist A. R. Luria suggested that portions of the parietal lobe constitute the aspect of cortical organization that is the most distinctly human.

But it is likely that just as there is more than one form of spatial experience so there is more than one form of consciousness, each with different neural representations. Thus, Edelman and Damasio distinguish between primary (or core) consciousness and higher-order (extended) consciousness. Primary consciousness is an awareness of objects in the world, of the ability to form mental images of them. Primary consciousness is not unique to humans but shared by nonhuman primates and perhaps by other vertebrate animals as well. By contrast, higher-order consciousness involves a consciousness of being conscious and is uniquely human. It allows for a concept of past and future and therefore the ability to think of the consequences of one's acts and feelings.

In their attempt to develop a coherent reductionist approach to the study of consciousness, Crick and Koch began with Sigmund Freud's view that most mental functions are unconscious, including much of thinking. We are only conscious of the sensory representation of mental activities. Freud wrote in 1923: "It dawns upon us like a new discovery that only something which has once been a perception can become conscious, and that anything arising from within [apart from feelings] that seeks to become conscious must try to transform itself into external perception."

To study consciousness one must rely on first-person reports of (subjective) perception. Thus an empirical definition of consciousness must take into account behavioral output (action), which is integral not only to the study but also to our concept of consciousness.

Intuitively we think that a conscious percept is one we can describe in words. What are words? They are sounds we associate with sensory percepts based on a set of rules for manipulating those sounds (ie, language). Thus, we might consider conscious percepts to be those percepts that can be flexibly linked with actions based on abstract rules.

If, while you are sleeping, a fly settles on your face and you wave it away, this action does not indicate consciousness. It is probably mediated by reflex pathways (similar to the pathways that mediate ocular convergence on rivalrous images). However, if asked to raise your right hand when sensing a light touch and your left hand when sensing a cold stimulus, you could perform that kind of action only if you were awake and conscious of the stimulus. Conscious percepts are those that can in principle support voluntary behavioral responses. This idea explains why correlates of consciousness show up in high-level areas that are also associated with action, such as parietal and prefrontal cortices.

Eric R. Kandel

Selected Readings

Beaumont JG. 1983. *Introduction to Neuropsychology.* New York: Guilford.

Block N, Flanagan O, Güzeldere G (eds). 1997. *The Nature of Consciousness: Philosophical Debates.* Cambridge, MA: MIT Press.

Crick F, Koch C. 2003. A framework for consciousness. Nat Neurosci 6:119–126.

Damasio AR. 1999. *The Feeling of What Happens: Body and Emotion in the Making of Consciousness.* New York: Harcourt Brace.

Edelman GM. 2004. *Wider Than the Sky: The Phenomenal Gift of Consciousness.* New Haven, CT: Yale University Press.

Farber IB, Churchland PS. 1995. Consciousness and the neurosciences: philosophical and theoretical issues. In: M Gazzaniga (ed). *The Cognitive Neurosciences,* pp. 1295–1306. Cambridge, MA: MIT Press.

Feinberg TE, Farah M. 2003. *Behavioral Neurology and Neuropsychology.* New York: McGraw-Hill.

Koch C. 2004. *The Quest for Consciousness: A Neurobiological Approach.* Englewood, CO: Roberts.

Kolb B, Whishaw IQ. 1995. *Fundamentals of Human Neuropsychology,* 4th ed. New York: Freeman.

Libet B, Gleason CA, Wright EW, Pearl DK. 1983. Time of conscious intention to act in relation to onset of cerebral activity (readiness-potential): the unconscious initiation of a freely voluntary act. Brain 106:623–642.

Lumer ED, Friston KJ, Rees G. 1998. Neural correlates of perceptual rivalry in the human brain. Science 280:1930–1934.

McCarthy RA, Warrington EK. 1990. *Cognitive Neuropsychology: A Clinical Introduction.* San Diego: Academic.

McGinn C. 1999. Can we ever understand consciousness? Review of *Mind, Language, and Society: Philosophy in the Real World,* JR Searle (New York: Basic Books) and *On the Contrary: Critical Essays,* 1987–1997, PM Churchland and PS Churchland (Bradford/MIT Press, Cambridge, MA.) NY Rev Books 46 (Jun 10, 1999):44–48. Available online at http://www.nybooks.com/articles/archives/1999/jun/10/can-we-ever-understand-consciousness/?pagination=false

Ramachandran VS, Blakeslee S. 1998. *Phantom in the Brain: Probing the Mysteries of the Human Mind.* New York: William Morrow.

Weiskrantz L. 1997. *Consciousness Lost and Found.* Oxford: Oxford Univ. Press.

References

Andersen RA. 1987. Inferior parietal lobule function in spatial perception and visuomotor integration. In: F Plum (ed). *Handbook of Physiology,* Sect. 1 *The Nervous System.* Vol. 5 *Higher Functions of the Brain,* Pt. 2, pp. 483–518. Bethesda, MD: American Physiological Society.

Bisiach E, Luzzatti C. 1978. Unilateral neglect of representational space. Cortex 14:129–133.

Bisley JW, Goldberg ME. 2010. Attention, intention, and priority in the parietal lobe. Annu Rev Neurosci 33: 1–21.

Bloom F, Lazerson A. 1988. *Brain, Mind and Behavior,* 2nd ed., p. 300. New York: Freeman.

Bushnell MC, Goldberg ME, Robinson DL, 1981. Behavioral enhancement of visual responses in monkey cerebral cortex: I. Modulation in posterior parietal cortex related to selective visual attention. J Neurophysiol 46:755–772.

Chomsky N. 1968. Language and the mind. Psychol Today 1:48–68.

Corbetta M, Miezin FM, Shulman GL, Petersen SE. 1993. A PET study of visuospatial attention. J Neurosci 13: 1202–1226.

Crick F, Koch C. 1990. Towards a neurobiological theory of consciousness. Semin Neurosci 2:263–275.

Darian-Smith I. 1982. Touch in primates. Annu Rev Psychol 33:155–194.

Dehaene S, Changeux J-P. 2011. Experimental and Theoretical Approaches to Conscious Processing. Neuron 70:201–227.

Dennett D. 1991. *Consciousness Explained.* Boston: Little Brown.

Fink GR, Halligan PW, Marshall JC, Frith CD, Frackowiak RS, Dolan RJ. 1996. Where in the brain does visual attention select the forest and the trees? Nature 382: 626–628.

Freud S. 1915. *The Unconscious.* [Standard Edition 14:159–204.] London: Hogarth Press.

Freud S. 1923. *The Ego and the Id.* [Standard Edition 19:1–59.] London: Hogarth Press.

Gardner EP, Hamalainen HA, Palmer CI, Warren S. 1989. Touching the outside world: representation of motion and direction within primary somatosensory cortex. In: JS Lund (ed). *Sensory Processing in the Mammalian Brain: Neural Substrates and Experimental Strategies,* pp. 49–66. New York: Oxford University Press.

Hyvärinen J, Poranen A. 1978. Movement-sensitive and direction and orientation-selective cutaneous receptive fields in the hand area of the post-central gyrus in monkeys. J Physiol 283:523–537.

Jackson JH. 1915. On affections of speech from diseases of the brain. Brain 38:107–174.

James W. [1890] 1950. *The Principles of Psychology.* New York: Dover.

Jenkins WM, Merzenich MM, Ochs MT, Allard T, Guic-Robles E. 1990. Functional reorganization of primary somatosensory cortex in adult owl monkeys after behaviorally controlled tactile stimulation. J Neurophysiol 63:83–104.

Jung R. 1974. Neuropsychologie und Neurophysiologie des Kontur und Formensehens in Zeichnerei und Malerei. In: Wieck HH (ed). *Psycho-pathologie Musischer Bestaltungen,* pp. 29–88. Stuttgart: Schaltauer.

Kaas JH, Nelson RJ, Sur M, Lin CS, Merzenich MM. 1979. Multiple representations of the body within the primary somatosensory cortex of primates. Science 204:521–523.

Kaas JH, Nelson RJ, Sur M, Merzenich MM. 1981. Organization of somatosensory cortex in primates. In: FO Schmitt, FG Worden, G Adelman, SG Dennis (eds). *Organization of the Cerebral Cortex: Proceedings of a Neurosciences Research Program Colloquium,* pp. 237–261. Cambridge, MA: MIT Press.

Kolb B, Whishaw IQ. 1990. *Fundamentals of Human Neuropsychology,* 3rd ed. New York: Freeman.

Luria A. 1980. *Higher Cortical Functions in Man.* New York: Basic Books.

Marshall JC, Halligan PW. 1995. Seeing the forest but only half the trees? Nature 373:521–523.

Marshall WH, Woolsey CN, Bard P. 1941. Observations on cortical somatic sensory mechanisms of cat and monkey. J Neurophysiol 4:1–24.

McGinn C. 1997. Consciousness. In: *The Character of Mind,* 2nd ed., pp. 40–48. Oxford: Oxford Univ. Press.

Mesulam M-M. 1985. *Principles of Behavioral Neurology.* Philadelphia, PA: F.A. Davis.

Mogilner A, Grossman JA, Ribraly V, Joliot M, Volkmann J, Rappaport D, Beasley RW, Llinas RR. 1993. Somato-sensory cortical plasticity in adult humans revealed by magnetoencephalography. Proc Natl Acad Sci U S A 9:3593–3597.

Mountcastle VB. 1984. Central nervous mechanisms in mechanoreceptive sensibility. In: I. Darian-Smith (ed). *Handbook of Physiology.* Sect. 1, Vol. III, Pt. 2, pp. 789–878. Bethesda, MD: American Physiological Society.

Nagel T. 1993. What is the mind-body problem? In: GR Block, J Marsh (eds). *Experimental and Theoretical Studies of Consciousness. (Ciba Foundation Symposium 174).* Chichester, United Kingdom: John Wiley.

Neisser U. 1967. *Cognitive Psychology,* p. 3. New York: Appleton-Century Crofts.

Pandya DN, Seltzer B. 1982. Association areas of the cerebral cortex. Trends Neurosci 5:386–390.

Penfield W, Rasmussen T. 1950. *The Cerebral Cortex of Man.* New York: Macmillan.

Pons TP, Garraghty PE, Friedman DP, Mishkin M. 1987. Physiological evidence for serial processing in somatosensory cortex. Science 237:417–420.

Posner MI, Dahaene S. 1994. Attentional networks. Trends Neurosci 17:75–79.

Ramachandran VS. 1993. Behavioral and magnetoencephalographic correlates of plasticity in the adult human brain. Proc Natl Acad Sci U S A 90:10413–10420.

Salzman CD, Belova MA, Paton JJ. 2005. Beetles, boxes and brain cells: neural mechanisms underlying valuation and learning. Curr Opin Neurobiol 6:721–729.

Searle JR. 1998. How to study consciousness scientifically. In: K Fuxe, S Grillner, T Hökfelt, L Olson, LF Agnati (eds). *Towards an Understanding of Integrative Brain Function,* pp. 379–387. Amsterdam: Elsevier.

Shadlen M. 1997. Look but don't touch or vice versa. Nature 386:122–123.

Skinner BF. 1938. *The Behavior of Organisms: An Experimental Analysis.* New York: Appleton-Century-Crofts.

Snyder LH, Batista AP, Anderson RA. 1997. Coding for intention in the posterior parietal cortex. Nature 386:167–170.

Thorndike EL. 1911. *Animal Intelligence: Experimental Studies.* New York: Macmillan.

Tolman EC. 1932. *Purposive Behavior in Animals and Men.* New York: Appleton-Century-Crofts.

Vallbo ÅB, Olsson KÅ, Westberg KG, Clark FJ. 1984. Microstimulation of single tactile afferents from the human hand: sensory attributes related to unit type and properties of receptive fields. Brain 107:727–749.

Watson JB. 1930. *Behaviorism.* New York: W.W. Norton, Chicago: University of Chicago Press.

Weinberg S. 1995. Reductionism redux. Review of *Nature's Imagination: The Frontiers of Scientific Vision,* J Cornwell, ed. NY Rev Books 42 (Oct 5, 1995):39–42. Available online at http://www.nybooks.com/articles/archives/1995/oct/05/reductionism-redux/?pagination=false

Wurtz RH, Goldberg ME, Robinson DL. 1982. Brain mechanisms of visual attention. Sci Am 246:124–135.

18

The Organization of Cognition

In the previous chapter we examined how the activity of single nerve cells can be related to the internal representations required for simple cognitive tasks. In this chapter we survey the anatomical and physiological organization of the cortex through which the activity of populations of neurons mediate complex aspects of cognition. For this purpose we draw on the insights that have emerged from studies of the neural mechanisms of cognition in monkeys and studies of cognitive impairment resulting from brain injury in humans. In the following chapter we extend this analysis to the premotor cortex and the control of voluntary movement. In Chapter 20 we discuss how neuroimaging studies of cognition in humans are consistent with the findings from these experimental and clinical studies.

Cognitive functions are mediated by specialized areas of neocortex distributed across the cerebral hemisphere in an orderly arrangement. This was already well established in 1962 when Alexander Luria published his landmark *Higher Cortical Functions in Man*. Neurologists of Luria's generation knew that lesions at neighboring sites on the cortical surface tend to produce related symptoms. For example, lesions of the occipital cortex give rise to lower-order visual deficits (cortical blindness), whereas lesions of adjacent temporal cortex result in higher-order visual deficits (object agnosia). Similarly, lesions in the posterior sector of the frontal lobe give rise to lower-order motor deficits (weakness and paralysis), whereas more anterior lesions give rise to higher-order deficits of executive control (the prefrontal syndrome). How can these observations be explained?

Luria proposed that sensory and motor cortex comprise multiple specialized subareas that are connected hierarchically. A primary sensory area lies next to a secondary sensory area that in turn borders a tertiary area. These areas have progressively more complex functions, culminating in the integration of multiple sensory modalities in the tertiary zones. Areas in the frontal lobe concerned with motor behavior are similarly organized. The primary motor cortex lies next to a secondary motor area (the premotor cortex) that in turn borders a tertiary area, the prefrontal cortex, concerned with the executive control of behavior. In Luria's scheme sensory information flows into the central nervous system through a series of synaptic relays from primary to secondary to tertiary sensory areas, whereas motor commands flow from tertiary to secondary to primary motor areas. The tertiary areas at the peak of these sensory and motor hierarchies interact and are the seats of cognitive function.

More than 45 years after publication of Luria's book these general principles are still accepted. However, our understanding of the neural systems of cognition is far richer than that of Luria and his contemporaries, in large part because of newer methodologies.

Functionally Related Areas of Cortex Lie Close Together

The cortex of each cerebral hemisphere is a continuous sheet of gray matter. At the coarsest level, it consists of five lobes as illustrated in Figure 18–1. Within each of these lobes the cortex is further subdivided into anatomically and functionally defined areas.

Functional areas are distinguished by cellular structure, connectivity, and the physiological response properties of neurons. Identification of the functions of a cortical area requires characterizing the behavioral conditions under which its neurons are electrically active (by means of single-neuron recording) and determining its anatomical connections with other areas (by means of neuroanatomical tracers).

These invasive methods cannot be used in humans except under rare circumstances in which there is some clinical benefit. Consequently the major advances in identifying the function of anatomically or physiologically discrete areas of cortex have come from studies of animals, in particular the rhesus monkey, a species of the macaque (*Macaca*), an Old World monkey. Old World monkeys are our closest living relatives aside from the apes; like us, they are able to carry out demanding tasks that require well-developed cognitive abilities such as attention, memory, and pattern discrimination.

In the macaque a region of cortex is defined as functionally distinct if neurons within it have similar functional properties (such as responding to similar types of visual stimulation) and common connections (such as receiving the same input from primary visual cortex). In addition, to qualify as an area of lower-order sensory or motor cortex the neurons in that area must be organized into a single, coherent neural map of the sensory or motor periphery. The number of functionally distinct areas identified by these criteria (Figure 18–1) is much greater than the number of areas defined cytoarchitecturally because an area with anatomically similar cells may contain several functionally and connectionally distinct areas.

A few simple precepts govern the organization of functional areas in the macaque cerebral cortex: (1) all areas fall into a few major functional categories; (2) areas in a given category occupy a discrete, continuous portion of the cortical sheet; and (3) areas that are functionally related occupy neighboring sites (Figure 18–2).

Sensory Information Is Processed in the Cortex in Serial Pathways

In analyzing how the areas of the cerebral cortex act together to produce behavior it is useful to ask, as in the study of social organizations, who talks to whom? Cortical areas communicate with each other by means of bundles of axons traveling together in identifiable tracts. As a result of neuro-anatomical tracing studies in the monkey, the neural tracts (or projections) running from area to area are now well understood. A dye injected into one population of neurons is carried by axonal transport to distant clusters of neurons that can be identified because they are labeled with the dye (see Box 4–2).

These tracing studies have confirmed Luria's idea that the sensory areas of cortex are organized hierarchically. Within each sensory system (visual, auditory, etc.) signals from the periphery arrive at a primary sensory area, such as the primary visual cortex (V1), primary auditory cortex (A1), or primary somatosensory cortex (S-I).

Primary sensory areas possess four properties characteristic of their role in the early stages of information processing.

1. Their input is from thalamic sensory relay nuclei. (The thalamus is the main subcortical source of input to all areas of cortex, but only some thalamic nuclei relay sensory signals).
2. The neurons in a primary sensory area have small receptive fields—the region on the receptor surface that must be stimulated in order for the neuron to fire—and are arranged to form a precise somatotopic map of the sensory receptor surface (retina, cochlea, or skin).
3. Injury to a part of the map causes a simple sensory loss confined to the corresponding part of the contralateral sensory receptor surface.
4. Connections to other cortical areas are limited, confined almost entirely to nearby areas that process information in the same modality.

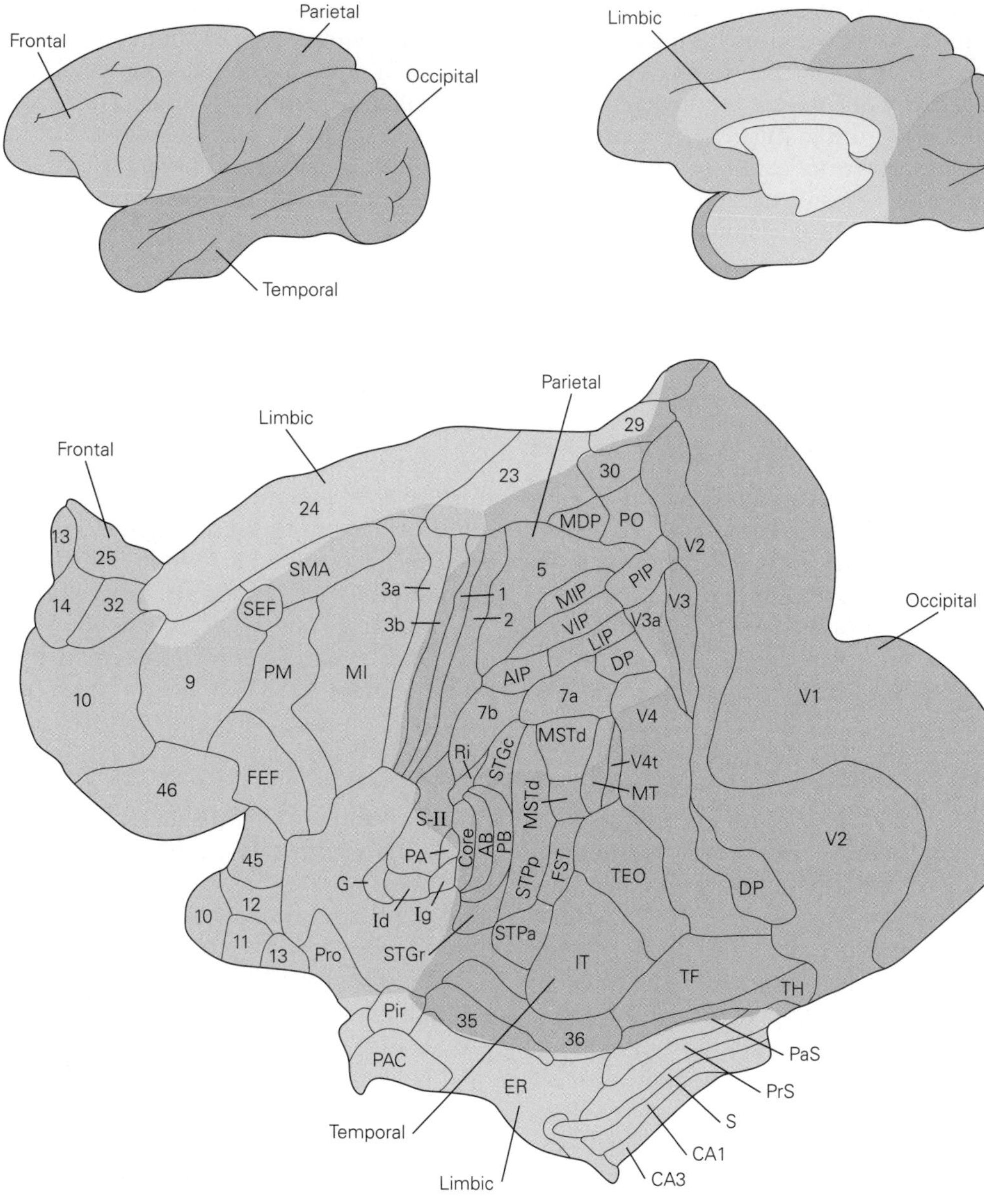

Figure 18–1 The cerebral cortex of the macaque monkey. Lateral and medial views show the location of five cortical lobes. The labeled areas on the unfolded hemisphere (lower panel) are those defined in physiological and anatomical studies. (Adapted, with permission, from Van Essen et al. 2001.)

The anatomical labels are as follows. The numbered areas are Brodmann's areas; **AB**, auditory belt; **AIP**, anterior intraparietal area; **CA_1**, **CA_3**, cornu ammonis fields of hippocampus; **Core**, primary auditory cortex; **DP**, dorsal prelunate area; **ER**, entorhinal cortex; **FEF**, frontal eye field; **FST**, floor of superior temporal sulcus; **G**, gustatory cortex; **Id**, **Ig**, insular cortex, dysgranular and granular divisions; **IT**, inferotemporal cortex; **LIP**, lateral intraparietal area; **MDP**, medial dorsal parietal area; **M1**, primary motor cortex; **MIP**, medial intraparietal area; **MSTd**, **MSTl**, medial superior temporal sulcus, dorsal and lateral divisions; **MT**, middle temporal area; **PA**, postauditory area; **PAC**, periamygdaloid cortex; **PaS**, parasubiculum; **PB**, auditory parabelt cortex; **PIP**, posterior intraparietal; **Pir**, piriform cortex; **PM**, premotor cortex; **PO**, parieto-occipital area; **Pro**, orbital proisocortex; **PrS**, presubiculum; **Ri**, retroinsular area; **S**, subiculum; **SEF**, supplementary eye field; **S-II**, secondary somatosensory area; **SMA**, supplementary motor and adjacent cingulate motor areas; **STGc**, **STGr**, superior temporal gyrus, caudal and rostral divisions of auditory cortex; **STPa**, **STPp**, superior temporal polysensory area, anterior and posterior divisions; **TEO**, temporo-occipital area; **TF**, **TH**, parahippocampal areas; **V_1**, **V_2**, **V_3**, **V_{3a}**, **V_4**, **V_{4t}**, visual areas; **VIP**, ventral intraparietal area.

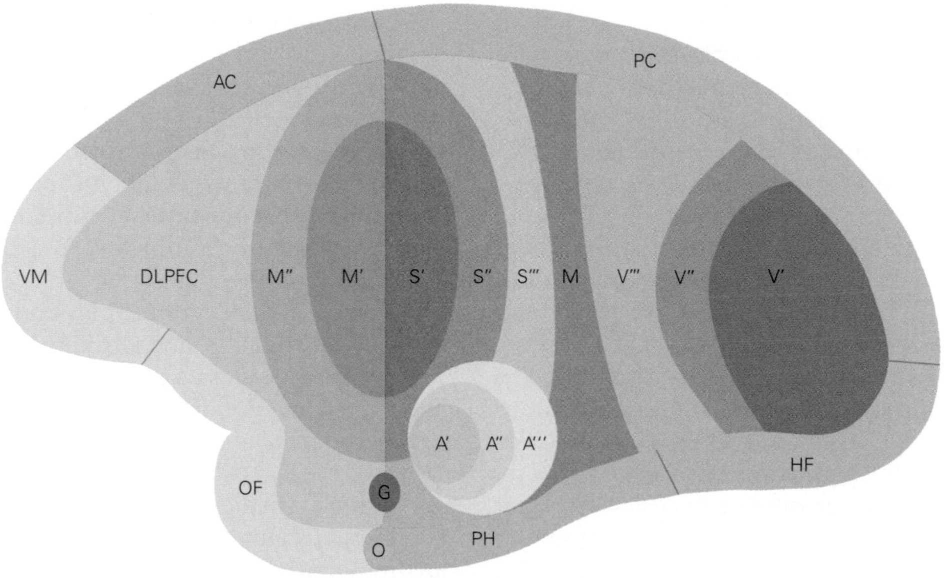

Category	Subcategory	Key	Figure 18-1
Visual	Primary	V′	V1
	Secondary	V″	V2, V3, V3a, PIP, PO, MT, V4
	Tertiary	V‴	MDP, LIP, 7a, MSTd, MSTl, FST, IT
Somatosensory	Primary	S′	3a, 3b
	Secondary	S″	1, 2, S-II
	Tertiary	S‴	5, MIP, AIP, 7b, Ri, Id, Ig
Auditory	Primary	A′	Core
	Secondary	A″	AB, PA
	Tertiary	A‴	PB, STGc, STGr
Multimodal		M	VIP, STPp, STPa
Gustatory		G	G
Olfactory		O	Pir, PAC
Motor	Primary	M′	M1
	Secondary	M″	PM, SMA, FEF, SEF, 24
Dorsolateral prefrontal	Dorsal		9, 10, 14
	Dorsolateral	DLPFC	46
	Ventral convexity		45
Orbital-ventromedial prefrontal	Orbital	OF	11, 12, 13, Pro
	Ventromedial	VM	25, 32
Limbic	Anterior cingulate	AC	24
	Posterior cingulate	PC	23, 29, 30
	Hippocampal	HF	CA1, CA3, S, PrS, PaS
	Parahippocampal	PH	ER, TF, TH, 35, 36

Figure 18–2 The cerebral cortex is divided into discrete functional categories. Cortical areas in each functional category occupy a continuous physical region of the cortical sheet, shown here in a schematic version of the unfolded hemisphere in Figure 18–1. The table indicates the functionally distinct areas within each category. Primary sensory areas send their outputs to multiple secondary sensory areas, which in turn provide inputs to tertiary (higher-order) areas. Multimodal areas are tertiary areas with significant input from more than one sensory system.

Higher-order sensory areas have a different set of properties that are important to their role in the later stages of information processing.

1. They receive little input from the sensory relay nuclei in the thalamus; instead, their input arises from other thalamic nuclei and lower-order areas of sensory cortex.
2. Their neurons have large receptive fields and are organized into imprecise maps of the array of receptors in the periphery.
3. Injury results in abnormalities of perception and of related cognitive functions but does not impair the ability to detect sensory stimuli.
4. They are connected not only to nearby unimodal sensory areas but also to distant areas in the frontal and limbic lobes.

Thus, sensory information is processed serially, with each area in the chain carrying out certain computations and conveying the results to the next area. For example, in the ventral pathway of the visual system, which is concerned with processing information about form, the pathway begins with neurons that respond to detailed features of a visual stimulus and proceeds to neurons that encode the overall form. Receptive fields of individual neurons in the primary visual cortex (V_1) span approximately 1 degree of visual angle; those of neurons in V_4 (a mid-order area) span approximately 10 degrees; and those in the inferotemporal cortex (a higher-order area) span up to 100 degrees. Thus an individual neuron in V_1 could be sensitive to a small detail in a face, such as an eyebrow aligned in a certain direction within its small receptive field, whereas a neuron in the inferotemporal cortex can respond to an entire face.

However, sensory pathways are not exclusively serial; in each functional pathway higher-order areas project back to the lower-order areas from which they receive input. In this way neurons in higher-order areas, sensitive to the global pattern of sensory input, can modulate the activity of neurons in lower-order areas that are sensitive to local detail. For example, top-down signals originating in the inferotemporal cortex might help neurons in V_1 to resolve a detail in a part of the face.

The hierarchical chain of sensory processing leads to areas with functions so complex that they cannot be described as simply sensory. In the late 19th century Santiago Ramón y Cajal proposed that areas with sensory functions were fundamentally distinct from those with cognitive functions, calling the latter the *association cortex*. This term is rooted in the idea that cognition depends upon our learning which of the myriad stimuli impinging on our senses are associated with one another. Modern neuroscientists apply the term *association cortex* to regions of cortex where injury causes cognitive deficits that cannot be explained by impairment of sensory or motor function alone.

Large regions of association cortex are contained within each of the four lobes and contribute to cognition in distinctive ways.

The *parietal association cortex* is critical for sensory guidance of motor behavior and spatial awareness.

The *temporal association cortex* is important for recognition of sensory stimuli and for storage of semantic (factual) knowledge.

The *frontal association cortex* plays a key role in organizing behavior and in working memory.

The *limbic association cortex* serves complex functions related to emotion and episodic (autobiographical) memory.

Association areas have much more extensive input and output connections than do lower-order sensory and motor areas. Some association areas have a variety of visual, auditory, somatosensory, and motor connections that permit them to integrate sensory modalities or to use sensory information to guide motor behavior (see Chapter 19). In addition, all association areas are interconnected by a dense network of pathways within and between the parietal, temporal, frontal, and limbic lobes.

Parallel Pathways in Each Sensory Modality Lead to Dorsal and Ventral Association Areas

In addition to serial processing another principle of cortical organization is that the same information is processed differently in parallel pathways. In the visual system for example, two major parallel pathways terminate in different higher-order areas of cortex. The dorsal stream processes spatial information (position, motion, speed) and projects to parietal association cortex. The ventral stream processes information about form (color, shape, texture) and projects to temporal association cortex.

Dorsal and ventral pathways exist in other sensory systems as well (Figure 18–3). In the auditory and somatosensory systems dorsal pathways serve motor and spatial functions, whereas ventral pathways serve recognition functions. The dorsal-ventral division extends into frontal association cortex.

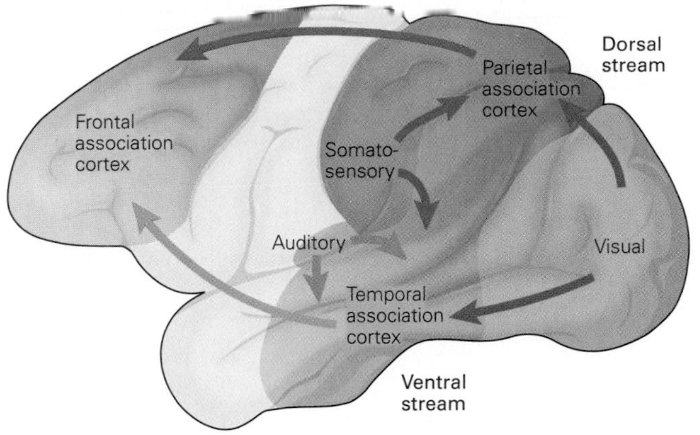

Figure 18–3 The dorsal and ventral systems of the cerebral cortex. Lower-order sensory areas send their output in parallel to the parietal (dorsal stream) and temporal (ventral stream) association cortices, which in turn send their output to the frontal association cortex. The parietal cortex projects primarily to dorsal areas of frontal cortex, areas that serve motor and executive control functions for which spatial information is important. The temporal cortex projects primarily to ventral regions of frontal cortex, including the orbital prefrontal cortex, areas that mediate emotional responses to things in the environment. Emotional significance can be assigned to an object only after the object has been recognized, an ability that depends on areas of the temporal lobe.

The Dorsal Visual Pathway Carries Spatial Information and Leads to Parietal Association Cortex

The parietal cortex plays a key role in the visual guidance of motor behavior and in spatial perception and cognition (and understanding where objects are relative to each other). These two functions are related because visuomotor control requires processing spatial information. Reaching for your coffee cup while you read the newspaper requires that the brain take into account where the image of the cup is on your retina and where your eyes are pointing so as to determine where the cup is relative to your hand.

The parietal cortex is ideally suited for such computations because it is connected to visual, somatosensory, and motor areas of cortex. Parietal cortex may have initially developed the capacity to represent where things are relative to the body to guide actions such as grasping, and then developed the ability to represent where things are relative to each other without reference to the body.

As we have learned in Chapter 17, injury to the parietal cortex in humans results in a wide range of behavioral impairments, which can be classified into two broad categories. In the first category are impairments of body awareness, motor control, and visual guidance of motor behavior. These deficits result from damage to dorsal parts of the parietal cortex close to and connected with the somatosensory cortex. In the second category are impairments of spatial perception and cognition. These deficits result from damage to ventral parts of parietal cortex close to and connected with the visual cortex. Thus the parietal cortex can be thought of as having two subdivisions: a dorsal component serving primarily motor functions and a ventral component serving primarily spatial functions.

Specific impairments in the first category include asomatognosia, a disorder of body awareness in which patients deny the existence of the arm or leg contralateral to the lesion or refuse to acknowledge that it belongs to them even when they can see it. Another is ideomotor apraxia, which arises from damage to the dominant hemisphere; patients are unable to execute certain movements such as waving goodbye, either on command or by imitation, although they may spontaneously make the same movement under circumstances that evoke it habitually. A third deficit in this category, optic ataxia, results from damage to the dorsomedial parietal cortex. Patients with this deficit have difficulty reaching for an object in the peripheral visual field (as when reaching for a coffee cup while reading the newspaper). The hand may go to the wrong location, or it may be misoriented when attempting to grasp the object (Figure 18–4). Patients can, however, perform a reaching task that does not depend on vision, for example touching one's knee in the dark, and can report the locations of visible objects correctly. This collection of symptoms cannot be explained by a purely motor or purely visual mechanism but instead reflects difficulty in coordinating visual input and motor output.

Specific impairments in the second category include hemispatial neglect. Patients with this defect are profoundly inattentive to events in the half of space opposite the injured side (see Chapter 17). Another is constructional apraxia, an inability to appreciate the structure and arrangement of things by looking at them. Patients suffering from constructional apraxia have difficulty arranging a set of tiles or matchsticks according to a model placed in plain view. They may also be deficient in tests of writing and drawing because these require putting marks on a page in a precise arrangement (Figure 18–5).

Injury to parietal cortex can impair cognitive tasks that require abstract spatial thinking. For example, patients with acalculia have trouble understanding and manipulating numbers, particularly multidigit numbers where the value of a digit depends on its place.

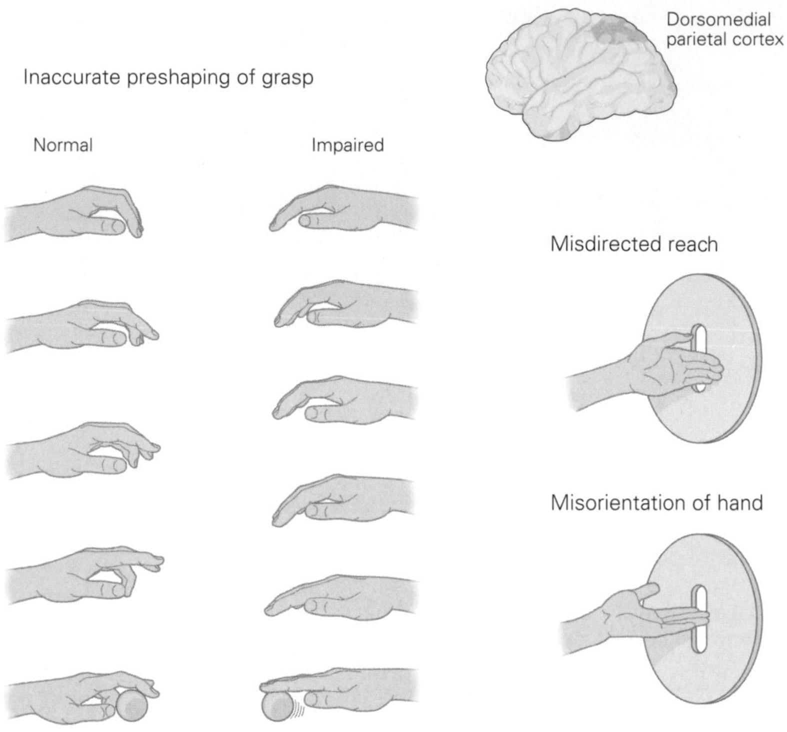

Figure 18–4 Patients with damage to the dorsomedial parietal cortex have difficulty with visually guided grasping and reaching (optic ataxia). When required to grasp an object, patients fail to shape their hand appropriately. When required to place their fingers through a slot in a plate, they reach to the wrong location and fail to orient the hand correctly. (Adapted, with permission, from Jeannerod 1986 [left panels]; and Perenin and Vighetto 1988 [right panels].)

Injury to the left angular gyrus, a region at the lateral edge of the parietal lobe, results in agraphia with alexia, a condition in which patients cannot read, write, or spell and cannot understand a word spelled out orally. Reading and writing involve spatial thinking in that they depend on the ability to perceive, remember, and reproduce the sequence of letters in a word.

Although clinical observations pinpoint the parietal cortex as important for many spatially based abilities, they do not tell us about the underlying neural mechanisms. Our understanding of these mechanisms comes in large part from studies of monkeys using single-neuron recording. Four areas in the monkey's intraparietal sulcus have been thoroughly studied: the lateral, ventral, medial, and anterior intraparietal areas. Neurons in all of these areas carry spatial information, signaling the location of an object to which the monkey is paying attention or is about to direct movement. Within a given area neurons respond to one or more specific kinds of sensory stimulation (somatosensory or visual), fire in conjunction with a specific kind of movement (looking, reaching, or grasping), and encode the location of a target relative to a specific part of the body (eye, head, or hand) or the environment.

The lateral intraparietal area encodes retina-centered information about points in the visual field that the monkey has selected for attention and is involved in visual attention and eye movements. Its neurons, like those in unimodal visual areas, have receptive fields for fixed points on the retina. Visual responses in these neurons increase when the monkey is paying attention to a stimulus in the receptive field (Figure 18–6A). This enhancement of the response occurs whether or not the monkey is planning an eye movement toward the stimulus. Neurons here also fire when the monkey is anticipating the appearance of a stimulus or remembering the location where a stimulus appeared, and some neurons fire around the time of an eye movement toward the receptive field.

The ventral intraparietal area encodes head-centered spatial information about visual and tactile stimuli and is involved in multisensory guidance of head and mouth movements. Individual neurons respond to both visual and somatosensory stimuli. Most neurons respond to tactile stimulation on the face or head and to visual stimuli presented near the receptive field. The match between somatosensory and visual receptive fields is maintained when the eyes move: The visual receptive fields are shifted so as to remain at a fixed position relative to the head (Figure 18–6B).

The medial intraparietal area encodes both retina-centered and body-centered spatial information and is involved with visually guided reaching. Neurons in this area respond to visual targets and are active when the monkey is planning and executing reaching movements. They are sensitive to the direction of reaching in relation both to where the monkey is looking (right or left of the gaze) and to the body (right or left of the trunk) (Figure 18–6C).

The anterior intraparietal area encodes object-centered and hand-centered spatial information and is involved with visually guided grasping. Individual neurons are selective for objects of particular shapes and for the hand shapes required to grasp them. A neuron that fires when the monkey sees a given object will also fire when it prepares to grasp that object (Figure 18–6D).

Clinical observations in humans and electrophysiological studies in monkeys lead to two general conclusions. First, the parietal cortex is specialized for the sensory guidance of motor behavior as well as for spatial perception and cognition. Second, different regions within the parietal cortex serve different functions: Dorsal regions close to the somatosensory cortex contribute to motor control of the body, whereas ventral regions close to the visual cortex contribute to spatial perception and cognition.

The Ventral Visual Pathway Processes Information About Form and Leads to Temporal Association Cortex

The temporal association cortex, like the parietal association cortex, is a region where higher-order areas of different sensory systems share borders and are interconnected. These association areas receive information about vision, sound, and touch from lower-order

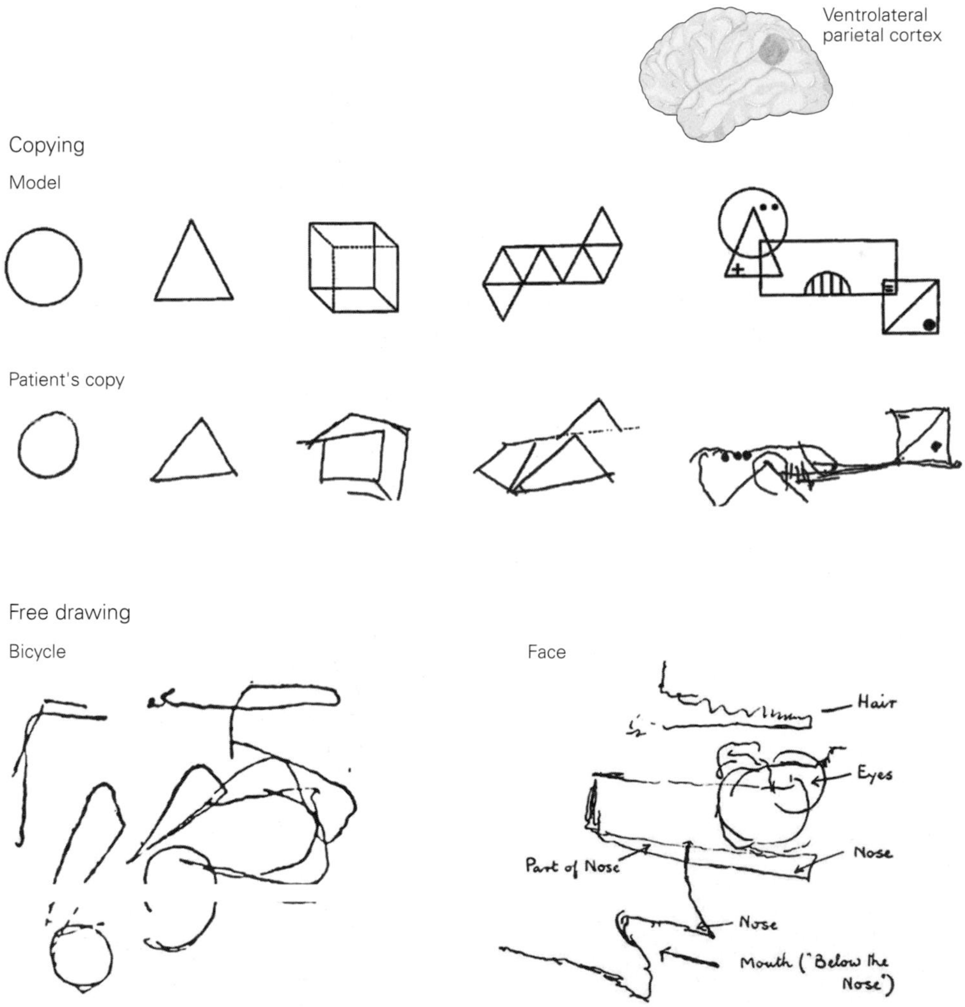

Figure 18–5 Disorders of copying and drawing result from damage to the parietal cortex. Drawings of complex figures are grossly inaccurate whether drawn from a model or from memory. The problem arises from an inability to perceive the spatial relations of the parts of an object. (Reproduced, with permission, from Critchley 1953; and Trojano and Grossi 1998.)

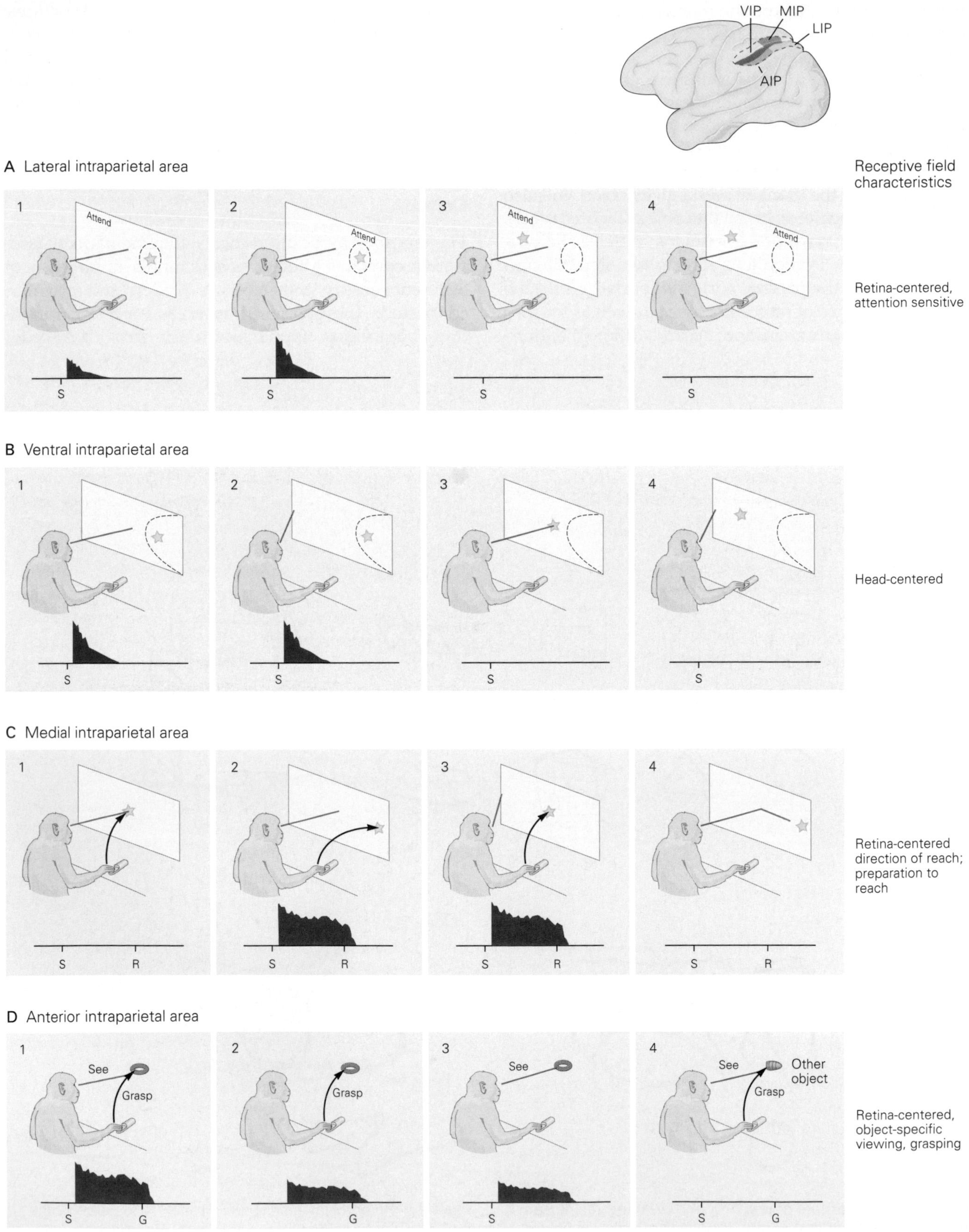
VIP
MIP
LIP
AIP
A Lateral intraparietal area
Receptive field characteristics
Attend
S
Retina-centered, attention sensitive
B Ventral intraparietal area
Head-centered
C Medial intraparietal area
R
Retina-centered direction of reach; preparation to reach
D Anterior intraparietal area
See
Grasp
Other object
G
Retina-centered, object-specific viewing, grasping

visual, auditory, and somatosensory areas. For example, the inferotemporal cortex receives information about the shape, color, and texture of visual images through the ventral visual pathway. The temporal association cortex uses this information to mediate the recognition of objects in the environment and, through projections to the ventral frontal cortex, trigger appropriate emotional responses to them (see Figure 18–3).

Injury to the visual and auditory association areas of the temporal lobe in humans impairs recognition of the significance of sensory stimuli, resulting in a variety of perceptual deficits termed *agnosias*. Patients with visual object agnosia, a result of injury to a medioventral part of the temporal cortex, cannot recognize things but can draw them (Figure 18–7). This deficit is a striking contrast to patients with parietal cortex injury, who can recognize things but often cannot draw them well (Figure 18–5). Patients with visual object agnosia may be unable to recognize objects in general or may be unable to make fine distinctions within a category of objects such as faces. An impairment in recognition specific to faces is called prosopagnosia.

Auditory agnosia has been described, although reports of it are rare, perhaps because the condition is associated with more disabling disorders of language comprehension. Patients with auditory agnosia, when asked to describe recordings of natural sounds, demonstrate that they are not deaf but that their ability to recognize the sounds is impaired.

By far the most debilitating of all conditions arising from damage to the human temporal lobe is Wernicke aphasia, a disorder in understanding spoken language. Wernicke aphasia arises from damage to the superior temporal gyrus of the left hemisphere, a region corresponding to Brodmann's area 22 (comparable in location to the auditory association cortex in the superior temporal gyrus in the monkey). In addition to the disorder of speech comprehension, the patient's own speech is severely garbled. This indicates that auditory forms of words stored in the temporal lobe serve not only as templates for speech recognition but also as guides for speech production.

Semantic dementia is a degenerative disorder typically arising from pathology of the temporal cortex. Studies of patients with this disorder indicate that this part of cortex is critical not only for object recognition but also for semantic memory. To have semantic knowledge of a thing means that one must be able to associate disparate pieces of information about it, for example, the sound, feel, appearance, and use of a telephone. These associations are forged through experience-dependent changes in the synaptic connections among the same temporal lobe areas on which recognition depends. A patient with semantic dementia shown pictures of an ostrich and a penguin may name them simply "bird" or even "animal." The loss of detailed knowledge about things in the world emerges even in tests requiring only nonverbal responses, such as placing together pictures of things that are semantically related.

Figure 18–6 (Opposite) **Neurons in the parietal cortex of the monkey are selective for the location of objects in the visual field relative to particular parts of the body.** Each histogram represents the firing rate of a representative neuron as a function of time following presentation of a stimulus. In each diagram the line emanating from the eyes indicates where the monkey is looking.

A. Neurons in the lateral intraparietal area (**LIP**) have *retina-centered* receptive fields. The strength of the visual response depends on whether the monkey is paying attention to the stimulus. The neuron fires when a light is flashed inside its receptive field (**dotted circle**) (**1**). The visual response is increased if the monkey is instructed to attend to the location of the stimulus (**2**). The neuron does not fire if the stimulus is presented outside the receptive field regardless of where attention is directed (**3, 4**).

B. In the ventral intraparietal area (**VIP**) some neurons have *head-centered* receptive fields. This is determined by keeping the head in a fixed position while the monkey is instructed to shift its gaze to various locations. This neuron fires when a light appears to the right of the midline of the head (**1, 2**). It does not fire when the light appears at another location relative to the head, as on the midline or to the left (**3, 4**). The critical contrast is between situations 1 and 4. The retinal location of the light is the same in both (slightly to the right of the fixation point) yet the neuron fires in 1, when the stimulus is to the right of the head, but not in 4, when the stimulus is to the left of the head.

C. In the medial intraparietal area (**MIP**) neurons fire when the monkey is preparing to reach for a visual target and are selective for the retina-centered direction of the reach. This neuron fires when the monkey reaches for a target to the right of where he is looking (**2, 3**). It does not fire when he reaches for a target at which he is looking (**1**) or when he moves only his eyes to the target at the right (**4**). The physical direction of the reach is not a factor in the neuron's firing: It is the same in 1 and 3 and yet the neuron fires only in 3.

D. In the anterior intraparietal area (**AIP**) neurons fire when the monkey is looking at or preparing to grasp an object and are selective for objects of particular shapes. This neuron fires when the monkey is viewing a ring (**3**) or making a memory-guided reach to it in the dark (**2**). It fires especially strongly when the monkey is grasping the ring under visual guidance (**1**). It does not fire during viewing or grasping of other objects (**4**).

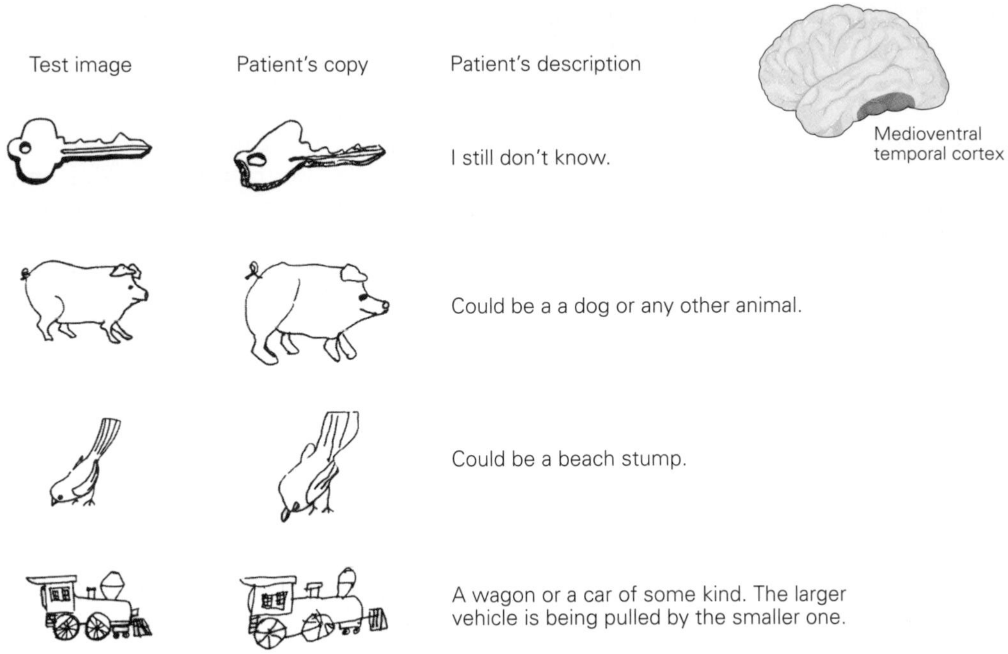
Test image
Patient's copy
Patient's description
Medioventral temporal cortex
I still don't know.
Could be a a dog or any other animal.
Could be a beach stump.
A wagon or a car of some kind. The larger vehicle is being pulled by the smaller one.

Figure 18–7 Injury to a medioventral region of temporal cortex results in visual object agnosia. When presented with the drawings shown in the left column, a patient with visual object agnosia was able to copy them but could not accurately identify the objects. (Reproduced, with permission, from Rubens and Benson 1971.)

Neurons in the temporal association cortex of monkeys become active under circumstances that suggest involvement in object recognition. The best understood area of temporal association cortex is the inferotemporal cortex, which occupies most of the inferior temporal gyrus and extends dorsally into the superior temporal sulcus. The activity of inferotemporal neurons, unlike neurons in the parietal cortex, is not influenced by the motor behavior of the animal. If a visual stimulus enters the neuron's receptive field and the monkey is paying attention to it, the neuron will fire at a virtually identical rate regardless of what the animal is doing or planning to do.

Inferotemporal neurons also differ from parietal neurons in that they are sensitive to the shape, color, and texture of an object in the visual receptive field. In one study individual inferotemporal neurons responded to only a few shapes out of a large test set (Figure 18–8). Because each neuron responded to different stimuli, it was possible by monitoring the activity of many neurons to determine reliably which stimulus was present on the screen. The pattern selectivity of inferotemporal neurons is largely unaffected by image size and location as long as the image falls somewhere in the neuron's typically large receptive field. This insensitivity to size and location is further evidence that the inferotemporal cortex plays a role in shape recognition (for which location and size are irrelevant) but not in motor guidance (for which they are crucial).

Just as neurons in the inferotemporal cortex are selective for visual shapes, neurons in the auditory association cortex of the superior temporal gyrus are selective for patterns of sound. Although little studied, this region is known to contain neurons selective for particular species-specific vocalizations. Overall, the temporal association cortex plays a critical role in recognizing things and in storing some kinds of knowledge. It is not involved in the guidance of movement or in spatial perception and cognition, functions that depend instead on parietal cortex.

Goal-Directed Motor Behavior Is Controlled in the Frontal Lobe

All areas of the frontal lobe participate in the control of motor behavior but in different ways. Just as in the posterior sensory cortex, frontal areas are connected in series in a functional hierarchy (Figure 18–9). At the lower end of the chain is the primary motor cortex (Brodmann's area 4), also referred to as M1. Neurons here are organized into a detailed map of the body.

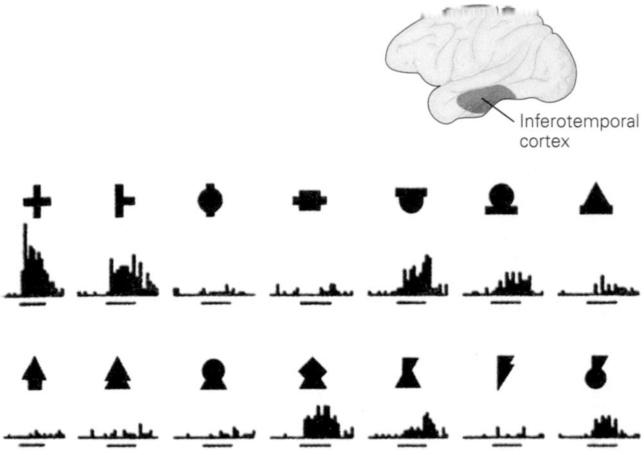

Figure 18–8 Neurons in the inferotemporal cortex of the monkey respond selectively to particular shapes. Shown are responses of a single inferotemporal neuron to 14 different silhouette shapes. The histogram under each shape represents the rate at which the neuron fired as a function of time during a 2-second trial. The bar under the histogram indicates the 1-second period during which the stimulus appeared. (Reproduced, with permission, from Kobatake et al. 1998.)

The primary motor cortex has numerous subregions that produce movement of different parts of the body.

Adjacent to the primary motor cortex and reciprocally connected to it are several higher-order motor areas collectively called the premotor cortex. Neurons in each of these areas are arranged in a comparatively coarse map of the body. Neuronal activity in the premotor areas reflects global aspects of motor behavior such as the combination of limbs to be used or the sequence of movements. In addition, the premotor cortex of the inferior frontal gyrus contains mirror neurons that respond to the movement of others (see Chapter 19). The premotor cortex is connected to the dorsolateral prefrontal cortex, which is important for cognitive control of motor behavior. This area is connected in turn to the orbital-ventromedial prefrontal cortex, an area involved in emotional processes associated with the executive control of behavior.

In contrast to the sensory systems, where information flows from the periphery into higher-order areas, in the motor systems signals flow from the higher-order areas of the frontal lobe to the primary motor cortex. Emotional processes in the orbital-ventromedial prefrontal cortex influence cognitive processes in the dorsolateral prefrontal cortex, which in turn act on spinal motor nerves through the premotor and primary motor cortex.

Prefrontal Cortex Is Important for the Executive Control of Behavior

Much of what we do in daily life depends on our ability to remember and act on intentions. Intentions can be simple or nested; they can concern particular actions or general plans, a small bit of mental arithmetic or a career path. The mental processes underlying the executive control of behavior are so diverse that it seems unlikely that they could be served by one area of the brain. Yet, remarkably, a single large region of the cerebral hemisphere, the prefrontal cortex, is implicated in many forms of executive control.

Patients with damage confined to the prefrontal cortex are typically normal in their perceptual ability and motor behavior and may perform normally on tests of intelligence. Yet they are unable to function effectively in daily life. Their emotional state is abnormal, and their behavior is disorganized because they lack concentration and thus are ineffective at carrying out plans. The physician John Harlow, writing in 1868, provided the first clear description of such a case. His patient, Phineas Gage, was a railroad worker who had suffered extensive prefrontal damage when blasting powder, exploding prematurely, drove a tamping iron through his head (Figure 18–10). Formerly "a shrewd, smart business man, very energetic and persistent in pursuing all his plans," Gage seemed transformed into another person altogether, "pertinaciously obstinate, yet capricious and vacillating, devising many plans of future operation, which are no sooner arranged than they are abandoned in turn for others appearing more feasible."

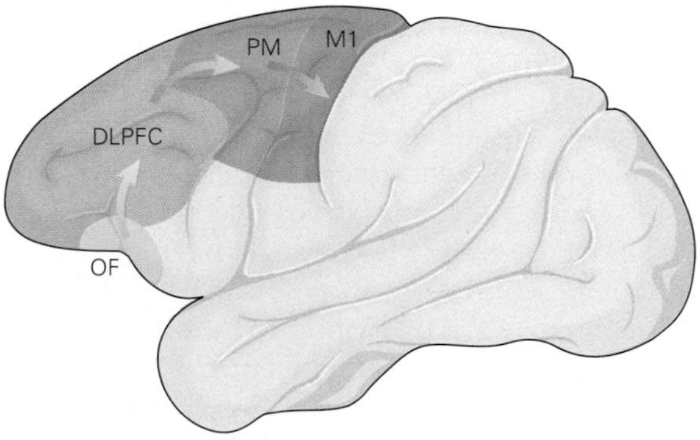

Figure 18–9 Regions of the frontal lobe are connected in series. Emotional and cognitive processes in the prefrontal cortex exert control over behavior through a pathway that begins in the orbitofrontal-ventromedial prefrontal cortex (**OF**) and from there projects to the dorsolateral prefrontal cortex (**DLPFC**), the premotor cortex (**PM**), and finally the primary motor cortex (**M1**).

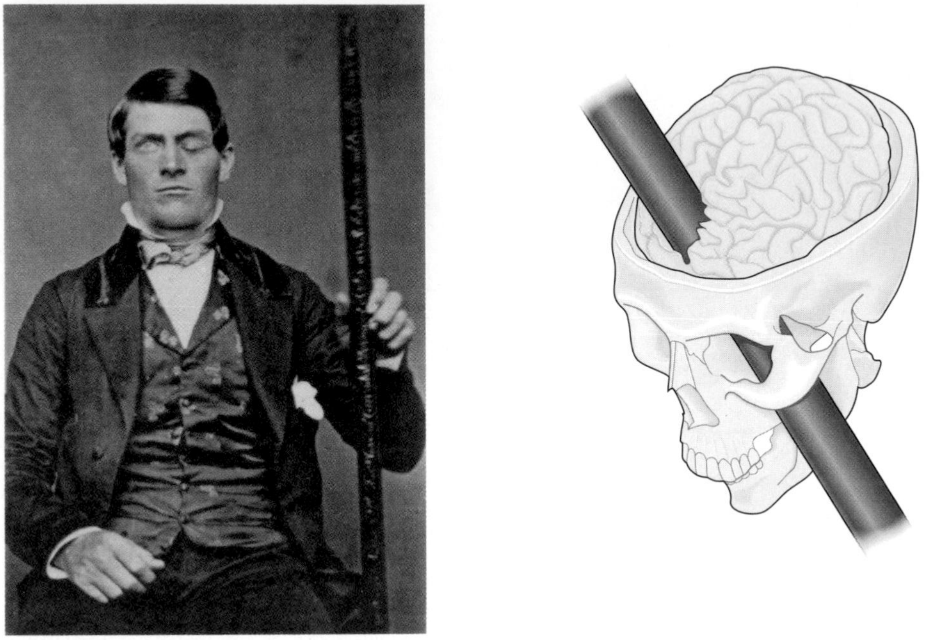

Figure 18–10 A 19th century case revealing the dependence of personality on prefrontal cortex.

Left: Phineas Gage with the 3-foot long tamping iron that was driven through his head by an explosion. (Adapted and reproduced, with permission, from the collection of Phyllis Gage Hartley.)

Right: A computer reconstruction of a drawing of the passage of the tamping iron through Gage's brain. This injury resulted in severe personality changes that added to our understanding of the function of the frontal lobes. (Adapted, with permission, from H. Damasio et al. 1994.)

Patients with prefrontal damage are unable to travel on their own because they will board whatever bus comes along first. They are unable to wait on tables in a restaurant because they lack the ability to respond to competing demands. One patient, an accomplished cook before sustaining brain damage, was able to use familiar recipes but could not follow new ones. If she went out to buy food she might be gone for hours, having coffee with a friend and forgetting all about the task at hand.

Emotional tone following prefrontal injury typically is characterized by flatness, shallowness, and indifference. This may take the form of loss of religious feeling, loss of appreciation for literature or music, insensitivity to the feelings of others, or indifference to the financial consequences of one's own actions.

Similar emotional changes occur in nonhuman primates. The observation by Charles Jacobsen that chimpanzees with prefrontal lesions no longer became upset when they failed to perform simple tasks led the Portuguese neurosurgeon Egas Moniz to introduce prefrontal lobotomy as a last-resort treatment for uncontrollable behavioral problems in patients with mental illness. This treatment was ultimately abandoned because of its devastating and irreversible damage to the patient's personality. Although cognitive and affective problems often occur together, cognitive deficits are especially pronounced after injury to dorsolateral prefrontal cortex, whereas emotional abnormalities are especially pronounced after orbital-ventromedial injury.

Dorsolateral Prefrontal Cortex Contributes to Cognitive Control of Behavior

Injury to the dorsolateral prefrontal cortex results in cognitive deficits that are manifested in a number of objective tests ranging from the very complex to the remarkably simple. An example of a complex test is to send patients on a shopping expedition with a set of specific instructions on where to go and what to buy. Typically, patients do not comply with the instructions, break accepted rules of social interaction, proceed inefficiently, and consequently fail to obtain all of the items specified.

A simple test that is highly sensitive to dorsolateral prefrontal damage is the Wisconsin Card Sort Test. Subjects are given a deck of cards printed with symbols and must select one card at a time and place it next to one of four samples. Told only whether each choice is correct or incorrect, they must discover by trial and error whether the correct choice is based on the number of symbols on the card, their shape, or their color (Figure 18–11). Patients with lesions of the dorsolateral prefrontal cortex persist in using an unsuccessful strategy, making so-called perseverative errors. They also make capricious errors, abandoning a successful rule unnecessarily. It is as if conscious oversight of behavior has been weakened, releasing habitual or random responses that are normally suppressed. It is easy to see how this condition could give rise to erratic behavior in everyday tasks.

Tests of verbal fluency are also sensitive indicators of dorsolateral prefrontal injury. When instructed to write down as many five-letter words as possible beginning with the letter "R" within a limited period of time, patients with prefrontal lesions produce relatively few words and sometimes break the rule by generating words with fewer or more letters than the required number. Asked about what it is like to perform this task, one patient said: "My brain becomes a blank. I completely run out of words. I can't think any more."

Studies of nonhuman primates have helped us understand the functions of the prefrontal cortex. Systematic study of prefrontal contributions to cognition began with Jacobsen's demonstration in the 1930s that chimpanzees with prefrontal lesions do poorly in delayed-response tasks. In a typical delayed-response task the animal is allowed to watch while food is placed under one of two objects and a curtain is drawn. After a delay the curtain is raised, and the animal is allowed to lift one of the two objects. If the animal chooses the object covering the piece of food, it is allowed to retrieve and eat the food. The success rate is lower in animals with prefrontal lesions than in normal controls, especially with long delays. Later studies in macaque monkeys showed that this deficit results specifically from injury to the dorsolateral prefrontal cortex in and around the principal sulcus, roughly coincident with Brodmann's area 46.

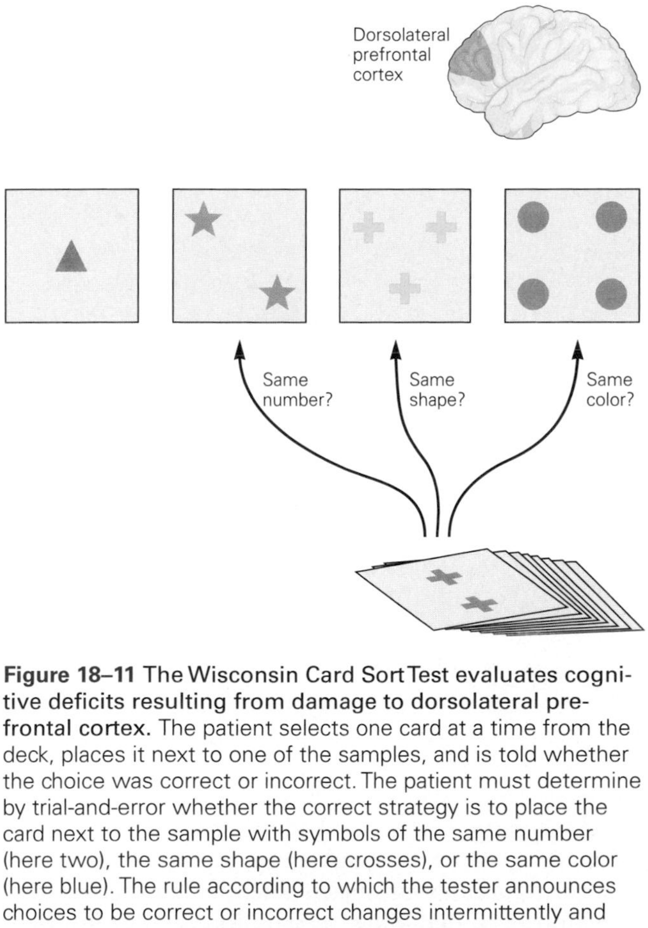

Figure 18–11 The Wisconsin Card Sort Test evaluates cognitive deficits resulting from damage to dorsolateral prefrontal cortex. The patient selects one card at a time from the deck, places it next to one of the samples, and is told whether the choice was correct or incorrect. The patient must determine by trial-and-error whether the correct strategy is to place the card next to the sample with symbols of the same number (here two), the same shape (here crosses), or the same color (here blue). The rule according to which the tester announces choices to be correct or incorrect changes intermittently and without warning. Healthy subjects rapidly adjust their strategy, but patients with prefrontal damage typically continue to use the old strategy long after it has ceased to be effective. (Reproduced, with permission, from Milner and Petrides 1984.)

Single-cell recordings in the prefrontal cortex of monkeys have cast light on why neuronal activity here is important to delayed-response performance. The ocular delayed-response task has been widely used in such investigations. Early in each trial, while the monkey is looking at a spot projected in the center of a screen, an image flashes briefly in the periphery of the screen. After the peripheral image has been extinguished the monkey must continue to fixate the central spot until it goes off, which is the instruction to look to the peripheral location where the image had appeared. During the delay period some neurons in the dorsolateral prefrontal cortex are active; these neurons are selective for specific locations. For example, a neuron may fire strongly when the monkey is planning to move to the left but only weakly when movement to the right is planned. This neuronal activity during the delay between a stimulus and the response maintains information on the location of the stimulus after it has vanished.

Is such activity in the prefrontal cortex related specifically to planning movements or to a more general function such as working memory? (Working memory is the ability to hold information in mind and manipulate it mentally, as when dialing a telephone number or doing mental arithmetic.) To answer this question, researchers carried out single-cell recordings in monkeys that had to remember information without planning a specific movement. Under these conditions some prefrontal neurons were active (Figure 18–12), indicating that prefrontal cortex is not concerned exclusively with planning movement. Nevertheless, working memory and executive control of movement may be related because both depend on the ability to retain information over time. Presumably a patient who is sent to buy food but ends up going off with a friend is unable to hold in her mind the plan with which she set out.

Orbital-Ventromedial Prefrontal Cortex Contributes to Emotional Control of Behavior

The orbital-ventromedial prefrontal cortex plays a critical role in goal-directed behavior because of its

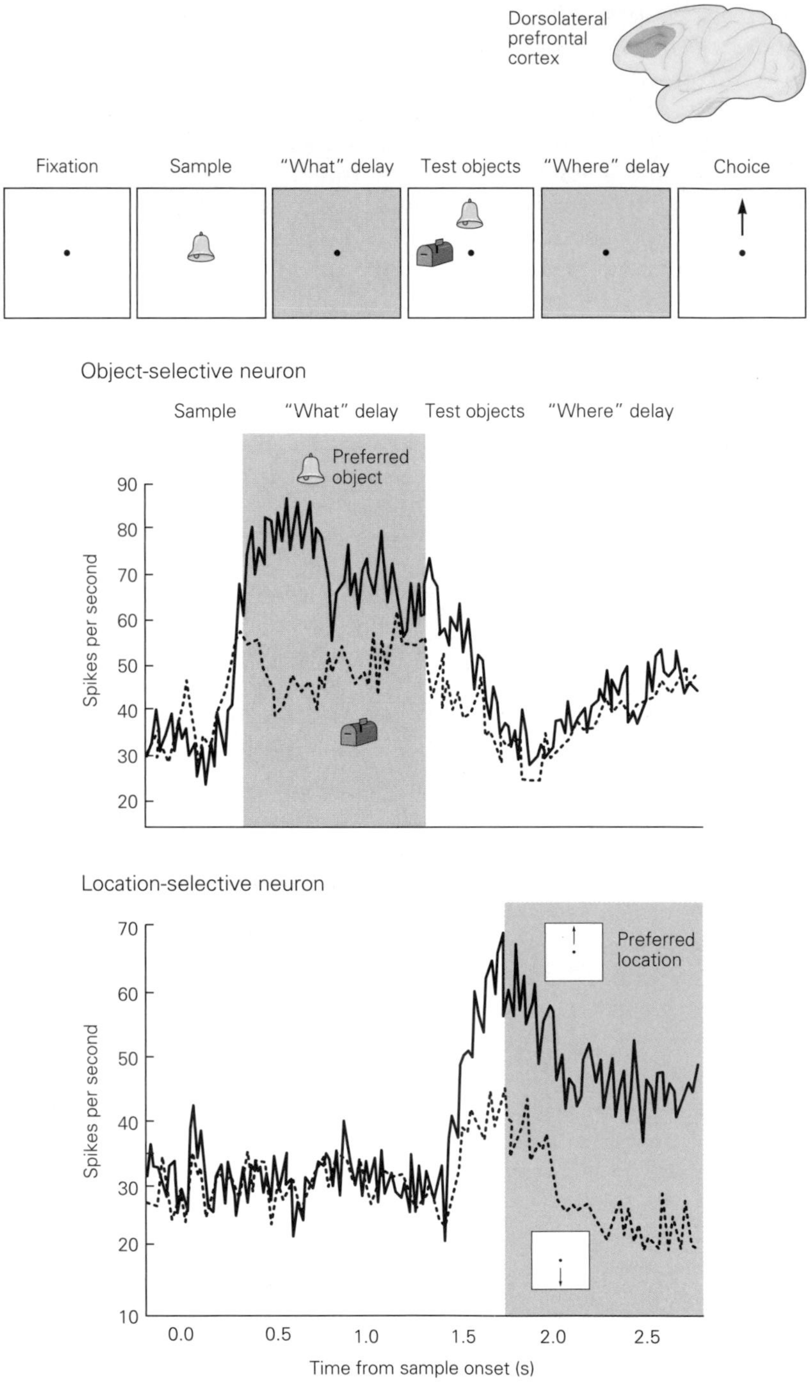

Figure 18–12 Neurons in the dorsolateral prefrontal cortex of a monkey are involved in holding information in working memory. In the experiment illustrated here a trial begins with the monkey looking at a small spot in the center of the screen. Then a sample object (in this case a bell) appears briefly. The screen is then left blank for a period during which the monkey has to fixate a central spot and remember what object was presented (the "what" delay). Two test objects are then displayed at different locations on the screen (in this case the bell at the screen's top and a mailbox at the screen's left). The monkey has to recognize the object matching the previous sample (the bell) and note its location (at the top of the screen). The display then vanishes and a second delay period ensues during which the monkey has to fixate the spot in the screen center and remember where the matching object was presented (the "where" delay). At the end of the delay four dots are displayed in the periphery and the fixation spot is extinguished. To complete the trial successfully the monkey has to make an eye movement to the dot at the location where the matching object appeared (the top of the screen in this example).

The firing rate of two neurons is shown as a function of time during the trial. During the "what" delay (requiring the monkey to remember what image had been presented) a typical object-selective prefrontal neuron was more active when the monkey was correctly remembering a bell rather than choosing the alternative object (in this trial a mailbox). During the "where" delay (requiring the monkey to remember where to make an eye movement) a typical location-sensitive neuron was more active when the monkey was preparing to shift his gaze upward than downward. (Reproduced, with permission, from Rao et al. 1997.)

connections to three neural systems. (1) It is linked strongly to the hypothalamus and amygdala, subcortical structures that mediate homeostatic drive states such as hunger and thirst and instinctual drive states such as those that underlie fear, aggression, and mating. Through these connections it has access to information about various drives. (2) It receives input from every sensory system including the gustatory and olfactory systems. Through these inputs it has access to information about objects such as their color, texture, and taste that allow recognition and appropriate emotional responses. (3) It projects to the dorsolateral prefrontal cortex, which in turn projects to premotor cortex. Through this pathway it is in a position to trigger appropriate behavior. For example, if hunger were strong and a nearby fruit had the color, texture, and taste of ripeness, then the orbital-ventromedial prefrontal cortex could trigger eating.

In some patients with injury to the orbital-ventromedial prefrontal cortex the emotional control of behavior is severely affected, although cognitive impairments are relatively minor. One such patient, EVR, performed at normal or above normal levels on numerous tests of cognitive ability, including the Wisconsin Card Sort Test. Yet in day-to-day life he was incapacitated in part by impaired decision making. His indecisiveness in selecting a restaurant exemplifies the problems that beset him. It could take him hours to choose a restaurant as he drove to each one and carefully considered the relative merits of the menu, seating plan, and atmosphere.

Patients like EVR fail in clinical tests of decision making as well. In the Gambling Task the participant selects at will one card at a time from any of four decks. With some selections the subject receives a reward, with others a penalty is imposed. The schedule of rewards and penalties is such that decks A and B deliver larger individual rewards but lower net returns. Healthy subjects learn by trial and error to avoid these bad decks and to select from decks C and D instead. EVR showed the opposite pattern, persisting in a losing strategy (Figure 18–13). Presumably he did so because he lacked

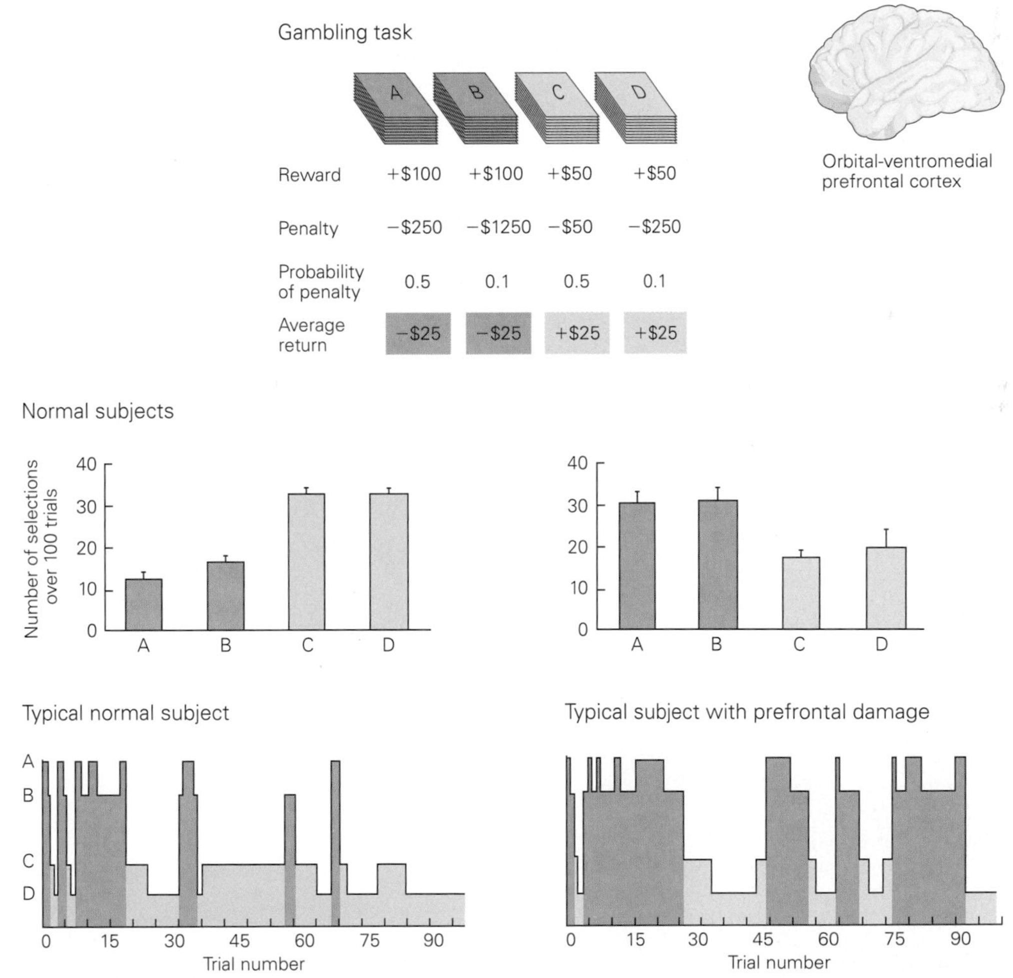

Figure 18–13 Injury to the orbital-ventromedial prefrontal cortex impairs anticipation of the consequences of decisions. This impairment is evident in a gambling task. Choosing cards from two stacks (A and B) leads to a net loss, whereas choosing from the other two (C and D) leads to a net gain. Healthy subjects learn by trial and error to make the majority of their choices from stacks C and D. Patients with damage to the orbital-ventromedial prefrontal cortex do not adjust their strategy over time to maximize the reward. (Reproduced, with permission, from Bechara et al. 1994.)

an aversive emotional response to the poor returns of decks A and B. Unlike healthy participants, who show apprehension by sweating when they prepare to take a card from a bad deck, EVR showed no skin conductance response before selecting a card.

Single-neuron recordings in monkeys have shown that orbitofrontal cortex activity reflects the value of anticipated rewards. In a typical testing situation the monkey is seated in front of a pair of levers. A cue presented above one lever tells the monkey what reward he will receive if he presses the lever. During the delay before the animal is permitted to respond, single neurons in the orbitofrontal cortex fire at a rate that reflects the monkey's preferences: If the animal likes raisins, most of the neurons will fire strongly when the monkey anticipates receiving a raisin (Figure 18–14).

When contextual factors alter the value the monkey attaches to a given food, the rate of neuronal firing in the orbitofrontal cortex shifts to reflect this fact. For example, neuronal responses decline as the monkey

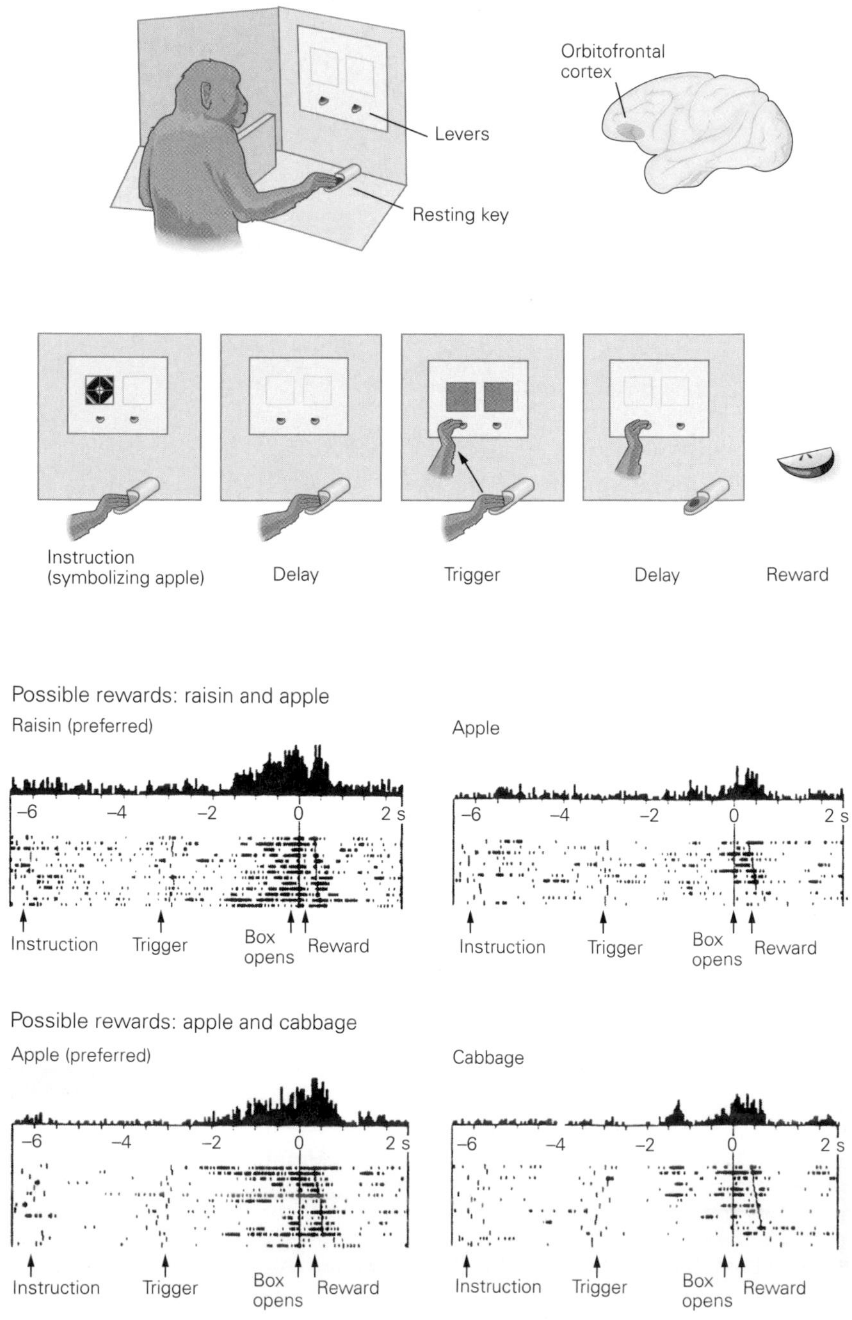

Figure 18–14 Neurons in the orbitofrontal cortex of a monkey signal the subjective value of an expected reward. In the experiment illustrated here the monkey sat facing a display screen with two buttons. He initiated a trial by depressing a key with his hand. A symbol then appeared above one of the two buttons indicating a particular food would be available by pressing that button (instruction). After a delay a pair of squares appeared (trigger), a cue to the monkey to push one button. After a further delay the door of a food box opened, giving him access to the predicted reward. The histograms are from an orbitofrontal neuron that fired as the time for reward approached but only if the expected reward was the preferred food of a pair of alternatives. The monkey preferred raisins over apples and apples over cabbage (determined by his choices on trials, not shown, when he was allowed to choose between alternatives). Each histogram indicates the average firing rate across many trials. The rows of dots underneath each histogram represent action potentials fired on individual trials. (Reproduced, with permission, from Tremblay and Schultz 1999.)

becomes satiated. They can also increase or decrease when the subjective value of a given food is increased or decreased by pairing it with alternatives that the monkey likes less or more. A typical neuron fires strongly or weakly when the monkey anticipates a piece of apple, depending on whether the alternative is a less preferred food (a piece of cabbage) or a more preferred food (a raisin). The relation between single-neuron studies in the monkey and clinical observations of patients with orbital-ventromedial prefrontal damage is clear. The loss of neurons that signal the appetitive value of anticipated rewards might well give rise to decision-making problems such as difficulty in selecting a restaurant.

Limbic Association Cortex Is a Gateway to the Hippocampal Memory System

The cortex at the edge of the cortical surface forms a ring that is visible in a medial view of the hemisphere. Because it coincides with the edge (or limbus) of the cortical surface this ring is termed the *limbic lobe* or *limbic association cortex* (Figure 18–15).

Several decades ago it was thought that the limbic lobe association cortex, together with a collection of subcortical structures including the amygdala and hypothalamus, formed a unitary system, the "limbic system," that served homeostatic and instinctual drives (see Chapters 47 and 48). This classic description certainly applies to the orbital and ventromedial prefrontal areas described in the preceding section. These two areas belong to the limbic lobe, are strongly connected to the amygdala and hypothalamus, and contribute to

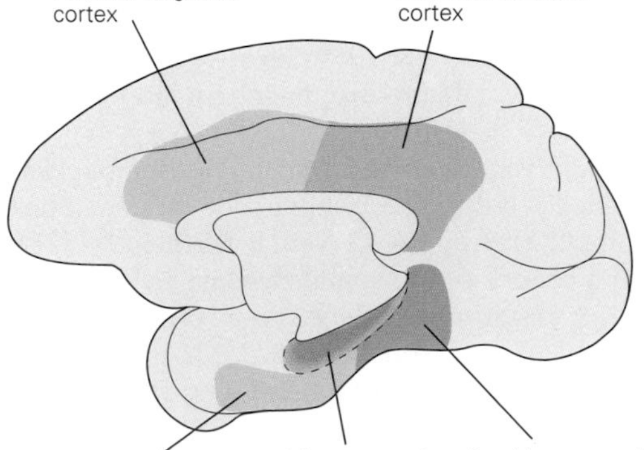

Figure 18–15 The limbic lobe includes the hippocampal formation. The hippocampal formation, including the hippocampus and subicular complex, plays a decisive role in forming long-term episodic memory. The functions of the other limbic areas on the medial surface are not well understood.

emotional processes. Other limbic lobe regions, however, are not primarily concerned with emotions. For example, the hippocampal formation which is part of the limbic lobe plays a critical role in episodic memory, the ability to remember past events including those with little or no emotional content.

The hippocampal formation consists of the hippocampus and the subiculum to which it is linked. The hippocampal formation mediates the formation of long-term memories and is critical for memory consolidation. Injury to it results in anterograde amnesia; patients are unable to form new memories but retain old memories. As we shall learn in Chapters 65 and 66, the hippocampus is thought to store memories temporarily through long-term synaptic plasticity. The hippocampus then transfers these memories to neocortex by inducing a replay in parietal, temporal, and frontal association cortex of activity patterns elicited by recent events. As a result, these cortical areas ultimately form their own stored representations of the events. Memories stored in the cortex are not dependent on the hippocampus and survive its loss.

The other divisions of the limbic lobe (Figure 18–15) serve as intermediaries between the hippocampal formation and the frontal, parietal, and temporal association areas. Their individual functions are not yet well understood.

An Overall View

The unimodal sensory and motor areas of the cerebral hemisphere occupy only a small part of the cortical sheet. Adjoining and surrounding them are large regions of association cortex where cognitive processes occur. Basic principles governing the organization and operation of association cortex have emerged from comparing the results of human clinical studies and physiological and anatomical studies in monkeys.

The two main principles of cortical organization are serial and parallel processing. In posterior cortex sensory information is extracted in a series of unimodal areas with increasingly complex functions. Each sensory modality (visual, auditory, or somatosensory) is processed in a chain of cortical areas leading outward from the primary sensory area. Parallel dorsal and ventral subdivisions of each modality process aspects of sensory information important for spatial behavior and for stimulus identification. Within each sensory modality, areas that process spatial information form a dorsal stream leading to parietal association cortex whereas areas that process feature information form a ventral stream leading to temporal association cortex.

The parietal association cortex, in addition to receiving convergent input from multiple sensory systems, is also strongly linked to motor areas in the dorsal frontal lobe. In humans injury to the parietal cortex results in disorders of body awareness, motor control, visual guidance of behavior, spatial vision, and spatial cognition. In monkeys parietal neurons fire in response to sensory stimuli and during motor behavior; their firing is selective for the spatial attributes of both objects and actions.

The temporal association cortex, in addition to receiving input from multiple sensory systems, is strongly linked to areas in the ventral frontal lobe concerned with emotion and cognition. In humans injury to the temporal lobe creates the agnosias (disorders of recognition), Wernicke aphasia (a disorder of speech comprehension), and the degradation of semantic memory. Thus the functions of temporal cortex include recognizing things and storing knowledge about them. In monkeys temporal neurons fire in response to sensory stimuli, and their firing is selective for the features of objects that are important for recognition.

The frontal association cortex consists of the dorsolateral and ventromedial prefrontal areas. These areas play a critical role in the executive control of behavior. The dorsolateral prefrontal cortex is important for maintaining intention. In humans injury to this region results in disorganized behavior and distractibility. In monkeys neuronal activity in this region represents working memory or plans of action.

The orbital-ventromedial prefrontal cortex contributes to motivational states by representing the emotional value of objects that might become targets of action. Injury to this cortex in humans results in a failure to properly value the expected consequences of an action. In monkeys neuronal activity in this region encodes the value of expected rewards.

The limbic association cortex, through its connections with the hippocampus, plays an important role in long-term episodic memory formation.

Carl R. Olson
Carol L. Colby

Selected Readings

Colby CL, Goldberg ME. 1999. Space and attention in parietal cortex. Annu Rev Neurosci 22:319–349.

Feinberg TE, Farah MJ. 2003. *Behavioral Neurology and Neuropsychology*. New York: McGraw-Hill.

Goldman-Rakic PS. 1996. The prefrontal landscape: implications of functional architecture for understanding human mentation and the central executive. Philos Trans R Soc Lond B Biol Sci 351:1445–1453.

Kolb B, Whishaw IQ. 2003. *Fundamentals of Human Neuropsychology*, 5th ed. New York: Worth.

Miller EK, Cohen JD. 2001. An integrative theory of prefrontal cortex function. Annu Rev Neurosci 24:167–202.

Olson CR. 2003. Brain representation of object-centered space in monkeys and humans. Annu Rev Neurosci 26:331–354.

Rolls ET. 1996. The orbitofrontal cortex. Philos Trans R Soc Lond B Biol Sci 351:1433–1443.

Squire LR, Stark CE, Clark RE. 2004. The medial temporal lobe. Annu Rev Neurosci 27:279–306.

Tanaka K. 1996. Inferotemporal cortex and object vision. Annu Rev Neurosci 19:109–139.

Van Essen DC. 2003. Organization of visual areas in macaque and human cerebral cortex. In: LM Chalupa, JS Werner (eds). *The Visual Neurosciences*, pp. 507–521. Cambridge, MA: MIT Press.

References

Barbas H. 2000. Connections underlying the synthesis of cognition, memory, and emotion in primate prefrontal cortices. Brain Res Bull 52:319–330.

Batista AP, Buneo CA, Snyder LH, Andersen RA. 1999. Reach plans in eye-centered coordinates. Science 285:257–260.

Bechara A, Damasio AR, Damasio H, Anderson SW. 1994. Insensitivity to future consequences following damage to human prefrontal cortex. Cognition 50:7–15.

Colby CL, Duhamel JR, Goldberg ME. 1996. Visual, presaccadic and cognitive activation of single neurons in monkey lateral intraparietal area. J Neurophysiol 76:2841–2852.

Critchley M. 1953. *The Parietal Lobes*. New York: Hafner.

Damasio H, Grabowski T, Frank R, Galaburda AM, Damasio AR. 1994. The return of Phineas Gage: clues about the brain from the skull of a famous patient. Science 264:1102–1105.

Duhamel JR, Colby CL, Goldberg ME. 1998. Ventral intraparietal area of the macaque: congruent visual and somatic response properties. J Neurophysiol 79:126–136.

Eslinger PJ, Damasio AR. 1985. Severe disturbance of higher cognition after bilateral frontal lobe ablation: patient EVR. Neurol 35:1731–1741.

Felleman DJ, van Essen DC. 1991. Distributed hierarchical processing in the primate cerebral cortex. Cereb Cortex 1:1–47.

Friedman DP, Murray EA, O'Neill B, Mishkin M. 1986. Cortical connections of the somatosensory fields of the lateral sulcus of macaques: evidence for a corticolimbic pathway for touch. J Comp Neurol 252:323–347.

Funahashi S, Bruce CJ, Goldman-Rakic PS. 1993. Dorsolateral prefrontal lesions and oculomotor delayed-response performance: evidence for mnemonic "scotomas." J Neurosci 13:1479–1497.

Harlow JM. 1868. Recovery from the passage of an iron bar through the head. Publications of the Massachusetts Medical Society 2:327–347.

Jacobsen CF. 1935. Function of the frontal association area in primates. Arch Neurol Psychiatry 33:558–569.

Jeannerod M. 1986. The formation of finger grip during prehension. A cortically mediated visuomotor pattern. Behav Brain Res 19:99–116.

Kaas JH, Hackett TA. 1999. "What" and "where" processing in auditory cortex. Nat Neurosci 2:1045–1047.

Kobatake E, Wang G, Tanaka K. 1998. Effects of shape-discrimination training on the selectivity of inferotemporal cells in adult monkeys. J Neurophysiol 80:324–330.

Luria AR. 1968. *Higher Cortical Functions in Man*. New York: Basic Books.

Milner B, Petrides M. 1984. Behavioural effects of frontal-lobe lesions in man. Trends Neurosci 7:403–407.

Murata A, Gallese V, Luppino G, Kaseda M, Sakata H. 2000. Selectivity for the shape, size, and orientation of objects for grasping in neurons of monkey parietal area AIP. J Neurophysiol 83:2580–2601.

Perenin MT, Vighetto A. 1988. Optic ataxia: a specific disruption in visuo-motor mechanisms. I: Different aspects of the deficit in reaching for objects. Brain 111(Pt. 3): 643–674.

Rao SC, Rainer G, Miller EK. 1997. Integration of what and where in the primate prefrontal cortex. Science 276:821–824.

Rondot P, de Recondo J, Dumas JL. 1977. Visuomotor ataxia. Brain 100:355–376.

Rubens AB, Benson DF. 1971. Associative visual agnosia. Arch Neurol 24:305–316.

Rylander G. 1948. Personality analysis before and after frontal lobotomy. In: *The Frontal Lobes,* Proceedings of the Association for Research in Nervous and Mental Disease, December 12 and 13, 1947, pp. 691–705. New York: Hafner.

Tian B, Reser D, Durham A, Kustov A, Rauschecker JP. 2001. Functional specialization in rhesus monkey auditory cortex. Science 292:290–293.

Tremblay L, Schultz W. 1999. Relative reward preference in primate orbitofrontal cortex. Nature 398:704–708.

Trojano L, Grossi D. 1998. "Pure" constructional apraxia—a cognitive analysis of a single case. Behav Neurol 11:43–49.

Ungerleider LG, Mishkin M. 1982. Two cortical visual systems. In: DJ Ingle, MA Goodale, RJW Mansfield (eds). *Analysis of Visual Behavior*, pp. 549–586. Cambridge, MA: MIT Press.

Vaina LM. 1994. Functional segregation of color and motion processing in the human visual cortex: clinical evidence. Cereb Cortex 4:555–572.

Van Essen DC, Drury HA, Dickson J, Harwell J, Hanlon D, Anderson CH. 2001. An integrated software suite for surface-based analyses of cerebral cortex. J Am Med Inform Assoc 8:443–459.

Wapner W, Judd T, Gardner H. 1978. Visual agnosia in an artist. Cortex 14:343–364.

19

Cognitive Functions of the Premotor Systems

In Chapter 18 we surveyed the higher-order organization of sensory systems. In this chapter we turn to the higher-order functioning of the motor systems, by examining how the brain represents behavioral goals and how voluntary actions are planned to achieve those goals. To illustrate how the motor systems generate goal-oriented behavior, we focus on reaching and grasping, actions that are possible because of the prehensile hand.

The evolution of the prehensile hand greatly enriched the development of cognitive capacities in primates. Indeed, the two are interdependent. As the German philosopher Friedrich Engels wrote: "Man alone has succeeded in impressing his stamp on nature. He has accomplished this primarily and essentially by means of the hand. But step by step with the development of the hand went that of the brain."

The prehensile hand radically changed the way in which primates relate to the external world; but the change occurred slowly, and required the evolution of cortical circuits for a variety of new specialized movements adapted to different objects. In his book *The Sensory Hand,* Vernon Mountcastle, one of the pioneers in the study of the connection between sensation and action, quotes Herbert Spencer (*Principles of Psychology,* 1885) on why the hand is so critical to understanding action:

> All that we need notice here is the extent to which in the human race a perfect tactual apparatus subserves the highest processes of the intellect. I do not mean merely that the tangible attributes of things rendered completely cognisable by the complex adjustments of the human hands, and the accompanying manipulative powers have made possible those populous societies in which alone a wide intelligence can be evolved. I mean the most far-reaching cognitions, and inferences (even those) most remote from perception, have their roots in the . . . impression which the human hands can receive.

The final neural pathway for all bodily actions, including movement of the hand, is through motor neurons in the ventral horn of the spinal cord. These motor neurons are not simply responding to independently generated sensory information, however. The sensory information needed for action is the product of interaction between the motor systems and sensory systems. Under many circumstances, therefore, action and perception are inseparable. Indeed, many sensory functions serve only to allow for the planning of motor acts. As we focus on and reach for a cup of coffee, our arm is controlled in a manner that is independent of conscious experience—we do not think about which movements to perform and which muscles to contract.

Perception of space, and even more complex cognitive acts, were once thought to be represented only in higher-order sensory and association areas of cerebral cortex. In a radical departure from previous thinking, we now believe that the premotor areas in the cortex may also have cognitive functions.

At the highest levels of sensory-motor interaction, neurons do not simply encode the physical features of the sensory stimulus or the force or direction of movement. Rather, they encode something more abstract that includes features of both the object and the movement: They encode the relationship between the body and the object with respect to a particular goal. For example, in anticipation of drinking they may represent a configuration of the hand in relation to graspable features of a cup.

Direct Connections Between the Cerebral Cortex and Spinal Cord Play a Fundamental Role in the Organization of Voluntary Movements

Although picking up a cup appears to be a simple mechanical action, the neural machinery underlying it is surprisingly complex, requiring a number of preparatory steps in the parietal and frontal premotor and motor cortex.

As discussed in Chapter 1, the discovery that electrical stimulation of different parts of the frontal lobe produces movements of the opposite side of the body had a major effect on thinking about localization of function in the brain. Brodmann's area 4, the area in the frontal lobe in which the lowest-intensity stimulation elicited movement, was designated the primary motor cortex (Figure 19–1). By systematically stimulating the primary motor cortex and attributing the movement elicited with each stimulus to the activation of neurons near the electrodes, researchers identified

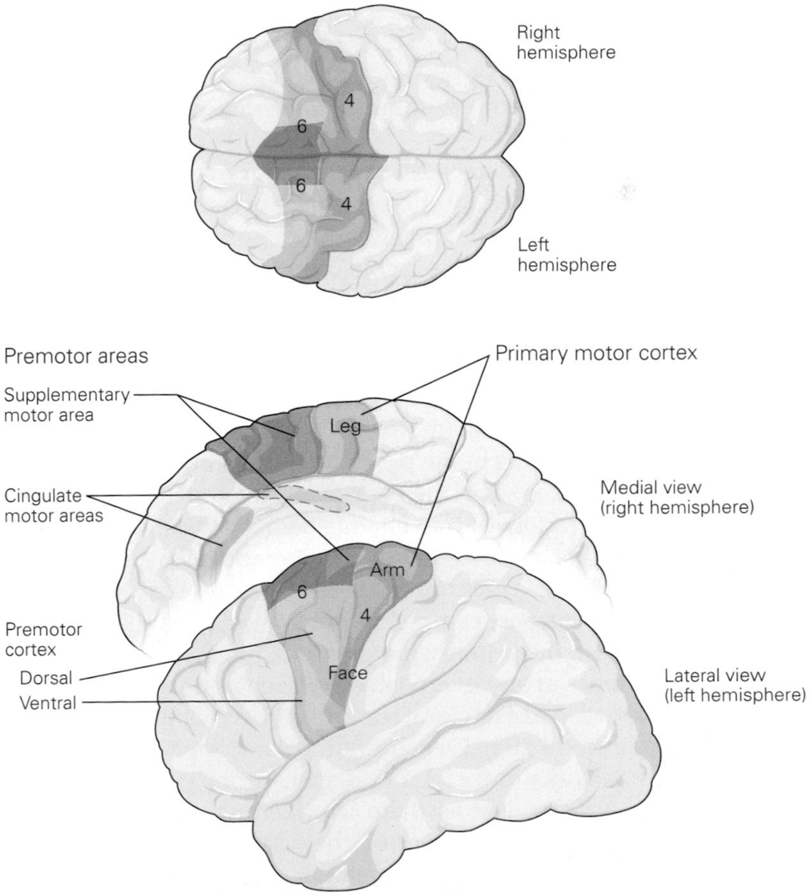

Figure 19–1 The cortical motor areas. The cortical motor areas lie largely in Brodmann's area 4 and area 6. Area 6 includes the supplementary motor area located largely on the medial brain surface, and the dorsal and ventral premotor areas located on the lateral surface. Area 4 includes the face, arm, and leg representations of the primary motor cortex. Additional motor areas are located in and around the banks of the cingulate sulcus.

groups of neurons that controlled movement of specific body parts and learned that these functional groups were distributed on the cortex in the form of a somatotopic map.

In recent years our understanding of the functional organization of the motor areas of the cerebral cortex has changed dramatically, and a new picture of the cortical control of movement is emerging. The functional organization of the primary motor cortex is not simply an isomorphic map of the body in which adjacent peripheral sites are represented in adjacent cortical sites. Instead, individual muscles and joints are represented in the cortex multiple times in a complex mosaic. This makes it possible for the cortex to organize combinations of elemental movements suitable to specific tasks.

Each muscle and joint is represented by a column of neurons whose axons branch and terminate in several functionally related spinal motor nuclei (this branching is minimal for cortical cells that control distal muscles because these muscles require more independent control). The cortical neurons also form synapses with interneurons in the spinal cord. These connections allow voluntary movements to switch on entire spinal circuits—the motor neurons, interneurons, and central pattern generators that execute reflex actions. These circuits are then able to integrate and convert local sensory input to motor output without further direction from cortical centers.

In the 1930s physiologists discovered that movement could also be elicited by stimulation of premotor areas. Brodmann's area 6 contains four main premotor areas that project directly to the spinal cord. Two areas lie on the lateral surface and two on the medial surface in Brodmann's area 6 (Figure 19–1.) Each of these four cortical areas may be viewed as a relay in a densely interconnected network that controls reaching and grasping by activating spinal motor circuits.

In contrast to neurons in the primary motor cortex, movement-related neurons in the premotor areas fire in connection with a variety of movements because these neurons encode a general goal-directed command such as "grasp the cup" or "pick up the raisin." Neurons called set-related neurons, common in premotor areas but relatively rare in the primary motor cortex, are more active in the absence of any overt behavior, such as during the delay between a behavioral cue and the behavior. Other neurons encode global sensorimotor transformations, such as "always move at 180 degrees from the visual stimulus." Thus, just as there is a hierarchy of spinal and supraspinal motor control, there is a hierarchy of representations of movement features within the different motor and premotor areas of the cortex.

To produce movement, signals from premotor and motor areas of the cortex must ultimately reach motor neurons in the spinal cord. The Dutch anatomist Hans Kuypers identified three motor pathways: a direct corticospinal pathway and two indirect pathways, the medial and lateral brain stem systems (Figure 19–2).

The historically well-known *corticospinal system* is involved in the control of all aspects of body and limb movement but has a special role in the fractionated movements necessary for skilled motor acts such as playing the piano or typing. Much of the control of fractionated movements is exercised by the primary motor cortex. Thus, a lesion of the primary motor cortex destroys the ability to oppose the thumb and first finger so as to pick up a raisin or grasp a cup. A patient with such damage is unable to move the fingers independently and can only grasp a cup clumsily.

In humans the corticospinal tract consists of approximately one million axons, of which 30% to 40% originate from neurons in the primary motor cortex. The rest of the axons have their origins mainly in the premotor and supplementary motor cortices, and in the parietal areas lying posterior to the precentral sulcus. Together, corticospinal axons from these various areas descend through the subcortical white matter, internal capsule, and cerebral peduncle. As the fibers of the corticospinal tract descend they form the medullary pyramids, prominent protuberances on the ventral surface of the medulla. Consequently the entire projection is sometimes called the pyramidal tract. Like the ascending somatosensory system, most fibers of the descending corticospinal tract cross the midline in the medulla, at the pyramidal decussation, to terminate in the spinal cord of the opposite side.

The motor information carried in the corticospinal tract is significantly modulated by a continuous stream of information from other motor regions as well as tactile, visual, and proprioceptive information needed to make voluntary movement both accurate and properly sequenced.

The *medial brain stem system* originates in portions of the reticular formation, vestibular nuclei, and superior colliculus. This system receives information from the cortex and other motor centers for the control of posture and locomotion. The *lateral brain stem system* originates from the red nucleus. It receives input from the cortex as well but is involved in the control of arm and hand movements.

Spinal motor circuits are not regulated solely by descending commands. Reflex circuits and pattern generators within the spinal cord can coordinate stereotyped movements such as stepping without

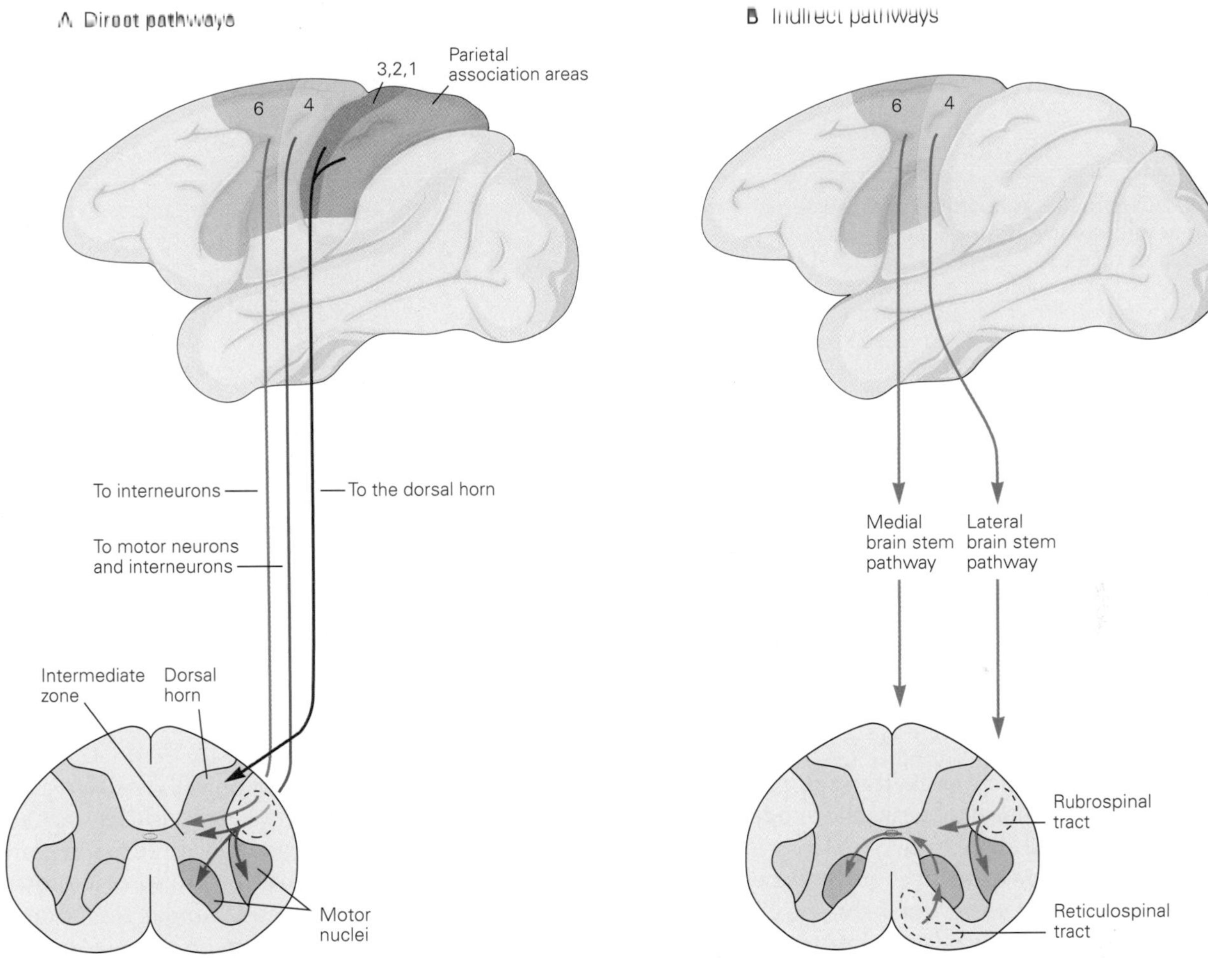

Figure 19–2 Direct and indirect motor pathways to the spinal cord. In the lateral view of the human brain; numbered areas are functional areas identified by Brodmann. The transverse section of the spinal cord shows three functional areas. The dorsal horn contains the sensory neurons of the spinal cord; the intermediate zone contains interneurons; and the motor nuclei zone contains the motor neurons that innervate the muscles.

A. The corticospinal tract, also called the pyramidal tract, originates in a vast region around the central sulcus that includes the parietal lobe and the posterior part of the frontal lobe (areas 4 and 6). Area 4, the primary motor cortex, is the only area of motor cortex that directly connects with spinal motor neurons. Area 6 comprises various subareas, most of which send fibers to interneurons in the intermediate zone of the spinal cord. The parietal lobe sends fibers to the dorsal horns.

B. Indirect pathways to spinal motor neurons originate in area 4 and area 6 and terminate in medial and lateral areas of the brain stem. The main components of the medial pathways are the reticulospinal, medial and lateral vestibulospinal, and tectospinal tracts; they descend in the ventral column and terminate in the ventromedial area of the spinal gray matter. The main lateral pathway is the rubrospinal tract, which originates in the magnocellular portion of the red nucleus, descends in the contralateral dorsolateral column, and terminates in the dorsolateral area of the spinal gray matter.

descending signals (see Chapter 35). A newborn infant, whose descending pathways cannot yet control the spinal cord, is able to execute stepping movements when lifted into the air. Descending systems coordinate reflex and patterned movements generated by spinal motor circuits and can even create new patterns of muscle activation through direct action on motor neurons. This cortical control enables greater flexibility of movements than is possible through exclusively local coordination among the spinal motor circuits.

The cortical motor areas and brain stem in turn receive input from two major subcortical structures: the cerebellum and basal ganglia (Figure 19–3, and see Figure 16–9). These two structures provide feedback essential for the smooth execution of skilled movements and thus are important for motor learning,

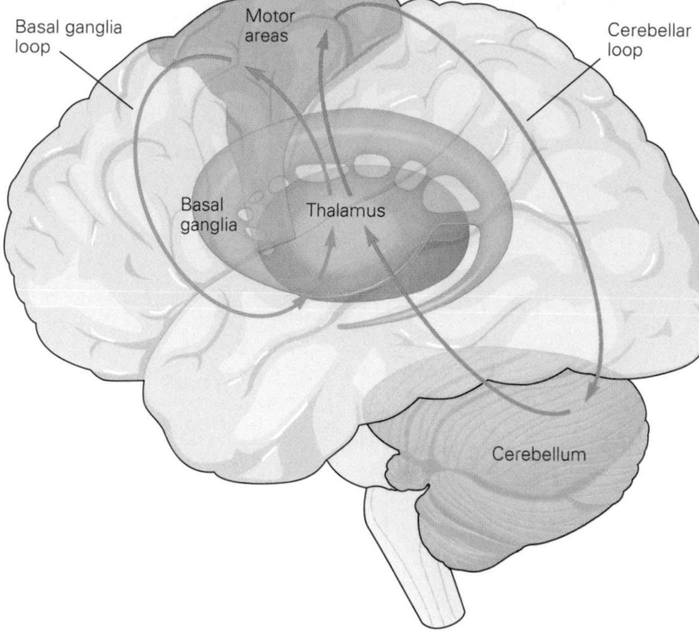

Figure 19–3 The major subcortical brain systems that initiate and control motor actions. Both the basal ganglia and cerebellum influence cortical motor circuits through connections in the thalamus. The motor cortex determines which muscle groups are activated and the magnitude of force to exert. Based on inputs from the motor cortex, basal ganglia, cerebellum, and other brain stem nuclei, the spinal cord initiates appropriate muscle contractions to accomplish purposeful movement.

the improvement in motor skills through practice. The cerebellum and the basal ganglia store memory for unconscious motor skills through pathways that are separate from those used to store factual memories of events that can be recalled consciously (see Chapter 66).

The cerebellum receives somatosensory information directly from primary afferent fibers arising in the spinal cord as well as information about movement from corticospinal axons descending from the neocortex. The basal ganglia receive direct projections from much of the neocortex, which supply both sensory information and information about movement (see Figure 16–9).

The Four Premotor Areas of the Primate Brain Also Have Direct Connections in the Spinal Cord

In primates four functionally distinct premotor areas also send direct connections to the spinal cord (see Figure 19–1).

The two areas on the lateral surface are the *lateral ventral premotor area* and *lateral dorsal premotor area.* As we shall see later, the ventral premotor cortex mostly controls mouth and hand movements. Most of its neurons do not discharge in association with simple movements toward an object. They only become active during goal-directed actions such as grasping, holding, or manipulating an object. The two areas on the medial surface are the *supplementary motor area,* which lies in the medial wall of Brodmann's area 6, and the *cingulate motor areas,* a group of motor areas buried in the cingulate sulcus. Similar premotor areas also exist in humans, but differences in size and sulcal patterns make it difficult to identify homologous areas with precision.

These four premotor areas are connected to the primary motor cortex. In addition, like the primary motor cortex, each premotor area has neurons that project to the brain stem as well as neurons that project directly to the spinal cord. Thus voluntary movements are controlled by descending signals from several cortical areas. For this reason, the task of generating limb movements is thought to be broken up into multiple subtasks, each managed in parallel by one of the several cortical motor areas.

These premotor areas also have dense reciprocal connections with the association areas in the posterior parietal cortex (Figure 19–4). These reciprocal connections constitute the visuomotor circuits that mediate different types of visually guided motor behavior such as mouth movements, arm reaching, and hand grasping.

Primates have remarkable visuomotor capacities. We can link the sight of an object with quite different actions. Seeing a cup of coffee, we can pick it up, drink from it, or throw it against the wall. As we shall learn in greater detail in the chapters on vision, some visual pathways are concerned only with perception, whereas some are concerned with planning motor acts. In fact, these two kinds of visual information are processed in separate pathways originating in different areas of cortex: the ventral (what) and dorsal (where) visual streams (Figure 19–5).

The *ventral stream* terminates ventrally in the inferotemporal lobe. It carries information that allows us to distinguish the visual properties of objects, an orange from a tennis ball, for example. Because the visual properties of the orange and the tennis ball are different, they are represented differently in the inferotemporal cortex, even though they may be the same size and occupy the same spatial location.

Charles Gross first demonstrated that the neurons in the inferotemporal cortex are highly selective for specific and complex visual stimuli. For example, some neurons are selective for individual faces, an extreme example of visual discrimination. Other neurons in the inferotemporal lobe near the superior temporal sulcus react selectively to the sight of movements of other individuals.

The *dorsal stream* terminates in the posterior parietal lobe and carries information that allows us to locate objects in space and to act on them. The dorsal stream has two branches: a dorsal (dorso-dorsal) branch and a ventral (ventro-dorsal) branch (Figure19–5B). The dorso-dorsal stream is involved in the control of movements. Damage of this pathway produces optic ataxia,

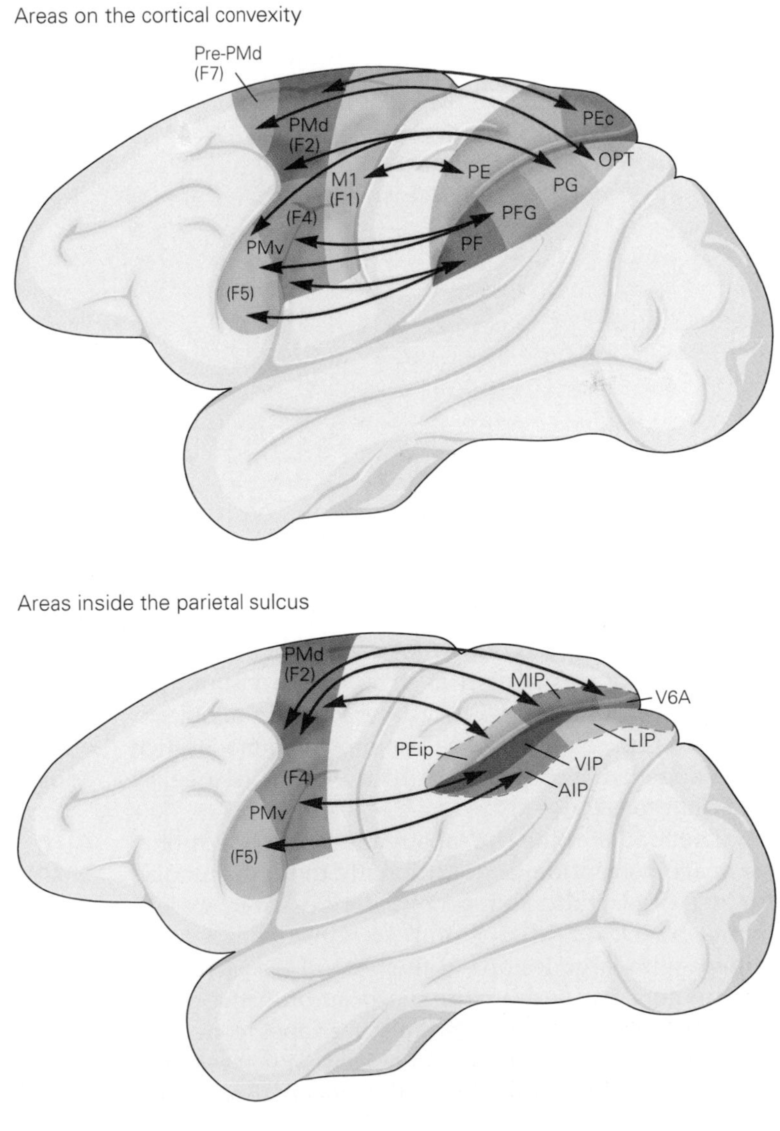

Figure 19–4 The premotor areas have rich connections with the association areas of the posterior parietal cortex. Functional areas in the posterior parietal lobe and motor areas of frontal cortex are shown in lateral views of the monkey brain. For illustration, the intraparietal sulcus is opened in the brain below. The new terms for frontal areas are indicated in parentheses. The new terminology, replacing that originally proposed by Brodmann, was advanced by Massimo Matelli and co-workers and derived from Constantino von Economo. It is based on gross anatomical location as well as cytoarchitectonic properties. The parietal areas are designated in von Economo's terminology by the letter P (parietal), followed by letters instead of numbers to indicate the cytoarchitectonically different areas. Areas **PF** and **PFG** roughly correspond to Brodmann's area 7b, areas **PG** and **OPT** to Brodmann's area 7a. Areas inside the intraparietal sulcus include the anterior, lateral, medial, and ventral intraparietal areas (**AIP**, **LIP**, **MIP**, **VIP**), as well as the PE intraparietal area (**PEip**) and visual area 6A (**V6A**).

F, frontal; **M1**, primary motor cortex; **OPT**, occipito-parieto-temporal; **P**, parietal; **PMd**, dorsal premotor cortex; **PMv**, ventral premotor cortex; **Pre-PMd**, predorsal premotor cortex.

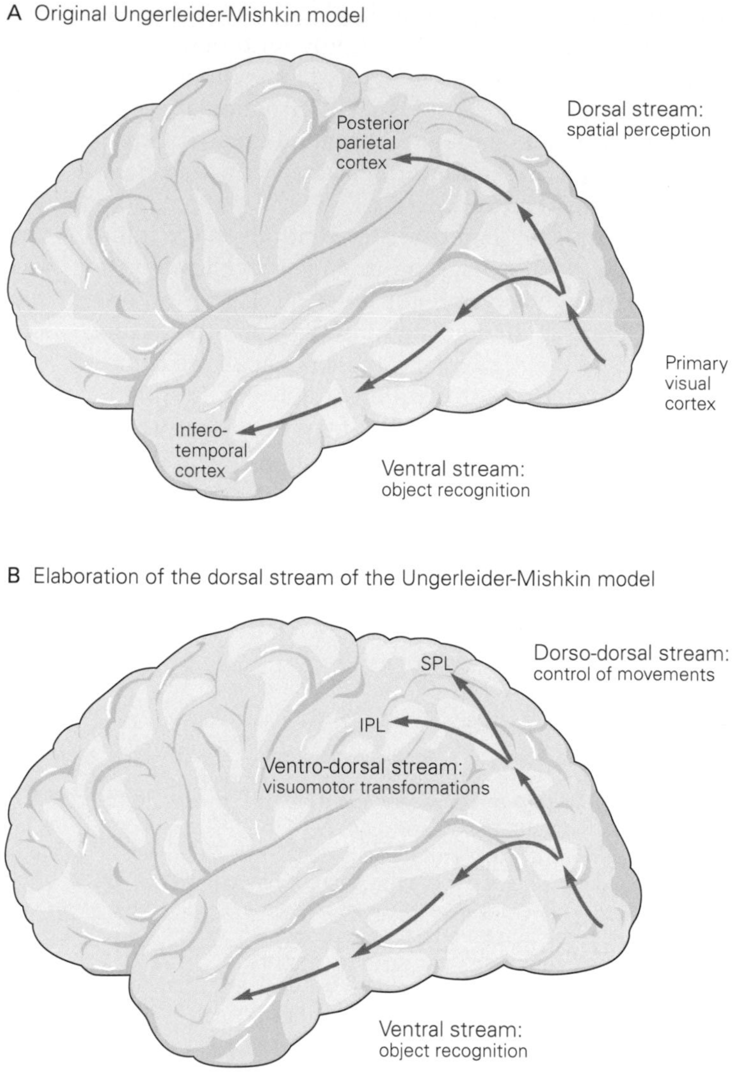

Figure 19–5 The ventral and dorsal streams of visual processing. The streams shown on a human brain are bidirectional but are shown as unidirectional for the sake of clarity. The original model of Leslie Ungerleider and Mortimer Mishkin (**A**) has been elaborated in a more recent model by Giacomo Rizzolatti and Massimo Matelli, which takes into account the subdivision of the dorsal stream into two branches (**B**). Of these two branches, the dorsal branch is involved in control of specific movements, as originally proposed by David Milner and Melvin Goodale, whereas the ventral one mediates the visuomotor transformations necessary for the organization of purposeful action, such as reaching and grasping, and perception of space and actions. The ventral branch also plays a role in interpreting the purpose of movements observed in others. (**SPL**, superior parietal lobe; **IPL**, inferior parietal lobe.)

a clinical syndrome in which the patient knows the location of objects but is unable to reach them properly. The ventro-dorsal stream is involved in visuomotor transformations necessary for interacting with objects, as well as space perception. The most common deficit following damage of this pathway is spatial neglect (see Chapter 17).

The idea that the dorsal stream is crucial not only for space perception, as traditionally thought, but also for the organization of action, derives from experiments by David Milner and Melvin Goodale on a patient with large lesions of the ventral visual stream. This patient had a dramatic dissociation between the capacity to distinguish geometric shapes conceptually and the capacity to act on objects. When asked to describe the orientation of a slot, the patient would respond virtually at chance. However, when asked to insert a card inside the slot, the patient performed the action well, moving the card toward the slot in the correct orientation and inserting it accurately (Figure 19–6). Thus the visuomotor circuits of the dorsal stream alone are capable of guiding behavior.

Motor Circuits Involved in Voluntary Actions Are Organized to Achieve Specific Goals

Voluntary initiation of movement is one of the defining characteristics of animal behavior. Reflex actions are more or less stereotypic responses to external or internal stimuli. Voluntary actions are manifestations of centrally generated intentions to move; the goal—reaching for a cup of hot coffee—determines a series of actions that will lead to its achievement.

Voluntary movements allow an animal to explore the world around it to satisfy not only immediate but also future needs. Unlike reflex behavior, the stimuli for voluntary behavior do not determine the response; they only set the occasion for it. Therefore, an animal may or may not respond to a stimulus, or it may respond to the same stimulus in different ways depending upon its needs. Under different conditions an animal may approach, avoid, or ignore the same stimulus.

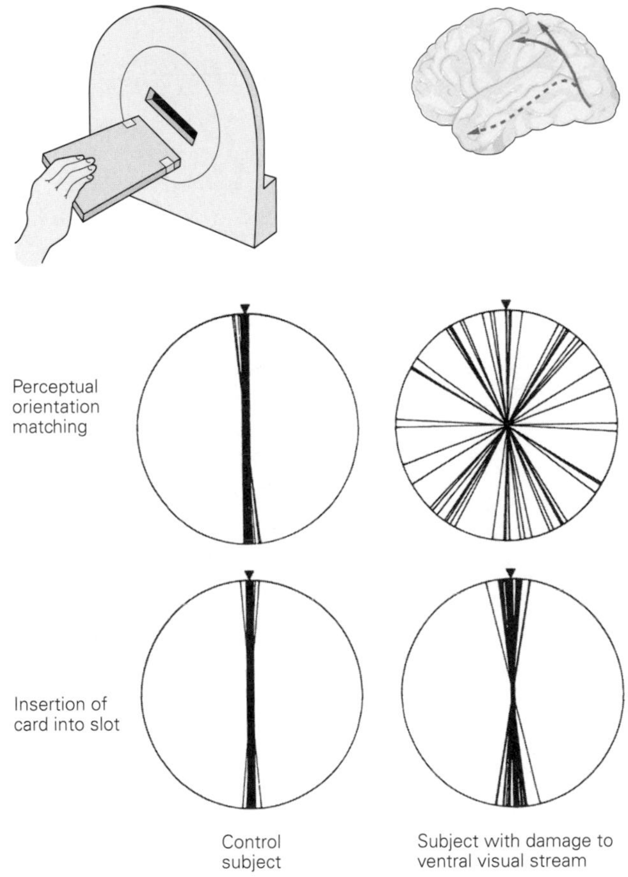

Figure 19–6 Damage to the ventral visual stream impairs conscious recognition of shape. A patient with visual agnosia caused by damage of the ventral visual stream (see Figure 19–5) and an age-matched control were tested on two tasks. Subjects were first asked to match the orientation of a hand-held card with that of a slot placed in front of them. Polar plots illustrate the variability in orientation of the card. They then were asked to insert the card into the slot. Polar plots illustrate the orientation of the card as it was brought to the slot; the correct orientation has been normalized to the vertical orientation. (Reproduced, with permission, from Milner and Goodale 2002.)

The primate brain, particularly the human brain, is characterized by an enormous expansion of the cerebral cortex. This expansion correlates with an extraordinary increase of sensory, motor, and cognitive capacities. A large part of the expansion has occurred in three regions: the rostral part of the frontal lobe (the prefrontal cortex) and two posterior regions of cortex, the posterior part of the parietal lobe and the inferotemporal cortex.

As discussed in the preceding chapters, the posterior part of the parietal lobe and the inferotemporal cortex are association areas that integrate information from different sensory modalities. This association is essential for the formation of percepts, like space and objects. Indeed, patients with lesions in the parietal cortex typically have deficits in spatial perception, whereas patients with damage in the inferotemporal cortex have problems recognizing objects and faces.

Prior to 1970 deficits in spatial perception following parietal damage were attributed to the destruction of an area that was thought to encode a single internal representation of the external world. However, a series of anatomical and functional studies have revealed that the parietal lobe contains more than one representation of space and each of these representations is strikingly dependent on motor activity.

Jaana Hyvärinen assessed the responses of individual neurons in the inferior parietal cortex to sensory stimuli and during motor behaviors. He found that most neurons respond to sensory stimuli that occur in specific locations and often to stimuli of different modalities, both visual and somatic stimuli for example. Other neurons discharge in association with motor acts. Actions carried out with different parts of the body are represented in different but overlapping zones.

This orderly representation of movements is similar to the somatotopic arrangement of somatosensory inputs in the postcentral gyrus (see Chapter 17). Neurons in the rostral part of the inferior parietal lobe discharge in relation to movements of the mouth; neurons in the central part of this lobe fire in association with hand and arm movements; those located more caudally fire in relation to eye movements. Some neurons in this region respond to objects that lie close to the subject, in the space within arm's reach (peripersonal space), without necessarily requiring that the movement actually occur. Other neurons prefer stimuli located far from an individual's body. Neurons that respond to objects in peripersonal space are located mostly in the part of the inferior parietal lobe where mouth and hand movements are represented, whereas neurons that respond preferentially to objects further away from the body are found mostly in the part of the parietal lobe where eye movements are represented.

The Hand Has a Critical Role in Primate Behavior

What are the critical steps involved in grasping? The neural control of grasping has been studied by Hideo Sakata and Giacomo Rizzolatti. Sakata investigated the anterior intraparietal area (AIP) (see Figure 19–4), the region where previous studies had identified neurons that discharge in association with grasping movements. Sakata and his colleagues recorded the activity of individual neurons in alert monkeys trained to grasp different types of objects, each requiring a specific type of grip. The monkeys carried out these tasks under normal light, using visual guidance, but also in the dark, using memory. In this way Sakata and his colleagues discovered that the neurons in this area fall into three main classes: motor-dominant, visual-dominant, and visual-and-motor neurons.

Motor-dominant neurons discharge equally well during movements performed in light and in the dark. Visual-dominant neurons discharge only during movement performed in light. Visual-and-motor neurons fire during movements performed in both light and dark but their discharge is stronger in the light. Most visual-dominant and visual-and-motor neurons also respond when the monkey looks at an object but does not reach for it. Neurons that discharge selectively during manipulation of an object also discharge selectively during visual fixation of that object without movement. Based on this finding Sakata proposed that neurons in the anterior intraparietal area are involved in transforming sensory representations of objects into motor representations of how to grasp them.

Rizzolatti and co-workers next recorded the activity of neurons in a sector of the ventral premotor cortex of monkeys—area F5 within Brodmann's area 6 (see Figure 19–4)—while the animals performed a variety of actions. They found sets of neurons that discharged in association with different types of hand actions: grasping, holding, and manipulating. Some were active regardless of how the object was grasped. Most, however, discharged only when the monkey used a specific type of grip. The most commonly represented grip types were the precision grip (grasping with the index finger and thumb, typically used for small objects), whole-hand grasp (clutching, used for large objects), and finger grasp.

Surprisingly, a considerable fraction of neurons in area F5, called *canonical neurons,* also discharged when the monkey simply observed an object, whether or not the object was subsequently grasped (Figure 19–7). Thus these neurons discharged in response to presentation of an object even though the neuron did not have anything to do with preparation to grasp the object.

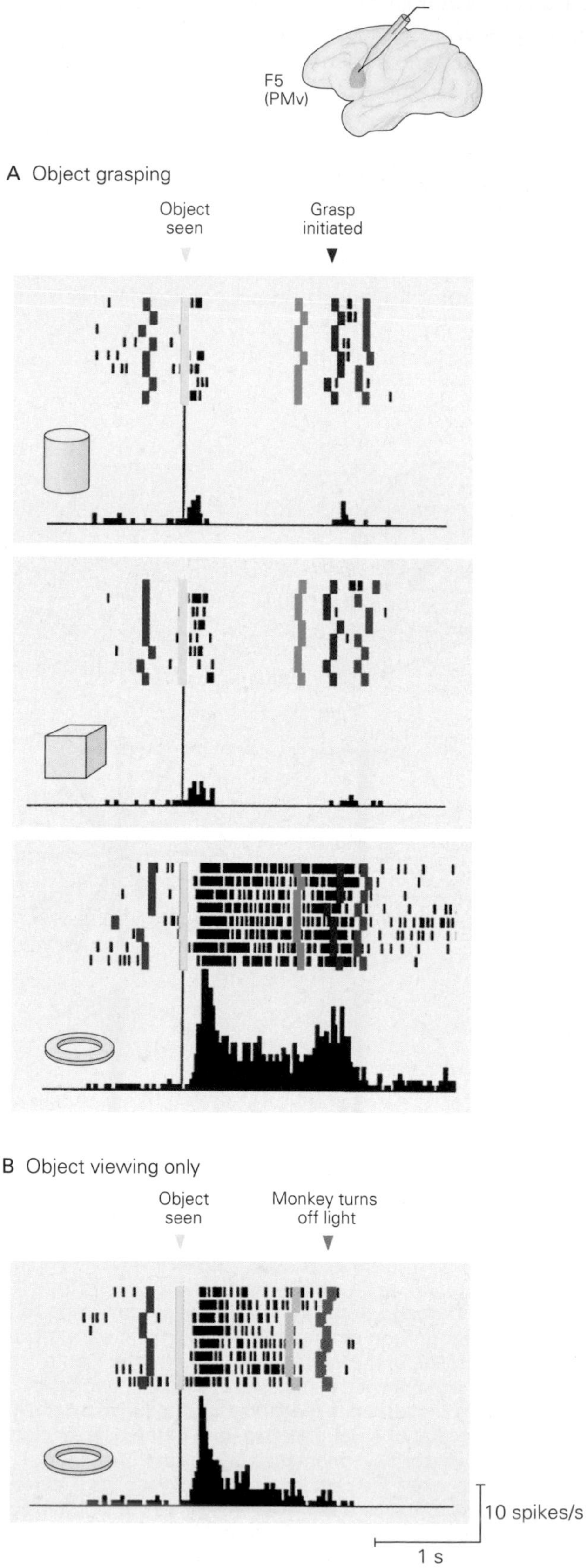

Most canonical neurons were selectively activated by the presentation of objects of a certain size, shape, and orientation. Neurons that discharged during a precision grip (performed with the index finger and thumb) also fired in response to the presentation of small objects, whereas neurons that discharged during whole-hand grasping also fired in response to the presentation of large objects.

What explains the behavior of canonical neurons? The fact that their activity is not related to motor planning and their responses are selective for certain objects and not others rules out nonspecific factors such as attention or intention, because nonspecific factors would have the same effect for all presented objects. Rather the presentation of an object seems to trigger the translation of the object's physical properties into a *potential motor act*.

The Joint Activity of Neurons in the Parietal and Premotor Cortex Encodes Potential Motor Acts

Some Neurons Encode the Possibilities for Interaction with an Object

The studies of the parietal and premotor canonical neurons led Michael Arbib, and subsequently Rizzolatti and Giuseppe Luppino, to formulate a new model of how sensory representations of objects are transformed into hand movements.

Figure 19–7 (Opposite) **Canonical neurons respond both when the animal is grasping and when it is simply viewing an object of a particular shape.** Recordings were made from a neuron in the F5 portion of the ventral premotor area while a monkey was presented with objects of different shapes. In the raster plots each row represents a separate trial and each tick in the row indicates the discharge of the neuron. Below each plot the neuronal activity is summarized in a histogram. The experimental protocol is as follows. A red light-emitting diode (LED) is turned on and the monkey fixates it (**red ticks**). The monkey then presses the key that turns on a light inside the training box (**yellow**), illuminating an object. The red LED turns green, cueing the monkey to grasp the object (**green**). The monkey releases the key and starts reaching (**violet**), and then finally grasps the object (**blue**). (Reproduced, with permission, from Murata et al. 1997.)

A. The response of the neuron to an image of a ring is more vigorous than its responses to a cube or a cylinder. Peaks in neuronal activity occur both when the monkey sees the object and when the monkey grasps it. After the object is grasped, the neuron's activity virtually ceases.

B. The neuron is also activated when the monkey views the object with no intention to act on it. In this part of the experiment the monkey again fixates the LED and turns on a light to make the object visible but then follows a cue (**light blue**) to simply turn off the light (**brown**).

Their model is based on the functional significance of the responses of visual-dominant and visual-and-motor neurons in the anterior intraparietal area to the presentation of three-dimensional objects. Their thinking about these responses was influenced by the notion of *affordance* introduced several years ago by the psychologist James J. Gibson. According to Gibson the sight of an object triggers an immediate and automatic selection of those properties of the object that allow one to interact with it. These properties, or affordances, are not the visual aspects of the object (shape, mass, color, etc.) but the *pragmatic opportunities* that the object affords the observer.

As we have seen, aspects of visual stimuli that are useful for action are analyzed in the dorsal stream of the visual system. Based on the extensive elaboration of an object's properties in the extrastriate visual areas of the dorsal stream beginning in V_2, the visual-dominant and visual-and-motor neurons in the anterior intraparietal cortex are able to encode the object's affordances. This information is then sent to F5 neurons that encode potential motor acts. An F5 neuron can transform a given affordance into an appropriate potential motor act because of the congruence of its response to the affordance and the motor act it controls. Object becomes action.

In real life objects usually have more than one affordance and may be grasped in several ways. How does the brain determine which is optimal? Behavioral analysis of grasping reveals that nonvisual factors determine the choice of affordance and thus how an object will actually be grasped. These factors relate both to what the object is for and the individual's intent at that moment. A cup is a simple example. The cup has three major affordances: the handle, the top, and the body. If the cup is recognized as a cup and the person wants to use it in the way a cup is commonly used, the person will grasp it by the handle. However, if the person wants to move the cup or give it to someone, the cup may be taken not by the handle but by its body or its rim (Figure 19–8).

Thus a more complete (and realistic) model of the grasping circuit involving the anterior intraparietal area and the premotor area F5 must assume that the circuit extracts automatically not one but all the affordances of an object. A specific affordance will be selected according to the information the circuit receives about the meaning of the object and the individual's intention.

As far as the *meaning* of the object is concerned, the ventral visual stream (Figure 19–8) is specifically dedicated to description of objects. This stream ends in the inferotemporal lobe, which is richly connected

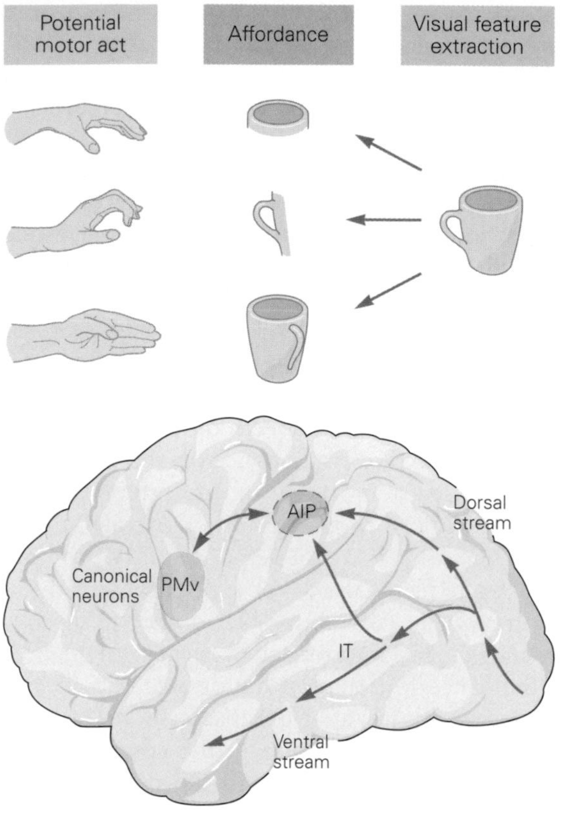

Figure 19–8 Neural control of grasping. The sight of a cup automatically triggers the motor act appropriate for grasping it. The brain centers involved in grasping are indicated below, and the operations carried out by them are summarized in the upper part of the figure. Affordances are not the visual aspects of the object (shape, size, color, etc.) but the *pragmatic opportunities* that the object affords the observer. (**AIP**, anterior intraparietal area; **PMv**, ventral premotor cortex; **IT**, inferotemporal cortex.)

reciprocally with the inferior parietal lobe, including the anterior intraparietal area. It is likely that these connections convey to the parietal lobe the semantic properties of an object; this information, as well as the motor use of the object specified in the premotor circuits, is the basis for the selection of an appropriate affordance consistent with the standard uses of the object.

The anatomical substrate for selecting affordances on the basis of the individual's current goal could be the input to the inferior parietal lobe from the prefrontal lobe, where long-term motor planning occurs. Thus when an unconventional use of an object is intended, the prefrontal input could override the selection of *standard* affordances and select those affordances that are congruent with the individual's intention. For example, if an individual wants to throw a cup instead of drinking from it, the affordances presented by the body of the cup or its top will be selected rather than the affordance presented by the handle.

Mirror Neurons Respond to the Motor Actions of Others

Canonical neurons discharge both when the monkey acts on an object and when it simply looks at the object without acting. In both cases these neurons fire in much the same manner and send the same signal to other neural centers. The firing of the neuron in the absence of an overt movement represents therefore a potential motor act: This activity occurs in a circuit that plans a movement but does not trigger a motor command. Potential motor acts afford an individual the freedom to choose whether or not to respond to a stimulus or simply hold it in memory.

Potential motor acts have an entirely different significance in a set of extremely interesting visuomotor neurons, the *mirror neurons*, in area F5. These neurons, like all neurons in F5, discharge during specific motor acts such as grasping, tearing, or holding. In addition, they also fire when the monkey observes another individual (human or monkey) performing the same motor act. They do not discharge in response to mere object presentation. In other words, these neurons represent the action done by another individual as a potential motor act.

What may be the function of these neurons? One attractive idea is that individuals know the outcome of the motor acts they plan. Thus, when the mirror neurons discharge in response to a motor act done by another individual, the observer understands what the other individual is doing because the observed action elicits in his premotor cortex a motor plan whose outcome is known to him.

At first glance it may seem strange that our motor faculties might be involved in understanding what others are doing, what their intentions are. But how else could we obtain this information? Although our visual system provides us with a description of the overt aspects of an action, it does not tell us what the action means, what its purpose is. Mirror neurons could in principle provide us with an experience-based understanding of observed actions, a basis for understanding the *intention* of others (see Chapter 38).

An essential step in the biological evolution of social cognition is our ability to interact with each other in a meaningful and constructive way. When you and I talk, you not only know the content of your own mind but also have a sense of what I am thinking and how I am reacting. A defect in social cognition may contribute to autism, a serious developmental disorder in which a child's ability to communicate socially is impaired. Normal communication requires, in addition to familiarity with language and the ability to express oneself, certain sensitivity to the thoughts and feelings of the person with whom one is communicating. One of the central features of autism is difficulty in understanding the perspectives, thoughts, ideas, and intentions of another person.

The mirror neurons are probably the most basic system the brain has for understanding others' intentions. Other cortical regions, such as the region near the superior temporal sulcus and some rostral medial cortical areas, also play a role in understanding another's intentions, especially when complex reasoning is required.

Potential Motor Acts Are Suppressed or Released by Motor Planning Centers

The representation of potential motor acts by the nervous system raises a further question. What prevents a potential motor act from being executed? Are there control mechanisms inhibiting or facilitating implementation? Damage to certain premotor cortical areas, or the motor cortex, results in neurological syndromes that strongly suggest that there are such controls. Some of these behavioral disorders include difficulty in initiating movements or making movements that are not consciously intended.

A particularly telling example is the *utilization behavior* syndrome. Individuals with this syndrome pick up objects in an almost compulsive way. Once they observe an object, they immediately grasp it, even if it belongs to another person or to the doctor examining them. This syndrome may result from impaired restraint of the potential motor acts elicited by objects.

A key feature of voluntary motor behavior is that certain motor acts are executed while others are restrained. Voluntary action depends on sequencing elementary movements to form purposeful action. This ability is the prerequisite for many of our daily actions such as typing, using a computer, playing a musical instrument, and even speech. Karl Lashley called the task of sequencing motor actions the "serial order problem" of motor behavior. The sequence of motor actions is thought to involve parallel computations in multiple cortical areas and subcortical nuclei, including the basal ganglia and the supplementary motor area.

Neurons in the supplementary motor area are involved in the planning, generation, and control of sequential motor actions. Thus, when monkeys were trained to perform different sequences of three simple elemental arm movements—push, pull, and turn—some neurons in the supplementary motor area were active before any movement occurred but only when a specific sequence was planned. For example, a neuron could be active prior to the performance of a pull-turn-push sequence but not before a pull-push-turn sequence. Other neurons were active while a particular movement was performed but only if the movement was preceded or followed by another specific movement.

An Overall View

The brain recognizes objects and carries out actions in ways no existing computer can even begin to approach. Recognizing a face and appreciating a landscape are amazing computational achievements that require sophisticated processing of complex information. Indeed, all our perceptions are analytical triumphs. However, even more amazing is how all this perceptual analysis is integrated with motor circuits for even the simplest voluntary actions such as picking up a cup of coffee.

The final neural pathway for any action that determines the force exerted by individual muscles is through the motor neurons in the ventral horn of the spinal cord. Nevertheless, in sophisticated animals like monkeys or humans, actions are not produced by the spinal cord alone. Several sensory and motor regions in the brain are also involved.

The planning and execution of voluntary movement relies on sensorimotor transformations in which representations of the external environment are integrated with intentions and motor programs. This integration is the product of premotor and primary motor areas operating in conjunction with sensory and association areas of the cerebral cortex. An example of this is the communication between parietal and motor areas during visually guided reaching.

In our everyday experience it seems we perceive an object before interacting with it; and thus intuitively we might expect the brain to work in this sequential way. According to this model perceptual mechanisms first generate a unified representation of the external world, cognitive processes use this replica of the world to decide on a course of action, and finally an action plan is relayed to the motor systems for implementation.

As we have seen, this intuitive view does not capture the reality of how the brain decides and executes movement. In fact, a novel behavior requires simultaneous processing in multiple motor and sensory areas because the behavioral action is continuously monitored for errors and modified. As the behavior becomes more accurate, the need for sampling of the sensory inflow and updating of the motor program decreases—the need for the computational power of large networks lessens. Thus, for example, the presupplementary motor area is active during the learning of a behavior but becomes less active as learning progresses. After long periods of practice, when the behavior becomes automatic, activity in the presupplementary motor area ceases.

Giacomo Rizzolatti
Peter L. Strick

Selected Readings

Arbib MA. 1981. Perceptual structures and distributed motor control. In: VB Brooks (ed). *Handbook of Physiology,* Sect. 1, Vol. 2, Pt. 2, pp. 1449–1480. Bethesda, MD: American Physiological Society.

Dum RP, Strick PL. 1996. The corticospinal system: a structural framework for the central control of movement. In: RB Rowell, JT Sheperd (eds). *Handbook of Physiology,* Vol. 12, pp. 217–254. New York: Oxford Univ. Press.

Houk JC, Wise SP. 1995. Distributed modular architectures linking basal ganglia, cerebellum and cerebral cortex: their role in planning and controlling actions. Cereb Cortex 5:95–110.

Hubel DH. 1988. *Eye, Brain, and Vision.* New York: WH Freeman.

Jeannerod M. 2006. *Motor Cognition.* Oxford: Oxford Univ. Press.

Milner AD, Goodale MA. 2002. The visual brain in action. In: A Noe, E Thompson (eds). *Vision and Mind: Selected Readings in the Philosophy of Perception.* Cambridge, MA: MIT Press.

Mountcastle VB, Lynch JC, Georgopoulos A, Sakata H, Acuna C. 1975. Posterior parietal association cortex of the monkey: command functions for operations within extrapersonal space. J Neurophysiol 38:871–908.

Rizzolatti G, Luppino G. 2001. The cortical motor system. Neuron 31:889–901.

Ungerleider LG, Mishkin M. 1982. Two cortical visual systems. In: DJ Ingle, MA Goodale, RJW Mansfield (eds). *Analysis of Visual Behavior,* pp. 549–586. Cambridge, MA: MIT Press.

References

Alexander GE, Crutcher MD, De Long MR. 1990. Basal ganglia-thalamocortical circuits: parallel substrates for motor, oculomotor, "prefrontal" and "limbic" functions. Prog Brain Res 85:119–146.

Andersen RA, Buneo CA. 2002. Intentional maps in posterior parietal cortex. Annu Rev Neurosci 25:189–220.

Berti A, Rizzolatti G. 1992. Visual processing without awareness: evidence from unilateral neglect. J Cogn Neurosci 4:345–351.

Berti A, Smania N, Allport A. 2001. Coding of far and near space in neglect patients. Neuroimage 14(1 Pt 2): S98–S102.

Colby CL. 1996. A neurophysiological distinction between attention and intention. In: T Inui, JL McClelland (eds). *Attention and Performance XVI. Information Integration in Perception and Communication,* pp. 157–178. Cambridge, MA: MIT Press.

De Renzi E. 1982. *Disorders of Space Exploration and Cognition.* New York: Wiley.

Fagg AH, Arbib MA. 1998. Modeling parietal-premotor interactions in primate control of grasping. Neural Netw 11:1277–1303.

Felleman DJ, Van Essen DC. 1991. Distributed hierarchical processing in the primate cerebral cortex. Cereb Cortex 1:1–47.

Fogassi L, Gallese V, Fadiga L, Luppino G, Matelli M, Rizzolatti G. 1996. Coding of peripersonal space in inferior premotor cortex (area F4). J Neurophysiol 76: 141–157.

Gallese V, Fadiga L, Fogassi L, Rizzolatti G. 1996. Action recognition in the premotor cortex. Brain 119:593–609.

Goodale MA, Milner AD. 1982. Fractioning orienting behavior in rodents. In: DJ Ingle, MA Goodale, RJW Mansfield (eds). *Analysis of Visual Behavior,* pp. 549–586. Cambridge, MA: MIT Press.

Graziano MSA, Gross CG. 1996. Multiple pathways for processing visual space. In: T Inui, Gopher D, JL McClelland, Koriat A (eds). *Attention and Performance XVI: Information Integration in Perception and Communication,* pp. 181–207. Cambridge, MA: MIT Press.

Gross CG, Rocha-Miranda CE, Bender DB. 1972. Visual properties of neurons in the inferotemporal cortex of the macaque. J Neuropysiol 35:96–111.

Gurfinkel VS. 1994. The mechanisms of the postural regulation in man. Soviet Scientific Reviews F Phys Gen Biol 4:59–89.

He SQ, Dum RP, Strick PL. 1993. Topographic organization of the corticospinal projections from the frontal lobe: motor areas on the lateral surface of the hemisphere. J Neurosci 13:952–980.

He SQ, Dum RP, Strick PL. 1995. Topographic organization of the corticospinal projections from the frontal lobe: motor areas on the medial surface of the hemisphere. J Neurosci 15:3284–3306.

Hyvarinen J. 1982. Posterior parietal lobe of the primate brain. Physiol Rev 62:1060–1129.

Ingle DJ. 1973. Two visual systems in the frog. Science 181:1053–1055.

Jeannerod M, Arbib MA, Rizzolatti G, Sakata H. 1995. Grasping objects: the cortical mechanisms of visuomotor transformation. Trends Neurosci 18:314–320.

Jenmalm P, Johansson RS. 1997. Visual and somatosensory information about object shape control manipulative fingertip forces. J Neurosci 17: 4486–4499.

Kuypers HGJM. 1981. Anatomy of the descending pathways. In: VB Brooks (ed). *Handbook of Physiology,* Sect. 1, Vol. 2, pp. 597–666. Bethesda, MD: American Physiological Society.

Lemon RN. 2008. Descending pathways in motor control. Ann Rev Neurosci 31:195–218.

Murata A, Fadiga L, Fogassi L, Gallese V, Raos V, Rizzolatti G. 1997. Object representation in the ventral premotor cortex (area F5) of the monkey. J Neurophysiol 78: 2226–2230.

Mussa-Ivaldi FA, Bizzi E. 2000. Motor learning through the combination of primitives. Phil Trans R Soc London B 355:1755–1769.

Penfield W, Rasmussen T. 1950. *The Cerebral Cortex of Man: A Clinical Study of Localization of Function.* New York: Macmillan.

Perrett DI, Harries MH, Bevan R, et al. 1989. Frameworks of analysis for the neural representation of animate objects and actions. J Exp Biol 146:87–113.

Porter R, Lemon RN. 1993. *Corticospinal Function and Voluntary Movement.* Oxford: Clarendon.

Rizzolatti G, Riggio L, Sheliga BM. 1994. Space and selective attention. In: C Umiltà, M Moscovitch (eds). *Attention and Performance XV: Conscious and Nonconscious Information Processing,* pp. 231–265. Cambridge, MA: MIT Press.

Rizzolatti G, Craighero L. 2004. The mirror-neuron system. Ann Rev Neurosci 27:169–192.

Rizzolatti G, Matelli M. 2003. Two different streams form the dorsal visual system. Exp Brain Res 153:146–157.

Sakata H, Taira M, Murata A, Mine S. 1995. Neural mechanisms of visual guidance of hand action in the parietal cortex of the monkey. Cereb Cortex 5:429–438.

Spencer H. 1855. *Principles of Psychology.* London: Longmans.

Tanaka K. 1996. Inferotemporal cortex and object vision. Annu Rev Neurosci 19:109–139.

20

Functional Imaging of Cognition

THE ABILITY OF NEURO-IMAGING to observe areas of the human brain that are active during cognitive processes has helped to stimulate the current interest in the biological underpinnings of cognitive functioning. Because invasive experiments cannot be done ethically on humans, research on the biological basis of cognitive function was until quite recently confined to laboratory animals and clinical studies of patients with cognitive disorders.

The development of techniques such as functional magnetic resonance imaging (fMRI) has made it possible to study human subjects, affording unprecedented views of the complexities of the intact working brain. Imaging of the living brain allows us to explore the behavioral significance of local neural circuits, such as cortical columns, as well as observe large-scale systems of interconnected brain regions concerned with specific mental processes such as seeing, hearing, feeling, moving, talking, and thinking.

Functional Imaging Reflects the Metabolic Demand of Neural Activity

Functional Imaging Emerged from Studies of Blood Flow

Functional imaging evolved out of seminal studies in the late 1940s by Seymour Kety and Carl F. Schmidt, who succeeded in measuring blood flow in the living brain. Although Charles S. Roy and Charles S. Sherrington earlier had found a relationship between blood flow and brain metabolism, Kety and Schmidt were the first to quantify cerebral blood flow noninvasively.

To accomplish this task, Kety and Schmidt measured the rate of cerebral blood flow by having subjects inhale nitrous oxide, a metabolically inert gas, and measuring its outflow concentration from the jugular vein (Box 20–1). In a series of landmark studies they evaluated how blood flow from the intact brain varied in different metabolic states, such as sleep and wakefulness, and in so doing they laid the foundations for modern functional imaging.

These early experiments measured only the total level of activity of the entire brain, however. They could not provide information about which parts of the brain were active, nor could they tell us whether some brain areas became more active while others became less active under set conditions.

A significant advance came in the 1970s with the introduction of positron emission tomography (PET) by Michel Ter-Pogossian, Michael Phelps, and Louis Sokoloff (Box 20–2). In the 1980s Marcus Raichle collaborated with Michael Posner to visualize the brain

Box 20–1 Application of the Fick Principle to Brain Metabolism

Devised as a technique for measuring cardiac output by Adolf Eugen Fick, the Fick principle states that an organ must receive blood at a rate that is equal to the rate at which the organ metabolizes a constituent of blood, divided by the concentration of that constituent.

The essence of the Fick principle is that blood flow to an organ can be calculated using a marker substance. The principle may be applied in many ways. For example, if blood flow to an organ is known, together with the arterial and venous concentrations of the marker substance, then the uptake or metabolism by the organ may be calculated.

Seymour Kety and Carl F. Schmidt adapted the Fick principle so that it could be applied to the brain and showed that it can be used to measure cerebral blood flow. The Fick Principle has also been used to explain BOLD (Blood Oxygen Level Dependent) fMRI. BOLD fMRI detects changes in deoxyhemoglobin content within a unit volume of brain. As can be derived from the Fick principle, deoxyhemoglobin concentration is proportional to the cerebral metabolic rate of oxygen ($CMRO_2$) divided by cerebral blood flow (CBF).

activity of subjects engaged in complex tasks of thought and language, thereby demonstrating that PET can be used to explore cognitive functioning.

A further advance in functional imaging occurred in 1990 when Seiji Ogawa and David Tank discovered that magnetic resonance imaging (MRI) can be made sensitive to changes in deoxyhemoglobin that are caused when neurons change their metabolic rates. They exploited the fact, first discovered in 1936 by Linus Pauling, that when oxyhemoglobin is converted to deoxyhemoglobin (by stripping hemoglobin of its four oxygen molecules), it becomes paramagnetic.

In particular, they showed that in MRI images of the hippocampal formation of anesthetized rodents areas of increased vascularity appeared darker than areas with less vascularity. When rodents breathed 100% oxygen, the image intensities in the hippocampus were brighter, thereby suggesting that these differences in intensity were caused by changes in blood oxygenation. Finally, Ogawa went on to link these differences in image intensity with metabolism. He found that systematic pharmacological alteration of basal brain metabolism in anesthetized animals induced a corresponding increase in the image intensity (Box 20–3).

In brain regions with increased metabolism the flow of oxygenated blood is greater than the consumption of oxygen, and thus leads to a relative decrease in deoxyhemoglobin. MRI areas with increased metabolism and flow of oxygenated blood appear brighter than regions that are not experiencing increased metabolism (Box 20–3). This form of functional MRI has been termed BOLD (blood oxygen level dependent) imaging.

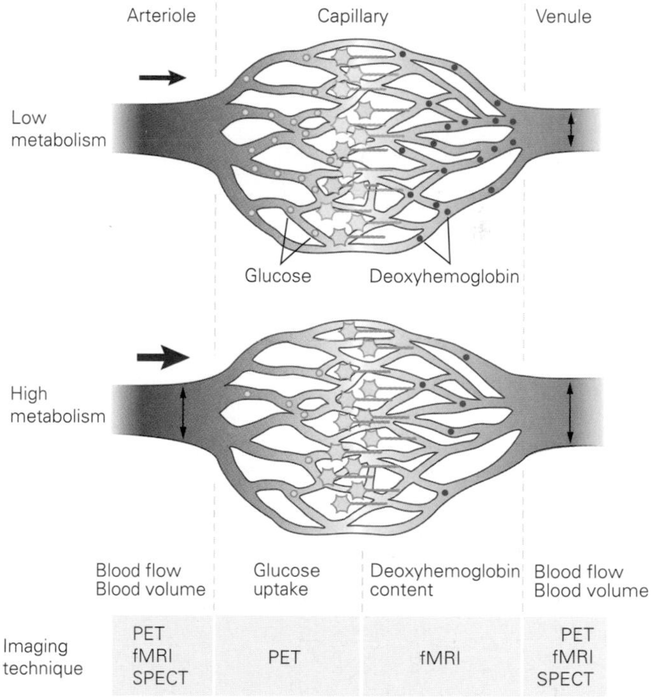

Figure 20–1 Relationship to brain metabolism. The energy metabolism of neurons is influenced by changes in synaptic activity or synaptic strength. Shifts in metabolism are associated with local increases in cerebral blood flow, glucose uptake, and cerebral blood volume, and a decrease in deoxyhemoglobin content. These different changes are detected with different techniques. Imaging techniques: **fMRI**, functional magnetic resonance imaging; **PET**, positron emission tomography; **SPECT**, single-photon emission computed tomography.

Box 20–2 Positron Emission Tomography

Positron emission tomography (PET) imaging requires the introduction into the brain of substances tagged with radionuclides that emit positrons (positively charged electrons). Commonly used substances are ^{11}C, ^{18}F, ^{15}O, and ^{13}N. The synthesis of compounds with these radionuclides does not result in the loss of biological activity; thus $H_2{}^{15}O$ behaves like $H_2{}^{16}O$ and ^{18}F-deoxyglucose like deoxyglucose.

The radionuclides are produced in a cyclotron, which adds protons into the nuclei of atoms. For example, bombarding oxygen with hydrogen ions makes ^{18}F. Incorporation of an extra proton into the nucleus produces an unstable nucleus.

These unstable radionuclides can be detected when the extra proton spontaneously breaks down into two particles: (1) a neutron, which remains within the nucleus because a stable nucleus can contain extra neutrons, and (2) a positron, a particle that travels away from the nucleus at the speed of light, dissipating energy as it goes. The positron eventually collides with an electron, and the collision leads to their mutual annihilation and the emission of two gamma rays (high-energy photons) in opposite directions (Figure 20–2A).

PET scanners contain arrays of gamma ray detectors (scintillation crystals coupled to photomultiplier tubes) encircling the subject's head (Figure 20–2B). The two gamma rays emitted by the annihilation of a positron and electron ultimately reach pairs of coincidence detectors that record an event when, and only when, two gamma rays are detected simultaneously.

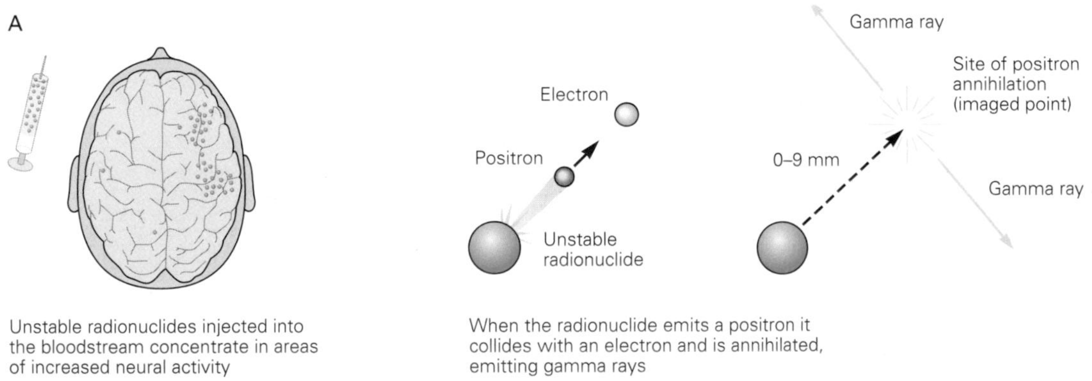

Figure 20–2A **Emission of gamma rays.** The nucleus of an unstable radionuclide emits a positron. The positron travels a certain distance before it collides with an electron and is annihilated, emitting two gamma rays that travel in precisely opposite directions. The site of positron annihilation that is imaged may be a few millimeters from the site of origin. For example, the average distance between the site of origin and annihilation is 2 mm for ^{18}F and 3 mm for ^{15}O. The distance between the emitting nucleus and the site where the positron is annihilated is an absolute limit on the spatial resolution of PET scan images. (Adapted, with permission, from Oldendorf 1980.)

Functional Imaging Reflects Energy Metabolism

As these discussions make clear, functional imaging does not measure neural activity but rather reflects energy metabolism, best defined as the rate at which mitochondria produce adenosine triphosphate (ATP). Because direct imaging of ATP production is difficult, functional imaging assesses correlates of energy metabolism that can be visualized with clinical imaging devices (Figure 20–1).

A surprisingly large amount of a neuron's total energy metabolism, approximately one-half, is devoted simply to maintaining the resting membrane potential—the electric potential across the cell membrane. Therefore any shift in the membrane potential will affect the rate of energy metabolism and influence functional imaging

A coincident pair of gamma ray emissions is detected along a line in one plane or slice. The site where the positron is annihilated is the site detected by the scanner. Multiple positron-electron annihilations are pinpointed by monitoring coincident gamma rays in multiple slices. Clusters of annihilations indicate increased neural activity, which is mapped onto the brain in the final PET image (Figure 20–2C).

The distance between the site of annihilation and the emitting nucleus, which can be several millimeters, limits the spatial resolution of the method, which is typically 6 to 8 mm. The temporal resolution of PET imaging is limited by the rate at which positrons are emitted, which ranges from minutes to hours depending on the radionuclide used and the compound in which it is incorporated.

B

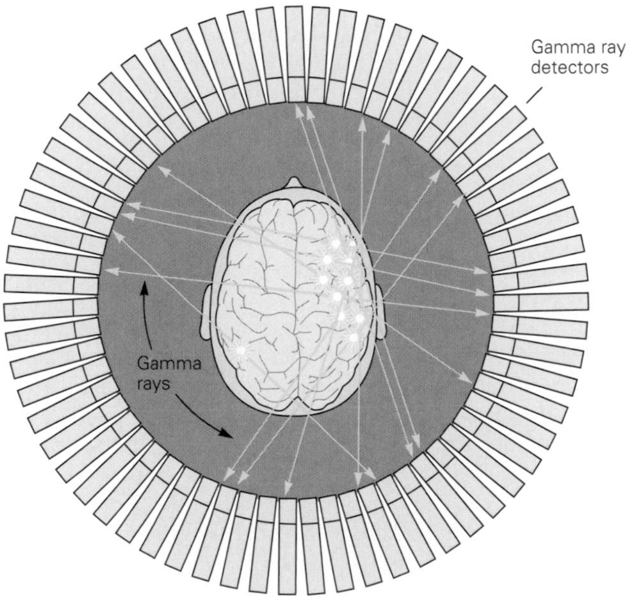

Figure 20–2B PET scanners contain an array of gamma ray detectors encircling the subject's head. Only gamma rays that are detected simultaneously by diagonally placed detectors are recorded. (Adapted, with permission, from Oldendorf 1980.)

C

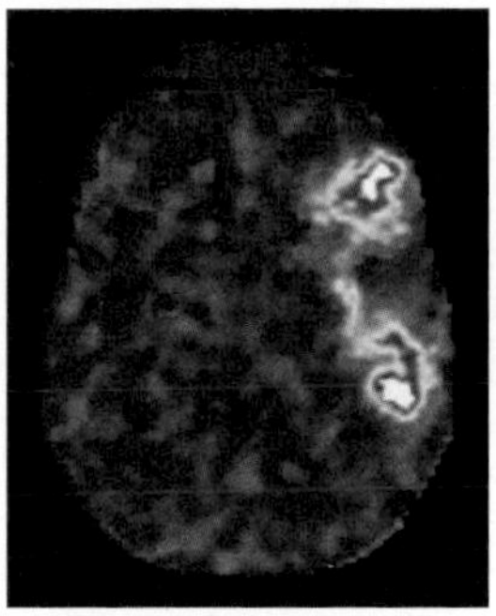

Figure 20–2C PET image. PET produces an image showing the areas of heightened neural activity as revealed by the radionuclides.

measures. The membrane potential changes when a cell fires an action potential and also in response to subthreshold excitatory or inhibitory synaptic potentials.

The remaining half of a neuron's energy metabolism is devoted to other biochemical processes, and alterations in these pathways also affect functional imaging measures, although typically on a slower time scale. These biochemical processes include all of the molecular reactions required for normal synaptic function: vesicle recycling, recruitment of second-messenger cascades, local protein synthesis, axonal transport, and transmitter release. Thus functional imaging in principle can measure the transient effect an external stimulus has on the electrical activity of neurons, as well as the more permanent effect of a disease process on neuronal biochemistry.

Box 20–3 Functional Magnetic Resonance Imaging

The development of functional magnetic resonance imaging (fMRI) emerged from a chain of discoveries that began in 1937 with the description of molecular beam magnetic resonance by Isidor Rabi and the discovery in 1945 of nuclear magnetic resonance (NMR), made independently by Edward Purcell and Felix Bloch. In 1949 Erwin Hahn observed that NMR decays differentially depending on the chemical makeup of an object, the key phenomenon that has made fMRI possible.

MRI scanners consist of several components. The first component is a superconducting magnet that provides a powerful and very uniform magnetic field (1.5 tesla for a standard clinical MRI scanner). Each water proton in the body rotates around its axis and acts like a small bar magnet. Water protons normally have random directions so the tissue essentially has no net magnetization. However, when placed in a magnetic field the protons become aligned (Figure 20–3A).

The second component is a *radio frequency coil* (or RF coil), a specially designed coil of wire placed near the subject. A brief, rapidly alternating electrical current in the RF coil generates a rapidly varying magnetic field because of Ampere's law. This second magnetic field is superimposed with the scanner's main magnetic field. The alternating electrical current in the RF coil is called a radio frequency pulse (or RF pulse) because it alternates at a frequency comparable to FM radio frequencies.

The magnetic field induced by the RF pulse causes the protons to start wobbling around their axes (Figure 20–3A), much as a spinning top wobbles around its axis when the force of gravity competes with its spin. This wobbling is called precession. The protons continue to precess after the RF pulse has been turned off.

Summed across all of the individual water protons, the precession creates a rotating magnetic field that changes in time (Figure 20–3A) and, according to Faraday's law, generates an alternating electric current back in the RF coil. It is this electric current that is measured in MRI (Figure 20–3B).

The amplitude of the measured electric current decays over time at a rate that is dependent upon a number of factors, including the type of tissue in which the protons are embedded. Thus, differences in tissue type appear as different intensities in the resulting images.

The third component of an MRI scanner is the *magnetic gradient coils*. One of the most important developments in MRI is the ability to make three-dimensional images of the body. This is accomplished by using magnetic gradients, magnetic fields in which the strength of the field changes gradually along an axis.

It is beyond the scope of this chapter to explain in detail how two-dimensional images (or three-dimensional volumes) are acquired with MRI, but the basic idea is that controlling the magnetic gradients allows one to measure the MRI signal (the electric current in the RF coil) at a large number of adjacent locations, each corresponding to a small volume (or voxel) of tissue.

Functional MRI primarily measures changes in the relative amount of deoxyhemoglobin within each voxel (Figure 20–4). When neurons are active, the supply of oxygenated blood to the active region increases. For reasons that are still unclear, the delivery of oxygenated hemoglobin is greater than local oxygen consumption, resulting in a greater proportion of oxygenated to deoxygenated hemoglobin.

Oxygenated and deoxygenated hemoglobin have different magnetic properties. Hemoglobin contains iron, which is exposed when oxygen is stripped from the hemoglobin molecule. The presence of deoxyhemoglobin introduces an inhomogeneity in the nearby magnetic field. Some water protons (those that are near a deoxyhemoglobin molecule) now experience a magnetic field strength that is slightly different from the other water protons.

Figure 20–3 (Opposite) Magnetic resonance imaging.

A. Water protons spin around their axes, creating individual magnetic fields with random directions (**1**). When a vertical magnetic field is applied to the tissue, the protons align with it to create a net magnetic field that is also vertical but very small and difficult to detect (**2**). A radio frequency pulse applied in a second (horizontal) direction makes the protons wobble, or precess, around their vertical axes (**3**). Summed across all of the individual water protons, this creates a net magnetic field that changes in time and gives rise to an electric current that is ultimately measured in MRI (**4**).

B. An MRI measurement begins by placing the subject in a vertical magnetic field. With the protons aligned vertically, a horizontal radio frequency pulse is applied to tip the protons so that they rotate in the horizontal plane synchronously, or "in phase" with one another (**1**). The horizontal pulse is then turned off (**2**), and the rotating protons begin to move out of phase with one another—they "dephase." Dephasing occurs relatively quickly and leads to a decrease or decay in the measured current. The time constant of this decay is called T_2* (approximately 30 ms). After withdrawal of the horizontal pulse the protons realign with the vertical magnetic field (**3–5**). This "righting" or recovery of the vertical magnetization occurs more slowly than the dephasing. The time constant of the recovery is called T_1 (several seconds). The entire process can be repeated many times to yield a time series of measurements that reflect changes in the rates of decay and recovery.

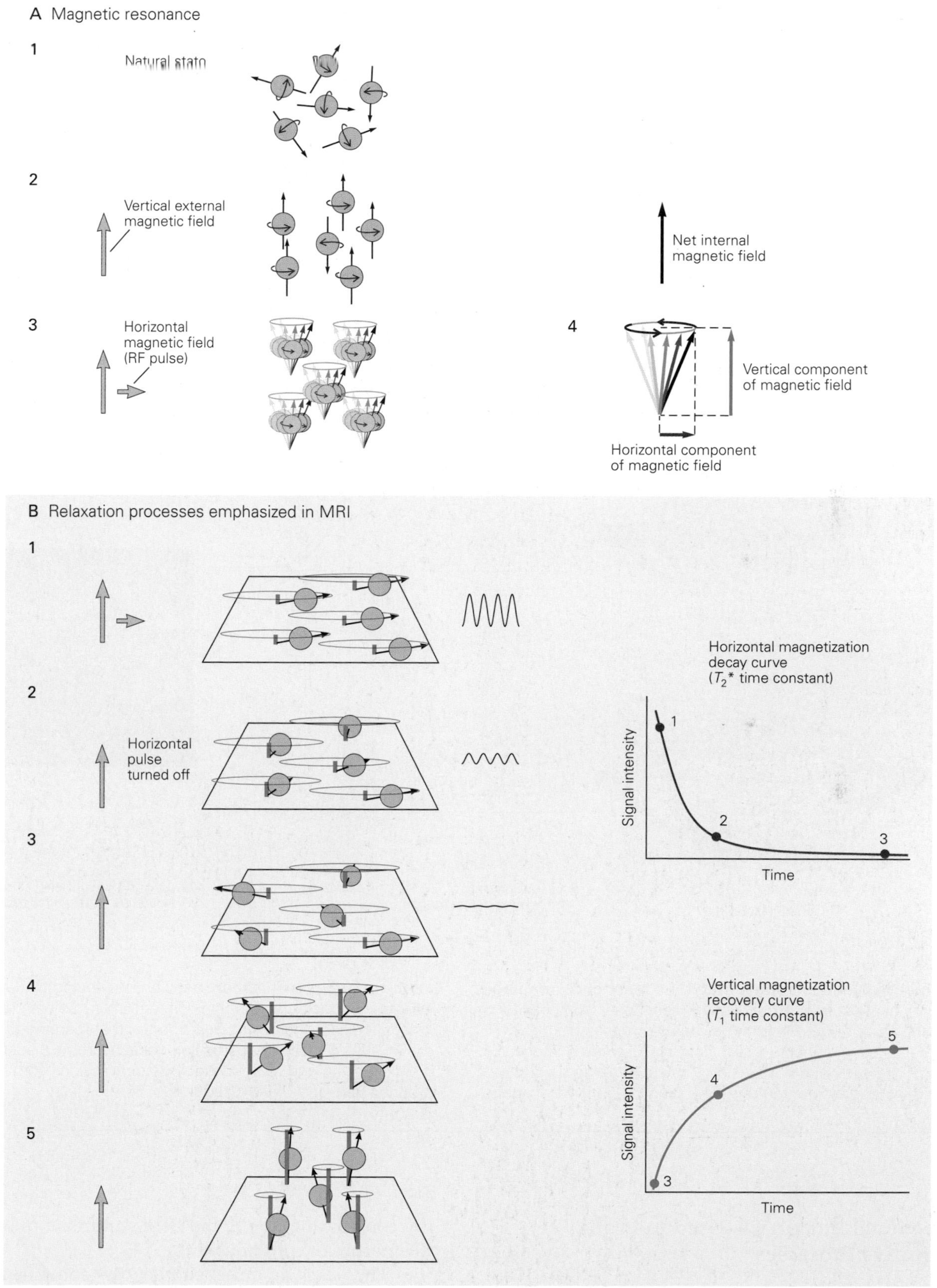
A Magnetic resonance
1
Natural state
2
Vertical external magnetic field
Net internal magnetic field
3
Horizontal magnetic field (RF pulse)
4
Vertical component of magnetic field
Horizontal component of magnetic field
B Relaxation processes emphasized in MRI
1
2
Horizontal pulse turned off
3
4
5
Horizontal magnetization decay curve (T_2* time constant)
Signal intensity
Time
Vertical magnetization recovery curve (T_1 time constant)
Signal intensity
Time

(continued)

Box 20–3 Functional Magnetic Resonance Imaging (continued)

Greater inhomogeneity causes the protons to desynchronize more rapidly resulting in a more rapid decay time (T_2*). When there is an increase in oxygenated blood in areas with greater neuronal activity, and hence a more homogeneous magnetic field, the result is a longer T_2* decay time, and brighter image intensity.

Like PET scanning, fMRI is sensitive to the increased blood flow associated with neural activity. This technique has several advantages over PET scanning, however. It requires no injection of foreign substances into the bloodstream (fMRI uses endogenous hemoglobin as its marker). It also offers finer spatial and temporal resolution than PET.

For example, fMRI has been used to visualize the ocular dominance columns in human V1, which requires a spatial resolution of less than a millimeter, and it has been used to estimate differences in the timing of neural activity with a temporal resolution of approximately 100 ms. Sub-millimeter and sub-millisecond resolutions are not yet routine practice but have been demonstrated convincingly. The fMRI image in Figure 20–4 was acquired with a spatial resolution of 1 mm.

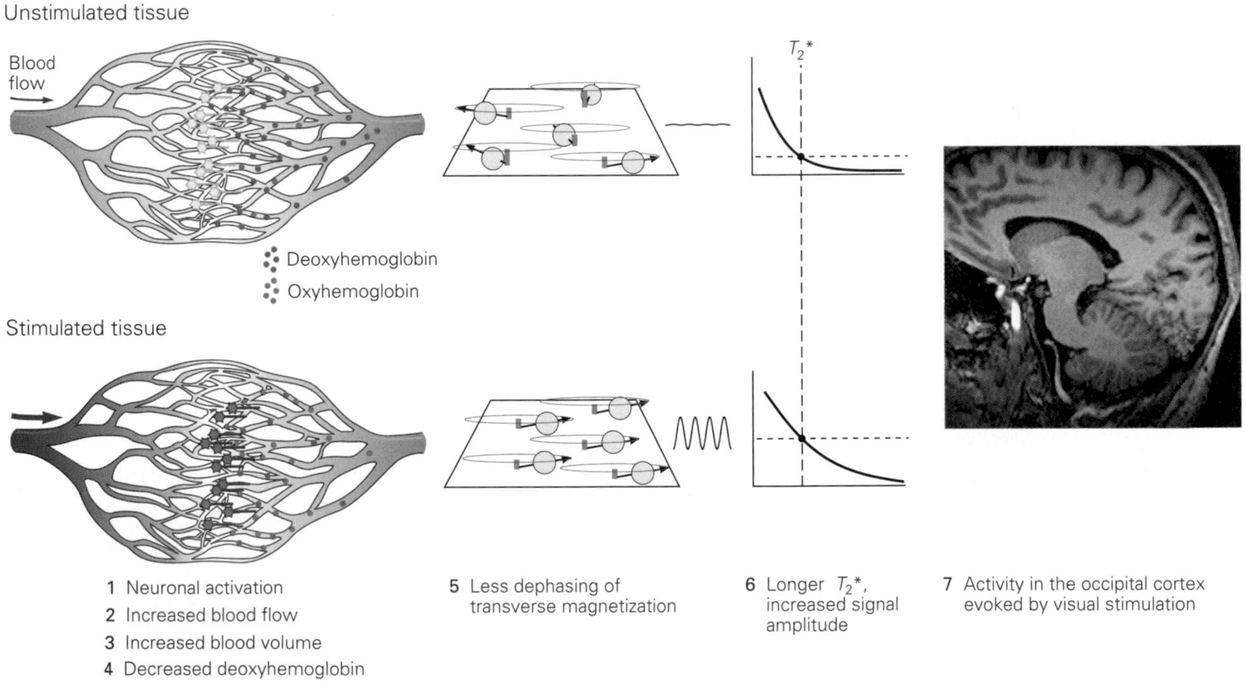

Figure 20-4 **Functional magnetic resonance imaging.** An increase in neuronal activity results in an increased supply of oxygenated blood. This decreases the deoxyhemoglobin concentration, causing dephasing to occur more slowly and hence slowing down the decay of the measured electric current. The result is an fMRI image of the locations of metabolic activity as revealed by the changes in deoxyhemoglobin concentration. Colors in the image indicate regions of visual cortex that responded to visual stimuli placed at particular locations in the visual field. (fMRI image reproduced, with permission, from Souheil Inati and David Heeger.)

Functional Imaging Is Used to Probe Cognitive Processes

By visualizing the brain at work, functional imaging has transformed cognitive neuroscience. We will illustrate some insights derived from functional imaging by considering one of the field's ultimate questions—the nature of consciousness.

The idea is quite simple: By comparing brain activity between conscious and unconscious states we should be able to identify brain regions in which the activity is correlated with consciousness. Because systematically manipulating consciousness is not trivial, translating this logic into a scientific experiment is difficult. To accomplish this task, scientists have relied on the fact that exposure to the identical external stimulus can alternately evoke a conscious or unconscious experience depending on other controllable factors. For example, as you read this chapter you have blinked numerous times; nevertheless, although your brain has recorded the flickered light caused by blinking, your consciousness has not. Now, once brought to your attention, you become aware of the perceptual effects of blinking (in fact, it is now difficult for you to suppress this awareness).

Just as sensory stimuli can be processed with and without conscious perception by the brain, the recall of objects from memory can also be conscious or unconscious. Consider running into someone you met once before. Viewing the person's face may activate conscious recall of the initial meeting—the place, the time, the person's name. Or, as is often the case, you might sense that the face is familiar, but you cannot quite connect it to a time or place—the face simply does not evoke conscious recall of the initial meeting. Even worse, you might not consciously recognize the face, even though (as can be demonstrated) some regions of your brain are responding unconsciously to the face (as if your brain remembers, but you do not).

By comparing the hemodynamic response associated with perception and recall, both with and without consciousness, functional imaging studies have begun to identify regions of the brain correlated with consciousness.

Imaging Perception with and Without Consciousness

Mapping of brain function began in the middle of the 19th century, fully 100 years before the advent of functional imaging of the brain. By correlating cognitive performance with the anatomical location of brain lesions, neurologists identified brain regions involved in specific cognitive functions (see Chapter 1). However, this approach has a number of important limitations that prevented many questions about function from being answered.

For example, just because an area of primary sensory cortex may be necessary for conscious perception, because it is involved in the initial processing of sensory information, does not mean it is responsible for the conscious experience. It may simply relay sensory information to higher-order cortex that is responsible for consciousness. In principle, functional imaging can help make these distinctions.

Indeed, neural correlates of conscious perception can be measured experimentally using visual illusions in which the percept is dissociated from the physical stimulus. One such illusion results from binocular rivalry, which occurs when different visual stimuli are presented simultaneously to each eye. Typically, awareness of one or the other stimulus is suppressed so that we are consciously aware of one stimulus at a time, never both. Thus one eye's view dominates consciousness for several seconds, only to be replaced by the other eye's view. What makes binocular rivalry so remarkable is that the perceptual experience fluctuates while the physical stimulus remains constant. Because of this dissociation, binocular rivalry presents a unique opportunity for studying the neural correlates of consciousness.

What systems are recruited when one eye's view becomes dominant? According to one idea, neurons in the early stages in visual processing respond to the physical stimulus of each eye, but in later stages the signals from these neurons are switched on and off, causing the perceptual alternations. That is, a later stage serves as a "gate" to visual consciousness.

Does such a gate exist? If so, what neurons in the brain have this gating function? Are the neurons localized in particular brain areas? Are they a particular cell type? Does the gating occur through modulation of the cells' firing rates or some other component of their responses (eg, spike timing, synchronous firing)? What are the neural circuits and neural computations that support the competition between the two stimuli?

Although we do not yet have firm answers to these questions, the evoked metabolic activity of the brain under conditions of binocular rivalry has been measured with fMRI. One fMRI experiment capitalized on an interesting aspect of this perceptual phenomenon; during an alternation one typically perceives a traveling wave in which one pattern emerges initially at one location and expands progressively as it renders the other pattern invisible. The physical stimulus does not change while this conscious perceptual change is taking place—it is all "in your brain." This experiment established that waves of activity in primary visual cortex (V1) accompanied the perceptual changes during binocular rivalry.

Because the primary visual cortex is topographically organized—adjacent neurons respond to adjacent locations in the visual field (see Chapter 27)—it was possible to show that neural activity propagated over subregions of primary visual cortex. The sequential activation of these subregions correlated with the dynamic perceptual changes experienced during binocular rivalry (Figure 20–6). Similar waves of activity propagated over the immediately adjacent secondary visual areas (V2 and V3).

Box 20–4 Diffusion Tensor Imaging

Diffusion tensor imaging (DTI) is another application of MRI, complementary to fMRI, for visualizing anatomical properties of the brain. DTI begins with measurements of how far water diffuses within the brain. The random displacements of molecules resulting from thermal agitation (Brownian motion) obey a statistical law that was described by Einstein in 1905.

In a homogeneous medium the average distance moved by the molecules increases linearly with the square root of time. For water at body temperature, 68% of the molecules will have moved less than 17 μm during 50 ms. Water diffusion in the presence of large molecules or cell membranes is impeded.

It has been known for decades that MRI can be used to measure differences in the extent of water diffusion, called diffusion MRI, that depend on brain anatomy. One of the most successful clinical applications of diffusion MRI has been in the management of stroke. Michael Moseley discovered in 1990 that water diffusion decreases considerably in ischemic brain tissue within minutes of a restriction in blood flow. Diffusion MRI has since become a standard diagnostic procedure for the evaluation and management of stroke patients.

Peter Basser realized in 1994 that MRI could be used to characterize the anisotropy of water diffusion (differences in diffusion in different directions), which led to the development of DTI. DTI can be used to characterize the local orientation of the fiber bundles at each location in the white matter of the brain. This is because white matter is made up of bundles of axons (fascicles), and diffusion of water is approximately three to six times faster in the direction of the white matter fiber bundles than in the perpendicular direction.

A DTI measurement begins like all MRI measurements, by placing the subject in a strong magnetic field. A radio frequency pulse is applied so that the water protons wobble in phase with one another (see Box 20–3). Next a gradient in the magnetic field is introduced along one axis for a brief period of time. Let's assume for the moment that this gradient is initially applied in the rostral-caudal direction so that the magnetic field is stronger at the front of the brain than at the back of the brain; but we will see that each of several gradient directions will be used in sequence.

Because of the gradient, the rate of precession is faster for the water protons in the front of the brain than for those in the back of the brain. Indeed, the rate is slightly faster for the water protons at the front of each voxel than for those at the back of each voxel. When the gradient is turned off, therefore, the water protons dephase, each by a fixed amount depending on its front-back location.

A reversed gradient is then introduced with the same amplitude and duration but with the opposite direction (caudal-rostral in this example). If nothing has moved in the front-back direction, then this reversed gradient will perfectly rephase all of the water protons so that they are once again precessing in perfect synchrony.

Because of diffusion, however, each of the water molecules will have moved by some amount during the time period between the first gradient application and the reversed gradient. If diffusion (in the front-back direction) is less in one voxel than in another, the result will be better resynchronization and a brighter MRI image intensity in the voxel with less diffusion. For this example with rostral and caudal gradients, diffusion only in the front-back direction matters. If a water molecule diffuses rightward or leftward, then the dephasing and rephasing caused by the two gradients will perfectly cancel.

The measurement is repeated for each of several directions to characterize the diffusion anisotropy. A separate image of the brain is reconstructed for each direction. A voxel in white matter will typically exhibit greater diffusion in the direction of the fiber tract (dimmer image intensity in the corresponding image) and less diffusion in the other directions (brighter image intensities). These separate images can then be combined to show the degree of anisotropy and the dominant direction of anisotropy (Figure 20–5A).

The most advanced application of DTI is fiber tracking, the only noninvasive method currently available to characterize anatomical connectivity in the living human brain. Fiber tracking is a computational analysis of the DTI measurements, the basic idea of which is to follow the path of anisotropy (and hence the fiber track) from one location in the brain to another (Figure 20–5B).

There are, however, important limitations to the accuracy and precision with which fiber tracking can be done with DTI. Unlike the use of retro- and anterograde tracers that label connections established by individual axons, DTI reflects the statistical average of axon trajectories through each voxel of white matter tissue.

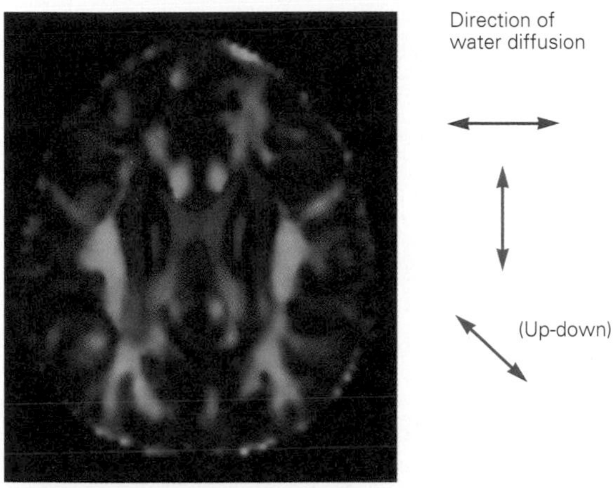

Figure 20–5A MRI measurement of diffusion anisotropy. Water diffusion in white matter is anisotropic, and the anisotropy can be measured with MRI. The color and brightness at each location in the image represents the diffusion of a small volume (or voxel) of tissue. Brightness corresponds to the degree of diffusion anisotropy. White matter mostly appears bright (diffusion is highly anisotropic), whereas gray matter and ventricles are dark (isotropic diffusion). Colors represent the dominant orientation of white matter fibers: **red** indicates that diffusion is greatest in the right–left direction, **green** indicates diffusion is greatest in the front–back direction, and **blue** indicates diffusion is greatest in the up–down direction. (Reproduced, with permission, from Ben-Shachar, Dougherty, and Wandall 2007.)

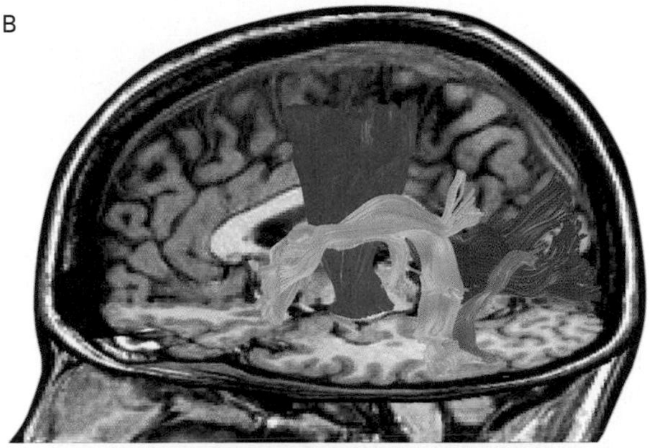

Figure 20–5B White matter fiber tracts reconstructed from DTI. Each "virtual fiber bundle" was computed from the DTI measurements by starting at one location in the brain and following the path of greatest anisotropy. Depicted are four fiber tracts that are believed to be important for reading. **Yellow** fibers are the superior longitudinal fasciculus that connects temporoparietal cortex (including Wernicke's area, which is critical for language comprehension) with lateral frontal cortex (including Broca's area, implicated in language production). The **purple** fibers are passing through the corpus callosum connecting regions of the two occipital lobes and regions of the two temporal lobes. **Blue** fibers are corona radiata fibers that pass through the posterior limb of the internal capsule. Finally, the **orange** fibers connect the posterior occipitotemporal cortex (including a region believed to be critical for letter recognition) with the lateral cortical surface at the border between the occipital and temporal lobes.

Specifically, the intensity in each voxel of each diffusion MRI image depends on the average diffusion of all of the water molecules within that voxel.

Hence, only white matter bundles composed of large numbers of axons are visible (current methods fail to detect tracts smaller than 5 mm in cross-section diameter). The many thin tendrils of white matter connecting nearby cortical areas are not reliably detectable, nor are intracortical connections that remain entirely within gray matter.

In some white matter regions fiber tracking is difficult because different fiber bundles cross, so there is no single dominant diffusion direction. In other regions different fiber bundles travel together over some distance and then separate, which can cause fiber tracking software to make errors.

Even so, DTI is being used in conjunction with fMRI to characterize the normal development of human brain connectivity, and to identify subtle anomalies in brain function and connectivity in a variety of neurological diseases (eg, multiple sclerosis, Alzheimer disease), developmental disabilities (eg, dyslexia), and mental illnesses (eg, schizophrenia).

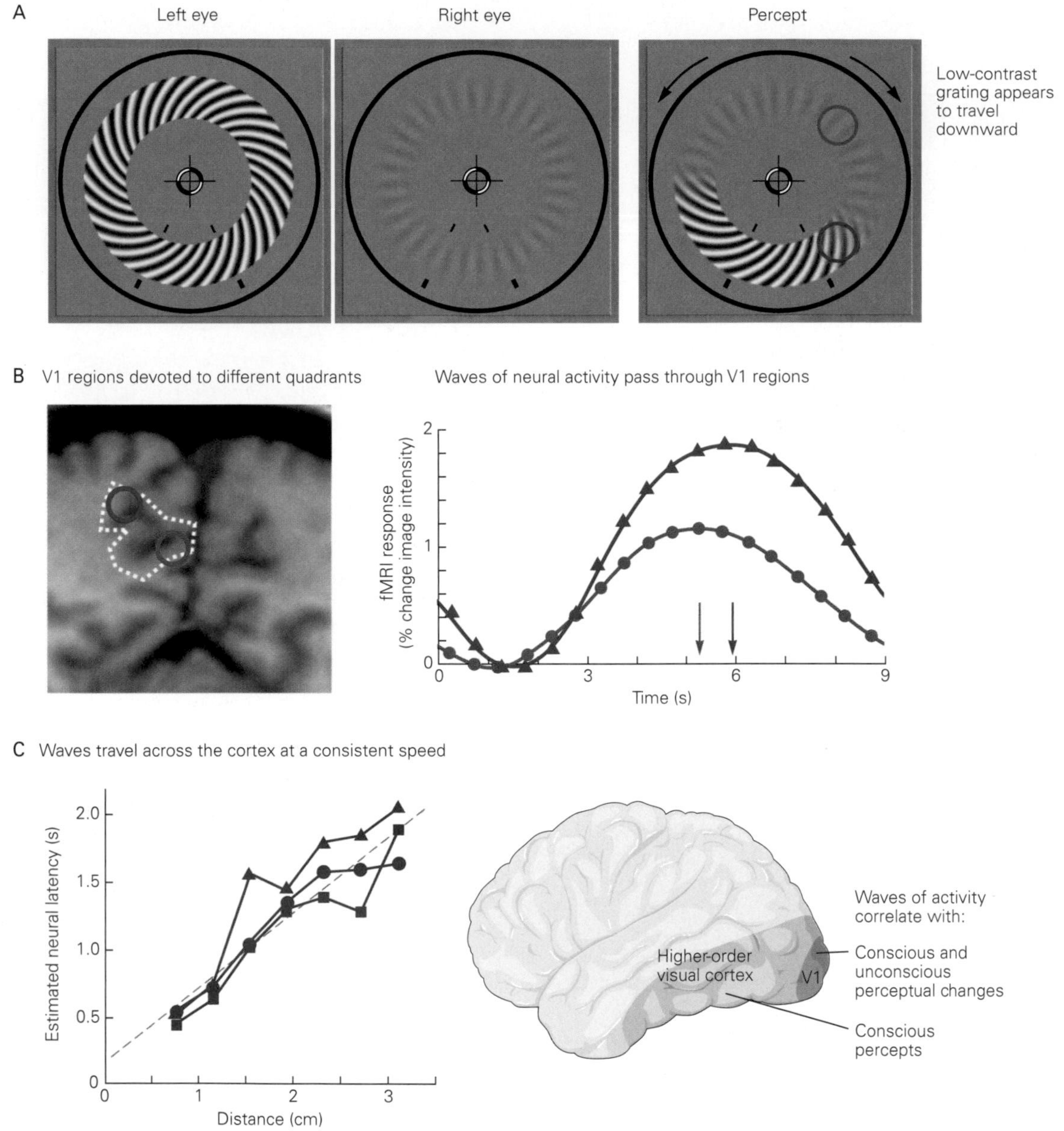

Figure 20–6 Neural correlates of conscious visual perception. (Reproduced, with permission, from Lee, Blake, and Heeger 2005.)

A. A subject is presented with a high-contrast spiral grating in the left eye and a low-contrast radial grating in the right, and each image is restricted to an annular region of the visual field. The subject perceives a traveling wave in which the low-contrast pattern is seen to spread around the annulus, starting at the top and progressively erasing the other image from awareness. (See part B for the explanation of the red and blue circles.)

B. An anatomical image cut through the posterior occipital lobe, perpendicular to the calcarine sulcus. The **red circle** identifies a subregion of primary visual cortex where cells represent the upper-right quadrant of the annular region of the visual field (depicted in part A). The **blue circle** identifies a subregion where cells represent the lower-right quadrant. The plot compares the fMRI measurements from these two subregions. Red and blue curves correspond to the red and blue outlined subregions; **arrows** indicate when these curves peak. The blue curve is delayed in time and larger in amplitude, as the high-contrast pattern remained visible for a longer period of time.

C. Propagation speed of the underlying neural activity, computed from the fMRI measurements of three subjects. Temporal latency of the neural activity is plotted as a function of cortical distance measured along the folded surface of the cerebral cortex. The **dashed slope** corresponds to a propagation speed of approximately 2 cm/s across the cortical surface.

Another experiment showed, however, that the activity waves in primary visual cortex are not themselves sufficient for conscious perception. In this experiment subjects were temporarily distracted (their attention was diverted) so that they did not perceive the rival stimulus patterns presented to the two eyes. Waves of activity were still clearly evident in primary visual cortex, even though subjects did not experience a corresponding traveling wave. However, waves of activity were not evident in V2 and V3.

Indeed, activity in a number of brain areas other than the primary visual cortex correlates with the perceptual alternations of binocular rivalry, including higher-order visual areas in the inferior temporal lobe and areas in parietal and prefrontal cortex. It is likely that these different higher-order cortical areas play distinctive roles in visual perception during binocular rivalry. Attention, mediated by feedback from areas in parietal and prefrontal cortex, is thought to play a crucial role in coordinating the activity across these brain areas to yield conscious perceptual states, as discussed in a later section.

Perceptions are typically made up of multiple sensations, not just a single sensation isolated in experimental conditions. An introduction to a person, for example, involves visual, auditory, and often somatosensory and olfactory information, so that the conscious experience likely reflects activity in several higher-order sensory cortices. Although a multimodal percept arises from activity in numerous brain regions, we sense the conscious experience as a unified, seamless whole. The linkage between discrete functional systems in the brain that gives rise to a unified experience of consciousness is sometimes called the "binding problem." According to one view, a conscious experience occurs when neural activity in disparate regions of the brain is time locked: The activity in these areas becomes temporarily synchronous.

Imaging Memory with and Without Consciousness

Conscious perception and conscious memories have long been linked. According to one view, conscious recall occurs when a stimulus reactivates the brain regions that first encoded the conscious percept being remembered. An fMRI experiment by Randy Buckner and colleagues provided the first empirical evidence in support of this idea.

Buckner trained subjects to associate pictures or sounds with a written word. For example, the word "dog" was associated either with a picture of a dog or the sound of a dog barking. Subjects were scanned with fMRI after they were shown the word and asked to recall the associated picture or sound, thereby mapping memory-storage regions. In addition, they were scanned during exposure to the picture or sound, thereby mapping regions involved in perception.

Remarkably, first hearing and later recalling a sound stimulated some of the same higher-order regions in the auditory cortex, and viewing and later recalling a picture stimulated some of the same higher-order regions in the visual cortex. However, conscious recall of sounds or pictures did not activate areas of primary sensory cortex. These results provide evidence that conscious memory recall used some of the same regions of the brain that were used for conscious perception.

The notion that higher-order sensory cortex is recruited for memory is reinforced by studies of different stages of sleep. Although dreams are not faithful recollections of the external world, they are remarkably vivid, comparable to conscious memory. Functional imaging studies of rapid-eye-movement sleep, during which dreaming occurs, and slow-wave sleep, characterized by the absence of dreams, have found that dreaming is associated with activity throughout higher-order sensory cortical areas. Just as in Buckner's experiment, primary sensory cortex is not activated during dreaming.

Other imaging studies have found that when a stimulus induces only a sense of familiarity, not a full-blown recollection, brain activity tends to be confined to specific sensory regions representing one, or at most, a very few modalities. Taken together these studies demonstrate that, just as with conscious perception, simultaneous activity in several higher-order sensory regions underlies recollection (conscious recall of the stimulus along with the associated details of the context, when and where the stimulus was initially perceived, what else happened at the same time, etc.).

Imaging Attentional Modulation of Conscious Perception

Our brain is constantly bombarded by external and internal stimulation, yet at any given moment we are only aware of a small fraction of this input. Attention is one factor that influences the focus and scope of our awareness. As we mentioned earlier in Chapter 17, the American psychologist William James defined attention as ". . . the taking possession by the mind, in clear and vivid form, of one out of what seem several simultaneous possible objects or trains of thought." James captured the key element of attention—when confronted with more than one input the brain does not process all inputs equally.

Performance on a wide variety of perceptual discrimination and identification tasks is faster and more accurate when subjects attend to the right place at the right time. Several investigators have developed experimental protocols to characterize the behavioral consequences of attention. For example, in a visual attention experiment the subject is asked to fixate a spot at the center of a computer screen while visual stimuli are shown on either side. The subject is instructed to shift attention to one side of the screen, without moving the eyes, when a visual cue, such as an arrow, indicates an upcoming stimulus at the side of the screen. Behavioral performance (speed or accuracy) in a visual discrimination task is enhanced when subjects shift their attention to the side of the screen containing the stimulus.

On the basis of studies of patients with attention deficits as a consequence of a neglect syndrome following a stroke, the parietal and frontal lobes have long been implicated in the control of visual attention (Chapter 17). Using PET imaging, Michael Posner and his colleagues have confirmed that frontal and parietal lobe regions contribute to the control of attention. Similarly, as we saw in Chapter 17, electrophysiological studies of attention by Michael Goldberg have identified neurons in areas of the parietal lobe that respond more strongly to attended stimuli than to unattended stimuli.

William James described two different kinds of attention. One is passive, automatic, stimulus-driven, and transient, whereas the other is active, voluntary, conceptually driven, and sustained. In "passive immediate sensorial attention the stimulus is a sense-impression, either very intense, voluminous, or sudden . . . big things, bright things, moving things . . . blood." We now refer to passive, nonvoluntary attention as exogenous attention, whereas active and voluntary attention is called endogenous attention.

Functional imaging has revealed that the two types of attention recruit different subregions of the brain. During voluntary attention certain parietal areas (within the intraparietal sulcus) and frontal areas (frontal eye fields) are active when subjects are instructed to shift or maintain attention. Shifts in attention are mediated by transient responses in the frontal and parietal regions immediately following the presentation of a cue. The maintenance of attention, critical for our ability to focus on a particular location in the visual field over an extended period of time, is mediated by sustained activity in the visual cortex as well as some of the same parietal and frontal brain regions. Additional brain areas become active when attention is diverted by a particularly significant or unexpected stimulus. For example, the amygdala is involved in diverting attention to emotionally salient (particularly fearful) stimuli such as a fearful face or a snake (see Chapter 48).

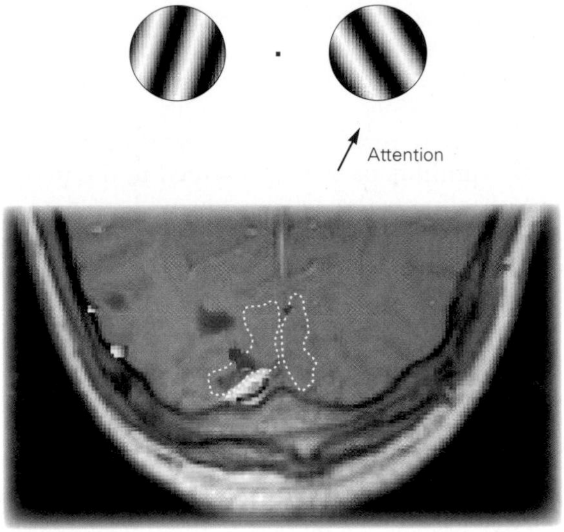

Figure 20–7 Neural correlate of attention. Subjects had to fixate on the center of a display (above) and were instructed to attend to one side or the other without moving their eyes. Here an axial (horizontal) slice through the occipital lobe of the brain (below) shows functional activity (**red** and **orange**) superimposed on the brain anatomy. The **dashed outlines** mark the boundaries of primary visual cortex. Activity in the left hemisphere increased when the subject attended to the right and vice versa (stimuli on the right are processed by neurons in the left hemisphere and vice versa). (Adapted, with permission, from Gandhi, Heeger, and Boynton 1999.)

Attention is believed to be controlled by a particular network of cortical and subcortical areas. But how does this give rise to the improved behavioral performance discussed above? One idea is that signals from higher-order cortical areas flow back down to sensory cortical areas to facilitate the sensory representation of an attended stimulus. Functional imaging experiments have found that in this way the neural representation of an attended stimulus is amplified. This amplification is correlated with, and is believed to cause, the improvements in behavioral performance that accompany attention (Figure 20–7).

Functional Imaging Has Limitations

Despite its remarkable abilities, functional imaging, like any tool, has some technical and conceptual limitations. Four variables that correlate with brain metabolism can be used in functional imaging: glucose uptake, cerebral blood flow, cerebral blood volume, and deoxyhemoglobin content. The latter is the basis of the BOLD response on which most fMRI measurements are based (see Box 20–3).

Deoxyhemoglobin content is the only one that cannot be measured in absolute terms and is in fact dependent on a complex and poorly understood interplay among cerebral blood flow, cerebral blood volume, and the basal (or "resting") state of the brain region under investigation. Two brain regions with differing basal states, therefore, may lead to different BOLD responses, even if a stimulus induces identical changes in oxygen metabolism in each region.

Thus, inferring that differences in the BOLD response necessarily reflect underlying differences in oxygen metabolism and neural activity can lead to false conclusions. For example, the amplitude of the BOLD response to visual stimuli measured in the primary visual cortex is typically larger than the BOLD response to motor stimuli measured in the primary motor cortex. One might conclude that the visual cortex is metabolically more responsive then the motor cortex, but this difference between the regions is more likely to reflect differences in basal deoxyhemoglobin. The BOLD response, therefore, can be similar in several areas of the brain stimulated by a particular stimulus, but this similarity cannot tell us which area of the brain is more metabolically active than another.

Moreover, because most disorders of the brain affect the basal state and deoxyhemoglobin of targeted brain regions, similar false conclusions might be drawn when comparing the BOLD responses of patients and healthy controls (Figure 20–8). This limitation has hampered the usefulness of BOLD fMRI in clinical populations but can be overcome by calibrating BOLD measurements. Moreover, new functional MRI techniques measure cerebral blood flow or cerebral blood volume in absolute terms.

What component of neuronal activity is most highly correlated with these measures of brain metabolism? Although it is known that the BOLD response (and the other functional imaging measures) is triggered by metabolic demands of increased neural activity, the details of this process are poorly understood. Considerable evidence suggests that increased blood flow follows from increased synaptic activity. Thus, fMRI responses may be most closely related to synaptic input and intracortical processing within a cortical area, not the spiking output, and there are some clear demonstrations that change in blood flow can be dissociated from spiking activity.

Cortical circuits are, however, dominated by massive local connectivity; most synaptic inputs originate from nearby neurons, while only a small minority originates from distant sites such as the thalamus or other cortical areas. Thus, synaptic inputs in the cerebral cortex are produced mostly by neighboring neurons, leading typically to a tight coupling of synaptic and spiking activity, as well as metabolic responses (including BOLD fMRI). It is not surprising, therefore, that fMRI responses have often been found to be highly correlated with neural spiking. The extent of decoupling of

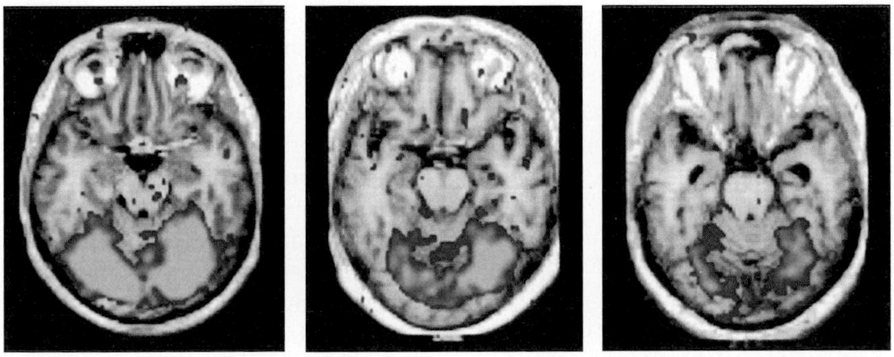

Young Old Alzheimer disease

Figure 20–8 A potential pitfall of functional magnetic resonance imaging. Deoxyhemoglobin content, which is the basis for blood oxygen level dependent (BOLD) fMRI, is the result of a complex interplay between blood flow, blood volume, and oxygen metabolism. For this reason it is a correlate of brain metabolism for which absolute measurements cannot be made. Imaging deoxyhemoglobin content, therefore, must be interpreted with caution. For example, as shown here, a simple visual stimulation experiment results in different BOLD signals in the visual cortex of young, old, and Alzheimer subjects with no apparent visual defects. These results may reflect differences in vascular physiology associated with aging and disease more than underlying differences in brain function. (Adapted, with permission, from Buckner et al. 2000.)

Box 20–5 Limitations of Functional Imaging

Another potential pitfall with functional imaging is the logic by which the results are interpreted. Research using functional imaging often begins by hypothesizing that a particular cognitive process occurs in a functionally specialized brain area. An experiment is then designed with two or more stimuli or tasks that differ in the demands they make on the hypothesized cognitive process. If there is such a cognitive process and if it is functionally localized in the brain, then the particular brain area would be expected to become more active with increased demand on that cognitive process.

If the brain region of interest is activated during the experiment, one is tempted to conclude that the hypothesis has been confirmed. This kind of reasoning is flawed and has led to a latter-day phrenology in which every bump in brain anatomy is assigned a function.

If subjects are asked to view two or more different stimuli or perform two or more different tasks, the brain will certainly respond differently to the different stimuli or different tasks. If no difference in brain activity is shown in the experiment, it may be because of a failure in the measurement technique (eg, insufficient spatial or temporal resolution, too much noise or artifact in the measurements, etc.).

In fact, finding a difference in brain activity merely confirms that the participant experienced two or more different stimuli or performed two or more different tasks. This one experiment cannot confirm or disprove that some cognitive process is localized in one area of the brain, but it may be a worthwhile starting point for further research. Further experiments can determine if the activity in the brain area changes systematically with parallel cellular–physiological studies of the homologous area in monkeys or with theoretical predictions based on a computational model of the hypothesized cognitive process.

It is also important to rule out alternative theories. Showing a correlation with the predictions of a theory provides only weak evidence in support of that theory. Showing a positive correlation with the predictions of one theory and negative correlations with the predictions of alternative hypotheses provides much stronger support.

synaptic and spiking activity depends on the nature of the cortical circuits, that is, whether the cortical activity is dominated by the local recurrent circuitry or by synaptic inputs (either feedforward or feedback) from other brain areas. Functional MRI measurements may be highly correlated with the spiking activity of a brain area under some circumstances, but with subthreshold modulatory input under other circumstances. One implication of this is that fMRI measurements must be interpreted with caution (Box 20–5).

An Overall View

Functional imaging provides a key bridge between behavioral studies of human cognition and electrophysiologic studies of neural function in intact experimental animals such as monkeys or genetically modified mice. Insofar as cognition emerges from a complex interplay across many regions of the brain, the ability to record brain activity simultaneously from multiple areas endows functional imaging with unique exploratory powers.

Functional imaging is expanding on three fronts. First, although it is clear that functional imaging can record meaningful signals from the brain at work, it is also clear that we do not yet have a complete understanding of what is causing these changes in signal, how they are generated, and what they are precisely telling us about underlying neural processes. Achieving a full understanding will require coupling functional imaging with invasive techniques. Accordingly, one of the important developments in the field is in the use of monkeys and transgenically engineered mice to investigate the physiological and molecular mechanisms underlying functional imaging.

Second, functional imaging studies are moving beyond establishing a catalog of the component parts of cognition toward an understanding of how the parts interact within large-scale networks. For example, investigators are beginning to explore how higher- and lower-order sensory areas interact with the medial temporal lobes and the parietal and prefrontal cortex to give rise to cognition or consciousness.

Third, studies are scaling down from the large-scale analysis of the whole brain to a more focused investigation of discrete brain areas, such as the numerous visual cortical areas, the olfactory bulb, and the hippocampal formation. These studies are designed not for human brain mapping but rather to test computational theories of the function and functional organization of predefined brain areas.

Scott A. Small
David J. Heeger

Selected Readings

Blake R, Logothetis NK. 2002. Visual competition. Nat Rev Neurosci 3:13–21.

Heeger DJ, Ress D. 2002. What does fMRI tell us about neuronal activity? Nat Rev Neurosci 3:142–151.

Logothetis NK, Wandell BA. 2004. Interpreting the BOLD signal. Annu Rev Physiol 66:735–769.

Ogawa S, Lee TM, Kay AR, Tank DW. 1990. Brain magnetic resonance imaging with contrast dependent on blood oxygenation. Proc Natl Acad Sci U S A 87:9868–9872.

Pauling L, Coryell CD. 1936. The magnetic properties of hemoglobin, oxyhemoglobin and carbonmonoxyhemoglobin. Proc Natl Acad Sci U S A 22:210–216.

Small SA. 2004. Quantifying cerebral blood flow; regional regulation with global implications. J Clin Invest 114:1046–1048.

References

Basser PJ, Mattiello J, LeBihan D. 1994. MR diffusion tensor spectroscopy and imaging. Biophys J 66:259–267.

Ben-Shachar M, Dougherty RF, Wandall BA. 2007. White matter pathways in reading. Curr Opin Neurobiol 17:258–270.

Boynton GM, Engel SA, Glover GH, Heeger DJ. 1996. Linear systems analysis of functional magnetic resonance imaging in human V1. J Neurosci 16:4207–4221.

Buckner RL, Bandettini PA, O'Craven KM, Savoy RL, Petersen SE, Raichle ME, Rosen BR. 1996. Detection of cortical activation during averaged single trials of a cognitive task using functional magnetic resonance imaging. Proc Natl Acad Sci U S A 93:14878–14883.

Buckner BL, Snyder AZ, Raichle ME, Morris JC. 2000. Functional brain imaging of young, nondemented, and demented older adults. J Cogn Neurosci 12(Suppl 2): 24–34.

Buxton RB, Wong EC, Frank LR. 1998. Dynamics of blood flow and oxygenation changes during brain activation: the balloon model. Magn Reson Med 39:855–864.

Cheng K, Waggoner RA, Tanaka K. 2001. Human ocular dominance columns as revealed by high-field functional magnetic resonance imaging. Neuron 32:359–374.

Corbetta M, Shulman GL. 2002. Control of goal-directed and stimulus-driven attention in the brain. Nat Rev Neurosci 3:201–215.

Crick F. 1995. *The Astonishing Hypothesis: The Scientific Search for the Soul*. New York: Touchstone/Simon & Schuster.

Crick F, Koch C. 1995. Are we aware of neural activity in primary visual cortex? Nature 375:121–123.

Fox PT, Raichle ME. 1986. Focal physiological uncoupling of cerebral blood flow and oxidative metabolism during somatosensory stimulation in human subjects. Proc Natl Acad Sci U S A 83:1140–1144.

Fox PT, Raichle ME, Mintun MA, Dence C. 1988. Nonoxidative glucose consumption during focal physiologic neural activity. Science 241:462–464.

Friston KJ, Jezzard P, Turner R. 1994. Analysis of functional MRI time-series. Hum Brain Mapp 1:153–171.

Gandhi SP, Heeger DJ, Boynton GM. 1999. Spatial attention affects brain activity in human primary visual cortex. Proc Natl Acad Sci U S A 96:3314–3319.

Kastner S, Ungerleider LG. 2000. Mechanisms of visual attention in the human cortex. Annu Rev Neurosci 23:315–341.

LeBihan D. 2003. Looking into the functional architecture of the brain with diffusion MRI. Nat Rev Neurosci 4: 469–480.

Lee SH, Blake R, Heeger DJ. 2005. Traveling waves of activity in primary visual cortex during binocular rivalry. Nat Neurosci 8:22–23.

Lee SH, Blake R, Heeger DJ. 2007. Hierarchy of cortical responses underlying binocular rivalry. Nat Neurosci 10:1048–1054.

Lennie P. 2003. The cost of cortical computation. Curr Biol 13:493–497.

Logothetis NK, Pauls J, Augath M, Trinath T, Oeltermann A. 2001. Neurophysiological investigation of the basis of the fMRI signal. Nature 412:150–157.

Lumer ED, Friston KJ, Rees G. 1998. Neural correlates of perceptual rivalry in the human brain. Science 280: 1930–1934.

Moseley ME, Kucharczyk J, Mintorovitch J, Cohen Y, Kurhanewicz J, Derugin N, Asgari H, Norman D. 1990. Diffusion-weighted MR imaging of acute stroke: correlation with T2-weighted and magnetic susceptibility-enhanced MR imaging in cats. AJNR Am J Neuroradiol 11:423–429.

Oldendorf WH. 1980. *The Quest for an Image of the Brain: Computerized Tomography in the Perspective of Past and Future Imaging Methods*. New York: Raven.

Posner MI. 1980. Orienting of attention. Q J Exp Psychol 32:3–25.

Posner M. 1994. Attention: the mechanisms of consciousness. Proc Natl Acad Sci U S A 91:7398–7403.

Rees G, Kreiman G, Koch C. 2002. Neural correlates of consciousness in humans. Nat Rev Neurosci 3:261–270.

Ress D, Backus BT, Heeger DJ. 2000. Activity in primary visual cortex predicts performance in a visual detection task. Nat Neurosci 3:940–945.

Schwartz WJ, Smith CB, Davidsen L, Savaki H, Sokoloff L, Mata M, Fink DJ, Gainer H. 1979. Metabolic mapping of functional activity in the hypothalamo-neurohypophysial system of the rat. Science 205:723–725.

Tong F. 2003. Primary visual cortex and visual awareness. Nat Rev Neurosci 4:219–229.

Treisman AM, Gelade G. 1980. A feature-integration theory of attention. Cogn Psychol 12:97–136.

Wagner AD, Schacter DL, Rotte M, Koutstaal W, Maril A, Dale AM, Rosen BR, Buckner RL. 1998. Building memories: remembering and forgetting of verbal experiences as predicted by brain activity. Science 281:1188–1191.

Wheatstone C. 1838. Contributions to the physiology of vision. Part the first: On some remarkable and unobserved phenomena of binocular vision. Phil Trans R Soc Lond 128:371–394.

Zeki S, Watson JD, Lueck CJ, Friston KJ, Kennard C, Frackowiak RS. 1991. A direct demonstration of functional specialization in human visual cortex. J Neurosci 11:641–649.

Part V

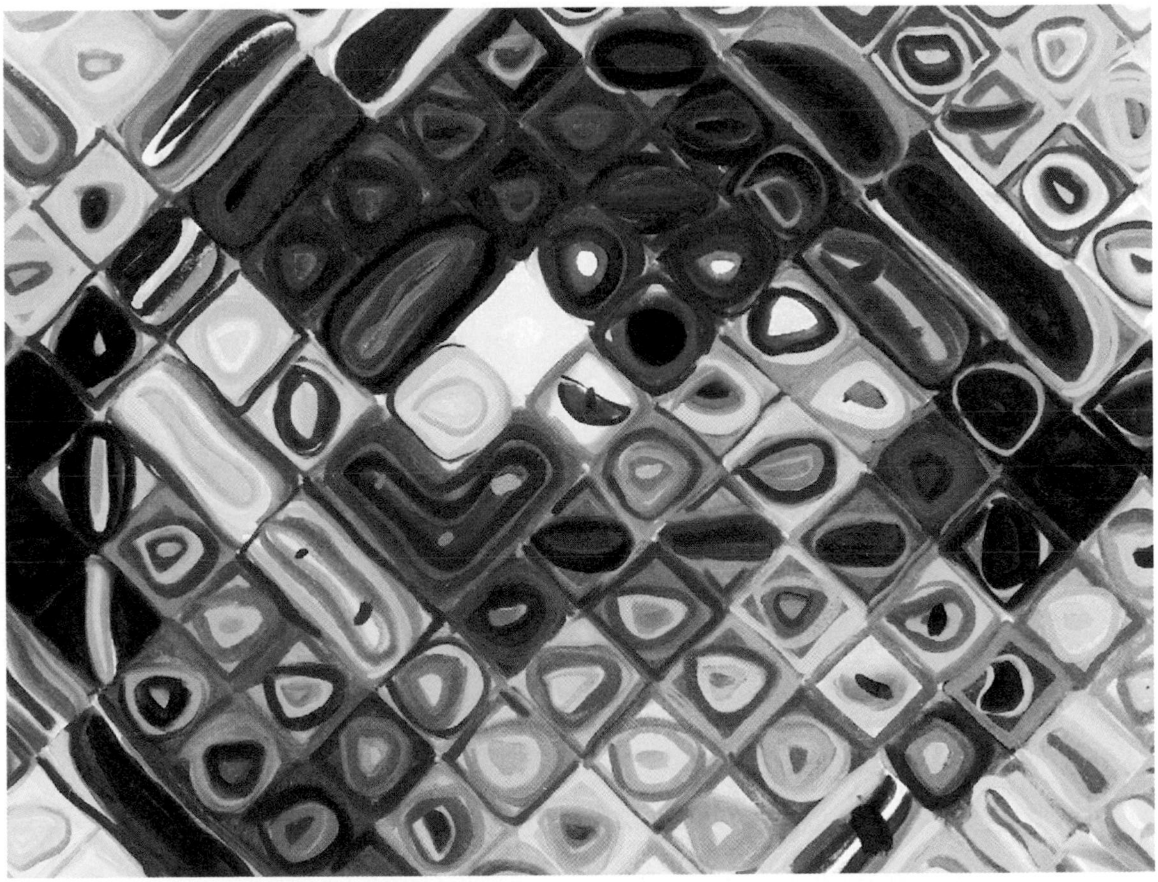

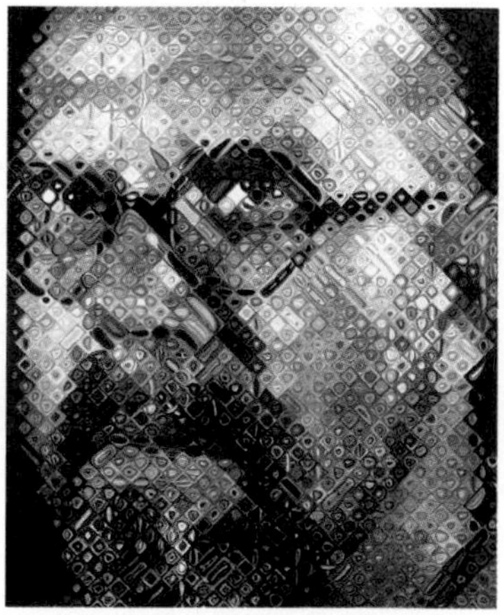

Preceding Page

Detail of a self-portrait by Chuck Close. Viewed from a short distance, this painting appears to be an abstract grid of vividly colored squares and ovals. But, when viewed from farther away, the local colors blend and we begin to perceive a spectacle-framed eye. The interplay between these local and global features, which are conveyed by discrete visual pathways, gives the portrait its particular dynamism.

Chuck Close has prosopagnosia, or difficulty in recognizing faces; his technique of flattening and subdividing an image into manageable elements enhances his ability to both perceive and portray the face. The complete painting is shown above. (Reproduced, with permission, from digital image: copyright the Museum of Modern Art/licensed by SCALA/Art Resource, NY; Copyright Chuck Close, courtesy of The Pace Gallery.)

V Perception

> . . . one day in winter, on my return home, my mother, seeing that I was cold, offered me some tea, a thing I did not ordinarily take. I declined at first, and then, for no particular reason, changed my mind. She sent for one of these squat, plump little cakes called "petites madeleines," which look as though they had been moulded in the fluted valve of a scallop shell. And soon, mechanically, dispirited after a dreary day with the prospect of a dreary morrow, I raised to my lips a spoonful of the tea in which I had soaked a morsel of the cake. No sooner had the warm liquid mixed with the crumbs touched my palate than a shudder ran through me and I stopped, intent upon the extraordinary thing that was happening to me. An exquisite pleasure had invaded my senses, something isolated, detached, with no suggestion of its origin. And at once the vicissitudes of life had become indifferent to me, its disasters innocuous, its brevity illusory—this new sensation having had on me the effect which love has of filling me with a precious essence; or rather this essence was not in me, it was me.*

THE TASTE OF THE MADELEINE dipped in tea is one of the most famous evocations of sensory experience in literature. Proust's description of the conscious nature of sensation and memory provides profound insights into some of the subjects that we shall explore in the next few chapters. His description of the shape of the pastries on the plate, the warmth of the tea, and the mingled flavors of tea and cake remind us that knowledge of the world arises through the senses.

Perceptions begin in receptor cells that are sensitive to one or another kind of stimulus energy. Most sensations are identified with a particular type of stimulus. Thus, light of short wavelength falling on the eye is seen as blue, and sugar on the tongue tastes sweet. How the quantitative aspects of physical stimuli correlate with the sensations they evoke is the subject of psychophysics. Additional information about perception can be obtained from studying the various sensory receptors and the stimuli to which they respond as well as the sensory pathways that carry information from these receptors to the cerebral cortex. Specific cells in the sensory system, both peripheral receptors and central neurons, encode certain critical attributes of sensations, such as location and intensity. Other attributes of sensation are represented by the pattern of activity in a population of sensory neurons. We know, for example, that taste depends greatly

---

*Proust, M. [1913] 1981. *Remembrance of Things Past. Volume 1: Swann's Way: Within a Budding Grove.* Pléiad edition translated by C.K. Scott Moncrieff and Terence Kilmartin. New York: Vintage. p. 48.

on receptor specificity. In contrast, the differentiation of sounds depends in large part on pattern coding. Determining the extent to which receptor specificity and patterns of neural activity are used in different sensory systems to encode information is a major task of current research in sensory physiology.

Each sensory modality is mediated by a distinct neural system with multiple components that contribute to perception. Sensory pathways include neurons that link the receptors at the periphery with the spinal cord, brain stem, thalamus, and cerebral cortex. The perception of a touch on the hand begins when cutaneous mechanoreceptors cause a population of afferent fibers to discharge action potentials, thus setting up a propagated response in the dorsal column nuclei and then in the thalamus. From the thalamus sensory information flows to several areas of the cerebral cortex, each of which analyzes particular aspects of the original stimulus. This cortical representation is closely correlated with our conscious perception. For example, an illusion of sensation in the hand, albeit a slightly blunted one, can be elicited by electrical stimulation of the cortical area that represents the hand.

In this part of the book, we examine the principles essential for understanding how perception occurs in the brain. Contrary to our intuitive understanding based on personal experience, perceptions are not direct copies of the world around us. The information available to sensory systems at any instant in time is imperfect and incomplete. So perceptual systems are not built like physical devices for making measurements, but instead are built to perform inferences about the world. Sensory data should not be thought of as giving answers, but as providing clues.

The brain, for example, is where seeing happens; it is the brain that figures out what the clues mean. Thus visual perception is a creation of the brain. It is based on the input extracted from the retinal image. But what is seen in the "mind's eye" goes far beyond what is presented in the input. The brain uses information it has extracted previously as the basis for educated guesses—perceptual inferences about the state of the world.

Sensory systems contain many representations that each specialize in different kinds of sensory information processing. Throughout each sensory system, from the peripheral receptors to the cerebral cortex, information about physical stimuli is transformed in stages according to computational rules that reflect the functional properties of the neurons and their interconnections at each stage.

The visual system, for example, transforms the stimulus energy that the retinal receptors receive into a neural code of action potentials like the dots and dashes of a Morse code. The brain solves the problem of computation by performing relatively simple operations in parallel in massive numbers of neurons, and by repeating these operations at multiple hierarchical stages. The great mystery of vision is how we respond to trains of action potentials in different neurons of the visual system by seeing an image—like a face.

A major goal of cognitive neural science is to determine how the information that reaches the cerebral cortex by means of parallel afferent pathways is bound together to form a unified conscious perception. Indeed, one of the hopes driving cognitive neural science is that progress in understanding the binding problem will yield our first insights into the biological basis of attention and ultimately consciousness.

Part V

21

Sensory Coding

SINCE ANCIENT TIMES HUMANS have been fascinated by the nature of sensory experience. The Greek philosopher Aristotle defined five senses—vision, hearing, touch, taste, and smell—each linked to specific sense organs in the body: the eyes, ears, skin, tongue, and nose (Figure 21–1). Pain was not considered to be a specific sensory modality but rather an affliction of the soul. Intuition, often referred to colloquially as a "sixth sense," was something beyond the experience of classic sensory systems. Today neurobiologists are more likely to describe intuition as inferences derived from previous experience and thus the result of cognitive rather than sensory processes.

In this chapter we consider the organizational principles and coding mechanisms universal to all sensory systems. We define *sensory* information as neural activity originating from stimulation of receptor cells in specific parts of the body. These senses include the classic five senses plus a variety of modalities not recognized by the ancients but essential to bodily function: the *somatic* sensations of proprioception (posture and movement of our own body), pain, itch, and temperature; *visceral* sensations (both conscious and unconscious) necessary for homeostasis; and the *vestibular* senses of balance (the position of the body in the gravitational field) and head movement.

The extent to which features of sensory processing have been conserved in the course of human evolution seems nothing short of astonishing. In each of the sensory systems receptors provide the first neural representation of the external world. This information flows centrally to regions of the brain involved in cognition. The sensory pathways have both serial and parallel components, consisting of fiber tracts with thousands or millions of axons interrupted by synaptic relays comprising millions of neurons. Along the way information is transformed from relatively simple forms to

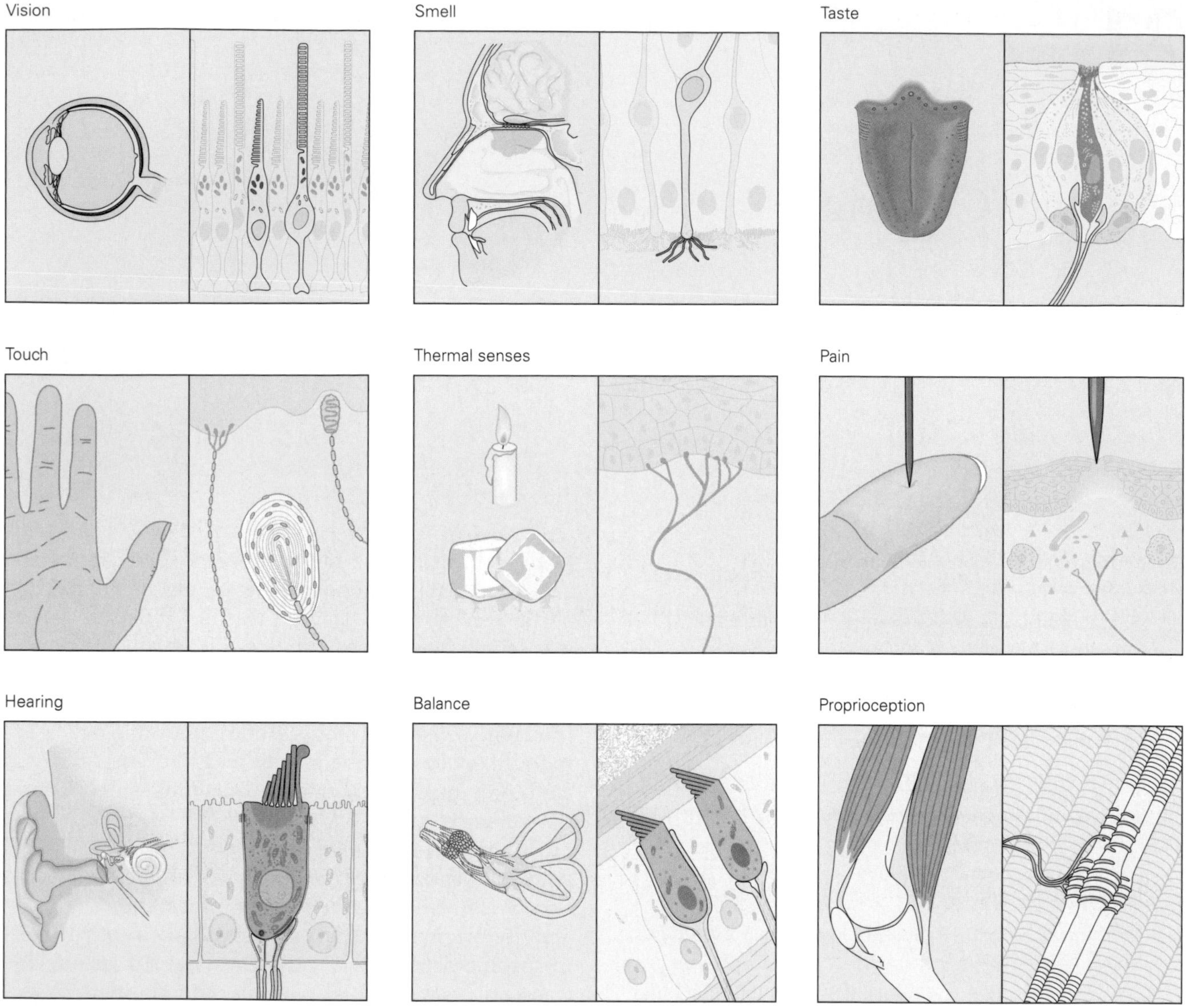

Figure 21–1 The major sensory modalities in humans are mediated by distinct classes of receptor neurons located in specific sense organs. Each class of receptor cell transforms one type of stimulus energy into electrical signals that are encoded as trains of action potentials. The principal receptor cells include photoreceptors (vision), chemoreceptors (smell, taste, and pain), thermal receptors, and mechanoreceptors (touch, hearing, balance, and proprioception). The classic five senses—vision, smell, taste, touch, and hearing—and the sense of balance are mediated by receptors in the eye, nose, mouth, skin, and inner ear, respectively. The other somatosensory modalities—thermal senses, pain, and proprioception—are mediated by receptors distributed throughout the body.

the complex forms that are the basis of cognition. Sensory pathways are also recursive. The higher centers in the brain modify and structure the incoming flow of sensory signals by feeding information back to earlier stages of processing; thus percepts are shaped by internal as well as environmental factors.

In each sensory modality a specific type of stimulus energy is transformed into electrical signals by specialized receptors. The sensory information is transmitted to the central nervous system by trains of action potentials that represent particular aspects of the stimulus. The question that has intrigued philosophers and scientists alike is whether experienced sensations accurately reflect the stimuli that produce them or whether our knowledge of the world is inherently subjective and imprecise.

Modern thought about how knowledge is represented in the brain began with European philosophers of the 17th, 18th, and 19th centuries whose interest in sensation and perception was related to the question of human nature itself. The major division was between the empiricists, represented by John Locke, George Berkeley, and David Hume, and the idealists, including René Descartes, Immanuel Kant, and Georg Wilhelm Friedrich Hegel. Locke, the preeminent empiricist, advanced the idea that the mind at birth is a blank slate, or *tabula rasa*, void of any ideas. Knowledge is obtained through sensory experience—what we see, hear, feel, taste, and smell. In fact, Berkeley questioned whether there was any sensory reality beyond the experiences and knowledge acquired through the senses. He asked the now-famous question: Does a falling tree make a sound if no one is near enough to hear it?

The idealists responded that the human mind possesses certain innate abilities, including logical reasoning itself. The 18th-century German philosopher Immanuel Kant classified the five senses as categories of human understanding. He argued that perceptions were not direct records of the world around us but rather were products of the brain and thus depended on the architecture of the nervous system. Kant referred to these brain properties as *a priori* knowledge.

Thus in Kant's view the mind was not the passive receiver of sense impressions envisaged by the empiricists. Rather the human mind had evolved to conform to certain universal conditions such as space, time, and causality. These conditions were independent of any physical stimuli detected by the body. For Kant and the idealists this meant that knowledge is based not only on sensory stimulation but also on the brain's properties that organize sensory experience. If sensory experience is inherently subjective and personal, they said, it may not be subject to scientific analysis.

Psychophysics Relates the Physical Properties of Stimuli to Sensations

The modern study of sensation and perception began in the 19th century with the emergence of experimental psychology as a scientific discipline. The first psychologists—Ernst Weber, Gustav Fechner, Hermann Helmholtz, and Wilhelm Wundt—focused their experimental study of mental processes on sensation, which they believed was the key to understanding the mind. Their findings gave rise to the fields of psychophysics and sensory physiology.

Psychophysics describes the relationship between the physical characteristics of a stimulus and the attributes of the sensory experience. *Sensory physiology* examines the neural consequences of a stimulus—how the stimulus is transduced by sensory receptors and processed in the brain. Some of the most exciting advances in our understanding of perception have come from merging these two approaches in both human and animal studies. For example, functional magnetic resonance imaging (fMRI) and positron emission tomography (PET) have been used in controlled experiments to identify regions of the human brain involved in the perception of pain.

Psychophysical Laws Govern the Perception of Stimulus Intensity

Early scientific studies of the mind focused not on the perception of complex qualities such as color or taste but on phenomena that could be isolated and measured precisely: the size, shape, amplitude, velocity, and timing of stimuli. Weber and Fechner developed simple experimental paradigms to study how and under what conditions humans are able to distinguish between two stimuli of different amplitudes. They quantified the intensity of sensations in the form of mathematical laws that allowed them to predict the relationship between stimulus magnitude and sensory discrimination.

For example, in 1834 Weber demonstrated that the sensitivity of a sensory system to differences in intensity depends on the absolute strength of the stimuli. We easily perceive that 1 kg is different from 2 kg, but it is difficult to distinguish 50 kg from 51 kg. Yet both sets differ by 1 kg. This relationship is expressed in the equation now known as Weber's law:

$$\Delta S = K \cdot S$$

where ΔS is the minimal difference in strength between a reference stimulus S and a second stimulus that can be discriminated, and K is a constant. This is termed the *just noticeable difference* or difference limen. It follows that the difference in magnitude necessary to discriminate between a reference stimulus and a second stimulus increases with the strength of the reference stimulus.

Fechner extended Weber's law to describe the relationship between the stimulus strength (S) and the intensity of the sensation (I) experienced by a subject:

$$I = K \log (S/S_0)$$

where S_0 is the threshold amplitude of the stimulus and K is a constant. Although Fechner's law was widely accepted for nearly a century after its publication in 1860, his assumption that the intensity of sensation could be equated with the sum of equal increments in "just noticeable differences" turned out to be incorrect.

In 1953 S. S. Stevens demonstrated that, over an extended range of stimulation, subjective experience of sensation intensity is best described by a power function rather than by a logarithmic relationship. Stevens' law states that:

$$I = K(S - S_0)^n$$

For some sensory experiences, such as the sense of pressure on the hand, the relationship between the stimulus magnitude and the perceived intensity is linear, that is, a power function with a unity exponent ($n = 1$).

The lowest stimulus strength a subject can detect is termed the *sensory threshold*. Thresholds are normally determined statistically by presenting a subject with a series of stimuli of random amplitude. The percentage of times the subject reports detecting the stimulus is plotted as a function of stimulus amplitude, forming a relation called the *psychometric function* (Figure 21–2). By convention, threshold is defined as the stimulus amplitude detected in half of the trials. Thresholds can also be determined by the method of limits, in which the subject reports the intensity at which a progressively decreasing stimulus is no longer detectable or an increasing stimulus is detectable. This technique is widely used in audiology to measure hearing thresholds.

The measurement of sensory thresholds is a useful diagnostic technique for determining sensory function in individual modalities. An elevated threshold may signal an abnormality in sensory receptors (such as loss of hair cells in the inner ear caused by aging or exposure to very loud noise), deficits in nerve conduction properties (as in multiple sclerosis), or a lesion in sensory-processing areas of the brain. Sensory thresholds may also be altered by emotional or psychological factors related to the conditions in which stimulus detection is measured.

Psychophysical Measurements of Sensation Magnitude Employ Standardized Protocols

The lasting importance of Fechner's work was the development of formal quantitative methods for measuring sensory performance and mathematical techniques to analyze them. Three of his methods are still widely used, either exactly as he formulated them or in a modified form: (1) the method of constant stimuli, in which a fixed set of stimuli is presented repeatedly to obtain a statistical characterization of the behavior associated with each stimulus; (2) the method of limits,

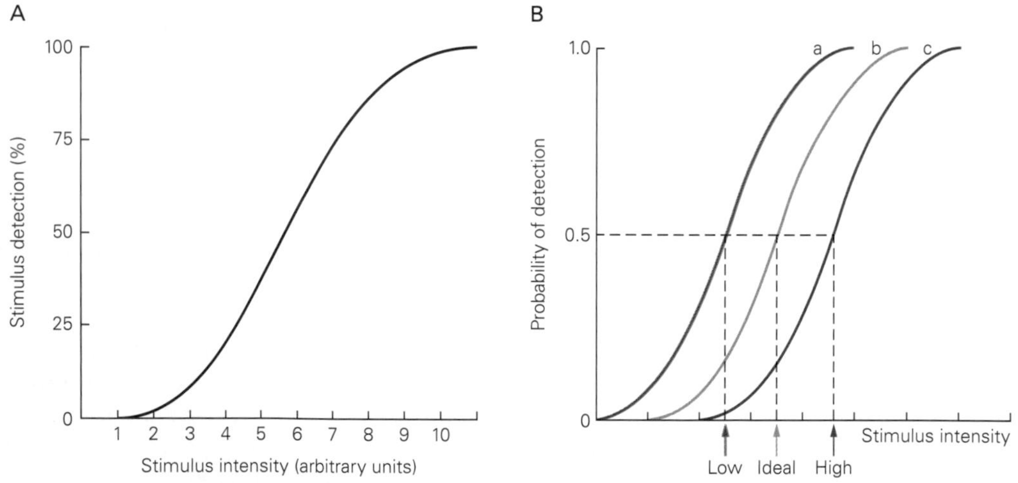

Figure 21–2 The psychometric function defines the mathematical relationship between the amplitude of a stimulus and the intensity of the sensation felt by the subject.

A. The psychometric function plots the percentage of stimuli detected by a human observer as a function of the stimulus magnitude. Threshold is defined as the stimulus intensity detected on 50% of the trials. Psychometric functions are also used to measure the just noticeable difference between stimuli that differ in intensity, frequency, or other parametric properties.

B. Detection and discrimination thresholds depend on the criteria used by individual subjects in psychophysical tasks. An ideal observer correctly detects the presence and absence of stimuli with equal probability (**curve b**). An observer who is told to respond to the slightest indication of a stimulus reports many false positives when no stimuli occur and has low sensory thresholds (**curve a**). An observer who is told to respond only when very certain that a stimulus has occurred reports more hits than false positives and has high sensory thresholds (**curve c**).

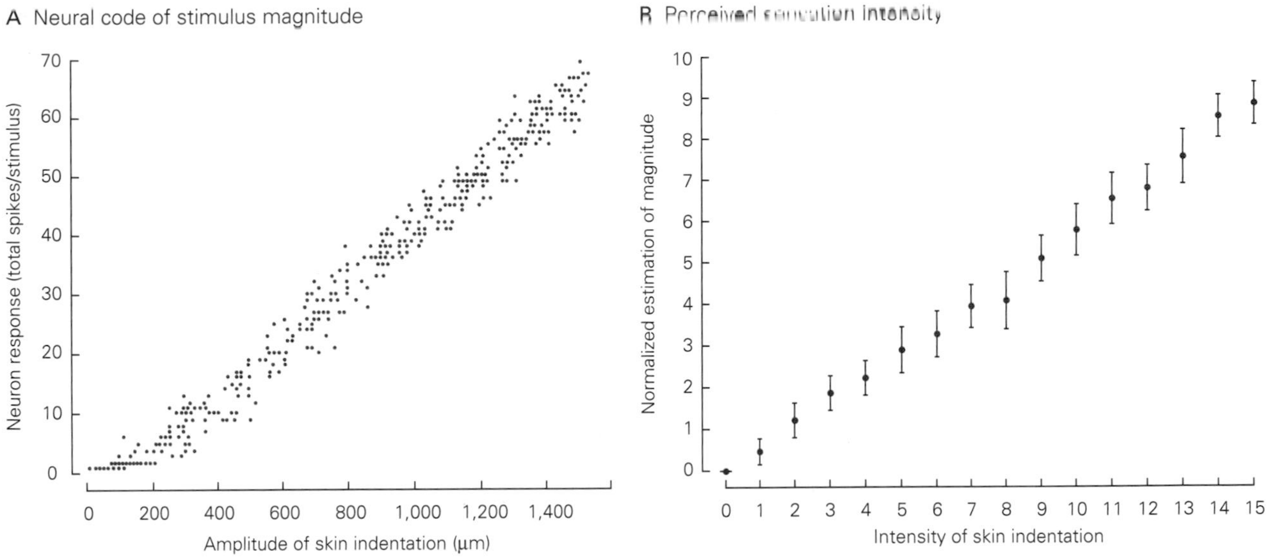

Figure 21–3 The firing rates of sensory nerves encode the stimulus magnitude. The data in the two plots suggest that the neural coding of stimulus intensity is faithfully transmitted from peripheral receptors to cortical centers that mediate conscious sensation. (Adapted, with permission, from Mountcastle, Talbot, and Kornhuber 1966.)

A. The number of action potentials per second recorded from a touch receptor in the hand is proportional to the amplitude of skin indentation. Each dot represents the response of the receptor to pressure applied by a small probe. The relationship between the neural firing rate and the pressure stimulus is linear. This receptor does not respond to stimuli weaker than 200 μm, its touch threshold.

B. Estimates made by human subjects of the magnitude of sensation produced by pressure on the hand increase linearly as a function of skin indentation. The relation between a subject's estimate of the intensity of the stimulus and its physical strength resembles the relation between the discharge frequency of the sensory neuron and the stimulus amplitude.

described earlier; and (3) the method of adjustment or reproduction, in which a subject adjusts a second stimulus to match or reproduce the intensity of the first one.

The next major methodological and conceptual developments in psychophysics came almost a century later when S. S. Stevens introduced the technique of *magnitude estimation,* whereby subjects use a numerical scale to rate the intensity of the sensations experienced by stimuli of different amplitude (Figure 21–3). Verbal reports of subjective experience are widely used because they are usually reliable and repeatable. *Reliability* is assessed by correlations between observers rating the same stimuli; *repeatability* is measured by correlations between responses from the same subject to similar stimuli.

Stevens generalized the method of direct verbal reporting by defining four scales of measurement—the nominal, ordinal, interval, and ratio scales—and specifying appropriate methods for analyzing data of each type. On *nominal scales* items have names but not rank; examples are names of colors, tastes, and smells. On *ordinal scales* items are ranked with a logical range and ordered relationship to each other, but the intervals between them cannot be compared meaningfully. Verbal descriptors of pain intensity are an example of an ordinal scale. When a clinician says, "On a scale from 1 to 10 in which 10 is the worst imaginable pain, how would you rate your pain?" there is no suggestion that the pain associated with an 8 is twice as intense as the pain associated with a 4 or that the difference between 5 and 6 equals the difference between 1 and 2.

On *interval scales* distances but not ratios between values have meaning. Counts of the number of stimuli delivered in a session or estimates of the position of an object on a grid map are examples of interval scales. In *ratio scales* the concepts of rank, interval, and ratio all have valid meanings. Estimates of the perceived intensity of a stimulus are treated as ratio scales. Subjects are instructed to assign a number proportional to the perceived intensity when a stimulus is detected, and to report "zero" when they feel no stimulus. Subjects typically choose their own numerical scale within a session. The values measured during an experiment are then normalized to allow comparisons of stimulus ratings between subjects. These scales permeate modern statistics and are used widely beyond the field of experimental psychology for which they were developed.

Sensations Are Quantified Using Probabilistic Statistics

Decision theory offers another approach to measurement of sensations by using statistical methods to explain the variability of subjects' responses or false reports. When subjects are pressed to detect the weakest possible stimuli, they give many false-positive responses; that is they respond affirmatively in catch trials in which no stimulus was presented. As a result, the psychophysical thresholds measured are very low (Figure 21–2B, blue curve). Conversely, when subjects are told to avoid false positives, their perceptual thresholds become quite elevated. Trials in which strict criteria are used yield higher than normal threshold values (Figure 21–2B, red curve).

In 1927 L. L. Thurstone proposed that the variability of sensations evoked by a stimulus could be represented as a normal or Gaussian probability function with a mean (m_s) and a standard deviation (σ_s):

$$F(x) = (2\pi\sigma_s^2)^{-1/2} \exp\,[-(x - m_s)^2/2\sigma_s^2].$$

This allowed him to use the mathematics of probability theory and statistical tables to predict the discriminability of pairs of stimuli that differed along a physical dimension such as intensity. He proposed to equate the physical distance between the amplitudes of two stimuli to a psychological scale value of inferred loudness called the *discrimination index* or *d′*. He equated the number of correct responses (hits) and error trials (false positives when one stimulus is confused with another) with the sensory overlap of the two stimuli. This allowed him to use statistical tables of the normal probability function to calculate *d′* values (Box 21–1).

Decision theory methods were first applied to psychophysical studies in 1954 by the psychologists Wilson Tanner and John Swets. They developed a series of experimental protocols for stimulus detection that allowed accurate calculation of *d′* as well as techniques for measurement of subjective bias during sensory testing. Their methods were initially developed for engineers studying the detection of very weak radar pulses reflected from distant airplanes. As the engineers lowered the threshold for detection they detected more radar pulses, but their apparatus gave more false positives because it was triggered more frequently by noise. Tanner and Swets hypothesized that subjects gave false-positive responses when the sensory noise exceeded their response threshold.

Signal detection theory has been widely applied in sensory discrimination tests that require the subject to make a binary choice. Threshold measurements are a good example. In a "yes-no" experiment the beginning and end of an observation interval are cued, and the subject is required to say whether or not a signal, such as a tone, was present. We can represent trial-to-trial fluctuations of the perceived stimulus intensity and that of the silent "noise" period as two overlapping Gaussian curves. The subject says "yes" when the signal exceeds a criterion (called a decision boundary) that has been set by the subject, and "no" when it does not. When the stimulus is very weak the neural signal it evokes is very small, and there is considerable overlap between the pure noise and the stimulus signal plus noise. Hence there is no decision boundary that allows error-free responses. Nevertheless, the mathematical formulation of the probability density function allows the experimenter to compensate for subjective differences in response criteria in calculations of *d′* (Box 21–1).

Sensory thresholds can also be measured using a *two-alternative forced-choice* protocol in which there are two observation intervals. The subject is asked whether the stimulus occurred in the first or second interval. The two-interval procedure is widely used for measuring relative intensity or sensory quality because the results obtained are more accurate than verbal judgments and the responses required are simple. Subjects can also provide nonverbal responses in such tests using levers, buttons, or other manipulanda that allow accurate measurement of decision times. Such instrumented behaviors allow neuroscientists to measure sensory processes in experimental animals by training them to use these tools to make easy sensory judgments. Such techniques can be used to probe the sensory capabilities of animal subjects as the discrimination tasks become more difficult and to investigate the underlying neural mechanisms when electrophysiological and behavioral studies are combined in the same experiment.

Decision Times Are Correlated with Cognitive Processes

Another important quantitative measure of psychophysical behavior is the *reaction time*, which is the time taken to perform a perceptual task. Franciscus Donders was the first, in 1865, to measure the time required to respond to stimuli. He and others found that reaction times elicited by strong stimuli are shorter than those elicited by weak stimuli. Similarly, in forced-choice tasks the time required for a decision is shorter when the stimuli are clearly distinctive in intensity or quality than when they are near the discrimination threshold. Reaction times are widely used as measures of certainty of responses in humans and animals. They are often correlated with neural activity in sensory areas of the brain and in studies of sensory-triggered motor behaviors.

Reaction times are also used to evaluate cognitive function. The tasks illustrated in Figure 21–5 were devised by Anne Treisman to investigate the mechanisms of visual pattern recognition. The subjects were asked to locate a blue cross within an array of symbols. With some patterns the blue cross seems to "pop out," but with others the array must be carefully examined to find the blue cross.

One explanation for this is that when the sought-after item differs from the other elements of the array in only one property we can scan quickly the entire array (a parallel search), but when it shares two or more properties we need to examine all of the elements one-by-one (a serial search). If this hypothesis is true, the reaction time should not depend on the *number* of elements in an array when the sought-after item differs in only one property, but it should increase in proportion to the number of elements if we must examine them individually. That is exactly the result obtained in such experiments. The same hypothesis also predicts that it should take twice as long to determine that an item is *absent* because we need to examine all elements in an array before concluding that a particular one is absent.

Subjects typically locate a sought-after item halfway through the search. The slope of the curve relating the search time to the number of elements in the array shows how long it takes to examine each element. Such experiments indicate that 30 to 50 ms is required to compare each element with the target item (Figure 21–5C). Knowing what kinds of visual features allow a parallel search and the reaction time for detecting features in a serial search provides important clues to the underlying neural mechanisms.

Physical Stimuli Are Represented in the Nervous System by Means of the Sensory Code

The psychophysical methods described in the previous section provide objective techniques for analyzing sensations evoked by particular stimuli. These quantitative measures have been combined with neurophysiological techniques to study the neural mechanisms that transform sensory signals into specific percepts.

This approach to the neural coding problem was pioneered by Vernon Mountcastle in the 1960s. He showed that neurophysiological recordings from individual sensory neurons in the peripheral and central nervous system provide a statistical description of the neural activity evoked by a physical stimulus. He then tested hypotheses to determine which quantitative aspects of the neural response might correspond to psychophysical measurements in sensory tasks, and just as important, which do not.

The study of neural coding of information is fundamental to understanding how the brain works. A neural code describes the relationship between the activity in a specified neural population and its functional consequences for the operations that follow. The sensory systems provide a useful avenue to the study of neural coding in the brain because both the input and output of these systems can be precisely defined and quantified. Experimenters can control the physical stimuli provided to sensory receptors and measure the resulting sensations evoked by them using a variety of psychophysical techniques. By recording neuronal activity at various stages of sensory processing, neuroscientists attempt to decipher the codes that convey information in peripheral nerves and in the brain, and analyze the transformation of signals along pathways in the cerebral cortex. Indeed, study of the details of neural coding may lead to insight into the coding principles that underlie cognition.

When analyzing sensory experience it is important to realize that our conscious sensations differ qualitatively from the physical properties of stimuli because, as Kant and the idealists predicted, the nervous system extracts only certain pieces of information from each stimulus while ignoring others. It then interprets this information within the constraints of the brain's intrinsic structure and previous experience. Thus we *receive* electromagnetic waves of different frequencies, but we *see* them as colors. We receive pressure waves from objects vibrating at different frequencies, but we hear sounds, words, and music. We encounter chemical compounds floating in the air or water, but we experience them as smells and tastes. Colors, tones, smells, and tastes are mental creations constructed by the brain out of sensory experience. They do not exist as such outside the brain.

The dominant research strategy in sensory neuroscience is to follow the flow of sensory information from receptors toward the cognitive centers of the brain, attempting to understand the processing mechanisms that occur at each synaptic relay and how they shape our internal representation of the external world. The neural coding of sensory information is better understood at the early stages of processing than at later stages.

Box 21–1 Signal Detection Theory

Signal detection theory is useful for quantitative analyses of sensations in both human and animal subjects. Such studies are designed to measure comparative judgments of a physical property of a stimulus such as its intensity, size, temporal frequency, or detection threshold. They usually employ a *two-alternative forced-choice* protocol with two observation intervals and a pair of stimuli.

Subjects are asked to report whether the second stimulus is stronger or weaker, higher or lower, larger or smaller, same or different than the first stimulus. In measurements of sensory thresholds the subject is asked whether the stimulus occurred during the first or second interval. Responses in each trial are tabulated in a four-cell stimulus-response matrix in which one of the choices is designated a hit (Figure 21–4A).

For example, when measuring sensory thresholds the statistical hypothesis tested is that the stimulus occurs in the first interval. Trials in which the stimulus occurs in the first interval are labeled *hits* if the subject responds "interval 1" and *misses* if the subject responds "interval 2." Trials in which the stimulus occurs in the second interval are labeled *correct rejections* if the subject responds "interval 2," and *false positives* if the subject responds "interval 1."

The subject is considered to be an ideal observer—without any bias—if the hit rate equals the rate of correct rejection (ie, the data in the matrix are symmetric along the diagonals). In most cases subjects display an innate preference or bias for one choice or another, such that the hit rate and correct rejection rate differ (Figure 21–4B).

One can get a rough approximation of the true discrimination performance by averaging these two values. However, the most accurate estimate is obtained by using the normal distribution tables to measure the distance between the means of the stimulus and noise distributions (d'). We use the intersection of the hit rate and false-positive rate to define the amount of overlap of the curves and to set the decision boundary (Figure 21–4B); summation of the matching z-scores provides the value of d'.

In the example shown in Figure 21–4B the subject had a very strict detection criterion and a low hit rate (65%). However, he rarely guessed that the stimulus occurred on blank trials and had a low false-positive rate (20%). As a result, the real performance is better than 65% correct. The matching percent correct calculated using signal detection methods (PC_{max}) is 73%.

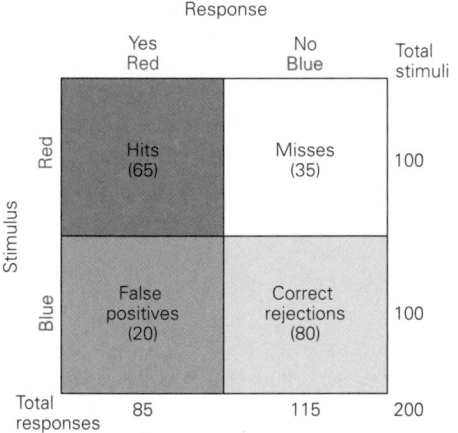

Figure 21–4A The stimulus-response matrix for a stimulus detection task (yes-no) or a categorical judgment task (red-blue). Although there are two possible stimuli and two possible responses, the data represent conditional probabilities in which the experimenter controls the stimuli and measures the subject's responses. The numbers provide examples of behavioral data obtained from a strict observer who responds "yes" less often than the actual frequency of occurrence of the stimulus. (Adapted, with permission, from Green and Swets 1966.)

Sensory Receptors Are Responsive to a Single Type of Stimulus Energy

It is often said that the power of the brain lies in the millions of neurons processing information in parallel. That formulation, however, does not capture the essential difference between the brain and all the other organs of the body. The power of a kidney or a muscle lies in the parallel action of many cells, each doing the same thing; if we understand a muscle cell, we essentially understand how a whole muscle works. The power of the brain lies in the parallel action of millions of cells, each doing something *different*; to understand the brain we need to understand how its tasks are organized and how individual neurons carry out those tasks.

Functional differences between sensory systems arise from the different stimulus energies that drive

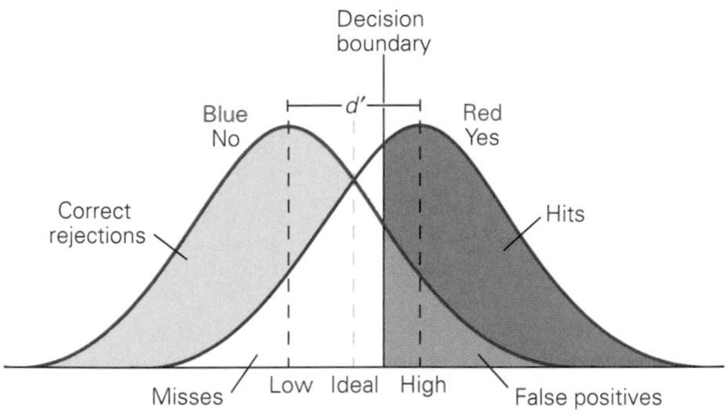

Figure 21–4B The stimuli tested in a discrimination task are represented by Gaussian curves with standard deviations that measure the fluctuation in sensations from trial to trial. The discriminability of a pair of stimuli is correlated with the distance between the peaks of the two curves (*d′*) and the amount of overlap between them. When two stimuli are similar in magnitude, the two Gaussian curves overlap and no single criterion allows error-free responses. The frequency of hits and false positives (and their complements, misses and correct rejections) is determined by the criteria used in the decision task. An ideal observer maximizes the number of correct responses and minimizes the total errors, setting the decision boundary at the intersection of the two curves (**orange dashed line**). A strict observer minimizes the number of false positives but also reduces the total hits, setting the decision boundary to the right (**solid line**). A lax observer maximizes the number of hits but also increases the total false positives, setting the decision boundary to the left of the ideal subject. Judgments are not always ideal because the observer must balance the benefits of correct choices (hits and correct rejections) and the consequences of errors (misses and false-positive responses). (Adapted, with permission, from Green and Swets 1966.)

Subjects' response criteria can be manipulated experimentally by altering the rewards and penalties for correct and incorrect responses. Signal detection theory predicts a progressive shift in the hit rate and false-positive responses as the payoffs increase. Similarly, alteration in the frequency of presentation of one or the other stimulus in a particular interval can also alter response probabilities.

Signal detection techniques are also used in studies of categorical judgments in which a series of stimuli are classified into groups with defined names. Categorical judgments are made of spatial attributes (left/right, horizontal/vertical), colors (blue/green, black/white), shapes (round/rectangle, A/B), or physical characteristics (male/female, plant/animal, house/object). Categorical judgments are often more difficult than comparative judgments, as the subject must identify and name each sample before making a decision.

Signal detection methods have been applied recently in studies of neural responses to visual stimuli that differ in orientation, spatial frequency, or coherence of motion in order to correlate changes in neural firing rates with sensory processing. Discriminability (*d′*) is measured with *receiver operating characteristic* (ROC) analyses that compare the neural firing rates evoked by pairs of stimuli that differ in some property. The assumption is that one of the two stimuli evokes higher firing rates than the other; *d′* is correlated with the difference in mean evoked rates and the overlap between the two distributions of activity.

ROC graphs of neural data plot the proportion of trials judged correctly (hits) and incorrectly (false positives) when the decision criteria are set at various firing levels. The area under the ROC curve provides an accurate estimate of *d′* for each stimulus pair. The neurometric function, plotting neural discriminability as a function of stimulus differences, corresponds closely to the psychometric function obtained in forced-choice paradigms testing the same stimuli, thereby providing a physiological basis for the observed behavioral responses.

them and the discrete pathways that comprise each system. Because of these characteristics each neuron performs a specific task, and the train of action potentials it produces has a specific functional significance for all postsynaptic neurons. This basic idea was expressed in the theory of specificity set forward by Charles Bell and Johannes Müller in the 19th century and remains one of the cornerstones of sensory neuroscience.

The richness of sensory experience begins with millions of highly specific sensory receptors. Each receptor responds to a specific kind of energy at specific locations on the body and sometimes only to energy with a particular temporal or spatial pattern. The receptor transforms the stimulus energy into electrical energy, thus establishing a common signaling mechanism in all sensory systems. The amplitude and duration of the electrical signal produced by the receptor, termed the

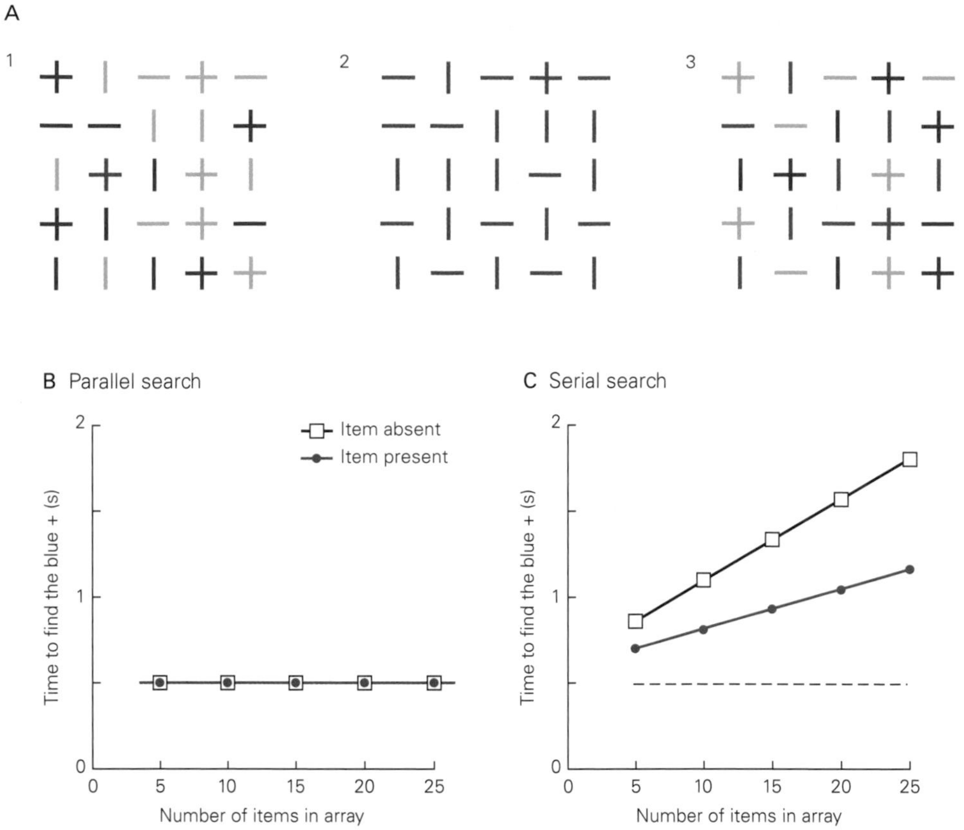

Figure 21–5 Reaction times are used to investigate the mechanisms of pattern recognition. (Modified, with permission, from Treisman 1991.)

A. Visual stimuli used to investigate the mechanisms of pattern recognition in humans. Subjects are asked to find the blue cross in each array. The task is easy with the array at left because the blue cross is the only blue item and therefore seems to "pop out." Detection is harder with the middle array because all of the items are the same color, but only one has two line segments. In the array at right, detection is difficult because the blue cross has the same shape as eight of the items and the same color as another eight. Each of the items must be examined individually to find the right one.

B. The time needed (reaction time) to detect the blue cross in arrays 1 and 2 is independent of the total number of objects because the items are similar in color or shape, allowing all of the objects to be scanned together (parallel search).

C. The time needed to detect the blue cross in an array of items that vary in shape or color (as in array 3) increases in proportion to the number of items when they share at least one property (color or shape in this example) because the search must examine each item (serial search). On average, the target item is found halfway through the search. It takes twice as long to determine that an item is *absent* because all of the objects must be examined.

receptor potential, are related to the intensity and time course of stimulation of the receptor. The process by which specific stimulus energy is converted into an electrical signal is called *stimulus transduction*.

Sensory receptors are morphologically specialized to transduce specific forms of energy, and each receptor has a specialized anatomical region where stimulus transduction occurs. Most receptors are optimally selective for a single type of stimulus energy, a property termed *receptor specificity*. We see particular colors, for example, because we have receptors that are selectively sensitive to photons with specific wavelengths, and we smell particular odors because we have receptors that bind specific odorant molecules (Figure 21–6).

Human sensory receptors are classified as mechanoreceptors, chemoreceptors, photoreceptors, or thermoreceptors (Table 21–1). Mechanoreceptors and chemoreceptors are the most widespread and the most varied in form and function.

Six different kinds of mechanoreceptors that sense skin deformation, motion, stretch, and vibration are responsible for the sense of touch. Muscles contain three kinds of mechanoreceptors that signal muscle length, velocity, and force, whereas other mechanoreceptors in the joint capsule signal joint angle. Hearing is based on two kinds of mechanoreceptors, inner and outer hair cells, that transduce motion of the basilar membrane in the inner ear. Other hair cells in the vestibular labyrinth sense motion and acceleration of the fluids of the inner ear to signal head motion and orientation. Visceral mechanoreceptors detect the distension of internal organs such as the bowel and bladder. Osmoreceptors in the brain, which sense the state of hydration, are activated when a cell swells. Certain mechanoreceptors report extreme distortion that threatens to damage tissue; their signals reach pain centers in the brain.

Chemoreceptors are responsible for olfaction, gustation, itch, pain, and many visceral sensations. A significant part of pain is due to chemoreceptors that detect molecules spilled into the extracellular fluid by tissue injury and molecules that are part of the inflammatory response. Several kinds of thermoreceptors in the skin sense skin warming and cooling. Another thermoreceptor, which monitors blood temperature in the hypothalamus, is mainly responsible for whether we feel warm or cold.

Vision is mediated by four kinds of photoreceptors in the retina. The light sensitivities of these receptors define the visible spectrum. The photopigments in rods and cones detect electromagnetic energy of wavelengths that span the range 390 to 670 nm (Figure 21–7A). Unlike some other species, such as birds or reptiles, humans do not detect ultraviolet light or infrared radiation because we lack receptors that detect the appropriate short or long wavelengths. Similarly, radio waves and microwave energy bands are not perceived because humans have not evolved receptors for these frequencies.

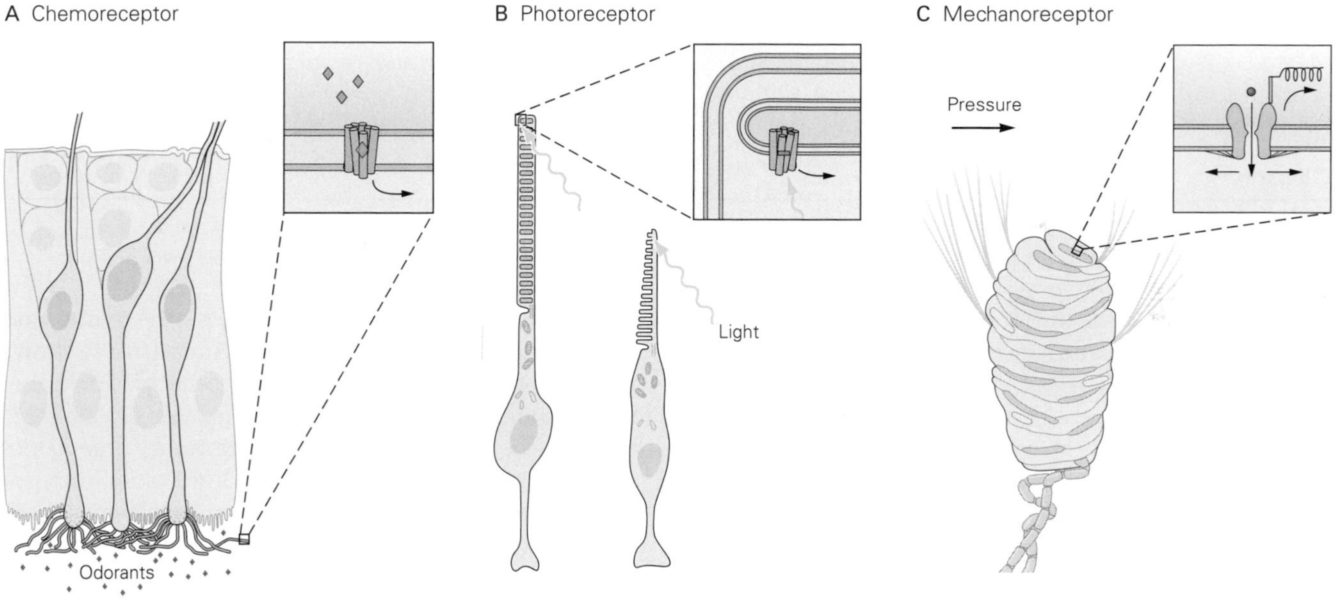

Figure 21–6 Sensory receptors are specialized to transduce a particular type of stimulus energy into electrical signals. Sensory receptors are classified as chemoreceptors, photoreceptors, or mechanoreceptors depending on the class of stimulus energy that excites them. They transform that energy into an electrical signal that is transmitted along pathways that serve one sensory modality. The insets in each panel illustrate the location of the ion channels that are activated by stimuli.

A. The olfactory hair cell responds to chemical molecules in the air. The olfactory cilia on the mucosal surface bind specific odorant molecules and depolarize the sensory nerve through a second-messenger system. The firing rate signals the concentration of odorant in the inspired air.

B. Rod and cone cells in the retina respond to light. The outer segment of both receptors contains the photopigment rhodopsin, which changes configuration when it absorbs light of particular wavelengths. Stimulation of the chromophore by light reduces the concentration of cyclic guanosine 3′, 5′-monophosphate (cGMP) in the cytoplasm, closing cation channels and thereby hyperpolarizing the photoreceptor. (Adapted, with permission, from Shepherd 1994.)

C. Meissner's corpuscles respond to mechanical pressure. The fluid-filled capsule (**blue**) surrounding the sensory nerve endings (**pink**) is linked to the fingerprint ridges by collagen fibers. Pressure or motion on the skin opens stretch-sensitive ion channels in the nerve fiber endings, thus depolarizing them. (Adapted, with permission, from Andres and von Düring 1973.)

Table 21-1 Classification of Sensory Receptors

Sensory system	Modality	Stimulus	Receptor class	Receptor cells
Visual	Vision	Light (photons)	Photoreceptor	Rods and cones
Auditory	Hearing	Sound (pressure waves)	Mechanoreceptor	Hair cells in cochlea
Vestibular	Head motion	Gravity, acceleration, and head motion	Mechanoreceptor	Hair cells in vestibular labyrinths
Somatosensory				Cranial and dorsal root ganglion cells with receptors in:
	Touch	Skin deformation and motion	Mechanoreceptor	Skin
	Proprioception	Muscle length, muscle force, and joint angle	Mechanoreceptor	Muscle spindles and joint capsules
	Pain	Noxious stimuli (thermal, mechanical, and chemical stimuli)	Thermoreceptor, mechanoreceptor, and chemoreceptor	All tissues except central nervous system
	Itch	Histamine	Chemoreceptor	Skin
	Visceral (not painful)	Wide range (thermal, mechanical, and chemical stimuli)	Thermoreceptor, mechanoreceptor, and chemoreceptor	Gastrointestinal tract, urinary bladder, and lungs
Gustatory	Taste	Chemicals	Chemoreceptor	Taste buds
Olfactory	Smell	Odorants	Chemoreceptor	Olfactory sensory neurons

Multiple Subclasses of Sensory Receptors Are Found in Each Sense Organ

Sensory receptors are found in specialized epithelia called sense organs, principally the eye, ear, nose, tongue, and skin. The arrangement of receptors in an organized structure allows further specialization of function within each sensory system.

Each major sensory system has several constituent qualities or *submodalities*. For example, taste can be sweet, sour, salty, or bitter; objects that we see differ in color; and touch has qualities of temperature, texture, and rigidity. Submodalities exist because each class of receptors contains a variety of specialized receptors that respond to limited ranges of stimulus energies.

The receptor behaves as a filter for a narrow range or bandwidth of energy. For example, an individual photoreceptor is not sensitive to all wavelengths of light but only to a small part of the spectrum. We say that a receptor is *tuned* to an optimal or best stimulus, the unique stimulus that activates the receptor at low energy and evokes the strongest response. As a result, we can plot a tuning curve for each receptor based on physiological experiments (the white and black curves in Figure 21–7A). The tuning curve shows the range of sensitivity of the receptor, including its threshold, the minimum stimulus intensity at which the receptor is activated. For example, blue cones in the retina are most sensitive to light of 437 nm; for that reason, they are also termed S or short-wavelength receptors. Green cones, termed M receptors for their sensitivity to middle wavelengths, respond best to 533 nm; red cones, the L or long-wavelength receptors, respond most vigorously to 564 nm wavelengths. The blue, green, and red cones respond to other wavelengths of light but these responses are weaker (see Chapter 26).

The graded sensitivity of photoreceptors means that each rod and cone responds to a wide spectrum of colors yet signals a specific wavelength by the amplitude of the evoked receptor potential. However, because the tuning curve is symmetric around the best frequency, wavelengths of greater or lesser values may evoke identical responses. For example, red cones respond equally well to light of 520 and 600 nm. How does the brain interpret these signals?

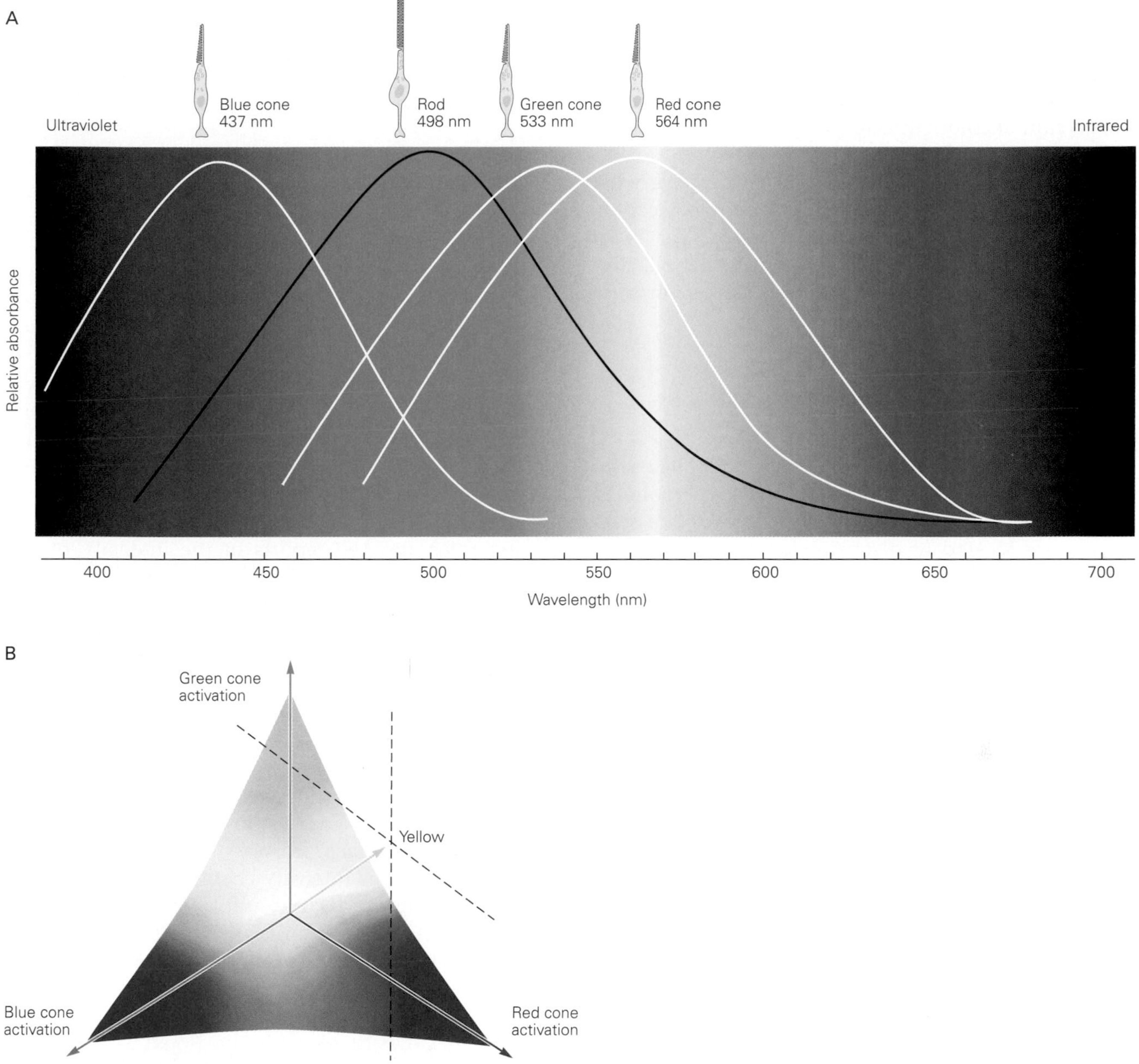

Figure 21–7 Human perception of colors results from the simultaneous activation of three different classes of photoreceptors in the retina.

A. The visible spectrum of light spans wavelengths of 390 to 670 nm. Individual rod or cone photoreceptors are sensitive to a broad range of wavelengths (**black** and **white curves**), but each is most responsive to light in a particular spectral band. As a result, cone photoreceptors are classified as red, green, and blue types. The specific colors perceived result from the relative activation of the three cone types. (Adapted, with permission, from Dowling 1987.)

B. The neural coding of color and brightness in the retina can be portrayed as a three-dimensional vector in which the strength of activation of each cone type is plotted along one of the three axes. Each point in this three-dimensional space represents a unique pattern of activation of the three cone types. The direction of the vector represents the relative activation of the three cone types and the color seen. In the example shown here strong activation of red cones, moderate stimulation of green cones, and weak activation of blue cones produces the perception of yellow. The length of the vector from the origin to the point represents the intensity or brightness of light in that region of the retina.

The answer lies with the green and blue cones. Green cones respond very strongly to light of 520 nm, as it is close to their preferred wavelength, but respond weakly to 600 nm light. Blue cones do not respond to 600 nm light and are barely activated at 520 nm. As a result, 520 nm light is perceived as green, whereas 600 nm is seen as orange. Thus we are able to perceive a spectrum of colors through varying combinations of photoreceptors.

Similarly, the complex flavors we perceive when eating are a result of combinations of chemoreceptors of varying affinities for natural ligands. The broad tuning curves of a large number of distinct olfactory and gustatory receptors afford endless combinatorial possibilities.

Neural Firing Patterns Transmit Sensory Information to the Brain

The receptor potential generated by an adequate stimulus produces a local depolarization or hyperpolarization of the sensory receptor cell. However, the sense organs are located at distances far enough from the central nervous system that passive propagation cannot suffice to convey signals there. To communicate sensory information to the brain a second step in neural coding must occur. The change in membrane potential produced by the sensory stimulus is transformed into action potentials that can be propagated over long distances.

Action potentials are generated in olfactory sensory neurons and dorsal root ganglion neurons of the somatosensory system whose axons project directly to the central nervous system. In the auditory, vestibular, and gustatory (taste) systems the receptor cells make synaptic contact with the peripheral branches of the sensory axons that form cranial nerves VIII, VII, and IX. The retina has the most elaborate neural network for processing sensory information. Photoreceptors send signals through a series of local interneurons to retinal ganglion cells that transform visual information into bursts of action potentials that travel to the brain through the optic nerve.

Sensory receptors encode the intensity of the stimulus in the amplitude of the receptor potential. This analog signal of intensity is transformed into a digital pulse code in which the frequency of action potentials is proportional to the intensity of the stimulus (see Figure 21–3A). The notion of an analog-to-digital transformation dates back to 1925 when Edgar Adrian and Yngve Zotterman discovered the all-or-none properties of the action potential in sensory neurons. Zotterman would later write:

> November 2, 1925, was a red letter day for both of us.... We were excited, both of us quite aware that what we now saw had never been observed before and that we were discovering a great secret of life, how the sensory nerves transmit their information to the brain.... We had found that the transmission in the nerve fiber occurred according to impulse frequency modulation (FM) twenty years before FM was introduced in teletechnique.

Despite the rather crude recording instruments available at that time, Adrian and Zotterman discovered that the frequency of firing—the number of action potentials per second—varies with the strength of the stimulus and the time over which it has been in action; stronger stimuli evoked larger receptor potentials that generated a greater number and a higher frequency of action potentials.

In later years, as recording technology improved and digital computers allowed precise quantification of the timing of action potentials, Mountcastle and his colleagues demonstrated a precise correlation between sensory thresholds and neural responses, as well as the parametric relationship between neural firing rates and self-reports of the intensity of sensations (see Figure 21–3). They also found that the dynamics of the spike train conveys important information about fluctuations of the stimulus, such as the frequency of vibration or a change in rate of movement. Humans can report changes in sensory experience that correspond to alterations in the firing patterns of sensory neurons in the range of a few milliseconds.

The temporal properties of a changing stimulus are encoded as changes in the pattern of sensory neuron activity. Many sensory neurons signal the rate at which stimulus intensity changes by rapidly altering their firing rates. For example, in slowly adapting mechanoreceptors the initial spike discharge when a probe touches the skin is proportional to both the speed at which the skin is indented and the total amount of pressure (Figure 21–8A). During steady pressure the firing rate slows to a level proportional to skin indentation. Firing stops when the probe is retracted. Thus, neurons signal important properties of stimuli not only when they fire but also when they stop firing.

The instantaneous firing patterns of sensory neurons are as important to sensory perception as the total number of spikes fired over long periods. Steady rhythmic firing in nerves innervating the skin is perceived as vibration or steady pressure. Bursting patterns may be perceived as motion. If a stimulus persists unchanged for several minutes without a change in position or amplitude, the neural response diminishes and sensation is lost, a condition called *receptor adaptation*.

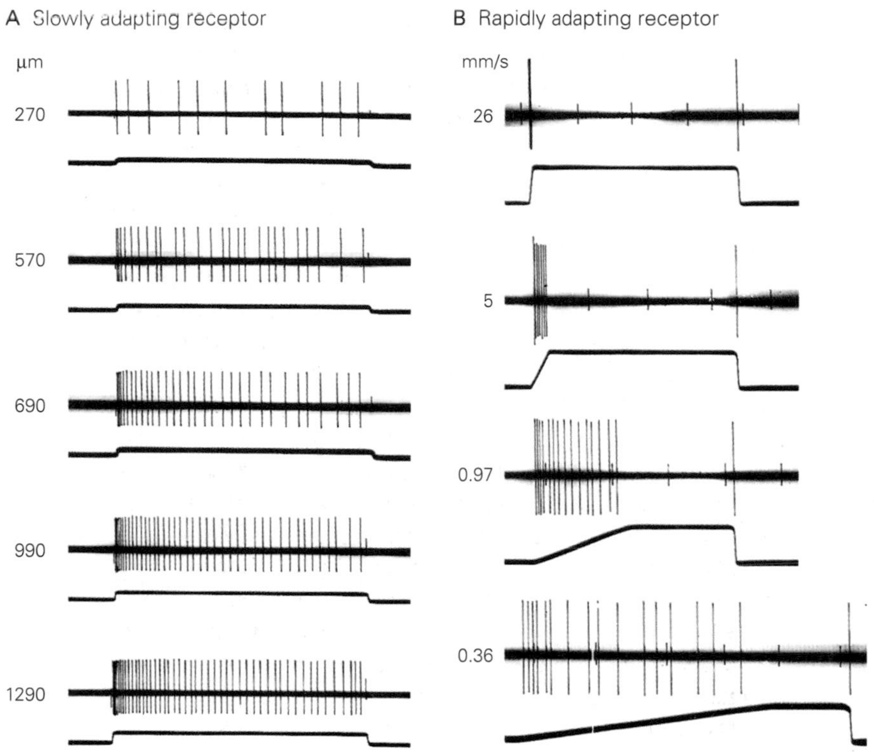

Figure 21–8 Firing rates of sensory neurons convey information about the stimulus intensity and time course. These records illustrate responses of two different classes of touch receptors to a probe pressed into the skin. The stimulus amplitude and time course are shown in the lower trace of each pair; the upper trace shows the action potentials recorded from the sensory nerve fiber in response to the stimulus.

A. A slowly adapting mechanoreceptor responds as long as pressure is applied to the skin. The total number of action potentials discharged during the stimulus is proportional to the amount of pressure applied to the skin. The firing rate is higher at the beginning of skin contact than during steady pressure, as this receptor also detects how rapidly pressure is applied to the skin. When the probe is removed from the skin, the spike activity ceases. (Adapted, with permission, from Mountcastle, Talbot, and Kornhuber 1966.)

B. A rapidly adapting mechanoreceptor responds at the beginning and end of the stimulus, signaling the rate at which the probe is applied and removed; it is silent when pressure is maintained at a fixed amplitude. Rapid motion evokes a brief burst of high-frequency spikes, whereas slow motion evokes a longer-lasting, low-frequency spike train. (Adapted, with permission, from Talbot et al. 1968.)

Receptor adaptation is thought to be an important neural basis of perceptual adaptation, whereby a constant stimulus fades from consciousness. Receptors that respond to prolonged and constant stimulation, known as slowly adapting receptors, encode stimulus duration by generating action potentials throughout the period of stimulation. In contrast, rapidly adapting receptors respond only at the beginning or end of a stimulus; they *cease* firing in response to constant amplitude stimulation and are active only when the stimulus intensity increases or decreases (Figure 21–8B).

The existence of two kinds of receptors—rapidly and slowly adapting sensors—illustrates another important principle of sensory coding. Sensory systems detect *contrasts* in discrete stimuli, changes in the temporal and spatial patterns of stimulation.

The intensity of a stimulus is also represented in the brain by the total number of active neurons in the receptor population. This type of *population code* depends on the fact that individual receptors in a sensory system differ in their sensory thresholds or in their affinity for particular molecules. Most sensory systems have low- and high-threshold receptors. When stimulus intensity changes from weak to strong, low-threshold receptors are first recruited, followed by high-threshold receptors. Parallel processing in low- and high-threshold pathways extends the dynamic range of a sensory system by overcoming the maximum firing rate of 1,000 spikes per second imposed by

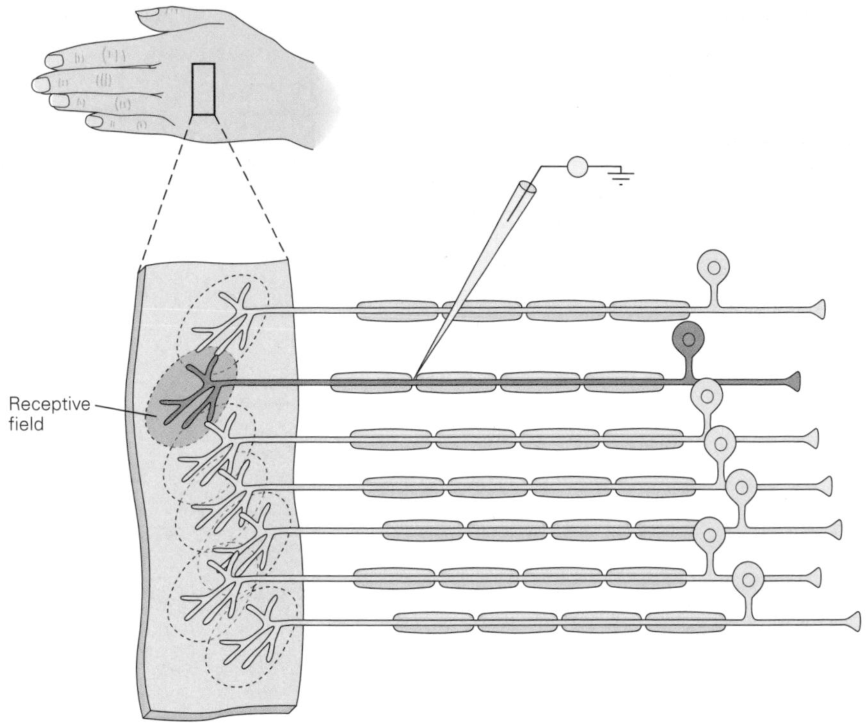

Figure 21–9 The receptive field of a sensory neuron is the spatial domain in the sense organ where stimulation excites or inhibits the neuron. The receptive field of a touch-sensitive neuron denotes the region of skin where gentle tactile stimuli evoke action potentials in that neuron. It encompasses all of the receptive endings and terminal branches of the sensory nerve fiber. If the fiber is stimulated electrically with a microelectrode, the subject experiences touch localized to the receptive field on the skin. The area from which the sensation arises is called the *perceptive field*. A patch of skin contains many overlapping receptive fields, allowing sensations to shift smoothly from one sensory neuron to the next in a continuous sweep. The axon terminals of sensory neurons in the central nervous system are arranged somatotopically, providing an orderly map of the innervated region of the body.

the absolute refractory period. For example, rod cells in the retina are activated in very dim light but reach their maximal receptor potentials in daylight. Cone cells do not respond in dim light but sense differences in brightness in daylight. The combination of the two types of photoreceptors allows us to perceive light intensity over several orders of magnitude.

As this discussion illustrates, the possibilities for information coding through temporal patterning within and between neurons in a population are enormous. For example, the timing of action potentials in the presynaptic cell can determine whether the postsynaptic cell fires. Two action potentials that arrive synchronously or nearly so will drive the postsynaptic neuron's membrane potential much further toward or away from the threshold for an action potential than would asynchronous action potentials. The timing of action potentials between neurons also has a profound effect on long-term potentiation and long-term depression at synapses (see Chapter 67).

The Receptive Field of a Sensory Neuron Conveys Spatial Information

Populations of neurons are also important for conveying the spatial properties of stimuli in a variety of modalities. The spatial attributes of visual, tactile, and auditory stimuli include the location, dimensions, shape, and tonal frequency of the stimuli. The spatial attributes of proprioceptive stimuli include the length of muscles, joint postures, and the body's orientation in the gravitational field. These properties are linked to the anatomical arrangement of receptors within each sense organ.

The position of a sensory neuron in the sense organ is a major element of the specific information conveyed by that neuron (Figure 21–9). The skin area or region of space or tonal domain in which stimuli can activate a sensory neuron is called its *receptive field*. The skin area or region of space from which a sensation seems to arise is called the neuron's *perceptive field*. The two usually coincide.

The dimensions of receptive fields play an important role in the ability of a sensory system to encode spatial information. The objects that we see with our eyes or hold in our hands are much larger than the receptive field of an individual sensory neuron, and therefore stimulate groups of adjacent receptors. The size of the stimulus therefore influences the total number of receptors that are activated. In this manner the spatial distribution of active and silent receptors provides a neural image of the size and contours of the stimulus. This pattern is called an *isomorphic representation* of the stimulus.

Each receptor in the active population encodes the type of energy applied to the receptive field, the local stimulus magnitude, and its temporal properties. For example, auditory codes describe the tonal frequency, loudness, and duration of sound-pressure waves hitting the ear, whereas visual codes describe the hue, brightness, and time course of light hitting the retina. The neural representation of an object or scene is therefore composed of a mosaic of individual receptors that collectively signal its size, contours, texture, color, and temperature.

A good way to visualize the neural activity of a population of neurons, and to grasp the range of possibilities for population coding, is to think of neurons as points in a visual display that flash brightly whenever an action potential occurs. If the action potentials occur at random times, one would perceive a disorganized pattern of flickering dots like the "snow" on old-style television screens without a signal. However, if groups of pixels are turned on and off synchronously, coherent spatial patterns appear. Similarly, when a horizontal bar of light stimulates a row of adjacent photoreceptors in the retina, action potentials are generated in neighboring ganglion cells. Although each photoreceptor simply registers light in its receptive field, the pattern of a bar emerges from the population of active ganglion cells. Neurons in the central nervous system decipher the image of a bar by responding preferentially to specific ensembles of active receptors.

Synchronous patterns of activity in sensory neuron populations convey the spatial dimensions of the stimulus but do not in themselves signal its intensity. The brightness and contours of a video image are created by modulation of the luminance of each pixel. Similarly, in neural codes signal strength is conveyed by the impulse rates of the individual neurons. This is called *rate coding*. The temporal integration of action potentials that occurs at synapses smooths the staccato on-off firing patterns into a continuous modulated signal analogous to the gray scale of a video monitor. High firing rates in this model yield white zones, intermediate rates produce gray zones, and silence gives a black region. Rate coding thereby allows the population of neurons to simultaneously transmit the spatial properties and intensity of stimuli.

The spatial resolution of a sensory system is proportional to the total number of receptor neurons and how their receptive fields are apportioned within the population (Figure 21–10). Regions of a sense organ with a high density of receptors, such as the central retina (the fovea), have small receptive fields because the terminals of each sensory neuron are confined to a local cluster of receptors. Each retinal ganglion cell in the fovea measures the average light intensity in a small spot of the visual field; but because there are so many of them, the population of cells in the fovea transmits a very detailed representation of the visual scene.

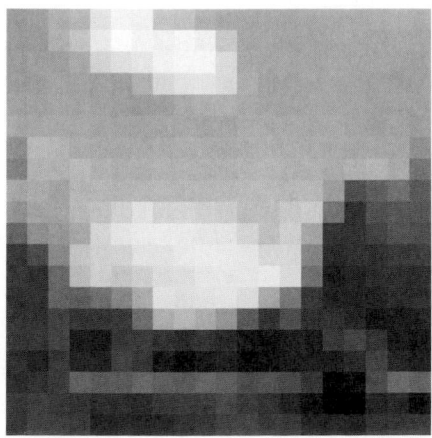

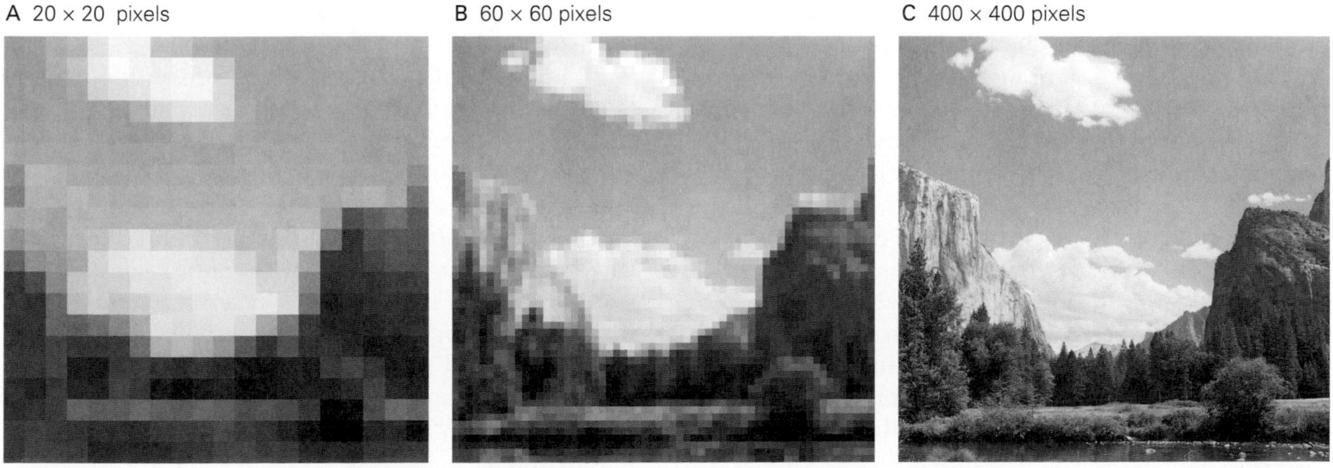

Figure 21–10 The spatial properties of scenes and objects are conveyed by populations of neurons, each of which represents a small component of the image. The resolution of detail is inversely correlated with the area of the receptive field of individual neurons. Each square or pixel in these images represents a receptive field. The gray scale in each pixel is proportional to the average light intensity in the corresponding receptive field. If there are a small number of neurons, and each spans a large area of the image, the result is a very schematic representation of the scene (**A**). As the density of neurons increases, and the size of each receptive field decreases, the spatial detail becomes clearer (**B**, **C**). The increased spatial resolution comes at the cost of larger populations of neurons required to transmit the information. (Photographs reproduced with permission of Daniel Gardner.)

Ganglion cells in the periphery of the retina have larger receptive fields because the receptor density is much lower. The dendrites of each ganglion cell receive information from a wider area of the retina, and thereby integrate light intensity over a greater portion of the visual field. This arrangement yields a less detailed image of the scene (Figure 21–10A). Similarly, the region of the body most often used to touch objects is the hand. Not surprisingly, mechanoreceptors for touch are concentrated in the fingertips, and the receptive fields on the hand are smaller than those on the arm or trunk.

Spatial coding is ubiquitous for two reasons. First, it takes advantage of the parallel architecture of the nervous system. The number of neurons in each unimodal area of sensory cortex is approximately 100 million. Thus the possible number of spatial patterns of neural activity greatly exceeds the number of atoms in the universe. Second, each neuron is a spatial as well as a temporal decoder: It fires only when many of its excitatory synapses receive action potentials and most of the inhibitory synapses do not. That is, it fires in response to some patterns of stimulation and not others. The fact that on average each cortical neuron has 10,000 synapses makes the number of spatial coding possibilities enormous.

Spatial codes are sometimes called vector codes from the mathematical idea of vector spaces. The firing rate of each neuron in a population can be plotted in a coordinate system with multiple axes such as modality, location, intensity, and time. The neural components along these axes combine to form a vector that represents the population's activity (see Figure 21–7B). The vector interpretation is useful because it makes available powerful mathematical techniques.

The fragmentation of a stimulus into components, each encoded by an individual neuron, is the initial step in sensory processing. Assembly of the components into an internal representation of an object occurs within neural networks in the brain. This process allows the brain to abstract certain features of an object, person, scene, or external event from the detailed receptor input. As a result, the internal representation formed in the brain may exaggerate some features that are important at the moment while ignoring others. In this sense our percepts are not perfect mirrors of the stimuli that evoke them but instead a creation of the mind.

Modality-Specific Pathways Extend to the Central Nervous System

Bell and Müller realized that the richness provided by the specificity of our receptors would be lost without connections to brain centers that are as rich and varied as the receptors themselves. A sensory neuron's action potentials have a specific effect on our sensory experience because of the neuron's central connections, not because of the stimulus that evokes the action potentials. Action potentials in nerve fibers of the cochlea, for example, evoke the sensation of a tone whether activated by sound waves or by electrical stimulation with a neural prosthesis.

Each class of sensory receptors makes connections with structures in the central nervous system that are dedicated to one sensory modality, at least in the early stages of information processing. Thus sight or touch is experienced because specific central nervous structures are activated. Each sensory modality is therefore represented by the ensemble of central neurons connected to a specific class of receptors. Such ensembles of neurons are referred to as *sensory systems*, which include the somatosensory, visual, auditory, vestibular, olfactory, and gustatory systems (see Table 21–1).

Sensory information flows through pathways dedicated to conveying stimulus information before ending in brain regions that are more clearly concerned with cognition and action than with sensory processing. However, synaptic relays in sensory pathways do more than simply pass on signals received. Each relay neuron receives convergent excitatory synaptic inputs from many neurons in the presynaptic pathway. Likewise, each receptor neuron excites a large number of postsynaptic neurons. In addition, inhibitory interneurons in the relay nucleus modulate the excitability of relay neurons, thereby regulating the amount of sensory information transmitted centrally to higher levels of the network (Figure 21–11).

Like the primary sensory neurons in the periphery, neurons in the central sensory pathways have specific receptive and perceptive fields. The specificity of a central neuron is determined by the receptive fields of the neurons that excite and inhibit it. The neuron responds optimally to stimuli that simultaneously activate a particular set of presynaptic excitatory neurons. The neuron's receptive field is also shaped by inhibitory input. The inhibitory region of a receptive field provides an important mechanism for enhancing the contrast between stimuli and thus gives the sensory systems additional power to resolve spatial detail.

The activity of sensory neurons in the brain is more variable from trial to trial than that of sensory neurons in the periphery. Central sensory neurons also fire irregularly before and after stimulation, and during periods when no stimuli are present. The variability of the evoked central responses is a result of several factors: the subject's state of alertness, whether

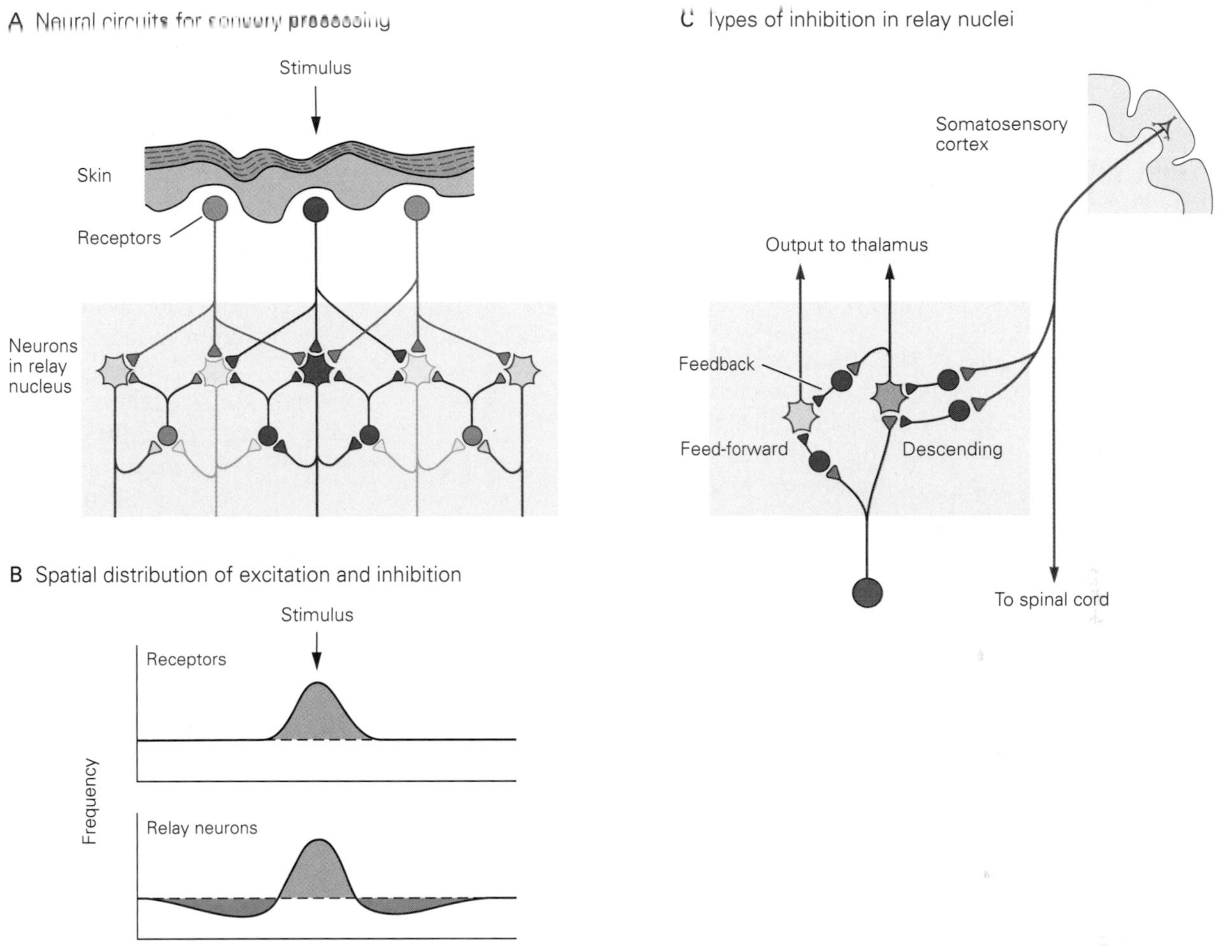

Figure 21–11 Neural networks in relay nuclei integrate sensory information from multiple receptors.

A. Sensory information is transmitted in the central nervous system through hierarchical processing networks. A stimulus to the skin is registered by a large group of postsynaptic neurons in relay nuclei in the brain stem and thalamus, but most strongly by neurons in the center of the array (**red neuron**). The receptive field of an individual relay neuron is larger than that of any of the presynaptic sensory neurons because of the convergent connections. (Adapted, with permission, from Dudel 1983.)

B. Inhibition (**gray areas**) mediated by local interneurons confines excitation (**orange area**) to the central zone where stimulation is strongest, enhancing the contrast between strongly and weakly stimulated relay neurons.

C. Inhibitory interneurons in a relay nucleus are activated by three distinct excitatory pathways. Feed-forward inhibition is produced by the afferent fibers of receptors that terminate on the inhibitory interneurons. Feedback inhibition is produced by recurrent collateral axons of neurons in the output pathway from the nucleus. The interneurons in turn inhibit nearby output neurons, creating sharply defined zones of excitatory and inhibitory activity in the nucleus. In this way the most active relay neurons reduce the output of adjacent, less active neurons, permitting a winner-take-all strategy that ensures that only one of two or more competing responses is expressed. Inhibitory interneurons are also activated by neurons in other brain regions such as the cerebral cortex. The descending pathways allow cortical neurons to control the relay of sensory information centrally, providing a mechanism by which attention can select sensory inputs.

his or her attention is engaged, previous experience of that stimulus, and recent activation of the pathway by similar stimuli. Similarly, behavioral conditions during stimulus presentation, subjective intentions, motor plans that may evoke feedback responses, or intrinsic oscillations of the neuron's membrane potential can all modify the incoming sensory information. For these reasons, neural responses to sensory stimulation or during motor behaviors are usually illustrated both by raster plots that depict the trial-to-trial variability of firing (see Figure 21–15) and by histograms that average neural activity across trials.

The Receptor Surface Is Represented Topographically in Central Nuclei

As we saw in Chapter 17, receptor axons terminate in the brain in an orderly manner forming maps of the receptor sheet. At all levels of a sensory system the stimulus sensitivity of individual neurons varies in an orderly way across a nucleus. Maps of primary specificity—the qualities to which neurons are most narrowly tuned—provide clues to the functional organization of a nucleus.

In the first relay nuclei of the somatosensory, visual, and auditory systems adjacent neurons represent adjacent areas of the body, retina, and cochlea, respectively. The organization of these nuclei is thus said to be somatotopic, retinotopic, or tonotopic. Nuclei in the auditory system are called tonotopic because the inputs from cochlear hair cells are arranged to create an orderly shift in frequency sensitivity from cell to cell, reflecting the functional organization of the hair cells in the cochlea (Figure 21–12). In other words, the firing of a particular neuron in a population signals the location of a stimulus on the receptor surface.

Neurons in the primary sensory areas of the cerebral cortex continue to represent location-specific features of a stimulus, and the functional maps of these areas are also somatotopic, retinotopic, or tonotopic. However, at higher levels within each sensory system neurons are more sharply selective of other stimulus features. Thus central auditory neurons are less selective for frequency and more selective for certain kinds of sound. For example, some neurons are specific for vocalizations by members of the same species. In each successive nucleus the spatial organization is progressively lost as neurons become less concerned with the descriptive features of stimuli and more concerned with properties of behavioral importance in that modality (Figure 21–13).

One of the most important insights into feature detection in the cortex arose from combined physiological and anatomical studies of the cortical visual pathways by Mortimer Mishkin and Leslie Ungerleider. They discovered that sensory information arriving in the primary visual areas is divided in two parallel pathways. One pathway conveys information needed for immediate action and the other information needed for classification of images. Visual features that identify *what* an object is are transmitted in a *ventral* pathway to the temporal lobe and eventually to the hippocampus and entorhinal cortex. Visual information about *where* the object is located and its size and shape is transmitted in a more *dorsal* pathway to the parietal lobe and eventually to the motor areas of frontal cortex (Figure 21–14).

The ventral and dorsal streams of sensory information are used as the basis of two major forms of memory: semantic memory, which allows us to talk about objects or persons, and procedural memory, which we use to interact with objects or persons.

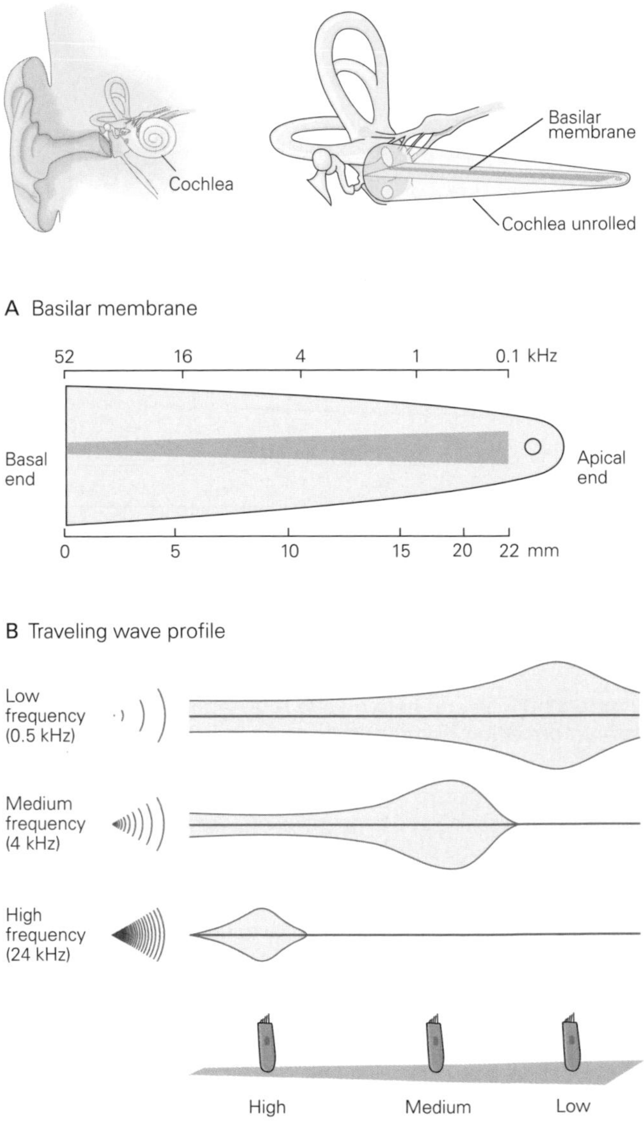

Figure 21–12 Receptors in the cochlea, the sense organ of the inner ear, are arranged tonotopically. (Adapted, with permission, from Shepherd 1994.)

A. The frequency selectivity of hair cell receptors in the cochlea is due in part to the change in dimensions along the length of the basilar membrane where the hair cells are embedded.

B. When sound is received at the cochlea, a traveling wave moves along the basilar membrane. The increasing width of the basilar membrane alters the amplitude of vibration: high frequencies evoke the greatest displacement toward the basal end, whereas low frequencies are strongest at the apical end.

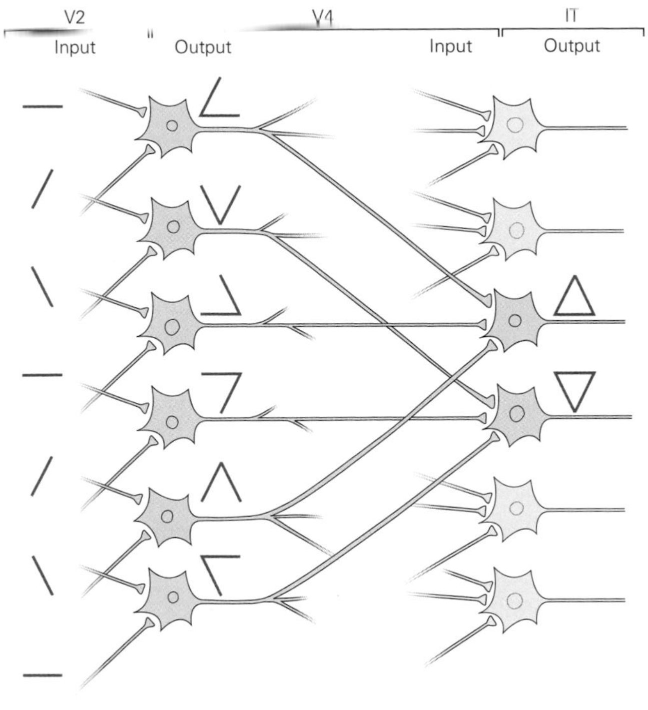

Figure 21–13 Convergent connections allow cortical neurons to abstract complex information from simple patterns. Individual neurons in primary (V1) and secondary visual cortex (V2) respond optimally to bars with specific orientations and locations in the visual field. Convergent inputs from different sets of V2 neurons enable V4 cells to signal an angle. In turn, the outputs of V4 neurons converge on neurons in the inferior temporal cortex (IT) that respond optimally to more complex shapes such as a triangle. Thus, stimulation of the retina creates fragmented representations of an object that are integrated into a recognizable form in higher cortical areas. (Adapted, with permission, from Brincat and Connor 2004.)

Ventral and dorsal streams are also evident in other sensory systems. In the auditory system acoustic information from speech is transmitted to Wernicke's area in the temporal lobe, which has a strong role in language comprehension, and to the Broca area in the frontal cortex, which is involved in speech production. In the somatosensory system information about an object's features such as size and shape is transmitted to ventral areas of parietal cortex for object recognition. Tactile information about object size, weight, and texture is also communicated to posterior parietal and frontal motor areas, where it is needed to plan handling of the object.

Feedback Regulates Sensory Coding

The sensory systems are not simply assembly lines that reassemble initial neural representations into ones that are more appropriate for cognition. That view is at odds with our own experience of sensation and perception. We have enormous control over perception and consciousness at high and low levels. At a high level, for example, we can switch our attention from the subject matter of a painting to the painter's use of form, color, and texture.

At a much lower level we can to some extent control the sensations that reach consciousness. We may, for example, watch television to take our minds off the pain of a sprained ankle. Direct, volitional control of the sensory information that reaches consciousness can be readily demonstrated by suddenly directing your attention to a body part, such as the fingers of your left hand, to which you were oblivious as you were attending to this text. Sensations from the fingers flood consciousness until attention is redirected to the text. Neural recordings in somatosensory and visual cortex indicate that neurons change their sensitivity, as reflected in their firing rates, but not their selectivity for stimuli (Figure 21–15).

Each of the sensory systems also has feedback projections. Each primary sensory cortex has extensive projections back to its principal relay nucleus in the thalamus. In fact, the number of feedback axons exceeds the number of afferent axons from the thalamus to the cortex. These projections have an important function that is not yet clear. One possibility is that they modulate the responsiveness of certain neurons when attention and vigilance change or during motor tasks.

Higher centers in the brain are also able to modulate the responsiveness of sensory receptors. For example, neurons in the motor cortex can alter the sensitivity of sensory receptors in skeletal muscle that signal muscle length. Activation of gamma motor neurons by corticospinal pathways enhances the sensory responses of muscle spindle afferents to stretch. Neurons in the brain stem can directly modulate the frequency sensitivity of hair cells in the cochlea. So even at the level of individual sensory receptors the information sent to the brain signals properties of both the stimulus and the subject who receives the information.

Top-Down Learning Mechanisms Influence Sensory Processing

What we perceive is always some combination of the sensory stimulus itself and the memories it evokes. The late coach of the Boston Celtics, Red Auerbach, once reflected that, in motivating a team, "It's not what you say to them, but what they hear that matters."

The relationship between perception and memory was originally developed by the empiricists, particularly

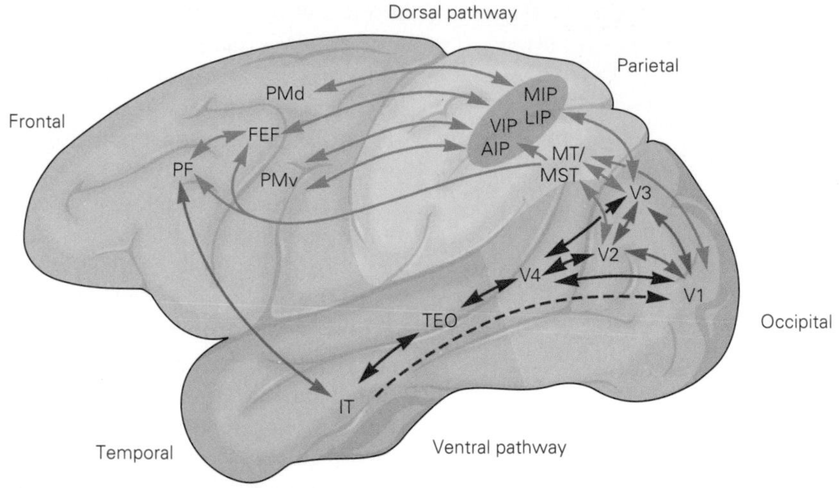

Figure 21–14 Visual stimuli are processed by serial and parallel networks in the cerebral cortex. When you read this text the spatial pattern of the letters is sent to the cerebral cortex through successive synaptic links comprising photoreceptors, bipolar cells of the retina, retinal ganglion cells, cells in the lateral geniculate nucleus of the thalamus, and layer IV neurons of the primary visual cortex (V1). Within the cortex there is a gradual divergence to successive processing areas called ventral and dorsal streams that are neither wholly serial nor parallel. The ventral stream in the temporal lobe (**burgundy arrows**) analyzes and encodes information about the form and structure of the visual scene and objects within it, delivering this information to the parahippocampal cortex (not shown) and prefrontal cortex (PF). The dorsal stream in the parietal lobe (**blue arrows**) analyzes and represents information about stimulus location and motion and delivers this information to motor areas of the frontal cortex that control movements of the eyes, hand, and arm. The anatomical connections between these areas are reciprocal, involving both feed-forward and feedback circuits. (**V1**, **V2**, **V3**, and **V4**, occipital visual areas; **MT**, middle temporal; **MST**, medial superior temporal; **AIP**, **VIP**, **LIP**, and **MIP**, anterior, ventral, lateral, and medial intraparietal; **TEO**, temporal-occipital; **IT**, inferior temporal; **PMd** and **PMv**, dorsal and ventral premotor; **FEF**, frontal eye fields.) (Adapted, with permission, from Albright and Stoner 2002.)

the associationist philosophers James Mill and his son John Stuart Mill. Their idea was that sensory and perceptual experiences that occur together or in close succession, particularly those that do so repeatedly, become associated so that one thereafter triggers the other. It is easy to see how associationism verges on a theory of knowledge, thought, intelligence, and even consciousness. Association is a powerful mechanism and much of learning consists of committing associations to memory through repeated exposure.

We understand in principle how a network of neurons can "recognize" a specific pattern of inputs from a population of presynaptic neurons. The mechanism is called *template matching*. Each neuron in the target population has a pattern of excitatory and inhibitory presynaptic connections. If the pattern of arriving action potentials fits the postsynaptic neuron's pattern of synaptic connections even approximately—activates many of its excitatory synapses but mostly avoids activating its inhibitory synapses—the target neuron fires.

This mechanism also contains the essential elements of association. Suppose the pattern of inputs is a representation of the letter A, and the pattern of action potentials evoked in the target population is the representation of the letter B; B then becomes associated with A. Exposure to A evokes the internal representation of B. If the representation of B is fed back to this same target population and it evokes the representation of a C, an associative chain has been established. Whether the brain uses a mechanism like this is not known, but the speed of recognition and association together with the parallel architecture of the brain suggest that something like this must occur.

This template-matching mechanism is very powerful and forms the basis of virtually all computer-based pattern-recognition schemes. Nonetheless, no artificial scheme comes close to the human ability to recognize patterns of many kinds because artificial systems cannot handle the extreme variability of sensory stimuli in the real world. In general, attempts to recognize stimuli by referring to stored records of earlier stimuli fail because of this variability; subsequent occurrences of the same or similar stimuli rarely match earlier occurrences. The general approach among computer scientists is to search for a way to separate information about the form and structure of a stimulus from information about the properties that vary from one exposure to the next.

Whether the brain solves the recognition problem in this way is uncertain. There is currently much evidence that the neural representation of a stimulus conveyed by a large population of receptor neurons in the initial pathways of sensory systems is an isomorphic representation of the stimulus. Successive synaptic regions transform these initial neural representations into abstracted representations of our environment

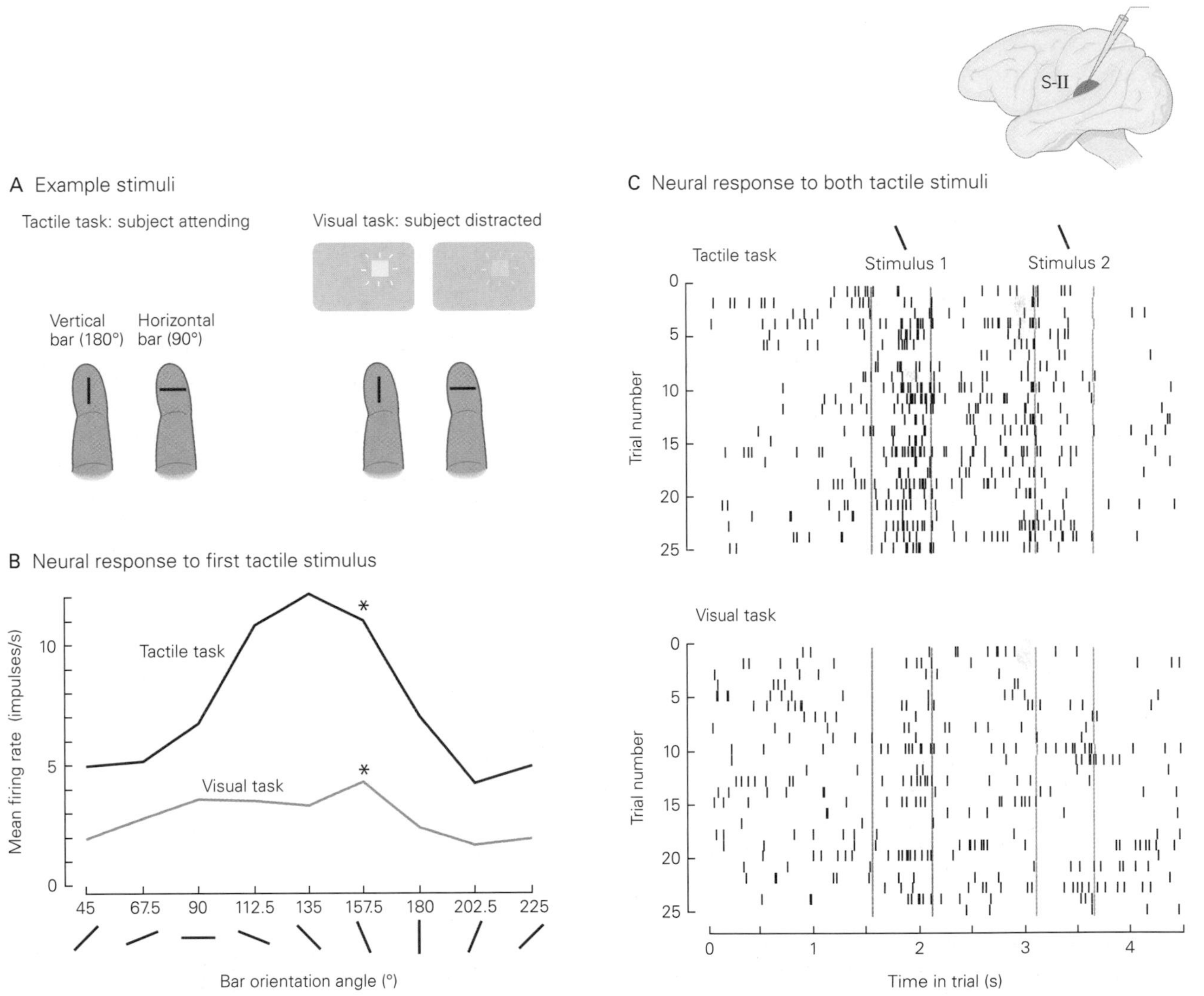

Figure 21–15 Attention to a stimulus enhances the responses of a neuron in the secondary somatosensory cortex. When we pay attention to a stimulus we are selecting certain sensory inputs for cognitive processing, and ignoring or suppressing other information. (Adapted, with permission, from Hsiao, Lane, and Fitzgerald 2002.)

A. A pair of bars was successively pressed against the skin of a monkey's fingertips while the animal performed a tactile or visual task. In the tactile task the animal was required to indicate whether the orientations of the bars were the same or different. In the visual task the animal had to detect a change in the brightness of a square displayed on a computer monitor while the bars were pressed against its fingertips.

B. The mean firing rate of the neuron was significantly higher for all bar orientations when the animal attended to the tactile stimulus (tactile task) than when the stimulus was ignored (visual task). The asterisks mark the firing rates evoked by stimulus 1 (shown in part C).

C. Raster plots of the spike trains of the neuron in response to a bar oriented at the most preferred orientation of 157.5°. Each vertical tick in the plots indicates an action potential; each row represents a single trial. Vertical lines indicate the beginning and end of each stimulus. The responses to stimulus 1 were stronger in the tactile task when the animal attended to the stimulus. Stimulus 2 evoked weaker responses than stimulus 1, and was followed by a period of inhibition after the animal had made its choice.

that we are beginning to decipher. In contrast, we barely understand the top-down mechanisms by which incoming sensory information invokes memories of past occurrences and activates our subjective prejudices and opinions. These topics are difficult to analyze experimentally, particularly in animal models. When we do understand these neural codes it is likely that we will be on the verge of understanding cognition, the way in which information is coded in memory. That is what makes the study of neural coding so challenging and exciting.

An Overall View

Our sensory systems provide the means by which we perceive the external world, remain alert, form a body image, and regulate our movements. Sensations arise when external stimuli interact with some of the billion sensory receptors that innervate every organ of the body. The information detected by these receptors is conveyed to the brain as trains of action potentials traveling along individual sensory axons.

These messages are analyzed centrally by several million sensory neurons performing different, specific functions in parallel. Each sensory neuron extracts highly specific and localized information about the external or internal environment and in turn has a specific effect on sensation and cognition because it projects to specific places in the brain that have specific sensory functions.

All sensory systems respond to four elementary features of stimuli—modality, location, intensity, and duration. The diverse sensations we experience—the sensory modalities—reflect different forms of energy that are transformed by receptors into depolarizing or hyperpolarizing electrical signals called receptor potentials. Receptors specialized for particular forms of energy, and sensitive to particular ranges of the energy bandwidth, allow humans to sense many kinds of mechanical, thermal, chemical, and electromagnetic events. To maintain the specificity of each modality within the nervous system, receptor axons are segregated into discrete anatomical pathways that terminate in unimodal nuclei. After about a dozen synaptic steps in each sensory system, neural activity converges on neuronal groups whose function is polymodal and more directly cognitive.

The location and spatial dimensions of a stimulus are conveyed through each receptor's receptive field, the precise area in the sensory domain in which stimulation activates the receptor. The identity of the active sensory neurons therefore signals not only the modality of a stimulus, but also the place where it occurs. The intensity and duration of stimulation are represented by the amplitude and time course of the receptor potential and by the total number of receptors activated. In the brain, intensity is encoded in the frequency of firing, which is proportional to the strength of the stimulus. The temporal features of a stimulus, such as duration and changes in magnitude, are signaled by the dynamics of the spike train.

The pattern of action potentials in peripheral nerves and in the brain gives rise to sensations whose qualities can be measured directly using a variety of psychophysical paradigms such as magnitude estimation and signal detection and discrimination tasks. Reaction times to stimuli also provide a means for measuring the intensity of stimulation and the ease of sensory discrimination in both human and animal subjects.

The richness of sensory experience—the complexity of sounds in a Mahler symphony, the subtle layering of color and texture in views of the Grand Canyon, or the multiple flavors of a salsa—requires the activation of large ensembles of receptors acting in parallel, each one signaling a particular aspect of a stimulus. The neural activity in a set of thousands or millions of neurons should be thought of as coordinated activity that conveys a "neural image" of specific properties of the external world.

Sensory information in the central nervous system is processed in stages, in the sequential relay nuclei of the spinal cord, brain stem, thalamus, and cerebral cortex. Each nucleus integrates sensory inputs from adjacent receptors and, using networks of inhibitory neurons, emphasizes the strongest signals. Processing of sensory information in the cerebral cortex occurs in multiple cortical areas in parallel, and is not strictly hierarchical. Feedback connections from areas of the brain involved in cognition, memory, and motor planning control the incoming stream of sensory information, allowing us to interpret sensory stimulation in the context of past experience and current goals.

Esther P. Gardner
Kenneth O. Johnson

Selected Readings

Adrian ED. 1928. *The Basis of Sensation*. London: Christophers.

Boring EG. 1942. *Sensation and Perception in the History of Experimental Psychology*. New York: Appleton-Century.

Dowling JE. 1987. *The Retina: An Approachable Part of the Brain*. Cambridge, MA: Belknap.

Green DM, Swets JA. 1966. *Signal Detection Theory and Psychophysics.* New York: Wiley; 1974. Reprint. Huntington, NY: Robert E. Krieger.

Johnson KO, Hsiao SS, Yoshioka T. 2002. Neural coding and the basic law of psychophysics. Neuroscientist 8:111–121.

Perkel DH, Gerstein GL, Moore GP. 1967a. Neuronal spike trains and stochastic point processes. I. The single spike train. Biophys J 7:391–418.

Perkel DH, Gerstein GL, Moore GP. 1967b. Neuronal spike trains and stochastic point processes. II. Simultaneous spike trains. Biophys J 7:419–440.

Shepherd GM. 1994. *Neurobiology*, 3rd ed. New York: Oxford Univ. Press.

Singer W. 1999. Neuronal synchrony: a versatile code for the definition of relations? Neuron 24:49–65.

Stevens SS. 1961. The psychophysics of sensory function. In: WA Rosenblith (ed). *Sensory Communication*, pp. 1–33. Cambridge, MA: MIT Press.

Stevens SS. 1975. *Psychophysics: Introduction to Its Perceptual, Neural, and Social Prospects*. New York: Wiley.

References

Adrian ED, Zotterman Y. 1926. The impulses produced by sensory nerve-endings. Part 2. The response of a single end-organ. J Physiol (Lond) 61:151–171.

Albright TD, Stoner GR. 2002. Contextual influences on visual processing. Annu Rev Neurosci 25:339–379.

Alitto HJ, Usrey WM. 2003. Corticothalamic feedback and sensory processing. Curr Opin Neurobiol 13:440–445.

Andres KH, von Düring M. 1973. Morphology of cutaneous receptors. In: A Iggo (ed). *Handbook of Sensory Physiology,* Vol. 2, *Somatosensory System*, pp. 3–28. Berlin: Springer-Verlag.

Berkeley G. [1710] 1957. *A Treatise Concerning the Principles of Human Knowledge*. K. Winkler (ed). Indianapolis: Bobbs-Merrill.

Bradley A, Skottun BC, Ohzawa I, Sclar G, Freeman RD. 1987. Visual orientation and spatial frequency discrimination: A comparison of single neurons and behavior. J Neurophysiol 57:755–772.

Brincat SL, Connor CE. 2004. Underlying principles of visual shape selectivity in posterior inferotemporal cortex. Nat Neurosci 7:880–886.

Britten KH, Shadlen MN, Newsome WT, Movshon JA. 1992. The analysis of visual motion: a comparison of neuronal and psychophysical performance. J Neurosci 12: 4745–4768.

Connor CE, Hsiao SS, Phillips JR, Johnson KO. 1990. Tactile roughness: neural codes that account for psychophysical magnitude estimates. J Neurosci 10:3823–3836

Dudel J. 1983. General sensory physiology. In: RF Schmitt, G Thews (eds). *Human Physiology*, pp. 177–192. Berlin: Springer-Verlag.

Egan JP, Clarke FR. 1956. Source and receiver behavior in the use of a criterion. J Acoust Soc Am 28:1267–1269.

Fechner G. [1860] 1966. In: DH Howes, EG Boring (eds). *Elements of Psychophysics*. Vol. 1. HE Adler (transl). New York: Holt, Rinehart and Winston.

Gerstein GL, Perkel DH, Dayhoff JE. 1985. Cooperative firing activity in simultaneously recorded populations of neurons: detection and measurement. J Neurosci 5:881–889.

Gochin PM, Colombo M, Dorfman GA, Gerstein GL, Gross CG. 1994. Neural ensemble coding in inferior temporal cortex. J Neurophysiol 71:2325–2337.

Hsiao SS, Lane J, Fitzgerald P. 2002. Representation of orientation in the somatosensory system. Behav Brain Res 135:93–103.

Hsiao SS, O'Shaughnessy DM, Johnson KO. 1993. Effects of selective attention on spatial form processing in monkey primary and secondary somatosensory cortex. J Neurophysiol 70:444–447.

Hubel DH, Wiesel TN. 1968. Receptive fields and functional architecture of monkey striate cortex. J Physiol 195: 215–243.

Hume D. [1739] 1984. *A Treatise of Human Nature*. EC Mossner (ed). New York: Penguin.

Johansson RS, Vallbo AB. 1979. Detection of tactile stimuli. Thresholds of afferent units related to psychophysical thresholds in the human hand. J Physiol 297:405–422.

Kant I. [1781/1787] 1961. *Critique of Pure Reason*. NK Smith (transl.). London: Macmillan.

Kirkland KL, Gerstein GL. 1999. A feedback model of attention and context dependence in visual cortical networks. J Comput Neurosci 7:255–267.

Kuffler SW. 1953. Discharge patterns and functional organization of mammalian retina. J Neurophysiol 16:37–68.

LaMotte RH, Mountcastle VB. 1975. Capacities of humans and monkeys to discriminate between vibratory stimuli of different frequency and amplitude: a correlation between neural events and psychophysical measurements. J Neurophysiol 38:539–559.

Livingstone MS, Hubel DH. 1987. Psychophysical evidence for separate channels for the perception of form, color, movement, and depth. J Neurosci 7:3416–3468.

Locke J. 1690. *An Essay Concerning Human Understanding: In Four Books*, Book 2, Chapter 1. London.

Moore GP, Perkel DH, Segundo JP. 1966. Statistical analysis and functional interpretation of neuronal spike data. Annu Rev Physiol 28:493–522.

Mountcastle VB, Powell TP. 1959. Neural mechanisms subserving cutaneous sensibility, with special reference to the role of afferent inhibition in sensory perception and discrimination. Bull Johns Hopkins Hosp 105: 201–232.

Mountcastle VB, Talbot WH, Kornhuber HH. 1966. The neural transformation of mechanical stimuli delivered to the monkey's hand. In: AVS de Reuck, J Knight (eds). *Ciba Foundation Symposium: Touch, Heat and Pain*, pp. 325–351. London: Churchill.

Müller J. 1838. *Handbuch der Physiologie des Menschen für Vorlesungen*, 2 vols. Coblenz: Hölscher.

Ochoa J, Torebjörk E. 1983. Sensations evoked by intraneural microstimulation of single mechanoreceptor units innervating the human hand. J Physiol 342:633–654.

Roy A, Steinmetz PN, Hsiao SS, Johnson KO, Niebur E. 2007. Synchrony: a neural correlate of somatosensory attention. J Neurophysiol 98:1645–1661.

Talbot WH, Darian-Smith I, Kornhuber HH, Mountcastle VB. 1968. The sense of flutter-vibration: comparison of the human capacity with response patterns of mechanoreceptive afferents from the monkey hand. J Neurophysiol 31:301–334.

Tanner WP, Birdsall TG. 1958. Definitions of *d′* and η as psychophysical measures. J Acoust Soc Am 30:922–928.

Tanner WP, Swets JA. 1954. A decision-making theory of visual detection. Psychol Rev 61:401–409.

Treisman A. 1991. Search, similarity and integration of features between and within dimensions. J Exp Psychol Hum Percept Perform 17:652–676.

Ungerleider LG, Mishkin M. 1982. Two cortical visual systems. In: DG Ingle, MA Goodale, RJW Mansfield (eds). *Analysis of Visual Behavior*, pp. 549–586. Cambridge, MA: MIT Press.

Yoshioka T, Gibb B, Dorsch AK, Hsiao SS, Johnson KO. 2001. Neural coding mechanisms underlying perceived roughness of finely textured surfaces. J Neurosci 21: 6905–6916.

Zotterman Y. 1978. How it started: a personal review. In: DR Kenshalo (ed). *Sensory Functions of the Skin of Humans*, pp. 5–22. New York: Plenum.

22

The Somatosensory System: Receptors and Central Pathways

WE BEGIN THE STUDY OF THE INDIVIDUAL sensory systems with the somatosensory system (Greek *soma*, the body), the system in which sensory coding was first studied electrophysiologically. Somatic information is provided by receptors distributed throughout the body. One of the earliest investigators of the bodily senses, Charles Sherrington, noted that the somatosensory system serves three major functions: proprioception, exteroception, and interoception.

Proprioception is the sense of oneself (Latin *proprius*, one's own). Receptors in skeletal muscle, joint capsules, and the skin enable us to have conscious awareness of the posture and movements of our own body, particularly the four limbs and the head. Although one can move parts of the body without sensory feedback from proprioceptors, the movements are often clumsy, poorly coordinated, and inadequately adapted to complex tasks, particularly if visual guidance is absent.

Exteroception is the sense of direct interaction with the external world as it impacts on the body. The principal mode of exteroception is the sense of touch, which includes sensations of contact, pressure, stroking, motion, and vibration, and is used to identify objects. Some touch involves an active motor component—stroking, tapping, grasping, or pressing—whereby a part of the body is moved against another surface or organism. The sensory and motor components of touch are intimately connected anatomically in the brain and are important in guiding behavior.

Exteroception also includes the thermal senses of heat and cold. Thermal sensations are important controllers of behavior and homeostatic mechanisms needed to maintain the body temperature near 37°C (98.6°F). Finally, exteroception includes the sense of pain, or nociception, a response to external events that damage or harm the body. Nociception is a prime motivator of actions necessary for survival, such as withdrawal or combat.

The third component of somatic sensation, *interoception*, is the sense of the function of the major organ systems of the body and its internal state. Although most of the events recorded by receptors in the viscera do not become conscious sensations, the information conveyed by these receptors is crucial for regulating autonomic functions, particularly in the cardiovascular, respiratory, digestive, and renal systems. Interoceptors are primarily chemoreceptors that monitor organ function through such indicators as blood gases and pH.

Abnormal function in major organ systems resulting from disease or trauma can evoke conscious sensations of pain. Much of our knowledge of the neural mechanisms of pain is derived from studies of cutaneous nociceptors because the mechanisms are easier to study in cutaneous nerves than in visceral nerves. Nevertheless, the neural mechanisms underlying visceral pain are similar to those for pain arising from the surface of the body.

This diverse group of sensory functions may seem an unlikely combination to form a sensory system. We treat all of the somatic senses in one introductory chapter because they are mediated by one class of sensory neurons, the dorsal root ganglion neurons. Individual neurons in a dorsal root ganglion respond selectively to specific types of stimuli because of morphological and molecular specialization of their peripheral terminals.

In this chapter we consider the principles common to all dorsal root ganglion neurons and those that distinguish their individual sensory function. We begin with a description of the peripheral nerves and their organization, followed by a survey of the receptors responsible for each of the major bodily senses. We then consider their sensory pathways in the spinal cord and brain stem. The chapter concludes with a discussion of the central processing centers for each submodality in the thalamus. The physiological function of touch, pain, proprioception, and autonomic regulation are described in more detail in separate chapters.

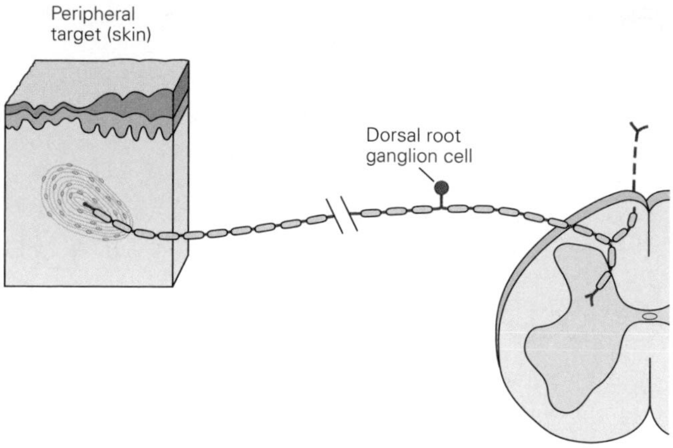

Figure 22–1 The dorsal root ganglion neuron is the primary sensory receptor cell of the somatosensory system. The neuron cell body is located in a dorsal root ganglion adjacent to the spinal cord. The axon has two branches, one projecting to the periphery, where its specialized terminal contains receptors for a particular form of stimulus energy, and one projecting to the spinal cord or brain stem, where the afferent signals are processed.

The Primary Sensory Neurons of the Somatosensory System Are Clustered in the Dorsal Root Ganglia

Somatosensory information from the skin, muscles, joint capsules, and viscera is conveyed by dorsal root ganglion neurons innervating the limbs and trunk or by trigeminal sensory neurons that innervate cranial structures (the face, lips, oral cavity, conjunctiva, and dura mater). These sensory neurons perform two major functions: the transduction and encoding of stimuli into electrical signals and the transmission of those signals to the central nervous system.

The cell body of a dorsal root ganglion neuron lies in a ganglion on the dorsal root of a spinal or cranial nerve. Dorsal root ganglion neurons originate from the neural crest and are intimately associated with the nearby segment of the spinal cord.

Dorsal root ganglion neurons are a type of bipolar cell, called pseudo-unipolar cells. The axon of a dorsal root ganglion neuron has two branches, one projecting to the periphery and one projecting to the central nervous system (Figure 22–1). The peripheral terminals of different neurons innervate the skin, muscle, joint capsules, or viscera and contain receptors specialized for particular kinds of stimuli. They differ in receptor morphology and stimulus selectivity. The central branches terminate in the spinal cord or brain stem, forming the first synapses in somatosensory pathways. Thus the axon of each dorsal root ganglion cell serves as a single transmission line with one polarity between the receptor terminal and the central nervous system. This axon is called the *primary afferent fiber*.

Individual primary afferent fibers innervating a particular region of the body, such as the thumb or fingers, are grouped together into bundles or fascicles of axons forming the *peripheral nerves*. They are guided during development to a specific location in the body by various trophic factors. The peripheral nerves also include motor axons innervating nearby muscles, blood vessels, glands, or viscera.

Damage to peripheral nerves or their targets in the brain may produce sensory deficits in more than one somatosensory submodality. Knowledge of where somatosensory modalities overlap morphologically, and where they diverge, facilitates diagnosis of neurological disorders and malfunction.

Peripheral Somatosensory Nerve Fibers Conduct Action Potentials at Different Rates

The diverse modalities of somatic sensation are mediated by peripheral nerve fibers that differ in diameter and conduction velocity. Mechanoreceptors for touch and proprioception are innervated by dorsal root ganglion neurons with large-diameter, myelinated axons that conduct action potentials rapidly. Thermal receptors, nociceptors, and other chemoreceptors have small-diameter axons that are either unmyelinated or thinly myelinated; these nerves conduct impulses more slowly. The difference in conduction velocity allows signals of touch and proprioception to reach the spinal cord and higher brain centers sooner than noxious or thermal signals.

Large-diameter fibers conduct action potentials more rapidly because the internal resistance to current flow along the axon is low, and the nodes of Ranvier are widely spaced along its length (see Chapter 6). The conduction velocity of large myelinated fibers (in meters per second) is approximately six times the axon diameter (in micrometers), whereas thinly myelinated fibers conduct at five times the axon diameter. For unmyelinated fibers, the factor for converting axon diameter to conduction velocity is 1.5 to 2.5.

Peripheral nerve fibers are classified into functional groups based on properties related to axon diameter and myelination, conduction velocity, and whether they are sensory or motor. The first classification scheme was devised in 1894 by Charles Sherrington, who measured the diameter of myelin-stained axons in sensory nerves, and subsequently codified by David Lloyd (Table 22–1). They found two or three overlapping groups of axonal diameters (Figure 22–2). It was later discovered that in muscle nerves these anatomical groupings are functionally important. Group I axons innervate muscle-spindle receptors and Golgi tendon organs, which signal muscle length and contractile force. Group II fibers innervate secondary spindle endings and receptors in joint capsules; these receptors also mediate proprioception. Group III fibers, the smallest myelinated muscle afferents, and the unmyelinated group IV afferents signal disorders in muscles and joints that can be sensed as painful.

Cutaneous nerves contain two sets of myelinated fibers: Group II fibers innervate cutaneous mechanoreceptors that respond to touch, and group III fibers mediate thermal and noxious stimuli. Unmyelinated group IV cutaneous afferents, like those in muscle, also mediate thermal and noxious stimuli.

Another method for classifying peripheral nerve fibers is based on electrical stimulation of whole nerves. In this widely used diagnostic technique nerve conduction velocities are measured between pairs of stimulating and recording electrodes placed on the skin above a peripheral nerve. When studying conduction in the median or ulnar nerve, for example, the stimulation electrode might be placed on the wrist and

Table 22–1 Classification of Sensory Fibers in Peripheral Nerves[1]

	Muscle nerve	Cutaneous nerve[2]	Fiber diameter (μm)	Conduction velocity (m/s)
Myelinated				
Large diameter	I	Aα	12–20	72–120
Medium diameter	II	Aβ	6–12	36–72
Small diameter	III	Aδ	1–6	4–36
Unmyelinated	IV	C	0.2–1.5	0.4–2.0

[1]Sensory fibers from muscle are classified according to their diameter, whereas those from the skin are classified by conduction velocity.
[2]The types of receptors innervated by each type of fiber are listed in Table 22–2.

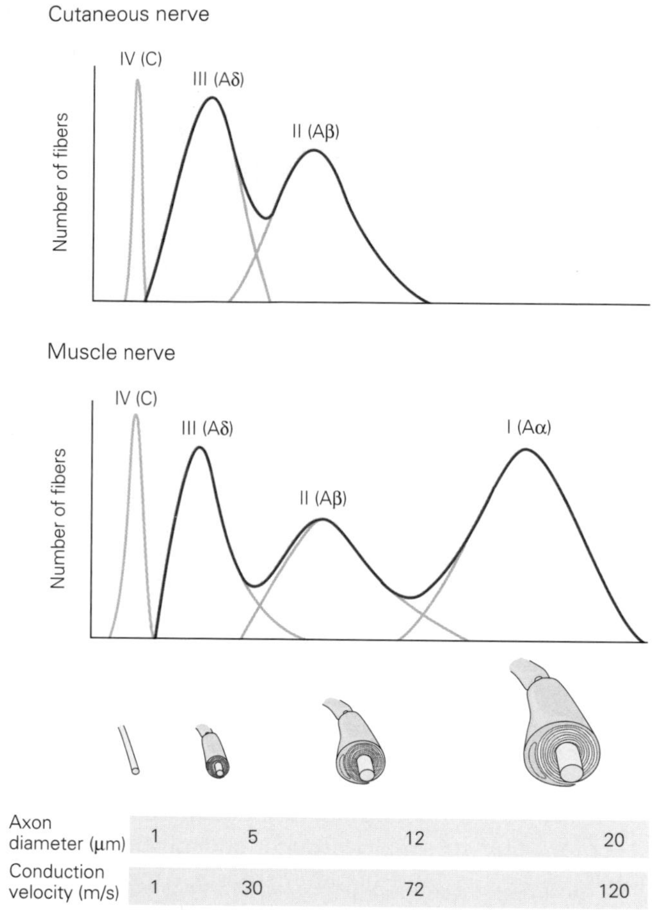

Figure 22–2 Peripheral nerves innervating skeletal muscle and the skin contain several types of sensory nerve fibers. The graphs illustrate the distribution of four groups of sensory nerve fibers innervating skeletal muscle and the skin. Each group has a characteristic axon diameter and conduction velocity. **Light blue lines** are the sum of fibers in each group in the zones of overlap. The conduction velocity of myelinated peripheral nerve fibers is approximately six times the fiber diameter. (Adapted, with permission, from Boyd and Davey 1968.)

the recording electrode on the upper arm. Brief electrical pulses applied through the stimulating electrode evoke action potentials in the nerve that are recorded a short time later in the arm. The recorded signal represents the summed action potentials of all of the nerve fibers excited by the stimulus pulse and is called the *compound action potential*. It increases in amplitude as more nerve fibers are stimulated; the summed activity is roughly proportional to the total number of active nerve fibers.

Electrical stimuli of increasing strength evoke action potentials in the largest axons first, for they have the lowest electrical resistance, and then in progressively smaller axons. The earliest signal recorded in the compound action potential occurs in fibers with conduction velocities greater than 90 m/s. Called the Aα wave (Figure 22–3), this signal reflects the action potentials generated in group I fibers and in motor neurons innervating skeletal muscle. The sensation is barely perceived by the subject in the region innervated.

A second signal, the Aβ wave, appears as more large fibers are recruited. This component corresponds to group II fibers in skin or muscle nerves and becomes larger as the shock intensity is increased. At higher voltages, when axons in the smaller Aδ range are recruited, the stimulus becomes painful, resembling an electric shock produced by static electricity. Voltages sufficient to activate unmyelinated C fibers evoke sensations of burning pain. Stimulation of motor neurons innervating muscle spindles evoke an intermediate wavelet called the Aγ wave, but this is usually difficult to discern because the conduction velocities of these motor neurons overlap those of Aβ and Aδ sensory axons.

The clinician takes advantage of the known distribution of the conduction velocities of afferent fibers in peripheral nerves to diagnose diseases that result in sensory-fiber degeneration or motor neuron loss. In certain conditions the loss of axons is selective; in the neuropathy characteristic of diabetes, for example, the large-diameter sensory fibers degenerate. Such a selective loss is reflected in a reduction in the appropriate peak of the compound action potential, a slowing of nerve conduction, and a corresponding diminution of sensory capacity. Similarly, in multiple sclerosis the myelin sheath of large-diameter fibers in the central nervous system degenerates, producing slowing of nerve conduction or failure of impulse transmission.

Rapid conduction in a peripheral nerve axon solves two problems. First, it provides the prompt sensory feedback required for motor control. The greatest velocities are in the afferent fibers from muscle that signal muscle length, contraction velocity, and force. Any delay in the feedback signal would cause instability, which probably explains why the fibers innervating spindles have the greatest diameters among peripheral axons.

Conduction-delay dispersion poses a second significant problem because conduction velocity varies among afferent fibers. Synchronous firing of a set of neurons becomes desynchronized by the time the action potentials reach the postsynaptic cells by an amount that is proportional to the mean conduction delay and the variation in conduction velocities. If the delay is great, either because the pathway is long or

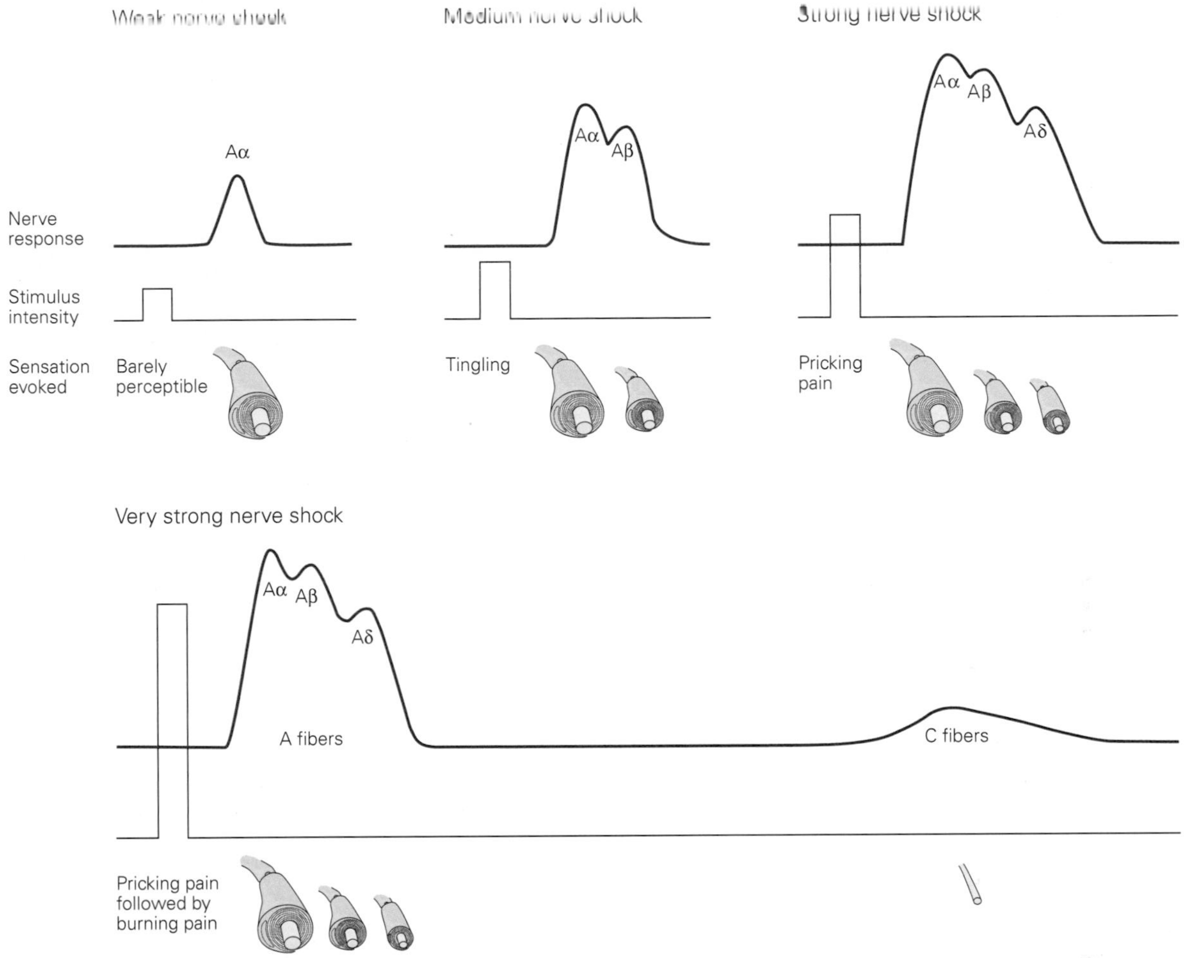

Figure 22–3 Conduction velocities of peripheral nerves are measured clinically from compound action potentials. Electrical stimulation of a peripheral nerve at varying intensities activates different types of nerve fibers. The action potentials of all the nerves stimulated by a particular amount of current are summed to create the compound action potential. The distinct conduction velocities of different classes of sensory and motor axons produce multiple deflections. (Adapted, with permission, from Erlanger and Gasser 1938.)

because the conduction velocities are low, the desynchronization can be substantial.

As a general rule, conduction velocity throughout the nervous system is correlated with the need to maintain synchrony. The disparity in conduction times from a fingertip to the spinal cord can be calculated from the conduction velocities in Table 22–1 and by considering that the distance is approximately 0.8 m. In C fibers delays range from 0.8 s to 1.8 s, the mean delay is about 1.3 s, and the spike arrival times are distributed over about 1 s; thus events occurring more often than once per second are smeared together. In Aα fibers delays range from 7.5 ms to 12.5 ms, the mean delay is 10 ms, and the arrival times vary by only 5 ms; events can therefore occur as often as 200 per second without smearing. The comparable limits for Aδ and Aβ fibers are approximately 8 Hz and 80 Hz. A blind person can scan his or her fingers across Braille dot patterns at remarkable rates of up to 100 mm/s with little loss of information because tactile information is conveyed by Aβ afferents, which maintain synchrony to within 12 ms.

Many Specialized Receptors Are Employed by the Somatosensory System

The particular receptor class expressed in the nerve terminal of a sensory neuron determines the type of stimulus detected by the neuron. The peripheral axons of the sensory neurons that mediate touch and proprioception terminate in a nonneural capsule. They sense mechanical stimuli that indent or otherwise physically deform the receptive surface. In contrast the peripheral axons of neurons that detect noxious, thermal, or chemical events have unsheathed endings with multiple branches.

When a somatic receptor is activated by an appropriate stimulus, the terminal of the sensory neuron is typically depolarized. Stimuli of sufficient strength produce action potentials that are transmitted along the peripheral branch of the neuron's axon and into the central branch that terminates in the spinal cord or brain stem.

A variety of morphologically specialized receptors underlie the various somatosensory submodalities. For example, the median nerve that innervates the skin of the hand and some of the muscles controlling the hand contains tens of thousands of nerve fibers that can be classified into 30 functional types. Of these, 22 types are afferent fibers (sensory axons conducting impulses toward the spinal cord), and eight types are efferent fibers (motor axons conducting impulses away from the spinal cord to skeletal muscle, blood vessels, and sweat glands). The afferent fibers convey signals from eight kinds of cutaneous mechanoreceptors that are sensitive to different kinds of skin deformation; five kinds of proprioceptors that signal information about muscle force, muscle length, and joint angle; four thermoreceptors that report the temperatures of objects touching the skin; four nociceptors that signal potentially injurious stimuli; and at least one kind of itch receptor. The major receptor groups within each submodality are listed in Table 22–2.

Mechanoreceptors Mediate Touch and Proprioception

Mechanoreceptors sense physical deformation of the tissue in which they reside. Mechanical distension,

Table 22–2 Receptor Types Active in Somatic Sensation

Receptor type	Fiber group[1]	Fiber name	Modality
Cutaneous and subcutaneous mechanoreceptors			Touch
Meissner corpuscle	Aα,β	RA1	Stroking, flutter
Merkel disk receptor	Aα,β	SA1	Pressure, texture
Pacinian corpuscle[2]	Aα,β	RA2	Vibration
Ruffini ending	Aα,β	SA2	Skin stretch
Hair-tylotrich, hair-guard	Aα,β	G1, G2	Stroking, fluttering
Hair-down	Aδ	D	Light stroking
Field	Aα,β	F	Skin stretch
C mechanoreceptor	C		Stroking, erotic touch
Thermal receptors			Temperature
Cool receptors	Aδ	III	Skin cooling (<25°C [77°F])
Warm receptors	C	IV	Skin warming (>35°C [95°F])
Heat nociceptors	Aδ	III	Hot temperature (>45°C [113°F])
Cold nociceptors	C	IV	Cold temperature (<5°C [41°F])
Nociceptors			Pain
Mechanical	Aδ	III	Sharp, pricking pain
Thermal-mechanical (heat)	Aδ	III	Burning pain
Thermal-mechanical (cold)	C	IV	Freezing pain
Polymodal	C	IV	Slow, burning pain
Muscle and skeletal mechanoreceptors			Limb proprioception
Muscle spindle primary	Aα	Ia	Muscle length and speed
Muscle spindle secondary	Aβ	II	Muscle stretch
Golgi tendon organ	Aα	Ib	Muscle contraction
Joint capsule receptors	Aβ	II	Joint angle
Stretch-sensitive free endings	Aδ	III	Excess stretch or force

[1]See Table 22–1.

[2]Pacinian corpuscles are also located in the mesentery, between layers of muscle, and on interosseous membranes.

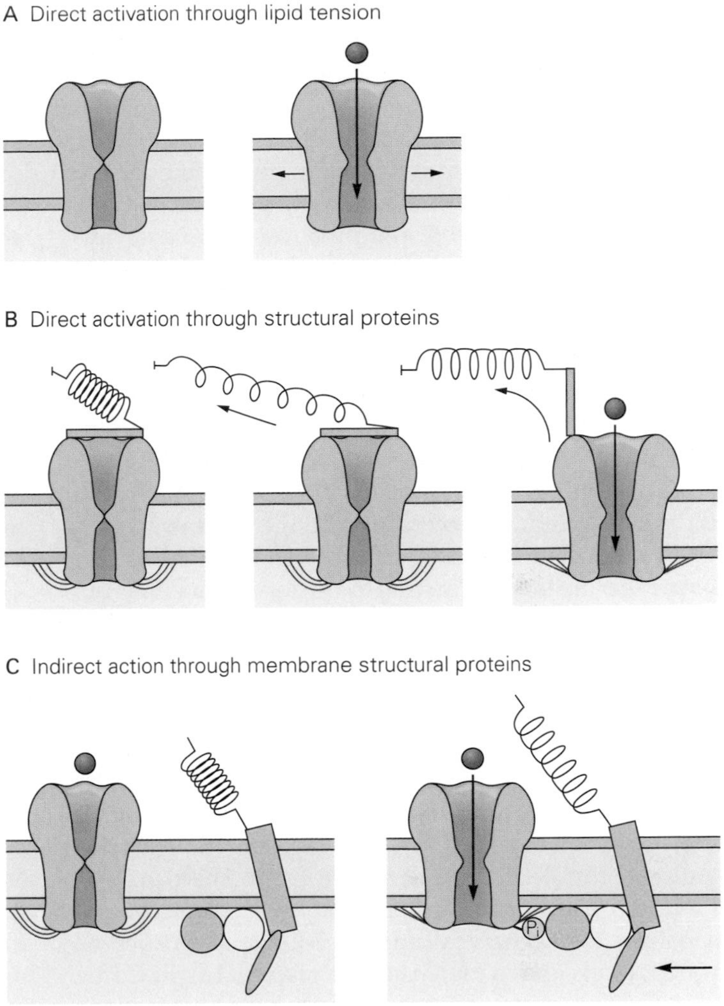

Figure 22–4 Ion channels in mechanoreceptor nerve terminals are activated by mechanical stimuli that stretch or deform the cell membrane. Mechanical displacement leads to channel opening, permitting the influx of cations. (Modified, with permission, from Lin and Corey 2005.)

A. Channels can be directly activated by forces conveyed through lipid tension in the cell membrane, such as osmotic swelling.

B. Forces conveyed through structural proteins linked to the ion channel can also directly activate channels. The linking proteins may be either extracellular (attached to the surrounding tissue) or intracellular (bound to the cytoskeleton) or both.

C. Channels can be indirectly activated by forces conveyed to a force sensor (a separate protein) in the membrane. An internal second messenger carries the sensory signal from the mechanosensitive protein to the channel.

such as pressure on the skin or stretch of muscles, is transduced into electrical energy by the physical action of the stimulus on cation channels in the membrane. Mechanical stimulation deforms the receptor protein, thus opening stretch-sensitive ion channels and increasing Na^+ and Ca^{2+} conductances that depolarize the receptor neuron. Removal of the stimulus relieves mechanical stress on the receptor and allows stretch-sensitive channels to close.

Some mechanoreceptor ion channels are activated directly by forces applied to the tissue, permitting rapid activation and inactivation. For example, Pacinian corpuscle receptors in the skin can respond to vibration at frequencies as high as 500 Hz, firing one impulse for each vibratory cycle. This means that the receptor is capable of firing an impulse every 2 ms for sustained periods.

Various mechanisms for direct activation of mechanoreceptor ion channels have been proposed. Some mechanoreceptors appear to respond to forces conveyed through tension in the lipids of the plasma membrane (Figure 22–4A). This may be the mechanism for detection of cellular swelling, which plays an important role in osmoregulation.

Another mechanism for direct activation of mechanoreceptors is linking the channel to the surrounding tissue of the skin or to muscle cell membranes through structural proteins. The extracellular linkage is elastic and often represented as a spring, whereas the intracellular portion of the channel is anchored directly to proteins of the cytoskeleton (Figure 22–4B). Direct channel gating in this model may be produced by forces perpendicular or parallel to the receptor cell membrane that stretch the extracellular linkage protein.

This type of direct channel gating may be used by hair cells of the inner ear. Similar mechanical linkages between the skin and cutaneous mechanoreceptors have been postulated.

Likewise, mechanical coupling of sensory nerve terminals to skeletal muscle or tendons is thought to underlie proprioception. Unfortunately, because these receptors are embedded in nonneural tissue and thus difficult to isolate for biochemical analysis, the proteins involved in transduction have not been identified in mammals. Studies of invertebrates suggest that the transduction molecules for mechanosensation in skin and muscle may belong to the degenerin superfamily, which includes ion channels related to vertebrate epithelial Na^+ channels.

Some mechanoreceptor ion channels are activated indirectly through second-messenger pathways. In this case the force sensor in the receptor's cell membrane is a protein distinct from the ion channel (Figure 22–4C). A variety of intracellular messengers signal stimulation of the sensor to the ion channel, causing the channel to open. Unlike direct activation, the indirect pathway is slow to activate and inactivate, often outlasting the stimulus. The great advantage of the second-messenger mechanism of course is that the sensory signal is amplified; the conductance of many ionic channels can be affected by the activation of a single sensor molecule in the receptor cell. These properties are consistent with the responses of pain receptors sensitive to mechanical damage of the skin, such as pinch, or excessive distension of viscera. David Corey and co-workers have suggested that these sensations are mediated by TRPV4 receptors, a class of transient receptor potential (TRP) receptors that are also involved in thermal senses (see below).

The specialized, nonneural end organ that surrounds the nerve terminal of a mechanoreceptor nerve must be deformed in specific ways to excite the nerve. For example, individual receptors may respond selectively to pressure or motion, and may detect the direction of force applied to the skin, joints, or muscle fibers. The end organ can also amplify or modulate the sensitivity of the receptor to mechanical displacement.

The skin has eight types of mechanoreceptors that are responsible for the sense of touch (see Table 22–2). They are described briefly here and in greater detail in Chapter 23. The glabrous skin of the hands and feet contains four kinds of mechanoreceptors: Meissner corpuscles, Merkel cells, Pacinian corpuscles, and Ruffini endings (Figure 22–5). Two of these receptors are classified as slowly adapting (SA) because they continue to fire in response to steady pressure on the skin. The other two receptors are rapidly adapting (RA), responding to motion on the skin but not to steady pressure. They also differ in receptor size and location within the skin.

Merkel cells are innervated by slowly adapting type 1 (SA1) fibers. They signal the amount of pressure applied to the skin and are particularly sensitive to edges, corners, and points. They distinguish textures and play key roles in the ability to read Braille. The Ruffini endings are innervated by slowly adapting type 2 (SA2) fibers. These receptors respond more vigorously to stretch than to indentation of skin, and consequently are particularly sensitive to the shape of large objects held in the hand. They also signal movements of the fingers and other joints that stretch the overlying skin.

Meissner corpuscles are innervated by rapidly adapting type 1 (RA1) fibers. These receptors detect the initial contact of the hand with objects, slippage of objects held in the hand, motion of the hand over textured surfaces, and low-frequency vibration. The Pacinian corpuscles are innervated by rapidly adapting type 2 (RA2) fibers. The receptor is a large, onion-like capsule that surrounds the axon terminal. It responds to motion in the nanometer range and mediates high-frequency vibration. The most important role of Pacinian corpuscles is detection of vibrations in tools, objects, or probes held in the hand.

The general hairy skin includes all of the mechanoreceptor organs of the glabrous skin except the Meissner corpuscle; the hair follicle afferents serve a function similar to that of Meissner corpuscles. Hair follicle afferents innervate 10 to 30 hairs spread over an area of 1 to 2 cm^2 and are sensitive to hair movement but not to static pressure. Other mechanoreceptors of the hairy skin include field receptors, which are very sensitive to skin movement, and low-threshold mechanoreceptors innervated by C fibers that respond to slow stroking of the skin and are thought to mediate erotic touch.

Proprioceptors Measure Muscle Activity and Joint Positions

Mechanoreceptors in muscles and joints convey information about the posture and movements of the body and thereby play an important role in proprioception and motor control. These receptors include two types of muscle-length sensors, the type Ia and II muscle-spindle endings; one muscle force sensor, the Golgi tendon organ; and joint-capsule receptors, which transduce tension in the joint capsule.

The muscle spindle consists of a bundle of thin muscle fibers, or intrafusal fibers, that are aligned parallel to the larger fibers of the muscle and enclosed within a capsule (Figure 22–6A). The intrafusal fibers

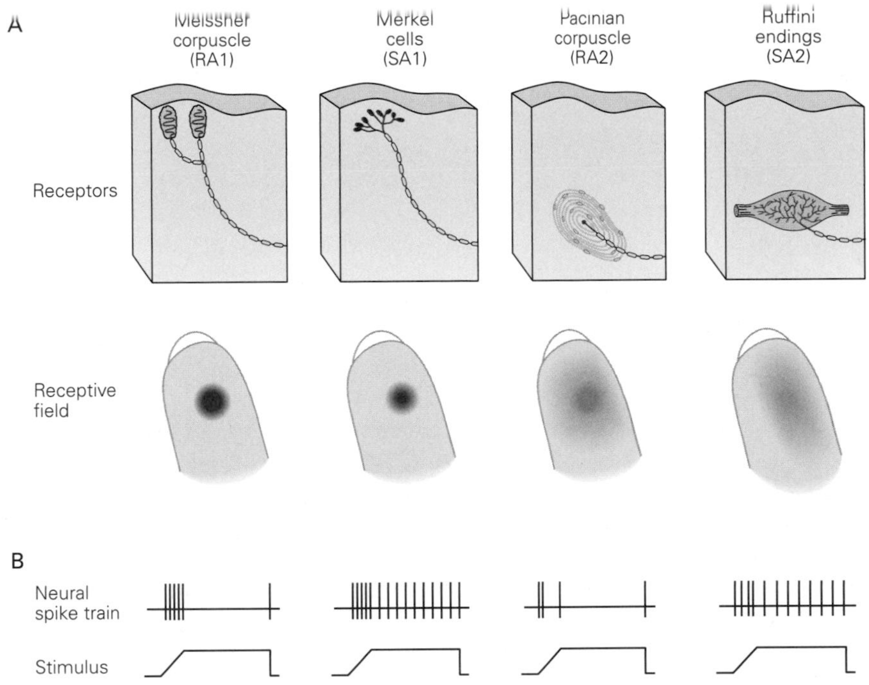

Figure 22–5 Touch is mediated by four types of mechanoreceptors in the human hand. The terminals of myelinated sensory nerves innervating the hand are surrounded by specialized structures that detect contact on the skin. The receptors differ in morphology, innervation patterns, location in the skin, receptive field size, and physiological responses to touch. (Adapted, with permission, from Johansson and Vallbo 1983.)

A. The superficial and deep layers of the glabrous (hairless) skin of the hand each contain distinct types of mechanoreceptors. The superficial layers contain small receptor cells: Meissner corpuscles and Merkel cells. The sensory nerve fibers innervating these receptors have branching terminals such that each fiber innervates multiple receptors of one type. The deep layers of the skin and subcutaneous tissue contain large receptors: Pacinian corpuscles and Ruffini endings. Each of these receptors is innervated by a single nerve fiber, and each fiber innervates only one receptor. The receptive field of a mechanoreceptor reflects the location and distribution of its terminals in the skin. Touch receptors in the superficial layers of the skin have smaller receptive fields than those in the deep layers. (**RA1**, rapidly adapting type 1; **RA2**, rapidly adapting type 2; **SA1**, slowly adapting type 1; **SA2**, slowly adapting type 2.)

B. The nerve fibers innervating each type of mechanoreceptor respond differently when activated. The spike trains show responses of each type of nerve when its receptor is activated by constant pressure against the skin. The RA type fibers that innervate Meissner and Pacinian corpuscles adapt rapidly to constant stimulation while the SA type nerves that innervate Merkel cells and Ruffini endings adapt slowly.

are entwined by a pair of sensory axons that detect muscle stretch because of mechanoreceptive ion channels in the nerve terminals. Intrafusal muscles are also innervated by motor neurons that determine contractile force. (See Box 35–1 for details on muscle spindles.)

Although the receptor potential and firing rates of the sensory axons are proportional to muscle length (Figure 22–6B), these responses can be modulated by higher centers in the brain that regulate contraction of intrafusal muscles. In this manner the spindle afferents are able to signal the amplitude and speed of internally generated voluntary movements as well as passive limb displacement by external forces.

Golgi tendon organs, located between skeletal muscle and tendons, measure the forces generated by muscle contraction. (See Box 35–3 for details on Golgi tendon organs.) Although these receptors play an important role in reflex circuits modulating muscle force, they appear to contribute little to conscious sensations of muscle activity. Psychophysical experiments in which muscles are fatigued or partially paralyzed have shown that perceived muscle force is mainly related to centrally generated effort rather than to actual muscle force.

Joint receptors play little if any role in postural sensations of joint angle. Instead, the perception of the angle of proximal joints such as the elbow or knee depends on afferent signals from muscle spindle receptors and efferent motor commands. Likewise, conscious sensations of finger position and hand shape

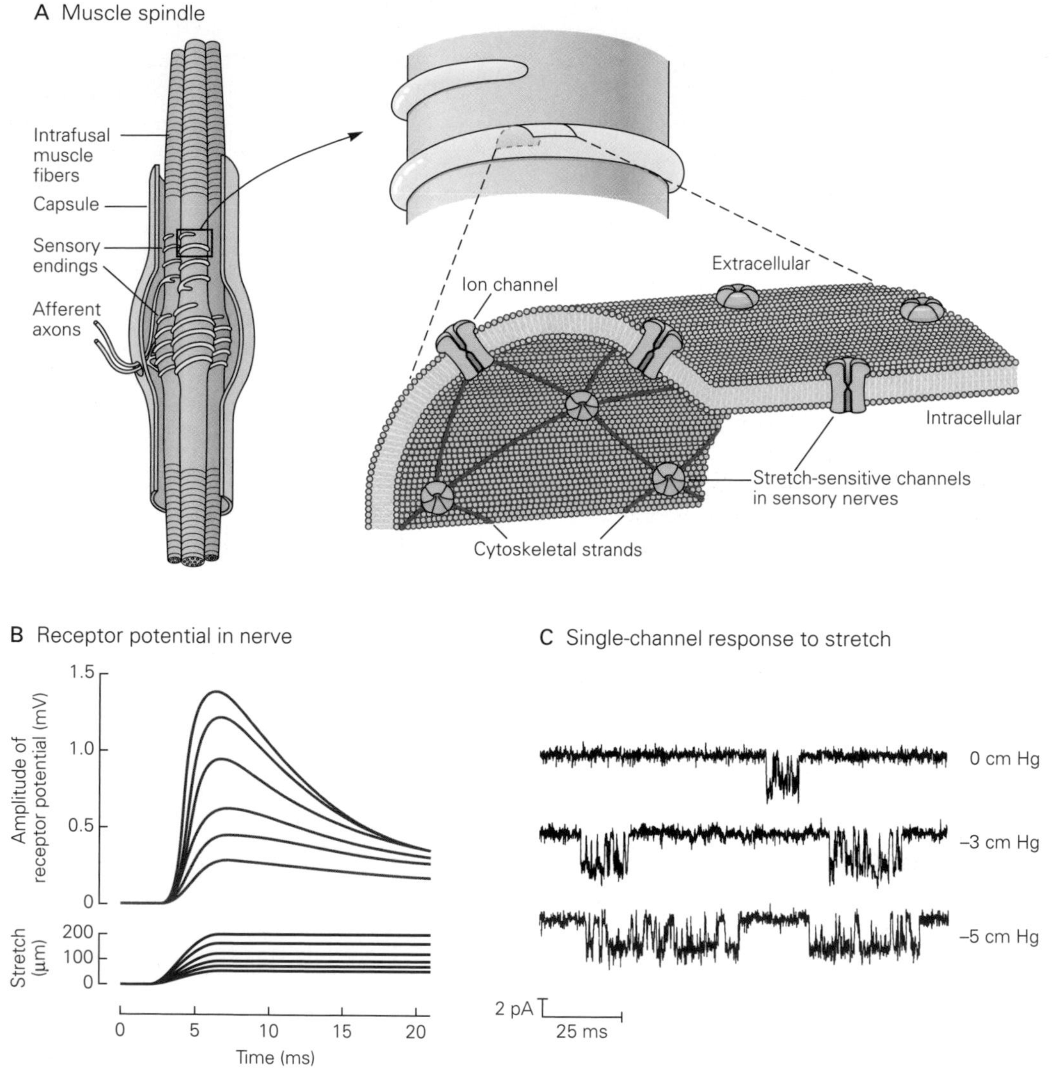

Figure 22–6 The muscle spindle is the principal receptor mediating proprioception.

A. The muscle spindle is located within skeletal muscle and is excited by stretch of the muscle. It consists of a bundle of thin (intrafusal) muscle fibers entwined by a pair of sensory axons, and is also innervated by several motor axons (not shown) that produce contraction of the intrafusal muscle fibers. Stretch-sensitive ion channels in the sensory nerve terminals are linked to the cytoskeleton by the protein spectrin. (Adapted, with permission, from Sachs 1990.)

B. The depolarizing receptor potential recorded in a group Ia fiber innervating the muscle spindle (**upper record**) is proportional to both the velocity and amplitude of muscle stretch parallel to the myofilaments (**lower record**). When stretch is maintained at a fixed length, the receptor potential decays to a lower value. (Adapted, with permission, from Ottoson and Shepherd 1971.)

C. Patch clamp recordings of a single stretch-sensitive channel in myocytes. Pressure is applied to the receptor cell membrane by suction. At rest (**top record**) the channel opens sporadically for short time intervals. As the pressure applied to the membrane increases (**lower records**) the channel opens more often and remains in the open state longer. This allows more current to flow into the receptor cell, resulting in higher levels of depolarization. (Adapted, with permission, from Sachs 1990.)

depend on stretch receptors in the skin as well as muscle spindles and possibly joint receptors.

Nociceptors Mediate Pain

The receptors that respond selectively to stimuli that can damage tissue are called *nociceptors* (Latin *nocere*, to injure). They respond directly to mechanical and thermal stimuli, and indirectly to other stimuli by means of chemicals released from cells in the traumatized tissue. Nociceptors signal impending tissue injury and, more importantly, they provide a constant reminder of tissues that are already injured and must be protected.

Nociceptors in the skin, muscle, joints, and visceral receptors fall into two broad classes based on the myelination of their afferent fibers. Nociceptors innervated by Aδ fibers produce short-latency pain that is described as sharp and pricking. The majority are called mechanical nociceptors because they are excited by sharp objects that penetrate, squeeze, or pinch the skin (Figure 22–7). Many of these Aδ fibers also respond to noxious heat that can burn the skin.

Nociceptors innervated by C fibers produce dull, burning pain that is diffusely localized and poorly tolerated. The most common type are polymodal nociceptors that respond to a variety of noxious mechanical, thermal, and chemical stimuli, such as pinch or puncture, noxious heat and cold, and irritant chemicals applied to the skin. Electrical stimulation of these fibers in humans evokes prolonged sensations of burning pain. In the viscera nociceptors are activated by distension or swelling, producing sensations of intense pain.

Thermal Receptors Detect Changes in Skin Temperature

Although the size, shape, and texture of objects held in the hand can be apprehended visually as well as by touch, the thermal qualities of objects are uniquely somatosensory. Humans recognize four distinct types of thermal sensation: cold, cool, warm, and hot. These sensations result from differences between the external temperature of the air or of objects contacting the body and the normal skin temperature of approximately 32°C (90°F).

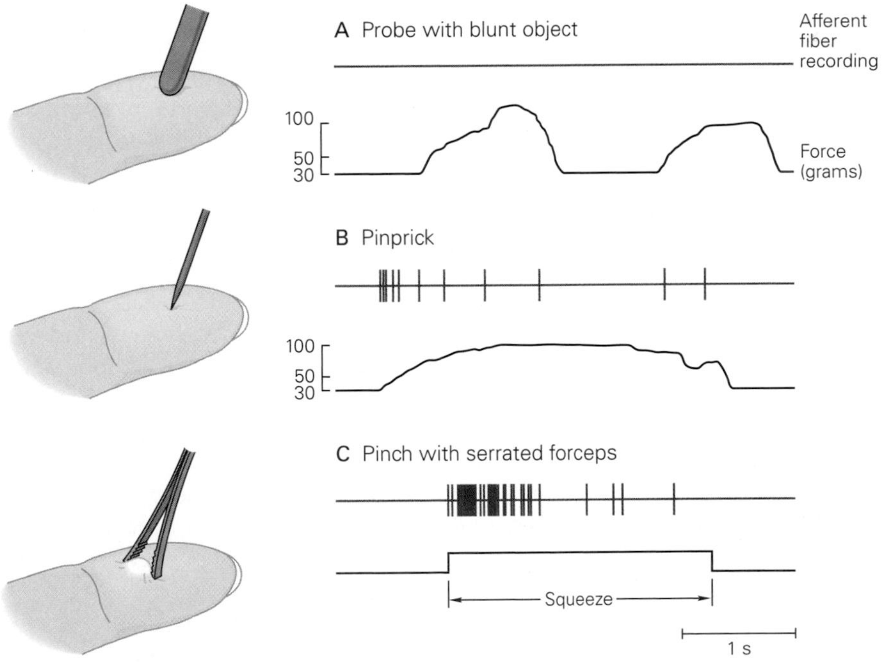

Figure 22–7 Mechanical nociceptors respond to stimuli that puncture, squeeze, or pinch the skin. Sensations of sharp, pricking pain result from stimulation of Aδ fibers with free nerve endings in the skin. These receptors respond to sharp objects that puncture the skin (**B**) but not to strong pressure from a blunt probe (**A**). The strongest responses are produced by pinching the skin with serrated forceps that damage the tissue in the region of contact (**C**). (Adapted, with permission, from Perl 1968.)

Although we are exquisitely sensitive to sudden changes in skin temperature, we are normally unaware of the wide swings in skin temperature that occur as our cutaneous blood vessels open and close to discharge or conserve body heat. If skin temperature changes slowly, we are unaware of changes in the range 31° to 36°C (88–97°F). Below 31°C (88°F) the sensation progresses from cool to cold and finally, beginning at 10° to 15°C (50–59°F), to pain. Above 36°C (97°F) the sensation progresses from warm to hot and then, beginning at 45°C (113°F), to pain.

Thermal sensations result from the combined activity of six types of afferent fibers: low-threshold and high-threshold cold receptors, warm receptors, and two classes of heat nociceptors. The low-threshold cold receptor fibers are small-diameter, myelinated Aδ fibers with unmyelinated endings within the epidermis. They are approximately 100 times more sensitive to sudden drops in skin temperature than to gradual changes. This extreme sensitivity to change allows humans to detect a draft from a distant open window. The high-threshold cold receptor fibers are much less sensitive to small cooling changes, but can signal rapid skin cooling even below 0°C (32°F).

The various qualities of cold sensations can be experienced by grasping an ice cube in a closed fist. Over the first five seconds or so the sensation progresses from cool to cold. After 10 seconds the sensation becomes progressively more painful. If the ice is held still longer, the sensation begins to include a deep, aching quality. The low-threshold and high-threshold receptors account for the initial sensations; the aching cold pain likely results from receptors within the veins.

Warm receptors are located in the terminals of C fibers that end in the dermis. Unlike the cold receptors, warm receptors act more like simple thermometers; their firing rates rise monotonically with increasing skin temperature up to the threshold of pain and then saturate at higher temperatures. Thus they cannot play a role in signaling heat pain. They are much less sensitive to rapid changes in skin temperature than are cold receptors. Consequently, humans are less responsive to warming than cooling; the threshold for detecting sudden skin warming, even in the most sensitive subject, is about 0.1 Centigrade degree.

Heat nociceptors are activated by temperatures exceeding 45°C (113°F) and inactivated by skin cooling. The burning pain caused by high temperatures is transmitted by both myelinated Aδ fibers and unmyelinated C fibers.

Recent studies by David Julius and his colleagues revealed that thermal stimuli activate specific classes of TRP ion channels in the membrane. These nonselective cation receptor-channels are similar in structure to voltage-gated channels. They have four protein subunits, each of which contains six transmembrane domains, with a pore between the fifth and sixth segments. Both the C and N terminals are located in the cytoplasm. Individual TRP receptor-channels are distinguished by their sensitivity to heat or cold, showing sharp increases in conductance to cations when their thermal threshold is exceeded (Figure 22–8). Their names specify the genetic subfamily of TRP receptors and the member number. Examples include TRPV1 (for TRP vanilloid-1), TRPM8 (for TRP melastatin-8), and TRPA1 (for TRP ankyrin-1).

Two classes of TRP receptors are activated by cold temperatures and inactivated by warming. TRPM8 receptors respond to temperatures below 25°C (77°F); such temperatures are perceived as cool or cold. TRPA1 receptors have thresholds below 17°C (63°F); this range is described as cold or frigid. Both TRPM8 and TRPA1 receptors are expressed in high-threshold cold receptor terminals, but only TRPM8 receptors are expressed in low-threshold cold receptor terminals.

Four types of TRP receptors are activated by warm or hot temperatures and inactivated by cooling. TRPV3 receptors are expressed in warm type fibers; they respond to warming of the skin above 35°C (95°F) and generate sensations ranging from warm to hot. TRPV1 and TRPV2 receptors respond to temperatures exceeding 45°C (113°F) and mediate sensations of burning pain; they are expressed in heat nociceptors. TRPV4 receptors are activated by temperatures above 27°C and respond to normal skin temperatures. They may play a role in touch sensation.

The role of TRP receptors in thermal sensation was originally discovered by analyses of natural substances such as capsaicin and menthol that produce burning or cooling sensations when applied to the skin or injected subcutaneously. Capsaicin, the active ingredient in chili peppers, has been used extensively to activate nociceptive afferents that mediate sensations of burning pain. These studies indicate that the various TRP receptors also bind other molecules that induce painful sensations, such as toxins, venoms, and substances released by diseased or injured tissue. These substances act by covalent modification of cysteines in the TRP channel protein.

Itch Is a Distinctive Cutaneous Sensation

Itch is a common sensory experience that is confined to the skin, the ocular conjunctiva, and the mucosa. Itch has some properties in common with pain and

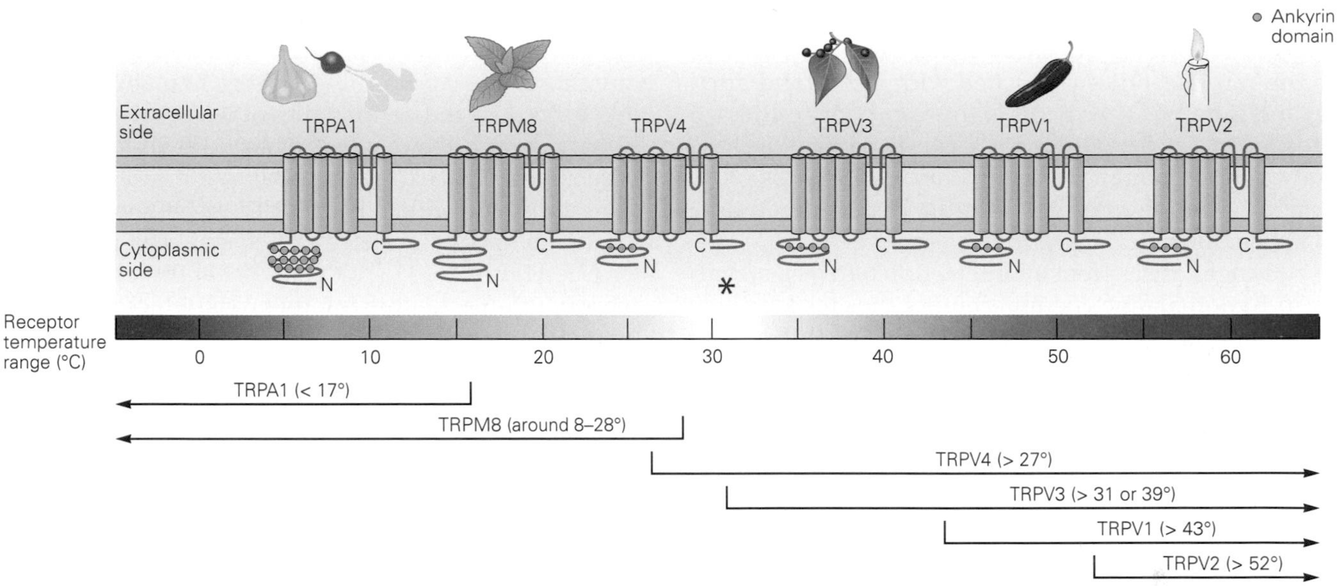

Figure 22–8 Transient receptor potential ion channels. Transient receptor potential (TRP) channels are membrane proteins with six transmembrane domains. A pore is formed between the fifth (S5) and sixth (S6) segments. Both C- and N-terminals are located in the cytoplasm. Most of these receptors contain ankyrin repeats in the N-terminal domains and a common 25-amino acid motif adjacent to S6 in the C-terminal domain. All TRP channels are gated by temperature and various chemical ligands, but different types respond to different temperature ranges and have different activation thresholds. At least six types of TRP receptors have been identified in sensory neurons; the thermal sensitivity of a neuron is determined by the particular TRP receptors expressed in its nerve terminals. At 32°C (90°F), the resting skin temperature (asterisk), only TRPV4 and some TRPV3 receptors are stimulated. TRPA1 and TRPM8 receptors are activated by cooling and cold stimuli. TRPM8 receptors also respond to menthol and various mints; TRPA1 receptors respond to alliums such as garlic and radishes. TRPV3 receptors are activated by warm stimuli and also bind camphor. TRPV1 and TRPV2 receptors respond to heat and produce burning pain sensations. TRPV1 but not TRPV2 receptors bind capsaicin, which mediates the burning sensations evoked by chili peppers. TRPV4 receptors are active at normal skin temperatures and respond to touch. (Adapted, with permission, from Jordt, McKemy, and Julius 2003; Dhaka, Viswanath, and Patapoutian 2006.)

until recently was thought to result from low firing rates in nociceptive fibers. Like pain, itch is inherently unpleasant whatever its intensity; even at the expense of inducing pain, we attempt to eliminate it by scratching. When nerve conduction is blocked with pressure, itch persists until the slowest unmyelinated fibers stop firing.

Itch can be induced either by the injection of histamine or by procedures that release endogenous histamine, which suggests that the transducers are coupled to histamine receptors. Intradermal injection of a large dose of histamine produces intense itch that persists for tens of minutes but only mild pain, a strong indication that itch is not the result of low-level firing in polymodal nociceptors. Instead, itch appears to be mediated by a recently discovered class of C fibers with very slow conduction velocities (0.5 m/s) and physiological properties paralleling the time course of histamine-evoked itch.

Visceral Sensations Represent the Status of Various Internal Organs

Visceral sensations are important physiologically because they drive several types of behavior that are critical for survival, such as respiration, hunger, thirst, sexual arousal, and copulation. After about a minute without breathing, hunger for air, feelings of suffocation, and the need to relieve those sensations become all-consuming behavioral goals. These sensations allow us to hold our breath when needed with the knowledge that an internal sensory signal will tell us when it is no longer safe to do so. Thirst and hunger likewise provide the motivation to drink and eat; they come to dominate our behavior when we have been without water or food for periods that threaten our survival.

Visceral sensations that are linked directly to survival result from both peripheral and central sensors. Sensations associated with the need to breathe, for example, arise from partial pressure of oxygen (PO_2) and partial pressure of carbon dioxide (PCO_2) sensors in the carotid bodies associated with the carotid arteries and from PCO_2 receptors in the respiratory centers of the medulla and hypothalamus (see Chapter 45). Damage to these medullary centers results in a loss of air hunger (Ondine's curse) and often death from failure of automatic breathing during sleep.

Hunger arises from an interaction between signals from hypothalamic chemoreceptors that respond to a variety of molecules in the blood and signals from the gut that indicate the presence or absence of food (see Chapter 49). Thirst results from central mechanisms whose site is uncertain and from peripheral signals from osmoreceptors in the liver and stretch receptors in the cardiopulmonary blood vessels that provide information on blood volume (see Chapter 49).

Nausea, which teaches animals—including us—which foods are unsafe to eat, depends on vagal serotonin receptors in the gut as well as the area postrema in the brain stem. Neurons within the area postrema are able to sense toxins in the blood and cerebrospinal fluid because the area lacks a blood-brain barrier (see Appendix D).

Sensations associated with sexual arousal and copulation, which are essential for survival of the species, arise from low-threshold mechanoreceptors in the genitalia and other body sites. Although the central component is not certain, functional imaging studies and experimental lesion studies suggest that the preoptic area and anterior hypothalamus are important components of arousal (see Chapter 47).

Somatosensory Information Enters the Central Nervous System Through Cranial and Spinal Nerves

Sensory information reaches the central nervous system either through the 31 spinal nerves, which enter through openings between the vertebrae of the spine, or through the 12 cranial nerves, which enter through openings in the cranium. The afferent and efferent axons within a spinal nerve arise from the dorsal and ventral roots of the spinal cord (see Figure 16–3), which are arrayed more or less continuously along the dorsal and ventral surfaces of each half of the cord (see Figure 16–2). To exit between the vertebrae, the roots gather into nerves that are named for the vertebrae below the foramen through which they pass (cervical nerves) or above (thoracic, lumbar, and sacral nerves).

The skin and deeper tissues innervated by the afferent fibers of a single spinal nerve constitute a *dermatome* (Figure 22–9); the muscles innervated by the same nerve constitute a *myotome*. These are the skin and muscle regions affected by damage to a single spinal nerve. Because the dermatomes overlap, three adjacent spinal nerves often have to be blocked to anesthetize a particular area of skin.

Individual spinal nerves terminate on neurons located in specific zones of the spinal cord gray matter (see Figure 16–1). The spinal neurons that receive sensory input are either interneurons, which terminate upon other spinal neurons within the same or neighboring segment, or projection neurons that serve as the cells of origin of major ascending pathways to higher centers in the brain.

All but one of the spinal nerves contain both afferent and efferent nerve fibers; the exception is C1, which usually has only efferent axons. In contrast, 8 of the 12 cranial nerves are either pure motor or pure sensory nerves serving the special senses (olfactory, optic, and vestibulocochlear). The remaining four nerves (trigeminal, facial, glossopharyngeal, and vagus) are mixed nerves that together serve the same range of bodily senses as do the spinal nerves. Like the spinal nerves, the cell bodies of cranial nerves lie in ganglia near the point of entry to the central nervous system.

Each of the mixed cranial nerves has a distinct pattern of termination within the central nervous system and each is devoted principally to sensory information either from the viscera or from the skin and muscles (see Figure 45–5). The trigeminal nerve conveys sensory information from muscles of mastication and skin on the anterior half of the head. The facial and glossopharyngeal nerves innervate the taste buds of the tongue, the skin of the ear, and some of the skin of the tongue and pharynx. The glossopharyngeal and vagus nerves provide some cutaneous information, but their main sensory role is visceral. Cutaneous and proprioceptive information from all four nerves enters the trigeminal nuclei; visceral information flows into the nucleus of the solitary tract.

Somatosensory Information Flows from the Spinal Cord to the Thalamus Through Parallel Pathways

The nerve fibers that convey the various somatosensory submodalities from each dermatome are bundled together in the peripheral nerves as they enter the dorsal root ganglia. However, as the fibers exit the ganglia and approach the spinal cord, the large- and small-diameter fibers separate into medial and lateral divisions.

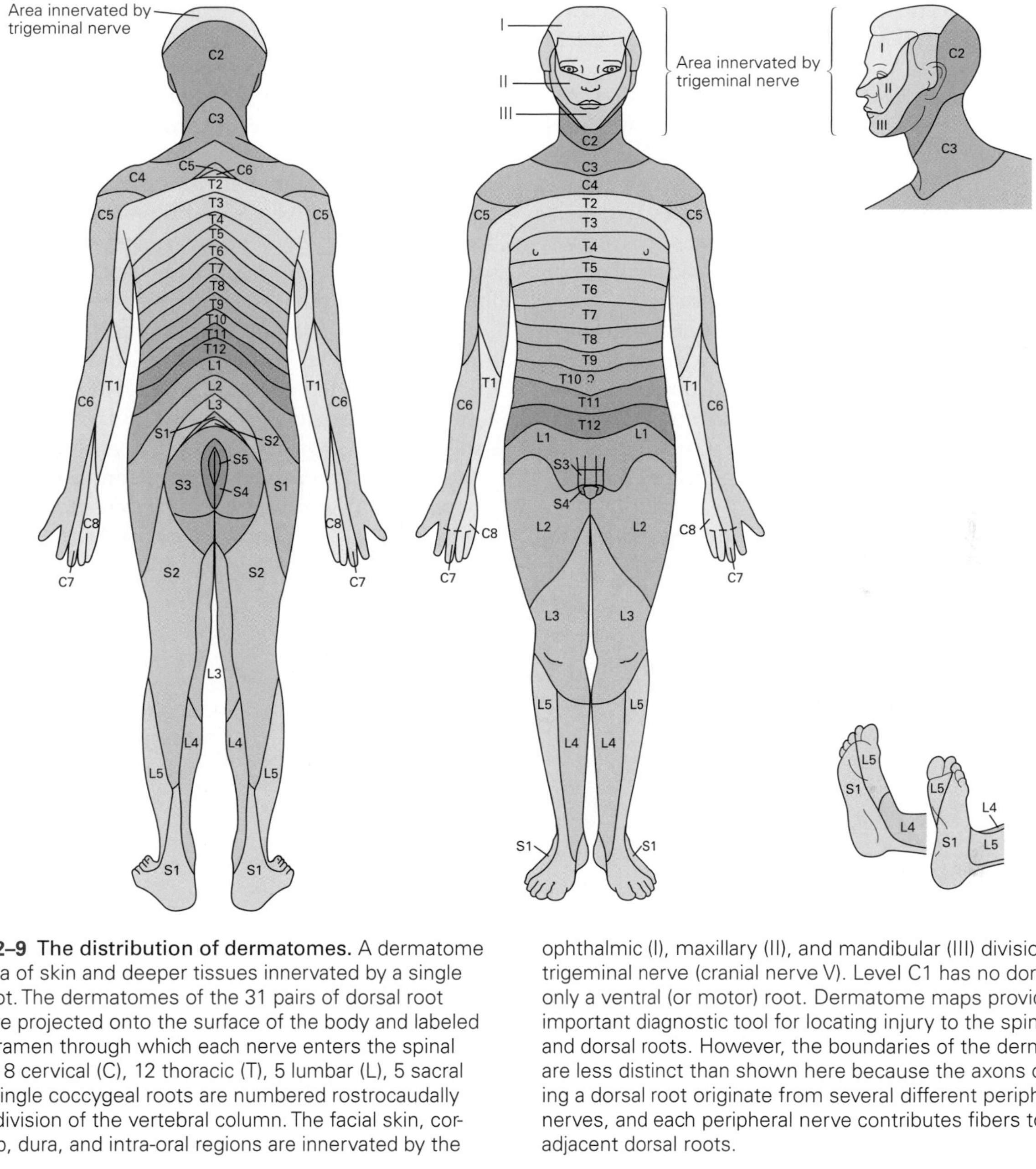

Figure 22–9 The distribution of dermatomes. A dermatome is the area of skin and deeper tissues innervated by a single dorsal root. The dermatomes of the 31 pairs of dorsal root nerves are projected onto the surface of the body and labeled by the foramen through which each nerve enters the spinal cord. The 8 cervical (C), 12 thoracic (T), 5 lumbar (L), 5 sacral (S), and single coccygeal roots are numbered rostrocaudally for each division of the vertebral column. The facial skin, cornea, scalp, dura, and intra-oral regions are innervated by the ophthalmic (I), maxillary (II), and mandibular (III) divisions of the trigeminal nerve (cranial nerve V). Level C1 has no dorsal root, only a ventral (or motor) root. Dermatome maps provide an important diagnostic tool for locating injury to the spinal cord and dorsal roots. However, the boundaries of the dermatomes are less distinct than shown here because the axons comprising a dorsal root originate from several different peripheral nerves, and each peripheral nerve contributes fibers to several adjacent dorsal roots.

The medial division includes large, myelinated $A\alpha$ and $A\beta$ fibers that transmit proprioceptive and cutaneous information from a dermatome. The lateral division includes small thinly myelinated $A\delta$ and unmyelinated C fibers that transmit noxious, thermal, and visceral information from the same dermatome. After entering the spinal cord the afferent fibers become further segregated according to modality and terminate on different functional sets of neurons in the gray matter of the same or adjacent spinal segments. In addition, the $A\alpha$ and $A\beta$ fibers send a major branch to the medulla through the dorsal columns.

The gray matter in each spinal segment is divided into three functionally distinct regions: the dorsal and ventral horns and an intermediate zone. As a general rule the largest fibers ($A\alpha$) terminate in or near the ventral horn, the medium-size fibers ($A\beta$) from the skin and muscle terminate in intermediate layers of the dorsal horn, and the smallest fibers (Aδ and C) terminate in the most dorsal portion of the spinal gray matter.

The spinal gray matter is further subdivided into 10 laminae (or layers), numbered I to X from dorsal to ventral, based on differences in cell and fiber composition. Lamina I consists of a thin layer of neurons capping the dorsal horn of the spinal cord and pars caudalis of the spinal trigeminal nucleus. Individual neurons of lamina I receive monosynaptic inputs from small myelinated fibers (Aδ) or unmyelinated C fibers of a single type (Figure 22–10) and therefore transmit information about noxious, thermal, or visceral stimuli. Inputs from warm, cold, itch, and pain receptors have been identified in lamina I, and some neurons have unique cellular morphologies. Lamina I neurons generally have small receptive fields localized to one dermatome.

Neurons in laminae II and III are interneurons that receive inputs from Aδ and C fibers, and make excitatory or inhibitory connections to neurons in lamina I, IV, and V that project to higher brain centers. The dendrites of neurons in laminae III to V are the main targets of the large myelinated sensory (Aβ) fibers from cutaneous mechanoreceptors (Figure 22–10). Neurons in lamina V typically respond to more than one modality—low-threshold mechanical stimuli, visceral stimuli, or noxious stimuli—and have therefore been named *wide-dynamic-range neurons*.

Visceral C fibers have widespread projections in the spinal cord that terminate ipsilaterally in laminae I, II, V, and X; some also cross the midline and terminate in lamina V and X of the contralateral gray matter. The extensive spinal distribution of visceral C fibers appears to be responsible for the poor localization of visceral pain sensations. Afferents from the pelvic viscera make important connections to cells in the central gray matter (lamina X) of spinal segments L5 and S1. Lamina X neurons in turn project their axons along the midline of the dorsal columns to

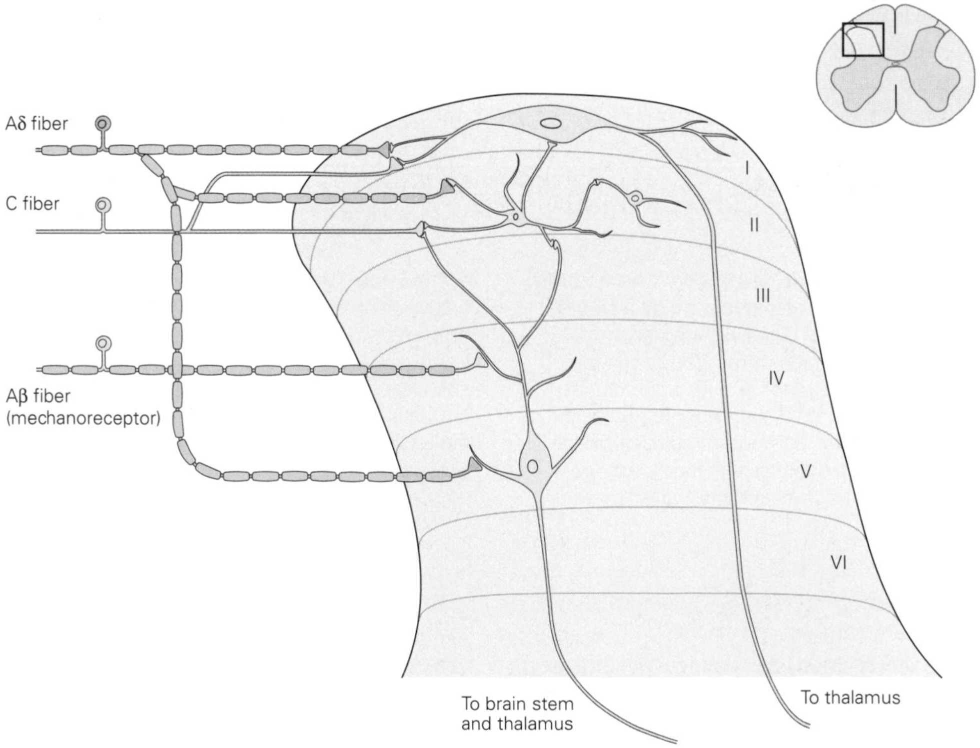

Figure 22–10 The spinal gray matter in the dorsal horn and intermediate zone is divided into six layers of cells (laminae I–VI) each with functionally distinct populations of neurons. The axons of neurons in laminae I and V make up the majority of fibers in the spinothalamic tract (see Figure 22–11). Neurons in lamina I receive nociceptive or thermal inputs from receptors innervated by Aδ or C fibers, and from interneurons in lamina II; their axons are the fastest conducting fibers in the spinothalamic tract. Neurons in lamina V respond to nociceptive and tactile information because they receive inputs from both Aβ and Aδ fibers as well as from interneurons in laminae II, III, and IV. (Adapted, with permission, from Fields 1987.)

the nucleus gracilis in a postsynaptic dorsal column pathway for visceral pain.

Primary afferent fibers that terminate in the deepest laminae in the ventral horn feed back information from proprioceptors that is required for somatic motor control, such as spinal reflexes (see Chapter 35).

Functional separation of sensory afferents is maintained in the pathways to higher centers in the brain. Somatosensory information is conveyed to the thalamus and cerebral cortex by two ascending pathways. The dorsal column–medial lemniscal system transmits tactile and proprioceptive information, and the spinothalamic tract pain and thermal information. A third pathway, the dorsolateral tract, conveys somatosensory information from the lower half of the body to the cerebellum.

The Dorsal Column–Medial Lemniscal System Relays Tactile and Proprioceptive Information

The dorsal column on each side contains the central branches of Aα and Aβ afferents as they ascend to the medulla and thus form the major ascending pathway for tactile and proprioceptive information to the brain stem nuclei from which somatosensory information is conveyed to the cerebral cortex. They represent the most prominent anatomical feature of the dorsal funiculus of the spinal cord.

Each dorsal column is bounded medially by the median septum and laterally by the dorsal horn of the gray matter (Figure 22–11). Each contains about a million fibers as it enters the brain stem and terminates within the ipsilateral dorsal column nuclei. Of these fibers 90% are axons of dorsal root ganglion cells, and the remaining 10% are axons of spinal neurons. The postsynaptic dorsal column axons that course along the midline adjacent to the medial septum provide a specialized rapid pathway for visceral pain.

Fibers from the spinal nerves are added successively to the medial edge of the dorsal column, beginning with the fibers from the upper cervical segment and ending with the most caudal spinal nerve in the layer next to the midline. This lateral-to-medial arrangement reflects the fact that during development the most rostral spinal segments are formed earlier than the more caudal ones. In this way the dorsal column is arranged in layers, one for each dermatome. Because the dermatomes overlap extensively, adjacent layers do not convey a continuous somatotopic representation of the skin. However, when the fibers reach the brain stem they are sorted into a coherent map of the receptor sheet, with the anogenital skin of the ipsilateral side of the body most medial and the skin of the ipsilateral neck and head most lateral.

Caudal to T7 the dorsal column on each side is called the *gracile* (slender) *fascicle*. At about T7 a sulcus appears, and the remaining spinal nerves contribute to a second column called the *cuneate* (wedge-shaped) *fascicle*. The division between gracile and cuneate fascicles is important only because they terminate in anatomically distinct nuclei in the caudal brain stem, the gracile and cuneate nuclei (Figure 22–11). Together with the external cuneate nucleus and other minor nuclei, they form the dorsal column nuclei.

The gracile and cuneate nuclei are shaped like sausages with a rostrocaudal orientation. Primary afferent fibers terminate on neurons throughout the rostrocaudal extent of each nucleus so that a rod-like collection of cells extending the length of the nucleus represents one small skin region, and the neurons in any cross section represent the entire body. The somatic representation in that neural map is of a headless homunculus lying on his back with his sacrum toward the midline and his hands and feet extended dorsally. Tactile and proprioceptive information from the head, face, and mouth is represented in the adjacent principal trigeminal nucleus.

Somatosensory submodalities are segregated in the dorsal column nuclei: Individual neurons receive synaptic inputs from afferents of a single type and neurons of distinct types are spatially separated. The rostral third of the dorsal column nuclei is dominated by neurons that process proprioceptive information; nearly 75% receive sensory information from muscle afferents. Tactile inputs predominate in the middle third where nearly 90% of the neurons process cutaneous information. The neurons in the caudal third are evenly divided between cutaneous and proprioceptive modalities.

There is also a dorsal-ventral gradient both in the dorsal columns and in the dorsal column nuclei; proprioceptive neurons are more common ventrally and cutaneous neurons more common dorsally. This division may simply reflect the fact that the hands and feet, which have dense cutaneous innervation but relatively little musculature, are represented dorsally, whereas the trunk and proximal limbs, with more muscle and less skin innervation, are represented ventrally.

Lateral and rostral to the cuneate nucleus proper is the external cuneate nucleus, which receives proprioceptive afferents from the arm and hand. The external cuneate nucleus projects to both the cerebellum and thalamus.

Axons of neurons in the dorsal column nuclei form the *medial lemniscus*, which crosses the midline in the medulla and is joined medially by the homologous projection from the trigeminal nuclei (Figure 22–11). In transit the somatotopic representation becomes inverted; within the thalamus the somatotopic map displays the head medially, the sacrum laterally, and the hands and feet ventrally. Because of the crossing of the fibers in the medial lemniscus, the left side of the brain receives somatosensory input from the mechanoreceptors on the right side of the body, and vice versa.

Cutaneous information from the dorsal column and trigeminal nuclei enters the lateral and medial ventral posterior nuclei of the thalamus, which form a single functional entity. Proprioceptive information enters the superior ventral posterior nucleus, which lies just above the other two (see Figure 16–5).

The Spinothalamic System Conveys Noxious, Thermal, and Visceral Information

The *spinothalamic tract* is the principal pathway transmitting noxious, thermal, and visceral information to the thalamus and cerebral cortex (Figure 22–11). It originates from neurons in laminae I, V, and VII, the main targets of the small-diameter fibers with sensory information destined for conscious perception. These neurons have distinctive physiological properties based on their sensory inputs.

More than 50% of spinal projections to the thalamus originate from neurons in lamina I, neurons that receive inputs from nociceptors, thermal receptors, visceral afferents, or itch receptors. Lamina I has the characteristics of a modality-segregated sensory relay nucleus for somatic and visceral information transmitted by small-diameter myelinated fibers (Aδ) or unmyelinated C fibers of a single type. The second major origin of fibers in the spinothalamic tract is wide-dynamic-range neurons in lamina V that respond to various combinations of tactile, visceral, thermal, and noxious stimuli.

It is reasonable to suppose, based on the neurophysiological responses of neurons in lamina I and V, that thermal sensations originate in fibers arising in lamina I whereas pain originates in fibers from either system. The pattern of sensation evoked by stimulation also reflects the projection patterns of spinothalamic tract neurons, for most but not all cross the midline to ascend in the contralateral tract (82% of the stimulus sites produced contralateral sensation, 12% ipsilateral, and 6% bilateral sensations).

The third major source of spinothalamic tract fibers is neurons in lamina VII and in deeper parts of the spinal gray matter. Lamina VII neurons receive inputs from large areas of the body, including the viscera, and therefore have very large receptive fields. This severely limits their ability to localize sensory stimuli. Further, they project to nuclei in the thalamus that are more involved in affective responses to stimuli than in identification and localization of stimuli.

The axons of most neurons in lamina I cross the midline, just ventral to the central canal, and ascend in the contralateral *lateral spinothalamic tract* located in the lateral funiculus. Axons of lamina V neurons cross the spinal cord and ascend in the contralateral *ventral spinothalamic tract*. They convey mixed information from visceroceptors, nociceptors, and low-threshold mechanoreceptors to the thalamus.

As in the medial lemniscus, fibers in the spinothalamic tract are arranged somatotopically. Fibers originating in the lumbar and sacral segments are located laterally, whereas those from the cervical spinal segments are positioned medially. The spinothalamic tract is joined by axons from the trigeminal nucleus caudalis.

As a result of the decussation of spinothalamic fibers in the spinal cord, noxious and thermal information from each dermatome is transmitted contralaterally in the anterolateral column, whereas touch and proprioception are transmitted ipsilaterally in the dorsal column. Unilateral injury to the spinal

Figure 22–11 (Opposite) Somatosensory information from the limbs and trunk is conveyed to the thalamus and cerebral cortex by two ascending pathways. Brain slices along the neuraxis from the spinal cord to the cerebrum illustrate the anatomy of the two principal pathways conveying somatosensory information to the cerebral cortex. The two pathways are separated until they reach the pons, where they are juxtaposed.

Dorsal column—medial lemniscal system. Tactile and limb proprioception signals are conveyed to the spinal cord and brain stem by large-diameter myelinated fibers and transmitted to the thalamus in this system. In the spinal cord the fibers for touch and proprioception divide, one branch going to the spinal gray matter and the other ascending in the ipsilateral dorsal column to the medulla. The second-order fibers from the dorsal column nuclei cross the midline in the medulla and ascend in the medial lemniscus toward the thalamus, where they terminate in the lateral and medial ventral posterior nuclei. These nuclei convey tactile and proprioceptive information to the primary somatic sensory cortex.

Anterolateral system. Pain, itch, temperature, and visceral information is conveyed to the spinal cord by small-diameter myelinated and unmyelinated fibers that terminate in the dorsal horn. This information is conveyed across the midline within the spinal cord and transmitted to the brain stem and the thalamus in the contralateral anterolateral system. Anterolateral fibers terminating in the brain stem comprise the spinoreticular and spinomesencephalic tracts; the remaining anterolateral fibers form the spinothalamic tract.

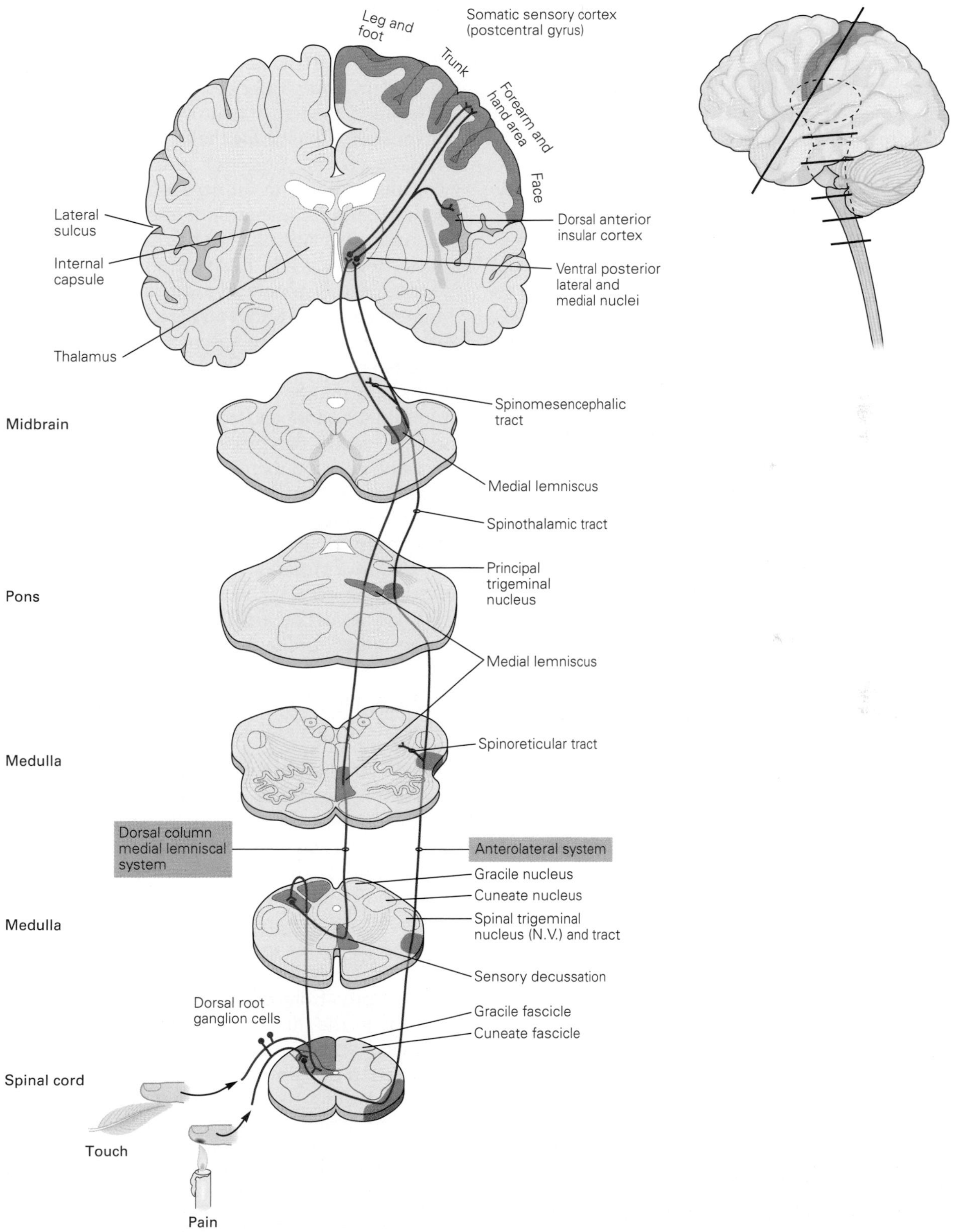

Leg and foot
Somatic sensory cortex (postcentral gyrus)
Trunk
Forearm and hand area
Face
Lateral sulcus
Internal capsule
Thalamus
Dorsal anterior insular cortex
Ventral posterior lateral and medial nuclei
Midbrain
Spinomesencephalic tract
Medial lemniscus
Spinothalamic tract
Pons
Principal trigeminal nucleus
Medial lemniscus
Medulla
Spinoreticular tract
Dorsal column medial lemniscal system
Anterolateral system
Gracile nucleus
Cuneate nucleus
Spinal trigeminal nucleus (N.V.) and tract
Medulla
Sensory decussation
Dorsal root ganglion cells
Gracile fascicle
Cuneate fascicle
Spinal cord
Touch
Pain

cord may therefore produce deficits in tactile and proprioceptive sensations on the same side of the body as the lesion, and impairments in thermal or painful sensations on the side opposite the lesion. The somatosensory submodalities of touch, proprioception, temperature, and pain are reunited on the contralateral side of the neuraxis higher in the brain stem as the medial lemniscus and spinothalamic tract approach the thalamus (Figure 22–11).

Information carried by small-diameter sensory fibers may also reach the cerebral cortex through several polysynaptic routes other than the spinothalamic tract. These paths include the spinomesencephalic, spinoreticular, and spinolimbic tracts that project to brain stem nuclei such as the parabrachial nucleus (Figure 22–11). These brain stem nuclei in turn project to the thalamus and to other sites that may have a sensory role, such as the hypothalamus and amygdala. Although many of these pathways originate from neurons in lamina I and V, and have physiological properties similar to spinothalamic tract neurons, they arise from a different group of neurons. Neurons that project to sites other than the thalamus may be involved in homeostasis and autonomic regulation.

Finally, as noted above, the most medial fibers in the dorsal column relay signals from nociceptors in the pelvic and abdominal viscera. We know that the postsynaptic dorsal column pathway originates with cells in the central gray matter of the sacral and midthoracic spinal cord and terminates in the gracile nucleus. Morphine infusion at these loci in animals blocks transmission of visceral pain signals. This pathway is important clinically because midline myelotomy at T10 relieves pelvic cancer pain in patients with colorectal distension.

The Thalamus Has a Number of Specialized Somatosensory Regions

The thalamus is an egg-shaped cluster of nuclei in the center of the brain that acts as a center of communication between many subcortical brain centers and the neocortex. The locations of nuclei within the thalamus correspond roughly with the hemispheric locations of the regions of the cerebral cortex with which they communicate (see Figure 16–5).

The Ventral Posterior Nucleus Relays Tactile and Proprioceptive Information

The fibers of the medial lemniscus, which convey tactile and proprioceptive signals, terminate in the ventral posterior nucleus of the thalamus. The medial zone of the nucleus receives trigeminal nerve fibers from the head and face. The lateral zone receives fibers from the dorsal column nuclei; these inputs are arranged somatotopically, with the forelimb medial and the trunk and legs lateral. Individual body parts are represented by rod-shaped clusters of neurons aligned along the anterior-posterior axis of the thalamus.

The ventral posterior nucleus—called nucleus ventralis caudalis in humans—has traditionally been thought of as a single nucleus in which the fibers carrying cutaneous signals terminate in a large central and caudal region while those conveying proprioceptive information terminate in a dorsal and rostral region. More recently, Jon Kaas and his colleagues have argued that the two regions represent separate nuclei: the ventral posterior nucleus proper, which receives the cutaneous information conveyed by medial lemniscal and trigeminal axons, and the ventral posterior superior nucleus, which processes proprioceptive information. These nuclei send their outputs to different subregions of the cerebral cortex. The ventral posterior nucleus transmits cutaneous information primarily to area 3b of the primary somatosensory cortex, whereas the ventral posterior superior nucleus conveys proprioceptive information principally to area 3a in the postcentral gyrus. (The cortical areas for touch and proprioception are described in Chapter 23.)

Noxious, Thermal, and Visceral Information Is Processed in Several Thalamic Nuclei

The information for pain, temperature, itch, and the visceral senses takes a more complex path through the thalamus. Because virtually all of the research on this subject is concerned with the pathways for pain (see Chapter 24), inferences about the pathways for the other bodily senses relayed by the laminae I and V systems are tentative and controversial.

The axons of neurons in lamina V terminate in the ventral posterior nucleus and overlap some of the tactile inputs from the same body region. Nociceptive neurons in the nucleus project primarily to area 3a in the postcentral gyrus and are thought to play a role in localization of painful sensations.

The lamina I system terminates heavily in a concentrated region of thalamus rich in neurons that are immunoreactive to calbindin, a calcium-binding protein found in some cortical and thalamic neurons. This region spans the posterior part of the ventral posterior nucleus and the posterior part of the adjacent ventral medial nucleus. The gustatory and visceral inputs from the nucleus of the solitary tract, which terminate in the parabrachial nuclei, also are arrayed topographically in the ventral medial nucleus.

Neurons in the ventral medial nucleus project to the insula, where they terminate in a topographic array. Functional imaging studies show that this region is a primary cortical region for thermal sensations. Because the insula also responds to visceral inputs arising from the spinal nucleus and nucleus of the solitary tract, it is sometimes called the interoceptive or visceral cortex.

An Overall View

The bodily senses mediate a wide range of experiences that are important for normal bodily function and for survival. Although diverse, they share common pathways and common principles of organization. The most important of those principles is specificity: Each of the bodily senses arises from a specific type of receptor distributed throughout the body.

Mechanoreceptors are sensitive to specific aspects of local tissue distortion, thermoreceptors to particular temperature ranges and shifts in temperature, and chemoreceptors to particular molecular structures.

The information from each type of somatosensory receptor is conveyed in discrete pathways that constitute submodalities. Information from all of the somatosensory submodalities is carried to the spinal cord or brain stem by the axons of neurons with cell bodies that generally lie in ganglia close to the point of entry. The axons are gathered together in nerves, which form the peripheral nervous system. Axon diameter and myelination, both of which determine the speed of action potential conduction, vary in different sensory pathways according to the need for speedy information.

When the axons enter the central nervous system they separate to form five separate sensory pathways with different properties. In three of those systems (the medial lemniscal, lamina I spinothalamic, and solitary tract systems) the pathways for submodalities appear to be segregated until they reach the cerebral cortex.

The medial lemniscal system includes the large myelinated axons and is organized for high-fidelity temporal and spatial information processing. Fibers from lamina I and the nucleus of the solitary tract convey information about temperature and impending and actual tissue damage, and a wide range of visceral stimuli from the small myelinated and unmyelinated axons. The lamina V spinothalamic system combines information from different submodalities at the first synapse in the pathway; the responses of neurons in lamina V correlate closely with reports of pain intensity. The lamina VII spinothalamic system gathers information from widespread parts of the body and apparently plays a significant role in emotional responses to sensory stimuli. These afferent systems terminate in different regions of the thalamus with different functions and different cortical targets.

As described in the next few chapters, afferent nerves conveying specific somatosensory submodalities remain segregated as they reach the cerebral cortex. Information carried by large-diameter axons is conveyed to the postcentral gyrus of the neocortex and then to cortical regions concerned with motor control and cognition. Information that originated in the small-diameter axons travels to the primary somatosensory cortex but also to cortical regions concerned with autonomic functions and the emotions, such as the insula and anterior cingulate cortex.

Esther P. Gardner
Kenneth O. Johnson

Selected Readings

Christensen AP, Corey DP. 2007. TRP channels in mechanosensation: direct or indirect activation? Nat Rev Neurosci 8:510–521.

Craig AD. 2003. Pain mechanisms: labeled lines versus convergence in central processing. Annu Rev Neurosci 26:1–30.

Dhaka A, Viswanath V, Patapoutian A. 2006. TRP ion channels and temperature sensation. Annu Rev Neurosci 29:135–161.

Iggo A, Andres KH. 1982. Morphology of cutaneous receptors. Annu Rev Neurosci 5:1–31.

Johnson KO. 2001. The roles and functions of cutaneous mechanoreceptors. Curr Opin Neurobiol 11:455–461.

Jones EG. 2007. *The Thalamus*. Cambridge: Cambridge Univ. Press.

Julius D, Basbaum AI. 2001. Molecular mechanisms of nociception. Nature 413:203–210.

Kaas JH, Gardner EP (eds). 2008. *The Senses: A Comprehensive Reference*, Vol. 6, *Somatosensation*. Oxford: Elsevier.

Lumpkin EA, Caterina MJ. 2007. Mechanisms of sensory transduction in the skin. Nature 445:858–865.

Mano T, Iwase S, Toma S. 2006. Microneurography as a tool in clinical neurophysiology to investigate peripheral neural traffic in humans. Clin Neurophysiol 117:2357–2384.

Matthews PBC. 1972. *Mammalian Muscle Receptors and Their Central Actions*. Baltimore: Williams and Wilkins.

Vallbo ÅB, Hagbarth KE, Torebjörk HE, Wallin BG. 1979. Somatosensory, proprioceptive, and sympathetic activity in human peripheral nerves. Physiol Rev 59:919–957.

Vallbo ÅB, Hagbarth KE, Wallin BG. 2004. Microneurography: how the technique developed and its role in the investigation of the sympathetic nervous system. J Appl Physiol 96:1262–1269.

Willis WD. 2007. The somatosensory system, with emphasis on structures important for pain. Brain Res Rev 55:297–313.

Willis WD, Coggeshall RE. 2004. *Sensory Mechanisms of the Spinal Cord*, 3rd ed. New York: Kluwer Academic/Plenum.

References

Al-Chaer ED, Lawand NB, Westlund KN, Willis WD. 1996. Visceral nociceptive input into the ventral posterolateral nucleus of the thalamus: a new function for the dorsal column pathway. J Neurophysiol 76:2661–2674.

Applebaum AE, Beall JE, Foreman RD, Willis WD. 1975. Organization and receptive fields of primate spinothalamic tract neurons. J Neurophysiol 38:572–586.

Bandell M, Macpherson LJ, Patapoutian A. 2007. From chills to chilis: mechanisms for thermosensation and chemesthesis via thermoTRPs. Curr Opin Neurobiol 17: 490–497.

Boyd IA, Davey MR. 1968. *Composition of Peripheral Nerves*. Edinburgh: Livingston.

Chung JM, Surmeier DJ, Lee KH, Sorkin LS, Honda CN, Tsong Y, Willis WD. 1986. Classification of primate spinothalamic and somatosensory thalamic neurons based on cluster analysis. J Neurophysiol 56:308–327.

Collins DF, Refshauge KM, Todd G, Gandevia SC. 2005. Cutaneous receptors contribute to kinesthesia at the index finger, elbow, and knee. J Neurophysiol 94:1699–7106.

Craig AD. 2002. How do you feel? Interoception: the sense of the physiological condition of the body. Nat Rev Neurosci 3:655–666.

Craig AD. 2004. Lamina I, but not lamina V, spinothalamic neurons exhibit responses that correspond with burning pain. J Neurophysiol 92:2604–2609.

Darian-Smith I, Johnson KO, Dykes R. 1973. "Cold" fiber population innervating palmar and digital skin of the monkey: responses to cooling pulses. J Neurophysiol 36:325–346.

Darian-Smith I, Johnson KO, LaMotte C, Shigenaga Y, Kenins P, Champness P. 1979. Warm fibers innervating palmar and digital skin of the monkey: responses to thermal stimuli. J Neurophysiol 42:1297–1315.

Dhaka A, Viswanath V, Patapoutian A. 2006. TRP ion channels and temperature sensation. Annu Rev Neurosci 29:135–161.

Edin BB, Vallbo AB. 1990. Dynamic response of human muscle spindle afferents to stretch. J Neurophysiol 63:1297–1306.

Erlanger J, Gasser HS. 1938. *Electrical Signs and Nervous Activity*. Philadelphia: Univ. of Pennsylvania Press.

Fields HL. 1987. *Pain*. New York: McGraw-Hill.

Gandevia SC, McCloskey DI, Burke D. 1992. Kinaesthetic signals and muscle contraction. Trends Neurosci 15:62–65.

Gandevia SC, Smith JL, Crawford M, Proske U, Taylor JL. 2006. Motor commands contribute to human position sense. J Physiol 571:703–710.

Han ZS, Zhang ET, Craig AD. 1998. Nociceptive and thermoreceptive lamina I neurons are anatomically distinct. Nat Neurosci 1:218–225.

Hensel H. 1973. Cutaneous thermoreceptors. In: A Iggo (ed). *Handbook of Sensory Physiology*, Vol. 2 *Somatosensory System*, pp. 79–110. Berlin: Springer.

Hodge CJ Jr, Apkarian AV. 1990. The spinothalamic tract. Crit Rev Neurobiol 5:363–397.

Iggo A. 1960. Cutaneous mechanoreceptors with afferent C fibres. J Physiol (Lond) 152:337–353.

Johanek LM, Meyer RA, Hartke T, Hobelmann JG, Maine DN, LaMotte RH, Ringkamp M. 2007. Psychophysical and physiological evidence for parallel afferent pathways mediating the sensation of itch. J Neurosci 27:7490–7497.

Johansson RS, Vallbo ÅB. 1983. Tactile sensory coding in the glabrous skin of the human hand. Trends Neurosci 6:27–32.

Johansson RS, Vallbo ÅB, Westling G. 1980. Thresholds of mechanosensitive afferents in the human hand as measured with von Frey hairs. Brain Res 184:343–351.

Johnson KO, Hsiao SS. 1992. Neural mechanisms of tactual form and texture perception. Annu Rev Neurosci 15: 227–250.

Jordt S-E, McKemy DD, Julius D. 2003. Lessons from peppers and peppermint: the molecular logic of thermosensation. Curr Opin Neurobiol 13:487–492.

Kaas JH. 2008. The somatosensory thalamus and associated pathways. In: JH Kaas, EP Gardner (eds). *The Senses: A Comprehensive Reference*, Vol. 6 *Somatosensation*, pp. 117–141. Oxford: Elsevier.

Light AR, Perl ER. 1979. Spinal termination of functionally identified primary afferent neurons with slowly conducting myelinated fibers. J Comp Neurol 186:133–150.

Light AR, Trevino DL, Perl ER. 1979. Morphological features of functionally defined neurons in the marginal zone and substantia gelatinosa of the spinal dorsal horn. J Comp Neurol 186:151–171.

Lin S-Y, Corey DP. 2005. TRP channels in mechanosensation. Curr Opin Neurobiol 15:350–357.

Macefield VG. 2005. Physiological characteristics of low-threshold mechanoreceptors in joints, muscle and skin in human subjects. Clin Exp Pharmacol Physiol 32:135–144.

Macefield G, Gandevia SC, Burke D. 1990. Perceptual responses to microstimulation of single afferents innervating joints, muscles and skin of the human hand. J Physiol 429:113–129.

Ochoa J, Torebjörk E. 1989. Sensations evoked by intraneural microstimulation of C nociceptor fibres in human skin nerves. J Physiol 415:583–599.

Ottoson D, Shepherd GM. 1971. Transducer properties and integrative mechanisms in the frog's muscle spindle. In: WR Lowenstein (ed). *Handbook of Sensory Physiology*, Vol. 1 *Principles of Receptor Physiology*, pp. 442–499. Berlin: Springer-Verlag.

Perl ER. 1968. Myelinated afferent fibers innervating the primate skin and their response to noxious stimuli. J Physiol (Lond) 197:593–615.

Perl ER. 1996. Cutaneous polymodal receptors: characteristics and plasticity. Prog Brain Res 113:21–37.

Proske U. 2005. What is the role of muscle receptors in proprioception? Muscle Nerve 31:780–787.

Ralston HJ. 2005. Pain and the primate thalamus. Prog Brain Res 149:1–10.

Refshauge KM, Kilbreath SL, Gandevia SC. 1998. Movement detection at the distal joint of the human thumb and fingers. Exp Brain Res 122:85–92.

Sachs F. 1990. Stretch-sensitive ion channels. Sem Neurosci 2:49–57.

Simone DA, Zhang X, Li J, Zhang JM, Honda CN, LaMotte RH, Giesler GJ Jr. 2004. Comparison of responses of primate spinothalamic tract neurons to pruritic and algogenic stimuli. J Neurophysiol 91:213–222.

Sugiura Y, Terui N, Hosoya Y. 1989. Difference in distribution of central terminals between visceral and somatic unmyelinated (C) primary afferent fibers. J Neurophysiol 62:834–840.

Torebjörk HE, Vallbo ÅB, Ochoa JL. 1987. Intraneural microstimulation in man. Its relation to specificity of tactile sensations. Brain 110:1509–1529.

Vallbo ÅB, Olausson H, Wessberg J, Kakuda N. 1995. Receptive field characteristics of tactile units with myelinated afferents in hairy skin of human subjects. J Physiol 483:783–795.

Vallbo ÅB, Olsson KA, Westberg KG, Clark FJ. 1984. Microstimulation of single tactile afferents from the human hand. Sensory attributes related to unit type and properties of receptive fields. Brain 107:727–749.

Wessberg J, Olausson H, Fernström KW, Vallbo ÅB. 2003. Receptive field properties of unmyelinated tactile afferents in the human skin. J Neurophysiol 89:1567–1575.

Wessberg J, Vallbo ÅB. 1995. Human muscle spindle afferent activity in relation to visual control in precision finger movements. J Physiol 482:225–233.

Willis WD, Al-Chaer ED, Quast MJ, Westlund KN. 1999. A visceral pain pathway in the dorsal column of the spinal cord. Proc Natl Acad Sci U S A 96:7675–7679.

Willis WD, Westlund KN. 1997. Neuroanatomy of the pain system and of the pathways that modulate pain. J Clin Neurophysiol 14:2–31.

23

Touch

In this chapter on the sense of touch, we focus on the hand because of its importance in the sensory appreciation of object properties and its role in skilled motor tasks. The hand is one of evolution's great creations. The fine manipulative capacity provided by our fingers is possible because of their fine sensory capacity; if we lose tactile sensation in our fingers we lose manual dexterity.

When we become skilled in the use of a tool, such as a scalpel or a pair of scissors, we feel conditions at the working surface of the tool as though our fingers were there because two groups of mechanoreceptors monitor the vibrations and forces produced by those distant conditions. When we scan our fingers across a surface we feel its form and texture because another group of mechanoreceptors has high spatial and temporal acuity. A blind person uses this capacity to read Braille at a hundred words per minute. When we grip and manipulate an object we do so delicately, with only as much force as is required, because yet another group of mechanoreceptors continually monitors slip and adjusts our grip appropriately.

We are also able to recognize objects placed in the hand from touch alone. When we are handed a baseball we recognize it instantly without having to look at it because of its shape, size, weight, density, and texture. We do not have to think about the information provided by each finger to deduce that the object must be a baseball; the information flows to memory and instantly matches previously stored representations of baseballs. Even if we have never previously handled a baseball, we perceive it as a single object, not as a collection of discrete features. The somatosensory pathways of the brain have the daunting task of integrating information from thousands of sensors in each hand and transforming it to a form suitable for cognition.

Sensory information is extracted for the purpose of motor control as well as cognition, and different kinds of information are extracted for those purposes. We can, for example, shift our attention from the baseball's shape to its location in the hand to readjust our grip for an effective throw. This selective attention to different aspects of the sensory information is brought about by cortical mechanisms.

Active and Passive Touch Evoke Similar Responses in Mechanoreceptors

Touch is defined as direct contact between two physical bodies. In neuroscience touch refers to the special sense by which contact with the body is perceived consciously. Touch can be active, as when you move your hand or some other part of the body against another surface, or passive, as when someone or something else touches you.

Active and passive modes of tactile stimulation excite the same population of receptors in the skin and evoke similar responses in afferent fibers. They differ somewhat in cognitive features that reflect attention and behavioral goals during the period of stimulation. Passive touch is used for naming objects or describing sensations; active touch is used when the hand manipulates objects. The sensory and motor components of touch are intimately connected anatomically in the brain and are important functionally in guiding motor behavior.

The distinction between active and passive touch is important clinically when patients have deficits in hand use. Motor deficits such as weakness, stiffness, or clumsiness may result from sensory loss, which is why passive sensory testing is important in the neurological examination (see Appendix B). Common neurological tests for touch include measurements of detection thresholds, vibration sense, two-point or texture discrimination, and the ability to recognize form through touch (stereognosis). The neural mechanisms underlying these tests are discussed in this chapter. Other common tests of somatosensory function—tendon reflexes, pinprick, and thermal tests—are discussed in other chapters.

Nearly all of these neurological tests involve passive touch; the clinician stimulates the body in a controlled and reproducible fashion. The tests measure the sensitivity and function of various receptors for touch. Deviations from the expected values may help diagnose the sensory deficits or lesions that underlie sensory dysfunction.

The Hand Has Four Types of Mechanoreceptors

The softness and compliance of the skin plays a major role in the sense of touch. When an object contacts the hand, the skin conforms to its contours, forming a mirror image of the object surface. The resultant displacement and indentation of the skin stretches the tissue, thereby stimulating the sensory endings of mechanoreceptors at or near the region of contact.

These receptors are highly sensitive and are continually active as we manipulate objects and explore the world with our hands. They provide information to the brain about the position of the stimulus on the skin, its shape and surface texture, the amount of force applied at the contact point, and how these features change over time when the hand or the object moves.

Tactile sensations in the human hand arise from four kinds of mechanoreceptors: Meissner corpuscles, Merkel cells, Pacinian corpuscles, and Ruffini endings (Figure 23–1). The sense of touch can be understood as the combined result of the information provided by these four systems acting in concert.

Each receptor responds in a distinctive manner depending on its morphology, innervation pattern, and depth in the skin. Receptors are innervated by either slowly adapting or rapidly adapting axons. Slowly adapting (SA) fibers respond to steady skin indentation with a sustained discharge, whereas rapidly adapting (RA) fibers stop firing as soon as the indentation is stationary. Sustained mechanical sensations from the hand must accordingly arise from the SA fibers. The sensation of motion across the skin is signaled by RA fibers. The receptors are further subdivided into two types based on size and location in the skin; each type includes both rapidly and slowly adapting fibers.

Thus tactile sensation in the hand is mediated by four functional units: rapidly adapting type 1 (RA1), slowly adapting type 1 (SA1), rapidly adapting type 2 (RA2), and slowly adapting type 2 (SA2). Each unit consists of an afferent fiber, the fiber's distal branches, and the receptor organ(s) that surround the axon terminals (Table 23–1).

Type 1 fibers terminate in clusters of small receptors in the superficial layers of the skin at the margin between the dermis and epidermis (Figure 23–1). RA1 fibers are the most numerous tactile afferents in the hand, reaching a density of approximately 2 per mm^2 at the fingertip in man and monkey. The RA1 receptor organ, the Meissner corpuscle, is a globular, fluid-filled structure that encloses a set of flattened, lamellar cells

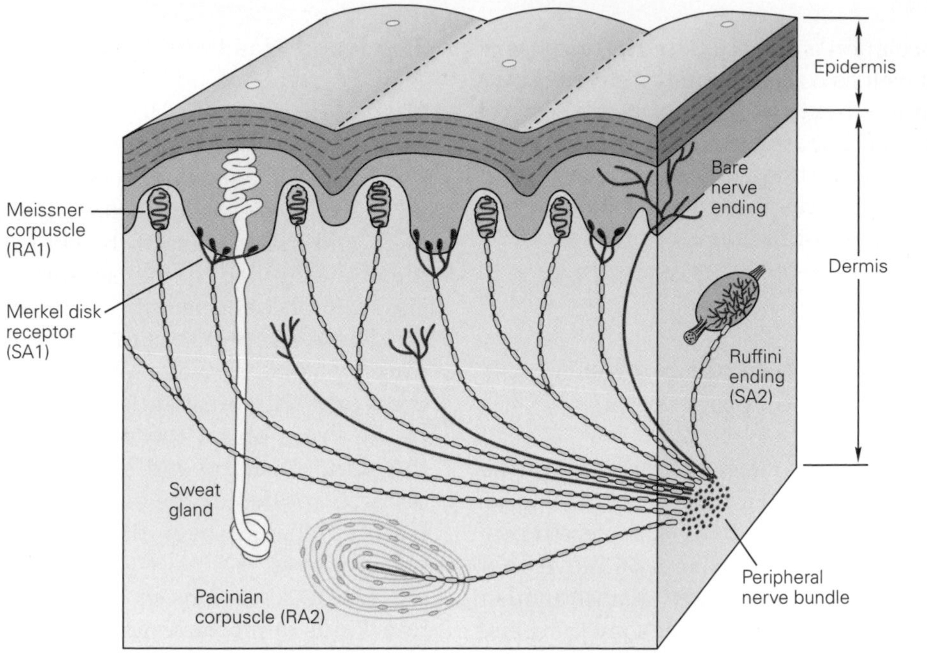

Figure 23–1 Four mechanoreceptors are responsible for the sense of touch. A cross section of the glabrous skin shows the principal receptors for touch. All of these receptors are innervated by large-diameter myelinated fibers. The Meissner corpuscles and Merkel cells lie in the superficial layers of the skin at the base of the epidermis, 0.5 to 1.0 mm below the skin surface. The Meissner corpuscles border the edges of each papillary ridge, whereas the Merkel cells form dense bands surrounding the sweat gland ducts along the center of the ridges. The RA1 and SA1 fibers that innervate these receptors branch at their terminals so that each fiber innervates several nearby receptor organs. The Pacinian and Ruffini corpuscles lie within the dermis (2–3 mm thick) and deeper tissues. The RA2 and SA2 fibers that innervate these receptors each innervate only one receptor organ. (**RA1**, rapidly adapting type 1; **RA2**, rapidly adapting type 2; **SA1**, slowly adapting type 1; **SA2**, slowly adapting type 2.)

Table 23–1 Cutaneous Mechanoreceptor Systems

	Type 1		Type 2	
	SA1	**RA1**[1]	**SA2**	**RA2**[2]
Receptor	Merkel cell	Meissner corpuscle	Ruffini ending	Pacinian corpuscle
Location	Tip of epidermal sweat ridges	Dermal papillae (close to skin surface)	Dermis	Dermis (deep tissue)
Axon diameter (μm)	7–11	6–12	6–12	6–12
Conduction velocity (ms)	40–65	35–70	35–70	35–70
Best stimulus	Edges, points	Lateral motion	Skin stretch	Vibration
Response to sustained indentation	Sustained with slow adaptation	None	Sustained with slow adaptation	None
Frequency range (Hz)	0–100	1–300		5–1,000
Best frequency (Hz)	5	50		200
Threshold for rapid indentation or vibration (best) (μm)	8	2	40	0.01

[1]Also called RA, QA, or FA1.
[2]Also called PC or FA2.
RA1, rapidly adapting type 1; **RA2**, rapidly adapting type 2; **SA1**, slowly adapting type 1; **SA2**, slowly adapting type 2.

originating from the myelin sheath (see Figure 21–6). The lamellae are coupled mechanically to the edge of the papillary ridge by collagen fibers, a relationship that confers fine mechanical sensitivity to frictional forces as the hand is moved across surfaces (Box 23–1). An RA1 axon typically innervates 10 to 20 Meissner corpuscles, integrating information from several adjacent papillary ridges. Each Meissner corpuscle is innervated by 2 to 5 RA1 axons (Figure 23–3A).

SA1 fibers are also widely distributed in the skin, particularly in the fingertips. The SA1 receptor organs, the Merkel cells, consist of small epithelial cells that surround the terminal branches of an axon. Each Merkel cell encloses a semirigid structure that transmits compressive strain to the sensory nerve ending. Because there are synapse-like junctions between the Merkel cells and the SA1 axon terminals, it has been proposed that the mechanosensitive ion channels reside in the Merkel cells rather than in the nerve endings. Merkel cells are densely clustered in the center of each papillary ridge in glabrous skin (Figure 23–3A), placing them in an excellent position

Box 23–1 Fingerprint Structure Enhances Touch Sensitivity in the Hand

The histological structure of glabrous skin—the smooth, hairless skin of the palm and fingertips—plays a crucial role in the hand's sensitivity to touch. The fingerprints are formed by a regular array of parallel ridges in the epidermis, the papillary ridges (Figure 23–2).

Each ridge is bordered by epidermal folds—the limiting ridges—that are visible as thin lines on the fingers and palm border. The limiting ridges increase the stiffness and rigidity of the skin, protecting it from damage when contacting objects or when walking barefooted.

The fingerprints give the glabrous skin a corrugated, rough structure that increases friction, allowing us to grasp objects without slippage. Frictional forces are augmented further when these ridges contact the textured surfaces of objects. Smooth surfaces slide easily underneath the fingers and thus require greater grip force to maintain stability in the hand; the screw caps on bottles are often ridged to make them easy to turn. Frictional forces between the limiting ridges and objects also amplify surface features when we palpate them, allowing us to detect small irregularities such as the grain of wood.

The regular spacing of the papillary ridges—and the precise localization of specific receptors within this grid—allow us to repeatedly scan surfaces with back and forth hand movements while preserving a constant spatial alignment of adjacent surface features.

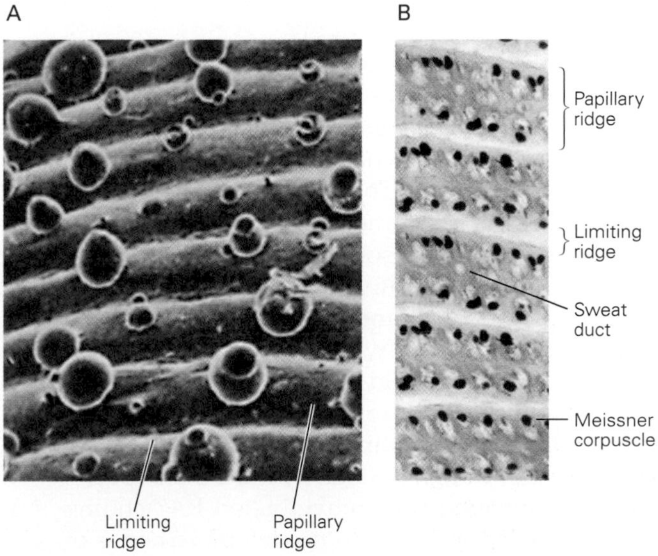

Figure 23–2 The skin of the finger.

A. Scanning electron micrograph of the fingerprints in the human index finger. The glabrous skin of the hand is structured as arrays of papillary ridges and intervening sulci (limiting ridges) that recur at regular intervals. Globules of sweat exude from ducts at the center of the papillary ridges, forming a grid-like pattern along each ridge. The Merkel cells are located in dense clusters along the center of the papillary ridges between the ducts (see Figure 23–1). (Adapted, with permission, from Quilliam 1978.)

B. Histological section of the glabrous skin cut parallel to the skin surface. The cholinesterase-stained Meissner corpuscles form regularly spaced chains along both sides of each papillary ridge. Thus Meissner corpuscles and Merkel cells form alternating bands of RA1 and slowly adapting type 1 (SA1) touch receptors that span each fingerprint ridge. (Adapted, with permission, from Bolanowski and Pawson 2003.)

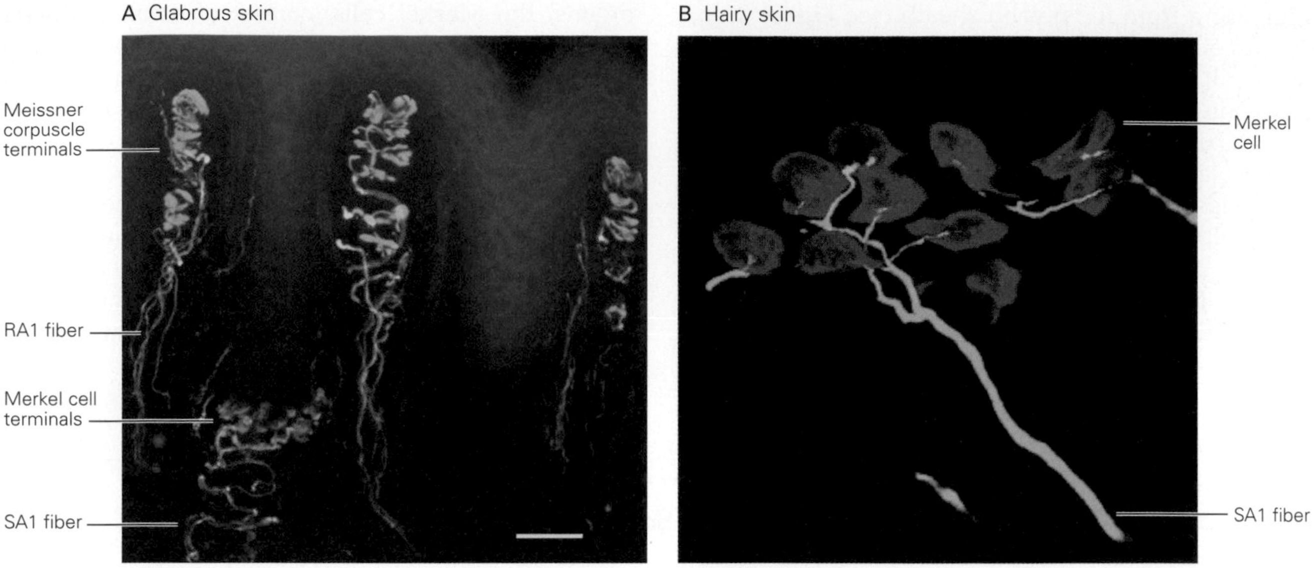

Figure 23–3 Innervation pattern of Meissner corpuscles and Merkel cells in hairy and glabrous skin.

A. A confocal transverse section of a papillary ridge in the human glabrous skin shows the innervation of mechanoreceptors in the fingertip. Meissner corpuscles are located just below the epidermis (**blue**) at the apex of the ridge, and are innervated by two or more rapidly adapting type 1 (RA1) fibers. The fibers lose their myelin sheaths (**orange**) when entering the receptor capsule, exposing broad terminal bulbs at which sensory transduction occurs (**green**). Individual slowly adapting type 1 (SA1) fibers innervate groups of Merkel cells clustered at the base of the intermediate ridge, providing localized signals of pressure applied to that ridge. Scale bar = 50 μm. (Adapted, with permission, from Nolano et al. 2003.)

B. A higher-magnification micrograph portrays antibody-labeled Merkel cells (**red**) innervated by an SA1 fiber (**green**). Each fiber extends multiple branches parallel to the surface of the skin that allow it to integrate tactile information from multiple receptor cells in a small zone of skin. The diameter of each Merkel cell is approximately 10 μm. (Adapted, with permission, from Snider 1998.)

to detect deformation of the overlying skin, either from pressure above or lateral stretch. In hairy skin Merkel cells are localized in small clusters called touch domes (Figure 23–3B).

Type 2 fibers innervate the skin sparsely and terminate in single large receptors in the deeper layers of the dermis or in the subcutaneous tissue (Figure 23–1). The receptors are larger and less numerous than the receptor organs of the type 1 fibers. The large size of these receptors allows them to sense mechanical displacement at some distance from the sensory nerve endings.

The RA2 fibers terminate in Pacinian corpuscles located in the subcutaneous tissue (Figure 23–1). Each RA2 axon terminates without branching in a single Pacinian corpuscle, and each Pacinian corpuscle receives but a single RA2 axon. Pacinian corpuscles are large onion-like structures in which successive layers of connective tissue are separated by fluid-filled spaces. These layers surround the unmyelinated RA2 ending and its myelinated axon up to one or more nodes of Ranvier. The capsule amplifies high-frequency vibration, a role that is important for tool use. Estimates of the number of Pacinian corpuscles in the human hand range from 2,400 in the young to 300 in the elderly.

The SA2 fibers innervate Ruffini endings concentrated at the finger and wrist joints and along the skin folds in the palm; they are relatively rare in the fingertips. The Ruffini endings are elongated fusiform structures that enclose collagen fibrils extending from the subcutaneous tissue to folds in the skin at the joints, in the palm, or in the fingernails. The SA2 nerve endings are intertwined between the collagen fibers in the capsule, and are excited by stimuli that stretch the receptor along its long axis.

Receptive Fields Define the Zone of Tactile Sensitivity

Individual mechanoreceptor fibers convey information from a limited area of skin called the receptive field. Tactile receptive fields have been determined in the human hand using microneurography.

Åke Vallbo and Roland Johansson inserted microelectrodes through the skin into the median or ulnar nerves in the human hand and recorded the responses of individual afferent fibers. They found that in humans, as in other primate species, there are important differences between touch receptors, both in their physiological responses and in the structure of their receptive fields.

Type 1 fibers have small, highly localized receptive fields with multiple spots of high sensitivity that reflect the branching patterns of their axons in the skin (Figure 23–4). Receptive fields on the fingertips are the smallest on the body, averaging 11 mm^2 for SA1 fibers and approximately 25 mm^2 for RA1 fibers. The fields are small because of the high density of receptors in the fingertips. Receptive fields become progressively larger on the proximal phalanges and the palm, consistent with the lower density of mechanoreceptors in these regions.

In contrast, type 2 fibers innervating the deep layers of skin are connected to only a single Pacinian corpuscle or Ruffini ending. Because these receptors are

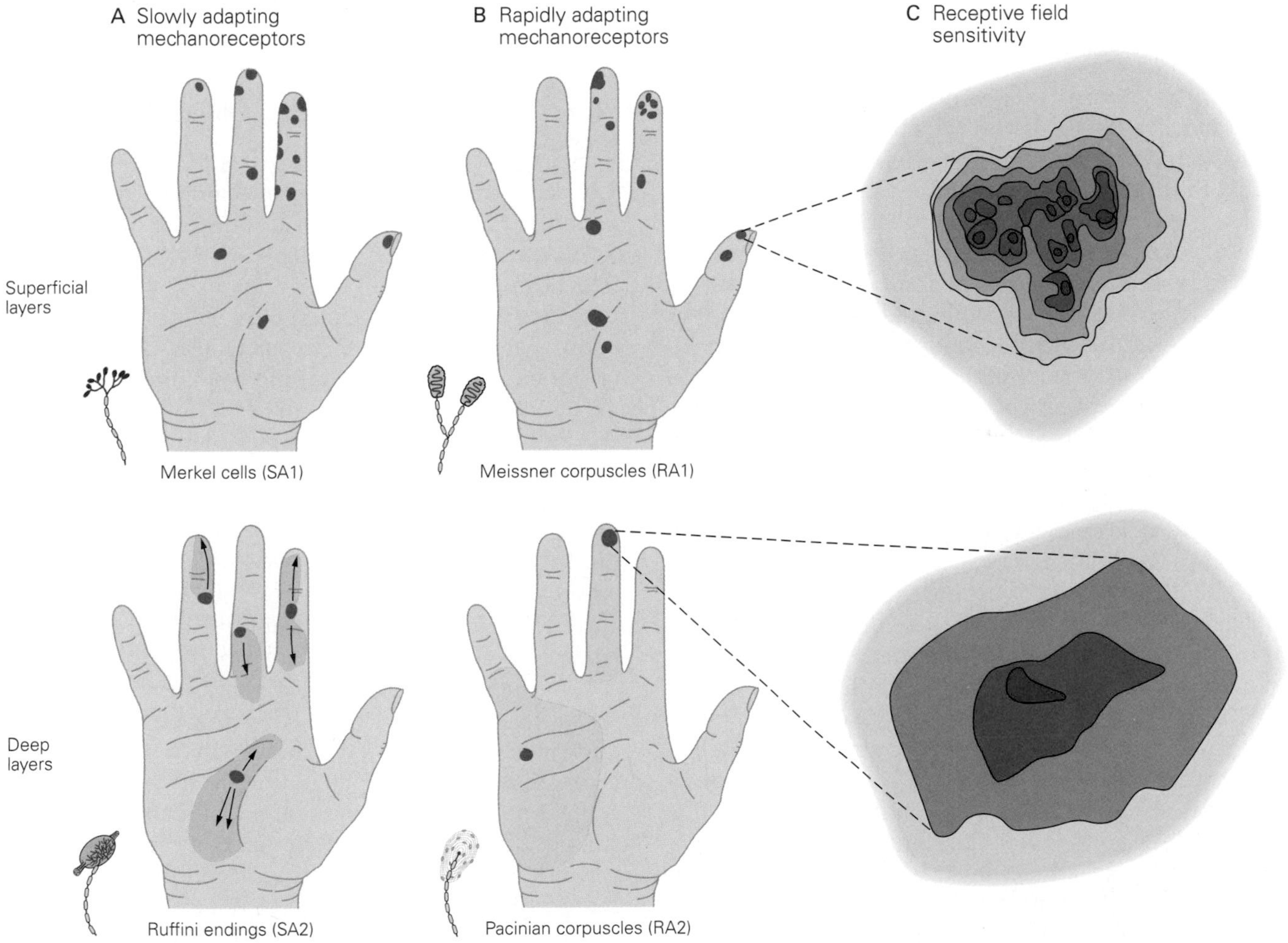

Figure 23–4 Receptive fields in the human hand are smallest at the fingertips. Each colored area on the hands indicates the receptive field of an individual sensory nerve fiber. (Adapted, with permission, from Johansson and Vallbo 1983.)

A–B. The receptive fields of receptors in the superficial layers of skin encompass spot-like patches of skin. Those of receptors in the deep layers extend across wide regions of skin (**light shading**), but responses are strongest in the skin directly over the receptor (**dark spots**). The arrows indicate the directions of skin stretch that activate SA2 fibers.

C. Pressure sensitivity throughout the receptive field is shown as a contour map. The most sensitive regions are indicated in red and the least sensitive areas in pale pink. The receptive field of an RA1 fiber (above) has many points of high sensitivity, marking the positions of the group of Meissner corpuscles innervated by the fiber. The receptive field of an RA2 fiber (below) has a single point of maximum sensitivity overlying the Pacinian corpuscle. The receptive field of SA1 fibers is similar to that of RA1 fibers. Likewise, the receptive field of SA2 fibers resembles that of RA2 fibers.

large they collect information from a broader area of skin. Their receptive fields contain a single "hot spot" where sensitivity to touch is greatest; this point is located directly above the receptor (Figure 23–4).

The receptive fields of type 1 fibers are significantly smaller than most objects that contact the hand. Thus RA1 and SA1 fibers detect small pieces of an object, signaling the properties of only a portion of its surface. As in the visual system, the spatial features of objects are distributed across a population of stimulated receptors with responses that are integrated in the brain to form a unified percept.

Two-Point Discrimination Tests Measure Texture Perception

The ability of humans to resolve spatial details of textured surfaces depends on which part of the body is contacted. Tactile acuity is highest on the fingertips and the lips, where receptive fields are smallest (Figure 23–5A). The separation that defines performance midway between chance and perfect discrimination, the threshold for spatial acuity, is approximately 1 mm on the fingertips of young adults; by the sixth or seventh decade of life it declines on average to approximately 2 mm. When we grasp an object we can discriminate features of its surface separated by as little as 0.5 mm. Humans are able to distinguish horizontal from vertical orientation of gratings with remarkably narrow spacing of the ridges (Figure 23–5B).

Tactile acuity is slightly greater in women than in men and varies between fingers but not between hands. The distal pad of the index finger has the keenest sensitivity; spatial acuity declines progressively from the index to the little finger and declines rapidly at locations proximal to the distal finger pads. Tactile spatial resolution is 50% poorer at the distal pad of the little finger and six to eight times coarser on the palm.

Tactile acuity on proximal parts of the body decreases in parallel with the growing size of receptive fields of SA1 and RA1 fibers (Figure 23–5A). When a pair of probes is spaced several millimeters apart on the hand, each of them is perceived as a distinct point because they produce separate dimples in the skin and stimulate nonoverlapping populations of SA1 and RA1 receptors. As the probes are moved closer together, the two sensations become blurred because both probes are contained within the same receptive field. The spatial interactions between tactile stimuli form the basis of neurological tests of two-point discrimination and texture recognition.

Blind individuals use the fine spatial sensitivity of SA1 and RA1 fibers to read Braille. The Braille alphabet represents letters as simple dot patterns that are easy to distinguish by touch (Figure 23–6). A blind person reads Braille by moving the fingers over the dot patterns. This hand movement enhances the sensations produced by the dots.

Because the Braille dots are spaced approximately 3 mm apart, a distance greater than the receptive field diameter of an SA1 fiber, each dot stimulates a different set of SA1 fibers. An SA1 fiber fires a burst of action potentials as a dot enters its receptive field and is silent once the dot leaves the field (Figure 23–6). Specific combinations of SA1 fibers that fire synchronously signal the spatial arrangement of the Braille dots. RA1 fibers also discriminate the dot patterns, enhancing the signals provided by SA1 fibers.

Slowly Adapting Fibers Detect Object Pressure and Form

The most important functional feature of the slowly adapting fibers (SA1 and SA2) is their ability to signal skin deformation and pressure. The sensitivity of an SA1 receptor to edges, corners, points, and curvature provides information about object shape, size, surface texture, and compliance. We perceive an object as hard or rigid if it indents the skin, and soft if the skin surface instead deforms the object.

Paradoxically, as an object's diameter increases, the responses of individual SA1 fibers become weaker and the sensation less distinct. For example, the tip of a pencil pressed 1 mm into the skin feels sharp, unpleasant, and highly localized at the contact point, whereas a 1 mm indentation by the eraser feels blunt and broad. The weakest sensation is evoked by a flat surface pressed against the finger pad (Figure 23–7).

To understand why these objects evoke different sensations, we need to consider the physical events that occur when the skin is touched. When a pencil tip is pressed against the skin it dimples the surface at the contact point and forms a shallow, sloped basin in the surrounding region (approximately 4 mm in radius). Although the indentation force is concentrated in the center, the surrounding region is also perturbed by local stretch, called tensile strain. SA1 receptors at both the center and the surrounding "hillsides" of skin are stimulated, firing spike trains proportional to the degree of local stretch.

If a second probe is pressed close to the first one, more SA1 fibers are stimulated but the neural response of each fiber is reduced because the force needed to displace the skin is shared between the two probes. Ken Johnson and his colleagues have shown that as more probes are added within the receptive field, the

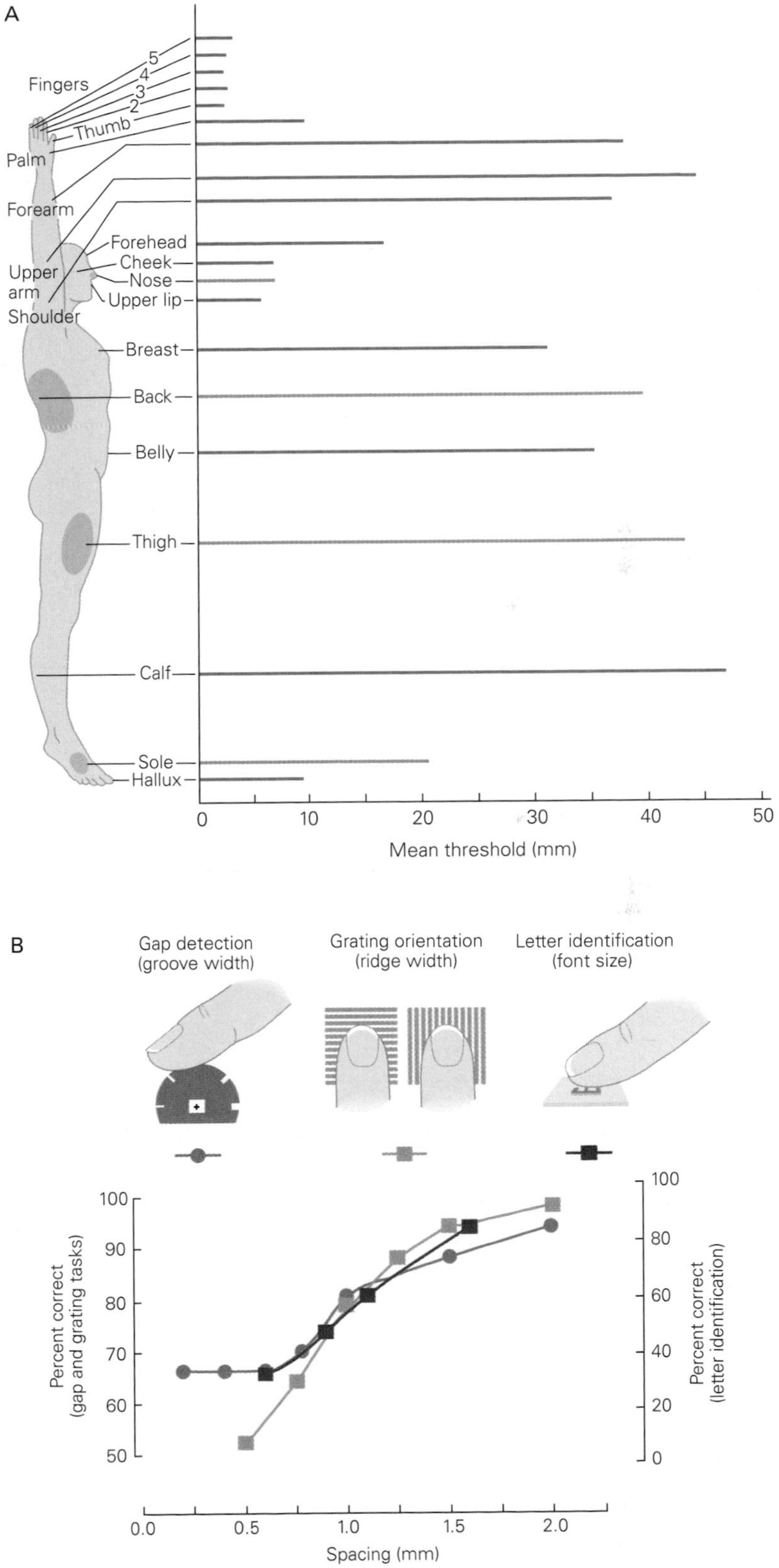

Figure 23–5 Tactile acuity in the human hand is highest on the fingertip.

A. The two-point threshold measures the minimum distance at which two stimuli are resolved as distinct. This distance varies for different body regions; it is approximately 2 mm on the fingers, but as much as 10 mm on the palm and 40 mm on the arm, thigh, and back. The two-point perceptual thresholds highlighted in **pink** match the diameters of the receptive fields of receptors in the pink zones on the body. The greatest discriminative capacity is afforded in the fingertips, lips, and tongue, which have the smallest receptive fields. (Adapted, with permission, from Weinstein 1968.)

B. Spatial acuity is measured in psychophysical experiments by having a blindfolded subject touch a variety of textured surfaces. As shown here, the subject is asked to determine whether the surface of a wheel is smooth or contains a gap, whether the ridges of a grating are oriented across the finger or parallel to its long axis, or which letters appear on raised type used in letterpress printing. The tactile acuity threshold is defined as the groove width, ridge width, or font size that yields 75% correct performance (detectable midway between chance and perfect accuracy). The threshold spacing on the human fingertip is 1.0 mm in each of these tests. (Adapted, with permission, from Johnson and Phillips 1981.)

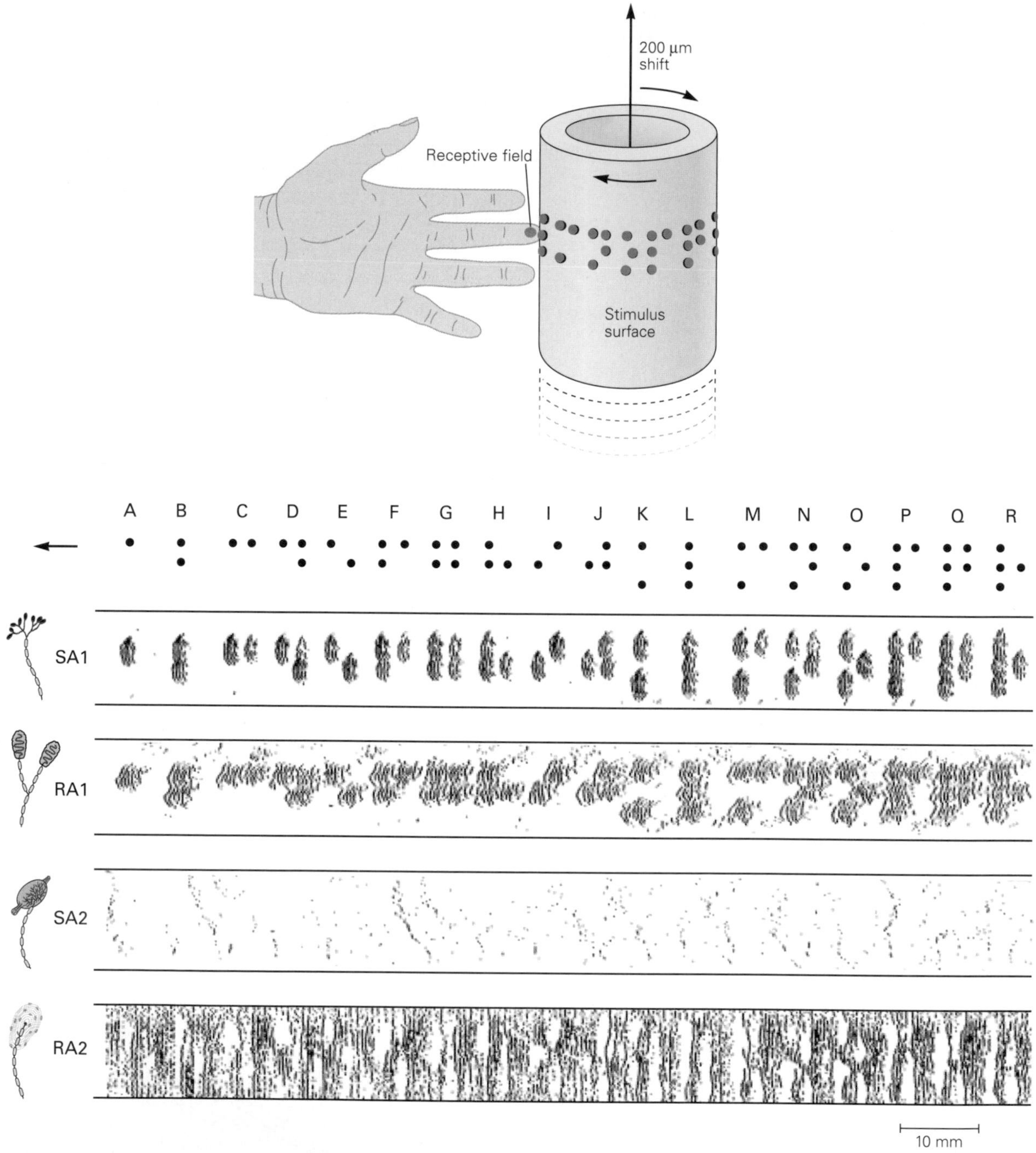

Figure 23–6 Responses of touch receptors to Braille dots scanned by the fingers. The Braille symbols for the letters A through R were mounted on a drum that was repeatedly rotated against the fingertip of a human subject. Following each revolution the drum was shifted upward so that another portion of the symbols was scanned across the finger. Microelectrodes placed in the median nerve of this subject recorded the responses of the mechanoreceptive fibers innervating the fingertip. The action potentials discharged by the nerve fibers as the Braille symbols were moved over the receptive field are represented in these records by small dots; each horizontal row of dots represents the responses of the fiber to a single revolution of the drum. The SA1 receptors register the sharpest image of the Braille symbols, representing each Braille dot with a series of action potentials and falling silent when the spaces between Braille symbols provide no stimulation. RA1 receptors provide a blurred image of the Braille symbols because their receptive fields are larger, but the individual dot patterns are still recognizable. Neither RA2 nor SA2 receptors are able to encode the Braille patterns because their receptive fields are larger than the dot spacing. The high firing rate of the RA2 fibers reflects the keen sensitivity of Pacinian corpuscles to vibration. (**RA1**, rapidly adapting type 1; **RA2**, rapidly adapting type 2; **SA1**, slowly adapting type 1; **SA2**, slowly adapting type 2.) (Reproduced, with permission, from Phillips, Johansson, and Johnson 1992.)

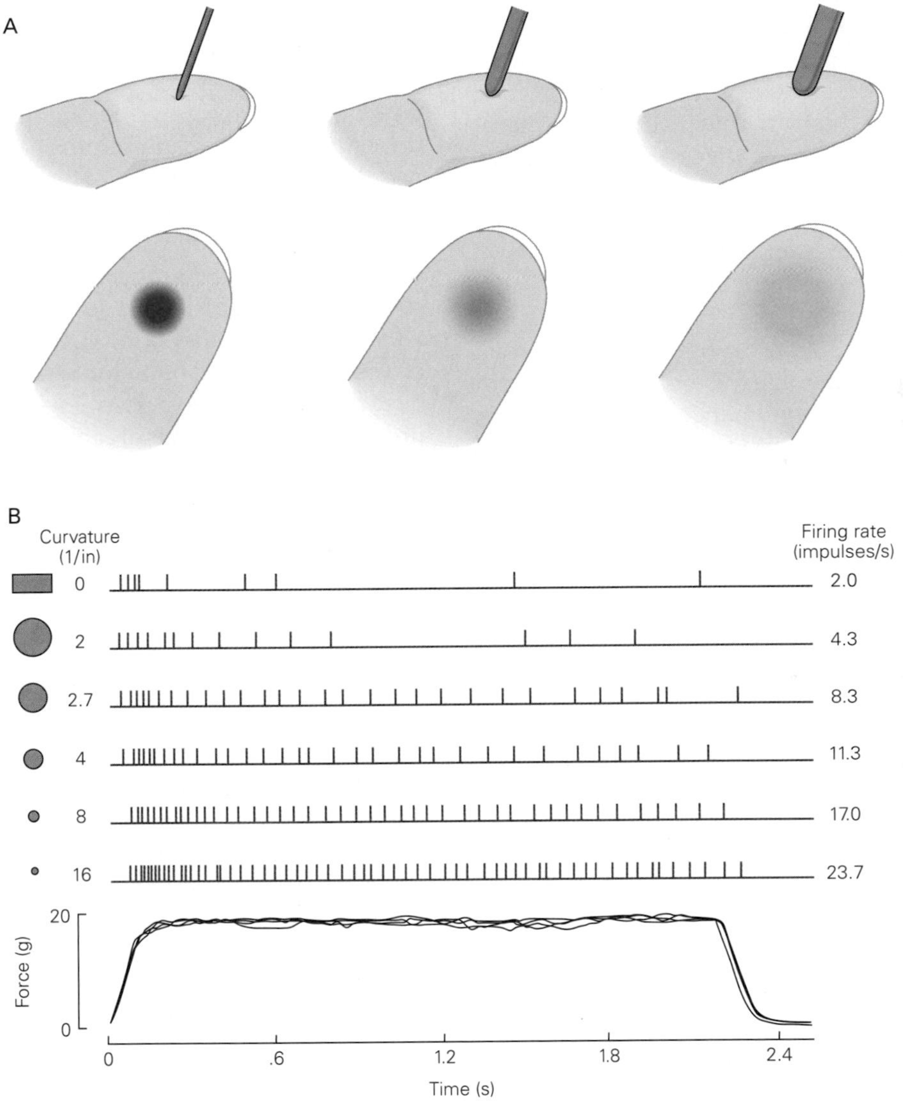

Figure 23–7 Slowly adapting type 1 (SA1) fibers encode the shape and size of objects touching the hand.

A. The area of contact on the skin determines the firing rate and total number of SA1 fibers stimulated. The **pink region** on the fingertip shows the spread of excitation when probes of different diameters are pressed upon the skin with constant force. The intensity of color is proportional to the firing rates of the stimulated receptors. A small-diameter, sharply pointed probe (left) activates a small population of SA1 receptors. The activated fibers fire intensely because all of the force is concentrated in a small area. A medium-size probe (middle) excites more receptors, but the spread of the force reduces peak firing rates. The probe does not feel as sharp as the small-diameter probe. A large round probe (right) stimulates a large population of SA1 receptors spread across the width of the finger. These fibers fire at low rates because the force is spread over a wide area of skin. The sensation of pressure is diffuse. (Adapted, with permission, from Goodwin, Browning, and Wheat 1995.)

B. The firing rate of an individual SA1 fiber is determined by the probe diameter. When a probe first contacts the skin, the SA1 response is strong regardless of probe diameter. During steady pressure the firing rate is proportional to the curvature of each probe. The highest firing rates are evoked by the smallest probe, while the weakest responses are produced by flat surfaces and gently rounded (large diameter) probes. The tip's curvature is expressed as the inverse of its spherical radius. (Adapted, with permission, from Srinivasan and LaMotte 1991.)

response intensity of each fiber becomes progressively weaker because the displacement forces on the skin are distributed across the entire contact zone. Thus the skin mechanics results in a case of "less is more." Individual SA1 fibers respond more vigorously to a small object than to a large one because the force needed to indent the skin is concentrated at a small contact point. In this manner each SA1 fiber integrates the local skin indentation profile within its receptive field.

The sensitivity of SA1 receptors to local stretch of the skin also enables them to detect edges, the places where an object's curvature changes abruptly. SA1 firing rates are many times greater when a finger touches an edge than when it touches a flat surface.

The indentation force of a flat or gently curved surface is distributed symmetrically within the central contact zone, whereas the force applied by an object boundary displaces the skin asymmetrically, beyond the edge as well as at the edge. This asymmetric distribution of force produces enhanced responses from receptive fields located along the edges of an object. As edges are often perceived as sharp, we tend to grasp objects on flat or gently curved surfaces rather than by their edges.

The SA2 fibers that innervate Ruffini endings respond more vigorously to stretch of the skin than to indentation because the receptors are located along the palmar folds or at the finger joints. The SA2 fibers therefore provide information about the shape of large objects grasped with the entire hand, the "power grasp" in which all five fingers press an object against the palm. They also provide information about hand shape and finger movements when the hand is empty. If the fingers are fully extended and abducted we feel the stretch in the palm and proximal phalanges as the glabrous skin is flattened. Similarly, if the fingers are fully flexed, forming a fist, we feel the stretch of the skin on the back of the hand, particularly over the metacarpal-phalangeal and proximal interphalangeal joints.

The SA2 system may play a central role in stereognosis—the recognition of three-dimensional objects using touch only—as well as other perceptual tasks in which skin stretch is a major cue. Benoni Edin has shown that SA2 innervation in the hairy skin plays a substantial role in the perception of hand shape and finger position. The SA2 fibers aid the perception of finger joint angle by detecting skin stretch around the knuckles. The Ruffini endings near these joints are aligned such that different groups of receptors are stimulated as the fingers move in specific directions (Figure 23–4A). In this manner the SA2 system provides a neural representation of skin stretch over the entire hand, a proprioceptive rather than exteroceptive function.

Rapidly Adapting Fibers Detect Motion and Vibration

The RA1 receptor organ, the Meissner corpuscle, detects events that produce low-frequency, low-amplitude skin motion. This includes hand motion over the surface of objects, the detection of microscopic surface features, and low-frequency vibration. RA1 fibers contribute to detection of Braille patterns because they sense the change in skin indentation as individual dots pass over their receptive fields (Figure 23–6). They can detect irregularities and bumps as small as 10 μm. We use the sensitivity of RA1 fibers to motion to adjust grip force when we grasp an object.

The RA2 receptor, the Pacinian corpuscle, is the most sensitive mechanoreceptor in the somatosensory system. It is exquisitely responsive to high-frequency (30–500 Hz) vibratory stimuli, and can detect vibration of 250 Hz in the nanometer range (Figure 23–8). The buzzing sensation experienced when a tuning fork is pressed against the skin in a neurological examination is mediated by the synchronized firing of RA2 units. It is a useful measurement of dynamic sensitivity to touch, particularly in cases of localized nerve damage.

The Pacinian corpuscle's filtering and amplifying of high-frequency vibration allows us to feel conditions at the working surface of a tool in our hand as if our fingers themselves were touching the object under the tool. The clinician uses this exquisite sensitivity to guide a needle into blood vessel and to probe tissue stiffness. The auto mechanic can use vibratory sense to position wrenches on unseen bolts. We can write in the dark because we feel the vibration of the pen as it contacts the paper and transmits the resulting frictional forces from the surface roughness to our fingers.

Both Slowly and Rapidly Adapting Fibers Are Important for Grip Control

In addition to their role sensing the size, shape, and texture of objects, mechanoreceptors provide important information concerning the actions of the hand during skilled movements. Roland Johansson and Gören Westling used microneurography to determine the role of mechanoreceptors when objects are grasped in the hand. By placing microelectrodes in the median nerve, they were able to record the firing patterns of individual mechanosensitive fibers as an object was initially contacted by the fingers, grasped between the thumb and index finger, lifted, held above a table, lowered, and returned to the rest position.

They found that all four classes respond to grasp and that each fiber type monitors a particular function.

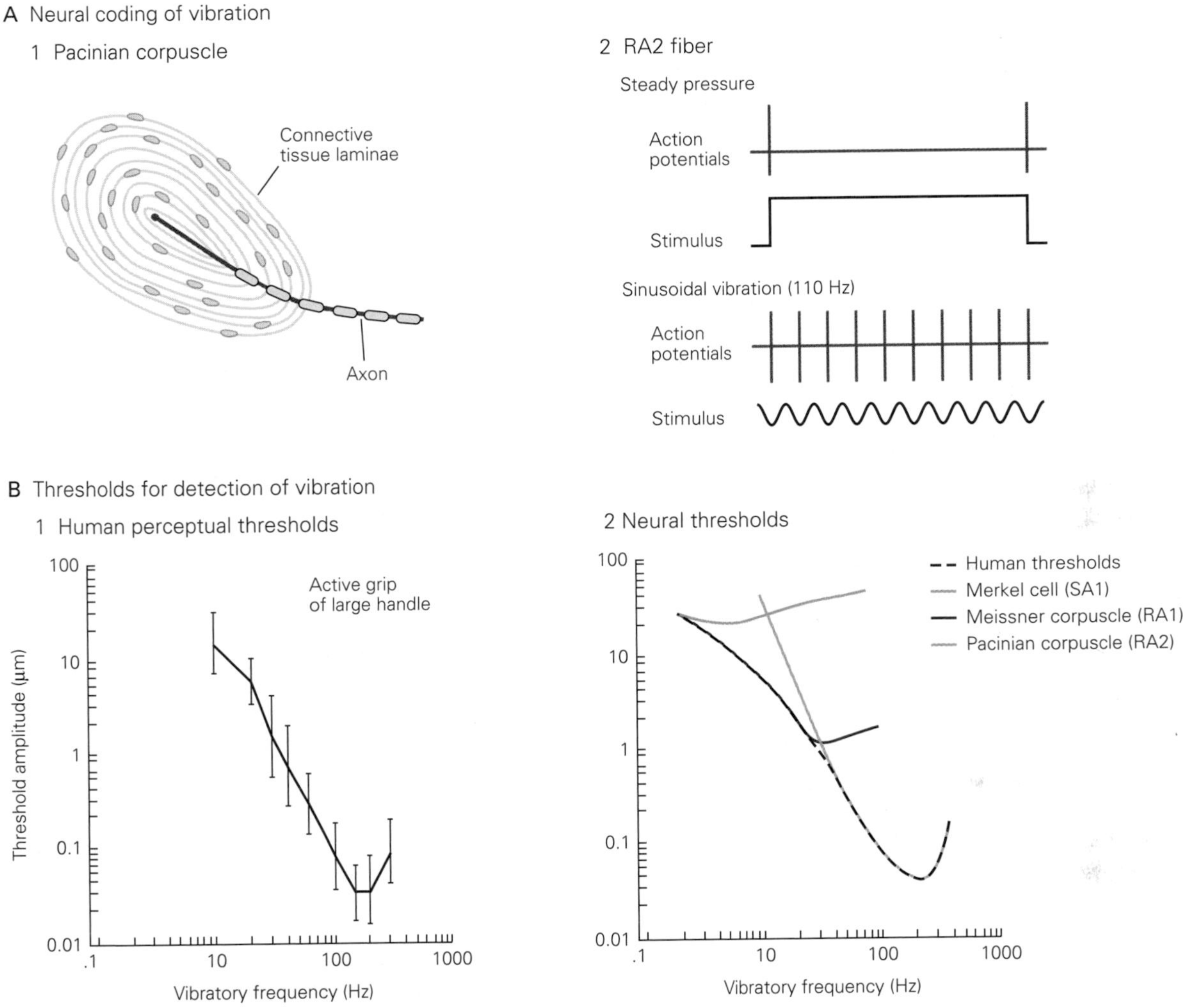

Figure 23–8 Rapidly adapting type 2 (RA2) fibers encode vibration. Vibration is the sensation produced by sinusoidal stimulation of the skin, as by the hum of an electric motor, the strings of a musical instrument, or the tuning fork used in the neurological examination.

A. 1. The Pacinian corpuscle consists of concentric, fluid-filled lamellae of connective tissue that encapsulate the terminal of an RA2 fiber. This structure is uniquely suited to the detection of motion. Sensory transduction in the RA2 fiber occurs in stretch-sensitive cation channels linked to the inner lamellae of the capsule. **2.** When steady pressure is applied to the skin the RA2 fiber fires a burst at the start and end of stimulation. In response to sinusoidal stimulation (vibration) the fiber fires at regular intervals such that each action potential signals one cycle of the stimulus. Our perception of vibration as a rhythmically repeating event results from the simultaneous activation of many RA2 units, which fire in synchrony.

B. 1. Psychophysical thresholds for detection of vibration depend on the stimulation frequency. As shown here, humans can detect vibrations as small as 10 nm at 200 Hz when grasping a large object; the threshold is higher at other frequencies and when tested with small probes. (Adapted, with permission, from Brisben, Hsiao, and Johnson 1999.) **2.** The neural threshold for detection of vibration is defined as the lowest stimulus intensity that evokes one action potential per cycle of the sinusoidal stimulus. Each type of mechanosensory fiber is most sensitive to a specific range of frequencies. Slowly adapting type 1 (SA1) fibers are most sensitive between 0.3 Hz and 3 Hz, rapidly adapting type 1 (RA1) fibers between 2 Hz and 50 Hz, and RA2 fibers between 30 Hz and 500 Hz. Human thresholds for vibration match those of the most sensitive touch fibers in each range. (Adapted, with permission, from Mountcastle, Lynch, and Carli 1972; Bolanowski et al. 1988.)

The RA1, RA2, and SA1 fibers detect contact when an object is first touched (Figure 23–9). The SA1 fibers signal the amount of grip force applied by each finger, and the RA1 fibers sense how quickly the grasp is applied. The RA2 fibers detect the small shock waves transmitted through the object when it is lifted from the table and placed on another surface. We know when an object makes contact with the table top because of these vibrations and therefore can manipulate the object without looking at it. The RA1 and RA2 fibers cease responding after grasp is established. The SA2 fibers signal flexion or extension of the fingers during grasp or release of the object and thereby monitor the hand posture as these movements proceed.

Signals from the hand that report on the shape, size, and texture of an object are important factors governing the application of force during grasping. Johansson and his colleagues have shown that we lift and manipulate an object with delicacy—with grip forces that just exceed the forces that result in overt slip—and that the grip force is adjusted automatically to compensate for differences in the friction coefficient between surfaces. Subjects predict how much force is required to grasp and lift an object and modify the grip force based on the tactile information provided by SA1 and RA1 afferents. Objects with smooth surfaces are grasped more firmly than those with rough textures, properties coded by RA1 afferents during initial contact of the hand with an object. The significance of the tactile information in grasping is seen in cases of nerve injury or during local anesthesia of the hand; patients apply unusually high grip forces, and the coordination between the grip and load forces applied by the fingers is poor.

The information supplied by the RA1 receptors to monitor grasping actions is critical for grip control, allowing us to hold on to objects when perturbations cause them to slip unexpectedly. RA1 fibers are silent during steady grasp and usually remain quiet until the object is returned to rest and the grasp released. However, if the object is unexpectedly heavy or jolted by external forces and begins to slip from the hand, the RA1 fibers fire in response to the small tangential movements of the object. The net result of this RA1 activity is that grip force is increased by signals from the motor cortex.

Tactile Information Is Processed in the Central Touch System

As described in Chapter 22, the central touch system comprises the dorsal column tracts of the spinal cord, relay nuclei in the brain stem and thalamus, and a hierarchy of regions in the cerebral cortex (see Figure 22–11). Tactile information enters the cerebral cortex through the primary somatosensory cortex (S-I) in the postcentral gyrus of the parietal lobe.

The neurons in S-I are at least three synapses beyond the receptors in the skin. Their inputs represent information processed in the dorsal column nuclei, the thalamus, and the cortex itself. Each cortical neuron receives inputs arising from receptors in a specific area of the skin, and these inputs together are its receptive field. We perceive that a particular location on the skin is touched because a specific population of neurons in the brain is activated. This experience can be experimentally induced by electrical stimulation of the same cortical neurons.

The primary somatic sensory cortex comprises four cytoarchitectural areas: Brodmann's areas 3a, 3b, 1, and 2 (Figure 23–10A). These areas are extensively interconnected such that processing of sensory information at this level involves both serial and parallel processing. Neurons in areas 3a and 3b receive inputs from the lateral and medial zones of the ventral posterior nucleus of the thalamus and project their axons to areas 1 and 2 (Figure 23–10B). Areas 3b and 1 receive information from receptors in the skin, whereas areas 3a and 2 receive proprioceptive information from receptors in muscles, joints, and the skin.

Somatosensory information is conveyed in parallel from the four areas of S-I to higher centers in the cortex, including the secondary somatosensory cortex (S-II), the posterior parietal cortex, and the primary motor cortex.

Cortical Receptive Fields Integrate Information from Neighboring Receptors

The receptive fields of cortical neurons are much larger than those of mechanoreceptive fibers in peripheral nerves. For example, the receptive fields of SA1 and RA1 fibers innervating the fingertip are tiny spots on the skin, whereas those of the cortical neurons receiving these inputs cover an entire fingertip or several adjacent fingers (Figure 23–11). The receptive field of a neuron in area 3b represents a composite of inputs from 300 to 400 sensory nerve fibers.

Receptive fields in higher cortical areas are even larger, spanning functional regions of skin that are activated simultaneously during motor activity. These include the tips of several adjacent fingers, or both the fingers and the palm. Receptive fields of neurons in the posterior parietal cortex and S-II are often bilateral, including symmetric positions on the contralateral and ipsilateral hands.

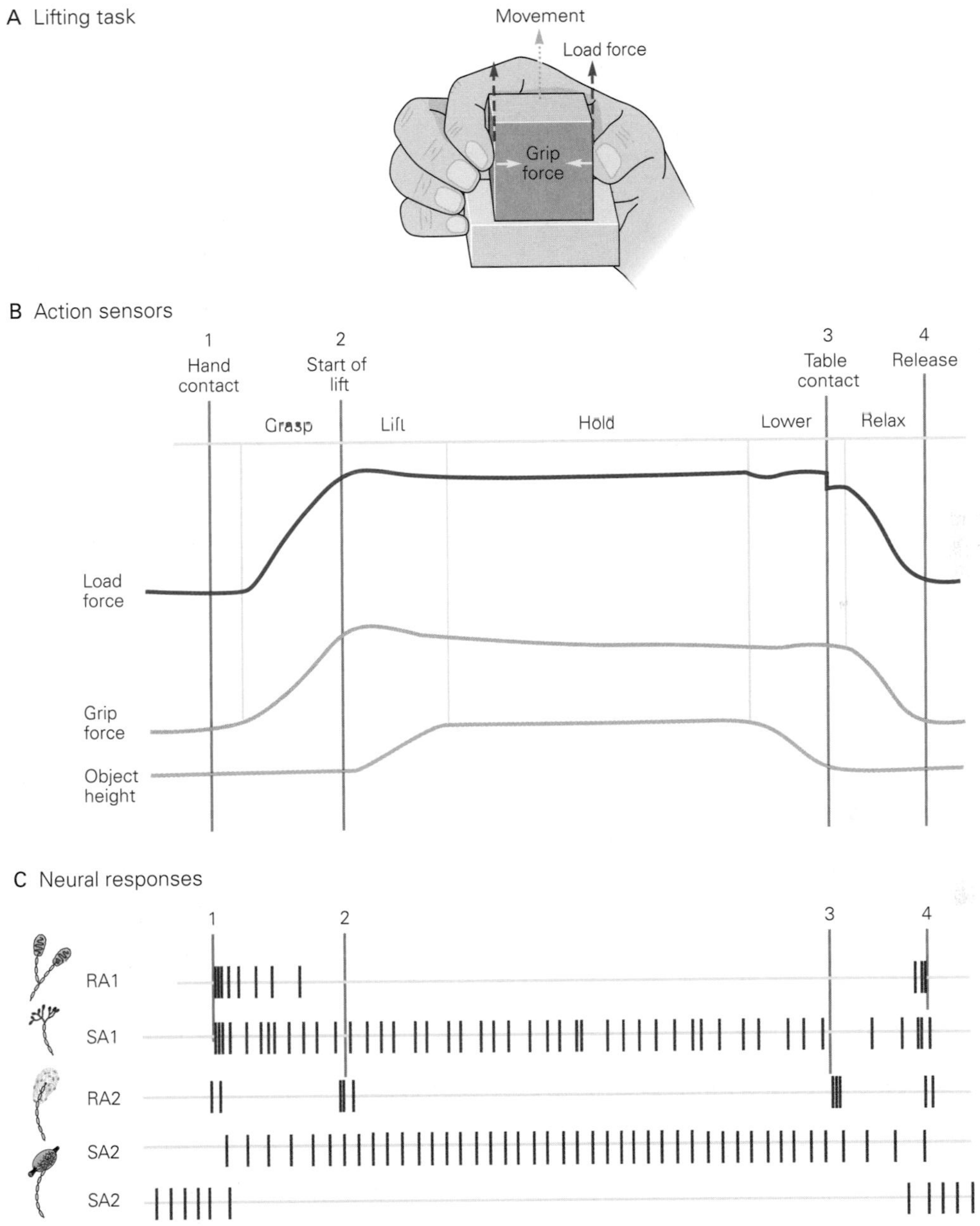

Figure 23–9 Sensory information from the hand during grasping and lifting. (Adapted, with permission, from Johansson 1996.)

A. The subject grasps and lifts a block between the thumb and fingertips, holds it above a table, and then returns it to the resting position. The normal (grip) force secures the object in the hand, and the tangential (load) force overcomes gravity. The grip force is adapted to the surface texture and weight of the object.

B. The grip and load forces are monitored with sensors in the object. These forces are coordinated following contact with the object, plateau as lift begins, and relax in concert after the object is returned to the table.

C. All four mechanoreceptors detect hand contact with the object but each monitors a different aspect of the action as the task progresses. SA1 fibers encode the grip force and SA2 fibers the hand posture. RA1 fibers encode the rate of force application and movement of the hand on the object. RA2 fibers sense vibrations in the object with each movement: at hand contact, lift-off, table contact, and release of grasp. (**RA1**, rapidly adapting type 1; **RA2**, rapidly adapting type 2; **SA1**, slowly adapting type 1; **SA2**, slowly adapting type 2.)

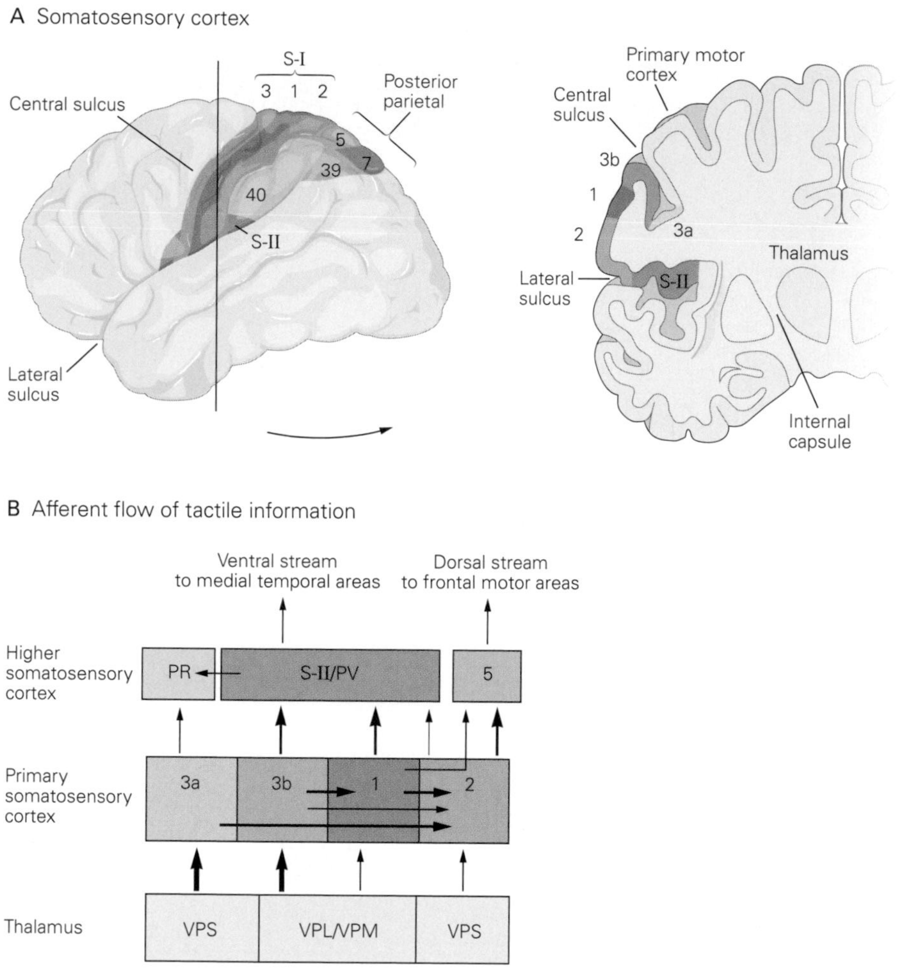

Figure 23–10 The somatosensory areas of the cerebral cortex.

A. The somatosensory areas of cortex lie in the parietal lobe and consist of three major divisions. The *primary somatosensory cortex* (S-I) forms the anterior part of the parietal lobe. It extends throughout the postcentral gyrus beginning at the bottom of the central sulcus, extending posteriorly to the postcentral sulcus, and into the medial wall of the hemisphere to the cingulate gyrus (not shown). The S-I comprises four distinct cytoarchitectonic regions: Brodmann's areas 3a, 3b, 1, and 2. The *secondary somatosensory cortex* (S-II) is located on the upper bank of the lateral sulcus (Sylvian fissure) and on the parietal operculum; it covers Brodmann's area 43. The *posterior parietal cortex* surrounds the intraparietal sulcus on the lateral surface of the hemisphere, extending from the postcentral sulcus to the parietal-occipital sulcus and medially to the precuneus. The superior parietal lobule (areas 5 and 7) is a somatosensory area; the inferior parietal lobule (areas 39 and 40) receives both somatosensory and visual inputs. A coronal section through the postcentral gyrus illustrates the anatomical relationship of S-I, S-II, and the primary motor cortex (area 4). S-II lies lateral to area 2 in S-I and extends medially along the upper bank of the lateral sulcus to the insular cortex. The primary motor cortex lies rostral to area 3a within the wall of the central sulcus.

B. Hierarchical connections to and from S-I. Neurons projecting from the thalamus send their axons mainly to areas 3a and 3b, but some thalamic neurons also project to areas 1 and 2. In turn, neurons in cortical areas 3a and 3b project to areas 1 and 2. Information from the four areas of S-I is conveyed to neurons in the posterior parietal cortex (area 5) and S-II. (**PR**, parietal rostroventral cortex; **PV**, parietal ventral cortex; **VPL**, ventral posterior lateral nuclei; **VPM**, ventral posterior medial nuclei; **VPS**, ventral posterior superior nuclei.) (Adapted, with permission, from Felleman and Van Essen 1991.)

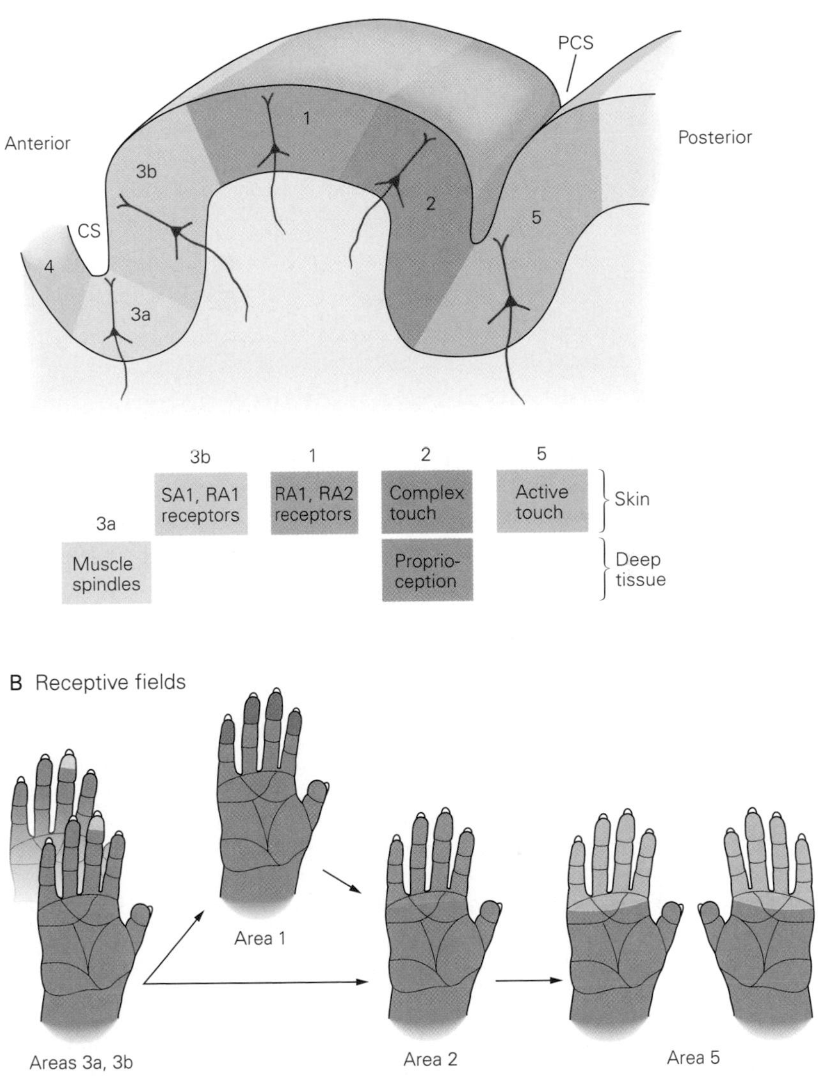

Figure 23–11 The receptive fields of neurons in the primary somatic sensory cortex.

A. This sagittal section illustrates the rostrocaudal anatomy of the four regions of S-I (areas 3a, 3b, 1, and 2) as well as the primary motor cortex (area 4) and the posterior parietal cortex (area 5). The four regions process different types of somatosensory information. Neurons in area 3a receive inputs from muscle spindles and other deep receptors. Neurons in area 3b receive inputs from specific classes of touch receptors in the skin. Neurons in areas 1 and 2 receive convergent inputs from multiple types of somatosensory receptors innervating the same body part. Neurons in area 5 are active mainly during active hand movements.

B. Typical receptive fields of neurons in each area of S-I in monkeys are shown in colors corresponding to those in A. (Receptive fields were measured by applying light touch to the skin.) The receptive fields are smallest in area 3b, where tactile information first enters the cortex. They are progressively larger in areas 1, 2, and 5, reflecting convergent inputs from neurons in area 3b that are stimulated together when we use the hand. Many neurons in area 5 and in S-II cortex have bilateral receptive fields because they respond to touch at mirror image locations on both the contralateral and ipsilateral hands. These neurons enable bilateral coordination when the two hands work synergistically. (**CS**, central sulcus; **PCS**, postcentral sulcus; **RA1**, rapidly adapting type 1; **RA2**, rapidly adapting type 2; **SA1**, slowly adapting type 1; **SA2**, slowly adapting type 2.) (Adapted, with permission, from Gardner 1988; Iwamura et al. 1993; Iwamura, Iriki, and Tanaka 1994.)

The size and position of receptive fields on the skin are not fixed permanently but can be modified by experience or by injury to sensory nerves (see Chapter 17). Cortical receptive fields appear to be formed during development and maintained by simultaneous activation of the input pathways.

The receptive fields of cortical neurons usually have an excitatory zone surrounded by or superimposed upon inhibitory zones (Figure 23–12). Stimulation of regions of skin outside the excitatory zone may reduce the neuron's responses to tactile stimulation within the receptive field. Similarly, repeated stimulation within the receptive field may also decrease neuronal responsiveness because the excitability of the pathway is diminished by inhibition.

Inhibitory receptive fields created by feed-forward and feedback connections through interneurons in the dorsal column nuclei, the thalamus, and the cortex itself limit the spread of excitation. Inhibition generated by strong activity in one circuit reduces the output of nearby neurons that are only weakly excited. The inhibitory networks ensure that the strongest of several competing responses is transmitted, permitting a winner-take-all strategy. These circuits prevent blurring of tactile details such as texture when large populations of touch neurons are stimulated. In addition, higher centers in the brain use inhibitory circuits to focus attention on relevant information from the hand when it is used in skilled tasks, by suppressing unwanted, distracting inputs during such behaviors.

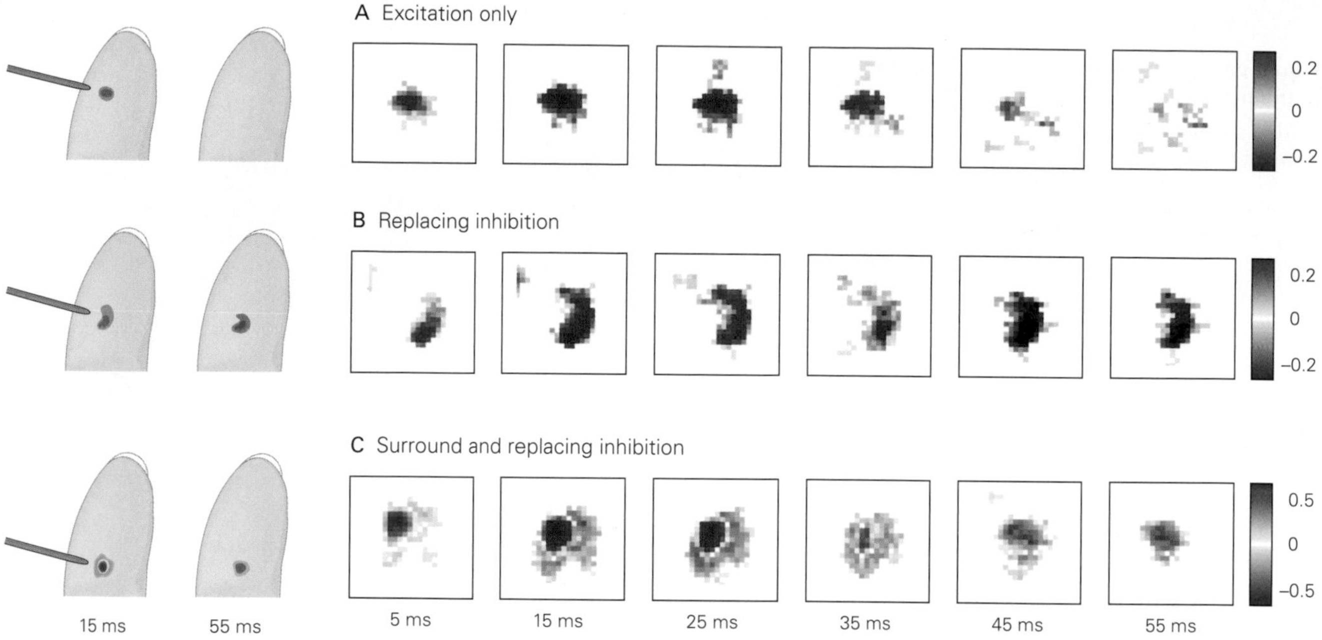

Figure 23–12 Excitatory and inhibitory zones of receptive fields of neurons in area 3b. The excitability of cortical neurons varies over time and as a function of the stimulus location on the skin. Peak excitation occurs in the middle of the receptive field 15 to 25 ms following brief taps on the skin. Inhibition occurs shortly thereafter and is strongest at 45 ms. Delayed inhibition allows each stimulus to be perceived as a distinct event when delivered at rates lower than 25 Hz. Each map indicates the intensity of excitation (**red**) and inhibition (**blue**) produced over 10 ms periods following brief taps to a small patch of skin on the fingertip. Cortical neurons vary in the relative strength and spatial location of excitatory and inhibitory fields. (Adapted, with permission, from Sripati et al. 2006.)

A. Purely excitatory responses occur in only 6% of area 3b neurons.

B. In 42% of neurons in area 3b initial excitation is replaced by inhibition in response to subsequent tactile stimulation of the same skin region.

C. The majority of neurons in area 3b (52%) are excited by stimulation in an excitatory zone and inhibited by stimulation in the surrounding inhibitory zone.

Neurons in the Somatosensory Cortex Are Organized into Functionally Specialized Columns

In a series of pioneering studies of the cerebral cortex, Vernon Mountcastle discovered that the cortex is organized into vertical columns or slabs. Each column is 300 to 600 μm wide and spans all six cortical layers from the surface to the white matter. All of the neurons within a column receive inputs from the same local area of the receptor sheet and respond to the same class or classes of receptors (Figure 23–13). A column is therefore an anatomical structure that, by organizing inputs that convey related information on location and modality, comprises an elementary functional module of the cortex.

Although the receptive fields of the neurons comprising a column in the somatosensory cortex are not precisely congruent, they share a common center that is most clearly evident in layer IV. In addition, the neurons in a column usually process only one submodality, such as pressure or vibration. This is not surprising, as the somatosensory submodalities are conveyed in anatomically separate pathways, and within these pathways the different types of mechanoreceptive fibers are also segregated (see Chapter 22).

The columnar organization of the cortex is a direct consequence of the intrinsic cortical circuitry and the migration pathway of neuroblasts during cortical development. The pattern of connections within the cerebral cortex is oriented vertically, perpendicular to the cortical surface. Thalamocortical axons terminate mainly on clusters of stellate cells neurons in layer IV, the axons of which project vertically toward the surface of the cortex (Figure 23–13B). The apical dendrites and axons of cortical pyramidal cells are also oriented vertically, parallel to the stellate cell axons. Thus the thalamocortical input is relayed to a narrow column of pyramidal cells with apical dendrites that are contacted by the stellate cell axons. This means that the same information is relayed up

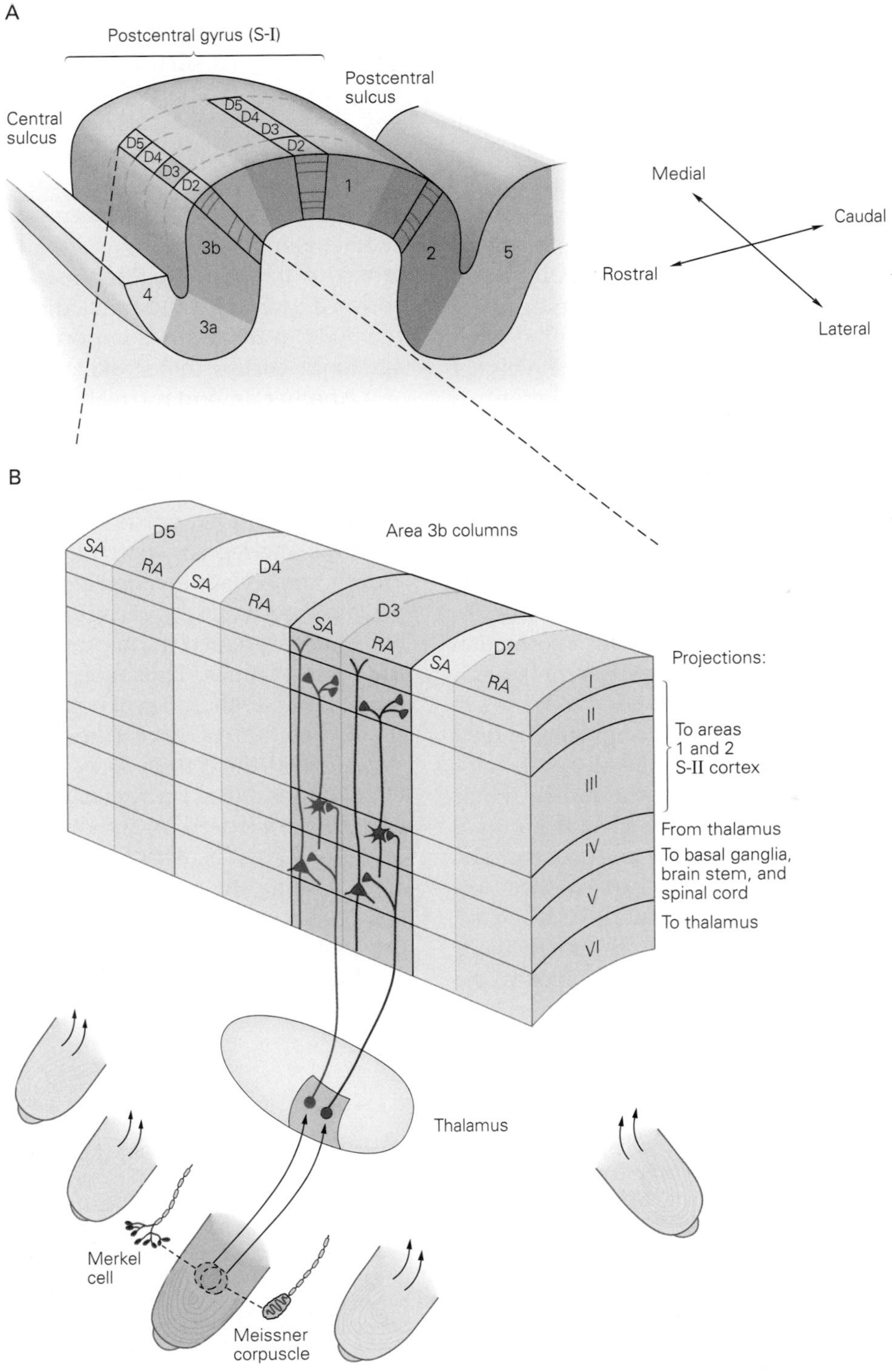

Figure 23–13 Columnar organization of the somatosensory cortex.

A. In each region of the somatic sensory cortex, inputs from the skin or deep tissue are organized in columns of neurons that run from the surface of the brain to the white matter. Each column receives input from one part of the body, here the individual fingers D2 to D5.

B. Details of the columnar organization of tactile inputs from the fingers in a portion of area 3b. Adjacent columns represent adjacent fingers, and for each finger alternating columns of neurons receive inputs from rapidly adapting (RA) and slowly adapting (SA) receptors. Neurons in each cortical layer send their output to specific regions of the brain. (Adapted, with permission, from Kaas et al. 1981; Sur, Wall, and Kaas 1984.)

and down through the thickness of the cortex in a columnar fashion.

The sensory properties computed in each column are output in parallel to multiple regions of the brain. Neurons in each of the six cortical layers project to specific targets. Horizontal connections within layers II and III link neurons in neighboring columns, allowing them to share information when activated simultaneously by the same stimulus. For this reason, neurons in these supragranular layers have larger receptive fields than neurons in layer IV. Neurons in layers II and III also project to other cortical regions, both on the same side of the brain and at mirror locations in the other hemisphere. These feed-forward connections to higher cortical areas allow complex signal integration, as detailed later in this chapter.

Neurons in layer V receive inputs from layers II and III in the same and adjacent columns; they project to subcortical structures, including the basal ganglia, the pontine and other brain stem nuclei, the spinal cord, and the dorsal column nuclei. Layer VI neurons project to the thalamus.

In addition to feed-forward signals of information from mechanoreceptors, recurrent signals from layers II and III of higher brain areas are provided to layer I in each column. These feedback signals originate not only in somatosensory areas of the brain, but also in sensorimotor areas of the posterior parietal cortex, frontal motor areas, limbic areas, and regions of the medial temporal lobe involved in memory formation and storage. The recurrent signals are thought to play a role in the selection of sensory information for cognitive processing (by the mechanisms of attention) and in short-term memory tasks. Feedback pathways may also be involved in the gating of sensory signals during motor activity.

Cortical Columns Are Organized Somatotopically

The columns within the primary somatic sensory cortex are arranged such that there is a complete somatotopic representation of the body in each of the four areas (3a, 3b, 1, and 2). The cortical map of the body corresponds roughly to the spinal dermatomes (see Figure 22–9). Sacral segments are represented medially, lumbar and thoracic segments centrally, cervical segments more laterally, and the trigeminal representation of the head at the most lateral portion of S-I cortex (Figure 23–14). Knowledge of the neural map of the body in the brain is important for localizing damage to the cortex from stroke or head trauma.

Another important feature of somatotopic maps is the amount of cerebral cortex devoted to each body part. A neural map of the body in the brain does not duplicate exactly the spatial topography of the skin. Rather, it has disproportionately large areas devoted to certain body regions, particularly the hand, foot, and mouth, and relatively smaller areas devoted to more proximal body parts (see Figure 16–6). Each part of the body is represented in proportion to its importance to the sense of touch. Thus more cortex is devoted to the fingers than to the entire trunk (Figure 23–14C).

The amount of cortical area devoted to a unit area of skin—called the *cortical magnification*—varies by more than a hundredfold across different body surfaces. It is closely correlated with the innervation density and thus the spatial acuity of the mechanoreceptors in an area of skin. The areas with greatest magnification—the lips, tongue, fingers, and toes—have tactile spatial thresholds of 0.5, 0.6, 1.0, and 4.5 mm, respectively.

Brain regions activated by tactile stimuli have been visualized with high-resolution optical imaging

Figure 23–14 (Opposite) **Each region of the primary somatosensory cortex contains a neural map of the entire body surface.** (Adapted, with permission, from Nelson et al. 1980; Pons et al. 1985.)

A. The primary somatosensory cortex in the macaque monkey lies caudal to the central sulcus as in the human brain. The colored areas correspond to the homologous Brodmann's areas of the human brain shown in Figure 23–10A. Area 5 in the macaque monkey is homologous to areas 5 and 7 in humans. Area 7 in the macaque monkey is homologous to areas 40 and 39 in humans.

B. Body maps in the postcentral gyrus of the primary somatosensory cortex of the macaque monkey obtained from microelectrode recordings. In the diagram the cortex is unfolded along the central sulcus (**dotted line** that parallels the border between areas 3b and 1). The upper part of the diagram includes cortex unfolded from the medial wall of the hemisphere. The body surface is mapped to columns within rostrocaudal bands arranged in the order of the spinal dermatomes. The maps in areas 3b and 1 form mirror images of the distal-proximal or dorsal-ventral axes of each dermatome. Each finger (D5–D1) has its own representation in areas 3b and 1, along the medial-lateral axis of the cortex, but inputs from several adjacent fingers converge in the receptive fields of neurons in area 2.

C. The finger-representation areas occupy a larger expanse of cortex than the trunk-representation areas. Although the trunk (**violet**) is covered by a greater area of skin than the fingers (**red**), the number of cortical columns responding to touch on the fingers is nearly three times the number activated by touching the trunk.

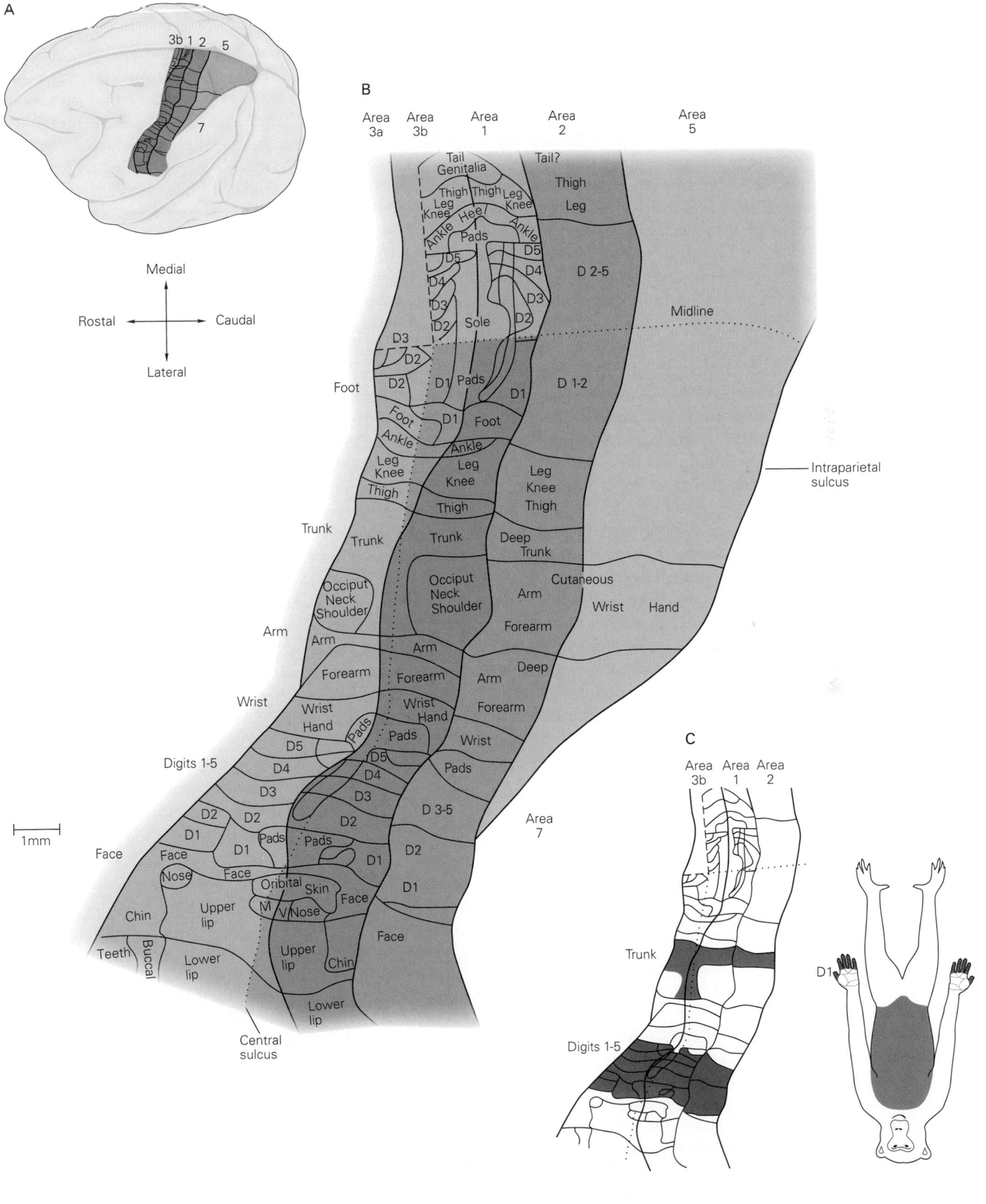
A
3b 1 2 5
7
Medial
Rostal
Caudal
Lateral
B
Area 3a
Area 3b
Area 1
Area 2
Area 5
Tail
Genitalia
Tail?
Thigh
Leg
Knee
Heel
Ankle
Pads
D5
D4
D3
D2
D1
Sole
D 2-5
Midline
D 1-2
Foot
Ankle
Leg
Knee
Thigh
Intraparietal sulcus
Trunk
Deep Trunk
Occiput
Neck
Shoulder
Cutaneous
Arm
Wrist
Hand
Forearm
Deep
Digits 1-5
D 3-5
Area 7
1mm
Face
Nose
Orbital
Skin
M
V
Chin
Upper lip
Lower lip
Teeth
Buccal
Central sulcus
C
Area 3b
Area 1
Area 2
Trunk
Digits 1-5
D1

of intrinsic signals generated by capillary blood flow. Cortical responses to air puffs applied to each finger of a monkey's hand are strongest in narrow transverse bands across areas 3b and 1 (Figure 23–15). Although inputs from neighboring fingers are organized in sequential bands, there is significant overlap between them, especially for the areas activated by digits 3 through 5, which are generally used in concert. The thumb and index finger, which often operate independently, have distinct territories and occupy a slightly larger cortical area, reflecting their importance in hand function.

Jon Kaas and his collaborators noted that somatotopic maps are important neurologically because they allow functionally related neurons to interconnect efficiently. For example, horizontal connections between cortical columns representing adjacent fingers enable us to perceive the surfaces contacted by different fingers as a continuous surface. The proximity of neurons representing the hand and mouth is likely to be useful in feeding behaviors, particularly in humans and other primates that bring food to the mouth with their hands.

The body surface has at least 10 distinct neural maps in the parietal lobe: four in S-I, four in S-II, and at least two in the posterior parietal cortex. Microelectrode mapping studies in monkeys have shown that the four areas of S-I (3a, 3b, 1, and 2) each have a complete, separate somatotopic representation of the body surface specific to a particular somatic sensory modality (Figure 23–14B). Area 3a receives input primarily from muscle stretch receptors; area 3b receives input from both SA1 and RA1 fibers; area 1 receives input primarily from RA1 and RA2 fibers; and area 2 contains a map of both touch and proprioception (Figure 23–11A).

As a result, these regions mediate different aspects of somatic sensation. Areas 3b and 1 are involved in sensing the details of surface texture, whereas area 2 is responsible for sensing the size and shape of objects. These attributes of somatic sensation are further elaborated in S-II and the posterior parietal cortex, where they form the basis of cognitive acts (object discrimination) and motor acts (object manipulation).

Touch Information Becomes Increasingly Abstract in Successive Central Synapses

As we have seen, the responses of mechanoreceptors to Braille dot patterns or embossed letters touched by the fingers faithfully encode the stimulus contours (see Figure 23–6) and specify precisely where on the hand touch occurs. The sharp sensory images encoded by receptors in the skin are preserved up to the first stage of cortical processing in area 3b.

As information flows toward higher-order cortical areas, specific combinations of stimuli or stimulus patterns are needed to excite individual neurons. Neurons in areas 1 and 2 of S-I are concerned with more abstract features than just the location of a tactile stimulus. Neurons with receptive fields that include more than one finger fire at higher rates when several fingers are touched, and thus are concerned with the size of objects held in the hand.

Signals from neighboring neurons are combined in higher cortical areas to discern global properties of objects such as their orientation on the hand, the direction of motion across the skin (Figure 23–16), and their shape. In general, cortical neurons are concerned with sensory features that are independent of the stimulus position in their receptive field, allowing the brain to represent patterns common to stimuli of a particular class.

A cortical neuron is able to detect the orientation of an edge or the direction of motion because of the spatial arrangement of the presynaptic receptive fields. The receptive fields of the excitatory presynaptic neurons are aligned along a preferred axis; a stimulus orientation that matches the alignment elicits a strong excitatory response. In addition, the receptive fields of inhibitory presynaptic neurons at one side of the excitatory fields reinforce the orientation and direction selectivity of the postsynaptic cell (Figure 23–17).

Convergent inputs from different sensory modalities allow neurons in higher cortical areas to detect the size and shape of objects. Whereas neurons in areas 3b and 1 respond only to touch, and neurons in area 3a respond to muscle stretch, many of the neurons in area 2 receive both inputs. Thus neurons in area 2 can integrate information on the hand posture used to grasp an object, the grip force applied by the hand, and the tactile stimulation produced by the object, and this integrated information allows us to recognize the object.

Cognitive Touch Is Mediated by Neurons in the Secondary Somatosensory Cortex

An S-I neuron's response to touch depends almost exclusively on input within the neuron's receptive field. This feed-forward pathway is often described as a *bottom-up* process because the receptors in the periphery are the principal source of excitation of S-I neurons.

Higher-order somatosensory areas receive information not only from peripheral receptors, but also are strongly influenced by top-down processes, such as goal setting and attentional modulation. Data obtained from single-neuron studies in monkeys, neuroimaging

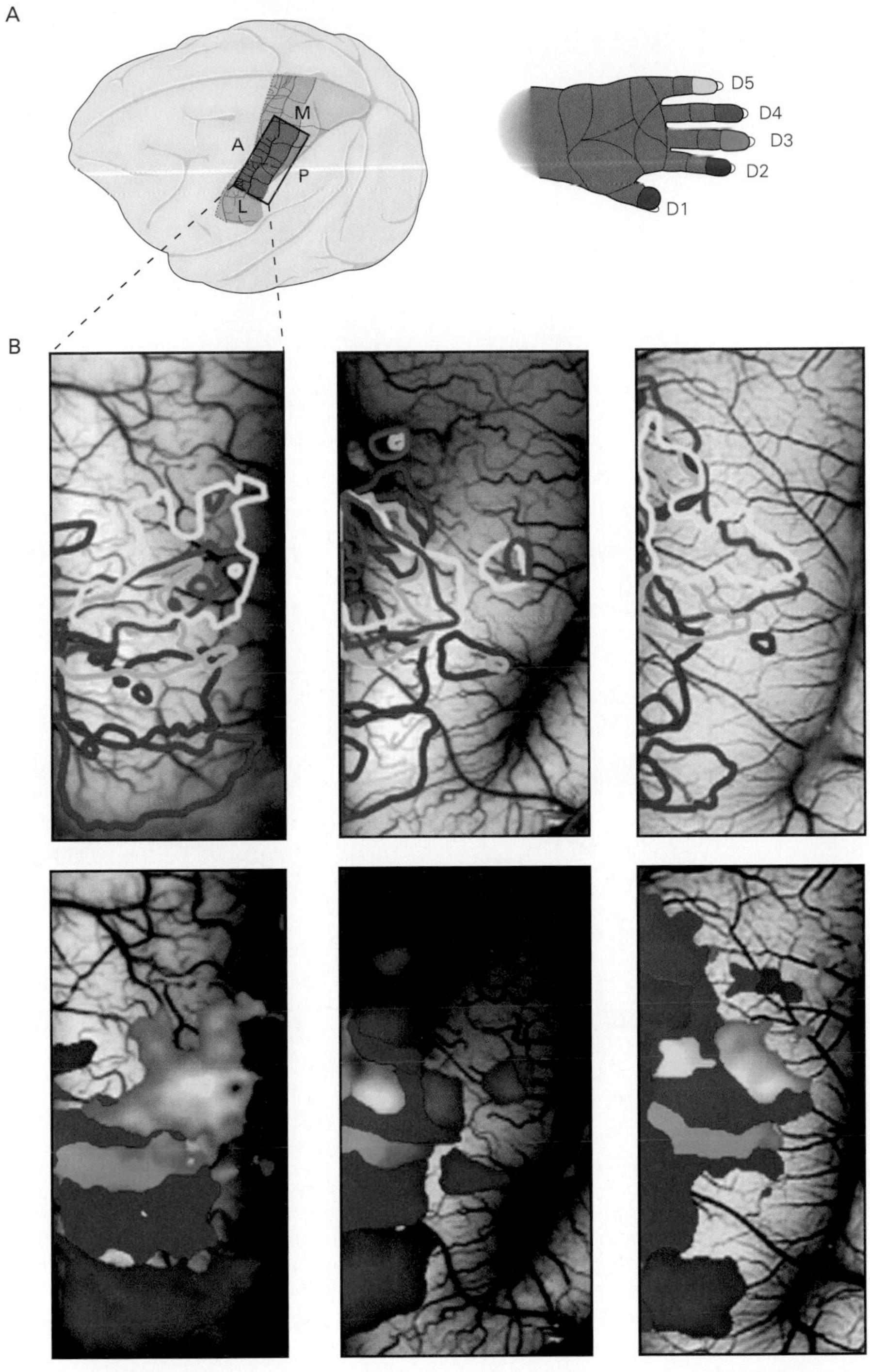

Figure 23–15 The representation of single fingers in S-I cortex follows a common plan. High-resolution optical imaging of intrinsic signals visualizes the areas of sensory cortex that represent each digit and allows one to identify precisely the neural representation of the hand. (Reproduced, with permission, from Shoham and Grinvald 2001.)

A. A schematic dorsal view of the macaque brain outlines the cortical territory explored with brain imaging.

B. The somatotopic organization of the hand area in three monkeys is superimposed on brain images of S-I cortex. The anterior part of each brain image shows Brodmann's area 1, and the posterior part shows areas 2 and 5. Although each animal has a distinctive map of the hand, all three have the same topographical organization.

Top: Outlines of the cortical regions activated by air puffs applied to individual digits are superimposed on the surface vasculature image. The outline colors correspond to the colors shown on each digit in part A. The regions stimulated by each digit are similar in total area. The regions responding to digits 3 to 5 overlap, whereas those activated by the thumb (**red**) and index finger (**blue**) do not.

Bottom: The information from the maps for each digit is integrated using a winner-take-all rule. The colors designate the digit that gave the strongest response; the intensity encodes the amplitude of the response to the "winning" digit. The domains of digits 3 to 5 appear as narrow stripes in the winner-take-all maps because of the larger overlap between their activated cortical areas.

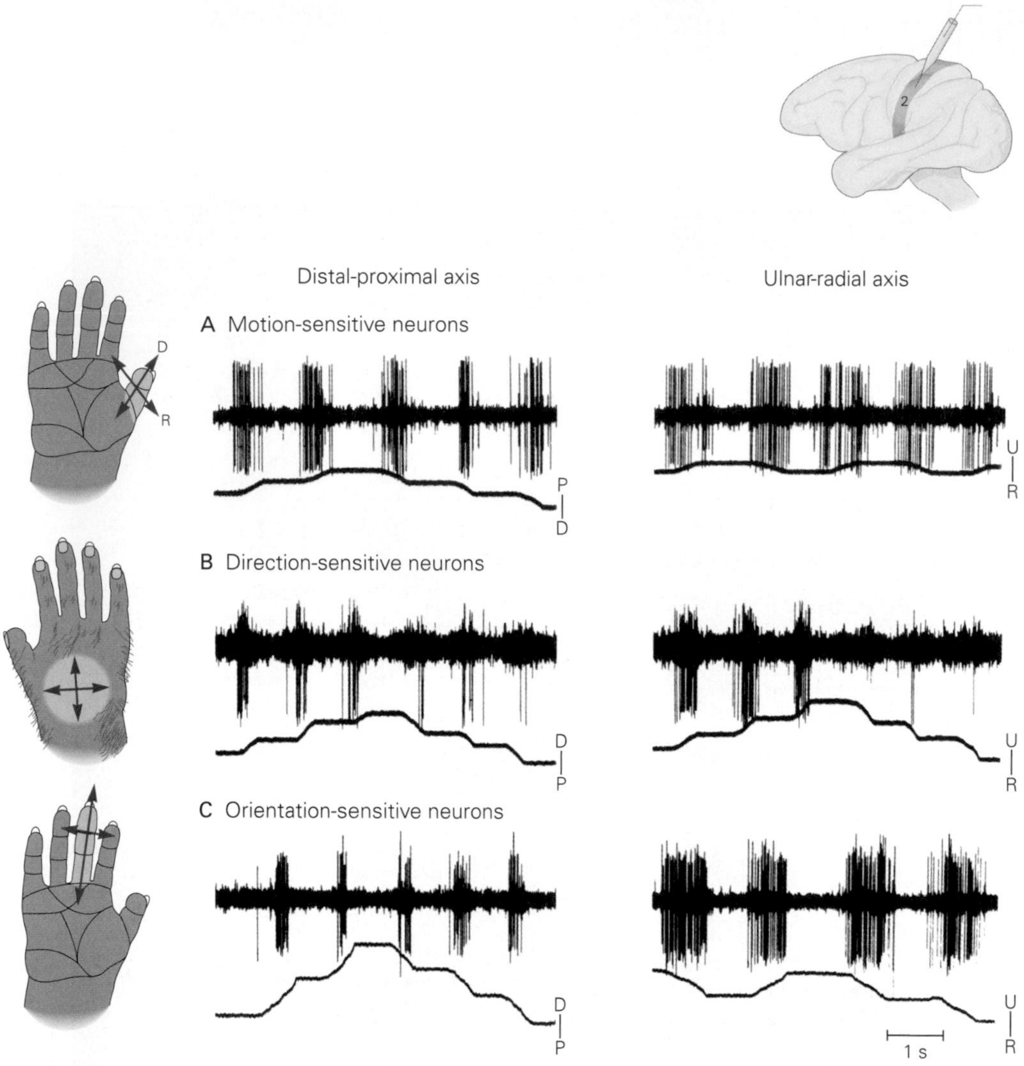

Figure 23–16 Neurons in area 2 encode complex tactile information. These neurons respond to motion of a probe across the receptive field but not to touch at a single point. The lower trace indicates the direction of motion by upward and downward deflections. (Adapted, with permission, from Warren, Hämäläinen, and Gardner 1986.)

A. A motion-sensitive neuron responds to stroking the skin in all directions.

B. A direction-sensitive neuron responds strongly to motion toward the ulnar side of the palm but fails to respond to motion in the opposite direction. Responses to distal or proximal movements are weaker.

C. An orientation-sensitive neuron responds better to motion across a finger (ulnar-radial) than to motion along the finger (distal-proximal), but does not distinguish ulnar from radial nor proximal from distal directions.

studies in humans, and clinical observations of patients with lesions in higher-order somatosensory areas suggest that the ventral and dorsal regions of the parietal lobe serve complementary functions in the touch system similar to the dorsal (what) and ventral (where) pathways of the visual system (see Chapter 25).

Like S-I, the S-II cortex contains four distinct anatomical subregions with separate maps of the body. In both humans and monkeys S-II is located on the upper bank and adjacent parietal operculum of the Sylvian or lateral fissure (see Figure 23–10A). The central zone—consisting of S-II proper and the adjacent parietal ventral area—receives its major input from areas 3b and 1, largely tactile information from the hand and face. A more rostral region, the parietal rostroventral area, receives information from area 3a about active hand movements (Figure 23–18). The most caudal somatosensory region of the lateral sulcus extends onto the parietal operculum. This region abuts the posterior parietal cortex and plays a role in integrating somatosensory and visual properties of objects.

Physiological studies indicate that S-II plays a key role in the use of touch to recognize objects placed in the hand. S-II neurons are essential for distinguishing spatial features such as shape and texture and temporal properties such as vibratory frequency. Although neurons in S-II respond to textures such as Braille dots, embossed letters, or gratings, their pattern of firing does not encode the spatial or temporal patterns of the stimuli. Instead, they simply fire at different rates for different patterns. Similarly, they do not represent vibration as periodic spike trains linked to the oscillatory frequency, as do the sensory fibers from the skin. Instead, their firing rates also depend on behavioral context or motivational state.

In an elegant study Ranulfo Romo and his colleagues compared responses of neurons in S-I, S-II, and various regions of the frontal lobe of monkeys while the animals performed a two-alternative forced-choice task (Figure 23–19). The animals were rewarded if they correctly recognized which of two vibratory stimuli was higher in frequency. Neurons in S-I faithfully represented the vibratory cycles each stimulus, firing a brief burst in response to each. In contrast, S-II neurons responded to the first stimulus with spike trains proportional to its frequency but responded to the second stimulus with a signal that combined the frequencies of both stimuli. Thus the same vibratory stimulus could evoke different firing rates in S-II, depending on whether the preceding stimulus was higher or lower in frequency.

Romo's group found that neurons in prefrontal and premotor cortex that receive inputs from S-II preserve a memory of the first stimulus, continuing to fire after it ends. They proposed that the memory signal is fed back to S-II from these higher brain regions, modifying the response of S-II neurons to the direct tactile signals from the hand. In this manner sensorimotor memories of previous stimuli influence sensory processing in the brain, allowing us to make cognitive judgments about newly arriving tactile stimuli.

S-II is the gateway to the temporal lobe via the insular cortex. Regions of the medial temporal lobe, particularly the hippocampus, are vital to the storage of explicit memory (see Chapter 67). We do not store in memory every scintilla of tactile information that enters the nervous system, only that which has some behavioral

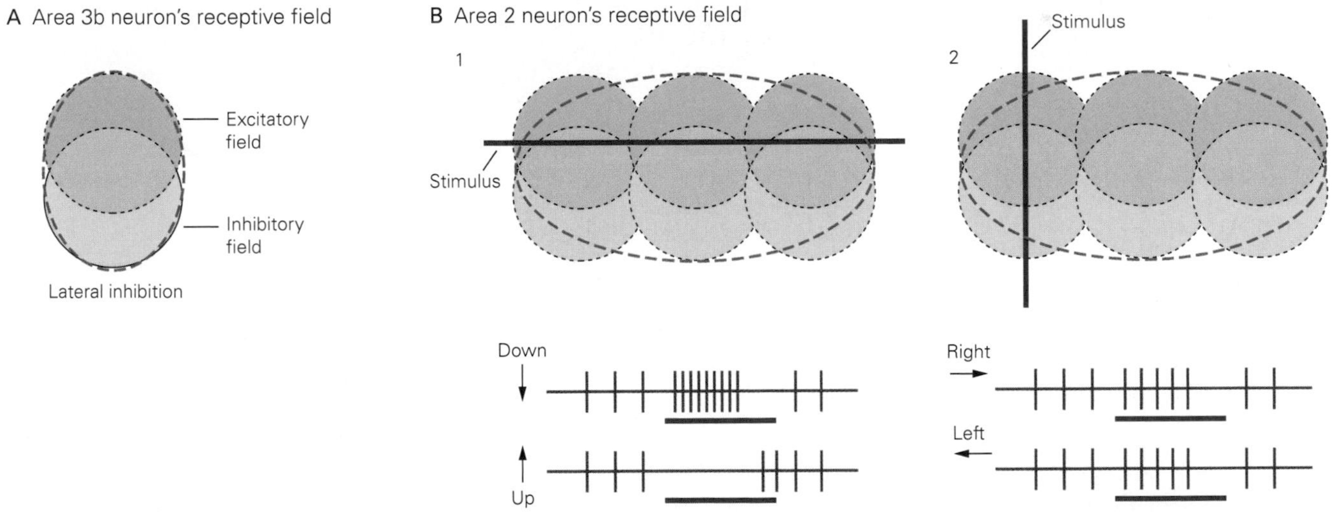

Figure 23–17 The spatial arrangement of excitatory and inhibitory inputs to a cortical neuron determines which features of a stimulus will be encoded by the neuron.

A. A neuron in area 3b of the primary somatosensory cortex has overlapping excitatory and inhibitory zones within its receptive field.

B. Convergence of three presynaptic neurons with the same arrangement of excitatory and inhibitory zones allows direction and orientation selectivity in a neuron in area 2. **1.** Downward motion of a horizontal bar across the receptive field of the postsynaptic cell produces a strong excitatory response because the excitatory fields of all three presynaptic neurons are contacted simultaneously. Upward motion of the bar strongly inhibits firing because it enters all three inhibitory fields first. The neuron responds poorly to upward motion through the excitatory field because the initial inhibition outlasts the stimulus. **2.** Motion of a vertical bar across the receptive field evokes a weak response because it simultaneously crosses the excitatory and inhibitory receptive fields of the input neurons. Motion to the left and right are not distinguished in this example.

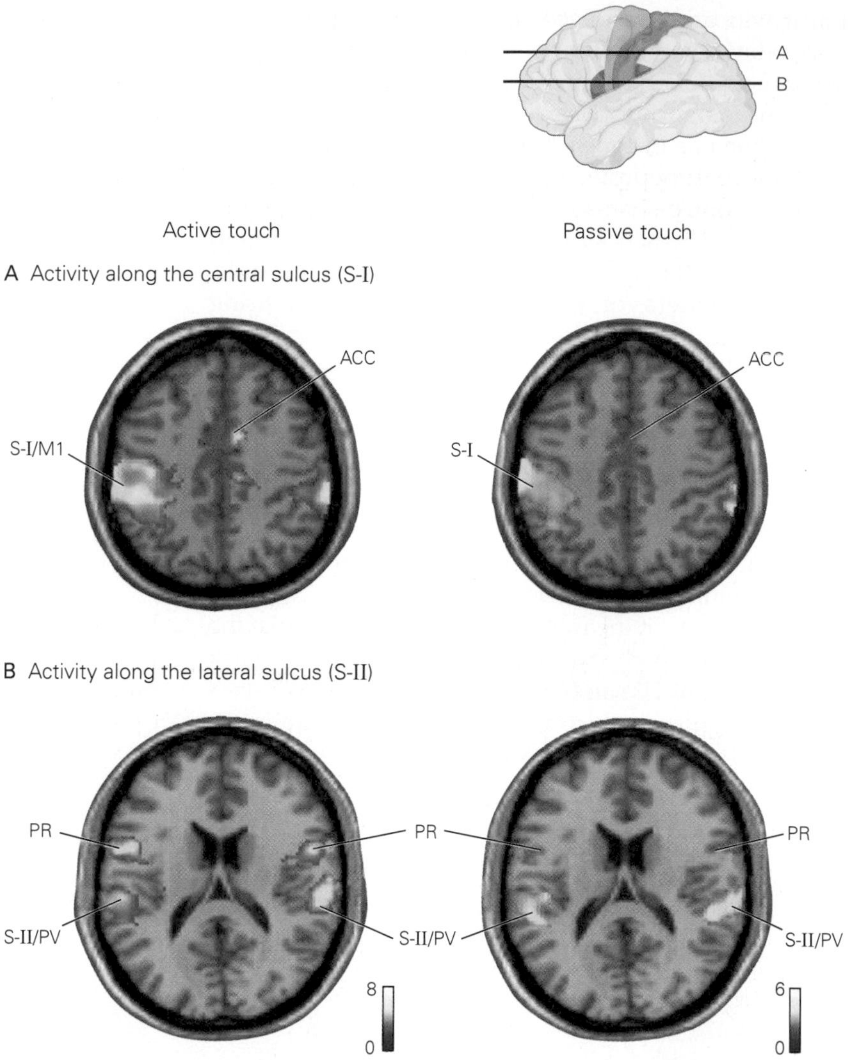

Figure 23–18 Active touch evokes more complex responses in S-I and S-II than passive touch. Cortical regions in the human brain stimulated by passive and active touch are localized using functional magnetic resonance imaging (fMRI). (Adapted, with permission, from Hinkley et al. 2007.)

A. Axial views of activity along the central sulcus during passive stroking of the right hand with a sponge (right panel) and during active touching of the sponge (left panel). Areas 3b and 1 are activated in the left hemisphere in both conditions. Active touch also engages the primary motor cortex (**M1**) in the left hemisphere, the anterior cingulate cortex (**ACC**), and evokes weak activity in the ipsilateral **S-I** (right hemisphere). These sites were confirmed independently using magnetoencephalography in the same subjects.

B. Axial views of activity along the Sylvian fissure in the same experiment. Bilateral activity occurs in **S-II** and the parietal ventral (**PV**) area during passive stroking and is stronger when the subject actively moves the hand. The parietal rostroventral area (**PR**) is active only during active touch. Magnetoencephalographic responses in S-II/PV and PR occur later than in S-I, reflecting serial processing of touch from S-I to S-II/PV, and from S-II/PV to PR.

significance. In light of the demonstration that the firing patterns of S-II neurons are modified by selective attention, S-II could make the decision whether a particular bit of tactile information is remembered.

Active Touch Engages Sensorimotor Circuits in the Posterior Parietal Cortex

The posterior parietal regions surrounding the intraparietal sulcus play an important role in the sensory guidance of movement rather than in discriminative touch. In monkeys these regions include areas 5 and 7 and in humans they include the superior parietal (Brodmann's areas 5 and 7) and inferior parietal cortex (areas 39 and 40).

Neurons in medial portions of area 5 receive postural information from SA2 fibers in the skin overlying the wrist, elbow, and shoulder, from receptors deep in these joints, and from muscle spindles that provide information about the movements of the arm. In monkeys these neurons are particularly sensitive when the animal extends its hand to grasp an object. Other cells located more laterally in area 5 integrate tactile and postural information from the hand. They respond most vigorously when the monkey shapes the hand in anticipation of grasping an object or plucks food morsels from a small container.

Neurons in area 7 of the monkey integrate tactile and visual stimuli that overlap in space and thus play an important role in eye-hand coordination. They respond more vigorously when the monkey is able to observe its hand while manipulating objects of interest than when simply looking at the object or handling it in the dark. Firing patterns in area 7 are also correlated with the hand posture used to grasp different objects.

It was originally believed that areas 5 and 7 were higher-order somatosensory areas that processed tactile information for object recognition and shape discrimination, and used proprioceptive signals for internal representations of integrated postures of the limbs. These theories were supported by anatomical data that showed that the principal sensory inputs to area 5 originate in area 2 of S-I cortex. However, these ideas about the role of areas 5 and 7 had to be altered following the discovery by Vernon Mountcastle, Juhani Hyvärinen, and others that these areas are involved in motor control.

In fact, during reaching and grasping, neural activity in the posterior parietal cortex coincides with activation of neurons in motor and premotor areas of

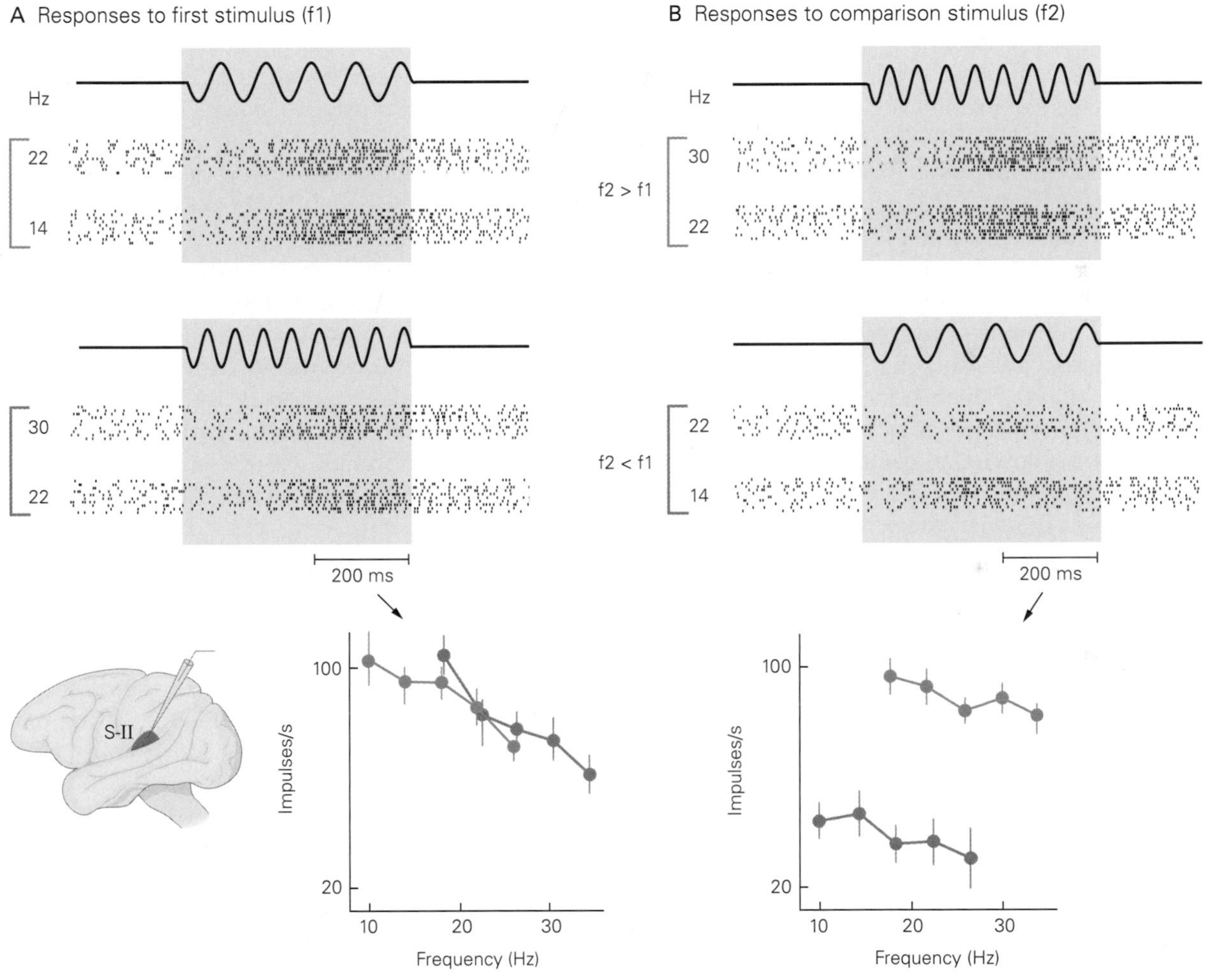

Figure 23–19 The sensitivity of an S-II neuron to vibratory stimuli is modulated by attention and behavioral conditions. A monkey was trained to compare two vibratory stimuli applied to the fingertips (f1 and f2) and to report which had the higher frequency. The plots show the mean firing rates of the neuron during each of the two stimuli. The animal's decision about which frequency is higher can be predicted from the neural data during each type of trial. The mean firing rates of this neuron are significantly higher at each stimulation frequency when f2 is greater than f1 (**blue**) than when f2 is less than f1 (**gold**). (Adapted, with permission, from Romo et al. 2002.)

A. Raster plots show the responses of an S-II neuron to various sample stimuli (f1). The vertical tick marks in each row denote action potentials, and individual rows are separate trials of the stimulus pairs. Trials are grouped according to the frequencies tested. The firing rate of the neuron encodes the vibratory frequency of the sample stimulus; it is higher for low-frequency vibration regardless of the subsequent events.

B. Each row in the raster plots illustrates responses to the comparison stimulus (f2) during the same trials shown in A. The neuron's response to f2 reflects the frequency of both f2 and f1. When f2 > f1 the neuron fires at high rates during f2 and the animal reports that f2 is the higher frequency. When f2 < f1 the neuron fires at low rates during f2 and the animal reports that f1 is the higher frequency. In this manner the responses of S-II neurons reflect the animal's memory of an earlier event.

the frontal cortex and precedes activity in S-I. There is strong evidence that area 5 receives convergent central and peripheral signals that allow it to compare central motor commands with peripheral sensory feedback during reaching and grasping behaviors. Sensory feedback from the hand to the posterior parietal cortex is used to confirm the goal of the planned action, thereby reinforcing a previously learned skill or correcting those plans when errors occur.

Predicting the sensory consequences of hand actions is an important component of active touch. For example, when we view an object and reach for it, we predict how heavy it should be and how it should feel in the hand; we use such predictions to initiate grasping. Daniel Wolpert and Randy Flanagan have proposed that during active touch the motor system controls the afferent flow of somatosensory information so that subjects can predict when tactile information should arrive in S-I and reach consciousness. Convergence of central and peripheral signals allows neurons to compare planned and actual movements. Corollary discharge from motor areas to somatosensory regions of the cortex may play a key role in active touch. It provides posterior parietal neurons with information on intended actions, allowing these neurons to compare planned and actual neural responses to tactile stimuli. Such mechanisms may explain why it is so difficult to tickle oneself.

Lesions in Somatosensory Areas of the Brain Produce Specific Tactile Deficits

Loss of tactile sensation in the hand produces significant motor as well as sensory deficits. Local anesthesia of the hand provides a direct way to appreciate the sensorimotor role of touch.

Loss of touch does not cause paralysis or weakness because much of skilled movement is predictive, relying on sensory feedback for adjustment if necessary. The motor system compensates for the absence of tactile information by generating more force than necessary. Under local anesthesia hand movements are clumsy and poorly coordinated, and force generation during grasping is abnormally slow. With the loss of tactile sensibility one is completely reliant on vision for directing the hand.

These motor problems are further exacerbated by long-term, chronic loss of tactile function because of injury to peripheral nerves or dorsal column lesions. Deafferentation produces major changes in the afferent connections in the brain (see Chapter 18), as do certain diseases. Myelinated afferent fibers in the dorsal columns degenerate in patients with demyelinating diseases, such as multiple sclerosis. In late-stage syphilis the large-diameter neurons in the dorsal root ganglia are destroyed (tabes dorsalis). These patients have severe chronic deficits in touch and proprioception but often little loss of temperature perception and nociception. The somatosensory losses are accompanied by motor deficits: clumsy and poorly coordinated movements and dystonia.

Similar impairments occur in patients with damage to S-I caused by stroke or head trauma, or following surgical excision of the postcentral gyrus. The severity and extent of the deficit depends on the site of the lesion. The sensory and motor deficits resulting from lesions in various parts of the parietal lobe have been compared in clinical studies.

Patients with lesions in the anterior parietal cortex have severe difficulties with simple tactile tests—touch thresholds, vibration and joint position sense, and two-point discrimination (Figure 23–20A). The patients also perform poorly on more complex tasks, such as texture discrimination, stereognosis, and visual-tactile matching tests. Motor deficits are less pronounced than sensory losses, particularly during tests of force and position control. Exploratory movements and skilled tasks, such as catching a ball or pinching small objects between the fingertips, are also somewhat abnormal.

In contrast, patients with lesions in the posterior parietal cortex have only mild difficulty with simple tactile tests. However, they have profound difficulty with complex tactile recognition tasks, and use few exploratory and skilled movements (Figure 23–20B). They display kinematic deficits when interacting with objects, failing to shape and orient the hand properly to grasp them, and misdirect the arm during reaching. They use too much grip force when an object is placed in their hand and are unable to direct the fingers properly when asked to evaluate its size and shape. These deficits are described clinically as the "useless hand" syndrome (tactile apraxia).

Humans with lesions localized to S-II also cannot perform complex tactile discrimination tasks such as stereognosis, but the deficits appear to be cognitive rather than sensorimotor. Mel Goodale and David Milner found that patients that are unable to discriminate the size of objects in clinical psychophysical tests are able to use visual information to match the shape of the hand to that of an object they must grasp. They propose that the dorsal parietal areas bordering the intraparietal sulcus serve a sensorimotor function, guiding hand movements in handling objects. The ventral somatosensory areas bordering the lateral sulcus serve a cognitive function, allowing us to recognize and name objects and thereby remember them.

Studies of sensory deficits in human patients are complicated by the fact that disease states or

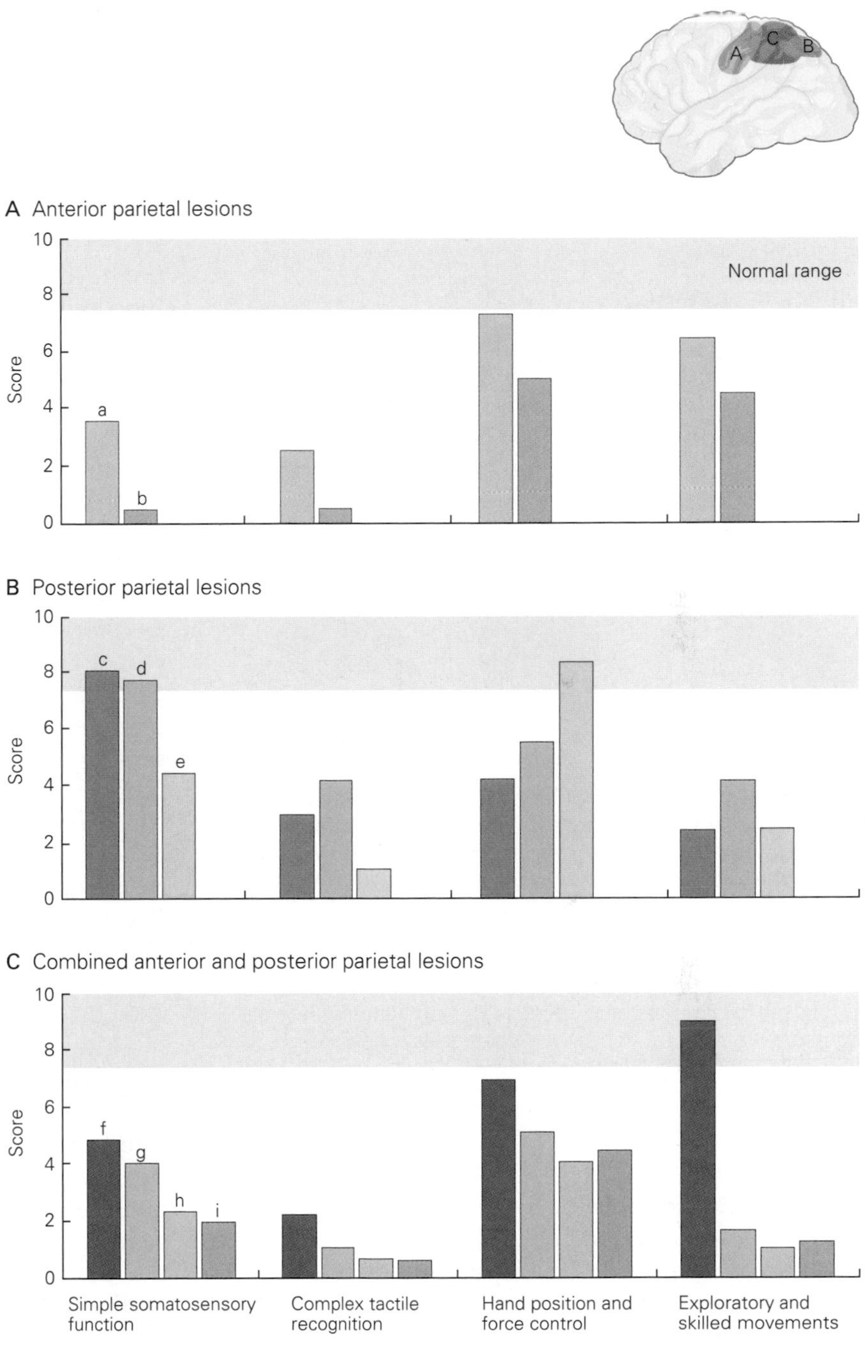

Figure 23–20 Lesions of anterior and posterior regions of the parietal lobe produce characteristic sensory and motor deficits of the hand. Bar graphs rank the performance of nine patients (a – i) on four sets of standardized tests of sensory and motor function of the hand. The behavioral scores are ranked from normal (10) to maximal deficit (0). The "normal range" shows the performance scores of these patients for the ipsilateral limb. Tests of *simple somatosensory function* include light touch from a 1 g force-calibrated probe, two-point discrimination on the finger and palm, vibration sense, and position sense of the index finger metacarpophalangeal joint. Tests of *complex tactile recognition* assess texture discrimination, form recognition, and size discrimination. Tests of *hand position and force control* measure grip force, tapping, and reaching to a target. Tests of *exploratory and skilled movements* evaluate insertion of pegs in slots, pincer grip of small objects, and exploratory movements when palpating objects. (Adapted, with permission, from Pause et al. 1989.)

A. Two patients with lesions to the anterior parietal lobe show severe impairment in both sets of tactile tests but only moderate impairment in the motor tasks.

B. Three patients with posterior parietal lesions show only minor deficits in simple somatosensory tests but severe impairment in complex tests of stereognosis and form. Motor deficits are greater in skilled tasks.

C. Four patients with combined lesions to anterior and posterior parietal cortex show severe impairment in all tests. Interestingly, the patient who showed the least impairment in this group (patient f) suffered brain damage at birth; the developing brain was able to compensate for the loss of major somatosensory areas. Lesions in the other patients resulted from strokes later in life.

trauma rarely produce a "clean" lesion confined to one localized brain area. For this reason analyses of experimentally controlled lesions in animals have been useful for understanding the etiology of the sensory deficits observed in human patients. For example, macaque monkeys with a lesion of the cuneate fascicle show chronic losses in tactile discrimination, such as higher touch thresholds, impaired vibration sense, and poor two-point discrimination. They also display major deficits in the control of fine finger movements during grooming, scratching, and manipulation of objects.

A similar deficit in the execution of skilled movements can be produced experimentally in monkeys by inhibiting the neurons in the hand-representation region of area 2. The animal has great difficulty coordinating movements of the fingers because tactile feedback is absent (Figure 23–21).

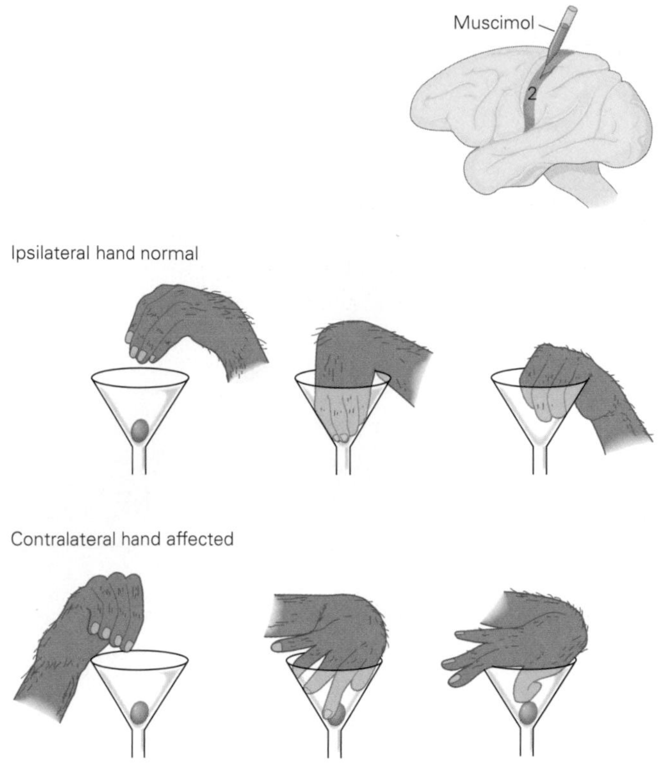

Figure 23–21 Finger coordination is disrupted when synaptic transmission in the somatic sensory cortex is inhibited in a monkey. Muscimol, a γ-aminobutyric acid (GABA) agonist that inhibits cortical cells, was injected into Brodmann's area 2 on the left side of a monkey's brain. Within minutes after injection the finger coordination of the right hand (contralateral) was severely disrupted; the monkey was unable to pick up a grape from a funnel. The injection effects are known to be specific to the injected hemisphere because the left hand (ipsilateral) continues to perform normally. (Adapted, with permission, from Hikosaka et al. 1985.)

Experimental ablation of somatosensory areas of the cortex has provided valuable information about the function of these areas. Small lesions limited to area 3b produce major deficits in touch sensation from a particular part of the body. Lesions in area 1 produce a defect in the assessment of the texture of objects, whereas lesions in area 2 alter the ability to differentiate the size and shape of objects. The resulting damage to tactile function is less severe when such lesions are made in infant animals, apparently because in the developing brain S-II cortex may take over functions normally assumed by S-I.

Removal of S-II cortex in monkeys causes severe impairment in the discrimination of both shape and texture and prevents the animals from learning new tactile discriminations. Ablation of area 5 produces deficits in roughness discrimination but few other alterations in passive touch. However, motor performance is severely compromised as these animals misdirect reaches to objects and fail to preshape the hand to grasp objects skillfully.

The similarity between the impairments observed in humans and monkeys is an important basis for understanding clinical losses of somatosensory function. We shall learn in later chapters that lesioning studies of other cortical areas in monkeys have also provided insight into higher-order sensory and motor functions of the brain.

An Overall View

When we explore an object with our hands a large part of the brain may become engaged by the sensory experience, by the thoughts and emotions it evokes, and by motor responses to it. These sensations result from the parallel actions of multiple cortical areas engaged in feed-forward and feedback networks.

At the first touch the peripheral sensory apparatus deconstructs the object into tiny segments, distributed over a large population of approximately 20,000 sensory nerve fibers. The SA1 system provides high-fidelity information about its spatial structure that is the basis of form and texture perception. The RA1 system conveys information about motion of the object in the hand, which enables us to manipulate it skillfully. The RA2 receptors transmit information about vibration of objects that allows us to use them as tools. The SA2 system provides information about the hand conformation and posture during grasping and other hand movements.

The information from these mechanoreceptors is conveyed to consciousness by the dorsal column fiber tracts of the spinal cord, relay nuclei in the brain stem and thalamus, and a hierarchy of intracortical pathways. By analyzing patterns of activity across the entire population, the brain constructs a neural representation of the object and the actions of the hand.

Central pathways have four important functions as they process the information from these mechanoreceptors. First, they convey the information provided by the receptors to the cognitive mechanisms responsible for perception. For this function the organization of these pathways is critical. A central theme is specificity: Computations of different kinds are kept separate by parallel pathways and by segregation of function at synaptic relays within single pathways.

Computations in these pathways are complex and accomplished serially, beginning in the dorsal column nuclei, progressing through the thalamus and several cortical stages, and terminating in regions of the medial temporal cortex concerned with memory and perception and in motor areas of the frontal lobe that mediate voluntary movements.

The brain's processing of touch is aided by the somatotopic organization of the neurons involved at each relay. Adjacent skin areas that are stimulated together are linked anatomically and functionally in central relays. Body parts that are especially sensitive to touch—the hands, feet, and mouth—are represented in large areas of the brain, reflecting the importance of tactile information conveyed from these regions.

The second function of the central pathways is transformation of the disaggregated representation of object properties in thousands of neurons to an integrated representation of complex object properties in a few neurons. Convergent excitatory connections between neurons representing neighboring skin areas and intracortical inhibitory circuits enable higher-order cortical cells to integrate global features of objects. In this manner the somatosensory areas of the brain represent properties common to particular classes of objects.

A third function is regulating the afferent flow of somatosensory information. The peripheral fibers deliver much more information than can be handled at any one moment; the central neural pathways compensate by selecting information for delivery to the mechanisms of perception and memory. Recurrent pathways from higher brain areas modify the ascending information provided by touch receptors, thus fitting the stream of sensory information to previous experience and task goals.

Finally, the touch system provides information necessary for the control and guidance of movement. Interactions between sensory and motor areas of parietal and frontal cortex provide a neural mechanism for predicting the sensory consequences of motor behaviors and for skill learning from repeated experience.

Esther P. Gardner
Kenneth O. Johnson

Selected Readings

Freund HJ. 2003. Somatosensory and motor disturbances in patients with parietal lobe lesions. Adv Neurol 93:179–193.

Hyvärinen J. 1982. Posterior parietal lobe of the primate brain. Physiol Rev 62:1060–1129.

Johnson KO. 2001. The roles and functions of cutaneous mechanoreceptors. Curr Opin Neurobiol 11:455–461.

Jones EG, Peters A (eds). 1986. *Cerebral Cortex.* Vol 5, *Sensory-Motor Areas and Aspects of Cortical Connectivity.* New York: Plenum Press.

Kaas JH, Gardner EP (eds). 2008. *The Senses: A Comprehensive Reference,* Vol. 6, *Somatosensation.* Oxford: Elsevier.

Kaas JH, Nelson RJ, Sur M, Merzenich MM. 1981. Organization of somatosensory cortex in primates. In: FO Schmitt, FG Worden, G Adelman, SG Dennis (eds). *The Organization of the Cerebral Cortex: Proceedings of a Neurosciences Research Program Colloquium,* pp. 237–261. Cambridge, MA: MIT Press.

Mountcastle VB. 1995. The parietal system and some higher brain functions. Cerebral Cortex 5:377–390.

Mountcastle VB. 2005. *The Sensory Hand: Neural Mechanisms of Somatic Sensation.* Cambridge MA: Harvard Univ. Press.

Romo R, Salinas E. 2001. Touch and go: decision-making mechanisms in somatosensation. Ann Rev Neurosci 24:107–137.

Wing AM, Haggard P, Flanagan JR (eds). 1996. *Hand and Brain.* San Diego CA: Academic Press.

References

Ageranioti-Bélanger SA, Chapman CE. 1992. Discharge properties of neurones in the hand area of primary somatosensory cortex in monkeys in relation to the performance of an active tactile discrimination task. II. Area 2 as compared to areas 3b and 1. Exp Brain Res 91:207–228.

Bell J, Bolanowski S, Holmes MH. 1994. The structure and function of Pacinian corpuscles: a review. Prog Neurobiol 42:79–128.

Bolanowski SJ, Gescheider GA, Verrillo RT, Checkosky CM. 1988. Four channels mediate the mechanical aspects of touch. J Acoust Soc Am 84:1680–1694.

Bolanowski SJ, Pawson L. 2003. Organization of Meissner corpuscles in the glabrous skin of monkey and cat. Somatosens Mot Res 20:223–231.

Brisben AJ, Hsiao SS, Johnson KO. 1999. Detection of vibration transmitted through an object grasped in the hand. J Neurophysiol 81:1548–1558.

Brochier T, Boudreau M-J, Paré M, Smith AM. 1999. The effects of muscimol inactivation of small regions of motor and somatosensory cortex on independent finger movements and force control in the precision grip. Exp Brain Res 128:31–40.

Carlson M. 1981. Characteristics of sensory deficits following lesions of Brodmann's areas 1 and 2 in the postcentral gyrus of *Macaca mulatta*. Brain Res 204:424–430.

Carlson M, Burton H. 1988. Recovery of tactile function after damage to primary or secondary somatic sensory cortex in infant *Macaca mulatta*. J Neurosci 8:833–859.

Chapman CE, Meftah el-M. 2005. Independent controls of attentional influences in primary and secondary somatosensory cortex. J Neurophysiol 94:4094–4107.

Chen LM, Turner GH, Friedman RM, Zhang N, Gore JC, Roe AW, Avison MJ. 2007. High-resolution maps of real and illusory tactile activation in primary somatosensory cortex in individual monkeys with functional magnetic resonance imaging and optical imaging. J Neurosci 27:9181–9191.

Costanzo RM, Gardner EP. 1980. A quantitative analysis of responses of direction-sensitive neurons in somatosensory cortex of alert monkeys. J Neurophysiol 43:1319–1341.

Culham JC, Valyear KF. 2006. Human parietal cortex in action. Curr Opin Neurobiol 16:205–212.

DiCarlo JJ, Johnson KO, Hsaio SS. 1998. Structure of receptive fields in area 3b of primary somatosensory cortex in the alert monkey. J Neurosci 18:2626–264.

Edin BB, Abbs JH. 1991. Finger movement responses of cutaneous mechanoreceptors in the dorsal skin of the human hand. J Neurophysiol 65:657–670.

Felleman DJ, Van Essen DC. 1991. Distributed hierarchical processing in the primate cerebral cortex. Cereb Cortex 1:1–47.

Fitzgerald PJ, Lane JW, Thakur PH, Hsiao SS. 2004. Receptive field properties of the macaque second somatosensory cortex: evidence for multiple functional representations. J Neurosci 24:11193–11204.

Flanagan JR, Vetter P, Johansson RS, Wolpert DM. 2003. Prediction precedes control in motor learning. Curr Biol 13:146–150.

Friedman DP, Murray EA, O'Neill JB, Mishkin M. 1986. Cortical connections of the lateral sulcus of macaques: evidence for a corticolimbic pathway for touch. J Comp Neurol 252:323–347.

Friedman RM, Chen LM, Roe AW. 2004. Modality maps within primate somatosensory cortex. Proc Natl Acad Sci U S A 101:12724–12729.

Gardner EP. 1988. Somatosensory cortical mechanisms of feature detection in tactile and kinesthetic discrimination. Can J Physiol Pharmacol 66:439–454.

Gardner EP. 2008. Dorsal and ventral streams in the sense of touch. In: JH Kaas, EP Gardner (eds). *The Senses: A Comprehensive Reference,* Vol. 6, *Somatosensation*, pp. 233–258. Oxford: Elsevier.

Gardner EP, Babu KS, Ghosh S, Sherwood A, Chen J. 2007. Neurophysiology of prehension: III. Representation of object features in posterior parietal cortex of the macaque monkey. J Neurophysiol 98:3708–3730.

Glendinning DS, Cooper BY, Vierck CJ, Leonard CM. 1992. Altered precision grasping in stumptail macaques after fasciculus cuneatus lesions. Somatosens Mot Res 9:61–73.

Goodwin AW, Browning AS, Wheat HE. 1995. Representation of curved surfaces in responses of mechanoreceptive afferent fibers innervating the monkey's fingerpad. J Neurosci 15:798–810.

Grinvald A, Shoham D, Shmuel A, Glaser DE, Vanzetta I, Shtoyerman E, Slovin H, et al. 1999. In-vivo optical imaging of cortical architecture and dynamics. In: U Windhorst, H Johansson (eds). *Modern Techniques in Neuroscience Research*, pp. 894–969. Heidelberg: Springer.

Hikosaka O, Tanaka M, Sakamoto M, Iwamura Y. 1985. Deficits in manipulative behaviors induced by local injections of muscimol in the first somatosensory cortex of the conscious monkey. Brain Res 325:375–380.

Hinkley LB, Krubitzer LA, Nagarajan SS, Disbrow EA. 2007. Sensorimotor integration in S2, PV, and parietal rostroventral areas of the human Sylvian fissure. J Neurophysiol 97:1288–1297.

Hsiao SS, O'Shaunessy DM, Johnson KO. 1993. Effects of selective attention on spatial form processing in monkey primary and secondary somatosensory cortex. J Neurophysiol 70:444–447.

Hyvärinen J, Poranen A. 1978. Movement-sensitive and direction and orientation-selective cutaneous receptive fields in the hand area of the post-central gyrus in monkeys. J Physiol (Lond) 283:523–537.

Iwamura Y, Iriki A, Tanaka M. 1994. Bilateral hand representation in the postcentral somatosensory cortex. Nature 369:554–556.

Iwamura Y, Tanaka M, Sakamoto M, Hikosaka O. 1993. Rostrocaudal gradients in neuronal receptive field complexity in the finger region of the alert monkey's postcentral gyrus. Exp Brain Res 92:360–368.

Jenmalm P, Birznieks I, Goodwin AW, Johansson RS. 2003. Influence of object shape on responses of human tactile afferents under conditions characteristic of manipulation. Eur J Neurosci 18:164–176.

Johansson RS. 1996. Sensory control of dexterous manipulation in humans. In: AM Wing, P Haggard, and JR Flanagan (eds). *Hand and Brain,* pp. 381–414. San Diego, CA: Academic Press.

Johansson RS, Vallbo ÅB. 1983. Tactile sensory coding in the glabrous skin of the human hand. Trends Neurosci 6: 27–32.

Johnson KO, Phillips JR. 1981. Tactile spatial resolution: I. Two-point discrimination, gap detection, grating resolution and letter recognition. J Neurophysiol 46: 1177–1191.

Jones EG, Friedman DP. 1982. Projection pattern of functional components of thalamic ventrobasal complex on monkey somatosensory cortex. J Neurophysiol 489:521–544.

Jones EG, Powell TPS. 1969. Connexions of the somatic sensory cortex of the rhesus monkey. I. Ipsilateral cortical connexions. Brain 92:477–502.

Khalsa PS, Friedman RM, Srinivasan MA, Lamotte RH. 1998. Encoding of shape and orientation of objects indented into the monkey fingerpad by populations of slowly and rapidly adapting mechanoreceptors. J Neurophysiol 79:3238–3251.

Klatzky RA, Lederman SJ, Metzger VA. 1985. Identifying objects by touch: an "expert system." Percept Psychophys 37:299–302.

Koch KW, Fuster JM. 1989. Unit activity in monkey parietal cortex related to haptic perception and temporary memory. Exp Brain Res 76:292–306.

LaMotte RH, Mountcastle VB. 1979. Disorders in somethesis following lesions of parietal lobe. J Neurophysiol 42: 400–419.

Milner AD, Goodale MA. 1995. *The Visual Brain in Action.* Oxford: Oxford Univ. Press.

Mountcastle VB. 1997. The columnar organization of the neocortex. Brain 120:701–722.

Mountcastle VB, LaMotte RH, Carli G. 1972. Detection thresholds for stimuli in humans and monkeys: comparison with threshold events in mechanoreceptive afferent fibers innervating the monkey hand. J Neurophysiol 35:122–136.

Mountcastle VB, Lynch JC, Georgopoulos AP, Sakata H, Acuna C. 1975. Posterior parietal association cortex of the monkey: command functions for operations within extrapersonal space. J Neurophysiol 38:871–908.

Murray EA, Mishkin M. 1984 Relative contributions of SII and area 5 to tactile discrimination in monkeys. Behav Brain Res 11:67–83.

Nelson RJ, Sur M, Felleman DJ, Kaas JH. 1980. Representations of the body surface in postcentral parietal cortex of *Macaca fascicularis.*J Comp Neurol 192:611–643.

Nolano M, Provitera V, Crisci C, Stancanelli A, Wendelschafer-Crabb G, Kennedy WR, Santoro L. 2003. Quantification of myelinated endings and mechanoreceptors in human digital skin. Ann Neurol 54:197–205.

Pandya DN, Seltzer B. 1982. Intrinsic connections and architectonics of posterior parietal cortex in the rhesus monkey. J Comp Neurol 204:196–210.

Pause M, Kunesch E, Binkofski F, Freund H-J. 1989. Sensorimotor disturbances in patients with lesions of the parietal cortex. Brain 112:1599–1625.

Phillips JR, Johansson RS, Johnson KO. 1992. Responses of human mechanoreceptive afferents to embossed dot arrays scanned across finger pad skin. J Neurosci 12: 827–839.

Pons TP, Garraghty PE, Cusick CG, Kaas JH. 1985. The somatotopic organization of area 2 in macaque monkeys. J Comp Neurol 241:445–466.

Pons TP, Garraghty PE, Mishkin M. 1992. Serial and parallel processing of tactual information in somatosensory cortex of rhesus monkeys. J Neurophysiol 68:518–527.

Quilliam TA. 1978. The structure of finger print skin. In: G Gordon (ed). *Active Touch,* pp. 1–18. Oxford: Pergamon Press.

Robinson CJ, Burton H. 1980. Somatic submodality distribution within the second somatosensory (SII), 7b, retroinsular, postauditory and granular insular cortical areas of *M. fascicularis.* J Comp Neurol 192:93–108.

Romo R, Hernandez A, Zainos A, Lemus L, Brody CD. 2002. Neuronal correlates of decision-making in secondary somatosensory cortex. Nat Neurosci 5:1217–1235.

Shoham D, Grinvald A. 2001. The cortical representation of the hand in macaque and human area S-I: high resolution optical imaging. J Neurosci 21:6820–6835.

Snider WD. 1998. How do you feel? Neurotrophins and mechanotransduction. Nat Neurosci 1(1):5–6.

Srinivasan MA, LaMotte RH. 1991. Encoding of shape in the responses of cutaneous mechanoreceptors. In: O Franzen, J Westman (eds). *Wenner Gren International Symposium Series: Information Processing in the Somatosensory System,* pp. 59–69. London: Macmillan.

Sripati AP, Yoshioka T, Denchev P, Hsiao SS, Johnson KO. 2006. Spatiotemporal receptive fields of peripheral afferents and cortical area 3b and 1 neurons in the primate somatosensory system. J Neurosci 26:2101–2114.

Sur M, Merzenich M, Kaas JH. 1980. Magnification, receptive-field area, and "hypercolumn" size in areas 3b and 1 of somatosensory cortex in owl monkeys. J Neurophysiol 44:295–311.

Sur M, Wall JT, Kaas JH. 1984. Modular distribution of neurons with slowly adapting and rapidly adapting responses in area 3b of somatosensory cortex in monkeys. J Neurophysiol 56:598–622.

Vega-Bermudez F, Johnson KO. 1999. Surround suppression in the responses of primate SA1 and RA mechanoreceptive afferents mapped with a probe array. J Neurophysiol 81:2711–2719.

Warren S, Hämäläinen HA, Gardner EP. 1986. Objective classification of motion- and direction-sensitive neurons in primary somatosensory cortex of awake monkeys. J Neurophysiol 56:598–622.

Weinstein S. 1968. Intensive and extensive aspects of tactile sensitivity as a function of body part, sex, and laterality. In: DR Kenshalo (ed). *The Skin Senses,* pp. 195–222. Springfield, IL: Thomas.

Westling G, Johansson RS. 1987. Responses in glabrous skin mechanoreceptors during precision grip in humans. Exp Brain Res 66:128–140.

24

Pain

PAIN DESCRIBES THE UNPLEASANT sensory and emotional experiences associated with actual or potential tissue damage. Pricking, burning, aching, stinging, and soreness are among the most distinctive of all the sensory modalities. As with the other somatic sensory modalities—touch, pressure, and position sense—pain serves an important protective function, alerting us to injuries that require evasion or treatment. In children born with insensitivity to pain, severe injuries often go unnoticed and can lead to permanent tissue damage. Yet pain is unlike other somatic sensory modalities, or vision, hearing, and smell in that it has an urgent and primitive quality, possessing both affective and emotional components.

The perception of pain is subjective and is influenced by many factors. An identical sensory stimulus can elicit quite distinct responses in the same individual under different conditions. Many wounded soldiers, for example, do not feel pain until they have been removed from the battlefield; injured athletes are often not aware of pain until a game is over. Simply put, there are no purely "painful" stimuli, sensory stimuli that invariably elicit the perception of pain in all individuals. The variability of the perception of pain is yet another example of a principle that we have encountered in earlier chapters: Pain is not the direct expression of a sensory event but rather the product of elaborate processing by the brain of a variety of neural signals.

When pain is experienced it can be acute, persistent, or in extreme cases chronic. Persistent pain characterizes many clinical conditions and is usually the reason that patients seek medical attention. In contrast, chronic pain appears to have no useful purpose; it only makes patients miserable. Pain's highly individual and subjective nature is one of the factors that make it so difficult to define objectively and to treat clinically.

In this chapter we discuss the neural processes that underlie the perception of pain in normal individuals and explain the origins of some of the abnormal pain states that are encountered clinically.

Noxious Insults Activate Nociceptors

Many organs in the periphery, including skin and subcutaneous structures such as joints and muscles, possess specialized sensory receptors that are activated by noxious insults. Unlike the specialized somatosensory receptors for light touch and pressure, most of these *nociceptors* are simply the free nerve endings of primary sensory neurons. There are three main classes of nociceptors—thermal, mechanical, and polymodal—as well as a more enigmatic fourth class, termed silent nociceptors.

Thermal nociceptors are activated by extremes in temperature, typically greater than 45°C (115°F) or less than 5°C (41°F). They are the peripheral endings of small-diameter, thinly myelinated Aδ axons that conduct action potentials at speeds of 5 to 30 m/s (Figure 24–1A). *Mechanical nociceptors* are activated optimally by intense pressure applied to the skin; they too are the endings of thinly myelinated Aδ axons. *Polymodal nociceptors* can be activated by high-intensity mechanical, chemical, or thermal (both hot and cold) stimuli. This class of nociceptors is found at the ends of small-diameter, unmyelinated C axons that conduct more slowly, at speeds less than 1.0 m/s (Figure 24–1A).

These three classes of nociceptors are widely distributed in skin and deep tissues and are often coactivated.

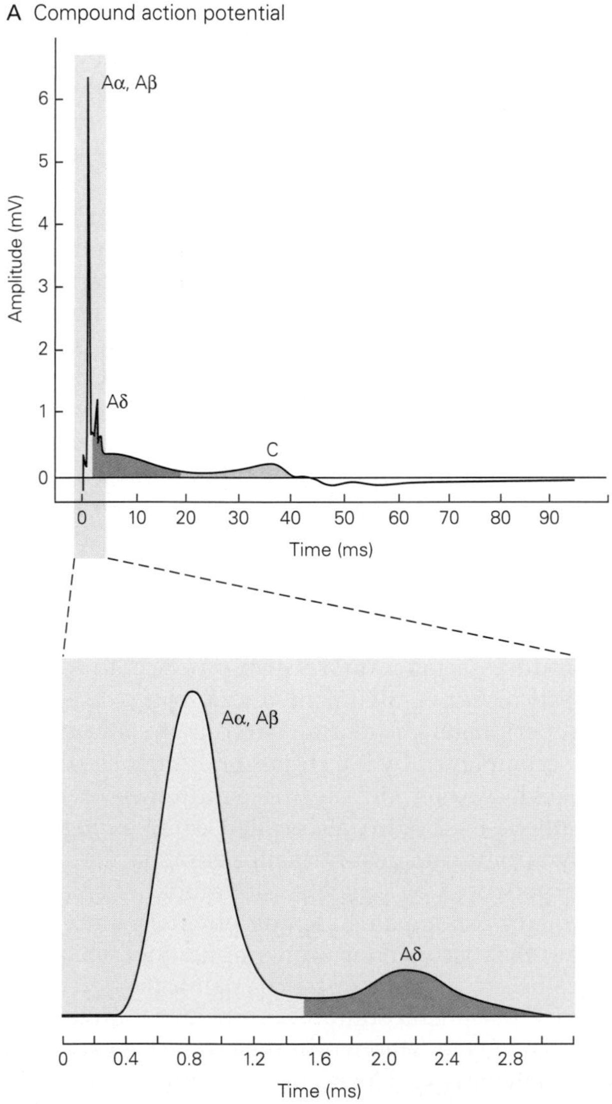

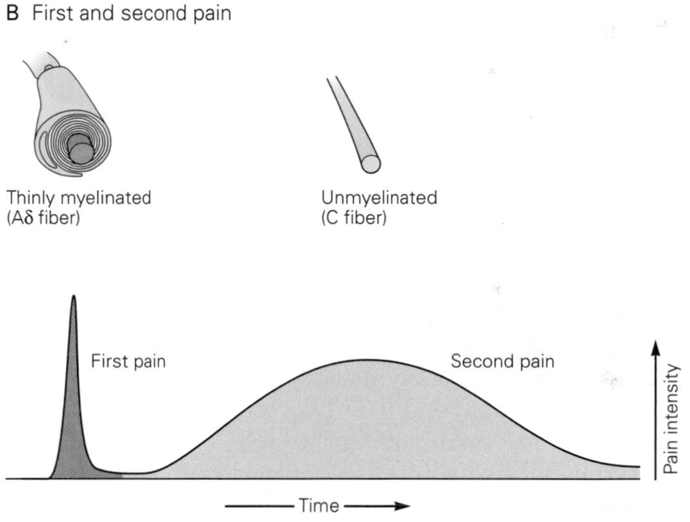

Figure 24–1 Propagation of action potentials in different classes of nociceptive fibers.

A. The speed at which action potentials are conducted is a function of each fiber's cross-sectional diameter. Wave peaks in the figure are labeled alphabetically in order of latency. The first peak and its subdivisions are the summed electrical activity of myelinated A fibers. A delayed (slowly conducting) deflection represents the summed action potentials of unmyelinated C fibers. The compound action potential of the A fibers is shown on a faster time-base to depict the summation of the action potentials of several fibers. (Modified, with permission, from Perl 2007.)

B. First and second pain are carried by two different primary afferent fibers. (Modified, with permission, from Fields 1987.)

When a hammer hits your thumb, you initially feel a sharp pain ("first pain") followed by a more prolonged aching and sometimes burning pain ("second pain") (Figure 24–1B). The fast sharp pain is transmitted by Aδ fibers that carry information from damaged thermal and mechanical nociceptors. The slow dull pain is transmitted by C fibers that convey signals from polymodal nociceptors.

Silent nociceptors are found in the viscera. This class of receptors is not normally activated by noxious stimulation; instead, inflammation and various chemical agents dramatically reduce their firing threshold. Their activation is thought to contribute to the emergence of secondary hyperalgesia and central sensitization, two prominent pain syndromes.

Noxious stimuli depolarize the bare nerve endings of afferent axons and generate action potentials that are propagated centrally. How is this achieved? The membrane of the nociceptor contains receptors that convert the thermal, mechanical, or chemical energy of noxious stimuli into a depolarizing electrical potential. One such protein is a member of a large family of so-called transient receptor potential (TRP) ion channels. This receptor-channel, TRPV1, is expressed selectively by nociceptive neurons and mediates the pain-producing actions of capsaicin, the active ingredient of hot peppers, and many other pungent chemicals. The TRPV1 channel is also activated by noxious thermal stimuli, which suggests that it normally transduces the sensation of painful heat. In addition, TRPV1-mediated membrane currents are enhanced by a reduction in pH, a characteristic of the chemical milieu of inflammation.

Additional members of the TRP channel family are expressed by nociceptive neurons, and the variety of TRP channels in nociceptors is thought to underlie the perception of a wide range of temperatures from extreme cold to intense heat. The TRPV2 channel is expressed predominantly in Aδ fiber terminals and is activated by very high temperatures, whereas the TRPM8 channel is activated by low temperatures and by chemicals such as menthol (Figure 24–2).

In addition to this constellation of TRP channels, other receptors and ion channels that participate in the transduction of peripheral stimuli are expressed in nociceptive sensory endings. Nociceptors selectively express tetrodotoxin-resistant Na^+ channels. One Na^+ channel (SCN9A, also called $Na_V1.7$) plays a key role in the perception of pain in humans, as revealed by the rare pain-insensitive individuals who possess mutations in the corresponding gene. One class of mutations inactivates the SCN9A channel and results in a complete inability to sense pain. But in all other respects these individuals are healthy and exhibit normal sensory responses to touch, mild temperature, proprioception, tickle, and pressure. A second class of mutations in the SCN9A gene changes the inactivation kinetics of this channel; individuals with these mutations exhibit an inherited condition called paroxysmal extreme pain disorder, characterized by rectal, ocular, and submandibular pain.

Nociceptors also express an ionotropic purinergic receptor, PTX3, that is activated by adenosine triphosphate (ATP) released from peripheral cells after tissue damage. In addition, they express members of the Mas-related G protein-coupled receptor (Mrg) family, which are activated by peptide ligands and serve to sensitize nociceptors to other chemicals released in their local environment (see Figure 24–7). These receptors and channels provide attractive targets for the development of drugs with actions selective for nociceptive sensory neurons.

The uncontrolled activation of nociceptors is associated with several pathological conditions. Allodynia and hyperalgesia are two common pain states that reflect changes in nociceptor activity. Patients with *allodynia* feel pain in response to stimuli that are normally innocuous: by a light stroking of sunburned skin, by the movement of joints in patients with rheumatoid arthritis, and even by the act of getting out of bed in the morning after a vigorous workout. Nevertheless, patients with allodynia do not feel pain constantly; in the absence of a peripheral stimulus there is no pain. In contrast, patients with *hyperalgesia*—an exaggerated response to noxious stimuli—typically report persistent pain in the absence of sensory stimulation.

Persistent pain can be subdivided into two broad classes, nociceptive and neuropathic. *Nociceptive pain* results from the activation of nociceptors in the skin or soft tissue in response to tissue injury, and it usually arises from an accompanying inflammation. Sprains and strains produce mild forms of nociceptive pain, whereas arthritis or a tumor that invades soft tissue produces a much more severe nociceptive pain. *Neuropathic pain* results from direct injury to nerves in the peripheral or central nervous system and is often accompanied by a burning or electric sensation. Neuropathic pains include the syndromes of reflex sympathetic dystrophy, also called complex regional pain syndrome, and post-herpetic neuralgia, the severe pain experienced by patients after a bout of shingles. Other neuropathic pains include phantom limb pain, the pain that occurs after limb amputation, which we discuss below. In some instances pain can even occur without a peripheral stimulus, a phenomenon termed *anesthesia dolorosa*. This syndrome can be triggered following attempts to block chronic pain, for example

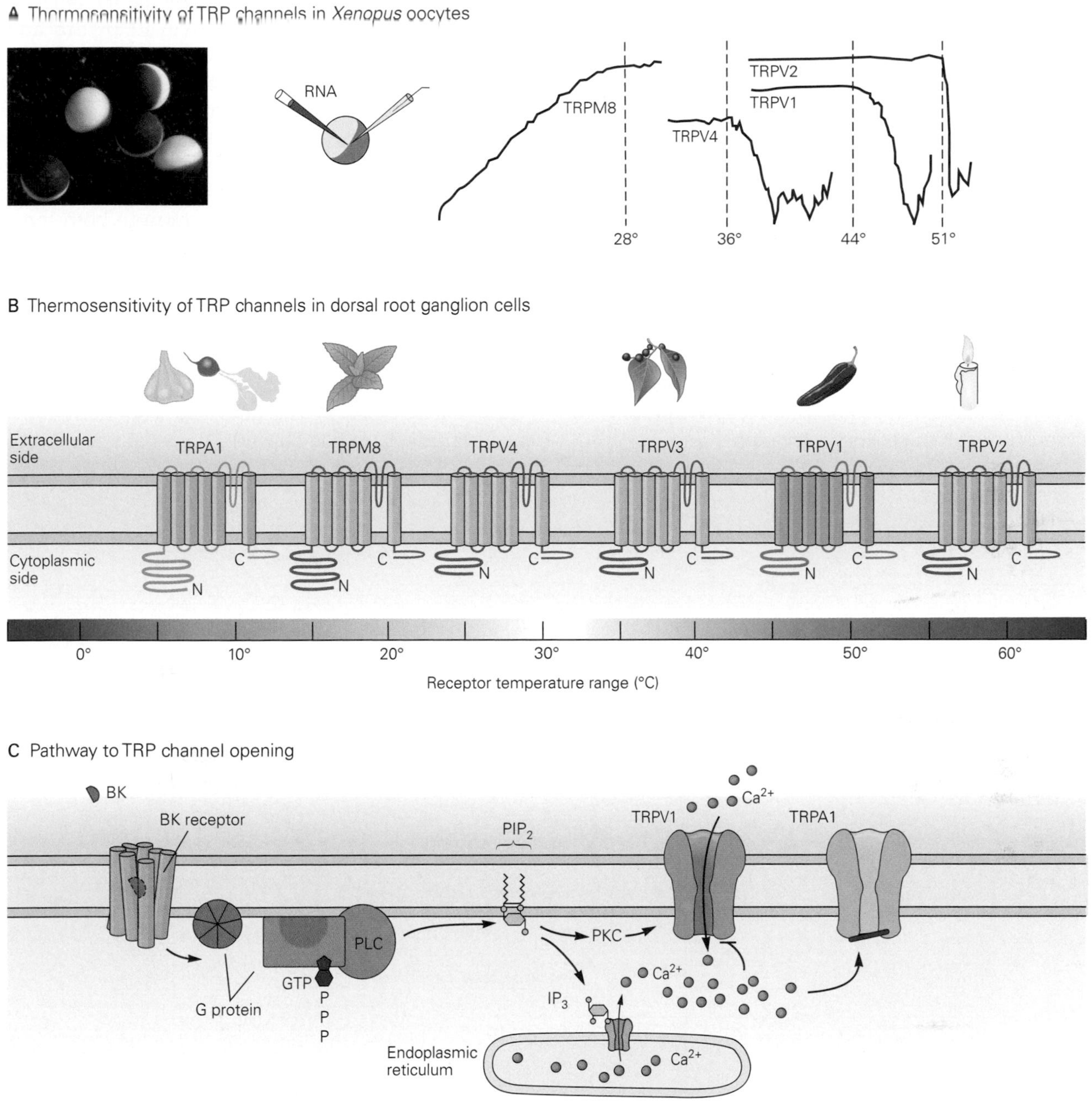

Figure 24–2 Transient receptor potential ion channels in nociceptive neurons.

A. *Xenopus* oocytes are injected with mRNA encoding transient receptor potential (TRP) channels. Electrophysiological recordings from the oocytes reveal the thermosensitivity of the channels. The temperature (centigrade) at which a specific TRP channel is activated is shown by the downward deflection of the recording. (Photograph on left reproduced, with permission, from Erwin Sigel 1987. Traces on the right reproduced, with permission, from Tominaga and Caterina 2004.)

B. Temperature response profiles of different TRP channels expressed by dorsal root ganglion neurons. (Modified, with permission, from Jordt, McKemy, and Julius 2003; Dhaka, Viswanath, and Patapoutian 2006.)

C. Bradykinin (BK) binds to G protein-coupled receptors on the surface of primary afferent neurons to activate phospholipase C (PLC), leading to the hydrolysis of membrane phosphatidylinositol bisphosphate (PIP_2), the production of inositol 1,4,5-trisphosphate (IP_3), and the release of Ca^{2+} from intracellular stores. Activation of protein kinase C (PKC) regulates TRP channel activity. The TRPV1 channel is sensitized, leading to channel opening and Ca^{2+} influx. (Modified, with permission, from Bautista et al. 2007.)

after therapeutic transection of sensory afferent fibers in the dorsal roots.

Signals from Nociceptors Are Conveyed to Neurons in the Dorsal Horn of the Spinal Cord

The perception of noxious stimuli arises from signals in the peripheral axonal branches of nociceptive sensory neurons whose cell bodies are located in dorsal root ganglia or the trigeminal ganglia. The central branches of these neurons terminate in the spinal cord in a highly orderly manner. Most terminate in the dorsal horn. Primary afferent neurons that convey distinct sensory modalities terminate in different laminae (Figure 24–3B). Thus there is a tight link between the anatomical organization of dorsal horn neurons, their receptive properties, and their function in sensory processing.

Many neurons in the most superficial lamina of the dorsal horn, termed *lamina I* or the *marginal layer*, respond to noxious stimuli conveyed by Aδ and C fibers. Because they respond selectively to noxious stimulation they have been called *nociception-specific neurons*. This set of neurons projects to higher brain centers, notably the thalamus. A second class of lamina I neurons receives input from C fibers that are activated selectively by intense cold. Other classes of lamina I neurons respond in a graded fashion to both innocuous and noxious mechanical stimulation and thus are termed *wide-dynamic-range neurons*.

Lamina II, the substantia gelatinosa, is a densely packed layer that contains many different classes of local interneurons, some excitatory and others inhibitory. Some of these interneurons respond selectively to nociceptive inputs, whereas others also respond to innocuous stimuli. Laminae III and IV contain a mixture of

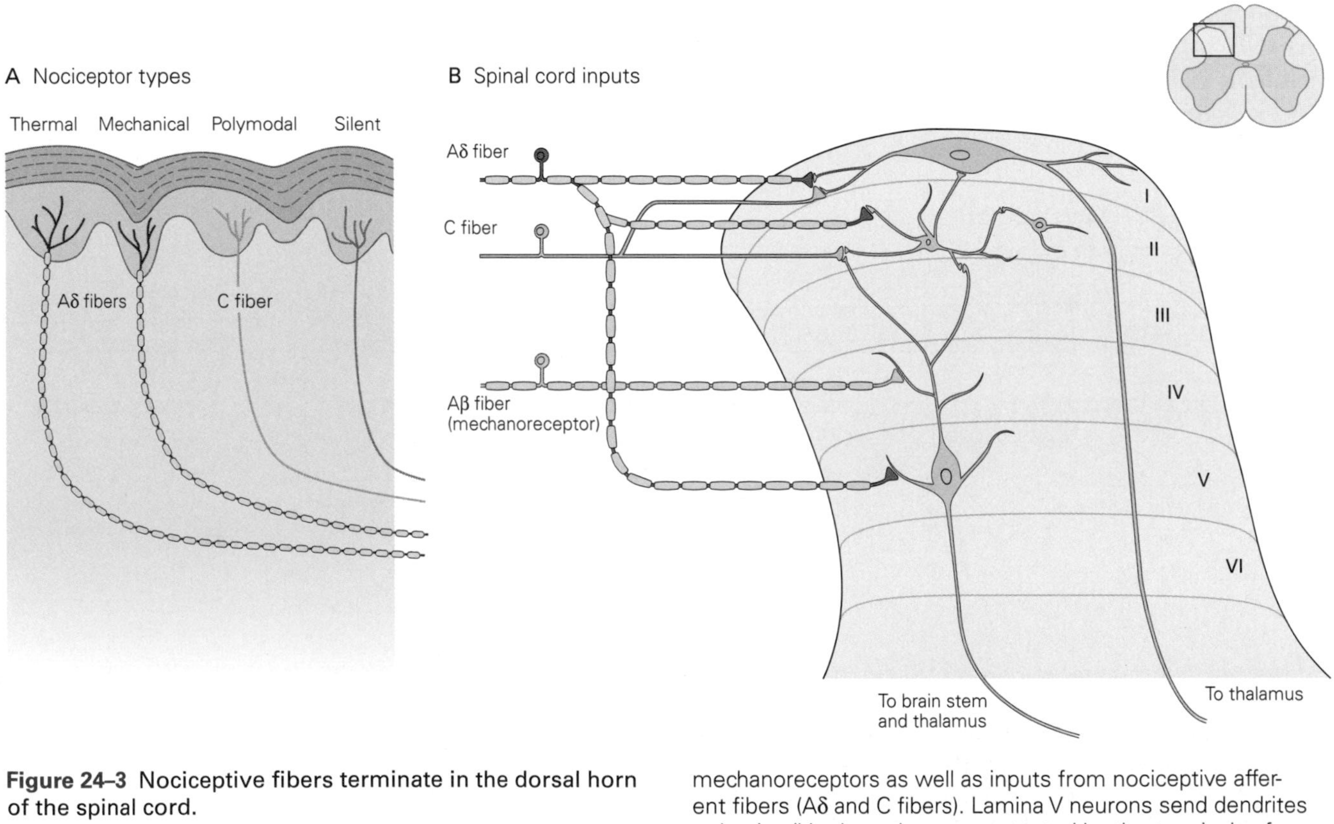

Figure 24–3 Nociceptive fibers terminate in the dorsal horn of the spinal cord.

A. Peripheral nociceptor classes.

B. Neurons in lamina I of the dorsal horn receive direct input from myelinated (Aδ) nociceptive fibers and both direct and indirect input from unmyelinated (C) nociceptive fibers via interneurons in lamina II. Lamina V neurons receive low-threshold input from large-diameter myelinated fibers (Aβ) of mechanoreceptors as well as inputs from nociceptive afferent fibers (Aδ and C fibers). Lamina V neurons send dendrites to lamina IV, where they are contacted by the terminals of Aβ primary afferents. Dendrites in lamina III arising from cells in lamina V are contacted by the axon terminals of lamina II interneurons. Aα fibers innervate motor neurons and interneurons in the ventral spinal cord (not shown). (Modified, with permission, from Fields 1987.)

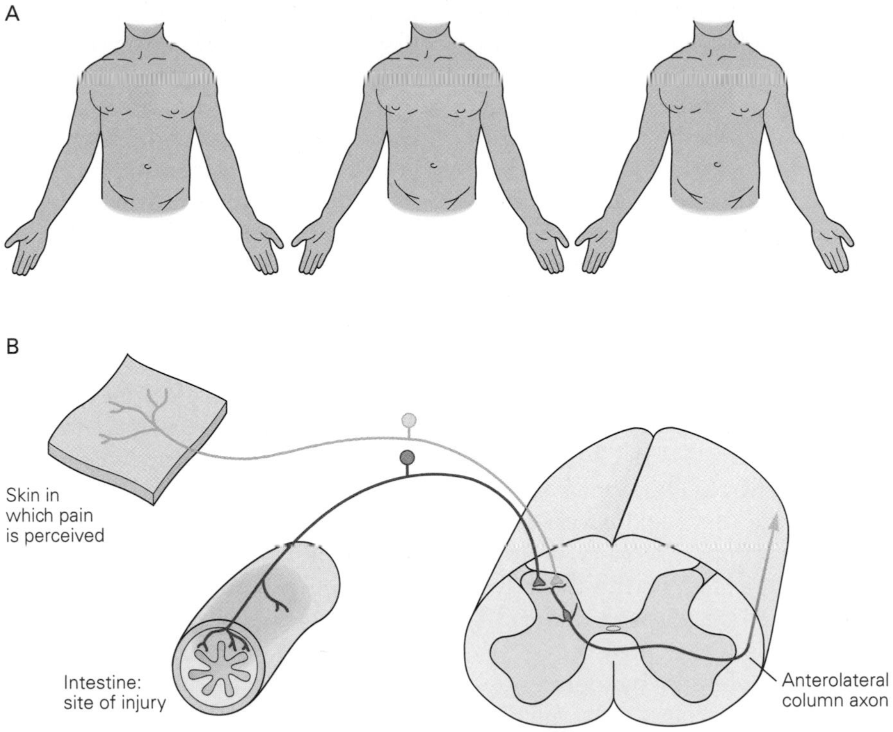

Figure 24–4 **Signals from nociceptors in the viscera can be felt as "referred pain" elsewhere in the body.**

A. Myocardial infarction and angina can be experienced as deep referred pain in the chest and left arm. The source of the pain can be readily predicted from the site of referred pain.

B. Convergence of visceral and somatic afferent fibers may account for referred pain. Nociceptive afferent fibers from the viscera and fibers from specific areas of the skin converge on the same projection neurons in the dorsal horn. The brain has no way of knowing the actual site of the noxious stimulus and mistakenly associates a signal from a visceral organ with an area of skin. (Adapted, with permission, from Fields 1987.)

local interneurons and supraspinal projection neurons. Many of these neurons receive input from Aβ afferent fibers that respond to innocuous cutaneous stimuli, such as the deflection of hairs and light pressure. Lamina V contains neurons that respond to a wide variety of noxious stimuli and project to the brain stem and thalamus. These neurons receive direct inputs from Aβ and Aδ fibers and, because their dendrites extend into lamina II, are also innervated by C fiber nociceptors (Figure 24–3B).

Neurons in lamina V also receive input from nociceptors in visceral tissues. The convergence of somatic and visceral nociceptive inputs onto individual lamina V neurons provides one explanation for a phenomenon called "referred pain," a condition in which pain from injury to a visceral tissue is perceived as originating from a region of the body surface. Patients with myocardial infarction, for example, frequently report pain from the left arm as well as the chest (Figure 24–4). This phenomenon occurs because a single lamina V neuron receives sensory input from both regions, and thus a signal from this neuron does not inform higher brain centers about the source of the input. As a consequence, the brain often incorrectly attributes the pain to the skin, possibly because cutaneous inputs predominate. Another anatomical explanation for instances of referred pain is that the axons of nociceptive sensory neurons branch in the periphery, innervating both skin and visceral targets.

Neurons in lamina VI receive inputs from large-diameter fibers that innervate muscles and joints. These neurons are activated by innocuous joint movement and do not contribute to the transmission of nociceptive information. In contrast, many neurons located in laminae VII and VIII, the intermediate and ventral regions of the spinal cord, do respond to noxious stimuli. These neurons typically have complex response properties because the inputs from nociceptors to these neurons are conveyed through many intervening synapses. Neurons in lamina VII often respond to stimulation of either side of the body, whereas most dorsal horn neurons receive unilateral input. The activation of lamina VII neurons is therefore thought to contribute to the diffuse quality of many pain conditions.

Nociceptive sensory neurons that activate neurons in the dorsal horn of the spinal cord release two major classes of neurotransmitters. Glutamate is the primary neurotransmitter of all primary sensory neurons, regardless of sensory modality. Neuropeptides are released as cotransmitters by many nociceptors with unmyelinated axons. These peptides include substance P, calcitonin gene–related peptide (CGRP), somatostatin, and galanin (Figure 24–5). Glutamate is stored in small, electron-lucent vesicles, whereas peptides are sequestered in large, dense-core vesicles at the central terminals of nociceptive sensory neurons (Figure 24–6). Separate storage sites permit these two classes of neurotransmitters to be released under different physiological conditions.

Of the neuropeptides expressed by nociceptive sensory neurons, the actions of substance P, a member of the neurokinin peptide family, have been studied in most detail. Substance P is released from the central terminals of nociceptive afferents in response to tissue injury or after intense stimulation of peripheral nerves. Its interaction with neurokinin receptors on dorsal horn neurons elicits slow excitatory postsynaptic potentials that prolong the depolarization elicited by glutamate. Although the physiological actions of glutamate and neuropeptides on dorsal horn neurons are different, these transmitters act coordinately to regulate the firing properties of dorsal horn neurons.

There is no efficient means for peptide reuptake into nerve terminals, so neuropeptides released from sensory terminals diffuse over a greater distance than glutamate and thus have excitatory influences on many dorsal horn neurons in the immediate vicinity of the release site. This diffuse signaling system may contribute to the poorly localized character of many pain conditions. In addition, the levels of neuropeptide expression in primary nociceptive neurons are elevated in some pathological conditions. Such reactive changes in peptide expression may contribute to the enhanced excitability of dorsal horn neurons that accompanies some chronic pain states.

Details of the interaction of neuropeptides with their receptors on dorsal horn neurons have suggested strategies for pain regulation. Infusion of substance P coupled to a neurotoxin into the dorsal horn of experimental animals results in selective destruction of neurons that express neurokinin receptors. Animals treated in this way fail to develop the central sensitization that is normally associated with peripheral injury. This method of neuronal ablation is more selective than traditional surgical interventions such as partial spinal cord transection (anterolateral cordotomy) and is being explored as a treatment for patients suffering from chronic pain syndrome.

Hyperalgesia Has Both Peripheral and Central Origins

Up to this point we have considered the mechanisms that convey noxious signals in the normal physiological state. But the normal process of sensory signaling can be dramatically altered when peripheral tissue is damaged, resulting in an increase in pain sensitivity or hyperalgesia. This condition can be elicited by sensitizing peripheral nociceptors through repetitive exposure to noxious mechanical stimuli (Figures 24–7).

The sensitization is triggered by a complex mix of chemicals released from damaged cells that accumulate at the site of tissue injury. This cocktail contains peptides and proteins such as bradykinin, substance P, and nerve growth factor, as well as molecules such as ATP, histamine, serotonin, prostaglandins, leukotrienes, and acetylcholine. Many of these chemical mediators are released from distinct cell types, but together they act to decrease the threshold of nociceptor activation.

Where do these chemicals come from and what exactly do they do? Histamine is released from mast cells after tissue injury and activates polymodal nociceptors. The lipid anandamide, an endogenous cannabinoid agonist, is released under conditions of inflammation, activates the TRPV1 channel, and may trigger pain associated with inflammation. ATP, acetylcholine, and serotonin are released from damaged endothelial cells and platelets; they act indirectly to sensitize nociceptors by triggering the release of chemical agents such as prostaglandins and bradykinin from peripheral cells. Bradykinin is one of the most active pain-producing agents. Its potency stems in part from the fact that it directly activates Aδ and C nociceptors as well as increasing the synthesis and release of prostaglandins from nearby cells.

Damaged cells also release prostaglandins, metabolites of arachidonic acid that are generated through the activity of cyclooxygenase (COX) enzymes that cleave arachidonic acid. The COX2 enzyme is preferentially induced under conditions of peripheral inflammation, contributing to enhanced pain sensitivity. The enzymatic pathways of prostaglandin synthesis are targets

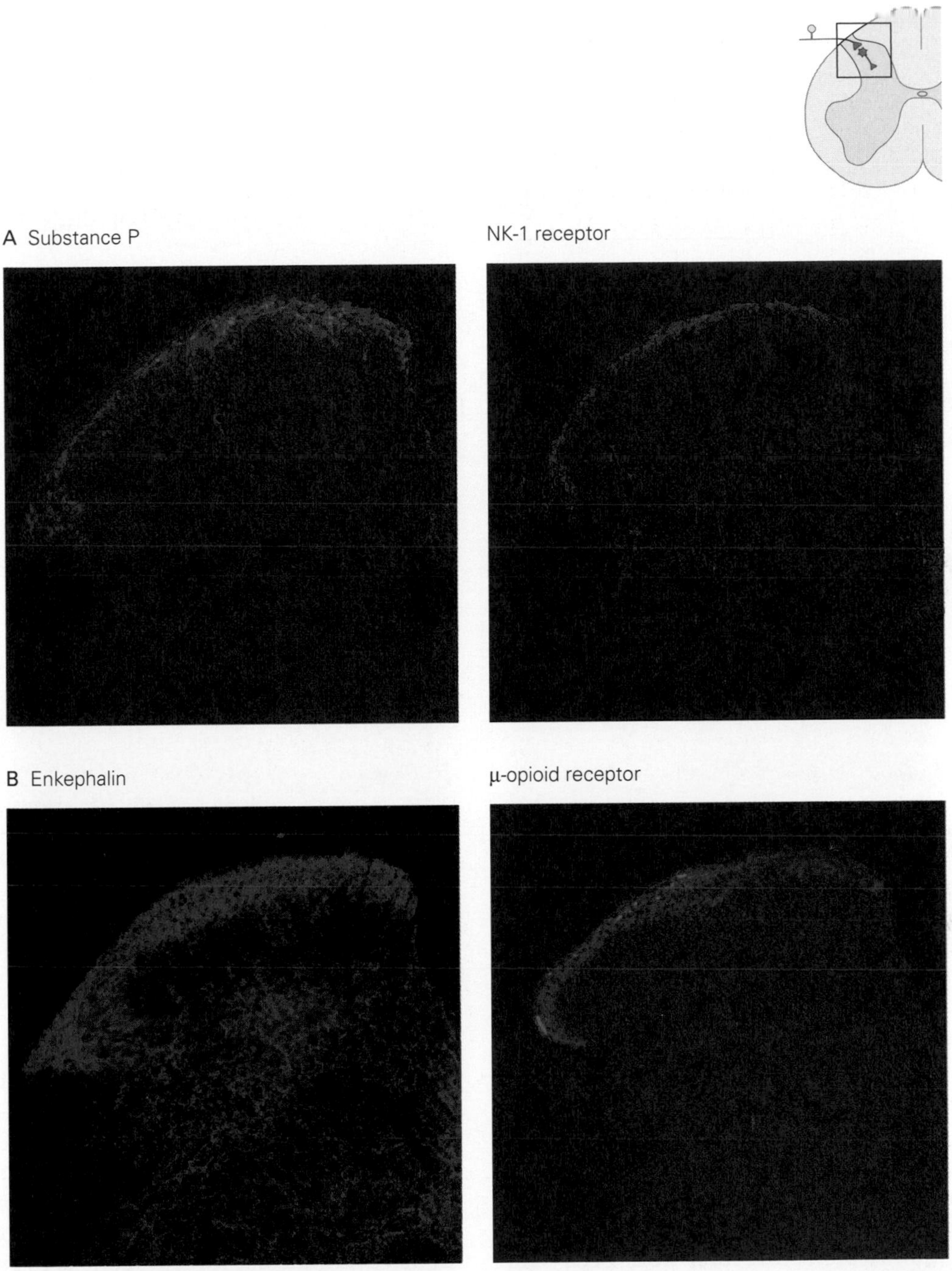

Figure 24–5 Neuropeptides and their receptors in the superficial dorsal horn of the rat spinal cord. (Images from A. Basbaum, reproduced with permission.)

A. Substance P is concentrated in the terminals of primary sensory neurons in the superficial dorsal horn. Its receptor, neurokinin-1 antagonist (NK1) is also expressed by neurons in the superficial dorsal horn.

B. Enkephalin is localized in interneurons and found in the same region of the dorsal horn as terminals containing substance P. The μ-opioid receptor for enkephalins is expressed by neurons in the superficial dorsal horn and also in sensory afferent terminals.

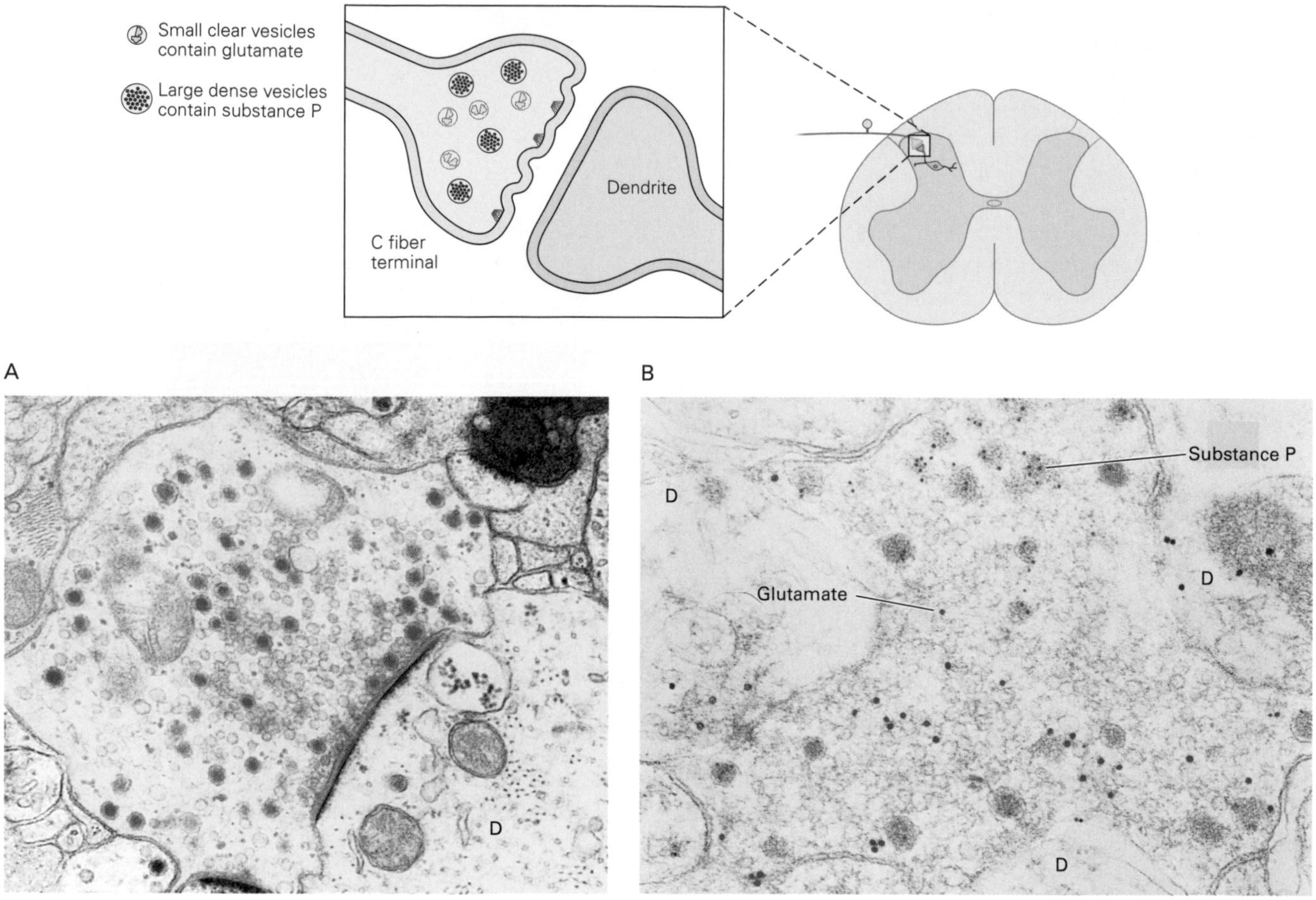

Figure 24–6 Transmitter storage in the synaptic terminals of primary nociceptive neurons in the dorsal spinal cord.

A. The terminal of a C fiber on the dendrite (**D**) of a dorsal horn neuron has two classes of synaptic vesicles that contain different transmitters. Small electron-lucent vesicles contain glutamate while large dense-cored vesicles hold neuropeptides. (Image from H. J. Ralston III, reproduced with permission.)

B. Glutamate and the peptide substance P are scattered in the axoplasm of a sensory terminal in lamina II of the dorsal horn. (Image from A. Rustioni, reproduced with permission.)

of commonly used analgesic drugs. Aspirin and other nonsteroidal anti-inflammatory analgesics are effective in controlling pain because they block the activity of most COX enzymes, reducing prostaglandin synthesis. The drug acetaminophen appears to exert its analgesic effects through selective inhibition of COX3.

Tissue inflammation also results from peripheral injury. The cardinal signs of inflammation are heat (calor), redness (rubor), and swelling (tumor). Heat and redness result from the dilation of peripheral blood vessels, whereas swelling results from plasma extravasation, a process in which proteins, cells, and fluids are able to penetrate post-capillary venules. Release of the neuropeptides substance P and CGRP from the peripheral terminals of C fibers can elicit each of these pathological responses. Because this form of inflammation depends on neural activity, it has been termed *neurogenic inflammation* (Figure 24–8).

The release of substance P and CGRP from the peripheral terminals of sensory neurons is also responsible for the *axon reflex*, a physiological process characterized by vasodilation in the vicinity of a cutaneous injury. Pharmacological antagonists of substance P are able to block neurogenic inflammation and vasodilation in humans; this discovery illustrates how knowledge of nociceptive mechanisms has relevance for improved clinical therapies for pain.

In addition to these small molecules and peptides, neurotrophins are causative agents in pain. Nerve growth factor (NGF) is particularly active in inflammatory pain states; the synthesis of NGF is upregulated in many inflamed peripheral tissues (Figure 24–9).

NGF-neutralizing molecules are effective analgesic agents in animal models of persistent pain. Indeed, inhibition of NGF function and signaling blocks pain sensation as effectively as COX inhibitors and opiates. The expression of brain derived neurotrophic factor (BDNF) is also elevated in nociceptive neurons under conditions of inflammatory and neuropathic pain. BDNF is transported to the central terminals of the primary afferents in the spinal dorsal horn, where its release enhances the response of dorsal horn neurons to painful stimuli (Figure 24–9). Drugs that block BDNF expression in nociceptive neurons may therefore be useful as analgesics.

What accounts for the enhanced sensitivity of dorsal horn neurons to nociceptor signals? Under conditions of persistent injury C fibers fire repetitively and the response of dorsal horn neurons increases progressively (Figure 24–10A). The gradual enhancement in the excitability of dorsal horn neurons has been termed "wind-up" and is thought to involve *N*-methyl-D-aspartate (NMDA)-type glutamate receptors (Figure 24–10B).

Repeated exposure to noxious stimuli therefore results in long-term changes in the response of dorsal horn neurons through mechanisms that are similar to those underlying the long-term potentiation of synaptic responses in many circuits in the brain. In essence these prolonged changes in the excitability of dorsal horn neurons constitute a "memory" of the state of C fiber input. This phenomenon has been termed *central sensitization* to distinguish it from sensitization at the peripheral terminals of the dorsal horn neurons, a process that involves activation of the enzymatic pathways of prostaglandin synthesis.

The sensitization of dorsal horn neurons also involves recruitment of second-messenger pathways and activation of protein kinases that have been implicated in memory storage in other regions of the central nervous system. One consequence of this enzymatic cascade is the expression of immediate-early genes that encode transcription factors such as *c-fos,* which are thought to activate effector proteins that sensitize dorsal horn neurons to sensory inputs.

In certain clinical conditions alterations in the excitability of dorsal horn neurons can decrease pain thresholds and lead to spontaneous pain. One dramatic illustration of this phenomenon is phantom limb pain, the persistent sensations of pain that appear to originate from the region of an amputated limb (Figure 24–11). Until recently limb amputation was performed solely with a general anesthetic on the assumption that this alone should be sufficient to eliminate memory of the traumatic surgical procedure. Surgeons found, however, that even under general anesthesia the spinal cord "experiences" the insult of the surgical procedure, presumably because of ongoing central sensitization. So to reduce the risk of phantom limb pain, amputation

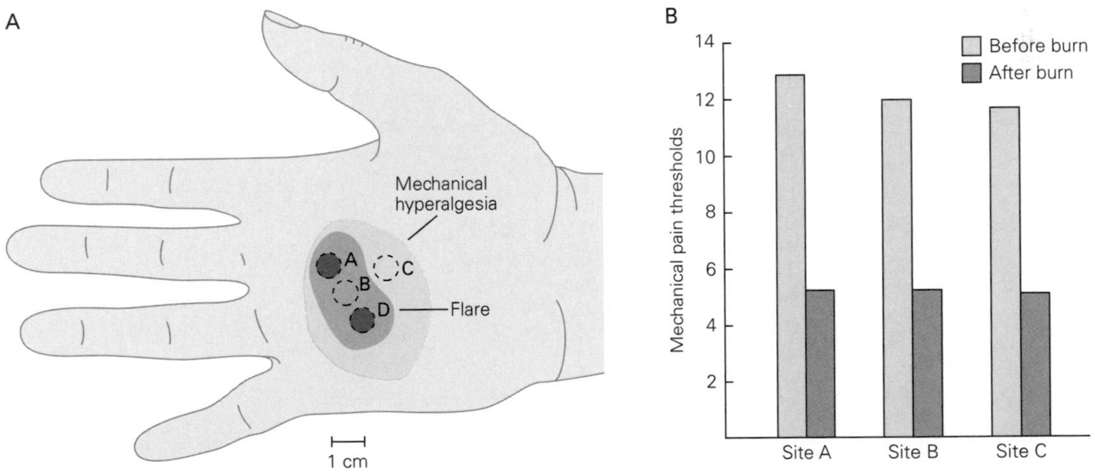

Figure 24–7 Hyperalgesia results from sensitization of nociceptors. (Reproduced, with permission, from Raja, Campbell, and Meyer 1984.)

A. Mechanical thresholds for pain were recorded at sites A, B, and C before and after burns at sites A and D. The areas of reddening (flare) and mechanical hyperalgesia resulting from the burns are shown on the hand of one subject. In all subjects the area of mechanical hyperalgesia was larger than the area of flare. Mechanical hyperalgesia was present even after the flare disappeared.

B. Mean mechanical pain thresholds before and after burns. The mechanical threshold for pain is significantly decreased after the burn.

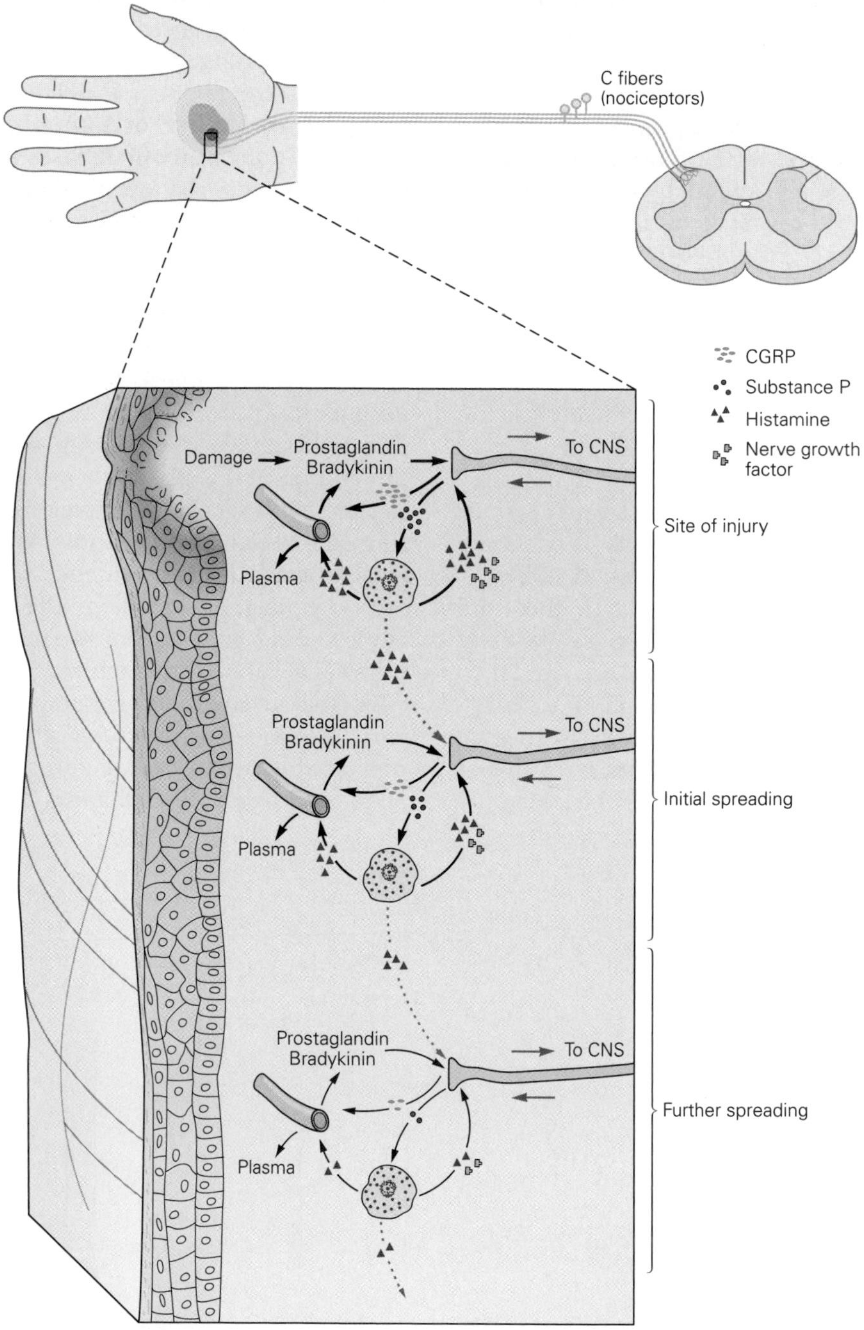

Figure 24–8 Neurogenic inflammation. Injury or tissue damage releases bradykinin and prostaglandins, which activate or sensitize nociceptors. Activation of nociceptors leads to the release of substance P and CGRP (calcitonin gene–related peptide). Substance P acts on mast cells in the vicinity of sensory endings to evoke degranulation and the release of histamine, which directly excites nociceptors. Substance P produces plasma extravasation, and CGRP produces dilation of peripheral blood vessels; the resultant edema causes additional liberation of bradykinin. These mechanisms also occur in healthy tissue, where they cause secondary or spreading hyperalgesia.

now includes interventions that block the central sensitization of dorsal horn neurons. General anesthesia is often supplemented with direct spinal administration of an analgesic agent or local administration of anesthetic at the injury site.

Nociceptive Information Is Transmitted from the Spinal Cord to the Thalamus

Five Major Ascending Pathways Convey Nociceptive Information

Five major ascending pathways—the spinothalamic, spinoreticular, spinomesencephalic, cervicothalamic, and spinohypothalamic tracts—contribute to the central processing of nociceptive information.

The *spinothalamic tract* is the most prominent ascending nociceptive pathway in the spinal cord. It includes the axons of nociception-specific, thermosensitive, and wide-dynamic-range neurons in laminae I and V through VII of the dorsal horn. These axons cross the midline of the spinal cord at their segment of origin and ascend in the anterolateral white matter before terminating in thalamic nuclei (Figure 24–12). The spinothalamic tract has a crucial role in the transmission of nociceptive information. Electrical stimulation of the tract is sufficient to elicit the sensation of pain; conversely, lesioning this tract (anterolateral cordotomy) can result in a marked reduction in pain sensation on the side of the body contralateral to that of the lesion.

The *spinoreticular tract* contains the axons of projection neurons in laminae VII and VIII. This tract ascends in the anterolateral quadrant of the spinal cord

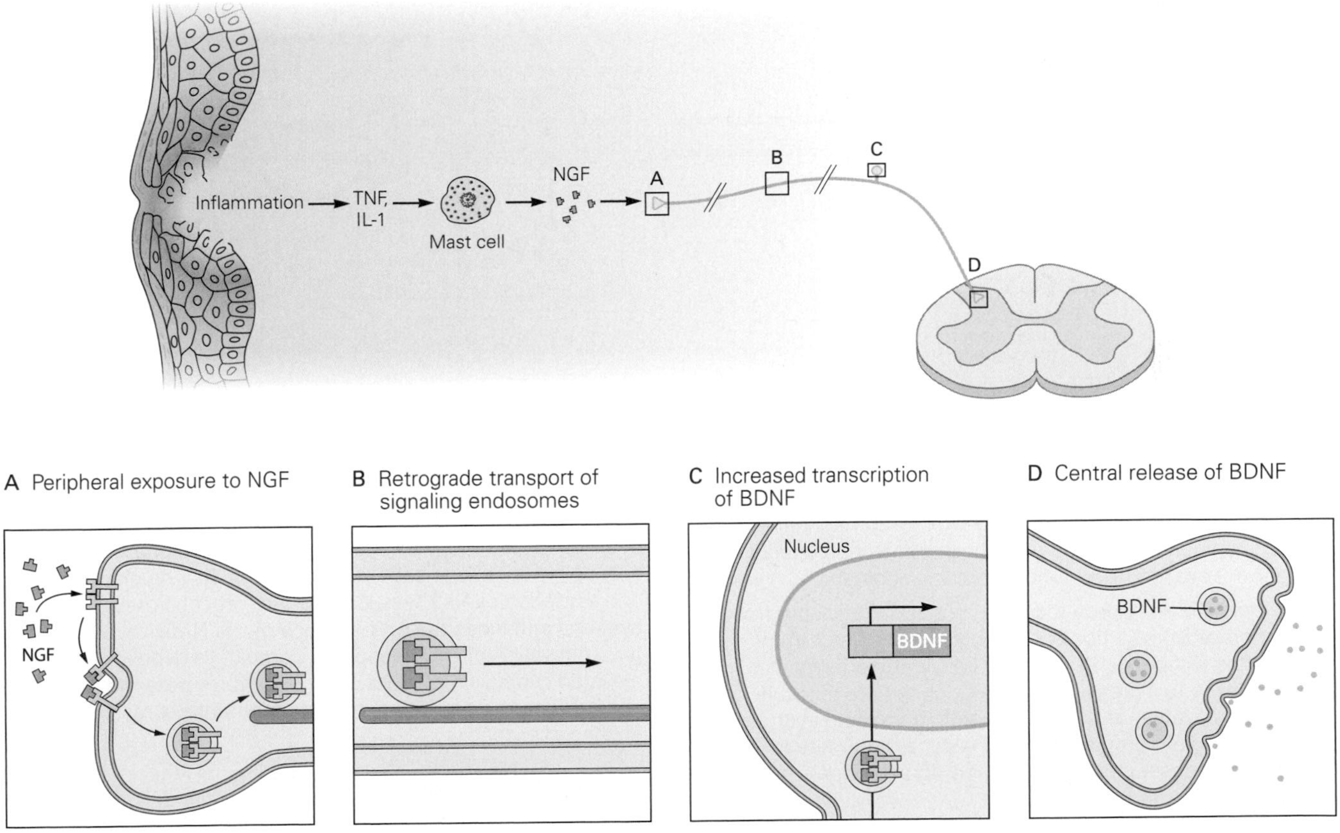

Figure 24–9 Neurotrophins are pain mediators. Local production of inflammatory cytokines such as interleukin-1 (IL-1) and tumor necrosis factor (TNF) promotes the synthesis and release of nerve growth factor (NGF) from several cell types in the periphery. NGF binds to TrkA receptors on primary nociceptive terminals (**A**), triggering localized post-transitional changes in expression of ion channels that increase nociceptor excitability. Retrograde transport of signaling endosomes to the cell body (**B**) results in enhanced expression of brain derived neurotrophic factor (BDNF) (**C**), and its release from sensory terminals in the spinal cord (**D**) further increases excitability and facilitates the activation of dorsal horn neurons.

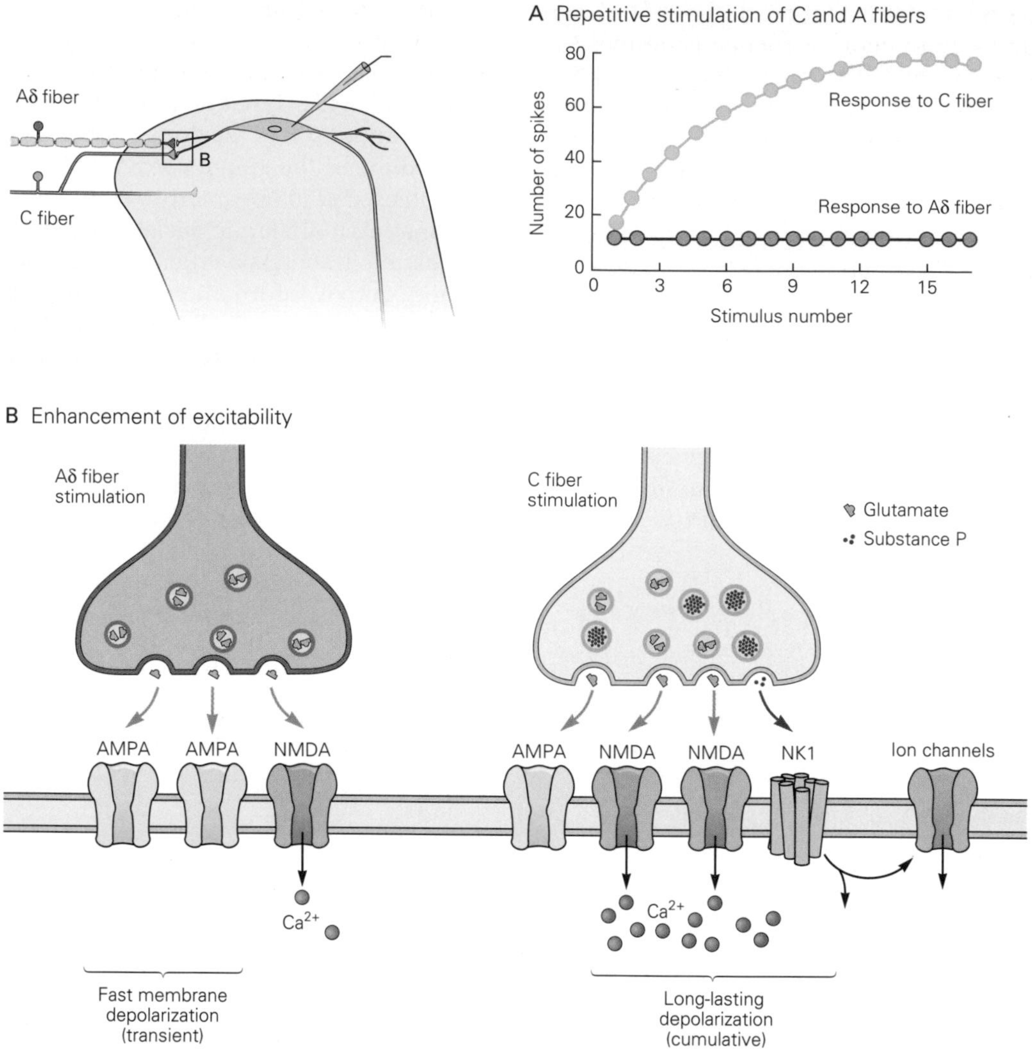

Figure 24–10 Mechanisms for enhanced excitability of dorsal horn neurons.

A. Typical responses of a dorsal horn neuron in the rat to electrical stimuli delivered transcutaneously at a frequency of 1 Hz. With repetitive stimulation the long-latency component evoked by a C fiber increases gradually, whereas the short-latency component evoked by an A fiber remains constant.

B. The dorsal horn neuron receives monosynaptic input from mechanoreceptors (A fibers) and polysynaptic input from nociceptors (C fibers). Elevation of Ca^{2+} in the presynaptic terminal leads to increased release of glutamate and substance P. Activation of the postsynaptic α-amino-3-hydroxy-5-methylisoxazole-4-propionate (AMPA)-type glutamate receptors by A fibers causes a fast transient membrane depolarization, which relieves the Mg^{2+} block of the *N*-methyl-D-aspartate (NMDA)-type receptors. Activation of the postsynaptic NMDA-type receptors and neurokinin-1 (NK1) antagonist receptors by C fibers generates a long-lasting cumulative depolarization. The cytosolic Ca^{2+} concentration in the dorsal horn neuron increases because of Ca^{2+} entry through the NMDA-type and AMPA-type channels and voltage-sensitive Ca^{2+} channels. The elevated Ca^{2+} and activation of NK1 receptors through second-messenger systems enhances the performance of the NMDA-type receptors. Activation of NK1 receptors, cumulative depolarization, elevated cytosolic Ca^{2+}, and other factors regulate the behavior of ion channels responsible for action potentials, resulting in enhanced excitability.

and terminates in both the reticular formation and the thalamus (Figure 24–12). The axons of spinoreticular tract neurons do not cross the midline.

The *spinomesencephalic* (or *spinoparabrachial*) *tract* contains the axons of projection neurons in laminae I and V. Information transmitted along this tract is thought to contribute to the affective component of pain. This tract projects in the anterolateral quadrant of the spinal cord to the mesencephalic reticular formation and periaqueductal gray matter (Figure 24–12).

Axons in this tract also project to the parabrachial nucleus. Neurons of the parabrachial nucleus project to the amygdala, a key nucleus of the limbic system that regulates emotional states. Many of the axons of this pathway course through the dorsal part of the lateral funiculus rather than in the anterolateral quadrant. In surgical procedures designed to relieve pain, such as anterolateral cordotomy, the sparing of these fibers may explain the persistence or recurrence of pain after surgery.

The *cervicothalamic tract* runs in the lateral white matter of the upper two cervical segments of the spinal cord and contains the axons of neurons of the lateral cervical nucleus, which receives input from neurons in laminae III and IV of the dorsal horn. Most axons in the cervicothalamic tract cross the midline and ascend in the medial lemniscus of the brain stem, terminating in midbrain nuclei and in the ventroposterior lateral and posteromedial nuclei of the thalamus. Other neurons in laminae III and IV send their axons directly into the

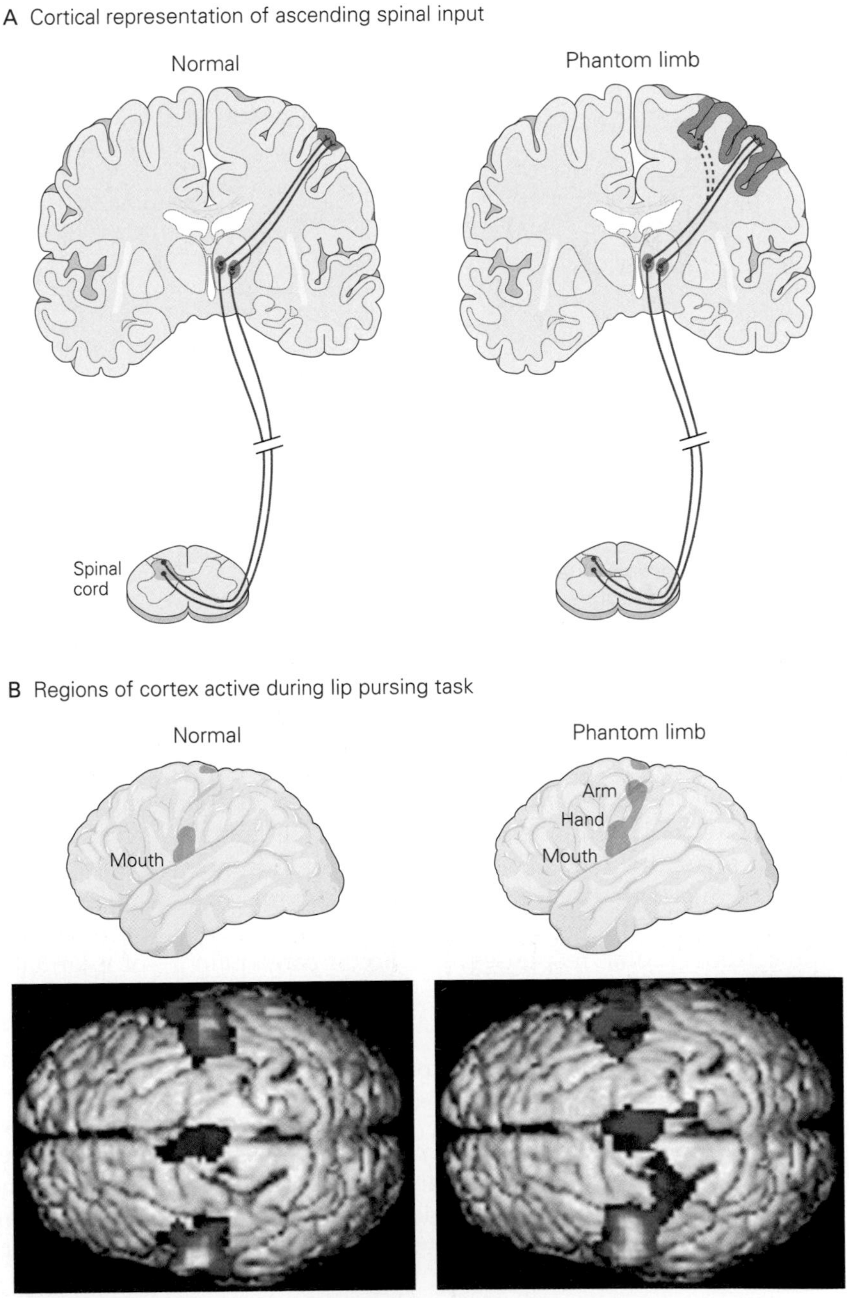

Figure 24–11 Changes in neural activation in phantom limb pain.

A. The domain of cerebral cortex activated by ascending spinal sensory inputs is expanded in patients with phantom limb pain.

B. Functional magnetic resonance imaging (fMRI) of patients with phantom limb pain and healthy controls during a lip pursing task. In amputees with phantom limb pain, cortical representation of the mouth has extended into the regions of the hand and arm. In amputees without pain, the areas of primary somatosensory and motor cortices that are activated are similar to those in healthy controls (image not shown). (Modified, with permission, from Flor, Nokolajsen, and Jensen 2006.)

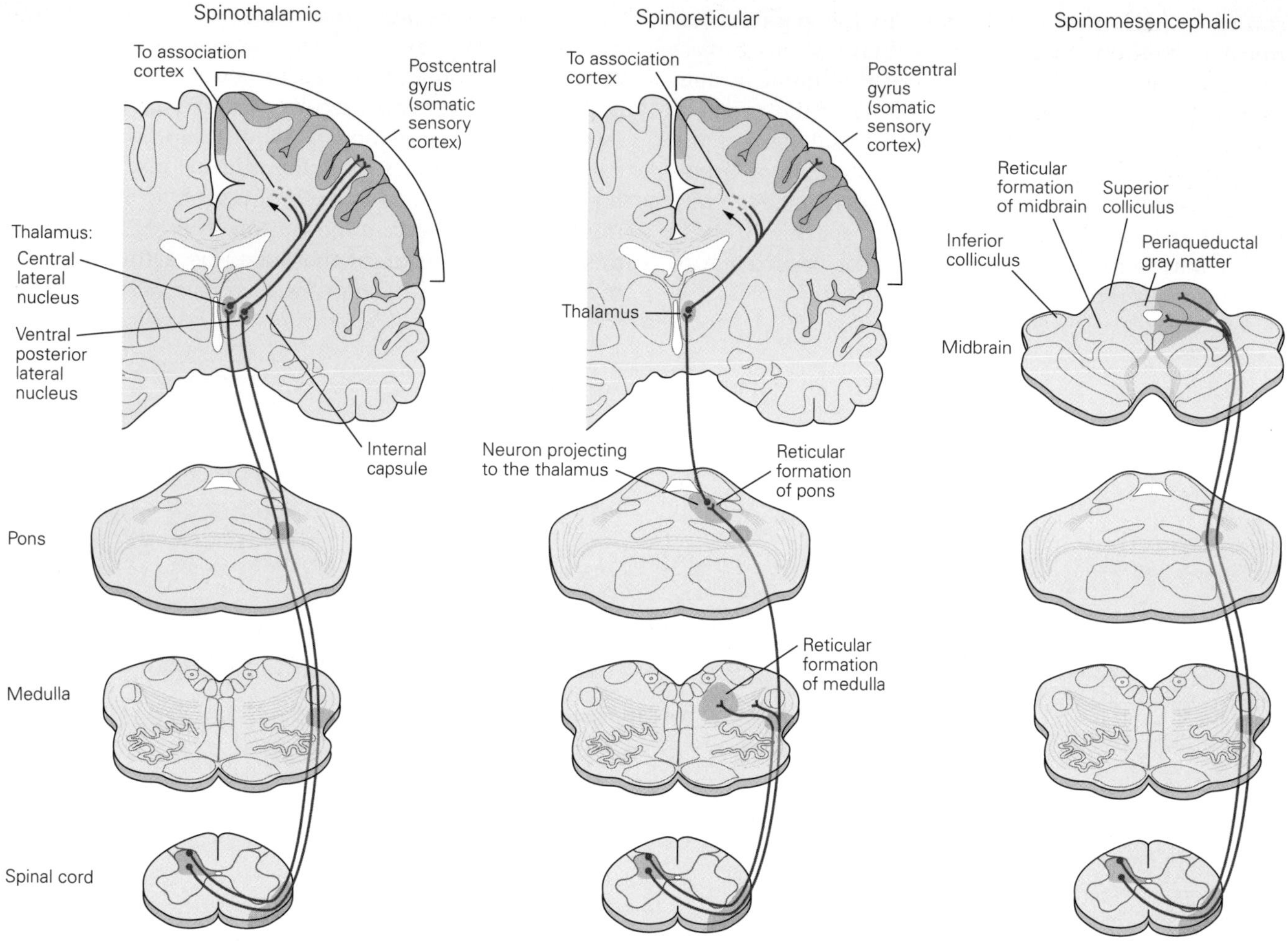

Figure 24–12 Three of the five ascending pathways that transmit nociceptive information from the spinal cord to higher centers. (Adapted, with permission, from Willis 1985.)

dorsal columns and terminate in the cuneate and gracile nuclei of the medulla.

The *spinohypothalamic tract* contains the axons of neurons found in laminae I, V, and VIII of the dorsal horn in the spinal cord. These axons project to hypothalamic nuclei that serve as autonomic control centers involved in the regulation of the neuroendocrine and cardiovascular responses that accompany pain syndromes.

Several Thalamic Nuclei Relay Nociceptive Information to the Cerebral Cortex

The thalamus contains several relay nuclei that participate in the central processing of nociceptive information. Two of the most important regions of the thalamus are the lateral and medial nuclear groups.

The *lateral nuclear group* comprises the ventroposterior medial nucleus, the ventroposterior lateral nucleus, and the posterior nucleus. These three nuclei receive inputs through the spinothalamic tract from nociception-specific and wide-dynamic-range neurons in laminae I and V of the dorsal horn. The lateral thalamus is thought to be concerned with the processing of information about the precise location of an injury, information usually conveyed to consciousness as acute pain. Consistent with this view, neurons in the lateral thalamic nuclei have small receptive fields, matching those of the presynaptic spinal neurons.

Injury to the spinothalamic tract and its thalamic targets causes a severe form of pain termed *central pain*. An infarct in a small region of the ventroposterolateral thalamus produces the perception of a spontaneous burning pain, together with other abnormal sensations (called dysesthesias) that are perceived as originating from diverse regions of the body. This constellation of abnormal percepts has been termed the Dejerine-Roussy syndrome. Electrical stimulation of the thalamus can also result in intense pain. In one dramatic clinical case, electrical stimulation of the thalamus rekindled sensations of angina pectoris that were so realistic that the anesthesiologist thought the patient was experiencing a heart attack. This and other clinical observations suggest that in chronic pain conditions there is a fundamental change in thalamic and cortical circuitry.

The *medial nuclear group* of the thalamus comprises the central lateral nucleus of the thalamus and the intralaminar complex. Its major input is from neurons in laminae VII and VIII of the dorsal horn. The pathway to the medial thalamus was the first spinothalamic projection evident in the evolution of mammals and is therefore known as the *paleospinothalamic tract.* It is also sometimes referred to as the spinoreticulothalamic tract because it includes indirect connections through the reticular formation of the brain stem. The projection from the lateral thalamus to the ventroposterior lateral and medial nuclei is most developed in primates, and is termed the *neospinothalamic tract.* Many neurons in the medial thalamus respond optimally to noxious stimuli and project widely to the basal ganglia and different cortical areas.

Pain Is Controlled by Cortical Mechanisms

Cingulate and Insular Areas Are Active During the Perception of Pain

Until recently research on the central processing of pain concentrated on the thalamus. But pain is a complex perception that involves many cortical areas whose activity is influenced critically by the context in which the noxious stimulus is presented, as well as by an individual's prior experience.

Neurons in several areas of the cerebral cortex respond to nociceptive input. In the somatosensory cortex neurons typically have small receptive fields and may not contribute greatly to the diffuse perception of aches and pains that characterize most clinical syndromes. The cingulate gyrus and insular cortex contain neurons that are activated strongly and selectively by nociceptive somatosensory stimuli (Box 24–1). The cingulate gyrus forms part of the limbic system and is thought to be involved in processing emotional states associated with pain. The insular cortex receives direct projections from the thalamus, specifically the medial nuclei and the ventroposterior medial nucleus. Neurons in the insular cortex process information about the internal state of the body and contribute to the autonomic component of pain responses.

Patients with lesions of the insular cortex present the striking syndrome of asymbolia for pain: They perceive noxious stimuli as painful and can distinguish sharp from dull pain but fail to display appropriate emotional responses. These observations implicate the insular cortex as an area in which the sensory, affective, and cognitive components of pain are integrated.

Pain Perception Is Regulated by a Balance of Activity in Nociceptive and Non-Nociceptive Afferent Fibers

Many projection neurons in the dorsal horn of the spinal cord respond selectively to noxious inputs, but others receive convergent inputs from both nociceptive and non-nociceptive afferents. The concept that the convergence of sensory inputs onto spinal projection neurons regulates pain processing first emerged in the 1960s.

Ronald Melzak and Patrick Wall proposed that the relative balance of activity in nociceptive and non-nociceptive afferents might influence the transmission and perception of pain. In particular, they proposed that activation of non-nociceptive sensory neurons closes a "gate" for central transmission of nociceptive signals that can be opened by the activation of nociceptive sensory neurons. In the original and simplest form of this gate-control theory the interaction between large and small fibers occurred at the first possible site of convergence on projection neurons in the dorsal horn of the spinal cord (Figure 24–14). We now know that such interactions can also occur at many supraspinal relay centers and the strict anatomical predictions of the gate-control theory remain to be established.

Nevertheless, the core concept of convergence of different sensory modalities has provided an important basis for the design of new pain therapies. Viewed in its broadest sense, the convergence of high- and low-threshold inputs at spinal or supraspinal sites provided a plausible explanation for several empirical observations about the perception of pain. The shaking of the hand that follows a hammer blow or burn is a reflexive behavior and may alleviate pain by activating large-diameter afferents that suppress the central transmission of noxious stimuli.

The idea of convergence also helped to promote the use of transcutaneous electrical nerve stimulation (TENS) and dorsal column stimulation for the relief of pain. With TENS, stimulating electrodes placed

Box 24–1 Localizing Illusory Pain in the Cerebral Cortex

Thunberg's illusion, first demonstrated in 1896, is a strong, often painful heat felt after placing the hand on a grill of alternating warm and cool bars (Figure 24–13A).

This illusory sensation occurs because two classes of neurons in the ascending spinothalamic tract, those sensitive to innocuous or noxious cold, respond differently to the grill. This finding has led to a model of pain perception based on a central disinhibition or unmasking process in the cerebral cortex (Figure 24–13B).

The model predicts perceptual similarities between grill-evoked and cold-evoked pain, a prediction that has been verified psychophysically. The thalamocortical integration of pain and temperature stimuli can explain the burning sensation felt when nociceptors are activated by cold.

To identify the anatomical site of the unmasking phenomenon described above, positron emission tomography (PET) was used to compare the cortical areas activated by Thunberg's grill with those activated by cool, warm, noxious cold, and noxious heat stimuli separately. All thermal stimuli activate the insula and somatosensory cortices. The anterior cingulate cortex is activated by Thunberg's grill and by noxious heat and cold, but not by discrete warm and cool stimuli (Figure 24–13C).

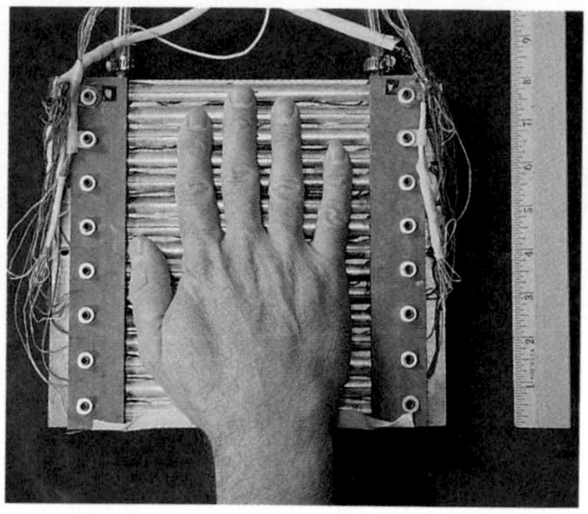

Figure 24–13A Thunberg's thermal grill. The stimulus surface (20 × 14 cm) is made of 15 sterling silver bars, each 1 cm wide, set approximately 3 mm apart. Underneath each bar are three longitudinally spaced thermoelectric (Peltier) elements (1 cm^2), and on top of each bar is a thermocouple. Alternate (even- and odd-numbered) bars can be controlled independently. (Adapted, with permission, from Craig and Bushnell 1994; Craig et al. 1996.)

at peripheral locations activate large-diameter afferent fibers that overlap the area of injury and pain. The region of the body in which pain is reduced maps to those segments of the spinal cord in which nociceptive and non-nociceptive afferents from that body region terminate. This makes intuitive sense: You do not shake your left leg to relieve pain in your right arm.

Electrical Stimulation of the Brain Produces Analgesia

Several sites of endogenous pain regulation are located in the brain. One effective means of suppressing nociception involves stimulation of the periaqueductal gray region, the area of the midbrain that surrounds the

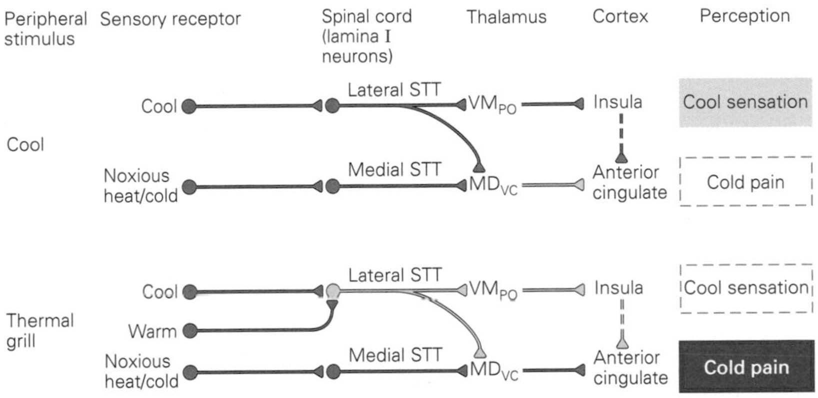

Figure 24–13B A model of regulation of pain perception. Excitation of nociceptive spinothalamic neurons by cool stimuli does not produce pain, presumably because cool-specific spinothalamic neurons exert a suppressive action on nociceptors. The grill stimulus has a similar effect but excites the cool-specific cells to a lesser extent, thus reducing their suppressive effect on cold pain. "Medial STT" refers to skin temperature test (STT) projections to the medial dorsal nucleus of the thalamus; "lateral STT" refers to spinothalamic axons in the middle of the lateral funiculus, as opposed to the ventral or anterior STT projections, which lie in the anterior funiculus. (MD_{VC}, ventral caudal part of medial dorsal nucleus; VM_{PO}, ventroposterior medial nucleus.) (Adapted, with permission, from Craig and Bushnell 1994; Craig et al. 1996.)

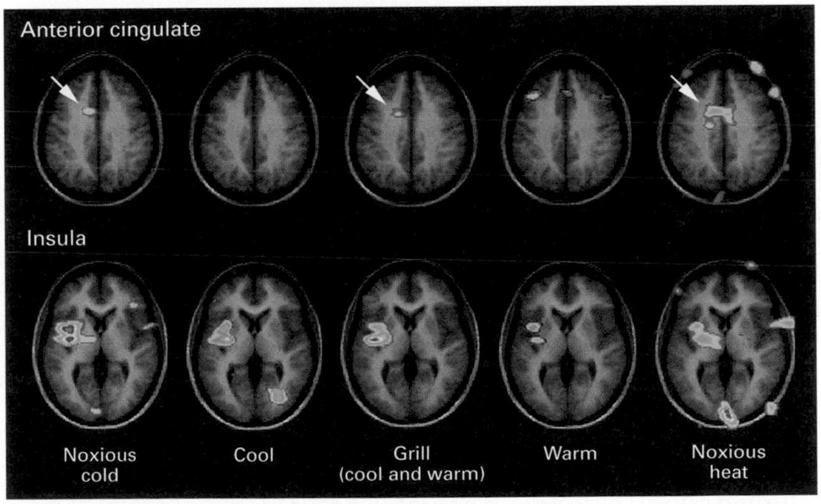

Figure 24–13C Cortical areas activated by Thunberg's grill. The anterior cingulate and insula regions of the cerebral cortex are activated when the hand is placed on the grill but not when warm and cool stimuli are applied separately. (Adapted, with permission, from Craig and Bushnell 1994; Craig et al. 1996.)

third ventricle and the cerebral aqueduct. In experimental animals stimulation of this region elicits a profound and selective analgesia. This *stimulation-produced analgesia* is remarkably specific; animals still respond to touch, pressure, and temperature within the body area that exhibits analgesia, but they feel less pain. Indeed, stimulation-evoked analgesia has proved to be an effective way of relieving pain in a limited number of human pain conditions.

Stimulation of the periaqueductal gray matter is able to block spinally mediated withdrawal reflexes that are normally evoked by noxious stimulation. Few of the neurons in the periaqueductal gray matter project directly to the dorsal horn of the spinal cord.

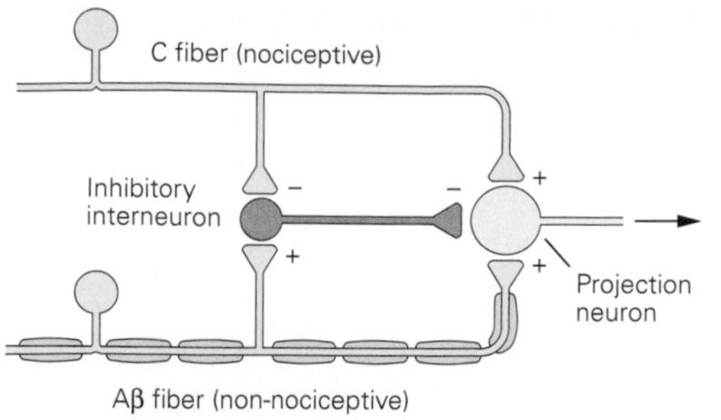

Figure 24–14 The gate-control theory of nociception. The gate-control hypothesis was proposed in the 1960s to account for the ability of low-threshold fiber activation to attenuate pain. The hypothesis focused on the interaction of neurons in the dorsal horn of the spinal cord: the nociceptive (C) and non-nociceptive (Aβ) sensory neurons, projection neurons, and inhibitory interneurons. In the original version of the model, as shown here, the projection neuron is excited by both classes of sensory neurons and inhibited by interneurons in the superficial dorsal horn. The two classes of sensory fibers also terminate on the inhibitory interneurons; the C-fibers inhibit the interneurons, thus increasing the activity of the projection neuron, while the Aβ fibers excite the interneurons, thus suppressing the output of the projection neurons.

Most make excitatory connections with neurons of the rostroventral medulla, including serotonergic neurons in a midline region called the nucleus raphe magnus, or neurons of the nuclei of the raphe complex. The axons of these serotonergic neurons project through the dorsal region of the lateral funiculus to the spinal cord, where they form inhibitory connections with neurons in laminae I, II, and V of the dorsal horn (Figure 24–15). Stimulation of the rostroventral medulla thus inhibits the firing of many classes of dorsal horn neurons, including projection neurons of the spinothalamic tract that convey afferent nociceptive signals.

A second major monoaminergic descending system can also suppress the activity of nociceptive neurons in the dorsal horn. This noradrenergic system originates in the locus ceruleus and other nuclei of the medulla and pons. These projections inhibit neurons in laminae I and V of the dorsal horn through direct and indirect synaptic actions.

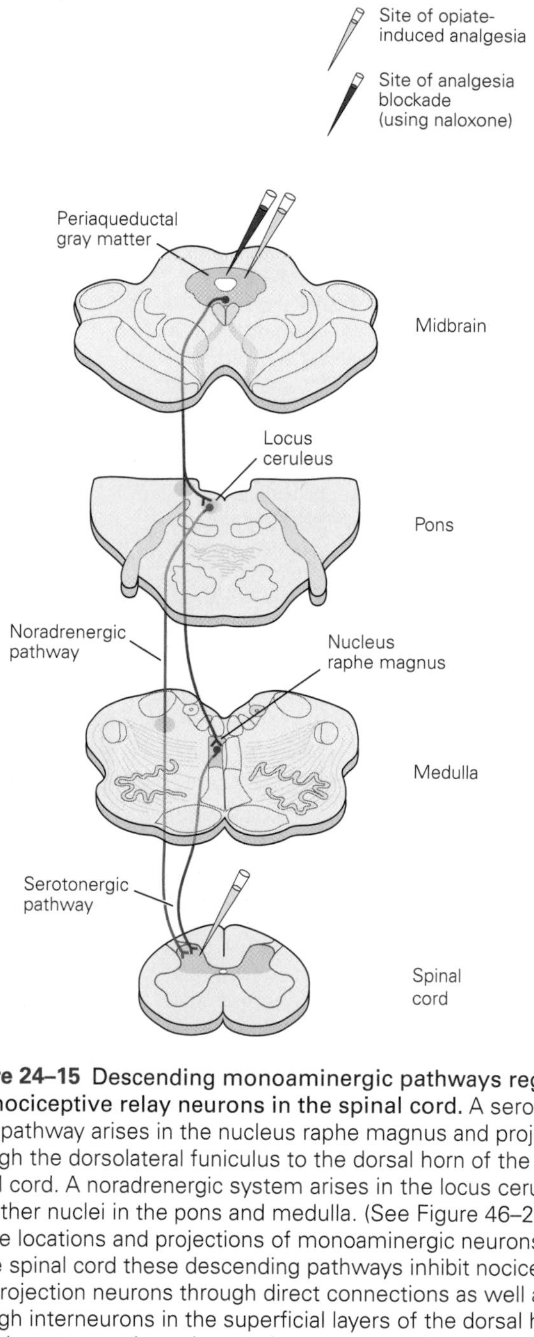

Figure 24–15 Descending monoaminergic pathways regulate nociceptive relay neurons in the spinal cord. A serotonergic pathway arises in the nucleus raphe magnus and projects through the dorsolateral funiculus to the dorsal horn of the spinal cord. A noradrenergic system arises in the locus ceruleus and other nuclei in the pons and medulla. (See Figure 46–2 for the locations and projections of monoaminergic neurons.) In the spinal cord these descending pathways inhibit nociceptive projection neurons through direct connections as well as through interneurons in the superficial layers of the dorsal horn. Both the sertonergic nucleus raphe magnus and noradrenergic nuclei receive input from neurons in the periaqueductal gray region. Sites of opioid peptide expression and actions of exogenously administered opioids are shown.

Opioid Peptides Contribute to Endogenous Pain Control

Since discovery by the Sumerians in 3300 BC, the opium poppy and its active ingredients, opiates such as morphine and codeine, have been recognized as powerful analgesic agents. Over the past two decades we have begun to understand many of the molecular mechanisms and neural circuits through which opiates exert their analgesic actions. In addition, we have come to realize that the neural networks involved in stimulation-produced and opiate-induced analgesia are intimately related.

Two key discoveries led to these advances. The first was the recognition that morphine and other opiates interact with specific receptors on neurons in the spinal cord and brain. The second was the isolation of endogenous neuropeptides with opiate-like activities at these receptors. The observation that the opiate antagonist naloxone blocks stimulation-produced analgesia provided the first clue that the brain contains endogenous opioids.

Table 24–1 Four Major Classes of Endogenous Opioid Peptides

Propeptide	Peptide(s)	Preferential receptor
POMC	β-endorphin	μ/δ
	Endomorphin-1	μ
	Endomorphin-2	μ
Proenkephalin	Met-enkephalin	δ
	Leu-enkephalin	δ
Prodynorphin	Dynorphin A	κ
	Dynorphin B	κ
Pro-orphanin FQ	Orphanin FQ	Orphan receptor

Endogenous Opioid Peptides and Their Receptors Are Distributed in Pain-Modulatory Systems

Opioid receptors fall into four major classes: mu (μ), delta (δ), kappa (κ), and orphanin FQ. The genes encoding each of these receptor types constitute a subfamily of G protein-coupled receptors. The μ receptors are particularly diverse; numerous μ receptor isoforms have been identified, many with different patterns of expression. This finding has prompted a search for analgesic drugs that target specific isoforms.

The opioid receptors were originally defined on the basis of the binding affinity of different agonist compounds. Morphine and other opioid alkaloids are potent agonists at μ receptors, and there is a tight correlation between the potency of an analgesic and its affinity of binding to μ receptors. Mice in which the gene for the μ receptor has been inactivated are insensitive to morphine and other opiate agonists. Many opiate antagonist drugs, such as naloxone, also bind to the μ receptor and compete with morphine for receptor occupancy without activating receptor signaling.

The μ receptors are highly concentrated in the superficial dorsal horn of the spinal cord, the ventral medulla, and the periaqueductal gray matter, important anatomical sites for the regulation of pain. Nevertheless, like other classes of opioid receptors, they are also found at many other sites in the central and peripheral nervous systems. Their widespread distribution explains why systemically administered morphine influences many physiological processes in addition to the perception of pain.

The discovery of opioid receptors and their expression by neurons in the central and peripheral nervous systems led to the definition of four major classes of endogenous opioid peptides, each interacting with a specific class of opioid receptors (Table 24–1).

Three classes—the enkephalins, β-endorphins, and dynorphins—are the best characterized. These peptides are formed from large polypeptide precursors by enzymatic cleavage (Figure 24–16) and encoded by distinct genes. Despite differences in amino acid sequence, each contains the sequence Tyr-Gly-Gly-Phe. There are two enkephalins, leucine and methionine enkephalin, which are closely related small peptides. β-endorphin is a cleavage product of a precursor that also generates the active peptide adrenocorticotropic hormone (ACTH). Both β-endorphin and ACTH are synthesized by cells in the pituitary and are released into the bloodstream in response to stress. Dynorphins are derived from the polyprotein product of the *dynorphin* gene. Enkephalins are active at both μ and δ receptors, whereas dynorphin is a relatively selective agonist of the κ receptor. The fourth endogenous opioid peptide is orphanin FQ or nociceptin (OFQ/N1–17). This 17-amino acid peptide is related in sequence to dynorphin and binds to the OFQ/N receptor.

Members of the four classes of opioid peptides are distributed widely in the central nervous system and individual peptides are located at sites associated with the processing or modulation of nociceptive information. Neuronal cell bodies and axon terminals containing enkephalin and dynorphin are found in the dorsal horn of the spinal cord, particularly in laminae I and II, as well as in the rostral ventral medulla and the periaqueductal gray matter. Neurons that synthesize β-endorphin are confined primarily to the hypothalamus; their axons terminate in the periaqueductal gray region and on noradrenergic neurons in the brain stem. Orphanin FQ appears to participate in a broad range of other physiological functions.

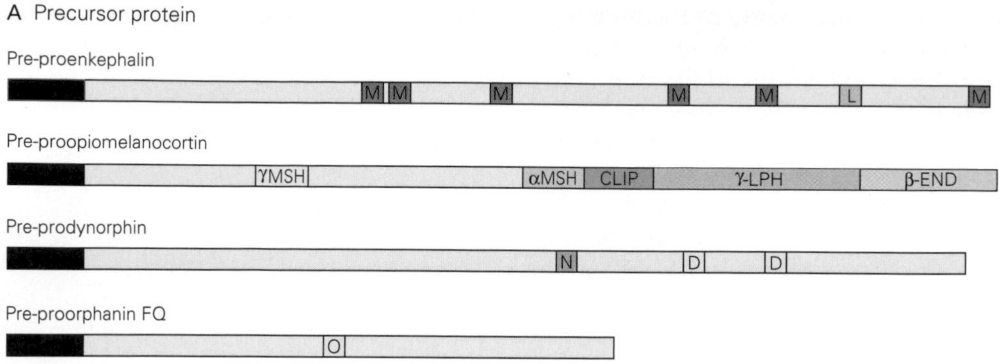

B Proteolytically processed opioid peptides

		Amino acid sequence
M	Methionine-enkephalin	**Tyr Gly Gly Phe** Met OH
L	Leucine-enkephalin	**Tyr Gly Gly Phe** Leu OH
β-END	β-Endorphin	**Tyr Gly Gly Phe** Met Thr Ser Glu Lys Ser Gln Thr Pro Leu Val Thr Leu Phe Lys Asn Ala Ile Val Lys Asn Ala His Lys Gly Gln OH
D	Dynorphin	**Tyr Gly Gly Phe** Leu Arg Arg Ile Arg Pro Lys Leu Lys Trp Asp Asn Gln OH
N	α-Neoendorphin	**Tyr Gly Gly Phe** Leu Arg Lys Tyr Pro Lys
O	Orphanin FQ	**Tyr Gly Gly Phe** Thr Gly Ala Arg Lys Ser Ala Arg Lys Leu Ala Asn Gln

Figure 24–16 Four families of endogenous opioid peptides arise from large precursor polyproteins.

A. Each of the precursor molecules is cleaved by proteolytic enzymes to generate shorter, biologically active peptides, some of which are shown in this diagram. The proenkephalin precursor protein contains multiple copies of methionine-enkephalin (M), leucine-enkephalin (L), and several extended enkephalins. Proopiomelanocortin (POMC) contains β-endorphin, melanocyte-stimulating hormone (MSH), adrenocorticotropic hormone (ACTH), and corticotropin-like intermediate-lobe peptide (CLIP). The prodynorphin precursor can produce dynorphin (D) and α-neoendorphin (N). The pro-orphanin precursor contains the orphanin FQ peptide (O). The black domains indicate a signal peptide.

B. Amino acid sequences of proteolytically processed bioactive peptides. The amino acid residues shown in bold type mediate interaction with opioid receptors. (Adapted, with permission, from Fields 1987.)

Morphine Controls Pain by Activating Opioid Receptors

Microinjection of low doses of morphine or other opiates directly into specific regions of the rat brain produces a powerful analgesia. The periaqueductal gray region is among the most sensitive sites, but local administration of morphine into other regions, including the spinal cord, also elicits a powerful analgesia.

Morphine-induced analgesia can be blocked by injection of the opiate antagonist naloxone into the periaqueductal gray region or the nucleus raphe magnus (Figure 24–15). In addition, bilateral transection of the dorsal lateral funiculus in the spinal cord blocks analgesia induced by central administration of morphine. Thus the central analgesic actions of morphine involve the activation of descending pathways to the spinal cord.

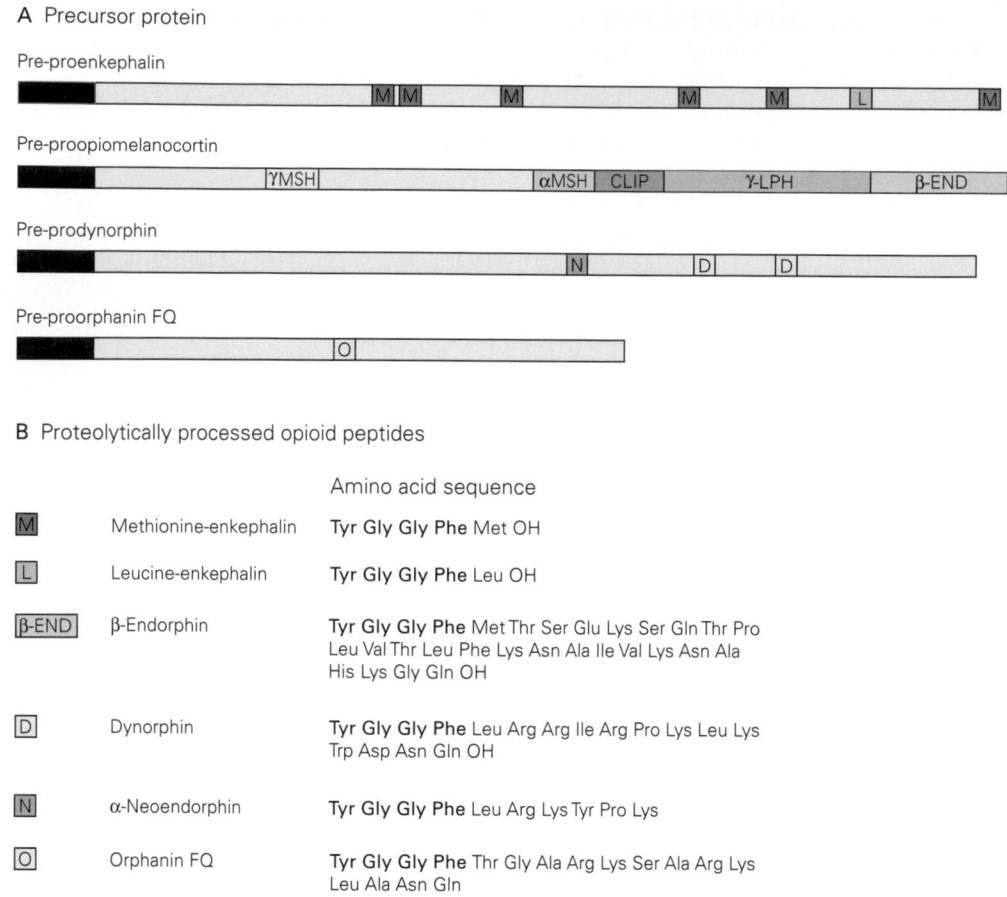

In the spinal cord, as elsewhere, morphine acts by mimicking the actions of endogenous opioid peptides. The superficial dorsal horn of the spinal cord contains interneurons that express enkephalin and dynorphin, and the terminals of these neurons lie close to synapses formed by nociceptive sensory neurons and spinal projection neurons (Figure 24–17A). Moreover, the μ, δ, and κ receptors are located on the terminals of the

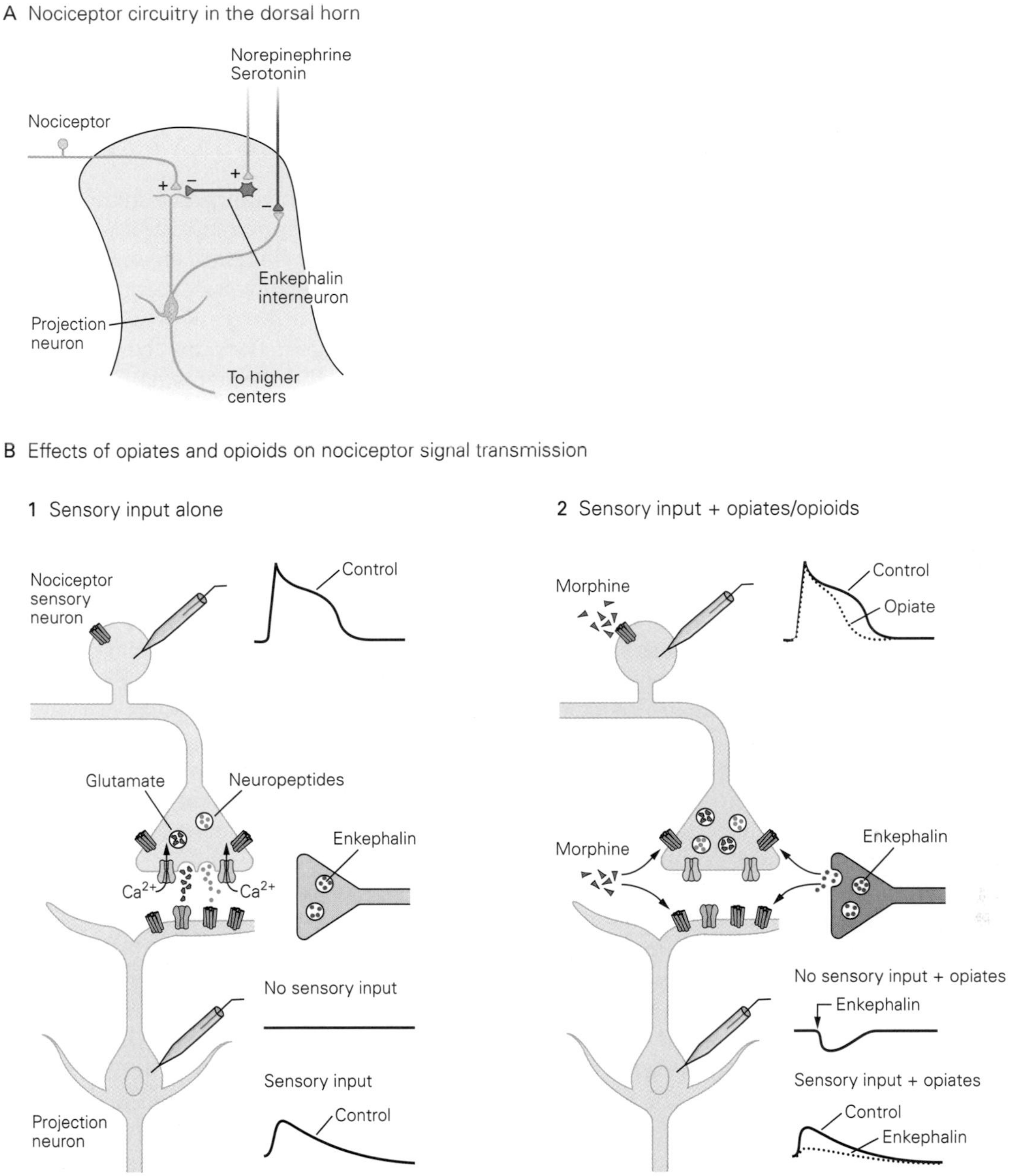

Figure 24–17 Local interneurons in the spinal cord integrate descending and afferent nociceptive pathways.

A. Nociceptive afferent fibers, local interneurons, and descending fibers interconnect in the dorsal horn of the spinal cord (see also Figure 24–3B). Nociceptive fibers terminate on second-order spinothalamic projection neurons. Local enkephalin-containing interneurons exert both pre- and postsynaptic inhibitory actions at these synapses. Serotonergic and noradrenergic neurons in the brain stem activate the local interneurons and also suppress the activity of the spinothalamic projection neurons.

B. Regulation of nociceptive signals at dorsal horn synapses. 1. Activation of a nociceptor leads to the release of glutamate and neuropeptides from the primary sensory neuron, producing an excitatory postsynaptic potential in the projection neuron. **2.** Opiates decrease the duration of the postsynaptic potential, probably by reducing Ca^{2+} influx and thus decreasing the release of transmitter from the primary sensory terminals. In addition, opiates hyperpolarize the dorsal horn neurons by activating a K^+ conductance and thus decrease the amplitude of the postsynaptic potential in the dorsal horn neuron.

nociceptive sensory neurons as well as on the dendrites of dorsal horn neurons that receive afferent nociceptive input, thus placing endogenous opioid peptides in a strategic position to regulate sensory afferent input. The number of μ receptors on Aδ nociceptors, which mediate fast and acute pain or "first pain", exceeds that on C fiber nociceptors, which mediate slow persistent pain or "second pain" (Figure 24–1). This may help to explain why morphine is more effective in the treatment of persistent rather than acute pains.

Opiates regulate nociceptive transmission at synapses in the dorsal horn through two main mechanisms. First, they increase membrane K^+ conductances in the dorsal horn neurons, hyperpolarizing the neurons and thus increasing the threshold for activation. Second, by binding to receptors on presynaptic sensory terminals opiates inhibit the release of neurotransmitter and thus decrease the extent of activation of the postsynaptic dorsal horn neurons. The decrease in neurotransmitter release appears to result from a decrease in Ca^{2+} conductance and consequent reduction of Ca^{2+} entry into the sensory nerve terminal (Figure 24–17B).

Many of the side effects of opiates are caused by the activation of opiate receptors within the brain and periphery. Opiate receptors are expressed by muscles of the bowel and anal sphincter; their activation contributes to constipation. The activation of opiate receptors in the nucleus of the solitary tract is responsible for respiratory depression and cardiovascular side effects. Confining drug administration to the spinal cord or to the periphery can minimize the side effects of systemic opiates. The release of endogenous opioid peptides from chromaffin cells of the adrenal medulla or from immune cells that migrate into injury sites may normally be involved in regulating the activation of nociceptors. The presence of peripheral opioid receptors has potential clinical relevance. Prolonged relief of pain after arthroscopic surgery can be achieved by injection of morphine into joints at doses that are ineffective when administered systemically. This peripheral route of opiate administration significantly reduces the side effects of opiate drugs.

Because the dorsal horn of the spinal cord has a high density of opioid receptors, morphine injected into the cerebrospinal fluid of the spinal cord subarachnoid space interacts with these receptors to elicit a profound and prolonged analgesia. Local administration of morphine is now commonly used in the treatment of postoperative pain, notably the pain associated with Caesarean section during childbirth. In addition to producing prolonged analgesia, intrathecal injection of morphine has fewer side effects because the drug does not diffuse far from its site of injection. Continuous local infusion of morphine to the spinal cord has also been used for the treatment of certain cancer pains.

Tolerance and Addiction to Opioids Are Distinct Phenomena

The chronic use of morphine invites major problems, most notably tolerance and addiction. The repeated use of morphine for pain relief can cause patients to develop resistance to the analgesic effects of the drug, with the consequence that progressively higher drug doses are required to achieve the same therapeutic effect.

What are the mechanisms underlying opiate tolerance? One theory holds that tolerance results from uncoupling of the opioid receptor from its G protein transducer. Nevertheless, the binding of naloxone to μ opiate receptors can precipitate withdrawal symptoms in tolerant subjects, suggesting that the opioid receptor is still active in the tolerant state. Tolerance may therefore also reflect a cellular response to the activation of opioid receptors, a response that counteracts the effects of the opiate and resets the system. Then, when the opiate is abruptly removed or naloxone is administered, this compensatory response is unmasked and withdrawal results.

Such physiological tolerance differs from addiction, a psychological craving for the drug. Psychological addiction almost never occurs when morphine is used to treat chronic pain.

An Overall View

Pain is a complex sensory state that reflects the integration of many sensory signals. More than most sensory modalities, its perception is influenced by emotional state and environmental contingency. Because pain is dependent on experience and varies so markedly from person to person, it remains notoriously difficult to treat.

Our understanding of the organization of central pain circuits, under both normal and pathological conditions, remains sadly incomplete. Nevertheless, over the past decade remarkable insights into the molecular mechanisms of peripheral pain transduction have developed, opening the way for new and more effective pain therapies.

First, human genetics and molecular biology have revealed that specific Na^+ channels are expressed selectively by nociceptive sensory neurons, and that mutation in the genes encoding one of these channels results in congenital insensitivity to pain while preserving other somatosensory modalities. These findings have prompted the search for small-molecule chemicals that can block nociceptor-specific Na^+ channels and thereby serve as selective peripheral analgesics. Second, the discovery that TRP channels encode sensory responses to a range of temperatures—from burning cold to scalding hot—and the knowledge that capsaicin and other small molecules activate these channels in a selective manner, has led to the development of many small-molecule TRP channel antagonists, some of which may prove to be effective in clinical pain syndromes.

How noxious mechanical stimuli are transduced remains a mystery, and defining the nature of the ion channels involved in the mechanotransduction of noxious stimuli remains an important challenge.

The classical finding that the balance of activity in small- and large-diameter sensory fibers modulates the perception of pain prompted the use of transcutaneous and dorsal-column electrical stimulation in the control of certain types of peripheral pain. This along with the observation that stimulation of specific sites in the brain stem produces profound analgesia has fostered efforts to control pain by activating endogenous modulatory systems. For example, the knowledge that opiates applied directly to the spinal cord elicit a potent analgesia led to the localized administration of opiates in certain clinical conditions by intrathecal and epidural routes.

Nevertheless, the uncertainties about the basic anatomy and functional organization of pain pathways mean that for most central pain syndromes there are still no effective pain therapies. Future progress in pain therapy will therefore depend on defining the logic of brain circuits that transmit nociceptive signals under normal and pathological conditions.

Allan I. Basbaum
Thomas M. Jessell

Selected Readings

Basbaum AI, Julius D. 2006. Toward better pain control. Sci Am 294:60–67.

Campbell JN, Meyer RA. 2006. Mechanisms of neuropathic pain. Neuron 52:77–92.

D'Mello R, Dickenson AH. 2008. Spinal cord mechanisms of pain. Br J Anaesth 101:8–16.

Fields HL, Basbaum AI. 1999. Central nervous system mechanisms of pain modulation. In: P Wall, R Melzack (eds). *Textbook of Pain*, pp. 243–57. Edinburgh: Churchill-Livingston.

Julius D. 2006. From peppers to peppermints: natural products as probes of the pain pathway. Harvey Lect 101: 89–115.

Marchand F, Perretti M, McMahon SB. 2005. Role of the immune system in chronic pain. Nat Rev Neurosci 6: 521–532.

Perl ER. 2007. Ideas about pain, a historical view. Nat Rev Neurosci 8:71–80.

Suzuki R, Rygh LJ, Dickenson AH. 2004. Bad news from the brain: descending 5-HT pathways that control spinal pain processing. Trends Pharmacol Sci 25:613–617.

Tracey I. 2008. Imaging pain. Br J Anaesth 101:32–39.

Wood JN. 2007. Ion channels in analgesia research. Handb Exp Pharmacol 177:329–358.

References

Akil H, Mayer DJ, Liebeskind JC. 1976. Antagonism of stimulation-produced analgesia by naloxone, a narcotic antagonist. Science 191:961–962.

Bautista DM, Siemens J, Glazer JM, Tsuruda PR, Basbaum AI, Stucky CL, Jordt SE, Julius D. 2007. The menthol receptor TRPM8 is the principal detector of environmental cold. Nature 44:204–208.

Bingham S, Beswick PJ, Blum DE, Gray NM, Chessell IP. 2006. The role of the cyclooxygenase pathway in nociception and pain. Semin Cell Dev Biol 17:544–554.

Brooks J, Tracey I. 2005. From nociception to pain perception: imaging the spinal and supraspinal pathways. J Anat 207:19–33.

Caterina MJ, Schumacher MA, Tominaga M, Rosen TA, Levine JD, Julius D. 1997. The capsaicin receptor: a heat-activated ion channel in the pain pathway. Nature 389: 816–824.

Cervero F, Iggo A. 1980. The substantia gelatinosa of the spinal cord. A critical review. Brain 103:717–772.

Coull JA, Beggs S, Boudreau D, Boivin D, Tsuda M, Inoue K, Gravel C, Salter MW, DeKonick Y. 2005. BDNF from microglia causes the shift in neuronal anion gradient underlying neuropathic pain. Nature 15:1017–1021.

Coutaux A, Adam F, Willer, J, LeBars D. 2005. Hyperalgesia and allodynia: peripheral mechanisms. Joint Bone Spine 72:359–371.

Cox JJ, Reimann F, Nicholas AK, Thornton G, Roberts E, Springell K, Karbani G, et al. 2006. An SCN9A channelopathy causes congenital inability to experience pain. Nature 444:894–898.

Craig AD. 2003. Pain mechanisms: labeled lines versus convergence in central processing. Annu Rev Neurosci 26:1–30.

Craig AD, Bushnell MC. 1994. The thermal grill illusion: unmasking the burn of cold pain. Science 265:252–255.

Craig AD, Reiman EM, Evans A, Bushnell MC. 1996. Functional imaging of an illusion of pain. Nature 384: 258–260.

Darland T, Heinricher MM, Grandy DK. 1988. Orphanin FQ/nociceptin: a role in pain and analgesia, but so much more. Trends Neurosci 21:215–221.

De Biasi S, Rustioni A. 1988. Glutamate and substance P co-exist in primary afferent terminals in the superficial laminae of spinal cord. Proc Natl Acad Sci U S A 85:7820–7824.

Dejerine J, Roussy G. 1906. Le syndrome thalamique. Rev Neurol 14:521–532.

Dhaka A, Viswanath V, Patapoutian A. 2006. TRP ion channels and temperature sensation. Annu Rev Neurosci 29:135–161.

Eide PK. 2000. Wind-up and the NMDA receptor complex from a clinical perspective. Eur J Pain 4:5–15.

Einarsdottir E, Carlsson A, Minde J, Toolanen G, Sevensson O, Solders G, Holmgren G, Holmberg D, Holmberg M. 2004. A mutation in the nerve growth factor beta gene causes loss of pain perception. Hum Mol Genet 13: 799–805.

Fertleman CR, Baker MD, Parker KA, Moffatt S, Elmslie FV, Abrahamsen B, Ostman J, et al. 2006. SCN9A mutations in paroxysmal extreme pain disorder: allelic variants underlie distinct channel defects and phenotypes. Neuron 52:767–774.

Fields H. 1987. *Pain*. New York: McGraw-Hill.

Flor H, Nikolajsen L, Staehelin Jensen TS. 2006. Phantom limb pain: a case of maladaptive CNS plasticity? Nature Rev Neurosci 7:873–881.

Foley KM. 1999. Advances in cancer pain. Arch Neurol 56:413–417.

Gold MS, Flake NM. 2005. Inflammation-mediated hyperexcitability of sensory neurons. Neurosignals 14:147–157.

Hefti FF, Rosenthal A, Walicke PA, Wyatt S, Vergara G, Shelton DL, Davies AM. 2006. Novel class of pain drugs based on antagonism of NGF. Trends Pharmacol Sci 27:85–91.

Heppenstall PA, Lewin GR. 2000. Neurotrophins, nociceptors and pain. Curr Opin Anaesthesiol 13:573–576.

Herrero JF, Laird JM, Lopez-Garcia JA. 2000. Wind-up of spinal cord neurons and pain sensation: much ado about something? Prog Neurobiol 61:169–203.

Hill RG, Oliver KR. 2007. Neuropeptide and kinin antagonists. Handb Exp Pharmacol 177:181–216.

Hosobuchi Y. 1986. Subcortical electrical stimulation for control of intractable pain in humans: report of 122 cases 1970–1984. J Neurosurg 64:543–553.

Huang J, Zhang X, McNaughton PA. 2006. Modulation of temperature-sensitive TRP channels. Semin Cell Dev Biol 17:638–645.

Ji RR, Strichartz G. 2004. Cell signaling and the genesis of neuropathic pain. Sci STKE 14:1–19.

Jones SL. 1992. Descending control of nociception. In: AR Light (ed). *Pain and Headache*, Vol. 12, *The Initial Processing of Pain and Its Descending Control: Spinal and Trigeminal Systems*, pp. 203-295. New York: Karger.

Jordt SE, McKemy DD, Julius D. 2003. Lessons from peppers and peppermint: the molecular basis of thermosensation. Curr Opin Neurobiol 13:487–492.

La Motte RH. 1984. Can the sensitization of nociceptors account for hyperalgesia after skin injury? Hum Neurobiol 3:47–52.

Levine JD, Fields HL, Basbaum A. 1993. Peptides and the primary afferent nociceptor. J Neurosci 13:2273–2286.

Lewin GR, Moshourab R. 2004. Mechanosensation and pain. J Neurobiol 61:30–44.

Light AR, Perl ER. 1984. Peripheral sensory systems. In: PJ Dyck, PK Thomas, EH Lambert, R Bunge (eds). *Peripheral Neuropathy* Vol. 1, 2nd ed, pp. 210–230. Philadelphia: Saunders.

Mason, P. 2001. Contributions of the medullary raphe and ventromedial reticular region to pain modulation and other homeostatic functions. Annu Rev Neurosci 24: 737–777.

Mantyh PW, Rogers SD, Honore P, Allen BJ, Gilardi JR, Li J, Daughters RS, Lappi DA, Wiley RG, Simone DA. 1997. Inhibition of hyperalgesia by ablation of lamina I spinal neurons expressing the substance P receptor. Science 278: 275–279.

Matthes HW, Maldonado R, Simonin F, Valverde O, Slowe S, Kitchen I, Befort K, et al. 1996. Loss of morphine-induced analgesia, reward effect and withdrawal symptoms in mice lacking the μ-opioid-receptor gene. Nature 383:819–823.

Melzack R, Wall PD. 1965. Pain mechanisms: a new theory. Science 150:971–979.

Milne RJ, Foreman RD, Giesler GJ Jr, Willis WD. 1981. Convergence of cutaneous and pelvic visceral nociceptive inputs onto primate spinothalamic neurons. Pain 11:163–183.

Minde JK. 2006. Norrbottnian congenital insensitivity to pain. Acta Orthop Suppl 77:2–32.

Pasternak GW. 2004. Multiple opiate receptors: déjà vu all over again. Neuropharmacology 47:312–323.

Pezet S, McMahon SB. 2006. Neurotrophins: mediators and modulators of pain. Annu Rev Neurosci 29:507–538.

Porreca F, Ossipov MH, Gebhart GF. 2002. Chronic pain and medullary descending facilitation. Trends Neurosci 25:319–325.

Raja SN, Campbell JN, Meyer RA. 1984. Evidence for different mechanisms of primary and secondary hyperalgesia following heat injury to the glabrous skin. Brain 107: 791–1188.

Reid G. 2005. ThermoTRP channels and cold sensing: what are they really up to? Eur J Physiol 451:250–263.

Silbert SC, Beacham DW, McCleskey EW. 2003. Quantitative single-cell differences in mu-opioid receptor mRNA distinguish myelinated and unmyelinated nociceptors. J Neurosci 23:34–42.

Strigo IA, Duncan GH, Boivin M, Bushnell MC. 2003. Differentiation of visceral and cutaneous pain in the human brain. J Neurophysiol 89:3294–3303.

Suzuki R, Dickenson A. 2005. Spinal and supraspinal contributions to central sensitization in peripheral neuropathy. Neurosignals 14:175–181.

Talbot JD, Marrett S, Evans AC, Meyer E, Bushnell MC, Duncan GH. 1991. Multiple representations of pain in human cerebral cortex. Science 251:1355–1358.

Terman GW, Shavit Y, Lewis JW, Cannon JT, Liebeskind JC. 1984. Intrinsic mechanisms of pain inhibition: activation by stress. Science 226:1270–1277.

Tominaga M, Caterina MJ. 2004. Thermosensation and pain. J Neurobiol 61:3–12.

Trafton JA, Basbaum AI. 2000. The contribution of spinal cord neurokinin-1 receptor signaling to pain. J Pain 1:57–65.

Willis WD. 1985. *The Pain System: The Neural Basis of Nociceptive Transmission in the Mammalian Nervous System.* Basel: Karger Press.

Yaksh TL, Noueihed R. 1985. The physiology and pharmacology of spinal opiates. Annu Rev Pharmacol Toxicol 25:433–462.

Yaksh TL, Rudy TA. 1976. Analgesia mediated by a direct spinal action of narcotics. Science 192:1357–1358.

Yotsumoto S, Setoyama M Hozumi H, Mizoguchi S, Fukumaru S, Kobayashi K, Saheki T, Kanzaki T. 1999. A novel point mutation affecting the tyrosine kinase domain of the TRKA gene in a family with congenital insensitivity to pain with anhidrosis. J Invest Dermatol 112:810–814.

Zeilhofer HU, Brune K. 2006. Analgesic strategies beyond the inhibition of cyclooxygenases. Trends Pharmacol Sci 27:467–4774.

25

The Constructive Nature of Visual Processing

We are so familiar with seeing, that it takes a leap of imagination to realize that there are problems to be solved. But consider it. We are given tiny distorted upside-down images in the eyes and we see separate solid objects in surrounding space. From the patterns of stimulation on the retina we perceive the world of objects and this is nothing short of a miracle.

—Richard L. Gregory, *Eye and Brain,* 1966

MOST OF OUR IMPRESSIONS of the world and our memories of it are based on sight. Yet the mechanisms that underlie vision are not at all obvious. How do we perceive form and movement? How do we distinguish colors? Identifying objects in complex visual environments is an extraordinary computational achievement that artificial vision systems have yet to duplicate. Vision is used not only for object recognition but also for guiding our movements, and these separate functions are mediated by at least two parallel and interacting pathways.

The existence of parallel pathways in the visual system raises one of the central questions of cognition, the binding problem. How are different types of information carried by discrete pathways brought together into a coherent visual image?

Visual Perception Is a Constructive Process

Vision is often incorrectly compared to the operation of a camera. Unlike a camera, however, the visual system is able to create a three-dimensional representation of the world from the two-dimensional images on the retina. In addition, an object is perceived as the same under strikingly different visual conditions.

A camera reproduces point-by-point the light intensities in one plane of the visual field. The brain, in contrast, parses scenes into distinct components, separating foreground from background, to determine which light stimuli belong to one object and which to others. In doing so it uses previously learned rules about the structure of the world. In analyzing the incoming stream of visual signals the brain guesses at the scene presented to the eyes based on past experience.

This *constructive* nature of visual perception has only recently been fully appreciated. Earlier thinking about sensory perception was greatly influenced by the British empiricist philosophers, notably John Locke, David Hume, and George Berkeley, who thought of perception as an atomistic process in which simple sensory elements, such as color, shape, and brightness, were assembled in an additive way, component by component. The modern view that perception is an active and creative process that involves more than just the information provided to the retina has its roots in the philosophy of Immanuel Kant and was developed in detail in the early 20th century by the German psychologists Max Wertheimer, Kurt Koffka, and Wolfgang Köhler, who founded the school of Gestalt psychology.

The German term *Gestalt* means configuration or form. The central idea of the Gestalt psychologists is that what we see about a stimulus—the perceptual interpretation we make of any visual object—depends not just on the properties of the stimulus but also on its context, on other features in the visual field. The Gestalt psychologists argued that the visual system processes sensory information about the shape, color, distance, and movement of objects according to computational rules inherent in the system. The brain has a way of looking at the world, a set of expectations that derives in part from experience and in part from built-in neural wiring.

Max Wertheimer wrote: "There are entities where the behavior of the whole cannot be derived from its individual elements nor from the way these elements fit together; rather the opposite is true: the properties of any of the parts are determined by the intrinsic structural laws of the whole." In the early part of the 20th century the Gestalt psychologists worked out the laws of perception that determine how we see, including similarity, proximity, and good continuation.

We see a uniform six-by-six array of dots as either rows or columns because of the brain's tendency to impose a pattern. Thus if the dots in each row are similar we are more likely to see a pattern of alternating rows (Figure 25–1A). If the dots in each column are closer together than those in the rows, we are more disposed to see a pattern of columns (Figure 25–1B). The principle of good continuation is an important basis for linking line elements into unified shapes (Figure 25–1C). It is also seen in the phenomenon of contour saliency, whereby smooth contours tend to pop out from complex backgrounds (Figure 25–1D).

An important step in object recognition is separating figure from background. At different moments the same elements in the visual field can be organized into a recognizable figure or serve as part of the background for other figures (Figure 25–2). Segmentation relies not only on certain geometric principles, but also on cognitive influences such as attention and expectation. Thus a priming stimulus or an internal representation of object shape can facilitate the association of visual elements into a unified percept (Figure 25–3).

The brain analyzes a visual scene at three levels: low, intermediate, and high (Figure 25–4). At the lowest level, which we consider in the next chapter, visual attributes such as local contrast, orientation, color, and movement are discriminated. The intermediate level involves analysis of the layout of scenes and of surface properties, parsing the visual image into surfaces and global contours, and distinguishing foreground from background (see Chapter 27). The highest level involves object recognition (see Chapter 28). Once a scene has been parsed by the brain and objects recognized, the objects can be matched with memories of shapes and their associated meanings. Vision also has an important role in guiding body movement, particularly hand movement (see Chapter 29).

In vision as in other cognitive operations, various features—motion, depth, form, and color—occur together in a unified percept. This unity is achieved not by one hierarchical neural system but by multiple areas in the brain that are fed by at least two major interacting neural pathways. Because distributed processing is one of the main organizational principles in the neurobiology of vision, one must have a grasp of the anatomical pathways of the visual system to understand fully the physiological description of visual processing in later chapters.

In this chapter we lay the foundation for understanding the neural circuitry and organizational principles of the visual pathways. These principles apply quite broadly and are relevant not only for the multiple areas of the brain concerned with vision but also for other types of information processing by the brain.

Visual Perception Is Mediated by the Geniculostriate Pathway

Visual processing begins in the two retinae (see Chapter 26). The axons of the retinal ganglion cells, the projection neurons of the retina, form the optic nerve that extends to a midline crossing point, the optic chiasm. Beyond the chiasm fibers from the temporal hemiretinas proceed to the ipsilateral hemisphere; fibers from the nasal hemiretinas cross to the contralateral hemisphere (Figure 25–5). Because the temporal hemiretina of one eye sees the same half of the visual field (hemifield) as the nasal hemiretina of the other, the partial decussation of fibers at the chiasm ensures that all the information about each hemifield is processed in the visual cortex of the contralateral hemisphere.

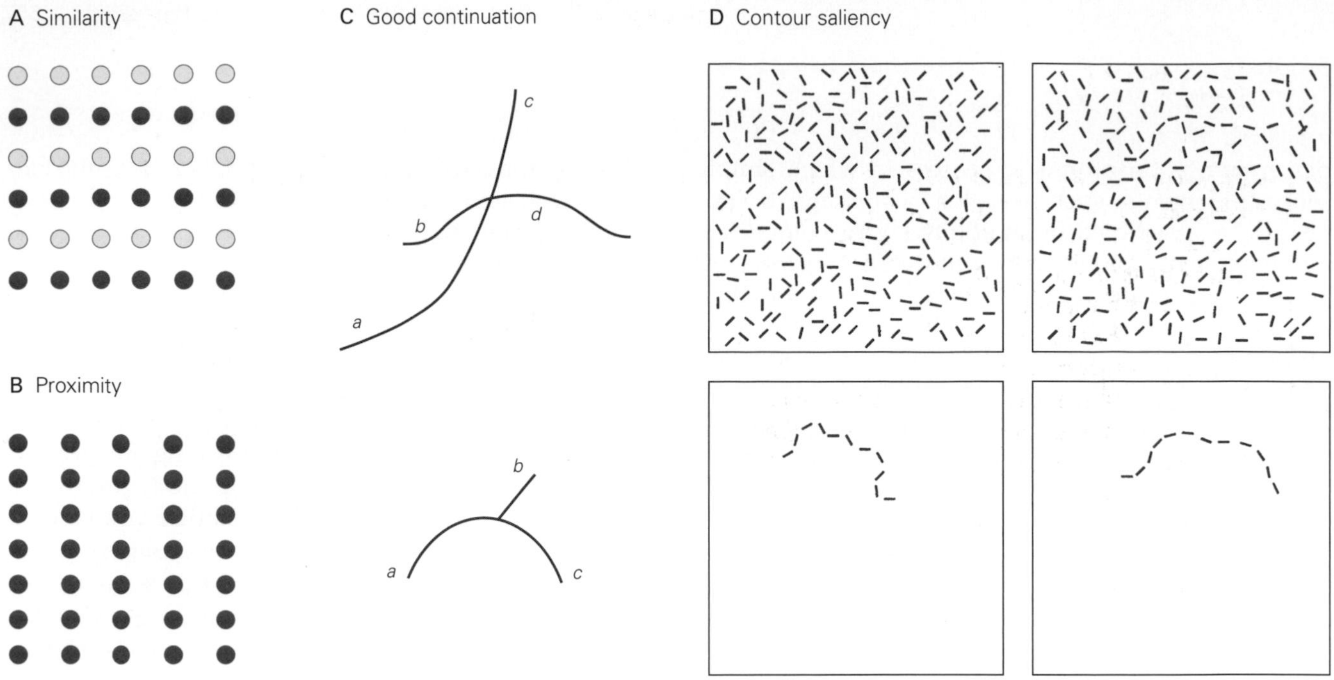

Figure 25–1 Organizational rules of visual perception. To link the elements of a visual scene into unified percepts, the visual system relies on organizational rules such as similarity, proximity, and good continuation.

A. The dots in each row have the same color, and thus, an overall pattern of alternating blue and white rows is perceived.

B. The dots in the columns are closer together than those in the rows, leading to the perception of columns.

C. Line segments are perceptually linked when they are collinear. In the top set of lines, one is more likely to see line segment **a** as belonging with **c** rather than **d**. In the bottom set **a** and **c** are perceptually linked because they maintain the same curvature, whereas **a** and **b** appear to be discontinuous.

D. The principle of good continuation is also seen in contour saliency. On the right a smooth contour of line elements pops out from the background, whereas the jagged contour on the left is lost in the background. (Adapted, with permission, from Field, Hayes, and Hess 1993.)

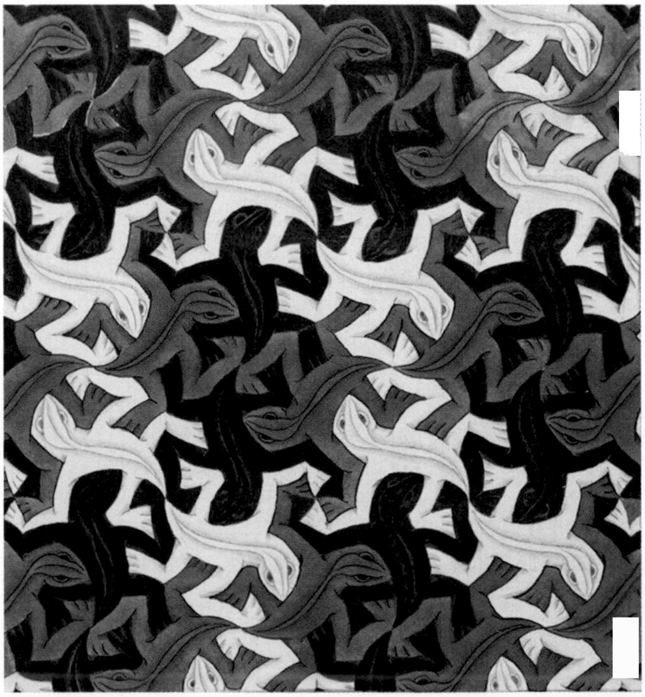

Figure 25–2 Object recognition depends on the separation of foreground and background in a scene. Recognition of the white salamanders in this image depends on the brain's segmentation of the image, situating the white salamanders in the foreground and the brown and black salamanders in the background. The image also illustrates the role of higher influences in segmentation: One can consciously select any of the three colors as the foreground. (Reproduced, with permission, from M.C. Escher's "Symmetry Drawing E56" © 2010 The M.C. Escher Company-Holland. All rights reserved. www.mcescher.com.)

Figure 25–3 Expectation and perceptual task play a critical role in what is seen. It is difficult to segment the dark and white patches in this figure into foreground and background without additional information. After viewing the priming image on page 561, this figure immediately becomes recognizable. In this example higher-order representations of shape guide lower-order processes of segmentation. (Reproduced, with permission, from Porter 1954.)

Beyond the optic chiasm the axons from nasal and temporal hemiretinas carrying input from one hemifield join in the optic tract, which extends to the lateral geniculate nucleus of the thalamus. The lateral geniculate nucleus in primates consists of six layers, each of which receives input from either the ipsilateral or the contralateral eye. Because each layer contains a map of the contralateral hemifield, six concordant maps are stacked atop one another. The thalamic neurons then relay retinal information to the primary visual cortex.

The primary visual pathway is also called the geniculostriate pathway because it passes through the lateral geniculate nucleus on its way to the primary visual cortex, also known as the striate cortex because of the myelin-rich stripe that runs through its middle layers. A second pathway from the retina runs to the superior colliculus and is important in controlling eye movements. This pathway continues to the pontine formation in the brain stem and then to the extraocular motor nuclei. A third pathway extends from the retina to the pretectal area of the midbrain, where neurons mediate the pupillary reflexes that control the amount of light entering the eyes.

Each lateral geniculate nucleus projects to the primary visual cortex through a pathway known as the optic radiation (Figure 25–6A). These afferent fibers form a complete neural map of the contralateral visual field in the primary visual cortex. Beyond the striate cortex lie the extrastriate areas, a set of higher-order visual areas that are also organized as neural maps of the visual field. The preservation of the spatial arrangement of inputs from the retina is called retinotopy, and a neural map of the visual field is described as retinotopic or having a retinotopic frame of reference.

The primary visual cortex constitutes the first level of cortical processing of visual information. From there information is transmitted over two major pathways. A ventral pathway into the temporal lobe carries information about what the stimulus is, and a dorsal pathway into the parietal lobe carries information about where the stimulus is, information that is critical for guiding movement.

A major fiber bundle called the corpus callosum connects the two hemispheres, transmitting information across the midline. The primary visual cortex in either hemisphere represents slightly more than half the visual field, with the two hemifield representations overlapping at the vertical meridian. One of the functions of the corpus callosum is to unify the perception of objects spanning the vertical meridian by linking the cortical areas that represent opposite hemifields.

Form, Color, Motion, and Depth Are Processed in Discrete Areas of the Cerebral Cortex

In the late 19th and early 20th centuries the cerebral cortex was differentiated by the anatomist Korbinian Brodmann and others using anatomical criteria. The criteria included the size, shape, and packing density of neurons in the cortical layers and the thickness and density of myelin. The functionally distinct cortical areas we have considered heretofore correspond only loosely to Brodmann's classification. The primary visual cortex (V1) is identical to Brodmann's area 17. In the extrastriate cortex the secondary visual area, V2, corresponds to area 18. Beyond that, however, area 19 contains several functionally distinct areas that generally cannot be defined by anatomical criteria.

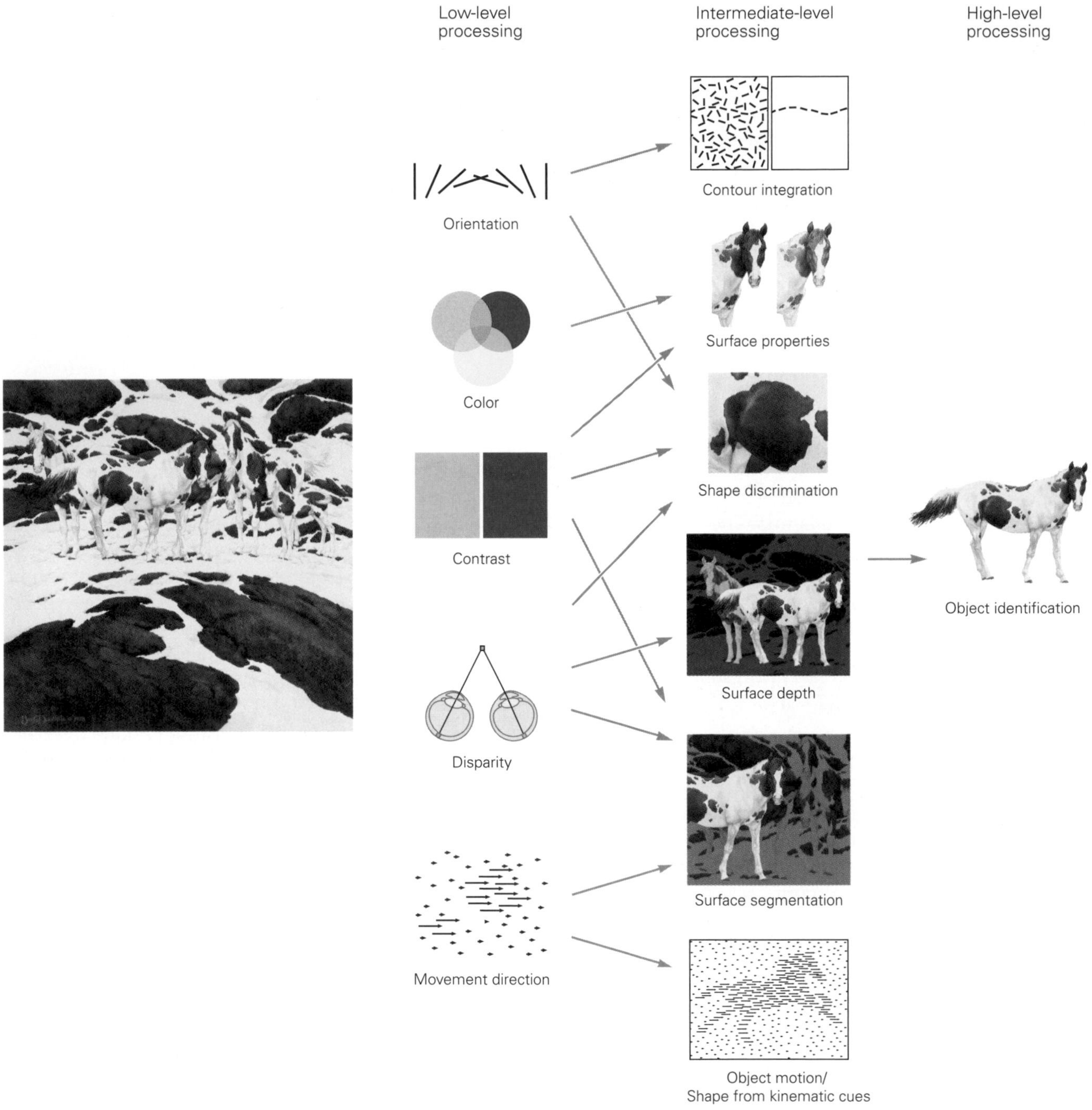

Figure 25–4 A visual scene is analyzed at three levels. First, simple attributes of the visual environment are analyzed (low-level processing). These low-level features are used to parse the visual scene (intermediate-level processing): Local visual features are assembled into surfaces, objects are segregated from background (surface segmentation), local orientation is integrated into global contours (contour integration), and surface shape is identified from shading and kinematic cues. Finally, surfaces and contours are used to identify the object (high-level processing). (Images of horses reproduced, with permission, from *Pintos*, © Bev Doolittle, courtesy of The Greenwich Workshop, Inc., www.greenwichworkshop.com.)

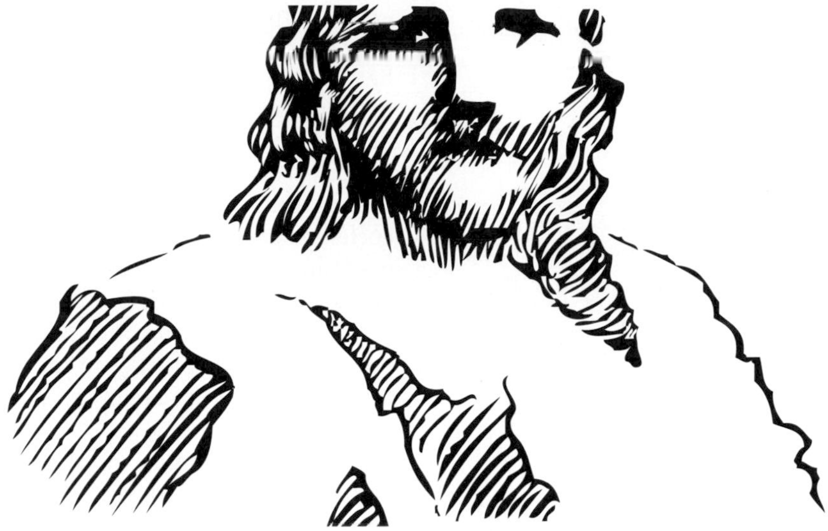

Priming image for Figure 25–3

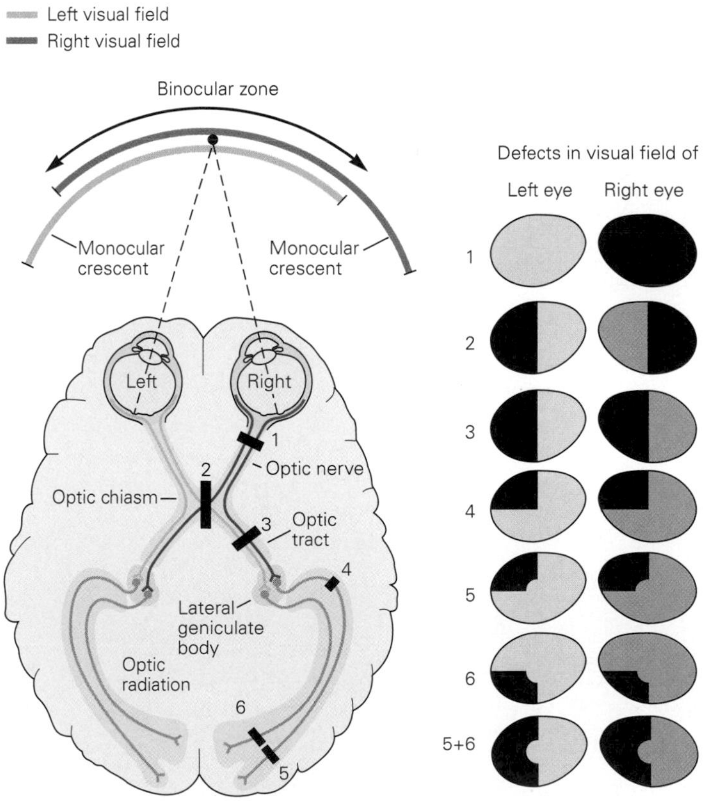

Figure 25–5 Representation of the visual field along the visual pathway. Each eye sees most of the visual field, with the exception of a portion of the peripheral visual field known as the monocular crescent. The axons of retinal neurons (ganglion cells) carry information from each visual hemifield along the optic nerve up to the optic chiasm, where fibers from the nasal hemiretina cross to the opposite hemisphere. Fibers from the temporal hemiretina stay on the same side, joining the fibers from the nasal hemiretina of the contralateral eye to form the optic tract. The optic tract carries information from the opposite visual hemifield originating in both eyes and projects into the lateral geniculate nucleus. Cells in this nucleus send their axons along the optic radiation to the primary visual cortex.

Lesions along the visual pathway produce specific visual field deficits, as shown on the right:

1. A lesion of an optic nerve causes a total loss of vision in one eye.

2. A lesion of the optic chiasm causes a loss of vision in the temporal half of each visual hemifield (bitemporal hemianopsia).

3. A lesion of the optic tract causes a loss of vision in the opposite half of the visual hemifield (contralateral hemianopsia).

4. A lesion of the optic radiation fibers that curve into the temporal lobe (Meyer's loop) causes loss of vision in the upper quadrant of the contralateral visual hemifield in both eyes (upper contralateral quadrantic anopsia).

5,6. Partial lesions of the visual cortex lead to deficits in portions of the contralateral visual hemifield. For example, a lesion in the upper bank of the calcarine sulcus (**5**) causes a partial deficit in the inferior quadrant, while a lesion in the lower bank (**6**) causes a partial deficit in the superior quadrant. The central area of the visual field tends to be unaffected by cortical lesions because of the extent of the representation of the fovea and the duplicate representation of the vertical meridian in the hemispheres.

The number of functionally discrete areas of visual cortex varies between species. Macaque monkeys have more than 30 areas. Although not all visual areas in humans have yet been identified, the number is likely to be at least as great as in the macaque. If one includes oculomotor areas and prefrontal areas contributing to visual memory, almost half of the cerebral cortex is involved with vision. Functional magnetic resonance imaging (fMRI) has made it possible to establish homologies between the visual areas of the macaque and human brains (Figure 25–7). Based on pathway tracing studies in monkeys, we now appreciate that these areas are organized in functional streams (Figure 25–7B).

The visual areas of cortex can be differentiated either by their representation of visual space, known as a visuotopic (or retinotopic) map, or by the functional properties of their neurons. Studies of these two differences have revealed that the visual areas are organized in two hierarchical pathways, a ventral pathway involved in object recognition and a dorsal pathway dedicated to the use of visual information for guiding movements. The ventral or object-recognition pathway extends from the primary visual cortex to the temporal lobe; it is described in detail in Chapter 28. The dorsal

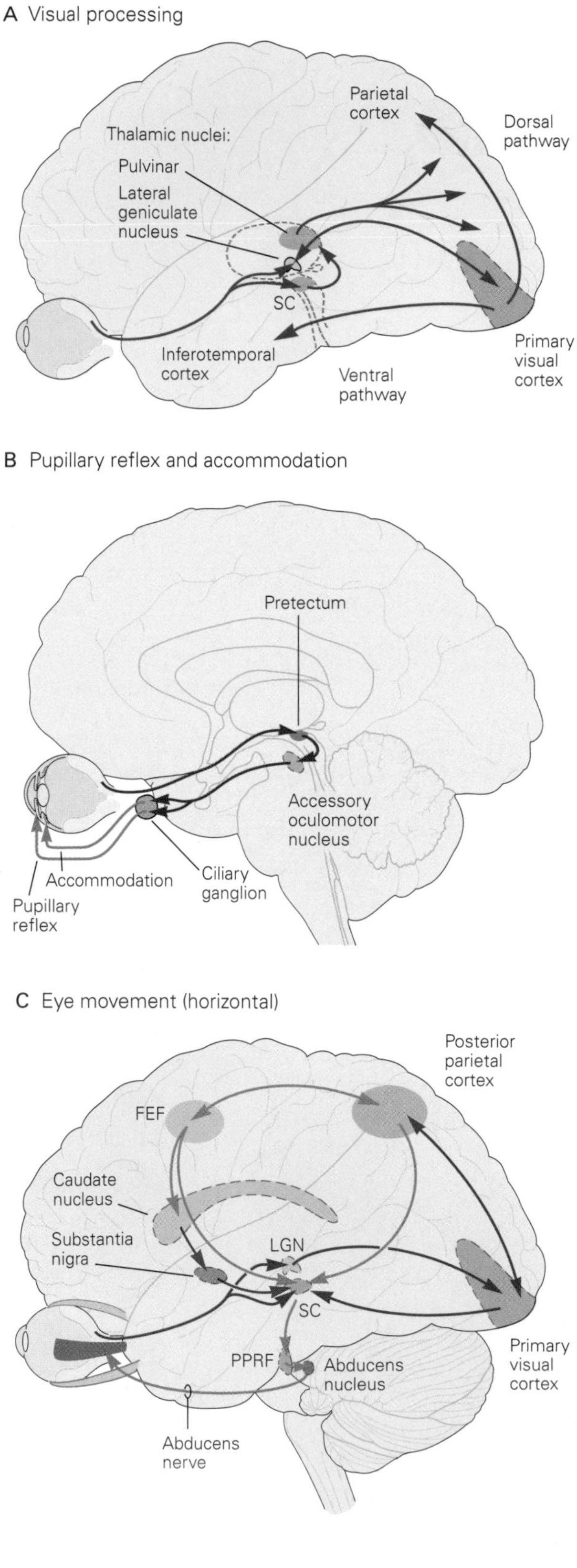

Figure 25–6 Pathways for visual processing, pupillary reflex and accommodation, and control of eye position.

A. *Visual processing.* The eye sends information first to thalamic nuclei, including the lateral geniculate nucleus and pulvinar, and from there to cortical areas. Cortical projections go forward from the primary visual cortex to areas in the parietal lobe (the dorsal pathway, which is concerned with visually guided movement) and areas in the temporal lobe (the ventral pathway, which is concerned with object recognition). The pulvinar also serves as a relay between cortical areas to supplement their direct connections.

B. *Pupillary reflex and accommodation.* Light signals are relayed through the midbrain pretectum, to preganglionic parasympathetic neurons in the Edinger-Westphal nucleus, and out through the parasympathetic outflow of the oculomotor nerve to the ciliary ganglion. Postganglionic neurons innervate the smooth muscle of the pupillary sphincter, as well as the muscles controlling the lens.

C. *Eye movement.* Information from the retina is sent to the superior colliculus (**SC**) directly along the optic nerve and indirectly through the geniculostriate pathway to cortical areas (primary visual cortex, posterior parietal cortex, and frontal eye fields) that project back to the superior colliculus. The colliculus projects to the pons (**PPRF**), which then sends control signals to oculomotor nuclei, including the abducens nucleus, which controls lateral movement of the eyes. (**FEF**, frontal eye field; **LGN**, lateral geniculate nucleus; **PPRF**, paramedian pontine reticular formation.)

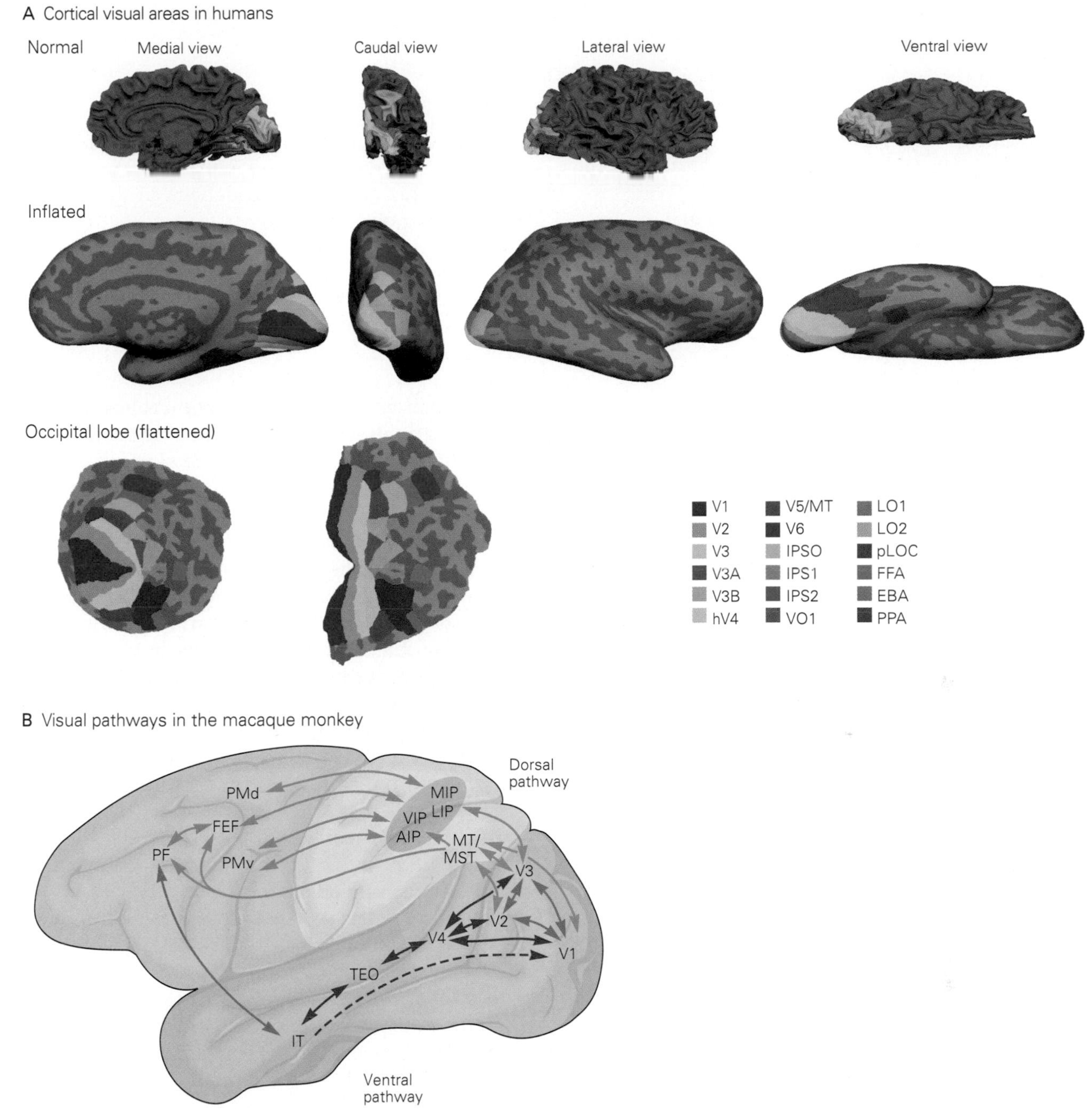

Figure 25–7 Visual pathways in the cerebral cortex.

A. Areas of the human cerebral cortex involved in visual processing as shown by fMRI. The **top row** shows areas on the gyri and sulci of a normal brain; the **middle row** shows inflated views of the brain, with light and dark grey regions representing gyri and sulci; the **bottom row** shows a two-dimensional representation of the occipital lobe (**left**) and a representation with less distortion by making a cut along the calcarine fissure. The areas are delineated by stimulus-based retinotopy (early visual areas V1, V2, and V3 converge at the representation of the fovea at the occipital pole, V3A, V3B, V6, V7, hV4, VO1, LO1, LO2, V5/MT), attention-based retinotopy (IPS1 and IPS2), or responsiveness to specific attributes or classes of objects (for less strictly retinotopic areas). Functional specificity has been demonstrated for a number of these areas: VO1 is implicated in color processing, the lateral occipital complex (LO2, pLOC) codes object shape, FFA (fusiform face area) codes faces, the parahippocampal place area (PPA) responds more strongly to places than to objects, the extrastriate body area (EBA) responds more strongly to body parts than objects, and V5/MT is involved in motion processing. Areas in the intraparietal sulcus (IPS1 and IPS2) are involved in control of spatial attention and saccadic eye movements. (Images from V. Piech, reproduced with permission.)

B. In the macaque monkey V1 is located on the surface of the occipital lobe and sends axons in two pathways. A dorsal pathway courses through a number of areas in the parietal lobe and into the frontal lobe, and a ventral pathway projects through V4 into areas of the inferior temporal cortex. In addition to feedforward pathways extending from primary visual cortex into the temporal, parietal, and frontal lobes, there are reciprocal or feedback pathways running in the opposite direction. (**AIP**, anterior intraparietal area; **FEF**, frontal eye field; **IT**, inferior temporal cortex; **LIP**, lateral intraparietal area; **MIP**, medial intraparietal area; **MT**, middle temporal area; **PF**, prefrontal cortex; **PMd**, dorsal premotor cortex; **PMv**, ventral premotor cortex; **V1**, primary visual cortex, Brodmann's area 17; **V2**, secondary visual area, Brodmann's area 18; **V3**, **V4**, third and fourth visual areas; **VIP**, ventral intraparietal area.)

or movement-guidance pathway connects the primary visual cortex with the parietal lobe and then with the frontal lobes.

The pathways are interconnected so that information is shared. For example, movement information in the dorsal pathway can contribute to object recognition through kinematic cues. Information about movements in space derived from areas in the dorsal pathway is therefore important for the perception of object shape and is fed into the ventral pathway.

Reciprocity is an important feature of the connectivity between cortical areas. All connections between cortical areas are reciprocal—each area sends information back to the areas from which it receives input. These feedback connections provide information about cognitive functions, including spatial attention, stimulus expectation, and emotional content, to earlier levels of visual processing. The pulvinar in the thalamus serves as a relay between cortical areas (see Figure 25–6A).

The dorsal pathway courses through the parietal cortex, a region that uses visual information to direct the movement of the eyes and limbs, that is, for visuomotor integration. One area, the lateral intraparietal area named for its location in the interparietal sulcus, is involved in representing points in space that are the targets of eye movements or reaching. Patients with lesions of parietal areas fail to attend to objects on one side of the body, a syndrome called *unilateral neglect* (see Chapter 17).

The ventral pathway extends into the temporal lobe. The inferior temporal cortex stores information about the shapes and identities of objects; one portion represents faces, for damage to that region results in the inability to recognize faces (*prosopagnosia*).

The dorsal and ventral pathways each comprise a hierarchical series of areas that can be delineated by several criteria. First, at many relays the array of inputs forms a map of the visual hemifield, and each such representation can be used to delineate a visual area. This is particularly useful at early levels of the pathway where the receptive fields of neurons are small and visuotopic maps are precisely organized. At higher levels, however, the receptive fields become larger, the maps less precise, and visuotopic organization is therefore a less reliable basis to delineate the boundaries of an area.

Another means to differentiate one area from another, as shown by experiments in monkeys, depends upon the distinctive functional properties exhibited by the neurons in each area. The clearest example of this is an area in the dorsal pathway, the middle temporal area (MT or V5), which contains neurons with a strong selectivity for the direction of movement across their receptive fields. Consistent with the idea that the middle temporal area is involved in the analysis of motion, lesions of this area produce deficits in the ability to track moving objects.

The Receptive Fields of Neurons at Successive Relays in an Afferent Pathway Provide Clues to How the Brain Analyzes Visual Form

In 1906 Charles Sherrington coined the term *receptive field* in his analysis of the scratch withdrawal reflex: "The whole collection of points of skin surface from which the scratch-reflex can be elicited is termed the receptive field of that reflex." When it became possible to record from single neurons in the eye, H. Keffer Hartline applied the concept of the receptive field in his study of the retina of the horseshoe crab, *Limulus:* "The region of the retina which must be illuminated in order to obtain a response in any given fiber . . . is termed the receptive field of that fiber." In the visual system a neuron's receptive field represents a small window on visual space (Figure 25–8).

But responses measured with only one spot of light yielded only a limited understanding of a cell's receptive field. Using two small spots of light, both Hartline and Stephen Kuffler, who studied the mammalian retina, found an inhibitory surround or lateral inhibitory region in the receptive field. In 1953 Kuffler observed that "not only the areas from which responses can actually be set up by retinal illumination may be included in a definition of the receptive field but also all areas which show a functional connection, by an inhibitory or excitatory effect on a ganglion cell." Kuffler thus revealed that the receptive fields of retinal ganglion cells have functionally distinct subareas. These receptive fields have a center-surround organization and fall into one of two categories: *on-center* and *off-center*. Later work demonstrated that neurons in the lateral geniculate nucleus have similar receptive fields.

The on-center cells fire when a spot of light is turned on within a circular central region. Off-center cells fire when a spot of light in the center of their receptive field is turned off. The surrounding annular region has the opposite sign. For on-center cells a light stimulus that does not include the center produces a response when the light is turned off, a response termed *on-center, off-surround*. The center and surround areas are mutually inhibitory (Figure 25–9). When both center and surround are illuminated with diffuse light there is little or no response. Conversely, a light-dark boundary across the receptive field produces a brisk response. Because these neurons are most sensitive to

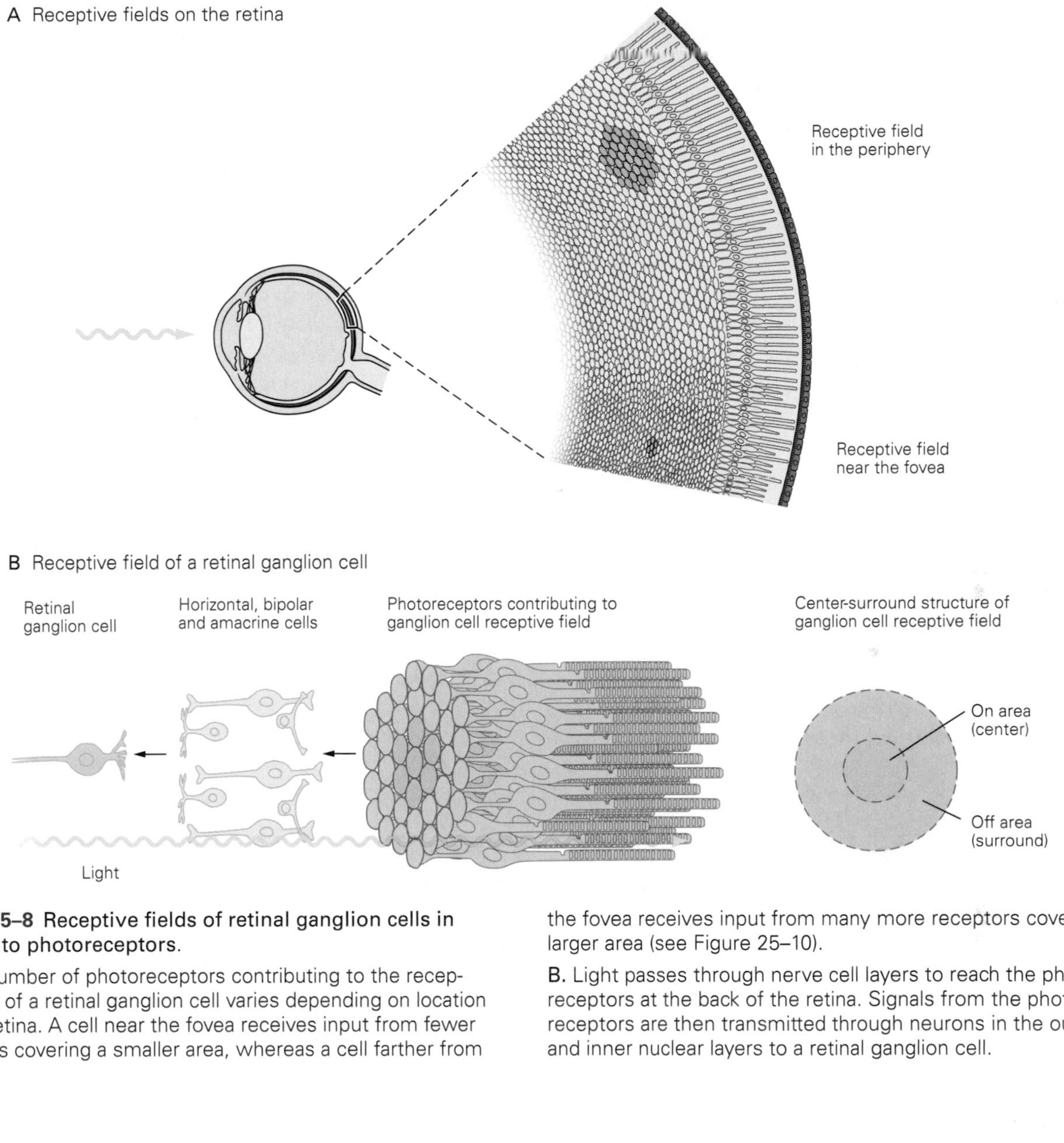

Figure 25–8 Receptive fields of retinal ganglion cells in relation to photoreceptors.

A. The number of photoreceptors contributing to the receptive field of a retinal ganglion cell varies depending on location on the retina. A cell near the fovea receives input from fewer receptors covering a smaller area, whereas a cell farther from the fovea receives input from many more receptors covering a larger area (see Figure 25–10).

B. Light passes through nerve cell layers to reach the photoreceptors at the back of the retina. Signals from the photoreceptors are then transmitted through neurons in the outer and inner nuclear layers to a retinal ganglion cell.

borders and contours—to differences in illumination as opposed to uniform surfaces—they encode information about contrast in the visual field.

The size on the retina of a receptive field varies both according to the field's *eccentricity*—its position relative to the fovea, the central part of the retina where visual acuity is highest—and the position of neurons along the visual pathway. Receptive fields with the same eccentricity are relatively small at early levels in visual processing and become progressively larger at later levels. The size of the receptive field is expressed in terms of degrees of visual angle; the entire visual field covers nearly 180° (Figure 25–10A). In early relays of visual processing the receptive fields near the fovea are the smallest. The receptive fields for retinal ganglion cells that monitor portions of the fovea subtend approximately 0.1°, whereas those in the visual periphery reach up to 10°.

The amount of cortex dedicated to a degree of visual space changes with eccentricity. More cortical space is dedicated to the central part of vision, where the receptive fields are smallest and the visual system has the greatest spatial resolution (Figure 25–10C).

Receptive-field properties change from relay to relay along a visual pathway. By determining these properties one can assay the function of each relay

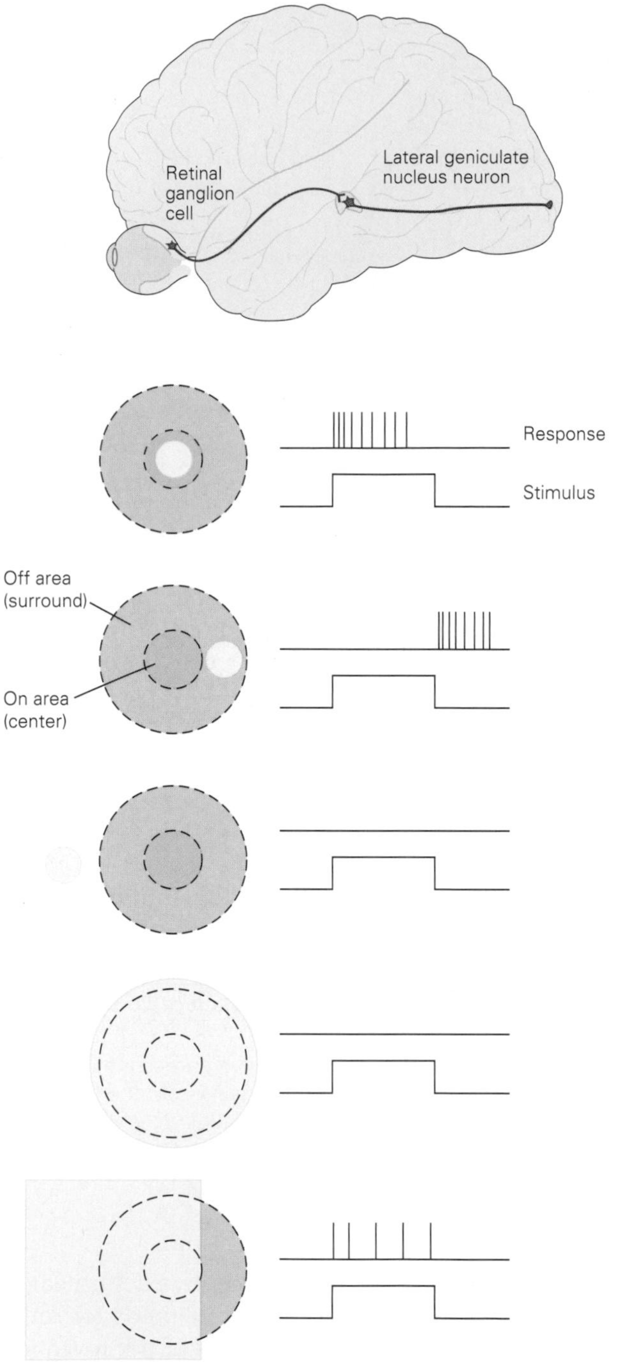

Figure 25–9 Receptive fields of neurons at early relays of visual pathways. A circular symmetric receptive field with mutually antagonistic center and surround is characteristic of retinal ganglion cells and neurons in the lateral geniculate nucleus of the thalamus. The center can respond to the onset or offset of a spot of light (**yellow**), and the surround has the opposite response. Outside the surround there is no response, thus defining the receptive field boundary. The response is weak when light covers both the center and surround, so these neurons respond optimally to contrast (a light-dark boundary) in the visual field.

nucleus and how visual information is progressively analyzed by the brain. For example, the change in receptive-field structure that occurs between the lateral geniculate nucleus and cerebral cortex reveals an important mechanism in the brain's analysis of visual form. The key property of the form pathway is selectivity for the orientation of contours in the visual field. This is an emergent property of signal processing in primary visual cortex; it is not a property of the cortical input but is generated within the cortex itself.

Whereas retinal ganglion cells and neurons in the lateral geniculate nucleus have concentric center-surround receptive fields, those in the cortex, although equally sensitive to contrast, also analyze contours. David Hubel and Torsten Wiesel discovered this characteristic in 1958 while studying what visual stimuli provoked activity in neurons in the primary visual cortex. While showing an anesthetized animal slides containing a variety of images, they recorded extracellularly from individual neurons in the visual cortex. As they switched from one slide to another they found a neuron that produced a brisk train of action potentials. The cell was responding not to the image on the slide but to the edge of the slide as it was moved into position.

The Visual Cortex Is Organized into Columns of Specialized Neurons

The dominant feature of the functional organization of the primary visual cortex is the visuotopic organization of its cells: the visual field is systematically represented across the surface of the cortex (Figure 25–11A).

In addition, cells in the primary visual cortex with similar functional properties are located close together in columns that extend from the cortical surface to the white matter. The columns are concerned with the functional properties that are analyzed in any given cortical area and thus reflect the functional role of that area in vision. The properties that are developed in the primary visual cortex include orientation specificity and the integration of inputs from the two eyes, which is measured as the relative strength of input from each eye, or ocular dominance.

Ocular-dominance columns reflect the segregation of thalamocortical inputs arriving from different layers of the lateral geniculate nucleus. Alternating layers of this nucleus receive input from retinal ganglion cells located in either the ipsilateral or contralateral retina (Figure 25–12). This segregation is maintained in the inputs from the lateral geniculate nucleus to the primary visual cortex, producing the alternating left-eye and right-eye ocular dominance bands (Figure 25–11B),

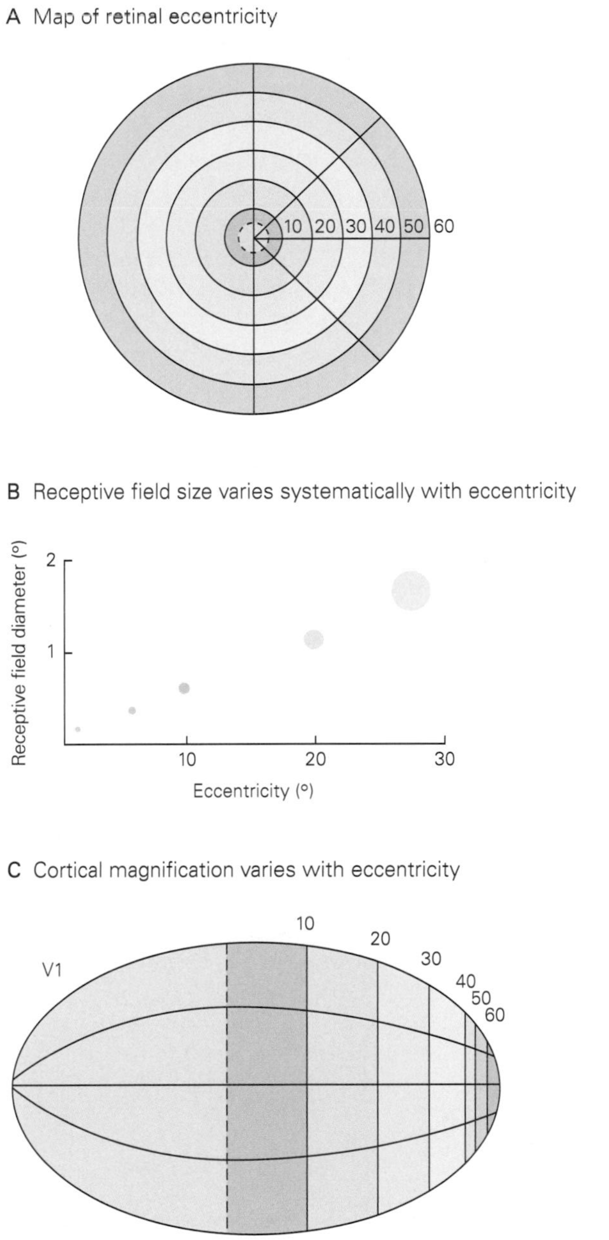

Figure 25–10 Receptive field size, eccentricity, retinotopic organization, and magnification factor. The color code refers to position in visual space or on the retina.

A. The distance of a receptive field from the fovea is referred to as the eccentricity of the receptive field.

B. Receptive field size varies with distance from the fovea. The smallest fields lie in the center of gaze, the fovea, where the visual resolution is highest; fields become progressively larger with distance from the fovea.

C. The amount of cortical area dedicated to inputs from within each degree of visual space, known as the magnification factor, also varies with eccentricity. The central part of the visual field commands the largest area of cortex. For example, in area V1 more area is dedicated to the central 10° of visual space than to all the rest. The map of V1 shows the cortical sheet unfolded.

which receive input from the respective layers of the lateral geniculate nucleus.

Cells with similar orientation preferences are also grouped into columns. Across the cortical surface there is a regular clockwise and counterclockwise cycling of orientation preference with the full 180° cycle repeating every 750 μm (Figure 25–11C). One full cycle of orientation columns is called a *hypercolumn*. Likewise, the left- and right-eye dominance columns alternate with a periodicity of 750 to 1,000 μm. The orientation and ocular dominance columns are crisscrossed over the cortical surface.

Both types of columns were first mapped by recording the responses of neurons at closely spaced electrode penetrations in the cortex. The ocular-dominance columns were also identified by making lesions or tracer injections in individual layers of the lateral geniculate nucleus. More recently a technique known as optical imaging has enabled researchers to visualize a surface representation of the orientation and ocular dominance columns in living animals. Developed for studies of cortical organization by Amiram Grinvald, this technique visualizes changes in surface reflectance associated with the metabolic requirements of active groups of neurons, known as intrinsic-signal optical imaging, or changes in fluorescence of voltage-sensitive dyes. Intrinsic-signal imaging depends on activity-associated changes in local blood flow and alterations in the oxidative state of hemoglobin and other intrinsic chromophores.

An experimenter can visualize the distribution of cells with left or right ocular dominance, for example, by subtracting the image obtained while stimulating one eye from that acquired while stimulating the other. When viewed in a plane tangential to the cortical surface, the ocular dominance columns appear as alternating left- and right-eye stripes, each approximately 750 μm in width (Figure 25–11B).

The cycles of orientation columns form various structures, from parallel stripes to pinwheels. Sharp jumps in orientation preference occur at the pinwheel centers and "fractures" in the orientation map (Figure 25–11C). Superimposed on these is a third columnar system of continuously changing directional preference.

Embedded within the orientation and ocular-dominance columns are clusters of neurons that have poor orientation selectivity but strong color preferences. These units of specialization, located within the superficial layers, were revealed by a histochemical label for the enzyme cytochrome oxidase, which is distributed in a regular patchy pattern of blobs and interblobs. In the primary visual cortex these blobs are

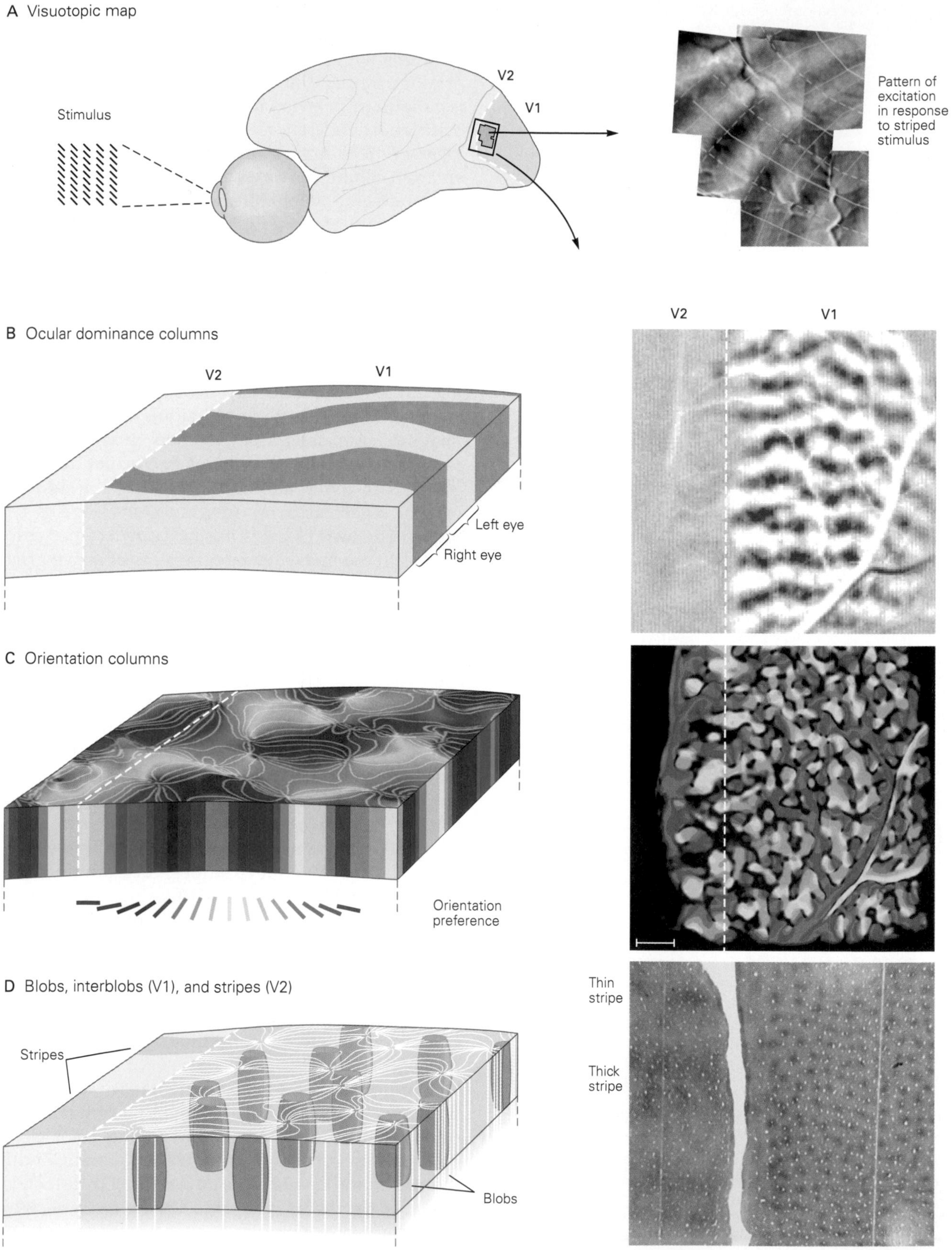
A Visuotopic map
Stimulus
V2
V1
Pattern of excitation in response to striped stimulus
B Ocular dominance columns
V2
V1
Left eye
Right eye
C Orientation columns
Orientation preference
D Blobs, interblobs (V1), and stripes (V2)
Stripes
Blobs
Thin stripe
Thick stripe

Figure 25–11 (Opposite) **Functional architecture of the primary visual cortex.** (Images from M. Kinoshita and A. Das, reproduced with permission.)

A. The surface of the primary visual cortex is functionally organized in a map of the visual field. The elevations and azimuths of visual space are organized in a regular grid that is distorted because of variation in the magnification factor (see Figure 25–10). The grid is visible here in the dark stripes (visualized with intrinsic-signal optical imaging), which reflect the pattern of neurons that responded to a series of vertical candy stripes. Within this surface map one finds repeated superimposed cycles of functionally specific columns of cells, as illustrated in B, C, and D.

B. The dark and light stripes represent the surface view of the left and right ocular dominance columns. These stripes intersect the border between areas V1 and V2, the representation of the vertical meridian, at right angles.

C. Some columns contain cells with similar selectivity for the orientation of stimuli. The different colors indicate the orientation preference of the columns. The orientation columns in surface view are best described as pinwheels surrounding singularities of sudden changes in orientation (the center of the pinwheel). The scale bar represents 1 mm. (Surface image of orientation columns on the left reproduced, with permission, from G. Blasdel.)

D. Patterns of blobs in V1 and stripes in V2 represent other modules of functional organization. These patterns are visualized with cytochrome oxidase.

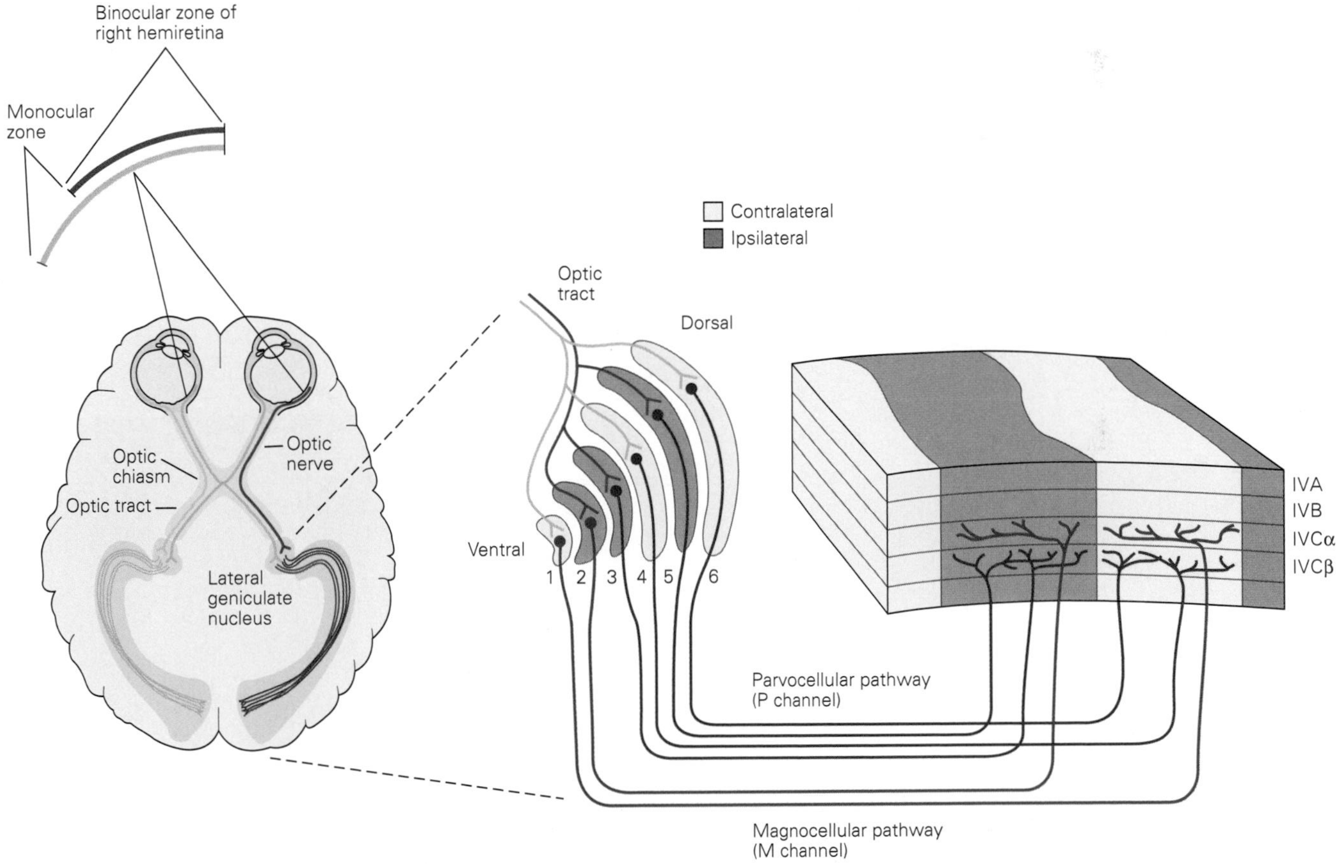

Figure 25–12 Projections from the lateral geniculate nucleus to the visual cortex. The lateral geniculate nucleus in each hemisphere receives input from the temporal retina of the ipsilateral eye and the nasal retina of the contralateral eye. The nucleus is a laminated structure comprising four parvocellular layers (layers 3 to 6) and two magnocellular layers (layers 1 and 2). The inputs from the two eyes terminate in different layers: The contralateral eye projects to layers 1, 4, and 6, whereas the ipsilateral eye sends input to layers 2, 3, and 5. The parvocellular and magnocellular inputs to the primary visual cortex arrive in separate sublayers. The parvocellular layers project to layer IVCβ and the magnocellular layers to layer IVCα. In addition, the afferents from the ipsilateral and contralateral layers of the lateral geniculate nucleus are segregated into alternating ocular-dominance columns.

a few hundred micrometers in diameter and 750 μm apart (Figure 25–11D). The blobs correspond to clusters of color-selective neurons. Because they are rich in cells with color selectivity and poor in cells with orientation selectivity, the blobs are specialized to provide information about surfaces rather than edges.

In area V2 thick and thin dark stripes separated by pale stripes are evident with cytochrome oxidase labeling (Figure 25–11D). The thick stripes contain neurons selective for direction of movement and for binocular disparity as well as cells that are responsive to illusory contours and global disparity cues. The thin stripes hold cells specialized for color. The pale stripes contain orientation-selective neurons.

For every visual attribute to be analyzed at each position in the visual field there must be adequate tiling, or coverage, of neurons with different functional properties. As one moves in any direction across the cortical surface, the progression of the visuotopic location of receptive fields is gradual, whereas the cycling of columns occurs more rapidly. Any given position in space can therefore be analyzed adequately in terms of the orientation of contours, the color and direction of movement of objects, and the stereoscopic depth. The small segment of visual cortex that deals with that particular part of the visual field represents all possible values of all the columnar systems (Figure 25–13).

The columnar systems serve as the substrate for two fundamental types of connectivity along the visual pathway. *Serial processing* occurs in the successive connections between cortical areas, connections that run from the back of the brain forward. At the same time *parallel processing* occurs simultaneously in subsets of fibers that process different submodalities such as form, color, and movement.

Many areas of visual cortex reflect this arrangement; for example, functionally specific cells in V1 communicate with cells of the same specificity in V2. These pathways are not absolutely segregated, however, for there is some mixing of information between different visual attributes (Figure 25–14).

Columnar organization confers several advantages. It minimizes the distance required for neurons with similar functional properties to communicate with one another and allows them to share inputs from discrete pathways that convey information about particular sensory attributes. This efficient connectivity economizes on the use of brain volume and maximizes processing speed. The clustering of neurons into functional groups, as in the columns of the cortex, allows the brain to minimize the number of neurons required for analyzing different attributes. If all neurons were tuned for every attribute, the resultant combinatorial explosion would require a prohibitive number of neurons.

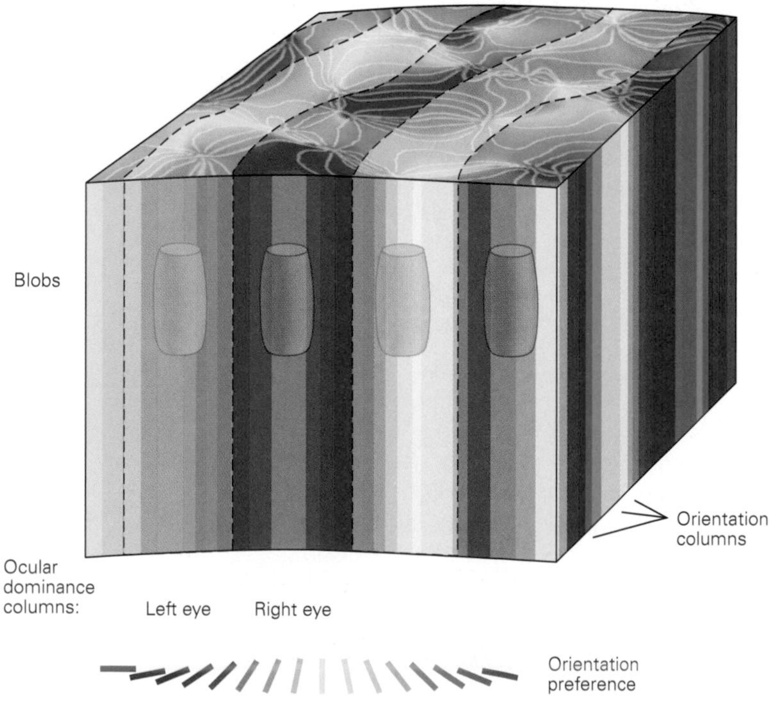

Figure 25–13 A cortical computational module. A chunk of cortical tissue roughly 1 mm in diameter contains an orientation hypercolumn (a full cycle of orientation columns), one cycle of left- and right-eye ocular-dominance columns, and blobs and interblobs. This module would presumably contain all of the functional and anatomical cell types of primary visual cortex, and would be repeated hundreds of times to cover the visual field. (Adapted, with permission, from Hubel 1988.)

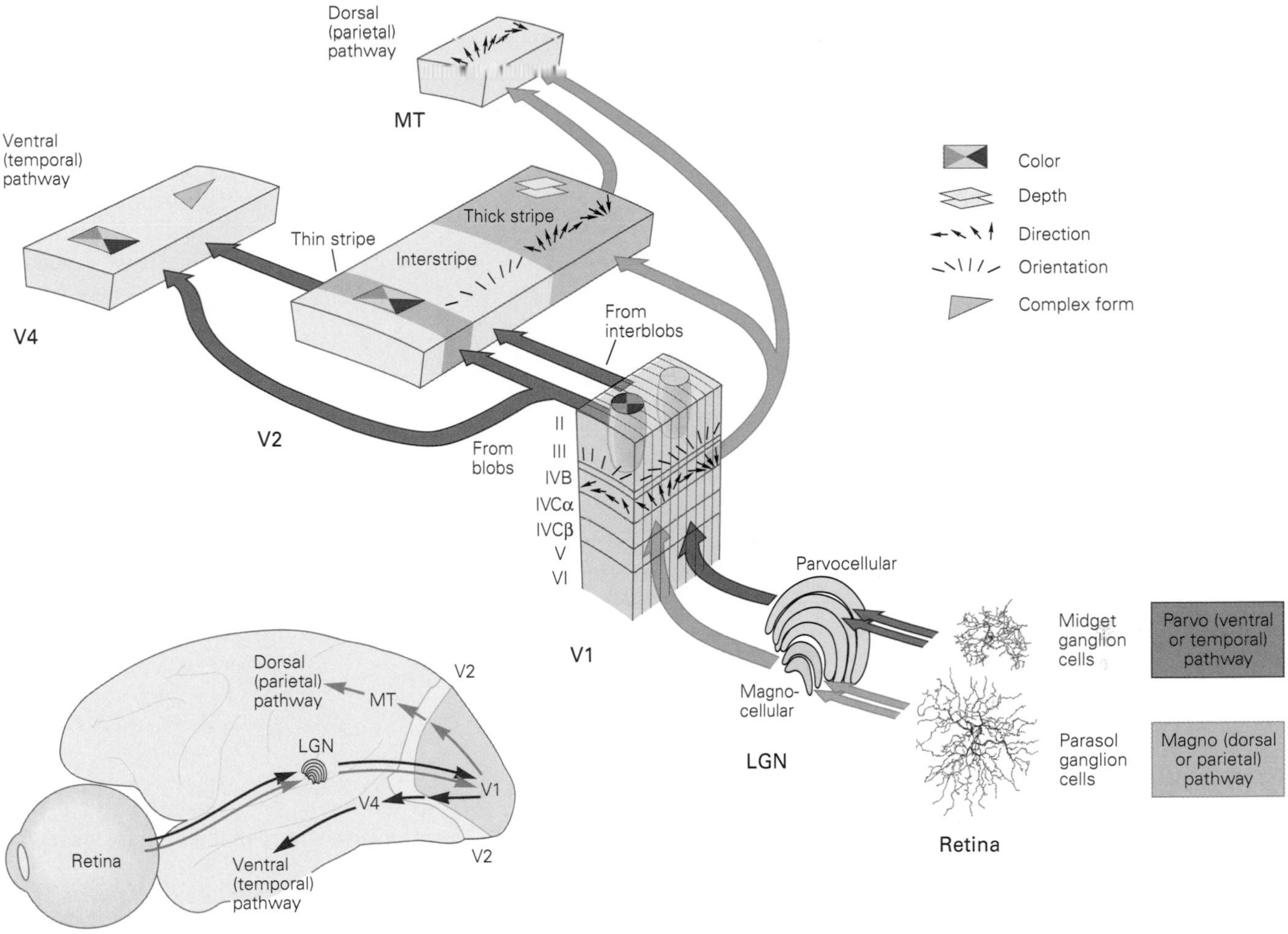

Figure 25–14 **Parallel processing in visual pathways.** The ventral stream is primarily concerned with object identification, carrying information about form and color. The dorsal pathway is dedicated to visually guided movement, with cells selective for direction of movement. These pathways are not strictly segregated, however, and there is substantial interconnection between them even in the primary visual cortex. (**LGN**, lateral geniculate nucleus; **MT**, middle temporal area.) (Retinal ganglion cell images from Dennis Dacey, reproduced with permission.)

Intrinsic Cortical Circuits Transform Neural Information

Each area of the visual cortex transforms information gathered by the eyes and processed at earlier synaptic relays into a signal that represents the visual scene. This transformation is accomplished by local circuits formed by excitatory and inhibitory neurons.

The principal input to the primary visual cortex comes from two parallel pathways that originate in the parvocellular and magnocellular layers of the lateral geniculate nucleus (see Figure 25–12). Neurons in the parvocellular layers project to cortical layer IVCβ, whereas those in the magnocellular layers project to layer IVCα. From there a sequence of interlaminar connections, mediated by the excitatory spiny stellate neurons, processes visual information over a stereotyped set of connections (Figure 25–15).

This characterization of parallel pathways is only an approximation, as there is considerable interaction between the pathways. This interaction is the means by which various visual features—color, form, depth, and movement—are linked, leading to a unified visual percept. One way this linkage, or binding, may be accomplished is through cells that are tuned to more than one attribute.

At each stage of cortical processing pyramidal neurons extend output to other brain areas. Superficial-layer

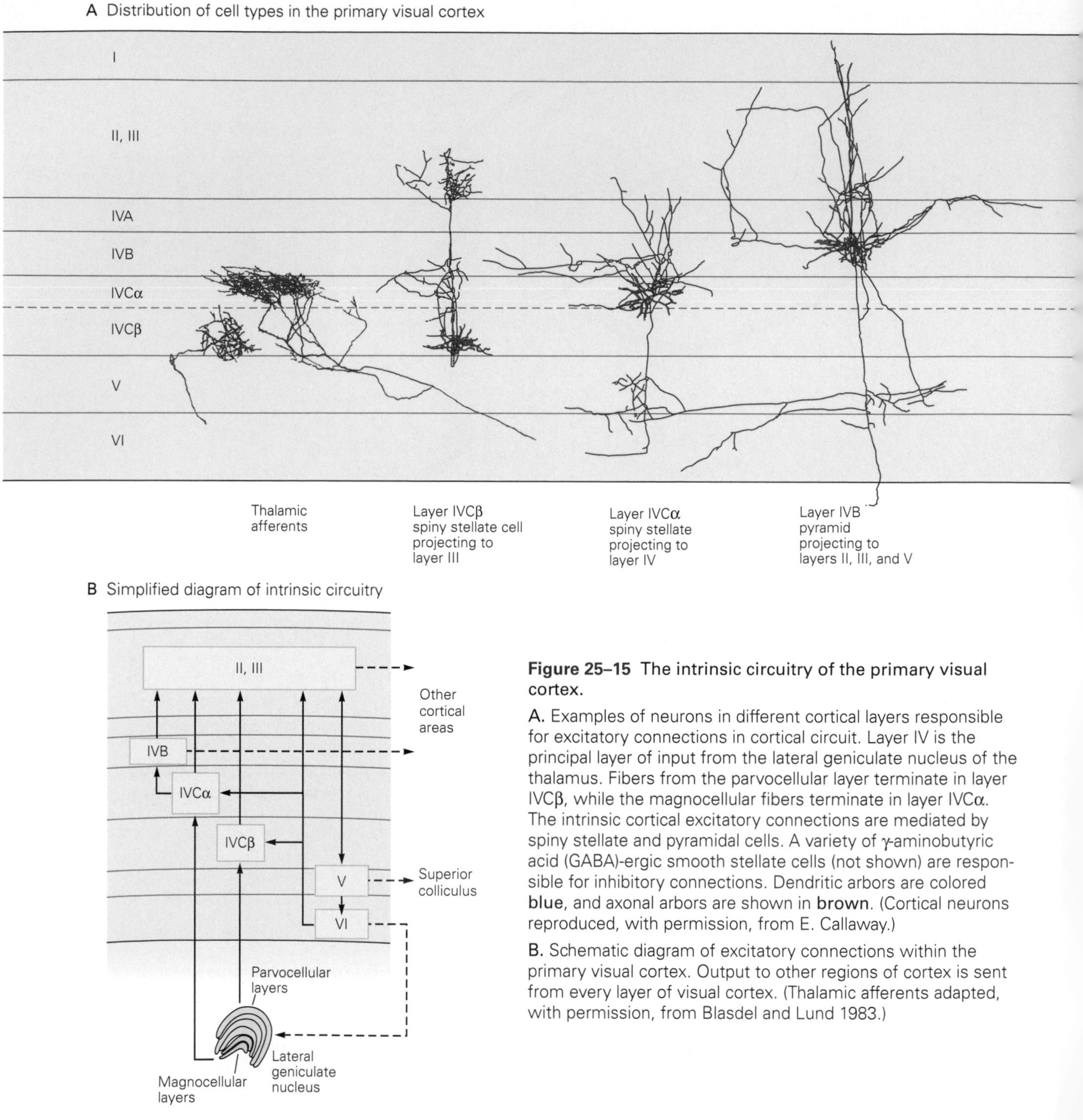

Figure 25–15 The intrinsic circuitry of the primary visual cortex.

A. Examples of neurons in different cortical layers responsible for excitatory connections in cortical circuit. Layer IV is the principal layer of input from the lateral geniculate nucleus of the thalamus. Fibers from the parvocellular layer terminate in layer IVCβ, while the magnocellular fibers terminate in layer IVCα. The intrinsic cortical excitatory connections are mediated by spiny stellate and pyramidal cells. A variety of γ-aminobutyric acid (GABA)-ergic smooth stellate cells (not shown) are responsible for inhibitory connections. Dendritic arbors are colored **blue**, and axonal arbors are shown in **brown**. (Cortical neurons reproduced, with permission, from E. Callaway.)

B. Schematic diagram of excitatory connections within the primary visual cortex. Output to other regions of cortex is sent from every layer of visual cortex. (Thalamic afferents adapted, with permission, from Blasdel and Lund 1983.)

cells are responsible for connections to higher-order areas of cortex. Layer V pyramidal neurons project to the superior colliculus and pons in the brain stem. Layer VI cells are responsible for feedback projections, both to the thalamus and to lower-order cortical areas.

Neurons in different layers have distinctive receptive-field properties. Neurons in the superficial layer of V1 have small receptive fields whereas deeper-layer neurons have large ones. The superficial-layer neurons are specialized for high-resolution pattern

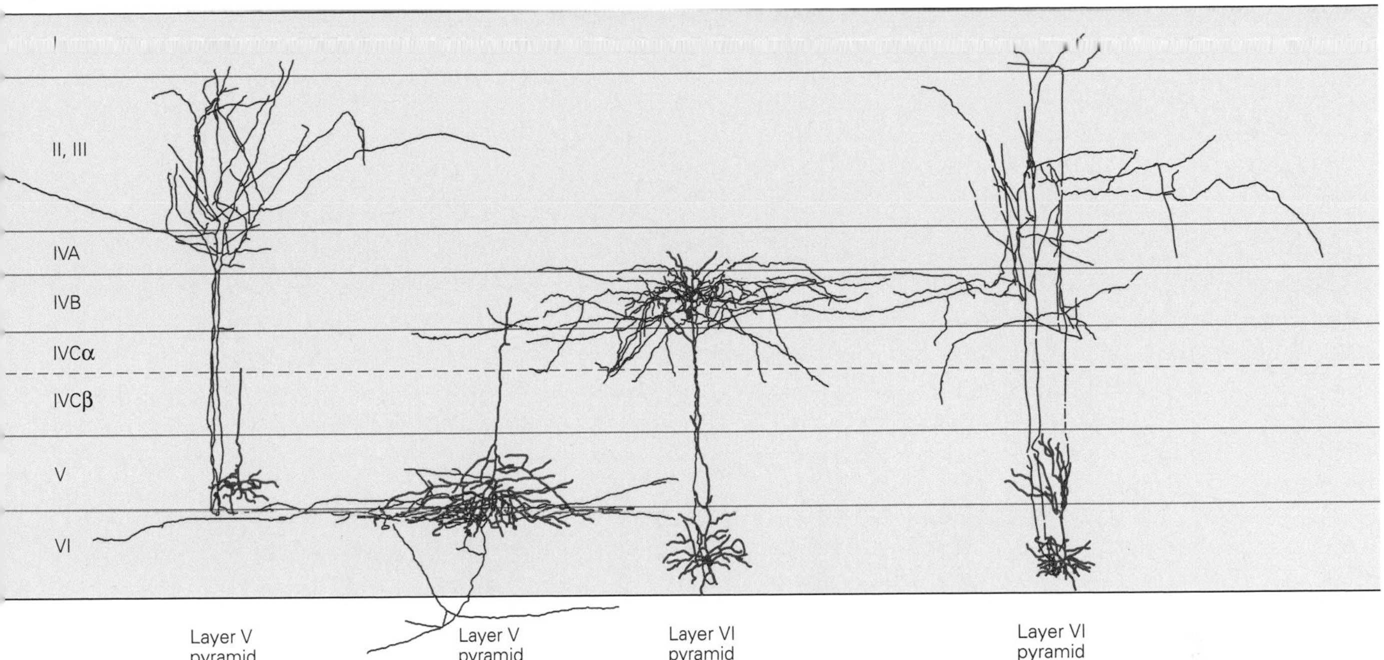

recognition. The deeper-layer neurons, such as those in layer V that are selective for the direction of movement, are specialized for the tracking of objects in space.

Feedback projections are thought to provide a means whereby higher centers in a pathway can influence lower ones. The number of neurons projecting from the cortex to the lateral geniculate nucleus is tenfold the number providing input to the cortex from the lateral geniculate nucleus. Although this feedback projection is obviously important, its function is largely unknown.

In addition to serial feed-forward and feedback connections, an important component of cortical circuits are the fibers that travel parallel to the cortical surface within each layer and provide long-range horizontal connections (Figure 25–16). These connections and their role in the functional architecture of cortex were analyzed by Charles Gilbert and Torsten Wiesel, who used intracellular recordings and dye injection to correlate anatomical features with cortical function. Because the visual cortex is organized visuotopically, the horizontal connections allow target neurons to integrate information over a relatively large area of the visual field and are therefore important in assembling the components of a visual image into a unified percept.

Integration can also be achieved by other means. The considerable convergence and divergence of connections at the synaptic relays of the afferent visual pathway imply that the receptive fields of neurons are larger and more complex at each successive relay and thus necessarily acquire an integrative function. Feedback connections may also support integration, both because of their divergence and because they originate from cells with larger receptive fields.

Visual Information Is Represented by a Variety of Neural Codes

Individual neurons in a sensory pathway respond to a range of stimulus values. For example, a neuron in a color-detection pathway is not limited to responding to one wavelength but is instead tuned to a range of wavelengths. A neuron's response peaks at a particular value and tails off on either side of that value, forming a bell-shaped tuning curve with a particular bandwidth. Thus a neuron with a peak response at 650 nm and a bandwidth of 100 nm might give identical responses at 600 nm and 700 nm.

To be able to determine the wavelength from neuronal signals one needs at least two neurons representing

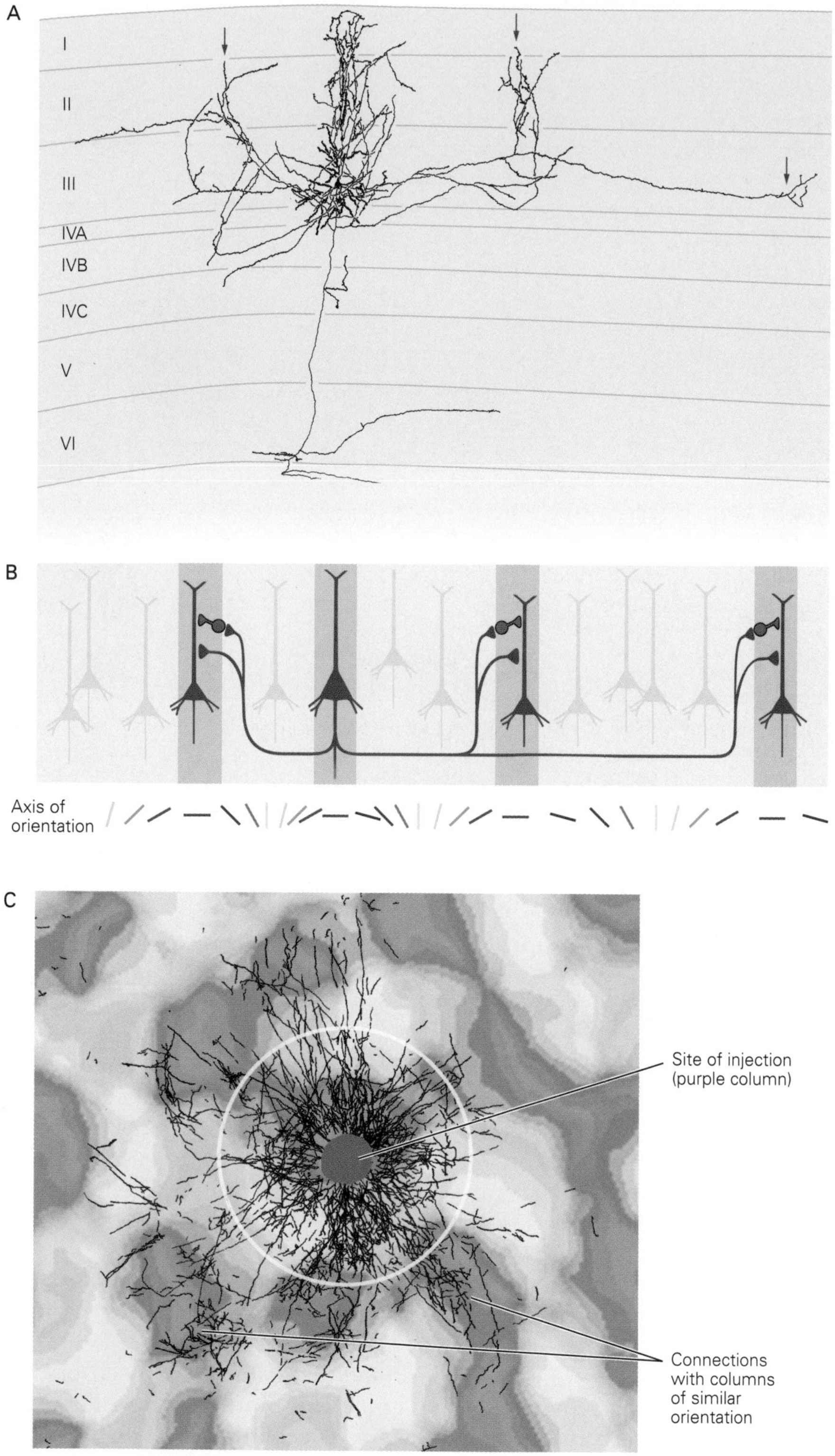

Figure 25–16 Long-range horizontal connections in each layer of the visual cortex integrate information from different parts of the visual field.

A. The axons of pyramidal cells extend for many millimeters parallel to the cortical surface. Axon collaterals form connections with other pyramidal cells as well as with inhibitory interneurons. This arrangement enables neurons to integrate information over large parts of the visual field. An important characteristic of these connections is their relationship to the functional columns. The axon collaterals are found in clusters (**arrows**) at distances greater than 0.5 mm from the cell body. (Reproduced, with permission, from Gilbert and Wiesel 1983.)

B. Horizontal connections link columns of cells with similar orientation specificity.

C. The pattern of horizontal connections is visualized by injecting an adenoviral vector containing the gene encoding green fluorescent protein into one orientation column and superimposing the labeled image (**black**) on an optically imaged map of the orientation columns in the vicinity of the injection. (Scale: diameter of white circle is 1 mm.) (Reproduced, with permission, from Stettler et al. 2002.)

filters centered at different wavelengths. Each neuron can be thought of as a *labeled line* in which activity signals a stimulus with a given value. When more than one such neuron fires, the convergent signals at the postsynaptic relay represent a stimulus with a wavelength that is the weighted average of the values represented by all the inputs.

A single visual percept is the product of the activity of a number of neurons operating in a specific combinatorial and interactive fashion called a *population code.* Population coding has been modeled in various ways. The most prevalent model is called *vector averaging.*

We can illustrate population coding with a population of orientation-selective cells, each of which responds optimally to a line with a specific orientation. Each neuron responds not just to the preferred stimulus but rather to any line that falls within a range of orientations described by a Gaussian tuning curve with a particular bandwidth. A stimulus of a particular orientation most strongly activates cells with tuning curves centered at that orientation; cells with tuning curves centered away from but overlapping that orientation are excited less strongly.

Each cell's preferred orientation, the line label, is represented as a vector pointing in the direction of that orientation. Each cell's firing is a "vote" for the cell's line label, and the cell's firing rate represents the weighting of the vote. The cell's signal can thus be represented by a vector pointing in the direction of the cell's preferred orientation with a length proportional to the strength of the cell's response. For all the activated cells one can calculate a vector sum with a direction that represents the value of the stimulus (Figure 25–17).

Another aspect of the population code is the variability of a neuron's response to the same stimulus. Repeated presentations of the same stimulus to a neuron sensitive to that stimulus will elicit a range of responses. The most sensitive part of a neuron's tuning curve lies not at the peak but along the flanks, where the tuning curve is steepest. Here small changes in the value of a stimulus produce the strongest change in response. Changes in stimulus value must, however, be sufficient to elicit a change in response that significantly exceeds the normal variability in the response of the neuron. One can compare that amount of change to the perceptual discrimination threshold. When many neurons contribute to the discrimination, the signal-to-noise ratio increases, a process known as probability summation, and the critical difference in stimulus value required for a significant change in neuronal response is less.

When the brain represents a piece of information, an important consideration is the number of neurons that participate in that representation. Although all information about a visual stimulus is present in the retina,

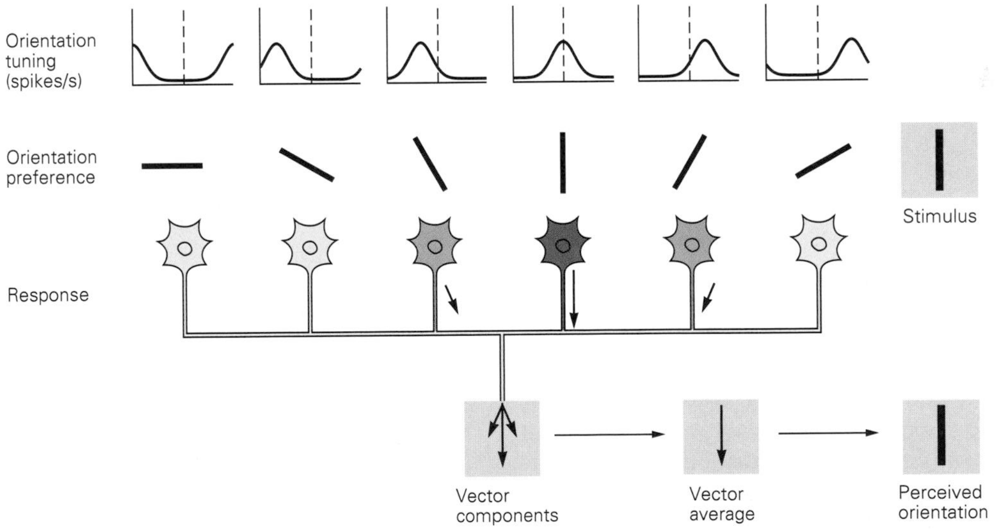

Figure 25–17 Vector averaging is one model for population coding in neural circuits. Vector averages describe the possible relationship between the responses in an ensemble of neurons, the tuning characteristics of individual neurons in the ensemble, and the resultant percept. Individual neurons respond optimally to a particular orientation of a stimulus in the visual field, but also respond at varying rates to a range of orientations. The stimulus orientation to which a neuron fires best can be thought of as a line label—when the cell fires briskly, its activity signifies the presence of a stimulus with that orientation. A number of neurons with different orientation preferences will respond to the same stimulus. Each neuron's response can be represented as a vector whose length indicates the strength of its response and whose direction represents its preferred orientation, or line label. (Adapted, with permission, from Kapadia, Westheimer, and Gilbert 2000.)

the retinal representation is not sufficient for object recognition. At the other end of the visual pathway some neurons in the temporal lobe are selective for complex objects, such as faces. Can an individual cell represent something as complex as a particular face? Such a hypothetical neuron has been dubbed a "grandmother cell" because it would represent exclusively a person's grandmother, or a "pontifical cell" because it would represent the apex of a hierarchical cognitive pathway.

The nervous system does not, however, represent entire objects by the activity of single neurons. Instead some cells represent parts of an object and an ensemble of neurons represents an entire object. Each member of the ensemble may participate in different ensembles that are activated by different objects. This arrangement is known as a *distributed code.* Distributed codes can involve a few neurons or many. In any case, a distributed code requires complex connectivity between the cells representing a face and those representing the name and experiences associated with that person.

The foregoing discussion assumes that neurons signal information by their firing rate and their line labels. An alternative hypothesis is that the timing of action potentials itself carries information in a kind of Morse code. The code might be read from the synchronous firing of different sets of neurons over time. At one instant one group of cells might fire together followed by the synchronous firing of another group. Over a single train of action potentials a single cell could participate in many such ensembles. Whether sensory information is represented this way, and whether the nervous system carries more information than that represented by firing rate alone, is not known.

An Overall View

Visual perception involves an interaction between the retina, thalamic nuclei, and multiple areas of the cerebral cortex. The retina defines the limits of vision: the ability to resolve fine details, the discrimination of tiny movements, and the capacity to detect subtle contrasts and differences in the wavelength of reflected light.

The visual cortex acquires information coming from complex scenes, parses it into the surfaces and contours belonging to individual objects, and segments those objects from their background. This process involves a simultaneous analysis of local properties, such as orientation, direction of movement, and color, as well as the integration of these properties across space.

The mechanisms of visual processing may be observed in the receptive-field properties of individual neurons and in the functional organization of the cortex. Certain aspects of vision are analyzed in parallel by distinct pathways, one of which is involved in object recognition and another in visually guided movements.

Charles D. Gilbert

Selected Readings

Hubel DH, Wiesel TN. 1962. Receptive fields, binocular interaction and functional architecture in the cat's visual cortex. J Physiol 160:106–154.

Hubel DH, Wiesel TN. 1977. Functional architecture of macaque monkey visual cortex. Proc R Soc Lond B Biol Sci 198:1–59.

Hubener M, Shohan D, Grinvald A, Bonhoeffer T. 1997. Spatial relationships among three columnar systems in cat area 17. J Neurosci 17:9270–9284.

VanEssen DC, Anderson CH, Felleman DJ. 1992. Information processing in the primate visual system: an integrated systems perspective. Science 255:419–423.

Wertheimer, M. 1938. *Laws of Organization in Perceptual Forms*. London: Harcourt, Brace & Jovanovitch.

Wiesel TN, Hubel DH. 1966. Spatial and chromatic interactions in the lateral geniculate body of the rhesus monkey. J Neurophysiol 29:1115–1156.

References

Blasdel GG, Lund JS. 1983. Termination of afferent axons in macaque striate cortex. J Neurosci 3:1389–1413.

Callaway EM. 1998. Local circuits in primary visual cortex of the macaque monkey. Annu Rev Neurosci 21:47–74.

Field DJ, Hayes A, Hess RF. 1993. Contour integration by the human visual system: evidence for a local "association field." Vision Res 33:173–193.

Gilbert CD, Wiesel TN. 1983. Clustered intrinsic connections in cat visual cortex. J Neurosci 3:1116–1133.

Hartline HK. 1941. The neural mechanisms of vision. Harvey Lect 37:39–68.

Hubel DH, Wiesel TN. 1974. Uniformity of monkey striate cortex. A parallel relationship between field size, scatter and magnification factor. J Comp Neurol 158:295–306.

Hubel DH. 1983. Eye, Brain and Vision. p. 131. New York: Scientific American Library.

Kapadia MK, Westheimer G, Gilbert CD. 2000. Spatial distribution of contextual interactions in primary visual cortex and in visual perception. J Neurophysiol 84:2048–2062.

Kuffler SF. 1953. Discharge patterns and functional organization of mammalian retina. J Neurophysiol 16:37–68.

Porter PB. 1954. Another puzzle-picture. Am J Psychol 67: 550–551.

Stettler DD, Das A, Bennett J, Gilbert CD. 2002. Lateral connectivity and contextual interactions in macaque primary visual cortex. Neuron 36:739–750.

26

Low-Level Visual Processing: The Retina

THE RETINA IS THE BRAIN'S WINDOW on the world. All visual experience is based on information processed by this neural circuit in the eye. The retina's output is conveyed to the brain by just one million optic nerve fibers, and yet almost half of the cerebral cortex is used to process these signals. Visual information lost in the retina—by design or deficiency—can never be recovered. Because retinal processing sets fundamental limits on what can be seen, there is great interest in understanding how the retina functions.

On the surface the vertebrate eye appears to act much like a camera. The pupil forms a variable diaphragm, and the cornea and lens provide the refractive optics that project a small image of the outside world onto the light-sensitive retina lining the back of the eyeball (Figure 26–1). But this is where the analogy ends. The retina is a thin sheet of neurons, a few hundred micrometers thick, composed of five major cell types that are arranged in three cellular layers separated by two synaptic layers (Figure 26–2).

The photoreceptor cells, in the outermost layer, absorb light and convert it into a neural signal, an essential process known as phototransduction.

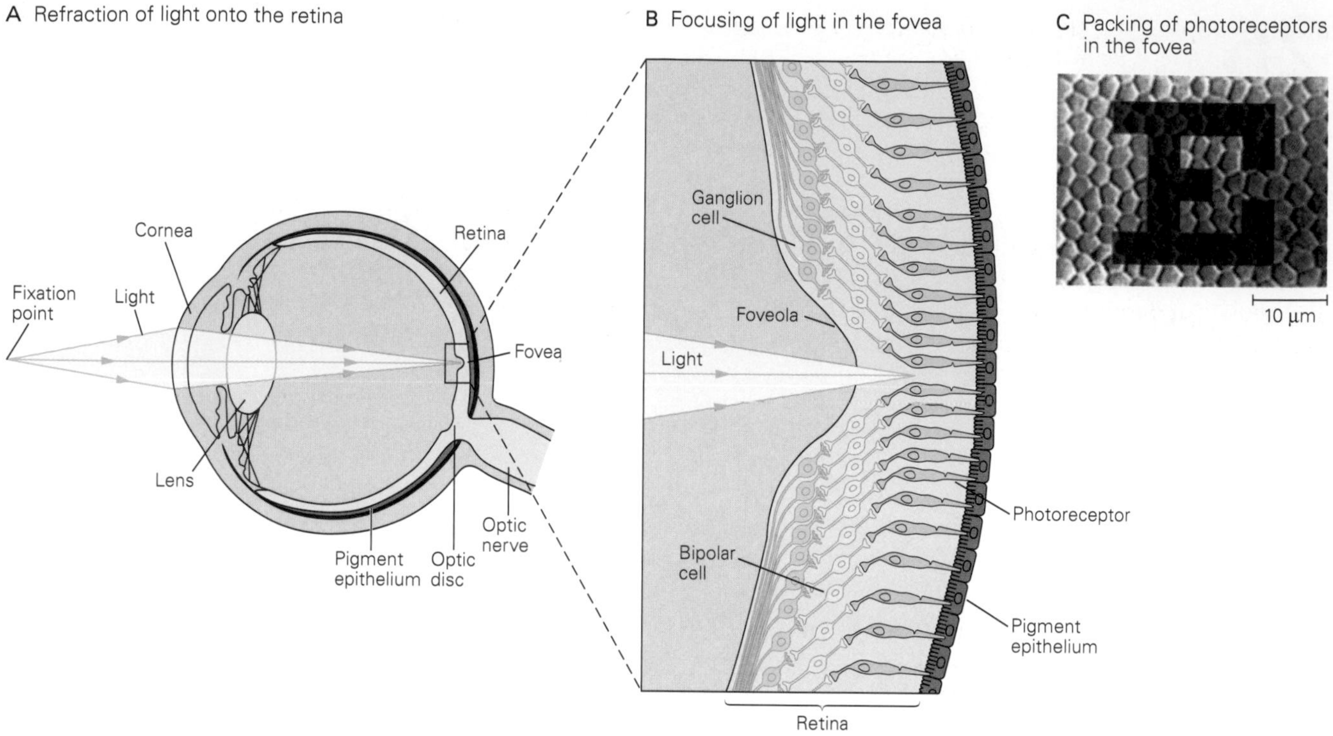

Figure 26–1 The eye projects the visual scene onto the retina's photoreceptors.

A. Light from an object in the visual field is refracted by the cornea and lens and focused onto the retina.

B. In the foveola, corresponding to the very center of gaze, the proximal neurons of the retina are shifted aside so light has direct access to the photoreceptors.

C. A letter from the eye chart for normal visual acuity is projected onto the densely packed photoreceptors in the fovea. Although less sharply focused than shown here as a result of diffraction by the eye's optics, the smallest discernible strokes of the letter are approximately one cone diameter in width. (Adapted, with permission, from Curcio and Hendrickson 1982.)

These signals are passed synaptically to bipolar cells, which in turn connect to retinal ganglion cells in the innermost layer. Retinal ganglion cells are the output neurons of the retina and their axons form the optic nerve. In addition to this vertical pathway from sensory to output neurons, the retinal circuit includes many lateral connections provided by horizontal cells in the outer synaptic layer and amacrine cells in the inner synaptic layer (Figure 26–3).

The retinal circuit performs low-level visual processing, the initial stage in the analysis of visual images. It extracts from the raw images in the left and right eyes certain spatial and temporal features and conveys them to higher visual centers. The rules of this processing are very plastic. In particular, the retina must adjust its sensitivity to ever-changing conditions of illumination. This adaptation allows our vision to remain more or less stable despite the vast range of light intensities encountered during the course of each day.

In this chapter we discuss in turn the three important aspects of retinal function: phototransduction, preprocessing, and adaptation. We will illustrate both the neural mechanisms by which they are achieved and their consequences for visual perception.

The Photoreceptor Layer Samples the Visual Image

Ocular Optics Limit the Quality of the Retinal Image

The sharpness of the retinal image is determined by several factors: diffraction at the pupil's aperture, refractive errors in the cornea and lens, and scattering due to material in the light path. A point in the outside world is generally focused into a small blurred circle on the retina. As in other optical devices this blur is smallest near the optical axis, where the image quality approaches the limit imposed by diffraction at the pupil. Away from the axis the image is degraded significantly owing to aberrations in the cornea and lens. The image may be degraded further by abnormal conditions such as light-scattering cataracts or refractive errors such as myopia.

The area of retina near the optical axis, the *fovea,* is where vision is sharpest and corresponds to the center of gaze that we direct toward the objects of our attention. The density of photoreceptors, bipolar cells, and ganglion cells is highest at the fovea. The spacing between photoreceptors there is well matched to the size of the optical blur circle, and thus samples the image in an ideal fashion. Light must generally traverse several layers of cells before reaching the photoreceptors, but in the center of the fovea, called the *foveola,* the other cellular layers are pushed aside to reduce additional blur from light scattering (Figure 26–1B). Finally, the back of the eye is lined by a black pigment epithelium that absorbs light and keeps it from scattering back into the eye.

The retina contains another special site, the optic disc, where the axons of retinal ganglion cells converge

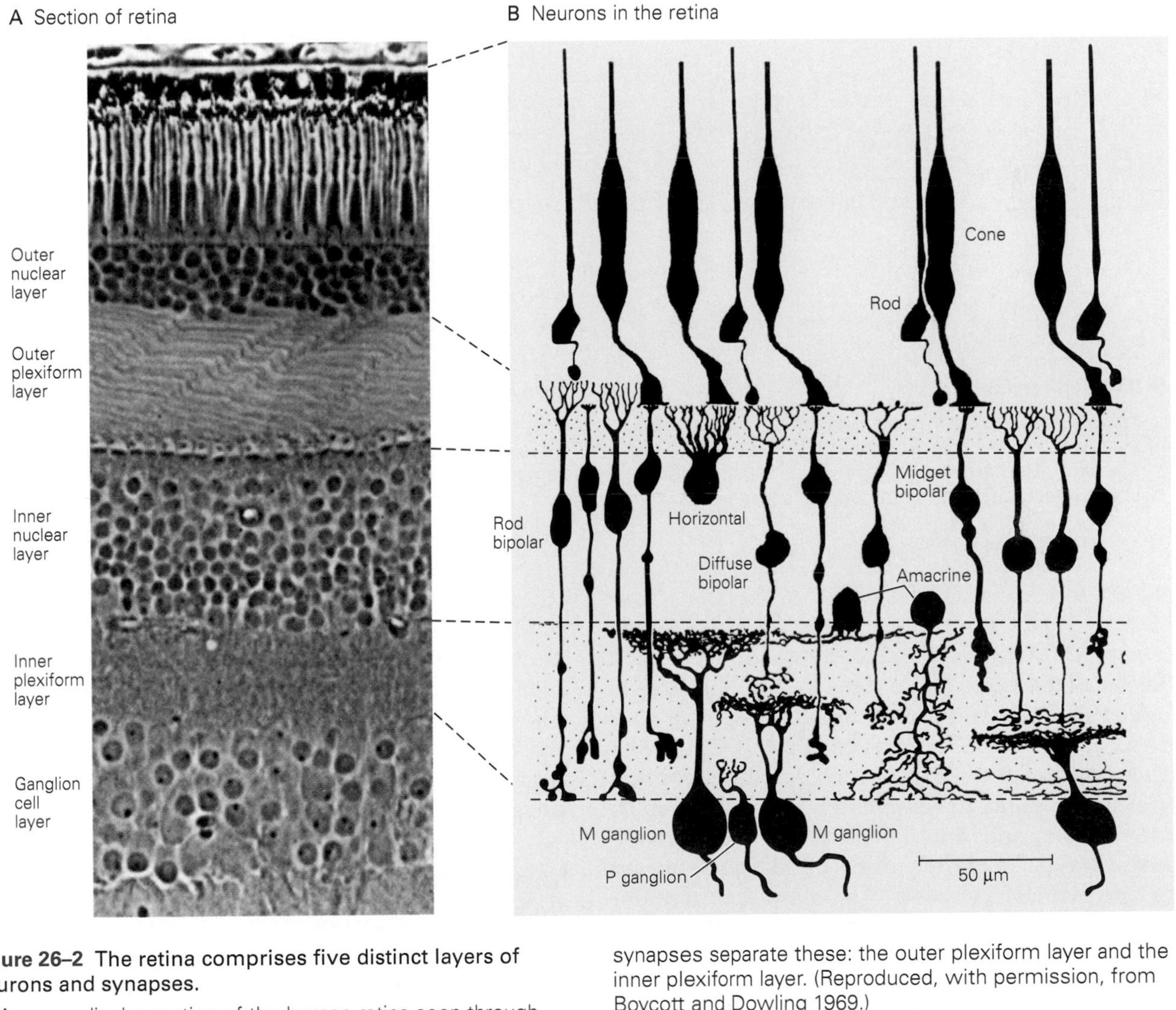

Figure 26–2 The retina comprises five distinct layers of neurons and synapses.

A. A perpendicular section of the human retina seen through the light microscope. Three layers of cell bodies are evident. The outer nuclear layer contains cell bodies of photoreceptors; the inner nuclear layer includes horizontal, bipolar, and amacrine cells; and the ganglion cell layer contains ganglion cells and some displaced amacrine cells. Two layers of fibers and synapses separate these: the outer plexiform layer and the inner plexiform layer. (Reproduced, with permission, from Boycott and Dowling 1969.)

B. Neurons in the retina of the macaque monkey based on Golgi staining. The cellular and synaptic layers are aligned with the image in part A. (**M ganglion**, magnocellular ganglion cell; **P ganglion**, parvocellular ganglion cell.) (Reproduced, with permission, from Polyak 1941.)

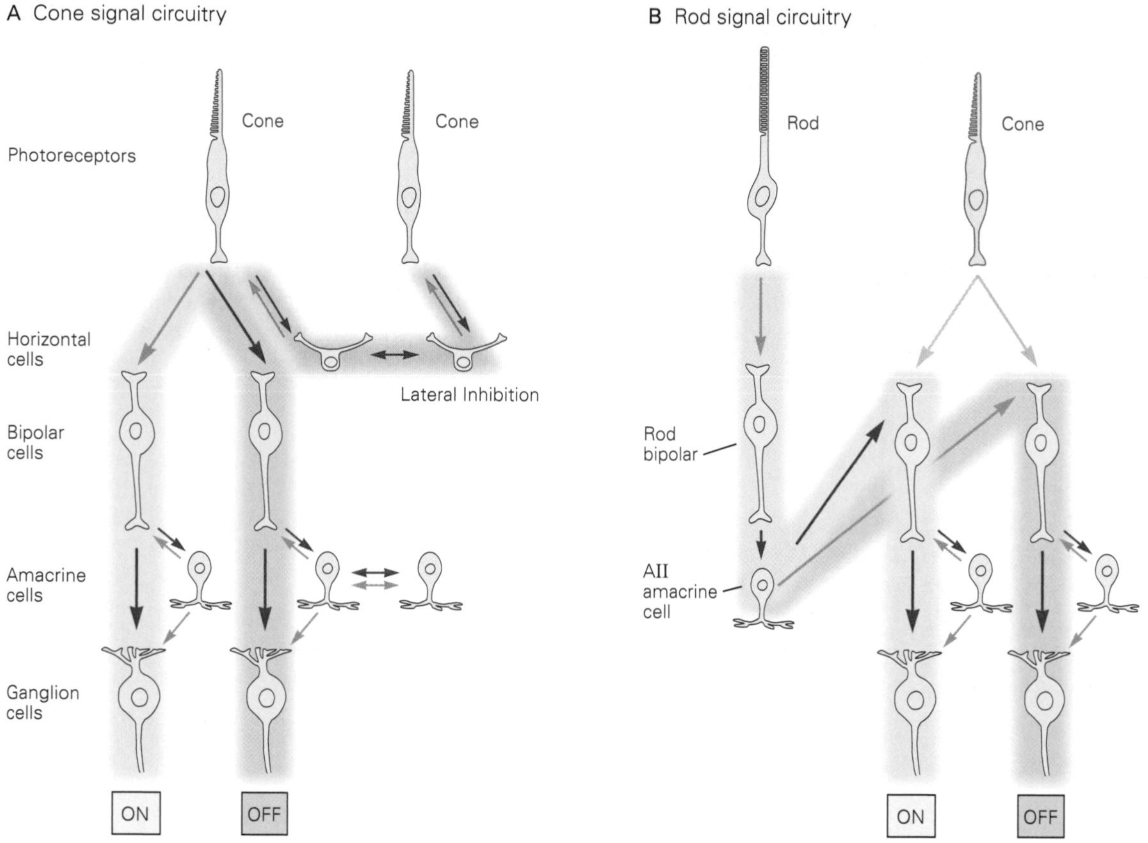

Figure 26–3 The retinal circuitry.

A. The circuitry for cone signals, highlighting the split into ON and OFF pathways as well as the pathway for lateral inhibition in the outer layer. **Red arrows** indicate sign-preserving connections through electrical or glutamatergic synapses. **Gray arrows** represent sign-inverting connections through GABA-ergic, glycinergic, or glutamatergic synapses.

B. Rod signals feed into the cone circuitry through the AII amacrine cell, which serves to split the ON and OFF pathways.

and extend through the retina to emerge from the back of the eye as the optic nerve. By necessity this area is devoid of photoreceptors and thus corresponds to a *blind spot* in the visual field of each eye. Because the disc lies nasal to the fovea of each eye, light coming from a single point never falls on both blind spots simultaneously, and thus normally we are unaware of them. We can experience the blind spot only by using one eye (Figure 26–4). The blind spot demonstrates what blind people experience—not blackness, but simply nothing. This explains why damage to the peripheral retina often goes unnoticed. It is usually through accidents, such as bumping into an unnoticed object, or through clinical testing that a deficit of sight is revealed.

The blind spot is a necessary consequence of the inside-out design of the retina, which has puzzled and amused biologists for generations. The purpose of this organization may be to enable the tight apposition of photoreceptors with the retinal pigment epithelium, which plays an essential role in the turnover of retinal pigment and recycles photoreceptor membranes by phagocytosis.

There Are Two Types of Photoreceptors: Rods and Cones

All photoreceptor cells have a common structure with four functional regions: the outer segment, located at the distal surface of the neural retina; the inner segment, located more proximally; the cell body; and the synaptic terminal (Figure 26–5A).

Most vertebrates have two types of photoreceptors, rods and cones, distinguished by their morphology.

Figure 26–4 The blind spot of the human retina. Locate the blind spot in your left eye by shutting the right eye and fixating the cross with the left eye. Hold the book about 12 inches from your eye and move it slightly nearer or farther until the circle on the left disappears. Now place a pencil vertically on the page and sweep it sideways over the circle. Note the pencil appears unbroken, even though no light can reach your retina from the region of the circle. Next move the pencil lengthwise and observe what happens when its tip enters the circle. (Adapted, with permission, from Hurvich 1981.)

A rod has a long, cylindrical outer segment within which the stacks of discs are separated from the plasma membrane, whereas a cone often has a shorter, tapered outer segment, and the discs are continuous with the outer membrane (Figure 26–5B).

Rods and cones also differ in function, most importantly in their sensitivity to light. Rods can signal the absorption of a single photon and are responsible for vision under dim illumination such as moonlight. But as the light level increases toward dawn, the electrical

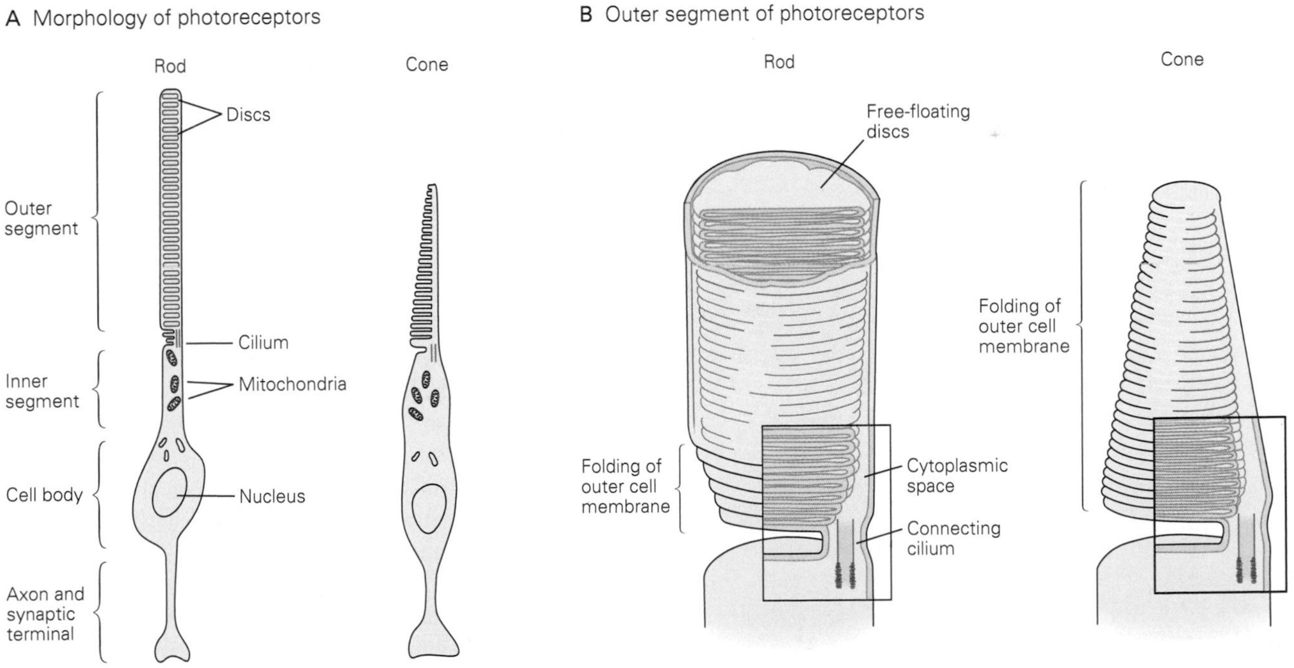

Figure 26–5 Rod and cone photoreceptors have similar structures.

A. Both rod and cone cells have specialized regions called the outer and inner segments. The outer segment, which is attached to the inner segment by a cilium, contains the light-transducing apparatus. The inner segment holds mitochondria and much of the machinery for protein synthesis.

B. The outer segment consists of a stack of membranous discs that contain the light-absorbing photopigments. In both types of cells these discs are formed by infolding of the plasma membrane. In rods, however, the folds pinch off from the membrane so that the discs are free-floating within the outer segment, whereas in cones the discs remain part of the plasma membrane. (Adapted, with permission, from O'Brien 1982; and Young 1970.)

response of rods becomes saturated and the cells cease to respond to variations in intensity. Cones are much less sensitive to light; they make no contribution to night vision, but are solely responsible for vision in daylight. Their response is considerably faster than that of rods. Primates have only one type of rod but three kinds of cone photoreceptors, distinguished by the range of wavelengths to which they respond: the L (long-wave), M (medium-wave), and S (short-wave) cones (Figure 26–6).

The human retina contains approximately 100 million rods and 6 million cones, but the two cell types are differently distributed. The central fovea contains no rods but is densely packed with small cones. A few millimeters outside the fovea rods greatly outnumber cones. All photoreceptors become larger and more widely spaced toward the periphery of the retina. The S cones make up only 10% of all cones and are absent from the central fovea.

The retinal center of gaze is clearly specialized for daytime vision. The dense packing of cone photoreceptors in the fovea sets the limits of our visual acuity. In fact, the smallest letters we can read on a doctor's eye chart have strokes whose images are just 1–2 cone diameters wide on the retina, a visual angle of about 1 minute of arc (Figure 26–1C). At night the central fovea is blind owing to the absence of rods. Astronomers know that one must look just to the side of a dim star to see it at all. During nighttime walks in the forest we nonastronomers tend to follow our daytime reflex of looking straight at the source of a suspicious sound. Mysteriously, the object disappears, only to jump back into our peripheral field of view as we avert our gaze.

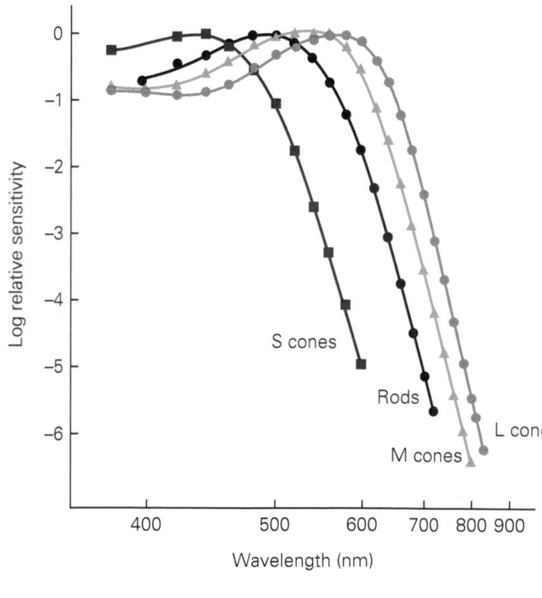

Figure 26–6 Sensitivity spectra for the three cones and the rod. At each wavelength the sensitivity is inversely proportional to the intensity of light required to elicit a criterion neural response. Sensitivity varies over a large range and thus is shown on a logarithmic scale. The different classes of photoreceptors are sensitive to broad and overlapping ranges of wavelengths. (Reproduced, with permission, from Schnapf et al. 1988.)

Phototransduction Links the Absorption of a Photon to a Change in Membrane Conductance

As in many other neurons the membrane potential of a photoreceptor is regulated by the balance of membrane conductances to Na^+ and K^+ ions, whose transmembrane gradients are maintained by metabolically active pumps (see Chapter 6). In the dark, Na^+ ions flow into the photoreceptor through nonselective cation channels that are activated by the second messenger cyclic guanosine 3′-5′ monophosphate (cGMP).

Absorption of a photon by the pigment protein sets in motion a biochemical cascade that ultimately lowers the concentration of cGMP, thus closing the cGMP-gated channels and moving the cell closer to the K^+ equilibrium potential. In this way light hyperpolarizes the photoreceptor (Figure 26–7). Here we describe this sequence of events in detail. Most of this knowledge derives from studies of rods, but the mechanism in cones is very similar.

Light Activates Pigment Molecules in the Photoreceptors

Rhodopsin, the visual pigment in rod cells, has two components. The protein portion, *opsin,* is embedded in the disc membrane and does not by itself absorb visible light. The light-absorbing moiety, *retinal,* is a small molecule whose 11-*cis* isomer is covalently linked to a lysine residue of opsin (Figure 26–8A). Absorption of a photon by retinal causes it to flip from the 11-*cis* to the all-*trans* configuration. This reaction is the only light-dependent step in vision.

The change in shape of the retinal molecule causes a conformational change in the opsin to an activated state called *metarhodopsin II,* which triggers the second step of phototransduction. Metarhodopsin II is unstable and splits within minutes, yielding opsin and free all-*trans* retinal. The all-*trans* retinal is then transported from rods to pigment epithelial cells, where it is reduced to all-*trans* retinol (vitamin A), the precursor of 11-*cis* retinal, which is subsequently transported back to rods.

All-*trans* retinal is thus a crucial compound in the visual system. Its precursors, such as vitamin A, cannot be synthesized by humans and so must be a regular part of the diet. Deficiencies of vitamin A can lead to night blindness and, if untreated, to deterioration of receptor outer segments and eventually to blindness.

Each type of cone in the human retina produces a variant of the opsin protein. These three cone pigments are distinguished by their *absorption spectrum*, the dependence on wavelength of the efficiency of light absorption (see Figure 26–6). The spectrum is determined by the protein sequence through the interaction between retinal and certain amino-acid side chains near the binding pocket. Red light excites L cones more than the M cones, whereas green light excites the M cones more. Therefore the relative degree of excitation in these cone types contains information about the spectrum of the light, independent of its intensity. The brain's comparison of signals from different cone types is the basis for color vision.

In night vision only the rods are active, so all functional photoreceptors have the same absorption spectrum. A green light consequently has exactly the same effect on the visual system as a red light of a greater intensity. Because a single-photoreceptor system cannot distinguish the spectrum of a light from its intensity, "at night all cats are gray." By comparing the sensitivity of a rod to different wavelengths of light, one obtains the absorption spectrum of rhodopsin. It is a remarkable fact that one can measure this molecular property accurately just by asking human subjects about the appearance of various colored lights (Figure 26–9). The quantitative study of perception, or psychophysics, provides similar insights into other mechanisms of brain processing.

Excited Rhodopsin Activates a Phosphodiesterase Through the G Protein Transducin

Activated rhodopsin, in the form of metarhodopsin II, diffuses within the disc membrane where it encounters transducin, a member of the G protein family (Chapter 11). As is the case for other G proteins, the inactive form of transducin binds a molecule of guanosine diphosphate (GDP). Interaction with metarhodopsin II promotes the exchange of GDP for guanosine triphosphate (GTP). This leads to dissociation of transducin's subunits into an active α subunit carrying the GTP (Tα-GTP) and the β and γ subunits (T$\beta\gamma$). Metarhodopsin II can activate hundreds of additional transducin molecules, thus significantly amplifying the cell's response.

The active transducin subunit Tα-GTP forms a complex with a cyclic nucleotide phosphodiesterase, another protein associated with the disc membrane. This interaction greatly increases the rate at which the enzyme hydrolyzes cGMP to 5′-GMP. Each phosphodiesterase molecule can hydrolyze more than 1,000 molecules of cGMP per second, thus increasing the degree of amplification.

The concentration of cGMP controls the activity of the cGMP-gated channels in the plasma membrane of the outer segment. In darkness, when the cGMP concentration is high, a sizeable Na^+ influx through the open channels maintains the cell at a depolarized level of approximately –40 mV. As a consequence, the cell's synaptic terminal continuously releases the transmitter glutamate. The light-evoked decrease in cGMP results in the closure of the cGMP-gated channels, thus reducing the inward flux of Na^+ ions and hyperpolarizing the cell (Figure 26–7B1). Hyperpolarization slows the release of neurotransmitter from the photoreceptor terminal, thereby initiating a neural signal.

Multiple Mechanisms Shut Off the Cascade

The photoreceptor's response to a single photon must be terminated so that the cell can respond to another photon. Metarhodopsin II is inactivated through phosphorylation by a specific rhodopsin kinase followed by binding of the soluble protein arrestin, which blocks the interaction with transducin.

Active transducin (Tα-GTP) has an intrinsic GTPase activity, which eventually converts bound GTP to GDP. Tα-GDP then releases phosphodiesterase and recombines with T$\beta\gamma$, ready again for excitation by rhodopsin. Once the phosphodiesterase has been inactivated, the cGMP concentration is restored by a guanylate cyclase that produces cGMP from GTP. At this point the membrane channels open, the Na^+ current resumes, and the photoreceptor depolarizes back to its dark potential.

In addition to these independent mechanisms that shut off individual elements of the cascade, an important feedback mechanism ensures that large responses are terminated more quickly. This is mediated by a change in the Ca^{2+} concentration in the cell. Calcium ions enter the cell through the cGMP-gated channels and are extruded by rapid cation exchangers. In the dark the intracellular Ca^{2+} concentration is high; but during the cell's light response when the cGMP-gated channels close, the Ca^{2+} level drops quickly to a few percent of the dark level.

This reduction in Ca^{2+} concentration modulates the biochemical reactions in many ways (Figure 26–7B2).

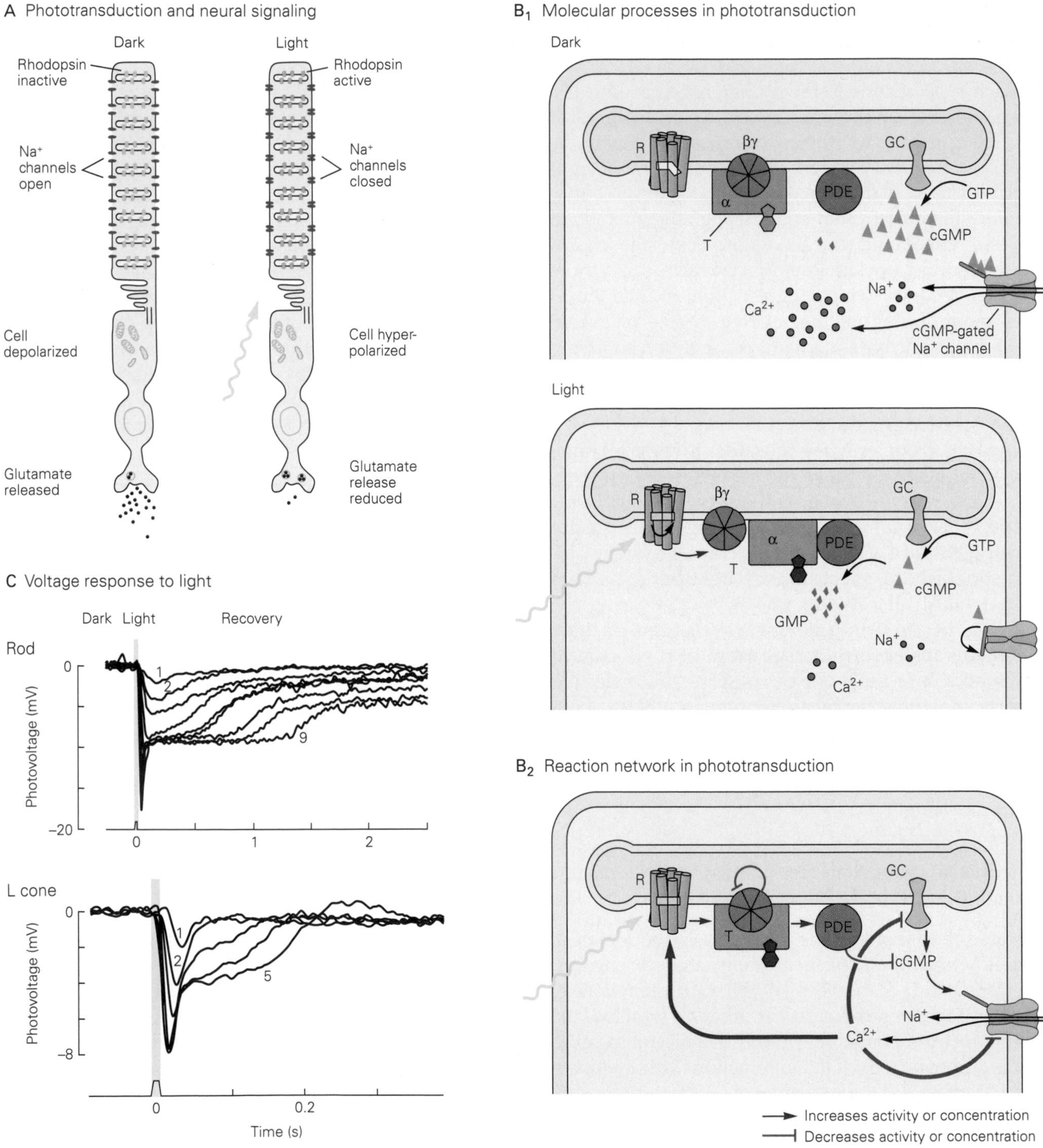
A Phototransduction and neural signaling
Dark
Light
Rhodopsin inactive
Rhodopsin active
Na+ channels open
Na+ channels closed
Cell depolarized
Cell hyper-polarized
Glutamate released
Glutamate release reduced
B1 Molecular processes in phototransduction
Dark
R
βγ
α
T
PDE
GC
GTP
cGMP
Na+
Ca2+
cGMP-gated Na+ channel
Light
R
βγ
α
T
PDE
GC
GTP
cGMP
GMP
Na+
Ca2+
B2 Reaction network in phototransduction
R
T
PDE
GC
cGMP
Na+
Ca2+
Increases activity or concentration
Decreases activity or concentration
C Voltage response to light
Dark
Light
Recovery
Rod
Photovoltage (mV)
0
–20
1
2
9
L cone
Photovoltage (mV)
0
–8
1
2
5
0
0.2
Time (s)

Rhodopsin phosphorylation is accelerated through the action of the Ca^{2+}-binding protein recoverin on rhodopsin kinase, thus reducing activation of transducin. The activity of guanylyl cyclase is accelerated by Ca^{2+}-dependent guanylyl cyclase-activating proteins. Finally, the affinity of the cGMP-gated channel is increased through the action of Ca^{2+}-calmodulin. All these effects promote the return of the photoreceptor to the dark state.

Defects in Phototransduction Cause Disease

Not surprisingly, defects in the phototransduction machinery have serious consequences. One prominent defect is color blindness, which results from loss or abnormality in the genes for cone pigments, as discussed below.

Stationary night blindness results when rod function has been lost but cone function remains intact. This disease is heritable, and mutations have been identified in many components of the phototransduction cascade: rhodopsin, rod transducin, rod phosphodiesterase, rhodopsin kinase, and arrestin. In some cases it appears that the rods are permanently activated, as if exposed to a constant blinding light.

Unfortunately, many defects in phototransduction lead to *retinitis pigmentosa,* a progressive degeneration of the retina that ultimately results in blindness. The disease has multiple forms, many of which have been associated with mutations that affect signal transduction in rods. Why these changes in function lead to death of the rods and subsequent degeneration of the cones is not understood.

Ganglion Cells Transmit Neural Images to the Brain

The photoreceptor layer produces a relatively simple neural representation of the visual scene: Neurons in bright regions are hyperpolarized, whereas those in dark regions are depolarized. Because the optic nerve has only about 1% as many axons as there are receptor cells, the retinal circuit must edit the information in the photoreceptors before it is conveyed to the brain.

This step constitutes *low-level visual processing,* the first stage in deriving visual percepts from the pattern of light falling on the retina. To understand this selective process we must first understand the neural image at the retina's output and how retinal ganglion cells respond to various patterns of light.

The Two Major Types of Ganglion Cells Are ON Cells and OFF Cells

Many retinal ganglion cells fire action potentials spontaneously even in darkness or constant illumination. If the light intensity is suddenly increased, so-called ON cells fire more rapidly. Other ganglion cells, the OFF cells, fire more slowly or cease firing altogether. When the intensity diminishes again, the ON cells fire less and OFF cells fire more. The retinal output thus includes two complementary representations that differ in the polarity of their response to light.

This arrangement serves to communicate rapidly both brightening and dimming in the visual scene. If the retina had only ON cells, a dark object would be

Figure 26–7 (Opposite) Phototransduction.

A. The rod cell responds to light. Rhodopsin molecules in the outer-segment discs absorb photons, which leads to the closure of cGMP-gated channels in the plasma membrane. This channel closure hyperpolarizes the membrane and reduces the rate of release of the neurotransmitter glutamate. (Adapted, with permission, from Alberts 2008.)

B. 1. Cyclic GMP (cyclic guanosine 3′-5′ monophosphate) is produced by a guanylate cyclase (**GC**) and hydrolyzed by a phosphodiesterase (**PDE**). In the dark the phosphodiesterase activity is low, the cGMP concentration is high, and the cGMP-gated channels are open, allowing the influx of Na^+ and Ca^{2+}. In the light rhodopsin (**R**) is excited by absorption of a photon, then activates transducin (**T**), which in turn activates the phosphodiesterase; the cGMP level drops, the membrane channels close, and less Na^+ and Ca^{2+} enter the cell. The transduction enzymes are all located in the internal membrane discs, and the soluble ligand cGMP serves as a messenger to the plasma membrane.

2. Calcium ions have a negative feedback role in the reaction cascade in phototransduction. Stimulation of the network by light leads to the closure of the cGMP-gated channels. This causes a drop in the intracellular concentration of Ca^{2+}. Because Ca^{2+} modulates the function of at least three components of the cascade—rhodopsin, guanylyl cyclase, and the cGMP-gated channel—the drop in Ca^{2+} counteracts the excitation caused by light.

C. Voltage response of a primate rod and cone to brief flashes of light of increasing intensity. Higher numbers on the traces indicate greater intensities of illumination (not all traces are labeled). For dim flashes the response amplitude increases linearly with intensity. At high intensities the receptor saturates and remains hyperpolarized steadily for some time after the flash; this leads to the afterimages that we perceive after a bright flash. Note that the response peaks earlier for brighter flashes and that cones respond faster than rods. (Reproduced, with permission, from Schneeweis and Schnapf 1995.)

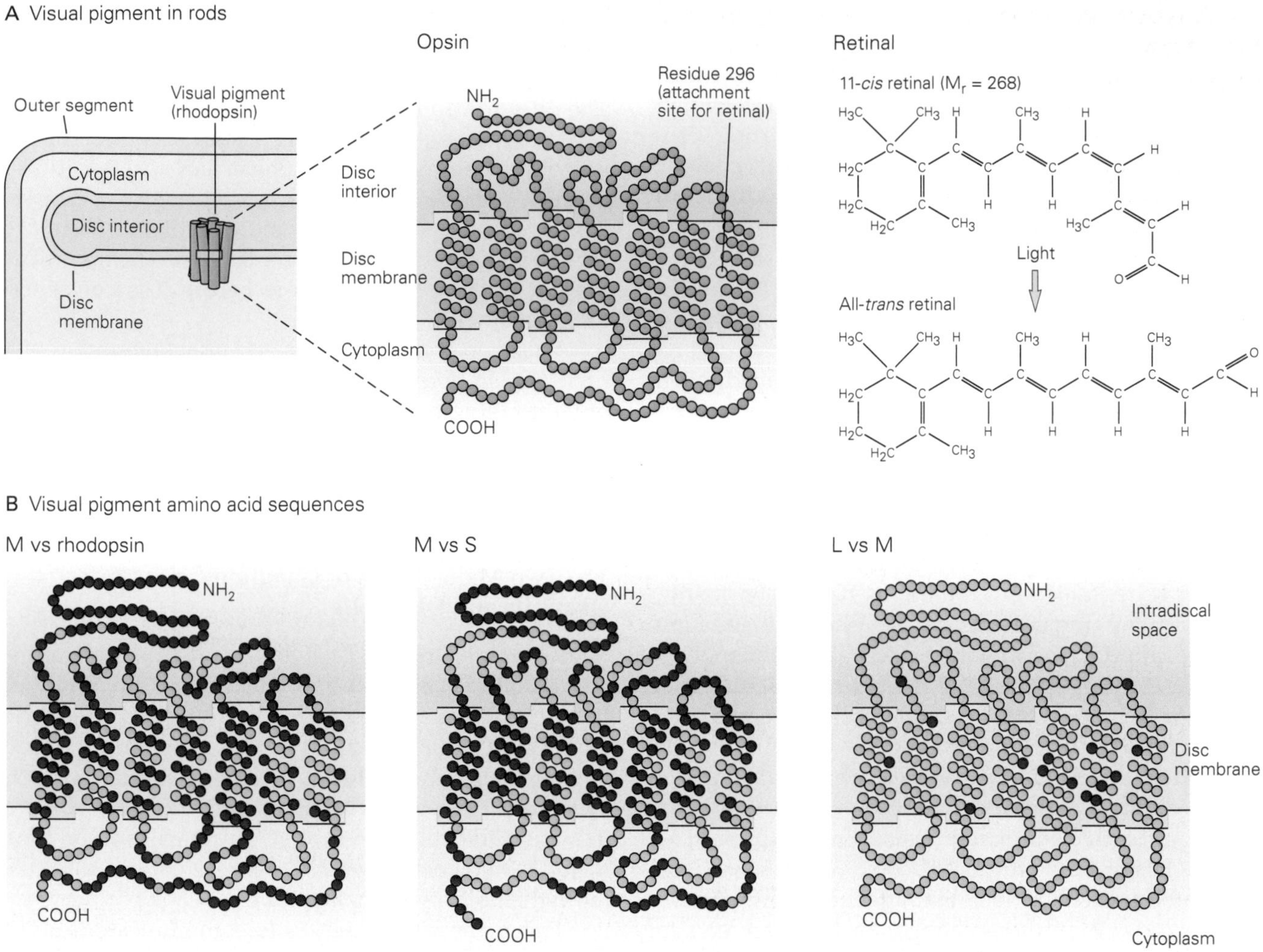

Figure 26–8 Structure of the visual pigments.

A. Rhodopsin, the visual pigment in rod cells, is the covalent complex of a large protein, opsin, and a small light-absorbing compound, retinal. Opsin has 348 amino acids and a molecular mass of approximately 40,000 daltons. It loops back and forth seven times across the membrane of the rod disc. Retinal is covalently attached to a side chain of lysine 296 in the protein's seventh membrane-spanning region. Absorption of light by 11-*cis* retinal causes a rotation around the double bond. As retinal adopts the more stable all-*trans* configuration, it causes a conformational change in the protein that triggers the subsequent events of visual transduction. (Adapted, with permission, from Nathans and Hogness 1984.)

B. Amino acid sequences of cone and rod pigments. **Blue circles** denote identical amino acids; **black circles** denote differences. The three types of cone opsins resemble each other and rhodopsin, suggesting that all four evolved from a common precursor by duplication and divergence. The L and M opsins are most closely related, with 96% identity in their amino acid sequences. They are thought to derive from a gene-duplication event approximately 30 million years ago, after Old World monkeys, which have three pigments, separated from New World monkeys, which generally have only two.

encoded by a decrease in firing rate. If the ganglion cell fired at a maintained rate of 10 spikes per second and then decreased its rate, it would take about 100 ms for the postsynaptic neuron to notice the change in frequency of action potentials. In contrast, an increase in firing rate to 200 spikes per second is noticeable within only 5 ms.

Many Ganglion Cells Respond Strongly to Edges in the Image

To probe the responses of a ganglion cell in more detail, one can focus a small spot of light on different portions of the retina to test how the cell's firing varies with the location and time course of the spot.

A typical ganglion cell is sensitive to light in a compact region of the retina near the cell body, called the cell's *receptive field*. Within that area one can often distinguish a *center* region and *surround* region in which light produces opposite responses. An ON cell, for example, fires faster when a bright spot shines on its receptive field's center but decreases its firing when the spot shines on the surround. If light covers both the center and the surround, the response is much weaker than for center-only illumination. A bright spot on the center combined with a dark annulus on the surround elicits very strong firing. For an OFF cell these relationships are reversed; the cell is strongly excited by a dark spot in a bright annulus (Figure 26–10).

The output produced by a population of retinal ganglion cells thus enhances regions of spatial contrast in the input, such as an edge between two areas of different intensity, and gives less emphasis to regions of homogeneous illumination.

The Output of Ganglion Cells Emphasizes Temporal Changes in Stimuli

When an effective light stimulus appears, a ganglion cell's firing typically increases sharply from the resting level to a peak and then relaxes to an intermediate rate. When the stimulus turns off, the firing rate drops sharply then gradually recovers to the resting level.

The rapidity of decline from the peak to the resting level varies among ganglion cell types. *Transient neurons* produce a burst of spikes only at the onset of the stimulus whereas *sustained neurons* maintain an almost steady firing rate for several seconds during stimulation (Figure 26–10).

In general, however, the output of ganglion cells emphasizes temporal changes in the visual input over periods of constant light intensity. In fact, when the image is stabilized on the retina with an eye-tracking device, it fades from view within seconds. Fortunately this never happens in normal vision; even when we attempt to fix our gaze, small automatic eye movements (saccades) continually scan the image across the retina and prevent the world from disappearing.

Retinal Output Emphasizes Moving Objects

Based on these observations we can understand more generally the response of ganglion cells to visual inputs. For example, a moving object elicits strong firing in the ganglion cell population near the edges of the object's image because these are the only regions of spatial contrast and the only regions where the light intensity changes over time (Figure 26–11).

We can imagine why the retina highlights these features. The outline of an object is particularly useful for inferring its shape and identity. Similarly, objects that move or change suddenly are more worthy of immediate attention than those that do not. Retinal processing thus extracts low-level features of the scene that are useful for guiding behavior and transmits those selectively to the brain. In fact, the rejection of features that are constant either in space or in time accounts for the spatiotemporal sensitivity of human perception (Box 26–1).

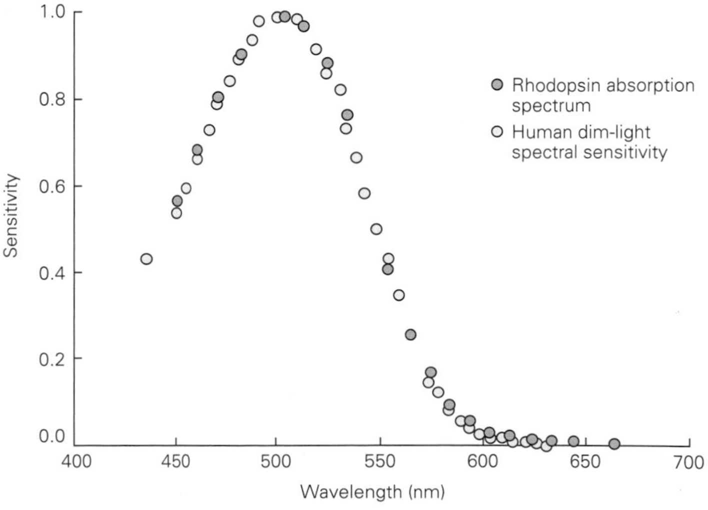

Figure 26–9 Absorption spectrum of rhodopsin. This plot compares the absorption spectrum of human rhodopsin measured in a cuvette and the spectral sensitivity of human observers to very dim light flashes. The psychophysical data have been corrected for absorption by the ocular media. (Reproduced, with permission, from Wald and Brown 1956.)

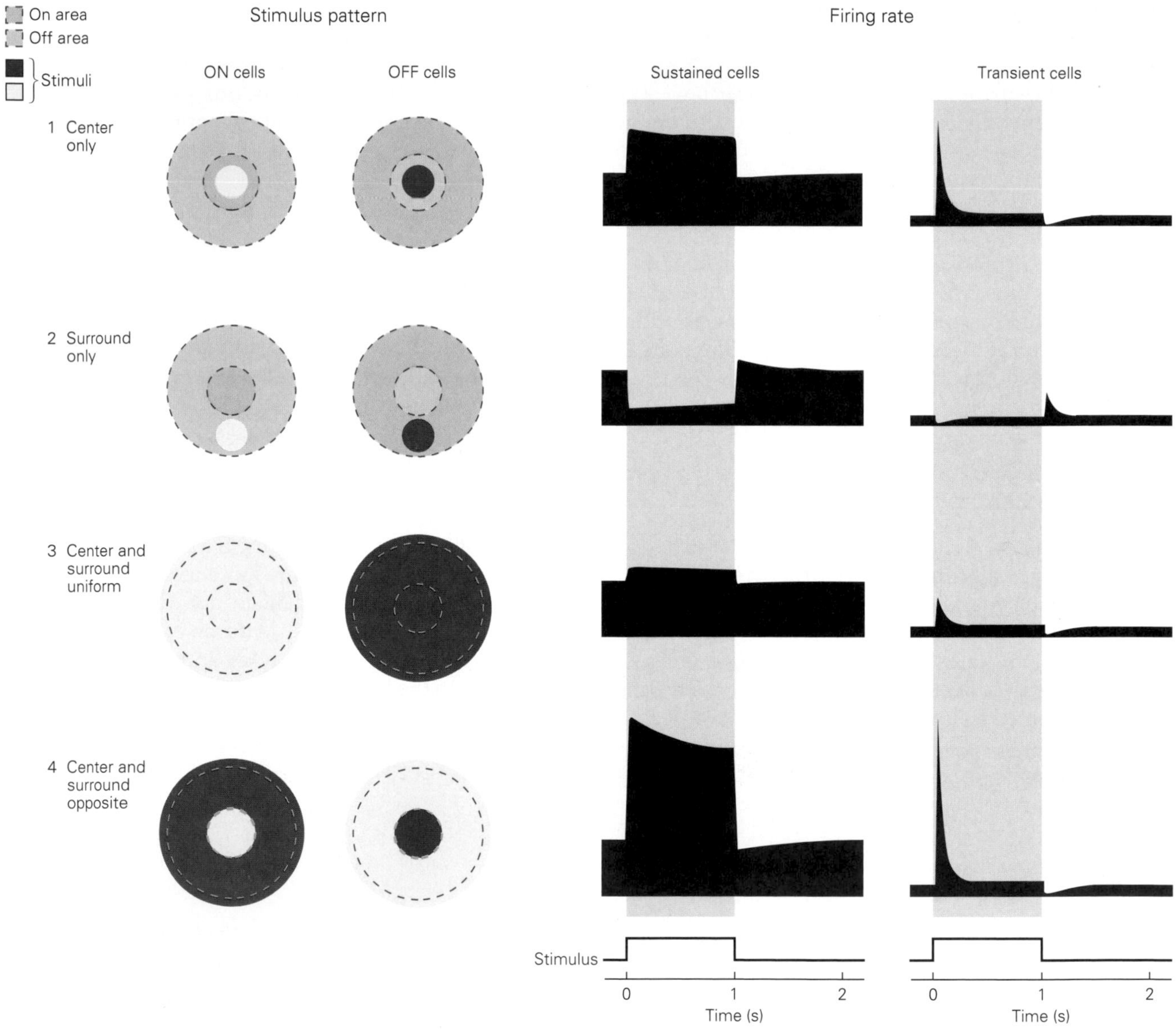

Figure 26–10 Responses of retinal ganglion cells with center-surround receptive fields. In these idealized experiments the stimulus changes from a uniform gray field to the pattern of bright (yellow) and dark (black) regions indicated on the left. **1.** ON cells are excited by a bright spot in the receptive field center, OFF cells by a dark spot. In *sustained cells* the excitation persists throughout stimulation, whereas in *transient cells* a brief burst of spikes occurs just after the onset of stimulation. **2.** If the same stimulus that excites the center is applied to the surround, firing is suppressed. **3.** Uniform stimulation of both center and surround elicits a response like that of the center, but much smaller in amplitude. **4.** Stimulation of the center combined with the opposite stimulus in the surround produces the strongest response.

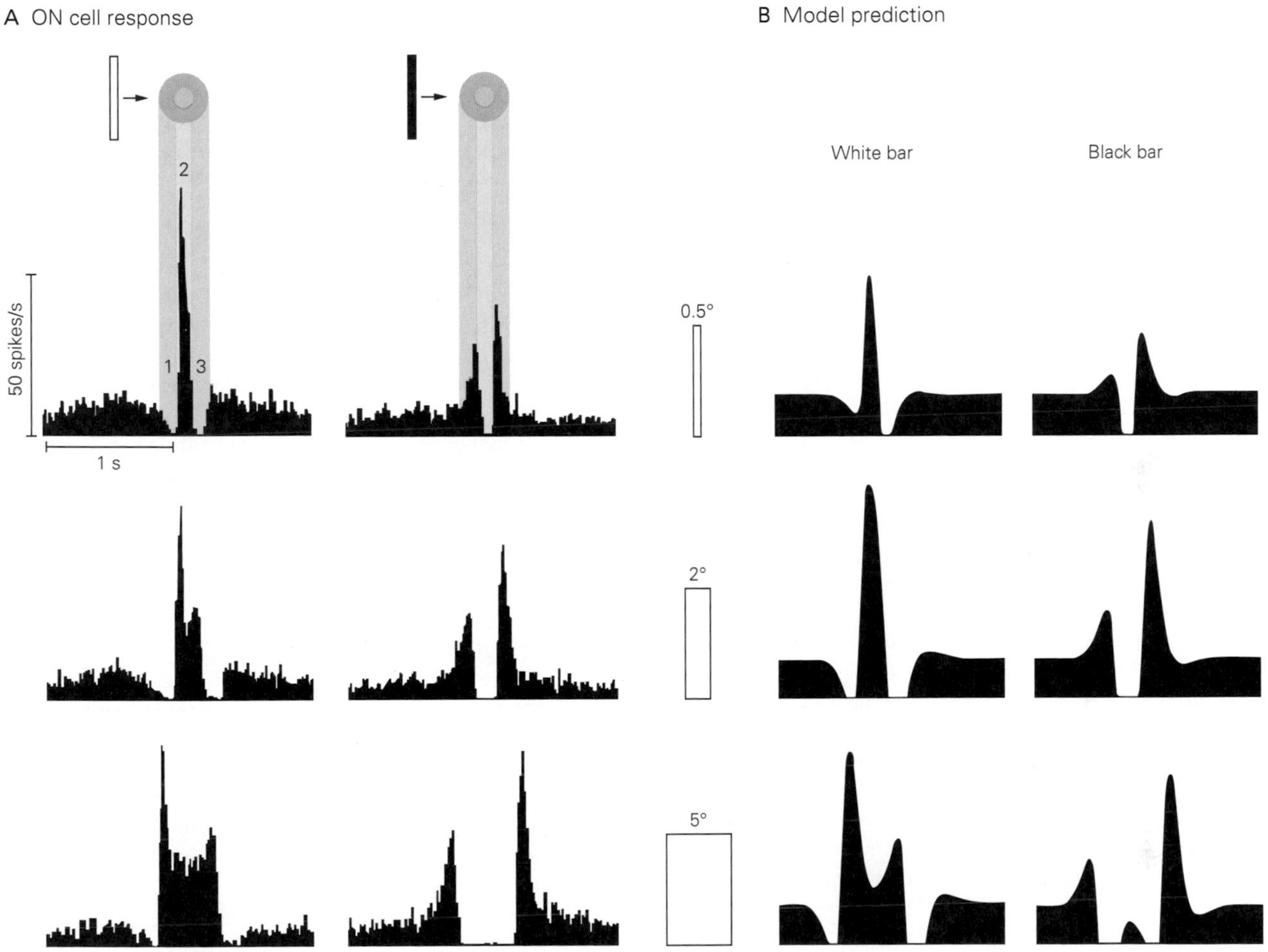

Figure 26–11 The representation of moving objects by retinal ganglion cells.

A. The firing rate of an ON ganglion cell in the cat's retina in response to a variety of bars (white or black, various widths) moving across the retina. Each bar moves at 10° per second; 1 degree corresponds to 180 μm on the retina. In response to the white bar the firing rate first decreases as the bar passes over the receptive-field surround (**1**), increases as the bar enters the center (**2**), and decreases again as the bar passes through the surround on the opposite side (**3**). The dark bar elicits responses of the opposite sign. Because retinal ganglion cells similar to this one are distributed throughout the retina, one can also interpret this curve as an instantaneous snapshot of activity in many different ganglion cells, plotting firing rate as a function of location on the retina. In effect this is the neural representation of the moving bar transmitted to the brain. A complementary population of OFF ganglion cells (not shown here) conveys another neural image in parallel. In this way both bright edges and dark edges can be signaled by a sharp increase in firing.

B. A simple model of retinal processing that incorporates center-surround antagonism and a transient temporal filter is used to predict ganglion-cell firing rates. The predictions match the essential features of the responses in part A. (Reproduced, with permission, from Rodieck 1965.)

Box 26–1 Spatiotemporal Sensitivity of Human Perception

Whereas small spots of light are useful for probing the receptive fields of single neurons, different stimuli are needed to learn about human visual perception. One method to probe how our visual system deals with spatial and temporal patterns uses *grating stimuli.*

The subject views a display in which the intensity varies about the mean as a sinusoidal function of space (Figure 26–12). Then the contrast of the display—defined as the peak-to-peak amplitude of the sinusoid divided by the mean—is reduced to a threshold at which the grating is barely visible. One then repeats this measurement for gratings of different spatial frequencies, measuring the threshold contrast in each case.

Plotting the inverse of this threshold against the spatial frequency, one obtains the *contrast sensitivity curve,* a measure of sensitivity of visual perception to patterns of different scales (Figure 26–13A). When measured at high light intensity, sensitivity declines sharply at high spatial frequencies, with an absolute threshold at approximately 50 cycles per degree. This sensitivity is limited fundamentally by the quality of the optical image and the spacing of cone cells in the fovea (see Figure 26–1C).

Interestingly, sensitivity also declines at low spatial frequencies. Patterns with a frequency of approximately 5 cycles per degree are most visible. The visual system is said to have *band-pass* behavior because it rejects all but a band of spatial frequencies.

One can measure the sensitivity of individual ganglion cells to spatial contrast by stimulating the primate retina with the same displays. The results resemble those for human visual perception (Figure 26–13A), suggesting that the perceptual effects originate in the retina.

The band-pass behavior can be understood on the basis of spatial antagonism in center-surround receptive fields (Figure 26–13B). A very fine grating presents many dark and bright stripes within the receptive-field center; their effects cancel one another and thus provide no net excitation. With a very coarse grating, a single stripe can cover both the center and surround of the receptive field, and their antagonism again provides the ganglion cell little net excitation. The strongest response is produced by a grating of intermediate spatial frequency that just covers the center with one stripe and most of the surround with stripes of the opposite polarity.

In dim light the visual system's contrast sensitivity declines, but more so at high than at low spatial frequencies (Figure 26–13A). Thus the peak sensitivity shifts to lower spatial frequencies, and eventually the curve loses its peak altogether. In this state the visual system has so-called *low-pass* behavior, for it selectively passes stimuli of low spatial frequency. It has been shown that the receptive fields of ganglion cell lose their antagonistic surrounds in dim light, which can explain this transition from band-pass to low-pass spatial filtering (Figure 26–13B).

Similar experiments can be done to test visual sensitivity to temporal patterns. Here the intensity of a test stimulus flickers sinusoidally in time, while the contrast is gradually brought to the threshold level of detection. For humans, contrast sensitivity declines sharply at very high flicker frequencies, but it also declines at very low frequencies (Figure 26–14A). Flicker at approximately 10 Hz is the most effective stimulus. One finds similar band-pass behavior in the flicker sensitivity of macaque retinal ganglion cells (Figure 26–14B).

Sensitivity to temporal contrast also depends on the mean light level. For human subjects the optimum flicker frequency shifts downward, and the peak in the curve becomes less and less prominent at lower stimulus intensities (Figure 26–14). The fact that primate retinal ganglion cells duplicate this behavior suggests that retinal processing limits visual perception in these simple tasks.

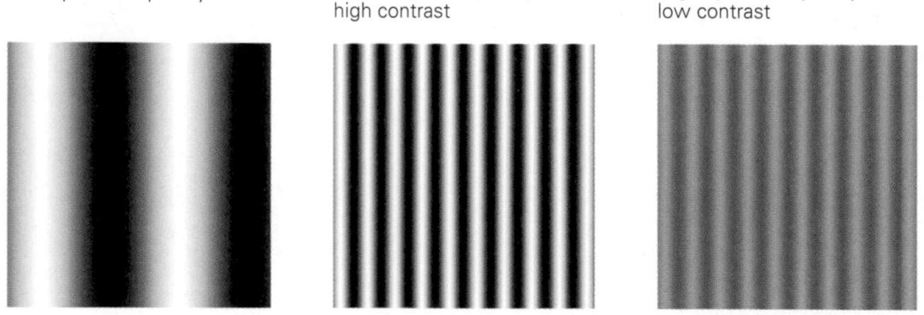

Figure 26–12 Sinusoid grating displays used in psychophysical experiments with human subjects. These stimuli are employed in the experiments discussed in Figure 26–13.

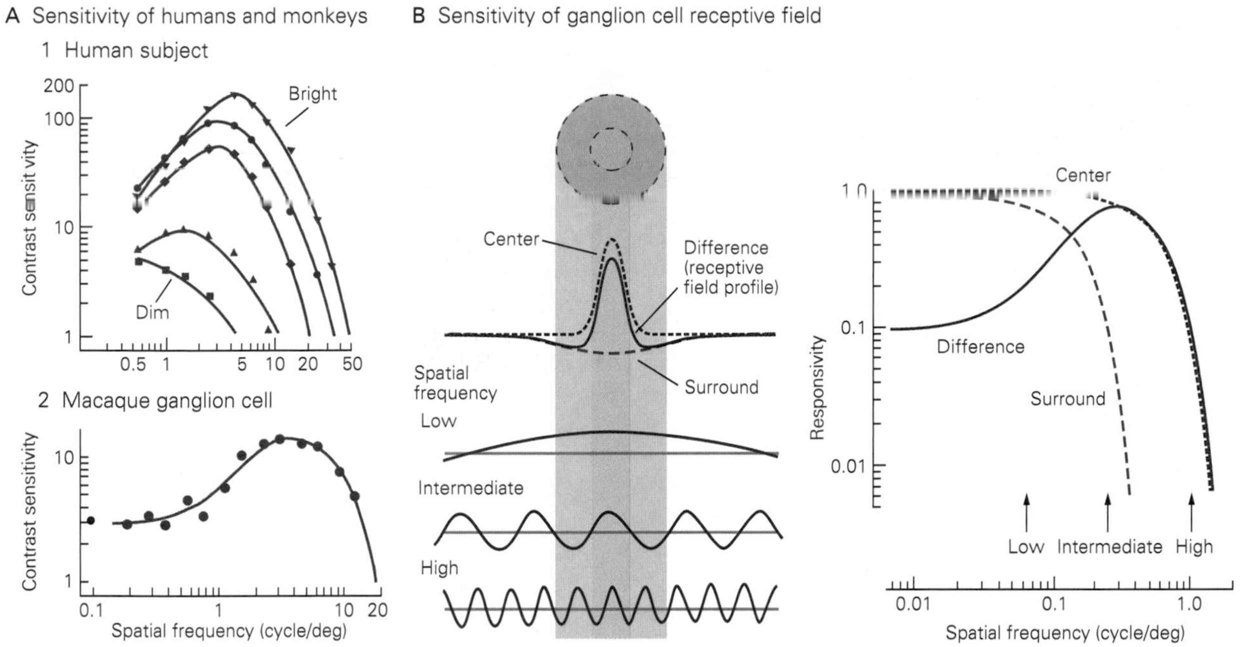

Figure 26–13 Spatial contrast sensitivity.

A. 1. Contrast sensitivity of human subjects. Using gratings at different spatial frequencies, the threshold contrast required for detection was measured and the inverse of that contrast value was plotted against spatial frequency. The curves were obtained at different mean intensities, decreasing by factors of 10 from the top to the bottom curve. (Reproduced, with permission, from DeValois, Morgan, and Snodderly 1974.) **2.** Contrast sensitivity of a P-type ganglion cell in the macaque retina measured at high intensity. At each spatial frequency the contrast was gradually increased until it produced detectable modulation of the neuron's firing rate. The inverse of that threshold contrast was plotted as in part A. The isolated dot at left marks the sensitivity at zero spatial frequency, a spatially uniform field. (Reproduced, with permission, from Derrington and Lennie 1984.)

B. Stimulation of a center-surround receptive field with sinusoid gratings. The neuron's sensitivity to light at different points on the retina is modeled as a "difference-of-Gaussians" receptive field, with a narrow positive Gaussian for the excitatory center and a broad negative Gaussian for the inhibitory surround. Multiplying the spatial frequency with the receptive-field profile and integrating over all space calculates the stimulus strength delivered by a particular grating. The resulting sensitivity of the receptive field to gratings of different frequency is shown in the plot on the right. At low spatial frequencies the negative contribution from the surround cancels the contribution from the center, leading to a drop in the difference curve. (Reproduced, with permission, from Enroth-Cugell and Robson 1984.)

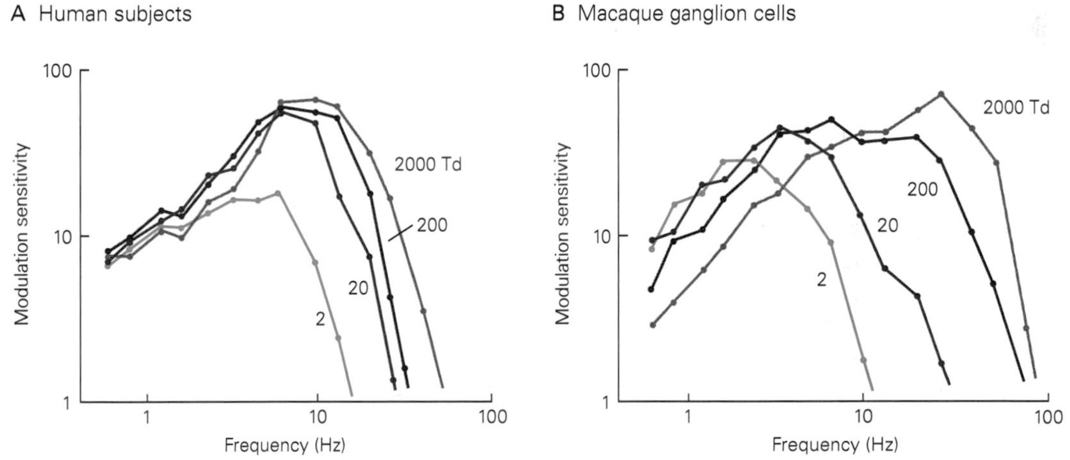

Figure 26–14 Temporal contrast sensitivity. (Reproduced, with permission, from Lee et al. 1990.)

A. Perceptual sensitivity of human observers. These measurements are similar to those in Figure 26–13, but the stimulus was a large spot, 4.6° in diameter, with an intensity that varied sinusoidally in time rather than space. The inverse of the minimal contrast required for detection is plotted against the flicker frequency. Sensitivity declines at both high and low frequencies. The mean light level varied, decreasing by factors of 10 from the top to the bottom trace.

B. Sensitivity of M-type ganglion cells in the macaque retina. These experiments were identical to those on human subjects in part A. The detection threshold for the neural response was defined as a variation of 20 spikes per second in the cell's firing rate in phase with the flicker.

Several Ganglion Cell Types Project to the Brain Through Parallel Pathways

Several different types of ganglion cells have been identified on the basis of their shapes and light responses. The ON and OFF cells occur in every vertebrate retina, and in the primate retina two major classes of cells, the P-cells and M-cells, each include ON and OFF types (see Figure 26–2B). At any given distance from the fovea the receptive fields of M-cells (Latin *magno*, large) are much larger than those of P-cells (Latin *parvo*, small). The M-cells also have faster and more transient responses than P-cells. A type of ganglion cell discovered recently is intrinsically light-sensitive owing to expression of the visual pigment melanopsin.

In total about 20 ganglion-cell types have been described. Each type covers the retina in a tiled fashion, such that any point on the retina lies within the receptive field center of at least one ganglion cell. One can envision each separate population as sending a distinct neural representation of the visual field to the brain, where the firing of an individual ganglion cell represents one pixel in the representation. In this view the optic nerve conveys about 20 neural representations of the world that differ in polarity (ON or OFF), spatial resolution (fine or coarse), temporal responsiveness (sustained or transient), spectral filtering (broadband or dominated by red, green, or blue), and selectivity for other image features such as motion.

These neural representations are directed to various visual centers in the brain, including the lateral geniculate nucleus of the thalamus, a relay to the visual cortex; the superior colliculus, a midbrain region involved in spatial attention and orienting movements; the pretectum, involved in control of the pupil; the accessory optic system, which analyzes self-motion to stabilize gaze; and the suprachiasmatic nucleus, a central clock that directs circadian rhythm and whose phase can be set by light cues (Chapter 51). In many cases the same ganglion-cell type sends axon collaterals to multiple target areas; M-cells, for example, project to the thalamus and the superior colliculus.

A Network of Interneurons Shapes the Retinal Output

We now consider in more detail the basic retinal circuit and how it accounts for the intricate response properties of retinal ganglion cells.

Parallel Pathways Originate in Bipolar Cells

The photoreceptor forms synapses with bipolar cells and horizontal cells (see Figure 26–3A). In the dark the cell's synaptic terminal releases glutamate continuously. On illumination the photoreceptor hyperpolarizes, less Ca^{2+} enters the terminal, and the terminal releases less glutamate. Photoreceptors do not fire action potentials; like bipolar cells they release neurotransmitter in a graded fashion using a specialized structure, the *ribbon synapse*. In fact, most retinal processing is accomplished with graded membrane potentials: Action potentials occur only in certain amacrine cells and in ganglion cells.

The two principal varieties of bipolar cells, ON and OFF cells, respond to glutamate at the synapse through distinct mechanisms. The OFF cells use ionotropic receptors, namely glutamate-gated cation channels of the AMPA-kainate variety (AMPA = α-amino-3-hydroxy-5-methylisoxazole-4-propionate). The glutamate released in darkness depolarizes these cells. The ON cells use metabotropic receptors that are linked to a G protein whose action ultimately closes cation channels. Glutamate activation of these receptors thus hyperpolarizes the cells in the dark.

Bipolar ON and OFF cells differ in shape and especially in the levels within the inner plexiform layer where their axons terminate. The axons of ON cells end in the proximal (lower) half, those of OFF cells in the distal (upper) half (Figure 26–15). There they form specific synaptic connections with amacrine and ganglion cells whose dendritic trees ramify in specific levels of the inner plexiform layer. The ON bipolar cells excite ON ganglion cells, while OFF bipolar cells excite OFF ganglion cells (see Figure 26–3A). Thus the two principal subdivisions of the retinal output signal, the ON and OFF pathways, are already established at the level of bipolar cells.

Bipolar cells can also be distinguished by the morphology of their dendrites (Figure 26–15). In the central region of the primate retina the *midget bipolar cell* receives input from a single cone and excites a P-type ganglion cell. This explains why the centers of P-cell receptive fields are so small. The *diffuse bipolar cell* receives input from many cones and excites an M-type ganglion cell. The receptive-field centers of M-cells are accordingly much larger. Thus stimulus representations in the ganglion cell population originate in dedicated bipolar cell pathways that are differentiated by their selective connections to photoreceptors and postsynaptic targets.

Spatial Filtering Is Accomplished by Lateral Inhibition

Signals in the parallel vertical pathways are modified by lateral interactions with horizontal and amacrine cells (see Figure 26–3A). Horizontal cells have broadly

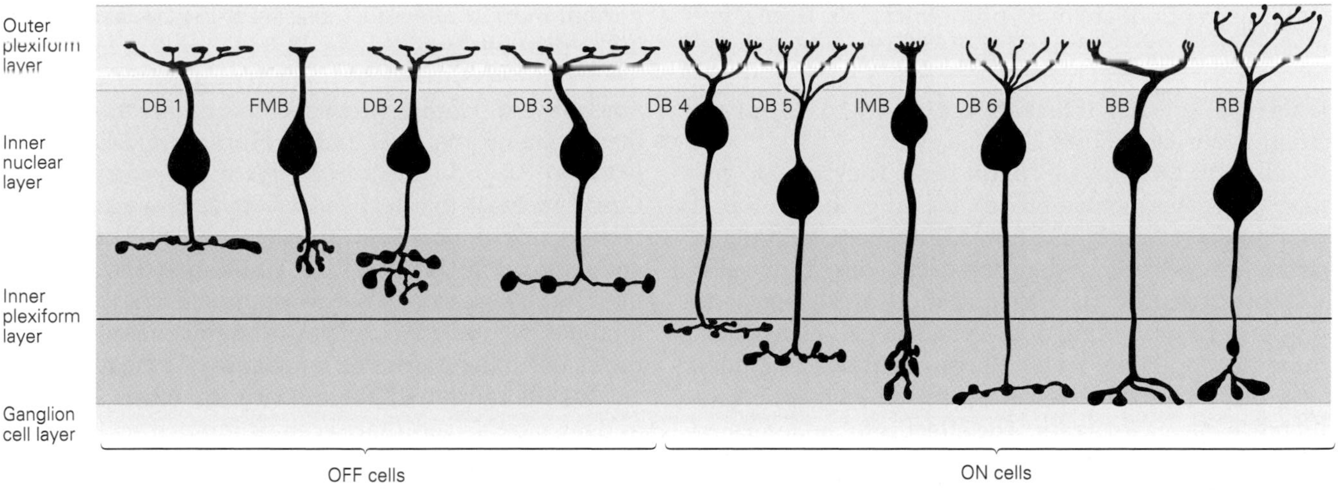

Figure 26–15 Bipolar cells in the macaque retina. The cells are arranged according to the depth of their terminal arbors in the inner plexiform layer. The horizontal line dividing the distal and proximal levels of this layer represents the border between the axonal terminals of OFF and ON types. Bipolar cells with axonal terminals in the upper (distal) half are presumed to be OFF cells, those in the lower (proximal) half ON cells. Cell types are diffuse bipolar cells (**DB**), ON and OFF midget bipolars (**IMB, FMB**), S-cone ON bipolar (**BB**), and rod bipolar (**RB**). (Reproduced, with permission, from Boycott and Wässle 1999.)

arborizing dendrites that spread laterally in the outer plexiform layer. The tips of these arbors contact photoreceptors at terminals shared with bipolar cells. Glutamate released by the photoreceptors excites the horizontal cell. In addition, horizontal cells are electrically coupled with each other through gap junctions.

A horizontal cell effectively measures the average level of excitation of the photoreceptor population over a broad region. This signal is fed back to the photoreceptor terminal through an inhibitory synapse. Thus the photoreceptor terminal is under two opposing influences: light falling on the receptor hyperpolarizes it, but light falling on the surrounding region depolarizes it through the sign-inverting synapses from horizontal cells. As a result, the bipolar cell, which shares the photoreceptor's glutamatergic terminals with the horizontal cells, has an antagonistic receptive field structure.

This spatial antagonism in the receptive field is enhanced by lateral inhibition from amacrine cells in the inner retina. Amacrine cells are axonless neurons with dendrites that ramify in the inner plexiform layer. Approximately 30 types of amacrine cells are known, some with small arbors only tens of micrometers across, and others with processes that extend all across the retina. Amacrine cells generally receive excitatory signals from bipolar cells at glutamatergic synapses. Some amacrine cells feed back directly to the presynaptic bipolar cell at a *reciprocal inhibitory synapse*. Some amacrine cells are electrically coupled to others of the same type, forming an electrical network much like that of the horizontal cells.

Through this inhibitory network a bipolar cell terminal can receive inhibition driven by other, distant bipolar cells, in a manner closely analogous to the lateral inhibition of photoreceptor terminals (see Figure 26–3A). Amacrine cells also inhibit retinal ganglion cells directly. These lateral inhibitory connections contribute substantially to the antagonistic receptive field component of retinal ganglion cells.

Temporal Filtering Occurs in Synapses and Feedback Circuits

For many ganglion cells a step change in light intensity produces a transient response, an initial peak in firing that declines to a smaller steady rate (see Figure 26–10). Part of this sensitivity originates in the negative-feedback circuits involving horizontal and amacrine cells.

For example, a sudden decrease in light intensity depolarizes the cone terminal, which excites the horizontal cell, which in turn repolarizes the cone terminal (see Figure 26–3A). Because this feedback loop involves a brief delay, the voltage response of the cone peaks abruptly and then settles to a smaller steady level. Similar processing occurs at the reciprocal synapses between bipolar and amacrine cells in the inner retina.

In both cases the delayed-inhibition circuit favors rapidly changing inputs over slowly changing inputs. The effects of this filtering, which can be observed in visual perception, are most pronounced for large stimuli that drive the horizontal cell and amacrine cell networks most effectively. For example, a large spot can be seen easily when it flickers at a rate of 10 Hz but not at a low rate (see Figure 26–14).

In addition to these circuit properties, certain cellular processes contribute to shaping the temporal response. For example, the AMPA-kainate type of glutamate receptor undergoes strong desensitization. A step increase in the concentration of glutamate at the dendrite of a bipolar or ganglion cell leads to an immediate opening of additional glutamate receptors. As these receptors desensitize, the postsynaptic conductance decreases again. The effect is to render a step response more transient.

Retinal circuits seem to go to great lengths to speed up their responses and emphasize temporal changes. One likely reason is that the very first neuron in the retinal circuit, the photoreceptor, is exceptionally slow (see Figure 26–7C). Following a flash of light a cone takes about 40 ms to reach the peak response, an intolerable delay for proper visual function. Through the various filtering mechanisms in retinal circuitry, subsequent neurons respond sensitively during the rising phase of the cone's response. Indeed, some ganglion cells have a response peak only 20 ms after the flash. Temporal processing in the retina clearly helps to reduce visual reaction times, a life-extending trait in highway traffic as on the savannas of our ancestors.

Color Vision Begins in Cone-Selective Circuits

Throughout recorded history philosophers and scientists have been fascinated by the perception of color. This interest was fueled by the relevance of color to art, later by its relation to the physical properties of light, and finally by commercial interests in television and photography. The 19th century witnessed a profusion of theories to explain color perception, of which two have survived modern scrutiny. They are based on careful psychophysics that placed strong constraints on the underlying neural mechanisms.

Early experiments on color matching showed that the percept of any given light could be matched by mixing together appropriate amounts of three primary lights. Thomas Young and Hermann von Helmholtz accordingly postulated the trichromatic theory of color perception based on absorption of light by three mechanisms, each with a different sensitivity spectrum. We now know that these correspond to the three cone types (see Figure 26–6), whose measured absorption spectra fully explain the color-matching results both in normal individuals and those with genetic anomalies in the pigment genes.

In an effort to explain our perception of different hues, Ewald Hering proposed the opponent-process theory, later formalized by Leo Hurvich and Dorothea Jameson. According to this theory, color vision involves three processes that respond in opposite ways to light of different colors: (y–b) would be stimulated by yellow and inhibited by blue light; (r–g) stimulated by red and inhibited by green; and (w–bk) stimulated by white and inhibited by black. We can now recognize some of these processes in the post-receptor circuitry of the retina.

In the central 10° of the human retina a single midget bipolar cell that receives input from a single cone excites each P-type ganglion cell. An L-ON ganglion cell, for example, has a receptive field center consisting of a single L cone and an antagonistic surround involving a mixture of L and M cones. When stimulated with a large spot that extends over both the center and the surround, this neuron is depolarized by red light and hyperpolarized by green light. Similar antagonism holds for the three other P-cells: L-OFF, M-ON, and M-OFF. These P-cells send their signals to the parvocellular layers of the lateral geniculate nucleus.

Although S cones are relatively rare, a dedicated type of S-ON bipolar cell collects their signals selectively and transmits them to ganglion cells of the small bistratified type. Because this ganglion cell also receives excitation from L-OFF and M-OFF bipolar cells, it is depolarized by blue light and hyperpolarized by yellow light. Another ganglion cell type shows the opposite signature: S-OFF and (L + M)-ON. These signals are transmitted to the koniocellular layers of the lateral geniculate nucleus.

The M cells are excited by diffuse bipolar cells, which in turn collect inputs from many cones regardless of pigment type. These ganglion cells therefore have large receptive fields with broad spectral sensitivity. Their axons project to the magnocellular layers of the lateral geniculate nucleus.

In this way chromatic signals are combined and formatted by the retina for transmission to the thalamus and cortex. In the primary visual cortex these signals are recombined in different ways, leading to a great variety of receptive field layouts. Note that only about 10% of cortical neurons are preferentially driven by color contrast rather than luminance contrast. This likely reflects the fact that color vision—despite its great esthetic appeal—makes only a small contribution to our overall fitness. As an illustration of this, recall that colorblind individuals, who in a sense have lost half of their color space, can grow up without noticing that defect.

Congenital Color Blindness Takes Several Forms

Few people are truly colorblind in the sense of being wholly unable to distinguish a change in color from a change in the intensity of light, but many individuals have impaired color vision and experience difficulties in making distinctions that for most of us are trivial, for example between red and green. Most such abnormalities of color vision are congenital and have been characterized in detail; some other abnormalities result from injury or disease of the visual pathway.

The study of inherited variation in color vision has contributed in important ways to our understanding of the mechanisms of normal color vision. The first major insight, well understood in the 19th century, is that some people have only two classes of receptors instead of the three in normal trichromatic vision. These dichromats find it difficult or impossible to distinguish some surfaces whose colors appear distinct to trichromats. The dichromat's problem is that every surface reflectance function is represented by a two-value description rather than a three-value one, and this reduced description causes dichromats to confuse many more surfaces than do trichromats. Simple tests for color-blindness exploit this fact. Figure 26–16 shows an example from the Ishihara test, in which the numerals defined by colored dots are seen by normal trichromats but not by most dichromats.

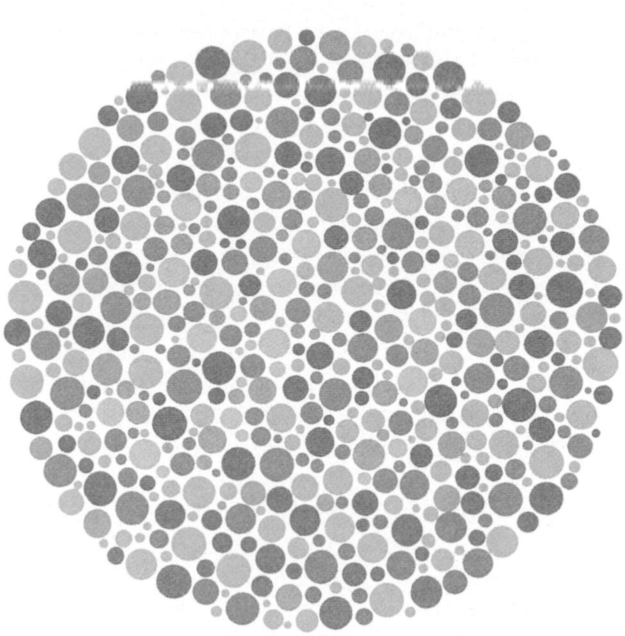

Figure 26–16 A test for some forms of color blindness. The numerals embedded in this color pattern can be distinguished by people with trichromatic vision but not by certain dichromats, including the Editor of this section of the book, who are weak in red–green discrimination. (Reproduced, with permission, from Ishihara 1993.)

When a person with normal color vision fails to distinguish two physically different surface reflectance functions, a dichromat will also fail to distinguish them. This failure means that each class of cone gives rise to the same signal when absorbing light reflected by either surface, so the fact that the dichromat is confused by the same surfaces that confuse a trichromat shows that the cones in the dichromat have normal pigments.

Although there are three forms of dichromacy, corresponding to the loss of each of the three types of cones, two kinds of dichromacy are much more common than the third. The common forms correspond to the loss of the L cones or M cones and are called *protanopia* and *deuteranopia*, respectively. Protanopia and deuteranopia almost always occur in males, each with a frequency of about 1%. The conditions are transmitted by women who are not themselves affected, and so implicate genes on the X chromosome. A third form of dichromacy, *tritanopia*, corresponds to the loss or dysfunction of the S cone. It affects only about 1 in 10,000 people, afflicts women and men with equal frequency and has a gene on chromosome 7.

Because the L and M cones exist in large numbers, one might think that the loss of one or the other type would impair vision more broadly than just weakening color vision. In fact, this does not happen because the total number of L and M cones in the dichromat retina is not altered. All cells destined to become L or M cones are probably converted to L cones in deuteranopes and to M cones in protanopes.

In addition to the relatively severe forms of colorblindness represented by dichromacy, there are milder forms, again affecting mostly males, that result in an impaired capacity to distinguish different reflectance functions that are readily distinguished by normal trichromats. People with these milder impairments are referred to as anomalous trichromats, for their cones provide three-value descriptions of the light reflected by surfaces. In contrast to dichromats, however, they do not see as identical the physically different spectral functions distinguished by a normal trichromat.

These anomalous trichromats have cones whose spectral sensitivities differ from those of cones in normal trichromats. Anomalous trichromacy occurs in different forms, corresponding to the replacement of one of the normal cone pigments by an altered protein with a different spectral sensitivity. Two common forms, protanomaly and deuteranomaly, together affect about

7% of males and represent respectively the replacement of the L or M cones by a pigment with some intermediate spectral sensitivity.

The occurrence of sex-linked inherited defects of color vision points to the X chromosome as the locus of genes that encode the visual pigments of L and M cones. These genes, and the amino acid sequences of the pigments they encode, have now been identified, largely through the work of Jeremy Nathans and his colleagues. Their discovery reveals some interesting complexities in the molecular organization underlying color vision. Molecular cloning of the genes for the L and M pigments shows the genes to be very similar and arranged head-to-tail on the X chromosome (Figure 26–17A). The pigments also have very similar structures, differing in only 4% of their amino acids.

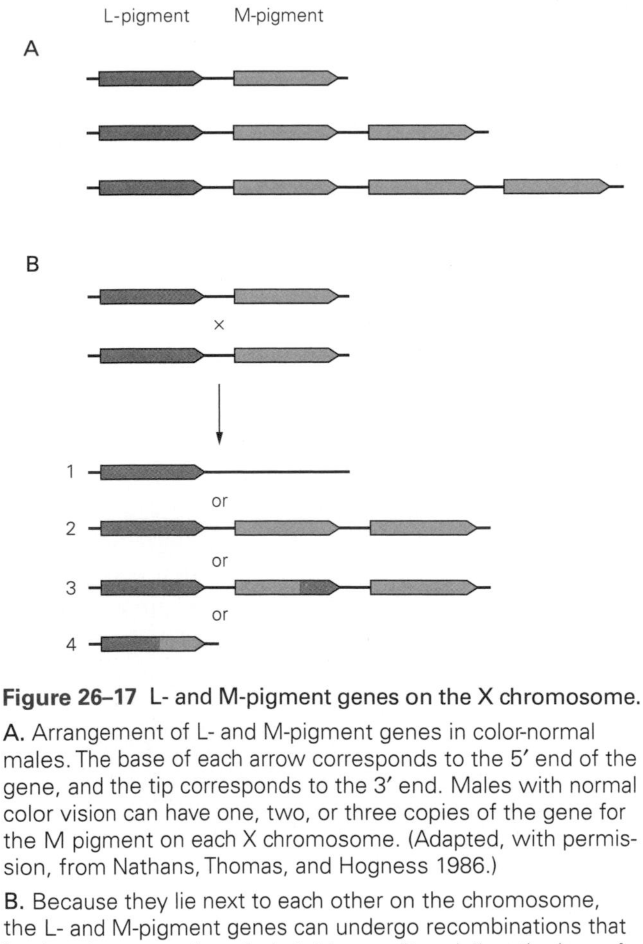

Figure 26–17 L- and M-pigment genes on the X chromosome.

A. Arrangement of L- and M-pigment genes in color-normal males. The base of each arrow corresponds to the 5′ end of the gene, and the tip corresponds to the 3′ end. Males with normal color vision can have one, two, or three copies of the gene for the M pigment on each X chromosome. (Adapted, with permission, from Nathans, Thomas, and Hogness 1986.)

B. Because they lie next to each other on the chromosome, the L- and M-pigment genes can undergo recombinations that lead to the generation of a hybrid gene (3 and 4) or the loss of a gene (1), the patterns observed in colorblind men. Spurious recombination can also cause gene duplication (2), a pattern observed in some people with normal color vision. (Adapted, with permission, from Stryer 1988.)

People with normal color vision possess a single copy of the gene for the L pigment and from one to three—occasionally as many as five—nearly identical copies of the gene for the M pigment.

The proximity and similarity of these genes is thought to predispose them to varied forms of recombination, leading either to the loss of a gene or to the formation of hybrid genes that account for the common forms of red-green defect (Figure 26–17B). Examination of these genes in dichromats reveals a loss of the L-pigment gene in protanopes and a loss of one or more M-pigment genes in deuteranopes. Anomalous trichromats have L-M or M-L hybrid genes that code for visual pigments with shifted spectral sensitivity, the extent of the shift depending on the point of recombination. In tritanopes, the loss of S-cone function arises from mutations in the S-pigment gene.

Rod and Cone Circuits Merge in the Inner Retina

For vision under low-light conditions the mammalian retina has an ON bipolar cell that is exclusively connected to rods (see Figure 26–3B). By collecting inputs from up to 50 rods, this rod bipolar cell can pool the effects of dispersed single-photon absorptions in a small patch of retina. This neuron is excited by light and there is no corresponding OFF bipolar cell dedicated to rods.

Unlike all other bipolar cells, the rod bipolar cell does not contact ganglion cells directly but instead excites a dedicated neuron called the AII amacrine cell. This amacrine cell receives inputs from several rod bipolar cells and conveys its output to cone bipolar cells. It sends excitatory signals to ON bipolar cells through gap junctions as well as glycinergic inhibitory signals to OFF bipolar cells. These cone bipolar cells in turn excite ON and OFF ganglion cells as described above. Thus the rod signal is fed into the cone system after a detour, involving the rod bipolar and AII amacrine cells, that produces the appropriate signal polarities for the ON and OFF pathways. The purpose of these added interneurons may be to allow greater pooling of rod signals than of cone signals.

Rod signals also enter the cone system through two other pathways. Rods can drive neighboring cones directly through electrical junctions, and they make connections with an OFF bipolar cell that services primarily cones. Once the rod signal has reached the cone bipolars through these pathways, it can take advantage of the same intricate circuitry of the inner retina. One gets the impression that the rod system of the mammalian retina is an evolutionary afterthought added to the cone circuits.

The Retina's Sensitivity Adapts to Changes in Illumination

Vision operates under many different lighting conditions. The intensity of the light coming from an object depends on the intensity of the illuminating light and the fraction of this light reflected by the object's surface, called the *reflectance*. The range of intensities encountered in a day is enormous, with variation spanning 10 orders of magnitude, but most of this variation is useless for the purpose of guiding behavior.

The illuminant intensity varies by about nine logarithmic units, mostly because our planet turns about its axis once a day, while the object reflectance varies much less, by about one order of magnitude in a typical scene. But this reflectance is the interesting quantity for vision, for it characterizes objects and distinguishes them from the background. In fact, our visual system is remarkably good at calculating surface reflectances independently of the illuminant intensity (Figure 26–18).

When illumination becomes stronger, all points in the retinal image increase in intensity by the same factor. If the retina could simply reduce its sensitivity by the same factor, the neural representation of the retinal image would remain unchanged at the level of the ganglion cells and could be processed by the rest of the brain in the same way as before the change in illumination. Moreover, the retinal ganglion cells would only need to encode the tenfold range of image intensities owing to the different object reflectances, instead of the 10-billionfold range that includes variations in illumination. In fact, the retina does perform such an automatic gain control, called *light adaptation*, that approaches the ideal normalization we have imagined here.

Light Adaptation Is Apparent in Retinal Processing and Visual Perception

The responses of a retinal ganglion cell to varying flashes of light with a steady background illumination fit a sigmoidal curve (Figure 26–19A). The weakest flashes elicit

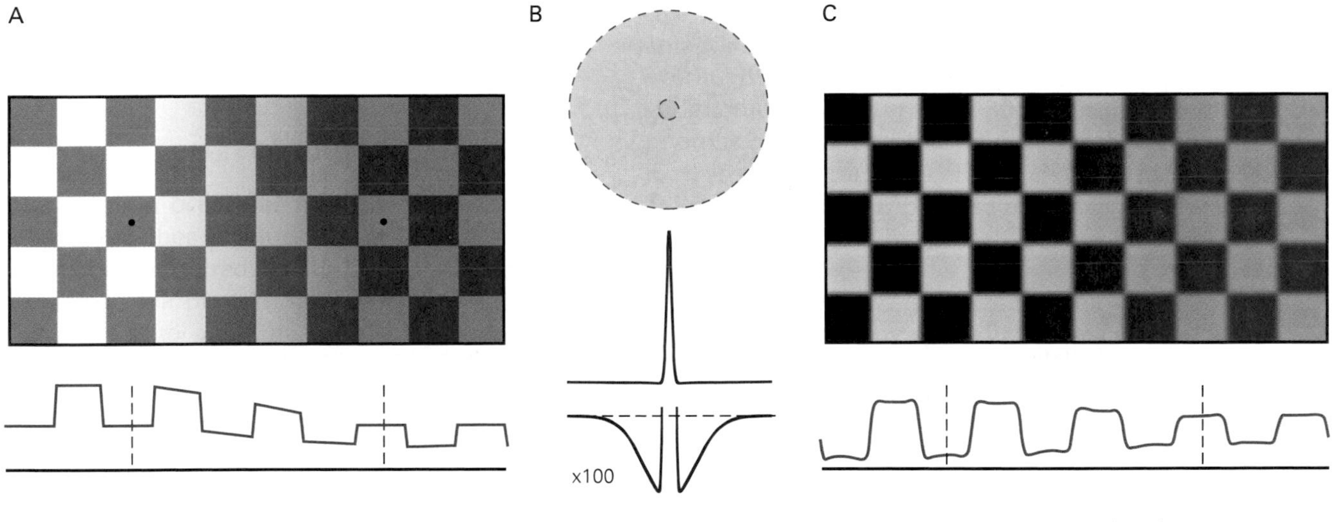

Figure 26–18 A brightness illusion.

A. The two tiles marked with small dots appear to have different brightness but actually reflect the same light intensity. (To see this, fold the page so they touch.) The trace underneath plots a profile of light intensity at the level of the arrowheads. Your visual system interprets this retinal image as a regular tile pattern under graded illumination with a diffuse shadow in the right half. Perceptual processing tries to discount this shadow to extract the underlying surface reflectance, and thus assigns a greater lightness to the right tile than the left. As you can see, this process is automatic and requires no conscious analysis.

B. Retinal processing contributes to the perception of "lightness" by discounting the shadow's smooth gradients of illumination and accentuating the sharp edges between checkerboard fields. The profile of the receptive field for a visual neuron with an excitatory center and an inhibitory surround is shown at the top. As shown in a hundredfold magnification at the bottom, the surround is weak but extends over a much larger area than the center.

C. The result when a population of visual neurons with receptive fields as in B processes the image in A. This operation—the convolution of the image in A with the profile in B—subtracts from each point in the input image the average intensity in a large surrounding region. The output image has largely lost the effects of shading, and the two tiles in question do indeed have different lightness values in this representation.

In fact, the crucial need for light adaptation may be why the neural circuitry resides in the eye and not in the brain at the other end of the optic nerve.

An Overall View

The retina transforms light patterns projected onto photoreceptors into neural signals that are conveyed through the optic nerve to specialized visual centers in the brain. Different populations of ganglion cells transmit multiple neural representations of the retinal image along parallel pathways.

In producing its output the retina discards much of the stimulus information available at the receptor level and extracts certain low-level features of the visual field useful to the central visual system. Fine spatial resolution is maintained only in a narrow region at the center of gaze. Intensity gradients in the image, such as object edges, are emphasized over spatially uniform portions; temporal changes are enhanced over unchanging parts of the scene.

The retina adapts flexibly to the changing conditions for vision, especially the large diurnal changes in illumination. With increases in average light level the retina becomes progressively less sensitive, so that the response to a fractional change in intensity is almost independent of the overall illumination. Information about the absolute light level is largely discarded, favoring the subsequent analysis of object reflectances within the scene.

The transduction of light stimuli begins in the outer segment of the photoreceptor cell when a pigment molecule absorbs a photon. This sets in motion an amplifying G protein cascade that ultimately reduces the membrane conductance, hyperpolarizes the photoreceptor, and decreases glutamate release at the synapse. Multiple feedback mechanisms, in which intracellular Ca^{2+} has an important role, serve to turn off the enzymes in the cascade and terminate the light response.

Rod photoreceptors are efficient collectors of light and serve nocturnal vision. Cones are much less sensitive and function throughout the day. Cones synapse onto bipolar cells that in turn excite ganglion cells. Rods connect to specialized rod bipolar cells whose signals are conveyed through amacrine cells to the cone bipolar cells. These vertical excitatory pathways are modulated by horizontal connections that are primarily inhibitory. Through these lateral networks light in the receptive-field surround of a ganglion cell counteracts the effect of light in the center. The same negative-feedback circuits also sharpen the transient response of ganglion cells.

As we shall see in subsequent chapters, the segregation of information into parallel pathways and the shaping of response properties by inhibitory lateral connections are pervasive organizational principles in the visual system.

Markus Meister
Marc Tessier-Lavigne

Selected Readings

Dacey DM. 2004. Origins of perception: retinal ganglion cell diversity and the creation of parallel visual pathways. In: MS Gazzaniga (ed). *The Cognitive Neurosciences,* pp. 281–301. Cambridge, MA: MIT Press.

Dowling JE. 1987. *The Retina: An Approachable Part of the Brain.* Cambridge, MA: Harvard Univ. Press.

Fain GL, Matthews HR, Cornwall MC, Koutalos Y. 2001. Adaptation in vertebrate photoreceptors. Physiol Rev 81:117–151.

Gollisch T, Meister M. 2010. Eye smarter than scientists believed: neural computations in circuits of the retina. Neuron 65:150–164.

Lee BB. 1996. Receptive field structure in the primate retina. Vision Res 36:631–644.

MacNeil MA, Brown SP, Rockhill RL, Masland RH. 2000. Retinal cell mosaics and neurotransmitters. In: DM Albert, FA Jakobiec (eds). *Principles and Practice of Ophthalmology,* pp. 1729–1745. Philadelphia: Saunders.

Meister M, Berry MJ. 1999. The neural code of the retina. Neuron 22:435–450.

Oyster CW. 1999. *The Human Eye: Structure and Function.* Sunderland, MA: Sinauer.

Roof DJ, Makino CL. 2000. The structure and function of retinal photoreceptors. In: DM Albert, FA Jakobiec (eds). *Principles and Practice of Ophthalmology,* pp. 1624–1673. Philadelphia: Saunders.

Shapley R, Enroth-Cugell C. 1984. Visual adaptation and retinal gain controls. Prog Retin Eye Res 3:263–346.

Wandell BA. 1995. *Foundations of Vision.* Sunderland, MA: Sinauer.

Wässle, H. 2004. Parallel processing in the mammalian retina. Nat Rev Neurosci 5:747–757.

References

Alberts B, Johnson A, Lewis J, Raff M, Roberts K, Walter P. 2008. *Molecular Biology of the Cell,* 5th ed. New York: Garland Science.

Boycott B, Wässle H. 1999. Parallel processing in the mammalian retina: the Proctor Lecture. Invest Ophthalmol Vis Sci 40:1313–1327.

Boycott BB, Dowling JE. 1969. Organization of the primate retina: light microscopy. Philos Trans R Soc Lond B Biol Sci 255:109–184.
Curcio CA, Hendrickson A. 1982. Organization and development of the primate photoreceptor mosaic. Prog Retinal Res 10:89–120.
De Valois RL, Morgan H, Snodderly DM. 1974. Psychophysical studies of monkey vision. 3. Spatial luminance contrast sensitivity tests of macaque and human observers. Vision Res 14:75–81.
Derrington AM, Lennie P. 1984. Spatial and temporal contrast sensitivities of neurones in lateral geniculate nucleus of macaque. J Physiol 357:219–240.
Enroth-Cugell C, Robson JG. 1984. Functional characteristics and diversity of cat retinal ganglion cells. Basic characteristics and quantitative description. Invest Ophthalmol Vis Sci 25:250–267.
Hurvich LM. 1981. *Color Vision.* Sunderland, MA: Sinauer.
Ishihara S. 1993. Ishihara's Tests for Colour-blindness. Tokyo: Kanehara & Co.
Lee BB, Pokorny J, Smith VC, Martin PR, Valberg A. 1990. Luminance and chromatic modulation sensitivity of macaque ganglion cells and human observers. J Opt Soc Am A 7:2223–2236.
Nathans J, Hogness DS. 1984. Isolation and nucleotide sequence of the gene encoding human rhodopsin. Proc Natl Acad Sci U S A 81:4851–4855.
Nathans J, Thomas D, Hogness DS. 1986. Molecular genetics of human color vision: the genes encoding blue, green, and red pigments. Science 232:193–202.
O'Brien DF. 1982. The chemistry of vision. Science 218: 961–966.
Polyak SL. 1941. *The Retina.* Chicago: Univ of Chicago Press.
Rodieck RW. 1965. Quantitative analysis of cat retinal ganglion cell response to visual stimuli. Vision Res 5:583–601.
Sakmann B, Creutzfeldt OD. 1969. Scotopic and mesopic light adaptation in the cat's retina. Pflügers Arch 313:168–185.
Schnapf JL, Kraft TW, Nunn BJ, Baylor DA. 1988. Spectral sensitivity of primate photoreceptors. Vis Neurosci 1:255–261.
Schneeweis DM, Schnapf JL. 1995. Photovoltage of rods and cones in the macaque retina. Science 268:1053–1056.
Schneeweis DM, Schnapf JL. 2000. Noise and light adaptation in rods of the macaque monkey. Vis Neurosci 17:659–666.
Solomon GS, Lennie P. 2007. The machinery of color vision. Nat Rev Neurosci 8:276–286.
Stryer L. 1988. *Biochemistry,* 3rd ed. New York: Freeman.
Wade NJ. 1998. *A Natural History of Vision.* Cambridge: MIT Press.
Wald G, Brown PK. 1956. Synthesis and bleaching of rhodopsin. Nature 177:174–176.
Wyszecki G, Stiles WS. 1982. *Color Science: Concepts and Methods, Quantitative Data and Formulas,* Chapter 7 "Visual Thresholds." New York: Wiley.
Young RW. 1970. Visual cells. Sci Am 223:80–91.

27

Intermediate-Level Visual Processing and Visual Primitives

WE HAVE SEEN IN THE PRECEDING chapter that the eye is not a mere camera but instead contains sophisticated retinal circuitry that decomposes the retinal image into signals representing contrast and movement. These data are conveyed through the optic nerve to the primary visual cortex, which uses this information to analyze the shape of objects. It first identifies the boundaries of objects, represented by numerous short line segments, each with a specific orientation. The cortex then integrates this information into a representation of specific objects, a process referred to as *contour integration.*

These two steps, local analysis of orientation and contour integration, exemplify two distinct stages of visual processing. Computation of local orientation is an example of low-level visual processing, which is concerned with identifying local elements of the light structure of the visual field. Contour integration is an example of intermediate-level visual processing, the first step in generating a representation of the unified visual field. At the earliest stages of analysis in the cerebral cortex these two levels of processing are accomplished together.

A visual scene comprises many thousands of line segments and surfaces. Intermediate-level visual processing is concerned with determining which boundaries and surfaces belong to specific objects and which are part of the background (see Figure 25–4). It is also involved in distinguishing the lightness and color of a surface from the intensity and wavelength of light reflected from that surface. The physical characteristics of reflected light result as much from the intensity and color balance of the light that illuminates a surface as from the color of that surface. Determining the actual surface color of a single object requires comparison of the wavelengths of light reflected from multiple surfaces in a scene.

Intermediate-level visual processing thus involves assembling local elements of an image into a unified percept of objects and background. Although determining which elements belong together in a single object is a highly complex problem with the potential for an astronomical number of solutions, the brain has built-in logic that allows it to make assumptions about the likely spatial relationships between elements. In certain cases these inherent rules can lead to the illusion of contours and surfaces that do not actually exist in the visual field (Figure 27–1).

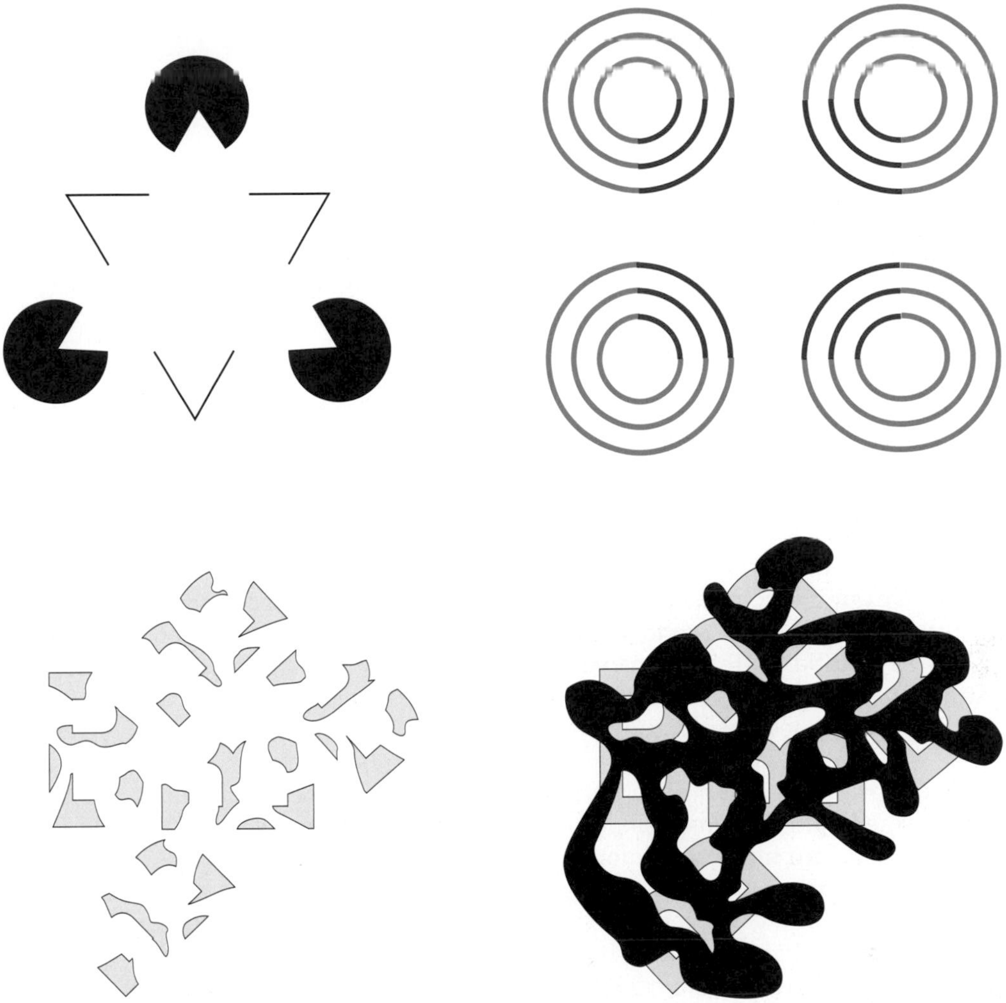

Figure 27–1 Illusory contours and perceptual fill-in. The visual system uses information about local orientation and contrast to construct the contours and surfaces of objects. This constructive process can lead to the perception of contours and surfaces that do not appear in the visual field, including those seen in illusory figures. In the Kanizsa triangle illusion (**top left**) one perceives continuous boundaries extending between the apices of a white triangle, even though the only real contour elements are those formed by the Pac-Man–like figures and the acute angles. The inside and outside of the illusory pink square (**top right**) are the same white color as the page, but a continuous transparent pink surface within the square is perceived. As seen in the lower figures, contour integration and surface segmentation can also occur through occluding surfaces. The irregular shapes on the left appear to be unrelated, but when a partially occluding black area is overlaid on them (**right**) they are easily seen as fragments of the letter B.

First, context plays an important role in overcoming ambiguity in the signals from the retina. The way in which a visual feature is perceived depends on everything that surrounds that feature. The perception of a point or a line depends on how that object is perceptually linked to other visual features. Thus the response of a neuron in the visual cortex is context-dependent: It depends as much on the presence of contours and surfaces outside the cell's receptive field as on the attributes within it. Second, the functional properties of neurons in the visual cortex are highly dynamic and can be altered by visual experience or perceptual learning. Finally, visual processing in the cortex is subject to the influence of cognitive functions, specifically attention, expectation, and "perceptual task," ie, the active engagement in visual discrimination or detection. The interaction between these three factors—visual context, experience-dependent changes in cortical circuitry, and expectation—is vital in the visual system's analysis of complex scenes.

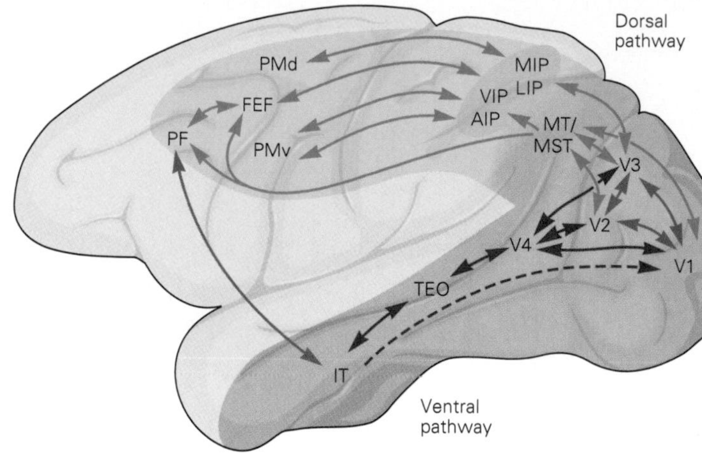

Figure 27–2 Cortical areas involved with intermediate-level visual processing. Many cortical areas in the macaque monkey, including V1, V2, V3, V4, and middle temporal area (**MT**), are involved with integrating local cues to construct contours and surfaces and segregating foreground from background. The shaded areas extend into the frontal and temporal lobes because cognitive output from these areas, including attention, expectation, and perceptual task, contribute to the process of scene segmentation. (**AIP**, anterior intraparietal cortex; **FEF**, frontal eye fields; **IT**, inferior temporal cortex; **LIP**, lateral intraparietal cortex; **MIP**, medial intraparietal cortex; **MST**, medial superior temporal cortex; **MT**, middle temporal cortex; **PF**, prefrontal cortex; **PMd**, dorsal premotor cortex; **PMv**, ventral premotor cortex; **TEO**, occipitotemporal cortex; **VIP**, ventral intraparietal cortex; **V1**, **V2**, **V3**, **V4**, primary, secondary, third, and fourth visual areas.)

In this chapter we examine how the brain's analysis of the local features in a visual scene, or *visual primitives,* proceeds in parallel with the analysis of more global features. Visual primitives include contrast, line orientation, brightness, color, movement, and depth.

Each type of visual primitive is subject to the integrative action of intermediate-level processing. Lines with particular orientations are integrated into object contours, local contrast information into surface lightness, wavelength selectivity into color constancy and surface segmentation, and directional selectivity into object motion. The analysis of visual primitives begins in the retina with the detection of brightness and color and continues in the primary visual cortex with the analysis of orientation, direction of movement, and stereoscopic depth. Properties related to intermediate-level visual processing are analyzed together with visual primitives in the visual cortex starting in the primary visual cortex (V1), which plays a role in contour integration and surface segmentation. Other areas of the visual cortex specialize in different aspects of this task: V2 analyzes properties related to object surfaces, V4 integrates information about color and object shape, and V5—the middle temporal area or MT—integrates motion signals across space (Figure 27–2).

Internal Models of Object Geometry Help the Brain Analyze Shapes

A first step in determining an object's contour is identification of the orientation of local parts of the contour. This step commences in V1, which plays a critical role in both local and global analysis of form.

Neurons in the visual cortex respond selectively to specific local features of the visual field, including orientation, binocular disparity or depth, and direction of movement, as well as to properties already analyzed in the retina and lateral geniculate nucleus, such as contrast and color. Orientation selectivity, the first emergent property identified in the receptive fields of cortical neurons, was discovered by David Hubel and Torsten Wiesel in 1959.

Neurons in the lateral geniculate nucleus have circular receptive fields with a center-surround organization (see Chapter 25). They respond to the light-dark contrasts of edges or lines in the visual field but are not selective for the orientations of those edges. In the visual cortex, however, neurons respond selectively to lines of particular orientations. Each neuron responds to a narrow range of orientations, approximately 40°, and different neurons respond optimally to distinct orientations. There is now good evidence for the idea, first proposed by Hubel and Wiesel, that this orientation selectivity reflects the arrangement of the inputs from cells in the lateral geniculate nucleus. Each V1 neuron receives input from several neighboring geniculate neurons whose center-surround receptive fields are aligned so as to represent a particular axis of orientation (Figure 27–3).

Two principal types of orientation-selective neurons have been identified. *Simple cells* have receptive fields divided into ON and OFF subregions (Figure 27–4). When a visual stimulus such as a bar of light enters the receptive field's ON subregion, the neuron fires; the cell also responds when the bar leaves the OFF subregion. Simple cells have a characteristic response to a moving bar; they discharge briskly when a bar of light leaves an OFF region and enters an ON region.

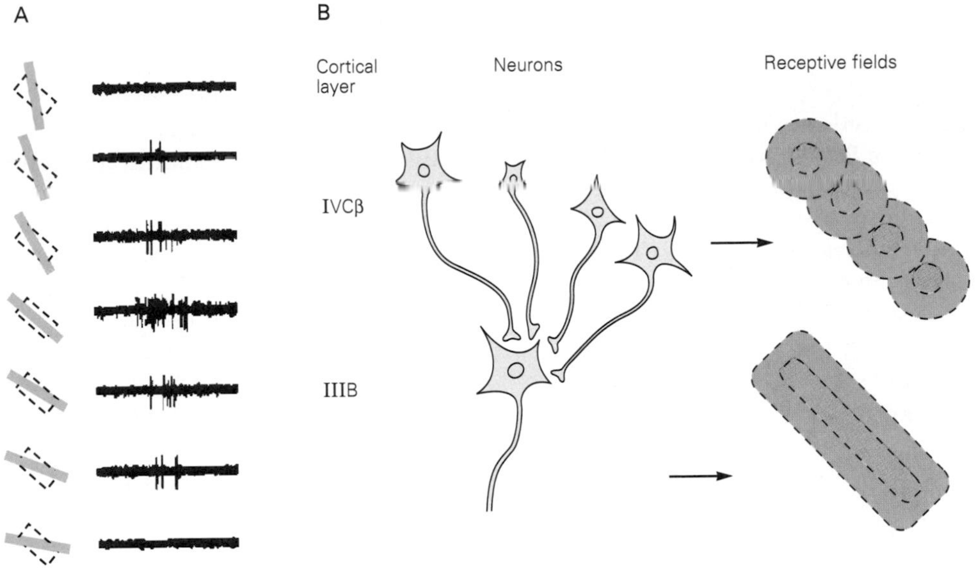

Figure 27–3 Orientation selectivity and mechanisms.

A. A neuron in the primary visual cortex responds selectively to line segments that fit the orientation of its receptive field. This selectivity is the first step in the brain's analysis of an object's form. (Reproduced, with permission, from Hubel and Wiesel 1968.)

B. The orientation of the receptive field is thought to result from the alignment of the circular center-surround receptive fields of several presynaptic cells in the lateral geniculate nucleus. In the monkey, neurons in layer IVCβ of V1 have unoriented receptive fields. However, the projections of neighboring IVCβ cells onto a neuron in layer IIIB create a receptive field with a specific orientation.

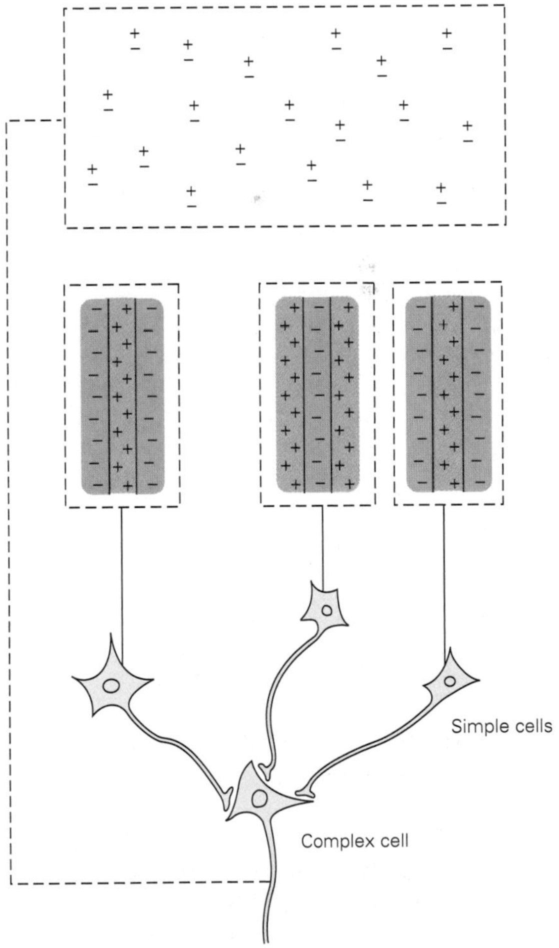

Figure 27–4 Simple and complex cells in the visual cortex. The receptive fields of simple cells are divided into subfields with opposite response properties. In an ON subfield, designated by "+," the onset of a light triggers a response in the neuron; in an OFF subfield, indicated by "–," the extinction of a bar of light triggers a response. Complex cells have overlapping ON and OFF regions and respond continuously as a line or edge traverses the receptive field along an axis perpendicular to the receptive-field orientation.

The responses of these cells are therefore highly selective for the position of a line or edge in space.

Complex cells, in contrast, are less selective for the position of object boundaries. They lack discrete ON and OFF subregions and respond similarly to light and dark at all locations across their receptive fields. They fire continuously as a line or edge stimulus traverses their receptive fields.

Moving stimuli are often used to study the receptive fields of visual cortex neurons, not only to simulate the conditions under which an object moving in space is detected but also to simulate the conditions under which stationary objects are tracked by the eyes, which constantly scan the visual environment and therefore move the boundaries of stationary objects across the retina. In fact, visual perception requires eye movement. Visual cortex neurons do not respond to an image that is stabilized on the retina because they require moving or flashing stimuli to be activated: They fire in response to transient stimulation.

Some visual cortex neurons have receptive fields in which an excitatory center is flanked by inhibitory regions. Inhibitory regions along the axis of orientation, a property known as *end-inhibition,* restrict a neuron's responses to lines of a certain length (Figure 27–5). End-inhibited neurons respond well to a line that does not extend into the inhibitory flanks but lies entirely within the excitatory part of the receptive field. Because the inhibitory regions share the orientation preference of the central excitatory region, end-inhibited cells are selective for line curvature and also respond well to corners.

To define the shape of the object as a whole, the visual system must integrate the information on local orientation and curvature into object contours. The way in which the visual system integrates contours reflects the geometrical relationships present in the natural world (Figure 27–6). As originally pointed out by Gestalt psychologists early in the 20th century, contours that are immediately recognizable tend to follow the rule of good continuation: Curved lines maintain a constant radius of curvature and straight lines stay straight. In a complex visual scene such smooth contours tend to "pop out," whereas more jagged contours are difficult to detect.

The responses of a visual cortex neuron can be modulated by stimuli that themselves do not activate the cell and therefore lie outside the receptive field's core. This *contextual modulation* endows a neuron with selectivity for more complex stimuli than would be predicted by placing the components of a stimulus at different positions in and around the receptive field. The same factors that facilitate the detection of an object in a complex scene (Figure 27–6A) also apply to contextual modulation. The properties of perceptible contours are reflected in the responses of neurons in the primary visual cortex, which are sensitive to the global characteristics of contours, even those that extend well outside their receptive fields.

Contextual influences over large regions of visual space are likely to be mediated by connections between multiple columns of neurons in the visual cortex that have similar orientation selectivity (Figure 27–6B). These connections are formed by pyramidal-cell axons that run parallel to the cortical surface (see Figure 25–16). The extent and orientation dependency of these horizontal connections provide the interactions that could mediate contour saliency (see Figure 25–14).

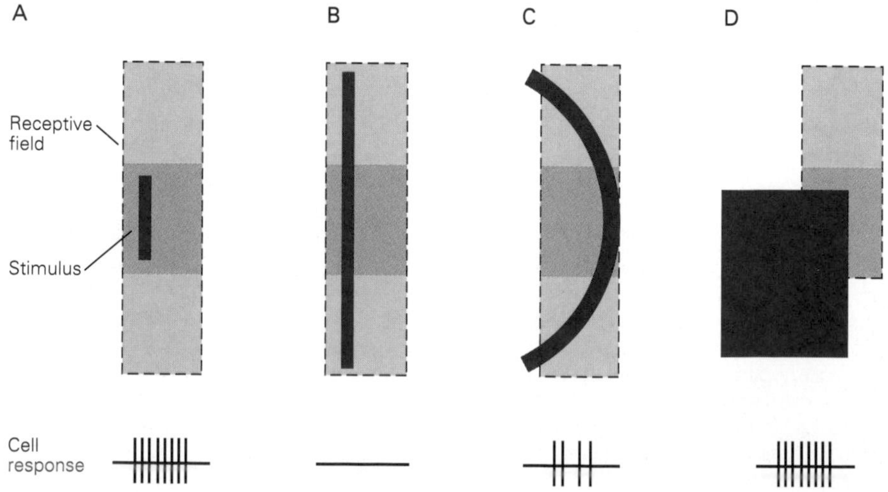

Figure 27–5 End-inhibited receptive fields. Some receptive fields have a central excitatory region flanked by inhibitory regions that have the same orientation selectivity. Thus a short line segment or a long curved line will activate the neuron (**A** and **C**) but a long straight line will not (**B**). A neuron with a receptive field that displays only one inhibitory region in addition to the excitatory region can signal the presence of corners (**D**).

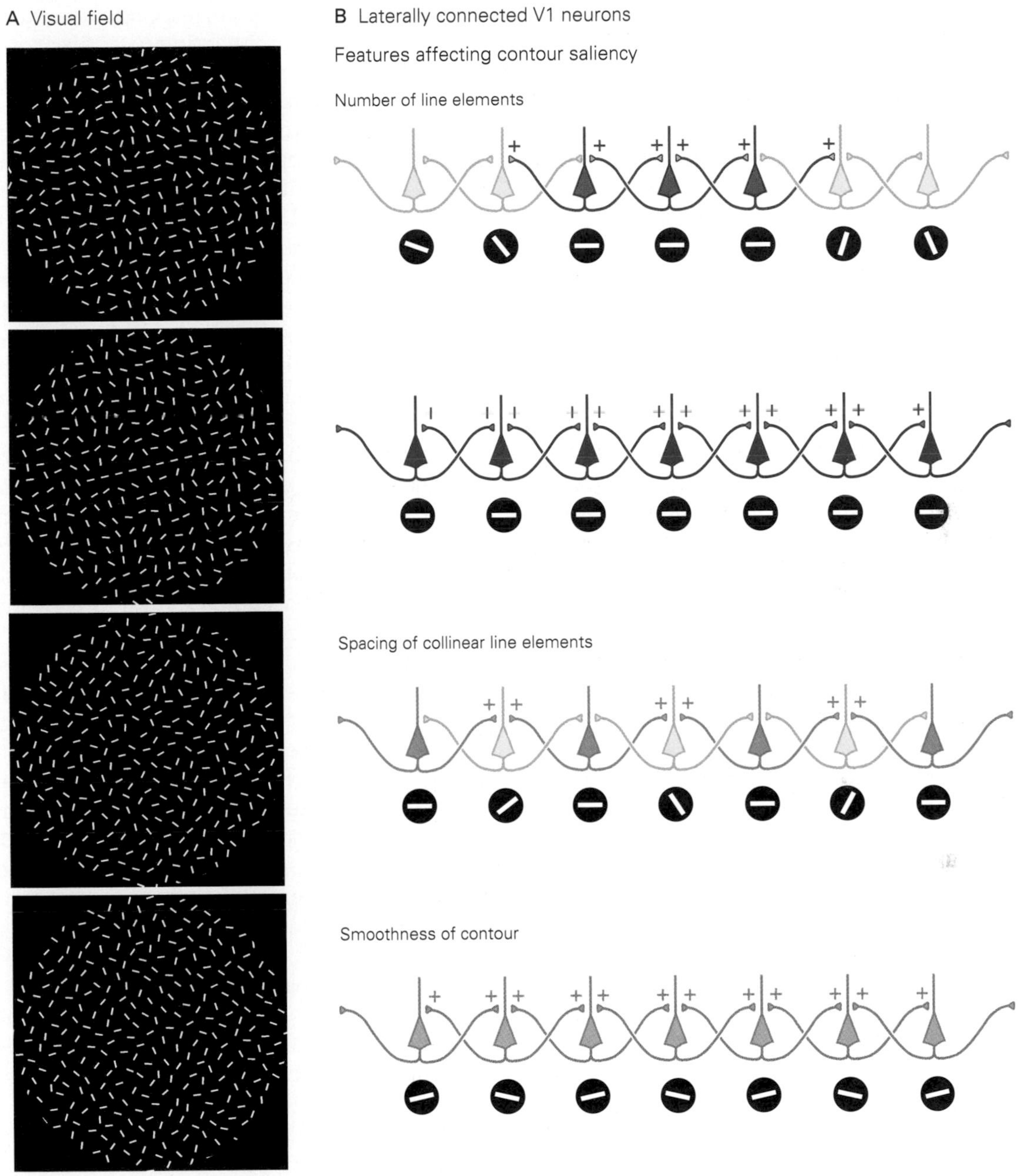

Figure 27–6 Contour integration. (Adapted, with permission, from Li W and Gilbert CD 2002.)

A. Contour integration reflects the perceptual rules of proximity and good continuation. Each of the four images here has a straight line in the center, and all four lines have the same oblique orientation. In some images the line pops out more or less immediately, without searching. Factors that contribute to contour saliency include the number of contour elements (compare the first and second frames), the spacing of the elements (third frame), and the smoothness of the contour (bottom frame). When the spacing between contour elements is too large or the orientation difference between them too great, one must search the image to find the contour.

B. These perceptual properties are reflected in the horizontal connections that connect columns of neurons in the primary visual cortex with similar orientation selectivity. As long as the contour elements are spaced sufficiently close together, excitation can propagate from cell to cell, thus facilitating the responses of V1 neurons. Each neuron in the network then augments the responses of neurons on either side and the facilitated responses propagate across the network.

Depth Perception Helps Segregate Objects from Background

Depth is another key feature in determining the shape of an object. An important cue for the perception of depth is the difference between the two eyes' views of the world, which must be computed and reconciled by the brain. The integration of binocular input begins in the primary visual cortex, the first level at which individual neurons receive signals from both eyes. The balance of input from the two eyes, a property known as ocular dominance, varies among cells in V1.

These neurons are also selective for depth, which is computed from the relative retinal positions of objects placed at different distances from the observer. An object that lies in the *plane of fixation* produces images at corresponding positions on the two retinas (Figure 27–7). The images of objects that lie in front of or behind the plane of fixation fall on slightly different locations in the two eyes. Individual visual cortex neurons are selective for a narrow range of such disparities. Some are selective for objects lying on the plane of fixation (tuned excitatory or inhibitory cells), whereas others respond only when objects lie in front of the plane of fixation (near cells) or behind that plane (far cells).

Depth plays an important role in the perception of object shape, in surface segmentation, and in establishing the three-dimensional properties of a scene. Objects that are placed near an observer can partially occlude those situated farther away. A surface passing behind an object is perceived as continuous even though its two-dimensional image on each retina represents two surfaces separated by the occluder. When the brain encounters a surface interrupted by gaps displaying appropriate alignment and contrast and lying in the near-depth plane, it fills in the gaps to create a continuous surface (Figure 27–8).

Although the depth of a single object can be established easily, determining the depths of multiple objects within a scene is a much more complex problem that requires linking the retinal images of all objects in the two eyes. The disparity calculation is therefore a global one: The calculation in one part of the visual image influences the calculation for other parts. When the assignment of depth is unambiguous in one part of an image, that information is applied to other parts of the image where there is insufficient information to determine depth, a phenomenon known as disparity capture.

Random-dot stereograms provide a dramatic demonstration of the global nature of disparity analysis. The image presented to each eye appears as noise, but when the images are viewed binocularly the disparity between the random array of dots in the two images allows an embedded shape to become visible (Figure 27–8C). The calculation underlying this percept is not simple, but requires determining which features shown to the left eye correspond to features seen by the right eye and propagating local disparity information across the image.

Neurons in area V2 display sensitivity to global disparity cues. Even when no contrast boundary exists in a neuron's receptive field, the neuron will respond to illusory contours formed by adjacent line elements (Figure 27–8B). The neuron's response is facilitated when collinear lines appear inside or outside the receptive field. When a perpendicular bar occludes the lines, indicating a break between them, the facilitation disappears. But when the bar is moved to a plane nearer than that of the collinear lines, as would occur if the lines were connected behind the occluder, the facilitation returns.

In addition to binocular disparity, the visual system also uses many monocular cues to discriminate depth. Depth determination through monocular cues, such as size, perspective, occlusion, brightness, and movement, is not difficult. Another cue that originates outside the visual system is vergence, the angle between the optical axes of the two eyes for objects at varying distances. Yet another binocular cue, known as DaVinci stereopsis, is the presence of features visible to one eye but occluded in the other eye's view.

Neurons in areas V1 and V2 also signal foreground-background relationships. A cell with its receptive field in the center of a textured field may respond even when the boundary of that field is distant from the receptive field. This response helps differentiate the object from its background. In parsing an image the brain must identify which edge belongs to which object and differentiate the edge from the background of the object. Some cells in area V2 have the property of "border ownership," firing only when a figure but not the background is to one side of the edge, even when the local edge information is identical in both instances (Figure 27–9).

Local Movement Cues Define Object Trajectory and Shape

The primary visual cortex determines the direction of movement of objects. Directional selectivity in neurons likely involves sequential activation of regions on different sides of the receptive field.

If an object moving at an appropriate velocity first encounters a region of a neuron's receptive field with long response latencies and then passes into regions with progressively shorter latencies, signals from throughout

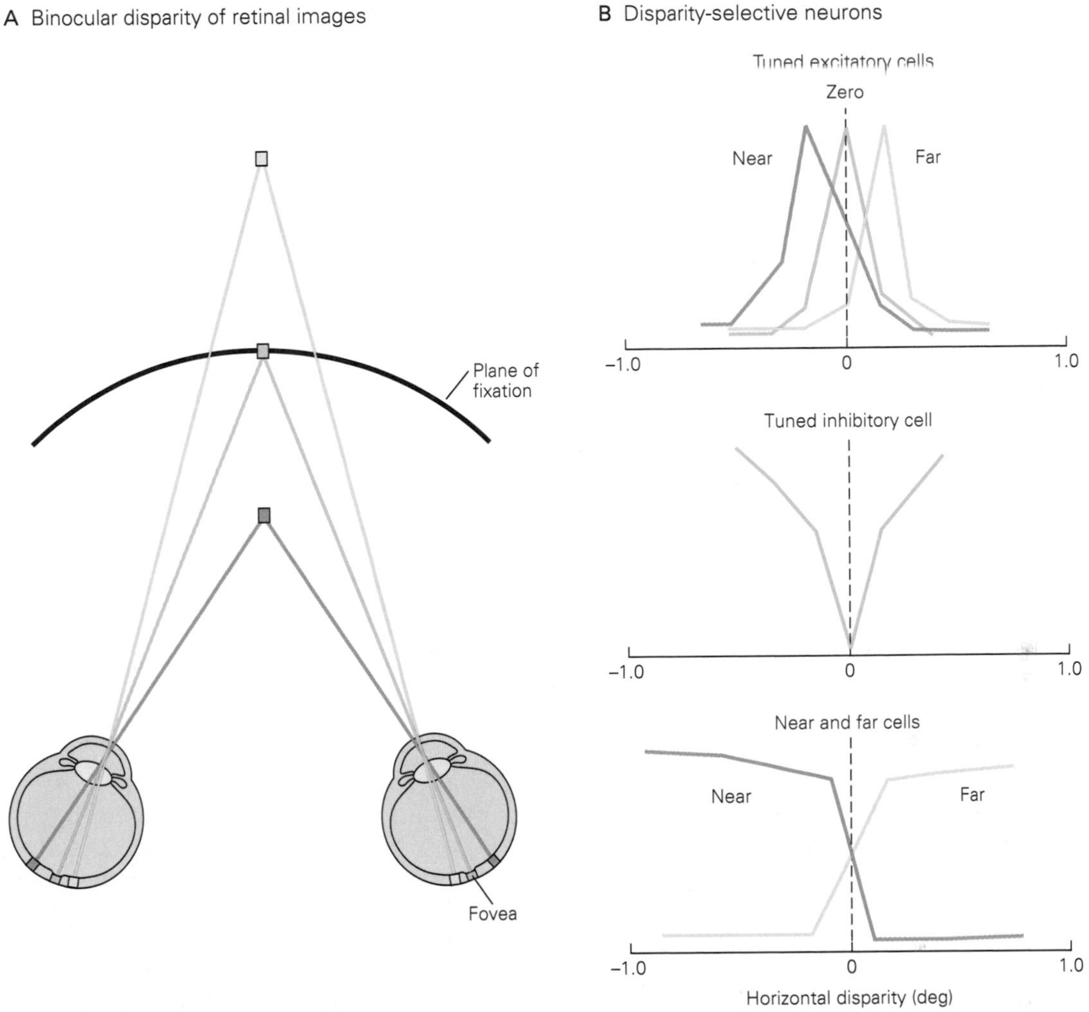

Figure 27–7 Stereopsis and binocular disparity.

A. Depth is computed from the positions at which images occur in the two eyes. The image of an object lying in the plane of fixation (**green**) falls on corresponding points on the two retinas. The images of objects lying in front of the plane of fixation (**blue**) or behind it (**yellow**) fall on noncorresponding locations on the two retinas, a phenomenon termed *binocular disparity*.

B. Visual cortex neurons are selective for particular ranges of disparity. Each plot shows the responses of a neuron to binocular stimuli with different disparities (abscissa). Some neurons are tuned to a narrow range of disparities and thus have particular disparity preferences (tuned excitatory or tuned inhibitory neurons), whereas others are tuned broadly for objects in front of the fixation plane (near cells) or beyond the plane (far cells). (Adapted, with permission, from Poggio 1995.)

the receptive field will arrive at the cell simultaneously and the neuron will fire vigorously. If the object instead moves in the opposite direction, signals from the different regions will not summate and the cell may never reach the threshold for firing (Figure 27–10).

Early in the visual pathways analysis of the movement of an object is limited by the size of the receptive fields of the sensory neurons. Even in the initial cortical areas V1 and V2 the receptive fields of neurons are small and might encompass only a fraction of an object. Eventually, however, information about the direction and speed of movement of discrete aspects of an object must be integrated into a computation of the movement of a whole object. This problem is more difficult than one might expect.

If one observes a complex shape moving through a small aperture, the part of the object's boundary within the aperture appears to move in a direction

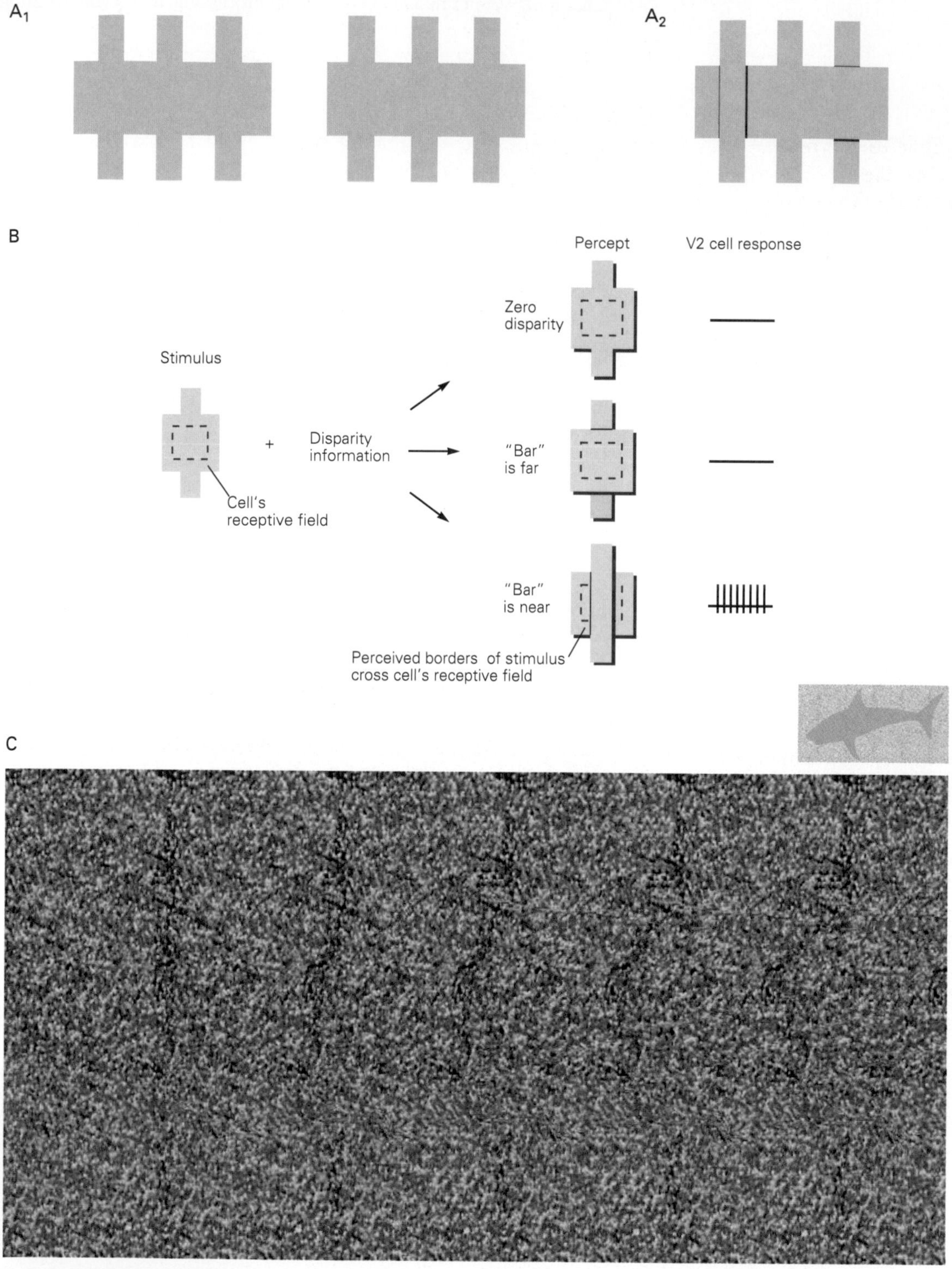

Figure 27–8 Global analysis of binocular disparity.

A. Depth cues contribute to surface segmentation. Viewing a single image of three gray vertical bars crossing a gray horizontal rectangle, you see a uniform gray area within the rectangle. However, if you fuse the two rectangles in A_1 with diverged eyes, the three vertical bars fall on the two retinas with near, zero, and far disparity, respectively, as portrayed in A_2. Thus the bar at left appears to hover in front of the rectangle with an illusory vertical edge crossing the rectangle, whereas the bar at right appears to lie behind the edges of the horizontal rectangle.

B. A neuron in area V2 responds to illusory edges formed by binocular disparity cues. When the cell's receptive field is centered in the gray square, the cell does not respond to a vertical bar that has far disparity or the same disparity as the square. When the vertical bar has near disparity, the cell responds as the illusory vertical edge crosses its receptive field. (Reproduced, with permission, from Bakin, Nakayama, and Gilbert 2000.)

C. A random-dot stereogram is seen as a random array of colored dots until one diverges or converges the eyes to bring the adjacent dark vertical stripes into register, producing a three-dimensional image of a shark hovering in front of the background noise. This effect stems from systematic disparity for selected sets of dots. (© Fred Hsu/Wikimedia Commons/CC-BY-SA-3.0.)

perpendicular to the boundary's orientation (Figure 27–11A). One cannot detect a line's true direction of movement if the line's ends are not visible. The image of a line appears the same if it is moving slowly along an axis perpendicular to its orientation or more quickly along an oblique axis. This is the quandary presented by the receptive field of a V1 neuron. The visual system's solution is to assume that the movement of a contour is perpendicular to its orientation. Thus an object is first presented to the visual system in countless small pieces with boundaries of different orientations, all of which appear to be moving in different directions and at different velocities (Figure 27–11A).

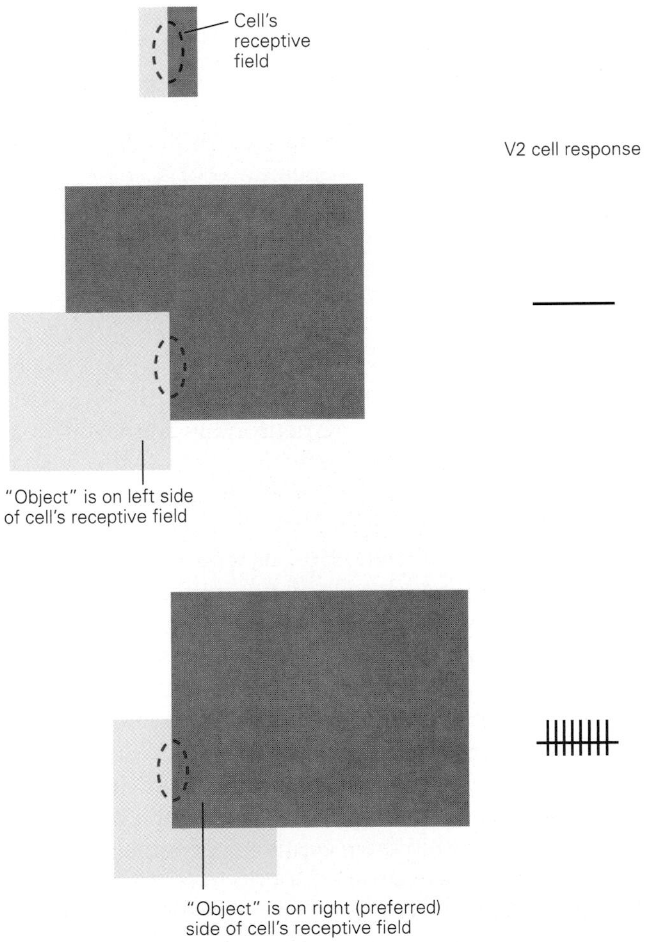

Figure 27–9 Border ownership. Cells in area V2 are sensitive to the boundaries of whole objects. Even though the local contrast is the same for the two rectangles within a cell's receptive field, the cell responds only when the boundary is part of a complete surface that lies on the preferred side of the receptive field. (Adapted, with permission, from Zhou, Friedman, and von der Heydt 2000.)

Determining the direction of motion of an object requires resolving multiple cues. This can be demonstrated readily by placing one grating on top of another and moving the two in different directions. The resulting checkerboard pattern appears to move in an intermediate direction between the trajectories of the individual gratings (Figure 27–11B). This percept depends on the relative contrast of the gratings and the area of grating overlap. With large relative contrasts the gratings appear to slide across each other, moving in their individual directions rather than together in a common direction.

An important determinant of perceived direction is scene segmentation, the separation of moving elements into foreground and background. In a scene with moving objects segmentation is not based on local cues of direction; instead, perception of direction depends on scene segmentation. The barber-pole illusion provides another example of the predominance of global relationships over the perception of simple attributes. The rotating stripes are perceived as moving vertically along the long axis of the pole (Figure 27–11C). The perception of motion in the visual field uses a complex algorithm that integrates the bottom-up analysis of local motion signals with top-down scene segmentation.

Integration of these local motion signals in monkeys has been observed in the middle temporal area (area MT or V5), an area specializing in motion. Remarkably this neural integration mirrors the perceptual effects. The neurons are selective for a particular direction of movement of an overall pattern, rather than to the motion of individual components of the pattern. Their responses also depend on transparency and display the barber-pole effect, sensitivity to the shape and dimensions of the aperture within which the movement is seen.

Context Determines the Perception of Visual Stimuli

Brightness and Color Perception Depend on Context

The visual system attempts to measure the surface characteristics of objects by comparing the light arriving from different parts of the visual field. As a result, the perception of brightness and color is highly dependent on context. In fact, perceived brightness and color can be quite different from what is expected from the physical properties of an object. At the same time, perceptual constancies make objects appear similar even when the brightness and wavelength distribution of

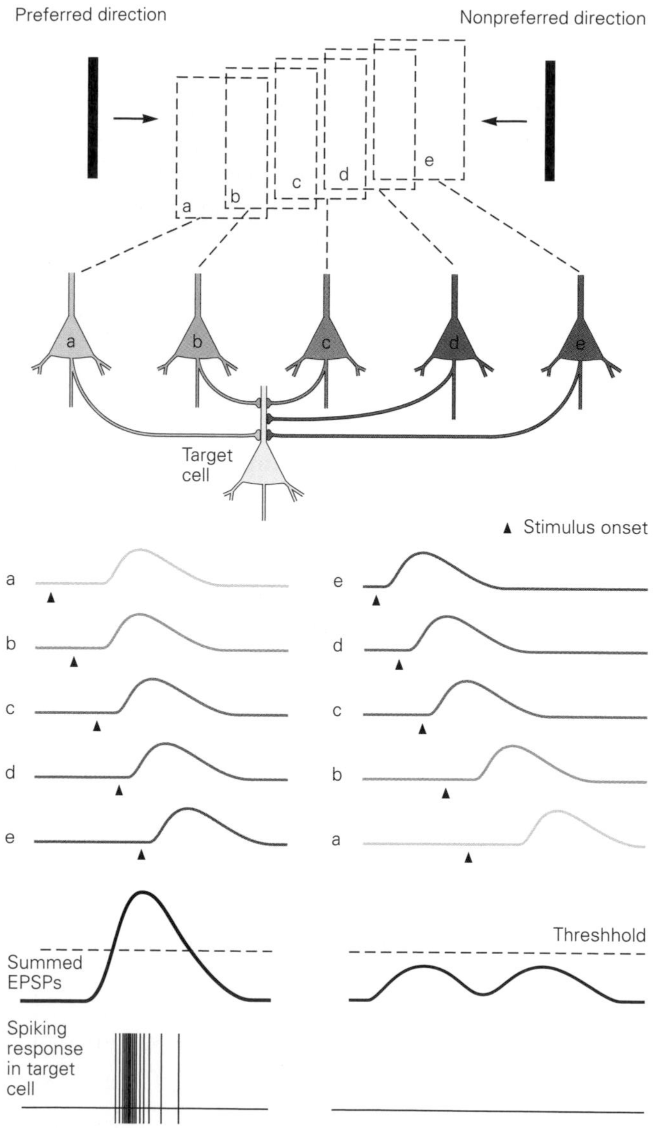

Figure 27–10 Directional selectivity of movement. The selectivity of a neuron to the direction of movement depends on the response latencies of presynaptic neurons. The response latencies of presynaptic neurons *a* and *b* relative to the onset of a stimulus are somewhat longer than those of neurons *d* and *e*. When a stimulus moves from left to right, neurons *a* and then *b* are activated first, but because their responses are delayed their inputs arrive simultaneously with inputs from neurons *d* and *e* and therefore sum at the target neuron, causing it to fire. In contrast, stimuli moving leftward produce responses that arrive at different times and therefore do not reach threshold. (**EPSP**, excitatory postsynaptic potential.) (Adapted, with permission, from Priebe and Ferster 2008.)

the light that illuminates them changes from natural to artificial light, from sunlight to shadow, or from dawn to midday (Figure 27–12A).

As we move about or as the ambient illumination changes, the retinal image of an object—its size, shape, and brightness—also changes. Yet under most conditions we do not perceive the object itself to be changing. As we move from a brightly lit garden into a dimly lit room, the intensity of light reaching the retina may vary a thousandfold. Both in the room's dim illumination and in the sun's glare we nevertheless see a white shirt as white and a red tie as red. Likewise, as a friend walks toward you she is seen as coming closer; you do not perceive her to be growing larger even though the image on your retina does expand. Our ability to perceive an object's size and color as constant illustrates again the fundamental principle of the visual system: It does not record images passively, like a camera, but instead uses transient and variable stimulation of the retina to construct representations of a stable, three-dimensional world.

Another example of contextual influence is color induction, whereby the appearance of a color in one region shifts toward that in an adjoining region. Shape also plays an important role in the perception of surface brightness. Because the visual system assumes that illumination comes from above, gray patches on a folded surface appear very different when they lie on the top or bottom of the surface, even when they are in fact the same shade of gray (Figure 27–12B).

The responses of some neurons in the visual cortex correlate with perceived brightness. Most visual neurons respond to surface boundaries; the center-surround structure of the receptive fields of retinal ganglion cells and geniculate neurons is suited to capturing boundaries. Most such cells do not respond to the interior parts of surfaces, for uniform interiors produce no contrast gradients across receptive fields. However, a small percentage of neurons do respond to the interiors of surfaces, signaling local brightness, texture, or color. Their responses are influenced by context: As the brightness of surfaces outside a cell's receptive field change, the cell's response changes, even when the brightness of the surface within the receptive field remains fixed.

Because most neurons respond to surface boundaries and not to areas of uniform brightness, the visual system calculates the brightness of surfaces from information about contrast at the edges of surfaces. The brain's analysis of surface qualities from boundary information is known as perceptual fill-in. If one fixates the boundary between a dark disk and a surrounding bright area for a few seconds, the disk will "fill in" with the same brightness as the surrounding area.

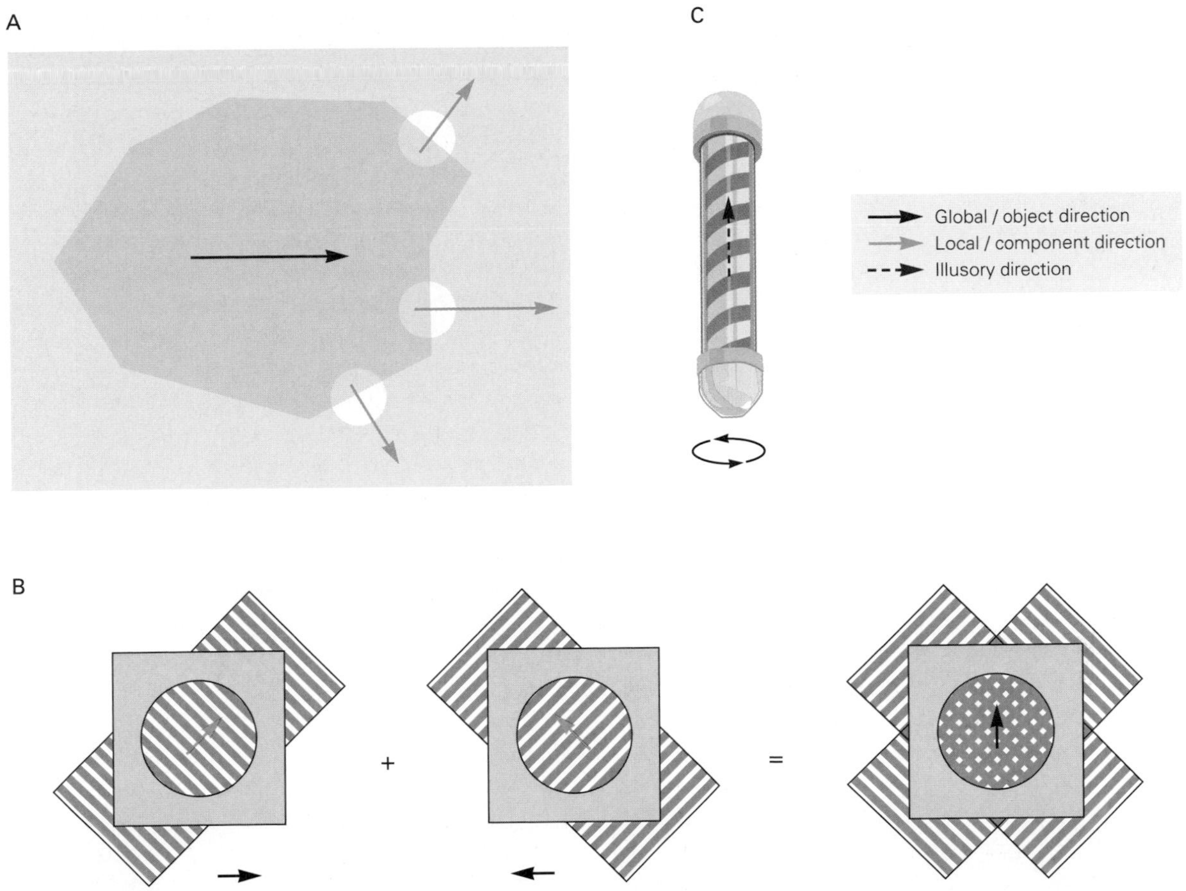

Figure 27–11 The aperture problem and barber-pole illusion.

A. Although an object moves in one direction, each component edge when viewed through a small aperture appears to move in a direction perpendicular to its orientation. The visual system must integrate such local motion signals into a unified percept of a moving object.

B. Gratings are used to test whether a neuron is sensitive to local or global motion signals. When the gratings are superimposed and moved independently in different directions, one does not see the two gratings sliding past each other but rather a plaid pattern moving in a single, intermediate direction. Neurons in the middle temporal area of monkeys are responsive to such global motion rather than to local motion.

C. Motion perception is influenced by surrounding segmentation cues, as seen in the barber-pole illusion. Even though the pole rotates around its axis, one perceives the stripes as moving vertically.

This occurs because the cells that respond to edges fire only when the eye or stimulus moves. They gradually cease to respond to a stabilized image and no longer signal the presence of the boundary. Neurons with receptive fields within the disk gradually begin to respond in a fashion similar to those with receptive fields in the surrounding area, demonstrating short-term plasticity in their receptive-field properties.

An object's color always appears more or less the same despite the fact that under different conditions of illumination the wavelength distribution of light reflected from the object varies widely. To identify an object we must know the properties of its surface rather than those of the reflected light, which are constantly changing. Computation of an object's color is therefore more complex than analyzing the spectrum of reflected light. To determine a surface's color the wavelength distribution of the incident light must be determined. In the absence of that information surface color can be estimated by determining the balance of wavelengths coming from different surfaces in a scene. Some neurons in V4 respond similarly to different illumination wavelengths if the perceived color remains constant. By being responsive to the light across an extensive surface, these neurons are selective for surface color rather than wavelength.

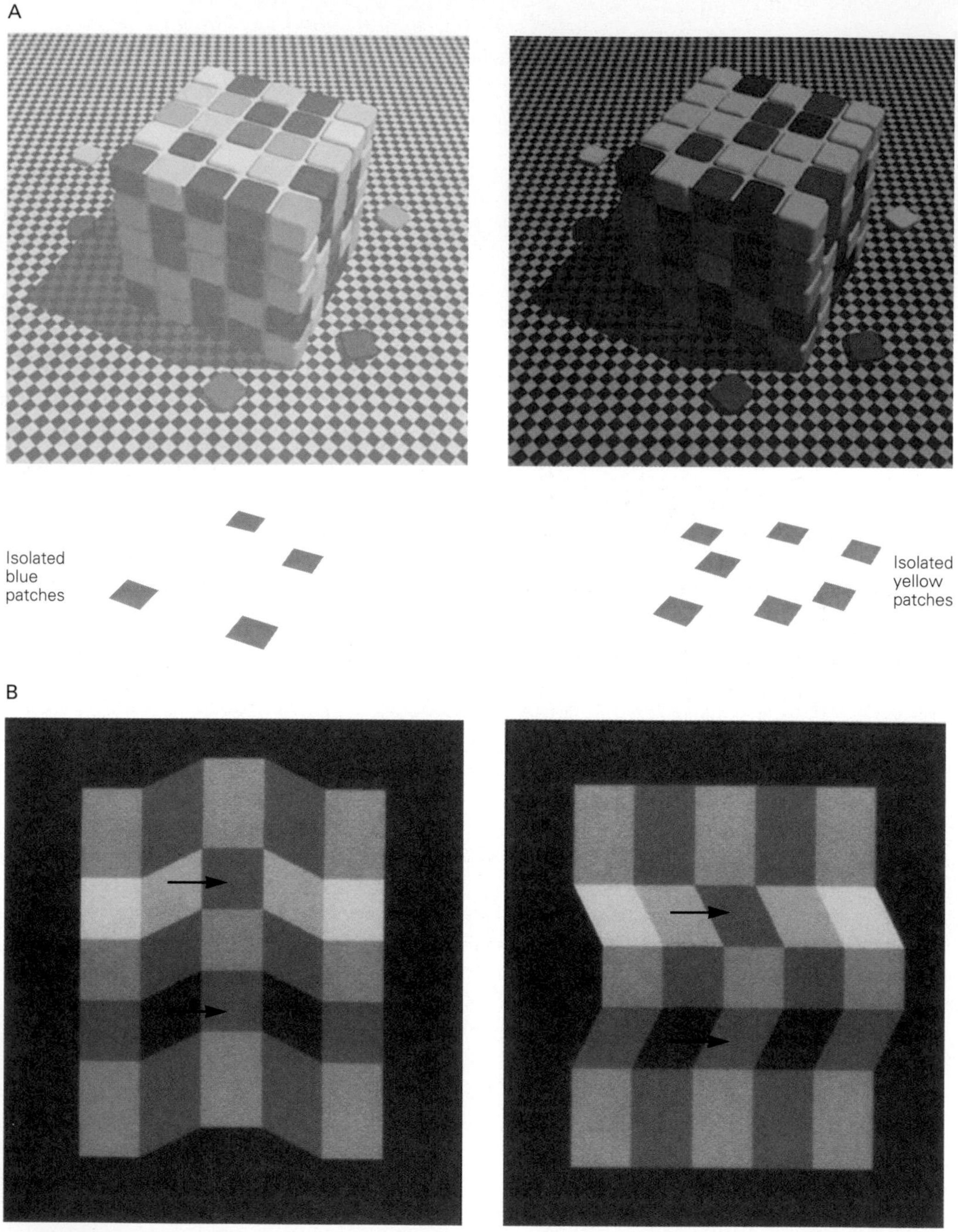

Figure 27–12 Color and brightness perception depend on contextual cues.

A. The perception of surface color remains relatively stable under different illumination conditions and the consequent changes in the wavelengths of light reflected from the surface. The yellow squares on the left and right cubes appear similar despite the fact that the wavelengths of light coming from the two sets of surfaces are very different. In fact, if the blue squares on the top of the left cube and the yellow squares on the top of the right cube are isolated from their contextual squares, their colors appear identical. (Reproduced, with permission, from R. Beau Lotto at www.lottolab.org.)

B. Brightness perception is also influenced by three-dimensional shape. The four gray squares indicated by arrows all have the same luminance. In the left illustration the apparent brightnesses are similar. At the right, however, the apparent brightnesses are different. The visual system has an inherent expectation that illumination comes from above (the position of the sun relative to us), which leads to the perception that the surface below the fold appears brighter than the surface of the same luminance that lies above. (Reproduced, with permission, from Adelson 1993.)

Receptive-Field Properties Depend on Context

The distinction between local and global effects—between stimuli that occur within a receptive field and those beyond—poses the problem of how the receptive field itself is defined. Because the original characterization of the receptive fields of visual cortex neurons did not take into account contextual influences, some investigators now distinguish between "classical" and "nonclassical" receptive fields.

However, even the earliest description of the sensory receptive field allowed for the possibility of influences from portions of the sensory surface outside the narrowly defined receptive field. In 1953 Steven Kuffler, in his pioneering observations on the receptive-field properties of retinal ganglion cells, noted that "not only the areas from which responses can actually be set up by retinal illumination may be included in a definition of the receptive field but also all areas which show a functional connection, by an inhibitory or excitatory effect on a ganglion cell. This may well involve areas which are somewhat remote from a ganglion cell and by themselves do not set up discharges."

A more useful distinction contrasts the response of a neuron to a simple stimulus, such as a short line segment, with its response to a stimulus with multiple components. Even in the primary visual cortex neurons are highly nonlinear; their response to a complex stimulus cannot be predicted from their responses to a simple stimulus placed in different positions around the visual field. Their responses to local features are instead dependent on the global context within which the features are embedded. Contextual influences are pervasive in intermediate-level visual processing, including contour integration, scene segmentation, and the determination of object shape and surface properties.

Cortical Connections, Functional Architecture, and Perception Are Intimately Related

Intermediate-level visual processing requires sharing of information from throughout the visual field. The interconnections within the primary visual cortex and the relationship of these connections to the functional architecture of this area suggest that they mediate contour integration.

Cortical circuits include a plexus of long-range horizontal connections, running parallel to the cortical surface, formed by the axons of pyramidal neurons. Horizontal connections exist in every area of the cerebral cortex, but their function varies from one area to the next depending on the functional architecture of each area. In the visual cortex these connections mediate interactions between orientation columns of similar specificity thus integrating information over a large area of visual cortex that represents a great expanse of the visual field (see Figure 25–14).

The combination of this like-to-like rule of connections and the fact that the horizontal connections link distant locations in the visual field suggest these connections have a role in contour integration. Contour integration and the related property of contour saliency reflect the Gestalt principle of good continuation. Contour integration and saliency are mediated by the horizontal connections in V1 (see Figure 27–6).

A final feature of cortical connectivity important for visuospatial integration is feedback projection from higher-order cortical areas. Feedback connections are as extensive as the feed-forward connections that originate in the thalamus or at earlier stages of cortical processing. Little is known about the function of these feedback projections. They likely play a role in mediating the top-down influences of attention, expectation, and perceptual task, all of which are known to affect early stages in cortical processing.

Perceptual Learning Requires Plasticity in Cortical Connections

The synaptic connections in ocular-dominance columns are adaptable to experience only during a critical period in development (see Chapter 57). This suggests that the functional properties of visual cortex neurons are fixed in adulthood. Nevertheless, many properties of cortical neurons remain mutable throughout life. For example, changes in the visual cortex can occur following retinal lesions.

When focal lesions occur in corresponding positions on the two retinas, the corresponding part of the cortical map, referred to as the lesion projection zone, is initially deprived of visual input. Over a period of several months, however, the receptive fields of cells within this region shift from the lesioned part of the retina to the functioning area surrounding the lesion. As a result, the cortical representation of the lesioned part of the retina shrinks while that of the surrounding region expands (Figure 27–13).

The plasticity of cortical maps and connections did not evolve as a response to lesions. Instead, plasticity is the neural mechanism for improving our perceptual skills. Many of the attributes analyzed by the visual cortex, including stereoscopic acuity, direction of movement, and orientation, become sharper with practice. Hermann von Helmholtz stated in 1866 that

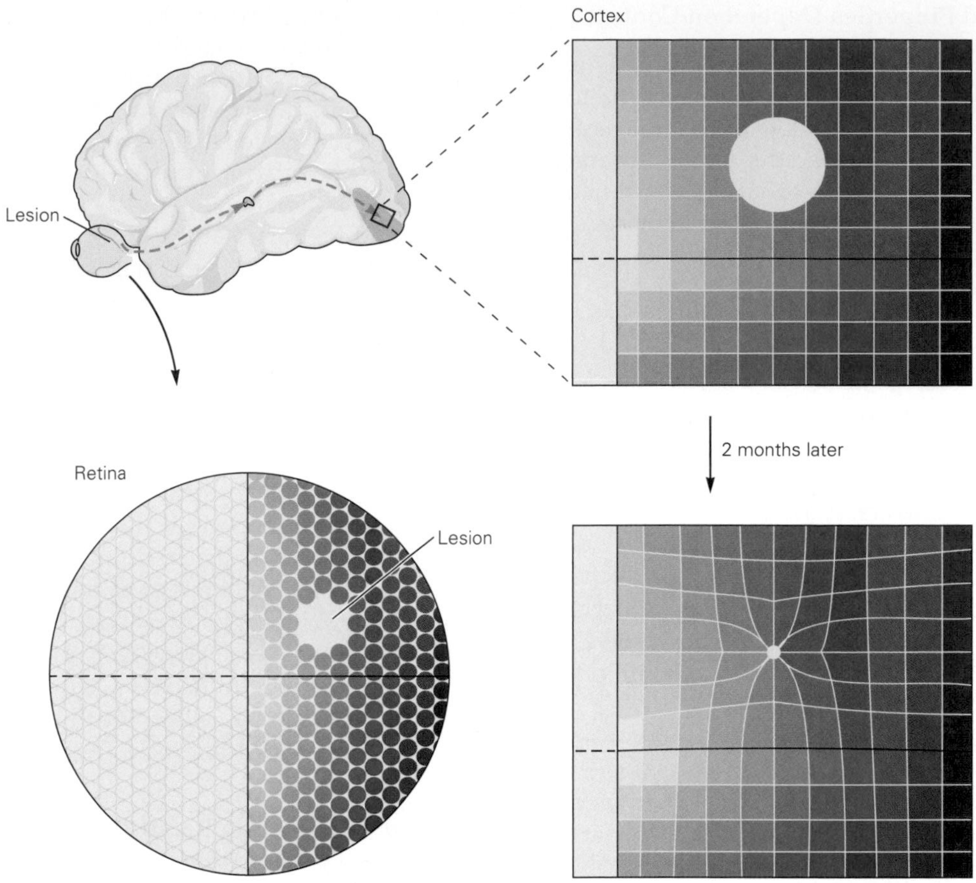

Figure 27-13 **Adult cortical plasticity.** When corresponding positions in both eyes are lesioned, the cortical area receiving input from the lesioned areas—the lesion projection zone—is initially silenced. The receptive fields of neurons in the lesion projection zone eventually shift from the area of the lesion to the surrounding, intact retina. This occurs because neurons surrounding the lesion projection zone sprout collaterals that form synaptic connections with neurons inside the zone. As a result, the cortical representation of the lesioned part of the retina shrinks while that of the surrounding retina expands.

"the judgment of the senses may be modified by experience and by training derived under various circumstances, and may be adapted to the new conditions. Thus, persons may learn in some measure to utilize details of the sensation which otherwise would escape notice and not contribute to obtaining any idea of the object." This perceptual learning is a variety of implicit learning that does not involve conscious processes (see Chapter 65).

Perceptual learning involves repeating a discrimination task many times and does not require error feedback to improve performance. Improvement manifests itself as a decrease in the threshold for discriminating small differences in the attributes of a target stimulus or in the ability to detect a target in a complex environment. Several areas of visual cortex, including the primary visual cortex, participate in perceptual learning.

An important aspect of perceptual learning is its specificity: Training on one task does not transfer to other tasks. For example, in a three-line bisection task the subject must determine whether the centermost of three parallel lines is closer to the line on the left or the one on the right. The amount of offset from the central position required for accurate responses decreases substantially after repeated practice (Figure 27–14A).

The learning in this task is specific to the location in the visual field and to the orientation of the lines. This specificity suggests that early stages of visual processing are responsible, for in the early stages receptive fields are smallest, visuotopic maps are most precise, and orientation tuning is sharpest. The learning is also

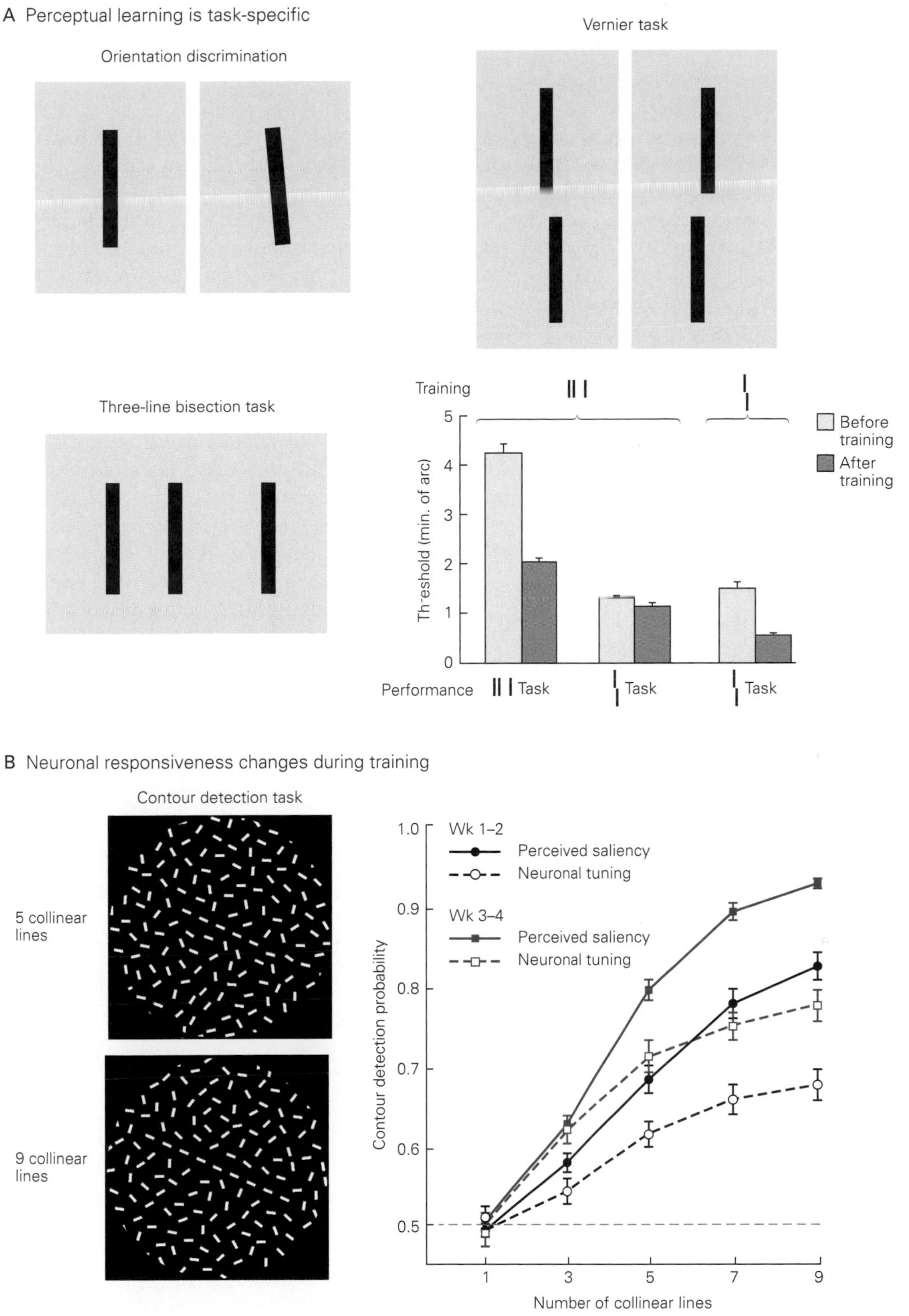

Figure 27–14 Perceptual learning. Perceptual learning is a form of implicit learning. With practice one can learn to discriminate smaller differences in orientation, position, depth, and direction of movement of objects.

A. The improvement is seen as a reduction in the amount of change required to reliably detect a tilted line or one positioned to the left or right of a nearly collinear line (vernier task). Perceptual learning is highly specific, so that training on a three-line bisection task leads to substantial improvement in that task (left pair of bars in the bar graph) without affecting performance on the vernier discrimination task (central pair of bars). However, training specifically on vernier discrimination does enhance performance on that task (right pair of bars).

B. The responses of neurons in V1 parallel perceptual learning. Subjects can detect collinear line segments embedded in a random background more easily as the number of segments is increased. The responses of neurons in V1 grow correspondingly stronger with the increase in the number of line segments. After practice, a line with fewer segments stands out more easily, and with this improvement the responses in V1 also increase. (Reproduced, with permission, from Crist et al. 2001; and Li et al. 2008.)

specific for the stimulus configuration. Training on three-line bisection does not transfer to a vernier discrimination task in which the context is a line that is collinear with the target line (see Figure 27–14A).

The response properties of neurons in the primary visual cortex change during the course of perceptual learning in a way that tracks the perceptual improvement. An example of this is seen in contour saliency. With practice, subjects can more easily detect contours embedded in complex backgrounds. Detection improves with contour length, and the responses of neurons in V1 increase as well. With practice, subjects improve their ability to detect shorter contours and V1 neurons become correspondingly more sensitive to shorter contours (see Figure 27–14B).

Visual Search Relies on the Cortical Representation of Visual Attributes and Shapes

The detectability of features such as color, orientation, and shape is related to the process of visual search. Certain objects emerge or "pop out" from others in a complex image because the visual system processes simultaneously, in parallel pathways, the features of the target and the surrounding distractors (Figure 27–15). When the features of a target are complex, the target can be identified only through careful inspection of an entire image or scene (see Figure 21–5).

The pop-out phenomenon can be influenced by training. A stimulus that initially cannot be found without effortful searching will pop out after training. The neuronal correlate of such a dramatic change is not certain. Parallel processing of the features of an object and its background is possible because feature information is encoded within retinotopically mapped areas at multiple locations in the visual cortex. Pop-out probably occurs early in the visual cortex. The pop-out of complex shapes such as numerals lends support to the idea that early in visual processing neurons can represent, and be selective for, shapes more complex than line segments with a particular orientation.

Cognitive Processes Influence Visual Perception

Scene segmentation—the parsing of a scene into different objects—involves a combination of bottom-up

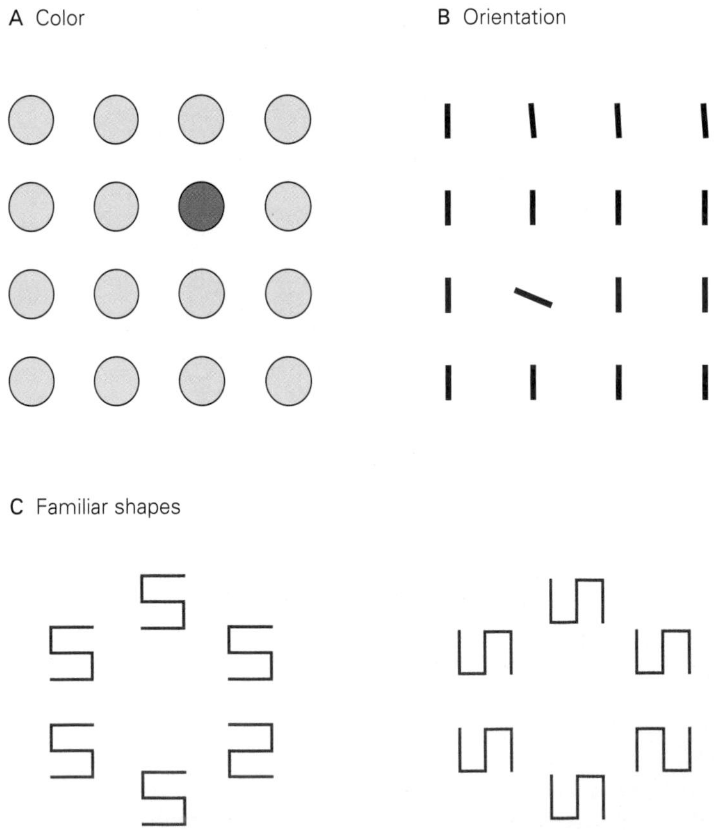

Figure 27-15 One object in a complex image stands out under certain conditions.

A. A differently colored object pops out.

B. A differently oriented line also pops out.

C. More complex shapes can pop out when they are very familiar, such as the numeral 2 embedded in a field of 5s. Rotating the image by 90° renders the elements of the figure less recognizable, making it more difficult to find the one figure that differs from the rest. (Reproduced, with permission, from Wang, Cavanagh, and Green 1994.)

processes that follow the Gestalt rule of good continuation and top-down processes that create object expectation.

One strong top-down influence is spatial attention, which can change focus without any movement of an observer's eyes. Spatial attention is object-oriented in that it is distributed over the area occupied by the attended object, allowing the visual cortex to analyze the shape and attributes of objects one at a time.

Attentional mechanisms can solve the superposition problem. For us to recognize an object in a scene that includes multiple objects, we must determine which features correspond to which objects. Our sense that we identify multiple objects simultaneously is illusory. Instead, we serially process objects in rapid succession by shifting attention from one to the next. The results of each analysis build up the perception of a complex environment populated with many distinct objects. A dramatic demonstration of the importance of attention in object recognition is *change blindness.* If a subject rapidly shifts between two slightly different views of the same scene, he will not be able to detect the absence of an important component of the scene in one view without considerable scrutiny (see Figure 29–3).

Another top-down influence is perceptual task. At early stages in visual processing the properties of the same neuron vary with the type of visual discrimination being performed. Object identification itself involves a process of hypothesis testing in which internal representations of objects are compared with information arriving from the retina. This process is reflected in studies of visual imagery: Early stages in processing such as the primary visual cortex are activated when one imagines scenes in the absence of visual input.

An Overall View

Intermediate-level visual processing is concerned with parsing the visual world into contours and surfaces that belong to objects and segregating these elements from the background. This is the most challenging job that the visual system must perform. When confronted with a complex visual environment, we could assemble local features into a potentially enormous number of distinct objects. Nonetheless, we quickly classify the local features into a set of objects that can be matched with internal representations of object shape and identity that are stored in the brain from earlier experiences.

This global integration is simplified by applying rules of perceptual grouping that were described by Gestalt psychologists and are apparently implemented by circuits beginning in the primary visual cortex. Global integration involves analysis of local attributes that depends on the properties of sensory neurons: Selectivity for local orientation supports the analysis of extended contours, directional sensitivity underlies the determination of object motion, disparity selectivity implements global stereopsis, and contrast sensitivity mediates color constancy. The process of integration is not simply a bottom-up one but is influenced by information arriving from higher-order areas of the visual cortex. Attention, expectation, and perceptual task influence how we segment the visual world.

Intermediate-level vision is a product of lateral connections between functional columns of neurons in a cortical area and the convergence of feed-forward signals with feedback information from higher-order areas. Vision therefore is not simply a feed-forward mechanism that assembles shapes in stages with increasing complexity. The underlying processes are highly dynamic on short time scales. The strategies that we use to interpret visual scenes also involve experience-dependent changes in the cortical circuits in which we constantly store information about shapes that we experience throughout life.

Charles D. Gilbert

Selected Readings

Albright TD, Stoner GR. 2002. Contextual influences on visual processing. Annu Rev Neurosci 25:339–379.

Gilbert CD, Sigman M. 2007. Brain states: top-down influences in sensory processing. Neuron 54:677–696.

Gilbert CD, Sigman M, Crist R. 2001. The neural basis of perceptual learning. Neuron 31:681–697.

Li W, Piech V, Gilbert CD. 2004. Perceptual learning and top-down influences in primary visual cortex. Nat Neurosci 7:651–657.

Li W, Piech V, Gilbert CD. 2006. Contour saliency in primary visual cortex. Neuron 50:951–962.

Priebe NJ, Ferster D. 2008. Inhibition, spike threshold, and stimulus selectivity in primary visual cortex. Neuron 57:482–497.

References

Adelson EH. 1993. Perceptual organization and the judgment of brightness. Science 262:2042–2044.

Bakin JS, Nakayama K, Gilbert CD. 2000. Visual responses in monkey areas V1 and V2 to three-dimensional surface configurations. J Neurosci 20:8188–8198.

Crist RE, Li W, Gilbert CD. 2001. Learning to see: experience and attention in primary visual cortex. Nat Neurosci 4:519–525.

Cumming BG, DeAngelis GC. 2001. The physiology of stereopsis. Annu Rev Neurosci 24:203–238.

Ferster D, Miller KD. 2000. Neural mechanisms of orientation selectivity in the visual cortex. Annu Rev Neurosci 23:441–471.

He ZJ, Nakayama K. 1994. Apparent motion determined by surface layout not be disparity or three-dimensional distance. Nature 367:173–175.

Hubel DH, Wiesel TN. 1968. Receptive fields and functional architecture of monkey striate cortex. J Physiol 195:215–243.

Li W, Gilbert CD. 2002. Global contour saliency and local colinear interations. J Neurophysiol 88:2846–56.

Li W, Piech V, Gilbert CD. 2008. Learning to link visual contours. Neuron 57:442–451.

Movshon JA, Adelson EH, Gizzi MS, Newsome WT. 1985. The analysis of moving visual patterns. In: C Chagas, R Gattass, CG Gross (eds.). *Study Group on Pattern Recognition Mechanisms* pp. 67–86, Vatican City: Pontifica Academia Scientiarum.

Nakayama K. 1996. Binocular visual surface perception. Proc Natl Acad Sci U S A 93:634–639.

Nakayama K, Joseph JS. 2000. Attention, pattern recognition and popout in visual search. In: R Parasuraman (ed.). *The Attentive Brain.* Cambridge, MA: MIT Press.

Poggio GE. 1995. Mechanisms of stereopsis in monkey visual cortex. Cereb Cortex 5:193–204.

Purves D, Lotto RB, Nundy S. 2002. Why we see what we do. Am Sci 90:236–243.

Wang Q, Cavanagh P, Green M. 1994. Familiarity and popout in visual search. Percept Psychophys 56:495–500.

Zhou H, Friedman HS, von der Heydt R. 2000. Coding of border ownership in monkey visual cortex. J Neurosci 20:6594–6611.

28

High-Level Visual Processing: Cognitive Influences

THE IMAGES PROJECTED ONTO THE retina are generally complex dynamic patterns of light of varying intensity and color. As we have seen, low-level visual processing is responsible for detection of various types of contrast in these images (see Chapters 25 and 26), whereas intermediate-level processing is involved in the identification of so-called visual primitives, such as contours and fields of motion, and the representation of surfaces (see Chapter 27). High-level visual processing integrates information from a variety of sources and is the final stage in the visual pathway leading to conscious visual experience.

In practice high-level visual processing depends on top-down signals that imbue bottom-up (afferent) sensory representations with semantic significance, such as that arising from short-term working memory, long-term memory, and behavioral goals. High-level visual processing thus selects behaviorally meaningful attributes of the visual environment (Figure 28–1).

High-Level Visual Processing Is Concerned with Object Identification

Our visual experience of the world is fundamentally object-centered. Objects are often visually complex, being composed of a large number of conjoined visual features. In addition, the features projected on the retina by an object vary greatly under different viewing conditions, such as lighting, angle, position, and distance.

Moreover, objects are commonly associated with specific experiences, other remembered objects, other sensations—such as the hum of the coffee grinder or the aroma of a lover's perfume—and a variety of emotions. Animate beings, which are objects to the visual

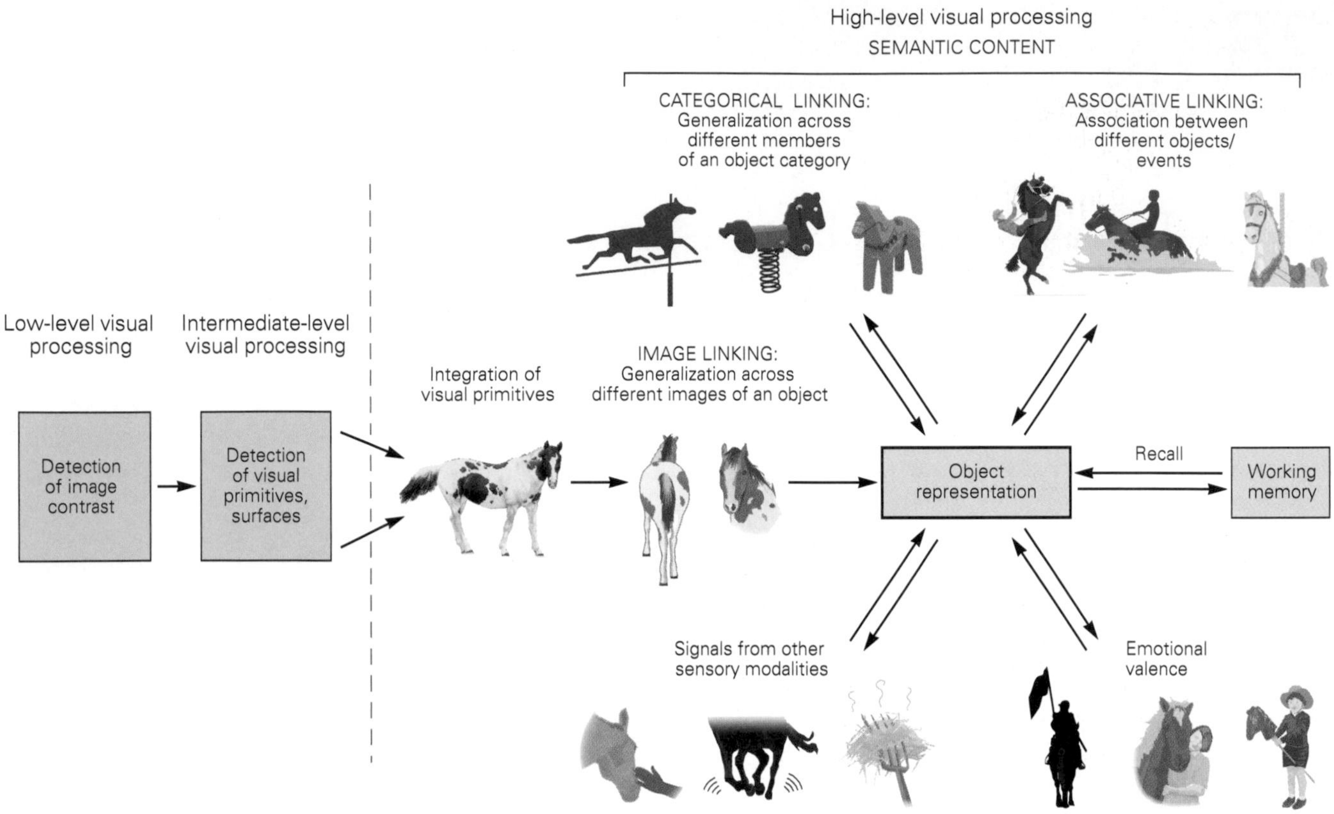

Figure 28–1 The neuronal representation of entire objects is central to high-level visual processing. Object representation involves integration of visual features extracted at earlier stages in the visual pathways. Ideally the resulting representation is a generalization of the numerous retinal images generated by the same object and of different members of an object category. The representation also incorporates information from other sensory modalities, attaches emotional valence, and associates the object with the memory of other objects or events. Object representations can be stored in working memory and recalled in association with other memories.

system, also direct intentions, desires, and actions at others and ourselves. In conjunction with our own behavioral goals, it is the behavioral saliency of individual objects, memories, and emotional valences as well as the real or implied actions of others that enables us to take action based on visual information. Object perception is thus the nexus between vision and cognition.

The Inferior Temporal Cortex Is the Primary Center for Object Perception

Primate studies implicate neocortical regions of the temporal lobe, principally the inferior temporal cortex, in object perception. Because the hierarchy of synaptic relays in the cortical visual system extends from the primary visual cortex to the temporal lobe, the temporal lobe is a site of convergence of many types of visual information.

As we shall later see, neuropsychological studies have found that damage to the inferior temporal cortex can produce specific failures of object recognition. Neurophysiological and brain-imaging studies have in turn yielded remarkable insights into the ways in which the activity of inferior temporal neurons represents objects, how these representations relate to perceptual and cognitive events, and how they are modified by experience.

Visual signals originating in the retina are processed in the lateral geniculate nucleus of the thalamus before reaching the primary visual cortex (V1). Thereafter ascending visual pathways follow two parallel and hierarchically organized streams: the ventral and dorsal streams (see Chapter 25). The ventral stream extends ventrally and anteriorly from V1 through

V2, V4, and the temporal-occipital junction before reaching the inferior temporal cortex, which comprises the lower bank of the superior temporal sulcus and the ventrolateral convexity of the temporal lobe (Figure 28–2). This pathway makes the inferior temporal cortex the seat of the highest stage of cortical visual processing. Neurons at each synaptic relay in this ventral stream receive convergent input from the preceding stage. Inferior temporal neurons are thus in a position to integrate a large and diverse quantity of visual information over a vast region of visual space.

The inferior temporal cortex is a large brain region. The patterns of anatomical connections to and from this area indicate that it comprises at least two main functional subdivisions: the posterior and anterior inferior temporal cortex. Anatomical evidence identifies the anterior subdivision as a higher processing stage than the posterior subdivision. As we shall see,

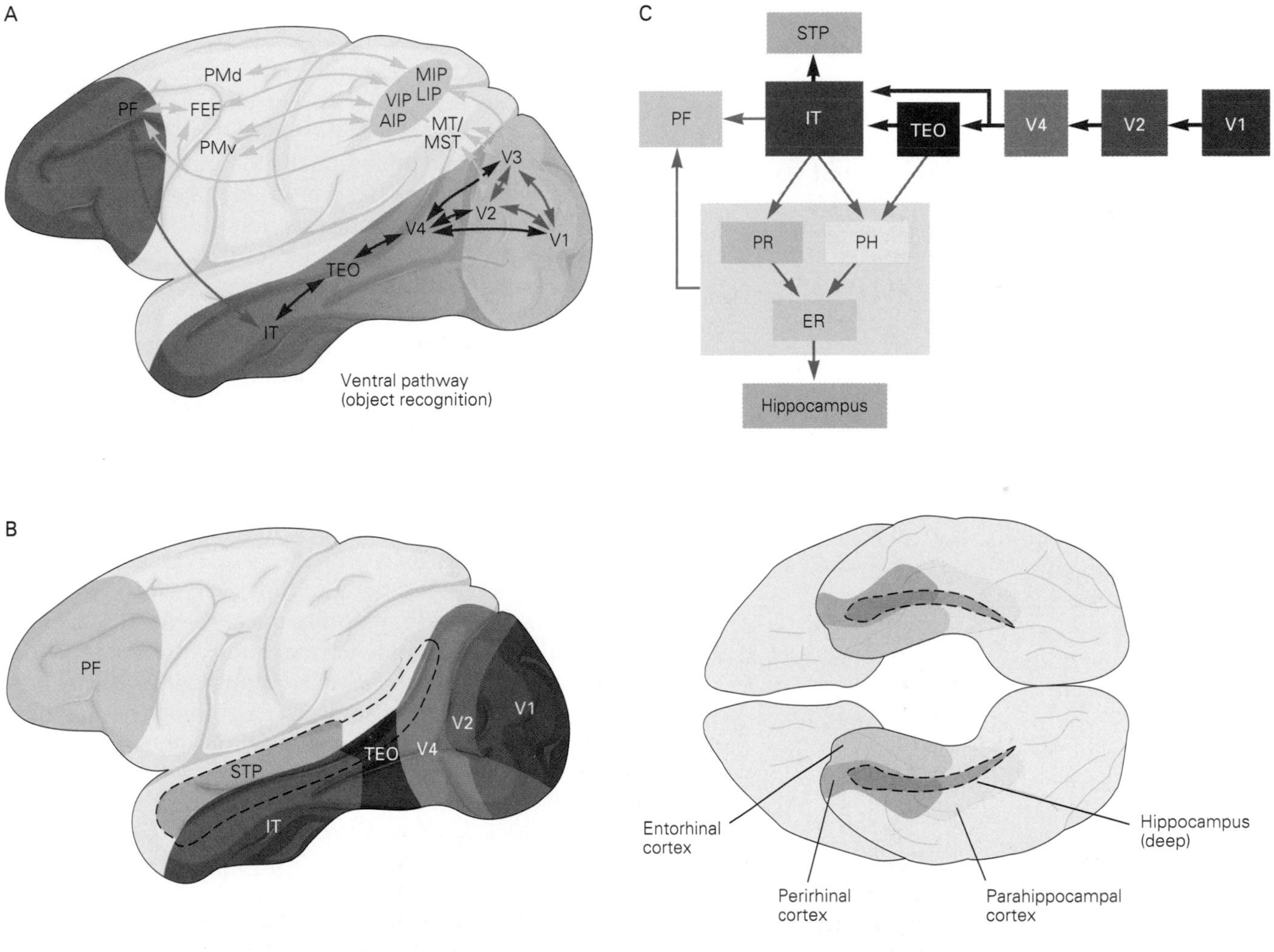

Figure 28–2 Cortical pathway for object recognition.

A. The pathway for object recognition (**red**) is identified in a lateral view of the brain showing the major pathways involved in visual processing. (**AIP**, anterior intraparietal cortex; **FEF**, frontal eye fields; **IT**, inferior temporal cortex; **LIP**, lateral intraparietal cortex; **MIP**, medial intraparietal cortex; **MST**, medial superior temporal cortex; **MT**, middle temporal cortex; **PF**, prefrontal cortex; **PMd**, dorsal premotor cortex; **PMv**, ventral premotor cortex; **TEO**, temporo-occipital cortex; **VIP**, ventral intraparietal cortex.)

B. Cortical areas involved in object recognition are shown on lateral and ventral views of the monkey brain.

C. The inferior temporal cortex (IT) is the end stage of the ventral stream (**red arrows**), and is reciprocally connected with neighboring areas of the medial temporal lobe and prefrontal cortex (**gray arrows**). This chart illustrates the main connections and predominant direction of information flow. (**ER**, entorhinal cortex; **PF**, prefrontal cortex; **PH**, parahippocampal cortex; **PR**, perirhinal cortex; **STP**, superior temporal polysensory area; **TEO**, temporo-occipital cortex.)

this distinction is supported by both neuropsychological and neurophysiological evidence.

Clinical Evidence Identifies the Inferior Temporal Cortex as Essential for Object Recognition

The first clear insight into the neural pathways mediating object recognition was obtained in the late 19th century when the American neurologist Sanger Brown and the British physiologist Edward Albert Schäfer found that experimental lesions of the temporal lobe in primates resulted in loss of the ability to recognize objects. This impairment is distinct from the deficits that accompany lesions of occipital cortical areas in that sensitivity to basic visual attributes, such as color, motion, and distance, remains intact. Because of the unusual type of visual loss, the impairment was originally called psychic blindness, but this term was later replaced by *visual agnosia* ("without visual knowledge"), a term coined by Sigmund Freud.

In humans there are two basic categories of visual agnosia, apperceptive and associative, the description of which led to a two-stage model of object recognition in the visual system (Figure 28–3). With apperceptive agnosia the ability to match or copy complex visual shapes or objects is impaired. This impairment is perceptual in nature, resulting from disruption of the first stage of object recognition: integration of visual features into sensory representations of entire objects. In contrast, patients with associative agnosia can match or copy complex objects, but their ability to identify the objects is impaired. This impairment results from disruption of the second stage of object recognition: association of the sensory representation of an object with knowledge of the object's meaning or function.

Consistent with this functional hierarchy, apperceptive agnosia is most common following damage to the posterior inferior temporal cortex, whereas associative agnosia, a higher-order perceptual deficit, is more common following damage to the anterior inferior temporal cortex, a later stage in the functional hierarchy. Neurons in the anterior subdivision exhibit a variety of memory-related properties not seen in the posterior area.

Neurons in the Inferior Temporal Cortex Encode Complex Visual Stimuli

The coding of visual information in the temporal lobe has been studied extensively using electrophysiological techniques, beginning with the work of Charles Gross and colleagues in the 1970s. Neurons in this region have distinctive response properties.

They are relatively insensitive to simple stimulus features such as orientation and color. Instead, the vast majority possess large, centrally located receptive fields and encode complex stimulus features. These selectivities often appear somewhat arbitrary. An individual neuron might, for example, respond strongly to a crescent-shaped pattern of a particular color and texture. Cells with such unique selectivities likely provide inputs to yet higher-order neuronal representations of meaningful objects.

Indeed, several small subpopulations of neurons encode objects that convey to the observer highly meaningful information, such as faces and hands (Figure 28–4). For cells that respond to the sight of a hand, individual fingers are particularly critical. Among cells that respond to faces, the most effective stimulus for some cells is the frontal view of the face, whereas for others it is the side view. Although some neurons respond preferentially to faces, others respond to facial expressions. It seems likely that such cells contribute directly to face recognition.

Damage to a small region of the human temporal lobe results in an inability to recognize faces, a form of associative agnosia known as *prosopagnosia*. Patients with prosopagnosia can identify a face as a face, recognize its parts, and even detect specific emotions expressed by the face, but they are unable to identify a particular face as belonging to a specific person.

Prosopagnosia is one example of "category-specific" agnosia, in which patients with temporal-lobe damage fail to recognize items within a specific semantic category. There are reported cases of category-specific agnosias for living things, fruits, vegetables, tools, or animals. Owing to the pronounced behavioral significance of faces and the normal ability of people to recognize an extraordinarily large number of items from this category, prosopagnosia may simply be the most common variety of category-specific agnosia.

Neurons in the Inferior Temporal Cortex Are Functionally Organized in Columns

Early relays in the cortical visual system are organized in columns of neurons that represent the same stimulus features, such as orientation or direction of motion, in different parts of the visual field. Cells within the inferior temporal cortex are also organized in columns of neurons representing the same or similar stimulus properties (Figure 28–5). These columns commonly extend throughout the cortical thickness and over a range of approximately 400 μm. Columnar patches in the inferior temporal cortex are arranged such that different stimuli that possess some similar features are

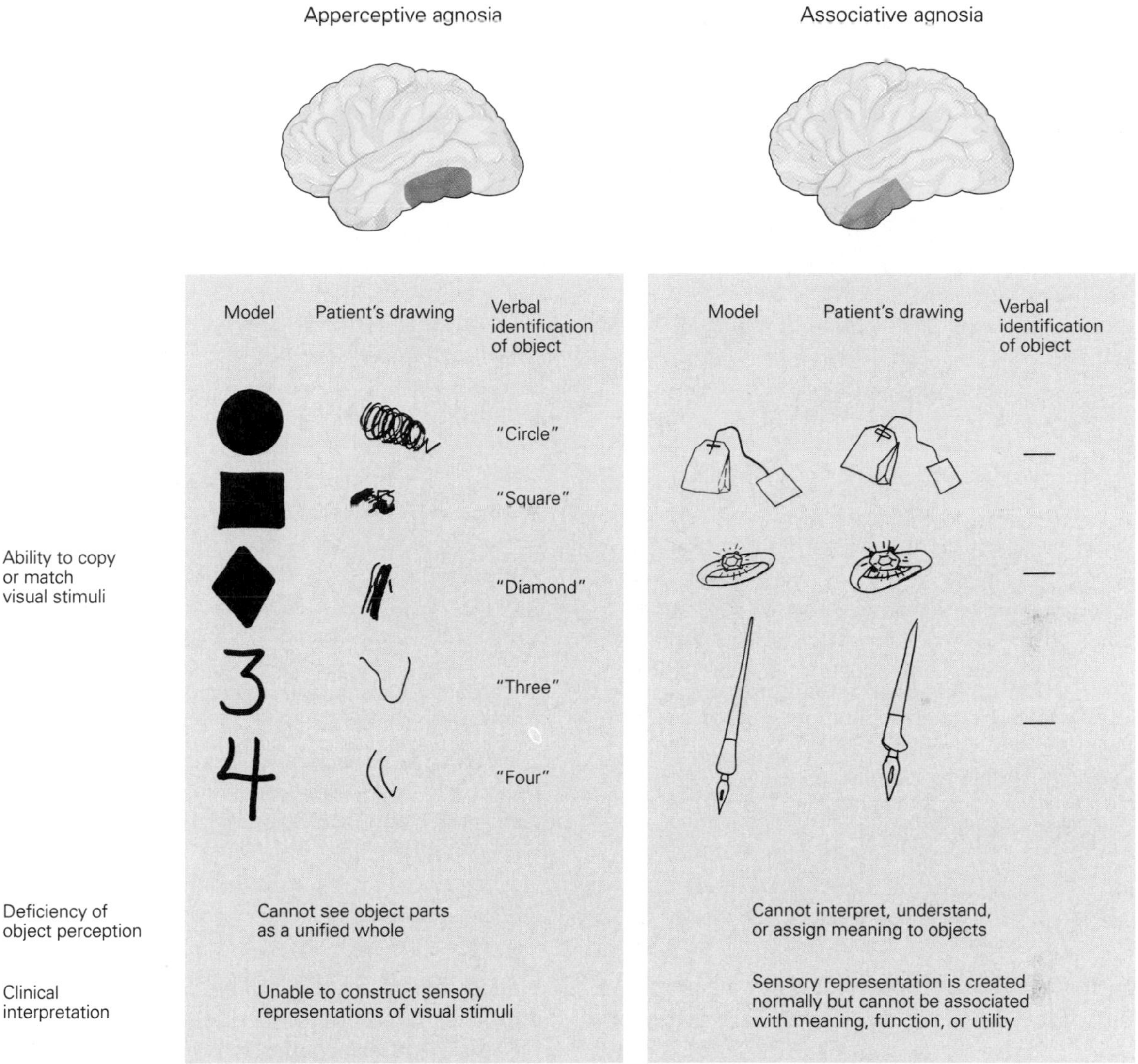

Figure 28–3 Neuropsychological evidence for the neuronal correlates of object recognition in the temporal lobe. Damage to inferior temporal cortex (IT) impairs the ability to recognize visual objects, a condition known as visual agnosia. There are two major categories of visual agnosia: apperceptive, a result of damage to the posterior region, and associative, resulting from damage of the anterior region. (Reproduced, with permission, from Farah 1990.)

represented in partially overlapping columns (Figure 28–5). Thus one stimulus can activate multiple patches within the cortex. Long-range horizontal connections within the cortex may serve to connect patches into distributed networks for object representation.

Face-selective cells constitute a highly specialized class of neurons. Indeed, the fact that prosopagnosia often occurs in the absence of any other form of agnosia suggests that face-selective neurons of the temporal lobe may be located in exclusive clusters. While many early studies of neuronal response properties offered circumstantial evidence for such clustering, in 2006 Doris Tsao and Margaret Livingstone obtained dramatic support for this hypothesis. Functional magnetic resonance images of monkeys that were viewing faces revealed large active zones in a region of cortex in the lower bank of the superior temporal sulcus. Neurophysiological recordings of neurons in these zones confirmed that face-recognition cells formed large, dense clusters (Figure 28–6). Winrich Freiwald and Tsao later found that the five face-representation areas in monkeys interconnect with one another and form a processing system, with each node apparently concerned with a different aspect of face recognition.

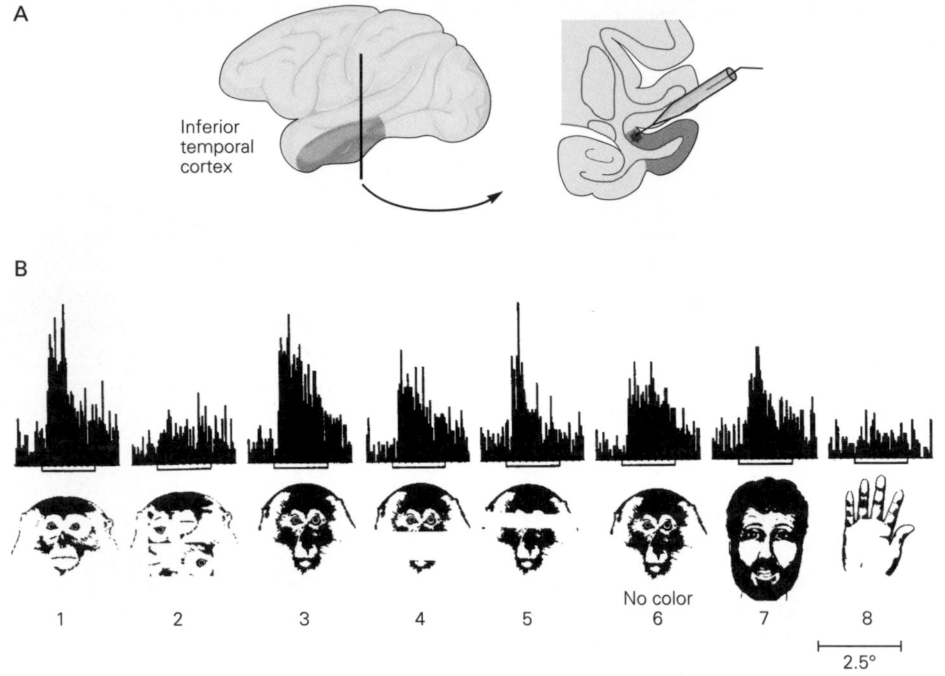

Figure 28–4 Neurons in the inferior temporal cortex of the monkey are involved in face recognition. (Reproduced, with permission, from Desimone et al. 1984.)

A. The location of the inferior temporal cortex of the monkey is shown in a lateral view and coronal section. The colored area is the location of the recorded neurons.

B. Peristimulus histograms illustrate the frequency of action potentials in a single neuron in response to the different images illustrated below. This neuron responded selectively to faces. Masking of critical features, such as the mouth or eyes (**4**, **5**), led to a substantial but not complete reduction in response. Scrambling the parts of the face (**2**) nearly eliminated the response.

The Inferior Temporal Cortex Is Part of a Network of Cortical Areas Involved in Object Recognition

Object recognition is intimately intertwined with visual categorization, visual memory, and emotion, and the outputs of the inferior temporal cortex contribute to these functions (see Figure 28–2).

Among the principal projections are those to the perirhinal and parahippocampal cortices, which lie medially adjacent to the ventral surface of the inferior temporal cortex (see Figure 28–2C). These regions project in turn to the entorhinal cortex and the hippocampal formation, both of which are involved in long-term memory storage and retrieval. A second major projection from the inferior temporal cortex is to the prefrontal cortex, which is increasingly recognized as an important contributor to high-level vision. As we shall see, prefrontal neurons play important roles in categorical visual perception, visual working memory, and recall of stored memories.

The inferior temporal cortex also provides input—directly and indirectly via the perirhinal cortex—to the amygdala, which is believed to apply emotional valence to sensory stimuli and to engage the cognitive and visceral components of emotion (see Chapter 48). Finally, the inferior temporal cortex is a major source of input to multimodal sensory areas of cortex such as the superior temporal polysensory area.

Object Recognition Relies on Perceptual Constancy

The ability to recognize objects as the same under different viewing conditions, despite the sometimes markedly different retinal images, is one of the most functionally important requirements of visual experience. The invariant attributes of an object—for example, the spatial and chromatic relationships between image features or characteristic features such as the stripes of a zebra—are cues to the identity and meaning of the objects.

For object recognition to take place, these invariant attributes must be represented independently of other image properties. The visual system does this with proficiency, and its behavioral manifestation is

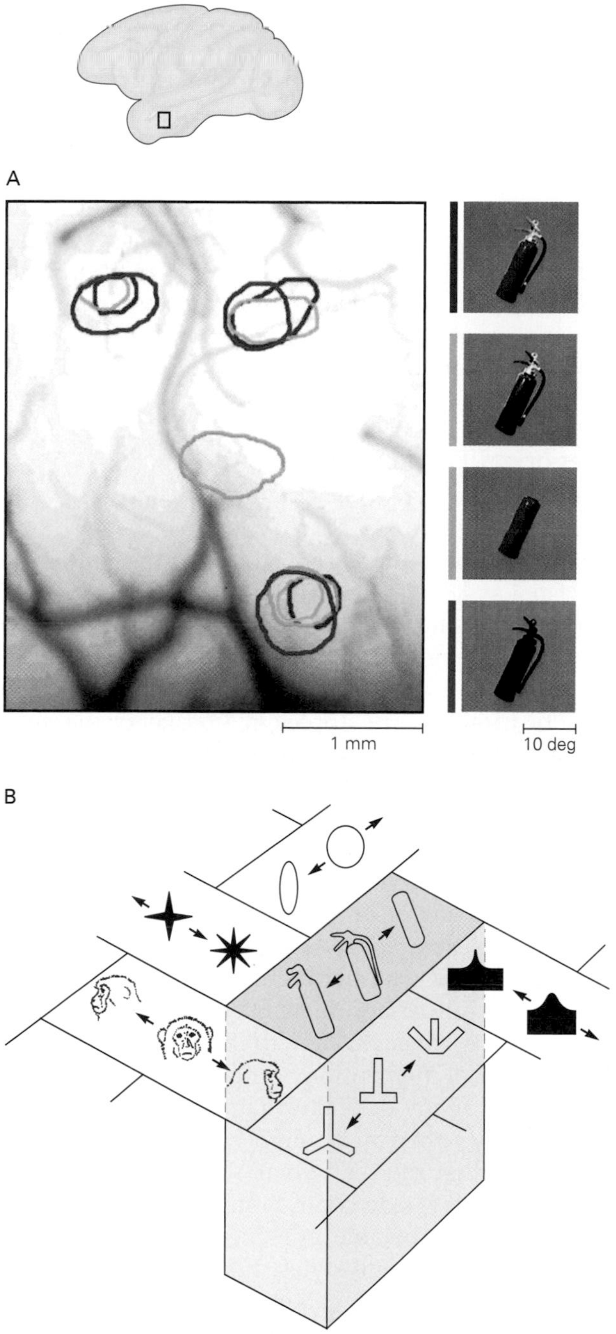

Figure 28–5 Neurons in the anterior portion of the inferior temporal cortex that represent complex visual stimuli are organized into columns. (Reproduced, with permission, from Tanaka 2003.)

A. Optical images of the surface of the anterior inferior temporal cortex illustrate regions selectively activated by the objects shown at the right.

B. In this schematic depiction of the columnar structure of the inferior temporal cortex the vertical axis represents cortical depth. According to this model each column includes neurons that represent a distinct complex pattern. Columns of neurons that represent variations of a pattern, such as the different faces or the different fire extinguishers, constitute a hypercolumn.

termed *perceptual constancy*. Perceptual constancy has many forms ranging from invariance across simple transformations of an object, such as size, position, and rotation, to the sameness of objects within a common category: All zebras look alike.

One of the best examples is *size constancy*. An object placed at different distances from an observer is perceived as having the same size, even though the object produces images of different absolute size on the retina. Size constancy has been recognized for centuries, but only in the past several decades has it been possible to identify the neural mechanisms responsible. An early study found that lesions of the inferior temporal cortex lead to failures of size constancy in monkeys, suggesting that neurons in this area play a critical role in size constancy. Indeed, one of the most striking and best-documented features of the response properties of individual inferior temporal neurons is the invariance of their pattern of selective responses to changes in stimulus size (Figure 28–7A).

Another relatively simple type of perceptual constancy is *position constancy*, in which objects are recognized as the same regardless of their location in the visual field. The pattern of selective responses of many inferior temporal neurons does not vary when the position of an object within their large receptive fields is changed (Figure 28–7B). *Form-cue invariance* refers to the constancy of a form when the cues that define the form change. The silhouette of Abraham Lincoln's head, for example, is readily recognizable whether it is black on white, white on black, or red on green. The responses of many inferior temporal neurons do not change with changes in contrast polarity (Figure 28–7C), color, or texture.

Viewpoint invariance refers to the perceptual constancy of three-dimensional objects observed from different angles. Despite the limitless range of retinal images that might be cast by a familiar object, an observer can readily recognize the object independently of the angle at which it is viewed. There are notable exceptions to this rule, which generally occur when an object is viewed from an angle that yields an uncharacteristic retinal image, such as a bucket viewed from directly above.

Investigators have looked for neurons whose response properties would account for viewpoint invariance but have found surprisingly little evidence. On the contrary, most neurons are tuned for specific viewing angles of a three-dimensional object. Although this tuning is often broad, thus reflecting partial viewpoint invariance, it appears that individual neurons do not generalize across inputs sufficiently to account for viewpoint invariance. Another possibility is that viewpoint invariance is the product of population coding by an ensemble of neurons each tuned to a different viewing angle. Finally, viewpoint invariance may be

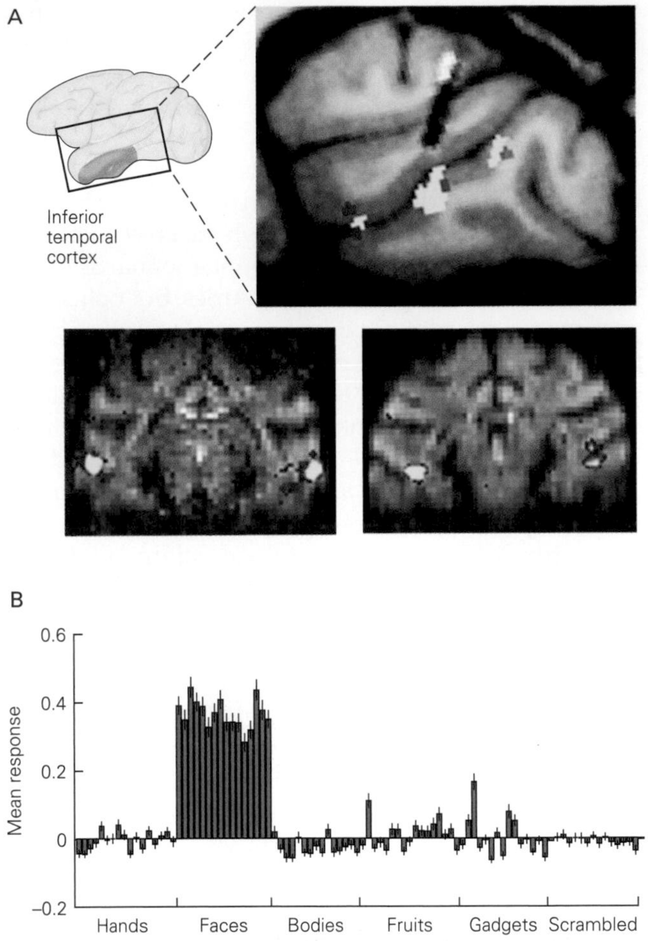

Figure 28–6 The inferior temporal cortex contains dense clusters of face-selective neurons. (Reproduced, with permission, from Tsao et al. 2006.)

A. Functional magnetic resonance imaging (fMRI) identifies three regions of the inferior temporal cortex that are selectively activated by faces. The upper image, a sagittal section, shows the three active zones along the lower bank of the superior temporal sulcus in one monkey. The two lower images are coronal sections through the face-representation areas in two monkeys.

B. Neurophysiological recordings reveal a preponderance of face-selective neurons in the middle face area identified by fMRI. The histogram plots the mean normalized response rate (minus baseline) of 182 neurons in the middle face area of one monkey. The monkey was shown 96 visual stimuli in six categories. Only faces elicited consistently vigorous responses.

achieved at a higher stage of cortical processing, such as the prefrontal cortex, through convergent inputs from neurons selective for specific viewpoints.

Studies of the conditions under which viewpoint invariance fails may lead to insights into the neural mechanisms of the behavior. One such condition is presentation of mirror images. Although mirror images are not identical, they are frequently perceived as the same, a confusion reflecting a false-positive identification by the system for viewpoint invariance. Carl Olson and colleagues examined the responses of neurons in the inferior temporal cortex to stimuli that were mirror images. Consistent with the perceptual confusion, many inferior temporal neurons responded similarly to both images. This result reinforces the conclusion that activity in the inferior temporal cortex reflects perceptual invariance, albeit incorrectly in this case, rather than the actual sensory information.

Categorical Perception of Objects Simplifies Behavior

All forms of perceptual constancy are the product of the visual system's attempts to generalize across different retinal images generated by a single object. A still more general type of constancy is the perception of individual objects as belonging to the same semantic category. The apples in a basket or the many appearances of the letter *A,* for example, are physically distinct but are effortlessly perceived as *categorically* identical under many behavioral conditions.

Categorical perception is classically defined by the ability to distinguish objects of different categories even when objects of the same category cannot be distinguished. For example, it is more difficult to discriminate between two red lights that differ in wavelength by 10 nm than to discriminate between red and orange lights with the same wavelength difference.

Categorical perception simplifies behavior. For example, it usually does not matter whether an apple is completely spherical or slightly mottled on the left side, or whether the seat we are offered is a Windsor or a Chippendale side chair. Similarly, reading ability requires that one be able to recognize the alphabet in a broad variety of type styles. Like the simpler forms of perceptual constancy, categorical perception reflects sensitivity to invariant visual attributes.

Is there a population of neurons that respond uniformly to objects within a category and differentially to objects of different categories? To test this Earl Miller and colleagues created a set of images in which features of dogs and cats were merged; the proportions of dog and cat in the composite images varied continuously from one extreme to the other. Monkeys were trained to identify these stimuli reliably as either dog or cat. Miller and colleagues then recorded from visually responsive neurons in the lateral prefrontal cortex, a region that receives direct input from the inferior

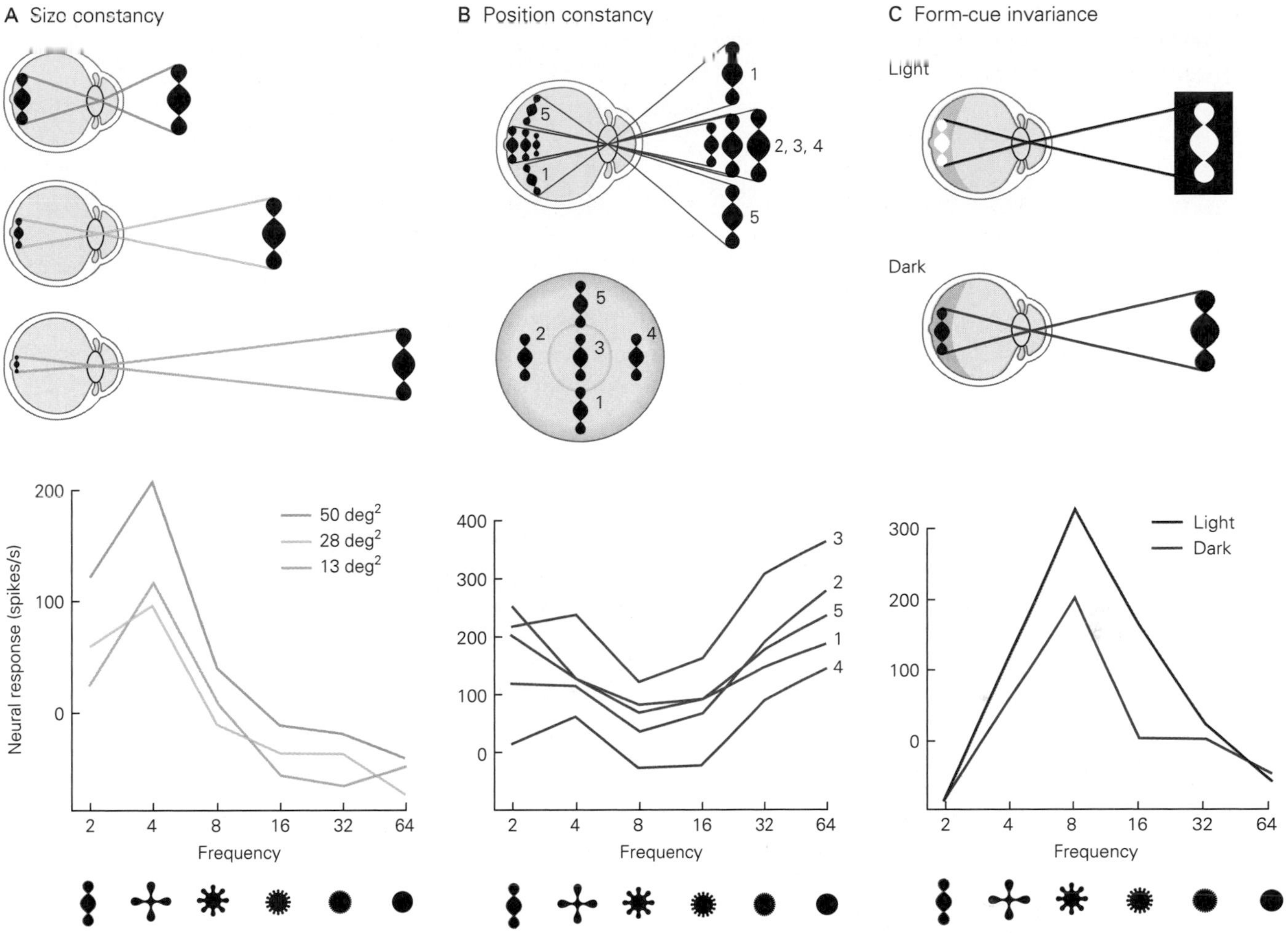

Figure 28–7 Perpetual constancy is reflected in the behavior of neurons in the inferior temporal cortex. The responses of many inferior temporal neurons are selective for stimuli with particular numbers or frequencies of lobes but invariant with regard to object size, position, and reflectance. (Reproduced, with permission, from Schwartz et al. 1983.)

A. *Size constancy.* An object is perceived to be the same even when the retinal image size decreases with the distance of the object in the visual field. The response of the vast majority of inferior temporal neurons to substantial changes in retinal image size is invariant, as illustrated here by the record of a single cell.

B. *Position constancy.* An object is perceived to be the same despite changes in position in the retinal image. Almost all inferior temporal neurons respond similarly to the same stimulus in different positions in the visual field, as illustrated here by the record of a single neuron.

C. *Form-cue invariance.* An object is perceived to be the same despite changes in reflectance. Most inferior temporal neurons respond similarly to the two viewing conditions illustrated, as shown in the record of the individual neuron.

temporal cortex. Not only did these neurons exhibit the predicted category-specific responses—responding well to cat but not dog, or *vice versa*—but the neuronal category boundary also corresponded to the behaviorally learned category boundary (Figure 28–8).

The fact that category-specific agnosias sometimes follow damage to the temporal lobe suggests there are neurons in the inferior temporal cortex that have category-specific responses similar to those of neurons in the prefrontal cortex. Face-recognition cells appear to meet this criterion, for their responses to a range of faces are often similar. Face-recognition cells may constitute a special case, however, for learned category-specific responses of the sort tested by Miller in the prefrontal cortex are rarely seen in the inferior temporal cortex. For most stimulus conditions category-specific

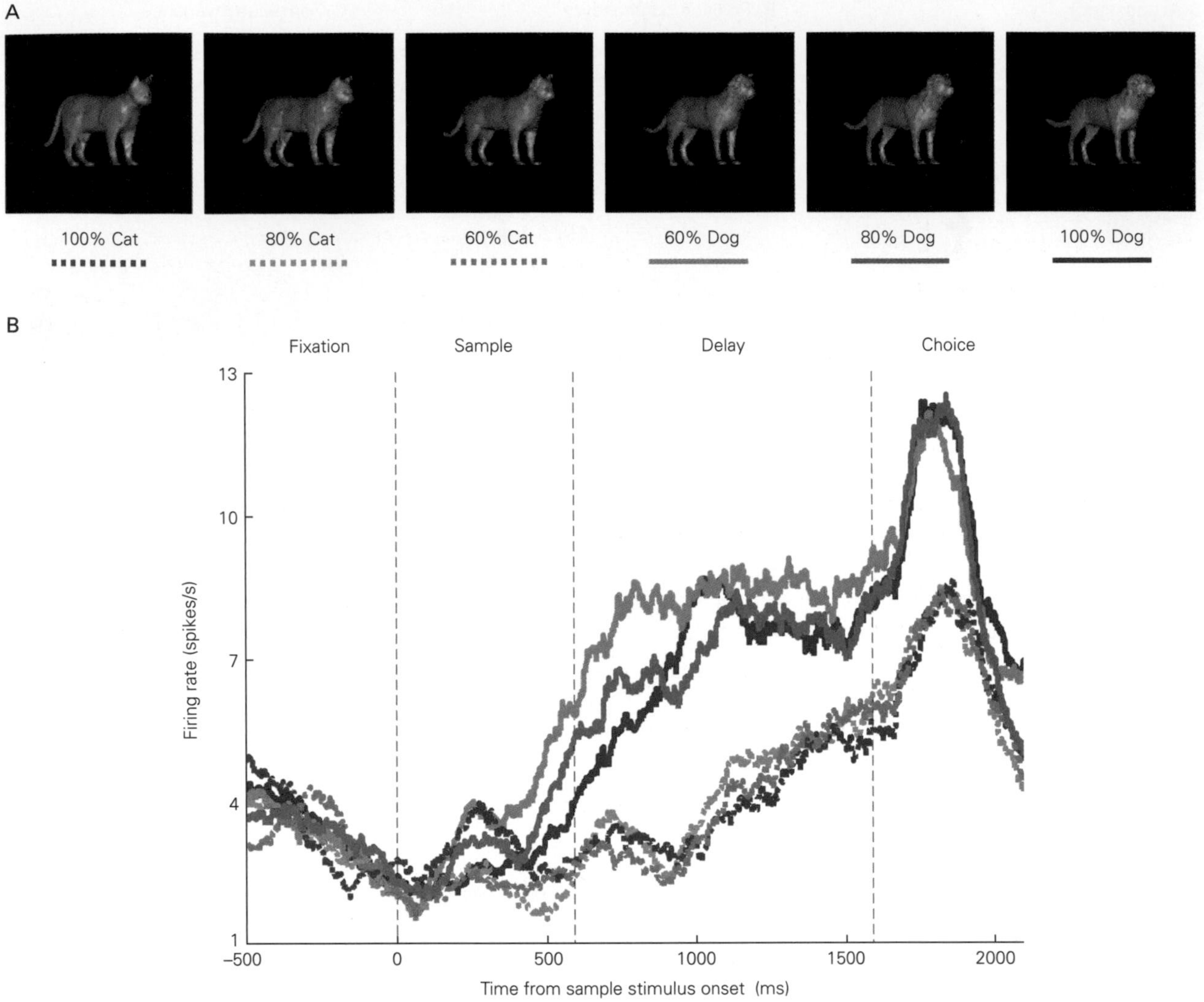

Figure 28–8 **Neural coding for categorical perception.** (Reproduced, with permission, from Freedman et al. 2002.)

A. The images combine cat and dog features in varying proportions. Monkeys were trained to identify an image as cat or dog if it had 50% or more features of that animal.

B. Peristimulus histograms illustrate the responses of a prefrontal cortex neuron to the images shown in part A. The neuron was selectively responsive to images of dogs. Despite the different retinal images, the responses to images within each category (dog or cat) are similar. By contrast, the responses to images in different categories (cat *versus* dog) differ significantly. Category-specific responses are common among visual neurons of the prefrontal cortex.

representations may be generated in the prefrontal cortex, where visual responses are more commonly linked to the behavioral significance of the stimuli.

Visual Memory Is a Component of High-Level Visual Processing

Visual experience can be stored as memory, and visual memory influences the processing of incoming visual information. Object recognition, in particular, relies on the observer's previous experiences with objects. Thus the contributions of the inferior temporal cortex to object recognition must be modifiable by experience.

Studies of the role of experience in visual perception have focused on two distinct types of experience-dependent plasticity in the visual system. One stems from repeated exposure or practice, which leads to improvements in visual discrimination and object-recognition ability. These experience-dependent changes constitute a form of implicit learning known as perceptual learning (see Chapter 27). The other occurs in connection with the storage of explicit learning, the learning of facts or events that can be recalled consciously (see Chapter 67).

Implicit Visual Learning Leads to Changes in the Selectivity of Neuronal Responses

The ability to resolve differences between complex visual stimuli is highly modifiable by experience. For example, individuals who attend to and examine fine differences between different models of automobiles or eyeglasses become far better at discriminating and recognizing such differences.

In the inferior temporal cortex neuronal selectivity for complex objects can undergo change that parallels changes in the ability to distinguish objects. For example, in one study monkeys were trained to identify novel three-dimensional objects, such as randomly bent wire forms, from two-dimensional views of the objects. Extensive training led to pronounced improvements in the ability to recognize the objects from two-dimensional views. Extracellular recordings from the inferior temporal cortex after training revealed a population of neurons that exhibited marked selectivity for the views seen earlier but not for other two-dimensional views of the same objects (Figure 28–9).

Other studies with monkeys have shown that familiarity with novel faces alters the tuning of many face-selective neurons in the inferior temporal cortex. Similarly, when an animal has experience with novel objects formed from simple features, inferior-temporal neurons become selective for those objects. Such neuronal changes can result from either active discrimination or passive viewing and are often manifested as a sharpening of stimulus selectivity rather than changes in absolute firing rate. Sharpening is precisely the sort of neuronal change that could underlie improvements in perceptual discrimination of visual stimuli.

Explicit Visual Learning Depends on Linkage of the Visual System and Declarative Memory Formation

Progress has been made in understanding the neurobiology of interaction between vision and memory, specifically in relation to two issues. First, how is visual sensory information maintained in short-term working memory? Working memory has a limited capacity, acting like a buffer in a computer operating system, and is susceptible to interference as when trying to remember the face of a person you have just met. Second, how are long-term visual memories and the associations between them stored and recalled?

Visual neurons in both the inferior temporal and prefrontal cortices continue firing during the delay in a visual delayed-response task (Box 28–1).

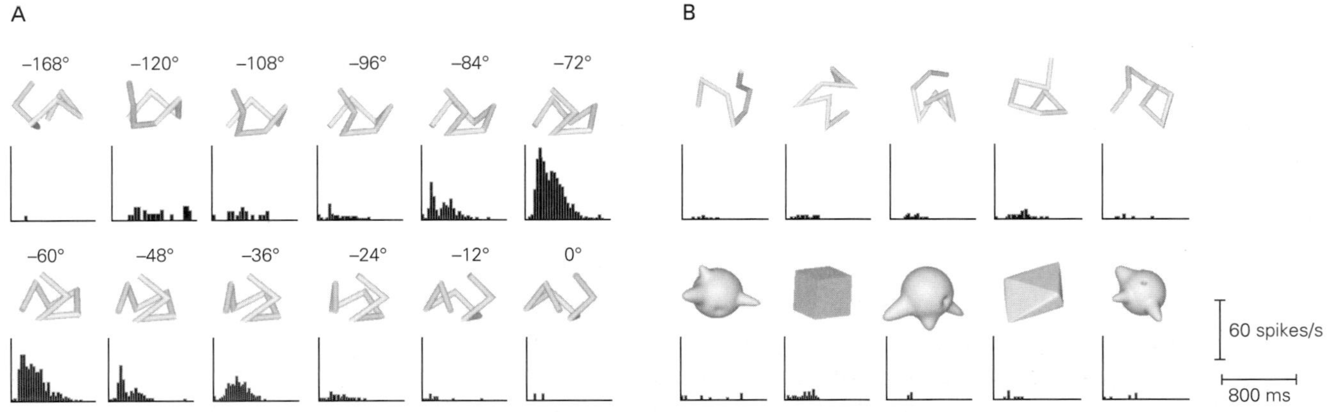

Figure 28–9 Familiarity with particular complex objects leads inferior temporal neurons to respond selectively for those objects. (Reproduced, with permission, from Logothetis and Pauls 1995.)

A. Monkeys were trained to recognize a randomly bent wire from a set of two-dimensional views of the wire. The wire form was rotated 12 degrees in each successive view. Once performance was stable at a high level, extracellular recordings were made from neurons in the inferior temporal cortex while each view was presented. The responses of a typical neuron to each view are plotted in the form of peristimulus histograms. This neuron responded selectively to views that represented a small range of rotation of the object.

B. The same neuron was tested with two sets of "distractor" stimuli that were unfamiliar to the monkey. It failed to respond to any of these stimuli.

Box 28–1 Investigating Interactions Between Vision and Memory

The relationship between vision and memory can be studied by combining a neuropsychological approach with single-cell electrophysiological methods.

One behavioral paradigm used to study memory is the *delayed-response task*. An animal is required to make a specific response based on information remembered during a brief delay. In one form of this task, known as *delayed match-to-sample,* the subject must indicate whether a visual stimulus is the same or different from a previously viewed sample (Figure 28–10A).

For example, the subject is shown a photograph of a tractor and then, after a brief delay, is shown several photographs of tractors, only one of which is identical to the sample tractor previously viewed. The task is to identify the tractor that matches the sample.

When used in conjunction with single-cell recording, this task allows the experimenter to isolate three key components of a neuronal response: (1) the sensory component, the response elicited by the sample stimulus; (2) the short-term or working-memory component, the response that occurs during the delay between the sample and the match; and (3) the recognition-memory or familiarity component, the difference between the response elicited by the match stimulus and the earlier response to the sample stimulus.

A second behavioral paradigm, known as the *visual paired-association task,* has been used in conjunction with electrophysiology to explore the cellular mechanisms underlying the long-term storage and recall of associations between visual stimuli (Figure 28–10B).

This task differs from the delayed match-to-sample task in that the match and sample are two different stimuli. The sample stimulus might consist of the letter *A* and the match stimulus the letter *B*. Through repeated temporal pairing and conditional reinforcement, subjects learn that *A* and *B* are predictive of one another: They are associated.

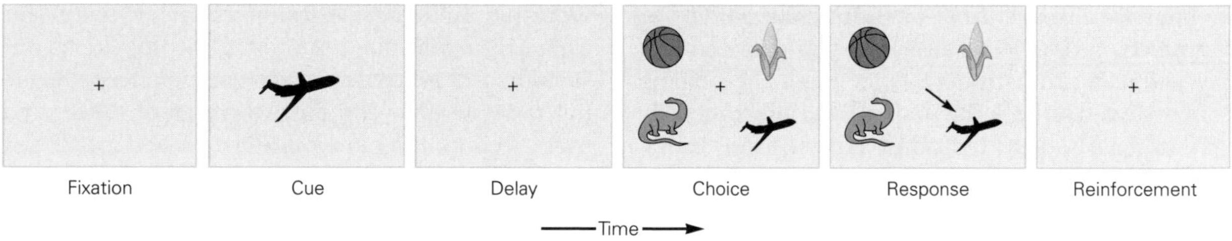

Figure 28–10A Delayed match-to-sample task. In this paradigm a trial begins with the appearance of a fixation spot that directs the subject's attention and gaze to the center of the computer screen. A sample image then appears briefly, typically for 500 ms, followed by a delay in which the display is blank. The delay can be varied to fit the experimental goals. Following the delay several test images, including the sample, are displayed. The monkey must choose the sample, typically either by pressing a button or by a saccade to the stimulus. If the animal chooses the sample, it receives a small juice reward. In the task illustrated here all of the test images appear at once (a simultaneous match-to-sample task). They can also be presented sequentially (a sequential match-to-sample task). Although the trial's duration may be longer for the sequential task, this paradigm can be advantageous for electrophysiological studies by limiting the visual stimuli present at any time.

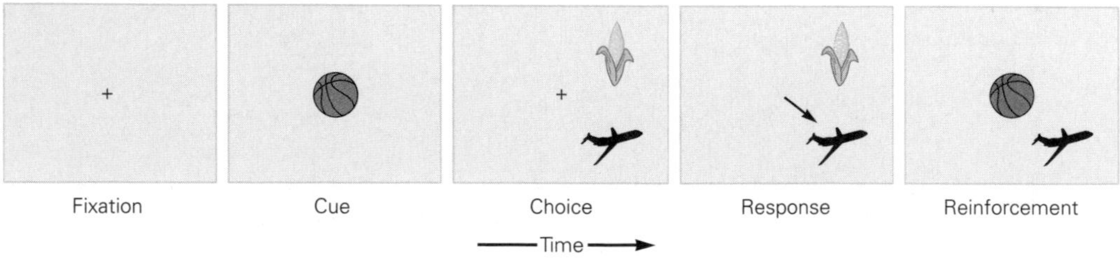

Figure 28–10B The paired-association task. This paradigm resembles the match-to-sample paradigm except that the sample and test stimuli are not the same. The subject must discover the correct association by trial-and-error learning. The task thus serves to build an association between stimuli. The paired-association task can also incorporate a delay between presentation of the sample and test stimuli, and it can be used in both simultaneous (shown) and sequential forms.

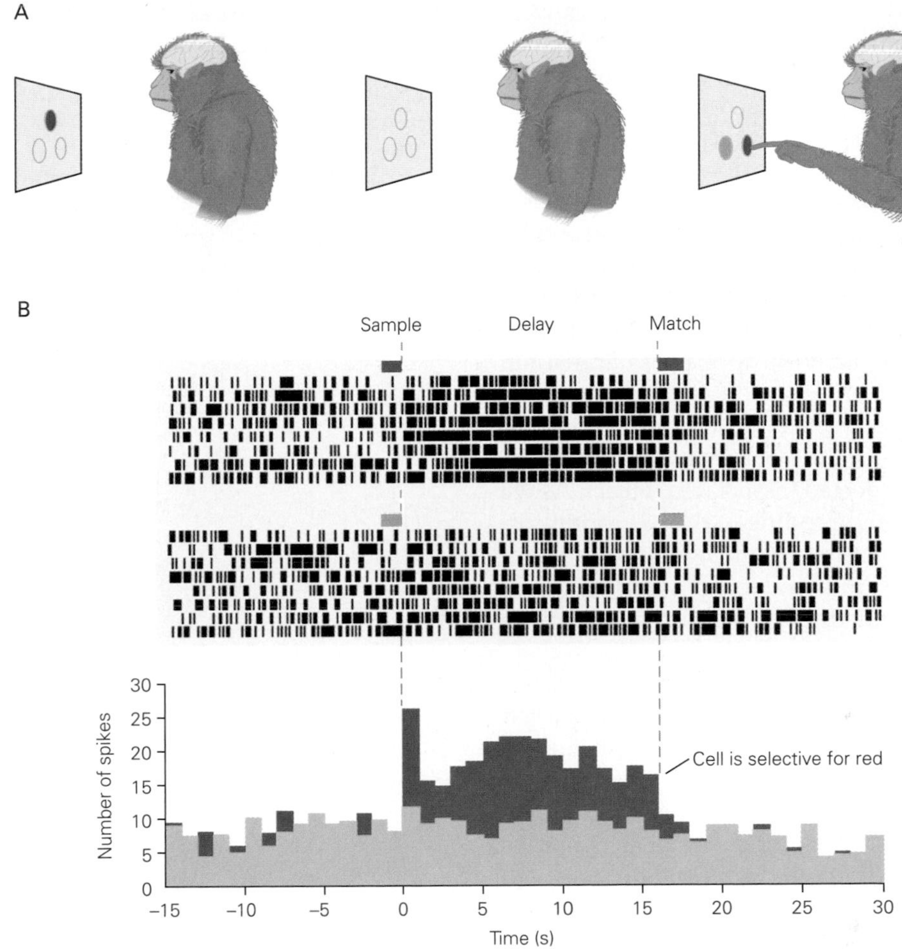

Figure 28–11 Neural activity representing an object is sustained while the object is held in working memory. (Reproduced, with permission, from Fuster and Jervey 1982.)

A. Monkeys were trained to perform a color match-to-sample task. For example, a red stimulus was first presented and the animal later had to choose a red stimulus from among many colored stimuli. The task incorporated a brief delay (1–2 seconds) between display of the sample and the match, during which information about the correct target color had to be maintained in working memory. The inferior temporal cortex is shown.

B. Peristimulus histograms and raster plots of action potentials illustrate responses of a single neuron in the inferior temporal cortex during the delayed match-to-sample task. The upper record is from trials in which the sample was red and the lower record from trials in which it was green. The recordings show that the cell responds preferentially to red stimuli. In trials with a green sample the activity of the neuron does not change, whereas in trials with a red sample the cell exhibited a brief burst of activity following presentation of the sample and continued firing throughout the delay. Many visual neurons in the inferior temporal and prefrontal cortices exhibit this kind of behavior.

This delay-period activity is thought to maintain information in short-term working memory. Delay-period activity in the inferior temporal and in prefrontal cortices differ in a number of ways. For one, the activity in the inferior temporal cortex is associated with the short-term storage of visual patterns and color information, whereas the activity in the prefrontal cortex encodes not only visual spatial information but also information about other sensory modalities. Delay-period activity in the inferior temporal cortex also appears to be closely attuned to visual experience, for it encodes the sample image and can be eliminated by the appearance of another image (Figure 28–11).

In the prefrontal cortex, by contrast, delay-period activity is more likely to depend on task requirements and is not terminated by later sensory inputs, suggesting that it may play a role in the recall of long-term memories. Experiments by Earl Miller and colleagues support this view. In these experiments monkeys were trained to associate multiple pairs of objects and then tested. Each behavioral test began with presentation of a single sample object. After a brief delay a monkey was shown a test object and asked to indicate whether it was the object paired with the sample during training.

There are two possible ways to solve this task. During the delay the animal could remember the sample object by retaining a sensory code or thinking ahead to the expected object—the one associated with the sample during training—using a "prospective code." Remarkably, neuronal activity appears to transition from one to the other during the delay. Neurons in the prefrontal cortex initially encode the sensory properties of the sample object—the one just seen—but later begin to encode the expected (associated) object. As we shall see, such prospective coding in the prefrontal cortex may be the source of top-down signals to the inferior temporal cortex, activating neurons that represent the expected object and thus giving rise to conscious recall of that object.

The relation between long-term declarative memory storage and visual processing has been explored extensively in the context of remembered associations between visual stimuli. A century ago William James, a founder of the American school of experimental psychology, suggested that learning of visual associations might be mediated by enhanced connectivity between the neurons encoding individual stimuli. To test this hypothesis monkeys were trained to associate pairs of objects that had no prior physical or semantic relatedness. The monkeys were later tested while extracellular recordings of neurons in the inferior temporal cortex were made. Objects that had been paired often elicited similar neuronal responses, as one would expect if functional connections had been enhanced, whereas responses elicited by unpaired objects were unrelated.

To determine whether this pattern of selectivity was indeed temporally and conditionally tied to learning, Thomas Albright and colleagues recorded from individual inferior temporal neurons while monkeys were learning new visual associations. They found that responses to paired objects became more similar over the course of training (Figure 28–12). Most importantly, the changes in neuronal activity occurred on the same timescale as the behavioral changes and were dependent on successful learning.

The learning-dependent changes in the stimulus selectivity of inferior temporal cortex neurons are long-lasting, suggesting that this cortical region is part of the neural circuitry for visual associative memories. The results also support the view that learned associations are implemented rapidly by highly specific changes in the strength of synaptic connections between neurons representing the associated stimuli.

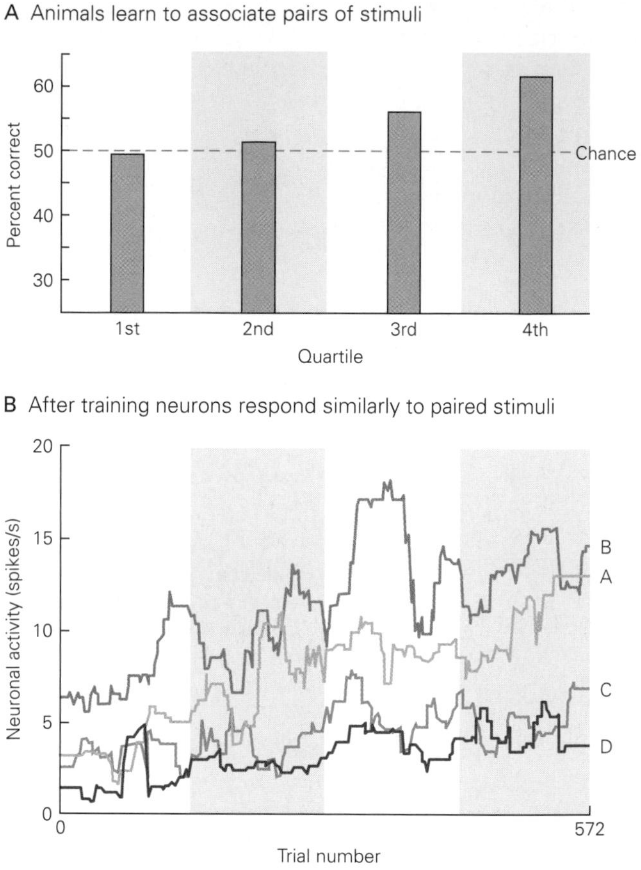

Figure 28–12 Object recognition is linked to associative memory. Monkeys learned associations between pairs of visual stimuli while activity was recorded from a neuron in the inferior temporal cortex. (Reproduced, with permission, from Messinger et al. 2001.)

A. Behavioral performance on a paired-association task is plotted for each quartile of a single training session (572 trials). The animal was presented with four novel stimuli and was required to learn two paired associations. As expected, performance began at chance (50% correct) and gradually climbed as the animal learned the associations.

B. Mean firing rates of an inferior temporal neuron recorded during the behavioral task described in part A. Each trace represents the firing rate during presentation of one of the four stimuli (A, B, C, or D). Although the responses to all stimuli were of similar magnitude at the outset, as the paired associations were learned the neuronal responses to the paired stimuli A and B began to cluster at a different level from responses to the paired stimuli C and D. The neuron's activity thus corresponded to the learned associations between the two pairs.

We know that the hippocampus and neocortical areas of the medial temporal lobe—the perirhinal, entorhinal, and parahippocampal cortices—are essential both for the acquisition of visual associative memories and for the functional plasticity of the inferior temporal cortex. The hippocampus and medial temporal lobe may facilitate the reorganization of local neuronal circuitry in the inferior temporal cortex as required to store visual associative memories. The reorganization itself may reflect a form of Hebbian plasticity, initiated by the temporal coincidence of the associated visual stimuli.

Associative Recall of Visual Memories Depends on Top-Down Activation of the Cortical Neurons That Process Visual Stimuli

One of the most intriguing features of high-level visual processing is the fact that the sensory experience of an image in one's visual field and the recall of the same image are subjectively similar. The former depends on the bottom-up flow of visual information and is what we traditionally regard as vision. The latter, by contrast, is a product of top-down information flow. This distinction is anatomically accurate but obscures the fact that under normal conditions afferent and descending signals collaborate to yield visual experience.

The study of visual associative memory has provided valuable insights into the cellular mechanisms underlying visual recall. As we have seen, visual associative memories are stored in the visual cortex through changes in the functional connectivity between neurons that independently represent the associated stimuli. The practical consequence of this change is that a neuron that responded only to stimulus *A* prior to learning will respond to both stimulus *A* and stimulus *B* after these stimuli have been associated (Figure 28–13). Activation of an *A*-responsive neuron by the associated stimulus *B* can be viewed as the neuronal correlate of top-down recall of stimulus *A*.

Neurons in the inferior temporal cortex exhibit precisely this behavior. The activity correlated with cued recall is nearly identical to the bottom-up activation by the stimulus. These neurophysiological findings

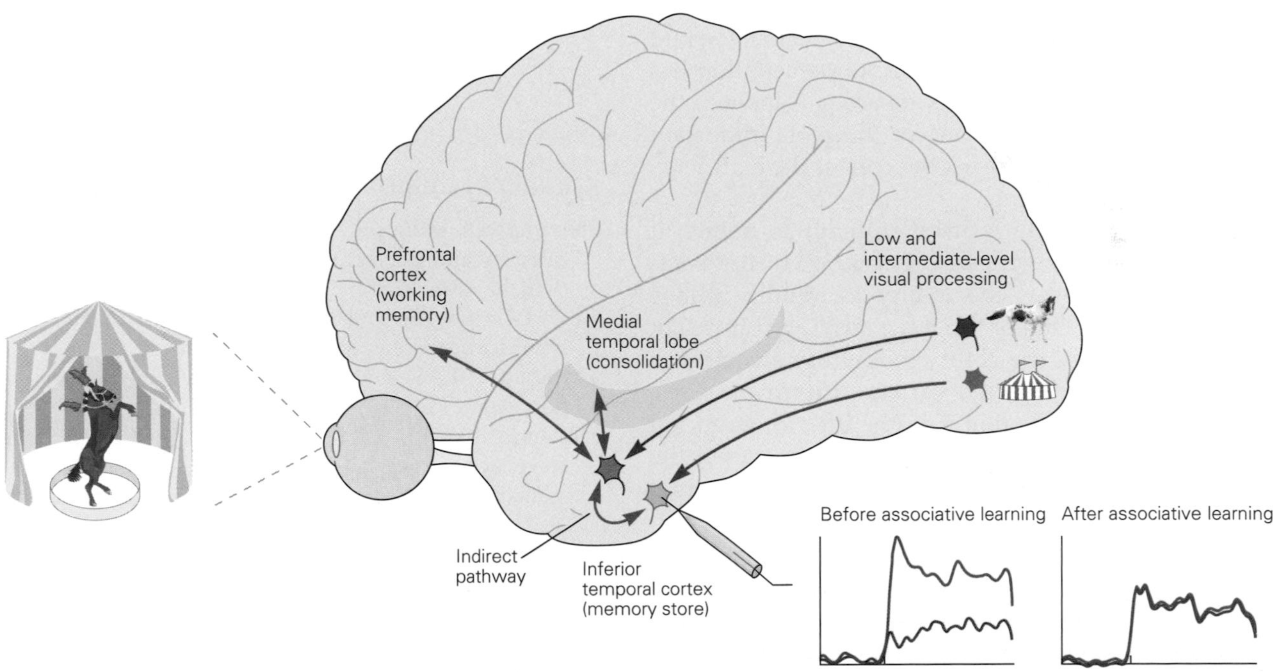

Figure 28–13 Circuits for visual association and recall. Bottom-up signals—afferent signals initiated by objects in the observer's visual field—lead to representation of those objects in the inferior temporal cortex. Before associative learning, a neuron (**light blue**) responds well to the circus tent but not to the horse. Learned associations between objects are consolidated in the inferior temporal cortex by strengthening connections between neurons representing each of the paired objects (the indirect pathway in the figure). That consolidation is mediated by memory structures of the medial temporal lobe. Thus recall of the circus tent following presentation of the horse is achieved by activating the indirect pathway. Indirect activation can also be triggered by the contents of working memory (feedback from the prefrontal cortex). Under normal conditions visual experience is the product of a combination of direct and indirect inputs to the inferior temporal cortex.

are supported by a number of brain-imaging studies that have identified selective activity in the visual cortex during cued and spontaneous recall of objects.

Although learned associations between images are likely to be stored through circuit changes in the inferior temporal cortex, the prefrontal cortex is essential for activating these circuits for conscious recall. The afferent signal for one of a pair of images might be received by the inferior temporal cortex and relayed to the prefrontal cortex, whereupon the information would be maintained in working memory. As we have seen, the signaling of many prefrontal neurons during the delay period of a delayed match-to-sample task initially encodes the sample image but changes to encode the associated image that is expected to follow. Signals from prefrontal cortex to the inferior temporal cortex would selectively activate neurons representing the associated image, and that activation would constitute visual recall.

An Overall View

The eminent neuropsychologist Hans-Lukas Teuber once wrote that failure of object recognition "would appear in its purest form as a normal percept that has somehow been stripped of its meaning." Indeed, the assignment of meaning is one of the most important processes in vision and forms the core of the high-level stage of visual processing.

Although meaning is itself difficult to define, it has generally acknowledged connotations. For example, meaning suggests the ability to identify things that are the same. One of the most striking features of object recognition is the ability to identify an object as the same despite an infinite variety of retinal images. This occurs because a neuron in the inferior temporal cortex is activated by the various retinal images of the same object. Similarly, visual neurons in the prefrontal cortex fire in response to objects that are physically different but semantically related.

Meaning may also connote function, utility, or intention. In the case of visual recognition meaning is formed by the observer's prior sensory experiences and the acquired associations between these experiences. These attributes are fundamental in high-level visual processing and include enhanced perceptual and neuronal selectivity for objects that are commonplace as well as associative links between neuronal representations of objects.

Although much is now known about the neuronal *correlates* of object recognition, very little is yet known about the circuits that *cause* these neuronal representations. Even less is known about the cellular and molecular mechanisms by which these circuits are modified by visual experience. Thus future experiments need to address a number of important questions.

How are categorical representations formed? What is the mechanism by which incoming sensory stimuli are compared with stored representations to achieve object recognition? If we accept that associative memories are stored as patterns of connections between neocortical neurons, what then are the specific contributions of the hippocampus and neocortical structures of the medial temporal lobe, and by what cellular mechanisms do they exert their influences? And how does reinforcement cement changes in the strength of the interconnections between neurons that are presumed to underlie associative memories?

The confluence of molecular-genetic, cellular, neurophysiological, and behavioral approaches in solving these and other problems promises a bright future for understanding of high-level visual processing.

Thomas D. Albright

Selected Readings

Freedman DJ, Miller EK. 2008. Neural mechanisms of visual categorization: insights from neurophysiology. Neurosci Biobehav Rev 32:311–329.

Gross CG. 1999. *Brain, Vision, Memory: Tales in the History of Neuroscience.* Cambridge, MA: MIT Press.

Logothetis NK, Sheinberg DL. 1996. Visual object recognition. Annu Rev Neurosci 19:577–621.

Messinger A, Squire LR, Zola SM, Albright TD. 2005. Neural correlates of knowledge: stable representation of stimulus associations across variations in behavioral performance. Neuron 48:359–371.

Miller EK, Li L, Desimone R. 1991. A neural mechanism for working and recognition memory in inferior temporal cortex. Science 254:1377–1379.

Miyashita Y. 1993. Inferior temporal cortex: where visual perception meets memory. Annu Rev Neurosci 16:245–263.

Schlack A, Albright TD. 2007. Remembering visual motion: neural correlates of associative plasticity and motion recall in cortical area MT. Neuron 53:881–890.

Squire LR, Zola-Morgan S. 1991. The medial temporal lobe memory system. Science 253:1380–1386.

Ungerleider LG, Courtney SM, Haxby JV. 1998. A neural system for human visual working memory. Proc Natl Acad Sci U S A 95:883–890.

References

Baker CI, Behrmann M, Olson CR. 2002. Impact of learning on representation of parts and wholes in monkey inferotemporal cortex. Nat Neurosci 5:1210–1216.

Brown S, Schafer ES. 1888. An investigation into the functions of the occipital and temporal lobes of the monkey's brain. Philos Trans R Soc Lond B Biol Sci 179:303–327.

Damasio AR, Damasio H, Van Hoesen GW. 1982. Prosopagnosia: anatomic basis and behavioral mechanisms. Neurology 32:331–341.

Desimone R, Albright TD, Gross CG, Bruce CJ. 1984. Stimulus selective properties of inferior temporal neurons in the macaque. J Neurosci 8:2051–2062.

Desimone R, Fleming J, Gross CG. 1980. Prestriate afferents to inferior temporal cortex: an HRP study. Brain Res 184:41–55.

Farah MJ. 1990. *Visual Agnosia: Disorders of Object Recognition and What They Tell Us about Normal Vision*. Cambridge, MA: MIT Press.

Felleman DJ, Van Essen DC. 1991. Distributed hierarchical processing in the primate cerebral cortex. Cereb Cortex 1:1–47.

Freedman DJ, Riesenhuber M, Poggio T, Miller EK. 2002. Visual categorization and the primate prefrontal cortex: neurophysiology and behavior. J Neurophysiol 88:929–941.

Fujita I, Tanaka K, Ito M, Cheng K. 1992. Columns for visual features of objects in monkey inferotemporal cortex. Nature 360:343–346.

Fuster JM, Jervey JP. 1982. Neuronal firing in the inferotemporal cortex of the monkey in a visual memory task. J Neurosci 2:361–375.

Gross CG, Bender DB, Rocha-Miranda CE. 1969. Visual receptive fields of neurons in inferotemporal cortex of the monkey. Science 166:1303–1306.

Kosslyn SM. 1994. *Image and Brain*. Cambridge, MA: MIT Press.

Logothetis NK, Pauls J. 1995. Psychophysical and physiological evidence for viewer-centered object representations in the primate. Cereb Cortex 5:270–288.

Messinger A, Squire LR, Zola SM, Albright TD. 2001. Neuronal representations of stimulus associations develop in the temporal lobe during learning. Proc Natl Acad Sci U S A 98:12239–12244.

Miyashita Y, Chang HS. 1988. Neuronal correlate of pictorial short-term memory in the primate temporal cortex. Nature 331:68–70.

Rainer G, Rao SC, Miller EK. 1999. Prospective coding for objects in primate prefrontal cortex. J Neurosci 19: 5493–5505.

Rollenhagen JE, Olson CR. 2000. Mirror-image confusion in single neurons of the macaque inferotemporal cortex. Science 287:1506–1508.

Sakai K, Miyashita Y. 1991. Neural organization for the long-term memory of paired associates. Nature 354:152–155.

Schwartz EL, Desimone R, Albright TD, Gross CG. 1983. Shape recognition and inferior temporal neurons. Proc Natl Acad Sci U S A 80:5776–5778.

Suzuki WA, Amaral DG. 2004. Functional neuroanatomy of the medial temporal lobe memory system. Cortex 40: 220–222.

Tanaka K. 2003. Columns for complex visual object features in the inferotemporal cortex: clustering of cells with similar but slightly different stimulus selectivities. Cereb Cortex 13:90–99.

Teuber HL. 1968. Disorders of memory following penetrating missile wounds of the brain. Neurology 18:287–288.

Tomita H, Ohbayashi M, Nakahara K, Hasegawa I, Miyashita Y. 1999. Top-down signal from prefrontal cortex in executive control of memory retrieval. Nature 401:699–703.

Tsao DY, Freiwald WA, Tootell RB, Livingstone MS. 2006. A cortical region consisting entirely of face-selective cells. Science 311:670–674.

Wheeler ME, Petersen SE, Buckner RL. 2000. Memory's echo: vivid remembering reactivates sensory-specific cortex. Proc Natl Acad Sci U S A 97:11125–11129.

29

Visual Processing and Action

VISION REQUIRES EYE MOVEMENTS. Small eye movements are essential for maintaining the contrast of objects that we are examining. Without these movements the perception of an object rapidly fades to a field of gray, a phenomenon correlated with the decreased response of neurons in area V1 (see Chapter 25). Large eye movements direct the fovea from one object to another. These movements or saccades bring the high resolution of the fovea to bear on different regions of the visual field, exploiting the high density of photoreceptors in the central fovea. Without saccades this high-resolution processing could be achieved only by moving the head or body.

The preceding chapters have described how visual images are constructed, beginning with the processing of intensity and contrast, then the integration of visual primitives, and finally the high-level processing that leads to the recognition of objects. But the visual system involves more than just object recognition. It must also support the brain's goal of assigning significance to objects in order to develop strategies for interacting with the environment. Thus the brain must be able to select some objects for greater examination while ignoring others.

In this chapter we consider how saccades support that goal. We first consider the essential benefits that saccades provide, shifting attention in the visual field and assisting with the preparation to grasp objects. We then consider the brain mechanisms that solve a major problem created by saccades—the fact that the retinal image is abruptly displaced with every saccade.

In shifting our attention from how the brain constructs a visual scene to how it uses visual information to plan actions, we now concentrate on the region of the brain referred to as the dorsal visual pathway (Figure 29–1). This pathway extends from V1 to the regions in parietal cortex that continue the intermediate level of visual processing, such as the middle temporal area, and then to other regions of parietal and frontal cortex. The regions particularly relevant to this chapter are in the parietal cortex, such as the lateral intraparietal area, but include also the frontal eye field region of the frontal cortex.

Successive Fixations Focus Our Attention in the Visual Field

A saccade usually lasts less than 40 ms and redirects the center of sight in the visual field. Saccades occur several times per second, and each intervening period

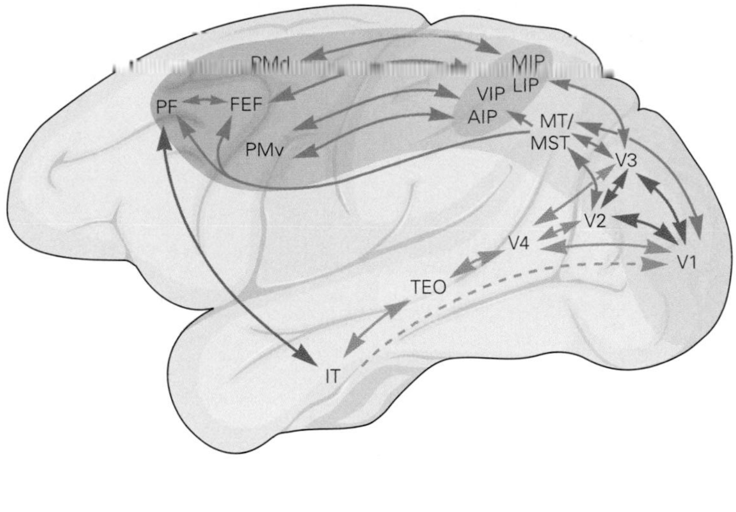

Figure 29–1 Pathways involved in visual processing for action. The dorsal visual pathway (**blue**) extends to the posterior parietal cortex and then to the frontal cortex. The ventral visual pathway (**pink**) is considered in Chapter 27. (**AIP**, anterior intraparietal cortex; **FEF**, frontal eye field; **IT**, inferior temporal cortex; **LIP**, lateral intraparietal cortex; **MIP**, medial intraparietal cortex; **MST**, medial superior temporal cortex; **MT**, middle temporal cortex; **PF**, prefrontal cortex; **PMd**, **PMv**, dorsal and ventral premotor cortices; **TEO**, occipitotemporal cortex; **VIP**, ventral intraparietal cortex; **V1–V4**, areas of visual cortex.)

of fixation lasts several hundred milliseconds. The Russian psychologist Alfred Yarbus was the first to show that the pattern of saccades made by a human looking at a picture reflected the cognitive purpose of vision. He found that saccades were not directed equally to all parts of a scene. Areas of apparent interest were fixated most frequently, whereas background objects were ignored. For example, the faces of people were fixated repeatedly (Figure 29–2).

The image on the fovea shifts with each saccade, yet we perceive a stable visual world. How does that come about? One possibility is that the brain creates a representation of the entire visual scene from a series of visual fixations across the scene and that what we see is this summed representation of the visual world. If that were so, we should have detailed knowledge of the entire visual scene at any given instant.

A series of experiments on change blindness showed that this is not the case. These experiments involved changing a picture during the brief time when the viewer made a saccade from one part of the scene to another. If there were a relatively complete internal representation of the scene before the saccade, then any substantial change made during the saccade should have been recognized. But even a large change frequently went unrecognized. This change blindness occurred even when there were no actual eye movements, as when two pictures were shown in succession with only a brief blank between them to simulate the effect of an eye movement (Figure 29–3).

The results of the change-blindness experiments are inconsistent with the hypothesis that we are continually updating a complete representation of the visual field from second to second. Instead we seem to pay attention to only certain fragments of the scene. This selective visual attention relies on the saccades that bring the images of desired parts of the visual field onto the fovea.

Attention Selects Objects for Further Visual Examination

In the 19th century William James described attention as "the taking possession by the mind in clear and vivid form, of one out of what seem several simultaneously possible objects or trains of thought. It implies withdrawal from some things in order to deal effectively with others." James went on to describe two kinds of attention: "It is either passive, reflex, nonvoluntary, effortless or active and voluntary. In passive immediate sensorial attention the stimulus is a sense-impression, either very intense, voluminous, or sudden ... big things, bright things, moving things ... blood."

More recently these two kinds of attention have been termed *involuntary* (exogenous) and *voluntary* (endogenous) attention, or bottom-up and top-down attention. Your attention to this page as you read it is an example of voluntary attention. If a bright light suddenly flashed, your attention would probably be pulled away involuntarily from the page.

Voluntary attention is closely linked to saccades because the fovea has a much denser array of cones than the peripheral retina (see Figure 26–1), and this permits a finer-grain analysis of objects than is possible with peripheral vision.

Attention, both voluntary and involuntary, has several measurable effects on human visual performance: It shortens reaction time and makes perception

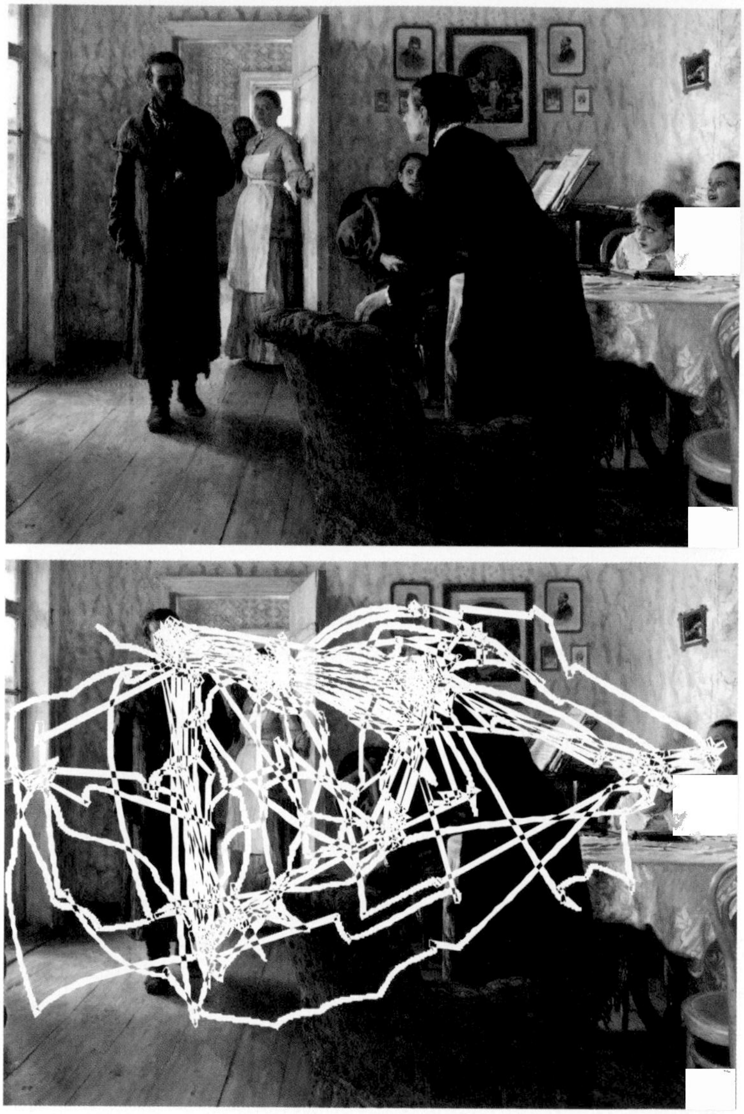

Figure 29–2 Eye movements during vision. A subject viewed this painting (*An Unexpected Visitor* by Ilya Repin) for several minutes, making saccades to selected fixation points—primarily faces—that presumably were of most interest. Lines indicate saccades, and spots indicate points at which the eyes fixated. (Reproduced, with permission, from Yarbus 1967.)

more sensitive. This increased sensitivity includes the abilities to detect objects at a lower contrast and ignore distracters close to an object. The abrupt appearance of a behaviorally irrelevant cue such as a light flash reduces the reaction time to a test stimulus presented 300 ms later in the same place, but increases reaction time when the test stimulus appears at a different place. The light flash involuntarily draws attention to itself, and attention to that location is maintained for a brief period, thus accelerating the visual response to the later test stimulus at the location. Similarly, if a subject plans a saccade to a particular part of the visual field, the contrast threshold at which any object there can be seen is lowered by 50%. The saccade, under voluntary control, draws attention to its goal.

Activity in the Parietal Lobe Correlates with Attention Paid to Objects

Clinical studies have long implicated the parietal lobe in the process of visual attention. Patients with lesions of the right parietal lobe have normal visual fields when their visual perception is studied with a single stimulus in an uncomplicated visual world. However, when presented with a more complicated world, with objects in the right (ipsilateral) and left (contralateral) visual hemifields, they tend to report more of what lies in the right visual hemifield.

This deficit, known as *neglect syndrome* (see Chapter 17), arises because attention is focused on the visual hemifield ipsilateral to the lesion. Even when

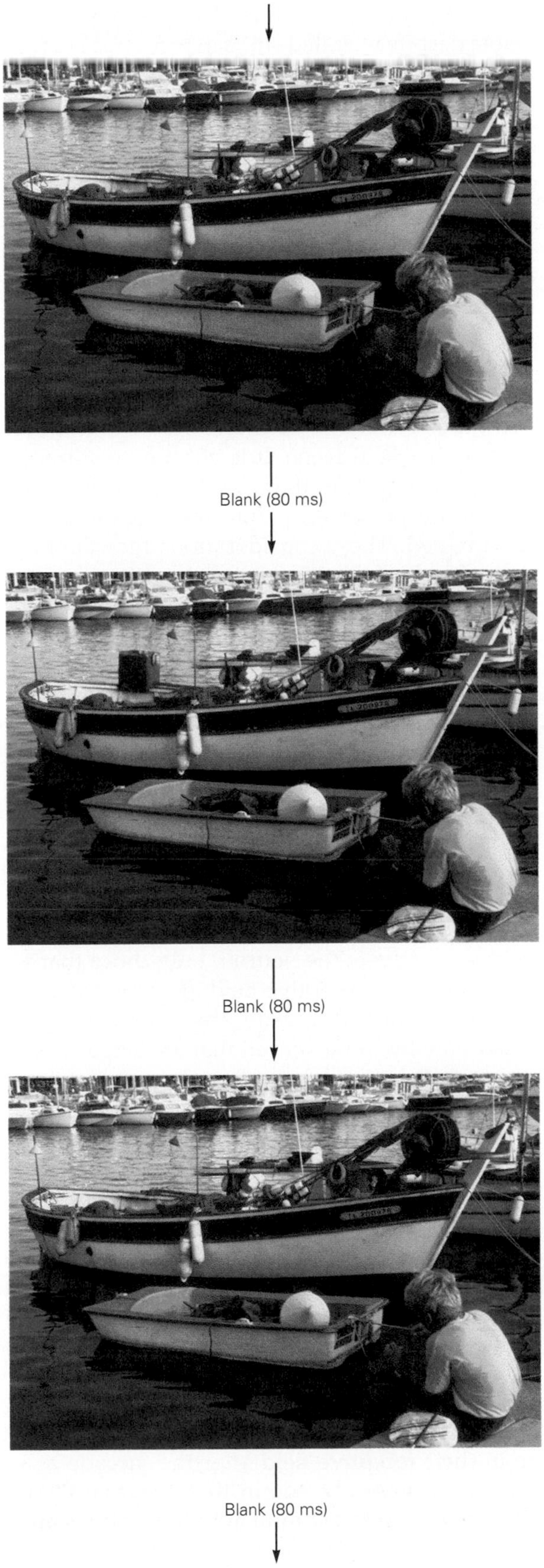

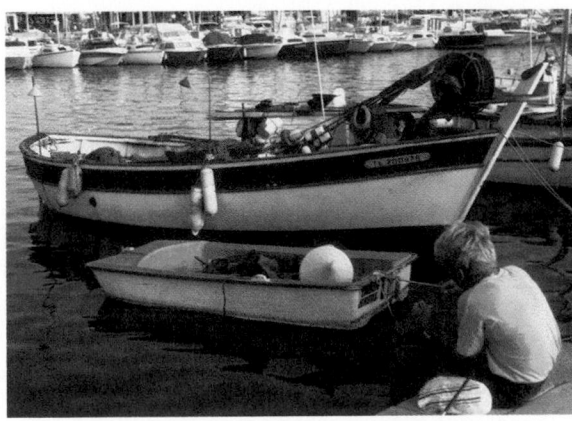

patients are presented with only two stimuli, one in each field, they report seeing only the stimulus in the ipsilateral hemifield. They do not have the ability to focus attention in the hemifield contralateral to the lesion, and as a result they may not see everything in that hemifield, even though the sensory pathway from the eye to the striate and prestriate cortex is intact.

This neglect of the contralateral visual hemifield extends to the neglect of the contralateral half of individual objects. Patients with right parietal deficits often have difficulty reproducing drawings. When asked to draw a clock, for example, they may force all of the numbers into the right side of the face (see Figure 17–11), or when asked to draw a candlestick they may draw only its right side (Figure 29–4).

The process of attentional selection is evident at the level of single parietal neurons in the monkey. The responses of neurons in the lateral intraparietal area to a visual stimulus depend not only on the physical properties of the stimulus but also on how the monkey behaves toward it. When a monkey fixates a spot, a stimulus in the neuron's receptive field evokes a moderate response. When the animal must attend to the same stimulus, the stimulus evokes a greater response, often by a factor of two. Conditions that evoke both involuntary and voluntary attention—the abrupt onset of a visual stimulus in the receptive field or the planning of a saccade to the receptive field of the neuron—evoke still greater responses (Box 29–1).

Neurons in the lateral intraparietal area collectively represent the entire visual hemifield, but the neurons active at any one moment represent only the important or salient objects in the hemifield. That is, a few salient objects—such as the goal of an eye movement or a recent flash—evoke responses in a subset of neurons, and the activity of these neurons is greater than the background activity of the entire population of cells. Both the attention mechanisms and saccades are directed to the peak of the map.

The absolute value of the response evoked by a salient stimulus does not determine whether the stimulus is the most likely saccade target or most highly attended stimulus. When a monkey plans a saccade to

Figure 29–3 Change blindness. In this example one picture is presented followed by a blank for 80 ms, followed by the second picture, another blank, and a repeat of the cycle. The subject is asked to report what changed in the scene. There is a substantial and, once perceived, obvious change between the two pictures. It takes multiple repetitions for most observers to detect the difference. (Reproduced, with permission, from Ronald Rensink.)

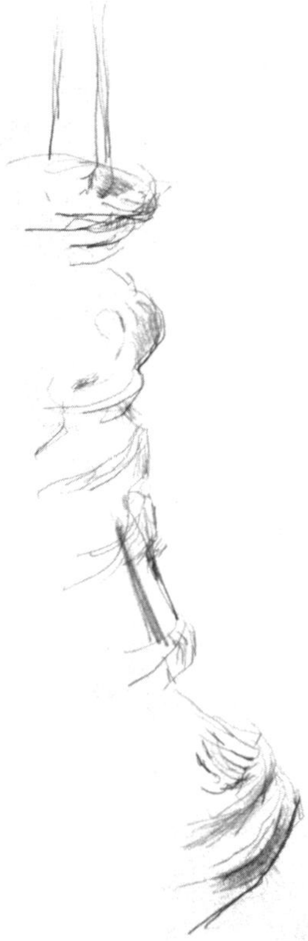

Figure 29–4 Drawing of a candlestick by a patient with a right parietal lesion. The patient neglects the left side of the candlestick, drawing only its right half. (Reproduced, with permission, from Peter Halligan.)

a stimulus in the visual field, attention is on the goal of the saccade, and the activity evoked by the saccade plan lies at the peak of the salience map. However, if a bright light appears elsewhere in the visual field, attention is involuntarily drawn to the bright light, which evokes more neuronal activity than does the saccade plan. Thus the locus of attention can be ascertained only by examining the entire salience map and choosing its peak; it cannot be identified by monitoring activity at one point alone.

The Visual Scene Remains Stable Despite Continual Shifts in the Retinal Image

Saccades create a major challenge for visual processing. Successive saccades produce a series of discrete images, each centered where the eye is looking (Figure 29–8). Although this result might be expected to resemble a home movie with the camera moving about in a jumpy fashion, it does not. How visual scenes remain stable despite repeated shifts in focus has been a source of speculation since the 1600s.

Although the basis of this stability is not understood, changes in perception at the time of a saccade offer clues. At the time of a saccade, objects in the perceived scene do not have exactly the same spatial arrangement as in the visual field. The perceived scene appears spatially compressed such that stimuli presented just before the saccade appear closer to the presaccade point of fixation, whereas stimuli presented after the saccade appear to be closer to the saccade's target (Figure 29–9).

This spatial compression is usually no larger than half the size of the saccade and occurs only when there is a larger visual scene. It is not due to stimuli falling on different parts of the retina because of the saccade, for stimuli presented before the saccade also appear compressed. These considerations indicate that some extravisual information is involved in the processing of saccade commands.

What neuronal mechanism might underlie this apparent shift in images at the time of saccades? Neurons in the parietal cortex alter their activity preceding saccades in ways that seem remarkably related to the perceptual phenomenon. When a monkey is about to make a saccade, a neuron becomes less sensitive to the stimulus already present in its receptive field and begins to respond to the stimulus that will be within the receptive field after the saccade (Figure 29–10).

This shift in selectivity can begin even before the saccade commences. Not every stimulus in the visual field will activate the neuron, only those that will fall in the neuron's receptive field after the saccade. After completion of the saccade, the neuron is again activated only by those stimuli that are actually within its receptive field.

These observations reveal two neuronal mechanisms that contribute to the stabilization of the visual scene during saccades. First, neurons shift their receptive fields from one part of the visual field to another before the saccade occurs. This shift in receptive field is comparable to the change in perceived location of stimuli before the saccade and might contribute to the compression in the perceived visual scene at the time of the saccade. The output of the parietal neurons is interpreted as indicating that stimuli are present in one part of the visual field, although at the time of the saccade the neurons are responding to stimuli that will be in their receptive field after the saccade as well as to stimuli presently within the receptive field. If the brain assumes that stimuli at both locations are joined together, this could account for the compression of the perceived scene.

Second, because the new receptive-field position after a saccade depends on the amplitude and direction of the saccade, the parietal neurons must have advance information about the saccade. There are only two potential sources of this information. One is the feedback to the brain from the peripheral proprioceptors in the eye muscles that could inform the brain that the eye is moving. This is unlikely because both the receptive field shifts and the perceptual compression begin even before the eye moves, and the cortical representation of eye position lags the eye movement by nearly 100 ms. The second potential source is the motor system that controls movement of the eyes (see Chapter 39). This system could send a copy of its signals, known as a corollary discharge or efference copy, to the parietal cortex to inform it that the saccade is about to occur. This signal would provide the information on the amplitude and direction of the impending saccade needed to compute the new receptive-field location before the saccade actually occurs.

The specific source of a corollary discharge to the parietal cortex remains unknown, but neurons in the frontal eye field that show shifts in receptive-field sensitivity similar to those in the lateral intraparietal area do receive an identified corollary discharge. The source of this corollary discharge is the saccade-generating neurons in the superior colliculus. Because the parietal cortex and frontal eye field have strong reciprocal connections, the same corollary discharge input could affect both structures.

The corollary discharge from the superior colliculus reaches the frontal eye field through a relay in a higher-order thalamic nucleus, the medial dorsal nucleus (Figure 29–11A). Neurons in this nucleus signal the amplitude and direction of an impending saccade and could therefore provide the information needed to shift the receptive fields of neurons in the frontal eye field and lateral intraparietal area before the saccade occurs. But do they? Inactivation of neurons in the thalamic relay greatly reduces the ability of frontal eye field neurons to shift their receptive fields prior to a saccade (Figure 29–11B), providing evidence that the shift does depend on an efferent copy of the saccade motor program.

Vision Lapses During Saccades

During a saccade the visual scene is not only displaced but also swept rapidly across the retina as the eye moves at high speed. Because we are unaware of this sweep, the American psychologist Edwin Holt at the beginning of the 20th century posited that there must be a central anesthesia during the eye movement.

But this cannot be true, for there are instances in which vision is quite clear during a saccade. An object can be seen during a saccade if it is moving as fast as the eye and in the same direction, as occurs for example during a saccade in the direction of a car passing the observer in a train. What may instead be the case is that much of the visual scene is ordinarily blurred by the speed of eye movement. But why does the blur not reach consciousness? Two underlying mechanisms in combination probably account for this perceptual omission.

The first mechanism is visual masking, which is the effect one image has on another when the two are presented in rapid succession. For example, a higher-contrast image reduces or eliminates the perception of a lower-contrast image. This happens during a saccade: The rapid movement of the eye over the scene produces a blurred, low-contrast image that is masked by the stable, high-contrast images before and after the saccade. This masking can be demonstrated by an experiment in which high-contrast images are not present before or after the saccade. Under these conditions a blurred image is seen. If a high-contrast image is present after the saccade, however, the blur vanishes (Figure 29–12A).

There are conditions, however, when extravisual input, such as a corollary discharge, also must be present. For example, a coarse grating can be seen even when it moves across the retina at the high speeds of saccades if the bars are oriented in the same direction as the saccade (Figure 29–12B). When the eyes are fixated, low- and middle-frequency gratings can be seen but very high-frequency gratings are not well seen. In contrast, during a saccade the detection of low-frequency gratings is markedly impaired but the highest-frequency gratings remain visible. Thus the reduction of sensitivity during the saccade, known as saccadic suppression, is specific for low-frequency gratings.

These low spatial frequencies are precisely those most likely to escape the effects of visual masking, so that a reduction in sensitivity to these stimuli must result from extravisual input such as a corollary discharge. They are also the best stimuli for the magnocellular component of the geniculostriate pathway, for the parvocellular pathway is more sensitive to high spatial frequencies. Both masking and corollary discharge must jointly act to produce the saccadic suppression that usually eliminates the intrusive motion of the scene during saccades.

Box 29–1 The Effect of Behavioral Significance on Neuronal Responses

The responses of neurons in the lateral intraparietal area to visual stimuli vary with the behavioral significance of stimuli as well as the physical characteristics of the stimuli. This can be demonstrated by recording from neurons while a monkey makes eye movements across a stable array.

Stable objects in the visual world are rarely the objects of attention. In the lateral intraparietal area, as in most other visual centers of the brain, neuronal receptive fields are retinoptic, that is, they are defined relative to the center of gaze. As a monkey scans the visual field, fixed objects enter and leave the receptive fields of neurons with every eye movement without attracting the animal's attention (Figure 29–5).

The abrupt appearance of a visual stimulus can evoke involuntary attention, however. When a light flashes in the receptive field of a lateral intraparietal neuron, that cell responds briskly (Figure 29–6A). In contrast, a stable, task-irrelevant stimulus evokes little response when eye movements bring it into the neuron's receptive field (Figure 29–6B).

When the stimulus appears abruptly outside the receptive field, a saccade brings the attention-commanding stimulus into the receptive field, evoking a large response from the neuron (Figure 29–6C). When the monkey makes the saccade, the objects in the visual field are identical in both cases. However, the stable stimulus is presumably unattended, whereas the light flash evokes attention and provokes a much larger response. Stable objects can evoke enhanced responses when they become relevant to the animal's current behavior.

In the experiment of Figure 29–7 the monkey begins by fixating one of several images outside the receptive field. A cue appears, also outside the receptive field, that tells the monkey which image it should fixate after a saccade to the center of the array of images. If this second target is already in the receptive field the stimulus evokes a large response. If it is not, the stimulus evokes little response when the saccade brings it into the receptive field. Thus attention modulates the activity of neurons in the lateral intraparietal cortex (LIP) regardless of how that attention is evoked.

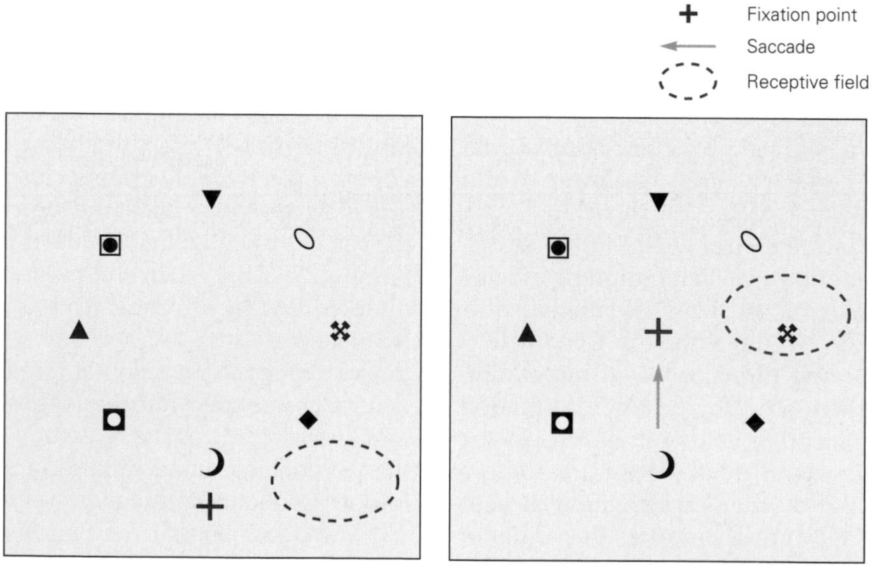

Figures 29–5 Exploring a stable array of objects. The monkey views a screen with a number of objects, which remain in place throughout the experiment. The monkey's gaze can be positioned so that none of the objects are included in the receptive field of a neuron (**left**), or the monkey can make a saccade that brings one of the objects into the receptive field (**right**). (Reproduced, with permission, from Kusunoki, Gottlieb, and Goldberg 2000.)

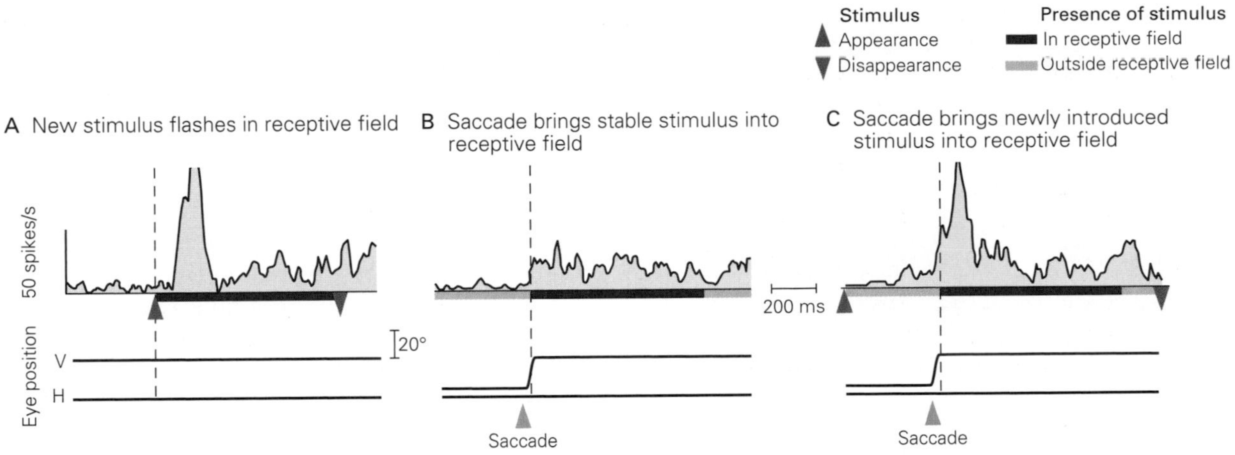

Figures 29–6 A neuron in the lateral intraparietal area fires only in response to salient stimuli. In each panel neuronal activity along with horizontal (**H**) and vertical (**V**) eye positions are plotted against time.

A. A stimulus flashes in the receptive field while the monkey fixates.

B. The monkey makes a saccade that brings a stable, task-irrelevant stimulus into the receptive field.

C. The monkey makes a saccade that brings the position of the recent light flash into the receptive field.

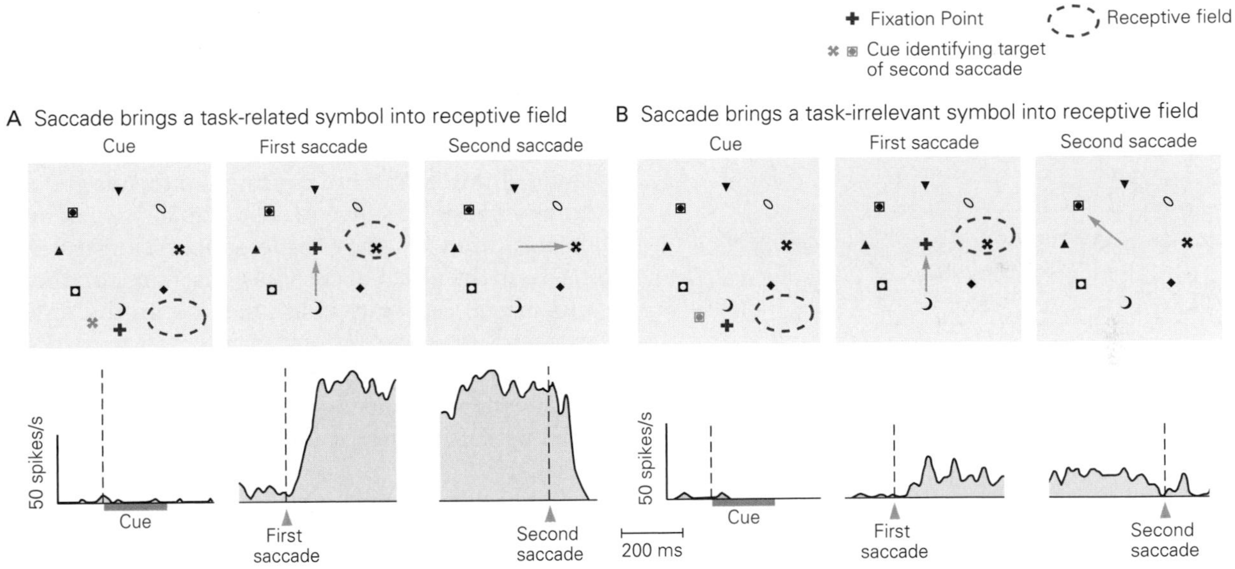

Figures 29–7 A neuron in the lateral intraparietal area fires before a saccade to a stable object. On each trial one object in a stable array becomes significant to the monkey because the monkey must make a saccade to it. The monkey fixates a point outside the array, and a cue that matches an object in the array appears outside the neuron's receptive field. The monkey must then make a saccade to the center of the array and a second saccade to the object that matches the cue. Two experiments are shown, each in three panels. The left panel shows the response to the cue when it appears outside the receptive field, the center panel shows the response after the first saccade that brings the cued object into the receptive field, and the right panel shows the response just before the saccade to the cued object. The cues are shown here in green for clarity but were black in the experiment.

A. The monkey is trained to make the second saccade to the cued object; the cell fires intensely when the first saccade brings the object into the receptive field.

B. The monkey is trained to make the second saccade to an object outside the receptive field; the cell fires much less when the saccade brings the task-irrelevant stimulus into the receptive field. The visual scene at the time of the saccade is identical in both experiments.

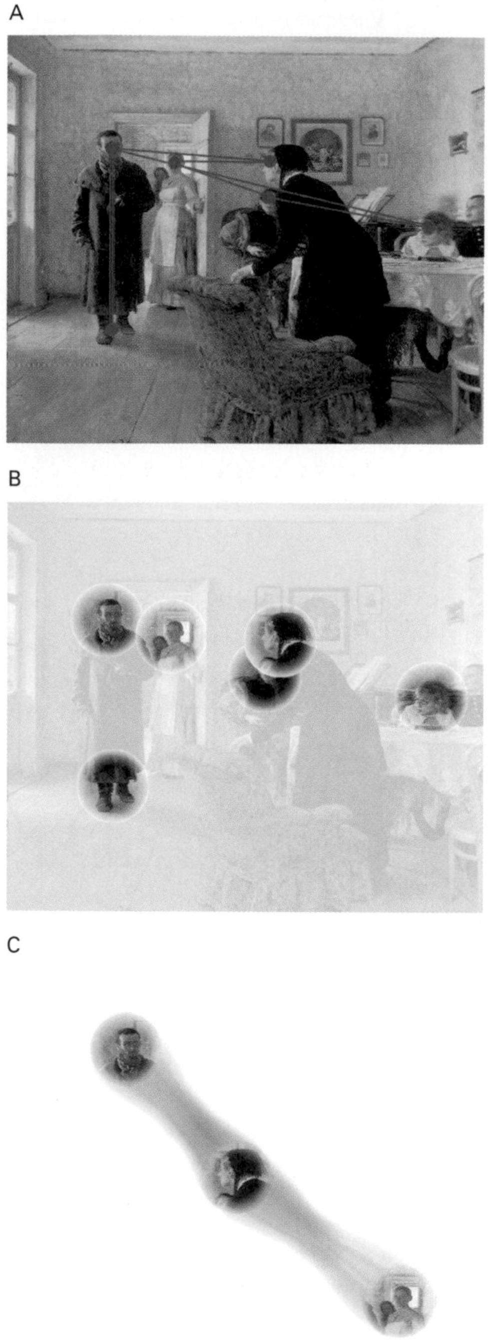

Figure 29–8 Saccades present the brain with rapid changes in the retinal image. (Reproduced, with permission, from Wurtz 2008.)

A. Saccades (**blue lines**) result in a series of fixations at various locations in the visual field (**blue dots**)

B. The successive fixations are represented here as isolated foveal images.

C. The sensory signals for successive fixations provide no information about the location of each fixation. The visual information from each fixation is interspersed with the blurs from the intervening saccades.

Changes in neuronal activity that are associated with a reduction of visual sensitivity have been found along the visual pathway and are probably due to both visual masking and corollary discharge. Neuronal correlates of visual masking are evident in the responses of neurons in the primary visual cortex. Many V1 neurons fire when eye movement sweeps a lone stimulus across their receptive fields but do not fire when another stimulus falls within their receptive fields just before the saccade (Figure 29–13A). The masking effect of the stimulus falling within the receptive fields before the saccade is analogous to the stationary visual scene before and after a saccade masking the blur of the scene during the saccade. The same masking occurs when moving stimuli sweep across the receptive fields at saccade speeds while the monkey continues to fixate. This neuronal masking effect therefore stems entirely from visual processing; no saccade is required.

Saccadic suppression due to corollary discharge is most pronounced for stimuli with low spatial frequency and high contrast, the stimuli that are most effective for activating neurons in the magnocellular pathway of the visual system. During saccades the activity of neurons in the lateral geniculate nucleus is altered and frequently reduced, but the suppression is limited and not confined to the magnocellular layers. In the absence of visual masking, neurons in cortical area V1 show little suppression during saccades so the effect of corollary discharge on the geniculocortical pathway is limited. But in the regions of extrastriate cortex devoted to motion processing, the middle temporal and medial superior temporal areas, there is clear suppression of visual stimuli during saccades that could result from a corollary discharge.

When eye movement sweeps the stimulus across the retina, neurons do not respond, but when the stimulus is moved at the same speed in front of the stationary eye, these same neurons fire robustly (Figure 29–13B). The likely explanation of this difference is that a corollary discharge of the saccade command reduces the response of the neurons to the stimulus. One possible source of this corollary discharge is the superior-collicular signal that shifts receptive fields in frontal and parietal cortex. This is a likely possibility because visual neurons in the superior colliculus are also suppressed during saccades and this suppression stems from corollary discharge.

At both the neuronal and behavioral levels, then, there is evidence that visual masking and corollary discharge act together to reduce the disruption of vision during saccades.

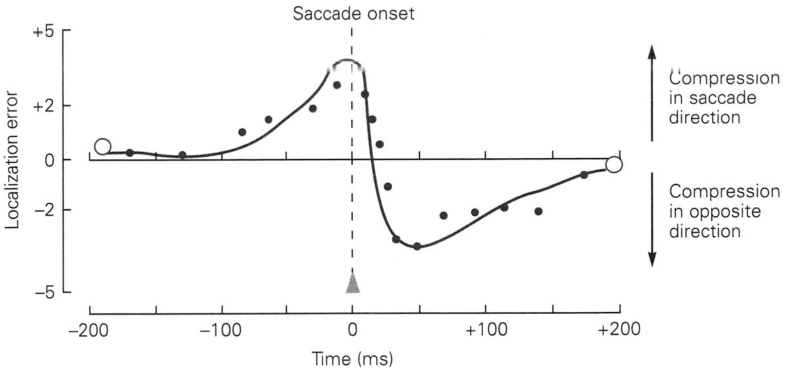

Figure 29–9 Compression of visual space at the time of a saccade. The perceived location of a stimulus presented just before or after a saccade is shifted toward the target of the saccade. (Reproduced, with permission, from Honda 1991.)

The Parietal Cortex Provides Visual Information to the Motor System

Vision interacts with the supplementary and premotor systems to prepare the hands for action. When you pick up a pencil your fingers are separated from your thumb by the width of a pencil; when you pick up a drink your fingers are separated from your thumb by the width of the glass. The visual system helps to adjust the grip width before your hand arrives at the

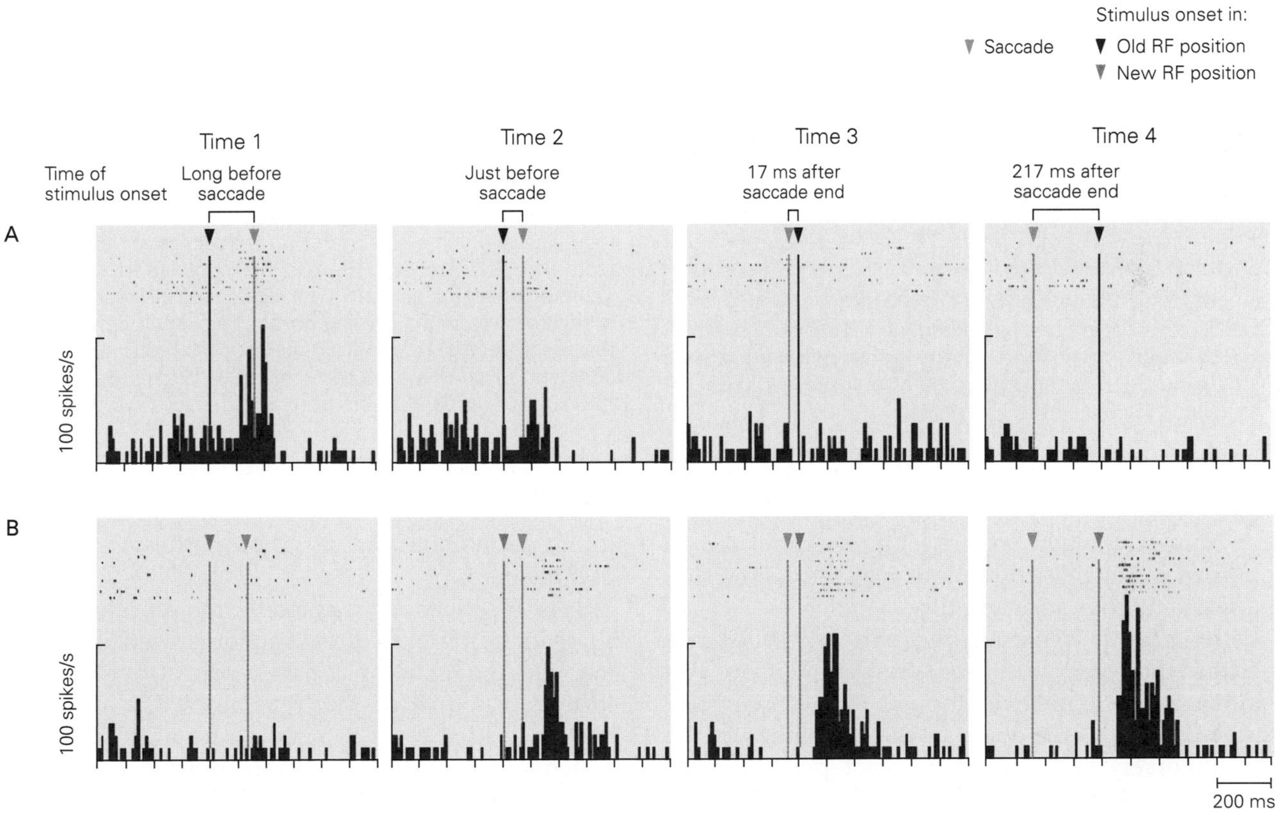

Figure 29–10 Activity in a parietal cortex neuron anticipates a change in position of its receptive field due to a saccade. Neuronal activity is aligned to the stimulus onset. The response of the cell to a stimulus in its receptive field decreases, even before the onset of the saccade (**A**), while its response to a stimulus in the anticipated postsaccade position of its receptive field increases (**B**). (Modified, with permission, from Nakamura and Colby 2002.)

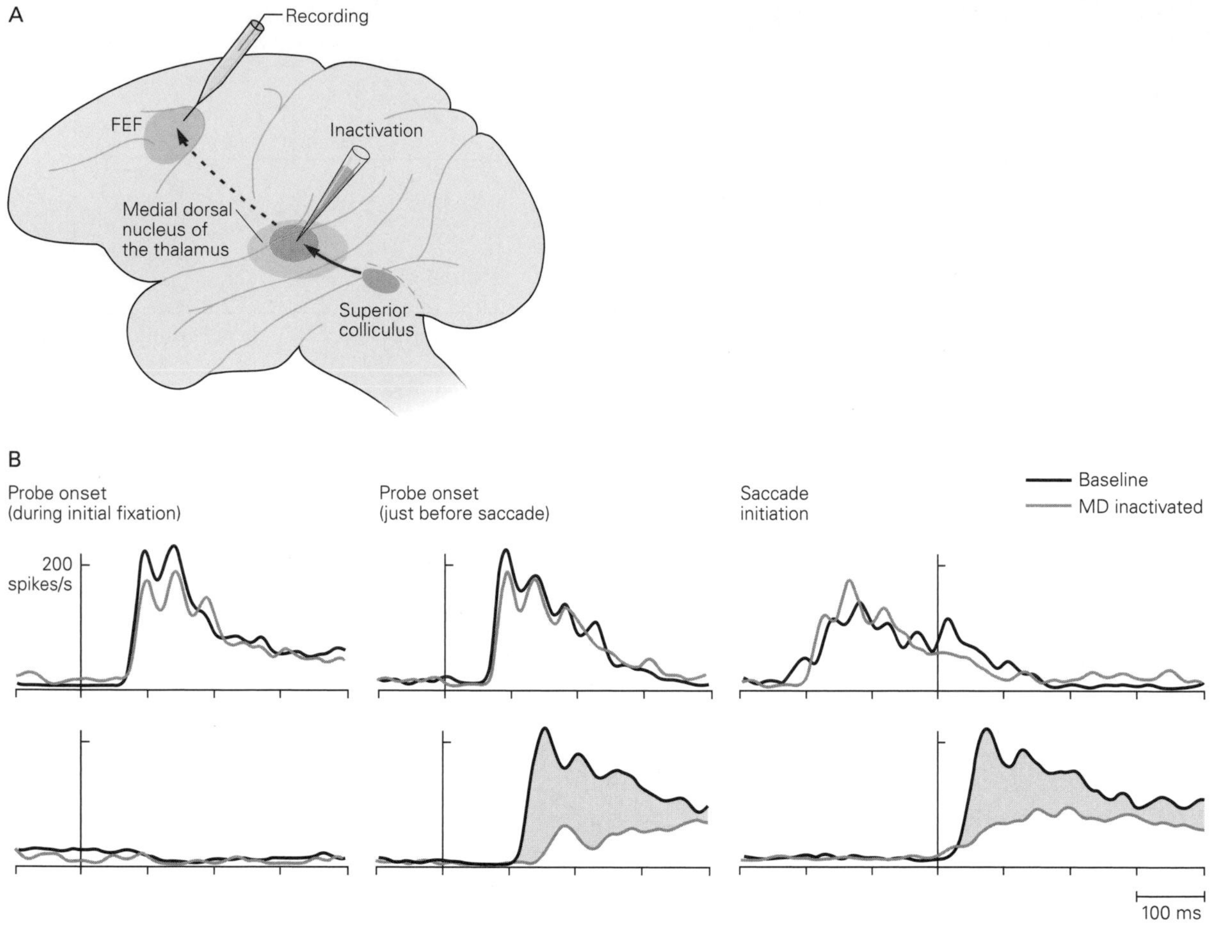

Figure 29–11 A corollary discharge from the motor program for saccades directs presaccade shifts in receptive-field location for frontal eye field neurons.

A. One possible pathway for a corollary discharge to the cerebral cortex originates in saccade-generating neurons in the superior colliculus, passes through the medial dorsal nucleus of the thalamus, and terminates in the frontal eye field (**FEF**) in the frontal cortex.

B. When the medial dorsal nucleus (**MD**) is inactivated, the response to a stimulus currently in the receptive field is unaffected (**upper records**), whereas the response to a stimulus in the prospective (postsaccade) location of the receptive field is severely impaired (**lower records**). This result demonstrates that a corollary discharge from the saccade motor program directs the shift in the neuron's receptive field properties. (Modified, with permission, from Sommer and Wurtz 2008.)

object. Similarly, when you insert a letter into a mail slot your hand is aligned to place the letter in the slot. If the slot is tilted, your hand tilts to match.

Patients with lesions of the parietal cortex cannot adjust their grip width or wrist angle using visual information alone, even though they can verbally describe the size of the object or the orientation of the slot. Conversely, patients with intact parietal lobes and deficits in the ventral stream cannot describe the size of an object or its orientation but can adjust their grip width and orient their hands as well as normal subjects can. The parietal lobe is a critical source of information about the visual properties of the targets of movement.

As described in Chapter 16, the representation of space in the parietal cortex is not organized into a single map like the retinotopic map in primary visual cortex. Instead it is divided into four areas that analyze the visual world in ways appropriate for individual motor systems and project to areas of premotor cortex that control individual movements (Figure 29–14).

The neural operations behind visually guided movements involve identifying targets, specifying their qualities, and ultimately generating a motor program

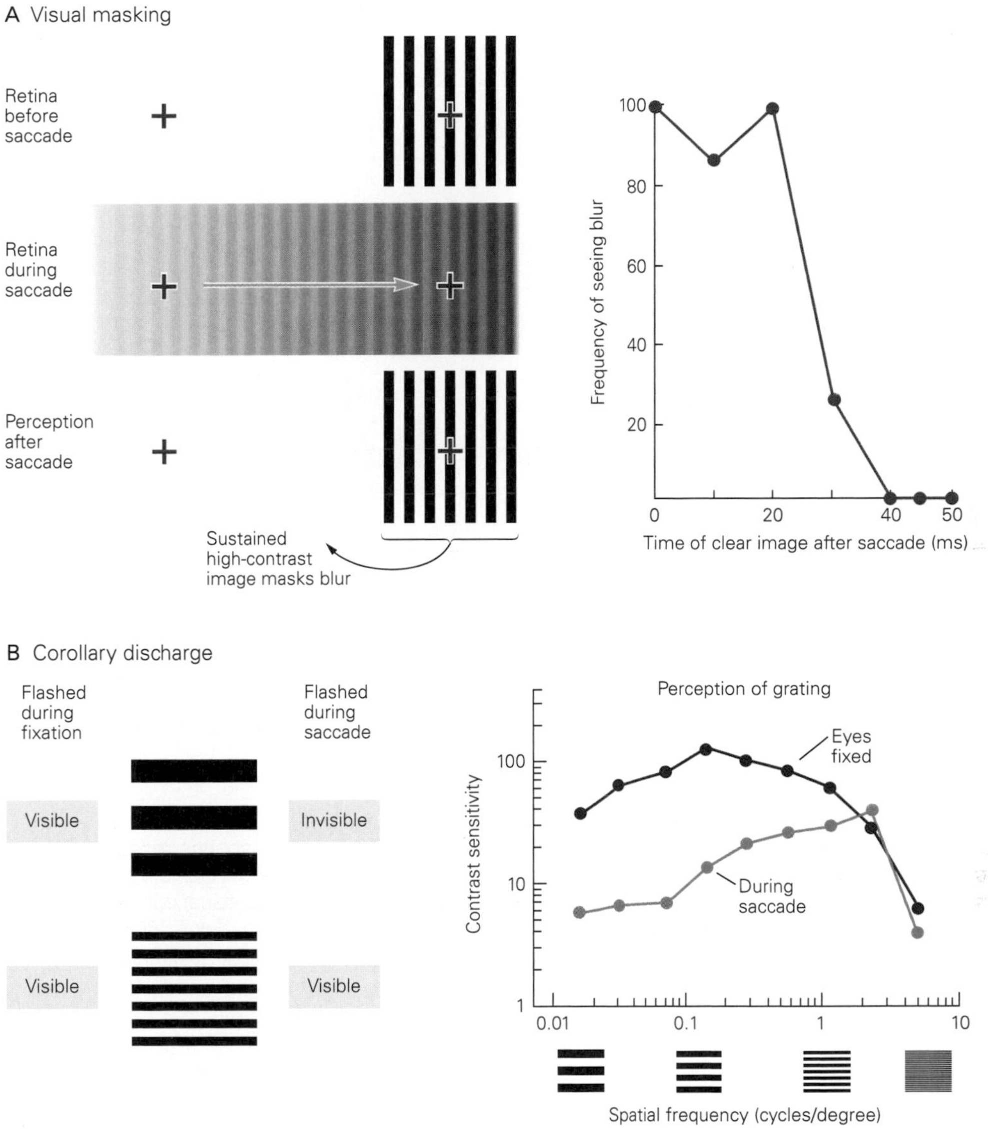

Figure 29–12 Saccadic suppression.

A. Visual masking. When a subject makes a saccade to a stable, high-contrast image (**top**), there is blurred image on the retina (**middle**) but the viewer sees only the high-contrast image after the saccade (**bottom**) and never a blur. If the high-contrast image is present only during the saccade or slightly after, the viewer sees a blur (zero on the horizontal axis of the graph). When the high-contrast image remains on the screen for a longer time after the saccade, the blurred image is no longer evident (40 ms on the graph): The high-contrast image after the saccade masks the low-contrast blur. (Reproduced, with permission, from Campbell and Wurtz 1978.)

B. Corollary discharge. A subject can see a coarse grating (low spatial frequency) much better when it is presented briefly during fixation than when it is presented during a saccade. A fine grating (high spatial frequency) is seen just as well during a saccade as during fixation (nearly superimposed **red** and **blue** data points at 2 cycles per degree). (Reproduced, with permission, from Burr, Morrone, and Ross 1994.)

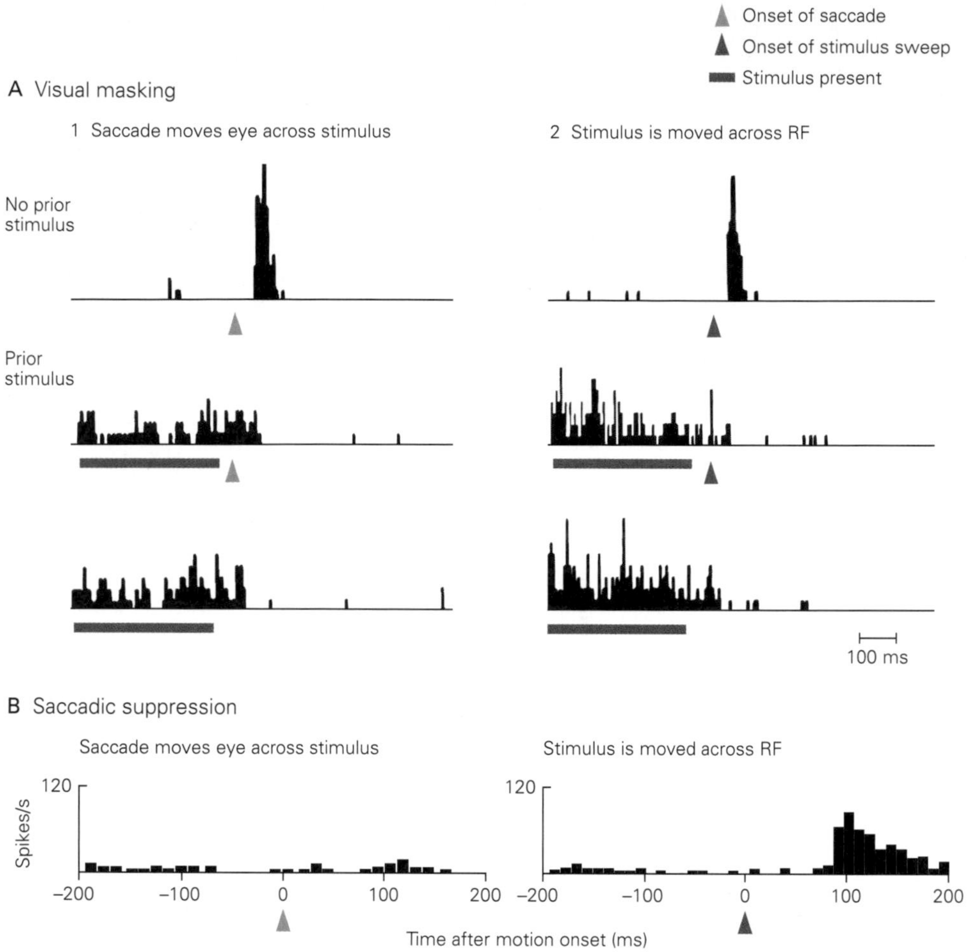

Figure 29–13 Neuronal correlates of saccadic suppression.

A. Visual masking. **1.** When a monkey makes a saccade across a stimulus on a blank screen, a neuron in V1 responds (**upper record**). However, if another stimulus falls in the neuron's receptive field before the saccade, the neuron does not respond to the stimulus flashed during the saccade (**middle record**), and the neuronal response resembles the response to the first stimulus alone (**lower record**). **2.** The same neuron responds if the stimulus is swept across its receptive field (RF) while the eye is stationary (**upper record**) but does not respond to the same stimulus motion when it is preceded by a stationary stimulus within the receptive field (**middle record**). Again the neuron's response resembles the response to the first stimulus alone. This lack of response is a correlate of the masking effect of one visual stimulus on another. (Modified, with permission, from Judge, Wurtz, and Richmond 1980.)

B. Saccadic suppression. A middle temporal area neuron does not fire during a saccade across a stationary stimulus (**left**) but does fire when the stimulus is moved at the same speed in front of the stationary eye (**right**). The difference is taken as evidence that a corollary discharge from the saccade motor system suppresses excitation of the neuron during the saccade. (Modified, with permission, from Thiele et al. 2002.)

to accomplish the movement. Neurons in the parietal cortex provide the visual information necessary for independent movements.

The anterior intraparietal cortex has neurons that signal the size, depth, and orientation of objects that can be grasped. Neurons in this area respond to stimuli that could be the targets for a grasping movement, and also respond when the animal makes the movement (Figure 29–15). Similarly, neurons in the medial intraparietal cortex represent the targets for reaching movements and project to the frontal area that generates the premotor signal for these movements.

The ventral intraparietal area has bimodal neurons that respond to both tactile and visual stimuli in the face (Figure 29–16). This area projects to the face area of premotor cortex. Finally, neurons in the lateral

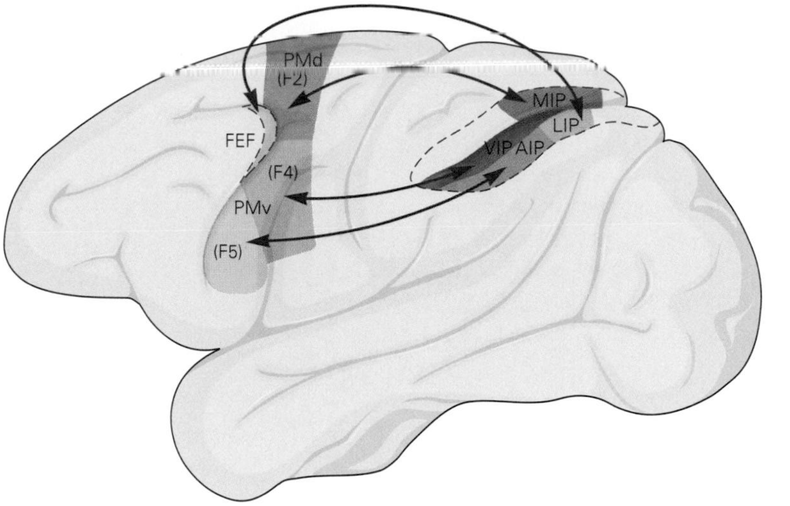

Figure 29–14 Four functionally discrete areas in the intraparietal sulcus project to areas in the premotor cortex. The medial intraparietal cortex (**MIP**) represents targets of arm movements and projects to the arm-control area of F2 in the dorsal premotor area (**PMd**). The lateral intraparietal cortex (**LIP**) represents targets of eye movements and projects to the frontal eye field (**FEF**). The anterior intraparietal cortex (**AIP**) represents targets for grasping and projects to the hand-control area of F5 in the ventral premotor area (**PMv**). The ventral intraparietal cortex (**VIP**) represents the face and projects to the face-control area of F4 in the ventral premotor area. (Reproduced, with permission, from Rizzolatti, Lupino, and Matelli 1998).

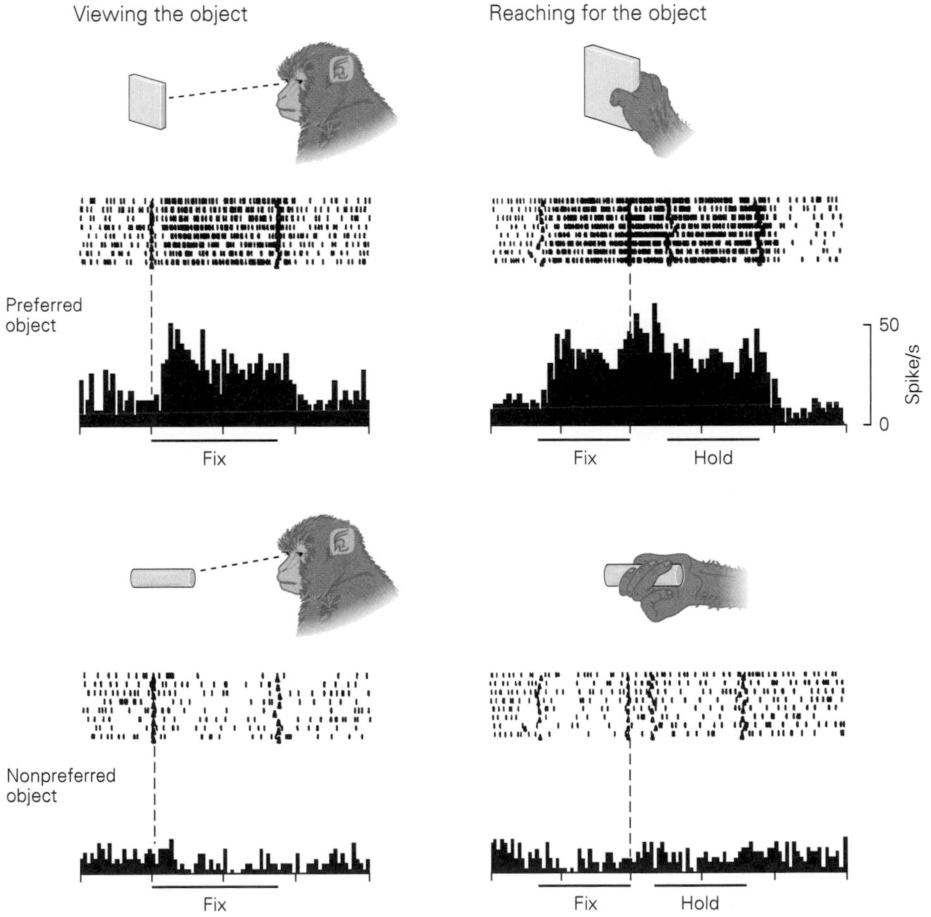

Figure 29–15 Neurons in the anterior intraparietal cortex respond selectively to specific shapes. The neuron shown here is selective for a rectangle, whether viewing the object or reaching for it. The neuron is not responsive to the cylinder in either case. (Reproduced, with permission, from Murata et al. 2000.)

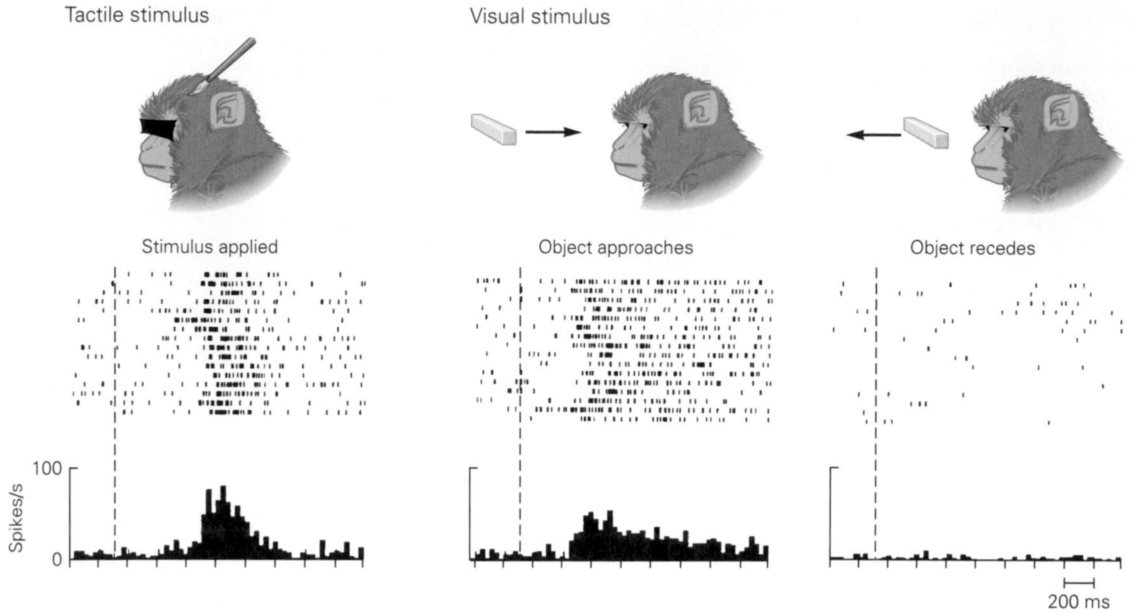

Figure 29–16 Bimodal neurons in the ventral intraparietal cortex of a monkey respond to both visual and tactile stimuli. The neuron shown here responds to tactile stimulation of the monkey's head or to a visual stimulus coming toward the head, but not to the same stimulus moving away from the head. (Reproduced, with permission, from Duhamel et al. 1997.)

intraparietal area describe the targets for saccadic eye movements and project to the frontal eye field.

An Overall View

The visual cortex is interconnected by ventral and dorsal streams of neuronal processing. The ventral stream provides information about the nature of the objects represented; the dorsal stream provides information that the oculomotor and skeletal motor system can use for movement.

A critical function of the dorsal stream is to mediate attention, which is necessary in order to select objects in the visual field for further analysis. Neurons in the parietal lobe of the monkey respond more vigorously to attended objects than to unattended ones, and the activity of neurons in the monkey's parietal lobe mirrors the attention paid to certain objects in the environment.

Because visual information enters the brain through eyes that are constantly moving, the brain requires a mechanism to compensate for eye movements, constructing a stable visual world from successive fixations. Information supplied by the motor system through corollary discharges is used to adjust the receptive fields of visual neurons to compensate for intervening eye movements. The parietal lobe has a number of distinct representations of the visual field, each of which provides information to a specific motor subsystem.

Michael E. Goldberg
Robert H. Wurtz

Selected Readings

Bisley JW, Goldberg ME. 2003. Neuronal activity in the lateral intraparietal area and spatial attention. Science 299:81–86.

Cohen YE, Andersen RA. 2002. A common reference frame for movement plans in the posterior parietal cortex. Nat Rev Neurosci 3:553–562.

Duhamel J-R, Colby CL, Goldberg ME. 1992. The updating of the representation of visual space in parietal cortex by intended eye movements. Science 255:90–92.

Henderson JM, Hollingworth A. 1999. High-level scene perception. Annu Rev Psychol 50:243–271.

Milner AD, Goodale MA. 1996. *The Visual Brain in Action.* Oxford: Oxford Univ. Press.

Morrone MC, Ross J, Burr DC. 1997. Apparent position of visual targets during real and simulated saccadic eye movements. J Neurosci 17:7941–7953.

Rensink RA. 2002. Change detection. Annu Rev Psychol 53:245–277.

Ross J, Concetta Morrone M, Goldberg ME, Burr DC. 2001. Changes in visual perception at the time of saccades. Trends Neurosci 24:113–121.

Ross J, Ma-Wyatt A. 2004. Saccades actively maintain perceptual continuity. Nat Neurosci 7:65–69.

Sommer MA, Wurtz RH. 2008. Brain circuits for the internal monitoring of movements. Annu Rev Neurosci 31: 317–338.

Wurtz RH. 2008. Neuronal mechanisms of visual stability. Vision Res 48:2070–2089.

References

Burr DC, Morrone MC, Ross J. 1994. Selective suppression of the magnocellular visual pathway during saccadic eye movements. Nature 371:511–513.

Burr DC, Ross J. 1982. Contrast sensitivity at high velocities. Vision Res 22:479–484.

Campbell FW, Wurtz RH. 1978. Saccadic omission: why we do not see a grey-out during a saccadic eye movement. Vision Res 18:1297–1303.

Duhamel J-R, Bremmer F, BenHamed S, Graf W. 1997. Spatial invariance of visual receptive fields in parietal cortex neurons. Nature 389:845–848.

Duhamel J-R, Colby CL, Goldberg ME. 1998. Ventral intraparietal area of the macaque: congruent visual and somatic response properties. J Neurophysiol 79: 126–136.

Duhamel J-R, Goldberg ME, FitzGibbon EJ, Sirigu A, Grafman J. 1992. Saccadic dysmetria in a patient with a right frontoparietal lesion: the importance of corollary discharge for accurate spatial behavior. Brain 115:1387–1402.

Goodale MA, Meenan JP, Bulthoff HH, Nicolle DA, Murphy KJ, Racicot CI. 1994. Separate neural pathways for the visual analysis of object shape in perception and prehension. Curr Biol 4:604–610.

Henderson JM, Hollingworth A. 2003. Global transsaccadic change blindness during scene perception. Psychol Sci 14:493–497.

Hollingworth A, Henderson JM. 2002. Accurate visual memory for previously attended objects in natural scenes. J Exp Psychol Hum Percept Perform 25:113–136.

Honda H. 1991. The time courses of visual mislocalization and of extraretinal eye position signals at the time of vertical saccades. Vision Res 31:1915–1921.

Judge SJ, Wurtz RH, Richmond BJ. 1980. Vision during saccadic eye movements. I. Visual interactions in striate cortex. J Neurophysiol 43:1133–1155.

Kusunoki M, Gottlieb J, Goldberg ME. 2000. The lateral intraparietal motion, and task relevance. Vision Res 40:1459–1468.

Murata A, Gallese V, Luppino G, Kaseda M, Sakata H. 2000. Selectivity for the shape, size, and orientation of objects for grasping in neurons of monkey parietal area AIP. J Neurophysiol 83:2580–2601.

Nakamura K, Colby CL. 2002. Updating of the visual representation in monkey striate and extrastriate cortex during saccades. Proc Natl Acad Sci U S A 99:4026–4031.

Perenin MT, Vighetto A. 1988. Optic ataxia: a specific disruption in visuomotor mechanisms. I. Different aspects of the deficit in reaching for objects. Brain 111:643–674.

Rizzolatti G, Luppino G, Matelli M. 1998. The organization of the cortical motor system: new concepts. Electroencephalogr Clin Neurophysiol 106:283–296.

Ross J, Morrone MC, Burr DC. 1997. Compression of visual space before saccades. Nature 386:598–601.

Snyder LH, Batista AP, Andersen RA. 1997. Coding of intention in the posterior parietal cortex. Nature 386:167–170.

Thiele A, Henning P, Kubischik M, Hoffmann KP. 2002. Neural mechanisms of saccadic suppression. Science 295:2460–2462.

Yarbus AL. 1967. *Eye Movements and Vision.* New York: Plenum.

30

The Inner Ear

HUMAN EXPERIENCE IS ENRICHED by our ability to distinguish a remarkable range of sounds—from the intimacy of a whisper to the warmth of a conversation, from the complexity of a symphony to the roar of a stadium. Hearing begins when the cochlea, the snail-shaped receptor organ of the inner ear, transduces sound energy into electrical signals and forwards them to the brain. Our ability to recognize small differences in sounds stems from the cochlea's capacity to distinguish among frequency components and to inform us of both the tones present and their amplitudes.

Deafness can be devastating. For the elderly, hearing loss can result in a painful and protracted estrangement from family, friends, and colleagues. Children may lack hearing as a result of pre- or perinatal infections and especially of genetic conditions, which affect one child in a thousand. Such children are often deprived of the normal avenue to the development of speech, and thus of reading and writing as well. It is for this reason that a modern pediatric examination must include an assessment of hearing. Many children thought to be cognitively impaired are found instead to be hard of hearing, and their intellectual development resumes its normal course when this problem is corrected.

Acute hearing loss in the intermediate years exacts an enormous price for two reasons. First, hearing plays an important, but often overlooked, role in our psychological well-being. Daily conversation with family and colleagues helps to establish our social context. The abrupt loss of such social intercourse as a result of sudden deafness leaves a person distressingly lonely and may lead to depression and even suicide. Hearing also serves us in another, more subtle way. Our auditory system is a remarkably efficient early warning system, subconsciously informing us about our environment. For example, when other people enter the room or approach us we often hear them before we see them. More obviously, awareness of fire alarms and the sirens of emergency vehicles can be lifesaving. Deafness may leave a person with an ominous sense of vulnerability to unheard changes in the environment.

Hearing loss is often accompanied by another distressing symptom, *tinnitus,* or ringing in the ears. By interfering with concentration and disrupting sleep, tinnitus can exasperate, depress, and even madden its victims. Because on rare occasions tinnitus stems from lesions to the auditory pathways, such as acoustic neuromas, it is important in neurological diagnosis to exclude such causes. Most tinnitus, however, is idiopathic: Its cause is uncertain. Some drugs trigger the condition; antimalarial drugs related to quinine and aspirin at the high dosages used in the treatment of rheumatoid arthritis are notorious for this. Often, however, tinnitus occurs at high frequencies to which a damaged ear is no longer sensitive. In these instances tinnitus may reflect hypersensitivity in the deafferented central nervous system, a phenomenon analogous to phantom-limb pain (see Chapter 24).

Hearing depends on the remarkable properties of hair cells, the receptors of the internal ear. Hair cells receive mechanical inputs that correspond to sounds and transduce these signals into electrical responses that are forwarded to the brain for interpretation. These cells can measure motions of atomic dimensions and transduce stimuli ranging from static inputs to those at frequencies of tens of kilohertz. Hair cells also serve as mechanical amplifiers that augment our auditory sensitivity. Each of the paired cochleas contains approximately 16,000 of these cells. Deterioration of hair cells accounts for most of the hearing loss that afflicts more than 30 million Americans.

The Ear Has Three Functional Parts

Sound consists of alternating compressions and rarefactions propagated by an elastic medium, the air, at a speed of approximately 340 m/s. As we are reminded on making the effort to shout, producing these pressure changes requires that work be done on the air by our vocal apparatus or some other sound source. Each of our ears must capture this mechanical energy, transmit it to the receptor organ, and transduce it into electrical signals suitable for neural analysis. These three tasks are the functions of, respectively, the external ear, the middle ear, and the inner ear (Figure 30–1).

The most obvious component of the human external ear is the auricle, a prominent fold of cartilage-supported skin. Much as a parabolic antenna collects

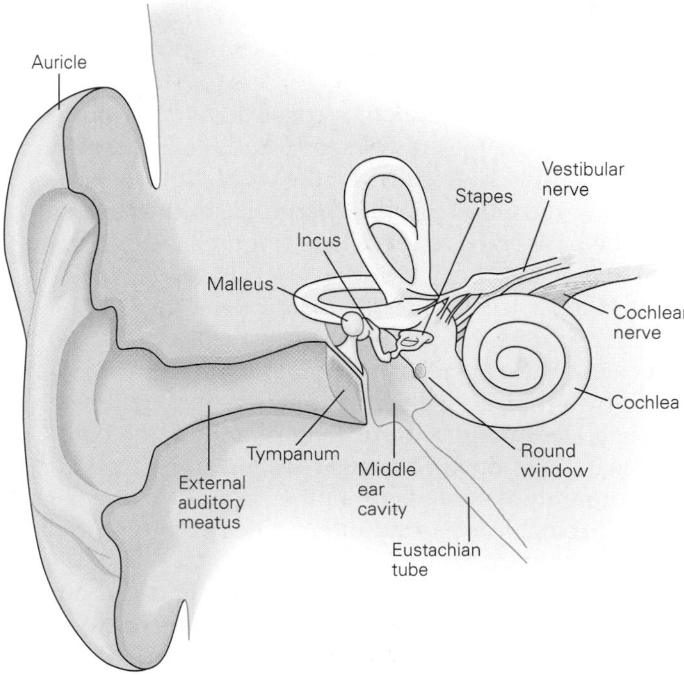

Figure 30–1 The structure of the human ear. The external ear, especially the prominent auricle, focuses sound into the external auditory meatus. Alternating increases and decreases in air pressure vibrate the tympanum. These vibrations are conveyed across the air-filled middle ear by three tiny, linked bones: the malleus, the incus, and the stapes. Vibration of the stapes stimulates the cochlea, the hearing organ of the inner ear.

electromagnetic radiation, the auricle acts as a reflector to capture sound efficiently and to focus it into the external auditory meatus, or ear canal. The external auditory meatus ends at the tympanum or eardrum, a thin diaphragm approximately 9 mm in diameter.

The external ear is not uniformly effective at capturing sound from any direction; the auricle's corrugated surface collects sounds best when they originate at different, but specific, positions with respect to the head. Our capacity to localize sounds in space, especially along the vertical axis, depends critically on the sound-gathering properties of the external ear.

The middle ear is an air-filled pouch connected to the pharynx by the Eustachian tube. Airborne sound traverses the middle ear as vibrations of three tiny ossicles, or bones: the malleus (hammer), incus (anvil), and stapes (stirrup). The base of the malleus is attached to the tympanic membrane; its other extreme makes a ligamentous connection to the incus, which is similarly connected to the stapes. The flattened termination of the stapes, the footplate, inserts in an opening—the oval window—in the bony covering of the cochlea. The first two ossicles are relics of evolution, for their antecedents served as components of the jaw in reptilian ancestors.

The inner ear, or cochlea (from the Greek *cochlos,* meaning snail), is a coiled structure of progressively diminishing diameter wound like a snail's shell around a conical bony core (Figure 30–1). It is approximately 9 mm across, the size of a chickpea. The cochlea is covered with a thin layer of laminar bone and embedded within the dense structure of the temporal bone. The inner and outer aspects of the cochlea's bony surface are lined with layers of connective tissue, the endosteum and periosteum.

The interior of the cochlea consists of three liquid-filled compartments termed *scalae* (Latin, meaning staircases). In a cross section of the cochlea at any position along its spiral course, the compartment farthest from the base is the *scala vestibuli* (Figure 30–2). At the basal end of this chamber is the oval window, an opening that is sealed by the footplate of the stapes. The chamber nearest the cochlear base is the *scala tympani;* it too has a basal aperture, the round window, which is closed by a thin, elastic diaphragm. The two chambers are separated along most of their length by the cochlear partition or duct. The scala vestibuli and scala tympani communicate with one another at the helicotrema, where the cochlear partition terminates slightly below the cochlear apex.

The third liquid-filled cavity, the *scala media,* lies within the cochlear partition. A pair of elastic structures separates the scala media from the other ducts (Figure 30–2). The thin Reissner's membrane, or vestibular membrane, divides the scala media from the scala vestibuli. The basilar membrane separates the scala media from the subjacent scala tympani; it is a complex structure involved in auditory transduction.

Hearing Commences with the Capture of Sound Energy by the Ear

Psychophysical experiments have established that we perceive an approximately equal increment in loudness for each tenfold increase in the amplitude of a sound stimulus. This type of relation is characteristic of many of our senses and is the basis of the Weber-Fechner law (see Chapter 21). A logarithmic scale is therefore useful in relating quantitatively sound intensity to perceived loudness. The sound-pressure level, L, of any sound may be expressed in decibels as

$$L = 20 \cdot \log_{10}(P/P_{REF}),$$

in which P, the magnitude of the stimulus, is the root-mean-square sound pressure (in units of pascals, abbreviated Pa, or newtons per square meter). For a sinusoidal stimulus the amplitude exceeds the root-mean-square value by a factor of $\sqrt{2}$. The reference level on this scale, 0 dB, corresponds to a root-mean-square sound pressure, P_{REF}, of 20 μPa. This level represents the approximate threshold of human hearing at 1 to 4 kHz, the frequency range in which our ears are most sensitive.

That sound consists of alternating changes in the local air pressure is evident when a loud noise rattles a window. The loudest sound tolerable to humans, with an intensity of approximately 120 dB, transiently alters the local atmospheric pressure by only ±0.01%. Acting on a window 1 m on each side, this oscillatory pressure nonetheless produces a force of ±14 newtons. To rattle the same window by pushing upon it, we would need to exert a comparable force, approximately ±3 lb. In contrast, a tone at the threshold level causes a fractional change in the local pressure of much less than one part in a billion.

Despite their small magnitude, sound-induced increases and decreases in air pressure push and pull effectively upon the tympanum, moving it inward and outward (Figure 30–3A, B). The subsequent motions of the ossicles are complex, depending on both the frequency and the intensity of sound. In simple terms, however, the actions of these bones may be understood as those of two interconnected levers (the malleus and incus) and a piston (the stapes). The vibration of the incus alternately drives the stapes deeper into the oval

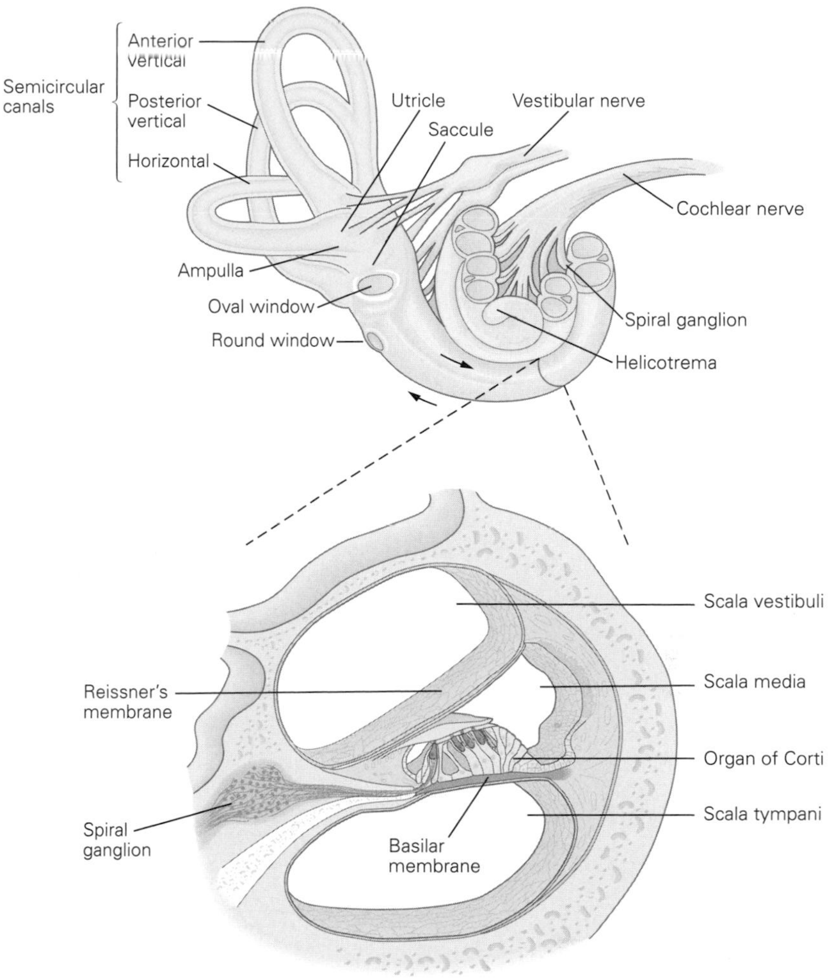

Figure 30–2 The structure of the cochlea. A cross section of the cochlea shows the arrangement of the three liquid-filled ducts or scalae, each of which is approximately 33 mm long. The scala vestibuli and scala tympani communicate through the helicotrema at the apex of the cochlea. At the base each duct is closed by a sealed aperture. The scala vestibuli is closed by the oval window, against which the stapes pushes in response to sound; the scala tympani is closed by the round window, a thin, flexible membrane. Between these two compartments lies the scala media, an endolymph-filled tube whose epithelial lining includes the 16,000 hair cells in the organ of Corti surmounting the basilar membrane. The cross section in the lower diagram has been rotated so that the cochlear apex is oriented toward the top.

window and retracts it. The footplate of the stapes thus serves as a piston that pushes and pulls cyclically upon the liquid in the scala vestibuli. The overall effect of the middle ear is to match the impedance of the air outside the ear to that of the cochlear partition, thus ensuring the efficient transfer of sound energy from the first medium to the second.

The action of the stapes at the oval window produces changes in pressure that propagate throughout the liquid of the scala vestibuli at the speed of sound. Because the aqueous perilymph is virtually incompressible, however, the primary effect of the stapes's motion is to displace the liquid in the scala vestibuli in the one direction that is not restricted by a rigid boundary: toward the elastic cochlear partition (Figure 30–3B). The deflection of the cochlear partition downward increases the pressure in the scala tympani. The enhanced pressure displaces a liquid mass that causes outward bowing of the round window. Each cycle of a sound stimulus thus evokes a cycle of up-and-down movement of a minuscule volume of liquid in each of the inner ear's three chambers.

Because the energy associated with acoustic signals is generally quite small, compromise of the middle ear's normal structure may lead to *conductive hearing loss,* of which two forms are especially common. First, scar tissue caused by middle-ear infection (otitis media) can immobilize the tympanum or ossicles. Second, a proliferation of bone in the ligamentous attachments of the ossicles can deprive the ossicles of their normal freedom of motion. This chronic condition of unknown origin, termed *otosclerosis,* can lead to severe deafness.

A clinician may test for conductive hearing loss by the simple Rinné test. A patient is asked to compare the loudness of a vibrating tuning fork held in the air near an affected ear with that perceived when the base of the tuning fork is pressed against the patient's head just

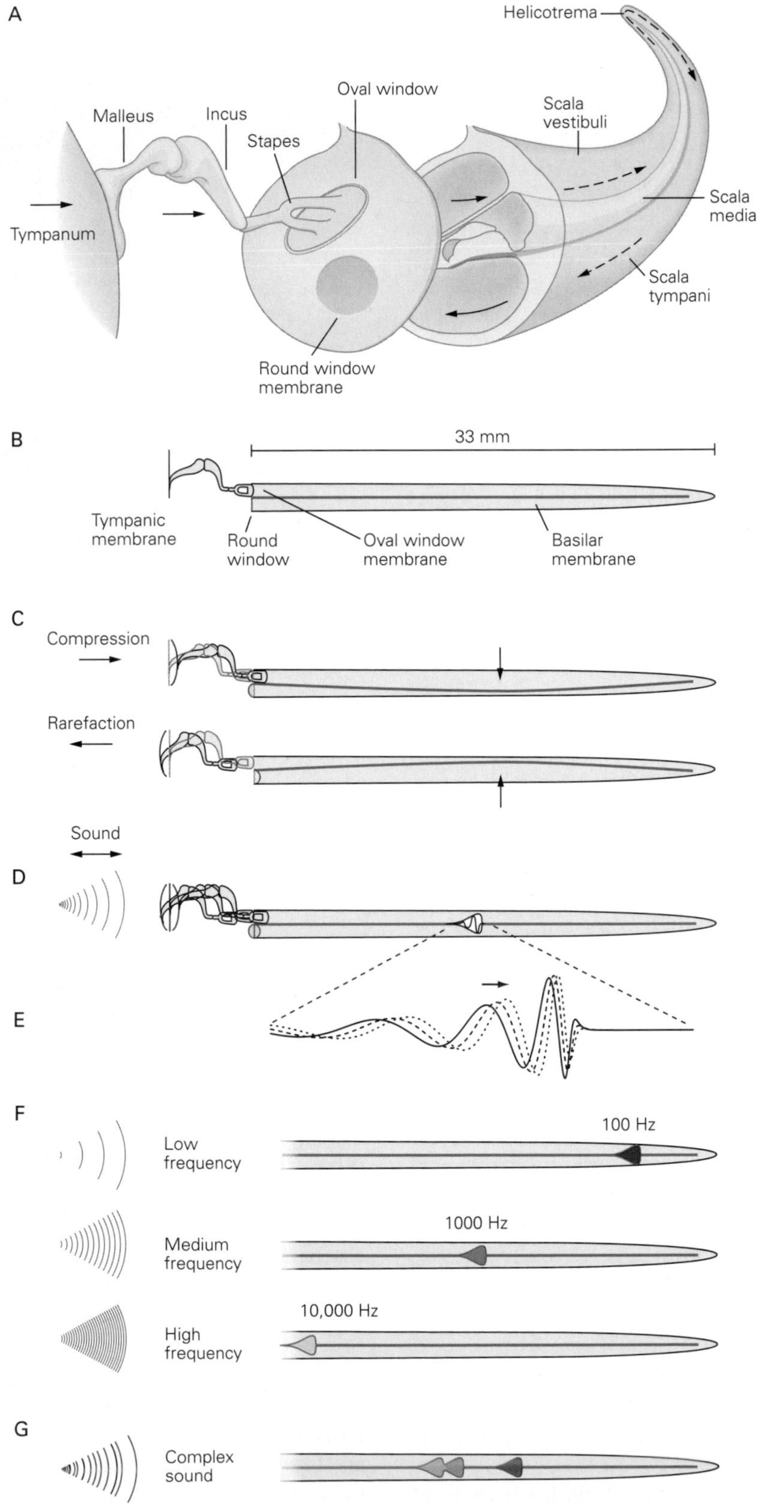
A
Helicotrema
Oval window
Malleus
Incus
Stapes
Scala vestibuli
Scala media
Tympanum
Scala tympani
Round window membrane
B
33 mm
Tympanic membrane
Round window
Oval window membrane
Basilar membrane
C
Compression
Rarefaction
Sound
D
E
F
100 Hz
Low frequency
1000 Hz
Medium frequency
10,000 Hz
High frequency
G
Complex sound

behind the auricle. If the latter stimulus is perceived to be louder, the patient's conductive pathway may be damaged but the internal ear is likely to be intact. In contrast, if bone conduction is not more efficient than airborne stimulation, the patient may have inner-ear damage, that is, sensorineural hearing loss. The diagnosis of conductive hearing loss is important because surgical intervention is highly effective: Removal of scar tissue or reconstitution of the conductive pathway with an inert prosthesis can in many instances restore excellent hearing.

The Hydrodynamic and Mechanical Apparatus of the Cochlea Delivers Mechanical Stimuli to the Receptor Cells

The Basilar Membrane Is a Mechanical Analyzer of Sound Frequency

The mechanical properties of the basilar membrane are key to the cochlea's operation. To appreciate this, suppose that the basilar membrane had uniform dimensions and mechanical properties along its entire length, approximately 33 mm. Under these conditions a fluctuating pressure difference between the scala vestibuli and the scala tympani would move the entire basilar membrane up and down with similar excursions at all points (Figure 30–3C).

This would occur regardless of the frequency of stimulation; any pressure difference between the scala vestibuli and the scala tympani would propagate throughout those chambers within microseconds, so the basilar membrane would be subjected to similar forces at any position along its length. This simple form of basilar-membrane motion in fact occurs in the auditory organs of some reptiles.

In reality, however, the mechanical properties of the mammalian basilar membrane vary continuously along the cochlea's length. The basilar membrane at the apex of the human cochlea is more than five times as broad as at the base. Thus, although the cochlear chambers become progressively larger from the organ's apex toward its base, the basilar membrane *decreases* in width. Moreover, the basilar membrane is

Figure 30–3 (Opposite) Motion of the basilar membrane.

A. An uncoiled cochlea, with its base displaced to show its relation to the scalae, indicates the flow of stimulus energy. Sound vibrates the tympanum, which sets the three ossicles of the middle ear in motion. The piston-like action of the stapes, a bone inserted partially into the elastic oval window, produces oscillatory pressure differences that rapidly propagate along the scala vestibuli and scala tympani. Low-frequency pressure differences are shunted through the helicotrema, where the two ducts communicate. The oval and round windows do not actually lie at the extreme base of the cochlea, but occur at oblique angles slightly toward the apex.

B. The functional properties of the cochlea are conceptually simplified if the cochlea is viewed as a linear structure with only two liquid-filled compartments separated by the elastic basilar membrane.

C. If the basilar membrane had uniform mechanical properties along its full extent, a compression would drive the tympanum and ossicles inward, increasing the pressure in the scala vestibuli and forcing the basilar membrane downward. Opposite movements would occur during a rarefaction. The pressure changes in the scala tympani are relieved by bowing of the round-window membrane. The movements of the tympanum, ossicles, and basilar membrane are greatly exaggerated.

D. In fact, the basilar membrane's mechanical properties vary continuously along its length. The oscillatory stimulation of a sound causes a traveling wave on the basilar membrane, shown here within the envelope of maximal displacement over an entire cycle. The magnitude of movement is grossly exaggerated in the vertical direction; the loudest tolerable sounds move the basilar membrane by only ±150 nm, a scaled distance less than one-hundredth the width of the lines representing the basilar membrane in these figures.

E. An enlargement of the active region in **D** demonstrates the motion of the basilar membrane in response to stimulation with sound of a single frequency. The continuous curve depicts a traveling wave at one instant; the vertical scale of basilar-membrane deflection is exaggerated about one-millionfold. The **dashed** and **dotted curves** portray the traveling wave at successively later times as it progresses from the cochlear base (left) toward the apex (right). As the wave approaches the characteristic place for the stimulus frequency, it slows and grows in amplitude. The stimulus energy is then transferred to hair cells at the position of the wave's peak.

F. Each frequency of stimulation excites maximal motion at a particular position along the basilar membrane. Low-frequency sounds produce basilar-membrane motion near the apex, where the membrane is relatively broad and flaccid. Mid-frequency sounds excite the membrane in its middle. The highest frequencies that we can hear excite the basilar membrane at its narrow, taut base. The mapping of sound frequency onto the basilar membrane is approximately logarithmic.

G. The basilar membrane performs spectral analysis of complex sounds. In this example a sound with three prominent frequencies, such as the three formants of a vowel sound, excites basilar-membrane motion in three regions, each of which represents a particular frequency. Hair cells in the corresponding positions transduce the basilar-membrane oscillations into receptor potentials, which in turn excite the nerve fibers that innervate these particular regions.

relatively thin and floppy at the apex of the cochlea but thicker and tauter toward the base. Because its mechanical properties vary along its length, the basilar membrane does not oscillate like a single string on a musical instrument; instead, it more resembles a panoply of strings that vary from the coarsest string on a bass viol to the finest string on a violin.

Stimulation with a pure tone evokes a complex and elegant movement of the basilar membrane. Over one complete cycle of a sound, each affected segment along the basilar membrane undergoes a single cycle of vibration (Figure 30–3D, E). The various parts of the membrane do not, however, oscillate in phase with one another; instead, some portions of the membrane move upward while others move downward. As first demonstrated by Georg von Békésy using stroboscopic illumination, the overall pattern of motion of the membrane is that of successive traveling waves.

Because mechanical stimulation is applied at the cochlear base as a pressure difference between scala vestibuli and scala tympani, the traveling wave progresses from the cochlear base toward the apex. Each wave reaches its maximal amplitude at a particular position appropriate for the frequency of stimulation, then declines rapidly in size as it advances toward the cochlear apex. A traveling wave ascending the basilar membrane resembles an ocean wave rolling toward the shore: As the wave nears the beach its crest grows to a maximal height, then breaks and rapidly fades away.

Although the analogy of an ocean wave gives some sense of the appearance of the basilar membrane's motion, the connection between the cochlear traveling wave and the movement of an ocean wave is only metaphorical—the physical bases of the two waves are quite distinct. An ocean wave is the result of the momentum of a wind-blown mass of water. In contrast, movement of the basilar membrane is the result of motion of the liquid masses above and below the membrane. These liquids are continuously driven up and down by the energy supplied by the stapes's piston-like movements at the oval window.

The variation in the mechanical properties of the mammalian basilar membrane explains why the membrane is tuned to different frequencies at each point along its length. In humans the membrane at the apex of the cochlea responds best to the lowest audible frequencies, down to approximately 20 Hz. At the cochlear base it responds to frequencies as great as 20 kHz. The intervening frequencies are represented along the basilar membrane in a continuous array (Figure 30–3F). In the 19th century the German physiologist Hermann von Helmholtz was the first to appreciate that the basilar membrane's operation is essentially the inverse of a piano's. The piano synthesizes a complex sound by combining the pure tones produced by numerous vibrating strings; the cochlea deconstructs a complex sound by isolating each component tone at a discrete segment of the basilar membrane.

The arrangement of vibration frequencies along the basilar membrane is an example of a *tonotopic map*. The relation between frequency and position on the basilar membrane varies smoothly and monotonically but is not linear. Instead, the logarithm of the best frequency is roughly proportional to the distance from the cochlea's apex. The frequencies from 20 Hz to 200 Hz, those between 200 Hz and 2 kHz, and those spanning 2 kHz to 20 kHz are each apportioned approximately one-third of the basilar membrane's extent.

Analysis of the response to a complex sound illustrates how the basilar membrane operates in daily life. A vowel sound in human speech, for example, ordinarily comprises three dominant frequency components termed formants. Measurement of the sound pressure outside an ear exposed to such a sound reveals a complex, seemingly chaotic signal. The movements of the tympanum and ossicles in response to a vowel sound likewise appear very complicated. The motion of the basilar membrane, however, is much simpler. Each frequency component of the stimulus establishes a traveling wave that, to a first approximation, is independent of the waves evoked by the others (Figure 30–3G). Each traveling wave reaches its peak excursion at a point on the basilar membrane appropriate for that frequency component. Moreover, the amplitude of each traveling wave is proportional, albeit in a complex way, to the intensity of the corresponding frequency component. The basilar membrane thus acts as a mechanical frequency analyzer by distributing specific stimulus energies to hair cells arrayed along its length, and in doing so begins the encoding of the frequencies and intensities in a sound.

The Organ of Corti Is the Site of Mechanoelectrical Transduction in the Cochlea

The organ of Corti, a ridge of epithelium extending along the basilar membrane, is the receptor organ of the inner ear. Each organ of Corti contains approximately 16,000 hair cells innervated by approximately 30,000 afferent nerve fibers, which carry information into the brain along the eighth cranial nerve. Like the basilar membrane itself, both the hair cells and the auditory nerve fibers are tonotopically organized: At any position along the basilar membrane the hair cells are most sensitive to a particular frequency, and these frequencies are logarithmically mapped in ascending order from the cochlea's apex to its base.

The organ of Corti includes a variety of cells, many of obscure function, but four types have obvious importance. First, there are two varieties of hair cells. The *inner hair cells* form a single row of approximately 3,500 cells, whereas approximately 12,000 *outer hair cells* lie in three rows farther from the central axis of the cochlear spiral (Figure 30–4). The outer hair cells are supported at their bases by the Deiters's (phalangeal) cells; the space between the inner and outer hair cells is delimited and mechanically supported by pillar cells.

A second epithelial ridge adjacent to the organ of Corti, but nearer the cochlea's central axis, gives rise to the tectorial membrane, a cantilevered gelatinous shelf that covers the organ of Corti (Figure 30–4). The tectorial membrane is anchored at its base by the interdental cells, which are also partly responsible for secreting

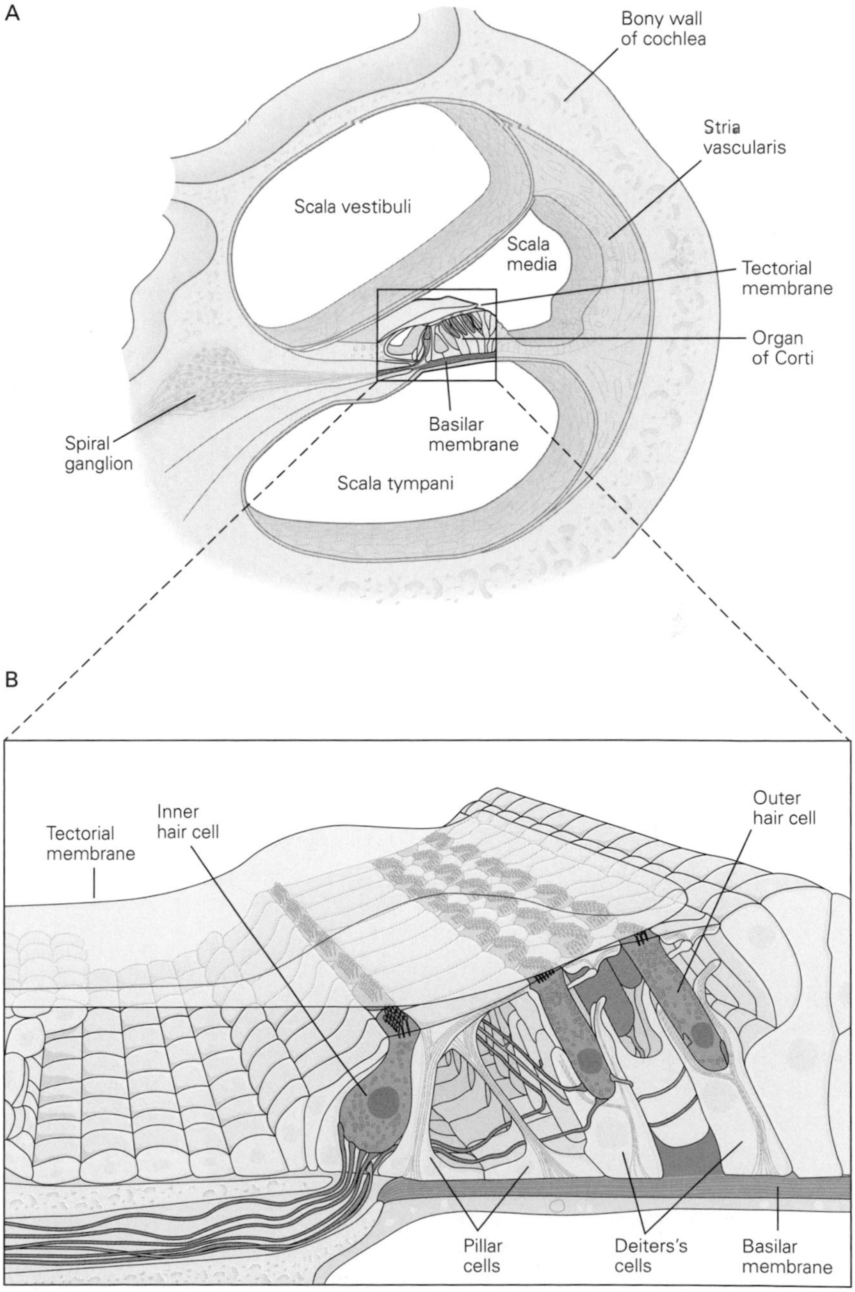

Figure 30–4 Cellular architecture of the human organ of Corti. Although there are differences among species, the basic plan is similar for all mammals.

A. The organ of Corti, the inner ear's receptor organ, is an epithelial strip that surmounts the elastic basilar membrane. The organ contains some 16,000 hair cells arrayed in four rows: a single row of inner hair cells and three rows of outer hair cells. The mechanically sensitive hair bundles of these receptor cells protrude into endolymph, the liquid within the scala media. Reissner's membrane, which provides the upper boundary of the scala media, separates the endolymph from the perilymph in the scala vestibuli. The hair bundles of outer hair cells are attached at their tops to the lower surface of the tectorial membrane, a gelatinous shelf that extends the full length of the basilar membrane.

B. The hair cells are separated and supported by pillar cells and Deiters's cells. One hair cell has been removed from the middle row of outer hair cells to reveal the three-dimensional relationship between supporting cells and hair cells. Efferent nerve endings at the bases of outer hair cells have been omitted from the drawing.

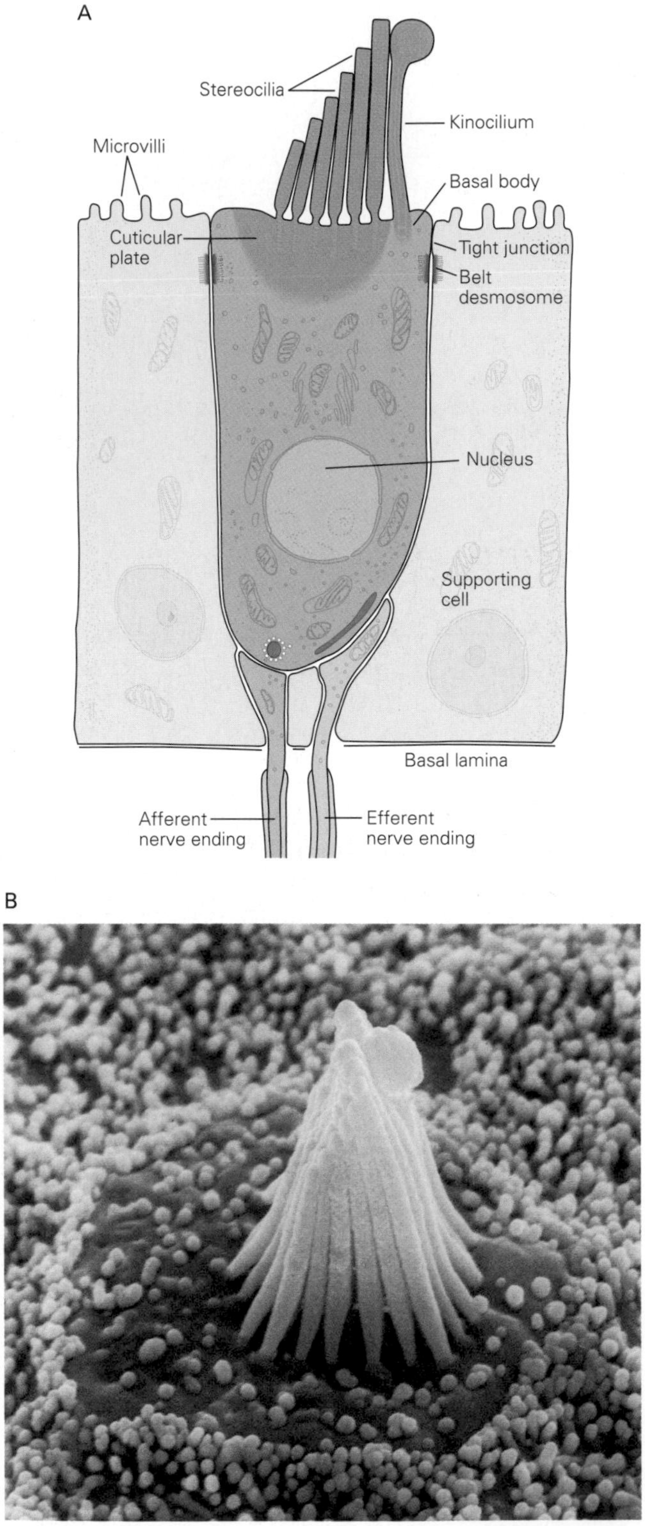

this extracellular structure. The tectorial membrane's tapered distal edge forms a fragile connection with the organ of Corti. When the basilar membrane vibrates in response to a sound, the organ of Corti and the overlying tectorial membrane move with it. Because the basilar and tectorial membranes pivot about different lines of insertion, their up-and-down motion is accompanied by back-and-forth shearing motion of the upper surface of the organ of Corti and the lower surface of the tectorial membrane. This motion is detected by hair cells.

Hair cells originate from the surface ectoderm of the embryo and retain an epithelial character. Columnar or flask-shaped, a hair cell lacks both dendrites and an axon (Figure 30–5A). Around its apex the hair cell is connected to nonsensory supporting cells. A special saline solution, the endolymph, bathes the cell's apical aspect. A tight junction separates this liquid from the ordinary extracellular fluid, or perilymph, that contacts the basolateral surface of the cell. Immediately below the tight junction an intermediate junction provides a strong mechanical attachment for the hair cell.

The hair bundle, which serves as a receptor for mechanical stimuli, projects from the flattened apical surface of the hair cell. Cochlear hair bundles comprise a few hundred cylindrical processes, the *stereocilia,* arranged in a hexagonal array and extending several micrometers from the cell surface. Because successive stereocilia across a cell's surface vary in length, a hair bundle is beveled like the tip of a hypodermic needle (Figure 30–5B). In the mammalian cochlea the inner hair cell bundles have a roughly linear cross-sectional form. Outer hair cell bundles, in contrast, have a V shape (Figure 30–6).

Figure 30–5 Structure of a vertebrate hair cell.

A. The epithelial character of the hair cell is evident in this drawing of the sensory epithelium from a frog's internal ear. The cylindrical hair cell is joined to adjacent supporting cells by a junctional complex around its apex. The hair bundle, a mechanically sensitive organelle, extends from the cell's apical surface. The bundle comprises some 60 stereocilia arranged in stepped rows of varying length. At the bundle's tall edge stands the single kinocilium, an axonemal structure with a bulbous swelling at its tip; in the mammalian cochlea this organelle degenerates around the time of birth. Deflection of the hair bundle's top to the right depolarizes the hair cell; movement in the opposite direction elicits hyperpolarization. The hair cell is surrounded by supporting cells, whose apical surfaces bear a stubble of microvilli. Afferent and efferent synapses contact the basolateral surface of the plasma membrane.

B. This scanning electron micrograph of a hair cell's apical surface reveals the hair bundle protruding approximately 8 μm into the endolymph.

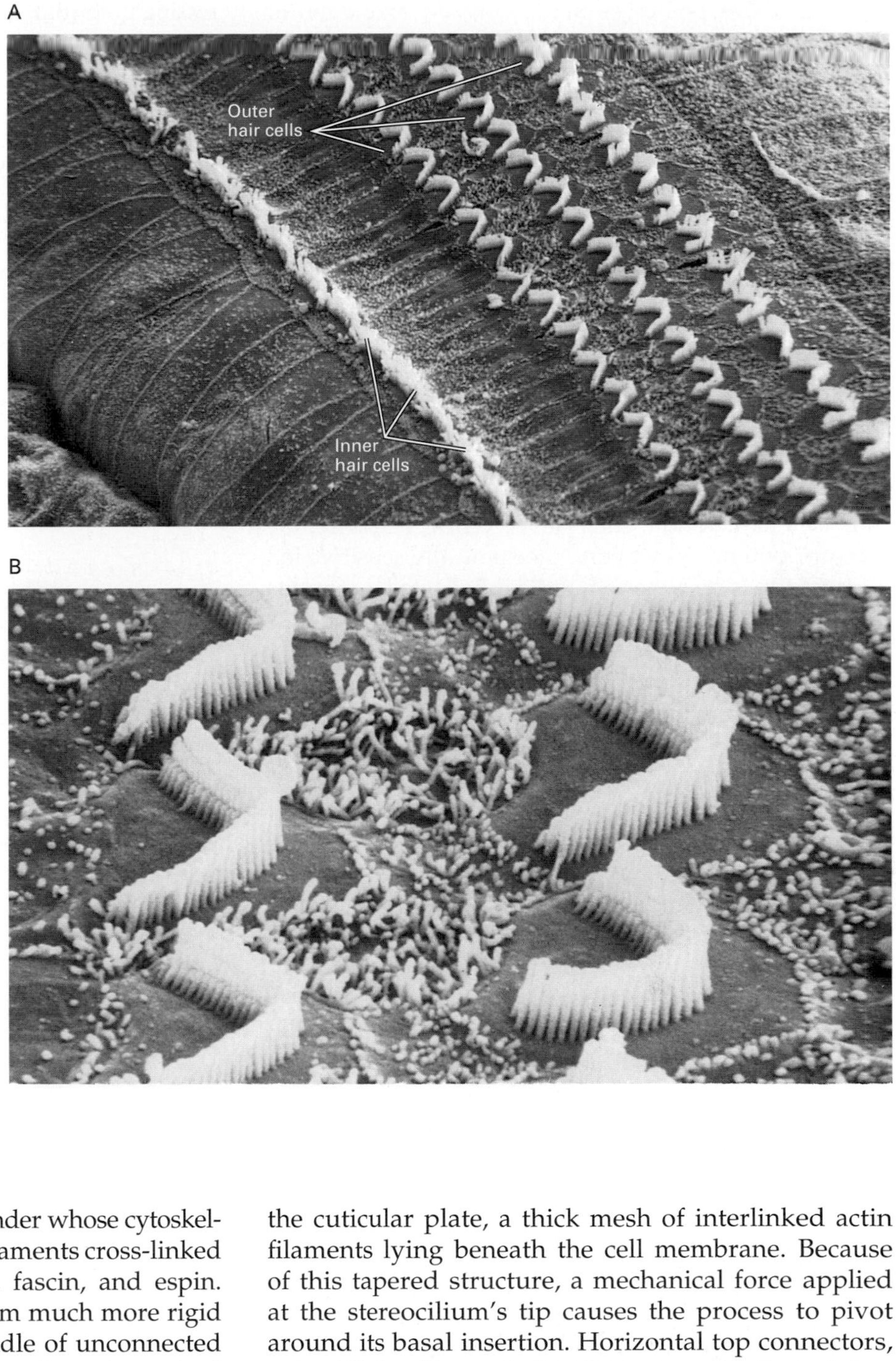

Figure 30–6 Arrangement of the hair cells in the organ of Corti.

A. Inner hair cells form a single row, and the stereocilia of each cell are arranged linearly. In contrast, outer hair cells are distributed in three rows, and the stereocilia of each cell are arranged in a V configuration. The apical surfaces of several other cells are visible: inner spiral sulcus cells, pillar cells, Deiters's cells, and Hensen's cells.

B. Higher magnification shows more clearly the V-shaped configuration of the hair bundle atop each outer hair cell. The hair-cell surface around the stereocilia is smooth, whereas the surfaces of supporting cells are endowed with microvilli.

Each stereocilium is a rigid cylinder whose cytoskeleton consists of a fascicle of actin filaments cross-linked by the proteins plastin (fimbrin), fascin, and espin. Cross-linking renders a stereocilium much more rigid than would be expected for a bundle of unconnected actin filaments. The core of the stereocilium is covered by a tubular sheath of plasma membrane. Although a stereocilium is of constant diameter along most of its length, it tapers over the micrometer or so just above its basal insertion. As the stereocilium narrows from approximately 0.4 μm to one-quarter that diameter, the number of actin filaments diminishes from several hundred to only a few dozen. This thin cluster of microfilaments anchors the stereocilium in the cuticular plate, a thick mesh of interlinked actin filaments lying beneath the cell membrane. Because of this tapered structure, a mechanical force applied at the stereocilium's tip causes the process to pivot around its basal insertion. Horizontal top connectors, extracellular filaments that interconnect adjacent stereocilia along each of the hair bundle's hexagonal axes, cause the bundle to move as a unit during stimulation at low frequencies. At high frequencies, the viscosity of the liquid between the stereocilia opposes their separation and again results in unitary motion of the hair bundle.

During its development every hair bundle includes at its tall edge a single true cilium, the *kinocilium*.

This structure possesses at its core an axoneme, or array of nine paired microtubules, and sometimes an additional central pair of microtubules. The kinocilium is not essential for mechanoelectrical transduction, for in mammalian cochlear hair cells it degenerates around the time of birth.

Hair Cells Transform Mechanical Energy into Neural Signals

Deflection of the Hair Bundle Initiates Mechanoelectrical Transduction

Just as in the human vestibular organs (see Chapter 40), mechanical deflection of the hair bundle is the stimulus that excites hair cells of the cochlea. A mechanical stimulus to a hair bundle elicits an electrical response, the receptor potential, by gating mechanically sensitive ion channels. In vitro, when a bundle is deflected by a probe attached near its top, the hair cell's response depends on the direction and magnitude of the stimulus.

In an unstimulated cell approximately 10% of the channels involved in stimulus transduction are open. As a result, the cell's resting potential, approximately –60 mV, is determined in part by the influx of cations through these channels. A stimulus that displaces the bundle toward its tall edge opens additional channels, thereby depolarizing the cell (Figure 30–7). In contrast, a stimulus that displaces the bundle toward its short edge shuts those transduction channels that are open at rest, thus hyperpolarizing the cell.

Hair cells respond only to stimuli parallel to the hair bundle's axis of morphological symmetry: Stimuli at right angles to the axis produce no change from the resting potential. An oblique stimulus elicits a response proportional to its vectorial projection along the axis of sensitivity.

A hair cell's receptor potential is graded. As the stimulus amplitude increases, the receptor potential grows progressively larger up to the point of saturation.

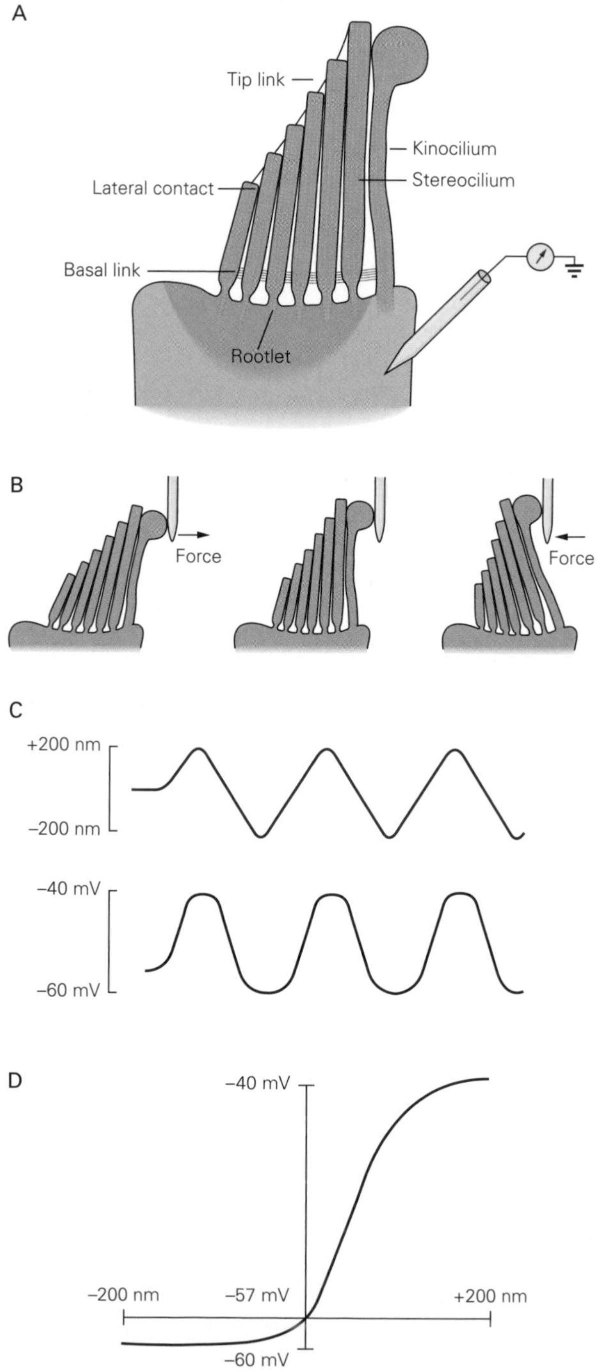

Figure 30–7 Mechanical sensitivity of a hair cell.

A. A recording electrode is inserted into a hair cell.

B. A probe attached to the bulbous tip of the stereocilium is moved by a piezoelectric stimulator, deflecting the elastic hair bundle from its resting position. The actual deflections are generally only one-tenth as large as those portrayed.

C. When the top of a hair bundle is displaced back-and-forth (**upper trace**), the opening and closing of mechanically sensitive ion channels produces an oscillatory receptor potential (**lower trace**) that may saturate in both the depolarizing and the hyperpolarizing directions.

D. The relation between hair-bundle deflection (abscissa) and receptor potential (ordinate) is sigmoidal. The entire operating range is only approximately 100 nm, less than the diameter of an individual stereocilium.

The receptor potential of an inner hair cell can be as great as 25 mV in peak to peak magnitude. The relation between a bundle's deflection and the resulting electrical response is sigmoidal (Figure 30–7D). A displacement of only ±100 nm represents approximately 90% of the response range. During normal stimulation a hair bundle moves through an angle of ±1 degree or so, that is, by much less than the diameter of one stereocilium.

Hair cells are so sensitive that their response threshold is probably set by brownian motion; still weaker stimuli are lost in the thermal clatter of the ear's components. When observed in vitro a hair bundle exhibits brownian motion of approximately ±3 nm. However, because the auditory system averages responses over several cycles to improve its signal-to-noise ratio, the threshold of hearing corresponds to hair-bundle deflection of as little as ±0.3 nm. A stimulus of this magnitude evokes a receptor potential near 100 μV in amplitude.

The ion channels in hair cells that are involved in stimulus transduction are relatively nonselective, cation-passing pores with a conductance near 100 pS. Because small organic cations can support measurable current, and small fluorescent molecules can traverse the channel, the transduction channel's pore is about 1.3 nm in diameter. Most of the transduction current is carried by K^+, the cation with the highest concentration in the endolymph bathing the hair bundle.

The large diameter and poor selectivity of the pore permit transduction channels to be blocked by aminoglycoside antibiotics, such as streptomycin, gentamicin, and tobramycin. When used in large doses to counter bacterial infections, these drugs have a toxic effect on hair cells; the antibiotics damage hair bundles and eventually kill hair cells. These drugs evidently insinuate themselves through transduction channels at a low rate and thus cause long-term toxic effects by interfering with protein synthesis on the mitochondrial ribosomes, which resemble prokaryotic ribosomes. Consistent with this hypothesis, human sensitivity to aminoglycosides is maternally inherited and in many instances reflects a single base change in the 12S ribosomal RNA gene of the mitochondrion.

Single-channel recordings and noise analysis suggest that each hair cell possesses only a few hundred transduction channels. Because the number of channels is about the same as the number of stereocilia in a hair bundle and because the magnitude of the receptor potential is roughly proportional to the number of stereocilia remaining in a microdissected bundle, there are probably only two active transduction channels per stereocilium. The paucity of channels along with the lack of high-affinity ligands with which to label them explains why the biochemical identity of the transduction channels remains uncertain. Genetic and physiological evidence suggests, however, that proteins of the transmembrane channel family, specifically TMC1 and TMC2, are involved in mechanoelectrical transduction.

Mechanical Force Directly Opens Transduction Channels

The mechanism for gating of transduction channels in hair cells differs fundamentally from the mechanisms used for such electrical signals as the action potential or postsynaptic potential. Many ion channels respond to changes in membrane potential or to specific ligands (see Chapters 5, 7, 9–11). In contrast, the mechanoelectrical transduction channels in the hair cell are activated by mechanical strain.

Two lines of evidence suggest that the opening and closing of transduction channels is regulated by tension in elastic structures within the hair bundle. First, a bundle is stiffer along its axis of morphological symmetry, and hence of mechanical sensitivity, than at a right angle. This observation suggests that a portion of the work done in deflecting a bundle goes into elastic elements, termed *gating springs,* that pull on the molecular gates of the transduction channels. Because the gating springs contribute over half of a hair bundle's stiffness, the transduction channels efficiently capture the energy supplied when a bundle is deflected. In addition, hair-bundle stiffness decreases during channel gating, a phenomenon expected if the channels are gated directly through a mechanical linkage to the hair bundle.

A second indication that transduction channels are directly controlled by gating springs is the rapidity with which hair cells respond. The response latency is so brief, only a few microseconds, that gating is more likely to be direct than to involve a second messenger (see Chapter 11). Moreover, the electrical responses of hair cells to a series of step stimuli of increasing magnitude become successively larger and faster. This behavior favors a kinetic scheme in which mechanical force controls the rate constant for channel gating. If the mechanical energy from a stimulus is stored in a spring attached to the channel's gate, the rates of channel opening and closing are determined by the probability that the stored energy of the spring exceeds the transition-state energy for channel gating.

Mechanoelectrical transduction occurs near the tips of the stereocilia, as demonstrated by three experimental techniques. First, the region where cations flow into a hair cell was inferred by measuring small differences in the extracellular potential around a stimulated hair bundle. The voltage signal is strongest at the bundle's top; cations flowing toward transduction channels converge near the stereociliary tips. Second, aminoglycoside antibiotics, which block these channels, have their greatest effect when applied from a microelectrode directed at the top of the hair bundle. Finally, Ca^{2+}-sensitive fluorescent indicators initially signal Ca^{2+} entry near the apex of a deflected hair bundle. Measurements from cochlear hair cells at high temporal resolution suggest that the channels occur precisely at the stereociliary tips. When transduction current enters the channels, the ensuing change in membrane potential must propagate axially down the stereocilia before it changes the potential at the base of the cell body and thus influences the rate of transmitter release. Because the stereocilia are short, however, their cable properties do not attenuate electrical signals significantly.

The *tip link* is a probable component of the gating spring. A tip link is a fine molecular braid joining the distal end of one stereocilium to the side of the longest adjacent process (Figure 30–8A). The upper two-thirds of the link consists of a parallel homodimer of cadherin-23 molecules; the lower third represents a parallel homodimer of protocadherin-15 chains. The two components are joined at their tips in a Ca^{2+}-sensitive manner. It is thought that each link is attached, probably at its lower end, to the molecular gates of two transduction channels. Deflection of a hair bundle toward its tall edge tenses the tip link and promotes channel opening; movement in the opposite direction slackens the link and allows the associated channels to close (Figure 30–8B).

Three experimental results suggest that the tip links are components of the gating springs. First, tip links are universal features of hair bundles and are situated at the site of transduction inferred from biophysical experiments. Second, the orientation of the links is consistent with the vectorial sensitivity of transduction. The links invariably interconnect stereocilia in a direction parallel with the hair bundle's plane of mirror symmetry. Stimulation at a right angle to the bundle's plane of symmetry, which would not be expected to alter the length of the links, elicits little or no response from a hair cell. Finally, when tip links are destroyed by exposing hair cells to Ca^{2+} chelators, transduction vanishes. As the tip links regenerate over the course of approximately 12 hours, a hair cell regains mechanosensitivity. It remains unclear whether the elasticity of gating springs resides primarily in the tip links or in the structures at their two insertions.

In the mammalian cochlea hair bundles are deflected through their linkage to the tectorial membrane. As the basilar membrane oscillates up and down, carrying the hair cells with it, a shearing motion occurs between the organ of Corti and the overlying tectorial membrane (Figure 30–9). The hair bundles of outer hair cells, whose tips are firmly attached to the tectorial membrane, are directly deflected by this movement. The hair bundles of inner hair cells, which do not contact the tectorial membrane, are deflected by movement of the liquid beneath the membrane. This mode of stimulation affords some mechanical amplification of the signals reaching hair bundles. At least for high-frequency stimuli, the movements of hair bundles are thought to be severalfold greater than that of the basilar membrane.

Direct Mechanoelectrical Transduction Is Rapid

In contrast to hair cells, many other sensory receptors, such as photoreceptors and olfactory neurons, use cyclic nucleotides or other second messengers in stimulus transduction. This strategy is advantageous in that the enzymatic pathway that generates a second messenger amplifies the signal, and feedback within the metabolic pathway readily permits adaptation and desensitization (see Chapter 11).

What is the advantage of transduction without the intervention of a second messenger? The answer probably lies in its speed. Hair cells operate much more quickly than do other sensory receptor cells of the vertebrate nervous system, and indeed more quickly than neurons themselves. To deal with the frequencies of biologically relevant sounds, transduction by hair cells must be rapid. Given the behavior of sound in air and the dimensions of sound-emitting and sound-absorbing organs such as vocal cords and eardrums, optimal auditory communication occurs in the frequency range of 10 Hz to 100 kHz. Much higher frequencies propagate poorly through air; much lower frequencies are inefficiently produced and captured by animals of moderate size.

Locating sound sources, one of the most important functions of hearing, sets even more stringent limits on the speed of transduction. A sound from a source directly to one side of a person reaches the nearer ear somewhat sooner than the farther. Although this delay is at most 700 μs, a human observer can locate sound sources on the basis of much smaller delays, about 10 μs. For this to occur, hair cells must be capable of detecting acoustic waveforms with microsecond-level resolution.

The ability of hair cells to discriminate high frequencies of stimulation implies that transduction channels are gated very rapidly. Even in animals sensitive

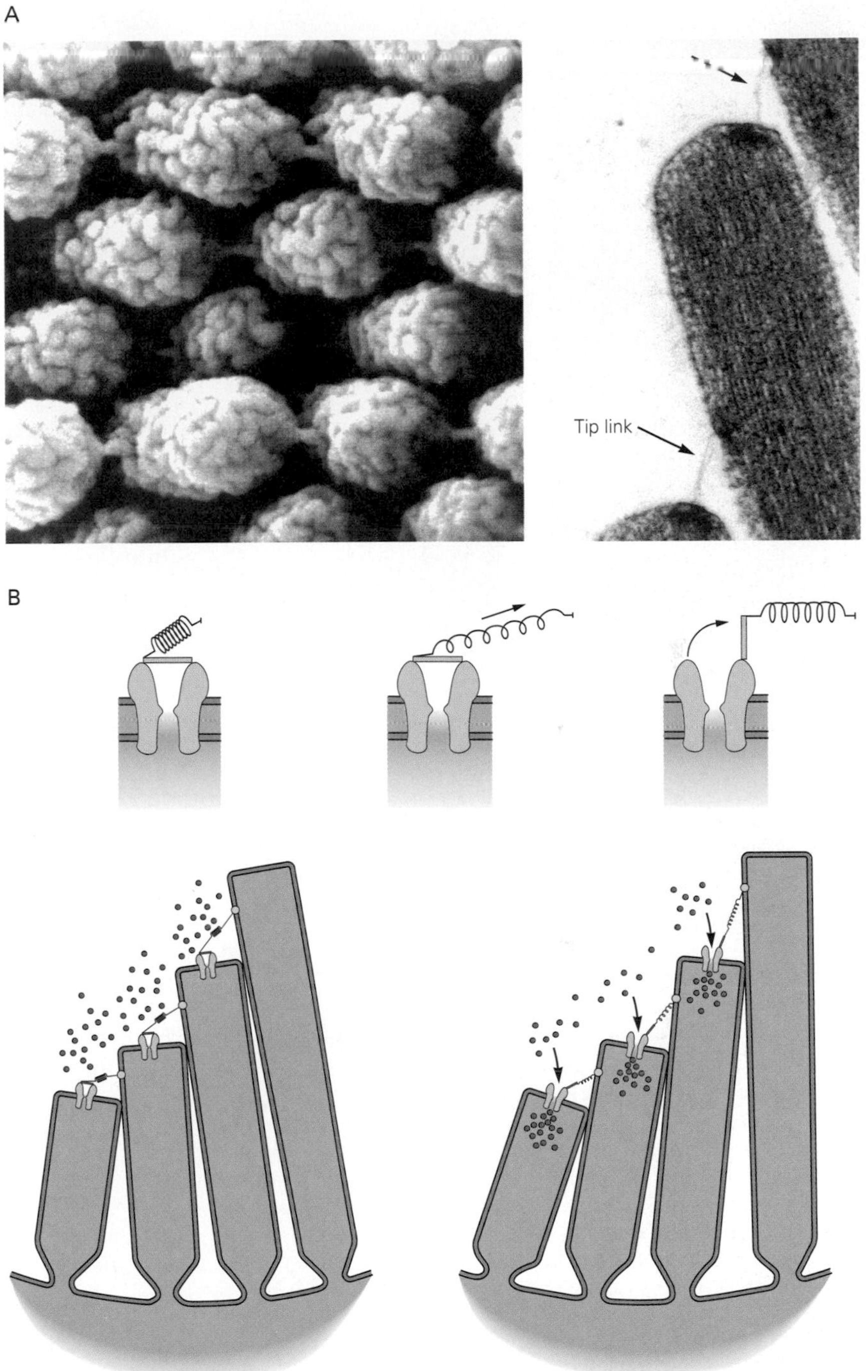

Figure 30–8 Mechanoelectrical transduction by hair cells.

A. A tip link connects each stereocilium to the side of the longest adjacent stereocilium, as seen in a scanning electron micrograph (**left**) and a transmission electron micrograph (**right**) of a hair bundle's top surface. Each tip link is only 3 nm in diameter. The links appear stouter in the illustration on the left because of metallic coating during specimen preparation. (Reproduced, with permission, from Assad, Shepherd, and Corey 1991; reproduced, with permission, from Hudspeth and Gillespie 1994.)

B. Top: Ion flux through the channel that underlies mechanoelectrical transduction in hair cells is regulated by a molecular gate. The opening and closing of the gate are controlled by the tension in an elastic element, the gating spring, that senses hair-bundle displacement. (Adapted, with permission, from Howard and Hudspeth 1988.)

Bottom: When the hair bundle is at rest each transduction channel clatters between closed and open states, spending most of its time shut. Displacement of the bundle in the positive direction increases the tension in the gating spring, here assumed to be in part a tip link, attached to each channel's molecular gate. The enhanced tension promotes channel opening and the influx of cations, thereby producing a depolarizing receptor potential. (Adapted, with permission, from Hudspeth 1989.)

to relatively low frequencies, the response to a stimulus of moderate intensity has a time constant of only 80 μs at room temperature. For mammals to be able to respond to frequencies greater than 100 kHz, the hair cells evidently display gating rates that are an order of magnitude greater.

The Temporal Responsiveness of Hair Cells Determines Their Sensitivity

The mechanical sensitivity of hair cells is not constant; responsiveness varies in such a way that a given cell best detects behaviorally relevant stimuli. When it is

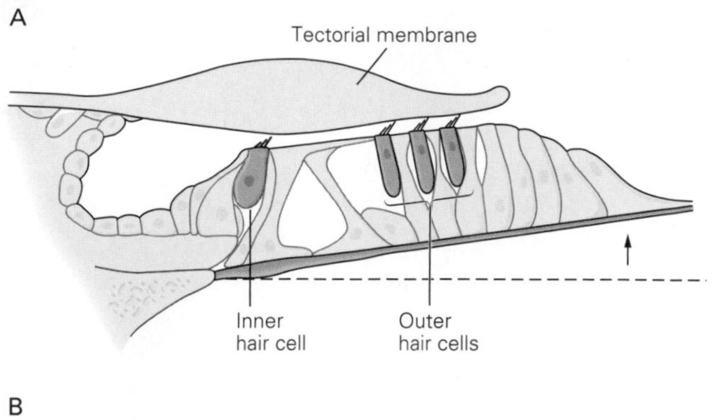

Figure 30–9 Forces acting on cochlear hair cells. Hair cells in the cochlea are stimulated when the basilar membrane is driven up and down by differences in the pressure between the scala vestibuli and scala tympani. This motion is accompanied by shearing movements between the tectorial membrane and organ of Corti. These motions deflect the hair bundles of outer hair cells, which are attached to the lower surface of the tectorial membrane. The hair bundles of inner hair cells, which are not attached to the tectorial membrane, are deflected by the movement of liquid in the space beneath that structure. In both instances the deflection initiates mechanoelectrical transduction of the stimulus.

A. When the basilar membrane is driven upward, shear between the hair cells and the tectorial membrane deflects hair bundles in the excitatory direction, toward their tall edge.

B. At the midpoint of an oscillation the hair bundles resume their resting position.

C. When the basilar membrane moves downward, the hair bundles are driven in the inhibitory direction.

appropriate that low-frequency inputs be disregarded, hair cells possess a unique mechanism of adaptation that acts as a high-pass filter. In addition, many hair cells in auditory systems display electrical resonance that tunes them to specific frequencies of stimulation. Finally, hair cells employ mechanical amplification that enhances and further tunes their mechanosensitivity.

Hair Cells Adapt to Sustained Stimulation

Despite the precision with which a hair bundle grows, it cannot develop in such a way that the sensitive transduction apparatus is perfectly poised at its position of greatest mechanosensitivity. Some mechanism must compensate for developmental irregularities, as well as for environmental changes, by adjusting the gating springs so that transduction channels are active at the bundle's resting position. An adaptation process that continuously resets the hair bundle's range of mechanical sensitivity does just that. Because of adaptation, a hair cell can maintain a high sensitivity to transient stimuli while rejecting static inputs a million times as large.

Adaptation manifests itself as a progressive decrease in the receptor potential during protracted deflection of the hair bundle (Figure 30–10). The process is not one of desensitization, for the sensitivity of the receptor persists. However, with prolonged stimulation the sensitivity shifts from that of the bundle's resting point to approximately 80% of its deflected position. Adaptation occurs on a time scale three orders of magnitude slower than mechanoelectrical transduction: The time constant of adaptation is approximately 20 ms when endolymph bathes the hair bundle. The rate and extent of adaptation increase with increasing concentration of Ca^{2+} in the liquid contacting the apical cell surface.

How does adaptation occur? Because the mechanical force exerted by a hair bundle changes as adaptation proceeds, the process evidently involves an adjustment in the tension borne by the gating springs. It appears likely that the structure anchoring the upper end of each tip link, the *insertional plaque,* is repositioned during adaptation by an active molecular motor. Hair bundles contain at least five isoforms of myosin, the motor molecule associated with motility along actin filaments (see Chapter 34). Immunohistochemical studies indicate that myosin-1c occurs in clusters at insertional plaques and near the stereociliary tips, and site-directed mutagenesis implicates this isozyme in adaptation. Several dozen such myosin molecules associated with each tip link are thought to maintain tension by ascending cytoskeletal actin filaments and pulling the link's insertion with them (Figure 30–11).

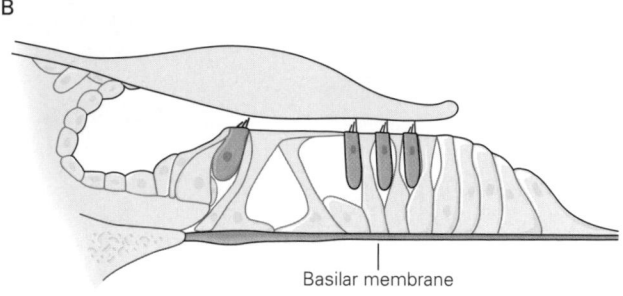

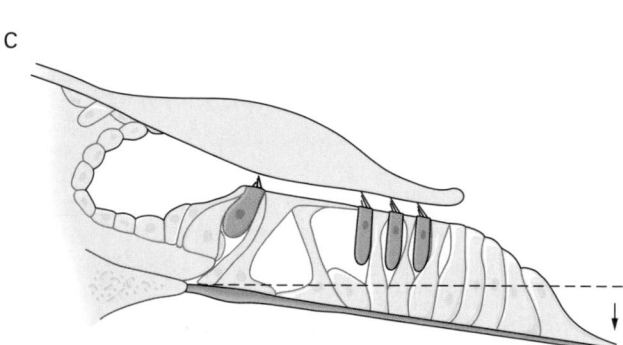

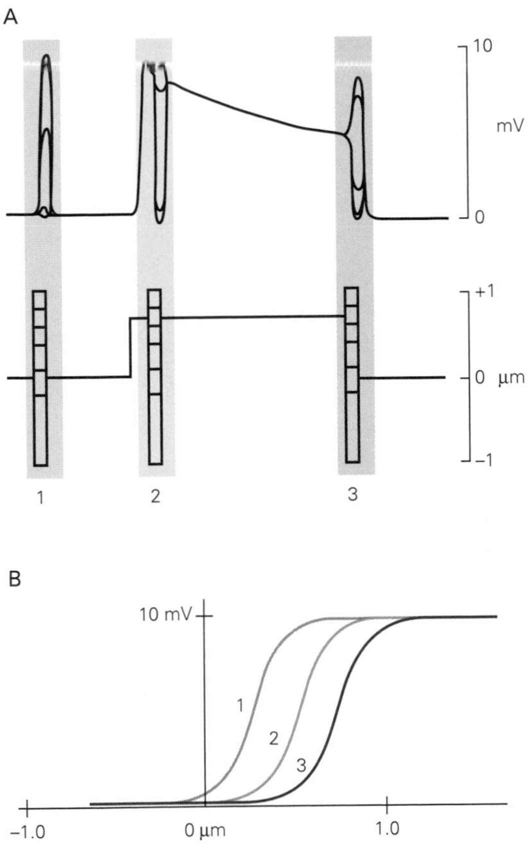

Figure 30–10 Adaptation of mechanoelectrical transduction in hair cells.

A. The **lower trace** shows mechanical test stimuli of various sizes applied before prolonged (100 ms) deflection of a hair bundle (**1**) and at two times during the deflection (**2**, **3**). As shown in the **upper trace**, the rapid depolarization at the onset of the deflection is followed by a gradual decline toward a plateau. Seven records, each with a different test stimulus, are superimposed.

B. Adaptation alters the relation between hair-bundle displacement and the receptor potential of the hair cell before and during displacement. Each of the three curves is generated by plotting the electrical responses to the seven test stimuli against the respective hair-bundle displacements. As adaptation proceeds the sigmoidal relation shifts to the right along the abscissa without substantial changes in the curve's shape or amplitude. This result implies that during adaptation to a protracted stimulus a hair bundle's range of mechanical sensitivity approaches the position at which the bundle is held.

When a stimulus step increases the tension in a gating spring, the associated transduction channel opens, permitting an influx of cations. As Ca^{2+} ions accumulate in the stereociliary cytoplasm, they bind to the calmodulin light chains that adorn the neck region of myosin-1c. The activation of calmodulin in turn reduces the upward force of the myosin-1c molecule, thereby shortening the gating spring. When the spring reaches its resting tension, closure of the channel reduces the Ca^{2+} influx to its original level, restoring a balance between the upward force of myosin and the downward tension in the spring.

Hair Cells Are Tuned to Specific Stimulus Frequencies

As a result of the tonotopic arrangement of the mammalian basilar membrane, every cochlear hair cell is most sensitive to stimulation at a specific frequency, termed its characteristic, natural, or best frequency. On average, the characteristic frequencies of adjacent inner hair cells differ by approximately 0.2%; adjacent piano strings, in comparison, are tuned to frequencies some 6% apart.

The sensitivity of a cochlear hair cell extends within a limited range above and below its characteristic frequency. This follows from the fact that the traveling wave evoked even by a pure sinusoidal stimulus spreads somewhat along the basilar membrane. The traveling wave of a stimulus tone with a pitch lower than the characteristic frequency of a particular hair cell passes that cell and peaks somewhat farther up the cochlear spiral. A higher-pitched tone causes a traveling wave that crests below the cell. Nevertheless, in either instance the basilar membrane undergoes some motion at the hair cell's site, so that the cell responds to the stimulus.

The frequency sensitivity of a hair cell may be displayed as a tuning curve. To construct a tuning curve, an experimenter stimulates the ear with pure tones at numerous frequencies below, at, and above the cell's characteristic frequency. The intensity of stimulation is adjusted for each frequency until the response reaches a predefined criterion magnitude. An investigator might, for example, ask what stimulus intensity is necessary at each frequency to produce a receptor potential 1 mV in peak-to-peak magnitude. The tuning curve is then a graph of sound level, presented logarithmically in decibels sound-pressure level, against stimulus frequency.

The tuning curve for an inner hair cell is typically V-shaped (Figure 30–12). The curve's tip represents the cell's characteristic frequency, the frequency that produces the criterion response for the lowest-intensity stimulus. Sounds of greater or lesser frequencies require higher intensities to excite the cell to the criterion response. As a consequence of the traveling

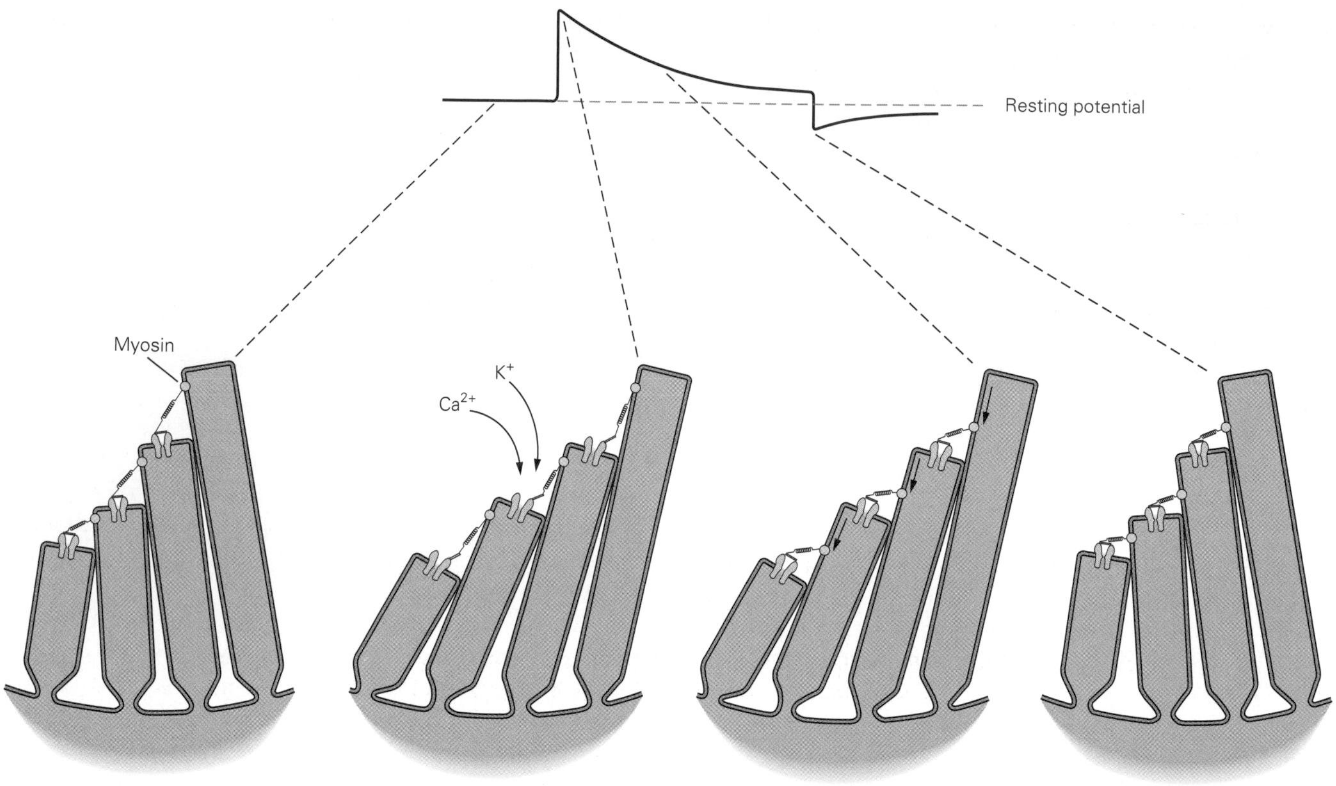

Figure 30–11 A model of adaptation by hair cells. Prolonged deflection of the hair bundle in the positive direction elicits an initial depolarization followed by a decline to a plateau and an undershoot at the cessation of the stimulus. Initially the stimulation increases tension in the tip link, thus opening transduction channels. As stimulation continues, however, a tip link's upper attachment is thought to slide down the stereocilium, allowing each channel to close during adaptation. Prolonged deflection of the hair bundle in the negative direction elicits a complementary response. The cell is slightly hyperpolarized at first but shows a rebound depolarization at the end of stimulation; tension is restored to the initially slack tip link as myosin molecules actively pull up the link's upper insertion.

wave's shape, the slope of a tuning curve is far steeper on its high-frequency flank than on its low-frequency flank.

Hair cells must contend with acoustic stimuli that have a very low energy content. If the stimulus consists of a periodic signal, such as the sinusoidal pressure of a pure tone, a detection system can increase the signal-to-noise ratio by enhancing selectively the response to a relevant frequency. At least two cellular mechanisms are known to accomplish this task, thereby supplementing the tuning accomplished by the basilar membrane.

First, the mechanical properties of a hair bundle help tune it to a particular frequency, in the same way a tuning fork's resonant frequency depends on the mechanical properties of its tines. These properties include the bundle's flexibility and mass. The flexible elements that restore a bundle to its resting upright position are the gating springs and the actin-filled rootlets at the base of the stereocilia. Because the bundle moves through a viscous medium, the mass relevant to the bundle's tuning includes that of a volume of water dragged along by the moving bundle. Viscosity also heavily dampens the motion.

In the auditory organs of many animals the lengths of the hair bundles vary systematically along the tonotopic axis. Hair cells that respond to low-frequency acoustic stimuli have the longest bundles, whereas those that respond to the highest-frequency signals bear the shortest bundles. In the human cochlea, for example, an inner hair cell with a characteristic frequency of 20 kHz bears a 4 μm hair bundle. At the opposite extreme, a cell sensitive to a 20 Hz stimulus has a bundle more than 7 μm high.

Computer modeling shows that the tuning-fork mechanism helps to tune cochlear hair cells with freestanding hair bundles, those that are not attached to a tectorial membrane. In humans these cells are the inner hair cells, the receptors that provide most of the information conveyed by the cochlear nerve. The length of the stereocilia may also affect the tuning of cells whose hair bundles are inserted into a tectorial membrane, for in these hair cells too there is an inverse relation between bundle length and characteristic frequency.

The second mechanism that tunes individual hair cells to specific frequencies is electrical in nature. In many fishes, amphibians, and reptiles including birds the membrane potential of each hair cell resonates at a particular frequency in response to an injected current pulse (Figure 30–13A). When a cell is stimulated with sounds of various frequencies but constant amplitude, it responds over a broad range of frequencies. However, when current is injected the cell responds most strongly to stimulation at the particular frequency at which the cell's membrane potential resonates. Whether electrical resonance contributes to frequency tuning in the ears of mammals, including humans, remains uncertain.

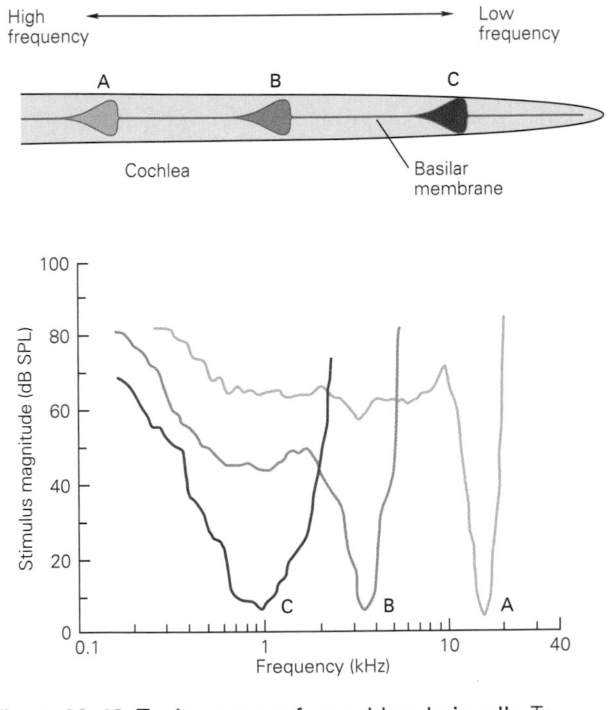

Figure 30–12 Tuning curves for cochlear hair cells. To construct a curve the experimenter presents sound at several frequencies. At each frequency the stimulus intensity is adjusted until the cell produces a criterion response, here 1 mV. The curve thus reflects the threshold of the cell for stimulation at a range of frequencies. Each cell is most sensitive to a specific frequency, its characteristic frequency. The threshold rises briskly—the sensitivity falls abruptly—as the stimulus frequency is raised or lowered. (Reproduced, with permission, from Pickles 1988.)

The basis of electrical resonance has been determined by voltage-clamp recordings from isolated hair cells. The depolarizing phase of an oscillation is driven by current carried into the cell through voltage-gated Ca^{2+} channels, whereas the repolarizing component results primarily from outward current through Ca^{2+}-sensitive K^+ channels (Figure 30–13B). Several factors establish the frequency and sharpness of the resonance, including the membrane capacitance, the numbers of Ca^{2+} and K^+ channels, and the time course of Ca^{2+} removal. In addition, variation in the K^+ channels along the cochlea is a factor in the differences in frequency selectivity of the hair cells. Alternative splicing of the mRNA encoding cochlear K^+ channels generates several channel isoforms that differ in their kinetics and their sensitivities to Ca^{2+} and voltage. Moreover, expression of the channel's auxiliary β subunit, which also regulates gating kinetics, displays a gradient along the tonotopic axis. How hair cells become tuned to their characteristic frequencies during development remains to be determined.

Sound Energy Is Mechanically Amplified in the Cochlea

The inner ear faces an important obstacle to efficient operation: A large portion of the energy in an acoustic stimulus goes into overcoming the damping effects of cochlear liquids on basilar-membrane motion rather than into excitation of hair cells. The sensitivity of the cochlea is too great, and auditory frequency selectivity too sharp, to result solely from the inner ear's passive mechanical properties. The cochlea must therefore possess some means of actively amplifying sound energy.

One indication that amplification occurs in the cochlea comes from measurements of the basilar membrane's movements with sensitive laser interferometers. In a preparation stimulated with low-intensity sound the motion of the membrane at any point is highly sensitive to frequency. As the sound intensity is increased, however, the membrane's sensitivity declines precipitously and its tuning becomes less sharp: The sensitivity of basilar-membrane motion to stimulation at 80 dB is less than 1% that for 10 dB excitation. The sensitivity predicted in modeling studies of a passive cochlea corresponds to that observed with high-intensity

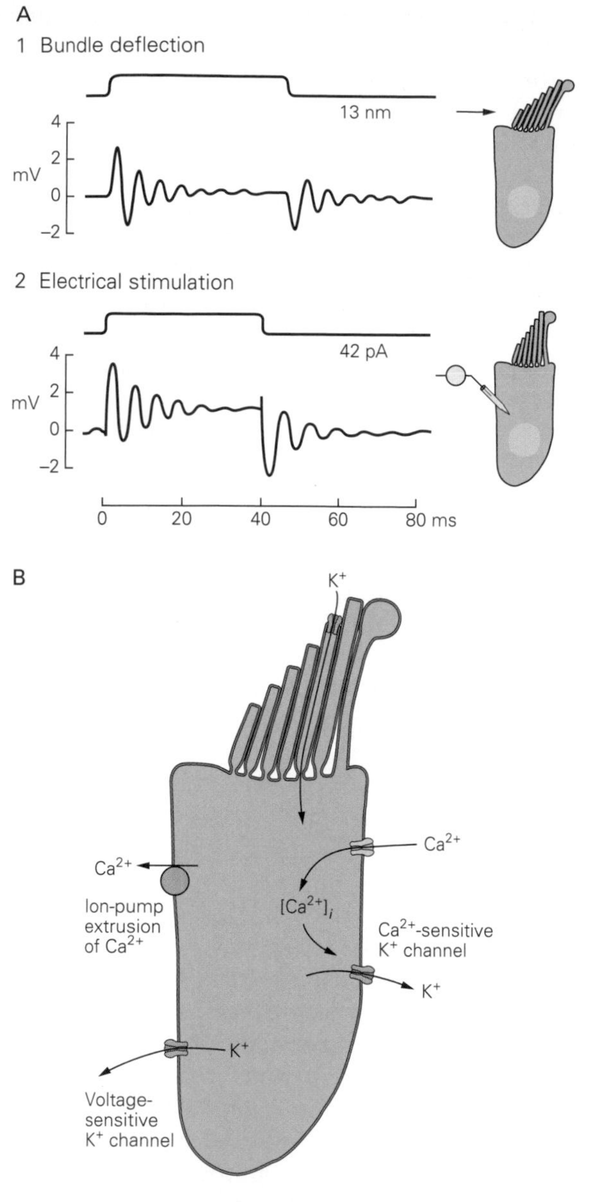

Figure 30–13 Electrical tuning of a hair cell.

A. 1. When the hair bundle is deflected, this hair cell's membrane potential oscillates at a frequency of approximately 180 Hz. **2.** Passing electrical current into the same hair cell through a microelectrode evokes oscillation of the membrane potential at a similar frequency, an indication that the cell is tuned to a specific stimulus frequency by an electrical resonator. (Reproduced, with permission, from Crawford and Fettiplace 1981.)

B. A model of electrical resonance in a hair cell. Positive deflection of the hair bundle opens mechanoelectrical transduction channels in the stereocilia, thus depolarizing the cell. The depolarization opens voltage-sensitive Ca^{2+} channels, and the resulting Ca^{2+} influx augments the depolarization. As Ca^{2+} accumulates in the cytoplasm, however, it activates Ca^{2+}-sensitive K^+ channels that, along with voltage-sensitive K^+ channels, allow K^+ efflux that repolarizes the cell. To maintain an appropriate cytoplasmic Ca^{2+} concentration the Ca^{2+} must be sequestered and eventually pumped from the cell.

stimuli. This result implies that the motion of the basilar membrane is augmented more than 100-fold during low-intensity stimulation but that amplification diminishes progressively as the stimulus grows in strength.

In addition to this circumstantial evidence, experimental observations support the idea that the cochlea contains a mechanical amplifier. When a normal human ear is stimulated with a click, that ear emits one to several measurable pulses of sound. Each pulse includes sound in a restricted frequency band. High-frequency sounds are emitted with the shortest latency, approximately 5 ms, whereas low-frequency emissions occur after a delay as great as 20 ms (Figure 30–14A). These so-called *evoked otoacoustic emissions* are not simply echoes; they represent the emission of mechanical energy by the cochlea, triggered by acoustic stimulation.

A still more compelling manifestation of the cochlea's active amplification is *spontaneous otoacoustic emission.* When a suitably sensitive microphone is used to measure sound pressure in the ear canals of subjects in a quiet environment, at least 70% of normal human ears continuously emit one or more pure tones (Figure 30–14B). Although these sounds are generally too faint to be directly audible by others, physicians have reported hearing sounds emanating from the ears of newborns! The ears of adults, too, occasionally emit audible sounds. The active process in the cochlea ordinarily serves to counter the viscous damping effects of cochlear fluids on the basilar membrane. However, if this cochlear amplifier is overly active the ear emits sound, just as a public-address system howls when its gain is excessive.

What is the source of evoked and spontaneous otoacoustic emissions, and presumably of cochlear amplification as well? Several lines of evidence implicate outer hair cells as the elements that enhance cochlear sensitivity and frequency selectivity and hence as the energy sources for amplification. The afferent nerve fibers that extensively innervate the inner hair cells make only minimal contacts with the outer hair cells. Instead, the outer hair cells receive an extensive efferent innervation that, when activated, decreases cochlear sensitivity and frequency discrimination. Pharmacological ablation of outer hair cells with selectively ototoxic drugs degrades the ear's responsiveness still more profoundly.

When stimulated electrically, an isolated outer hair cell displays the unique phenomenon of electromotility: The cell body shortens when depolarized and elongates when hyperpolarized (Figure 30–15). This response can occur at frequencies exceeding 80 kHz, an attractive feature for a process postulated to assist high-frequency hearing.

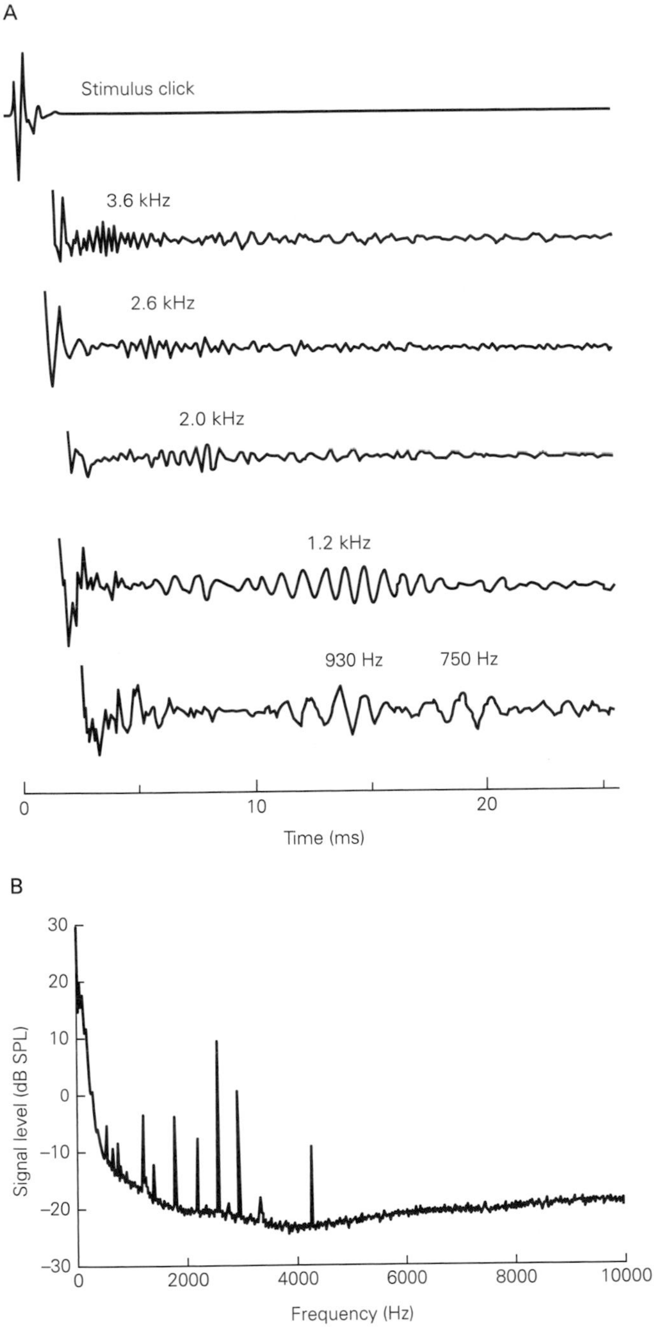

Figure 30–14 The cochlea actively emits sounds.

A. The records display evoked otoacoustic emissions from the ears of five human subjects. A brief click was played into each ear through a miniature speaker. A few milliseconds later a tiny microphone in the external auditory meatus detected one or more bursts of sound emission from the ear. (Reproduced, with permission, from Wilson 1980.)

B. Under suitably quiet recording conditions, spontaneous otoacoustic emissions occur in most normal human ears. This spectrum displays the acoustic power of six prominent emissions and several smaller ones. (Reproduced, with permission, from Murphy et al. 1995.)

The energy for these movements is drawn from the experimentally imposed electrical field rather than from hydrolysis of an energy-rich substrate such as adenosine triphosphate (ATP). Movement occurs when changes in the electric field across the membrane reorient molecules of the protein prestin. The concerted movement of several million of these molecules changes the membrane's area and thus the cell's length. When an outer hair cell transduces mechanical stimulation of its hair bundle into receptor potentials, cochlear amplification might then occur as voltage-induced movement of the cell body augments basilar-membrane motion. Consistent with this hypothesis, mutation of certain amino-acid residues required for

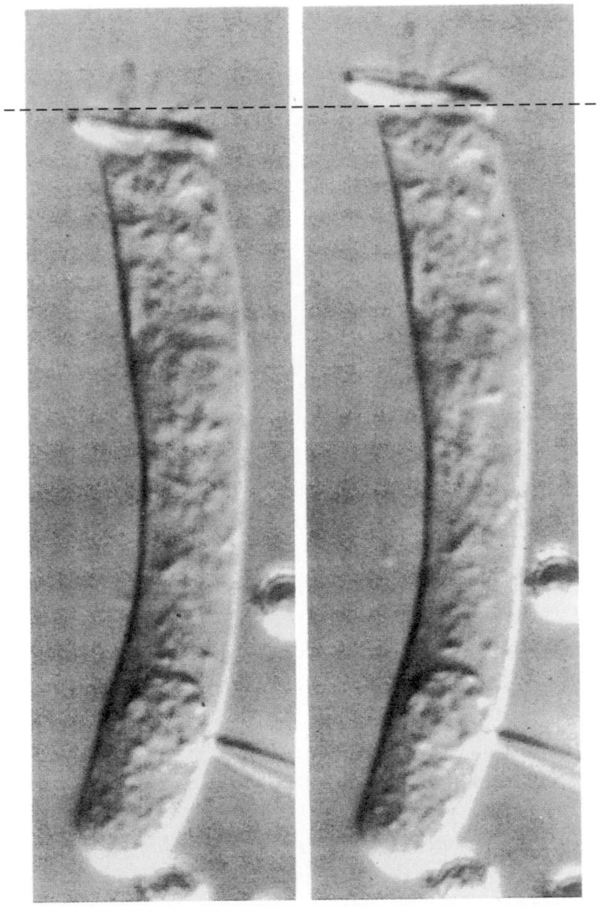

Figure 30–15 Voltage-induced motion of an outer hair cell. Depolarization of an isolated outer hair cell through the electrode at its base causes the cell body to shorten (**left**); hyperpolarization causes it to lengthen (**right**). The oscillatory motions of outer hair cells may provide the mechanical energy that amplifies basilar-membrane motion and thus enhances the sensitivity of human hearing. (Reproduced, with permission, from Holley and Ashmore 1988.)

the voltage sensitivity of prestin abolishes the active process in mice.

Because sharp tuning, high sensitivity, and otoacoustic emissions are also observed in animals that lack outer hair cells, electromotility cannot be the only form of mechanical amplification by hair cells. In addition to detecting stimuli, hair bundles are also mechanically active and contribute to amplification. Hair bundles can make spontaneous back-and-forth movements that might underlie spontaneous otoacoustic emissions. Under experimental conditions bundles can exert force against stimulus probes, performing mechanical work and thereby amplifying the input. In vitro experiments indicate that active hair-bundle motility contributes to the cochlear active process even in the mammalian ear.

Several features of auditory responsiveness suggest that cochlear hair cells operate on the verge of an instability termed the Hopf bifurcation. This phenomenon explains hair cells' amplification and frequency selectivity, their nonlinear sensitivity to stimulus intensity, and their capacity to become unstable and spontaneously emit sound. The fact that active hair-bundle motility demonstrates a Hopf bifurcation in vitro provides further evidence that this mechanism contributes to cochlear amplification.

Although active hair-bundle movements have been demonstrated at sound frequencies as high as a few kilohertz, it remains uncertain whether bundles can generate forces at the very high frequencies at which sharp frequency selectivity and otoacoustic emissions are observed in the mammalian cochlea. Active hair-bundle motility and electromotility may function synergistically, with the former serving metaphorically as a tuner and preamplifier and the latter as a power amplifier. Alternatively, hair-bundle motility may operate at relatively low frequencies but be superseded by electromotility at the highest frequencies.

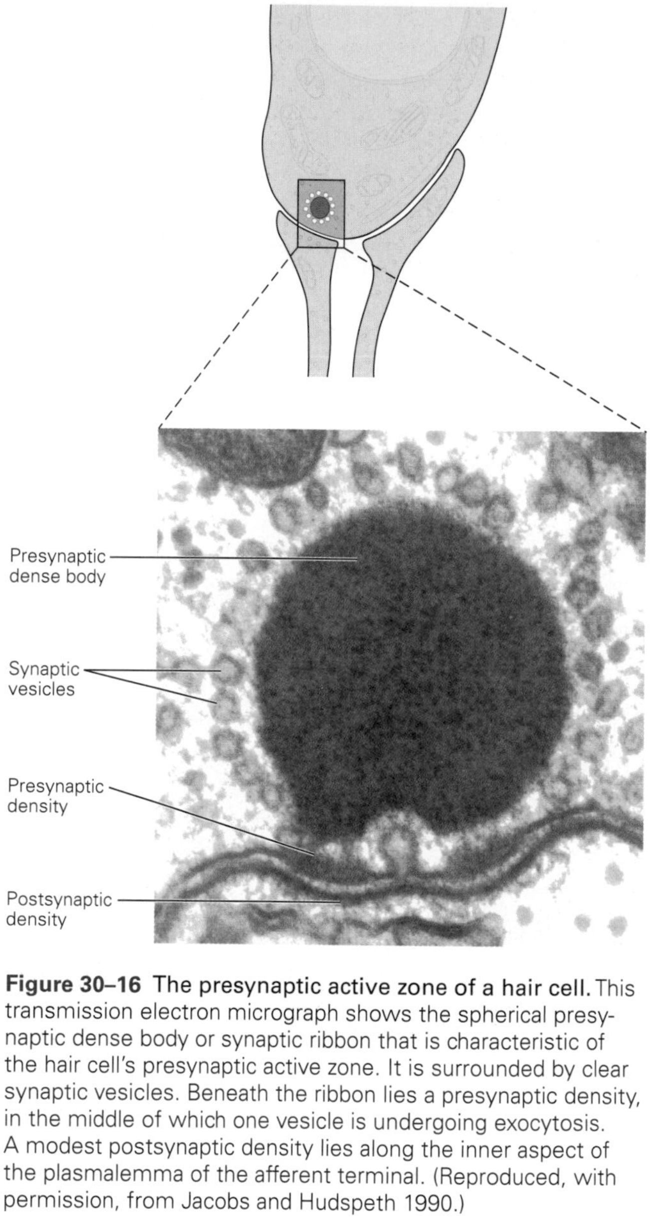

Figure 30–16 The presynaptic active zone of a hair cell. This transmission electron micrograph shows the spherical presynaptic dense body or synaptic ribbon that is characteristic of the hair cell's presynaptic active zone. It is surrounded by clear synaptic vesicles. Beneath the ribbon lies a presynaptic density, in the middle of which one vesicle is undergoing exocytosis. A modest postsynaptic density lies along the inner aspect of the plasmalemma of the afferent terminal. (Reproduced, with permission, from Jacobs and Hudspeth 1990.)

Hair Cells Use Specialized Ribbon Synapses

In addition to being sensory receptors, hair cells also form synapses with sensory neurons. The basolateral membrane of each cell contains several presynaptic active zones at which chemical neurotransmitter is released. An active zone is characterized by four prominent morphological features (Figure 30–16).

A presynaptic dense body or synaptic ribbon lies in the cytoplasm adjacent to the release site. This fibrillar, osmiophilic structure may be spherical, ovoidal, or flattened, and usually measures a few hundred nanometers across. The dense body resembles the synaptic ribbon of a photoreceptor cell and represents a specialized elaboration of the smaller presynaptic densities found at the neuromuscular junction and at central nervous system synapses. In addition to molecular components shared with conventional synapses, ribbon synapses contain large amounts of the protein ribeye.

The presynaptic ribbon is surrounded by clear synaptic vesicles, each 35 nm to 40 nm in diameter, which are attached to the dense body by tenuous filaments. Between the dense body and the presynaptic plasma membrane lies a striking presynaptic density that comprises several short rows of fuzzy material. Within the plasmalemma rows of large particles are aligned with the strips of presynaptic density. These particles are thought to include the Ca^{2+} channels involved in the release of transmitter as well as the K^+ channels that participate in electrical resonance.

Studies of nonmammalian experimental models show that, as with most other synapses (see Chapter 12), the release of transmitter by hair cells is evoked by presynaptic depolarization and requires Ca^{2+} from the extracellular medium. Hair cells lack synaptotagmins 1 and 2, however, and the role of those proteins as rapid Ca^{2+} sensors has probably been assumed by the protein otoferlin, which also promotes the replenishment of synaptic vesicles. Postsynaptic recordings indicate that the release of the hair cell's synaptic transmitter is quantal in nature, resembling that of the neuromuscular junction. Although glutamate is the principal afferent neurotransmitter, other substances are released as well.

The presynaptic apparatus of hair cells has several unusual features that underlie the signaling abilities of these cells. Hair cells release synaptic transmitter continuously at rest. The rate of transmitter release can then be modulated upward or downward, depending on whether the hair cell is respectively depolarized or hyperpolarized. Consistent with this observation, the Ca^{2+} channels of hair cells are activated at the resting potential, providing a steady leak of Ca^{2+} that evokes transmitter release from unstimulated cells. Another unusual feature of the hair cell's synapses is that, like those of photoreceptors, they must be able to release neurotransmitter reliably in response to a threshold receptor potential of only 100 μV or so. This feature, too, results from the fact that the presynaptic Ca^{2+} channels are activated at the resting potential.

Most hair cells receive inputs from neurons in the brain stem at large boutons on the basolateral cell surface. These efferent terminals contain numerous clear synaptic vesicles about 50 nm in diameter as well as a smaller number of larger, dense-core vesicles. The principal transmitter at these synapses is acetylcholine (ACh); calcitonin gene–related peptide (CGRP) also occurs in efferent terminals and may be co-released with ACh. ACh binds nicotinic ionotropic receptors consisting of α9 and α10 subunits. These receptor-channels have a substantial permeability to Ca^{2+} as well as Na^+ and K^+. The Ca^{2+} that enters through these channels activates small-conductance Ca^{2+}-sensitive K^+ channels (SK channels), whose opening leads to a protracted hyperpolarization. The cytoplasm of a hair cell immediately beneath each efferent terminal holds a single cisterna of smooth endoplasmic reticulum. This structure may be involved in the reuptake of the Ca^{2+} that enters in response to efferent stimulation.

The best-understood role of efferent input in the cochlea is its effect on hair cells that employ electrical resonance for frequency tuning. Stimulation of the efferent nerve fibers hyperpolarizes a hair cell. The associated increase in membrane conductance perturbs the critically tuned resonance circuit in the cell's membrane, thus decreasing both the sharpness of frequency selectivity and the gain of electrical amplification. In the mammalian cochlea, where efferent fibers contact outer hair cells, the efferent system desensitizes the cochlea by turning down the active process.

Auditory Information Flows Initially Through the Cochlear Nerve

Bipolar Neurons in the Spiral Ganglion Innervate Cochlear Hair Cells

Information flows from cochlear hair cells to primary sensory neurons whose cell bodies lie in the cochlear ganglion. The central processes of these bipolar neurons form the cochlear division of the vestibulocochlear nerve (cranial nerve VIII). Because this ganglion follows a spiral course within the bony core of the cochlea, it is also called the *spiral ganglion.* Approximately 30,000 ganglion cells innervate the hair cells of each inner ear.

The afferent pathways from the human cochlea reflect the functional distinction between inner and outer hair cells. At least 90% of the spiral ganglion cells terminate on inner hair cells (Figure 30–17). Each axon contacts only a single inner hair cell, but each cell directs its output to several nerve fibers, on average nearly 10. This arrangement has three important consequences.

First, the neural information from which hearing arises originates almost entirely at inner hair cells. Second, because the output of each inner hair cell is sampled by many afferent nerve fibers, the information from one receptor is encoded independently in several parallel channels. Third, at any point along the cochlear spiral, or at any position within the spiral ganglion, each ganglion cell responds best to stimulation at the characteristic frequency of the presynaptic hair cell. The tonotopic organization of the auditory

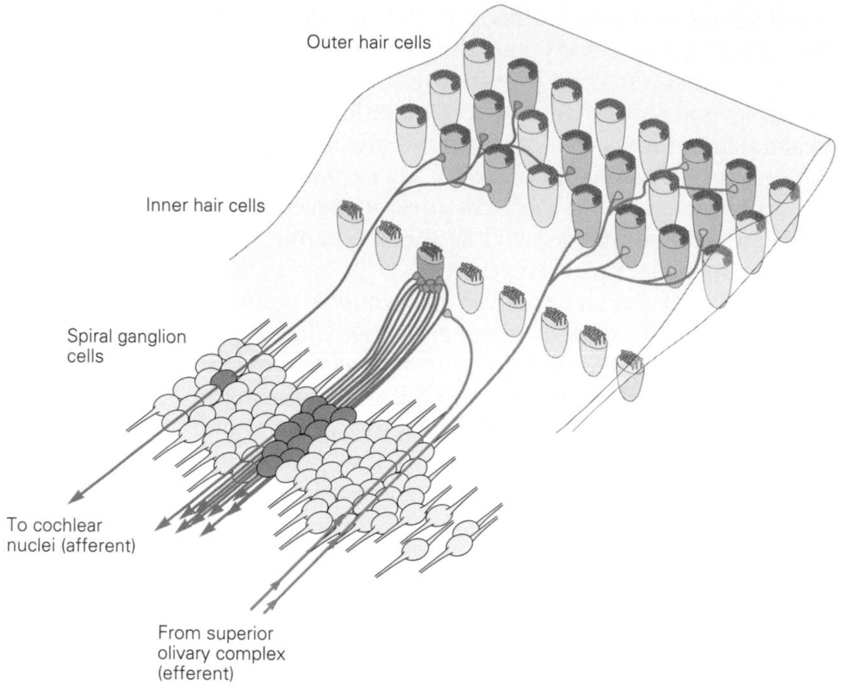

Figure 30–17 Innervation of cochlear hair cells. The great majority of sensory axons in the cochlea carry signals from inner hair cells, each of which constitutes the sole input to an average of 10 axons. A few sensory axons of small caliber transmit information from the outer hair cells. Efferent axons largely innervate the outer hair cells and do so directly. In contrast, efferent innervation of inner hair cells is sparse and occurs on the sensory axon terminals. (Adapted, with permission, from Spoendlin 1974.)

neural pathways thus begins at the earliest possible site, immediately postsynaptic to inner hair cells.

Relatively few cochlear ganglion cells contact outer hair cells, and each such neuron extends branching terminals to numerous outer hair cells. Although the ganglion cells that receive input from outer hair cells are known to project into the central nervous system, these neurons are so few that it is not certain whether their projections contribute significantly to the analysis of sound.

The patterns of efferent and afferent connections of cochlear hair cells are complementary. Mature inner hair cells do not receive efferent input; just beneath these cells, however, are extensive axo-axonic synaptic contacts between efferent axon terminals and the endings of afferent nerve fibers. In contrast, efferent nerves have extensive connections with outer hair cells on their basolateral surfaces. Each outer hair cell receives input from several large efferent terminals, which fill the space between the cell's base and the associated Deiters's cell.

Cochlear Nerve Fibers Encode Stimulus Frequency and Intensity

The acoustic sensitivity of axons in the cochlear nerve mirrors the connection pattern of the spiral ganglion cells. Each axon is most responsive to a characteristic frequency. Stimuli of lower or higher frequency also evoke responses but only when presented at greater intensities. An axon's responsiveness may be characterized by a tuning curve, which is V-shaped like the curves for basilar-membrane motion and hair-cell sensitivity (Figure 30–12). The tuning curves for nerve fibers with different characteristic frequencies resemble one another but are shifted along the abscissa.

The relation between sound-pressure level and firing rate in each fiber of the cochlear nerve is approximately linear. Because of the dependence of level on sound pressure, this relation implies that sound pressure is logarithmically encoded by neuronal activity. Very loud sounds saturate a neuron's response. Because an action potential and the subsequent refractory period last almost 1 ms, the greatest sustainable firing rate is somewhat above 500 spikes per second.

Even among nerve fibers with the same characteristic frequency, the threshold of responsiveness varies from axon to axon. The most sensitive fibers, whose response thresholds extend down to approximately 0 dB, characteristically have high rates of spontaneous activity and produce saturating responses for stimulation at moderate intensities, approximately 40 dB. At the opposite extreme, the least sensitive afferent fibers have less spontaneous activity and much higher thresholds but respond in graded fashion to intensities in excess of 100 dB. The activity patterns of most fibers range between these extremes.

The afferent neurons of lowest sensitivity contact the surface of an inner hair cell nearest the axis of the cochlear spiral. The most sensitive afferent neurons contact the hair cell's opposite side. The multiple innervation of each inner hair cell is therefore not wholly redundant. Instead, the output from a given hair cell is directed into several parallel channels of differing sensitivity and dynamic range.

The firing pattern of fibers in the eighth cranial nerve has both phasic and tonic components. Brisk firing occurs at the onset of a tone presented for a few seconds. As adaptation occurs, however, the firing rate declines to a plateau level over a few tens of milliseconds. When stimulation ceases there is usually a transitory cessation of activity with a similar time course before resumption of the spontaneous firing rate (Figure 30–18).

When a periodic stimulus such as a pure tone is presented, the firing pattern of a cochlear nerve fiber encodes information about the periodicity of the stimulus. For example, a relatively low-frequency tone at a moderate intensity might produce one spike in a nerve fiber during each cycle of stimulation. The phase of firing is also stereotyped. Each action potential might occur, for example, during the compressive phase of the stimulus. As the stimulation frequency rises, the stimuli eventually become so rapid that the nerve fiber can no longer produce action potentials on a cycle-by-cycle basis. Up to a frequency in excess of 4 kHz, however, phase-locking persists; a fiber may produce an action potential only every few cycles of the stimulus, but its firing continues to occur at a particular phase in the stimulus cycle.

Periodicity in neuronal firing enhances the information about the stimulus frequency. Any pure tone of sufficient intensity evokes firing in numerous cochlear nerve fibers. Those fibers whose characteristic frequency coincides with the frequency of the stimulus respond at the lowest stimulus level, but respond still more briskly for stimuli of moderate intensity. Other nerve fibers with characteristic frequencies close to the stimulus also respond, although somewhat less vigorously. Regardless of their characteristic frequencies, however, all the responsive fibers display phase locking: Each tends to fire during a particular part of the stimulus cycle.

The central nervous system can therefore gain information about stimulus frequency in two ways. First, there is a *place code;* the fibers are arrayed in a tonotopic map in which the position is related to characteristic frequency. Second, there is a *frequency code;* the fibers fire at a rate that signals the frequency of the stimulus. Frequency coding is of particular importance

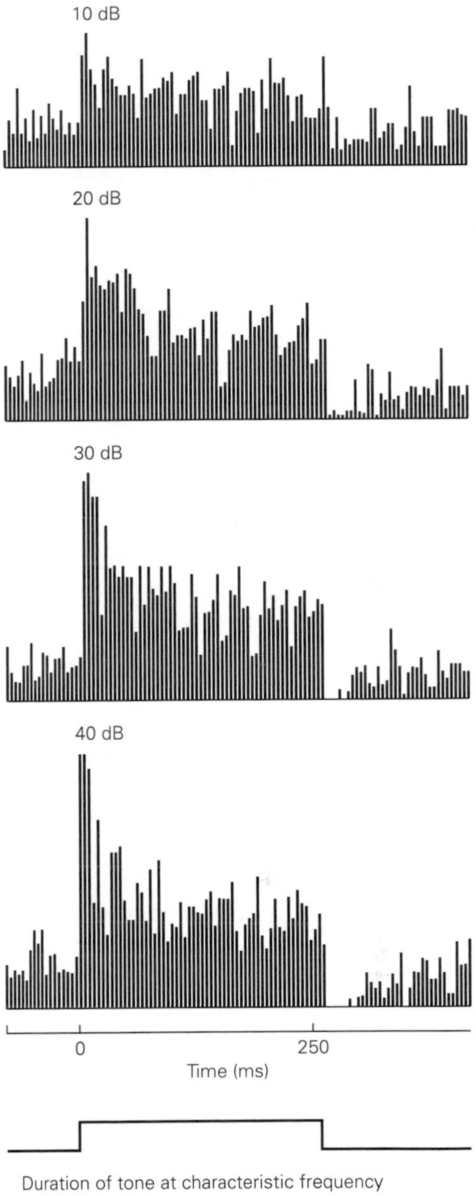

Figure 30–18 The firing pattern of a cochlear nerve fiber. A cochlear nerve fiber is stimulated for somewhat more than 250 ms with a tone burst at about 5 kHz, the cell's characteristic frequency. After a quiet period the stimulus is repeated. Histograms show the average response patterns of the fiber as a function of stimulus intensity. The sample period is divided into discrete temporal bins, and the number of spikes occurring in each bin is displayed. An initial, phasic increase in firing is correlated with the onset of the stimulus. The discharge continues during the remainder of the stimulus following adaptation, but decreases following termination. This pattern is evident when the stimulus is 20 dB or more above threshold. Activity gradually returns to baseline during the interval between stimuli. (Adapted, with permission, from Kiang 1965.)

when a sound is loud enough to saturate the neuronal firing rate. Although fibers with different characteristic frequencies respond to such a stimulus, each provides information about the stimulus frequency in its firing pattern.

Sensorineural Hearing Loss Is Common but Treatable

Whether mild or profound, most deafness falls into the category of *sensorineural hearing loss,* often misnamed "nerve deafness." Although hearing loss can result from damage to the eighth cranial nerve, for example from an acoustic neuroma (see Chapter 45), deafness stems primarily from the loss of cochlear hair cells.

The 16,000 hair cells in each human cochlea are not replaced by cell division but must last a lifetime. However, in amphibians and birds supporting cells can be experimentally induced to divide and their progeny to produce new hair cells. In the zebrafish some hair cell populations are regenerated continually by the activity of stem cells. Researchers have recently succeeded in replenishing mammalian hair cells in vitro. Until we understand how hair cells can be restored to the organ of Corti, however, we must cope with hearing loss, which is becoming more prevalent because of our aging population and increasingly noisy environment.

The last few decades have brought remarkable advances in our ability to treat deafness. For the majority of patients who have significant residual hearing, hearing aids can amplify sounds to a level sufficient to activate the surviving hair cells. A modern aid is custom-tailored to compensate for each individual's hearing loss, so that the device most amplifies sounds at frequencies to which the wearer is least sensitive while providing little or no enhancement to those that can still be heard well. To the credit of our society, the stigma formerly associated with wearing a hearing aid is dissipating rapidly; using such an aid is now regarded as unremarkable as wearing eyeglasses.

When most or all of a person's cochlear hair cells have degenerated, no amount of amplification can assist hearing. However, hearing can be restored by bypassing the damaged cochlea with a cochlear prosthesis. A user wears a compact unit that picks up sounds, decomposes them into their frequency components, and forwards electronic signals representing these constituents along separate wires to small antennas situated just behind the auricle. The signals are then transmitted transdermally to receiving antennas implanted in the temporal bone. From there, fine wires bear the signals to appropriate electrodes implanted at various positions along the scala tympani. Activation of the electrodes excites action potentials in nearby axons (Figure 30–19).

The cochlear prosthesis takes advantage of the tonotopic representation of stimulus frequency along the cochlea. Because the axons innervating each segment of the cochlea are concerned with a specific, narrow range of frequencies, each electrode in a prosthesis can excite a cluster of nerve fibers that are sensitive to similar frequencies. The stimulated neurons then forward their outputs along the intact eighth nerve to the central nervous system, where these signals are interpreted as a sound of the frequency represented at that position on the basilar membrane. An array of approximately 20 electrodes can mimic a complex sound by appropriately stimulating several clusters of neurons.

Cochlear prostheses have now been implanted in more than 100,000 patients worldwide. Their effectiveness varies widely from person to person. In the best outcome an individual can understand speech nearly as well as a normally hearing person and can even conduct telephone conversations. At the other extreme are patients who derive little benefit from prostheses, presumably because of extensive degeneration of the nerve fibers near the electrode array. Most patients find their prostheses of great value. Even if hearing is not completely restored, the devices help in lip reading and alert patients to noises in the environment.

The other way to overcome deafness relies not on high technology but on the efforts of generations of deaf individuals and their teachers. Sign languages have probably existed for as long as humans have spoken, and perhaps even longer. Many such languages represent attempts to translate spoken language into a system of hand signs. Signed English, for example, provides an effective means of communication that largely obeys the rules of English speech.

However, sign languages that diverge more radically from spoken languages are far more effective. Freed from the constraint of mirroring English, American Sign Language, or ASL, has become an elegant and eloquent language in its own right. Linguists now recognize American Sign Language as a distinct language whose range of expressiveness generally matches—and sometimes exceeds—that of spoken English.

An Overall View

Hearing, a key sense in human communication, begins with capture of sound by the ear. Mechanical energy captured by the outer ear flows through the middle

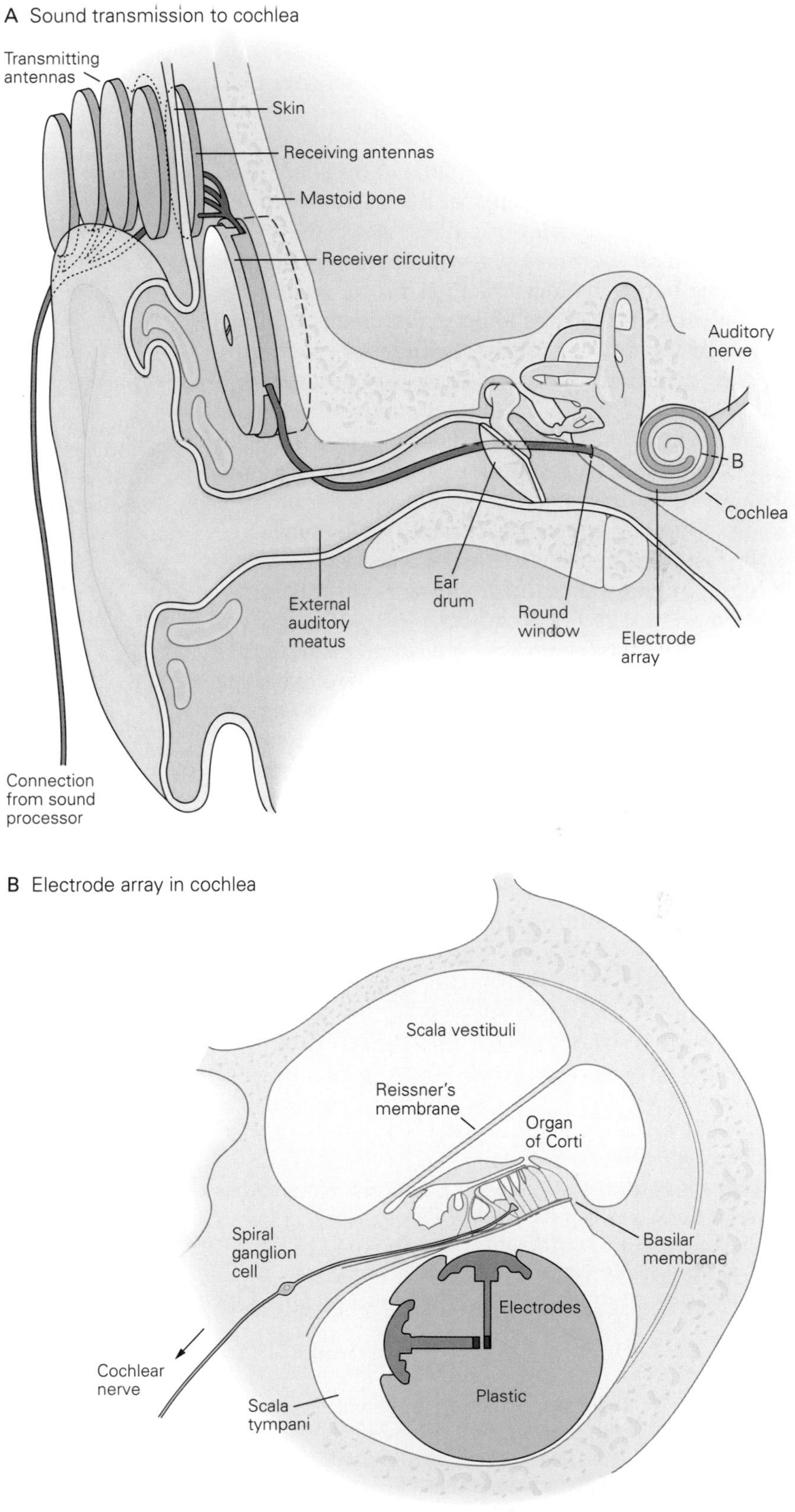

Figure 30–19 A cochlear prosthesis. (Reproduced, with permission, from Loeb et al. 1983.)

A. Transmitting antennas receive electrical signals from a sound processor, located behind the subject's auricle or on the frame of his eyeglasses, and forward them across the skin to receiving antennas implanted subdermally behind the auricle. The signals are then conveyed in a fine cable to an electrode array in the cochlea.

B. This cross section of the cochlea shows the placement of pairs of electrodes in the scala tympani. A portion of the extracellular current passed between an electrode pair is intercepted by nearby cochlear nerve fibers, which are thus excited and send action potentials to the brain.

ear to the cochlea, where it causes the elastic basilar membrane to oscillate. Aligned along the basilar membrane in a tonotopic array, 16,000 hair cells detect the frequency components of a stimulus and transduce them into receptor potentials that cause sensory neurons to fire.

As the population ages and as society becomes more concerned about hearing loss, physicians will increasingly confront patients and families who are experiencing the social difficulties associated with deafness. This subject is at present politically charged. On the one hand, the rapid technical improvement in cochlear prostheses leads their developers to advocate use of the devices whenever practical, including for young children. Many members of the deaf community, on the other hand, believe that widespread implantation of cochlear prostheses, particularly in children, will foster a generation of individuals whose ability to communicate is dependent on technological support of as yet unproved durability. The extensive use of prostheses might also diminish the use of American Sign Language and thus reverse the deaf community's remarkable recent advances.

Although this debate will not soon subside, it is worthwhile to emphasize the most positive aspect of the issue. A few decades ago there were no widely effective ways of coping with profound deafness; now there are two. Moreover, these solutions are not mutually exclusive; with a cochlear prosthesis a deaf individual can benefit from bilingualism in spoken English and American Sign Language.

A. J. Hudspeth

Selected Readings

Crawford AC, Fettiplace R. 1981. An electrical tuning mechanism in turtle cochlear hair cells. J Physiol 312:377–412.

Holt JR, Gillespie SKH, Provance DW, Jr., Shah K, Shokat KM, Corey DP, Mercer JA, Gillespie PG. 2002. A chemical-genetic strategy implicates myosin-1c in adaptation by hair cells. Cell 108:371–381.

Hudspeth AJ. 1989. How the ear's works work. Nature 341:397–404.

Hudspeth AJ. 2008. Making an effort to listen: mechanical amplification in the ear. Neuron 59:530–545.

Hudspeth, AJ, Jülicher F, Martin P. 2010. A critique of the critical cochlea: Hopf—a bifurcation—is better than none. J Neurophysiol 104:1219–1229.

Kazmierczak P, Sakaguchi H, Tokita J, Wilson-Kubalek EM, Milligan RA, Müller U, Kachar B. 2007. Cadherin 23 and protocadherin 15 interact to form tip-link filaments in sensory hair cells. Nature 449:87–91.

Loeb GE. 1985. The functional replacement of the ear. Sci Am 252:104–111.

Pickles JO. 2008. *An Introduction to the Physiology of Hearing*, 3rd ed. New York: Academic.

References

Art JJ, Crawford AC, Fettiplace R, Fuchs PA. 1985. Efferent modulation of hair cell tuning in the cochlea of the turtle. J Physiol 360:397–421.

Ashmore JF. 1987. A fast motile response in guinea-pig outer hair cells: the cellular basis of the cochlear amplifier. J Physiol 388:323–347.

Assad JA, Shepherd GM, Corey DP. 1991. Tip-link integrity and mechanical transduction in vertebrate hair cells. Neuron 7:985–994.

Beurg M, Fettiplace R, Nam J-H, Ricci AJ. 2009. Localization of inner hair cell mechanotransducer channels using high-speed calcium imaging. Nat Neurosci 12:553–558.

Chan DK, Hudspeth AJ. 2005. Ca^{2+} current-driven nonlinear amplification by the mammalian cochlea in vitro. Nat Neurosci 8:149–155.

Crawford AC, Fettiplace R. 1985. The mechanical properties of ciliary bundles of turtle cochlear hair cells. J Physiol 364:359–379.

Dallos P, Harris D. 1978. Properties of auditory nerve responses in absence of outer hair cells. J Neurophysiol 41:365–383.

Dallos P, Wu X, Cheatham MA, Gao J, Zheng J, Anderson CT, Jia S, et al. 2008. Prestin-based outer hair cell motility is necessary for mammalian cochlear amplification. Neuron 58:333–339.

Helmholtz HLF. [1877] 1954. *On the Sensations of Tone as a Physiological Basis for the Theory of Music.* New York: Dover.

Holley MC, Ashmore JF. 1988. On the mechanism of a high-frequency force generator in outer hair cells isolated from the guinea pig cochlea. Proc R Soc Lond B Biol Sci 232:413–429.

Howard J, Hudspeth AJ. 1988. Compliance of the hair bundle associated with gating of mechanoelectrical transduction channels in the bullfrog's saccular hair cell. Neuron 1:189–199.

Hudspeth AJ. 1982. Extracellular current flow and the site of transduction by vertebrate hair cells. J Neurosci 2:1–10.

Hudspeth AJ, Gillespie PG. 1994. Pulling springs to tune transduction: adaptation by hair cells. Neuron 12:1–9.

Jacobs RA, Hudspeth AJ. 1990. Ultrastructural correlates of mechanoelectrical transduction in hair cells of the bullfrog's internal ear. Cold Spring Harbor Symp Quant Biol 55:547–561.

Johnson SL, Beurg M, Marcotti W, Fettiplace R. 2011. Prestin-driven cochlear amplification is not limited by the outer hair cell membrane time constant. Neuron 70:1143–1154.

Kawashima Y, Géléoc GS, Kurima K, Labay V, Lelli A, Asai Y, Makishima T, et al. 2011. Mechanotransduction in mouse inner ear hair cells requires transmembrane channel-like genes. J Clin Invest 2011 121:4796–4809.

Kiang NY-S. 1965. *Discharge Patterns of Single Fibers in the Cat's Auditory Nerve.* Cambridge, MA: MIT Press.

Kozlov AS, Baumgart J, Risler T, Versteegh CPC, Hudspeth AJ. 2011. Forces between clustered stereocilia minimize friction in the ear on a subnanometre scale. Nature 474:376–379.

Liberman MC. 1982. Single-neuron labeling in the cat auditory nerve. Science 216:1239–1241.

Loeb GE, Byers CL, Rebscher SJ, Casey DE, Fong MM, Schindler RA, Gray RF, Merzenich MM. 1983. Design and fabrication of an experimental cochlear prosthesis. Med Biol Eng Comput 21:241–254.

Lumpkin EA, Hudspeth AJ. 1998. Regulation of free Ca^{2+} concentration in hair-cell stereocilia. J Neurosci 18:6300–6318.

Martin P, Hudspeth AJ. 1999. Active hair-bundle movements can amplify a hair cell's response to oscillatory mechanical stimuli. Proc Natl Acad Sci U S A 96:14306–14311.

Murphy WJ, Tubis A, Talmadge CL, Long GR. 1995. Relaxation dynamics of spontaneous otoacoustic emissions perturbed by external forces. II. Suppression of interacting emissions. J Acoust Soc Am 97:3711–3720.

Rosenblatt KP, Sun Z-P, Heller S, Hudspeth AJ. 1997. Distribution of Ca^{2+} activated K^+ channel isoforms along the tonotopic gradient of the chicken's cochlea. Neuron 19:1061–1075.

Roux I, Safieddine S, Nouvian R, Grati M, Simmle M-C, Bahloul A, Perfettii I, et al. 2006. Otoferlin, defective in a human deafness form, is essential for exocytosis at the auditory ribbon synapse. Cell 127:277–289.

Ruggero MA. 1992. Responses to sound of the basilar membrane of the mammalian cochlea. Curr Opin Neurobiol 2:449–456.

Rzadzinska AK, Schneider ME, Davies C, Riordan GP, Kachar B. 2004. An actin molecular treadmill and myosins maintain stereocilia functional architecture and self-renewal. J Cell Biol 164:887–897.

Spoendlin H. 1974. Neuroanatomy of the cochlea. In: E Zwicker, E Terhardt (eds.). *Facts and Models in Hearing,* pp. 18–32. New York: Springer-Verlag.

Stauffer EA, Scarborough JD, Hirono M, Miller ED, Shah K, Mercer JA, Holt JR, Gillespie PG. 2005. Fast adaptation in vestibular hair cells requires myosin-1c activity. Neuron 47:541–553.

Tilney LG, Tilney MS, Saunders JS, DeRosier DJ. 1986. Actin filaments, stereocilia, and hair cells of the bird cochlea. III. The development and differentiation of hair cells and stereocilia. Dev Biol 116:100–118.

von Békésy G. 1960. *Experiments in Hearing.* EG Wever (ed, transl). New York: McGraw-Hill.

Wilson JP. 1980. Evidence for a cochlear origin for acoustic re-emissions, threshold fine-structure and tonal tinnitus. Hear Res 2:233–252.

Zhang DS, Piazza V, Perrin BJ, Rzadzinska AK, Poczatek JC, Wang M, Prosser HM, et al. 2012. Multi-isotope imaging mass spectrometry reveals slow protein turnover in hair-cell stereocilia. Nature 481:520-524.

Zheng J, Shen W, He DZZ, Long KB, Madison LD, Dallos P. 2000. Prestin is the motor protein of cochlear outer hair cells. Nature 405:149–155.

31

The Auditory Central Nervous System

BECAUSE OF ITS ROLE IN THE UNDERSTANDING and production of speech, auditory perception is one of the most important sensory modalities in humans. In most animals hearing is crucial for localizing and identifying sounds; for some species, hearing additionally guides the learning of vocal behavior.

Once sounds have been transformed into electrical responses in the cochlea, a rich hierarchy of auditory circuits analyzes and processes these signals to give rise to auditory perception. The auditory system differs from most other sensory systems in that the location of stimuli in space is not conveyed by the spatial arrangement of the afferent pathways. Instead, the localization and identification of sounds is constructed from patterns of frequencies mapped at the two ears as well as from their relative intensity and timing. The auditory system is also notable for its temporal sensitivity; time differences as small as 10 μs can be detected. Auditory pathways resemble other sensory systems, however, in that different features of acoustic information are processed in discrete circuits that eventually converge to form complex representations of sound.

In addition to studies of primates and mammals such as cats and rodents, research on animals with especially acute or specialized auditory capacities—frogs, bats, barn owls, and songbirds—has provided a wealth of information about auditory processing. Many of the principles learned from the study of such auditory specialists have proven to be generally applicable. They are simply easier to detect in animals with specialized mechanisms.

Multiple Types of Information Are Present in Sounds

Hearing helps to alert animals to the presence of unseen dangers or opportunities, and in many species also serves as a basis for communication. Information about where sounds arise and what they mean must be extracted from the representations of the physical characteristics of sound at each of the ears. To understand how animals process sound, it is useful first to consider what cues are available.

Most vertebrates take advantage of having two ears for localizing sounds in the horizontal plane. Sound sources at different positions in that plane affect the two ears differentially: Sound arrives earlier and is more intense at the ear nearer the source (Figure 31–1A). The size of the head determines how interaural time delays are related to the location of sound sources; the neuronal circuitry determines the precision with which time delays are resolved. Because sound travels at roughly 340 m/s in air, the maximal interaural delay in humans is approximately 600 μs; in small birds the greatest delay is only 35 μs. Humans can resolve the location of a sound source directly ahead to within approximately 1 degree, corresponding to an interaural time difference of 10 μs. Interaural time differences are particularly well conveyed by neurons that encode relatively low frequencies, for groups of these neurons can fire at the same position in every cycle of the sound and in this way encode the interaural time difference as an interaural phase difference.

Sounds of high frequencies produce *sound shadows* or intensity differences between the two ears. For many mammals with small heads, high-frequency sounds provide the primary cue for localizing sound in the horizontal plane.

Spectral filtering in mammals allows sounds to be localized in the vertical plane and with a single ear (Figure 31–1B). High-frequency sounds, with wavelengths that are close to or smaller than the dimensions of the head, shoulders, and external ears, interact with those parts of the body to produce constructive and destructive interference, introducing broad spectral peaks and narrow, deep spectral notches whose frequency changes with the location of the sound. High-frequency sounds from different origins are filtered differently because in mammals the shape of the external ear differs back-to-front as well as top-to-bottom. Animals learn to use these spectral cues to locate sound sources. If the shape of the ear is experimentally altered, even adult humans can learn to make use of a new pattern of spectral cues. If animals lose hearing in one ear, they lose interaural timing and intensity cues and must depend completely on spectral cues for localizing sounds.

How do we make sense of the sounds that we hear? Most natural sounds contain energy over a wide range of frequencies and change rapidly over time. The information used to recognize sounds varies among animal species, and depends on listening conditions and experience. Human speech, for example, can be understood in the midst of noise, over electronic devices that distort sounds, and even through cochlear implants. One reason for its robustness is that speech contains redundant cues: The vocal apparatus produces sounds in which multiple parameters covary. At the same time, this makes the task of understanding how animals recognize patterns a complicated one. It is not clear which cues are used by animals under what conditions.

Music is a source of pleasure to human beings. Musical instruments and human voices produce sounds that have energy at the fundamental frequency that corresponds to the perceived pitch as well as at multiples of that frequency that give sounds a quality that allows us, for example, to distinguish a flute from a violin when their pitch is the same. Musical pitches are largely in the low frequency range in which auditory nerve fibers fire in phase with sounds. Musical sounds when combined simultaneously produce chords, and chord progressions produce melodies. Euphonious, pleasant chords elicit regular, periodic firing in the auditory nerve in which the most common interval between action potentials corresponds to the period of the perceived pitch. In dissonant sounds there is less regularity both in the sound itself and in the firing of auditory nerve fibers; the component frequencies are so close that they interfere with one another instead of periodically reinforcing one another.

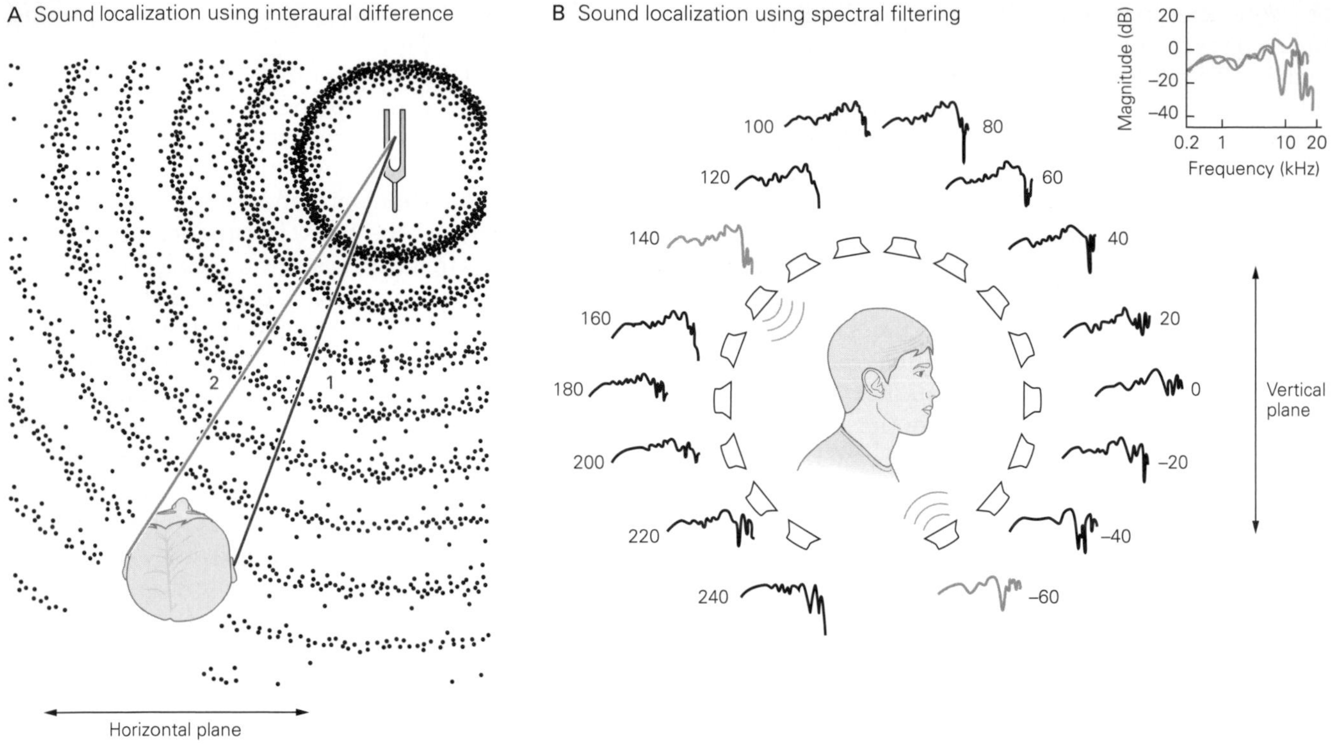

Figure 31–1 Cues for localizing sound sources.

A. A sound arising in the horizontal plane arrives differently at the two ears. Sounds arrive earlier and are louder at the ear nearer the source. Interaural time and intensity differences are cues for localizing sound sources in the horizontal plane, or azimuth. A sound that arises directly in the front or back travels the same distance to the right and left ears and thus arrives at both ears simultaneously. A sound that arises from the side travels a shorter distance to the near ear than to the far ear and thus arrives at the near ear before it arrives at the far ear. In humans the maximal interaural time difference is approximately 600 μs. High-frequency sounds, with short wavelengths, are deflected by the head, producing a sound shadow on the far side. Interaural intensity differences are used by mammals as an additional cue for localizing sounds in the horizontal plane. Interaural time and intensity do not vary with the movement of sound sources in the vertical plane, so it is impossible to localize a pure sinusoidal tone in the vertical plane. (Adapted, with permission, from Geisler 1998.)

B. Mammals can localize broadband sounds in both the vertical and horizontal planes on the basis of spectral filtering. When a noise that has equal energy at all frequencies over the human hearing range (*white noise*) is presented through a speaker, the ear, head, and shoulders cancel energy at some frequencies and enhance others. The amount of sound energy at each frequency at the ear canal is shown by the traces beside each speaker, which plot in decibels the power spectrum of sound that reaches the eardrum relative to the white noise that is produced by the speakers. For a white noise the power spectrum is flat. Note that by the time the noise has reached the bottom of the ear canal its spectrum is no longer flat. The small plot in the upper right compares spectral filtering of sounds coming from low in the front (**blue**) with sounds coming from behind and above the listener's head (**brown**). At high frequencies filtering by the ear introduces deep notches into spectra that vary depending on where the sounds arose. Sounds that lack energy at high frequencies and narrowband sounds are difficult to localize in the vertical plane. Spectral filtering also varies in the horizontal plane and provides the only location cue to animals that have lost hearing in one ear. You can test the salience of these spectral cues with a simple experiment. Close your eyes as a friend jingles keys directly in front of you at various elevations. Compare your ability to localize sounds under normal conditions and when you distort the shape of both ears by pushing them with your fingers from the back. The numerical values of the sound waves are measured in degrees beginning in front of the listener(–60 degrees) and moving in 20-degree increments in a vertical arc until the sound is broadcast behind the listener at 240 degrees. (Data reproduced, with permission, from D. Kistler and F. Wightman.)

The Neural Representation of Sound Begins in the Cochlear Nuclei

The neural pathways that process acoustic information extend from the ear to the brain stem, through the midbrain and thalamus, to the cerebral cortex (Figure 31–2). Acoustic information is conveyed from the cochlea by the central processes of cochlear ganglion cells (see Figure 30–17) that terminate in the cochlear nuclei in the brain stem. There information is relayed to several different types of neurons, most of which are arrayed tonotopically.

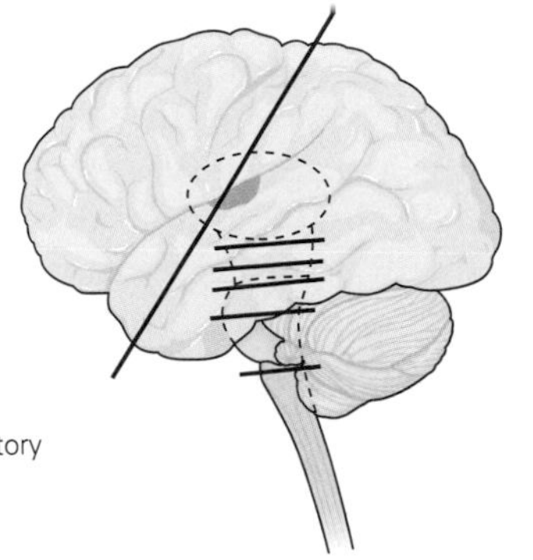

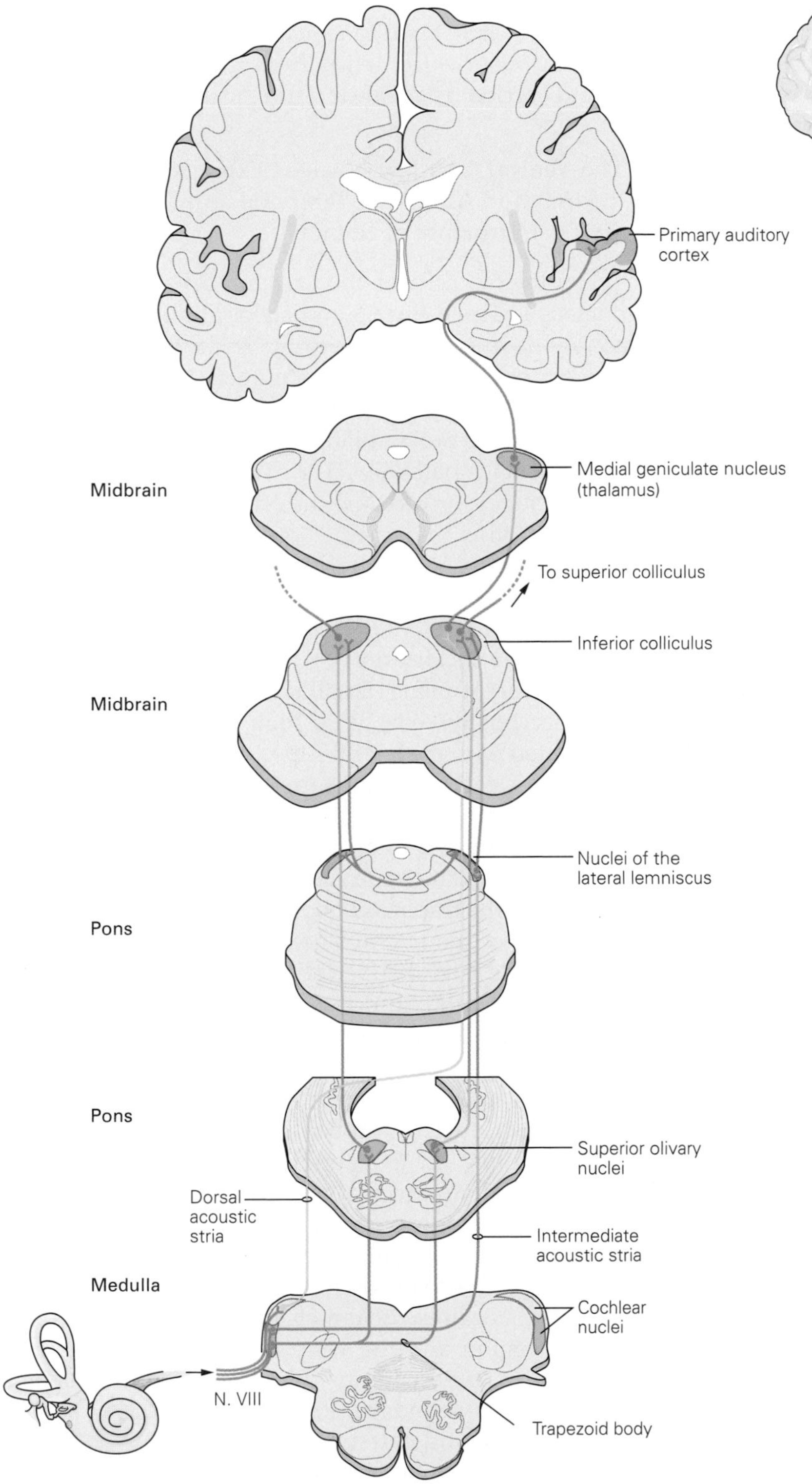

Figure 31–2 The central auditory pathways extend from the brain stem through the midbrain and thalamus to the auditory cortex. All cochlear (eighth cranial) nerve fibers terminate in the cochlear nuclei of the brain stem. The neurons of these nuclei project in several parallel pathways to the inferior colliculus. Their axons exit through the trapezoid body, intermediate acoustic stria, or dorsal acoustic stria. Some cells terminate directly in the inferior colliculus. Others contact cells in the superior olivary complex and in the nuclei of the lateral lemniscus, which in turn project to the inferior colliculus. Neurons of the inferior colliculus project to the superior colliculus and to the medial geniculate nucleus of the thalamus. Thalamic neurons project to the auditory cortex. Only the cochlear nuclei and the ventral nuclei of the lateral lemniscus receive monaural input. (Adapted, with permission, from Brodal 1981.)

The axons of each of these types of neurons take a different route and terminate on separate targets in the brain stem and midbrain, ultimately bringing acoustic information mainly to the contralateral inferior colliculus. Some of the pathways from the cochlear nuclei to the inferior colliculus are direct; others involve one or two synaptic stages in brain stem auditory nuclei. From the inferior colliculi acoustic information flows two ways: to the ipsilateral superior colliculus, where it participates in orienting the head and eyes in response to sounds, and to the ipsilateral thalamus, the relay to auditory areas of the cerebral cortex. The afferent auditory pathways from the periphery to higher brain regions include efferent feedback at many levels.

The Cochlear Nerve Imposes a Tonotopic Organization on the Cochlear Nuclei and Distributes Acoustic Information into Parallel Pathways

The afferent nerve fibers from cochlear ganglion cells are bundled in the cochlear or auditory component of the vestibulocochlear (eighth cranial) nerve and terminate exclusively in the cochlear nuclei. The cochlear nerve in mammals contains two groups of fibers: a large contingent (95%) of myelinated fibers that receives input from inner hair cells, and a small number (5%) of unmyelinated fibers that receives input from outer hair cells.

The larger, more numerous, myelinated fibers are much better understood than the unmyelinated fibers. Each myelinated fiber detects energy over a narrow range of frequencies; together these fibers carry information about the moment-to-monent variation in the frequency content of sounds. The unmyelinated fibers terminate on the large neurons in the ventral cochlear nuclei and on the small granule cells that surround the ventral cochlear nuclei. These fibers integrate information from a relatively wide region of the cochlea and are therefore unlikely to be as sharply tuned as the myelinated fibers. Because it is difficult to record from these tiny fibers, the information they convey to the brain is unknown. Indirect evidence suggests that they encode the intensity of sounds over a wide dynamic range.

Two features of the cochlear nuclei are important. First, the cochlear nerve fibers terminate in these nuclei in a tonotopic organization. Fibers that carry information from the apical end of the cochlea, which detects low frequencies, terminate ventrally in the ventral and dorsal cochlear nuclei; those that carry information from the basal end of the cochlea, which detects high frequencies, terminate dorsally (Figure 31–3). Second, each cochlear nerve fiber innervates several different areas within the cochlear nuclei, contacting various types of neurons that have distinct projection patterns to higher auditory centers. As a result, the auditory pathway is split into at least four parallel ascending pathways that simultaneously extract different facets of acoustic information from the representation of sound carried by cochlear nerve fibers.

The Ventral Cochlear Nucleus Extracts Information About the Temporal and Spectral Structure of Sounds

The principal cells of the unlayered ventral cochlear nucleus sharpen timing and spectral information and convey it to other auditory nuclei in the brain stem. Three types of neurons are intermingled and form separate pathways through the brain stem.

Bushy cells project bilaterally to the superior olivary complex. This pathway has two parts, one through the medial superior olive and the other through the lateral superior olive and medial nucleus of the trapezoid body. Large spherical bushy cells sense low frequencies and project bilaterally to the medial superior olive, forming a circuit that detects interaural time delay and permits the localization of low-frequency sounds in the horizontal plane. Small spherical bushy cells and globular bushy cells sense high frequencies and are associated with the lateral superior olive. Small spherical bushy cells probably excite the lateral superior olive ipsilaterally. The globular bushy cells, through calyceal axonal endings that surround the postsynaptic neurons, excite neurons in the contralateral medial nucleus of the trapezoid body that in turn inhibit principal cells of the lateral superior olive. The pathways through the lateral superior olive are involved in the detection of interaural intensity differences and contribute to the localization of high-frequency sounds in the horizontal plane.

Stellate cells excite neurons in the ipsilateral dorsal cochlear nucleus, probably in the ipsilateral lateral superior olive, in the periolivary nuclei, and in the contralateral ventral nucleus of the lateral lemniscus through collaterals of axons that project to the contralateral inferior colliculus. The tonotopic array of stellate cells encodes the spectra of sounds.

Octopus cells excite targets in the contralateral periolivary region and the ventral nucleus of the lateral lemniscus. These neurons detect onset transients and periodicity in sounds and may be involved in the recognition of sound patterns.

The differences in the integrative tasks performed by these pathways are evident in the synaptic structures and shapes of the three types of neurons.

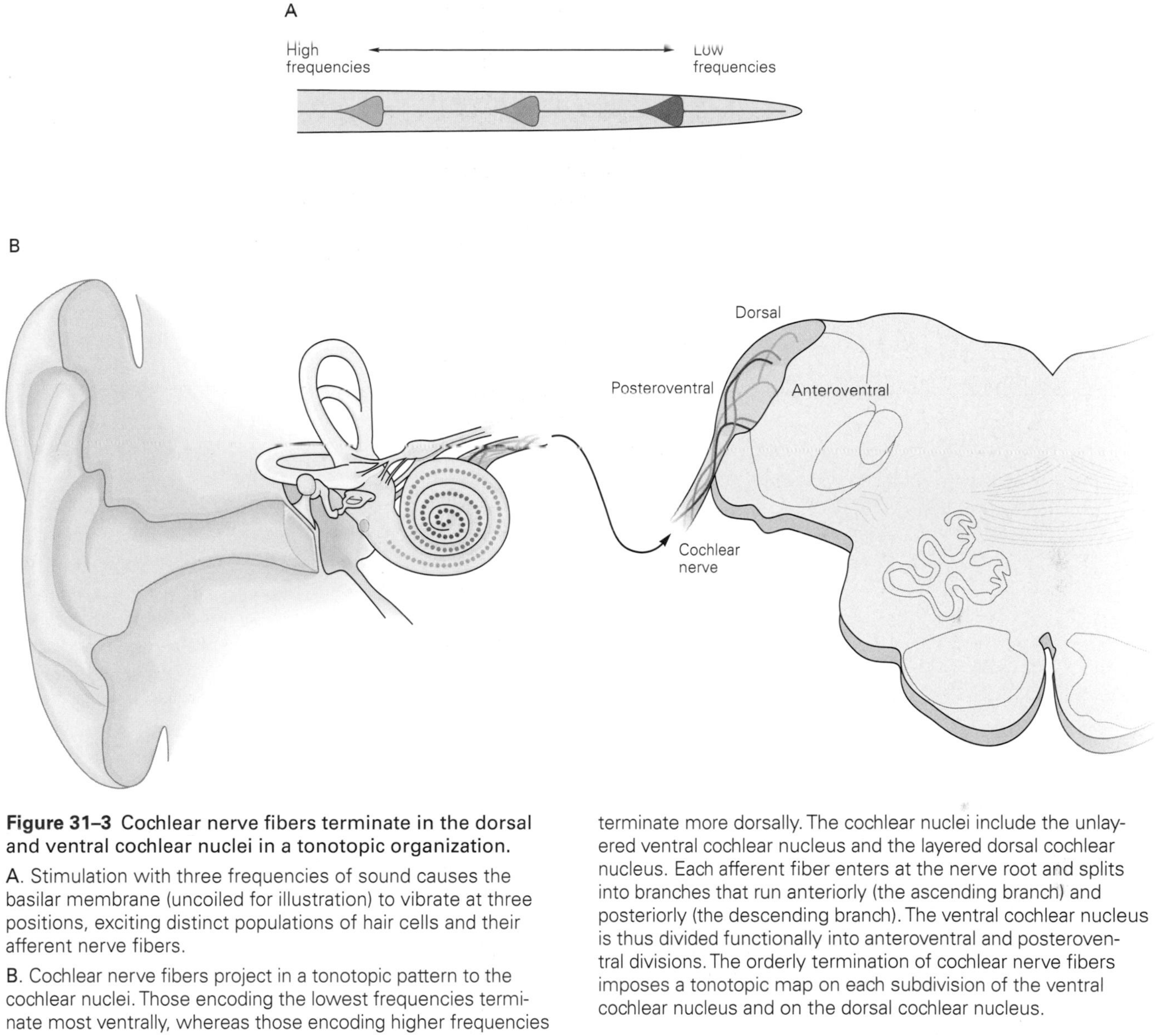

Figure 31–3 Cochlear nerve fibers terminate in the dorsal and ventral cochlear nuclei in a tonotopic organization.

A. Stimulation with three frequencies of sound causes the basilar membrane (uncoiled for illustration) to vibrate at three positions, exciting distinct populations of hair cells and their afferent nerve fibers.

B. Cochlear nerve fibers project in a tonotopic pattern to the cochlear nuclei. Those encoding the lowest frequencies terminate most ventrally, whereas those encoding higher frequencies terminate more dorsally. The cochlear nuclei include the unlayered ventral cochlear nucleus and the layered dorsal cochlear nucleus. Each afferent fiber enters at the nerve root and splits into branches that run anteriorly (the ascending branch) and posteriorly (the descending branch). The ventral cochlear nucleus is thus divided functionally into anteroventral and posteroventral divisions. The orderly termination of cochlear nerve fibers imposes a tonotopic map on each subdivision of the ventral cochlear nucleus and on the dorsal cochlear nucleus.

The shapes of their dendrites differ, reflecting differences in the way they collect information from cochlear nerve fibers (Figure 31–4A,B). The dendrites of bushy and stellate cells span only a small range of the tonotopic array of auditory nerve fibers, receive input from relatively few auditory nerve fibers, and are consequently sharply tuned. Many of the inputs to bushy cells are from unusually large terminals that surround the cell bodies, meeting the need for large synaptic currents. Octopus cells, in contrast, have dendrites that span a large proportion of the array of afferent fibers, receiving input from many cochlear nerve fibers, and thus are broadly tuned. Their need for large synaptic currents is met by summing inputs from large numbers of small terminals.

The biophysical properties of neurons determine how synaptic currents are converted to voltage changes and over how long a time synaptic inputs are integrated. Octopus and bushy cells in the ventral cochlear nucleus are able to respond with exceptionally rapid and precisely timed synaptic potentials. These neurons have a prominent, low-voltage-activated K^+ conductance that confers a low input resistance and rapid responsiveness and prevents repetitive firing (Figure

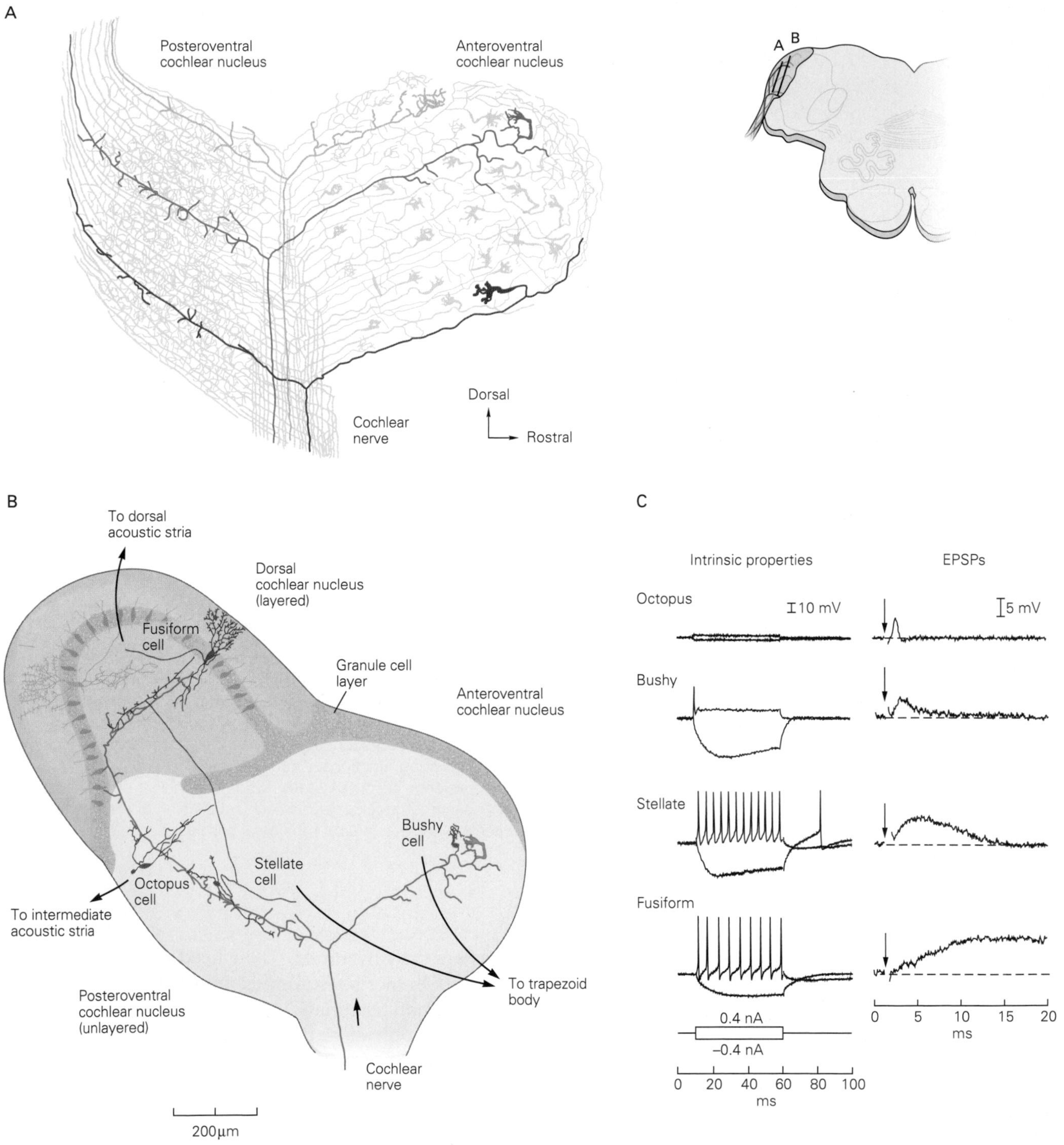
A
Posteroventral
cochlear nucleus
Anteroventral
cochlear nucleus
Cochlear
nerve
Dorsal
Rostral
A B
B
To dorsal
acoustic stria
Dorsal
cochlear nucleus
(layered)
Fusiform
cell
Granule cell
layer
Anteroventral
cochlear nucleus
Bushy
cell
Stellate
cell
Octopus
cell
To intermediate
acoustic stria
To trapezoid
body
Posteroventral
cochlear nucleus
(unlayered)
Cochlear
nerve
200μm
C
Intrinsic properties
EPSPs
Octopus
10 mV
5 mV
Bushy
Stellate
Fusiform
0.4 nA
–0.4 nA
0 20 40 60 80 100
ms
0 5 10 15 20
ms

31–4C). The large synaptic currents that are required to trigger action potentials in these leaky cells are delivered through rapidly gated, high-conductance, AMPA-type (α-amino-3-hydroxy-5-methylisoxazole-4-propionate) glutamate receptors found at many synaptic release sites. In contrast, stellate cells, in which even relatively small depolarizing currents produce large, protracted voltage changes, generate slower excitatory postsynaptic potentials (EPSPs) in response to synaptic currents. NMDA-type (*N*-methyl-D-aspartate) glutamate receptors enhance the slow responses.

Neurons in the ventral cochlear nucleus are able to encode different features of sounds because of differences in the pattern of input and their biophysical properties. Octopus cells detect synchronous firing in cochlear nerve fibers with exceptional temporal precision. Large, low-voltage-activated K^+ and hyperpolarization-activated conductances give octopus cells exceptionally low input resistances so that individual cochlear nerve fibers can produce synaptic responses of only approximately 1 mV and only 1 ms in duration. To fire action potentials octopus cells require summation of the rising phases of numerous synaptic inputs. Individual octopus cells detect coincident firing in the relatively large number of cochlear nerve fibers (more than 60) that contact them. Coincident firing in large numbers of cochlear nerve fibers is produced by periodic sounds such as vowels and musical sounds and by the onset of broadband sounds found in consonants or clicks.

Compared to octopus cells, bushy cells convey a more sharply tuned but less temporally precise version of the firing patterns of cochlear nerve fibers. The roughly 10 cochlear nerve fibers that terminate on each bushy cell deliver relatively large synaptic currents that require summation of only a few inputs to trigger an action potential. Two properties of bushy cells enable these neurons to encode with precision the detailed temporal structure of sounds. The cells' low input resistance shortens the voltage changes produced by the incoming synaptic currents; their need to summate several inputs removes variability in the timing of firing in cochlear nerve fibers by averaging.

The temporal fine structure of sounds that bushy cells encode provides information about the relative time of arrival of inputs to the two ears and is used at the next synaptic stage to form a map of the interaural time differences that underlie the ability to localize sound sources in the horizontal plane. The detection of musical pitch also requires the encoding of the temporal fine structure of sounds, but whether that information is carried through octopus or bushy cells or through a combination of pathways is not known.

Individual stellate cells detect intensity over a narrow frequency range and as a population they provide a continuous representation of the spectrum of sound energy. They are sharply tuned, being driven by only approximately 10 cochlear nerve fibers. Feedforward excitation through other, similarly tuned stellate cells and enhancement of inputs through NMDA-type receptors compensates for adaptation and obscures the fine structure of sound, encoded by cochlear nerve inputs, but allows the tonic firing rate of the cells to reflect the intensity of sounds to which they are tuned. Sideband inhibition enhances the cells' encoding of spectral peaks and troughs. Stellate cells track

Figure 31–4 **(Opposite) Cells in the cochlear nuclei extract acoustic information from the distinct electrophysiological properties of individual cochlear nerve fibers.**

A. The terminals along the length of each cochlear nerve fiber in the ventral cochlear nucleus differ in size and shape, reflecting differences in their targets. Large end bulbs form synapses on bushy cells; smaller boutons contact stellate and octopus cells. The nerve fibers are color-coded as in Figure 30–3: The **yellow fiber** encodes the highest frequencies and the **red fiber** the lowest. (Adapted, with permission, from Cajal 1909.)

B. A layer of granule cells separates the unlayered ventral cochlear nucleus (**beige**) from the layered dorsal nucleus (**brown**). In the dorsal cochlear nucleus the cell bodies of fusiform and granule cells are intermingled in a region between the outermost molecular layer and the deep layer. Cochlear nerve fibers, color-coded for frequency as in part A, terminate in both nuclei but with different patterns of convergence on the principal cells. Bushy, stellate, and fusiform cells each receive input from a few auditory nerve fibers and are sharply tuned, whereas individual octopus cells are contacted by many auditory nerve fibers and are broadly tuned.

C. Differences in the intrinsic electrical properties of the principal cells of the cochlear nuclei are reflected in the patterns of voltage change in the cells. When steadily depolarized, stellate and fusiform cells fire repetitive action potentials, whereas low-voltage-activated conductances prevent repetitive firing in bushy and octopus cells. The low input resistance of bushy and octopus cells in the depolarizing voltage range makes voltage changes rapid but also small; the rise and fall of voltage changes in stellate and fusiform cells is slower. Synaptic currents, too, produce different synaptic potentials. The synaptic potentials are brief in octopus and bushy cells but longer-lasting in stellate and fusiform cells. The brief synaptic responses in bushy and octopus cells require larger synaptic currents but encode the timing of auditory nerve inputs more faithfully than do the longer-lasting responses of stellate or fusiform cells. (Reproduced, with permission, from N. Golding.)

modulations in intensity on a timescale of tens of milliseconds that is known to be important for understanding speech.

The Dorsal Cochlear Nucleus Integrates Acoustic with Somatosensory Information in Making Use of Spectral Cues for Localizing Sounds

In mammals cochlear nerve fibers extend into a layered dorsal cochlear nucleus (Figure 31–4A,B). The dorsal cochlear nucleus receives input from two systems of neurons that project to different layers.

The outermost molecular layer is the terminus of a system of parallel fibers, the unmyelinated axons of granule cells that are scattered in and around the cochlear nuclei. The parallel fibers terminate on interneurons that bear a strong resemblance to those in the cerebellum. This system transmits somatosensory, vestibular, and auditory information from widespread regions of the brain to the molecular layer.

The deep layer is the terminus of cochlear nerve fibers, which convey acoustic information directly and indirectly through stellate cells of the ventral cochlear nucleus. The cochlear nerve inputs are tonotopically organized in isofrequency laminae that run at right angles to parallel fibers.

Inputs from both systems of fibers are combined in the principal neurons of the dorsal cochlear nucleus, the fusiform cells. Parallel fibers excite fusiform cells on their spiny apical dendrites in the molecular layer at plastic synapses, whereas cochlear nerve fibers and stellate cells of the ventral cochlear nucleus excite fusiform cells on their smooth basal dendrites in the deep layer at synapses that show little plasticity. Both fiber systems also inhibit fusiform cells through inhibitory interneurons.

Eric Young and his colleagues proposed that the dorsal cochlear nucleus helps mammals interpret spectral cues for localization of sound sources. When animals move their head or ears or walk, they affect the angle of incidence of sounds to the ears even when a sound source stays in one place. To make full use of spectral cues, animals must differentiate the predictable cues that are produced by their own movements from the more interesting, unpredictable ones that inform them about the location of external sound sources. The somatosensory and vestibular information about the position of the head and ears, as well as descending information from higher levels of the nervous system about the animal's own movements, can serve to identify the predictable cues. Fusiform cells thus relate the spectral cues they receive through the deep layer with predictable cues received through the molecular layer.

Among vertebrates only mammals have dorsal cochlear nuclei and only mammals have been shown to make use of spectral cues. Most birds and other reptiles hear to only 5 kHz, which corresponds to a wavelength of 6.8 cm. Sounds with wavelengths that exceed 7 cm do not interact with heads whose diameters are less than 2 cm wide and thus do not provide spectral cues. Conversely, humans hear to 20 kHz, corresponding to a wavelength of 1.7 cm; cats and dogs hear to approximately 50 kHz; and mice and bats hear to 100 kHz. The wavelengths of these high-frequency sounds are small with respect to the dimensions of the heads and ears and therefore provide useful spectral cues.

The Superior Olivary Complex of Mammals Contains Separate Circuits for Detecting Interaural Time and Intensity Differences

In many vertebrates, including mammals and birds, neurons in the superior olivary complex compare the activity of cells in the bilateral cochlear nuclei to locate sound sources. Separate circuits detect interaural time and intensity differences.

The Medial Superior Olive Generates a Map of Interaural Time Differences

Differences in arrival times at the ears are not represented at the cochlea. Instead, a map of interaural phase is created in the medial superior olive by a comparison of the timing of firing in responses to sounds from the two ears. Sounds arrive at the near ear before they arrive at the far ear, with interaural time differences being directly related to the location of sound sources in the horizontal plane.

Cochlear nerve fibers tuned to frequencies below 4 kHz and their bushy cell targets encode sounds by firing in phase with the pressure waves. This property is known as *phase-locking*. Although individual neurons may fail to fire at some cycles, the population of neurons represents the fine structure of sound waves by firing with every cycle. In so doing, these neurons carry information about the timing of inputs with every cycle of the sound. Sounds arriving from the side evoke phase-locked firing that is consistently earlier at the near ear than at the far ear, resulting in consistent interaural phase differences (Figure 31–5A).

In 1948 Lloyd Jeffress suggested that an array of detectors of coincident inputs from the two ears, transmitted through *delay lines* comprising axons with systematically differing lengths, could form a map of interaural time differences and thus a map of the location of sound sources (Figure 31–5B). In such a circuit conduction delays compensate for the early arrival at the near ear. Interaural time delays increase systematically as sounds move from the midline to the side, resulting in coincident firing further toward the edge of the neuronal array.

Such neuronal arrays have indeed been found in the barn owl in the homolog of the medial superior olivary nucleus. Mammals and chickens use a variant of this neuronal arrangement. The principal neurons of the medial superior olive form a sheet of one or a few cells' thickness on each side of the midline. Each neuron has two tufts of dendrites, one extending to the lateral face of the sheet, the other projecting to the medial face of the sheet (Figure 31–5C). The dendrites at the lateral face are contacted by large spherical bushy cells from the ipsilateral cochlear nucleus, whereas the dendrites at the medial face are contacted by large spherical bushy cells of matching best frequency from the contralateral cochlear nucleus. The axons of bushy cells terminate in the contralateral medial superior olive with delay lines just as Jeffress had suggested, but the branches that innervate the ipsilateral medial superior olive are of equal length (see Figure 31–5C).

Each medial superior olive receives coincident inputs from the two ears only when sounds come from the contralateral half of space. As sound sources move from the midline to the most lateral point on the contralateral side of the head, the earlier arrival of sounds at the contralateral ear needs to be compensated by successively longer delay lines. This results in inputs from the two ears coinciding at increasingly posterior regions of the medial superior olive, thereby forming a map of interaural phase. Recent findings indicate that inhibition that is superimposed on these excitatory inputs plays a significant role in sharpening the map of interaural phase.

In responding to interaural phase, individual neurons in the medial superior olive provide ambiguous information about interaural time differences. Phase ambiguities are resolved when sounds have energy at multiple frequencies, as natural sounds almost always do. The sheet of neurons of the medial superior olive forms a representation of interaural phase along the rostrocaudal dimension but its tonotopic innervation by bushy cells imposes a tonotopic organization in the dorsoventral dimension. Sounds that contain energy at multiple frequencies evoke maximal coincident firing in a single dorsoventral column of neurons that localizes sound sources unambiguously.

Each medial superior olive thus forms a map of the location of sound sources in the contralateral hemifield. The striking difference between this spatial map and those in other sensory systems is that this map is not the result of the spatial arrangement of inputs, like retinotopic or somatosensory maps, but is inferred by the brain from computations made in the afferent pathways.

The Lateral Superior Olive Detects Interaural Intensity Differences

Sounds with wavelengths that are similar to or smaller than the head are deflected by the head, causing the intensity at the near ear to be greater than that at the far ear. In humans interaural intensities can differ in sounds that have frequencies greater than about 2 kHz. Interaural intensity differences produced by such *head shadowing* are detected by a neuronal circuit that includes the medial nucleus of the trapezoid body and the lateral superior olive.

Although the lateral superior olive does not form a map of the location of sounds in the horizontal plane, it performs the first of several integrative steps that use interaural intensity differences to localize sounds. Neurons in this nucleus balance excitatory input from small spherical bushy cells and stellate cells in the ipsilateral ventral cochlear nucleus with inhibitory input from a disynaptic pathway that includes globular bushy cells in the contralateral ventral cochlear nucleus and principal neurons of the ipsilateral medial nucleus of the trapezoid body (Figure 31–6). Sounds that arise ipsilaterally generate relatively strong excitation and relatively weak inhibition whereas those that arise contralaterally generate stronger inhibition than excitation. Differences in the location of the sound sources that generate differences in the balance between excitation and inhibition are reflected in the firing rates of neurons in the lateral superior olive. Neurons in the lateral superior olive are thus activated more strongly by sounds from the ipsilateral than from the contralateral hemifield.

The relative strength of inhibitory and excitatory inputs varies in the population of cells in the lateral superior olive, and thus in the degree of interaural level difference that causes them to stop firing. Although no individual neuron is sharply tuned to a particular interaural intensity difference, the combination of firing from a variety of neurons with different cutoffs conveys the necessary information through a population code.

In order to balance excitation and inhibition stimulated by the same sound, the ipsilateral excitation and contralateral inhibition must arrive at neurons in the lateral superior olive at the same time. Thus excitation that arises monosynaptically from the ipsilateral ventral cochlear nucleus must arrive at the same time as inhibition that arises disynaptically from the contralateral cochlear nucleus. It is probably for this reason that the

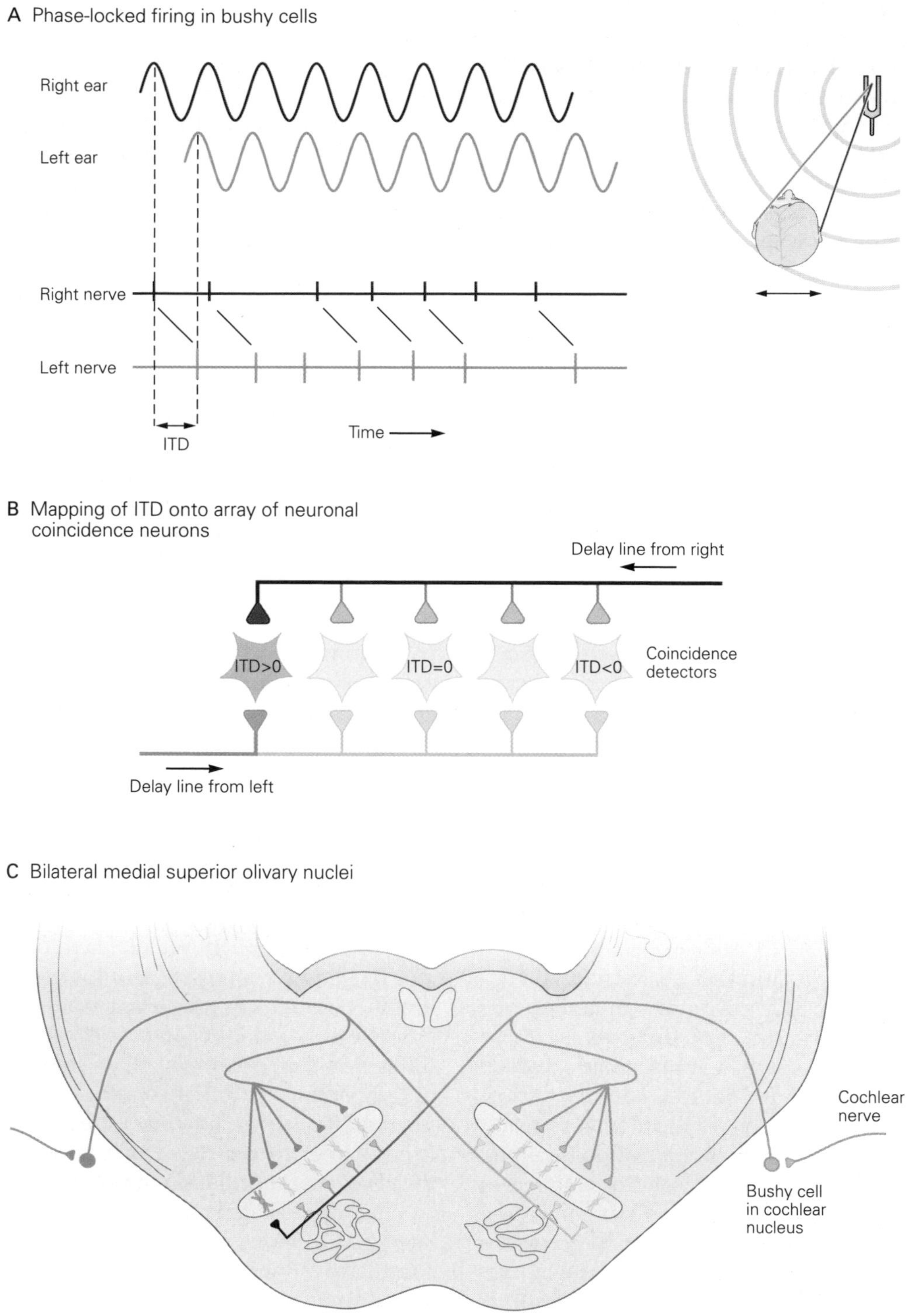
A Phase-locked firing in bushy cells
Right ear
Left ear
Right nerve
Left nerve
ITD
Time
B Mapping of ITD onto array of neuronal coincidence neurons
Delay line from right
ITD>0
ITD=0
ITD<0
Coincidence detectors
Delay line from left
C Bilateral medial superior olivary nuclei
Cochlear nerve
Bushy cell in cochlear nucleus

axons of globular bushy cells are exceptionally large; their synapses with the principal cells of the medial nucleus of the trapezoid body are the large calyces of Held that produce synaptic responses with short and consistently timed delays. The axons of small spherical bushy cells and cochlear nuclear stellate cells that carry ipsilateral excitation are smaller than those of globular bushy cells and thus conduct more slowly.

The terminals of the globular bushy cells, the calyces of Held, engulf the cell bodies of trapezoid-body neurons so dramatically that they caught the attention of early anatomists and modern biophysicists. A single somatic terminal releases neurotransmitter at numerous release sites and generates large synaptic currents. The capability of making reliable recordings pre- and postsynaptically has allowed the mechanisms of synaptic transmission to be studied in detail at this synapse (see Chapter 12).

Efferent Signals from the Superior Olivary Complex Provide Feedback to the Cochlea

Although sensory systems are largely afferent, bringing sensory information to the brain, recent studies have led to an appreciation of the importance of efferent regulation at many levels of the auditory system, including even efferent signaling to the cochlea from the superior olivary complex in the brain stem.

Olivocochlear neurons form a feedback loop from the superior olivary complex to hair cells in the cochlea. Their cell bodies lie around the major dense clusters of cell bodies in the olivary nuclei. In mammals two groups of olivocochlear neurons have been distinguished. The medial olivocochlear neurons have myelinated axons that terminate on the outer hair cells bilaterally; the lateral olivocochlear neurons have unmyelinated axons that terminate ipsilaterally on the afferent fibers associated with inner hair cells.

Most medial olivocochlear neurons, with cell bodies that lie ventral and medial within the olivary complex, send their axons to the contralateral cochlea (Figure 31–7), but many also innervate the ipsilateral cochlea. These cholinergic neurons act on hair cells through a special class of nicotinic acetylcholine receptor-channels formed from $\alpha9$ and $\alpha10$ subunits. Calcium ions that enter through these channels activate K^+ channels that hyperpolarize outer hair cells. These neurons thus mediate negative feedback and are binaural, being driven predominantly but not exclusively by stellate cells of the contralateral ventral cochlear nucleus. Collateral branches of olivocochlear neurons terminate on stellate cells in the cochlear nucleus, acting on conventional nicotinic and muscarinic acetylcholine receptors, forming an excitatory feedback loop. Activity in these efferent fibers increases the representation of signals in noise, reduces the sensitivity of the cochlea, and protects it from damage by loud sounds.

Figure 31–5 (Opposite) **Interaural time differences localize sound sources in the horizontal plane.**

A. When a sound, such as a pure tone, arises from the right, the right ear detects the sound earlier than the left ear. The difference in the time of arrival at the two ears is the interaural time delay (**ITD**). Cochlear nerve fibers and their bushy cell targets fire in phase with changes in sound pressure. Although individual neurons sometimes skip cycles, the population of bushy cells encodes the timing of low-frequency sounds and its frequency with every cycle. Comparison of the timing of action potentials of bushy cells at the two sides reveals the ITDs (**slanted black lines**).

B. Interaural time differences can be detected with delay lines. If axons have systematically differing lengths, their action potentials reach the nearest terminals before they reach the farthest ones. An array of neurons that detects coincident inputs from delay lines can produce a map of ITDs. When sounds come from the right, action potentials from the right ear must be delayed to compensate for the fact that they arrive earlier than those from the left and to allow the signals from right and left to coincide at one side of the array (**mustard-colored cell**). Such an arrangement of delay lines has been found in the nucleus laminaris of the barn owl, the homolog of the medial superior olivary nucleus.

C. Mammals use delay lines on the contralateral side only to form a map of interaural time differences. The bitufted neurons of the medial superior olivary nucleus form a sheet that is contacted on the lateral face by bushy cells from the ipsilateral cochlear nucleus and on the medial face by bushy cells from the contralateral cochlear nucleus. On the ipsilateral side the branches of the bushy cell axon are of equal length and thus deliver synaptic currents to their targets in the medial superior olive simultaneously. On the contralateral side the branches deliver synaptic currents first to the anterior regions, closest to the midline, and then to progressively more posterior regions. The postsynaptic neurons can detect synchronous excitation only when sounds arise from the contralateral half of space. When sounds arise from the right side, their early arrival at the right ear is compensated by progressively later arrival at neurons in the posterior region of the left medial superior olive (the **mustard-colored cell** is activated by a sound from the far right, as in part B). When sounds arise from the front and there is no interaural time difference, neurons in the anterior end of the medial superior olive are activated synchronously from both sides. Thus each medial superior olive forms a map of where sounds arise in the contralateral hemifield. (Adapted, with permission, from Yin 2002.)

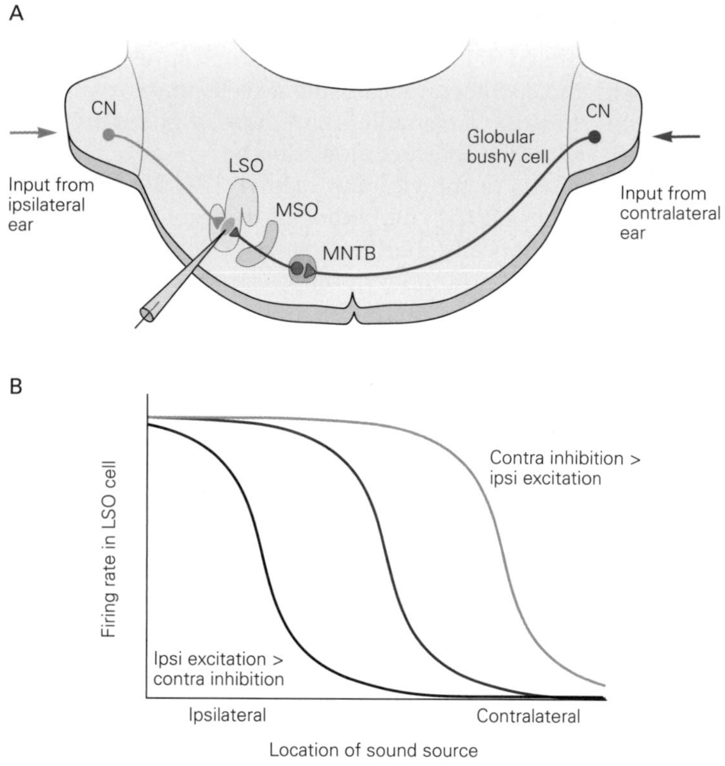

Figure 31–6 Interaural intensity differences localize sound sources in the horizontal plane.

A. Principal cells of the lateral superior olivary nucleus (**LSO**) receive excitatory input from the ipsilateral cochlear nucleus (**CN**) and inhibitory input from the contralateral cochlear nucleus. A coronal section through the brain stem of a cat illustrates the anatomical connections. Small spherical bushy cells and stellate cells in the ipsilateral ventral cochlear nucleus provide direct excitation. Globular bushy cells in the contralateral ventral cochlear nucleus project across the midline and excite neurons in the medial nucleus of the trapezoid body (**MNTB**) through large terminals, the calyces of Held. Cells of the medial nucleus of the trapezoid body inhibit neurons in both the lateral superior olive and medial superior olive (**MSO**). For neurons of the lateral superior olive to compare intensities of the same sound, the timing of the ipsilateral excitatory input must be matched with the timing of the contralateral inhibitory input. To this end globular bushy cells have particularly large axons and synaptic transmission through a calyx of Held in the medial nucleus of the trapezoid body is strong so that the synaptic delay is short and invariant in its timing.

B. The firing of neurons in the lateral superior olive reflects a balance of ipsilateral excitation and contralateral inhibition. For any particular neuron, when sounds arise from the ipsilateral side, excitation is relatively stronger and inhibition is relatively weaker than when sounds arise from the contralateral side. The transition between the dominance of excitation and inhibition varies between neurons (**black, red, blue**) so that firing in the population of neurons reflects the location of the sound source.

Lateral olivocochlear neurons, with cell bodies that lie in and around the lateral superior olive, send their unmyelinated axons exclusively to the ipsilateral cochlea, where they terminate on the afferent fibers from inner hair cells. These efferents balance the excitability of cochlear nerve fibers at the two ears.

Brain Stem Pathways Converge in the Inferior Colliculus

The inferior colliculus occupies a central position in the auditory pathway of all vertebrate animals because all auditory pathways ascending through the brain stem converge there (Figure 31–7). The most important sources of excitation are stellate cells of the contralateral ventral cochlear nucleus, fusiform cells of the contralateral dorsal cochlear nucleus, principal cells of the ipsilateral medial superior olive and contralateral lateral superior olive, principal cells of ipsi- and contralateral dorsal nuclei of the lateral lemniscus, commissural connections from the contralateral inferior colliculus, and pyramidal cells in layer V of the auditory cortex. Important sources of inhibition include the nuclei of the lateral lemniscus, the ipsilateral lateral superior olive, the superior paraolivary nucleus, and the contralateral inferior colliculus.

The inferior colliculus of mammals is subdivided into the central nucleus, dorsal cortex, and external cortex. The central nucleus is tonotopically organized. All neurons in each lamina have similar best frequencies. Low frequencies are represented dorsolaterally and high frequencies ventromedially. Fine mapping has shown that the tonotopic organization is discontinuous; the separation between best frequencies corresponds to psychophysically measured critical bands of approximately one-third octave. Although the central nucleus is organized tonotopically, the spectral range of inputs to these neurons is broader than at earlier stages in the auditory pathway. Inhibition sharpens the frequency tuning of inferior colliculus excitatory neurons, and tuning can be further modulated by descending inputs from the cortex.

Many neurons in the central nucleus carry information about the location of sound sources. The majority of these cells are sensitive to interaural time and intensity differences, which are known to be essential cues for localizing sounds in the azimuth. Neurons are also sensitive to spectral cues that localize sounds in the vertical plane (see Figure 31–1B). To localize sounds accurately, animals must ignore the reflections of sounds from surrounding surfaces that arrive after the initial direct wave front. Psychophysical experiments have shown that mammals suppress all but the earliest versions, a phenomenon termed the *precedence effect*. Physiological correlates of the precedence effect have been measured in the inferior colliculus, where inhibition suppresses simulated reflections of sounds.

Sound Location Information from the Inferior Colliculus Creates a Spatial Map of Sound in the Superior Colliculus

The inferior colliculus is not only a convergence point but also a branch point for ascending or outflow pathways.

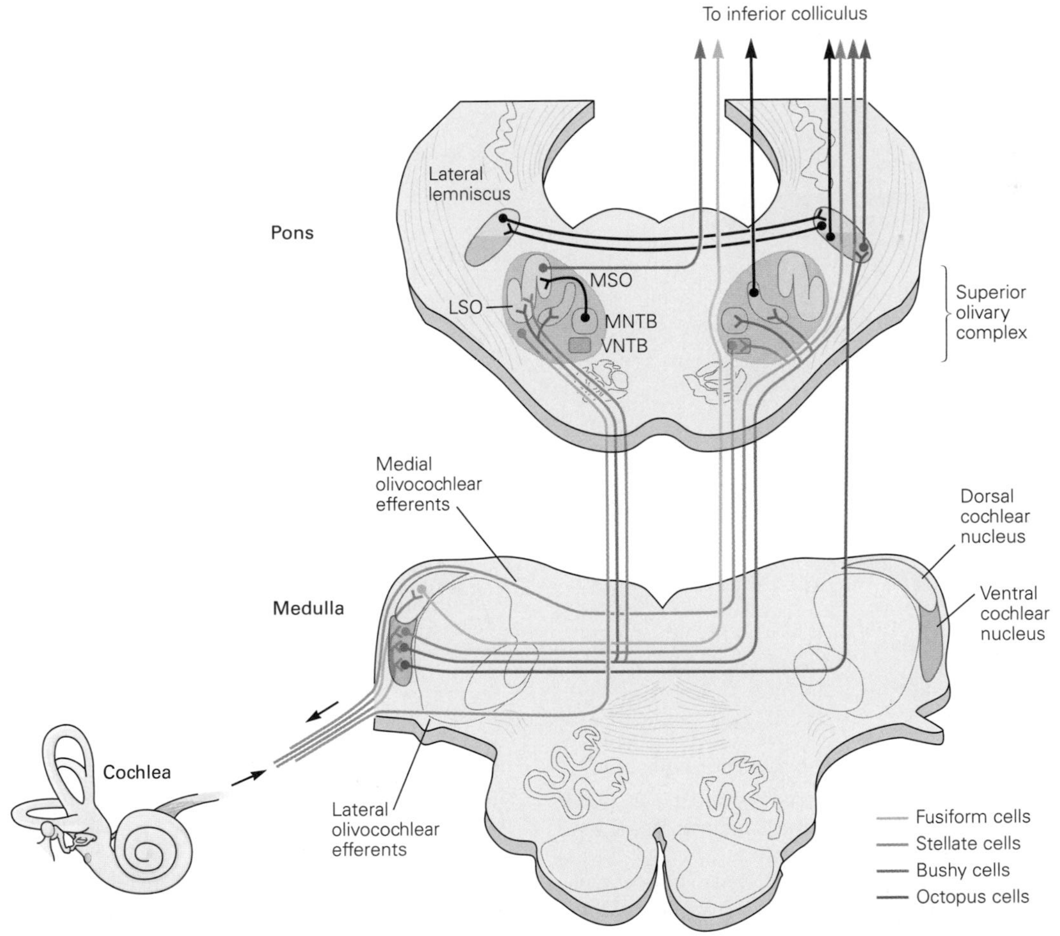

Figure 31–7 Major components of the ascending and descending auditory pathways. The major connections among the nuclei that form the early auditory pathway are shown; because the auditory pathway is bilaterally symmetrical, only one side is illustrated. The ascending pathway begins in the cochlea and progresses through several parallel pathways through the brain stem cochlear nuclei: the cochlear nuclei, the superior olivary nuclei, and the ventral and dorsal nuclei of the lateral lemniscus. These signals converge in the inferior colliculus, which projects to the medial geniculate body of the thalamus and thence to the cerebral cortex (see Figure 31–2). Some of the connections are excitatory pathways (**colored lines**) and others inhibitory pathways (**black lines**). These same nuclei are also interconnected through descending pathways (**blue lines**) and through commissural projections. (**LSO,** lateral superior olivary nucleus; **MNTB,** medial nucleus of the trapezoid body; **MSO,** medial superior olive; **VNTB,** ventral nucleus of the trapezoid body.)

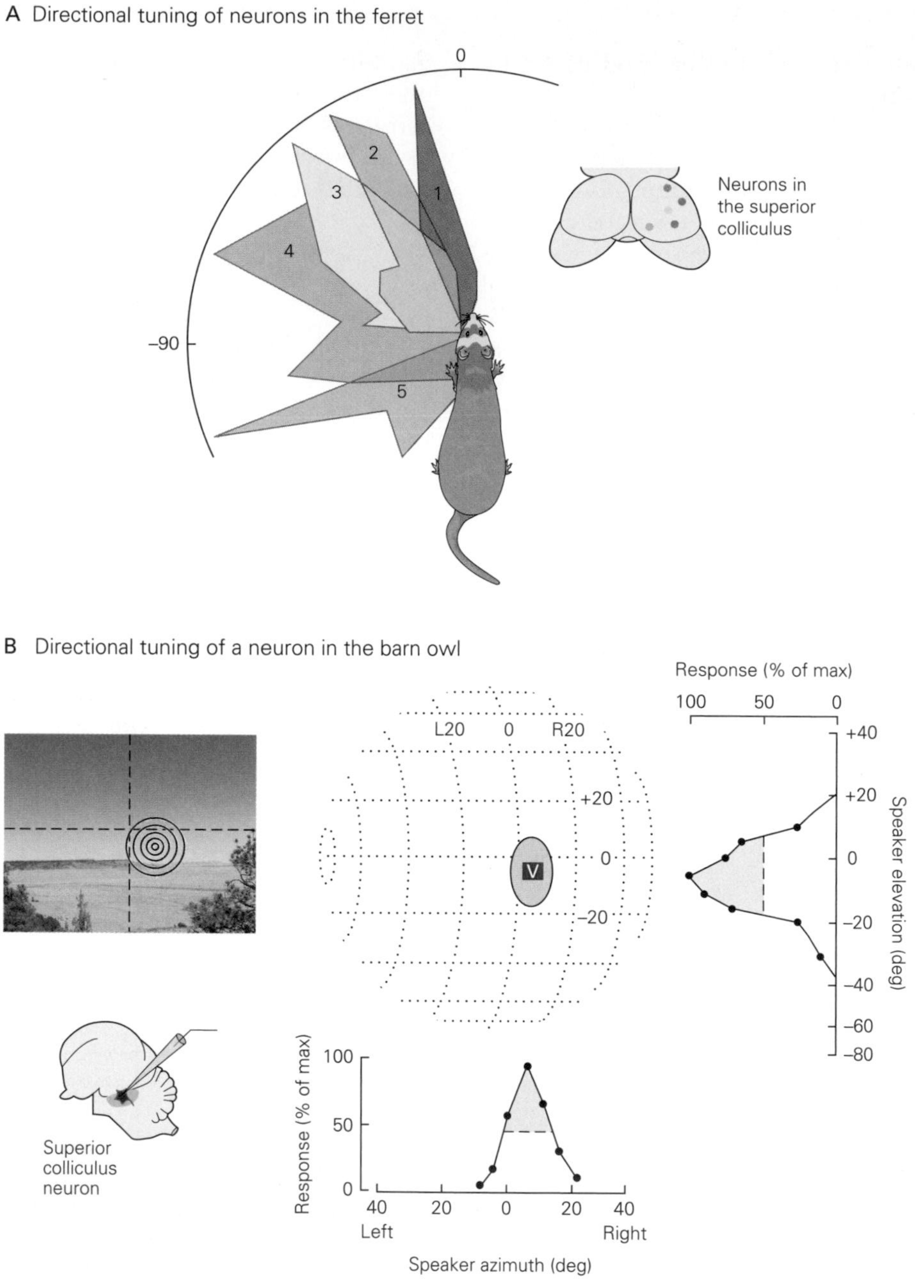

Figure 31–8 Sound localization in the superior colliculus.

A. Neurons in the ferret's superior colliculus are directionally tuned to sound in the horizontal plane. The colored areas represent the firing rate response profiles of collicular neurons 1 through 5 as a function of where the sounds are located, plotted in polar coordinates centered on the head. The inset shows the location of the recorded neurons in the colliculus. Note that neuron 1 responds best to sounds in front of the animal, whereas the responses of neurons that are located progressively more caudally in the colliculus shift correspondingly to sounds that originate farther contralaterally. The location of the sound begins in front of the animal at 0 degrees and moves contralaterally to a point beyond −90 degrees. (Modified, with permission, from King 1999.)

B. The normalized responses of a neuron in the barn owl's superior colliculus to noise bursts presented at various locations along the horizon or at various elevations are plotted below and at the right, respectively. The yellow areas in these tuning curves indicate where responses exceed 50% of the maximum. The sensitivity of the neuron to a particular location along the horizon as well as a particular elevation creates a discrete best auditory area in space for this neuron, shown as the ellipse labeled "V" on a plot of spatial locations with respect to a point straight in front of the owl. The neuron also responds to visual cues from the same area in space. The photograph illustrates the neuron's best area in space with respect to the position of the head; the intersection of the dashed lines indicates where the owl's head is pointing; photo reproduced, with permission, from Malia Jensen (Modified, with permission, from Cohen and Knudsen 1999.)

Central nucleus neurons project to the thalamus and also to the external cortex of the inferior colliculus and the nucleus of the brachium of the inferior colliculus, both of which then project to the superior colliculus (or the optic tectum in birds).

The superior colliculus is critical for reflexive orienting movements of the head and eyes to acoustic and visual cues in space. By the time they reach the superior colliculus, binaural sound cues and the monaural spectral cues that underlie mammalian sound localization merge to create a spatial map of sound, an auditory map, in which neurons are unambiguously tuned to specific sound directions. This convergence is critical, for the binaural level and timing differences alone cannot unambiguously code for a single position in space. The spectral cues that provide information about vertical location are essential. Different locations in the vertical plane can give rise to identical interaural time or intensity differences. Such a spatial map is formed both in birds and in some mammals (Figure 31–8). In ferrets and guinea pigs topographic representations of the location of sound in the horizontal plane are found in the external cortex and the nucleus of the brachium of the inferior colliculus.

Within the superior colliculus the auditory map is congruent with maps of visual space and the body surface. Unlike the visual and somatosensory maps, the auditory map is computed from a combination of cues that identify the specific position of a sound source in space, and is not based on the peripheral receptor surface.

Auditory, visual, and somatosensory neurons in the superior colliculus all converge on output pathways in the same structure that controls orienting movements of the eyes, head, and external ears. The motor circuits of the superior colliculus are mapped with respect to motor targets in space, and are aligned with the sensory maps. Such sensory-motor correspondence facilitates the sensory guiding of movements.

Midbrain Sound-Localization Pathways Are Sensitive to Experience in Early Life

Cues for sound localization vary both within and across individuals as a result of differences in the size and shape of the head and ears. Moreover, the neural representation of these cues can also vary during development and with changes of the brain as a result of aging. The neural system for sound localization, especially in barn owls, has become an important model for the study of synaptic plasticity in the brain.

In addition to studies of normal development of sound localization, artificial manipulations of sensory experience have been particularly revealing. In adult mammals and birds occlusion of one ear alters the binaural acoustic cues and causes mislocalization of sounds toward the open ear. When such manipulations of sound cues are conducted in young owls, the animals initially misorient but recover accurate orienting responses over a period of weeks. This is accompanied by a shift in the tuning of auditory neurons in the colliculi toward the abnormal cues that result from use of the earplug. If the earplug is removed after adaptation, owls initially make orienting errors in the opposite direction, but gradually recover accurate behavior as well as a normal spatial map of sound in the brain.

Because visual and auditory cues are normally in alignment in the external world, their representations are also congruent in the superior colliculus (Figure 31–8B). Alterations of visual inputs, and thus of the normal match between acoustic and visual cues, also affect sound localization. When carried out early in development, such visual manipulations cause striking changes in the spatial mapping of sound in the colliculi. For example, when an eye is deviated laterally in a young ferret by removal of an extraocular muscle, the auditory map in the contralateral superior colliculus undergoes a shift so that the visual and auditory maps remain in alignment.

In barn owls, which cannot move their eyes, the visual field has been experimentally misaligned by raising owls with prisms that shift the visual world horizontally (Figure 31–9A). Over the course of weeks owls adjust their auditory orienting responses so that their movements correspond to the location of a target in the shifted visual space. Although the response to sounds is incorrect in terms of purely auditory cues, this is an adaptive response because it causes the animal to look at the source of the sound. In parallel with the changes in behavior, neurons in the colliculi gradually shift their response to interaural time differences by the amount of displacement in the visual field (Figure 31–9B).

The mechanisms of this plasticity, which may be very general, have been extensively studied by Eric Knudsen and his colleagues. The auditory map in the central nucleus of the inferior colliculus does not change in young owls reared with prisms. However, orderly axonal connections from the central nucleus to the external nucleus gradually sprout, forming a pathway that represents the newly learned interaural timing difference (Figure 31–10). The original inputs from the central nucleus persist but are actively suppressed by GABA-ergic inhibitory inputs. The retention of the old functional connections likely underlies the rapid

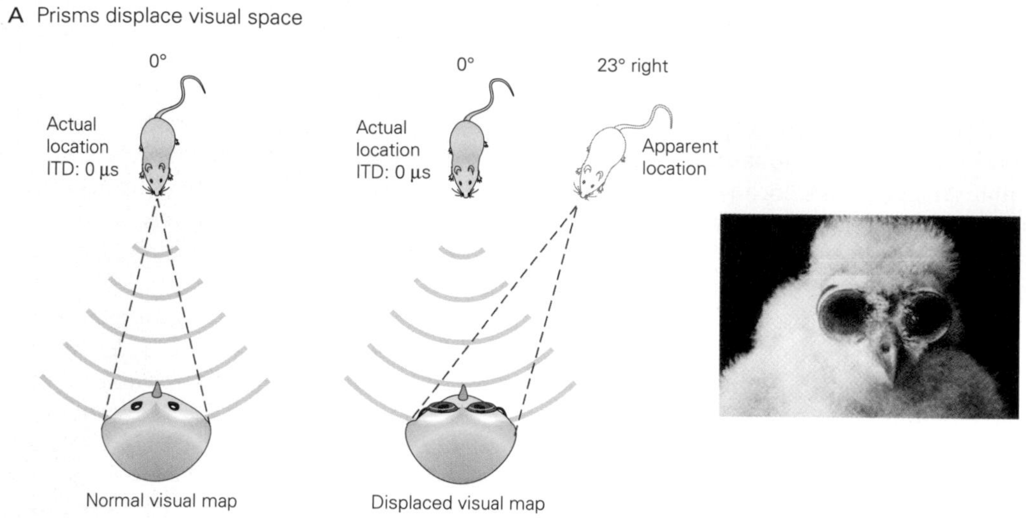

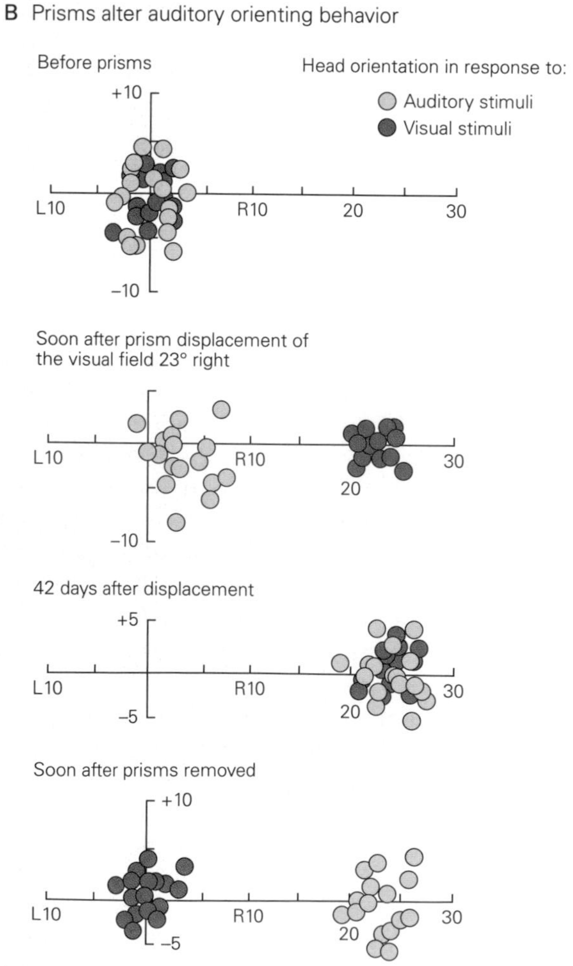

Figure 31–9 The sensitivity of sound localization to experience.

A. The diagrams show the normal relationship of sounds and visual cues for a juvenile barn owl and the disturbance of this correspondence by prisms that shift the visual field 23 degrees. Normally when a mouse is at the center of the visual field the sounds arrive at the two ears simultaneously; with the prisms, when the mouse is seen 23 degrees to the right of the visual-field center, the sounds nevertheless are perceived to originate at the true location of the rodent (0 degrees) and are therefore mismatched with visual perception. Reinterpreting the sound cues as being shifted to the right reestablishes the correspondence between visual and auditory cues. (**ITD**, interaural time delay.) (Modified, with permission, from Brainard and Knudsen 1993.)

B. Plots of a barn owl's head movements in response to visual and auditory cues before and after wearing prisms. Normally sounds and sights from the center of the visual field (0°,0°) make the animal point its head at that location. When the animal is fitted with prisms that shift the visual field 23 degrees to the right, it turns its head to the central location in response to sound but looks 23 degrees to the right (the shifted location) for a centrally located visual cue. In time the owl shifts its head movements to the right by 23 degrees when it hears a centrally located sound, so that they correspond with head movements made in response to the shifted visual cues. A plot of head movements shortly after the prisms are removed, when both visual and auditory cues are again veridical, reveals the locus of plasticity: The animal's mapping of sounds has shifted, whereas the map of visual cues is unchanged.

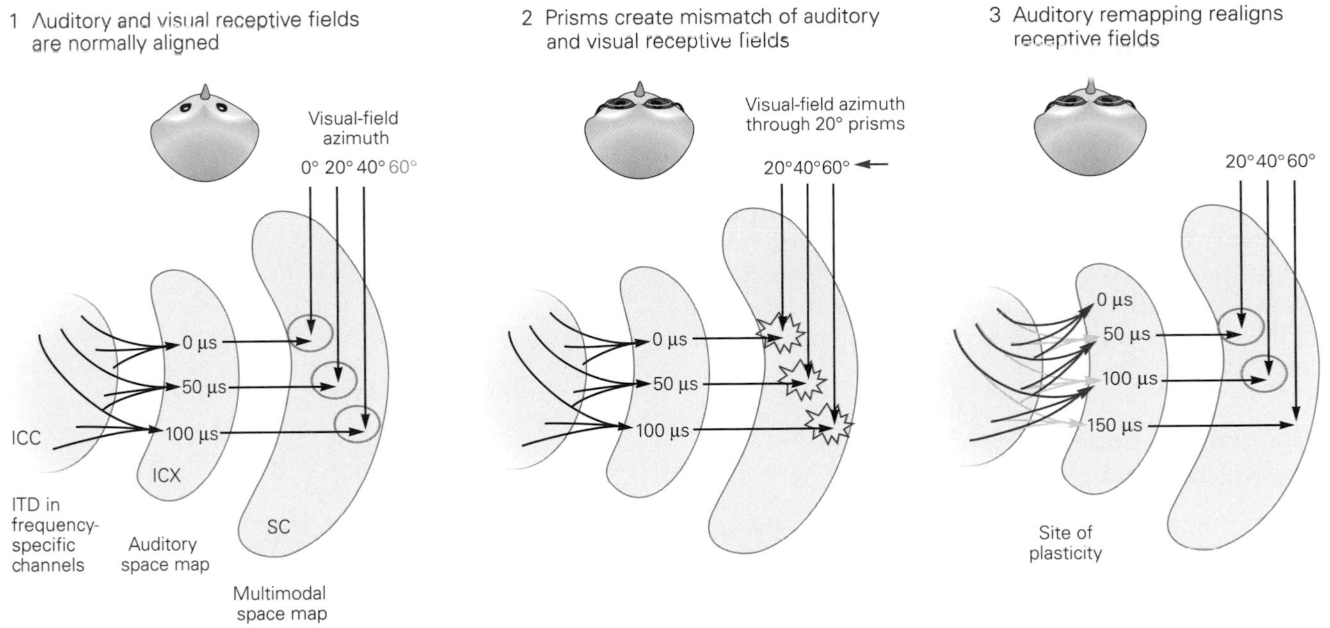

Figure 31–10 The neural locus of plasticity in sound localization. The neural pathway for sound localization originates in the central nucleus of the inferior colliculus (**ICC**), extends to the external nucleus of the inferior colliculus (**ICX**), and from there to the superior colliculus (**SC**), also known as the optic tectum. (Modified, with permission, from Knudsen 1999.)
1. Neurons tuned to interaural time delays (**ITDs**) from many different frequency bands in the central nucleus normally converge on the external nucleus in a topographic manner to create a systematic map of space based on sound cues (here only the map from 0 µs to 100 µs is shown for simplicity). This map is then relayed to the superior colliculus, where it is in register with the visual map (**circles**). **2**. In the prism-reared owl the shift in the visual field initially creates a mismatch in the superior colliculus between the auditory and visual maps. **3**. In time the inferior colliculus axons sprout collaterals (**burgundy**) that create a shifted map of space within the external nucleus. This shifted map, when relayed to the superior colliculus, is now in register with the shifted visual map. The original projections persist but are actively suppressed.

restoration of normal tuning after the prisms have been removed.

The prism experiments illustrate that vision plays a dominant role in changes in synaptic function in the auditory system. As further evidence for this idea, a small lesion in the superior colliculus prevents synaptic changes in the corresponding area of the inferior colliculus to accommodate prism displacement. Presumably the same instructive signals from the superior colliculus guide the transformation of auditory cues into a well-aligned spatial map of sounds during normal development.

A striking aspect of plasticity in both birds and mammals is the sensitivity of the spatial map to an animal's age. As in many other systems there is a critical period in which altered sensory experience can alter the brain and behavior. Marked adaptive changes in orienting behavior are seen in juvenile owls, ferrets, and guinea pigs but ordinarily not in adults. However, learning in young animals increases the capacity for plasticity in adults. If juvenile owls are subjected to a period of prism displacement but then returned to normal vision, they are capable of reacquiring the shifted map and the corresponding behavior when exposed to the same prism displacement as adults. However, their inferior colliculus cannot acquire a map to which they were not exposed to as juveniles. The period of early learning thus leaves a specific and permanent trace in the nervous system.

An animal's motivational state is also important in how malleable its brain is. If adult barn owls fitted with prisms are allowed to hunt for live mice, a more arousing situation than typical laboratory conditions, they display behavioral and neural plasticity intermediate between that of normally housed adults and juveniles. Similar increases in sensory plasticity have been seen in mammals actively involved in tasks that require specific sensory information. This suggests the clinically important point that more plasticity can be elicited from the adult brain if attention and motivation can be engaged appropriately.

The Inferior Colliculus Transmits Auditory Information to the Cerebral Cortex

Auditory information ascends to the cerebral cortex through the thalamus. Neurons of the inferior colliculus project to the medial geniculate body, where principal cells in turn project to the auditory cortex. The pathways from the inferior colliculus include a lemniscal or core pathway and extralemniscal or belt pathways. Descending projections from the auditory cortex to the medial geniculate body are prominent both anatomically and functionally.

The Auditory Cortex Maps Numerous Aspects of Sound

Ascending auditory pathways terminate in the auditory cortex, which includes multiple distinct areas on the dorsal surface of the temporal lobe. The most prominent projection is from the ventral division of the medial geniculate nucleus to the primary auditory cortex (A1, or Brodmann area 41). As in the lower relays of auditory processing, this cytoarchitectonically distinct region contains a tonotopic representation of characteristic frequencies: Neurons are arrayed in a systematic map reflecting the frequencies that best stimulate them. Neurons tuned to low frequencies are found at the rostral end of A1, and those responsive to high frequencies in the caudal region (Figure 31–11). Thus, like the visual and somatosensory cortices, the primary auditory cortex contains a map reflecting the pattern of peripheral sensors.

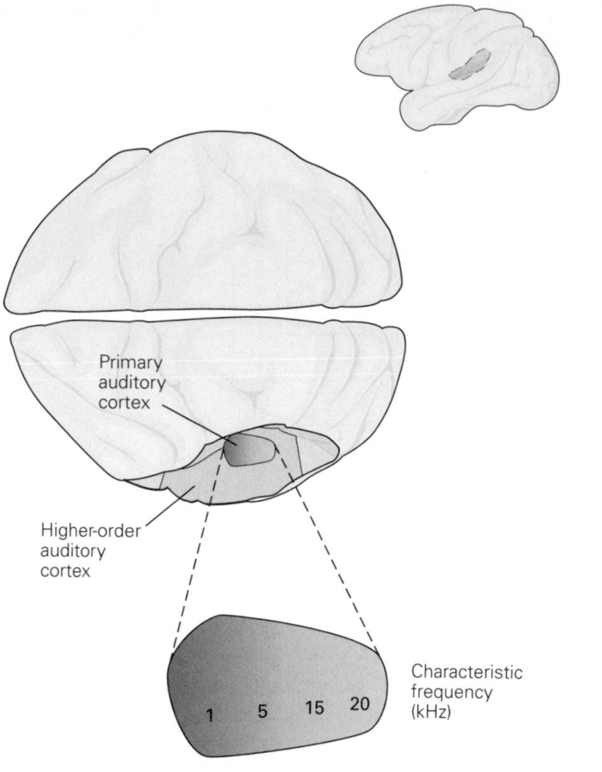

Figure 31–11 The auditory cortex of primates has multiple primary and secondary areas. The expanded figure shows the major tonotopic map of the primary auditory cortex. The primary areas are surrounded by higher-order areas (see Figure 31–13).

Because the cochlea encodes only frequency, however, a one-dimensional map from the periphery is spread across the two-dimensional surface of the cortex, with a smooth frequency gradient in one direction and iso-frequency contours along the other direction. In many animals subregions of the auditory cortex representing biologically significant frequencies are enlarged because of extensive inputs, similar to the large area in the primary visual cortex devoted to inputs from the fovea.

In addition to frequency, other features of auditory stimuli are mapped in the primary auditory cortex, although the overall organization is less clear and precise than for vision. Auditory neurons in A1 are excited by input from both ears (EE), with the contralateral input usually stronger than the ipsilateral contribution, or by unilateral input (EI). The EI neurons are inhibited by stimulation of the opposite ear. Summation columns of EE neurons alternate with suppression columns of EI neurons, especially in the high-frequency portion of A1, creating a map of interaural interactions at right angles to the axis of tonotopic mapping. This partitions the auditory cortex into columns responsive to every audible frequency and each type of binaural interaction.

Certain neurons in A1 also seem to be organized according to bandwidth, that is, according to their responsiveness to a narrow or broad range of frequencies. Distinct subregions of A1 form clusters of cells with narrow or broadband tuning within individual iso-frequency contours. Synaptic connections within the cortex respect these clusters, with neurons receiving intracortical input primarily from neurons with similar bandwidths and characteristic frequencies. This modular organization of bandwidth selectivity may allow redundant processing of incoming signals through neuronal filters of varying bandwidths as well as center frequencies, which could be useful for the analysis of spectrally complex sounds such as species-specific vocalizations, including speech.

Several other parameters are mapped on the surface of A1. These include neuronal response latency, loudness, modulation of loudness, and the rate and direction of frequency modulation. Although it remains to be seen how these various maps intersect, this array of parameters clearly endows each neuron and each location in A1 with the ability to represent many independent variables of sound and generates a great diversity of neuronal selectivity.

As is true for visual and somatosensory areas of the cortex, sensory representation in A1 can change in response to altered input. After peripheral hearing loss, tonotopic mapping can be altered so that neurons originally responsive to sounds within the range of the hearing loss begin to respond to adjacent frequencies. The work of Michael Merzenich and others has shown that behavioral training of adult animals can also result in large-scale reorganization of auditory cortex, so that the most behaviorally relevant frequencies—those specifically associated with attention or reinforcement—come to be overrepresented.

The auditory areas of young animals are particularly plastic. In rodents the frequency organization of A1 emerges gradually during development from an early, crude frequency map. Raising animals in acoustic environments in which they are exposed to repeated tone pulses of a particular frequency results in a persistent expansion of cortical areas devoted to that frequency, accompanied by a general deterioration and broadening of the tonotopic map. This result not only suggests that the development of A1 is experience-dependent, but raises the possibility that early exposure to abnormal sound environments can create long-term disruptions of high-level sensory processing. A greater understanding of how this happens and whether it is also true for human fetuses and infants may provide insights into the origin and remediation of disorders in which auditory processing is centrally impaired, such as many forms of dyslexia. Moreover, the ability to induce synaptic changes in adult auditory cortex by engaging attention or reward raises new hopes for brain repair even in adulthood.

Auditory Information Is Processed in Multiple Cortical Areas

The primary auditory area of mammals is surrounded by multiple distinct regions, many of which are tonotopic. These highly tonotopic areas resemble A1 in that they receive direct input from the ventral division of the medial geniculate nucleus. Like the major thalamocortical visual projection, this input primarily contacts cortical layers IIIb and IV. Adjacent tonotopic fields have mirror-image tonotopy: The direction of tonotopy reverses at the boundary between fields.

As many as 7 to 10 secondary (belt) areas surround 3 to 4 primary or primary-like (core) areas (see Figure 31–13). These cortical areas receive input from the core areas of auditory cortex and in some cases from thalamic nuclei. Electrophysiological and imaging studies have confirmed that the primary auditory cortex in humans lies on Heschl's gyrus, in the temporal lobe, medial to the sylvian fissure. In addition, recent functional magnetic-resonance imaging studies have revealed that in humans, just as in monkeys, pure tones activate primarily core regions, whereas the neurons of belt areas prefer complex sounds such as narrow-band noise bursts.

Insectivorous Bats Have Cortical Areas Specialized for Behaviorally Relevant Features of Sound

Although it is generally assumed that the upstream auditory areas perform increasingly specialized functions related to hearing, our knowledge about the functions of serial relays is much less in the auditory system than the visual system. In humans one of the most important aspects of audition is its role in processing language, but we know relatively little about how speech sounds are analyzed by neural circuits. New techniques for imaging the human brain are gradually providing insights into the localization of cortical areas associated with language (see Chapter 60).

The best evidence for specialized analysis of complex auditory signals in auditory cortical areas comes from studies of insectivorous bats. These animals find their prey almost entirely through *echolocation*, emitting ultrasonic pulses of sound that are reflected by flying insects. Bats analyze the timing and structure of the echoes to help locate and identify the targets, and discrete auditory areas are devoted to processing different aspects of the echoes.

Many bats, such as the mustached bat studied by Nobuo Suga and his collaborators, emit echolocating pulses with two components. An initial *constant-frequency* (CF) component consists of several harmonically related sounds or *harmonics*. These harmonics are emitted stably for tens to hundred of milliseconds, akin to human vowel sounds. The constant-frequency component is followed by a sound that steeply decreases in frequency, the *frequency-modulated* (FM) component, which resembles the rapidly changing frequencies of human consonants (Figure 31–12A).

The FM sounds are used to determine the distance to the target. The bat measures the interval between the emitted sound and the returning echo, which corresponds to a particular distance, based on the relatively constant speed of sound. Neurons in the FM-FM area

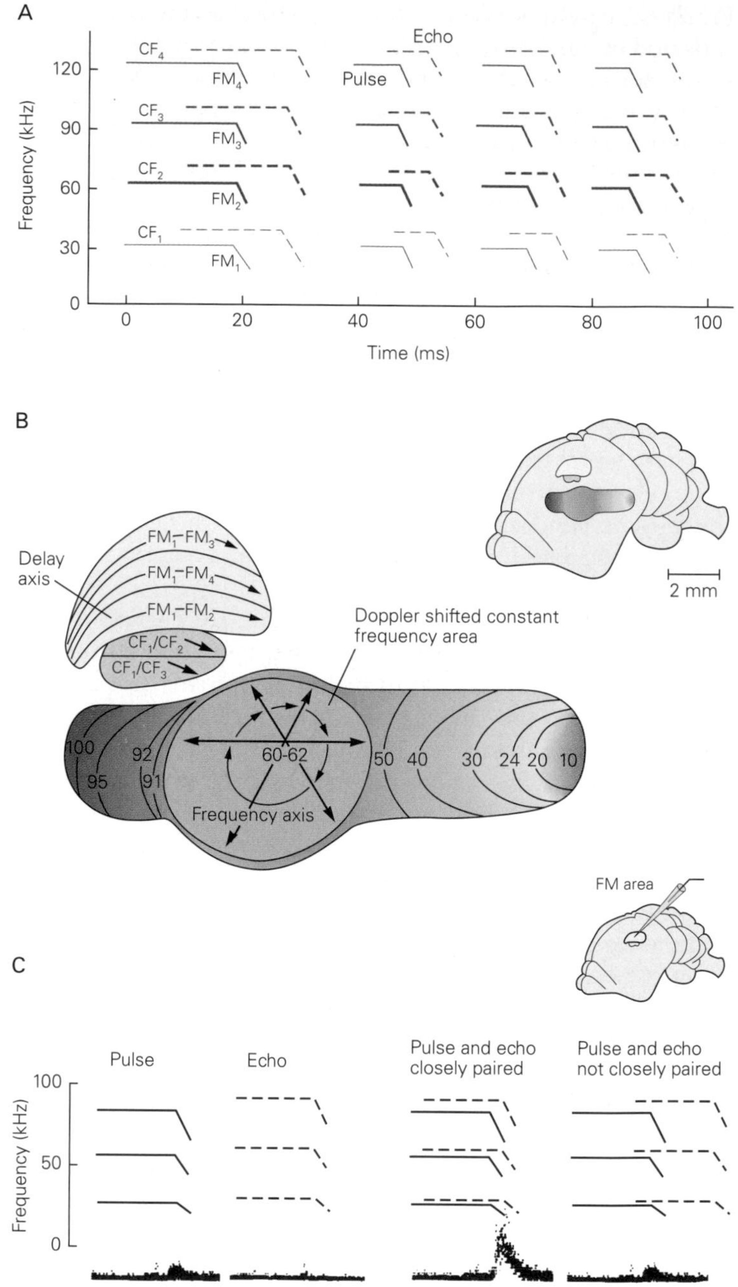

Figure 31–12 The auditory system of the bat has specialized areas for locating sounds.

A. A sonogram of an animal's calls (**solid lines**) and the resultant echoes (**dashed lines**) illustrates the two components of the call: the protracted, harmonically related constant-frequency (**CF**) signal and the briefer frequency-modulated (**FM**) signal. The duration of the calls decreases as the animal approaches its target.

B. A view of the cerebral hemisphere of the mustached bat shows three of the functional areas within the auditory cortex. The FM area is where the distance from the target is computed; the CF area is where the velocity of the target is computed; and the Doppler-shifted CF area is specialized for the identification of small fluttering objects. The expanded cortical representation of Doppler-shifted CFs near the second harmonic of the call frequency (60 to 62 kHz) forms the acoustic "fovea."

C. An FM-FM combination-sensitive neuron does not respond significantly to either pulses or echoes alone, but responds very strongly to a closely paired pulse and echo. However, the neuron is also sensitive to the time difference between the pulse and echo, as seen in the record on the right, where the neuron fails to respond to a pulse-echo combination that is not closely paired. (Modified, with permission, from Suga et al. 1983).

of auditory cortex (Figure 31–12B) respond preferentially to pulse-echo pairs separated by a specific delay. Moreover, these neurons respond better to particular combinations of sounds than to the individual sounds in isolation; such neurons are called *feature detectors* (Figure 31–12C). The FM-FM area contains an array of such detectors, with preferred delays systematically ranging from 0.4 ms to 18 ms, corresponding to target ranges of 7 cm to 310 cm, mapped along the cortical surface (see Figure 31–12B). These neurons are organized in columns, each of which is responsive to a particular combination of stimulus frequency and delay. In this way the bat, like the barn owl in its inferior colliculus, is able to represent an acoustic feature that is not directly represented by sensory receptors.

The CF components of bat calls are used to determine the relative speed of the target with respect to the bat and the acoustic image of the target. When an echolocating bat is flying toward an insect, the sounds reflected from the insect are Doppler-shifted to a higher frequency at the bat's ear, for the bat is moving toward the returning sound waves from the target, causing a relative speeding up of these waves at its ear. Similarly, a receding insect yields reflections of lowered frequency at the bat's ear. Neurons in the CF-CF area (see Figure 31–12B) are sharply tuned to a combination of frequencies close to the emitted frequency or its harmonics. Each neuron responds best to a combination of a pulse of a particular fundamental frequency and an echo corresponding to the first or second harmonic of the pulse, Doppler-shifted to a specific extent. As in the FM-FM area, neurons do not respond to the pulse or echo alone, but rather to the combination of the two CF signals.

CF-CF neurons are arranged in columns, each encoding a particular combination of frequencies. These columns are arranged regularly along the cortical surface, with the fundamental frequency along one axis and the echo harmonics along a perpendicular axis. This dual-frequency coordinate system creates a map wherein a specific location corresponds to a particular Doppler shift and thus a particular target velocity, ranging systematically from −2 m/s to 9 m/s.

The CF components of returning echoes are also used for detailed frequency analysis of the acoustic image, presumably important in its identification. The Doppler-shifted constant-frequency area (DSCF) of the mustached bat is a dramatic expansion of the primary auditory cortex's representation of frequencies between 60 kHz and 62 kHz, corresponding well to the set of returning echoes from the major CF component of the bat's call (see Figure 31–12B). Within the DSCF area individual neurons are extremely sharply tuned to frequency, so that the tiny changes in frequency created by fluttering moth wings are easily detected.

Transient inactivation of some of these specialized cortical areas, while the bat performs a discrimination task, strikingly supports the importance of their functional specialization in behavior. Silencing of the DSCF selectively impairs fine frequency discrimination while leaving time perception intact. Conversely, inactivation of the FM-FM area impairs the bat's ability to detect small differences in the time of arrival of two echoes, while leaving frequency perception unchanged.

Investigation of this auditory system was greatly facilitated by knowledge of the stimuli relevant to bats. It remains to be seen whether these cortical areas are functionally or anatomically analogous to particular fields in cats, monkeys, and humans. Regardless, ethologically significant stimuli are likely to be as useful in studying these other species as they have been in studies of bats.

A Second Sound-Localization Pathway from the Inferior Colliculus Involves the Cerebral Cortex in Gaze Control

Many auditory neurons in the cerebral cortex are sensitive to interaural time and level differences and therefore to the location of sounds in space. Most of these cells have large receptive fields and broad tuning. In contrast to the auditory relays in the midbrain, however, there is no evidence for an organized spatial map of sound in any of the cortical areas sensitive to sound location.

The sound-localization pathways in the cortex originate in the central nucleus of the inferior colliculus and ascend through the auditory thalamus, area A1, and cortical association areas, eventually reaching the frontal eye fields involved in gaze control. Eye or head movements can be elicited by stimulating the frontal eye fields, which connect directly to brain stem tegmentum premotor nuclei that mediate gaze changes, as well as to the superior colliculus. But the midbrain pathway from location-sensitive neurons in the inferior colliculus to the superior colliculus to gaze-control circuitry can directly regulate orientation movements of the head, eyes, and ears. Why should there be a second sound-localization pathway connected to gaze-control circuitry?

Behavioral experiments shed light on this question. Although lesions of A1 can result in profound sound-localization deficits in a monkey, no deficiency is seen when the task is simply to indicate the side of the sound source by pushing a lever. The deficit becomes apparent only when the animal must approach the location of a brief sound source, that is, when the task is the more complex one of forming an image of the source, remembering it, and moving toward it.

Experiments in barn owls have produced particularly compelling evidence. The ability of owls to orient to sounds in space is unaffected by inactivation of the avian equivalent of the frontal eye fields. Similarly, when the midbrain localization pathway is disrupted by pharmacological inactivation of the superior colliculus, the probability of an accurate head turn is decreased but animals still respond correctly more than half of the time. In contrast, when both structures are inactivated, animals are completely unable to orient accurately to acoustic stimuli on the contralateral side. Thus cortical and subcortical sound-localization pathways have parallel access to gaze control centers, perhaps providing some redundancy. Moreover, when only the frontal eye fields are inactivated, birds lose their ability to orient their gaze toward a target that has been extinguished and must be remembered, just as is seen with mammalian A1 lesions. Thus in both mammals and birds cortical pathways are required for more complex sound-localization tasks.

This appears to be a general difference between cortical and subcortical pathways. Subcortical circuits are important for rapid and reliable performance of behaviors that are critical to survival. Cortical circuitry allows for working memory, complex recognition tasks, and selection of stimuli and evaluation of their significance, resulting in slower but more differentiated performance. Examples of this also exist in auditory pathways not involved in localization. Conditioned fear responses to simple auditory stimuli are mediated by direct rapid pathways from the auditory thalamus to the amygdala; they can be elicited after cortical inactivation. However, fear responses that require more complex discrimination of auditory stimuli require pathways through the cortex, and are accordingly slower but more specific.

Auditory Circuits in the Cerebral Cortex Are Segregated into Separate Processing Streams

In the visual system the output from the primary visual cortex is segregated into separate dorsal and ventral streams concerned respectively with object location in space and object identification. A similar division of labor is thought to exist in the somatosensory cortex, and recent evidence suggests that the auditory cortex follows this plan.

Anatomical tracing studies of the three most accessible belt areas in primates show that the more rostral and ventral areas connect primarily to the more rostral and ventral areas of the temporal lobe, whereas the more caudal area projects to the dorsal and caudal temporal lobe. In addition, these belt areas and their temporal lobe targets both project to largely different areas of the frontal lobes (Figure 31–13).

The frontal areas receiving anterior auditory projections are generally implicated in nonspatial functions, whereas those that are targets of posterior auditory areas are implicated in spatial processing.

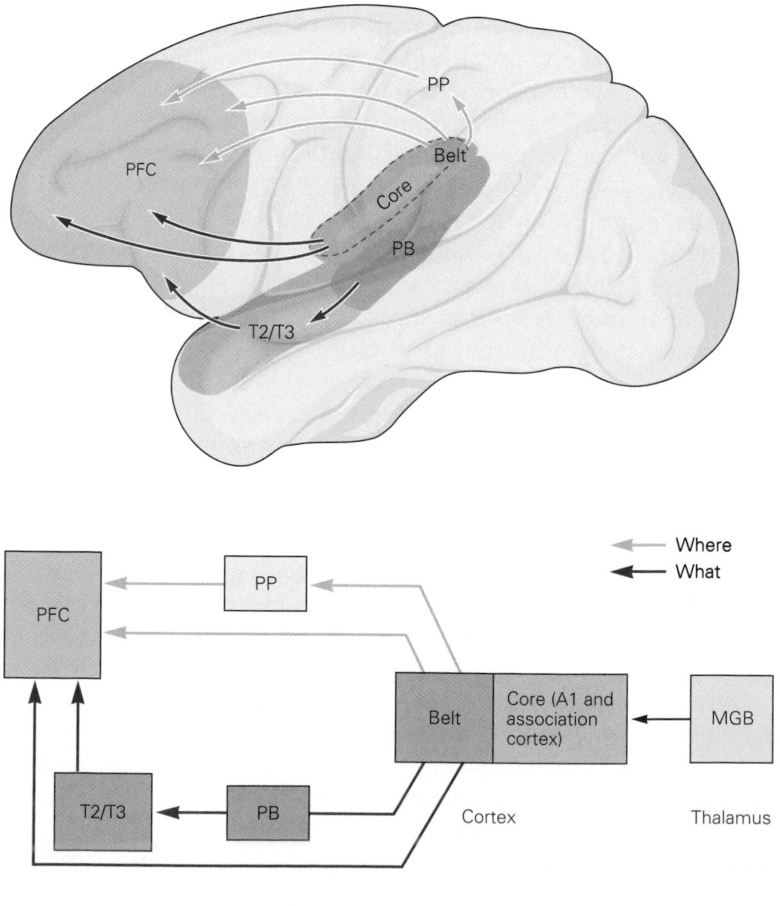

Figure 31–13 The "what" and "where" streams in the auditory cortical system of primates. The ventral "what" stream and dorsal "where" stream originate in different parts of primary and belt cortex and ultimately project to distinct regions of prefrontal cortex through independent paths. (**MGB**, medial geniculate body of the thalamus; **PB**, parabelt cortex; **PFC**, prefrontal cortex; **PP**, posterior parietal cortex; **T2/T3**, areas of temporal cortex.) (Modified, with permission, from Rauschecker 2000 and from Romanski and Averbeck 2009.)

Electrophysiological and imaging studies provide support for this. Caudal and parietal areas are more active when a sound must be located or moves, and ventral areas are more active during identification of the same stimulus or analysis of its pitch. Consistent with this segregation, inactivation of the posterior auditory field in cats impairs performance of a sound-localization task, whereas inactivation of the anterior auditory field interferes with a pattern-discrimination task, but not vice versa. Thus anterior-ventral pathways may identify auditory objects by analyzing spectral and temporal characteristics of sounds, whereas the more dorsal-posterior pathways may specialize in sound-source location, detection of sound-source motion, and spatial segregation of sources.

Although the idea that all sensory areas of the cerebral cortex initially segregate object identification and location is attractive, it is likely an oversimplification. It is clear that the medial-belt areas of the auditory cortex project to both dorsal and ventral frontal cortices, and neurons with broad spatial responsiveness are distributed throughout caudal and anterior areas. Imaging studies with more complex stimuli suggest that parietal pathways are involved in additional functions, including analysis of the temporal properties of acoustic stimuli such as spectral motion. The latter property might explain the clear role of the posterior pathway in speech perception in humans. Nonetheless, although the details may differ between systems, the basic concept holds that sensory systems decompose stimuli into features and analyze these in discrete pathways.

The Cerebral Cortex Modulates Processing in Subcortical Auditory Areas

An intriguing feature of all mammalian cortical areas, and one shared by the auditory system, is the massive projection from the cortex back to lower areas. There are almost 10-fold as many corticofugal fibers entering the sensory thalamus as there are axons projecting from the thalamus to the cortex. Projections from the auditory cortex also innervate the inferior colliculus, olivocochlear neurons, some basal ganglionic structures, and even the dorsal cochlear nucleus.

Insights into possible functions of this feedback have come from the bat's auditory system. Silencing of frequency-specific cortical areas leads to decreased thalamic and collicular responses, whereas activation of cortical projections increases and sharpens the responses of some neurons. The auditory cortex can therefore actively adjust and improve auditory signal processing in subcortical structures.

A variety of evidence suggests that cortical feedback also occurs in the visual and somatosensory components of the thalamus. This challenges the view that ascending sensory pathways are purely feedforward circuits, and suggests that we should regard the thalamus and cortex as reciprocally and highly interconnected circuits in which the cortex exercises some top-down control of perception.

Hearing Is Crucial for Vocal Learning and Production in Both Humans and Songbirds

Virtually all animals use hearing for localization and recognition of sounds, including behaviorally important communication sounds of individuals of the same species (conspecifics), such as mating and warning calls. For animals known as vocal learners, hearing is also necessary for learning to mimic sounds produced by others.

Humans are consummate vocal learners. Human speech involves fantastically complex and variable communication sounds, and we depend critically on hearing the speech both of ourselves and of others for normal speech development. Much is being learned about the auditory areas associated with human speech recognition and production from imaging and electrophysiological techniques. To understand basic brain mechanisms of vocal learning and its disorders, however, it is important to study animals with related behaviors. Surprisingly, there are relatively few other vocal learners.

Although the vocalizations of nonhuman primates can be complex, none have been shown to be learned. Among other mammals there is evidence for vocal learning only in cetaceans (whales and dolphins) and some bats. In striking contrast to this paucity of mammalian vocal learners, the many thousands of songbird species, as well as the parrot and hummingbird groups, all must learn to produce their complex songs. Songbirds have provided a particularly useful model, and there is a wealth of information on their vocal behavior and the underlying brain substrates, with some striking parallels to human speech learning.

Normal Vocal Behavior Cannot Be Learned in Isolation

What do we mean by vocal learning, and how can we demonstrate it? One indication of vocal learning is great variation in the vocal output of a species, such as the multitude of human languages and dialects. Similarly, many songbird species have local dialects (Figure 31–14A), and songs also vary between individual songbirds.

Because such variability could in theory be genetically encoded, a critical test of vocal learning is whether animals develop normal vocal behavior in the absence of hearing other individuals. It is well established that deaf children do not learn to speak normally. In addition, the rare cases of so-called wild children raised without exposure to human speech, such as the girl called Genie, show that speech does not develop normally when hearing is intact but no speech has been heard. In songbirds as well deafness early in life prevents normal song learning and production. Birds reared without exposure to conspecific songs sing highly simplified *isolate* songs, which nevertheless display some features characteristic of the species (Figure 31–14B, C). In contrast, monkeys reared without exposure to the vocalizations of other monkeys display essentially normal vocal behavior, as do non-songbirds, such as chickens or flycatchers, deafened or raised in isolation. Clearly both birdsong and speech are learned, with a strong dependence on hearing.

Hearing serves two independent functions in vocal learning. For one, hearing the vocalizations of others allows imitation. This aspect of learning is perceptual in both humans and birds; in songbirds a sensory memory of the tutor's song, often called the template, is rapidly formed and stored during a period called the *sensory learning phase.* However, neither humans nor songbirds can directly translate their sensory memory of others into a faithful vocal copy. Rather, they initially produce rambling and immature vocalizations, called babbling in humans and subsong in songbirds. They must then be able to hear these vocalizations to gradually refine them and make them match their desired vocal output during a process of *sensorimotor learning.*

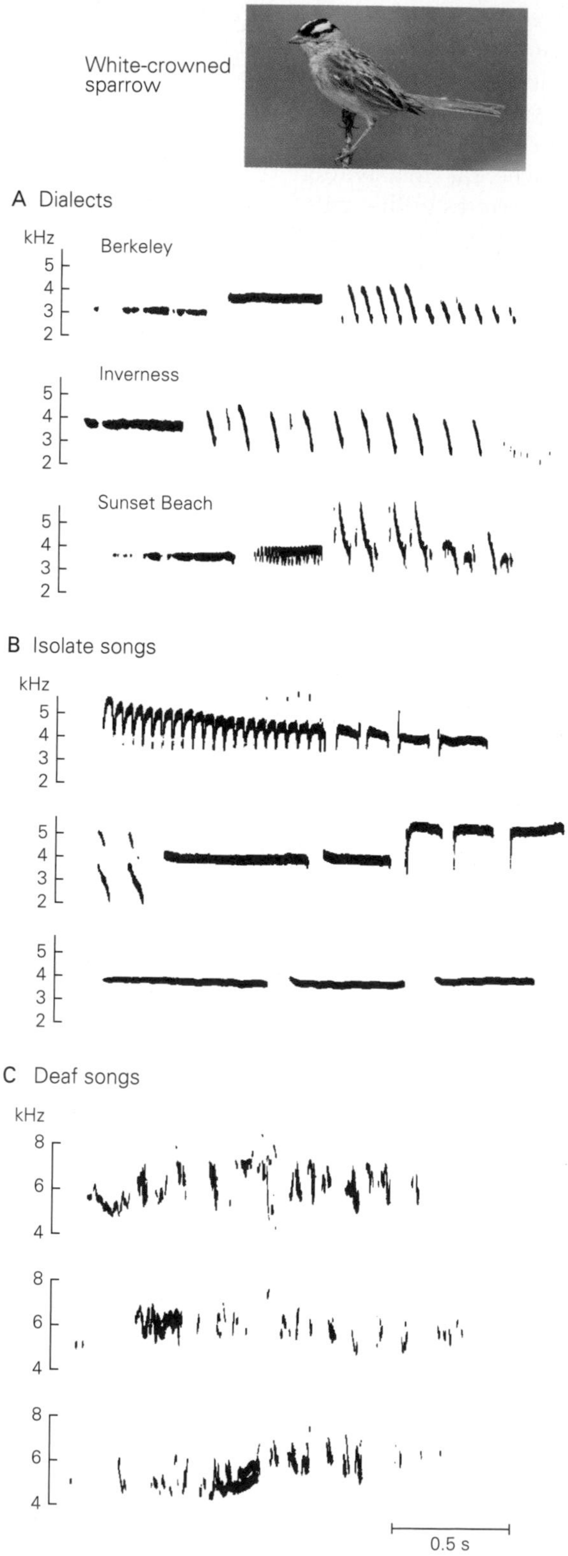

Figure 31–14 Birdsong is learned through mimicry.

A. Distinct dialects of white-crowned sparrow song are recognizable in these sonograms of recordings from three locations on the northern California coast. Sonograms plot sound frequency against time, with amplitude indicated by density. Common structural elements such as whistles, buzzes, and trills differ in length and frequency in the dialects. Birds learn their dialect early in life from a local tutor, and develop some individual song features as well.

B. White-crowned sparrows raised without tutors sing isolate songs, which resemble normal sparrow song in duration and whistle-like features but are otherwise much simpler.

C. Songs of birds that were deaf before sensorimotor learning of song are even more abnormal than isolate songs. This is true whether the animals were tutored or not, so the abnormal song reflects the lack of auditory feedback as birds attempt to produce sounds. (Modified, with permission, from Marler 1970; modified, with permission, from Konishi 1985).

Second, hearing provides vocal learners with sensory information about the accuracy of their motor performance, in the form of auditory feedback. This is especially clear in songbirds. They can memorize adult tutor songs with a relatively small amount of song exposure, and if isolated after such exposure will nevertheless produce a good copy of the tutor song so long as they are able to hear themselves. In contrast, if they are deafened after sensory learning, they produce highly abnormal songs, without even the innate structure usually present in isolate songs (Figure 31–14C). The same dependence on hearing of one's own voice is evident in humans. For instance, the speech of children who become deaf during childhood, even after significant speech learning, deteriorates markedly.

Of course, some aspects of birdsong are clearly not analogous to human speech. Although birdsong is used for communication, it does not seem to be language in the sense of conveying complex meaning. What it shares with speech is the learned sensorimotor control of an elaborate vocal system, with a pronounced dependence on hearing.

Vocal Learning Is Optimal During a Sensitive Period

A variety of evidence makes it clear that neither human nor avian vocal learners are born as "blank slates." Human babies as early as 3 weeks of age can make perceptual distinctions between categories of sounds in languages to which they have never been exposed. For instance, newborn babies in both the United States and Japan can distinguish the sounds "r" and "l," a distinction that does not exist in Japanese and is not well perceived by adult monolingual Japanese speakers (see Chapter 60). Similarly, newly hatched songbirds show innate recognition of and preference for all songs of their own species, relative to other species.

Acoustic experience quickly shapes the nervous system after birth. By 1 year of age children exposed only to Japanese no longer distinguish "r" and "l" sounds, and children being raised in English no longer distinguish the several classes of "h"-like sounds in Hindi or "shi"-like sounds in Mandarin. Similarly, young songbirds quickly begin to learn the songs to which they are actually exposed.

The ability of sensory experience to alter perceptual ability varies with age, as we saw earlier in connection with sound localization. During sensitive or critical periods for learning young children exposed to a language are able to speak the language fluently and without accent. However, their ability to do so decreases as they grow older. If not exposed to a foreign language by adolescence, most humans cannot learn to speak that language in a manner that is indistinguishable from native speakers, primarily in accent and grammatical usage. This inability seems to reflect decreased perceptual abilities, and not simply limits on the ability to produce the sounds of speech. Songbirds also have clear sensitive periods. In most species birds not exposed to song in the first several months of life go on to sing isolate song even if subsequently exposed to normal adult song; such birds are known as closed learners.

An animal model with sensitive periods for vocal learning like our own can provide insights into the factors that control the synaptic changes, and ultimately the neural mechanisms involved and thus potentially into remediation. For instance, the sensitive period for song learning does not have a strict age limit. Rather, experience itself is centrally involved in closing the sensitive period. Songbirds tutored only with songs from birds of other species (heterospecifics) can incorporate new songs from their own species at a time when birds raised with conspecifics no longer can. In some species birds reared in complete isolation can still incorporate new song elements as adults. Thus a lack of normal experience leaves the brain open to be shaped by the appropriate input for a longer than usual period.

Attentional or motivational factors also influence the timing of the sensitive period. Birds learn from live tutors for longer than they learn from taped tutors. Hormonal factors may play a role as well. Manipulations that delay the onset of singing and decrease testosterone levels appear to extend the sensitive period. In light of this it is intriguing that the human critical period for speech appears to end in adolescence.

Both Humans and Songbirds Possess Specialized Neural Networks for Vocalization

Along with the many behavioral similarities between speech and song learning, both humans and songbirds have evolved specialized neural systems for vocal learning and production. At first glance the very different organization in birds and humans, especially of forebrain areas, seems to make drawing any direct parallels between the two brain systems difficult.

One major difference between birds and humans is that birds do not have the multilayered cortex seen in all mammals, including humans. Rather, the evolutionarily related avian forebrain areas—derived like mammalian cortex from the embryonic region known as the pallium—are organized in nuclei, just as many lower areas are in both mammals and birds. A closer look at the vocal control systems of humans and songbirds, however, reveals numerous anatomical and functional similarities in the organization of neural pathways for vocal production and processing.

All primates and birds, and many mammals as well, have pathways from midbrain areas to lower respiratory and vocal motor centers as well as medullary centers that integrate respiratory and vocal tract control. Stimulation in these midbrain areas, such as the periaqueductal grey in primates and the dorsomedial intercollicular area in birds, can elicit well-formed vocalizations. However, a critical evolutionary step in the adaptation of learned vocalizations was the development of high-level forebrain areas that control the lower motor pathways for vocalization; both songbirds and humans have such areas whereas nonlearners do not.

In humans numerous perisylvian and parietotemporal cortical areas are critical for speech production, as shown by the effects of lesions and the fact that stimulation of many of these areas can elicit vocalizations or disrupt ongoing speech. In striking contrast, there are no neocortical areas in monkeys from which vocalizations can be elicited by stimulation or whose ablation affects calls. Among birds, only songbirds and other vocal learners such as parrots have evolved an elaborate forebrain system, often called the song system, for control of the lower brain areas involved in vocalization (Figure 31–15A).

The motor control portion of this circuit consists of a chain of nuclei, including in part the premotor nucleus HVC, an erstwhile acronym used as a proper name, which contains a central pattern generator for song. HVC projects to a motor cortex-like area called the robust nucleus of the arcopallium (RA), which then connects to all the lower nuclei involved with vocal motor and respiratory control. Just as in the analogous human areas, stimulation or ablation of HVC or RA dramatically affects song. Moreover, neural recordings demonstrate directly the sequential premotor activity of neurons in these areas during singing.

It has become apparent that, in addition to neocortex or its avian equivalents, the thalamus, basal ganglia, and cerebellum are important in vocal production. Lesion, stimulation, and imaging studies of humans suggest that these areas are involved in fluency, volume, articulation, and rhythm of speech. Whether the cerebellum contributes to birdsong is still unknown, but it is very clear that a specialized loop known as the anterior forebrain pathway connects HVC and RA and is critical for song learning and plasticity throughout life. Numerous recent studies of this circuit are providing insights into the function of the basal ganglia not only in song plasticity but also in motor learning more generally. These functions include acting as a source of motor variability and biasing signals important for trial-and-error learning and modulating motor output in response to social cues.

Finally, both humans and songbirds have numerous high-level auditory areas associated with processing and recognition of complex vocalizations. Many of the areas described earlier receive such auditory inputs and in fact encompass sensorimotor rather than purely motor circuits. A crucial step in the evolution of specialized vocal control areas may have been the acquisition of auditory input by preexisting motor control areas in the forebrain, giving those auditory inputs the ability to change the vocal motor map. The close relatives of songbirds, the suboscine birds such as flycatchers and phoebes, can sing but display no vocal learning; these birds also show no evidence of a specialized forebrain song-control system. In humans the capacity to learn speech and the development of specialized cortical systems for its control may have resulted from close interaction of motor control areas for orofacial movements with a variety of areas involved in processing and memorizing complex sounds.

Songbirds Have Feature Detectors for Learned Vocalizations

Reflecting the critical importance of hearing in song learning, the song system contains some of the most complex auditory neurons known. The use of behaviorally relevant stimuli, such as the bird's own song and the songs of conspecifics, was critical to the discovery of these remarkable neurons. Song-selective neurons are found throughout the adult male song system and respond more strongly to an animal's own song, and in some cases to the tutor's song, than to other equally complex auditory stimuli, such as conspecific songs or the animal's own song played in reverse or with the syllables out of order (Figure 31–15B).

In addition, many of these neurons are combination-sensitive: They show a highly nonlinear increase in firing when the component sounds of the bird's own song are combined and played in the correct sequence, compared to those sounds played alone (Figure 31–15C). Feature detectors with such marked spectral and temporal sensitivity could provide feedback to song motor areas, in the form of their firing rate or pattern, about how well sounds match the bird's goal and when the correct sequence has been sung. It is tempting to speculate that analogous neurons with responsiveness to well-learned speech sequences exist in humans.

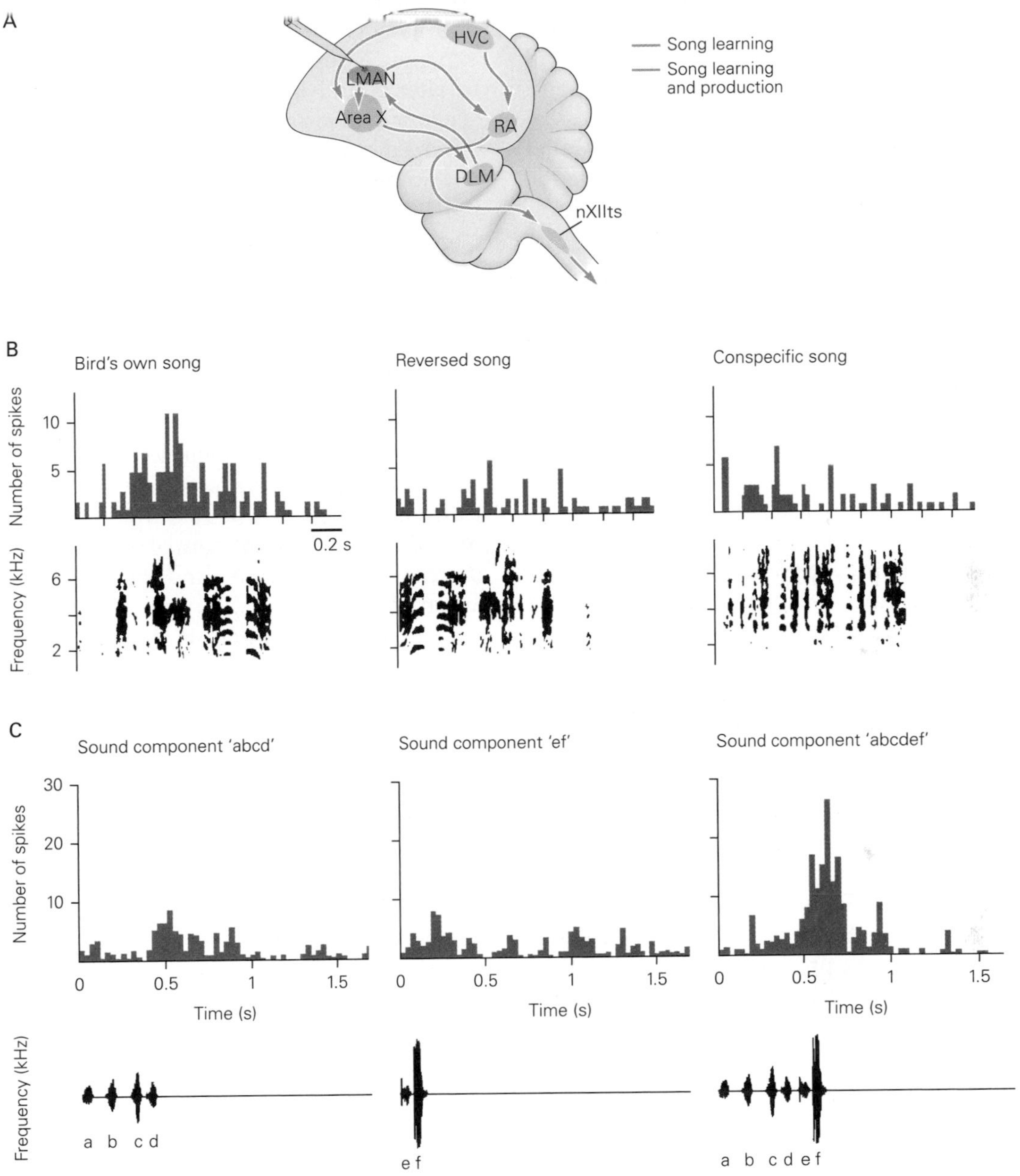

Figure 31–15 Song-selective neurons in the songbird brain.

A. A side view of the songbird brain illustrates some of the major components of the song system. The premotor nucleus HVC and robust nucleus of the arcopallium (RA) form the motor pathway for producing song. The RA motor nucleus projects to peripheral effectors that include the hypoglossal nucleus (nXIIts). The anterior forebrain pathway connects the HVC and RA through the rostral part of the brain, and includes the basal ganglionic nucleus area X, the medial nucleus of the dorsolateral thalamus (DLM), and the lateral magnocellular nucleus of the anterior nidopallium (LMAN), an outflow region that connects back to RA.

B. Peristimulus time histograms of recordings from an LMAN neuron in an adult zebra finch show that the neuron responds more vigorously to the bird's own song than to a reversed version of the song or even to a conspecific song. The song is displayed beneath each histogram as a sonogram, or plot of frequency against time. Such song-selective neurons are found throughout the song system.

C. An LMAN neuron is much more sensitive to a complete song "abcdef" than to isolated components "abcd" or "ef". In this panel the song is portrayed as an oscillogram, or plot of sound pressure against time. (Modified, with permission, from Doupe 1997.)

The song selectivity of these songbird neurons is not present in young birds, but emerges during the course of song learning. Early in the sensory learning phase the neurons respond equally well to all conspecific song stimuli. Over time their response to the bird's own song increases while responsiveness to other stimuli declines. In this way the neurons parallel the initial broad acoustic sensitivity of human infants, which is subsequently narrowed and shaped by individual auditory experience.

Song-selective neurons not only respond to complex sensory signals, but can also be active during motor production. For instance, the same neurons that respond to a particular song are also active during singing of the song. These neurons are thus another example of mirror neurons (Chapter 38). Because adult song is such a stereotyped motor act, song neurons may provide insight into the function of mirror neurons. For instance, there is a remarkable correspondence between these song neurons' auditory responses and their premotor activity: playback of one set of syllables triggers an auditory response that resembles the premotor activity for the next syllable in the song. Thus the auditory response could be considered a prediction of the motor command for the following syllable.

The sensorimotor, mirror properties of song-selective neurons raise the possibility that they are critically involved in linking sensory and motor representations in the song system; such action-perception coupling may be the function of mirror neurons more generally. In this intermixing of sensory and motor processing, birdsong is again reminiscent of human speech. Electrical stimulation of a single language area in humans can affect both production and perception of speech, and some cortical neurons respond differently to the same word depending on whether it is spoken by the subject or by someone else. In songbirds it should be possible to explore the mechanisms underlying this sensory-motor interaction.

An Overall View

The central auditory system transforms the firing patterns of eighth-nerve fibers into the neural signals required for the localization and recognition of sounds, and in some animals for shaping vocal output. As in other sensory systems, this processing is accomplished by detecting and extracting different features of sound and analyzing these in separate pathways, only later merging the results.

Sound localization, which is best understood, involves representing information about interaural timing and level differences and about the amplitude spectrum of sounds that reflects filtering by the ear, and associating these with locations in space in an experience-dependent way. The ability of visual cues to alter sound localization is a potent reminder that sensory systems evolved together to guide behavior: Animals localize sounds in order to find their sources.

Sound recognition is much less understood, and the multiplicity of cortical auditory areas involved suggests that analyzing it will be a challenge. The study of auditory specialists such as bats and their use of natural auditory stimuli has, however, taught us a great deal about what different auditory areas accomplish. This suggests that the continuing use of specialized animals and behaviorally relevant stimuli will be important in future discoveries. For primates, including humans, this will include the study of their own vocalizations. Songbirds, which show complex vocal learning with similarities to human speech acquisition, provide an additional source of insights into neural mechanisms of learning and the developmental regulation of plasticity.

The auditory system is the site of several critical periods, likely including that for speech learning, but can be coaxed into plasticity in adult animals. Demonstrated originally in experimental animals but now applied in humans as well, this result raises hope for new strategies to remediate deficits in human brain function.

Donata Oertel
Allison J. Doupe

Selected Readings

Brainard MS, Doupe AJ. 2002. What songbirds teach us about learning. Nature 417:351–358.

Chase SM, Young ED. 2006. Spike-timing codes enhance the representation of multiple simultaneous sound-localization cues in the inferior colliculus. J Neurosci 26:3889–3898.

Gao E, Suga N. 2000. Experience-dependent plasticity in the auditory cortex and the inferior colliculus of bats: role of the corticofugal system. Proc Natl Acad Sci U S A 97:8081–8086.

Hofman PM, Van Riswick JG, Van Opstal AJ. 1998. Relearning sound localization with new ears. Nat Neurosci 1:417–421.

Joris PX, Yin TCT. 2007. A matter of time: internal delays in binaural processing. Trends Neurosci 30:70–78.

Knudsen EI. 2002. Instructed learning in the auditory localization pathway of the barn owl. Nature 417:322–328.

Konishi M. 1990. Similar algorithms in different sensory systems and animals. Cold Spring Harb Symp Quant Biol 55:575–584.

Lomber SG, Malhotra S. 2008. Double dissociation of "what" and "where" processing in auditory cortex. Nat Neurosci 11:609–616.

Oertel D, Young ED. 2004. What's a cerebellar circuit doing in the auditory system? Trends Neurosci 27:104–110.

Suga N. 1990. Cortical computational maps for auditory imaging. Neural Netw 3:3–21.

Zhang LI, Bao S, Merzenich MM. 2001. Persistent and specific influences of early acoustic environments on primary auditory cortex. Nat Neurosci 4:1123–1130.

References

Brainard MS, Knudsen EI. 1993. Experience-dependent plasticity in the inferior colliculus: a site for visual calibration of the neural representation of auditory space in the barn owl. J Neurosci 13:4589–4608.

Brodal A. 1981. *Neurological Anatomy in Relation to Clinical Medicine*. New York: Oxford Univ. Press.

Cajal SR. 1909. *Histologie du Systeme Nerveux de l'Homme et des Vertebres*. Paris: A. Maloine.

Cariani PA, Delgutte B. 1996. Neural correlates of the pitch of complex tones. I. Pitch and pitch salience. J Neurophysiol 76:1698–1716.

Cohen YE, Knudsen EI. 1999. Maps versus clusters: different representations of auditory space in the midbrain and forebrain. Trends Neurosci 22:97–142.

Darrow KN, Maison SF, Liberman MC. 2006. Cochlear efferent feedback balances interaural sensitivity. Nat Neurosci 9:1474–1476.

Dave AS, Margoliash D. 2000. Song replay during sleep and computational rules for sensorimotor vocal learning. Science 290:812–816

Doupe AJ. 1997. Song- and order-selective neurons in the songbird anterior forebrain and their emergence during vocal development. J Neurosci 17:1147–1167.

Doupe AJ, Kuhl PK. 1999. Birdsong and human speech: common themes and mechanisms. Annu Rev Neurosci 22:567–631.

Geisler CD. 1998. *From Sound to Synapse, Physiology of the Mammalian Ear*. New York: Oxford Univ. Press.

Kanold PO, Young ED. 2001. Proprioceptive information from the pinna provides somatosensory input to cat dorsal cochlear nucleus. J Neurosci 21:7848–7858.

King AJ. 1999. Sensory experience and the formation of a computational map of auditory space in the brain. BioEssays 21:900–911.

Knudsen EI. 1999. Mechanisms of experience-dependent plasticity in the auditory localization pathway of the barn owl. J Comp Physiol A 185:305–321.

Konishi M. 1985. Birdsong: from behavior to neuron. Annu Rev Neurosci 8:125–170.

Konishi M. 1990. Similar algorithms in different sensory systems and animals. Cold Spring Harb Symp Quant Biol 55:575–584.

Liberman MC. 1978. Auditory-nerve response from cats raised in a low-noise chamber. J Acoust Soc Am 63:442–455.

Marler P. 1970. Birdsong and speech development: could there be parallels? Am Sci 58:669–673.

Musicant AD, Chan JCK, Hind JE. 1990. Direction-dependent spectral properties of cat external ear: new data and cross-species comparisons. J Acoust Soc Am 87:757–781.

Oertel D, Bal R, Gardner SM, Smith PH, Joris PX. 2000. Detection of synchrony in the activity of auditory nerve fibers by octopus cells of the mammalian cochlear nucleus. Proc Nat Acad Sci USA 97:11773–11779.

Prather JF, Peters S, Nowicki S, Mooney R. 2008. Precise auditory-vocal mirroring in neurons for learned vocal communication. Nature 451:305–310.

Rauschecker JP, Tian B. 2000. Mechanisms and streams for processing of "what" and "where" in auditory cortex. Proc Nat Acad Sci U S A 97:11800–11806.

Riquimaroux H, Gaioni SJ, Suga N. 1991. Cortical computational maps control auditory perception. Science 251: 565–568.

Romanski LM, Averbeck BB. 2009. The primate cortical auditory system and neural representation of conspecific vocalizations. Annu Rev Neurosci 32:315–346.

Schnupp JW, King AJ. 1997. Coding for auditory space in the nucleus of the brachium of the inferior colliculus in the ferret. J Neurophysiol 78:2717–2731.

Schreiner CE, Winer JA. 2007. Auditory cortex mapmaking: principles, projections, and plasticity. Neuron 56:356–65.

Scott LL, Mathews PJ, Golding NL. 2005. Posthearing developmental refinement of temporal processing in principal neurons of the medial superior olive. J Neurosci 25:7887–7895.

Suga N, O'Neill WE, Kujirai K, Manabe T. 1983. Specificity of combination-sensitive neurons for processing of complex biosonar signals in auditory cortex of the mustached bat. J Neurophysiol 49:1573–626.

Tollin DJ, Yin TC. 2002. The coding of spatial location by single units in the lateral superior olive of the cat. II. The determinants of spatial receptive fields in azimuth. J Neurosci 22:1468–1479.

Warr WB. 1992. Organization of olivocochlear efferent systems in mammals. In: DB Webster, AN Popper, RR Fay (eds). *The Mammalian Auditory Pathway: Neuroanatomy*, pp. 410–448. New York: Springer.

Winer JA, Saint Marie RL, Larue DT, Oliver DL. 1996. GABAergic feedforward projections from the inferior colliculus to the medial geniculate body. Proc Natl Acad Sci U S A 93:8005–8010.

Yin TCT. 2002. Neural mechanisms of encoding binaural localization cues in the auditory brainstem. In: D Oertel, RR Fay, AN Popper (eds). *Integrative Functions in the Mammalian Auditory Pathway*, pp. 238–318. New York: Springer.

32

Smell and Taste: The Chemical Senses

THROUGH THE SENSES OF SMELL and taste we are able to perceive a staggering number and variety of chemicals in the external world. These chemical senses inform us about the availability of foods and their potential pleasure or danger. Smell and taste also initiate physiological changes required for the digestion and utilization of food. In many animals the olfactory system also serves an important social function by detecting pheromones that elicit innate behavioral or physiological responses.

Although the discriminatory ability of humans is somewhat limited compared with that of many other animals, odor chemists estimate that the human olfactory system may be capable of detecting more than 10,000 different volatile chemicals. Perfumers who are highly trained to discriminate odorants can distinguish as many as 5,000 different types of odorants, and wine tasters can discern more than 100 different components of taste based on combinations of flavor and aroma.

In this chapter we consider how odor and taste stimuli are detected and how they are encoded in patterns of neural signals transmitted to the brain. In recent years much has been learned about the mechanisms underlying chemosensation in a variety of animal species. Certain features of chemosensation have been conserved through evolution, whereas others are specialized adaptations of individual species.

A Large Number of Olfactory Receptor Proteins Initiate the Sense of Smell

Odorants—volatile chemicals that are perceived as odors—are detected by olfactory sensory neurons in the nose. The sensory neurons are embedded in a specialized olfactory epithelium that lines part of nasal cavity, approximately 5 cm^2 in area in humans (Figure 32–1), and are interspersed with glia-like supporting cells (Figure 32–2). They are relatively short-lived, with a life span of only 30 to 60 days, and are continuously replaced from a layer of basal stem cells in the epithelium.

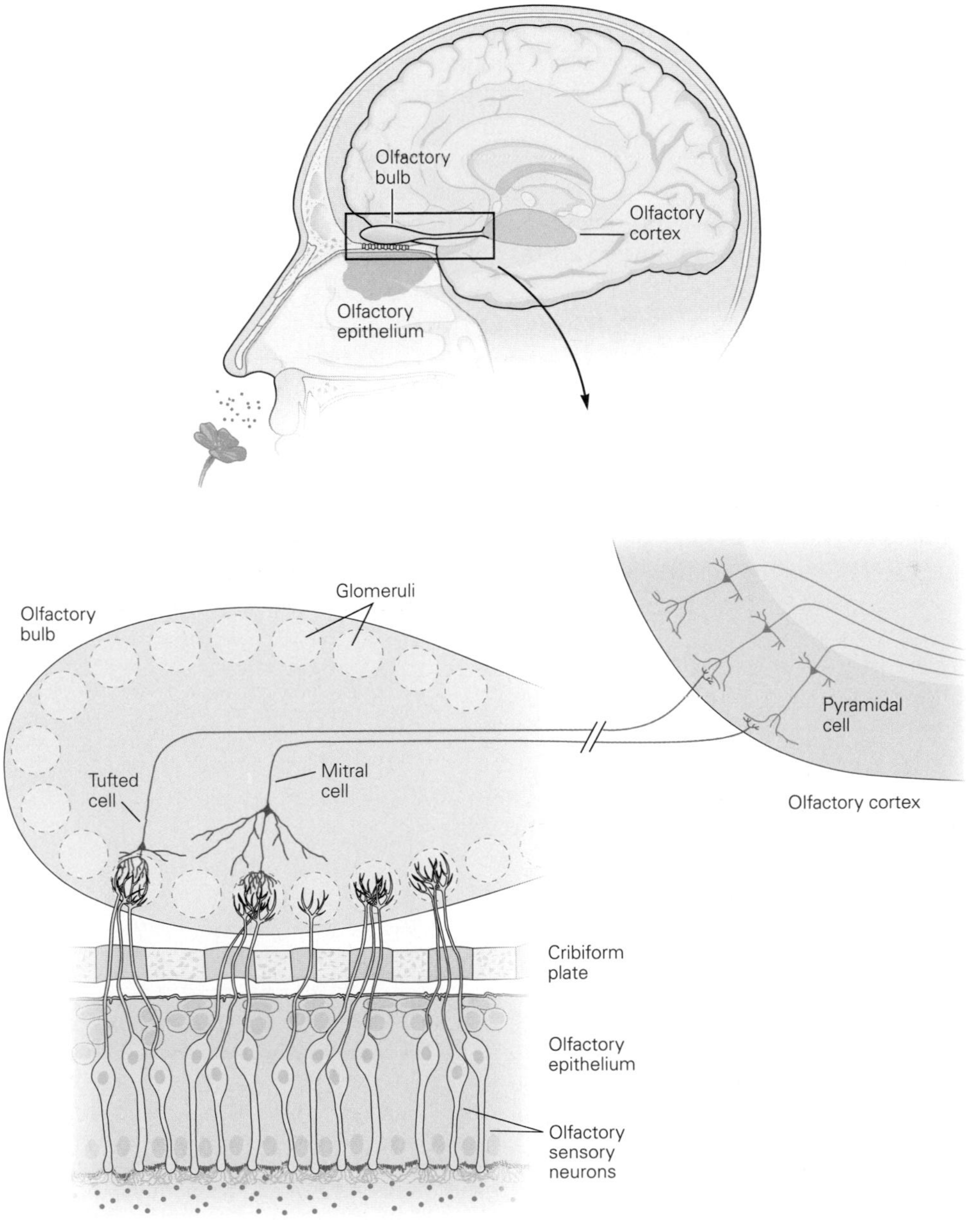

Figure 32–1 The olfactory system. Odorants are detected by olfactory sensory neurons in the olfactory epithelium, which lines part of the nasal cavity. The axons of these neurons project to the olfactory bulb where they terminate on mitral and tufted cell relay neurons within glomeruli. The relay neuron axons project to the olfactory cortex where they terminate on the dendrites of pyramidal neurons whose axons project to other brain areas.

The olfactory sensory neuron is a bipolar nerve cell. A single dendrite extends from the apical end to the epithelial surface, where it gives rise to numerous thin cilia that protrude into the mucus that coats the nasal cavity (Figure 32–2). The cilia have receptors that recognize odorants as well as the transduction machinery needed to amplify the sensory signals and transform them into electrical signals in the neuron's axon, which projects from the basal pole of the neuron to the brain. The axons of olfactory sensory neurons pass through the cribriform plate, a perforated region in the skull above the nasal cavity. The axons then synapse in the olfactory bulb, the first relay in the olfactory pathway (see Figure 32–1).

Mammals Share a Large Family of Odorant Receptors

Odorant receptors are proteins encoded by a multigene family that is evolutionarily conserved and found in all vertebrate species. Humans have approximately 350 different odorant receptors, whereas mice have approximately 1,000. Although odorant receptors belong to the G protein-coupled receptor superfamily, they share sequence motifs not seen in other superfamily members. Significantly, the odorant receptors vary considerably in amino acid sequence (Figure 32–3A).

Like other G protein-coupled receptors, odorant receptors have seven hydrophobic regions that are likely to serve as transmembrane domains (Figure 32–3A). Detailed studies of other G protein-coupled receptors, such as the β-adrenergic receptor, suggest that odorant binding occurs in a pocket in the transmembrane region formed by a combination of the transmembrane domains. The amino acid sequences of odorant receptors are especially variable in several transmembrane domains, providing a possible basis for variability in the odorant binding pocket that could account for the ability of different receptors to recognize structurally diverse ligands.

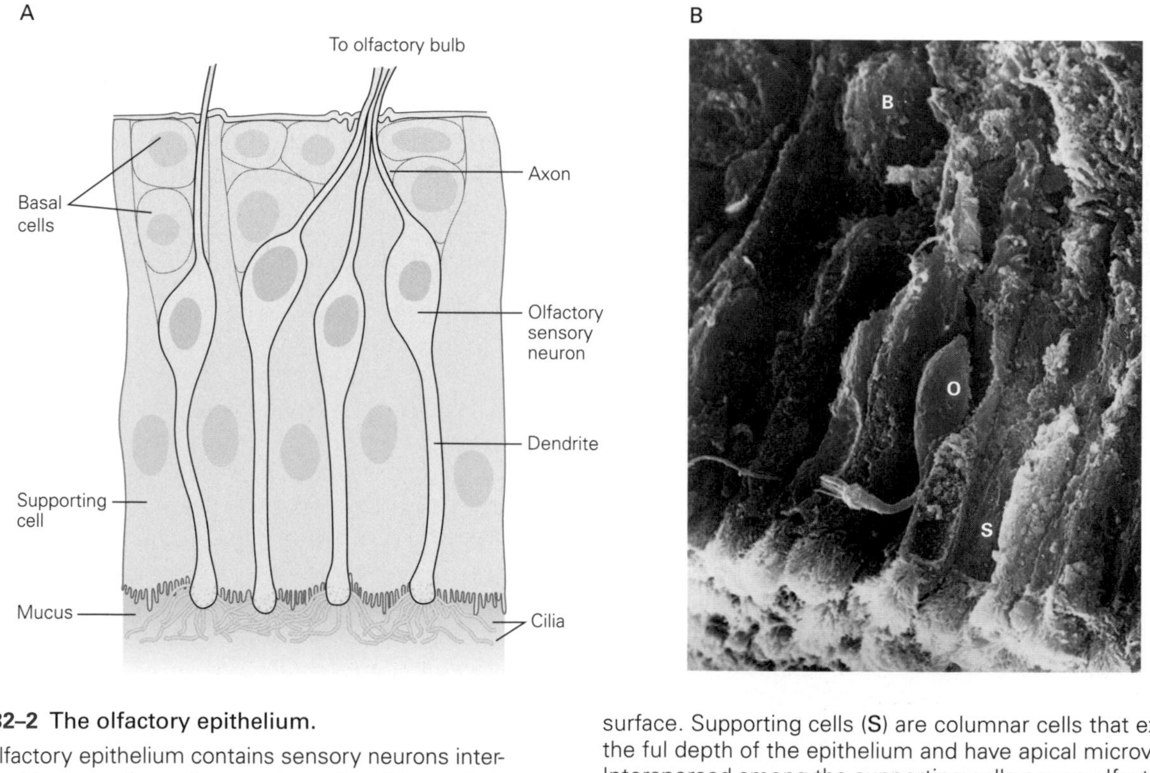

Figure 32–2 The olfactory epithelium.

A. The olfactory epithelium contains sensory neurons interspersed with supporting cells as well as a basal layer of stem cells. Cilia extend from the dendrite of each neuron into the mucus lining the nasal cavity. An axon extends from the basal end of each neuron to the olfactory bulb.

B. A scanning electron micrograph of the olfactory epithelium shows the dense mat of sensory cilia at the epithelial surface. Supporting cells (**S**) are columnar cells that extend the ful depth of the epithelium and have apical microvilli. Interspersed among the supporting cells are an olfactory sensory neuron (**O**) with its dendrite and cilia and a basal stem cell (**B**). (Reproduced, with permission, from Morrison and Costanzo 1990.)

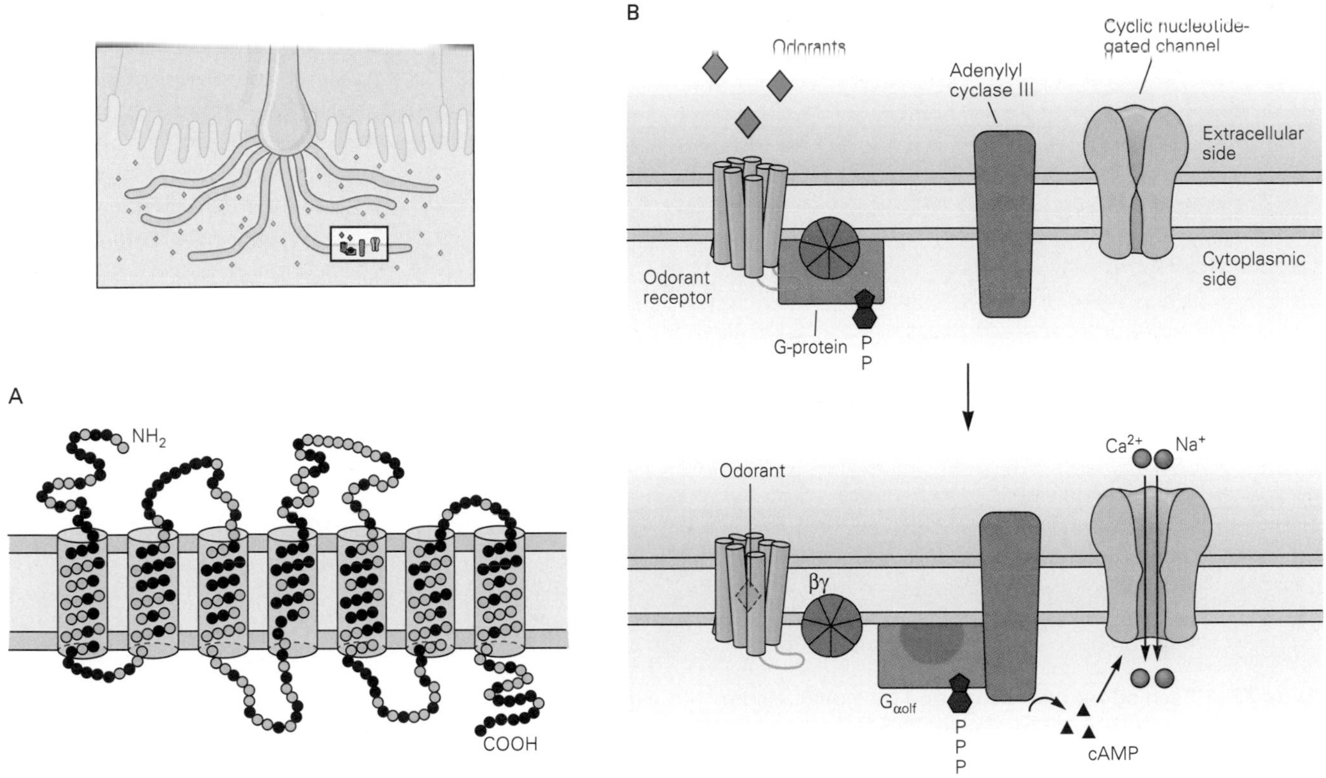

Figure 32–3 Odorant receptors.

A. Odorant receptors have the seven transmembrane domains characteristic of G protein-coupled receptors. They are related to one another but vary in amino acid sequence (positions of highest variability are shown here as **black balls**). Humans have approximately 350 different odorant receptors, and mice have approximately 1,000. (Reproduced, with permission, from Buck and Axel 1991.)

B. Binding of an odorant causes the odorant receptor to interact with $G_{\alpha olf}$, the α-subunit of a heterotrimeric G protein. This causes the release of a GTP-coupled $G_{\alpha olf}$, which stimulates adenylyl cyclase III, leading to an increase in cAMP. The elevated cAMP in turn induces the opening of cyclic nucleotide-gated cation channels, causing cation influx and a change in membrane potential in the ciliary membrane. (**cAMP**, cyclic adenosine monophosphate; **GTP**, guanosine triphosphate.)

A second, smaller family of chemosensory receptors is also expressed in the olfactory epithelium. These receptors, called trace amine-associated receptors (TAARs), are G protein-coupled, but their protein sequence is unrelated to that of odorant receptors. They are encoded by a small family of genes present in humans and mice as well as fish. Studies in mice, which have 14 different olfactory TAARs, indicate that TAARs recognize volatile amines, some of which are enriched in the urine of males compared to that of females. It is possible that this small receptor family has a function distinct from that of the other odorant receptors, perhaps one associated with the detection of social cues.

The binding of an odorant to its receptor induces a cascade of intracellular signaling events that depolarize the olfactory sensory neuron (Figure 32–3B). The depolarization spreads passively to the cell body of the olfactory sensory neuron, causing action potentials that are actively conducted in the axon to the olfactory bulb.

Humans and other animals rapidly accommodate to odors, as witnessed by the weakening of an unpleasant odor when it is continuously present. The ability to sense an odorant rapidly recovers when the odorant is temporarily removed. The adaptation to odorants is caused in part by modulation of the cyclic nucleotide-gated ion channel, but the mechanism by which sensitivity is speedily restored is not yet understood.

Different Combinations of Receptors Encode Different Odorants

To be distinguished perceptually, different odorants must cause different signals to be transmitted from the nose to the brain. This is accomplished in two ways.

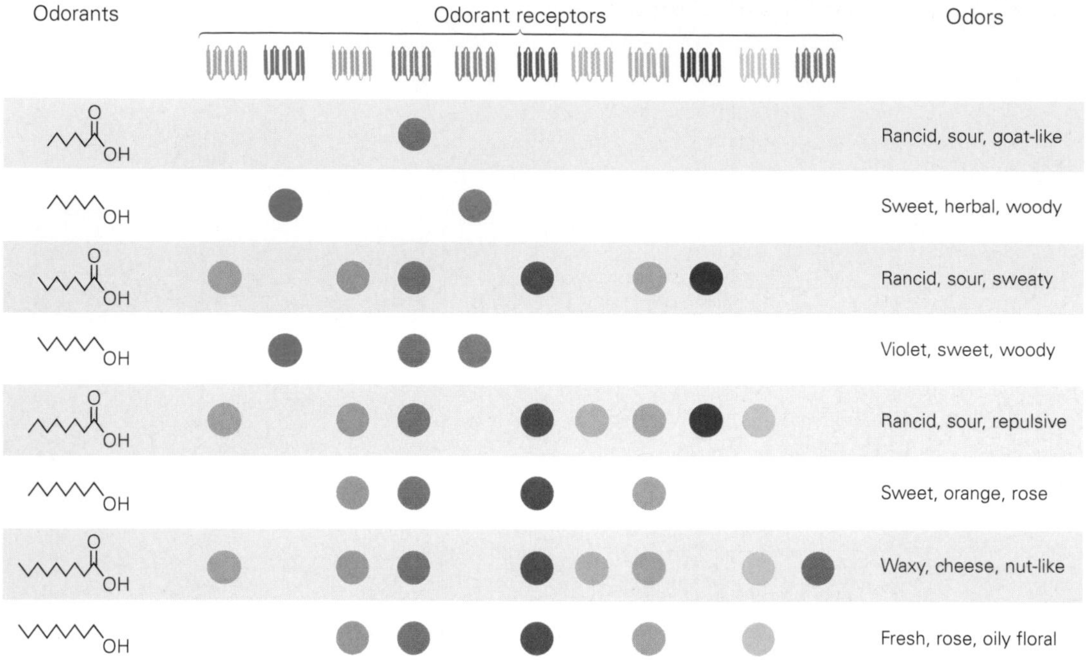

Figure 32–4 Each odorant is recognized by a unique combination of receptors. A single odorant receptor can recognize multiple odorants, and one odorant is recognized by a specific combination of different receptors. That is, different odorants are detected by different combinations of receptors. This combinatorial coding of specific odorants explains how mammals can distinguish odorants with similar chemical structures. The data in the figure were obtained by testing mouse olfactory sensory neurons with different odorants and then determining the odorant receptor gene expressed by each responsive neuron. The perceived qualities of these odorants in humans are shown on the right. (Adapted, with permission, from Malnic et al. 1999.)

First, each olfactory sensory neuron expresses only one odorant receptor gene and therefore one type of receptor. Second, each receptor recognizes multiple odorants, and conversely each odorant is detected by different types of receptors. Importantly, however, each odorant is detected by a unique constellation of receptors and thus causes a distinctive pattern of signals to be transmitted to the brain.

The combinatorial coding of odorants greatly expands the discriminatory power of the olfactory system. If each odorant were detected by only three different receptors, this strategy could in theory generate millions of different receptor combinations—and an equivalently vast number of different signaling patterns. Interestingly, even odorants with nearly identical structures are recognized by different combinations of receptors (Figure 32–4). The fact that highly related odorants have different receptor codes explains why a slight change in the structure of an odorant can alter its perceived odor. In some cases the result is dramatic, for example changing the perception of a chemical from rose to sour.

A change in concentration of an odorant can also change the perceived odor. For example, a low concentration of thio terpineol smells like tropical fruit, a higher concentration smells like grapefruit, and an even higher concentration smells putrid. As the concentration of an odorant is increased, additional receptors with lower affinity for the odorant are recruited into the response and change the receptor code, providing an explanation for the effects of odorant concentration on perception.

Olfactory Information Is Transformed Along the Pathway to the Brain

Odorants Are Encoded in the Nose by Dispersed Neurons

How is a large array of different odorant receptors organized to generate diverse odor perceptions? This question has been investigated in the mouse. Studies in mice have revealed that olfactory information undergoes a series of spatial transformations as it travels from the olfactory epithelium to the olfactory bulb and then to the olfactory cortex.

Different types of odorant receptors are expressed in several coarse zones of the olfactory epithelium of the mouse (Figure 32–5). Each receptor type is expressed in approximately 5,000 neurons that are confined to one zone. (Recall that each neuron expresses only one odorant receptor gene.) Neurons with the same receptor are randomly scattered within the zone so that neurons with different receptors are interspersed. Although one zone may have more receptors for a particular odorant compared to other zones, all zones contain a variety of receptors, so that a specific odorant may be recognized by receptors in several different zones. The evolutionary significance of the zones is unclear, but, as we shall see, the fact that neurons within different epithelial zones project axons to distinct parts of the olfactory bulb suggests that the arrangement of receptors into discrete zones contributes to the establishment of precise information pathways.

Because each odorant is detected by an ensemble of neurons that is widely dispersed across the epithelial sheet, some receptors detecting a particular odorant will remain functional when part of the epithelium is damaged by respiratory infection.

Sensory Inputs in the Olfactory Bulb Are Arranged by Receptor Type

The axons of olfactory sensory neurons project to the ipsilateral olfactory bulb, whose rostral end lies just above the olfactory epithelium. The sensory axons terminate on the dendrites of olfactory bulb neurons within bundles of neuropil called glomeruli that are arrayed over the bulb's surface (Figure 32–6). In each glomerulus the sensory axons make synaptic connections with three types of neurons: mitral and tufted relay neurons, which project axons to the olfactory cortex, and periglomerular interneurons, which encircle the glomerulus.

The axon of an olfactory sensory neuron terminates in only one glomerulus. Similarly, the primary dendrite of each mitral and tufted relay neuron is confined to a single glomerulus. In each glomerulus the axons of several thousand sensory neurons converge on the dendrites of approximately 40 to 50 relay neurons. This convergence results in approximately a 100-fold decrease in the number of neurons transmitting olfactory signals.

The organization of sensory information in the olfactory bulb is dramatically different from that of the epithelium. Whereas olfactory sensory neurons with the same odorant receptor are randomly

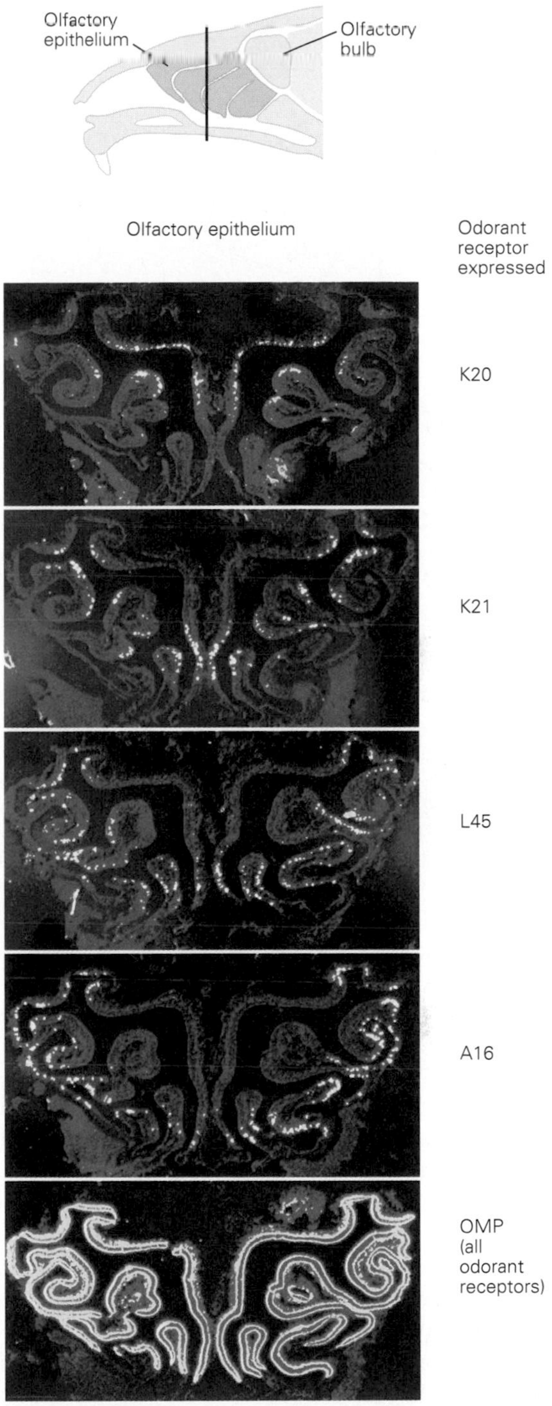

Figure 32–5 Organization of sensory inputs in the olfactory epithelium. Sensory neurons in the olfactory epithelium are distributed in discrete areas known as zones, and each odorant receptor gene is expressed by a small subset of neurons within a single zone. Neurons labeled by four different receptor probes are shown here in different zones in sections through the mouse nose. An olfactory marker protein (OMP) probe labels all neurons expressing odorant receptors. (Adapted, with permission, from Ressler, Sullivan, and Buck 1993; adapted, with permission, from Sullivan et al. 1996.)

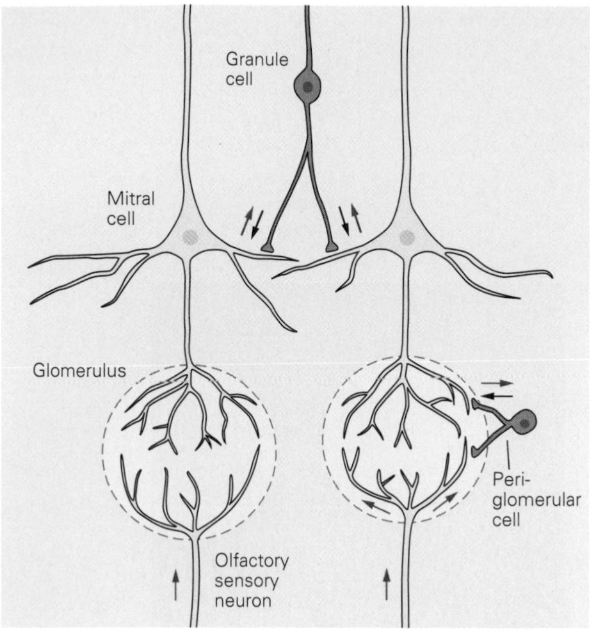

Figure 32–6 Olfactory bulb interneurons. Within the glomerulus, the dendrites of GABAergic periglomerular cells receive excitatory input from olfactory sensory neurons and have reciprocal synapses with the primary dendrites of mitral and tufted relay neurons, suggesting a possible role in signal modification. The dendrites of GABAergic granule cells deeper in the bulb have reciprocal excitatory-inhibitory synapses with the secondary dendrites of the relay neurons and are thought to provide negative feedback to relay neurons that shapes the odor response. (Adapted, with permission, from Shepherd and Greer 1998.)

scattered in one epithelial zone, their axons converge in a few glomeruli at two spots, one on either side of the olfactory bulb (Figure 32–7). Each glomerulus, and each mitral and tufted relay neuron connected to it, receives input from just one type of odorant receptor. The result is a precise arrangement of inputs from different odorant receptors, which is similar between individuals.

Because each odorant is recognized by a unique combination of receptor types, each odorant also activates a particular combination of glomeruli in the olfactory bulb (Figure 32–7B). At the same time, just as an odorant receptor recognizes multiple odorants, a single glomerulus—or a given mitral or tufted cell—is activated by more than one odorant. Closely related odorants can stimulate glomeruli in the same subregion of the bulb, suggesting that the organization of inputs is related to odorant structure. Owing to the nearly stereotyped pattern of receptor inputs in the olfactory bulb, the patterns of glomerular activation elicited by individual odorants are similar in all individuals and are bilaterally symmetrical in the two adjacent bulbs.

This organization of sensory information in the olfactory bulb is likely to be advantageous in two respects. First, the fact that signals from thousands of sensory neurons with the same odorant receptor type always converge on the same few glomeruli and relay neurons in the olfactory bulb may optimize the detection of odorants present at low concentrations. Second, although olfactory sensory neurons with the same receptor type are dispersed and are continually replaced, the arrangement of inputs in the olfactory bulb remains unaltered. As a result, the neural code for an odorant in the brain is maintained over time, assuring that an odorant encountered previously can be recognized years later.

One mystery that remains unsolved is how all the axons of olfactory sensory neurons with the same type of receptor are directed to the same glomeruli. Studies using transgenic mice indicate that the odorant receptor itself somehow determines the target of the axon, but how it does so is unclear.

Sensory information is processed and possibly refined in the olfactory bulb before it is forwarded to the olfactory cortex. Each glomerulus is encircled by periglomerular interneurons that receive excitatory input from sensory axons and form inhibitory dendrodendritic synapses with mitral and tufted cell dendrites in that glomerulus and perhaps adjacent glomeruli. The periglomerular interneurons may therefore have a role in signal modulation. In addition, granule cell interneurons deep in the bulb provide negative feedback onto mitral and tufted cells. The granule cell interneurons are excited by the basal dendrites of mitral and tufted cells and in turn inhibit those postsynaptic relay neurons and others with which they are connected. The lateral inhibition afforded by these connections is thought to dampen signals from glomeruli and relay neurons that respond to an odorant only weakly, thereby sharpening the contrast between important and irrelevant sensory information before its transmission to the cortex.

Other potential sources of signal refinement are the retrograde projections to the olfactory bulb from the olfactory cortex, basal forebrain (horizontal limb of the diagonal band), and midbrain (locus ceruleus and raphe nuclei). These connections may modulate olfactory bulb output according to the physiological state of an animal. When the animal is hungry, for example, some centrifugal projections might heighten the perception of the aroma of foods.

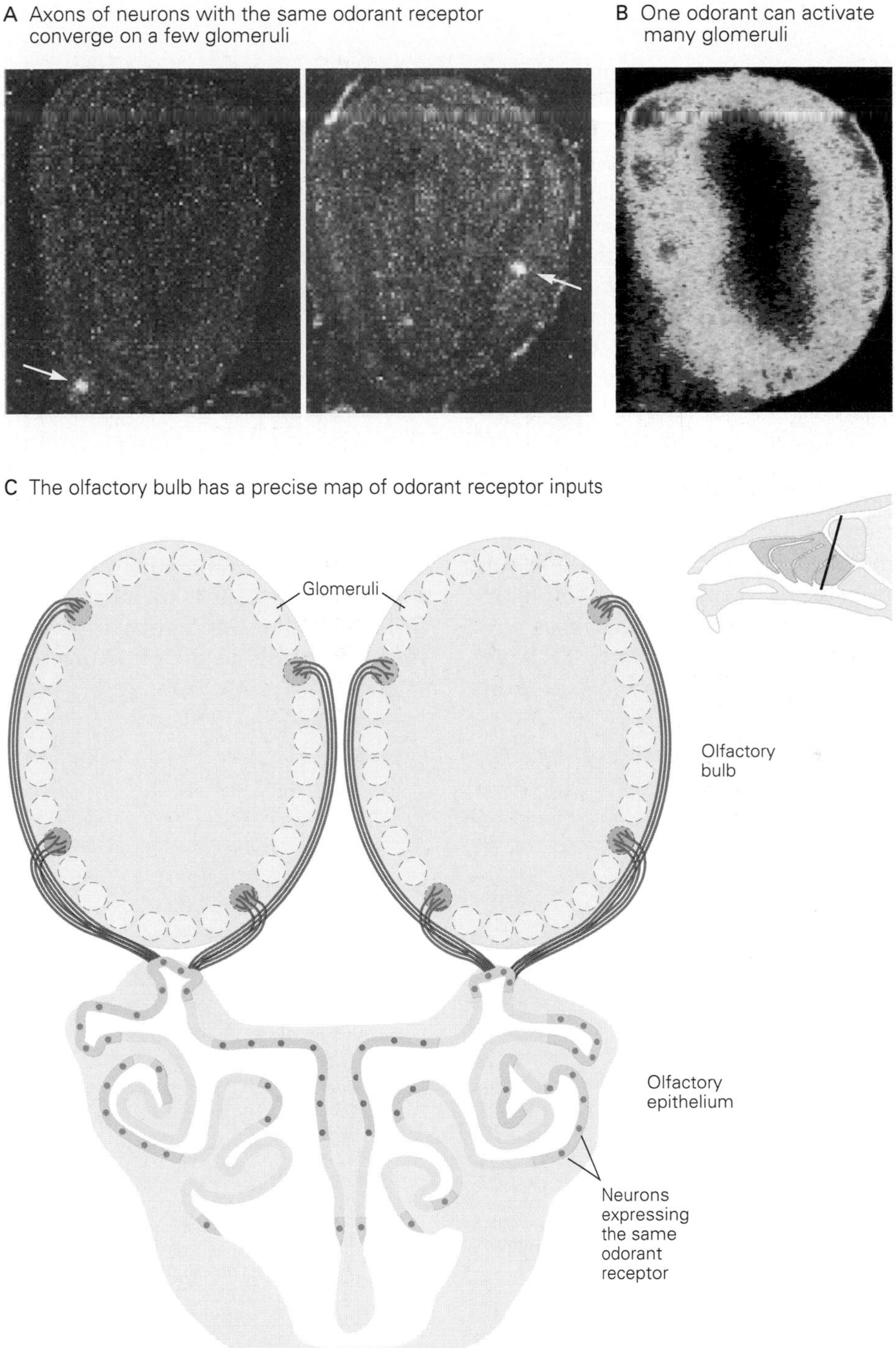
A Axons of neurons with the same odorant receptor converge on a few glomeruli
B One odorant can activate many glomeruli
C The olfactory bulb has a precise map of odorant receptor inputs
Glomeruli
Olfactory bulb
Olfactory epithelium
Neurons expressing the same odorant receptor

Figure 32–7 Odor responses in the olfactory bulb.

A. The axons from neurons in one epithelial zone with the same odorant receptor type usually converge to two glomeruli, one on each side of the olfactory bulb. Here a probe specific for one odorant receptor gene labeled a glomerulus on the medial side (**left**) and lateral side (**right**) of a mouse olfactory bulb. The probe hybridized to receptor messenger RNAs present in sensory axons in these coronal sections. (Adapted from Ressler, Sullivan, and Buck 1994.)

B. This section of a rat olfactory bulb shows the uptake of radiolabeled 2-deoxglucose at multiple foci (**red**) following exposure of the animal to the odorant methyl benzoate. The labeled foci correspond to numerous glomeruli at different locations in the olfactory bulb. (Reproduced, with permission, from Johnson, Farahbod, and Leon 2005.)

C. The olfactory bulb has a precise map of odorant receptor inputs because each glomerulus is dedicated to only one type of receptor. The maps in the two olfactory bulbs are bilaterally symmetrical and are nearly identical across individuals. The maps on the medial and lateral sides of each bulb are similar, but slightly displaced along the dorsal-ventral and anterior-posterior axes.

The Olfactory Bulb Transmits Information to the Olfactory Cortex

The axons of the mitral and tufted relay neurons of the olfactory bulb project through the lateral olfactory tract to the olfactory cortex (Figure 32–8 and see Figure 32–1). The olfactory cortex, defined roughly as that portion of the cortex that receives a direct projection from the olfactory bulb, comprises five main areas: (1) the anterior olfactory nucleus, which connects the two olfactory bulbs through a portion of the anterior commissure; (2) the anterior and posterior cortical nuclei of the amygdala; (3) the olfactory tubercle; (4) part of the entorhinal cortex; and (5) the piriform cortex, the largest and considered the major olfactory cortical area.

In the piriform cortex the axons of olfactory bulb mitral and tufted cells leave the lateral olfactory tract to form excitatory glutamatergic synapses with pyramidal neurons, the projection neurons of the cortex. Signal transmission by the pyramidal neurons appears to be modulated by inhibitory inputs from local GABA-ergic interneurons as well as by excitatory inputs from neighboring pyramidal neurons and the piriform cortex of the other hemisphere. The piriform cortex also receives centrifugal inputs from modulatory brain areas, suggesting that its activity may be adjusted according to behavioral state. Finally, the olfactory cortex projects to the olfactory bulb, providing yet another possible means of signal modulation.

As with the olfactory bulb relay neurons, individual pyramidal neurons can be activated by more than one odorant. However, the pyramidal neurons activated by a particular odorant are scattered across the piriform cortex, an arrangement different from that of the olfactory bulb. Mitral cells in different parts of the olfactory bulb can project axons to the same subregion of the piriform cortex, further indicating that the highly organized map of odorant receptor inputs in the olfactory bulb is not recapitulated in the cortex.

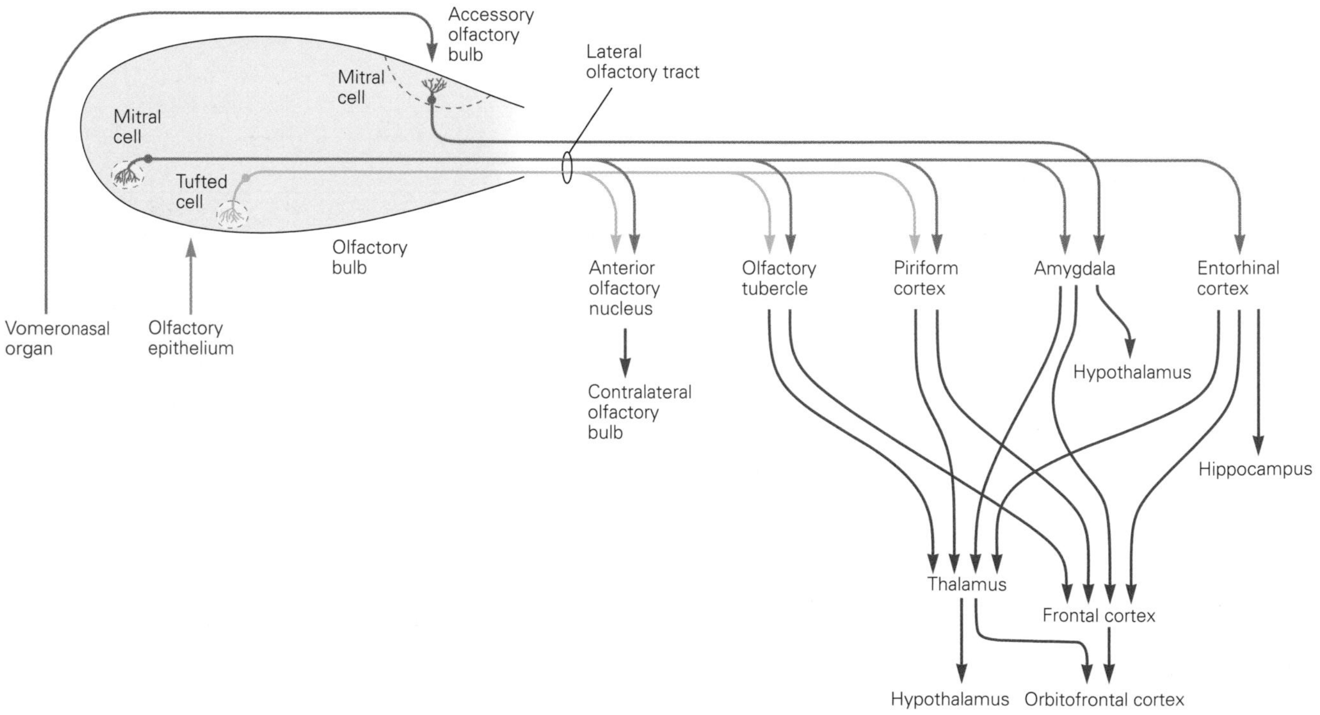

Figure 32–8 The olfactory cortex. The axons of mitral and tufted relay neurons of the olfactory bulb project through the lateral olfactory tract to the olfactory cortex. The olfactory cortex consists of a number of distinct areas, the largest of which is the piriform cortex. From these areas olfactory information is transmitted directly to other brain areas as well as indirectly via the thalamus. Targets include frontal and orbitofrontal areas of the neocortex, which are thought to be important for odor discrimination, and the amygdala and hypothalamus, which may be involved in emotional and physiological responses to odors. Mitral cells in the accessory olfactory bulb project to specific areas of the amygdala that transmit signals to the hypothalamus.

Output from the Olfactory Cortex Reaches Higher Cortical and Limbic Areas

Pyramidal neurons in the olfactory cortex transmit information indirectly to the orbitofrontal cortex through the thalamus and directly to the frontal cortex. These pathways to higher cortical areas are thought to be important in odor discrimination. In fact, people with lesions of the orbitofrontal cortex are unable to discriminate odors. Interestingly, recordings in the orbitofrontal cortex suggest that some individual neurons in that area receive multimodal input and can respond, for example, to the smell, sight, and taste of a banana.

Most areas of the olfactory cortex also relay information to the lateral hypothalamus, an area important in appetite. In addition, studies of rodents indicate that one part of the olfactory cortex, the anterior cortical nucleus of the amygdala, transmits information to other areas of the amygdala and to more anterior regions of the hypothalamus, including those involved in reproduction. These limbic areas are thought to mediate the emotional and motivational aspects of smell as well as many of the behavioral and physiological effects of odorants. In animals they may be important in the generation of stereotyped behavioral and physiological responses to odors of predators or to pheromones that are detected in the olfactory epithelium.

Olfactory Acuity Varies in Humans

Olfactory acuity can vary as much as 1,000-fold among humans, even among people with no obvious abnormality. The most common olfactory aberration is *specific anosmia*. An individual with a specific anosmia has lowered sensitivity to a specific odorant even though sensitivity to other odorants appears normal. Specific anosmias to some odorants are common, a few occurring in 1 to 20% of people. For example, 12% of individuals tested in one study exhibited a specific anosmia for musk. Recent studies indicate that specific anosmias can be caused by mutations in particular odorant receptors.

Far rarer abnormalities of olfaction, such as *general anosmia* (complete lack of olfactory sensation) or *hyposmia* (diminished sense of smell), are often transient and can derive from respiratory infections. Chronic anosmia or hyposmia can result from damage to the olfactory epithelium caused by infections; from particular diseases, such as Parkinson disease; or from head trauma that severs the olfactory nerves passing through holes in the cribriform plate, which then become blocked by scar tissue. Olfactory hallucinations of repugnant smells (*cacosmia*) can occur as a consequence of epileptic seizures.

Odors Elicit Characteristic Innate Behaviors

Pheromones Are Detected in Two Olfactory Structures

In many animals the olfactory system detects not only odors but also pheromones, chemicals that are released from animals and influence the behavior or physiology of members of the same species. Pheromones play important roles in a variety of mammals, although they have not been compellingly demonstrated in humans. Often contained in urine or glandular secretions, some pheromones modulate the levels of reproductive hormones or stimulate sexual behavior or aggression. Pheromones are detected by two separate structures: the nasal olfactory epithelium, where odorants are detected, and the vomeronasal organ, an accessory olfactory organ thought to be specialized for pheromone detection.

The vomeronasal organ is present in many mammals although not in humans. It is a tubular structure in the nasal septum that has a duct opening into the nasal cavity and one inner wall lined by a sensory epithelium (Figure 32–9). Signals generated by sensory neurons in the epithelium of the vomeronasal organ follow a distinct pathway. They travel through the accessory olfactory bulb to the medial amygdala and from there to the hypothalamus, which controls a variety of physiological and behavioral responses.

Sensory detection in the vomeronasal organ differs from that in the olfactory epithelium. The vomeronasal organ has two different families of chemosensory receptors, the V1R and V2R families. In the mouse each family has more than one hundred members. Variation in amino acid sequence between members of each receptor family suggests that each family may recognize a variety of different ligands. Like odorant receptors, V1R and V2R receptors have the seven transmembrane domains typical of G protein-coupled receptors. The V2R receptor differs from both V1R and odorant receptors in having a large extracellular domain at the N-terminal end (Figure 32–9A). By analogy with receptors with similar structures, ligands may bind V1Rs in a membrane pocket formed by a combination of transmembrane domains, whereas binding of V2Rs may occur in the large extracellular domain.

The V1R and V2R families are each localized in one of two zones in the vomeronasal organ that express

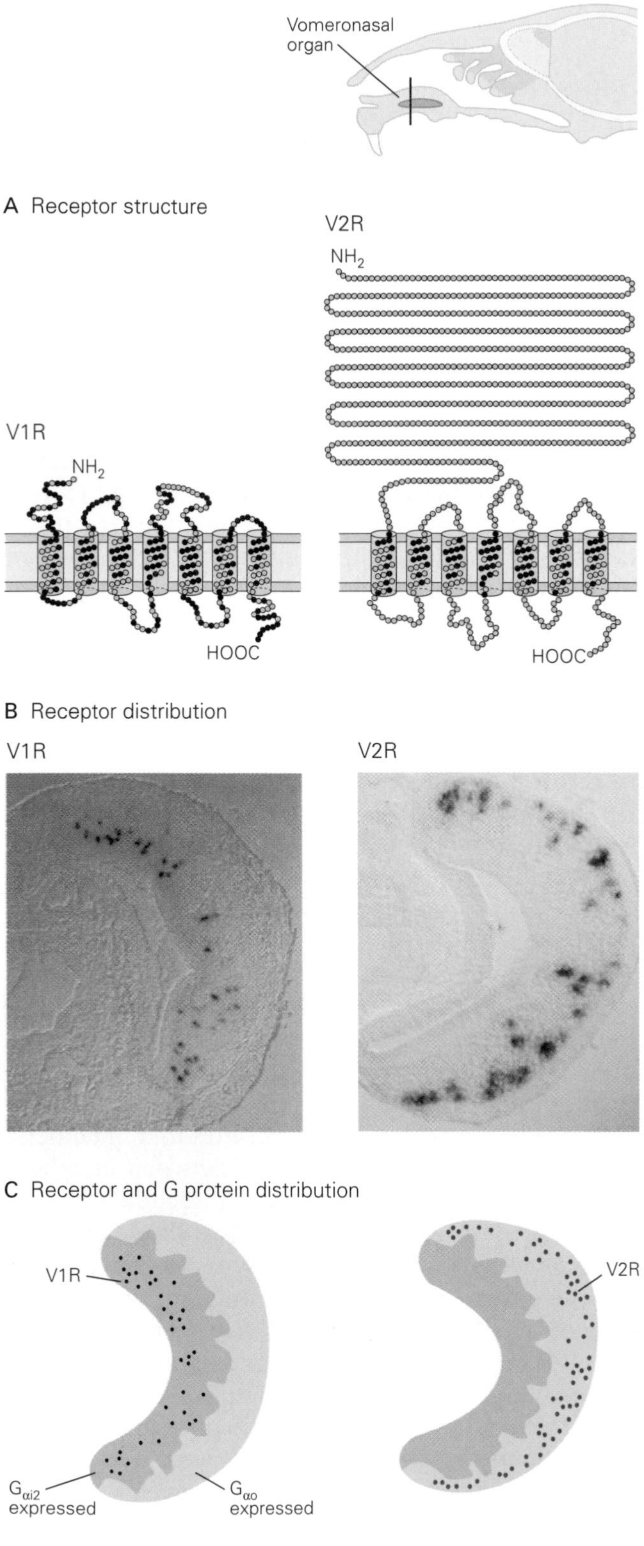

different G proteins (Figure 32–9B and C). The *V1R* and *V2R* genes are each expressed in a small percentage of neurons scattered throughout one zone, an arrangement similar to that of odorant receptors in the olfactory epithelium. Similar to the main olfactory bulb, the vomeronasal neurons with the same receptor type project to the same glomeruli in the accessory olfactory bulb, although the glomeruli for each receptor type are more numerous and their distribution less stereotyped than in the main olfactory bulb.

Invertebrate Olfactory Systems Can Be Used to Study Odor Coding and Behavior

Because invertebrates have simple nervous systems and often respond to olfactory stimuli with stereotyped behaviors, they are useful for understanding the relationship between the neural representation of odor and behavior.

Certain features of chemosensory systems are highly conserved in evolution. First, all metazoan animals can detect a variety of organic molecules using specialized chemosensory neurons with cilia or microvilli that contact the external environment. Second, the initial events of odor detection are mediated by families of transmembrane receptors with specific expression patterns in peripheral sensory neurons. Other features of the olfactory system differ between species, reflecting selection pressures and evolutionary histories of the animals.

The Anatomy of the Insect Olfactory System Resembles That of Vertebrates

The primary sensory organs of insects are the antennae and appendages known as maxillary palps near the mouth (Figure 32–10A). Whereas mammals have

Figure 32–9 Candidate pheromone receptors in the vomeronasal organ.

A. The V1R and V2R families of receptors are expressed in the vomeronasal organ. In the mouse each family has more than 100 members, which vary in protein sequence. Members of both families have the seven transmembrane domains of G protein-coupled receptors, but V2R receptors also have a large extracellular domain at the N-terminal end that may be the site of ligand binding.

B. Sections through the vomeronasal organ show individual V1R and V2R probes hybridized to subsets of neurons in two distinct zones. (Micrographs reproduced, with permission, from Dulac and Axel 1995 and from Matsunami and Buck 1997.)

C. The two zones express high levels of different G proteins, $G_{\alpha i2}$ and $G_{\alpha o}$.

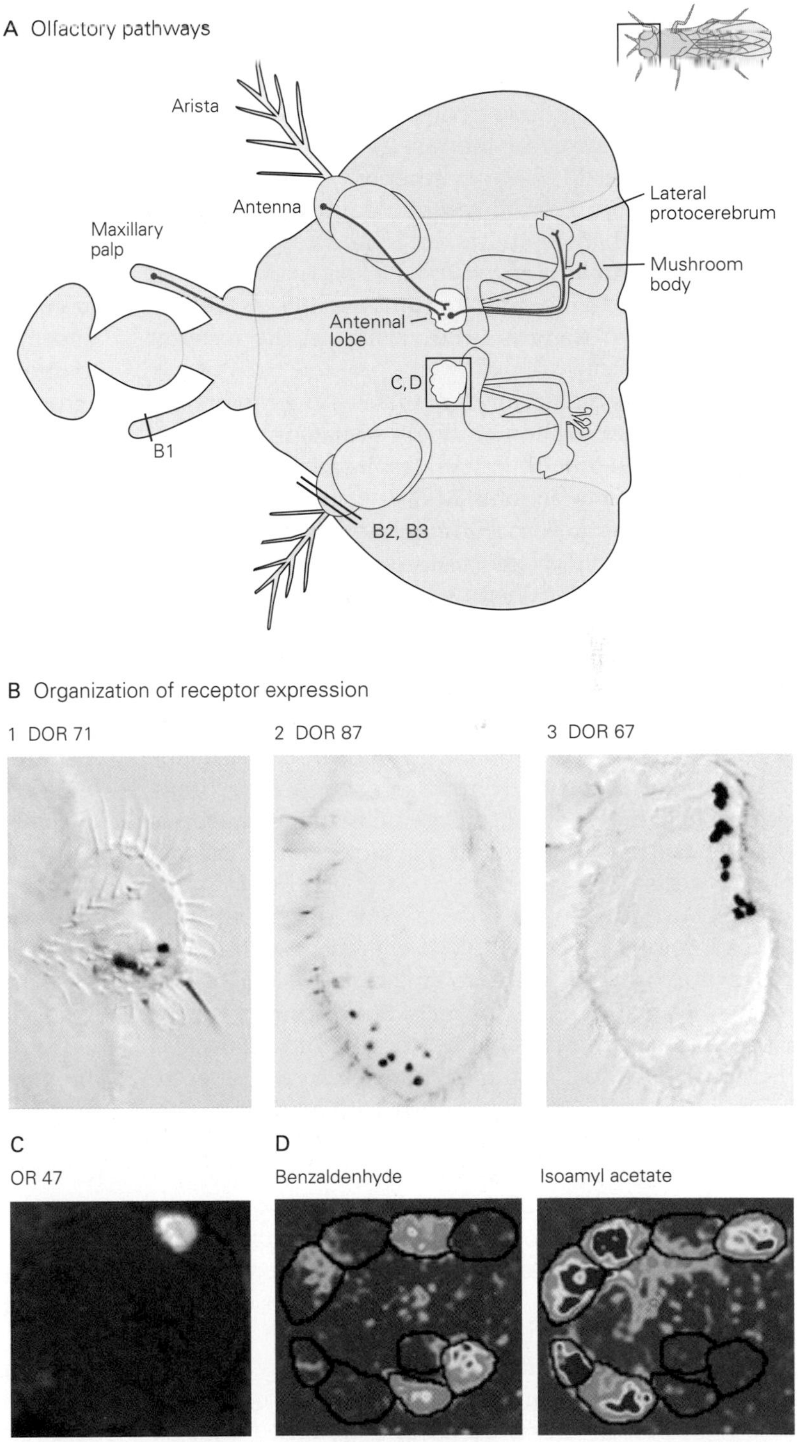

Figure 32–10 Olfactory pathways from the antenna to the brain in *Drosophila*.

A. Olfactory neurons with cell bodies and dendrites in the antenna and maxillary palp project axons to the antennal lobe. Projection neurons in the antennal lobe then project to two regions of the fly brain, the mushroom body and lateral protocerebrum. (Reproduced, with permission, from Takaki Komiyama and Liqun Luo.)

B. The neurons that express one type of olfactory receptor gene, detected by RNA in situ hybridization, are scattered in the maxillary palp (1) or antenna (2, 3).

C. All neurons that express the olfactory receptor gene *OR47* converge on a glomerulus in the antennal lobe. (Reproduced, with permission, from Vosshall et al. 1999 and from Vosshall, Wong, and Axel 2000.)

D. Each odorant elicits a physiological response from a subset of glomeruli in the antennal lobe. Two-photon calcium imaging was used to detect odor-evoked signals. (Reproduced, with permission, from Wang et al. 2003.)

millions of olfactory neurons, insects have a much smaller number. There are approximately 2,600 olfactory neurons in the simple fruit fly *Drosophila* and approximately 60,000 in a complex insect, the honeybee.

The insect odorant receptors were discovered by finding multigene receptor families in the *Drosophila* genome, and these genes have now been examined in other insect genomes as well. Remarkably, they have little similarity to mammalian odorant receptors save for the presence of many transmembrane domains. Indeed, insect receptors appear to have an independent evolutionary origin from mammalian receptors, and may not even be G protein-coupled receptors—an extreme example of the fast evolutionary change observed across all olfactory receptor systems. In *Drosophila* the main odorant receptor family has only 60 genes rather than the hundreds characteristic of vertebrates. The malaria mosquito *Anopheles gambiae* and the honeybee have similar numbers (85–95 genes), suggesting that there is little variety in the receptor families of insects.

Despite the molecular dissimilarity in receptors, the anatomical organization of the fly's olfactory system is quite similar to that of vertebrates. Each olfactory neuron expresses one or sometimes two functional odorant receptor genes. The neurons expressing a particular gene are loosely localized to a region of the antenna, but interspersed with neurons expressing other genes (Figure 32–10B). This scattered distribution is not the case at the next level of organization, the antennal lobe. Axons from sensory neurons that express one type of receptor converge on two invariant glomeruli in the antennal lobe, one each on the left and right sides of the animal (Figure 32–10C). This organization is strikingly similar to that of the first sensory relay in the vertebrate olfactory bulb and is found in the moth, honeybee, and other insects.

Because there are only a few dozen receptor genes in insects, it is possible to characterize the entire repertory of odorant-receptor interactions, a goal that is not yet attainable in mammals. Sophisticated genetic methods can be used to label and record from a *Drosophila* neuron expressing a single known odorant receptor gene. By repeating this experiment with many receptors and odors, the receptive fields of the odorant receptors have been defined, and shown to be quite diverse.

In insects individual odorant receptors can detect large numbers of odorants, including odorants with very different chemical structures. This broad recognition of odorants by "generalist" receptors is necessary if only a small number of receptors is available to detect all biologically significant odorants. A single insect receptor protein that detects many odors can be stimulated by some odors and inhibited by others, often with distinct temporal patterns. A subset of insect odorant receptors is more selective in its recognition, and conveys information about pheromones or other unusual odors like carbon dioxide. Thus the coding potential of each olfactory neuron can be broad or narrow, and arises from a combination of stimulatory and inhibitory signals delivered to its receptors.

Information from the olfactory neurons is relayed to the first processing station, the antennal lobe (Figure 32–10A). Sensory neurons expressing the same odorant receptor converge onto a small number of projection neurons in one glomerulus of the antennal lobe. Because *Drosophila* glomeruli are stereotyped in position and have one type of odorant receptor input, the transformation of information across the synapse can be described. Convergence leads to a great increase in signal-to-noise ratios of olfactory signals, so projection neurons are much more sensitive to odor than individual olfactory neurons. Within the antennal lobe most information from an individual olfactory neuron goes to one glomerulus, but information is also distributed across the entire antennal lobe and processed by excitatory and inhibitory interneurons that connect many glomeruli. Excitatory interneurons distribute signals to projection neurons at distal locations, and inhibitory interneurons feed back onto the olfactory sensory neurons to dampen their input.

The projection neurons from the antennal lobe extend to higher brain centers called mushroom bodies and lateral protocerebrum (Figure 32–10A). These structures may represent insect equivalents of the olfactory cortex. The mushroom bodies are sites of olfactory associative learning and multimodal associative learning; the lateral protocerebrum is important for innate olfactory avoidance responses. At this stage projection neurons form complex connections with a large number of downstream neurons. Neurons in higher brain centers in *Drosophila* have the potential to integrate information from many receptors. Because they respond to only a small number of odors, their tuning to odors appears to be far more specific than that of the sensory neurons or antennal projection neurons. Even this higher-order pattern in the lateral protocerebrum seems highly reproducible from fly to fly, suggesting that a detailed higher-order map of insect odor representation can be defined.

Olfactory Cues Elicit Stereotyped Behaviors and Physiological Responses in the Nematode

The nematode roundworm *Caenorhabditis elegans* has one of the simplest nervous systems in the animal kingdom, with only 302 neurons in the entire animal. Of these, 32 are ciliated chemosensory neurons. Because *C. elegans* has strong behavioral responses to a wide variety of chemicals it has been a useful animal for relating olfactory signals to behavior. Each chemosensory neuron detects a specific set of chemicals and activation of the neuron is required for the behavioral responses to those substances. The neuron for a particular response, such as attraction to a specific odor, occurs in the same position in all individuals.

The molecular mechanisms of olfaction in *C. elegans* were elucidated through genetic screens for anosmic worm mutants. The G protein-coupled receptor for the volatile odorant diacetyl emerged from these screens (Figure 32–11). This receptor is one of approximately 1,700 predicted G protein-coupled chemoreceptor genes in *C. elegans*, the largest number of chemoreceptors among known genomes. Other kinds of chemosensory receptors are also present; for example, *C. elegans* senses external oxygen levels indirectly by detecting soluble guanylate cyclases that bind directly to oxygen. With so many chemoreceptors, nematodes are able to recognize a large variety of odors with great sensitivity. Downstream of the receptors some chemosensory neurons use G proteins to regulate cyclic guanosine 3′–5′ monophosphate (cGMP) and a cGMP-gated channel, a signal transduction pathway like that of vertebrate photoreceptors. Other chemosensory neurons signal through a transient receptor potential vanilloid (TRPV) channel, like vertebrate nociceptive neurons.

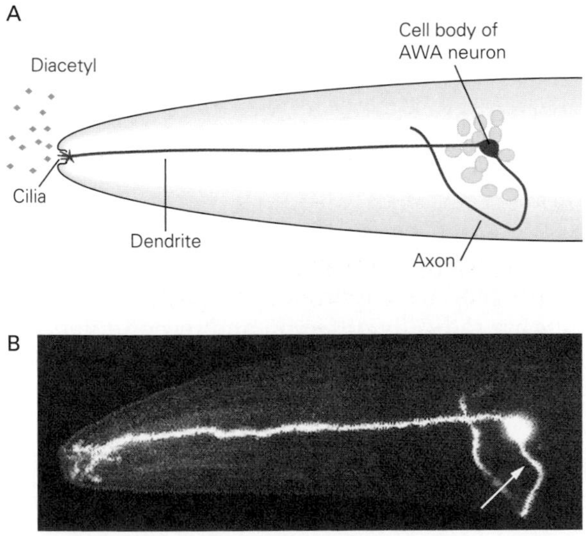

Figure 32–11 The receptor for diacetyl is expressed in a specific chemosensory neuron in the nematode worm *C. elegans*.

A. A lateral view of the worm's anterior end shows the cell body and processes of the AWA chemosensory neuron. The dendritic process terminates in cilia that are exposed to environmental chemicals. The neuron detects the volatile chemical diacetyl; animals with a mutation in the *odr-10* gene are unable to sense diacetyl.

B. The *odr-10* gene product, marked with a fusion to a fluorescent reporter protein, is seen only in the AWA neuron, whose axon is marked with an arrow. (Reproduced, with permission, from Sarafi-Reinach and Sengupta 2000.)

The "one neuron, one receptor" principle observed in vertebrates and insects does not operate in nematodes as the number of neurons is much smaller than the number of receptors. Each of the many chemoreceptor genes is typically expressed in only one pair of chemosensory neurons, but each neuron expresses many receptor genes. The small size of its nervous system limits the olfactory computations that *C. elegans* can perform. For example, a single neuron responds to many odors, but odors can be distinguished efficiently only if they are sensed by different primary sensory neurons.

The relationship between odor detection and behavior has been explored in *C. elegans* through genetic manipulations. For example, diacetyl is normally attractive to worms, but when the diacetyl receptor is experimentally expressed in an olfactory neuron that normally senses repellents, the animals are instead repelled by diacetyl. This observation indicates that specific sensory neurons encode the hardwired behavioral responses of attraction or repulsion, and that a "labeled line" connects specific odors to specific behaviors. Similar ideas have emerged from genetic manipulations of taste systems in mice and flies, where sweet and bitter preference pathways appear to be encoded by different sets of sensory cells.

Olfactory cues are linked to physiological responses as well as behavioral responses in nematodes. Food and pheromone cues that regulate development are detected by specific sensory neurons through G protein-coupled receptors. At low pheromone and high food levels animals rapidly develop to adulthood, whereas high pheromone levels and scarce food drive entry into a long-lived arrested larval stage called a *dauer larva* (Figure 32–12). Activation of these sensory neurons ultimately regulates the activity of an insulin signaling pathway that controls physiology and growth, as well as life span, of the nematode. It is an open question whether the chemosensory systems and physiological systems of other animals are as entangled as they are in nematodes.

Strategies for Olfaction Have Evolved Rapidly

Why have independent families of odorant receptors evolved in mammals, nematodes, and insects? And why have the families changed so rapidly compared to genes involved in other important biological processes? The answer lies in a fundamental difference between olfaction and other senses such as vision, touch, and hearing.

Most senses are designed to detect physical entities with reliable physical properties: photons, pressure, or sound waves. By contrast, olfactory systems are designed

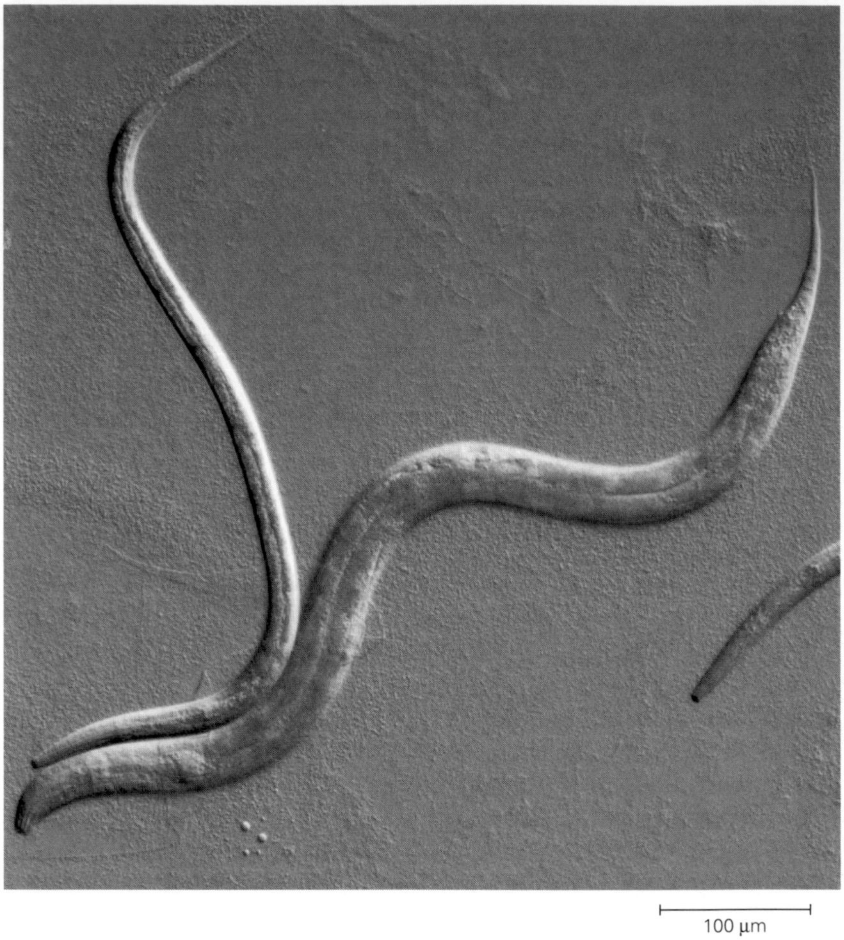

Figure 32–12 Chemosensory cues regulate the development of *C. elegans.* When exposed to different chemosensory cues, two larvae of the same age adopt distinct fates. At the left is a dauer larva, a small, slender animal that forms under stressful conditions of low food and high animal density. The dauer larva is a nonfeeding, nonreproductive, stress-resistant form. At the right is a fourth-larval-stage animal in a rich environment favoring reproductive growth. (Reproduced, with permission, from Manuel Zimmer.)

to detect organic molecules that are infinitely variable and do not fit into a simple continuum of properties. Moreover, the organic molecules that are detected are produced by other living organisms, which evolve far more rapidly than the world of light, pressure, and sound.

An ancient olfactory system was present in the common ancestors of all animals that exist today. That ancestor lived in the ocean, where it gave rise to different lineages for mammals, insects, and nematodes. Those three phyla of animals came onto land hundreds of millions of years after the phyla diverged. Each phylum independently modified its olfactory system to detect airborne odors, leading to diversification of the receptors.

A consideration of the natural history of dipteran and hymenopteran insects, which have evolved in the last 200 million years, helps explain the rapid diversification of the odorant receptors. These insects include honeybees that pollinate flowers, fruit flies that feed on rotting fruit, flesh flies that arrive within minutes of death, and mosquitoes that seek animal prey. The odorants that are important for the survival of these insects are radically different, and receptor genes that are tuned to those odorants have evolved accordingly.

The Gustatory System Controls the Sense of Taste

Taste Has Five Submodalities or Qualities

The primary function of the gustatory system is nutritional. Humans and other mammals can distinguish five different taste qualities: sweet, bitter, salty, sour, and umami, the taste associated with amino acids. Taste chemicals (tastants) perceived as sweet are associated with food high in caloric content, while those sensed as umami are indicative of protein.

Consistent with the nutritional importance of carbohydrates and proteins, both sweet and umami tastants elicit pleasurable sensations in humans and are attractants for animals. In contrast, bitter tastants, which are often found in poisonous plants, elicit an aversive response that is innate in animals as well as human infants and likely prevents the ingestion of toxic substances.

Taste is often thought to be synonymous with flavor. However, taste refers strictly to the five qualities encoded in the gustatory system, whereas flavor, with its rich and varied qualities, actually stems from a combination of inputs from the gustatory, olfactory, and somatosensory systems.

Taste Detection Occurs in Taste Buds

In the gustatory system sensory signals generated in the mouth are relayed through the brain stem and thalamus to the gustatory cortex (Figure 32–13). Tastants are detected by taste receptor cells that are clustered in taste buds. Although the majority of taste buds in humans are located on the tongue, some can also be found on the palate, pharynx, epiglottis, and upper third of the esophagus.

Taste buds on the tongue occur in structures called papillae, of which there are three types based on morphology and location. *Fungiform papillae*, located on the anterior two-thirds of the tongue, are peg-like structures that are topped with taste buds. Both the *foliate papillae*, situated on the posterior edge of the tongue, and the *circumvallate papillae*, of which there are only a few in the posterior area of the tongue, are structures surrounded by grooves lined with taste buds (Figure 32–14A). Each fungiform papilla contains one to five taste buds, while each circumvallate or foliate papilla contains hundreds.

The taste bud is a garlic-shaped structure embedded in the epithelium. A small opening at the epithelial

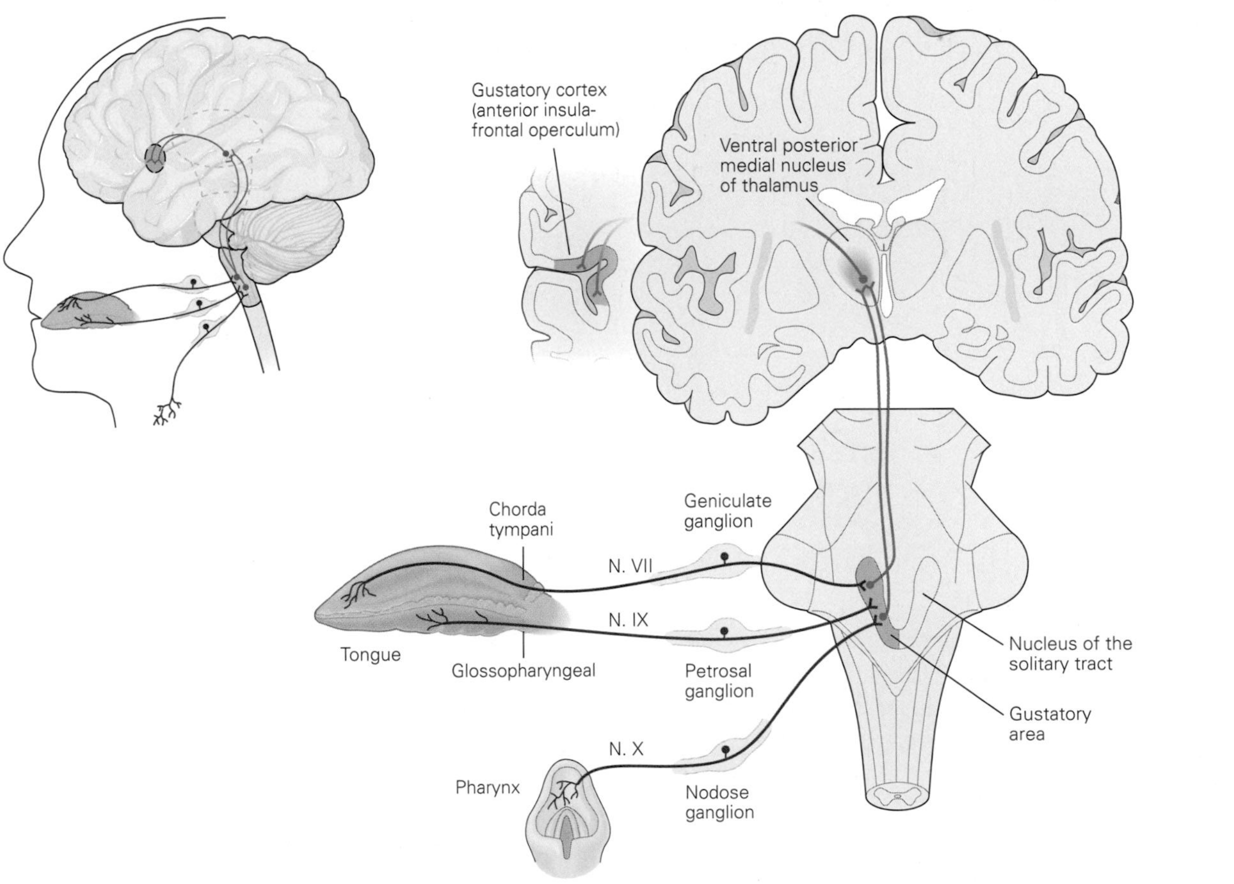

Figure 32–13 The gustatory system. Tastants are detected in taste buds in the oral cavity. Taste buds on the tongue are innervated by the peripheral fibers of gustatory sensory neurons, which travel in the glossopharyngeal and chorda tympani nerves and terminate in the nucleus of the solitary tract in the brain stem. From there taste information is relayed through the thalamus to the gustatory cortex as well as to the hypothalamus.

surface, the taste pore, is the point of contact with tastants (Figure 32–14B). Each taste bud contains approximately 100 taste receptor cells (taste cells), elongated cells that stretch from the taste pore to the basal area of the bud. The taste bud also contains other elongated cells that are thought to serve a supporting function, as well as a small number of round cells at the base, which are thought to serve as stem cells. Taste cells are short-lived and appear to be continually replaced from the stem cell population.

Each taste cell extends microvilli into the taste pore, allowing the cell to contact chemicals dissolved in saliva at the epithelial surface. At its basal end the taste cell contacts the afferent fibers of gustatory sensory neurons, whose cell bodies reside in specific sensory ganglia (Figures 32–13 and 32–14). Although taste cells are nonneural, their contacts with the gustatory sensory neurons have the morphological characteristics of chemical synapses, including clustered presynaptic vesicles. Taste cells also resemble neurons in that they are electrically excitable; they have voltage-gated Na^+, K^+, and Ca^{2+} channels and are capable of generating action potentials.

Each Taste Is Detected by a Distinct Sensory Transduction Mechanism and Distinct Population of Taste Cells

Each of the five taste qualities involves a different sensory transduction mechanism in the microvilli of taste cells. There are, however, two general types. Bitter, sweet, and umami tastants interact with G protein-coupled receptors, whereas salty and sour tastants appear to involve specific ion channels (Figure 32–15). These interactions depolarize the taste cell, leading to the generation of action potentials in the afferent gustatory fibers.

Sweet Taste

Compounds that humans perceive as sweet include sugars, artificial sweeteners such as saccharin and

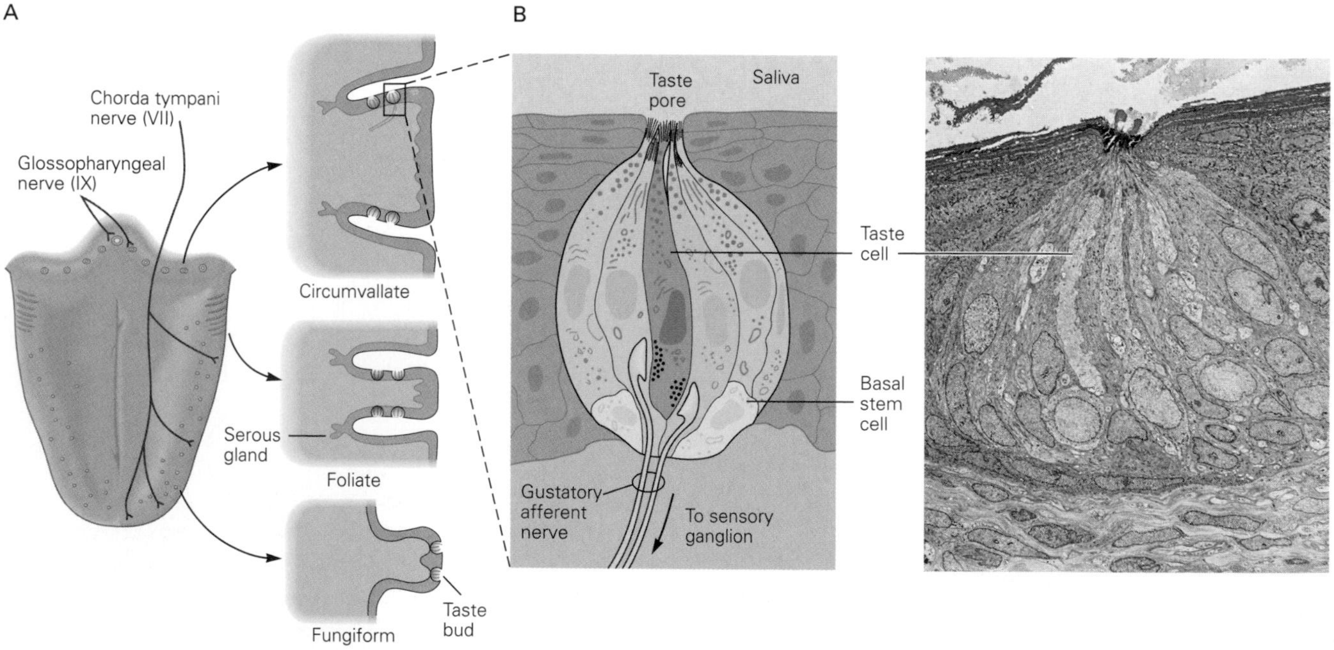

Figure 32–14 Taste buds are clustered in papillae on the tongue.

A. The three types of papillae—circumvallate, foliate, and fungiform—differ in morphology and location on the tongue and are differentially innervated by the chorda tympani and glossopharyngeal nerves.

B. Each taste bud contains 50 to 150 elongated taste receptor cells, as well as supporting cells and a small population of basal stem cells. The taste cell extends microvilli into the taste pore, allowing it to detect tastants dissolved in saliva. At its basal end the taste cell contacts gustatory sensory neurons that transmit stimulus signals to the brain. The scanning electron micrograph shows a taste bud in a foliate papilla in a rabbit. (Reproduced, with permission, from Royer and Kinnamon 1991.)

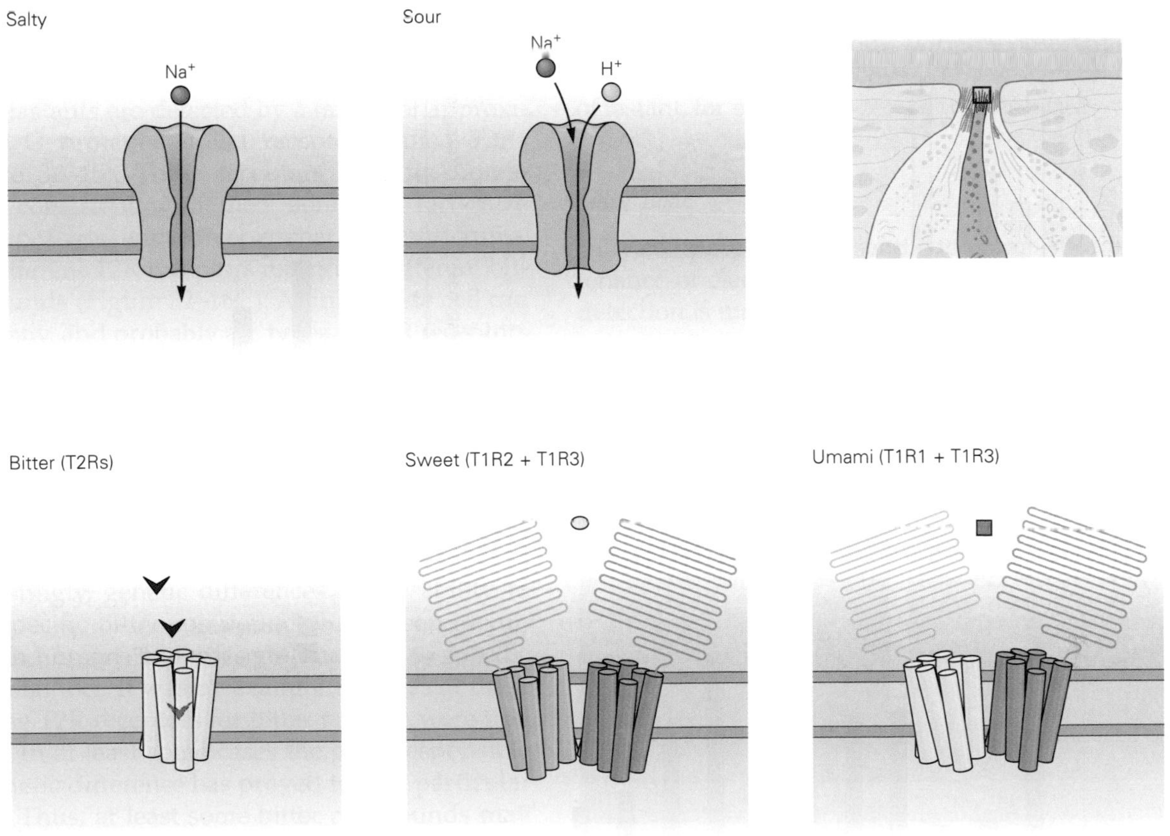

Figure 32–15 Sensory transduction in taste cells. Different taste qualities involve different detection mechanisms in the microvilli at the apical taste pore of taste cells (see Figure 32–14B). Salty and sour tastants activate ion channels, whereas tastants perceived as bitter, sweet, or umami activate G protein-coupled receptors. Bitter tastants are detected by T2R receptors, whereas sweet tastants are detected by a combination of T1R2 and T1R3 and umami tastants by a combination of T1R1 and T1R3.

aspartame, a few proteins such as monellin and thaumatin, and some D-amino acids. All of these sweet-tasting compounds are detected by a complex of two related G protein-coupled receptors, T1R2 and T1R3 (Figure 32–16).

T1R receptors have a large N-terminal extracellular domain (Figure 32–15) like the V2R receptors of vomeronasal neurons. Changing a single amino acid in this domain in mice can alter an animal's sensitivity to sweet compounds. Indeed, T1R3 was initially discovered by examining genes at the mouse saccharin preference (Sac) locus, a chromosomal region that governs sensitivity to saccharin, sucrose, and other sweet compounds.

In mice, taste cells with T1R2 receptors are found mostly in foliate and circumvallate papillae; almost invariably those cells also possess T1R3 receptors (Figure 32–17A). Gene knockout experiments in mice indicate that the T1R2/T1R3 complex mediates the detection of all sweet compounds except for high concentrations of sugars, which can also be detected by T1R3 alone.

Umami Taste

Umami is the name given to the savory taste of monosodium glutamate, an amino acid widely used as a flavor enhancer. It is believed that the pleasurable sensation associated with umami taste encourages the ingestion of proteins and is thus important to nutrition.

The taste cell receptor responsible for umami taste is a complex of two related G protein-coupled receptors: T1R1 and T1R3 (Figure 32–15). In both humans and mice the T1R1/T1R3 complex can interact with all L-amino acids (Figure 32–16B), but in humans it is preferentially activated by glutamate. Purine nucleotides, such as inosine 5′-monophosphate (IMP), are often added to monosodium glutamate to enhance its

underlying mechanisms are not yet known (see Figure 32–15). Detection of sodium chloride (NaCl), for example, might result from a diffusion of Na^+ ions down an electrochemical gradient through Na^+ channels on taste cell microvilli, or it might involve ion channels that are opened by Na^+ ions.

Sour Taste

Sour taste is associated with acidic food or drink. As with bitter compounds, animals are innately averse to sour substances, prompting the suggestion that the adaptive advantage of sour taste is avoidance of spoiled foods.

The molecular mechanisms underlying sour stimulus transduction in the taste cell have not been identified. Detection of sour tastants may involve ion channels that are opened by H^+ ions or that allow an influx of those ions that results in a depolarization of the taste cell (Figure 32–15). However, as with salty taste, the proteins responsible for sour taste transduction have not yet been defined.

Molecular-genetic studies indicate that bitter, sweet, and umami tastants are each detected by a distinct subset of taste cells. As already discussed, a combination of T1R1 and T1R3 is responsible for all umami taste, while a combination of T1R2 and T1R3 is needed for all sweet taste detection except for the detection of high concentrations of sugars, which can be mediated by T1R3 alone. T1R1 and T1R2 are expressed by separate subsets of taste cells, indicating that the detection of sweet and umami tastants is segregated.

In mice a transduction protein (PLCb2) is required for detection of bitter, sweet, and umami tastants. When this protein is expressed only in cells with bitter receptors, the cells are responsive to bitter compounds but not to sweet compounds or amino acids. This result confirms that taste cells that detect bitter compounds are distinct from those that detect sweet and umami tastants. Taste cells that detect salty and sour tastants may form two additional subsets of cells.

Studies in mice further indicate that it is the taste cells rather than the receptors that determine the animal's response to a tastant. The human bitter receptor T2R16 recognizes a bitter tastant that mice cannot detect. When this receptor was expressed in mouse taste cells that express the T1R2/T1R3 sweet complex, the human T2R ligand elicited an attractive response; when it was expressed in mouse cells that express T2R bitter receptors, the same ligand instead caused aversion. These findings suggest that innate responses of mice to sweet and bitter compounds result from specific gustatory pathways (labeled lines) that link the activation of different subsets of taste cells to different behavioral outcomes.

Sensory Neurons Carry Taste Information from the Taste Buds to the Brain

Each taste cell is innervated at its base by the peripheral branches of the axons of primary sensory neurons (Figure 32–14). Each sensory fiber branches many times, innervating several taste cells within numerous taste buds. The release of neurotransmitter from taste cells onto the sensory fibers induces action potentials in the fibers and the transmission of signals to the sensory cell body.

The cell bodies of gustatory sensory neurons lie in the geniculate, petrosal, and nodose ganglia. The peripheral branches of gustatory sensory neurons in these three ganglia travel in cranial nerves VII, IX, and X (Figure 32–13).

The central branches of axons of the gustatory sensory neurons enter the medulla, where they terminate on neurons in the gustatory area of the nucleus of the solitary tract (Figure 32–13). In most mammals neurons in this nucleus transmit signals to the parabrachial nucleus of the pons, which in turn sends gustatory information to the ventroposterior medial nucleus of the thalamus. In primates, however, these neurons transmit gustatory information directly to the taste area of the thalamus.

Taste Information Is Transmitted from the Thalamus to the Gustatory Cortex

From the thalamus taste information is transmitted to the gustatory cortex, a region of the cerebral cortex located along the border between the anterior insula and the frontal operculum (Figure 32–13). The gustatory cortex is believed to mediate the conscious perception and discrimination of taste stimuli. The taste area of the thalamus also transmits information both directly and indirectly to the hypothalamus, a structure that controls feeding behavior and autonomic responses.

Recordings made from neurons in the gustatory cortex indicate that some neurons respond to different classes of tastants, whereas others respond to only one, such as bitter or sweet. It might be that neurons responsive to more than one class of tastants encode information about blends whereas those in gustatory cortex or other areas that respond to single taste categories are involved in innate responses, such as attraction to sweet tastants or aversion to bitter tastants.

Perception of Flavor Depends on Gustatory, Olfactory, and Somatosensory Inputs

Much of what we think of as the flavor of foods derives from information provided by the olfactory system. Volatile molecules released from foods or beverages in the mouth are pumped into the back of the nasal cavity by the tongue, cheek, and throat movements that accompany chewing and swallowing. Although the olfactory epithelium of the nose clearly makes a major contribution to sensations of flavor, such sensations are localized in the mouth rather than in the nose.

The somatosensory system is thought to be involved in this localization of flavors. The coincidence between somatosensory stimulation of the tongue and the retronasal passage of odorants into the nose is assumed to cause odorants to be perceived as flavors in the mouth. Sensations of flavor also frequently have a somatosensory component that includes the texture of food as well as sensations evoked by spicy and minty foods and by carbonation.

Insect Taste Organs Are Distributed Widely on the Body

Like vertebrates, insects have specialized organs for taste. Some of the taste neurons occur in internal mouth parts. Others lie near the mouth on the proboscis, or are scattered on the leg, wing, and oviposition organs.

The gustatory receptors of *Drosophila* are membrane-spanning receptors that are very distantly related to the odorant receptors of the fly. The fly has approximately 60 gustatory receptor genes, a surprisingly large number considering it has approximately 60 olfactory receptor genes. Members of the gustatory receptor gene family are expressed in all of the different kinds of taste organs. Some occur in particular cell types, whereas others are present in many parts of the body.

As in vertebrates, in flies numerous taste receptor genes appear to be expressed in a single neuron. Sweet-sensing and bitter-sensing neurons in the labial palp mediate food acceptance or rejection, respectively. Other neurons have distinct functions. For example, neurons in the male leg express gustatory receptors that are involved in recognizing females during courtship.

An Overall View

The senses of smell and taste allow us to evaluate volatile molecules in our environment and both volatile and nonvolatile components of foodstuffs. Humans can perceive a vast number of volatile chemicals as having a distinct odor and distinguish odorants with nearly identical structures.

The basic design and functional capacities of olfactory systems are highly conserved across vertebrate species and to some extent in invertebrates. In addition to providing a means of distinguishing between appropriate and potentially harmful substances prior to ingestion, the sense of smell also plays an important role in predator-prey relationships as well as the regulation of social relationships critical to reproduction and the rearing of offspring.

Odorant detection in the nose is mediated by hundreds of different odorant receptors, each expressed by a subset of neurons. Different combinations of odorant receptors detect specific odorants and encode their identities. In the olfactory epithelium neurons with the same receptor are randomly distributed throughout one spatial zone. In the olfactory bulb the axons of neurons with the same type of receptor all converge in a few glomeruli, such that each glomerulus and its associated relay neurons are dedicated to one type of odorant receptor. Thus in the nose the code for an odorant is dispersed across an ensemble of neurons, each expressing one receptor component of the odorant's code, whereas in the olfactory bulb a specific combination of glomeruli receives input from those receptors, an arrangement that is similar in different individuals.

In the olfactory cortex neurons responsive to a given odorant are distributed broadly, but the underlying organization of sensory inputs is unknown. The olfactory cortex transmits information to a variety of other brain areas, including higher cortical areas involved in perception and the hypothalamus, which controls appetite and other basic drives.

Pheromones that elicit innate behavioral or physiological responses are detected in the nasal olfactory epithelium as well as in the vomeronasal organ, an olfactory structure present in most mammals, although not in humans. The vomeronasal organ has two different families of chemosensory receptors. The organization of inputs from these receptors resembles that seen for odorant receptors, but vomeronasal signals travel through a separate neural pathway that targets the hypothalamus but not cortical brain areas.

Humans can distinguish five taste qualities: bitter, salty, sweet, sour, and umami. Salty and sour taste detection is thought to involve specific ion channels, whereas the other three taste qualities derive from G protein-coupled receptors. Three classes of receptors are expressed by separate subsets of taste cells, but a single taste cell expresses many or all of the T2R bitter receptors. Studies in transgenic mice indicate that innate attraction to sweet tastants and aversion to bitter tastants involve hardwired neural pathways that link different subsets of taste cells on the tongue to different behavioral outcomes. The perception of blends of tastants may involve the gustatory cortex, where some neurons can respond to more than one class of tastants.

Studies of flies and worms have revealed a striking similarity to mammals in the strategies used to detect and distinguish chemicals in the external environment. In the fruit fly *Drosophila* and the nematode *C. elegans*, large families of receptors mediate the detection of environmental chemicals. Although the neural circuits that carry inputs from these receptors differ from those in mammals, they have certain features in common with mammals, suggesting that studies of these relatively simple organisms could provide insight into mechanisms underlying chemosensation in vertebrates as well as invertebrates. Because odors and tastes often elicit innate behaviors in these organisms, they also provide a means of exploring neural circuits that mediate instinctive behaviors.

Linda B. Buck
Cornelia I. Bargmann

Selected Readings

Bargmann CI. 2006. Comparative chemosensation from receptors to ecology. Nature 444:295–301.

Chandrashekar J, Hoon MA, Ryba NJ, Zuker CS. 2006. The receptors and cells for mammalian taste. Nature 444: 288–294.

Dulac C, Torello AT. 2003. Molecular detection of pheromone signals in mammals: from genes to behaviour. Nat Rev Neurosci 4:551–562.

Halpern M, Martinez-Marcos A. 2003. Structure and function of the vomeronasal system: an update. Prog Neurobiol 70:245–328.

Mori K, Takahashi YK, Igarashi KM, Yamaguchi M. 2006. Maps of odorant molecular features in the mammalian olfactory bulb. Physiol Rev 86:409–433.

Neville KR, Haberly LB. 2004. The olfactory cortex. In: GM Shepherd (ed). *The Synaptic Organization of the Brain*, pp. 415–454, New York: Oxford Univ. Press.

Vosshall LB, Stocker RF. 2007. Molecular architecture of smell and taste in *Drosophila*. Annu Rev Neurosci 30:505–533.

Yamamoto T. 2006. Neural substrates for the processing of cognitive and affective aspects of taste in the brain. Arch Histol Cytol 69:243–255.

References

Adler E, Hoon MA, Mueller KL, Chandrashekar J, Ryba NJ, Zuker CS. 2000. A novel family of mammalian taste receptors. Cell 100:693–702.

Berghard A, Buck LB. 1996. Sensory transduction in vomeronasal neurons: evidence for G alpha o, G alpha i2, and adenylyl cyclase II as major components of a pheromone signaling cascade. J Neurosci 16:909–918.

Buck L. 1996. Information coding in the vertebrate olfactory system. Annu Rev Neurosci 19:517–544.

Buck L, Axel R. 1991. A novel multigene family may encode odorant receptors: a molecular basis for odor recognition. Cell 65:175–187.

Chandrashekar J, Hoon MA, Ryba NJ, Zuker CS. 2006. The receptors and cells for mammalian taste. Nature 444: 288–294.

Chandrashekar J, Mueller KL, Hoon MA, Adler E, Feng L, Guo W, Zuker CS, Ryba NJ. 2000. T2Rs function as bitter taste receptors. Cell 100:703–711.

Dulac C, Axel R. 1995. A novel family of genes encoding putative pheromone receptors in mammals. Cell 83:195–206.

Dulac C, Torello AT. 2003. Molecular detection of pheromone signals in mammals: from genes to behaviour. Nat Rev Neurosci 4:551–562.

Glusman G, Yanai I, Rubin I, Lancet D. 2001. The complete human olfactory subgenome. Genome Res 11:685–702.

Godfrey PA, Malnic B, Buck LB. 2004. The mouse olfactory receptor gene family. Proc Natl Acad Sci U S A 101:2156–2161.

Hallem EA, Carlson JR. 2006. Coding of odors by a receptor repertoire. Cell 125:143–160.

Halpern M, Martinez-Marcos A. 2003. Structure and function of the vomeronasal system: an update. Prog Neurobiol 70:245–328.

Herrada G, Dulac C. 1997. A novel family of putative pheromone receptors in mammals with a topographically organized and sexually dimorphic distribution. Cell 90:763–773.

Hoon MA, Adler E, Lindemeier J, Battey JF, Ryba NJ, Zuker CS. 1999. Putative mammalian taste receptors: a class of taste-specific GPCRs with distinct topographic selectivity. Cell 96:541–551.

Johnson BA, Farahbod H, Leon M. 2005. Interactions between odorant functional group and hydrocarbon structure influence activity in glomerular response modules in the rat olfactory bulb. J Comp Neurol 483:205–216.

Keller A, Zhuang H, Chi Q, Vosshall LB, Matsunami H. 2007. Genetic variation in a human odorant receptor alters odour perception. Nature 449:468–472.

Kitagawa M, Kusakabe Y, Miura H, Ninomiya Y, Hino A. 2001. Molecular genetic identification of a candidate receptor gene for sweet taste. Biochem Biophys Res Commun 283:236–242.

Leinders-Zufall T, Lane AP, Puche AC, Ma W, Novotny MV, Shipley MT, Zufall F. 2000. Ultrasensitive pheromone detection by mammalian vomeronasal neurons. Nature 405:792–796.

Liberles SD, Buck LB. 2006. A second class of chemosensory receptors in the olfactory epithelium. Nature 442:645–650.

Malnic B, Godfrey PA, Buck LB. 2004. The human olfactory receptor gene family. Proc Natl Acad Sci U S A 101:7205.

Malnic B, Hirono J, Sato T, Buck LB. 1999. Combinatorial receptor codes for odors. Cell 96:713–723.

Matsunami H, Buck LB. 1997. A multigene family encoding a diverse array of putative pheromone receptors in mammals. Cell 90:775–784.

Matsunami H, Montmayeur JP, Buck LB. 2000. A family of candidate taste receptors in human and mouse. Nature 404:601–604.

Max M, Shanker YG, Huang L, Rong M, Liu Z, Campagne F, Weinstein H, Damak S, Margolskee RF. 2001. *Tas1r3,* encoding a new candidate taste receptor, is allelic to the sweet responsiveness locus *Sac.* Nat Genet 28:58–63.

Mombaerts P, Wang F, Dulac C, Chao SK, Nemes A, Mendelsohn M, Edmondson J, Axel R. 1996. Visualizing an olfactory sensory map. Cell 87:675–686.

Montmayeur JP, Liberles SD, Matsunami H, Buck LB. 2001. A candidate taste receptor gene near a sweet taste locus. Nat Neurosci 4:492–498.

Morrison EE, Costanzo RM. 1990. Morphology of the human olfactory epithelium. J Comp Neurol 297:1–13.

Mueller KL, Hoon MA, Erlenbach I, Chandrashekar J, Zuker CS, Ryba NJ. 2005. The receptors and coding logic for bitter taste. Nature 434:225–229.

Nelson G, Chandrashekar J, Hoon MA, Feng L, Zhao G, Ryba NJ, Zuker CS. 2002. An amino-acid taste receptor. Nature 416:199–202.

Nelson G, Hoon MA, Chandrashekar J, Zhang Y, Ryba NJ, Zuker CS. 2001. Mammalian sweet taste receptors. Cell 106:381–390.

Northcutt RG. 2004. Taste buds: development and evolution. Brain Behav Evol 64:198–206.

Rennaker RL, Chen CF, Ruyle AM, Sloan AM, Wilson DA. 2007. Spatial and temporal distribution of odorant-evoked activity in the piriform cortex. J Neurosci 27:1534–1542.

Ressler KJ, Sullivan SL, Buck LB. 1993. A zonal organization of odorant receptor gene expression in the olfactory epithelium. Cell 73:597–609.

Ressler KJ, Sullivan SL, Buck LB. 1994. Information coding in the olfactory system: evidence for a stereotyped and highly organized epitope map in the olfactory bulb. Cell 79:1245–1255.

Royer SM, Kinnamon JC. 1991. HVEM serial-section analysis of rabbit foliate taste buds. I. Type III cells and their synapses. J Comp Neurol 306:49–72.

Sarafi-Reinach TR, Sengupta P. 2000. The forkhead domain gene *unc*-130 generates chemosensory neuron diversity in *C. elegans*. Genes Dev 14:2472–2485.

Shepherd GM, Greer CA. 1998. The olfactory bulb. In: GM Shepherd (ed). *The Synaptic Organization of the Brain*, 4th ed., pp. 159–203 Oxford Univ. Press.

Stapleton JR, Lavine ML, Wolpert R, Nicolelis MA, Simon SA. 2006. Rapid taste responses in the gustatory cortex during licking. J Neurosci 26:4126–4138.

Sullivan SL, Adamson MC, Ressler KJ, Kozak CA, Buck LB. 1996. The chromosomal distribution of mouse odorant receptor genes. Proc Natl Acad Sci U S A 93:884–888.

Troemel ER, Kimmel BE, Bargmann CI. 1997. Reprogramming chemotaxis responses: sensory neurons define olfactory preferences in *C. elegans*. Cell 91:161–169.

Vassar R, Ngai J, Axel R. 1993. Spatial segregation of odorant receptor expression in the mammalian olfactory epithelium. Cell 74:309–328.

Vosshall L, Amrein H, Morozov PS, Rzhetsky A, Axel R. 1999. A spatial map of olfactory receptor expression in the *Drosophila* antenna. Cell 96:725–736.

Vosshall LB, Wong AM, Axel R. 2000. An olfactory sensory map in the fly brain. Cell 102:147–159.

Wang JW, Wong AM, Flores J, Vosshall LB, Axel R. 2003. Two-photon calcium imaging reveals an odor-evoked map of activity in the fly brain. Cell 112:271–282.

Wong AM, Wang JW, Axel R. 2002. Spatial representation of the glomerular map in the *Drosophila* protocerebrum. Cell 109:229–241.

Zhang X, Firestein S. 2002. The olfactory receptor gene superfamily of the mouse. Nat Neurosci 5:124–133.

Zhang Y, Hoon MA, Chandrashekar J, Mueller KL, Cook B, Wu D, Zuker CS, Ryba NJ. 2003. Coding of sweet, bitter, and umami tastes: different receptor cells sharing similar signaling pathways. Cell 112:293–301.

Zhao GQ, Zhang Y, Hoon MA, Chandrashekar J, Erlenbach I, Ryba NJ, Zuker CS. 2003. The receptors for mammalian sweet and umami taste. Cell 115:255–266.

Part VI

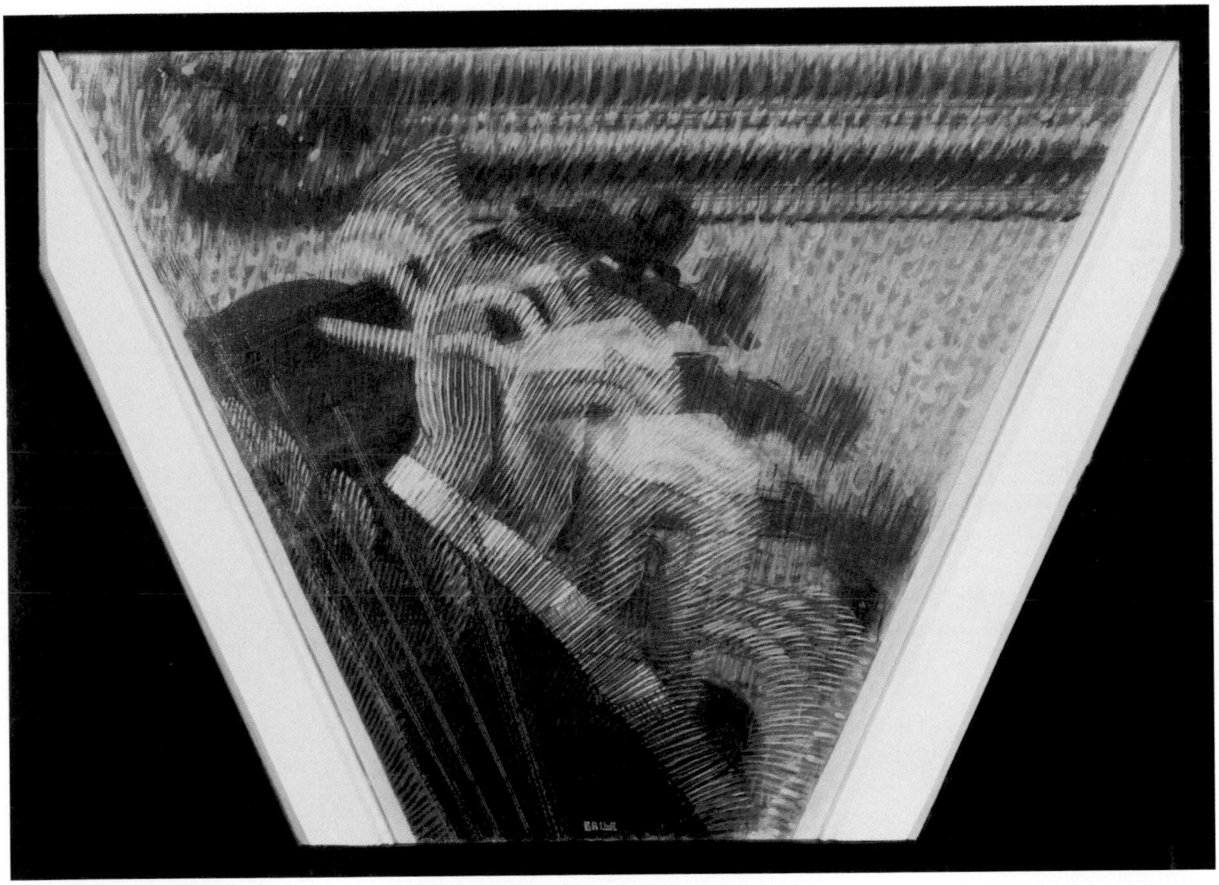

Preceding Page

The characteristic movement of a musician's hand is captured in a painting by Giacomo Balla from 1912, "The Hand of the Violinist". Balla studied violin as a boy and, like his contemporaries in the Futurist movement, was interested in depicting motion and speed. The rhythmic brushstrokes evoke the energy of the performer and the vibrations of the music. (Reproduced, with permission, from the Copyright 2011 Artists Rights Society (ARS), New York/SIAE, Rome; and the Bridgeman Art Library International, NY.)

VI Movement

THE CAPACITY FOR MOVEMENT, as many dictionaries remind us, is a defining feature of animal life. As Sherrington, who pioneered the study of the motor system pointed out, "to move things is all that mankind can do, for such the sole executant is muscle, whether in whispering a syllable or in felling a forest."*

The immense repertoire of motions that humans are capable of stems from the activity of some 640 skeletal muscles—all under the control of the central nervous system. After processing sensory information about the body and its surroundings, the motor centers of the brain and spinal cord issue neural commands that effect coordinated, purposeful movements.

The task of the motor systems is the reverse of the task of the sensory systems. Sensory processing generates an internal representation in the brain of the outside world or of the state of the body. Motor processing begins with an internal representation: the desired purpose of movement. Critically, however, this internal representation needs to be continuously updated by internal (efference copy) and external sensory information to maintain accuracy as the movement unfolds.

Just as psychophysical analysis of sensory processing tells us about the capabilities and limitations of the sensory systems, psychophysical analyses of motor performance reveal regularities and invariances in the control rules used by the motor system.

Because many of the motor acts of daily life are unconscious, we are often unaware of their complexity. Simply standing upright, for example, requires continual adjustments of numerous postural muscles in response to the vestibular signals evoked by miniscule swaying. Walking, running, and other forms of locomotion involve the combined action of central pattern generators, gated sensory information, and descending commands, which together generate the complex patterns of alternating excitation and inhibition to the appropriate sets of muscles. Many actions, such as serving a tennis ball or executing an arpeggio on a piano, occur far too quickly to be shaped by sensory feedback. Instead, centers, such as the cerebellum, make use of predictive models that simulate the consequences of the outgoing commands and allow very short latency corrections. Motor learning provides one of the most fruitful subjects for studies of neural plasticity.

Motor systems are organized in a functional hierarchy, with each level concerned with a different decision. The highest and most abstract level,

*Sherrington CS. 1979. 1924 Linacre lecture. In: JC Eccles, WC Gibson (eds). *Sherrington: His Life and Thought*, p. 59. New York: Springer-Verlag.

likely requiring the prefrontal cortex, deals with the purpose of a movement. The next level, which is concerned with the formation of a motor plan, involves interactions between the posterior parietal and premotor areas of the cerebral cortex. The premotor cortex specifies the spatial characteristics of a movement based on sensory information from the posterior parietal cortex about the environment and about the position of the body in space. The lowest level of the hierarchy coordinates the spatiotemporal details of the muscle contractions needed to execute the planned movement. This coordination is executed by the primary motor cortex, brain stem, and spinal cord. This serial view has heuristic value, but evidence suggests that many of these processes can occur in parallel.

Some functions of the motor systems and their disturbance by disease have now been described at the level of the biochemistry of specific transmitter systems. In fact, the discovery that neurons in the basal ganglia of parkinsonian patients are deficient in dopamine was the first important clue that neurological disorders can result from altered chemical transmission. Imaging techniques can provide information as to how local transmitter abnormalities can lead to widespread changes in the networks involved in the selection and control of movements.

Understanding the functional properties of the motor system is not only fundamental in its own right, but it is of further importance in helping us to understand disorders of this system and explore the possibilities for recovery. As would be expected for such a complex apparatus, the motor system is subject to various malfunctions. Lesions at different levels in the motor hierarchy produce distinctive symptoms, including the movement-slowing characteristic of disorders of the basal ganglia, such as parkinsonism, the incoordination seen with cerebellar disease, and the spasticity and weakness typical of spinal damage. For this reason, the neurological examination of a patient inevitably includes tests of reflexes, gait, and dexterity, all of which provide information about the status of the nervous system. In addition to pharmacological therapies, the treatment of neurological disease has recently been augmented by two new approaches. First, focal stimulation of the basal ganglia has been discovered to restore motility to certain patients with Parkinson disease; such deep-brain stimulation is also being tested in the context of other neurological conditions. And second, the motor systems have become a target for the application of neural prosthetics; neural signals are decoded and used to drive mechanical devices that aid patients with paralysis caused by spinal cord injury and stroke.

Part VI

33

The Organization and Planning of Movement

IN THE PRECEDING PART OF THIS BOOK we considered how the brain constructs internal representations of the world around us. These internal representations have no intrinsic value and are behaviorally meaningful only when used to guide movement, whether foraging for food or attracting a waiter's attention. Thus the ultimate function of the sensory representations is to shape the actions of the motor systems. Sensory representations are the framework in which the motor systems plan, coordinate, and execute the motor programs responsible for purposeful movement.

In this part of the book we describe the principles of motor control that allow the brain and spinal cord to maintain balance and posture; to move our body, limbs, and eyes; and to communicate through speech and gesture.

Although movements are often classified according to function—eye movements, prehension (reach and grasp), posture, locomotion, breathing, and speech—many of these functions are subserved by overlapping groups of muscles. In addition, the same groups of muscles can be controlled voluntarily, rhythmically, or reflexively. For example, the muscles that control respiration can be used to take a deep breath voluntarily before diving under water, to breathe automatically and rhythmically in a regular cycle of inspiration and expiration, or to act reflexively in response to a noxious stimulus in the throat, producing a cough.

Voluntary movements are those that are under conscious control by the brain. Rhythmic movements can also be controlled voluntarily, but many such movements differ from voluntary movements in that their timing and spatial organization is to a large extent controlled autonomously by spinal or brain stem circuitry. Reflexes are stereotyped responses to specific stimuli that are generated by simple neural circuits in the spinal cord or brain stem. Although reflexes are highly adaptable to changes in behavioral goals, mainly because several different circuits exist to connect sensory and motor neurons, they cannot be directly controlled voluntarily.

In this chapter we focus on voluntary movements, using arm and hand movements to illustrate principles of sensorimotor control. Reflexes and rhythmic movements are discussed in detail in Chapters 35 and 36.

Conscious processes are not necessary for moment-to-moment control of movement. Although we may be aware of the intent to perform a task or of planning certain sequences of actions and at times are aware of deciding to move at a particular moment, movements generally seem to occur automatically. We carry out the most complicated movements without a thought to the actual joint motions or muscle contractions required. The tennis player does not consciously decide which muscles to use to return a serve with a backhand or which body parts must be moved to intercept the ball. In fact, thinking about each body movement before it takes place can disrupt the player's performance.

In this chapter we review the principles that govern the neural control of movement using concepts derived from behavioral studies and from computational models that are used both to understand the brain and to control the movements of robots. First, we look at how the brain transforms sensory inputs into motor outputs through a cascade of sensorimotor transformations. Second, we examine how sensory feedback can be used to correct errors that arise during movement. Finally, we see how motor learning allows us to improve our performance; to adapt to new mechanical conditions, as when using a tool; or to adapt to novel correspondences between sensory and motor events, for example when learning to use a computer mouse to control a cursor.

Motor Commands Arise Through Sensorimotor Transformations

Motor outputs are neural commands that act on the muscles, causing them to contract and generate movement. These outputs are derived from sensory inputs in circuits that represent *sensorimotor transformations.* Sensory inputs include extrinsic information about the state of world as well as intrinsic information about our body. Extrinsic information, for example the spatial location of a target, can be provided by auditory and visual inputs. Intrinsic information includes both kinematic and kinetic information about our body.

Kinematic information includes the position, velocity, and acceleration of the hand, joint angles, and lengths of muscles without reference to the forces that cause them. *Kinetic information* is concerned with the forces generated or experienced by our body. These different forms of intrinsic information are provided by different sensors. For example, information about muscle lengths and their rate of change is provided mainly by muscle spindles, whereas Golgi tendon organs in the muscles and mechanoreceptors in our skin provide information about the force we are exerting.

Simple reflexes, such as a tendon-jerk reflex, involve a simple sensorimotor transformation: Sensory inputs cause motor output directly without the intervention of higher brain centers. However, voluntary movement requires multistage sensorimotor transformations. The involvement of multiple processing centers actually simplifies processing: Higher levels plan more general goals, whereas lower levels concern themselves with how these goals can be implemented.

Such a hierarchy accounts for the fact that a specific motor action, such as writing, can be performed in different ways with more or less the same result. Handwriting is structurally similar regardless of the size of the letters or the limb or body segment used to produce it (Figure 33–1). This phenomenon, termed *motor equivalence,* suggests that purposeful movements are represented in the brain abstractly rather than as sets of specific joint motions or muscle contractions. Such abstract representations of movement, able to drive different effectors, provide a degree of flexibility of action not practical with preset motor programs.

How do sensorimotor transformations generate movement to a desired location? For a person to reach toward an object, sensory information about the target's location must be converted into a sequence of muscle actions leading to joint rotations that will bring the hand to the target.

First, the target is localized in space relative to some part of the body such as the head or arm (*egocentric space*). Several sources of information are combined in this process. For example, the location of the target relative to the head is computed from the location of the target on each retina together with the direction of gaze of the eyes (Figure 33–2A). A person also needs to know the initial location of his hand or the tip of the tool that he wishes to place on the target (the end-effector or *endpoint*). The initial location of the endpoint can be estimated by combining visual inputs, proprioceptive signals, and tactile sensations, each of which can provide location information. Once the current configuration of the arm and location of the target are calculated, a movement can be planned. A plan typically has to specify both a particular *path,* the successive spatial positions of the endpoint, and also the

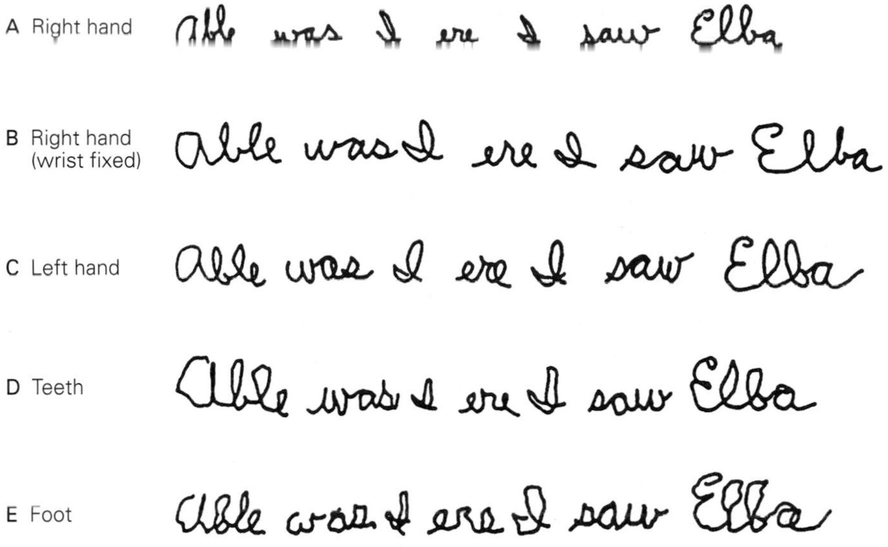

Figure 33–1 Motor equivalence. The ability of different motor systems to achieve the same behavior is called motor equivalence. For example, writing can be performed using different parts of the body. The examples here were written by the same person using the right (dominant) hand (**A**), the right hand with the wrist immobilized (**B**), the left hand (**C**), the pen gripped between the teeth (**D**), and the pen attached to the foot (**E**). (Reproduced, with permission, from Raibert 1977.)

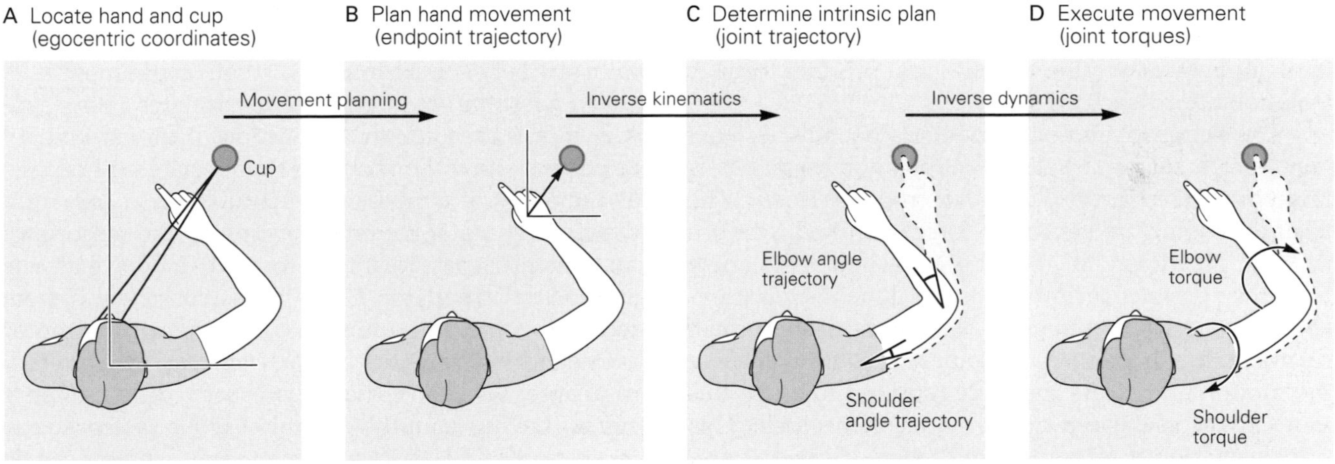

Figure 33–2 Sensorimotor transformations used to generate a particular movement. The task of generating a goal-directed movement is often broken down into a set of sequential stages, the details of which are still being elucidated. The figure shows one possible set of stages to generate a reaching movement, and the arrows indicate the processes required to move between the stages.

A. Spatial orientation. To reach for an object, the object and hand are first located visually in a coordinate system relative to the head (egocentric coordinates).

B. Movement planning. The direction and distance the hand must move to reach the object (the endpoint trajectory) are determined based on visual and proprioceptive information about the current locations of the arm and object.

C. Inverse kinematic transformation. The joint trajectories that will achieve the hand path are determined. The transformation from a desired hand movement to the joint trajectory depends on the kinematic properties of the arm, such as the lengths of the arm's segments.

D. Inverse dynamic transformation. The joint torques or muscle activities that are necessary to achieve the desired joint trajectories are determined. The joint torques required to achieve a desired change in joint angles depend on the dynamic properties of the arm such as the mass of the segments.

trajectory, the time course over which these positions will be covered, and thus the accelerations and speeds of the movement (Figure 33–2B).

In a hierarchical model of planning the goal can be expressed in kinematic terms, such as the desired positions and velocities of the hand, or in kinetic terms, such as the force exerted by the hand. Movement can be planned as an *endpoint trajectory,* a desired change in the configuration of the limb expressed in coordinates intrinsic to the limb. Such a coordinate system could determine the change in joint angles or be based on a desired change in proprioceptive feedback. For example, the endpoint trajectory could be defined kinematically as the distance and direction the hand has to move to reach the target, as well as the speed along the path to the target.

Transformations can be expressed as changes in kinematic variables, such as the position of the hand and the joint angles that place the hand at that position. The calculation of an endpoint from a set of joint angles is termed *forward kinematic transformation,* whereas calculation of a set of joint angles that can reach an endpoint is termed *inverse kinematic transformation* (Figure 33–2C). This transformation must take into account the geometric parameters of the arm, such as the lengths of the upper arm and forearm (recall that kinematics considers motion without reference to the forces that cause it). The motor system controls joint angle by activating muscles that produce torques (rotational forces) at the joint.

The action of motor commands on muscles that results in a set of angular positions and velocities is known as the *forward dynamic transformation.* The term "dynamic" refers to the forces required to cause motion. However, to generate a desired joint angle trajectory the system must convert kinematic parameters into motor commands. That is, the system must calculate the torques at each joint necessary to achieve the motion and relate the force required to cause this motion to the desired acceleration of the limb. This transformation is known as the *inverse dynamic transformation* (Figure 33–2D). In general, to cause any acceleration the forces applied must exceed any resistive forces arising from the viscosity or stiffness of the limb, from gravity, and from external loads. The force not required to overcome the total resistive force will cause an angular acceleration, with the acceleration being dependant on the limb's inertia; the lower the inertia, the higher the acceleration.

Thus through a series of sensorimotor transformations, sensory input is finally converted into muscle contractions that generate movement. Although we have described one possible series of transformations that can achieve a movement, the actual computations used by the central nervous system are still under active investigation.

The Central Nervous System Forms Internal Models of Sensorimotor Transformations

We know from cellular studies that the central nervous system contains internal representations ("neural maps") of the various sensory receptor arrays and the musculature. Experimental and modeling studies strongly suggest that the central nervous system also maintains internal representations that relate motor commands to the sensory signals expected as a result of movement.

Given the fixed lengths of our limb segments, there is a mathematical relationship between the joint angles of the arm and the location of the hand in space. A neural representation of this relationship allows the central nervous system to estimate hand position if it knows the joint angles and segment lengths. The neural circuits that compute such sensorimotor transformations are examples of *internal models* (Box 33–1). Such neural representations may not exactly match true relationships because of structural differences (the models only approximate the true relationship between joint angles and hand position) or errors in the model's parameters (incorrect estimates of segment lengths).

An internal model that represents the causal relationship between actions and their consequences is called a *forward model* because it estimates future sensory inputs based on motor outputs. A forward model anticipates how the motor system's state will change as the result of a motor command. Thus, a copy of a descending motor command acting on the sensorimotor system is passed into a forward model that acts as a neural simulator of the musculoskeletal system moving in the environment. This copy of the motor command is known as an *efference copy* (or corollary discharge) to signify that it is a copy of the efferent signal flowing from the central nervous system to the muscles. We will see later how such simulations can be learned and used in sensorimotor control.

An internal model that calculates motor outputs from sensory inputs is known as an *inverse model.* Such a model can determine what motor commands are needed to produce the particular movements necessary to achieve a desired sensory consequence.

Forward and inverse models can be better understood if we place the two in series. If the structure and parameter values of each model are correct, the output of the forward model (the predicted behavior) will be the same as the input to the inverse model (the desired behavior) (Figure 33–3).

Box 33–1 Internal Models

The utility of numerical models in the physical sciences has a long history. Numerical models are abstract quantitative representations of complex physical systems. Some start with equations and parameters that represent initial conditions and run *forward*, either in time or space, to generate physical variables at some future state. For example, we can construct a model of the weather that predicts wind speed and temperature two weeks from now. In general, the algorithms and parameters of the model should lead to one correct answer.

Other models start with a state, a set of physical variables with specific values, and operate in the *inverse* direction to determine what parameters in the system account for that state. When we fit a straight line to a set of data points, we are constructing an inverse model that estimates slope and intercept based on the equations of the system being linear. An inverse model may thus inform us how to set the parameters of the system to obtain desired outcomes.

Over the last 50 years the idea that the nervous system has similar predictive models of the physical world to guide behavior has become a major issue in neuroscience. The idea originated in Kenneth Craik's notion of *internal models* for cognitive function. In his 1943 book, *The Nature of Explanation*, Craik was perhaps the first to suggest that organisms make use of internal representations of the external world:

"If the organism carries a 'small scale model' of external reality and of its own possible actions within its head, it is able to try out various alternatives, conclude which is the best of them, react to future situations before they arise, utilize the knowledge of past events in dealing with the present and future, and in every way to react in a much fuller, safer, and more competent manner to the emergencies which face it."

In this view an internal model allows an organism to contemplate the consequences of current actions without actually committing itself to those actions.

Considering the human body from the viewpoint of sensorimotor control, we should ask two fundamental questions. First, how can we generate actions on the system so as to control its behavior? Second, how can we predict the consequences of our actions?

The central nervous system must exercise both control and prediction to achieve skilled motor performance. Prediction and control are two sides of the same coin, and the two processes map exactly onto forward and inverse models. Prediction turns motor commands into expected sensory consequences, whereas control turns desired sensory consequences into motor commands.

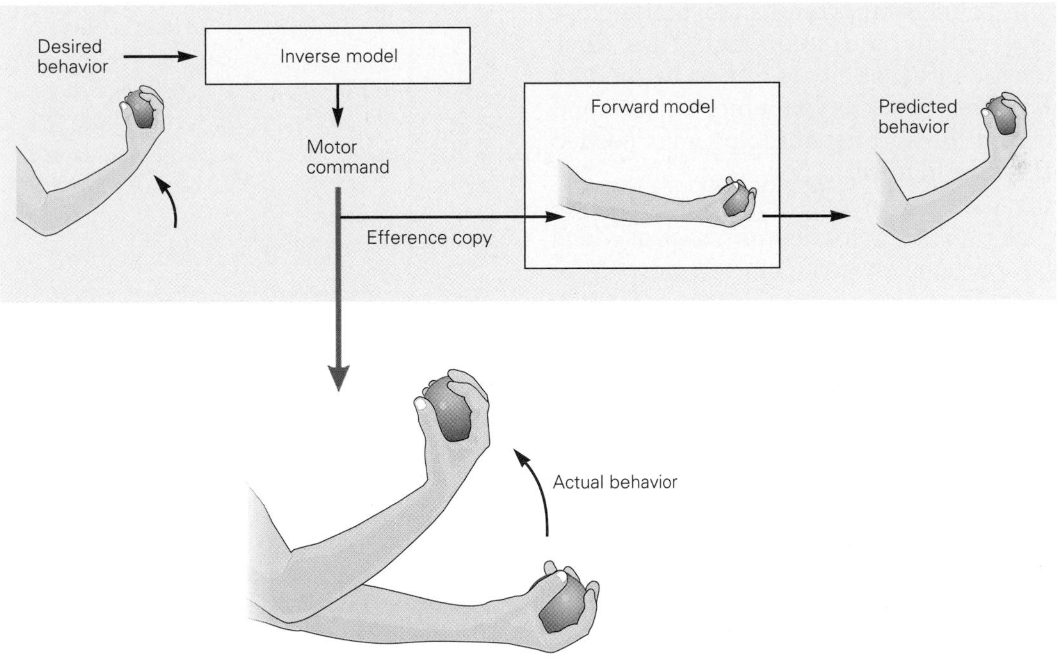

Figure 33–3 Internal models represent relationships of the body and external world. The inverse model determines the motor commands that will produce a behavioral goal, such as raising the arm while holding a ball. A descending motor command acts on the musculoskeletal system to produce the movement. A copy of the motor command is passed to a forward model that simulates the interaction of the motor system and the world and can therefore predict behaviors. If both forward and inverse models are accurate, the output of the forward model (the predicted behavior) will be the same as the input to the inverse model (the desired behavior).

Movement Inaccuracies Arise from Errors and Variability in the Transformations

Motor control is often imprecise. Indeed, society celebrates those who can throw a dart into a small area of a board or hit a small white ball into a hole with a club. However, even the movements of the most skilled players show some degree of variability. In the 1890s the psychologist Robert Woodworth showed that fast movements are less accurate than slow ones. People slow their movements when accuracy is demanded. Inaccuracy can arise either from variability in the sensory inputs and motor outputs or from errors in the internal representations of this information.

An important component of sensorimotor variability is the intrinsic variability of our sensors and motor neurons because of fluctuations in their membrane potential. Because of these fluctuations, known as neural noise, the level of input signals required to trigger postsynaptic action potentials also varies. On the input side, neural noise limits the *accuracy* of estimates of the location of a target or limb (how near an estimate is to the true value) as well as their *precision* (how accurate the estimate is when repeated). On the output side, neural noise limits the accuracy and precision with which we contract our muscles. Moreover, the amount of noise in motor commands tends to increase with larger motor commands, limiting our ability to move rapidly and accurately at the same time. This increase in variability is caused by random variation in both the excitability of motor neurons and the recruitment of the additional motor units needed to produce increases in force.

Incremental increases in force are produced by progressively smaller sets of motor neurons, each of which produces disproportionately greater increments of force (see Chapter 34). Therefore, as force increases, fluctuations in the number of motor neurons lead to greater fluctuations in force. The consequences of this can be observed experimentally by asking subjects to generate a constant force or a force pulse of fixed amplitude. Not only are subjects unable to maintain constant force, but the variability of force also increases with the level of the force. Over a large range this increase in variability is captured by a constant coefficient of variation (the standard deviation divided by the mean force). This dependence of variability on force corresponds to the increase in the variability of pointing movements with the average speed of movement. The decrease in accuracy of movement with increasing speed is known as the *speed-accuracy trade-off* (Figure 33–4).

Errors can also arise from inaccuracy in the internal models that compute sensorimotor transformations. Neural representations of the musculature cannot easily capture the complex biomechanical properties of the musculoskeletal system, and this in turn significantly complicates the ability of the brain to compute accurate sensorimotor transformations. Indeed, the dependence of muscle force on the motor command is itself highly complex. A model prescribing motion in a system with just a single joint must not only estimate the muscle

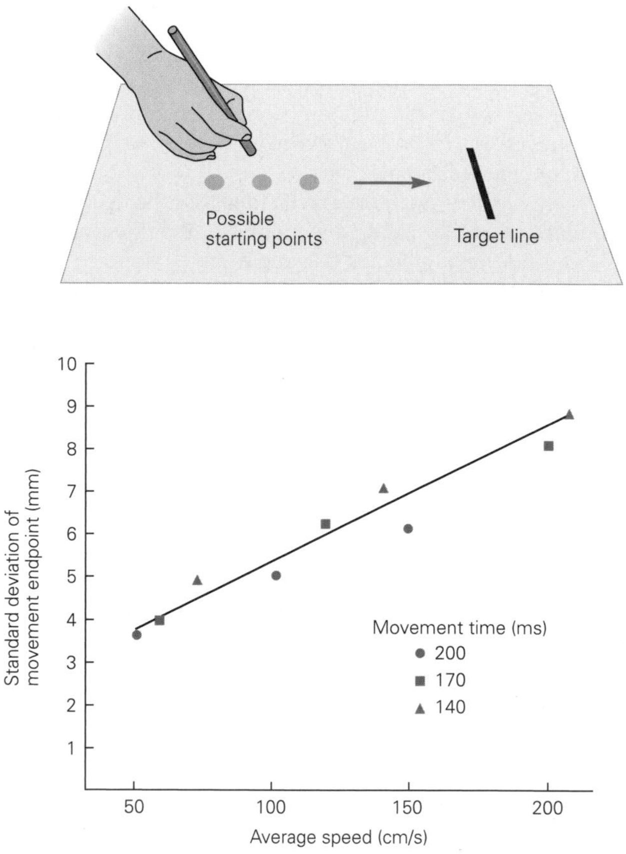

Figure 33–4 Accuracy of movement varies in direct proportion to its speed. Subjects held a stylus and were required to try and hit a target line lying perpendicular to the direction in which they moved. Each subject started from three different initial positions and was required to complete the movement within three different times (140, 170, or 200 ms). A successful trial was one in which the subject completed the movement within 10% of the required time. Only successful trials were used for analysis. Subjects were informed if their movements were more than 10% different from the required duration. The plot shows the variability in the motion of the subjects' arm movements as the standard deviation of the extent of movement versus average speed (for each of three movement starting points and three movement times, giving nine data points). The variability in movement increases in proportion to the speed and therefore to the force producing the movement. (Reproduced, with permission, from Schmidt et al. 1979.)

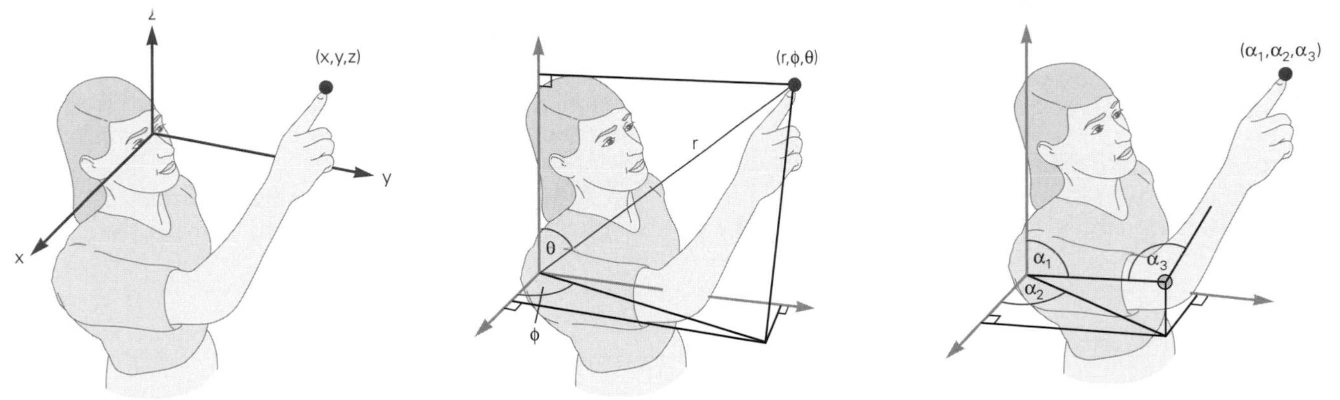

Figure 33–5 The location of the finger in space can be specified in different egocentric coordinate systems.

A. Cartesian coordinates centered on the eyes.

B. Spherical polar coordinates centered on the shoulder (distance *r*, azimuth ϕ, and elevation θ).

C. An intrinsic coordinate system based on shoulder angles (α_1 and α_2), which relate the orientation of the upper arm to the Cartesian axes, and elbow angle (α_3), which specifies the angle between the upper and lower arm.

force (or torque) but also take into account inertia (the mass resisting acceleration), viscosity (resistive forces proportional to velocity), stiffness (elastic forces proportional to displacement) produced by the muscles and tendons opposing movement, and gravity.

The dynamic relationship between segments of limbs further complicates sensorimotor transformations. The motion of each segment produces torques, and potentially motions, at all other segments through mechanical interactions. For example, flexion of the upper arm through shoulder rotation can lead to either extension or flexion of the elbow depending on the initial elbow angle. In general, because of the interactions between linked segments, the torques needed to produce a specific change in angle at a particular joint depend not only on the muscles acting directly at this joint but also on the configurations and the motions of all other joints, and especially their acceleration. The brain develops an internal model of these complex mechanical interactions through learning early in childhood. We will see later that this learning is updated throughout life and depends critically on proprioception, which provides the brain with information about changes in muscle length and joint angles.

Different Coordinate Systems May Be Employed at Different Stages of Sensorimotor Transformations

Different coordinate systems are used in sensorimotor transformations and are encoded in several brain regions. Coordinate systems are either extrinsic or intrinsic to the body. Extrinsic coordinate systems relate objects in the outside world to other objects (allocentric coordinates) or to our body (egocentric coordinates) using exteroceptive information, usually visual or auditory (Figures 33–5A and B). Intrinsic coordinate systems, such as the set of muscle lengths or set of joint angles (Figure 33–5C), are based on information provided primarily by proprioceptive systems.

Elucidating the coordinate systems used in sensorimotor transformations is a major endeavor in neuroscience. We will see in later chapters that this issue can be fruitfully studied by examining how the firing patterns of neurons in different parts of the brain encode task features or movement parameters. Such studies aim to determine the variables (such as position or velocity) or type of coordinate system (such as allocentric or egocentric) that the neurons encode.

Behavioral studies also have used a variety of methods to examine the coordinate systems used in directing movement. One way has been to examine the details of the errors made during movement in different tasks. When subjects are asked to reach rapidly and repeatedly to a target, the error in the movements can be measured in different ways. If we average the final location of the hand across many trials, we may find a constant error or bias in the movement. We can examine the distribution of the final locations of the hand about this average position and infer from the patterns of constant and variable error the coordinate system used in the movement (Box 33–2).

Stereotypical Patterns Are Employed in Many Movements

Given a task, motor plans are underconstrained. For example, the hand can move to a target along an infinite number of possible paths, and for each path there is an infinite number of trajectories. Having specified the path and velocity, each point along the path could be reached by any number of combinations of arm joint angles and, owing to the overlapping actions of muscles and the ability to co-contract, each arm configuration could be achieved by many different combinations of muscles.

Although we have described different types of sensorimotor transformations, in general the inverse

Box 33–2 The Brain's Choice of Spatial Coordinate System Depends on the Task

When subjects are shown a visual target and asked to reach for it repeatedly, the pattern of errors they make varies with the circumstance of the task. By examining these errors it is possible to assess which coordinate system is used to represent the target position under different conditions.

For example, when subjects are required to move their hands on a horizontal surface and can estimate the starting position of their hands before movement, the pattern of errors indicates planning in "hand-centered" coordinates. The distributions of the endpoints of the movements demonstrate that, under the conditions of the task, errors in distance and direction are independent of each other (Figure 33–6) and thus that errors in the extent of a movement cannot be predicted from errors in direction. The independence of the two types of errors suggests that for this type of task subjects estimate distance and direction relative to a specific starting location (that is a movement vector) in Cartesian coordinates.

Conversely, when subjects make large three-dimensional movements to remembered visual targets in the dark, a different pattern of error is observed.

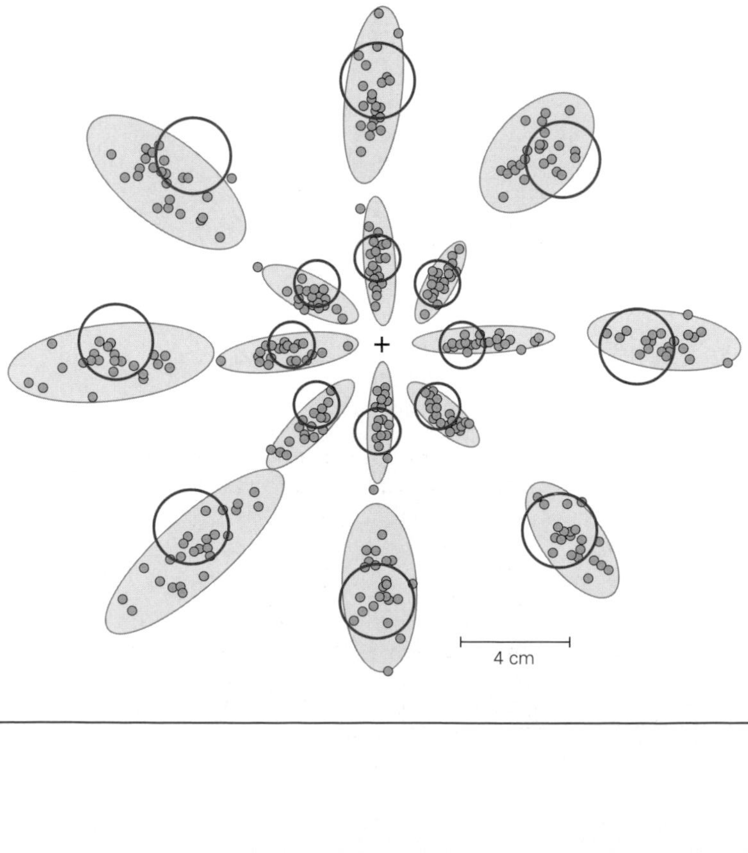

Figure 33–6 Errors in distance and direction of movement are independent of each other. Distribution of endpoints for reaching movements to 16 targets (eight directions and two distances) by one subject. Targets (**red circles**) were presented 24 times in random order, and each time the subject was asked to place a finger on the target. All movements begin from a central starting position (designated +). Endpoints for individual movements are represented by **blue dots**. The endpoints for the reaches to each target are fitted with an ellipse, demonstrating that errors in distance and direction are independent of each other. (Adapted, with permission, from Gordon, Ghilardi, and Ghez 1994.)

transformations cannot be uniquely specified. For example, the inverse kinematic transformation that transforms hand positions into joint angles can have many outputs based on the same input. This is because many different combinations of joint angles will put the hand in the same place. The ability of the motor systems to achieve a task in many different ways is called *redundancy.* If one way of achieving a task is not practical, there is usually an alternative.

Some of the earliest studies of movement examined how the brain determines the duration of a movement. Fitts's law describes the relationship between the amplitude, accuracy, and duration of a movement. This law relates the duration of a movement to the accuracy required of the task, as determined by the target width and amplitude of the movement, and applies to a variety of tasks such as reaching, placing pegs in holes, and picking up objects (Figure 33–8).

When the target and finger locations at the end of the reach are plotted against each other in terms of spherical coordinates centered on the shoulder, angular errors (elevation and azimuth) are small, whereas errors in the radial extent of the movement are significant (Figure 33–7). Moreover, the two types of errors are not correlated. However, if the target and finger locations are plotted in terms of spherical coordinates centered on the head, the errors are correlated.

The fact that the spherical coordinate system centered on the shoulder produces uncorrelated errors suggests that at some stage in the sensorimotor transformation the target is represented in shoulder-centered coordinates. Recent work suggests that this pattern of errors reflects planning for a final hand position rather than a particular hand trajectory.

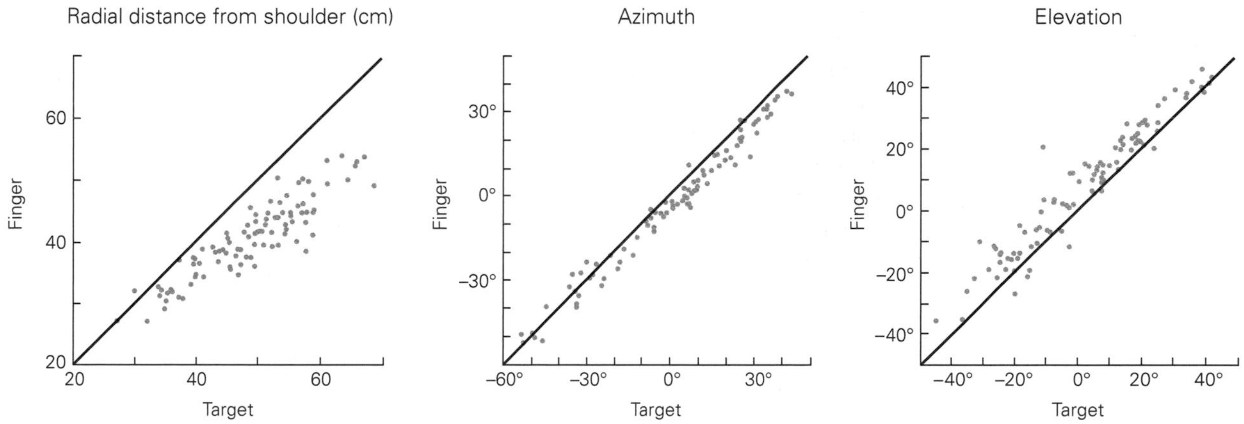

Figure 33–7 Distance errors are greater than direction errors for movements in the dark. A subject was asked to place a finger on the remembered location of a target in the dark. Final finger position and target location are plotted in spherical coordinates centered on the shoulder (see Figure 33–5B). The straight line represents perfect performance and the dots individual reaching movements. Radial distance errors and angular errors (azimuth and elevation) are plotted separately. (Adapted, with permission, from Soechting and Flanders 1989.)

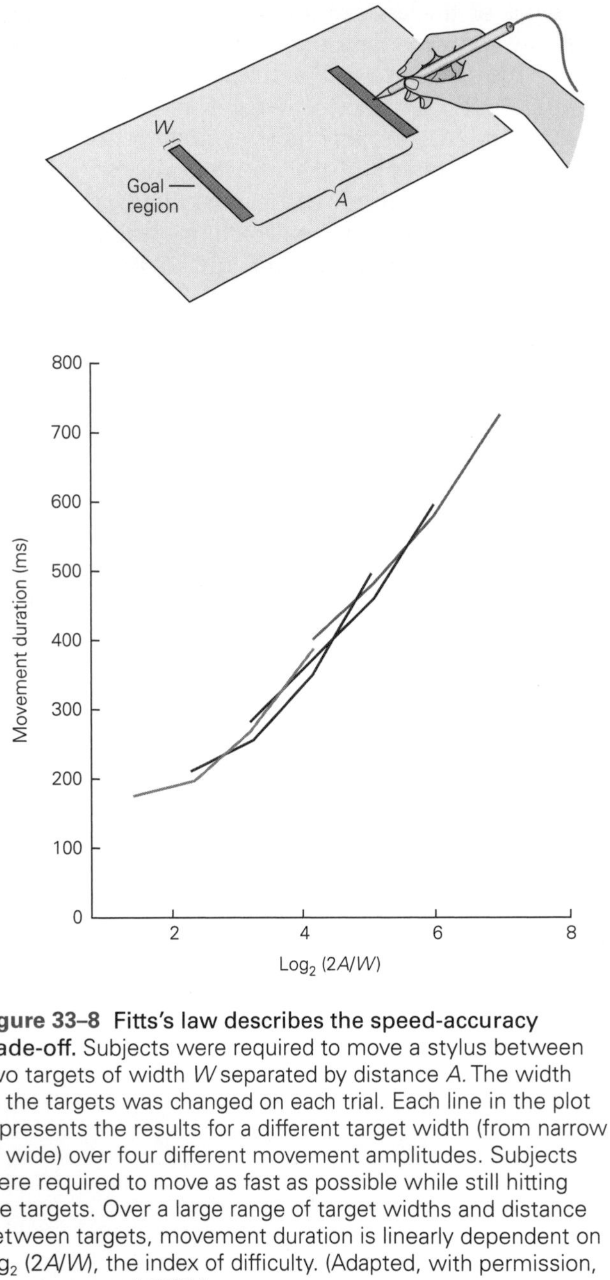

Figure 33–8 Fitts's law describes the speed-accuracy trade-off. Subjects were required to move a stylus between two targets of width *W* separated by distance *A*. The width of the targets was changed on each trial. Each line in the plot represents the results for a different target width (from narrow to wide) over four different movement amplitudes. Subjects were required to move as fast as possible while still hitting the targets. Over a large range of target widths and distance between targets, movement duration is linearly dependent on $\log_2(2A/W)$, the index of difficulty. (Adapted, with permission, from Jeannerod 1988.)

Despite variations in movement direction, speed, and location, several aspects of reaching movements are stereotypical or invariant. First, the hand tends to follow roughly a straight path (Figure 33–9A), although significant curvature is observed for certain movements, particularly vertical movements and movements near the boundaries of the reachable space. The tendency to make straight-line movements characterizes a large class of movements and is surprising given that the muscles act to rotate joints. Second, a plot of hand speed over time is typically smooth, unimodal, and roughly symmetric (bell-shaped) (Figure 33–9B). This is not the case when movement accuracy requirements are high or corrections to the movement are made.

In contrast, the motions of the joints in series (such as the shoulder, elbow, and wrist) are complicated and vary greatly with different initial and final positions. Because rotation at a single joint would produce an arc at the hand, both elbow and shoulder joints must be rotated concurrently to produce a straight path. In some directions the elbow moves more than the shoulder; in others, the reverse occurs. When the hand is moved from one side of the body to the other (see Figure 33–9A, movement from T2 to T5) one or both joints may have to reverse direction in midcourse. The fact that hand trajectories are more invariant than joint trajectories suggests that the motor system typically controls the hand by adjusting joint rotations and torques to achieve desired hand trajectories.

Invariances can also be seen in more complex movements. The nervous system puts together complex actions from elemental movements that have highly stereotyped spatial and temporal characteristics. For example, the seemingly continuous motion of drawing a figure eight actually consists of several discrete movements that are roughly constant in duration, regardless of their size. Moreover, there is a relationship between the curvature of each elemental movement and speed: Subjects tend to slow the hand as the curvature of the path increases. Empirical studies have shown that for many tasks a power law relation, the two-thirds power law, governs the relationship between hand speed and path curvature (Figure 33–10).

The simple spatiotemporal elements of a complex movement are called movement primitives or *movement schemas*. Like the simple lines, ovals, or squares in computer graphics programs, movement schemas can be scaled in size or time. The neural representations of complex actions, such as prehension, writing, typing, or drawing, are thought to be stored sets of these simple spatiotemporal elements.

Recent computational studies of a variety of tasks suggest that a repertory of movement schemas is the result of a process in which all possible ways of moving are ranked and the best is selected. This idea implies that either through evolution or motor learning our movements improve progressively until some limit is reached.

To quantify how good or bad a movement the brain assigns a cost to each possible movement, and the movement with the lowest cost is executed. The cost is specified as some function of the movement and task, and the challenge to researchers has been to determine, from observed movement patterns and perturbation studies, the form of this function.

The cost may be kinematic; for example, lack of smoothness in a movement can be corrected by minimizing the rate of change of hand acceleration summed over a movement. Alternatively, the cost may be dynamic. For example, because the variability in the motor output is proportional to the magnitude of the motor command, repetition of the same sequence of intended motor commands many times will lead to a distribution of actual movements. Modifying the sequence of motor commands can control aspects of this distribution, such as the spread of positions of the hand at the end of the movement. In a simple aiming movement the cost is the final error, as measured by the variability about the target. A model that minimizes this cost would accurately predict the trajectories of both eye and arm movements.

Motor Signals Are Subject to Feedforward and Feedback Control

So far we have focused on how sensory inputs are used to plan a movement and why the resulting movements

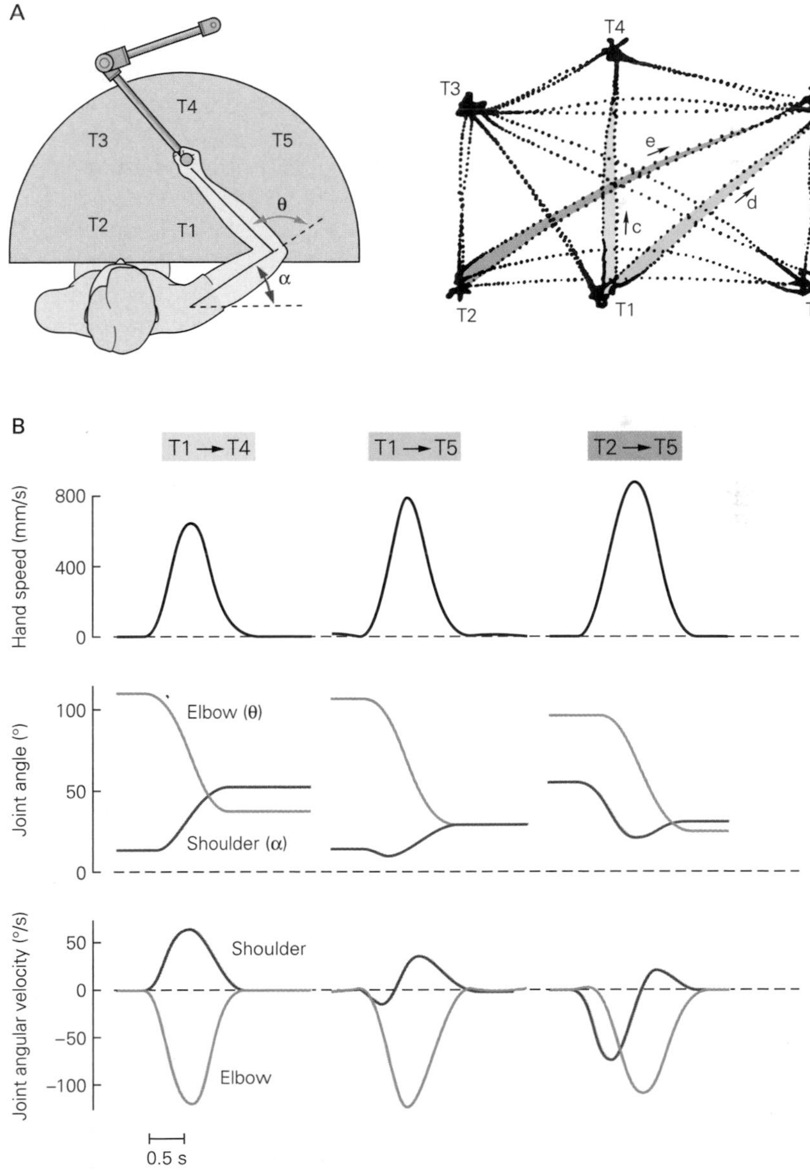

Figure 33–9 Hand path and velocity have stereotypical features. (Adapted, with permission, from Morasso 1981.)

A. The subject sits in front of a semicircular plate and grasps the handle of a two-jointed apparatus that moves in one plane and records hand position. The subject is instructed to move the hand between various targets (T1–T6). The record on the right shows the paths traced by one subject.

B. Kinematic data for three hand paths shown in part A (**c**, **d**, and **e**). All paths are roughly straight, and all hand speed profiles have the same shape and scale in proportion to the distance covered. In contrast, the profiles for the angular velocity of the elbow and shoulder for the three hand paths differ. The straight hand paths and common profiles for speed suggest that planning is done with reference to the hand because these parameters can be linearly scaled. Planning with reference to joints would require computing nonlinear combinations of joint angles.

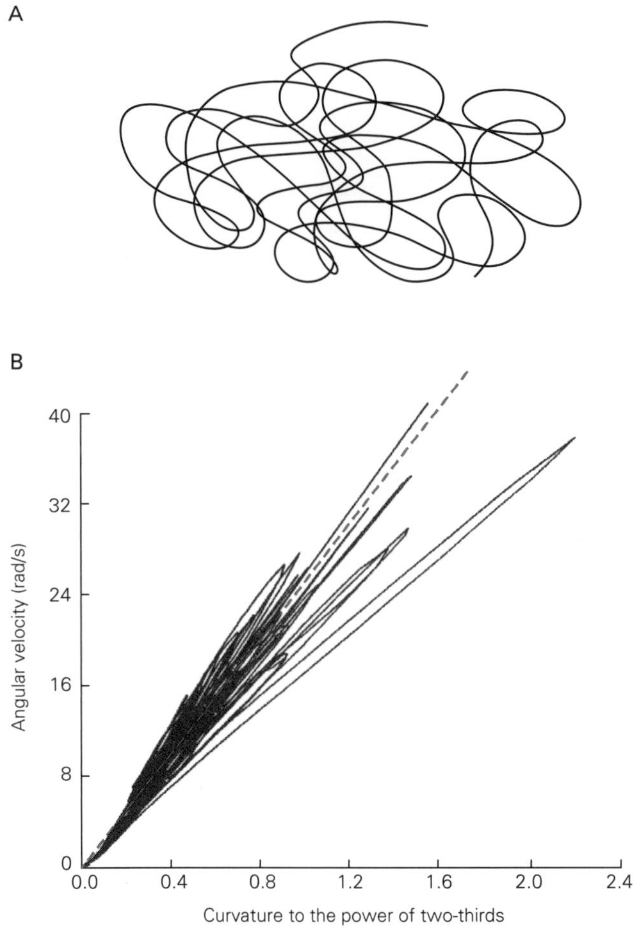

Figure 33–10 Complex movements obey the two-thirds power law. (Reproduced, with permission, from Lacquaniti, Terzuolo, and Viviani 1983.)

A. Nondirected scribbling is a complex movement.

B. Instantaneous values of the angular velocity of the hand while scribbling are plotted against the curvature of the hand's path raised to the power of two-thirds. The relation between the two variables is piecewise linear. Each segment in the bundle, corresponding to nonoverlapping segments of the trajectory, has a different slope. The slopes cluster around the average (**dashed line**), a typical result for this type of experiment. Therefore the relationship between the speed of hand motion and the degree of curvature of the hand path is roughly constant: Velocity varies as a continuous function of the curvature raised to the power of two-thirds. This two-thirds power law governs virtually all movements and expresses an obligatory slowing of the hand during movement segments that are more curved and a speeding up during segments that are straight. Because angular velocity is the speed of the hand multiplied by the path curvature, in the plot an increase in angular velocity represents a decrease in hand speed.

can have errors. Sensory inputs to the motor systems during a movement provide information about errors that arise from neural noise, from inaccuracies in the motor commands as a result of flaws in the internal models, or from changes in the outside world, such as the unexpected motion of a target. We now examine what part these errors play in two forms of motor control, feedforward and feedback control.

Feedforward Control Does Not Use Sensory Feedback

Movements that are not correctible during the movement are often termed *ballistic*. This term is ordinarily applied to the trajectory of unpowered projectiles (such as ballistic missiles) that, once launched, can no longer be controlled and are subject only to gravity. Because arm movements can potentially be controlled throughout their course, however, the term *feedforward control* more accurately describes the trajectory. Feedforward commands are generated without regard to the consequences. Such commands are also termed *open-loop* because the sensorimotor loop is not completed by sensory feedback (Figure 33–11A).

Open-loop control is advantageous if we consider the delays inherent in the sensorimotor system. Both conversion of stimulus energy into neural signals by stimulus receptors and conveyance of the sensory signals to central neurons take time. For example, visual feedback can take approximately 100 ms to be processed in the retina and transmitted to the visual cortex. In addition to delays in the peripheral sensory system, there are also delays in central processing, in the transmission of efferent signals to motor neurons, and in the response of muscles. In all, the combined sensorimotor loop delay is appreciable, approximately 200 ms for a response to a visual stimulus. This delay means that rapid movements, such as the saccades of the eye that last less than 100 ms, cannot use sensory feedback to guide the eye onto a target.

Even with slower movements, such as deliberate reaching, which can take approximately 500 ms, sensory information cannot be used to guide the initial part of a movement, so open-loop control must be used. This open-loop component can be clearly demonstrated. Both the initial speed and the acceleration of the hand during reaching are proportional to the distance of the target. This and the straightness of hand paths mean that the extent of a movement is planned before the movement is initiated, and the movement is generated in a feedforward manner (Figure 33–12).

Open-loop control also has disadvantages. Any movement errors caused by inaccuracies in planning

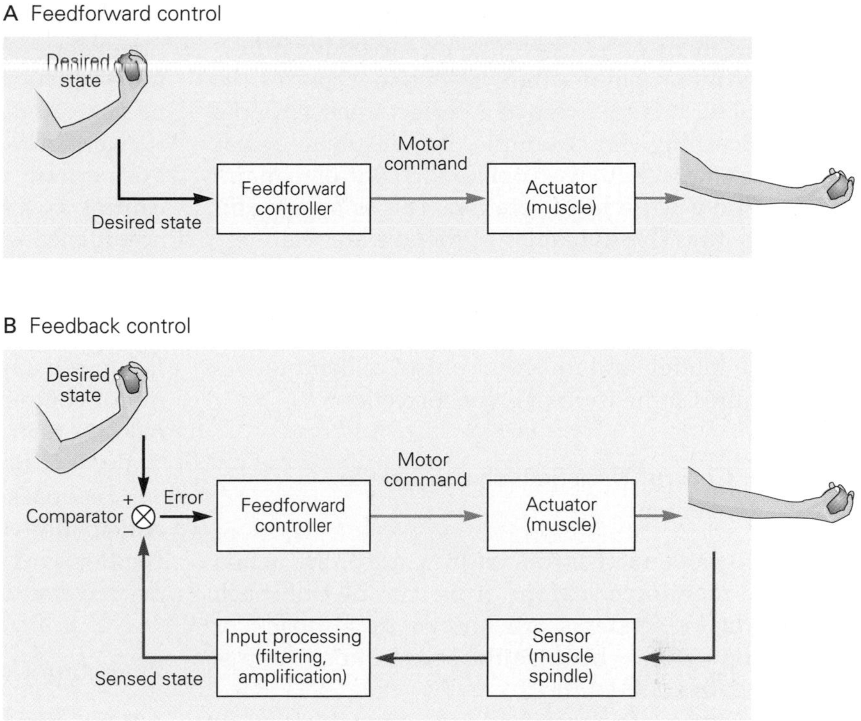

Figure 33–11 Feedforward and feedback control.

A. A feedforward controller generates a motor command based on a desired state. Any errors that arise during the movement are not monitored.

B. With feedback control the desired and sensed states are compared (at the comparator) to generate an error signal, which helps shape the motor command. There can be considerable delay in the feedback of sensory information to the comparator.

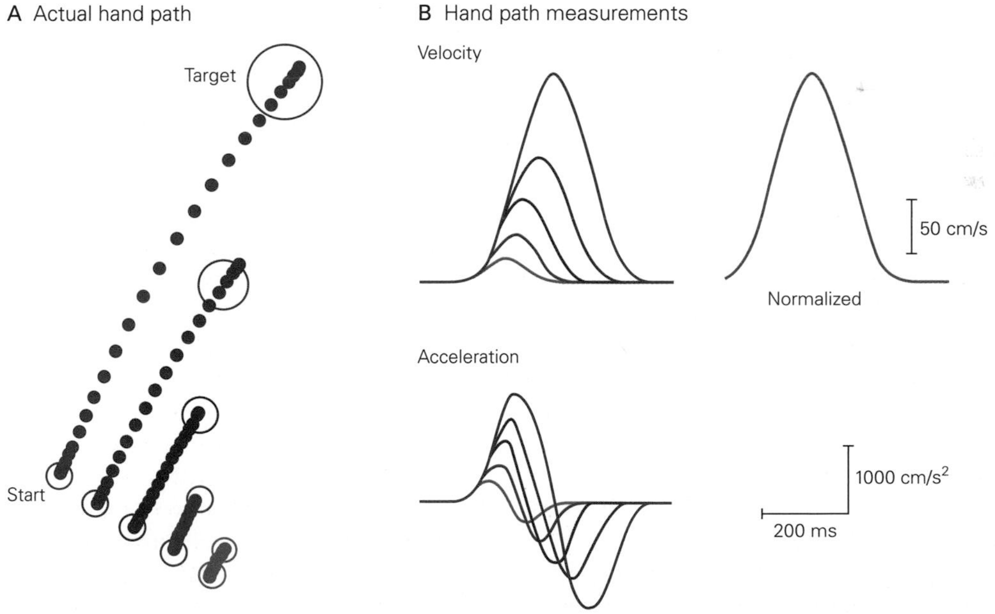

Figure 33–12 Acceleration and velocity of reaching are a function of target distance. (Modified, with permission, from Gordon et al. 1994.)

A. Hand paths measured to targets located 2.5, 5, 10, 20, and 30 cm from the starting position.

B. Average velocity and acceleration of the hand movements shown in part A. The acceleration and velocity profiles scale linearly as a function of the distance to the target. All the velocity profiles are self-similar and when normalized in time and amplitude are nearly identical. The single peaks indicate that the extent of movement is specified prior to actual movement. If it were not, the first peak would be the same for all target distances, and secondary peaks representing feedback adjustment would be seen.

or execution will not be corrected, and therefore will compound themselves over time or successive movements. The more complex the system under control, the more difficult it is to arrive at a perfect inverse model through learning. For example, the vestibulo-ocular reflex (see Chapter 40) uses open-loop control to maintain fixation during head rotation. This is a very efficient system as the dynamics of the eye are relatively simple, and the rotation of the head can be directly sensed by the vestibular labyrinth. The complexity of the arm, however, makes it very difficult to optimize an inverse model, and thus the control of hand movement requires some form of error correction.

Feedback Control Uses Sensory Signals to Correct Movements

To correct movement errors as they arise, the action must be monitored before it is completed. Such error-correcting systems are known as feedback or closed-loop systems because the sensorimotor loop is complete (Figure 33–11B).

The simplest form of feedback control is one in which the control system generates a fixed response when the error exceeds some threshold. Such a system is seen in most central heating systems in which a thermostat is set to a desired temperature. When the house temperature falls below the specified level, the heating is turned on until the temperature reaches that level. Although such a system is simple and can be effective, it has the drawback that the amount of heat being put into the house does not relate to the discrepancy between the actual and desired temperature (the error). A better system is one in which the control signal is proportional to the error.

Such proportional control of movement involves sensing the error between the actual and desired position of, for example, the hand. The size of the corrective motor command is in proportion to the size of the error and in a direction to reduce the error. The amount by which the corrective motor command is increased or decreased per unit of positional error is called the *gain* (Figure 33–13). By continuously correcting a movement, feedback control can be robust both to noise in the sensorimotor system and to environmental perturbations.

In most motor systems movement control is achieved through both feedforward and feedback processes. Because sensory feedback is not available for the first portion of a movement, feedforward processes generate the initial motor command only. As the movement progresses, information on performance becomes available, allowing feedback control to play a role.

When lifting an object between thumb and index finger, for example, sufficient grip force (perpendicular force between the digits and the object's surface) must be generated to prevent slippage owing to load force (tangential force between the digit and object surface arising from the object's weight). We use feedforward control to set our grip force and the lifting force in accordance with the expected slipperiness and weight of the object. If cutaneous receptors indicate that slippage is occurring, our grip force is increased immediately through rapid feedback control (Figure 33–14). Because cutaneous information on slippage evokes a motor command to increase grip force only when the object is being lifted, this feedback circuit is said to be "gated" during lifting.

Feedback control cannot generate a command in anticipation of an error: It is always driven by an error. Feedforward control, conversely, is based only on a desired state and can therefore null the error.

Prediction Compensates for Sensorimotor Delays

Accurate feedback control of movement requires information on the body's current state, for example, the positions and velocities of our body segments. However, sensory feedback from the periphery is both noisy and slow. Delays in feedback can lead to problems during a movement, as the delayed information does not reflect the present state of the body and world. Two strategies can compensate for such delays and thus increase the accuracy of sensory feedback during movement: intermittency of movement and prediction of changes in body states due to movement. With intermittency, movement is momentarily interrupted by rest, as in eye saccades and manual tracking. Provided the interval of rest is greater than the time delay of the sensorimotor loop, intermittency fosters more accurate sensory feedback.

Prediction is a better strategy and can form a major component of a state estimator. Although sensory signals provide necessary information about the body, the motor command also provides useful information. If both the current state of the body and the descending motor command are known, the next state of the body can be estimated. This estimate is derived from a forward model that predicts how the body will change in response to the motor command. Because this estimate is predictive, it is time-advanced, thereby compensating for the feedback delays. However, this estimate will tend to drift over time if the forward model is not perfectly accurate.

The drawbacks of using only sensory feedback or only motor prediction can be ameliorated by monitoring

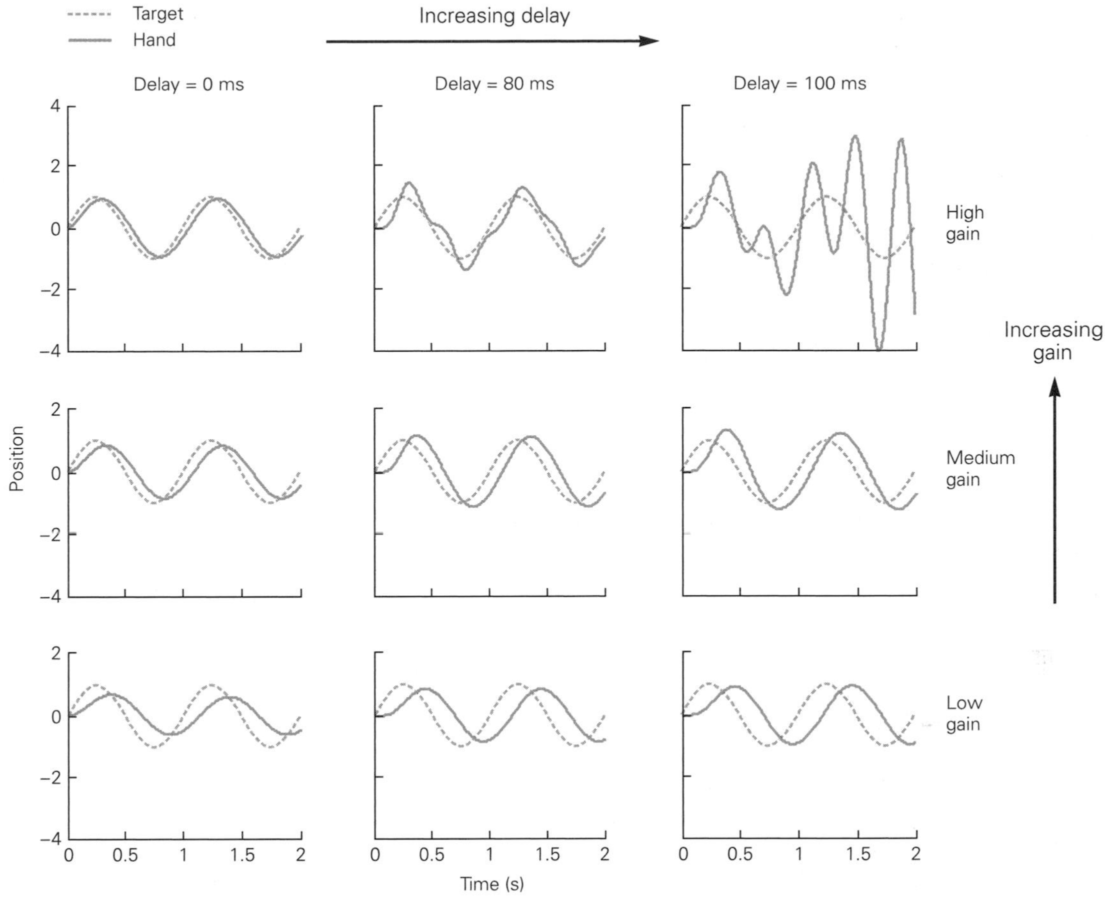

Figure 33–13 The interplay of gain and delay in feedback control. Subjects use a controller to track a target moving sinusoidally in one dimension. The sensory feedback signal that conveys error in the hand's position arrives after some period of time (the delay), and the motor system tries to correct for the error by increasing or decreasing the size of its command relative to the error (the gain).

The plots show the performance of a subject tracking a sinusoidal target in which there is either instantaneous feedback of error (**left column**) or feedback with a delay (**middle** and **right columns**). When the gain is high, and the delay is low, tracking is very good. However, as the delay increases, the motor system corrects for error inappropriately, and this leads to oscillations and large errors. To maintain stability, the gain can be lowered, but tracking is not perfect.

At low gain (**bottom row**) the feedback controller corrects errors only slowly and tracking is inaccurate. As the gain increases (**middle row**) the feedback controller corrects errors more rapidly and tracking performance improves. At high gain (**top row**) the system corrects rapidly but is prone to overcorrect, leading to instability when the time delay in feedback is on the order of physiological time delays (**top right**). Because the controller is compensating for errors that existed 100 ms earlier, the correction may therefore be inappropriate for the current error. This overcorrection leads to oscillations and is one mechanism proposed to account for some forms of oscillatory tremor seen in neurological disease.

both and using a forward model to estimate the current state of the body. A neural apparatus that does this is known as an *observer model*. The major objectives of the observer model are to compensate for sensorimotor delays and to reduce uncertainty in the estimate of the state of the body owing to noise in both the sensory and motor signals (Figure 33–15). Such a model has been supported by empirical studies of how the nervous system estimates hand position, posture, and head orientation.

The nervous system has several different internal models of control that use prediction and sensory feedback to different extents. The comparative advantages of these various models are nicely illustrated

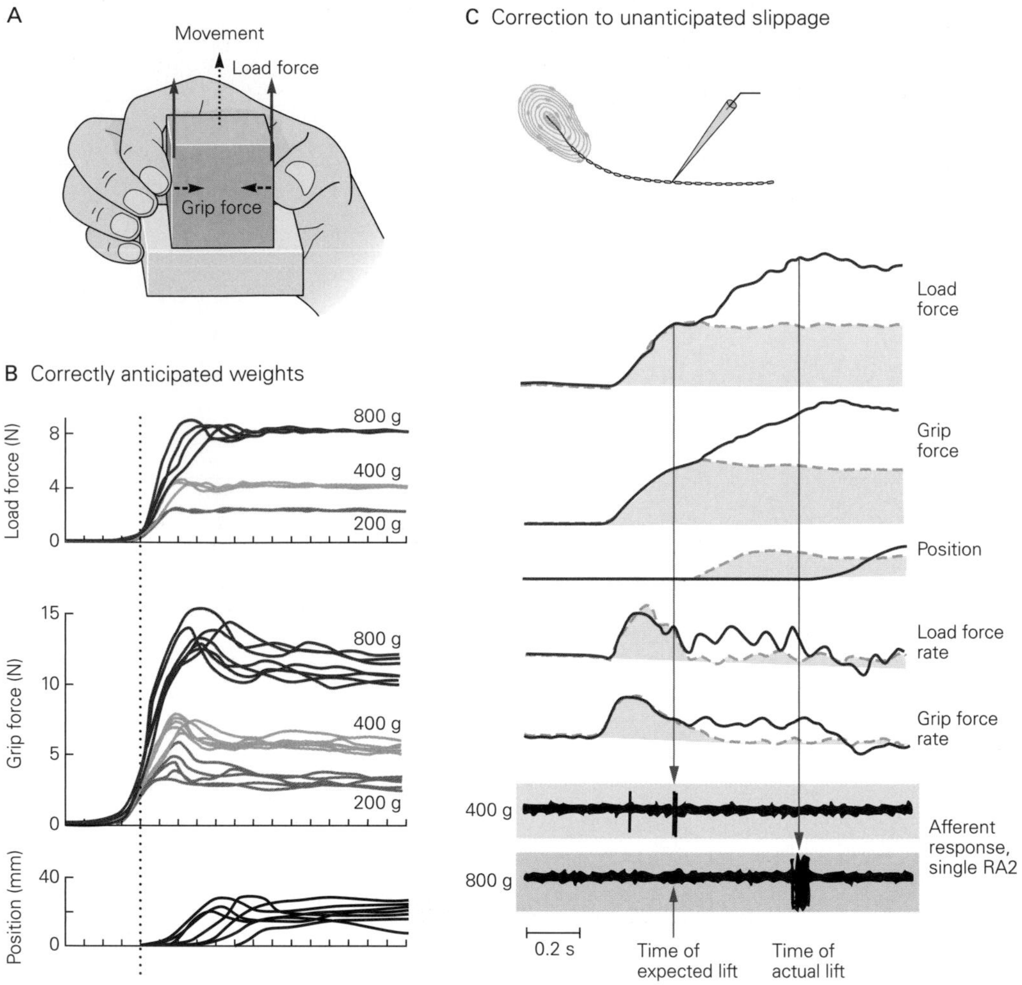

Figure 33–14 Both feedback and feedforward controls are used when lifting an object.

A. The subject lifts an object from the table. Sensory receptors measure vertical motion, grip force, and the load force applied to the object to overcome gravity and inertia. The discharge of different sensory receptors is recorded by microelectrodes inserted within identified sensory axons of the peripheral nerve, a procedure called microneurography.

B. When the subject knows the weight of the object in advance, the applied forces are adequate to lift the object. Three sets of traces (24 trials superimposed) show load force, grip force, and position as subjects lifted three objects of different weights (200, 400, and 800 g). The grip force increases in proportion to the weight of the object. This is done by scaling a preprogrammed force profile (the profiles have the same shape but different amplitudes).

C. When the weight is larger than expected, the object slips initially, but force is increased before lifting begins. When the subject begins to lift a 400 g object, Pacinian corpuscles in the skin are activated and a burst of action potentials occurs in the afferent RA2 fibers, signaling the beginning of the hold phase during which the grip force is constant. After being presented with the 400 g object for several trials (**dashed lines**), the subject is given an 800 g object (**solid lines**). When the subject begins to lift the 800 g object, the object slips, and the RA2 fibers are not activated. The absence of RA2 signals triggers a slow increase in force that is terminated when lifting begins. (Reproduced, with permission, from Johansson et al. 1991.)

by differences in object manipulation under different conditions. When the object's behavior is unpredictable, sensory feedback provides the most useful signal for estimating load. For example, when flying a kite we need to adjust our grip almost continuously in response to unpredictable motions of the kite. When dealing with such unpredictability, grip force needs to be high to prevent slippage because it tends to lag behind load force (Figure 33–16A).

However, when handling objects with stable properties, predictive control mechanisms can be effective. For example, when the load is increased by a self-generated action, such as moving the arm, the grip force increases instantaneously with load force (Figure 33–16B). Sensory detection of the load would be too slow to account for this rapid increase in grip force. Such predictive control is essential for the rapid movements commonly observed in dexterous behavior.

The discrepancy between actual and predicted sensory feedback is also essential in motor control. For example, when we pick up an object, we anticipate when the object will lift off. The brain is particularly

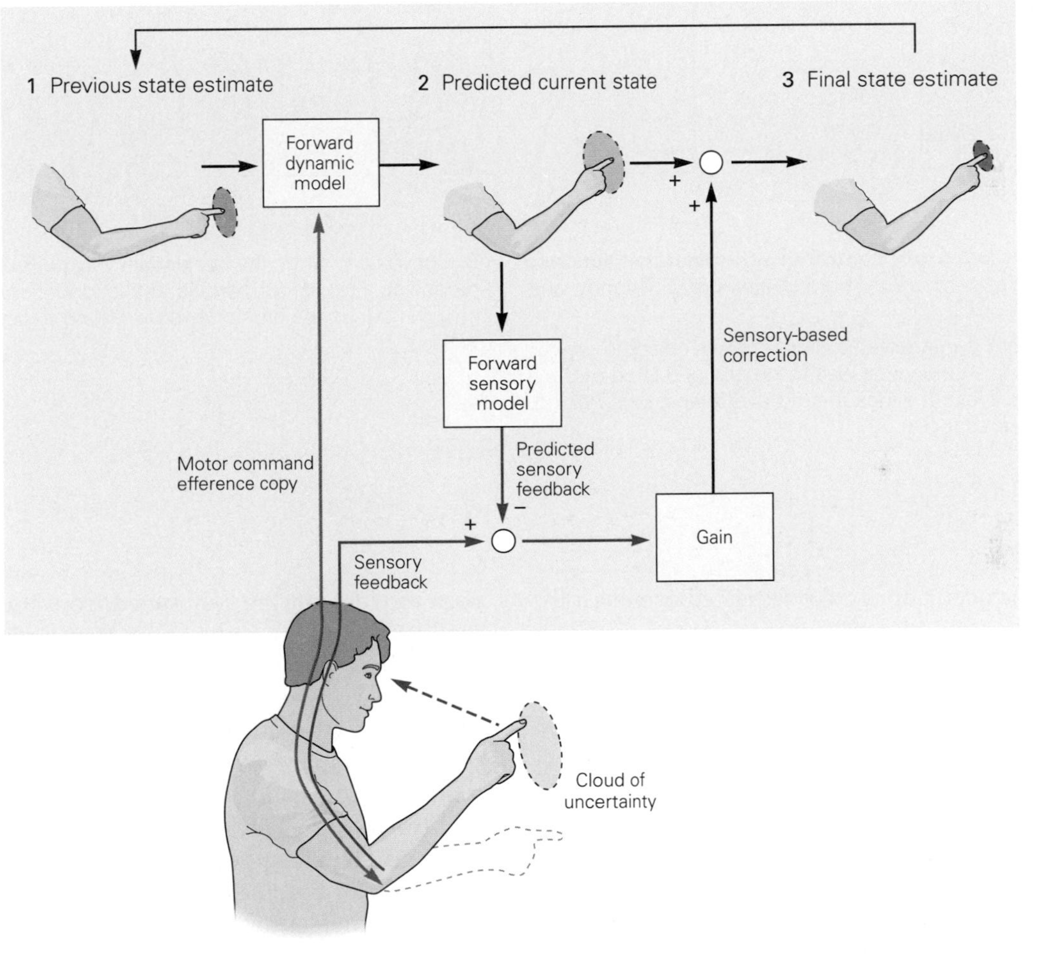

Figure 33–15 An observer model. The drawing shows how the finger's location can be estimated during movement of the arm. A previous estimate of the distribution of possible finger positions (**1**) is the basis for a new estimate (**2**). This estimation uses an efference copy of the motor command and a model of the dynamics. The new distribution of estimated finger positions (the "cloud of uncertainty") is larger than that of the previous estimate. The model then predicts the sensory feedback that would occur for these new finger positions, and the error between the predicted and actual sensory feedback is used to correct the estimate of current finger position. This correction changes the sensory error into state errors and also determines the relative reliance on the efference copy and sensory feedback. The final estimate of current finger position (**3**) has less uncertainty. This estimate becomes the new previous estimate for subsequent movement as this sequence is repeated many times. Delays in sensory feedback that must be compensated have been omitted from the diagram for clarity.

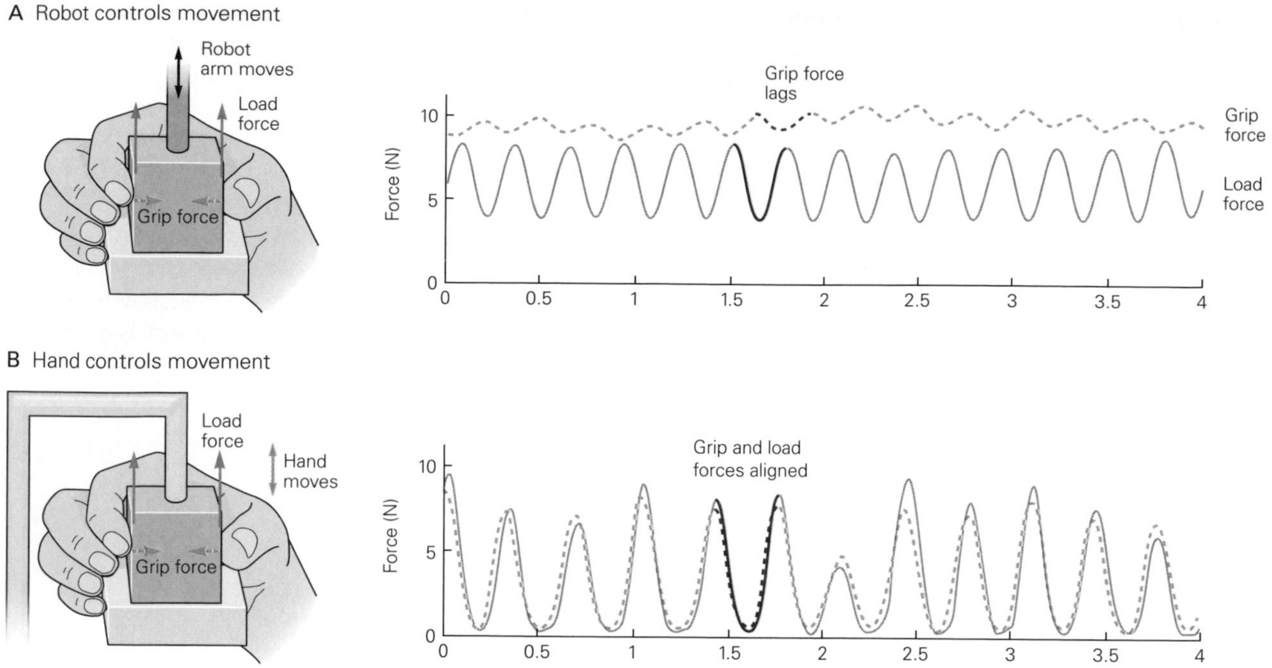

Figure 33–16 **Anticipatory control of self-generated actions.** (Reproduced, with permission, from Blakemore, Goodbody, and Wolpert 1998.)

A. When a subject is instructed to hold onto an object to which a robot is applying a sinusoidal load force, the grip force of the fingers is high to prevent slippage but nevertheless lags behind the increases in load force.

B. Conversely, when the subject actively pulls down the object, producing a similar load profile, the load force can be anticipated and thus the grip force is lower and tracks the load force without delay.

sensitive to the occurrence of unexpected events or the nonoccurrence of an expected event. Thus if an object is lighter or heavier than expected, and therefore is lifted too early or cannot be lifted, reactive responses are evoked. The brain seems to pay particular attention to these critical moments to determine whether the subsequent actions that are part of the task should proceed.

In addition to its use in compensating for sensory feedback delays, prediction is a key element in perceptual processing. Sensory feedback can originate from two sources: either external sources or our own movement. In the sensory receptor these two sources are not distinguished, however, and sensory signals do not carry a label "external stimulus" or "internal stimulus."

Sensitivity to external events can be amplified by reducing the feedback from our own movement. Thus predictions of sensory signals that arise from our own movements are subtracted from the total sensory feedback, thereby enhancing the signals that carry information about external events. Such a predictive mechanism is responsible for the fact that tickling oneself is a less intense experience than tickling by another. When participants are asked to tickle themselves with a time delay introduced between the motor command and the resulting tickle, the greater the time delay the more ticklish the sensation. As the time delay increases, the predictor becomes more inaccurate, thereby failing to cancel the sensory feedback resulting in the tickle sensation.

Sensory Processing Is Different for Action and Perception

A growing body of research supports the idea that the sensory information used to control actions is processed in neural pathways that are distinct from the afferent pathways that contribute to perception. Mel Goodale and David Milner have proposed that visual information flows in two streams in the brain (see Chapter 25). A dorsal stream projects to the posterior parietal cortex and is particularly involved in the use of vision for action (see Chapter 38). Conversely, a ventral stream projects to the inferotemporal cortex and is involved in conscious visual perception (see Chapter 28).

This distinction between the uses of vision for action and perception is based on a double-dissociation seen in patient studies. For example, the patient D. F. developed visual agnosia after damage to her ventral stream. She is unable, for example, to explain the orientation of a slot either verbally or with her hand. However, when asked to perform a simple action, such as putting a card through the slot, she has no difficulty orienting her hand appropriately to put the card through the slot. Conversely, patients with damage to the dorsal stream can develop optic ataxia in which perception is intact, but control is affected.

Although the distinction between perception and action arose from clinical observations, it can also be seen in normal people, as in the size–weight illusion. When lifting two objects of different size but equal weight, people report that the smaller object feels heavier. This illusion, first documented more than 100 years ago, is both powerful and robust. It does not lessen when a person is informed that the objects are of equal weight and does not weaken with repeated lifting.

When subjects begin to lift large and small objects that weigh the same, they generate larger grip and load forces for the larger object because they assume that larger objects are heavier. After alternating between the two objects, they rapidly learn to scale their fingertip forces precisely for the true object weight (Figure 33–17). This shows that the sensorimotor system recognizes that the two weights are equal. Nevertheless, the size–weight illusion persists, suggesting not only that the illusion is a result of high-level cognitive centers in the brain but also that the sensorimotor system can operate independently of these centers.

Motor Systems Must Adapt to Development and Experience

Animals have a remarkable capacity for learning new motor skills through their interaction with the environment. This learning is distinct from and independent of the development of skills through

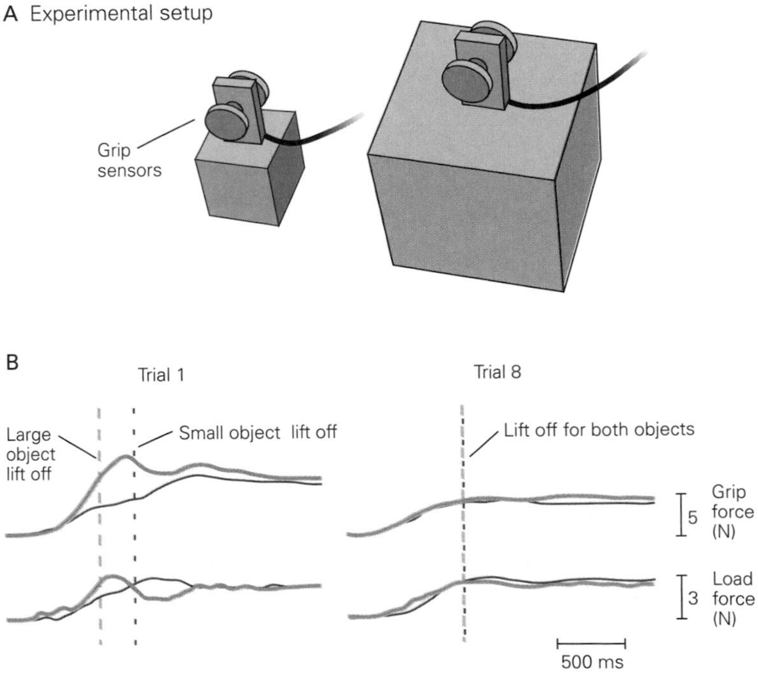

Figure 33–17 The size–weight illusion. (Reproduced, with permission, from Flanagan and Beltzner 2000.)

A. In each trial subjects lifted first a large object and then a small object that weighed the same. Subjects thought the smaller object felt heavier than it actually was.

B. In the first trial subjects generated greater grip and load forces for the bigger object (**orange traces**) as it was expected to be heavier than the small object. In the eighth trial the grip and load forces are the same for the two objects, showing that the sensorimotor system generates grip and load forces appropriate to the weights of the two objects despite the conscious perception of a difference in weight.

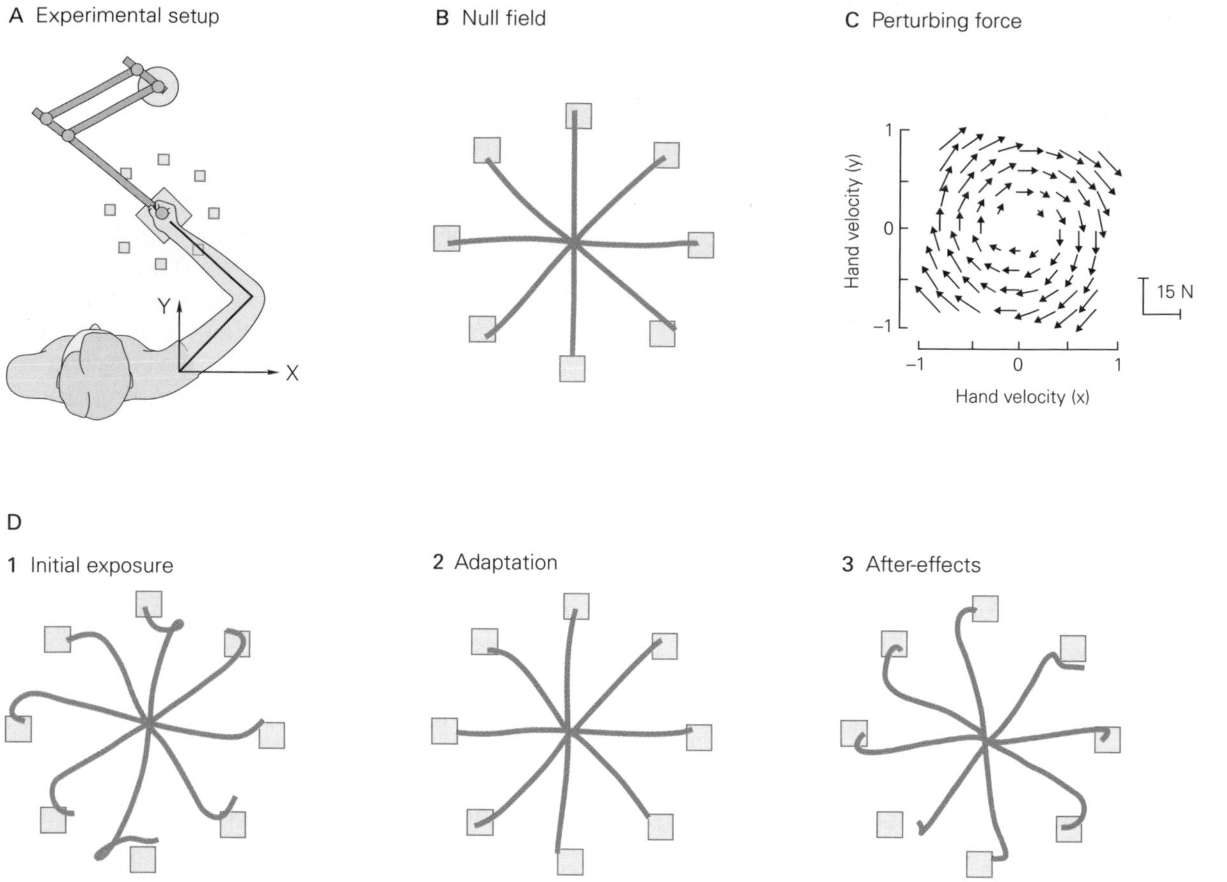

Figure 33–18 Learning improves the accuracy of reaching in a novel dynamic environment.

A. A subject holds an apparatus that measures the position and velocity of the hand and applies forces to the hand. (Reproduced, with permission, from Brashers-Krug, Shadmehr, and Bizzi 1996.)

B. When the motors are off (null field) the subject makes approximately straight movements from the center of the workspace to targets arrayed in a circle.

C. A clockwise force is then applied to the hand, shown as a function of hand velocity. This field produces a force proportional to the speed of the hand that always acts at right angles to the current direction of motion.

D. Initially the hand paths are severely perturbed in response to the perturbing force (**1**). After some time the subject adapts and can again follow a straight path during the entire movement (**2**). When the motors are then turned off, movement is again perturbed but in a direction opposite to the earlier perturbation (**3**).

maturation. Although evolution can hard-wire some motor behaviors, such as the ability of a foal to stand, motor behavior in general must adapt to new and varying environments.

New motor skills cannot be acquired by a fixed neural control system. Sensorimotor control systems must constantly adapt over a lifetime as body size and proportions change, thereby maintaining an appropriate relationship between motor commands and body mechanics. In addition, learning is the only way to acquire motor skills that are defined by social convention, such as writing or dancing.

Most forms of motor learning involve *procedural* or *implicit* learning, so-called because subjects are generally unable to express what it is they have learned. Implicit learning often takes place without consciously thinking about it and can be retained for extended periods of time without practice (see Chapter 66). Typical examples of procedural learning are learning to ride a bicycle or play the piano. In contrast, *explicit* or *declarative* learning involves the acquisition of knowledge that can be expressed in statements about the world and is available to introspection (see Chapter 67). Memorizing the names and routes of the cranial nerves or directions to the local hospital are examples of explicit learning. Declarative memory tends to be easily forgotten, although repeated exposure can lead to long-lasting retention.

Motor learning can occur more or less immediately or require some time. One learns to pick up an object of unknown weight almost immediately and learns to ride a bicycle after a little practice, but mastering the piano requires years. These different timescales may reflect the intrinsic difficulty of the task as well as evolutionary constraints that have to be unlearned to perform the task. For example, piano playing requires learning precise control of the fingers, whereas in normal movements, such as reaching and grasping, individuated finger movements are rare.

Motor Learning Involves Adapting Internal Models for Novel Kinematic and Dynamic Conditions

Sensorimotor transformations have kinematic and dynamic components. Kinematic transformations relate events in different spatial coordinate systems, such as joint angles of the arm and the position of the hand in space. To control a computer mouse, for example, we must learn the kinematic transformation between the handheld mouse and the image of the cursor on the screen. Dynamic transformations relate forces acting at the joints to the motion of the system. We must relate the forces we apply to the mouse to the resulting movement, a transformation that depends on the inertia of the mouse and the friction between the mouse and pad. The kinematics and dynamics of movement vary greatly as we grow and interact with new objects. The brain adapts by reorganizing or adjusting motor commands to generate new actions.

As we saw earlier, we normally move the hand in a straight line to reach an object. Unexpected dynamic interactions may produce curved paths, but subjects learn to anticipate these effects. This learning is conveniently studied by having subjects make pointing movements with an apparatus through which novel forces can be applied to the arm (Figure 33–18A). For example, applying a force that is proportional to the speed of the hand but which acts at right angles to the direction of movement forces the hand into a brief curving movement before reaching the target. Over time the subject adapts to this perturbation and is able to maintain a straight-line movement (Figure 33–18D).

Subjects might adapt to such a situation in two possible ways. First, they could co-contract the muscles in their arm, thereby stiffening the arm and reducing the impact of the perturbation. Alternatively, they could learn an internal model that compensates for the expected forces, one that uses a new set of motor commands. By examining the subjects' movements after the force is turned off, we can distinguish between these two forms of learning. If the arm simply stiffens, it should continue to move in a straight path. If a new internal model is learned, the new model should compensate for a force that no longer exists, thereby producing a path in the direction opposite from the earlier perturbation. In fact, when the force is turned off, subjects show a large after-effect in the opposite direction, demonstrating that they had learned to compensate for the perturbation (Figure 33–18D).

Although motor learning often takes much practice, once a task is no longer performed de-adaptation is typically quite swift. The context of the movement, that is the sensory inputs associated with a particular task, can be enough to switch behavior. When subjects wear prismatic glasses that rotate visual space, for example, they initially misreach targets but soon learn to reach correctly. After repeated trials the contextual cue of the feel of the glasses, without the prisms in place, is sufficient to switch subjects into behavior suitable with the prisms.

Kinematic and Dynamic Motor Learning Rely on Different Sensory Modalities

Not all sensory modalities are equally important in learning motor tasks. In learning dynamic tasks, proprioception is more important than vision. We normally learn dynamic tasks equally well with or without vision. Patients who have lost proprioception have particular difficulty controlling the dynamic properties of their limbs (Box 33–3) or learning new dynamic tasks without vision.

However, the same patients are easily able to adapt to drastic kinematic changes, such as tracing a drawing while viewing their hand in a mirror. In fact these subjects perform better than normal subjects at such a task, perhaps because they have learned to guide their movements visually and, because of the lack of proprioception, do not experience any conflict between vision and proprioception.

Box 33–3 Proprioception Is Critical for Planning Hand Trajectories and Controlling Dynamics

Sensory neuropathies selectively damage the large-diameter sensory fibers in peripheral nerves and dorsal roots that carry most proprioceptive information. Impairments in motor control resulting from loss of proprioception have fascinated neurologists and physiologists for well over a century. Studies of patients with sensory neuropathies provide invaluable insight into the interactions between sensation and movement planning.

As expected, such patients lose joint position sense and vibration and fine tactile sensations (as well as tendon reflexes), but the sense of pain and temperature are fully preserved. These patients are unable to maintain a steady posture, for example while holding a cup or standing, with the eyes closed. Movements also become clumsy, uncoordinated, and inaccurate.

Some recovery of function may occur over many months as the patient learns to use vision as a substitute for proprioception, but this compensation leaves patients completely incapacitated in the dark. Some of this difficulty reflects an inability to detect errors that develop during unseen movements, as occurs if the weight of an object or resistance differs from expectation.

However, this is not all. When the limb cannot be seen, errors in feedforward control of movements

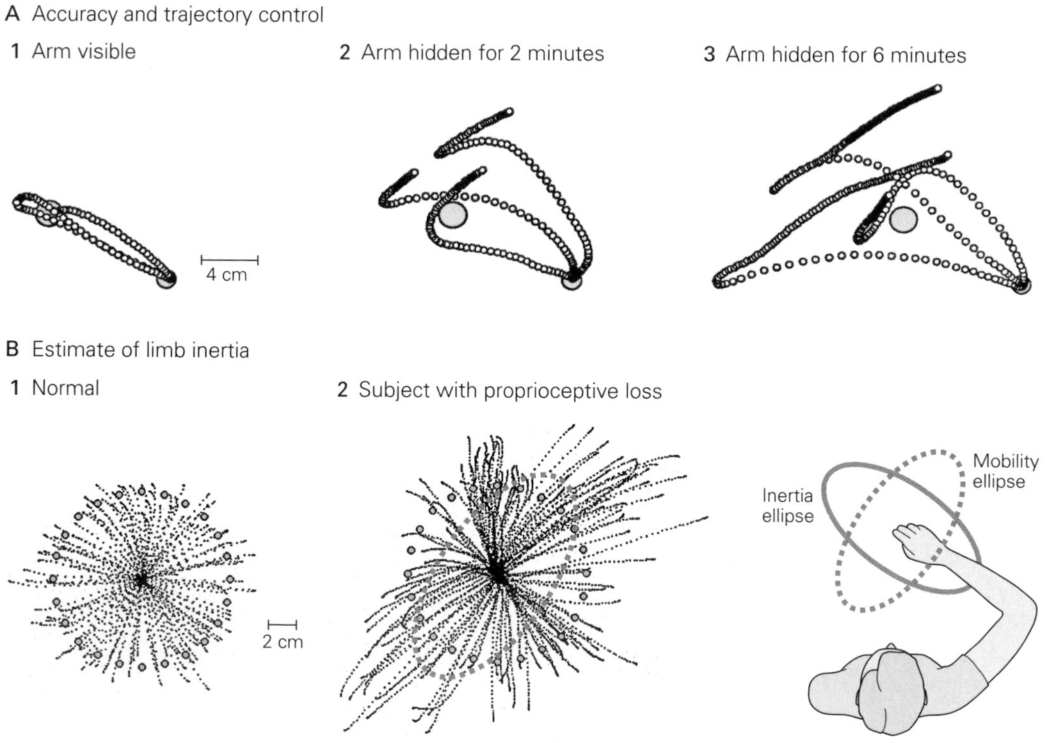

Figure 33–19 Patients lacking proprioception cannot maintain internal models of limb inertia.

A. Accuracy and trajectory control decay rapidly when patients cannot see their limbs. A patient with large-fiber sensory neuropathy, with no sense of position in the arm for several years, moved a mouse-like cursor repeatedly from a starting position to a target displayed on a computer screen in front of her. When the patient was able to see the screen cursor and her hand, movements were straight and reasonably accurate (**1**). Movements become increasingly curved and inaccurate after vision of her arm was removed for 2 minutes (**2**) and 6 minutes (**3**). (Reproduced, with permission, from Ghez, Gordon, and Ghilardi 1995.)

B. A patient without proprioception plans movement without taking account of variations in limb inertia. Patients and normal subjects were instructed to move a finger to 22 targets arranged concentrically. Subjects were prevented from seeing their limb. (**1**) Movements made by a control subject are straight and evenly distributed throughout the workspace. (**2**) Movements made by a patient with loss of limb proprioception vary in extent in different directions. The variation in extent is explained by the fact that directional changes in inertia vary with movement direction according to an elliptical contour (inertia ellipse). This means that a constant initial force at the hand will accelerate the limb differently in different directions (mobility ellipse); high acceleration occurs in directions that have low inertia. The mobility computed for the subject's arm plotted over the hand paths shown at left closely matches the variations in movement extent. (Reproduced, with permission, from Gordon, Ghilardi, and Ghez 1995.)

increase over a few minutes and patients become uncertain of where their hands actually move. This is seen clearly in the succession of movements in Figure 33–19A. Movements that are straight and accurate with vision become increasingly curved; instead of stopping, movements drift off to one side or another without the subject's awareness. Thus proprioception is needed to update both inverse models used to control movement and forward models used to estimate body positions resulting from motor commands.

The defects in these models are revealed by examining the errors that occur when the hand moves to targets in different directions (Figure 33–19B). In moving to equidistant targets in many directions, a normal subject moves his hand approximately the same distance in all directions. For patients with proprioceptive loss, the distance moved varies with the direction of movement; movements along the 45-degree axis, perpendicular to the forearm, overshoot the target.

These variations match changes in the inertial resistance of the arm. When the hand moves in the direction of the forearm (moving both arm and forearm), inertia is two to three times greater than when the hand moves perpendicular to the forearm (moving the forearm alone). Changes in inertia with movement direction fit an elliptical contour. This means that a constant force applied perpendicularly would accelerate the forearm two to three times faster than one applied in the same direction as the forearm.

In all subjects acceleration does indeed vary with movement in different directions, but normal subjects plan movements of shorter duration in directions with lower inertia. In contrast, patients without proprioception are unable to vary the duration (unless they see their limb before moving). Errors therefore reflect the rapid decay of the patient's internal model of limb inertia.

Another form of error occurs in movements with rapid direction reversals. Analyses of the joint torques during these movements show that subjects with intact sensation anticipate intersegmental torques, whereas those without proprioception fail to do so (Figure 33–20).

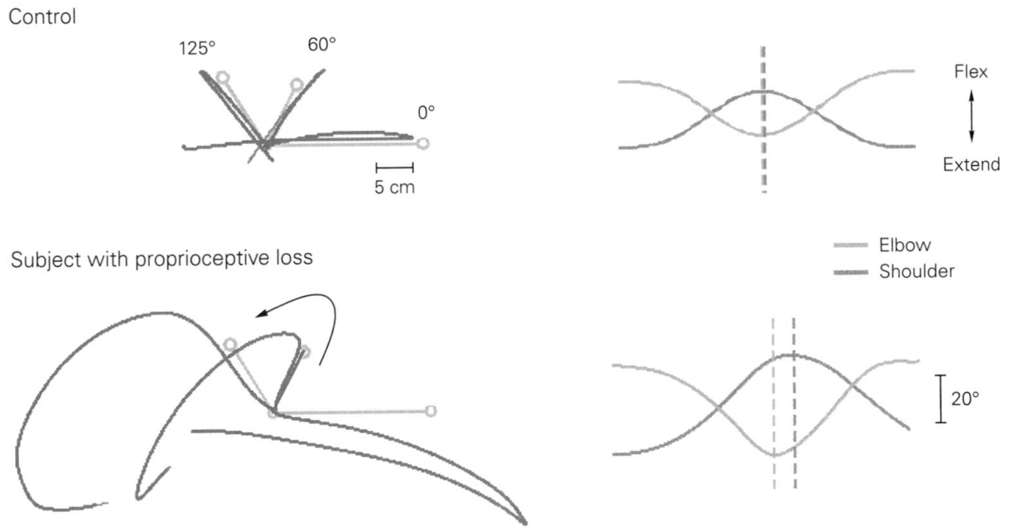

Figure 33–20 Patients lacking proprioception cannot make an accurate movement that requires a rapid reversal in path. In normal subjects the joint angles for the elbow and shoulder show good alignment, leading to an accurate reversal. In subjects who lack proprioceptive input the timing of the joint reversal is poor, leading to large errors in the path. These patients cannot anticipate and correct for the intersegmental dynamics that occur around the path reversal. (Reproduced, with permission, from Sainburg et al. 1995.)

An Overall View

The primary purpose of the elaborate information processing and storage that occurs in the brain is to enable us to interact with our environment. Our infinitely varied and purposeful motor behaviors are governed by the integrated actions of the brain's several motor systems.

To control action the central nervous system uses a sequence of sensorimotor transformations that convert incoming sensory information into motor outputs. The brain uses internal models at each stage in the sensorimotor transformation. Variability in the inputs and outputs of these transformations and inaccuracies in their representation underlie the errors and variability in movement and lead to the ubiquitous trade-off between speed and accuracy.

The motor systems generate commands using feedforward circuits or error-correcting feedback circuits; most movement involves both types of control. The adverse effects of delays in feedback are reduced through the use of predictive processes.

Finally, motor control circuits are not static but undergo continual modification and recalibration throughout life. Motor learning improves motor control in novel situations, and different forms of sensory information are vital for learning.

The ease with which we conduct ordinary movements masks the true complexity of the control processes involved. Many factors inherent in sensorimotor control are responsible for this complexity, which becomes clearly evident when we try to build machines that can perform human-like control of movement. Although computers can beat grandmasters at chess, no computer can yet control a robot to manipulate a chess piece with the dexterity of a six-year-old child.

Daniel M. Wolpert
Keir G. Pearson
Claude P.J. Ghez

Selected Readings

Jeannerod M. 1997. *Cognitive Neuroscience of Action.* Cambridge: Blackwell.

Rosenbaum DA. 2009. *Human Motor Control,* San Diego: Academic Press.

Scott S. 2004. Optimal feedback control and the neural basis of volitional motor control. Nat Rev Neurosci 5:532–546.

Shadmehr R, Wise SP. 2005. *Computational Neurobiology of Reaching and Pointing: A Foundation for Motor Learning.* Cambridge, MA: MIT Press.

Wolpert DM, Diedrichsen J, Flanagan JR. 2011. Principles of sensorimotor learning. Nat Rev Neurosci 12:739–751.

References

Blakemore SJ, Frith CD, Wolpert DM. 1999. Perceptual modulation of self-produced stimuli: the role of spatio-temporal prediction. J Cogn Neurosci 11:551–559.

Blakemore SJ, Goodbody SJ, Wolpert DM. 1998. Predicting the consequences of our own actions: the role of sensorimotor context estimation. J Neurosci 18:7511–7518.

Brashers-Krug T, Shadmehr R, Bizzi E. 1996. Consolidation in human motor memory. Nature 382:252–255.

Craik, KJW. 1943. *The Nature of Explanation.* Cambridge: Cambridge Univ. Press.

Flanagan JR, Beltzner MA. 2000. Independence of perceptual and sensorimotor predictions in the size-weight illusion. Nat Neurosci 3:737–741.

Flash T, Hogan N. 1985. The coordination of arm movements: an experimentally confirmed mathematical model. J Neurosci 5:1688–1703.

Ghez C, Gordon J, Ghilardi MF. 1995. Impairments of reaching movements in patients without proprioception. II. Effects of visual information on accuracy. J Neurophysiol 73:361–372.

Goodale MA, Milner AD. 1992. Separate visual pathways for perception and action. Trends Neurosci 15:20–25.

Gordon J, Ghilardi MF, Cooper SE, Ghez C. 1994. Accuracy of planar reaching movements. II. Systematic extent errors resulting from inertial anisotropy. Exp Brain Res 99: 112–130.

Gordon J, Ghilardi MF, Ghez C. 1994. Accuracy of planar reaching movements. I. Independence of direction and extent variability. Exp Brain Res 99:97–111.

Gordon J, Ghilardi MF, Ghez C. 1995. Impairments of reaching movements in patients without proprioception. I. Spatial errors. J Neurophysiol 73:347–360.

Harris CM, Wolpert DM. 1998. Signal-dependent noise determines motor planning. Nature 394:780–784.

Hebb DO. 1949. *Organization of Behavior.* New York: Wiley.

Jeannerod M. 1988. *The Neural and Behavioural Organization of Goal-Directed Movements.* Oxford: Clarendon Press.

Johansson RS, Westling G. 1991. Afferent signals during manipulative tasks in man. In: O Franzen, J Westman (eds). *Somatosensory Mechanisms,* pp. 25–48. London: Macmillan.

Lacquaniti P, Terzuolo C, Viviani P. 1983. The law relating the kinematic and figural aspects of drawing movements. Acta Psychol (Amst) 54:115–130.

Miall RC, Weir DJ, Stein JF. 1986. Manual tracking of visual targets by trained monkeys. Behav Brain Res 20:185–201.

Morasso P. 1981. Spatial control of arm movements. Exp Brain Res 42:223–227.

Raibert MH. 1977. *Motor Control and Learning by a State-Space Model*. Technical Report no. AI-TR-439. Artificial Intelligence Laboratory, MIT.

Rothwell JC, Traub MM, Day BL, Obeso JA, Thomas PK, Marsden CD. 1982. Manual motor performance in a de-afferented man. Brain 105:515–542.

Sainburg R, Ghilardi MF, Poizner H, Ghez C. 1995. The control of limb dynamics in normal subjects and patients without proprioception. J Neurophysiol 73:820–835.

Schmidt RA, Zelaznik H, Hawkins B, Franks JS, Quinn JTJ. 1979. Motor output variability: a theory for the accuracy of rapid motor acts. Psychol Rev 86:415–451.

Soechting JF, Flanders M. 1989. Sensorimotor representations for pointing to targets in three-dimensional space. J Neurophysiol 62:582–594.

Woodworth RS. 1899. The accuracy of voluntary movement. Psychol Rev 3:1–114.

34

The Motor Unit and Muscle Action

Any action—ascending a flight of stairs, typing on a keyboard, even holding a pose—requires coordinating the movement of body parts. This is accomplished by the interaction of the nervous system with muscle. The role of the nervous system is to activate just those muscles that will exert the force needed to move in a particular way. This is not a simple task: Not only must the nervous system decide which muscles to activate and how much to activate them in order to move one part of the body, but it must also control muscle forces on other body parts and maintain posture.

This chapter examines how the nervous system controls muscle force and how the force exerted by a limb depends on muscle structure. We also describe how muscle activation differs with different types of movement.

The Motor Unit Is the Elementary Unit of Motor Control

A Motor Unit Consists of a Motor Neuron and Multiple Muscle Fibers

The nervous system controls muscle force with signals sent from motor neurons in the spinal cord to the muscle fibers. A motor neuron and the muscle fibers it innervates are known as a motor unit, the basic functional unit by which the nervous system controls movement, a concept proposed by Charles Sherrington in 1925.

A typical muscle is controlled by a few hundred motor neurons whose cell bodies are clustered in a motor nucleus in the spinal cord or brain stem (Figure 34–1). The axon of each motor neuron exits the spinal cord through the ventral root or through a cranial nerve in the brain stem and runs in a peripheral nerve to the muscle. When the axon reaches the muscle, it branches and innervates from a few to several thousand muscle fibers.

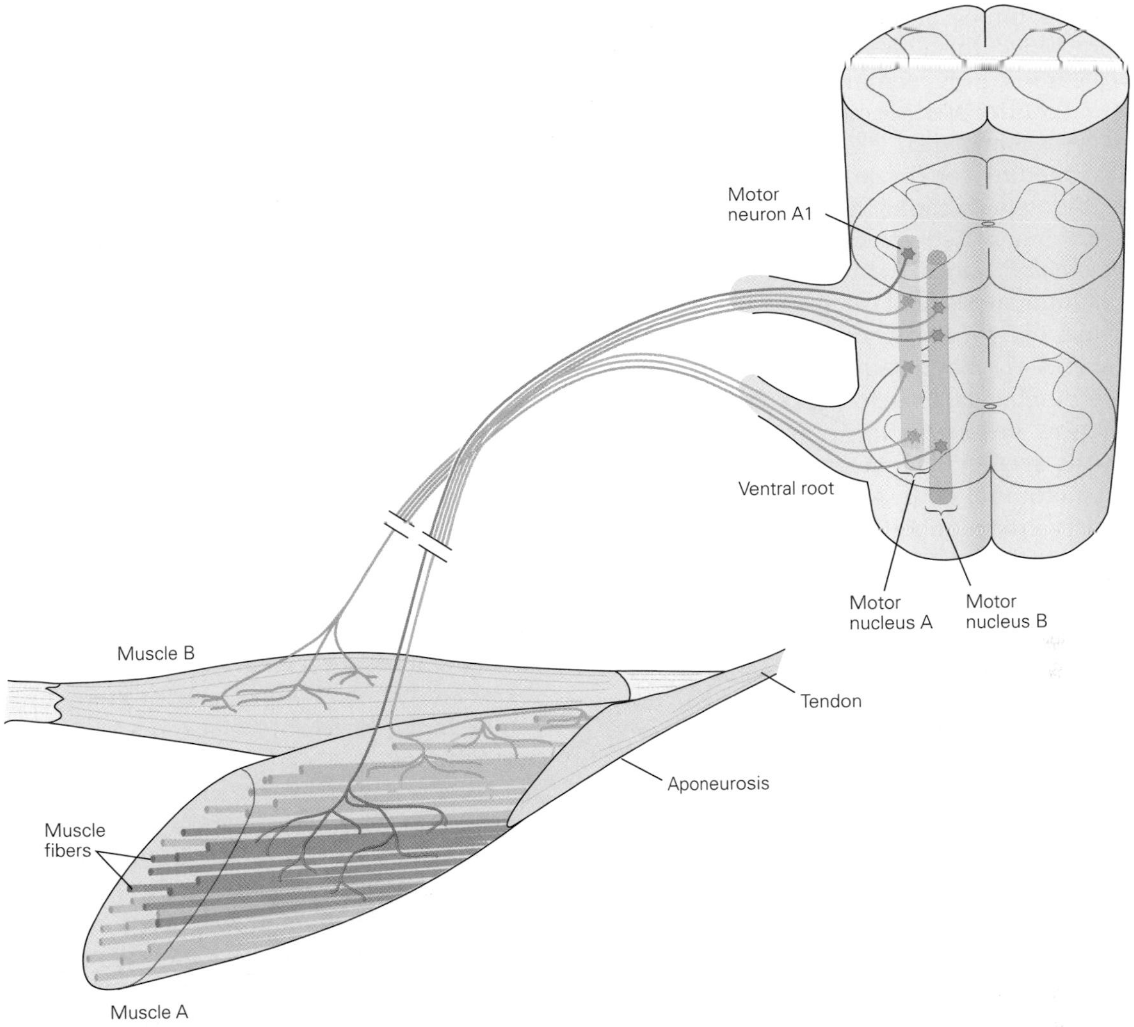

Figure 34–1 A typical muscle consists of many thousands of muscle fibers working in parallel and organized into a smaller number of motor units. A motor unit consists of a motor neuron and the muscle fibers that it innervates, illustrated here by motor neuron A1. The motor neurons innervating one muscle are usually clustered into an elongated motor nucleus that may extend over one to four segments within the ventral spinal cord. The axons from a motor nucleus exit the spinal cord in several ventral roots and peripheral nerves but are collected into one nerve bundle near the target muscle. In the figure, motor nucleus A includes all those motor neurons innervating muscle A; muscle B is innervated by motor neurons lying in motor nucleus B. The extensively branched dendrites of one motor neuron tend to intermingle with those of motor neurons from other nuclei.

Once synaptic input depolarizes the membrane potential of a motor neuron above threshold, the neuron generates an action potential that is propagated along the axon to its terminal in the muscle. The action potential releases neurotransmitter at the neuromuscular synapse, and this causes an action potential in the sarcolemma of the muscle fibers. A muscle fiber has electrical properties similar to those of a large-diameter, unmyelinated axon, and thus action potentials propagate along the sarcolemma, although more slowly owing to the fiber's higher capacitance. Because the action potentials in all the muscle fibers of a motor unit occur at approximately the same time, they contribute to extracellular currents that sum to generate a field potential near the active muscle fibers.

Most muscle contractions involve the activation of many motor units, whose currents sum to produce signals detected by electromyography. In many instances the electromyogram (EMG) signal is large and can be easily recorded with electrodes placed on the skin over the muscle. The timing and amplitude of EMG activity, therefore, reflect the activation of muscle fibers by the motor neurons. EMG signals are useful for studying the neural control of movement and for diagnosing pathology (see Chapter 14).

In most mature vertebrate muscles each fiber is innervated by a single motor neuron. The number of muscle fibers innervated by one motor neuron, the *innervation number*, varies with the muscle type and function. In human skeletal muscles it ranges from average values of 5 for an eye muscle to 1,800 for a leg muscle (Table 34–1). Because the innervation number denotes the number of muscle fibers within a motor unit, differences in innervation number indicate differences in the average increment in force that occurs each time a motor unit in the same muscle is activated. Thus the innervation number also indicates the fineness of control of the muscle; the smaller the innervation number, the finer the control achieved by varying the number of activated motor units.

Table 34–1 Innervation Numbers in Human Skeletal Muscles

Muscle	Alpha motor axons	Muscle fibers	Innervation number
Biceps brachii	774	580,000	750
Brachioradialis	333	>129,200	>410
Cricothyroid	112	18,550	155
Gastrocnemius (medial)	579	1,042,000	1,800
Interossei dorsales (1)	119	40,500	340
Lumbricales (1)	96	10,269	107
Masseter	1,452	929,000	640
Opponens pollicis	133	79,000	595
Platysma	1,096	27,100	25
Posterior cricoarytenoid	140	16,200	116
Rectus lateralis	4,150	22,000	5
Temporalis	1,331	1,247,000	936
Tensor tympani	146	1,100	8
Tibialis anterior	445	272,850	613
Transverse arytenoid	139	34,470	247

(Adapted, with permission, from Enoka 2008.)

Not all motor units in a muscle have the same innervation number. Indeed, the differences can be substantial. For example, motor units of the first dorsal interosseous muscle of the hand have innervation numbers ranging from approximately 21 to 1,770. Consequently, the strongest motor unit in the hand's first dorsal interosseous muscle can exert about the same force as the average motor unit in the leg's medial gastrocnemius muscle.

The muscle fibers of a single motor unit are distributed throughout the muscle and intermingle with fibers innervated by other motor neurons. The muscle fibers of a single motor unit can occupy from 8% to as much as 75% of the volume in a limb muscle, with 2 to 5 muscle fibers per 100 belonging to the same motor unit. Therefore the muscle fibers in a given volume of muscle belong to 20 to 50 different motor units. This distribution changes with age and with some neuromuscular disorders. For example, muscle fibers lose their innervation after the death of a motor neuron and can be reinnervated by collateral sprouts from neighboring axons.

In some muscles the fibers of motor units are confined to discrete compartments that correspond to the regions of the muscle supplied by the primary branches of the muscle nerve. Selective activation of different compartments that exert forces in different directions provides a biomechanical advantage. Branches of the median and ulnar nerves in the forearm, for example, innervate distinct compartments in three multitendon extrinsic hand muscles that enable the fingers to be moved relatively independently. A muscle can therefore consist of several functionally distinct regions.

The Properties of Motor Units Vary

The force exerted by a muscle depends not only on the number of motor units that are activated during a contraction but also on three properties of those motor units: contraction speed, maximal force, and fatigability. These properties are assessed by examining the force exerted by individual motor units in response to variations in the number and rate of evoked action potentials.

The response to a single action potential is known as a *twitch contraction*. The time it takes the twitch to reach its peak force, the *contraction time*, is one measure of the contraction speed of the muscle fibers that comprise a motor unit. Slow-twitch motor units have long contraction times; fast-twitch units have shorter

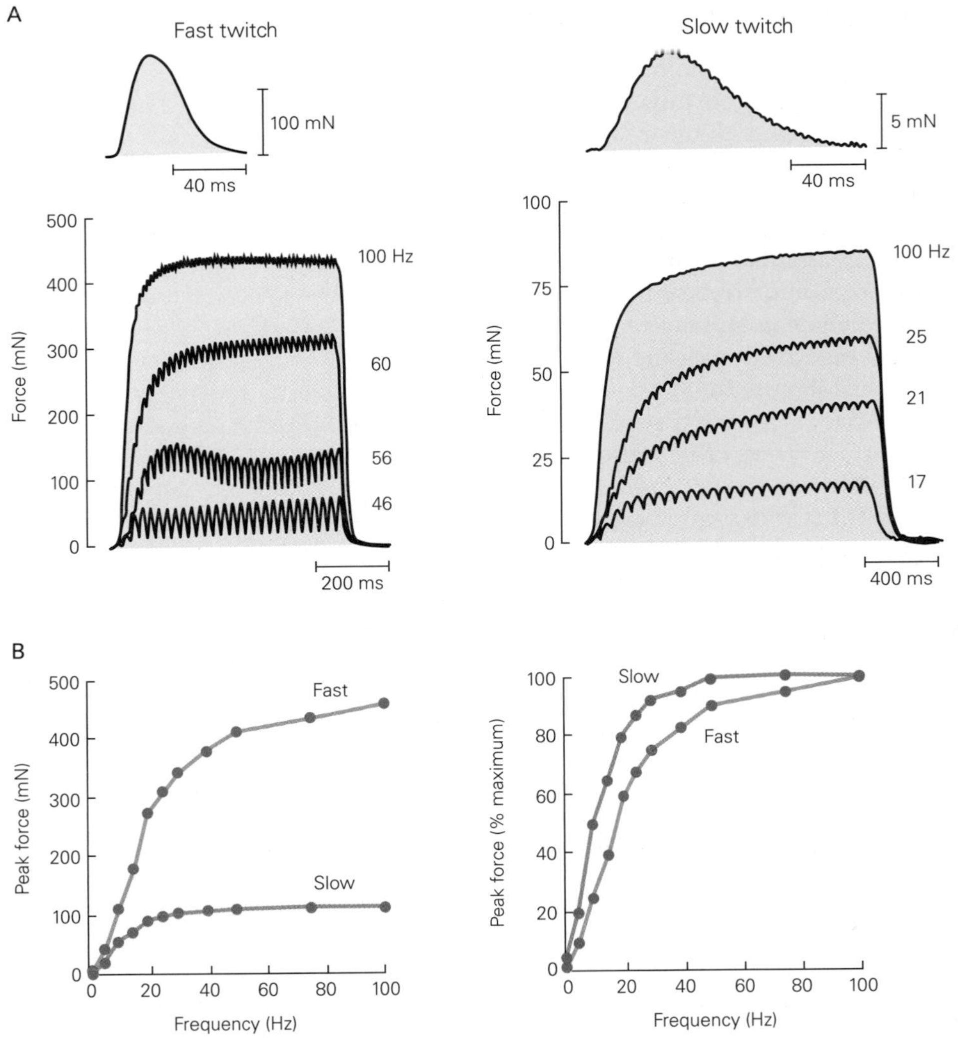

Figure 34–2 The force exerted by a motor unit varies with the rate of the action potentials.

A. Traces show the forces exerted by fast- and slow-twitch motor units in response to a single action potential (top trace) and a series of action potentials (set of four traces below). The time to the peak twitch force, or contraction time, is briefer in the fast-twitch unit. The rates of the action potentials used to evoke the tetanic contractions ranged from 17 to 100 Hz in the slow-twitch unit to 46 to 100 Hz in the fast-twitch unit. The peak force for the 100 Hz tetanus is greater in the fast-twitch unit. Note the different force scales for the two sets of traces. (Adapted with permission from Botterman et al. 1986; Fuglevand, Macefield, and Bigland-Ritchie 1999; and Macefield, Fuglevand, and Bigland-Ritchie 1996.)

B. Relation between peak force and the rate of action potentials for fast- and slow-twitch motor units. The absolute force (left plot) is greater for the fast-twitch motor unit at all frequencies. At lower stimulus rates (right plot) the force evoked in the slow-twitch motor unit summed to a greater relative force (longer contraction time) than in the fast-twitch motor unit (briefer contraction time).

contraction times. A rapid series of action potentials elicits superimposed twitches known as a *tetanic contraction* or *tetanus*.

The force exerted during a tetanic contraction depends on the extent to which the twitches overlap and summate: The force varies with the contraction time of the motor unit and the rate at which the action potentials are evoked. At lower rates of stimulation the ripples in the tetanus denote the peaks of individual twitches (Figure 34–2A). The peak force achieved during a tetanus varies as a sigmoidal function of action potential rate, with the shape of the curve depending on the contraction time of the motor unit (Figure 34–2B). Maximal force is reached at different action potential rates for fast-twitch and slow-twitch motor units and is often greater in fast-twitch units.

The functional properties of motor units vary across the population and between muscles. At one end of the distribution motor units have long twitch contraction times and produce small forces, but are difficult to fatigue. These motor units are the first activated during a voluntary contraction. In contrast, the last motor units activated have short contraction times, produce large forces, and are easy to fatigue. As observed by Jacques Duchateau and colleagues, most human motor units produce low forces and have intermediate contraction times (Figure 34–3).

Because these contractile properties of a motor unit depend on the characteristics of its muscle fibers, we can distinguish different types of muscle fibers. This distinction stems from structural specializations and differences in the metabolic properties of muscle fibers. All muscle fibers belonging to a motor unit have similar biochemical and histochemical properties.

One commonly used scheme distinguishes muscle fibers by their reactivity to histochemical assays for the enzyme myosin adenosine triphosphatase (ATPase), which is used as an index of contractile speed. Based on histochemical stains for myosin ATPase, it is possible to identify type I and type II muscle fibers. Slow contracting motor units contain type I muscle fibers, and fast contracting units include type II fibers. The type II fibers can be further classified into the least fatigable (type IIa) and most fatigable (type IIb, IIx, or IId). Another commonly used scheme distinguishes muscle fibers on the basis of genetically defined isoforms of the myosin heavy chain. Those in slow contracting motor units express myosin heavy chain-I, those in fast contracting and least fatigable units express myosin heavy chain-IIa, and fibers in fast contracting and most fatigable units express myosin heavy chain-IIb or -IIx. There is a high degree of correspondence between the two classification schemes for muscle fibers.

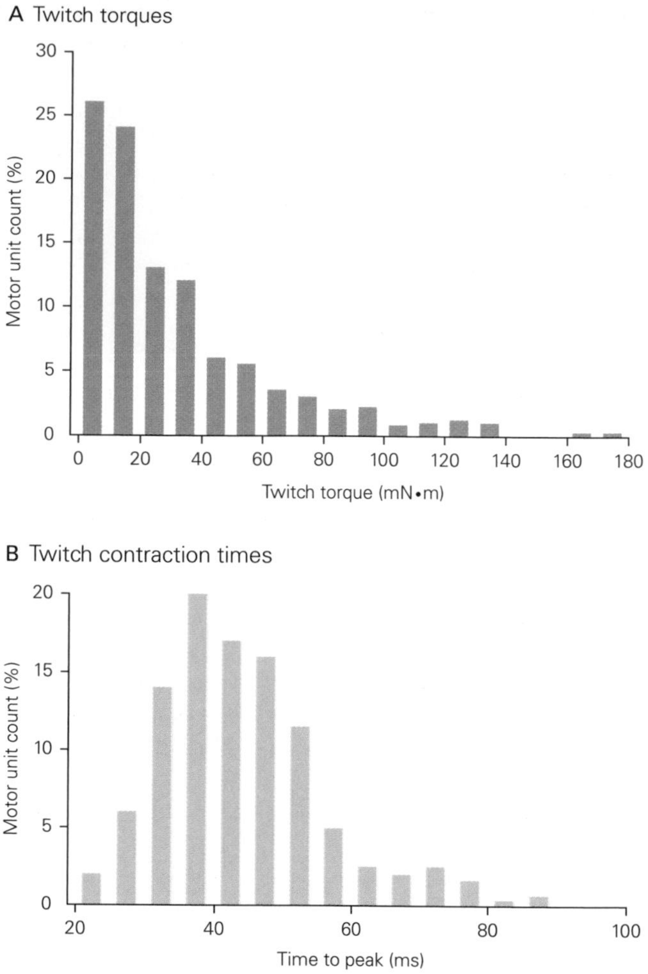

Figure 34–3 Distributions of motor unit properties. (Reproduced, with permission, from Van Cutsem et al. 1997.)

A. Distribution of twitch torques for 528 motor units in the tibialis anterior muscle.

B. Distribution of twitch contraction times for 528 motor units in the tibialis anterior muscle.

Physical Activity Can Alter Motor Unit Properties

Alterations in habitual levels of physical activity can influence the three contractile properties of motor units (contraction speed, maximal force, and fatigability). A decrease in muscle activity, such as occurs with aging, bed rest, limb immobilization, or space flight, reduces the maximal capabilities of all three properties. The effects of increased physical activity depend on the intensity and duration of the activity. Brief sets of high-intensity contractions performed a few times each week can increase contraction speed and motor unit force, whereas prolonged periods of low-intensity contractions can reduce motor unit fatigability. Physical activity regimens that involve such differences are often described as strength training and endurance training, respectively.

Changes in the contractile properties of motor units involve adaptations in the structural specializations and biochemical properties of muscle fibers. The improvement in contraction speed caused by strength training, for example, is associated with an increase in the maximal shortening velocity of a muscle fiber caused by the enhanced capabilities of the myosin molecules in the fiber. Similarly, the increase in maximal force is associated with the enlarged size and increased intrinsic force capacity of the muscle fibers produced by an increase in the number and density of the contractile proteins.

In contrast, alterations in the fatigability of a muscle fiber can be caused by many different adaptations, such as changes in capillary density, the number of mitochondria, excitation-contraction coupling, and the metabolic capabilities of the muscle fibers. Endurance exercise can promote the biogenesis of mitochondria and enhance the oxidative capacity of a muscle fiber, thereby reducing its fatigability. Although the adaptive capabilities of muscle fibers decline with age, the muscles remain responsive to exercise even at 90 years of age.

Despite the efficacy of strength and endurance training in altering the contractile properties of muscle fibers, these training regimens have little effect on the composition of a muscle's fibers. Although several weeks of exercise can change the proportion of type IIa and IIx fibers, there is no change in the proportion of type I fibers. All fiber types adapt in response to exercise, although to varying extents depending on the type of exercise. For example, strength training of leg muscles for 2 to 3 months can increase the cross-sectional area of type I fibers by 0% to 20% and of type II fibers by 20% to 60%, increase the proportion of type IIa fibers by approximately 10%, and decrease the proportion of type IIx fibers by a similar amount. Furthermore, endurance training may increase the enzyme activities of oxidative metabolic pathways without noticeable changes in the proportions of fiber types, but the relative proportions of type IIa and IIx fibers do change as a function of the duration of each exercise session. Conversely, several weeks of bed rest or limb immobilization do not change the proportions of fiber types in a muscle, but they do decrease the size and intrinsic force capacity of muscle fibers.

Although physical activity has little influence on the proportion of type I fibers in a muscle, more substantial interventions can have an effect. Space flight, for example, exposes muscles to a sustained decrease in gravity, reducing the proportion of type I fibers in leg muscles. A few weeks of continuous electrical stimulation at a low frequency causes a marked increase in the proportion of type I fibers and a substantial decrease in fiber size. Similarly, surgically changing the nerve that innervates a muscle alters the pattern of activation; eventually the muscle exhibits properties similar to those of the muscle that was originally innervated by the transplanted nerve. Connecting a nerve that originally innervated a rapidly contracting leg muscle to a slowly contracting leg muscle, for example, will cause the slower muscle to become more like a faster muscle.

Muscle Force Is Controlled by the Recruitment and Discharge Rate of Motor Units

The force exerted by a muscle during a contraction depends on the number of motor units that are activated and the rate at which each of the active motor neurons discharges action potentials. Force is increased during a muscle contraction by the activation of additional motor units, which are recruited progressively from the weakest to the strongest (Figure 34–4). A motor unit's recruitment threshold is the force during the contraction at which the motor unit is activated. Muscle force decreases gradually by terminating the activity of motor units in the reverse order from strongest to weakest.

The order in which motor units are recruited is highly correlated with several indices of motor unit size, including the size of the motor neuron cell bodies, the diameter and conduction velocity of the axons, and the amount of force that the muscle fibers can exert. Because the recruitment threshold of a motor unit depends on the membrane resistance of the motor neuron, which is inversely related to its surface area, a given synaptic current will produce larger changes in the membrane potential of small-diameter motor neurons. Consequently, increases in the net excitatory input to a motor nucleus cause the levels of depolarization to reach threshold in an ascending order of motor neuron size: The smallest motor neuron is recruited first and the largest motor neuron last (Figure 34–5). This effect is known as the size principle of motor neuron recruitment, a principle enunciated by Elwood Henneman in 1957.

The size principle has two important consequences for the control of movement by the nervous system. First, the sequence of motor-neuron recruitment is determined by spinal mechanisms and not by higher regions of the nervous system. This means that the brain cannot selectively activate specific motor units. Second, motor units are activated in order of increasing fatigability, so the least fatigable motor units available produce the initial force required for a specific task.

As suggested by Edgar Adrian in the 1920s, the muscle force at which the last motor unit in a motor nucleus is recruited varies between muscles. In some hand muscles all the motor units have been recruited when the force reaches approximately 60% of maximum during a slow muscle contraction. In the biceps brachii, deltoid, and tibialis anterior muscles, recruitment continues up to approximately 85% of the maximal force. However, because the recruitment threshold of motor units decreases with contraction speed, during a rapid contraction most motor units in a muscle are recruited

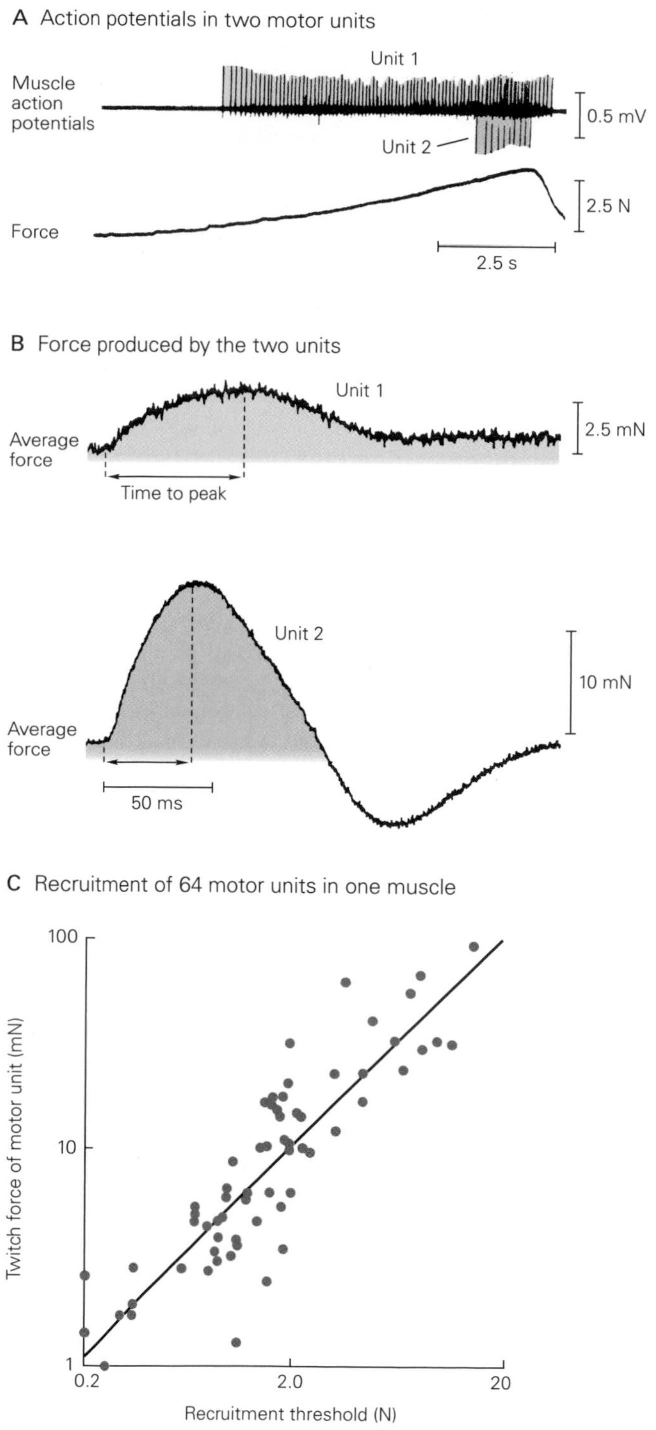

with a load of approximately 33% of maximum. Beyond the upper limit of motor unit recruitment, muscle force can still be increased by varying the rate of action potentials in the motor neurons. Below the upper limit of recruitment, the rate of firing can also be varied in addition to increasing the number of active motor units (Figure 34–6). In fact, beneath the upper recruitment limit variation in discharge rate can have the greater influence on muscle force.

The Input–Output Properties of Motor Neurons Are Modified by Input from the Brain Stem

The discharge rate of motor neurons depends on the magnitude of the depolarization generated by excitatory inputs and the intrinsic membrane properties of the motor neurons in the spinal cord. These properties can be profoundly modified by input from monoaminergic neurons in the brain stem. In the absence of this input, the dendrites of motor neurons passively transmit synaptic current to the cell body, resulting in a modest depolarization that immediately ceases when the input stops. Under these conditions the relation between input current and discharge rate is linear over a wide range.

The input–output relation becomes nonlinear, however, when the monoamines serotonin and norepinephrine activate L-type Ca^{2+} channels on the dendrites of the motor neurons. The resulting inward Ca^{2+} currents can enhance synaptic currents by five- to tenfold (Figure 34–7). In an active motor neuron this enhanced current can sustain an elevated discharge rate after a brief depolarizing input, a behavior known as *self-sustained firing*. A subsequent brief inhibitory

Figure 34–4 Motor units that exert low forces are recruited before those that exert greater forces. (Adapted, with permission, from Desmedt and Godaux 1977 and from Milner-Brown, Stein, and Yemm 1973.)

A. Action potentials in two motor units were recorded concurrently with a single intramuscular electrode while the subject gradually increased muscle force. Motor unit 1 began discharging action potentials near the beginning of the voluntary contraction, and its discharge rate increased during the contraction. Motor unit 2 began discharging action potentials near the end of the contraction.

B. Average twitch forces for motor units 1 and 2 as extracted with an averaging procedure during the voluntary contraction.

C. The plot shows the forces at which 64 motor units in a hand muscle of one person were recruited (recruitment threshold) during a voluntary contraction versus the twitch forces of the motor units.

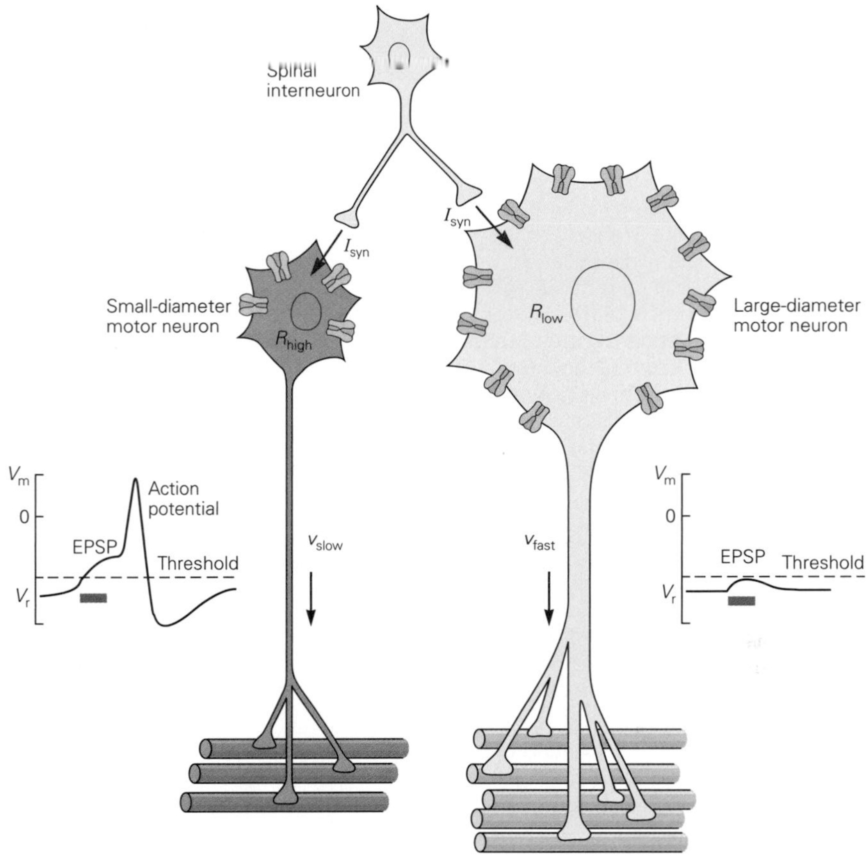

Figure 34–5 The response of a motor neuron to synaptic input depends on its size. Two motor neurons of different sizes have the same resting membrane potential (V_r) and receive the same excitatory synaptic current (I_{syn}) from a spinal interneuron. Because the small motor neuron has a smaller surface area, it has fewer parallel ion channels and therefore a higher resistance (R_{high}). According to Ohm's law ($V = IR$), I_{syn} in the small neuron produces a large excitatory postsynaptic potential (EPSP) that reaches threshold, resulting in the discharge of an action potential. The small motor neuron has a small-diameter axon that conducts the action potential at a low velocity (v_{slow}) to fewer muscle fibers. In contrast, the large motor neuron has a larger surface area, which results in a lower transmembrane resistance (R_{low}) and a smaller EPSP that does not reach threshold in response to I_{syn}.

input at a low velocity returns the discharge rate to its original value.

Because the properties of motor neurons are strongly influenced by monoamines, the excitability of the pool of motor neurons innervating a single muscle is under control of the brain stem. Moderate monoaminergic input to the motor neurons of slow contracting motor units promotes self-sustained firing. This is probably the source of the sustained force exerted by slower motor units to maintain posture. During sleep,

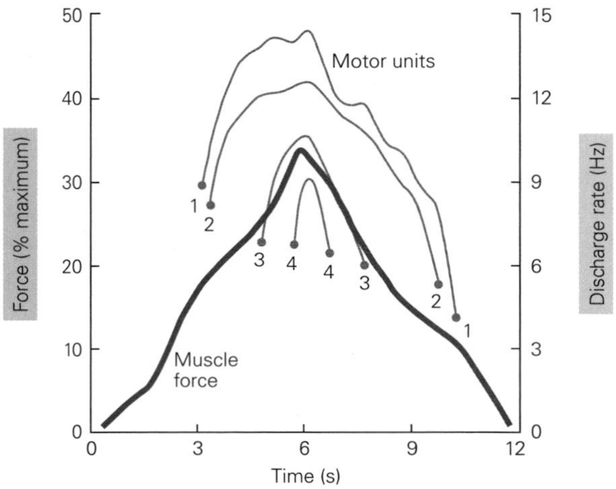

Figure 34–6 Muscle force can be adjusted by varying the number of active motor units and their discharge rate. A gradual increase and then a decrease in the force (**blue line**) exerted by the knee extensor muscles involved the concurrent activation of four (out of many) motor units. The muscle force was changed by varying both the number of motor units that were active and the rate at which the motor neurons discharged action potentials. Motor unit 1 was activated when muscle force reached 20% of maximum. Initially the motor neuron discharged action potentials at a rate of 9 Hz. As force increased, the discharge rate increased up to 15 Hz, when both the force and discharge rate declined, and the motor unit was inactivated at 14% of maximal force. Motor units 2, 3, and 4 were activated at greater forces but discharge rate was modulated similarly. (Reproduced, with permission, from Person and Kudina 1972.)

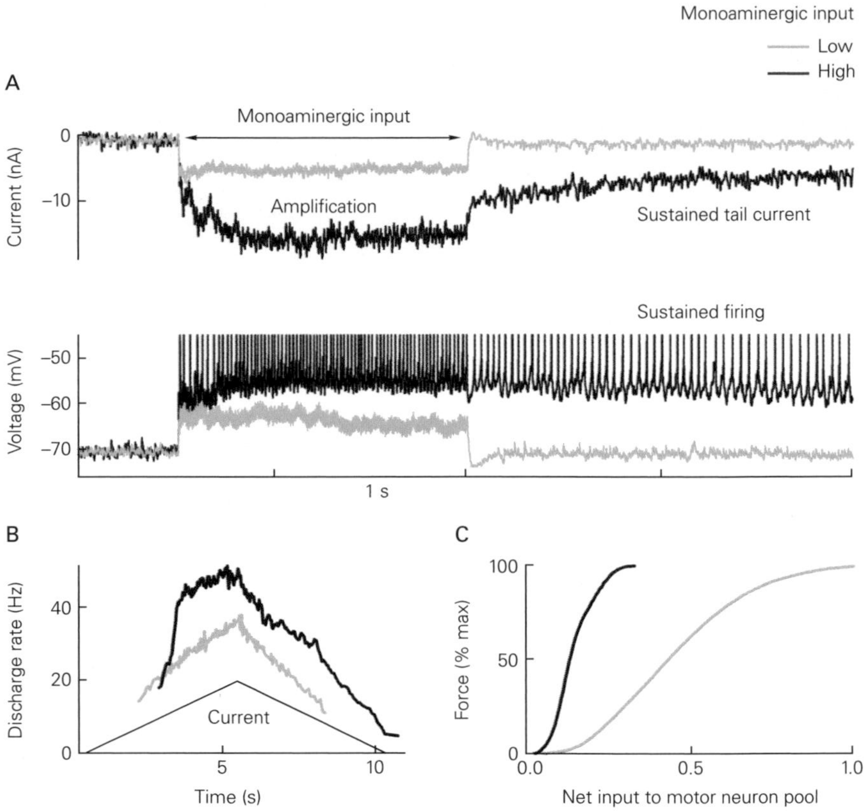

Figure 34–7 Effects of monoaminergic input on motor neurons. (Data from C. J. Heckman.)

A. Membrane currents and potentials in spinal motor neurons of adult cats that were either deeply anesthetized (low monoaminergic drive) or decerebrate (moderate monoaminergic drive). When monoaminergic input is absent or low, a brief excitatory input produces an equally brief synaptic current during voltage clamp (**upper record**). This current is not sufficient to bring the membrane potential of the cell to threshold for discharging action potentials (**lower record**). During high levels of monoaminergic input the same brief excitatory input activates a persistent inward current in the dendrites, which amplifies the synaptic current and generates a long-lasting tail current (**upper record**). This persistent inward current causes a high discharge rate during the input and the tail current sustains the discharge after the input ceases (**lower record**). A brief inhibition will return the cell to the resting state.

B. With high levels of monoaminergic input the persistent inward current produces a much higher discharge rate for a given amount of current.

C. When the entire motor pool innervating a muscle is considered, the monoamine-induced increase in the rate of motor neuron discharge produces a much larger force for a given amount of input and maximal force is achieved with less input to the motor neuron pool.

when monoaminergic drive is withdrawn, excitability decreases, thus helping to ensure a relaxed motor state. Monoaminergic input from the brain stem can adjust the gain of the motor unit pool to suit the demands of different tasks. This flexibility does not compromise the size principle of orderly recruitment because the threshold for activation of the persistent inward currents is lowest in the motor neurons of slower motor units, which are the first recruited even in the absence of monoamines.

Muscle Force Depends on the Structure of Muscle

Muscle force depends not only on the amount of motor unit activity but also on the arrangement of the fibers in the muscle. Because movement involves the controlled variation of muscle force, the nervous system must take into account the structure of muscle to achieve specific movements.

The Sarcomere Contains the Contractile Proteins

Individual muscles contain thousands of fibers that vary from 1 to 500 mm in length and from 10 to 60 μm in diameter. The variation in fiber dimensions reflects differences in the quantity of contractile protein. Despite this quantitative variation, the organization of contractile proteins is similar in all muscle fibers. The proteins are arranged in repeating sets of thick and thin filaments, each set known as a *sarcomere* (Figure 34–8). The physiological length of a sarcomere, which is bounded by Z disks, ranges from 1.5 μm to 3.5 μm. Sarcomeres are arranged in series to form a *myofibril,* and the myofibrils are aligned in parallel to form a muscle fiber.

The force that each sarcomere can generate arises from the interaction of the contractile thick and thin filaments. The thick filament consists of a few hundred myosin molecules arranged in a structured sequence. Each myosin molecule comprises paired coiled-coil domains that terminate in two globular heads. The myosin molecules in the two halves of a thick filament point in opposite directions and are progressively displaced so that the heads, which extend away from the filament, protrude from the entire thick filament (Figure 34–8C). To maximize the interaction between the globular heads and the thin filaments, six thin filaments surround each thick filament.

The primary components of the thin filament are two helical strands of fibrous F-actin, each of which contains approximately 200 actin monomers. Superimposed on F-actin are tropomyosin and troponin, proteins that control the interaction between actin and myosin. Tropomyosin consists of two coiled strands that lie in the groove of the F-actin helix; troponin is a small molecular complex that is attached to tropomyosin at regular intervals (Figure 34–8C).

The thin filaments are anchored to the Z disk at each end of the sarcomere, whereas the thick filaments occupy the middle of the sarcomere (Figure 34–8B). This organization accounts for the alternating light and dark bands of striated muscle (Figure 34–8A). The light band contains only thin filaments, whereas the dark band contains both thick and thin filaments. When a muscle is activated, the width of the light band decreases, but the width of the dark band does not change, suggesting that the thick and thin filaments slide relative to one another during a contraction. This led to the *sliding filament hypothesis* of muscle contraction proposed by A. F. Huxley and H. E. Huxley in the 1950s.

The sliding of the thick and thin filaments is triggered by the release of Ca^{2+} within the sarcoplasm of a muscle fiber in response to an action potential at the fiber's membrane, the sarcolemma. Varying the amount of Ca^{2+} in the sarcoplasm controls the interaction between the thick and thin filaments. Under resting conditions the Ca^{2+} concentration in the sarcoplasm is kept low by active pumping of Ca^{2+} into the sarcoplasmic reticulum, a network of longitudinal tubules and chambers of smooth endoplasmic reticulum (Figure 34–8A). Calcium is stored in the terminal cisternae, which are located next to intracellular extensions of the sarcolemma known as transverse tubules. The transverse tubules, terminal cisternae, and sarcoplasmic reticulum constitute an activation system that transforms an action potential into the sliding of the filaments.

As an action potential propagates along the sarcolemma it invades the transverse tubules and causes the rapid release of Ca^{2+} from the terminal cisternae into the sarcoplasm. Once in the sarcoplasm Ca^{2+} diffuses among the filaments and binds reversibly to troponin, which results in the displacement of the troponin-tropomyosin complex and activates the sliding of the thick and thin filaments. Because a single action potential is insufficient to release enough Ca^{2+} to bind all available troponin sites in skeletal muscle, the strength of a contraction increases with the action potential rate.

The sliding of the filaments depends on mechanical work performed by the globular heads of myosin, work that uses chemical energy contained in adenosine triphosphate (ATP). The actions of the myosin heads are regulated by the *cross bridge cycle,* a sequence of detachment, activation, and attachment (Figure 34–9). In each cycle a globular head undergoes a displacement of 5 to 10 nm. Contractile activity continues as long as Ca^{2+} and ATP are present in the cytoplasm in sufficient amounts.

Noncontractile Elements Provide Essential Structural Support

Structural elements of the muscle fiber maintain the alignment of the contractile proteins within the fiber and facilitate the transmission of force from the sarcomeres to the skeleton. A network of proteins (nebulin, titin) maintains the orientation of the thick and thin filaments within the sarcomere, whereas other proteins (desmin, skelemins) constrain the lateral alignment of the myofibrils (Figure 34–8B). These proteins contribute to the elasticity of muscle and maintain the appropriate alignment of cellular structures when the muscle is loaded.

Although some of the force generated by the cross bridges is transmitted along the sarcomeres in series, some travels laterally from the thin filaments to an extracellular matrix that surrounds each muscle fiber, through a group of transmembrane and membrane-associated proteins called a *costamere* (Figure 34–8B). The lateral transmission of force follows two pathways through the costamere, one through a dystrophin-glycoprotein complex and the other through vinculin and members of the integrin family. Mutations of genes that encode components of the dystrophin-glycoprotein complex cause muscular dystrophies in humans.

Contractile Force Depends on Muscle Fiber Activation, Length, and Velocity

The force that a muscle fiber can exert depends on the number of cross bridges formed and the force

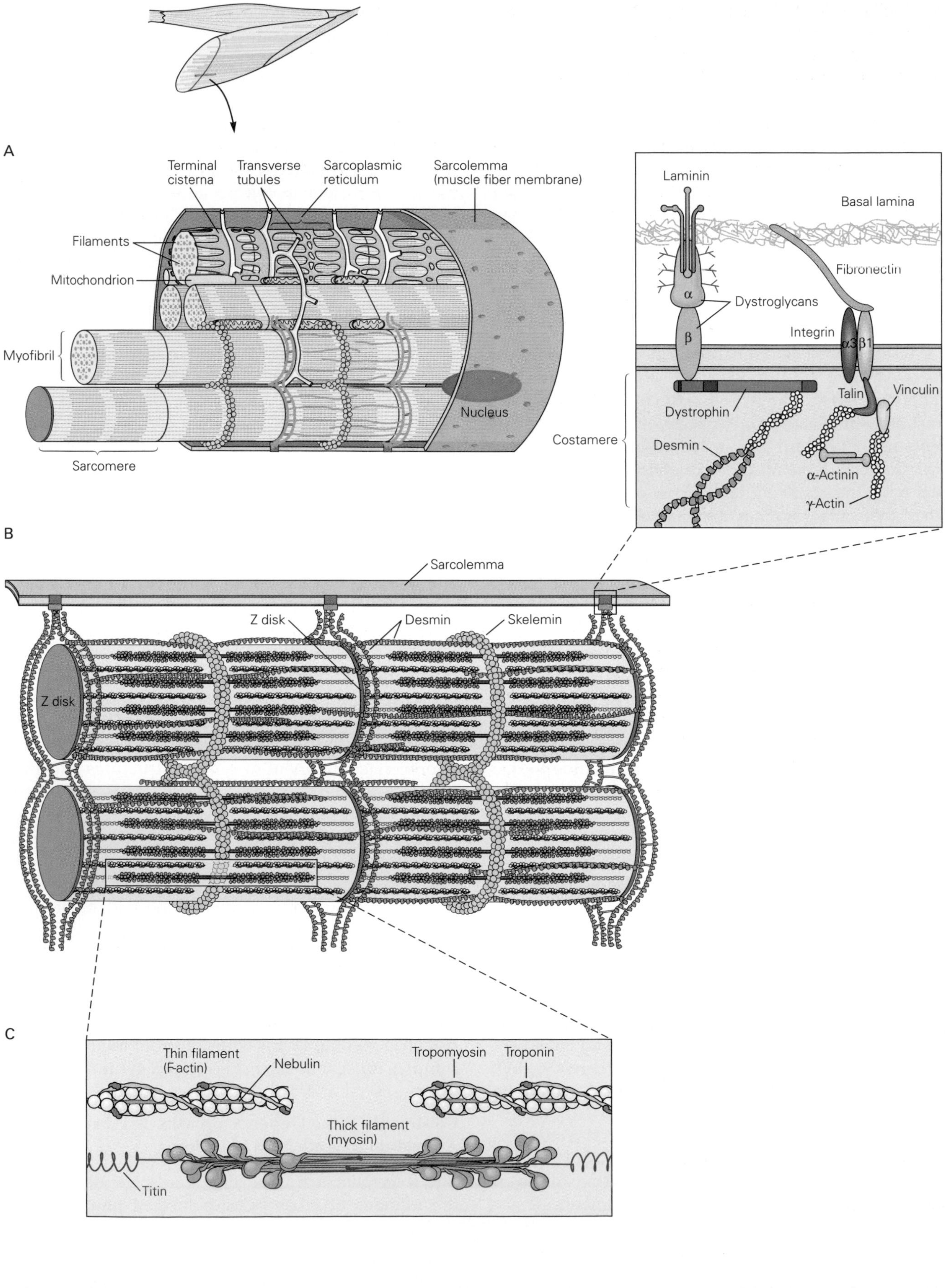
A
Terminal cisterna
Transverse tubules
Sarcoplasmic reticulum
Sarcolemma (muscle fiber membrane)
Filaments
Mitochondrion
Myofibril
Sarcomere
Nucleus
Laminin
Basal lamina
Fibronectin
α
β
Dystroglycans
Integrin
α3β1
Talin
Vinculin
Dystrophin
Costamere
Desmin
α-Actinin
γ-Actin
B
Sarcolemma
Z disk
Desmin
Skelemin
Z disk
C
Thin filament (F-actin)
Nebulin
Tropomyosin
Troponin
Thick filament (myosin)
Titin

produced by each cross bridge. These two factors are influenced by the Ca^{2+} concentration in the sarcoplasm, the amount of overlap between the thick and thin filaments, and the velocity with which the thick and thin filaments slide past one another. The influx of Ca^{2+} that activates formation of the cross bridges is transitory because continuous pump activity quickly returns Ca^{2+} to the sarcoplasmic reticulum. The release and reuptake of Ca^{2+} in response to a single action potential occurs so quickly that only some of the potential cross bridges are formed. This explains why the peak force of a twitch is less than the maximal force of the muscle fiber (see Figure 34–2A). Maximal force can be achieved only with a series of action potentials that sustains the Ca^{2+} concentration in the sarcoplasm, thus maximizing cross bridge formation.

Although Ca^{2+} activates formation of the cross bridges, cross bridges can be formed only when the thick and thin filaments overlap. This overlap varies as the filaments slide relative to one another (Figure 34–10A). At an intermediate sarcomere length (L_o) the amount of overlap between actin and myosin is optimal, and the relative force is maximal. Increases in sarcomere length reduce the overlap between actin and myosin and the force that can be developed. Decreases in sarcomere length cause the thin filaments to overlap, reducing the number of binding sites available to the myosin heads. Although many muscles operate over a narrow range of sarcomere lengths (approximately 94 ± 13% L_o, mean ± SD), among muscles there is considerable diversity in sarcomere lengths during movement.

Because structures that connect the contractile proteins to the skeleton also influence the force that a muscle can exert, muscle force increases with length over its operating range. This property enables muscle to function like a spring and to resist changes in length. Muscle stiffness, which corresponds to the slope of the relation between muscle force and muscle length (N/m), depends on the structure of the muscle. A stiffer muscle, like a stronger spring, is more resistant to changes in length.

Once activated, cross bridges perform work and cause the thick and thin filaments to slide relative to one another. Because of the elasticity of intermediate-length filaments and the extracellular matrix, sarcomeres can shorten even when the length of the muscle fiber is held fixed. The direction and rate of change in sarcomere length depend on the amount of force relative to the magnitude of the load against which the sarcomere acts. Sarcomere length decreases when the force exceeds the load (*shortening contraction*) but increases when the force is less than the load (*lengthening contraction*). The maximal force that a muscle fiber can exert decreases as shortening velocity increases but increases as lengthening velocity increases (Figure 34–10B).

The maximal rate at which a muscle fiber can shorten is limited by the peak rate at which cross bridges can form. The variation in fiber force as contraction velocity changes is largely caused by differences in the average force exerted by each cross bridge. For example, the decrease in force during a shortening contraction is attributable to a reduction in cross bridge displacement during each power stroke and the failure of some myosin heads to find attachment sites. Conversely, the increase in force during a lengthening contraction reflects the stretching of incompletely activated sarcomeres and the more rapid reattachment of cross bridges after they have been pulled apart.

The rate of cross bridge cycling not only depends on contraction velocity, but also on the preceding activity of the muscle. For example, after a brief isometric contraction the rate increases. When a muscle is stretched while in this state, such as would occur

Figure 34–8 (Opposite) **The sarcomere is the basic functional unit of muscle.** (Adapted, with permission, from Bloom and Fawcett 1975 and from Patel and Lieber 1997.)

A. This section of a muscle fiber shows its anatomical organization. Several myofibrils lie side-by-side in a fiber, and each myofibril is made up of sarcomeres arranged end-to-end and separated by Z disks (see part B). The myofibrils are surrounded by an activation system that includes the transverse tubules, terminal cisternae, and sarcoplasmic reticulum.

B. Sarcomeres are connected to one another and to the muscle fiber membrane by the cytoskeletal lattice. The cytoskeleton influences the length of the contractile thick and thin filaments, maintains the alignment of these filaments within a sarcomere, connects adjacent myofibrils, and transmits force to the extracellular matrix of connective tissue through costameres. One consequence of this organization is that the force exerted by the contractile elements in a sarcomere can be transmitted along and across sarcomeres (through desmin and skelemin), within and between sarcomeres (through nebulin and titin), and to the costameres. The Z disk is a focal point for many of these connections.

C. The thick and thin filaments consist of various contractile proteins. The thin filament includes polymerized actin along with the regulatory proteins tropomyosin and troponin. The thick filament is an array of myosin molecules; each molecule includes a stem that terminates in a double globular head, which extends away from the filament.

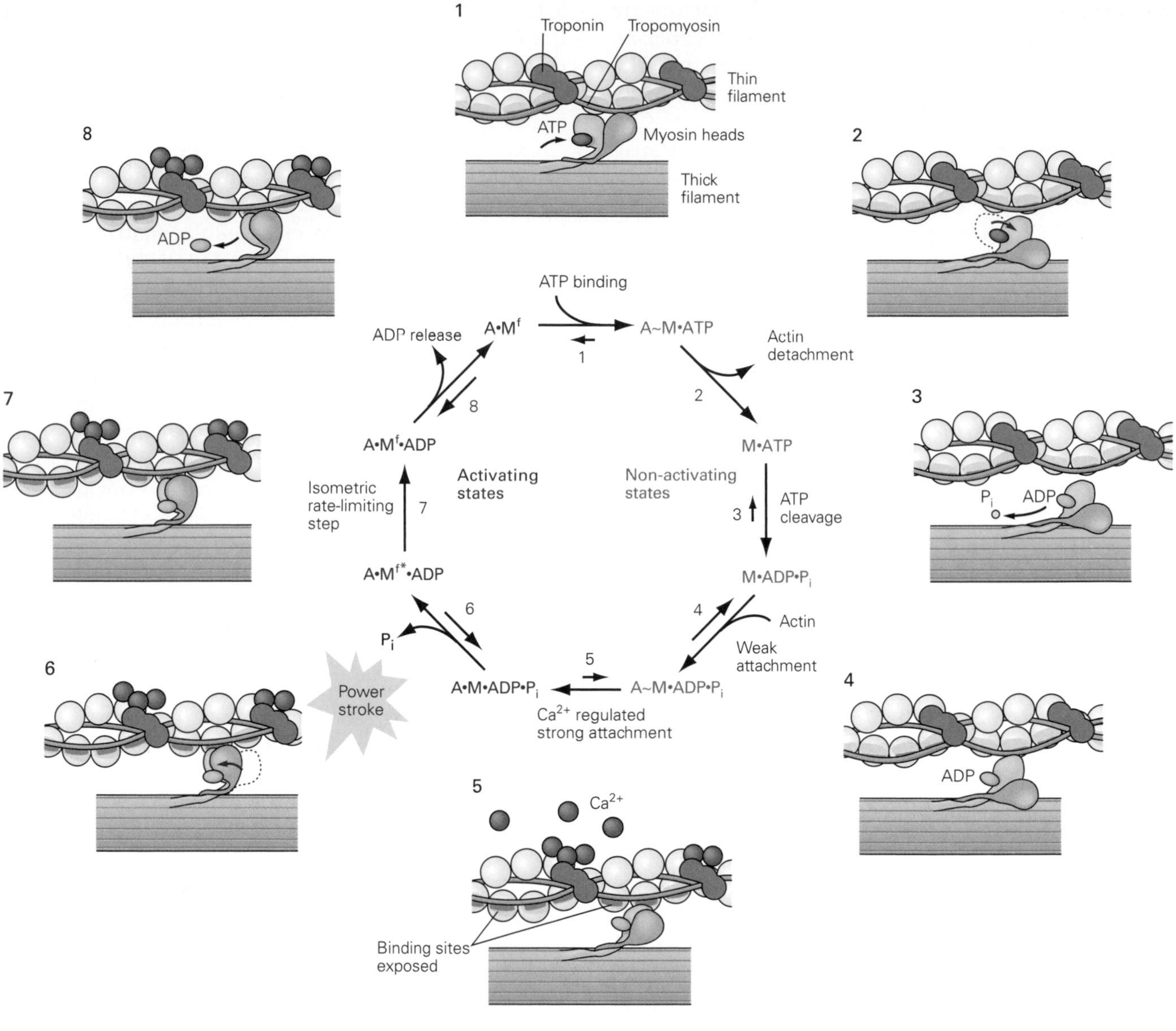

Figure 34–9 The cross bridge cycle. Several nonactivating states are followed by several activating states triggered by Ca^{2+}. The cycle begins at the top (**step 1**) with the binding of adenosine triphosphate (ATP) to the myosin head. The myosin head detaches from actin (**step 2**), ATP is hydrolyzed to phosphate (P_i) and ADP (**step 3**), and the myosin becomes weakly bound to actin (**step 4**). The binding of Ca^{2+} to troponin causes tropomyosin to slide over actin and enables the two myosin heads to close (**step 5**). This results in the release of P_i and the extension of the myosin neck, the power stroke of the cross bridge cycle (**step 6**). Each cross bridge exerts a force of about 2 pN during a structural change (**step 7**) and the release of adenosine diphosphate (ADP) (**step 8**). (**•**, strong binding; ~, weak binding; $\mathbf{M^f}$, cross bridge force of myosin; and $\mathbf{M^{f}*}$, force-bearing state of myosin.) (Adapted, with permission, from Gordon, Regnier, and Homsher 2001.)

during a postural disturbance, muscle stiffness is enhanced, and the muscle is more effective at resisting the change in length. This property is known as *short-range stiffness*. Conversely, the cross bridge cycling rate decreases after shortening contractions, and the muscle does not exhibit short-range stiffness.

Muscle Torque Depends on Musculoskeletal Geometry

The anatomy of a muscle has a pronounced effect on its force capacity, range of motion, and shortening velocity. The anatomical features that influence function include

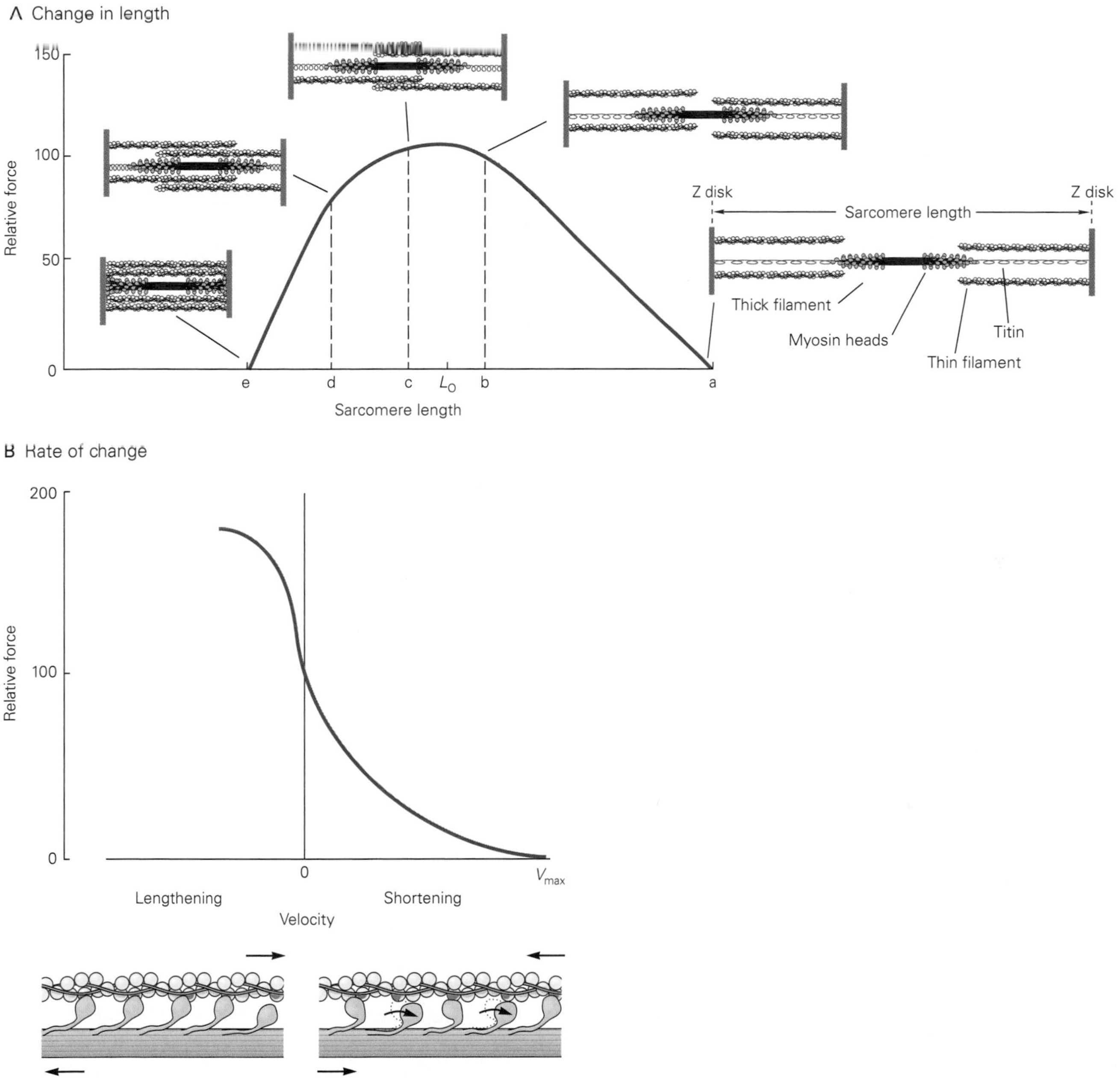

Figure 34–10 Contractile force varies with the change in sarcomere length and velocity.

A. Change in length. At an intermediate sarcomere length, L_o, the amount of overlap between actin and myosin is optimal and the relative force is maximal. When the sarcomere is stretched beyond the length at which the thick and thin filaments overlap (length **a**), cross bridges cannot form and no force is exerted. As sarcomere length decreases and the overlap of the thick and thin filaments increases (between lengths **a** and **b**), the force increases because the number of cross bridges increases. With further reductions in length (between lengths **c** and **e**) the extreme overlap of the thin filaments with each other occludes potential attachment sites and the force decreases.

B. Rate of change. Contractile force varies with the rate of change in sarcomere length. Relative to the force that a sarcomere can exert during an isometric contraction (zero velocity), the peak force declines as the rate of shortening increases. At the maximal shortening velocity (V_{max}) muscle force reaches a minimum. In contrast, when the sarcomere is lengthened while being activated, the peak force increases to values greater than those during an isometric contraction. Shortening causes the myosin heads to spend more time near the end of their power stroke, where they produce less contractile force, and more time detaching, recocking, and reattaching, during which they produce no force. When the muscle is actively lengthened the myosin heads spend more time stretched beyond their angle of attachment and little time unattached because they do not need to be recocked after being pulled away from the actin in this manner.

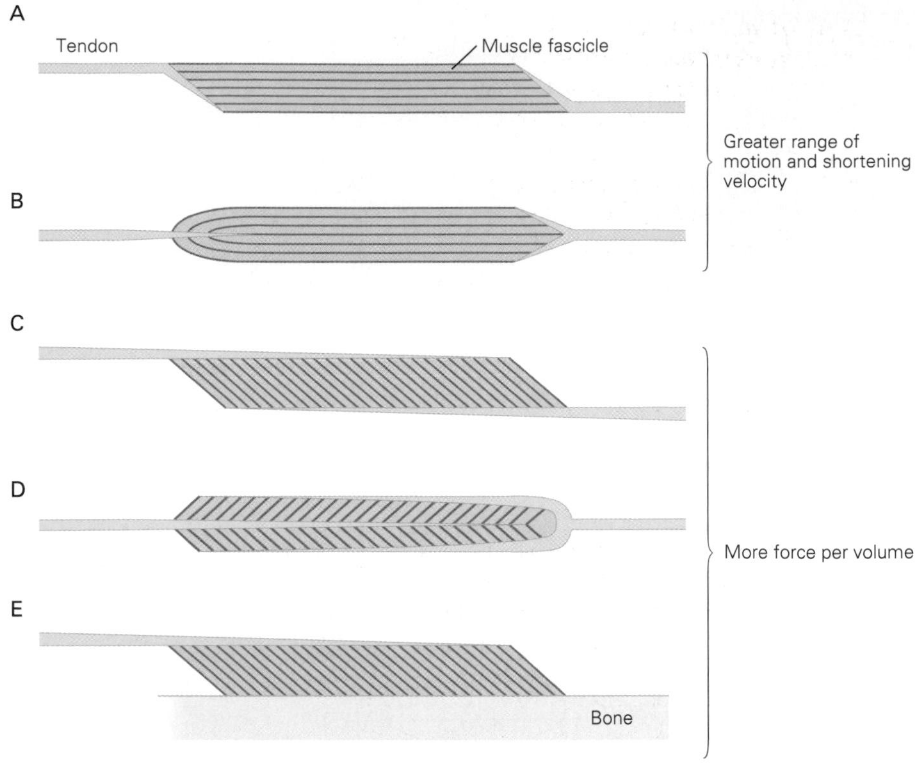

Figure 34–11 Five common arrangements of tendon and muscle. (Reproduced, with permission, from Alexander and Ker 1990.)

the arrangement of the sarcomeres in each muscle fiber, the organization of the muscle fibers within the muscle, and the location of the muscle on the skeleton. These features vary widely among muscles (Figure 34–11).

At the level of the single muscle fiber the number of sarcomeres in series and in parallel can vary. The number of sarcomeres in series determines the length of the myofibril and thus the length of the muscle fiber. Because one sarcomere can shorten by a certain length with a given maximal velocity, both the range of motion and the maximal shortening velocity of a muscle fiber are proportional to the number of sarcomeres in series. The force that a myofibril can exert is equal to the average sarcomere force and is not influenced by the number of sarcomeres in series. The force capacity of a fiber, however, depends on the number of sarcomeres in parallel and hence on the diameter or cross-sectional area of the fiber.

At the level of the muscle, the functional attributes of the fibers are modified by the orientation of the fascicles to the line of pull of the muscle and the length of the fiber relative to the muscle length. In most muscles the fascicles are not parallel to the line of pull but fan out in feather-like (pennate) arrangements (Figure 34–11). The relative orientation, or pennation angle of the fascicles, ranges from 0 degrees (biceps brachii, sartorius) to approximately 30 degrees (soleus). Because more fibers can fit into a given volume as the pennation angle increases, muscles with large pennation angles typically have more myofibrils in parallel and hence large cross-sectional areas. Given the linear relation between cross-sectional area and maximal force ($\sim 0.25\ \text{N}\cdot\text{mm}^{-2}$), these muscles are capable of a greater maximal force. However, the fibers in pennate muscles are generally short and have a lesser maximal shortening velocity than those in nonpennate muscles.

The functional consequences of this anatomical arrangement can be seen by comparing the contractile properties of two muscles with different numbers of fibers and fiber lengths. If the two muscles have identical fiber lengths, but one has twice as many fibers, the range of motion of the two muscles will be similar because it is a function of fiber length, but the maximal force capacity will vary in proportion to the number of muscle fibers. If the two muscles have identical numbers of fibers but the fibers in one muscle are twice as long, the muscle with the longer fibers will have a greater range of motion and a greater maximal shortening velocity, even though the two muscles have a similar force capacity. Because of this effect, the muscle with longer fibers is able to exert more force and produce more power (the product of force and velocity) at a given absolute shortening velocity (Figure 34–12).

Muscle fiber lengths and cross-sectional areas vary substantially throughout the human body, which suggests that the contractile properties of individual muscles also differ markedly. In the leg, for example, fiber length ranges from 20 mm (soleus) to 460 mm (sartorius), and cross-sectional area ranges from 200 mm^2 (sartorius) to 5,800 mm^2 (soleus). Functionally coupled muscles tend to have complementary combinations of these properties. For example, muscles characterized by large pennation angles, large cross-sectional areas, and short fibers (quadriceps femoris) are often functionally coupled with those that have smaller cross-sectional areas and longer fibers (hamstrings).

Movement is the muscle-controlled rotation of adjacent body segments, which means that the capacity of a muscle to contribute to a movement also depends on its location relative to the joint that it spans. The rotary force exerted by a muscle about a joint is referred to as *muscle torque* and is calculated as the product of the muscle force and the *moment arm*, the shortest perpendicular distance from the line of pull of the muscle to the joint's center (Figure 34–13).

The moment arm usually changes as a joint rotates through its range of motion; the amount of change depends on where the muscle is attached to the skeleton relative to the joint. If the force exerted by a muscle remains relatively constant throughout the joint's range of motion, muscle torque varies in direct proportion to the change in the moment arm. For many muscles the moment arm is maximal in the middle of the range of motion, which usually corresponds to the position of maximal muscle force and hence greatest muscle torque.

Different Movements Require Different Activation Strategies

The human body has approximately 600 muscles, each with a distinct torque profile about one or more joints. To perform a desired movement the nervous system must activate an appropriate combination of muscles with adequate intensity and timing of activity. The activation must be appropriate for the contractile properties and musculoskeletal geometry of many muscles, as well as the mechanical interactions between body segments. As a result of these demands, activation strategies differ with the details of the movement.

Contraction Velocity Can Vary in Magnitude and Direction

Movement speed depends on the contraction velocity of a muscle. The only ways to vary contraction velocity are to alter either the number of motor units recruited or the rates at which they discharge action potentials. The velocity of a contraction can vary in both magnitude and direction (see Figure 34–10B). To control the velocity of a contraction the nervous system must scale the magnitude of the net muscle torque relative to the load torque, which includes both the weight of the body segment and any load applied externally to the body.

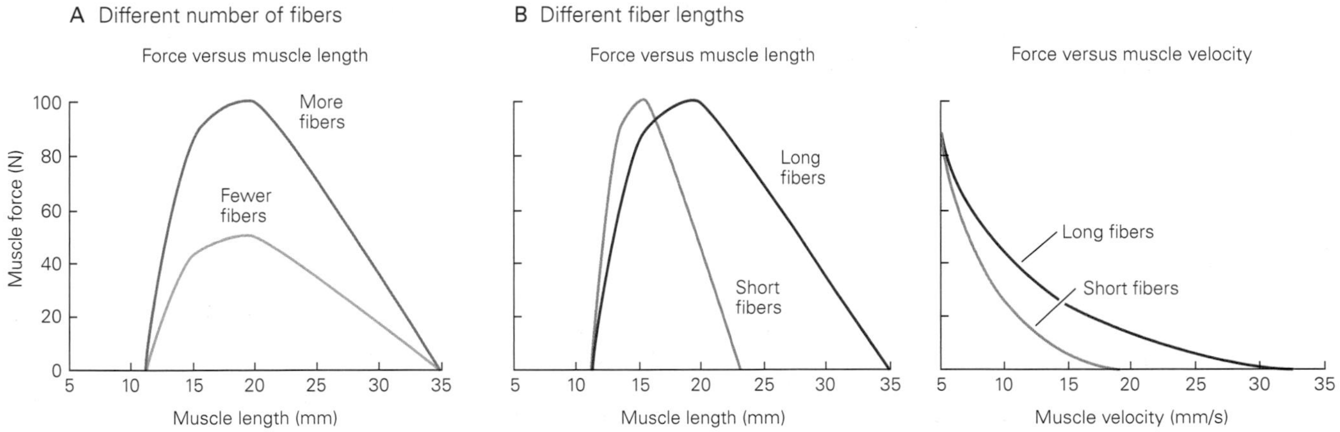

Figure 34–12 Muscle dimensions influence the peak force and maximal shortening velocity. (Reproduced, with permission, from Lieber and Fridén 2000.)

A. Muscle force at various muscle lengths for two muscles with similar fiber lengths but different numbers of muscle fibers (different cross-sectional area). The muscle with twice as many fibers exerts greater force.

B. Muscle force at various muscle lengths for two muscles with the same cross-sectional area but different fiber lengths. The muscle with longer fibers (about twice as long as those of the other muscle) has an increased range of motion (left plot). It also has a greater maximal shortening velocity and exerts greater force at a given absolute velocity (right plot).

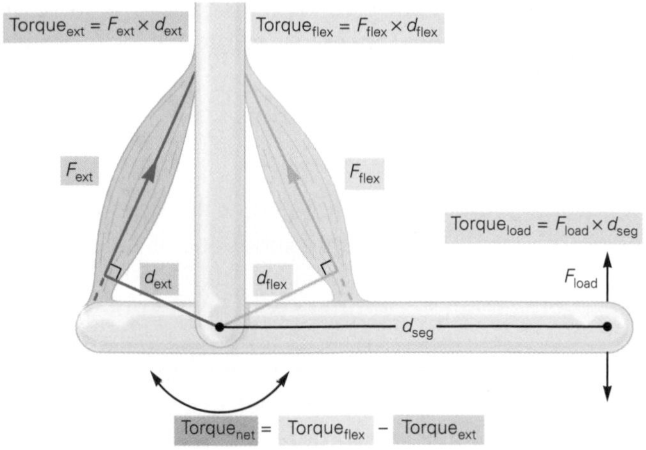

Figure 34–13 Muscle torque varies over a joint's range of motion. A muscle exerts a torque about a joint that is the product of its contractile force (*F*) and its moment arm at the joint (*d*). The moment arm is the shortest perpendicular distance from the line of pull of the muscle to the joint's center of rotation. Because the moment arm changes when the joint rotates, muscle torque varies with angular displacement about the joint. The net torque about a joint, which determines the mechanical action, is the difference in the torques exerted by opposing muscles, such as extensors (ext) and flexors (flex). Similarly, a force applied to the limb (F_{load}) will exert a torque about the joint that depends on F_{load} and its distance from the joint (d_{seg}).

When muscle torque exceeds load torque, the muscle shortens as it performs a shortening contraction. When muscle torque is less than load torque, the muscle lengthens as it performs a lengthening contraction. For the example shown in Figure 34–13, the load is lifted with a shortening contraction of the flexor and lowered with a lengthening contraction. Both types of contractions are common in daily activities.

Shortening and lengthening contractions are not simply the result of adjusting motor unit activity so that the net muscle torque is greater or less than the load torque. When the task involves lifting a load with a prescribed trajectory, activation of the motor units must be aligned so that the summed rise times match the desired trajectory during the shortening contraction, whereas the lengthening contraction requires that the summed decay times be matched. The nervous system accomplishes this by varying the descending input and sensory feedback during the two contractions. Because of these differences, some people, such as older adults and persons performing rehabilitation exercises after an orthopedic procedure, have greater difficulty performing lengthening contractions.

The amount of motor-unit activity relative to the load also influences the contraction velocity. This effect depends on both the number of motor units recruited and the maximal rates at which the motor units can discharge action potentials. For example, the maximal rate of increase in muscle torque during a submaximal contraction increases after several weeks of physical training and is associated with a marked increase in the initial discharge rates of the activated motor units. Physical training increases the rate at which motor units can discharge trains of action potentials, an effect that can be mimicked by the rapid injection of current into a motor neuron. Changes in the maximal shortening velocity of a muscle after a change in the habitual level of physical activity are the result, at least partly, of factors that influence the ability of motor units to discharge action potentials at high rates.

Movements Involve the Coordination of Many Muscles

To achieve a prescribed trajectory the nervous system must activate not only the muscles that produce the desired displacement but also muscles that prevent unintended actions. For example, the elbow flexor muscles are used to rapidly rotate the forearm about the elbow joint. But unless the muscles that cross the wrist are also activated to stabilize the wrist joint, rotation of the forearm would cause the hand to flail about the wrist joint.

In the simplest case muscles span a single joint and cause the attached body segments to accelerate about a single axis of rotation (Figure 34–14A). Because muscles can exert only a pulling force, motion about a single axis of rotation requires at least two muscles or groups of muscles. Thus, the flexion-extension motion about the knee joint involves the hamstring muscles to exert force in the direction of flexion and the quadriceps to exert force in the direction of extension.

However, many muscles attach to the skeleton slightly off center and can cause movement about more than one axis of rotation. If one of the actions is not required, the nervous system must activate other muscles to control the unwanted movement. For example, activation of the radial flexor muscle of the wrist can cause the wrist to flex and abduct. If the intended action is only wrist flexion, then the abduction action must be opposed by another muscle, such as the ulnar flexor muscle, which causes wrist flexion and adduction. Depending on the geometry of the articulating surfaces and the attachment sites of the muscles, the multiple muscles that span a joint are capable of producing movements about one to three axes of rotation. Furthermore, some structures can be displaced linearly (eg, the scapula on the trunk), adding to the degrees of freedom about a joint.

This organization enhances the flexibility of the skeletal motor system, for the same movement can be achieved by activating different combinations of muscles. However, this additional flexibility comes with a cost in the corresponding variation in the unwanted actions that must be controlled. A solution used by the nervous system is to organize relations among selected muscles to produce specific actions. A particular balance of muscle activations that changes over time is known as a *muscle synergy*, and movement is produced through the coordinated activation of these synergies. For example, electromyographic recordings suggest that a range of human movements, such as grasping objects with the hand, reaching and pointing in different directions, and walking and running at several speeds, are controlled by approximately five muscle synergies.

The number of muscles that participate in a movement also varies with the speed of the movement. For example, slow lifting of the load shown in Figure 34–13 requires only that the muscle torque slightly exceed the load torque, and thus only the flexor muscle is activated. This strategy is used when lifting a handheld weight with the elbow flexor muscles. In contrast, to perform this movement rapidly with an abrupt termination, both the flexor and extensor muscles must be activated. First the flexor muscle is activated to accelerate the limb in the direction of flexion, followed by activation of the extensor muscle to accelerate the limb in the direction of extension, and finally a burst of activity by the flexor muscle to reduce the angular momentum of the limb and the handheld weight in the direction of flexion so that it arrives at the desired joint angle (Figure 34–14B). The amount of extensor activity increases with the speed of the movement.

Increases in movement speed introduce another factor that the nervous system must control: unwanted accelerations in other body segments. Because body segments are interconnected, motion in one segment can induce motion in another. At the beginning of the swing phase in running, for example, the hip flexor muscles are activated and accelerate the thigh in a forward direction (Figure 34–15A). The motion of the thigh causes the lower leg to rotate backward about the knee joint. To control the backward displacement

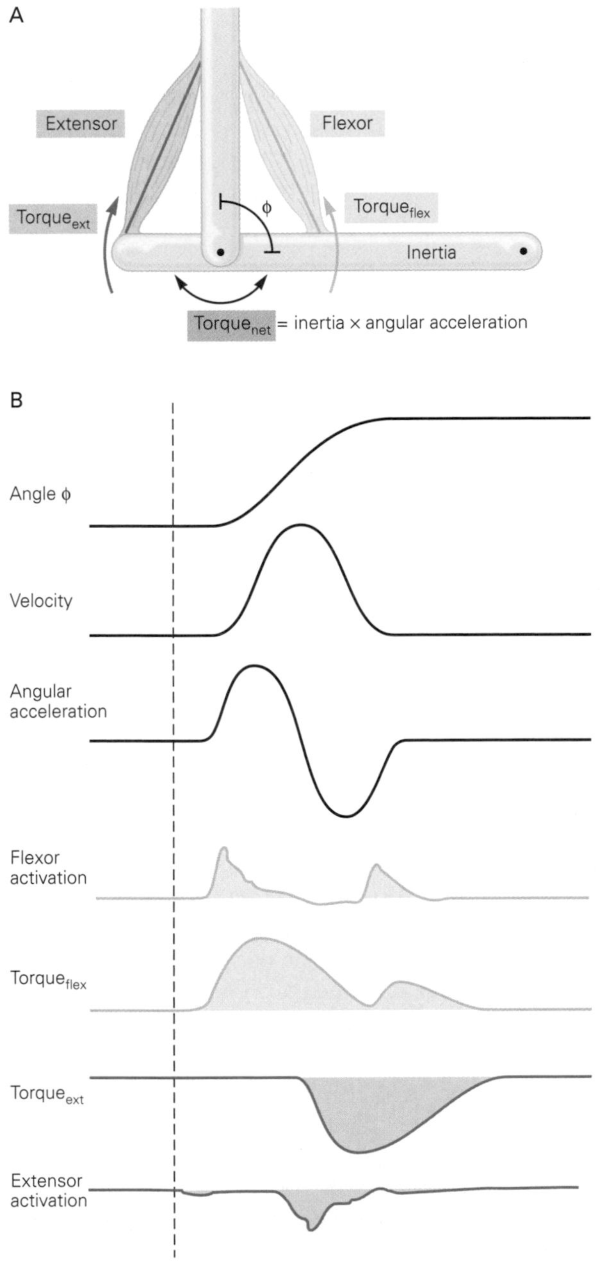

Figure 34–14 Muscle torque must overcome inertia when a movement is started and stopped.

A. According to Newton's law of acceleration (force = mass × acceleration), force is required to change the velocity of a mass. Muscles exert a torque to accelerate the inertial mass of the skeletal segment around a joint. For angular motion, Newton's law is written as torque = rotational inertia × angular acceleration.

B. The angular velocity for movement of a limb from one position to another has a bell-shaped profile reflecting Newton's law of acceleration. Acceleration in one direction is followed by acceleration in the opposite direction—the flexor and extensor muscles are activated in succession. The records here show the activation profiles and associated muscle torques for an elbow flexion movement. Because contractile force decays relatively slowly, the flexor muscle is usually activated a second time to counter the prolonged acceleration generated by the extensor muscle and to stop the limb exactly on target.

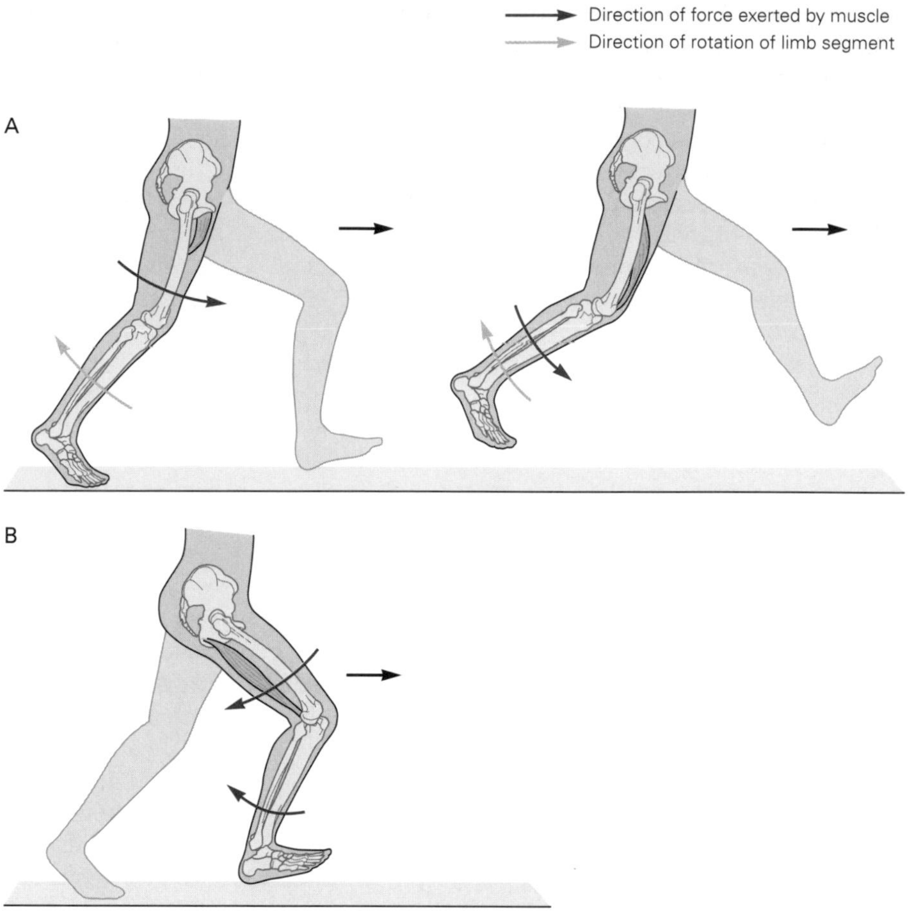

Figure 34–15 A single muscle can influence the motion about many joints.

A. Muscles that cross one joint can accelerate an adjacent body segment. For example, at the beginning of the swing phase while running, the hip flexor muscles are activated to accelerate the thigh forward (**red arrow**). This action causes the lower leg to rotate backward (**blue arrow**) and the knee joint to flex. To control the knee joint flexion during the first part of the swing phase, the knee extensor muscles are activated and undergo a lengthening contraction to accelerate the lower leg forward (**red arrow**) while it continues to rotate backward (**blue arrow**).

B. Many muscles cross more than one joint to exert an effect on more than one body segment. For example, the hamstring muscles of the leg accelerate the hip in the direction of extension and the knee in the direction of flexion (**red arrows**). At the end of the swing phase during running, the hamstring muscles are activated and undergo lengthening contractions to control the forward rotation of the leg (hip flexion and knee extension). This strategy is more economical than activating individual muscles at the hip and knee joints to control the forward rotation of the leg.

of the lower leg, the quadriceps muscles are activated to accelerate the lower leg in the forward direction. As the lower leg rotates backward, the quadriceps muscles perform a lengthening contraction that becomes a shortening contraction to rotate the lower leg forward in the middle of the swing phase.

Muscles that span more than one joint can be used to control the motion-dependent interactions between body segments. At the end of the swing phase in running, activation of the hamstring muscles causes both the thigh and lower leg to accelerate backward (Figure 34–15B). If a hip extensor muscle was used to accelerate the thigh backward instead of the hamstring muscles, the lower leg would accelerate forward, requiring activation of a knee flexor muscle to control the unwanted motion so that the foot could be placed on the ground. Use of the two-joint hamstring muscles is a more economical strategy, but one that can subject the hamstrings to high stresses during fast movements, such as sprinting. The control of such motion-dependent interactions often involves lengthening contractions, which maximize muscle stiffness and the ability of muscle to resist changes in length.

For most movements the nervous system must establish rigid connections between some body segments for two reasons. First, as expressed in Newton's law of action and reaction, a reaction force must provide a foundation for the acceleration of a body segment. For example, in a reaching movement performed by a person standing upright, the ground must provide a reaction force against the feet. The muscle actions that produce the arm movement exert forces that are transmitted through the body to the feet and are opposed by the ground. Different substrates provide different amounts of reaction force, so ice or sand substantially alter movement capabilities.

Second, uncertain conditions are usually accommodated by stiffening the joints through concurrent activation of the muscles that produce force in opposite directions. Coactivation of opposing muscles occurs often when a support surface is unsteady, when the body might experience an unexpected perturbation, or when lifting a heavy load. Because coactivation increases the energetic cost of performing a task, one characteristic of skilled performance is the ability to accomplish a task with minimal activation of muscles that span associated joints.

Muscle Work Depends on the Pattern of Activation

Limb muscles in healthy young adults are active 10% to 20% of the time during waking hours. For much of this time the muscles perform constant-length (*isometric*) contractions to maintain a variety of static body postures. In contrast, muscle length has to change during a movement so that the muscle can perform work to displace body segments. A muscle performs positive work and produces power during a shortening contraction, whereas it performs negative work and absorbs power during a lengthening contraction. The capacity of muscle to do positive work establishes performance capabilities, such as the maximal height that can be jumped.

The nervous system enhances the work capacity of muscle by commanding a brief period of negative work before positive work. This activation sequence, the *stretch-shorten cycle,* occurs in many movements. When a person jumps in place on two feet, for example, the support phase involves an initial stretch and subsequent shortening of the ankle extensor and knee extensor muscles (Figure 34–16A). The forces in the Achilles

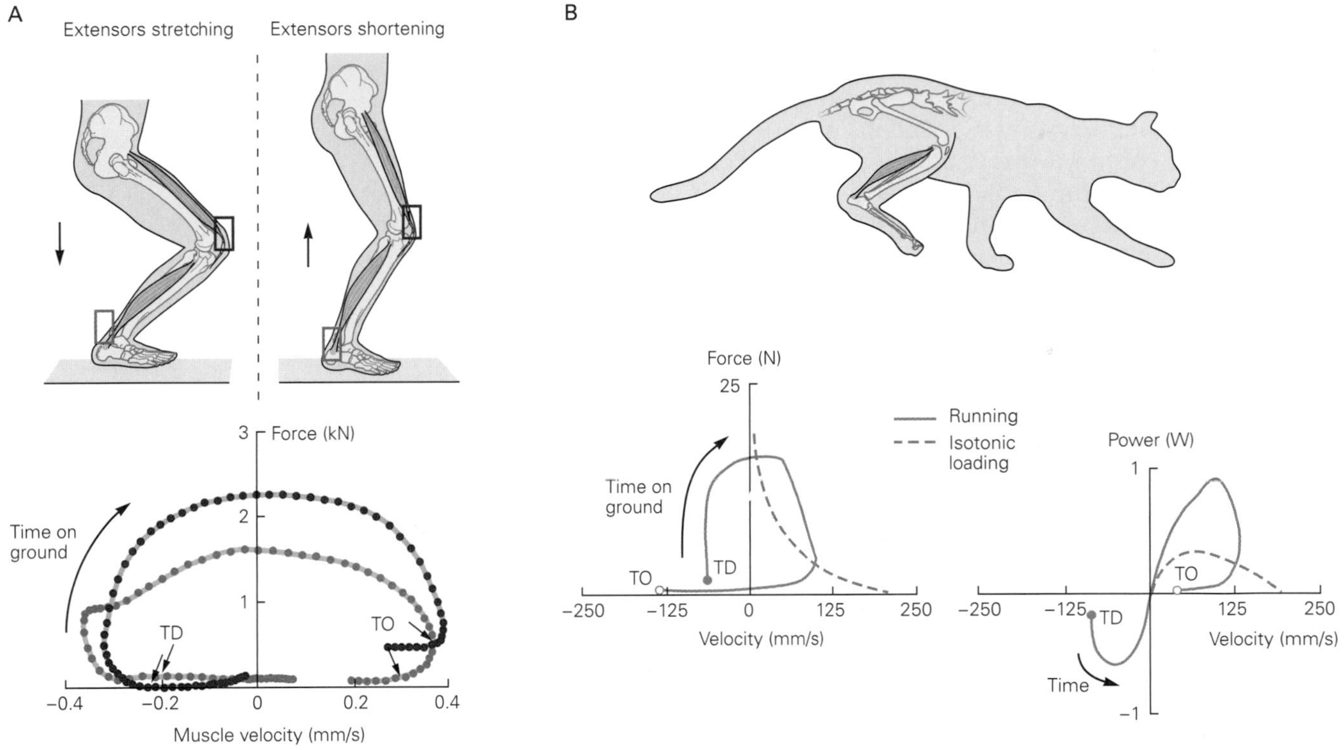

Figure 34–16 An initial phase of negative work enhances subsequent positive work performed by the muscle. (Reproduced, with permission, from Finni, Komi, and Lepola 2000 and from Gregor et al. 1988.)

A. The force in the Achilles tendon and patellar tendon vary during the ground-contact phase of two-legged hopping. The feet contact the ground at touchdown (TD) and leave the ground at toe-off (TO). For approximately the first half of the movement the quadriceps and triceps surae muscles lengthen, performing negative work (negative velocity). The muscles perform positive work when they shorten (positive velocity).

B. The force exerted by the soleus muscle of a cat running at moderate speed varies from the instant the paw touches the ground (TD) until it leaves the ground (TO). The force exerted by the muscle during the shortening contraction is greater than the peak forces measured when the muscle contracts maximally against various constant loads (isotonic loading). Negative velocity reflects a lengthening contraction in the soleus muscle. The power produced by the soleus muscle of the cat during running is greater than that produced in an isolated-muscle experiment (**dashed line**). The phase of negative power corresponds to the lengthening contraction just after the paw is placed on the ground (TD), when the muscle performs negative work.

and patellar tendons increase during the stretch and reach a maximum at the onset of the shortening phase. As a result, the muscles can perform more positive work and produce more power during the shortening contraction (Figure 34–16B).

Although negative work involves an increase in the length of the muscle, the length of the fascicles in the muscle often remains relatively constant, which indicates that the connective-tissue structures are stretched prior to the shortening contraction. Thus the capacity of the muscle to perform more positive work comes from strain energy that can be stored in the tendon during the stretch phase and released during the subsequent shortening phase. The ability of a muscle to benefit from this strategy depends on its morphological characteristics and is greatest in muscles with long tendons.

An Overall View

Movement involves the coordinated interaction of the nervous system and muscle. The basic functional unit of motor control is the motor unit, which consists of a motor neuron and the muscle fibers that it innervates. The force exerted by a muscle depends in part on the number and properties of the motor units that are activated. These properties include contraction speed, maximal force, and fatigability, all of which can be altered by physical activity. The rate of firing in each active motor neuron is also a factor in muscle force. Motor units tend to be activated in a stereotypical order that is highly correlated with motor-neuron size.

Muscle force depends not only on the characteristics of motor-unit activity, but also on the arrangement of the muscle fibers. The sarcomere is the smallest element of muscle to include a complete set of contractile proteins. A transient connection between the contractile proteins myosin and actin, known as the cross bridge cycle, enables muscle to exert a force. The organization of the sarcomeres within a muscle varies substantially and has a major effect on the contractile properties of the muscle.

For a given arrangement of sarcomeres, the force a muscle can exert depends on the activation of the cross bridges by Ca^{2+}, the amount of overlap between the thick and thin filaments, and the velocity of the moving filaments. The functional capability of a muscle depends on the torque that it can exert, which is influenced both by its contractile properties and by the location of its attachments on the skeleton relative to the joint that it spans.

To perform a movement the nervous system activates multiple muscles and controls the torque exerted about the involved joints. The nervous system can vary the magnitude and direction of a movement by altering the amount of motor unit activity, and hence muscle torque, relative to the load acting on the body. Increases in movement speed, however, enhance motion-dependent interactions between body segments, producing unwanted accelerations that must be controlled by the nervous system. Furthermore, the nervous system must coordinate the activity of multiple muscles to provide a mechanical link between moving body segments and the required support from the surroundings. The patterns of muscle activity vary substantially between movements and often include strategies that augment the work capacity of muscles.

Roger M. Enoka
Keir G. Pearson

Selected Readings

Dounskaia N. 2010. Control of human limb movements: the leading joint hypothesis and its practical applications. Exerc Sport Sci Rev 38:201–208.

Duchateau J, Semmler JG, Enoka RM. 2006. Training adaptations in the behavior of human motor units. J Appl Physiol 101:1766–1775.

Enoka RM. 2008. *Neuromechanics of Human Movement*. Champaign, IL: Human Kinetics.

Faulkner JA, Larkin LM, Claflin DR, Brooks SV. 2007. Age-related changes in the structure and function of skeletal muscles. Clin Exp Pharmacol Physiol 34:1091–1096.

Fitts RH. 2003. Effects of regular exercise training on skeletal muscle contractile function. Am J Phys Med Rehabil 82:320–331.

Gordon AM, Regnier M, Homsher E. 2001. Skeletal and cardiac muscle contractile activation: tropomyosin "rocks and rolls." News Physiol Sci 16:49–55.

Huxley AF. 2000. Mechanics and models of the myosin motor. Philos Trans R Soc Lond B Biol Sci 355:433–440.

Kernell D. 2006. *The Motoneurone and Its Muscle Fibres*. New York: Oxford Univ. Press.

Latash ML. 2010. Motor synergies and the equilibrium-point hypothesis. Motor Control 14:294–322.

Lieber RL, Ward SR. 2011. Skeletal muscle design to meet functional demands. Philos Trans R Soc Lond B Biol Sci 366:1466–1476.

Monti RJ, Roy RR, Edgerton VR. 2001. Role of motor unit structure in defining function. Muscle Nerve 24:848–866.

References

Alexander RM, Ker RF. 1990. The architecture of leg muscles. In: JM Winters, SL-Y Woo (eds). *Multiple Muscle Systems: Biomechanics and Movement Organization*, pp. 568–577. New York: Springer-Verlag.

Bloch RJ, Gonzalez-Serratos H. 2003. Lateral force transmission across costameres in skeletal muscle. Exerc Sport Sci Rev 31:73–78.

Bloom W, Fawcett DW. 1975. *A Textbook of Histology*, 10th ed. Philadelphia, PA: Saunders.

Botterman BR, Iwamoto GA, Gonyea WJ. 1986. Gradation of isometric tension by different activation rates in motor units of cat flexor carpi radialis muscle. J Neurophysiol 56:494–506

Burkholder TJ, Lieber RL. 2001. Sarcomere length operating range of vertebrate muscles during movement. J Exp Biol 204:1529–1536.

Cavagna GA, Citterio G. 1974. Effect of stretching on the elastic characteristics of the contractile component of the frog striated muscle. J Physiol 239:1–14.

Desmedt JE, Godaux E. 1977. Ballistic contractions in man: characteristic recruitment pattern of single motor units of the tibialis anterior muscle. J Physiol 264:673–693.

Duchateau J, Enoka RM. 2008. Neural control of shortening and lengthening contractions: influence of task constraints. J Physiol 586:5853–5864.

Duchateau J, Semmler JG, Enoka RM. 2006. Training adaptations in motor unit behavior. J Appl Physiol 101: 1766–1775.

Enoka RM. 2008. *Neuromechanics of Human Movement*. Chapter 6: Muscle and motor units, p. 218. Champaign, IL: Human Kinetics.

Enoka RM. 2012. Muscle fatigue - from motor units to clinical symptoms. J Biomech 45:427–433.

Enoka RM, Fuglevand AJ. 2001. Motor unit physiology: some unresolved issues. Muscle Nerve 24:4–17.

Farina D, Holobar A, Merletti R, Enoka RM. 2004. Decoding the neural drive to muscles from the surface electromyogram. Clin Neurophysiol 121:1616–1623.

Finni T, Komi PV, Lepola V. 2000. In vivo human triceps surae and quadriceps muscle function in a squat jump and counter movement jump. Eur J Appl Physiol 83:416–426.

Fuglevand AJ, Macefield VG, Bigland-Ritchie B. 1999. Force-frequency and fatigue properties of motor units in muscles that control digits of the human hand. J Neurophysiol 81:1718–1729.

Fukunaga T, Kawakami Y, Kubo K, Kanehisa H. 2002. Muscle and tendon interactions during human movement. Exerc Sport Sci Rev 30:106–110.

Gardiner PF. 2006. Changes in α-motoneuron properties with altered physical activity levels. Exerc Sport Sci Rev 34:54–58.

Gordon AM, Regnier M, Homsher R. 2001. Skeletal and cardiac muscle contractile activation: tropomyosin "rocks and rolls." News Physiol Sci 16:49–55.

Gregor RJ, Roy RR, Whiting WC, Lovely RG, Hodgson JA, Edgerton VR. 1988. Mechanical output of the cat soleus during treadmill locomotion: *in vivo* vs *in situ* characteristics. J Biomech 21:721–732.

Hamilton MT, Booth FW. 2000. Skeletal muscle adaptation to exercise: a century of progress. J Appl Physiol 88:327–331.

Heckman CJ, Mottram CJ, Quinlan K, Theiss R, Schuster J. 2009. Motoneuron excitability: the importance of neuromodulatory inputs. Clin Neurophysiol 120:2040–2054.

Henneman E, Somjen G, Carpenter DO. 1965. Functional significance of cell size in spinal motoneurons. J Neurophysiol 28:560–580.

Huxley AF, Simmons RM. 1971. Proposed mechanism of force generation in striated muscle. Nature 233:533–538.

Lieber RL, Fridén J. 2000. Functional and clinical significance of skeletal muscle architecture. Muscle Nerve 23:1647–1666.

Liddell EGT, Sherrington CS. 1925. Recruitment and some other factors of reflex inhibition. Proc R Soc Lond B Biol Sci 97:488–518.

Lombardi V, Piazzesi G. 1990. The contractile response during lengthening of stimulated frog muscle fibres. J Physiol 431:141–171.

Macefield VG, Fuglevand AJ, Bigland-Ritchie B. 1996. Contractile properties of single motor units in human toe extensors assessed by intraneural motor axon stimulation. J Neurophysiol 75:2509–2519.

Milner-Brown HS, Stein RB, Yemm R. 1973. The orderly recruitment of human motor units during voluntary isometric contraction. J Physiol 230:359–370.

Nichols TR. 2002. The contribution of muscles and reflexes to the regulation of joint and limb mechanics. Clin Orthop Related Res 402 Suppl:S43-50.

Patel TJ, Lieber RL. 1997. Force transmission in skeletal muscle: from actomyosin to external tendons. Exerc Sport Sci Rev 25:321–363.

Person RS, Kudina LP. 1972. Discharge frequency and discharge pattern of human motor units during voluntary contraction of muscle. Electroencephalogr Clin Neurophysiol 32:471–483.

Rassier DE, MacIntosh BR, Herzog W. 1999. Length dependence of active force production in skeletal muscle. J Appl Physiol 86:1445–1457.

Roberts TJ. 2002. The integrated function of muscles and tendons during locomotion. Comp Biochem Physiol A Mol Integr Physiol 133:1987–1099.

Sherrington CS. 1925. Remarks on some aspects of reflex inhibition. Proc R Soc Lond B Biol Sci 97:519–545.

Van Cutsem M, Duchateau J, Hainaut K. 1998. Changes in single motor unit behaviour contribute to the increase in contraction speed after dynamic training in humans. J Physiol 513:295–305.

Van Cutsem M, Feiereisen P, Duchateau J, Hainaut K. 1997. Mechanical properties and behaviour of motor units in the tibialis anterior during voluntary contractions. Can J Appl Physiol 22:585–597.

Ward SR, Eng CM, Smallwood LH, Lieber RL. 2009. Are current measurements of lower extremity muscle architecture accurate? Clin Orthop Relat Res 467:1074–1081.

35

Spinal Reflexes

During purposeful movements the central nervous system uses information from a vast array of sensory receptors to ensure that the pattern of muscle activity suits the purpose. Without this sensory information movements tend to be imprecise, and tasks requiring fine coordination in the hands, such as buttoning one's shirt, are impossible.

Charles Sherrington was among the first to recognize the importance of sensory information in regulating movements. In 1906 he proposed that simple reflexes—stereotyped movements elicited by activation of receptors in skin or muscle—are the basic units for movement. He further posited that complex sequences of movements can be produced by combining simple reflexes. This view guided motor physiology for much of the 20th century.

The view that reflexes are automatic, stereotyped movements in response to stimulation of peripheral receptors arose primarily from laboratory studies of reflexes in animals with central nervous system lesions. Once investigators began to measure reflexes in intact animals engaged in normal behavior, ideas about reflexes changed. We now know that reflexes are flexible, that under normal conditions they can be adapted to a task. The prevalent view today is that reflexes are integrated by centrally generated motor commands into complex adaptive movements.

In this chapter we consider the principles underlying the organization and function of reflexes, focusing on spinal reflexes. The sensory stimuli for spinal reflexes arise from receptors in muscles, joints, and skin, and the neural circuitry responsible for the motor response is entirely contained within the spinal cord.

Reflexes Are Adaptable to Particular Motor Tasks

A good example of the adaptability of reflexes is how certain reflexes change in response to stretching the wrist muscles. When a person is kneeling or standing the stretched muscles contract, but muscles in other limbs also contract to prevent a loss of balance. Interestingly, the reflex response of the elbow extensor of the *opposite* arm depends on how that arm is being used. If the arm is used to stabilize the body by holding the edge of a table, a large excitatory response in the elbow extensor muscle resists the forward sway of the body. If the arm is instead holding an unsteady object such as a cup of tea, reflex inhibition of the elbow extensors prevents movement of the cup (Figure 35–1A).

Another example of adaptability is the reflex of finger and thumb flexor muscles in response to stretching thumb muscles. If a subject rhythmically taps the tips of the index finger and thumb to each other, and flexion of the thumb is resisted, a short-latency reflex response is produced in *both* the finger and thumb flexor muscles. As a result, the reflex in the finger flexor muscle produces a larger flexion movement of the finger to compensate for the reduced flexion of the thumb and ensure the performance of the intended task (Figure 35–1B). If the subject is simply making rhythmic thumb movements, a reflex response is produced only in the thumb flexor muscle.

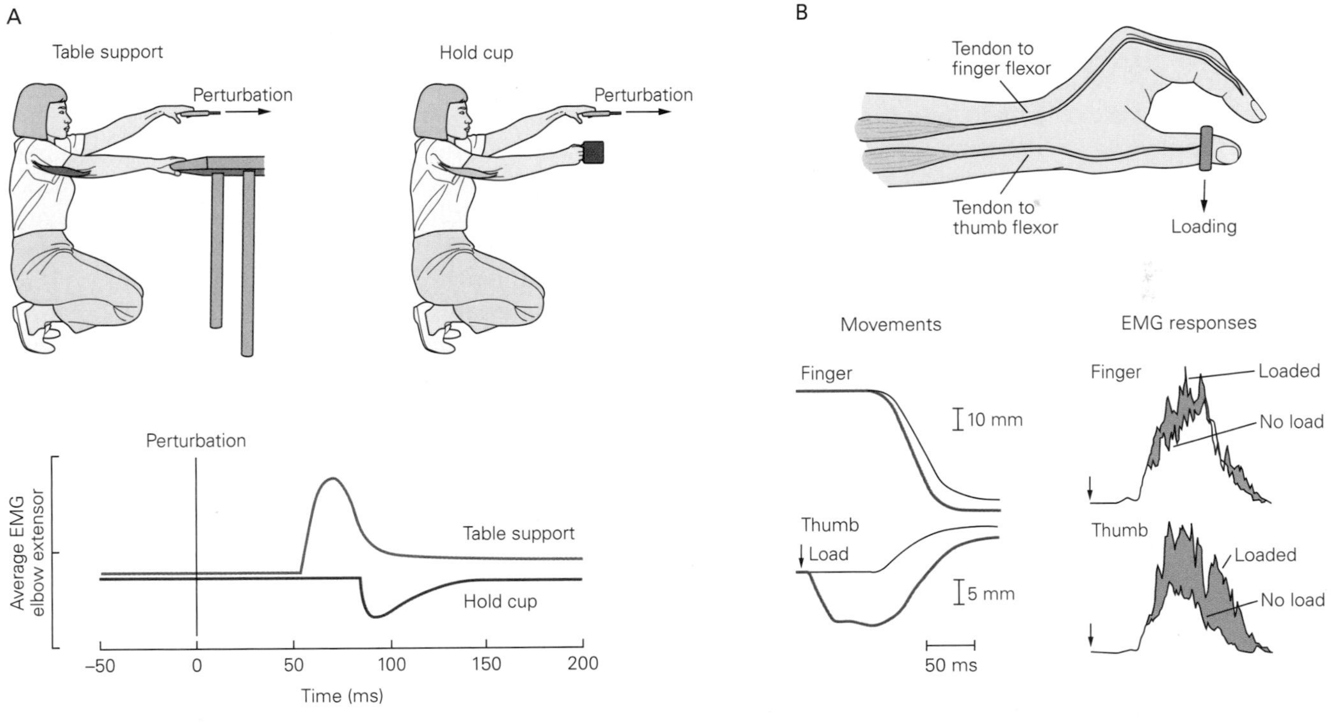

Figure 35–1 Reflex responses are often complex and can change depending on the task.

A. Perturbation of one arm causes an excitatory reflex response in the contralateral elbow extensor muscle when the contralateral limb is used to prevent the body from moving forward by grasping a table. The same stimulus produces an inhibitory response in the muscle when the contralateral hand holds a filled cup. (Adapted, with permission, from Marsden et al. 1981.)

B. Loading the thumb during a rhythmic sequence of finger-to-thumb pinching movements produces a reflex response in the finger muscle as well as the thumb muscle. The additional movement of the finger ensures that the pinching movement remains accurate. The blue area in the electromyogram (EMG) records indicates the reflex response. (Adapted, with permission, from Cole et al. 1984.)

A third example of adaptability is the conditioning of the flexion-withdrawal reflex. Flexion-withdrawal can be associated with an auditory tone by classical conditioning (see Chapter 65). A subject is asked to place the palmar surface of an index finger on an electrode. A mild electrical shock is then paired with an audible tone. As expected, after only a few pairings the tone alone will elicit the withdrawal reflex. What exactly has been conditioned? Is it the contraction of a fixed group of muscles or the behavioral *act* that withdraws the finger from the noxious stimulus?

This question can be answered by having the subject turn his or her hands over after conditioning is complete, so that now the dorsal surface of the finger is in contact with the electrode. Most subjects will withdraw their fingers from the electrode when the tone is played, even though this means that the opposite muscles now contract. Thus, the conditioned response is not merely a stereotyped set of muscle contractions but the elicitation of an appropriate behavior.

Three important principles are illustrated by these examples. First, neural signaling in reflex pathways is adjusted according to the motor task. The state of the reflex pathways for any task is referred to as the *functional set.* Exactly how a functional set is established for most motor tasks is largely unknown, and unraveling the underlying mechanisms is one of the challenging areas of contemporary research on motor systems. Second, sensory input from a localized source generally produces coordinated reflex responses in several muscles at once, some of which may be distant from the stimulus. Third, supraspinal centers play an important role in modulating and adapting spinal reflexes, even to the extent of reversing movements when appropriate.

To understand the neural basis for reflexes and how they are modified for a particular task, we must first have a thorough knowledge of how reflex pathways are organized in the spinal cord. Although under normal conditions descending central commands directly shape spinal reflexes, many qualitative features of spinal reflexes are maintained after complete transection of the spinal cord, a condition that isolates the spinal circuits from the brain.

Spinal Reflexes Produce Coordinated Patterns of Muscle Contraction

Cutaneous Reflexes Produce Complex Movements That Serve Protective and Postural Functions

A familiar example of a spinal reflex is the flexion-withdrawal reflex, in which a limb is quickly withdrawn from a painful stimulus. Flexion-withdrawal is a protective reflex in which a discrete stimulus causes all the flexor muscles in that limb to contract coordinately. We know that this is a spinal reflex because it persists after complete transection of the spinal cord.

The sensory signal activates divergent polysynaptic reflex pathways. One excites motor neurons that innervate flexor muscles of the stimulated limb, whereas another inhibits motor neurons that innervate the limb's extensor muscles (Figure 35–2A). Excitation of one group of muscles and inhibition of their antagonists—those that act in the opposite direction—is what Sherrington called *reciprocal innervation,* a key principle of motor organization that is discussed later in this chapter.

The reflex can produce an opposite effect in the contralateral limb, that is, excitation of extensor motor neurons and inhibition of flexor motor neurons. This *crossed-extension reflex* serves to enhance postural support during withdrawal of a foot from a painful stimulus. Activation of the extensor muscles in the opposite leg counteracts the increased load caused by lifting the stimulated limb. Thus, flexion-withdrawal is a complete, albeit simple, motor act.

Although flexion reflexes are relatively stereotyped, both the spatial extent and the force of muscle contraction depend on stimulus intensity. Touching a stove that is slightly hot may produce moderately fast withdrawal only at the wrist and elbow, whereas touching a very hot stove invariably leads to a forceful contraction at all joints, leading to a rapid withdrawal of the entire limb. The duration of the reflex usually increases with stimulus intensity, and the contractions produced in a flexion reflex always outlast the stimulus.

Because of the similarity of the flexion-withdrawal reflex to stepping, it was once thought that the flexion reflex is important in producing contractions of flexor muscles during walking. We now know, however, that a major component of the neural control system for walking is a set of intrinsic spinal circuits that do not require sensory stimuli (see Chapter 36). Nevertheless, in mammals the intrinsic spinal circuits that control walking share many of the interneurons that are involved in flexion reflexes.

The Stretch Reflex Resists the Lengthening of a Muscle

Perhaps the most important—certainly the most studied—spinal reflex is the *stretch reflex,* a lengthening contraction of a muscle. Stretch reflexes were originally thought to be an intrinsic property of muscles. But early in the last century Liddell and Sherrington showed that they could be abolished by cutting either the dorsal or the ventral root, thus establishing that

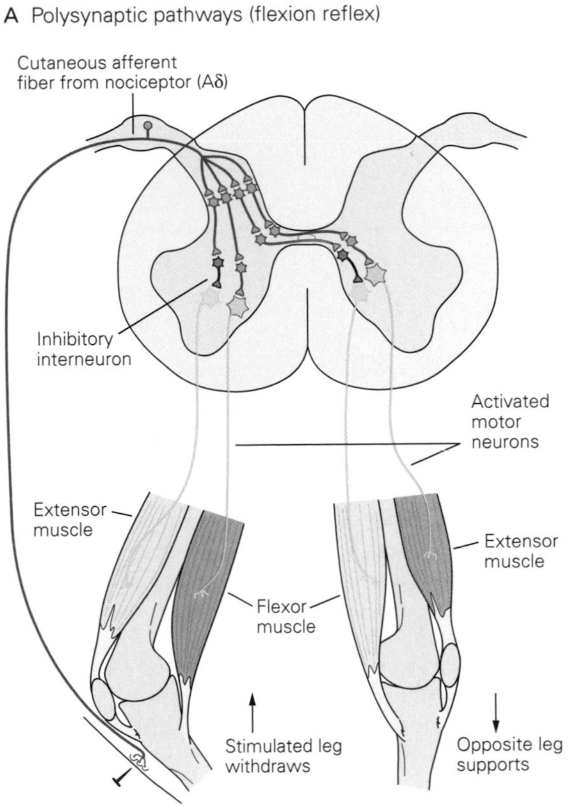

Figure 35–2 Spinal reflexes involve coordinated contractions of numerous muscles in the limbs.

A. Polysynaptic pathways in the spinal cord mediate flexion and crossed-extension reflexes. One excitatory pathway activates motor neurons that innervate ipsilateral flexor muscles, which withdraw the limb from noxious stimuli. Another pathway simultaneously excites motor neurons that innervate contralateral extensor muscles, providing support during withdrawal of the limb. Inhibitory interneurons ensure that the motor neurons supplying antagonist muscles are inactive during the reflex response. (Adapted, with permission, from Schmidt 1983.)

B. Monosynaptic pathways mediate stretch reflexes. Afferent axons from muscle spindles make excitatory connections on two sets of motor neurons: alpha motor neurons that innervate the same (homonymous) muscle from which they arise and motor neurons that innervate synergist muscles. They also act through interneurons to inhibit the motor neurons that innervate antagonist muscles. When a muscle is stretched by a tap with a reflex hammer, the firing rate in the afferent fiber from the spindle increases. This leads to contraction of the same muscle and its synergists and relaxation of the antagonist. The reflex therefore tends to counteract the stretch, enhancing the spring-like properties of the muscles. The records on the right demonstrate the reflex nature of contractions produced by muscle stretch in a decerebrate cat. When an extensor muscle is stretched it normally produces a large force, but it produces a very small force (**dashed line**) after the sensory afferents in the dorsal roots have been severed. (Adapted, with permission, from Liddell and Sherrington 1924.)

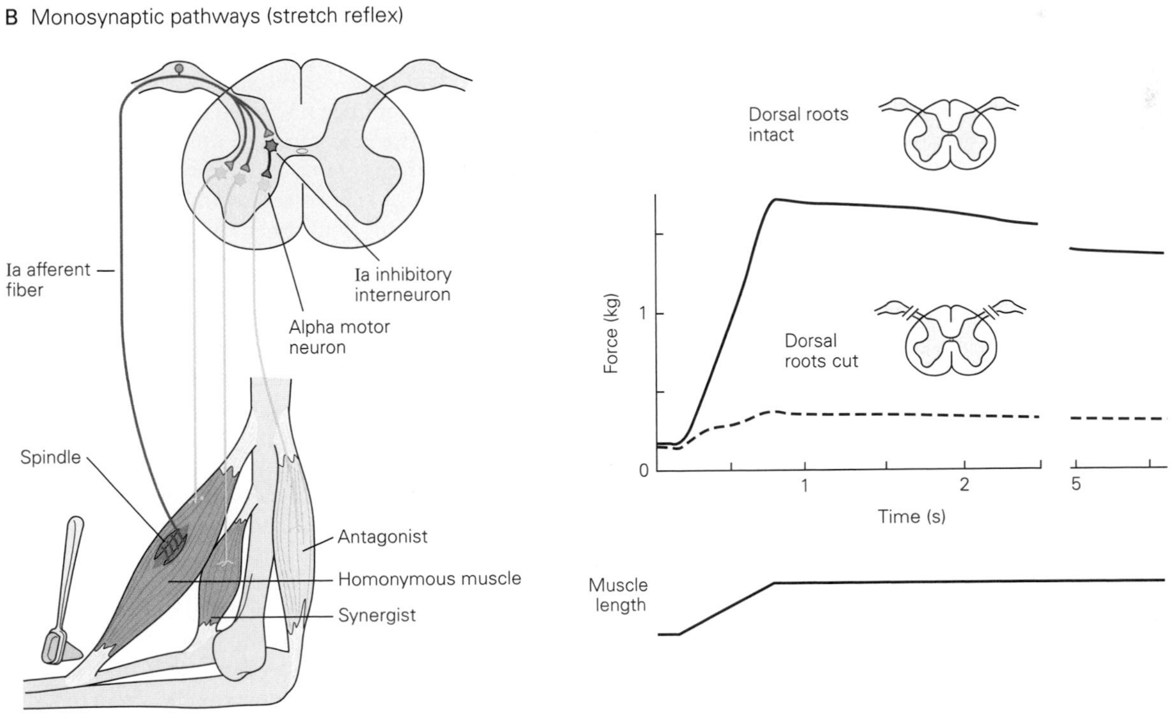

these reflexes require sensory input from muscle to spinal cord and a return path to muscle (Figure 35–2B).

We now know that the receptor that senses the change of length is the muscle spindle (Box 35–1) and that the type Ia axon from this receptor makes direct excitatory connections with motor neurons. (The classification and nomenclature of sensory fibers from muscle are discussed in Box 35–2.) The afferent axon also connects to interneurons that inhibit the motor neurons that innervate antagonist muscles, another

Box 35–1 Muscle Spindles

Muscle spindles are small encapsulated sensory receptors that have a spindle-like or fusiform shape and are located within the fleshy part of a muscle. Their main function is to signal changes in the length of the muscle within which they reside. Changes in length of muscles are closely associated with changes in the angles of the joints that the muscles cross. Thus muscle spindles are used by the central nervous system to sense relative positions of the body segments.

Each spindle has three main components: (1) a group of specialized *intrafusal* muscle fibers with central regions that are noncontractile; (2) sensory fibers that terminate in the noncontractile central regions of the intrafusal fibers; and (3) motor axons that terminate in the polar contractile regions of the intrafusal fibers (Figure 35–3A).

When the intrafusal fibers are stretched, often referred to as "loading the spindle," the sensory nerve endings are also stretched and increase their firing rate. Because muscle spindles are arranged in parallel with the *extrafusal* muscle fibers that make up the main body of the muscle, the intrafusal fibers change in length as the whole muscle changes. Thus, when a muscle is stretched, activity in the sensory endings of muscle spindles increases. When a muscle shortens, the spindle is unloaded and the activity decreases.

The intrafusal muscle fibers are innervated by *gamma* motor neurons, which have small-diameter myelinated axons, whereas the extrafusal muscle fibers are innervated by *alpha* motor neurons, with large-diameter myelinated axons. Activation of gamma motor neurons causes shortening of the polar regions of the intrafusal fibers. This in turn stretches the central region from both ends, leading to an increase in firing rate of the sensory endings or to a greater likelihood that the sensory endings will fire in response to stretch of the muscle. Thus the gamma motor neurons adjust the sensitivity of the muscle spindles. Contraction of the intrafusal muscle fibers does not contribute significantly to the force of muscle contraction.

The structure and functional behavior of muscle spindles is considerably more complex than this simple description implies. When a muscle is stretched the change in length has two phases: a dynamic phase, the period during which length is changing, and a static or steady-state phase, when the muscle has stabilized at a new length. Structural specializations within each component of the muscle spindles allow spindle afferents to signal aspects of each phase separately.

There are two types of intrafusal muscle fibers: nuclear bag fibers and nuclear chain fibers. The bag fibers can be divided into two groups, dynamic and static. A typical spindle has two or three bag fibers and a variable number of chain fibers, usually about five. Furthermore, the intrafusal fibers receive two types of sensory endings. A single Ia (large diameter) axon spirals around the central region of all intrafusal muscle fibers and serves as the primary sensory ending (Figure 35–3B). A variable number of type II (medium diameter) axons, located adjacent to the central regions of the static bag and chain fibers, serve as secondary sensory endings.

The gamma motor neurons can also be divided into two classes: Dynamic gamma motor neurons innervate the dynamic bag fibers, whereas the static gamma motor neurons innervate the static bag fibers and the chain fibers.

This duality of structure is reflected in a duality of function. The tonic discharge of both primary and secondary sensory endings signals the steady-state length of the muscle. The primary sensory endings are, in addition, highly sensitive to the velocity of stretch, allowing them to provide information about the speed of movements. Because they are highly sensitive to small changes, the primary endings rapidly provide information about sudden unexpected changes in length, which can be used to generate quick corrective reactions.

Increases in the firing rate of dynamic gamma motor neurons increase the dynamic sensitivity of primary sensory endings but have no influence on secondary sensory endings. Increases in the firing rate of static gamma motor neurons increase the tonic level of activity in both primary and secondary sensory endings, decrease the dynamic sensitivity of primary endings (Figure 35–3C), and can prevent the silencing of primary endings when a muscle is released from stretch. Thus the central nervous system can independently adjust the dynamic and static sensitivity of the different sensory endings in muscle spindles.

instance of reciprocal innervation. This inhibition prevents muscle contractions that might otherwise resist the movements produced by the stretch reflexes.

Sherrington developed an experimental model for investigating spinal circuitry that is especially valuable in the study of stretch reflexes. He conducted his experiments on cats whose brain stems had been surgically transected at the level of the midbrain, between the superior and inferior colliculi. This is referred to as a *decerebrate preparation*. The effect of this procedure is to

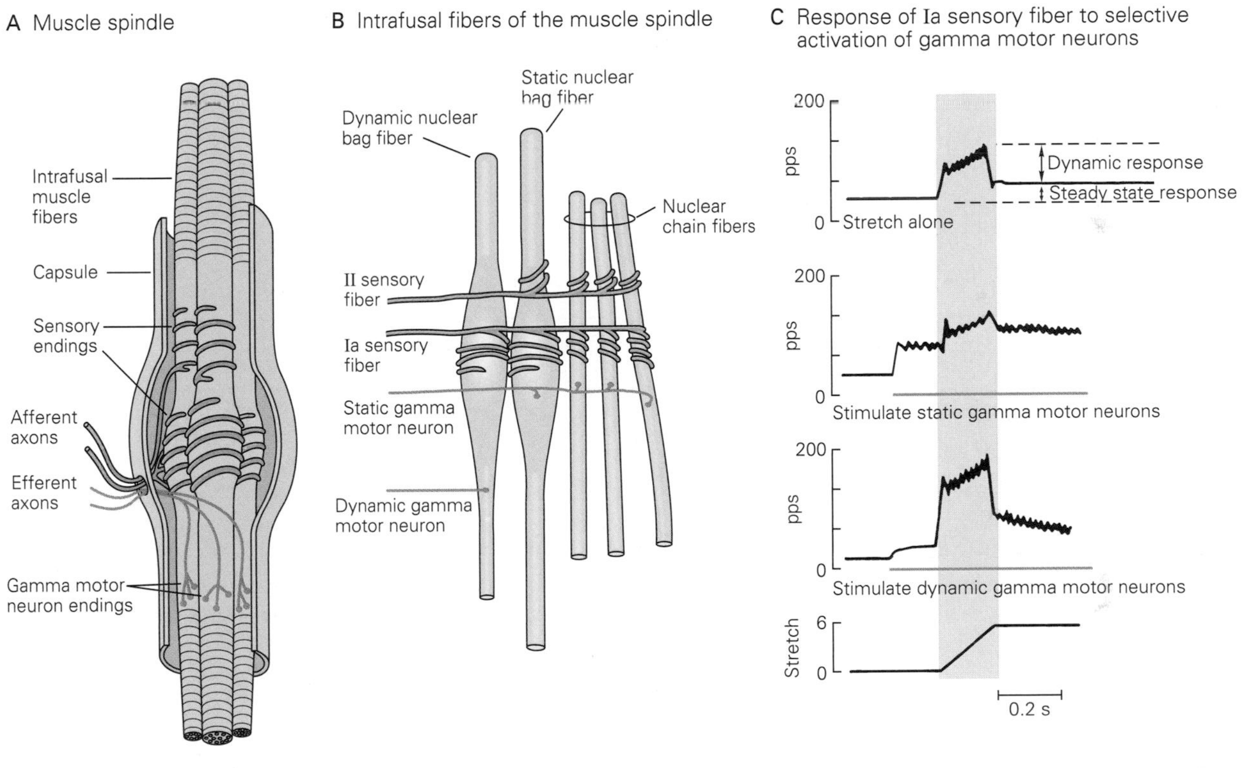

Figure 35–3 The muscle spindle detects changes in muscle length.

A. The main components of the muscle spindle are intrafusal muscle fibers, afferent sensory endings, and efferent motor endings. The intrafusal fibers are specialized muscle fibers with central regions that are not contractile. Gamma motor neurons innervate the contractile polar regions of the intrafusal fibers. Contraction of the polar regions pulls on the central regions of the intrafusal fiber from both ends. The sensory endings spiral around the central regions of the intrafusal fibers and are responsive to stretch of these fibers. (Adapted, with permission, from Hulliger 1984.)

B. The muscle spindle contains three types of intrafusal fibers: dynamic nuclear bag, static nuclear bag, and nuclear chain fibers. A single Ia sensory axon innervates all three types of fibers, forming a primary sensory ending. Type II sensory axons innervate the nuclear chain fibers and static bag fibers, forming a secondary sensory ending. Two types of motor neurons innervate different intrafusal fibers. Dynamic gamma motor neurons innervate only dynamic bag fibers; static gamma motor neurons innervate various combinations of chain and static bag fibers. (Adapted, with permission, from Boyd 1980.)

C. Selective stimulation of the two types of gamma motor neurons has different effects on the firing of the Ia fibers from the spindle. Without gamma stimulation the Ia fiber shows a small dynamic response to muscle stretch and a modest increase in steady-state firing. When a static gamma motor neuron is stimulated, the steady-state response of the Ia fiber increases, but there is a decrease in the dynamic response. When a dynamic gamma motor neuron is stimulated, the dynamic response of the Ia fiber is markedly enhanced, but the steady-state response gradually returns to its original level. (Adapted, with permission, from Brown and Matthews 1966.)

Box 35–2 Classification of Sensory Fibers from Muscle

Sensory fibers are classified according to their diameter. Axons with larger diameters conduct action potentials more rapidly than do fibers of smaller diameters. Because each class of sensory receptors is innervated by fibers with diameters within a restricted range, this method of classification distinguishes to some extent the fibers that arise from the different types of receptor organs. The main groups of sensory fibers from muscle are listed in Table 35–1.

The organization of reflex pathways in the spinal cord has been established primarily by electrically stimulating the sensory fibers and recording evoked responses in different classes of neurons in the spinal cord. This method of activation has three advantages over natural stimulation. The timing of afferent input can be precisely established; the responses evoked in motor neurons and other neurons by different classes of sensory fibers can be assessed by grading the strength of the electrical stimulus; and certain classes of receptors can be selectively activated.

The strength of the electrical stimulus required to activate a sensory fiber is measured relative to the strength required to activate the afferent fibers with the largest diameter because these fibers have the lowest threshold for electrical activation. The threshold of type I fibers is usually one to two times that of the largest afferents (with Ia fibers having, on average, a slightly lower threshold than Ib fibers). For most type II fibers the threshold is 2 to 5 times higher, whereas type III and IV have thresholds in the range of 10 to 50 times that of the largest afferents.

Table 35–1 Classification of Sensory Fibers from Muscle

Type	Axon	Receptor	Sensitive to
Ia	12–20 μm myelinated	Primary spindle ending	Muscle length and rate of change of length
Ib	12–20 μm myelinated	Golgi tendon organ	Muscle tension
II	6–12 μm myelinated	Secondary spindle ending	Muscle length (little rate sensitivity)
II	6–12 μm myelinated	Nonspindle endings	Deep pressure
III	2–6 μm myelinated	Free nerve endings	Pain, chemical stimuli, and temperature (important for physiological responses to exercise)
IV	0.5–2 μm nonmyelinated	Free nerve endings	Pain, chemical stimuli, and temperature

disconnect the rest of the brain from the spinal cord, thus blocking sensations of pain as well as interrupting normal modulation of reflexes by higher brain centers. A decerebrate animal has stereotyped and usually heightened stretch reflexes, making it is easier to examine the factors controlling their expression.

Without control by higher brain centers, descending pathways from the brain stem powerfully facilitate the neuronal circuits involved in the stretch reflexes of extensor muscles. This results in a dramatic increase in extensor muscle tone that sometimes suffices to support the animal in a standing position. In normal animals, owing to the balance between facilitation and inhibition, stretch reflexes are weaker and considerably more variable in strength than those in decerebrate animals.

Local Spinal Circuits Contribute to the Coordination of Reflex Responses

The Stretch Reflex Involves a Monosynaptic Pathway

The neural circuit responsible for the stretch reflex was one of the first reflex pathways to be examined in detail. The physiological basis of this reflex was examined by measuring the latency of the response in ventral roots to electrical stimulation of dorsal roots. When the Ia sensory axons innervating the muscle spindles were selectively activated, the reflex latency through the spinal cord was less than 1 ms. This demonstrated that the Ia fibers make direct connections on the alpha motor neurons, for the delay at a single synapse is typically 0.5 ms to 0.9 ms (Figure 35–4B).

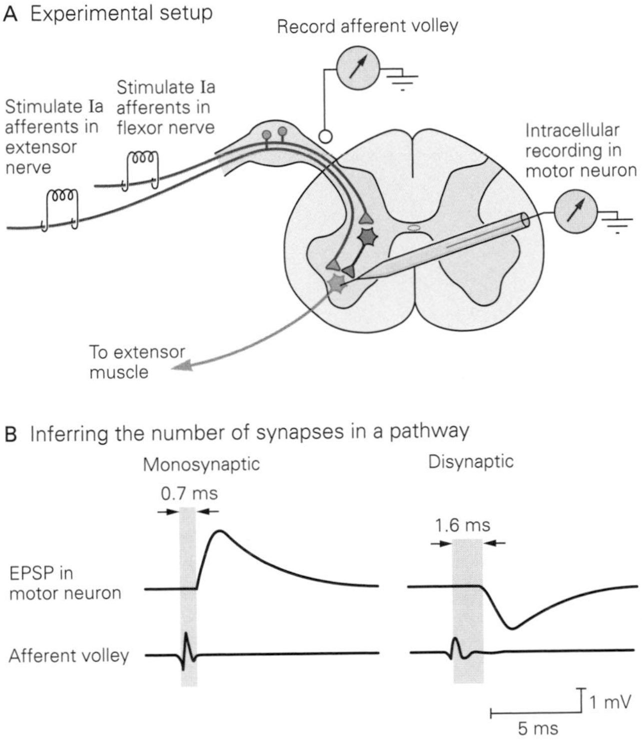

Figure 35–4 The number of synapses in a reflex pathway can be inferred from intracellular recordings.

A. An intracellular recording electrode is inserted into the cell body of a spinal motor neuron that innervates an extensor muscle. Stimulation of Ia sensory fibers from flexor or extensor muscles produces a volley of action potentials at the dorsal root.

B. Left: When Ia fibers from an extensor muscle are stimulated, the latency between the recording of the afferent volley and the excitatory postsynaptic potential in the motor neuron is only 0.7 ms. Because this is approximately equal to the duration of signal transmission across a single synapse, it can be inferred that the excitatory action of the stretch reflex pathway is monosynaptic. **Right:** When Ia fibers from an antagonist flexor muscle are stimulated, the latency between the recording of the afferent volley and the inhibitory postsynaptic potential in the motor neuron is 1.6 ms. Because this is approximately twice the duration of signal transmission across a single synapse, it can be inferred that the inhibitory action of the stretch reflex pathway is disynaptic.

The pattern of connections of Ia fibers to motor neurons can be shown directly by intracellular recording. Ia fibers from a muscle excite not only the motor neurons innervating the same (*homonymous*) muscle, but also those innervating other (*heteronymous*) muscles with a similar mechanical action. The Ia fibers also form inhibitory connections with the alpha motor neurons innervating antagonistic muscles through the *Ia inhibitory interneurons.* This disynaptic inhibitory pathway is the basis for reciprocal innervation: When a muscle is stretched, its antagonists relax.

Ia Inhibitory Interneurons Coordinate the Muscles Surrounding a Joint

Reciprocal innervation is useful not only in stretch reflexes but also in voluntary movements. Relaxation of the antagonist muscle during a movement enhances speed and efficiency because the muscles that act as prime movers are not working against the contraction of opposing muscles.

The Ia inhibitory interneurons involved in the stretch reflex are also used to coordinate muscle contraction during voluntary movements. These interneurons receive inputs from collaterals of axons descending from neurons in the motor cortex that make direct excitatory connections with spinal motor neurons. This organizational feature simplifies the control of voluntary movements, for higher centers do not have to send separate commands to the opposing muscles.

Sometimes it is advantageous to contract the prime mover and the antagonist at the same time. Such *co-contraction* has the effect of stiffening the joint and is most useful when precision and joint stabilization are critical. An example of this phenomenon is the co-contraction of flexor and extensor muscles of the elbow immediately before catching a ball. The Ia inhibitory interneurons receive both excitatory and inhibitory signals from all of the major descending pathways (Figure 35–5A). By changing the balance of excitatory and inhibitory inputs onto these interneurons, supraspinal centers can reduce reciprocal inhibition of muscles and enable co-contraction, thus controlling the relative amount of joint stiffness to meet the requirements of the motor act.

The activity of spinal motor neurons is also regulated by another important class of inhibitory interneurons, the *Renshaw cells.* Excited by collaterals of the axons of motor neurons, Renshaw cells make inhibitory synaptic connections with several populations of motor neurons, including the motor neurons that excite them and the Ia inhibitory interneurons (Figure 35–5B). The connections with motor neurons form a negative

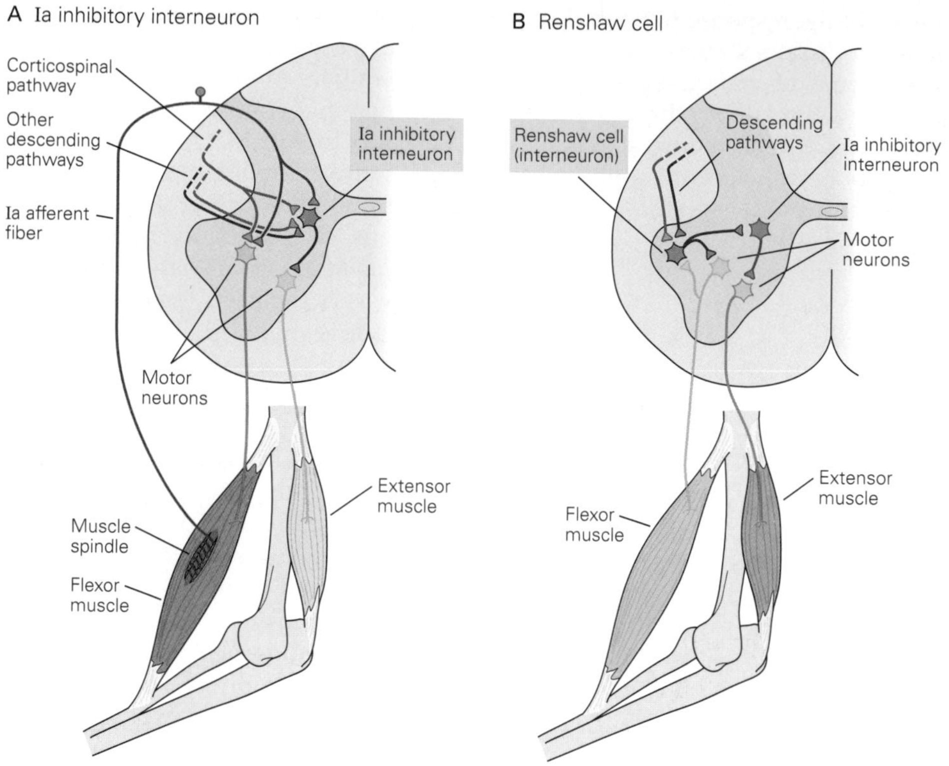

Figure 35–5 Inhibitory spinal interneurons coordinate reflex actions.

A. The Ia inhibitory interneuron regulates contraction in antagonist muscles in stretch-reflex circuits through its divergent contacts with motor neurons. In addition, the interneuron receives excitatory and inhibitory inputs from corticospinal and other descending pathways. A change in the balance of these supraspinal signals allows the interneuron to coordinate co-contractions in antagonist muscles at a joint.

B. Renshaw cells are spinal interneurons that produce recurrent inhibition of motor neurons. These interneurons are excited by collaterals from motor neurons and inhibit those same motor neurons. This negative feedback system regulates motor neuron excitability and stabilizes firing rates. Renshaw cells also send collaterals to synergist motor neurons (not shown) and Ia inhibitory interneurons that synapse on antagonist motor neurons. Thus, descending inputs that modulate the excitability of the Renshaw cells adjust the excitability of all the motor neurons around a joint.

feedback system that may help stabilize the firing rate of the motor neurons, whereas the connections with the Ia inhibitory interneurons may regulate the strength of inhibition of antagonistic motor neurons. In addition, Renshaw cells also receive significant synaptic input from descending pathways and distribute inhibition to task-related groups of motor neurons and Ia interneurons. It is therefore likely that Renshaw cells help establish the pattern of signaling in divergent Ia sensory pathways according to the motor task.

Divergence in Reflex Pathways Amplifies Sensory Inputs and Coordinates Muscle Contractions

In all reflex pathways in the spinal cord the sensory neurons form divergent connections with a large number of target neurons through extensive axonal branching. The flexion-withdrawal reflex, for example, involves extensive divergence within the spinal cord. Stimulation of a small number of sensory axons from a small area of skin is sufficient to cause contractions of widely distributed muscles and thus to produce a coordinated motor pattern.

Lorne Mendell and Elwood Henneman used a computer enhancement technique called *spike-triggered averaging* to determine the extent to which the action potentials in single Ia fibers are transmitted to a population of spinal motor neurons. They found that individual Ia axons make excitatory synapses with all homonymous motor neurons innervating the medial gastrocnemius of the cat. This widespread divergence effectively amplifies the signals of individual Ia fibers, leading to a strong excitatory drive to the muscle from which they originate (*autogenic excitation*).

The Ia axons in reflex pathways also provide excitatory inputs to many of the motor neurons innervating synergist muscles (up to 60% of the motor neurons of some synergists). Although widespread, these connections are not as strong as the connections to homonymous motor neurons. The strength of these connections varies from muscle to muscle in a complex way according to the similarity of the mechanical actions of the synergists. We have already noted that, in the control of voluntary movements, descending pathways make use of reciprocal inhibition of antagonists in the stretch reflex. A similar convergence principle holds for the activation of motor neurons innervating synergist muscles. Thus stretch reflex pathways provide a principal mechanism by which the contractions of different muscles can be linked in voluntary as well as reflex actions.

Convergence of Inputs on Ib Interneurons Increases the Flexibility of Reflex Responses

Thus far we have considered reflex pathways as though each included only one type of sensory fiber. But an enormous diversity of sensory information converges on interneurons in the spinal cord.

The *Ib inhibitory interneuron* is one of the best-studied interneurons that receive extensive convergent input. Its principal input is from Golgi tendon organs, sensory receptors that signal the tension in a muscle (Box 35–3), and it makes inhibitory connections with homonymous motor neurons. As one might expect from this connectivity, stimulation of tendon organs or their Ib afferent fibers in passive animals produces disynaptic inhibition of homonymous motor neurons (*autogenic inhibition*). However, stimulation of Ib afferents in active animals does not always inhibit homonymous motor neurons. Indeed, we shall see in the next section that stimulation of tendon organs may in certain conditions excite homonymous motor neurons.

One reason that the reflex actions of the sensory axons from tendon organs are complex in natural situations is that the Ib inhibitory interneurons also receive input from the muscle spindles, cutaneous receptors, and joints (Figure 35–7A). In addition, they receive both excitatory and inhibitory input from various descending pathways.

Golgi tendon organs were first thought to have a protective function, preventing damage to muscle, for it was assumed that they always inhibited homonymous motor neurons and that they fired only when tension in the muscle was high. But we now know that these receptors signal minute changes in muscle tension, thus providing the nervous system with precise information about the state of a muscle's contraction.

The convergence of sensory input from tendon organs, cutaneous receptors, and joint receptors onto interneurons that inhibit motor neurons may allow for precise spinal control of muscle force in activities such as grasping a delicate object. Additional input from cutaneous receptors may facilitate activity in the Ib inhibitory interneurons when the hand reaches an object, thus reducing the level of muscle contraction and permitting a soft grasp.

Finally, like the Ia fibers from muscle spindles, the Ib fibers from tendon organs form widespread connections with motor neurons that innervate muscles acting at different joints. Therefore the connections of the afferent fibers from tendon organs with the Ib inhibitory interneurons are part of spinal reflex networks that regulate movements of whole limbs.

Central Motor Commands and Cognitive Processes Can Alter Synaptic Transmission in Spinal Reflex Pathways

Both the strength and the sign of synaptic transmission in spinal reflex pathways can be altered during behavioral acts. For example, in humans the strength of the monosynaptic reflex declines as we progress from standing to walking to running. It does so because stiffness increases naturally as muscle force increases, and thus reflexes are not needed.

Another example of a change in sign occurs in the activity of Ib sensory axons during walking. As we have seen, in passive animals the Ib fibers from extensor muscles have an inhibitory effect on homonymous motor neurons. During locomotion they produce an excitatory effect on those same motor neurons because transmission in the disynaptic inhibitory pathway is depressed (Figure 35–7B). This phenomenon is called *state-dependent reflex reversal.*

Transmission in spinal reflex pathways can also be modified in association with higher cognitive functions. Examples are increases in the tendon jerk reflex in the soleus muscle of humans while imagining pressing a foot pedal, and modulation of the Hoffmann reflex in arm and leg muscles when subjects observe grasping and walking movements, respectively. The latter findings indicate that the mirror-neuron system identified in cortical networks (see Chapter 38) influences neuronal systems in the spinal cord. Furthermore, intracellular recordings from monkeys engaged in normal behavior have demonstrated that the intention

Box 35–3 Golgi Tendon Organs

Golgi tendon organs are slender encapsulated structures approximately 1 mm long and 0.1 mm in diameter located at the junction between skeletal muscle fibers and tendon. Each capsule encloses several braided collagen fibers connected in series to a group of muscle fibers.

Each tendon organ is innervated by a single Ib axon that branches into many fine endings inside the capsule; these endings become intertwined with the collagen fascicles (Figure 35–6A).

Stretching of the tendon organ straightens the collagen fibers, thus compressing the Ib nerve endings and causing them to fire. Because the nerve endings are so closely associated with the collagen fibers, even very small stretches of the tendons can compress the nerve endings.

Whereas muscle spindles are most sensitive to changes in length of a muscle, tendon organs are most sensitive to changes in muscle tension. Contraction of the muscle fibers connected to the collagen fiber bundle containing the receptor is a particularly potent stimulus to a tendon organ. The tendon organs are thus readily activated during normal movements. This has been demonstrated by recordings from single Ib axons in humans making voluntary finger movements and in cats walking normally.

Studies in anesthetized animal preparations have shown that the average level of activity in the population of tendon organs in a muscle is a good index of the total force in a contracting muscle (Figure 35–6B). This close agreement between firing frequency and force is consistent with the view that the tendon organs continuously measure the force in a contracting muscle.

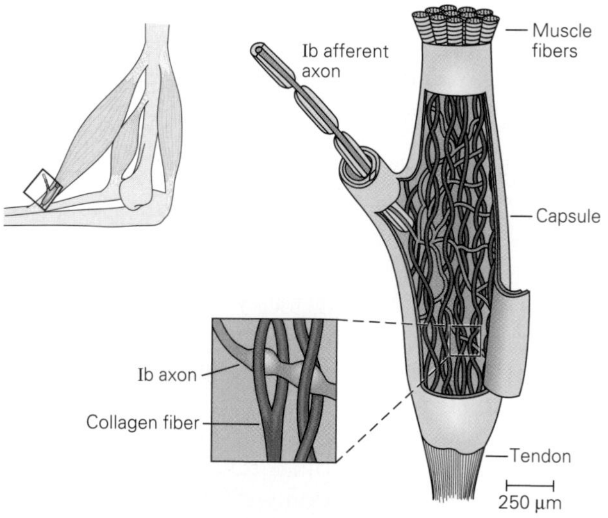

Figure 35–6A When the Golgi tendon organ is stretched (usually because of contraction of the muscle), the Ib afferent axon is compressed by collagen fibers (see inset) and its rate of firing increases. (Adapted, with permission, from Schmidt 1983; inset adapted, with permission, from Swett and Schoultz 1975.)

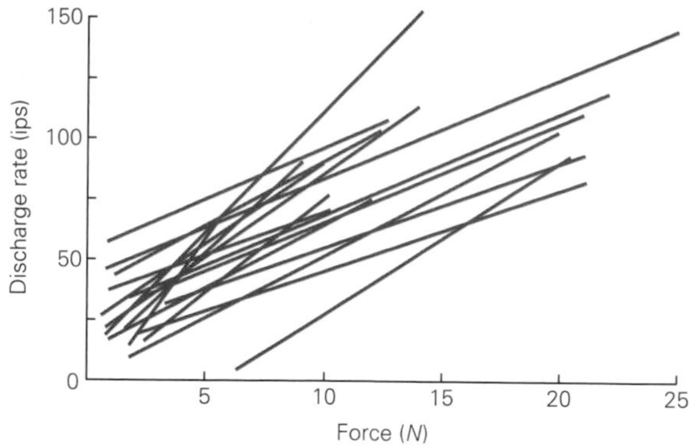

Figure 35–6B The discharge rate of a population of Golgi tendon organs signals the force in a muscle. Linear regression lines show the relationship between discharge rate and force for Golgi tendon organs of the soleus muscle of the cat. (Adapted, with permission, from Crago et al. 1982.)

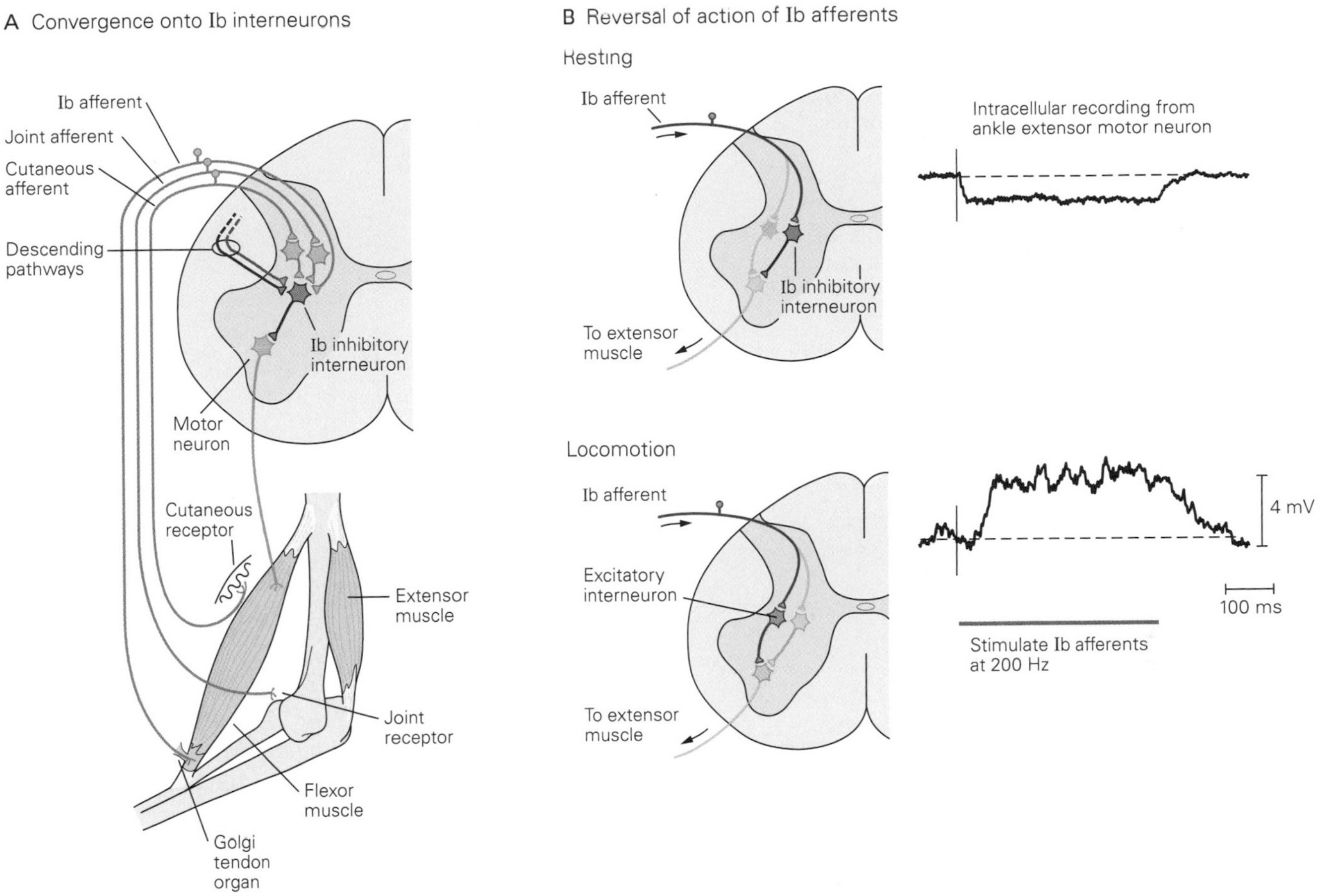

Figure 35–7 The reflex actions of Ib afferent fibers from Golgi tendon organs.

A. The Ib inhibitory interneuron receives input from tendon organs, muscle spindles (not shown), joint and cutaneous receptors, and descending pathways.

B. The action of Ib sensory fibers on extensor motor neurons is reversed from inhibition to excitation when walking is initiated. When the animal is resting, stimulation of Ib fibers from the ankle extensor muscle inhibits ankle extensor motor neurons through Ib inhibitory interneurons, as shown by the hyperpolarization in the record. During walking the Ib inhibitory interneurons are inhibited while excitatory interneurons that receive input from Ib sensory fibers are facilitated by the command system for walking, thus opening a Ib excitatory pathway from the Golgi tendon organs to motor neurons.

to make a movement modifies activity in interneurons in the spinal cord and alters the transmission in spinal reflex pathways.

Central Neurons Can Regulate the Strength of Spinal Reflexes at Three Sites in the Reflex Pathway

As noted earlier, the force of a reflex can vary, although the sensory stimulus remains constant. This variability in reflex strength is possible because synaptic transmission in spinal reflex pathways can be modified at three possible sites: alpha motor neurons, interneurons in all reflex circuits except monosynaptic pathways with Ia afferent fibers, and the presynaptic terminals of the afferent fibers (Figure 35–8A).

All three sites receive inputs from neurons in motor centers in the brain stem and cerebral cortex as well as other regions of the spinal cord. Signals from these higher-level neurons regulate the strength of reflexes by changing the background (tonic) level of activity at any of the three sites in the spinal reflex pathway. For example, an increase in tonic excitatory input to the alpha motor neurons moves the membrane potential of these cells closer to threshold so that

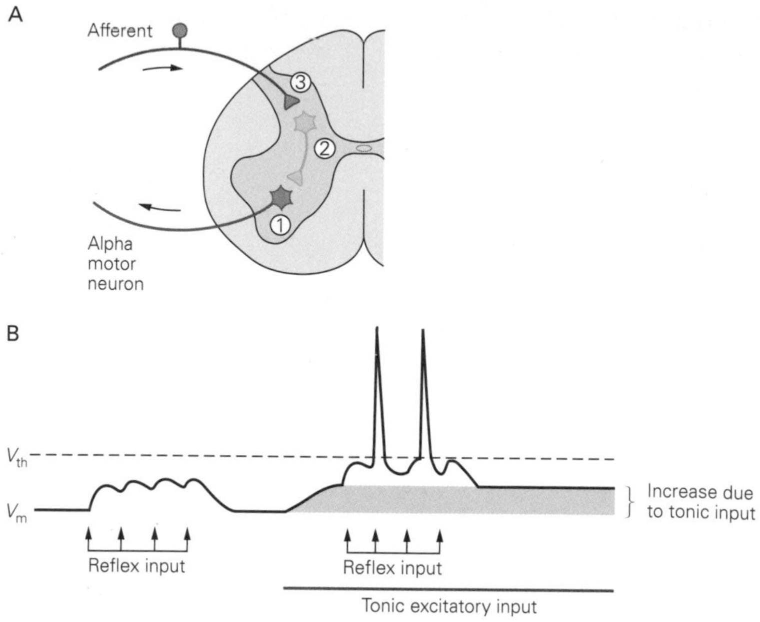

Figure 35–8 The strength of a spinal reflex can be modulated by changes in synaptic transmission in the reflex pathway.

A. A reflex pathway can be modified at three sites: alpha motor neurons (**1**), interneurons in polysynaptic pathways (**2**), and afferent axon terminals (**3**). Transmitter release from the primary afferent fibers is regulated by presynaptic inhibition (see Figure 12–16).

B. An increase in tonic (background) excitatory input to a motor neuron depolarizes the neuron to a level that enables an otherwise ineffective reflex input (**left**) to initiate action potentials. The reflex input is represented by a series of excitatory postsynaptic potentials. (V_{th}, threshold voltage; V_m, membrane potential.)

even the slightest reflex input will more easily activate the motor neurons (Figure 35–8B). Another mechanism for modulating the strength of reflexes is to change the physiological properties of motor neurons and perhaps interneurons. Activity in descending monoaminergic systems can alter the properties of motor neurons so they either discharge at a much higher rate in response to the same synaptic input or remain active following a brief excitatory input (see Chapter 34).

Reflex strength can be changed quickly to adapt to the requirements of specific tasks. Intracellular recordings suggest that presynaptic inhibition of the Ia fibers from muscle spindles is particularly important for producing these changes. For example, during locomotion the level of presynaptic inhibition is rhythmically modulated; this action presumably modulates the strength of reflexes during the different phases of the gait cycle (see Chapter 36).

Gamma Motor Neurons Adjust the Sensitivity of Muscle Spindles

Activity of muscle spindles may be modulated by changing the level of activity in the gamma motor neurons, which innervate the intrafusal muscle fibers of muscle spindles (see Box 35–1). This function of gamma motor neurons, often referred to as the fusimotor system, can be demonstrated by selectively stimulating the alpha and gamma motor neurons under experimental conditions.

When only alpha motor neurons are stimulated, the firing of the Ia fiber from the muscle spindle pauses during contraction of the muscle because the muscle is shortening and therefore unloading (slackening) the spindle. However, if gamma motor neurons are activated at the same time as alpha motor neurons, the pause is eliminated. The contraction of the intrafusal fibers by the gamma motor neurons keeps the spindle under tension, thus maintaining the firing rate of the Ia fibers within an optimal range for signaling changes in length, whatever the actual length of the muscle (Figure 35–9). This *alpha-gamma co-activation* thus stabilizes the sensitivity of the muscle spindles and is used in many voluntary movements.

In addition to the axons of gamma motor neurons, axon collaterals of alpha motor neurons sometimes innervate the intrafusal fibers. Axons that innervate both intrafusal and extrafusal muscle fibers are referred to as *beta* axons. Beta axon collaterals provide the equivalent of alpha-gamma coactivation. Beta innervation in spindles exists in both cats and humans, although it is unquantified for most muscles.

The beta fusimotor system's forced linkage of extrafusal and intrafusal contraction highlights the importance of the independent fusimotor system (the gamma motor neurons). Indeed, in lower vertebrates, such as amphibians, beta efferents are the only source of intrafusal innervation. Mammals have evolved a mechanism that frees muscle spindles from complete dependence on the behavior of their parent muscles. In principle this uncoupling allows greater flexibility in controlling spindle sensitivity for different types of motor tasks.

This conclusion is supported by recordings in spindle sensory afferents during a variety of natural movements in cats. The amount and type of activity in gamma motor neurons are set at steady levels, which vary according to the specific task or context. In general, activity levels in both static and dynamic gamma motor neurons (see Figure 35–3B) are set at progressively higher levels as the speed and difficulty of the movement increase. Unpredictable conditions, such as when the cat is picked up or handled, lead to marked increases in activity in dynamic gamma motor neurons and thus increased spindle responsiveness when muscles are stretched. When an animal is performing a difficult task, such as walking across a narrow beam,

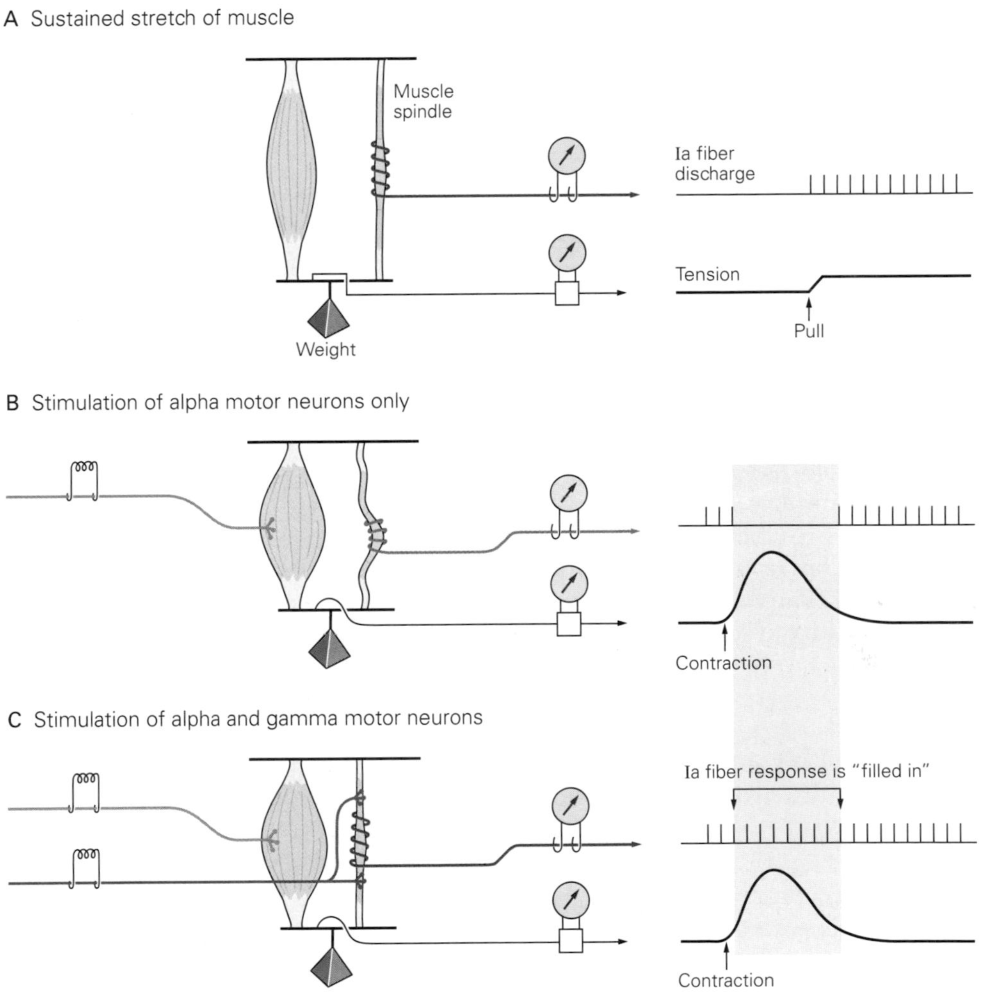

Figure 35–9 Activation of gamma motor neurons during active muscle contraction maintains muscle spindle sensitivity to muscle length. (Adapted, with permission, from Hunt and Kuffler 1951.)

A. Sustained tension elicits steady firing in the Ia sensory fiber from the muscle spindle (the two muscle fibers are shown separately for illustration only).

B. A characteristic pause occurs in the discharge of the Ia fiber when the alpha motor neuron is stimulated, causing a brief contraction of the muscle. The Ia fiber stops firing because the spindle is unloaded by the contraction.

C. Gamma motor neurons innervate the contractile polar regions of the intrafusal fibers of muscle spindles (see Figure 35–3A). If a gamma motor neuron is stimulated at the same time as the alpha motor neuron, the spindle is not unloaded during the contraction. As a result, the pause in discharge of the Ia sensory fiber that occurs when only the alpha motor neuron is stimulated is "filled in" by the response of the fiber to stimulation of the gamma motor neuron.

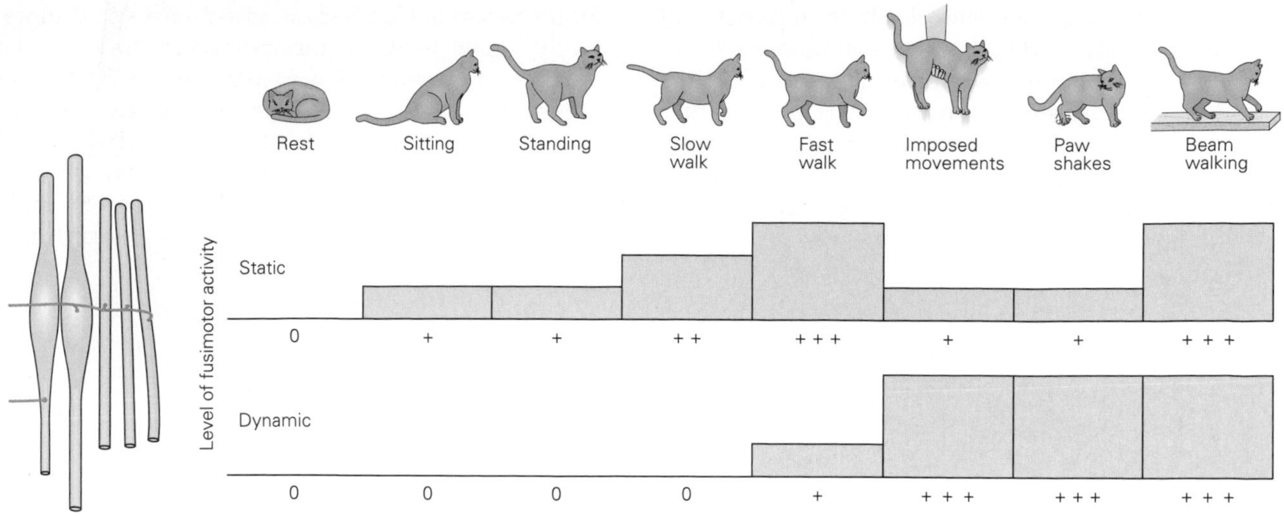

Figure 35–10 The level of activity in the fusimotor system varies with the type of behavior. Only static gamma motor neurons are active during activities in which muscle length changes slowly and predictably. Dynamic gamma motor neurons are activated during behaviors in which muscle length may change rapidly and unpredictably. (Adapted, with permission, from Prochazka et al. 1988.)

both static and dynamic gamma activation are at high levels (Figure 35–10).

Thus the nervous system uses the fusimotor system to fine-tune muscle spindles so that the ensemble output of the spindles provides information most appropriate for a task. The task conditions under which independent control of alpha and gamma motor neurons occurs in humans have not yet been clearly established.

Proprioceptive Reflexes Play an Important Role in Regulating Both Voluntary and Automatic Movements

All movements activate receptors in muscles, joints, and skin. Sensory signals generated by the body's own movements were termed *proprioceptive* by Sherrington, who proposed that they control important aspects of normal movements. A good example is the Hering-Breuer reflex, which regulates the amplitude of inspiration. Stretch receptors in the lungs are activated during inspiration, and the Hering-Breuer reflex eventually triggers the transition from inspiration to expiration when the lungs are expanded.

A similar situation exists in the walking systems of many animals; sensory signals generated near the end of the stance phase initiate the onset of the swing phase (see Chapter 36). Proprioceptive signals can also contribute to the regulation of motor activity during voluntary movements, as has been shown in recent studies of individuals with sensory neuropathy of the arms. These patients display abnormal reaching movements and have difficulty in positioning the limb accurately because the lack of proprioception results in a failure to compensate for the complex inertial properties of the human arm.

Therefore, a primary function of proprioceptive reflexes in regulating voluntary movements is to adjust the motor output according to the changing biomechanical state of the body and limbs. This adjustment ensures a coordinated pattern of motor activity during an evolving movement and compensates for the intrinsic variability of motor output.

Reflexes Involving Limb Muscles Are Mediated Through Spinal and Supraspinal Pathways

Reflexes involving the limbs are mediated by multiple pathways acting in parallel through spinal and supraspinal pathways. Consider the response evoked by a sudden stretch of a flexor muscle of the thumb. This response has two discrete components. The first, the M1 response, is generated by the monosynaptic connection of muscle spindle afferents to the spinal motor neurons. The second, the M2 response, is also a reflex because its latency is shorter than the voluntary reaction time (Figure 35–11A).

The M2 response has been observed in virtually all limb muscles. In the distal muscles the M2 responses are mediated by pathways that include the motor cortex, as shown in studies of patients with Klippel-Feil syndrome. In this unusual condition axons descending from neurons in the motor cortex bifurcate and make connections to homologous motor neurons on both sides of the body. Thus, when the individual voluntarily moves the fingers of one hand, these movements are mirrored by movements of the fingers of the other (Figure 35–11B). Similarly, when the M2 component is evoked by stretching muscles of one hand, a response with the same latency is evoked in the corresponding muscle of the other hand, even though no

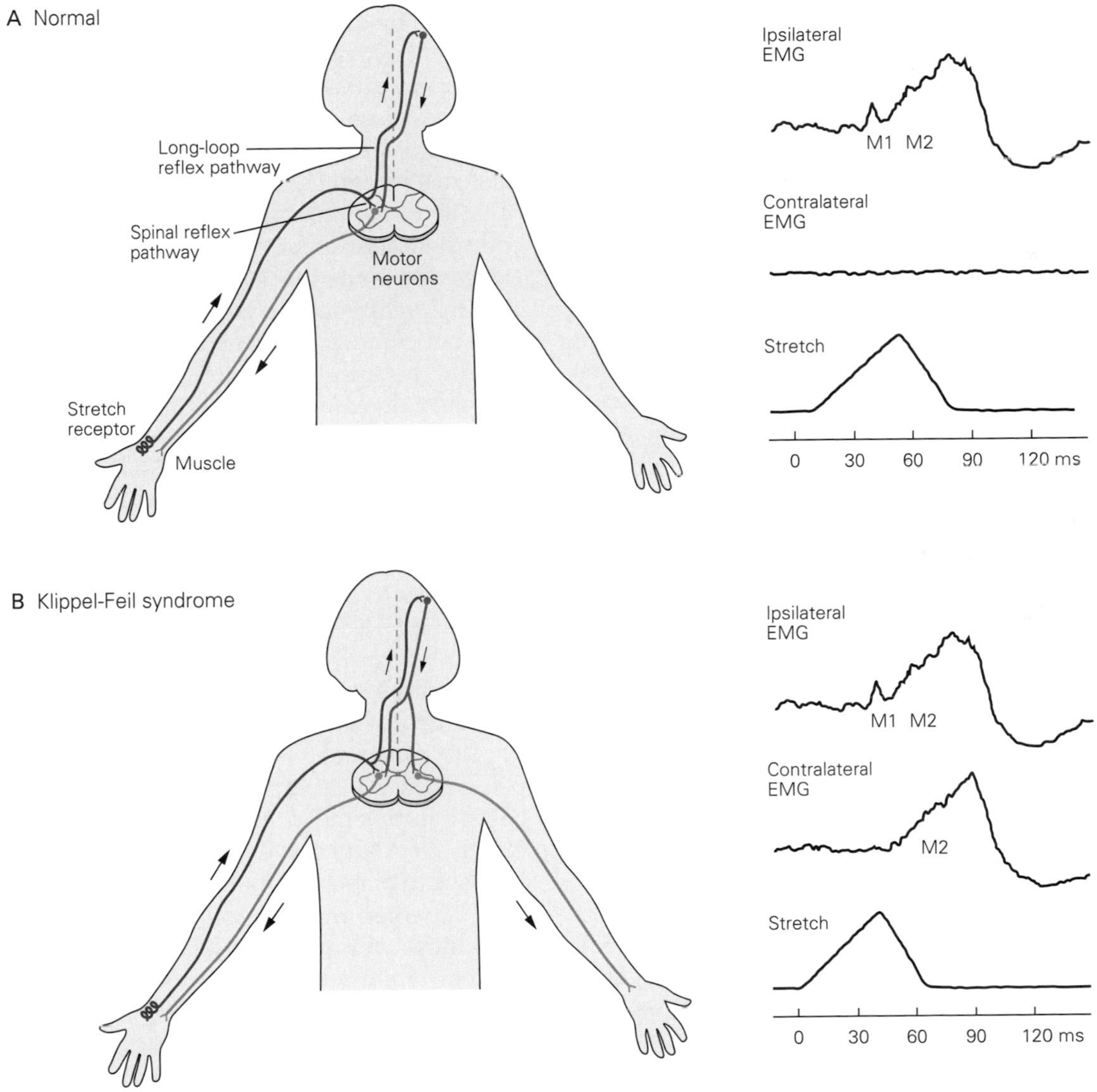

Figure 35–11 Reflexes of the limbs are mediated by spinal reflex pathways and long-loop pathways that involve the motor cortex. (Adapted, with permission, from Matthews 1991.)

A. In normal individuals a brief stretch of a thumb muscle produces a response that has two components. A short-latency response (M1) in the stretched muscle is controlled by the spinal reflex pathway, the monosynaptic connection between muscle spindle afferents and spinal motor neurons. This is followed by a long-latency response (M2) controlled by a pathway that loops through the motor cortex.

B. In individuals with Klippel-Feil syndrome the M2 response is evoked bilaterally because neurons in the motor cortex activate motor neurons bilaterally.

M1 response has occurred in the other hand. The reflex pathway responsible for the M2 response must therefore traverse the motor cortex (Figure 35–11B).

Reflex responses mediated through the motor cortex and other supraspinal structures, the *long-loop reflexes,* have been investigated in numerous muscles in humans and other animals. The general conclusion is that long-loop reflexes via the cortex are of primary importance in regulating contractions in distal muscles, whereas subcortical reflex pathways are largely responsible for regulating the contractions of proximal muscles.

This type of organization is related to functional demands. Many tasks involving distal muscles require precise regulation by voluntary commands. By transmitting sensory signals to regions of cortex most involved in controlling voluntary movements, motor commands can be quickly adapted to the evolving needs of a task. More automatic motor functions, such as maintaining balance and producing gross bodily movements, can be efficiently executed largely through subcortical and spinal pathways.

Pioneering studies by Edward Evarts in the 1960s revealed that activity in approximately 50% of neurons in the motor cortex is modified in response to loading muscles during the voluntary maintenance of wrist position and during simple movements at the wrist. This early finding was initially interpreted as evidence that long-loop cortical reflexes are involved in compensating for change in loading conditions by functioning as online negative feedback controllers. However, subsequent studies on multijoint movements revealed complex response patterns in cortical neurons, many of which are not consistent with this concept. Moreover, the long delays in transmission in long-loop reflexes make these reflexes inappropriate for a direct role in load compensation because the potential delays would create instabilities.

Currently the function of proprioceptive input to the motor cortex in the volitional control of movement remains a puzzle. One contemporary notion is that proprioceptive input is integrated into internal models for estimating the state of the system (see Chapter 33). Another hypothesis is that proprioceptive inputs play a key role in motor cortical circuits that function as optimal feedback controllers, which use only those sensory signals that are required for attaining a specific goal.

Stretch Reflexes Reinforce Central Commands for Movements

Stretch-reflex pathways can contribute to regulation of motor neurons during voluntary movements and maintenance of posture because they form closed feedback loops. For example, stretching a muscle increases activity in spindle sensory afferents, leading to muscle contraction and consequent shortening of the muscle. Muscle shortening in turn leads to decreased activity in spindle afferents, reduction of muscle contraction, and lengthening of the muscle.

The stretch reflex loop thus acts continuously—the output of the system, a change in muscle length, becomes the input—tending to keep the muscle close to a desired or reference length. The stretch reflex is a negative feedback system, or *servomechanism,* because it tends to counteract or reduce deviations from the reference value of the regulated variable.

In 1963 Ragnar Granit proposed that the reference value in voluntary movements is set by descending signals that act on both alpha and gamma motor neurons. The rate of firing of alpha motor neurons is set to produce the desired shortening of the muscle, and the rate of firing of gamma motor neurons is set to produce an equivalent shortening of the intrafusal fibers of the muscle spindle. If the shortening of the whole muscle is less than that required by a task, as when the load is greater than anticipated, the sensory fibers increase their firing rate because the contracting intrafusal fibers are stretched (loaded) by the relatively greater length of the whole muscle. If shortening is greater than necessary, the sensory fibers decrease their firing rate because the intrafusal fibers are relatively slackened (unloaded) (Figure 35–12A).

In theory this mechanism could permit the nervous system to produce a movement of a given distance without having to know in advance the actual load or weight being moved. In practice, however, the stretch-reflex pathways do not have sufficient control over motor neurons to overcome large unexpected loads. This is immediately obvious if we consider what happens when we attempt to lift a heavy suitcase that we believe to be empty. Automatic compensation for the greater-than-anticipated load does not occur. Instead, we have to pause briefly to plan a new movement with much greater muscle activation. Thus, rather than providing compensation for large unexpected loads, monosynaptic and long-loop stretch reflex pathways may compensate for small changes in load and intrinsic irregularities in the muscle contraction, with the relative contribution of each pathway dependent on the muscle and the task.

Strong evidence that alpha and gamma motor neurons are co-activated during voluntary human movement has come from direct measurements of the activity of muscle spindles. In the late 1960s Åke Vallbo and Karl-Erik Hagbarth developed microneurography, a technique for recording from the largest afferent fibers

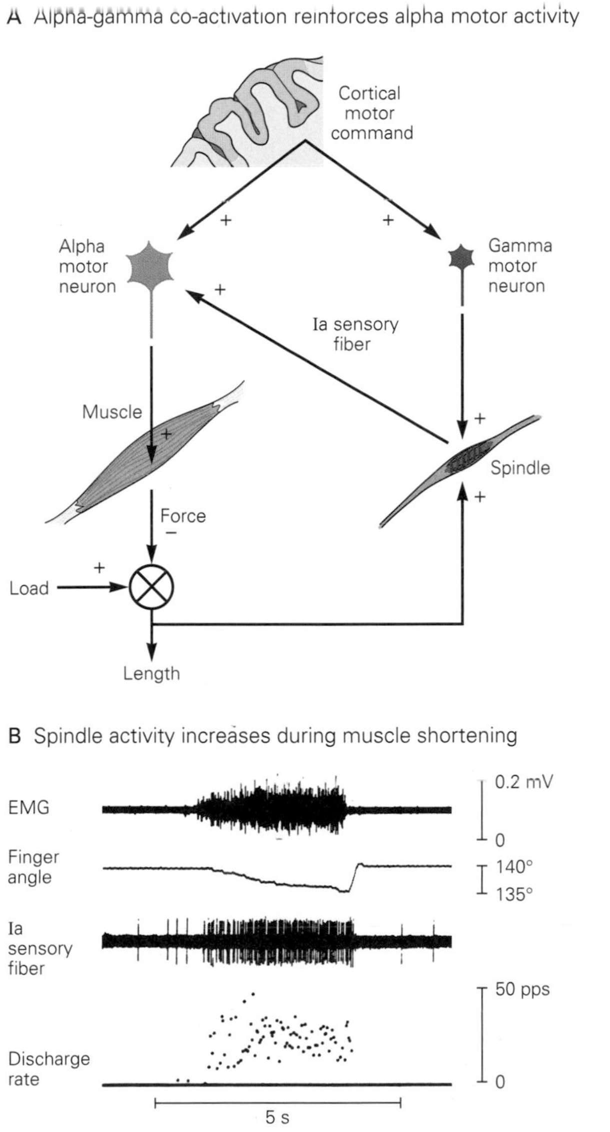

Figure 35–12 Alpha and gamma motor neurons are co-activated during voluntary movements.

A. Co-activation of alpha and gamma motor neurons by a cortical motor command allows feedback from muscle spindles to reinforce activation in the alpha motor neurons. Because any disturbance during a movement alters the length of the muscle and changes the activity in the muscle spindles, altering the spindle input to the alpha motor neuron compensates for the disturbance.

B. The discharge rate in the Ia sensory fiber of a spindle increases during slow flexion of a finger. This increase depends on alpha-gamma co-activation. If the gamma motor neurons were not active, the spindle would slacken, and its discharge rate would decrease as the muscle shortened (see Figure 35–9C). (Adapted, with permission, from Vallbo 1981.)

in peripheral nerves. Vallbo later showed that during slow movements of the fingers the large-diameter Ia fibers from spindles in the contracting muscles increase their rate of firing even when the muscle shortens as it contracts (Figure 35–12B). This occurs because the gamma motor neurons, which have direct excitatory connections with spindles, are co-activated with alpha motor neurons.

Furthermore, when subjects attempt to make slow movements at a constant velocity, the firing of the Ia fibers mirrors small deviations in velocity in the trajectory of the movements (sometimes the muscle shortens quickly and other times more slowly). When the velocity of flexion increases transiently, the rate of firing in the fibers decreases because the muscle is shortening more rapidly and therefore exerts less tension on the intrafusal fibers. When the velocity decreases, firing increases because the muscle is shortening more slowly, and therefore the relative tension on the intrafusal fibers increases. This information can be used by the nervous system to compensate for irregularities in the movement trajectory by exciting the alpha motor neurons.

Damage to the Central Nervous System Produces Characteristic Alterations in Reflex Response and Muscle Tone

Stretch reflexes can be evoked in many muscles throughout the body and are routinely used in clinical examinations of patients with neurological disorders. They are typically elicited by sharply tapping the tendon of a muscle with a reflex hammer.

Although the responses are often called tendon reflexes or tendon jerks, the receptor that is stimulated, the muscle spindle, actually lies in the muscle rather than the tendon. Only the primary sensory fibers in the spindle participate in the tendon reflex, for these are selectively activated by a rapid stretch of the muscle produced by the tendon tap. An electrical analog of the tendon jerk is the Hoffmann reflex (Box 35–4).

Measuring alterations in the strength of the stretch reflex can assist in the diagnosis of certain conditions and in localizing injury or disease in the central nervous system. Absent or hypoactive stretch reflexes often indicate a disorder of one or more of the components of the peripheral reflex pathway: sensory or motor axons, the cell bodies of motor neurons, or the muscle itself. Nevertheless, because the excitability of motor neurons is dependent on descending excitatory and inhibitory signals, absent or hypoactive stretch reflexes can also result from lesions of the central nervous system.

Box 35–4 The Hoffmann Reflex

The characteristics of the monosynaptic connections from Ia sensory fibers to spinal motor neurons in humans can be studied using an important technique introduced in the 1950s and based on early work by Paul Hoffmann. This technique involves electrically stimulating the Ia fibers in a peripheral nerve and recording the reflex response in the homonymous muscle. The response is known as the *Hoffmann reflex,* or H-reflex (Figure 35–13A).

The H-reflex is readily measured in the soleus muscle, an ankle extensor. The Ia fibers from the soleus and its synergists are excited by an electrode placed above the tibial nerve behind the knee. The response recorded from the soleus muscle depends on stimulus strength. At low stimulus strengths a pure H-reflex is evoked, for the threshold for activation of the Ia fibers is lower than the threshold for motor axons. Increasing the stimulus strength excites the motor axons innervating the soleus, producing two successive responses.

The first results from direct activation of the motor axons, and the second is the H-reflex evoked by stimulation of the Ia fibers (Figure 35–13B). These two components of the evoked electromyogram are called the M-wave and H-wave. The H-wave occurs later because it results from signals that travel to the spinal cord, across a synapse, and back again to the muscle. The M-wave, in contrast, results from direct stimulation of the motor axon innervating the muscle.

As the stimulus strength is increased still further, the M-wave continues to become larger and the H-wave progressively declines (Figure 35–13C). The decline in the H-wave amplitude occurs because action potentials in the motor axons propagate toward the cell body (antidromic conduction) and cancel reflexively evoked action potentials in the same motor axons. At very high stimulus strengths only the M-wave persists.

An interesting feature of the H-reflex is that its magnitude depends on motor experience. For example, it is low in highly trained ballet dancers and varies among different kinds of athletes. This strongly suggests that modification of spinal reflexes is an important process in learning motor skills.

Extensive studies of humans, monkeys, and rats by Jonathan Wolpaw and his colleagues have demonstrated that H-reflexes can be operantly conditioned to either increase or decrease. The mechanisms underlying these changes are complex and involve alterations at multiple sites including changes in motor neuron properties. For down-conditioning they are dependent on corticospinal signals.

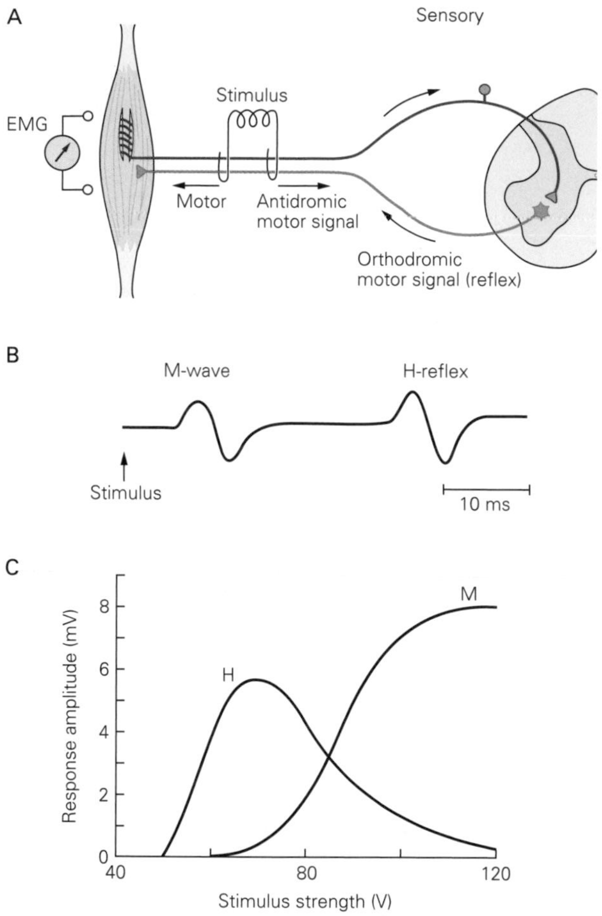

Figure 35–13 The Hoffmann reflex.

A. The Hoffmann reflex (H-reflex) is evoked by electrically stimulating Ia sensory fibers from muscle spindles in mixed nerves. The sensory fibers excite alpha motor neurons, which in turn activate the muscle. Muscle activation is detected by the electromyogram (EMG).

B. At intermediate stimulus strengths motor axons in the mixed nerve are excited in addition to the spindle afferents. Excitation of the motor neurons produces an M-wave that precedes the H-wave (H-reflex) in the EMG.

C. At low stimulus strengths only an H-wave is produced because only the spindle afferents are excited. As the stimulus strength increases, the magnitude of the H-reflex also increases, then declines, because the orthodromic motor signals generated reflexively by the spindle afferents are cancelled by antidromic signals initiated by the electrical stimulus in the same motor axons. At very high stimulus strengths only an M-wave is evoked. (Adapted, with permission, from Schieppati 1987.)

Hyperactive stretch reflexes, conversely, always indicate that the lesion is in the central nervous system.

Interruption of Descending Pathways to the Spinal Cord Frequently Produces Spasticity

Muscle tone, the force with which a muscle resists being lengthened, depends on the muscle's intrinsic elasticity, or stiffness. Because a muscle has elastic elements in series and parallel that resist lengthening, it behaves like a spring. However, there is also a neural contribution to muscle tone; the feedback loop inherent in the stretch reflex pathway acts to resist lengthening of the muscle. The local neural circuits responsible for stretch reflexes provide the brain with a mechanism for adjusting muscle tone to suit different circumstances.

Because the strength of stretch reflexes is controlled by higher brain centers, disorders of muscle tone are frequently associated with lesions of the motor system, especially those that interfere with descending motor pathways. These conditions may involve either an abnormal increase in tone (*hypertonus*) or a decrease (*hypotonus*). The most common form of hypertonus is spasticity, which is characterized by hyperactive tendon jerks and an increase in resistance to rapid stretching of the muscle. A slowly applied stretch in a patient with spasticity elicits little resistance; as the speed of the stretch is increased, resistance to the stretch also rises progressively.

Thus spasticity is primarily a phasic phenomenon. An active reflex contraction occurs only during a rapid stretch; when the muscle is held in a lengthened position the reflex contraction subsides. In some patients, however, the hypertonus also has a tonic component; that is, the reflex contraction continues even after the muscle is no longer being lengthened.

The pathophysiology of spasticity is still unclear. It was long thought that hyperactivity of stretch reflexes in spasticity resulted from overactivity of the gamma motor neurons. Recent experiments have cast doubt on this explanation. Although gamma motor neurons may be overactive in some cases, changes in the background activity of alpha motor neurons and interneurons are probably more important. Especially important may be modifications in the properties of motor neurons that enable sustained firing in response to brief excitatory input (see Chapter 34).

Whatever the precise mechanism that produces spasticity, the effect is a strong facilitation of synaptic transmission in the Ia sensory fibers in the monosynaptic reflex pathway. Indeed, this can provide a mechanism for treatment. A common therapeutic procedure today is to mimic presynaptic inhibition in the terminals of the Ia fibers by intrathecally administering the drug baclofen to the spinal cord. Baclofen is an agonist of $GABA_B$ (γ-aminobutyric acid) receptors; binding of the drug to these receptors decreases the influx of Ca^{2+} into presynaptic terminals, reducing transmitter release.

Transection of the Spinal Cord in Humans Leads to a Period of Spinal Shock Followed by Hyperreflexia

Damage to the spinal cord can cause large changes in the strength of spinal reflexes. Each year approximately 11,000 Americans sustain spinal cord injuries. More than half of these injuries produce permanent disability, including impairment of motor and sensory functions and loss of voluntary bowel and bladder control. Approximately 250,000 people in the United States today have some permanent disability from spinal cord injury.

When the spinal cord is completely transected, there is usually a period immediately after the injury when all spinal reflexes below the level of the transection are reduced or completely suppressed. This condition is known as *spinal shock*. During the course of weeks and months spinal reflexes gradually return, often greatly exaggerated. For example, a light touch to the skin of the foot may elicit strong flexion withdrawal of the leg.

The mechanisms underlying spinal shock and recovery are poorly understood. The initial shock is thought to result from the sudden withdrawal of tonic facilitatory influence from the brain. Several mechanisms may contribute to the recovery, including sprouting of afferent sensory terminals and denervation supersensitivity owing to increased numbers of postsynaptic receptors.

Interestingly, the period of recovery from spinal shock is much shorter in animals than in humans. In nonhuman primates the recovery period is rarely more than a week; in cats and dogs it is only a few hours. The longer recovery period for humans presumably reflects the greater influence of supraspinal centers on spinal reflex circuits. This may in turn reflect the increased complexity of upright bipedal locomotion. Indeed, as we shall see in the next chapter, in humans with spinal cord injury the recovery of automatic locomotor patterns is slight compared with that of quadrupedal mammals.

An Overall View

Reflexes are coordinated, involuntary motor responses initiated by a stimulus applied to peripheral receptors. Some reflexes initiate movements to avoid potentially hazardous situations, whereas others automatically adapt motor patterns to achieve or maintain a behavioral goal. The actual response evoked by a reflex depends on mechanisms that set the strength and pattern of responses according to the task and the behavioral state, or functional set. We know little about the details of these mechanisms, except that modification of synaptic transmission in spinal reflex pathways by descending signals from the brain is thought to be an important factor.

Many groups of interneurons in spinal reflex pathways are also involved in producing complex movements such as walking and transmitting voluntary commands from the brain. In addition, some components of reflex responses, particularly those involving the limbs, are mediated by supraspinal centers, such as brain stem nuclei, the cerebellum, and the motor cortex. Reflexes can be smoothly integrated into centrally generated motor commands because of the convergence of sensory signals onto spinal and supraspinal interneuronal systems involved in initiating movements. Establishing the details of these integrative events is one of the major challenges of contemporary research on reflex regulation of movement.

Because of the role of supraspinal centers in spinal reflex pathways, injury to or disease of the central nervous system often results in significant alterations in the strength of spinal reflexes. The pattern of changes provides an important aid to diagnosis of patients with neurological disorders.

Keir G. Pearson
James E. Gordon

Selected Readings

Baldissera F, Hultborn H, Illert M. 1981. Integration in spinal neuronal systems. In: JM Brookhart, VB Mountcastle, VB Brooks, SR Geiger (eds). *Handbook of Physiology: The Nervous System,* pp. 509–595. Bethesda, MD: American Physiological Society.

Boyd IA. 1980. The isolated mammalian muscle spindle. Trends Neurosci 3:258–265.

Dietz V. 1992. Human neuronal control of automatic functional movements: interaction between central programs and afferent input. Physiol Rev 72:33–61.

Fetz EE, Perlmutter SI, Orut Y. 2000. Functions of spinal interneurons during movement. Curr Opin Neurobiol 10:699–707.

Jankowska E. 1992. Interneuronal relay in spinal pathways from proprioceptors. Prog Neurobiol 38:335–378.

Matthews PBC. 1991. The human stretch reflex and the motor cortex. Trends Neurosci 14:87–90.

Prochazka A. 1996. Proprioceptive feedback and movement regulation. In: L Rowell, JT Sheperd (eds). *Handbook of Physiology: Regulation and Integration of Multiple Systems,* pp. 89–127. New York: American Physiological Society.

Scott SH. 2008. Inconvenient truths about neural processing in primary motor cortex. J Physiol 586:1217–1224.

Windhorst U. 2007. Muscle proprioceptive feedback and spinal networks. Brain Res Bull 73:155–202.

Wolpaw JR. 2007. Spinal cord plasticity in acquisition and maintenance of motor skills. Acta Physiol (Oxf) 189: 155–169.

References

Appenteng K, Prochazka A. 1984. Tendon organ firing during active muscle lengthening in normal cats. J Physiol (Lond) 353:81–92.

Brown MC, Matthews PBC. 1966. On the sub-division of the efferent fibres to muscle spindles into static and dynamic fusimotor fibres. In: BL Andrew (ed). *Control and Innervation of Skeletal Muscle,* pp. 18–31. Dundee, Scotland: University of St. Andrews.

Cole KJ, Gracco VL, Abbs JH. 1984. Autogenetic and nonautogenetic sensorimotor actions in the control of multiarticulate hand movements. Exp Brain Res 56:582–585.

Crago A, Houk JC, Rymer WZ. 1982. Sampling of total muscle force by tendon organs. J Neurophysiol 47:1069–1083.

Ghez C, Gordon J, Ghilardi MF. 1995. Impairments of reaching movements in patients without proprioception. II. Effects of visual information on accuracy. J Neurophysiol 73:361–372.

Gossard JP, Brownstone RM, Barajon I, Hultborn H. 1994. Transmission in a locomotor-related group Ib pathway from hind limb extensor muscles in the cat. Exp Brain Res 98:213–228.

Granit R. 1970. *Basis of Motor Control.* London: Academic.

Hagbarth KE, Kunesch EJ, Nordin M, Schmidt R, Wallin EU. 1986. Gamma loop contributing to maximal voluntary contractions in man. J Physiol (Lond) 380:575–591.

Hoffmann P. 1922. *Untersuchungen über die Eigenreflexe (Sehnenreflexe) menschlicher Muskeln.* Berlin: Springer.

Hulliger M. 1984. The mammalian muscle spindle and its central control. Rev Physiol Biochem Pharmacol 101: 1–110.

Hunt CC, Kuffler SW. 1951. Stretch receptor discharges during muscle contraction. J Physiol (Lond) 113:298–315.

Liddell EGT, Sherrington C. 1924. Reflexes in response to stretch (myotatic reflexes). Proc R Soc Lond B Biol Sci 96:212–242.

Marsden CD, Merton PA, Morton HB. 1981. Human postural responses. Brain 104:513–534.

Matthews PBC. 1972. *Muscle Receptors.* London: Edward Arnold.

Mendell LM, Henneman E. 1971. Terminals of single Ia fibers: location, density, and distribution within a pool of 300 homonymous motoneurons. J Neurophysiol 34:171–187.

Pearson KG, Collins DF. 1993. Reversal of the influence of group Ib afferents from plantaris on activity in model gastrocnemius activity during locomotor activity. J Neurophysiol 70:1009–1017.

Prochazka A, Hulliger M, Trend P, Dürmüller N. 1988. Dynamic and static fusimotor set in various behavioural contexts. In: P Hnik, T Soukup, R Vejsada, J Zelena (eds). *Mechanoreceptors: Development, Structure and Function,* pp. 417–430. New York: Plenum.

Schieppati M. 1987. The Hoffmann reflex: a means of assessing spinal reflex excitability and its descending control in man. Prog Neurobiol 28:345–376.

Schmidt RF. 1983. Motor systems. In: RF Schmidt, G Thews (eds), MA Biederman-Thorson (transl). *Human Physiology,* pp. 81–110. Berlin: Springer.

Sherrington CS. 1906. *Integrative Actions of the Nervous System.* New Haven, CT: Yale Univ. Press.

Swett JE, Schoultz TW. 1975. Mechanical transduction in the Golgi tendon organ: a hypothesis. Arch Ital Biol 113: 374–382.

Vallbo ÅB. 1981. Basic patterns of muscle spindle discharge in man. In: A Taylor, A Prochazka (eds). *Muscle Receptors and Movement,* pp. 263–275. London: Macmillan.

Vallbo ÅB, Hagbarth KE, Torebjörk HE, Wallin BG. 1979. Somatosensory, proprioceptive, and sympathetic activity in human peripheral nerves. Physiol Rev 59:919–957.

Wickens DD. 1938. The transference of conditioned excitation and conditioned inhibition form one muscle group to the antagonist muscle group. J Exp Psychol 22:101–123.

36

Locomotion

THE ABILITY TO MOVE IS ESSENTIAL for the survival of animals. Although many forms of locomotion have evolved—swimming, flying, crawling, and walking—all use rhythmic and alternating movements of the body or appendages. This rhythmicity makes locomotion appear to be repetitive and stereotyped. Indeed, locomotion is controlled automatically at relatively low levels of the central nervous system without intervention by higher centers. Nevertheless, locomotion often takes place in environments that are either unfamiliar or present unpredictable conditions. Locomotor movements must therefore be continually modified, usually in a subtle fashion, to adapt otherwise stereotyped movement patterns to the immediate surroundings.

The study of the neural control of locomotion must address two fundamental questions. First, how do assemblies of nerve cells generate the rhythmic motor patterns associated with locomotor movements? Second, how does sensory information adjust locomotion to both anticipated and unexpected events in the environment? In this chapter we address both of these questions by examining the neural mechanisms controlling walking.

Although most information on neural control of walking has come from studying the cat's stepping movements, important insights have also come from studies of other animals as well as rhythmic behaviors other than locomotion. Therefore, we shall also consider the more general question of how rhythmic motor activity can be generated and sustained by networks of neurons.

Several critical insights into the neural mechanisms controlling quadrupedal stepping were obtained nearly a century ago when it was found that removing the cerebral hemispheres in dogs did not abolish walking—decerebrate animals are still able to walk spontaneously. One animal was observed to rear itself up in order to rest its forepaws on a gate at feeding time. It was soon discovered that stepping of the hind legs could be induced in cats and dogs after complete transection of the spinal cord. The stepping movements in these *spinal preparations* (Box 36–1) are similar to normal stepping. Nonrhythmic electrical stimulation of the cut cord elicits stepping at a rate related to the intensity of the stimulating current. Another important early observation was that passive movement of a limb by the experimenter could initiate stepping movements in spinal cats and dogs, suggesting that proprioceptive reflexes are crucial in regulating the movements.

Finally, in 1911 Thomas Graham Brown discovered that rhythmic, alternating contractions could be evoked in deafferented hind leg muscles immediately after transection of the spinal cord. He therefore proposed the concept of the half-center, whereby flexors and extensors inhibit each other reciprocally, giving rise to alternating stepping movements. Four conclusions can be drawn from these early studies.

1. Supraspinal commands are not necessary for producing the basic motor pattern for stepping.
2. The basic rhythmicity of stepping is produced by neuronal circuits contained entirely within the spinal cord.
3. The spinal circuits can be modulated by tonic descending signals from the brain.
4. The spinal pattern-generating networks do not require sensory input but nevertheless are strongly regulated by input from limb proprioceptors.

For almost half a century following these early studies few investigations were aimed at establishing the neural mechanisms for walking. Instead, research on motor systems focused on the organization of spinal reflex pathways and the mechanisms of synaptic integration within the spinal cord (see Chapter 35). Modern research on the neural control of locomotion dates from the 1960s and two major experimental successes. First, rhythmic patterns of motor activity were elicited in spinal animals by the application of adrenergic drugs. Second, walking on a treadmill was evoked in decerebrate cats by electrical stimulation of a small region in the brain stem.

At about the same time electromyographic recordings from numerous hind leg muscles in intact cats during unrestrained walking revealed the complexity of the locomotor pattern and brought to prominence the question of how spinal reflexes are integrated with intrinsic spinal circuits to produce the locomotor pattern. Soon thereafter, investigations of stepping in spinal cats demonstrated the similarity of locomotor patterns in spinal preparations and intact animals, thus firmly establishing the idea that the motor output for locomotion is produced primarily by a neuronal system in the spinal cord.

A Complex Sequence of Muscle Contractions Is Required for Stepping

For the purpose of examining the patterns of muscle contraction during locomotion, the step cycle in cats and humans can be divided into four distinct phases: flexion (F), first extension (E_1), second extension (E_2), and third extension (E_3) (Figure 36–2A). The F and E_1 phases occur during the time the foot is off the ground (*swing*), whereas E_2 and E_3 occur when the foot is in contact with the ground (*stance*).

Swing commences with flexion at the hip, knee, and ankle (the F phase). Approximately midway through swing the knee and ankle begin to extend while the hip continues to flex (the E_1 phase). Extension at the knee and ankle during E_1 moves the foot ahead of the body and prepares the leg to accept weight in anticipation of foot contact at the onset of stance. During early stance (the E_2 phase) the knee and ankle joints flex, even though extensor muscles are contracting strongly. A lengthening contraction of ankle and knee extensor muscles occurs because weight is being transferred to the leg. The spring-like yielding of these muscles as weight is accepted allows the body to move smoothly over the foot, and is essential for establishing an efficient gait. During late stance (the E_3 phase) the hip, knee, and ankle all extend to provide a propulsive force to move the body forward.

The rhythmic movements of the legs during stepping are produced by contractions of many muscles. In general, contractions of flexor muscles occur during the F phase, whereas contractions of extensor muscles occur during one or more of the E phases. However, the timing and amounts of activity are different in different muscles (Figure 36–2B). For example, a hip flexor muscle (iliopsoas) contracts continuously during the F and E_1 phases, whereas a knee flexor muscle (semitendinosus) contracts briefly at the beginning of the F and E_2 phases. Another complexity is that some

Box 36–1 Preparations Used to Study the Neural Control of Stepping

The literature on the neural control of quadrupedal stepping can be confusing because different experimental preparations are used in different studies. In addition to intact animals, spinal and decerebrate cats are commonly used in studies of the neural mechanisms of locomotor rhythmicity. Moreover, each of these preparations may be used in two experimental strategies, deafferentation and immobilization, depending on what is being investigated. Finally, neonatal rat and mouse preparations have proven useful for analyzing the cellular properties of neurons generating the locomotor rhythm.

Spinal Preparations

In spinal preparations the spinal cord is transected at the lower thoracic level (Figure 36–1A), thus isolating the spinal segments that control the hind limb musculature from the rest of the central nervous system. This allows investigations of the role of spinal circuits in generating rhythmic locomotor patterns.

In *acute* spinal preparations adrenergic drugs such as L-DOPA (L-dihydroxyphenylalanine) and nialamide are administered immediately after the transection. These drugs elevate the level of norepinephrine in the spinal cord and lead to the spontaneous generation of locomotor activity approximately 30 minutes after administration. Clonidine, another adrenergic drug, enables locomotor activity to be generated in acute spinal preparations but only if the skin of the perineal region is also stimulated.

In *chronic* spinal preparations animals are studied for weeks or months after transection. Without drug treatment locomotor activity can return within a few weeks of cord transection. Locomotor function returns spontaneously in kittens, but in adult cats daily training is usually required.

Decerebrate Preparations

In decerebrate preparations the brain stem is completely transected at the level of the midbrain, disconnecting rostral brain centers, especially the cerebral cortex, from the spinal centers where the locomotor pattern is generated. Because brain stem centers remain connected to the spinal cord, these preparations allow investigation of the role of the cerebellum and brain stem structures in controlling locomotion.

Two decerebrate preparations are commonly used. In one the locomotor rhythm is generated spontaneously, whereas in the other it is evoked by electrical stimulation of the mesencephalic locomotor region. This difference depends on the level of decerebration. Spontaneous walking occurs in *premammillary preparations,* in which the brain stem is transected from the rostral margin of the superior colliculi to a point immediately rostral to the mammillary bodies. When the transection is made caudal to the mammillary bodies *postmammillary or mesencephalic preparation*, spontaneous stepping does not occur; rather, electrical stimulation of the mesencephalic locomotor region is required to evoke walking (Figure 36–1B).

When supported on a motorized treadmill, both preparations walk with a coordinated stepping pattern in all four limbs and the rate of stepping is matched to the treadmill speed. The motor activity can be recorded during stepping, and sensory nerves can be stimulated with implanted electrodes to examine the reflex mechanisms that regulate stepping.

Deafferented Preparations

An early view of the neural control of locomotion was that it involved a "chaining" of reflexes: Successive stretch reflexes in flexor and extensor muscles were thought to produce the basic rhythm of walking. This view was disproved by Graham Brown, who showed that rhythmic locomotor patterns were generated even after complete removal of all sensory input (deafferentation) from the moving limbs.

Deafferentation is accomplished by transection of all the dorsal roots that innervate the limbs. Because the dorsal roots carry only sensory axons, motor innervation of the muscles remains intact. Deafferented preparations were once useful for demonstrating the capabilities of the isolated spinal cord but are rarely used today, principally because the loss of all tonic sensory input drastically reduces the excitability of interneurons and motor neurons in the spinal cord. Thus, changes in the locomotor pattern after deafferentation might result from the artificial reduction in excitability of neurons rather than from the loss of specific sensory inputs.

Immobilized Preparations

The role of proprioceptive input from the limbs can be more systematically investigated by preventing activity in motor neurons from actually causing any movement. This is typically accomplished by paralyzing the muscles with *d*-tubocurarine, a competitive inhibitor of acetylcholine that blocks synaptic transmission at the neuromuscular junction.

When locomotion is initiated in such an immobilized preparation, often referred to as fictive locomotion, the motor nerves to flexor and extensor muscles fire alternately but no actual movement takes place and the proprioceptive afferents are not phasically excited. Thus the effect of proprioceptive reflexes is removed whereas tonic sensory input is preserved.

Because immobilized preparations allow intracellular and extracellular recording from neurons in the spinal cord, they are used to examine the synaptic events associated with locomotor activity and the organization of central and reflex pathways controlling locomotion.

Neonatal Rodent Preparation

The spinal cord is removed from a neonatal rat or mouse (0–5 days after birth) and placed in a saline bath, where it will generate coordinated bursts of activity in leg motor neurons when exposed to NMDA and serotonin (Figure 36–1C). This preparation allows more detailed analysis of the locations and roles of the specific neurons involved in rhythm generation, as well as pharmacological studies on the rhythm-generating network.

The ability to genetically modify neurons in the spinal cord of mice allows studies on the function of identified classes of neurons in these animals.

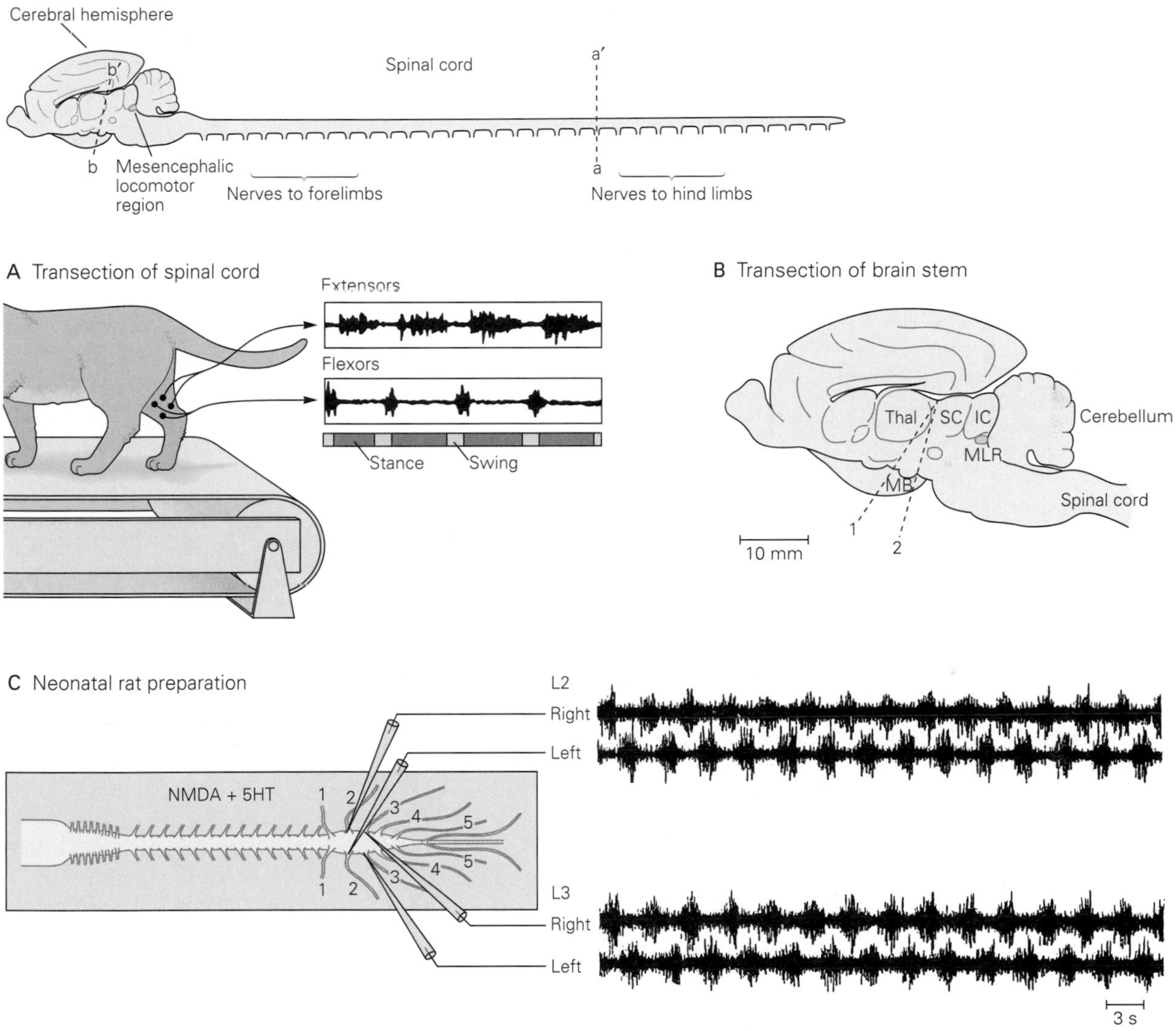

Figure 36–1 **A.** Transection of the spinal cord of a cat at the level a-a′ isolates the segments of the cord with nerves that project to the hind limbs. The hind limbs are still able to step on a treadmill either immediately after recovery from surgery if adrenergic drugs are administered or a few weeks after surgery if the animal is exercised regularly on the treadmill. Transection of the brain stem at the level b-b′ isolates the spinal cord and lower brain stem from the cerebral hemispheres.

B. Depending on the exact level of the transection of the brain stem, locomotion occurs spontaneously (1) or can be initiated by electrical stimulation of the mesencephalic locomotor region (**MLR**) (2). The mesencephalic locomotor region is a small region of the brain stem close to the cuneiform nucleus approximately 6 mm below the surface of the inferior colliculus (**IC**). (**Thal**, thalamus; **SC**, superior colliculus; **MB**, mammillary body.)

C. The spinal cord is removed from a neonatal rat and placed in a saline bath. Addition of *N*-methyl-D-aspartate (NMDA) and serotonin (5-hydroxytryptamine, or 5-HT) to the bath elicits rhythmic bursting in the motor neurons supplying leg muscles, as shown in recordings from nerve roots of the second (L2) and third (L3) lumbar segments. Intracellular or tight-seal recordings can also be made from lumbar neurons during periods of rhythmic activity. (Adapted, with permission, from Cazalets, Borde, and Clarac 1995.)

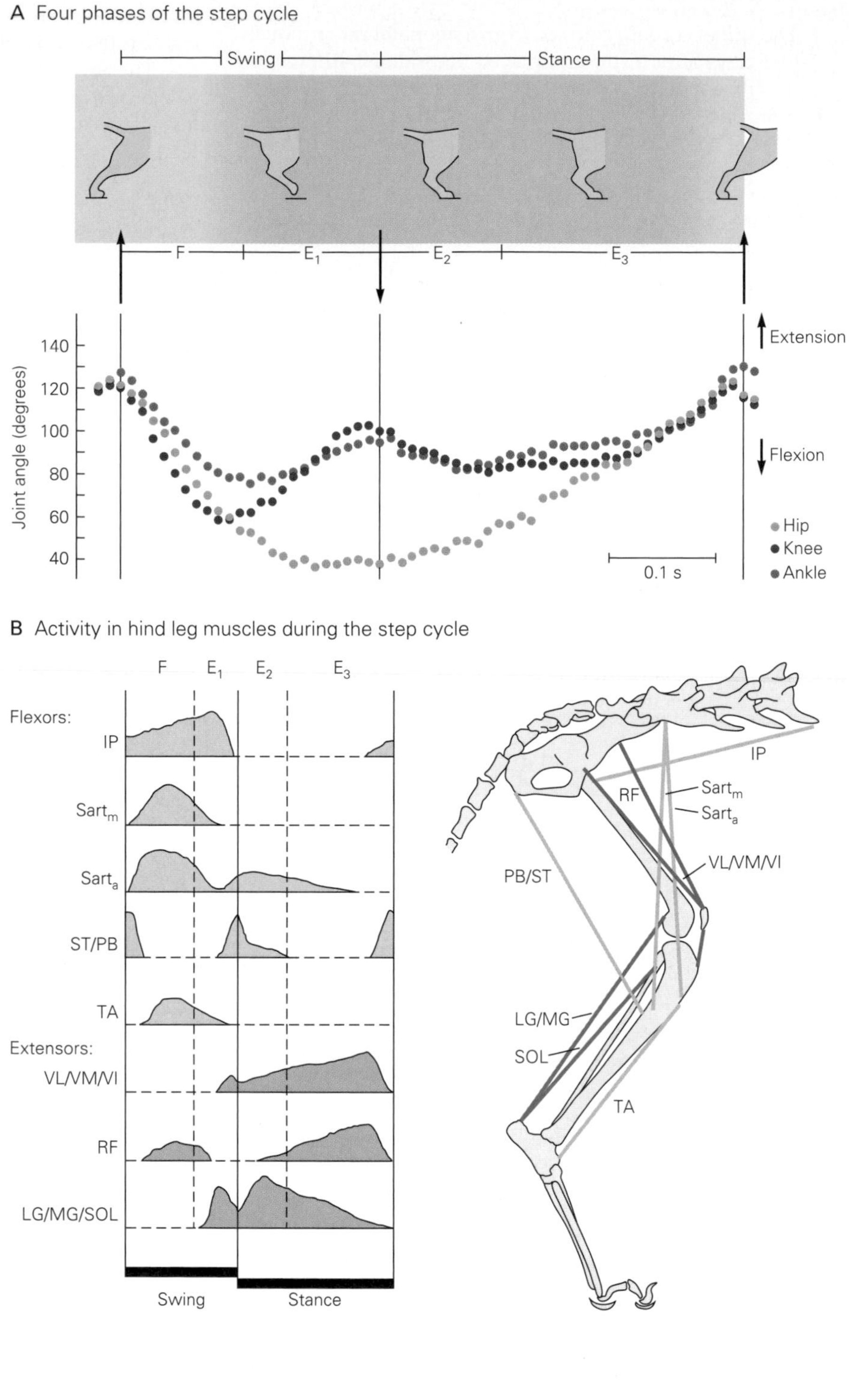

Figure 36–2 Stepping is produced by complex patterns of contractions in leg muscles.

A. The step cycle is divided into four phases: the flexion (F) and first extension (E_1) phases occur during swing, when the foot is off the ground, whereas second extension (E_2) and third extension (E_3) occur during stance, when the foot contacts the ground. Second extension is characterized by flexion at the knee and ankle as the leg begins to bear the animal's weight. The contracting knee and ankle extensor muscles lengthen during this phase. (Adapted, with permission, from Engberg and Lundberg 1969.)

B. Profiles of electrical activity in some of the hind leg flexor and extensor muscles in the cat during stepping. Although flexor and extensor muscles are generally active during swing and stance, respectively, the overall pattern of activity is complex in both timing and amplitude. (**IP**, iliopsoas; **LG** and **MG**, lateral and medial gastrocnemius; **PB**, posterior biceps; **RF**, rectus femoris; **$Sart_m$** and **$Sart_a$**, medial and anterior sartorius; **SOL**, soleus; **ST**, semitendinosus; **TA**, tibialis anterior; **VL**, **VM**, and **VI**, vastus lateralis, medialis, and intermedialis.)

muscles contract during both swing and stance. Thus the motor pattern for stepping is not merely alternating flexion and extension at each joint, but a complex sequence of muscle contractions, each precisely timed and scaled to achieve a specific task in the act of locomotion.

The Motor Pattern for Stepping Is Organized at the Spinal Level

Transection of the spinal cord of quadrupeds initially causes complete paralysis of the hind legs. It does not, however, permanently abolish the capacity of hind legs to make stepping movements: Hind leg stepping often recovers spontaneously over a period of a few weeks, particularly if the transection is made in young animals. Recovery of stepping in adult cats can be facilitated by daily training on a treadmill evoked by nonspecific cutaneous stimulation of the perineal region.

Electromyographic records of the hind leg muscles of chronic spinal cats during stepping are quite similar to those of normally walking animals. Many of the reflex responses that occur in normal animals can also be evoked in spinal animals. Spinal animals are not, however, able to maintain balance on the treadmill. Adequate control of balance requires descending signals from brain stem centers, such as the vestibular nuclei.

Contraction in Flexor and Extensor Muscles of the Hind Legs Is Controlled by Mutually Inhibiting Networks

From the studies by Graham Brown early in the 20th century we know that the isolated spinal cord can generate rhythmic bursts of reciprocal activity in flexor and extensor motor neurons of the hind legs even in the absence of sensory input (Figure 36–3). Graham Brown proposed that contractions in the flexor and extensor muscles are controlled by two systems of neurons, or *half-centers,* that mutually inhibit each other (Figure 36–4B).

According to Graham Brown, activity alternates between half-centers because of fatigue of the inhibitory connections. For example, if two half-centers receive tonic excitatory input, and the flexor half-center receives the stronger input, the flexor muscles will contract while the extensor half-center is inhibited. Then, as the inhibitory output fatigues, the extensor half-center's output will increase, causing inhibition of the flexor half-center and contraction of the extensor muscles until its inhibitory output fatigues. Thus the flexor and extensor muscles controlled by the two half-centers will alternately contract and relax as long as the half-centers receive sufficient tonic excitatory input.

The half-center hypothesis was supported by studies in the 1960s on the effects in spinal cats of the drug L-dihydroxyphenylalanine (L-DOPA), a precursor of the monoamine transmitters dopamine and norepinephrine. After the cats were treated with L-DOPA, brief

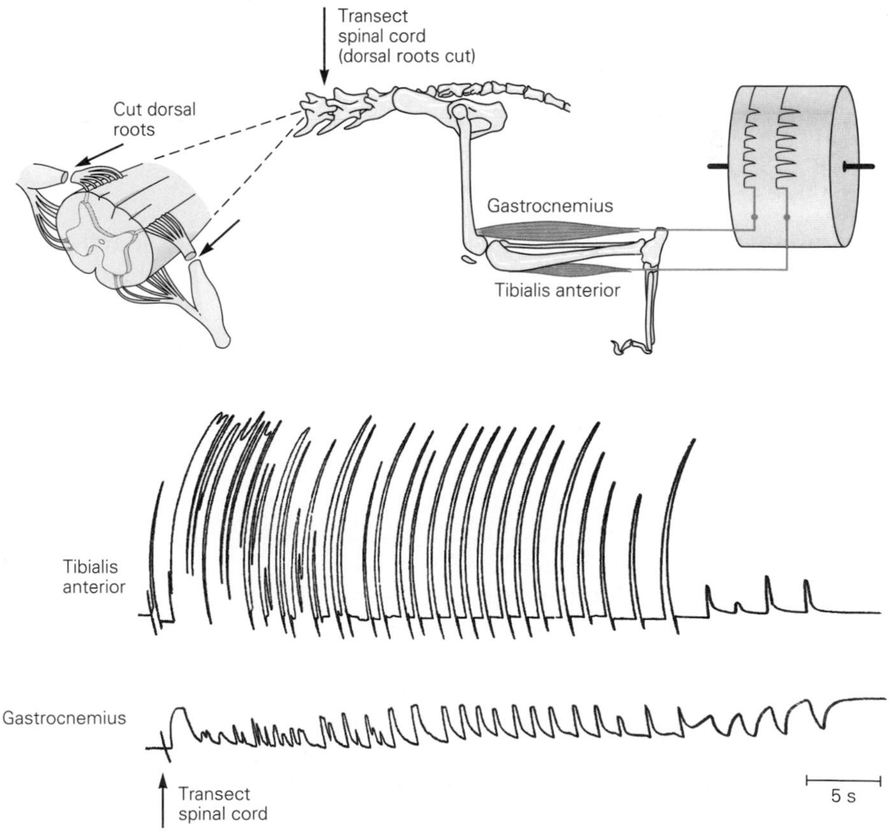

Figure 36–3 Rhythmic activity for stepping is generated by networks of neurons in the spinal cord. The existence of such spinal networks was first demonstrated by Thomas Graham Brown in 1911. Graham Brown developed an experimental preparation system in which dorsal roots were cut so that sensory information from the limbs could not reach the spinal cord. An original record from Graham Brown's study shows that rhythmic alternating contractions of ankle flexor (tibialis anterior) and extensor (gastrocnemius) muscles begin immediately after transection of the spinal cord.

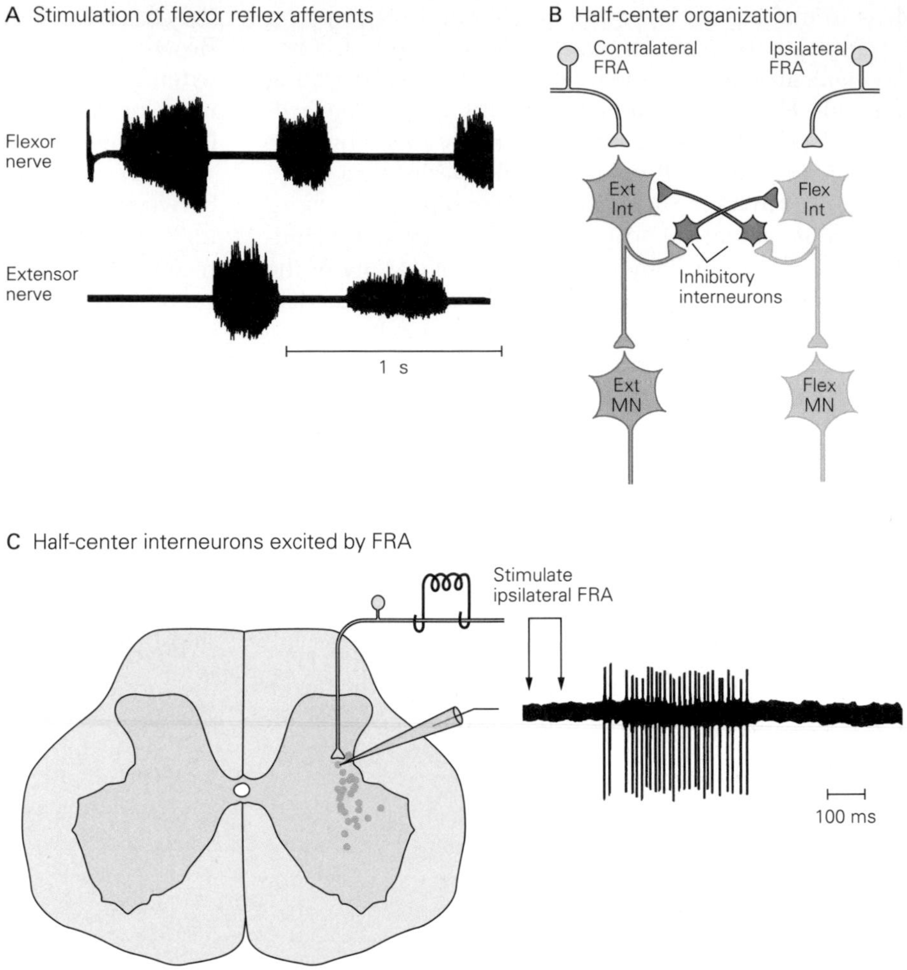

Figure 36–4 Reciprocal activity in flexor and extensor motor neurons.

A. High-threshold cutaneous and muscle afferents called flexor reflex afferents (FRA) were electrically stimulated in spinal cats treated with L-DOPA (L-dihydroxyphenylalanine) and nialamide. Brief stimulation of ipsilateral FRAs evoked a short sequence of rhythmic activity in flexor and extensor motor neurons. (Adapted, with permission, from Jankowska et al. 1967a.)

B. Interneurons in the pathways mediating long-latency reflexes from the ipsilateral and contralateral FRAs mutually inhibit one another. This "half-center" organization of the flexor and extensor interneurons likely mediates rhythmic stepping.

C. Stimulation of the ipsilateral FRA evokes a delayed, long-lasting burst of activity in the half-center interneurons located in the intermediate region of the gray matter. (Adapted, with permission, from Jankowska et al. 1967b.)

trains of electrical stimuli were applied to small-diameter sensory fibers from skin and muscle. These trains of stimuli evoked long-lasting bursts of activity in either flexor or extensor motor neurons, depending on whether ipsilateral or contralateral nerves were stimulated. The afferents producing these effects are collectively termed *flexor reflex afferents.* Additional administration of nialamide, a drug that prolongs the action of norepinephrine released in the spinal cord, often resulted in short sequences of rhythmic reciprocal activity in flexor and extensor motor neurons (Figure 36–4A).

The system of interneurons generating flexor bursts was found to inhibit the system of interneurons generating the extensor bursts, and vice versa (Figure 36–4B). This organizational feature is consistent with Graham Brown's theory that mutually inhibiting "half-centers" produce the alternating burst activity in flexor and extensor motor neurons. The interneurons mediating the burst patterns arising from stimulation of the flexor reflex afferents have not been fully identified but they may include interneurons in the intermediate region of the gray matter in the sixth lumbar segment. Interneurons in this region produce prolonged bursts of activity in response to brief stimulation of either ipsilateral or contralateral flexor reflex afferents in spinal cats treated with L-DOPA (Figure 36–4C).

Central Pattern Generators Are Not Driven by Sensory Input

Neuronal spinal networks capable of generating rhythmic motor activity in the absence of rhythmic input from peripheral receptors are termed *central pattern generators* (Box 36–2). Largely because the mammalian nervous system is so complex, we lack detailed information on the neuronal circuitry and mechanisms for rhythm generation by central pattern generators in the mammalian spinal cord. However, we have considerable knowledge

Box 36–2 Central Pattern Generators

A central pattern generator (CPG) is a neuronal network within the central nervous system that is capable of generating a rhythmic pattern of motor activity without phasic sensory input from peripheral receptors. CPGs have been identified and analyzed in more than 50 rhythmic motor systems, including those controlling such diverse behaviors as walking, swimming, feeding, respiration, and flying.

The motor pattern generated by a CPG under experimental conditions is sometimes very similar to the motor pattern produced during natural behavior, as in lamprey swimming (see Box 36–3), but there are often significant differences. In nature the basic pattern produced by a CPG is usually modified by sensory information and signals from other regions of the central nervous system.

The rhythmic motor activity generated by CPGs depends on three factors: (1) the cellular properties of individual nerve cells within the network, (2) the properties of the synaptic junctions between neurons, and (3) the pattern of interconnections between neurons (Table 36–1). Modulatory substances, usually amines or peptides, can alter cellular and synaptic properties, thereby enabling a CPG to generate a variety of motor patterns.

The simplest CPGs contain neurons that burst spontaneously. Such endogenous bursters can drive motor neurons, and some motor neurons are themselves endogenous bursters. Bursters are common in CPGs that produce continuous rhythms, such as those for respiration. They are also found in locomotor systems. Locomotion, however, is an episodic behavior, so bursters in locomotor systems must be regulated.

Bursting is often induced by modulatory input from neurons projecting to the rhythm generating system. Neuromodulatory inputs can also alter the cellular properties of neurons so that brief depolarizations lead to maintained depolarizations (plateau potentials) that long outlast the initial depolarization. Neurons with the capacity to generate plateau potentials have been found in a large number of CPGs, and in some systems they are essential for rhythm generation.

Rhythmicity does not always depend on bursting or plateau potentials. A simple network can generate rhythmic activity if the firing of some neurons can be enhanced or reduced according to some temporal pattern. One process is postinhibitory rebound, a brief increase in excitability of a neuron after the termination of inhibitory input. Two neurons that mutually inhibit each other can oscillate in an alternating fashion if each neuron has the property of postinhibitory rebound.

Other time-dependent processes include synaptic depression, delayed onset of activity after a depolarization (delayed excitation), and differences in the time course of synaptic actions through parallel pathways connecting two neurons.

Most CPGs produce a complex temporal pattern of activation of different groups of motor neurons. Sometimes the pattern can be divided into a number of distinct phases; even within a phase the activity of different motor neurons can be timed separately. The sequencing of activity in motor neurons is regulated by a number of mechanisms. Perhaps the simplest mechanism is mutual inhibition; interneurons that fire out of phase with each other are usually reciprocally coupled by inhibitory connections

Another mechanism is the rate of recovery from inhibition, which can influence the relative time of onset of activity in two neurons simultaneously released from inhibition. Finally, mutual excitation is an important mechanism for establishing synchronous firing in a group of neurons. Electrical synapses are often employed for mutual excitation, particularly when a rapid high-intensity burst within a group of neurons is needed.

Table 36–1 Building Blocks of Rhythm-Generating Networks

Cellular properties	Synaptic properties	Patterns of connection
Threshold	Sign	Reciprocal inhibition
Frequency-current relationship	Strength	Recurrent inhibition
Spike frequency adaptation	Time course	Parallel excitation and inhibition
Post-burst hyperpolarization	Transmission (electrical, chemical)	Mutual excitation
Delayed excitation	Release mechanisms (spike, graded signal)	
Post-inhibitory rebound		
Plateau potentials	Multicomponent postsynaptic potentials	
Bursting (endogenous, conditional)	Facilitation/depression (short-term, long-term)	

about the cellular, synaptic, and network properties of central pattern generators in invertebrates and lower vertebrates, which have less complex nervous systems than mammals. For example, the analysis by Sten Grillner of the central pattern generator controlling swimming in the lamprey has provided considerable insight into the mechanisms of rhythm generation in vertebrate motor systems (Box 36–3).

Recent studies using the spinal cord of the neonatal rat have identified several classes of rhythmically active interneurons and demonstrated that some of these interneurons can generate sustained membrane

Box 36–3 Lamprey Swimming

One of the best-analyzed central pattern generators is that for lamprey swimming. Lampreys swim by alternating muscle contrations on the two sides of each body segment (Figure 36–5). Each segment contains a neural network capable of generating rhythmic, alternating activity in motor neurons on the two sides (Figure 36–6).

On each side of the network excitatory interneurons drive the motor neurons and two classes of inhibitory interneurons, commissural and local. The axons of the commissural interneurons cross the midline and inhibit all neurons in the contralateral half of the network, ensuring that when muscles on one side of the network are active, muscles on the other side are silent. The local inhibitory interneurons inhibit the commissural interneurons on the same side.

A number of cellular and synaptic mechanisms are involved in the initiation and termination of activity on one side of the network. One important mechanism in the initiation of activity is the opening of NMDA-type glutamate receptor-channels. Once the inhibition from contralateral commissural interneurons is terminated, the NMDA-type receptor-channels in all ipsilateral neurons are opened by a brief depolarization (post-inhibitory rebound) and the voltage-dependency of the channels leads to plateau potentials.

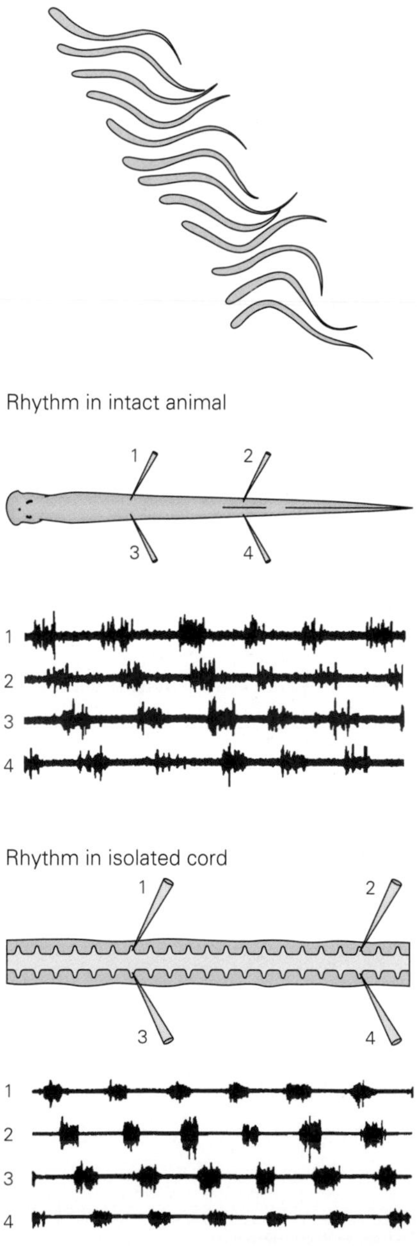

Figure 36–5 The lamprey swims by means of a wave of muscle contractions traveling down one side of the body 180 degrees out of phase with a similar traveling wave on the opposite side. This pattern is evident in electromyogram recordings from four locations along the animal during normal swimming. A similar pattern is recorded from four spinal roots in an isolated cord. (Adapted, with permission, from Grillner et al. 1987.)

depolarizations (*plateau potentials*) in response to weak synaptic input. Because this active membrane property is known to be important for rhythm generation in simpler systems, it is likely that it also contributes to rhythm generation in the mammalian spinal cord.

Spinal Networks Can Generate Complex Locomotor Patterns

The locomotor patterns generated in deafferented or immobilized spinal animals are generally much simpler than normal stepping patterns. Usually they

Activation of low-voltage Ca^{2+} channels further strengthens the depolarization. The influx of Ca^{2+} through these channels and the NMDA-type receptor-channels activates calcium-dependent K^+ channels. The resultant increase in K^+ conductance terminates the plateau potentials and so contributes to the termination of activity.

Two additional mechanisms contribute to the termination of activity in each half of the network. One is a progressive decline in the discharge rate of the neurons resulting from the summation of slow afterhyperpolarizations. The other is delayed excitation of the local inhibitory interneurons. When excited, these interneurons inhibit the commissural interneurons (Figure 36–6), thereby removing inhibition from the contralateral half of the network and enabling it to become active.

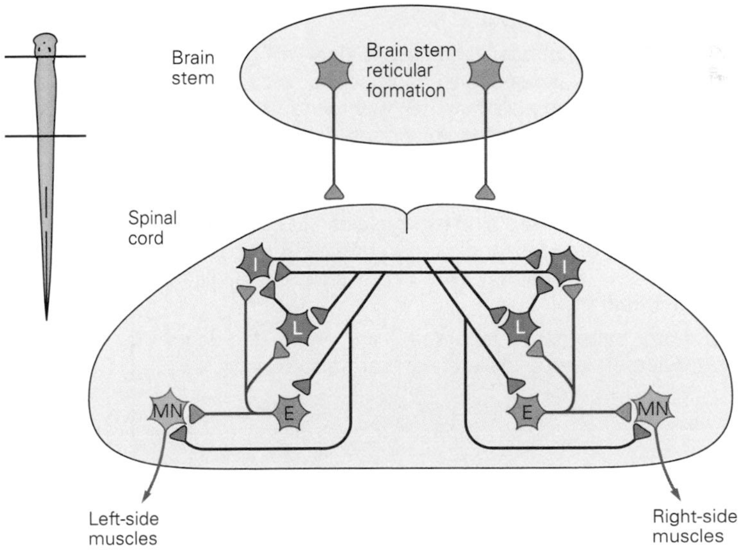

Figure 36–6 **Each body segment of the lamprey contains a neuronal network responsible for the motor pattern in that segment.** Activity in each segmental network is initiated by activity in glutamatergic axons descending from the brain stem reticular formation. The reticulospinal neurons increase the excitability of all neurons in a segmental network by activation of both NMDA-type and non–NMDA-type glutamate receptors. On each side of the network excitatory interneurons (**E**) drive the motor neurons (**MN**) and two classes of inhibitory interneurons, commissural (**I**) and local (**L**). (Adapted, with permission, from Grillner et al. 1995.)

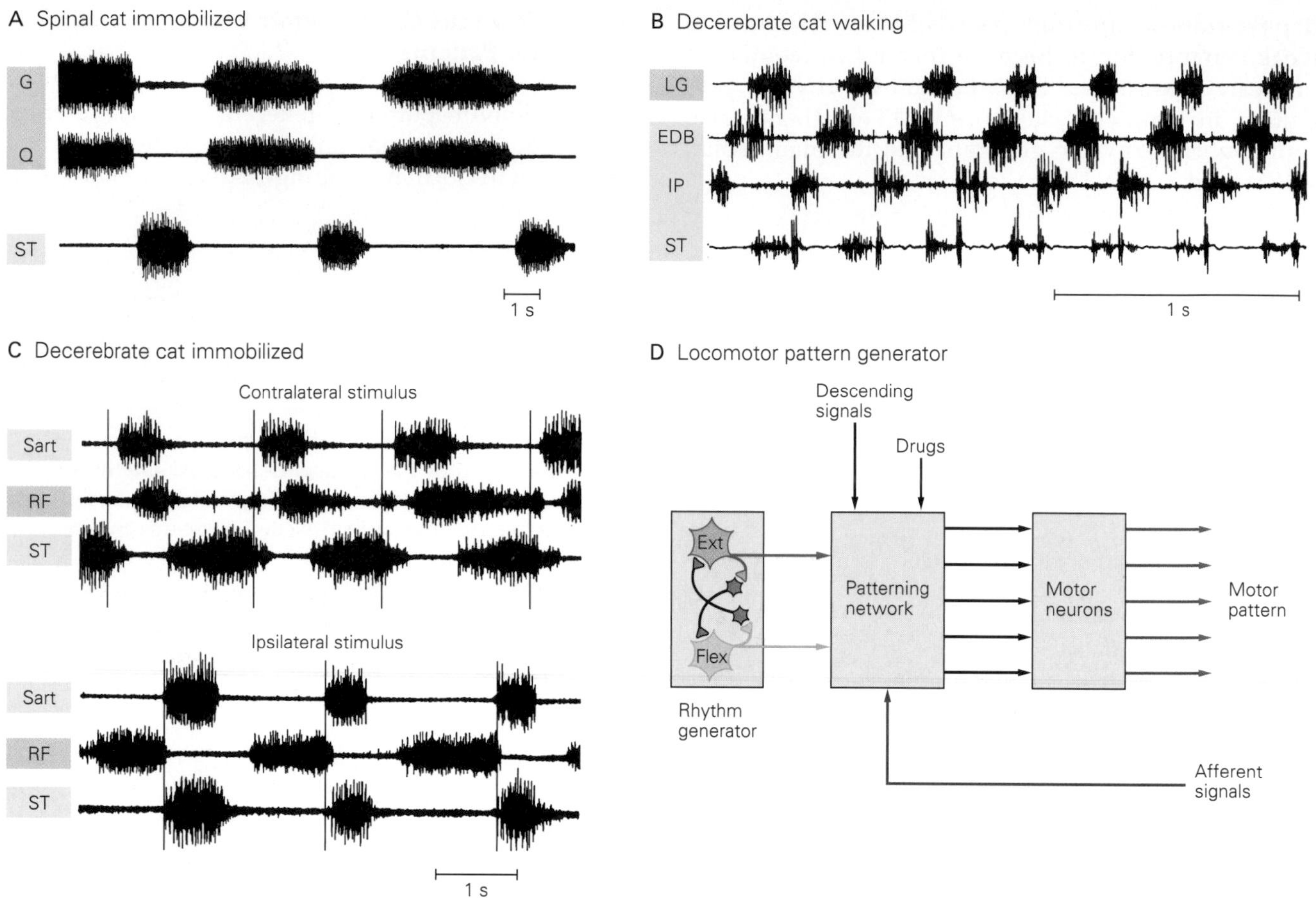

Figure 36–7 A variety of motor patterns can be generated without phasic sensory input.

A. A reciprocal pattern of activity in nerves innervating flexor and extensor muscles is seen in an immobilized spinal cat treated with L-DOPA and nialamide. (**G**, gastrocnemius; **Q**, quadriceps; **ST**, semitendinosus.) (Adapted, with permission, from Edgerton et al. 1976.)

B. A complex motor pattern is recorded from a walking decerebrate cat with deafferented hind-leg muscles. (**LG**, lateral gastrocnemius; **EDB**, extensor digitorum brevis; **IP**, iliopsoas; **ST**, semitendinosus.) (Adapted, with permission, from Grillner and Zangger 1984.)

C. Fictive motor patterns are recorded in an immobilized decorticate cat when either the ipsilateral or contralateral paw is squeezed. The patterns are radically different. (**Sart**, sartorius; **RF**, rectus femoris; **ST**, semitendinosus.) (Adapted, with permission, from Perret and Cabelguen 1980.)

D. This schematic description of a locomotor pattern generator is based on recent studies on fictive locomotion in decerebrate cats. The basic rhythmic pattern is produced by mutually inhibiting flexor and extensor half-centers. The interneurons of these half-centers drive the motor neurons through an intermediate system of interneurons (patterning network) that control the timing of activation of different classes of motor neurons. Descending signals, drugs, or afferent signals can modify the temporal motor activity pattern by altering the functioning of interneurons in the patterning network. (Adapted, with permission, from Rybak et al. 2006.)

consist of alternating bursts of activity in flexor and extensor motor neurons (Figure 36–7A). More complex locomotor patterns can be generated in immobilized spinal animals after a period of training or through the application of additional drugs such as 4-aminopyridine. Moreover, in decerebrate animals elaborate locomotor patterns can be produced in hind limb motor neurons after deafferentation (Figure 36–7B). These patterns resemble those recorded in the same animals before deafferentation. Finally, a variety of patterns can be generated in immobilized decerebrate animals, and these patterns can be altered significantly by changing the level of tonic sensory input (Figure 36–7C).

From these observations it is clear that the spinal pattern-generating network for each leg can produce a variety of motor patterns. Which pattern is generated depends on many factors, such as the supraspinal and tonic sensory inputs to the spinal pattern generators as well as the drugs used to experimentally initiate rhythmicity. This functional flexibility may be explained by a scheme in which mutually inhibiting half-centers produce the basic rhythmicity and establish a general pattern of reciprocal activity in flexor and extensor motor neurons, whereas the details of the temporal pattern are established by a network of interneurons (the patterning network) connecting the half-centers and motor neurons (Figure 36–7D).

Sensory Input from Moving Limbs Regulates Stepping

Although normal walking is automatic, it is not necessarily stereotyped. Mammals constantly use sensory input to adjust their stepping patterns to variations in terrain and to anticipated and unexpected conditions. This input is provided predominantly by three sensory systems: the visual, vestibular, and somatosensory systems. Proprioceptors in muscles and joints provide information about body movements and are involved in the automatic regulation of stepping. Cutaneous receptors in the skin, sometimes referred to as exteroceptors, adjust stepping to external stimuli and can also provide important feedback about body movements.

Proprioception Regulates the Timing and Amplitude of Stepping

One of the clearest indications that somatosensory signals from the limbs regulate the step cycle is that the rate of stepping in spinal and decerebrate cats matches the speed of the motorized treadmill belt on which they tread. Specifically, afferent input regulates the duration of the stance phase. As the stepping rate increases, the stance phase becomes shorter while the swing phase remains relatively constant. This observation suggests that some form of sensory input signals the end of stance and thus leads to the initiation of swing.

Sherrington was the first to propose that proprioceptors in muscles acting at the hip are primarily responsible for regulating the stance phase. He noticed that rapid extension at the hip joint, but not at the knee and ankle joints, led to contractions in the hip flexor muscles of chronic spinal cats and dogs. More recent studies have found that preventing hip extension in a limb suppresses stepping in that limb, whereas rhythmically moving the hip can entrain the locomotor rhythm, that is, cause the timing of the neural output to match the rhythm of the externally imposed movements.

During entrainment a burst of activity in hip flexor motor neurons is initiated in synchrony with hip extension (Figure 36–8A). The afferent fibers that signal hip angle for swing initiation arise from muscle spindles in the hip flexor muscles. In decerebrate animals stretching these muscles to mimic the lengthening that occurs at the end of the stance phase inhibits the extensor half-center and thus facilitates the initiation of burst activity in flexor motor neurons during walking (Figure 36–8B).

Other important proprioceptive signals for regulating the step cycle arise from proprioceptors in extensor muscles. Electrical stimulation of sensory fibers from Golgi tendon organs and muscle spindles prolongs the stance phase, often delaying the onset of swing until the stimulus has ended (Figure 36–9A). Sensory fibers from both types of receptors are active during stance.

The intensity of the signal from the Golgi tendon organs is related to the load carried by the leg. Golgi tendon organs have an excitatory action on ankle extensor motor neurons during walking but an inhibitory action when the body is at rest (see Chapter 35). The functional consequence of this reflex reversal is that the swing phase is not initiated until the extensor muscles are unloaded and the forces exerted by these muscles are low, as signaled by a decrease in activity from the Golgi tendon organs. Unloading of extensor muscles normally occurs near the end of stance, when the animal's weight is borne by the other legs and the extensor muscles are shortened and thus unable to produce high forces.

In addition to regulating the transition from stance to swing, proprioceptive information from muscle spindles and Golgi tendon organs contributes significantly to the generation of burst activity in extensor motor neurons. Reducing this sensory input in cats diminishes the level of extensor activity by more than half; in humans it has been estimated that up to 30% of the activity of ankle extensor motor neurons is caused by feedback from the extensor muscles.

At least three excitatory pathways transmit sensory information from extensor muscles to extensor motor neurons: a monosynaptic pathway from primary muscle spindles (group Ia afferents), a disynaptic pathway from primary muscle spindles and Golgi tendon organs (group Ia and Ib afferents), and a polysynaptic pathway from primary muscle spindles and Golgi tendon organs that includes interneurons in the central pattern generator (Figure 36–9B). The continuous regulation of the

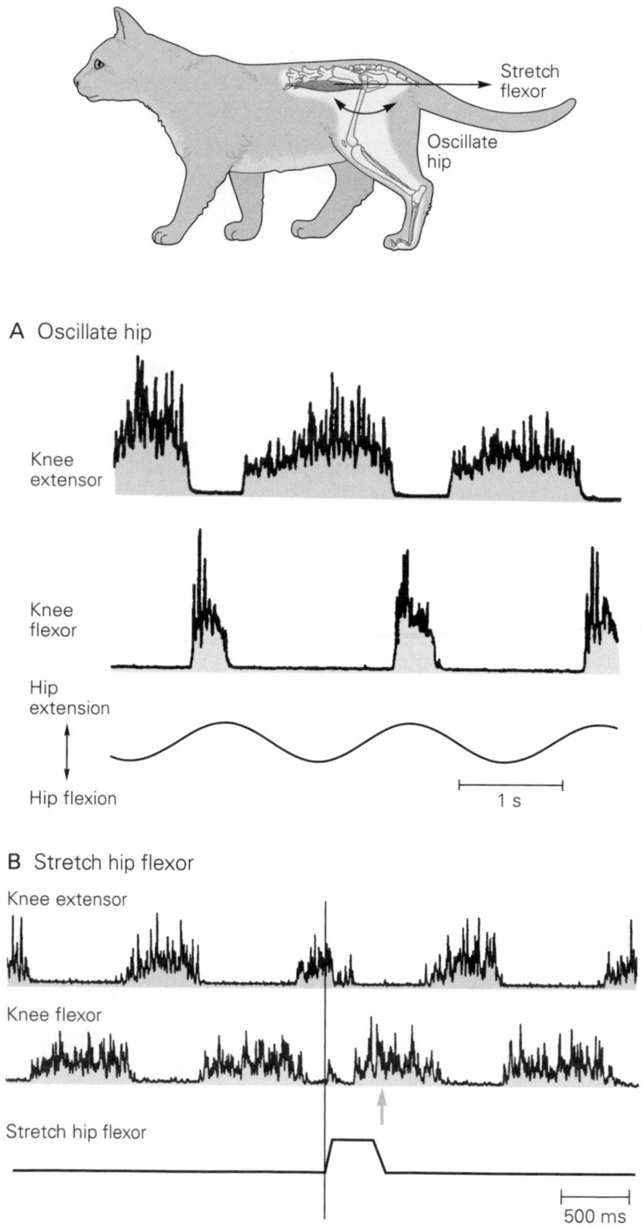

Figure 36–8 Information on hip extension controls the transition from stance to swing.

A. In an immobilized decerebrate cat oscillating movement around the hip joint entrains the fictive locomotor pattern in knee extensor and flexor motor neurons. The flexor bursts, corresponding to the swing phase, are generated when the hip is extended. (Adapted, with permission, from Kriellaars et al. 1994.)

B. In a walking decerebrate cat stretching of the hip flexor muscle (iliopsoas) inhibits knee extensor activity allowing knee flexor activity to begin earlier. The **arrow** in the knee-flexor record indicates the expected onset of knee flexor activity had the hip flexor muscle not been stretched. Activation of sensory fibers from muscle spindles in the hip flexor muscle is responsible for this effect. (Adapted, with permission, from Hiebert et al. 1996.)

level of extensor activity by proprioceptive feedback presumably allows automatic adjustment of force and length in extensor muscles in response to unexpected unloading and loading of the leg.

Sensory Input from the Skin Allows Stepping to Adjust to Unexpected Obstacles

Sensory receptors in the skin have a powerful influence on the central pattern generator for walking. One important function of these receptors is to detect obstacles and adjust stepping movements to avoid them. A well-studied example is the stumbling-corrective reaction in cats. A mild mechanical stimulus applied to the dorsal part of the paw during the swing phase produces excitation of flexor motor neurons and inhibition of extensor motor neurons, leading to rapid flexion of the paw away from the stimulus and elevation of the leg in an attempt to step over the object. Because this corrective response is readily observed in spinal cats, it must be produced to a large extent by circuits entirely contained within the spinal cord.

One of the interesting features of the stumbling-corrective reaction is that corrective flexion movements are produced only if the paw is stimulated during the swing phase. An identical stimulus applied during the stance phase produces the opposite response, excitation of extensor muscles that reinforces the ongoing extensor activity. This extensor action is appropriate; if a flexion reflex were produced during the stance phase the animal might collapse because it is being supported by the limb. This is an example of a *phase-dependent reflex reversal:* The same stimulus excites one group of motor neurons during one phase of locomotion but activates the antagonist motor neurons during another phase.

Descending Pathways Are Necessary for Initiation and Adaptive Control of Stepping

Although the basic motor pattern for stepping is generated in the spinal cord, fine control of stepping movements involves many regions of the brain, including the motor cortex, cerebellum, and various sites within the brain stem. Many neurons in each of these regions are rhythmically active during locomotor activity and hence participate in the production of the normal motor pattern. Each region, however, plays a different role in the regulation of locomotor function.

Supraspinal regulation of stepping can be divided into three functional systems. One activates the spinal locomotor system, initiates walking, and controls the

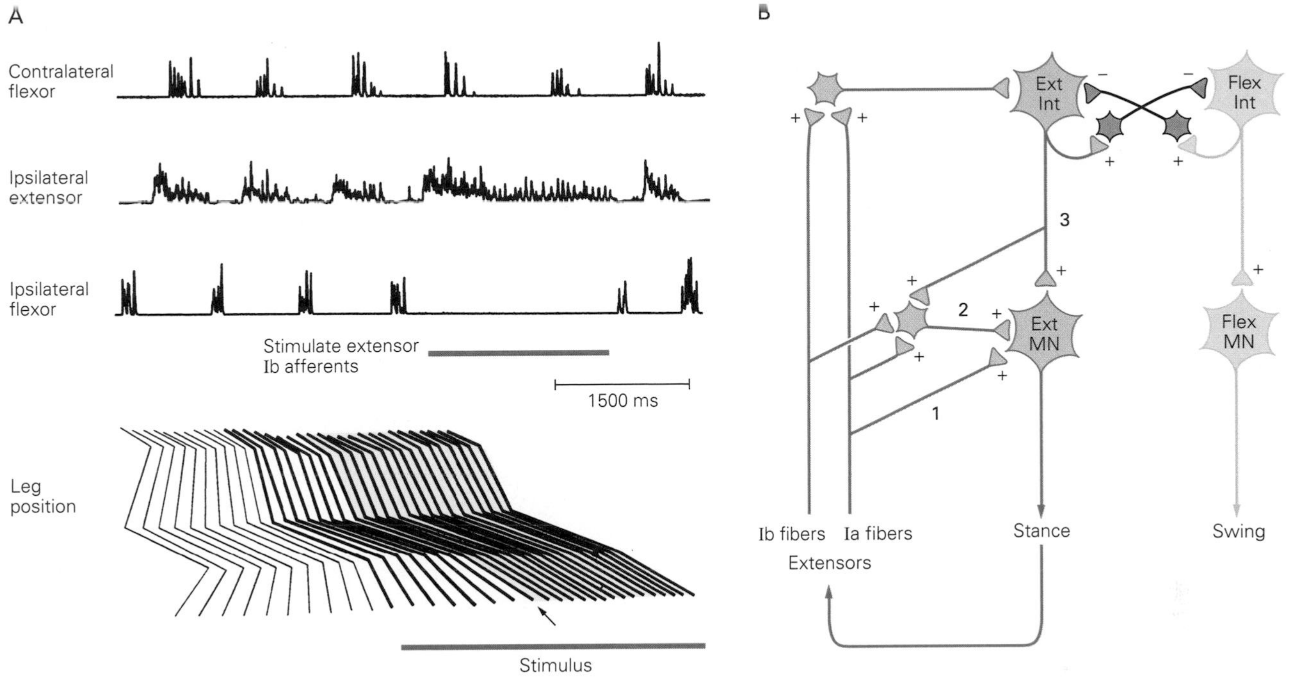

Figure 36–9 The swing phase of walking is initiated by sensory feedback from extensor muscles.

A. In a decerebrate cat electrical stimulation of group I sensory fibers from ankle extensor muscles inhibits bursting in ipsilateral flexors and prolongs the burst in the ipsilateral extensors during walking. The timing of contralateral flexor activity is not altered. Stimulating group I fibers from the extensors prevents initiation of the swing phase, as can be seen in the position of the leg during the time the fibers were stimulated. The **arrow** shows the point at which the swing phase would normally have occurred had the extensor afferents not been stimulated. (Adapted, with permission, from Whelan, Hiebert, and Pearson 1995.)

B. Afferent pathway from extensor muscles regulating stance. Two mutually inhibiting groups of extensor and flexor interneurons constitute a central pattern generator. Feedback from extensor muscles increases the level of activity in extensor motor neurons during stance and maintains extensor activity when the extensor muscles are loaded. The feedback is relayed through three excitatory (+) pathways: monosynaptic connections from Ia fibers to extensor motor neurons (**1**); disynaptic connections from Ia and Ib fibers (**2**); and a polysynaptic excitatory pathway through the extensor interneurons (**3**).

overall speed of locomotion; another refines the motor pattern in response to feedback from the limbs; and the third visually guides limb movement (Figure 36–10).

Pathways from the Brain Stem Initiate Walking and Control Its Speed

In their seminal studies of decerebrate cats, Mark Shik, Fidor Severin, and Grigori Orlovsky found that tonic electrical stimulation of the mesencephalic locomotor region initiates stepping when decerebrate animals are placed on a treadmill. The mesencephalic locomotor region is situated approximately 6 mm ventral to the inferior colliculus (Figure 36–11A), close to the cuneiform nucleus. The rhythm of the locomotor pattern is related only to the intensity of electrical stimulation, not to its pattern. Weak stimulation produces a slow walking gait, which accelerates as the intensity increases; progressively stronger stimulation produces trotting and finally galloping (Figure 36–11B).

The transition from trotting to galloping is especially interesting for it involves a shift from an out-of-phase relationship between left and right legs in trotting to an in-phase relationship in galloping. This shift in interlimb coordination is also observed in spinal cats walking on a motorized treadmill as the speed is increased. Therefore it is most likely implemented by local circuits in the spinal cord.

In addition to the mesencephalic locomotor region, several other motor regions of the brain can produce locomotion when stimulated electrically. These include a subthalamic locomotor region and a nucleus

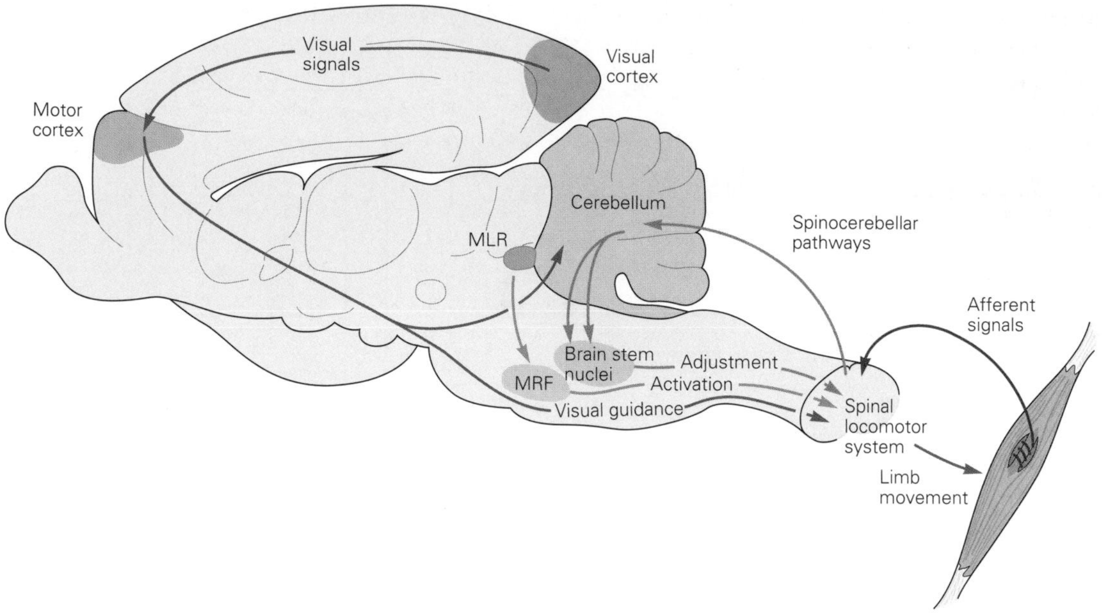

Figure 36–10 The brain stem and motor cortex control locomotion. The spinal locomotor system is activated by signals from the mesencephalic locomotor region (**MLR**) relayed by neurons in the medial reticular formation (**MRF**). The cerebellum receives signals from both peripheral receptors and spinal central pattern generators and adjusts the locomotor pattern through connections in brain stem nuclei. Visual information conveyed to the motor cortex can also modify stepping movements.

in the pontine reticular formation (pontine peduncular nucleus). How these different brain stem regions interact in the normal control of locomotion is not yet known.

How are signals from locomotor regions of the brain stem transmitted to patterning networks in the spinal cord? Because application of adrenergic drugs is often sufficient to initiate stepping in acute spinal animals, an early hypothesis was that the initiation and maintenance of locomotor activity depends on activity in the descending noradrenergic pathway from the locus ceruleus or the descending serotonergic pathway from the raphe nucleus. However, because locomotor activity can be evoked after depletion of norepinephrine and serotonin, neither of these aminergic pathways is essential for locomotion. The current view is that these transmitters are modulators that regulate the magnitude and timing of motor neuron activity in the locomotor networks in the spinal cord. Although adrenergic drugs can initiate stepping movements in the spinal animal, aminergic neurons may not serve this function in nature.

Clues about the identity of the descending system that initiates locomotor activity came first from studies on the neonatal rat and lamprey. Administration of glutamate receptor agonists to the isolated spinal cord was found to initiate locomotor activity. In decerebrate cats administration of agonists to the NMDA-type glutamate receptors in the spinal cord initiates locomotor activity similar to that evoked by electrical stimulation of the mesencephalic locomotor region. The application of glutamate receptor antagonists prevents this response. These observations suggest that glutamatergic pathways are involved in initiating locomotor activity.

Considerable research has been devoted to identifying the origin and course of the descending pathways that initiate locomotor activity. The central pattern generators in the spinal cord cannot be directly activated by neurons in the nuclei near the mesencephalic locomotor region, for the axons of these neurons do not descend directly to the cord. Instead, the mesencephalic motor neurons form connections with neurons in the medullary reticular formation, whose axons descend in the ventrolateral region of the spinal cord (Figure 36–11A). These neurons are excited by stimulation of the mesencephalic locomotor region, and transection of their axons in the ventrolateral funiculus of the spinal cord prevents stimulation of the mesencephalic locomotor region from initiating locomotor activity. Thus current evidence indicates that the signals that activate locomotion and control its speed are transmitted to the spinal cord by glutamatergic neurons with axons that travel in ventral reticulospinal pathways.

The Cerebellum Fine-Tunes Locomotor Patterns by Regulating the Timing and Intensity of Descending Signals

Damage to the cerebellum results in marked abnormalities in locomotor movements, including a widened base of support, impaired coordination of joints, and abnormal coupling between limbs during stepping. These symptoms are called *ataxia* (see Chapter 42). Ataxic walking resembles a drunken gait. Because ataxic gait is apparent in patients with cerebellar lesions even when they are walking on level surfaces, we can conclude that the cerebellum is involved in regulating all stepping movements.

The cerebellum receives sensory information about the actual stepping movements as well as information on the state of the central pattern generators through

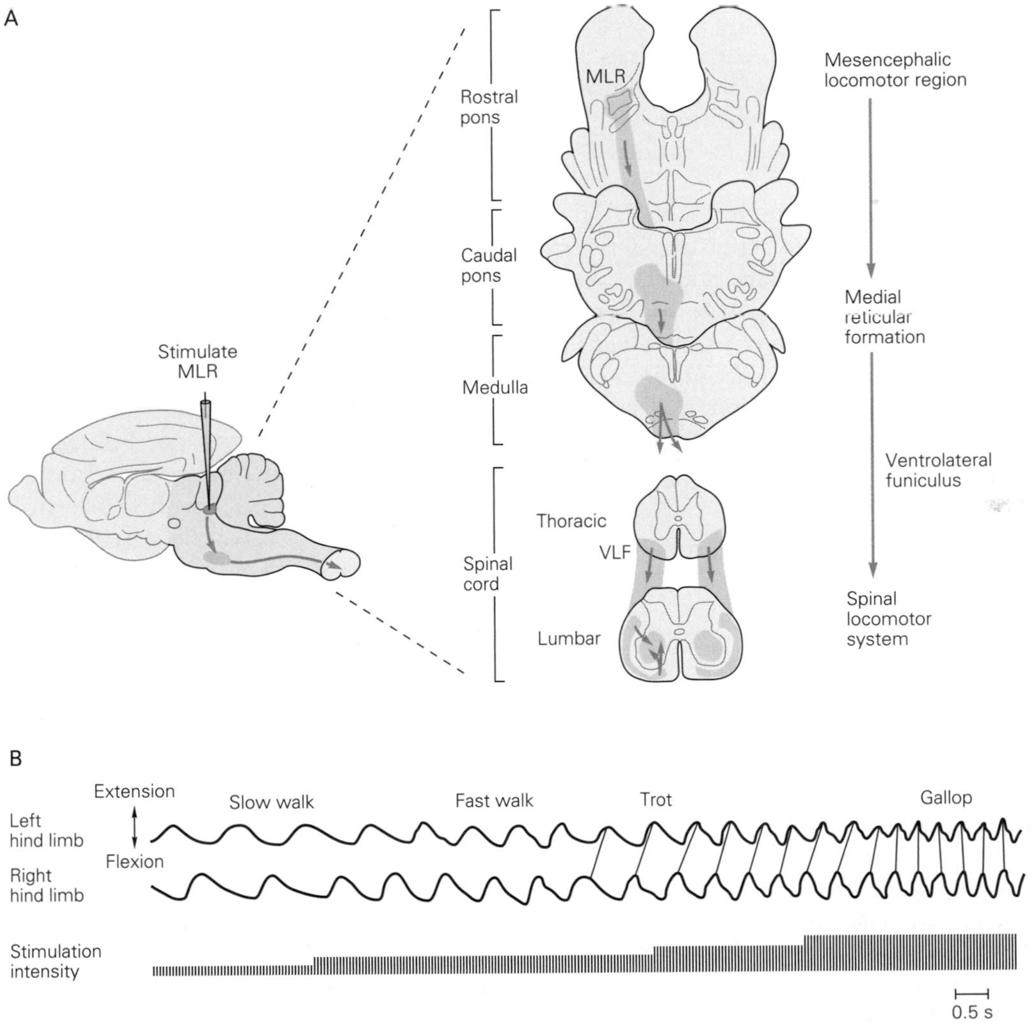

Figure 36–11 The mesencephalic locomotor region modifies stepping patterns.

A. Stimulation of the mesencephalic locomotor region (**MLR**) excites interneurons in the medial reticular formation whose axons descend in the ventrolateral funiculus (**VLF**) to the spinal locomotor system. (Adapted, with permission, from Mori et al. 1992.)

B. When the strength of stimulation of the mesencephalic locomotor region in a decerebrate cat walking on a treadmill is gradually increased, the gait and rate of stepping change from slow walking to trotting and finally to galloping. As the cat progresses from trotting to galloping, the hind limbs shift from alternating to simultaneous flexion and extension.

two ascending pathways. For the hind legs of the cat these are the dorsal and ventral spinocerebellar tracts. Neurons in the dorsal tract are strongly activated by numerous leg proprioceptors and thus provide the cerebellum with detailed information about the mechanical state of the hind legs. In contrast, neurons in the ventral tract are activated primarily by interneurons in the central pattern generator, thus providing the cerebellum with information about the state of the spinal locomotor network. The cerebellum also receives input from the motor cortex and other forebrain regions related to locomotor function.

It is thought that the cerebellum compares actual movements of the legs—proprioceptive signals in the dorsal spinocerebellar tract—with intended movements—the central commands conveyed in the ventral spinocerebellar tract and collaterals of corticospinal tract neurons. When these two types of information differ, representing an error, the cerebellum computes corrective signals and sends these to various brain stem nuclei.

During walking the cerebellum influences several brain stem nuclei, including the vestibular nuclei, red nucleus, and nuclei in the medullary reticular formation. The signals from the cerebellum to the vestibular nuclei during walking are likely used to regulate balance by integrating information about the position and movement of the head derived from the vestibular system with proprioceptive information about movements of the legs.

The Motor Cortex Uses Visual Information to Control Precise Stepping Movements

Normal walking is often guided by vision, and the motor cortex is essential for visually guided movement. Experimental lesions of the motor cortex do not prevent animals from walking on a smooth floor or even on smooth inclines, but they severely impair tasks requiring a high degree of visuomotor coordination, such as walking on the rungs of a horizontal ladder, stepping over a series of barriers, and stepping over single objects placed on a treadmill belt. Such "skilled walking" is associated with considerable modulation in the activity of a large number of neurons in the motor cortex (Figure 36–12).

Many of these neurons project directly to the spinal cord and thus may regulate the activity of interneurons in the central pattern generator for locomotion, thereby adapting the timing and magnitude of motor activity to a specific task. Electrical stimulation of either the motor cortex or the corticospinal tract in normal walking cats influences the timing of locomotor activity; these effects are generally stronger than those elicited by stimulation of brain stem regions.

Planning and Coordination of Visually Guided Movements Involves the Posterior Parietal Cortex

When humans and animals approach an obstacle in their pathway they must adjust their stepping to either move around the obstacle or step over it. These adjustments begin two or three steps before the obstacle is reached. Recent studies by Trevor Drew and his colleagues have shown that the posterior parietal cortex has an essential role in planning these adjustments.

Small lesions in this region cause walking cats to misplace the positioning of their paws as they approach an obstacle, and to increase the probability that one or more legs contact the obstacle as they step over it. Recordings in the parietal cortex have identified sets of neurons that could be involved in the planning and coordination of stepping movements. Some neurons increase their activity as an animal approaches an obstacle, whereas others maintain their activity when an obstacle passes under the animal (Figure 36–13).

Visual information about the size and location of an obstacle is registered as the obstacle is approached, and this information is stored in working memory, a form of short-term memory, to guide the legs. In humans obstructing vision one stride before an obstacle is encountered does not influence foot clearance over the obstacle. In quadrupeds, however, such working memory is necessary because an obstacle is no longer within the visual field by the time the hind legs are stepping over it.

Many of the features of the working memory for guiding the legs have recently been established in cats. The main features are that the forelegs must step over the obstacle in order for the memory to be established, the trajectories of the hind legs are scaled appropriately for the height of the obstacle and for the relative positions of the hind paws and the obstacle, and the memory persists for many minutes without declining.

The neurobiological mechanisms underlying this form of memory remain to be established, but the persistence of the memory appears to depend upon neuronal systems in the posterior parietal cortex. With bilateral lesions of the medial posterior parietal cortex the memory is completely abolished after a few seconds (Figure 36–14). Complementing this observation is the recent identification by Trevor Drew and colleagues of neurons in the posterior parietal cortex whose activity is elevated while the cat straddles an obstacle with the forelegs on one side and the hind legs on the other side.

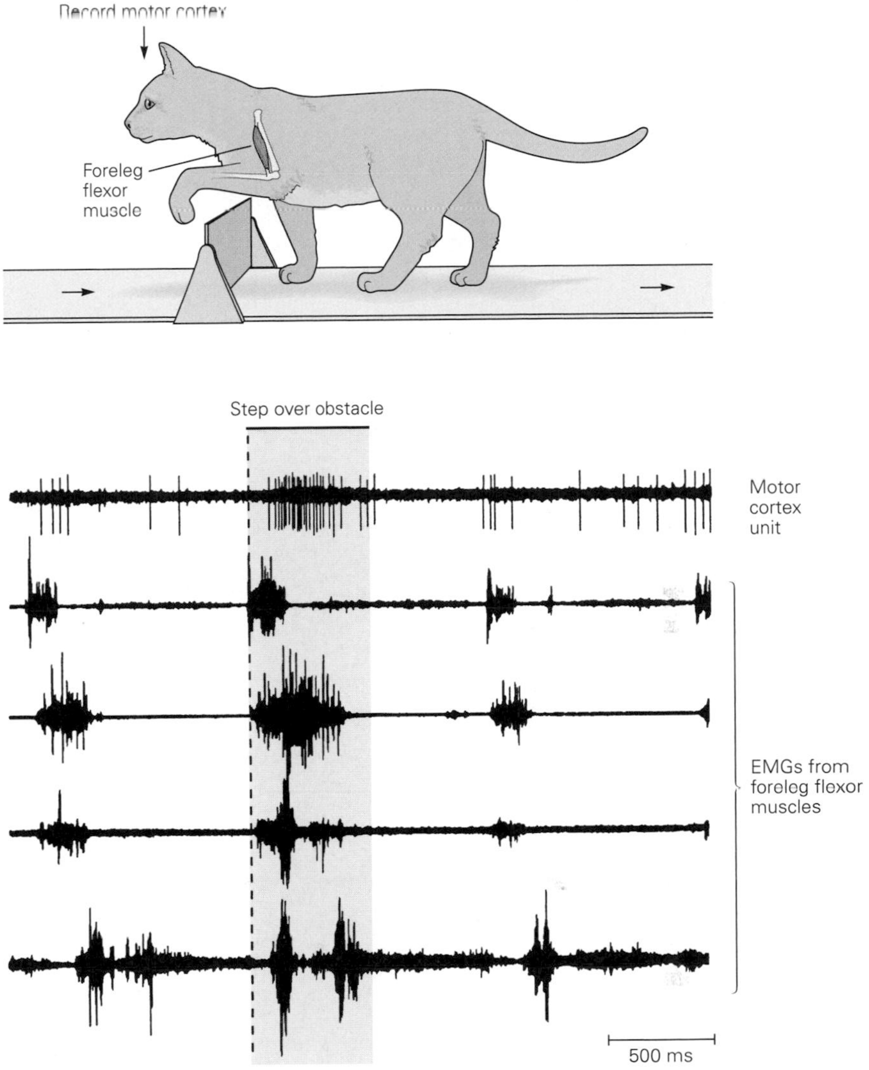

Figure 36–12 Stepping movements are adapted by visual input in the motor cortex. When a normal cat steps over a visible object fixed to the belt of a treadmill, neurons in the motor cortex increase in activity. This increase in cortical activity is associated with enhanced activity in foreleg muscles, as seen in the electromyograms (**EMG**). (Adapted, with permission, from Drew 1988.)

Human Walking May Involve Spinal Pattern Generators

Unlike spinal cats and other quadrupeds, humans with spinal cord transection generally are not able to walk spontaneously. Nevertheless, some observations of patients with spinal cord injury parallel the findings from studies of spinal cats. In one striking case a patient with nearly complete transection of the spinal cord showed uncontrollable, spontaneous, rhythmic movements of the legs when the hips were extended. This behavior closely parallels the rhythmic stepping movements in chronic spinal cats. In another study on a few patients with severe spinal cord injury, stepping on a treadmill was improved by clonidine, a drug influencing biogenic amines.

Compelling evidence for the existence of spinal rhythm-generating networks in humans comes from studies of development. Human infants make rhythmic stepping movements immediately after birth if held upright and moved over a horizontal surface. This strongly suggests that some of the basic neuronal circuits for locomotion are innate. Because stepping can occur in infants who lack cerebral hemispheres (anencephaly), these circuits must be located at or below the brain stem, perhaps entirely within the spinal cord.

During the first year of life, as automatic stepping is transformed into functional walking, these basic circuits are thought to be brought under supraspinal control in two ways. First, the infant develops voluntary control of locomotion. From what we know about the neuronal mechanisms in the cat, this ability could depend on the

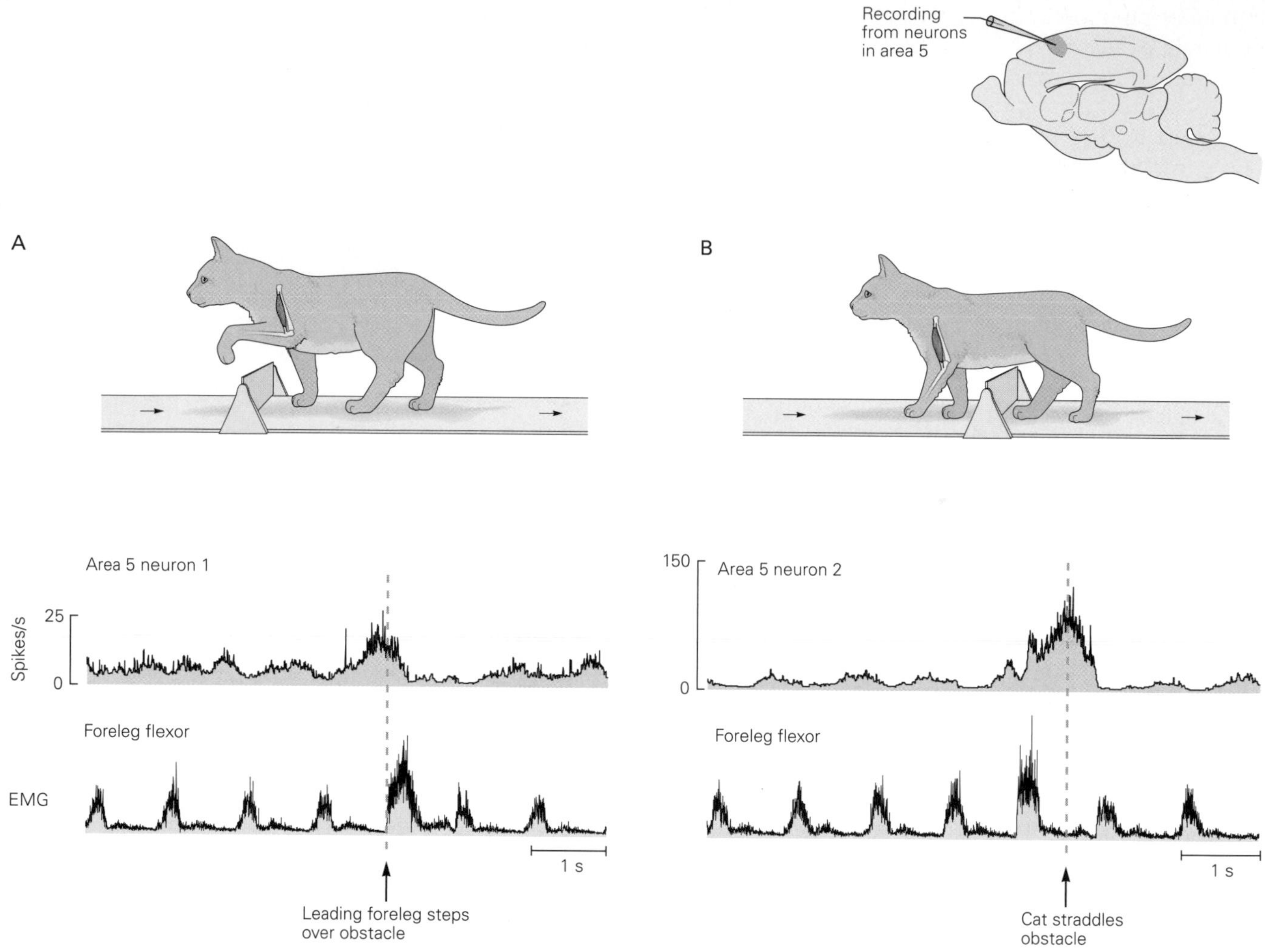

Figure 36–13 Neurons in area 5 of the posterior parietal cortex of the cat are involved in visuomotor transformations of walking. (Adapted, with permission, from Drew et al. 2008.)

A. The activity of a neuron increases as the animal approaches an obstacle and then declines the instant the leading foreleg begins to step over the obstacle.

B. Activity in a different neuron increases after the leading foreleg begins to step over an obstacle and is maximally active when the cat straddles the obstacle.

maturation of reticulospinal pathways and regions of the brain stem that project to reticulospinal neurons, such as the mesencephalic locomotor region. Second, the stepping pattern gradually develops from a primitive flexion-extension pattern that generates little effective forward movement to the mature pattern of complex movements. Again based on studies of cats, it is plausible that this adaptation reflects maturation of descending systems that originate in the motor cortex and brain stem nuclei and which are modulated by the cerebellum.

Parallels between human and quadrupedal walking have also been found in patients trained after spinal cord injury. Daily training restores stepping in spinal cats and improves stepping in patients with chronic spinal injuries. In patients with complete spinal cord injury motor patterns evoked in response to rhythmic leg movements can also be modified by daily therapy (Box 36–4). Thus the spinal networks for locomotion in humans and cats can adapt.

In light of these findings there is reason to believe that human walking relies on the same general principles of neuronal organization as quadrupedal walking: Intrinsic oscillatory networks are activated and modulated by other brain structures and by afferent input. Nevertheless, human bipedal locomotion differs from most animal locomotion in that it places significantly greater demands on descending systems that control balance during walking. Indeed, maturation of the systems that control balance and stepping patterns is necessary for the infant to begin walking independently at the end of the first year. In contrast, horses can stand and walk within hours after birth. It is therefore likely that the locomotor spinal networks in humans are more dependent on supraspinal centers than those in quadrupeds. This dependence may explain in part the relatively few observations of spontaneous stepping movements in humans with complete spinal cord injury.

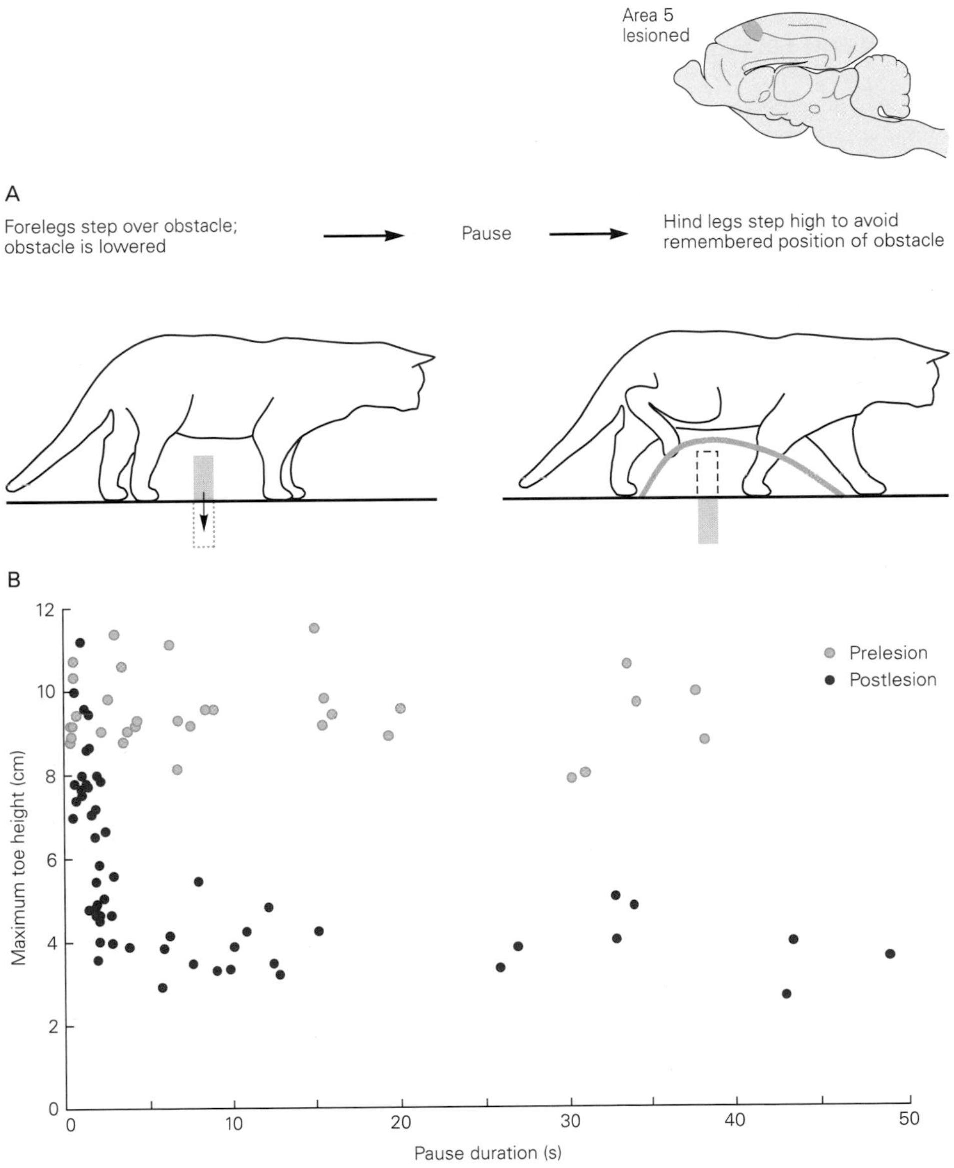

Figure 36–14 A walking cat's working memory of an obstacle is impaired following bilateral lesions of area 5 in the posterior parietal cortex.

A. A normal animal walks forward, steps over an obstacle, and pauses. While the animal pauses, the obstacle is removed. When walking resumes, the hind legs step high to avoid the remembered obstacle. The **blue line** traces the elevated trajectory of one toe.

B. The maximum toe heights of the hind legs are plotted against pause duration before and a few days after bilateral lesions of area 5 of posterior parietal cortex. The impairment of memory is indicated by the decline in maximum toe height for pause durations greater than a few seconds. (Adapted, with permission, from McVea et al. 2009.)

Box 36–4 Improving Walking After Spinal Cord Injury

Every year approximately 11,000 people in the United States injure their spinal cords, and for many this results in permanent loss of sensation, movement, and autonomic function. The devastating loss of functional abilities, together with the enormous cost of treatment and care, creates an urgent need for effective methods to repair the injured spinal cord and to facilitate functional recovery.

Over the past decade considerable progress has been made in animal research aimed at repairing the axons of damaged neurons in the spinal cord and promoting the regeneration of severed axons through and beyond the site of injury. In many instances the regeneration of axons has been associated with modest recovery of locomotor function. However, none of these strategies has reached the point where it can be confidently used in humans with spinal cord injury.

Therefore, rehabilitative training is the preferred treatment for patients with spinal cord injury. One especially successful technique for enhancing walking in patients with partial damage to the spinal cord is repetitive, weight-supported stepping on a treadmill (Figure 36–15). This technique is firmly based on the observation that spinal cats can be trained to step with their hind leg on a moving treadmill (see Box 36–1).

For humans partial support of the body weight through a harness system is critical to the success of training; presumably it facilitates the training of spinal cord circuits by reducing the requirements for supraspinal control of posture and balance.

Although the neural basis for the improvement in locomotor function with treadmill training has not been established, it is thought to depend on synaptic plasticity in local spinal circuits as well as successful transmission of at least some command signals from the brain through preserved descending pathways.

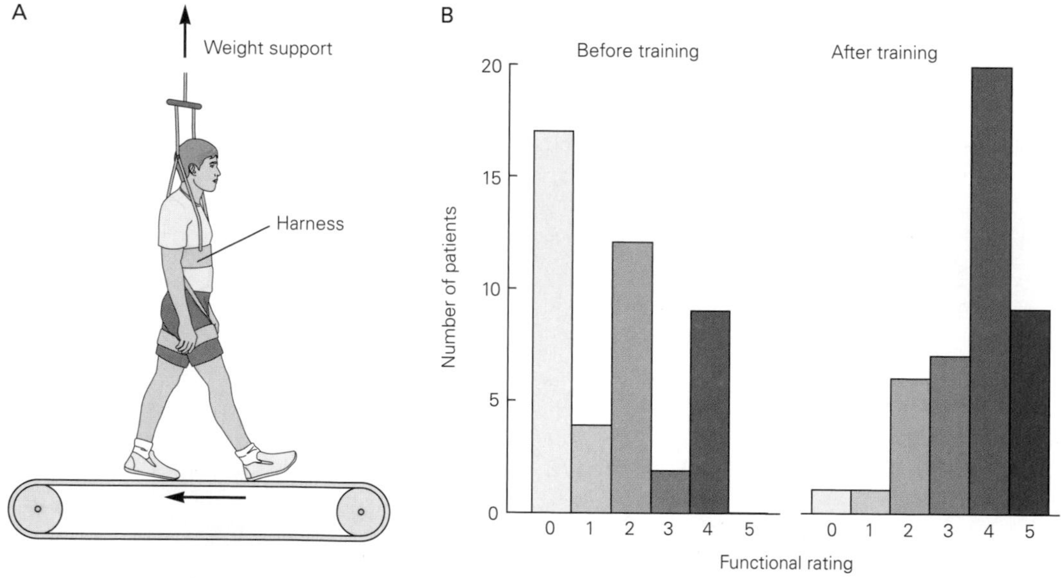

Figure 36–15 Treadmill training improves locomotor function in patients with partial spinal cord injury. (Adapted, with permission, from Wernig et al. 1995.)

A. A patient is partially supported on a moving treadmill by a harness, and stepping movements are assisted by therapists.

B. Locomotor function improved in 44 patients with chronic spinal cord injury after they received daily training lasting from 3 to 20 weeks. The functional rating ranges from 0 (unable to stand or walk) to 5 (walking without devices for more than five steps).

An Overall View

Locomotion in mammals typically involves rhythmic movements of the body and one or more limbs. These movements depend on precise regulation of the timing and strength of contractions in numerous muscles. Local spinal circuits, known as central pattern generators, can produce the basic motor pattern for locomotion even without sensory information from peripheral receptors. Numerous examples of central pattern generators have been analyzed at the cellular level, and it is clear that a wide variety of cellular, synaptic, and network properties are involved in these local networks.

Central pattern generators are extremely flexible; their cellular and synaptic properties can be modified by modulatory signals at chemical synapses. Their functioning depends on how they are activated and the pattern of afferent input they receive.

Modern research on mammalian locomotion dates from the 1960s, when two important experimental animal preparations were introduced. In the decerebrate animal stepping can be initiated by electrical stimulation of a site in the brain stem, the mesencephalic locomotor region. In the spinal preparation centrally generated locomotor activity can be evoked after the administration of adrenergic drugs.

Using these preparations, investigators have confirmed and extended fundamental observations made at the beginning of the 20th century, namely that the basic rhythm for locomotion is generated centrally in spinal networks, that the transition from stance to swing is regulated by afferent signals from leg flexor and extensor muscles, and that descending signals from the brain regulate the intensity of locomotion and modify stepping movements according to the terrain on which the animal is walking.

Keir G. Pearson
James E. Gordon

Selected Readings

Burke RE. 1999. The use of state-dependent modulation of spinal reflexes as a tool to investigate the organization of spinal interneurons. Exp Brain Res 128:263–277.

Clarac F, Pearlstein E, Pflieger J-F, Vinay L. 2005. The in-vitro neonatal rat spinal cord preparation: a new insight into mammalian locomotor mechanisms. J Comp Physiol A Neuroethol Sens Neural Behav Physiol 190:343–357.

Drew T, Andujar J-E, Lajoie K, Yakovenko S. 2008. Cortical mechanisms involved in visuomotor coordination during precision walking. Brain Res Rev 57:199–211.

Fetz EE, Perlmutter SI, Orut Y. 2000. Functions of spinal interneurons during movement. Curr Opin Neurobiol 10:699–707.

Grillner S. 1981. Control of locomotion in bipeds, tetrapods and fish. In: VB Brooks (ed). *Handbook of Physiology,* Sect 1 *The Nervous System*, Vol. 2 *Motor Control,* pp. 1179–1236. Bethesda, MD: American Physiological Society.

Grillner S, Wallen P. 2002. Cellular bases of a vertebrate locomotor system—steering, intersegmental and segmental coordination and sensory control. Brain Res Rev 40: 92–106.

Marder E, Calabrese R. 1996. Principles of rhythmic motor pattern generation. Physiol Rev 76:687–717.

Pearson KG. 1993. Common principles of motor control in vertebrates and invertebrates. Annu Rev Neurosci 16: 265–297.

Pearson KG. 2003. Generating the walking gait: role of sensory feedback. Prog Brain Res 143:123–129.

Rossignol S, Dubuc R, Gossard J-P. 2006. Dynamic sensorimotor interactions in locomotion. Physiol Rev 86:89–154.

Scott SH. 2008. Inconvenient truths about neural processing in primary motor cortex. J Physiol 586:1217–1224.

Wolpaw JR. 2007. Spinal cord plasticity in acquisition and maintenance of motor skills. Acta Physiol (Oxf) 189: 155–169.

References

Belanger M, Drew T, Provencher J, Rossignol S. 1996. A comparison of treadmill locomotion in adult cats before and after spinal transection. J Neurophysiol 76:471–491.

Calancie B, Needham-Shropshire B, Jacobs P, Willer K, Zych G, Green BA. 1994. Involuntary stepping after chronic spinal cord injury: evidence for a central rhythm generator for locomotion in man. Brain 117:1143–1159.

Cazalets J-R, Borde M, Clarac F. 1995. Localization and organization of the central pattern generator for hindlimb locomotion in newborn rat. J Neurosci 15:4943–4951.

Douglas JR, Noga BR, Dai X, Jordan LM. 1993. The effects of intrathecal administration of excitatory amino acid agonists and antagonists on the initiation of locomotion in the adult cat. J Neurosci 13:990–1000.

Drew T. 1988. Motor cortical cell discharge during voluntary gait modification. Brain Res 457:181–187.

Edgerton VR, Grillner S, Sjüström A, Zangger P. 1976. Central generation of locomotion in vertebrates. In: RM Herman, S Grillner, PSG Stein, DG Stuart (eds). *Neural Control of Locomotion,* pp. 439–467. New York: Plenum.

Eide AL, Kjaerulff O, Kiehn O. 1999. Characterization of commissural interneurons in the lumbar region of the neonatal rat spinal cord. J Comp Neurol 403:332–345.

Engberg I, Lundberg A. 1969. An electromyographic analysis of muscular activity in the hindlimb of the cat during un-restrained locomotion. Acta Physiol Scand 75:614–630.

Forssberg H. 1985. Ontogeny of human locomotor control. I. Infant stepping, supported locomotion and transition to independent locomotion. Exp Brain Res 57:480–493.

Forssberg H. 1979. Stumbling corrective reaction: a phase dependent compensatory reaction during locomotion. J Neurophysiol 42:936–953.

Graham Brown T. 1911. The intrinsic factors in the act of progression in the mammal. Proc R Soc Lond B Biol Sci 84:308–319.

Graham Brown T. 1914. On the nature of the fundamental activity of the nervous centres; together with an analysis of the conditioning of rhythmic activity in progression, and a theory of the evolution of function in the nervous system. J Physiol (Lond) 48:18–46.

Grillner S, Deliagina T, Ekebuerg Ö, El Manira A, Hill RH, Lansner A, Orlovsky GN, Wallen P. 1995. Neural networks that coordinate locomotion and body orientation in lamprey. Trends Neurosci 18:270–280.

Grillner S, Wallén P, Dale N, Brodin L, Buchanan J, Hill R. 1987. Transmitters, membrane properties and network circuitry in the control of locomotion in the lamprey. Trends Neurosci 10:34–41.

Grillner S, Zangger P. 1984. The effect of dorsal root transection on the efferent motor pattern in the cat's hindlimb during locomotion. Acta Physiol Scand 120:393–405.

Hiebert GW, Whelan PJ, Prochazka A, Pearson KG. 1996. Contribution of hindlimb flexor muscle afferents to the timing of phase transitions in the cat step cycle. J Neurophysiol 75:1126–1137.

Jankowska E, Jukes MGM, Lund S, Lundberg A. 1967a. The effect of DOPA on the spinal cord. 5. Reciprocal organization of pathways transmitting excitatory action to alpha motoneurones of flexors and extensors. Acta Physiol Scand 70:369–388.

Jankowska E, Jukes MGM, Lund S, Lundberg A. 1967b. The effect of DOPA on the spinal cord. VI. Half-centre organization of interneurons transmitting effects from flexor reflex afferents. Acta Physiol Scand 70:389–402.

Kriellaars DJ, Brownstone RM, Noga BR, Jordan LM. 1994. Mechanical entrainment of fictive locomotion in the decerebrate cat. J Neurophysiol 71:2074–2086.

Lajoie K, Andujar J-E, Pearson K, Drew T. 2010. Neurons in area 5 of the posterior parietal cortex in the cat contribute to interlimb coordination during visually guided locomotion: a role in working memory. J Neurophysiol 103: 2234–2254.

McVea DA, Pearson KG. 2006. Long-lasting memories of obstacles guide leg movements in the walking cat. J Neurosci 26:1175–1178.

McVea DA, Taylor AJ, Pearson KG. 2009. Long-lasting working memories of obstacles established by foreleg stepping in walking cats require area 5 of the posterior parietal cortex. J Neurosci 29:9396–9494.

Mori S, Matsuyama K, Kohyama J, Kobayashi Y, Takakusaki K. 1992. Neuronal constituents of postural and locomotor control systems and their interactions in cats. Brain Dev 14:S109–S120.

Noga BR, Kriellaars DJ, Jordan LM. 1991. The effect of selective brain stem or spinal cord lesions on treadmill locomotion evoked by stimulation of the mesencephalic or ponto-medullary locomotor region. J Neurosci 11: 1691–1700.

Perret C, Cabelguen JM. 1980. Main characteristics of the hindlimb locomotor cycle in the decorticate cat with special reference to bifunctional muscles. Brain Res 187: 333–352.

Rybak IA, Shevtzova NA, Lafreniere-Roula M, McCrea DA. 2006. Modelling spinal circuitry involved in locomotion pattern generation: insights from deletions during fictive locomotion. J Physiol (Lond) 577:617–639.

Sherrington CS. 1910. Flexor-reflex of the limb, crossed extension reflex, and reflex stepping and standing (cat and dog). J Physiol (Lond) 40:28–121.

Shik ML, Severin FV, Orlovsky GN. 1966. Control of walking and running by means of electrical stimulation of the midbrain. Biophysics (Oxf) 11:756–765.

Thelen E. 1985. Developmental origins of motor coordination: leg movements in human infants. Dev Psychobiol 18:1–22.

Wernig A, Muller S, Nanassy A, Cagol E. 1995. Laufband therapy based on "rules of spinal locomotion" is effective in spinal cord injured persons. Eur J Neurosci 7:823–829.

Whelan PJ, Hiebert GW, Pearson KG. 1995. Stimulation of the group I extensor afferents prolongs the stance phase in walking cats. Exp Brain Res 103:20–30.

37

Voluntary Movement: The Primary Motor Cortex

"…. The physiology of movements is basically a study of the purposive activity of the nervous system as a whole."

— Gelfand et al., 1966

One of the main functions of the brain is to direct the body's purposeful interaction with the environment. Understanding how the brain fulfils this role is one of the great challenges in neural science. Because large areas of the cerebral cortex are implicated in voluntary motor control, the study of the cortical control of voluntary movement provides important insights into the functional organization of the cerebral cortex as a whole.

Evolution has endowed mammals with adaptive neural circuitry that allows them to interact in sophisticated ways with the complex environments in which they live. Adaptive patterning of voluntary movements gives mammals a distinct advantage in locating food, finding mates, and avoiding predators, all of which enhance the survival potential of the individual and a species.

The ability to use fingers, hands, and arms in voluntary actions independent of locomotion further helps primates, and especially humans, exploit their environment. Most animals must search their environment for food when hungry. In contrast, humans can also "forage" by using their hands to cook a meal or simply punch a few buttons on a telephone and order takeout. The central neural circuits responsible for such nonlocomotor behavior emerged from and remain intimately associated with the phylogenetically older circuits that control the forelimb during locomotor behaviors.

In this and the following chapter we focus on the control of voluntary movements of the hand and arm in primates. In this chapter we describe the cortical networks that control voluntary movement, particularly the role of the primary motor cortex in the generation of motor commands. In the next chapter we address broader questions about cortical control of voluntary motor behavior, in particular how the cerebral cortex organizes the stream of incoming sensory information to guide voluntary movement.

Voluntary movements differ from reflexes and basic locomotor rhythms in several important ways. By definition they are intentional—they are initiated by an internal decision to act—whereas reflexes are automatically triggered by external stimuli. Even when a voluntary action is directed toward an object, such as reaching for a cup, the cause of action is not the object but an internal decision to interact with the object. The presence of the object provides only the opportunity for acting. Voluntary actions involve choices between alternatives, including the choice not to act. Furthermore, they are organized to achieve some goal in the near or distant future.

Voluntary movements often have a labile, context-dependent association with sensory inputs. The same object can evoke different voluntary actions or no response at all depending on the context in which it appears. That is, the neural circuits controlling voluntary behavior are able to differentiate between an object's physical properties and its behavioral salience.

The nature and effectiveness of voluntary movements often improve with experience. The motor system can learn new behavioral strategies or new reactions to familiar stimuli to improve behavioral outcomes, and it can learn new skills to cope with predictable variations and perturbations of the environment.

Thus the neural control of voluntary movement involves far more than simply generating a particular pattern of muscle activity. It also involves processes that are usually considered to be more sensory, perceptual, and cognitive in nature. As we shall see, these processes are not rigidly compartmentalized into different neural structures or neural populations.

Motor Functions Are Localized within the Cerebral Cortex

For centuries it was believed that the human cerebral cortex was responsible for only higher-order, conscious mental functions. In the middle of the 19th century the English neurologist John Hughlings Jackson made the controversial proposal that a specific part of the cerebral cortex anterior to the central sulcus has a causal role in movement. He reached this conclusion from treating patients with epileptic seizures that were characterized by repeated spasmodic involuntary movements that sometimes resembled fragments of purposive voluntary actions.

During each episode the seizures always spread to different body parts in a fixed temporal sequence that varied from patient to patient, a pattern called *Jacksonian march.* Jackson concluded that paroxysmal neural activity generated by epileptic foci located near the central sulcus caused the involuntary seizures. He speculated that the progression of seizures across the body resulted from the spread of paroxysmal activity across small clusters of neurons lying along the central sulcus, each of which controlled movement of a different body part. Jackson's proposal that a discrete cortical region is involved in the control of movement was a strong argument for the localization of different functions in distinct parts of the cerebral cortex. His observations, along with contemporaneous studies by Pierre Paul Broca and Karl Wernicke on the language deficits resulting from specific cortical lesions, laid the foundation for the modern scientific study of cortical function.

It was not until later in the 19th century, however, when improved anesthesia and aseptic surgical techniques allowed direct experimental study of the cerebral cortex in live subjects, that conclusive experimental evidence for a discrete region of the cerebral cortex devoted to motor function was possible. Gustav Fritsch and Eduard Hitzig in Berlin and David Ferrier in England showed that electrical stimulation of the surface of a limited area of cortex of different surgically anesthetized mammals evoked movements of parts of the contralateral body. The electric currents needed to evoke movements were lowest in a narrow strip along the rostral bank of the central sulcus.

Their experiments demonstrated that, even within this strip of tissue, discrete sites contained neurons with distinctive functions. Stimulation of adjacent sites evoked movements in adjacent body parts, starting with the foot, leg, and tail medially, and proceeding to the trunk, arm, hand, face, mouth, and tongue more laterally. When they lesioned a cortical site at which stimulation had evoked movements of a part of the body, motor control of that body part was perturbed or lost after the animal recovered from surgery. These early experiments showed that the motor strip contains an orderly motor map of the contralateral body and that the integrity of the motor map is necessary for voluntary control of the corresponding body parts.

In the first half of the 20th century more focal electrical stimulation allowed the motor map to be defined in greater detail. Clinton Woolsey and his colleagues tested the functional organization of the motor cortex in several species of mammals, whereas Wilder Penfield and co-workers tested discrete sites in human neurosurgical patients (Figure 37–1). Their findings

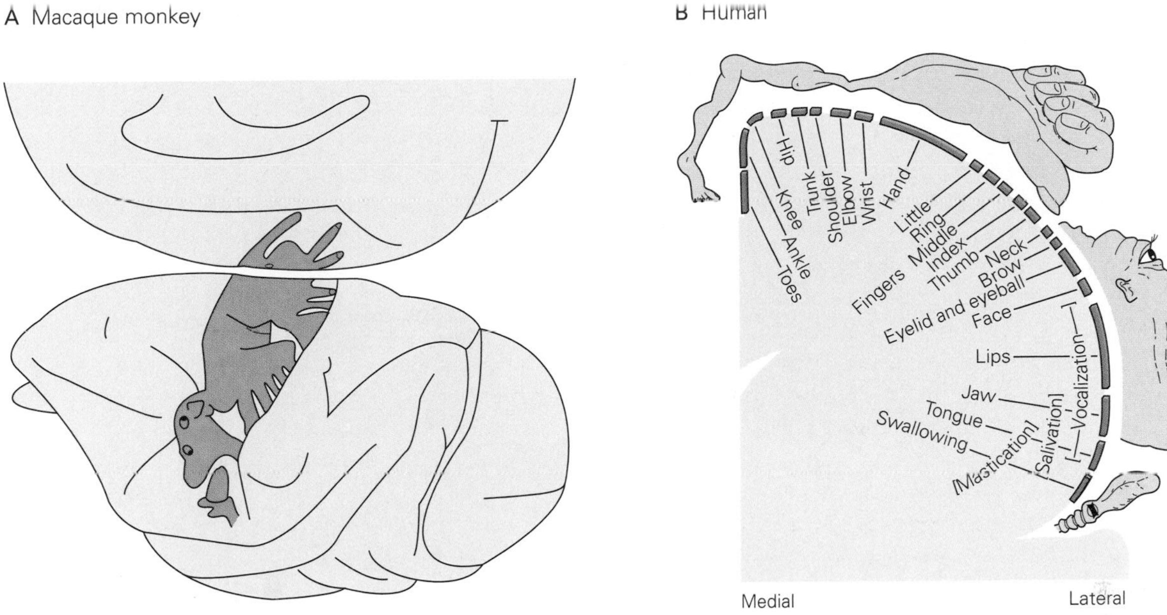

Figure 37–1 The motor cortex contains a topographic map of motor output to different parts of the body.

A. Studies by Clinton Woolsey and colleagues confirmed that the representation of different body parts in the monkey follows an orderly plan: Motor output to the foot and leg is medial, whereas the arm, face, and mouth areas are more lateral. The areas of cortex controlling the foot, hand, and mouth are much larger than the regions controlling other parts of the body.

B. Wilder Penfield and colleagues showed that the human motor cortex motor map has the same general mediolateral organization as in the monkey. However, the areas controlling the hand and mouth are even larger than in monkeys, whereas the area controlling the foot is much smaller. Penfield emphasized that this cartoon illustrated the relative size of the representation of each body part in the motor map; he did not claim that each body part was controlled by a single separate part of the motor map.

demonstrated that the same general topographic organization is conserved across many species. One important discovery was that the motor map is not a point-to-point representation of the body. Instead, the most finely controlled body parts, such as the fingers, face, and mouth, are represented in the motor map by disproportionately large areas, reflecting the larger number of neurons needed for fine motor control.

Woolsey and Penfield both recognized, however, that their simple motor map masked a deeper complexity. Today the best-studied regions of the map are those parts controlling the arm and hand. Recent mapping studies have revealed that the neurons controlling the muscles of the digits, hand, and distal arm tend to be concentrated within a central zone, whereas those controlling more proximal arm muscles are located in a horseshoe-shaped ring around the central core (Figure 37–2A). Furthermore, across the concentrically organized areas of the arm motor map there is extensive overlap of stimulation sites that causes contractions of muscles acting across different joints; conversely, each muscle can be activated by stimulating many widely dispersed sites (Figure 37–2B). Moreover, different combinations of muscle contractions and joint motions can be evoked by stimulating different sites. Finally, local horizontal axonal connections link different sites, allowing neural activity at multiple output sites in the map to be coordinated during the formation of motor commands.

To date, studies have not revealed any repeating functional elements in the fine details of the motor map for the arm and hand analogous to the ocular-dominance bands and orientation pinwheels in the visual cortex. However, the complex, extensively overlapped organization of the arm motor map and the network of local horizontal connections likely provide a mechanism to coordinate whole-limb actions such as reaching to grasp and manipulate an object.

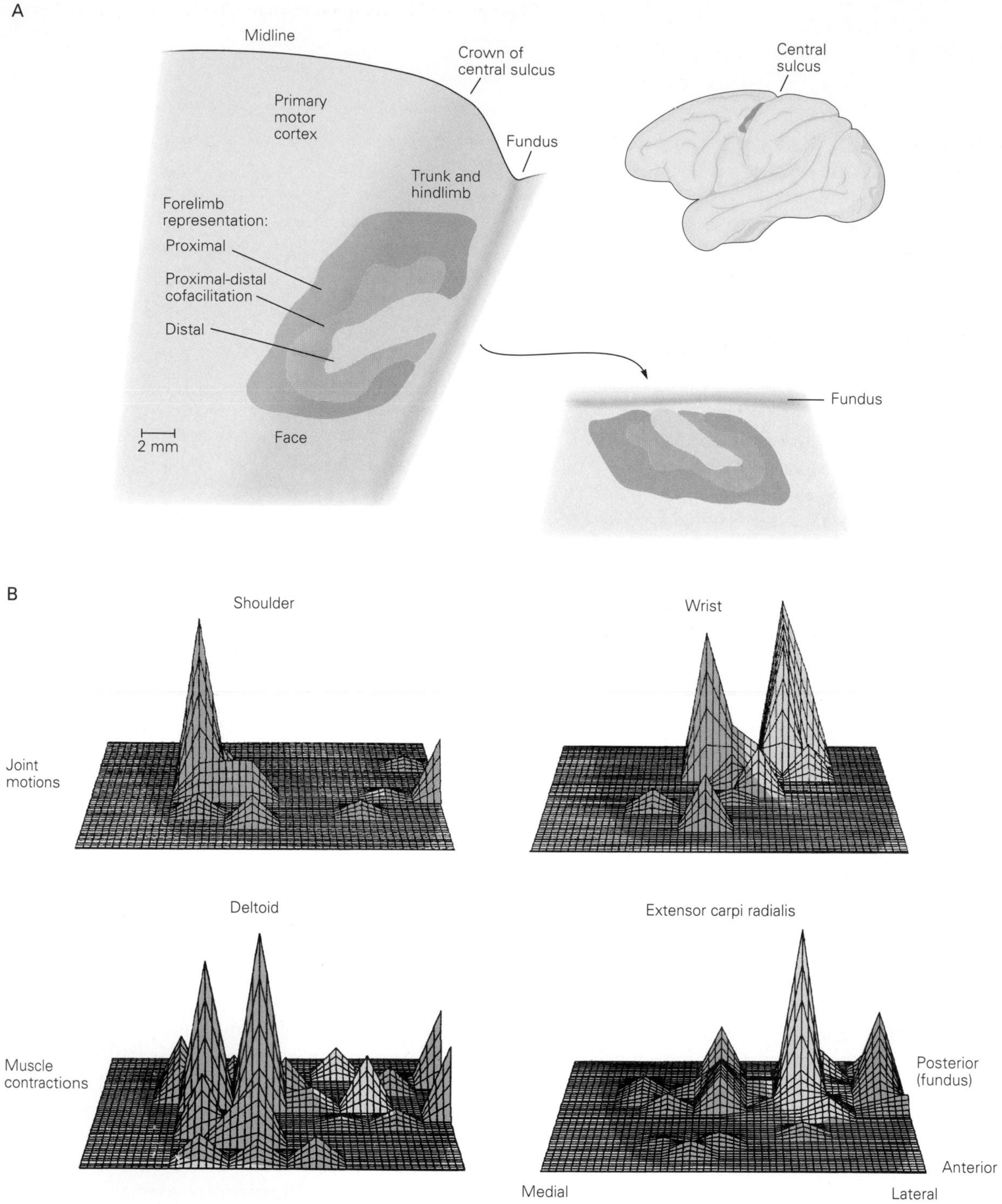

Figure 37–2 Internal organization of the motor map of the arm in the motor cortex.

A. The arm motor map in monkeys has a concentric, horseshoe-shaped organization: Neurons that control the distal arm (digits and wrist) are concentrated in a central core (**yellow**) surrounded by neurons that control the proximal arm (elbow and shoulder; **blue**). The neuron populations that control the distal and proximal parts of the arm overlap extensively in a zone of proximal-distal cofacilitation (**green**). The arm motor representation is seen in its normal anatomical location in the anterior bank of the central sulcus (**left**), and also after flattening and rotation to bring it into approximate alignment with the microstimulation maps in part B. (Reproduced, with permission, from Park et al. 2001.)

B. Microstimulation of several sites in the arm motor map can produce rotations of the same joint. Neurons that control wrist movements are concentrated in the central core whereas those that regulate shoulder movements are distributed around the core, with some overlap between the two populations. In these maps, the height of each peak is scaled to the inverse of the stimulation current: the higher the peak, the lower the current necessary to produce a response. The distribution and overlap of stimulation sites that evoke contractions of muscles in the shoulder (deltoid) and wrist (extensor carpi radialis) are even more extensive than that of sites for joint rotations. The yellow, green, and blue color zones on these maps correspond only approximately to the functional zones identified in the motor map of part A. (Reproduced, with permission, from Humphrey and Tanji 1991.)

Many Cortical Areas Contribute to the Control of Voluntary Movements

Voluntary Motor Control Appears to Require Serial Processing

Much of what we do in everyday life involves a sequence of actions. One normally does not take a shower after getting dressed or put cake ingredients into the oven to bake before blending them into a batter. It seems logical that most brain functions are also serial.

Largely on the basis of indirect psychological studies, the neural processes by which the brain controls voluntary behavior are commonly divided into three sequential stages. First, perceptual mechanisms generate a unified sensory representation of the external world and the individual within it. Next, cognitive processes use this internal replica of the world to decide on a course of action. Finally, the selected motor plan is relayed to action systems for implementation (Figure 37–3A).

The final stage, execution of the chosen motor plan, also appears to be serial in nature. It has often been modeled as a series of sensorimotor transformations of representations of a movement into different coordinate frameworks, progressing from a general description of the overall form of the movement to increasingly specific details, culminating in patterns of muscle activity (Figure 37–3B).

According to this serial scheme, each sequential operation is encoded by a different neuronal population. Each population encodes specific features or parameters of the intended movement in a particular coordinate system, such as the direction of movement of the hand through space or the patterns of muscle contractions and forces. These several populations are connected serially and only the last population in the chain projects to the spinal cord.

As we shall see in this and the next chapter, this model has some heuristic value for describing how the brain is organized to control voluntary movement,

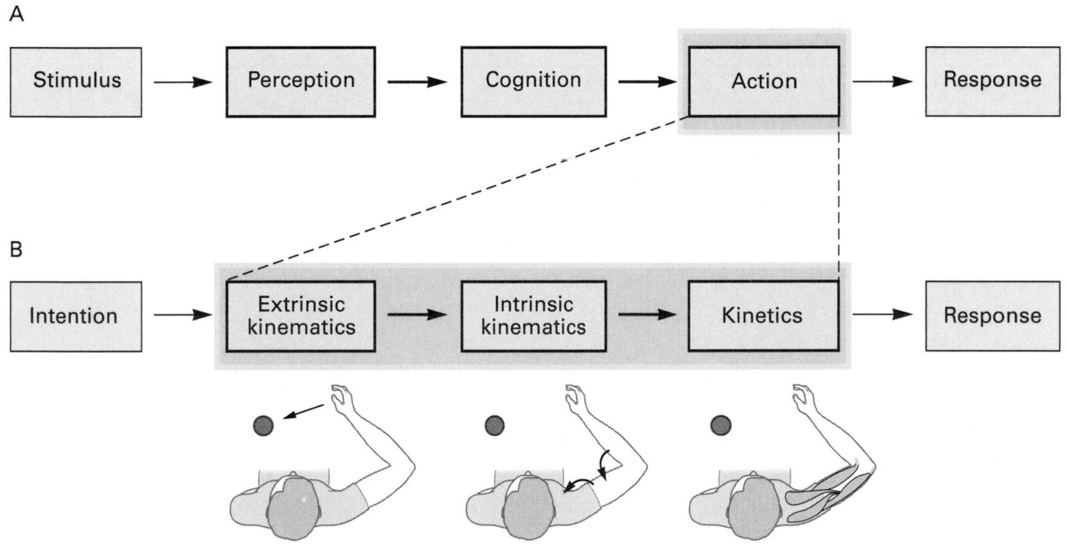

Figure 37–3 Cortical control of voluntary behavior appears to be organized in a hierarchical series of operations.

A. The brain's control of voluntary behavior has often been divided into three main operational stages, in which perception generates an internal neuronal image of the world, cognition analyzes and reflects on this image to decide what to do, and the final decision is relayed to action systems for execution. However, this three-stage serial organization was largely based on introspective psychological studies rather than on direct neurophysiological study of neural mechanisms.

B. Each of the three main operational stages is presumed to involve its own serial processes. For example, the "action" stage that converts an intention into a physical movement is often presumed to involve a hierarchy of operations that transform a general plan into progressively more detailed instructions about its implementation. The model shown here, inspired by early controller designs for multijoint robots, suggests that the brain plans a chosen reaching movement by first calculating the extrinsic kinematics of the movement (eg, target location, trajectory of hand displacement from the starting location to the target location), then calculating the required intrinsic kinematics (eg, joint rotations) and finally the causal kinetics or dynamics of movement (eg, forces, torques, and muscle activity). (See also Figure 33–2.)

but direct neurophysiological studies of neural mechanisms show that a strict adherence to serial processing is simplistic and incorrect. We know now for instance that the brain does not have a single, unified perceptual representation of the world (see Chapter 38). The serial scheme also wrongly implies that the only role of the motor system is to determine which muscles to contract, when, and by how much. We now know that several cortical motor areas also play a critical role in the actual choice of what action to take, a process that is usually considered more "cognitive" than "motor." This is described in more detail in Chapter 38.

The Functional Anatomy of Precentral Motor Areas is Complex

In the early 20th century Alfred Campbell and Korbinian Brodmann divided the human cerebral cortex into a large number of cytoarchitectonic areas with distinct anatomical features. They noted that the *precentral cortex* in the gyri immediately rostral to the central sulcus lacks the six layers characteristic of most cerebral cortex. It lacks a distinct internal granule cell layer and thus is often called *agranular cortex.* Campbell and Brodmann subdivided the precentral cortex into caudal and rostral parts, which Brodmann designated cytoarchitectonic areas 4 and 6 (Figure 37–4).

Campbell proposed that these two regions were functionally distinct motor areas. He thought that the caudal region, or *primary motor cortex,* controlled the motor apparatus in the spinal cord and generated simple movements. The rostral region, he argued, was specialized for higher-order aspects of motor control and for movements that are more complex, conditional, and voluntary in nature. He thought that these areas influenced movement indirectly by projecting to the primary motor cortex and so he named them the *premotor cortex.*

Some years later, while mapping motor areas of cortex with electrical stimuli, Clinton Woolsey and

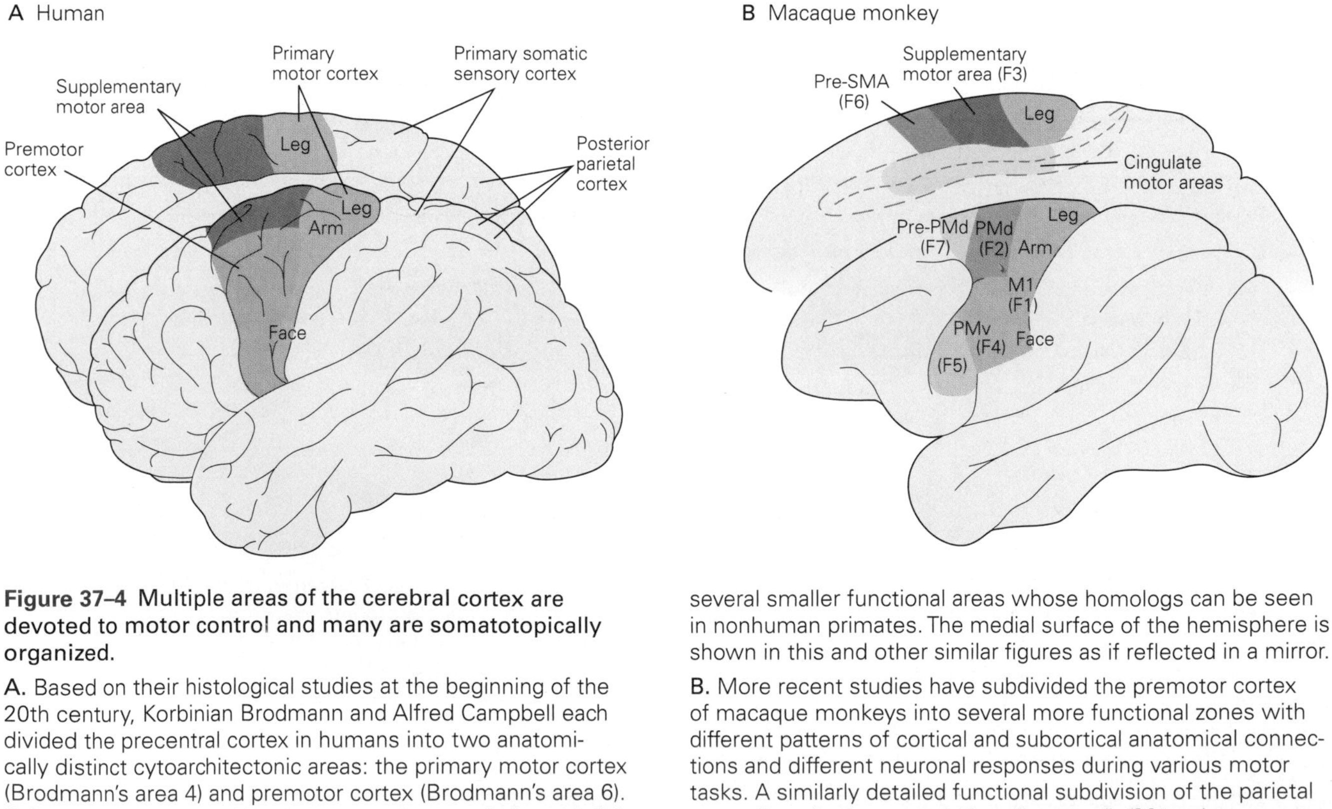

Figure 37–4 Multiple areas of the cerebral cortex are devoted to motor control and many are somatotopically organized.

A. Based on their histological studies at the beginning of the 20th century, Korbinian Brodmann and Alfred Campbell each divided the precentral cortex in humans into two anatomically distinct cytoarchitectonic areas: the primary motor cortex (Brodmann's area 4) and premotor cortex (Brodmann's area 6). Subsequent studies by Woolsey and colleagues led to subdivision of the premotor cortex into medial and lateral halves, the supplementary motor area and lateral premotor cortex, respectively. Since those pioneering studies the human premotor cortex and supplementary motor area have been subdivided into several smaller functional areas whose homologs can be seen in nonhuman primates. The medial surface of the hemisphere is shown in this and other similar figures as if reflected in a mirror.

B. More recent studies have subdivided the premotor cortex of macaque monkeys into several more functional zones with different patterns of cortical and subcortical anatomical connections and different neuronal responses during various motor tasks. A similarly detailed functional subdivision of the parietal cortex has also been made (not illustrated). (**M1**, primary motor cortex; **Pre-SMA**, pre-supplementary motor area; **PMd**, dorsal premotor cortex; **Pre-PMd**, pre-dorsal premotor cortex; **PMv**, ventral premotor cortex.)

his colleagues discovered that movements of the contralateral body can be evoked not only by electrical stimulation of the primary motor cortex, but also by stimulating a second region in a part of the premotor cortex on the medial surface of the cerebral hemisphere now known as the *supplementary motor area* (Figure 37–4B). The motor map of different body parts evoked by stimulation of the supplementary motor area is less detailed than that of the primary motor cortex and lacks the enlarged distal arm and hand representation seen in the primary motor cortex. Stimulation of the supplementary motor area can evoke movements on both sides of the body or halt ongoing voluntary movements, effects that rarely result from stimulation of the primary motor cortex.

Anatomical and functional studies in humans and nonhuman primates over the past 25 years have radically changed the view of how the precentral cortex is organized functionally. First, architectonic studies demonstrated that Brodmann's area 6 is not homogeneous but consists of several distinct subareas. Second, these subareas have specific connections among themselves and with the rest of the cerebral cortex. Third, functional studies found that each subarea separately controls movements of some or all parts of the body and that the properties of neurons in each subarea differ in important ways. These areas are identified by two different nomenclatures in the literature.

As a result, in current maps of the precentral cortex Brodmann's area 6 is usually divided into five or six functional areas in addition to the *primary motor cortex* (or area F1) in Brodmann's area 4 (Figure 37–4B). The classical supplementary motor area originally identified by Woolsey on the medial cortical surface is now split into two functional regions. The more caudal part is called the *supplementary motor area proper* (area F3), whereas the more rostral part is the *pre-supplementary motor area* (F6). The caudal and rostral parts of the dorsal convexity of area 6 are called the *dorsal premotor cortex (F2)* and *pre-dorsal premotor cortex* (F7), respectively. The ventral convexity of Brodmann's area 6 has also been identified as a separate functional area called the *ventral premotor cortex*, and has been further subdivided into two subareas called F4 and F5 (Figure 37–4B). Finally, three additional motor areas outside Brodmann's area 6, in the rostral cingulate cortex, have been delineated recently.

The multiplicity of cortical motor areas would seem redundant if their only role was to initiate or coordinate muscle activity. However, we now know that neurons in these areas have unique properties and interact to perform diverse operations that select, plan, and generate actions appropriate to external and internal needs and context.

The Anatomical Connections of the Precentral Motor Areas Do Not Validate a Strictly Serial Organization

To understand the roles of these multiple precentral motor areas in voluntary motor control, it is important to know their connections with one another, their connections with other cortical areas, and their descending projections.

The cortical motor areas are interconnected by complex patterns of reciprocal, convergent, and divergent projections rather than simple serial pathways. The supplementary motor area, dorsal premotor cortex, and ventral premotor cortex have somatotopically organized reciprocal connections not only with the primary motor cortex but also with each other. The primary motor cortex and supplementary motor area receive somatotopically organized input from the primary somatosensory cortex and the rostral parietal cortex, whereas the dorsal and ventral premotor areas are reciprocally connected with progressively more caudal, medial, and lateral parts of the parietal cortex. These somatosensory and parietal inputs provide the primary motor cortex and caudal premotor regions with sensory information to organize and guide motor acts.

In contrast, the pre-supplementary and pre-dorsal premotor areas do not project to the primary motor cortex and are only weakly connected with the parietal lobe. They receive higher-order cognitive information through reciprocal connections with the prefrontal cortex and so may impose more arbitrary context-dependent control over voluntary behavior.

Several cortical motor regions project in multiple parallel tracts to subcortical areas of the brain as well as the spinal cord. The best studied output path is the *pyramidal tract,* which originates in cortical layer V in a number of precentral and parietal cortical areas. Precentral areas include not only primary motor cortex but also the supplementary motor and dorsal and ventral premotor areas. The pre-supplementary motor and pre-dorsal premotor areas do not send axons to the spinal cord; their descending output reaches the spinal cord indirectly through projections to other subcortical structures. Parietal areas that contribute descending axons to the pyramidal tract include the primary somatosensory cortex and adjacent rostral parts of the superior and inferior parietal lobules.

Many pyramidal tract axons decussate at the pyramid and project to the spinal cord itself, forming the *corticospinal tract* (Figure 37–5A). Because several cortical areas contribute axons to the corticospinal tract, the traditional view that the primary motor cortex is the "final common path" from the cerebral cortex to the

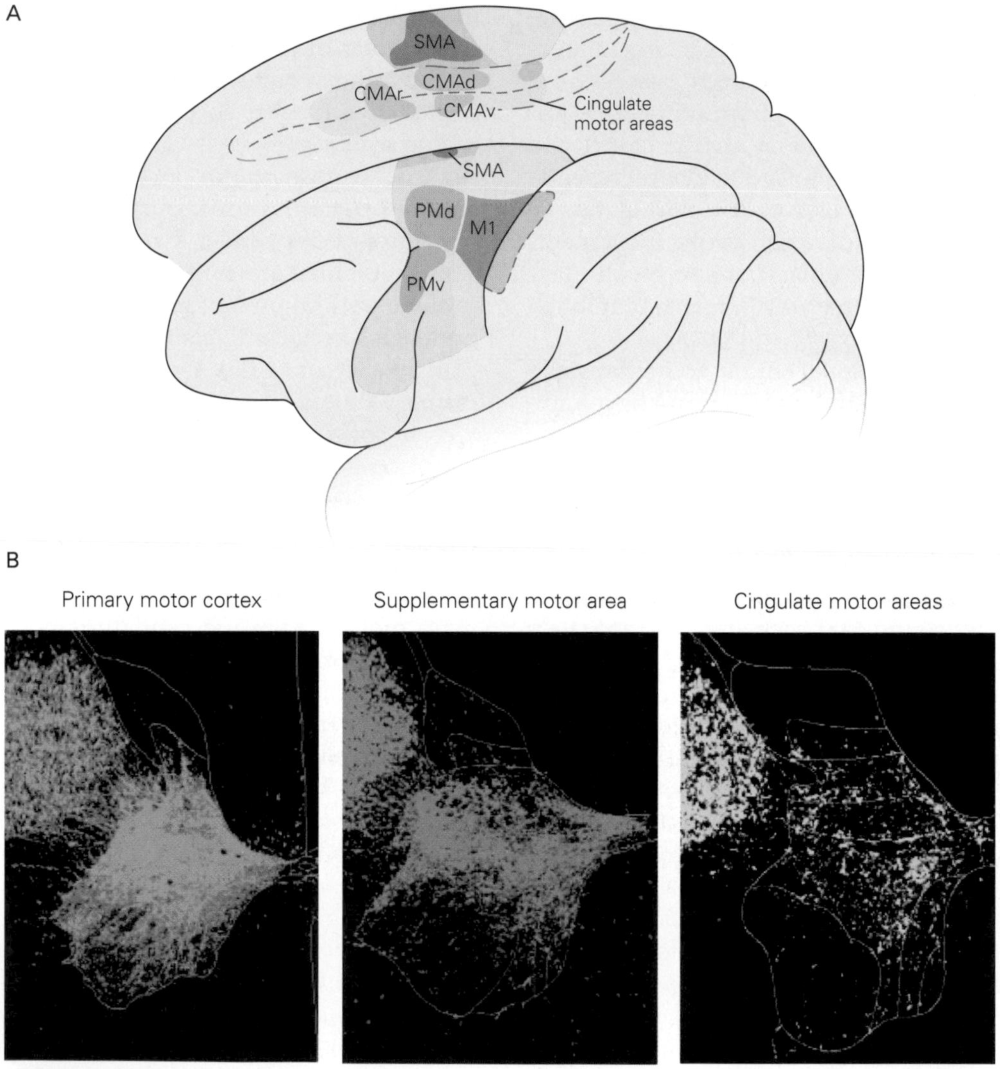

Figure 37–5 Cortical origins of the corticospinal tract. (Reproduced, with permission, from Dum and Strick 2002.)

A. Neurons that modulate muscle activity in the contralateral arm and hand originate in the primary motor cortex (**M1**) and many subdivisions of the premotor cortex (**PMd, PMv, SMA**) and project their axons into the spinal cord cervical enlargement. Corticospinal fibers projecting to the leg, trunk, and other somatotopic parts of the brain stem and spinal motor system originate in the other parts of the motor and premotor cortex. (**M1**, primary motor cortex; **SMA**, supplementary motor area; **PMd**, dorsal premotor cortex; **PMv**, ventral premotor cortex; **CMAd**, dorsal cingulate motor area; **CMAv**, ventral cingulate motor area; **CMAr**, rostral cingulate motor area.)

B. The axons of corticospinal fibers from the primary motor cortex, supplementary motor area, and cingulate motor areas terminate on interneuronal networks in the intermediate laminae (VI, VII, and VIII) of the spinal cord. Only the primary motor cortex contains neurons whose axons terminate directly on spinal motor neurons in the most ventral and lateral part of the spinal ventral horn. Rexed's laminae I to IX of the dorsal and ventral horns are shown in faint outline. The dense cluster of labeled axons adjacent to the dorsal horn (upper left) in each section are the corticospinal axons descending in the dorsolateral funiculus, before entering the spinal intermediate and ventral laminae.

spinal cord is incorrect. Instead, several premotor and parietal areas of cortex can also influence spinal motor function through their own corticospinal projections.

Many corticospinal axons from the primary motor cortex and premotor areas in primates, and virtually all corticospinal axons in other mammals, terminate on spinal interneurons in the intermediate region of the spinal cord (Figure 37–5B). These interneurons are components of reflex and pattern-generating circuits that produce stereotypical motor synergies and locomotor rhythms (see Chapter 36). In primates much of the control exerted by the primary motor cortex on spinal motor circuits and all of the control from premotor areas is mediated indirectly through these descending cortical projections to spinal interneurons.

In primates the terminals of some corticospinal axons also extend into the ventral horn of the spinal cord (lamina IX) where they arborize and contact the dendrites of spinal motor neurons (Figure 37–6B; Figure 37–5B). These monosynaptically projecting cortical neurons are called *corticomotoneurons.* The axons of these neurons become a progressively larger component of the corticospinal tract in primate phylogeny from prosimians to monkeys, great apes, and humans.

In monkeys corticomotoneurons are found only in the most caudal part of the primary motor cortex that lies within the anterior bank of the central sulcus. There is extensive overlap in the distribution of the corticomotoneurons that project to the spinal motor neuron pools innervating different muscles (Figure 37–6A). In monkeys more corticomotoneurons project to the motor neuron pools for muscles of the digits, hand, and wrist than to those for more proximal parts of the arm.

The terminal of a single corticomotoneuron axon often branches and terminates on spinal motor neurons for several different agonist muscles, and can also influence the contractile activity of still more muscles through synapses on spinal interneurons (Figure 37–6B, C). This termination pattern is functionally organized to produce coordinated patterns of activity in a *muscle field* of agonist and antagonist muscles. Most frequently, a single corticomotoneuron axon directly excites the spinal motor neurons for several agonist muscles and indirectly suppresses the activity of some antagonist muscles through local inhibitory interneurons (Figure 37–6C). The fact that corticomotoneurons are more prominent in humans than in monkeys may be one of the reasons why lesions of the primary motor cortex have such a devastating effect on motor control in humans compared to lower mammals (Box 37–1).

Although neurons in several motor-cortical areas send axons into the corticospinal tract, the primary motor cortex has the most direct access to spinal motor neurons, including the monosynaptic projections of corticomotoneurons. However, the corticospinal tract is not the only pathway for descending control signals to spinal motor circuits. The spinal cord also receives inputs from the rubrospinal, reticulospinal, and vestibulospinal tracts. These pathways influence movement through monosynaptic terminations onto spinal interneurons and spinal motor neurons.

In summary, a strictly serial organization of voluntary movement would require a pattern of serial connections between cortical areas, ending at the primary motor cortex, which then projects to the spinal cord. In reality, however, the multiple precentral and parietal cortical motor areas are interconnected by a complex network of reciprocal, divergent, and convergent axonal projections. Moreover, several cortical areas project to the spinal cord in parallel with projections from the primary motor cortex. Finally, the spinal motor circuits receive inputs from several subcortical motor centers in addition to those from the cerebral cortex.

The Primary Motor Cortex Plays an Important Role in the Generation of Motor Commands

In the 1950s Herbert Jasper and colleagues pioneered chronic microelectrode recordings from alert animals engaged in natural behaviors. This approach, which allows researchers to study the activity of single neurons while animals perform a controlled behavioral task, has made enormous contributions to our knowledge of the neuronal mechanisms underlying many brain functions. A microelectrode can also be used to deliver weak electrical currents to a small volume of tissue around its tip. When used in the cerebral cortex, this technique is called *intracortical microstimulation.*

These methods have been complemented more recently by techniques that can be used in human subjects, such as functional imaging and transcranial magnetic stimulation. Nearly every insight that will be described in the rest of this chapter and in Chapter 38 has been derived from these techniques.

Edward Evarts, the first to use chronic microelectrode recordings to study the primary motor cortex in behaving monkeys, made several discoveries of fundamental importance. He found that single neurons in this area discharge during movements of a limited part of the contralateral body, such as one or two adjacent joints in the hand, arm, or leg (Figure 37–9). Some neurons discharge during flexion of a particular

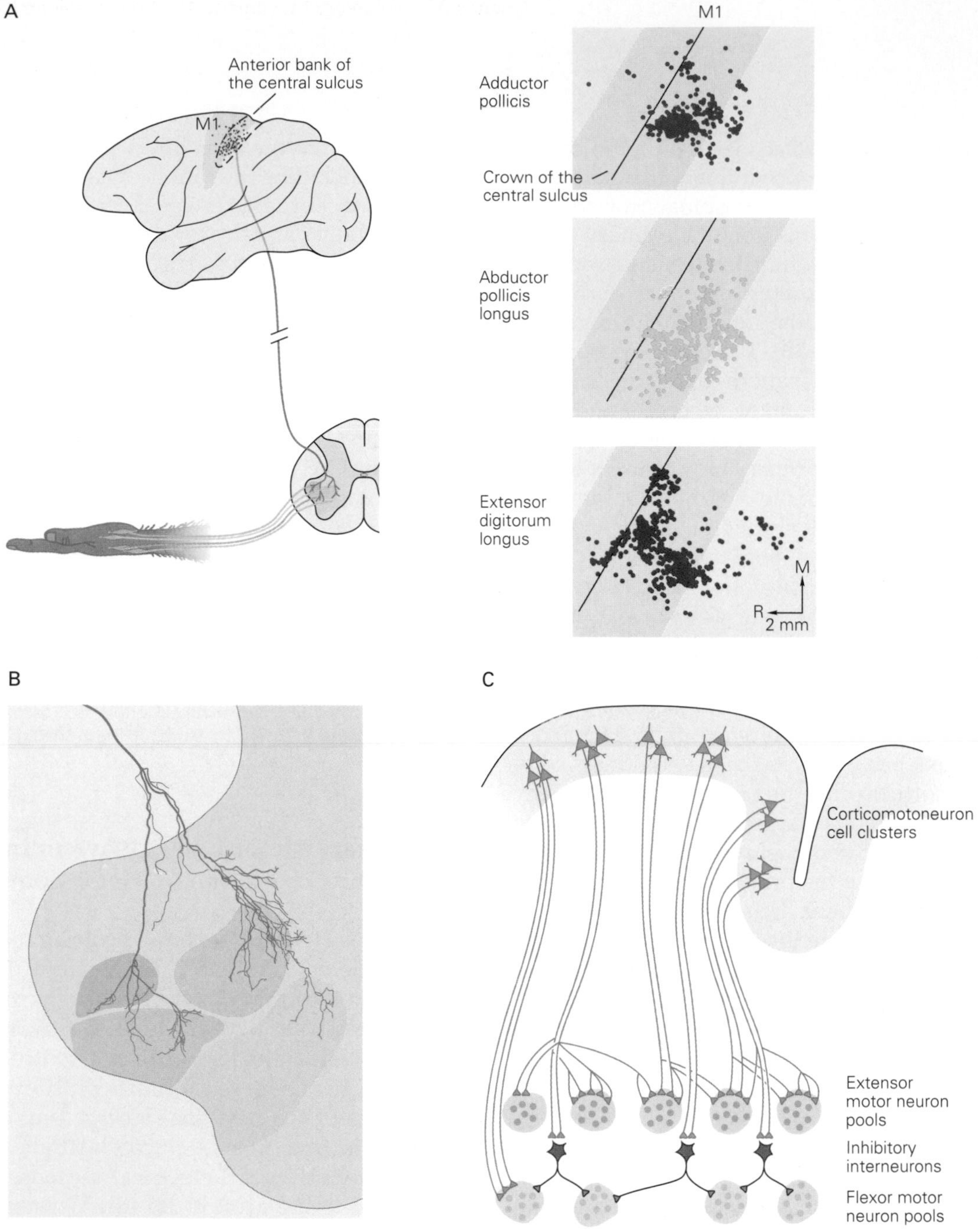

Figure 37–6 Corticomotoneurons activate complex muscle patterns through divergent connections with spinal motor neurons that innervate different arm muscles.

A. Corticomotoneurons, which project monosynaptically to spinal motor neurons, are located almost exclusively in the caudal part of the primary motor cortex (**M1**), within the anterior bank of the central sulcus. The corticomotoneurons that control a single hand muscle are widely distributed throughout the arm motor map, and there is extensive overlap of the distribution of neurons projecting to different hand muscles. The distributions of the cell bodies of corticomotoneurons that project to the spinal motor neuron pools that innervate the adductor pollicis, abductor pollicis longus, and extensor digitorum communis (shown on the right), illustrate this pattern. (**R**, rostral; **M** medial.) (Reproduced, with permission, from Rathelot and Strick 2006.)

B. A single corticomotoneuron axon terminal is shown arborized in the ventral horn of one segment of the spinal cord. It forms synapses with the spinal motor neuron pools of four different intrinsic hand muscles (**yellow** and **blue** zones) as well as with surrounding interneuronal networks. Each axon has several such terminal arborizations distributed along several spinal segments. (Reproduced, with permission, from Shinoda, Yokata, and Futami 1981.)

C. Different colonies of corticomotoneurons in the primary motor cortex terminate on different combinations of spinal interneuron networks and spinal motor neuron pools, thus activating different combinations of agonist and antagonist muscles. Many other corticospinal axons terminate only on spinal interneurons (not shown). The figure shows corticomotoneuronal projections largely onto extensor motor neuron pools. Flexor motor pools receive similar complex projections (not shown). (Modified, with permission, from Cheney, Fetz, and Palmer 1985.)

Box 37–1 Lesion Studies of Voluntary Motor Control

Naturally occurring or experimentally induced lesions have long been used to infer the roles of different neural structures in motor control. However, the effects of lesions must always be interpreted with caution.

It is often incorrect to conclude that the function perturbed by an insult to a part of the motor system resides uniquely in the damaged structure, or that the injured neurons explicitly perform that function. Furthermore, the effects of lesions can be masked or altered by compensatory mechanisms in remaining, intact structures. Nevertheless, lesion experiments have been fundamental in differentiating the functional roles of cortical motor areas as well as the pyramidal tract.

Focal lesions of the primary motor cortex typically result in such symptoms as muscle weakness, slowing and imprecision of movements, and discoordination of multijoint motions, perhaps as a result of selective perturbations of the control circuitry for specific muscles (Figure 37–7). Larger lesions lead to temporary or permanent paralysis.

If the lesion is limited to a part of the motor map, the paralysis affects primarily the movements represented in that sector, such as the contralateral arm, leg, or face. There is diminished use of the affected body parts, and movements of the distal extremities are much more affected than those of the proximal arm and trunk.

The severity of the deficit as a result of focal lesions also depends on the degree of required skill. Control of fine motor skills, such as independent movements of the fingers and hand and precision grip, is abolished. Any residual control of the fingers and the hand is usually reduced to clumsy, claw-like, synchronous flexion and extension motions of all fingers, not unlike the unskilled grasps of young infants. Even remaining motor functions, such as postural activity, locomotion, reaching, and grasping objects with the whole hand, are often clumsy and lack refinement.

Large lesions of the motor cortex or its descending pathways (for example the internal capsule) often produce a suite of symptoms known as the pyramidal syndrome (Figure 37–8). This condition is characterized by contralateral paralysis; increase of muscular tone (spasticity), often preceded by a transient phase of flaccid paralysis with decreased muscle tone; increase of deep reflexes (such as the patellar reflex); disappearance of superficial reflexes (such as the abdominal reflex); and appearance of the Babinski reflex (dorsiflexion of the great toe and fanning of the other toes when a blunt needle is drawn along the lateral edge of the sole). The increase in muscle tone alters the patient's posture, such that the arm contralateral to the lesion is flexed and adducted whereas the leg is extended.

The term "pyramidal syndrome" is a misnomer. In fact, the symptoms result from lesions of descending cortical projections to several subcortical sites, not just the pyramidal tract. Spasticity, for instance, results from damage to nonpyramidal fibers, specifically those that innervate the brain stem centers involved in the control of muscular tone. Clear evidence for this comes from observation of the behavior of monkeys following surgical transection of the medullary pyramid, an anatomical structure that contains only pyramidal tract fibers. Transection at this level produces contralateral hypotonia rather than spasticity.

Lesions of the primary motor cortex in humans perturb the dexterous execution of movements, with deficits ranging from weakness and discoordination to complete paralysis. Lesions of other cortical regions, in contrast, do not result in paralysis and have less impact on the execution of movements than on the organization of action. One effect is difficulty in suppressing the natural motor response to a stimulus in favor of other actions that would be more appropriate to accomplish a goal.

For example, when a normal monkey sees a tasty food treat behind a small transparent barrier, it readily reaches around the barrier to grasp it. However, after a large premotor cortex lesion the monkey persistently tries to reach directly toward the treat rather than making a detour around the barrier, and thus repeatedly strikes the barrier with its hand.

Focal lesions of premotor areas cause a variety of more selective deficits that do not result from an inability to perform individual actions but rather an inability to choose the appropriate course of action. Lesions or inactivation of the ventral premotor cortex perturb the ability to use visual information about an object to shape the hand appropriately for the object's size, shape, and orientation before grasping it. Lesions of the dorsal premotor cortex or supplementary motor area impact the ability to learn and recall arbitrary sensorimotor mappings such as visuomotor rotations, conditional stimulus-response associations, and temporal sequences of movement.

The effects of motor cortex lesions also differ across species. Large lesions in cats do not cause paralysis; the animals can move and walk on a flat surface. However, they have severe difficulties using visual information to navigate within a complex environment, avoid obstacles, or climb the rungs of a ladder. Trevor Drew and col-

(continued)

Box 37–1 Lesion Studies of Voluntary Motor Control (continued)

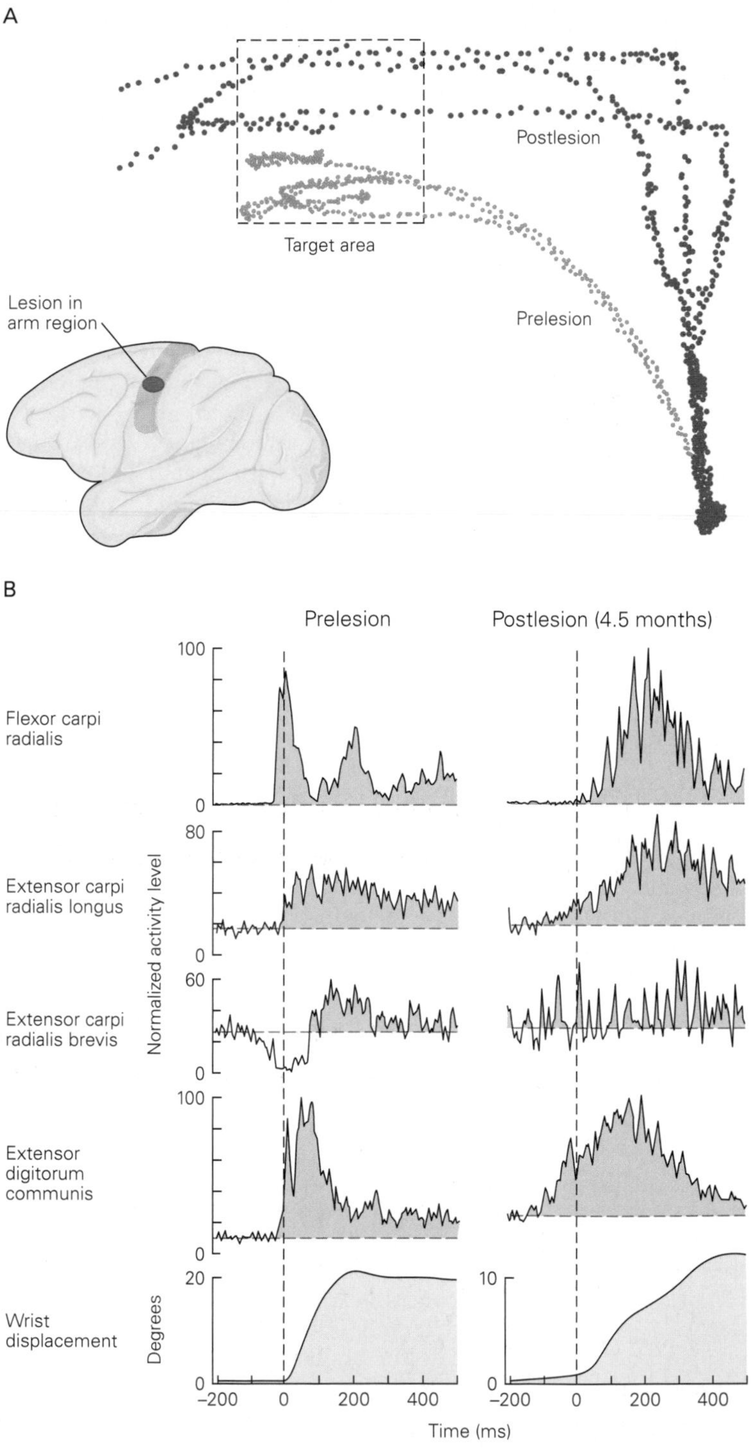

Figure 37–7 Fractionated control of muscle activity patterns requires cortical input.

A. A monkey can readily make diagonal movements of the wrist that require complex coordinated muscle patterns before a motor cortical lesion ("prelesion"). After a large lesion of the arm region of the motor cortex, the monkey shows major deficits in the ability to make diagonal movements even after lengthy rehabilitation.

B. The movement deficit is accompanied by a severe loss of the ability to make precisely timed fractionated muscle contractions of different agonist and antagonist muscles. (Reproduced, with permission, from Hoffman and Strick 1995.)

leagues have shown that pyramidal tract neurons in the motor cortex of cats are much more strongly activated when the cats must modify their normal stepping to clear an obstacle under visual guidance than during normal, unimpeded locomotion over a flat, featureless surface.

Similar lesions of motor cortex in monkeys have more drastic consequences, including initial paralysis and usually the permanent loss of independent, fractionated movements of the thumb and fingers. Monkeys nevertheless recover some ability to make clumsy movements of the hands and arms and to walk and climb, even after large lesions (Figure 37–8). In humans large lesions of the motor cortex are particularly devastating, often resulting in flaccid or spastic paralysis with a limited potential for recovery.

These differences in primates and man presumably reflect the increased importance in man of descending signals from motor cortex and a correspondingly diminished capacity of subcortical motor structures to compensate for the loss of those descending signals.

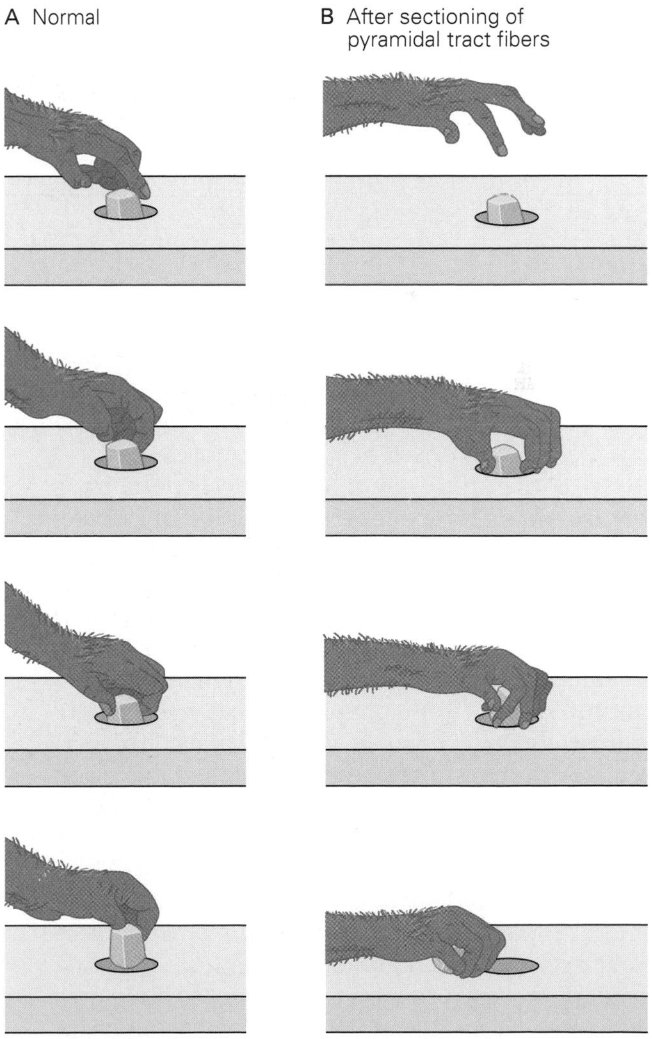

Figure 37–8 A lesion of the pyramidal tract abolishes fine grasping movements.

A. A monkey is normally able to make individuated movements of the wrist, fingers, and thumb in order to pick up food in a small well.

B. After bilateral sectioning of the pyramidal tract the monkey can remove the food only by grabbing it clumsily with the whole hand. This change results mainly from the loss of direct inputs from corticomotoneurons onto spinal motor neurons. A pyramidal tract transection is not equivalent to a motor cortex lesion, however, because not all pyramidal tract axons terminate in the spinal cord. The axons that do project to the spinal cord originate in several cortical areas, including the motor cortex, and the corticospinal tract is only one of several parallel output pathways of the motor cortex. (Reproduced, with permission, from Lawrence and Kuypers 1968.)

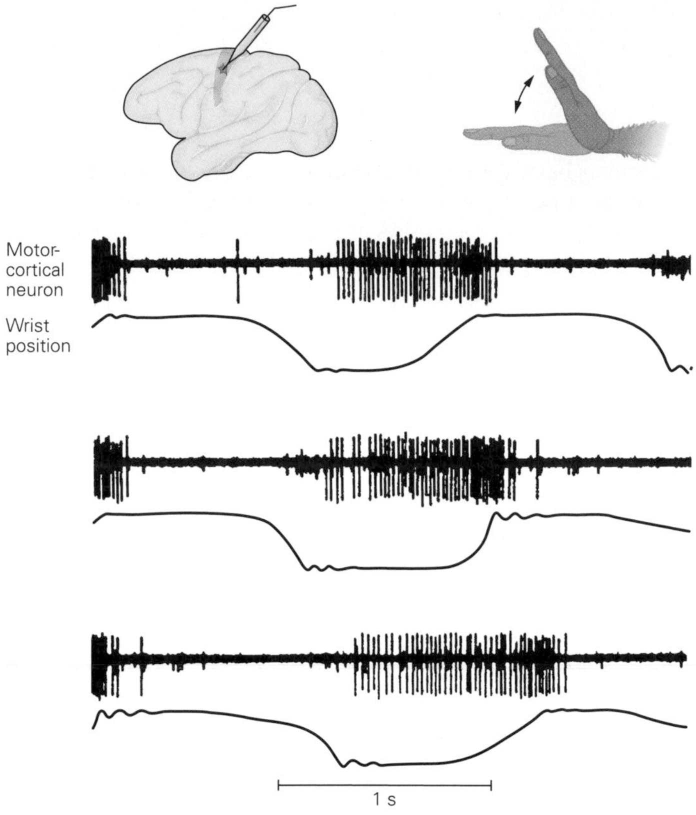

Figure 37–9 The discharge of individual pyramidal tract neurons varies with particular movements of specific parts of the body. The discharge of a motor cortex neuron with an axon that projects down the pyramidal tract is recorded while a monkey makes a sequence of flexion and extension movements of the wrist. The three parts of the figure show three consecutive flexion-extension cycles, proceeding from top to bottom. In the trace showing wrist position the direction of flexion is down and extension up. The pyramidal tract neuron discharges before and during extensions and is reciprocally silent during flexion movements. It does not discharge during movements of other body parts. Other motor cortex neurons show the opposite pattern of activity, discharging before and during flexion movements. (Reproduced, with permission, from Evarts 1968.)

joint and are reciprocally suppressed during extension, whereas other cells display the opposite pattern. This movement-related activity typically begins 50 to 150 ms before the onset of agonist muscle activity. These pioneering studies suggested that single neurons in primary motor cortex generate signals that provide specific information about movements of specific parts of the body before those movements are executed.

Many subsequent studies have provided further insight into the contribution of different cortical motor areas to the control of voluntary movements. In general, the output signals from premotor areas are strongly dependent on the context in which the action is performed, such as the stimulus-response associations and the rules that guide which movement to make. In contrast, the commands generated by the primary motor cortex are more closely related to the mechanical details of the movement and are usually less influenced by the behavioral context. However, the relative role of these different areas to voluntary motor control, including the primary motor cortex itself, continues to be an area of active research and controversy. The rest of this chapter and Chapter 38 describe our current understanding of the different roles of cortical motor areas.

Columnar arrays of neurons with similar response properties are a prominent feature of many sensory areas of cortex. It is surprising therefore that there is only weak evidence for such functional columns in the primary motor cortex. The cell bodies and apical dendrites of primary motor cortex neurons tend to form radially oriented columns. The terminal arbors of thalamocortical and corticocortical axons form localized columns or bands and corticomotoneurons tend to cluster in small groups with similar muscle fields. Motor cortex neurons recorded successively as a microelectrode descends perpendicularly through the neuronal layers between the pial surface and the white matter typically discharge during movements of the same part of body and can have similar preferred movement directions. Nevertheless, adjacent cells often show very different response patterns.

Motor Commands Are Population Codes

The complex overlapping organization of the motor map for the arm and hand suggests at least two different ways to generate the motor command for a given movement. The map could function as a *look-up table* within which a desired movement is generated by selective activation of a few sites whose combined output produces all the required muscle activity and joint motions. Or it could be a distributed *functional map* in which many sites contribute to each motor command.

Apostolos Georgopoulos and colleagues recorded from the primary motor cortex while a monkey reached in different directions from a central starting position toward targets arrayed on a circle in the horizontal plane. Individual neurons responded during many movements, not just a single one (Figure 37–10A). Each neuron's activity was strongest for a *preferred* direction and often weakest for the opposite direction, as Evarts had found for single-joint movements. However, each cell also responded in a graded fashion to directions of movement between the preferred and the opposite directions. Its activity pattern thus formed a broad directional tuning curve, maximal at the preferred direction and decreasing gradually with increasing difference between the preferred direction and the target direction.

Different cells had different preferred directions, and their tuning curves overlapped extensively.

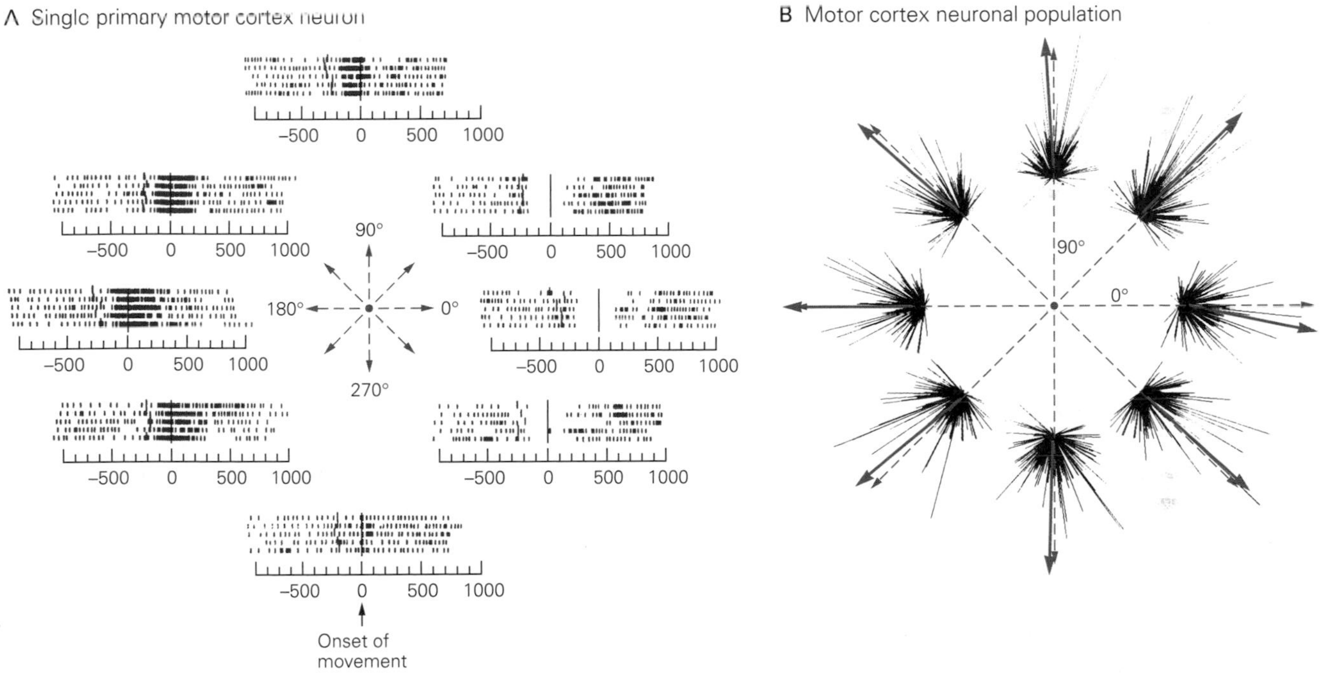

Figure 37–10 A reaching movement is coded by a population of neurons in the arm motor map.

A. Raster plots show the firing pattern of a single primary motor cortex neuron during movements in eight directions. The neuron discharges at the maximal rate for movements near 135 degrees and 180 degrees and at lesser intensities for movements in other directions. The cell's lowest firing rate is for movements opposite the cell's preferred direction. Different cells have different preferred directions, and their broad directional tuning curves overlap extensively. The plots are from a study in which a monkey was trained to move a handle to eight targets arranged radially on a horizontal plane around a central starting position. Each row of tics in each raster plot represents the activity in a single trial, aligned at the time of movement onset (time zero). (Reproduced, with permission, from Georgopoulos et al. 1982.)

B. Many primary motor cortex neurons with a broad range of preferred movement directions respond at different intensities during reaching movements in a particular direction. The overall directional bias of the activity within the population of neurons shifts systematically with movement direction so that the vectorial sum of the activity of all cells is a population vector that closely matches that of the direction of movement. This shows that the motor command for a movement is generated by a widely distributed population of cells throughout the arm motor map, each of which fires at a different intensity for movement in a particular direction.

The eight single-neuron vector clusters and the population vectors shown here represent the activity of the same population of cells during reaching movements in eight different directions. The activity of each neuron during each reaching movement is represented by a thin black vector that points in the neuron's preferred movement direction and whose length is proportional to the discharge of the neuron during that movement. **Blue arrows** are the population vectors, calculated by vectorial addition of all the single-cell vectors in each cluster; **dashed arrows** represent the direction of movement of the arm. (Reproduced, with permission, from Georgopoulos et al. 1983.)

All directions were represented in the neuronal population. Cells with similar preferred directions were located at several different sites in the arm motor map, and nearby cells often had different preferred directions. As a result, many cells with a broad range of preferred directions discharged at different intensities at many locations across the arm motor map during each reaching movement.

Despite the apparent complexity of the response properties of single neurons, Georgopoulos found that the global pattern of activity of the entire population provided a clear signal for each movement. He represented each cell's activity by a vector pointing in the cell's preferred direction. The vector's length for each direction of movement was proportional to the mean level of activity of that cell averaged over the duration of the movement (Figure 37–10B). This vectorial representation implied that an increase of activity of a given cell is a signal that the arm should move in the cell's preferred direction, and that the strength of this directional influence varies continuously for different reach directions as a function of the neuron's directional tuning.

Vectorial addition of all of the single-cell contributions to each output command produces a *population vector* that corresponds closely to the actual movement direction. That is, an unambiguous signal about the desired motor output is encoded by the summed activity of a large population of active neurons throughout the arm motor map in the primary motor cortex. As a result, neurons in all parts of the arm motor map contribute to the motor command for each reaching movement, and the pattern of activity across the motor map changes continuously as a function of the intended direction of the reaching movement.

Andrew Schwartz and colleagues used the same population-vector analysis to represent temporal variations in the activity of populations of primary motor cortex neurons every 25 ms while monkeys performed continuous arm movements. In the resulting time sequence of population vectors, each vector predicts the instantaneous direction and speed of the motion of the monkey's arm approximately 100 ms later (Figure 37–11). These results show that the pattern of neural activity distributed across the arm motor map varies continuously in time during complex arm movements, signaling the moment-to-moment details of the desired movement.

Further studies have confirmed that similar population-coding mechanisms are used in all cortical motor areas. This common coding mechanism undoubtedly facilitates the communication of movement-related information between the multiple areas of motor cortex during voluntary behavior.

The Motor Cortex Encodes Both the Kinematics and Kinetics of Movement

Population-vector analyses show that neural activity in the primary motor cortex contains information about the trajectory of hand motions during reaching and drawing movements. However, to execute those movements the motor system must implement the desired motions by generating particular patterns of muscle activity.

Electrical stimulation of the primary motor cortex readily evokes muscle contractions, and some cells in this region have direct access to spinal motor neurons. Indeed, it was long assumed that the major role of the primary motor cortex was to specify the muscle activity that generates voluntary movements. Because muscle contractions generate the forces that displace a joint or limb in a particular direction, a critical question is whether primary motor cortex neurons signal the desired spatiotemporal form of a behavior or the forces and muscle activity required to generate the movement. That is, do these neurons encode the kinematics or the kinetics of an intended movement (Box 37–2)?

Kinematics refers to the parameters that describe the spatiotemporal form of movement, such as direction, amplitude, speed, and path. *Kinetics* concerns the causal forces and muscle activity. It is also useful to distinguish the *dynamic* forces that cause movements from the *static* forces required to maintain a given posture against constant external forces such as gravity.

Evarts was the first to address this question with single-neuron recordings. Using a system of pulleys and weights, he applied a load to the wrist of a monkey to pull the wrist in the direction of flexion or extension. To make a particular movement the animal had to alter its level of muscle activity to compensate for the load. As a result, the kinematics (direction and amplitude) of wrist movements remained constant but the kinetics (forces and muscle activity) changed with the load. The activity of many primary motor cortex neurons associated with movements of the hand and wrist increased during movements in their preferred direction when the load opposed that movement but decreased when the load assisted it (Figure 37–12). These changes in neural activity paralleled the changes in muscle activity required to compensate for the external loads. This was the first study to show that the activity of many primary motor cortex neurons is more closely related to *how* a movement is performed, the kinetics of motion, than to *what* movement is performed, the corresponding kinematics.

A later study confirmed this property of motor cortex activity during whole-arm reaching movements.

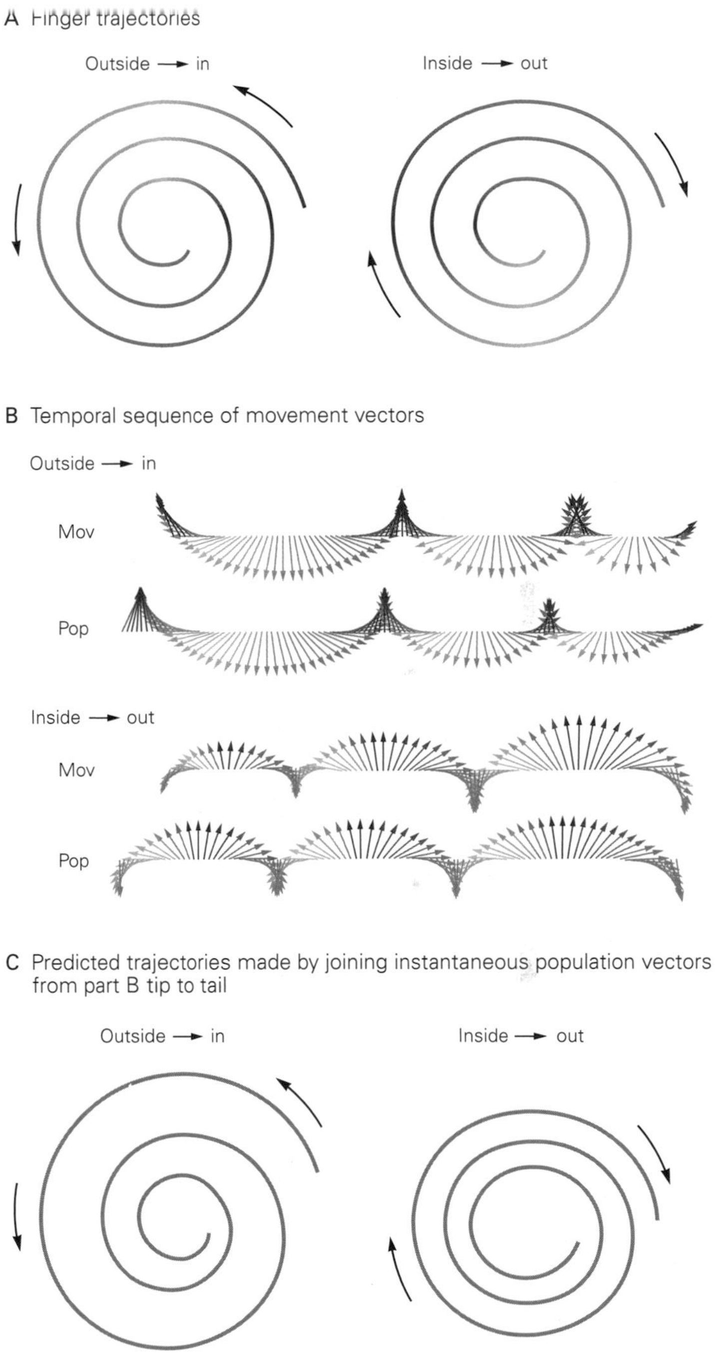

Figure 37–11 The moment-to-moment activity of a population of motor cortex neurons predicts arm movements over time. (Reproduced, with permission, from Moran and Schwartz 1999.)

A. A monkey uses its arm to trace spirals with its finger.

B. Temporal sequences of vectors, reading left to right, illustrate the instantaneous direction and speed of movement of the finger (**Mov**) and the net population vector signal (**Pop**) of the activity of 241 motor cortex neurons every 25 ms during the drawing movements. The population vectors precede the hand displacement vectors by approximately 100 ms.

C. Joining the instantaneous population vectors tip to tail produces "neural trajectories" that predict the spatial trajectory of movement of the finger along the spiral path approximately 100 ms in the future.

A monkey made arm movements exactly as in the task used by Georgopoulos (Figure 37–10), but additional external loads pulled the arm in different directions. To continue to move the arm along the same path, the monkey had to change the activity of its arm muscles to counteract the external loads. The level of activity of many motor cortex neurons changed systematically with the direction of the external load even though the movement path did not change. When the load opposed the direction of reach, the single-cell and total population activity increased. When the load assisted the reaching direction, the neural activity decreased

Box 37–2 The Equilibrium-Point Hypothesis of Movement

Most theoretical and neurophysiological studies of neural control of movement are based on variants of the force-control hypothesis, which states that the motor system controls a movement by planning and controlling its causal dynamic forces or muscle activity.

The *position-control* or *equilibrium-point hypothesis*, however, argues that cortical motor centers do not compute inverse kinematics or dynamics to specify the necessary muscle activity. Instead, this model proposes that the output from the motor cortex signals the desired spatial endpoints and equilibrium configurations of the arm and body, that is, the posture in which all external and internal (muscular) forces are at balance and no further movement occurs.

According to the equilibrium-point hypothesis, the motor cortex causes a movement of part or all of the body by generating a signal specifying a particular equilibrium or *referent configuration*. This descending signal exploits spinal reflex circuits and the spring-like biomechanical properties of muscles to change muscle activity and create an imbalance between external and internal forces, causing the limb to move until equilibrium is restored.

If no external force is applied to the limb, the desired, signaled, and actual equilibrium configurations should all correspond. If the motor system is confronted with an external force, however, it must signal a different referent configuration whose internal forces compensate for the external forces. Thus, according to the equilibrium-point hypothesis, the motor cortex commands the desired movement without computing the complex transformations required to encode the required forces and muscle activities. According to the hypothesis, the inverse-kinematics and inverse-dynamics transformations occur implicitly at the local spinal cord circuits and in the motor periphery itself.

in a manner that signaled the change in muscle activity and output forces required to make the movement (Figure 37–13).

Other studies have examined the issue whether the primary motor cortex organizes the kinematics or kinetics of movement by using tasks in which subjects generate isometric forces against immovable objects rather than moving the arm. The activity of many primary motor cortex neurons varies with the direction and level of static isometric output forces generated across a single joint, such as the wrist or elbow, as well as during precise pinches with the thumb and index finger (Figure 37–14A). At least over part of the tested range these responses vary linearly with the level of static force. When a monkey uses its whole arm to exert isometric force in different directions, the activity of many motor cortex neurons varies systematically with force direction, and the directional tuning curves resemble those for activity associated with reaching movements (Figure 37–14B). Because no movement is intended or produced in isometric tasks, this strongly suggests that the primary motor cortex contributes to the control of static and dynamic output forces during many motor actions.

Finally, several studies have found that the activity of some motor cortex neurons can be correlated with the detailed contraction patterns of specific muscles during such diverse tasks as isometric force generation, precision pinching of objects between the thumb and index finger, and complex reaching and grasping actions (Figure 37–15).

These findings show that some neurons in the primary motor cortex can provide information about the causal forces and muscle activity of motor outputs. Nevertheless, the activity of other neurons in the primary motor cortex appears to signal the desired kinematics of arm and hand movements rather than their kinetics, or the desired direction of isometric force but not its magnitude. Perhaps most surprisingly, the activity of some corticomotoneurons does not always correlate with the contraction of their target muscles. For instance, some corticomotoneurons discharge strongly while a monkey generates weak contractions of the target muscles to make carefully controlled delicate movements of the hand and fingers, but are nearly silent when the monkey generates powerful contractions of the same muscles to make brisk, forceful movements.

How can we reconcile these apparently contradictory findings about the role of the primary motor cortex in the control of movement? According to the serial model of motor control all of the neurons in the primary motor cortex should have similar properties and so should represent either the kinematics or kinetics of the desired movement, but not both.

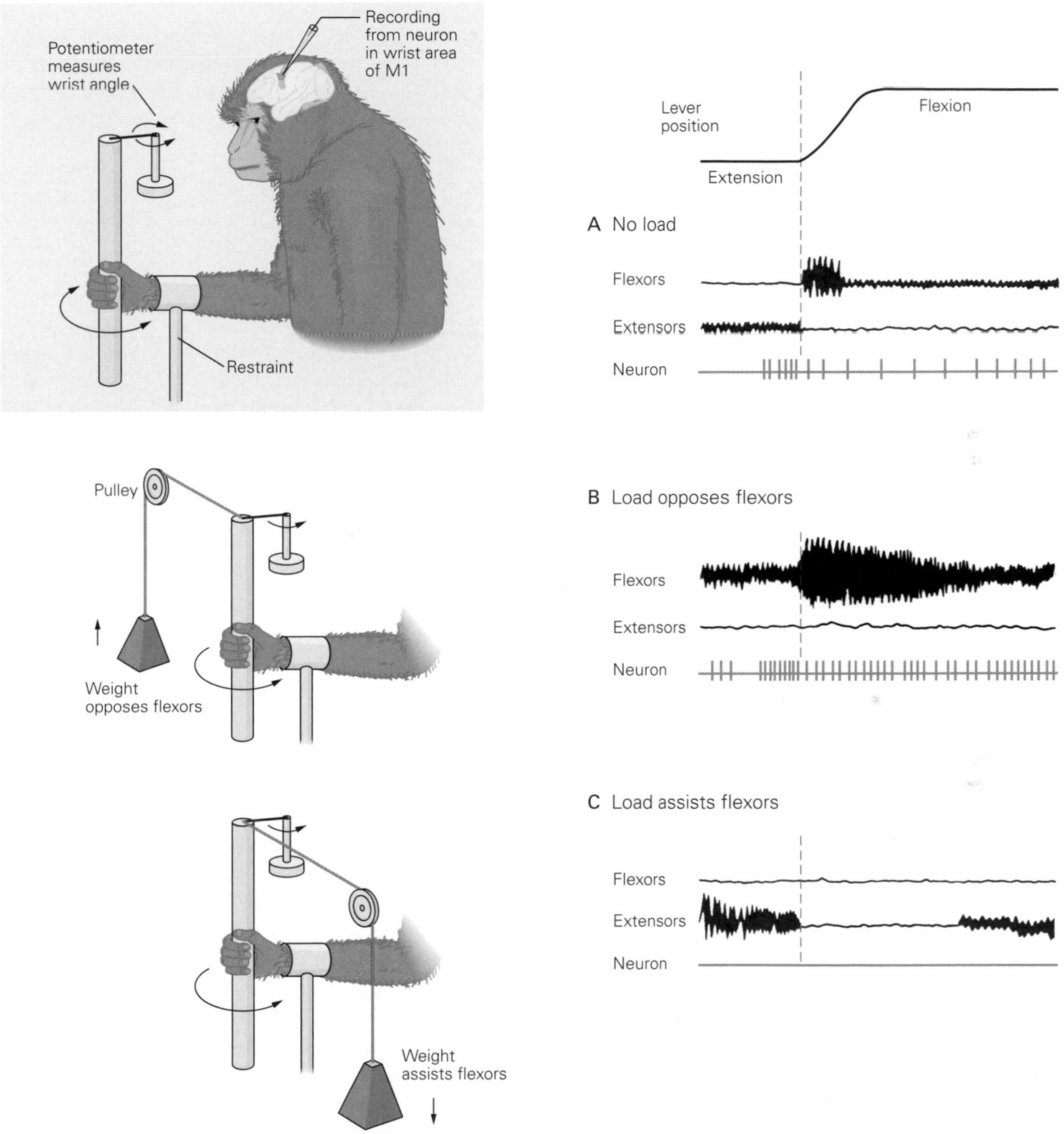

Figure 37–12 Activity of a motor cortex neuron correlates with changes in the direction and amplitude of muscle forces during wrist movements. The records are from a primary motor cortex (**M1**) neuron with an axon that projected down the pyramidal tract. The monkey flexes its wrist under three load conditions. When no load is applied to the wrist, the neuron fires before and during flexion (**A**). When a load opposing flexion is applied, the activity of the flexor muscles and the neuron increases (**B**). When a load assisting wrist flexion is applied, the flexor muscles and neuron fall silent (**C**). In all three conditions the wrist displacement is the same, but the neuronal activity changes as the loads and compensatory muscle activity change. Thus the activity of this motor cortex neuron is better related to the direction and level of forces and muscle activity exerted during the movement than to the direction of wrist displacement. (Reproduced, with permission, from Evarts 1968.)

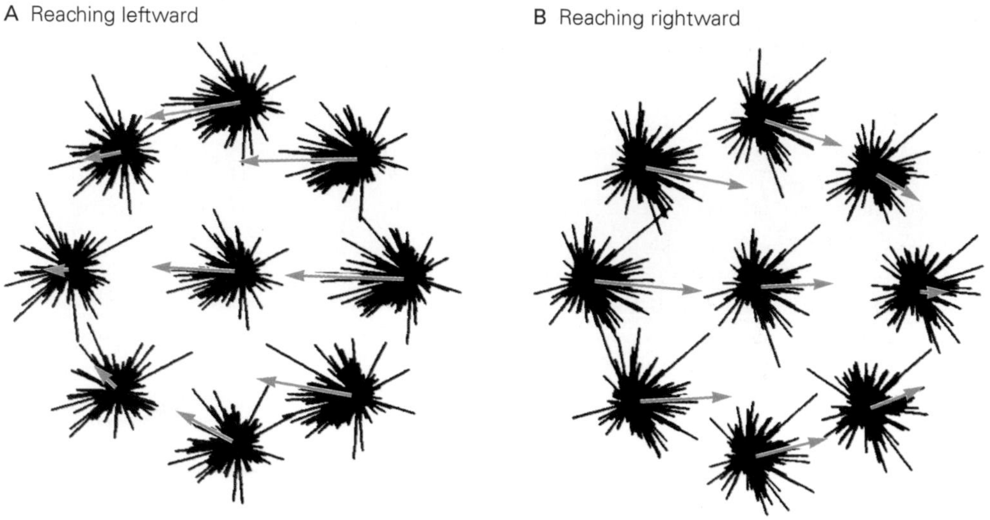

Figure 37–13 Activity of primary motor cortex neurons varies with the forces required to maintain the direction of reaching movements against external loads. A vectorial representation of the directional activity of approximately 260 motor cortex neurons (**black lines**) when a monkey makes reaching movements to the left and right. The vectors in the center represent activity when no external load is applied to the arm, whereas the vector clusters around the center represent the activity of the same 260 neurons when an external load pulls the arm in different directions. The location of each vector cluster relative to the central cluster corresponds to the direction in which the external load pulls on the arm. The change in population vectors (**blue arrows**) for the vector clusters around the center indicates that the strength and overall directional bias of the activity of the neural population vary systematically with the direction of the external load, in order to counteract its effect, even though the trajectory of the movement does not change. (Reproduced, with permission, from Kalaska et al. 1989.)

However, the experimental evidence suggests that a strictly serial model is too simplistic. The response properties of primary motor cortex neurons are not homogeneous. Signals about both the desired kinematics and required kinetics of movements may be generated simultaneously in different, or possibly even overlapping, populations of primary motor cortex neurons. Rather than representing only what movement to make (kinematics) or how to make it (kinetics), the true role of the motor cortex may be to perform the transformation between these two representations of voluntary movements.

Delineating the movement-related information encoded in motor cortex activity is increasingly important for the development of brain-controlled interfaces and neuroprosthetic controllers that allow patients with severe motor deficits to control remote devices such as a computer cursor, a wheelchair, or a robotic limb by neural activity alone (Box 37–3).

Hand and Finger Movements Are Directly Controlled by the Motor Cortex

The monosynaptic projection from the primary motor cortex onto spinal motor neurons is most dense for muscles of the distal arm, hand, and fingers. This arrangement allows the primary motor cortex to regulate the activity of those muscles directly, in contrast to its indirect regulation of muscles through the reflex and pattern-generating functions of the spinal circuits. It also provides primates and humans with a greatly enhanced capacity for individuated control of hand and finger movements. Large lesions of the primary motor cortex permanently destroy this capacity.

Although monkeys and humans can make isolated movements of the thumb and fingers, most hand and finger actions involve combinations of stereotypical hand and finger configurations and coordinated wrist and digit movements. This has led to the hypothesis that separate cortical circuits selectively control these different stereotypical hand actions, and that the primary motor cortex converts these signals into more specific motor commands (see Chapter 38).

The anatomy of the muscles of the wrist and fingers further complicates the commands for individuated finger and hand movements. Several muscles have long, bifurcating tendons that act across several joints and even act on several fingers rather than just one. As a consequence, individuated control of hand

and finger movements requires highly specific patterns of activation and inhibition of multiple muscles.

Cortical neurons controlling the hand and digits occupy the large central core of the primary motor cortex motor map but also overlap extensively with populations of neurons controlling more proximal parts of the arm (see Figure 37–2A). Some neurons within the central core discharge preferentially during movements of a single digit, but many discharge during coordinated movements of several digits, and even of the wrist and more proximal joints. Neurons that discharge during movements of different digits are distributed throughout the motor map in an extensively overlapping fashion. As a result, neural activity required to generate an individuated action of the hand and digits is distributed broadly across the distal arm and hand areas of the motor map, as is also the case for the output to more proximal parts of the arm.

This highly intermixed organization of the hand and digit motor map stands in striking contrast to the much more highly ordered representation of tactile sensory inputs from different parts of the hand and digits in the primary somatosensory cortex. This difference likely reflects differences in the cortical mechanisms

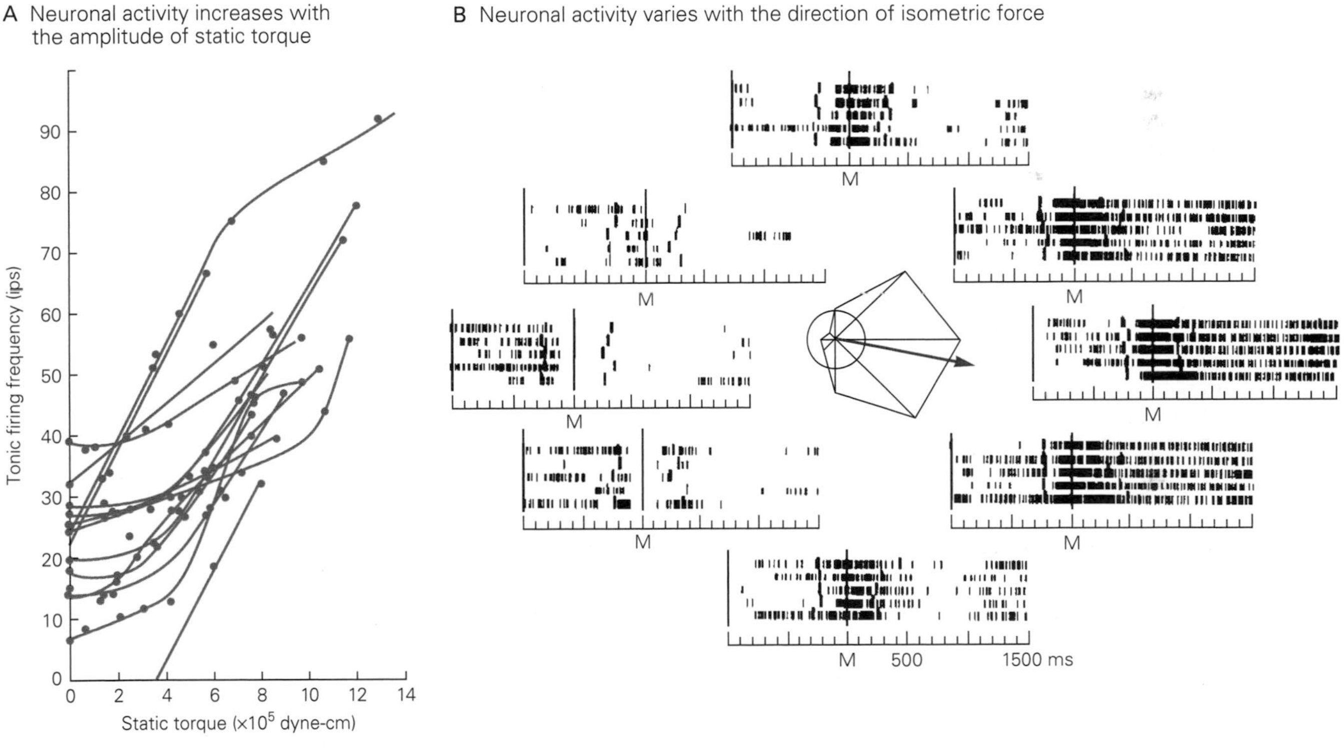

Figure 37–14 The firing rates of many primary motor cortex neurons correlate with the level and direction of force exerted in an isometric task.

A. The activity of many primary motor cortex neurons increases with the amplitude of static torque generated across a single joint. The plot shows the tonic firing rates of several different corticomotoneurons at different levels of static torque exerted in the direction of wrist extension. Other motor cortex neurons show increasing activity with torque exerted in the direction of wrist flexion, and so would show response functions with the opposite slope (not shown). (Reproduced, with permission, from Fetz and Cheney 1980.)

B. When a monkey uses its whole arm to push on an immovable handle in its hand, the activity of some primary motor cortex neurons varies with the direction of isometric forces. Each of the eight raster plots shows the activity of the same primary motor cortex neuron during five repeated force ramps in one direction. Each row shows the pattern of spikes during a single trial of the task. The position of each raster of activity corresponds to the direction in which the monkey is generating isometric forces on the handle. The onset of the force ramp is indicated by the vertical line labeled **M**. The thick ticks to the left of that line in each row indicate when the target appeared on a computer monitor, telling the monkey the direction in which it should push on the handle. The central polar plot illustrates the directional tuning function of the neuron as a function of the direction of isometric forces. Note the similarity of the shapes of the tuning function for the direction of whole-arm isometric forces here and for whole-arm reaching movements in Figure 37–10A. (Reproduced, with permission, from Sergio and Kalaska 2003.)

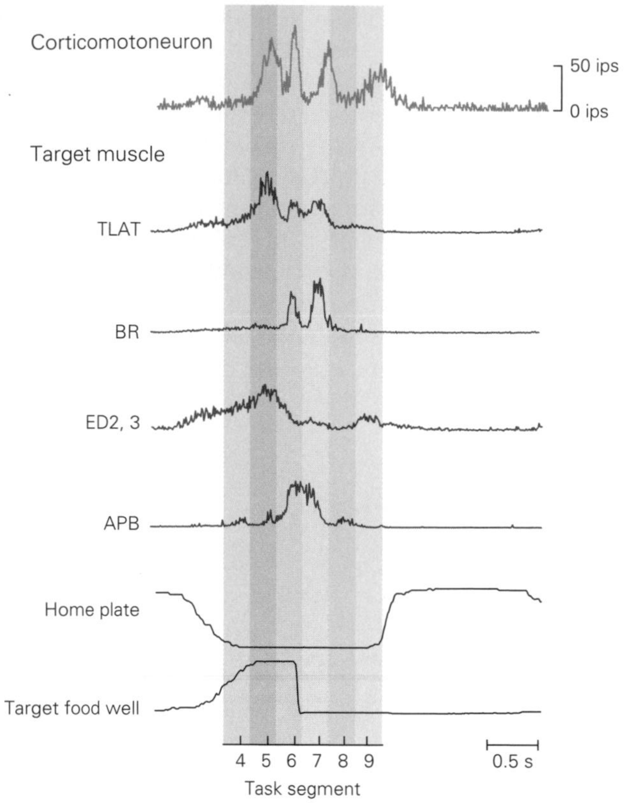

Figure 37–15 The activity of some primary motor cortex neurons can be correlated with particular patterns of muscle activity. The bursts of activity in a single corticomotoneuron during a reach-and-grasp movement to retrieve food pellets from a small well are correlated with bursts of contractile activity in several of its target muscles at different times during the movement. (**APB**, abductor pollicis brevis; **BR**, brachioradialis; **ED2, 3**, extensor digitorum 2, 3; **TLAT**, lateral triceps.) (Reproduced, with permission, from Griffin et al. 2008.)

required to analyze the spatiotemporal distribution of tactile input on the hand and digits versus those needed to coordinate individuated movements of the digits and hand.

Sensory Inputs from Somatic Mechanoreceptors Have Feedback, Feed-Forward, and Adaptive Learning Roles

Many primary motor cortex neurons receive sensory input from proprioceptors or cutaneous mechanoreceptors. The tactile input is particularly prominent on neurons implicated in the control of hand and digit movements. These inputs inform the motor system about the current state of the body, such as the position, posture, and movement of the arm and hand and their interactions with the environment. This information can play at least three functional roles: in feedback control of ongoing movements, in feed-forward control of intended movements, and as a teaching signal during motor learning.

Sensory feedback from the arm provides information about both the progress of an ongoing arm movement and deviations from the intended path that should be corrected. Feedback corrections during movement are implemented by neural circuits at many levels of the motor system, ranging from reflex responses in the spinal cord to corrective adjustments of voluntary motor commands from the motor cortex. Similarly, the activity of many neurons in the primary motor cortex that control hand movements is strongly influenced by tactile stimuli on the glabrous surface of the digits and palm of the hand. This tactile input helps adjust the output signal from hand-related neurons to ensure that the subject applies enough force to the surface of an object to grasp and manipulate it, but not to crush it or let it slip.

Sensory feed-forward control involves continuously adjusting the level and distribution of neuronal activity throughout the cortical motor map to reflect the limb's current state of posture and movement. By pretuning the pattern of activity in the motor-cortical map and spinal motor apparatus as a function of the limb's motor state before the onset of a movement, somatic sensory input helps to assure that the appropriate motor command is generated in the motor cortex and converted into the appropriate patterns of muscle activity at the spinal level.

Finally, sensory input can provide information about errors experienced during movement that could be used by adaptive motor circuits to make changes to future motor commands, thus facilitating motor learning.

The Motor Map Is Dynamic and Adaptable

The mediolateral sequence of major body segments in the motor map is highly consistent across individuals, but the details in each functional subregion can vary. This suggests that the motor map is continually shaped by an individual's motor experience. The dynamic nature of the map has been demonstrated in several ways. For instance, functional reorganization often occurs after a focal lesion so that some of the movements that had been evoked by the injured tissue are now generated by the adjacent cortex. This reorganization likely contributes to the recovery of function after local infarcts.

Learning a motor skill can also induce reorganization. Randy Nudo and colleagues trained monkeys to

Box 37–3 Enhancing the Quality of Life of Neurological Patients: Brain-Machine Interfaces

Every year thousands of people suffer severe spinal cord trauma, subcortical strokes, or degenerative neuromuscular diseases such as multiple sclerosis and amyotrophic lateral sclerosis. Although their cortical motor systems remain largely intact and they try strenuously to move, they cannot convert their willful intentions into physical action.

These patients must depend on caregivers to attend to even their most basic needs. One of the greatest quality-of-life issues for these patients is the loss of autonomy resulting from the inability to move and sometimes even to communicate. Several technological solutions have been sought to enhance the autonomy of such patients.

One approach has been to use electroencephalographic activity recorded by scalp electrodes as a control signal for remote devices such as computer cursors or robotic tools. An alternative approach has been to record the eye movements of subjects and to use them as the control signals.

However, both methods have significant limitations. Electroencephalographic control often takes months to master because the subjects must learn how to synchronize the activity of large populations of neurons within a cortical region to generate an electrical signal that is recordable and discriminable in real time and without extensive averaging of multiple repetitions.

Eye-movement methods are much easier to implement and learn, but they prevent subjects from looking toward other objects of interest while attempting to perform a task. Moreover, both approaches require intense concentration and the focused attention of the subjects to the virtual exclusion of all other activities.

A major recent advance has been the development of brain-machine interfaces (also often called brain-computer, brain-controlled, or neuroprosthetic interfaces). This technology records neural activity reflecting the motor intentions of the individual and converts this activity into control signals for external devices. It exploits the discovery that information about static arm postures and the direction and velocity of arm movements can be extracted from the activity patterns of neuronal populations in the primary motor cortex and other arm movement-related areas of the cerebral cortex.

Brain-machine interfaces include four basic components:

1. Implantable electrode arrays and associated hardware to record the activity of neuronal populations in a cortical area.
2. Computer algorithms to extract signals about the motor intentions of the individual.
3. Interfaces to convert the extracted signals into control signals to generate the desired action by an external effector.
4. Sensory feedback signals to improve performance.

Originally tested in experimental animals, brain-machine interfaces are now undergoing clinical trials in human neurological patients. Severely paralyzed patients with multi-electrode arrays in the primary motor cortex are quickly able to learn to control a cursor on a computer monitor so as to operate computer programs, compose messages, track the random motions of a moving target, and control a simple robotic arm. The subjects are able to control the remote effectors merely by thinking about making the corresponding movements.

The centrally generated intentions activate motor cortex neurons in a manner similar to that during normal movements. The subjects can control the devices while at the same time engaged in other activities such as looking around the laboratory or even engaging in conversations. This ability dramatically illustrates the fact that much of the cortical activity that converts a motor intention into overt action occurs in the subconscious.

The initial studies using this technology demonstrated that electrodes implanted in different cortical areas yield different types of neural signals. Electrodes in the primary motor cortex provide the best signals for continuous control of the time-varying details of the kinematics and kinetics of the trajectory of a robotic device. Such control is particularly useful for tasks like manipulating objects and for making complex movements as in drawing or writing.

In contrast, signals from the premotor cortex and posterior parietal cortex may be more appropriate for specifying the overall goals and desired outcome of an action, such as the final target location, without elaborating the details of how to accomplish the goal.

A brain-controlled interface that uses a combination of signals from different cortical areas might afford a level of context-dependent control that resembles the normal voluntary control of behavior.

use precise movements of the thumb, index finger, and wrist to extract treats from a small well. After a monkey had become adept at the task, the area of its motor map in which intracortical microstimulation could evoke the skilled movements was larger than before training (Figure 37–16). If the monkey did not practice the task for a lengthy period, its skill level decreased, as did the cortical area from which the relevant movements could be elicited. Similar modifications of the representation of practiced actions have also been demonstrated in human motor cortex by functional imaging and transcranial magnetic stimulation.

John Donoghue and colleagues demonstrated that these adaptive changes depend on horizontal connections and local inhibitory circuits. They found two adjacent sites in the rat's motor map at which intracortical microstimulation caused contractions of muscles in the upper lips or forearm (Figure 37–17A). Within minutes after transection of the facial nerve innervating the lip muscles, stimulation of the lip-muscle site began to evoke contractions of forearm muscles.

In a related experiment they injected bicuculline into a forearm-muscle site in the motor cortex of an intact rat without a facial nerve transection to block the neurotransmitter GABA (γ-aminobutyric acid). Within minutes stimulation of the lip-muscle site evoked contractions of both lip and forearm muscles. They concluded that stimulation of the lip-muscle site activated local horizontal axons that projected into the forearm-muscle site, activity that was normally suppressed by GABAergic inhibitory interneurons (Figure 37–17B).

The Motor Cortex Contributes to Motor Skill Learning

One of the most remarkable properties of the brain is the adaptability of its circuitry to changes in the environment—the capacity to learn from experience and store the acquired knowledge as memories. When human subjects practice a motor skill their performance improves. Important advances have been made in understanding the mechanisms underlying the learning of motor skills, also known as procedural learning (see Chapter 66). For instance, Donoghue and colleagues found an increase in the synaptic strength of local horizontal connections between different parts of the arm motor map in rats that became increasingly skilled at reaching through a small hole in a transparent barrier to grasp, retrieve, and eat small food pellets.

Adaptation to perturbations of movement caused by external forces has been studied extensively in human subjects. One type of force field pushes on the arm in a direction perpendicular to the direction of the arm's movement; the strength of this force increases with movement speed. Although such *viscous curl* fields may seem odd, they are exactly the kind of forces that act on an arm when a person reaches out while simultaneously turning his or her body. Normally, these coriolis forces do not deflect the arm movement from its intended path because your motor system has learned to predict that these forces will arise during this natural behavior and generates a motor command that corrects for them in advance.

However, when a subject is stationary and unexpectedly encounters an experimentally generated viscous curl field for the first time during an arm movement, the arm is deflected sideways from its usual, nearly straight path and the hand path becomes curved. When the subject makes repeated movements in the same field, the movement paths become incrementally straighter until they are indistinguishable from movements without the curl field. If the force field is then unexpectedly turned off, the path of movement curves strongly in the opposite direction (Figure 37–18A). This *after-effect* demonstrates that the subject has changed the motor command required to produce the desired straight movement in anticipation of the perturbing effect of the force field.

As a subject adapts to the force field, motor behavior changes from feedback correction for actual perturbations to predictive feed-forward compensation for expected perturbation. Motor-learning theory suggests that this adaptive process may involve at least two distinct learning mechanisms, known as feedback-error learning and supervised learning.

In *feedback-error learning* sensory signals about the experienced error both guide the correction for the immediate perturbation and alter adaptive feedback control circuits to permit more efficient compensation for expected perturbation. In *supervised learning* the motor system gradually adapts internal models, neural circuits that learn the relationship between desired movements and required motor commands in that environment (see Chapter 33). An internal *forward model* estimates the state of the limb in the near future based on an efference copy of the motor command and sensory feedback of the ongoing movement, and uses this estimate to generate an error signal proportional to the deviation of the estimated movement from its desired kinematics. An internal *inverse model* uses this and other error signals to learn how to generate the motor command that will produce a desired movement by compensating in a predictive manner for the anticipated perturbation. Neural circuits that constitute these internal forward and inverse models are thought

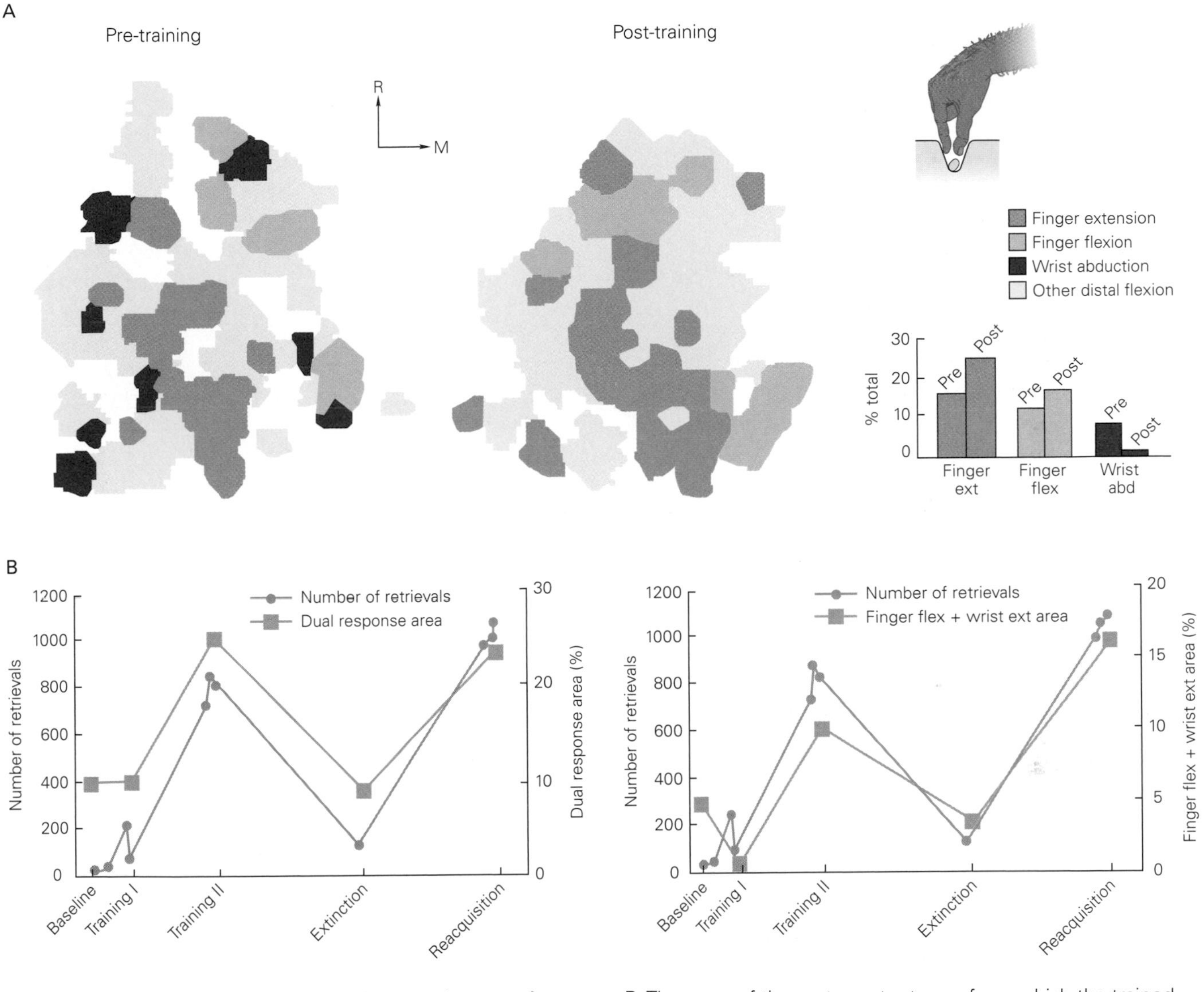

Figure 37–16 Learning a motor skill changes the organization of the motor map. (Reproduced, with permission, from Nudo et al. 1996.)

A. Motor maps for the hand in a monkey before and after training on retrieval of treats from a small well. Before training output sites that generate index finger and wrist movements occupy less than half of a monkey's motor map. After training the area from which those trained movements can be evoked by intracortical microstimulation expands substantially. The area of the map from which one could elicit individuated movements such as finger extension and flexion has expanded considerably, while the areas controlling wrist abduction, which this monkey used less in the new skill, became less prominent. (**R**, rostral; **M**, medial.)

B. The areas of the motor output map from which the trained movements can be evoked parallel the level of performance (number of successful pellet retrievals) during acquisition of the motor skill and extinction (due to lack of practice). Two areas were tested: a "dual response" area (**left plot**), from which any combination of finger and wrist motions could be evoked, and an area from which the specific combination of finger flexion and wrist extension could be evoked (**right plot**). Both areas increased as the monkey's skill improved with practice and decreased as the monkey's skill was extinguished through lack of practice. These data are from a different monkey than the one in part A but one that was trained in the same task.

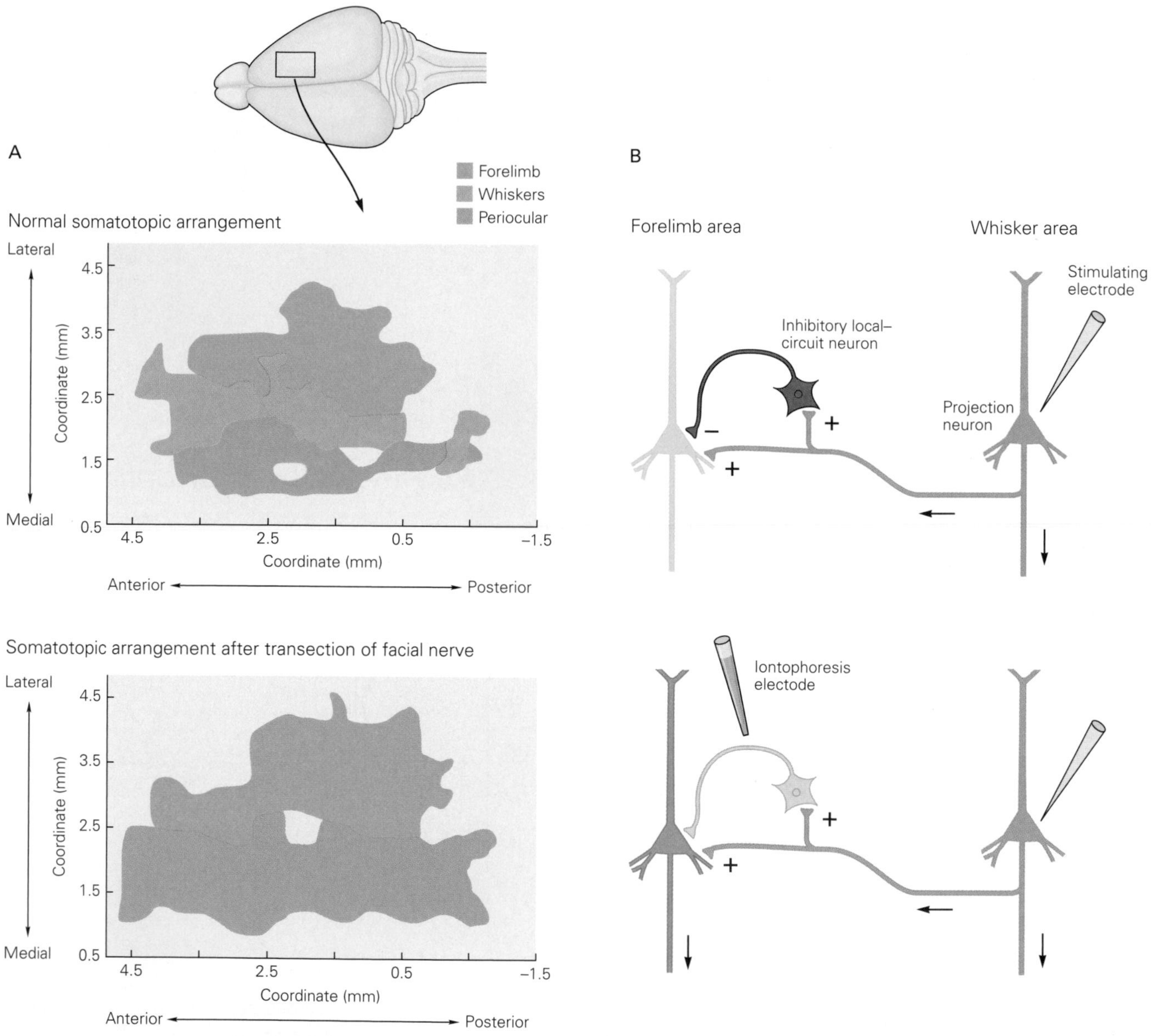

Figure 37–17 The functional organization of the motor map of a rat changes rapidly after transection of the facial nerve. (Reproduced, with permission, from Sanes et al. 1988 and from Jacobs and Donoghue 1991.)

A. A surface view of the rat's frontal cortex shows the normal somatotopic arrangement of areas representing forelimb, whisker, and periocular muscles. Within minutes after transection of the branches of the facial nerve that innervate whiskers, stimulation of cortical sites that formerly activated whisker muscles causes contraction of forelimb and periocular muscles.

B. Elimination of the sensory inputs after transection of the facial nerve may lead to rapid changes in the balance of local inhibitory circuits in the motor cortex. Under normal conditions (**top**) the excitatory effect of horizontal axonal projections between different parts of the motor map is subject to inhibition mediated by local inhibitory interneurons, so that electrical stimulation of a whisker site evokes contractions of only whisker muscles and not forelimb muscles. Iontophoretic injection of bicuculline into a forelimb site in the motor map blocks local GABA-mediated inhibition (**bottom**). As a result, stimulation of whisker sites can excite output neurons in forelimb and periocular sites through horizontal axonal collaterals whose influence is normally restricted by inhibitory interneurons.

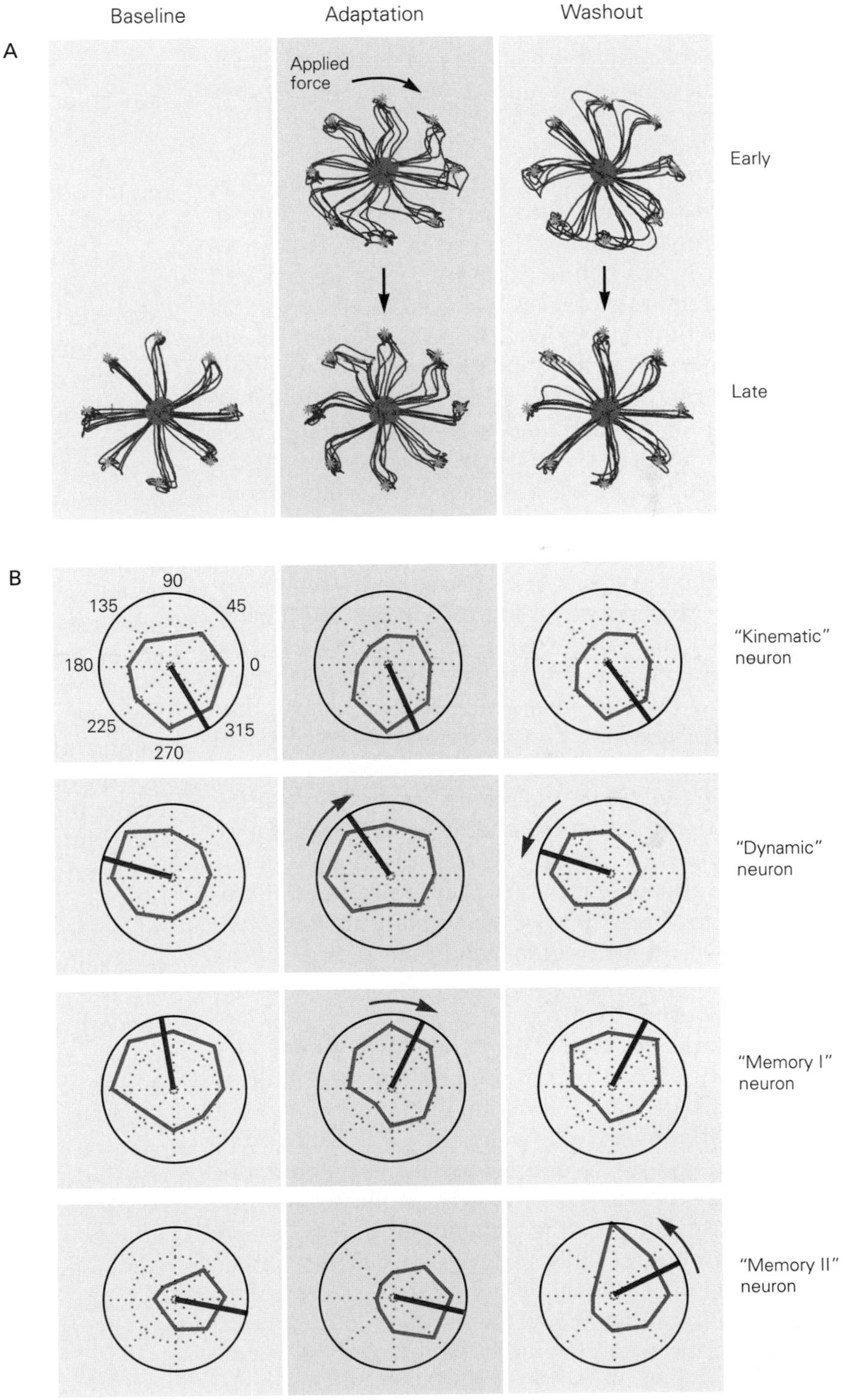

Figure 37–18 Different motor cortex neurons may contribute to different aspects of adaptation to an external force field.

A. The records depict the hand paths of reaching movements from a central position to eight peripheral targets prior to and during adaptation to an external force field and then during the return to original baseline conditions. Paths are generally straight when no external force field is applied during reaching to the targets (**late baseline**). When a viscous curl field pushes the arm in the clockwise direction (**arrow**) hand paths are initially curved in the clockwise direction (**early adaptation**). After approximately 150 trials the paths become much straighter, indicating that the subject has learned to correct for the perturbing effect of the external force field (**late adaptation**). When the external field is abruptly removed, the paths in the first few trials are curved in the opposite direction (**early washout**), indicating that the exposure to the force field had led to a change in the subject's internal model of the environment to reflect the presence of the field. It takes several trials in the original conditions before the after-effect of the learning episode is no longer evident in hand kinematics (**late washout**). (Adapted, with permission, from Padoa-Schioppa, Li, and Bizzi 2004.)

B. Response patterns of four motor cortex neurons during and after adaptation to arm movement in a viscous curl field. All four neurons were directionally tuned in the baseline conditions (**left column**). The tuning of some neurons changed only during adaptation ("memory I" neuron); only during washout, that is, readaptation to the baseline conditions ("memory II" neuron); or both ("dynamic" neuron). Muscles showed the same pattern of responses as the "dynamic" neuron, implicating this neuron in the control of the forces needed to compensate for the field. (Adapted, with permission, from Li, Padoa-Schioppa, and Bizzi 2001.)

to be located in several brain structures, including the cerebellum, superior parietal cortex, premotor cortex, and primary motor cortex.

Emilio Bizzi and colleagues recorded the activity of the same primary motor cortex neurons over several hours in monkeys as the animals first made arm movements without an external force field, then while they made many movements to adapt to a viscous curl field, and finally while they readapted to the baseline condition (the "washout" period). As the monkeys adapted to the force field the directional tuning of many neurons gradually changed by 15 to 20 degrees from what it was before exposure to the viscous curl field, and then rotated back to the baseline during the washout period (Figure 37–18B). Arm muscles showed similar changes during adaptation and washout, implicating those neurons in the incremental adaptation of the motor command to the external curl field. Other neurons did not change directionality during either adaptation or washout, as if their signals communicated the desired movement kinematics across all force-field conditions.

Two other groups of neurons showed special properties. The directional tuning of one group changed when the monkeys switched from the null field to the curl field but did not return to baseline during washout (Figure 37–18B). The other group did not change during the original adaptation from null field to curl field but changed during washout. Bizzi proposed that these two groups of neurons retain the memory of one or the other of the successive learning episodes—adaptation and washout—in the task. That is, even though the motor performance of the monkeys returned to baseline, the functional state of the primary motor cortex did not revert to its original condition—a trace of the recent learning history persisted in the altered tuning properties of some neurons.

These and similar findings from other studies suggest that the motor map of the primary motor cortex is not static. Instead, the neuronal circuitry creates a dynamic, adaptive map that generates the motor commands required to accomplish desired actions under different conditions. This strongly implicates the primary motor cortex in the acquisition, retention, and recall of procedural skills, but does not clarify whether it functions primarily as part of a feedback controller, as an inverse internal model for task dynamics, or both.

Furthermore, recent studies have found that adaptive changes in motor cortex activity lag the improvement in motor performance by several trials during adaptation. This suggests that learning-related adjustments to motor commands are initially made elsewhere, with the cerebellum as one strong candidate. The primary motor cortex may thus be more strongly involved in the slower processes of long-term retention and recall of motor skills rather than the initial phase of learning a new skill.

An Overall View

The discovery of a topographically organized map of motor outputs to different parts of the body within a limited area of the cerebral cortex provided the first compelling experimental evidence for the cortical localization of motor function. For many years thereafter the role of the motor cortex was relegated to that of a simple map of muscles and muscle activity patterns by which the rest of the cerebral cortex controlled spinal motor neurons. Terms such as "upper-motor-neuron disease" were common in the clinical literature of an earlier era, but this view of motor cortex function is simplistic and incorrect.

Although the motor cortex does play a critical role in the control of voluntary movements, its neurons do not function like spinal motor neurons whose sole role is to encode muscle activity patterns. Instead, the motor cortex contains a heterogeneous population of neurons that contribute to the several operations required to convert a plan of action into the motor commands that execute the plan. The novel evolutionary development in primates of a direct, monosynaptic projection onto spinal motor neurons enables the primary motor cortex to control movements of the hand and fingers in a uniquely skillful way. This feature has been critical in the acquisition of dexterous hand movements that only higher primates and especially humans possess.

The primary motor cortex is part of a distributed network of cortical motor areas, each with its own role in voluntary motor control. The primary motor cortex should be regarded as a dynamic computational map whose internal organization and spinal connections convert central signals about motor intentions and sensory feedback about the current state of the limb into motor output commands, rather than as a static map of specific muscles or movements of body parts. The motor cortex also provides a substrate for adaptive alterations during the acquisition of motor skills and the recovery of function after lesions.

John F. Kalaska
Giacomo Rizzolatti

Selected Readings

Ashe J. 1997. Force and the motor cortex. Behav Brain Res 87:255–269.

Dum RP, Strick PL. 2002. Motor areas in the frontal lobe of the primate. Physiol Behav 77:677–682.

Kalaska JF. 2009. From intention to action: motor cortex and the control of reaching movements. Adv Exp Med Biol 629:139–178.

Lemon RN. 2008. Descending pathways in motor control. Annu Rev Neurosci 31:195–218.

Porter R, Lemon R. 1993. *Corticospinal Function and Voluntary Movement.* Oxford: Clarendon.

Rizzolatti G, Luppino G. 2001. The cortical motor system. Neuron 31:889–901.

Schieber M. 2001. Constraints on somatotopic organization in the primary motor cortex. J Neurophysiol 86:2125–2143.

Taylor CSR, Gross CG. 2003. Twitches versus movements: a story of motor cortex. Neuroscientist 9:332–342.

References

Arce F, Novick I, Mandelblat-Cerf Y, Israel Z, Ghez C, Vaadia E. 2010. Combined adaptiveness of specific motor cortical ensembles underlies learning. J Neurosci 30:5415–5525.

Asanuma H, Rosén I. 1972. Topographical organization of cortical efferent zones projecting to distal forelimb muscles in the monkey. Exp Brain Res 14:243–256.

Ashe J, Georgopoulos AP. 1994. Movement parameters and neural activity in motor cortex and area 5. Cereb Cortex 4:590–600.

Caminiti R, Johnson PB, Urbana A. 1990. Making arm movements within different parts of space: dynamic aspects in the primate motor cortex. J Neurosci 10:2039–2058.

Carmena JM, Lebedev MA, Crist RE, O'Doherty JE, Santucci DM, Dimitrov D, Patti PG, Henriquez CS, Nicolelis MA. 2003. Learning to control a brain-machine interface for reaching and grasping by primates. PLoS Biol 1:193–208.

Cheney PD, Fetz EE. 1980. Functional classes of primate corticomotoneuronal cells and their relation to active force. J Neurophysiol 44:773–791.

Cheney PD, Fetz EE. 1985. Comparable patterns of muscle facilitation evoked by individual corticomotoneuronal (CM) cells and by single intracortical microstimuli in primates: evidence of functional groups of CM cells. J Neurophysiol 53:786–804.

Cheney PD, Fetz EE, Palmer SS. 1985. Patterns of facilitation and suppression of antagonist forelimb muscles from motor cortex sites in the awake monkey. J Neurophysiol 53:805–820.

Evarts EV. 1968. Relation of pyramidal tract activity to force exerted during voluntary movement. J Neurophysiol 31:14–27.

Evarts EV, Fromm C, Kröller J, Jennings VA. 1983. Motor cortex and control of finely graded forces. J Neurophysiol 49:1199–1215.

Fetz EE, Cheney PD. 1980. Postspike facilitation of forelimb muscle activity by primate corticomotoneuronal cells. J Neurophysiol 44:751–772.

Fetz EE, Finocchio DV. 1975. Correlations between activity of motor cortex neurons and arm muscles during operantly conditioned response patterns. Exp Brain Res 23:217–240.

Georgopoulos AP, Ashe J, Smyrnis N, Taira M. 1992. The motor cortex and the coding of force. Science 256:1692–1695.

Georgopoulos AP, Caminiti R, Kalaska JF, Massey JT. 1983. Spatial coding of movement: A hypothesis concerning the coding of movement direction by motor cortical populations. Exp Brain Res Suppl 7:327–336.

Georgopoulos AP, Kalaska JF, Caminiti R, Massey JT. 1982. On the relations between the direction of two-dimensional arm movements and cell discharge in primate motor cortex. J Neurosci 2:1527–1537.

Georgopoulos PA, Merchant H, Naselaris T, Amirikian B. 2007. Mapping of the preferred direction in the motor cortex. Proc Natl Acad Sci U S A 104:11068–11072.

Gribble PL, Scott SH. 2002. Overlap of internal models in motor cortex for mechanical loads during reaching. Nature 417:938–941.

Griffin DM, Hudson HM, Belhaj-Saïf A, Cheney PD. 2009. Stability of output effects from motor cortex to forelimb muscles in primates. J Neurosci 29:1915–1927.

Griffin DM, Hudson HM, Belhaj-Saïf A, McKiernan BJ, Cheney PD. 2008. Do corticomotoneuronal cells predict target muscle EMG activity? J Neurophysiol 99:1169–1186.

He SQ, Dum RP, Strick PL. 1993. Topographic organization of corticospinal projections from the frontal lobe: motor areas on the lateral surface of the hemisphere. J Neurosci 13:952–980.

Hochberg, LR, Serruya, MD, Friehs GM, Mukand JA, Saleh M, Caplan AH, Branner A, Chen D, Penn RD, Donohgue JP. 2006 Neuronal ensemble control of prosthetic devices by a human with tetraplegia. Nature 442:164–171.

Hoffman DS, Strick PL. 1995. Effects of a primary motor cortex lesion on step-tracking movements of the wrist. J Neurophysiol 73:891–895.

Humphrey DR, Schmidt EM, Thompson WD. 1970. Predicting measures of motor performance from multiple cortical spike trains. Science 170:758–762.

Humphrey DR, Tanji J. 1991. What features of voluntary motor control are encoded in the neuronal discharge of different cortical areas? In: DR Humphrey, H-J Freund (eds). *Motor Control: Concepts and Issues*, pp 413–443. New York: Wiley.

Jackson A, Mavoori J, Fetz EE. 2007. Correlations between the same motor cortex cells and arm muscles during a trained task, free behavior, and natural sleep in the macaque monkey. J Neurophysiol 97:360–374.

Jacobs KM, Donoghue JP. 1991. Reshaping the cortical motor map by unmasking latent intracortical connections. Science 251:944–947.

Kakei S, Hoffman DS, Strick PL. 1999. Muscle and movement representations in the primary motor cortex. Science 285:2136–2139.

Kalaska JF, Cohen DA, Hyde ML, Prud'Homme M. 1989. A comparison of movement direction-related versus load direction-related activity in primate motor cortex, using a two-dimensional reaching task. J Neurosci 9:2080–2102.

Lawrence DG, Kuypers HG. 1968. The functional organization of the motor system in the monkey. I. The effects of bilateral pyramidal lesions. Brain 91:1–14.

Lemon RN. 1981. Functional properties of monkey motor cortex neurones receiving afferent input from the hand and fingers. J Physiol 311:497–519.

Li CS, Padoa-Schioppa C, Bizzi E. 2001. Neuronal correlates of motor performance and motor learning in the primary motor cortex of monkeys adapting to an external force field. Neuron 30:593–607.

Maier MA, Bennett KM, Hepp-Reymond MC, Lemon RN. 1993. Contribution of the monkey corticomotoneuronal system to the control of force in precision grip. J Neurophysiol 69:772–785.

McKiernan BJ, Marcario JK, Kerrer JH, Cheney PD. 2000. Correlations between corticomotoneuronal (CM) cell postspike effects and cell-target muscle covariation. J Neurophysiol 83:99–115.

Moran DW, Schwartz AB. 1999. Motor cortical activity during drawing movements: population representation during spiral tracing. J Neurophysiol 82:2693–2704.

Morrow MM, Jordan LR, Miller LE. 2007. Direct comparison of the task-dependent discharge of M1 in hand space and muscle space. J Neurophysiol 97:1786–1798.

Muir RB, Lemon RN. 1983. Corticospinal neurons with a special role in precision grip. Brain Res 261:312–316.

Murphy JT, Kwan MC, MacKay WA, Wong YC. 1978. Spatial organization of precentral cortex in awake primates. III. Input-output coupling. J Neurophysiol 41:1132–1139.

Musallam S, Corneil BD, Greger B, Scherberger H, Andersen RA. 2004. Cognitive control signals for neural prosthetics. Science 305:258–262.

Nudo RJ, Milliken GW, Jenkins WM, Merzenich MM. 1996. Use-dependent alterations of movement representations in primary motor cortex of adult squirrel monkeys. J Neurosci 16:785–807.

Li C-SR, Padoa-Schioppa C, Bizzi E. 2001. Neuronal correlates of motor performance and motor learning in the primary motor cortex of monkeys adapting to an external force field. Neuron 30:593–607.

Padoa-Schioppa C, Li CS, Bizzi E. 2004. Neuronal activity in the supplementary motor area of monkeys adapting to a new dynamic environment. J Neurophysiol 91:449–473.

Paninski L, Fellows MR, Hatsopoulos NG, Donoghue JP. 2004. Spatiotemporal tuning of motor cortical neurons for hand position and velocity. J Neurophysiol 91:515–532.

Park MC, Belhaj- Saïf A, Cheney PD. 2004. Properties of primary motor cortex output to forelimb muscles in rhesus macaques. J Neurophysiol 92:2968–2984.

Park MC, Belhaj-Saïf A, Gordon M, Cheney PD. 2001. Consistent features in the forelimb representation of primary motor cortex in rhesus macaques. J Neurosci 21: 2784–2792.

Paz R, Boraud T, Natan, Bergman H, Vaadia E. 2003. Preparatory activity in motor cortex reflects learning of local visuomotor skills. Nat Neurosci 6:882–890.

Rathelot JA, Strick PL. 2006. Muscle representation in the macaque motor cortex: an anatomical perspective. Proc Natl Acad Sci U S A 103:8257–8262.

Rioult-Pedotti MS, Friedman D, Hess G, Donoghue JP. 1998. Strengthening of horizontal cortical connections following skill learning. Nat Neurosci 1:230–234.

Rosén I, Asanuma H. 1972. Peripheral afferent inputs to the forelimb area of the monkey motor cortex: input-output relations. Exp Brain Res 14:257–273.

Sanes JN, Suner S, Lando JF, Donoghue JP. 1988. Rapid reorganization of adult rat motor cortex somatic representation patterns after motor nerve injury. Proc Natl Acad Sci U S A 85:2003–2007.

Schwartz AB. 1993. Motor cortical activity during drawing movements: population representation during sinusoidal tracing. J Neurophysiol 70:28–36.

Schwartz AB, Kettner RE, Georgopoulos AP. 1988. Primate motor cortex and free arm movements to visual targets in three-dimensional space. I. Relations between single cell discharge and direction of movement. J Neurosci 8:2928–2937.

Scott SH, Kalaska JF. 1997. Reaching movements with similar hand paths but different arm orientations. I. Activity of individual cells in motor cortex. J Neurophysiol 77: 826–852.

Sergio LE, Kalaska JF. 2003. Systematic changes in motor cortex cell activity with arm posture during directional isometric force generation. J Neurophysiol 89:212–228.

Sergio LE, Hamel-Pâquet C, Kalaska JF. 2005. Motor cortex neural correlates of output kinematics and kinetics during isometric-force and arm-reaching tasks. J Neurophysiol 94:2353–2378.

Shen L, Alexander GE. 1997. Neural correlates of a spatial sensory-to-motor transformation in primary motor cortex. J Neurophysiol 77:1171–1194.

Shinoda Y, Yokota J, Futami T. 1981. Divergent projections of individual corticospinal axons to motoneurons of multiple muscles in the monkey. Neurosci Lett 23:7–12.

Smith AM, Hepp-Reymond MC, Wyss UR. 1975. Relation of activity in precentral cortical neurons to force and rate of force change during isometric contractions of finger muscles. Exp Brain Res 23:315–332.

Thach WT. 1978. Correlation of neural discharge with pattern and force of muscular activity, joint position, and direction of intended next arm movement in motor cortex and cerebellum. J Neurophysiol 41:654–476.

Townsend BR, Paninski L, Lemon RN. 2006. Linear coding of muscle activity in primary motor cortex and cerebellum. J Neurophysiol. 96:2578–2592.

Velliste M, Perel S, Spalding MC, Whitford AS, Schwartz AB. 2008. Cortical control of a prosthetic arm for self-feeding. Nature 453:1098–1101.

Wise SP, Moody SL, Blomstrom KJ, Mitz AR. 1998. Changes in motor cortical activity during visuomotor adaptation. Exp Brain Res 121:285–299.

38

Voluntary Movement: The Parietal and Premotor Cortex

In this chapter we describe how the cerebral cortex uses sensory information about the external world in deciding on which actions to take and how to organize voluntary movements to accomplish those actions. Studies over the past 25 years have shown that the cortical motor system is not an unthinking, passive circuit controlled by more intelligent parts of the brain. Instead, it is intimately involved in the many interrelated neural processes required to choose a plan of action, including processes that appear to be more perceptual and cognitive than motor in nature. The motor system also contributes to cognitive processes that appear unrelated to motor control, such as understanding the actions of others and the potential outcomes of observed events.

Voluntary Movement Expresses an Intention to Act

Voluntary behavior is the physical expression of an intention to act on the environment to achieve a goal. Let us say you want a cup of coffee. There may be many reasons why: You may wish to enjoy the stimulating effect of caffeine or may simply be thirsty. Whatever its origin, your behavioral goal is established by your motivational state but is fulfilled by voluntary motor behavior. The motor system has to transform your intention into action.

How you achieve your goal depends on the circumstances in which you find yourself. If the cup of coffee is already prepared and sitting in front of you, you can simply reach out, grasp the cup, and bring it to your lips. Often, however, the situation is more complex. The coffee might not be ready, or you might not have any coffee at home. In this case, to satisfy your craving for coffee you must organize and perform a complex series of actions to fulfill your goal of drinking coffee. You may go out to buy the coffee and return home, or you may go to a café, order a coffee, and drink it there. Alternatively, if it is too late in the evening or if the weather is inclement, you may alter your goal, such as drinking tea instead of coffee.

Each of these different voluntary behaviors is an action that serves an intermediate goal. However, only the entire series of actions can achieve your ultimate goal. The capacity to maintain a behavioral goal during a series of actions, and to develop alternative behavioral strategies and action sequences to fulfill the goal, are hallmarks of voluntary behavior. The prefrontal cortex located rostral to the motor areas plays a critical role in the organization of voluntary behavior. Here we focus on the neuronal mechanisms in the parietal and premotor cortex that mediate voluntary behaviors.

Voluntary behavior often involves physical interaction with objects in the external world. This requires the brain to convert sensory inputs about the state of the world and the individual's internal state into motor commands. As described in Chapter 33, the transformation involves a sequence of neural operations in many cortical and subcortical areas. No single area is responsible for all the steps between intention and action, or indeed for any one particular operation. This distributed organization is characteristic of all aspects of the neural control of voluntary behavior.

Another important feature of voluntary behavior is that once an intention is formed, action can be delayed or not performed at all. One is not irrevocably compelled to act on an intention the moment it is formed. A reflex, by contrast, is evoked immediately by a stimulus. Without self-control over whether, how, and when to act, behavior would be driven by the moment—impulsive, compulsive, and even antisocial. These considerations suggest that the motor system operates in at least two stages: movement planning and execution. Planning involves deciding what action or series of actions to perform to fulfill an intention, whereas execution orchestrates actual movement.

Studies of nearly every cortical area involved in arm movement have attempted to identify the neural pathways specific to planning or execution. This is often done by imposing a delay between the instruction about what movement to make and the cue to execute it. These studies show that none of the cortical areas contains a homogeneous population of neurons dedicated only to planning or execution. Instead, a broad range of neuronal function is evident in each area. Some neurons respond only during the planning phase of the task, whereas others discharge during the execution phase. Still others show activity changes during both stages (Figure 38–1).

The major difference between cortical areas is whether the predominant neural activity is correlated with planning or execution. Whereas many primary motor cortex neurons discharge mainly during execution, premotor and parietal cortices contain more neurons that are strongly activated during the planning stage.

Neural activity during the planning stage also provides information about the intended act. The activity of single neurons and populations during the delay period of reach-to-grasp tasks conveys such information as the location of the target, the direction of arm movement, and the configuration of the hand required to grasp an object. This activity even encodes information about higher-order aspects of the action, such as its goal and expected reward value.

Even when a well-trained monkey makes the wrong movement in response to an instruction, the neural activity during the delay period before movement onset generally predicts the erroneous response. This is compelling evidence that the activity is a neural correlate of the intended motor act, not a passive sensory response to the stimulus that instructed it.

Further evidence of motor planning in the cortex comes from comparing the neural activity in a monkey when it has been instructed to make a reaching movement and when it has been instructed to withhold reaching. Many neurons in the premotor cortex generate directionally tuned activity during the delay period when the monkey is instructed to move, but not when it is instructed to refrain from moving. This differential activity represents an unequivocal signal about the monkey's intention either to reach in different directions or not to move in response to an instructional cue seconds before the action is executed (Figure 38–2).

These studies demonstrate that activity in several movement-related cortical areas signals information about the nature of an intended motor act

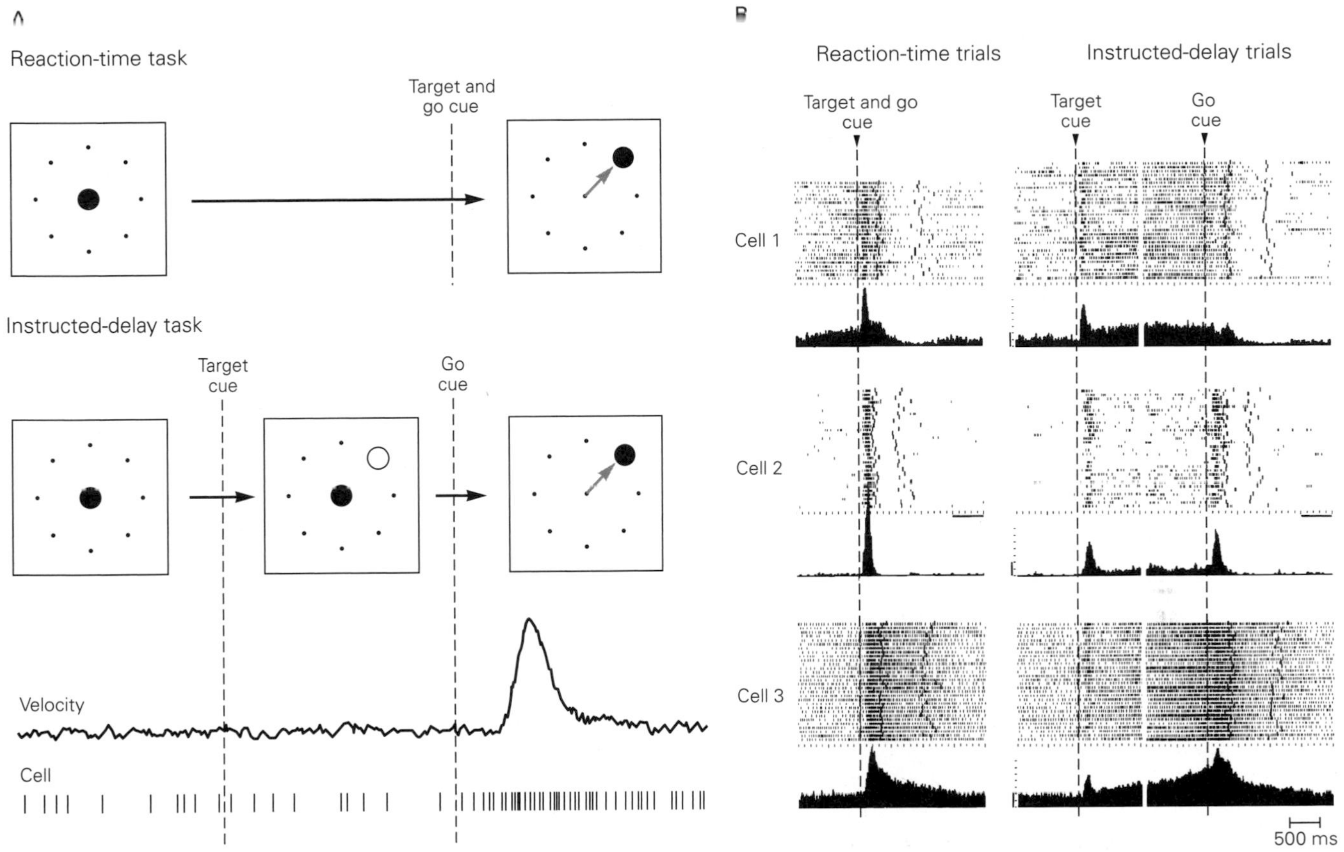

Figure 38–1 Neural processes related to movement planning and movement execution can be dissociated in time. (Reproduced, with permission, from Crammond and Kalaska 2000.)

A. In a *reaction-time task* a sensory cue instructs the subject both where to move (target cue) and when to move (go cue). All neuronal operations required to plan and initiate the execution of the movement are performed in the brief time between the appearance of the cue and the onset of movement. In an *instructed-delay task* an initial cue tells the subject where to move and only later is the cue given to start movement. The knowledge provided by the first cue permits the subject to plan the upcoming movement. Any changes in activity that occur after the first cue but before the second are presumed to be neuronal correlates of the planning stage.

B. Movement planning and execution are not completely segregated at the level of single neurons or neuronal populations in a given cortical area. Raster plots and cumulative histograms show the responses of three premotor cortex neurons to movements in each cell's preferred direction during reaction-time trials and instructed-delay trials. In the raster plots each row represents activity in a single trial. The thin tics represent action potentials, and the two thicker tics show the time of movement onset and end. In reaction-time trials the monkey does not know in which direction to move until the target appears. In contrast, in instructed-delay trials an initial cue informs the monkey where the target lies well in advance of the appearance of a second signal to initiate the movement. During the delay period many premotor cells show directionally tuned changes in activity that signal the direction of the impending delayed movement. The activity in cell 1 appears to be strictly related to the planning phase of the task, for there is no execution-related activity after the go signal in the instructed-delay task. The other two cells show different degrees of activity related to both planning and execution.

well before execution of the act. Many neurons in the same cortical areas also discharge during movement execution, implicating those areas in the control of movement. Given this close anatomical proximity of planning- and execution-related activity, even at the level of individual neurons, a major unresolved question is why planning-related neural activity does not immediately initiate the movement. There must exist a mechanism that either prevents movement execution during the delayed planning stage or permits the start of movement at a later time (see Box 38–2).

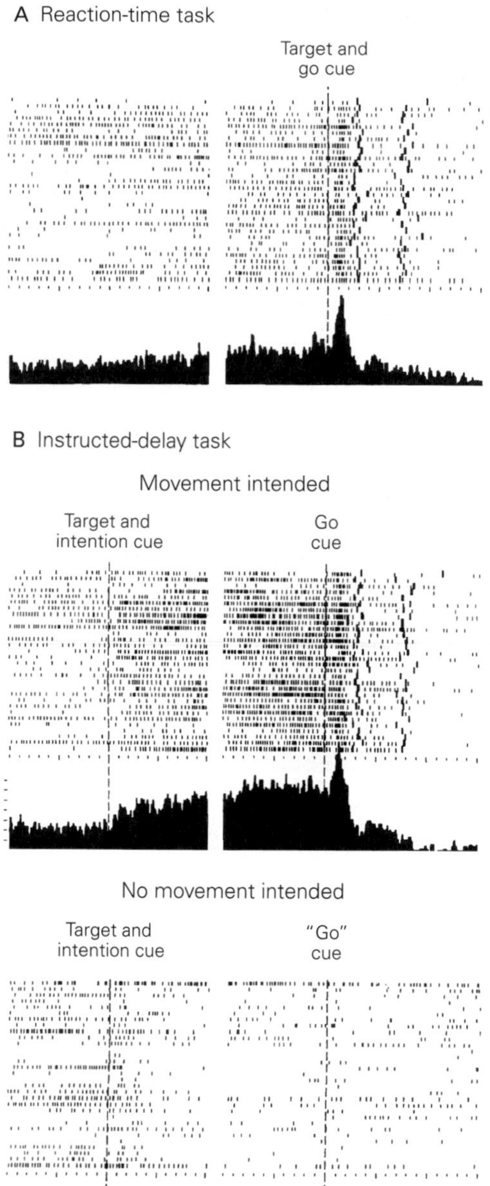

Figure 38–2 Decisions about response choices are evident in the activity of premotor cortex neurons. (Reproduced, with permission, from Crammond and Kalaska 2000.)

A. In a reaction-time task (reaching) a cell exhibits gradually increasing, nondirectional, tonic firing while waiting for the appearance of a target. When the target appears (**go cue**) the cell generates a directionally tuned response.

B. In an instructed-delay task, when a monkey is shown the target and instructed to move once the go cue appears, the cell generates a strong, directionally tuned signal for the duration of the delay period before the go cue. When the monkey is shown the target but is instructed not to move when the go cue appears, the cell's activity decreases.

Voluntary Movement Requires Sensory Information About the World and the Body

Let us return to the action of getting a cup of coffee. The deceptively simple action of drinking from a cup represents not a single motor act but a series of motor acts, each with a specific goal: reaching for the cup, grasping, lifting, holding, and bringing the cup to the mouth. The sequence of acts must be coordinated so that the arm and hand can interact physically with the cup in an efficient manner to achieve the desired goal.

To reach out and grasp the cup the motor system must solve two basic problems. First, it has to localize the cup in space and transform this location into a reaching movement of the arm to bring the hand to the cup. Second, it must encode the physical properties of the cup, such as its size and shape, and transform them into a particular grip. One might suppose that reaching and grasping are conducted sequentially. However, recordings of hand and arm kinematics show that this is not so: The two acts occur largely simultaneously. As the arm reaches toward the cup, the hand starts to rotate and open to match the size, shape, and orientation of the target. The hand and fingers then begin to close even before the hand contacts the cup. Furthermore, although the two processes occur in parallel, they can influence each other. Both the velocity and acceleration of grasping and reaching, for example, can depend on the location, distance, orientation, size, and shape of the object to be lifted.

Along with information about the target object the motor system requires information about the current status of the arm, including its posture and motion and the position of the hand relative to the target. The various brain operations required to plan and guide arm movements are implemented in part by interconnected populations of neurons in the primary motor cortex, premotor cortex, and parietal cortex.

The parietal lobe is the principal target of the dorsal visual stream. It has long been implicated in a variety of functions such as the perception of the spatial structure of the world and the control of directed attention. As a result, the dorsal visual stream is often called the "where" pathway to distinguish it from the "what" pathway, the ventral visual stream that projects from the primary visual cortex into the temporal lobe and is involved in the recognition of objects.

Pioneering neurophysiological studies of the parietal lobe in active monkeys conducted independently by Vernon Mountcastle and Juhani Hyvärinen and their colleagues in the 1970s showed that many parietal neurons also discharge during eye, arm, or hand movements when an animal attentively explores and interacts with its environment. One striking property that both groups observed is that the discharge of many parietal neurons is highly dependent on the goal of the behavior. Neurons discharge strongly when a monkey reaches to grasp an object, searches for an object in a box, or manipulates an object with its hand, but are much less active when the monkey makes other arm and hand movements.

More recently, behavioral studies by Mel Goodale and David Milner and their collaborators have led to an important and still controversial hypothesis about the role of the dorsal visual stream. They propose that a primary function of the parietal lobe is to extract sensory information about the external world and one's own body that is useful for the planning and guidance of movements. This sensory guidance of action may operate in parallel with and independently of perceptual processes evoked by the same sensory inputs. For instance, whereas our perception of the size and orientation of objects can be deceived by certain visual illusions, the motor system often behaves as if it is not fooled and makes accurate movements (Figure 38–3). As a result, the dorsal visual stream is also called the "how" pathway (see Chapter 18).

This does not mean, however, that the parietal lobe has no role in spatial perception or attention. On the contrary, we now recognize that its contributions to spatial perception, attention, and sensorimotor transformations are intimately intertwined. This interconnectedness of function is clear in an examination of how different parts of the parietal lobe and associated precentral motor areas contribute to the planning and execution of the reach-to-grasp action required to drink a cup of coffee.

Reaching for an Object Requires Sensory Information About the Object's Location in Space

Although we describe the neural processes underlying reach and grasp separately, the two actions are usually coordinated. Coordination is achieved through reciprocal axonal connections between reach- and grasp-related populations both within the same cortical areas and between different areas and through populations of neurons that discharge in connection with components of both reach and grasp.

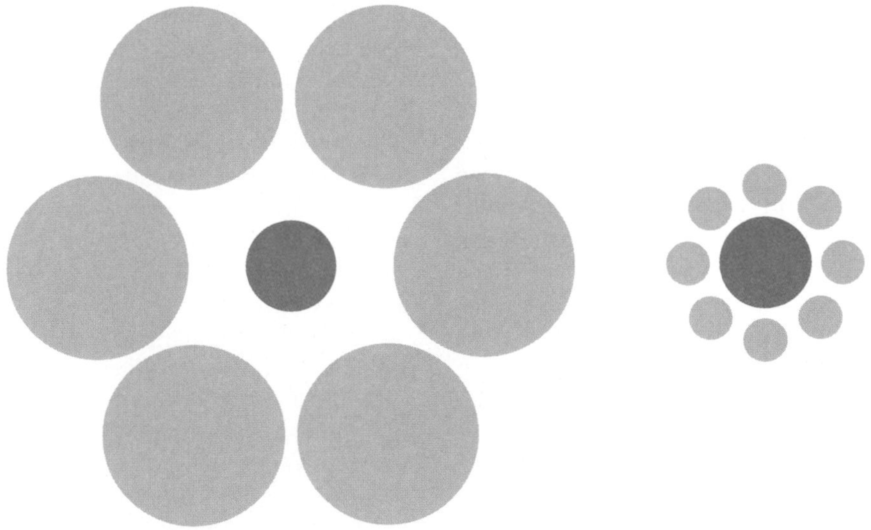

Figure 38–3 The visual information that serves object perception and movement may be processed in distinct, parallel pathways. In the Ebbinghaus illusion two orange disks of identical diameter appear to be of different size because one is surrounded by large disks and the other by small disks. Mel Goodale and collaborators reported that when subjects were asked to indicate the size of the central disks with their thumb and index finger, the separation between finger and thumb was significantly larger for the disk on the right. However, when subjects reached out to grasp the identical disks surrounded by larger or smaller disks, their thumb-finger separation was nearly the same in both cases. This and similar evidence suggests that visual pathways to the parietal lobe are distinct from those that support object perception and that the parietal inputs are not solely the output of the perceptual pathways.

Space Is Represented in Several Cortical Areas with Different Sensory and Motor Properties

The planning of a reaching movement is usually defined as the neural process by which the location of an object in space is translated into an arm movement that brings the hand into contact with the object. Our intuitive conception of space as a single continuous expanse—one that extends in all directions and within which objects have locations relative to one another and to ourselves—has long influenced neuroscience.

According to classical neurology the neural counterpart of the space that we experience is a single map in the parietal lobe constructed by inputs from different sensory modalities. This unified, multimodal neural replica of the world is assumed to provide all the information necessary for acting on an object and is shared by the different motor circuits that control the eyes, arm, hand, and other effectors.

An alternative view is that there are many maps each related to a different motor effector and adapted to its specific needs. These spatial representations are created when the individual interacts with its environment, defining a series of motor relations determined by the properties of a particular effector. For example, a rodent has a locomotion map in the hippocampus and adjacent entorhinal cortex representing the animal's current location and direction of motion. This alternative hypothesis suggests that our intuitive sense of space arises at least in part from our motor interactions with the world.

Evidence collected in recent years clearly does not support the notion of a single topographically organized representation of space in the parietal cortex. First, the parietal cortex is organized as a series of areas working in parallel. Second, *near space* or *peripersonal space,* the space within our reach, is encoded in areas different from those that represent *far space,* the space beyond our reach. Third, the functional properties of the neurons in parietal and frontal areas of cortex involved in spatial coding vary depending on the body part controlled, such as the eyes versus the arm.

These findings support the idea there are many spatial maps, some located in the parietal cortex and others in the frontal cortex, whose properties are tuned to the motor requirements of different effectors. Moreover, the spatial maps in each cortical area are not maps in the usual sense of a faithful point-to-point representation of surrounding space, but rather dynamic maps that may expand or shrink according to the motor requirements necessary to interact with a given stationary or moving object.

The Inferior Parietal and Ventral Premotor Cortex Contain Representations of Peripersonal Space

In monkeys several areas in the inferior parietal cortex and interconnected parts of the premotor cortex contain representations of peripersonal space. One such area, the ventral intraparietal area, is located in the fundus of the intraparietal sulcus (Figure 38–4A). It receives visual projections from components of the dorsal visual stream, including areas MST (medial superior temporal cortex) and MT (medial temporal cortex), that are involved in the analysis of optic flow and visual motion.

Some ventral intraparietal neurons respond only to visual stimuli and respond preferentially either to expanding (looming) or contracting (receding) stimuli or to stimuli moving in the horizontal or vertical plane. Others have polymodal receptive fields within which inputs from different sensory modalities lie in spatial register (Figure 38–5A). These neurons respond to tactile stimuli, most often near the mouth or on the face but also on the arm or trunk, as well as to visual stimuli located immediately adjacent to the tactile receptive field. Some even respond to auditory stimuli in the same spatial location. Certain polymodal neurons respond to both visual and tactile stimuli moving in the same direction whereas others are strongly activated by visual stimuli that move toward their tactile receptive field but only if the path of motion will eventually intersect the tactile receptive field.

Ventral intraparietal neurons appear to represent an early stage in the construction of a peripersonal spatial map that is more fully expressed in a caudal part of the ventral premotor cortex, area F4, with which it is strongly interconnected. Virtually all neurons in area F4 respond to somatosensory inputs, especially tactile stimuli. The tactile receptive fields are located primarily on the face, neck, arms, and hands. Half of the neurons also respond to visual stimuli and a few to auditory stimuli.

As with ventral intraparietal neurons, the modality-specific receptive fields in area F4 lie in register (Figure 38–5B). This suggests that the visual receptive fields are not defined by the location of the visual stimulus on the retina, as in most neurons in the visual cortex, but are anchored to specific parts of the individual's body. One striking feature of such a polymodal neuron, especially in the ventral premotor cortex, is that its visual receptive field remains aligned with the tactile receptive field when the monkey looks in different directions, but moves with the tactile receptive field to a different part of peripersonal space when the monkey moves the corresponding part of its body.

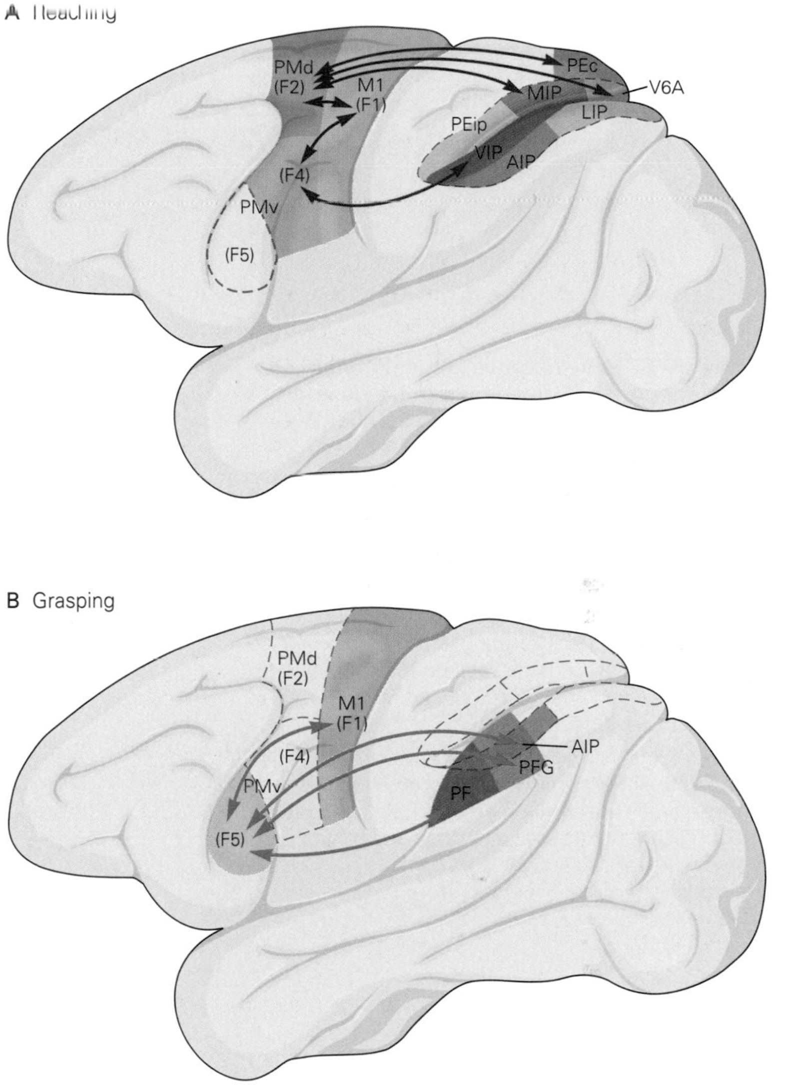

Figure 38–4 Separate parietofrontal pathways are involved in the visuomotor transformations for reaching and grasping.

A. The visuomotor transformation necessary for reaching is mediated by the parietofrontal network shown here. The areas located within the intraparietal sulcus are shown in an unfolded view of the sulcus. Two serial pathways are involved in the organization of reaching movements. The *ventral stream* has its principal nodes in the ventral intraparietal area (**VIP**) and area F4 of the ventral premotor cortex, whereas the *dorsal stream* has synaptic relays in the superior parietal lobe (**MIP, V6A**) and the dorsal premotor cortex (**PMd**), which includes area F2. (Parietal areas include **AIP**, anterior intraparietal area; **LIP**, lateral intraparietal area; and **V6A**, the parietal portion of the parieto-occipital area.) PEc and PEip are parietal areas according to the nomenclature of von Economo. Somatosensory areas 1, 2, and 3 and area PE, which provide somatosensory input to M1 (**F1**), are not shown in the figure. Precentral areas include F5, a subdivision of PMv, the ventral premotor cortex, and the primary motor cortex (**M1, F1**).

B. The visuomotor transformation necessary for grasping is mediated by the parietofrontal network shown here. The AIP and PFG areas are concerned mostly with hand movements, whereas area PF is concerned with mouth movements. PF and PFG are parietal areas according to the nomenclature of von Economo. Area F5 in PMv is concerned with both hand and mouth motor acts. Some grasping neurons have been found in F2, the ventral part of PMd. Area M1 (or F1) contains a large sector that controls the fingers, hand, and wrist (see Figure 37–2A). Other abbreviations are explained in part A.

Nevertheless, area F4 is a motor area and its neurons also discharge in association with movements, most often of the arm, wrist, neck, and face. The neurons in this area control movements of the head and arm toward different parts of the body, or toward objects close to the body, to permit the animal to grasp them with its mouth or hand. Some neurons discharge during the entire action of bringing the hand to the mouth and opening the mouth to ingest food, as well as during arm reaching and associated neck- and trunk-orienting movements. Activity in other neurons is correlated not only with reaching but also with other behaviors such as the avoidance of threatening stimuli. The sensory representation of peripersonal space in area F4 contributes to the planning and execution of those behaviors.

The Superior Parietal Cortex Uses Sensory Information to Guide Arm Movements Toward Objects in Peripersonal Space

A key requirement for efficient reaching is knowledge of where the arm is before and during the action. Lesion studies suggest that this information is represented in Brodmann's area 2, the primary somatosensory area (S-I), and in the superior parietal lobule. Patients with lesions of these regions are unable to reach toward objects efficiently, even though they do not have the deficits of spatial perception, such as spatial neglect, that are typical of lesions in the inferior parietal lobe (see Chapter 19).

Although single-neuron studies confirm the role of these areas in providing information about arm

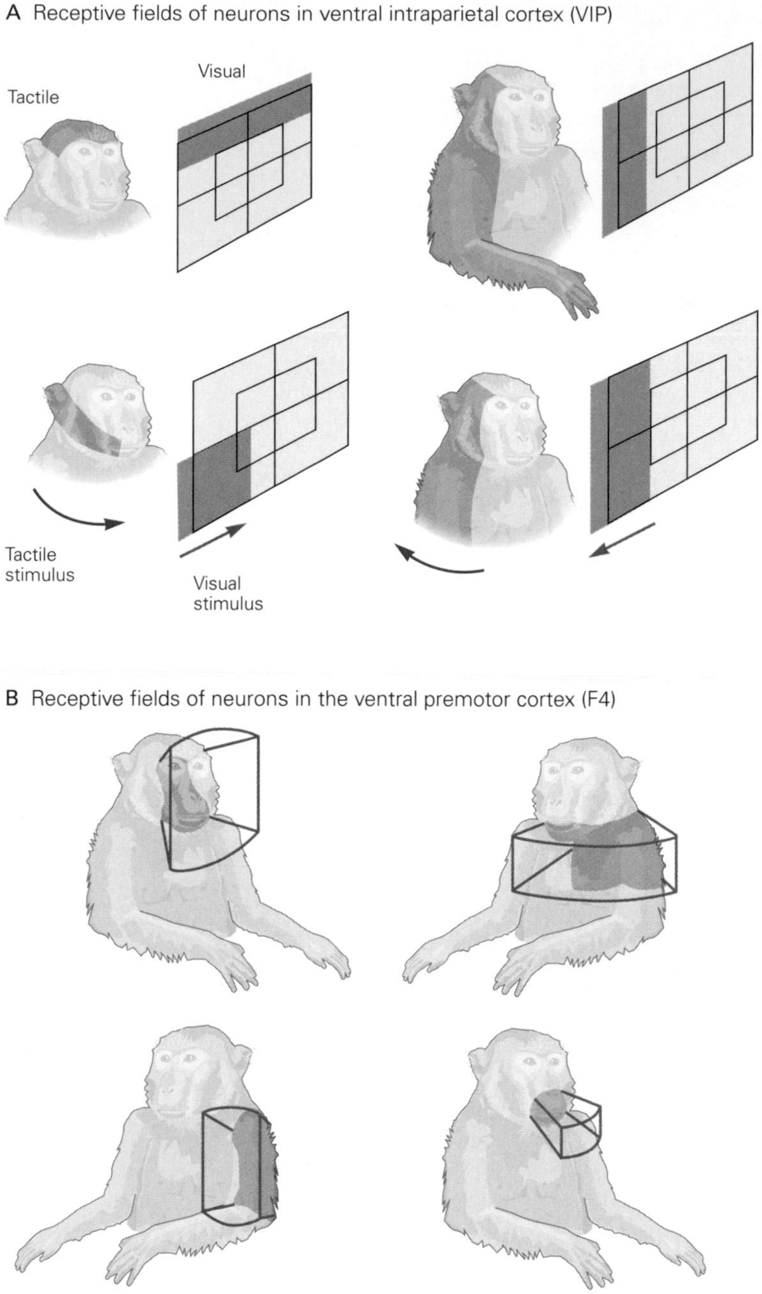

Figure 38–5 Some neurons in the parietal and premotor cortex respond to both tactile and visual stimuli within receptive fields that are spatially in register.

A. Some neurons in the ventral intraparietal cortex have tactile and visual receptive fields that are aligned in a congruent manner. **Orange** areas on the monkey represent tactile receptive fields; **purple** areas on the screen in front of the monkey's face and centered on its nose represent visual receptive fields. Many of the neurons also share directional preferences for movement of tactile and visual stimuli (**arrows**). (Reproduced, with permission, from Duhamel, Colby, and Goldberg 1998.)

B. Neurons in ventral premotor cortex area F4 respond to either tactile or visual stimulation. **Orange** areas are tactile receptive fields; **purple lines** indicate the three-dimensional receptive fields within which visual stimuli activate the neuron. (Reproduced, with permission, from Fogassi et al. 1996.)

location, there are clear functional differences between the two areas. Neurons in area 2 usually respond to tactile input from a limited part of the body or to movements of a single joint or a few adjacent joints in specific directions and most commonly on the contralateral side of the body. In contrast, many neurons in the superior parietal lobule discharge during combined movements of multiple joints, the assumption of specific postures, or movements of the limbs and the body. Some cells also respond during combined movements of the arms and hind limbs or bilateral movements of both arms.

These findings indicate that, unlike neurons in area 2 that encode the positions and movements of specific parts of the body, neurons in the superior parietal lobe integrate information on the positions of individual joints as well as the positions of limb segments with respect to the body. This integration creates a body schema that provides information on where the arm is located with respect to the body and how the different arm segments are positioned with respect to one another. This schema provides fundamental information for the proprioceptive guidance of arm movements.

More posterior and medial sectors of the superior parietal cortex also receive input from areas V2 and V3 of the extrastriate visual cortex. Important nodes in this network include areas V6A and PEc and an area of parietal cortex involved in reaching described by Richard Andersen and colleagues and which most likely corresponds to the medial intraparietal area (MIP) and nearby parts of the superior and inferior parietal cortex (see Figure 38–4A). In these areas the spatial representation for reaching is not based on body-centered coordinates. For example, neurons in V6A and PEc often signal the retinal location of possible targets for reaching, but their activity is also strongly modulated by complex combinations of inputs related to the direction of gaze and the current arm posture and hand position.

Andersen and his associates propose that the reach-related region of parietal cortex is particularly important for specifying the goal or target of reaching but not how the action should be performed. The activity of many neurons in this area varies with the location of the target relative to the hand. Remarkably, however, this motor error signal is not centered on the current location of the hand or target but rather on the current direction of gaze. Each time the monkey looks in a different direction the reach-related activity in the neurons changes (Figure 38–6). In contrast, the reach-related activity of many neurons in area PEip is less gaze-centered and more related to the current hand position and arm posture.

Another important property of neurons in the parietal reach region is that they respond not only to passive sensory inputs but also before the onset of movements and during the planning period of delayed-reaching tasks. This behavior indicates that these neurons receive centrally generated signals about motor intentions prior to movement onset, likely through their reciprocal connections with precentral motor areas. Recent theoretical and experimental findings suggest that this combination of peripheral sensory and central motor inputs permits the parietal reach region to integrate sensory input with efference copies of outgoing motor commands to compute a continuously updated estimate of the current arm state and a prediction about how the arm will respond to the motor command. This forward internal model of the arm could be used to make rapid corrections for errors in ongoing arm movements and to acquire motor skills.

The functional properties of areas in the superior parietal cortex concerned with reaching suggest an intriguing explanation of the clinical phenomenon of *optic ataxia*. Patients with a lesion of the superior parietal cortex have difficulty with visually guided arm movements toward an object. Making errors in the frontal or sagittal plane, the arm gropes for the target until it encounters the object almost by chance. The deficit is severe when the target is in the peripheral part of the visual field, less when the target lies in the parafoveal region, and negligible when the patient fixates the target. The symptoms of optic ataxia may result from failure of the neural circuits that convert sensory information about targets and the arm into motor plans or from failure of the circuits that contribute to a predictive forward model of the arm's current state.

Premotor and Primary Motor Cortex Formulate More Specific Motor Plans About Intended Reaching Movements

The reach-related areas of the parietal cortex are reciprocally connected to several precentral motor areas, including the primary motor cortex, dorsal and ventral premotor cortex, and supplementary motor area. Neurons in all of these areas contribute to sensorimotor transformations that provide increasingly detailed information about the desired spatial kinematics and causal mechanical details of the movements.

For example, the reach-related neurons in the dorsal premotor cortex are much less strongly influenced by the direction of gaze than are neurons in the parietal reach area. Instead they are driven by the direction of the intended reaching movements during the planning period of delayed-reaching tasks and during the reaching movement itself. Furthermore, during the planning period many dorsal premotor neurons signal the direction of movement to the target whether the left or right arm is used to reach for the target (Figure 38–7). This finding suggests that the premotor neurons represent the appropriate extrinsic spatial kinematics of the reaching movement independent of the arm that will perform it. In contrast, the activity of most reach-related neurons in the primary motor cortex is related to movement of the contralateral arm.

In other studies a monkey was trained to make arm movements to move a cursor on a computer monitor. In some trials the motions of the arm and cursor were collinear. In other trials they were decoupled in

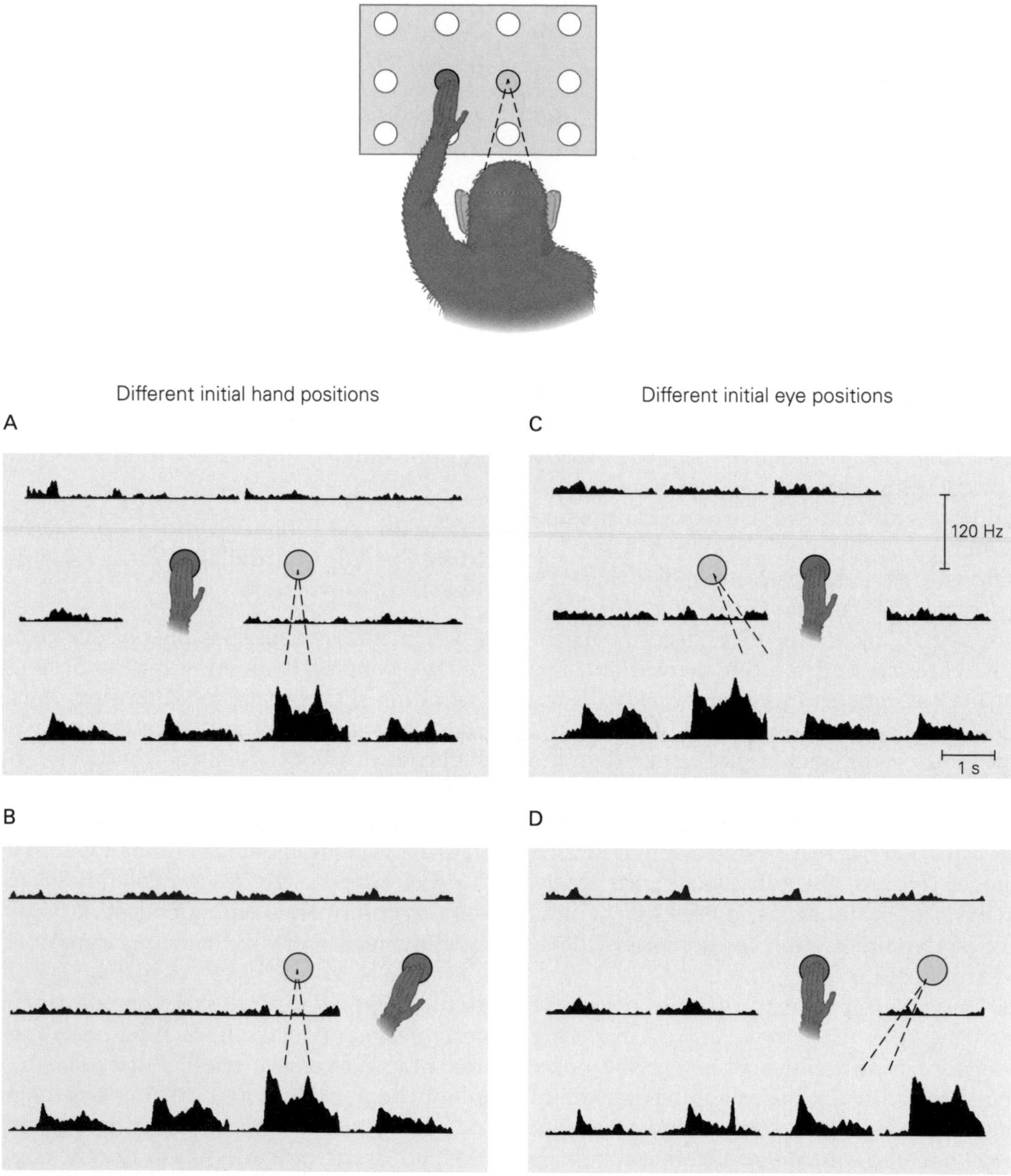

Figure 38–6 Neurons in the parietal reach area encode target location in eye-centered coordinates. An upright board contains an array of pushbuttons. The four panels show the possible behavioral conditions at the beginning of a trial. The initial hand position and point of visual fixation are indicated by the **green** and **orange buttons**, respectively. Histograms of activity in a single neuron are arranged to correspond to the locations of the buttons on the board that serve as the target of a reaching movement from the start position in different trials. The firing pattern of this neuron does not vary with changes in initial limb position (**A, B**), but shifts with a change in the initial direction of gaze (**C, D**). The neuron thus signals the target location relative to the current direction of gaze, independent of the direction of arm movement required to reach the target. (Modified, with permission, from Andersen and Buneo 2002.)

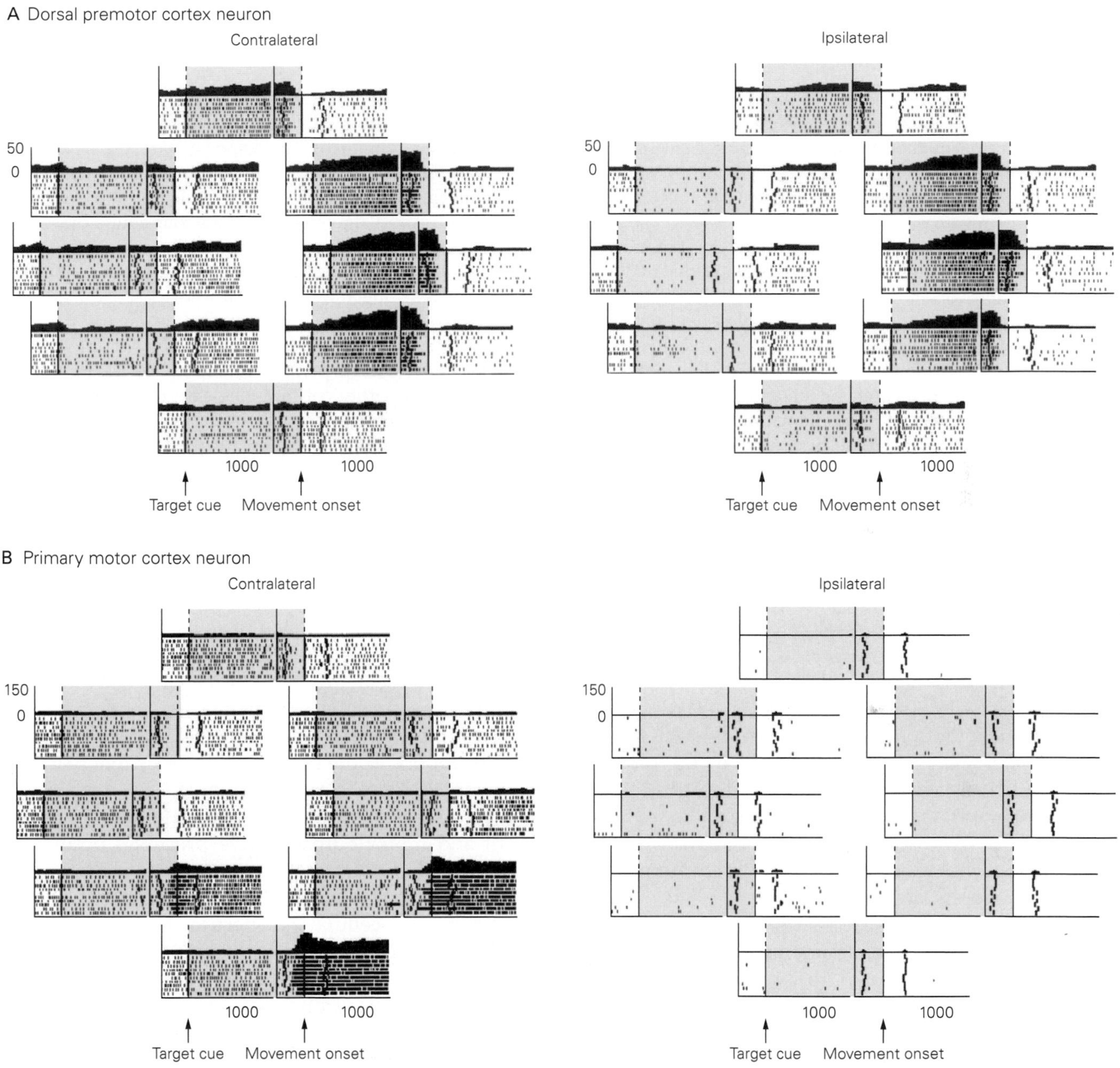

Figure 38–7 Reaching movement is represented differently in the premotor and primary motor cortex during planning and execution of the movement. (Modified, with permission, from Cisek, Crammond, and Kalaska 2003.)

A. Activity of a dorsal premotor cortex neuron in a monkey during an instructed-delay reaching task. The animal is trained to reach for targets in eight directions from a central starting position using either arm. During testing one arm is contralateral and one arm is ipsilateral to the recording site. During the planning period—the time between the presentation of the target cue and the delayed onset of movement—the neuron is directionally tuned with a preference for rightward movements. The directional tuning is identical whether the left or right arm is used. The neuron is relatively inactive during movement execution. In each raster plot the left vertical line indicates presentation of the target cue, and the right vertical line indicates the onset of arm movement. The thick tics to the left and right of the movement-onset line in each trial indicate, respectively, presentation of the go cue and the end of movement.

B. Activity of a primary motor cortex neuron during the same task as in part A. The neuron is strongly active and directionally tuned toward the lower targets when the contralateral arm is used but only during the execution phase. It is essentially inactive when the ipsilateral arm is used.

Box 38–1 The Cortical Motor System Does Not Solve Newtonian Equations

Understanding the cortical mechanisms underlying the planning and execution of reaching movements requires insight into how single neurons and neuronal populations encode different properties of intended movements and how they transform that information into motor commands.

For many years the study of the cerebral cortical mechanisms of motor control has been guided by terminology and concepts borrowed from physics, engineering, and control theory. Many studies have therefore sought and found statistical correlations between the activity of neurons in movement-related cortical areas and such movement-related parameters as target location, the velocities of hand displacement and reach trajectory, motor output force, and joint torque.

It is unlikely, however, that the motor system controls movements by encoding them in the familiar but arbitrary terms of Newtonian mechanics or by solving equations derived from the Newtonian laws of motion. Even though neural responses are consistent with a sequence of sensorimotor transformations, it is improbable that neural circuits explicitly solve the trigonometric and algebraic equations that define those transformations.

The cortical mechanisms for the planning and control of reaching movements are not based on the formalisms and first principles of physics, mechanics, and mathematics. They are determined by the stream of signals provided by peripheral sensors, by the force-generating properties of muscles, by the emergent dynamic mechanical properties of the arm, and by the properties of the spinal motor circuitry that converts the descending motor commands into muscle activity and movements.

one of three ways: by rotating the cursor motion at a 90 degree angle to the arm movement, applying a mirror-image transformation, or requiring the monkey to make elliptical motions of its arm to draw a circle with the cursor. Some neurons, especially in the primary motor cortex, signaled the motions of the arm in both the collinear and decoupled conditions. Other neurons concentrated in the dorsal and ventral premotor cortex signaled the desired motions of the cursor under the different visuomotor conditions.

These findings indicate that premotor cortex neurons can generate an abstract representation of the goal of the motor output, in this case the motion of the cursor that the monkey was moving, independent of the arm movements that control the cursor's motion. Other neurons in the premotor and primary motor cortex translate that abstract representation into signals about what the arm must do to produce the desired cursor movements.

Although these results suggest that the motor system initially plans reaching movements in extrinsic spatial coordinates, we move by contracting muscles. Many neurophysiological studies have therefore sought the neural correlates of the transformation of a desired spatiotemporal movement pattern into its causal forces and muscle activity. The consensus is that the primary motor cortex plays an important role in that transformation (see Chapter 37). However, the final motor command for the muscle-activity patterns required to execute the desired reaching movement is probably generated by spinal motor circuits.

In summary, neurophysiological studies have provided support for the general hypothesis that reaching movements involve neuronal processes that implement a sequence of transformations between sensory input and motor output. These processes occur in a dynamic, distributed network of cortical areas rather than in a strictly serial pathway. There are no abrupt transitions of cellular properties between cortical areas; instead there is a progression. Neural correlates of each putative transformation can be seen in both parietal and precentral areas, whose true nature and functions are still not fully known (Box 38–1).

Grasping an Object Requires Sensory Information About Its Physical Properties

At the same time as neural populations in several areas of the parietal and precentral cortex are controlling the reaching movement to bring your hand into proximity with a coffee cup, neural populations in several other overlapping and adjacent parietal and precentral areas are preparing the hand to grasp and lift the cup. These areas include the anterior intraparietal area (AIP) and area PFG of the rostral inferior parietal cortex, the ventral premotor cortex, and the large central core of the arm's motor map in the primary motor cortex (see Figure 38–4B).

We have seen how the planning and control of the reaching movement involves a sequence of sensorimotor transformations that convert input about the spatial location of the coffee cup into a motor command to move the hand to the cup. The sensorimotor transformation involved in grasping the coffee cup is somewhat different. The sensorimotor system for the hand must possess a mechanism that can match the configuration of the hand and fingers and the grip forces exerted by the fingers to the physical properties of the cup. These include properties that you can see, such as the size, shape, and spatial orientation of the coffee cup. They can also include physical properties that have been learned through experience, such as the cup's expected weight and fragility and whether it contains hot or cold liquid. All of these factors influence how you use your hand to grasp and lift the cup.

To help understand how visual information about an object is transformed into specific movements to grasp and manipulate it, we shall speak of the *affordances* of an object, a concept introduced by James Gibson. When we observe an object our visual system automatically identifies the parts of it that allow for efficient manipulation of it. Those parts are not necessarily the features that permit recognition of the object, but rather those that afford specific opportunities for action. For example, the handle, body, and top of the coffee cup afford opportunities to grasp it. Any one affordance may be more appropriate in particular circumstances. If the cup is hot, for example, you will likely prefer to use the handle. If the handle is large, you may be able to insert all four fingers into it, but if it is small you may be able to use only one or two. If the coffee is not too hot, you may just as likely grasp the cup by its body or top.

Neurons in the Inferior Parietal Cortex Associate the Physical Properties of an Object with Specific Motor Acts

Beside being involved in the representation of space and the sensory guidance of reaching movements, the dorsal visual stream also provides the inferior parietal cortex with the visual information necessary for coding object affordances. The cortical processes that extract the affordances of observed objects and associate them with specific actions begin in the lateral and rostral part of the inferior parietal cortex, especially in the AIP and PFG areas (see Figure 38–4B).

The functional properties of neurons in AIP of the monkey have been investigated by Hideo Sakata and co-workers. They recorded the responses of neurons under three conditions: grasping objects in the light when they can be seen or in the dark when they cannot be seen, and merely observing the objects. The experiments showed that the neurons fall into three major categories: visually dominant, visuomotor, and motor-dominant neurons. Together these three classes of neurons contribute to neural operations that use visual input to encode the affordances of observed objects and associate them with appropriate motor acts.

Visual-dominant neurons discharge when the monkey fixates an object or grasps it in the light, but not when the monkey grasps an object in the dark (Figure 38–8). In contrast, *motor-dominant neurons* are active during grasping both in the light and in darkness. They are not active, however, during object fixation, indicating that they signal primarily the motor act of grasping, independent of visual input. Many visual-dominant and motor-dominant neurons respond selectively to objects of particular shapes such as spheres, rings, and flat disks, each of which requires a different type of grip.

Visuomotor neurons discharge when the monkey grasps objects, whether in the dark or in the light, but also during visual fixation. Individual visuomotor neurons additionally respond preferentially to shape: A neuron that becomes active when the monkey looks at a small disk also discharges when the monkey grasps the disk, but not when it grasps a sphere. This specificity to the shape of viewed objects indicates that these neurons link the affordances of an object to particular motor actions.

The Activity of Neurons of the Inferior Parietal Cortex Is Influenced by the Purpose of an Action

We often perform similar motor acts for different purposes. We pick up a coffee cup to drink from it or to wash it. The motor act of grasping is the same, but the objective is different.

As already noted, Mountcastle and Hyvärinen reported that the activation of many parietal neurons depends on the goal of the act being performed. More recently, Leonardo Fogassi and co-workers compared the firing patterns of grasp-related inferior parietal neurons under two conditions. In one the monkey grasped a piece of food and brought it to its mouth; in the other it placed the food into a container. The activity of many of the neurons varied with the task. Some were strongly active when the monkey picked up food

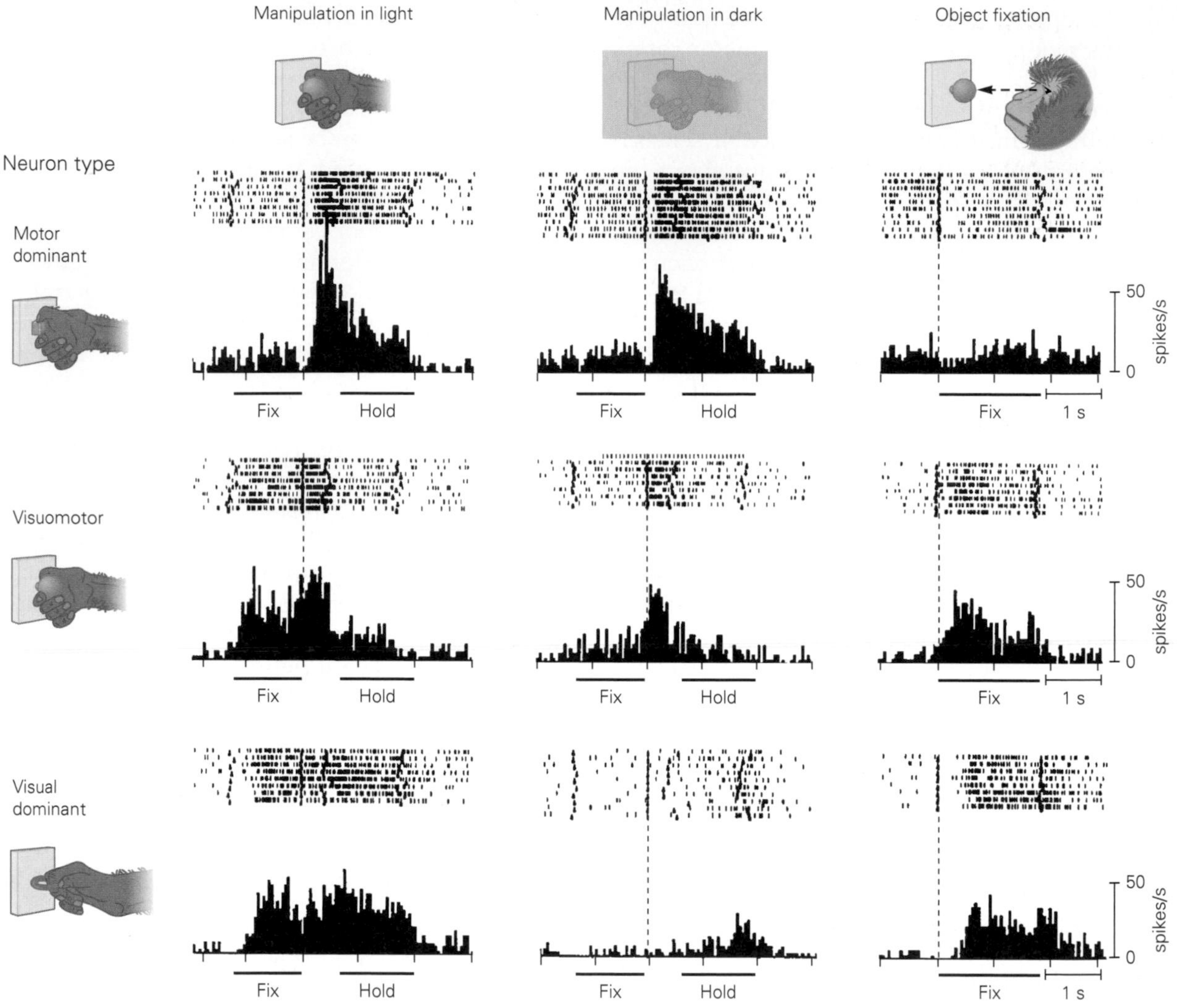

Figure 38–8 The three major categories of neurons in the anterior intraparietal area. A monkey sits in front of a dark box housing six distinct objects that are presented one at a time in a random order. Neural activity is tested during three behaviors: manipulation of the object in light, manipulation in the dark, and object fixation. The protocol for the manipulation in light begins with a red spot of light projected onto the object. The monkey fixates the spot of light and presses a lever that turns on a light inside the box that illuminates the object. After the monkey has held the lever for 1.0–1.2 s, the light changes to green, cuing the monkey to release the lever and grasp the object. In the records shown here trials are aligned at the end of the visual fixation period and beginning of the reach-to-grasp period. The protocol for manipulation in the dark is similar except that all trials after the first are executed in darkness. In the object fixation protocol the green light cues the monkey to fixate the red spot of light and press the lever to illuminate the object; the animal then releases the lever but does not grasp the object. Trials are aligned at the beginning of the fixation period. The activity of different anterior intraparietal neurons shows differing degrees of dependence on the visual and motor components of this task. (Modified, with permission, from Murata et al. 2000.)

to bring it to the mouth, but only weakly excited when it picked up food to put it into a container. Others showed the opposite response (Figure 38–9). Factors such as grasping force, kinematics of reaching movements, and type of stimulus could not account for the context-specific activation of the neurons.

The Activity of Neurons in the Ventral Premotor Cortex Correlates with Motor Acts

The rostral part of the ventral premotor cortex, often called area F5, is reciprocally connected with the anterior intraparietal area, the rostral part of the inferior parietal cortex, and the secondary somatosensory area. Functional mapping of area F5 based on electrical stimulation shows that this area contains representations of hand and mouth movements that overlap considerably.

Recording studies in monkeys indicate that the response properties of F5 neurons are elaborations of the properties of neurons in the parietal regions that project into area F5. Unlike the anterior intraparietal area, however, F5 contains few or no visually dominant neurons. Murata and colleagues found that many neurons in area F5 discharge exclusively during the execution of certain motor acts, both in the light and in the dark. About 20% of the neurons, called *canonical neurons*, also

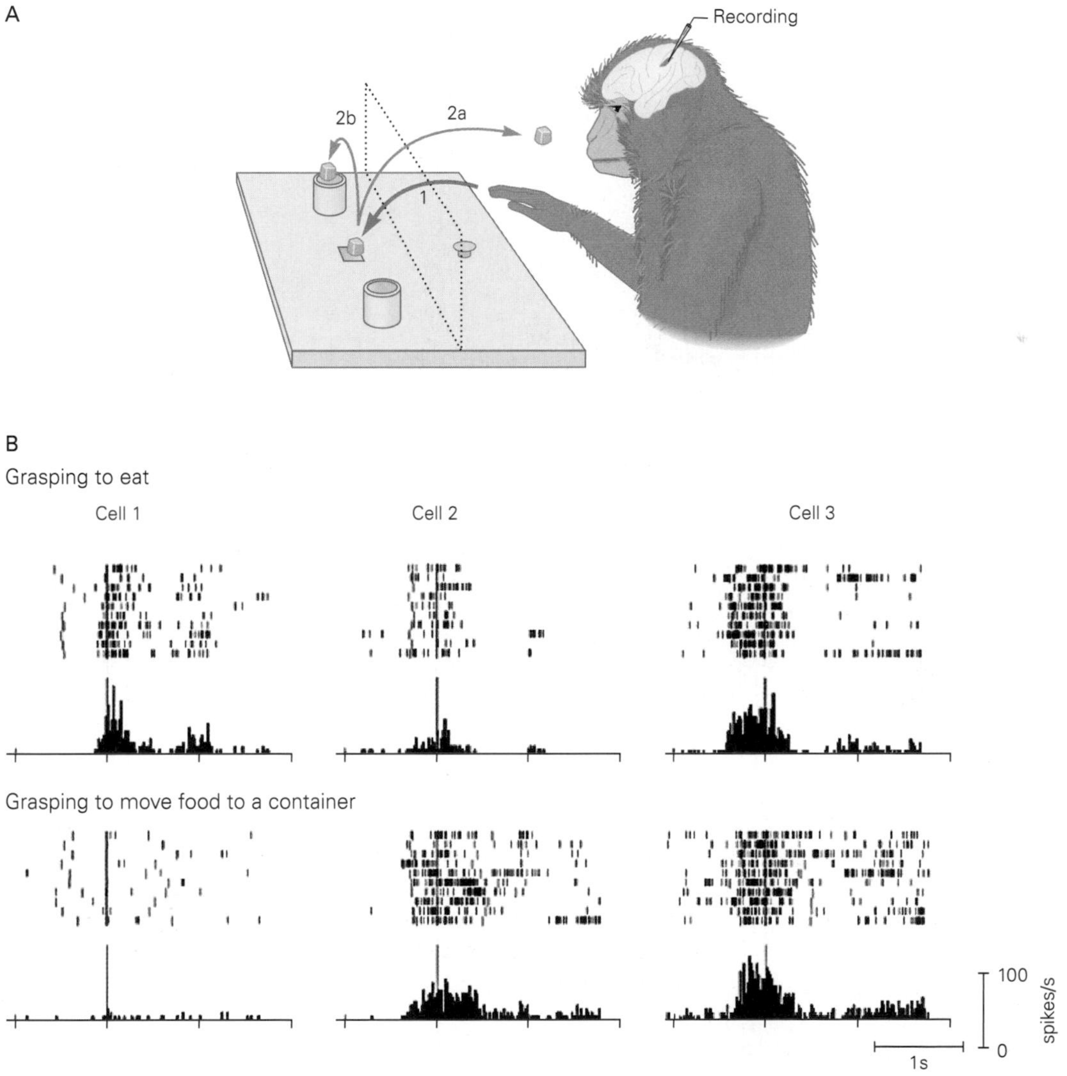

Figure 38–9 The activity of functionally distinct parietal motor neurons varies with the purpose of a grasping action. (Modified, with permission, from Fogassi et al. 2005.)

A. Apparatus and protocol for the experiment. A monkey is trained to press a button (start position) and reach and grasp a piece of food (**1**) either to bring it to the mouth (**2a**) or to place it into a container (**2b**). In the first condition the monkey eats the food brought to the mouth, whereas in the second it receives a food reward after the correct response.

B. Activity of three neurons in the inferior parietal cortex during the two actions. Cell 1 discharges more strongly when the monkey grasps the food to eat it than when it grasps the food simply to move it. The behavior of cell 2 is the opposite. Cell 3 shows no difference between the two actions. Raster plots and histograms are aligned with the moment when the monkey touches the object to be grasped. **Orange tics** indicate when the monkey releases its hand from the button at the starting position; **green tics** indicate when the hand touches the container.

respond to the sight of three-dimensional objects. They thus discharge whether the animal grasps an object or simply observes it and they show a preference for a particular type of grip (Figure 38–10).

The signal from a canonical neuron is identical whether the monkey observes or grasps an object. Thus when the cell is activated by the sight of an object, its activity signifies how to interact with the object. The activation of a canonical neuron does not automatically lead to overt action, for inhibitory control is exerted by other neural circuits. Only when that inhibition is released does the internal representation become an overt action.

Another fundamental property of area F5 neurons is that their discharge correlates with the goal of a motor act and not with the individual movements forming it. Thus many neurons in F5 discharge when grasping is executed with effectors as different as the right hand, the left hand, and even the mouth. Conversely, an area F5 neuron may be active when an

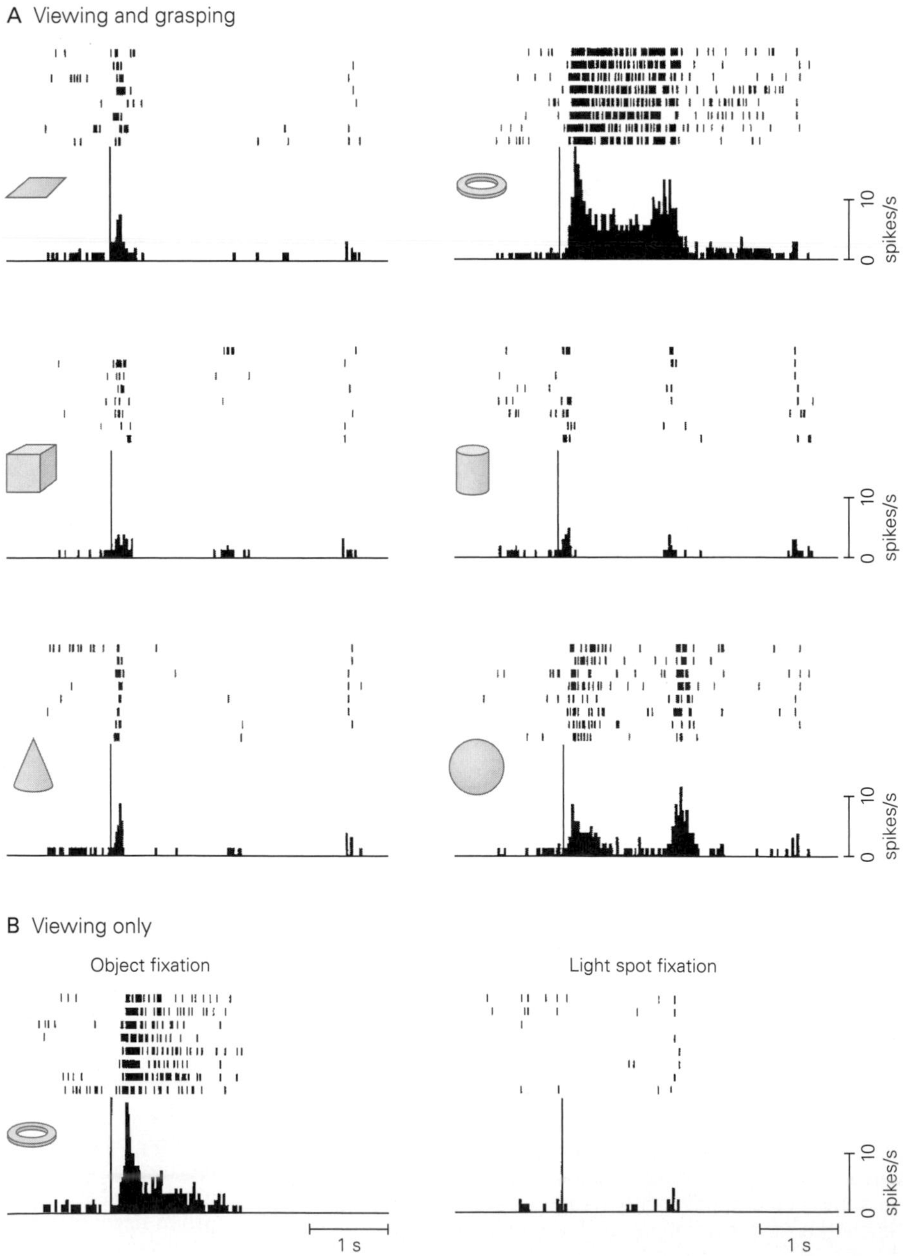

Figure 38–10 A canonical neuron in the ventral premotor cortex (area F5) of a monkey. (Reproduced, with permission, from Murata et al. 1997.)

A. The neuron's responses to viewing and grasping of six objects vary with the shape of the objects. The cell is more strongly activated by a ring-shaped object than by other shapes.

B. The neuron responds when the animal fixates a ring-shaped object but not when the animal fixates a light spot. Raster plots and histograms are aligned (**vertical bar**) with the moment when the object becomes visible.

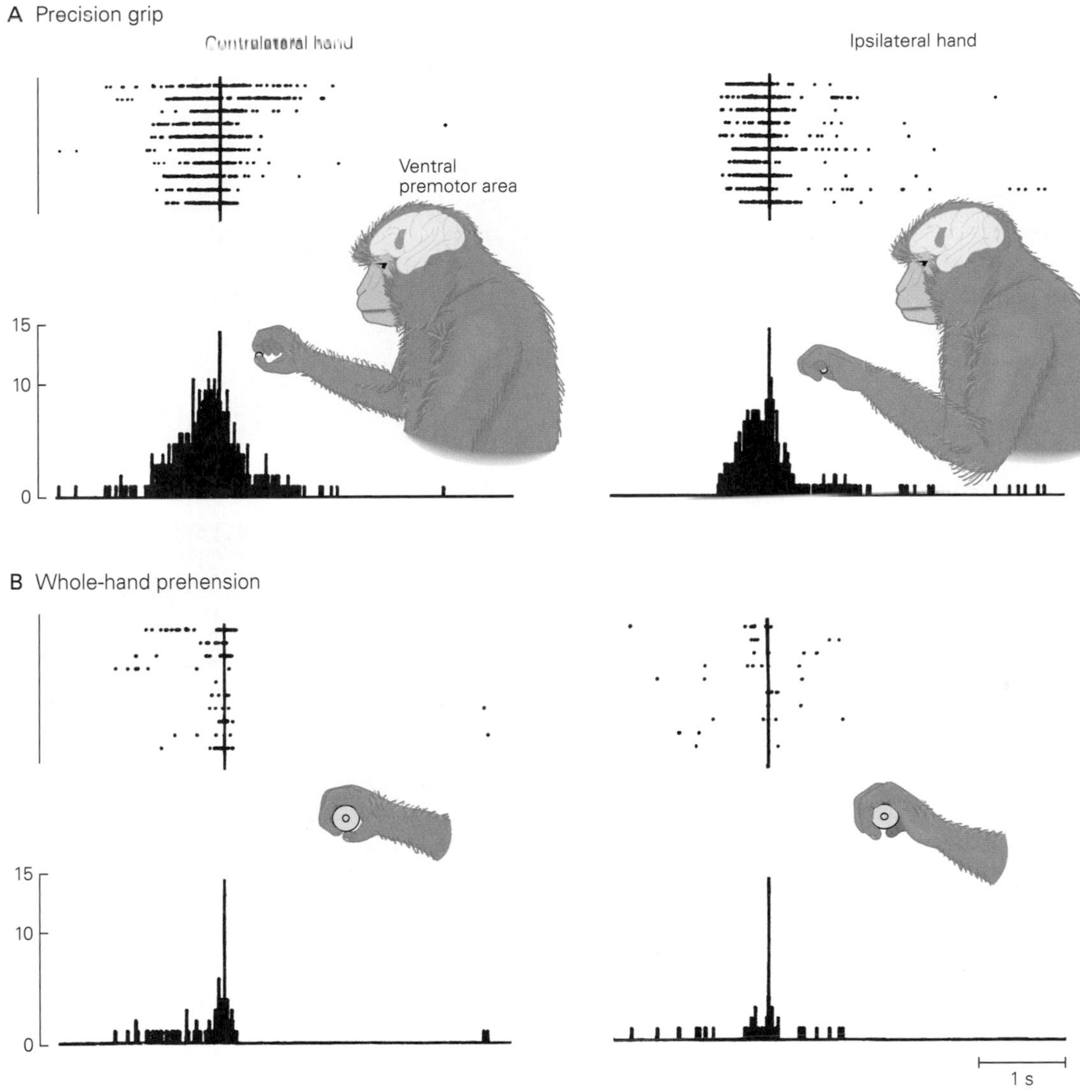

Figure 38–11 Some individual neurons in the ventral premotor cortex (area F5) of a monkey discharge selectively during one type of grasping. This neuron discharges vigorously during precision grip with either the right or the left hand but barely at all during whole-hand prehension with either hand. Raster plots and histograms are aligned (vertical line) with the moment the monkey touches the food (**A**) or grasps the handle (**B**). (Reproduced, with permission, from Rizzolatti et al. 1988.)

index finger is flexed to grasp an object but not when the animal flexes the same finger to scratch itself. This property of grasp-related neurons in area F5 resembles that of many reach-related neurons in the dorsal premotor cortex.

Based on these properties, Giacomo Rizzolatti and co-workers subdivided F5 neurons into several functional classes that discharge preferentially during certain stereotypical hand actions, such as grasping, holding, tearing, or manipulating objects. In each of these classes many neurons discharge only if the monkey uses a specific type of grip, such as precision grip, whole-hand prehension, or finger prehension (Figure 38–11). Precision grip is the type most represented. Moreover, individual F5 neurons may discharge selectively at particular stages of one type of prehension. Some discharge throughout the entire action, others during the opening of the fingers, and still others during finger closure.

The view that the organization of area F5 is based on a repertory of motor acts has important implications. First, the existence of neurons that encode a limited range of specific motor acts is consistent with and may account for the fact that we repeatedly interact with a particular object in a specific way. There exists in principle a very large number of possible ways to grasp an object, but we typically use only a few of them. We almost never use the fourth and fifth fingers to lift a cup of coffee, for example. The organization of area F5 allows the object affordances extracted by the anterior intraparietal area to be associated with appropriate motor actions. As we shall see later, this organization may also underlie the ability to recognize the goals of actions performed by others.

The Primary Motor Cortex Transforms a Grasping Action Plan into Appropriate Finger Movements

The ventral premotor cortex, including areas F4 and F5, projects to the hand and arm fields of the primary motor cortex. The primary motor cortex contains the largest and most detailed representation of finger and hand movements of all cortical motor areas (see Chapter 37).

Although some hand-related neurons in the primary motor cortex discharge in relation to the goal of a motor act rather than to specific movements, many others are active during finger or wrist movements across a broad range of grasping motions and object manipulation as well as during other activities. The grasp-selective input from premotor areas could facilitate the recruitment and organization of a set of neurons distributed across the motor map that controls a particular grasping action and matches it to an object's shape (Figure 38–12).

A

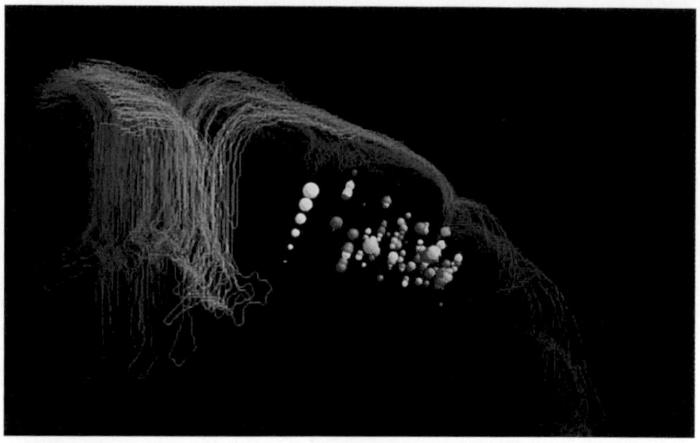

B

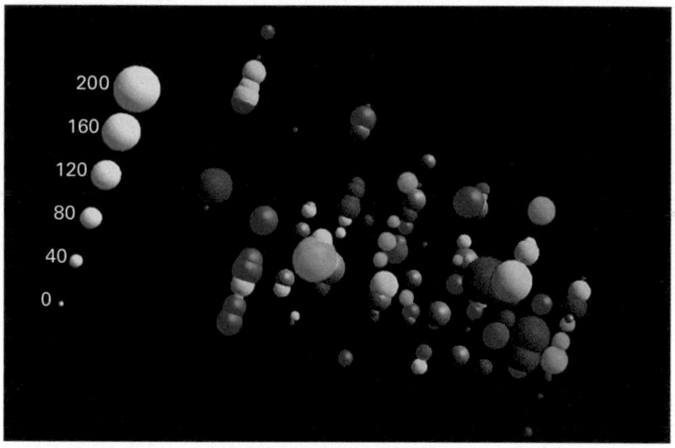

Figure 38–12 Neurons that control the movement of individual fingers are distributed throughout the hand-control area of the primary motor cortex. (Reproduced, with permission, from Schieber and Hibbard 1993.)

A. A view of the frontal pole of the monkey's cerebral cortex shows the interhemispheric fissure and lateral convexity. The colored spheres represent the locations of single neurons in the hand-control region of the primary motor cortex from which recordings were made.

B. The same data at a higher magnification. Neurons that discharge preferentially during isolated movements of individual digits and the wrist are represented by different colors. As shown by the scale at the left, the diameter of a sphere indicates a neuron's change in firing frequency (spikes per second). Neurons that are most active for a particular digit or for the wrist are not grouped together but instead are distributed throughout the hand-control area of the primary motor cortex.

During grasping, hand muscles must exert gripping forces perpendicular to the surface of the object to secure it between the fingers without slippage and to overcome the load forces imposed by gravity. Many neurons in the primary motor cortex are very sensitive to sensory feedback from somatic receptors in the hand that signal deformations of the skin perpendicular to the skin's surface. These cells are ideally organized to provide feedback control of grip and load forces during grasping and manipulation of an object.

In summary, when you look at your cup of coffee, neurons in the inferior parietal cortex, especially in the anterior intraparietal area, begin signaling the cup's affordances. These affordances are linked with specific grip representations in the parietal cortex and in the ventral premotor cortex. This activity is not sufficient to initiate grasping. Other areas controlling the initiation of action must also become active to allow the action represented in area F5 to be executed. When this occurs F5 neurons activate primary motor cortex neurons that control independent finger movements and spinal motor neurons and interneurons involved in hand opening and closing. Finally, as your hand touches the cup's handle, sensory feedback provides the somatosensory information necessary for forming and maintaining a stable grip.

This picture of grip generation is very schematic. It does not take into consideration the activity of reciprocal connections from the primary motor cortex to premotor areas and from there to the associated parietal areas. Even more important, we have focused exclusively on the cortical mechanisms responsible for action generation, leaving aside the important contributions of the cerebellum and basal ganglia (see Chapters 42 and 43).

The Supplementary Motor Complex Plays a Crucial Role in Selecting and Executing Appropriate Voluntary Actions

Classical electrical-stimulation studies of motor regions of the cortex showed that the medial wall of the frontal cortex contains a map of contralateral body movements (see Chapter 37). This region was initially called the supplementary motor area. Today there is agreement that this region contains two areas that have distinct cytoarchitectonic characteristics, connections, and functional properties: a more caudal supplementary motor area (SMA) proper and a more rostral presupplementary motor area (pre-SMA), which we will collectively call the supplementary motor complex (SMC).

The motor map in SMA covers the entire contralateral body but is not as detailed as the motor map in the primary motor cortex. Neurons in SMA require strong stimulus currents to evoke movements, which are often complex actions such as postural adjustments or stepping and climbing and can involve both sides of the body. Such movements are rarely evoked by stimulation of the primary motor cortex. In humans stimulation of the SMC below the threshold for movement initiation sometimes evokes an urge to move. Lesions of the SMC do not result in paralysis but do produce problems initiating or suppressing movement (Box 38–2).

The results of stimulation and lesion studies of the SMC indicate that motor centers outside of the primary motor cortex have a role in motor control. Further support for this idea emerged from studies of humans using evoked potentials. Recordings of slow cortical potentials from motor areas during the execution of self-generated movements showed that a slow potential arises in the frontal cortex 0.8 s to 1.0 s before the onset of movement. This signal, named the *readiness potential,* has its peak in the medial part of the precentral motor region over the SMC. Because it occurs well before movement, the readiness potential provides evidence that this region is involved in forming the intention to move, not just in movement execution.

Neurons in both the SMA and pre-SMA discharge before and during voluntary movements. There is a gradient in response properties across each area. Recent studies have indicated that much of the higher-order control of motor behavior originally attributed to SMA proper actually reflects the contribution of the

Box 38–2 Neurological Disorders Affect the Initiation and Suppression of Voluntary Behavior

Lesions of the supplementary motor area, presupplementary motor area, and prefrontal areas connected with them produce deficiencies in the initiation and release of movements.

Initiation deficits manifest themselves as loss of self-initiated arm movements, even though the patient can move when adequately prompted. This deficit can involve contralesional parts of the body (*akinesia*) and speech (*mutism*).

Release phenomena, in contrast, include a large variety of behaviors that patients cannot suppress when inappropriate. These include compulsive grasping of a stimulus when the hand touches it (*forced grasping*), irrepressible reaching and searching movements aimed at an object that has been presented visually (*groping movement*), and impulsive arm and hand movements to grab nearby objects and even people without conscious awareness of the intention to do so (*alien-* or *anarchic-hand* syndromes).

Particularly interesting is the syndrome known as *utilization behavior,* in which a patient compulsively grabs objects and uses them without consideration of need or the social situation. Examples are picking up and putting on multiple pairs of glasses or reaching for and eating food even when the individual is not hungry or when the food is clearly part of someone else's meal.

These deficits in the initiation and suppression of actions may represent opposite facets of the same functional role for the supplementary motor area and especially the presupplementary motor area in the conditional control of voluntary behavior.

pre-SMA. Unlike neurons in the primary motor cortex, the activity of most SMA neurons is less tightly coupled to particular actions of a specific part of the body and instead appears to be associated with more complex, coordinated motor acts of the hand, arm, head, or trunk.

In contrast, pre-SMA neurons often begin to discharge long before movement onset, are less tightly coupled to the execution of movements, and show an even more context-dependent relation to impending movements. For example, when tested in the same conditions used to study reach- and grasp-related activity in the parietal and ventral premotor cortex, the activity of pre-SMA neurons is less coupled to distinct actions of the hand or arm than neurons in the other regions, but is instead related to the overall act of reaching to grasp and manipulate objects.

Some pre-SMA neurons begin to discharge when a graspable object appears anywhere in the monkey's field of view and increase firing as the object moves within reach. Others are initially inhibited when the object appears but begin to discharge as soon as it moves within reach. Some neurons discharge during the actual reach-to-grasp movement, whereas others are inhibited. Although the patterns of response may vary, what remains constant is that changes in firing rate depend on whether an object can or cannot be acted upon. The pre-SMA may therefore contain a system that controls the execution of motor acts that are encoded in more lateral parietal-precentral circuits.

Many different roles in voluntary behavior have been attributed to the SMC, and its contribution remains controversial. One popular hypothesis was that the SMC is concerned with self-generated or internally guided behavior, whereas the dorsal and ventral premotor cortex primarily controls externally guided behavior. However, recent single-neuron studies do not support that functional dichotomy.

The SMC has been implicated in the organization and execution of movement sequences. Tanji and coworkers showed that some SMC neurons discharge before the performance of a particular sequence of three movements but not before a different sequence of the same movements (Figure 38–13). Other neurons discharge when a particular movement occurs in a specific position in a sequence or when a particular pair of consecutive movements occurs regardless of their order. Some SMC neurons encode the position of a movement in a sequence independently of the nature of the act or of how many movements remain to be executed before a reward is delivered.

Still other studies have suggested that the SMC is primarily concerned with the acquisition of certain motor skills and less with their performance. Finally, the SMC has been implicated in the so-called *executive control* of behavior, such as the operations that are required to switch between different actions, plans, and strategies. For example, some SMC neurons discharge strongly when a subject receives a sensory cue instructing it to change movement targets or to suppress a previously intended movement.

These seemingly disparate behaviors may reflect a more general role of the SMC in *contextual control* of voluntary behavior. Contextual control is concerned with selecting and executing actions deemed appropriate on the basis of different combinations of internal and external cues as well as withholding inappropriate actions. Such control also situates a particular action in a goal-directed sequence or in a specific environmental and social context.

The Cortical Motor System Is Involved in Planning Action

So far we have focused on the role of cortical motor areas in the sensorimotor transformations required to reach for and grasp an object. However, voluntary behavior is not always directed specifically at objects or shaped by their physical properties. It is often determined by long-term goals and social conventions and may involve choosing from among alternative actions.

Furthermore, like the supplementary motor complex, many cortical areas implicated in the sensorimotor control of reaching and grasping also contribute to the choice of action. Neurons in these areas are involved not only in choosing particular actions but even in setting and applying the rules on which those choices are based.

Cortical Motor Areas Apply the Rules That Govern Behavior

Behavior is often guided by rules that link specific symbolic cues to particular actions. When driving your car you must perform different actions depending on whether a traffic light is green, yellow, or red. In monkeys that have learned to associate arbitrary cues with specific movements, many cells in the motor and premotor cortices respond selectively to specific cues.

This activity is dependent on the nature of the selection rule. In monkeys that have been trained to choose between several possible movements based on a spatial rule (an icon's location) or a semantic rule (an icon's designated meaning), many neurons in

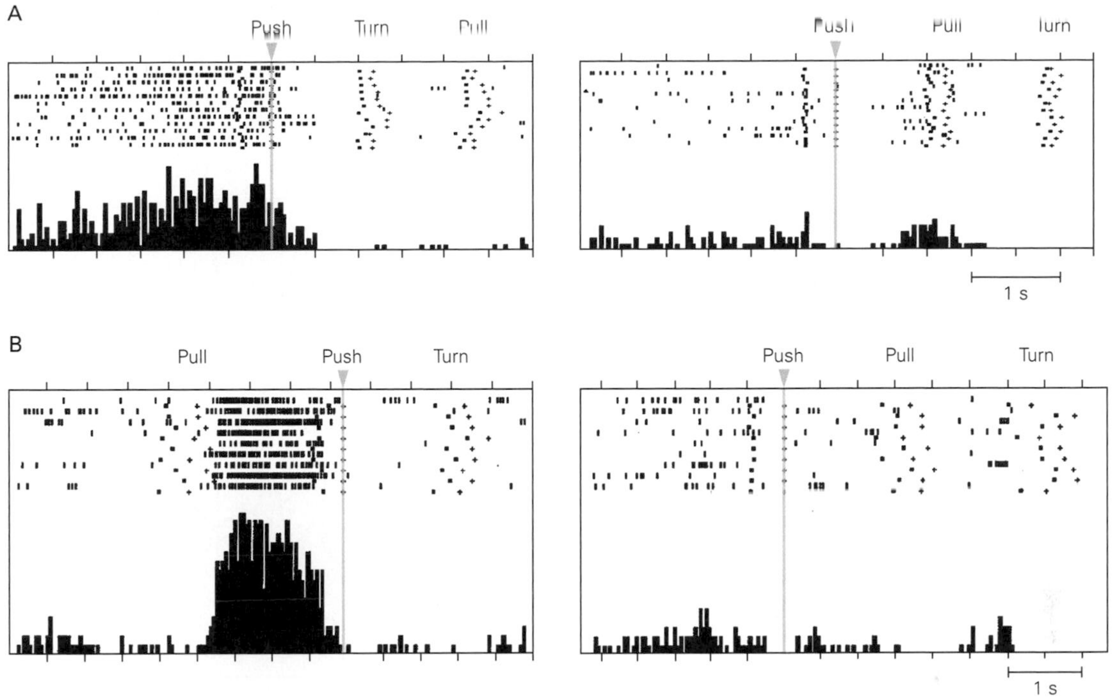

Figure 38–13 Some neurons in the supplementary motor complex encode a specific sequence of motor acts. (Modified, with permission, from Tanji 2001.)

A. A neuron discharges selectively during the waiting period before the first movement of the memorized sequence push-turn-pull (left panel). The cell remains relatively silent, however, when the sequence is push-pull-turn (right panel), even though the first movement in both sequences is the same. Triangles at the top of each raster plot indicate the start of the first movement.

B. Records of a neuron whose activity increases selectively during the interval between completion of one motor act, a pull, and the initiation of another act, a push. The cell is not active when a push is the first movement in the sequence, or when pull is followed by turn.

both prefrontal and premotor cortices are more active when the animal chooses a movement using one rule but not the other. This strong correlation of neuronal responses with the selection rule shows that both prefrontal and premotor cortices use concrete rules to interpret behaviorally salient sensory inputs and associate them with appropriate actions. Such neuronal activity is related not to the identity of the sensory input or the chosen action but to the association between them.

Cortical motor areas are involved in the implementation of even very abstract rules. Jonathan Wallis and Earl Miller trained monkeys to decide whether to make a particular hand movement (a *go/no-go decision*). In each trial the monkey first had to make a perceptual decision whether the two images were the same or different. In some trials the animal was required to move its hand if the images were identical and to refrain from movement if they differed; in other trials the rule was reversed (a *match/nonmatch decision*) after viewing sequential pairs of complex images. The animal therefore had to make two decisions, one perceptual and the other behavioral, neither of which had any a priori significance.

Neural populations in both the prefrontal and dorsal premotor cortices generated activity that correlated with either the perceptual or the behavioral decision (Figure 38–14). Neuronal correlates of the perceptual decision were more prominent in the prefrontal cortex, whereas correlates of the behavioral decision were stronger in the dorsal premotor cortex. Most strikingly, however, activity correlated with the perceptual choice was stronger and occurred earlier in the dorsal premotor cortex than in the prefrontal cortex. These results suggest that the dorsal premotor cortex has a major role in applying rules that govern the appropriateness of a behavior and in making decisions about movement according to the prevailing rules.

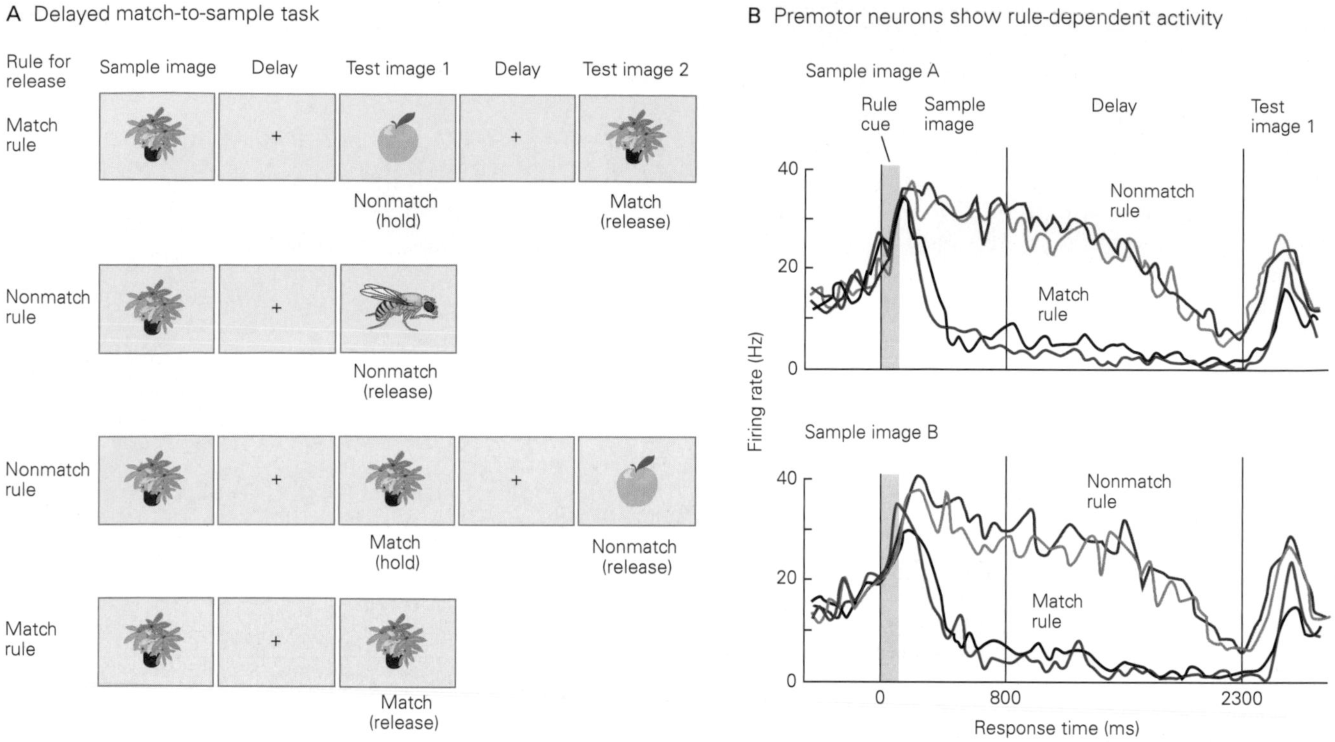

Figure 38–14 Premotor cortex neurons choose particular voluntary behaviors based on decisional rules. (Reproduced, with permission, from Wallis and Miller 2003.)

A. A monkey must make a decision about whether to release a lever or keep holding it based on two prior decisions: a perceptual choice, whether a test image is the same as or different from a sample image presented earlier, and a behavioral choice, whether the current rule is to release the lever when the test image is the same as the sample (match rule) or when it is different (nonmatch rule). The monkey is informed of the behavioral rule that applies in each trial by a rule cue, such as an auditory tone or juice drops, which is presented for 100 ms at the same time as the onset of the sample image.

B. A neuron in the dorsal premotor cortex has a higher discharge rate whenever the nonmatch rule is in effect during the delay between the presentation of the first and second images. The top and bottom sets of responses were recorded from the same cell in trials with different sample images, indicating that the rule-dependent activity is not altered by changing the images. Nor, as shown by the pairs of differently colored histograms associated with each rule, does activity depend on the type of rule cue (auditory tone or juice drops). Other dorsal premotor cortex cells (not shown) respond preferentially to the match rule over the nonmatch rule. The differential activity of the neuron up to presentation of the test image reflects the nature of the rule that will guide the animal's motor response to the test image, not the physical nature of the visual stimuli or the motor response.

The Premotor Cortex Contributes to Perceptual Decisions That Guide Motor Behavior

An elegant series of studies by Ranulfo Romo and his colleagues provides further evidence that cortical motor areas contain not only representations of the sensory information that guides voluntary movements but also the neuronal operations necessary to act on perceptual decisions. Although intuitively it may seem that perceptual processes are completely outside the domain of motor control, Romo's results indicate otherwise.

A monkey was trained to discriminate the difference in frequency between two brief vibratory stimuli applied to one finger and separated in time by a few seconds. The animal had to decide whether the frequency of the second stimulus was higher or lower than the first and to report the perceptual decision by making one of two movements with the other hand.

The decision-making process in this task can be conceived as a chain of neural operations: encode the first stimulus frequency (f1) when it is presented; maintain a representation of f1 in working memory during the interval between the two stimuli; encode the second stimulus frequency (f2) when it is presented; compare f2 to the memory trace of f1; decide whether the frequency of f2 is higher or lower than that of f1; and, finally, use that decision to choose the appropriate movement of the other hand. Everything prior to the last step would appear to fall entirely within the domain of sensory processing.

While the monkeys performed the task, neurons in the primary (S-I) and secondary (S-II) somatosensory cortices encoded the frequencies of the stimuli as they were presented. During the interval between f1 and f2 there was no sustained activity in S-I representing the memorized f1 and only a transient representation in S-II that vanished before f2 was presented.

Strikingly, however, many neurons in the prefrontal cortex, supplementary motor complex, and ventral premotor cortex encoded the f1 and f2 frequencies. Furthermore, some of the prefrontal and premotor neurons that encoded the frequency of f1 sustained their activity during the delay period between f1 and f2 (Figure 38–15). Most remarkably, many neurons in those areas, especially the ventral premotor cortex, encoded the *difference* in frequency between f2 and f1 independently of their actual frequencies. This centrally generated signal is appropriate to mediate the perceptual discrimination that determined the corresponding motor response. Neurons that encoded the f2–f1 difference were absent in S-I and were far more common in the supplementary motor complex and ventral premotor cortex than in S-II.

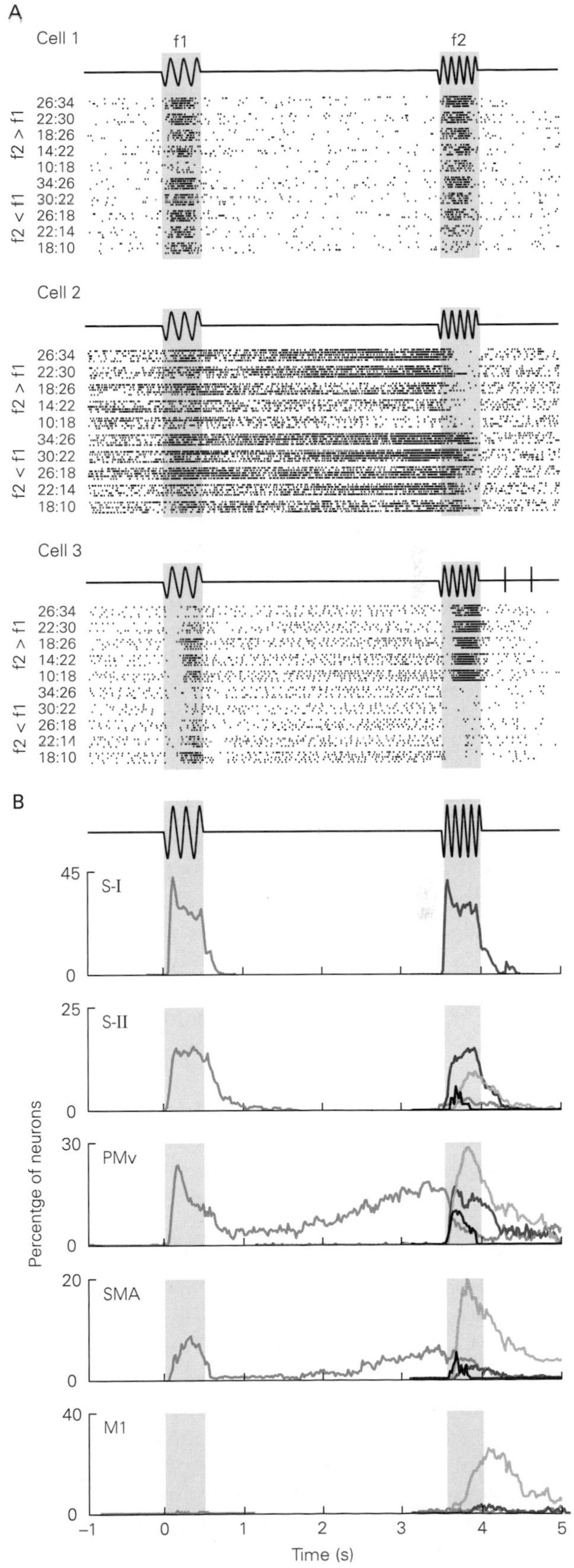

Figure 38–15 The ventral premotor cortex contains the operations required to choose a motor response based on sensory information. (Modified, with permission, from Romo, Hernandez, and Zainos 2004.)

A. These records of three neurons in the ventral premotor cortex of a monkey were made while the animal performed a task in which it had to decide whether the second of two vibration stimuli (f1 and f2, applied to the index finger of one hand) was of higher or lower frequency than the first. The choice was signaled by pushing one of two buttons with the nonstimulated hand. The frequencies of f1 and f2 are indicated by the numbers on the left of each set of raster plots. Cell 1 encoded the frequencies of both f1 and f2 while the stimuli were being presented but was not active at any other time. This response profile resembles that of many neurons in the primary somatosensory cortex. Cell 2 encoded the frequency of f1 and sustained its response during the delay period. During the presentation of f2 the neuron's response was enhanced when f1 exceeded f2 and suppressed when f2 exceeded f1. Cell 3 responded to f1 during stimulation and was weakly active during the delay period. However, during exposure to f2 the cell's activity explicitly signaled the difference f2–f1 independently of the specific frequencies f1 and f2.

B. The histograms show the percentage of neurons in different cortical areas whose activity correlated at each instant with different parameters during the tactile discrimination task. **Green** shows the correlation with f1, **red** the correlation with f2, **black** the interaction between f1and f2, and **blue** the correlation with the difference between f2–f1. (**S-I**, primary somatosensory cortex; **S-II**, secondary somatosensory cortex; **PMv**, ventral premotor cortex; **SMA**, supplementary motor area; **M1**, primary motor cortex.)

The premotor cortex activity that encodes, stores, and compares f1 and f2 does not necessarily contribute to the sensations evoked by the tactile stimuli. Nevertheless, these experiments show dramatically that premotor cortex contains prominent representations of selected sensory information and the neuronal operations required to make a perceptual decision prior to choosing a motor action.

The Premotor Cortex Is Involved in Learning Motor Skills

The premotor cortex has been implicated in the acquisition of new motor skills. Steven Wise and his colleagues recorded from neurons in the dorsal premotor cortex of a monkey while the animal learned a rule for associating unfamiliar visual cues with different directions of movement. Although an experienced monkey's choices were initially random, the animal could learn the rules within a few dozen trials.

Even though the monkey made an arm movement in response to each cue, many dorsal premotor neurons were only weakly active during the early, guessing phase of learning. Their activity gradually increased as the animal learned which cue signaled which movement. Other neurons showed a reciprocal decline in activity as the rules were acquired. These changes in activity reflected not only the movement choices but also the knowledge of the rule linking cues with actions.

These findings demonstrate that different cortical areas are involved in the acquisition of new motor skills and the recall of well-practiced skills. The role of cortical areas can change as new skills become motor habits that presumably require less attention, monitoring of performance, and feedback control.

Cortical Motor Areas Contribute to Understanding the Observed Actions of Others

Premotor and parietal areas may be active when no overt action is intended, such as when an individual is asked to imagine performing a certain motor act or when he observes someone else performing an action.

The first condition, termed *motor imagery,* has been demonstrated in humans by functional brain imaging. When an individual follows the instruction "imagine yourself performing a specific action," the premotor and parietal cortex and even the primary motor cortices become active even though no overt act occurs. If the instruction is "imagine observing yourself performing an action as in a picture and not as an acting individual," the motor system is only weakly activated and activation of visual centers prevails. Motor imagery is interpreted by the brain as preparation to act disassociated from motor execution.

The second condition in which cortical motor circuits are activated is when an individual observes another individual performing motor acts that belong to his own motor repertory. The control of behavior and social interaction depends greatly on the ability to recognize and understand what others are doing and why they are doing it. Such understanding could of course come from visual analysis of the stimuli and subsequent inferential reasoning. An alternative interpretation of actions done by others is the *direct matching hypothesis,* according to which observation of the actions of others activates the motor circuits responsible for similar motor actions by the observer. This empathetic activation of motor circuits would provide a link between the observed actions and the observer's stored knowledge of the nature, motives, and consequences of his own corresponding actions.

Compelling evidence in support of the direct-matching hypothesis was provided when Rizzolatti and colleagues discovered a remarkable population of neurons in area F5 of the ventral premotor cortex. These so-called *mirror neurons* discharge both when the monkey performs a motor act and when it observes a similar act performed by another monkey or by the experimenter (Figure 38–16).

Mirror neurons do not respond when a monkey simply observes an object or when it observes mimed arm and hand actions without a target object. Because each of us understands the causes and outcomes of our own motor acts, the direct-matching hypothesis proposes that the activity of mirror neurons during observation of the actions of others provides a mechanism of transforming complex visual inputs into a high-level understanding of the observed actions.

Other experiments with monkeys have provided further evidence that mirror neurons become active whenever an individual recognizes and understands the motor acts of others. For example, a noisy action such as ripping paper or cracking open a peanut can be recognized from its sound without direct visual observation. Many area F5 mirror neurons respond to such sounds in the absence of visual input. Some F5 neurons selectively discharge when the monkey observes the act of grasping an object with the hand. When the target object is obscured by a screen, some of those mirror neurons discharge as the hand approaches the hidden object and continue to respond while the hand is behind the screen. If the monkey is first shown that there is no object behind the screen, however, those same neurons remain silent when the hand disappears

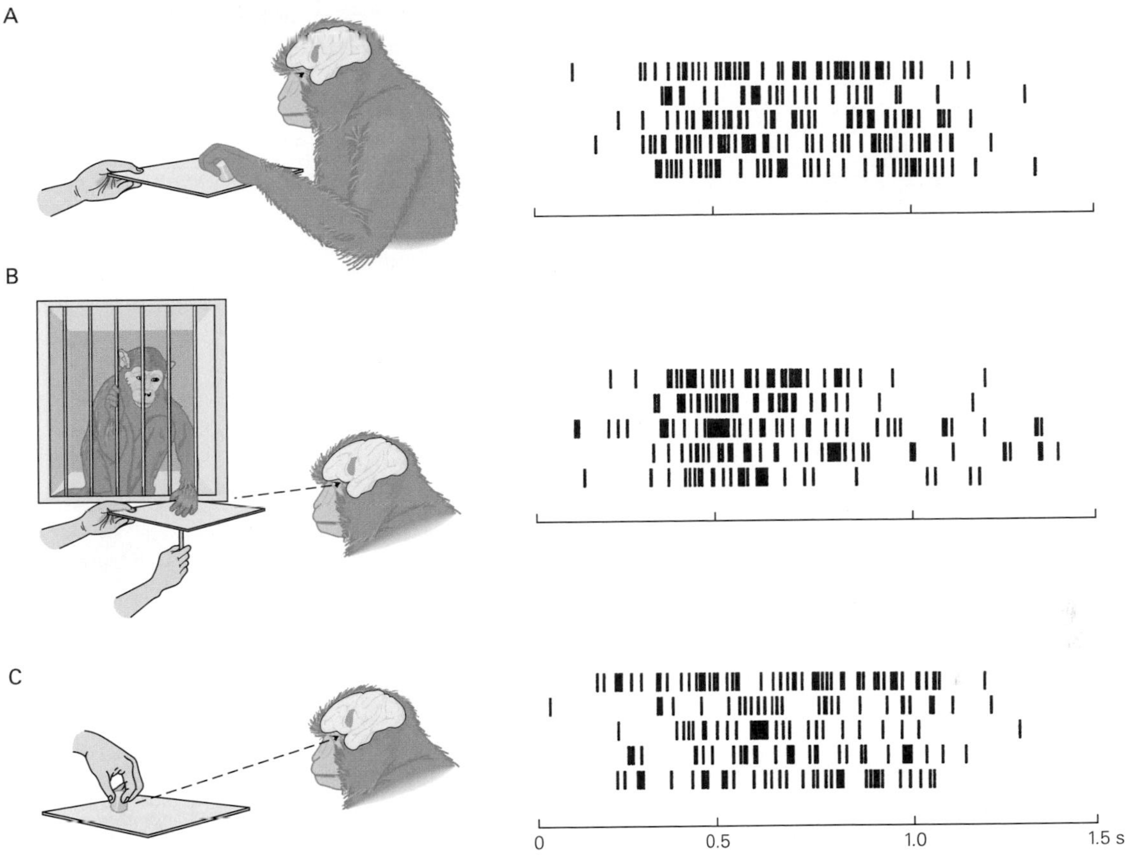

Figure 38–16 A mirror neuron in the ventral premotor cortex (area F5). (Reproduced, with permission, from Rizzolatti et al. 1996.)

A. The neuron is active when the monkey grasps an object.

B. The same neuron is also excited when the monkey observes another monkey grasping the object.

C. The neuron is similarly activated when the monkey observes the human experimenter grasping the object.

behind the screen. This result suggests that mirror neurons generate an internal representation of the action even when it is not visible.

Although area F5 receives no direct input from visual areas, the rostral intraparietal cortex that projects to it receives visual input from the superior temporal sulcus, a region that encodes high-level visual information but is devoid of motor signals. Some neurons in the rostral intraparietal lobule have properties similar to F5 mirror neurons. They discharge more strongly when the monkey observes motor acts that have a particular goal, for example grasping food to eat it but not simply to move it (Figure 38–17). This type of coding indicates that when the monkey understands the intention behind an observed action, it is able to predict the next motor action.

Neurophysiological and brain-imaging studies show that humans too are endowed with the mirror mechanism, matching observed actions with actions encoded in their motor system. This mechanism is located in various areas including the rostral inferior parietal lobule, intraparietal sulcus, ventral premotor cortex, and the posterior sector of the inferior frontal gyrus. Recent studies suggest that defects in the human mirror-neuron system contribute to some of the symptoms of autism. Whereas the motor system of a normally developing child is activated when he observes another person performing an action, this activation is lacking in children with autism. As a result, autistic children may lack the neuronal mechanism that normally mediates direct, experiential understanding of the intentions of others. Autistic children who are able to understand the behavior of others are thought to use cognitive inferential processes to compensate for the lack of a functional mirror-neuron system.

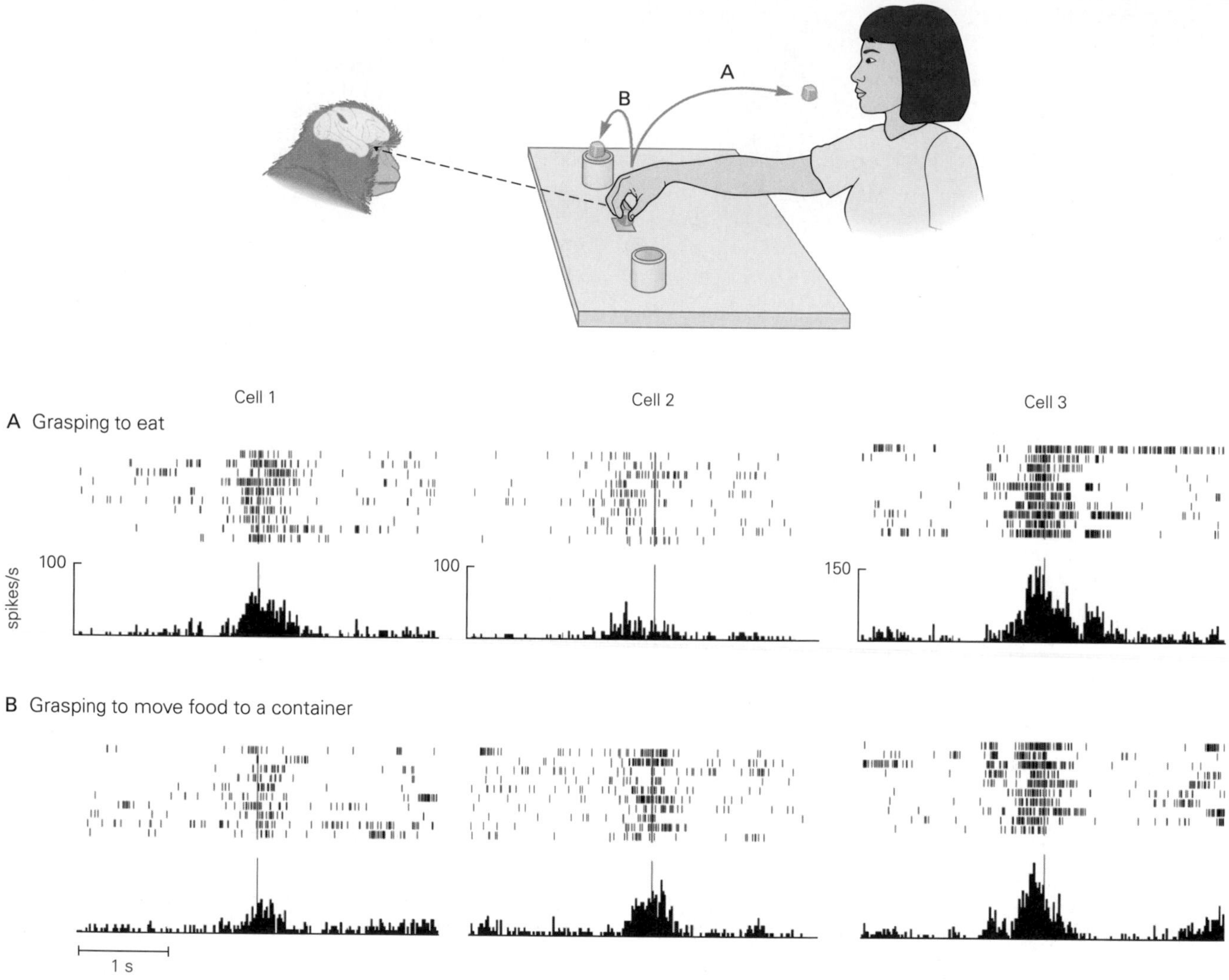

Figure 38–17 Mirror neurons in the inferior parietal cortex of a monkey are activated when the monkey observes a motor act. A monkey observes the experimenter perform the same grasping action to bring food to the mouth (**A**) or to place it into a container (**B**). Cell 1 discharges more strongly when the monkey observes the experimenter grasp the food to eat it, whereas cell 2 discharges more briskly when the monkey observes the experimenter grasp the food to put it into another container. Cell 3 shows no difference in activity between the two conditions. Raster plots and histograms are aligned with the instant when the experimenter touches the food to be grasped. (Modified, with permission, from Fogassi et al. 2005.)

The involvement of cortical motor circuits in understanding and predicting the outcomes of observed events may not be limited to the mirror-neuron mechanism in the parietal and ventral premotor cortex. Recent experiments have revealed similar processes in the dorsal premotor cortex. Cisek and Kalaska found many neurons in the dorsal premotor cortex that showed directionally tuned activity when a monkey used visual cues to select the correct target for arm and cursor movements from among eight possibilities. The animal watched the cues and cursor motions on a monitor; the cursor was moved by an unseen party. The monkey received a juice reward when the cursor approached the correct target but not if the cursor moved in the wrong direction. The monkey began to lick the reward tube shortly after the cursor started to move in the correct direction but long before the juice was actually delivered. When the cursor moved in the wrong direction, however, the monkey quickly removed its mouth from the tube. This behavior showed that the monkey correctly interpreted what it saw and predicted the consequences.

Remarkably, activity in the majority of dorsal premotor neurons was strikingly similar whether the monkey used visual cues to plan and make arm movements or simply observed and predicted the outcome. Those neurons stopped responding during observation if no reward was delivered after correct trials or if the animal became sated and was no longer interested in receiving rewards. This showed that the neurons were not simply responding to the sensory inputs, but instead were processing the observed sensory events to predict their ultimate outcome for the subject, namely the likelihood of a free reward.

The Relationship between Motor Acts, the Sense of Volition, and Free Will Is Uncertain

At the beginning of the previous chapter we stated that voluntary behavior is willful: An action is considered voluntary if it is intentionally initiated by the actor following a decision to act, including a rejection of the alternative of doing nothing. This concept is a fundamental tenet of our legal system: A person is subject to criminal prosecution or civil liability for his actions if he performs them voluntarily and with full knowledge of their implications.

The subjective experience associated with a voluntary movement is different from that evoked when the movement is passively imposed; it includes a sense of ownership of the action. Our everyday experience also leaves us with the sense that our voluntary behavior is under conscious control and that intention precedes action. However, many skilled voluntary movements can be performed with minimal levels of conscious attention; we can, for example, ride a bicycle or drive a car while simultaneously engaged in conversation.

The relationship between behavior, intention, sense of volition, and free will has long been the subject of intense debate in philosophy and psychology. Some investigators propose that, contrary to our everyday impression, our subjective experience that intention and volition are mental processes that precede action is in fact a post hoc construct of the brain. According to this hypothesis, whenever the brain detects a temporal correlation between a motor command and subsequent sensory events, including feedback from the moving limb, it retrospectively infers that the motor command caused those events and therefore that the action was intended and that the individual was the causal agent.

Benjamin Libet and his colleagues explored this issue in the early 1980s by examining electroencephalographic activity during a self-paced movement task. They asked subjects to make a hand movement at a time of their choosing and then to use a clock-like visual time scale to report when they first became aware of his or her intention to move. Their surprising finding was that the subjects reported that they first recognized the intention to move only about 200 ms before the onset of muscle activity, as much as a second after the onset of the readiness potential, a bilateral signal arising in the frontal cortex and associated with the volitional preparation for movement. Libet concluded that neural processes leading to the initiation of a voluntary movement begin long before the subject reports any awareness of the intention to move and thus that consciousness and free will have little role in the early processes related to the control of voluntary behavior.

Libet's findings have been corroborated by other studies that show that the timing of the awareness of intention is better correlated with the onset of a later electroencephalographic event, the *lateralized readiness potential,* recorded over the motor cortex contralateral to the active limb about 200 ms before movement. The lateralized readiness potential is generally assumed to reflect the end of the decision making process and the onset of the formation of the motor command in the motor cortex.

Although the issue remains controversial, the consensus from these studies is that conscious awareness that one is about to perform a voluntary action is temporally coupled to neural activity in the brain areas associated with the planning and control of the movements. The sense that one is the causal agent of an impending action and that the action is an act of free will may be linked to neural activity in movement-related areas of the brain, rather than activity in separate, higher-order cortical areas that supposedly instruct motor areas what to do.

An Overall View

Not long ago the motor system was viewed as a passive apparatus used by more "intelligent" parts of the brain to implement their plans. Experimental results in recent years have required a profound reevaluation of the role of the motor system in the totality of brain function.

Theoretical and behavioral investigations suggest that the control of motor behavior involves a sequence of neuronal operations that select, plan, and execute a movement. Neurophysiological studies identify those operations in populations of neurons in the parietal, premotor, prefrontal, and primary motor regions of the cerebral cortex. Neurons do not encode motor acts in terms of conventional coordinate systems and motor parameters derived from first principles of physics and engineering. Instead their activity reflects empirical solutions shaped by evolution.

Functions are distributed throughout the cortical motor system without a fixed serial order. A given neuronal operation is spread across multiple cortical areas and related operations occur in parallel in several areas. The particular distribution of activity across this network varies from moment to moment as a function of changing combinations of information and neuronal operations required to learn, plan, and execute the desired behavior in different situations.

Perception, cognition, and action have traditionally been considered distinct and serially ordered functions: An individual perceives the world, reflects on the resultant internal image of the world, and finally acts. This perspective relegates the motor system to the role of a passive apparatus that implements the decisions made by cleverer parts of the brain. Contemporary research indicates that perception, cognition, and action are neither functionally independent nor anatomically segregated. Neural correlates of the decision-making operations involved in voluntary behavior are distributed across cortical areas responsible for the motor control of the effectors that implement those decisions. No single area is responsible for general decisions about action that are then relayed to appropriate output systems for execution.

The complex behavior of higher primates is often regarded as a consequence of the development of sophisticated and adaptive perceptual and cognitive systems. This point of view may invert the evolutionary relationship. The most sophisticated cognitive processes have no inherent survival value without the means to translate them into action. The evolution of increasingly complex motor interactions with the world may have provided the evolutionary driving force that led to the development of more sophisticated perceptual and cognitive capacities to serve the needs of action.

Giacomo Rizzolatti
John F. Kalaska

Selected Readings

Andersen RA, Buneo CA. 2002. Intentional maps in posterior parietal cortex. Ann Rev Neurosci 25:189–220.

Buneo CA, Andersen RA. 2006. The posterior parietal cortex: sensorimotor interface for the planning and online control of visually guided movements. Neuropsychologia 44:2594–2606.

Cisek P, Kalaska JF. 2010. Neural mechanisms for interacting with a world full of action choices. Annu Rev Neurosci 33:269–298.

Colby CL, Duhamel JR. 1996. Spatial representations for action in parietal cortex. Cogn Brain Res 5:105–115.

Colby CL, Goldberg ME. 1999. Space and attention in parietal cortex. Annu Rev Neurosci 22:319–349.

Fabbri-Destro M, Rizzolatti G. 2008. Mirror neurons and mirror systems in monkeys and humans. Physiology 23: 171–179.

Gibson JJ. 1979. *The Ecological Approach to Visual Perception.* Boston: Houghton Mifflin.

Haggard P. 2009. Human volition: towards a neuroscience of will. Nat Rev Neurosci 9:934–946.

Hyvärinen J. 1982. Posterior parietal lobe of the primate brain. Physiol Rev 62:1060–1129.

Jeannerod M. 1988. *The Neural and Behavioral Organisation of Goal-Directed Movements.* Oxford: Clarendon Press.

Jeannerod M, Arbib MA, Rizzolatti G, Sakata H. 1995. Grasping objects: the cortical mechanisms of visuomotor transformation. Trends Neurosci 18:314–320.

Mountcastle VB, Lynch JC, Georgopoulos A, Sakata H, Acuna C. 1975. Posterior parietal association cortex of the monkey: command functions for operations with extrapersonal space. J Neurophysiol 38:871–908.

Nachev P, Kennard C, Husain M. 2008. Functional role of the supplementary and pre-supplementary motor areas. Nat Rev Neurosci 9:856–869.

Rizzolatti G, Luppino G. 2001. The cortical motor system. Neuron 31:889–901.

Rizzolatti G, Sinigaglia C. 2010. The functional role of the of the parieto-frontal mirror circuit: interpretations and misinterpretations. Nat Rev Neurosci 11:264–274.

Tanji J. 2001. Sequential organization of multiple movements: Involvement of cortical motor areas. Ann Rev Neurosci 24:631–651.

References

Ajemian R, Green A, Bullock D, Sergio L, Kalaska J, Grossberg S. 2008. Assessing the function of motor cortex: single-neuron models of how neural response is modulated by limb biomechanics. Neuron 58:414–28.

Buch ER, Brasted PJ, Wise SP. 2006. Comparison of population activity in dorsal premotor cortex and putamen during the learning of arbitrary visuomotor mappings. Exp Brain Res 169:69–84.

Cattaneo L, Fabbri-Destro M, Boria S, Pieraccini C, Monti A, Cossu G, Rizzolatti G. 2007. Impairment of actions chains in autism and its possible role in intention understanding. Proc Natl Acad Sci U S A 104:17825– 17830.

Cisek P, Crammond DJ, Kalaska JF. 2003 Neural activity in primary motor and dorsal premotor cortex in reaching tasks with the contralateral versus ipsilateral arm. J Neurophysiol 89:922–942.

Cisek P, Kalaska JF. 2005. Neural correlates of reaching decisions in dorsal premotor cortex: specification of multiple direction choices and final selection of action. Neuron 45:801–814.

Cisek P, Kalaska JF. 2004. Neural correlates of mental rehearsal in dorsal premotor cortex. Nature 431:993–996.

Crammond DJ, Kalaska JF. 2000. Prior information in motor and premotor cortex: activity in the delay period and effect on pre-movement activity. J Neurophysiol 84:986–1005.

Cui H, Andersen RA. 2007. Posterior parietal cortex encodes autonomously selected motor plans. Neuron 56:552–559.

Deecke L, Kornhuber HH. 1969. Distribution of readiness potential, pre-motion positivity, and motor potential of the human cerebral cortex preceding voluntary finger movements. Exp Brain Res 7:158–168.

Duhamel JR, Bremmer F, BenHamed S, Graf W. 1997. Spatial invariance of visual receptive fields in parietal cortex neurons. Nature 389:845–848.

Duhamel JR, Colby CL, Goldberg ME. 1998. Ventral intraparietal area of the macaque: congruent visual and somatic response properties. J Neurophysiol 79:126–136.

Fattori P, Kutz DF, Breveglieri R, Marzocchi N, Galletti C. 2005. Spatial tuning of reaching activity in the medial parieto-occipital cortex (area V6A) of macaque monkey. Eur J Neurosci 22:956–972.

Fogassi L, Ferrari PF, Gesierich B, Rozzi S, Chersi F, Rizzolatti G. 2005. Parietal lobe: from action organization to intention understanding. Science 308:662–667.

Fogassi L, Gallese V, Fadiga L, Luppino G, Matelli M, Rizzolatti G. 1996. Coding of peripersonal space in inferior premotor cortex (area F4). J Neurophysiol 76:141–157.

Gallese V, Fadiga L, Fogassi L, Rizzolatti G. 1996. Action recognition in the premotor cortex. Brain 119:593–609

Graziano MSA, Yap GS, Gross CG. 1994. Coding of visual space by premotor neurons. Science 266:1054–1057.

Hikosaka O, Sakai K, Nakahara H, Lu X, Miyachi S, Nakamura K, Rand MK. 1999. Neural mechanisms for learning of sequential procedures. In: MS Gazzaniga (ed). *The New Cognitive Neurosciences,* pp. 553–572. Cambridge, MA: MIT Press.

Hoshi E, Tanji J. 2006. Differential involvement of neurons in the dorsal and ventral premotor cortex during processing of visual signals for action planning. J Neurophysiol 95: 3596–3616.

Hoshi E, Tanji J. 2004. Differential roles of neuronal activity in the supplementary and presupplementary motor areas: from information retrieval to motor planning and execution. J Neurophysiol 92:3482–3499.

Jeannerod M, Arbib MA, Rizzolatti G, Sakata H. 1995. Grasping objects: the cortical mechanisms of visuomotor transformation. Trends Neurosci 18:314–320.

Jeannerod M, Decety J. 1995. Mental motor imagery: a window into the representational stages of action. Curr Opin Neurobiol 5:727–732.

Kakei S, Hoffman DS, Strick PL. 2001. Direction of action is represented in the ventral premotor cortex. Nat Neurosci 4:1020–1025.

Kalaska JF, Crammond DJ. 1995. Deciding not to go: neuronal correlates of response selection in a GO/NOGO task in primate premotor and parietal cortex. Cereb Cortex 5:410–428.

Libet B. 2004. *Mind Time: The Temporal Factor in Consciousness.* Cambridge, MA: Harvard Univ Press.

Luppino G, Matelli M, Camarda RM, Gallese V, Rizzolatti G. 1991. Multiple representations of body movements in mesial area 6 and the adjacent cingulate cortex: an intracortical microstimulation study in the macaque monkey. J Comp Neurol 311:463–482.

Massion J. 1992. Movement, posture and equilibrium: interaction and coordination. Prog Neurobiol 38:35–56.

Mitz AR, Godschalk M, Wise SP. 1991. Learning-dependent neuronal activity in the premotor cortex: activity during the acquisition of conditional motor associations. J Neurosci 11:1855–1872.

Murata A, Fadiga L, Fogassi L, Gallese V, Raos V, Rizzolatti G. 1997. Object representation in the ventral premotor cortex (area F5) of the monkey. J Neurophysiol 78:2226–30.

Murata A, Gallese V, Luppino G, Kaseda M, Sakata H. 2000. Selectivity for the shape, size, and orientation of objects for grasping in neurons of monkey parietal area AIP. J Neurophysiol 83:2580–2601.

Nakayama Y, Yamagata T, Tanji J, Hoshi E. 2008. Transformation of a virtual action plan into a motor plan in the premotor cortex. J Neurosci 28:10287–10297.

Ochia T, Muchiake H, Tanji J. 2005. Involvement of the ventral premotor cortex in controlling image motion of the hand during performance of a target-capturing task. Cereb Cortex 15:929–937.

Rizzolatti G, Camarda R, Fogassi L, Gentilucci M, Luppino G, Matelli M. 1988. Functional organization of inferior area 6 in the macaque monkey. II. Area F5 and the control of distal movement. Exp Brain Res 71:491–507.

Rizzolatti G, Gentilucci M, Camarda RM, Gallese V, Luppino G, Matelli M, Fogassi L. 1990. Neurons related to reaching-grasping arm movements in the rostral part of area 6 (area 6ab). Exp Brain Res 82:337–350.

Rizzolatti G, Fadiga L, Gallese V, Fogassi L. 1996. Premotor cortex and the recognition of motor actions. Brain Res Cogn Brain Res 3:131–141.

Romo R, Hernández A, Zainos A. 2004. Neuronal correlates of a perceptual decision in ventral premotor cortex. Neuron 41:165–173.

Sakata H, Taira M, Murata A, Mine S. 1995. Neural mechanism of visual guidance of hand action in the parietal cortex of the monkey. Cereb Cortex 5:429–438.

Schieber MH, Hibbard LS. 1993. How somatotopic is the motor cortex hand area? Science 261:489–492.

Wallis JD, Miller EK. 2003. From rule to response: neuronal processes in the premotor and prefrontal cortex. J Neurophysiol 90:1790–1806.

Yamagata T, Nakayama Y, Tanji J, Hoshi E. 2009. Processing of visual signals for direct specification of motor targets and for conceptual representation of action targets in the dorsal and ventral premotor cortex. J Neurophysiol 102:3280–3294.

39

The Control of Gaze

In preceding chapters we learned about the motor systems that control the movements of the body in space. In this and the next two chapters we consider the motor systems concerned with gaze, balance, and posture. As we explore the world around us, these motor systems act to stabilize our body, particularly our eyes. In examining these motor systems we shall be concerned with how these systems have resolved three biological challenges to knowing where we are in space: How do we visually explore our environment quickly and efficiently? How do we compensate for planned and unplanned movements of the head? How do we stay upright?

The gaze system stabilizes the image of an object on the retina when the object moves in the world or the head moves and keeps the eyes still when the image remains stationary. It has two components: the oculomotor system and the head-movement system. The oculomotor system moves the eyes in the orbits; the head-movement system moves the eye sockets.

In this chapter we describe the oculomotor system and how visual information guides eye movements. It is one of the simplest motor systems, requiring the coordination of only the 12 muscles that move the two eyes. In humans and primates the main job of the oculomotor system is to control the position of the fovea, the central, most sensitive part of the retina. The fovea is less than 1 mm in diameter and covers a tiny fraction of the visual field. When we want to examine an object, we must move its image onto the fovea.

Six Neuronal Control Systems Keep the Eyes on Target

Hermann Helmholtz and other 19th-century psychophysicists who first studied visual perception systematically were particularly interested in eye movements. They appreciated that an analysis of eye movements was essential for understanding visual perception, but they did not realize that there is more than one kind of eye movement. In 1890 Edwin Landott discovered a second type of eye movement. When reading, the eyes do not move smoothly along a line of text but make fast, intermittent movements—saccades—each followed by a short pause (see Chapter 29).

By 1902 Raymond Dodge was able to outline five distinct types of eye movement that direct the fovea to a visual target and keep it there. All of these eye movements share an effector pathway originating in the three bilateral groups of oculomotor neurons in the brain stem.

- Saccadic eye movements shift the fovea rapidly to a new visual target.
- Smooth-pursuit movements keep the image of a moving target on the fovea.
- Vergence movements move the eyes in opposite directions so that the image is positioned on both foveae.
- Vestibulo-ocular reflexes hold images still on the retina during brief head movements.
- Optokinetic movements hold images stationary during sustained head rotation or translation.

A sixth system, the fixation system, holds the eye stationary during intent gaze when the head is not moving. This requires active suppression of eye movement. The optokinetic and vestibular systems are discussed in Chapter 40; we consider the remaining four systems here.

An Active Fixation System Keeps the Fovea on a Stationary Target

Vision is most accurate when the eyes are still. The gaze system actively prevents the eyes from moving when we examine an object of interest. It is not as active in suppressing movement when we are doing something that does not require vision, such as mental arithmetic. Patients with disorders of the fixation system—for example, some individuals with congenital nystagmus—have poor vision not because their visual acuity is deficient but because they cannot hold their eyes still enough for the visual system to work correctly.

The Saccadic System Points the Fovea Toward Objects of Interest

Our eyes explore the world in a series of very quick saccades that move the fovea from one fixation point to another (Figure 39–1). Saccades allow us to scan the environment quickly and to read. They are highly stereotyped; they have a standard waveform with a single smooth increase and decrease of eye velocity. They are also extremely fast, occurring within a fraction of a second at angular speeds up to 900 degrees per second (Figure 39–2A). The velocity of a saccade is determined by only the distance of the target from the fovea. We can change the amplitude and direction of saccades voluntarily but not their speed.

Ordinarily there is no time for visual feedback to modify the course of a saccade; corrections to the direction of movement are made in successive saccades. Only fatigue, drugs, or pathological states can slow saccades. Accurate saccades can be made not only to visual targets but also to sounds, tactile stimuli, memories of locations in space, and even verbal commands ("look left").

The Smooth-Pursuit System Keeps Moving Targets on the Fovea

The smooth-pursuit system holds the image of a moving target on the fovea by calculating how fast the target is moving and moving the eyes at the same speed. Smooth-pursuit movements have a maximum angular velocity of approximately 100 degrees per second, much

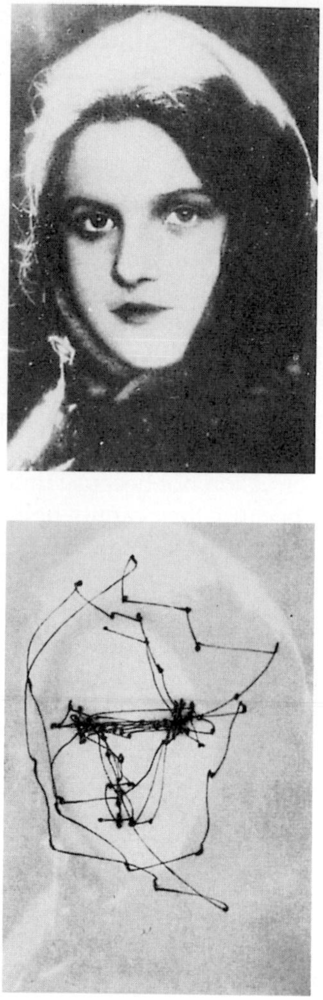

Figure 39–1 Eye movements track the outline of an object of attention. An observer looks at a picture of a woman for 1 minute. The resulting eye positions are then superimposed on the picture. As shown here, the observer concentrated on certain features of the face, lingering over the woman's eyes and mouth (*fixations*) and spending less time over intermediate positions. The rapid movements between fixation points are *saccades*. (Reproduced, with permission, from Yarbus 1967.)

slower than saccades. Drugs, fatigue, alcohol, and even distraction degrade the quality of these movements.

Smooth pursuit and saccades have very different central control systems. This is best seen when a target jumps away from the center of gaze and then slowly moves back toward it. A smooth-pursuit movement is initiated first because the smooth-pursuit system has a shorter latency and responds to target motion on the peripheral retina as well as on the fovea. As the target moves back toward the center of gaze, the eye briefly moves away from the target before the saccade is initiated (Figure 39–2B). The subsequent saccade then brings the eye to the target.

The Vergence System Aligns the Eyes to Look at Targets at Different Depths

The smooth-pursuit and saccade systems produce conjugate eye movements: Both eyes move in the same direction and at the same speed. In contrast, the vergence system produces disconjugate movements of the eyes. When we look at an object that is close to us, our eyes rotate toward each other, or *converge;* when we look at an object that is farther away, they rotate away from each other, or *diverge* (Figure 39–3). These disconjugate movements ensure that the image of the object falls on the foveae of both retinas. Whereas the visual system uses slight differences in left and right retinal positions, or *retinal disparity,* to create a sense of depth, the vergence system drives disconjugate movements to eliminate retinal disparity at the fovea.

Vergence is a function of the horizontal rectus muscles only. Near-field viewing is accomplished by simultaneously increasing the tone of the medial recti muscles and decreasing the tone of the lateral recti muscles. Distance viewing is accomplished by reducing medial-rectus tone and increasing lateral-rectus tone. Accommodation and vergence are controlled by midbrain neurons in the region of the oculomotor nucleus. Neurons in this region discharge during vergence, accommodation, or both.

At any given time the entire visual field is not in focus on the retina. When we look at something close by, distant objects are blurred. When we look at something far away, near objects are blurred. When we wish to focus on an object in a closer plane in the visual field, the oculomotor system contracts the ciliary muscle, thereby changing the radius of curvature of the lens. This process is called *accommodation.* In older individuals accommodation declines owing to increased rigidity of the lens; reading glasses are then needed to focus images at short distances.

Accommodation and vergence are linked. Accommodation is elicited by the blurring of an image, and whenever accommodation occurs the eyes also converge. Conversely, retinal disparity induces vergence, and whenever the eyes converge, accommodation also takes place. At the same time, the pupils transiently constrict to increase the depth of field of the focus. The linked phenomena of accommodation, vergence, and pupillary constriction comprise the *near response.*

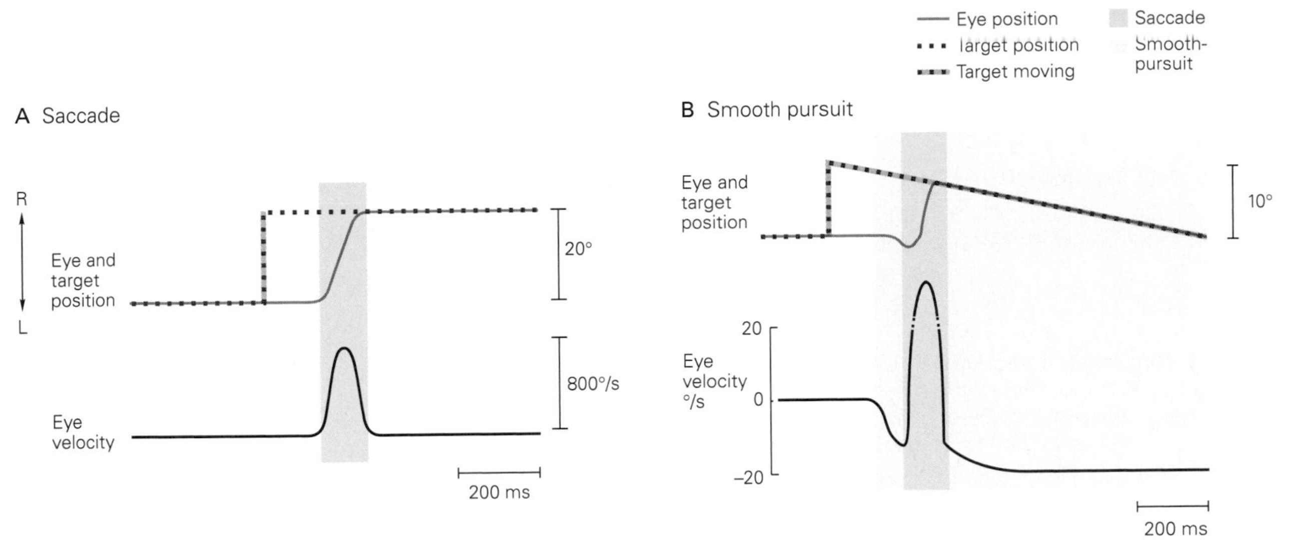

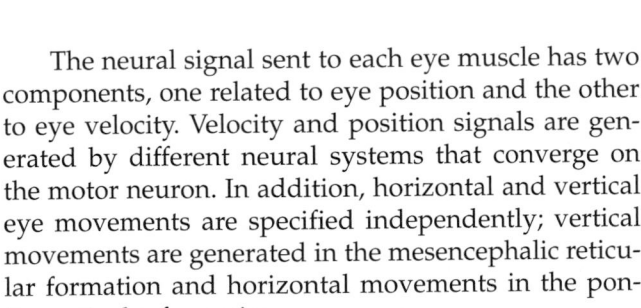

Figure 39–2 Saccadic and smooth-pursuit eye movements. Eye position, target position, and eye velocity are plotted against time.

A. The human saccade. At the beginning of the plot the eye is on the target (the traces representing eye and target positions are superimposed). Suddenly the target jumps to the right, and within 200 ms the eye moves to bring the target back to the fovea. Note the smooth, symmetric velocity profile. Because eye movements are rotations of the eye in the orbit, they are described by the angle of rotation. Similarly, objects in the visual field are described by the angle of arc they subtend at the eye. Viewed at arm's length, a thumb subtends an angle of approximately 1 degree. A saccade from one edge of the thumb to the other therefore traverses 1 degree of arc.

B. Human smooth pursuit. In this example the subject is asked to make a saccade to a target that jumps away from the center of gaze and then slowly moves back to center. The first movement seen in the position and velocity traces is a smooth-pursuit movement in the same direction as the target movement. The eye briefly moves *away* from the target before a saccade is initiated because the latency of the pursuit system is shorter than that of the saccade system. The smooth-pursuit system is activated by the target moving back toward the center of gaze, the saccade adjusts the eye's position to catch the target, and thereafter smooth pursuit keeps the eye on the target. The recording of saccade velocity is clipped so that the movement can be shown on the scale of the pursuit movement, an order of magnitude slower than the saccade.

The neural signal sent to each eye muscle has two components, one related to eye position and the other to eye velocity. Velocity and position signals are generated by different neural systems that converge on the motor neuron. In addition, horizontal and vertical eye movements are specified independently; vertical movements are generated in the mesencephalic reticular formation and horizontal movements in the pontine reticular formation.

Inhibitory neurons suppress unwanted eye movements. Omnipause neurons in the pontine reticular formation prevent excitatory neurons in the brain stem from stimulating the motor neurons. Fixation neurons in the rostral superior colliculus inhibit movement-related neurons in the colliculus while exciting omnipause neurons in the pons. Inhibitory neurons in the substantia nigra inhibit these same movement-related neurons from firing except during saccades.

The Eye Is Moved by the Six Extraocular Muscles

Eye Movements Rotate the Eye in the Orbit

To a good approximation, the eye is a sphere that sits in a socket, the orbit. Eye movements are simply rotations of the eye in the orbit. The eye's orientation can be defined by three axes of rotation—horizontal, vertical, and torsional—that intersect at the center of the eyeball, and eye movements are described as rotations around these axes. Horizontal and vertical eye movements change the line of sight by redirecting the fovea; torsional eye movements rotate the eye around the line of sight but do not change gaze.

Horizontal rotation of the eye away from the nose is called *abduction* and rotation toward the nose is *adduction*. Vertical movements are referred to as *elevation*

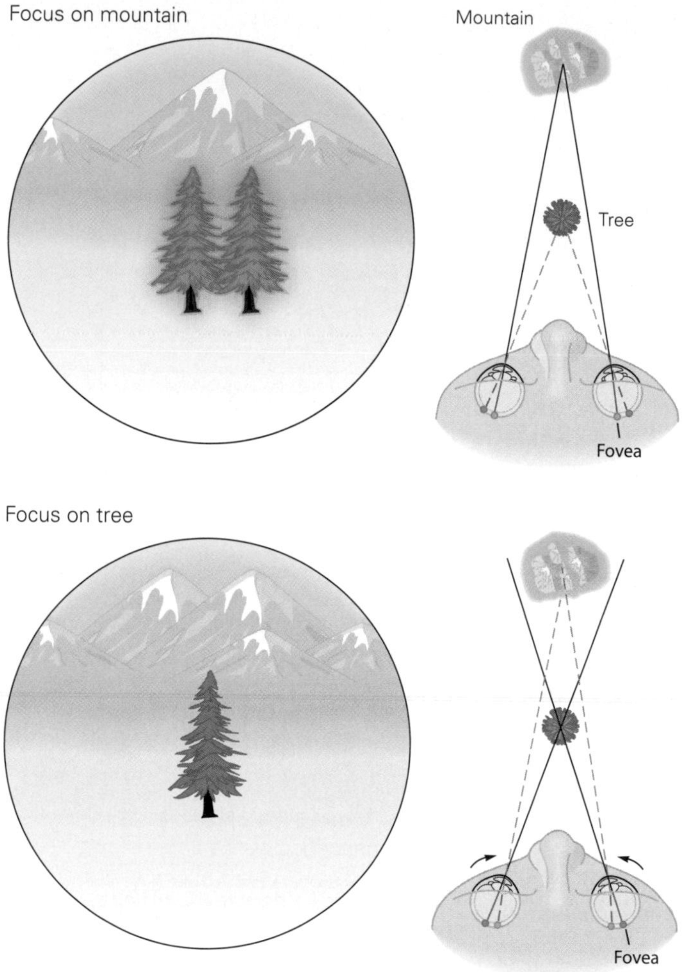

Figure 39–3 Vergence movements. When the eyes focus on a distant mountain, images of the mountain lie on the foveae, whereas those of the nearer tree occupy different retinal positions relative to the two foveae, yielding the percept of a double image. When the viewer looks instead at the tree (**below**), the vergence system must rotate each eye inward. Now the tree's image occupies similar positions on the foveae of both retinas and is seen as one object, but the mountain's images occupy different locations on the retinas and appear double. (Reproduced, with permission, from F. A. Miles.)

(upward rotation) and *depression* (downward rotation). Finally, torsional movements include *intorsion* (rotation of the top of the cornea toward the nose) and *extorsion* (rotation away from the nose).

Except for vergence, most eye movements are conjugate. For example, during gaze to the right the right eye abducts and the left eye adducts. Similarly, if the right eye extorts, the left eye intorts.

The Six Extraocular Muscles Form Three Agonist–Antagonist Pairs

Each eye is rotated by six extraocular muscles arranged in three agonist–antagonist pairs (Figure 39–4). The four rectus muscles (lateral, medial, superior, and inferior) share a common origin, the annulus of Zinn, at the apex of the orbit. They insert on the surface of the eye, or sclera, anterior to the eye's equator. The origin of the inferior oblique muscle is on the medial wall of the orbit; the superior oblique muscle's tendon passes through the trochlea, or pulley, before inserting on the globe, so that its effective origin is also on the medial wall of the orbit. The oblique muscles insert on the posterior globe.

Each muscle has a dual insertion. The part of the muscle farthest from the eye inserts on a soft-tissue pulley through which the rest of the muscle passes on its way to the eye. When the extraocular muscles contract, they not only rotate the eye but also change their pulling directions.

The actions of the extraocular muscles are determined by their geometry and by the position of the eye in the orbit. The medial and lateral recti rotate the eye horizontally; the medial rectus adducts, whereas the lateral rectus abducts. The superior and inferior recti and the obliques rotate the eye both vertically and torsionally. The superior rectus and inferior oblique elevate the eye, and the inferior rectus and superior oblique depress it. The superior rectus and superior oblique intort the eye, whereas the inferior rectus and inferior oblique extort it.

The relative amounts of vertical and torsional rotation produced by the superior and inferior recti and the obliques depend on eye position. The superior and inferior recti exert their maximal vertical action when the eye is abducted, that is, when the line of sight is parallel to the muscles' pulling directions. Conversely, the oblique muscles exert their maximal vertical action when the eye is adducted (Figure 39–5).

Movements of the Two Eyes Are Coordinated

Humans and other animals with eyes in front have binocular vision. This facilitates stereopsis, the ability to perceive a visual scene in three dimensions, as well as depth perception. At the same time, binocular vision requires precise coordination of the movements of the two eyes so that both foveae are always directed at the target of interest. For most eye movements both eyes must move by the same amount and in the same direction. This is accomplished, in large part, through the pairing of eye muscles in the two eyes.

Just as each eye muscle is paired with its antagonist in the same orbit (eg, the medial and lateral recti), it is also paired with the muscle that moves the opposite eye in the same direction. For example, coupling of the left lateral rectus and right medial rectus moves both eyes to the left during a leftward saccade. The orientations of the vertical muscles are such that each pair consists of one rectus muscle and one oblique muscle. For example, the left superior rectus and the right inferior oblique both move the eyes upward in left gaze. The binocular muscle pairs are listed in Table 39–1.

The Extraocular Muscles Are Controlled by Three Cranial Nerves

The extraocular muscles are innervated by groups of motor neurons whose cell bodies are clustered in three

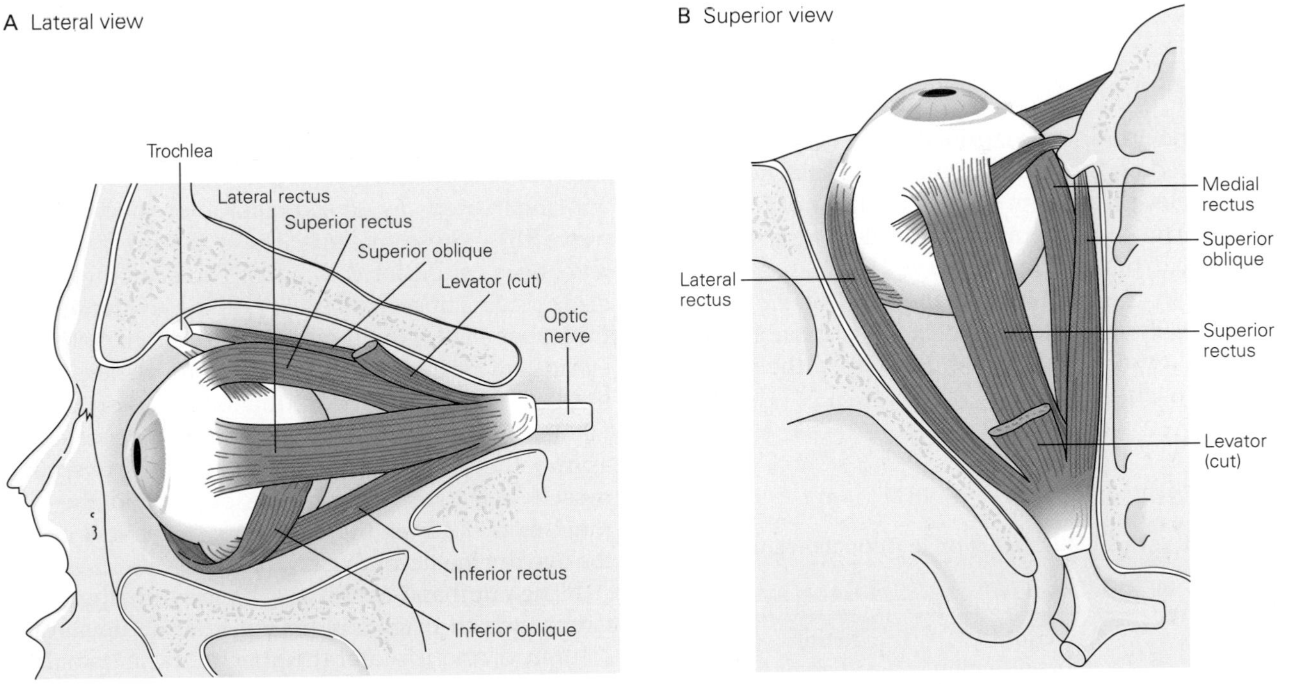

Figure 39–4 The origins and insertions of the extraocular muscles.

A. Lateral view of the left eye with the orbital wall cut away. Each rectus muscle inserts in front of the equator of the globe so that contraction rotates the cornea toward the muscle. Conversely, the oblique muscles insert behind the equator and contraction rotates the cornea away from the insertion. The superior oblique muscle passes through a bony pulley, the trochlea, before it inserts on the globe. The levator muscle of the upper eyelid raises the lid.

B. Superior view of the left eye with the roof of the orbit and the levator muscle cut away. The superior rectus passes over the superior oblique and inserts in front of it on the globe.

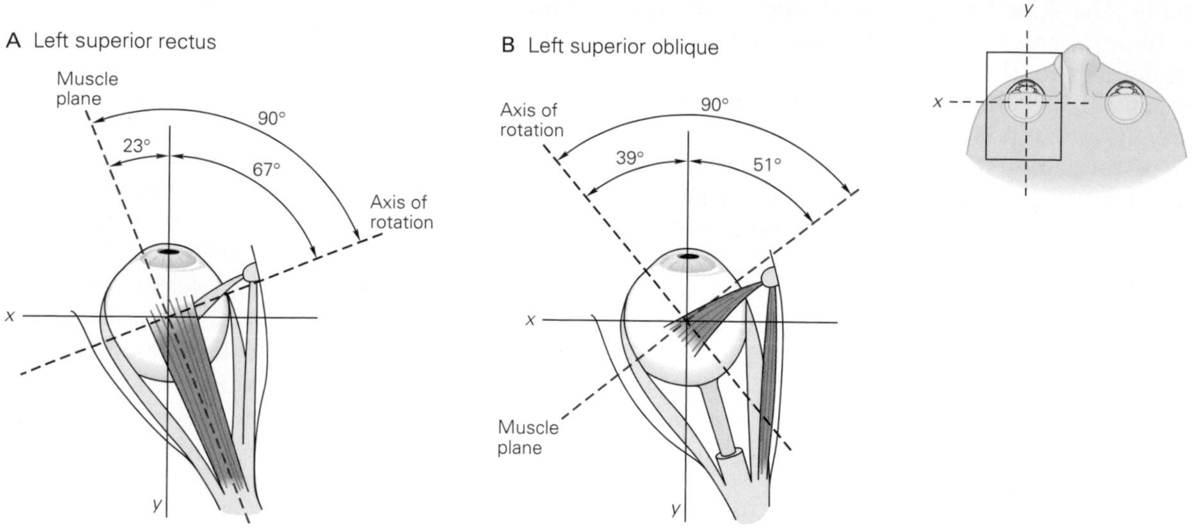

Figure 39–5 Each superior rectus and oblique muscle has both torsional and elevational actions. How much elevation and torsion each muscle provides depends on the position of the eye. (Adapted, with permission, from von Noorden 1980.)

A. When eye position is in the primary visual axis (the *y* axis in the diagram) or lateral to it (*abduction*), elevation is provided by the superior rectus and all of the intorsion is from the superior oblique muscle. When the eye is positioned completely medial to the visual axis (*adduction*), intorsion comes predominantly from the superior rectus and most of the elevation comes from the inferior oblique.

B. When the eye is positioned 16 degrees or more laterally from the primary visual axis, the superior oblique intorts the eye and depression comes from the inferior rectus. When it is completely medial to the visual axis, the superior oblique rotates the eye vertically downward and all of the intorsion comes from the superior rectus.

nuclei in the brain stem (Figure 39–6). The lateral rectus is innervated by the abducens nerve (cranial nerve VI), whose nucleus lies in the pons in the floor of the fourth ventricle. The superior oblique muscle is innervated by the trochlear nerve (cranial nerve IV), whose nucleus is located in the midbrain at the level of the inferior colliculus. (The trochlear nerve gets its name from the trochlea, the bony pulley through which the superior oblique muscle travels.)

Figure 39–6 Vertical Muscle Action in Adduction and Abduction

Muscle	Action in adduction	Action in abduction
Superior rectus	Intorsion	Elevation
Inferior rectus	Extorsion	Depression
Superior oblique	Depression	Intorsion
Inferior oblique	Elevation	Extorsion

All the other extraocular muscles—the medial, inferior, and superior recti and the inferior oblique—are innervated by the oculomotor nerve (cranial nerve III), whose nucleus lies in the midbrain at the level of the superior colliculus. The oculomotor nerve also contains fibers that innervate the levator muscle of the upper eyelid. Cell bodies of axons innervating both eyelids are located in the central caudal nucleus, a single midline structure within the oculomotor complex. Finally, traveling with the oculomotor nerve are parasympathetic fibers that innervate the iris sphincter muscle, the constrictor of the pupil, and the ciliary muscles that adjust the curvature of the lens to focus the eye during accommodation.

The pupil and eyelid also have sympathetic innervation, which originates in the intermediolateral cell column of the ipsilateral upper thoracic spinal cord. Fibers of these neurons synapse on cells in the superior cervical ganglion in the upper neck. Axons of these postganglionic cells travel along the carotid artery to the carotid sinus and then into the orbit. Sympathetic pupillary fibers innervate the iris dilator muscle, causing the pupil to dilate and thus providing the pupillary component of the so-called "fight or flight" response.

Sympathetic fibers also innervate Müller's muscle, a secondary elevator of the upper eyelid. The sympathetic control of pupillary dilatation and lid elevation is responsible for the "wide-eyed" look of excitement and sympathetic overload.

The best way to understand the actions of the extraocular muscles is to consider the eye movements that remain after a lesion of a specific nerve (Box 39–1).

Extraocular Motor Neurons Encode Eye Position and Velocity

We can illustrate how the gaze system generates eye movements by considering the activity of an oculomotor neuron during a saccade. To move the eye quickly to a new position in the orbit and keep it there, two passive forces must be overcome: the elastic force of the orbit, which tends to restore the eye to a central position in the orbit, and a velocity-dependent viscous force that opposes rapid movement. Thus the motor signal must include information about tonic position, which opposes the elastic force, and velocity, which overcomes orbital viscosity and moves the eye quickly to a new position.

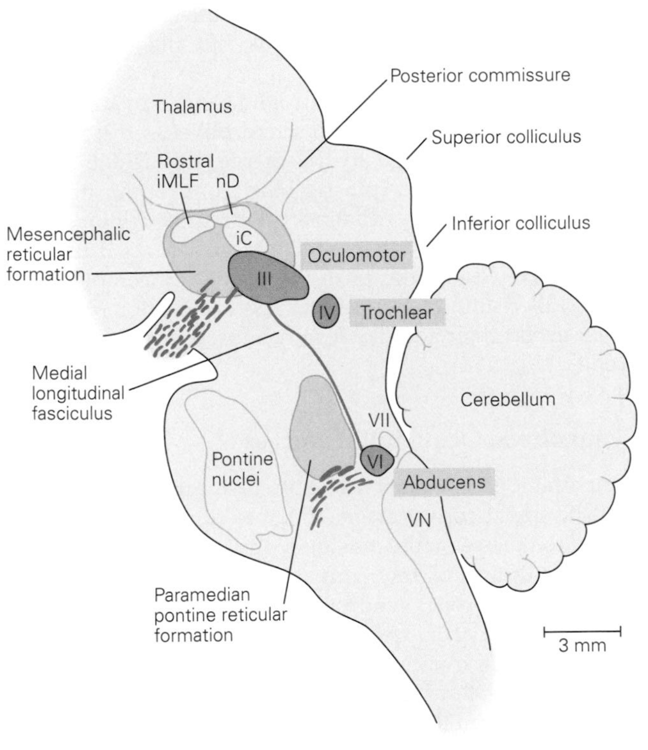

Figure 39–6 The ocular motor nuclei in the brain stem. The nuclei are shown in a parasagittal section through the thalamus, pons, midbrain, and cerebellum of a rhesus monkey. The oculomotor nucleus (cranial nerve III) lies in the midbrain at the level of the mesencephalic reticular formation. The trochlear nucleus (nerve IV) is slightly caudal, and the abducens nucleus (nerve VI) lies in the pons at the level of the paramedian pontine reticular formation, adjacent to the fasciculus of the facial nerve (VII). Compare Figure 45–5. (**iC**, interstitial nucleus of Cajal; **iMLF**, interstitial nucleus of the medial longitudinal fasciculus; **nD**, nucleus of Darkshevich; **VN**, vestibular nuclei.) (Adapted, with permission, from Henn et al. 1984.)

Information about the position and velocity of the eye is conveyed by the discharge frequency of an oculomotor neuron (Figure 39–8). The firing rate of the neuron rises rapidly as the eye's velocity increases from 0 degrees to 900 degrees per second; this is called the *saccadic pulse*. The frequency of this pulse determines the speed of the saccade, whereas the duration of the pulse controls the duration of the saccade. The difference in the firing rates before and after the saccade is called the *saccadic step*. As described below, the pulse and step are generated by different brain stem structures.

Oculomotor neurons differ from skeletal motor neurons in several ways. Although the extraocular muscles are rich in sensors resembling the muscle spindles of skeletal muscles, there are no ocular stretch reflexes. Oculomotor neurons do not have recurrent inhibitory connections. All oculomotor neurons participate equally in all types of eye movements; no motor neurons are specialized for saccades or smooth pursuit.

However, like skeletal motor units, eye motor units are recruited in a fixed sequence (see Chapter 38). Regardless of the type of eye movement, the specific ocular motor neurons recruited depend on the position of the eye in the orbit and the desired eye velocity. For example, as the eye moves laterally the number of active abducens neurons increases, causing more muscle fibers in the lateral rectus to contract.

The Motor Circuits for Saccades Lie in the Brain Stem

How are the motor signals for velocity and position of the eye determined? The higher centers that control gaze specify only a desired change in eye position. The activity of neurons in these centers specifies a target location in the visual field. This location signal must be transformed into a motor signal that encodes the velocity and position of eye movement.

Horizontal Saccades Are Generated in the Pontine Reticular Formation

The signal for horizontal saccades originates in the paramedian pontine reticular formation, adjacent to the

Box 39–1 Extraocular Muscle or Nerve Lesions

Patients with lesions of the extraocular muscles or their nerves complain of double vision (diplopia) because the images of the object of gaze no longer fall on the corresponding retinal locations in both eyes. Lesions of each nerve produce characteristic symptoms that depend on which extraocular muscles are affected. In general, double vision increases when the patient tries to look in the direction of the weak muscle.

Abducens Nerve

A lesion of the abducens nerve (VI) causes weakness of the lateral rectus. When the lesion is complete the eye cannot abduct beyond the midline, such that a horizontal diplopia increases when the subject looks in the direction of the affected eye.

Trochlear Nerve

A lesion of the trochlear nerve (IV) affects both torsional and vertical eye movements. When the patient looks straight ahead, the affected eye is above the normal eye (Figure 39–7A). The difference increases when the patient looks to the right, adducting the eye with the weak muscle (Figure 39–7B left), and decreases when the patient looks to the left, abducting the eye (Figure 39–7B right), because the superior oblique predominantly depresses the eye in adduction.

The deficit is worse when patients attempt to depress and adduct the eye, but improves when they elevate the adducted eye (Figure 39–7C). Patients with superior oblique paresis often keep their heads tilted away from the affected eye. A tilt of the head to one side, such that one ear is pointed downward, induces a small torsion of the eye in the opposite direction, known as ocular counter-roll.

When the head tilts to the left, the left eye is ordinarily intorted by the left superior rectus and left superior oblique, while the right eye is extorted by the right superior rectus and right inferior oblique. The elevation action of the superior rectus is canceled by the depression action of the superior oblique, so the eye only rotates. When the head tilts to the right, the inferior oblique and inferior rectus extort the left eye and the superior oblique relaxes.

With paresis of the left superior oblique, when the head tilts to the left the elevation of the superior rectus is unopposed and the eye moves upward (Figure 39–7D right). The diplopia can be minimized by tilting the head to the right (Figure 39–7D left).

Oculomotor Nerve

A lesion of the oculomotor nerve (III) has complex effects because this nerve innervates multiple muscles. A complete lesion spares only the lateral rectus and superior oblique muscles. Thus the paretic eye is typically deviated downward and abducted at rest, and it cannot move medially or upward from a middle position. Downward movement is partially affected because the inferior rectus muscle is weak but the superior oblique is preserved.

Because the fibers that control lid elevation, accommodation, and pupillary constriction travel in the oculomotor nerve, damage to this nerve also results in drooping of the eyelid (ptosis), blurred vision for near objects, and pupillary dilation (mydriasis). Although sympathetic innervation is still intact with an oculomotor nerve lesion, the ptosis is essentially complete, since Müller's muscle contributes less to elevation of the upper eyelid than does the levator muscle of the upper eyelid.

Sympathetic Oculomotor Nerves

Sympathetic fibers innervating the eye arise from the thoracic spinal cord, traverse the apex of the lung, and ascend to the eye on the outside of the carotid artery.

Interruption of the sympathetic pathways to the eye yields Horner syndrome, whose characteristic features are a partial ipsilateral ptosis owing to weakness of Müller's muscle and a relative constriction (miosis) of the ipsilateral pupil. The pupillary asymmetry is most pronounced in low light because the normal pupil is able to dilate but the pupil affected by Horner syndrome is not.

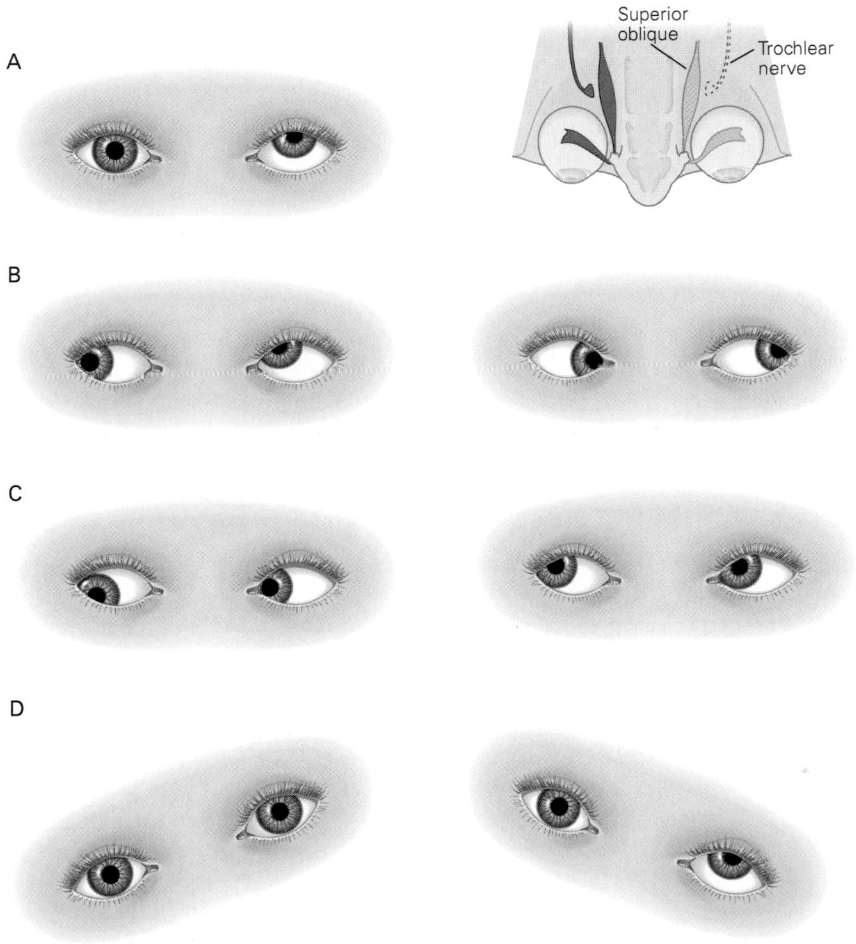

Figure 39–7 Effect of a left trochlear nerve palsy. The trochlear nerve innervates the superior oblique muscle, which inserts behind the equator of the eye. It depresses the eye when it is adducted and intorts the eye when it is abducted.

A. Hypertropia occurs when the eye is in the center of the orbit and the left eye is slightly above the right eye.

B. The hypertropia is worse when the eye is adducted because the unopposed inferior oblique pushes the eye higher (**left**). The condition is improved when the eye is abducted (**right**) because the superior oblique contributes less to depression than to intorsion.

C. When the patient looks to the right the hypertropia is worse on downward gaze (**left**) than it is on upward gaze (**right**).

D. The hypertropia is improved by head tilt to the right (**left**) and worsened by tilt to the left (**right**). The ocular counter-rolling reflex induces intorsion of the left eye on leftward head tilt, and extorsion of the eye on rightward head tilt (see Chapter 40). With leftward head tilt, intorsion requires increased activity of the superior rectus, whose elevating activity is unopposed by the weak superior oblique, causing increased hypertropia. With rightward head tilt and extorsion of the left eye, the unopposed superior rectus muscle is less active, and the hypertropia decreases.

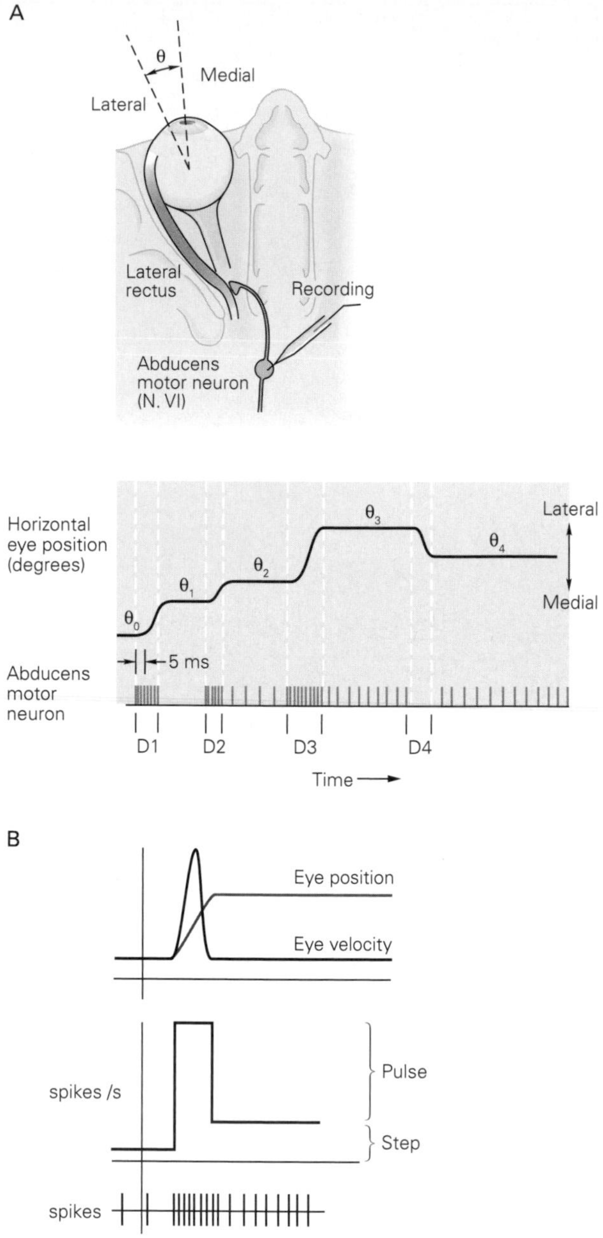

Figure 39–8 Oculomotor neurons signal eye position and velocity.

A. The record is from an abducens neuron of a monkey. When the eye is positioned in the medial side of the orbit the cell is silent (**position** θ_0). As the monkey makes a lateral saccade there is a burst of firing (**D1**), but in the new position (θ_1) the eye is still too far medial for the cell to discharge continually. During the next saccade there is a burst (**D2**), and at the new position (θ_2) there is a tonic position-related discharge. Before and during the next saccade (**D3**) there is again a pulse of activity and a higher tonic discharge when the eye is at the new position (θ_4). When the eye makes a medial movement there is a period of silence during the saccade (**D4**) even though the eye ends up at a position associated with a tonic discharge. (Adapted, with permission, from A. Fuchs 1970.)

B. Saccades are associated with a step of activity, which signals the change in eye position, and a pulse of activity, which signals eye velocity. The neural activity corresponding to eye position and velocity is illustrated both as a train of individual spikes and as an estimate of the instantaneous firing rate (spikes per second).

abducens nucleus to which it projects (Figure 39–9A). The paramedian pontine reticular formation contains a family of *burst neurons* that gives rise to the saccadic pulse. These cells fire at a high frequency just before and during ipsiversive saccades, and their activity resembles the pulse component of ocular motor neuron discharge (Figure 39–9B).

There are several types of burst neurons. Medium-lead burst neurons make direct excitatory connections to motor neurons and interneurons in the ipsilateral abducens nucleus. Long-lead burst neurons drive the medium-lead burst cells and receive excitatory input from higher centers. Inhibitory burst neurons suppress the activity of contralateral abducens neurons and contralateral excitatory burst neurons and are themselves excited by medium-lead burst neurons.

A second class of pontine cells, *omnipause neurons,* fire continuously except around the time of a saccade; firing ceases shortly before and during all saccades (Figure 39–9B). Omnipause neurons are located in the nucleus of the dorsal raphe in the midline (Figure 39–9A). They are GABA-ergic (γ-aminobutyric acid) inhibitory neurons that project to contralateral pontine and mesencephalic burst neurons. Electrical stimulation of omnipause neurons arrests a saccade, which resumes when the stimulation stops. Making a saccade requires simultaneous excitation of burst neurons and inhibition of omnipause cells; this provides the system with additional stability, such that unwanted saccades are infrequent.

If the motor neurons received signals from only the burst cells, the eyes would drift back to the starting position because there would be no new position signal to hold the eyes against elastic restorative forces. David A. Robinson first pointed out that the tonic position signal, the saccadic step, can be generated from

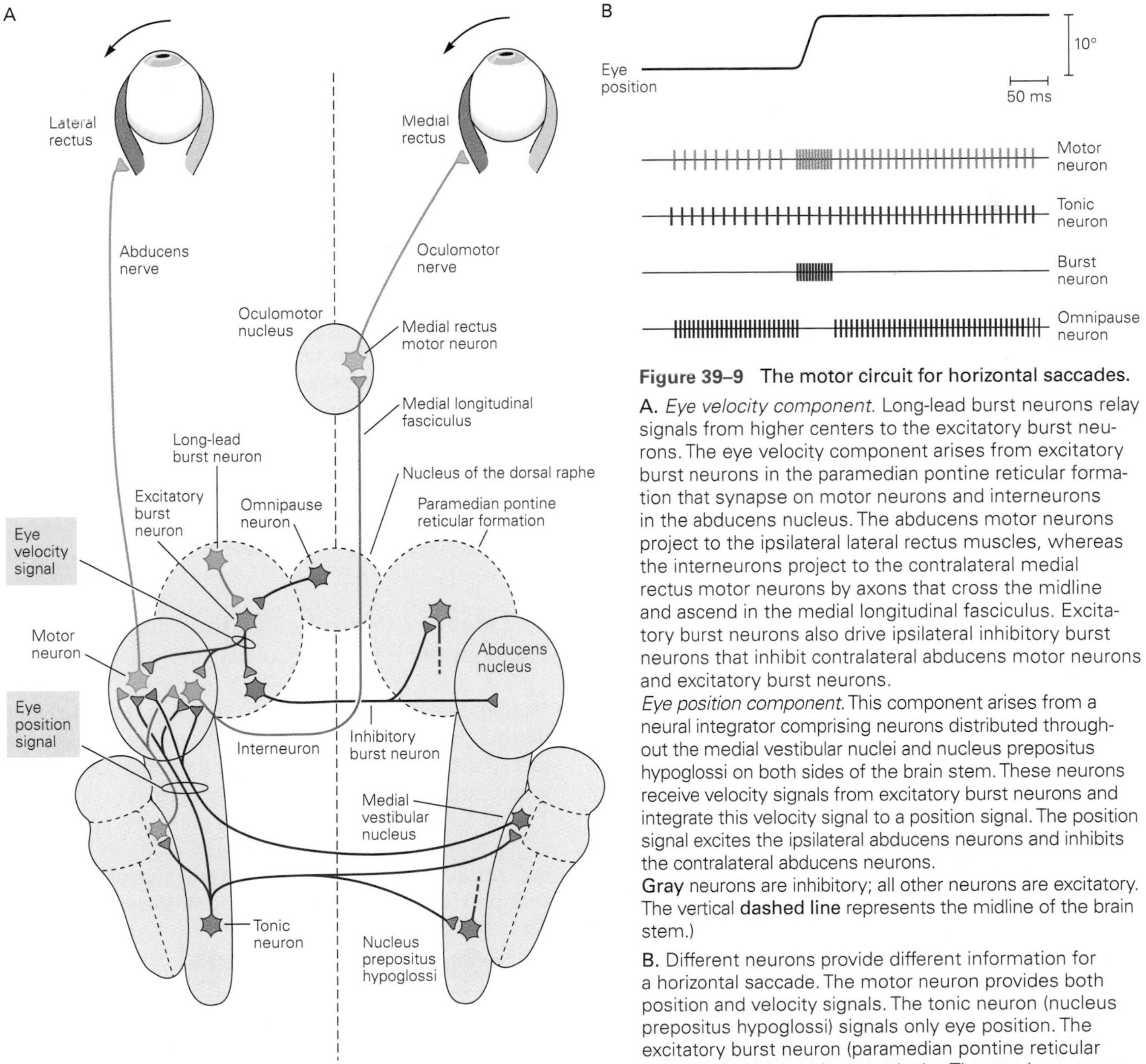

Figure 39–9 The motor circuit for horizontal saccades.

A. *Eye velocity component.* Long-lead burst neurons relay signals from higher centers to the excitatory burst neurons. The eye velocity component arises from excitatory burst neurons in the paramedian pontine reticular formation that synapse on motor neurons and interneurons in the abducens nucleus. The abducens motor neurons project to the ipsilateral lateral rectus muscles, whereas the interneurons project to the contralateral medial rectus motor neurons by axons that cross the midline and ascend in the medial longitudinal fasciculus. Excitatory burst neurons also drive ipsilateral inhibitory burst neurons that inhibit contralateral abducens motor neurons and excitatory burst neurons.
Eye position component. This component arises from a neural integrator comprising neurons distributed throughout the medial vestibular nuclei and nucleus prepositus hypoglossi on both sides of the brain stem. These neurons receive velocity signals from excitatory burst neurons and integrate this velocity signal to a position signal. The position signal excites the ipsilateral abducens neurons and inhibits the contralateral abducens neurons.
Gray neurons are inhibitory; all other neurons are excitatory. The vertical **dashed line** represents the midline of the brain stem.)

B. Different neurons provide different information for a horizontal saccade. The motor neuron provides both position and velocity signals. The tonic neuron (nucleus prepositus hypoglossi) signals only eye position. The excitatory burst neuron (paramedian pontine reticular formation) signals only eye velocity. The omnipause neuron discharges at a high rate except immediately before, during, and just after the saccade.

the velocity burst signal by the neural equivalent of the mathematical process of integration. Velocity can be computed by differentiating position with respect to time; conversely, position can be computed by integrating velocity with respect to time.

For horizontal eye movements, neural integration of the velocity signal is performed by the medial vestibular nucleus and the nucleus prepositus hypoglossi in conjunction with the flocculus of the cerebellum. As expected, animals with lesions of these areas make normal horizontal saccades but the eyes drift back to a middle position after a saccade. Integration of the horizontal saccadic burst requires coordination of the bilateral nuclei propositi hypoglossi and medial vestibular nuclei through commissural connections. A midline lesion of these connections causes failure of the neural integrator.

Medium-lead burst neurons in the paramedian pontine reticular formation and neurons of the medial vestibular nucleus and nucleus prepositus hypoglossi project to the ipsilateral abducens nucleus and deliver respectively the pulse and step components of the motor signal. Two populations of neurons in the abducens nucleus receive this signal. One is a group of motor neurons that innervate the ipsilateral lateral rectus muscle. The second group consists of interneurons whose axons cross the midline and ascend in the medial longitudinal fasciculus to the motor neurons for the contralateral medial rectus, which lie in the oculomotor nucleus (Figure 39–9A).

Thus, medial rectus motor neurons do not receive the pulse and step signals directly. This arrangement allows for precise coordination of corresponding movements of both eyes during horizontal saccades and other conjugate eye movements. The length of the medial longitudinal fasciculus and its vulnerability to demyelination and ischemia make it clinically important.

Vertical Saccades Are Generated in the Mesencephalic Reticular Formation

The burst neurons responsible for vertical saccades are found in the rostral interstitial nucleus of the medial longitudinal fasciculus in the mesencephalic reticular formation (see Figure 39–6). Vertical and torsional neural integration are performed in the nearby interstitial nucleus of Cajal. Both the pontine and mesencephalic systems participate in the generation of oblique saccades, which have both horizontal and vertical components.

Purely vertical saccades require activity on both sides of the mesencephalic reticular formation, and communication between the two sides occurs in the posterior commissure. In contrast, there are not separate omnipause neurons for horizontal and vertical saccades; pontine omnipause cells inhibit both pontine and mesencephalic burst neurons.

Brain Stem Lesions Result in Characteristic Deficits in Eye Movements

We can now understand how different brain stem lesions cause characteristic syndromes. Lesions that include the paramedian pontine reticular formation result in paralysis of ipsiversive horizontal gaze of both eyes but spare vertical saccades. A lesion of the abducens nucleus has a similar effect, for both abducens motor neurons and interneurons are affected. Lesions that include the midbrain gaze centers cause paralysis of vertical gaze. Certain neurological disorders cause degeneration of burst neurons and impair their function, leading to a progressive slowing of saccades.

Lesions of the medial longitudinal fasciculus disconnect the medial rectus motor neurons from the abducens interneurons (Figure 39–9A). Thus during conjugate horizontal eye movements, such as saccades and pursuit, the abducting eye moves normally but adduction of the other eye is impeded. Despite this paralysis in version movements, the medial rectus acts normally in vergence movements because the motor neurons for vergence lie in the midbrain, as will be discussed later. This syndrome, called an *internuclear ophthalmoplegia*, is a consequence of a brain stem stroke or demyelinating diseases such as multiple sclerosis.

Saccades Are Controlled by the Cerebral Cortex Through the Superior Colliculus

The pontine and mesencephalic burst circuits provide the motor signals necessary to drive the muscles for saccades. However, among higher mammals eye movements are ultimately driven by cognitive behavior. The decision when and where to make a saccade that is behaviorally important is usually made in the cerebral cortex. A network of cortical and subcortical areas controls the saccadic system through the superior colliculus (Figure 39–10).

The Superior Colliculus Integrates Visual and Motor Information into Oculomotor Signals to the Brain Stem

The superior colliculus in the midbrain is a major visuomotor integration region, the mammalian homolog

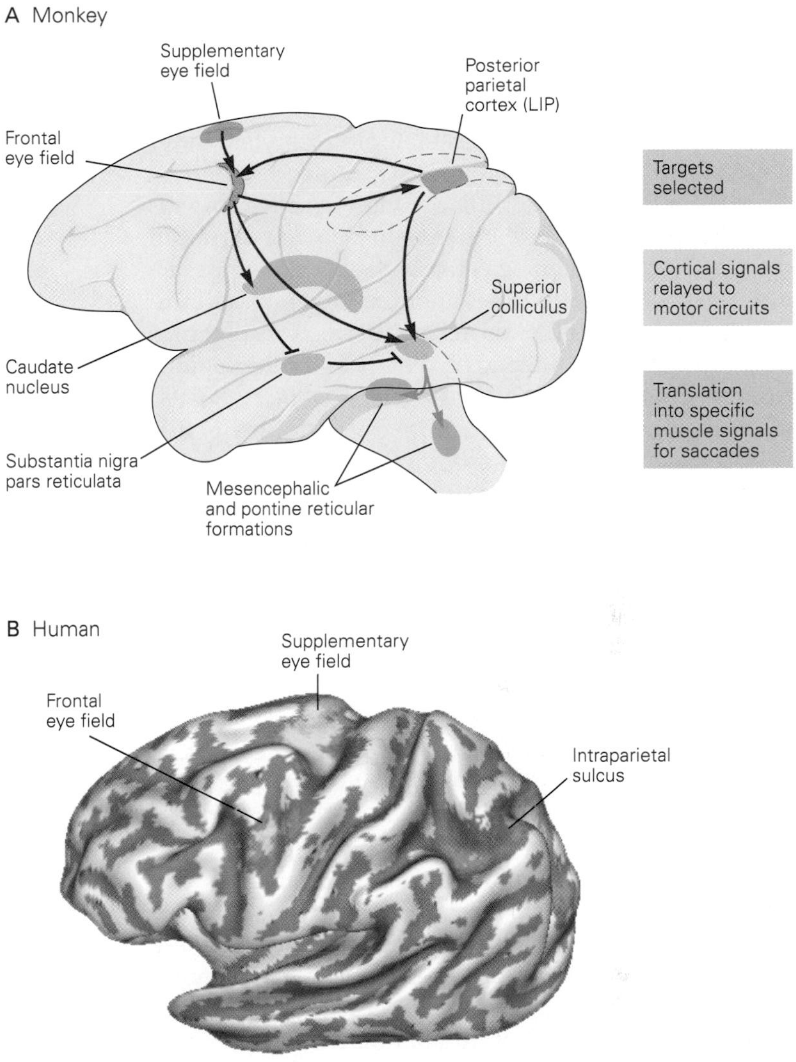

Figure 39–10 Cortical pathways for saccades. **A.** In the monkey the saccade generator in the brain stem receives a command from the superior colliculus. The colliculus receives direct excitatory projections from the frontal eye fields and the lateral intraparietal area (**LIP**) and an inhibitory projection from the substantia nigra. The substantia nigra is suppressed by the caudate nucleus, which in turn is excited by the frontal eye fields. Thus the frontal eye fields directly excite the colliculus and indirectly release it from suppression by the substantia nigra by exciting the caudate nucleus, which inhibits the substantia nigra. (Reproduced, with permission, from R. J. Krausliz.)

B. This lateral scan of a human brain shows areas of cortex activated during saccades. (Reproduced, with permission, from Curtis and Connelly 2010.)

of the optic tectum in nonmammalian vertebrates. It can be divided into two functional regions: the superficial layers and the intermediate and deep layers.

The three superficial layers receive both direct input from the retina and a projection from the striate cortex representing the entire contralateral visual hemifield. Neurons in the superficial layers respond to visual stimuli. In monkeys the responses of half of these vision-related neurons are quantitatively enhanced when an animal prepares to make a saccade to a stimulus in the cell's receptive field. This enhancement is specific for saccades. If the monkey attends to the stimulus without making a saccade to it—for example, by making a hand movement in response to a brightness change—the neuron's response is not augmented.

Neuronal activity in the two intermediate and deep layers is primarily related to oculomotor actions. The movement-related neurons in these layers receive visual information from the prestriate, middle temporal, and parietal cortices and motor information from the frontal eye field. The intermediate and deep layers also contain somatotopic, tonotopic, and retinotopic maps of sensory inputs, all in register with one another. For example, the image of a bird will excite a vision-related neuron, whereas the bird's chirp will excite an adjacent audition-related neuron, and both will excite a bimodal neuron. Polymodal spatial maps enable us to shift our eyes toward auditory or somatosensory stimuli as well as visual ones.

Much of the early research describing the sensory responsiveness of neurons in the intermediate layer was done in anesthetized animals. To understand how the brain generates movement, however, the activity of neurons needs to be studied in alert animals while they behave normally. Edward Evarts pioneered this approach in studies of the skeletomotor system, after which it was extended to the ocular motor system.

One of the earliest cellular studies in active animals revealed that individual movement-related neurons in the superior colliculus selectively discharge before saccades of specific amplitudes and directions, just as individual vision-related neurons in the superior colliculus respond to stimuli at specific distances and directions from the fovea (Figure 39–11A). The movement-related neurons form a map of potential eye movements that is in register with the visuotopic and tonotopic arrays of sensory inputs, so that the neurons that control eye movements to a particular target are found in the same region as the cells excited by the sounds and image of that target. Each movement-related neuron in the superior colliculus has a *movement field*, a region of the visual field that is the target for saccades controlled by that neuron. Electrical stimulation of the intermediate layers of the superior colliculus evokes saccades into the movement fields of the stimulated neurons.

Movement fields are large, so each superior colliculus cell fires before a wide range of saccades, although each cell fires most intensely before saccades of a specific direction and amplitude. A large population of cells is thus active before each saccade, and eye movement is encoded by the entire ensemble of these broadly tuned cells. Because each cell makes only a small contribution to the direction and amplitude of the movement, any variability or noise in the discharge of a given cell is minimized. Similar population coding is found in the olfactory system (see Chapter 32) and skeletal motor system (see Chapter 37).

Activity in the superficial and intermediate layers of the superior colliculus can occur independently: Sensory activity in the superficial layers does not always lead to motor output, and motor output can occur without sensory activity in the superficial layers. In fact, the neurons in the superficial layers do not provide a large projection directly to the intermediate layers. Instead, their axons terminate on neurons in the pulvinar and lateral posterior nuclei of the thalamus, which relay the signals from the superficial layers of the superior colliculus to cortical regions that project back to the intermediate layers.

Lesions of a small part of the colliculus affect the latency, accuracy, and velocity of saccades. Destruction of the entire colliculus renders a monkey unable to make any contralateral saccades, although with time this ability is recovered.

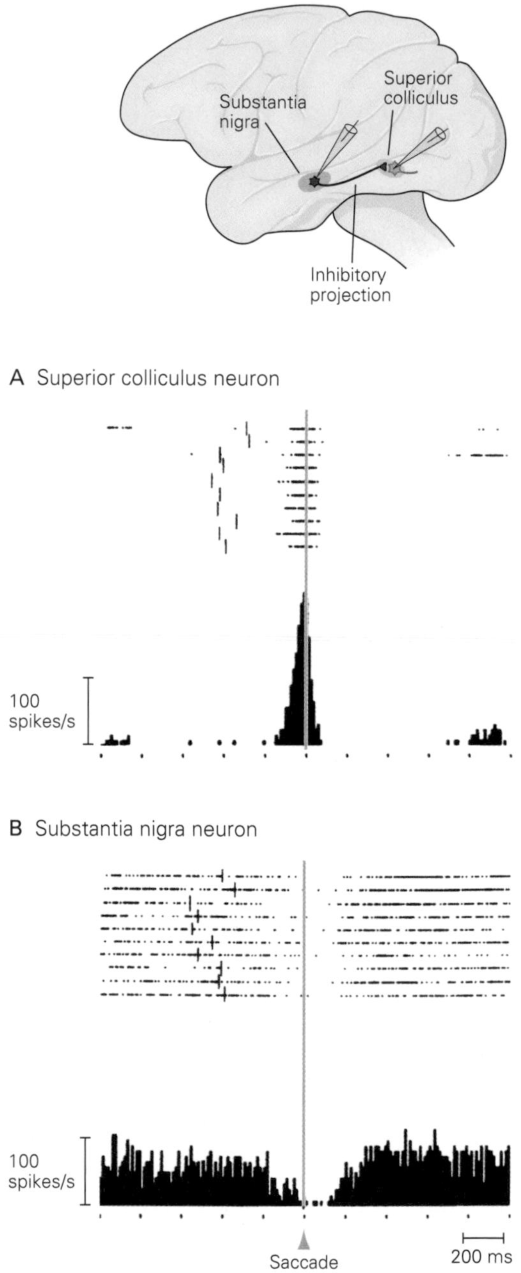

Figure 39–11 Neurons in the superior colliculus and substantia nigra are active around the time of a saccade. The two neurons were recorded simultaneously. (Reproduced, with permission, from Hikosaka and Wurtz 1989.)

A. A neuron in the superior colliculus fires in a burst immediately before the saccade. Raster plots of activity in successive trials of the same task are summed to form the histogram below.

B. A neuron in the substantia nigra pars reticulata is tonically active, becomes quiet just before the saccade, and resumes activity after the saccade. This type of neuron inhibits neurons in the intermediate layers of the superior colliculus.

The Rostral Superior Colliculus Facilitates Visual Fixation

The most rostral portion of the superior colliculus contains a representation of the fovea. Neurons in the intermediate layers in this region discharge strongly during active visual fixation and before small saccades to the contralateral visual field. Because the neurons are active during visual fixation, this area of the superior colliculus is often called the fixation zone.

Neurons here inhibit the movement-related neurons in the more caudal parts of the colliculus and also project directly to the nucleus of the dorsal raphe, where they inhibit saccade generation by exciting the omnipause neurons. With lesions in the fixation zone an animal is more likely to make saccades to distracting stimuli.

The Basal Ganglia Inhibit the Superior Colliculus

The substantia nigra pars reticulata sends a powerful GABAergic inhibitory projection to the superior colliculus. Neurons in the substantia nigra fire spontaneously with high frequency; this discharge is suppressed at the time of voluntary eye movements to the contralateral visual field (see Figure 39–11B). Suppression is mediated by inhibitory input from neurons in the caudate nucleus, which fire before saccades to the contralateral visual field.

Two Regions of Cerebral Cortex Control the Superior Colliculus

The superior colliculus is controlled by two regions of the cerebral cortex that have overlapping but distinct functions: the lateral intraparietal area of the posterior parietal cortex (part of Brodmann's area 7) and the frontal eye field (part of Brodmann's area 8). Each of these areas contributes to the generation of saccades and the control of visual attention.

Perception is better at an attended place in the visual field than at an unattended place, as measured either by a subject's reaction time to an object suddenly appearing in the visual field or by the subject's ability to perceive a stimulus that is just noticeable. Saccadic eye movements and visual attention are closely intertwined (see Figure 39–1).

The lateral intraparietal area in the monkey is important in the generation of both visual attention and saccades. The role of this area in the processing of eye movements is best illustrated by a memory-guided saccade. To demonstrate this saccade, a monkey first fixates a spot of light. An object (the stimulus) appears in the receptive field of a neuron and then disappears; then the spot of light is extinguished. After a delay the monkey must make a saccade to the location of the vanished stimulus. Neurons in the lateral intraparietal area respond at the onset of the stimulus and continue firing during the delay until the saccade begins (Figure 39–12A), but their activity can be also dissociated from saccade planning. If the monkey is planning a saccade to a target outside the receptive field of a neuron, and a distractor appears in the field during the delay period, the neuron responds as vigorously to the distractor as it does to the target of a saccade (Figure 39–12B).

Lesioning of a monkey's posterior parietal cortex, which includes the lateral intraparietal area, increases the latency of saccades and reduces their accuracy. Such a lesion also produces selective neglect: A monkey with a unilateral parietal lesion preferentially attends to stimuli in the contralateral visual hemifield. In humans as well, parietal lesions—especially right parietal lesions—initially cause dramatic attentional deficits. Patients act as if the objects in the neglected field do not exist, and they have difficulty making eye movements into that field (see Chapter 17).

Patients with Balint syndrome, which is usually the result of bilateral lesions of the posterior parietal and prestriate cortex, tend to see and describe only one object at a time in their visual environment. These patients make few saccades, as if they are unable to shift the focus of their attention from the fovea, and can therefore describe only a foveal target. Even after these patients have recovered from most of their deficits, their saccades are delayed and inaccurate.

Compared to the neurons in the parietal cortex, neurons in the frontal eye field are more closely associated with saccades. Three different types of neurons in the frontal eye field discharge before saccades.

Visual neurons respond to visual stimuli and half of these neurons respond more vigorously to stimuli that are the targets of saccades (Figure 39–13A). Activity in these cells is not enhanced when an animal responds to the stimulus without making a saccade to it. Likewise, these cells are not activated before saccades that are made without visual targets; monkeys can be trained to make saccades of a specific direction and amplitude in total darkness.

Movement-related neurons fire before and during all saccades to their movement fields, whether or not they are made to a visual target. These cells do not respond to stimuli in their movement fields that are not targets of saccades. Unlike the movement-related cells in the superior colliculus, which fire before all saccades, movement-related neurons of the frontal eye field fire only before saccades that are relevant to the monkey's

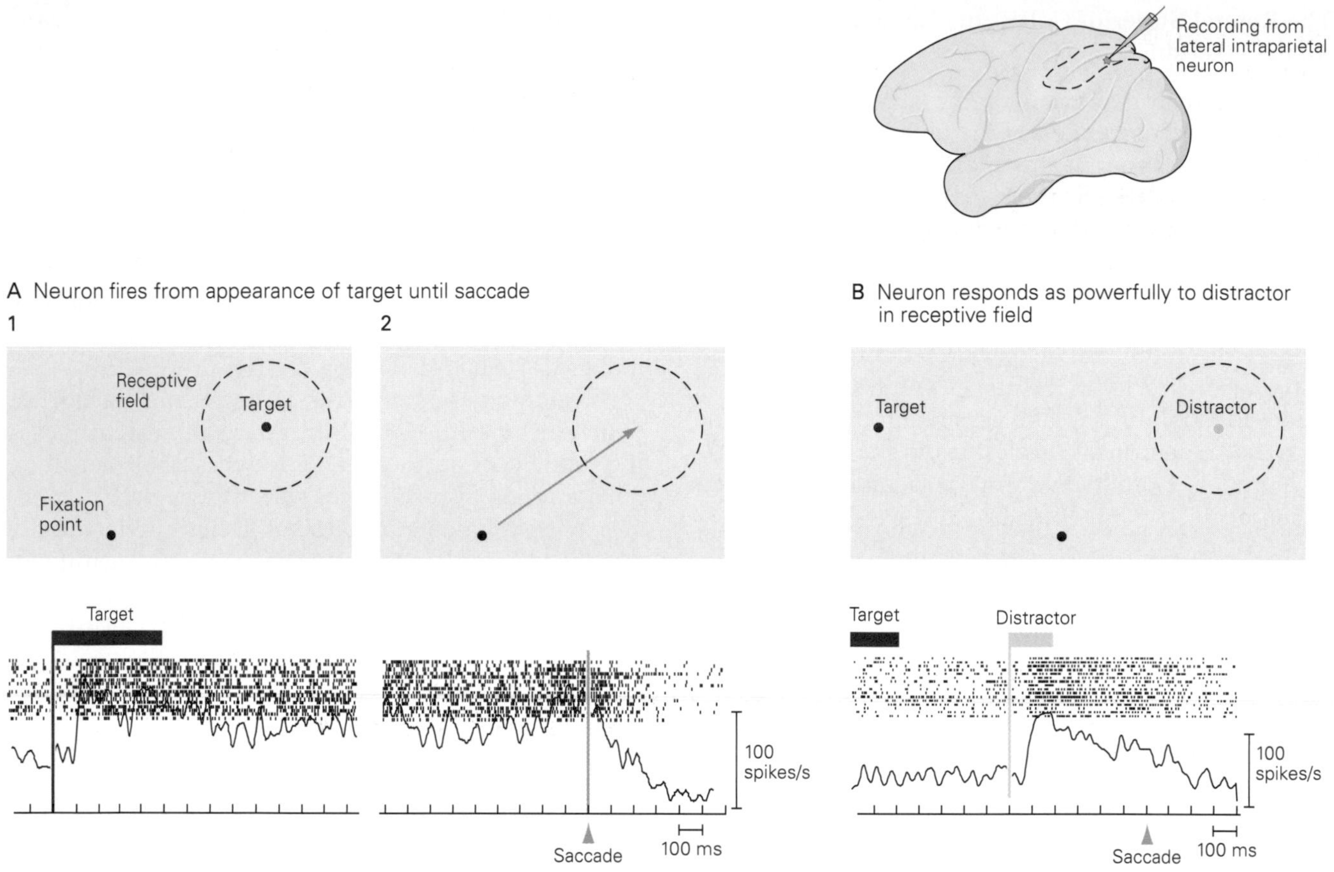

Figure 39–12 A parietal neuron is active before memory-guided saccades. Traces are aligned at events indicated by vertical lines. (Reproduced, with permission, from Powell and Goldberg 2000.)

A. The monkey plans a saccade from a fixation point to a target in the receptive field of a neuron in the lateral intraparietal cortex. The neuron responds to the appearance of the target (**1**). It continues to fire after the target has disappeared but before the signal to make the saccade, and stops firing after the onset of the saccade (**2**).

B. The monkey plans a saccade to a target outside the receptive field. The neuron responds to a distractor in the receptive field as strongly as it did to the target of a saccade.

behavior (Figure 39–13B). These neurons, especially those whose receptive fields lie in the visual periphery, project more strongly to the superior colliculus than do the visual neurons.

Visuomovement neurons have both visual and movement-related activity and discharge most strongly before visually guided saccades. Electrical stimulation of the frontal eye field evokes saccades to the movement fields of the stimulated cells. Bilateral stimulation of the frontal eye field evokes vertical saccades.

The frontal eye field controls the superior colliculus through two pathways (see Figure 39–10). First, the movement-related neurons project directly to the intermediate layers of the superior colliculus, exciting movement-related neurons there. Second, movement-related neurons form excitatory synapses on neurons in the caudate nucleus that inhibit the substantia nigra pars reticulata. Thus, activity of movement-related cells in the frontal eye field simultaneously excites the superior colliculus and releases it from the inhibitory influence of the substantia nigra. The frontal eye field also projects to the pontine and mesencephalic reticular formations, although not directly to the burst cells.

Two other cortical regions with inputs to the frontal eye field are thought to be important in the cognitive aspects of saccades. The *supplementary eye field* at the most rostral part of the supplementary motor area contains neurons that encode saccades in terms of spatial referents other than direction. For example, a neuron in the left supplementary eye field that ordinarily fires before rightward eye movements will fire before a leftward saccade if that saccade is to the right side of

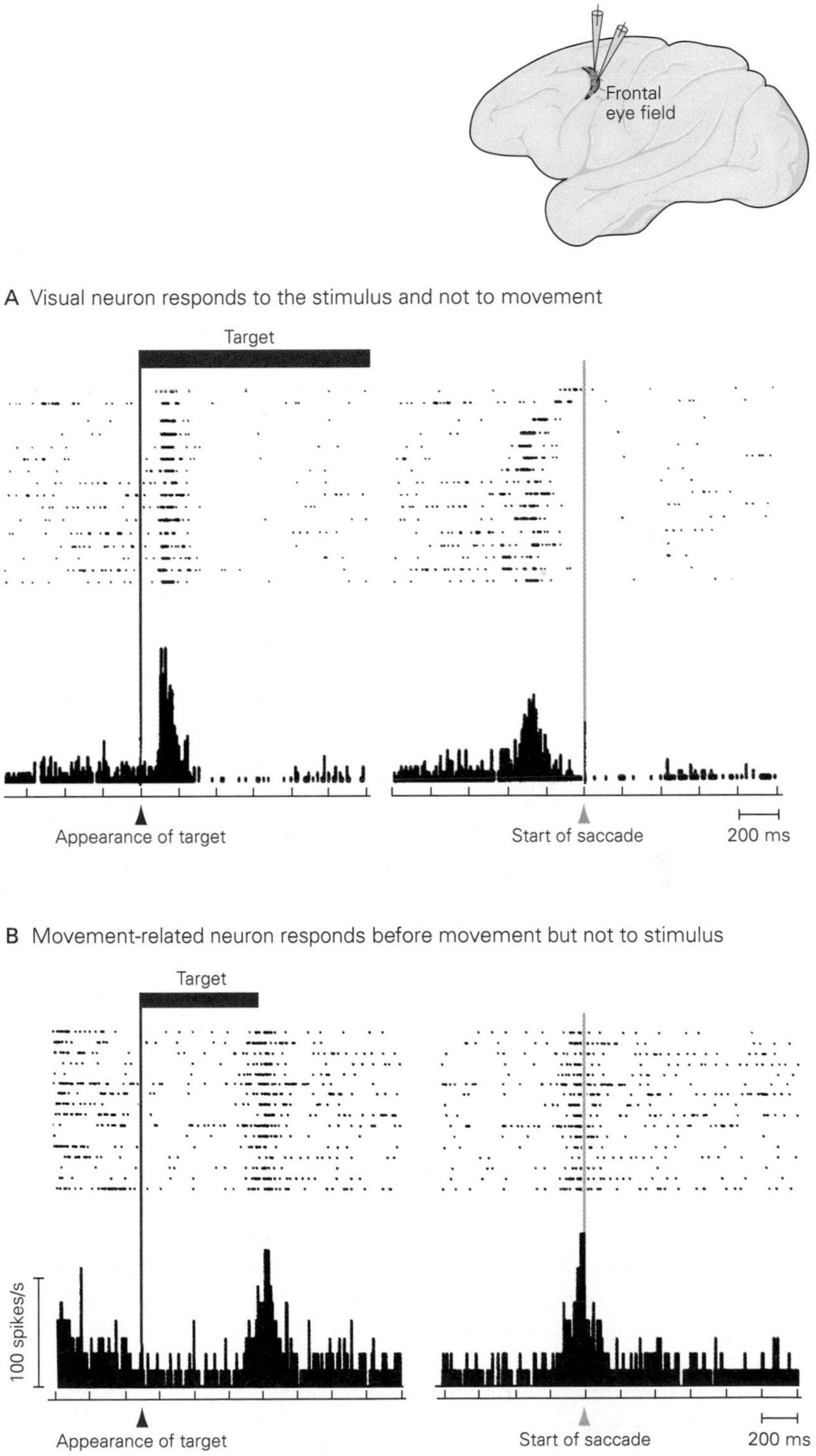

Figure 39–13 Visual and movement-related neurons in the frontal eye field. (Reproduced, with permission, from Bruce and Goldberg 1985.)

A. Activity of a visual neuron in the frontal eye field as a monkey makes a saccade to a target in its visual field. Raster plots of activity in successive trials of the same task are summed to form the histogram below. In the record on the left the individual trials are aligned at the appearance of the stimulus. A burst of firing is closely time-locked to the stimulus. In the record on the right the trials are aligned at the beginning of the saccade. Activity is not well aligned with the beginning of the saccade and stops before the saccade itself commences.

B. Activity of a movement-related neuron in the frontal eye field. The records of each trial are aligned as in part A. The cell does not respond to appearance of the saccade target (**left**). However, it is active at the time of the saccade (**right**).

the target. The *dorsolateral prefrontal cortex* has neurons that discharge when a monkey makes a saccade to a remembered target. The activity commences with the appearance of the stimulus and continues throughout the interval during which the monkey must remember the location of the target.

We can now understand the effects of lesions of these regions on the generation of saccades. Lesions of the superior colliculus in monkeys produce only transient damage to the saccade system because the projection from the frontal eye field to the brain stem remains intact. Animals can likewise recover from cortical lesions if the superior colliculus is intact. However, when both the frontal eye field and the colliculus are damaged, the ability to make saccades is permanently compromised. The predominant effect of a parietal lesion is an attentional deficit. After recovery, however, the system can function normally because the frontal eye field signals are sufficient to suppress the substantia nigra and stimulate the colliculus.

Damage to the frontal eye field alone causes more subtle deficits. Lesions of the frontal eye field in monkeys cause transient contralateral neglect and paresis of contralateral gaze that rapidly recover. The latter deficit may reflect the loss of frontal eye field control of the substantia nigra; this loss of control means that the constant inhibitory input from the substantia nigra to the colliculus does not get suppressed, and the colliculus is unable to generate any saccades. Eventually the system adapts, and the colliculus responds to the remaining parietal signal. After recovery the animals have no trouble producing saccades to targets in the visual field but have great difficulty with memory-guided saccades. Bilateral lesions of both the frontal eye fields and the superior colliculus render monkeys unable to make saccades at all.

Humans with lesions of the frontal cortex have difficulty suppressing unwanted saccades to attended stimuli. This is easily shown by asking subjects to make an eye movement away from a stimulus. When the stimulus appears the subject must attend to it, without turning the eyes toward it, and use its location to calculate the desired saccade. Patients with frontal lesions cannot suppress the saccade to the stimulus, even though they can make normal saccades to visual targets.

As we have seen, neurons in the lateral intraparietal area of monkeys are active when the animal attends to a visual stimulus whether or not the animal makes a saccade to the stimulus. In the absence of frontal eye field signals this undifferentiated signal is the only one to reach the superior colliculus. In humans the failure to suppress a saccade is therefore to be expected if the superior colliculus responds to a parietal signal that generates attention to the stimulus, without the frontal-nigral control that normally prevents saccades in response to parietal signals.

The Control of Saccades Can Be Modified by Experience

Quantitative study of the neural control of movement is possible because the discharge rate of a motor neuron has a predictable effect on a movement. For example, a certain frequency of firing in the abducens motor neuron has a predictable effect on eye position and velocity.

This relationship can change, however, if the muscle becomes weak through disease. The brain can compensate to some degree for such changes. For example, a diabetic patient may have an abducens-nerve lesion affecting one eye and a retinal hemorrhage in the other. He is forced to use the eye with the weak lateral rectus muscle because he experiences poor vision in the eye with the normal abducens nerve. If the latter eye is patched to prevent double vision, the influence of the weak eye increases, such that the weak eye is eventually able to make accurate saccades. The influence of the patched eye also increases, causing that eye to make excessively large saccades. This is of little importance to vision, however, because the patched eye does not contribute to vision. This change in the motor response depends on the fastigial nucleus and vermis of the cerebellum.

Smooth Pursuit Involves the Cerebral Cortex, Cerebellum, and Pons

The task of the smooth-pursuit system differs from that of the saccade system. Instead of driving the eyes as rapidly as possible to a point in space, it must match the velocity of the eyes to that of a target in space. Neurons that signal eye velocity for smooth pursuit are found in the medial vestibular nucleus and the nucleus prepositus hypoglossi. They project to the abducens nucleus as well as the ocular motor nuclei in the midbrain and receive projections from the flocculus of the cerebellum.

Neurons in both the vermis and flocculus transmit an eye-velocity signal that correlates with smooth pursuit (Figure 39–14). These areas receive signals from the cerebral cortex relayed by the dorsolateral pontine nucleus. Thus lesions in the dorsolateral pons disrupt ipsilateral smooth pursuit.

There are two major cortical inputs to the smooth-pursuit system in monkeys. One arises from motion-sensitive regions in the superior temporal sulcus and the middle temporal and medial superior temporal areas. The other arises from the frontal eye field.

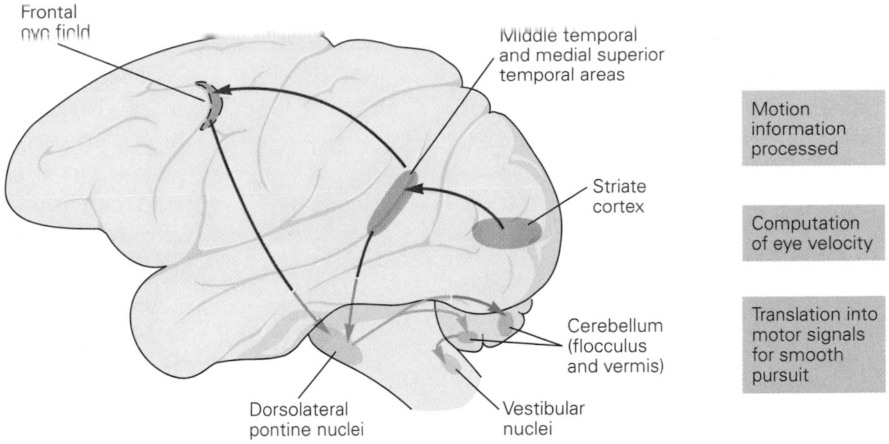

Figure 39–14 Pathways for smooth-pursuit eye movements in the monkey. The cerebral cortex processes information about motion in the visual field and sends it to the ocular motor neurons via the dorsolateral pontine nuclei, the vermis and flocculus of the cerebellum, and the vestibular nuclei. The initiation signal for smooth pursuit may originate in part from the frontal eye field. (Reproduced, with permission, from R. J. Krausliz.)

Neurons in both the middle temporal and medial superior temporal areas calculate the velocity of the target. When the eye accelerates to match the target's speed, the rate of the target's motion across the retina decreases. As the speed of the retinal image decreases, neurons in the middle temporal area, which describe retinal-image motion, stop firing, even though the target continues to move in space. Neurons in the medial superior temporal area continue to fire even if the target disappears briefly. These neurons have access to a process that adds the speeds of the moving eye and the target moving on the retina to compute the speed of the target in space.

Lesions of either the middle temporal or medial superior temporal area disrupt the ability of a subject to respond to targets moving in regions of the visual field represented in the damaged cortical area. Lesions of the latter area also diminish smooth-pursuit movements toward the side of the lesion, no matter where the target lies on the retina.

The temporal cortex provides the sensory information to guide pursuit movements but may not be able to initiate them. Electrical stimulation of either temporal area does not initiate smooth pursuit but can affect pursuit movement, accelerating ipsilateral pursuit and slowing contralateral pursuit. The frontal eye field may be more important for initiating pursuit. This area has neurons that fire in association with ipsilateral smooth pursuit. Electrical stimulation of the frontal eye field initiates ipsilateral pursuit, whereas lesions of the frontal eye field diminish, but do not eliminate, smooth pursuit.

In humans, disruption of the pursuit pathway anywhere along its course, including lesions at the level of cortical, cerebellar, and brain stem areas, prevents adequate smooth-pursuit eye movements. Instead, moving targets are tracked using a combination of defective smooth-pursuit movements, whose velocity is less than that of the target, and small saccades. Patients with brain stem and cerebellar lesions cannot pursue targets moving toward the side of the lesion.

Patients with parietal deficits have two different types of deficit. The first is a directional deficit that resembles that of monkeys with lesions of the middle superior temporal area: Targets moving toward the side of the lesion cannot be tracked. The second is a retinotopic deficit that resembles the deficit of monkeys with lesions of the medial temporal area. Normal subjects can generate smooth-pursuit eye velocity to match the velocity of a stimulus in the periphery (see Figure 39–2). Most patients cannot generate smooth pursuit of a stimulus limited to the visual hemifield opposite the lesion, regardless of the direction of motion.

Some Gaze Shifts Require Coordinated Head and Eye Movements

So far we have described how the eyes are moved when the head is still. When we look around, however, our head is moving as well. Head and eye movements must be coordinated to direct the fovea to a target.

Because the head has a much greater inertia than the eyes, a small shift in gaze drives the fovea to its target before the head begins to move. A small gaze shift usually consists of a saccade followed by a small head movement during which the vestibulo-ocular reflex moves the eyes back to the center of the orbit in the new head position (Figure 39–15). For larger gaze shifts, the eyes and the head move simultaneously in the same direction. Because the vestibulo-ocular reflex ordinarily moves the eyes in the direction opposite

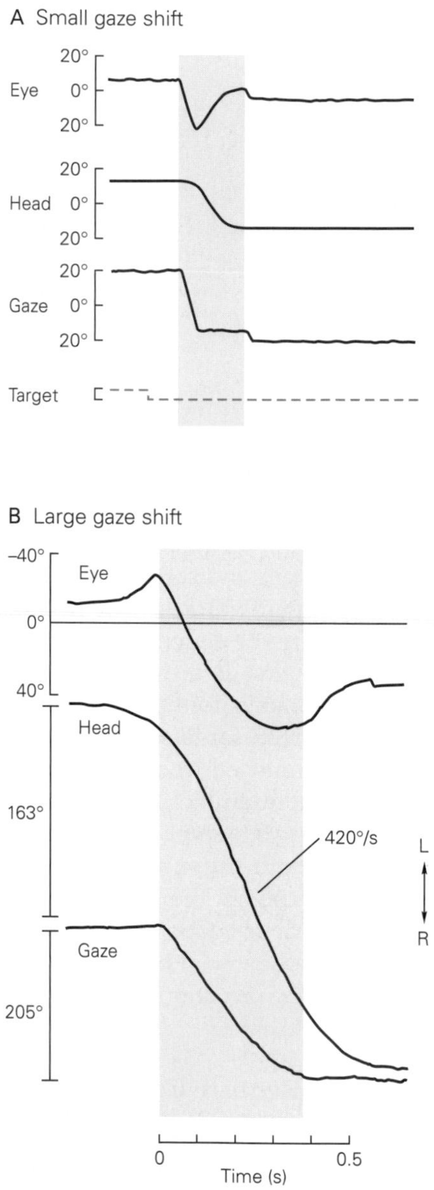

Figure 39–15 Directing the fovea to an object when the head is moving requires coordinated head and eye movements.

A. For a small gaze shift, the eye and head move in sequence. The eye begins to move 300 ms after the target appears. Near the end of the eye movement, the head begins to move as well. The eye then rotates back to the center of the orbit to compensate for the head movement. The gaze record is the sum of eye and head movements. (Reproduced, with permission, from Zee 1977.)

B. For a large gaze shift the eye and head move in the same direction simultaneously. Near the end of the gaze shift the vestibulo-ocular reflex returns, the eye begins to compensate for head movement as in A, and gaze becomes still. (Reproduced, with permission, from Laurutis and Robinson 1986.)

that of the head, the reflex must be temporarily suppressed for the eyes and head to move simultaneously.

Many of the neural centers that control simple saccades also control gaze shift. Electrical stimulation of the superior colliculus in a monkey with its head fixed evokes saccades, but stimulation of an animal whose head can move freely results in saccades combined with head movement. Neurons in the superior colliculus that carry eye-movement signals also project to neurons in the reticular formation that drive the neck muscles, presumably enabling a combined head and eye movement to position the fovea on an object of interest.

An Overall View

The oculomotor system provides a valuable window into the nervous system for both the clinician and the scientist. Patients with oculomotor deficits experience double vision, an alarming symptom that quickly sends them to seek medical help. A physician with a thorough knowledge of the oculomotor system can describe and diagnose most oculomotor deficits at the bedside and localize the site of the lesion within the brain based on the neuroanatomy and neurophysiology of eye movements. Much of our understanding of neural processes arises from our knowledge of the oculomotor system as a microcosm of human behavior.

The cerebral cortex chooses significant objects in the environment as targets for eye movements. Cortical signals are relayed to motor circuits in the brain stem by the superior colliculus. The cortical and collicular signals do not specify the contribution of each muscle to the movement. Instead, the motor programming for eye movements is performed in the brain stem, which translates the signals from higher centers into signals appropriate for each muscle. The cerebellum plays an important role in calibrating eye-muscle movement.

Michael E. Goldberg
Mark F. Walker

Selected Readings

Becker W. 1989. Metrics. In: RH Wurtz, ME Goldberg (eds). *The Neurobiology of Saccadic Eye Movements,* Vol. 3 *Reviews of Oculomotor Research.* Amsterdam: Elsevier.

Colby CL, Duhamel J-R, Goldberg ME. 1996. Visual, presaccadic and cognitive activation of single neurons in monkey lateral intraparietal area. J Neurophysiol 76:2841–2852.

Colby CL, Goldberg ME. 1999. Space and attention in parietal cortex. Annu Rev Neurosci 23:319–349.

Hepp K, Henn V, Vilis T, Cohen B. 1989. Brainstem regions related to saccade generation. In: RH Wurtz, ME Goldberg (eds). *The Neurobiology of Saccadic Eye Movements,* Vol. 3 *Reviews of Oculomotor Research,* pp. 105–212. Amsterdam: Elsevier.

Hikosaka O, Wurtz RH. 1989. The basal ganglia. In: RH Wurtz, ME Goldberg (eds). *The Neurobiology of Saccadic Eye Movements,* Vol. 3 *Reviews of Oculomotor Research,* pp. 257–284. Amsterdam: Elsevier.

Leigh RJ, Zee DS. 2006. *The Neurology of Eye Movements,* 4th ed. Philadelphia, PA: FA Davis.

Sparks DL, Mays LE. 1990. Signal transformations required for the generation of saccadic eye movements. Annu Rev Neurosci 13:309–336.

Wurtz RH, Komatsu H, Dürsteler MR, Yamasaki DSG. 1990. Motion to movement: cerebral cortical visual processing for pursuit eye movements. In: G Edelman, WE Gall, WM Cowan (eds). *Signal and Sense: Local and Global Order in Perceptual Maps,* pp. 233–260. New York: Wiley.

Yarbus AL. 1967. *Eye Movements and Vision.* New York: Plenum.

References

Andersen RA, Asanuma C, Essick G, Siegel RM. 1990. Corticocortical connections of anatomically and physiologically defined subdivisions within the inferior parietal lobule. J Comp Neurol 296:65–113.

Baker R, Highstein SM. 1975. Physiological identification of interneurons and motoneurons in the abducens nucleus. Brain Res 91:292–298.

Bisley JW, Goldberg ME. 2003. The role of the parietal cortex in the neural processing of saccadic eye movements. Adv Neurol 93:141–157.

Bisley JW, Goldberg ME. 2006. Neural correlates of attention and distractibility in the lateral intraparietal area. J Neurophysiol 95:1696–717.

Bruce CJ, Goldberg ME. 1985. Primate frontal eye fields. I. Single neurons discharging before saccades. J Neurophysiol 53:603–635.

Bruce CJ, Goldberg ME, Stanton GB, Bushnell MC. 1985. Primate frontal eye fields. II. Physiological and anatomical correlates of electrically evoked eye movements. J Neurophysiol 54:714–734.

Bushnell MC, Goldberg ME, Robinson DL. 1981. Behavioral enhancement of visual responses in monkey cerebral cortex. I. Modulation in posterior parietal cortex related to selective visual attention. J Neurophysiol 46:755–772.

Büttner-Ennever JA, Büttner U, Cohen B, Baumgartner G. 1982. Vertical gaze paralysis and the rostral interstitial nucleus of the medial longitudinal fasciculus. Brain 105:125–149.

Büttner-Ennever JA, Cohen B, Pause M, Fries W. 1988. Raphe nucleus of the pons containing omnipause neurons of the oculomotor system in the monkey, and its homologue in man. J Comp Neurol 267:307–321.

Cohen B, Henn V. 1972. Unit activity in the pontine reticular formation associated with eye movements. Brain Res 46:403–410.

Colby CL, Duhamel J-R, Goldberg ME. 1996. Visual, presaccadic and cognitive activation of single neurons in monkey lateral intraparietal area. J Neurophysiol 76:2841–2852.

Cumming BG, Judge SJ. 1986. Disparity-induced and blur-induced convergence eye movement and accommodation in the monkey. J Neurophysiol 55:896–914.

Curtis C, Connolly JD. 2008. Saccade preparation signals in the human frontal and parietal cortices. J Neurophysiol 99:133–145.

Demer JL, Miller JM, Poukens V, Vinters HV, Glasgow BJ. 1995. Evidence for fibromuscular pulleys of the recti extraocular muscles. Invest Ophthalmol Vis Sci 36:1125–1136.

Deng S-Y, Goldberg ME, Segraves MA, Ungerleider LG, Mishkin M. 1986. The effect of unilateral ablation of the frontal eye fields on saccadic performance in the monkey. In: E Keller, DS Zee (eds). *Adaptive Processes in the Visual and Oculomotor Systems,* pp. 201–208. Oxford: Pergamon.

Duhamel J-R, Colby CL, Goldberg ME. 1992. The updating of the representation of visual space in parietal cortex by intended eye movements. Science 255:90–92.

Dürsteler MR, Wurtz RH, Newsome WT. 1987. Directional pursuit deficits following lesions of the foveal representation within the superior temporal sulcus of the macaque monkey. J Neurophysiol 57:1262–1287.

Evarts EV. 1966. Methods for recording activity of individual neurons in moving animals. In: RF Rushmer (ed). *Methods in Medical Research,* pp. 241–250. Chicago: Year Book.

Fuchs AF, Luschei ES. 1970. Firing patterns of abducens neurons of alert monkeys in relationship to horizontal eye movement. J Neurophysiol 33:382–392.

Funahashi S, Bruce CJ, Goldman-Rakic PS. 1993. Dorsolateral prefrontal lesions and oculomotor delayed-response performance: evidence for mnemonic "scotomas." J Neurosci 13:1479–1497.

Funahashi S, Bruce CJ, Goldman-Rakic PS. 1989. Mnemonic coding of visual space in the monkey's dorsolateral prefrontal cortex. J Neurophysiol 61:331–349.

Goldberg ME, Bushnell MC. 1981. Behavioral enhancement of visual responses in monkey cerebral cortex. II. Modulation in frontal eye fields specifically related to saccades. J Neurophysiol 46:773–787.

Goldberg ME, Wurtz RH. 1972a. Activity of superior colliculus in behaving monkey. I. Visual receptive fields of single neurons. J Neurophysiol 35:542–559.

Goldberg ME, Wurtz RH. 1972b. Activity of superior colliculus in behaving monkeys. II. Effect of attention on neuronal responses. J Neurophysiol 35:560–574.

Gottlieb JP, MacAvoy MG, Bruce CJ. 1994. Neural responses related to smooth-pursuit eye movements and their correspondence with electrically elicited smooth eye movements in the primate frontal eye field. J Neurophysiol 74:1634–1653.

Hécaen J, de Ajuriaguerra J. 1954. Balint's syndrome (psychic paralysis of visual fixation). Brain 77:373–400.

Henn V, Hepp K, Büttner-Ennever JA. 1984. The primate oculomotor system. II. Premotor system. Hum Neurobiol 1:87–95.

Henn V, Lang W, Hepp K, Resine H. 1984. Experimental gaze palsies in monkeys and their relation to human pathology. Brain 107:619–636.

Highstein SM, Baker R. 1978. Excitatory termination of abducens internuclear neurons on medial rectus motoneurons: relationship to syndrome of internuclear ophthalmoplegia. J Neurophysiol 41:1647–1661.

Hikosaka O, Sakamoto M, Usui S. 1989. Functional properties of monkey caudate neurons. I. Activities related to saccadic eye movements. J Neurophysiol 61:780–798.

Horn AK, Büttner-Ennever JA, PW, Reichenberger I. 1994. Neurotransmitter profile of saccadic omnipause neurons in nucleus raphe interpositus. J Neurosci 4:2032–2046.

Judge SJ, Cumming BG. 1986. Neurons in the monkey midbrain with activity related to vergence eye movement and accommodation. J Neurophysiol 55:915–930.

Kanaseki T, Sprague JM. 1974. Anatomical organization of pretectal and tectal laminae in the cat. J Comp Neurol 158:319–337.

Keller EL. 1974. Participation of medial pontine reticular formation in eye movement generation in monkey. J Neurophysiol 37:316–332.

Komatsu H, Wurtz RH. 1989. Modulation of pursuit eye movements by stimulation of cortical areas MT and MST. J Neurophysiol 62:31–47.

Laurutis VP, Robinson DA. 1986. The vestibular-ocular reflex during human saccadic eye movements. J Physiol 373:209–233.

Lee C, Rohrer WH, Sparks DL. 1988. Population coding of saccadic eye movements by neurons in the superior colliculus. Nature 332:357–360.

Luschei ES, Fuchs AF. 1972. Activity of brain stem neurons during eye movements of alert monkeys. J Neurophysiol 35:445–461.

Lynch JC, Graybiel AM, Lobeck LJ. 1985. The differential projection of two cytoarchitectonic subregions of the inferior parietal lobule of macaque upon the deep layers of the superior colliculus. J Comp Neurol 235:241–254.

Lynch JC, McLaren JW. 1989. Deficits of visual attention and saccadic eye movements after lesions of parieto-occipital cortex in monkeys. J Neurophysiol 61:74–90.

Lynch JC, Mountcastle VB, Talbot WH, Yin TCT. 1977. Parietal lobe mechanisms for directed visual attention. J Neurophysiol 40:362–389.

May JG, Keller EL, Suzuki DA. 1988. Smooth-pursuit eye movement deficits with chemical lesions in the dorsolateral pontine nucleus of the monkey. J Neurophysiol 59:952–977.

McFarland JL, Fuchs AF. 1992. Discharge patterns in nucleus prepositus hypoglossi and adjacent medial vestibular nucleus during horizontal eye movement in behaving macaques. J Neurophysiol 68:319–332.

Morrow MJ, Sharpe JA. 1993. Retinotopic and directional deficits of smooth pursuit initiation after posterior cerebral hemispheric lesions. J Neurol 43:595–603.

Munoz DP, Wurtz RH. 1993a. Fixation cells in monkey superior colliculus. I. Characteristics of cell discharge. J Neurophysiol 70:559–575.

Munoz DP, Wurtz RH. 1993b. Fixation cells in monkey superior colliculus. II. Reversible activation and deactivation. J Neurophysiol 70:576–589.

Mustari MJ, Fuchs AF, Wallman J. 1988. Response properties of dorsolateral pontine units during smooth pursuit in the rhesus macaque. J Neurophysiol 60:664–686.

Newsome WT, Wurtz RH, Dürsteler MR, Mikami A. 1985. Deficits in visual motion processing following ibotenic acid lesions of the middle temporal visual area of the macaque monkey. J Neurosci 5:825–840.

Newsome WT, Wurtz RH, Komatsu H. 1988. Relation of cortical areas MT and MST to pursuit eye movements. II. Differentiation of retinal from extraretinal inputs. J Neurophysiol 60:604–620.

Olson CR, Gettner SN. 1995. Object-centered direction selectivity in the macaque supplementary eye field. Science 269:985–988.

Powell KD, Goldberg ME. 2000. The response of neurons in the lateral intraparietal area to a stimulus flashed during the delay period of a memory-guided saccade. J Neurophysiol 84:301–310.

Raybourn MS, Keller EL. 1977. Colliculo-reticular organization in primate oculomotor system. J Neurophysiol 269:985–988.

Robinson DA. 1975. Oculomotor control signals. In: G Lennerstrand, P Bach-y-Rita (eds). *Basic Mechanisms of Ocular Motility and Their Clinical Implications*, pp. 337–374. Oxford: Pergamon.

Robinson DA. 1970. Oculomotor unit behavior in the monkey. J Neurophysiol 33:393–404.

Schall JD. 1995. Neural basis of saccade target selection. Rev Neurosci 6:63–85.

Schiller PH, Koerner F. 1971. Discharge characteristics of single units in superior colliculus of the alert rhesus monkey. J Neurophysiol 34:920–936.

Schiller PH, True SD, Conway JL. 1980. Deficits in eye movements following frontal eye field and superior colliculus ablations. J Neurophysiol 44:1175–1189.

Segraves MA, Goldberg ME. 1987. Functional properties of corticotectal neurons in the monkey's frontal eye field. J Neurophysiol 58:1387–1419.

Suzuki DA, Keller EL. 1984. Visual signals in the dorsolateral pontine nucleus of the alert monkey: their relationship to smooth-pursuit eye movements. Exp Brain Res 53: 473–478.

Tyler HR. 1968. Abnormalities of perception with defective eye movements (Balint's syndrome). Cortex 4:154–171.

von Noorden GK. 1980. *Burian-Von Noorden's Binocular Vision and Ocular Motility.* St. Louis, MO: Mosby.

Wurtz RH, Goldberg ME. 1972. Activity of superior colliculus in behaving monkey. III. Cells discharging before eye movements. J Neurophysiol 35:575–586.

Zee DS. 1977. Disorders of eye-head coordination. In: BA Brooks, FJ Bajandas. *Eye Movements*, pp. 9–39. New York: Plenum.

40

The Vestibular System

Airplanes and submarines navigate in three dimensions using sophisticated guidance systems that register every acceleration and turn. Laser gyroscopes and computers make these navigational aids extremely precise. Yet the principles of inertial guidance are ancient: Vertebrates have used analogous systems for 500 million years and invertebrates for still longer.

In vertebrates the inertial guidance system is the vestibular system, comprising five sensory organs in the internal ear that measure linear and angular acceleration of the head. Acceleration of the head deflects hair bundles protruding from the hair cells in the inner ear; this distortion changes the cells' membrane potential, altering the synaptic transmission between the cells and the sensory neurons that innervate them. The signals from these vestibular neurons convey information on head velocity and acceleration to vestibular nuclei in the brain stem.

This information keeps the eyes still when the head moves, helps to maintain upright posture, and influences how we perceive our own movement and the space around us by providing a measure of the gravitational field in which we live. In this chapter we describe how the hair cells of the inner ear generate the signals for head acceleration and how these signals are integrated with other sensory information in the brain.

The Vestibular Apparatus in the Inner Ear Contains Five Receptor Organs

Vestibular signals originate in the labyrinths of the internal ear (Figure 40–1). The *bony labyrinth* is a hollow structure within the petrous portion of the temporal

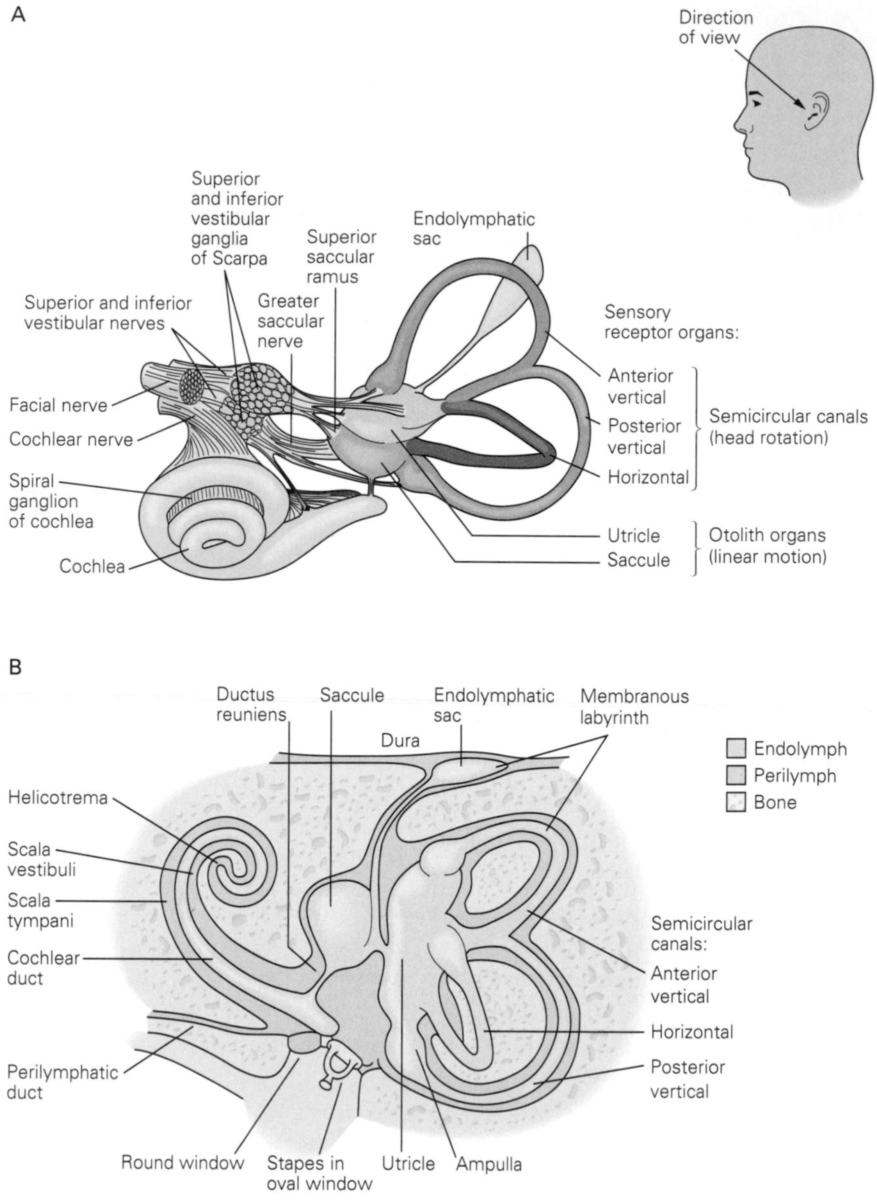

Figure 40–1 The vestibular apparatus of the inner ear.

A. The orientations of the vestibular and cochlear divisions of the inner ear are shown with respect to the head.

B. The inner ear is divided into bony and membranous labyrinths. The bony labyrinth is bounded by the petrous portion of the temporal bone. Lying within this structure is the membranous labyrinth, which contains the receptor organs for hearing (the cochlea) and equilibrium (the utricle, saccule, and semicircular canals). The space between bone and membrane is filled with perilymph, whereas the membranous labyrinth is filled with endolymph. Sensory cells in the utricle, saccule, and ampullae of the semicircular canals respond to motion of the head. (Adapted, with permission, from Iurato 1967.)

bone. Within it lies the *membranous labyrinth,* which contains sensors for both the vestibular and auditory systems.

The membranous labyrinth is filled with *endolymph,* a Na^+-poor, K^+-rich fluid whose composition is maintained by the action of ion pumps in specialized cells. Surrounding the membranous labyrinth, in the space between the membranous labyrinth and the wall of the bony labyrinth, is *perilymph.* Perilymph is a high-Na^+, low-K^+ fluid similar in composition to cerebrospinal fluid, with which it is in communication through the cochlear aqueduct. The endolymph and perilymph are kept separate by a junctional complex that girdles the apex of each cell.

During development the labyrinth progresses from a simple sac to a complex of interconnected sensory organs but retains the same fundamental topological organization. Each organ originates as an epithelium-lined pouch that buds from the otic cyst, and the endolymphatic spaces within the several organs remain continuous in the adult. The endolymphatic spaces of the vestibular labyrinth are also connected to the cochlear duct through the ductus reuniens (Figure 40–1B).

The vestibular portion of the labyrinth, or vestibular apparatus, lies posterior to the cochlea and consists of five sensory structures. Three *semicircular canals* (*horizontal*, also called lateral; *anterior*, also called superior; and *posterior*) sense head rotations, whereas two otolith organs (*utricle* and *saccule*) sense linear motion (also called translation). Because gravity is a linear acceleration, the otolith organs also sense the orientation, or tilt, of the head relative to gravity.

Hair Cells Transduce Mechanical Stimuli into Receptor Potentials

Each of the five receptor organs has a cluster of hair cells responsible for transducing head motion into vestibular signals. Angular or linear acceleration of the head leads to a deflection of the hair bundles in a particular group of hair cells of the appropriate receptor organ (Figure 40–2).

Vestibular signals are carried from the hair cells to the brain stem by branches of the vestibulocochlear nerve (cranial nerve VIII). Cell bodies of the vestibular nerve are located in the vestibular ganglia of Scarpa within the internal auditory canal (Figure 40–1A). The *superior vestibular nerve* innervates the horizontal and anterior canals and the utricle, whereas the *inferior vestibular nerve* innervates the posterior canal and the saccule. The labyrinth's vascular supply, which arises from the anterior inferior cerebellar artery, mirrors its innervation: The anterior vestibular artery supplies the structures innervated by the superior vestibular nerve, and the posterior vestibular artery supplies the structures innervated by the inferior vestibular nerve.

Like most other hair cells, those of the human vestibular system receive efferent inputs from the brain stem. Although the effect of these inputs has not been extensively studied by recording from hair cells in situ, stimulation of the fibers from the brain stem changes the sensitivity of the afferent axons from the hair cells. Stimulation decreases the excitability of some hair cells, as would be expected if activation of the efferent fibers elicited inhibitory postsynaptic potentials in hair cells. In other hair cells, however, activation of the efferent fibers increases excitability.

Given that hair cells are essentially strain gauges (see Chapter 30), the key to grasping how the vestibular organs operate is to understand how mechanical stimuli are delivered to the constituent hair cells. Distinctive mechanical linkages in the otolith organs and semicircular canals account for the contrasting sensitivities of the two types of vestibular organs.

The Semicircular Canals Sense Head Rotation

An object undergoes angular acceleration when its rate of rotation about an axis changes. The head therefore undergoes angular acceleration when it turns or tilts, when the body rotates, and during active or passive locomotion. The three semicircular canals of each vestibular labyrinth detect these angular accelerations and report their magnitudes and orientations to the brain.

Each semicircular canal is a roughly semicircular tube of membranous labyrinth extending from the utricle. One end of each canal is open to the utricle whereas at the other end, the ampulla, the entire lumen of the canal is traversed by a gelatinous diaphragm, the cupula. The cupula is attached to the epithelium along the perimeter and numerous hair bundles insert into the cupula (Figure 40–3).

The vestibular organs detect accelerations of the head because the inertia of their internal contents

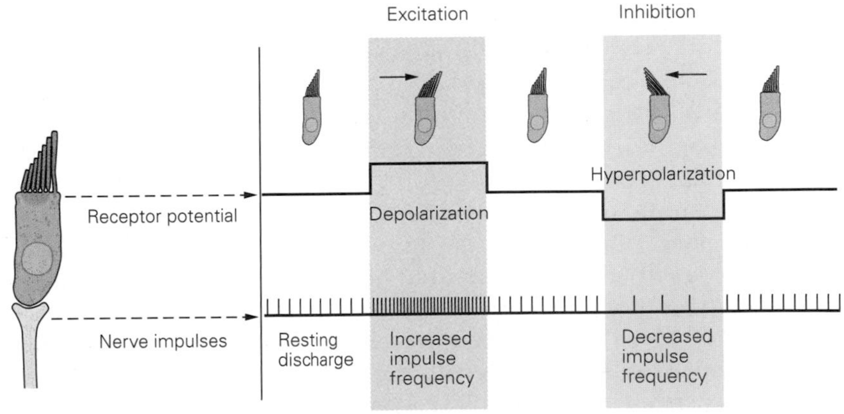

Figure 40–2 Hair cells in the vestibular labyrinth transduce mechanical stimuli into neural signals. At the apex of each cell is a hair bundle, the stereocilia of which increase in length toward a single kinocilium. The membrane potential of the receptor cell depends on the direction in which the hair bundle is bent. Deflection toward the kinocilium causes the cell to depolarize and thus increases the rate of firing in the afferent fiber. Bending away from the kinocilium causes the cell to hyperpolarize, thus decreasing the afferent firing rate. (Adapted, with permission, from Flock 1965.)

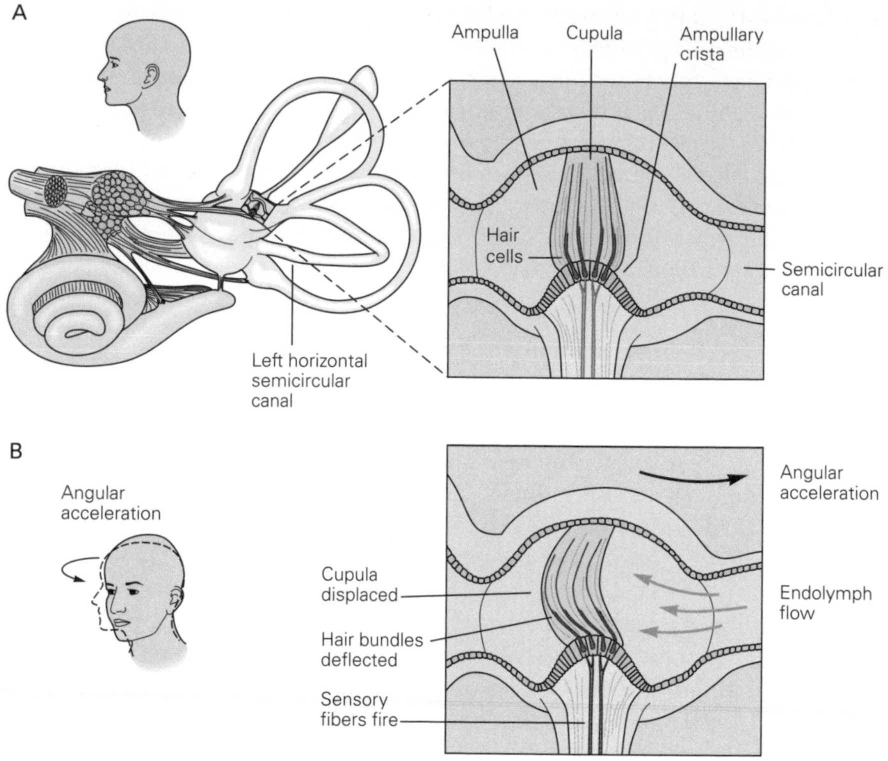

Figure 40–3 The ampulla of a semicircular canal.

A. A thickened zone of epithelium, the ampullary crista, contains the hair cells. The hair bundles of the hair cells extend into a gelatinous diaphragm, the cupula, which stretches from the crista to the roof of the ampulla.

B. The cupula is displaced by the flow of endolymph when the head moves. As a result, the hair bundles are also displaced. Their movement is greatly exaggerated in the diagram.

results in forces on their hair cells. Consider the simplest situation, a rotation in the plane of a semicircular canal. When the head begins to rotate, the membranous and bony labyrinths move along with it. Because of its inertia, however, the endolymph lags behind the surrounding membranous labyrinth, thus rotating within the canal in a direction opposite that of the head.

The motion of endolymph in a semicircular canal can be demonstrated with a cup of coffee. While gently twisting the cup about its vertical axis, observe a particular bubble near the fluid's outer boundary. As the cup begins to turn, the coffee tends to maintain its initial orientation in space and thus counter-rotates in the vessel. If you continue rotating the cup at the same speed, the coffee (and the bubble) eventually catch up to the cup and rotate with it. When the cup decelerates and stops, the coffee keeps rotating, moving in the opposite direction relative to the cup.

In the ampulla this relative motion of the endolymph creates pressure on the cupula, bending it toward or away from the adjacent utricle, depending on the direction of endolymph flow. The resulting deflection of the stereocilia alters the membrane potential of the hair cells, thereby changing the firing rates of the associated sensory fibers. The stereocilia are arranged so that endolymph flow toward the cupula is excitatory for the horizontal canals, whereas flow away from the cupula is excitatory for the anterior and posterior vertical canals.

Each semicircular canal is maximally sensitive to rotations in its plane. The horizontal canal is oriented roughly in the horizontal plane, rising slightly from posterior to anterior, and thus is most sensitive to rotations in the horizontal plane. The anterior and posterior canals are oriented more vertically, approximately 45 degrees from the sagittal plane (Figure 40–4).

Because there is approximate mirror symmetry of the left and right labyrinths, the six canals effectively operate as three coplanar pairs. The two horizontal canals form one pair; each of the other pairs consists of one anterior canal and the contralateral posterior canal. The canal planes are also roughly the pulling planes of the eye muscles. The pair of horizontal canals lies in the pulling plane of the lateral and medial rectus muscles. The left anterior and right posterior pair lies in the pulling plane of the left superior and inferior rectus and right superior and inferior oblique muscles. The right anterior and left posterior pair occupies the pulling plane of the left superior and inferior oblique and right superior and inferior rectus muscles.

The Otolith Organs Sense Linear Accelerations

The vestibular system must compensate not only for head rotations but also for linear motion. The two otolith organs, the utricle and saccule, detect linear motion as well as the static orientation of the head relative to gravity, which is itself a linear acceleration. Each organ consists of a sac of membranous labyrinth approximately 3 mm in the longest dimension. The hair cells of each organ are arranged in a roughly elliptical patch called the *macula*. The human utricle contains approximately 30,000 hair cells, whereas the saccule contains some 16,000.

The hair bundles of the otolithic hair cells extend into a gelatinous sheet, the *otolithic membrane*, that covers the entire macula (Figure 40–5). Embedded on the surface of this membrane are fine, dense particles of calcium carbonate called *otoconia* ("ear dust"), which give the otolith ("ear stone") organs their name. Otoconia are typically 0.5 to 10 μm long; millions of these particles are attached to the otolithic membranes of the utricle and saccule.

Gravity and other linear accelerations exert shear forces on the otoconial matrix and the gelatinous otolithic membrane, which can move relative to the membranous labyrinth. This results in a deflection of the hair bundles, altering activity in the vestibular nerve to signal linear acceleration owing to translational motion or gravity. The orientations of the otolith organs and the directional sensitivity of individual hair cells are such that a linear acceleration along any axis can be sensed. For example, with the head in its normal position, the macula of each utricle is approximately horizontal. Any substantial acceleration in the horizontal plane excites some hair cells in each utricle and inhibits others, according to their orientations (Figure 40–6).

In some instances the vestibular input from a receptor may be ambiguous. For example, acceleration signals from the otolith organs do not distinguish between linear acceleration owing to translation and acceleration owing to gravity (Figure 40–7). The brain, however, integrates inputs from the semicircular canals, otolith organs, and visual and somatosensory systems to properly interpret head and body motions.

The operation of the paired saccules resembles that of the utricles. The hair cells represent all possible orientations within the plane of each macula, but the maculae are oriented vertically in nearly parasagittal planes. The saccules are therefore especially sensitive to vertical accelerations including gravity. Certain saccular hair cells also respond to accelerations in the horizontal plane, in particular those along the anterior–posterior axis.

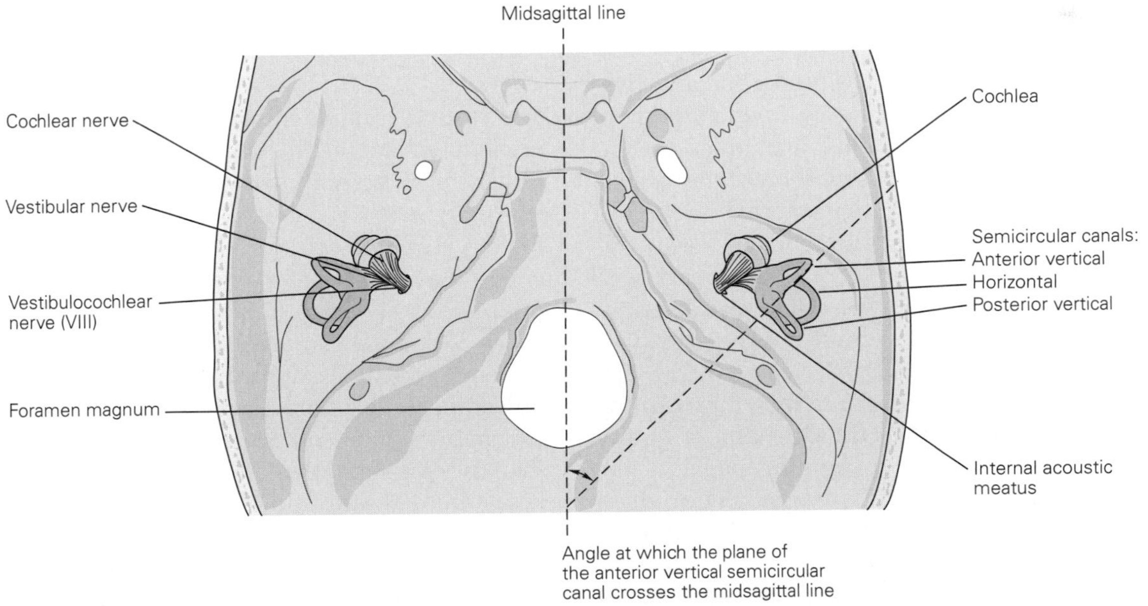

Figure 40–4 The bilateral symmetry of the semicircular canals. The horizontal canals on both sides lie in approximately the same plane and therefore are functional pairs. The bilateral vertical canals have a more complex relationship. The anterior canal on one side and the posterior canal on the opposite side lie in parallel planes and therefore constitute a functional pair.

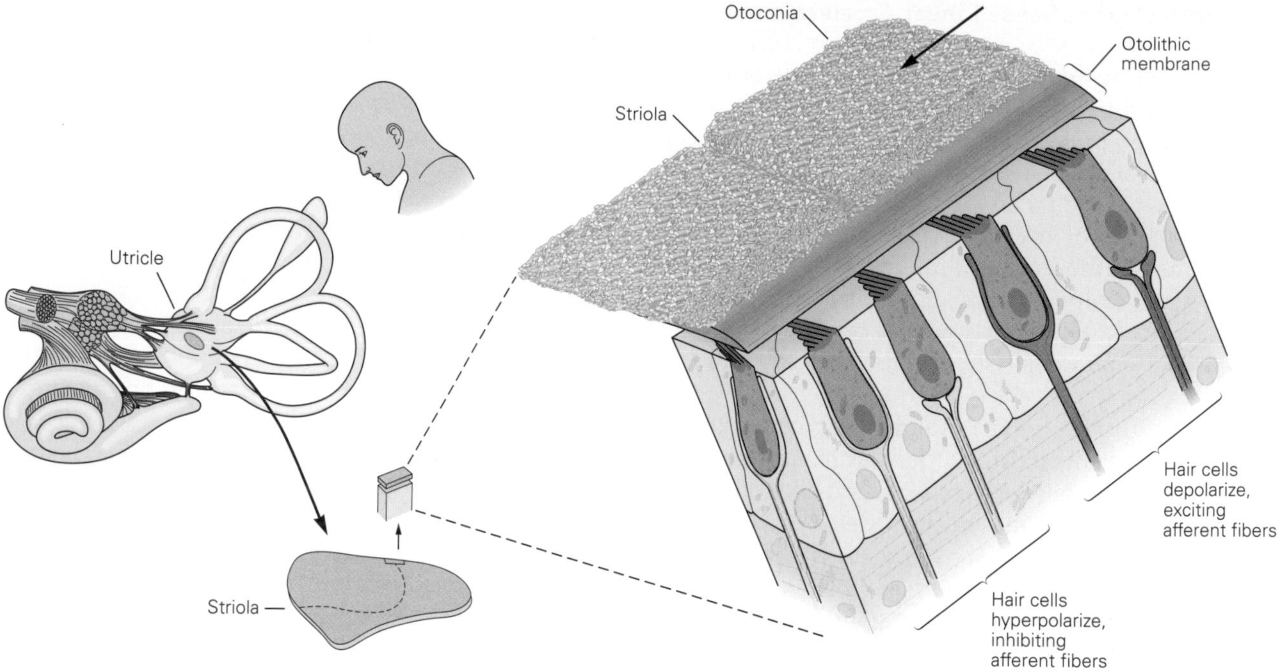

Figure 40–5 The utricle is organized to detect tilt of the head. Hair cells in the epithelium of the utricle have apical hair bundles that project into the otolithic membrane, a gelatinous material that is covered by millions of calcium carbonate particles (otoconia). The hair bundles are polarized but are oriented in different directions (see Figure 40–6). Thus when the head is tilted, the gravitational force on the otoconia bends each hair bundle in a particular direction. When the head is tilted in the direction of a hair cell's axis of polarity, that cell depolarizes and excites the afferent fiber. When the head is tilted in the opposite direction, the same cell hyperpolarizes and inhibits the afferent fiber. (Adapted, with permission, from Iurato 1967.)

Most Movements Elicit Complex Patterns of Vestibular Stimulation

Although the actions of the vestibular organs may be separated conceptually and experimentally, actual human movements generally elicit a complex pattern of excitation and inhibition in several receptor organs in both labyrinths. Consider, for example, the act of leaving the driver's seat of an automobile.

As you begin to swivel toward the door, both horizontal semicircular canals are stimulated strongly. The simultaneous lateral movement out the car's door stimulates hair cells in both utricles in a pattern that changes continuously as the orientation of the turning head changes with respect to the direction of bodily movement. When rising to a standing position, the vertical acceleration excites an appropriately oriented complement of hair cells in each of the saccules while inhibiting an oppositely oriented group. Finally, the maneuver's conclusion involves linear and angular accelerations opposite to those when you started to leave the car.

Vestibulo-Ocular Reflexes Stabilize the Eyes and Body When the Head Moves

The vestibular nerve transmits information about head acceleration to the vestibular nuclei in the medulla, which then distribute it to higher centers. This central network of vestibular connections is responsible for the vestibulo-ocular reflexes that the body uses to compensate for head movement. These neurons also determine the perception of the body's motion in space. Vestibular signals also enable the skeletal motor system to compensate for head movement. The vestibulospinal reflexes are discussed in Chapter 41.

Stable images on the retina are perceived better than moving ones. When the head moves, the eyes are kept still by the vestibulo-ocular reflexes. If you shake your head while reading you can still discern words because of the vestibulo-ocular reflexes. If instead you move the book at a similar speed, however, you can no longer read the words. In the latter instance vision is the brain's only cue for stabilization of the image on the retina, and visual processing is much slower and less effective than vestibular processing for image stabilization. The vestibular apparatus signals how fast the head is rotating, and the oculomotor system uses this information to stabilize the eyes to fix visual images on the retina.

There are three different vestibulo-ocular reflexes. The *rotational vestibulo-ocular reflex* compensates for head rotation and receives its input predominantly from the semicircular canals. The *translational vestibulo-ocular reflex* compensates for linear head movement. The *ocular counter-rolling response* compensates for head tilt in the vertical plane.

The Rotational Vestibulo-Ocular Reflex Compensates for Head Rotation

When the semicircular canals sense head rotation in one direction, the eyes usually begin to rotate in the opposite direction in the orbits. Ideally, eye velocity is matched to head velocity, minimizing retinal motion. This compensatory eye rotation is called the *vestibular slow phase,* although it is not necessarily slow: The eyes may reach speeds of more than 200 degrees per second if the head's rotation is fast. With continued head rotation the eyes would eventually reach the limit of their orbital range and stop moving. To prevent this, a rapid saccade-like movement called a *quick phase* displaces the eyes to a new point of fixation in the direction of head rotation.

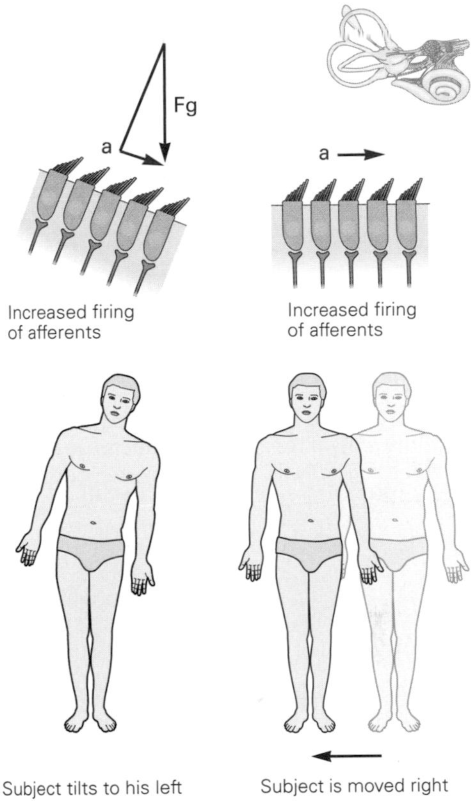

Figure 40–7 Vestibular inputs signalling body posture and motion can be ambiguous. The postural system cannot distinguish between tilt and linear acceleration of the body based on otolithic inputs alone. The same shearing force acting on vestibular hair cells can result from tilting of the head (**left**), which exposes the hair cells to a portion of the acceleration (**a**) owing to gravity (**Fg**), or from horizontal linear acceleration of the body (**right**).

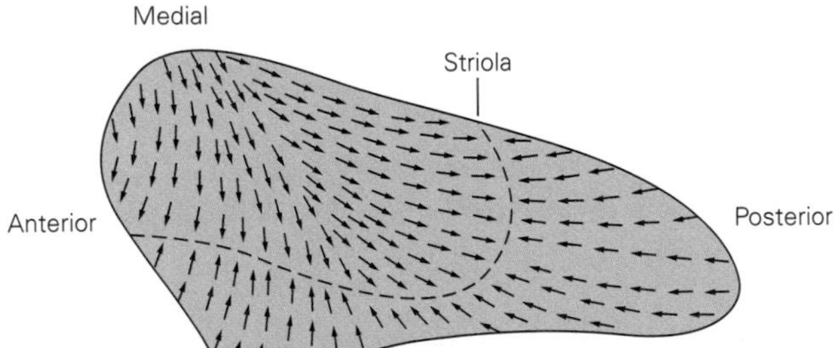

Figure 40–6 The axis of mechanical sensitivity of each hair cell in the utricle is oriented toward the striola. The striola curves across the surface of the macula, resulting in a characteristic variation in the axes of mechanosensitivity (**arrows**) in the population of hair cells. Because of this arrangement, tilt in any direction depolarizes some cells and hyperpolarizes others, while having no effect on the remainder. (Adapted, with permission, from Spoendlin 1966.)

If rotation is prolonged, the eyes execute alternating slow and quick phases called *nystagmus* (Greek *nod*), so called because a nod has a slow phase as the head drops and a quick phase as the head snaps back to an erect position (Figure 40–8). Although the slow phase is the primary response of the rotational vestibulo-ocular reflex, the direction of nystagmus is defined in clinical practice by the direction of its quick phase. Thus, rightward rotation excites the right horizontal canal and inhibits the left horizontal canal. This leads to leftward slow phases and a *right-beating nystagmus.*

If the angular velocity of the head remains constant, the inertia of the endolymph is eventually overcome, as in the coffee cup example earlier: The cupula relaxes and vestibular nerve discharge returns to its

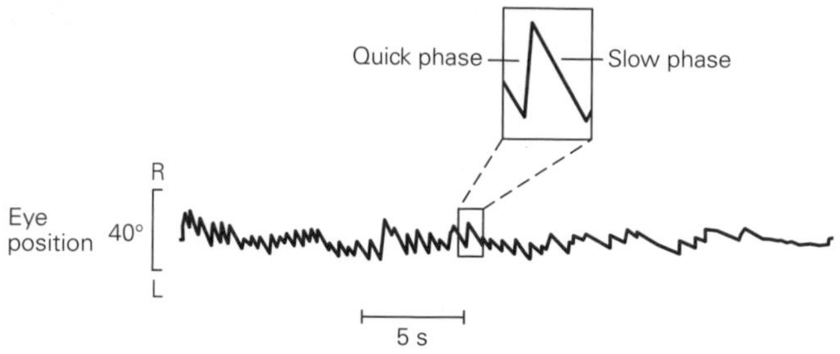

Figure 40–8 Vestibular nystagmus. The trace shows the eye position of a subject in a chair rotated counterclockwise at a constant rate in the dark. At the beginning of the trace the eye moves slowly at the same speed as the chair (slow phase) and occasionally makes rapid resetting movements (quick phase). The speed of the slow phase gradually decreases until the eye no longer moves regularly. (Reproduced, with permission, from Leigh and Zee 1991.)

baseline rate. As a consequence, slow-phase velocity decays and the nystagmus stops, although the head is still rotating.

In fact, the nystagmus lasts longer than would be expected based on cupular deflection. By a process called *velocity storage,* a brain stem network provides a velocity signal to the oculomotor system, although the vestibular nerve no longer signals head movement. Eventually, however, the nystagmus does decay and the sense of motion vanishes.

If head rotation stops abruptly, the endolymph continues to move in the same direction that the head had formerly rotated. With rightward rotation this inhibits the right horizontal canal and excites the left horizontal canal, resulting in a sensation of leftward rotation and a corresponding left-beating nystagmus. However, this occurs only in darkness. In the light, optokinetic reflexes maintain nystagmus as vestibular input diminishes, as long as the head continues to rotate. Correspondingly, optokinetic reflexes suppress post-rotatory nystagmus in the light.

The Otolithic Reflexes Compensate for Linear Motion and Head Deviations

The semicircular canals detect only head rotation; linear motion is sensed by the otolith organs. Linear movement presents the vestibular system with a more complex geometrical problem than does rotation.

When the head rotates, all images move with the same velocity on the retina. When the head moves sideways, however, the image of a close object moves more rapidly across the retina than does the image of a distant object. This can be understood easily by considering what happens when a person looks out the side window of a moving car: Objects near the side of the road move out of view almost with the speed of the car, whereas distant objects disappear more slowly. To compensate for linear head movement the vestibular system must take into account the distance to the object being viewed—the more distant the object, the smaller the eye movement.

Because gravity exerts a constant linear acceleration force on the head, the otolith organs also sense the orientation of the head relative to gravity. When the head tilts away from the vertical in the roll plane—around the axis running from the occiput to the nose—the eyes rotate in the opposite direction, along the axis of torsion, to reduce the tilt of the retinal image. This torsional eye rotation in response to head tilt is the ocular counter-rolling reflex.

Vestibulo-Ocular Reflexes Are Supplemented by Optokinetic Responses

The vestibulo-ocular reflexes represent movement imperfectly. They are best at sensing the onset or abrupt change of motion; they compensate poorly for sustained motion at constant speed during translation or constant angular velocity during rotation. In addition, they are insensitive to very slow rotations or linear accelerations.

Thus vestibular responses during prolonged motion in the light are supplemented by two visual following reflexes that maintain nystagmus when there is no longer any vestibular input. *Optokinetic nystagmus* refers to the response to full-field visual motion; *pursuit* involves the fovea following a small target. Although the two reflexes are distinct, their pathways overlap.

Central Connections of the Vestibular Apparatus Integrate Vestibular, Visual, and Motor Signals

The Vestibular Nerve Carries Information on Head Velocity to the Vestibular Nuclei

When the head is at rest there is a spontaneous tonic discharge in the bilateral vestibular nerves that is equal on both sides. That there is no imbalance in the firing rates indicates to the brain that the head is not moving. When the head rotates, the horizontal canal toward which the head is turning is excited whereas the opposite canal is inhibited, resulting in phasic increases and

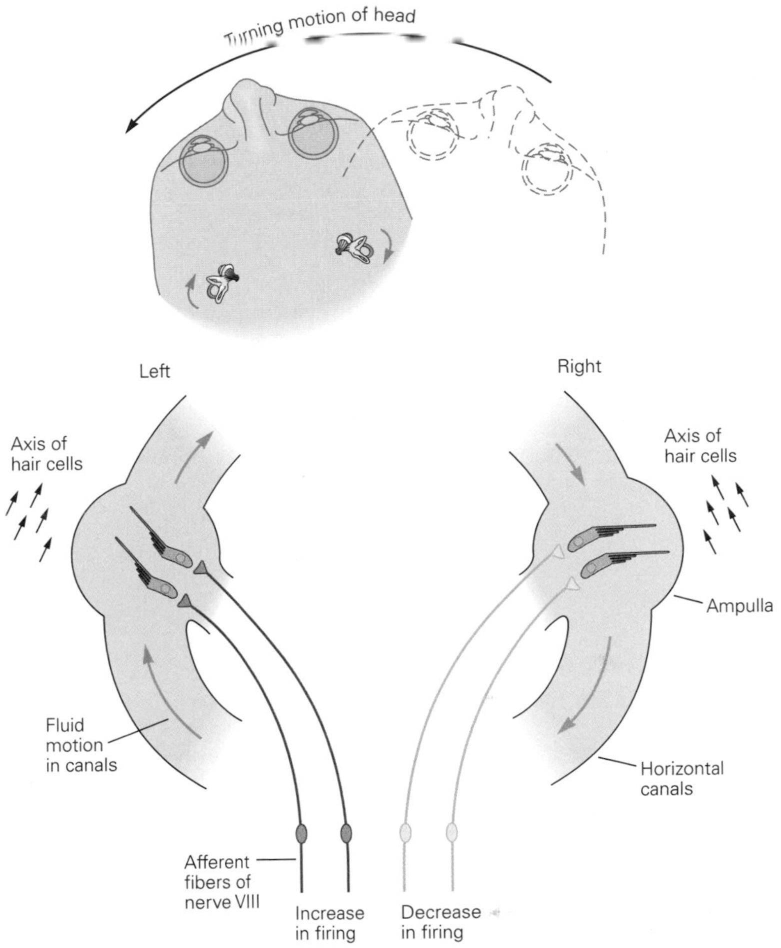

Figure 40–9 The left and right horizontal semicircular canals work together to signal head movement. Because of inertia, rotation of the head in a counterclockwise direction causes endolymph to move clockwise with respect to the canals. This deflects the stereocilia in the left canal in the excitatory direction, thereby exciting the afferent fibers on this side. In the right canal the afferent fibers are hyperpolarized so that firing decreases.

decreases in the vestibular signal (Figure 40–9). The phasic signal correlates with head velocity.

The vestibular nerve projects ipsilaterally from the vestibular ganglion to four *vestibular nuclei* in the dorsal part of the pons and medulla, in the floor of the fourth ventricle. These nuclei integrate signals from the vestibular organs with signals from the spinal cord, cerebellum, and visual system. They project in turn to several central targets: the oculomotor nuclei, reticular and spinal centers concerned with skeletal movement, the vestibular regions of the cerebellum (flocculus, nodulus, ventral paraflocculus, and ventral uvula), and the thalamus. In addition, each vestibular nucleus projects to other vestibular nuclei, both ipsilateral and contralateral.

The vestibular nuclei—medial, lateral, superior, and descending—were originally distinguished by their cytoarchitecture. Their anatomical differences correspond approximately to functional differences (Figure 40–10).

The superior and medial vestibular nuclei receive fibers predominantly from the semicircular canals. They send fibers to oculomotor centers and to the spinal cord. Neurons in the medial vestibular nucleus are predominantly excitatory, whereas those in the superior vestibular nucleus are chiefly inhibitory. These nuclei are concerned primarily with reflexes that control gaze (see Chapter 39).

The lateral vestibular nucleus (Deiters' nucleus) receives fibers from the semicircular canals and otolith organs and projects mostly into the lateral vestibulospinal tract. This nucleus is concerned principally with postural reflexes. The descending vestibular nucleus receives predominantly otolithic input and projects to the cerebellum and reticular formation as well as to the contralateral vestibular nuclei and the spinal cord. This nucleus is thought to be involved in integrating vestibular signals with central motor information. Vestibular projections to the spinal systems are discussed in Chapter 41.

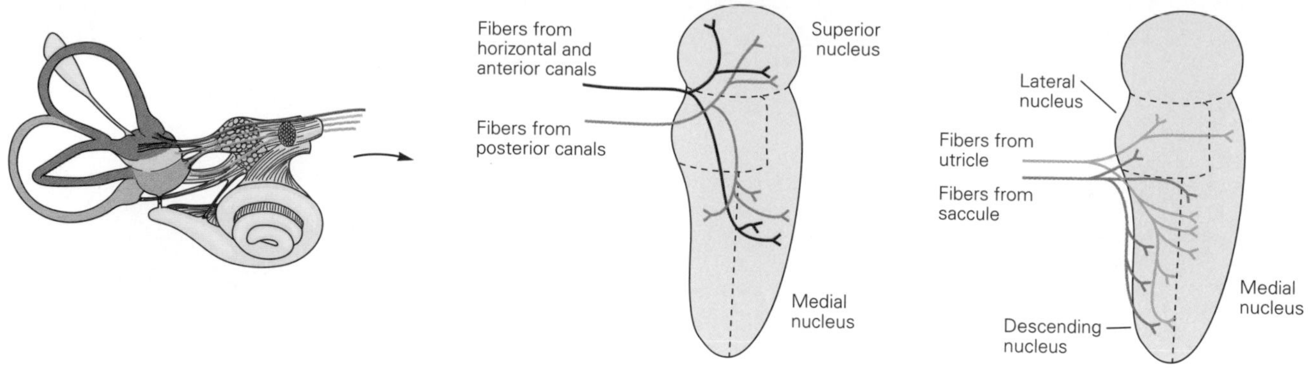

Figure 40–10 Sensory inputs to the vestibular nuclei. Neurons in the superior and medial vestibular nuclei receive input predominantly from the semicircular canals but also from the otolith organs. Neurons in the lateral vestibular nucleus (Deiters' nucleus) receive input from the semicircular canals and otolith organs. This nucleus is concerned predominantly with postural reflexes. The descending vestibular nucleus receives input predominantly from the otolith organs. (Adapted, with permission, from Gacek and Lyon 1974.)

A Brain Stem Network Connects the Vestibular System with the Oculomotor System

During fast head movements the vestibulo-ocular reflex must act quickly to maintain stable gaze. A disynaptic brain stem pathway, the three-neuron arc, connects each semicircular canal to the appropriate eye muscle (Figure 40–11). A direct pathway for the horizontal vestibulo-ocular reflex, the ascending tract of Deiters, is anatomically significant but may not be physiologically important. Even when Deiters' tract is intact, lesions of the medial longitudinal fasciculus impair the contribution of the medial rectus muscle to the horizontal vestibulo-ocular reflex.

The oculomotor centers for vertical and torsional movements lie in the mesencephalic reticular formation (see Chapter 39). Networks similar to those for the horizontal canals connect the vertical canals to their oculomotor targets.

These excitatory and inhibitory pathways of the vestibulo-ocular reflex connect each of the three pairs of semicircular canals to the four extraocular muscles, two for each eye, whose pulling directions are in roughly the same plane. For example, a leftward and downward head motion, such as tilting the head toward the front of the left shoulder, excites the left anterior canal and inhibits the right posterior canal. In turn, the left anterior canal excites the left superior rectus and right inferior oblique muscles, which move the eyes upward and to the right, and inhibits the left inferior rectus and right superior oblique muscles, which move the eyes downward and to the left. Simultaneously, the inhibited right posterior canal decreases its excitation of the left inferior rectus and right superior oblique, which move the eyes downward and to the left, and decreases its inhibition of the left superior rectus and right inferior oblique, which move the eyes upward and to the left. The primary muscle targets of the three canals are listed in Table 40–1.

Less is known of the central pathways mediating otolithic reflexes (translational vestibulo-ocular reflexes). Patients with cerebellar disease often have diminished vestibulo-ocular responses to linear motion but not rotation of the head, suggesting that the cerebellum is essential for the translational vestibulo-ocular reflexes.

Two Visual Pathways Drive the Optokinetic Reflexes

As we have seen, movement of images on the retina or head movement can induce nystagmus and the perception of self-motion. This perception occurs because vision-related neurons project to the vestibular nuclei. Retinal neurons project to the accessory optic system and the nucleus of the optic tract in the pretectum, which project to the same medial vestibular nucleus that receives signals from vestibular organs. Vestibular neurons that receive this visual input cannot distinguish between visual and vestibular signals (Figure 40–12). They respond identically to head movement and to motion of an image across the retina, which is presumably why people sometimes cannot distinguish the two.

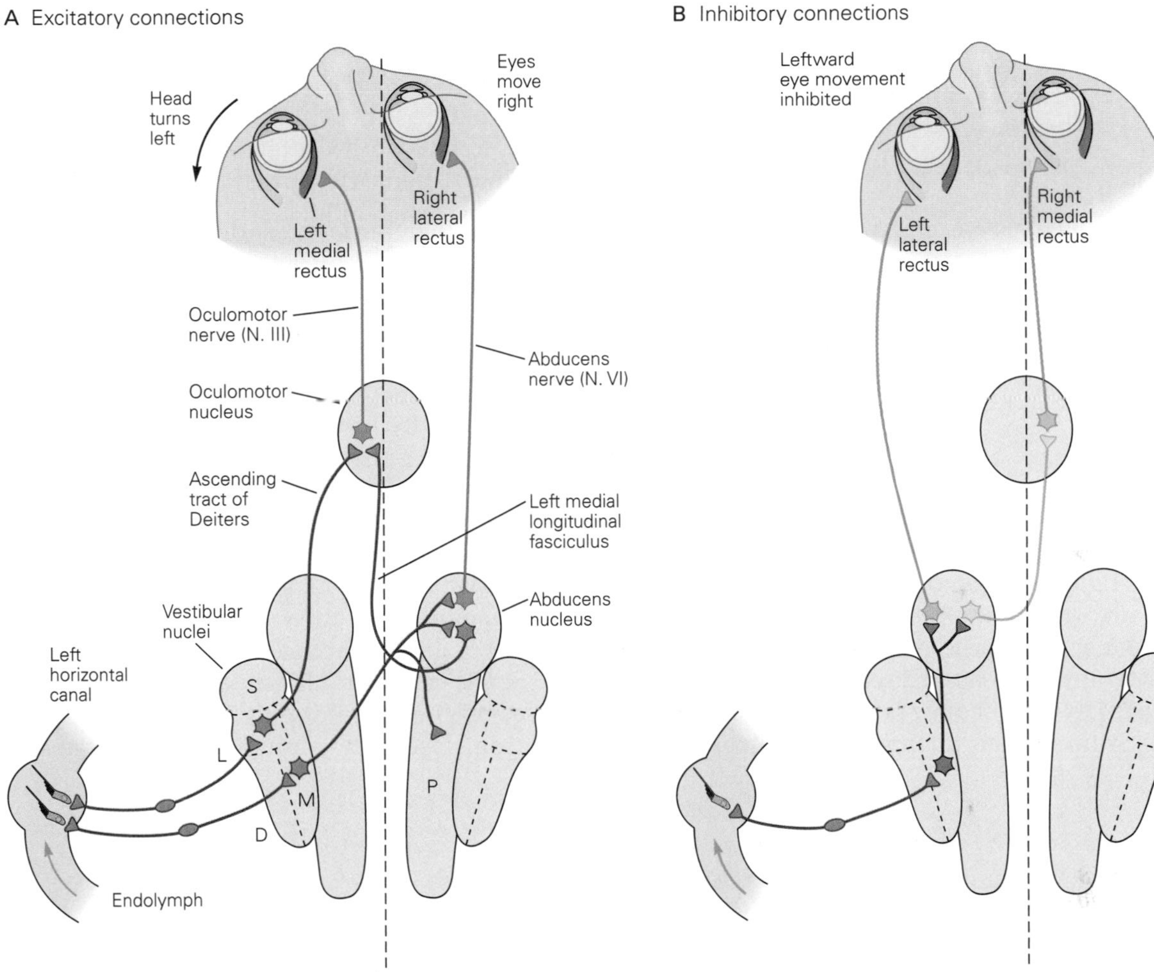

Figure 40–11 The horizontal vestibulo-ocular reflex. Similar pathways connect the anterior and posterior canals to the vertical recti and oblique muscles.

A. Leftward head rotation excites hair cells in the left horizontal canal, thus exciting neurons that evoke rightward eye movement. The vestibular nuclei include two populations of first-order neurons. One lies in the medial vestibular nucleus (**M**); its axons cross the midline and excite neurons in the right abducens nucleus and nucleus prepositus hypoglossi (**P**). The other population is in the lateral vestibular nucleus (**L**); its axons ascend ipsilaterally in the tract of Deiters and excite neurons in the left oculomotor nucleus, which project in the oculomotor nerve to the left medial rectus muscle.

The right abducens nucleus has two populations of neurons. A set of motor neurons projects in the abducens nerve and excites the right lateral rectus muscle. The axons of a set of interneurons cross the midline and ascend in the left medial longitudinal fasciculus to the oculomotor nucleus, where they excite the neurons that project to the left medial rectus muscle. These connections facilitate the rightward horizontal eye movement that compensates for leftward head movement. Other nuclei shown are the superior (**S**) and descending (**D**) vestibular nuclei.

B. During counterclockwise head movement, leftward eye movement is inhibited by sensory fibers from the left horizontal canal. These afferent fibers excite neurons in the medial vestibular nucleus that inhibit motor neurons and interneurons in the left abducens nucleus. This action reduces the excitation of the motor neurons for the left lateral and right medial rectus muscles. The same head movement results in a decreased signal in the right horizontal canal (not shown), which has similar connections. The weakened signal results in decreased inhibition of the right lateral and left medial rectus muscles and decreased excitation of the left lateral and right medial rectus muscles. (Adapted, with permission, from Suguichi et al. 2005.)

Table 40–1 Primary Muscle Targets of the Semicircular Canals

Canal	Ipsilateral muscles	Contralateral muscles
Horizontal	Excite medial rectus Inhibit lateral rectus	Excite lateral rectus Inhibit medial rectus
Anterior	Excite superior rectus Inhibit inferior rectus	Excite inferior oblique Inhibit superior oblique
Posterior	Excite superior oblique Inhibit inferior oblique	Excite inferior rectus Inhibit superior rectus

In rabbits, which are lateral-eyed and afoveate, optokinetic reflexes depend primarily on brain stem pathways involving the pretectal visual system. The rabbit optokinetic response is stronger when the image moves in a temporal-to-nasal direction and is relatively more efficient at low image speeds. The same asymmetry is seen in human infants and in patients with certain abnormalities of visual development, such as hereditary achromatopsia. Such asymmetries disappear in adult humans and nonhuman primates, which have well-developed binocular vision and thus a powerful cortical projection to the pretectum.

The Cerebral Cortex Integrates Vestibular, Visual, and Somatosensory Inputs

All vestibular nuclei project to the ventral posterior and ventral lateral nuclei of the thalamus, which then project to two regions in the primary somatosensory cortex (S-I): the vestibular regions of areas 2 and 3a (Figure 40–13). Vernon Mountcastle first showed that electrical stimulation of the vestibular nerve in the cat evoked activity in the primary somatosensory cortex (S-I) and in a parietal association cortex (area 7). Otto-Joachim Grüsser described neurons in areas 2 and 3a of the monkey that respond to head rotation. Vestibular activity has also been found in the monkey in the parieto-insular vestibular cortex, which is near the secondary somatosensory area (S-II), and in the periarcuate regions of the frontal lobe.

Single-cell recordings in animals have shown that these areas receive not only vestibular but also visual and somatosensory inputs. This arrangement likely

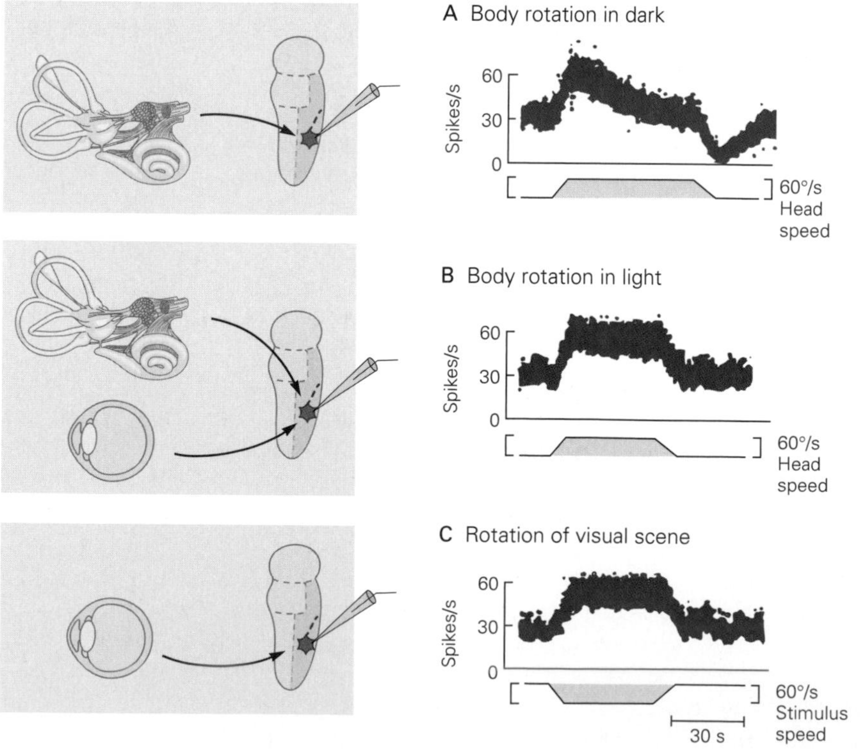

Figure 40–12 Individual neurons in the medial vestibular nucleus of a monkey receive both visual and vestibular signals. Each panel shows the spike rate of a single neuron over time. The angular velocity of the turntable used to rotate the subject or visual scene is shown below the plot. (Adapted, with permission, from Waespe and Henn 1977.)

A. When the animal is rotated in the dark, the activity of the neuron gradually falls to the baseline even while the animal is still rotating.

B. When the animal is rotated in the light, the discharge is maintained throughout rotation.

C. When the animal is still while the visual scene rotates around it, the neuron in the steady state responds as if the animal were rotating in the light, although it takes somewhat longer for the neuron to reach a constant level of activity. The similarity of response between body rotation in the light and rotation of the visual scene may explain why people sometimes feel they are moving when in fact the visual scene is moving.

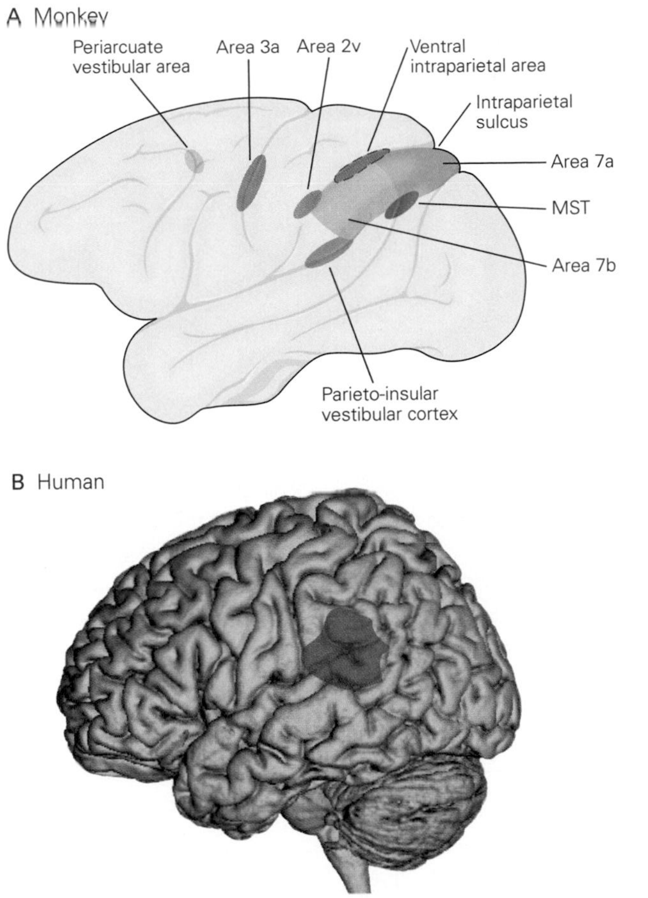

Figure 40–13 The vestibular cortex.

A. This lateral view of a monkey's brain shows the areas of cerebral cortex in which vestibular responses have been recorded. (MST, medial superior temporal area.)

B. Areas of human cortex that respond selectively to galvanic stimulation of the vestibular system. (Adapted, with permission, from Brandt and Dietrich 1999.)

facilitates the integration of all relevant sensory information for the perception of motion and orientation. In addition, vestibular and visual areas of cortex have reciprocal connections that may be involved in the resolution of contradictory vestibular and visual inputs. For example, motion of an object in the visual field of a person riding in a train or car moving at constant speed is correctly interpreted as self-motion, even though there is no corresponding vestibular signal. An undesired consequence of this is that motion in the visual field is often interpreted as self-motion even when a person is not moving, as when the observer has stopped at a red light and the adjacent vehicle accelerates.

Although the vestibular apparatus measures how one accelerates and tilts, the cerebral cortex employs this information to generate a subjective measure of self-movement in relation to the external world. Otolithic inputs are used by the vestibular cortex to determine the gravitational vertical axis in the visual field. Patients with lesions in this area may perceive themselves or objects in the environment to be tilted away from the side of the lesion. A few patients with parietal lesions perceive their visual environments to be rotated by 90 or 180 degrees.

The Cerebellum Adjusts the Vestibulo-Ocular Reflex

As we have seen, the vestibulo-ocular reflex keeps the gaze constant when the head moves. There are times, however, when the reflex is inappropriate. For example, when you turn your head while walking, you want your gaze to follow; the rotational vestibulo-ocular reflex, however, would prevent your eyes from turning with your head. To prevent this sort of biologically inappropriate response, the reflex is under the control of the cerebellum, which permits visual suppression of the vestibulo-ocular reflex.

In addition, the vestibulo-ocular reflex must be continuously calibrated to maintain its accuracy in the face of changes within the motor system (fatigue, injury to vestibular organs or pathways, eye-muscle weakness, or aging) and differing visual requirements (wearing corrective lenses). This is accomplished by sensory feedback that modifies the motor output. If the reflex is not working properly, the image moves across the retina. The motor command to the eye muscles must be adjusted until the gaze is again stable, retinal image motion is zero, and there is no error.

Anyone who wears eyeglasses depends on this plasticity of the vestibulo-ocular reflex. Because lenses for nearsightedness shrink the visual image, a smaller eye rotation is needed to compensate for a given head rotation, and the gain of the vestibulo-ocular reflex must be reduced. Conversely, glasses for farsightedness magnify the image, so the vestibulo-ocular reflex gain must increase during their use. More complicated is the instance of bifocal spectacles, in which the vestibulo-ocular reflex must use different gains for the two lenses. In the laboratory the vestibulo-ocular reflex can be conditioned by altering the visual consequences of head motion. For example, if a subject is rotated for a period of time while wearing magnifying glasses, the vestibulo-ocular reflex gain gradually increases (Figure 40–14A).

This process requires changes in synaptic transmission in both the cerebellum and the brain stem.

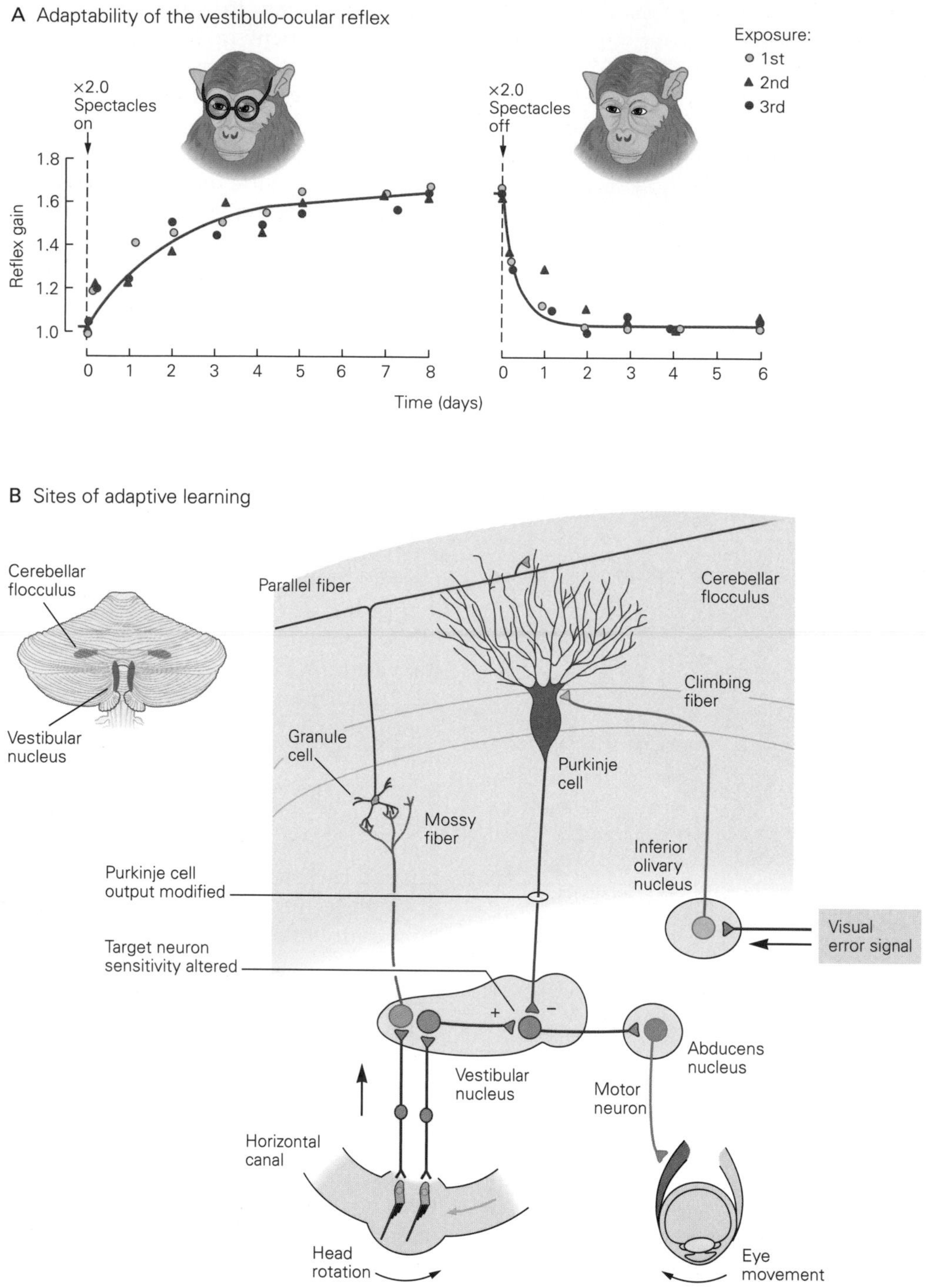

Figure 40–14 The vestibulo-ocular reflex is adaptable.

A. For several days the monkey continuously wears magnifying spectacles that double the speed of the retinal-image motion evoked by head movement. Each day the gain of the vestibulo-ocular reflex—the amount the eyes move for a given head movement—is tested in the dark so that the monkey cannot use retinal motion as a clue to modify the reflex. Over a period of 4 days the gain increases gradually (**left**). It quickly returns to normal when the spectacles are removed (**right**). (Adapted, with permission, from Miles and Eighmy 1980.)

B. Adaptation of the vestibulo-ocular reflex occurs in cerebellar and brain stem circuits. A visual error signal, triggered by motion of the retinal image during head movement, reaches the inferior olivary nucleus. The climbing fiber transmits this error signal to the Purkinje cell, affecting the parallel fiber–Purkinje cell synapse. The Purkinje cell transmits changed information to the floccular target cell in the vestibular nucleus, changing its sensitivity to the vestibular input. After the reflex has been adapted, the Purkinje cell input is no longer necessary.

If the flocculus and paraflocculus of the cerebellum are lesioned, the gain of the vestibulo-ocular reflex can no longer be modulated. Mossy fibers carry vestibular, visual, and motor signals from the pontine nuclei to the cerebellar cortex; the granule cells, with their parallel-fiber axons, relay these signals to the Purkinje cells (Figure 40–14B). David Marr suggested that the synaptic efficacy of parallel fiber input to a Purkinje cell could be modified by the concurrent action of climbing fiber input. Masao Ito showed that the climbing fiber input to the cerebellum did indeed carry a suitable visual error signal and postulated that this was the "teaching line" enabling the cerebellum to correct the error in the vestibulo-ocular reflex. This adaptation requires long-term depression of the Purkinje cell synapses (see Chapter 42). Transgenic mice lacking long-term synaptic depression in these neurons cannot adapt their vestibulo-ocular reflexes in a few hours, as can normal mice.

The Purkinje cell is not the only locus of change. Frederick Miles and Steven Lisberger showed that there is a class of neurons in the vestibular nucleus, the *flocculus target neurons,* that receive GABA-ergic inhibitory input from Purkinje cells in the flocculus as well as direct inputs from vestibular sensory fibers. During adaptation of the vestibulo-ocular reflex these neurons change their sensitivity to the vestibular inputs in the appropriate way, and after adaptation they can maintain those changes without further input from the cerebellum.

The importance of the cerebellum in calibrating eye movements is also evident in patients with cerebellar disease. Although the vestibulo-ocular reflex is still present, it may have an abnormal amplitude or direction. In many cases the translational vestibulo-ocular reflex is also poor.

Clinical Syndromes Elucidate Normal Vestibular Function

Unilateral Vestibular Hypofunction Causes Pathological Nystagmus

As we have seen, rotation excites hair cells in the semicircular canal whose hair bundles are oriented in the direction of motion and inhibits those whose hair bundles are oriented away from the motion. This imbalance in vestibular signals is responsible for the compensatory eye movements and the sensation of rotation that accompanies head movement. It can also originate from disease of one labyrinth or vestibular nerve, which results in a pattern of afferent vestibular signaling analogous to that stemming from rotation away from the side of the lesion, that is, more discharge from the intact side. There is accordingly a strong feeling of spinning, called vertigo.

The vestibulo-ocular reflex responds by generating eye movements in an attempt to compensate for this perceived rotation. The slow phases (see Figure 40–8) are directed away from the intact side and toward the lesioned side, and the intervening quick phases produce a nystagmus that beats toward the intact side. For example, an acute loss of left vestibular function causes a right-beating nystagmus, as if there were a prolonged rightward acceleration. Unlike physiological nystagmus, which stabilizes gaze, the pathological nystagmus causes retinal slip and a corresponding sensation that the visual world is moving, called *oscillopsia.*

The vertigo and nystagmus resulting from an acute vestibular lesion typically subside over several days, even if peripheral function does not recover. First, nystagmus can be suppressed by visual fixation, just as post-rotatory nystagmus is suppressed in the light. Second, central compensatory mechanisms restore the balance in vestibular signals in the brain stem, even when peripheral input is permanently lost.

The loss of input from one labyrinth also means that all vestibular reflexes must be driven by a single labyrinth. For the vestibulo-ocular reflex this condition is quite effective at low speeds because the intact labyrinth can be both excited and inhibited. However, during rapid, high-frequency rotations inhibition is not sufficient, such that the gain of the reflex is reduced when the head rotates toward the lesioned side. This is the basis of an important clinical test of canal function, the head-impulse test. In this test the head is moved rapidly one time along the axis of rotation of a single canal. If there is a significant decrease in gain owing to canal dysfunction, the movement of the eyes will lag behind that of the head, and there will be a visible catch-up saccade (Figure 40–15).

Bilateral Vestibular Hypofunction Interferes with Normal Vision

Vestibular function is sometimes lost simultaneously on both sides, for example from ototoxicity owing to aminoglycoside antibiotics such as gentamicin. The symptoms of bilateral vestibular hypofunction are different from those of unilateral loss. First, there is no vertigo because there is no imbalance in vestibular signals; input is reduced equally from both sides. For the same reason there is no spontaneous nystagmus. In fact, these patients may have no symptoms when they are at rest and the head is still.

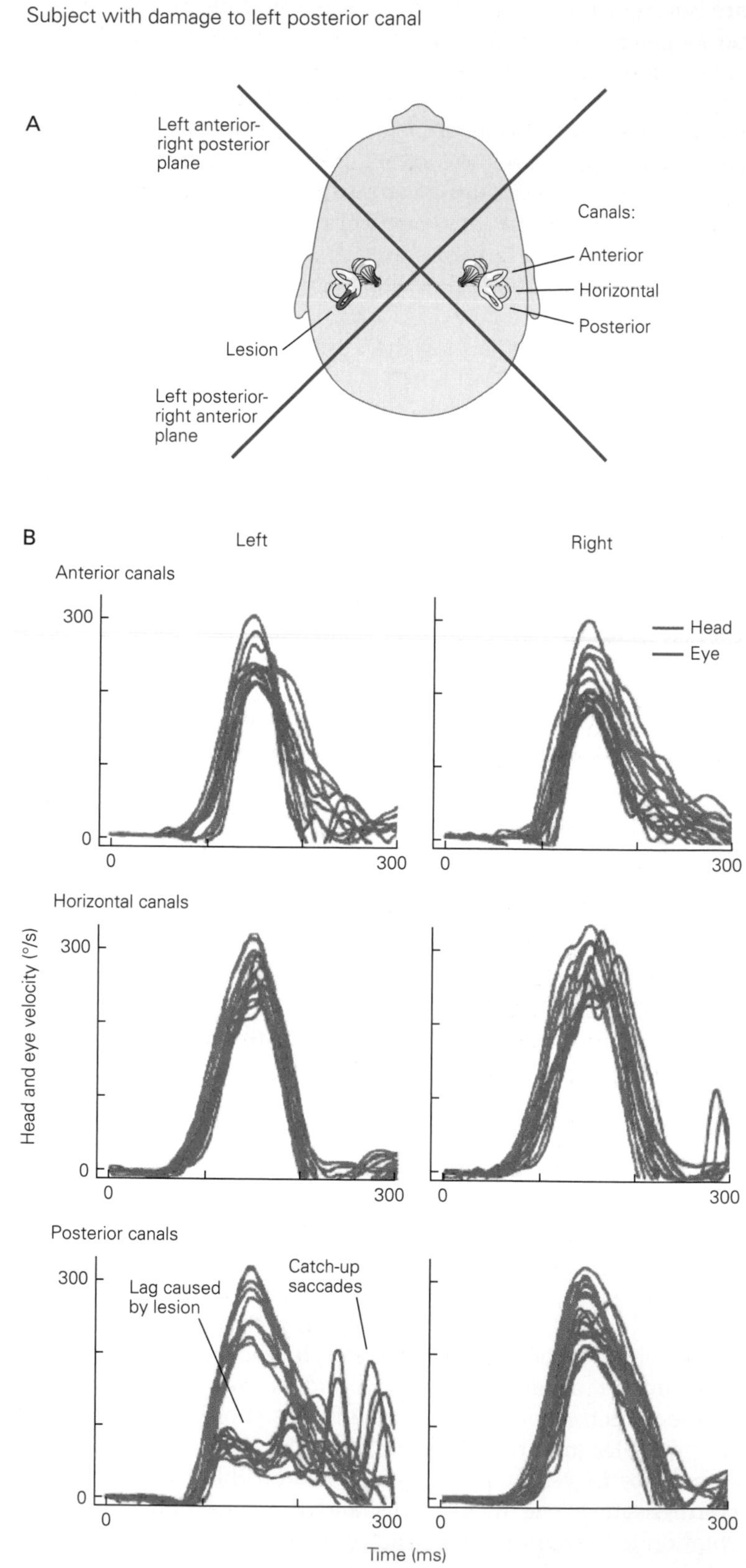

Figure 40–15 Clinical testing of the vestibulo-ocular reflex.

A. The examiner rotates the patient's head rapidly in the optimum direction for each canal while the subject fixates. This stimulus is termed a *head impulse*. If the canal and oculomotor systems are normal, eye velocity matches head velocity and the eyes maintain gaze—they do not move relative to the external environment. If there is a canal deficit, the eyes lag behind the head and make catch-up saccades after the head movement is finished.

B. The records are the results of impulse testing in a patient with a lesion of the left posterior canal. In the record for the left posterior canal (rotation in the left posterior–right anterior plane), eye velocity fails to track the head velocity during the most rapid parts of the head movement. After the head movement is over, pulses of eye velocity correspond to the catch-up saccades induced by the visual error.

Nevertheless, the loss of vestibular reflexes is devastating. A physician who lost his vestibular hair cells because of a toxic reaction to streptomycin wrote a dramatic account of this loss. Immediately after the onset of streptomycin toxicity he could not read in bed without steadying his head to keep it motionless. Even after partial recovery he could not read street signs or recognize friends while walking in the street; he had to stop to see clearly. Some patients may even "see" their heartbeat if the vestibulo-ocular reflex fails to compensate for the miniscule head movements that accompany each arterial pulse.

An Overall View

The vestibular system evolved to answer two of the questions basic to human life: "Which way is up?" and "Where am I going?" The system provides the brain with a rapid estimate of head motion. Although this estimate could be derived from vision and neck proprioception, those sensory mechanisms are slow and cumbersome. In contrast, the hair cells of the vestibular system sense head acceleration directly, and this responsiveness in turn allows those reflexes that require information about head motion to act efficiently and quickly.

There are two distinct sets of vestibular organs. The three semicircular canals sense head rotation, whereas the otolith organs—the utricle and saccule—detect linear acceleration. Signals from the canals and otolith organs are carried in the vestibular nerve to the ipsilateral vestibular nuclei.

Projections from the vestibular nuclei to the oculomotor system allow eye muscles to compensate for head movement by moving in such a way as to hold the image of the external world motionless on the retina. Sustained rotation results in a pattern of alternating slow and fast eye movements called nystagmus. The slow eye movement is equal and opposite to the head movement, whereas the fast eye movement represents a resetting movement in the opposite direction. Nystagmus in the absence of sustained head rotation is a sign of disease of the vestibular apparatus or its central connections. Vestibular signals habituate during sustained rotation and are relatively insensitive to very slow head movements.

Head movement evokes motion of the entire visual image on the retina as the moving eyes sweep across a stable visual field. This visual signal supplements the vestibular signal in the brain and compensates for the tendency of the vestibular signal to adapt during prolonged rotation. The optokinetic system provides the visual input to the central vestibular system. The motion of the retinal image induced by head movement enables the optokinetic system to induce eye movements and perceptions that are equivalent to those induced by actual head movement.

The vestibulo-ocular reflex is adaptable. If a process such as muscle weakness or visual distortion alters the relationship between the visual input and the motor output, the brain compensates for that change. This compensation requires activity in both the cerebellum and the vestibular nuclei.

Michael E. Goldberg
Mark F. Walker
A. J. Hudspeth

Selected Readings

Baloh RW, Honrubia V. 1990. *Clinical Neurology of the Vestibular System,* 2nd ed. Philadelphia: FA Davis.

Highstein SM, Holstein GR. 2005. The anatomy of the vestibular nuclei. Prog Brain Res 151:157–203.

Leigh RJ, Zee DS. 2006. *The Neurology of Eye Movements,* 4th ed. New York: Oxford Univ. Press.

References

Benser ME, Issa NP, Hudspeth AJ. 1993. Hair bundle stiffness dominates the elastic reactance to otolithic-membrane shear. Hear Res 68:243–252.

Bergström B. 1973. Morphology of the vestibular nerve. II. The number of myelinated vestibular nerve fibers in man at various ages. Acta Otolaryngol (Stockh) 76:173–179.

Brandt T, Dieterich M. 1994. Vestibular syndromes in the roll plane: topographic diagnosis from brainstem to cortex. Ann Neurol 36:337–347.

Brandt T, Dieterich M. 1999. The vestibular cortex. Its locations, functions, and disorders. Ann N Y Acad Sci 871:293–312.

Crèmer PD, Halmagyi GM, et al. 1998. Semicircular canal plane head impulses detect absent function of individual semicircular canals. Brain 121:699–716.

Crèmer PD, Migliaccio AA, Halmagyi GM, Curthoys IS. 1999. Vestibulo-ocular reflex pathways in internuclear ophthalmoplegia. Ann Neurol 45:529–533.

Dieterich M, Brandt T. 1995. Vestibulo-ocular reflex. Curr Opin Neurol 8:83–88.

Distler C, Mustari MJ, Hoffmann KP. 2002. Cortical projections to the nucleus of the optic tract and dorsal terminal nucleus and to the dorsolateral pontine nucleus in macaques: a dual retrograde tracing study. J Comp Neurol 444:144–158.

Fernandez C, Goldberg JM. 1976a. Physiology of peripheral neurons innervating otolith organs of the squirrel monkey. I. Response to static tilts and to long-duration centrifugal force. J Neurophysiol 39:970–984.

Fernandez C, Goldberg JM. 1976b. Physiology of peripheral neurons innervating otolith organs of the squirrel monkey. II. Directional selectivity and force-response relations. J Neurophysiol 39:985–995.

Fernandez C, Goldberg JM. 1971. Physiology of peripheral neurons innervating semicircular canals of the squirrel monkey. II. Response to sinusoidal stimulation and dynamics of peripheral vestibular system. J Neurophysiol 34:661–675.

Fernandez C, Goldberg JM, Abend WK. 1972. Response to static tilts of peripheral neurons innervating otolith organs of the squirrel monkey. J Neurophysiol 35:978–997.

Flock Å. 1965. Transducing mechanisms in the lateral line canal organ receptors. Cold Spring Harbor Symp Quant Biol 30:133–145.

Fukushima K. 1997. Corticovestibular interactions: anatomy, electrophysiology, and functional considerations. Exp Brain Res 117:1–16.

Gacek RR, Lyon M. 1974. The localization of vestibular efferent neurons in the kitten with horseradish peroxidase. Acta Otolaryngol (Stockh) 77:92–101.

Goldberg JM, Fernández C. 1971. Physiology of peripheral neurons innervating semicircular canals of the squirrel monkey. I. Resting discharge and response to constant angular accelerations. J Neurophysiol 34:635–660.

Grüsser OJ, Pause M, Schreiter U. 1990. Localization and responses of neurons in the parieto-insular vestibular cortex of awake monkeys (*Macaca fascicularis*). J Physiol (Lond) 430:537–557.

Hillman DE, McLaren JW. 1979. Displacement configuration of semicircular canal cupulae. Neuroscience 4:1989–2000.

Ito M. 2002. Historical review of the significance of the cerebellum and the role of Purkinje cells in motor learning. Ann N Y Acad Sci 978:273–288.

Iurato S. 1967. *Submicroscopic Structure of the Inner Ear.* Oxford: Pergamon Press.

Lisberger SG. 1998. Physiologic basis for motor learning in the vestibulo-ocular reflex. Otolaryngol Head Neck Surg 119:43–48.

Miles FA, Eighmy BB. 1980. Long-term adaptive changes in primate vestibuloocular reflex. I. Behavioral observations. J Neurophysiol 43:1406–1425.

Mustari MJ, Fuchs AF. 1990. Discharge patterns of neurons in the pretectal nucleus of the optic tract (NOT) in the behaving primate. J Neurophysiol 64:77–90.

Mustari MJ, Fuchs AF, Kaneko CRS, Robinson F. 1994. Anatomical connections of the primate pretectal nucleus of the optic tract. J Comp Neurol 349:111–128.

Shutoh F, Katoh A, Kitazawa H, Aiba A, Itohara S, Nagao S. 2002. Loss of adaptability of horizontal optokinetic response eye movements in mGluR1 knockout mice. Neurosci Res 42:141–145.

Spoendlin H. 1966. Ultrastructure of the vestibular sense organ. In: RJ Wolfson (ed). *The Vestibular System and Its Diseases*, pp. 39–68. Philadelphia: Univ. of Pennsylvania Press.

Sugiuchi Y, Izawa Y, Ebata S, Shinoda Y. 2005. Vestibular cortical areas in the periarcuate cortex: its afferent and efferent projections. Ann N Y Acad Sci 1039:111–123.

van Alphen AM, De Zeeuw CI. 2002. Cerebellar LTD facilitates but is not essential for long-term adaptation of the vestibulo-ocular reflex. Eur J Neurosci 16:486–490.

Waespe W, Henn V. 1977. Neuronal activity in the vestibular nuclei of the alert monkey during vestibular and optokinetic stimulation. Exp Brain Res 27:523–538.

Watanuki K, Schuknecht HF. 1976. A morphological study of human vestibular sensory epithelia. Arch Otolaryngol Head Neck Surg 102:583–588.

Yee RD, Baloh RW, Honrubia V. 1981. Eye movement abnormalities in rod monochromacy. Ophthalmology 88:1010–1018.

41

Posture

The control of posture is crucial for most tasks of daily living. The two components of posture, orientation and balance, require continual adjustment and involve several sensory systems.

To appreciate the complexity of maintaining balance and orientation, imagine that you are waiting tables on a tour boat. You have a tray full of drinks to be delivered to a table on the other side of the rolling deck. Even as your mind is occupied with remembering customer orders, unconscious processes allow you to move about in a smooth and coordinated manner.

The apparently simple task of delivering drinks is supported by a truly complex sensorimotor process for controlling postural orientation and balance. As you cross the deck your brain rapidly processes sensory information and adjusts motor output to maintain your balance, the upright orientation of your head and trunk, and stable arms supporting the tray of full glasses. Before you reach out to place a glass on the table, your nervous system makes anticipatory postural adjustments to maintain your balance. Sudden unexpected motions of the boat evoke automatic postural responses that prevent falls. Somatosensory, vestibular, and visual information is integrated to provide a coherent picture of the position and velocity of the body in space and to generate and update motor commands that maintain balance and orientation.

Postural Equilibrium and Orientation Are Distinct Sensorimotor Processes

Postural equilibrium, or balance, involves active resistance to external forces acting on the body. The dominant external force affecting equilibrium on earth is gravity. Postural orientation is the positioning of body segments with respect to each other and to the environment. Depending on the particular task or behavior, body segments may be aligned with respect to gravitational vertical, visual vertical, or the support surface.

The biomechanical requirements of postural control depend on anatomy and postural orientation and thus vary with the animal. Nevertheless, in a variety of species the control mechanisms for postural equilibrium and orientation have many common features. The sensorimotor mechanisms for postural control are quite similar in humans and quadrupedal mammals even though their habitual stance is different.

Postural Equilibrium Requires Control of the Body's Center of Mass

With many segments linked by joints, the body is mechanically unstable. To maintain balance the nervous system must control the position and motion of the body's *center of mass* as well as the body's rotation about its center of mass. The center of mass is a point that represents the average position of the body's total mass. In the standing cat, for example, the center of mass is located in the trunk just rostral to the midpoint between forelimbs and hind limbs.

Although gravity pulls on all body segments, the net effect on the body acts through the center of mass. The force of gravity is opposed by the *ground reaction force*, which pushes upward against each foot. The net ground reaction force occurs at an imaginary point on the ground called the *center of pressure* (Box 41–1).

The location of the center of mass in the body is not fixed but depends on postural orientation. When you are standing upright, for example, your center of mass is located in the abdomen approximately 20 mm in front of the second lumbar vertebra. When you flex at the hips, however, the center of mass moves forward to a position outside the body.

Maintaining balance while standing requires keeping the downward projection of the center of mass within the base of support, an imaginary area defined by those parts of the body in contact with the environment. For example, the four paws of a standing cat define a rectangular base of support (see Figure 41–1). When a standing person leans against a wall, the base of support extends from the ground under the feet to the contact point between the body and the wall. Because the body is always in motion, even during stable stance, the center of mass continually moves about with respect to the base of support. Postural instability is determined by how fast the center of mass is moving toward the boundary of its base of support and how close the downward projection of the body's center of mass is to the boundary.

Balance During Stance Requires Muscle Activation

Upright stance requires two actions: (1) maintaining support against gravity (keeping the center of mass at some height) and (2) maintaining balance (controlling the trajectory of the center of mass in the horizontal plane). Balance and antigravity support are controlled separately by the nervous system and may be differentially affected in certain pathological conditions.

Antigravity support, or postural tone, represents the tonic activation of muscles that generate force against the ground to keep the limbs extended and the center of mass at the appropriate height. A cat stands with its limbs in a semiflexed posture (see Figure 41–1) and its extensor muscles are tonically activated to prevent the joints from collapsing into flexion. In humans much of the support against gravity is provided by passive bone-on-bone forces in joints such as the knees, which are fully extended during stance, and in stretched ligaments such as those at the front of the hips. Nevertheless, antigravity support in humans also requires active muscle contraction, for example in ankle, trunk, and neck extensors. Tonic activation of antigravity muscles is not sufficient, however, for maintaining balance.

Both bipeds and quadrupeds are inherently unstable, and their bodies sway during quiet stance. Actively contracting muscles exhibit a spring-like stiffness that helps to resist body sway, but muscle stiffness alone is insufficient for maintaining balance. Likewise, stiffening of the limbs through muscle co-contraction is not sufficient for balance control. Instead, complex patterns of muscle activation produce direction-specific forces to control the body's center of mass. Body sway caused by even subtle movements, such as the motion of the chest during breathing, is actively counteracted by the posture control system.

Automatic Postural Responses Counteract Unexpected Disturbances

When a sudden disturbance causes the body to sway, various motor strategies are used to maintain the center

Box 41–1 Center of Pressure

The center of pressure is defined as the origin of the ground reaction force vector on the support surface. For the body to be in static equilibrium, the force caused by gravity and the ground reaction force must be equal and opposite, and the center of pressure must be directly under the center of mass.

Misalignment of the center of pressure and center of mass causes motion of the center of mass. If the center of pressure is behind and to the left of the center of mass projection onto the base of support, for example, the body will sway forward and to the right (Figure 41–1).

When no external forces other than gravity are present, the center of pressure and ground reaction force reflect the net effect of muscles activated by the postural system to actively control the center of mass position and therefore balance.

Standing is never truly static. The center of pressure and center of mass are continually in motion and are rarely aligned, although when averaged over time during quiet stance they are coincident. The actual sway of the body during quiet stance is described by the trajectory of the center of mass, not the center of pressure.

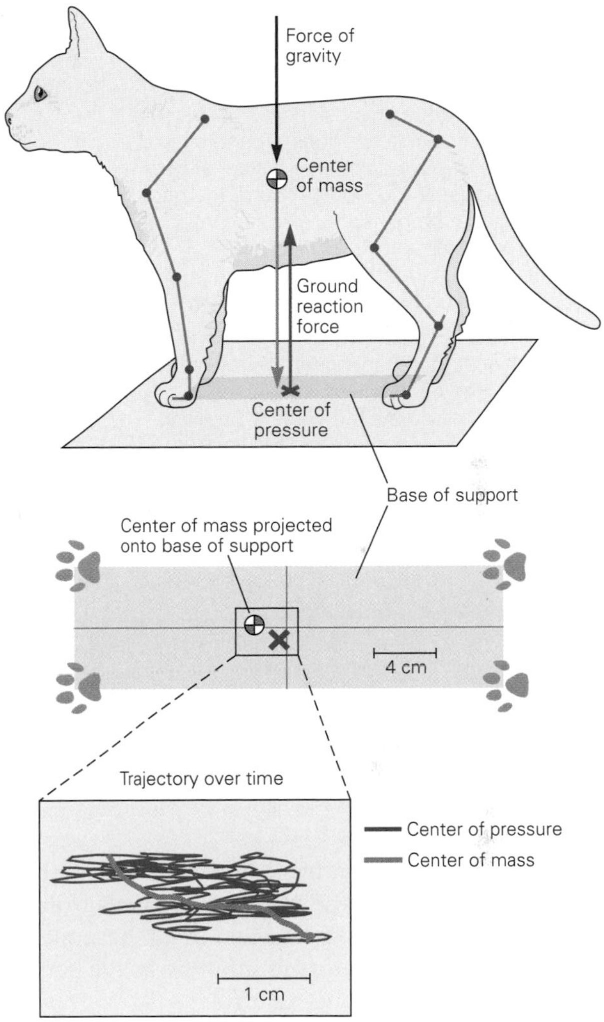

Figure 41–1 The center of mass moves during stance but remains within the base of support. The base of support of the standing cat is defined by the points of contact of the paws on the support surface. The force caused by gravity passes through the center of mass in the trunk. The surface exerts an upward force against each paw, such that the ground reaction force vector originates in the center of pressure on the support surface. Although the paws remain in place, the centers of pressure and mass are always in motion as the cat sways.

of mass within the base of support. In one strategy the base of support remains fixed relative to the support surface. While the feet remain in place the body rotates about the ankles back to the upright position (Figure 41–2A). In other strategies the base of support is moved or enlarged, for example by taking a step or by grabbing a support with the hand (Figure 41–2B).

Older views of motor control focused on trunk and proximal limb muscles as the main postural effectors. Recent behavioral studies show that any group of muscles from the neck and trunk, legs and arms, or feet and hands can act as postural muscles depending on the body parts in contact with the environment and the biomechanical requirements of equilibrium.

When studying the posture control system, scientists disrupt balance in a controlled manner to determine the subject's automatic postural response. This response is described by the ground reaction force vector under each foot, the motion of the center of pressure, and the movements of the body segments. The electrical activity of many muscles is recorded by electromyography (EMG), which reflects the firing of alpha

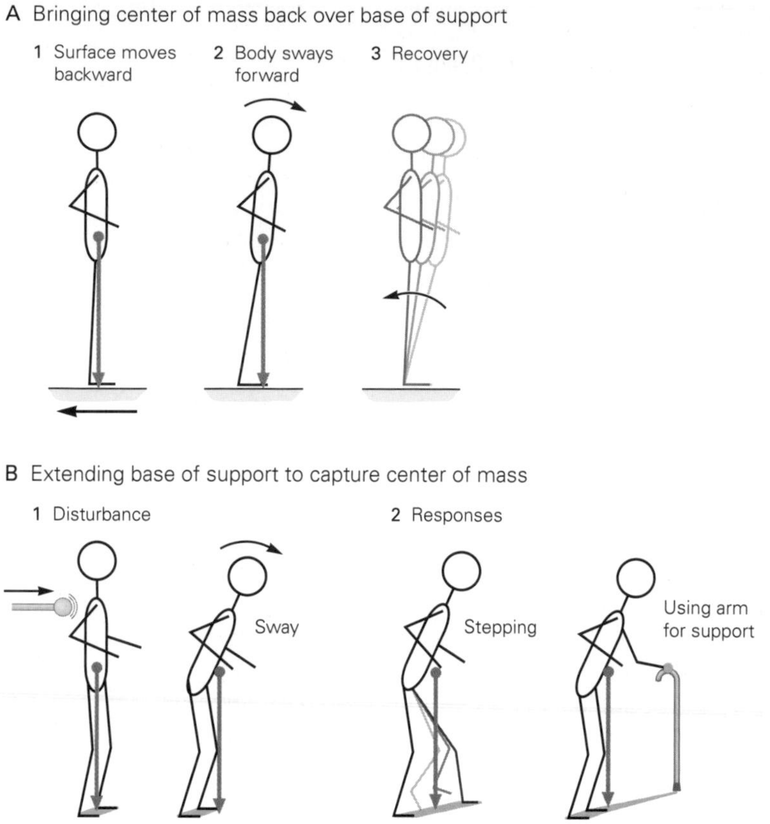

Figure 41–2 Automatic postural responses keep the downward projection of the center of mass within the boundaries of the base of support.

A. One strategy for regaining balance is to bring the center of mass back to its origin on the base of support. When the platform on which a subject is standing is suddenly moved backward, the body sways forward and the projection of the center of mass moves toward the toes. During recovery the body actively rotates about the ankles, bringing the center of mass back to the original position with respect to the feet.

B. An alternative strategy enlarges the base of support to keep the center of mass within the base. A disturbance causes the subject to sway forward and the center of mass moves toward the boundary of the base of support. The base can be enlarged in two ways: taking a step and placing the foot in front of the center of mass to decelerate the body's motion, or grabbing a support and thereby extending the base to include the contact point between the hand and support.

motor neurons that innervate skeletal muscle and thus provides a window into the nervous system's output for balance control. The combination of all these measurements allows investigators to infer the active neural processes underlying balance control.

An automatic postural response to a sudden disturbance is not a simple reflex but rather the synergistic activation of a group of muscles in a characteristic sequence with the goal of maintaining equilibrium. The recruitment of a muscle during a postural response reflects the requirements of equilibrium rather than the change in the muscle's length caused by the disturbance. For example, when the surface under a person is rotated in the toes-up direction, the ankle extensor (gastrocnemius) is lengthened and a small stretch reflex may occur. The postural response for balance recruits the antagonist ankle flexor (tibialis anterior), which itself is shortened by the surface rotation, while suppressing the stretch response in the gastrocnemius. In contrast, when the platform is moved backward the gastrocnemius is again lengthened but now it is recruited for the postural response, as evidenced by a second burst of EMG activity after the stretch reflex. Thus the initial change in length of a muscle induced by perturbation does not determine whether that muscle is recruited for postural control, and stretch reflexes are not the basis for postural control.

Automatic postural responses to sudden disturbances have characteristic temporal and spatial features. A postural response in muscles must be recruited rapidly following the onset of a disturbance. Sudden movement of the support surface under a standing cat evokes EMG activity within 40–60 ms (Figure 41–3). Humans have longer latencies of postural response (80–120 ms); the increased delay is attributed to the larger body size of humans and thus the greater signal conduction distances from sensory receptors to the central nervous system and thence to leg muscles. The latency of automatic postural responses is shorter than voluntary reaction time but longer than the stretch reflex.

Postural responses involving a change in support base, such as stepping, have longer latencies than those that occur when the feet remain in place.

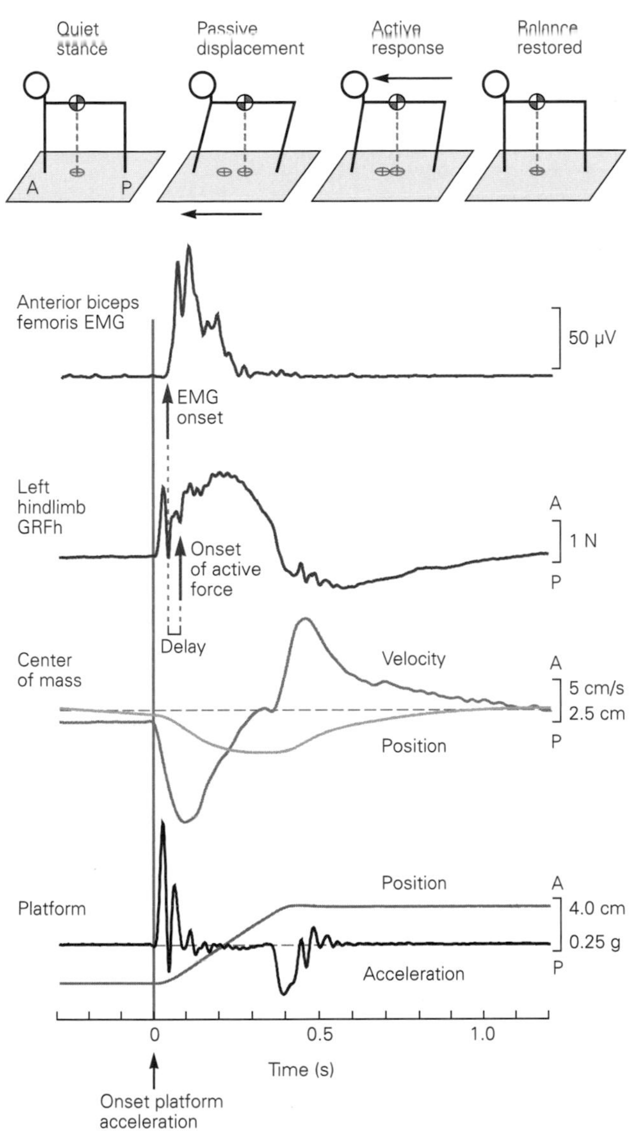

Figure 41–3 Automatic postural responses have stereotypical temporal characteristics. Electromyographic (EMG) activity has a characteristic latency. Anterior motion of the platform evokes an EMG response in the hip extensor muscle (anterior biceps femoris) approximately 40 ms after the onset of platform acceleration. This latency is stereotyped and repeatable across subjects and is approximately four times as long as that of the monosynaptic stretch reflex. As the platform moves, the paws are carried forward and the trunk remains behind owing to inertia, causing the center of mass of the cat to move backward with increasing velocity with respect to the platform. The velocity of the center of mass peaks and then decreases as the horizontal component of the ground reaction force (**GRFh**) increases following muscle activation. The delay of approximately 30 ms between the onset of EMG activity and the onset of the active response reflects excitation-contraction coupling and body compliance. The automatic postural response extends the hind limb, propelling the trunk forward and restoring the position of the center of mass with respect to the paws.

The longer time presumably affords greater flexibility in the response, for example the choice of foot to begin the step, the direction of the step, and the path of the step around obstacles.

Activation of postural muscles results in contraction and the development of force in the muscles, leading to torque (rotational force) at the joints. The net result is an active response, the ground reaction force, that restores the center of mass to its original position over the base of support (Figure 41–3). The delay between EMG activation and the active response, approximately 30 ms in the cat, reflects the excitation-contraction coupling time of each muscle as well as the compliance of the musculoskeletal system.

The amplitude of EMG activity in a particular muscle depends on both the speed and direction of postural disturbance. The amplitude increases as the speed of a platform under a standing human or cat increases, and it varies in a monotonic fashion as the direction of platform motion is varied systematically. Each muscle responds to a limited set of perturbation directions with a characteristic tuning curve (Figure 41–4).

Although individual muscles have unique directional tuning curves, muscles are not activated independently but instead are coactivated in synergies. The muscles within a synergy receive a common command signal during postural responses. In this way the many muscles of the body are controlled by just a few signals, reducing the time needed to compute the appropriate postural response (Box 41–2).

Automatic Postural Responses Adapt to Changes in the Requirements for Support

The set of muscles recruited in a postural response to a disturbance depends on the body's initial stance. The same disturbance elicits very different postural responses in someone standing unaided, standing while grasping a stable support, or crouching on all four limbs. For example, forward sway activates muscles at the back of the legs and trunk during upright free stance. When the subject is holding onto a stable support, muscles of the arms rather than those of the legs are activated. When the subject is crouched on toes and fingers, muscles at the front of the legs and in the arms are activated (Figure 41–6A).

Because postural responses are influenced by recent experience, they adapt only gradually to new biomechanical conditions. When forward sway is induced by backward motion of a platform on which a subject is standing, the posterior muscles of the ankle, knee, and hip are activated in sequence beginning

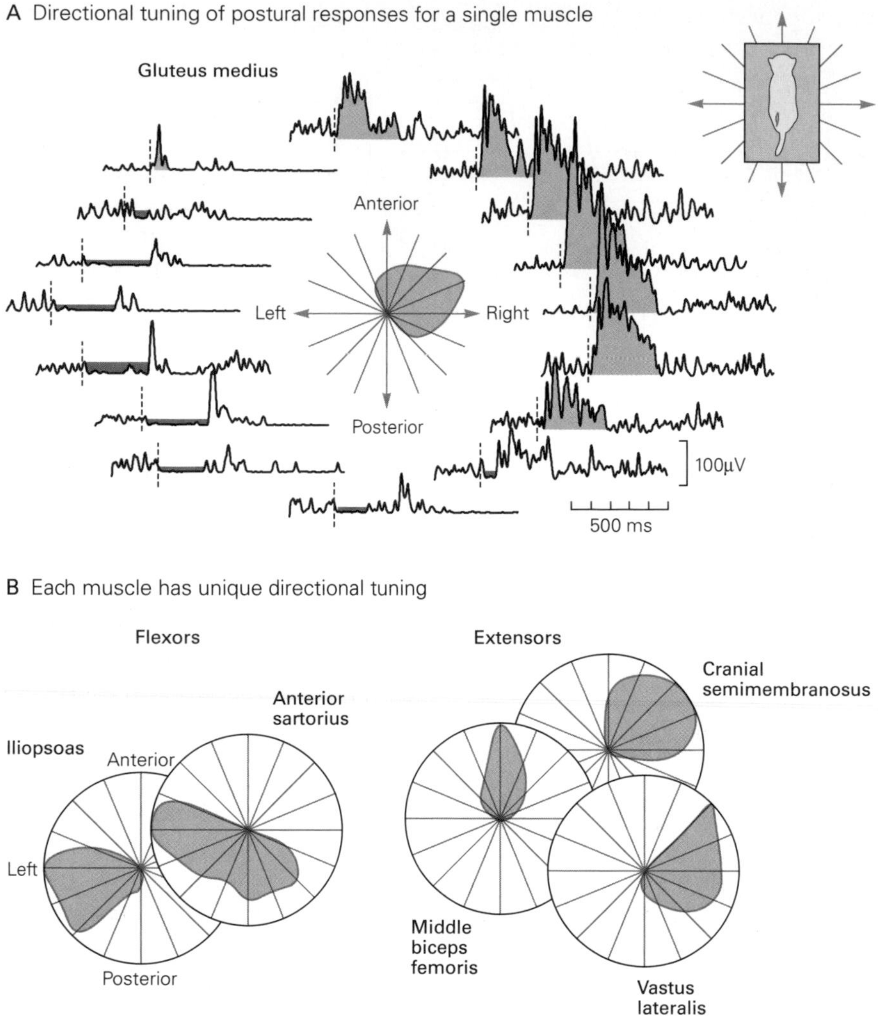

Figure 41–4 Automatic postural responses have stereotypical directional characteristics. (Adapted, with permission, from Macpherson 1988.)

A. The gluteus medius muscle in the cat, a hip extensor and abductor, responds to a range of directions of motion in the horizontal plane. The EMG records shown here are from a cat standing on a platform that was moved in the horizontal plane in each of 16 evenly spaced directions. The gluteus medius muscle of the left hind limb was activated by motion in several directions (**pink**) and inhibited in the remaining directions (**gray**). The dashed vertical lines indicate the onset of platform acceleration. In the center is a polar plot of the amplitude of EMG activity during the automatic postural response versus the direction of motion; it represents a directional tuning curve for the muscle. EMG amplitude was computed from the area under the curve during the first 80 ms of the response.

B. Every muscle has a characteristic directional tuning curve that differs from that of other muscles, even if they have similar actions. The middle biceps femoris and cranial semimembranosus, for example, are both extensors of the hip.

90 ms after the platform starts moving. This postural response, the *ankle strategy*, restores balance primarily by rotating the body about the ankle joints. However, when forward sway is induced by backward motion of a narrow beam, the anterior muscles of the hip and trunk are activated. This postural pattern, the *hip strategy*, restores the body's center of mass by bending forward at the hip joints and counter-rotating at the ankles (Figure 41–6B).

When a subject moves from the wide platform to the narrow beam, he persists in using the ankle strategy in the first few trials. This strategy does not work when standing on the beam, and the subject falls. He then gradually, over several trials, switches to the hip strategy. Similarly, moving from the beam back to the platform requires several trials to adapt the postural response (Figure 41–6C).

Although sensory stimulation changes immediately after subjects move from the beam to the floor, the postural response adjusts gradually as it is tuned for optimal behavior by trial and error. Trial-to-trial changes in postural behavior generally occur at the subconscious level and involve updating of the body schema.

Anticipatory Postural Adjustments Compensate for Voluntary Movements

Voluntary movements themselves can destabilize postural orientation and equilibrium. Rapidly lifting the arms forward while standing, for example, produces forces that extend the hips, flex the knees, and dorsiflex the ankles, moving the body's center of mass forward relative to the feet. The nervous system has advance knowledge of the effects of voluntary movement on postural alignment and stability and activates *anticipatory postural adjustments*, often in advance of the primary movement (Figure 41–7A).

Anticipatory postural adjustments are specific to biomechanical conditions. When a freely standing subject rapidly pulls on a handle fixed to the wall, the leg muscles (gastrocnemius and hamstrings) are activated before the arm muscles (Figure 41–7B). When the subject performs the same pull while his shoulders are propped against a rigid bar, no anticipatory leg muscle activity occurs because the nervous system relies on the support of the bar to prevent the body from moving forward. When the handle is pulled in response to an external cue, the arm muscles are activated faster in the supported condition than in the freestanding condition. Thus voluntary arm muscle activation is normally delayed when the task requires active postural stability.

Another common preparatory postural adjustment occurs when one begins to walk. The center of mass is accelerated forward and laterally by the unweighting of one leg. This postural adjustment appears to be independent of the stepping program that underlies ongoing locomotion. Similarly, a forward shift of the center of mass precedes the act of standing on the toes. A subject is unable to remain standing on his toes if he simply activates the calf muscles without moving his center of mass forward; he rises onto his toes only momentarily before gravity restores a flat-footed stance. Moving the center of mass forward over the toes before activating the calf muscles aligns it over the anticipated base of support and thus stabilizes the toe stance.

Locomotion, too, has an important postural component. During walking and running the body is in a constant state of falling as the center of mass moves forward and laterally toward the leg that is in the swing phase. The center of mass is within the base of support during walking only when both feet are on the ground, the double stance phase, and not at all during running. When one foot is supporting the body, the center of mass moves forward in front of the foot, always medial to the base of support. Falling is prevented during walking and running by moving the base of support forward and laterally under the falling center of mass. Postural equilibrium during gait relies on the appropriate placement of each step to control the speed and trajectory of the center of mass (Figure 41–7C). The nervous system plans foot placement several steps in advance using visual information about the terrain and surrounding environment (see Chapter 36).

Postural equilibrium during voluntary movement requires control not only of the position and motion of the body's center of mass but also of the angular momentum about the center of mass. A diver can perform elaborate rolls and twists of the body about the center of mass while airborne although the trajectory of his center of mass is fixed once he leaves the board. During swimming and flying the water or air currents in addition to the body's own movements may cause the body to pitch or roll about the center of mass. During voluntary movements postural adjustments control the body's angular momentum by anticipating rotational forces.

Postural Orientation Is Important for Optimizing Execution of Tasks, Interpreting Sensations, and Anticipating Disturbances to Balance

Animals arrange their body parts to accomplish specific tasks efficiently. Although this postural orientation interacts with balance control, the two systems can act independently.

The energy needed to maintain body position over a period of time can influence postural orientation. In humans, for example, the upright orientation of the trunk with respect to gravity minimizes the forces and thus the energy required to hold the body's center of mass over the base of support. Standing cats adopt a characteristic distance between front and back paws that minimizes the energy needed for remaining upright.

Task requirements also affect postural orientation. For some tasks it is important to stabilize the position of a body part in space, whereas for others it is necessary to stabilize one body part with respect to another. When walking while carrying a full glass, for example, it is important to stabilize the hand against gravity to prevent spillage. When walking while reading a book, the hand must be stabilized with respect to the head and eyes.

Subjects may adopt a particular postural orientation to optimize the accuracy of sensory signals regarding body motion, especially while on unstable or moving surfaces. In activities such as skiing and windsurfing, in which the substrate is unstable, information about earth vertical is derived primarily from vestibular and visual inputs. A person often aligns his head with respect to gravitational vertical because the perception of vertical is most accurate in this position and decreases in accuracy as the head is tilted. The vestibular and visual information regarding the external world, representing an extrinsic coordinate system,

Box 41–2 Synergistic Activation of Muscles

Coordinated movements require precise control of the many joints and muscles in the body. Maintaining control is biomechanically complex, in part because different combinations of joint rotations can achieve the same goal. Such redundancy confers great flexibility, for example in modifying stepping patterns to negotiate obstacles in our path, but comes at the cost of increased complexity in the brain's computation of movement trajectories and forces.

Many factors must be included in the computation of movement commands, including the effect of external forces such as gravity and the forces that one body segment exerts on another during motion. All these factors come into play when the brain computes postural responses to sudden disturbances, but with the added constraint of a time limit on computation: Responses must occur within a certain time or balance will be lost.

It has long been believed that the brain simplifies the control of movement by grouping control variables, for example activating several muscles together. In older concepts of synergy the same muscles are always recruited together. This kind of synergy cannot apply to balance responses because each muscle has a unique directional tuning curve and the tuning curves overlap imperfectly (see Figure 41–4B).

Using mathematical techniques that parse complex data into a small number of components, Lena Ting and Jane Macpherson showed that only four or five synergies are needed to account for the activation patterns of 15 hind limb muscles of the cat during automatic postural responses to many directions of platform motion (Figure 41–5). Activation of each synergy produces a unique direction of force against the ground, suggesting that postural control is based on task-related variables such as the force between foot and ground rather than the contraction force of individual muscles.

Like the arrangement of notes in a musical chord, each muscle synergy specifies how a particular muscle should be activated together with others. Just as one note belongs to several different chords, each muscle belongs to more than one synergy. When several chords are played simultaneously, the chord structure is no longer evident in the multitude of notes. Similarly, when several synergies are activated concurrently, the observed muscle pattern gives the appearance of unstructured complexity. Concurrent activation of synergies nevertheless simplifies the neural command signals for movement while allowing flexibility and adaptability.

Figure 41–5 Postural commands activate synergies rather than individual muscles.

A. The flow chart illustrates two hypothetical synergies that are recruited during the postural response to one direction of translation in the horizontal plane. A posture controller computes the appropriate force vector response for restoring center of mass position and then specifies how much to activate each synergy. Each muscle synergy activates the muscles in a fixed proportion. The height of each bar represents the relative amount of activation, or weighting, for each muscle M1 to M3. Synergy 1 produces a downward force vector by activating M1 strongly, M2 not at all, and M3 moderately. Synergy 2 produces a downward and posterior force vector using the same muscles but with different levels of activation: M1 slightly, M2 strongly, and M3 moderately. When synergy 1 is activated with an amplitude of 2 and synergy 2 an amplitude of 1, the desired force vector response is achieved. Signals from the two muscle synergies are summated in the population of motor neurons innervating each muscle. The contribution of each synergy to the total electromyogram (EMG) activation can be determined.

B. The two hypothetical synergies in part A can generate the unique tuning curves for muscles M1 to M3 in response to all 16 directions of translation in the horizontal plane. The posture controller generates a command signal to each synergy that is tuned to direction of translation (synergy tuning curves). Muscle synergy weightings are multiplied by the synergy amplitudes. Signals from the two synergies are summated at the motor neurons, resulting in EMG activity that is tuned to a direction (the EMG tuning curve). The tuning curve for each of the three muscles is different even though only two synergy commands are used. The contribution of each synergy to the EMG tuning curve of a muscle can also be determined. The **black dots** indicate the amplitudes of the two synergies and resulting EMG activity of the three muscles for the direction illustrated in part A.

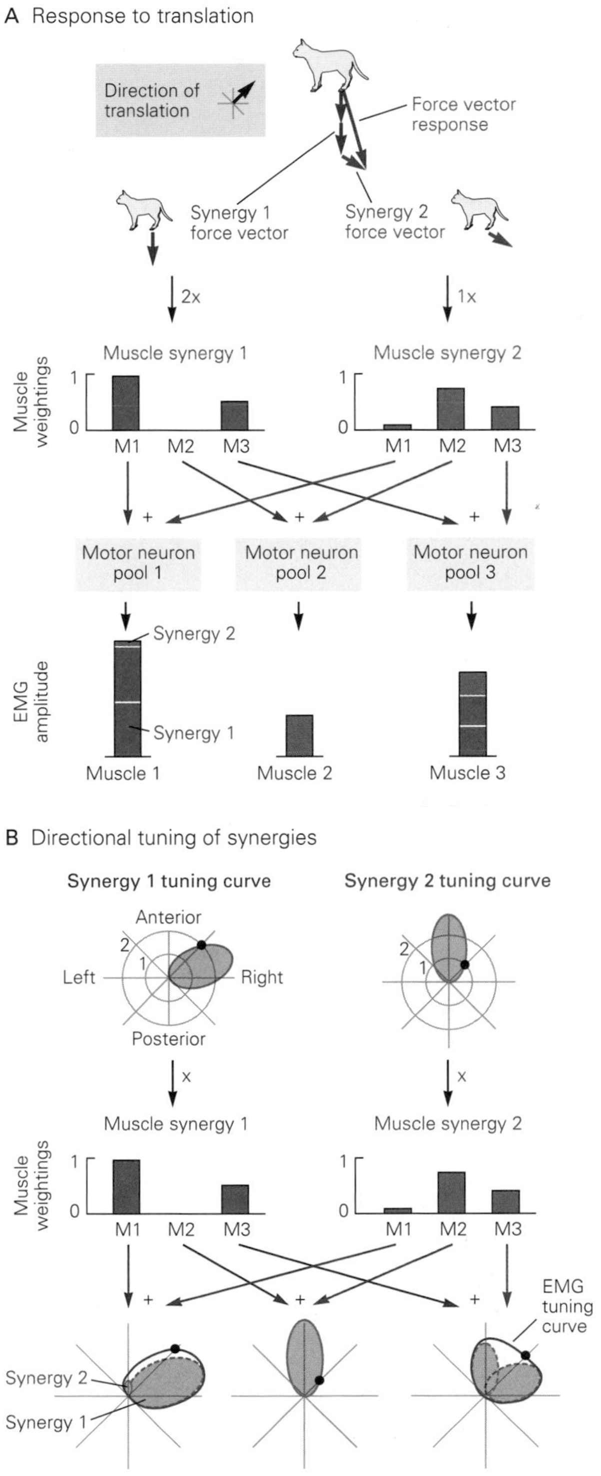

is integrated with proprioceptive information, representing an intrinsic coordinate system, to determine the position of the body in space (see Chapter 38). The accuracy of the transformation from intrinsic to extrinsic coordinates may be enhanced if at least one sensory input is aligned with the extrinsic system.

Anticipatory alterations of habitual body orientation can minimize the effect of a possible disturbance. For example, people often lean in the direction of an anticipated external force, or they flex their knees, widen their stance, and extend their arms when anticipating that surface stability will be compromised.

Sensory Information from Several Modalities Must Be Integrated to Maintain Equilibrium and Orientation

Information about motion from any one sensory system may be ambiguous. Thus multiple sources of sensory information must be integrated in postural centers to determine what orientation and motion of the body in space are appropriate. The influence of any one modality on the postural control system varies according to the task and biomechanical conditions.

According to the prevailing theory, sensory modalities are integrated to form an internal representation of the body that the nervous system uses to plan and execute motor behaviors. Over time this internal representation must adapt to changes associated with early development, aging, and injury.

Somatosensory Afferents Are Important for Timing and Direction of Automatic Postural Responses

Large-diameter, fast somatosensory fibers are critical for maintaining balance during stance. When these axons die, as occurs in some forms of peripheral neuropathy, postural responses to movement of the support surface are delayed, retarding the ground reaction force. As a result, the center of mass moves faster and farther from the initial position and takes longer to return (Figure 41–8). Because it is more likely that the center of mass will move outside the base of support, balance is precarious and a fall may occur. Individuals with large-fiber peripheral neuropathy in the legs accordingly experience ataxia and difficulties with balance.

The somatosensory fibers that give rise to the automatic postural response have not been identified. The largest fibers, those in group I (12–20 μm in diameter), appear to be essential for normal response latencies.

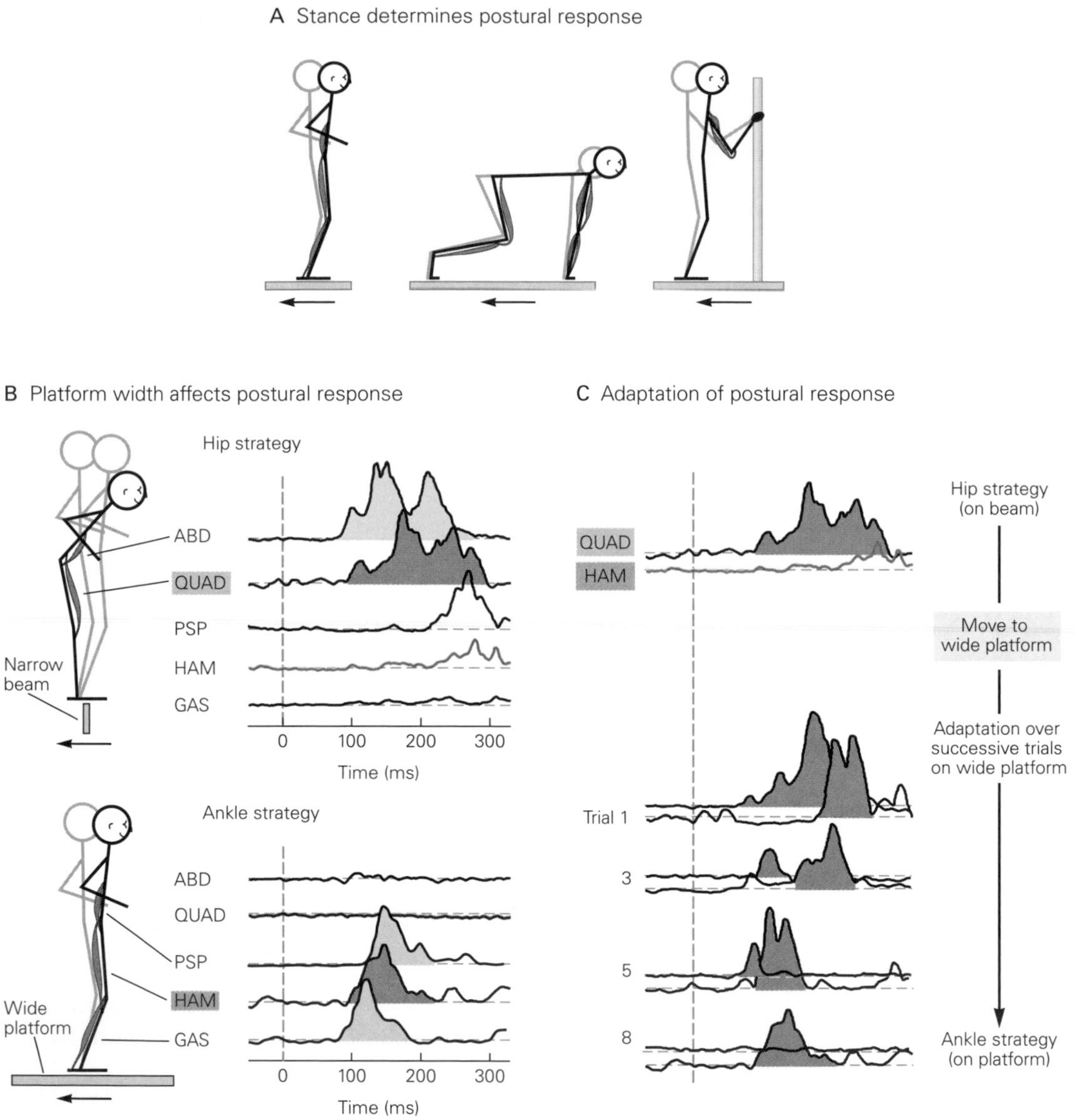

Figure 41–6 Automatic postural responses change with biomechanical conditions.

A. The backward movement of a platform activates different groups of muscles depending on initial stance. **Gray stick figures** show initial positions (upright unsupported, quadrupedal, or upright supported). The muscles activated in each postural response are shown in **red**. (Adapted, with permission, from Dunbar et al. 1986.)

B. When a subject stands on a narrow beam that is abruptly moved backward, the anterior muscles—abdominals (**ABD**) and quadriceps (**QUAD**)—are recruited to flex the trunk and extend the ankles, moving the hips backward (the hip strategy). When the subject instead stands on a wide platform that is moved backward, his posterior muscles—paraspinals (**PSP**), hamstrings (**HAM**), and gastrocnemius (**GAS**)—are activated to bring the body back to the erect position by rotating at the ankles (the ankle strategy). Muscles representative of different postural responses are highlighted in color. **Dashed vertical line** indicates onset of platform (or beam) acceleration.

C. Postural strategy adapts after the subject moves from the narrow beam onto the wide platform. On the beam the quadriceps are activated and the hamstrings are silent; after adaptation to the wide platform the reverse is observed. The transition from quadriceps to hamstrings occurs over a series of trials; the quadriceps activity gradually decreases in amplitude, whereas the hamstrings are activated earlier and earlier, until by trial eight quadriceps activity disappears altogether. Ankle and trunk muscles show similar patterns of adaptation. (Adapted, with permission, from Horak and Nashner 1986.)

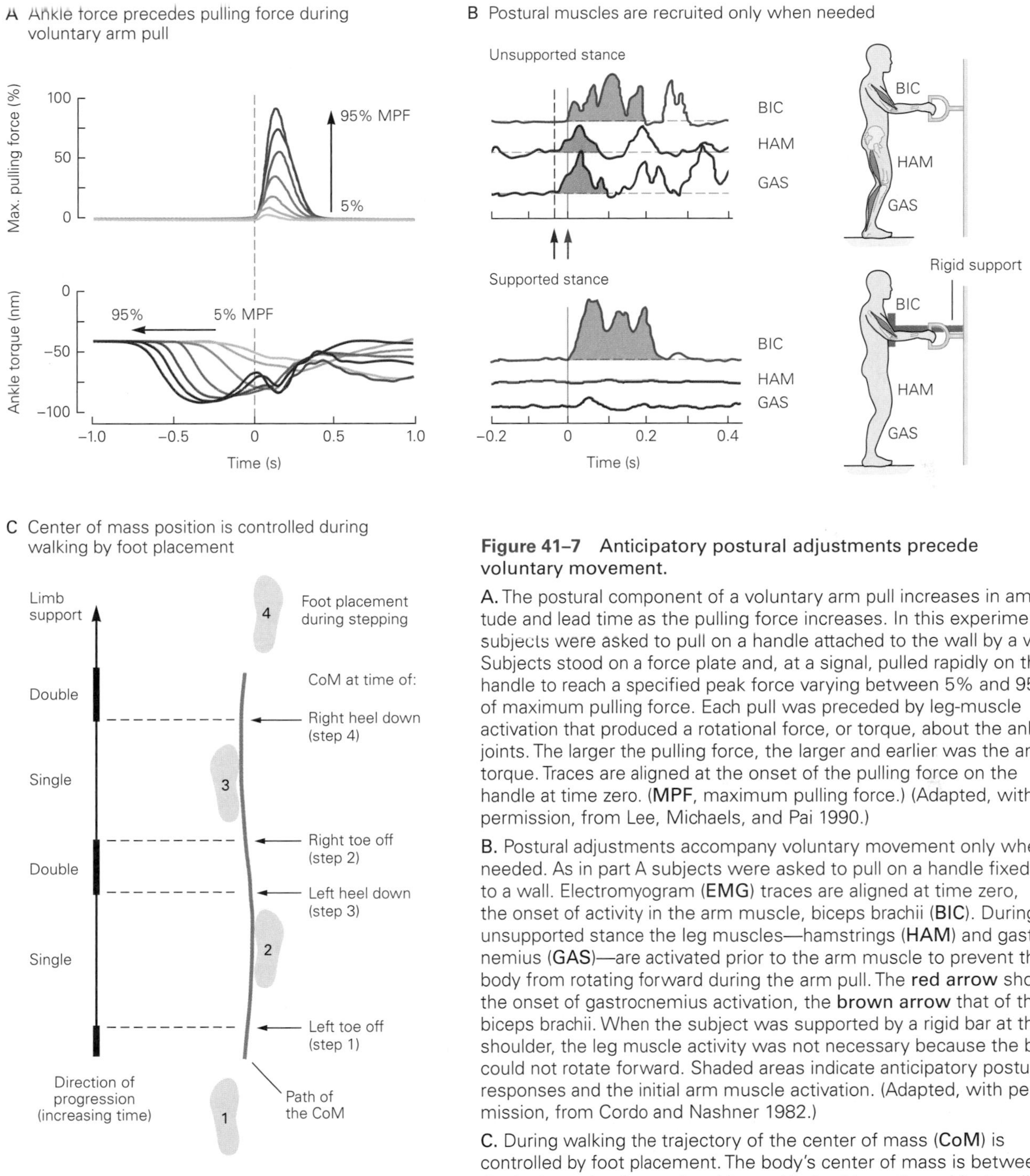

Figure 41–7 Anticipatory postural adjustments precede voluntary movement.

A. The postural component of a voluntary arm pull increases in amplitude and lead time as the pulling force increases. In this experiment subjects were asked to pull on a handle attached to the wall by a wire. Subjects stood on a force plate and, at a signal, pulled rapidly on the handle to reach a specified peak force varying between 5% and 95% of maximum pulling force. Each pull was preceded by leg-muscle activation that produced a rotational force, or torque, about the ankle joints. The larger the pulling force, the larger and earlier was the ankle torque. Traces are aligned at the onset of the pulling force on the handle at time zero. (**MPF**, maximum pulling force.) (Adapted, with permission, from Lee, Michaels, and Pai 1990.)

B. Postural adjustments accompany voluntary movement only when needed. As in part A subjects were asked to pull on a handle fixed to a wall. Electromyogram (**EMG**) traces are aligned at time zero, the onset of activity in the arm muscle, biceps brachii (**BIC**). During unsupported stance the leg muscles—hamstrings (**HAM**) and gastrocnemius (**GAS**)—are activated prior to the arm muscle to prevent the body from rotating forward during the arm pull. The **red arrow** shows the onset of gastrocnemius activation, the **brown arrow** that of the biceps brachii. When the subject was supported by a rigid bar at the shoulder, the leg muscle activity was not necessary because the body could not rotate forward. Shaded areas indicate anticipatory postural responses and the initial arm muscle activation. (Adapted, with permission, from Cordo and Nashner 1982.)

C. During walking the trajectory of the center of mass (**CoM**) is controlled by foot placement. The body's center of mass is between the feet, moving forward and from side to side as the subject walks forward. When the body is supported by only one leg, the center of mass is outside the base of support and moves toward the lifting limb. People do not fall while walking because the placement of the foot on the next step decelerates the center of mass and propels it back toward the midline. (Adapted, with permission, from MacKinnon and Winter 1993.)

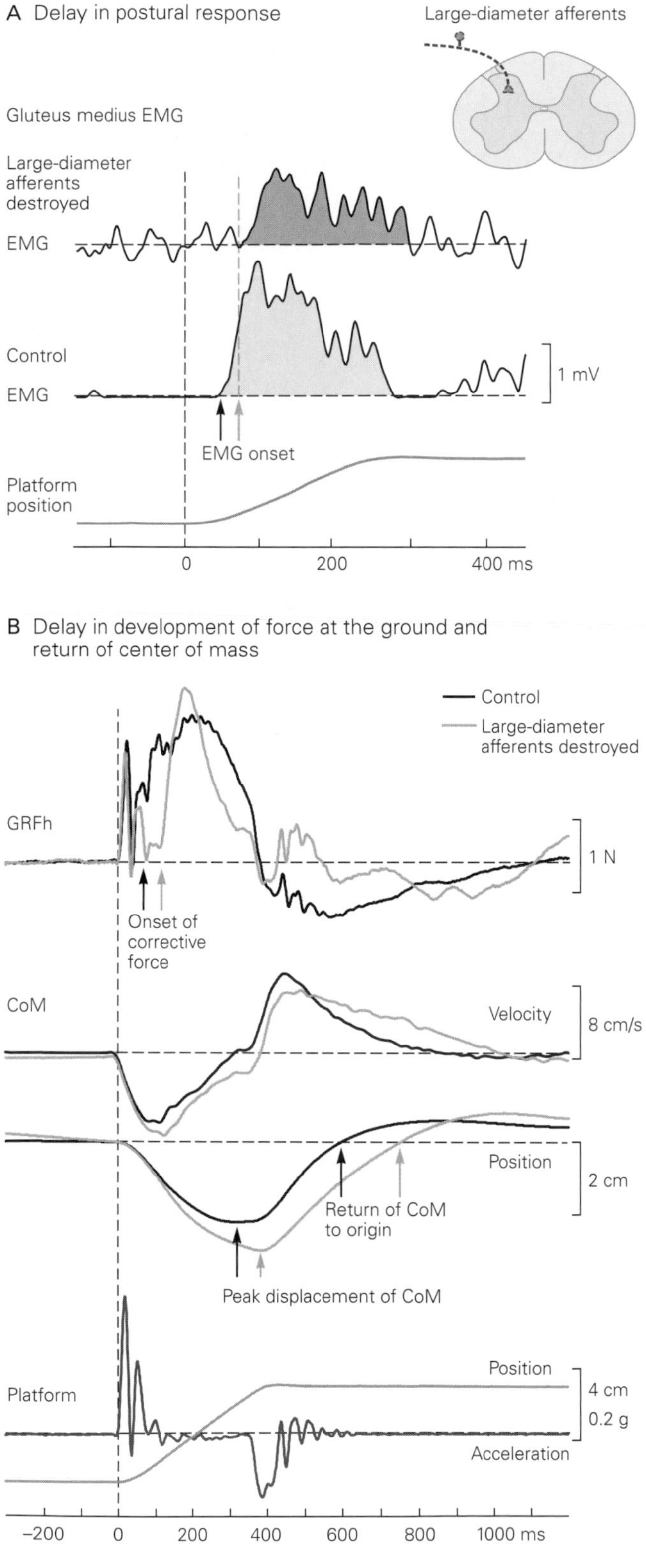

Figure 41–8 Loss of large-diameter somatosensory fibers delays automatic postural responses. Electromyograms **EMG** of postural responses to horizontal motion were recorded in a cat before and after destruction of the large-diameter (group I) somatosensory fibers throughout the body by vitamin B6 intoxication. Motor neurons and muscle strength are not affected by the loss of the somatosensory fibers, but afferent information about muscle length and force is diminished. (Reproduced, with permission, from J. Macpherson.)

A. The postural response in the gluteus medius evoked by horizontal motion of the support platform is significantly delayed after B6 intoxication. This delay of approximately 20 ms induces ataxia and difficulty in maintaining balance.

B. Destruction of group I fibers delays activation of the hind limb. This delay slows the restoration of the center of mass (**CoM**) and the recovery of balance following platform displacement. The delay in onset of the horizontal component of the ground reaction force (**GRFh**) results in a greater peak displacement of the center of mass and a delay in return of the center of mass to its origin relative to the paws.

The largest and most rapidly conducting sensory fibers are the Ia afferents from muscle spindles and Ib afferents from Golgi tendon organs as well as some fibers from cutaneous mechanoreceptors (see Chapter 22). Group I fibers provide rapid information about the biomechanics of the body including responses to muscle stretch, muscle force, and directionally specific pressure on the foot soles. Although group II fibers from muscle spindles and cutaneous receptors may also play a role in shaping automatic postural responses, they may be too slow to generate the earliest part of the response.

Lena Ting and co-workers showed that the temporal features of postural EMG in both quadrupeds and bipeds could be explained by a linear combination of position, velocity, and acceleration of the body's center of mass with a time delay. This suggests that information about the displacement of the center of mass is used in a feedback manner to sculpt the activation of postural muscles over time. According to this model the longer latency, slower rise time, and lower amplitude of the EMG response following destruction of group I fibers reflect a loss of acceleration information such as that encoded by muscle spindle primary receptors (Figure 41–8A). Thus center of mass acceleration may be signaled mainly by group I somatosensory fibers and center of mass velocity and position in part by the slower group II fibers.

Both proprioceptive and cutaneous inputs provide cues about postural orientation. During upright stance, for example, muscles lengthen and shorten as the body sways under the force of gravity, generating proprioceptive signals related to load, muscle length, and velocity of stretch. Joint receptors may detect compressive forces on the joints, whereas cutaneous receptors in the sole of the foot respond to motion of the center of pressure and to changes in ground reaction force angle as the body sways. Pressure receptors near the kidneys may be sensitive to gravity and used by the nervous system to help detect upright or tilted postures. All of these signals contribute to the neural map of the position of body segments with respect to each other and the support surface, and may contribute to the neural computation of center of mass motion.

Vestibular Information Is Important for Balance on Unstable Surfaces and During Head Movements

The otolithic organs of the vestibular apparatus provide information about the direction of gravity, whereas the semicircular canals measure the velocity of head rotation (see Chapter 40). Vestibular information can therefore inform the nervous system about how much the body is tilted with respect to gravity as well as whether it is swaying forward, backward, or sideways.

Somatosensory and vestibular information about the gravitational angle of the body is combined to orient the body with respect to gravity and other inertial forces. To maintain balance while riding a bike in a circular path at high speed, for example, the body and bike must be oriented with respect to a combination of gravitational and centripetal forces (Figure 41–9A).

Unlike somatosensory inputs, vestibular signals are not essential for the normal timing of balance reactions. Instead they influence the directional tuning of a postural response by providing information about the orientation of the body relative to gravity. In humans and experimental animals lacking vestibular signals, the postural response to *angular* motion or tilt of the support surface is opposite to the normal response. Instead of resisting the tilt, subjects lacking vestibular signals actively push themselves downhill (Figure 41–10). In contrast, the response to *linear*

A Orienting to gravito-inertial force

B Orienting to rotating visual field

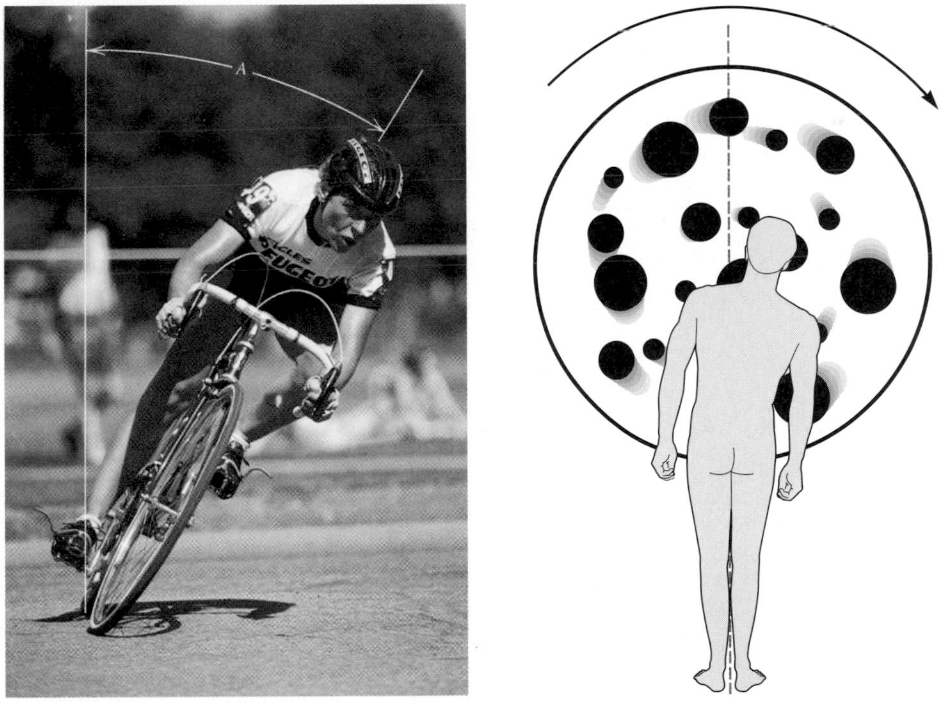

Figure 41–9 The postural system orients the body to various external reference frames.

A. When traveling at high speed along a curved path a cyclist orients to the gravito-inertial force (**angle A**), the vector sum of the force caused by gravity and the centripetal force caused by acceleration along the curved path. (Reproduced, with permission, from McMahon and Bonner 1983.)

B. The postural system can interpret rightward rotation of objects occupying a large region of the visual field as the body tilting to the left. In compensation for this illusion of motion the subject tilts to the right, adopting a new postural vertical that is driven by the visual system. Gravitational vertical is indicated by the **red dashed line**. (Adapted, with permission, from Brandt, Paulus, and Straube 1986.)

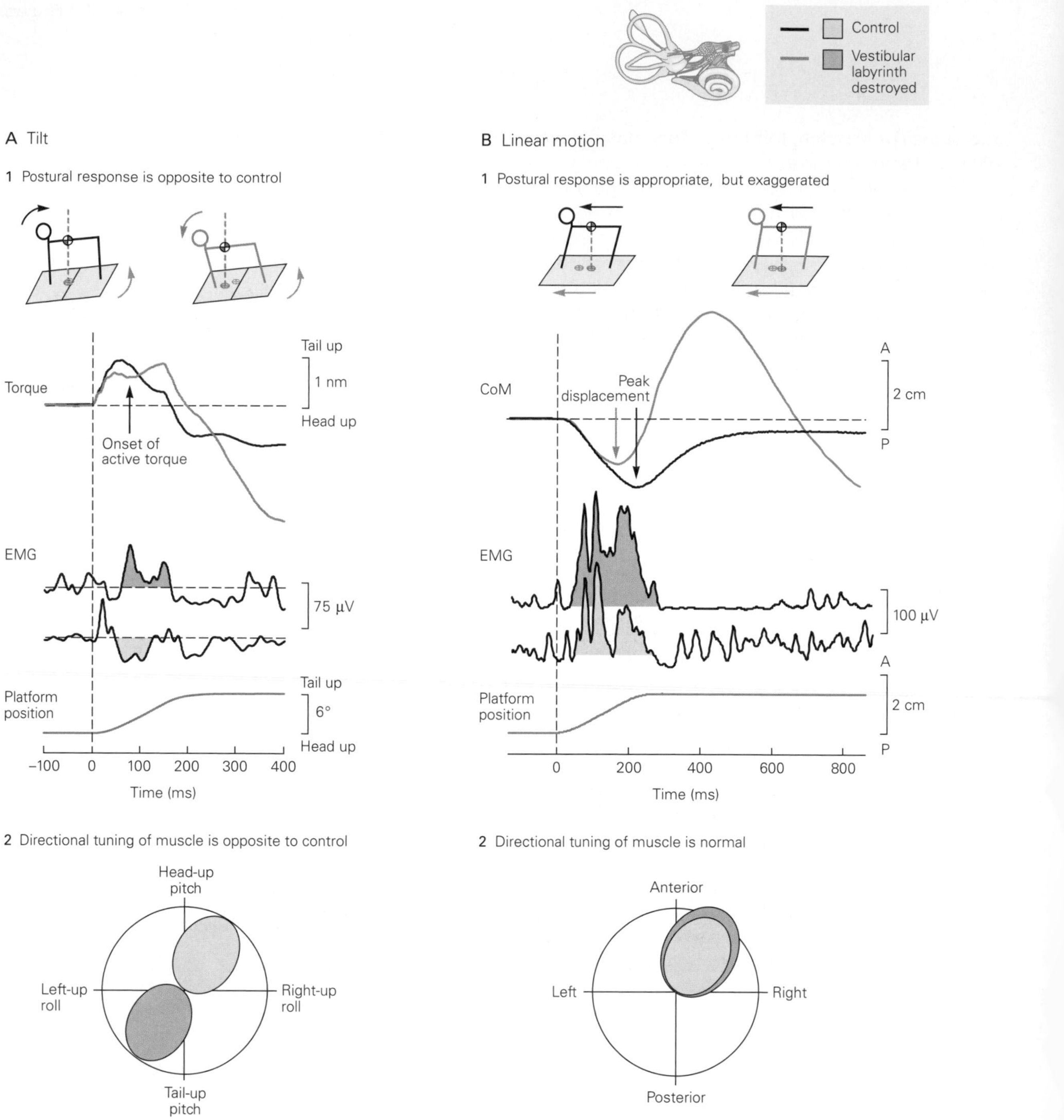

Figure 41–10 Loss of vestibular input disrupts the directional tuning of the automatic postural response to tilt of the support surface. The electromyogram (**EMG**) records are from cats standing on a movable platform before and after bilateral labyrinthectomy. (Adapted, with permission, from Macpherson et al. 2007.)

A. Without vestibular inputs the postural response to tilt of the platform is opposite to normal. **1.** The lateral gastrocnemius, an ankle extensor, is normally inhibited in response to a tail-up tilt, reducing the downhill torque (rotational force) and reducing body tilt relative to gravity. With vestibular loss the muscle is activated, which increases the downhill torque and increases body tilt, causing loss of balance. Platform displacement begins at time zero. **2.** The directional tuning of a left hip extensor muscle to platform tilt switches to the opposite quadrant after vestibular loss.

B. Immediately after vestibular loss the postural response to horizontal motion of the platform is appropriate but exceeds that of control trials. **1.** The response of the gluteus medius, a hip extensor and abductor, has normal latency but larger amplitude. In the control condition the center of mass (**CoM**) moves away from the origin and returns in a smooth trajectory. After vestibular loss the CoM displacement follows a trajectory similar to that of the control trace, but because of the larger muscle activation it peaks earlier in time. In the return phase the center of mass overshoots the origin and oscillates. Platform movement begins at time zero. (**A**, anterior; **P**, posterior.) **2.** The directional tuning of a left hip extensor muscle is the same with and without vestibular function when activated by linear motion of the platform. The amplitude of activation of the muscle is somewhat larger when vestibular function is lost.

motion of the support surface has the appropriate directional tuning and latency, even in the acute stage prior to vestibular compensation.

Why does the absence of vestibular signals cause difficulty with tilt but not with linear motion? The answer lies in how the nervous system determines the direction of vertical. Gravity is the main force that causes the body to fall. As the support surface tilts, healthy subjects orient to gravity using vestibular information to remain upright. In contrast, subjects without vestibular function use somatosensory inputs to orient themselves to the support surface and consequently fall downhill as the surface tilts. During linear motion, however, gravitational and surface vertical are collinear, and somatosensory signals are sufficient to compute the correct postural response. Although visual inputs also provide a vertical reference, visual processing is too slow to participate in the automatic postural response to rapid tilt, especially soon after the loss of vestibular function.

Without vestibular information the response to linear motion of the support surface is larger than normal (*hypermetria*), leading to overbalancing and instability (Figure 41–10B). Hypermetria is a major cause of ataxia when vestibular information is lost. Vestibular hypermetria may result from reduced cerebellar inhibition of the motor system, for the loss of vestibular inputs reduces the drive to the inhibitory Purkinje cells.

Humans and cats are quite ataxic immediately after loss of the vestibular apparatus. The head and trunk show marked instability, stance and gait are broad-based, and walking follows a weaving path with frequent falling. Instability is especially great on turning the head, probably because trunk motion cannot be distinguished from head motion using somatosensory information alone. Paul Stapley and colleagues showed that cats lacking vestibular inputs actively push themselves toward the side of a voluntary head turn, likely because somatosensory inputs that encode trunk and head motion are misinterpreted in the absence of vestibular inputs. The postural system erroneously senses that the body is falling to the side away from the head turn and generates a response in the opposite direction, resulting in imbalance.

Immediately following vestibular loss, neck muscles are abnormally activated during ordinary movements and often the head and trunk are moved together as a unit. After several months routine movement becomes more normal through vestibular compensation, which may involve greater reliance on the remaining sensory information. However, more challenging tasks are hampered by a residual hypermetria, stiffness in head-trunk control, and instability, especially when visual and somatosensory information is unavailable for postural orientation. Vestibular information is critical for balance when visual information is reduced and the support surface is not stable, for example at night, on a sandy beach, or on a boat's deck.

Visual Information Provides Advance Knowledge of Potentially Destabilizing Situations and Assists in Orienting to the Environment

Visual inputs provide the postural system with orientation and motion information from both near and far. Vision reduces body sway when standing still and provides stabilizing cues, especially when a new balancing task is attempted or balance is precarious. Skaters and dancers maintain stability while spinning by fixing their gaze on a point in the visual field. However, visual processing is too slow to significantly affect the postural response to a sudden disturbance of balance. Vision does play an important role in anticipatory postural adjustments during voluntary movements, such as planning where to place the feet when walking over obstacles.

Vision can have a powerful influence on postural orientation, as anyone can attest who has seen a movie filmed from the perspective of a moving viewer and projected on a large screen. Simulated rides in a roller coaster or plane, for example, can induce strong sensations of motion along with activation of postural muscles. An illusion of movement is induced when sufficiently large regions of the visual field are stimulated, as when a large disk in front of a standing subject is rotated. The subject responds to this illusion by tilting his body; clockwise rotation of the visual field is interpreted by the postural system as the body falling to the left, to which the subject compensates by leaning to the right (Figure 41–9B). The rate and direction of optic flow—the flow of images across the retina as people move about—provide clues about body orientation and movement.

Information from a Single Sensory Modality Can Be Ambiguous

Any one sensory modality alone may provide ambiguous information about postural orientation and body motion. The visual system, for example, cannot distinguish self-motion from object motion. We have all experienced the fleeting sensation while sitting in a stationary vehicle of not knowing whether we are moving or the adjacent vehicle is moving.

Vestibular information can also be ambiguous for two reasons. First, vestibular receptors are located in the head and therefore provide information about acceleration of the head but not about the rest of the body. The postural control system cannot use vestibular information alone to distinguish between the head tilting on a stationary trunk and the whole body tilting by rotation at the ankles, both of which activate the semicircular canals and otolith organs. Additional information from somatosensory receptors is required to resolve this ambiguity. The otolith organs also cannot distinguish between acceleration owing to gravity and linear acceleration of the head. Tilting to the left, for example, can produce the same otolithic stimulation as acceleration of the body to the right (Figure 41–11).

Studies of vestibulo-ocular reflexes suggest there are neural circuits that can disambiguate the head-tilt component of a linear acceleration by using a combination of canal and otolith inputs. Output from this circuit may allow the postural system to determine the orientation of gravity relative to the head regardless of head position and motion. The distinction between tilt and linear motion is especially important while standing on an unstable or a tilting surface.

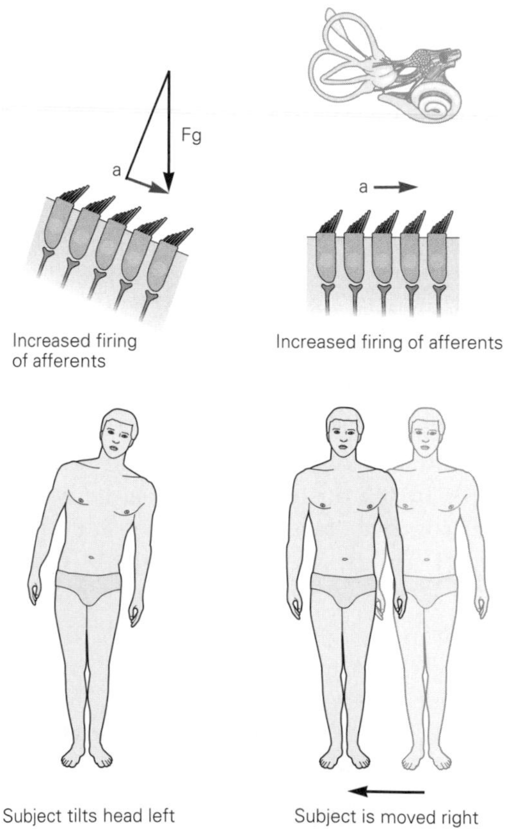

Figure 41–11 Vestibular inputs regarding body posture and motion can be ambiguous. The postural system cannot distinguish between tilt and linear acceleration of the body based on otolithic inputs alone. The mechanoreceptors of the vestibular system are hair bundles that bend in response to shearing forces, thus changing the firing rate of the tonically active sensory afferents. The same shearing force can result from tilting of the head (**left**), which exposes the hair cells to a portion of the acceleration (**a**) owing to gravity (**Fg**), or from horizontal linear acceleration of the body (**right**).

Somatosensory inputs may also provide ambiguous information about body orientation and motion. When we stand upright mechanoreceptors in the soles of our feet and proprioceptors in muscles and joints signal the motion of our body relative to the support surface. But somatosensory inputs alone cannot distinguish between body and surface motion, for example whether ankle flexion stems from forward body sway or tilting of the surface. Our common experience is that the ground beneath us is stable and that somatosensory inputs reflect movements of the body's center of mass as we sway. But surfaces may move relative to the earth, such as a boat's deck, or may be pliant under our weight, like a soft or spongy surface. Therefore, somatosensory information must be integrated with vestibular and visual inputs to give the nervous system an accurate picture of the stability and inclination of the support surface and of our body's relationship to earth vertical.

The Postural Control System Uses a Body Schema that Incorporates Internal Models for Balance

Because of the mechanical complexity of the body, with its many skeletal segments and muscles, the nervous system requires a coherent representation of the body and its interaction with the environment. To execute the simple movement of raising your hand and touching your nose with your index finger while your eyes are closed, your nervous system must know the characteristics (length, mass, and connections) of each segment of the arm, the shoulder, and head as well as the orientation of your arm with respect to the gravity vector and your nose. Thus information from multiple sensory systems is integrated into a central representation of the body and its environment, often called the body schema.

The body schema for postural control, as developed by Viktor Gurfinkel, is not simply a sensory map like the somatotopic representation of the skin in primary sensory cortex. Instead, it incorporates internal models of the body's relationship with the environment (see Chapter 33). This representation is used to compute appropriate anticipatory and automatic postural reactions to maintain balance and postural orientation.

A simplified example of such an internal model is one in which the body is represented as a single segment hinged at the foot (Figure 41–12A). The internal model generates an estimate of the orientation of the foot in space, which also serves as an estimate of the orientation of the support surface, a variable that cannot be directly sensed.

Henry Head, a neurologist working in the early part of the 20th century, described the body schema as a dynamic system in which both spatial and temporal features are continually updated, a concept that remains current. To allow adequate planning of movement strategies, the body schema must incorporate not only the relationship of body segments to space and to each other but also the mass and inertia of each segment and an estimate of the external forces acting on the body including gravity.

Another component of the body schema is a model of the sensory information expected as a result of a movement. Disorientation or motion sickness may result when the actual sensory information received by the nervous system does not match the expected sensory information, as in the microgravity environment of space flight. With continued exposure to the new environment, however, the model is gradually updated until expected and actual sensory information agree and the person is no longer spatially disoriented.

The internal model for balance control must be continually updated, both in the short term, as we use experience to improve our balance strategies, and in the long term, as we age and our bodies change in shape and size. One way the body schema is updated is by changing the weighting of each of the sensory modalities.

The Influence of Each Sensory Modality on Balance and Orientation Changes According to Task Requirements

The postural control system must be able to change the relative sensitivity or weighting of different sensory modalities to accommodate changes in the environment and movement goals. Subjects on a firm, stable surface tend to rely primarily on somatosensory information for postural orientation. When the support surface is unstable subjects depend more on vestibular and visual information. However, even when the support surface is not stable, light touch with a fingertip on a stable object is more effective than vision in maintaining postural orientation and balance. Vestibular information is particularly critical when visual and somatosensory information is ambiguous or absent, such as when skiing downhill or walking below deck on a ship.

The weighting of each sensory system changes with the type of task and with the characteristics of the environment. This change can be demonstrated in an experiment in which subjects are blindfolded and asked to stand quietly on a surface that is slowly tilted by varying amounts, up to 8 degrees in magnitude. For tilts of less than 2 degrees all subjects sway with the platform, suggesting that they use somatosensory information to orient their body to the support surface. At larger tilts healthy subjects attenuate their sway and orient their posture more with respect to gravitational vertical than to the surface, as if relying more on vestibular information. In contrast, patients who have lost vestibular function persist in swaying along with the platform and subsequently fall (Figure 41–12B). This behavior accords with the patients' inappropriate automatic postural response to rapid platform tilts.

Studies such as these suggest that when people are standing on moving or unstable surfaces, the weighting of vestibular and visual information increases whereas that of somatosensory information decreases. Any sensory modality may dominate at a particular time, depending on the conditions of postural support and the specific motor behavior to be performed.

Control of Posture Is Distributed in the Nervous System

Postural orientation and balance are achieved through the dynamic and context-dependent interplay among all levels of the central nervous system, from the spinal cord to cerebral cortex.

Spinal Cord Circuits Are Sufficient for Maintaining Antigravity Support but Not Balance

Adult cats with complete spinal transection at the thoracic level can be trained to support the weight of their hindquarters with fairly normal hind limb and trunk postural orientation, but they have little control of balance. These animals do not exhibit normal postural responses in their hind limbs when the support surface moves. Their response to horizontal motion consists of small, random, and highly variable bursts of activity in extensor muscles that are considerably delayed compared to normal activity, whereas postural activity in flexor muscles is absent (Figure 41–13). Active balance is absent despite the fact that extensors and flexors can be recruited for other movements such as stepping on a treadmill.

An adult cat with a spinal transection can stand independently for only short periods of time and within a narrow range of stability; head turns in particular cause the animal to lose balance. What stability

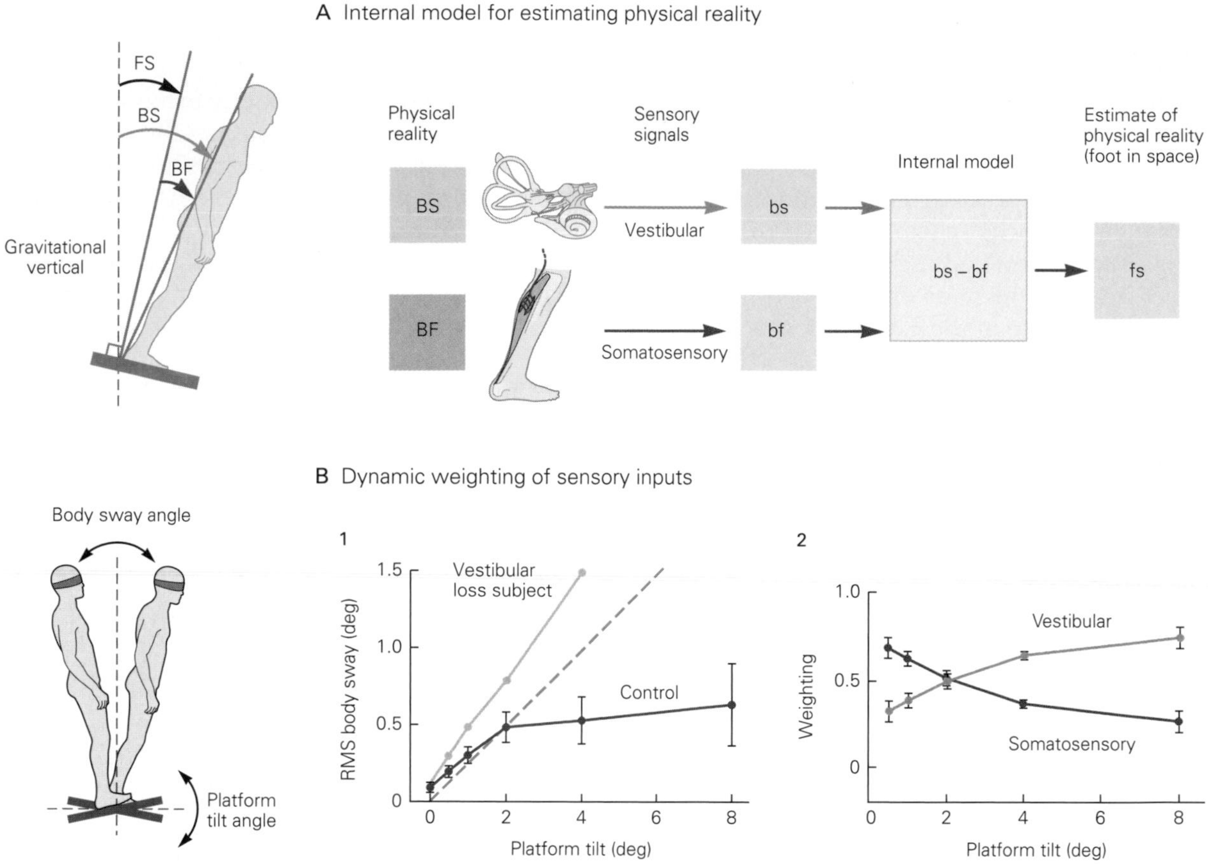

Figure 41–12 Many types of sensory signals are integrated and weighted in an internal model that optimizes balance and orientation. (Adapted, with permission, from Peterka 2002.)

A. The simple example of a person standing on a tilted surface illustrates how the nervous system might estimate physical variables that are not sensed directly. The physical variables are body tilt with respect to earth vertical or space (**BS**), and body angle relative to the foot (**BF**). The angle of the foot in space (**FS**) is simply the difference BS – BF. The neural estimate of body in space (**bs**) comes from vestibular and other receptors that detect tilt of the body relative to gravity. The neural estimate of body angle to foot (**bf**) comes from somatosensory signals related to ankle joint angle. The internal model for estimating physical reality, bs – bf, produces a neural estimate of the foot in space (**fs**). Such estimates of the physical world are continually updated based on experience.

B. Sensory information is weighted dynamically to maintain balance and orientation under varying conditions. The figure illustrates findings from an experiment in which human subjects stood blindfolded on a platform that slowly rotated continuously in the toes-up or toes-down direction at amplitudes of up to 8 degrees (peak to peak). **1.** Body-sway angle is measured relative to gravitational vertical during platform tilt and expressed as root mean square (**RMS**) sway in degrees. The **dashed line** represents equal platform and body sway; for example, for a platform tilt of 4 degrees an equal amount of body sway is 1 degree RMS. In control subjects the body and platform sway are equal for small platform tilts up to 2 degrees, suggesting that people normally use somatosensory signals to remain perpendicular to the platform (minimizing changes in ankle angle). With larger platform tilts, body sway does not increase much beyond 0.5 degree RMS. In contrast, subjects with vestibular loss sway even more than the platform (1.5 degrees RMS of body tilt at 4 degrees of platform tilt) and cannot remain standing at platform tilts above 4 degrees. Thus, when both vestibular and visual signals are absent, a person orients only to the support surface and has difficulty maintaining balance. **2.** In control subjects the influence of somatosensory input decreases with increasing platform tilt while the influence of vestibular input increases. At larger tilt angles the greater influence of vestibular input minimizes the degree of body sway away from gravitational vertical.

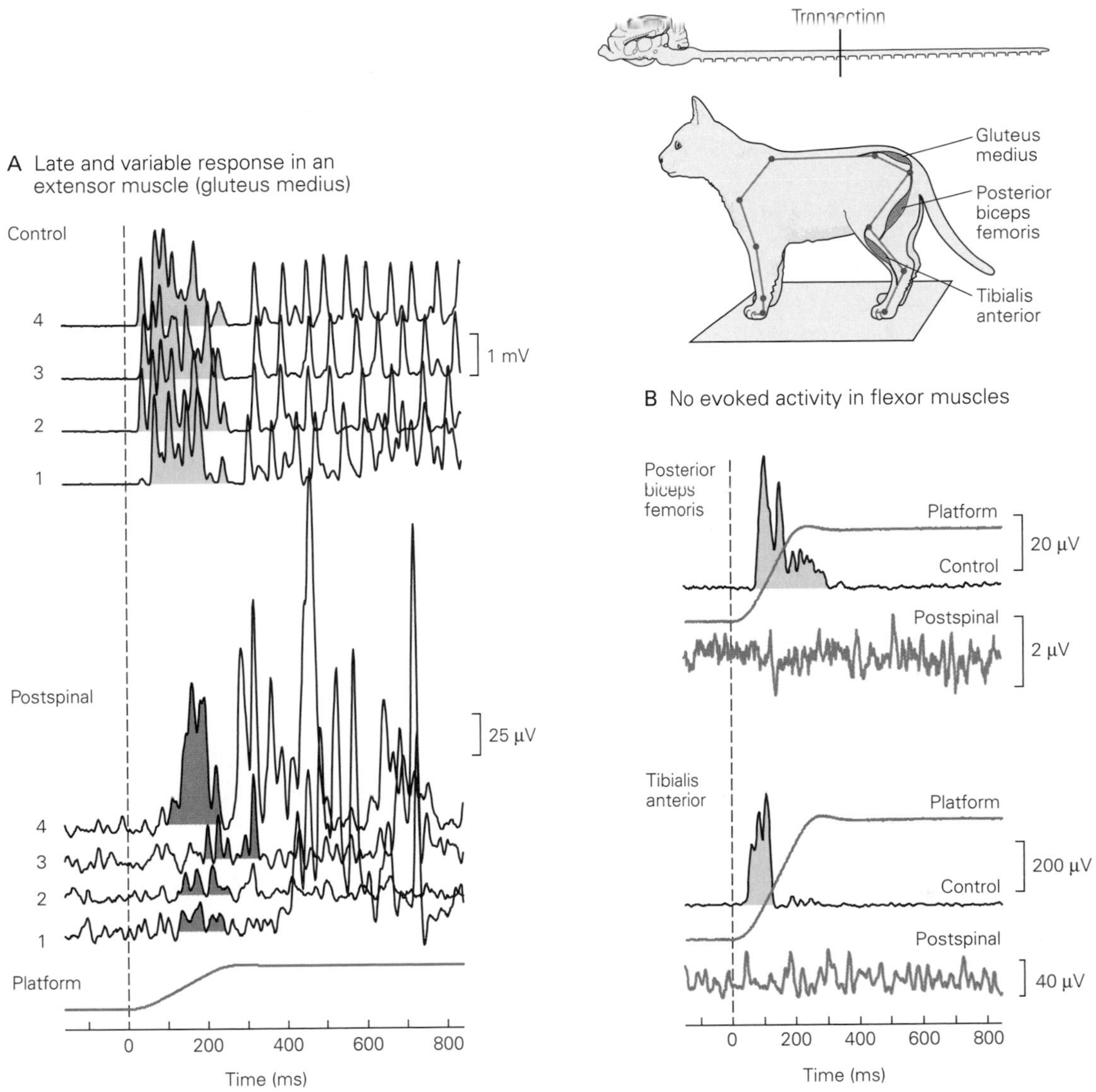

Figure 41–13 Spinal circuits alone do not generate automatic postural responses for balance. In this experiment automatic postural responses to horizontal motion are recorded before and after complete transection of the spinal cord at the level of the sixth thoracic vertebra. This transection leaves the lumbar spinal cord intact but isolated from higher neural centers. (Adapted, with permission, from Macpherson and Fung 1999.)

A. Electromyogram (EMG) records from a left hind limb extensor are disorganized after spinal transection. In four trials after transection the response amplitude of the left gluteus medius is greatly reduced following forward and rightward motion of the platform. In addition, the amplitude and onset time vary greatly between trials. Note that the scale of the postspinal records is considerably smaller than that of the control records.

B. Flexor muscles in the left hind limb are normally activated by platform motion in the backward and leftward direction. After spinal transection the flexors do not respond to translation. The posterior biceps femoris is a knee flexor; tibialis anterior is an ankle dorsiflexor.

there is likely results from the broad base of support afforded by quadrupedal stance, the stiffness of the tonically contracting hind limb extensors that support the weight of the hindquarters, and active compensation by forelimbs that continue to produce postural responses. Humans with spinal cord injuries have various amounts of antigravity muscle tonus but lack automatic postural responses below the level of the lesion. These results emphasize that antigravity support and balance control are distinct mechanisms and that the control of balance requires the involvement of supraspinal circuits.

The Brain Stem and Cerebellum Integrate Sensory Signals for Posture

If spinal circuits alone are not capable of producing automatic postural responses, what supraspinal centers are responsible for these responses? Although the answer to this question remains unknown, good candidates include the brain stem and cerebellum, which are highly interconnected and work together to modulate the descending commands to spinal motor centers of the limbs and trunk. These regions have the input-output structure that would be expected of centers for postural control.

Muscle synergies for automatic postural responses may be organized in the brain stem, perhaps the reticular formation. However, adaptation of postural synergies to changes in the environment and task demands may require cerebellar influence.

Two regions of the cerebellum influence orientation and balance: the vestibulocerebellum (nodulus, uvula, and fastigial nucleus) and the spinocerebellum (anterior lobe and interpositus nucleus). These regions are interconnected with the vestibular nuclei and reticular formation of the pons and medulla (see Figure 42–3). Lesions of the brain stem and vestibulocerebellum produce a variety of deficits in head and trunk control and a tendency to tilt from vertical, even with eyes open, suggesting a deficit in the internal representation of postural orientation. Lesions of the spinocerebellum result in excessive postural sway that is worse with the eyes closed, ataxia during walking, and hypermetric postural responses, suggesting deficits in balance reactions. Certain regions in the pons and medulla facilitate or depress extensor tonus and could thereby influence antigravity support.

The brain stem and cerebellum are sites of integration of sensory inputs, perhaps generating the internal model of body orientation and balance. Vestibular and visual inputs are distributed to brain stem centers (see Chapter 45) and the vestibulocerebellum. The spinocerebellum receives signals from rapidly conducting proprioceptive and cutaneous fibers. More slowly conducting somatosensory fibers project to the vestibular nuclei and reticular formation.

Two major descending systems carry signals from the brain stem and cerebellum to the spinal cord and could therefore trigger the automatic postural response for balance and orientation. The medial and lateral vestibulospinal tracts originate from the vestibular nuclei, and the medial and lateral reticulospinal tracts originate from the reticular formation of the pons and medulla (see Figure 42–7). Lesions of these tracts result in profound ataxia and postural instability. In contrast, lesions of the corticospinal and rubrospinal tracts have minimal effect on balance even though they produce profound disturbance of voluntary limb movements.

The Spinocerebellum and Basal Ganglia Are Important in Adaptation of Posture

Patients with spinocerebellar disorders, such as alcoholic anterior-lobe syndrome, and basal-ganglion deficits, such as Parkinson disease, experience postural difficulties. This suggests that the spinocerebellum and basal ganglia play complementary roles in adapting postural responses to changing conditions.

The spinocerebellum is where the magnitude of postural responses is adapted based on experience. The basal ganglia are important for quickly adjusting the postural set when conditions suddenly change, to ensure that postural responses are approximately correct. Both the spinocerebellum and the basal ganglia regulate muscle tone and force for voluntary postural adjustments. They are not necessary, however, for triggering or constructing the basic postural patterns.

Patients with disorders of the spinocerebellum have difficulty adjusting the magnitude of balance adjustments over the course of repeated trials but can readily adapt postural responses immediately after a change in conditions. For example, a patient standing on a movable platform exhibits appropriate postural responses when platform velocity is increased with each trial. These postural adjustments rely on velocity information, which is encoded by somatosensory inputs at the beginning of platform movement.

In contrast, when the amplitude of platform movement can be predicted on the basis of repeated presentation, a patient is unable to adjust the amplitude of his response to that of the anticipated perturbation. Because the amplitude of platform movement is not known until the platform has stopped moving, well after the initial postural response is complete, a subject must use his experience from one trial to modify his response in a subsequent trial of the same amplitude. Whereas a healthy subject does this quite readily, a patient with spinocerebellar disorders is unable to efficiently adapt his postural responses based on recent experience (Figure 41–14A).

In a healthy subject muscle activity during sudden backward motion of the support surface is appropriately scaled to counteract the forward sway induced by the perturbation. A subject with spinocerebellar disease always over-responds, although the timing of muscle activation is normal (Figure 41–14B). As a result, this individual returns beyond the upright

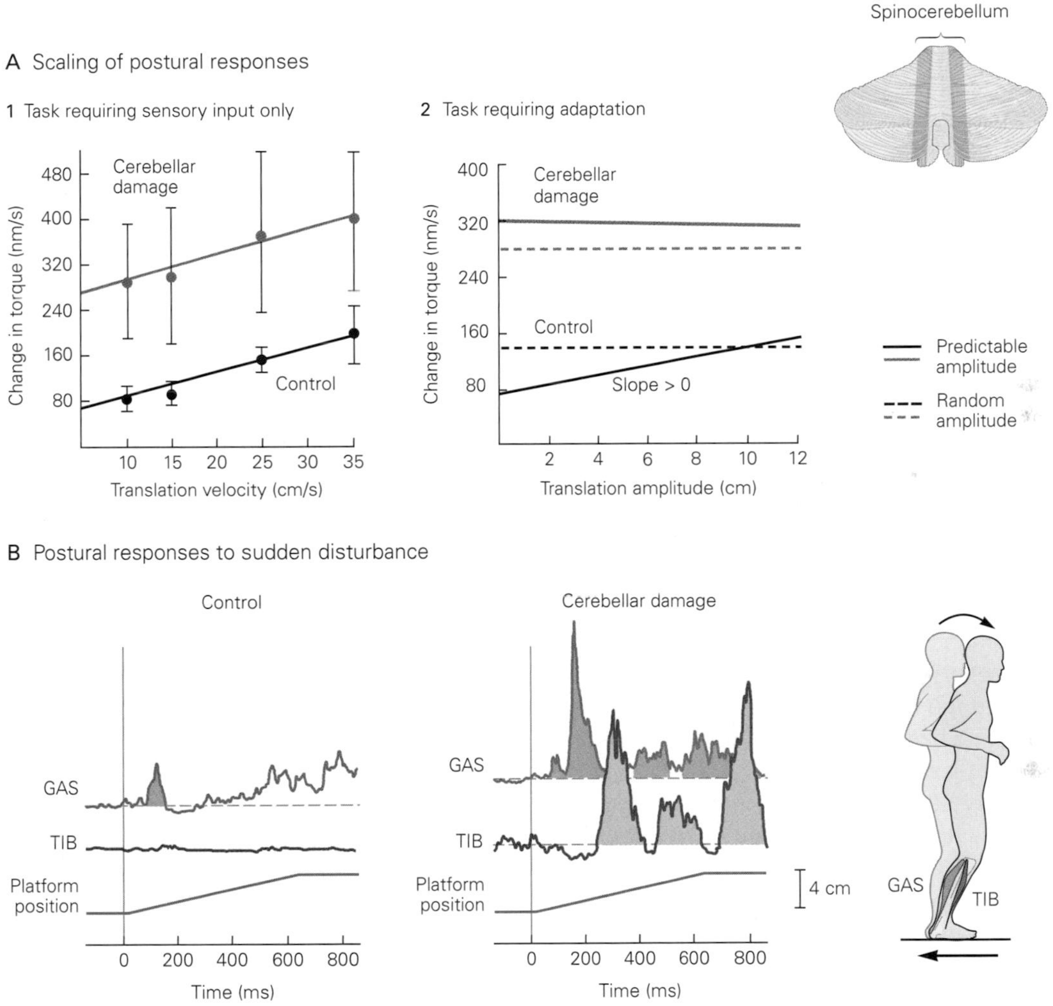

Figure 41–14 The spinocerebellum has a role in adapting postural responses to changing conditions. The spinocerebellum is important for adapting postural responses based on experience. Patients with a spinocerebellar disorder can use immediate sensory input but not experience to adjust automatic postural responses. (Adapted, with permission, from Horak and Diener 1994.)

A. 1. A subject stands on a platform that is moved horizontally; the velocity is increased on each trial. Maintaining balance requires scaling responses to the velocity of the platform using sensory feedback. The adjustments in a subject with a spinocerebellar disorder have the same regression coefficient (slope) as those of a control subject, even though in each trial the responses are larger and more variable than those of the control subject. **2.** When subjects are required to anticipate and adapt to platform translation, the postural adjustments in the spinocerebellar subject are compromised. When translation amplitude is random, responses are large, as if the subject expected a large translation. When trials with the same amplitude are repeated, a control subject learns to predict the amplitude of the disturbance and adjust his response. In contrast, a spinocerebellar subject shows no improvement in performance; he cannot use his experience in one trial to adjust his responses in subsequent trials. The responses are large, as if the subject always expected the large translation.

B. Postural responses to sudden disturbances are hypermetric in spinocerebellar patients. In this experiment subjects stand on a platform that is moved backward (6 cm amplitude at 10 cm/s). In a control subject the onset of movement evokes a small burst of activity in the gastrocnemius (**GAS**), an ankle extensor. In a subject with damage to the anterior lobe of the cerebellum the muscle responses are overly large, with bursts of activity alternating between the gastrocnemius and its antagonist, the tibialis anterior (**TIB**).

position and oscillates back and forth. Reminiscent of the hypermetria observed immediately after labyrinthectomy, cerebellar hypermetria may also result from loss of Purkinje-cell inhibition on spinal motor centers.

A patient with Parkinson disease can, with sufficient practice, gradually modify his postural responses but has difficulty changing responses when conditions change suddenly. Such postural inflexibility is seen when initial posture changes. For example, when a normal subject on a movable platform switches from standing upright to sitting on a stool, the pattern of his automatic postural response to backward movement of the platform changes immediately. Because leg-muscle activity is no longer necessary after the switch from standing to sitting, this component ceases to be recruited.

In contrast, a patient with Parkinson disease employs the same muscle activation pattern for both sitting and standing (Figure 41–15). L-DOPA replacement therapy does not improve the patient's ability to switch postural set. With repetition of trials in the seated posture, however, the leg-muscle activity eventually disappears, showing that enough experience permits adaptation of postural responses. A patient with Parkinson disease also has difficulty when instructed to increase or decrease the magnitude of a postural response, a difficulty that is consistent with the inability to change cognitive sets quickly.

A patient with a basal ganglion disorder has problems with postural tone and force generation in addition to an inability to adapt to changing conditions. The bradykinesia (slowness of movement) of Parkinson disease is reflected in slow development of force in postural responses and the disease's rigidity is manifested in co-contraction and stiffness. L-DOPA replacement greatly improves a patient's ability to generate not only forceful voluntary movements but also the accompanying postural adjustments, such as rising onto the toes and gait. However, neither the automatic postural response to an unexpected disturbance nor postural adaptation is improved by L-DOPA, suggesting that these functions involve the nondopaminergic pathways affected by Parkinson disease.

Cerebral Cortex Centers Contribute to Postural Control

Centers in the cerebral cortex influence postural orientation and equilibrium, including both anticipatory and automatic postural responses. Most voluntary movements, which are initiated in the cerebral cortex, require postural adjustments that must be integrated with the primary goal of the movement in both timing and amplitude. Where this integration occurs is not clear.

The cerebral cortex has more control over anticipatory postural adjustments than automatic postural reactions. However, recent electroencephalographic (EEG) studies show that areas of cerebral cortex are activated by anticipation of a postural disturbance before an automatic postural response is initiated. This finding is consistent with the idea that the cortex optimizes balance control as part of motor planning.

The supplementary motor area and temporoparietal cortex have both been implicated in postural control. The supplementary motor area (see Chapter 38) is likely involved with anticipatory postural adjustments that accompany voluntary movements. The temporoparietal cortex appears to integrate sensory information and may contain internal models for perception of body verticality. Lesions of insular cortex can impair perception of the visual vertical whereas lesions of superior parietal cortex impair perception of postural vertical, and either of these defects may impair balance when standing on an unstable support.

Sensorimotor cortex receives somatosensory inputs signaling balance disturbances and postural responses. However, this region is not essential for automatic postural adjustments. Jean Massion and colleagues have shown that lesioning the motor cortex in cats impairs the lifting of the forelimb evoked by light touch during stance, but does not abolish the accompanying postural adjustment in the contralateral forelimb. Although the sensorimotor cortex is not responsible for postural adjustments, it may have a role in the process.

Behavioral studies, too, have implicated cortical processes in postural control. Control of posture, like control of voluntary movement, requires attention. When subjects must press a button following a visual or auditory cue while also maintaining balance, their reaction time increases with the difficulty of the task (balancing on one foot versus sitting, for example). Moreover, when subjects try to perform a cognitive task while actively maintaining posture, the performance of either or both can degrade. For example, when a subject is asked to count backward by threes while standing on one foot, both the cognitive task and postural adjustment deteriorate. The timing of automatic postural responses to unexpected disturbances is little affected by cognitive interference.

Balance control is also influenced by emotional state, thus implicating the limbic system in posture control. Fear of falling, for example, can increase postural tone and stiffness, reduce sway area, increase sway velocity, and alter balancing strategies in response to disturbances.

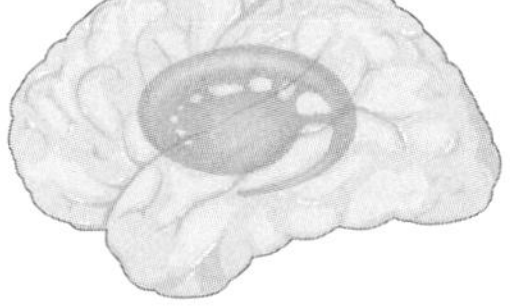

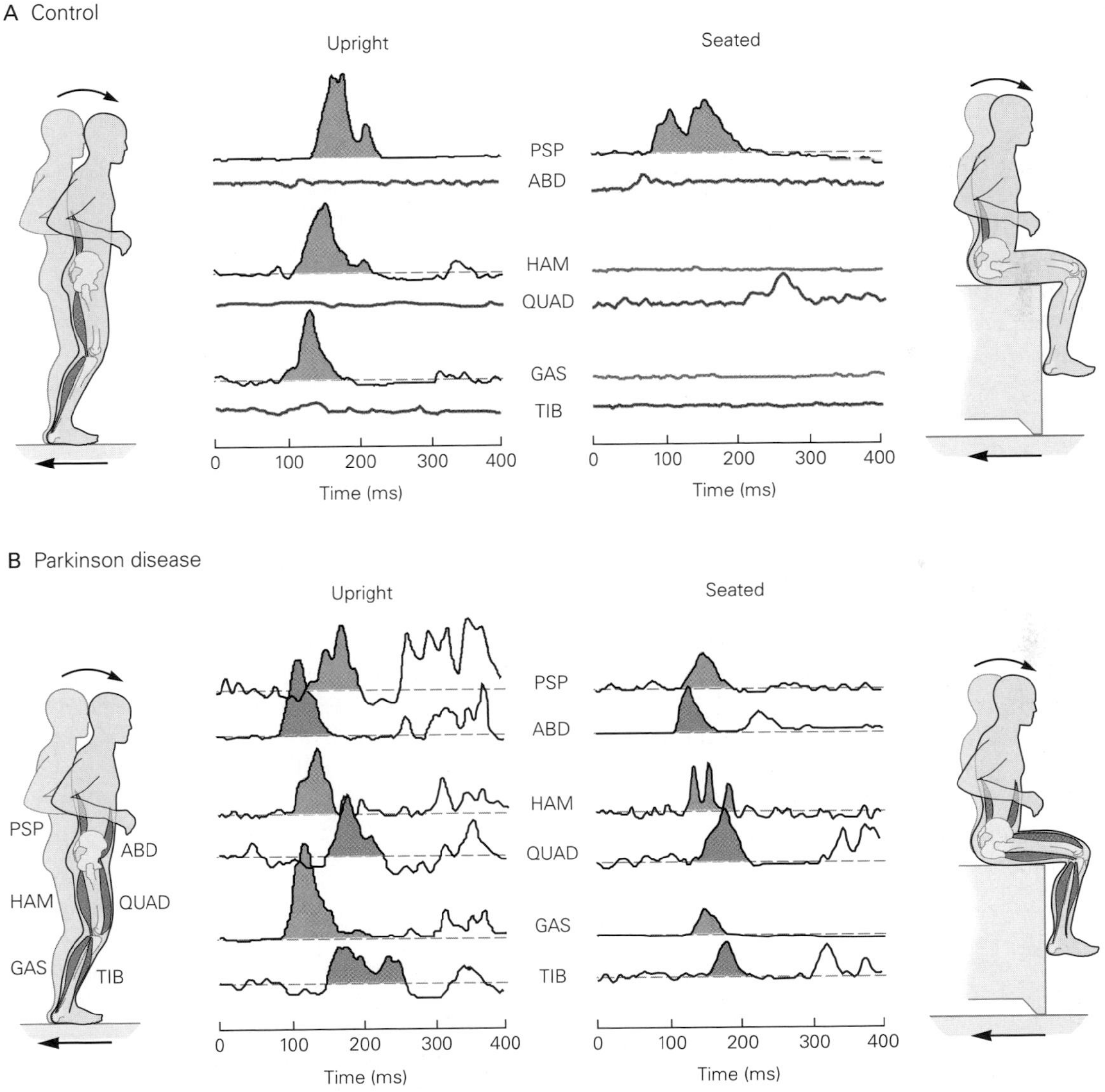

Figure 41–15 The basal ganglia are important for adapting postural responses to a sudden change in initial conditions. (Adapted, with permission, from Horak, Nutt, and Nashner 1992.)

A. When a normal subject switches from upright stance to sitting he immediately modifies his response to backward movement of the support platform. The postural response to movement while seated does not involve the leg muscles—the gastrocnemius (**GAS**) and hamstrings (**HAM**)—but does activate the paraspinal muscles (**PSP**) and with shorter latency than in the response to movement while standing. (**ABD**, abdominals; **QUAD**, quadriceps; **TIB**, tibialis anterior.)

B. A patient with Parkinson disease does not suppress the leg-muscle response in the first trial after switching from standing to sitting. The postural response of this subject is similar for both initial positions: antagonist muscles (**purple**) are activated along with agonists (**pink**).

Although the roles of specific areas of cerebral cortex in postural control are largely undefined, there is no doubt that the cortex is important for learning new, complex postural strategies. The cortex must be involved in the amazing improvement in balance and postural orientation of athletes and dancers who use cognitive information and advice from coaches. In fact, the cerebral cortex is involved in postural control each time we consciously maintain our balance while walking across a slippery floor, standing on a moving bus, or waiting tables on a rocking ship.

An Overall View

Although we are usually unaware of it, the posture control system is active during most of the activities we perform daily. Automatic postural adjustments prevent falling when some external force disrupts our balance. These responses are not simple reflexes but are highly organized, flexible, and adaptive patterns of muscle activation. Anticipatory postural adjustments accompany our voluntary movements to maintain balance and orientation.

Somatosensory, vestibular, and visual inputs all contribute to postural control for balance and orientation with differing degrees of influence as our environment changes. Many areas of the nervous system integrate sensory inputs to form a unified representation of the body's orientation and motion and of the environment. This body schema is used to compute the appropriate postural adjustments to maintain balance.

The postural system is highly adaptive, both in the short term to optimize postural behavior to a continually changing environment, and in the long term to accommodate changes in body morphology and mechanics caused by growth and development, aging, disease, and injury.

Jane M. Macpherson
Fay B. Horak

Suggested Readings

Brandt T. 1991. Man in motion—historical and clinical aspects of vestibular function—a review. Brain 114:2159–2174.

Dietz V. 1992. Human neuronal control of automatic functional movements—interaction between central programs and afferent input. Physiol Rev 72:33–69.

Horak FB, Macpherson JM. 1996. Postural orientation and equilibrium. In: LB Rowell and JT Shepherd (eds). *Handbook of Physiology,* Section 12 *Exercise: Regulation and Integration of Multiple Systems*, pp. 255–292. New York: Oxford Univ. Press.

Horak FB, Shupert CL, Mirka A. 1989. Components of postural dyscontrol in the elderly: a review. Neurobiol Aging 10:727–738.

Macpherson JM, Deliagina TG, Orlovsky GN. 1997. Control of body orientation and equilibrium in vertebrates. In: PSG Stein, S Grillner, AI Selverston, DG Stuart (eds). *Neurons Networks and Motor Behavior*, pp. 257–267. Cambridge, MA: MIT Press.

Massion J. 1994. Postural control system. Curr Opin Neurobiol 4:877–887.

Woollacott M, Shumway-Cook A. 2002. Attention and the control of posture and gait: a review of an emerging area of research. Gait Posture 16:1–14.

Zajac FE, Gordon ME. 1989. Determining muscle's force and action in multi-articular movement. Exer Sport Sci Rev 17:187–230.

References

Brandt T, Paulus W, Straube A. 1986. Vision and posture. In: W Bles, T Brandt (eds). *Disorders of Posture and Gait*, pp. 157–175. Amsterdam: Elsevier.

Burleigh AL, Horak FB, Malouin F. 1994. Modification of postural responses and step initiation: evidence for goal directed postural interactions. J Neurophysiol 72:2892–2902.

Cordo PJ, Nashner LM. 1982. Properties of postural adjustments associated with rapid arm movements. J Neurophysiol 47:287–302.

Dunbar DC, Horak FB, Macpherson JM, Rushmer DS. 1986. Neural control of quadrupedal and bipedal stance: implications for the evolution of erect posture. Am J Phys Anthropol 69:93–105.

Gurfinkel VS, Levick YS. 1991. Perceptual and automatic aspects of the postural body scheme. In: J Paillard (ed). *Brain and Space*, pp. 147–162. Oxford: Oxford Univ Press.

Horak FB, Diener HC. 1994. Cerebellar control of postural scaling and central set in stance. J Neurophysiol 72: 479–493.

Horak FB, Nashner LM. 1986. Central programming of postural movements: adaptation to altered support-surface configurations. J Neurophysiol 55:1369–1381.

Horak FB, Nutt J, Nashner LM. 1992. Postural inflexibility in parkinsonian subjects. J Neurol Sci 111:46–58.

Inglis JT, Horak FB, Shupert CL, Jones-Rycewicz C. 1994. The importance of somatosensory information in triggering and scaling automatic postural responses in humans. Exp Brain Res 101:159–164.

Inglis JT, Macpherson JM. 1995. Bilateral labyrinthectomy in the cat: effects on the postural response to translation. J Neurophysiol 73:1181–1191.

Lee WA, Michaels CF, Pai YC. 1990. The organization of torque and EMG activity during bilateral handle pulls by standing humans. Exp Brain Res 82:304–314.

MacKinnon CD, Winter DA. 1993. Control of whole body balance in the frontal plane during human walking. J Biomech 26:633–644.

Macpherson JM. 1988. Strategies that simplify the control of quadrupedal stance. 2. Electromyographic activity. J Neurophysiol 60:218–231.

Macpherson JM, Everaert DG, Stapley PJ, Ting LH. 2007. Bilateral vestibular loss in cats leads to active destabilization of balance during pitch and roll rotations of the support surface. J Neurophysiol 97:4357–4367.

Macpherson JM, Fung J. 1999. Weight support and balance during perturbed stance in the chronic spinal cat. J Neurophysiol 82:3066–3081.

Macpherson JM, Inglis JT. 1993. Stance and balance following bilateral labyrinthectomy. In: JHJ Allum, D Allum-Mecklenburg, F Harris, R Probst (eds). *Natural and Artificial Control of Hearing and Balance*, pp. 219–228. New York: Elsevier Science.

Maki BE, McIlroy WE, Fernie GR. 2003. Change-in-support reactions for balance recovery. IEEE Eng Med Biol Mag 22:20–26.

Massion J. 1979. Role of motor cortex in postural adjustments associated with movement. In: H Asanuma, V Wilson (eds). *Integration in the Nervous System*, pp. 239–260. Tokyo: Igaku-Shoin.

McMahon TA, Bonner JT. 1983. *On Size and Life*. New York: W.H. Freeman.

Mittelstaedt H. 1998. Origin and processing of postural information. Neurosci Biobehav Rev 22:473–478.

Mori S, Sakamoto T, Ohta Y, Takakusaki K, Matsuyama K. 1989. Site-specific postural and locomotor changes evoked in awake, freely moving intact cats by stimulating the brainstem. Brain Res 505:66–74.

Peterka RJ. 2002. Sensorimotor integration in human postural control. J Neurophysiol 88:1097–1118.

Stapley PJ, Ting LH, Hulliger M, Macpherson JM. 2002. Automatic postural responses are delayed by pyridoxine-induced somatosensory loss. J Neurosci 22:5803–5807.

Stapley PJ, Ting LH, Kuifu C, Everaert DG, Macpherson JM. 2006. Bilateral vestibular loss leads to active destabilization of balance during voluntary head turns in the standing cat. J Neurophysiol 95:3783–3797.

Ting LH, Macpherson JM. 2005. A limited set of muscle synergies for force control during a postural task. J Neurophysiol 93:609–613.

42

The Cerebellum

THE CEREBELLUM CONSTITUTES ONLY 10% of the total volume of the brain but contains more than one-half of its neurons. The structure comprises a series of highly regular, repeating units, each of which contains the same basic microcircuit. Different regions of the cerebellum receive projections from different parts of the brain and spinal cord and project to different motor systems. Nonetheless, the similarity of the architecture and physiology in all regions of the cerebellum implies that different regions of the cerebellum perform similar computational operations on different inputs.

The symptoms of cerebellar damage in humans and experimental animals give the clear impression that the cerebellum participates in the control of movement. Thus we describe these symptoms because knowledge of them, in addition to being critical for the clinician, constrains conjecture about the exact role of the cerebellum in controlling behavior. The goal of cerebellar research is to understand how the connections and physiology of cerebellar neurons define the function of the cerebellum. Thus a major part of this chapter covers the fundamentals of cerebellar physiology and anatomy.

Finally, there is a relationship between cerebellar operation and more theoretical concepts of "internal models" in motor control (see Chapter 33). A fundamental precept of modern cerebellar research is that these internal representations of the external world are implemented in the cerebellum. The cerebellum could adjust motor performance by using its learning capabilities to alter the internal models to match any changes in the motor effectors of the external world. Thus at the conclusion of this chapter we discuss cerebellar learning and its possible relationship to internal models.

Cerebellar Diseases Have Distinctive Symptoms and Signs

Disorders of the human cerebellum result in disruptions of normal movement, described originally by Joseph Babinski in 1899 and by Gordon Holmes in the 1920s. These disruptions are in stark contrast to the paralysis caused by damage to the cerebral cortex. We cannot yet link normal cerebellar structure and function to the symptoms of cerebellar damage in humans, but the fact that movements are disrupted rather than abolished and the nature of the disruptions are important clues about cerebellar function.

Cerebellar disorders are manifested in four symptoms. The first is *hypotonia*, a diminished resistance to passive limb displacements. Hypotonia is also thought to be related to so-called "pendular reflexes." The leg normally comes to rest immediately after a knee jerk produced by a tap on the patellar tendon with a reflex hammer. In patients who have cerebellar disease, however, the leg may oscillate like a pendulum as many as eight times before coming to rest.

The second symptom is *astasia-abasia*, an inability to stand or walk. Astasia is loss of the ability to maintain a steady limb or body posture across multiple joints. Abasia is loss of the ability to maintain upright stance against gravity. When sitting or standing, many cerebellar patients compensate by spreading their feet, an attempt to stabilize balance by increasing the base of support (see Chapter 41). They move their legs irregularly and often fall.

The third symptom is *ataxia*, the abnormal execution of multi-jointed voluntary movements, characterized by lack of coordination. Patients have problems initiating responses with the affected limb and controlling the size of a movement (dysmetria) and the rate and regularity of repeated movements (Figure 42–1). This last deficit, first described by Babinski, is most readily demonstrated when a patient attempts to perform rapid alternating movements, such as alternately touching

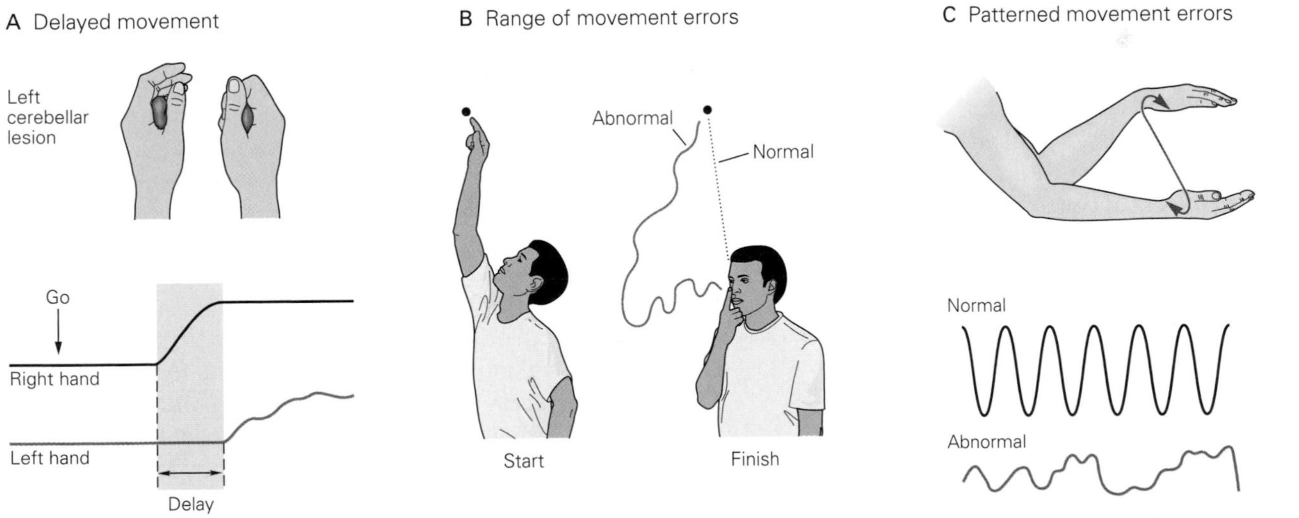

Figure 42–1 Typical defects observed in cerebellar diseases.

A. A lesion in the left cerebellar hemisphere delays the initiation of movement. The patient is told to clench both hands at the same time on a "go" signal. The left hand is clenched later than the right, as is evident in the recordings from a pressure bulb transducer squeezed by the patient.

B. A patient moving his arm from a raised position to touch the tip of his nose exhibits inaccuracy in range and direction (dysmetria) and moves his shoulder and elbow separately (decomposition of movement). Tremor increases as the finger approaches the nose.

C. A subject was asked to alternately pronate and supinate the forearm while flexing and extending at the elbow as rapidly as possible. Position traces of the hand and forearm show the normal pattern of alternating movements and the irregular pattern (dysdiadochokinesia) typical of cerebellar disorder.

the back and the palm of one hand with the palm of the other. Patients cannot sustain a regular rhythm or produce an even amount of force, a sign referred to as *dysdiadochokinesia* (Greek, impaired alternating movement). Holmes also noted that patients made errors in the timing of the components of complex multi-joint movements (decomposition of movement) and frequently failed to brace proximal joints against the forces generated by the movement of more distal joints.

The fourth symptom of cerebellar disease is a form of tremor at the end of a movement, when the patient attempts to stop the movement by using antagonist muscles. This *action* (or *intention*) *tremor* is the result of a series of erroneous corrections of the movement. Once a movement is clearly headed in the wrong direction, attempts to make corrections fail repeatedly and the hand oscillates irregularly around the target in a characteristic *terminal tremor*. This behavior clearly suggests that the cerebellum normally is responsible for the properly timed sequence of activation in agonist and antagonist muscles and that loss of proper timing causes movements that, although initiated in the correct direction, cannot be controlled or brought to an accurate endpoint.

One conspicuous feature of cerebellar disorders is a loss of the automatic, unconscious nature of most movements, especially for motor acts made up of multiple sequential movements. One of Holmes's patients, who had a lesion of his right cerebellar hemisphere, reported that "movements of my left arm are done subconsciously, but I have to think out each movement of the right arm. I come to a dead stop in turning and have to think before I start again." Normally movement is controlled seamlessly by cerebellar inputs and outputs; with a malfunctioning cerebellum it seems that the cerebral cortex needs to play a more active role in programming the details of motor actions.

The Cerebellum Has Several Functionally Distinct Regions

The cerebellum occupies most of the posterior cranial fossa. It is composed of an outer mantle of gray matter (the cerebellar cortex), internal white matter, and three pairs of deep nuclei: the fastigial nucleus, the interposed nucleus (itself comprising the emboliform and globose nuclei), and the dentate nucleus (Figure 42–2A).

The cerebellum is connected to the dorsal aspect of the brain stem by three symmetrical pairs of peduncles: the *inferior cerebellar peduncle* (also called the restiform body), the *middle cerebellar peduncle* (or brachium pontis), and the *superior cerebellar peduncle* (or brachium conjunctivum). Most of the output axons of the cerebellum arise from the deep nuclei and project through the superior cerebellar peduncle. The main exception is a group of Purkinje cells in the flocculonodular lobe that projects to vestibular nuclei in the brain stem.

The surface of the cerebellum is highly convoluted, with many parallel folds called *folia* (Latin, leaves). Two deep transverse fissures divide the cerebellum into three lobes. The primary fissure on the dorsal surface separates the anterior and posterior lobes, which together form the body of the cerebellum (Figure 42–2A). The posterolateral fissure on the ventral surface separates the body of the cerebellum from the smaller flocculonodular lobe (Figure 42–2B). Each lobe extends across the cerebellum from the midline to the most lateral tip.

In the orthogonal, anterior-posterior direction two longitudinal furrows divide three regions: the midline *vermis* (Latin, worm) and the *cerebellar hemispheres*, each of which is split into intermediate and lateral regions (Figure 42–2A).

The cerebellum is also divisible into three areas that have distinctive roles in different kinds of movements: the vestibulocerebellum, spinocerebellum, and cerebrocerebellum (Figure 42–3). The *vestibulocerebellum* consists of the flocculonodular lobe and is the most primitive part of the cerebellum, appearing first in fishes. It receives vestibular and visual inputs, projects to the vestibular nuclei in the brain stem, and participates in balance, other vestibular reflexes, and eye movements.

The *spinocerebellum* comprises the vermis and intermediate parts of the hemispheres and appears later in phylogeny. It is so named because it receives somatosensory and proprioceptive inputs from the spinal cord. The vermis receives visual, auditory, and vestibular input as well as somatic sensory input from the head and proximal parts of the body. It projects by way of the *fastigial nucleus* to cortical and brain stem regions that give rise to the medial descending systems controlling proximal muscles of the body and limbs. The vermis governs posture and locomotion as well as eye movements. The adjacent intermediate parts of the hemispheres also receive somatosensory input from the limbs. Neurons here project to the interposed nucleus, which provides inputs to lateral corticospinal and rubrospinal systems and controls the more distal muscles of the limbs and digits.

The *cerebrocerebellum* comprises the lateral parts of the hemispheres. These areas are phylogenetically most recent and are much larger in humans and apes than in monkeys and cats. Almost all of the inputs to and outputs from this region involve connections with the cerebral cortex. The output is transmitted through the *dentate nucleus*, which projects to motor, premotor, and prefrontal cortices. The lateral hemispheres have

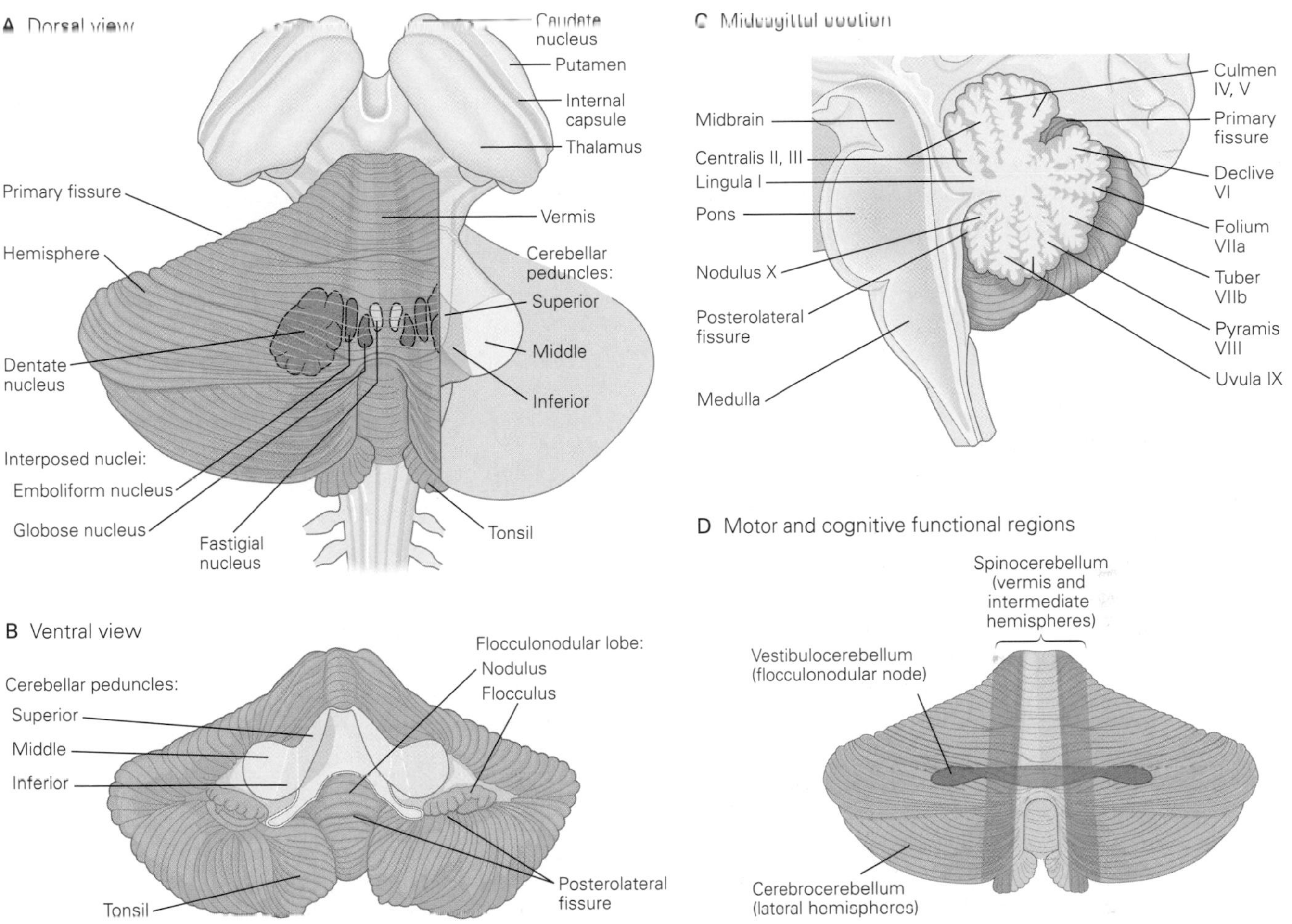

Figure 42–2 Gross features of the cerebellum. (Adapted, with permission, from Nieuwenhuys, Voogd, and van Huijzen 1988.)

A. Part of the right hemisphere has been cut away to reveal the underlying cerebellar peduncles.

B. The cerebellum is shown detached from the brain stem.

C. A midsagittal section through the brain stem and cerebellum shows the branching structure of the cerebellum. The cerebellar lobules are labeled with their Latin names and Larsell Roman numerals. (Reproduced, with permission, from Larsell and Jansen 1972.)

D. Functional regions of the cerebellum. (see also Figure 42–3.)

many functions but seem to participate most extensively in planning and executing movement. They may also have a role in certain cognitive functions unconnected with motor planning, such as working memory. There is now some correlative evidence implicating the cerebellar hemispheres in aspects of schizophrenia (see Chapter 62) and autism (see Chapter 64).

The Cerebellar Microcircuit Has a Distinct and Regular Organization

The cellular organization of the cerebellar microcircuit is striking, and one of the premises of cerebellar research has been that the details of the microcircuit are an important clue to how the cerebellum works. Four major features of the microcircuit are described in the next four subsections.

Neurons in the Cerebellar Cortex Are Organized into Three Layers

The three layers of the cerebellar cortex possess distinct kinds of neurons and perform different operations (Figure 42–4).

The deepest or *granular layer* is the input layer. It contains a vast number of granule cells, estimated at 100 billion, which appear in histological sections

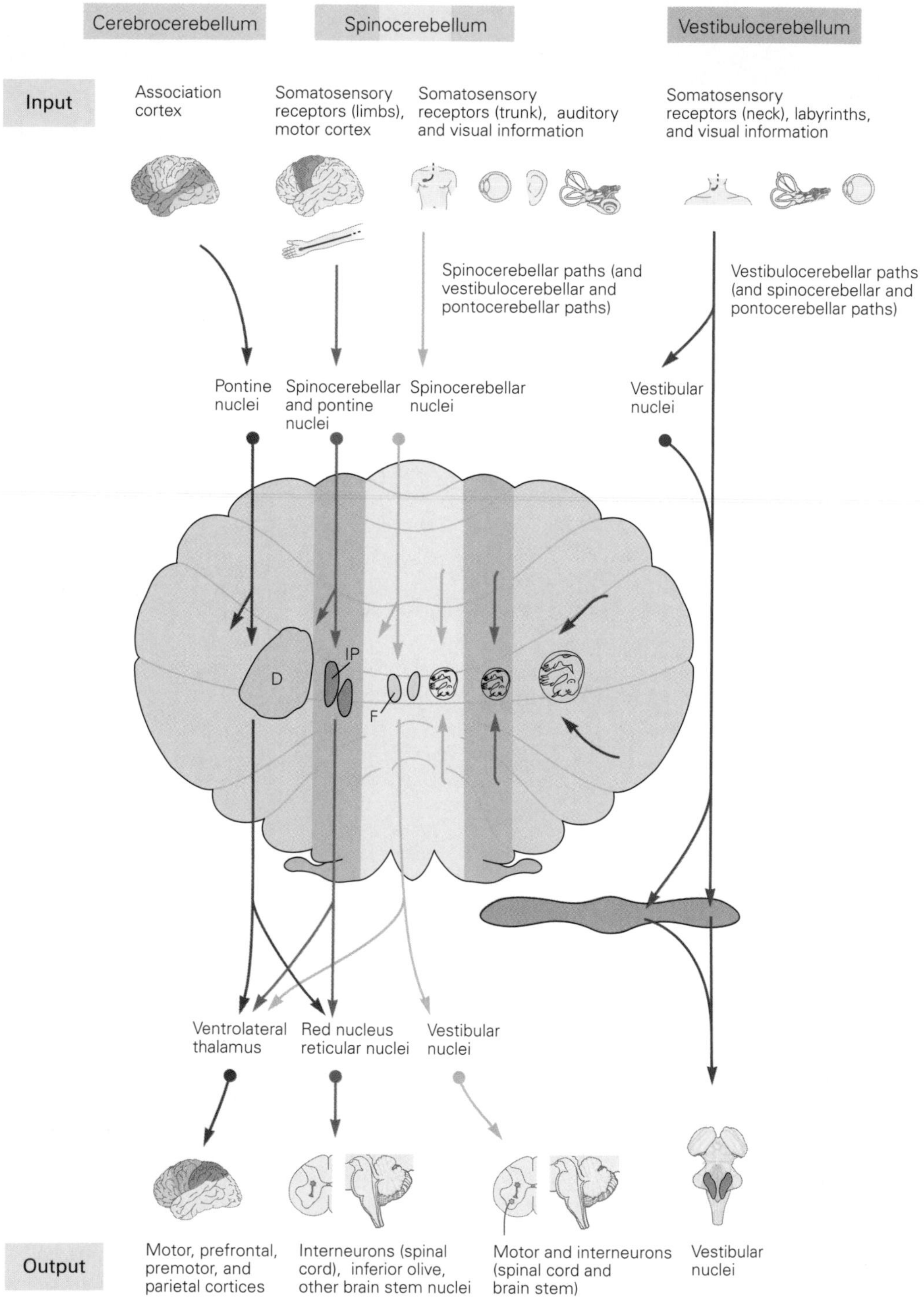

Figure 42–3 The three functional regions of the cerebellum have different inputs and different output targets. In the figure the cerebellum is unfolded, and arrows show the inputs and outputs of the different functional areas. The body maps in the deep nuclei are based on anatomical tracing and single-cell recordings in nonhuman primates. (**D**, dentate nucleus; **IP**, interposed nucleus; **F**, fastigial nucleus.) (Adapted, with permission, from Thach 1980.)

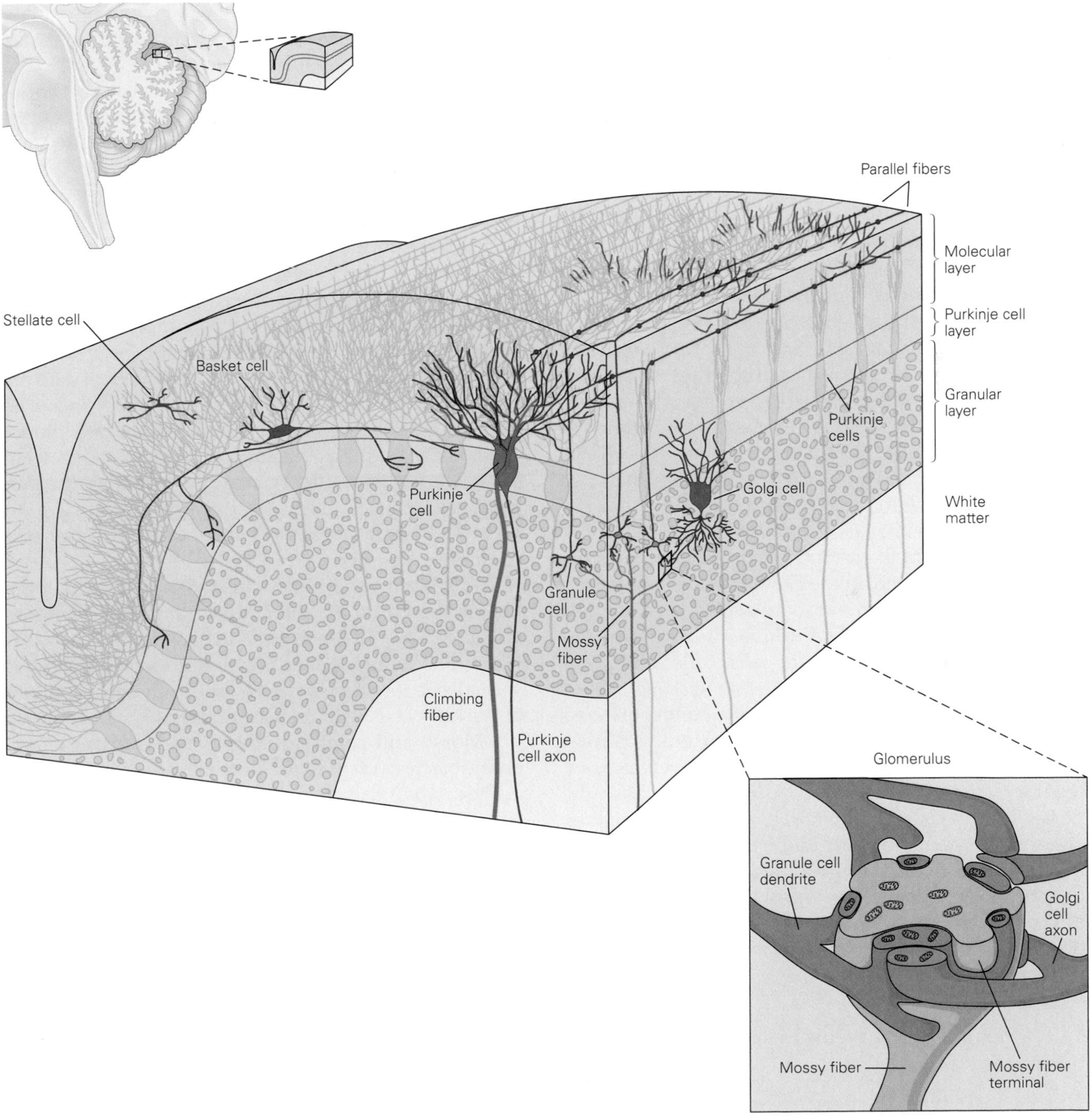

Figure 42–4 The cerebellar cortex contains five types of neurons organized into three layers. A vertical section of a single cerebellar folium illustrates the general organization of the cerebellar cortex. The detail of a cerebellar glomerulus in the granular layer is also shown. A glomerulus is the synaptic complex formed by the bulbous axon terminal of a mossy fiber and the dendrites of several Golgi and granule cells. Mitochondria are present in all of the structures in the glomerulus, consistent with their high metabolic activity.

as small, densely packed, darkly stained nuclei. This layer also contains a few larger Golgi interneurons and, in some cerebellar regions, a smattering of other neurons such as cells of Lugaro, unipolar brush cells, and chandelier cells. The mossy fibers, one of the two principal afferent inputs to the cerebellum, terminate in this layer. The bulbous terminals of the mossy fibers excite granule cells and Golgi neurons in synaptic complexes called *cerebellar glomeruli* (Figure 42–4). As we will see later when discussing recurrent circuits in the cerebellum, Golgi cells inhibit granule cells.

The middle, or *Purkinje cell layer*, is the output layer of the cerebellar cortex. This layer consists of a single sheet of Purkinje cells bodies, which are 50 to 80 μm in diameter. The fan-like dendrites of Purkinje cells extend upward into the molecular layer where they receive inputs from the second major type of afferent fiber in the cerebellum, the climbing fibers, as well as from inhibitory and excitatory interneurons. Purkinje cell axons conduct the entire output of the cerebellar cortex, projecting to the deep nuclei in the underlying white matter or to the vestibular nuclei in the brain stem where the GABA (γ-aminobutyric acid) released by their terminals has an inhibitory action.

The outermost, or *molecular layer*, is an important processing layer of the cerebellar cortex. It contains the cell bodies and dendrites of two types of inhibitory interneurons, the stellate and basket cells, as well as the extensive dendrites of Purkinje cells. It also contains the axons of the granule cells, called the *parallel fibers* because they run parallel to the long axis of the folia (see Figure 42–4). The spatially polarized dendrites of Purkinje neurons cover extensive terrain in the anterior-posterior direction, but a very narrow territory in the medial-lateral direction. Because the parallel fibers run in the medial-lateral direction, they are oriented perpendicular to the dendritic trees of the Purkinje cells. Thus each granule cell has the potential to form a few synapses with each of a large number of Purkinje neurons, while making denser connections on a few Purkinje neurons as its axon ascends into the molecular layer.

Two Afferent Fiber Systems Encode Information Differently

The two main types of afferent fibers in the cerebellum, the mossy fibers and climbing fibers, both form excitatory synapses with cerebellar neurons but terminate in different layers of the cerebellar cortex, produce different patterns of firing in the Purkinje neurons, and thus probably mediate different functions.

Mossy fibers originate from cell bodies in the spinal cord and brain stem and carry sensory information from the periphery as well as information from the cerebral cortex. They form excitatory synapses on the dendrites of granule cells in the granular layer (Figure 42–5). Each granule cell receives inputs from just a few mossy fibers, but the architecture of the granule cell axons distributes information widely from each mossy fiber to a large number of Purkinje cells. The mossy fiber input is highly convergent; each Purkinje neuron is contacted by axons from somewhere between 200,000 and 1 million granule cells.

Climbing fibers originate in the inferior olivary nucleus and convey sensory information to the cerebellum from both the periphery and the cerebral cortex. The climbing fiber is so named because each enwraps the cell body and proximal dendrites of a Purkinje neuron like a vine on a tree, making numerous synaptic contacts (Figure 42–5). Each climbing fiber contacts 1 to 10 Purkinje neurons, but each Purkinje neuron receives synaptic input from only a single climbing fiber. The terminals of the climbing fibers are arranged topographically in the cerebellar cortex; the axons from clusters of related olivary neurons terminate in thin parasagittal strips that extend across several folia. In turn, the Purkinje neurons within one strip project to a common group of deep nuclear neurons.

The highly specific connectivity of the climbing fiber system contrasts markedly with the massive convergence and divergence of the mossy and parallel fibers, and suggests that the climbing fiber system is specialized for precise control of the electrical activity of Purkinje cells with related functions.

Mossy and climbing fibers have different effects on the electrical activity of Purkinje cells. Climbing fibers have an unusually powerful influence. Each action potential in a climbing fiber generates a protracted, voltage-gated Ca^{2+} conductance in the soma and dendrites of the postsynaptic Purkinje cell. This results in prolonged depolarization that produces a complex spike: an initial large-amplitude action potential followed by a high-frequency burst of smaller-amplitude action potentials (Figure 42–5). Whether these smaller spikes are transmitted down the Purkinje cell's axon is not clear. In awake animals the climbing fibers spontaneously generate complex spikes at low rates, rarely more than one to three per second. When stimulated they fire single action potentials in temporal relation with specific sensory events.

The climbing-fiber system therefore seems specialized for event detection; the firing rate carries little or no information. Although climbing fibers fire only infrequently, synchronous firing in multiple climbing

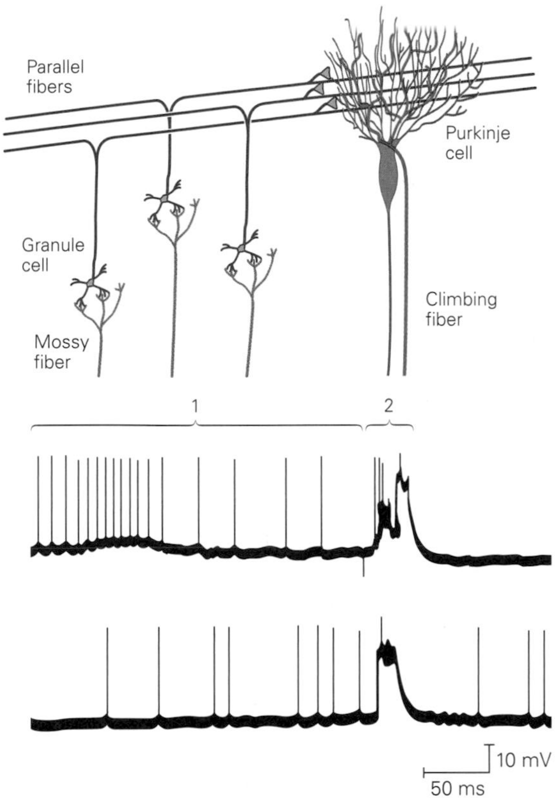

Figure 42–5 Simple and complex spikes recorded intracellularly from a cerebellar Purkinje cell. Simple spikes are produced by mossy fiber input (**1**), whereas complex spikes are evoked by climbing fiber synapses (**2**). (Reproduced, with permission, from Martinez, Crill, and Kennedy 1971.)

fibers enables them to signal important events. Synchrony seems to arise partly because neurons in the inferior olivary nucleus often are connected to one another electrotonically.

In contrast, parallel fibers produce only brief, small excitatory potentials in Purkinje neurons. These potentials spread to the initial segment of the axon where they generate simple spikes that propagate down the axon. However, inputs from many parallel fibers are needed to have a substantial effect on the frequency of simple spikes, for each postsynaptic potential is tiny. In awake animals Purkinje neurons emit a steady stream of simple spikes, with spontaneous firing rates as high as 100 per second even when an animal is sitting quietly. Purkinje neurons fire at rates as high as several hundred spikes per second during active eye, arm, and face movements, presumably because of somatosensory, vestibular, and other sensory signals that converge on granule cells through the mossy fibers. Thus the mossy-fiber system encodes the magnitude and duration of peripheral stimuli or centrally generated behaviors by controlling the firing rate of simple spikes in Purkinje cells.

Parallel Pathways Compare Excitatory and Inhibitory Signals

An important feature of the cerebellar circuit is that excitatory and inhibitory inputs are compared in both the cerebellar cortex and the deep nuclei. In the deep nuclei inhibitory inputs from Purkinje cells converge with excitatory inputs from mossy and climbing fibers (Figure 42–6).

The cerebellum is organized as a series of small, similar modules with close relationships among all the elements of each module. Within a given module a mossy fiber affects target neurons in the deep nuclei

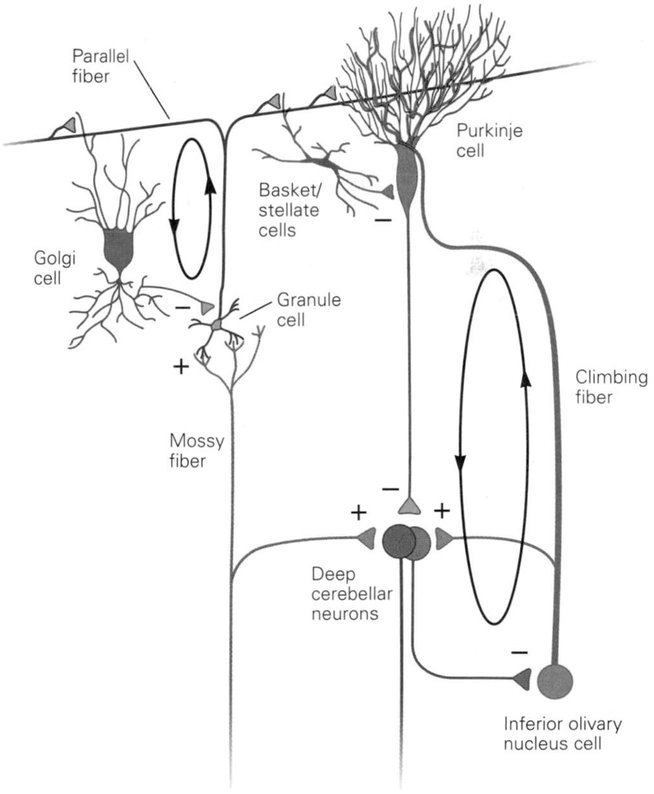

Figure 42–6 Synaptic organization of the cerebellar microcircuit. Excitation and inhibition converge both in the cerebellar cortex and in the deep nuclei. Recurrent loops involve Golgi cells within the cerebellar cortex and the inferior olive outside the cerebellum. (Adapted, with permission, from Raymond, Lisberger, and Mauk 1996.)

in two ways: directly by excitatory synapses and indirectly by pathways through the cortex and the inhibitory Purkinje cells. Thus the inhibitory output of the Purkinje cells modulates or sculpts the excitatory signals transmitted from mossy fibers to the deep nuclei. In almost all parts of the cerebellum the climbing fibers also give off collaterals that excite neurons in the deep nuclei.

In the cerebellar cortex excitatory and inhibitory inputs converge on Purkinje cells. Parallel fibers directly excite Purkinje neurons but also indirectly inhibit them through disynaptic connections from the stellate, basket, and Golgi interneurons. The short axons of stellate cells contact the nearby dendrites of Purkinje cells, whereas the long axons of basket cells run perpendicular to the parallel fibers and form synapses on the Purkinje cell bodies (Figure 42–4). The stellate cells have an inhibitory regulatory effect on the Purkinje cells that is local in that a stellate cell and the Purkinje cell it contacts are both excited by the same parallel fibers. In contrast, the basket cells create flanks of inhibition of Purkinje cells that are excited by flanking beams of parallel fibers other than the central beam that causes the lateral inhibition.

Recurrent Loops Occur at Several Levels

At the broadest level many parts of the cerebellum form recurrent loops with the cerebral cortex. The cerebral cortex projects to the lateral cerebellum through relays in the pontine nuclei. In turn, the lateral cerebellum projects back to the cerebral cortex through relays in the thalamus. This recurrent circuit is organized as a series of parallel closed loops, such that a given part of the cerebellum connects reciprocally with a given part of the cerebral cortex. Figure 42–7 shows how the cerebellum fits into the greater motor circuits from the cerebral cortex to the spinal cord.

Another recurrent loop involves the cerebellum and the inferior olivary nucleus, the source of all climbing fibers. The deep cerebellar nuclei contain GABAergic inhibitory neurons that project to the inferior olive. If inhibitory inputs from the deep nuclei increase then the firing frequency in inferior olive cells decreases, reducing the amount of excitatory climbing fiber input to cerebellar nuclear and Purkinje cells. This provides each part of the cerebellum a way to regulate its own climbing fiber inputs (see Figure 42–6), another in the many checks and balances built into cerebellar circuitry. Interestingly, the GABAergic fibers from the deep nuclei can regulate the electrotonic coupling between olivary neurons. By selectively disconnecting olivary neurons through inhibition, the nervous system

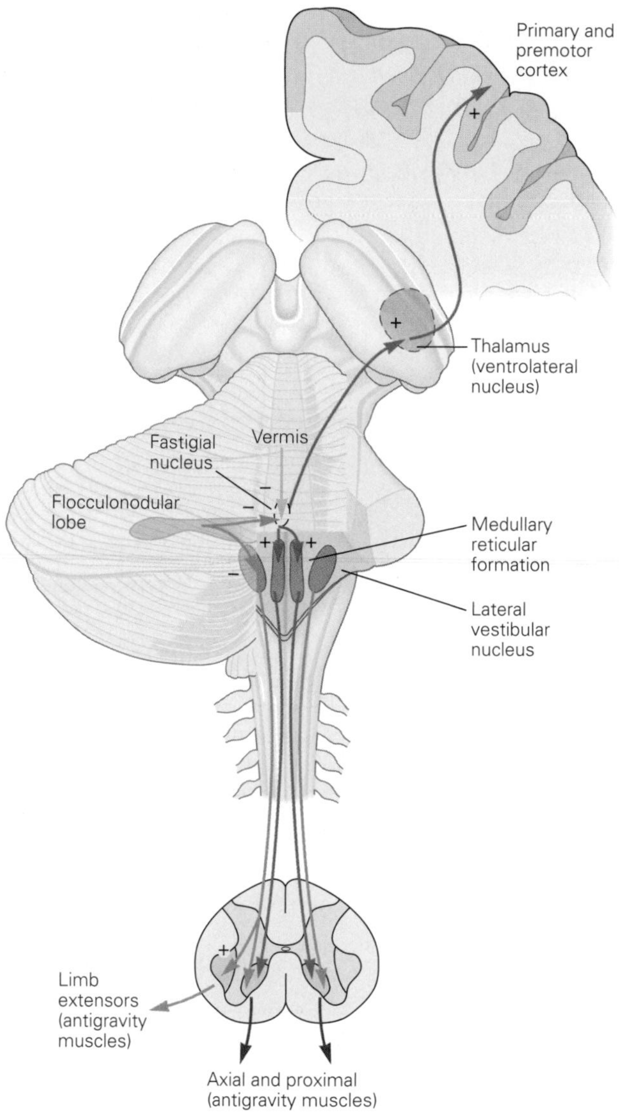

Figure 42–7 The vestibulocerebellum and the vermis control proximal muscles and limb extensors. The vestibulocerebellum (flocculonodular lobe) receives input from the vestibular labyrinth and projects directly to the vestibular nuclei. The vermis receives input from the neck and trunk, the vestibular labyrinth, and retinal and extraocular muscles. Its output is focused on the ventromedial descending systems of the brain stem, mainly the reticulospinal and vestibulospinal tracts and the corticospinal fibers acting on medial motor neurons. The oculomotor connections of the vestibular nuclei have been omitted for clarity.

can activate a specific array of Purkinje neurons synchronously.

The final recurrent loop is contained entirely within the cerebellar cortex and involves Golgi cells. Each Golgi cell receives excitatory inputs from parallel fibers; in turn, its GABAergic terminals provide inhibitory input to the granule cells (Figure 42–6). Golgi cell firing thus suppresses mossy fiber excitation of the granule cells and regulates the firing of the parallel fibers. This loop may shorten the duration of bursts in granule cells. Alternatively, it could limit the magnitude of the excitatory response of granule cells to their mossy fiber inputs. For example, the responses of granule cells could occur only when a certain number of mossy fiber inputs are active, or only when they achieve a threshold frequency of firing. One current idea is that the Golgi cells ensure that only a small number of granule cells are active at any given time, creating a *sparse code* in the input layer of the cerebellar cortex.

The Vestibulocerebellum Regulates Balance and Eye Movements

The vestibulocerebellum, or flocculonodular lobe, receives information from the semicircular canals and the otolith organs, which sense the head's motion and its position relative to gravity (Figure 42–3). Most of this vestibular input arises from the vestibular nuclei in the brain stem. The vestibulocerebellum also receives mossy fiber visual input, both from pretectal nuclei that lie deep in the midbrain beneath the superior colliculus and from the primary and secondary visual cortex through the pontine and pretectal nuclei.

The vestibulocerebellum is unique in that its output bypasses the deep cerebellar nuclei and proceeds directly to the vestibular nuclei in the brain stem. Purkinje cells in the midline parts of the vestibulocerebellum project to the lateral vestibular nucleus to modulate the lateral and medial vestibulospinal tracts, which predominantly control axial muscles and limb extensors to assure balance during stance and gait. Disruption of these projections through lesions or disease impairs equilibrium.

Purkinje neurons in the lateral parts of the vestibulocerebellum project to the medial vestibular nucleus to control eye movements and coordinate movements of the head and eyes (see Chapter 39). Interestingly, this ancient part of the cerebellum has been co-opted in more recent phylogeny by visual guidance of eye movements. In fact, the most striking deficits following lesions of the lateral vestibulocerebellum are in smooth-pursuit eye movement toward the side of the lesion. A patient with a lesion of the left lateral vestibulocerebellum can smoothly track a target that is moving to the right, but only poorly tracks motion to the left using predominantly saccades (Figure 42–8A).

Patients with lesions of the lateral vestibulocerebellum have normal ocular responses to head turns, but the responses cannot be suppressed by fixation (Figure 42–8B). If, for example, a patient seated in a barber's chair is rotated to the right in the dark, the vestibulo-ocular reflex causes smooth eye rotation to the left and resetting saccades to the right. If the patient is placed in the light and views an object attached to the chair, he or she can use fixation to suppress the smooth eye movements of the reflex. For leftward head rotation, however, the patient cannot do so. These deficits occur commonly if the lateral vestibulocerebellum is compressed by an acoustic neuroma, a benign tumor that grows on the eighth cranial nerve as it courses directly beneath the lateral vestibulocerebellum.

The Spinocerebellum Regulates Body and Limb Movements

The spinocerebellum comprises the vermis and intermediate parts of the cerebellar hemispheres (see Figure 42–2A).

Somatosensory Information Reaches the Spinocerebellum Through Direct and Indirect Mossy Fiber Pathways

The spinocerebellum receives extensive sensory input from the spinal cord, mainly from somatosensory receptors conveying information about touch, pressure, and limb position, through several direct and indirect pathways. This input provides the cerebellum with different reports of the changing state of the organism and its environment and permit comparisons between the two.

Direct pathways originate from interneurons in the spinal gray matter and terminate as mossy fibers in the vermis or spinocerebellum. Indirect pathways from the spinal cord to the cerebellum terminate first on neurons in one of several precerebellar nuclei in the brain stem reticular formation: the lateral reticular nucleus, reticularis tegmenti pontis, and paramedian reticular nucleus.

One fundamental principle of cerebellar operation can be appreciated on the basis of two important pathways from the spinal interneurons. The ventral and dorsal spinocerebellar tracts both transmit signals

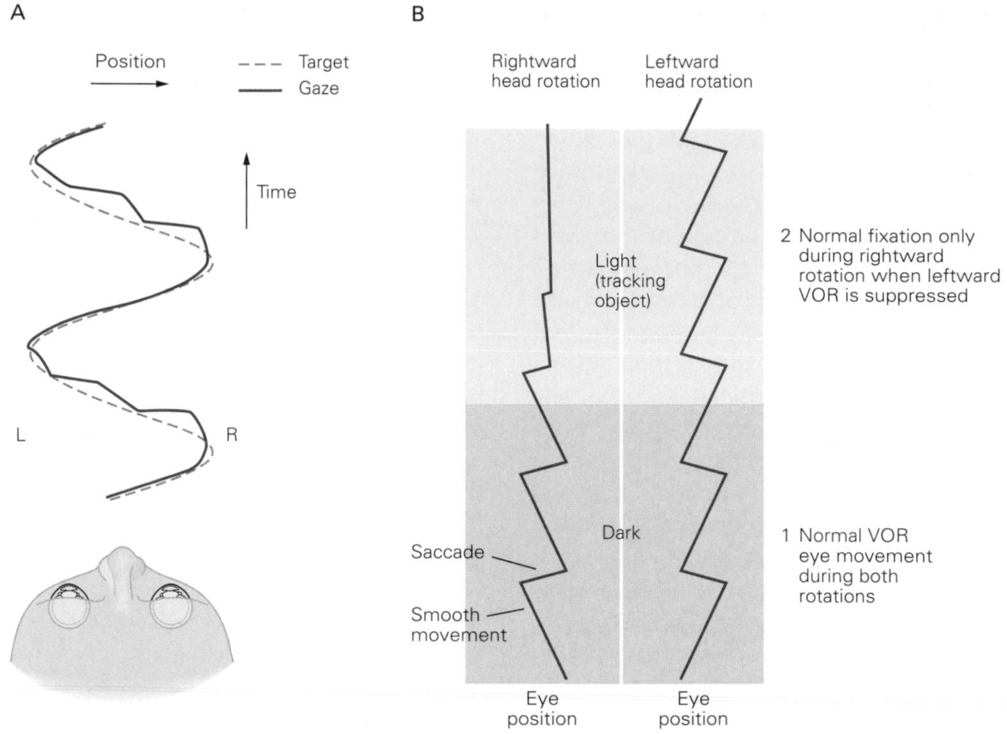

Figure 42–8 Lesions in the vestibulocerebellum have large effects on smooth-pursuit eye movements.

A. Sinusoidal target motion is tracked with smooth-pursuit eye movements as the target moves from left (L) to right (R). With a lesion of the left vestibulocerebellum, smooth pursuit is punctuated by saccades when the target moves from right to left.

B. In the same patient responses to vestibular stimulation are normal, whereas object fixation is disrupted during leftward rotation. Each trace shows the eye movements evoked by head rotation while the patient fixates on a target that moves along with him, first in the dark and then in the light. (1) In the dark the eyes show a normal vestibulo-ocular reflex (VOR) during rotation in both directions: The eyes move smoothly in the direction opposite to the head's rotation, then reset with saccades in the direction of head rotation. (2) In the light the eye position during rightward head rotation is normal: Fixation on the target is excellent and the vestibulo-ocular reflex is suppressed. During leftward head rotation, however, the subject is unable to fixate on the object and the vestibulo-ocular reflex cannot be suppressed.

from the spinal cord directly to the cerebellar cortex but convey two different kinds of information.

The *dorsal spinocerebellar tract* conveys somatosensory information from muscle and joint receptors, providing the cerebellum with sensory feedback about the consequences of the movement. This information flows whether the limbs are moved passively or voluntarily.

In contrast, the *ventral spinocerebellar tract* is active only during active movements. Its cells of origin receive the same inputs as spinal motor neurons and interneurons, and it transmits an efference copy or corollary discharge of spinal motor neuron activity that informs the cerebellum about the movement commands assembled at the spinal cord. The cerebellum is thought to compare this information on planned movement with the actual movement reported by the dorsal spinocerebellar tract in order to determine whether the motor command must be modified to achieve the desired movement. The dorsal and ventral spinocerebellar tracts provide inputs from the hind limbs, whereas the cuneocerebellar and rostral spinocerebellar tracts provide similar inputs from more rostral body parts.

The idea that the cerebellum compares the actual and expected sensory consequences of movements is supported by studies of a number of movement systems. As a decerebrated cat walks on a treadmill, for example, the firing rate of neurons in the dorsal and ventral spinocerebellar tracts is rhythmically modulated in phase with the step cycle. However, when the dorsal roots are cut, preventing spinal neurons from receiving peripheral inputs that modulate with the step cycle, neurons of the dorsal spinocerebellar tract fall silent, whereas the firing of neurons of the ventral spinocerebellar tract continues to be modulated.

Recordings from the vestibulocerebellum of monkeys show that Purkinje neurons compare vestibular sensory inputs related to head velocity with corollary inputs related to eye velocity. The simple-spike output from these Purkinje neurons is modulated only when the eye movements are different from those expected from the vestibulo-ocular reflex. The cerebellum participates in the control of smooth eye movement only when the brain stem reflex pathways alone cannot produce the desired motor outputs.

The Spinocerebellum Modulates the Descending Motor Systems

Purkinje neurons in the spinocerebellum project somatotopically to different deep nuclei that control various components of the descending motor pathways. Neurons in the vermis of both the anterior and posterior lobes send axons to the fastigial nucleus. The fastigial nucleus projects bilaterally to the brain stem reticular formation and lateral vestibular nuclei, which in turn project directly to the spinal cord (Figure 42–7).

The spinocerebellum therefore provides important inputs to the brain stem components of the medial descending systems. Its outputs are important for movements of the neck, trunk, and proximal parts of the arm, rather than the wrist and digits, for balance and postural control during voluntary motor tasks. Because these brain stem systems also receive large inputs from descending pathways and from sensory inputs, we think that the cerebellum modulates and initiates, rather than controls, the descending commands to the spinal cord.

Purkinje neurons in the intermediate part of the cerebellar hemispheres project to the interposed nucleus. Some axons of the interposed nucleus exit through the superior cerebellar peduncle and cross to the contralateral side of the brain to terminate in the magnocellular portion of the red nucleus. Axons from the red nucleus cross the midline again and descend to the spinal cord (Figure 42–9). Other axons from the interposed nucleus continue rostrally and terminate in the ventrolateral nucleus of the thalamus. Neurons in the ventrolateral nucleus project to the limb control areas of the primary motor cortex.

By acting on the neurons that give rise to the rubrospinal and corticospinal systems, the intermediate cerebellum focuses its action on limb and axial musculature. Because cerebellar outputs cross the midline twice before reaching the spinal cord, cerebellar lesions disrupt ipsilateral limb movements.

The Vermis Controls Saccadic and Smooth-Pursuit Eye Movements

The vermis is involved in the control of saccades and smooth-pursuit eye movements through Purkinje cells in lobules V, VI, and VII (Figure 42–2C). The cells discharge prior to and during such movements, and lesions of these areas cause deficits in the accuracy of both kinds of movements.

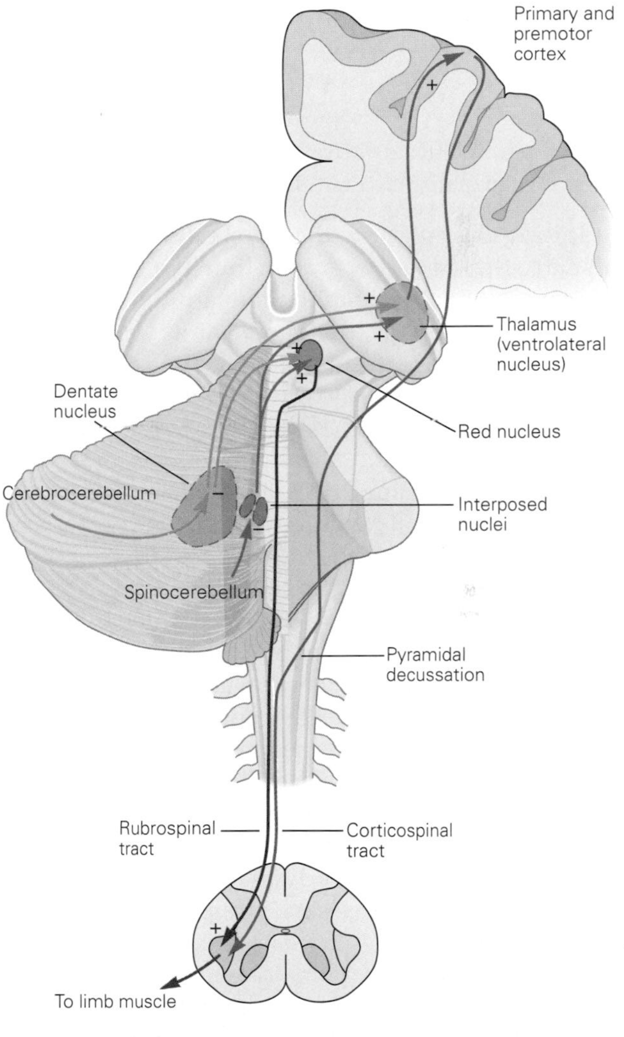

Figure 42–9 Neurons in the intermediate and lateral parts of the cerebellar hemispheres control limb and axial muscles. The intermediate part of each hemisphere (spinocerebellum) receives sensory information from the limbs and controls the dorsolateral descending systems (rubrospinal and corticospinal tracts) acting on the ipsilateral limbs. The lateral area of each hemisphere (cerebrocerebellum) receives cortical input via the pontine nuclei and influences the motor and premotor cortices via the ventrolateral nucleus of the thalamus.

The vermis may be the only area of the cerebellum responsible for saccades, but it seems to share responsibility for smooth pursuit with the lateral part of the flocculonodular lobe. The outputs from neurons of the vermis concerned with saccades are transmitted through a very small region of the caudal fastigial nucleus to the saccade generator in the reticular formation. The exact neural pathways for guidance of pursuit by the vermis are not known, but they involve more synaptic relays than the outputs from the lateral part of the flocculonodular lobe, which reach extraocular motor neurons through two intervening synapses. One idea currently being explored is that the vermis also plays a role in motor learning that corrects errors in saccades and smooth-pursuit movements.

Spinocerebellar Regulation of Movement Follows Three Organizational Principles

In addition to confirming that cerebellar lesions in animals have the same effects as in humans, animal studies have provided an initial understanding of what the cerebellum does in healthy people and why lesions of the cerebellum have the effects they do.

Many experiments using monkeys have recorded the action potentials of single neurons in the interposed and dentate nuclei and the intermediate and lateral cerebellar cortex during arm movements. Other experiments have used cooling probes or substances that temporarily inactivate neurons to compare specific aspects of motor behavior in an active and inactive cerebellum. From these experiments we can draw three basic conclusions regarding the function of the spinocerebellum.

First, both Purkinje neurons and deep cerebellar nucleus neurons discharge vigorously in relation to voluntary movements. Cerebellar output is related to the direction and speed of movement. The deep nuclei are somatopically organized into maps of different limbs and joints, as in the motor cortex. Moreover, the interval between the onset of modulation of the firing of cerebellar neurons and movement is remarkably similar to that for neurons in the motor cortex. This result emphasizes the cerebellum's participation in recurrent circuits that operate synchronously with the cerebral cortex.

Second, the cerebellum provides feed-forward control of muscle contractions to regulate the timing of movements. Rather than awaiting sensory feedback, cerebellar output anticipates the muscular contractions that will be needed to bring a movement smoothly, accurately, and quickly to its desired endpoint. Failure of these mechanisms causes the intention tremor of cerebellar disorders.

Normally a rapid single-joint movement is initiated by the contraction of an agonist muscle and terminated by an appropriately timed contraction of the antagonist. The contraction of the antagonist starts early in the movement, well before there has been time for sensory feedback to reach the brain, and therefore must be programmed as part of the movement. When the dentate and interposed nuclei are experimentally inactivated, however, contraction of the antagonist muscle is delayed until the limb has overshot its target. The programmed contraction seen in normal movements is replaced by a feedback correction driven by sensory input. This correction is itself dysmetric and results in another error, necessitating a new adjustment (Figure 42–10).

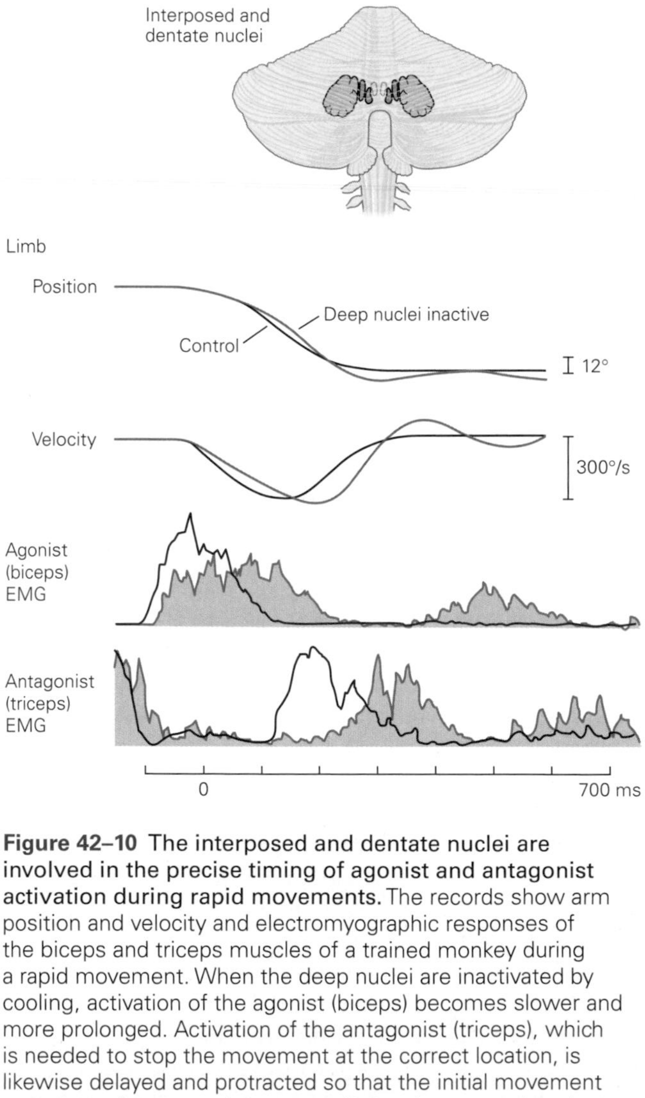

Figure 42–10 The interposed and dentate nuclei are involved in the precise timing of agonist and antagonist activation during rapid movements. The records show arm position and velocity and electromyographic responses of the biceps and triceps muscles of a trained monkey during a rapid movement. When the deep nuclei are inactivated by cooling, activation of the agonist (biceps) becomes slower and more prolonged. Activation of the antagonist (triceps), which is needed to stop the movement at the correct location, is likewise delayed and protracted so that the initial movement overshoots its appropriate extent. Delays in successive phases of the movement produce oscillations similar to the terminal tremor seen in patients with cerebellar damage.

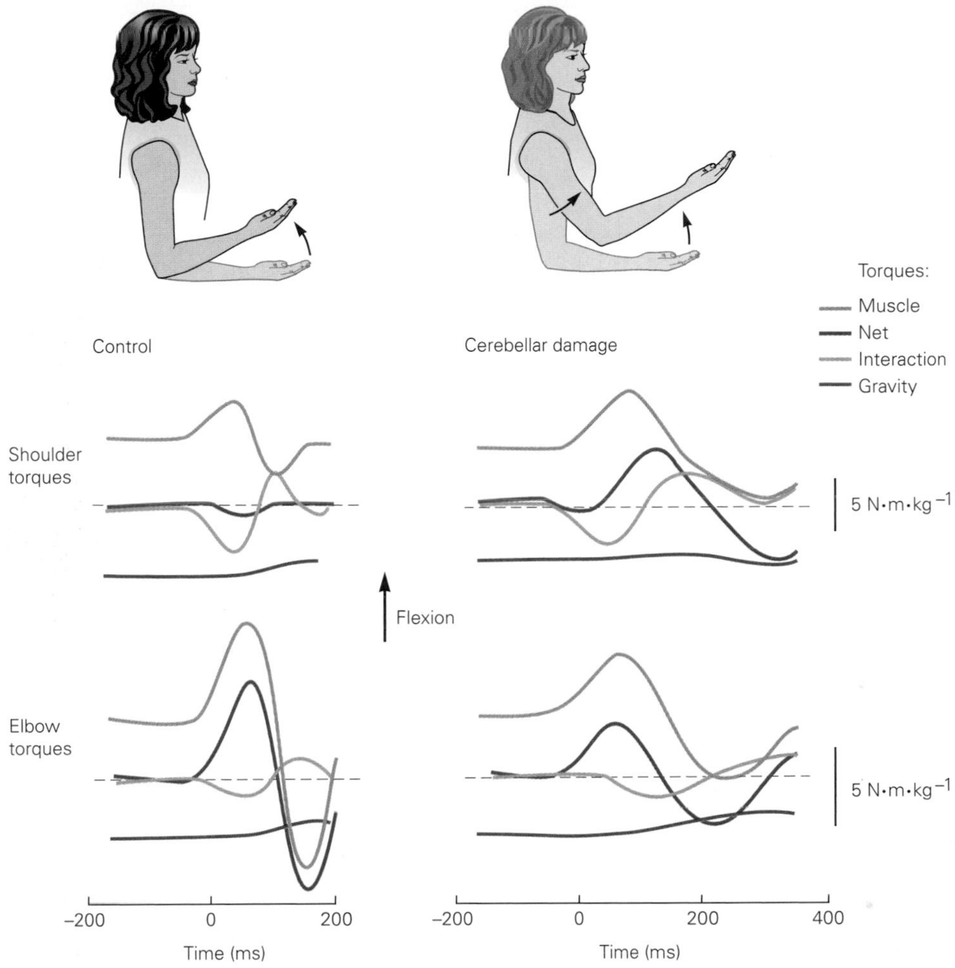

Figure 42–11 Failure of compensation for interaction torques can account for cerebellar ataxia. Subjects flex their elbows while keeping their shoulder stable. In both the control subject and the cerebellar patient the net elbow torque is large because the elbow is moved. In the control subject there is relatively little net shoulder torque because the interaction torques are automatically cancelled by muscle torques. In the cerebellar patient this compensation fails; the muscle torques are present but are inappropriate to cancel the interaction torques. As a result, the patient cannot flex her elbow without causing a large perturbation of her shoulder position. (Adapted, with permission, from Bastian, Zackowski, and Thach 2000.)

Third, the cerebellum has internal models of the limbs that automatically take account of limb structure. (See Chapter 33 for a discussion of internal models.) An accurate dynamic model of the arm, for example, can convert a desired final endpoint into a sequence of properly timed and scaled commands for muscular contraction. At the same time, an accurate kinematic model of the relationship between joint angles and finger position can specify the joint angles that are needed to achieve an endpoint. Recordings of the output of the cerebellum have provided evidence compatible with the idea that the cerebellum contains kinematic and dynamic models of both arm and eye movements.

Studies of the movements of patients with cerebellar disorders suggest that the interaction torques of a multi-segment limb are represented by an internal model in the cerebellum. Because of the structure of the arm and the momentum it develops when moving, movement of the forearm alone causes forces that move the upper arm. If a subject wants to flex or extend the elbow without simultaneously moving the shoulder, then muscles acting at the shoulder must contract to prevent its movement. These stabilizing contractions of the shoulder joint occur almost perfectly in control subjects but not in patients with cerebellar damage (Figure 42–11). Patients with cerebellar ataxia are unable to compensate for interaction torques.

They experience difficulty controlling the inertial interactions among multiple segments of a limb accounts and greater inaccuracy of multi-joint versus single-joint movements.

In conclusion, the cerebellum uses internal models to anticipate the forces that result from the mechanical properties of a moving limb and may use its learning capabilities to customize internal models to anticipate those forces accurately.

Recent research suggests that excessive variability of Purkinje-cell output can lead to ataxia, suggesting that the regularity of cerebellar activity must be closely regulated to achieve normal movement. In animal models cerebellar symptoms result when deletion of certain ion channels causes the firing of Purkinje cells to become excessively variable even though the mean firing rate is entirely normal when averaged across many repetitions of a movement.

Are the Parallel Fibers a Mechanism for Motor Coordination?

A conspicuous feature of cerebellar structure is the medial-lateral parallel fiber "beam." Parallel fibers extend up to 6 mm through the molecular layer and excite the dendrites of Purkinje, basket, stellate, and Golgi cells along their course (see Figure 42–4). Basket and stellate axons create inhibitory flanks along the sides of the parallel fiber beam.

One current idea is that the great extent of the parallel fibers allows them to tie together the activity of different cerebellar compartments. Purkinje cells project topographically onto the deep cerebellar nuclei, each of which contains a complete map of body parts and muscles. In each map the representation of the tail is located anteriorly and that of the head posteriorly, with the limbs medially and the trunk laterally. The long trajectory of the parallel fibers could link different body parts in a medial-lateral dimension in different combinations.

In rats trained to reach to a target, for example, Purkinje cells along the medial-lateral parallel fiber beam fire simple spikes simultaneously and in precise synchrony with the movement. Pairs of Purkinje cells that are not situated along the same excitatory beam show no such synchrony. The synchrony may link muscles for multi-muscle movements and synchronize their contractions.

Finally, sagittal splitting of the posterior vermis in children, an operation performed to remove tumors in the fourth ventricle, creates surprisingly little functional deficit. The children can walk and climb stairs without assistance or obvious abnormality, and they can hop on one leg repeatedly almost as well as healthy children. Nevertheless, a striking deficit occurs when they attempt heel-to-toe tandem gait. Without support they fall after three steps. The discrepancy between the large deficit in tandem gait and the normal one-legged hopping is striking because both require the integration of vestibular, somesthetic, and visual sensation. These observations imply that the severed parallel fibers crossing in the vermis are essential to coordination of the projections to the bilateral fastigial nuclei.

The Cerebrocerebellum Is Involved in Planning Movement

The Cerebrocerebellum Is Part of a High-Level Internal Feedback Circuit That Plans Movement and Regulates Cortical Motor Programs

Clinical observations by neurologists and neurosurgeons initially suggested that, like the rest of the cerebellum, the lateral hemispheres (the cerebrocerebellum) are primarily concerned with motor function. However, recent clinical and experimental studies indicate that the lateral hemispheres in humans also have perceptual and cognitive functions. Indeed, the lateral hemispheres are much larger in humans than in monkeys, just as in humans the frontal regions of the cerebral cortex are greatly expanded.

In contrast to other regions of the cerebellum, which receive sensory information more directly from the spinal cord, the lateral hemispheres receive input exclusively from the cerebral cortex. This cortical input is transmitted through the pontine nuclei and through the middle cerebellar peduncle to the contralateral dentate nucleus and lateral hemisphere (see Figure 42–3).

Purkinje neurons in the lateral hemisphere project to the dentate nucleus. Most dentate axons exit the cerebellum through the superior cerebellar peduncle and terminate in two main sites. One terminus is an area of the contralateral ventrolateral thalamus that also receives input from the interposed nucleus. These thalamic cells project to premotor and primary motor cortex (see Figure 42–9).

The second principal terminus of dentate neurons is the contralateral red nucleus, specifically a portion of the parvocellular area of the nucleus distinct from that which receives input from the interposed nucleus. These neurons project to the inferior olivary nucleus, which in turn projects back to the contralateral cerebellum as climbing fibers, thus forming a recurrent loop (see Figure 42–6). Neurons in the parvocellular portion of the red nucleus, in addition to receiving input from the dentate nucleus, also receive input from the lateral premotor areas. On the basis of brain imaging, the intriguing suggestion has been made that this loop involving the premotor cortex, lateral cerebellum, and rubrocerebellar tract participates in the mental rehearsal of movements and perhaps in motor learning (see Chapter 33).

Lesions of the Cerebrocerebellum Disrupt Motor Planning and Prolong Reaction Time

In the first half of the 20th century, neurologists identified two characteristic motor disturbances in patients with localized damage in the cerebrocerebellum: variable delays in initiating movements and irregularities in the timing of movement components. The same defects are seen in primates with lesions of the dentate nucleus.

Clinical observations suggest that the cerebrocerebellum has a role in the planning and programming of hand movements, and recordings of the activity of neurons in the dentate nucleus in primates support this idea. Some neurons in the dentate nucleus fire some 100 ms before a movement begins and even before the discharge of neurons in either the primary motor cortex or interposed nuclei, which are more directly concerned with the execution of movement. The onset of firing in the primary motor cortex, and thus the onset of movement, can be delayed experimentally by inactivating the dentate nucleus (Figure 42–10). Nevertheless, movement is simply delayed, not prevented, demonstrating that the dentate nucleus is not absolutely necessary for the initiation of movement.

The Cerebrocerebellum May Have Cognitive Functions Unconnected with Motor Control

When patients with cerebellar lesions attempt to make regular tapping movements with their hands or fingers, the rhythm is irregular, and the motions are variable in duration and force. Based on a theoretical model of how tapping movements are generated, Richard Ivry and Steven Keele inferred that medial cerebellar lesions interfere only with accurate execution of the response, whereas lateral cerebellar lesions interfere with the timing of serial events. This timing defect was not limited to motor events. It also affected the patient's ability to judge elapsed time in purely mental or cognitive tasks, as in the ability to distinguish whether one tone was longer or shorter than another or whether the speed of one moving object was greater or less than that of another.

This demonstration that the cerebellum is responsible for a cognitive computation independent of motor execution prompted other researchers to investigate purely cognitive functions of the cerebellum. For example, Steve Petersen, Julie Fiez, and Marcus Raichle used positron emission tomography to image the brain activity of people during silent reading, reading aloud, and speech. As expected, areas of the cerebellum involved in the control of mouth movements were more active when subjects read aloud than when they read silently.

In a task with greater cognitive load subjects were asked to name a verb associated with a noun; a subject might respond with "bark" if he or she saw the word "dog." Compared with simply reading aloud, the word-association task produced a pronounced increase in activity within the right lateral cerebellum. In agreement with this study, a patient with damage in the right cerebellum could not learn a word-association task.

Functional magnetic resonance imaging provides evidence that the lateral cerebellum has a role in other cognitive activities. For example, solving a pegboard puzzle involves greater activity in the dentate nucleus and lateral cerebellum than does the simple motor task of moving the pegs on the board. Interestingly, the active area of the dentate nucleus is the area that receives input from the part of the cerebral cortex (area 46) involved in working memory. The dentate nucleus appears to be particularly important in processing sensory information for tasks that require complex spatial and temporal judgments, which are essential for complex motor actions and sequences of movements.

The Cerebellum Participates in Motor Learning

Climbing-Fiber Activity Produces Long-Lasting Effects on the Synaptic Efficacy of Parallel Fibers

On the basis of mathematical modeling of cerebellar function and the striking features of the cerebellar microcircuit described earlier in the chapter, David Marr and James Albus independently suggested in the early 1970s that the cerebellum might be involved in learning motor skills. Along with Masao Ito, they proposed that the climbing-fiber input to Purkinje neurons modifies the response of the neurons to mossy-fiber inputs and does so for a prolonged period of time.

Subsequent experimental evidence has supported the theory. Despite the low frequency of their discharge, climbing fibers modulate the input of parallel fibers to Purkinje cells. In particular, climbing fibers can selectively induce *long-term depression* in the synapses between Purkinje neurons and parallel fibers that are activated concurrently with the climbing fibers. Long-term depression has been analyzed in slices and cultures of cerebellum, where it is possible to record the postsynaptic potentials of Purkinje cells following stimulation of climbing fibers and parallel fibers. Many studies have found that concurrent stimulation of climbing fibers and parallel fibers depresses the Purkinje cell responses to subsequent stimulation of the same parallel fibers but not to stimulation of parallel fibers that had not been stimulated earlier along with climbing fibers (Figure 42–12A). The resulting depression can last for minutes to hours.

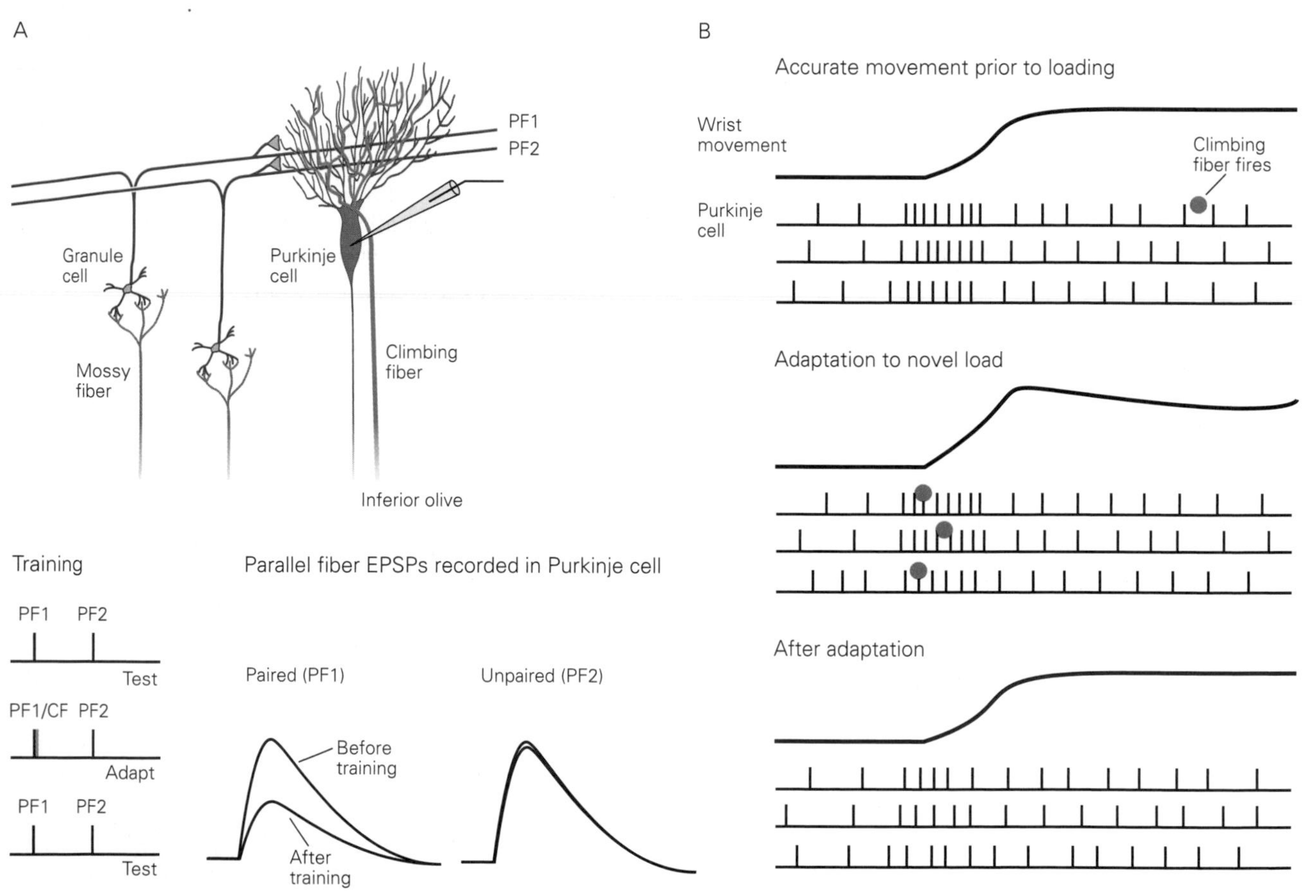

Figure 42–12 Long-term depression of the synaptic input from parallel fibers to Purkinje cells is one plausible mechanism for cerebellar learning.

A. Two different groups of parallel fibers and the presynaptic climbing fibers are electrically stimulated in vitro. Repeated stimulation of one set of parallel fibers (**PF1**) at the same time as the climbing fibers produces a long-term reduction in the responses of those parallel fibers to later stimulation. The responses of a second set of parallel fibers (**PF2**) are not depressed because they are not stimulated simultaneously with the presynaptic climbing fibers. (**CF**, climbing fiber; **EPSP**, excitatory postsynaptic potential.) (Adapted, with permission, from Ito et al. 1982.)

B. **Top**: An accurate wrist movement by a monkey is accompanied by a burst of simple spikes in a Purkinje cell, followed later by discharge of a single climbing fiber in one trial. **Middle**: When the monkey must make the same movement against a novel resistance (adaptation), climbing-fiber activity occurs during movement in every trial and the movement itself overshoots the target. **Bottom**: After adaptation the frequency of simple spikes during movement is quite attenuated, and the climbing fiber is not active during movement or later. This is the sequence of events expected if long-term depression in the cerebellar cortex plays a role in learning. Climbing fiber activity is usually low (1/s) but increases during adaptation to a novel load. (Adapted, with permission, from Gilbert and Thach 1977.)

What functional effects might this long-term depression have? According to the theories of Marr and Albus, altering the strength of certain synapses between parallel fibers and Purkinje cells shapes or corrects eye and limb movements. During an inaccurate movement the climbing fibers respond to specific movement errors and depress the synaptic strength of parallel fibers involved with those errors, namely those that had been activated with the climbing fiber (Figure 42–12B). With successive movements the parallel fiber inputs conveying the flawed central command are increasingly suppressed, a more appropriate pattern of simple-spike activity emerges, and eventually the climbing-fiber error signal disappears.

Learning Occurs at Multiple Sites in the Cerebellar Microcircuit

Initial studies of cerebellar learning focused on the vestibulo-ocular reflex, a coordinated response that keeps the eyes fixed on a target when the head is rotated (see Chapter 40). Motion of the head in one direction is sensed by the vestibular labyrinth, which initiates eye movements in the opposite direction to maintain the image in the same position on the retina.

When humans and experimental animals wear glasses that change the size of a visual scene, the vestibulo-ocular reflex initially fails to keep images stable on the retina because the amplitude of the reflex is inappropriate to the new conditions. After the glasses have been worn continuously for several days, however, the size of the reflex becomes progressively reduced (for miniaturizing glasses) or increased (for magnifying glasses). Adaptation of the vestibulo-ocular reflex can be blocked in experimental animals by lesions of the lateral part of the vestibulocerebellum, indicating that the cerebellum also has an important role in this form of learning, as discussed below.

Classical conditioning of the eye-blink response also depends on an intact cerebellum. In this form of associative learning a neutral stimulus such as a tone is played while a puff of air is directed at the cornea, causing the eye to blink just before the end of the tone. If this paradigm is repeated many times, the brain learns the tone's predictive power and the tone alone is sufficient to cause a blink. Michael Mauk and his colleagues have shown that the brain also can learn about the timing of the stimulus so that the eye blink occurs at the right time. It is even possible to learn to blink at different times in response to tones of different frequencies.

The cerebellum is also involved in learning limb movements that depend on eye-hand coordination. Adaptation of such movements can be demonstrated by having people wear prisms that deflect the light path sideways. When a person plays darts while wearing prisms that displace the entire visual field to the right, the initial dart throw lands to the left side of the target by an amount proportional to the strength of the prism. The subject gradually adapts to the distortion through practice, so that the darts land on target within 10 to 30 throws (Figure 42–13). When the prisms are removed, the adaptation persists, and the darts hit the right side of the target by roughly the same distance as the initial prism-induced error. Patients with a damaged cerebellar cortex or inferior olive are severely impaired or unable to adapt at all in this task.

Extensive analysis of the cerebellum during adaptation of the vestibulo-ocular reflex, classical conditioning of the eye-blink response, and voluntary arm movements has led to a coherent theory about the cerebellum's role in motor learning. Learning occurs not only in the cerebellar cortex, as postulated by Marr, Albus, and Ito, but also in the deep cerebellar nuclei (Figure 42–14). Available evidence is compatible with the long-standing suggestion that inputs from climbing fibers provide instructive signals that lead to changes in synaptic strength within the cerebellar cortex.

The original hypothesis of learning in the cerebellum focused on long-term depression of the synapses from parallel fibers to Purkinje cells, one of a group of possible sites where climbing fibers cause plasticity. But there are additional sites of synaptic and cellular plasticity throughout the microcircuit, notably in the deep cerebellar nuclei. Learning seems to be implemented through complementary synaptic changes in the cerebellar cortex and deep nuclei. The cerebellum appears to be the learning machine envisioned by the earliest investigators, but its learning capabilities may be even greater and more widely localized than imagined.

As outlined in Chapter 33 and earlier in this chapter, many operations performed by the motor system may be based on internal models. If the brain has accurate internal models of the dynamics and kinematics of the arm, for example, then it can compute signals that generate accurate movements. Synaptic plasticity could be the mechanism that creates and maintains accurate internal models. One important function of learning in the cerebellum may be to provide continuous tuning of internal models in the cerebellum. By using sensory feedback to adjust synaptic and cellular function, cerebellar internal models can be tuned to create commands for movements that are rapid, accurate, and smooth.

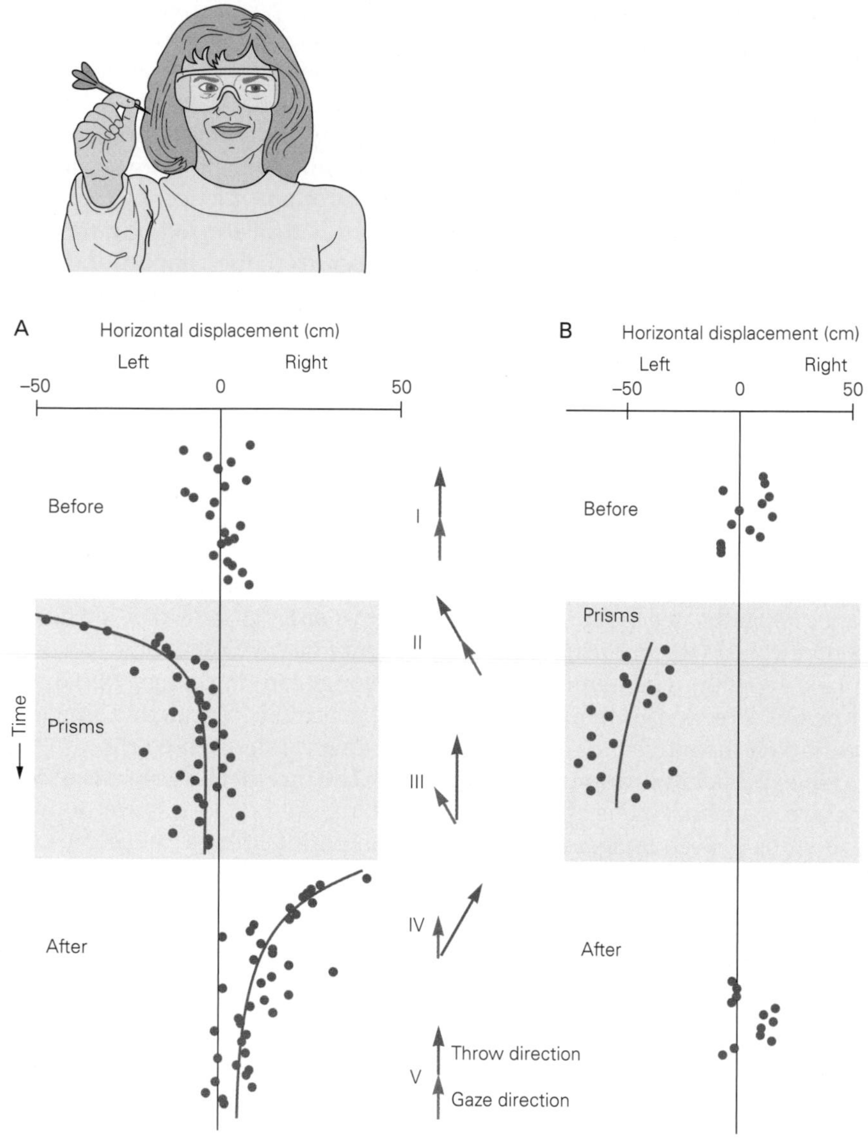

Figure 42–13 Adjustment of eye-hand coordination to a change in optical conditions. The subject wears prisms that bend the optic path to her right. She must look to her left along the bent light path to see the target directly ahead. (Adapted, with permission, from Martin et al. 1996a, 1996b.)

A. Without prisms the subject throws with good accuracy. The first hit after the prisms have been put in place is displaced left of center because the hand throws where the eyes are directed. Thereafter hits trend rightward toward the target, away from where the eyes are looking. After removal of the prisms the subject fixes her gaze in the center of the target; the first throw hits to the right of center, away from where the eyes are directed. Thereafter hits trend toward the target. Data during and after prism use have been fit with exponential curves. Gaze and throw directions are indicated by the **blue** and **brown arrows**, respectively, on the right. The inferred gaze direction assumes that the subject is fixating the target.

Before donning the prisms the subject looks at and throws toward the target (**I**). Just after donning prisms, when her gaze is directed along the bent light path away from the target, she throws in the direction of gaze, away from the target (**II**). After adapting to the prisms she directs her gaze along the bent light path away from the target but directs her throw toward the target (**III**). Immediately after removing the prisms she directs her gaze toward the target; her adapted throw is to the right of the direction of gaze and to the right of the target (**IV**). After recovery from adaptation she again looks at and throws toward the target (**V**).

B. Adaptation fails in a patient with unilateral infarctions in the territory of the posterior inferior cerebellar artery that involve the inferior cerebellar peduncle and inferior lateral posterior cerebellar cortex.

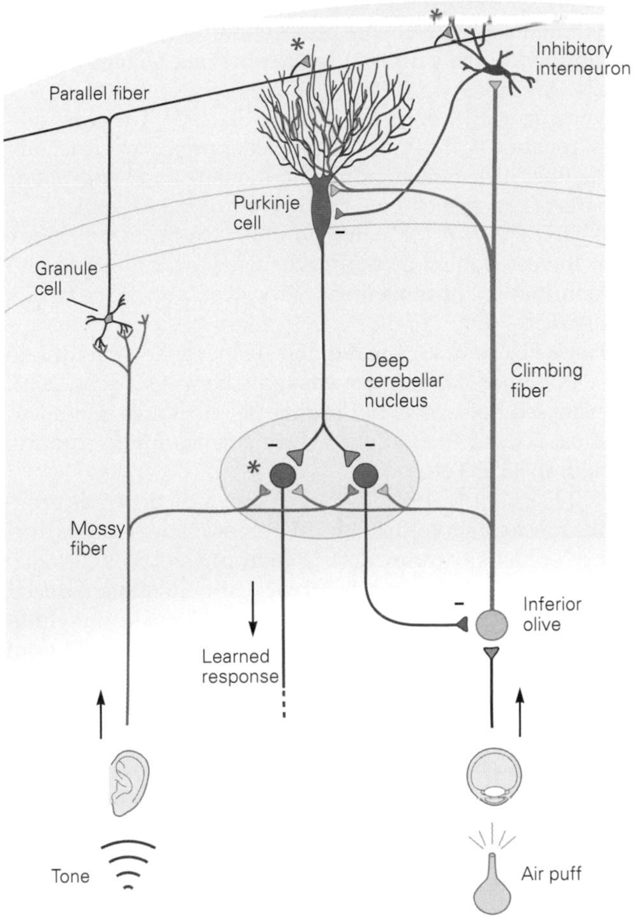

Figure 42–14 Learning can occur in the cerebellar microcircuit both in the cerebellar cortex and in the deep cerebellar nuclei. The diagram is based on classical conditioning of the eyelid response (combining a tone and air puff), but describes equally well adaptation of the vestibulo-ocular reflex when head turns are associated with image motion on the retina (see Chapter 40). Sites of learning are denoted by asterisks. (Adapted, with permission, from Carey and Lisberger 2002.)

An Overall View

Whereas lesions of other motor processing centers result in paralysis of voluntary movements, lesions of the cerebellum result in large errors in movements. How do these errors occur?

The organization of the inputs and outputs of the cerebellum indicates that the cerebellum compares internal feedback signals that report the intended movement with external feedback signals that report the actual motion. On a very short time scale during the execution of the movement, the cerebellum is able to generate corrective signals that help to make movements accurate. These corrective signals are feed-forward or anticipatory actions that operate on the descending motor systems of the brain stem and cerebral cortex. When these mechanisms fail because of lesions of the cerebellum, movement develops characteristic oscillations and tremors.

The corrective control of movement by the cerebellum is complemented by important cerebellar contributions to motor learning. Although some aspects of a movement can be adjusted "on-the-fly" during the movement, much about the movement must be well planned in advance, and planning necessarily incorporates adjustments of motor programs based on learning. The cerebellum may have a role in motor learning through the ability of the climbing fibers to depress activity in the parallel fibers. Because of their low firing frequencies, climbing fibers have only a modest capacity for transmitting moment-to-moment changes in sensory information. Instead, they may be involved in detecting error in a movement and changing the program for the next movement.

Finally, the cerebellum seems to have a role in some purely mental operations. In many respects these operations appear to be similar to the cerebellum's motor functions. For example, the different regions of the lateral hemisphere appear to be particularly important for forms of both motor and cognitive learning that depend on repeated practice.

Stephen G. Lisberger
W. Thomas Thach

Selected Readings

Adams RD, Victor M. 1989. *Principles of Neurology*, 4th ed. New York: McGraw-Hill.

Ito M. 1984. *The Cerebellum and Neural Control*. New York: Raven.

Jansen J, Brodal A (eds). 1954. *Aspects of Cerebellar Anatomy*. Oslo: Grundt Tanum.

Kelly RM, Strick PL. 2003. Cerebellar loops with motor cortex and prefrontal cortex of a nonhuman primate. J Neurosci 23:8432–8444.

Raymond JL, Lisberger SG, Mauk MD. 1996. The cerebellum: a neuronal learning machine? Science 272:1126–1131.

References

Adrian ED. 1943. Afferent areas in the cerebellum connected with the limbs. Brain 66:289–315.

Albus JS. 1971. A theory of cerebellar function. Math Biosci 10:25–61.

Arshavsky YI, Berkenblit MB, Fukson OI, Gelfand IM, Orlovsky GN. 1972. Recordings of neurones of the dorsal spinocerebellar tract during evoked locomotion. Brain Res 43:272–275.

Arshavsky YI, Berkenblit MB, Fukson OI, Gelfand IM, Orlovsky GN. 1972. Origin of modulation in neurones of the ventral spinocerebellar tract during locomotion. Brain Res 43:276–279.

Barbour B. 1993. Synaptic currents evoked in Purkinje cells by stimulating individual granule cells. Neuron 11: 749–769.

Bastian AJ, Martin TA, Keating JG, Thach WT. 1996. Cerebellar ataxia: abnormal control of interaction torques across multiple joints. J Neurophysiol 176: 492–509.

Bastian AJ, Mink JW, Kaufman BA, Thach WT. 1998. Posterior vermal split syndrome. Ann Neurol 44:601–610.

Bastian AJ, Zackowski KM, Thach WT. 2000. Cerebellar ataxia: torque deficiency or torque mismatch between joints? J Neurophys 83:3019–3030.

Botterell EH, Fulton JF. 1938. Functional localization in the cerebellum of primates. II. Lesions of midline structures (vermis) and deep nuclei. J Comp Neurol 69:47–62.

Botterell EH, Fulton JF. 1938. Functional localization in the cerebellum of primates. III. Lesions of hemispheres (neocerebellum). J Comp Neurol 69:63–87.

Carey M, Lisberger SG. 2002. Embarrassed but not depressed: eye opening lessons for cerebellar learning. Neuron 35: 223–226.

Courchesne E, Yeung-Courchesne R, Press GA, Hesselink JR, Jernigan TL. 1988. Hypoplasia of cerebellar vermal lobules VI and VII in autism. N Engl J Med 318:1349–1354.

Eccles JC, Ito M, Szentagothai J. 1967. *The Cerebellum as a Neuronal Machine*. New York: Springer.

Fiez JA, Petersen SE, Cheney MK, Raichle ME. 1992. Impaired non-motor learning and error detection associated with cerebellar damage. Brain 115:155–178.

Flament D, Hore J. 1986. Movement and electromyographic disorders associated with cerebellar dysmetria. J Neurophysiol 55:1221–1233.

Fortier PA, Kalaska JL, Smith AM. 1989. Cerebellar neuronal activity related to whole-arm reaching movements in the monkey. J Neurophysiol 62:198–211.

Frings M, Maschke M, Timmann D. 2007. Cerebellum and cognition—viewed from philosophy of mind. Cerebellum 12:1–7.

Gebhart AG, Petersen SE, Thach WT. 2002. The role of the posterolateral cerebellum in language. In SW Highstein and WT Thach (eds). *The Cerebellum: Recent Developments in Cerebellar Research*, pp. 318–333. New York: New York Academy of Sciences.

Ghasia FF, Meng H, Angelaki DE. 2008. Neural correlates of forward and inverse models for eye movements: evidence from three-dimensional kinematics. J Neurosci 28: 5082–5087.

Gilbert PFC, Thach WT. 1977. Purkinje cell activity during motor learning. Brain Res 128:309–328.

Groenewegen HJ, Voogd J. 1977. The parasagittal zonation within the olivocerebellar projection. I. Climbing fiber distribution in the vermis of cat cerebellum. J Comp Neurol 174:417–488.

Groenewegen HJ, Voogd J, Freedman SL. 1979. The parasagittal zonation within the olivocerebellar projection. II. Climbing fiber distribution in the intermediate and hemispheric parts of cat cerebellum. J Comp Neurol 183:551–601.

Heck DH, Thach WT, Keating JG. 2007. On-beam synchrony in the cerebellum as the mechanism for the timing and coordination of movement. Proc Natl Acad Sci U S A 104:7658–7663.

Hoebeek FE, Stahl JS, van Alphen AM, Schonewille M, Luo C, Rutteman M, van den Maagdenberg AM, et al. 2005. Increased noise level of Purkinje cell activities minimizes impact of their modulation during sensorimotor control. Neuron 45:953–965.

Hore J, Flament D. 1986. Evidence that a disordered servo-like mechanism contributes to tremor in movements during cerebellar dysfunction. J Neurophysiol 56:123–136.

Ito M, Sakurai M, Tongroach P. 1982. Climbing fibre induced depression of both mossy fibre responsiveness and glutamate sensitivity of cerebellar Purkinje cells. J Physiol Lond 324:113–134.

Ivry RB, Keele SW. 1989. Timing functions of the cerebellum. J Cogn Neurosci 1:136–152.

Kim SG, Ugurbil K, Strick PL. 1994. Activation of a cerebellar output nucleus during cognitive processing. Science 265:949–951.

Larsell O, Jansen J. 1972. *The Comparative Anatomy and Histology of the Cerebellum: The Human Cerebellum, Cerebellar Connection and Cerebellar Cortex*. pp. 111–119. Minneapolis, MN: University of Minnesota Press.

Lisberger SG. 1994. Neural basis for motor learning in the vestibulo-ocular reflex of primates III. Computational and behavioral analysis of the sites of learning. J Neurophysiol 72:974–998.

Lisberger SG, Fuchs AF. 1978. Role of primate flocculus during rapid behavioral modification of vestibulo-ocular reflex. I. Purkinje cell activity during visually guided horizontal smooth-pursuit eye movements and passive head rotation. J Neurophysiol 41:733–763.

Marr D. 1969. A theory of cerebellar cortex. J Physiol 202: 437–470.

Martin TA, Keating JG, Goodkin HP, Bastian AJ, Thach WT. 1996a. Throwing while looking through prisms. I. Focal olivocerebellar lesions impair adaptation. Brain 119:1183–1198.

Martin TA, Keating JG, Goodkin HP, Bastian AJ, Thach WT. 1996b. Throwing while looking through prisms. II. Specificity and storage of multiple gaze-throw calibrations. Brain 119:1199–1211.

Martinez FE, Crill WE, Kennedy TT. 1971. Electrogenesis of the cerebellar Purkinje cell response in cats. J Neurophysiol 34:348–356.

McCormick DA, Thompson RF. 1984. Cerebellum: essential involvement in the classically conditioned eyelid response. Science 223:296–299.

Medina JF, Lisberger SG. 2008. Links from complex spikes to local plasticity and motor learning in the cerebellum of awake-behaving monkeys. Nat Neurosci 11:1185–1192.

Nieuwenhuys T, Voogd J, van Huijzen C. 1988. *The Human Central Nervous System: A Synopsis and Atlas*, 3rd rev. ed. Berlin: Springer.

Ohyama T, Nores WL, Medina JF, Riusech FA, Mauk MD. 2006. Learning-induced plasticity in deep cerebellar nucleus. J Neurosci 26:12656–12663.

Pasalar S, Roitman AV, Durfee WK, Ebner TJ. 2006. Force field effects on cerebellar Purkinje cell discharge with implications for internal models. Nat Neurosci 9:1404–1411.

Robinson DA. 1976. Adaptive gain control of vestibuloocular reflex by the cerebellum. J Neurophysiol 39:954–969.

Ryding E, Decety J, Sjöholm H, Stenberg G, Ingvar DH. 1993. Motor imagery activates the cerebellum regionally. A SPECT rCBF study with 99mTc-HMPAO. Brain Res Cogn Brain Res 1:94–99.

Strata P, Montarolo PG. 1982. Functional aspects of the inferior olive. Arch Ital Biol 120:321–329.

Thach WT. 1968. Discharge of Purkinje and cerebellar nuclear neurons during rapidly alternating arm movements in the monkey. J Neurophysiol 31:785–797.

Thach WT. 1975. Timing of activity in cerebellar dentate nucleus and cerebral motor cortex during prompt volitional movement. Brain Res 88:233–241.

Thach WT. 1980. The cerebellum In: Mountcastle, V (ed). *Medical Physiology*. pp. 837–858. St. Louis: C.V. Mosby Co.

Thach WT, Perry JG, Kane SA, Goodkin HP. 1993. Cerebellar nuclei: rapid alternating movement, motor somatotopy, and a mechanism for the control of muscle synergy. Rev Neurol 149:607–628.

Tseng YW, Diedrichsen J, Krakauer JW, Shadmehr R, Bastian AJ. 2007. Sensory prediction errors drive cerebellum-dependent adaptation of reaching. J Neurophysiol 98:54–62.

Vilis T, Hore J. 1977. Effects of changes in mechanical state of limb on cerebellar intention tremor. J Neurophysiol 40:1214–1224.

Voogd J, Bigar F. 1980. Topographical distribution of olivary and cortico nuclear fibers in the cerebellum: a review. In: J Courville, C de Montigny, Y Lamarre (eds). *The Inferior Olivary Nucleus: Anatomy and Physiology*, pp. 207–234. New York: Raven.

Yeo CH, Hardiman MJ, Glickstein M. 1984. Discrete lesions of the cerebellar cortex abolish the classically conditioned nictitating membrane response of the rabbit. Behav Brain Res 13:261–266.

43

The Basal Ganglia

THE TRADITIONAL VIEW THAT THE BASAL ganglia play a role in movement stems largely from the fact that diseases of the basal ganglia, such as Parkinson and Huntington disease, are associated with prominent disturbances of movement and from the earlier belief that basal ganglia neurons send their output exclusively to the motor cortex by way of the thalamus. However, we now know that the basal ganglia also project to nonmotor areas of the cerebral cortex, providing a mechanism whereby they may participate in a wide variety of nonmotor functions, and that diseases of the basal ganglia are associated with complex behavioral and neuropsychiatric disturbances.

In this chapter we first describe the individual nuclei of the basal ganglia anatomically and then discuss their function in the context of the larger networks in which they participate. The delineation of brain circuits into which the basal ganglia are incorporated has enabled researchers to better understand the pathophysiology of some of the major diseases affecting basal ganglia functions. These disease states are described at the end of the chapter.

The Basal Ganglia Consist of Several Interconnected Nuclei

The basal ganglia comprise four principal structures: the striatum, globus pallidus, substantia nigra, and subthalamic nucleus (Figure 43–1).

The *striatum* is separated by the internal capsule into the caudate nucleus and the putamen. The striatum is the major input structure of the basal ganglia, receiving prominent projections from the cerebral cortex, brain stem, and thalamus. The *globus pallidus* consists of two separate nuclei, the external and internal segments, each with different connectivity and

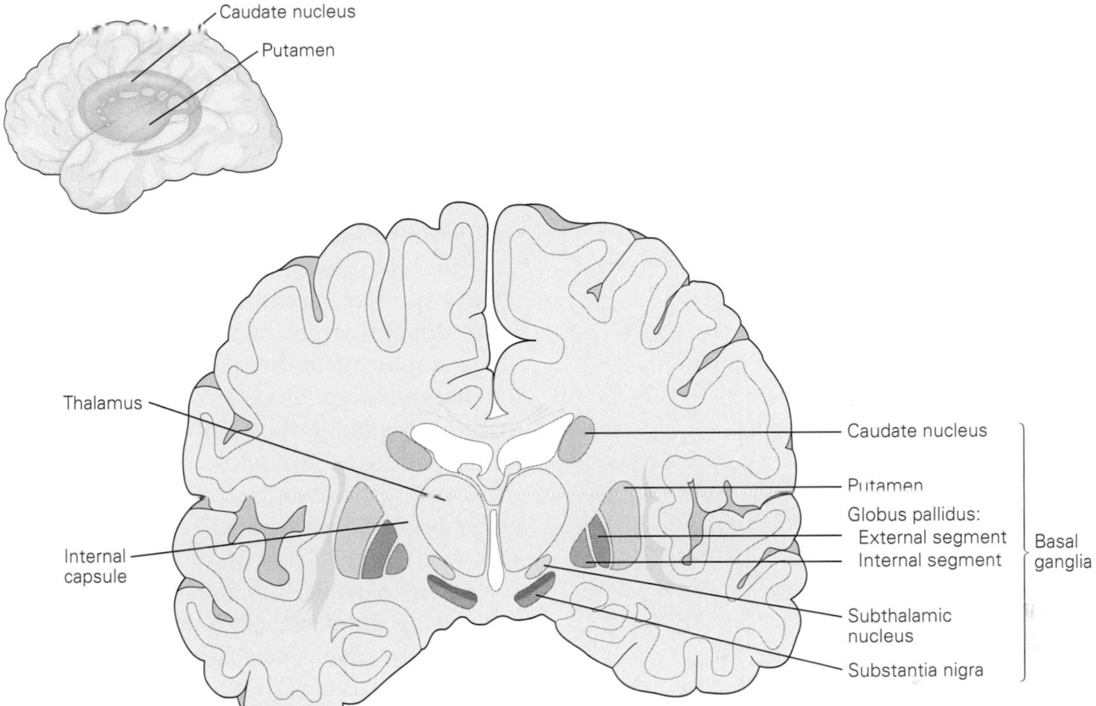

Figure 43–1 The basal ganglia and surrounding structures. The nuclei of the basal ganglia are identified on right in this coronal section. (Adapted, with permission, from Nieuwenhuys, Voogd, and van Huijzen 1981.)

functions. The internal segment is one of the major output structures of the basal ganglia, whereas the external segment is part of their intrinsic circuitry.

The *substantia nigra* includes two separate nuclei, the pars compacta and pars reticulata. Along with portions of the ventral tegmental area and other midbrain areas, the pars compacta, or mediodorsal portion of the substantia nigra, contains dopaminergic cells that project heavily to the striatum and to the other nuclei of the basal ganglia. The pars reticulata, or ventrolateral portion of the substantia nigra, is the other major output nucleus of the basal ganglia. In fact, the pars reticulata of the substantia nigra and the internal segment of the globus pallidus can be viewed as a single output structure divided by the internal capsule.

The fourth principal structure of the basal ganglia, the *subthalamic nucleus*, is a small nucleus situated between the thalamus and the substantia nigra. This nucleus receives projections from the external segment of the globus pallidus, the cerebral cortex, thalamus, and brain stem, and sends output to both segments of the globus pallidus and to the substantia nigra pars reticulata. The cortical inputs to the subthalamic nucleus and the related subthalamopallidal projections are referred to as the *hyperdirect* pathway (Figure 43–2).

The striatum, the main input nucleus of the basal ganglia, projects to the two basal ganglia output nuclei, the internal pallidal segment and the substantia nigra pars reticulata. The axons from the striatum follow two different pathways: a *direct* monosynaptic connection, and an *indirect* polysynaptic pathway that passes first to the external pallidal segment and from there to both output nuclei, either directly or via the intercalated subthalamic nucleus.

The output nuclei project to specific thalamic and brain stem areas. Projections to the thalamus are directed to the ventral anterior, the ventrolateral, and the intralaminar nuclei. Thalamic projections to the frontal lobe then transmit the output of the basal ganglia to the same areas of frontal cortex that provide input to the basal ganglia. In addition, descending pallidal and nigral projections to the brain stem, such as those to the pedunculopontine nucleus and superior colliculus, provide pathways by which the basal ganglia may directly influence brain stem and spinal

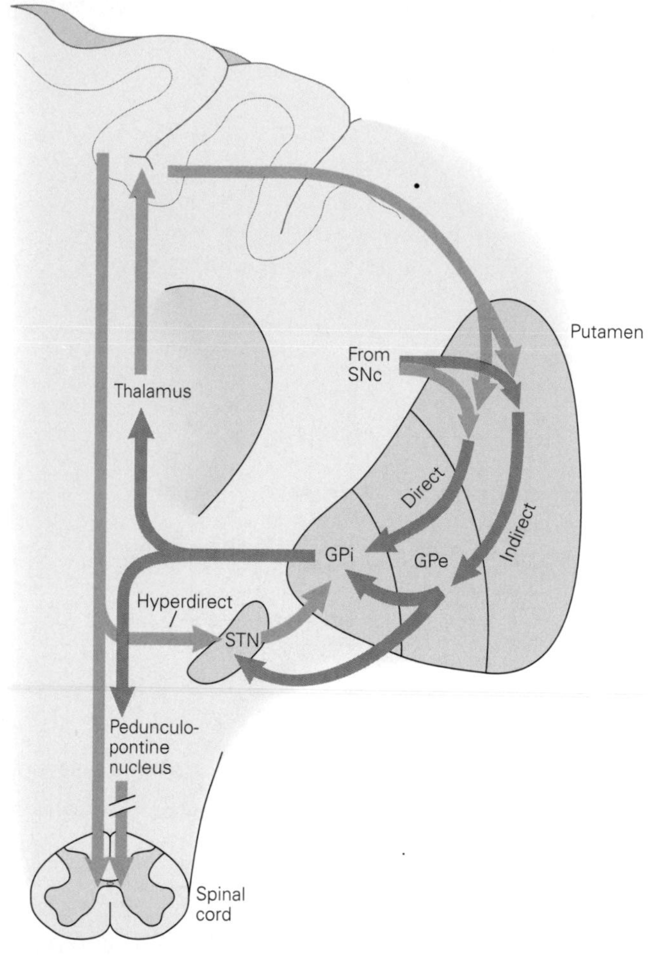

Figure 43–2 The basal ganglia–thalamocortical circuitry. The circuitry of the basal ganglia includes the striatum (here represented by one of its components, the putamen), the external and internal segments of the globus pallidus (**GPe** and **GPi**, respectively), the substantia nigra pars reticulata (not shown) and pars compacta (**SNc**), and the subthalamic nucleus (**STN**). Cortical input enters the striatum and subthalamic nucleus. Basal ganglia output is conveyed to several thalamic nuclei (the centromedian and parafascicular nuclei and the ventral anterior and ventral lateral nuclei) and the pedunculopontine nucleus. Excitatory connections are shown in **red**, inhibitory pathways in **gray**. The dopaminergic SNc projection to the striatum regulates corticostriatal transmission along direct and indirect pathways.

motor circuits, especially those related to gait and balance. The brain stem nuclei may integrate basal ganglia inputs with cerebellar inputs. The pedunculopontine nucleus is part of several feedback circuits through its projections back to the basal ganglia and thalamus. Output of the substantia nigra pars reticulata is also directed to the superior colliculus, which is involved in the control of head and eye movements.

In the striatum the most common neuronal cell type is the GABAergic (γ-aminobutyric acid) medium spiny neuron. These cells are so named because of the abundance of spines on their dendrites. They receive inputs from the cerebral cortex and thalamus as well as from several classes of local interneurons in the striatum, including large cholinergic interneurons and smaller GABAergic interneurons.

The activities of medium spiny neurons are modulated by other neurotransmitters, specifically inputs from dopaminergic neurons in the substantia nigra pars compacta and the ventral tegmental area. Some of the dopaminergic fibers terminate on the necks of dendritic spines of medium spiny neurons, where they are in a position to influence corticostriatal transmission (Figure 43–3). Dopamine released from terminals close to the dendritic spines may have similar effects through spillover and diffusion of the neurotransmitter.

The cytoarchitecture of the other basal ganglia nuclei is distinctly different from that of the striatum. Both segments of the globus pallidus consist of large GABAergic neurons that receive input from the striatum. The substantia nigra pars reticulata is histologically similar to the internal pallidal segment, containing GABAergic neurons that interdigitate with the more dorsal dopaminergic cells of the substantia nigra pars compacta. The subthalamic nucleus is a densely packed structure whose projection neurons, unlike those in the other basal ganglia nuclei, are glutamatergic.

A Family of Cortico–Basal Ganglia–Thalamocortical Circuits Subserves Skeletomotor, Oculomotor, Associative, and Limbic Functions

Areas of the cerebral cortex project in a highly topographic manner onto the striatum.

The topographic termination pattern establishes functional domains that are replicated throughout the basal ganglia–thalamocortical circuits by virtue of highly topographic projections at each synaptic relay. The different pathways that pass through the basal ganglia are named after the presumed functions of the regions of the frontal cortex from which they originate: the skeletomotor, oculomotor, prefrontal (associative), and limbic circuits. The frontal lobe origins of these circuits in the cerebral cortex are shown in Figure 43–4 and the synaptic relays are depicted in Figure 43–5.

Additional projections from the parietal, temporal, and occipital lobes that are reciprocally interconnected with the frontal areas converge onto the same areas in the striatum. Importantly, however, although each circuit receives both pre- and postcentral cortical inputs, output of the different circuits terminates only in the frontal lobe areas of their respective origin.

Ascending output in each functional pathway is projected in a somatotopical manner to the thalamus and from there to the frontal cortical area from which the circuit originated, thus partially closing a system of cortico-subcortical loops. The subcortical segregation of the functionally distinct circuits may allow different aspects of behavior to be processed in parallel.

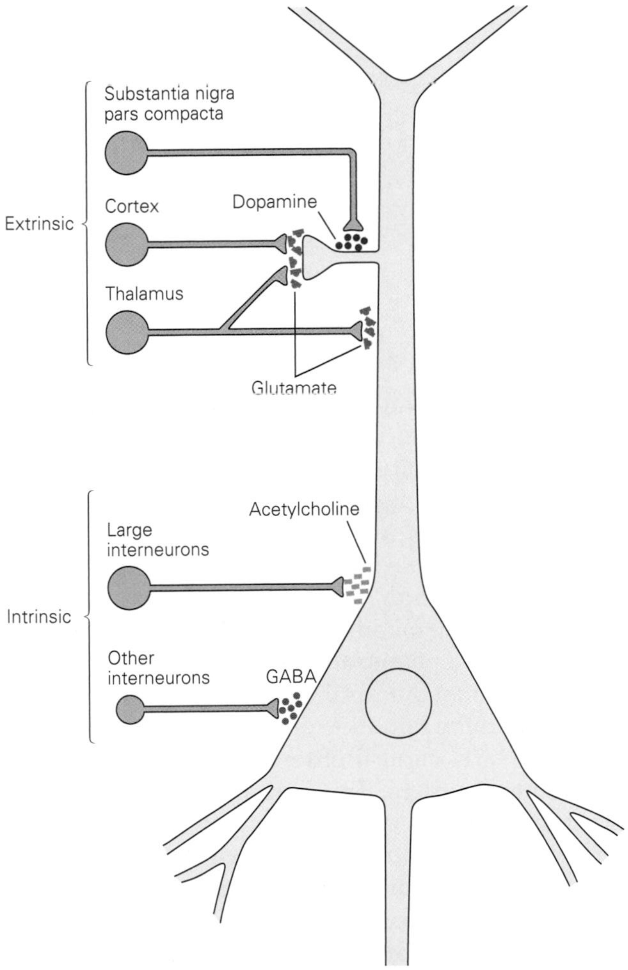

Figure 43–3 The medium spiny neurons in the striatum have extrinsic and intrinsic inputs. Glutamatergic inputs from the cerebral cortex and dopaminergic inputs from the substantia nigra pars compacta terminate on dendritic spines of medium spiny neurons. The reward-related dopaminergic inputs are thought to modulate the strength of cortical inputs and to play a role in synaptic changes and reinforcement learning in the striatum. Glutamatergic inputs from the thalamus end on the spines and shafts of dendrites of medium spiny neurons. Medium spiny neurons also receive cholinergic and GABAergic input from interneurons in the striatum.

The Cortico–Basal Ganglia–Thalamocortical Motor Circuit Originates and Terminates in Cortical Areas Related to Movement

Most of our knowledge about the anatomy and physiological functions of the basal ganglia–thalamocortical circuits comes from studies of the motor circuit. This circuit has attracted the attention of researchers because pathology within its anatomical elements has been implicated in several major disorders of movement.

The motor circuit originates in the pre- and postcentral sensorimotor cortical fields, which project to the putamen in a somatotopical manner. This arrangement has been demonstrated not only with anatomical methods but also with electrophysiological recordings of neuronal activity while animals were subjected to passive movements or carried out active movements of individual body parts. These studies showed that neurons responding to leg movements are found in a dorsolateral zone of the putamen, neurons responding to orofacial movements are located ventromedially, and neurons responding to arm movement are found in a zone between the leg and orofacial areas.

Neurons in the putamen project to the caudoventral portions of both segments of the pallidum and to the lateral portions of the substantia nigra pars reticulata. In turn, the motor portions of the internal pallidal segment and the substantia nigra pars reticulata project to specific motor-related areas of the ventral lateral, ventral anterior, and centromedian nucleus of the thalamus. The motor circuit is then closed by projections from the ventral lateral and ventral anterior nuclei to the motor cortex, supplementary motor area, and premotor cortex. The centromedian nucleus, one of the intralaminar nuclei of the thalamus, projects largely to the putamen as part of a subcortical feedback loop.

The larger motor circuit consists of segregated subcircuits, each centered on an individual precentral motor field. These subcircuits are believed to be responsible for different aspects of motor processing, such as motor planning, coordination of sequences of movement, or movement execution. Evidence for the subcircuit organization comes from anatomical studies. Several stages of the basal ganglia circuitry in the same animal have been traced by Peter Strick and his colleagues using small intracerebral injections of herpes and rabies viruses. Taken up by neurons and transported transsynaptically, the virus particles can be stained in anatomical slices. Using this technique at different time points after the injection, one may visualize circuit elements that lie two or more synapses away from the injection site.

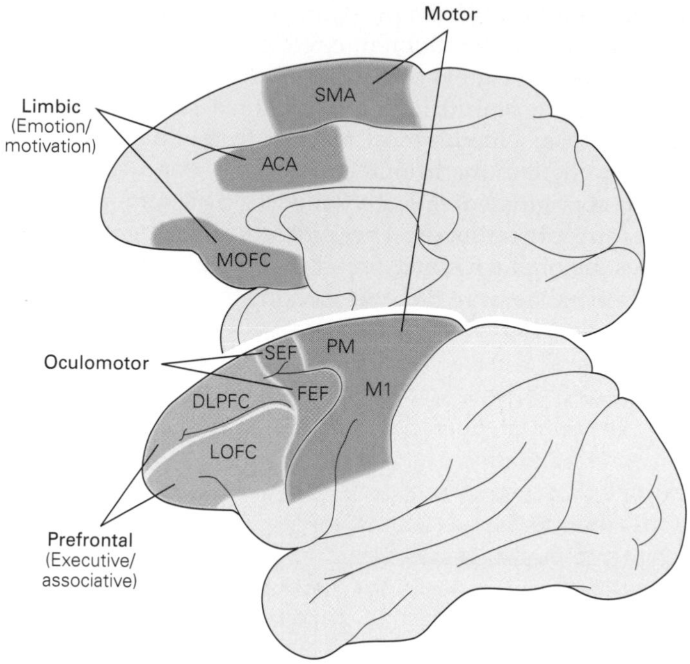

Figure 43–4 Four basal ganglia–thalamocortical circuits originate in four functionally distinct areas of frontal cortex. (**ACA**, anterior cingulate area; **DLPFC**, dorsolateral prefrontal cortex; **FEF**, frontal eye field; **LOFC**, lateral orbitofrontal cortex; **M1**, primary motor cortex; **MOFC**, medial orbitofrontal cortex; **PM**, premotor cortex; **SEF**, supplementary eye field; **SMA**, supplementary motor area.) (Adapted, with permission, from Alexander and Crutcher 1990.)

Separate injections of the primary motor cortex, supplementary motor area, and lateral premotor area produces retrograde labeling of separate populations of neurons in specific areas of the ventral lateral nucleus in the thalamus and separate populations of neurons in the internal pallidal segment, demonstrating that the separate cortical domains remain segregated throughout the basal ganglia networks. Segregated anterograde transsynaptic transport of input from cortical areas to the striatum and pallidum has likewise been shown, providing further support for the segregated circuit concept.

Because axons of cortical neurons terminate on a far smaller number of striatal neurons, there is considerable convergence of cortical information in the striatum. Similarly, the number of neurons in the pallidum and substantia nigra is smaller than that in the striatum, allowing further convergence along the direct and indirect pathways. However, given the somatotopic arrangement of striatopallidal and pallido-subthalamic projections, it appears that convergence occurs largely within rather than between the different basal ganglia–thalamocortical circuits and subcircuits.

The Motor Circuit Plays a Role in Multiple Aspects of Movement

The motor circuit has been examined in experimental studies in which portions of the basal ganglia were activated or inactivated, in studies using extracellular electrophysiological recordings of the activity of single neurons, as well as imaging and behavioral studies. Based on these investigations the motor circuit has been implicated in a wide range of motor behaviors including action selection, preparation for movement, movement execution, sequencing of movement, self-initiated or remembered movements, the control of movement parameters, and reinforcement learning.

The idea that the basal ganglia have a role in action selection and the initiation of movement was first suggested by early clinical observations in patients with movement disorders. The concept that the basal ganglia play a role in action selection, in the broadest sense, implies that they also participate in the acquisition of behaviors that lead to a reward or reinforcement and the avoidance of acts that lead to punishment or adverse outcomes. Reward may be simply the delivery of a pleasurable stimulus such as food, but may also involve the successful reaching of a goal or intended action. By modulating the strength of specific corticostriatal synapses, dopamine is widely implicated in this action selection function, as described below.

The general concept that the basal ganglia play a role in the acquisition and selection of beneficial behaviors later evolved into the idea that the basal ganglia act to focus specific movements through interactions between the direct (permissive) and indirect (inhibitory) pathways at the level of the internal pallidal segment, somewhat equivalent to the center-surround inhibition in a sensory system. This "focusing model" stems from the observation that the basal ganglia provide sustained inhibitory output to thalamocortical neurons. According to the model, cortical phasic activation of striatal neurons that contribute to the direct pathway transiently suppresses the high spontaneous discharge rate of movement-related neurons in the output nuclei of the basal ganglia. This in turn removes inhibition from specific thalamocortical neurons and allows cortical areas to become active, thus facilitating the selected movement. In contrast, phasic activation of striatal neurons that contribute to the indirect pathway, or of cortical neurons that project to the subthalamic nucleus, transiently increases inhibition of thalamocortical neurons and thereby inhibits movement. If the direct pathway is activated in anticipation of intended movements, and the indirect pathway is activated simultaneously to broadly inhibit pallidal inhibitory output, the combination facilitates intended movements and suppresses competing ones.

Although this focusing model is attractive, there are several strong arguments against it. For instance, the hypothesis would require that axons in the indirect and hyperdirect pathways diffusely target large areas of the pallidum in order to prevent unwanted movements, whereas the direct pathway would act on small areas of the internal pallidal segment to selectively facilitate the selected movement. Neither of these anatomical prerequisites is supported by anatomic studies, which indicate instead that inputs of the indirect pathway to the internal pallidal segment from the subthalamic nucleus are highly topographic. Furthermore, pallidal activation during movement initiation is generally considered to occur too late to play a significant role in the selection of movement.

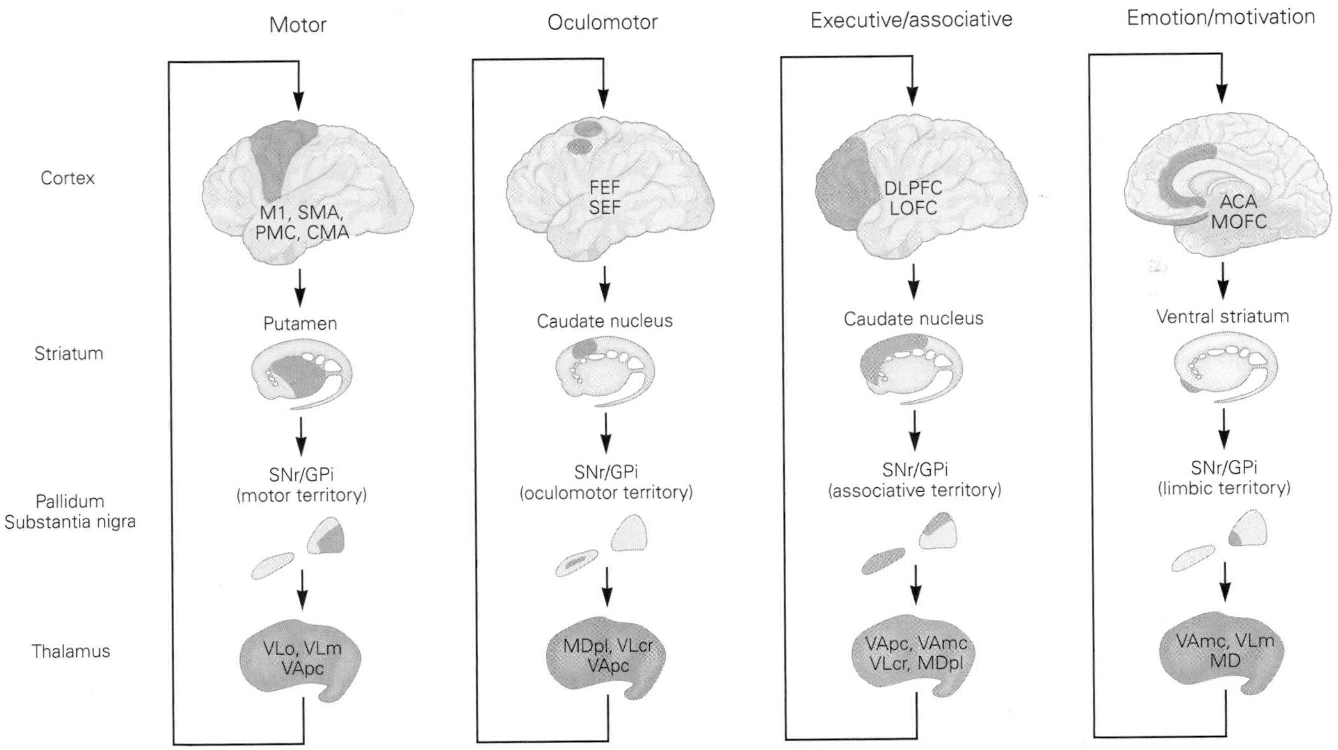

Figure 43–5 Global anatomy of cortico–basal ganglia–thalamocortical circuits. (**ACA**, anterior cingulate area; **CMA**, cingulate motor area; **DLPFC**, dorsolateral prefrontal cortex; **FEF**, frontal eye field; **GPi**, internal segment of the globus pallidus; **LOFC**, lateral orbitofrontal cortex; **M1**, primary motor cortex; **MDpl**, mediodorsal nucleus of thalamus, lateral part; **MOFC**, medial orbitofrontal cortex; **PMC**, premotor cortex; **SEF**, supplementary eye field; **SMA**, supplementary motor area; **SNr**, substantia nigra pars reticulata; **VAmc**, ventral anterior nucleus of thalamus, magnocellular part; **VApc**, ventral anterior nucleus of thalamus, parvocellular part; **VLcr**, ventrolateral nucleus of thalamus, caudal part, rostral division; **VLm**, ventrolateral nucleus of thalamus, medial part; **VLo**, ventrolateral nucleus of thalamus, pars oralis.) (Adapted, with permission, from Wichmann and DeLong 2006.)

Evidence that the motor circuit has a role in the preparation of movement comes from single-neuron recordings in monkeys performing delayed-response motor tasks. The animals were required to move an arm to a specified target after a delay period. In such studies the firing frequency of neurons in frontal and prefrontal cortical areas changed after animals were presented with a visual cue that specified the desired direction of movement (see Chapter 38). Changes similar to those found in the cortex are also found in the motor portions of the putamen, the internal segment of the globus pallidus, and the substantia nigra pars reticulata. These changes in activity occur while the animal is preparing the movement but not during the execution of the movement itself. Such changes are interpreted as involvement in a preparatory stage of motor control referred to as *motor set.*

Other basal ganglia neurons change their firing frequency phasically in relation to the onset of a movement, suggesting that they may be concerned with movement execution. As mentioned above, these changes in neural activity in a variety of stimulus-triggered movement tasks occur well *after* movement-related activities in the cerebral cortex or cerebellum, indicating that the basal ganglia do not participate in the initiation of such movements. This conclusion is reinforced by the results of a study with primates trained on a simple reaction time task: Pallidal lesions involving the motor circuit did not alter the reaction time between a cue and the movement triggered by that cue.

Changes in the activity of movement-related neurons in the internal pallidal segment correlate with the amplitude and velocity of arm movement, suggesting a role in the scaling of movement. In monkeys the activity of 30% to 50% of all movement-related neurons in the supplementary motor area, motor cortex, putamen, and pallidum is correlated with the direction of limb movement, but not with the activity of individual muscles. This suggests a role in the higher-level aspects of movement. The finding that individual neurons in the basal ganglia tend to be concerned with either the preparation or the execution of motor action suggests that these functions are mediated by separate subcircuits in the motor circuit.

Positron emission tomography and functional magnetic resonance imaging of humans have demonstrated that during simple finger or arm movements the peak activation of the basal ganglia occurs in the postcommissural putamen, and that changes in fundamental kinematic parameters, such as movement velocity, correlates with activity in the posteroventral pallidum, an area that has been identified as part of the motor territory of the basal ganglia in nonhuman primates (Figure 43–6). By contrast, in cognitively demanding tasks—for example, tasks that require subjects to generate novel sequences of movement or to imagine hand movements—anterior portions of the striatum (caudate nucleus and putamen rostral to the anterior commissure) are activated, along with the prefrontal cortex and the anterior cingulate area.

Dopamine has opposite actions in the direct and indirect pathways. Direct-pathway neurons are facilitated by dopamine through the activation of dopamine D_1 receptors, whereas indirect-pathway neurons are inhibited by dopamine, possibly by means of the activation of dopamine D_2 receptors. By virtue of the different polarities of connections between the basal ganglia nuclei, dopamine release in the striatum reduces activity in the output nuclei, thereby leading to disinhibition of thalamocortical neurons and perhaps facilitation of movement. These effects of dopamine have significant implications for our understanding of the pathophysiology of movement disorders.

Mechanistic models of motor circuit function are attractive because of their relative simplicity, because they provide researchers with testable hypotheses, and because they may help us understand how disorders of dopaminergic input in the striatum affect motor performance. However, these models are largely speculative; there is little direct experimental support for an important role of the basal ganglia in the online-control of movements. As noted, lesions of the motor circuit in the internal pallidal segment have little or no effect on reaction time or movement time.

Dopaminergic and Cholinergic Inputs to the Striatum Are Implicated in Reinforcement Motor Learning

Given the potential function of dopamine in regulating the balance between direct and indirect pathways, it is perhaps surprising that dopaminergic neurons in the substantia nigra pars compacta that project to the striatum are not activated in relation to specific aspects of movement. Instead, many of these neurons are activated in connection with behavioral reinforcement cues (Figure 43–7). This finding has resulted in the development of a highly specific hypothesis regarding the role of dopaminergic neurons in reinforcement learning.

The specific interpretation is that changes in the activity of the dopaminergic cells during behavioral tasks signal a discrepancy, the reward prediction error, between the expectation of a reward and its delivery. This signal triggers the release of dopamine that helps to shape the animal's behavior by strengthening synapses that are involved in generating the rewarded

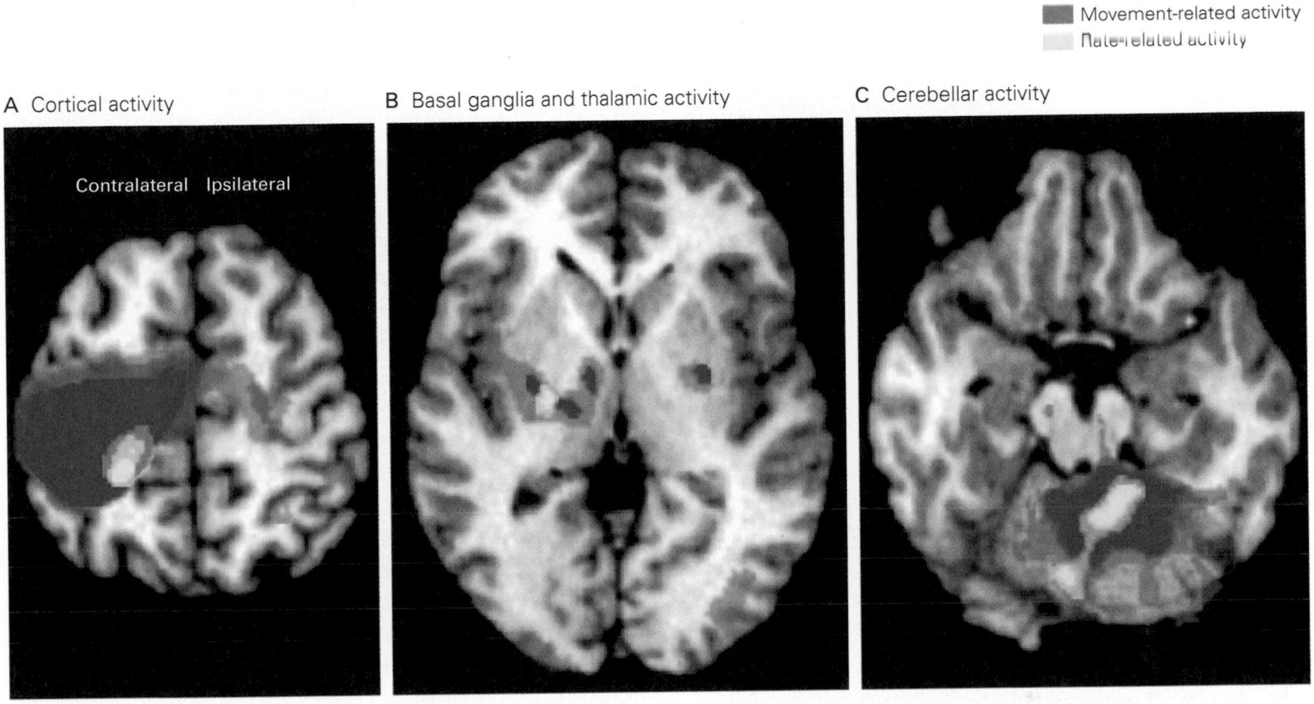

Figure 43–6 Areas of the brain with movement-related activity. PET images show significant levels of activity in human volunteers performing a sinusoidal arm movement. The images are shown superimposed on corresponding structural MRI images. The "ipsilateral" and "contralateral" hemispheres are in relation to the moving arm. (Adapted, with permission, from Turner et al. 1998.)

A. Movement-related activity in the cortex covers large portions of the primary sensorimotor, dorsolateral and mesial premotor, and dorsal parietal cortices, predominately contralateral to the moving extremity. Activity related to the rate of movement is restricted to a small band of cortex surrounding the contralateral central sulcus.

B. Movement-related activity in the basal ganglia and thalamus is seen in motor-related portions of the basal ganglia and thalamus primarily on the side contralateral to the moving arm. Rate-related activity is restricted to the posterior globus pallidus.

C. A large portion of the anterior cerebellum ipsilateral to the moving arm is active during movement. Movement-related activity is seen in a band covering the mesial portions of the cerebellum.

behavior. To effectively fulfill this role, dopaminergic neurons signal the presence of reinforcing or salient cues with very short latency. The sources of this information have not been identified, but they may include subcortical areas such as the superior colliculus, the pedunculopontine nucleus, the raphe nuclei, the lateral habenular nucleus, the amygdala, or limbic areas of cortex.

In addition to dopaminergic neurons in the substantia nigra pars compacta, cholinergic interneurons in the striatum are also activated in rewarded behavioral tasks. These cells are highly interconnected and tonically active. Their discharge is briefly reduced in response to rewards, reinforcements, noxious stimuli, and other behaviorally salient stimuli. Such responses are shaped in part by input to these neurons from the centromedian nucleus of the thalamus. Recent studies of the timing of cholinergic and dopaminergic inputs to the striatum suggest that the cholinergic interneurons may inform the medium spiny neurons in the striatum about the occurrence of salient stimuli (irrespective of their function as rewards), whereas the dopaminergic inputs may provide information about the behavioral value of the stimuli.

Chronic extracellular recordings have demonstrated that the striatal projection neurons alter their activity in the process of learning. Because the activity of striatal medium-sized spiny neurons is almost entirely driven by their excitatory cortical and thalamic inputs, such changes may reflect changes in these inputs to the striatum or in the strength of cortico- or thalamostriatal synapses through modification of the efficacy of synaptic transmission in the form of long-term potentiation (LTP), long-term depression

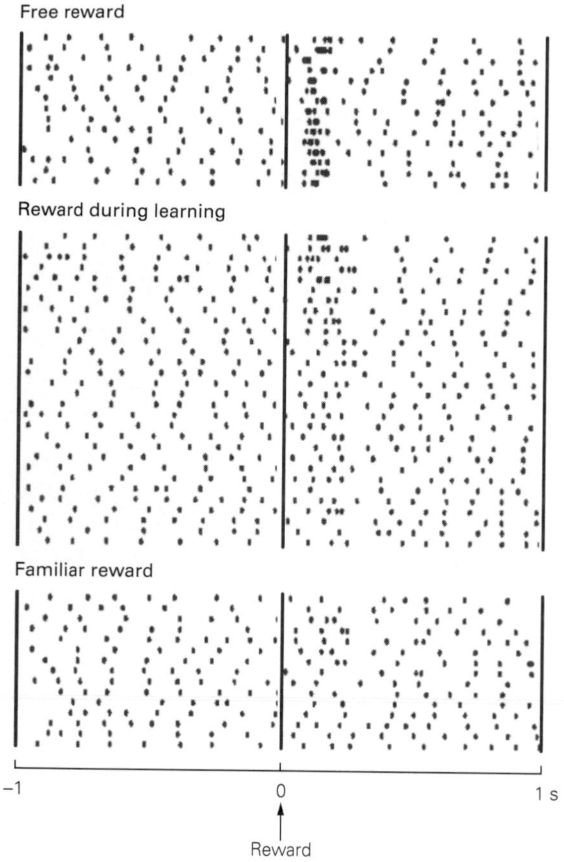

Figure 43–7 Dopaminergic neurons respond to behavioral rewards or reinforcements. Raster plots show the discharge of a dopaminergic neuron in a monkey. All trials are aligned to the time of presentation of a reward. The neuron responds each time a reward is given at random times (**top**). The responses to rewards decrease during learning of the association between a novel stimulus and a reward (**middle**). Once the reward has become familiar and predictable (**lower**), the neuron no longer responds to it. (Adapted, with permission, from Hollerman and Schultz 1998.)

(LTD), or spike-time dependent modulation of synaptic strength, brought about by the joint actions of the dopaminergic and cholinergic inputs. The striatum seems to be specifically involved with motor learning and the formation of habitual movement patterns (procedural memory). Storing such motor patterns in the form of larger behavioral units may be computationally advantageous to the brain—programmed sequences avoid the cost of repeatedly having to sequence individual movements.

The formation and execution of habitual movements appear to involve different areas of the striatum. During early stages of procedural learning the ventral striatum and caudate nucleus seem to be the primary sites of activity, whereas during later stages of learning and the execution of learned movements the dorsolateral striatum is more active. For example, experimental inactivation of the caudate nucleus in primates disrupts the acquisition of sequences of movement, whereas inactivation of the putamen interferes with the performance of previously learned sequences. As discussed earlier, however, lesions of the output from the motor circuit do not appear to have a significant effect on the execution of learned motor sequences.

Studies in songbirds also provide evidence that the basal ganglia are involved in motor learning. In some bird species lesions of the anterior forebrain pathway, the equivalent of the basal ganglia–forebrain circuitry in mammals, abolish the bird's ability to learn species-specific songs during its critical period for learning. Lesioning after the critical period does not interfere with song production but does prevent adaptive changes that may shape the bird's song in different acoustic environments, and the learned song may deteriorate over time.

Other Basal Ganglia Circuits Are Involved in the Regulation of Eye Movements, Mood, Reward, and Executive Functions

Because the patterns of connectivity of nonmotor circuits in the basal ganglia resemble those for the motor circuit, the fundamental processing in these different circuits is believed to be similar. For example, the role of the basal ganglia in the control of eye movements mirrors their role within the skeletomotor system. The *oculomotor* circuit originates from the frontal eye field and supplementary eye field, and engages oculomotor regions in the posterior caudate nucleus and precommissural putamen, oculomotor neurons in the external segment of the globus pallidus, the subthalamic nucleus and substantia nigra pars reticulata, and the mediodorsal, ventral anterior, and ventrolateral nuclei of the thalamus. In addition to this reentrant pathway that links the basal ganglia with the cerebral cortex, the substantia nigra pars reticulata provides descending projections to the superior colliculus that may be involved in the initiation and facilitation of saccadic eye movements (see Chapter 39).

The function of the descending nigrotectal pathway has been studied in detail, starting with seminal studies by Okihide Hikosaka and Robert Wurtz in the early 1980s. The available evidence indicates that voluntary saccades are initiated within the frontal eye fields of the cerebral cortex. Cortical neuronal discharge activates the GABA-ergic medium spiny neurons in the oculomotor region of the caudate nucleus, which in turn inhibit the tonic activity of GABA-ergic neurons in the substantia nigra, via the direct pathway. The resulting pause in nigral activity results in a transient disinhibition of the neurons in the superior colliculus that drive the brain stem saccade-generating machinery, resulting in a saccade. The circuit may also have a role in cognitive events associated with movement, such as memory-guided saccades.

In a general sense the oculomotor circuit appears to function in a manner similar to that originally proposed for limb movements by the motor circuit. However, the effects of manipulation of the nigro-collicular pathway have no clear parallel in the motor circuit. Whereas inactivation of the substantia nigra results in a disruption of saccades and the emergence of irrepressible involuntary saccades, inactivation of the basal ganglia output site of the motor circuit does not result in excessive limb movements.

Two prefrontal circuits involved in different aspects of cognitive and executive function have been identified. The larger *prefrontal circuit* is divided into the dorsolateral prefrontal and lateral orbitofrontal circuits. The *dorsolateral prefrontal circuit* originates in Brodmann's areas 9 and 10 of the cerebral cortex and projects to the head of the caudate nucleus, which in turn projects directly and indirectly to the dorsomedial portion of the internal pallidal segment and the rostral substantia nigra pars reticulata. Projections from these regions terminate in the ventral anterior and mediodorsal nuclei of the thalamus and in the dorsolateral area of prefrontal cortex. The dorsolateral prefrontal circuit has been implicated in executive functions such as organizing behavioral responses to complex problems and using verbal skills in problem solving.

The *lateral orbitofrontal circuit* arises in the lateral prefrontal cortex and projects to the ventromedial caudate nucleus. It engages portions of the basal ganglia output structures and thalamus and then returns to the orbitofrontal cortex. It appears to play a major role in the mediation of empathic and socially appropriate behavior.

The *limbic circuit* begins with projections from the anterior cingulate and medial orbitofrontal cortices to the ventral striatum, which also receives input from the hippocampus, amygdala, and entorhinal cortices. The ventral striatum projects to the ventral and rostromedial pallidum and rostrodorsal substantia nigra pars reticulata. From there the pathway continues to neurons in the paramedian portion of the mediodorsal nucleus of the thalamus, which projects back to the anterior cingulate cortex. The anterior cingulate circuit plays an important role in motivated behavior. Through inputs to the ventral tegmental areas and substantia nigra pars compacta, it may reinforce stimuli to diffuse areas of the basal ganglia and cerebral cortex.

Diseases of the Basal Ganglia Are Associated with Disturbances of Movement, Executive Function, Behavior, and Mood

Abnormalities in the Basal Ganglia Motor Circuit Result in a Wide Spectrum of Movement Disorders

Movement disorders arise from dysfunction of the basal ganglia–thalamocortical motor circuit, ranging from hypokinetic disorders, of which Parkinson disease is the best-known example, to hyperkinetic disorders, exemplified by Huntington disease, dystonia, and hemiballism.

Pathological changes in specific regions of the basal ganglia strongly affect neuronal activity throughout the entire basal ganglia–thalamocortical network and the activity of descending projections to the brain stem. The most severe and disruptive movement disturbances result from dysfunction in the striatum and subthalamic nucleus. By contrast, interruption of the major output nucleus of the basal ganglia, the internal segment of the globus pallidus, has little or no effect on movement. The reasons for these different effects are not understood. It seems, however, that the clinical features of specific disorders depend on unique combinations of changes in discharge rates and patterns, synchronization of discharge, and varying degrees of involvement of individual motor subcircuits.

Hypokinetic disorders are characterized by impairments of movement initiation (*akinesia*), reduction in the amplitude and velocity of voluntary movements (*bradykinesia*), muscular rigidity (increased resistance to passive displacements), and a 4–6 Hz tremor at rest and flexed posture. Hyperkinetic disorders, in contrast, are characterized by involuntary movements, such as *chorea* (random fragmented movements of individual body parts), *ballism* (large-amplitude movements particularly of the proximal limbs), and *dystonia* (slower, twisting movements and sustained abnormal postures).

A Deficiency of Dopamine in the Basal Ganglia Leads to Parkinsonism

Parkinson disease, first described by James Parkinson in 1817, affects over one million people in North America alone. In addition to the cardinal features of this condition—akinesia, bradykinesia, muscular rigidity, and tremor—other prominent motor features include a shuffling gait, flexed posture, reduced facial expression, decreased blinking, and small handwriting. These motor features are summarily referred to as parkinsonism.

Another clinical aspect of Parkinson disease is a loss of the automaticity of movement and the need for increased voluntary control manifested as difficulty carrying out simultaneous movements. The disruption of automatic and well-learned movements is believed to reflect a loss of the basal ganglia's role in procedural learning.

The salient pathological feature of idiopathic Parkinson disease is degeneration of the dopaminergic cells in the substantia nigra pars compacta that project to the striatum and to a lesser extent to other basal ganglia nuclei. Dopamine loss in these areas is considered to cause most of the movement abnormalities in this disorder, since they respond to dopamine replacement therapies. Nonmotor features of the disease include depression and anxiety, cognitive impairment, sleep disturbances, and autonomic dysfunction. These nonmotor signs and symptoms respond poorly or not at all to dopamine replacement therapy.

According to recent studies these features may be caused by additional pathological changes that affect widespread areas of the brain, with a slowly progressive ascending involvement of the lower brain stem nuclei, including the dorsal motor nucleus of the vagus nerve, locus ceruleus, nucleus gigantocellularis, raphe nuclei, amygdala, and thalamus, as well as portions of the cerebral cortex. Because little is known about the specific physiologic changes produced by these nonmotor signs, we focus here on the better-known causes and effects of dopaminergic cell loss in Parkinson disease.

The etiology of Parkinson disease is uncertain in most patients, who are said to suffer from "sporadic" Parkinson disease. Nevertheless, the disorder is believed to result from a combination of environmental and genetic factors. Exposure to environmental toxins, such as pesticides, is thought to underlie the association of Parkinson disease with rural living and consumption of well water. Several such compounds are mitochondrial toxins that may damage dopaminergic cells by interfering with their energy metabolism. Other environmental factors, such as a history of smoking or caffeine consumption, are known to *lower* the risk of developing Parkinson disease.

Single-gene mutations may also result in parkinsonism. For example, in several families with autosomal dominant parkinsonism the disorder is linked to a defect in the gene on chromosome 4 encoding α-synuclein or to duplication or triplication of the gene. This protein is one of the major components of eosinophilic inclusions (Lewy bodies) that are found in degenerating neurons in the substantia nigra pars compacta. In both sporadic and hereditary forms of Parkinson disease the accumulation of α-synuclein appears to be a major factor accounting for neuronal dysfunction and cell death. More common than mutations in the α-synuclein gene are parkinsonism-causing defects in the *parkin* gene on chromosome 6, or the more recently identified LRRK2 gene mutation. The pathogenetic mechanisms triggered by these mutations are not clear. However, it appears that factors such as oxidative damage, dysfunction of cellular mechanisms involved in the removal of toxic metabolites, and abnormal cellular calcium handling may contribute to the loss of dopaminergic cells in parkinsonism.

Direct evidence for the reduction of dopaminergic inputs to the striatum comes from postmortem biochemical analyses and from PET studies in humans with Parkinson disease (Figure 43–8). With PET the dopaminergic system can be visualized in vivo. Such studies have demonstrated that the reduction of dopamine is most severe in the caudal putamen, the portion of the striatum containing the motor circuit. This result is consistent with the observation that the earliest and most prominent manifestations of the disease involve the development of motor signs and symptoms.

Postmortem studies that have compared the brains of parkinsonian and control patients, as well as studies in experimental animals, have shown that the first overt motor signs of the disease occur when 70% or more of striatal dopamine are lost, attesting to a significant capacity of the basal ganglia–thalamocortical network to compensate for changes in dopamine levels. The presymptomatic compensation for dopamine loss may occur within the dopaminergic system itself, through increased activity of healthy dopaminergic neurons, sprouting of remaining dopaminergic fibers, and changes in the synthesis, release, or metabolism or receptor sensitivity. Mechanisms independent of dopamine, such as synaptic changes in the thalamus or cortex, may also play a role.

Dopamine loss in other nuclei of the basal ganglia (specifically the subthalamic nucleus, the internal pallidal segment, and the substantia nigra pars reticulata) may also contribute to the manifestations of Parkinson disease. Whether dopamine loss in regions outside the basal ganglia, such as the thalamus and frontal cortex, is a factor in the development of parkinsonism has not been examined in detail.

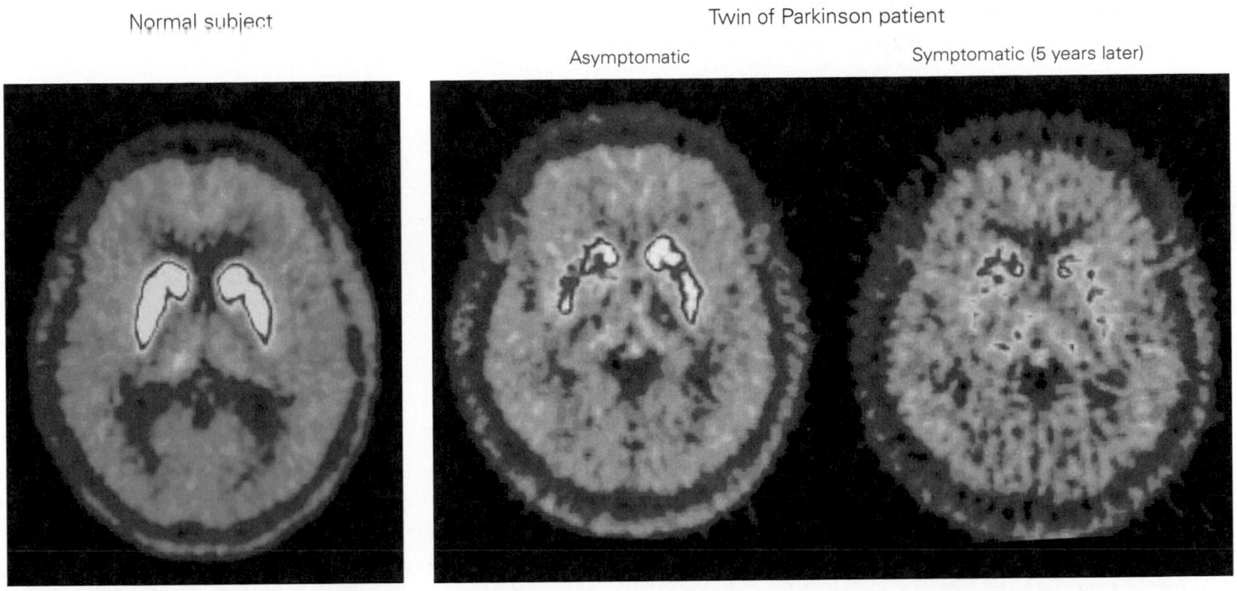

Figure 43–8 Loss of dopamine in the striatum in Parkinson disease. Positron emission tomography (PET) images of ^{18}F-DOPA uptake in the striatum in a normal subject and in a twin of a Parkinson patient show the extent of dopamine metabolism. In the twin, ^{18}F-DOPA uptake in the putamen was reduced when the subject was asymptomatic and more severely reduced five years later when symptomatic. (Adapted, with permission, from Brooks 2000.)

In the early 1980s a group of drug addicts injected themselves with a synthetic opioid that was contaminated with the meperidine analog MPTP (1-methyl-4-phenyl-1,2,3,6-tetrahydropyridine), a potent mitochondrial toxin. Soon after the exposure some of these individuals developed profound and irreversible parkinsonism. Investigations by William Langston and others revealed that MPTP is a potent neurotoxin able to destroy selectively the dopaminergic neurons in the midbrain. An important consequence of this discovery was that it allowed researchers to develop a phenotypically and anatomically convincing animal model of dopamine depletion, the MPTP-treated primate. Anatomical and electrophysiological studies in these animals have contributed greatly to circuit models of the pathophysiology of Parkinson disease.

Early microelectrode recordings and neuroimaging studies in MPTP-treated primates demonstrated that induction of parkinsonism is accompanied by a decrease in the discharge rates of neurons in the external pallidal segment and an increase in activity the subthalamic nucleus and internal pallidal segment. These changes, along with the motor signs of parkinsonism, can be reversed by systemic administration of dopamine receptor agonists. These findings led to the development of a highly influential pathophysiologic model in which loss of dopaminergic input to the striatum led to increased activity in the indirect pathway and decreased activity in the direct pathway. Both of these changes are thought to lead to a net increase of the activity of neurons in the internal segment of the globus pallidus and the substantia nigra pars reticulata. This increase in basal ganglia output would result in increased inhibition of thalamocortical and midbrain tegmental neurons and account for the hypokinetic features of the disease.

This so-called "rate model" of Parkinson disease has now been largely supplanted by models that place greater emphasis on changes in neuronal firing pattern and synchrony. The rate model cannot account for the lack of akinesia following thalamic lesions and of involuntary movements following lesions of the internal pallidum, as demonstrated in both experimental animal models and surgically treated patients.

Electrophysiological recordings from the basal ganglia in parkinsonian animals and in humans undergoing neurosurgical procedures have shown obvious abnormalities of firing patterns (Figure 43–9). Abnormal burst discharges and synchronized oscillatory neuronal activity throughout the basal ganglia–thalamocortical circuitry are now thought to be at least as important for the development of parkinsonian akinesia and tremor as the changes in discharge rates. It is important to emphasize that the abnormalities that

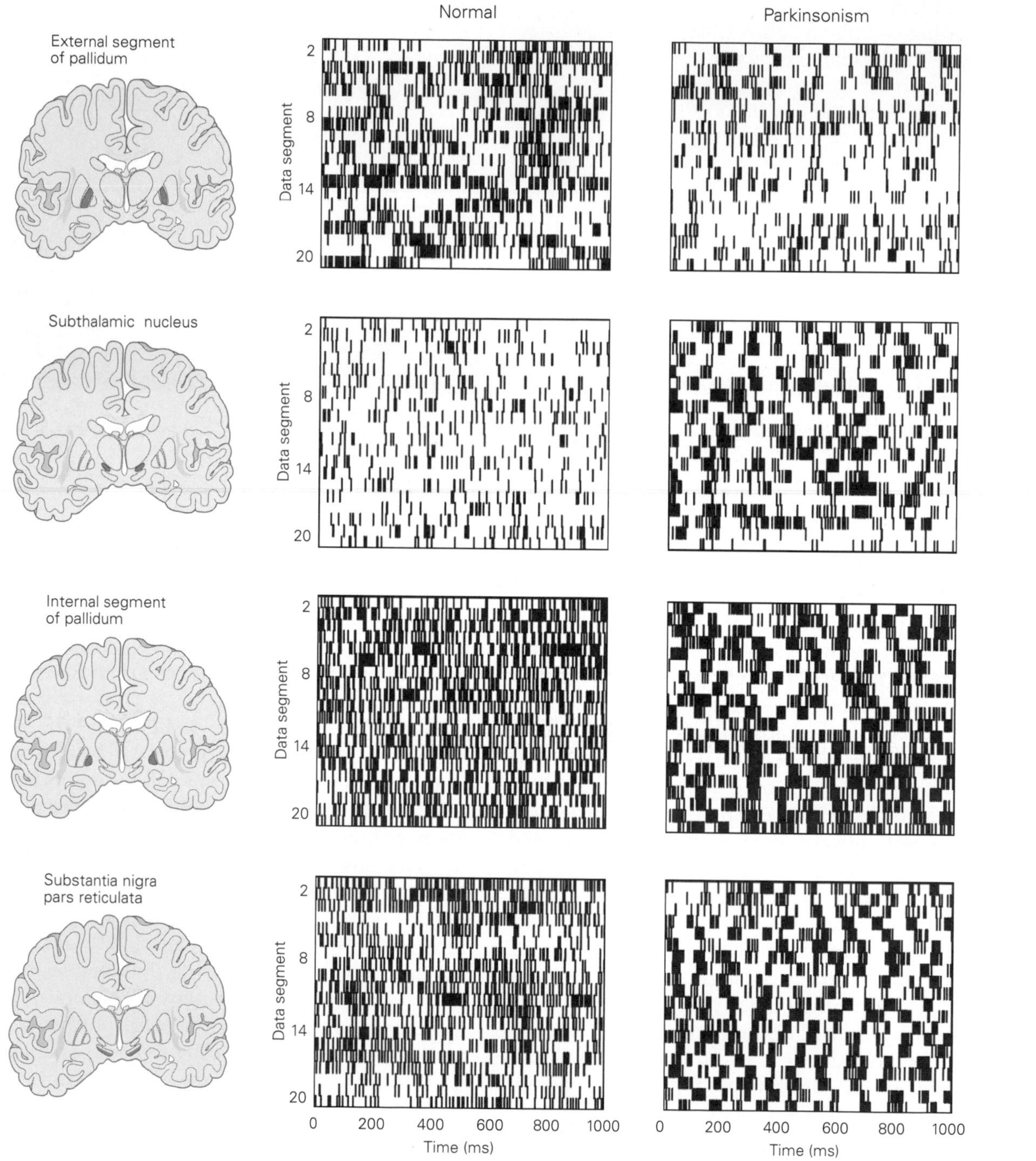

Figure 43–9 Abnormalities in the pattern of neuronal firing in the basal ganglia of parkinsonian monkeys. Raster plots show continuous data recordings from selected representative neurons situated in the structures portrayed at the left.

result in parkinsonism in the earlier rate model as well as in the newer models that emphasize pattern abnormalities are primarily found in the indirect pathway of the basal ganglia.

Recording of cells in vitro and related neural network modeling studies have elucidated some of the mechanisms that may underlie these abnormal patterns of activity in the basal ganglia. Because most pathways in the basal ganglia are GABAergic, the role of *rebound bursting*, triggered by prolonged and pathological GABAergic inhibition of basal ganglia cells, has been extensively studied. One of the connections studied in detail is the interaction between the external segment of the globus pallidus and the subthalamic nucleus. Subthalamic nucleus neurons fire spontaneously as a result of the interplay between a persistent depolarizing Na^+ current and after hyperpolarization, both of which follow each action potential and are in part caused by a K^+ current that is activated by Ca^{2+} entry into the cell associated with the action potential. These normal oscillations are reset by single inhibitory postsynaptic potentials evoked by pallidal inputs. In the presence of stronger inhibition, as may occur when the synchronicity of pallidal activity is increased in parkinsonism, the hyperpolarization may be sufficient to trigger rebound depolarization, a phenomenon that appears to be central to the generation of bursts of action potentials in subthalamic nucleus neurons.

In recent years oscillatory activity in the basal ganglia has also been assessed by recording of local field potentials. Such recordings, reflecting the activity of larger ensembles of neurons and their synaptic inputs, can be made in parkinsonian patients implanted with macroelectrodes. It was found that parkinsonism is associated with high-amplitude oscillation in the high alpha and beta frequencies (10–30 Hz) in the subthalamic nucleus, internal pallidal segment, and cerebral cortex. Such oscillation may prevent the circuitry (specifically in the cortex) from engaging in oscillations at higher (gamma-band) frequencies. Gamma-band oscillatory activity in frontal cortex and related areas is seen as a prerequisite for normal movement, and lack of gamma-band oscillations may contribute to akinesia and bradykinesia.

Changes in the cortical activity of parkinsonian patients that may result from disordered subcortical inputs have also been evaluated by functional imaging. The time resolution of such imaging is too low to show directly any changes in firing patterns. However, PET scans of patients performing a movement show decreases in synaptic activity in the anterior cingulate, supplementary motor area, and dorsolateral prefrontal cortex. In addition, brain areas that are not normally activated are recruited when patients perform visuomotor tracking. These changes may be compensatory or they may be part of the motor problem, as normal function in the newly recruited areas may be disrupted.

Progress in understanding the pathophysiology of Parkinson disease, and the finding that lesioning of motor circuit structures in parkinsonian animals has strong antiparkinsonian effects, has contributed to the resurgence of neurosurgical procedures to treat patients with advanced Parkinson disease. Initially, surgical lesioning of basal ganglia and thalamic targets was used to interrupt abnormal activity in the motor circuit, but these (irreversible) procedures have now been largely replaced by chronic high-frequency deep brain stimulation. In this less invasive and reversible procedure a programmable pulse generator, similar to a cardiac pacemaker, is placed subcutaneously and connected to a stimulating electrode inserted into the subthalamic nucleus or internal segment of the globus pallidus. Although the mechanisms of action of deep brain stimulation remain controversial, it is likely that chronic high-frequency stimulation in patients with Parkinson disease acts primarily by replacing the irregular, abnormal basal ganglia output to the cortex with a more regular and better-tolerated pattern that may then allow the cerebral cortex to function more normally. Alternatively, chronic stimulation may disrupt the abnormal and disruptive beta-frequency oscillations.

Reduced and Abnormally Patterned Basal Ganglia Output Results in Hyperkinetic Disorders

Lesions of the basal ganglia or imbalances in their neurotransmitter systems may result in involuntary movements such as hemiballism, Huntington disease, dystonia, and drug-induced involuntary movements.

Hemiballism is a hyperkinetic disorder characterized by spontaneous involuntary movements of the contralateral proximal limbs. Hemiballism most often results from lesions restricted to the subthalamic nucleus, usually as the result of small strokes. Experimental lesioning of the subthalamic nucleus in monkeys shows that involuntary movements result only when the lesion is confined to the nucleus and 20% or more of the nucleus is damaged. Such experimental lesions significantly reduce the tonic discharge of neurons in the internal segment of the globus pallidus and decrease the phasic responses of these neurons to limb displacement.

The reduced inhibitory input from the internal segment may permit thalamocortical neurons to respond in an exaggerated or abnormal manner to cortical or other inputs. If the basal ganglia inhibit planned or ongoing movements under physiological conditions, loss of this function could conceivably result in excessive movements, particularly involuntary movements. However, the finding that lesions of the internal segment relieve rather than worsen ballism and other hyperkinetic disorders argues strongly that this view is too simplistic, and that not only global activity changes but also altered patterns and synchrony of neuronal discharge in the thalamus and cortex play a major role in the generation and manifestation of hyperkinetic disorders.

Huntington disease is a hereditary disorder that affects men and women equally at a frequency of 5 to 10 per 100,000 individuals. The onset of the disease occurs most often after the third decade of life. The disease is characterized by the gradual development of motor symptoms, including chorea and eye-movement abnormalities. Nonmotor disturbances such as depression, behavioral disturbances, and cognitive impairment are also very common. Death occurs as the result of medical complications of the underlying neurological disease, in most cases 15 to 20 years after onset.

Huntington disease results from a defect on chromosome 4, affecting the gene that codes for the protein huntingtin, and is inherited in an autosomal dominant fashion. The disease is a prime example of a disorder resulting from trinucleotide repeats in a small portion of a gene (see Chapter 44). Higher numbers of trinucleotide repeats are associated with an earlier onset of the disease (anticipation).

Because of the lack of suitable animal models of Huntington disease, the pathophysiologic changes that underlie the clinical signs and symptoms in this disease are not as well established as those in Parkinson disease. The available evidence suggests that neuronal degeneration early in the disease process occurs primarily in the striatum, affecting strongly those output neurons that give rise to the indirect pathway. This reduces inhibition of neurons in the external segment of the globus pallidus leading to excessive inhibition of subthalamic nucleus neurons and a subsequent reduction in basal ganglia output. The functional inactivation of the subthalamic nucleus could explain the appearance of involuntary movements, which are similar to those seen in cases of hemiballism.

In later stages of Huntington disease a rigid and akinetic phenotype develops in most cases, possibly as the result of additional loss of the striatal neurons that project to the internal segment of the globus pallidus and substantia nigra pars reticulata. The resulting removal of inhibition from neurons of the internal segment may convert the hyperkinetic movement disorder into a hypokinetic problem with increasing rigidity and akinesia.

The gradual loss of brain stem and cortical neurons may also contribute to some aspects of the movement disorder. The profound behavioral, psychiatric, and cognitive problems seen in Huntington disease reflect the fact that nonmotor areas of the cortex and basal ganglia are involved in the pathology.

Dystonia is distinguished clinically from chorea and hemiballism by the presence of slower, twisting movements, often resulting in abnormal postures. Dystonic movements are triggered by voluntary movements. Typically, patients show co-contraction of agonist-antagonist muscle groups and an inability to restrict movements to a single body part (overflow).

Most of the pathological conditions that result in dystonia affect the functioning of the basal ganglia–thalamocortical network. Dystonia may result from genetic defects, focal lesions of the basal ganglia or other structures, or disorders of dopamine metabolism. Whereas most cases of dystonia in adults are focal and nonfamilial, dystonia starting in childhood (or in young adults) is often generalized and genetic in origin. These genetic forms of dystonia do not feature prominent neuronal degeneration. A common autosomal dominant form of generalized dystonia originates from a trinucleotide deletion on chromosome 9, leading to the formation of a mutant variant of a normal protein (torsinA). Another interesting form of dystonia is dopamine-responsive dystonia, resulting from mutations in genes involved in the production of tetrahydrobiopterin, an essential cofactor in the biosynthesis of dopamine and other biogenic amines (see Chapter 13). Similar to Parkinson disease, this disorder can be treated with dopamine replacement.

The exact role of the basal ganglia in dystonia remains poorly defined, at least in part because existing animal models of the disease do not fully replicate the phenotype. Some of the evidence regarding the role of the basal ganglia in dystonia comes from recordings in a small number of human patients undergoing neurosurgical procedures and from PET scans of dystonic patients. These studies have found that the average discharge rate in both segments of the globus pallidus is low. As in the other movement disorders, abnormally patterned or synchronized activity of the basal ganglia output neurons may play an important role in the pathophysiology of dystonia. In some cases dopaminergic dysfunction may also contribute to the development of dystonia. This view is supported by the findings that alterations in striatal dopamine transmission are seen in some forms of dystonia, that dystonia may occur in untreated Parkinson disease, and that dystonia can be seen in some patients receiving dopamine receptor-blocking drugs.

Dystonia has also been interpreted as a disorder of abnormal synaptic plasticity in the basal ganglia. A key finding supporting this view is that sensorimotor maps in the basal ganglia–thalamocortical circuits are less defined in patients with focal hand dystonia than in controls. Because focal hand dystonia is often seen in the hands of patients with writer's cramp or musician's dystonia, it is interpreted as the end product of pathological synaptic plasticity in subcortical or cortical regions. Evidence for disordered plasticity in the cortico–basal ganglia–thalamocortical circuits also comes from the finding that the beneficial effects of surgical treatments such as lesioning or chronic electrical stimulation of the globus pallidus require weeks or months to develop.

Abnormal Neuronal Activity in Nonmotor Circuits Is Associated with Several Neuropsychiatric Disorders

Disturbances of the nonmotor basal ganglia–thalamocortical circuits may contribute to the development of cognitive and behavioral problems accompanying movement disorders and to primary psychiatric disorders, such as obsessive-compulsive disorder, Tourette syndrome, and depression. Although processes outside the basal ganglia–thalamocortical loop systems may also contribute to the psychiatric disturbances, we concentrate here on the possible involvement of the basal ganglia circuitry.

The evidence for the functional relevance of the nonmotor areas comes mostly from clinical observations. In addition, animal studies employing microinjections of a GABA receptor antagonist, bicuculline, into motor, associative, and limbic portions of the external pallidal segment in primates have provided evidence for the notion that different neurobehavioral syndromes arise from dysfunction of different basal ganglia–thalamocortical circuits. Injections in the limbic part of the external segment of the globus pallidus induced stereotypic movements, whereas injections in the associative part induced hyperactivity. As predicted, abnormal movements were observed only when bicuculline was injected into the motor territory. These studies provide experimental support for the proposed behavioral domains in the basal ganglia and their role in abnormal motor and nonmotor behaviors.

Damage to the dorsolateral prefrontal cortex or subcortical portions of the prefrontal circuit results in a variety of abnormalities related to cognitive or executive functions, whereas damage to the lateral orbitofrontal circuit (for example, in stroke patients) is associated with lack of empathy, emotional lability, irritability, and failure to respond to social cues.

One of the best-studied psychiatric disorders arising from pathology in a nonmotor circuit is obsessive-compulsive disorder. The stereotypic behaviors (rigid behavioral patterns) and compulsions that are characteristic of this disorder have been interpreted as evidence for dysfunctional procedural learning. Functional imaging studies of patients with this disorder have demonstrated abnormalities in activity in the basal ganglia–thalamocortical limbic circuits that originate in portions of the orbitofrontal and anterior cingulate cortices. The most prominent changes are seen in the ventral striatum, specifically in the nucleus accumbens and ventromedial caudate nucleus, and in the midbrain. The beneficial outcome of neurosurgical treatments directed at the limbic circuitry, such as lesioning or stimulation of the anterior limb of the internal capsule and the ventral striatum, or lesions involving fibers emanating from orbitofrontal or anterior cingulate cortex, is evidence that the limbic circuit is involved in obsessive-compulsive disorder.

Tourette syndrome, in which obsessive-compulsive symptoms are associated with motor or vocal tics (brief involuntary movements or vocalizations), is also characterized by abnormalities in the limbic circuit. The fact that dopamine receptor-blocking drugs suppress tics implicates the basal ganglia in these disorders. Additional changes in brain activity occur in cortical areas associated with motor functions, particularly in the sensorimotor cortex and supplementary motor area. Chronic stimulation of the limbic and motor circuit at the pallidal and thalamic levels is now being explored as a treatment of severe, refractory Tourette syndrome.

An Overall View

It is now clear that the basal ganglia, together with the thalamus and cerebral cortex, participate in a family of neuronal networks that are involved not only in motor functions, but also in the higher-order aspects of behavior, linking emotion, reward, executive function, and mood, and that they may have specific relevance for adaptive shaping of behavior and action selection.

Basal ganglia disturbances are a factor in many major movement, behavioral, and psychiatric disorders that appear to result from dysfunction in specific basal ganglia–thalamocortical circuits. The existing models of basal ganglia function and dysfunction have stimulated research on the role of the basal ganglia in health and disease and contributed to the development of successful new treatments for these disorders.

Nevertheless, the present models are not fully satisfactory because they are too strongly based on disease considerations and the outcome of inactivation and disruptive manipulations that have remote effects, that do not necessarily reflect the actual functions of the basal ganglia, and that do not fully incorporate the adaptive properties of the circuits involved. Accordingly, future versions of functional models will need to take into account many of the more recent findings, including the close interactions of the basal ganglia with the brain stem and other structures and the role of abnormal neuronal activity patterns and synchrony in the pathophysiology of movement, cognitive, behavioral, and psychiatric disorders.

Thomas Wichmann
Mahlon R. DeLong

Selected Readings

Bonelli RM, Cummings JL. 2007. Frontal-subcortical circuitry and behavior. Dialogues Clin Neurosci 9:141–151.

Breakefield XO, Blood AJ, Li Y, Hallett M, Hanson PI, Standaert DG. 2008. The pathophysiological basis of dystonias. Nat Rev Neurosci 9:222–234.

DeLong MR, Wichmann T. 2007. Circuits and circuit disorders of the basal ganglia. Arch Neurol 64:20–24.

Eidelberg D. 2009. Metabolic brain networks in neurodegenerative disorders: a functional imaging approach. Trends Neurosci 32:548–557.

Galvan A, Wichmann T. 2008. Pathophysiology of parkinsonism. Clin Neurophysiol 119:1459–1474.

Graybiel AM. 2008. Habits, rituals, and the evaluative brain. Ann Rev Neurosci 31:359–387.

Hikosaka O. 2007. Basal ganglia mechanisms of reward-oriented eye movement. Ann NY Acad Sci 1104:229–249.

Kelly RM, Strick PL. 2004. Macro-architecture of basal ganglia loops with the cerebral cortex: use of rabies virus to reveal multisynaptic circuits. Prog Brain Res 143:449–459.

Kopell BH, Greenberg BD. 2008. Anatomy and physiology of the basal ganglia: implications for DBS in psychiatry. Neurosci Biobehav Rev 32:408–422.

Lees AJ, Hardy J, Revesz T. 2009. Parkinson's disease. Lancet 373:2055–2066.

Schultz W. 2007. Multiple dopamine functions at different time courses. Annu Rev Neurosci 30:259–288.

Surmeier DJ, Plotkin J, Shen W. 2009. Dopamine and synaptic plasticity in dorsal striatal circuits controlling action selection. Curr Opin Neurobiol 19:621–628.

References

Alexander GE, Crutcher MD, Delong MR. 1990. Functional architecture of basal ganglia circuits: neural substrates of parallel processing. Trends in Neurosci 13:226–271.

Brooks DJ. 2000. Morphological and functional imaging studies on the diagnosis and progression of Parkinson disease. J Neurology 247:II11–II18 (suppl).

Hollerman JR, Schultz W. 1998. Dopamine neurons report an error in the temporal prediction of reward during learning. Nat Neurosci 1:304–309.

Hoover JE, Strick PL. 1993. Multiple output channels in the basal ganglia. Science 259:819–821.

Nieuwenhuys R, Voogd J, van Huijzen C. 1981. *The Human Central Nervous System: A Synopsis and Atlas,* 2nd ed. Berlin: Springer.

Turner, RS, Grafton, ST, Votaw, JR, Delong, MR Hoffman, JM. 1998. Motor subcircuits mediating the control of movement velocity: a PET study. J Neurophysiol 80:2162–2176.

Wichmann T, Delong MR. 2006. Deep brain stimulation for neurologic and neuropsychiatric disorders. Neuron 52:197–204.

44

Genetic Mechanisms in Degenerative Diseases of the Nervous System

THE MAJOR DEGENERATIVE DISEASES of the nervous system—Alzheimer, Parkinson, and the triplet-repeat diseases (Huntington and the spinocerebellar ataxias)—afflict nearly 5 million people in the United States alone, and more than 25 million people throughout the world. Although this is a relatively small percentage of the population, these diseases bring a disproportionate amount of suffering and economic loss, not only to their victims but also to the families and friends of the afflicted.

Most of these disorders strike in mid-life or later; aging itself may in fact contribute to susceptibility. With the exception of Alzheimer disease, the first symptoms to appear usually involve loss of control of fine motor movements, although Huntington disease can first manifest itself in cognitive deficits. Nevertheless, the end result is the same. After a lengthy period of progressive deterioration, usually 10 to 20 years, the affected individual dies a terrible, helpless death.

The late-onset neurodegenerative diseases can be grouped conceptually into two categories: sporadic (unknown etiology) and inherited. Alzheimer disease and Parkinson disease are predominantly sporadic; inherited forms afflict a small number of patients. The triplet-repeat diseases, however, are notable for their dominant pattern of inheritance and the dynamic nature of the pathological mutation, an elongation of a CAG repeat tract that is subject to further expansion. Among the triplet-repeat neurodegenerative diseases are Huntington disease, the spinocerebellar ataxias, dentatorubropallidoluysian atrophy, and spinobulbar muscular atrophy. Identification of the molecular basis of some of these disorders has facilitated diagnosis and classification and provides hope for eventual treatment.

Expanded Trinucleotide Repeats Characterize Several Neurodegenerative Diseases

Huntington Disease Involves Degeneration of the Striatum

Huntington disease usually strikes in early or middle adulthood and affects 5 to 10 people per 100,000. The clinical presentation includes loss of motor control, cognitive impairment, and affective disturbance. Motor-control problems most commonly manifest themselves early as chorea, involuntary jerky movement that involves the small joints at first but then gradually creates instability of gait as the trunk and legs are affected. Fast, fluid movements are replaced by rigidity and bradykinesia (difficulty initiating action and unusually slow movements).

Cognitive impairment—such as difficulty in planning and executing complex functions—typically appears along with the involuntary movements but may be detected by formal neuropsychological testing even prior to motor dysfunction. Affective disturbances (psychiatric and behavioral features) include depression, irritability, social withdrawal, and disordered sleep. Hypomania and increased energy occur in 10% of the patients, whereas frank psychosis with delusions occurs in a smaller subset.

In adult patients the disease progresses inexorably to death some 17 to 20 years after onset. Juvenile-onset cases suffer a more rapid course of the disease and within only a few years typically develop bradykinesia, dystonia (spasm of the neck, shoulders, and trunk), rigidity (resistance to the passive motion of a limb), seizures, and severe dementia.

The pathological hallmark of Huntington disease is degeneration of the striatum, with the caudate nucleus being more affected than the putamen. Loss of a class of inhibitory interneurons in the striatum, the medium spiny neurons, reduces inhibition of neurons in the external pallidum (see Chapter 43). The resulting excessive activity of the pallidal neurons inhibits the subthalamic nucleus, which could account for the choreiform movements. As the disease progresses and striatal neurons projecting to the internal pallidum degenerate, rigidity replaces chorea. Abnormalities in corticostriatal projections are thought to contribute to pathogenesis. Juvenile cases suffer a more severe and generalized pathology that often includes cerebellar Purkinje cells.

Huntington disease is an autosomal dominant disorder and one of the first human diseases to have its gene mapped using polymorphic DNA markers. It is caused by expansion of a translated CAG repeat that encodes a glutamine tract in the huntingtin protein. Normal or wild-type alleles have 6 to 34 repeats, whereas disease-associated alleles typically have 36 or more repeats and are quite unstable when transmitted from one generation to the next, especially through paternal germ cells.

The dynamic nature of the mutation, expanding in successive generations, accounts for the greater severity of the disease in juvenile-onset cases, a phenomenon known as anticipation. The length of the repeat correlates inversely with the age of onset, one of the many common features of neurodegenerative diseases caused by CAG-repeat expansions (Figure 44–1). Huntington disease-like 2 (HDL2), a rare neurodegenerative disorder that is clinically similar to Huntington disease, is caused by CTG expansion in junctophilin 3.

Huntington disease appears to be a true dominant disease in that patients homozygous for the condition do not differ significantly from their heterozygous siblings. The expanded glutamine tract causes the huntingtin protein to gain toxic function in addition to its normal function. Huntingtin is expressed throughout the brain in the cytoplasm, where it associates with microtubules, with a minor fraction present in cell nuclei. Although its precise functions are unknown, huntingtin is an essential protein in normal embryonic

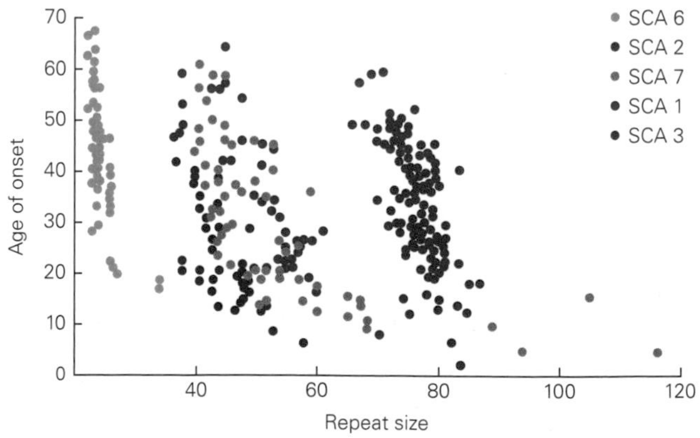

Figure 44–1 The length of the CAG repeat and age of onset in spinocerebellar ataxia are inversely correlated. The longer the CAG tract, the earlier the onset for a given disease. Specific repeat lengths, however, have different results depending on the host protein. For example, a 52-repeat of CAG causes juvenile onset of symptoms in spinocerebellar ataxia type 2 (**SCA2**), adult onset in spinocerebellar ataxia type 1 (**SCA1**), and no disease in spinocerebellar ataxia type 3 (**SCA3**).

development as shown by mouse knock-out studies; it is also essential for neuronal integrity in the postnatal brain.

Spinobulbar Muscular Atrophy Is Due to Abnormal Function of the Androgen Receptor

Spinobulbar muscular atrophy (Kennedy disease), the only X-linked disorder among the neurodegenerative diseases discussed in this chapter, is caused by expansion of a translated CAG repeat in the androgen receptor protein, a member of the steroid hormone receptor family. Only males manifest symptoms; the mutant androgen receptor is toxic when in the nucleus, and such localization requires the male hormone androgen. Proximal muscle weakness is usually the presenting symptom; eventually the distal and facial muscles weaken as well. Muscle wasting is prominent, secondary to degeneration of motor neurons.

Bulbar dysfunction results from loss of brain stem motor neurons. Many patients also develop gynecomastia, late hypogonadism, and sterility, indicating the loss of androgen receptor function. Individuals lacking androgen receptor function without expansion of CAG repeats do not, however, develop motor neuron degeneration. It thus appears that the glutamine expansion causes a partial loss of function that accounts for the secondary sexual characteristics and a partial gain of function that affects neurons and produces the neurological phenotype.

Hereditary Spinocerebellar Ataxias Include Several Diseases with Similar Symptoms but Distinct Etiologies

The spinocerebellar ataxias and dentatorubropallidoluysian atrophy are dominantly inherited neurodegenerative diseases that, for all their heterogeneity, are characterized predominantly by dysfunction of the cerebellum, spinal tracts, and various brain stem nuclei. The basal ganglia, cerebral cortex, and peripheral nervous system are also affected in some subtypes or in isolated cases (Table 44–1).

The two clinical features common to all the spinocerebellar ataxias are ataxia and dysarthria. These typically appear in mid-adulthood and gradually worsen, making walking impossible and speech incomprehensible. The brain stem dysfunction manifests itself through difficulties in swallowing and breathing and eventually causes death.

Features such as chorea or dementia are associated more strongly with one spinocerebellar ataxia than others, but these symptoms are so variable that they cannot be reliably used to refine the diagnosis. Even individuals within the same family can present a quite different clinical picture. Thus, although the spinocerebellar ataxias are single-gene Mendelian disorders, individual genetic makeup and environmental influences clearly affect the clinical-pathological situation.

For example, Machado-Joseph disease and spinocerebellar ataxia type 3 (SCA3) had been regarded clinically as distinct diseases before it was discovered that they are caused by mutations in the same gene. The clinical confusion arose by historical accident. The most prominent features of the Portuguese families first studied by Machado and Joseph were bulging eyes, faciolingual fasciculations, parkinsonism, and dystonia, whereas the first SCA3 patients had features more reminiscent of SCA1 (hypermetric saccades and brisk reflexes in addition to the characteristic ataxia and dysarthria). We now know that these apparent clinical differences are at least partially attributable to differences in length of the CAG repeats. Nonetheless, differences in the activity of other proteins caused by genetic variations are probably also at play.

Although the age of onset within each type of ataxia depends on the number of CAG repeats in the gene (Figure 44–1), the toxicity of the abnormally long glutamine tract in the protein product depends on the protein: Expanded glutamine tracts have different effects in different proteins. For example, very short repeat lengths that are detrimental to Purkinje cells in SCA6 are nonpathogenic in other SCAs. In fact, the CAG expansion in SCA6 is the shortest of all the spinocerebellar ataxias: 21 to 33 repeats in mutants compared to fewer than 18 in normal alleles. In contrast, the gene responsible for SCA7 normally tolerates a few dozen CAG repeats, and in the disease state undergoes some of the largest expansions seen in any spinocerebellar ataxia (hundreds of CAGs). (Table 44–2.)

Besides tolerating different CAG repeat lengths, the gene products of mutated genes in polyglutamine diseases vary widely in function. The affected gene product in SCA1, ataxin-1, seems to be important for learning and memory; it is predominantly a nuclear protein that shuttles to the cytoplasm and can bind RNA in vitro, which suggests that it might play a role in RNA transport and processing. The affected gene product in SCA6, CACNA1A, is the α_{1A} subunit of the voltage-gated Ca^{2+} channel; interestingly enough, loss-of-function mutations in the gene (not caused by CAG repeats) have been reported in patients with episodic ataxia and familial hemiplegic migraine. In SCA17 the affected gene product is the TATA box-binding protein, an essential transcription factor.

Table 44–1 Pattern of Inheritance and Main Clinical Features of Neurodegenerative Diseases Caused by Unstable Trinucleotide Repeats

Disease	Inheritance	Typical presenting features	Principal regions affected
SBMA	X-linked recessive	Muscle cramps, weakness, gynecomastia	Lower motor neurons and anterior horn cells
Huntington	AD	Cognitive impairment, chorea, depression, irritability	Striatum, cortex
Huntington-like 2	AD	Cognitive impairment, chorea, depression, irritability	Striatum, cortex
SCA1	AD	Hypermetric saccades, ataxia, dysarthria, ophthalmoparesis	Purkinje cells, dentate nucleus, inferior olive
SCA2	AD	Ataxia, hyporeflexia, slow saccades	Purkinje cells, granule cells, inferior olive
SCA3	AD	Ataxia, gaze-evoked nystagmus, bulging eyes, dystonia, spasticity	Pontine neurons, substantia nigra, anterior horn cells
SCA6	AD	Ataxia, late onset (>50 years of age)	Purkinje cells, granule cells
SCA7	AD	Ataxia, visual loss due to retinal degeneration, hearing loss	Purkinje cells, retina (cone and rod degeneration)
SCA8	AD	Scanning dysarthria, ataxia	Purkinje cells
SCA10	AD	Ataxia and seizures	Purkinje cells
SCA12	AD	Early arm tremor, hyperreflexia, ataxia	Purkinje cells (cortical and cerebellar atrophy)
SCA17	AD	Dysphagia, intellectual deterioration, ataxia, absence seizures	Purkinje cells, granule layer, upper motor neurons
DRPLA	AD	Dementia, ataxia, choreoathetosis	Dentate nucleus, red nucleus, globus pallidus, subthalamic nucleus, cerebellar cortex, cortex

AD, autosomal dominant; DRPLA, dentatorubropallidoluysian atrophy; SBMA, spinobulbar muscular atrophy; SCA, spinocerebellar ataxia.

The affected product in dentatorubropallidoluysian atrophy, atrophin-1, is thought to be a corepressor based on functional studies of its probable ortholog in *Drosophila*. Despite these differences, some pathogenetic mechanisms may be common to the polyglutamine diseases, as discussed later in this chapter.

A few spinocerebellar ataxias are caused by unstable trinucleotide repeats other than CAG (Table 44–2). Spinocerebellar ataxia type 8 is caused by an expansion of a CTG repeat in the 3′ untranslated region of a transcribed RNA with no open reading frames. The mutation responsible for SCA12 is a CAG repeat, but it occurs in a noncoding region upstream of a brain-specific regulatory subunit of the protein phosphatase 2A. Spinocerebellar ataxia type 10 is unique in that it is caused by massive expansion of a pentanucleotide (ATTCT) repeat in the intron of a novel gene. The pathogenic mechanisms accounting for the dominant phenotypes in spinocerebellar ataxia types 8, 10, and 12 are not yet known.

Parkinson Disease Is a Common Degenerative Disorder of the Elderly

Parkinson disease, one of the more common neurodegenerative disorders, affects 1% to 2% of the population older than 65 years of age. Patients with Parkinson disease suffer from a resting tremor, bradykinesia, rigidity, and impairment in their ability to initiate and sustain movements. Affected individuals walk with a distinctive shuffling gait, and their balance is often precarious. Spontaneous facial movements are greatly diminished, such that the face has a mask-like, expressionless appearance. The pathological hallmark of Parkinson disease is progressive loss of dopaminergic neurons, mainly in the substantia nigra (see Chapter 43).

Although the majority of parkinsonian cases are sporadic, studies of rare familial cases have provided insight into the genetic factors that predispose individuals to this disorder. Here we focus on how the genetic bases of some forms of Parkinson disease provides insights into sporadic Parkinson disease and link the pathogenic mechanism of parkinsonism to that seen in the polyglutamine disorders.

Both autosomal dominant and recessive inheritance patterns have been documented in familial parkinsonism. To date, several genetic loci have been mapped (designated PARK1–PARK8, PARK10, and PARK11), and the genes for all but three of these loci (PARK3, PARK10, and PARK11) have been identified (Table 44–3).

Parkinson disease type 1 (PARK1) is the locus for the dominantly inherited Parkinson disease caused by mutations in the gene *α-synuclein*. Two mutations in *α-synuclein* have been identified: A53T has been described in several Greek families, whereas A30P has been identified in one German family. Mutations in *α-synuclein* have not been identified in sporadic Parkinson disease. However, because the α-synuclein protein is a primary component of the Lewy bodies in the substantia nigra of patients with sporadic disease as well as those with PARK1, *α-synuclein* mutations could play an important role in the pathogenesis of the sporadic disease.

The function of the α-synuclein protein is not yet known, but its abundance in presynaptic terminals suggests a role in presynaptic function and perhaps synaptic plasticity. Patients with *α-synuclein* mutations differ from those with sporadic Parkinson disease in that the age of onset is earlier (a mean of 45 years), and they exhibit fewer tremors and more rigidity, cognitive decline, myoclonus, central hypoventilation, orthostatic hypotension, and urinary incontinence.

Parkinson disease type 2 (PARK2) is an autosomal recessive disease characterized by early onset (as young as three years of age), dystonia, brisk deep-tendon

Table 44–2 Hereditary Ataxias Caused by Expansion of Unstable Trinucleotide Repeats

					Repeat lengths	
Disease	**Gene**	**Locus**	**Protein**	**Mutation**	**Normal**	**Disease**
SCA1	SCA1	6p23	Ataxin-1	CAG repeat in coding region	6–44*	36–121
SCA2	SCA2	12q24.1	Ataxin-2	CAG repeat in coding region	15–31	36–63
SCA3 (Machado-Joseph disease)	SCA3, MJD1	14q32.1	Ataxin-3	CAG repeat in coding region	12–40	55–84
SCA6	SCA6	19p13	α_{1A} subunit of voltage-gated Ca^{2+} channel	CAG repeat in coding region	4–18	21–33
SCA7	SCA7	3p12-13	Ataxin-7	CAG repeat in coding region	4–35	37–306
SCA8	SCA8	13q21	None	CTG repeat in the 3′ terminal exon (antisense)	16–37	110–250
SCA10	SCA10	22q13ter	Ataxin-10	Pentanucleotide (ATTCT) repeat in the intron	10–20	500–4500
SCA12	SCA12	5q31-33	Protein phosphatase 2A	CAG repeat in 5′ UTR	7–28	66–78
SCA17	TBP	6qter	TATA-binding protein	CAG repeat in coding region	29–42	47–55
DRPLA	DRPLA	12q	Atrophin-1	CAG repeat in coding region	6–35	49–88
FXTAS	FMR1	Xq27.3	FMRP	CGG repeat in 5′ UTR	6–60	60–200

*Alleles with 21 or more repeats are interrupted by 1–3 CAT units; disease alleles contain pure CAG tracts.DRPLA, dentatorubropallidoluysian atrophy; FXTAS, fragile X-associated tremor ataxia syndrome; SCA, spinocerebellar ataxia.

Table 44–3 Genetics and Main Clinical Features of Inherited Parkinson Disease

Disease	Locus map	Inheritance pattern	Protein	Main features
PARK1, PARK4	4q21	AD	α-synuclein	Early onset, rigidity, and cognitive impairment
PARK2	6q25.2-q27	AR	Parkin	Juvenile onset, dystonia
PARK3	2p13	AD	Unknown	Adult onset, dementia
PARK5	4p14	Probably AD	UCH-L1	Adult onset
PARK6	1p36	AR	PINK1	Early onset, dystonia
PARK7	1p36	AR	DJ-1	Early onset, behavioral disturbance, dystonia
PARK8	12q12	AD	LRRK2	Classic PD
PARK10	1p32	Unknown	Unknown	Classic PD
PARK11	2q36-q37	Unknown	Unknown	Classic PD

AD, autosomal dominant; AR, autosomal recessive; PARK, PD, Parkinson disease.

reflexes, and cerebellar signs in addition to the classic Parkinson disease phenotype. More than 60 different mutations have been identified in the gene *PARK2*, and most are clearly inactivating, demonstrating that this form of the disease is caused by loss of function of the gene product, parkin. Whereas *α-synuclein* mutations have not been detected in the sporadic disease, mutations in the *parkin* gene have been found in isolated cases of early-onset Parkinson disease and in one patient with onset at 65 years of age. Loss of dopaminergic neurons in the substantia nigra is typical of this form of the disease, but Lewy bodies are not as common as in sporadic or PARK1 cases.

The *parkin* gene encodes an E3 ubiquitin ligase of the RING-finger family that transfers activated ubiquitin to lysine residues in proteins destined for degradation by proteasomes. The ligase is quite specific and transfers ubiquitin to only a few substrates. Some substrates for parkin have been identified, including a putative transmembrane G protein-coupled receptor named parkin-associated endothelin receptor-like receptor (Pael-R), the synaptic vesicle protein CDCrel-1, the O-glycosylated form of α-synuclein, the α-synuclein interactor synphilin-1, and parkin itself.

A missense mutation, I93M, in the gene encoding ubiquitin C-terminal hydrolase-L1 (UCH-L1) has been identified in a family with an apparently autosomal dominant Parkinson disease, PARK5. UCH-L1 is an abundant protein in the brain and is thought to cleave polyubiquitin chains as the ubiquitinated proteins are being degraded by the proteasome. This activity is decreased in individuals with the 193M mutant. A homologous protein is necessary for the formation of memory in the marine mollusk *Aplysia*.

Parkinson disease type 6 (PARK6) is caused by mutations in a gene that encodes a PTEN-induced putative kinase 1 (PINK1), a mitochondrial protein kinase, whereas Parkinson disease type 7 (PARK7) is caused by mutations in a gene that encodes DJ-1, a protein that may function as a sensor of oxidative stress. Mutations in the gene encoding the leucine-rich repeat kinase 2 (LRRK2) cause Parkinson disease type 8 (PARK8) as well as a small percentage of sporadic Parkinson disease cases.

Selective Neuronal Loss Occurs After Damage to Ubiquitously Expressed Genes

A perplexing aspect of these neurodegenerative diseases is that the altered gene products are widely and abundantly expressed not only in the nervous system but also in other tissues, yet the phenotypes are predominantly neurological. Moreover, the phenotypes reflect dysfunction in only specific groups of neurons (Figure 44–2), a phenomenon referred to as neuronal selectivity.

Why are striatal neurons the most vulnerable in Huntington disease, whereas the Purkinje cells are targeted in the spinocerebellar ataxias (SCA)? Why are the dopaminergic neurons in the substantia nigra primarily affected in Parkinson disease even though α-synuclein, parkin, DJ-1, PINK1, LRRK2, and UCH-L1 are abundant in many other neuronal groups? Although definitive answers are not yet available, there are some clues.

In the polyglutamine diseases the selectivity of the cellular pathology diminishes as the length of the glutamine tract increases: the more severe the mutation, the greater the number of neuronal groups affected. This is especially evident in the early-onset forms characterized by extremely long repeats. Juvenile SCA1 patients suffer from dystonia, rigidity, and cognitive impairment, features that overlap with Huntington disease and dentatorubropallidoluysian atrophy. Juvenile SCA7 patients can suffer seizures, delusions, and auditory hallucinations, and infantile cases also develop somatic features, including short stature and congestive heart failure. Spinocerebellar ataxia type 7 also causes progressive blindness owing to dystrophy of both rods and cones; interestingly, cases of infants with SCA2 who also suffer retinal degeneration have recently been reported.

These and similar observations suggest that various cell types have different thresholds of vulnerability to toxic proteins with expanded glutamine tracts. Retinal cells, for example, seem more resistant to polyglutamine toxicity than cerebellar neurons, but more

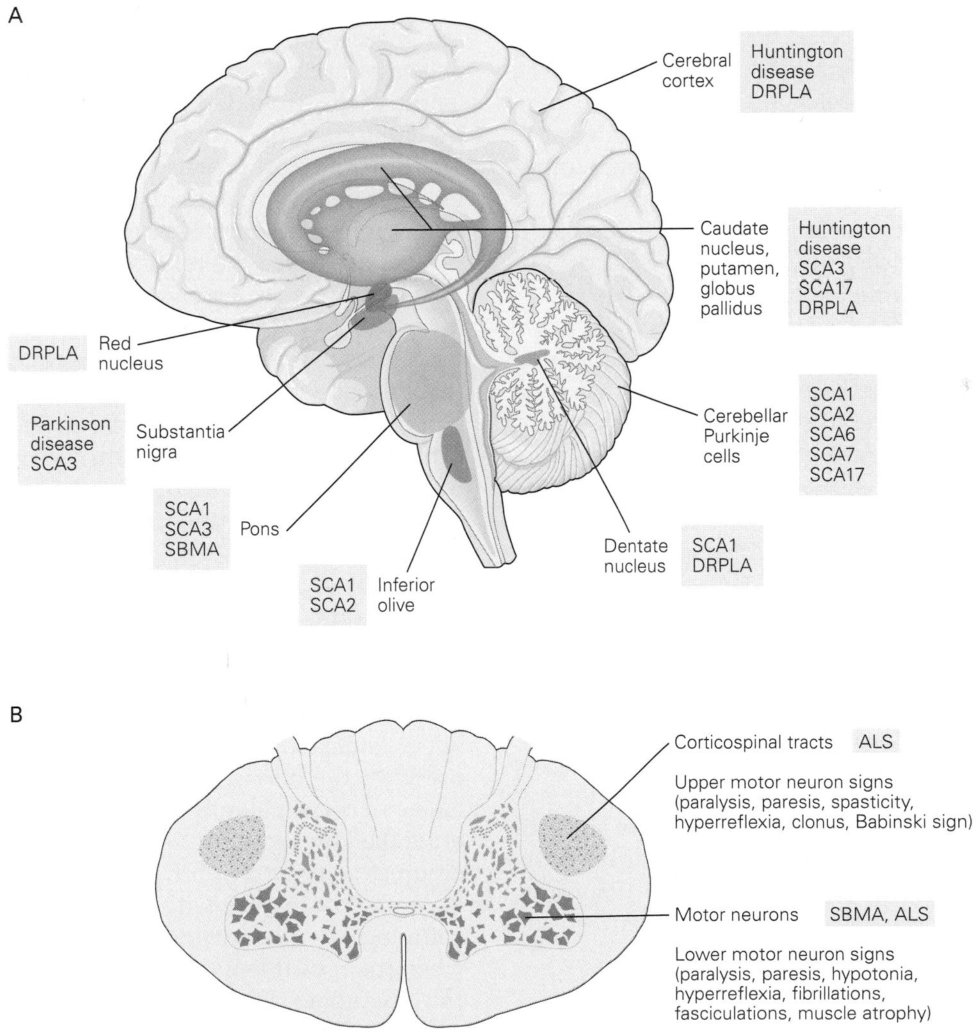

Figure 44–2 Primary sites of neuronal degeneration in the trinucleotide repeat diseases and Parkinson disease.

A. Brain regions most typically affected by adult-onset disease (see Table 44–1).

B. Comparison of neuropathology of amyotrophic lateral sclerosis (**ALS**) and spinobulbar muscular atrophy (**SBMA**).

vulnerable than cardiac myocytes. Once the number of glutamines in the tract expands beyond a certain length—which varies from one protein to the next—no cell is safe.

Studies using mouse models suggest that protein misfolding is responsible for polyglutamine disorders. The longer the glutamine tract, the more severe the misfolding and protein accumulation. As the tracts become very long, even cells with lower concentrations of disordered gene product become vulnerable. Indeed, studies of animal models show that even a doubling in concentration can be the difference between phenotypic manifestation and apparent normality. It is therefore conceivable that the neurons affected in each disease have more mutant protein than do the less vulnerable neurons. Although not detectable by current immunolabeling techniques, this increment would nevertheless be sufficient to interfere with cellular function if the neuron was exposed to the toxic mutant protein over decades.

Other major contributors to selective vulnerability might be variations in the levels of proteins that interact with or help dispose of the mutant proteins. Variations in the genes encoding such proteins could contribute to the clinical variability that is so prominent among ataxia families.

Why are neurons affected before other cells? As the organism ages, slight insults that have small detrimental effects could be exacerbated by the extra challenge the mutant protein presents to the protein-folding machinery. Because neurons are post-mitotic, they might be especially sensitive to perturbations in the balance of intracellular factors. If the organism could survive the neurological assault long enough, other tissues might also eventually show signs of distress.

Animal Models Are Powerful Tools for Studying Neurodegenerative Diseases

Animal models have proven extremely valuable for probing the pathogenesis of various neurodegenerative diseases and investigating therapies. Because of the ease in making mutations, the mouse has been the favored animal for modeling neurological disorders, but *Drosophila* models also have proven useful in the delineation of genetic pathways.

Mouse Models Reproduce Many Features of Neurodegenerative Diseases

With the exception of PARK2, the neurodegenerative diseases discussed here are caused mostly by a gain of function rather than loss of function. Thus most of the genetically engineered mice that model these diseases are created using two techniques. In transgene experiments an allele harboring the mutant gene is overexpressed, whereas in knock-in experiments a human mutation, such as an expanded CAG tract, is inserted into an endogenous mouse locus to control expression of the gene product temporally and spatially (see Box 3–2). In some mutants, such as spinocerebellar ataxia types 1, 2, 3, and 7, dentatorubropallidoluysian atrophy, and some Huntington disease models, a full-length cDNA with either wild-type or expanded alleles is overexpressed either in a particular class of neurons or in a larger population of cells. In other mutants, such as SCA3, Huntington disease, and spinobulbar muscular atrophy, truncated versions of the coding regions are expressed.

Knock-in mice have been generated for Huntington disease and spinocerebellar ataxia types 1 and 7. These models confirm that features other than the length of the expanded glutamine tract affect the toxicity of the tract. As noted above, the same expansion in two different host proteins affects cells differently. For example, in human patients 37 repeats cause SCA2 but not SCA3 (see Figure 44–1 and Table 44–2). In mouse models, however, the relationship of the length of the tract to the rest of a given host protein is a good predictor of toxicity.

Severe, widespread, nonselective neuronal dysfunction occurs in both transgenic mice in which the glutamine tract constitutes a major portion of the protein and mice bearing a truncated protein with a relatively large glutamine tract. In contrast, mice that express full-length proteins containing a CAG repeat develop a neurological syndrome that progresses more slowly. Similarly, weakly expressing promoters generally produce more selective neuronal dysfunction (Figure 44–3). In some cases expression of the full-length protein with even a moderately large expansion does not cause neurological dysfunction, but a truncated version bearing a similar repeat size produces the disease phenotype. In sum, a glutamine tract of a certain length is more toxic when in isolation or flanked by short peptide sequences, that is, when it occupies a larger proportion of the protein.

In knock-in mice with 80 to 111 glutamine repeats, neurological dysfunction is barely detectable; only when the repeat length is expanded to approximately 150 glutamines does a neurological phenotype become apparent. Because polyglutamine toxicity takes time to exert its effects, longer repeats are necessary to see a phenotype during the short life span of a mouse. However, massive overproduction of the mutant protein, as in transgenic mice, can compensate for a moderate

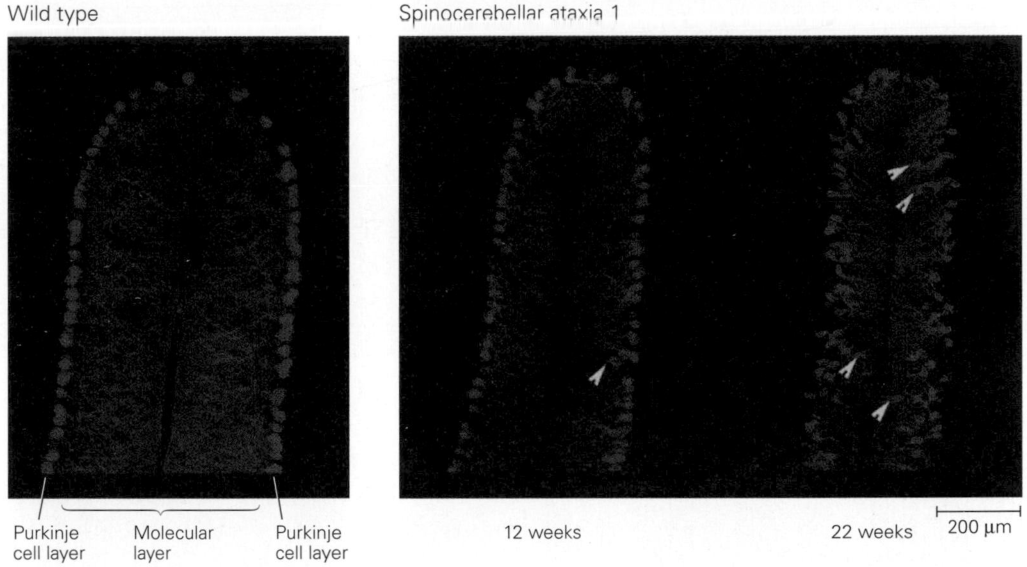

Figure 44–3 Progressive Purkinje cell pathology in a mouse model of spinocerebellar ataxia type 1. Cerebellar sections from a wild-type mouse and mice expressing a spinocerebellar ataxia type 1 (SCA1) transgene with 82 glutamines in Purkinje cells at 12 and 22 weeks of age. Calbindin immunofluorescence staining marks the Purkinje cells and their extensive dendritic arbors. In spinocerebellar ataxia type 1 there is progressive loss of dendrites, thinning of the molecular layer, and Purkinje cell displacement (**yellow arrowheads**). (Images, used with permission, by H.T. Orr.)

repeat length and brevity of exposure to the toxic repeat. Indeed, overproduction of wild-type ataxin 1 or α-synuclein in mice results in mild neurological dysfunction.

Analysis of brain tissue from patients and experimental mice reveals that misfolded proteins tend to accumulate in various neurons, sometimes forming visible aggregates (Figure 44–4). Lewy bodies and abnormal accumulation of α-synuclein, as observed for years in patients, develop in mouse models of Parkinson disease. Although protein accumulation is common to all these neurodegenerative disorders in humans and their respective mouse models, the localization of the accumulated protein in the cell varies, and location within the cell is a factor in the protein's pathogenicity. For example, mutant ataxin 1 that remains in the cytoplasm because of a mutant nuclear-localization signal exerts no detectable toxic effects.

The fact that mutated proteins accumulate in mouse models that do not overproduce the proteins as well as in human patients who carry a single mutant allele suggests that neurons have difficulty clearing the proteins. Support for this hypothesis comes from the finding that ubiquitin and proteasome components, the machinery of protein degradation, localize to the site of protein aggregates in both human and mouse tissues.

Invertebrate Models Manifest Progressive Neurodegeneration

Several invertebrate models have been used to study polyglutamine proteins and α-synuclein. The similarities in the pathogenic effects of these proteins across species are remarkable.

Flies with high levels of human α-synuclein develop age-dependent, progressive degeneration of dopaminergic neurons and have α-synuclein–immunoreactive cytoplasmic aggregates reminiscent of Lewy bodies. As in the mouse model, high levels of either wild-type or mutant α-synuclein in flies induce this phenotype, and the toxic effect of the expanded glutamine tract is reduced as more amino- or carboxyl-terminal amino acids are added to the polypeptide. Overproduction of wild-type or mutant ataxin-1 in flies induces progressive neuronal degeneration that is dependent on protein levels but is more severe for the mutant when protein levels are similar.

Polyglutamine toxicity has also been evaluated in the nematode *Caenorhabditis elegans* by expressing an amino terminal fragment of huntingtin containing glutamine tracts of different length. Neuronal dysfunction and cell death occur in worms expressing expanded alleles.

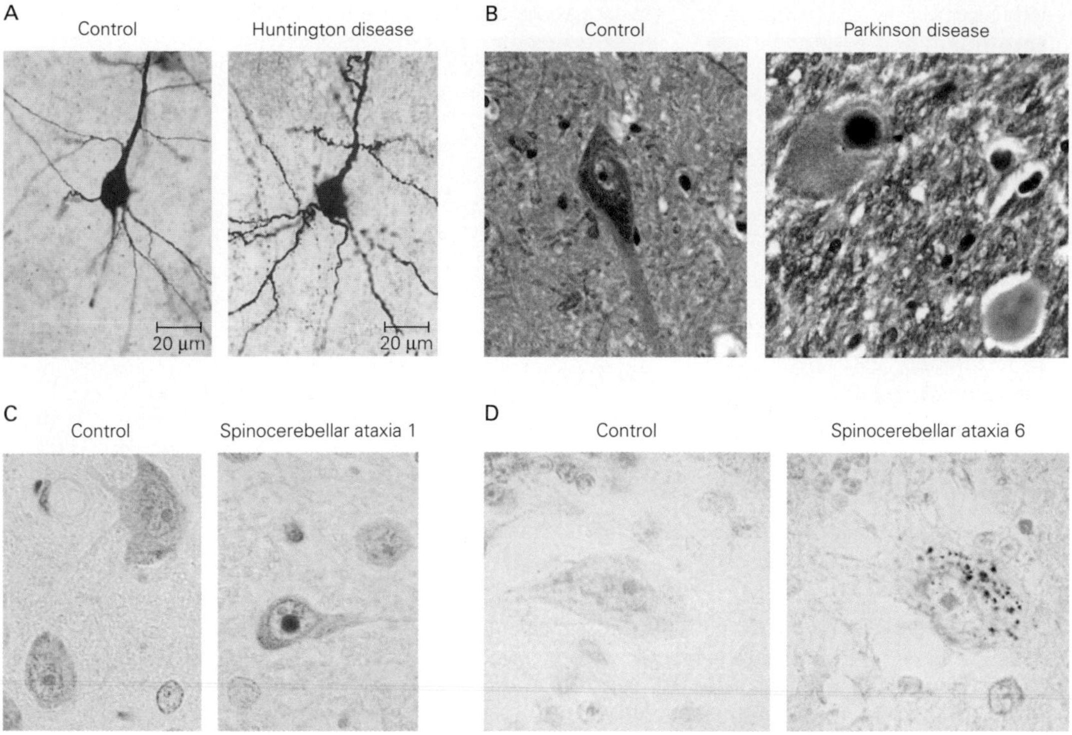

Figure 44–4 Neuropathological features of selected neurodegenerative disorders. (Control images in A, B, C, and D are used, with permission, from J-P Vonsattel. Huntington image (A), used with permission, from M. Di Figlia and J-P. Vonsattel. SCA1 image (C), used with permission, from H. Zoghbi.)

A. Comparison of a normal spiny neuron from the caudate nucleus and a spiny neuron affected by Huntington disease. Note the marked recurving of terminal dendritic branches in the diseased neuron.

B. A pigmented dopaminergic neuron in the substantia nigra with a classic cytoplasmic inclusion (Lewy body). The circular cytoplasmic inclusion is surrounded by a clear halo. Recent electron-microscopic and biochemical evidence indicates that the primary components of Lewy bodies are α-synuclein, ubiquitin, and abnormally phosphorylated neurofilaments that form a nonmembrane-bounded compacted skein in the cell body. Extracellular Lewy bodies occur following neuronal cell death and disintegration.

C. A neuron with a typical nuclear inclusion almost as large as the nucleolus.

D. Because spinocerebellar ataxia type 6 results from a repeat expansion in *CACNA1A,* the gene encoding a calcium channel, it is not surprising that affected neurons do not accumulate nuclear inclusions. *CACNA1A* labeling instead occurs diffusely throughout the cytoplasm.

Several Pathways Underlie the Pathogenesis of Neurodegenerative Diseases

Protein Misfolding and Degradation Contribute to Parkinson Disease

Proteins with expanded glutamine tracts and mutant α-synuclein accumulate in the neurons of patients and various animal models, indicating that these abnormal proteins are not degraded efficiently. Molecular chaperones, which facilitate cell protein refolding and degradation (see Chapter 4), are redistributed to the site of these protein aggregates.

The gradual accumulation of proteins with expanded glutamine tracts along with chaperones and components of the ubiquitin-proteasome degradation pathway, suggests that the glutamine tract expansion alters the folding state of the native protein, which in turn recruits the activity of the protein-folding and degradation machinery. When that machinery cannot process the protein, the protein molecules accumulate, eventually forming aggregates. Wild-type α-synuclein and ataxin-1 may have some tendency to misfold even in the absence of a mutation; when they are produced at sufficiently high levels the number of misfolded molecules increases, and their toxicity becomes apparent.

Evidence in support of this idea first came from studies in cell culture in which overproduction of chaperones both reduces protein aggregation and mitigates the toxicity of expanded glutamine tracts in proteins. In contrast, blocking the proteasome inhibits protein degradation and thus enhances aggregation and toxicity. Genetic studies in flies and mice provide even more compelling evidence. Overproduction of at least one chaperone, such as Hsp70, Hsp40, or tetratricopeptide protein 2, suppresses polyglutamine toxicity in *Drosophila* and mouse models of Parkinson disease and several different ataxias, whereas loss of chaperone function aggravates neurodegeneration (Figure 44–5).

The importance of the ubiquitin-proteasome pathway and protein degradation in the spinocerebellar ataxias is further supported by genetic modification in animal models. In a *Drosophila* model of SCA1, haploinsufficiency for ubiquitin, ubiquitin carrier enzymes, or a ubiquitin carboxyl-terminal hydrolase aggravates neurodegeneration. Loss of function of the E3 ubiquitin ligase Ube3a in mice exacerbates ataxin-1–induced neurodegeneration, even though the Purkinje cells develop no nuclear inclusions. It appears that inclusions are part of the cell's attempt to sequester the mutant protein and thereby limit its toxic effects. Cells that are unable to form aggregates of the mutated proteins suffer the worst damage from polyglutamine toxicity. Indeed, the knock-in mouse models of spinocerebellar ataxia types 1 and 7 show conclusively that cells that form aggregates survive longer; cerebellar Purkinje cells, the prime targets in this disease, are the last to form nuclear aggregates.

Studies of Parkinson disease further underscore the importance of the ubiquitin-proteasome pathway and reveal additional parallels with the polyglutamine diseases. The *parkin* gene, mutated in Parkinson disease type 2, encodes an E3 ubiquitin ligase that has among its targets the O-glycosylated form of α-synuclein. Levels of this glycosylated form of α-synuclein are increased in brains of patients with deformed parkin despite the absence of Lewy bodies. This suggests that Lewy-body formation requires ubiquitination of α-synuclein, and again indicates that the misfolded protein is sequestered when it is not completely degraded.

How do misfolded α-synuclein or expanded glutamine tracts disrupt neuronal function? A protein that resists degradation or has an aberrant conformation might have its normal function in the cell enhanced, as happens with glutamine-expanded ataxin-1. Part of the gain of toxic function involves alterations in gene expression.

Protein Misfolding Triggers Pathological Alterations in Gene Expression

One of the key consequences of misfolding as a result of expanded glutamine tracts is alteration in gene expression. This was first suspected when it was real-

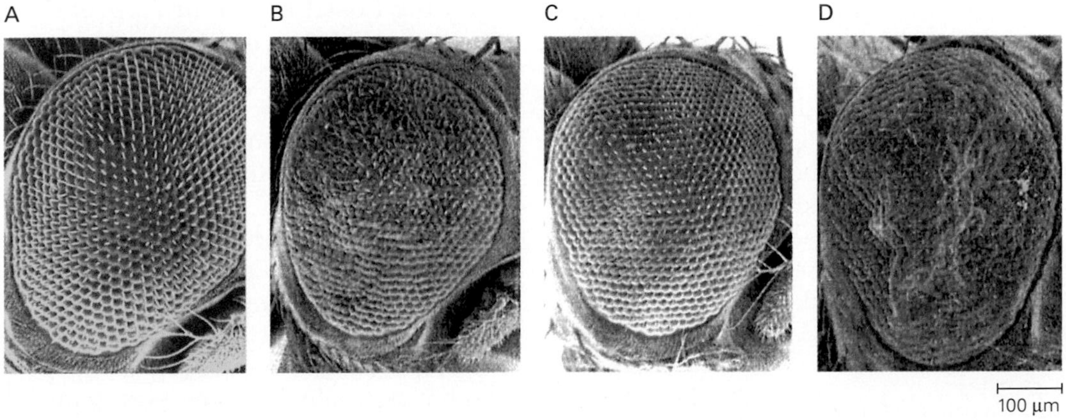

Figure 44–5 Polyglutamine-induced degeneration in the *Drosophila* eye and the effect of modifiers. (Images, used with permission, by J. Botas.)

A. A scanning electron micrograph depicts the eye of a fly with normal ommatidia.

B. Ommatidia of a transgenic fly bearing a protein with expanded glutamine repeats.

C. Owing to the mitigating effect of a heat-shock protein on the polyglutamine-induced phenotype, the ommatidia appear almost normal.

D. Absence of another heat-shock protein aggravates the polyglutamine-induced phenotype.

ized not only that most of the mutant proteins accumulate in the cell nucleus, but also that they interact with or affect the function of key transcriptional regulators. For example, CREB-binding protein interacts with huntingtin exon 1. Moreover, overproduction of polyglutamine proteins reduces levels of histone acetylation in cells, an effect that can be reversed by overproduction of CREB-binding protein.

Alterations in gene expression are among the earliest events in pathogenesis, occurring within days of expression of the mutant transgene in mouse models of SCA1 and Huntington disease. Many of the genes whose expression is altered are involved in Ca^{2+} homeostasis, synaptic transmission, and transduction of sensory events into neural signals. In fly models of SCA1 several modifiers of the neurodegenerative phenotype are transcriptional cofactors. Alterations in gene expression may also occur because of altered RNA processing or stability. Ataxin-1 binds RNAs in vitro, and several genetic modifiers in fly models of SCA1 encode proteins involved in RNA binding or processing.

Mitochondrial Dysfunction Exacerbates Neurodegenerative Disease

Evidence for mitochondrial dysfunction in polyglutamine disorders and Parkinson disease comes from morphological and functional studies. Lymphoblast mitochondria from patients with Huntington disease as well as brain mitochondria from a transgenic mouse model for Huntington disease have a lower membrane potential and depolarize at lower Ca^{2+} loads than do control mitochondria.

Several proteins implicated in Parkinson disease affect mitochondrial function and integrity. For example, in *Drosophila* the loss of PINK1 leads to mitochondrial dysfunction that can be rescued by parkin. LRRK2, which interacts with parkin, is localized in part to the outer mitochondrial membrane. Thus, given the functions and interactions of these proteins, mitochondrial dysfunction is likely to be a key contributor to the Parkinson disease phenotype.

Apoptosis and Caspase Modify the Severity of Neurodegeneration

Although animal studies of most neurodegenerative diseases have demonstrated that symptoms appear long before detectable cell death, loss of neurons is a hallmark of the end stage of all these disorders. Although many factors are implicated in the death of neurons, such as altered Ca^{2+} homeostasis and decreased induction of neuronal survival factors (eg, brain-derived neurotrophic factor in Huntington disease), there is specific evidence that the caspase activity critical for apoptosis is a contributing factor in neurodegenerative diseases. Some of the polyglutamine proteins, such as huntingtin, AR, ataxin-3, and atrophin-1, are substrates for caspases in vitro. This raises the possibility that the proteases liberate the fragments of these proteins with expanded glutamine tracts. As discussed earlier, such fragments are even more damaging than the full-length protein.

Intranuclear huntingtin increases production of caspase-1 in cells; this could lead to apoptosis and caspase-3 activation. Hip-1, a protein that interacts with huntingtin, forms a complex that activates caspase-8. This process might be enhanced by the glutamine expansion in huntingtin, because Hip-1 binds less avidly to mutant huntingtin than to the wild-type protein. In *Drosophila* production of the anti-apoptotic protein p35 results in partial rescue of the pigment loss induced by mutant ataxin-3.

In summary, expansions of polyglutamine tracts as well as several missense mutations in proteins implicated in neurodegenerative diseases alter the host protein, leading to its accumulation or abnormal interactions. The neuronal dysfunction results from the downstream effects of such abnormal interactions (Figure 44–6).

Advances in Understanding the Molecular Basis of Neurodegenerative Diseases Are Opening Possibilities for Approaches to Therapeutic Intervention

The discovery of the genetic bases and pathogenic mechanisms of various neurodegenerative diseases gives us hope that therapies for these diseases will soon emerge.

Dopamine replacement therapy has so far been the only option for Parkinson disease and other conditions with parkinsonian features, but it is not ideal. Patients tend to develop tolerance and require higher and higher doses of the drugs. Side effects therefore become as troubling as the symptoms being treated. Patients with Huntington disease and spinocerebellar ataxia are in a worse state: There are no treatments that slow the progressive loss of motor coordination.

The identification of protein misfolding as a key step in pathogenesis has led investigators to search for drugs that safely induce chaperone activity and that can be tested in the various animal models. Geldanamycin, a drug known to activate heat-shock

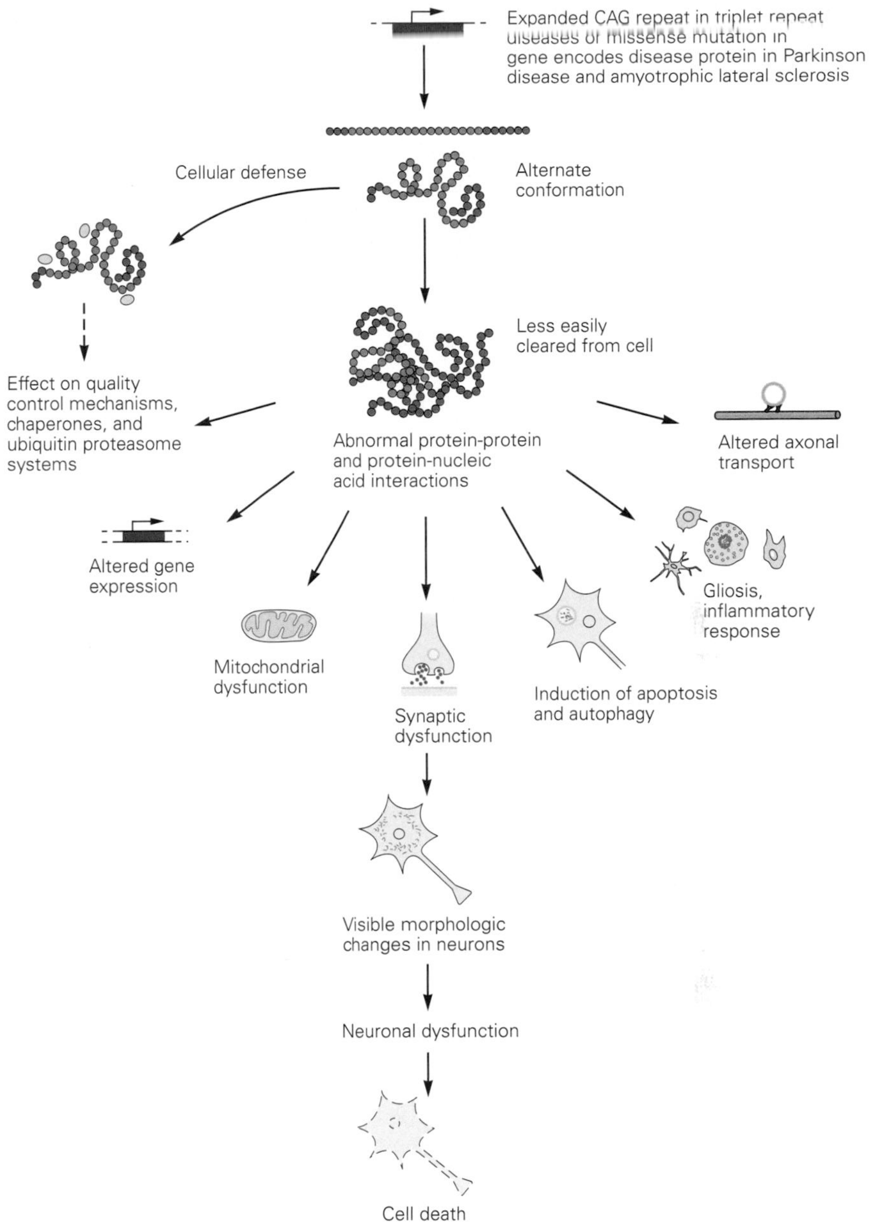

Figure 44–6 Current model for pathogenesis of the proteinopathies. The disease-causing protein adopts an alternative conformation that changes its interactions with other proteins, DNA, or RNA, altering gene expression and perhaps generating an inflammatory response. These early events in pathogenesis occur years before symptoms appear. This alternative conformation is also more difficult for the cell to refold or degrade; the mutant protein accumulates slowly, over a period of decades. As levels of the mutant protein rise, aggregates form. These protein deposits represent the cell's attempt at sequestering the mutant protein, but as the disease progresses they may themselves affect protein interactions or compromise the protein quality-control system.

chaperones, suppresses polyglutamine-induced protein aggregation and toxicity in cell culture. Because some glutamine-expanded proteins interact with or sequester CREB-binding protein, a protein with histone acetylase activity, inhibitors of histone deacetylase such as sodium butyrate and suberoylanilide hydroxamic acid have been used in mammalian cells, yeast cells, and *Drosophila* models expressing a polypeptide with an expanded glutamine tract. These treatments suppress cell death and improve the viability of cells of fruit flies—a very promising finding.

Cystamine, an inhibitor of the transglutaminase that is thought to promote protein aggregation, improves neuronal function. Moreover, caspase inhibitors enhance the survival of mice expressing an expanded glutamine tract in huntingtin exon 1. These results suggest that several pathways can be targeted for therapeutic intervention. Ideally, therapies would be targeted at some of the earliest pathogenic stages, at which neuronal dysfunction rather than cell death causes the neurological phenotype. Intervention at an early stage could prove beneficial clinically, for it might halt the disease and even allow recovery of function. Indeed, in mouse models of Huntington disease and SCA1 in which expression of the mutant gene can be turned on and off, neuronal dysfunction is reversible. When expression of the transgene is turned off, the neurons have a chance to clear the mutant polyglutamine protein and regain normal activity.

Because most neurodegenerative diseases progress over a period of decades, pharmacological interventions that even slightly modulate one or more of the pathways described earlier could delay disease progression or modestly improve function, which would greatly enhance the quality of life for patients suffering from these devastating disorders.

An Overall View

The identification of genes causing several forms of Parkinson disease and the various polyglutamine neurodegenerative diseases has allowed the accurate diagnosis and classification of these clinically heterogeneous disorders. More importantly, studies in cell culture and model organisms have revealed a pathogenic mechanism common to all of these diseases: protein misfolding. Mutations that cause the respective proteins to adopt an altered conformation gradually induce neuronal dysfunction either because of abnormal protein interactions or because of intracellular protein accumulation and altered activity. The identification of pathways that mediate some of the pathogenic effects is likely to lead to the discovery of drugs that can first be tested in model animals and then applied in humans.

Huda Y. Zoghbi

Selected Readings

Gatchel JR, Zoghbi HY. 2005. Diseases of unstable repeat expansion: mechanisms and common principles. Nat Rev Genet 6:743–755.

Giasson BI, Lee VM. 2001. Parkin and the molecular pathways of Parkinson's disease. Neuron 31:885–888.

Gusella JF, MacDonald ME. 2000. Molecular genetics: unmasking polyglutamine triggers in neurodegenerative disease. Nat Rev Neurosci 1:109–115.

Laforet GA, Sapp E, Chase K, McIntyre C, Boyce FM, Campbell M, Cadigan BA, et al. 2001. Changes in cortical and striatal neurons predict behavioral and electrophysiological abnormalities in a transgenic murine model of Huntington's disease. J Neurosci 21:9112–9123.

Moore DJ, West AB, Dawson VL, Dawson TM. 2005. Molecular pathophysiology of Parkinson's disease. Annu Rev Neurosci 28:57–87.

Orr HT. 2001. Beyond the Qs in the polyglutamine diseases. Genes Dev 15:8 925–932.

Sherman MY, Goldberg AL. 2001. Cellular defenses against unfolded proteins: a cell biologist thinks about neurodegenerative diseases. Neuron 1:15–32.

Steffan JS, Bodai L, Pallos J, Poelman M, McCampbell A, Apostol BL, Kazantsev A, et al. 2001. Histone deacetylase inhibitors arrest polyglutamine-dependent neurodegeneration in *Drosophila*. Nature 413:739–743.

Zoghbi HY, Botas J. 2002. Mouse and fly models of neurodegeneration. Trends Genet 18:463–471.

References

Auluck PK, Chan HY, Trojanowski JQ, Lee VM, Bonini NM. 2002. Chaperone suppression of α-synuclein toxicity in a *Drosophila* model for Parkinson's disease. Science 295:865–888.

Bonifati V, Oostra BA, Heutink P. 2004. Linking DJ-1 to neurodegeneration offers novel insights for understanding the pathogenesis of Parkinson's disease. J Mol Med 82:163–74.

Chai Y, Koppenhafer SL, Bonini NM, Paulson HL. 1999. Analysis of the role of heat shock protein (Hsp) molecular chaperones in polyglutamine disease. J Neurosci 19:10338–10347.

Chung KK, Zhang Y, Lim KL, Tanaka Y, Huang H, Gao J, Ross CA, Dawson VL, Dawson TM. 2001. Parkin ubiquitinates the α-synuclein-interacting protein, synphilin-1: implications for Lewy-body formation in Parkinson disease. Nat Med 7:1144–1150.

Clark IE, Dodson MW, Jiang C, Cao JH, Huh JR, Seol JH, Yoo SJ, Hay BA, Guo M. 2006. *Drosophila* pink1 is required for mitochondrial function and interacts genetically with parkin. Nature 441:1162–1166.

Cummings CJ, Mancini MA, Antalffy B, DeFranco DB, Orr HT, Zoghbi H. 1998. Chaperone suppression of ataxin-1 aggregation and altered subcellular proteasome localization imply protein misfolding in SCA1. Nat Genet 19:148–154.

Cummings CJ, Reinstein E, Sun Y, Antalffy B, Jiang Y-h, Ciechanover A, Orr HT, Beaudet AL, Zoghbi HY. 1999. Mutation of the E6-AP ubiquitin ligase reduces nuclear inclusion frequency while accelerating polyglutamine-induced pathology in SCA1 transgenic mice. Neuron 24:879–892.

Cummings CJ, Sun Y, Opal P, Antalffy B, Mestril R, Orr HT, Dillmann WH, Zoghbi HY. 2001. Over-expression of inducible HSP70 chaperone suppresses neuropathology and improves motor function in *SCA1* mice. Hum Mol Genet 10:1511–1518.

Feany MB, Bender WW. 2000. A *Drosophila* model of Parkinson's disease. Nature 404:394–398.

Fernandez-Funez P, Nino-Rosales ML, de Gouyon B, She WC, Luchak JM, Martinez P, Turiegano E, et al. 2000. Identification of genes that modify ataxin-1-induced neurodegeneration. Nature 408:101–106.

Funayama M, Hasegawa K, Kowa H, Saito M, Tsuji S, Obata F. 2002. A new locus for Parkinson's disease (PARK8) maps to chromosome 12p11.2-q13.1. Ann Neurol 51:296–301.

Hagerman RJ, Hagerman PJ. 2002. The fragile X premutation: into the phenotypic fold. Curr Opin Genet Dev 12:278–283.

Hegde AN, Inokuchi K, Pei W, Casadio A, Ghirardi M, Chain DG, Martin KC, Kandel ER, Schwartz JH. 1997. Ubiquitin C-terminal hydrolase is an immediate-early gene essential for long-term facilitation in *Aplysia*. Cell 89:115–126.

Holmes SE, O'Hearn EE, McInnis MG, Gorelick-Feldman DA, Kleiderlein JJ, Callahan C, Kwak NG, et al. 1999. Expansion of a novel CAG trinucleotide repeat in the 5′ region of PPP2R2B is associated with SCA12. Nat Genet 23:391–392.

Holmes SE, O'Hearn E, Rosenblatt A, Callahan C, Hwang HS, Ingersoll-Ashworth RG, Fleisher A, et al. 2001. A repeat expansion in the gene encoding junctophilin-3 is associated with Huntington disease-like 2. Nat Genet 29:377–378. (Erratum in: Nat Genet 2002 30:123.)

Huynh DP, Del Bigio MR, Ho DH, Pulst SM. 1999. Expression of ataxin-2 in brains from normal individuals and patients with Alzheimer's disease and spinocerebellar ataxia 2. Ann Neurol 45:232–241.

Huynh DP, Figueroa K, Hoang N, Pulst SM. 2000. Nuclear localization or inclusion body formation of ataxin-2 are not necessary for SCA2 pathogenesis in mouse or human. Nat Genet 26:44–50.

Imai Y, Soda M, Inoue H, Hattori N, Mizuno Y, Takahashi R. 2001. An unfolded putative transmembrane polypeptide, which can lead to endoplasmic reticulum stress, is a substrate of Parkin. Cell 105:891–902.

Karpuj MV, Becher MW, Springer JE, Chabas D, Youssef S, Pedotti R, Mitchell D, Steinman L. 2002. Prolonged survival and decreased abnormal movements in transgenic model of Huntington disease, with administration of the transglutaminase inhibitor cystamine. Nat Med 8: 143–149.

Kazemi-Esfarjani P, Benzer S. 2000. Genetic suppression of polyglutamine toxicity in *Drosophila*. Science 287: 1837–1840.

Kitada T, Asakawa S, Hattori N, Matsumine H, Yamamura Y, Minoshima S, Yokochi M, Mizuno Y, Shimizu N. 1998. Mutations in the *parkin* gene cause autosomal recessive juvenile parkinsonism. Nature 392:605–608.

Koob MD, Moseley ML, Schut LJ, Benzow KA, Bird TD, Day JW, Ranum LP. 1999. An untranslated CTG expansion causes a novel form of spinocerebellar ataxia (SCA8). Nat Genet 21:379–384.

Kruger R, Kuhn W, Muller T, Woitalla D, Graeber M, Kosel S, Przuntek H, Epplen JT, Schols L, Riess O. 1998. Ala30Pro mutation in the gene encoding α-synuclein in Parkinson's disease. Nat Genet 18:106–108.

La Spada AR, Fu YH, Sopher BL, Libby RT, Wang X, Li LY, Einum DD, et al. 2001. Polyglutamine-expanded ataxin-7 antagonizes CRX function and induces cone-rod dystrophy in a mouse model of SCA7. Neuron 31:913–927.

Leroy E, Boyer R, Auburger G, Leube B, Ulm G, Mezey E, Harta G, et al. 1998. The ubiquitin pathway in Parkinson's disease. Nature 395:451–452.

Lin X, Antalffy B, Kang D, Orr HT, Zoghbi HY. 2000. Polyglutamine expansion down-regulates specific neuronal genes before pathologic changes in SCA1. Nat Neurosci 3:157–163.

Lucking CB, Durr A, Bonifati V, Vaughan J, De Michele G, Gasser T, Harhangi BS, et al. 2000. Association between early-onset Parkinson's disease and mutations in the *parkin* gene. French Parkinson's Disease Genetics Study Group. N Engl J Med 342:1560–1567.

Luthi-Carter R, Strand A, Peters NL, Solano SM, Hollingsworth ZR, Menon AS, Frey AS, et al. 2000. Decreased expression of striatal signaling genes in a mouse model of Huntington's disease. Hum Mol Genet 9:1259–1271.

Masliah E, Rockenstein E, Veinbergs I, Mallory M, Hashimoto M, Takeda A, Sagara Y, Sisk A, Mucke L. 2000. Dopaminergic loss and inclusion body formation in α-synuclein mice: implications for neurodegenerative disorders. Science 287:1265–1269.

Matsuura T, Yamagata T, Burgess DL, Rasmussen A, Grewal RP, Watase K, Khajavi M, et al. 2000. Large expansion of the ATTCT pentanucleotide repeat in spinocerebellar ataxia type 10. Nat Genet 26:191–194.

McCampbell A, Taye AA, Whitty L, Penney E, Steffan JS, Fischbeck KH. 2001. Histone deacetylase inhibitors reduce polyglutamine toxicity. Proc Natl Acad Sci U S A 98:15179–15184.

Nakamura K, Jeong SY, Uchihara T, Anno M, Nagashima K, Nagashima T, Ikeda S, Tsuji S, Kanazawa I. 2001. SCA17, a novel autosomal dominant cerebellar ataxia caused by an expanded polyglutamine in TATA-binding protein. Hum Mol Genet 10:1441–1448.

Nucifora FC, Sasaki M, Peters MF, Huang H, Cooper JK, Yamada M, Takahashi H, et al. 2001. Interference by huntingtin and atrophin-1 with cbp-mediated transcription leading to cellular toxicity. Science 291:2423–2428.

Orr HT, Zoghbi HY. 2007. Trinucleotide repeat disorders. In Annu Rev Neurosci 30:575–621.

Panov AV, Gutekunst CA, Leavitt BR, Hayden MR, Burke JR, Strittmatter WJ, Greenamyre JT. 2002. Early mitochondrial calcium defects in Huntington's disease are a direct effect of polyglutamines. Nat Neurosci 5:731–736.

Park J, Lee SB, Lee S, Kim Y, Song S, Kim S, Bae E, et al. 2006. Mitochondrial dysfunction in *Drosophila* pink1 mutants is complemented by parkin. Nature 441:1157–1161.

Piedras-Renteria ES, Watase K, Harata N, Zhuchenko O, Zoghbi HY, Lee CC, Tsien RW. 2001. Increased expression of alpha 1A Ca^{2+} channel currents arising from expanded trinucleotide repeats in spinocerebellar ataxia type 6. J Neurosci 21:9185–9193.

Polymeropoulos MH, Lavedan C, Leroy E, Ide SE, Dehejia A, Dutra A, Pike B, et al. 1997. Mutation in the *α-synuclein* gene identified in families with Parkinson's disease. Science 276:2045–2047.

Shimura H, Schlossmacher MG, Hattori N, Frosch MP, Trockenbacher A, Schneider R, Mizuno Y, Kosik KS, Selkoe DJ. 2001. Ubiquitination of a new form of α-synuclein by parkin from human brain: implications for Parkinson's disease. Science 293:263–269.

Singleton AB, Farrer M, Johnson J, Singleton A, Hague S, Kachergus J, Hulihan M, et al. 2003. *α-Synuclein* locus triplication causes Parkinson's disease. Science 302:841.

Sittler A, Lurz R, Lueder G, Priller J, Lehrach H, Hayer-Hartl MK, Hartl FU, Wanker EE. 2001. Geldanamycin activates a heat shock response and inhibits huntingtin aggregation in a cell culture model of Huntington's disease. Hum Mol Genet 10:1307–1315.

Smith WW, Pei Z, Jiang H, Moore DJ, Liang Y, WestAB, Dawson VL, Dawson TM, Ross CA. 2005. Leucine-rich repeat kinase 2 (LRRK2) interacts with parkin, and mutant LRRK2 induces neuronal degeneration. Proc Natl Acad Sci U S A 102:18676–18681.

Valente EM, Abou-Sleiman PM, Caputo V, Muqit MM, Harvey K, Gispert S, Ali Z, et al. 2004. Hereditary early-onset Parkinson's disease caused by mutations in PINK1. Science. 304:1158–60.

van der Putten H, Wiederhold KH, Probst A, Barbieri S, Mistl C, Danner S, Kauffmann S, et al. 2000. Neuropathology in mice expressing human α-synuclein. J Neurosci 20: 6021–6029.

Vonsattel JP, DiFiglia M. 1998. Huntington disease. J Neuropathol Exp Neurol 57:369–384.

Warrick JM, Chan HY, Gray-Board GL, Chai Y, Paulson HL, Bonini NM. 1999. Suppression of polyglutamine-mediated neurodegeneration in *Drosophila* by the molecular chaperone HSP70. Nat Genet 23:425–428.

Zhang S, Xu L, Lee J, Xu T. 2002. *Drosophila* atrophin homolog functions as a transcriptional corepressor in multiple developmental processes. Cell 108:45–56.

Zhang Y, Gao J, Chung KK, Huang H, Dawson VL, Dawson TM. 2000. Parkin functions as an E2-dependent ubiquitin- protein ligase and promotes the degradation of the synaptic vesicle-associated protein, CDCrel-1. Proc Natl Acad Sci U S A 97:13354–13359.

Zu T, Duvick LA, Kaytor MD, Berlinger MS, Zoghbi HY, Clark HB, Orr HT. 2004. Recovery from polyglutamine-induced neurodegeneration in conditional SCA1 transgenic mice. J Neurosci 24:8853–8861.

Zuccato C, Ciammola A, Rigamonti D, Leavitt BR, Goffredo D, Conti L, MacDonald ME, et al. 2001. Loss of huntingtin-mediated BDNF gene transcription in Huntington's disease. Science 293:493–498.

Part VII

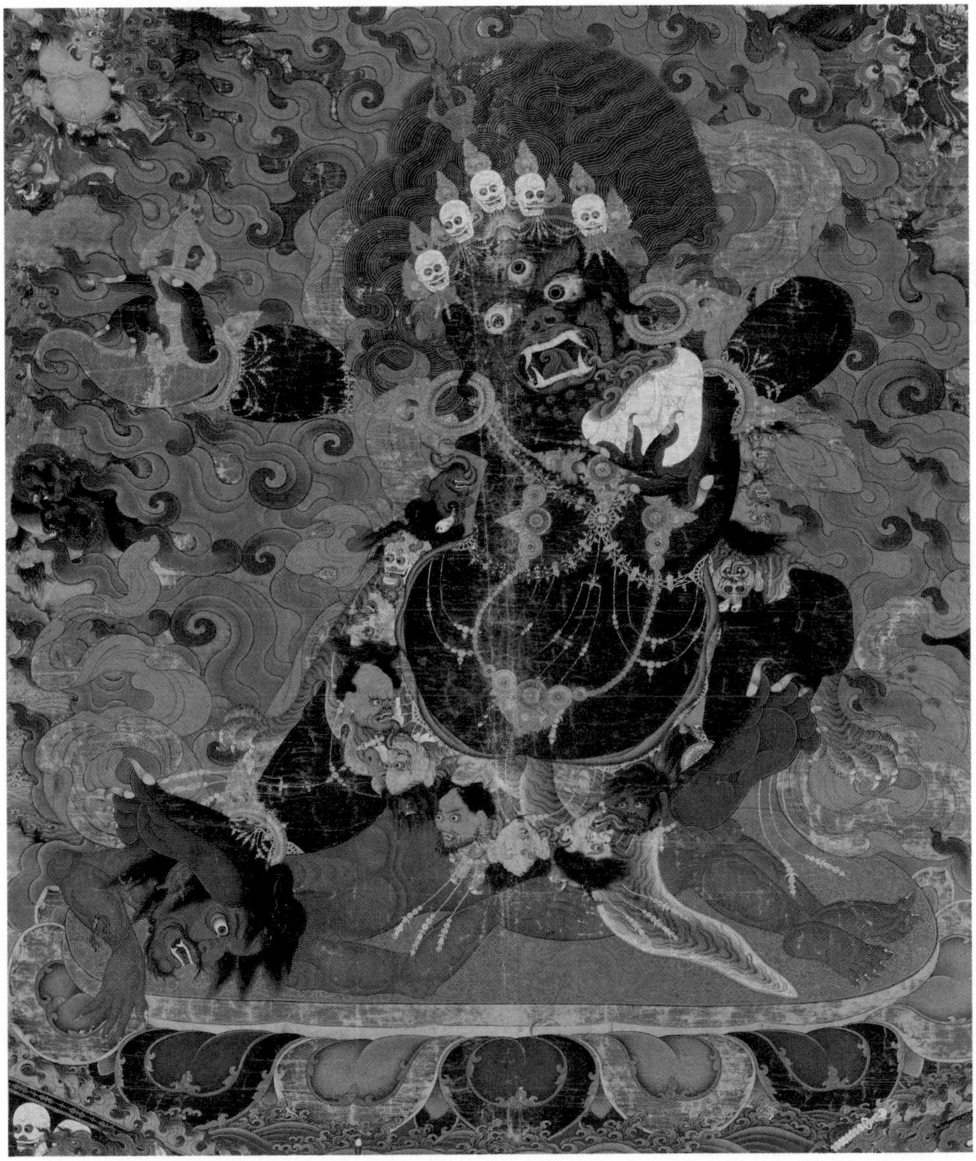

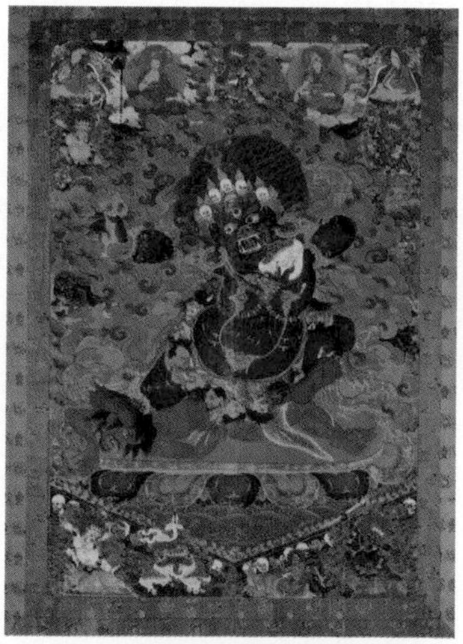

Preceding Page

Painting of Yama, the Indian God of death, made in Tibet around the 17th century. In Tibetan Buddhism Yama protects people against emotional addictions such as lust and hate. While religion, mythology, and medicine have been invoked throughout history to explain our emotions and control our appetites, Buddhism has articulated particularly well the perils of human craving and the benefits of expanding the scope of the conscious mind. This is a detail of the full painting shown above. (Reproduced, with permission, from image copyright: the Metropolitan Museum of Art; image source: Art Resource, NY.)

VII The Unconscious and Conscious Processing of Neural Information

MANY ASPECTS OF BEHAVIOR, ESPECIALLY EMOTIONAL and homeostatic behaviors, are unconscious and instinctive. They are mediated almost reflexively by systems in subcortical brain regions that are concerned with feeding, drinking, temperature regulation, and sex.

Thus, as Sigmund Freud first pointed out in 1900, we experience emotional states not only consciously but also unconsciously. Many of these emotional states, particularly those involving fear, depend on the amygdala, a subcortical region of the limbic system. The cognitive elements in emotions, which we call *feeling states*, are thought to be mediated by pathways to the cerebral cortex that originate from the musculature of the body and the internal organs, on the one hand, and from the amygdala, on the other hand. In contrast, unconscious emotional states are thought to depend on autonomic, endocrine, and skeletal motor responses in subcortical parts of the nervous system, especially connections between the nuclei of the amygdala, the hypothalamus, and the brain stem. These unconscious responses can prepare the body for action and communicate internal emotional states to other individuals. An emerging realization in the neurobiology of emotion is that an unconscious representation of our emotional state by the amygdala can lead to a somatic response that often precedes our cognitive awareness—our feeling—of an emotional state. This conscious feeling state presumably involves the cerebral cortex, the outer layer of the brain. When the function of the cerebral cortex is temporarily disrupted, as in an epileptic convulsion, we lose all sense of emotion and feeling, and commonly, we lose consciousness.

We begin our consideration of these systems with the brain stem, a structure critical for wakefulness and conscious attention on the one hand and sleep on the other. Thus, the significance of this small region of the central nervous system—located between the spinal cord and the diencephalon—is disproportionate to its size. Damage to the brain stem can profoundly affect motor and sensory processes because the brain stem contains all of the ascending tracts that bring sensory information from the surface of the body to the cerebral cortex and all the descending tracts from the cerebral cortex that deliver motor commands to the spinal cord. Damage to the brain stem also can affect consciousness and sleep because the brain stem contains the locus ceruleus, a center thought to be crucial for attention and therefore for many cognitive functions. In fact, fully half of all noradrenergic neurons of the brain are clustered together in this small nucleus. Finally, the brain stem contains neurons that control respiration and heartbeat as well as nuclei that give rise to most of the cranial nerves that innervate the head and neck.

Six neurochemical modulatory systems in the brain stem regulate sensory, motor, and arousal systems. The dopaminergic pathways that connect the midbrain to the limbic system and cortex are particularly important because they are involved in reinforcement of behavior and therefore contribute to motivational state and learning. Addictive drugs such as nicotine, alcohol, opiates, and cocaine are thought to produce their actions by co-opting the same neural pathways that positively reinforce behaviors essential for survival. Other modulatory transmitters regulate sleep and wakefulness, in part by controlling information flow between the thalamus and cortex. Disorders of electrical excitation in corticothalamic circuits can result in seizures and epilepsy.

Rostral to the brain stem lies the hypothalamus, one of whose functions is to maintain the stability of the internal environment by keeping physiological variables within the limits favorable to vital bodily processes. Homeostatic processes in the nervous system have profound consequences for behavior that have intrigued many of the founders of modern physiology, including Claude Bernard, Walter B. Cannon, and Walter Hess. Neurons controlling the internal environment are concentrated in the hypothalamus, a small area of the diencephalon that comprises less than 1% of the total volume of the brain. The hypothalamus, with closely linked structures in the brain stem and limbic system, acts directly on the internal environment through its control of the endocrine system and autonomic nervous system to achieve goal-directed behavior. It acts indirectly through its connections to higher brain regions to control emotional and motivational states. In addition to regulating specific motivated behaviors, the hypothalamus, together with the brain stem below and the cerebral cortex above, maintains a general state of arousal, which ranges from excitement and vigilance to drowsiness and stupor.

Part VII

45

The Sensory, Motor, and Reflex Functions of the Brain Stem

In primitive vertebrates—reptiles, amphibians, and fish—the forebrain is only a small part of the brain and is devoted mainly to olfactory processing and to the integration of autonomic and endocrine function with the basic behaviors necessary for survival. These basic behaviors include feeding, drinking, sexual reproduction, sleep, and emergency responses. Although we are accustomed to thinking that human behavior originates mainly in the forebrain, many complex responses, such as feeding—the coordination of chewing, licking, and swallowing—are actually made up of relatively simple, stereotypic motor responses governed by ensembles of neurons in the brain stem.

The importance of this pattern of organization in human behavior is clear from observing infants born without a forebrain (hydrancephaly). Hydrancephalic infants are surprisingly difficult to distinguish from normal babies. They cry, smile, suckle, and move their eyes, face, arms, and legs. As these sad cases illustrate, the brain stem can organize virtually all of the behavior of the newborn.

In this chapter we examine the role of the brain stem in reflex behavior. We also review the cranial nerves, their origin in the brain stem, as well as the ensembles of local circuit neurons that organize the simple behaviors of the face and head.

The brain stem is the rostral continuation of the spinal cord and its motor and sensory components are similar in structure to that of the spinal cord. But the portions of the brain stem that control the cranial nerves are much more complex than the corresponding parts of the spinal cord that control the spinal nerves because cranial nerves mediate more complex behaviors. The core of the brain stem, the *reticular formation,* is homologous to the intermediate gray matter of the spinal cord but is also more complex. Like the spinal cord, the reticular formation contains ensembles of local-circuit interneurons that generate motor and autonomic patterns and coordinate reflexes and simple behaviors. In addition, it contains clusters of dopaminergic, noradrenergic, and other modulatory neurons that act to optimize the functions of the nervous system. The modulatory actions of these nuclei are described in the next chapter.

The Cranial Nerves Are Homologous to the Spinal Nerves

Because the spinal nerves reach only as high as the first cervical vertebra, the cranial nerves provide the somatic and visceral sensory and motor innervation for the head. Two cranial nerves, the glossopharyngeal and vagus nerves, also supply visceral sensory and motor innervation of the neck, chest, and most of the abdominal organs with the exception of the pelvis. Unlike the spinal nerves, which supply all sensory and motor functions for specific body segments, each cranial nerve is associated with one or more functions and may therefore overlap the physical territory of another cranial nerve.

Assessment of the cranial nerves is an important part of the neurological examination (see Appendix B) because abnormalities of function can pinpoint a site in the brain stem that has been damaged. Therefore, it is important to know the origins of the cranial nerves, their intracranial course, and where they exit from the skull.

The cranial nerves are traditionally numbered I through XII in rostrocaudal sequence. Cranial nerves I and II enter at the base of the forebrain. The other cranial nerves arise from the brain stem at characteristic locations (Figure 45–1). All but one exit from the ventral surface of the brain stem. The exception is the trochlear (IV) nerve, which leaves the midbrain from its dorsal surface just behind the inferior colliculus and wraps around the lateral surface of the brain stem to join the other cranial nerves concerned with eye movements. The cranial nerves with sensory functions (V, VII, VIII, IX, and X) have associated sensory ganglia that operate much as dorsal root ganglia do for spinal nerves. These ganglia are located along the course of individual nerves as they enter the skull.

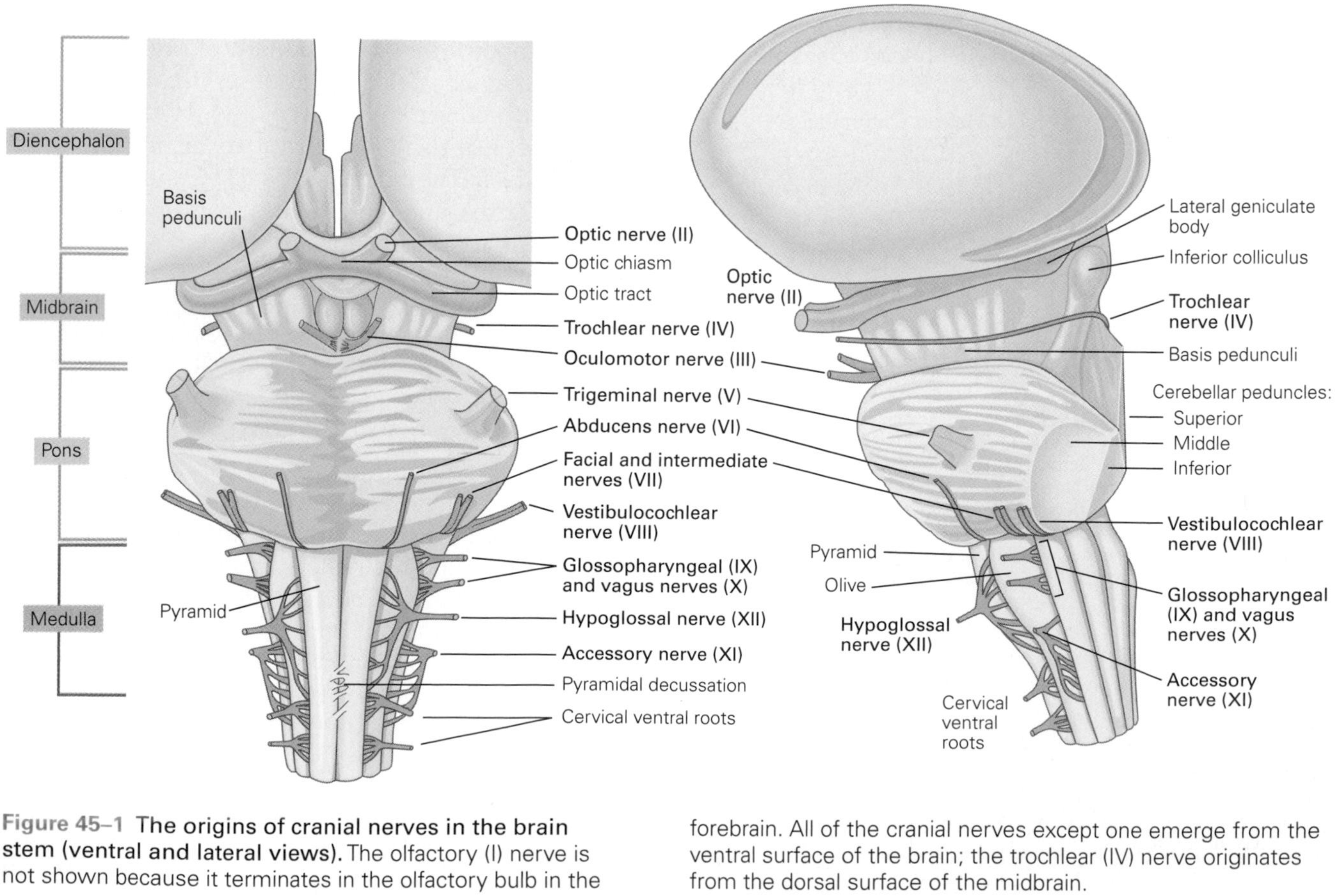

Figure 45–1 The origins of cranial nerves in the brain stem (ventral and lateral views). The olfactory (I) nerve is not shown because it terminates in the olfactory bulb in the forebrain. All of the cranial nerves except one emerge from the ventral surface of the brain; the trochlear (IV) nerve originates from the dorsal surface of the midbrain.

The olfactory (I) nerve, which is associated with the forebrain, is described in detail in Chapter 32; the optic (II) nerve, which is associated with the diencephalon, is described in Chapters 25 and 26. The spinal accessory (XI) nerve can be considered a cranial nerve anatomically but actually is a spinal nerve originating from the higher cervical motor rootlets. It runs up into the skull before exiting through the jugular foramen to innervate the trapezius and sternocleidomastoid muscles in the neck.

Cranial Nerves Mediate the Sensory and Motor Functions of the Face and Head and the Autonomic Functions of the Body

The *ocular motor nerves*—the oculomotor (III), trochlear (IV), and abducens (VI) nerves—control movements of the eyes. The abducens nerve has the simplest action; it contracts the lateral rectus muscle to move the globe laterally. The trochlear nerve also innervates a single muscle, the superior oblique, but its action both depresses the eye and rotates it inward, depending on the eye's position. The oculomotor nerve supplies all of the other muscles of the orbit, including the retractor of the lid. It also provides the parasympathetic innervation responsible for pupillary constriction in response to light and accommodation of the lens for near vision. The ocular motor system is considered in detail in Chapter 39.

The *trigeminal* (V) *nerve* is a mixed nerve (containing both sensory and motor axons) that leaves the brain stem in two roots. The motor root innervates the muscles of mastication (the masseter, temporalis, and pterygoids) and a few muscles of the palate (tensor veli palatini), inner ear (tensor tympani), and upper neck (mylohyoid and anterior belly of the digastric muscle).

The sensory fibers arise from neurons in the trigeminal ganglion, located at the floor of the skull in the middle cranial fossa, the central division of the skull, adjacent to the sella turcica, which houses the pituitary gland.

Three branches emerge from the trigeminal ganglion. The *ophthalmic division* (V_1) runs with the ocular motor nerves through the superior orbital fissure (Figure 45–2A) to innervate the orbit, nose, and forehead and scalp back to the vertex of the skull (Figure 45–3). Some fibers from this division also innervate the meninges and blood vessels of the anterior and middle intracranial fossas. The *maxillary division* (V_2) runs through the round foramen of the sphenoid bone to innervate the skin over the cheek and the upper portion of the oral cavity. The *mandibular division* (V_3), which also contains the motor axons of the trigeminal nerve, leaves the skull through the oval foramen of the sphenoid bone. It innervates the skin over the jaw, the area above the ear, and the lower part of the oral cavity, including the tongue.

Complete trigeminal sensory loss results in numbness of the entire face and the inside of the mouth. One-sided trigeminal motor weakness does not cause much weakness of jaw closure because the muscles of mastication on either side are sufficient to close the jaw. Nevertheless, the jaw tends to deviate toward the side of the lesion when the mouth is opened because the internal pterygoid muscle on the opposite side, when unopposed, pulls the jaw toward the weak side.

The *facial* (VII) *nerve* is also a mixed nerve. Its motor root supplies the muscles of facial expression as well as the stapedius muscle in the inner ear, stylohyoid muscle, and posterior belly of the digastric muscle in the upper neck. The sensory root runs as a separate bundle, the nervus intermedius, through the internal auditory canal and arises from neurons in the geniculate ganglion, located near the middle ear. Distal to the geniculate ganglion the sensory fibers diverge from the motor branch. Some innervate skin of the external auditory canal whereas others form the chorda tympani, which joins the lingual nerve and conveys taste sensation from the anterior two-thirds of the tongue. The *autonomic component* of the facial nerve includes parasympathetic fibers that travel through the motor root to the sphenopalatine and submandibular ganglia, which innervate lacrimal and salivary glands (except the parotid gland) and the cerebral vasculature.

The facial nerve may suffer isolated injury in Bell's palsy, a common complication of certain viral infections. Early on the patient may complain mainly of the face pulling toward the unaffected side because of the weakness of the muscles on the side of the lesion. Later the ipsilateral corner of the mouth droops, food falls out of the mouth, and the eyelids no longer close on that side. Loss of blinking may result in drying and injury to the cornea. The patient may complain that sound has a booming quality in the ipsilateral ear because the stapedius muscle fails to tense the ossicles in response to a loud sound (the stapedial reflex). Taste may also be lost on the anterior two-thirds of the tongue on the ipsilateral side. If the Bell's palsy is caused by a herpes zoster infection of the geniculate ganglion, small blisters may form in the outer ear canal, the ganglion's cutaneous sensory field.

The *vestibulocochlear* (VIII) *nerve* contains two main bundles of sensory axons from two ganglia. Fibers from the vestibular ganglion relay sensation of angular and linear acceleration from the semicircular canals, utricle, and saccule in the inner ear. Fibers from

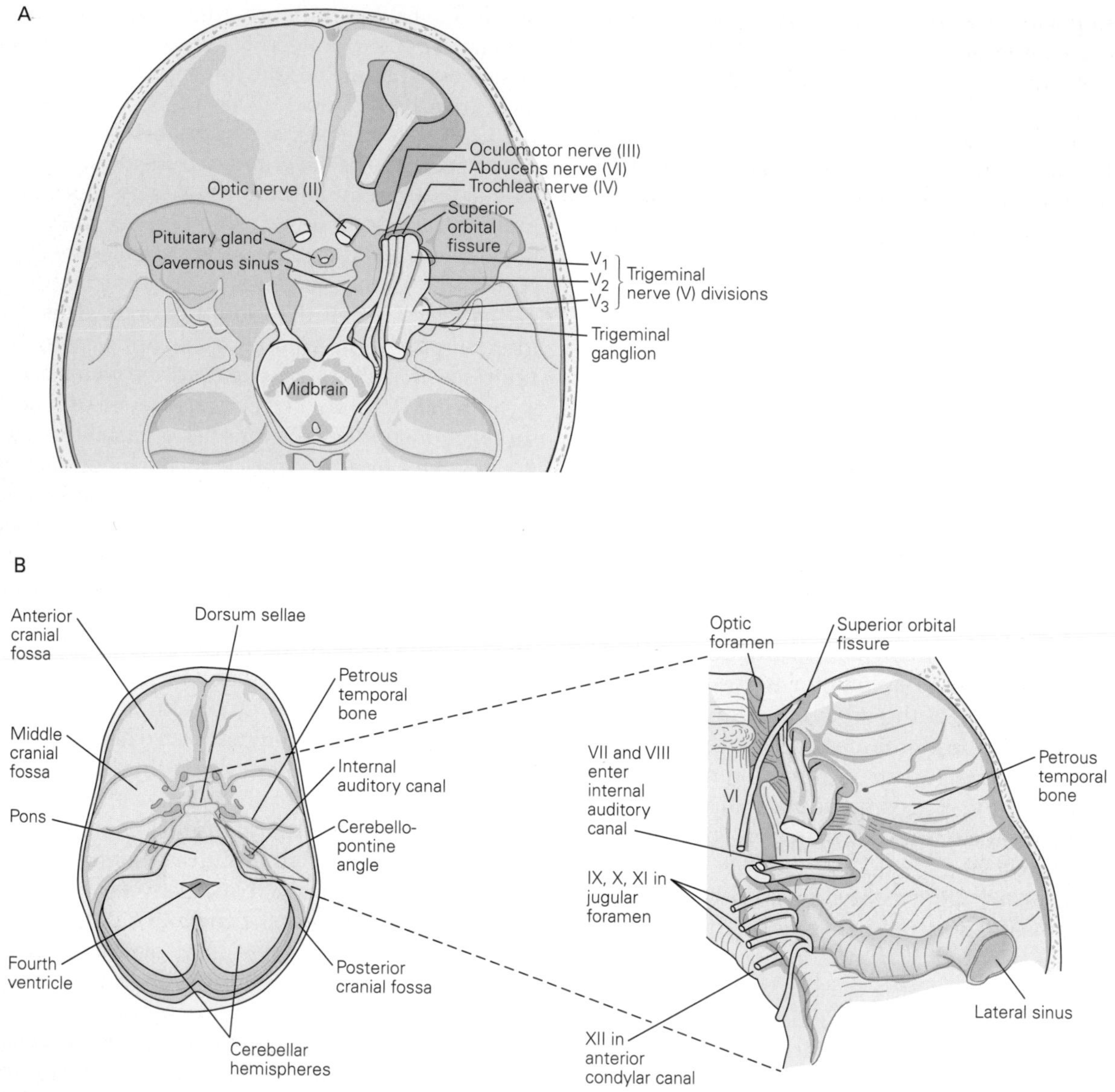

Figure 45–2 The cranial nerves exit the skull in groups.

A. Cranial nerves II, III, IV, V, and VI exit the skull near the pituitary fossa. The optic (II) nerve enters the optic foramen, but the oculomotor (III), trochlear (IV), and abducens (VI) nerves, and the first division of the trigeminal (V) nerve leave through the superior orbital fissure. The second and third divisions of the trigeminal nerve exit through the round and oval foramina, respectively.

B. In the posterior fossa the facial (VII) and vestibulocochlear (VIII) nerves exit through the internal auditory canal, whereas the glossopharyngeal (IX), vagus (X), and accessory (XI) nerves leave through the jugular foramen. The hypoglossal nerve (XII) has its own foramen.

the cochlear ganglion relay information from the cochlea concerning sound. A vestibular schwannoma, one of the most common intracranial tumors, may form along the vestibular component of cranial nerve VIII as it runs within the internal auditory meatus. Most patients complain only about hearing loss, as the brain is usually able to adapt to the gradual loss of vestibular input from one side.

The *glossopharyngeal* (IX) *nerve* and *vagus* (X) *nerve* are mixed but are predominantly autonomic. These closely related nerves transmit sensory information from the pharynx and upper airway as well as taste from the posterior third of the tongue and oral cavity. The glossopharyngeal nerve transmits visceral information from the neck (for example, information on blood oxygen and carbon dioxide from the carotid body, and arterial pressure from the carotid sinus), whereas the vagus nerve transmits visceral information from the thoracic and abdominal organs except for the distal colon and pelvic organs. Both nerves include parasympathetic motor fibers. The glossopharyngeal nerve provides parasympathetic control of the parotid salivary gland, whereas the vagus nerve innervates the rest of the internal organs of the neck, thorax, and abdomen. The glossopharyngeal nerve innervates only one muscle of the palate, the stylopharyngeus, which raises and dilates the pharynx. The remaining striated muscles of the larynx and pharynx are under control of the vagus nerve.

Because many of the functions of nerves IX and X are bilateral and partially overlapping, unilateral injury of nerve IX may be difficult to detect. Patients with unilateral cranial nerve X injury are hoarse, because one vocal cord is paralyzed, and may have some difficulty swallowing. Examination of the oropharynx shows weakness and numbness of the palate on one side.

The *spinal accessory* (XI) *nerve* is purely motor and originates from motor neurons in the upper cervical spinal cord. It innervates the trapezius and sternocleidomastoid muscles on the same side of the body. Because the mechanical effect of the sternocleidomastoid is to turn the head toward the opposite side, an injury of the left nerve causes weakness in turning the head to the right. A lesion of the cerebral cortex on the left will cause weakness of muscles on the entire right side of the body except for the sternocleidomastoid; instead, the ipsilateral sternocleidomastoid will be weak (because the left cerebral cortex is concerned with interactions with the right side of the world).

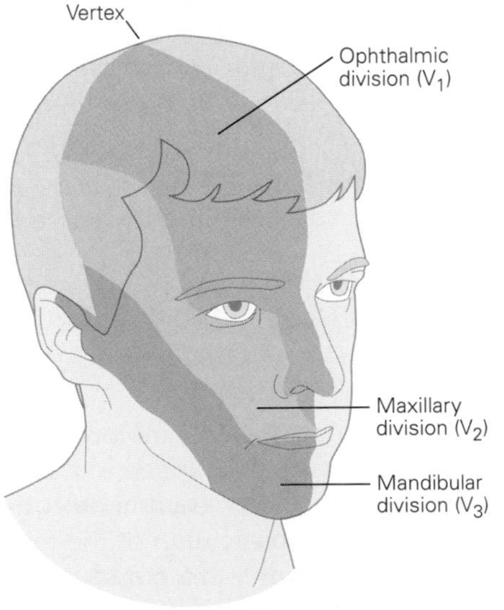

Figure 45–3 The three sensory divisions of the trigeminal (V) nerve innervate the face and scalp.

The *hypoglossal* (XII) *nerve* is also purely motor, innervating the muscles of the tongue. When the nerve is injured, for example during surgery for head and neck cancer, the tongue atrophies on that side. The muscle fibers exhibit twitches of muscle fascicles (fasciculations), which may be seen clearly through the thin mucosa of the tongue.

Cranial Nerves Leave the Skull in Groups and Often Are Injured Together

In assessing dysfunction of the cranial nerves it is important to determine whether the injury is within the brain or further along the course of the nerve. As cranial nerves leave the skull in groups through specific foramina, damage at these locations can affect several nerves.

The cranial nerves concerned with orbital sensation and movement of the eyes (III, IV, VI, and the ophthalmic division of the trigeminal nerve, V_1) are gathered together in the *cavernous sinus*, along the lateral margins of the sella turcica, and then exit the skull through the *superior orbital fissure* adjacent to the optic foramen (Figure 45–2A). Tumors in this region, such as those arising from the pituitary gland, often make their presence known first by pressure on these nerves or the adjacent optic chiasm.

Cranial nerves VII and VIII exit the brain stem at the *cerebellopontine angle*, the lateral corner of the brain stem at the juncture of the pons, medulla, and cerebellum (Figure 45–2B), and then leave the skull through the internal auditory meatus. A common tumor of the cerebellopontine angle is the vestibular schwannoma (sometimes erroneously called an "acoustic neuroma"), which derives from Schwann cells in the vestibular component of nerve VIII. If the tumor is large, it may not only impair the function of nerves VII and VIII but may also press on nerve V near its site of emergence from the middle cerebellar peduncle, causing facial numbness, or compress the cerebellum or its peduncles on the same side, causing ipsilateral clumsiness.

The lower cranial nerves (IX, X, and XI) exit through the *jugular foramen* (Figure 45–2B) and are vulnerable to compression by tumors at that site. Nerve XII leaves the skull through its own (hypoglossal) foramen and is generally not affected by tumors located in the adjacent jugular foramen, unless the tumor becomes quite large. If nerve XI is spared, the injury is generally within or near the brain stem rather than near the jugular foramen.

Cranial Nerve Nuclei in the Brain Stem Are Organized on the Same Basic Plan As Are Sensory and Motor Regions of the Spinal Cord

Cranial nerve nuclei are organized in rostrocaudal columns that are homologous to the sensory and motor laminae of the spinal cord (see Chapters 22 and 34). This pattern is best understood from the developmental plan of the caudal neural tube that gives rise to the brain stem and spinal cord.

The transverse axis of the embryonic caudal neural tube is subdivided into alar (dorsal) and basal (ventral) plates by the sulcus limitans, a longitudinal groove along the lateral walls of the central canal, fourth ventricle, and cerebral aqueduct (Figure 45–4). The alar plate forms the sensory components of the dorsal horn of the spinal cord, whereas the basal plate forms the motor components of the ventral horn. The intermediate gray matter is made up primarily of the interneurons that coordinate spinal reflexes and motor responses.

The brain stem shares this basic plan. As the central canal of the spinal cord opens into the fourth ventricle, the walls of the neural tube are splayed outward so that the dorsal sensory structures (derived from the alar plate) are displaced laterally whereas the ventral motor structures (derived from the basal plate) remain more medial. The nuclei of the brain stem are divided into *general nuclei*, which serve functions similar to those of the spinal cord laminae, and *special nuclei*, which serve functions unique to the head (such as hearing, balance, taste, and control of the branchial musculature).

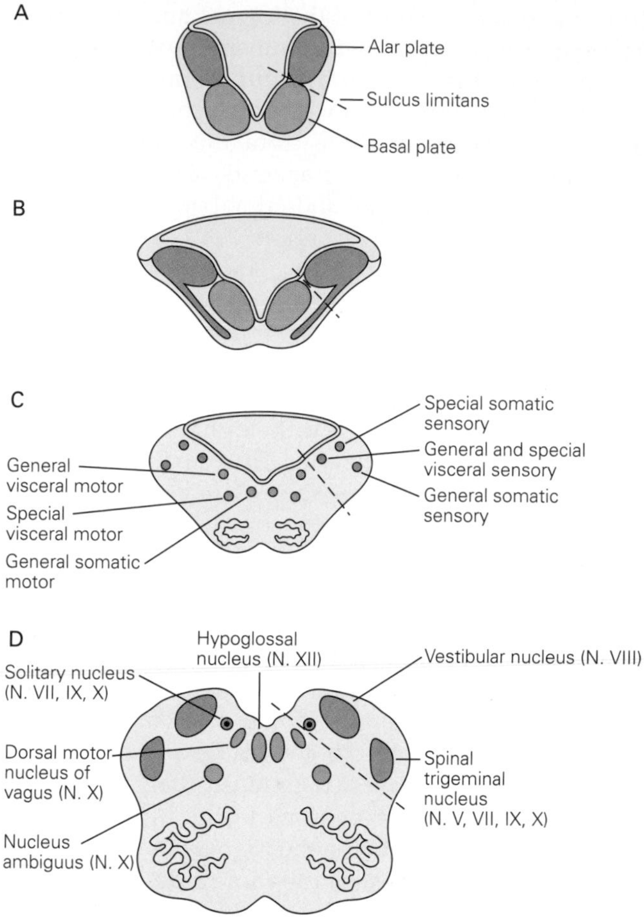

Figure 45–4 The developmental plan of the brain stem is the same general plan as that of the spinal cord.

A. The neural tube is divided into a dorsal sensory portion (the alar plate) and a ventral motor portion (the basal plate) by a longitudinal groove, the sulcus limitans.

B–D. During development the sensory and motor cell groups migrate into their adult positions, but largely retain their relative locations. In maturity (**D**) the sulcus limitans (**dashed line**) is still recognizable in the walls of the fourth ventricle and the cerebral aqueduct, demarcating the border between dorsal sensory structures (**orange**) and ventral motor structures (**green**). The section in D is from the rostral medulla.

Adult Cranial Nerve Nuclei Have a Columnar Organization

Overall, the brain stem nuclei on each side are organized in six rostrocaudal columns, three of sensory nuclei and three of motor nuclei (Figure 45–5). These are considered below, in dorsolateral to ventromedial sequence. The columns are discontinuous—the nuclei are not packed solidly along the rostrocaudal axis of the brain stem. Nuclei with similar functions (sensory or motor, somatic or visceral) have similar dorsolateral-ventromedial positions at each level of the brain stem.

Within each motor nucleus, motor neurons for an individual muscle are also arranged in a cigar-shaped longitudinal column. Thus each motor nucleus in cross section forms a mosaic map of the territory that is innervated. For example, in a cross section through the facial nucleus the clusters of neurons that innervate the different facial muscles form a topographic map of the face.

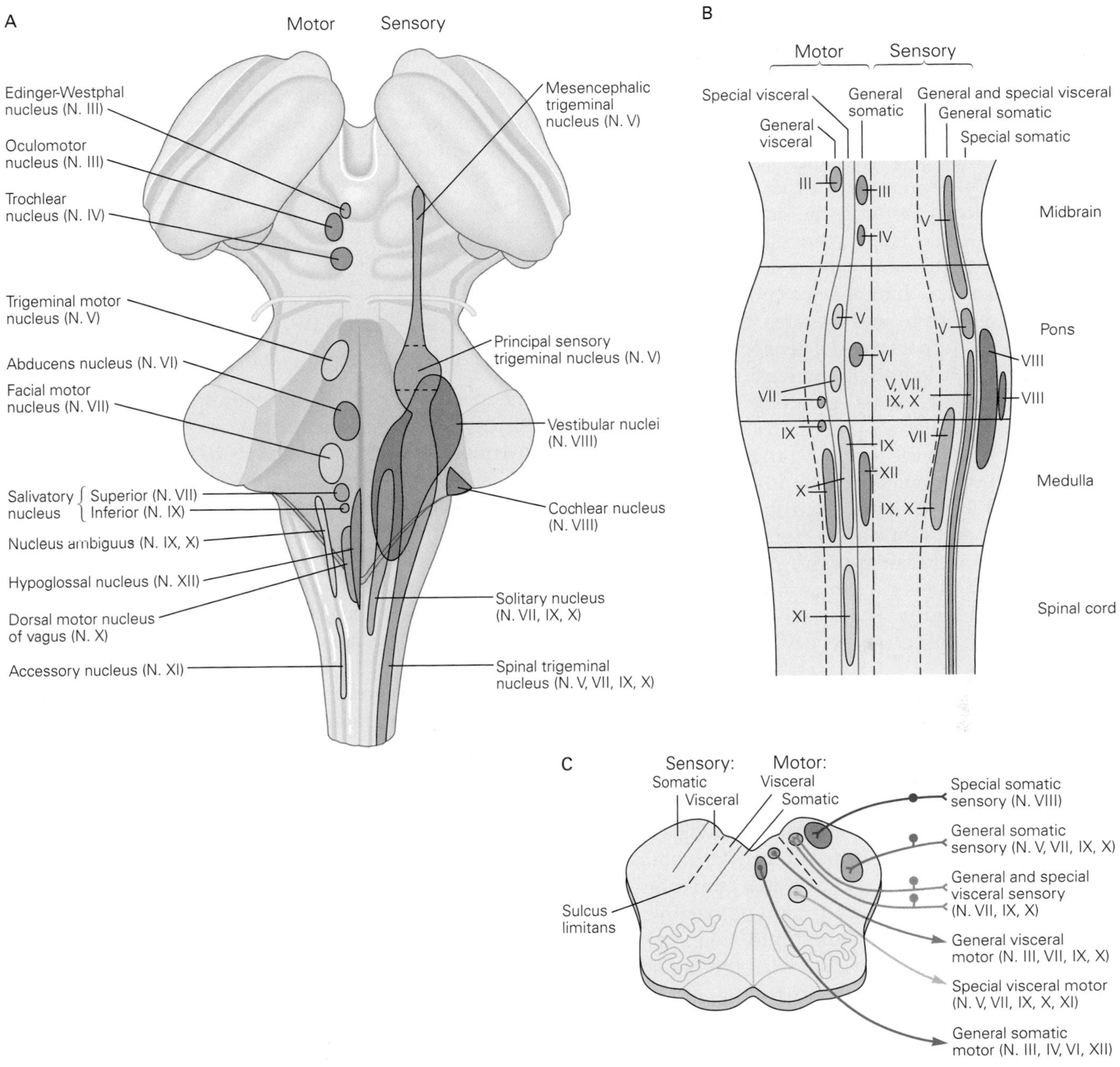

Figure 45–5 Adult cranial nerve nuclei are organized in six functional columns on the rostrocaudal axis of the brain stem.

A. This dorsal view of the human brain stem shows the location of the cranial nerve sensory nuclei (**right**) and motor nuclei (**left**).

B. A schematic view of the functional organization of the motor and sensory columns.

C. The medial-lateral arrangement of the cranial nerve nuclei is shown in a cross section at the level of the medulla (compare with Figure 45–4).

General Somatic Sensory Column

The general somatic sensory column occupies the most lateral region of the alar plate and includes the trigeminal sensory nuclei (N. V). The *spinal trigeminal nucleus* is a continuation of the dorsal-most laminae of the spinal dorsal horn (Figure 45–5A) and is sometimes called the medullary dorsal horn. Its outer surface is covered by the spinal trigeminal tract, a direct continuation of Lissauer's tract of the spinal cord (see Chapter 24), thus allowing some cervical sensory fibers to reach the trigeminal nuclei and some trigeminal sensory axons to reach the dorsal horn in upper cervical segments. This arrangement allows dorsal horn sensory neurons to have a range of inputs that are much broader than that of individual spinal or trigeminal segments, and ensures the integration of trigeminal and upper cervical sensory maps.

The spinal trigeminal nucleus receives sensory axons from the trigeminal ganglion (N. V) and from all cranial nerve sensory ganglia concerned with pain and temperature in the head, including geniculate ganglion (N. VII) neurons that relay information from the external auditory meatus, petrosal ganglion (N. IX) cells that convey information from the posterior part of the palate and tonsillar fossa, and nodose ganglion (N. X) axons that relay information from the posterior wall of the pharynx. The spinal trigeminal nucleus thus represents the entire oral cavity as well as the surface of the face.

The somatotopic organization of the afferent fibers is inverted: The forehead is represented ventrally and the oral region dorsally. Axons from the spinal trigeminal nucleus descend on the same side of the brain stem into the upper spinal cord, where they cross the midline in the anterior commissure with spinothalamic axons and join the opposite spinothalamic tract. (For this reason, upper cervical spinal cord injury may cause facial numbness.) The trigeminothalamic axons then ascend back through the brain stem, providing inputs to brain stem nuclei for reflex motor and autonomic responses in addition to carrying pain and temperature information to the thalamus.

The *principal sensory trigeminal nucleus* lies in the mid pons just lateral to the trigeminal motor nucleus. It receives the axons of neurons in the trigeminal ganglion concerned with position sense and fine touch discrimination, the same types of sensory information carried from the rest of the body by the dorsal columns. The axons from this nucleus are bundled with those from the dorsal column nuclei in the medial lemniscus, through which they ascend to the ventroposterior medial thalamus.

An additional component of the trigeminal sensory system, located at the midbrain level in the lateral surface of the periaqueductal gray matter, is the *mesencephalic trigeminal nucleus,* which relays mechanosensory information from the muscles of mastication and the periodontal ligaments. The large cells of this nucleus are not central neurons but primary sensory ganglion cells that derive from the neural crest and, unlike their relatives in the trigeminal ganglion, migrate into the brain during development. The central branches of the axons of these pseudo-unipolar cells contact motor neurons in the trigeminal motor nucleus, providing monosynaptic feedback to the jaw musculature, critical for the precise control of chewing movements.

Special Somatic Sensory Column

The special somatic sensory column has inputs from the acoustic and vestibular nerves and develops from the intermediate region of the alar plate. The *cochlear nuclei* (N. VIII), which lie at the lateral margin of the brain stem at the pontomedullary junction, receive auditory afferents from the spiral ganglion of the cochlea. The output of these nuclei is relayed through the pons to the superior olivary and trapezoid nuclei and bilaterally on to the inferior colliculus (see Chapter 31). The *vestibular nuclei* (N. VIII) are more complex. They include four distinct cell groups that relay information from the vestibular ganglion to various motor sites in the brain stem, cerebellum, and spinal cord concerned with maintaining balance and coordination of eye and head movements (see Chapter 40).

Visceral Sensory Column

The visceral sensory column is concerned with special visceral information (taste) and general visceral information from the facial (VII), glossopharyngeal (IX), and vagus nerves (X). It is derived from the most medial tier of neurons in the alar plate. All of the afferent axons terminate in the *nucleus of the solitary tract.* The solitary tract is analogous to the spinal trigeminal tract or Lissauer's tract, bundling afferents from different cranial nerves as they course rostrocaudally along the length of the nucleus. As a result, visceral sensory information from different afferent nerves produces a unified visceral sensory map of the body in the nucleus.

Special visceral afferents carrying taste information from the anterior two-thirds of the tongue reach the nucleus of the solitary tract through the chorda tympani branch of the facial nerve, whereas those from the posterior parts of the tongue and oral cavity arrive through the glossopharyngeal and vagus nerves. These afferents terminate in roughly somatotopic fashion in the anterior third of the nucleus of the solitary tract. General visceral afferents are relayed through the glossopharyngeal and vagus nerves. Those from the rest of the gastrointestinal tract (down to the transverse colon) terminate in the middle portion of the solitary nucleus in topographic order, whereas those from the cardiovascular and respiratory systems terminate in the caudal and lateral portions.

The solitary nucleus projects directly to parasympathetic and sympathetic preganglionic motor neurons in the medulla and spinal cord that mediate various autonomic reflexes, as well as to parts of the reticular formation that coordinate autonomic and respiratory responses. Most ascending projections from the viscera to the forebrain are relayed through the parabrachial nucleus in the pons, although some reach the forebrain directly from the solitary nucleus. Together the solitary and parabrachial nuclei supply visceral sensory information to the hypothalamus, basal forebrain, amygdala, thalamus, and cerebral cortex.

General Visceral Motor Column

All motor neurons initially develop adjacent to the floor plate, a longitudinal strip of non-neuronal cells at the ventral midline of the neural tube (see Chapter 52). Neurons fated to become the three types of brain stem motor neurons migrate dorsolaterally, settling in three distinct rostrocaudal columns. The neurons that form the general visceral motor column migrate to the most lateral region of the basal plate, just medial to the sulcus limitans.

The *Edinger-Westphal nucleus* (N. III) lies next to the oculomotor complex just below the floor of the cerebral aqueduct. It contains preganglionic neurons that control pupillary constriction and lens accommodation through the ciliary ganglion.

The *superior salivatory nucleus* (N. VII) lies just dorsal to the facial motor nucleus and comprises parasympathetic preganglionic neurons that innervate the sublingual and submandibular salivary glands and the lacrimal glands and intracranial circulation through the sphenopalatine and submandibular parasympathetic ganglia.

Parasympathetic preganglionic neurons associated with the gastrointestinal tract form a column at the level of the medulla just dorsal to the hypoglossal nucleus and ventral to the nucleus of the solitary tract. At the most rostral end of this column is the *inferior salivatory nucleus* (N. IX) comprising the preganglionic neurons that innervate the parotid gland through the otic ganglion. The rest of this column constitutes the *dorsal motor vagal nucleus* (N. X). Most of the preganglionic neurons in this nucleus innervate the gastrointestinal tract below the diaphragm; a few are cardiomotor neurons.

The *nucleus ambiguus* (N. X) is a cluster of neurons that runs the rostrocaudal length of the ventrolateral medulla and contains parasympathetic preganglionic neurons that innervate thoracic organs, including the esophagus, heart, and respiratory system, as well as special visceral motor neurons that innervate the striated muscle of the larynx and pharynx, and neurons that generate respiratory motor patterns (see below). The parasympathetic preganglionic neurons are organized in topographic fashion, with the esophagus represented most rostrally and dorsally.

Special Visceral Motor Column

The special visceral motor column includes motor nuclei that innervate muscles derived from the branchial (pharyngeal) arches. Because these arches are homologous to the gills in fish, the muscles are considered special visceral muscles, even though they are striated in mammals. During development these cell groups migrate to an intermediate position in the basal plate and are eventually located ventrolaterally in the tegmentum. The *trigeminal motor nucleus* (N. V) lies at midpontine levels and innervates the muscles of mastication. Associated with it are the *accessory trigeminal nuclei* that innervate the tensor tympani, tensor veli palatini, and mylohyoid muscles, and the anterior belly of the digastric muscle.

The facial motor nucleus (N. VII) lies caudal to the trigeminal motor nucleus at the level of the caudal pons and innervates the muscles of facial expression. During development facial motor neurons migrate medially and rostrally around the medial margin of the abducens nucleus before turning laterally, ventrally, and caudally toward their definitive location at the pontomedullary junction (Figure 45–6A). This sinuous course of the axons forms the *internal genu of the facial nerve*. The adjacent *accessory facial motor nuclei* innervate the stylohyoid and stapedius muscles and the posterior belly of the digastric muscle.

The nucleus ambiguus contains branchial motor neurons with axons that run in the glossopharyngeal and vagus nerves. These neurons innervate the striated muscles of the larynx and pharynx. During development these motor neurons migrate into the ventrolateral medulla, and as a consequence their axons form a hairpin loop within the medulla, similar to those of the facial motor axons.

General Somatic Motor Column

The neurons of the somatic motor column migrate the least during development, remaining close to the ventral midline. The *oculomotor nucleus* (N. III) lies at the midbrain level; it consists of five rostrocaudal columns of motor neurons innervating the medial, superior, and inferior rectus muscles, the inferior oblique muscle, and the levator of the eyelids. The motor neurons for the medial and inferior rectus and inferior oblique muscles are on the same side of the brain stem as the nerve exits, whereas those for the superior rectus are on the opposite side. The levator motor neurons are bilateral.

The *trochlear nucleus* (N. IV), which innervates the trochlear muscle, lies at the midbrain/rostral pontine level also on the opposite side of the brain stem from which the nerve exits. The *abducens nucleus* (N. VI), which innervates the lateral rectus muscle, is located at the midpontine level. The *hypoglossal nucleus* (N. XII) at the caudal end of the medulla consists of several columns of neurons, each of which innervates a single muscle of the tongue.

Embryonic Cranial Nerve Nuclei Have a Segmental Organization

Although the sensory and motor nuclei in the adult hindbrain are organized rostrocaudally, the arrangement of neurons at each level derives from a strikingly segmental pattern in the early embryo. Before neurons appear, the future hindbrain region of the neural plate becomes subdivided into a series of eight segments of approximately equal size, known as *rhombomeres* (Figure 45–6A).

Each rhombomere develops a similar set of differentiated neurons, as if the hindbrain is made up of series of modules. The even-numbered rhombomeres differentiate ahead of the odd-numbered ones. This is most clearly seen in the branchial (special visceral) motor neurons, which are readily identified early in development. Rhombomeres 2, 4, and 6 form the branchial motor nuclei of the trigeminal, facial, and glossopharyngeal nerves, respectively. Later, rhombomeres 3, 5, and 7 contribute motor neurons to these nuclei; in each case the axons of individual motor neurons extend rostrally as they join those of their even-numbered neighbor. At this developmental stage each of these nuclei is composed of homologous neurons derived from two adjacent segments. This early transverse segmental organization changes as rhombomere boundaries disappear and the dorsolateral migration of the cell bodies aligns the cells into rostrocaudal columns. The migration of the facial motor neurons of rhombomere 4 around the abducens nucleus (Figure 45–6A) generates the internal genu of the facial nerve.

The combination of the neurons of two rhombomeres into a single cranial nerve nucleus also corresponds to the relationship of the rhombomeres with the branchial arch muscles that are the targets of these motor neurons. For example, rhombomeres 2 and 3 (trigeminal) register with branchial arch 1 (mandibular), which forms the muscles of mastication; rhombomeres 4 and 5 (facial) register with branchial arch 2 (hyoid), which forms the muscles of facial expression (Figure 45–6A). Furthermore, neural crest cells from each rhombomere migrate into the corresponding branchial arches where they provide positional cues that determine the development and identity of the arch muscles.

The Organization of the Brain Stem and Spinal Cord Differs in Three Important Ways

One major difference between the organization of the brain stem and that of the spinal cord is that the long ascending and descending sensory tracts that run along the outside of the spinal cord are incorporated within the interior of the brain stem. Thus the ascending sensory tracts (the medial lemniscus and spinothalamic tract) run through the reticular formation of the brain stem as do the auditory, vestibular, and visceral sensory pathways.

A second major difference is that, in the brain stem, the cerebellum and its associated pathways form additional structures that are superimposed on the basic plan of the spinal cord. Fibers of the cerebellar tracts and nuclei are bundled with those of the pyramidal and extrapyramidal motor systems to form a large ventral portion of the brain stem. Thus, from the midbrain to the medulla the brain stem is divided into a dorsal portion, the tegmentum, which follows the basic segmental plan of the spinal cord, and a ventral portion, which contains the structures associated with the cerebellum and the descending motor pathways. At the level of the midbrain the ventral (motor) portion includes the cerebral peduncles, substantia nigra, and red nuclei. The base of the pons includes the pontine nuclei, corticospinal tract, and middle cerebellar peduncle. In the medulla the ventral motor structures include the pyramidal tracts and inferior olivary nuclei.

A

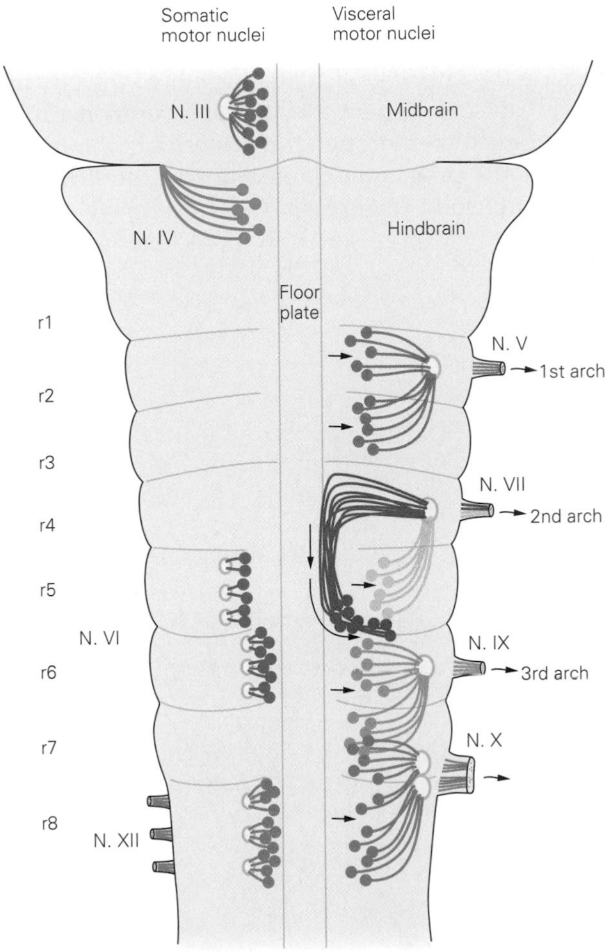

B

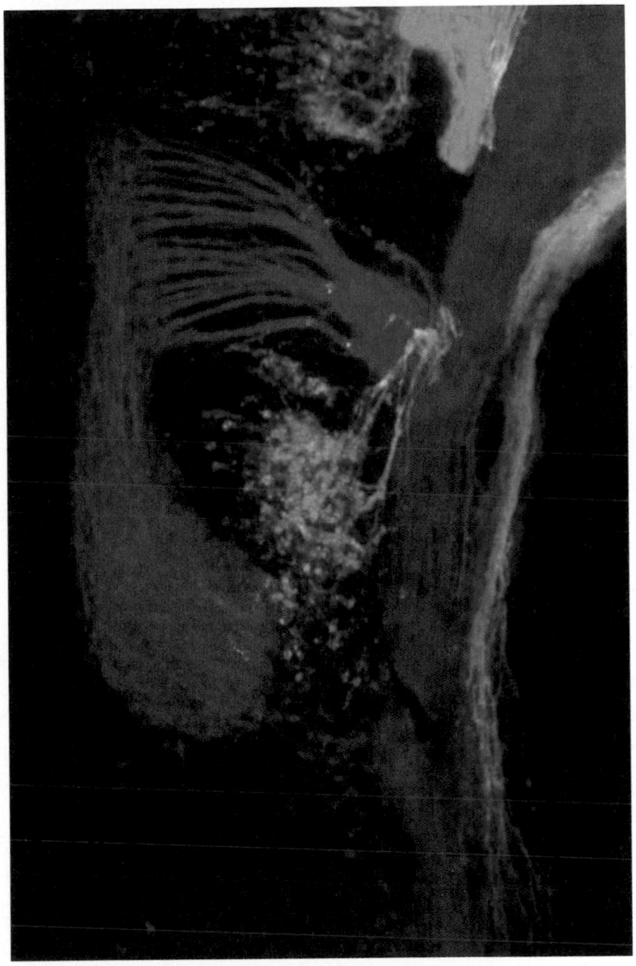

Figure 45–6 Embryonic cranial nerve nuclei are organized segmentally.

A. In the developing hindbrain (seen here from the ventral side) special and general visceral motor neurons form in each hindbrain segment (rhombomere) except rhombomere 1 (r1). Each special visceral motor nucleus comprises neurons in two rhombomeres: the trigeminal nucleus is formed by neurons in r2 and r3, the facial nucleus by neurons in r4 and r5, the glossopharyngeal nucleus by neurons in r6 and r7, and the motor nuclei of the vagus by neurons in r7 and r8. Axons of neurons in each of these nuclei course laterally within the brain, leaving the brain through exit points in the lateral neuroepithelium (of r2, r4, r6, and r7) and running together outside the brain to form the respective cranial motor nerves (V, VII, IX, X). The trigeminal (V) nerve innervates muscles in the 1st branchial arch, the facial (VII) nerve innervates muscles in the 2nd branchial arch, and the glossopharyngeal (IX) nerve innervates muscles in the 3rd branchial arch.

All of the visceral motor neurons (**green**) develop initially next to the floor plate at the ventral midline; after extending their axons toward their respective exit points, the cell bodies then migrate laterally (**arrows**). Exceptions are the facial motor neurons formed in r4 (**red**); the cell bodies, after extending their axons toward the exit point, migrate caudally to the axial level of r6 before migrating laterally.

General somatic motor neurons (**blue**) are formed in r1 (trochlear nucleus), r5 and r6 (abducens nucleus), and r8 (hypoglossal nucleus). The cell bodies of these neurons remain close to their place of birth, next to the floor plate. The axons of abducens and hypoglossal neurons exit the brain directly, without coursing laterally. The axons of trochlear neurons (**light blue**) extend laterally and dorsally within the brain until, caudal to the inferior colliculus, they turn medially, decussate, and exit near the midline of the opposite side.

B. The brain stem of a mouse embryo in which fluorescent dyes label cranial nerve VII motor neurons. A red-fluorescing dye fills the cell bodies of facial motor neurons via retrograde transport from the motor root of the facial nerve. These neurons develop initially in r4 and then migrate posteriorly, alongside the floor plate, to r6 (see red neurons in part A). A green-fluorescing dye fills the cell bodies of general visceral motor neurons in r5 (see light green neurons in part A) via retrograde transport from the root of the intermediate nerve (sensory and preganglionic general visceral motor axons). (Micrograph reproduced, with permission, from Dr. Ian McKay.)

A third major difference is that, although the hindbrain is segmented into rhombomeres during development, there is no clear repeating pattern in the adult brain. In contrast, the spinal cord is not segmented during development but the final pattern consists of repeating segments. The prominent ladder-like arrays of ventral root axons and dorsal root ganglia suggest that segmentation is imposed by a polarizing effect of the adjacent somites into which they migrate—in each somite the rostral part attracts axonal growth cones and neural crest cells, whereas the caudal part is repulsive (see Figure 52–1). In the head such patterning is lacking as the cranial mesoderm is not segmented into somites but rather develops under the influence of the rhombomeres.

Neuronal Ensembles in the Brain Stem Reticular Formation Coordinate Reflexes and Simple Behaviors Necessary for Homeostasis and Survival

A variety of reflexes and simple behaviors are mediated by the cranial nerves. These range from simple autonomic and motor responses to more complex patterns of facial expression and more complex behaviors such as breathing and eating, which in turn come under voluntary control by the forebrain. The stereotypic motor responses that make up these behaviors are controlled by neurons in the brain stem reticular formation. Impairment of cranial nerve reflexes and motor patterns in patients with neurological disease can be used to identify the precise site of brain stem damage.

Cranial Nerve Reflexes Involve Mono- and Polysynaptic Brain Stem Relays

The response of the pupils to light (*pupillary light reflexes*) are determined by the balance between sympathetic tone in the pupillodilator muscles and parasympathetic tone in the pupilloconstrictor muscles of the iris. Sympathetic tone is maintained by postganglionic neurons in the superior cervical ganglion, which in turn are innervated by preganglionic neurons in the first and second thoracic spinal segments. Parasympathetic tone is supplied by postganglionic ciliary ganglion cells under the control of preganglionic neurons in the Edinger-Westphal nucleus and adjacent areas of the midbrain.

Light impinging on the retina activates a special class of retinal ganglion cells that act as brightness detectors. These ganglion cells receive inputs from rhodopsin-containing rods and cones, but also have their own photopigment, melanopsin, which allows them to respond to light even in patients who have degeneration of the rods and cones. These cells send their axons through the optic nerve, chiasm, and tract, bypassing the lateral geniculate nucleus to the olivary pretectal nucleus, where they synapse onto neurons whose axons travel through the posterior commissure to contact the preganglionic neurons in the Edinger-Westphal nucleus (Figure 45–7). Thus injury to the

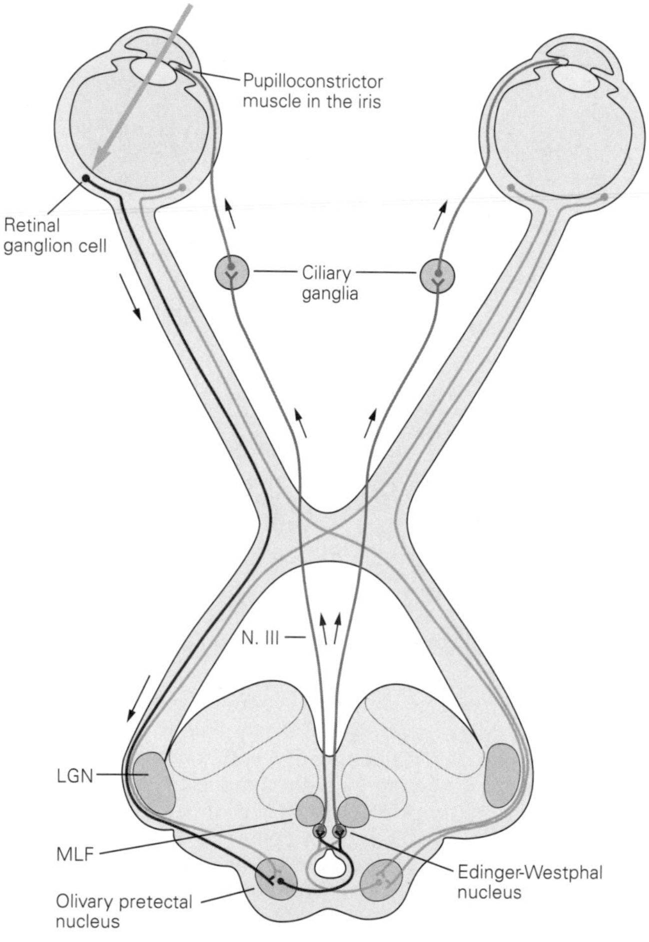

Figure 45–7 The pupillary response to light is mediated by the parasympathetic innervation of the iris. Retinal ganglion cells acting as luminance detectors send their axons through the optic tract to the olivary pretectal nucleus, at the junction of the midbrain and the thalamus. Neurons in this nucleus project through the posterior commissure to parasympathetic preganglionic neurons in and around the Edinger-Westphal nucleus. The axons of the preganglionic cells exit with the oculomotor (III) nerve and contact the ciliary ganglion cells, which control the pupilloconstrictor muscle in the iris. (**LGN**, lateral geniculate nucleus; **MLF**, medial longitudinal fasciculus.)

dorsal midbrain in the region of the posterior commissure can prevent pupillary light responses (midposition, fixed pupils), whereas injury to the oculomotor nerve eliminates parasympathetic tone to that pupil (fixed and dilated pupil). The melanopsin-containing retinal ganglion cells also project to the suprachiasmatic nucleus of the hypothalamus, where they entrain circadian rhythms to the day-night cycle.

Vestibulo-ocular reflexes stabilize the image on the retina during head movement by rotating the eyeballs counter to the direction of rotation of the head. These reflexes are activated by pathways from the vestibular ganglion and nerve to the medial, superior, and lateral vestibular nuclei, and from there to neurons in the reticular formation and ocular motor nuclei that coordinate eye movements. The reflex movements are seen most clearly in comatose patients, in whom turning the head will elicit counter-rotational movements of the eyes (so-called doll's eye movements). Damage to these pathways in the pons impairs these movements.

The *corneal reflex* involves closure of both eyelids as well as upward turning of the eyes (Bell's phenomenon) when the cornea is gently stimulated (eg, with a wisp of cotton). The sensory axons from the first division of the trigeminal nerve terminate in the spinal trigeminal nucleus, which relays the sensory signals to pattern generator neurons in the reticular formation adjacent to the facial motor nucleus. The pattern generator neurons provide bilateral inputs to the motor neurons that innervate the orbicularis oculi, which controls eye closure, and to the oculomotor nuclei, causing the elevation of the eyes. Because the output of the pattern generator is bilateral, damage along the sensory pathway prevents the reflex in both eyes, whereas damage to the facial nerve prevents closure on the same side only.

The *stapedial reflex* contracts the stapedius muscle in response to a loud sound, thus damping movement of the ossicles. The sensory pathway is through the cochlear nerve and nucleus to the reticular formation adjacent to the facial motor nucleus, and from there to the stapedial motor neurons, which run in the facial nerve. In patients with injury to the facial nerve (eg, Bell's palsy) the stapedial reflex is impaired, and the patient complains that sounds in that ear have a "booming" quality (hyperacusis).

A variety of gastrointestinal reflexes are controlled by multisynaptic brain stem relays. For example, the taste of food causes neurons in the solitary nucleus that project to the reticular formation adjacent to the nerve VII and IX nuclei to stimulate the preganglionic salivary neurons. The taste of food can also elicit gastric contractions and acid secretion, presumably through inputs from the solitary nucleus directly to parasympathetic preganglionic gastric neurons in the dorsal motor vagal nucleus.

The *gag reflex* protects the airway in response to stimulation of the posterior oropharynx. The afferent sensory fibers in the glossopharyngeal and vagus nerves terminate in the spinal trigeminal nucleus, whose axons project to the reticular formation adjacent to the nucleus ambiguus. Branchial motor neurons in the nucleus ambiguus innervate the posterior pharyngeal muscles, resulting in elevation of the palate, constriction of pharyngeal muscles (to expel the offending stimulus), and closure of the airway. Loss of the gag reflex on one side of the throat indicates injury to the medulla or to cranial nerves IX and X on that side.

Pattern Generator Neurons Coordinate Stereotypic and Autonomic Behaviors

Reflex responses such as the corneal or gag reflex are mediated by complex spatial and temporal patterns of activity in multiple motor nuclei. These patterns of activity are coordinated by *pattern generator neurons* in the adjacent reticular formation. Similar mechanisms control a variety of simple, stereotypic behaviors. For example, pools of pattern generator neurons in the reticular formation adjacent to the facial nucleus control facial expressions through stereotypic patterns of contraction of facial muscles simultaneously on the two sides of the face.

The patterns are so characteristic that Charles Darwin in his book on *Expression of the Emotions in Man and Animals* claimed that he could identify emotional states in animals like dogs and monkeys on the basis of contraction of homologous groups of facial muscles. Pattern generator neurons on each side of the brain stem project to the facial motor neurons on both sides of the brain, so that spontaneous facial expressions are virtually always symmetric. Even patients who have had major strokes in the cerebral hemispheres and cannot voluntarily move the contralateral orofacial muscles still tend to smile symmetrically when they hear a joke and can raise their eyebrows symmetrically.

Many orofacial movements involved in eating are produced by pattern generator neurons in the reticular formation near the cranial motor nuclei that mediate the behaviors. Licking movements are organized in the reticular formation near the hypoglossal nucleus, chewing movements near the trigeminal motor nucleus, sucking movements near the facial nucleus, and swallowing near the nucleus ambiguus. Not surprisingly, neurons in these reticular areas are closely interconnected with each other and receive inputs from the part of the nucleus of the solitary tract concerned with taste and the part of the spinal trigeminal nucleus concerned with tongue and oral sensation.

A variety of responses organized by the brain stem require coordination of cranial motor patterns with autonomic and sometimes endocrine responses. A good example is the baroreceptor reflex, which insures an adequate blood flow to the brain (see Chapter 47). The nucleus of the solitary tract receives information about stretch of the aortic arch through the vagus (X) nerve and stretch of the carotid sinus through the glossopharyngeal (IX) nerve. This information is relayed to neurons in the ventrolateral medulla that produce a coordinated response that protects the brain against a fall in blood pressure.

Reduced stretch of the aortic arch and carotid sinus reduces drive to the parasympathetic preganglionic cardiac-vagal neurons in the nucleus ambiguus, resulting in reduced vagal tone and increased heart rate. Simultaneously, increased firing of neurons in the rostral ventrolateral medulla drives sympathetic preganglionic vasoconstrictor and cardioaccelerator neurons. This combination of increased cardiac output and increased vascular resistance elevates blood pressure. Meanwhile, other neurons in the ventrolateral medulla increase the firing of hypothalamic neurons that secrete vasopressin from their terminals in the posterior pituitary gland. Vasopressin also has a direct vasoconstrictor effect, and it maintains blood volume by reducing water excretion through the kidney.

Vomiting is another example of a coordinated response mediated by pattern generator neurons. Toxic substances that enter the blood stream can be detected by nerve cells in the area postrema, a small region adjacent to the nucleus of the solitary tract along the floor of the fourth ventricle. Unlike most of the brain, which is protected by a blood–brain barrier (see Appendix D), the area postrema contains fenestrated capillaries that allow its neurons to sample the contents of the blood stream. When these neurons detect a toxin, they activate a pool of neurons in the ventrolateral medulla that control a pattern of responses that clears the digestive tract of any poisonous substances. These responses include reversal of peristalsis in the stomach and esophagus, increased abdominal muscle contraction, and activation of the same motor patterns used in the gag reflex to clear the oropharynx of unwanted material.

A Complex Pattern Generator Regulates Breathing

One of the most important functions of the brain stem is control of breathing. The brain stem automatically generates breathing movements beginning in utero at 11 to 13 weeks of gestation in humans, and continues nonstop from birth until death. This behavior does not require any conscious effort, and in fact it is rare for us to even think about the need to breathe. The primary purpose of breathing is to ventilate the lungs to control blood levels of oxygen, carbon dioxide, and hydrogen ions (pH), normal levels of which are essential for survival. (These are often measured together clinically and referred to as "blood gases.") Breathing movements involve contraction of the diaphragm, which is achieved by activating the phrenic nerve. The diaphragm is assisted when necessary by accessory muscles of respiration, including the intercostal muscles, pharyngeal muscles (to change airway diameter), some neck muscles (which help expand the chest), the tongue protruder muscles (to open the airway), and even some facial muscles (which flare the nares).

Respiratory activity can be generated by the medulla even when it is isolated from the rest of the nervous system. Within the medulla many neurons have patterns of firing that correlate with inspiration or expiration (Figure 45–8A). Some neurons have more complicated patterns, such as firing only during early inspiration or late inspiration. These respiratory neurons are concentrated in two regions. The *dorsal respiratory group*, located bilaterally in and around the ventrolateral part of the nucleus of the solitary tract, receives respiratory sensory input, including afferents from stretch receptors in the lungs and peripheral chemoreceptors. Neurons in the dorsal respiratory group contribute to reflexes such as limitation of lung inflation at high volume (the Hering-Breuer reflex) and the response to low oxygen (hypoxia). The *ventral respiratory group*, a column of neurons in and around the nucleus ambiguus, coordinates respiratory motor output. Some of these neurons are motor neurons with axons that leave the brain through the vagus nerve and innervate accessory muscles of respiration.

Respiratory neurons within the medulla in the rostral part of the ventral respiratory group, in an area called the *pre-Bötzinger complex*, are important components in the network that generates the respiratory rhythm. When transverse brain slices are prepared from the rostral medulla, neurons in the pre-Bötzinger complex are able independently to generate a respiratory rhythm that can be recorded in the XII cranial nerve rootlets that emerge from the ventral surface of the slices (Figure 45–8B). When neurons in this cell group are selectively killed acutely in intact animals, the animals are unable to maintain a normal respiratory rhythm. However, other areas of the medulla, such as the parafacial respiratory group, also contribute to

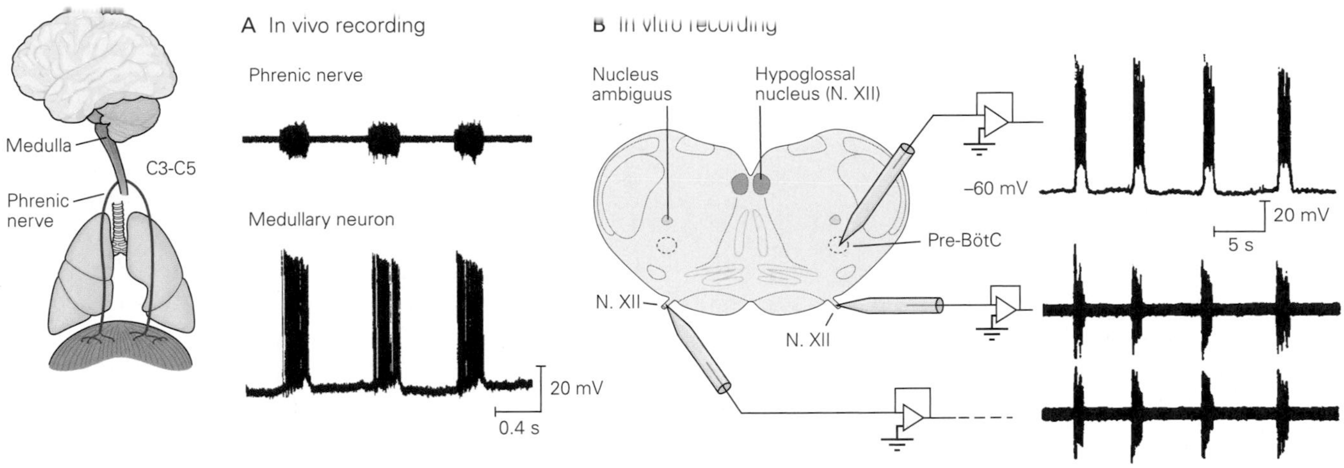

Figure 45–8 Rhythmic breathing is generated within the medulla.

A. Rhythmic motor activity in the phrenic nerve of a guinea pig is phase-locked to bursts of firing by neurons in the medulla. Each burst of firing in the phrenic nerve causes contraction of the diaphragm. Activity in the medullary neuron was recorded intracellularly. Neurons like this one project to the phrenic motor nucleus and contribute to the pattern of respiratory movement. (Reproduced, with permission, from Richerson and Getting 1987.)

B. Similar rhythmic firing can be recorded in vitro from accessory respiratory nerves, such as the hypoglossal (XII) nerve. The minimal tissue necessary to support this rhythm is a slice about 0.5 mm thick at the level of the rostral medulla. Neurons in the pre-Bötzinger complex (pre-BötC) near the nucleus ambiguus fire bursts that are phase-locked to the motor rhythm. Lesions of the pre-Bötzinger complex in vivo disrupt the normal respiratory rhythm, suggesting that its neurons are critical for producing the normal ventilatory motor pattern. (Reproduced, with permission, from Smith et al. 1991.)

respiratory rhythm generation. The exact roles of each of these areas, and their contributions to normal breathing, remain an active area of investigation.

The most important input into the respiratory pattern generator comes from chemoreceptors that sense oxygen (O_2) and carbon dioxide (CO_2). Under normal conditions ventilation is primarily regulated by the levels of CO_2 rather than O_2 (Figure 45–9A). However, breathing is strongly stimulated if O_2 becomes sufficiently low, such as at high altitude or in people with lung disease. The peripheral chemoreceptors in the carotid and aortic bodies respond primarily to a decrease in blood oxygen. During hypoxia they also respond to the increased acidity that results from an increase in CO_2 (water and CO_2 combine to form bicarbonate and hydrogen ions). Afferent fibers from peripheral chemoreceptors travel in the glossopharyngeal and vagus nerves and contact neurons in the dorsal respiratory group.

Central chemoreceptors in the brain stem respond to the decrease in pH induced by an increase in CO_2 (hypercapnia) but do not respond to hypoxia. Breathing increases when acidic solution is applied to the ventral surface of the medulla lateral to the pyramidal tract. Within this region and within the midline raphe nuclei are serotonergic neurons that are sensitive to acidosis (Figure 45–9B). Because these neurons surround large arteries (Figure 45–9C) and project to respiratory neurons, they are thought to be central chemoreceptors that sense hypercapnia in the blood. Indeed, genetic deletion or silencing of all central serotonergic neurons in mice reduces the ventilatory response to hypercapnia by 50%. Glutamatergic neurons in the nearby retrotrapezoid nucleus of the rostral ventrolateral medulla, as well as in other areas of the brain stem, are also central chemoreceptors, and current work is aimed at determining the relative importance of each of these chemoreceptor pools to the overall ventilatory response to hypercapnia.

Breathing must be coordinated with many motor actions that share the same muscles. To accomplish this coordination, respiratory neurons in the medulla receive input from neuronal networks concerned with vocalization, swallowing, sniffing, vomiting, and pain. For example, the ventral respiratory group is connected with a part of the parabrachial complex in the pons termed the *pontine respiratory group* or *pneumotaxic center*. These pontine neurons coordinate breathing with behaviors such as chewing and swallowing. They can cause holding of the breath at full inspiration (called

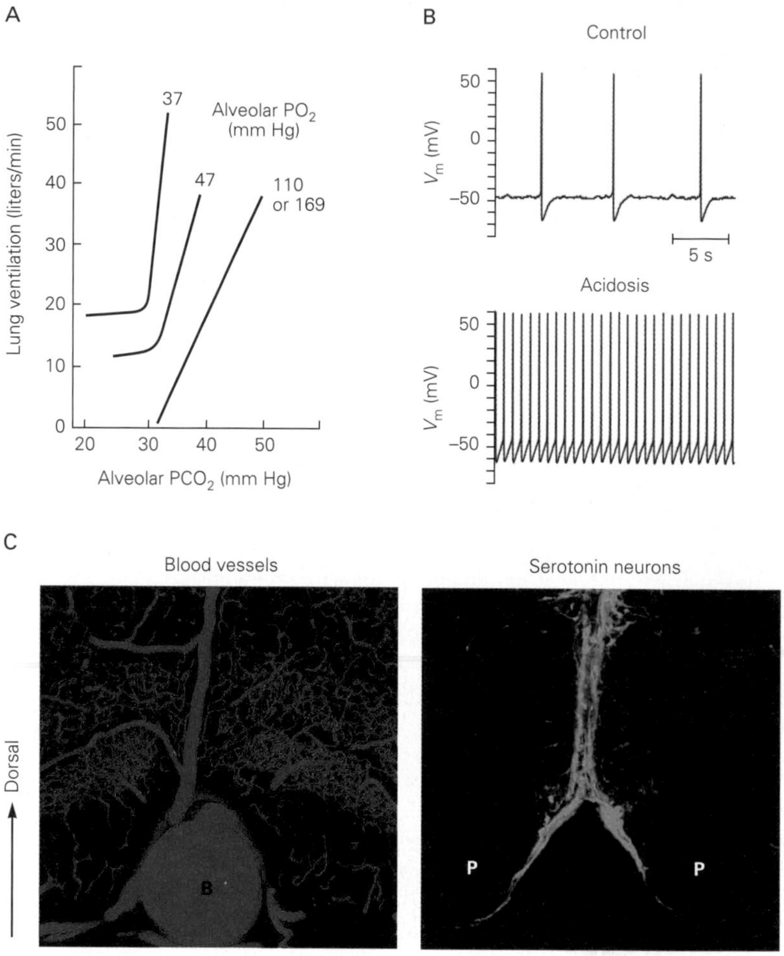

Figure 45–9 Respiratory motor output is regulated by carbon dioxide in the blood.

A. Lung ventilation (determined by the rate and depth of breathing) in humans is steeply dependent on the partial pressure of carbon dioxide (PCO_2) at normal levels of the partial pressure of oxygen (PO_2) (> 100 mmHg). When PO_2 drops to very low values (< 50 mmHg) breathing is stimulated directly and also becomes more sensitive to an increase in PCO_2 (seen here as an increase in the slope of the curves for alveolar PO_2 of 37 and 47 mmHg). (Reproduced, with permission, from Nielsen and Smith 1952.)

B. Central chemoreceptors in the medulla control ventilatory motor output to maintain normal blood CO_2. Serotonergic neurons within the raphe nuclei of the medulla may play this role by increasing the firing rate of the motor neurons when pH decreases (because of an increase in PCO_2). The records shown here are from in vitro recordings of a neuron in the raphe nuclei of a rat at two different levels of pH (7.4, control, and 7.2, acidosis). (Reproduced, with permission, from Wang et al. 2002.)

C. Serotonergic neurons are closely associated with large arteries in the ventral medulla where they can monitor local changes in PCO_2. Two images of the same transverse section of the rat medulla show blood vessels after injection of a fluorescent dye into the arterial system (left) and antibody staining for tryptophan hydroxylase, the enzyme that synthesizes serotonin (right). The basilar artery (**B**) is on the ventral surface of the medulla between the pyramidal tracts (**P**). (Reproduced, with permission, from Bradley et al. 2002.)

apneusis) during eating and drinking. The reserve of air in the lungs permits a cough, if necessary, to expel any food or drink that may enter the airway. Other neurons in the intertrigeminal zone, between the motor and principal sensory trigeminal nuclei, receive facial and upper airway sensory fibers and project to the ventrolateral medulla to temporarily stop breathing to protect against accidental inspiration of dust or water.

The motor pattern generated by the respiratory centers is remarkably stable in normal people, but a variety of abnormal patterns can emerge under some conditions (eg, during disease). One of the most easily recognized is the Cheyne-Stokes respiratory pattern, which is characterized by repeated cycles of gradually increasing then decreasing ventilation, alternating with cessation of breathing (apnea). At the peak of each cycle a high CO_2 level at the central chemoreceptors causes hyperventilation. The hyperventilation leads to a decrease in CO_2 in the capillaries of the lung, but it takes several breaths before this blood reaches the central chemoreceptors. By this time the subject has overcompensated, so that the CO_2 in the pulmonary capillaries is now too low. When that blood finally reaches the chemoreceptors, the low CO_2 causes apnea (Figure 45–10). This in turn causes an increase in CO_2 in the lung capillaries, and when this blood reaches the chemoreceptors it initiates another cycle.

Cheyne-Stokes breathing can be seen in patients with congestive heart failure in whom a decrease in cardiac output causes an increase in the delay between gas exchange in the lungs and the change in CO_2 at the central chemoreceptors in the brain stem. It is commonly seen in hospitalized patients. Although not dangerous in itself, it can indicate that there is a serious underlying cardiorespiratory problem that needs to be corrected. In normal healthy individuals this cycle does not occur because it is suppressed by other sensory afferents to the ventral respiratory group.

Conversely, at altitudes greater than 10,000 feet even normal individuals experience Cheyne-Stokes breathing, particularly during sleep, probably because the relative hypoxia sensitizes the CO_2 receptors. A variety of other symptoms (headaches, insomnia, breathlessness, nausea) also result from the hypoxia at high altitude. Many of these symptoms can be prevented by taking acetazolamide, which causes a decrease in brain pH. The decrease in pH stimulates central chemoreceptors, which increase ventilation and maintain blood O_2 levels closer to normal. When severe, the best treatment is to breathe oxygen or to return to lower altitude.

A variety of descending inputs can influence the brain stem respiratory system. Voluntary motor pathways can take over the control of breathing during talking, eating, swimming, or playing a musical instrument. Descending inputs cause hyperventilation at the onset of exercise, in anticipation of an increase in oxygen demand. In fact, this leads to a sustained drop in blood CO_2 during exercise—the opposite of what would be expected for a negative feedback control system. Other descending inputs from the limbic system produce hyperventilation in connection with pain or anxiety, and in some people may be responsible for causing spontaneous panic attacks, characterized by hyperventilation and a feeling of suffocation. These various descending inputs allow seamless integration of breathing with other brain functions, but they are superseded by the need to maintain blood gas homeostasis, as even a small increase in CO_2 produces severe air hunger or dyspnea. Thus the respiratory control system is a fascinating example of a brain stem pattern generator that must be sufficiently stable to insure survival yet flexible enough to accommodate a wide variety of behaviors.

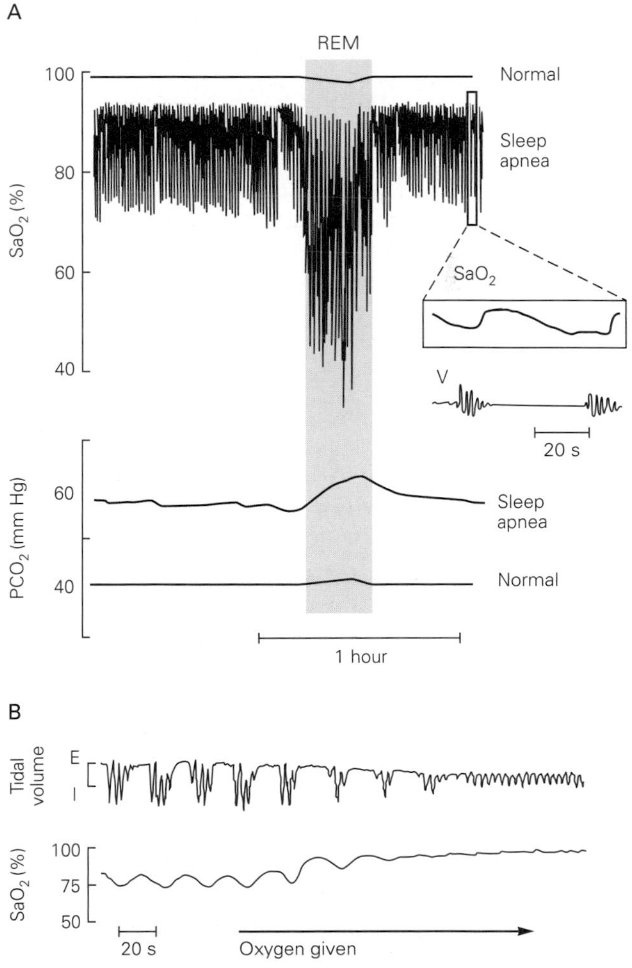

Figure 45–10 Breathing may become unstable during sleep.

A. Sleep apnea (cessation of breathing) is a common problem that often goes undetected. The records here show blood oxygen saturation (SaO_2) and CO_2 partial pressure (PCO_2) during sleep in a normal person (**black trace**) and a patient with obstructive sleep apnea (**purple traces**). In the normal person SaO_2 remains near 100%, and (PCO_2) remains near 40 mmHg during both rapid eye movement (REM) and non-REM sleep. In the patient with sleep apnea, reduced muscle tone during sleep allows collapse of the upper airway, resulting in obstruction and apnea. The repetitive attacks of apnea at the rate of approximately one per minute cause the patient's SaO_2 to fall repetitively and dramatically. (The inset shows a period of approximately 80 seconds on an expanded scale. Ventilation (**V**) begins at the nadir of the SaO_2 and again ceases when the blood oxygen increases.) During non-REM sleep the patient's PCO_2 increases to near 60 mm Hg. During REM sleep the SaO_2 and PCO_2 become even more abnormal, as worsening airway hypotonia causes greater obstruction. Many people with sleep apnea wake up repeatedly during the night because of the apnea, but the arousals are too brief for them to be aware that their sleep is interrupted. (Modified, with permission, from Grunstein and Sullivan 1990.)

B. Breathing becomes unstable during sleep at high altitudes in most normal individuals. The upper trace shows an example of a Cheyne-Stokes breathing pattern in a healthy person, during the first night after arriving at an altitude of 17,700 feet, where the low partial pressure of oxygen in the air reduces the blood SaO_2 to approximately 75 to 80%. Repeated cycles of waxing and waning ventilation are separated by periods of apnea. Administration of supplemental oxygen results in a rapid return to a normal respiratory pattern. This abnormal pattern disappears in most people after they have acclimated to the altitude. (Reproduced, with permission, from Lahiri et al. 1984.)

An Overall View

The plan for the brain stem and the cranial nerves unfolds early in development, as neurons assemble into clusters that come, in time, to assume their functional organization. Building on the basic plan of the spinal cord, motor and sensory neurons concerned with the face, head, neck and internal viscera form into discrete nuclei with specific functions and territories of innervation.

Neurons in the reticular formation surrounding these cranial nerve nuclei develop into ensembles of neurons that can generate patterns of autonomic and motor response that subserve simple, stereotyped, coordinated functions ranging from facial expression to feeding and breathing. These behavior patterns are sufficiently complex and flexible to represent the entire behavioral repertory of a newborn baby. As the forebrain develops and exerts its control over these brain stem pattern generators, a variety of more complex responses and ultimately volitional control of behavior evolves.

Even a skilled actor, however, finds it difficult to produce the facial expressions associated with specific emotions unless he recreates the emotional states internally, thereby triggering the pre-patterned facial expressions associated with those feeling states. Thus, some of the most complex human emotions and behaviors are played out unconsciously by means of stereotypic patterns of motor and autonomic responses in the brain stem.

Clifford B. Saper
Andrew G.S. Lumsden
George B. Richerson

Selected Readings

Coleridge HM, Coleridge JC. 1994. Pulmonary reflexes: neural mechanisms of pulmonary defense. Annu Rev Physiol 56:69–91.

Feldman JL. 1986. Neurophysiology of breathing in mammals. In: FE Bloom (ed). *Handbook of Physiology,* Sect 1: *The Nervous System*, Vol. IV: *Intrinsic Regulatory System of the Brain*, pp. 463–524. Bethesda, MD: American Physiological Society.

Grunstein RR, Sullivan CE. 1990. Neural control of respiration during sleep. In: MJ Thorpy (ed). *Handbook of Sleep Disorders,* pp. 77–102. New York: Marcel Dekker.

Leigh RJ, Zee DS. 1982. The diagnostic value of abnormal eye movements: a pathophysiological approach. Johns Hopkins Med J 151:122–135.

Lumsden A, Keynes R. 1989. Segmental patterns of neuronal development in the chick hindbrain. Nature 337 (6206):424–428.

Martin JH. 1996. General organization of the cranial nerve nuclei and the trigeminal system, and the somatic and visceral motor functions of the cranial nerves. In JH Martin: *Neuroanatomy, Text and Atlas,* pp. 291–347. New York: Elsevier.

Miller NR. 1985. The autonomic nervous system: pupillary function, accommodation and lacrimation, and the ocular motor system: embryology, anatomy, physiology, and topographic diagnosis. In: *Walsh and Hoyt's Clinical Neuro-Ophthalmology,* Vol 2, 4th ed., pp. 385–995. Baltimore: Lippincott-Williams & Wilkins.

Patten JP. 1995. *Neurological Differential Diagnosis,* 2nd ed. London: Springer.

Plum F, Posner JB. 1980. *The Diagnosis of Stupor and Coma,* 3rd ed. Philadelphia: Davis.

Rekling JC, Feldman JL. 1998. Pre-Botzinger complex and pacemaker neurons: hypothesized site and kernel for respiratory rhythm generation. Annu Rev Physiol 60:385–405.

Saper CB. 2002. The central autonomic nervous system: conscious visceral perception and autonomic pattern generation. Annu Rev Neurosci 25:433–469.

Saper CB. 2004. The central autonomic system. In: G Paxinos (ed). *The Rat Nervous System,* 3rd ed., pp. 759–794. San Diego: Academic.

References

Berlit P. 1991. Isolated and combined pareses of cranial nerves III, IV, and VI. A retrospective study of 412 patients. J Neurol Sci 103:10–15.

Bieger D, Hopkins DA. 1987. Viscerotropic representation of the upper alimentary tract in the medulla oblongata in the rat: the nucleus ambiguus. J Comp Neurol 262:546–562.

Blessing WW, Li Y-W. 1989. Inhibitory vasomotor neurons in the caudal ventrolateral region of the medulla oblongata. Prog Brain Res 81:83–97.

Bradley SR, Pieribone VA, Wang W, Severson CA, Jacobs RA, Richerson GB. 2002. Chemosensitive serotonergic neurons are closely associated with large medullary arteries. Nat Neurosci 5:401–402.

Chamberlin NL, Saper CB. 1998. A brainstem network mediating apneic reflexes in the rat. J Neurosci 18:6048–6056.

Gray PA, Janczewski WA, Mellen N, McCrimmon DR, Feldman JL. 2001. Normal breathing requires pre-Bötzinger complex neurokinin-1 receptor-expressing neurons. Nat Neurosci 4:927–930.

Grunstein RR, Sullivan CE. 1990. Neural control of respiration during sleep. In: MJ Thorpy (ed). *Handbook of Sleep Disorders*. New York: Marcel Dekker.

Jenny AB, Saper CB. 1987. Organization of the facial nucleus and cortico-facial projection in the monkey: a reconsideration of the upper motor neuron facial palsy. Neurol 37:930–939.

Lahiri S, Maret K, Sherpa M, Peters R Jr. 1984. Sleep and periodic breathing at high altitude: Sherpa natives vs. sojourners. In: J West, S Lahiri (eds). *High Altitude and Man,* pp. 73–90. Bethesda: American Physiological Society.

McKay IJ, Lewis J, Lumsden A. 1997. Organization and development of the facial motor neurons in the *kreisler* mutant mouse. Eur J Neurosci 9:1499–1506.

Morecraft RJ, Louie JL, Herrick JL, Stilwell-Morecraft KS. 2001. Cortical innervation of the facial nucleus in the non-human primate: a new interpretation of the effects of stroke and related subtotal brain trauma on the muscles of facial expression. Brain 124 (Pt 1):176–208.

Mulkey DK, Stornetta RL, Weston MC, Simmons JR, Parker A, Bayliss DA, Guyenet PG. 2004. Respiratory control by ventral surface chemoreceptor neurons in rats. Nat Neurosci 7:1360–1369.

Nielsen M, Smith H. 1952. Studies on the regulation of respiration in acute hypoxia; with an appendix on respiratory control during prolonged hypoxia. Acta Physiol Scand 24:293–313.

Richerson GB. 2004. Serotonergic neurons as carbon dioxide sensors that maintain pH homeostasis. Nat Rev Neurosci 5:449–461.

Richerson GB, Getting PA. 1987. Maintenance of complex neural function during perfusion of the mammalian brain. Brain Res 409:128–132.

Rinaman L, Card JP, Schwaber JS, Miselis RR. 1989. Ultrastructural demonstration of a gastric monosynaptic vagal circuit in the nucleus of the solitary tract in rat. J Neurosci 9:1985–1996.

Smith JC, Ellenberger HH, Ballanyi K, Richter DW, Feldman JL. 1991. Pre-Bötzinger complex: a brainstem region that may generate respiratory rhythm in mammals. Science 254:726–729.

Wang W, Bradley SR, Richerson GB. 2002. Quantification of the response of rat medullary raphé neurones to independent changes in pH_o and PCO_2. J Physiol 540:951–970.

46

The Modulatory Functions of the Brain Stem

As we learned in the previous chapter, the brain stem can respond independently to the environment with stereotypic actions. We have also seen, in discussing the sensory and motor systems, that the brain stem is the conduit for all ascending and descending pathways between the forebrain, spinal cord, and peripheral nervous system. In this chapter we examine still a third role of the brain stem, as the modulatory center that orchestrates the activity of the rest of the central nervous system, ensuring that its activity is optimized.

This modulatory function is mediated by several small groups of neurons in the brain stem. These neurons project widely, using as neurotransmitters acetylcholine and the monoamines (norepinephrine, epinephrine, serotonin, dopamine, and histamine). Many of the monoaminergic groups modify pain and help regulate the autonomic nervous system to maintain internal homeostasis. Some are essential for controlling the level of behavioral arousal; and together they influence attention, mood, and memory. Because they are involved in the pathophysiology of many human diseases and are targets of many commonly used drugs, these monoaminergic and cholinergic neurons are also important for clinical care.

Behaviors we regard as uniquely human, such as memory, language, and compassion, depend heavily on modulation of forebrain function by the ascending cholinergic and monoaminergic systems. This dependence is seen clinically in the links between Alzheimer's disease and the acetylcholine system, schizophrenia and the dopaminergic system, and alleviation of depression with drugs that affect serotonergic and noradrenergic synapses. Thus, although the brain stem is phylogenetically primitive, the modulatory systems that project from this region enable and modulate many of the higher-order behaviors that we regard as most human.

Ascending Monoaminergic and Cholinergic Projections from the Brain Stem Maintain Arousal

Some neurons in the brain stem that project to the forebrain control wakefulness and sleep. In the mid-1930s

Frederic Bremer found that transection of the cat's brain stem at the midbrain level produced a continuous sleep-like state, whereas transections that separated the medulla from the spinal cord did not (Figure 46–1). These experiments demonstrate that the portion of the brain stem from the midbrain to the medulla keeps the forebrain awake.

Consistent with this view, experiments in 1949 by Guiseppi Moruzzi and Horace Magoun found that damage to the brain stem reticular formation in cats led to loss of wakefulness. Conversely, stimulating the reticular formation immediately converted the electroencephalogram (EEG) of a sleeping cat to a waking EEG. Transection of the brain stem at the level of the midpons or lower did not cause loss of wakefulness, indicating that the critical structures that need to be connected to the forebrain for wakefulness are located in the rostral pons and caudal midbrain.

Moruzzi and Magoun proposed that this part of the brain stem provides a general activation energy for the entire brain and therefore called it the reticular activating system. Today this system is more accurately called the ascending arousal system, because we know it is not confined to the reticular formation. As we shall learn in Chapter 51, sleep and waking are regulated by interactions between this ascending arousal system and sleep-promoting regions in other parts of the brain. Damage to the ascending arousal system or its projections in the thalamus and hypothalamus leads to coma

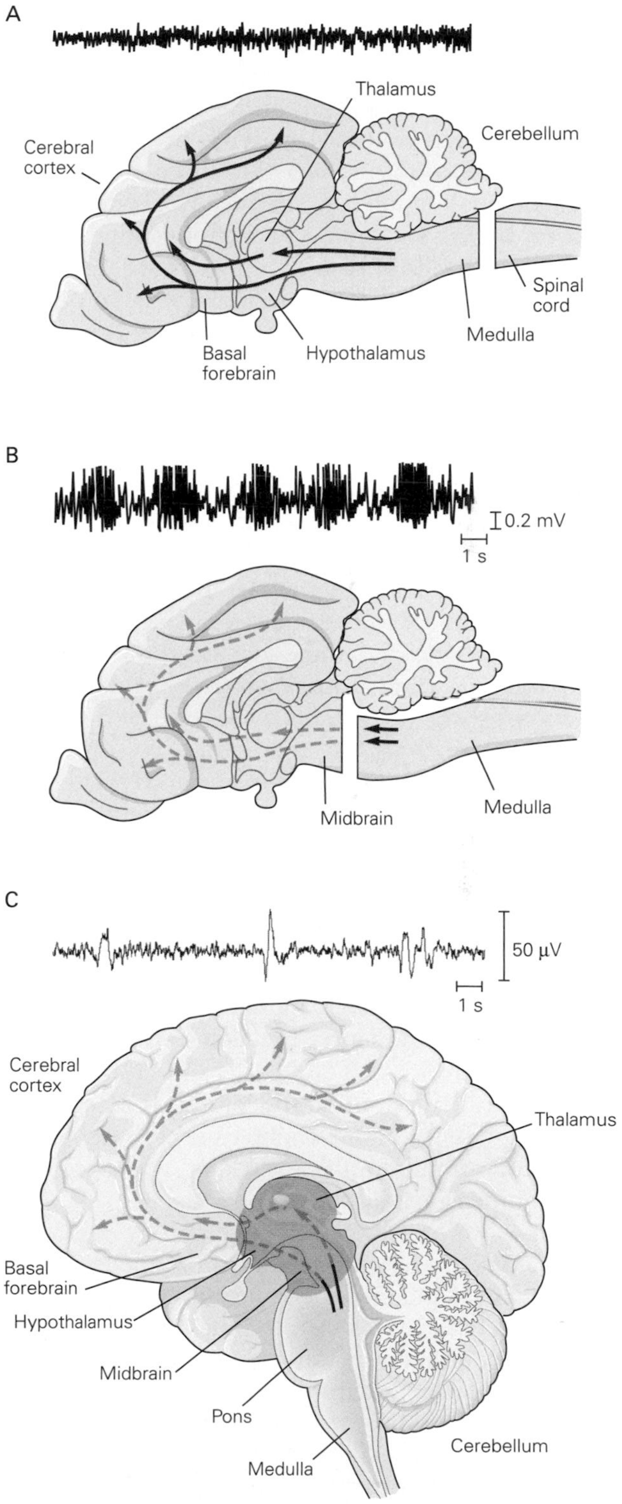

Figure 46–1 **Ascending projections from the rostral brain stem are necessary for maintaining arousal of the cortex.**

A. Transection of the brain stem in the lower medulla of a cat causes low-amplitude, fast electroencephalogram (EEG) activity characteristic of wakefulness. Animals appear awake and respond to sensory input from cranial nerves, but the muscles innervated by the spinal cord, including the diaphragm (which is required for breathing), are paralyzed.

B. Transection of the brain stem of a cat between the superior and inferior colliculi in the midbrain causes a sleep-like state from which the animal cannot be aroused. The EEG shows periods of slow delta waves (1–3 Hz) alternating with spindles (bursts of 8–11 Hz activity that wax and wane over a few seconds and are generated by the intact thalamus).

C. In humans injury to the rostral pons, the midbrain, or the thalamus and hypothalamus (shaded areas) causes impairment of consciousness. As shown here, the EEG of a drowsy patient consists of theta activity (4–7 Hz waves) and some larger delta waves. As the patient becomes less arousable, the amount of delta activity increases. Spindles similar to the cat appear as humans enter slow wave sleep but may not occur in coma if the thalamus is impaired.

(Figure 46–1C, and see the postscript, "Evaluation of the Comatose Patient," at the end of this chapter).

The ascending arousal system was originally viewed as a heterogeneous collection of neurons distributed diffusely throughout the brain stem reticular formation, which had widespread projections. This view changed radically in the early 1960s when Nils-Åke Hillarp and his students in Sweden used histofluorescence to discover that the neurons in this brain stem system fall into chemically distinct groups based on their monoamine neurotransmitter content. In a brilliant series of histochemical experiments they defined the location and projections of these neurons based on differences in the fluorescence signals produced by the different monoamines: norepinephrine, dopamine, and serotonin (Figure 46–2).

These findings were later expanded in studies that used antibodies against the synthetic enzymes for the monoamine neurotransmitters (which also allowed visualization of histamine and epinephrine) and acetylcholine. The connectivity of these cell groups is remarkable. Whereas most nuclei in the central nervous system project to specific regions or to a limited set of nuclei, the monoaminergic and cholinergic neurons of the ascending arousal system have widespread projections, some to virtually every part of the central nervous system.

A major part of the ascending arousal system consists of monoaminergic and cholinergic neurons in the brain stem. These neurons are found primarily in four regions (Figure 46–3A):

1. The locus ceruleus, which contains noradrenergic neurons
2. The dorsal and median raphe nuclei, which contain primarily serotonergic, but also some dopaminergic neurons
3. The pedunculopontine and laterodorsal tegmental nuclei, which contain cholinergic neurons
4. The tuberomammillary nucleus, which contains histaminergic neurons

The monoaminergic pathways from the locus ceruleus, and dorsal and median raphe nuclei, are thought to regulate sleep and waking. Other neurons in the parabrachial nucleus in the rostral pons and caudal midbrain, which largely use glutamate as a neurotransmitter, are also thought to contribute to the regulation of wakefulness and sleep. In addition to these reticular neurons, neurons in the lateral hypothalamus that contain the peptide neurotransmitters orexin and melanin-concentrating hormone are important for sleep and waking. Finally, cholinergic and GABA-ergic (γ-aminobutyric acid) neurons in the basal forebrain contribute to arousal through diffuse cortical projections.

Stimulation of noradrenergic neurons in the locus ceruleus or histaminergic cells in the tuberomammillary nucleus causes increases in EEG arousal (Figure 46–3B), indicating that these systems play an important role in cortical and behavioral arousal. However, lesions restricted to one biogenic amine cell group do not cause profound loss of wakefulness, suggesting that the various cell groups probably have overlapping and at least partly redundant roles in sleep/wake regulation. As we will see, the monoaminergic pathways alter specific cellular properties of postsynaptic neurons in the thalamus and cerebral cortex, enhancing alertness and interaction with environmental stimuli.

At the junction of the midbrain and diencephalon the projections from the ascending arousal system split into two major branches, dorsal and ventral. The dorsal branch terminates in the thalamus. The ventral branch travels through the lateral hypothalamic area and is joined by ascending projections from the hypothalamus and the basal forebrain before terminating throughout the cerebral cortex. Lesions that disrupt either of these two branches impair consciousness.

Monoaminergic and Cholinergic Neurons Share Many Properties and Functions

Monoamines are biochemical compounds with an aromatic ring that are synthesized from aromatic amino acids. They include the catecholamines (epinephrine, norepinephrine, and dopamine), serotonin, and histamine. Neurons that use monamines as neurotransmitters share many cellular properties. For example, most continue to fire spontaneous action potentials in a highly regular pattern when isolated from their synaptic inputs in brain slice preparations. Their action potentials typically are followed by a slow membrane depolarization that leads to the next spike (Figure 46–4A).

The spontaneous regular firing pattern of monoaminergic neurons is regulated by intrinsic pacemaker currents. Tonic firing in vivo may be important for ensuring the continuous delivery of monoamines to targets. For example, the basal ganglia depend on continuous exposure to dopamine from the neurons of the substantia nigra to facilitate motor responses.

The properties of monoaminergic neurons are suited to their unique and widespread modulatory roles in brain function. Indeed, some axon terminals of monoaminergic cells do not even form conventional synaptic connections, instead releasing neurotransmitter diffusely to many targets at once (Figure 46–4B).

Most monoamine neurotransmission occurs by means of metabotropic synaptic actions through G protein-coupled receptors. Many monoaminergic neurons co-release neuropeptides, which have slow effects through other G protein-coupled receptors. Thus, although some monoamine responses are mediated through fast synaptic mechanisms (see Chapter 10), many involve slower metabotropic and neuromodulatory actions as well (see Chapter 11).

Some cholinergic neurons in the brain stem share certain of these properties. For example, cholinergic neurons in the pedunculopontine and laterodorsal tegmental nuclei have widespread projections, providing the bulk of the cholinergic input to the thalamus, particularly to its relay and reticular nuclei. Many effects of cholinergic neurons also are mediated by G protein-coupled muscarinic receptors.

Many Monoaminergic and Cholinergic Neurons Are Linked to the Sleep-Wake Cycle

Most central neurons fire maximally during waking, decrease firing in a phase of sleep called slow-wave sleep, and then increase firing again during a phase of sleep called rapid eye movement (REM) sleep, the phase of the sleep cycle in which dreams are particularly likely to occur (see Chapter 51). Motor neurons are an exception; they have their lowest firing frequency during REM sleep because they are actively inhibited to prevent the acting out of dreams.

Noradrenergic, serotonergic, and histaminergic neurons are unlike most central neurons and more like motor neurons. They are maximally active during waking, their firing rates progressively decrease with increasing depth of non-REM sleep, and they stop almost completely during REM sleep (Figure 46–4A). Dopaminergic neurons within the dorsal raphe region also are most active during waking, but it has not yet been possible to distinguish their activity patterns during non-REM and REM sleep from those of the serotonergic neurons with which they intermingle.

In contrast to monoaminergic neurons, the firing rates of cholinergic neurons in the pedunculopontine and laterodorsal tegmental nuclei decrease during non-REM sleep but increase during REM sleep (Figure 46–4A). These and other properties indicate that the role of acetylcholine in controlling arousal is different from that of the monoamines.

The sleep-wake cycle has a strong circadian rhythm. The pacemaker for this rhythm is the suprachiasmatic nucleus in the hypothalamus (see Chapter 51). The suprachiasmatic nucleus regulates the circadian rhythm of sleep and waking primarily through connections with other hypothalamic areas, such as the dorsomedial nucleus. The dorsomedial nucleus in turn contacts both sleep- and wake-promoting cell groups in the hypothalamus and brain stem. As a result, the ascending arousal system entrains to the circadian rhythm (Figure 46–4A).

Monoaminergic and Cholinergic Neurons Maintain Arousal by Modulating Neurons in the Thalamus and Cortex

The monoaminergic and cholinergic neurons induce arousal by activating cortical neurons both directly and indirectly. They do this, in part, by modulating the activity of neurons in the hypothalamus, basal forebrain, and thalamus that activate the cerebral cortex.

Ionic mechanisms produce different modes of firing in thalamic neurons during sleep and wakefulness; during sleep the neurons fire in bursts, and during wakefulness they fire single spikes (see Chapter 51). Thalamic relay neurons exhibit activity in vitro that is similar to that seen in the intact brain during slow-wave sleep. When these neurons in brain slices are depolarized by injection of current, their firing pattern converts from burst mode to single-spike mode (like waking activity). Similarly, the firing pattern of thalamic and cortical neurons in brain slices changes from burst mode to single-spike mode when the cells are depolarized following application of acetylcholine, norepinephrine, serotonin and histamine (Figure 46–5A). Thus these neurotransmitters of the ascending arousal system regulate cortical activity in part by altering the firing of thalamic neurons.

Many pharmacological agents that target monoamines and acetylcholine influence arousal. For example, antihistamines cause drowsiness, serotonin reuptake blockers decrease the amount of REM sleep, and nicotine is a powerful stimulant. In addition, arousal is induced by amphetamines, cocaine, and other drugs that block dopamine reuptake; mice lacking the dopamine transporter are insensitive to such drugs.

Patients with Parkinson disease, who lose dopaminergic neurons in the substantia nigra, also lose noradrenergic neurons in the ascending arousal system and tend to be abnormally sleepy during the day. Some drugs used to treat Parkinson disease activate the D_2 dopamine receptor on presynaptic terminals of the remaining dopaminergic arousal neurons, which results in presynaptic inhibition, thus reducing dopamine release. As a result, although these drugs may make the movement disorder better (through their effects on postsynaptic D_2 receptors on neurons in the striatum), the inhibitory effect on remaining dopaminergic cells in the arousal system may exacerbate daytime sleepiness.

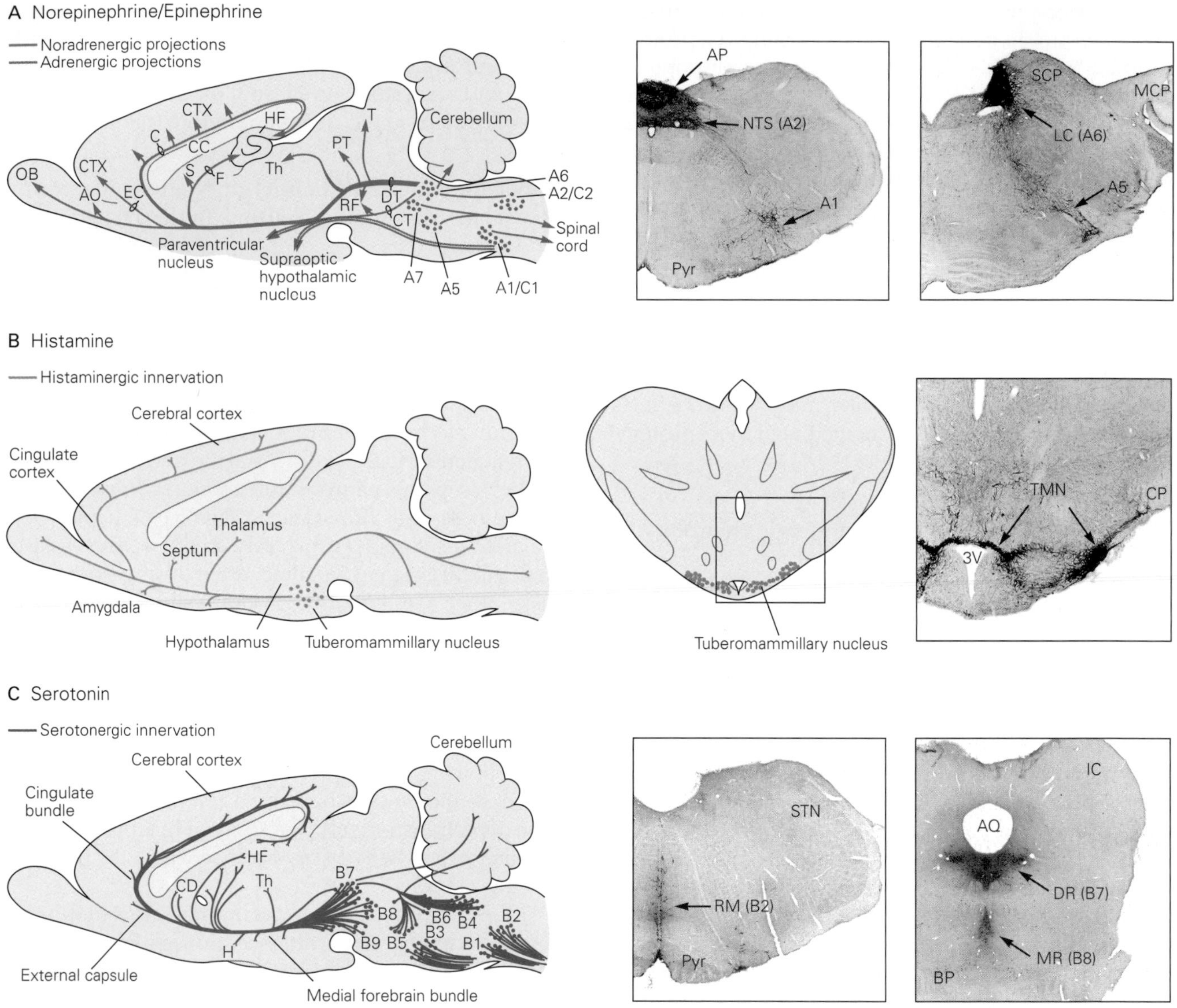

Figure 46–2 Locations and projections of monoaminergic and cholinergic neurons in the rat brain. (**3V**, third ventricle; **AC**, anterior commissure; **AP**, area postrema; **AQ**, Sylvian aqueduct; **ARC**, arcuate nucleus; **BM**, nucleus basalis of Meynert; **BP**, brachium pontis; **CD**, caudate; **CP**, cerebral peduncle; **DBh**, horizontal limb of the diagonal band; **DR**, dorsal raphe; **FX**, fornix; **IC**, inferior colliculus; **LC**, locus ceruleus; **LDT**, laterodorsal tegmental nucleus; **MCP**, middle cerebellar peduncle; **MGN**, medial geniculate nucleus; **MR**, median raphe; **MS**, medial septum; **MTT**, mammillothalamic tract; **NTS**, nucleus tractus solitarius; **OC**, optic chiasm; **PPT**, pedunculopontine tegmental nucleus; **PUT**, putamen; **Pyr**, pyramidal tract; **RM**, raphe magnus; **SC**, superior colliculus; **SCP**, superior cerebellar peduncle; **SN**, substantia nigra; **STN**, spinal trigeminal nucleus; **TMN**, tuberomammillary nucleus; **VTA**, ventral tegmental area.)

A. Noradrenergic neurons (A groups) and adrenergic neurons (C groups) are located in the medulla and pons (shaded). The A2 and C2 groups in the dorsal medulla are part of the nucleus of the solitary tract. The A1 and C1 groups in the ventral medulla are located near the nucleus ambiguus. Both groups project to the hypothalamus; some C1 neurons project to sympathetic preganglionic neurons in the spinal cord and control cardiovascular and endocrine functions. The A5, A6 (locus ceruleus), and A7 cell groups in the pons project to the spinal cord and modulate autonomic reflexes and pain sensation. The locus ceruleus also projects rostrally to the forebrain and plays an important role in arousal and attention.

B. All histaminergic neurons are located in the posterior lateral hypothalamus, mostly within the tuberomammillary nucleus. These neurons project to virtually every part of the neuraxis and play a major role in arousal.

C. Serotonergic neurons (B groups) are found within the medulla, pons, and midbrain, mostly near the midline in the raphe nuclei. Those within the medulla (the B1–B4 groups corresponding to the raphe magnus, raphe obscurus, and raphe pallidus) project throughout the medulla and spinal cord and modulate afferent pain signals, thermoregulation, cardiovascular control, and breathing. Those within the pons and midbrain (the B5–B9 groups in the raphe pontis, median raphe, and dorsal raphe) project throughout the forebrain and contribute to arousal, mood, and cognition.

D Acetylcholine

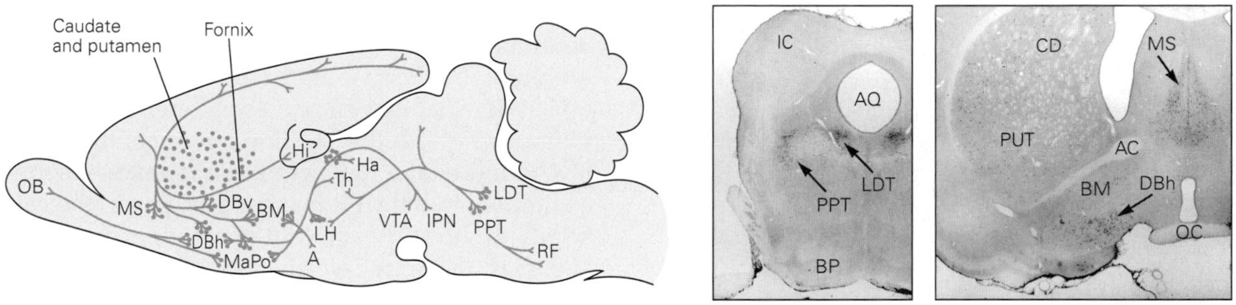

E Dopamine

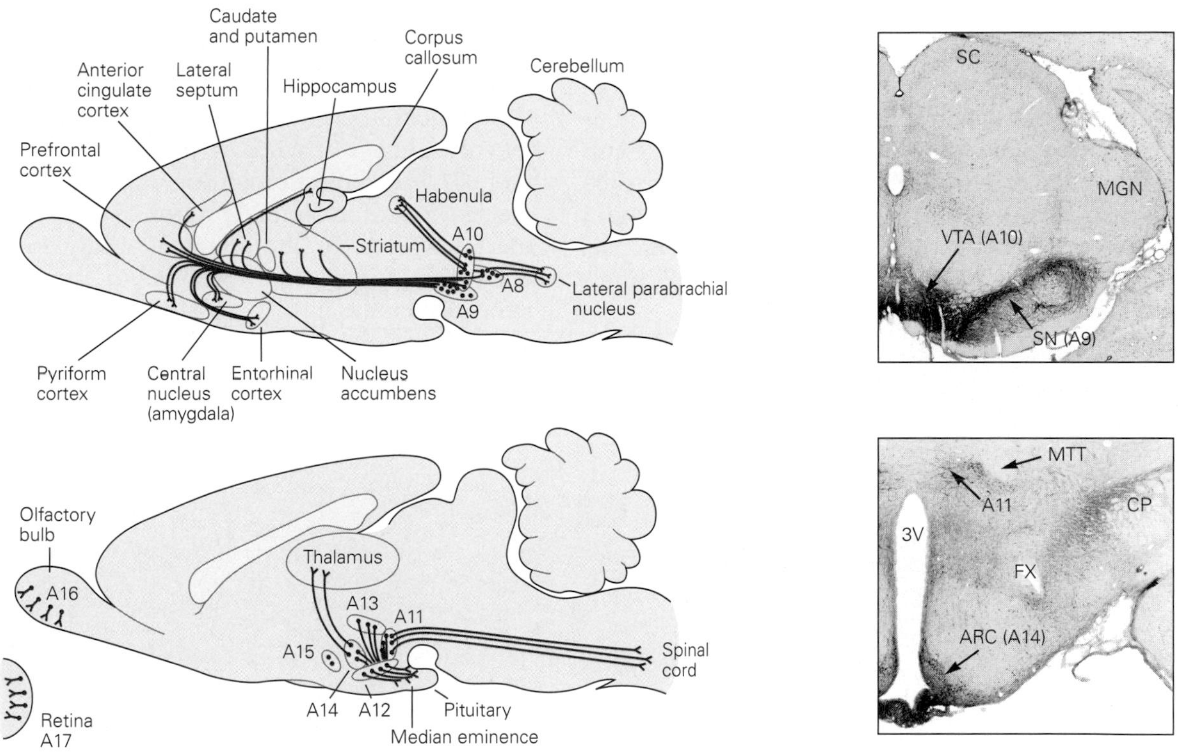

D. Cholinergic neurons (Ch groups) are located in the pons, midbrain, and basal forebrain. Those in the pons and midbrain (mesopontine groups) are divided into a ventrolateral cluster (pedunculopontine nucleus) and the dorsomedial cluster (laterodorsal tegmental nucleus). The mesopontine cholinergic neurons project to the brain stem reticular formation and the thalamus. Those in the basal forebrain are found in the medial septum, the nuclei of the vertical and horizontal limbs of the diagonal band, and the nucleus basalis of Meynert. These neurons project throughout the cerebral cortex, hippocampus, and amygdala. Both groups play an important role in arousal, and the basal forebrain groups are also involved in attention.

E. Dopaminergic neurons are located in the midbrain and hypothalamus. The dopaminergic cell groups were originally included with the noradrenergic lettering system and are still labeled as A groups. The A9 cell group is located in the substantia nigra pars compacta. The A8 group is in a region of the midbrain tegmentum, dorsally adjacent to the substantia nigra. These two groups of neurons project to the striatum and play an important role in initiation of movement. The A10 group is located in the ventral tegmental area just medial to the substantia nigra. These cells project to the frontal and temporal cortex and limbic structures of the basal forebrain and play a role in emotion and memory. The A11 and A13 cell groups in the zona incerta of the hypothalamus project to the lower brain stem and spinal cord and regulate sympathetic preganglionic neurons. The A12, A14, and A15 cell groups are components of the neuroendocrine system. Some of them inhibit release of prolactin into the hypophysial portal circulation, and others control gonadotrophin secretion. Dopaminergic neurons are also found in the olfactory bulb (A16) and the retina (A17).

Monoamines Regulate Many Brain Functions Other Than Arousal

In addition to their well-defined role in regulating arousal, monoaminergic neurons also regulate cognitive performance during waking and affect a variety of other central nervous system functions. We illustrate these effects with four examples.

Cognitive Performance Is Optimized by Ascending Projections from Monoaminergic Neurons

Although the monoamines and acetylcholine each induce arousal, they have different effects on cognitive function during waking. This occurs in part because each of the monoamines, and acetylcholine, uses distinct intracellular signaling pathways that act on different complements of ion channels (Figure 46–5B). Thus, in addition to differences in regional distribution, each type of monoamine receptor has a unique cellular and subcellular distribution (Figure 46–6). Hence each part of the brain and each type of neuron is affected differently by monoamines and acetylcholine.

Neurons of the locus ceruleus, which release norepinephrine, play an important role in attention. These neurons have a low baseline level of activity in drowsy monkeys. In alert monkeys the cells have two modes of activity that correspond to differences in behavior. In the *phasic mode* the baseline activity of the neurons is low to moderate. Just before the monkey responds to a stimulus to which it has been attentive, the cells are briefly excited. This pattern of activity correlates with and may facilitate selective attention. In contrast, in the *tonic mode* the baseline level of activity is elevated and does not change in response to external stimuli. This mode of firing may disrupt the ability to maintain attention on a single task and help to search for a new behavioral and attentional goal when the current task is no longer rewarding (Figure 46–7).

Monoaminergic inputs to the dorsolateral prefrontal cortex improve working memory (see Chapters 65 and 67). Microinjection of dopamine-receptor antagonists into the dorsolateral prefrontal cortex of monkeys markedly reduces the animals' ability to remember a location for several seconds. In functional magnetic resonance imaging (fMRI) studies of humans,

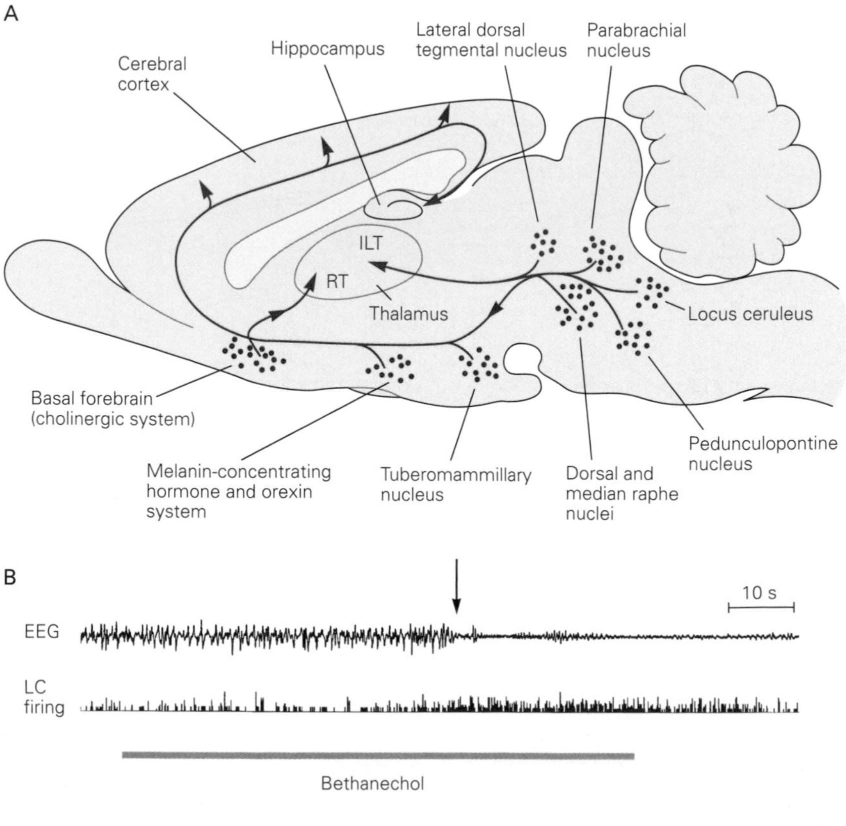

Figure 46–3 Major cell groups in the ascending arousal system in the rat brain.

A. Neurons using the neurotransmitters norepinephrine, serotonin, dopamine, histamine, and acetylcholine have widespread forebrain projections, but there are important differences in the distributions. They all contribute to arousal, but effects on other brain functions vary. Other groups of neurons that play an important role in arousal include the glutamatergic parabrachial nucleus and hypothalamic neurons that secrete orexin and melanin-concentrating hormone.

B. Stimulation of noradrenergic neurons in the locus ceruleus (LC) induces arousal. The cholinergic agonist bethanechol was microinjected directly into the locus ceruleus of a lightly anesthetized (halothane) rat. Arousal, which shows up in the EEG as low voltage, fast activity (**arrow**), coincides in time with the bethanechol-induced increase in firing of the locus ceruleus neurons. (**EEG**, electroencephalogram; **ILT**, intralaminar thalamic nuclei; **RT**, reticular nucleus of the thalamus.) (Reproduced, with permission, from Berridge and Foote 1991.)

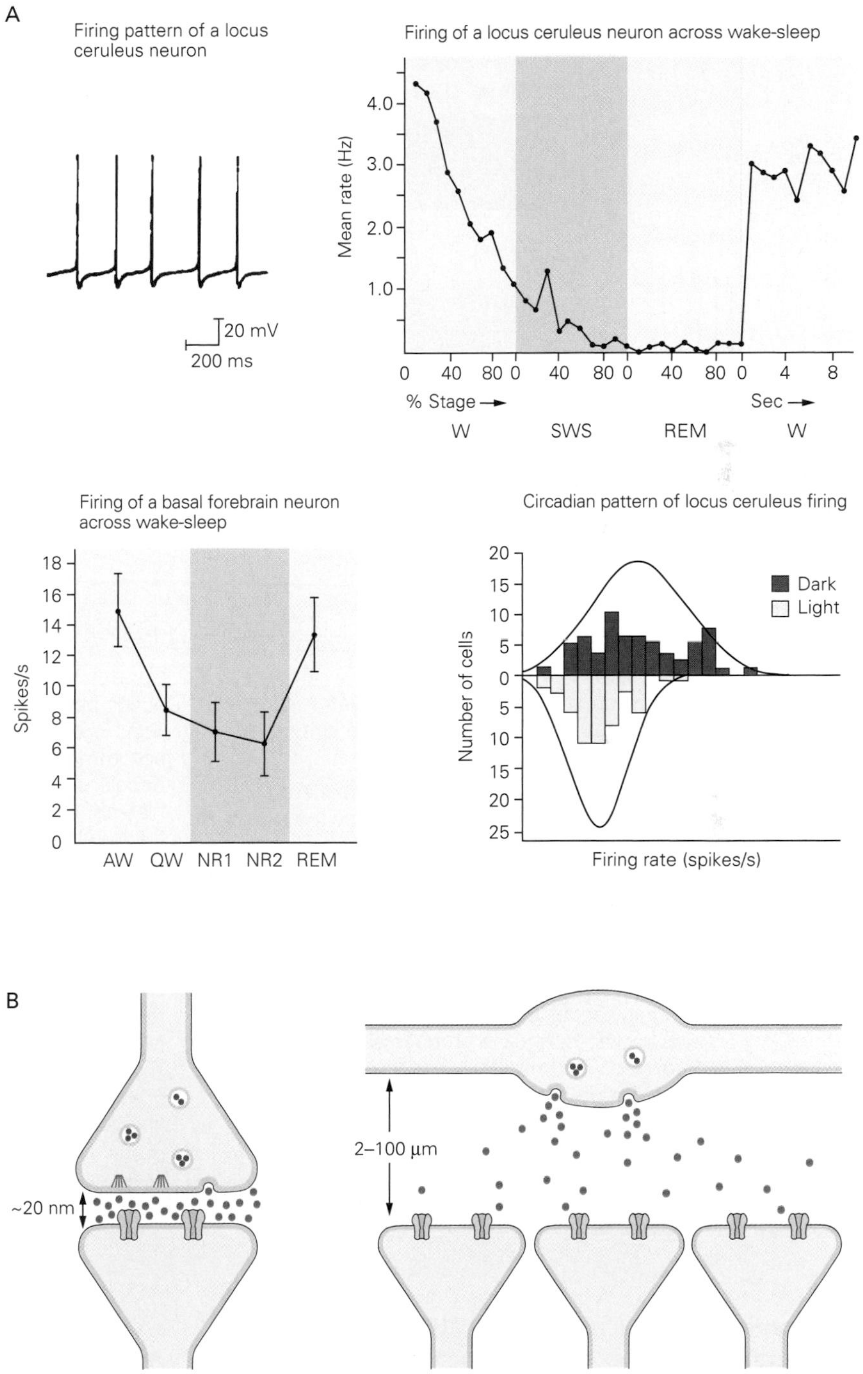

Figure 46–4 Monoaminergic neurons have common properties.

A. The baseline electrophysiological properties of all monoaminergic neurons are similar. The slow, regular firing pattern of a noradrenergic neuron in the locus ceruleus is shown at the upper left. Serotonergic and histaminergic neurons are similar. The upper right shows the average impulse activity of noradrenergic cells in the locus ceruleus in a behaving rat shown during different stages of sleep and waking. Histaminergic and serotonergic neurons exhibit a similar pattern of activity over the sleep-wake cycle. The bottom left shows the average activity of presumptive cholinergic neurons in the basal forebrain. Note decreased activity from waking to slow sleep (NR1 and NR2) but increased activity during REM sleep. The lower right shows that firing of neurons in the locus ceruleus follows a circadian rhythm. Histograms show the distributions of firing rates of the neurons during dark and light periods of the circadian cycle. Lesions of the dorsomedial nucleus of the hypothalamus eliminate the difference in locus ceruleus firing rates during the dark and light periods. (**REM**, rapid eye movement sleep; **SWS**, slow-wave sleep; **W**, wakefulness; **AW**, active wakefulness; **QW**, quiet wakefulness; **NR1**, lighter stages of non-REM sleep; **NR2**, deeper stages of non-REM sleep.) (Upper right reproduced, with permission, from Aston-Jones and Bloom 1981; lower left modified, with permission, from Szymusiak et al. 2000; lower right reproduced, with permission, from Aston-Jones et al. 2001.)

B. At conventional synapses the presynaptic terminal is closely aligned with the postsynaptic membrane (left). In contrast, the *en passant* terminal diffusely releases a transmitter that can affect several synapses within the immediate area (right). Acetylcholine and each of the monoamines can be released using this so-called paracrine mechanism.

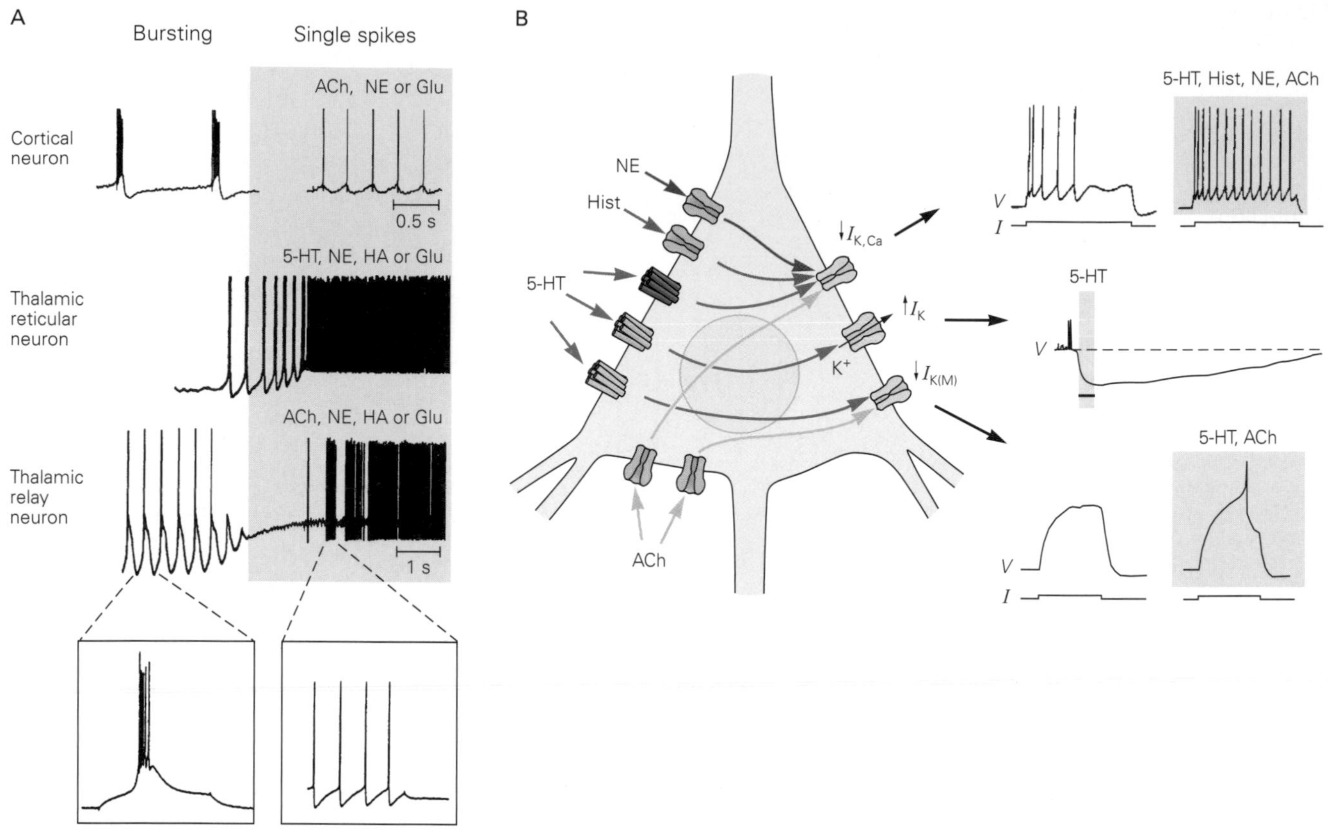

Figure 46–5 Monoaminergic and cholinergic systems induce and maintain arousal by modulating the activity of thalamic and cortical neurons.

A. The firing patterns of cortical and thalamic neurons are converted from burst mode to single-spike mode by the action of acetylcholine or monoamines. Recordings are from neurons in brain slices. (Reproduced, with permission, from Steriade, McCormick, and Sejnowski 1993.)

B. The effects of monoamines and acetylcholine on single neurons are complementary, not identical. In a cortical pyramidal neuron serotonin (5-HT) produces different effects on three different ion channels by acting on three types of receptors. Other monoamines and acetylcholine produce some but not all the responses observed with serotonin. The tops of the action potentials have been cut off in the middle and bottom traces. (Modified, with permission, from McCormick 1992.)

Top: *Left trace.* Depolarization elicits a train of action potentials that shows a gradual decrease in firing rate (spike accommodation) caused by entry of Ca^{2+} into the neuron during a burst of action potentials turning on a calcium-activated K^+ current, $I_{K,Ca}$. **Top:** *Right trace.* Serotonin inhibits $I_{K,Ca}$ and thus blocks spike accommodation, permitting the neuron to sustain firing during depolarization. The second-messenger pathways activated by histamine (acting on H2 receptors), norepinephrine (acting on β-adrenergic receptors), and acetylcholine (acting on muscarinic receptors) converge to also inhibit $I_{K,Ca}$.

Middle: A different type of serotonin receptor activates a different K^+ current, causing sustained hyperpolarization and inhibition of firing.

Bottom: *Left trace.* A third type of serotonin receptor inhibits the M-type K^+ current. A small depolarizing pulse activates the M-type K^+ current, which prevents the neuron from firing. *Right trace.* When the M-type current is inhibited by serotonin or acetylcholine, a small depolarizing pulse is able to produce an action potential (right).

(**5-HT**, serotonin; **ACh**, acetylcholine; **Glu**, glutamate; **Hist**, histamine; **HA**, hydroxyapatite; **NE**, norepinephrine.)

D_1 agonist drugs increased activation of the dorsolateral prefrontal cortex during a memory task. Injection of agonists of the α_2-adrenergic receptor into the dorsolateral prefrontal cortex of aging monkeys can also improve performance on working memory tasks.

Dopamine also has been linked to reward-based learning. Rewards are objects or events for which an animal will work (see Chapter 49) and are useful in reinforcing behavior. Activity of dopaminergic neurons increases when a reward (such as food or juice) is unexpectedly given. But after animals are trained to expect that a reward will follow a conditioned stimulus, the activity of the neurons increases immediately after the conditioned stimulus rather than after the reward.

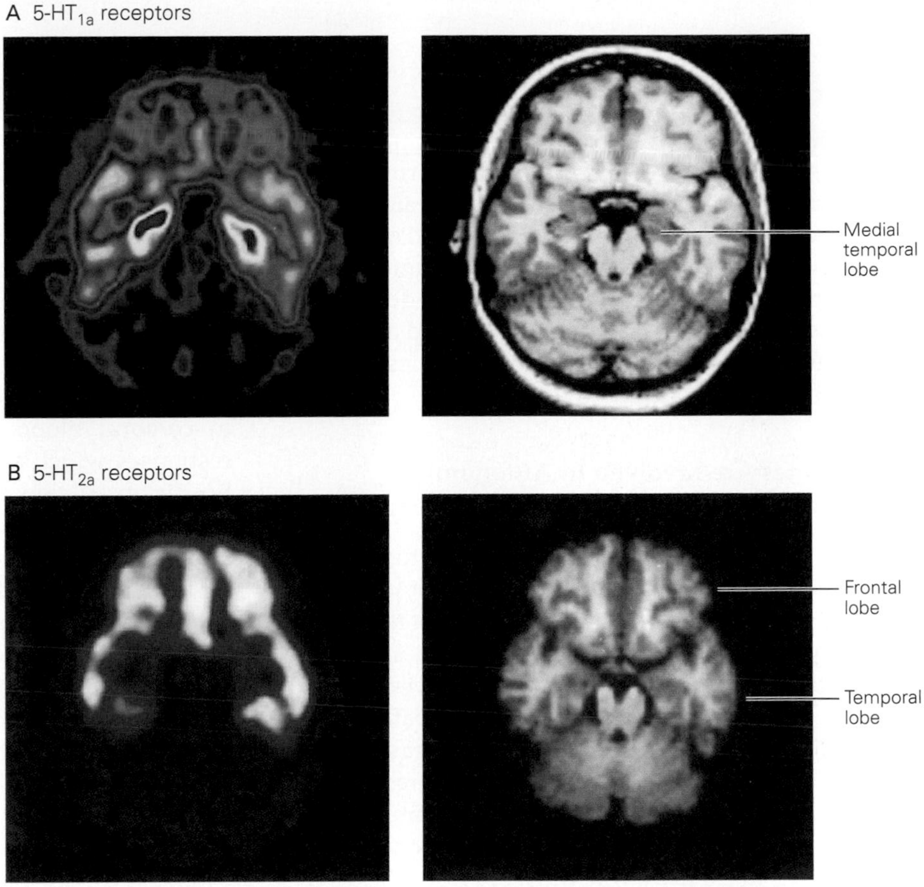

Figure 46–6 Different types of serotonin receptors are distributed differently within the brain. The left images are positron emission tomography (PET) scans showing the density of two types of serotonin (**5-HT**) receptors in the brain of a normal person, and the right images are magnetic resonance imaging (MRI) scans showing the anatomy at the same level.

A. The 5-HT$_{1a}$ receptors are concentrated mainly in the medial temporal lobe (**red**), and less so in the neocortex (**blue**). (Modified, with permission, from Plenevaux et al. 2000.)

B. At the same level, 5-HT$_{2a}$ receptors are concentrated mostly in the frontal and temporal neocortex and less so in the medial temporal lobe. (Modified, with permission, from Smith et al. 1998.)

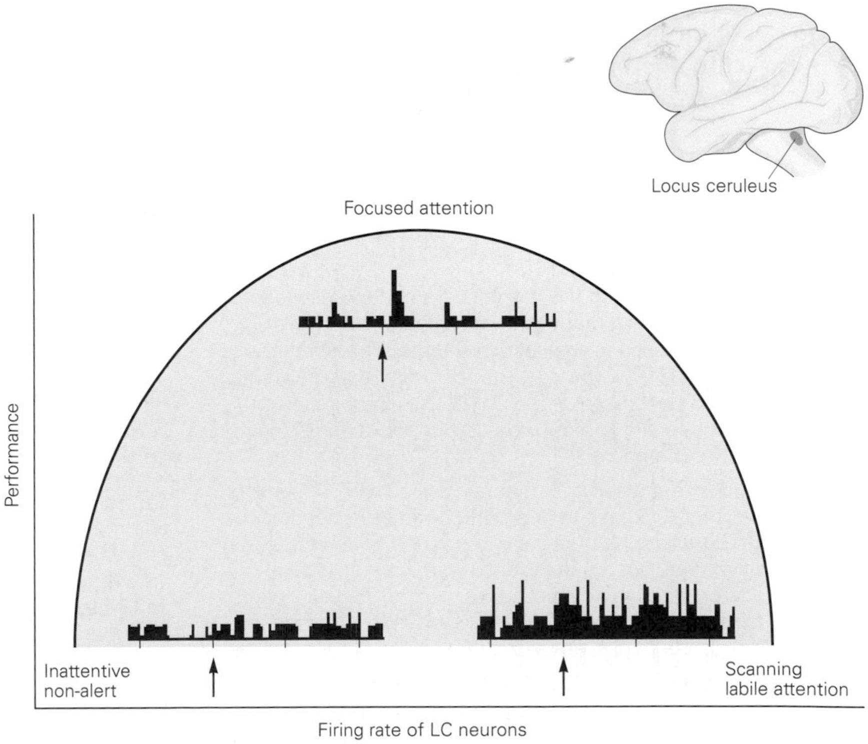

Figure 46–7 Locus ceruleus neurons exhibit different patterns of activity with different levels of attentiveness and task performance. Inverted U curve shows the relationship between a monkey's performance on a target detection task and the level of locus ceruleus (LC) activity. Histograms show the responses of LC neurons to presentation of the target during different levels of task performance. Performance is poor at low levels of LC activity because the animals are not alert. Performance is also poor when baseline activity is high because the higher baseline is incompatible with focusing on the assigned task. Performance is optimal when baseline activity is moderate and phasic activation follows presentation of the target (**arrow**). The tonic mode (with high baseline activity) might be optimal for tasks (or contexts) that require behavioral flexibility instead of focused attention. If so, the LC could regulate the balance between focused and flexible behavior. (Reproduced, with permission, from Aston-Jones and Cohen 2005.)

This pattern of activity indicates that dopaminergic neurons provide a reward-prediction error signal, an important element in reinforcement learning. The importance of dopamine in learning is also supported by observations that lesions of dopaminergic systems prevent reward-based learning. The same dopaminergic pathways that are important for reward and learning are involved in addiction to many drugs of abuse (see Chapter 49)

Monoamines Are Involved in Autonomic Regulation and Breathing

Neurons in the adrenergic C1 group in the rostral ventrolateral medulla play a key role in maintaining resting vascular tone as well as adjusting vasomotor tone necessitated by various behaviors. For example, an upright posture disinhibits neurons in the rostral ventrolateral medulla that directly innervate the sympathetic preganglionic vasomotor neurons, thus increasing vasomotor tone to prevent a drop in blood pressure (the baroreceptor reflex). Neurons in the noradrenergic A5 group in the pons inhibit the sympathetic preganglionic neurons and play a role in depressor reflexes (eg, the fall in blood pressure in response to deep pain).

Serotonin regulates many different autonomic functions including gastrointestinal peristalsis, thermoregulation, cardiovascular control, and breathing. Electrical stimulation of serotonergic neurons within the medullary raphe nuclei increases heart rate and blood pressure. Serotonergic neurons in the medulla also project to neurons in the medulla and spinal cord that regulate breathing (Figure 46–8A), and stimulation of the medullary raphe nuclei increases respiratory motor output (see Chapter 45). Some serotonergic neurons in the medulla are central chemoreceptors (CO_2 sensors), firing faster in response to an increase in CO_2 and in turn stimulating breathing to restore arterial acid/base homeostasis. Serotonergic neurons in the midbrain also sense arterial CO_2 (Figure 46–8B). These neurons may induce arousal, anxiety, and changes in cerebral blood flow when blood CO_2 increases, responses which are important for survival when airflow is obstructed. Consistent with these ideas, genetic deletion of all serotonergic neurons in mice leads to a large decrease in the ventilatory response to breathing air with increased CO_2 (hypercapnia) and these mice no longer wake up when presented with the same stimulus while asleep.

The role of serotonergic neurons as CO_2 receptors may explain why defects in the serotonergic system have been linked to sudden infant death syndrome (SIDS). SIDS is the leading cause of postneonatal mortality in the Western world, responsible for six infant deaths every day in the United States. It was defined by an expert panel of pathologists and pediatricians as "the sudden and unexpected death of an infant under one year of age that remains unexplained after a complete clinical review, autopsy, and death scene investigation and occurs in seemingly healthy infants usually during a sleep period" (Figure 46–8C).

A widely held theory holds that some SIDS cases are due to defective CO_2 chemoreception, breathing, and arousal. An increase in the number of serotonergic

Figure 46–8 (Opposite) **Serotonergic neurons have a role in the response to a rise in CO_2 levels as well as sudden infant death syndrome (SIDS).**

A. Serotonergic neurons in the medulla are central respiratory chemoreceptors that are thought to stimulate breathing in response to an increase in arterial blood PCO_2. The dendrites of these neurons wrap around large arteries and are stimulated by an increase in partial pressure of CO_2 (PCO_2) (see Figure 45–9). They project to and excite neurons in the medulla and spinal cord that control breathing.

B. Serotonergic neurons in the midbrain are also PCO_2 sensors. Shown here is the increase in firing rate of a serotonergic neuron from the dorsal raphe nucleus in response to an increase in PCO_2 (monitored by the resultant decrease in external pH). This increase in firing rate may convert thalamic and cortical neurons to single-spike mode and thus cause wakening from sleep, an important response to prevent airway obstruction during sleep when the airway is obstructed.

C. 1. Infants are at risk of death from SIDS when three conditions coincide (triple risk hypothesis). First, the infant must be vulnerable because of an underlying abnormality of the brain stem, such as a genetic predisposition or an environmental insult (eg, exposure to cigarette smoke). Second, the baby must be in the stage of development (usually less than 1 year of age) when it may be difficult to change position to escape airway obstruction. Third, there also must be an exogenous stressor (eg, lying face down in a pillow). (Reproduced, with permission, from Filiano and Kinney 1994.) **2.** One proposed mechanism of SIDS is that the combination of abnormal serotonergic neurons (eg, caused by exposure to cigarette smoke) and postnatal immaturity of neurons involved in respiratory control may lead to the inability to respond effectively to airway obstruction. The infant then does not wake up and turn its head or breathe faster, either of which would correct the problem. As a result, severe decreases in blood oxygenation (hypoxia) and elevation of blood carbon dioxide (hypercapnia) occur. (Reproduced, with permission, from Richerson 2004.)

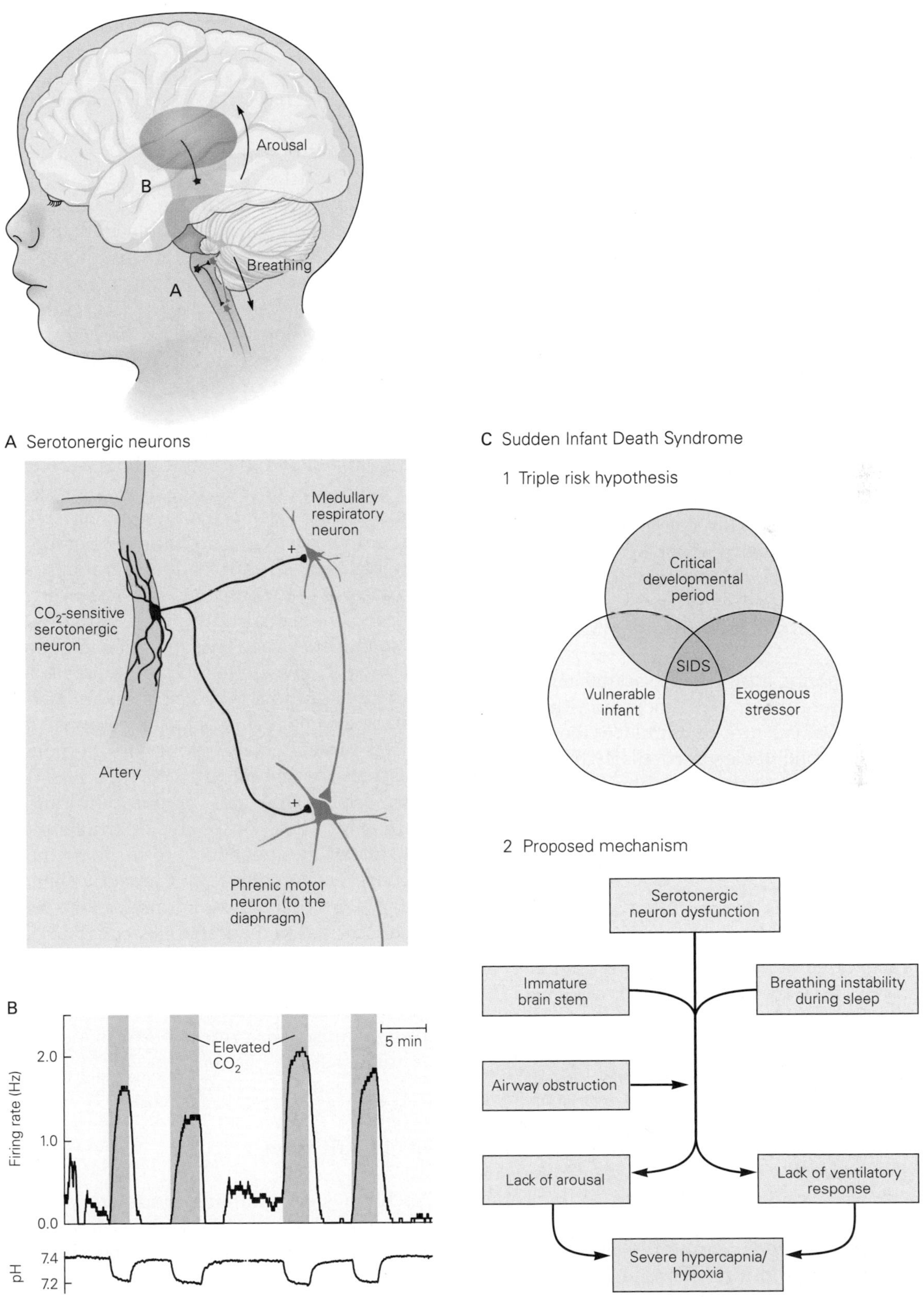
Arousal
B
Breathing
A
A Serotonergic neurons
Medullary respiratory neuron
CO_2-sensitive serotonergic neuron
Artery
Phrenic motor neuron (to the diaphragm)
B
Elevated CO_2
5 min
Firing rate (Hz)
2.0
1.0
0.0
pH
7.4
7.2
C Sudden Infant Death Syndrome
1 Triple risk hypothesis
Critical developmental period
SIDS
Vulnerable infant
Exogenous stressor
2 Proposed mechanism
Serotonergic neuron dysfunction
Immature brain stem
Breathing instability during sleep
Airway obstruction
Lack of arousal
Lack of ventilatory response
Severe hypercapnia/ hypoxia

neurons with an immature morphology, a decrease in serotonin levels, and changes in serotonergic receptor density are found in the raphe nuclei of infants who die of SIDS. A plausible neurobiological mechanism for SIDS is that a defect in development of serotonergic neurons leads to reduced ability to detect a rise in partial pressure of CO_2 when airflow is obstructed during sleep, thus blunting the normal protective response which should include arousal and increased ventilation (Figure 46–8C). Infants sleeping face down would be unable to arouse sufficiently to change position when bedding blocks the airway. This mechanism could explain the success of the Back to Sleep campaign that encourages mothers to place infants on their backs when put to sleep and has reduced the incidence of SIDS by 50%.

Pain and Anti-nociceptive Pathways Are Modulated by Monoamines

Although pain is necessary for an animal to avoid injury, continued pain following an injury may be maladaptive (eg, if the pain prevents vigorous escape from a predator). Hence the monoaminergic systems include important descending projections to the dorsal horn of the spinal cord that modulate pain perception (see Chapter 24).

The noradrenergic inputs to the spinal cord originate from pontine cell groups, including the locus ceruleus, A5, and A7 cell groups. Similarly, the serotonergic medullary raphe nuclei, particularly the nucleus raphe magnus, project to the dorsal horn where they modulate the processing of information about noxious stimuli. Direct application of serotonin to dorsal horn neurons inhibits their response to noxious stimuli, and intrathecal administration of serotonin attenuates the defensive withdrawal of the paw evoked by noxious stimuli. In addition, intrathecal administration of antagonists of serotonin receptors blocks the pain inhibition evoked by stimulation of the raphe nuclei.

Insight into the role of serotonin in pain processing has been used in treating migraine headaches. In particular, agonists to the 5-HT_{1D} receptors, the triptans have been found to be therapeutically effective. One of the possible mechanisms of action of this family of tryptamine-based drugs includes presynaptic inhibition of pain afferents from the meninges, preventing sensitization of central neurons. Drugs that block monoamine reuptake, including both traditional antidepressants and selective serotonin reuptake inhibitors, are effective in limiting pain in patients with chronic pain and migraine headaches.

Monoamines Facilitate Motor Activity

The dopaminergic system is critical for normal motor performance. A massive projection ascends from the substantia nigra pars compacta to the striatum. As described in Chapter 43, dopaminergic fibers act on striatal neurons via D_1 and D_2 receptors to release inhibition on motor responses.

As would be expected, patients with Parkinson disease in whom midbrain dopaminergic neurons have degenerated have trouble initiating movement and difficulty sustaining their movements. Such patients speak softly, write with small letters, and take small steps. Conversely, drugs that facilitate dopaminergic transmission in the striatum can result in unintended behaviors ranging from motor tics (small muscle twitches), to chorea (large scale, jerky limb movements), to complex cognitive behaviors (such as compulsive gambling or sexual activity).

As first shown by Sten Grillner, serotonergic neurons play an important role in generating motor programs. Drugs that activate serotonin receptors can induce hyperactivity, myoclonus, tremor, and rigidity, which are all part of the "serotonin syndrome." Increases in the firing of raphe neurons have been observed in animals during repetitive motor activities such as feeding, grooming, locomotion, and deep breathing. Conversely, the atonia and lack of movement that occur during REM sleep are associated with near cessation of firing of raphe neurons.

Noradrenergic cell groups in the pons also send extensive projections to motor neurons. This modulatory input facilitates excitatory inputs to motor neurons by acting on β- and α_1-adrenergic receptors. The sum of these effects is to facilitate motor neuron responses in stereotypic and repetitive behaviors such as rhythmic chewing, swimming, or locomotion. Conversely, increased β-adrenergic activation during stress can exaggerate motor responses and produce tremor. Drugs that block β-adrenergic receptors are used clinically to reduce certain types of tremor and are often taken by musicians prior to performances to minimize tremulousness.

An Overall View

The brain stem contains modulatory neurons with long axons that either ascend to the forebrain where they control various aspects of mood and cognition, or descend to the spinal cord where they regulate autonomic, somatosensory, or motor functions. These monoaminergic and cholinergic systems are also essential components of the ascending arousal system.

The dual roles of the brain stem as a conduit for information flow to and from the forebrain and a modulator of forebrain activity is illustrated poignantly in patients with injury of the midpons. Because the ascending arousal system begins at the upper pontine level, patients remain awake; but the intact and awake forebrain is unable to interact with the external world other than with eye movements, a condition described clinically as the locked-in syndrome. In contrast, patients in a persistent vegetative state have intact brain stems but in most cases have extensive forebrain damage (such as from hypoxia). These patients appear to be alternately awake and asleep but have no outward signs of consciousness.

Hence, normal conscious behavior requires close interaction between the brain stem and the forebrain. The monoaminergic and cholinergic regulatory systems are very important in clinical medicine because their various components are dysfunctional in a variety of neurological and psychiatric diseases, including depression, dementia, migraine, psychosis, and SIDS. They are the targets of a large number of clinically useful drugs.

These neurons play a disproportionately important role in normal brain function and a better understanding of them has great potential for treating neuropsychiatric disease.

Postscript: Evaluation of the Comatose Patient

Nowhere is knowledge of brain stem anatomy and function more important in clinical neurology than when caring for the comatose patient. Coma is a state of profound unconsciousness from which the patient cannot be aroused by external stimuli. Two neurological principles are important for determining the cause of coma.

First, any decrease in the level of consciousness (decreased arousal) implies dysfunction of either both cerebral hemispheres or of the ascending arousal system (or its projections in the thalamus or hypothalamus). Second, one can pinpoint the levels of the brain stem that are damaged by determining abnormalities of reflexes mediated by cranial nerves, which often accompany coma.

The keys to successful care of a comatose patient are, first, to provide life support if needed, and then to identify the specific etiology of the coma. The cause of coma can usually be determined by obtaining a history from witnesses, an examination focused on brain stem function, and use of targeted laboratory tests. Dysfunction of the ascending arousal system can result either from diffuse impairment of the brain, usually from a pharmacologic, toxic, or metabolic cause, or from a focal lesion that impinges on the upper brain stem, diencephalon, or both cerebral hemispheres.

In the case of coma from diffuse impairment, there are few if any signs of focal brain stem defects. In the case of focal injuries to the upper brain stem or forebrain there are generally locally restricted changes, and the neurological examination can pinpoint the location and give clues to the cause of the problem.

Thus the neurological examination is the critical first step in determining the cause and severity of coma, and its primary purpose is to determine whether there is any evidence of a focal lesion and, if so, at what levels of the brain stem. The neurological examination of comatose patients is much simpler than that of conscious patients because it is not possible to do many portions of a full exam that require patient cooperation. This abbreviated neurological exam is sometimes called the *coma exam* or the *brain stem exam* and includes the following.

The *level of consciousness* is assessed by observing the motor response to external stimuli. If the patient is unable to respond to verbal stimuli or gentle shaking, it may be necessary to apply a local painful stimulus (eg, pressing on a nail bed). The level of consciousness is assessed by the vigor with which the patient responds to the stimulus. Terms used to describe responsiveness include *comatose, semi-comatose, obtunded, somnolent, lethargic,* and *alert,* in increasing order of preservation of arousal. However, it is generally more reproducible to describe how the patient responds to a stimulus rather than to use these inexact terms.

Asymmetric motor responses suggest a focal impairment of either the sensory or motor systems responsible for the side of the body that is less responsive but does not help identify the level of the lesion (Figure 46–9). Flexion of both arms at the elbow and extension of both legs, occurring spontaneously or in response to pain, is called decorticate posturing and usually indicates a lesion above the midbrain. Extension of both arms and both legs is called decerebrate posturing and usually indicates a more severe lesion that often affects the upper part of the brain stem.

Abnormal respiratory patterns can help localize lesions and are important to recognize because they can predict whether a patient may later require mechanical ventilation (Figure 46–10). Periodic waxing and waning

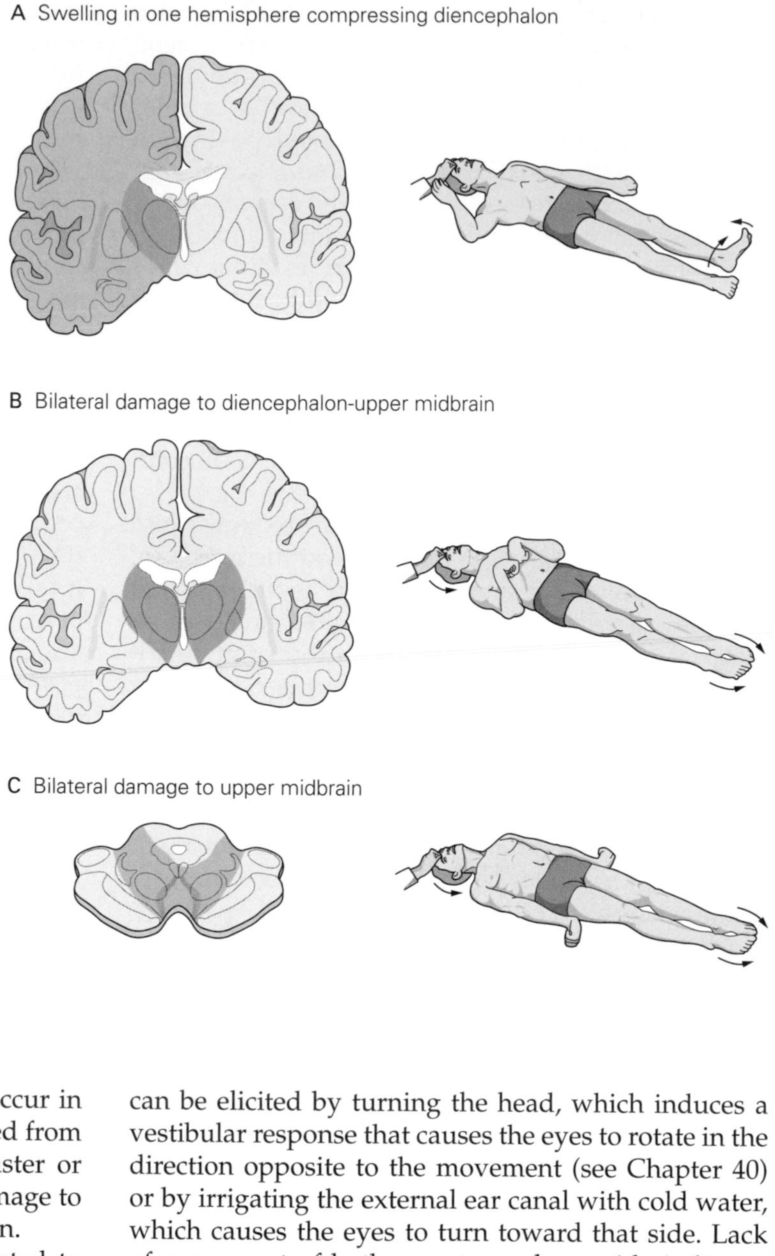

Figure 46–9 The motor response to painful stimulation is a key localizing sign of brain damage in coma. Shown are the movements of the arms and legs in response to pressure on the supraorbital ridge, just above the eye.

A. A patient with a diffuse metabolic encephalopathy (such as induced by high ammonia levels in the blood caused by liver failure) may respond to painful stimulation by trying to brush the examiner away. If there is a tumor or subdural hematoma in one hemisphere, the motor response may be asymmetric. The contralateral arm may not respond, the leg may be externally rotated, and stimulation of the sole of the foot may cause the big toe to flex upward (the Babinski reflex).

B. Decorticate posturing is caused by damage at the junction of the diencephalon and the upper midbrain: the upper extremities flex, the lower extremities extend, and the toes extend downward.

C. Decerebrate posturing is caused by more extensive damage often extending into the midbrain, and results in extension of both the upper and lower extremities. Progression from decorticate to decerebrate posturing heralds rostrocaudal deterioration of the brain stem, which may progress rapidly to respiratory arrest because of involvement of the medulla.

of respiration (Cheyne-Stokes breathing) can occur in forebrain depression. This must be differentiated from other irregular breathing patterns such as cluster or ataxic breathing, because the latter indicate damage to the lower brain stem and may require intubation.

Examination of cranial nerve function related to the pupillary light response and eye movements can be informative, because these pathways are closely adjacent to the structures of the ascending arousal system in the upper brain stem. The pupillary light reflex is tested by shining a bright light into one eye. Lesions at various levels of the brain stem produce characteristic changes in pupillary light responses that often can pinpoint the location of an injury (Figure 46–11).

Eye movements can also be equally helpful. Slow, roving eye movements are seen in patients with diffuse forebrain impairment but normal brain stem activity. In a more deeply comatose patient, eye movements can be elicited by turning the head, which induces a vestibular response that causes the eyes to rotate in the direction opposite to the movement (see Chapter 40) or by irrigating the external ear canal with cold water, which causes the eyes to turn toward that side. Lack of movement of both eyes toward one side indicates injury to the lower pons, where vestibular inputs reach the medial pontine circuitry that controls lateral gaze. Selective loss of abduction of one eye indicates damage to the abducens nerve, at the lower pontine level, whereas selective loss of conjugate adduction reflects injury to the medial longitudinal fasciculus, which travels in the medial part of the pons to the midbrain to connect the abducens and oculomotor nuclei. Selective loss of vertical eye movements implies an injury to the dorsal midbrain.

This brief explanation of the coma exam illustrates how it can often make it possible to determine

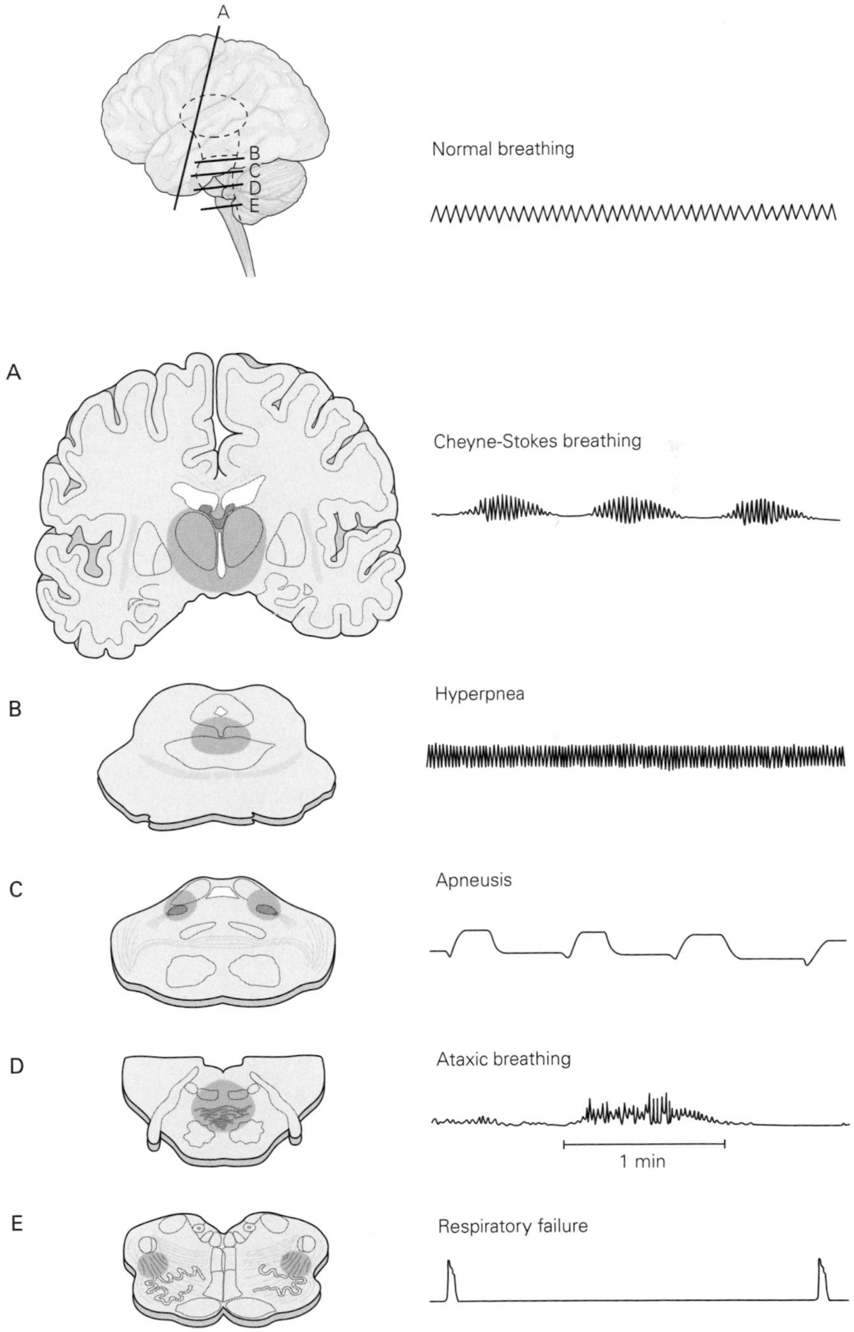

Figure 46–10 The respiratory pattern is a key indicator of the level of the brain that is not functioning properly in a comatose patient and provides a warning of impending respiratory arrest. The normal breathing pattern in an adult is regular, with approximately 14 to 16 breaths per minute while sitting quietly.

A. Cheyne-Stokes breathing is a waxing and waning pattern of breaths interspersed with periods of apnea. This pattern can occur with bilateral cortical or diencephalic dysfunction, caused by either structural damage or depression by drugs or metabolic problems. Cheyne-Stokes breathing also occurs in patients with cardiac failure and is seen in most normal individuals while sleeping at moderately high altitude (see Chapter 45).

B. Hyperpnea, or hyperventilation with deep, regular breaths, in comatose patients is most commonly caused by underlying medical problems (eg, liver failure, sepsis, or pulmonary edema). Rarely does it indicate a lesion in the central nervous system. Occasionally, central neurogenic hyperventilation is observed in patients with tumors of the brain stem (see Chapter 45).

C. Apneusis is a pattern of deep, prolonged inspirations. This pattern occurs with lesions of the rostral pons in the region of the parabrachial complex (also known as the pneumotaxic center).

D. Ataxic breathing is a pattern of breaths that are irregular in frequency, duration, and depth. It occurs with lesions of the pontomedullary junction and often heralds respiratory failure. It is important to recognize the difference between this pattern and Cheyne-Stokes breathing.

E. Lesions of the rostral ventrolateral medulla cause respiratory failure. There may be occasional gasping breaths separated by long periods of apnea, until respiration ceases entirely.

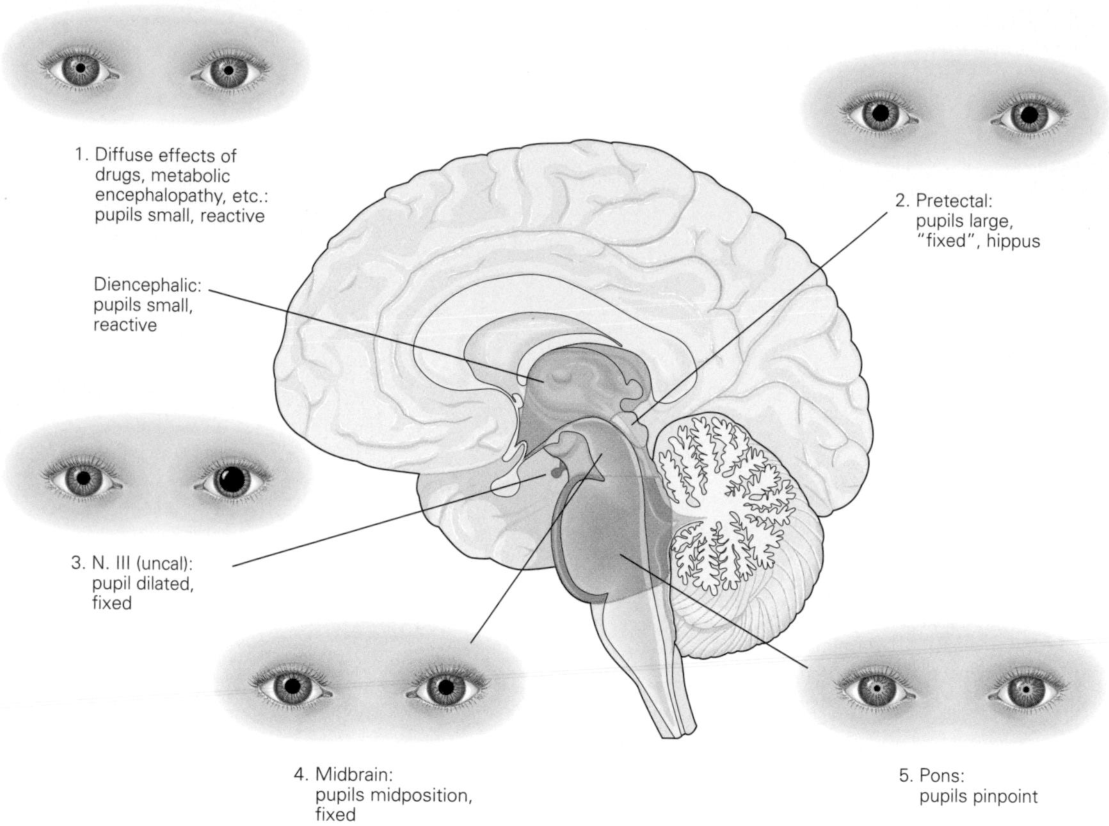

Figure 46–11 The pupillary light reflex is an important sign for determining the level of a brain stem lesion. In patients with depressed consciousness caused by metabolic encephalopathy, drug ingestion, or diffuse pressure on the diencephalon, the pupils are slightly smaller than normal but respond vigorously to light (**1**). Pressure on the pretectal area (eg, from a pineal tumor) prevents light from causing pupillary constriction and results in large, unreactive pupils (**2**). Injury to the oculomotor nerve (N. III) can occur because of swelling in the ipsilateral cerebrum (eg, from a brain tumor), which causes the uncus (the medial edge of the temporal lobe) to herniate through the tentorial opening and crush the oculomotor nerve. This first leads to a large, unreactive pupil in the affected eye (**3**). It can also later cause the affected eye to deviate laterally. This *blown pupil* is an ominous sign that the brain stem is about to be compressed from above. Damage to the midbrain tegmentum causes complete loss of pupillary response to light (**4**), but the pupils may dilate if a painful stimulus (eg, pinching the neck) is applied because of a sympathetic response (the ciliospinal response). Injury to the pons results in pinpoint pupils (**5**), which can be seen with a magnifying lens to respond slightly to light. Pontine injury not only disrupts the descending hypothalamic pupillodilator pathway but also interrupts ascending inputs to the Edinger-Westphal nucleus that inhibit its tone.

the precise level of the affected brain stem. Such information provides important clues as to the type of the injury and the kind of immediate treatment and further evaluation that may be required.

George B. Richerson
Gary Aston-Jones
Clifford B. Saper

Selected Readings

Aston-Jones G, Cohen JD. 2005. Adaptive gain and the role of the locus ceruleus-norepinephrine system in optimal performance. J Comp Neurol 493:99–110.

Fisch BJ. 1999. *Fisch & Spehlmann's EEG Primer: Basic Principles of Digital and Analog EEG,* 3rd ed. Amsterdam: Elsevier Science.

Hökfelt T, Johansson O, Goldstein M. 1984. Chemical anatomy of the brain. Science 225:1326–1334.

Jacobs BL, Azmitia EC. 1992. Structure and function of the brain serotonin system. Physiol Rev 72:165–229.

Mason P. 2001. Contributions of the medullary raphe and ventromedial reticular region to pain modulation and other homeostatic functions. Annu Rev Neurosci 24:737–777.

McCormick DA. 1992. Neurotransmitter actions in the thalamus and cerebral cortex and their role in neuromodulation of thalamocortical activity. Prog Neurobiol 39:337–388.

Posner JB, Saper CB, Schiff ND, Plum F. 2007. *Plum and Posner's Diagnosis of Stupor and Coma,* 4th ed. New York: Oxford Univ. Press.

Richerson GB. 2004. Serotonin neurons as CO_2 sensors that maintain pH homeostasis. Nat Rev Neurosci 5:449–461.

Saper CB, Scammell TE, Lu J. 2005. Hypothalamic regulation of sleep and circadian rhythms. Nature 437:1257–1263.

Schultz W. 2001. Reward signaling by dopamine neurons. Neuroscientist 7:293–302.

Wijdicks EF. 2001. Current concepts: the diagnosis of brain death. N Engl J Med 344:1215–1221.

References

Alreja M, Aghajanian GK. 1991. Pacemaker activity of locus coeruleus neurons: whole-cell recordings in brain slices show dependence on cAMP and protein kinase A. Brain Res 556:339–343.

Aston-Jones G, Bloom F. 1981. Activity of norepinephrine-containing locus ceruleus neurons in behaving rats anticipates fluctuations in the sleep-waking cycle. J Neurosci 1:876–886.

Aston-Jones G, Chen S, Zhu Y, Oshinsky M. 2001. A neural circuit for circadian regulation of arousal and performance. Nat Neurosci 4:732–738.

Aston-Jones G, Cohen JD. 2005. An integrative theory of locus coeruleus-norepinephrine function: adaptive gain and optimal performance. Annu Rev Neurosci 28:403–450.

Berridge CW, Foote SL. 1991. Effects of locus coeruleus activation on electroencephalographic activity in neocortex and hippocampus. J Neurosci 11:3135–3145.

Bradley SR, Pieribone VA, Wang W, Severson CA, Jacobs RA, Richerson GB. 2002. Chemosensitive serotonergic neurons are closely associated with large medullary arteries. Nat Neurosci 5:401–402.

Chou TC, Scammell TE, Gooley JJ, Gaus SE, Saper CB, Lu J. 2003. Critical role of the dorsomedial nucleus in a wide range of behavioral circadian rhythms. J Neurosci 23:10691–10702.

Delfs JM, Zhu Y, Druhan JP, Aston-Jones G. 2000. Noradrenaline in the ventral forebrain is critical for opiate withdrawal-induced aversion. Nature 403:430–434.

Filiano JJ, Kinney HC. 1994. A perspective on neuropathologic findings in victims of the sudden infant death syndrome: the triple-risk model. Biol Neonate 65:194–197.

Haas HL, Reiner PB. 1988. Membrane properties of histaminergic tuberomammillary neurones of the rat hypothalamus *in vitro.* J Physiol 399:633–646.

Harris GC, Aston-Jones G. 2000. Augmented accumbal serotonin levels decrease the preference for a morphine associated environment during withdrawal. Neuropsychopharmacology 24:75–85.

Harris GC, Altomare K, Aston-Jones G. 2001. Preference for a cocaine-associated environment is attenuated by augmented accumbal serotonin in cocaine withdrawn rats. Psychopharmacology (Berl) 156:14–22.

Hendricks TJ, Fyodorov DV, Wegman LJ, Lelutiu NB, Pehek EA, Yamamoto B, Silver J, Weeber EJ, Sweatt JD, Deneris ES. 2003. Pet-1 ETS gene plays a critical role in 5-HT neuron development and is required for normal anxiety-like and aggressive behavior. Neuron 37:233–247.

Jacobs BL, Fornal CA. 1999. Activity of serotonergic neurons in behaving animals. Neuropsychopharmacology 21:9S–15S.

Krous HF, Beckwith JB, Byard RW, Rognum TO, Bajanowski T, Corey T, Cutz E, Hanzlick R, Keens TG, Mitchell EA. 2004. Sudden infant death syndrome and unclassified sudden infant deaths: a definitional and diagnostic approach. Pediatrics 114:234–38.

Lu J, Jhou TC, Saper CB. 2006. Identification of wake-active dopaminergic neurons in the ventral periaqueductal gray matter. J Neurosci 26:193–202.

MacDermott AB, Role LW, Siegelbaum SA. 1999. Presynaptic ionotropic receptors and the control of transmitter release. Annu Rev Neurosci 22:443–485.

Maquet P, Degueldre C, Delfiore G, Aerts J, Peters JM, Luxen A, Franck G. 1997. Functional neuroanatomy of human slow wave sleep. J Neurosci 17:2807–2812.

McCormick DA, Bat T. 1997. Sleep and arousal: thalamocortical mechanisms. Annu Rev Neurosci 20:185–215.

Panigrahy A, Filiano J, Sleeper LA, Mandell F, Valdes-Dapena M, Krous HF, Rava LA, Foley E, White WF, Kinney HC. 2000. Decreased serotonergic receptor binding in rhombic lip-derived regions of the medulla oblongata in the sudden infant death syndrome. J Neuropathol Exp Neurol 59:377–384.

Plenevaux A, Lemaire C, Aerts J, Lacan G, Rubins D, Melega WP, Brihaye C, et al. 2000. [$^{(18)}$F]p-MPPF: a radiolabeled antagonist for the study of 5-$HT_{(1A)}$ receptors with PET. Nucl Med Biol 27:467–471.

Richerson GB, Wang W, Tiwari J, Bradley SR. 2001. Chemosensitivity of serotonergic neurons in the rostral ventral medulla. Respir Physiol 129:175–189.

Severson CA, Wang W, Pieribone VA, Dohle CI, Richerson GB. 2003. Midbrain serotonergic neurons are central pH chemoreceptors. Nat Neurosci 6:1139–1140.

Smith GS, Price JC, Lopresti BJ, Huang Y, Simpson N, Holt D, Mason NS, et al. 1998. Test-retest variability of serotonin 5-HT_{2A} receptor binding measured with positron emission tomography and [^{18}F] altanserin in the human brain. Synapse 30:380–392.

Steriade M, McCormick DA, Sejnowski TJ. 1993. Thalamocortical oscillations in the slweeping and aroused brain. Science 262:679-685.

Wang W, Zaykin RV, Bradley SR, Tiwari JK, Richerson GB. 2001. Acidosis-stimulated neurons of the medullary raphe are serotonergic. J Neurophysiol 85:2224–2235.

Wolfart J, Neuhoff H, Franz O, Roeper J. 2001. Differential expression of the small-conductance, calcium-activated potassium channel SK3 is critical for pacemaker control in dopaminergic midbrain neurons. J Neurosci 21:3443–3456.

47

The Autonomic Motor System and the Hypothalamus

When we are frightened our heart races, our breathing becomes rapid and shallow, our mouth becomes dry, our muscles tense, our palms become sweaty, and we may want to run. These bodily changes accompanying fear are mediated by the autonomic motor system, which controls heart muscle, smooth muscle, and exocrine glands. The autonomic motor system is controlled by a central neuronal network that includes the hypothalamus.

As we shall learn in this and the next two chapters, the hypothalamus regulates the autonomic circuits so as to recruit appropriate physiological responses for specific emotions and to coordinate these physiological and emotional responses with other aspects of behavior to insure constancy of the internal environment (homeostasis). The hypothalamus contributes to the maintenance of homeostasis by acting on three major systems: the autonomic motor system, the endocrine system, and an ill-defined neural system concerned with motivation.

The autonomic motor system is distinct from the somatic motor system, which controls skeletal muscle. Nevertheless, to produce behaviors the somatic and autonomic motor systems must work together. Whereas neurons in the somatic motor system regulate contractions of striated muscles (see Chapter 34), the autonomic motor system regulates gland cells as well as smooth and cardiac muscle, maintains constant body temperature, and controls eating, drinking, and sexual behavior.

Although the autonomic motor system is largely involuntary, the behaviors controlled by it are tightly integrated with voluntary movements controlled by the somatic motor system. Running, climbing, and lifting are voluntary actions with metabolic requirements and thermoregulatory consequences that are automatically met by the autonomic system through changes in cardiorespiratory drive, cardiac output, regional blood flow, and ventilation. Autonomic behaviors similarly are linked to emotional arousal, stress, motivation, and defensive reactions. Feelings of fear, anger, happiness, and sadness have characteristic autonomic manifestations.

In this chapter we first examine the peripheral components of the autonomic system and then their role in mediating behaviors. We then explore how these "autonomic behaviors" are orchestrated through a central autonomic network in the brain stem and hypothalamus. We conclude by considering the role of the amygdala and specialized areas of cerebral cortex in coordinating autonomic function with motivation, volition, and emotion. The autonomic and hypothalamic mechanisms involved in emotion and motivation are examined in more detail in the next two chapters.

The Autonomic Motor System Mediates Homeostasis

In the middle of the 19th century Claude Bernard in Paris drew attention to the stability of the body's internal environment, which includes the "fluid that surrounds and bathes all tissues," during a broad range of behavioral states and external conditions. Bernard wrote: "The internal environment (*le milieu interior*) is a necessary condition for a free life." Building on this idea, in the 1930s Walter B. Cannon introduced the concept of homeostasis to describe the mechanisms that maintain within a narrow physiological range the constancy of composition of the bodily fluids, body temperature, blood pressure, and other physiological variables.

As envisioned by Cannon, homeostatic mechanisms are adaptive because they extend the range of human behavior. For example, during exercise healthy people can increase their cardiac output four- to fivefold while maintaining blood pressure within a much narrower range. In the absence of these normal compensatory changes, blood pressure would increase in direct proportion to cardiac output, and the resulting increase in pressure would rupture blood vessels, perturb fluid composition, and alter the balance among the vascular, interstitial, and intracellular compartments. Increases in pressure of that proportion do not normally happen because the increase during exercise is curbed by an increase in diameter of the arteries that supply the working muscles and a resulting reduction of total vascular resistance to blood flow.

All homeostatic behavior, including control of the circulation, arises from neural modulation of the physiological properties of organ systems, mediated by hypothalamic control of the autonomic motor system and the endocrine system. We begin the discussion of these mechanisms by considering the peripheral components: the autonomic ganglia. The circuits of the ganglia connect with the spinal cord and brain stem and mediate simple reflexes that are the components of more complex behaviors.

The Autonomic System Contains Visceral Motor Neurons That Are Organized into Ganglia

Unlike the somatic motor system, in which the motor neurons are located in the ventral spinal cord and brain stem, the cell bodies of autonomic motor neurons are found in enlargements of peripheral nerves called *ganglia*.[1] The autonomic ganglia contain motor neurons that innervate the secretory epithelial cells in glands or smooth and cardiac muscle.

Overall, the nervous system has many more autonomic than somatic motor neurons. In humans the entire spinal cord contains only approximately 120,000 somatic motor nerve cells, whereas the superior cervical ganglion alone contains approximately 900,000 autonomic motor neurons. Although the significance of this difference in numbers is uncertain, it may reflect the great diversity and complexity of autonomically controlled target tissues—the stomach, intestine, bladder, heart, lungs, and vasculature—as compared to the relative uniformity of skeletal muscle controlled by the somatic motor system. Most autonomic ganglia contain far fewer cells. For example, in the lungs and gastrointestinal tract of humans there are many microscopic ganglia, each with only tens to hundreds of neurons. These differences in number of cells are thought to reflect differences in the degree of control and the size of peripheral target fields.

Efforts to understand the principles of organization of autonomic ganglia began in 1880 in England with the work of Walter Gaskell and were later continued by John N. Langley. Their pioneering studies determined how individual autonomic ganglia are functionally regulated by central nerves, and in turn how the different ganglia regulate different peripheral

[1]The peripheral nerves also have sensory ganglia, located on the dorsal roots of the spinal cord and on five of the cranial nerves: trigeminal (V), facial (VII), vestibulocochlear (VIII), glossopharyngeal (IX), and vagus (X) (see Chapter 45).

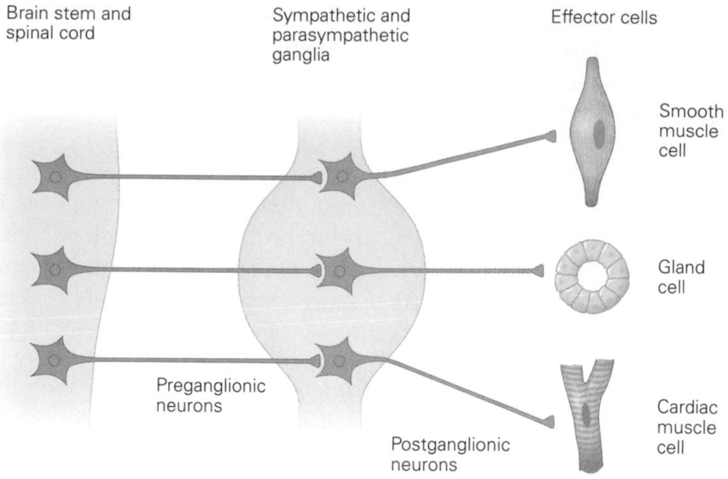

Figure 47–1 Autonomic pathways have three basic cell types. Autonomic motor neurons lie outside the central nervous system in clusters or ganglia and are controlled by preganglionic neurons in the spinal cord and brain stem. Specialized neurons in ganglia regulate specific types of effector cells, such as smooth muscle, gland cells, and cardiac muscle.

targets. Gaskell and Langley stimulated autonomic nerves and observed the responses of end-organs (eg, vasoconstriction, piloerection, sweating, pupillary constriction). They used nicotine to block signals from individual ganglia to test interactions between ganglia. In the course of these studies Langley proposed that specific chemical substances must be released by neurons of the autonomic ganglia and that these substances act by binding to receptors on the target cells. These ideas set the stage for the later investigations of chemical synaptic transmission. Langley also distinguished the autonomic and somatic motor systems and in so doing created much of our current nomenclature.

Langley divided the autonomic system into three divisions: sympathetic, parasympathetic, and enteric. All neurons in sympathetic and parasympathetic ganglia are controlled by *preganglionic* neurons whose cell bodies lie in the spinal cord and brain stem. The pre-ganglionic neurons synthesize and release the neurotransmitter acetylcholine (ACh), which acts on nicotinic ACh receptors in *postganglionic* neurons, producing fast excitatory postsynaptic potentials and initiating action potentials that propagate to synapses with effector cells in *end-organs* (Figure 47–1). The sympathetic and parasympathetic systems are distinguished by five criteria:

1. The segmental organization of their preganglionic neurons in the spinal cord and brain stem
2. The peripheral locations of their ganglia
3. The types and locations of end-organs they innervate
4. The effects they produce on end-organs
5. The neurotransmitters employed by their postganglionic neurons

Preganglionic Neurons Are Localized in Three Regions Along the Brain Stem and Spinal Cord

The parasympathetic pathways arise from a cranial nerve zone in the brain stem and a second zone in sacral segments of the spinal cord (Figure 47–2). These parasympathetic zones surround a sympathetic zone that extends continuously in thoracic and lumbar segments of the cord.

The cranial parasympathetic pathways arise from preganglionic neurons in the general visceral motor nuclei of four cranial nerves: the oculomotor nerve (N. III) in the midbrain and the facial (N. VII), glossopharyngeal (N. IX), and vagus (N. X) nerves in the medulla. The cranial parasympathetic nuclei are described in Chapter 45 together with the mixed cranial nerves (such as the facial, glossopharyngeal, and vagus). The spinal parasympathetic pathway originates in preganglionic neurons in sacral segments two to four (S2–S4). The cell bodies of most of these neurons are located in intermediate regions of the gray matter, and their axons project in peripheral nerves through the ventral roots.

The sympathetic preganglionic cell column extends between the cervical and lumbosacral enlargements of the spinal cord, corresponding to the first thoracic segment (T1) and third lumbar segment (L3) in humans (Figure 47–2). Most of the cell bodies of sympathetic preganglionic neurons are located in the intermediolateral cell column, near the lateral margin of the spinal gray matter at the level of the central canal (Figure 47–3). Others are found in the central autonomic area surrounding the central canal and in a band connecting the central area with the intermediolateral cell column. The axons of preganglionic sympathetic neurons project from the spinal cord through the nearest ventral root and then run with small connecting nerves known as *rami communicantes* before terminating on postganglionic cells in the paravertebral sympathetic chain (Figure 47–3).

Sympathetic Ganglia Project to Many Targets Throughout the Body

The sympathetic motor system regulates systemic physiological parameters such as blood pressure and body temperature by influencing target cells within virtually every tissue throughout the body (Figure 47–2). This regulation depends on afferent pathways from the spinal cord and from supraspinal structures that control the activity of the preganglionic neurons. Preganglionic neurons form synapses with neurons in paravertebral and prevertebral sympathetic ganglia (Figure 47–3) that in turn form synapses with a variety of end-organs, including blood vessels, heart, bronchial airways, piloerector muscles, and salivary and sweat glands. The preganglionic neurons also synapse on chromaffin cells in the medulla of the adrenal gland

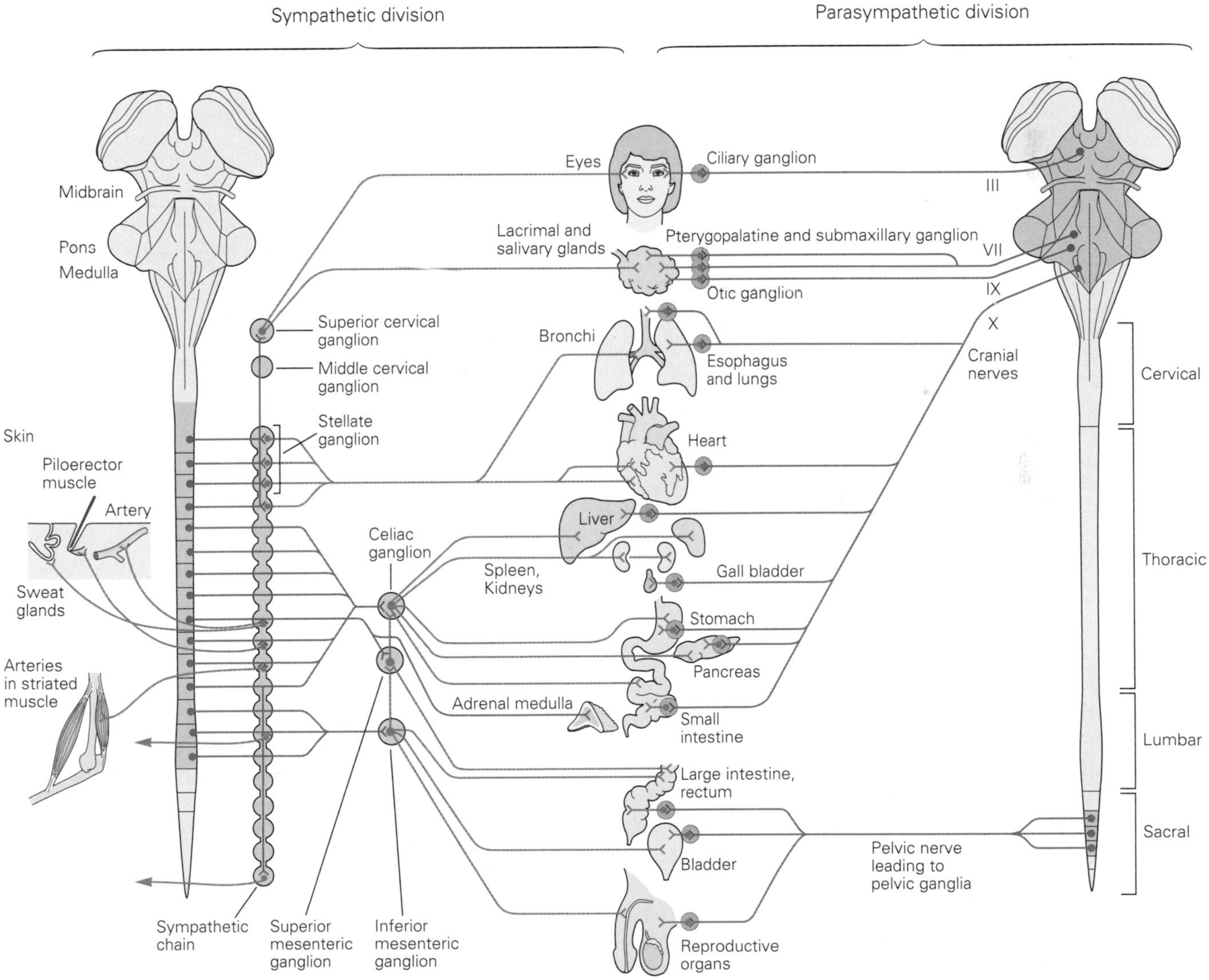

Figure 47–2 Sympathetic and parasympathetic divisions of the autonomic motor system. The sympathetic ganglia lie close to the spinal column and supply virtually every tissue in the body. Some tissues, such as skeletal muscle, are regulated only indirectly through their arterial blood supply. The parasympathetic ganglia are found in close apposition with their targets, which do not include the skin or skeletal muscle.

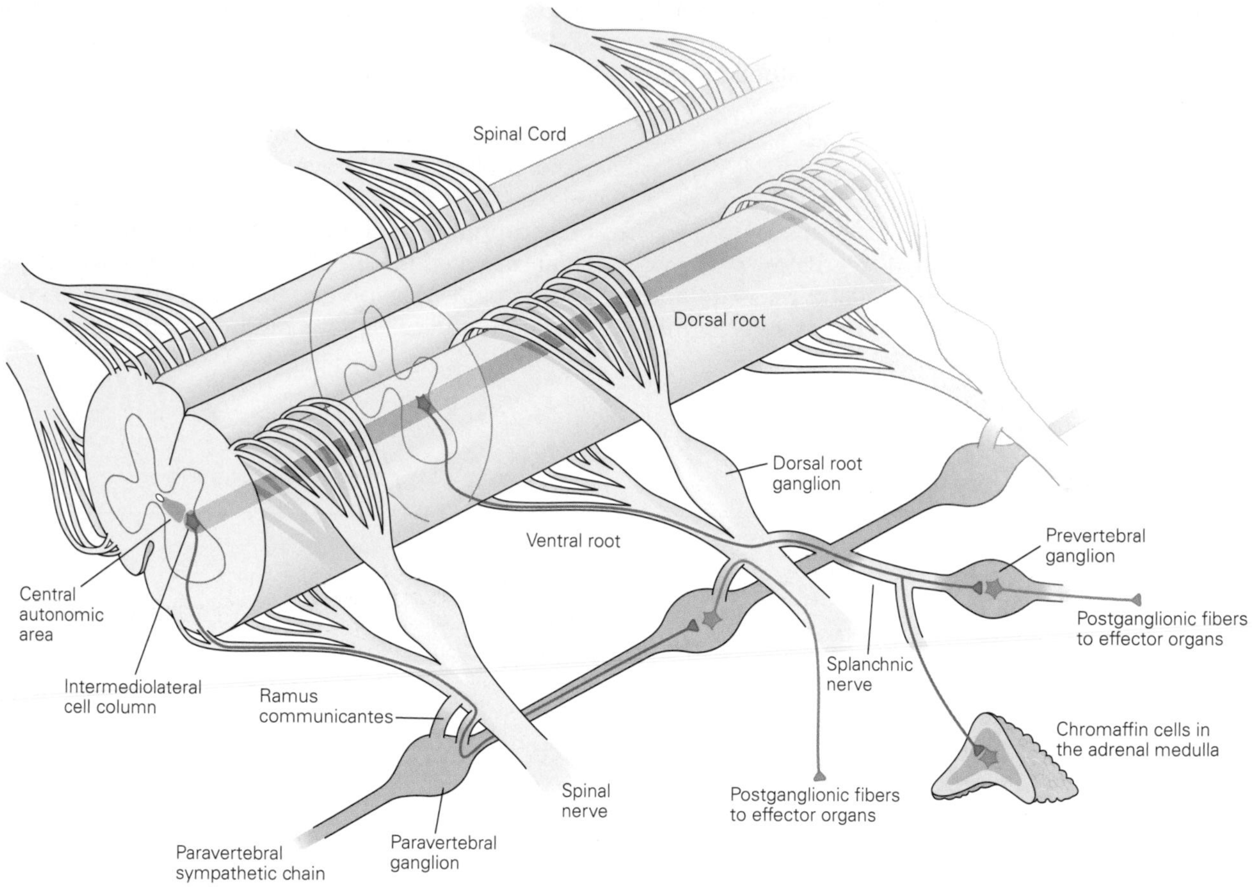

Figure 47–3 The sympathetic outflow is organized into groups of paravertebral and prevertebral ganglia. The axons of preganglionic cells in the spinal cord reach postganglionic neurons by way of ventral roots and the paravertebral sympathetic chain. The axons either form synapses on postganglionic neurons in paravertebral ganglia or project out of the chain into splanchnic nerves. Preganglionic axons in the splanchnic nerves form synapses with postganglionic neurons in prevertebral ganglia and with chromaffin cells in the adrenal medulla.

(Figure 47–3), which secrete epinephrine (adrenaline) and norepinephrine (noradrenaline) into the circulation as hormones to act on distant targets.

The paravertebral and prevertebral sympathetic ganglia differ both in location and organization. Paravertebral ganglia are distributed segmentally, extending bilaterally as two chains from the first cervical segment to the last sacral segment. The chains lie lateral to the vertebral column at its ventral margin and generally contain one ganglion per segment (Figures 47–2 and 47–3). Two important exceptions are the superior cervical and stellate ganglia. The superior cervical ganglion is a coalescence of several cervical ganglia and supplies sympathetic innervation to the entire head, including the cerebral vasculature. The stellate ganglion, which innervates the heart and lungs, is a coalescence of ganglia from lower cervical segments and the first thoracic segment. These sympathetic pathways have an orderly somatotopic relation to one another, from their segmental origin in preganglionic neurons to their terminus in peripheral targets.

The prevertebral ganglia are midline structures that lie close to the arteries for which they are named (Figures 47–2 and 47–3). In addition to sending sympathetic signals to visceral organs in the abdomen and pelvis, these ganglia also receive sensory feedback from their end-organs.

Parasympathetic Ganglia Innervate Single Organs

In contrast to sympathetic ganglia, which regulate many targets and lie some distance from their targets close to the spinal cord, parasympathetic ganglia generally innervate single end-organs and lie near to or within the end-organs they regulate (Figure 47–2). In addition, the parasympathetic system does not influence skin or skeletal muscle except in the head, where it regulates vascular beds in the jaw, lip, and tongue.

The cranial and sacral parasympathetic ganglia innervate different targets. The cranial outflow includes four ganglia in the head. The oculomotor (III) nerve projects to the ciliary ganglion, which controls pupillary size and focus by innervating the iris and ciliary muscles. The facial (VII) nerve and a small component of the glossopharyngeal (IX) nerve project to the pterygopalatine (or sphenopalatine) ganglion, which promotes production of tears by the lacrimal glands and mucus by the nasal and palatine glands. Cranial nerve IX and a small component of nerve VII project to the otic ganglion, which innervates the parotid, the largest salivary gland. Nerve VII also projects to the submandibular ganglion, which controls secretion of saliva by the submaxillary and sublingual glands.

The vagus (X) nerve projects broadly to parasympathetic ganglia in the heart, lungs, liver, gall bladder, and pancreas. It also projects to the stomach, small intestine, and more rostral segments of the gastrointestinal tract. The caudal parasympathetic outflow supplies the large intestine, rectum, bladder, and reproductive organs.

The Enteric Ganglia Regulate the Gastrointestinal Tract

The entire gastrointestinal tract, from the esophagus to the rectum—and including the pancreas and gall bladder—is controlled by the system of enteric ganglia. This system, by far the largest and most complex division of the autonomic nervous system, contains as many as 100 million neurons in humans.

The enteric system has been studied most extensively in the small intestine of the guinea pig, where the diversity of enteric neurons and their organization has been analyzed in two interconnected plexuses, small islands of interconnected neurons. The myenteric plexus controls smooth muscle movements of the gastrointestinal tract; the submucous plexus controls mucosal function (Figure 47–4). Working together, this distributed network of ganglia coordinates the orderly peristaltic propulsion of gastrointestinal contents and controls the secretions of the stomach and intestines and other components of digestion. In addition, the enteric system regulates local blood flow and is modulated by external inputs from sympathetic prevertebral ganglia and from parasympathetic components of the vagus nerve.

Unlike the sympathetic and parasympathetic divisions of the autonomic nervous system, the enteric ganglia contain interneurons and sensory neurons in addition to motor neurons. This intrinsic neural circuitry can maintain the basic functions of the gut even after the splanchnic sympathetic and vagal parasympathetic pathways are cut. Through splanchnic nerves and the vagus nerve the gastrointestinal tract also sends sensory information about the physiological states of the tract to the spinal cord and brain stem.

Both the Pre- and Postsynaptic Neurons of the Autonomic Motor System Use Co-Transmission at Their Synaptic Connections

Synaptic transmission in the peripheral autonomic nervous system was originally thought to be a simple tale of two neurotransmitters, ACh and norepinephrine. According to this idea, all preganglionic neurons in the sympathetic and parasympathetic systems use ACh as their neurotransmitter, binding and exciting ionotropic nicotinic ACh receptors on ganglionic neurons and thus opening nonselective cation channels similar to the nicotinic ACh receptors at the neuromuscular junction. The resulting action potentials propagate to postganglionic synapses with end-organs in the periphery. At these synapses parasympathetic neurons release ACh that activates muscarinic receptors whereas sympathetic neurons release norepinephrine that activates α- and β-adrenergic G protein-coupled receptors. The consequences can be either excitatory or inhibitory, depending on the type of target cell and its receptors (Table 47–1).

In addition to acting on different receptors in different postsynaptic cells, one transmitter can activate two or more receptor types in the same postsynaptic cell. This principle was first discovered in sympathetic ganglia where ACh activates both nicotinic and muscarinic postsynaptic receptors to produce both a fast and slow excitatory postsynaptic potential (EPSP) (Figure 47–5A, and see Chapter 13). In some cases one transmitter can activate both a postsynaptic receptor as well as a receptor on the presynaptic terminals from which the transmitter was released. Such presynaptic responses can either reduce transmitter release (presynaptic inhibition) or enhance it (presynaptic facilitation). This mechanism, also widespread, was discovered at autonomic junctions with blood vessels where different types of α-adrenergic receptors are expressed by some pre- and postsynaptic cells (Figure 47–5B). This specialization of synaptic transmission

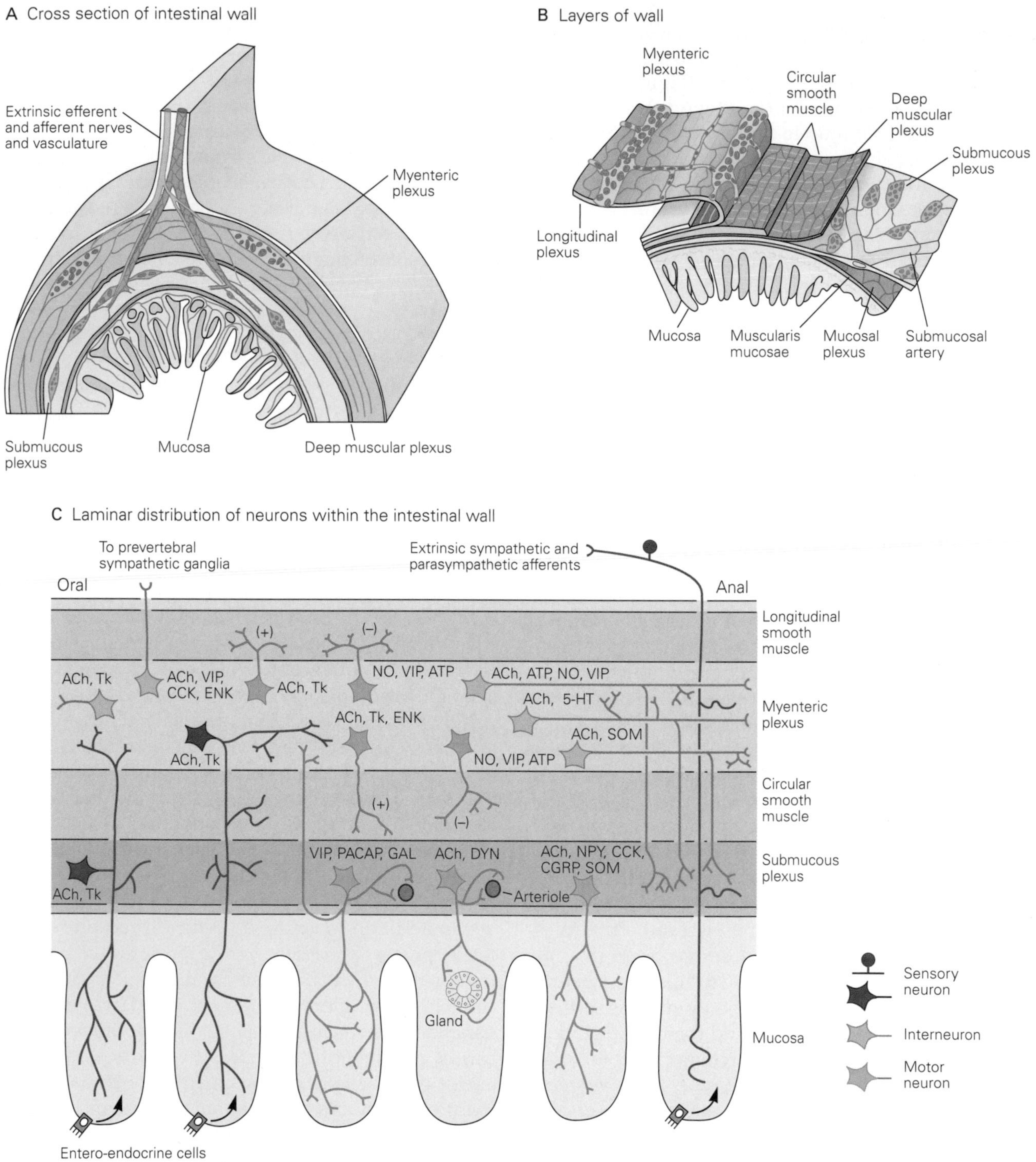

Figure 47–4 Organization of the enteric plexuses in the guinea pig. The myenteric plexus and submucous plexus lie between the layers of intestinal wall (A and B). At least 14 types of neurons have been identified within the enteric system based on morphology, chemical coding, and functional properties (C). Four sets of motor neurons provide excitatory (+) and inhibitory (–) inputs to two smooth muscle layers. Three additional groups of motor neurons control secretions from the mucosa and produce vasodilation. The network also includes two major classes of intrinsic sensory neurons. (**ACh**, acetylcholine; **ATP**, adenosine triphosphate; **CCK**, cholecystokinin; **CGRP**, calcitonin gene-related polypeptide; **DYN**, dynorphin; **ENK**, enkephalin; **GAL**, galanin; **NPY**, neuropeptide Y; **NO**, nitric oxide; **PACAP**, pituitary adenylate cyclase-activating peptide; **SOM**, somatostatin; **Tk**, tachykinin; **VIP**, vasoactive intestinal peptide; **5-HT**, serotonin.) (Parts A and B adapted, with permission, from Furness and Costa 1980; Part C reproduced, with permission, from Furness et al. 2004.)

Table 47–1 Autonomic Neurotransmitters and Their Receptors

Transmitter	Receptor	Responses
Norepinephrine	α_1	Stimulates smooth muscle contraction in arteries, urethra, gastrointestinal tract, iris (pupillary dilation), uterine contractions during pregnancy, ejaculation; glycogenolysis in liver; glandular secretion (salivary glands, lacrimal glands)
	α_2	Presynaptic inhibition of transmitter release from sympathetic and parasympathetic nerve terminals; stimulates contraction in some arterial smooth muscle
	β_1	Increases heart rate and strength of contraction
	β_2	Relaxes smooth muscle in airways and gastrointestinal tract; stimulates glycogenolysis in liver
	β_3	Stimulates lipolysis in fat cells; inhibits bladder contraction
Acetylcholine	Nicotinic	Fast EPSP in autonomic ganglion cells
	Muscarinic: M_1, M_2, M_3	Glandular secretion; ocular circular muscle (pupillary constriction); ciliary muscles (focus of lens); stimulates endothelial production of NO and vasodilation; slow EPSP in sympathetic neurons; slows heart rate; presynaptic inhibition at cholinergic nerve terminals; bladder contraction; salivary gland secretion
Neuropeptide Y	Y_1, Y_2	Stimulates arterial contraction and potentiates responses mediated by α_1-adrenergic receptors; presynaptic inhibition of transmitter release from some postganglionic sympathetic nerve terminals
Nitric oxide	Diffuses through membranes; often acts to stimulate intracellular soluble guanylate cyclase	Vasodilation, penile erection, urethral relaxation
Vasoactive intestinal peptide	VIPAC1, VIPAC2	Glandular secretion and dilation of blood vessels supplying glands
ATP	P_{2X}, P_{2Y}	Fast and slow excitation of smooth muscle in bladder, vas deferens, and arteries

ATP, adenosine triphosphate; EPSP, excitatory postsynaptic potential; NO, nitric oxide.

in sympathetic and parasympathetic neurons leads to functional diversity in the regulation of end-organ function.

Today we know that many transmitters are co-released at a single synapse, activating multiple receptor types and contributing to functional diversity. Many autonomic neurons release co-transmitters, often together with ACh or norepinephrine.

The cellular principles of co-transmission have been elucidated in part in a series of studies of paravertebral sympathetic ganglia in the bullfrog. These ganglia contain two major groups of neurons. Secretomotor B neurons selectively innervate mucous glands in the skin, whereas vasomotor C neurons selectively innervate arteries that supply striated muscle and skin. In addition, each cell group receives input from a distinct group of preganglionic neurons in the spinal cord. These cell types differ from one another in part by expressing different neuropeptides. Preganglionic B cells selectively express calcitonin gene-related peptide (CGRP). Preganglionic C neurons express luteinizing hormone-releasing hormone (LHRH), also known as gonadotropin-releasing hormone (GnRH), and their postganglionic target cells express neuropeptide Y (Figure 47–6A).

The co-release of LHRH and ACh by the preganglionic C neurons was discovered in 1979 by Stephen Kuffler with Lily Jan and Yuh Nung Jan. This discovery

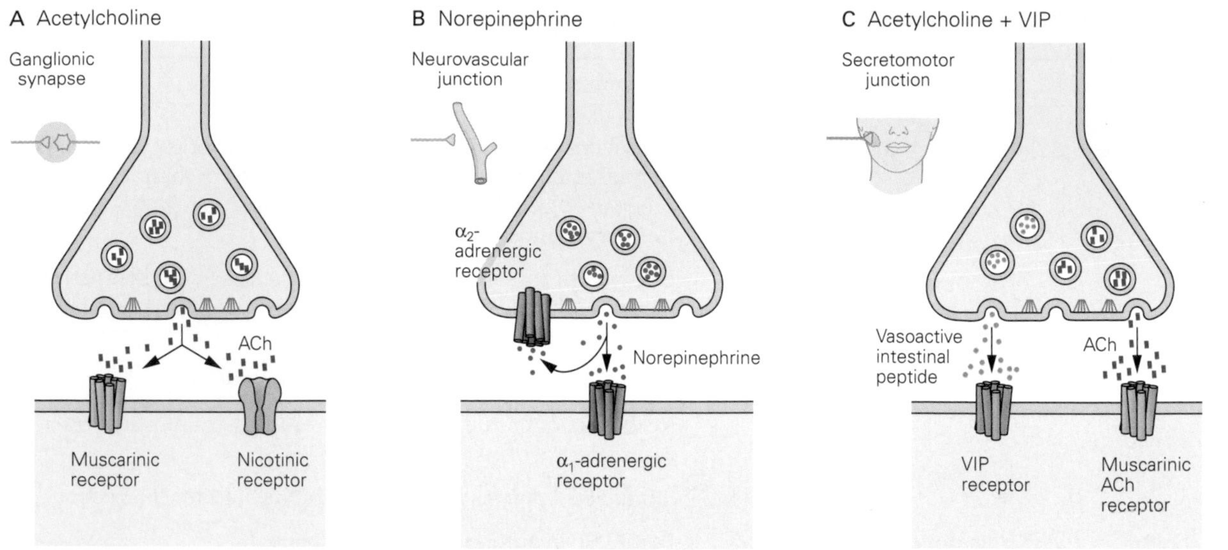

Figure 47–5 Synaptic transmission in the peripheral autonomic system.

A. In sympathetic ganglia ACh can activate both nicotinic and muscarinic receptors to produce fast and slow postsynaptic potentials, respectively.

B. At neurovascular junctions norepinephrine can simultaneously activate postsynaptic α_1-adrenergic receptors to produce vasoconstriction and presynaptic α_2-adrenergic receptors to inhibit further transmitter release.

C. Co-transmission involves the co-activation of more than one type of receptor by more than one transmitter. Parasympathetic postganglionic nerve terminals in the salivary glands release both ACh and vasoactive intestinal peptide (**VIP**) to control secretion. Autonomic synapses with end-organs sometimes employ more elaborate combinations, activating three or more receptor types.

Figure 47–6 (Opposite) **Synaptic organization of the paravertebral sympathetic system in the bullfrog.** The synaptic specialization of neurons that control different peripheral targets have been studied in paravertebral sympathetic ganglia associated with spinal segments 9 and 10. These amphibian ganglia are also a model system for analyzing synaptic co-transmission and its role in synaptic integration in the autonomic ganglia.

A. The secretomotor B and vasomotor C circuits originate in separate spinal segments, traverse the same ganglia, and then control different targets. In addition to their unique projection patterns, the two cell types co-release different neuropeptides along with acetylcholine (**ACh**). (**CGRP**, calcitonin gene-related peptide; **GIRK**, G protein-coupled inward-rectifying K^+ channel; **LHRH**, luteinizing hormone-releasing hormone.) (Adapted, with permission, from Horn and Stofer 1989.)

B. Synaptic events span a 3,000-fold range of time scales and differ in the stimulus patterns that are effective. **1.** The nicotinic excitatory postsynaptic potential (**EPSP**) in all ganglionic neurons is readily evoked by a single presynaptic stimulus and lasts for 50 ms. **2.** The muscarinic inhibitory postsynaptic potential (**IPSP**) in C neurons is caused by activation of G protein-coupled inward-rectifying K^+ channels (**GIRK**), is 50 times slower than the fast EPSP, and summates during repetitive stimulation. **3.** The neuropeptide luteinizing hormone releasing hormone (**LHRH**) is released by preganglionic C neurons and evokes a very slow EPSP in postganglionic B and C neurons due to its diffusion throughout the ganglion. Note the different time scales in 1–3. Neuropeptide release is greatly enhanced by high-frequency repetitive stimulation and produces a slow EPSP that is 60 times slower than the muscarinic IPSP. **4.** The muscarinic EPSP in B neurons is also slow and optimally elicited by repetitive stimulation. **5.** Finally, ACh released by preganglionic B neurons can bind presynaptic receptors. The operation of these presynaptic receptors can be demonstrated by activating them with the drug muscarine and recording the effect on fast nicotinic excitatory postsynaptic currents (**EPSCs**) under voltage-clamp elicited by stimulating the preganglionic nerve. The muscarine produces two effects. The upper trace shows the downward deflection of the baseline caused by activation of a slow excitatory inward postsynaptic current; the lower records show the reduction in amplitude of the EPSC caused by inhibition of the ACh released by the preganglionic B neurons. (Reproduced, with permission, from Adams and Brown 1982; reproduced, with permission, from Dodd and Horn 1983; reproduced, with permission, from Karila and Horn 2000; reproduced, with permission, from Peng and Horn 1991; reproduced, with permission, from Shen and Horn 1996.)

C. The consequences of synaptic integration in ganglia 9 and 10 can be studied by selectively stimulating preganglionic inputs to B or C neurons and observing the responses of mucous glands in the skin and of the abdominal aorta. A single preganglionic stimulus applied to the B pathway activates the mucous glands (measured by voltage drop across the skin). Multiple preganglionic stimuli applied to the C pathway evoke vasoconstriction (measured here by muscle tension). (Reproduced, with permission, from Jobling and Horn 1996; reproduced, with permission, from Thorne and Horn 1997.)

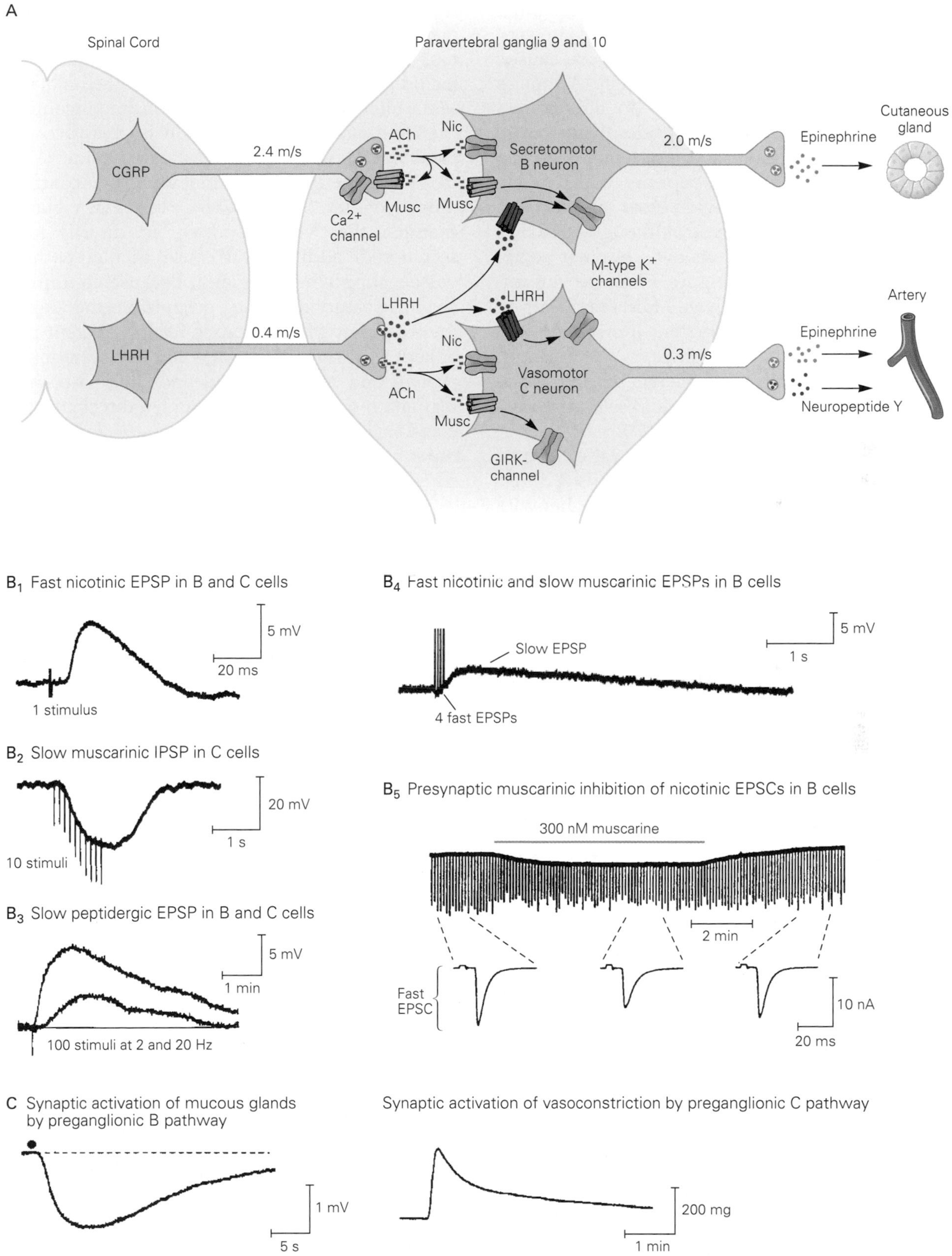
A
Spinal Cord
Paravertebral ganglia 9 and 10
CGRP
2.4 m/s
ACh
Nic
Secretomotor
B neuron
2.0 m/s
Epinephrine
Cutaneous
gland
Musc
Musc
Ca2+
channel
M-type K+
channels
LHRH
LHRH
LHRH
0.4 m/s
Nic
Vasomotor
C neuron
0.3 m/s
Artery
Epinephrine
Neuropeptide Y
ACh
Musc
GIRK-
channel
B1 Fast nicotinic EPSP in B and C cells
5 mV
20 ms
1 stimulus
B2 Slow muscarinic IPSP in C cells
20 mV
1 s
10 stimuli
B3 Slow peptidergic EPSP in B and C cells
5 mV
1 min
100 stimuli at 2 and 20 Hz
B4 Fast nicotinic and slow muscarinic EPSPs in B cells
Slow EPSP
5 mV
1 s
4 fast EPSPs
B5 Presynaptic muscarinic inhibition of nicotinic EPSCs in B cells
300 nM muscarine
2 min
Fast
EPSC
10 nA
20 ms
C Synaptic activation of mucous glands
by preganglionic B pathway
1 mV
5 s
Synaptic activation of vasoconstriction by preganglionic C pathway
200 mg
1 min

illustrated three general principles, establishing LHRH-mediated synaptic transmission as a model for other neuropeptide actions. First, peptides can mediate very slow synaptic events, even slower than those caused by muscarinic ACh receptor stimulation. Although mammalian preganglionic neurons do not express LHRH, they release other neuropeptides that produce slow synaptic actions similar to those seen in bullfrog sympathetic ganglia. Second, peptides act diffusely at a distance and thereby provide cross talk between different sympathetic cell types. Although LHRH is released by preganglionic inputs to C cells that do not form synapses with B cells (Figure 47–6A), it can diffuse many micrometers to activate LHRH receptors on adjacent B neurons. Finally, different transmitters can share intracellular signaling pathways. For example, the actions of LHRH both resemble and block the excitatory, muscarinic response to ACh in B cells (a process called *cross-desensitization*).

Studies of bullfrog sympathetic ganglia also illustrate how preganglionic release of ACh can co-activate different forms of muscarinic (slow) responses together with the nicotinic (fast) EPSP. The muscarinic responses include a slow EPSP in B neurons, a slow inhibitory postsynaptic potential (IPSP) in C neurons, and inhibition of ACh release from preganglionic nerve terminals in the B cell system (Figure 47–6B). Each of these events arises through regulation of different ion channels. In both mammalian and amphibian sympathetic neurons the slow EPSP is mediated by suppression of the voltage-gated M-type K^+ channel belonging to the KCNQ (K_v9) family. The slow IPSP is produced by activation of G protein-coupled, inward-rectifying K^+ channels (GIRKs) ($K_{ir}3$), and presynaptic inhibition by inhibition of N-type voltage-gated Ca^{2+} channels ($Ca_v2.2$).

The time courses of the fast and slow synaptic events reflect fundamental differences in synaptic signaling mechanisms. The EPSPs initiated by the nicotinic ACh receptors are brief, lasting 10 to 50 ms because ionotropic receptor-channels are directly gated by ligand binding (see Figure 8–9). In contrast, synaptic events initiated at metabotropic receptors—the muscarinic ACh, peptide, and epinephrine receptors as well as a type of adenosine triphosphate (ATP) receptor (P_{2Y})—are slow, with time courses lasting hundreds of milliseconds to minutes, because the receptor and ion channel are coupled by a multistep signaling cascade (see Chapter 11).

The final motor responses elicited by all three divisions of the autonomic system also depend on the properties of synaptic transmission at neuro-effector junctions. In particular they depend on the identity of postganglionic neurotransmitters and the pre- and postsynaptic receptors (Table 47–1). Understanding the pharmacology of these receptors and the second-messenger signaling pathways they control is important in the treatment of numerous medical conditions, including hypertension, heart failure, asthma, emphysema, allergies, sexual dysfunction, and incontinence.

Here again co-transmission is operative. Acetylcholine and vasoactive intestinal peptide (VIP) are frequently co-released from neurons that control glandular secretion (Figure 47–5C). In salivary glands, for example, the two transmitters act directly to evoke secretion. In addition, VIP causes dilation of the blood vessels supplying the gland. Because co-transmitters can be released in varying proportions that depend on the frequency of presynaptic firing, different patterns of activity can regulate the volume of secretions, their protein and water content, and their viscosity. This regulation operates both through a direct effect on the gland cells and through indirect effects on the glandular blood flow that provides the water contained in secretions.

Autonomic Behavior Is the Product of Cooperation Between All Three Autonomic Divisions

To survive, animals and humans must have a "fight-or-flight" response that prepares an animal to stand and fight a predator or run away and live to see another day. Walter Cannon, in addition to introducing the concept of homeostasis, also appreciated that this "fight-or-flight" response is a critical sympathetic function.

Two important ideas underlie this insight. First, the sympathetic and parasympathetic systems play complementary, even antagonistic, roles; the sympathetic system promotes arousal, defense, and escape, whereas the parasympathetic system promotes eating and procreation. Second, actions of the sympathetic system are diffuse; they influence all parts of the body and once turned on can persist for some time. These ideas are behind the popular notion of the "adrenaline rush" produced by excitement, as by a roller coaster ride.

We now know that extreme sympathetic responses such as the "fight-or-flight" response can have long-term pathological consequences resulting in the syndrome known as *post-traumatic stress disorder* (see Chapter 63). This disorder was first recognized in soldiers during World War I when it was referred to as "shell shock." A variety of life-threatening experiences, ranging from sexual abuse and domestic violence to aircraft disasters, can also induce post-traumatic stress disorder, a disorder that affects millions of people in the United States alone.

Because the fight-or-flight model assumes antagonistic roles for the sympathetic and parasympathetic systems, Cannon's model led to an overemphasis on the extremes of autonomic behavior. Actually during everyday life the different divisions of the autonomic system are tightly integrated. In addition, we now know that the sympathetic system is less diffusely organized than first envisioned by Cannon. Subsets of neurons even within the sympathetic division control specific targets, and these pathways can be activated independently.

As in the somatic motor system, reflexes in the autonomic motor system are elicited through sensory pathways and are hierarchically organized. The simplest feedback loops are confined to the periphery and spinal cord, whereas more complex loops extend to higher centers. An important feature of this organization is that it allows for coordination between the different divisions of the autonomic system. The interplay between different systems in simple autonomic behaviors is analogous to the role of antagonist muscles in locomotion. To walk, one must alternately contract antagonist muscles that flex and extend a joint. Similarly, the sympathetic and parasympathetic systems are often partners in the regulation of end-organs. In most cases, ranging from the simplest reflexes to more complex behaviors, all three peripheral divisions of the autonomic system work together.

We illustrate this organization with three examples: contractions of the gut (peristalsis), control of the bladder (micturition reflex), and regulation of blood pressure.

Peristalsis

Peristalsis of circular smooth muscle normally propels the contents of the gastrointestinal tract in the oral–anal direction. This coordinated motor program is generated locally by the enteric neural network (Figure 47–4C) and can be elicited as a simple reflex by passive distension of the gut wall. The reflex activates excitatory motor neurons located rostral (oral) to the stimulus and inhibitory motor neurons located caudal (anal) to the stimulus. The synaptic connections between antagonistic motor neurons and sensory neurons are so arranged that the enteric network can build a cycle of contraction and relaxation that propagates in unidirectional waves of contractions.

The sensory information required to initiate the basic reflex originates in and is integrated locally within the enteric network. Two groups of sensory neurons in the system provide additional feedback to higher centers. One group lies in the dorsal root ganglia and projects from the gut to the prevertebral sympathetic ganglia and into the spinal cord and ascending pathways. The other group projects through the vagus nerve to sensory neurons in the brain stem. These pathways signal hunger and satiety. In response, the central nervous system can enhance or inhibit digestion through excitatory parasympathetic efferents in the vagus nerve and inhibitory sympathetic efferents in prevertebral splanchnic nerves.

Micturition Reflex

The micturition reflex is another example of a physiological cycle resulting from coordination between sympathetic and parasympathetic systems. In this cycle the bladder is emptied by the parasympathetic pathway, which contracts the bladder and relaxes the urethra. The sympathetic system allows the bladder to fill by stimulating the urethra and inhibiting the parasympathetic pathway, thus inhibiting the reflex for bladder emptying. The sensory feedback required for this behavior is integrated with the motor outflow at both spinal and supraspinal levels.

Spinal components of the reflex are most influential during the storage phase of the micturition cycle, when sympathetic and somatic motor effects predominate. When the bladder is full, its distension triggers a sensory signal sufficient to activate the pontine micturition center. Parasympathetic mechanisms then predominate to empty the bladder. Somatic control of the external urinary sphincter, which consists of striated muscle, contributes to both phases of the micturition cycle and is a voluntary behavior that originates through forebrain mechanisms (Figure 47–7). Patients with spinal cord injuries at the cervical or thoracic levels retain the reflex but not voluntary control of urination because the connections between the bladder and the pons are severed.

Baroreceptor Reflex

The baroreceptor reflex is one of the simplest mechanisms for regulating blood pressure and an example of homeostatic control by antagonist sympathetic and parasympathetic pathways. It prevents orthostatic hypotension and fainting by compensating for rapid hydrostatic effects produced by changes in posture.

When a recumbent person stands up, the sudden elevation of the head above the heart causes a transient decrease of cerebral blood pressure that is rapidly sensed by baroreceptors in the carotid sinus in

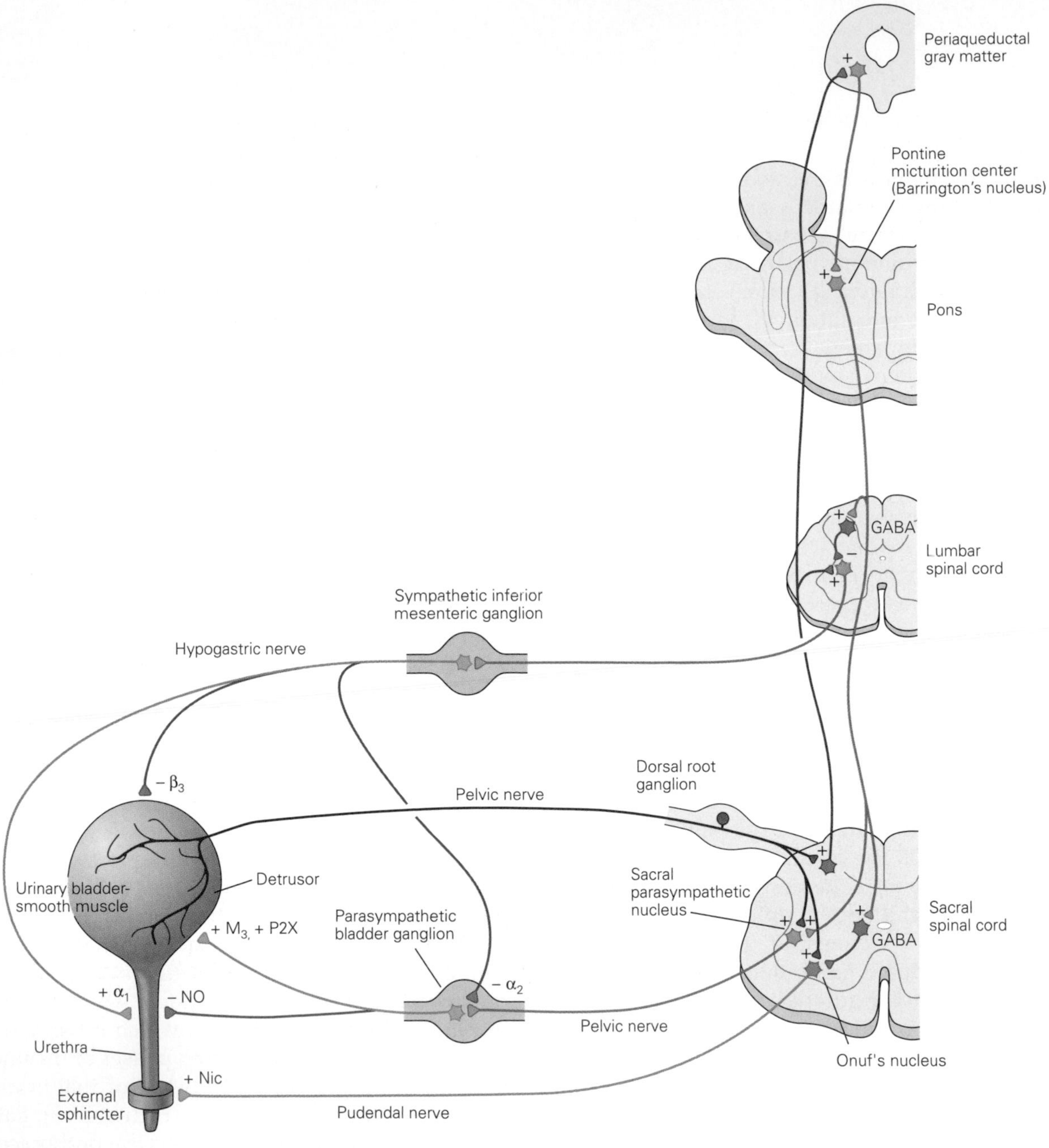

Figure 47–7 The micturition reflex requires interplay between the parasympathetic and sympathetic divisions of the autonomic system. When bladder volume is low, urinary outflow is inhibited because activity in sympathetic pathway is greater than activity in parasympathetic pathway. Mild distension of the detrusor (storage portion of the bladder) initiates a low level of sensory activity, which reflexively activates spinal preganglionic neurons. The resulting low level of preganglionic activity is effectively transmitted and amplified by the sympathetic inferior mesenteric ganglion but filtered out by the parasympathetic bladder ganglion because of differences in patterns of synaptic convergence in the two ganglia. The resulting predominance of sympathetic tone keeps the detrusor relaxed and the urethra constricted. Sympathetic postganglionic fibers also reduce parasympathetic activity by inhibiting preganglionic release of acetylcholine. In addition to their effects on the autonomic outflow, the sensory signals are sufficient to keep the external urinary sphincter closed.

When filling causes the bladder to reach a critical volume, the associated increase in sensory activity reaches a threshold that allows for impulses to pass through the pontine micturition center (Barrington's nucleus). Descending activity from this nucleus then further excites the parasympathetic outflow. The resulting increase in parasympathetic preganglionic firing promotes summation of fast EPSPs and initiation of postsynaptic action potentials in the bladder ganglion as it switches to its "on" state. During the emptying process descending pathways also inhibit the sympathetic and somatic outflows through inhibitory spinal interneurons. Inhibition of somatic motor neurons in Onuf's nucleus causes relaxation and opening of the external sphincter. In this figure the sacral spinal cord is enlarged relative to the other slices. (**GABA**, γ-aminobutyric acid; **NO**, nitric oxide; **M_3**, muscarinic ACh receptor 3; **nic**, nicotinic receptor; **P2X**, purinergic receptor.) (Adapted, with permission, from DeGroat et al. 1993.)

the neck. Other important pressure sensors are located in the aortic arch and in the pulmonary circulation. When neurons in the ventrolateral medulla detect the decrease in afferent baroreceptor activity produced by low blood pressure, they produce a reflexive suppression of parasympathetic activity and stimulation of sympathetic activity. These changes in autonomic tone restore blood pressure by increasing heart rate, the strength of cardiac contractions, and the overall vascular resistance to blood flow through arterial vasoconstriction.

Under the converse condition of elevated arterial pressure, the increase in baroreceptor activity enhances parasympathetic inhibition of the heart and decreases sympathetic stimulation of cardiac function and vascular resistance. In general, the parasympathetic component of the baroreceptor reflex has a more rapid onset and is briefer than the sympathetic component. Consequently, parasympathetic activity is critical for the rapid response of baroreceptor reflexes but less important than sympathetic activity for long-term blood pressure regulation.

Homeostatic control of physiological functions such as blood pressure and body temperature often involves negative feedback loops. In the baroreceptor reflex, for example, the firing of sensory neurons conveys information about arterial pressure that medullary circuits use as feedback to control descending commands and thereby regulate preganglionic sympathetic neurons. This feedback is said to be negative because of the inverse relation between sensory input and functional motor output: An increase in blood pressure increases sensory activity that decreases sympathetic motor tone, which then reduces pressure.

Set point and gain are critical components of this type of control, as they are in regulating motivational state. The set point is the target for regulation and is analogous to thermostat settings on home heating systems. Gain, as we will see in Chapter 49, is the amplification generated by the feedback loop. The mathematics of control theory shows that the accuracy and speed of regulation through negative feedback are established by the gain of the loop. At a higher gain the reflex loop will control pressure more effectively and more quickly (Figure 47–8B). The overall gain of the baroreceptor reflex is regulated by cellular mechanisms in the sensory transduction process, in the medulla, in paravertebral sympathetic ganglia where integration of nicotinic EPSPs can produce activity-dependent gain, and at the neurovascular junctions where co-release of neuropeptide Y can potentiate the actions of norepinephrine on arteries.

Autonomic and Endocrine Function Is Coordinated by a Central Autonomic Network Centered in the Hypothalamus

Sympathetic and parasympathetic response are coordinated by a central autonomic network, a network of brain regions that interacts with two other brain systems to support homeostasis, the "fight-or-flight" response, and reproduction. These other two systems control endocrine responses, especially from the pituitary gland, and the expression of eating and drinking behavior and defensive and reproductive (sexual and parental) behaviors common to all animals. Like the central autonomic network, these two systems are widely distributed in the brain, and their critical control elements are centered in the hypothalamus.

General visceral sensory information reaches the central autonomic network mainly through two cranial nerves (IX and X), which end in the nucleus of the solitary tract, and through the abdominal splanchnic nerves, which end in the spinal cord (see Chapter 45). Splanchnic information is transmitted to the brain through the spinothalamic tract (see Chapter 22), which branches out along the way to several parts of the central autonomic network, including the nucleus of the solitary tract (Figure 47–9A).

The nucleus of the solitary tract has two basic functions. First, it projects to networks in the brain stem and spinal cord that control and coordinate autonomic reflexes. For example, visceral sensory signals relayed through the nucleus regulate vagal motor control of the heart and gastrointestinal tract directly. Some neurons in the nucleus project to neurons in the ventrolateral medullary reticular formation that control blood pressure by regulating blood flow in particular vascular beds differentially (Figure 47–9B). Second, the nucleus has ascending projections that integrate autonomic with neuroendocrine and behavioral responses. As we will see, the forebrain plays an important role in this higher-order coordination.

The nucleus of the solitary tract has direct and indirect projections to the forebrain. A major indirect target is the pontine *parabrachial nucleus*, which is important for behavioral responses to visceral information as well as taste. Lesions of the nucleus prevent behavioral conditioning with gustatory stimuli. The general pattern of ascending projections from the nucleus is remarkably similar to that from the nucleus of the solitary tract. Furthermore, both nuclei receive inputs from many central autonomic centers in the forebrain.

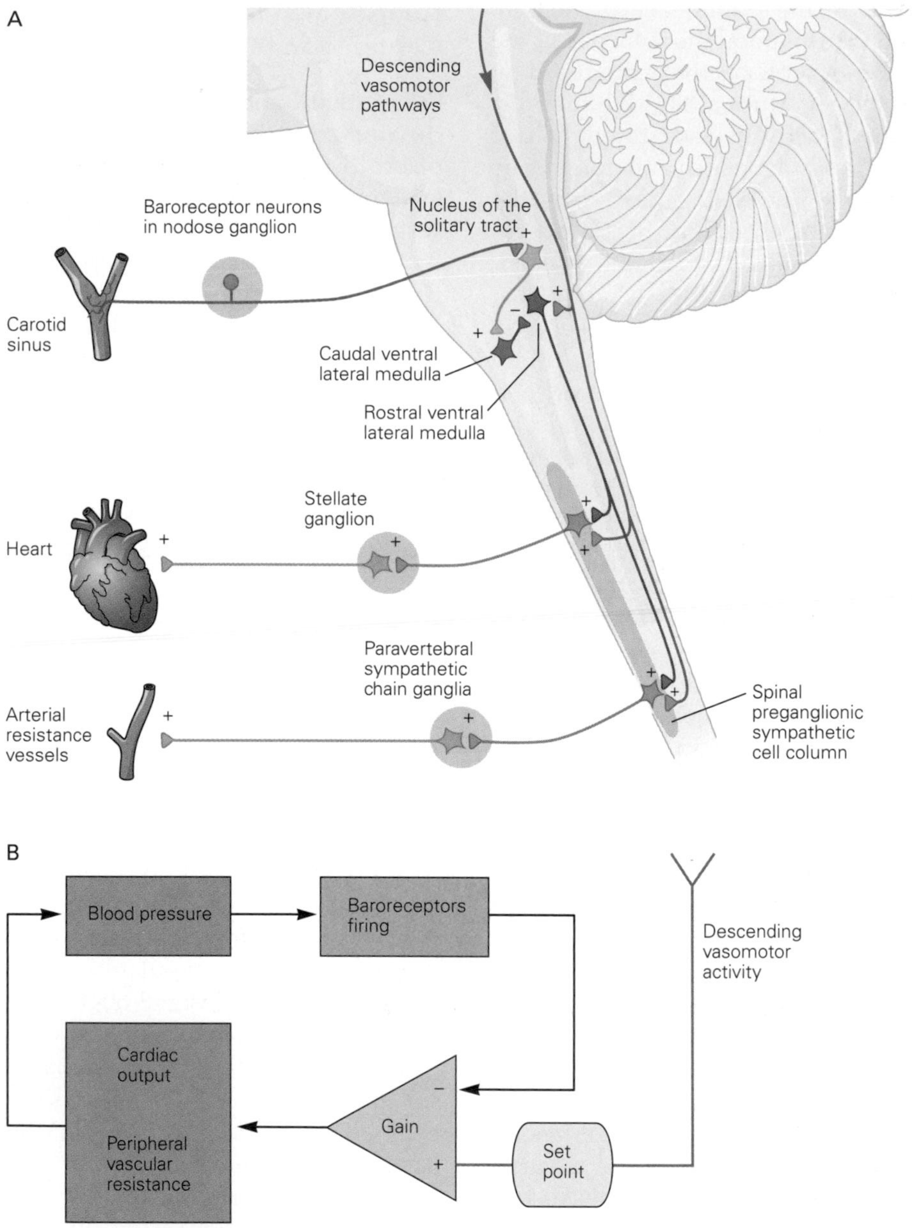

Figure 47–8 The baroreceptor reflex behaves as a negative feedback loop with gain.

A. Arterial blood pressure is sensed by baroreceptors, a type of stretch receptor neuron, in the carotid sinus near the base of the brain. After integration in the medulla this information provides negative feedback control of the cardiovascular system. The sympathetic component of the circuit includes outputs that stimulate the heart's pumping capacity (cardiac output) by increasing heart rate and the strength of contractions. In addition, sympathetic stimulation causes arteries to contract, which raises the hydraulic resistance to blood flow. Together the effects of increased cardiac output and increased vascular resistance raise mean arterial blood pressure. Importantly, inhibitory projections from the caudal to the rostral ventral lateral medulla create negative feedback so that an increase in blood pressure inhibits sympathetic activity, whereas a decrease raises sympathetic activity. Although omitted for simplicity, parasympathetic neurons in the cardiac ganglion also contribute to the reflex by creating an inhibitory cardiac input that is functionally antagonistic to the sympathetic pathway (see Figure 49–9B). During baroreceptor reflexes parasympathetic activity within the heart is therefore increased by hypertension and reduced by hypotension.

B. The neurons mediating the baroreceptor reflex behave as a negative feedback loop with gain. By amplifying the activity that provides the signals for cardiovascular control, neurons in this circuit can accurately control blood pressure. In a healthy individual with reflex gain of 8, systemic blood pressure can be maintained within 10% of its set point.

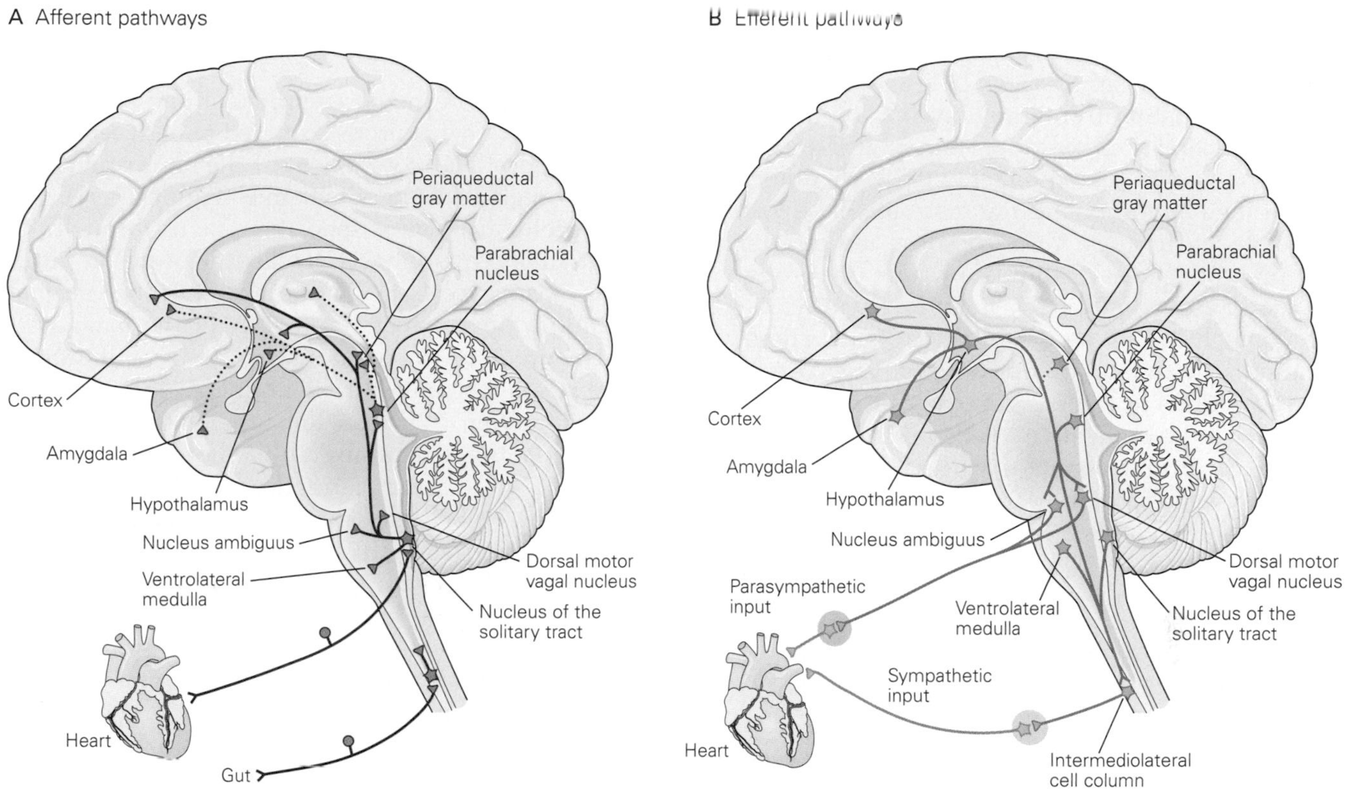

Figure 47–9 The central autonomic network. Nearly all of the cell groups illustrated here are interconnected with one another, forming the central autonomic network.

A. *Main afferent pathways.* Visceral information (**solid lines**) is distributed to the brain from the nucleus of the solitary tract and from ascending spinal pathways activated by the splanchnic nerves (from the gut, for example). The nucleus of the solitary tract distributes this information to preganglionic parasympathetic neurons (the dorsal motor vagal nucleus and nucleus ambiguus), to regions of the ventrolateral medulla that coordinate autonomic and respiratory reflexes, and to more rostral parts of the central autonomic network in the pons (parabrachial nucleus), midbrain (periaqueductal gray), and forebrain. The parabrachial nucleus also projects to many of the more rostral components of the central autonomic network, including visceral and gustatory nuclei of the thalamus (**dashed lines**). Other pathways from the spinal cord (not shown) also transmit visceral information to many parts of the central autonomic network, including the nucleus of the solitary tract, parabrachial nucleus, periaqueductal gray, hypothalamus, amygdala, and cortex. The spinal cord also projects to the main somatosensory nucleus of the thalamus (ventral posterolateral nucleus).

B. *Main efferent pathways.* All of the pathways shown here (except perhaps for the periaqueductal gray) project directly to autonomic preganglionic neurons. In the hypothalamus the descending division of the paraventricular nucleus and three cell clusters in the lateral zone project heavily to both parasympathetic and sympathetic preganglionic neurons. Other pathways (not shown) arise from certain monoaminergic cell groups in the brain stem, including noradrenergic neurons in the A5 region and serotonergic neurons in the raphe nuclei.

The periaqueductal gray, surrounds the cerebral aqueduct in the midbrain, which also receives inputs from most parts of the central autonomic network and projects to the medullary reticular formation to initiate integrated behavioral and autonomic responses. For example, in the defensive "fight-or-flight" response the periaqueductal gray helps redirect blood flow from the digestive system to the hind limbs, thus enhancing running.

Viscerosensory and gustatory information is relayed from the nucleus of the solitary tract and parabrachial nucleus in axons that end topographically in a specialized part of the thalamus, the parvicellular (small-cell) part of the ventral posterior nucleus. The parvicellular projections to viscerosensory and gustatory areas in the rostral half of the insular cortex relay information related to hunger, abdominal fullness, dry throat, and holding your breath. Information from the splanchnic nerves is transmitted to the main part of the ventral posterior nucleus, which receives somatosensory information (see Chapter 22).

The medial prefrontal region of the cerebral cortex is a visceral sensory-motor region. It includes two functional areas that interact with each other: the rostral insular cortex and the rostromedial tip of the cingulate gyrus (also referred to as the infralimbic and prelimbic areas). Stimulation here can produce a variety of autonomic effects including contractions of the stomach and changes in blood pressure. These visceral sensory and motor areas of cortex send descending projections to the parts of the central autonomic network in the brain stem already discussed. Lesions here may produce loss of visceral sensations and taste, as well as a condition known as abulia, where patients show blunted emotional responses to external stimuli.

Finally, visceral regions of cortex, along with many subcortical parts of the central autonomic network, interact with the amygdala. Complex pathways between certain amygdalar cell groups underlie conditioned emotional responses—learned associations between specific stimuli and behaviors with accompanying autonomic responses. When a rat learns that a mild electric shock follows an auditory cue, the auditory cue alone produces an elevated heart rate and the freezing reaction originally elicited by the shock alone (see Chapter 48). Such learned responses are prevented by selective lesions of the amygdalar region, which projects to the hypothalamus and lower brain stem parts of the central autonomic network (including the motor nucleus of the vagus nerve).

The Hypothalamus Integrates Autonomic, Endocrine, and Behavioral Responses

Transection of the brain axis roughly between the midbrain and diencephalon (hypothalamus), without lesioning the hypothalamus, eliminates all spontaneous behavior. In contrast, removal of the entire cerebral hemisphere (cortex and basal nuclei) and thalamus, sparing the hypothalamus, leaves animals able to eat and drink enough to maintain body weight and blood pressure, bear offspring (females only), defend against environmental threats with coordinated behavioral responses, and maintain a constant body temperature. The only difference in the two procedures is whether or not the hypothalamus is left intact (Figure 47–10). The functions of the hypothalamus (Table 47–2) can be enhanced or eliminated when particular sites are experimentally manipulated.

Magnocellular Neuroendocrine Neurons Control the Pituitary Gland Directly

Large neurons in the paraventricular and supraoptic nuclei (and a few neurons scattered in between) form the magnocellular component of the neuroendocrine motor system of the hypothalamus (Figure 47–11). The magnocellular neurons send their axons through the hypothalamo-hypophysial tract to the posterior pituitary or *neurohypophysis* (Figure 47–12). Under normal conditions approximately one-half of the magnocellular neuroendocrine neurons synthesize and secrete vasopressin (the antidiuretic hormone) into the general circulation, whereas the other half synthesize and secrete the structurally similar hormone oxytocin (Figure 47–11). These hormones circulate to organs that control blood pressure, water balance, uterine smooth muscle, and milk release.

In the 1950s Vincent DuVigneaud discovered that vasopressin and oxytocin are peptide hormones, each containing nine amino acid residues (Table 47–3). We later learned that, like other peptide hormones, they are synthesized in the cell body as larger prohormones (see Chapter 13) and then cleaved within Golgi transport vesicles before traveling down the axon to release sites in the posterior pituitary. The genes for these peptides are similar and probably arose by duplication.

Parvicellular Neuroendocrine Neurons Control the Pituitary Gland Indirectly

In the 1950s Geoffrey Harris proposed that the anterior pituitary or *adenohypophysis* is regulated indirectly by the hypothalamus. He showed that the hypophysial portal veins, which carry blood from the hypothalamic median eminence to the anterior pituitary, transport signals released from hypothalamic neurons that control anterior pituitary hormone secretion (Figure 47–12).

In the 1970s Andrew Schally, Roger Guillemin, and Wylie Vale determined the structure of a group of hypothalamic peptide hormones that control pituitary hormone secretion from five classic endocrine cell types in the anterior pituitary. These hormones fall into two classes: releasing hormones and release-inhibiting hormones (Table 47–4). Only one anterior pituitary hormone, prolactin, is under predominantly inhibitory control. Thus transection of the pituitary stalk increases prolactin secretion but causes insufficiency of adrenal cortical, thyroid, gonadal, and growth hormones.

The parvicellular neuroendocrine motor zone is centered along the wall of the third ventricle (Figure 47–10A). One population of parvicellular neurons releases

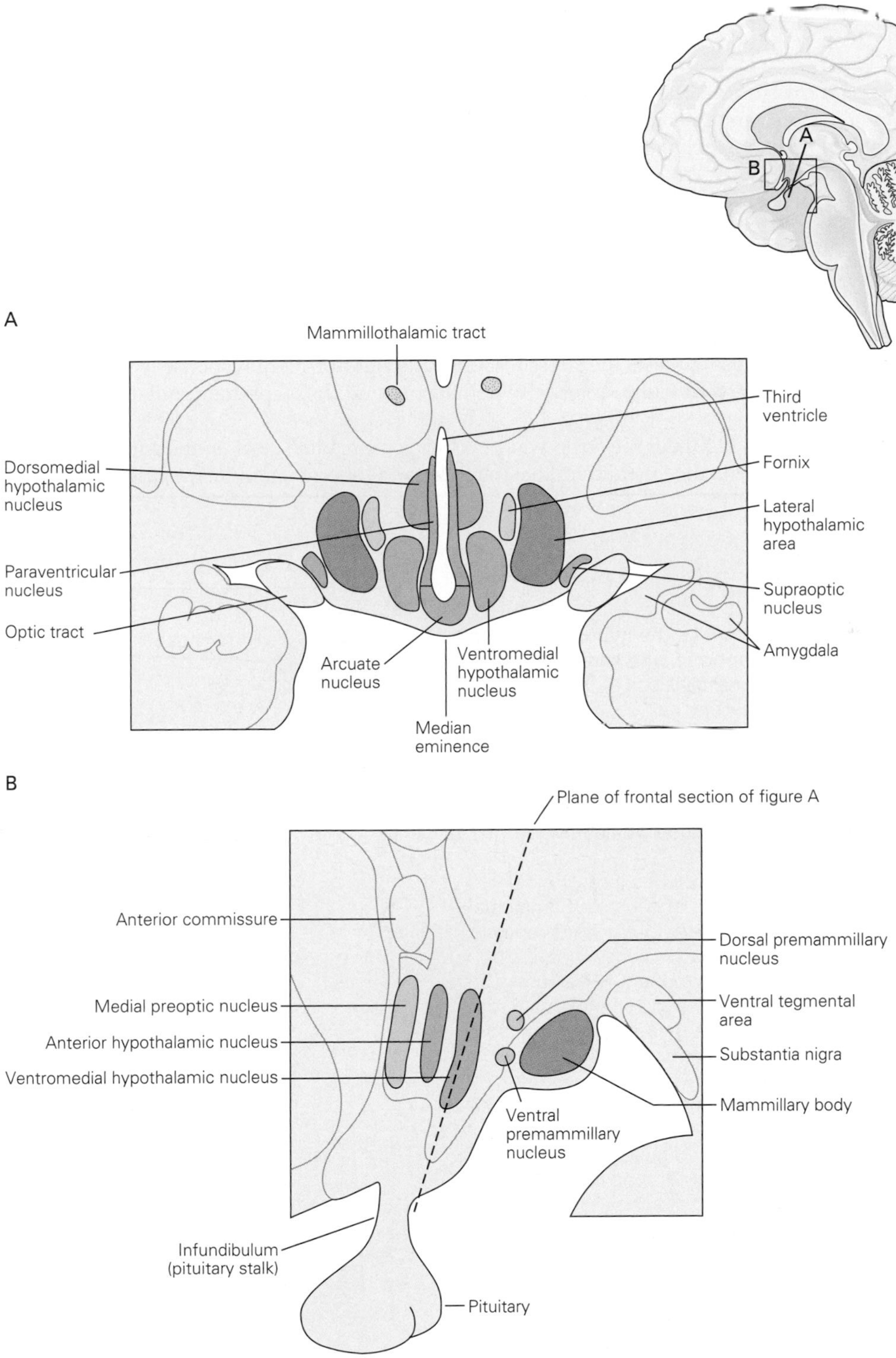

Figure 47–10 The structure of the hypothalamus.

A. Frontal view of the hypothalamus (section along plane A shown in the sagittal view of the brain, upper right). The third ventricle is in the midline; the paraventricular, dorsomedial, and arcuate nuclei adjacent to the ventricle form the neuroendocrine motor zone and periventricular region at this level. The ventromedial nucleus is part of the medial column of hypothalamic nuclei, and the lateral hypothalamic area is the lateral zone component represented in the part of the hypothalamus shown here.

B. Sagittal (rostrocaudal) view of the medial column of hypothalamic nuclei, showing the adjacent (caudal) substantia nigra and ventral tegmental area of the midbrain. The functional significance of key hypothalamic nuclei is summarized in Table 47–2.

Table 47–2 The Hypothalamus Integrates Behavioral (Somatomotor), Autonomic, and Neuroendocrine Responses Involved in Six Vital Functions

1. *Blood pressure and electrolyte composition*. The hypothalamus regulates thirst, salt appetite, and drinking behavior, autonomic control of vasomotor tone, and the release of hormones like vasopressin (via the paraventricular nucleus).
2. *Energy metabolism*. The hypothalamus regulates hunger and feeding behavior, the autonomic control of digestion, and the release of hormones such as glucocorticoids, growth hormone, and thyroid-stimulating hormone (via the arcuate and paraventricular nuclei and the lateral hypothalamic area).
3. *Reproductive (sexual and parental) behaviors*. The hypothalamus controls autonomic modulation of the reproductive organs and endocrine regulation of the gonads (via the medial preoptic, ventromedial, and ventral premammillary nuclei).
4. *Body temperature*. The hypothalamus influences thermoregulatory behavior (seeking a warmer or cooler environment), controls autonomic body heat conservation/loss mechanisms, and controls secretion of hormones that influence metabolic rate (via the preoptic region).
5. *Defensive behavior*. The hypothalamus regulates the stress response and fight-or-flight response to threats in the environment such as predators (via the paraventricular, anterior hypothalamic, and dorsal premammillary nuclei, and the lateral hypothalamic area).
6. *Sleep-wake cycle*. The hypothalamus regulates the sleep-wake cycle (via a circadian clock in the suprachiasmatic nucleus) and levels of arousal when awake (via the lateral hypothalamic area and tuberomammillary nucleus).

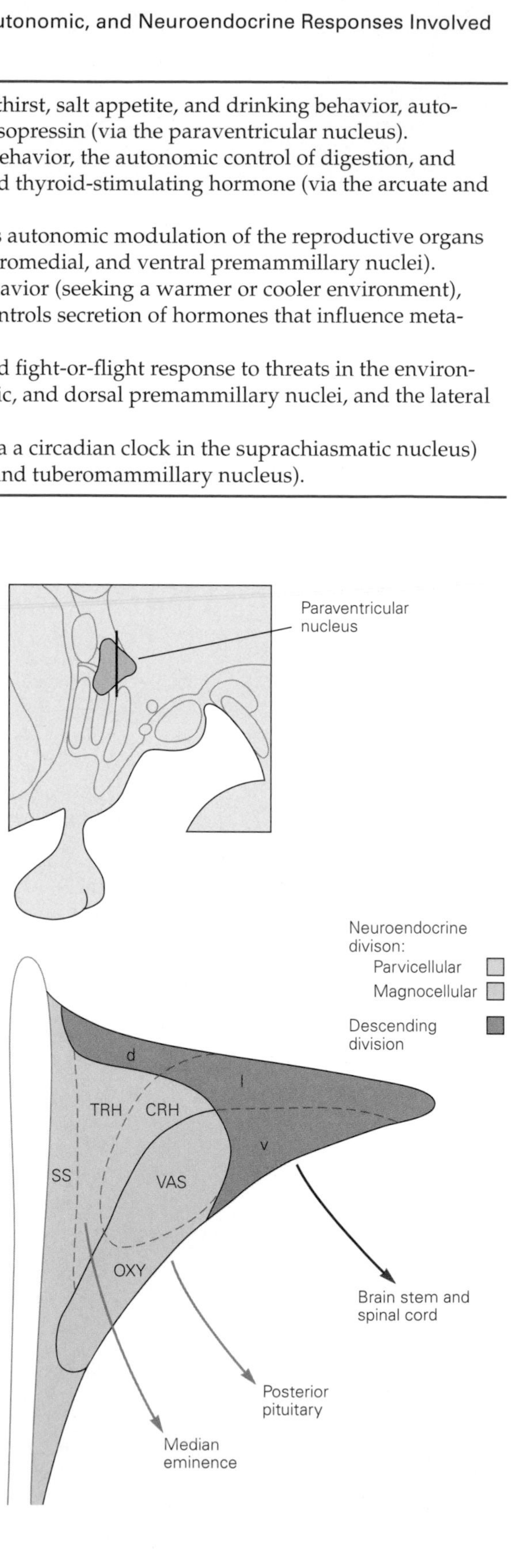

Figure 47–11 The paraventricular nucleus in the hypothalamus is a microcosm of neuroendocrine, autonomic, and sensory-motor integration. The three structural-functional divisions of the paraventricular nucleus are shown. The *magnocellular neuroendocrine division* comprises two distinct although partly interdigitated pools of neurons. These neurons normally synthesize vasopressin (**VAS**) and oxytocin (**OXY**) and release them from axons that course through the internal zone of the median eminence and terminate in the posterior pituitary. Another population of magnocellular neuroendocrine neurons lies in the supraoptic nucleus along the base of the brain.

The *parvicellular neuroendocrine division* includes three major, separate (although partly interdigitated) pools of neurons. Somatostatin (**SS**) neurons are concentrated along the wall of the third ventricle; thyrotropin-releasing hormone (**TRH**) neurons are concentrated a bit more laterally; and corticotropin-releasing hormone (**CRH**) neurons are concentrated even more laterally. Their axons end in the external zone of the median eminence, where they release their peptide neurotransmitters into the hypophysial portal veins to control anterior pituitary hormone secretion.

The *descending division* has three parts (dorsal, lateral, and ventral) with topographically organized projections to the brain stem and spinal cord. Axons terminate in many parts of the central autonomic network in the brain stem (see Figure 47–9), the marginal zone (lamina I) of the spinal cord and spinal trigeminal nucleus, and a number of regions in the brain stem reticular formation and periaqueductal gray matter. The descending division modulates autonomic outflow (and inflow), the inflow of nociceptive information, and eating and drinking behaviors. Appropriate integration of magnocellular neuroendocrine, parvicellular neuroendocrine, autonomic, and behavioral responses is mediated primarily by external inputs rather than by interneurons or extensive recurrent axon collaterals of projection neurons. All carefully studied inputs diverge to more than one functional division of the paraventricular nucleus, thus terminating on multiple types of neurons in the nucleus. Circulating steroid and thyroid hormones also produce selective effects on particular types of neurons in the paraventricular nucleus.

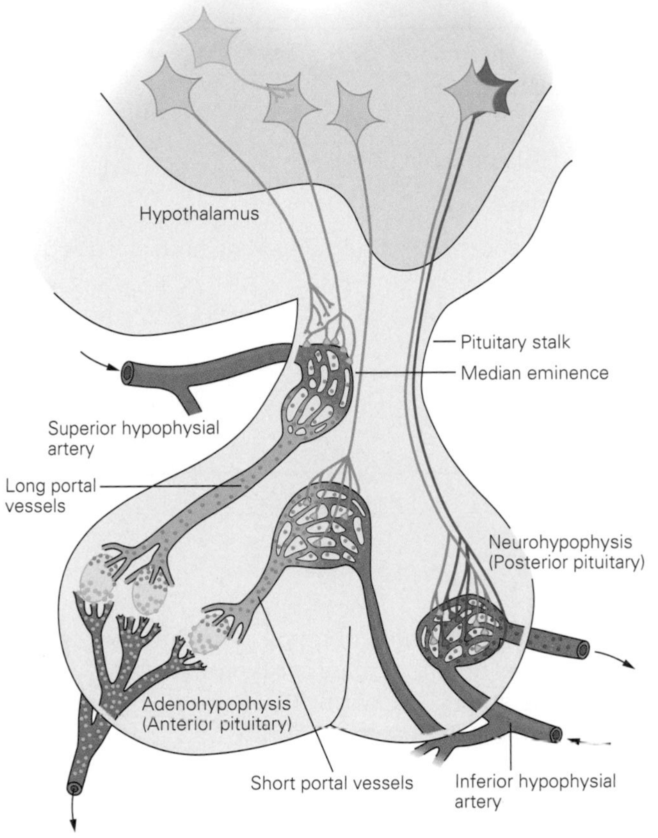

Figure 47–12 The hypothalamus controls the pituitary gland both directly and indirectly through hormone-releasing neurons. Neurons in the *magnocellular neuroendocrine system* (**blue**) send their axons directly to the posterior pituitary (neurohypophysis) where they release the peptides vasopressin and oxytocin into the general circulation. Neurons in the *parvicellular neuroendocrine system* (**yellow**) send their axons to a venous portal system in the median eminence and pituitary stalk. Long and short portal veins transport hypothalamic hormones (peptides and dopamine) to the anterior pituitary (adenohypophysis) where they bind to five classic types of endocrine cells and influence the release of their hormones (see Figure 47–11). The output of neuroendocrine neurons is regulated in large part by inputs from other regions of the brain. (Reproduced, with permission, from Reichlin 1978; and Gay 1972.)

GnRH. During embryogenesis these neurons arise in a specialized region of the olfactory placode or epithelium and then migrate along the terminal nerves to enter the base of the brain and eventually surround the rostral end of the third ventricle. Remarkably, only about a thousand GnRH neurons control all aspects of reproductive physiology and behavior.

Most of the remaining parvicellular neuroendocrine neurons are exceptionally important for the regulation of metabolism. This population lies within the paraventricular and arcuate nuclei and the short periventricular region between them (Figures 47–10 and 47–12). Distinct pools of neurons release corticotropin-releasing hormone (CRH), thyrotropin-releasing hormone (TRH), or somatostatin (or growth hormone release-inhibiting hormone). The pool of CRH neurons in the paraventricular nucleus controls the release of anterior pituitary adrenocorticotropic hormone (ACTH), which in turn controls the release of cortisol (glucocorticoids) from the adrenal cortex. Thus this pool of CRH neurons is the "final common pathway" for all centrally mediated stress responses.

The arcuate nucleus contains two critical pools of parvicellular neuroendocrine neurons. One group releases growth hormone-releasing hormone (GRH) and the other dopamine, which inhibits prolactin secretion. Some of the dopaminergic neurons are distributed dorsally as far as the paraventricular nucleus.

The axons of all these parvicellular neuroendocrine neurons travel in the hypothalamo-hypophysial tract and end in the specialized proximal end of the pituitary stalk, the median eminence (Figure 47–12). There, in a region of fenestrated capillary loops in the external zone of the median eminence, the axon terminals release the various hypophysiotrophic factors. The capillary loops are the proximal end of the hypophysial portal system of veins that carry the factors to the anterior pituitary, where they act on cognate receptors on the five types of endocrine cells (Figure 47–11).

Table 47–3 Hormones of the Posterior Pituitary Gland

Name	Structure	Function
Vasopressin	H-Cys-Tyr-Phe-Gln-Asn-Cys-Pro-Arg-Gly-NH_2-S-S	Vasoconstriction, water resorption by the kidney
Oxytocin	H-Cys-Tyr-Ile-Glu-Asn-Cys-Pro-Leu-Gly-NH_2-S-S	Uterine contraction and milk ejection

Table 47–4 Hypothalamic Substances That Release or Inhibit the Release of Anterior Pituitary Hormones

Hypothalamic substance	Anterior pituitary hormone
Releasing:	
Thyrotropin-releasing hormone (TRH)	Thyrotropin (TSH), prolactin (PRL)
Corticotropin-releasing hormone (CRH)	Adrenocorticotropin (ACTH), β-lipotropin
Gonadotropin-releasing hormone (GnRH)	Luteinizing hormone (LH), follicle-stimulating hormone (FSH)
Growth hormone-releasing hormone (GHRH or GRH)	Growth hormone (GH)
Inhibiting:	
Prolactin release-inhibiting hormone (PIH), dopamine	Prolactin
Growth hormone release-inhibiting hormone (GIH or GHRIH; somatostatin)	Growth hormone, thyrotropin

An Overall View

The three divisions of the autonomic nervous system form an integrated motor system that acts in parallel with the somatic and neuroendocrine motor systems to maintain homeostasis. Although once viewed as a system that exerts a diffuse control over its targets, recent work has made clear that autonomic neurons are exquisitely specialized to control different targets and that during different behaviors functional subsets of autonomic neurons can be selectively activated.

Synaptic convergence and co-transmission allow autonomic ganglia to operate in different modes: as relays, filters, or amplifiers of preganglionic activity. Even the simplest reflexes in the gut, bladder, or cardiovascular system involve the integration of sensory information and coordination of antagonistic functions.

Visceral sensory afferents are important regulators of motor outflow, and the nucleus of the solitary tract in the medulla is the most important relay station for this sensory information to reach the rest of the central autonomic control network. The hypothalamus integrates autonomic, neuroendocrine, and somatic behavioral responses, which are modulated by inputs from virtually all parts of the nervous system.

Looking back over the past 100 years, autonomic neuroscience has been very influential in shaping general concepts of synaptic transmission—from the first discoveries of neurotransmitters to the first discoveries of co-transmitters—while also having broad impact in the field of medicine. Many of the most commonly prescribed drugs act on the autonomic system and its target tissues.

In this present time of aging populations it is also important to note that many of the physical signs and symptoms associated with old age are autonomic in origin. Think how many people are affected by cardiovascular disease, metabolic and digestive disease, and problems with urogenital function.

One very exciting challenge for the future will therefore be to understand in greater detail how the central autonomic network can be manipulated therapeutically to counteract the loss of peripheral autonomic function. This will require closer interaction between the communities of scientists who study peripheral and central autonomic mechanisms. A second exciting challenge will be to unravel the still mysterious links between motivation, emotion, autonomic function, stress, and neuropsychiatric disorders. By combining current advances in molecular biology, genetics, and computational modeling, meeting all of these challenges now seems possible.

John P. Horn
Larry W. Swanson

Selected Readings

Canteras NS. 2002. The medial hypothalamic defensive system: hodological organization and functional implications. Pharmacol Biochem Behav 71:481–491.

Fadel PJ. 2008. Arterial baroreflex control of the peripheral vasculature in humans: rest and exercise. Med Sci Sports Exerc 40:2055–2062.

Grill HJ, Norgren R. 1978. Neurological tests and behavioral deficits in chronic thalamic and chronic decerebrate rats. Brain Res 143:299–312.

Guillemin R. 1978. Control of adenohypophysial functions by peptides of the central nervous system. Harvey Lect 71:71–131.

Guyenet PG. 2006. The sympathetic control of blood pressure. Nat Rev Neurosci 7:335–346.

Jan LY, Jan YN. 1982. Peptidergic transmission in sympathetic ganglia of the frog. J Physiol (London) 327:219–246.

Jänig W. 2006. *The Integrative Action of the Autonomic Nervous System*. New York: Cambridge University Press.

Saper CB, Chou TC, Scammell TE. 2001. The sleep switch: hypothalamic control of sleep and wakefulness. Trends Neurosci 24:726–731.

Sawchenko PE. 1998. Toward a new neurobiology of energy balance, appetite, and obesity: the anatomists weigh in. J Comp Neurol 420:435–441.

Swanson LW. 1986. Organization of mammalian neuroendocrine system. In: FE Bloom (ed). *Handbook of Physiology, The Nervous System*, Vol IV, pp. 317–363. Baltimore: Waverly Press.

Wheeler DW, Kullmann PHM, Horn JP. 2004. Estimating use-dependent synaptic gain in autonomic ganglia by computational simulation and dynamic-clamp analysis. J Neurophysiol 92:2659–2671.

References

Adams PR, Brown DA. 1982. Synaptic inhibition of the M-current: slow excitatory post-synaptic potential mechanism in bullfrog sympathetic neurones. J Physiol 332:263–272.

Andersson PO, Bloom SR, Edwards AV, Jarhult J. 1982. Effects of stimulation of the chorda tympani in bursts on submaxillary responses in the cat. J Physiol 322:469–483.

Bernard C. 1957. *An Introduction to the Study of Experimental Medicine*. New York: Dover.

Blessing WW. 1997. *The Lower Brainstem and Bodily Homeostasis*. New York: Oxford University Press.

Brookes SJ. 2001. Classes of enteric nerve cells in the guinea-pig small intestine. Anat Rec 262:58–70.

Burnstock G. 2006. Historical review: ATP as a neurotransmitter. Trends Pharmacol Sci 27:166–176.

Cannon WB. 1939. *The Wisdom of the Body*. New York: Norton.

DeGroat WC, Booth AM, Yoshimura N. 1993. Neurophysiology of micturition and its modification in animal models of human disease. In: CA Maggi (ed). *Nervous Control of the Urogenital System*, pp. 227–348. Chur, Switzerland: Harwood Academic Publishers.

Dodd J, Horn JP. 1983. Muscarinic inhibition of sympathetic C neurons in the bullfrog. J Physiol 334:271–291.

Ebbesson SO. 1968. Quantitative studies of superior cervical sympathetic ganglia in a variety of primates including man. I. The ratio of preganglionic fibers to ganglionic neurons. J Morphol 124:117–132.

Forger NC, Breedlove SM. 1987. Motoneuronal death during human fetal development. J Comp Neurol 264:118–122.

Furness JB, Costa M. 1980. Types of nerves in the enteric nervous system. Neurosci 5:1–20.

Furness JB, Jones C, Nurgali K, Clerc N. 2004. Intrinsic primary afferent neurons and nerve circuits within the intestine. Prog Neurobiol 72:143–164.

Gay VL. 1972. The hypothalamus: physiology and clinical use of releasing factors. Fertil Steril 23:50–63.

Gershon M. 1998. *The Second Brain*. New York: Harper Collins.

Gibbins I. 2003. Peripheral autonomic pathways. In: G Paxinos, JK Mai (eds). *The Human Nervous System*, pp. 134–189. San Diego, CA: Academic Press.

Horn JP, Stofer WD. 1988. Spinal origins of preganglionic B and C neurons that innervate paravertebral sympathetic ganglia nine and ten of the bullfrog. J Comp Neurol 268:71–83.

Horn JP, Stofer WD. 1989. Preganglionic and sensory origins of calcitonin gene-related peptide-like and substance P-like immunoreactivities in bullfrog sympathetic ganglia. J Neurosci 9:2543–2561.

Karila P, Horn JP. 2000. Secondary nicotinic synapses on sympathetic B neurons and their putative role in ganglionic amplification of activity. J Neurosci 20:908–918.

Jänig W, McLachlan EM. 1992. Specialized functional pathways are the building blocks of the autonomic nervous system. J Auton Nerv Syst 41:3–13.

Jobling P, Horn JP. 1996. In vitro relation between preganglionic sympathetic stimulation and activity of cutaneous glands in the bullfrog. J Physiol 494:287–296.

Kilduff TS, Peyron C. 2000. The hypocretin/orexin ligand-receptor system: implications for sleep and sleep disorders. Trends Neurosci 23:359–365.

Kullmann PH, Horn JP. 2006. Excitatory muscarinic modulation strengthens virtual nicotinic synapses on sympathetic neurons and thereby enhances synaptic gain. J Neurophysiol 96:3104–3113.

Langley JN. 1921. *The Autonomic Nervous System*. Cambridge: W Heffer.

Lichtman JW. 1980. On the predominantly single innervation of submandibular ganglion cells in the rat. J Physiol 302:121–130.

Loewy AD, Spyer KM. 1990. *Central Regulation of Autonomic Functions*. New York: Oxford University Press.

Lundberg JM, Rudehill A, Sollevi A, Fried G, Wallin G. 1989. Co-release of neuropeptide Y and noradrenaline from pig spleen in vivo: importance of subcellular storage, nerve impulse frequency and pattern, feedback regulation and resupply by axonal transport. Neurosci 28:475–486.

McLachlan E. 1995. *Autonomic Ganglia*. Chur, Switzerland: Harwood Academic Publishers.

McLachlan EM, Davies PJ, Häbler HJ, Jamieson J. 1997. On-going and reflex synaptic events in rat superior cervical ganglion cells. J Physiol 501:165–181.

McLachlan EM, Meckler RL. 1989. Characteristics of synaptic input to three classes of sympathetic neurone in the coeliac ganglion of the guinea pig. J Physiol 415: 109–129.

Peng Y-y, Horn JP. 1991. Continuous repetitive stimuli are more effective than bursts for evoking LHRH release in bullfrog sympathetic ganglia. J Neurosci 11:85–95.

Petrovich GD, Canteras NS, Swanson LW. 2001. Combinatorial amygdalar inputs to hippocampal domains and hypothalamic behavior systems. Brain Res Rev 38:247–289.

Reichlin S. 1978. The hypothalamus: introduction. Res Publ Assoc Res Nerv Ment Dis 56:1–14.

Ricardo JA, Koh ET. 1978. Anatomical evidence of direct projections from the nucleus of the solitary tract to the hypothalamus, amygdala, and other forebrain structures in the rat. Brain Res 153:1–26.

Scher AM, O'Leary DS, Sheriff DD. 1991. Arterial baroreceptor regulation of peripheral resistance and of cardiac performance. In: PB Persson, HR Kirchheim (eds). *Baroreceptor Reflexes: Integrative Functions and Clinical Aspects*, pp. 75–125. Berlin: Springer-Verlag.

Shen WX, Horn JP. 1996. Presynaptic muscarinic inhibition in bullfrog sympathetic ganglia. J Physiol 491:413–421.

Simerly RB. 2002. Wired for reproduction: organization and development of sexually dimorphic circuits in the mammalian forebrain. Annu Rev Neurosci 25:507–536.

Swanson LW. 2000. Cerebral hemisphere regulation of motivated behavior. Brain Res 886:113–164.

Tanev K. 2003. Neuroimaging and neurocircuitry in post-traumatic stress disorder: what is currently known? Curr Psychiatry Rep 5:369–383.

Thorne R, Horn JP. 1997. Role of ganglionic cotransmission in sympathetic control of the isolated bullfrog aorta. J Physiol 498:201–214.

Tompkins JD, Ardell JL, Hoover DB, Parsons RL. 2007. Neurally released pituitary adenylate cyclase-activating polypeptide enhances guinea pig intrinsic cardiac neuron excitability. J Physiol 582:87–93.

Tucker P, Trautman R. 2000. Understanding and treating PTSD: past, present and future. Bull Menninger Clin 64:A37–A51.

Wang FB, Holst MC, Powley TL. 1995. The ratio of pre- to postganglionic neurons and related issues in the autonomic nervous system. Brain Res Rev 21:93–115.

Zhang H, Craciun LC, Mirshahi T, Rohacs T, Lopes CM, Jin T, Logothetis DE. 2003. PIP(2) activates KCNQ channels, and its hydrolysis underlies receptor-mediated inhibition of M currents. Neuron 37:963–975.

48

Emotions and Feelings

ELATION, COMPASSION, SADNESS, FEAR, and anger are examples of emotions. These states have an enormous impact on our behavior. But what exactly is an emotion? Unfortunately, the term *emotion* is commonly and confusingly used in two ways. Sometimes it refers to physiological responses to certain kinds of stimuli; when in danger, your muscles tense and your heart pounds, and you may also feel afraid. But it also refers to conscious experiences, called *feelings*, that often (but not always) accompany these bodily responses. We need to consistently distinguish between these two states.

In this chapter we use the term *emotion* to refer to the first of the two states: The set of physiological responses that occur more or less unconsciously when the brain detects certain challenging situations. These automatic physiological responses occur within both the brain and the body proper. In the brain they involve changes in arousal levels and in cognitive functions such as attention, memory processing, and decision strategy. In the body proper they involve endocrine, autonomic, and musculoskeletal responses (see Chapter 47). We use the term *feeling* to refer to the conscious experience of these somatic and cognitive changes. In a certain sense feelings are accounts our brain creates to represent the physiological phenomena generated by the emotional state.

In sum, emotions are automatic, largely unconscious behavioral and cognitive responses triggered when the brain detects a positively or negatively charged significant stimulus. Feelings are the conscious perceptions of emotional responses.

Emotional reactions have been conserved throughout the evolution of species. Behavioral responses that we typically call emotional responses are found in very simple organisms that may not have consciousness and thus not have feelings. A bacterial cell can detect harmful and useful chemicals and respond to these in adaptive ways. Indeed, all organisms must have such capacities to survive and thrive.

Some stimuli—objects, animals, or situations—trigger emotions automatically, even in the absence of experience. These stimuli are said to have *emotional competence*. In addition, some otherwise insignificant objects and events that occur in conjunction with

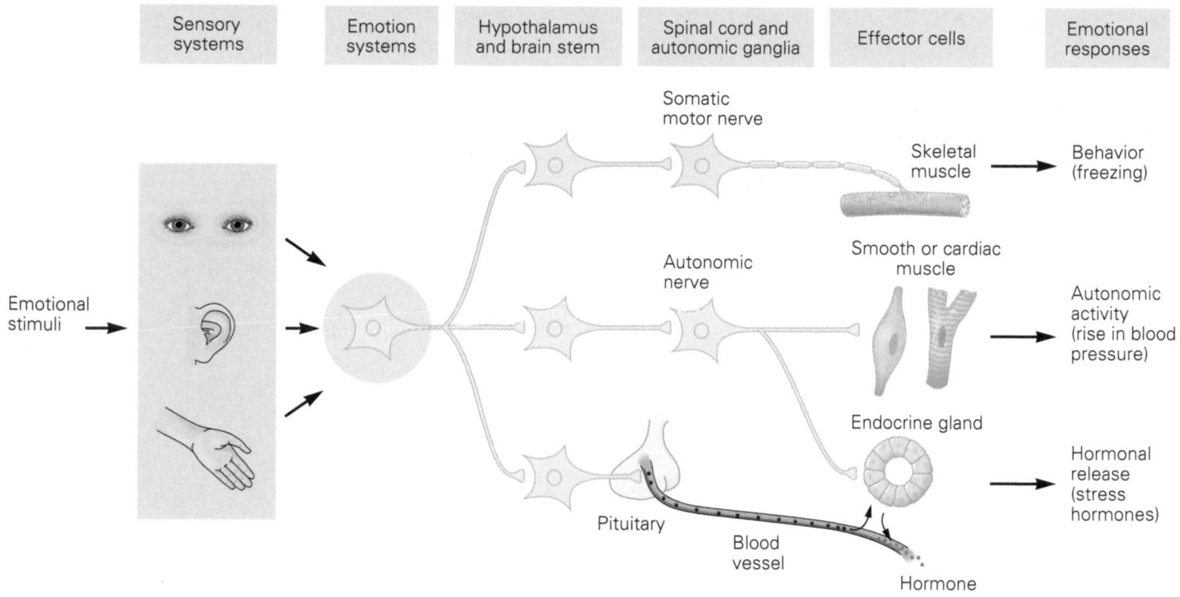

Figure 48–1 Neural control of emotional responses to external stimuli. External stimuli processed by sensory systems converge on emotional processing systems. If the stimuli are emotionally salient, emotion systems such as the amygdala are activated. Outputs of the emotion processing systems to hypothalamic and brain stem regions activate effector cells that control the expression of physiological responses, including skeletomuscular action, autonomic nervous system activity, and hormonal release. The figure shows some responses associated with fear.

emotionally competent stimuli can acquire emotional significance through associative learning. Thus, whereas emotionally competent stimuli are naturally significant (eg, painful or delicious), other objects and events acquire emotional competence by their association with emotionally competent stimuli.

When the brain detects emotionally competent stimuli, it sends commands to networks that control the endocrine glands, the autonomic motor system, and the musculoskeletal system (Figure 48–1). The endocrine system is responsible for the secretion and regulation of hormones into the bloodstream that affect bodily tissues and the brain. The autonomic system mediates changes in the physiological control systems of the body, including the cardiovascular system and the visceral organs and tissues in the body cavity (see Chapter 47). The skeletal motor system mediates overt behaviors such as freezing, fight-or-flight, and particular facial expressions. Together these three systems control the physiological expression of emotional states.

The autonomic and endocrine changes involved in emotional states are part of the body's homeostatic regulatory mechanisms, which are engaged whenever the body is confronted by an intrinsically charged stimulus. In fact, the body's response to strong emotion is not that different from its response to changes in other drive states or alterations in other bodily regulatory processes such as hunger, thirst, sex, and sleep, or its response to pain or changes in body metabolism that occur during vigorous exercise. These regulatory mechanisms are mediated mostly by subcortical structures—the amygdala, striatum, hypothalamus, and brain stem (see Chapter 47).

Most emotional states are observable either directly (for example, in facial expressions or other overt behaviors) or indirectly with psychophysiological or neurophysiological tests or endocrine assays. Thus many emotional responses are measurable and their neurobiological underpinnings can be investigated objectively in both human beings and experimental animals. On the other hand, measuring subjective feelings is more of a challenge and is only practical in humans.

We begin the chapter with a discussion of the historical antecedents of modern neural science research on emotion. We then describe the neural circuits and cellular mechanisms that underlie the most thoroughly studied emotion, fear. Finally, we consider how the brain processes complex social emotions and conscious feelings.

The Modern Search for the Emotional Brain Began in the Late 19th Century

The modern attempt to understand emotions began in 1890 when William James, the founder of American psychology, asked: What is the nature of fear? Do we run from the bear because we are afraid, or are we afraid because we run? James proposed that the conscious feeling of fear is a consequence of emotions, of the bodily changes that occur during the act of running away—we are afraid because we run.

According to James, each feeling (fear, joy, anger) results from its own unique pattern of emotional expression, or bodily signature, controlled by descending connections from the cerebral cortex. A feeling comes about when the bodily expression of that emotional response enters consciousness. James's *peripheral feedback theory* drew on the knowledge of the brain at the time, namely, that the cortex had areas devoted to movement and sensation (Figure 48–2). Little was known about specific areas of the brain responsible for emotion and feeling.

At the turn of the 20th century researchers found that animals were still capable of emotional responses after the total removal of the cerebral hemispheres, suggesting that some aspects of emotion are mediated by subcortical regions. The fact that electrical stimulation of the hypothalamus could elicit autonomic responses similar to those that occur as emotional responses in the intact animal suggested to Walter B. Cannon that the hypothalamus might be a key region in the control of fight-or-flight responses and other emotions.

In the 1920s Cannon showed that transection of the brain above the level of the hypothalamus (by means of a cut that separates the cortex and thalamus from the hypothalamus and lower brain areas) left an animal that was still capable of showing rage. But a transection below the hypothalamus, leaving only the brain stem and spinal cord, eliminated the coordinated reactions of natural rage. This clearly implicated the hypothalamus in emotional reactions. Cannon called these hypothalamically mediated reactions "sham rage" as they lacked input from cortical areas, which he assumed were critical for the emotional experience (Figure 48–3).

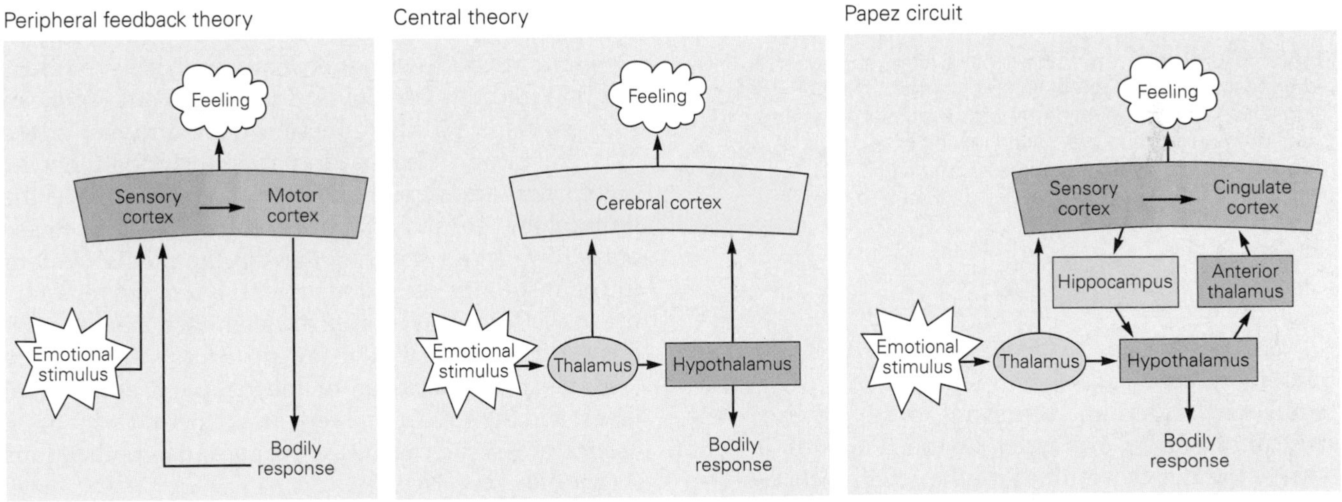

Figure 48–2 Early theories of the emotional brain. (Adapted, with permission, from LeDoux 1996.)

William James's peripheral feedback theory. James proposed that emotionally competent stimuli processed in sensory systems are transmitted to the motor cortex to produce emotional responses in the body. Feedback signals to the cortex convey sensory information about the body responses. The cortical processing of this sensory feedback is the "feeling," according to James.

The Cannon-Bard central theory. Walter Cannon and Philip Bard proposed that emotions are explained by processes within the central nervous system. In their model sensory information is transmitted to the thalamus where it is then relayed to both the hypothalamus and the cerebral cortex. The hypothalamus evaluates the emotional qualities of the stimulus, and its descending connections to the brain stem and spinal cord give rise to emotional responses. The thalamocortical pathways give rise to conscious feelings.

The Papez circuit. James Papez extended the Cannon-Bard theory by adding additional anatomical specificity. The cortical region that receives hypothalamic output in the creation of feelings is the cingulate cortex. The outputs of the hypothalamus reach the cingulate via the anterior thalamus, and the outputs of the cingulate reach the hypothalamus via the hippocampus.

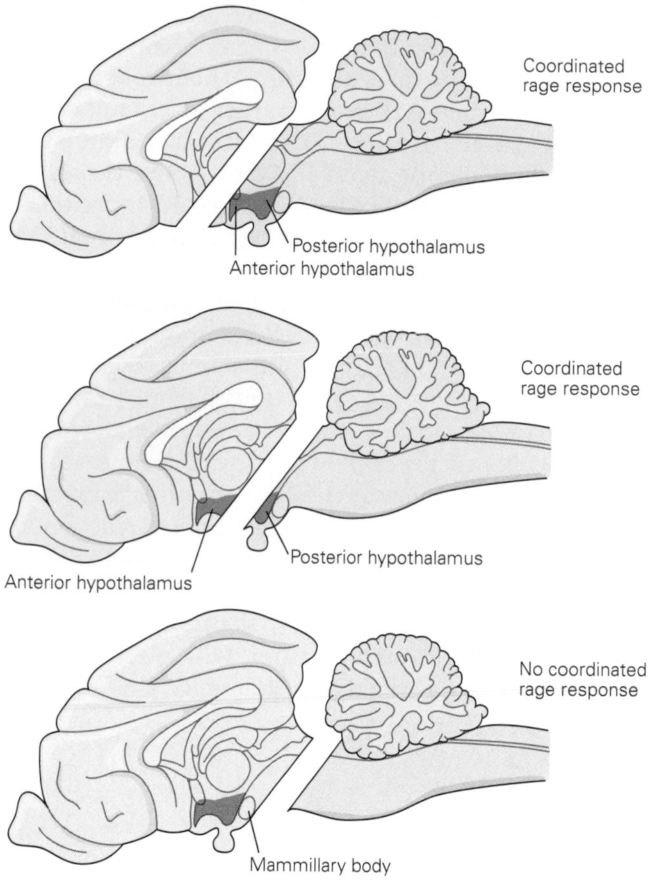

Figure 48–3 Sham rage. An animal exhibits sham rage following transection of the forebrain and the disconnection of everything above the transection (**top**) or transection at the level of the hypothalamus and the disconnection of everything above it (**middle**). Only isolated elements of rage can be elicited if the posterior hypothalamus also is disconnected (**bottom**).

Cannon and his student Phillip Bard proposed an influential theory of emotion centered on the hypothalamus and thalamus. According to their theory, sensory information processed in the thalamus is sent both to the hypothalamus and the cerebral cortex. The projections to the hypothalamus produce emotional responses (through connections to the brain stem and spinal cord) while the projections to the cerebral cortex produce conscious feelings (Figure 48–2). This theory implied that the hypothalamus is responsible for the brain's evaluation of the emotional significance of external stimuli and that emotional reactions depend on this appraisal.

In 1937 James Papez extended the Cannon-Bard theory. Like Cannon and Bard, Papez proposed that sensory information from the thalamus is sent to the hypothalamus. From there, descending connections to the brain stem and spinal cord give rise to emotional responses and ascending connections to the cerebral cortex give rise to feelings. But Papez expanded the neural circuitry of feelings considerably beyond the Cannon-Bard theory by interposing a new set of structures between the hypothalamus and the cerebral cortex. He argued that signals from the hypothalamus go first to the anterior thalamus and then to the cingulate cortex, where signals from the hypothalamus and sensory cortex converge. This convergence accounts for the conscious experience of feeling. The sensory cortex then projects to both the cingulate cortex and the hippocampus, which in turn makes connections with the mammillary bodies of the hypothalamus, thus completing the loop (Figure 48–2).

In the late 1930s Henrich Klüver and Paul Bucy removed the temporal lobes of monkeys bilaterally and found a variety of psychological disturbances, including alterations in feeding habits (the monkeys put inedible objects in their mouth) and sexual behavior (they attempted to have sex with inappropriate partners, like members of other species). In addition, the monkeys had a striking lack of concern for previously feared objects (eg, humans and snakes). This remarkable set of findings came to be known as the Klüver-Bucy syndrome.

Building on the Cannon-Bard and Papez models, and the findings of Klüver and Bucy, Paul MacLean suggested in 1950 that emotion is the product of the "visceral brain." The visceral brain included the various cortical areas that had long been referred to as the limbic lobe, so named by Paul Broca because these areas form a rim (Latin *limbus*) in the medial wall of the hemispheres. Later the visceral brain was renamed the *limbic system*. The limbic system includes the various cortical areas that make up Broca's limbic lobe (especially medial areas of the temporal and frontal lobes) and the subcortical regions connected with these cortical areas, such as the amgydala and hypothalamus (Figure 48–4).

MacLean intended his theory to be an elaboration of Papez's ideas. Indeed, many areas of MacLean's limbic system are parts of the Papez circuit. However, MacLean did not share Papez's idea that the cingulate cortex was the seat of feelings. Instead he thought of the hippocampus as the part of the brain where the external world (represented in sensory regions of the lateral cortex) converged with the internal world (represented in the medial cortex and hypothalamus), allowing internal signals to give emotional weight to external stimuli and thereby giving rise to conscious feelings. For MacLean the hippocampus was involved both in the expression of emotional responses in the body and in the conscious experience of feelings.

Subsequent findings raised problems for MacLean's limbic system theory. In 1957 it was found that damage to the hippocampus, the keystone of the limbic system, produced deficits in converting short- to long-term memory, a distinctly cognitive function. In addition, animals with damage to the hippocampus are able to express emotions, and humans with hippocampal lesions express and feel emotions normally. In general, damage to areas of the limbic system did not have the expected effects on emotional behavior.

Several of MacLean's other ideas on emotion are nevertheless still relevant. MacLean thought that emotional responses are essential for survival and therefore involve relatively primitive circuits that have been conserved in evolution, and this notion is key to an evolutionary perspective of emotion. Further, his idea that emotional states and cognitive processes involve somewhat distinct circuits and can function relatively independent of one another, as implied by Cannon and Bard and all subsequent theories of the emotional brain, also has some merit.

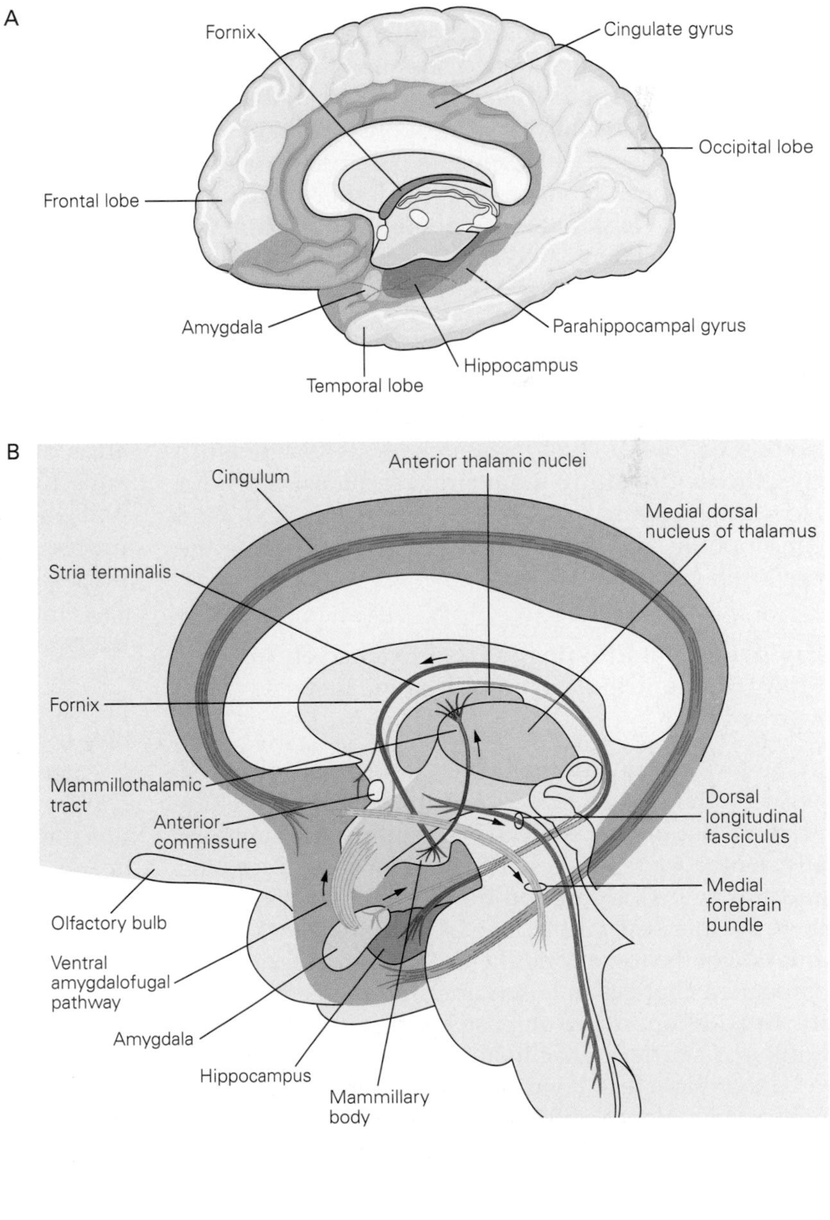

Figure 48–4 The limbic system consists of the limbic lobe and deep-lying structures.

A. This medial view of the brain shows the prefrontal limbic cortex and the limbic lobe. The limbic lobe consists of primitive cortical tissue (**blue**) that encircles the upper brain stem as well as underlying cortical structures (hippocampus and amygdala).

B. Interconnections of the deep-lying structures included in the limbic system. The arrows indicate the predominant direction of neural activity in each tract, although these tracts are typically bidirectional. (Adapted, with permission, from Nieuwenhuys et al. 1988.)

The Amygdala Emerged as a Critical Regulatory Site in Circuits of Emotions

Although damage to most limbic areas does not have the effects on emotional behavior predicted by the limbic system theory, one limbic area was consistently shown to be involved in emotion. This area is the amygdala.

Studies of Avoidance Conditioning First Implicated the Amygdala in Fear Responses

In the mid-1950s Lawrence Weiskrantz sought to understand which region of the temporal lobe was responsible for the emotional changes characteristic of the Klüver-Bucy syndrome. To do this, he used avoidance conditioning, a form of instrumental conditioning.

In avoidance conditioning an animal learns to perform responses that successfully avoid an aversive shock, the unconditioned stimulus (US). Successful avoidance of shock reinforces the response, ie, it increases the probability of the response. Normal monkeys learn instrumental responses (ie, pressing a lever) to avoid the shock, but monkeys with lesions of the amygdala do not. Weiskrantz concluded that a key function of the amgydala was to connect external stimuli with their aversive (punishing) or rewarding consequences.

Fear has been a popular emotion in neuroscience research because it is so important for survival and also because excellent behavioral protocols are available for studying fear in animals. Following Weiskrantz's discovery, many researchers used avoidance conditioning to study the neural mechanisms of fear. However fear can also be studied using Pavlovian conditioning and by the early 1980s had become the preferred protocol.

Pavlovian Conditioning Is Used Extensively to Study the Contribution of the Amygdala to Learned Fear

In Pavlovian fear conditioning an association is learned between the US (eg, shock) and the conditioned stimuli (CS) that predict the US. For example, an emotionally neutral CS (a tone) is presented for several seconds and the animal is shocked during the final second of the CS. After several pairings of tone and shock, presentation of the tone alone elicits defensive freezing and associated changes in autonomic and endocrine activity. In addition, many defensive reflexes, such as eyeblink and startle, are facilitated by the tone alone.

Pavlovian fear conditioning is actually the first phase of avoidance conditioning. The pairing of US and CS initially results in the conditioning of a response, but in the second phase the animal learns to perform an instrumental response to avoid the shock. By the early 1980s neuroscientists began to realize that a more efficient way to study fear learning is to focus on the first stage of avoidance conditioning—Pavlovian fear conditioning—and not extend the experimental design to the second phase.

Research carried out in a variety of laboratories established that lesions of the amygdala prevent Pavlovian fear conditioning from occurring. Animals with amygdala damage fail to learn the association between the CS and the US and thus do not express fear when the CS is later presented alone.

The amygdala consists of approximately 12 nuclei, but the lateral and central nuclei are especially important in fear conditioning (Figure 48–5). Damage to either nucleus, but not other regions, prevents fear conditioning. The lateral nucleus is the input nucleus receiving information about the CS (eg, a tone) from the thalamus. The central nucleus is the output region; neurons here project to brain stem areas involved in the control of defensive behaviors and associated autonomic and humoral responses (see Chapter 47). The lateral and central nuclei are connected by way of several intra-amygdala circuits, including connections in the basal and intercalated nuclei.

Sensory inputs reach the lateral nucleus from the thalamus both directly and indirectly. Much as predicted by the Cannon-Bard hypothesis, sensory signals from thalamic relay nuclei are conveyed to sensory areas of cortex. As a result the amygdala and cortex are activated simultaneously. However, the amygdala is able to respond to a danger cue before the cortex can process the stimulus information. Given that cortical processing is required to consciously experience fear, the emotional state triggered by thalamic inputs is likely to be initiated before we consciously feel fear.

The lateral nucleus is thought to be a site of synaptic change during fear conditioning. The CS and US signals converge in the lateral nucleus; when the CS and US are paired, the effectiveness of the CS is enhanced (Figure 48–6). The lateral nucleus appears to be functionally divided. Neurons in the most dorsal part of the dorsal division appear to initiate learning when the CS and US are paired, whereas neurons in an adjacent ventral part of the dorsal division are thought to mediate the long-term memory of the CS–US association. Recent studies have also shown that synaptic plasticity occurs in specific central amygdala circuits. The central amygdala thus does not simply drive motor outputs but is also part of the circuitry through which fear associations are formed and stored, very likely by transmitting information about the CS and US from the lateral nucleus.

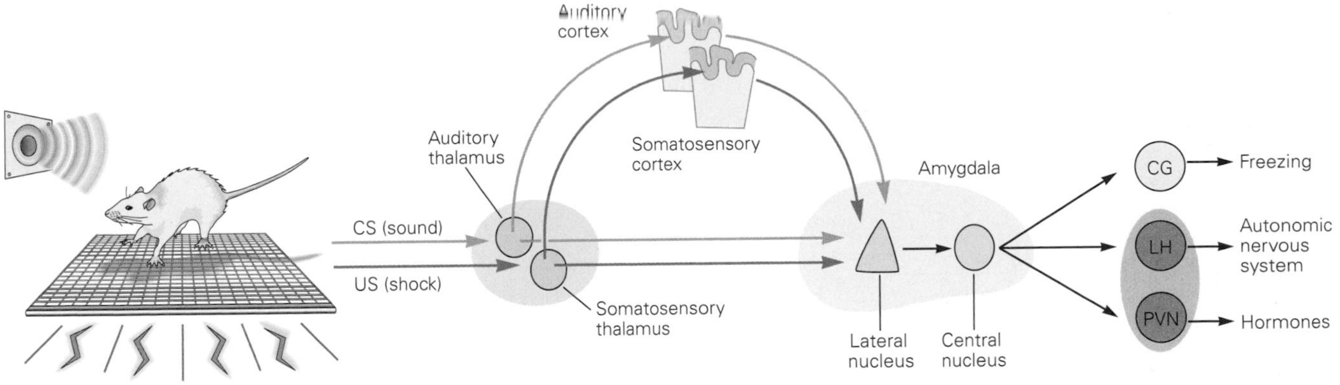

Figure 48–5 Neural circuits engaged during fear conditioning. The conditioned stimulus (**CS**) and unconditioned stimulus (**US**) are relayed to the lateral nucleus of the amygdala from the auditory and somatosensory regions of the thalamus and cerebral cortex. Convergence of the CS and US pathways in the lateral nucleus is believed to underlie the synaptic changes that mediate learning (see Figure 48–6). The lateral nucleus communicates with the central nucleus both directly and through intra-amygdala pathways (not shown) involving the basal and intercalated nuclei. The central nucleus then connects with regions that control various motor responses, including the central gray region (**CG**), which controls freezing behavior, the lateral hypothalamus (**LH**), which controls autonomic responses, and the paraventricular hypothalamus (**PVN**), which controls stress hormone secretion by the pituitary-adrenal axis. (Reproduced, with permission, from Medina et al. 2002.)

The emotional charge of a stimulus is evaluated by the amygdala to determine whether danger is present. If the amygdala detects danger, it orchestrates the expression of behavioral and physiological responses by way of connections to the hypothalamus and brain stem. For example, freezing behavior is mediated by connections from the central nucleus to the ventral periaqueductal gray region. But in addition, the amygdala has a variety of connections that allow it to also influence other cognitive functions. For example, through its widespread projections to cortical areas it can modulate attention, perception, memory, and decision-making. Its connections with the modulatory dopaminergic, noradrenergic, serotonergic, and cholinergic nuclei that project to cortical areas also influence cognitive processing (see Chapter 46).

The cellular and molecular mechanisms within the amygdala that underlie learned fear, especially in the lateral nucleus, have been elucidated in great detail (see Chapter 66). The findings support the view that the lateral nucleus is a site of memory storage in fear conditioning.

The Amygdala Has Been Implicated in Unconditioned (Innate) Fear in Animals

Many animals rely on innate (unconditioned) olfactory signals in the detection of threats, mates, food, and so forth. For example, rodents exhibit freezing and other defensive behaviors when fox urine is detected.

Recent studies have made considerable progress in uncovering the circuits underlying innate fear (see Chapter 47). In mammals unconditioned threats involving predator or conspecific odors are transmitted from the vermonasal component of the olfactory system (see Chapter 32) to medial amygdala. Outputs of the medial amygdala reach the ventromedial hypothalamus, which connects with the premammillary hypothalamic nucleus. In contrast to learned fear, which depends on the ventral periaqueductal gray region, unconditioned fear responses depend on connections from the hypothalamus to the dorsal periaqueductal gray region.

The Amygdala Is Also Important for Fear in Humans

The basic findings in animals regarding the role of the amygdala in emotion have been confirmed in studies of humans. Thus patients with damage to the amygdala fail to undergo fear conditioning when presented with a neutral CS paired with a US (electric shock or loud noise). Patients with damage to the amygdala also fail to recognize facial expressions of fear and do not generate autonomic fear responses to these.

In normal human subjects activity in the amygdala increases during CS–US pairing (Figure 48–7). This activity is especially strong when the stimuli are presented subliminally. In normal subjects fearful facial

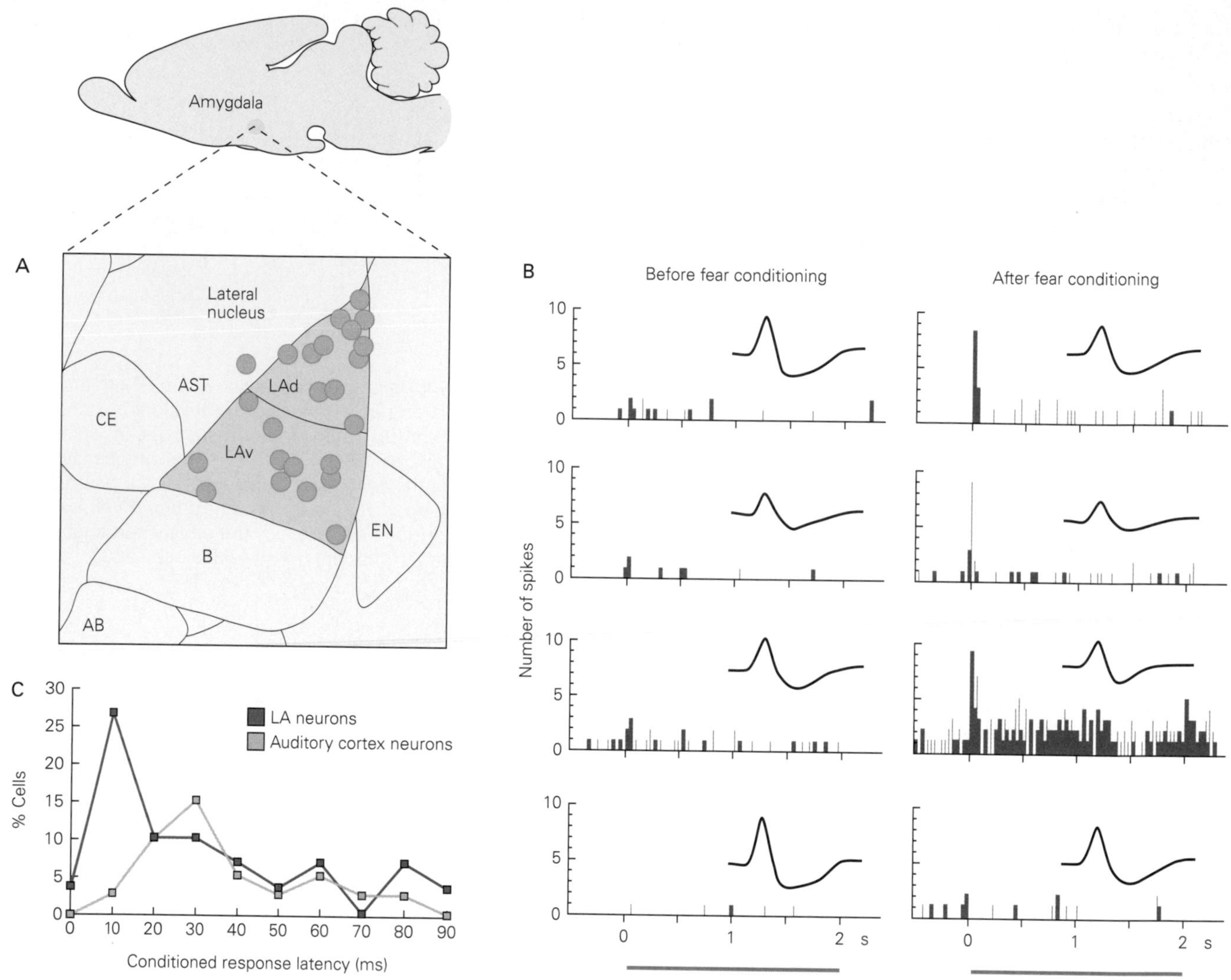

Figure 48–6 The responses of the lateral nucleus of the amygdala are enhanced by fear conditioning.

A. The blue dots indicate the placement of extracellular electrodes in the lateral nucleus. (**AST**, amygdalo-striatal transition area; **AB**, accessory basal nucleus of the amygdala; **B**, basal nucleus of the amygdala; **CE**, central nucleus of the amygdala; **EN**, endopiriform cortex; **LAd**, dorsal lateral nucleus; **LAv**, ventral lateral nucleus.)

B. Histograms show activity in four simultaneously recorded neurons in the lateral nucleus before and after conditioning. Each histogram represents the sum of 10 presentations of the conditioned stimulus (**black bar**). Representative spike waveforms are shown in insets.

C. After conditioning, the neurons in the dorsal lateral nucleus fire at shorter latencies than do neurons in the auditory cortex. They also fire at higher frequencies (not shown).

expressions also activate the amygdala, even when presented subliminally. These findings emphasize the importance of the amygdala as a subconscious evaluator of the meaning of a stimulus.

Certain forms of fear processing are unique to humans. For example, simply telling a human subject that the CS may be followed by a shock is enough to allow the CS to elicit fear responses. The CS elicits characteristic autonomic responses even though it was never associated with the delivery of the shock. Humans can also be conditioned by allowing them to observe someone else being conditioned—the observer learns to fear the CS even though the CS or US were never directly presented to the observing subject.

The emotional learning and memory capacities of the human amygdala fall into the category of *implicit learning* and memory (unconscious recall of perceptual and motor skills (see Chapter 65)). In situations of danger, however, the hippocampus and other components of the medial temporal lobe system concerned with *explicit learning* and memory (the conscious recall of people, places, and things) will encode the learning such that learned indicators of danger can also be recalled consciously.

Studies of patients with bilateral damage to the amygdala or hippocampus illustrate the separate contributions of the amygdala and the hippocampus to implicit and explicit memory, respectively. Patients with damage to the amygdala show no physiological responses to a CS (indicating no implicit learning) but have good memory of the conditioning experience (indicating explicit learning), whereas patients with hippocampal damage respond normally to the CS but have no conscious memory of the conditioning experience.

Amygdala function is altered in a number of psychiatric disorders in humans, especially disorders

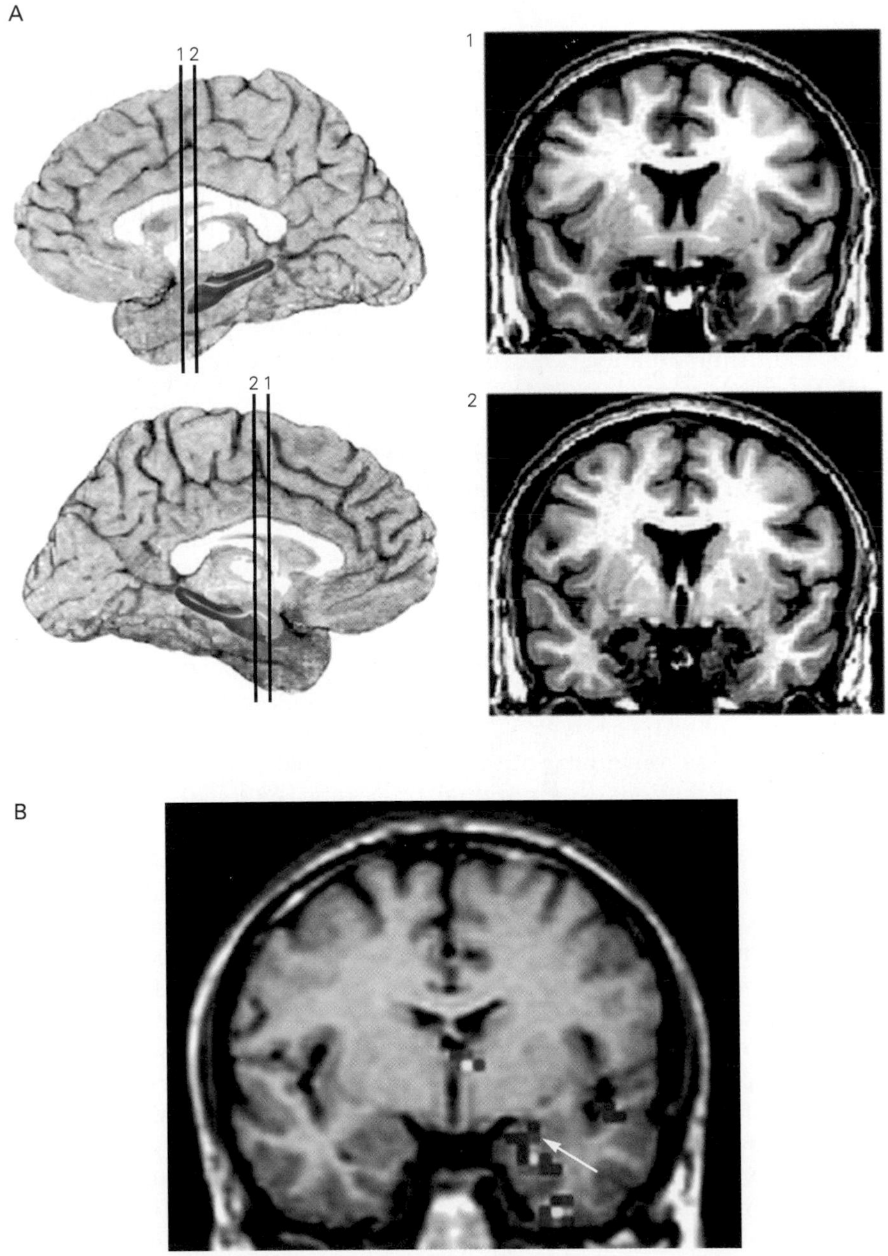

Figure 48–7 Lesion and imaging results implicate the human amygdala in conditioned fear.

A. Left side: Three-dimensional magnetic resonance imaging (MRI) reconstructions of a normal brain seen from a medial perspective (right hemisphere on top, left hemisphere below). The amygdala (**light blue**) and the hippocampus (**dark blue**), normally hidden by the parahippocampal gyrus, were traced and colored. **Right side:** Two coronal slices through the damaged amygdala of a patient with Urbach-Wiethe disease at the levels shown on the three-dimensional reconstruction. In such patients damage to the amygdala impairs fear responses and blocks fear conditioning. (Reproduced, with permission, from Hanna Damasio and Joel Bruss.)

B. Conditioned fear stimuli activate the human amygdala (**arrow**). Healthy volunteers underwent fear conditioning while their brains were scanned using functional MRI. Conditioning involved two conditioned stimuli, one paired with the unconditioned stimulus (CS+) and one not (CS–). Selective activation was assessed by subtracting the CS– scans from the CS+ scans. (Adapted, with permission, from LaBar et al. 1998.)

of fear and anxiety (see Chapter 63). In addition, the amygdala plays an important role in processing cues related to addictive drugs (see Chapter 49).

The Amygdala Is Involved in Positive Emotions in Animals and Humans

Although most work on the neural basis of emotion during the last half century has focused on aversive responses, especially fear, other studies have shown that the amygdala is also involved in positive emotions, in particular the processing of rewards. In monkeys and rats the amygdala is required for associating neutral stimuli with rewards.

Studies in nonhuman primates and rodents have followed up on Weiskrantz's suggestion that the amygdala connects stimulus rewards as well as punishers. For example, in a recent study monkeys were trained to associate abstract visual images with a reward or punisher. The meaning was then reversed (eg, by pairing a punisher with a stimulus that had previously been associated with a reward). In this way it was possible to separate the contributions of the amygdala to visual and value processing. Changes in the value of the images modulated neural activity in the amygdala, and the modulation occurred rapidly enough to account for behavioral learning.

A growing number of functional imaging studies of humans have also shown that the amygdala is involved in emotions. For example, the human amgydala is activated when subjects observe pictures of stimuli associated with food, sex, and money, or when people make decisions based on the reward value of stimuli.

Other Brain Areas Contribute to Emotional Processing

In addition to the amygdala, other brain areas make important contributions to emotional processing As seen in the case of conditioned and unconditioned fear, the amygdala contributes to emotional processing as part of a larger circuit that includes regions of the hypothalamus and brain stem, eg, the periaqueductal gray region in the brain stem.

Cortical areas are also important. A number of studies in humans have implicated the ventral region of the anterior cingulate cortex, the insular cortex, and the ventromedial prefrontal cortex in various aspects of emotional processing. These cortical circuits are especially important in complex emotional states.

Complex feelings are associated with social interaction, and range from empathy and pride to embarrassment and guilt. As in the primary emotions such as fear, pleasure, or sadness, social emotions consist of specific bodily changes and behaviors and are experienced consciously as distinct feelings. These feelings make important contributions to normal social interactions.

Studies of patients with neurological disease and focal brain lesions have advanced the understanding of the neural basis of social emotions. For example, damage to some sectors of the prefrontal cortex markedly impairs social emotions and related feelings. In addition, these patients show marked changes in social behavior that resemble the behavior of patients with developmental sociopathic personalities. Patients with damage to some sectors of the prefrontal cortex are unable to hold jobs, cannot maintain stable social relationships, are prone to violate social conventions, and cannot maintain financial independence. It is common for family ties and friendships to break after the onset of this condition. Recent studies reveal that, under controlled experimental conditions, the moral judgments of these patients can be flawed.

Unlike patients with parietal or parieto-frontal damage, patients with frontal damage do not have motor defects such as limb paralysis or speech defects and thus may appear at first to be neurologically normal. Their perceptual abilities, attention, learning, recall, language, and motor abilities do not show signs of disturbance. Some patients have IQ scores in the superior range. For these reasons they return to their work and social activities after their initial recovery from brain damage. Only when they start to interact with others are their defects noticed.

In the prefrontal cortex the ventromedial sector is particularly important. In most patients with impaired social emotions this sector is damaged bilaterally (Figure 48–8), although damage restricted to the right side is sufficient to cause antisocial symptoms. The critical region encompasses Brodmann's areas 12, 11, 10, 25, and 32, which receive extensive projections from the dorsolateral and dorsomedial sectors of the prefrontal cortex. Some of these areas project extensively to subcortical areas related to emotions: the amygdala, hypothalamus, and periaqueductal gray region in the brain stem tegmentum.

Patients with these frontal lesions do not exhibit changes in heart rate or degree of palm sweating when shown stimuli that normally cause emotions, although they can describe flawlessly the pictures. Normal subjects are equally proficient at describing the pictures but also have psychophysiological responses to the pictures. Unlike normal subjects, patients with frontal lesions do not show detectable skin conductance changes, a sign of sympathetic activation, during the

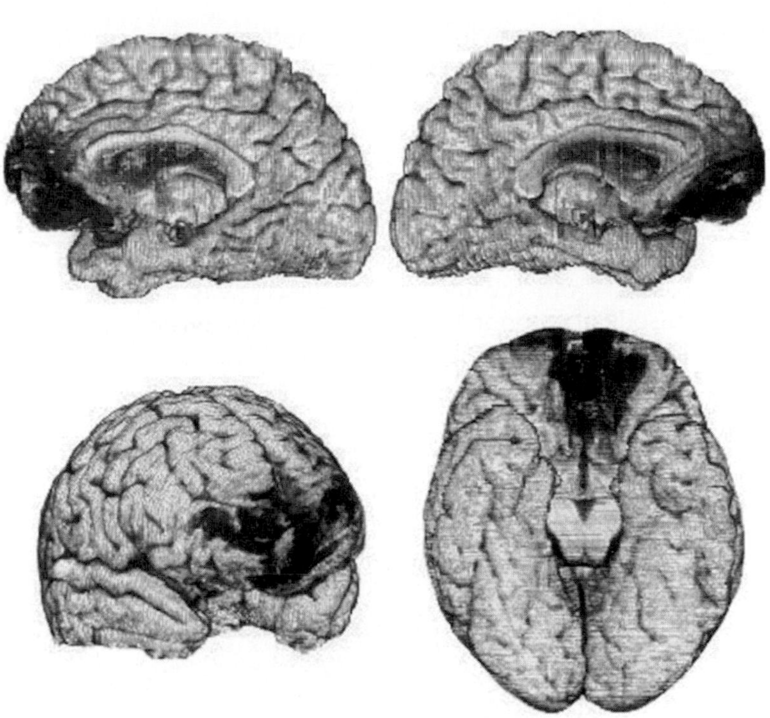

Figure 48–8 Prefrontal lesions can lead to a form of acquired sociopathy. This three-dimensional (MRI) reconstruction of a human brain shows damage centered in the ventral and medial region of the prefrontal cortex in both cerebral hemispheres. Such damage markedly impairs emotional responses, especially in the domain of social emotions and decision making. (Images, reproduced with permission, from Hanna Damasio.)

period that precedes making risky and disadvantageous decisions, suggesting that their emotional memory is not engaged during that critical period. Also unlike normal subjects, these patients fail in tasks in which they have to make a decision under conditions of uncertainty, and in which reward and punishment are important factors.

Interestingly, when asked about punishment, reward, or responsibility, adult patients with prefrontal damage respond as if they still have the basic knowledge of the rules, but their actions indicate that they fail to use them in real situations. This dissociation suggests that their behavioral defects are not caused by a loss of factual knowledge but rather by a difficulty in accessing that knowledge, perhaps because of defective emotional processing.

Functional imaging of normal human subjects shows that the ventromedial frontal cortex is activated during the period before a decision. That same region is activated by tasks involving punishment and reward, supporting the notion that the emotional significance of punishment and reward is relevant for decision making. Punishment and reward are frequently featured in experiments involving economic and moral decisions.

The prefrontal cortex, especially areas in the ventromedial sector, operates in parallel with the amygdala. During an emotional response ventromedial areas govern the attention accorded to certain stimuli, influence the content retrieved from memory, and help shape mental plans conceived as a response to the triggering stimulus. By influencing attention, both the amygdala and the ventromedial prefrontal cortex are also likely to alter cognitive processes, for example by speeding up or slowing down the flow of sensory representations (see Chapter 17). All of these changes are eventually incorporated in the circuitry of working memory in the dorsolateral prefrontal cortex, which contributes to the processing of conscious feelings.

The Neural Correlates of Feeling Are Beginning to Be Understood

We have defined feeling as the conscious experience of an emotion. Thus attempts to study the neural correlates of feelings in experimental animals are difficult because feelings are inherently subjective. Evidence for the neural correlates of feeling comes primarily from functional imaging studies of humans and from neuropsychological testing of patients with specific brain lesions.

One functional imaging study used positron emission tomography (PET) to test the idea that feelings are correlated with activity in cortical and subcortical somatosensory regions that specifically receive inputs related to the internal environment—the viscera, the endocrine glands, and the musculoskeletal system. Normal subjects were asked to recall personal episodes involving four different emotions—sadness, happiness, anger, and fear—and to attempt to reexperience as closely as possible the emotion that accompanied those events. From the moment a subject was told which episode or emotion to reexperience until the end of the scanning, the activity level in a number of cortical and subcortical regions was analyzed continuously, along with several psychophysiological parameters, such as skin conductance.

Activity changed in the insular cortex, secondary somatosensory cortex (S-II), cingulate cortex, hypothalamus, and upper brain stem, and the pattern of change differed with each emotion (Figure 48–9). Patterns of activation did not overlap. These results support the idea that at least a part of the neural substrate for feelings corresponds to the changes in the pattern of activity caused by the emotion being elicited.

When, for example, subjects experienced sadness, the subgenual sector of the cingulate cortex was

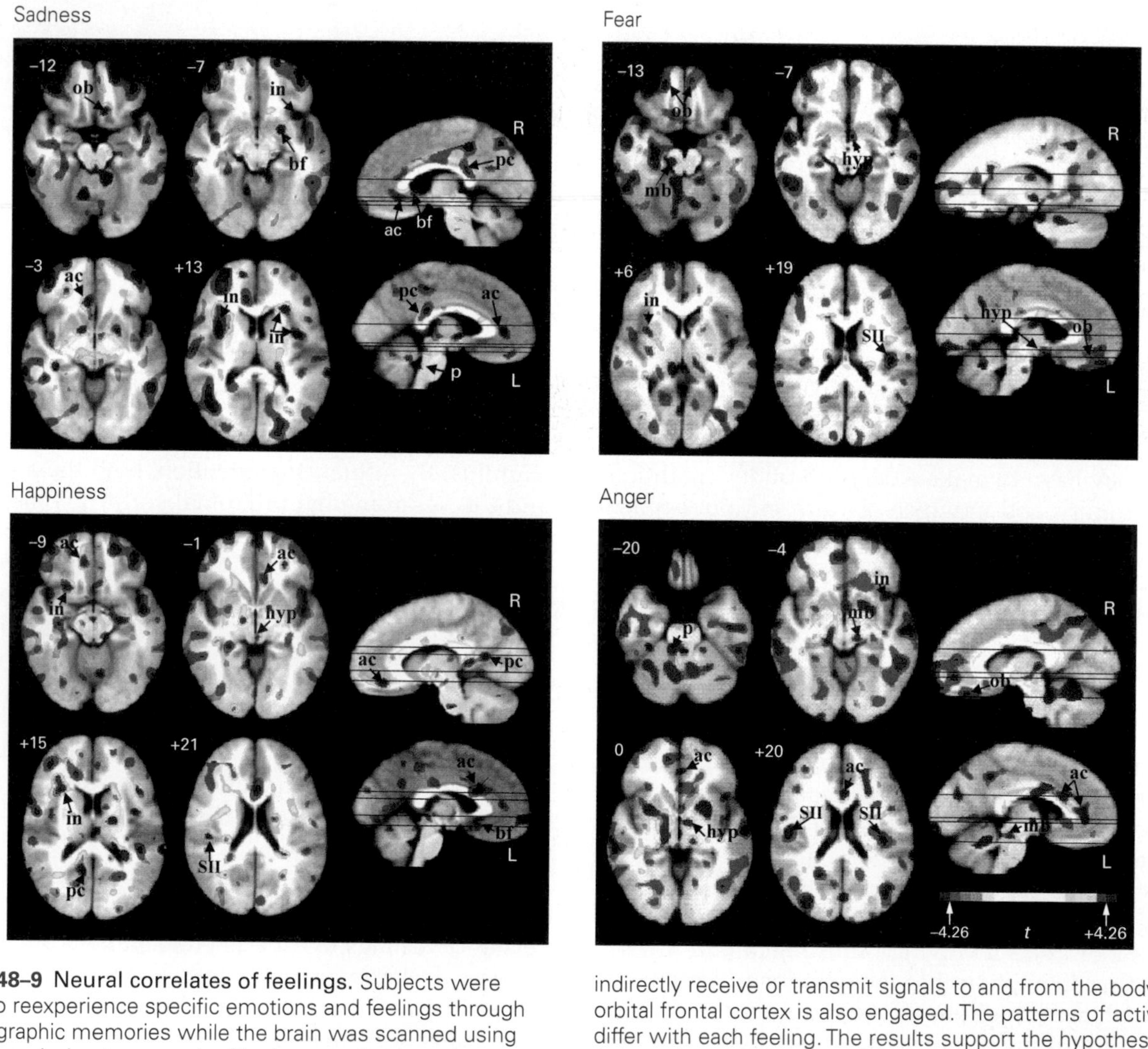

Figure 48–9 Neural correlates of feelings. Subjects were asked to reexperience specific emotions and feelings through autobiographic memories while the brain was scanned using positron emission tomography. The four panels show the brain regions activated or deactivated during different feelings. Significant increases of activity are shown in **orange** and **red**; significant decreases in **blue** and **purple**. The level of activity changes significantly in several brain regions that directly or indirectly receive or transmit signals to and from the body. The orbital frontal cortex is also engaged. The patterns of activity differ with each feeling. The results support the hypothesis that feelings are correlated with activity in brain regions concerned with representing and monitoring body states. (**in**, insular cortex; **S-II**, secondary somatosensory area; **hyp**, hypothalamus; **ac**, anterior cingulate cortex; **pc**, posterior cingulate cortex; **bf**, basal forebrain; **mb**, midbrain; **p**, pons; **ob**, orbitofrontal cortex.)

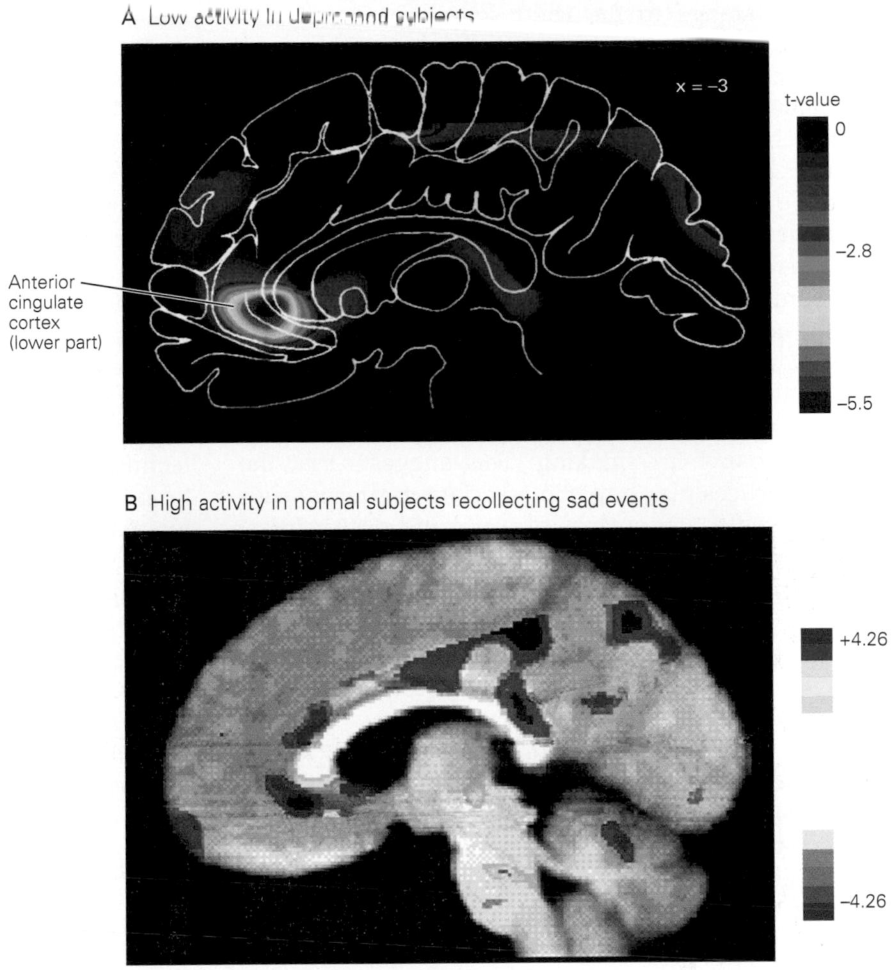

Figure 48–10 Activity in an area of the anterior cingulate cortex is differentially active in patients with depression when they recall sad events. The t-value indicates significance of activity. (In part A **red** denotes decreased activity, whereas in part B it denotes increased activity.)

A. In PET scans of patients with depression an area in the lower sector ion the anterior cingulate cortex shows low activity. This area, the subgenual sector, is Brodmann's area 25. In MRI studies of patients with chronic depression the same area is thinned out. (Reproduced, with permission, from Wayne Drevets.)

B. The same sector is intensely active in normal subjects recalling sad events from their own life. Helen Mayberg has found that electrical stimulation of this cortical region in patients with severe and refractory depression relieves the depressive symptoms rapidly and dramatically. (Reproduced, with permission, from Damasio et al. 2000.)

activated. This region is of special interest because it is also differentially activated in patients with bipolar depression. Moreover, this region appears thinned in structural MRI scans of patients with chronic depression (Figure 48–10). The amygdala is not activated during conscious feeling, evidence that it deals mainly with unconscious emotional states.

In humans, sectors of the insular cortex that are activated during recall of feelings are also activated during the conscious sensation of pain and temperature. The insular cortex receives homeostatic information (temperature and pain signals, changes in blood pH, carbon dioxide, and oxygen) through pathways that originate in peripheral nerve fibers. These afferent fibers include, for example, the C and Aδ fibers. Those fibers form synapses with neurons in lamina I of the spinal cord's posterior horn or the pars caudalis of the trigeminal nerve nucleus in the brain stem. The pathways from lamina I and the trigeminal nucleus project to brain stem nuclei (nucleus of the solitary tract and parabrachial nucleus); from there to the thalamus and then to the insular cortex. The identification of this functional system is further support for the idea that signals in the afferent somatosensory pathways play a role in the processing of feelings. Moreover, in patients with pure autonomic failure, a disease in which visceral afferent information is severely compromised, functional imaging studies reveal a blunting of emotional processes *and* attenuation of activity in the somatosensory areas that contribute to feelings.

Like other feelings, social feelings engage the insular cortices and the primary and secondary somatosensory cortices (S-I and S-II), as has been shown in functional neuroimaging experiments evaluating empathy for pain and, separately, admiration and compassion.

Insights about the neural correlates of feeling also have come from examination of patients with focal lesions. Damage to the right somatosensory cortex (S-II, S-I, and insula) impairs social feelings such as empathy. Consistent with this finding, patients with lesions in the right somatosensory cortex fail to guess accurately the feelings behind the facial expressions of other individuals. This ability to read faces is not impaired in patients with comparable lesions of the left somatosensory cortex, indicating that the right cerebral hemisphere is dominant in the processing of at least some feelings. Body feelings such as pain and itch remain intact as do feelings of basic emotions such as fear, joy, and sadness.

On the other hand, damage to the human insular cortex, especially on the left, can suspend addictive behaviors, such as smoking. This suggests that the insular cortices play a role in associating external cues with internal states such as pleasure and desire. Interestingly, complete bilateral damage to the human insular cortices, as caused by herpes simplex encephalitis, does not preclude emotional feelings or body feelings, suggesting that the somatosensory cortices and subcortical nuclei in the hypothalamus and brainstem are also involved in generating feeling states.

Finally, the neural basis for the hedonic component or pleasure aspect of feeling states is being elucidated in animal studies by Kent Berridge and his colleagues. These studies consistently implicate the nucleus accumbens and other nuclei of the basal ganglia, especially in the ventral striatum and ventral pallidum. A growing number of functional imaging studies of humans—especially in the field of neuroeconomics, which combines research methods from neuroscience, experimental and behavioral economics, and cognitive and social psychology to explore decision-making in humans—point in the same direction.

An Overall View

In the overall physiology of life regulation emotional states sit between the simple processes of reflexes and homeostatic regulation, on the one hand, and cognitive processes on the other.

Emotions serve as cues to appropriate behavior in response to challenges and opportunities in the environment, allowing an organism to deploy specific advantageous behaviors rapidly. The neural processing responsible for emotional states and their effect on behavior is largely unconscious, much as Freud had predicted. Indeed, functional imaging studies show that the amygdala is readily activated by stimuli that are prevented from entering awareness. But even though the initial neural processing of emotionally competent stimuli may be unconscious, that process can lead to feelings, the conscious awareness of the brain's response to the stimuli.

What might the adaptive role of feelings be? Given that emotional states can arise automatically and effectively, what would be the advantage of bringing to consciousness the physiological changes that constitute emotions? The observation of brain-damaged patients in whom feelings are severely compromised gives one possible answer: The loss or impairment of the neural processes responsible for feelings diminishes the ability to anticipate and plan behavior.

Conscious feelings facilitate learning about objects and situations that cause emotional responses. Thus feelings enhance the behavioral significance of emotions and orient the imaginative process necessary for planning of future actions. In brief, unconscious emotional states are automatic signals of danger and advantage, whereas conscious feelings, by recruiting cognitive abilities, give us greater adaptability in responding to dangerous and advantageous situations. Indeed, both emotions and feelings also play a major role in social behavior, including the formation of moral judgments and the framing of economic decisions.

Joseph E. LeDoux
Antonio R. Damasio

Selected Readings

Amaral DG. 2002. The primate amygdala and the neurobiology of social behavior: implications for understanding social anxiety. Biol Psych 51:11–17.

Bechara A, Damasio H, Damasio AR. 2000. Emotion, decision-making and the orbitofrontal cortex. Cereb Cortex 10:295–307.

Bechara A, Tranel D, Damasio H, Adolphs R, Rockland C, Damasio AR. 1995. A double dissociation of conditioning and declarative knowledge relative to the amygdala and hippocampus in humans. Science 269:1115–1118.

Craig AD. 2002. How do you feel? Interoception: the sense of the physiological condition of the body. Nat Rev Neurosci 3:655–666.

Damasio AR. 1994. *Descartes's Error: Emotion, Reason, and the Human Brain.* New York: Penguin Books.

Damasio AR. 1996. The somatic marker hypothesis and the possible functions of the prefrontal cortex. Philos Trans R Soc Lond B Biol Sci 351:1413–1420.

Damasio AR, Damasio H, Tranel D. 2012. Persistence of feelings and sentience after bilateral damage of the insula. Cer Cor doi: 10.1089.

Damasio AR, Grabowski TJ, Bechara A, Damasio H, Ponto LLB, Parvizi J, Hichwa RD. 2000. Subcortical and cortical brain activity during the feeling of self-generated emotions. Nat Neurosci 3:1049–1056.

Dolan RJ. 2002. Emotion, cognition, and behavior. Science 298:1191–1194.

Drevets WC, Price JL, Simpson JR Jr, Todd RD, Reich T, Vannier M, Raichle ME. 1997. Subgenual prefrontal cortex abnormalities in mood disorders. Nature 386:769–770.

Everitt BJ, Cardinal RN, Parkinson JA, Robbins TW. 2003. Appetitive behavior: impact of amygdala-dependent mechanisms of emotional learning. Ann N Y Acad Sci 985:233–250.

Kringelbach ML, Berridge KC (eds). 2010. *Pleasures of the Brain*. New York: Oxford.

LaBar KS, Cabeza R. 2006. Cognitive neuroscience of emotional memory. Nat Rev Neurosci 7:54–64.

LeDoux, JE. 1996. *The Emotional Brain*. 1996. New York: Simon & Schuster.

McGaugh JL, Cahill L, Roozendaal B. 1996. Involvement of the amygdala in memory storage: interaction with other brain systems. Proc Natl Acad Sci U S A 93:13508–13514.

Ohman A. 2005. The role of the amygdala in human fear: automatic detection of threat. Psychoneuroendocrinol 10:953–958.

Panksepp J. 1998. *Affective Neuroscience: The Foundations of Human and Animal Emotions*. New York: Oxford Univ. Press.

Phelps EA, LeDoux JE. 2005. Contributions of the amygdala to emotion processing: from animal models to human behavior. Neuron 48:175–187.

Quirk GJ, Gehlert DR. 2003. Inhibition of the amygdala: key to pathological states? Ann N Y Acad Sci 985:263–272.

Rolls E. 1999. *The Brain and Emotion*. New York: Oxford Univ. Press.

Smith KS, Berridge KC. 2005. The ventral pallidum and hedonic reward: neuromechanical maps of sucrose "liking" and food intake. J Neurosci. 25:8637–8649.

Whalen PJ, Phelps EA. 2009. *The Human Amygdala*. New York: Guilford Press.

References

Adolphs R, Damasio H, Tranel D, Cooper G, Damasio AR. 2000. A role for somatosensory cortices in the visual recognition of emotion as revealed by three-dimensional lesion mapping. J Neurosci 20:2683–2690.

Adolphs R, Gosselin F, Buchanan T, Tranel D, Schyns P, Damasio A. 2005. A mechanism for impaired fear recognition in amygdala damage. Nature 433:68–72.

Anderson SW, Bechara A, Damasio H, Tranel D, Damasio AR. 1999. Impairment of social and moral behavior related to early damage in human prefrontal cortex. Nat Neurosci 2:1032–1037.

Bechara A, Damasio H, Tranel D, Damasio AR. 1997. Deciding advantageously before knowing the advantageous strategy. Science 275:1293–1295.

Breiter HC, Aharon I, Kahneman D, Dale A, Shizgal P. 2001. Functional imaging of neural responses to expectancy and experience of monetary gains and losses. Neuron 30:619–639.

Cahill L, McGaugh JL. 1998. Mechanisms of emotional arousal and lasting declarative memory. Trends Neurosci 21:294–299.

Choi GB, Dong HW, Hurphy AJ, Valenzula DM, Yancopoulos, GD, Swanson LW, Anderson DJ. 2005. Lhx6 delineates a pathway mediating innate reproductive behaviors from the amygdala to the hypothalamus. Neuron 19:647–660.

Christopoulos GI, Tobler PN, Bossaerts P, Dolan RJ, Schultz W. 2009. Neural correlates of value, risk, and risk aversion contributing to decision making under risk. J Neurosci 29:12574–12583.

Craig AD. 2009. How do you feel—now? The anterior insula and human awareness. Nat Rev Neurosci 10:59–70.

Critchley HD. 2005. Neural mechanisms of autonomic, affective, and cognitive integration. J Comp Neurol 493: 154–166.

Damasio A. 2010. *Self Comes to Mind*. New York: Pantheon.

Damasio H, Grabowski T, Frank R, Galaburda AM, Damasio AR. 1994. The return of Phineas Gage: clues about the brain from the skull of a famous patient. Science 264:1102–1105.

Davis M, Whalen PJ. 2001. The amygdala: vigilance and emotion. Mol Psychiatry 6:13–34.

Everitt BJ, Cardinal RN, Parkinson JA, Robbins TW. 2003. Appetitive behavior: impact of amygdala dependent mechanisms of emotional learning. Ann NY Acad Sci 985:233–250.

Fanselow MS, Poulos AM. 2005. The neuroscience of mammalian associative learning. Annu Rev Psychol 56: 207–234.

Harrison NA, Gray MA, Gianaros PJ, Critchley HD. 2010. The embodiment of emotional feelings in the brain. J Neurosci 30:12878–12884.

Holland PC, Gallagher M. 2004. Amygdala-frontal interactions and reward expectancy. Curr Opin Neurobiol 14:148–155.

Immordino-Yang MH, McColl A, Damasio H, Damasio A. 2009. Neural correlates of admiration and compassion. Proc Natl Acad Sci USA 106:8021–8026.

Koenigs M, Young L, Adolphs R, Tranel D, Cushman F, Hauser M, Damasio A. 2007. Damage to the prefrontal cortex increases utilitarian moral judgments. Nature 446:908–911.

Kuhnen CM, Knutson B. 2005. The neural basis of financial risk taking. Neuron 47:763–770.

LaBar KS, Gatenby JC, Gore JC, LeDoux JE, Phelps EA. 1998. Human amygdala activation during conditioned fear acquisition and extinction: a mixed trial fMRI study. Neuron 20:937–945.

LaBar KS, LeDoux JE, Spencer DD, Phelps EA. 1995. Impaired fear conditioning following unilateral temporal lobectomy in humans. J Neurosci 15:6846–6855.

LeDoux JE. 1996. *The Emotional Brain*. 1996. New York: Simon & Schuster.

LeDoux JE. 2000. Emotion circuits in the brain. Annu Rev Neurosci 23:155–184.

Lin D, Boyle MP, Dollar P, Lee H, Perona P, Anderson DJ. 2011. Functional identification of an aggression locus in the mouse hypothalamus. Nature 470:221–226.

MacLean PD. 1990. *The Triune Brain in Evolution*. New York: Plenum.

Maren S. 2005. Synaptic mechanisms of associative memory in the amygdala. Neuron 47:783–786.

Mayberg HS, Liotti M, Brannan SK, McGinnis S, Mahurin RK, Jerabek PA, Silva JA, et al. 1999. Reciprocal limbic-cortical function and negative mood: converging PET findings in depression and normal sadness. Am J Psychiat 156:675–682.

McDonald AJ. 1998. Cortical pathways to the mammalian amygdala. Prog Neurobiol 55:257–332.

McGaugh JL. 2003. *Memory and Emotions: The Making of Lasting Memories*. New York: Columbia Univ Press.

Medina JF, Repa CJ, Mauk MD, LeDoux JE. 2002. Parallels between cerebellum- and amygdala-dependent conditioning. Nat Rev Neurosci 3:122–131.

Mishkin M, Aggleton J. 1981. Multiple functional contributions of the amygdala in the monkey. In: Y Ben-Ari (ed). *The Amygdalaloid Complex*, pp. 409–420. Amsterdam: Elsevier/North Holland.

Moll J, Krueger F, Zahn R, Pardini M, Oliveira-Souza RD, Grafman J. 2006. Human fronto-mesolimbic networks guide decisions about charitable donation. Proc Natl Acad Sci USA 103:15623–15628.

Morris JS, Frith CD, Perrett DI, et al. 1996. A different neural response in the human amygdala to fearful and happy facial expressions. Nature 383:812–815.

Motta SC, Goto M, Gouveia FV, Baldo MV, Canteras NS, Swanson LW. 2009. Dissecting the brain's fear system reveals the hypothalamus is critical for responding in subordinate conspecific intruders. Proc Natl Acad Sci USA 106:4870–4875.

Naqvi NH, Rudrauf D, Damasio H, Bechara A. 2007. Damage to the insula disrupts addiction to cigarette smoking. Science 315:531–534.

Nieuwenhuys R, Voogd J, van Huijzen Chr. 1988. *The Human Central Nervous System: A Synopsis and Atlas*, 3rd ed. Berlin: Springer-Verlag.

Pare D. 2003. Role of the basolateral amygdala in memory consolidation. Prog Neurobiol 70:409–420.

Paton JJ, Belova MA, Morrison SE, Salzman CD. 2006. The primate amygdala represents the positive and negative value of visual stimuli during learning. Nature 439: 865–870.

Petrovich GD. 2011. Learning and the motivation to eat: forebrain circuitry. Physiol Behav 104:582–589.

Phelps EA. 2006. Emotion and cognition: insights from studies of the human amygdala. Annu Rev Psychol 57:27–53.

Pitkänen A, Savander V, LeDoux JE. 1997. Organization of intra-amygdaloid circuitries in the rat: an emerging framework for understanding functions of the amygdala. Trends Neurosci 20:517–523.

Quirk GJ, Gehlert DR. 2003. Inhibition of the amygdala: key to pathological states? Ann N Y Acad Sci 985:263–272.

Rauch SL, Shin LM, Phelps EA. 2006. Neurocircuitry models of posttraumatic stress disorder and extinction: human neuroimaging research—past, present, and future. Biol Psychiat 60:376–382.

Repa JC, Muller J, Apergis J, Desrochers TM, Zhou Y, LeDoux JE. 2001. Two different lateral amygdala cell populations contribute to the initiation and storage of memory. Nat Neurosci 4:724–731.

Rodrigues SM, Schafe GE, LeDoux JE. 2004. Molecular mechanisms underlying emotional learning and memory in the lateral amygdala. Neuron 44:75–91.

Saver JL, Damasio AR. 1991. Preserved access and processing of social knowledge in a patient with acquired sociopathy due to ventromedial frontal damage. Neuropsychol 29:1241–1249.

Seymour B, Daw N, Dayan P, Singer T, Dolan R. 2007. Differential encoding of losses and gains in the human striatum. J Neurosci 27:4826–4831.

Singer T, Seymour B, O'Doherty J, Kaube H, Dolan RJ, Frith CD. 2004. Empathy for pain involves the affective but not sensory components of pain. Science 303:1157–1162.

Swanson LW, Petrovich GD. 1998. What is the amygdala? Trends Neurosci 21:323–331.

Vuilleumier P, Armony JL, Clarke K, Husain M, Driver J, Dolan RJ. 2002. Neural response to emotional faces with and without awareness: event-related fMRI in a parietal patient with visual extinction and spatial neglect. Neuropsychologia 40:2156–2166.

Walker DL, Toufexis DJ, Davis M. 2003. Role of the bed nucleus of the stria terminalis versus the amygdala in fear, stress, and anxiety. Eur J Pharmacol 463:199–216.

Weiskrantz L. 1956. Behavioral changes associated with ablation of the amygdaloid complex in monkeys. J Comp Physiol Psychol 49:381–391.

Whalen PJ, Kagan J, Cook RG, Davis FC, Kim H, Polis S, McLaren DL, et al. 2004. Human amygdala responsivity to masked fearful eye whites. Science 306:2061–2066.

Young L, Bechara A, Tranel D, Damasio H, Hauser M, Damasio A. 2010. Damage to ventromedial prefrontal cortex impairs judgment of harmful intent. Neuron 65: 845–851.

49

Homeostasis, Motivation, and Addictive States

The temperature of the air at higher latitudes can fluctuate by 70°C (158°F) or more over the year, yet some birds and mammals live year round in such environments without hibernating or estivating. These animals keep their core temperatures within a narrow range, on the order of a few degrees, during both the fierce blizzards of winter and the sultry days of summer. This regulatory feat is just one of many that keep key physiological variables within limits favorable to vital processes of the body, such as cell division, energy metabolism, macromolecular synthesis, and cell signaling.

The active maintenance of a relatively constant internal environment is called *homeostasis*. Constancy of the internal environment is the basis of the freedom of action we and other animals enjoy because it partially decouples our physiology from immediate external conditions and greatly extends the range of available habitats. For example, salmon are able to live in both fresh and salt water because they can regulate the osmolality of their extracellular fluid. Hagfish, conversely, are confined to marine habitats because they cannot regulate the osmolality of their extracellular fluid, which reflects that of the external environment.

In climates with wide variation in temperature the budget-minded homeowner may set the thermostat to a lower value during the winter and a higher one during the summer; more sharply contrasting daytime and nighttime settings may be chosen when heating or air-conditioning costs are high. Similarly, in physiological systems the means and variances of regulated variables may be adjusted over the course of the day, the seasons, and the life cycle. For example, a dehydrated camel conserves water by letting its temperature increase above normal before beginning to sweat; at night it lets its temperature decrease below normal, thus starting the day cooler and delaying the onset of sweating. The zoologist Nicholas Mrosovsky has coined the term *rheostasis* to refer to the linkage of regulatory targets and ranges to chronobiological and life-cycle events.

Regulation is achieved through interlinked control systems with both physiological and behavioral outputs (Box 49–1). A key feature of these control systems is *motivational states* such as hunger and thirst. These states arise as responses to internal stimuli, such as signals from detectors of core temperature, and external stimuli, such as the sight of a shaded refuge from the sun. Motivational states influence the

Box 49–1 What Is a Regulated System?

A simple regulated system is illustrated in Figure 49–1A. Water pours into a reservoir from a supply pipe and leaks out through a drain pipe. A float provides information about the water level. A shaft links the float to two valves. One controls the inflow through the supply pipe. This linkage is called *negative feedback* because raising the water level decreases flow through the supply pipe, and the linkage extends back from the float to an upstream stage of the system. The other valve controls outflow through the drain pipe. Such a linkage is called *positive feed-forward*

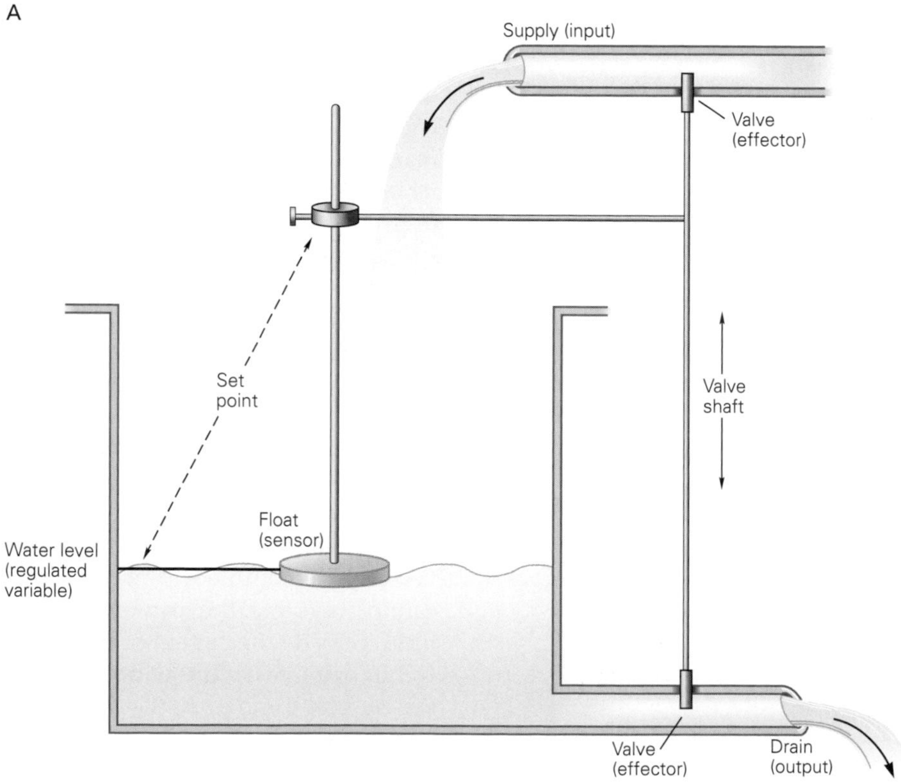

Figure 49–1A A simple regulated system. Changes in the position of the float alter the state of the valves in the supply and drain pipes so as to oppose changes in the water level. (Adapted, with permission, from Cabanac and Russek 2000.)

direction and vigor of behavior, steering the animal toward regions of the environment where conditions promote maintenance of normal body temperature and where resources essential to homeostasis, such as food and water, can be found. These states also influence the frequency and vigor of nonregulatory activities such as exploration and reproduction.

In this chapter we first look at homeostasis by focusing on the control systems responsible for the regulation of fluid and energy balance. We then explore motivational states, focusing on the brain's reward circuitry. Finally, we examine how motivational states and related homeostatic processes are co-opted by drugs of abuse and result in addictive behavior.

because raising the water level increases flow through the drain pipe, and the linkage extends forward from the float to a downstream stage of the system.

The feedback and feed-forward linkages between the float and the valves regulate the water level. Even if the flow rate in the supply or drain pipe is altered by adding a booster pump or a partial blockage, the valves will compensate, and the water level will be confined to a narrow range. The two valves are called *effectors* because they bring about the adjustments that regulate the water level.

Physiological regulation is often achieved by means of a combination of negative feedback control over inputs and positive feed-forward control over outputs. For example, to maintain body weight after consuming a large meal, it is useful both to reduce subsequent food intake and to increase energy expenditure.

Figure 49–1B shows a control diagram of the regulated system in Figure 49–1A. The float is called a *sensor* because it monitors the regulated variable, the water level, within a *regulated compartment*, the reservoir. The output of the sensor is compared to a reference value or *set point*, a water level determined by the height on the float shaft at which the valve shaft is attached. Movement of the waterline away from the set point drives the two effectors to oppose the deviation, thus holding the water level close to the set point; the deviation of the regulated variable from the set point is called an *error signal*.

Some physiologists prefer the concept of a *settling point* to a set point. A settling point requires neither comparison to a fixed reference nor a physiological embodiment of the error signal. The settling point is simply the value of the regulated variable at which the input and output subsystems are balanced. For example, in the system in Figure 49–1A the settling point is the water level at which inflow equals outflow.

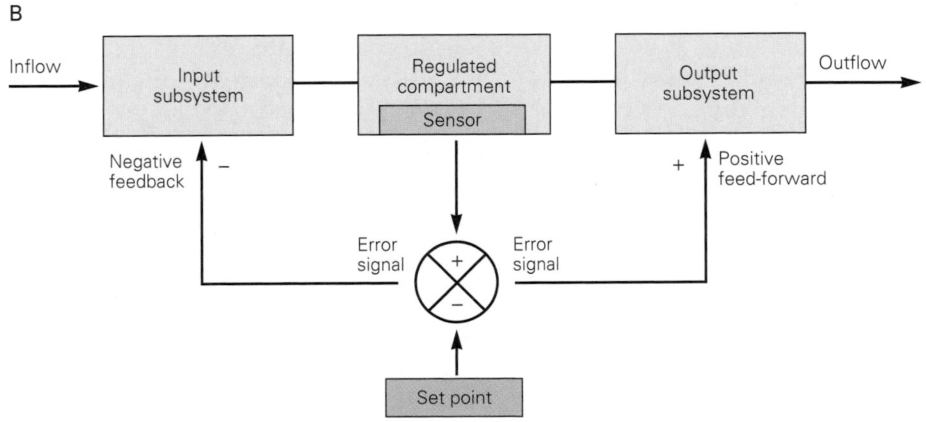

Figure 49–1B Control diagram of the simple regulated system. (Adapted, with permission, from Cabanac and Russek 2000.)

Drinking Occurs Both in Response to and in Anticipation of Dehydration

Severe dehydration generates an overwhelmingly powerful motivational state that focuses thought and action on procuring and consuming water while damping other needs and desires. A dehydrated animal will go to great extremes to find relief from the insistent discomfort of thirst. The behaviors associated with this tightly focused state are classified as *primary drinking* and can be construed as responses to an error signal (Figure 49–1B).

The control system underlying primary drinking enables the animal to respond to a physiological imbalance that would become life threatening if left uncorrected. But additional control over drinking is needed. If water were sought only when the animal was dehydrated, the animal could find itself in an inhospitable environment in which it would have to procure water while in a weakened and deteriorating state. Instead, behavior is programmed so as to avoid severe dehydration. When conditions allow, water is consumed in excess, even in the absence of an error signal, and the kidneys eliminate the surplus. Such *secondary drinking* often coincides with feeding.

In contrast to the simple system in Figure 49–1, physiological systems often comprise several compartmentalized subsystems that are separately regulated. A variety of sensors monitor these separate compartments, and different subsets of effectors are deployed to keep conditions constant within them. Fluid balance provides a case in point. Body water is partitioned between intracellular and extracellular compartments.

Body Fluids in the Intracellular and Extracellular Compartments Are Regulated Differentially

Intracellular and extracellular fluids must be separately regulated because of their different compositions. The principal extracellular cation is Na^+, whereas the principal intracellular cation is K^+. Fluctuation in the level of Na^+ is generally more pronounced than that of K^+. The fluctuations of these cations establish osmolality gradients that move water between the two compartments.

Loss of sodium and water from the extracellular compartment usually occurs with events that lead to decreased vascular volume (hypovolemia), such as hemorrhage or diarrhea. To offset the deficit, both water and sodium must be consumed. Thus primary drinking and sodium intake play essential roles in regulating vascular volume. These behaviors complement the physiological and endocrine mechanisms that maintain blood pressure while conserving water and sodium.

The Intravascular Compartment Is Monitored by Parallel Endocrine and Neural Sensors

Sensors for hypovolemia include detectors of arterial blood flow to the kidney that send information to the brain through two pathways: an endocrine signaling mechanism and a neural route. The neural pathway originates in vascular stretch receptors on the low-pressure side of the circulation, in the heart, great veins, and pulmonary circulation (baroreceptors). Visceral receptors monitoring the extracellular concentration of Na^+ and arterial blood pressure are also thought to contribute to fluid homeostasis.

The brain circuitry that controls the behavioral, physiological, and endocrine responses to hypovolemia is distributed along the central nervous system and includes both local and long-loop pathways (Figure 49–2). Baroreceptors project primarily to the nucleus of the solitary tract. A decrease in stimulation of these receptors activates sympathetic output neurons in the caudal brain stem that maintain both blood pressure and cardiac output by increasing heart rate and triggering peripheral vasoconstriction.

Through connections between the caudal brain stem and the hypothalamus, decreased baroreceptor input also drives release of the peptide vasopressin from the posterior pituitary. Vasopressin increases blood pressure and increases reabsorption of water in the kidney (thus its alternate name, *antidiuretic hormone*). Because the kidneys filter an enormous volume of fluid each day—approximately 60 times the plasma volume—adjustment of urinary output has a large and rapid impact on the volume of fluid in the vascular system. This is an example of feed-forward control (Figure 49–1B).

Whereas a decrease of cardiopulmonary baroreceptor firing may stimulate primary drinking, the high-pressure side of the circulation exerts an opposing influence. The nucleus of the solitary tract receives input from peripheral detectors of arterial blood pressure. As the arterial blood pressure increases (eg, during *hyper*volemia), noradrenergic projections from this nucleus to the median preoptic area, a small midline nucleus in the basal forebrain, reduce drinking. This is an example of negative feedback control (Figure 49–1B).

The endocrine signaling mechanism that monitors arterial blood flow functions in parallel with the neural pathway. The reduction in arterial blood flow to the kidneys during hypovolemia causes the release of the protease renin into the circulation. The substrate

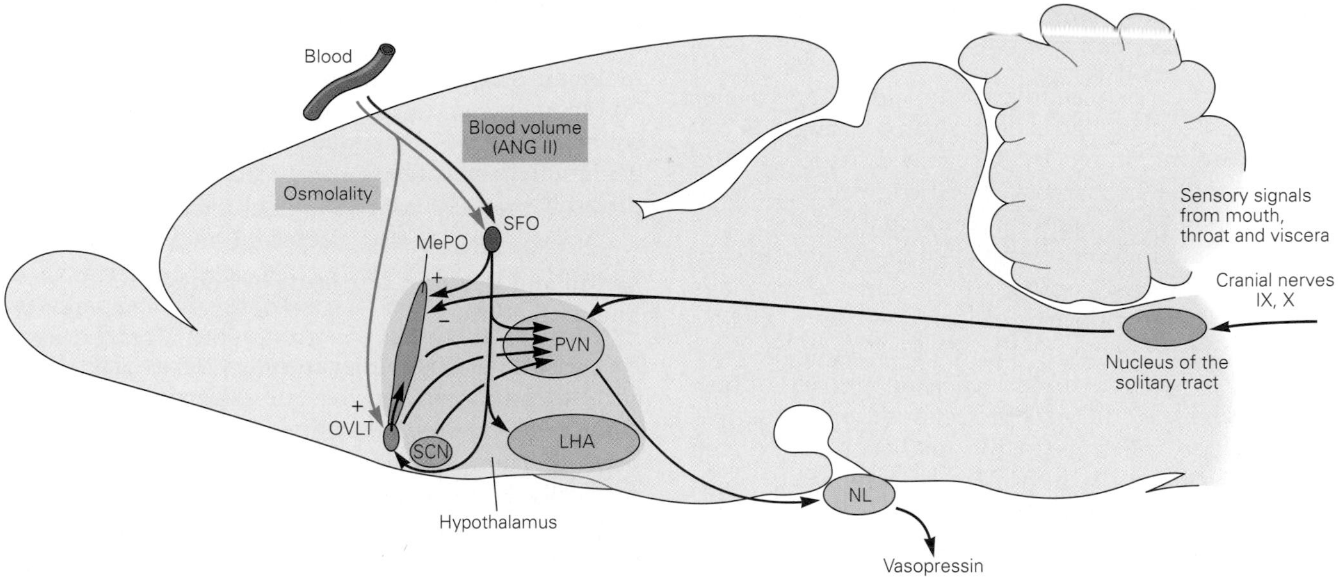

Figure 49–2 Components of the neural circuitry controlling fluid balance. The circuitry is shown in a stylized sagittal section through the rat brain. Information from baroreceptors in the circulatory system and from sensory receptors in the mouth, throat, and viscera is conveyed to the nucleus of the solitary tract and neighboring structures in the caudal brain stem through the glossopharyngeal (IX) and vagal (X) nerves (**right side**). The hormone angiotensin II (**ANG II**) provides the brain with an additional signal concerning low blood volume (**left side**). Circulating angiotensin II is sensed by receptors in the subfornical organ (**SFO**); SFO neurons project to and release angiotensin II in the median preoptic area (**MePO**), paraventricular nucleus of the hypothalamus (**PVN**), vascular organ of the lamina terminalis (**OVLT**), and adjacent lateral hypothalamic area (**LHA**). High arterial pressure is detected by baroreceptors that project to the caudal brain stem; when arterial pressure is too high, drinking is suppressed by an inhibitory input to the median preoptic area from the nucleus of the solitary tract. The osmolality of the blood is sensed by receptors in and near the OVLT that project to the median preoptic area and paraventricular nucleus of the hypothalamus. The latter nucleus is positioned to integrate inputs concerning both blood volume and osmolality and is believed to play a key role in triggering drinking. Neurosecretory cells in this nucleus (and in the supraoptic nucleus) trigger release of vasopressin from the neural lobe (**NL**) of the pituitary, thus decreasing urinary output. Input to the paraventricular nucleus from the suprachiasmatic nucleus (**SCN**) brings the fluid-regulatory system under the influence of the internal day/night clock (see Chapter 51). (Adapted, with permission, from Swanson 2000.)

for this protease is the circulating prohormone angiotensinogen, which is cleaved by renin to produce a decapeptide, angiotensin I. In turn, the angiotensin-converting enzyme transforms angiotensin I into angiotensin II, its active octapeptide derivative. The potent vasoconstricting effect of angiotensin II helps maintain blood pressure in the face of decreased vascular volume. Angiotensin II also stimulates aldosterone release from the adrenal cortex. Aldosterone increases reabsorption of Na^+ in the kidney while favoring K^+ excretion; these complementary effects shift fluid from the capacious intracellular compartment to the depleted intravascular compartment.

Peptide hormones, such as angiotensin II, do not cross the blood–brain barrier freely. However, the brain is able to monitor the circulation directly through specialized, densely vascularized structures, the circumventricular organs, which lack a normal blood–brain barrier and thus provide circulating peptides access to receptors on central neurons. In two of these circumventricular organs, the subfornical organ and vascular organ of the lamina terminalis, angiotensin II acts as a powerful stimulus of drinking and vasopressin release.

Neurons in the subfornical organ project to the median preoptic area and the paraventricular nucleus of the hypothalamus where they release angiotensin II. Injection of angiotensin II into these two nuclei elicits vigorous drinking, whereas cutting the input from the subfornical organ blocks the drinking response to circulating angiotensin II. Thus angiotensin II acts first as a hormone (in the subfornical organ) and then as a neurotransmitter (in the median preoptic area and paraventricular nucleus of the hypothalamus).

The Intracellular Compartment Is Monitored by Osmoreceptors

An increase in extracellular osmolality draws water out of cells, causing the cells to shrink. Changes in cell volume are monitored by specialized neurons called *osmoreceptors*, which translate cell shrinkage or swelling into changes in membrane potential.

A population of central osmoreceptive sensory neurons in the vascular organ of the lamina terminalis projects to neuroendocrine cells in the paraventricular and supraoptic nuclei of the hypothalamus to drive vasopressin release, thus decreasing urinary output (Figure 49–2). Additional projections from these primary sensory neurons to the median preoptic area carry signals that drive drinking in response to cellular dehydration. These latter signals are relayed to the paraventricular nucleus of the hypothalamus, where they converge with inputs from the system that regulates the intravascular compartment.

Motivational Systems Anticipate the Appearance and Disappearance of Error Signals

Changes in intake or expenditure are not immediately registered in physiological systems. For example, water that has been swallowed by an animal undergoing cellular dehydration must be absorbed from the gut and distributed before osmoreceptors of the brain can detect a return toward homeostasis. If consumption continued until the error signal disappeared, the system would overshoot its target. Wastefulness and instability are avoided by terminating drinking well before plasma osmolality is restored.

Thus the regulatory system acts as if it anticipates the cellular rehydration that will eventually follow fluid ingestion, perhaps by using information supplied by peripheral osmoreceptors or visceral Na^+ receptors. Such anticipatory control is a common feature of motivational systems. For example, migratory birds and whales gain prodigious amounts of weight prior to setting off on their journeys. Unlike the simple regulatory system shown in Box 49–1, the input and output subsystems of motivational systems can be adjusted in anticipation of the appearance and disappearance of error signals.

Energy Stores Are Precisely Regulated

Dieters need little convincing that long-term energy stores are regulated, for they have learned how difficult it is to maintain hard-won weight losses. If we are plump when we are young, we usually remain so. That is, our adiposity relative to the norm for our age tends to remain stable throughout our lives. Recent research on the neural, endocrine, and autonomic mechanisms controlling food intake and energy expenditure is beginning to reveal how energy stores are regulated so precisely.

Leptin and Insulin Contribute to Long-Term Energy Balance

Fat constitutes the long-term energy depot of the body and the brain monitors its state. Elegant experiments in mice first showed that a humoral signal is involved. The circulatory systems of pairs of mice were joined surgically (parabiosis). A normal mouse was paired with a mutant one carrying a recessive homozygous mutation of a gene called *obesity* (*ob*), which produces morbid obesity and hypothermia. This surgical linkage normalized the body weight and temperature of the mutant mouse. The *ob/ob* mouse lacks a circulating signal from energy stores that produces feedback control over food intake and feed-forward control over energy expenditure; the normal partner supplies this signal, correcting the deficits.

Mice with homozygous mutation of the *diabetes* (*db*) gene also are obese. Linking the circulatory system of these mice to that of a normal or *ob/ob* mouse not only failed to correct the diabetes and hypoglycemia, it also caused emaciation and death of the normal or *ob/ob* partner. In contrast to the *ob/ob* mouse, the *db/db* mouse produces the circulating signal but lacks a functional receptor. The signal is elevated in the obese *db/db* mouse, thus decreasing the food intake and increasing the energy expenditures of its unfortunate surgically joined partner.

Some 25 years after the first parabiosis studies, the circulating signal, the mutated receptor, and their genes were identified. The circulating signal was identified by Jeffrey Friedman and his colleagues as a peptide hormone called leptin. It is produced principally by white adipocytes (fat-storing cells) in amounts positively correlated with the level of stored fat. Leptin is transported across the blood–brain barrier and acts in the brain and in the periphery at receptors that are members of the cytokine-receptor superfamily.

In normal-weight individuals leptin reduces food intake while increasing energy expenditure, lipolysis, and thermogenesis. Most obese humans have very high levels of leptin, suggesting that they have become insensitive to this key hormone. The rare humans who lack leptin because of mutation of the *ob* gene are morbidly obese and hypothermic; the body weight and temperature of such individuals can be normalized by exogenous administration of leptin.

Levels of the pancreatic hormone insulin are also positively correlated with fat mass. Like leptin, insulin reduces food intake and increases thermogenesis. During fasting leptin and insulin levels decrease before the fat stores fall, and thus fat stores are rapidly replenished once eating is resumed.

Circulating leptin and insulin bind to receptors on two populations of neurons in the arcuate nucleus of the medial hypothalamus. These two populations have opposite responses to leptin and insulin and opposite influences on energy balance.

One population of arcuate neurons secretes two anabolic signaling molecules (signals that promote energy storage): neuropeptide Y and agouti-related peptide. The second population secretes two catabolic signaling molecules (signals that promote use of energy stores): α-melanocyte–stimulating hormone and cocaine- and amphetamine-related transcript (Figure 49–3B).

The antagonism between anabolic and catabolic signals from the arcuate nucleus is illustrated by the action of agouti-related peptide. This molecule is an endogenous antagonist of the melanocortin receptors MC3 and MC4. The endogenous agonist at these receptors is the α-melanocyte-stimulating hormone released from arcuate neurons when the organism is in a catabolic state. Agouti-related peptide blocks the ability of the hormone to reduce food intake, increase energy expenditure, and decrease fat storage. Injection of neuropeptide Y into the hypothalamus triggers feeding and promotes lipogenesis while decreasing energy expenditure. Thus release of either peptide produces anabolic feedback and feed-forward effects that promote weight gain while suppressing signaling in the antagonistic catabolic pathway.

Projections from the arcuate nucleus to the paraventricular and lateral regions of the hypothalamus relay signals carried by circulating leptin and insulin (Figure 49–3C). Neurons in these areas have long been implicated in energy balance. For example, bilateral lesions of the paraventricular nucleus increase food intake and body weight, whereas lesions in the lateral hypothalamic area produce opposite effects. Neuropeptides that decrease food intake or increase energy expenditure are released by different subgroups of neurons in the paraventricular nucleus. Neuropeptides that increase food intake are found in separate subgroups of neurons in the lateral and perifornical regions of the hypothalamus.

As with fluid balance, the neural circuitry responsible for energy balance is broadly distributed. This circuitry includes important components in the dorsal vagal complex of the caudal brain stem in addition to the hypothalamic cell groups described above.

Long-Term and Short-Term Signals Interact to Control Feeding

The gastrointestinal tract plays a role in short-term control of ingestive behavior. Two of the gastrointestinal hormones that inform the brain about the state of the gut are cholecystokinin and ghrelin (Figure 49–3A). Cholecystokinin is secreted from the gut during meals. It promotes the termination of the meal by slowing gastric emptying and by stimulating vagal inputs to the lower brain stem circuitry involved in the patterning of meals.

Ghrelin is implicated in the initiation rather than the termination of meals. In contrast to cholecystokinin, release of ghrelin from the stomach peaks prior to a meal, when the stomach is still empty. Ghrelin receptors are found in numerous brain sites; eating has been elicited by direct administration of ghrelin into the arcuate and paraventricular hypothalamic nuclei and the dorsal vagal complex.

To alter food intake, signals such as leptin and insulin, which reflect the state of long-term energy stores, must interact with the short-term signals that determine the composition and patterning of meals. These interactions occur at many levels. For example, leptin promotes the release of cholecystokinin from the duodenum; leptin and ghrelin exert opposing influences on arcuate neurons containing neuropeptide Y and agouti-related peptide. Leptin, insulin, and ghrelin all interact with the 5′-adenosine monophosphate-activated protein kinase (AMPK), a molecular sensor of short-term energy status. To fuel vital physiological processes, cells must maintain a high ratio of adenosine triphosphate (ATP) to 5′-adenosine monophosphate (AMP); AMPK is activated when this ratio falls below a critical threshold. Activation of AMPK stimulates catabolism while suppressing anabolism, thus restoring the ATP/AMP ratio. In hypothalamic neurons implicated in energy balance, leptin, insulin, and high glucose levels all inhibit AMPK activity whereas fasting and ghrelin activate it.

Motivational States Influence Goal-Directed Behavior

So far we have reviewed physiological, neuroendocrine, and neuroanatomical components of the control systems for fluid and energy homeostasis. We now

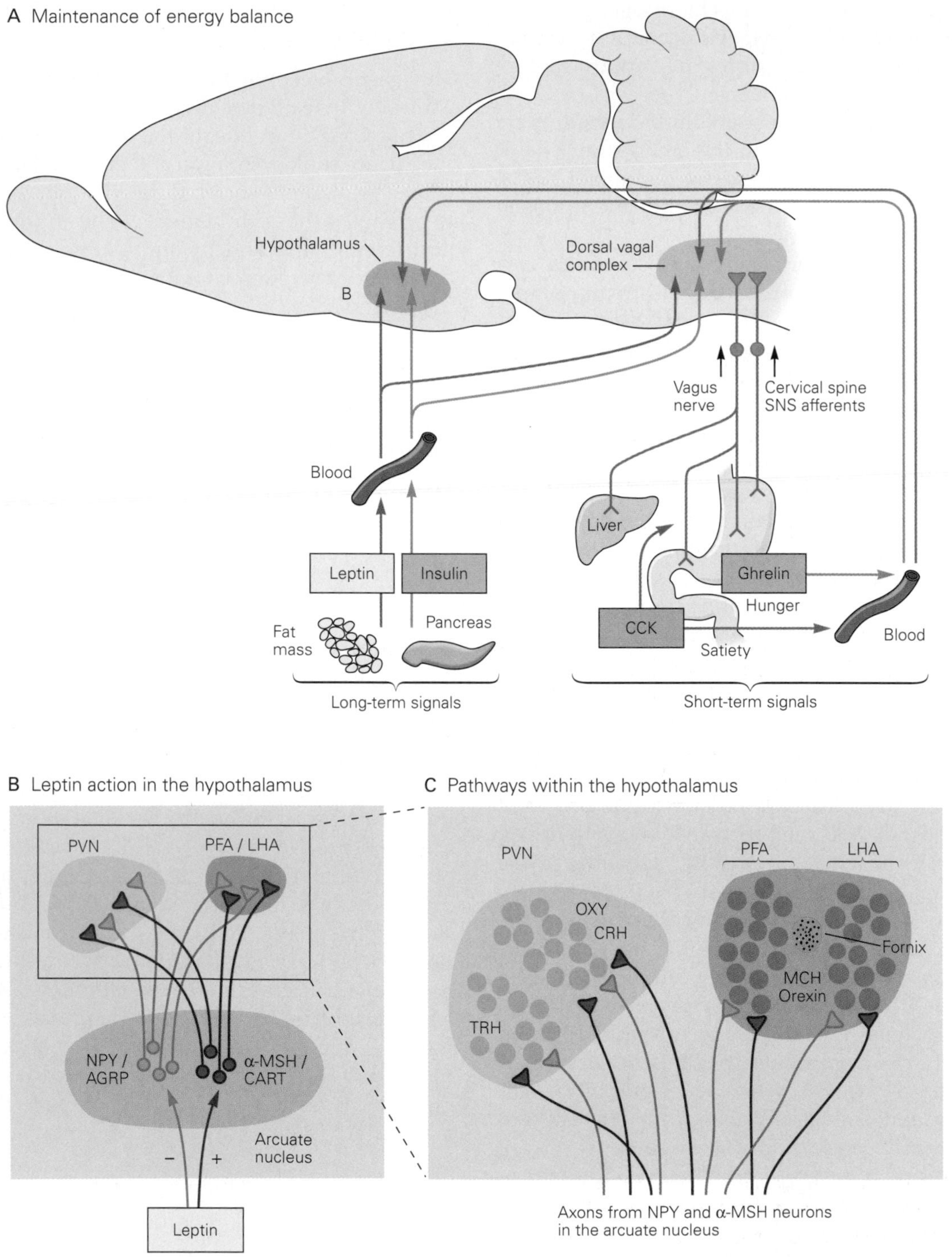
A Maintenance of energy balance
Hypothalamus
B
Dorsal vagal complex
Vagus nerve
Cervical spine SNS afferents
Blood
Liver
Leptin
Insulin
Ghrelin
Hunger
Fat mass
Pancreas
CCK
Satiety
Blood
Long-term signals
Short-term signals
B Leptin action in the hypothalamus
PVN
PFA / LHA
NPY / AGRP
α-MSH / CART
Arcuate nucleus
–
+
Leptin
C Pathways within the hypothalamus
PVN
PFA
LHA
OXY
CRH
TRH
Fornix
MCH
Orexin
Axons from NPY and α-MSH neurons in the arcuate nucleus

turn to another feature of homeostatic control systems: the motivational states governing the behaviors that provide the needed inputs, such as food and water.

A cheetah that has taken refuge from the mid-day sun in the shade of a tree greets the sight of a distant antelope with apparent indifference. In contrast, the sighting of an antelope toward the end of the afternoon provokes immediate orientation and stalking. The stimulus is the same, but the behavioral responses are very different. What has changed during the interval, separating the two sightings, is the motivational state of the animal.

Both Internal and External Stimuli Contribute to Motivational States

Motivational states influence attentiveness, goal selection, investment of effort in the pursuit of goals, and responsiveness to stimuli. The psychologist Dalbir Bindra proposed that motivational states arise from the interaction of internal and external inputs.

Internal inputs include physiological error signals and the circadian clock. For example, the frequency and duration of foraging varies with the time of day, the time since the cheetah has last eaten, and whether or not she is lactating. External inputs include *incentive stimuli* arising from the goal of the motivational state. For example, when a dehydrated cheetah comes across a water hole during a search for antelopes, the sight of the water may serve as an incentive stimulus, tipping the balance between hunger and thirst and driving the animal to interrupt its quest for food to drink.

There is positive feedback between incentive stimuli and motivational states; the more the animal interacts with the stimulus, the stronger the motivational state that promotes further contact. This positive feedback relationship helps ensure that complex behavioral sequences are completed. For example, the cheetah must stalk, chase, run down, and kill the antelope, and then drag the carcass to a refuge before beginning to feed.

Motivational States Serve Both Regulatory and Nonregulatory Needs

Feeding, drinking, and thermoregulatory behaviors and their underlying motivational states typically arise in response to or in anticipation of a physiological imbalance. In contrast, some motivational states such as sexual arousal serve biological imperatives other than homeostasis. Functionally, these non-regulatory states resemble those arising from physiological error signals. For example, some behaviors influenced by nonregulatory motivational states may be compensatory responses to deprivation, such as when a mammal that has been confined shows heightened motivation to explore once released from captivity.

Brain Reward Circuitry May Provide a Common Logic for Goal Selection

Goal-directed behaviors entail risks, costs, and benefits. Straying from the herd may offer an antelope better opportunities for foraging but at the risk of becoming an easier target for a lurking cheetah. Attacking the

Figure 49–3 (Opposite) Neural and endocrine mechanisms of energy balance.

A. Short- and long-term maintenance of energy balance. *Short-term signals*: During meals cholecystokinin (**CCK**) from the intestinal tract stimulates sensory fibers of the vagus nerve, thus promoting satiety; CCK is also secreted into the bloodstream. The vagal sensory fibers, along with sympathetic fibers from the gut and orosensory information, converge in the dorsal vagal complex, a set of structures in the caudal brain stem that includes the nucleus of the solitary tract, area postrema, and dorsal motor nucleus of the vagus nerve. Prior to mealtime, release of ghrelin from the stomach peaks, providing a blood-borne signal to neurons in the brain. Whereas CCK promotes satiety, ghrelin promotes eating.
Long-term signals: Leptin and insulin are among the humoral signals that inform the brain about the status of the fat stores. Leptin is produced in fat-storing cells, whereas insulin is produced in the pancreas. Both hormones are sensed by receptors in the arcuate nucleus of the hypothalamus as well as by receptors in the dorsal vagal complex. Leptin and insulin reduce food intake and increase energy expenditure.

B. Leptin has opposing influences on two populations of arcuate neurons. It inhibits cells that release neuropeptide Y (**NPY**) and agouti-related peptide (**AGRP**) but stimulates cells that release α-melanocyte–stimulating hormone (**α-MSH**) and cocaine- and amphetamine-regulated transcript (**CART**). Activation of arcuate neurons that release NPY and AGRP increases food intake and fat storage while decreasing energy expenditure. Activation of arcuate neurons that release α-MSH and CART decreases food intake and fat storage while increasing energy expenditure.

C. The arcuate neurons shown in part B project to multiple regions of the hypothalamus. The paraventricular nucleus (**PVN**) is a convergence zone for many signals involved in energy (and fluid) balance. Neurons in this nucleus synthesize several peptides that decrease food intake, including corticotropin-releasing hormone (**CRH**), thyrotropin-releasing hormone (**TRH**), and oxytocin (**OXY**). The perifornical area (**PFA**) and lateral hypothalamic area (**LHA**) contain neurons that synthesize orexins and melanin concentrating hormone (**MCH**), peptides that stimulate food intake. (Adapted, with permission, from Schwartz et al. 2000.)

venturesome antelope offers the cheetah the promise of a meal with the risk that energetic and hydromineral resources will be depleted if the antelope gets away. Thus the neural mechanisms responsible for goal selection must weigh anticipated risks, costs, and benefits of behaviors that are likely to attain a specific goal.

Many studies of these neural mechanisms have used electrical brain stimulation as a goal. Rats and other vertebrates ranging from goldfish to humans will work for electrical stimulation of certain brain regions. The avidity and persistence of this self-stimulation is remarkable. For example, rats will cross electrified grids, run uphill while leaping over hurdles, or press a lever for hours on end in order to trigger the electrical stimulation. The phenomenon that leads the animal to work for the stimulation is called *brain stimulation reward*.

Rewards are objects, stimuli, or activities that have positive value. Rewards can incite an animal to switch from one behavior to another or to resist interruption of ongoing action. For example, a rat that encounters a seed while scouting the environment may cease exploring to eat the food or carry it to a safe place; while nibbling the seed the rat will resist the efforts of another rat to steal the food from its paws. If seeds are made available only at a particular location and time, the rat will go to that location as the expected moment of reward delivery approaches. Much contemporary work in the neurosciences is directed at unraveling the neural mechanisms that mediate reward, how they shape behavior to meet physiological needs and environmental challenges and opportunities, and how they go awry in the case of behavioral pathologies such as drug addiction.

Although electrical stimulation is an artificial goal, it can mimic some of the rewarding properties of natural goal objects. For example, rewarding stimulation of the medial forebrain bundle can compete with, summate with, or substitute for hedonic stimuli such as sucrose solutions. The effectiveness of the reward produced by stimulating certain lateral hypothalamic sites is increased by weight loss and decreased by leptin, suggesting that the neural circuitry responsible for the rewarding effect plays a role in energy balance.

The circuitry that mediates brain stimulation reward is broadly distributed. Rewarding effects can be produced by electrical stimulation of sites at all levels of the brain, from the olfactory bulb to the nucleus of the solitary tract. Particularly effective sites lie along the course of the medial forebrain bundle and along longitudinally oriented fiber bundles coursing near the midline of the brain stem. Stimulation of both these pathways transsynaptically activates dopaminergic neurons in the ventral tegmental area of the midbrain; these neurons project to the nucleus accumbens (the major component of the ventral striatum), the ventromedial portion of the head of the caudate nucleus (in the dorsal striatum), the basal forebrain, and regions of the prefrontal cortex (Figure 49–4).

The midbrain dopaminergic neurons are activated by incentive stimuli and play a crucial role in brain stimulation reward. Pursuit of this reward is strengthened by increases in dopaminergic synaptic transmission and weakened by decreases. The dopaminergic neurons receive excitatory signals from cholinergic cells in the laterodorsal tegmental and pedunculopontine nuclei of the hindbrain. Stimulation of the medial forebrain bundle and caudal brain stem activates these cholinergic neurons. In turn, blockade of the cholinergic input to the midbrain dopaminergic neurons reduces the rewarding effects of the electrical stimulation.

Starving rats provided with brief daily access to food will forego eating to press a lever for brain stimulation. Such heedless pursuit of an artificial goal to the detriment of a biological need is one of many parallels between self-stimulation and drug abuse. More direct evidence comes from the fact that the animal will work even harder to self-stimulate when given a drug such as cocaine, amphetamine, heroin, and nicotine. As these results suggest, the midbrain dopaminergic neurons involved in the rewarding effect of brain stimulation also play a critical role in the rewarding effects of drugs.

Drug Abuse and Addiction Are Goal-Directed Behaviors

Before humans began farming, our species foraged for safe and nutritious plants. Among the many plants that humans sampled, a small number produced changes in perception, mood, cognition, or arousal. Of these, a smaller subset—opium poppies, coca, tobacco, hemp, and products of fermented plant matter—contained substances that proved strongly rewarding, even though they lacked any nutritional value. Humans learned to purify these substances and later to synthesize related compounds for use as medicines.

For example, morphine, purified from the opium poppy, was chemically modified in attempts to produce compounds with greater specificity for analgesia. Among these was diacetylmorphine, or heroin, which was mistakenly marketed as a nonaddictive treatment for pain and cough. Other drugs, such as the amphetamines and sedative-hypnotics, are wholly synthetic compounds developed for a variety of medical indications.

Addictive drugs include some with approved medical uses (eg, morphine, amphetamines, and benzodiazepines), some that are legal but lacking in medical

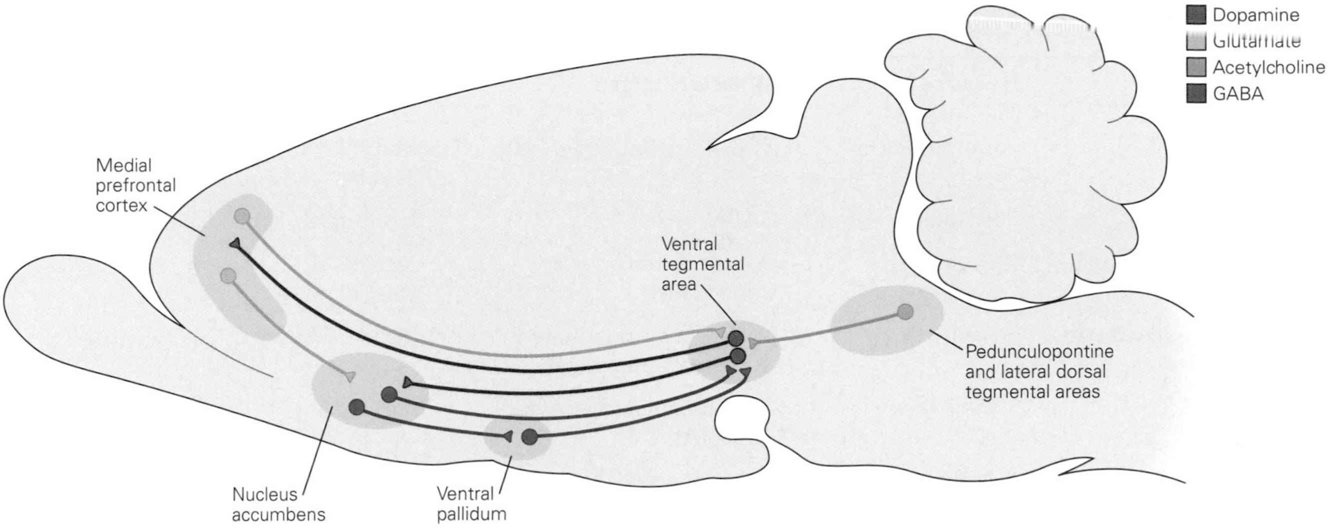

Figure 49–4 Neural pathways and structures implicated in reward. The dopaminergic pathways from the ventral tegmental area to the nucleus accumbens, medial prefrontal cortex, and other forebrain structures are a central component of reward circuitry. The neurons in the ventral tegmental area are regulated by cholinergic neurons in the brain stem, by inhibitory GABA-ergic (γ-aminobutyric acid) neurons in the nucleus accumbens and ventral pallidum, and by excitatory glutamatergic neurons in the prefrontal cortex.

usefulness (eg, alcohol and tobacco), and some that are illegal in many countries (eg, marijuana). The term *drug abuse* refers to the use of drugs outside of medical supervision and in a manner that is potentially harmful or illegal. The addictive drugs listed in Table 49–1 produce reward; thus, individuals willingly use them and tend to take them repetitively. Herein lies the central danger of these drugs. When used repetitively they initiate molecular changes in the brain that promote continued drug-taking, behavior that becomes increasingly difficult to control. Individuals who regularly use these drugs impair their health and their ability to function.

In people who are vulnerable as a result of genetic and nongenetic risk factors, drug use may progress to *addiction*, which is defined as compulsive drug use despite significantly negative consequences. The addicted person loses control over drug use—obtaining and using drugs come to dominate all other life goals. Addiction tends to persist despite attempts to limit drug use and despite serious negative consequences for the user, his family, and society.

Perhaps the most challenging and frustrating aspect of addiction is its persistence. Not only is it difficult to interrupt active drug use, but even when a person has successfully stopped using drugs the risk of relapse remains high for many years and in some cases for a lifetime. Even after long periods of abstinence, exposure to reminders (cues) of drug use, such as drug paraphernalia or people or places associated with prior drug use, may trigger intense drug urges and relapse into use. Cue-initiated relapses may occur even in individuals who have strongly resolved never to use drugs again, illustrating that addiction impairs the voluntary control of behavior.

In the laboratory, drug-associated cues elicit drug urges that correlate with physiologic responses, for example, activation of the sympathetic nervous system. Functional brain imaging has revealed that cue-conditioned drug responses activate medial regions of the prefrontal cortex; the amygdala, a structure that is thought to play a role in the consolidation of emotionally charged stimulus-reward associations (see Chapters 48 and 66); and the nucleus accumbens, a component of the brain reward circuitry (Figure 49–5).

Addictive Drugs Recruit the Brain's Reward Circuitry

As discussed above, the dopaminergic projections from the ventral tegmental area to the nucleus accumbens and other forebrain structures (Figure 49–4) are a central component of reward circuitry. The major dopamine receptor types in both the dorsal striatum and nucleus accumbens are the D_1 and D_2 G protein-coupled receptors. The D_1 receptors predominate in the prefrontal cortex. A dopamine transporter located

Table 49–1 Major Classes of Addictive Drugs

Class	Source	Molecular target	Examples
Opiates	Opium poppy	μ opioid receptor (agonist)	Morphine, methadone, oxycodone, heroin
Sedative-hypnotics	Synthetic	$GABA_A$ receptor (agonist)	Barbiturates, benzodiazepines
Psychomotor stimulants	Coca leaf Synthetic	Dopamine transporter (antagonist)	Cocaine Amphetamines
Phencyclidine-like drugs	Synthetic	NMDA-type glutamate receptor (antagonist)	Phencyclidine (PCP, "angel dust")
Cannabinoids	Cannabis	CB1 cannabinoid receptors (agonist)	Marijuana
Nicotine	Tobacco	Nicotinic acetylcholine receptor (agonist)	Tobacco
Ethyl alcohol	Fermentation	$GABA_A$ receptor (agonist), NMDA-type glutamate receptor (antagonist), and multiple other targets	Various beverage products

GABA, γ-aminobutyric acid; NMDA, *N*-methyl-D-aspartate.
Note: Caffeine can produce mild physical dependence but does not result in compulsive use. Some illegal drugs that are abused can be harmful but do not generally produce addiction; these include the hallucinogens lysergic acid diethylamide (LSD), mescaline, psilocybin, and 3,4-methylenedioxymethamphetamine (MDMA), popularly known as ecstasy.

on presynaptic neurons terminates the actions of the synaptically released dopamine by pumping it back into the presynaptic terminal (Figure 49–6).

Both pharmacological studies and analyses of lesions in animals confirm the importance of dopaminergic pathways in brain reward. Behavioral studies of the rewarding properties of drugs, using such paradigms as conditioned place preference or self-administration of drugs (Box 49–2), have found that drugs that block D_1 and D_2 dopamine receptors diminish the incentive properties of natural rewards and drugs. Similar conclusions have been reached in studies using other experimental disruptions of dopaminergic pathways.

Changes in extracellular dopamine levels within the nucleus accumbens and other brain structures can be measured in vivo using a microdialysis catheter. Although this method cannot measure dopamine within individual synapses, it can yield quantitative estimates that are thought to correlate with synaptic release of dopamine. This method demonstrates that all addictive drugs increase extracellular dopamine levels in the nucleus accumbens. Thus psychotropic drugs that do not produce significant dopamine release in the nucleus accumbens are not addictive.

There is one important caveat to what is often called the dopamine hypothesis of reward. Some drugs such as opiates also have receptors in reward pathways that are either parallel with or downstream of dopaminergic synapses. Thus opiates produce reward by both dopamine-dependent and dopamine-independent mechanisms. Mice that are genetically engineered to lack dopamine do not find cocaine to be rewarding but appear to gain significant residual reward from morphine.

Although the ability to increase synaptic dopamine is a shared property of all addictive drugs, they do so by different mechanisms. Psychostimulants, which include cocaine and amphetamines, act on the presynaptic terminals of dopaminergic neurons, and they do so in two different ways. Cocaine binds to and blocks the dopamine transporter on the membrane of presynaptic terminals, causing extracellular dopamine to accumulate to high levels following release. Amphetamines enter the presynaptic terminals of dopaminergic neurons through the dopamine transporter. Once in the cytoplasm they cause reverse transport of dopamine out of storage vesicles through the vesicular transporter and out of the neuron into the synapse through the membrane transporter. Thus the action of cocaine depends on normal vesicular release of dopamine by neurons of the ventral tegmental area, whereas the action of amphetamine does not.

Cocaine and amphetamines have analogous actions on the norepinephrine and serotonin transporters, causing increases in extracellular levels of those neurotransmitters as well. However, pharmacologic blockade and lesion experiments demonstrate that dopamine, not these other neurotransmitters, plays the key role in the rewarding properties of these drugs.

The effects of opiates on reward are more complex than those of the psychostimulants because opiates use both dopamine-dependent and dopamine-independent mechanisms. There are three classes of opioid receptors, μ, δ, and κ, and a structurally related receptor, ORL-1. The morphine-like opiates, including heroin (which is metabolized into morphine), methadone, and oxycodone, bind with highest affinity to μ receptors. The μ receptors are found in several regions of the brain and spinal cord where they serve different functions. In the brain stem and spinal cord they play a critical role in modulating pain information (Chapter 24). In other brain stem regions they play a role in controlling respiration, which is why opiates can cause respiratory arrest in overdose.

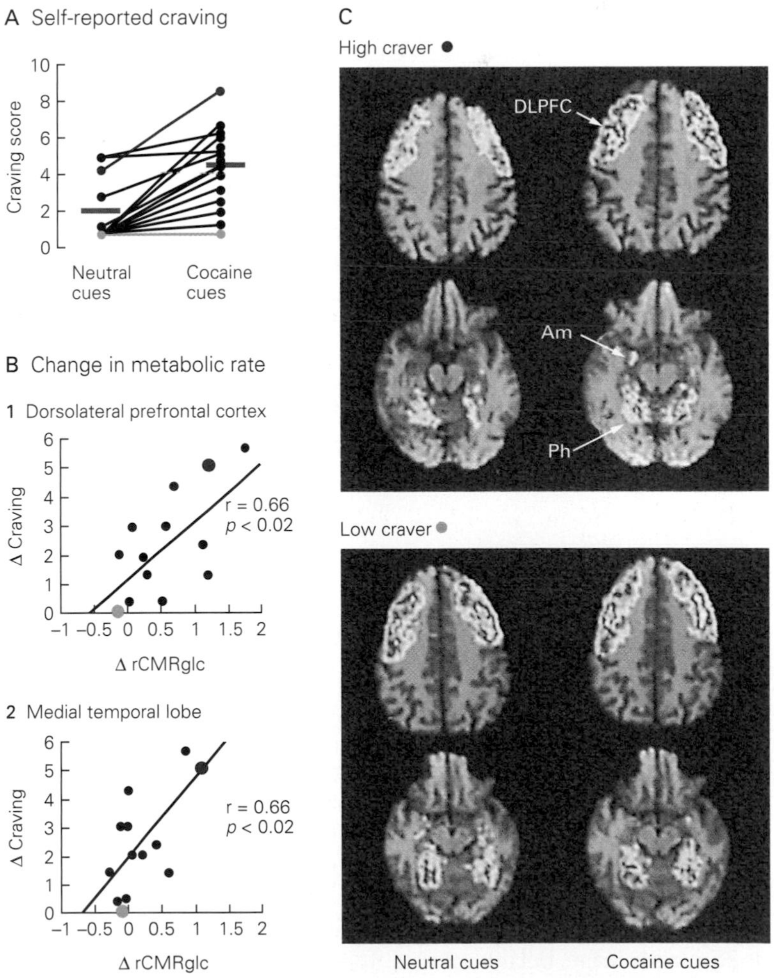

Figure 49–5 PET imaging reveals neural correlates of cue-induced cocaine craving.

A. Subjects were shown neutral or cocaine-related cues and asked, "Do you have a craving or urge for cocaine?" The mean score (**horizontal bar**) is significantly higher for exposure to cocaine-related cues than for exposure to neutral stimuli, even though the magnitude of the response across individuals varies considerably. Two subjects identified by red and blue dots represent high-level and low-level craving, respectively.

B. Changes in self-reported craving are correlated with changes in metabolic rate in the dorsolateral prefrontal cortex and medial temporal lobe during exposure to cocaine-related cues. Metabolic rate is measured as the regional cerebral metabolic rate for glucose (**rCMRglc**). The ordinate represents the difference between the average of the responses to the question, "Do you have a craving or urge for cocaine?" in separate sessions with neutral and cocaine-related cues. (Each session lasted 30 minutes, and in each session the question was asked three times.) The abscissa represents the difference in metabolic rate between the two sessions (activity with cocaine cues minus activity with neutral cues).

C. When subjects report a craving for cocaine metabolic activity increases in the dorsolateral prefrontal cortex (**DLPFC**) and in two medial temporal lobe structures, the amygdala (**Am**) and parahippocampal gyrus (**Ph**). Pseudocolored PET images of metabolic activity are spatially aligned with high-resolution structural magnetic resonance images. Metabolic rate markedly increased in the amygdala and parahippocampal gyrus in one subject who reported a large increase in craving during presentation of cocaine-related cues (**red dot** in parts A and B). This effect is not evident in a subject who reported no increase in craving while exposed to the cocaine-related cues (**blue dot** in parts A and B). Metabolic activity outside the dorsolateral prefrontal cortex and medial temporal lobe is not shown. (Adapted, with permission, from Grant et al. 1996.)

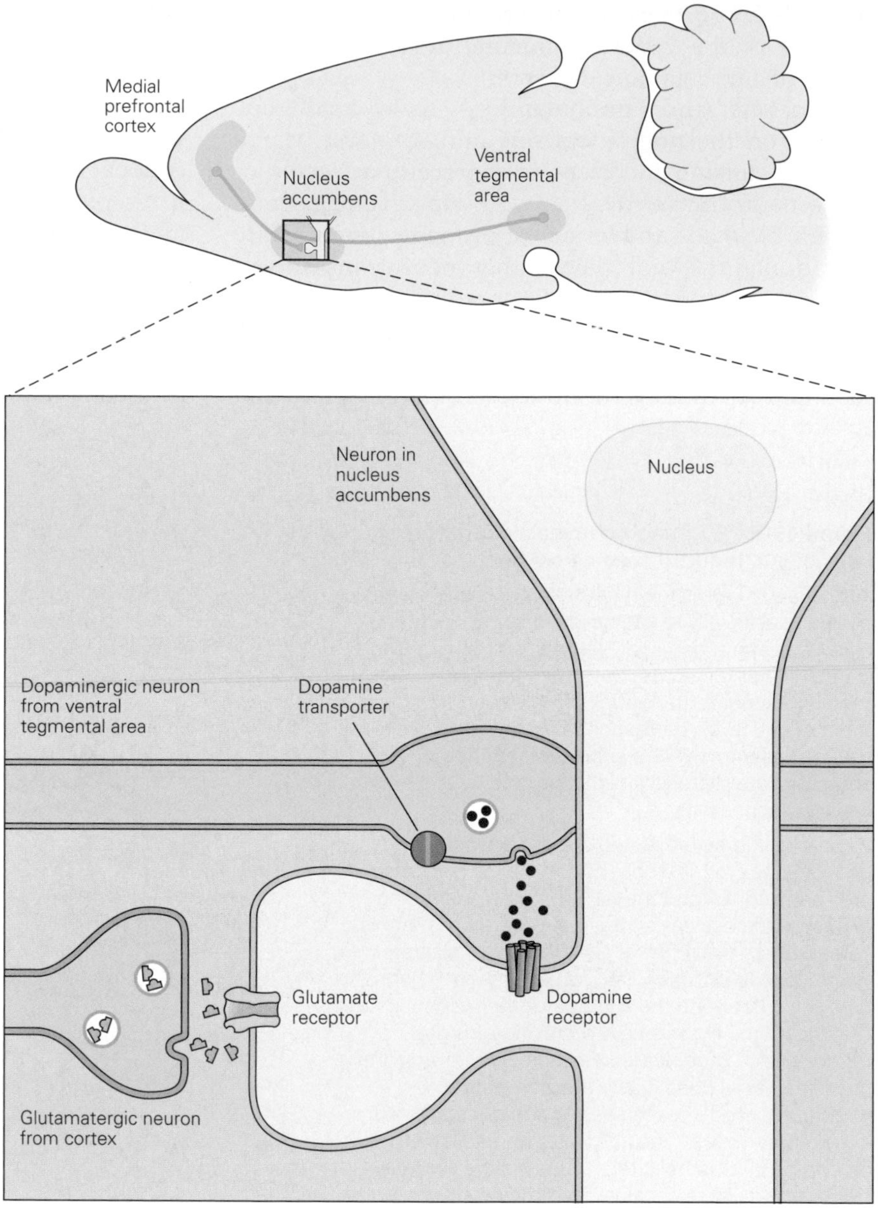

Figure 49–6 Dopamine and glutamate interact at synaptic spines in nucleus accumbens neurons. Glutamatergic neurons carrying sensorimotor information from the cerebral cortex and dopaminergic neurons carrying reward-related information from the ventral tegmental area form connections with the same medium spiny neurons in the dorsal striatum and nucleus accumbens. The glutamatergic neurons make excitatory synapses on the heads of dendritic spines and the dopaminergic neurons make en passant connections at the necks of spines.

The μ receptors are also found throughout brain reward circuitry. In the ventral tegmental area they are found on GABA-ergic interneurons that tonically inhibit the dopaminergic neurons that project to the nucleus accumbens and prefrontal cortex. Opiate binding to these μ receptors inhibits the interneurons, resulting in disinhibition of the dopaminergic neurons and dopamine release. Because μ receptors are also expressed by nucleus accumbens neurons, opiates can also exert rewarding effects independent of dopamine inputs.

Microdialysis demonstrates that nicotine, ethyl alcohol, tetrahydrocannabinol, and phencyclidine all cause dopamine to be released in the nucleus accumbens. In addition to their shared effect—increasing synaptic dopamine in the nucleus accumbens—each family of addictive drugs has unique properties based on the receptors with which they interact (Table 49–1). For example, both morphine and cocaine are rewarding and addictive, morphine-like opiates are analgesic and sedating, and cocaine stimulates arousal.

Addictive Drugs Alter the Long-Term Functioning of the Nervous System

In addition to producing short-term reward and other acute pharmacologic effects, addictive drugs can produce long-term alterations in the functioning of the nervous system. Repeated use of addictive drugs can produce tolerance, dependence, withdrawal, and sensitization to differing degrees, as well as addiction. In humans tolerance, dependence, and withdrawal can all contribute to altered behavior. The behavioral consequences of sensitization, a phenomenon well established in animal models, are less clear for human drug users. None of these states is equivalent to addiction, which is defined as compulsive drug use despite significant negative consequences.

Tolerance refers to the diminishing effect of a drug after repeated ingestion of the drug at a constant dose, or alternatively the need to increase the dose to produce a constant effect. For example, the amount of alcohol needed to get drunk increases with regular use. Tolerance results from homeostatic responses of cells to excessive drug stimulation—molecular and cellular adaptations alter normal physiology to counterbalance the effects of the drug. One mechanism of tolerance is *pharmacokinetic*, in which induction of hepatic metabolic enzymes increase the rate of metabolic clearance of a drug. Pharmacokinetic adaptation plays almost no role in tolerance for addictive drugs other than alcohol. A second mechanism is *pharmacodynamic*: The action of a drug within the brain that produces habituation.

Dependence is inferred when withdrawal symptoms occur after drug use is curtailed. Whereas tolerance results from homeostatic mechanisms those associated with dependence alter the basal physiological state of cells and circuits. As long as drug use continues, this altered physiology is masked and symptoms do not occur. Cessation of drug use unmasks the abnormal physiological state, resulting in withdrawal symptoms.

When effects grow stronger with repeated drug use they are said to undergo *sensitization*. For example, the locomotor activity produced by amphetamine or cocaine increases with repeated use of the drug. In general the stimulant effects of a drug are more likely to increase (sensitization), whereas depressant effects tend to diminish (tolerance).

The mechanisms by which opiates produce tolerance, dependence, and a withdrawal syndrome have been elucidated in studies of the behavior of neurons in the locus ceruleus, the major noradrenergic nucleus

Box 49–2 Animal Models of Drug Addiction

Animal models have played an important role in understanding how addictive drugs produce reward. Two of the most commonly used in research are conditioned place preference and self-administration.

Conditioned Place Preference

Animals learn to associate a particular environment with passive exposure to drugs; for example, a rodent may spend more time on the side of a box where it was given cocaine than on the side where it received saline. In experiments using this paradigm animals learn to associate a neutral cue, such as the features of one side of a box, with a reward. This paradigm is believed to demonstrate the strong cue-conditioned effects of addictive drugs and to provide an indirect measure of drug reward.

Self-Administration of Drugs

The reinforcing effects of a drug can be demonstrated in experiments in which a specific behavior produces the drug. For example, an animal may be taught that it will receive an injection of a drug every time it presses a particular lever in its cage. The drug acts as a reinforcer if it increases the occurrence of the behavior (pressing the lever) that leads to acquisition of the drug.

In this paradigm the amount of work an animal does to gain access to a given amount of drug indicates the reinforcing strength of the drug. The strength with which different drugs reinforce behavior in animals correlates well with the tendency of each drug to reinforce drug-seeking behavior in humans. Laboratory animals exposed to cocaine readily learn behaviors necessary to self-administer this drug and some of them will give up necessities, such as food and water, or work excessively, even to the point of death, to gain access to cocaine.

in the brain. Acute administration of opiates to rats or mice slows the basal firing rate of locus ceruleus neurons because μ opioid receptors activate a K^+ channel that reduces the firing rate. Over time, however, the neurons develop tolerance; their firing rate becomes more normal as the μ receptors become partly uncoupled from channel activation.

Chronic opiate administration also produces dependence that sets the stage for withdrawal. Following chronic opiate administration, blockade of μ receptors by the opioid receptor antagonist naloxone produces a dramatic withdrawal syndrome. (This is observed in laboratory rats, which exhibit such withdrawal symptoms as "wet dog" shakes, as well as in opiate-dependent humans given naloxone to reverse respiratory arrest.) One mechanism that contributes to dependence is the strengthening of a Na^+ conductance in locus ceruleus neurons; this adaptation can act to balance the efflux of K^+ produced by μ receptor stimulation. The relative excess of Na^+ influx following naloxone inhibition of μ receptor-mediated K^+ efflux renders the neurons hyperexcitable. This results in burst firing that correlates with withdrawal behaviors.

Historically, dependence and physical withdrawal were thought to be cardinal features of addiction. We now know that they are neither necessary nor sufficient. First, some drugs such as cocaine and amphetamines that readily cause compulsive, "out of control" use may produce little or no dependence and do not produce physical withdrawal. More importantly, the risk of relapse into drugs that can produce physical withdrawal, such as opiates and alcohol, can persist for years after drug use has stopped and withdrawal symptoms have resolved.

If dependence and withdrawal were the central mechanisms of addiction, we could successfully treat addicted people by sequestering them until they were well past the period of withdrawal. Unfortunately this is not the case, as stress or drug-related cues can readily cause relapse. Based on the important role of drug-associated cues in drug-seeking and relapse, some clinical investigators have emphasized the need to consider the neural mechanisms of associative learning as central to addiction.

Dopamine May Act As a Learning Signal

An earlier view of the function of dopamine was that it conveyed "hedonic signals" in the brain and that in humans it was directly responsible for subjective pleasure. From this point of view addiction would reflect the habitual choice of short-term pleasure despite a host of long-term life problems. However, the hedonic principle cannot easily explain the persistence of drug use by addicted persons as negative consequences mount.

In fact, the effects of dopamine have proven to be far more complex than was first thought. Dopamine can be released by stressful as well as by rewarding stimuli. Moreover, rodents lacking dopamine—rats in which dopamine is depleted by 6-hydroxydopamine and mice genetically engineered so that they cannot produce dopamine—continue to exhibit hedonic responses to sucrose.

Wolfram Schultz and his colleagues discovered that dopaminergic neurons have a complex and changing pattern of responses to rewards during learning. In one experiment Schultz trained monkeys to expect juice at a fixed interval after a visual or auditory cue. Before the monkeys learned the predictive cues, the appearance of the juice was unexpected and produced a transient increase above basal levels of firing in dopaminergic neurons. As the monkeys learned that certain cues predict the juice, the timing of the firing changed. The neurons no longer fired in response to presentation of the juice—the reward—but earlier, in response to the predictive visual or auditory cue. If a cue was presented but the reward was withheld, firing paused at the time the reward would have been presented. In contrast, if a reward exceeded expectation or was unexpected, because it appeared without a prior cue, firing was enhanced (Figure 49–7).

These observations suggest that dopamine release in the forebrain serves not as a pleasure signal but as a *prediction-error* signal. A burst of dopamine would signify a reward or reward-related stimulus that had not been predicted; pauses would signify that the predicted reward is less than expected or absent. If a reward is just as expected based on environmental cues, dopaminergic neurons would maintain their tonic (baseline) firing rates. Alterations in dopamine release are thought to modify future responses to stimuli to maximize the likelihood of obtaining rewards and to minimize fruitless pursuits. For natural rewards, like the sweet juice consumed by the monkeys in Schultz's experiments, once the environmental cues for a reward are learned, dopaminergic neuron firing returns toward baseline levels. Schultz has interpreted this to mean that as long as nothing changes in the environment, there is nothing more to learn and therefore no need to alter behavioral responses.

Addictive drugs differ from natural rewards in that they cause dopamine release in the reward circuitry no matter how often they are consumed. Dopamine is released even when these drugs do not produce subjective pleasure. To the brain, consumption of addictive drugs would thus always signal "better than expected" and in this way would continue to influence behavior to maximize drug-seeking and drug-taking.

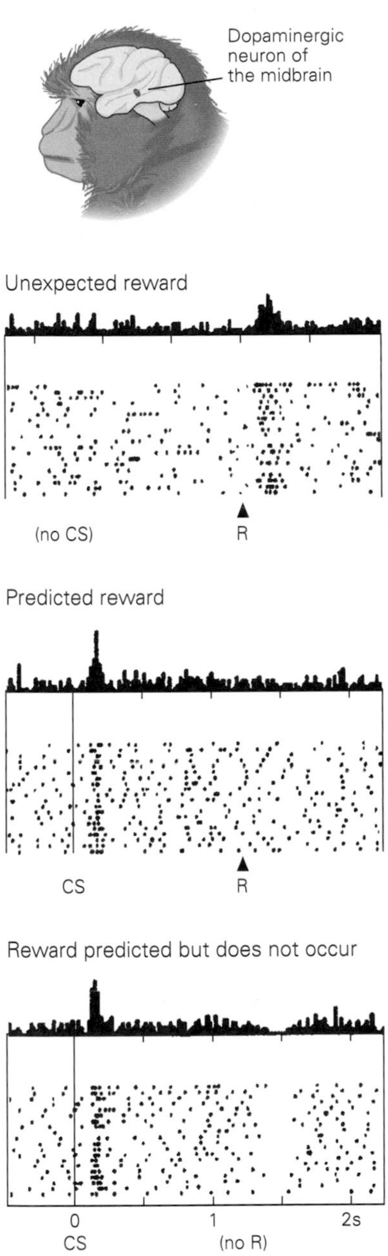

Figure 49–7 Dopaminergic neurons report an error in reward prediction. Graphs show firing rates recorded from midbrain dopaminergic neurons in awake, active monkeys. **Top:** A drop of sweet liquid is delivered without warning to a monkey. The unexpected reward (**R**) elicits a response in the neurons. The reward can thus be construed as a positive error in reward prediction. **Middle:** The monkey has been trained that a conditioned stimulus (**CS**) predicts a reward. In this record the reward occurs according to the prediction and does not elicit a response in the neurons because there is no error in the prediction of reward. The neurons are activated by the first appearance of a predicting stimulus but not by the reward. **Bottom:** A conditioned stimulus predicts a reward that fails to occur. The dopaminergic neurons show a decrease in firing at the time the reward would have occurred. (Reproduced, with permission, from Schultz et al. 1997.)

If this idea is correct, it might explain why drug-seeking and consumption become compulsive and why the life of the addicted person becomes focused on drug-taking at the expense of all other pursuits.

These experiments, combined with the importance of cues in promoting drug taking, have suggested that learning and memory might play a central role in addiction. For example, drug-seeking is often initiated by drug-related cues—the people, paraphernalia, bodily sensations, and smells associated with prior drug use. Such cues must, of course, be stored in memory and associated with specific behaviors. Interestingly, dopamine has been implicated in the formation of long-term memories in hippocampal and cerebral cortical circuits (Chapters 66 and 67).

These considerations have led to the idea that when someone uses addictive drugs the release of dopamine strengthens the associative memories that bind drug-related cues to drug urges and drug-seeking. The brain reward circuitry that normally reinforces the pursuit of goals with positive survival value is usurped by drug-related goals.

If dopamine-dependent associative memory processes are involved in the pathogenesis of addiction, what cellular and molecular mechanisms might be involved? Long-term change in synaptic function is a fundamental property of neural circuits involved in learning. The best characterized physiologic mechanisms of such long-term changes in the mammalian brain are long-term potentiation and long-term depression (Chapters 66 and 67). These mechanisms are thought to underlie many different types of learning and memory. Indeed, drug use can lead to synaptic changes similar to long-term potentiation and depression in the striatum and nucleus accumbens, as well as in the midbrain dopaminergic neurons themselves.

Activation of the dopaminergic pathways also resembles learning in that these pathways are capable of initiating many changes in gene expression. Relating these changes to learning-related alterations in synaptic connections and circuit function remains an important challenge. For example, dopamine action at the D_1 receptors leads to the activation of the transcription factor cyclic AMP response element binding protein (CREB). CREB has been implicated in diverse memory processes in a variety of species, including the *Drosophila* fly, the marine snail *Aplysia*, and mice (Figure 49–8, and see Chapters 66 and 67). In the dorsal striatum and nucleus accumbens, psychostimulants produce phosphorylation of CREB through activation of the D_1 receptors and the second messenger cyclic AMP. This leads to activation of the cAMP-dependent protein kinase, which then phosphorylates CREB, leading to its activation. A large number of

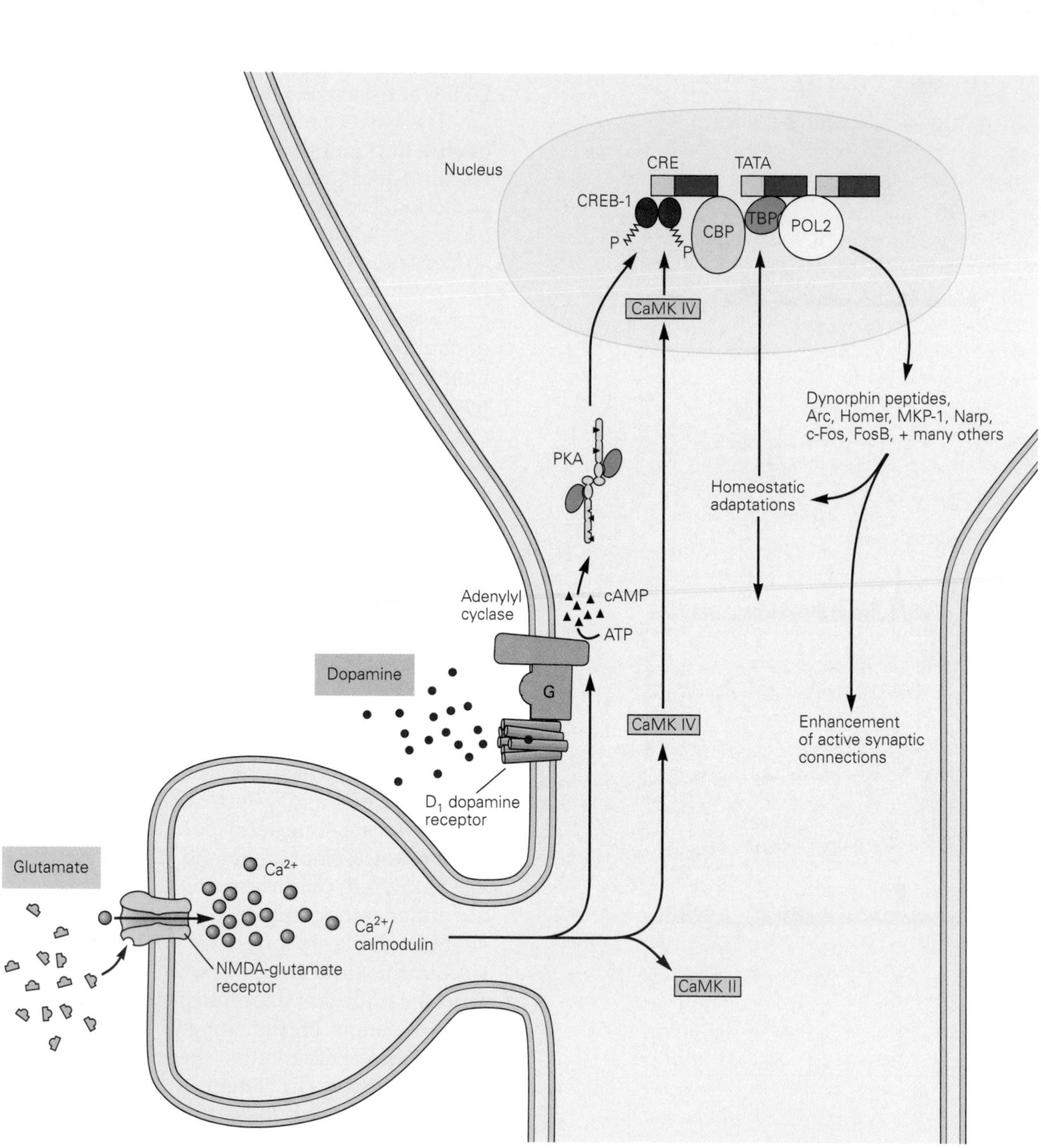

Figure 49–8 Intracellular signaling pathways activated by dopamine and glutamate. NMDA-type glutamate receptors permit Ca^{2+} entry, which binds calmodulin. The Ca^{2+}/calmodulin complex activates two Ca^{2+}/calmodulin-dependent protein kinases, CaMKII in the cytoplasm and CaMKIV in the cell nucleus. D_1 dopamine receptors activate a stimulatory G protein that in turn activates the adenylyl cyclase to produce cyclic adenosine monophosphate (**AMP**). The cyclic AMP-dependent protein kinase (protein kinase A or **PKA**) catalytic subunit can enter the nucleus. In this diagram PKA and CaMKIV phosphorylate and thus activate the cyclic AMP response element binding protein (**CREB**). CREB recruits CREB-binding protein (**CBP**) and thus activates the RNA polymerase II-dependent transcription of many genes, giving rise to proteins that can alter cellular function. Arc and Homer are localized in synaptic regions; Fos and FosB are transcription factors; and dynorphin gives rise to a family of endogenous opioid peptides. These proteins are thought to contribute both to homeostatic responses to excessive dopamine stimulation and to the remodeling of synapses associated with memory formation. (**NMDA**, *N*-methyl-D-aspartate; **POL 2**, RNA polymerase 2; **TBP**, TATA binding protein.)

CREB-regulated genes are thus induced by dopamine and psychostimulants.

An Overall View

The ability of cells, organs, and organisms to survive and function in the face of changing conditions such as alterations in temperature or nutrient availability depends on mechanisms that maintain a relatively constant internal milieu. Complex brain circuits orchestrate the physiological processes that redistribute and transform internal resources such as water, electrolytes, and energy stores to correct and anticipate deviations from homeostasis. Tightly integrated with these circuits are the neural systems mediating behaviors that procure vital resources from the environment and help to conserve scarce supplies or expend surpluses.

Motivational states adjust the vigor and incidence of these behaviors according to biological needs, both those stemming from regulatory imperatives such as the maintenance of blood volume and those stemming from nonregulatory imperatives such as reproduction. The strength of a motivational state depends not only on internal conditions but also on external incentive stimuli such as food or estrus odors.

Choosing between competing incentives requires that the current and predicted benefit of each incentive be assessed, a task attributed to brain reward circuitry. Activation of this circuitry creates resistance to interruption of ongoing actions and promotes behaviors that anticipate or procure rewards.

The dopaminergic projection from the ventral tegmental area to the nucleus accumbens powerfully influences goal-directed behavior. All addictive drugs increase synaptic dopaminergic transmission in this pathway, an effect that may mimic and ultimately overwhelm the influence of natural stimuli and motivational states. Dopamine facilitates the cellular and molecular mechanisms of learning and memory. In vulnerable individuals drug-associated cues may be transformed into powerful incentive stimuli. Thus reminders of prior drug use may precipitate relapses to drug-seeking despite the disastrous consequences that a return to drug use might bring. Such a state of addiction is not easily abolished, and relapse remains a serious risk even after many years of abstinence.

Peter B. Shizgal
Steven E. Hyman

Selected Readings

Berridge K, Robinson TE. 1998. What is the role of dopamine in reward: hedonic impact, reward learning, or incentive salience? Brain Res Rev 28:309–369.

Cabanac M, Russek M. 2000. Regulated biological systems. J Biol Sys 8:141–149.

Dagher A, Robbins TW. 2009. Personality, addiction, dopamine: insights from Parkinson's disease. Neuron 61:503–501.

Di Chiara G. 1998. A motivational learning hypothesis of the role of mesolimbic dopamine in compulsive drug use. J Psychopharmacol 12:54–67.

Fitzsimons JT. 1998. Angiotensin, thirst, and sodium appetite. Physiol Rev 78:583–686.

Grill HJ, Kaplan JM. 2002. The neuroanatomical axis for control of energy balance. Neuroendocrinol 23:2–40.

Hyman SE, Malenka RC, Nestler EJ. 2006. Neural mechanisms of addiction: the role of reward-related learning and memory. Annu Rev Neurosci 29:565–598.

Johnson AK, Thunhorst RL. 1997. The neuroendocrinology of thirst and salt appetite: visceral sensory signals and mechanisms of central integration. Front Neuroendocrinol 18:292–353.

Kelley AE, Berridge KC. 2002. The neuroscience of natural rewards: relevance to addictive drugs. J Neurosci 22:3306–3311.

Montague PR, Hyman SE, Cohen JD. 2004. Computational roles for dopamine in behavioural control. Nature 31: 760–767.

O'Brien CP, Childress AR, Ehrman R, Robbins SJ. 1998. Conditioning factors in drug abuse: can they explain compulsion? J Psychopharmacol 12:15–22.

Robinson TE, Berridge KC. 2000. The psychology and neurobiology of addiction: an incentive-sensitization view. Addiction 95:S91–117. Suppl 2.

Schwartz MW, Woods SC, Porte D Jr, Seeley RJ, Baskin DG. 2000. Central nervous system control of food intake. Nature 404:661–671.

Shizgal P. 1997. Neural basis of utility estimation. Curr Opin Neurobiol 7:198–208.

Stricker EM, Sved AF. 2000. Thirst. Nutrition 16:821–826.

Watts A, Swanson L. 2004. Anatomy of motivation. In: H. Pashler and R. Gallistel (eds). *Stevens' Handbook of Experimental Psychology*. Vol 3 *Learning, Motivation, and Emotion*, 3rd ed. New York: Wiley.

Zhang Y, Proenca R, Maffei M, Barone M, Leopold L, Friedman JM. 1994. Positional cloning of the mouse obese gene and its human homologue. Nature 372:425–432.

References

Ahima RS, Flier JS. 2000. Leptin. Annu Rev Physiol 62: 413–437.

Aghajanian GK. 1978. Tolerance of locus coeruleus neurones to morphine and suppression of withdrawal response by clonidine. Nature 276:186–188.

Arnold M, Mura A, Langhans W, Geary N. 2006. Gut vagal afferents are not necessary for the eating-stimulatory effect of intraperitoneally injected ghrelin in the rat. J Neurosci 26:11052–11060.

Bernard C. [1878] 1974. Lectures on the phenomena of life common to animals and plants. [Lecons sur les phénomènes de la vie communs aux animaux et aux végétaux.] Springfield, Illinois: Thomas Publishing.

Bindra D. 1968. Neuropsychological interpretation of the effects of drive and incentive-motivation on general activity and instrumental behavior. Psych Rev 75:1–22.

Bourque CW, Oliet SH. 1997. Osmoreceptors in the central nervous system. Annu Rev Physiol 59:601–619.

Breiter HC, Gollub RL, Weisskoff RM, Kennedy DN, Makris N, Nurke JD, Goodman JM, et al. 1997. Acute effects of cocaine on human brain activity and emotion. Neuron 19:591–611.

Breiter HC, Aharon I, Kahneman D, Dale A, Shizgal P. 2001. Functional imaging of neural responses to expectancy and experience of monetary gains and losses. Neuron 30:619–639.

Cannon WB. 1932. *The Wisdom of the Body*. New York: Norton.

Childress AR, Mozley PD, McElgin W, Fitzgerald J, Reivich M, O'Brien CP. 1999. Limbic activation during cue-induced cocaine craving. Am J Psych 156:11–18.

Coleman DL. 1973. Effects of parabiosis of obese mice with diabetes and normal mice. Diabetologia 9:294–298.

Craig W. 1917. Appetites and aversions as constituents of instincts. Proc Natl Acad Sci U S A 3:685–688.

Davis JD, Wirtshafter D. 1978. Set points or settling points for body weight? A reply to Mrosovsky and Powley. Behav Biol 24:405–411.

Everitt BJ, Robbins TW. 2005. Neural systems of reinforcement for drug addiction: from actions to habits to compulsion. Nature Neurosci 8:1481–89.

Fulton S, Woodside B, Shizgal P. 2000. Modulation of brain reward circuitry by leptin. Science 287:125–128.

Giros B, Jaber M, Jones SR, Wightman RM, Caron MG. 1996. Hyperlocomotion and indifference to cocaine and amphetamine in mice lacking the dopamine transporter. Nature 379:606–612.

Grant S, London ED, Newlin DB, Villemagne V, Liu X, Contoreggi C, Phillips R, Margolin A. 1996. Activation of memory circuits during cue-elicited cocaine cravings. Proc Natl Acad Sci U S A 93:12040–12045.

Heinrichs SC, Richard D. 1999. The role of corticotropin-releasing factor and urocortin in the modulation of ingestive behavior. Neuropeptides 33:350–359.

Hernandez G, Breton Y, Conover K. Shizgal, P. 2010. At what stage of neural processing does cocaine act to boost pursuit of rewards? PLoS ONE 5: e15081.

Huang YY, Kandel ER. 1995. D1/D5 receptor agonists induce a protein synthesis-dependent late potentiation in the CA1 region of the hippocampus. Proc Natl Acad Sci U S A 92:2446–2450.

Jequier E, Tappy L. 1999. Regulation of body weight in humans. Physiol Rev 79:451–480.

Johnson SW, North RA. 1992. Opioids excite dopamine neurons by hyperpolarization of local interneurons. J Neurosci 12:483–488.

Keesey RE, Hirvonen MD. 1997. Body weight set-points: determination and adjustment. J Nutr 127:1875S–1883S.

Kelz MB, Chen J, Carleson, WA Jr, Whisler K, Gilden L, Beckmann AM, Steffen C, et al. 1999. Expression of the transcription factor deltaFosB in the brain controls sensitivity to cocaine. Nature 401:272–276.

Kendler KS, Karkowski LM, Neale MC, Prescott CA. 2000. Illicit psychoactive substance use, heavy use, abuse, and dependence in a US population-based sample of male twins. Arch Gen Psychiatry 57:261–269.

Kilts CD, Schweitzer JB, Quinn, CK et al. 2001. Neural activity related to drug craving in cocaine addiction. Arch Gen Psychiatry 58:334–341.

Li TK, Yin SJ, Crabb DW, O'Connor S, Ramchandani VA. 2001. Genetic and environmental influences on alcohol metabolism in humans. Alcohol Clin Exp Res 25: 136–144.

Markou A, Koob GF. 1991. Postcocaine anhedonia. An animal model of cocaine withdrawal. Neuropsychopharmacology 4:17–26.

Merikangas KR, Stolar M, Stevens DE, Foulet H, Preisig MA, Fenton B, Shang H et al. 1998. Familial transmission of substance use disorders. Arch Gen Psychiatry 55:973–979.

Mrosovsky N. 1990. *Rheostasis: The Physiology of Change*. New York: Oxford Univ. Press.

Mrosovsky N, Powley TL. 1977. Set points for body weight and fat. Behav Biol 20:205–223.

O'Brien CP, Childress AR, McLellan T, Ehrman R. 1990. Integrating systemic cue exposure with standard treatment in recovering drug dependent patients. Addict Behav 15:355–365.

Olds J, Milner PM. 1954. Positive reinforcement produced by electrical stimulation of septal area and other regions of rat brain. J Comp Physiol Psych 47:419–427.

Piazza PV, Le Moal ML. 1996. Pathophysiological basis of vulnerability to drug abuse: role of an interaction between stress, glucocorticoids, and dopaminergic neurons. Annu Rev Pharmacol Toxicol 36:359–378.

Robinson TE, Kolb B. 1997. Persistent structural modifications in nucleus accumbens and prefrontal cortex neurons produced by previous experience with amphetamine. J Neurosci 17:8491–8497.

Schultz W, Dayan P, Montague PR. 1997. A neural substrate of prediction and reward. Science 275:1593–1599.

Schwartz GJ, Moran TH. 1996. Sub-diaphragmatic vagal afferent integration of meal-related gastrointestinal signals. Neurosci Biobehav Rev 20:47–56.

Shizgal P, Murray B. 1989. Neuronal basis of intracranial self-stimulation. In: JM Liebman, SJ Cooper (eds). *The Neuropharmacological Basis of Reward*, pp. 106–163. New York: Oxford Univ. Press.

Shizgal P, Fulton S, Woodside B. 2001. Brain reward circuitry and the regulation of energy balance. Int J Obes Relat Metab Disord 25:S17-S21. Suppl 5.

Sigvardsson S, Bohman M, Cloninger, CR. 1996. Replication of the Stockholm Adoption Study of Alcoholism Confirmatory Cross-Fostering Analysis. Arch Gen Psychiatry 53:681–687.

Swanson LW. 2000. Cerebral hemisphere regulation of motivated behavior. Brain Res 886(1–2):113–164.

Tsuang MT, Lyons MJ, Eisen SA, Goldberg H, True W, Lin N, Meyer JM, Toomey R, Faraone SV, Eaves L. 1996. Genetic influences on DSM-III-R drug abuse and dependence: a study of 3,372 twin pairs. Am J Med Genet 67:473–477.

Willie JT, Chemelli RM, Sinton CM, Yanagisawa M. 2001. To eat or to sleep? Orexin in the regulation of feeding and wakefulness. Annu Rev Neurosci 24:429–458.

Wirtshafter D, Davis JD. 1977. Set points, settling points, and the control of body weight. Physiol Behav 19:75–78.

Wise RA. 1996. Addictive drugs and brain stimulation reward. Annu Rev Neurosci 19:319–340.

Woods SC, Schwartz MW, Baskin DG, Seeley RJ. 2000. Food intake and the regulation of body weight. Annu Rev Psychol 51:255–277.

Yeomans JS, Mathur A, Tampakeras M. 1993. Rewarding brain stimulation: role of tegmental cholinergic neurons that activate dopamine neurons. Behav Neurosci 107:1077–1087.

Yeomans JS, Takeuchi J, Baptista M, Flynn D, Lepik K, Nobrega J, Fulton J, Ralph MR. 2000. Brain-stimulation reward thresholds raised by an antisense oligonucleotide for the M5 muscarinic receptor infused near dopamine cells. J Neurosci 20:8861–8867.

50

Seizures and Epilepsy

UNTIL QUITE RECENTLY THE FUNCTION and organization of the human cerebral cortex—the structure of the brain concerned with perceptual, motor, and cognitive functions—has eluded both clinicians and neuroscientists. In the past the analysis of brain function relied in large part on observations of the behavioral consequences of brain damage caused by strokes or trauma. These natural experiments provided much of the early evidence that distinct brain regions serve specific functions (see Chapter 1).

Observation of patients with seizures and epilepsy has been equally important in the study of brain function because the behavioral consequences of these disorders vary with the brain regions from which they originate. *Seizures* are temporary disruptions of brain function resulting from abnormal, excessive neuronal activity; *epilepsy* is a chronic condition of repeated seizures. For centuries understanding the neurological origins of seizures was confounded by the dramatic, sometimes bizarre behaviors associated with seizures. Epilepsy was widely associated with possession by evil spirits, while seizures were thought to reflect oracular, prescient, or special creative powers.

The Greeks in the time of Hippocrates (circa 400 BC) were aware that head injuries to one side of the brain could cause seizure activity on the opposite side of the body. In those earlier times the diagnosis of epilepsy was probably much broader than the contemporary definition. Other causes of episodic unconsciousness, such as syncope as well as mass hysteria and psychogenic seizures, were almost certainly classified with epilepsy. Moreover, historical writings typically describe generalized convulsive seizures involving both cerebral hemispheres. Thus it is likely that focal seizures involving a limited area of the brain were misdiagnosed or never diagnosed at all. Even today it can be difficult for physicians to distinguish between episodic loss of consciousness and the various types of seizures. Nevertheless, as our ability to treat and even cure epilepsy continues to improve, these diagnostic distinctions take on increasing significance.

The modern neurobiological analysis of epilepsy began with John Hughlings Jackson's work in London in the 1860s. Jackson realized that seizures need not involve loss of consciousness but could be associated with localized symptoms such as the jerking of an arm. His observation was the first formal recognition of what we now call *focal* (or *partial*) *seizures.* Jackson also observed patients whose seizures began with focal neurological symptoms and progressed to convulsions with loss of consciousness (the so-called Jacksonian march).

Another early development that presaged modern therapy was the first surgical treatment for epilepsy in 1886 by Victor Horsley. Horsley resected cerebral cortex adjacent to a depressed skull fracture and cured a patient with focal motor seizures. The modern surgical treatment for epilepsy dates to the work of Wilder Penfield and Herbert Jasper in Montreal in the early 1950s. Medical innovations include the first use of phenobarbital as an anticonvulsant in 1912 by Alfred Hauptmann, the development of electroencephalography by Hans Berger in 1929, and the discovery of the anticonvulsant properties of phenytoin (Dilantin) by Houston Merritt and Tracey Putnam in 1937.

As in any chronic disease, the physiological features of seizures are not the only consideration in the care and management of patients with epilepsy. Psychosocial factors are also extremely important. The diagnosis of epilepsy has consequences that can affect all aspects of everyday life, including educational opportunities, driving, and employment. Although many limitations imposed on epileptics are appropriate—most would agree that patients with epilepsy should not be commercial pilots—a diagnosis of epilepsy can have inappropriate, negative effects on educational opportunities and employment. To improve this situation, physicians have a duty to educate themselves and the public.

Classification of Seizures and the Epilepsies Is Important for Pathogenesis and Treatment

Not all seizures are the same. Thus the pathology of seizures must take into account their clinical features. Seizures, and the chronic condition of repetitive seizures (epilepsy), are common. Based on epidemiological studies in the United States, somewhere around 3% of all individuals living to the age of 80 years are diagnosed with epilepsy. The highest incidence occurs in young children and the elderly.

In many respects seizures represent a prototypic neurological disease in that the symptoms include both positive and negative sensory or motor manifestations. Examples of positive signs that can occur during a seizure include the perception of flashing lights or the jerking of an arm. Negative signs such as impairment of consciousness and self-awareness or even transient blindness or paralysis reflect impairment of normal brain function. These examples underscore a general feature of seizures: The signs and symptoms depend on the location and extent of brain regions that are affected. Finally, the manifestations of seizures result in part from the activity in normal tissue with normal cellular and network properties. The latter is particularly important in the spread of a focal or partial seizure beyond its original boundaries. Seizures quite literally hijack the normal functions of the brain.

Seizures Are Temporary Disruptions of Brain Function

Seizures can be classified conceptually into two categories: focal (or partial) and generalized (Table 50–1). Although the details of seizure classification are under continuous discussion, this simple dichotomy has proven extremely useful to clinicians because anticonvulsant medications often target preferentially to

Table 50–1 International League Against Epilepsy (ILAE) Classification of Seizures

Generalized seizures
Tonic-clonic (in any combination)
Absence (including typical, atypical, and absence with special features)
Myoclonic
Clonic
Tonic
Atonic
Focal seizures (formerly called simple partial and complex partial)
Unknown

Reproduced, with permission, from Berg et al., 2010.

one or the other type of seizure. The terms "focal" and "partial" are used interchangeably in this chapter.

Focal seizures originate in a small group of neurons (the seizure focus) and thus the symptoms depend on the location of the focus within the brain. Focal seizures were formerly classified as simple partial when there is no alteration of consciousness, or complex partial when there is an alteration of consciousness. A typical focal seizure might begin with jerking in the right hand and progress to clonic movements (ie, jerks) of the entire right arm. This seizure could also be called a *focal motor seizure.* If a focal seizure progresses further the patient may lose consciousness, fall to the ground, rigidly extend all extremities (tonic phase), then have jerking in all extremities (clonic phase). In this case, the focal seizure has secondarily generalized.

The onset of a focal seizure is often preceded by symptoms called *auras.* Common auras include abnormal sensations such as a sense of fear, a rising feeling in the abdomen, or even a specific odor. The aura is caused by electrical activity originating from the seizure focus and thus represents the earliest manifestations of a focal seizure. The time after a seizure but before the patient returns to his or her normal level of neurological function is called the *postictal period.*

Generalized seizures constitute the second main category. They begin without an aura or focal seizure and involve both hemispheres from the onset. Thus they are sometimes called *primary generalized seizures* to avoid confusion with seizures that begin from a focus and then generalize secondarily. Primary generalized seizures can be further divided into convulsive or nonconvulsive types depending on whether the seizure is associated with tonic or clonic movements.

The prototypic nonconvulsive generalized seizure is the *typical absence seizure* in children (formerly called petit mal). These seizures begin abruptly, usually last less than 10 seconds, are associated with cessation of all motor activity, and result in loss of consciousness but not loss of posture. The patients appear as if in a trance, but the episodes are so brief that their occurrence can be missed by a casual observer. Unlike a focal seizure there is no aura before the seizure or confusion after the seizure (the postictal period). Patients may exhibit mild motor manifestations such as eye blinking but do not fall or have tonic-clonic movements. Typical absence seizures have very distinctive electrical characteristics on the electroencephalogram (EEG).

Other types of generalized seizures can involve only abnormal movements (myoclonic, clonic, or tonic) or a sudden loss of motor tone (atonic). The most common convulsive generalized seizure is the tonic-clonic (formerly called grand mal seizure). Such seizures begin abruptly, often with a grunt or cry, as tonic contraction of the diaphragm and thorax forces expiration. During the tonic phase the patient may fall to the ground in a rigid posture with clenched jaw, lose bladder or bowel control, and become blue (cyanotic). The tonic phase typically lasts 30 seconds before evolving into clonic jerking of the extremities lasting 1 to 2 minutes. This active phase is followed by a postictal phase during which the patient is sleepy and may complain of a headache and muscle soreness.

A primary generalized tonic-clonic seizure can be difficult to distinguish on purely clinical grounds from a secondarily generalized tonic-clonic seizure with a brief aura. This distinction is not simply academic; it can be vital to choosing proper treatment as well as pinpointing the underlying cause.

Epilepsy Is the Chronic Condition of Recurrent Seizures

Recurrent seizures constitute the minimal criterion for the diagnosis of epilepsy. The oft-quoted clinical rule emphasizes this point: "A single seizure does not epilepsy make." Various factors that contribute to a clinical pattern of recurrent seizures—the underlying etiology of the seizures, the age of onset, or family history—are ignored in the seizure classification scheme in Table 50–1. The classification of the epilepsies initially evolved primarily based upon clinical observation rather than a precise cellular, molecular, or genetic understanding of the disorder. The factors influencing seizure type and severity were sometimes recognized as patterns of symptoms, referred to as the *epilepsy syndromes.*

In the 1989, according to the International League Against Epilepsy (ILAE) classification of the epilepsies, the primary variables were whether or not a focal brain abnormality could be identified (localization-related versus generalized epilepsies), and whether or not a cause could be identified (symptomatic versus idiopathic). Most adult-onset epilepsies could be classified as symptomatic localization-related epilepsy, a category that included such causes as trauma, stroke, tumors, and infections. However, many patients have adult-onset epilepsies without a clearly defined cause. Thus, despite the usefulness of this scheme, many types of epilepsy did not fit neatly into its categories. In 2010 the ILAE recommended focusing on the underlying causes of epilepsies based on three broad variables—genetic, structural/metabolic, and unknown—as well as a list of electroclinical syndromes. One expects and hopes that these classifications will be elaborated as knowledge of the underlying causes increases.

The Electroencephalogram Represents the Collective Behavior of Cortical Neurons

Because neurons are excitable cells, it should not be surprising that seizures result either directly or indirectly from a change in the excitability of single neurons or groups of neurons. This view dominated early experimental studies of seizures. Electrical recordings of brain activity can be made with intracellular or extracellular electrodes. Extracellular electrodes sense action potentials in nearby neurons and can detect the synchronized activity of ensembles of cells called *field potentials.*

At the slow time resolution of extracellular recording (hundreds of milliseconds to seconds) field potentials can appear as single transient changes called *spikes.* These spikes reflect action potentials in many neurons and should not be confused with spikes in single neurons, which are individual action potentials that last only 1 or 2 milliseconds. The EEG thus represents a set of field potentials as recorded by multiple electrodes on the surface of the scalp (Figure 50–1).

Because the electrical activity originates in neurons in the underlying brain tissue, the waveform recorded by the surface electrode depends on the orientation and distance of the electrical source with respect to the electrode. The EEG signal is inevitably distorted by the filtering and attenuation caused by intervening layers of tissue and bone that act in the same way as resistors and capacitors in an electric circuit. Thus the amplitude of EEG signals (measured in microvolts) is much smaller than the voltage changes in a single neuron (measured in millivolts). High-frequency activity in single cells, such as action potentials, is filtered out by the EEG signal, which primarily reflects slower voltage changes across the cell membrane, such as synaptic potentials.

Although the EEG signal is a measure of the extracellular current caused by the summated electrical activity of many neurons, not all cells contribute equally to the EEG. The surface EEG reflects predominantly the activity of cortical neurons in close proximity to the EEG electrode. Thus deep structures such as the hippocampus, thalamus, or brain stem do not contribute directly to the surface EEG. The contributions of individual nerve cells to the EEG are discussed in Box 50–1.

The surface EEG shows patterns of activity—characterized by the frequency and amplitude of the electrical activity—that correlate with various stages of sleep and wakefulness (see Chapter 51), and with some pathophysiological processes such as seizures. The normal human EEG shows activity over the range of 1 to 30 Hz with amplitudes in the range of 20 to 100 μV. The observed frequencies have been divided into several groups: alpha (8–13 Hz), beta (13–30 Hz), delta (0.5–4 Hz), and theta (4–7 Hz).

Alpha waves of moderate amplitude are typical of relaxed wakefulness and are most prominent over parietal and occipital sites. During intense mental activity, beta waves of lower amplitude are more prominent in frontal areas and over other regions. Alerting relaxed subjects by asking them to open their eyes results in so-called desynchronization of the EEG with a reduction in alpha activity and an increase in beta activity (Figure 50–1B). Theta and delta waves are normal during drowsiness and early slow-wave sleep; if present during wakefulness, these waves are a sign of brain dysfunction.

As neuronal ensembles become synchronized, as when a subject relaxes or becomes drowsy, the summated currents become larger and can be seen as abrupt changes from the baseline activity. Such *paroxysmal* activity can be normal; for example, episodes of high-amplitude activity (1–2 s, 7–15 Hz) occur during sleep (sleep spindles). However, a sharp wave or EEG spike can also provide a clue to the location of a seizure focus in a patient with epilepsy (Figure 50–4).

Focal Seizures Originate Within a Small Group of Neurons Known as a Seizure Focus

Despite the variety of clinically defined seizures, important insights into the generation of seizure activity can largely be understood by comparing the electrographic patterns of focal and primary generalized seizures. The defining feature of focal (and secondarily generalized) seizures is that the abnormal electrical activity originates from a *seizure focus.* The seizure focus is nothing more than a small group of neurons, perhaps 1,000 or so, which have enhanced excitability and the ability to occasionally spread that activity to neighboring regions and thereby cause a seizure.

The enhanced excitability (epileptiform activity) may result from many different factors such as altered cellular properties or altered synaptic connections caused by a local scar, blood clot, or tumor. A discrete focus in the primary motor cortex may cause twitching of a finger or jerking of a limb (sometimes called simple partial seizure), whereas a seizure focus in the limbic system is frequently associated with unusual behaviors or an alteration of consciousness (sometimes called complex partial seizure).

The development of a focal seizure can be arbitrarily divided into four phases: (1) the *interictal period* between seizures followed by (2) synchronization of activity

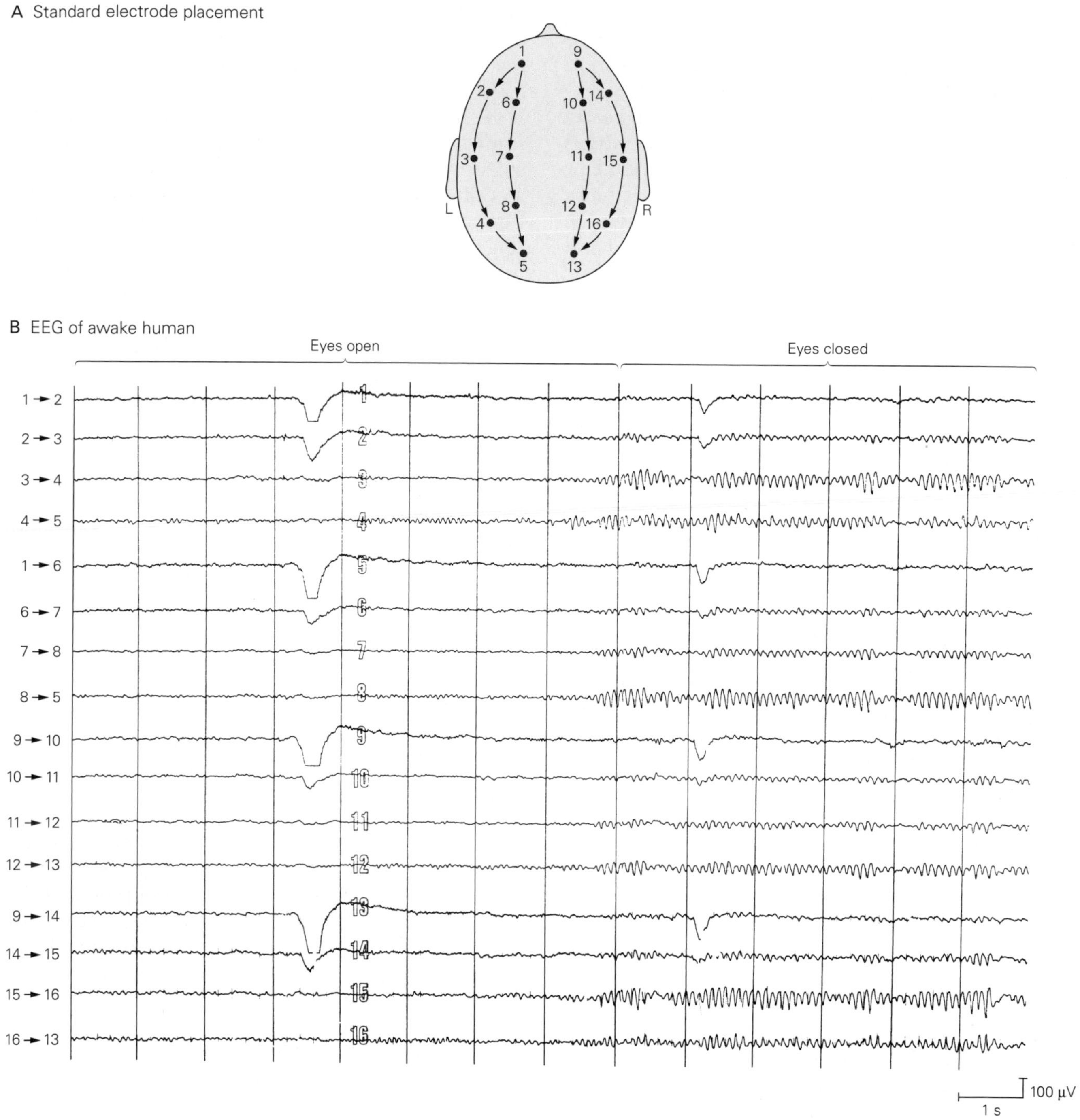

Figure 50–1 The normal electroencephalogram (EEG) in an awake human subject.

A. A standard set of placements (or montage) of electrodes on the surface of the scalp. The electrical response at each site reflects the activity between two of the electrodes.

B. At the beginning of the recording the EEG shows low-voltage activity (circa 20 μV) over the surface of the scalp. The vertical lines are placed at 1 second intervals. During the first 8 seconds the subject was resting quietly with eyes open, then the subject was asked to close his eyes. With the eyes closed, larger-amplitude activity (8–10 Hz) develops over the occipital region (sites 3, 4, 8, 12, 15, 16). This is the normal alpha rhythm characteristic of the relaxed, wakeful state. Slow large-amplitude artifacts occur at 3.5 seconds when the eyes blink and at 9 seconds when the eyes close.

within the seizure focus (Figure 50–4), (3) seizure spread, and finally (4) secondary generalization. Phases 2 to 4 represent the *ictal phase* of the seizure. Different factors contribute to each phase.

Much of our knowledge about the electrical events during seizures comes from studies of animal models of focal seizures. A seizure is induced in an animal by focal electrical stimulation or by acute injection of a convulsant agent. This approach and the development of in vitro brain slice preparations (Box 50–2) have provided a good understanding of electrical events within the focus during a seizure as well as during the interictal period

Neurons in a Seizure Focus Have Characteristic Activity

How does electrical activity in a single neuron or group of neurons lead to a seizure? Each neuron within a seizure focus has a stereotypic and synchronized electrical response called the *paroxysmal depolarizing shift*, an intracellular depolarization that is sudden, large (20–40 mV), and long-lasting (50–200 ms), and triggers a train of action potentials at its peak (Figure 50–7B). The paroxysmal depolarizing shift is followed by an afterhyperpolarization.

The paroxysmal depolarizing shift and afterhyperpolarization are shaped by the intrinsic membrane properties of the neuron (eg, voltage-gated Na^+, K^+, and Ca^{2+} channels) and by synaptic inputs from excitatory and inhibitory neurons (primarily glutaminergic and GABAergic, respectively). The depolarizing phase results primarily from activation of AMPA- and NMDA-type glutamate receptor-channels (Figure 50–8A), as well as voltage-gated Na^+ and Ca^{2+} channels. The NMDA-type receptor-channels are particularly suited to enhancing excitability because depolarization relieves Mg^{2+} blockage of the channel. Once unblocked, excitatory current through the channel increases, thus enhancing the depolarization and allowing extra Ca^{2+} to enter the neuron (see Chapter 10).

The normal response of a cortical pyramidal neuron to excitatory input consists of an excitatory postsynaptic potential (EPSP) followed by an inhibitory postsynaptic potential (IPSP) (because of the basic circuitry shown in Figure 50–8B). Thus the paroxysmal depolarizing shift can be viewed as a massive enhancement of the normal depolarizing and hyperpolarizing synaptic components. The afterhyperpolarization is generated by several types of K^+ channels as well as a GABA receptor-mediated Cl^- conductance (ionotropic $GABA_A$ receptors) and K^+ conductance (metabotropic $GABA_B$ receptors) (Figure 50–8A). The Ca^{2+} entry through voltage-dependent Ca^{2+} channels and NMDA-type receptor-channels triggers the opening of calcium-activated channels, particularly K^+ channels. The afterhyperpolarization limits the duration of the paroxysmal depolarizing shift; its gradual disappearance is an important factor in the onset of a focal seizure, as discussed later.

Thus it is not surprising that many convulsants act by enhancing excitation or blocking inhibition. Conversely, anticonvulsants act by blocking excitation or enhancing inhibition. For example, the benzodiazepines diazepam (Valium) and lorazepam (Ativan) enhance $GABA_A$-mediated inhibition and are used in the emergency treatment of prolonged repetitive seizures. The commonly used anticonvulsants phenytoin (Dilantin) and carbamazepine (Tegretol) cause reduction in the opening of the voltage-gated Na^+ channels that underlie the action potential. The ability of these drugs to block the Na^+ channels is enhanced by repetitive activity associated with seizures.

The Breakdown of Surround Inhibition Leads to Synchronization

As long as the abnormal electrical activity is restricted to a small group of neurons, there are no clinical manifestations. The synchronization of neurons in the focus is dependent not only on the intrinsic properties of each individual cell but also on the connections between neurons. During the interictal period the abnormal activity is confined to the seizure focus by inhibitory effects of the excited region on surrounding tissue. This *inhibitory surround* is particularly dependent on feed-forward and feedback inhibition by GABA-ergic inhibitory interneurons (Figure 50–9A).

During the development of a focal seizure the inhibitory surround is overcome and the afterhyperpolarization in the neurons of the original focus gradually disappears. As a result, the seizure begins to spread beyond the original focus and a nearly continuous high-frequency train of action potentials is generated (Figure 50–10).

An important factor in the spread of focal seizures appears to be that the intense firing of the pyramidal neurons results in a relative decrease in synaptic transmission from the inhibitory GABAergic interneurons. This decrease may result from a change in the release of GABA (presynaptic mechanisms), a change in the chloride gradient responsible for the $GABA_A$ receptor-mediated ion flux, or a change in GABA receptor activity (postsynaptic mechanism). Other factors that may contribute to the loss of the inhibitory surround include changes in dendritic morphology, changes in the density of receptors or channels, or changes

Box 50–1 The Contribution of Individual Neurons to the Electroencephalogram

The contribution of the activity of single neurons to the electroencephalogram (EEG) can be understood by examining a simplified cortical circuit and some basic electrical principles. Pyramidal neurons are the major projection neurons in the cortex (see Chapter 2). The apical dendrites of these cells, which are oriented perpendicular to the cell surface, receive a variety of synaptic inputs. Thus synaptic activity in the pyramidal cells is the principal source of EEG activity.

To understand the contribution of a single neuron to the EEG, consider the flow of charge produced by an excitatory synaptic potential (EPSP) on the apical dendrite of a cortical pyramidal neuron (Figure 50–2). Positive charge enters the dendrite at the site of generation of the EPSP, creating what is commonly called a *current sink*. It then must complete a loop by flowing down the dendrite and back out across the membrane at other sites, creating a current source.

The voltage signal created by a synaptic current is approximately predicted by the Ohm's law ($V = IR$, where V is voltage, I is current, and R is resistance). Because the resistance of the membrane (R_m) is much

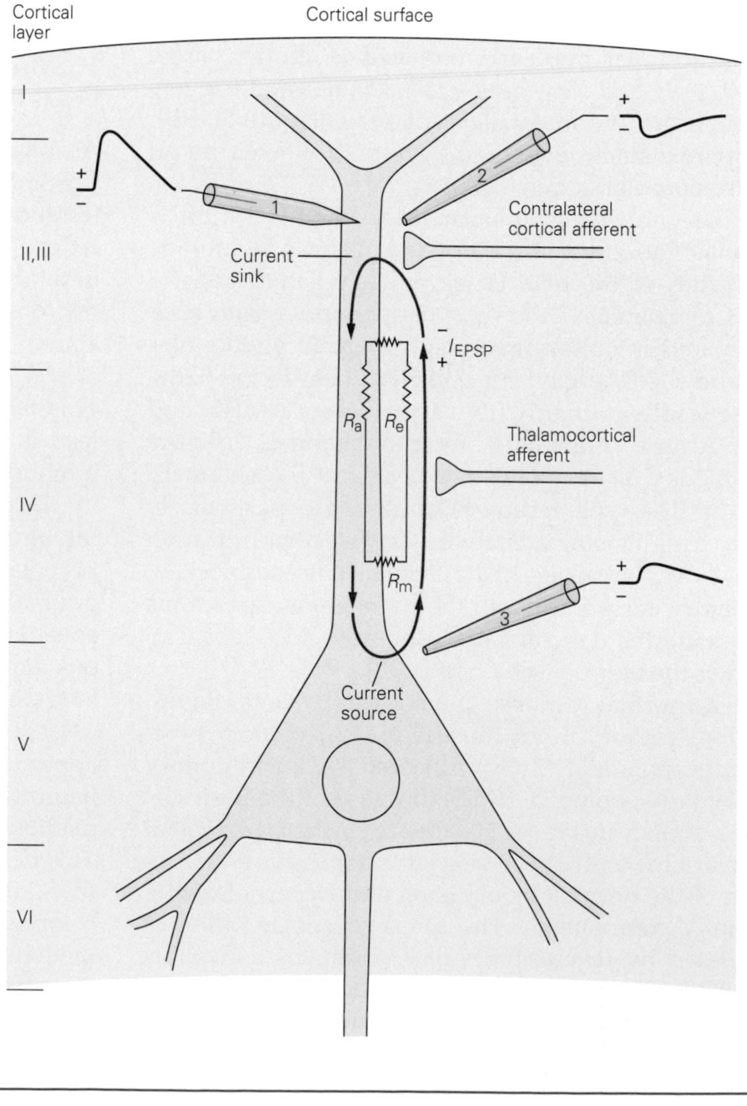

Figure 50–2 The pattern of electrical current flow for an excitatory postsynaptic potential (EPSP) initiated at the apical dendrite of a pyramidal neuron in the cerebral cortex. Activity is detected by three electrodes: an intracellular electrode inserted in the apical dendrite (**1**), an extracellular electrode positioned near the site of the EPSP in layer II of the cortex (**2**), and an extracellular electrode near the cell body in layer V (**3**). At the site of the EPSP (current sink) positive charge flows across the cell membrane (I_{EPSP}) into the cytoplasm, down the dendritic cytoplasm, and then completes the loop by exiting through the membrane near the cell body (current source). The potentials recorded by the extracellular electrodes at the sink and at the source have opposite polarity; the potentials recorded by the intracellular electrode have the same polarity regardless of the site. R_m, R_a, and R_e are the resistances of the membrane, cytoplasm, and extracellular space, respectively.

larger than that of the salt solution that constitutes the extracellular medium (R_e), the voltage recorded across the membrane with an intracellular electrode (V_m) is also larger than the voltage at an extracellular electrode positioned near the current sink (V_e).

At the site of generation of an EPSP the extracellular electrode detects the voltage change caused by charge flowing away from the electrode into the cytoplasm as a negative voltage deflection. However, an extracellular electrode near the current source records a signal of opposite polarity (compare electrodes 2 and 3 in Figure 50–2). The situation is reversed if the site of the EPSP generation is on the basal segment of the apical dendrites.

In the cerebral cortex excitatory axons from the contralateral hemisphere terminate primarily on dendrites in layers II and III, whereas thalamocortical axons terminate in layer IV (Figure 50–3). As a result, the activity measured by a surface EEG electrode will have opposite polarities for these two inputs even though the basic electrical event, membrane depolarization, is the same.

Similarly, the origin or polarity of cortical synaptic events cannot be unambiguously determined from surface EEG recordings alone. EPSPs in superficial layers and inhibitory postsynaptic potentials (IPSPs) in deeper layers both appear as upward (negative) potentials, whereas EPSPs in deeper layers and IPSPs in superficial layers have downward (positive) potentials (Figure 50–3).

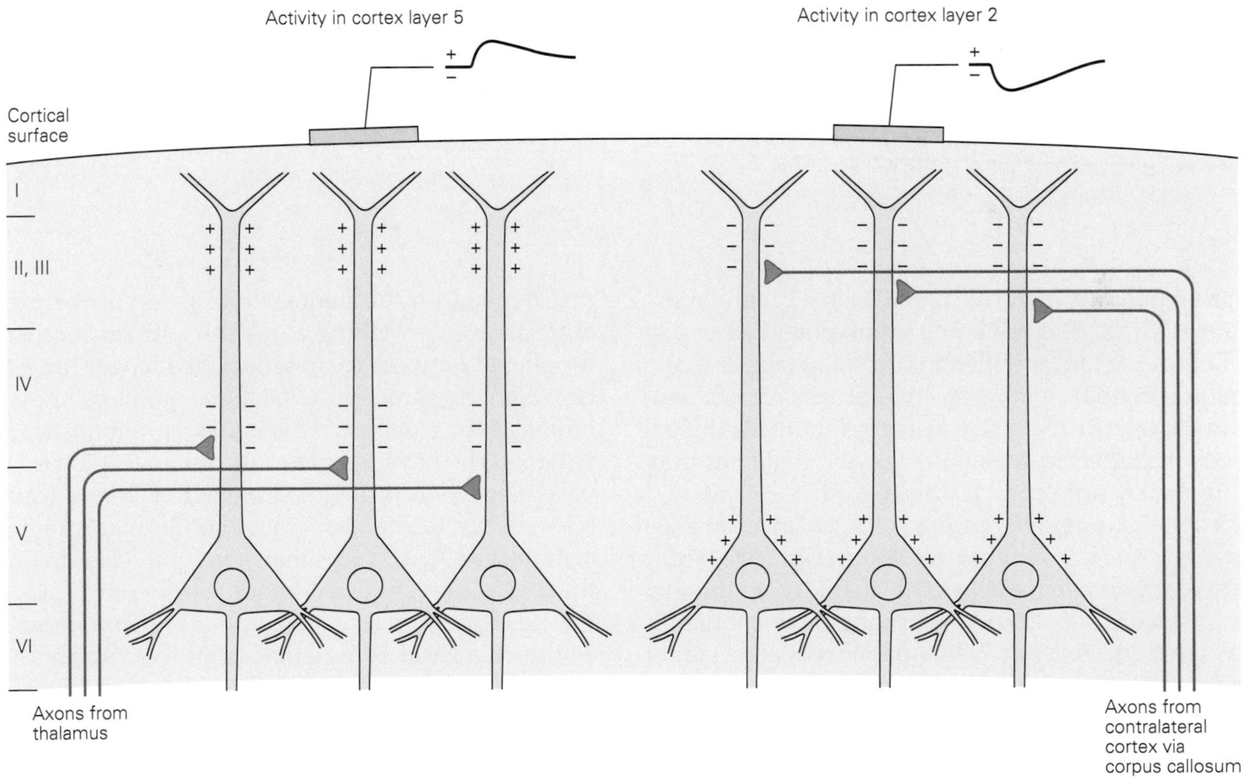

Figure 50–3 Surface electroencephalogram (EEG) recordings do not unambiguously indicate the polarity of synaptic events. The polarity of the surface EEG depends on the location of the synaptic activity within the cortex. A thalamocortical excitatory signal in layer V causes a upward voltage deflection at the surface EEG electrode because the electrode is nearer the current source. In contrast, an excitatory signal from the contralateral hemisphere in layer II causes an downward deflection because the electrode is nearer the sink.

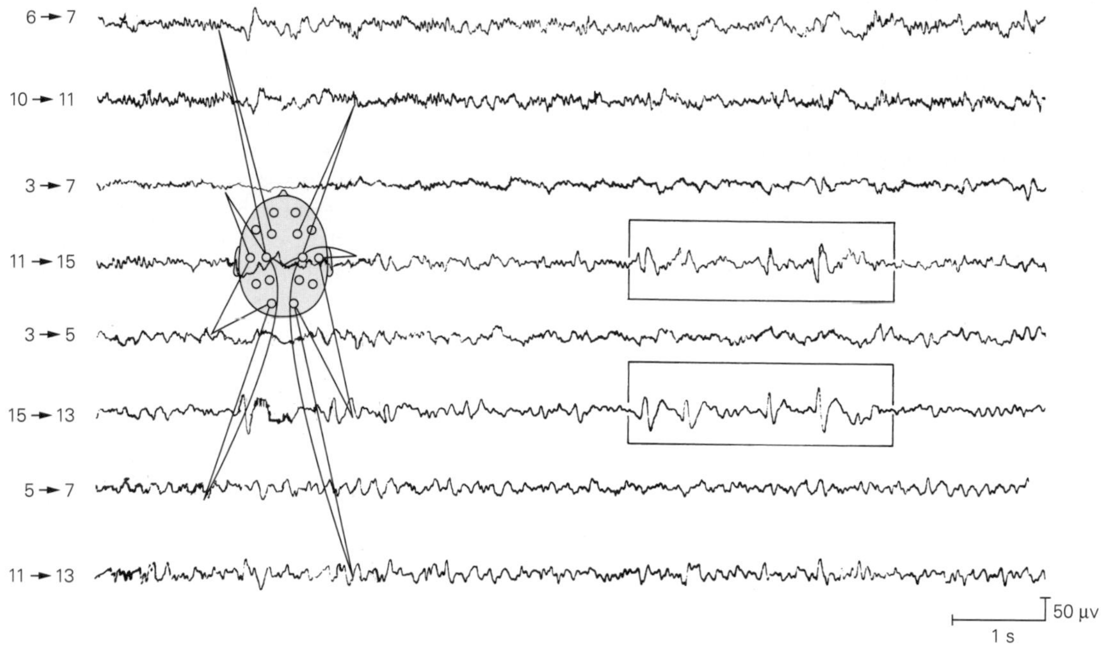

Figure 50–4 The EEG can provide clues to the location of a seizure focus. Each trace represents the electrical activity between pairs of scalp electrodes as indicated in the electrode map. For example, electrode pairs 11–15 and 15–13 measure activity from the right temporal area. In the EEG record shown here, from a patient with epilepsy, sharp waves occur over the right temporal area (records enclosed in boxes). Such paroxysmal activity arises suddenly and disrupts the normal background EEG pattern. The focal abnormality may indicate that the seizure focus in this patient is in the right temporal lobe. Because the patient had no clinical seizures during the recording, these are interictal spikes (see Figure 50–7). (Adapted, with permission, from Lothman and Collins 1990.)

in the amount of extracellular K^+ ion accumulation. Prolonged firing also transmits action potentials to distant sites in the brain, which in turn may trigger trains of action potentials in neurons that project back to neurons in the seizure focus (backpropagation). Reciprocal connections between the neocortex and thalamus may be particularly important in this regard.

Despite our understanding of such mechanisms, we still do not know what causes a seizure to occur at any particular moment. The inability to predict when a seizure will occur is perhaps the most debilitating aspect of epilepsy. Some patients become adept at adjusting their lifestyle to avoid circumstances that can increase the likelihood of a seizure, such as sleep deprivation or stress. But in many individuals seizures do not follow a predictable pattern. In a few patients sensory stimuli such as flashing lights can trigger seizures, suggesting that repetitive excitation of some circuits causes a change in excitability that is dependent on the frequency of neuronal firing.

Both NMDA-type glutamate receptor activity and GABAergic inhibition undergo changes in sensitivity that depend on the frequency of firing of the presynaptic neuron, providing a possible cellular mechanism for altered network excitability. On a longer time scale, circadian rhythms and hormonal patterns may also influence the likelihood of seizures, as demonstrated by patients who have seizures only while sleeping (nocturnal epilepsy) or during their menstrual period (catamenial epilepsy). New devices for continuous monitoring at or near a seizure focus may allow clinicians to predict the timing of seizure generation. Such approaches offer the possibility of acute therapeutic intervention such as direct cortical stimulation to prevent seizures. The modest success of implanted vagal nerve stimulators in epilepsy that does not respond to other treatments provides one example of such an approach.

The Spread of Focal Seizures Involves Normal Cortical Circuitry

If activity in the seizure focus is sufficiently intense, the electrical activity begins to spread to other brain regions. Spread of seizure activity from a focus generally

Box 50–2 Mammalian Brain Slice Preparation

The ability to record electrical activity in tissue slices revolutionized the study of the electrophysiological properties of mammalian neurons. Brain slices, which range from 70 to 400 μm thick, are prepared by quickly removing the brain and immersing it into chilled saline and then sectioning the tissue with a special type of microtome. This technique preserves the basic circuitry of neurons in the slice. The slice is placed in a recording chamber (Figure 50–5) through which oxygenated saline solution is circulated.

There are two principal advantages to recording from neurons in tissue slices. First, more stable electrophysiological recordings can be made because there are no mechanical pulsations resulting from respiration or the pumping of blood. This allows recording from very fine neuronal processes, such as dendrites.

Second, the tissue can be seen under a microscope. When the microscope is equipped with special optics, such as Nomarski differential interference contrast optics, one can actually see unstained living neurons. Direct observation of neurons allows them to be identified from their morphology or by genetic tagging of specific molecules or cell types with green fluorescent protein (Figure 50–6). Direct observation also facilitates patch clamping of individual neurons.

Recording from brain slices has been used to investigate various aspects of the function of mammalian neurons. Through the use of tissue slice techniques, cell- and molecular-biological approaches can be applied to virtually any part of the mammalian brain. Information obtained from recordings made in brain slices has provided important insights into such problems as synaptic plasticity, the mechanisms of epilepsy, and the actions of drugs on the brain.

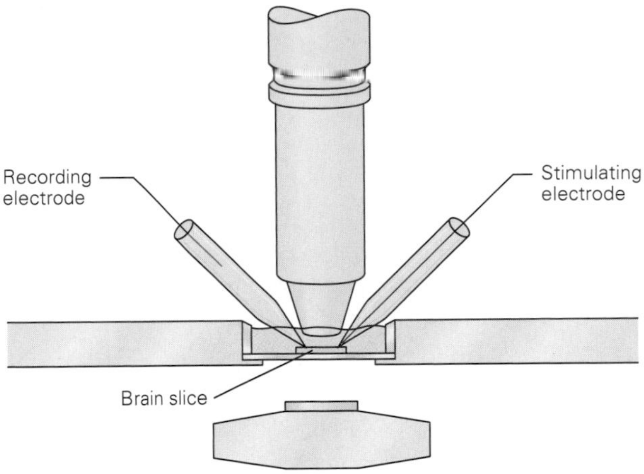

Figure 50–5 Set-up for recording from neurons in a brain slice. The slice is mounted in a chamber attached to the X-Y stage of a microscope. A water-immersion objective allows the slice to be viewed at high power through the saline solution. In this way, separate stimulation and recording electrodes can be placed in the tissue. (Adapted, with permission, from Konnerth 1990.)

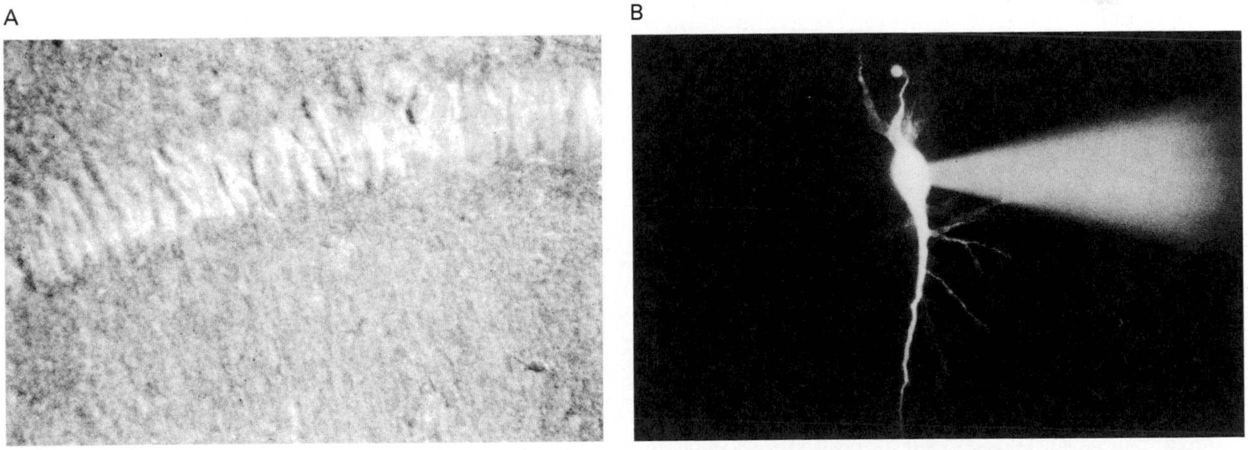

Figure 50–6 Photographs of a rat hippocampal slice. (Reproduced, with permission, from A. Konnerth.)

A. This light microscope image from the cut surface of the slice reveals the pyramidal cell layer in the CA1 region of the hippocampus. The contrast is enhanced using differential interference contrast (Nomarski) optics.

B. A single pyramidal cell has been filled with the fluorescent dye Lucifer yellow through a pipette directed at the cell body. The large apical dendrite projects toward the bottom of the photograph and the basilar dendrites toward the top.

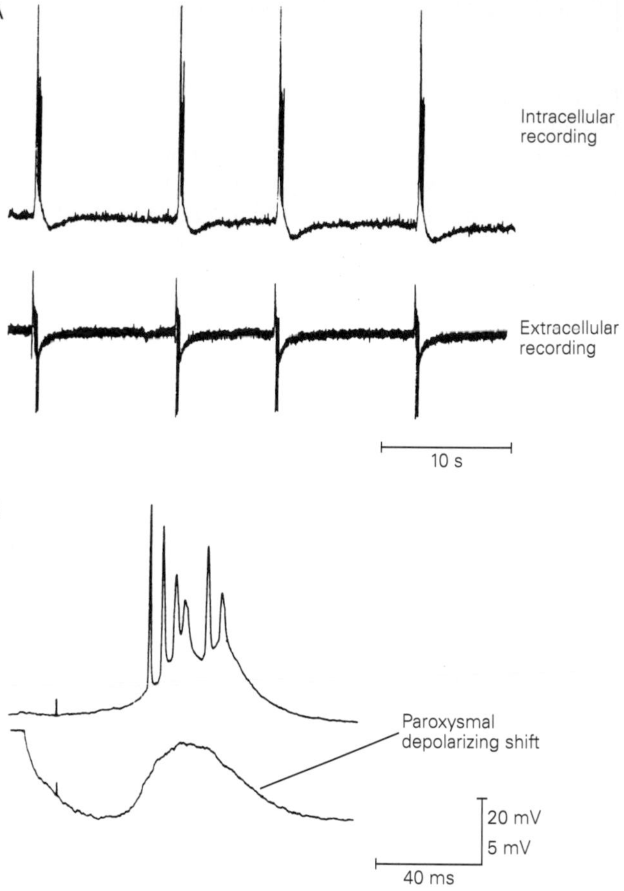

Figure 50–7 Interictal spikes as measured in the EEG result from the synchronized discharges of a group of hippocampal neurons. (Adapted, with permission, from Wong, Miles, and Traub 1984.)

A. Rhythmic firing is evident in an intracellular recording from a pyramidal cell in a hippocampal slice. An extracellular recording from the same slice shows the synchronized discharge of many neurons. This type of synchronized activity underlies interictal spikes in the EEG.

B. The hippocampal slice was perfused with bicuculline, which blocks the inhibition mediated by $GABA_A$ receptors in pyramidal cells and increases the occurrence of seizure-like activity. An intracellular recording from the slice shows several action potentials in one cell (**top trace**). On the next trial (**lower trace**) a hyperpolarizing current was injected to prevent the cell from firing, revealing the large paroxysmal depolarization shift that produces the sudden and long-lasting firing of neurons in a seizure focus.

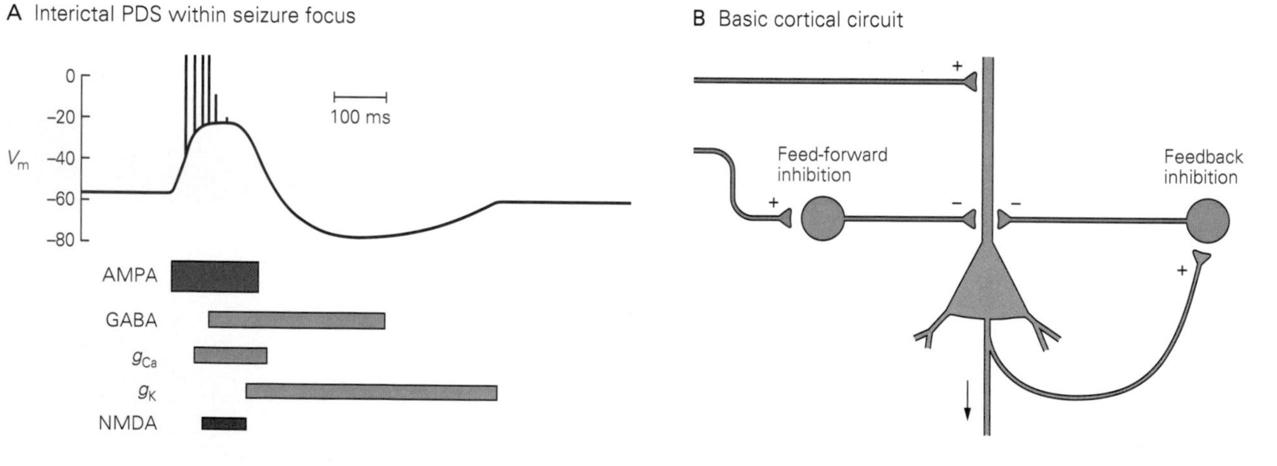

Figure 50–8 The conductances that underlie the paroxysmal depolarizing shift (PDS) of a neuron in a seizure focus.

A. The paroxysmal depolarizing shift is largely dependent on AMPA- and NMDA-type glutamate receptor-channels. The effectiveness of the NMDA-type is enhanced by the opening of voltage-gated Ca^{2+} channels (g_{Ca}). Following the depolarization the cell is hyperpolarized by activation of GABA receptors (both ionotropic $GABA_A$ and metabotropic $GABA_B$) as well as by voltage-gated and calcium-activated K^+ channels (g_K). (**AMPA**, α-amino-3-hydroxy-5-methylisoxazole-4-propionate; **GABA**, γ-aminobutyric acid; **NMDA**, *N*-methyl-D-aspartate.) (Adapted, with permission, from Lothman 1993a.)

B. A simplified version of the inputs to a cortical pyramidal neuron. The **orange** terminals are excitatory, whereas the **gray** terminals are inhibitory. Recurrent axon branches activate inhibitory neurons, causing feedback inhibition of the pyramidal neuron. Extrinsic excitatory inputs can also activate feed-forward inhibition.

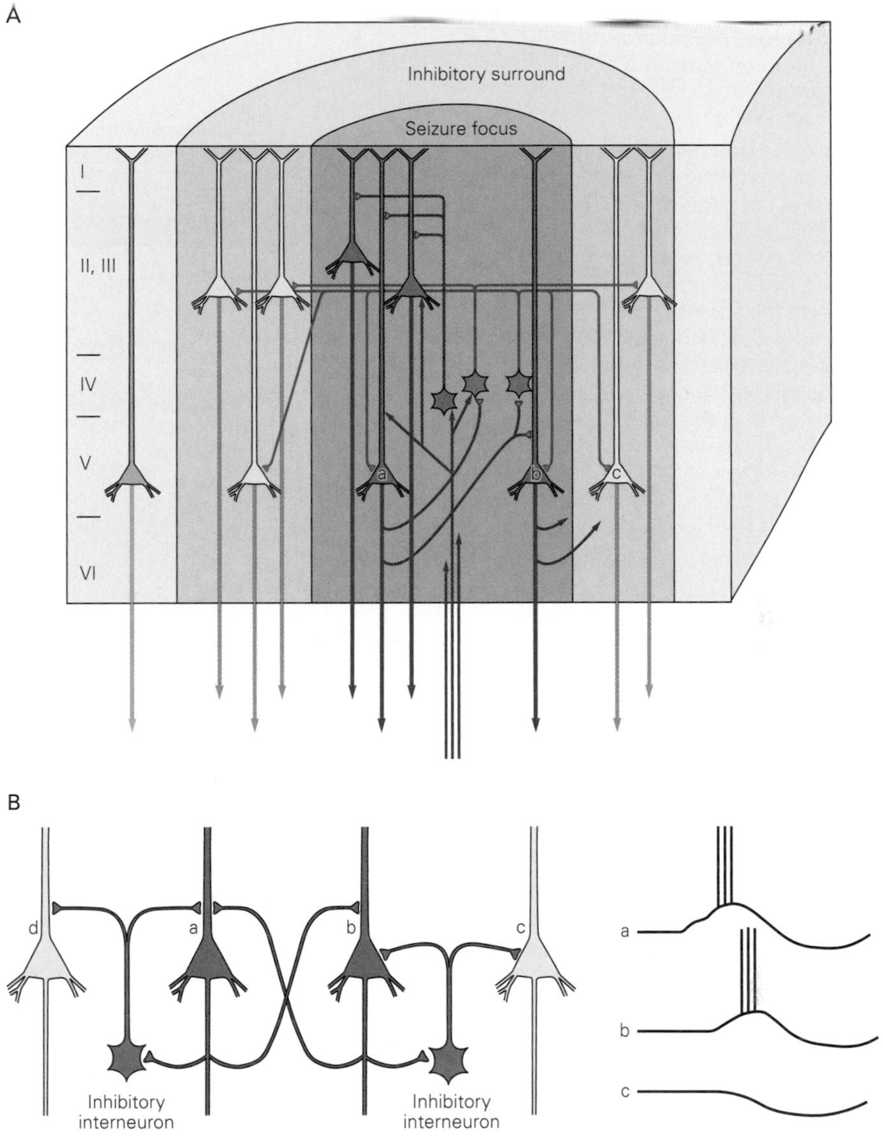

Figure 50–9 The spatial and temporal organization of a seizure focus depends on the interplay between excitation and inhibition of neurons in the focus.

A. In this hypothetical seizure focus in the neocortex, the pyramidal cell *a* shows the typical electrical properties of neurons in a focus (see part B). Activity in cell *a* activates another pyramidal cell (*b*), and when many such cells fire synchronously a spike is recorded on the EEG. However, cell *a* also activates GABAergic inhibitory interneurons (**gray**). These interneurons can reduce the activity of cells *a* and *b* through feedback inhibition, thus limiting the seizure focus temporally, as well as prevent the firing of cells outside the focus, represented here by cell *c*. This latter phenomenon creates an *inhibitory surround* that contains the seizure focus spatially. When extrinsic or intrinsic factors alter this balance of excitation and inhibition, the inhibitory surround begins to break down and the seizure activity spreads. (Reproduced, with permission, from Lothman and Collins 1990.)

B. The synaptic connections and activity patterns for cells *a*, *b*, and *c*. Cells *a* and *b* within the seizure focus undergo a paroxysmal depolarizing shift (see Figure 50–7B). However, cell *c* in the region surrounding the seizure focus is hyperpolarized because of input from GABAergic inhibitory interneurons.

follows the same axonal pathways as does normal cortical activity. For example, the neurons in the primary motor and sensory cortex are organized functionally into vertical columns that run from the pial surface to the underlying white matter (see Chapter 15). The major input to sensory cortex comes from the thalamus and terminates in layer IV, whereas the output cells are in layer V. Reciprocal thalamocortical pathways connect the thalamus and cortex. Intracortical connections occur via short U fibers between adjacent sulci and via the corpus callosum, the major connection between the cerebral hemispheres. These thalamocortical, subcortical, and interhemispheric pathways can all become involved in seizure spread.

Focal seizure activity can spread from the seizure focus to other areas of the same hemisphere or across the corpus callosum to the contralateral hemisphere (Figure 50–11A). Once both hemispheres become involved, the seizure has become secondarily generalized. At this point the patient generally experiences loss of consciousness. The spread of a focal seizure usually occurs within a few seconds but can also take many minutes.

As the focal seizure begins to spread, the patient may experience some warning symptoms (an aura). If the seizure spreads slowly across the cortex, it may lead to a progression of clinical symptoms—a Jacksonian march in the case of a focal seizure involving the motor cortex.

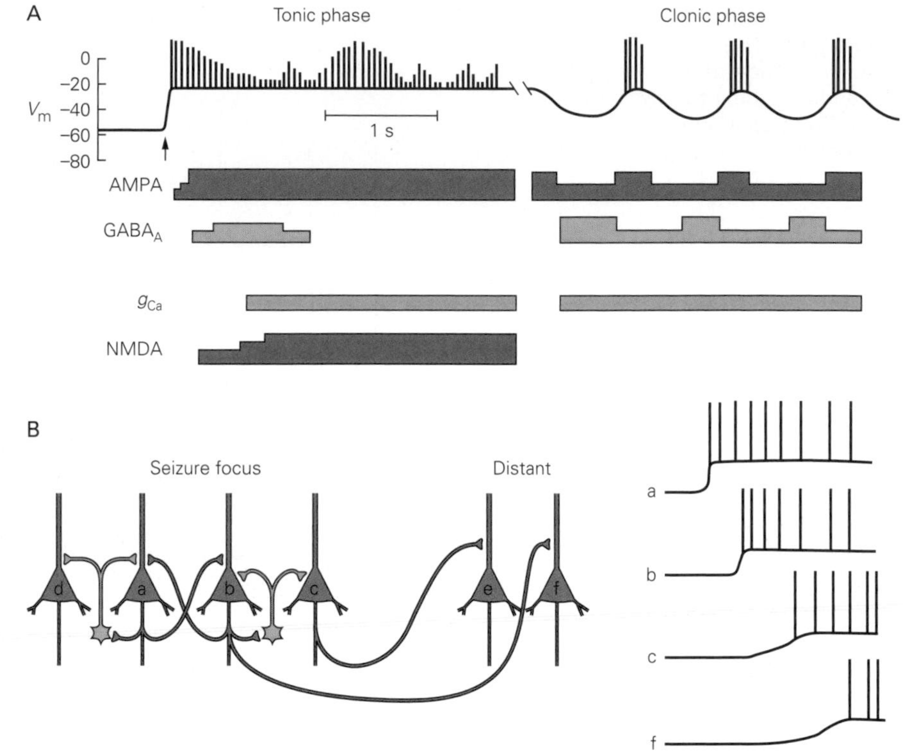

Figure 50–10 A focal seizure begins with the loss of the afterhyperpolarization and surround inhibition. (Adapted, with permission, from Lothman 1993a.)

A. At the onset of a seizure (**arrow**) neurons in the seizure focus depolarize as in the first phase of a paroxysmal depolarizing shift. However, unlike the interictal period, the depolarization persists for seconds or minutes. The GABA-mediated inhibition fails, whereas excitatory activity in the AMPA- and NMDA-type glutamate receptors is functionally enhanced. This activity corresponds to the tonic phase of a secondarily generalized tonic-clonic seizure. As the GABA-mediated inhibition gradually returns, the neurons in the seizure focus enter the clonic phase, a period of oscillation.

B. As the surround inhibition mediated by GABAergic interneurons breaks down, neurons in the seizure focus become synchronously excited and send trains of action potentials to distant neurons, thus spreading the abnormal activity from the focus. Compare the pattern of activity in cells *a* to *c* here with that during the interictal period in Figure 50–9B.

Focal seizures that quickly undergo secondary generalization provide little or no warning. Rapid secondary generalization is more likely if the seizure begins in the neocortex than if it begins in the limbic system (in particular, the hippocampus and amygdala).

An interesting unanswered question is what terminates a seizure. The only definitive conclusion at this point is that termination is not caused by metabolic exhaustion. During the initial 30 seconds or so of a typical secondarily generalized tonic-clonic seizure, neurons in the involved areas undergo prolonged depolarization and continuously fire action potentials (caused by loss of the afterhyperpolarization that normally follows a paroxysmal depolarizing shift). As the seizure evolves, the neurons begin to repolarize and the afterhyperpolarization reappears. The cycles of depolarization and repolarization correspond to the clonic phase of the seizure (Figure 50–10A).

The seizure is often followed by a period of decreased electrical activity, the postictal period, that may be accompanied by confusion, drowsiness, or even focal neurological deficits such as a hemiparesis (Todd paralysis). A neurological exam in the postictal period can lead to insights about the locus of the seizure focus.

Primary Generalized Seizures Are Driven by Thalamocortical Circuits

Unlike the focal seizure a primary generalized seizure disrupts normal brain activity in both cerebral hemispheres simultaneously (Figure 50–11B). Generalized seizures and their associated epilepsies vary both in their manifestations and etiologies. Although the cellular mechanisms of primary generalized seizures differ in a number of interesting respects from those of focal or secondarily generalized focal seizures, a primary generalized seizure can be difficult to distinguish from a focal seizure that rapidly generalizes.

The most studied type of primary generalized seizure is the typical absence seizure (petit mal), whose characteristic EEG pattern (the 3 Hz spike-wave pattern in Figure 50–12A) was first identified by Hans Berger in 1933. F.A. Gibbs recognized the relationship

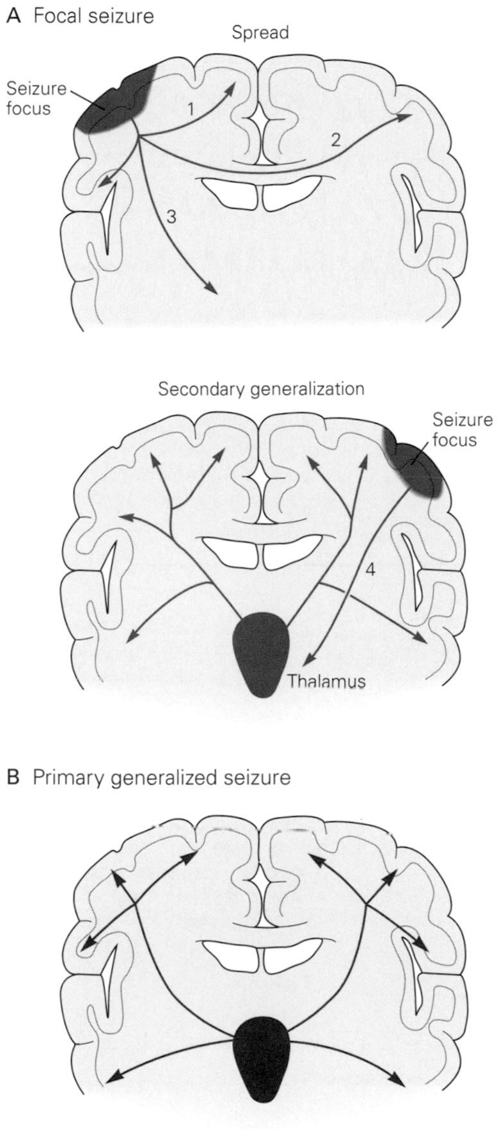

Figure 50–11 Seizures propagate via several pathways. (Reproduced, with permission, from Lothman 1993b.)

A. Focal seizures can spread locally from a focus via intrahemispheric fibers (**1**) and more remotely to homotopic contralateral cortex (**2**) and subcortical centers (**3**). The secondary generalization of focal seizure activity spreads to subcortical centers via projections to the thalamus (**4**). Widespread thalamocortical interconnections then contribute to rapid activation of both hemispheres.

B. Primary generalized seizures, such as a typical absence seizure, spread primarily through interconnections between the thalamus and cortex.

of this EEG pattern to typical absence seizures (he aptly described the pattern as "dart and dome") and he attributed the mechanism to generalized cortical disturbance. The distinctive clinical features of typical absence seizures are clearly correlated with the EEG activity.

The typical absence seizure begins suddenly, lasts 10 to 30 seconds, and produces loss of awareness and only minor motor manifestations such as blinking or lip smacking. Unlike secondarily generalized seizures, primary generalized seizures are not preceded by an aura or followed by postictal symptoms. The spike-wave EEG pattern can be seen in all cerebral areas simultaneously and is immediately preceded and followed by normal background activity. Brief (1–5 s) runs of 3 Hz EEG activity without apparent clinical symptoms are common in patients with childhood absence seizures.

In contrast to Gibbs's hypothesis of diffuse cortical hyperexcitability, Penfield and Jasper noted that the EEG in typical absence seizures is similar to rhythmic EEG activity in sleep, so-called sleep spindles (see Figure 51–1). They proposed a "centrencephalic" hypothesis in which rapid generalization was attributed to rhythmic activity (pacing) by neuronal aggregates in the upper brain stem or thalamus that project diffusely to the cortex.

Research on animal models of generalized seizures and recent studies on the genetics of generalized epilepsy suggest that elements of both hypotheses are correct. In cats parenteral injections of penicillin, a weak $GABA_A$ antagonist, produce behavioral unresponsiveness associated with an EEG pattern of bilateral synchronous slow waves (generalized penicillin epilepsy). During such a seizure thalamic and cortical cells become synchronized through the same reciprocal thalamocortical connections that contribute to normal sleep spindles during slow wave sleep.

Such seizures could in theory represent a form of diffuse hyperexcitability in the cortex. Recordings from individual cortical neurons show an increase in the rate of firing during a depolarizing burst that in turn produces a powerful GABAergic inhibitory feedback that hyperpolarizes the cell for approximately 200 ms after each burst (Figure 50–12C). This depolarization followed by inhibition differs fundamentally from the paroxysmal depolarizing shift in focal seizures in that GABAergic inhibition is preserved. In the typical absence seizure the summated activity of the bursts produces the spike while the summated inhibition produces the wave of the spike-wave EEG pattern.

What are the properties of cells and networks that facilitate this generalized and synchronous activity?

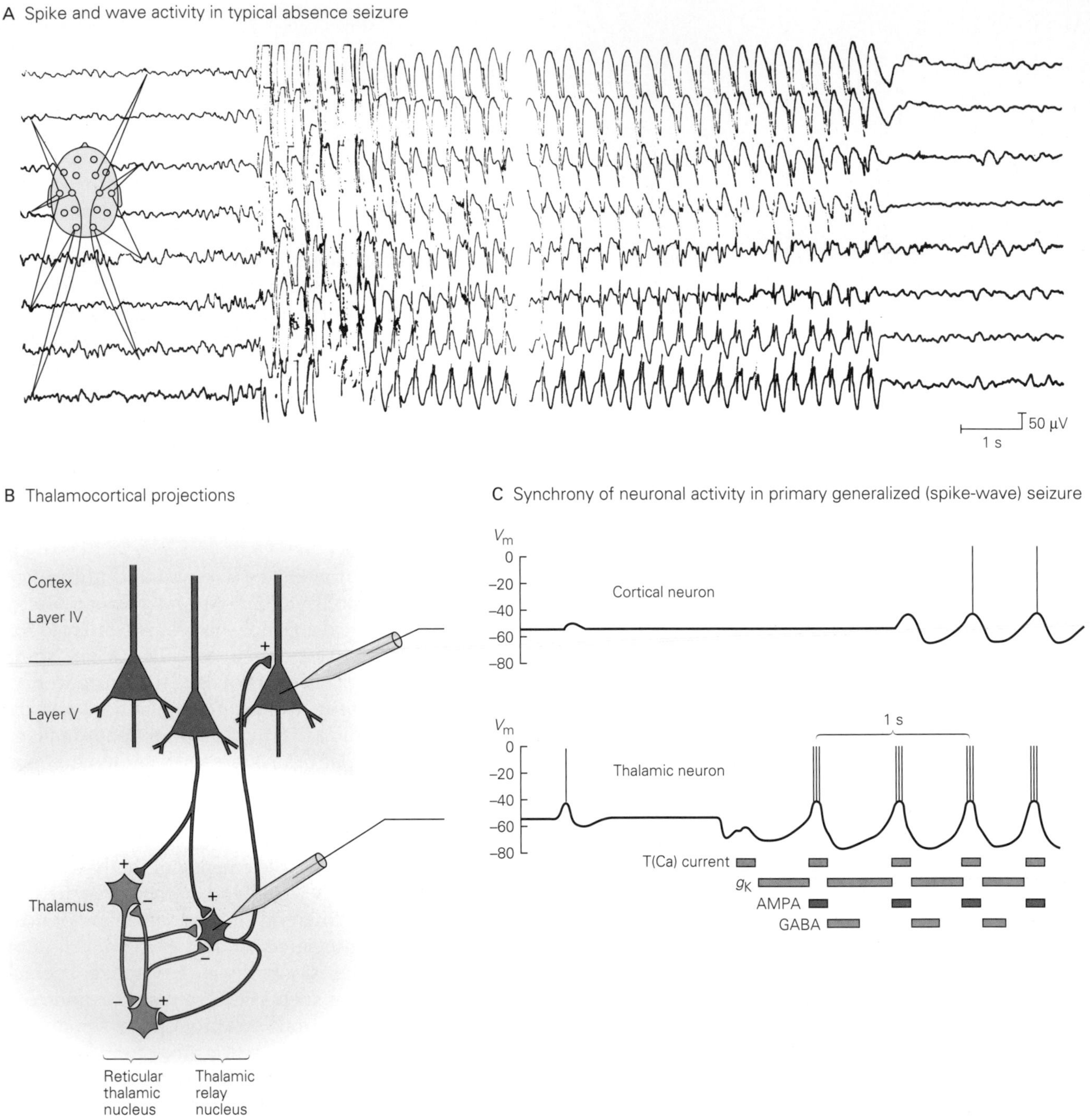

Figure 50–12 The generation of primary generalized seizures.

A. This EEG from a 12-year-old patient with typical absence (petit mal) seizures shows the sudden onset of synchronous spikes at a frequency of 3 per second and wave activity lasting approximately 14 seconds. The seizure was clinically manifest as a staring spell with occasional eye blinks. Unlike a focal seizure there is no buildup of activity preceding the seizure and the electrical activity returns abruptly to the normal background level following the seizure. Discontinuity in the trace is the result of removal of a 3 second period of recording. (Reproduced, with permission, from Lothman and Collins 1990.)

B. The thalamocortical connections that participate in the generation of sleep spindles (see Chapter 51) are thought to be essential for the generation of primary generalized seizures. Pyramidal cells in the cortex are reciprocally connected by excitatory synapses with thalamic relay neurons. GABAergic interneurons in the reticular thalamic nucleus are excited by pyramidal cells in the cortex and thalamic relay neurons, and inhibit the thalamic relay cells. The interneurons are also reciprocally connected.

C. Neuronal activity of cortical and thalamic neurons becomes synchronized during a primary generalized seizure. The depolarization is dependent on conductances in AMPA-type glutamate receptor-channels and T-type voltage-gated Ca^{2+} channels. The repolarization is caused by GABA-mediated inhibition as well as voltage- and calcium-dependent K^+ conductances (g_K). (Reproduced, with permission, from Lothman 1993a.)

An early clue came from studies of the intrinsic bursting of thalamic relay neurons. Henrik Jahnsen and Rodolfo Llinas found that these neurons robustly express the T-type voltage-gated Ca^{2+} channel that is inactivated at the resting membrane potential but becomes available for activation when the cell is hyperpolarized. A subsequent depolarization then transiently opens the Ca^{2+} channel (thus the name T-type) and the Ca^{2+} influx generates low-threshold Ca^{2+} spikes. Consistent with the hypothesis that T-type channels contribute to absence seizures, certain anticonvulsant agents that block absence seizures, such as ethosuximide (Zarontin) and valproic acid (Depakote), also block T-type channels. T-type channels are encoded by three related genes (*Cav3.1–Cav3.3*), with *Cav3.1* the predominant type in the thalamus.

The circuitry of the thalamus seems ideally suited to the generation of primary generalized seizures. The pattern of thalamic neuron activity during sleep spindles suggests a reciprocal interaction between thalamic relay neurons and GABAergic interneurons in the thalamic reticular nucleus and perigeniculate nucleus (Figure 50–12B). Studies of thalamic brain slices by David McCormick and his colleagues indicate that the interneurons hyperpolarize the relay neurons, thus removing the inactivation of T-type Ca^{2+} channels. This action leads to an oscillatory response: T-type Ca^{2+} channels drive rebound firing in the relay neurons, which stimulates GABAergic interneurons and leads to another round of rebound firing. The relay neurons also excite cortical neurons, as manifested in the EEG by a spindle wave (see Chapter 51). Both the T-type Ca^{2+} channel and the $GABA_B$ receptor-channel play an important role in the generation of this activity that resembles human absence seizures.

Mutations in voltage-gated Ca^{2+} channels have produced several mouse models of generalized epilepsy, including the so-called *totterer* mouse. Studies of these mutants by Jeffrey Noebels and his colleagues have revealed that the animals develop primary generalized seizures when they reach adolescence. EEGs in these animals show a paroxysmal spike-wave discharge and seizures that are characterized by an arrest of behavior, similar to typical absence seizures.

Locating the Seizure Focus Is Critical to the Surgical Treatment of Epilepsy

The pioneering studies of the surgeon Wilder Penfield in Montreal in the early 1950s led to the recognition that removal of the temporal lobe in certain patients with focal seizures of hippocampal origin could reduce or cure epilepsy. As surgical treatment for difficult-to-control (so-called intractable) focal seizures became more common, it became clear that the surgical outcome is directly related to the adequacy of the resection. Thus precise localization of the seizure focus is essential.

Electrical mapping of seizure foci originally relied on the surface EEG, which we have seen is biased toward particular sets of neurons in the cortex immediately adjacent to the skull. However, intractable seizures often begin in deep structures that show little or no abnormality on the surface EEG at the onset of the seizure. Thus the surface EEG is somewhat limited in identifying the location of the seizure focus.

The development of magnetic resonance imaging (MRI) has markedly improved the noninvasive anatomical mapping of seizure foci. This technique is now routine in the evaluation of seizure foci in the temporal lobe and increasingly promising for identifying seizure foci in other locations. Anatomical mapping of seizure foci by MRI has shown that most patients with intractable temporal lobe seizures have atrophy and cell loss in the mesial portions of the hippocampal formation. There is a dramatic loss of neurons within the hippocampus (mesial temporal sclerosis), changes in dendritic morphology of surviving cells, and collateral sprouting of some axons. The anatomical resolution of MRI provides a noninvasive, quantitative assessment of the size of the hippocampus in epilepsy patients. Loss of volume of the hippocampus on one or another side of the brain generally correlates well with the localization of seizure foci in the hippocampus by electrical criteria.

Patients with mesial temporal lobe epilepsy often have unilateral disease, which leads to shrinkage of the hippocampus on one side. This is apparent in brain imaging as an apparent dilatation of the temporal horn of the lateral ventricle (Box 50–3). However, in many patients abnormalities cannot be detected using anatomical MRI; thus several functional imaging methods have been used as well.

Metabolic mapping takes advantage of the changes in cerebral metabolism and blood flow that occur in the seizure focus during the ictal and interictal periods. The electrical activity associated with a seizure places a large metabolic demand on brain tissue. During a focal seizure there is an approximately threefold increase in glucose and oxygen use. Between seizures the seizure focus often shows decreased metabolism. Despite the increased metabolic demands, the brain is able to maintain normal adenosine triphosphate (ATP) levels during a focal seizure. Conversely, the transient interruption of breathing during a generalized

Box 50–3 Surgical Treatment of Temporal Lobe Epilepsy

A 27-year-old woman had episodes of decreased responsiveness beginning at age 19 years. At first she would stare off and appear confused during the episodes. Later she developed an aura consisting of a feeling of fear. This fear was followed by altered consciousness, a wide-eyed stare, tightening of the left arm, and a scream that lasted for 14 to 20 seconds (Figure 50–13).

These spells were diagnosed as complex partial seizures. The seizures occurred several times a week despite treatment with several antiepileptic drugs. She was unable to work or drive because of frequent seizures. She had a history of meningitis at age 6 months, and throughout childhood she had experienced brief episodes of altered perception described as "like someone threw a switch."

Based on an evaluation summarized in Figures 50–14 and 50–15, the right amygdala and hippocampus (amygdalohippocampectomy) were resected. The patient was seizure-free following the operation and returned to full-time employment.

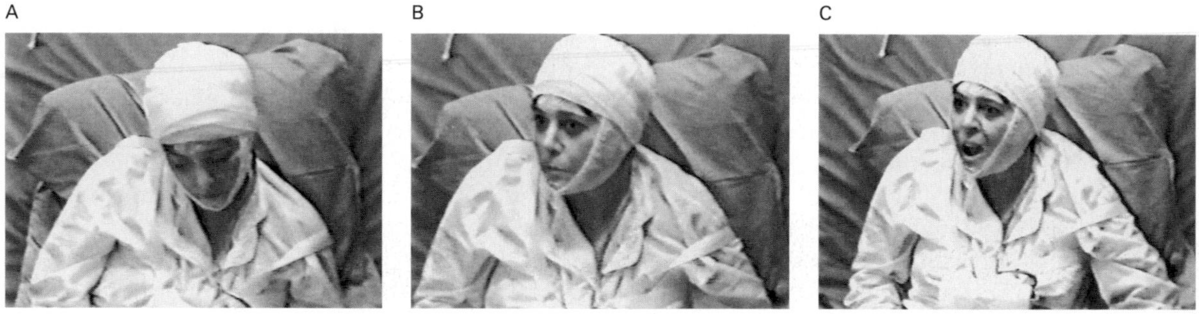

Figure 50–13 The patient is shown reading quietly in the period preceding the seizure (**A**), during the period when she reported a feeling of fear (**B**), and during the period when there was alteration of consciousness and an audible scream (**C**). (Reproduced, with permission, from Dr. Martin Salinsky.)

convulsive seizure causes a decrease in oxygen levels in the blood. This results in a drop in ATP concentration and an increase in anaerobic metabolism as indicated by rising lactate levels. This oxygen debt is quickly replenished in the postictal period, and no permanent damage to brain tissue results from a single generalized seizure.

Positron emission tomography (PET) scans of patients with focal seizures originating in the mesial temporal lobe frequently show interictal hypometabolism, with metabolic changes extending to the lateral temporal lobe, ipsilateral thalamus, basal ganglia, and frontal cortex. PET scans using nonhydrolyzable glucose analogs have been particularly helpful in identifying seizure foci in patients with normal MRI scans and in some early childhood epilepsies.

Unfortunately, for unclear reasons PET has been less reliable in localizing seizure foci in extratemporal areas such as the frontal lobe. An additional limitation is the expense of the PET scan and the short half-life of the isotopes (a nearby cyclotron is required). PET scanning can also be used to look for functional changes

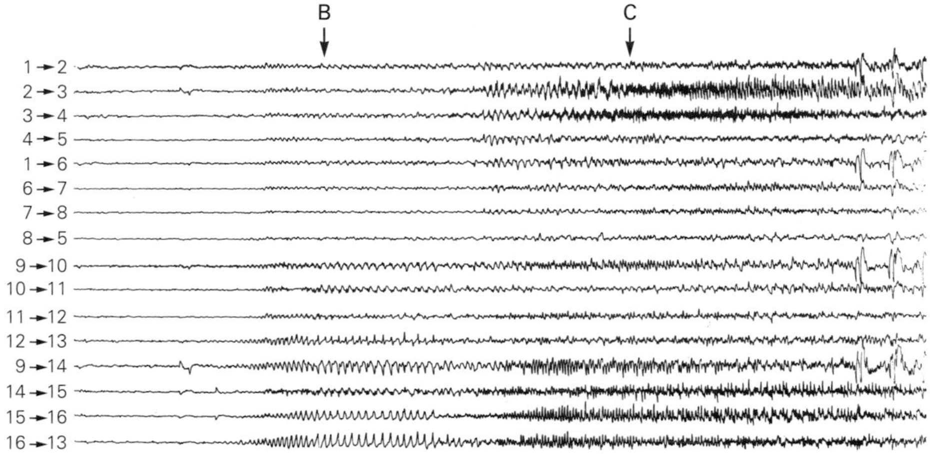

Figure 50–14 The EEG at the time of the photographs in Figure 50–13. Low-amplitude background rhythms occur at the beginning (**left**). At the point when the patient reported fear (**B**), there is a buildup of EEG activity at the onset of a complex partial seizure, but this activity is confined to the EEG electrodes over the right hemisphere (electrodes 9–16). At the point consciousness is altered (**C**) the seizure activity has spread to the left hemisphere (electrodes 1–8). EEG spike-waves are particularly prominent in leads 9–10 and 9–14 over the right anterior temporal region. (Reproduced, with permission, from Dr. Martin Salinsky.)

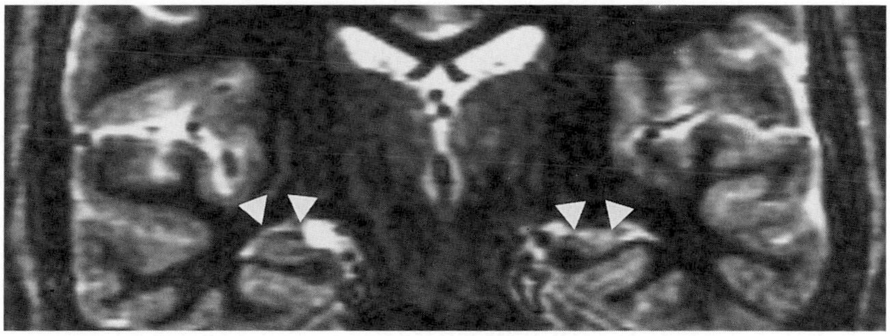

Figure 50–15 Enhanced MRI reveals atrophy of the right hippocampus (**arrowheads on right**) and a normal left hippocampus (**arrowheads on left**). (Reproduced, with permission, from Dr. Martin Salinsky.)

in neurotransmitter receptor binding and transport related to seizure activity.

A related technique that measures cerebral blood flow, single photon emission computed tomography (SPECT), has been used more frequently than PET. SPECT does not have the resolution of PET but can be performed in the nuclear medicine department of many large hospitals. Injection of radioisotopes and SPECT imaging at the time of a seizure (ictal SPECT) reveals a pattern of hypermetabolism followed by hypometabolism in the seizure focus and surrounding tissue. The use of magnetoencephalography and functional MRI may offer further advantages in the mapping of seizure foci.

With rigorous selection of patients for epilepsy surgery, the cure rate for seizures originating in the temporal lobe can approach 80%. Patients with complicating factors (eg, multiple foci) have lower success rates. However, even among these patients the number or severity of seizures is reduced. Patients who have been *cured* of seizures still experience cognitive problems such as memory loss and social problems such as adjustments to more independent living and limited employment opportunities. These factors emphasize the need for treatment as early in life as feasible.

Prolonged Seizures Can Cause Brain Damage

Repeated Convulsive Seizures Are a Medical Emergency

As noted earlier, brain tissue can compensate for the metabolic stress of a focal seizure or the transient decrease in oxygen delivery during a single generalized seizure. In a generalized seizure, stimulation of the hypothalamus leads to massive activation of the stress response of the sympathetic nervous system. The increased systemic blood pressure and serum glucose initially compensate for increased metabolic demand, but these homeostatic mechanisms fail during prolonged seizures, particularly seizures that are convulsive. The resulting systemic metabolic derangements, including hypoxia, hypotension, hypoglycemia, and acidemia, lead to a reduction in high-energy phosphates (ATP and phosphocreatine) in the brain and thus can be devastating to brain tissue.

Systemic complications such as cardiac arrhythmias, pulmonary edema, hyperthermia, and muscle breakdown can also occur. Repeated generalized seizures without return to full consciousness between seizures, called *status epilepticus,* is a true medical emergency. This condition requires aggressive seizure management and general medical support because 30 or more minutes of continuous convulsive seizures leads to brain injury or even death. Status epilepticus can involve nonconvulsive seizures (focal or primary generalized) for which the metabolic consequences are much less severe.

Excitotoxicity Underlies Seizure-Related Brain Damage

Repeated seizures can damage the brain independently of cardiopulmonary or systemic metabolic changes, suggesting that local factors in the brain can result in neuronal death. The immature brain appears particularly vulnerable to such damage, perhaps because of greater electrotonic coupling between neurons in the developing brain, less effective potassium buffering by immature glia, and decreased glucose transport across the blood-brain barrier.

Wilhelm Sommer in 1880 first noted the vulnerability of the hippocampus to such insults, with preferential loss of the pyramidal neurons in the CA1 and CA3 regions. This pattern has been duplicated in experimental animals by electrical stimulation of afferents to the hippocampus or by injection of excitatory amino acid analogs such as kainic acid. Interestingly, kainic acid causes local damage at the site of injection and also at the site of termination of afferents originating at the injection site.

These observations indicate that release of the excitatory transmitter L-glutamate during excessive stimulation such as a seizure can itself cause neuronal damage, a condition that has been termed *excitotoxicity.* Excitotoxicity following seizures probably is caused more by excessive stimulation of synaptically-activated glutamate receptors than by tonic increases in extracellular glutamate. The histological appearance of acute excitotoxicity includes massive swelling of cell bodies and dendrites, which is consistent with the predominant locations of glutamate receptors and excitatory synapses.

Although the cellular and molecular mechanisms of excitotoxicity are still not fully understood, several features are clear. Overactivation of glutamate receptors leads to an excessive increase in intracellular Ca^{2+} that can activate a self-destructive cellular cascade involving many calcium-dependent enzymes, such as phosphatases, proteases, and lipases. Lipid peroxidation can also cause production of free radicals that damage vital cellular proteins and lead to cell death. The role of mitochondria in Ca^{2+} homeostasis and in control of free radicals may also be important. The pattern of cell death was first thought to reflect necrosis because of the autolysis of critical cellular proteins. However, *death genes,* characteristic of programmed cell death or apoptosis, may also be involved.

Seizure-related brain damage or excitotoxicity can be specific to certain types of cells in particular brain regions, perhaps because of protective factors, such as calcium-binding proteins in some cells, and sensitizing factors, such as the expression of calcium-permeable glutamate receptors in other cells. For example, excitotoxicity induced in vitro by activation of AMPA-type glutamate receptors preferentially affects interneurons that express AMPA-type receptors that have high Ca^{2+} permeability, providing a possible mechanism for their selective vulnerability.

Several outbreaks of *amnestic* shellfish poisoning provide a vivid example of the consequences of overactivation of glutamate receptors. Domoic acid, a glutamate analog not present in the brain, is a natural product of certain species of marine algae that flourish during appropriate ocean conditions. Domoic acid can be concentrated by filter feeders such as shellfish. Ingestion of domoic acid contaminated shellfish sporadically causes outbreaks of neurological damage, including severe seizures and memory loss (amnesia). The area most sensitive to damage is the hippocampus, providing further support for the excitotoxicity hypothesis and the critical role of the hippocampus in learning and memory (see Chapter 65).

The Factors Leading to Development of Epilepsy Are an Unfolding Mystery

A single seizure does not warrant a diagnosis of epilepsy. Normal people can have a seizure under extenuating circumstances, such as following drug ingestion or extreme sleep deprivation. Clinicians look for possible causes of seizures in such cases but usually do not begin treatment with anticonvulsants following a single seizure. Unfortunately, our understanding of what factors contribute to susceptibility to epilepsy is still rudimentary.

Some forms of epilepsy are caused in part by a genetic predisposition. For example, infants with febrile seizures often have a family history of similar seizures. The role of genetics in epilepsy is supported by the existence of familial epileptic syndromes in humans as well as seizure-prone animal models with such exotic names as *Papio papio* (a baboon with photosensitive seizures), audiogenic mice (in which loud sounds induce seizures), and *reeler* and *totterer* mice (names alluding to the clinical manifestations of cerebellar mutations in these animals). Even with a genetic predisposition or a structural lesion, the evolution of the epileptic phenotype often involves maladaptive changes in brain structure and function.

Among the Genetic Causes of Epilepsy Are Ion Channel Mutations

Recent studies have provided a wealth of new information concerning the molecular genetics of epilepsy. At present more than 70 genes have been linked to an epileptic phenotype; approximately half of these were discovered in humans and the others in animals, mostly mice. The affected proteins include ion channel subunits, proteins involved in synaptic transmission such as transporters, vesicle proteins, synaptic receptors, and molecules involved in Ca^{2+} signaling. For example, seizures in the *totterer* mutant mouse are due to a spontaneous mutation in the gene that encodes the $Ca_V2.1$-subunit or α_{1A}-subunit of the P/Q-type voltage-gated Ca^{2+} channel. That mutations in these classes of proteins can cause epilepsy is perhaps not unexpected given the dependence of seizures on synaptic transmission and neuronal excitability. Some of the other genes linked to epilepsy in mice have been more surprising, such as the genes for Centromere BP-B, a DNA-binding protein, and the sodium/hydrogen exchanger, which is affected in the slow-wave epilepsy mouse.

A wide variety of human gene mutations cause neurological disorders of which epilepsy is only one manifestation. For example, Rett syndrome, a disease associated with mental retardation, autism, and seizures, is caused by mutations in the gene that codes for MECP2 (methyl-CpG-binding protein-2), a regulator of gene transcription. Although the exact links are unknown, it is clear that mutations in many different genes may result in epilepsy.

Most genetic epilepsy syndromes in humans have complex rather than simple (Mendelian) inheritance patterns, suggesting the involvement of many rather than single genes. Nevertheless, a number of *monogenic* epilepsies have been identified in studies of families with epilepsy. Ortrud Steinlein and colleagues reported in 1995 that a mutation in the α_4-subunit of the nicotinic acetylcholine receptor-channel is responsible for autosomal dominant nocturnal frontal lobe epilepsy (ADNFLE), the first example of an autosomal gene defect in human epilepsy. Since then other voltage- and ligand-gated channel proteins have been identified as critical genes for epilepsy. Mutations in ion channel genes (channelopathies) constitute a major cause of known monogenic epilepsies (Figure 50–16).

In voltage-gated channels, mutations largely affect the main pore-forming subunit(s), but there are also examples of epilepsy-causing mutations in regulatory subunits. When examined in vitro, the mutant channel proteins are most commonly associated with either reductions in the expression of the channel on the surface of the plasma membrane (caused by reduced targeting to the membrane or premature degradation) or altered kinetics of the channels. The problem of how changes in ion channel gating might affect the excitability of neurons and their synchronization during seizure generation is straight-forward. However, mutations in ion channel genes may also affect neuronal development and thus exert their epileptogenic effects through a secondary action on cell migration, network formation, or patterns of gene expression.

In the early days of research on epilepsy genes it was widely expected that the genes would underlie generalized epilepsies, based on the idea that a gene mutation (eg, in an ion channel) would be expected to affect most neurons. However, the first autosomal dominant epilepsy gene discovered by Steinlein and colleagues causes focal seizures. In retrospect this should not be so surprising because channel subunits are rarely expressed uniformly in the brain, and some brain regions are more likely to generate seizures than other regions. For example, *totterer* mice with mutations in the pore-forming $Ca_V2.1$-subunit of P/Q-type Ca^{2+} channels show spike-wave type seizures. The seizures occur principally in immature mice, presumably

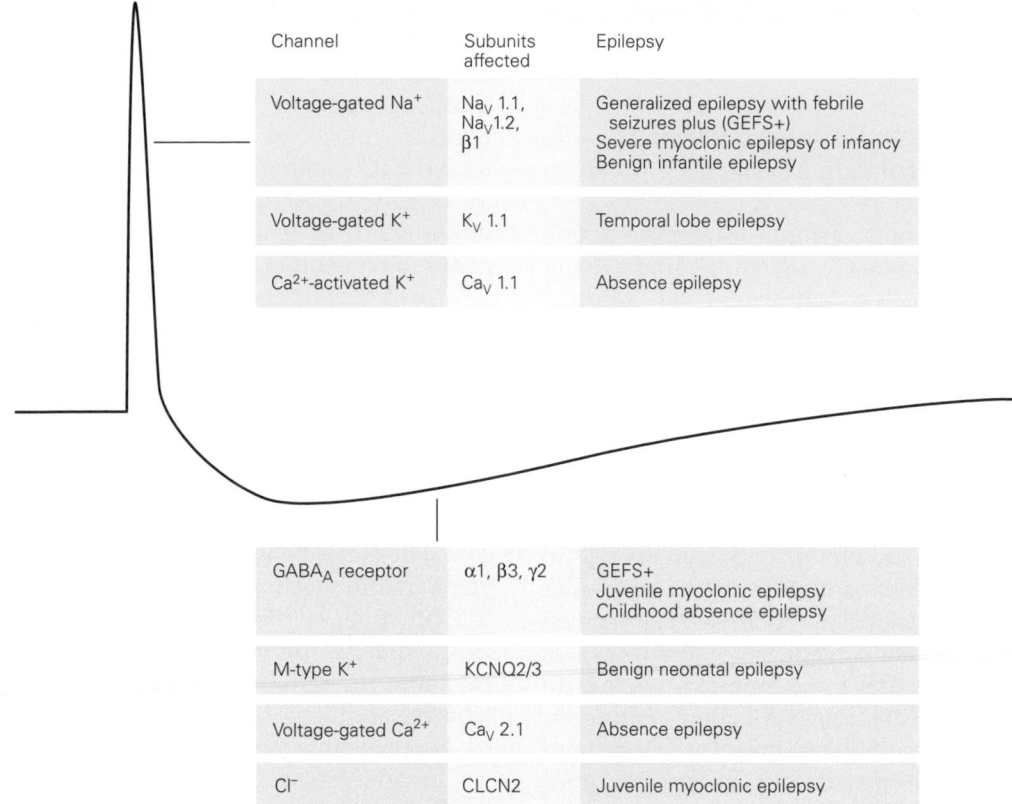

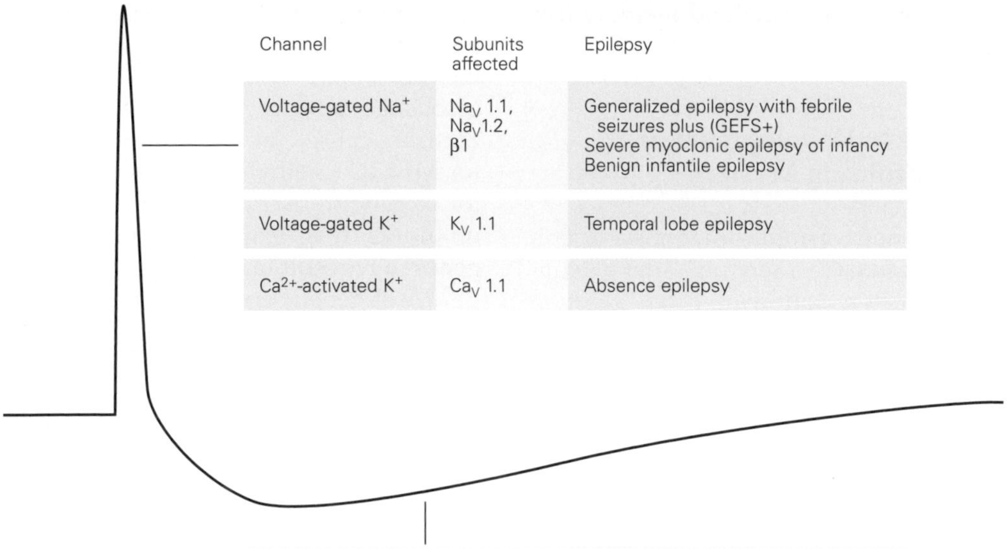

Channel	Subunits affected	Epilepsy
Voltage-gated Na^+	Na_V 1.1, Na_V1.2, β1	Generalized epilepsy with febrile seizures plus (GEFS+) Severe myoclonic epilepsy of infancy Benign infantile epilepsy
Voltage-gated K^+	K_V 1.1	Temporal lobe epilepsy
Ca^{2+}-activated K^+	Ca_V 1.1	Absence epilepsy

Channel	Subunits affected	Epilepsy
$GABA_A$ receptor	α1, β3, γ2	GEFS+ Juvenile myoclonic epilepsy Childhood absence epilepsy
M-type K^+	KCNQ2/3	Benign neonatal epilepsy
Voltage-gated Ca^{2+}	Ca_V 2.1	Absence epilepsy
Cl^-	CLCN2	Juvenile myoclonic epilepsy

Figure 50–16 Gene mutations that affect ion channel function are a major cause of monogenic human epilepsies. The human epilepsy genes discovered in the past 10 years can affect multiple phases of neuronal excitability, from the shape of the action potential to the afterpotentials and synaptic events that follow. In the figure the mutations listed near the spike affect the repolarization of the action potential; those listed below affect either the afterhyperpolarization, synaptic conductances, or interspike interval. (Adapted, with permission, from Jeffrey Noebels, unpublished data.)

because P/Q-type Ca^{2+} channels are the predominant isoform early in development, whereas N-type Ca^{2+} channels predominate later.

Moreover, one mutant gene can give rise to different epilepsy phenotypes, whereas different mutant genes can cause the same epilepsy phenotype. As an example of the latter, the ADNFLE syndrome, first discovered as a mutation in the α_4-subunit of the nicotinic acetylcholine receptor, can also be caused by a mutation in the α_2-subunit. But not all family members who carry this autosomal dominant mutation have epilepsy, indicating that even in monogenic epilepsy other, perhaps nongenetic, factors can influence the phenotype.

The GEFS+ syndrome (generalized epilepsy with febrile seizures plus) is a good example of this heterogeneity. It can involve different seizure types in different family members and has been seen in families with mutations in the genes for three different Na^+ channel subunits and two $GABA_A$ receptors. Family studies of primary generalized epilepsy suggest that seizure types may be heritable within families. These issues indicate that monogenic epilepsies are likely modified by other genes, environmental influences, and even experience-dependent changes in synapses.

Altered cortical development may be a common cause of epilepsy. The higher resolution of MRI scans has revealed an unexpectedly large number of cortical malformations and localized areas of abnormal cortical folding in patients with epilepsy. Thus mutations that disturb the normal formation of the cortex or network wiring are candidate genes for epilepsy. This idea is supported by the mapping of two X-linked cortical malformations with epileptic phenotypes: familial periventricular heterotopia and familial subcortical band heterotopia. The genes responsible for these two disorders, *filamin A* and *doublecortin*, are presumably important in neuronal migration. Small focal cortical dysplasias can function as seizure foci that give rise to focal and secondarily generalized seizures, whereas more extensive cortical malformations can cause a variety of seizure types and usually are associated with other neurological problems.

Unfortunately, most cases of epilepsy cannot be explained by even the recent surge in the identification of epilepsy genes. The identification of large numbers of patients through online registries, such as the Epilepsy Phenome/Genome Project, may provide the population sample needed to evaluate susceptibility genes that underlie complex inheritance patterns.

Epilepsies Involving Focal Seizures May Be a Maladaptive Response to Injury

Epilepsies involving repeated focal seizures often develop following a discrete cortical injury such as a penetrating head wound. This injury serves as the nidus for a seizure focus, leading at some later point to seizures. This has led to the idea that the early insult triggers a set of progressive physiological or anatomical changes that lead to chronic seizures. That is, the characteristic *silent* interval (usually months or years) between the insult and the onset of recurrent seizures may be a period of maladaptive changes that might be amenable to therapeutic manipulation. Although an attractive hypothesis, a unified picture of this process has yet to emerge. The most promising evidence has come from studies of tissue removed from patients undergoing temporal lobectomy and rodent models of limbic seizures.

In one experimental model hyperexcitability is induced by repeated stimulation of limbic structures, such as the amygdala or hippocampus. The initial stimulus is followed by an electrical response (the afterdischarge) that becomes more extensive and prolonged with repeated stimuli until a generalized seizure occurs. This process, called *kindling,* can be induced by electrical or chemical stimuli. Many investigators believe that kindling may contribute to the development of epilepsy in humans.

Kindling is thought to involve synaptic changes that resemble those important in learning and memory (see Chapter 65). These include short-term changes in excitability and persistent morphological changes, including axonal sprouting. Rearrangements of synaptic connections have been observed in the dentate gyrus of patients with long-standing focal seizures of hippocampal origin as well as following kindling in experimental animals (Figure 50–17). In addition

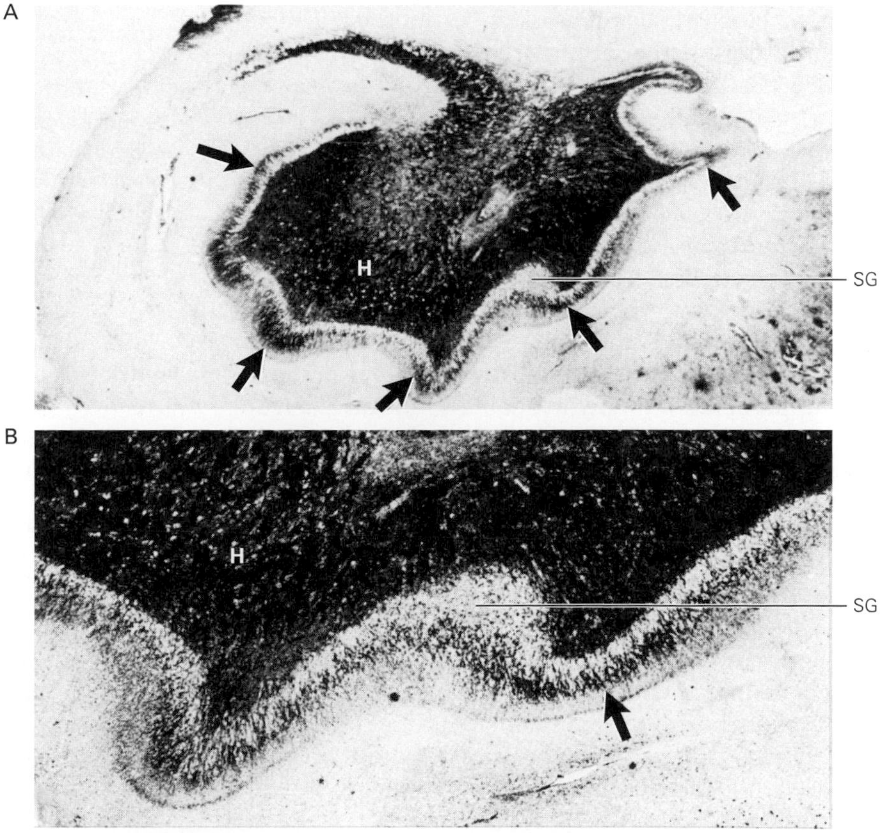

Figure 50–17 Mossy fiber synaptic reorganization (sprouting) in the human temporal lobe may cause hyperexcitability. (Reproduced, with permission, from Sutula et al. 1989.)

A. Timm stain of a transverse section of hippocampus removed from a patient at the time the temporal lobe was resected to control epilepsy. The stain appears black in the axons of the dentate granule cells (mossy fibers) because of the presence of zinc in these axons. The mossy fibers normally pass through the dentate hilus (**H**) on their way to synapse on CA3 pyramidal cells. In the epileptic tissue shown here stained fibers appear in the supragranular layer of the dentate gyrus (**SG**), which now contains not only the granule cell dendrites but also newly sprouted mossy fibers. These aberrant sprouts form new recurrent excitatory synapses on dentate granule cells.

B. This high magnification of a segment of the supragranular layer shows the Timm-stained mossy fibers in greater detail.

to axonal sprouting, changes include alterations in dendritic structure, control of transmitter release, and expression of ion channels and pumps.

The long-term changes that lead to epilepsy also are likely to involve specific patterns of gene expression. For example, the proto-oncogene c-*fos* and other immediate early genes as well as growth factors can be activated by seizures. Because many immediate early genes encode transcription factors that control other genes, the gene products that result from epileptiform activity could initiate a cascade of changes that contribute to the development of epilepsy by altering such mechanisms as cell fate, axon targeting, dendritic outgrowth, and synapse formation.

An Overall View

Seizures are one of the most dramatic examples of the collective electrical behavior of the mammalian brain. The distinctive clinical patterns of focal seizures and primary generalized seizures can be attributed to the different patterns of activity of cortical neurons. Studies of focal seizures in animals reveal a series of events—from the activity of neurons in the seizure focus to synchronization and subsequent spread of epileptiform activity throughout the cortex. The gradual loss of GABAergic surround inhibition is critical to the early steps in this progression. In contrast, generalized seizures are thought to arise from activity in thalamocortical circuits, perhaps combined with a general abnormality in the membrane excitability of cortical neurons.

The EEG has long provided a window on the electrical activity of the cortex, both in normal phases of arousal and during abnormal activities such as seizures. The EEG can be used to identify certain electrical activity patterns associated with seizures, but it provides limited insight into the pathophysiology of seizures. Several much more powerful and noninvasive approaches are now available to locate a seizure focus. These advances have led to the widespread and successful use of epilepsy surgery for selected patients, particularly those with focal seizures that originate in the hippocampus.

The increasing power of genetic, molecular, and modern cell-physiological techniques applied to the study of seizures and epilepsy gives new hope that this research will provide new therapeutic options for patients afflicted with epilepsy as well as new insights into the function of the mammalian brain. Further neurobiological studies of the progression from an acute seizure to the development of epilepsy should provide alternative strategies for treatment beyond the standard options of anticonvulsants or epilepsy surgery.

Gary L. Westbrook

Selected Readings

Berg AT, Berkovic SF, Brodie MJ, Buchhalter J, Cross JH, van Emde Boas W, Engel J, et al. 2010. Revised terminology and concepts for organization of seizures and epilepsy: report of the ILAE commission on classification and terminology, 2005-2009. Epilepsia 51:676–685.

Cascino GD. 2004. Surgical treatment for epilepsy. Epilepsy Res 60:179–186.

Chang BS, Lowenstein DH. 2003. Epilepsy. N Engl J Med 349:1257–1266.

Engel J. 1989. *Seizures and Epilepsy.* Philadelphia: Davis.

Jacobs MP, Fischbach GD, Davis MR, Dichter MA, Dingledine R, Lowenstein DH, Morrell MJ., et al. 2001. Future directions for epilepsy research. Neurology 57:1536–1542.

Lennox WG, Lennox MA. 1960. *Epilepsy and Related Disorders.* Boston: Little, Brown.

Lennox WG, Mattson RH. 2003. Overview: idiopathic generalized epilepsies. Epilepsia 44 Suppl 2:2–6.

Morrell MJ. 2011. Responsive cortical stimulation for the treatment of medically intractable partial epilepsy. Neurology 77:1729–1304.

Noebels JL. 2003. The biology of epilepsy genes. Annu Rev Neurosci 26:599–625.

Penfield W, Jasper H. 1954. *Epilepsy and the Functional Anatomy of the Human Brain.* Boston: Little, Brown.

Stables JP, Bertram EH, White HS, Coulter DA, Dichter MA, Jacobs MP, Loscher W, et al. 2002. Models for epilepsy and epileptogenesis: report from the NIH workshop. Epilepsia 43:1410–1420.

References

Biervert C, Schroeder BC, Kubisch C, Berkovic SF, Propping P, Jentsch TJ, Steinlein OK. 1998. A potassium channel mutation in neonatal human epilepsy. Science 279: 403–406.

Commission on Classification and Terminology of the International League Against Epilepsy. 1981. Proposal for revised clinical and electroencephalographic classification of epileptic seizures. Epilepsia 22:489–501.

Commission on the Classification and Terminology of the International League Against Epilepsy. 1985. Proposal for classification of epilepsies and epileptic syndromes. Epilepsia 26:268–278.

Epilepsy Phenome/Genome Project. Available at http://www.epgp.org.

George AL. 2004. Molecular basis of inherited epilepsy. Arch Neurol 61:473–478.

Haug K, Warnstedt M, Alekov AK, Sander T, Ramírez A, Poser B, Maljevic S, et al. 2003. Mutations in CLCN2 encoding a voltage-gated chloride channel are associated with idiopathic generalized epilepsies. Nat Genet 33:527–532.

Konnerth A. 1990. Patch-clamping in slices of mammalian CNS. Trends Neurosci 13:321–323.

Lothman EW. 1993a. The neurobiology of epileptiform discharges. Am J EEG Technol 33:93–112.

Lothman EW. 1993b. Pathophysiology of seizures and epilepsy in the mature and immature brain: cells, synapses and circuits. In: WE Dodson, JM Pellock (eds), *Pediatric Epilepsy: Diagnosis and Therapy,* pp. 1–15, New York: Demos Publications.

Lothman EW, Collins RC. 1990. Seizures and epilepsy. In: AL Pearlman, RC Collins (eds), *Neurobiology of Disease,* pp. 276–298, New York: Oxford Univ. Press.

Mulley JC, Scheffer IE, Harkin LA, Berkovic SF, Dibbens LM. 2005. Susceptibility genes for complex epilepsy. Hum Mol Genet 14:R243–R249.

Santhakumar V, Aradi S, Soltesz I. 2005. Role of mossy fiber sprouting and mossy cell loss in hyperexcitability: a network model of the dentate gyrus incorporating cell types and axonal topography. J Neurophysiol 93:437–463.

Spencer WA, Kandel ER. 1968. Cellular and integrative properties of the hippocampal pyramidal cell and the comparative electrophysiology of cortical neurons. Int J Neurol 6:266–296.

Steinlein OK, Mulley JC, Propping P, Wallace RH, Phillips HA, Sutherland GR, Scheffer IE, Berkovic SF. 1995. A missense mutation in the neuronal nicotinic acetylcholine receptor alpha 4 subunit is associated with autosomal dominant nocturnal frontal lobe epilepsy. Nat Genet 11:201–203.

Sutula T, Cascino G, Cavazos J, Parada I, Ramirez L. 1989. Mossy fiber synaptic reorganization in the epileptic human temporal lobe. Ann Neurol 26:321–330.

Teitelbaum J, Zatorre RJ, Carpenter S, Gendron S, Evans AC, Gjedde A, Cashman NR. 1990. Neurologic sequelae of domoic acid intoxication due to ingestion of contaminated mussels. N Engl J Med 322:1781–1787.

von Krosigk M, Bal T, McCormick DA. 1993. Cellular mechanisms of a synchronized oscillation in the thalamus. Science 261:361–364.

Walsh CA. 1999. Genetic malformations of the human cerebral cortex. Neuron 23:19–29.

Wiebe S, Blume WT, Girvin JP, Eliasziw M. 2001. Effectiveness and efficiency of surgery for temporal lobe epilepsy study. A randomized, controlled trial of surgery for temporal lobe epilepsy. N Engl J Med 14:211–216.

Winawer MR, Marini C, Grinton BE, Rabinowitz D, Berkovic SF, Scheffer IE, Ottman R. 2005. Familial clustering of seizure types within the idiopathic generalized epilepsies. Neurology 65:523–528.

Wong RKS, Miles R, Traub RD. 1984. Local circuit interactions in synchronization of cortical neurones. J Exp Biol 112:169–178.

51

Sleep and Dreaming

SLEEP IS A REMARKABLE STATE. It consumes fully a third of our lives—approximately 25 years in the average lifetime—yet most of us know little about this daily excursion into our inner world. Perhaps even more surprising, we are still hard pressed to give a *raison d'etre* for sleep.

The exact functions of sleep and of dreaming, one of the more spectacular components of sleep, have been debated over the ages and are still not known. Do dreams reveal some inner psychological functioning of unconscious mental processes, as Sigmund Freud first suggested, or are they merely the consequence of random firing of neurons in the brain? The psychic content of dreams has been a rich subject of speculation throughout history. Plato, anticipating Sigmund Freud, thought that all of us have a "terrible, fierce, and lawless blood of desires, which it seems are revealed in our sleep," whereas Aristotle believed that dreams are merely afterthoughts of the day's activities and experiences.

Although we have only limited understanding of the functions of sleep, our insight into its mechanisms has increased greatly over the past 50 years. We have moved away from the intuitively appealing but incorrect notion that sleep is a period of relative inactivity and rest—one that occurs reflexively in response to reduction of sensory input—to the current view that sleep is a highly organized state generated by the cooperative interplay of many behavioral and neural components. Although in many respects the biological function of sleep remains a mystery, we have begun to understand the cellular and molecular processes underlying sleep.

Sleep Consists of Alternating REM and Non-REM Periods

Sleep affects all of our bodily and mental functions, from the regulation of hormonal levels to muscle tone, from the regulation of respiration rate to the content of our thought processes. Given these important behavioral changes, it is not surprising that the brain's overall electrical activity changes significantly with sleep. During wakefulness the electroencephalogram (EEG) shows relatively low-voltage, high-frequency, fast activity, reflecting an active cerebral cortex busy with perception and cognition. Slow synchronized oscillatory activity is either at a minimum or occurs only transiently in small groups of neurons (Figure 51–1). Relaxing or closing the eyes may produce alpha waves, especially over the visual cortex, indicating relatively synchronous rhythmic activity in the underlying cortical networks.

To describe sleep quantitatively and to distinguish its stages, sleep researchers routinely use three measures: brain activity measured by the EEG (see Chapter 50), eye movements recorded by the electro-oculogram (EOG), and muscle tone measured by the electromyogram (EMG). These three measures are used because of their reliability, ease of recording, and discriminatory power.

Non-REM Sleep Has Four Stages

Based on these measures, sleep is subdivided into five stages. Stages 1 to 4 comprise non-rapid eye movement (REM) sleep, while stage 5 is REM sleep. *Stage 1 sleep* is the transition between waking and sleep, the period in which sleep is thought to be imminent but not yet developed. During stage 1 the EEG exhibits a decrease in the high-frequency activity that characterizes the waking state. *Stage 2*, the first true stage of sleep, is marked in the EEG by the onset of spindle waves, 7–15 Hz oscillations over a period of 1–2 seconds that resemble a spindle of thread, and K-complexes (Figure 51–1). Spindle waves and K-complexes reflect slow, synchronized oscillations of neuronal and synaptic activity within the thalamus and cerebral cortex. This state is the result of the relaxation and general hyperpolarization of neurons and neuronal networks that follow gradual inactivation of the brain mechanisms of arousal. During stage 2 sleep muscle tone decreases, and the eyes slowly roll back and forth. Respiration becomes more regular and slows (Figure 51–2), and body temperature begins to fall.

Stage 3 sleep is heralded in the EEG by the appearance of a significant fraction of delta wave oscillations (0.5–4 Hz). These signal a further reduction in arousal processes in the brain and increased synchronization of cortical and thalamic activity. A predominance of delta waves (> 50% of the time in the EEG) indicates that the person is in *stage 4 sleep*, the deepest stage. During stages 3 and 4 respiration continues to be slow and regular, heart rate slows, muscles relax, and temperature slowly drifts downward (Figure 51–2).

The progression from waking to stage 4 sleep at the beginning of the night typically occurs relatively quickly—over the first 30 minutes (Figure 51–1). After approximately 30 minutes in stage 4 sleep the sleeper ascends quickly through all four stages of sleep. Instead of waking, however, the sleeper now enters a unique stage known as rapid eye movement or REM sleep, a period in which dreams can become vivid, even bizarre.

Rapid eye movement (REM) sleep was discovered in 1953 when Eugene Aserinsky and Nathaniel Kleitman first recorded the EEG and EOG of sleeping adults and observed that during sleep these tests showed changes in activity approximately four to five times per night (changing to a state of higher frequency and lower amplitude similar to that of the waking state). During this "activated" period the eyes dart back and forth, thus giving this stage its name. Sleepers roused from REM sleep report experiencing vivid dreams approximately 80% to 95% of the time.

Interestingly, REM sleep is associated with an almost complete loss of muscle tone, owing to inhibition of the spinal motor neurons by descending pathways. Apparently the motor neurons in the brain stem that control eye movements are not inhibited, because the eyes move during REM sleep. During REM sleep temperature regulation is at a low point, and body temperature begins to fall further still.

Although sleep can be segregated into five stages, the REM stage is so distinctive that sleep is often separated into two phases, referred to simply as REM and non-REM (or NREM) sleep. The cycle of sleep—the non-REM sequence from stage 1 to stage 4 and the reverse sequence followed by a brief period of REM sleep—occurs repeatedly during the night, in a pattern that is best described as a damped oscillation. As the night progresses, the depth of non-REM sleep decreases and the duration spent in REM sleep increases (Figure 51–1). As a result of this pattern, and the fact that it is necessary to wake up to remember your dreams, the dreams that take place in the morning are the ones most often remembered.

REM and Non-REM Dreams Are Different

In adults REM sleep occupies approximately 25% of the total sleep time. Most people would be surprised

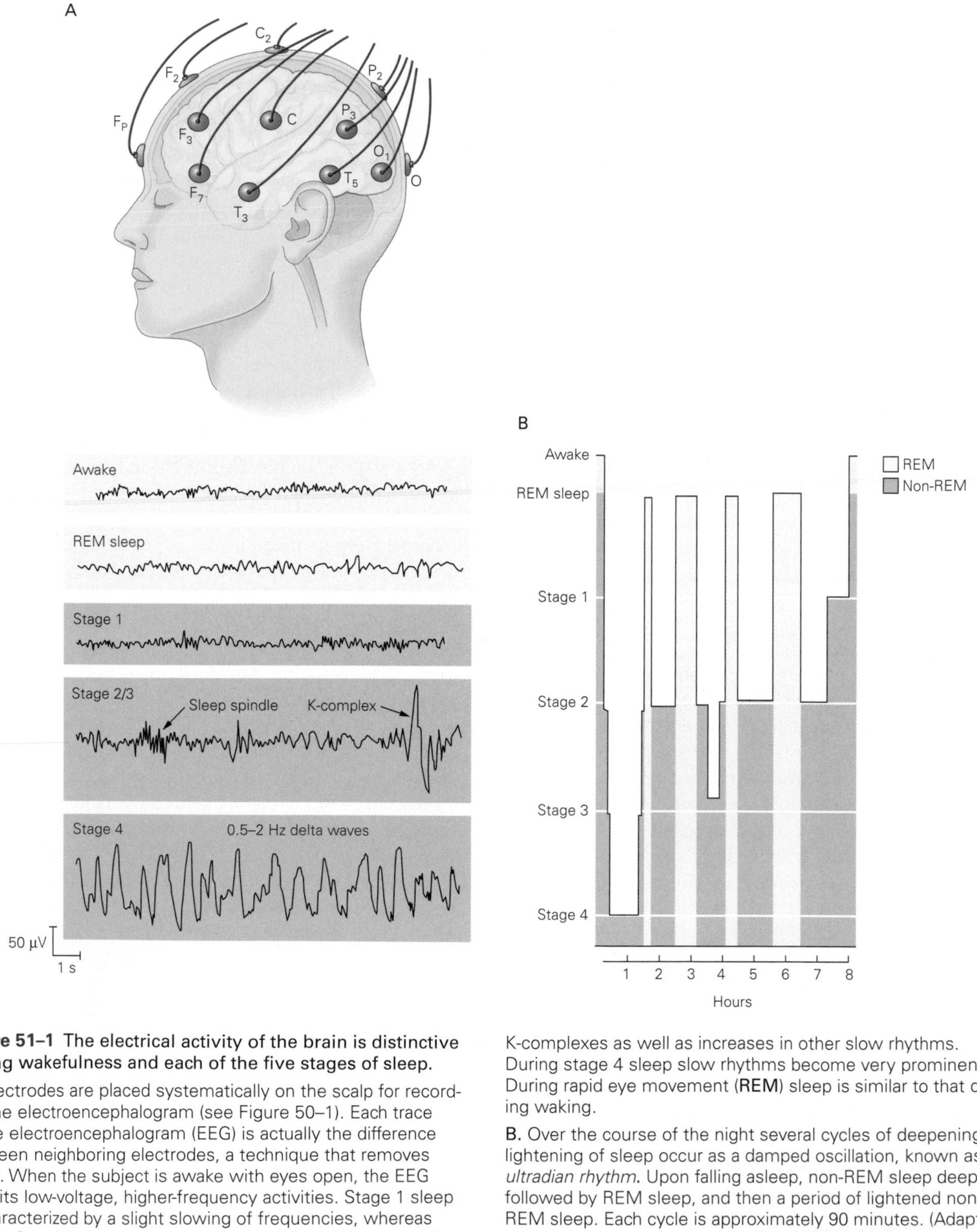

Figure 51–1 The electrical activity of the brain is distinctive during wakefulness and each of the five stages of sleep.

A. Electrodes are placed systematically on the scalp for recording the electroencephalogram (see Figure 50–1). Each trace of the electroencephalogram (EEG) is actually the difference between neighboring electrodes, a technique that removes noise. When the subject is awake with eyes open, the EEG exhibits low-voltage, higher-frequency activities. Stage 1 sleep is characterized by a slight slowing of frequencies, whereas stages 2 and 3 sleep are characterized by spindle waves and K-complexes as well as increases in other slow rhythms. During stage 4 sleep slow rhythms become very prominent. During rapid eye movement (**REM**) sleep is similar to that during waking.

B. Over the course of the night several cycles of deepening and lightening of sleep occur as a damped oscillation, known as the *ultradian rhythm*. Upon falling asleep, non-REM sleep deepens, followed by REM sleep, and then a period of lightened non-REM sleep. Each cycle is approximately 90 minutes. (Adapted, with permission, from Purves et al. 1997 and 2004.)

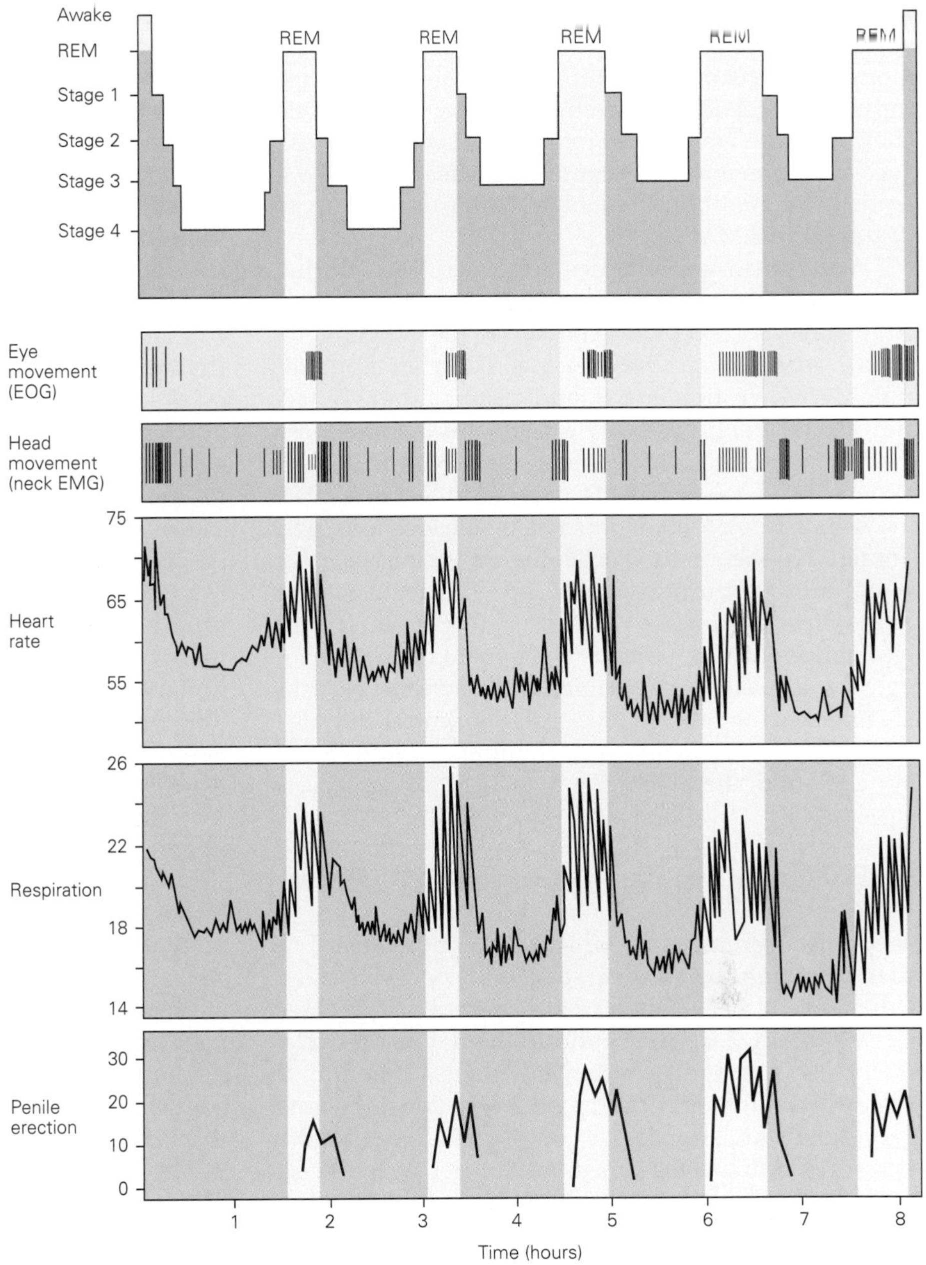

Figure 51–2 Physiological changes during sleep. Sleep consists of several cycles between stages 1 and 4 and rapid eye movement (**REM**) sleep. As sleep deepens, eye movements become less prominent; movements of the head, heart rate, and respiration all decrease. As the level of sleep lightens, these trends reverse. During REM sleep heart rate and respiration increase, as does penile erection. Neck movements can occur just before and after an episode of REM sleep, whereas during REM sleep muscle tone is very low. (**EOG**, electrooculogram; **EMG**, electromyogram.) (Adapted, with permission, from Purves et al. 2004.)

to find that they had vivid dreams for approximately 2 hours every night. Indeed, the inability to remember dreams (unless awakened) is one of the great mysteries of sleep.

Analysis of dreams and their content have revealed some surprising results. Most people believe that dreams are only occasional and fleeting occurrences of highly bizarre or emotional content, in which the entire scenario is dreamt in an instant. In reality, specific dreams recur with a regular and predictable periodicity, and mostly reflect everyday events. Even the fleeting nature of dreams is a misperception. Events in dreams occur over a period of time that is about as long as they would in real time. Only a small percentage of dreams contain bizarre and fantastic elements.

Dreams occur in both REM and non-REM sleep but the characteristics of REM and non-REM dreams differ. REM dreams are relatively long, primarily visual, somewhat emotional, and usually not connected to the immediate events of the everyday life of the dreamer. These resemble what Freud referred to as the latent content of the dream. Non-REM dreams are shorter, less visual, less emotional, more conceptual, and usually related to the current life of the dreamer. They resemble what Freud referred to as the day's residues, or the manifest content of the dream. This conceptual, "thought-like" mentation can occupy up to 50% of non-REM sleep.

What sensory modalities are experienced during dreams in REM sleep? Vision is preeminent, occurring in all dreams (except, of course, in the congenitally blind), whereas auditory events occur in approximately 65%, vestibular 8%, and temperature 4%; tactile, olfactory, and gustatory experiences are rare (only 1% each). The emotional content of dreams varies from anxiety (14%), to surprise (9%), joy (7%), sadness (5%), and shame (2%). Men experience penile erections, and women experience the physiological counterparts of sexual arousal during REM sleep. The regularity of penile erection during REM sleep (Figure 51–2) can help determine if impotence in a patient has a psychological or physiological origin. The emotional content is organized at several levels of the central nervous system but is, for the most part, unrelated to the specific content of the dream.

Sleep Obeys Circadian and Ultradian Rhythms

Sleep is a circadian behavior that is composed of cyclical or ultradian stages. In all species the period of sleep is dictated by the rotation of the earth and time clues (German, *zeitgebers*) that indicate the day-night cycle. The principal zeitgeber is the daily rising of the sun. It was once thought that the circadian rhythms of plants and animals are strongly or completely driven by the rising and setting of the sun. However, in 1729 the Swiss astronomer Jean-Jacques d'Ortous de Mairan observed that even in the dark the leaves of plants move according to a diurnal cycle. Since then endogenous rhythms of about 24 hours (ie, circadian rhythms) have been found to be prevalent throughout the plant and animal kingdoms. Circadian rhythms seem to have evolved so as to maximize the use of the day-night cycle by anticipating the rising and setting of the sun, even without clear signals from sunlight or other zeitgebers.

The features of the circadian rhythm of sleep in human beings, in the absence of zeitgebers, has been documented by a few brave individuals willing to live in isolation in specially constructed rooms in labs or caves. These rooms contain no clues as to the time of day in the outside world—no clocks, windows, radios, televisions, e-mail, Internet, or sounds that would tell subjects the time in the outside world. Under these conditions subjects were allowed to sleep and be active whenever their body dictated. Interestingly, the circadian rhythm persists, but its duration varies among subjects and is typically slightly longer (eg, 25 hours) than that of the normal day-night cycle, causing each person in isolation to slowly drift out of phase with the outside environment. Reexposure to the external day-night cycle rapidly resets the sleep-wake cycles (Figure 51–3A).

The sleep-wake cycle is not the only circadian rhythm in the body. Many other physiological processes also exhibit daily maximums and minimums. The level of arousal, the ability to do cognitive tasks such as math problems, body temperature, hormone release, and kidney function all follow endogenous 24-hour rhythms that normally are synchronized to the day-night cycle.

How do sleep and other circadian rhythms become synchronized to the day-night cycle? A small number of retinal ganglion cells (see Chapter 26) respond directly to light and project to the suprachiasmatic nucleus in the hypothalamus (Figure 51–3B). It is this pathway, described in detail later, that synchronizes the circadian rhythmicity with the day-night cycle. Although rare, some people with tumors or lesions of the hypothalamus lose the circadian rhythmicity of their sleep-wake cycle and therefore sleep for short periods throughout the day. Other people, equally rare, have a normal circadian rhythm in their sleep-wake cycle but are unable to synchronize it with the day-night cycle of their environment. The phase relationship between their own endogenous need to sleep, and the time of day, changes continually. Perhaps in these people the neural path conveying light information to the suprachiasmatic nucleus is defective.

Jet lag demonstrates other properties of our circadian rhythm. Travel to a distant time zone disrupts the synchrony of one's circadian rhythm with the day-night cycle. One may temporarily experience excessive sleepiness during the day, hunger at the wrong times, cold despite being in a warm environment, and awakenings in the middle of the night despite sleep deprivation. This feeling of being "out of phase" is common and has a physiological basis. Flying west is generally easier than flying east, presumably because our endogenous rhythm is approximately 25 hours. When flying west we take advantage of this long rhythm by staying up late and sleeping in. Indeed, many individuals practice this on a weekly basis—staying up late and sleeping in on the weekend. The jarring experience of the "Monday morning blues" results from a rapid shift in the

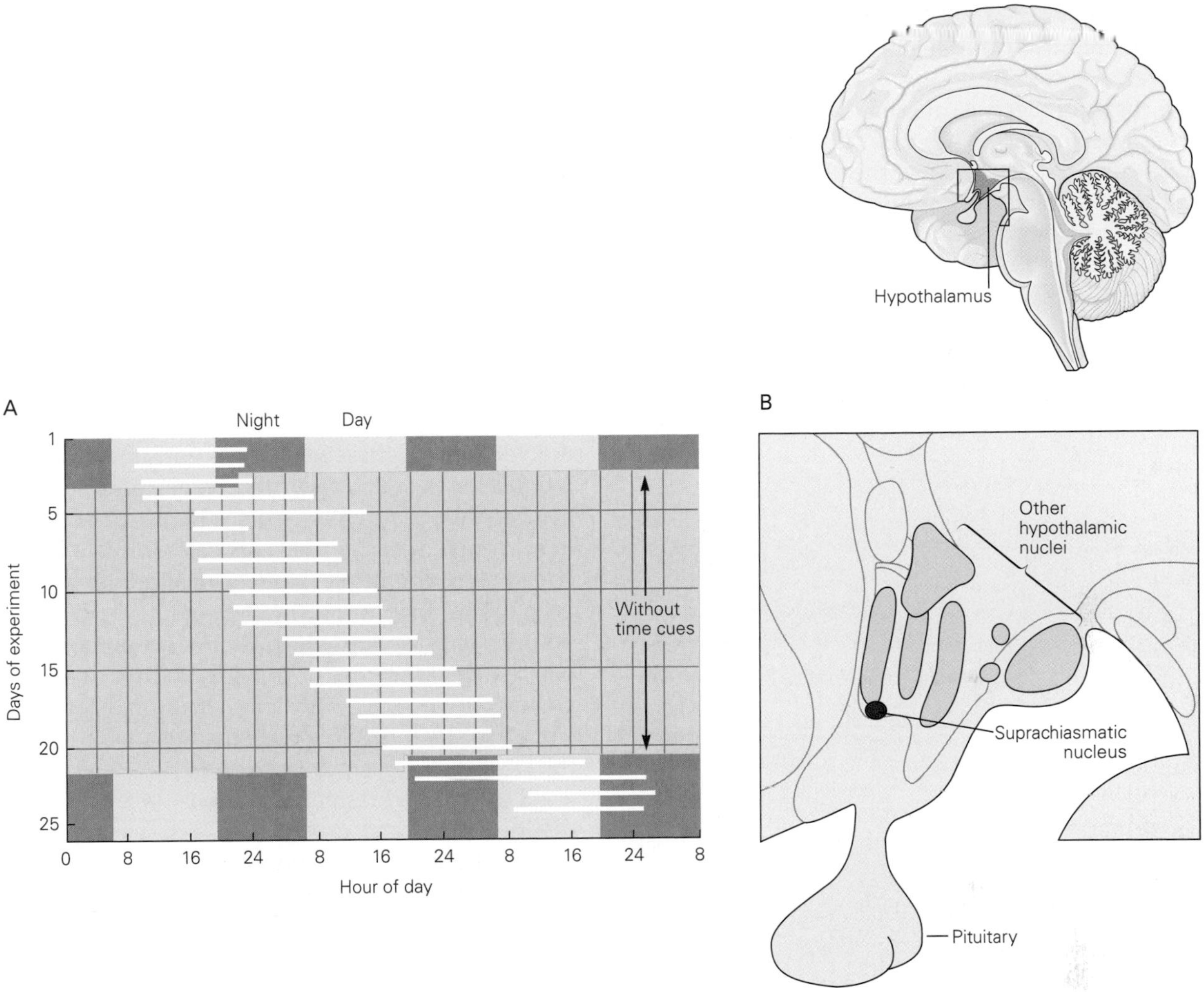

Figure 51–3 The endogenous circadian rhythm of sleep in humans.

A. A human volunteer isolated in an underground bunker is initially exposed to a normal day-night cycle and exhibits a circadian period of wakefulness (**white bar**) that is synchronized with the day-night cycle. However, following removal of external cues (after day 3) the volunteer's circadian cycle lengthens from 24 hours to approximately 26 hours (days 4–21). Because the endogenous cycle of the volunteer is longer than that of the normal day-night cycle, the period of wakefulness slowly drifts out of phase. Following reintroduction of environmental cues to the normal day-night cycle, the subject's periods of wakefulness once again become synchronized to the day-night cycle. (Adapted, with permission, from Aschoff 1965.)

B. The suprachiasmatic nucleus in the hypothalamus is the master circadian clock of the nervous system. (Adapted, with permission, from Purves et al. 1997.)

circadian cycle and perhaps a bit of sleep deprivation thrown in as well.

Sleepiness—the drive to sleep—depends on several factors. Two of the strongest are the time since the last full period of sleep and the circadian rhythm. We therefore can think of the drive to sleep as two separate processes: a "sleep deficit" that slowly builds up without sleep and dissipates with sleep, and a circadian rhythmicity in arousal. The difference between these processes reflects the sleep drive. After a full night of sleep the sleep deficit should be very low. In the morning our level of arousal slowly increases as does our sleep deficit. Because sleep deficit and alertness increase together, the difference between these two processes—the drive to sleep—is small and therefore weak. Toward evening, however, our sleep deficit continues to increase, and the circadian rhythm of arousal begins to wane, resulting in a larger and larger sleep drive (Figure 51–4A). Sleeping a full night once again removes the sleep debt, and the process starts over.

If a night of sleep is missed, one is likely to find that at approximately 3–4 a.m. it is nearly impossible to stay awake. This is because the sleep deficit is high and continues to increase, while the circadian rhythm in arousal (and other body functions such as temperature) is at a low point. Thus the sleep drive is high (Figure 51–4B). Sleep once again restores the balance, relieving this built-up sleep pressure.

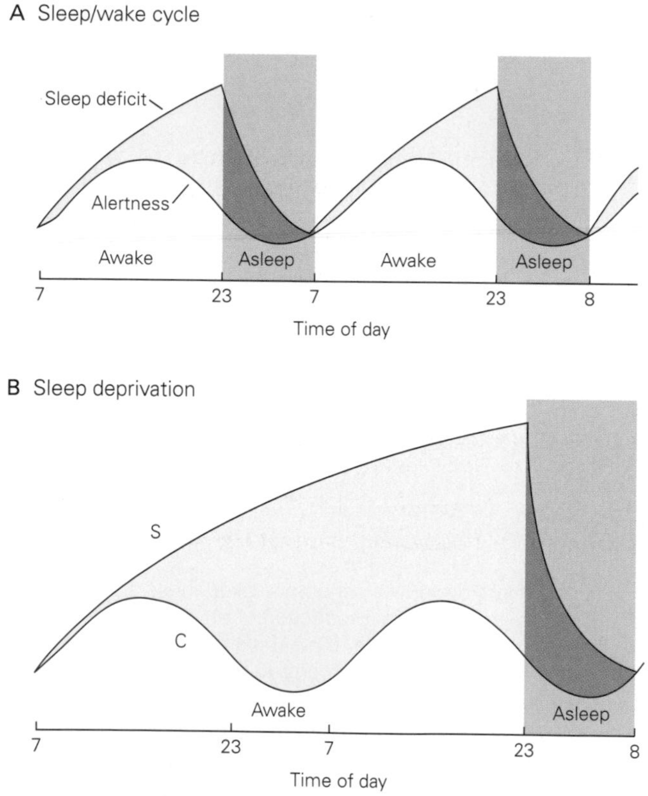

Figure 51–4 Hypothetical model of the circadian rhythmicity of the sleep drive. The difference between two interacting circadian processes—alertness and sleep deficit—determines sleep drive. (Adapted, with permission, from Daan et al. 1984.)

A. During a normal sleep-wake cycle the drive to sleep (**yellow**) accumulates during the day and declines during sleep (**blue**) such that the desire to sleep is greatest at bedtime and least on wakening.

B. Missing a night of sleep results in a continual build up of the sleep deficit (**curve S**) while the endogenous circadian rhythm of arousal (**curve C**) persists. As a result, over the period of wakefulness the sleep drive (the difference between S and C curves) varies. It is greatest in the middle of the night of missed sleep as well as at normal bedtime on the second evening.

The Circadian Rhythm Clock Is Based on a Cyclic Production of Nuclear Transcription Factors

The search for the neural basis of circadian rhythmicity of sleep has led to one site, the suprachiasmatic nucleus (Figure 51–3B), so named because of its location just above the optic chiasm, the place where the optic nerves cross underneath the hypothalamus.

The firing frequency of neurons in the suprachiasmatic nucleus follows an endogenous circadian rhythm (see Figure 51–6C). Thus the 20,000 neurons in the suprachiasmatic nucleus make up the master clock for circadian rhythms. They are the critical pacemaker for organizing sleep into a circadian pattern. The circadian activity of these neurons is entrained by environmental stimuli such as light, as measured by release of the transmitter vasopressin (see Figure 51–6C). Lesioning this nucleus in animals causes complete loss of the circadian rhythmicity of sleep-wake cycles. Animals with these lesions continue to have a normal daily amount of sleep, but sleep occurs randomly throughout the day and night. Transplantation of the suprachiasmatic nucleus from another animal can restore a circadian sleep rhythm, with the host animal adopting the sleep-wake cycle of the donor.

The suprachiasmatic nucleus is organized into distinct functional groups and acts as the controller for the rhythmic oscillations of clocks located in other organs in the body. These "peripheral" clocks are capable of maintaining their own circadian rhythms for only a few days without input from the suprachiasmatic nucleus.

Like a grandfather clock, the biological clocks that control circadian rhythms have many parts: A complex set of transcription factors, proteins, kinases, phosphatases, and regulatory molecules that have been remarkably conserved throughout the evolution of species. A number of molecules that play key roles in the clock mechanism have been identified over the last 20 years, largely from experiments in the fruit fly *Drosophila* and the mouse. The essence of the clock mechanism in the suprachiasmatic nucleus, as well as in other organs, is a pair of transcriptional feedback loops; one forms the core circadian mechanism whereas a second forms a modulatory loop that stabilizes the circadian rhythm. Such interlocking feedback loops are quite similar in flies and mammals (see Chapter 3).

At the center of the two loops are two transcriptional activators, CLOCK and BMAL1. These transcription factors bind to each other and form a heterodimer that enhances transcription of the mouse gene *per* (*mPer1–3*) and cryptochrome genes (*mCry1–2*), thereby increasing the cytoplasmic concentrations of the PER and CRY proteins. PER and CRY form heterodimers, reenter the nucleus, and inhibit CLOCK and BMAL1, thus repressing PER and CRY transcription. This sequence creates the core circadian mechanism in which *Bmal1* RNA reaches a peak 12 hours out of phase with *mPer* and *mCry* RNA. CLOCK and BMAL1 are also at the center of the modulatory loop that modifies the levels of CLOCK/BMAL1 heterodimers. Mutations in genes in the stabilizing loop do not disrupt circadian rhythms to the same degree as those in the core loop.

Once the central clock in the suprachiasmatic nucleus generates the rhythm and the environmental light-dark cycle synchronizes it, this information must be communicated to various systems through humoral or electrical signals. To achieve this, the rhythmic molecular signal is transduced into electrical activity in suprachiasmatic nucleus neurons and then transmitted to other brain regions through action potentials.

A number of areas in the hypothalamus receive input from the suprachiasmatic nucleus and play a role in integrating the output of the suprachiasmatic nucleus. For example, a large number of axons from the suprachiasmatic nucleus terminate in the dorsal and ventral subparaventricular zones of the hypothalamus. The dorsal subparaventricular zone appears to project to areas that are important for circadian rhythms of body temperature, whereas the ventral subparaventricular zone and the downstream dorsomedial nucleus of the hypothalamus are important in the sleep-wake cycle. The dorsomedial nucleus may serve as a common final pathway for a number of circadian rhythms as lesions of this nucleus interrupt circadian rhythms for feeding, locomotion, and corticosteroid secretion as well as the sleep-wake cycle.

The Ultradian Rhythm of Sleep Is Controlled by the Brain Stem

Our level of arousal can best be described by a circadian cycle of sleep and wakefulness, and an ultradian rhythm in the sleep period consisting of a damped oscillation between non-REM and REM periods (Figure 51–1B). Although the suprachiasmatic nucleus is critical to the generation and synchronization of circadian rhythms, it is not the generator of sleep and arousal, for animals without a functional suprachiasmatic nucleus continue to exhibit these states.

The search for brain structures essential for arousal and for the ultradian rhythm of sleep focused on the brain stem and hypothalamus. In 1949 Horace Magoun and Giuseppe Moruzzi demonstrated that electrical stimulation of anterior portions of the brain stem results in arousal of the forebrain (see Chapter 46). They dubbed this afferent pathway the "ascending activating system." This pathway in concert with portions of the hypothalamus appears to be responsible for maintaining the waking state. By cutting the brain at different levels, Michel Jouvet in France and others localized the neuronal groups needed to generate the brain activation, muscle atonia, and rapid eye movements of REM sleep to a restricted region of the pons and medulla.

Putting the two findings together it became clear that the brain stem is a central organizer for the control of arousal as well as the other components of REM sleep. For example, chemical stimulation of particular portions of the brain stem can cause a state similar to REM sleep, complete with activation of the EEG and muscle atonia (because of descending inhibition of spinal motor neurons). Lesions of the same region can result in an animal that lacks the muscle atonia of naturally occurring REM sleep, resulting in an animal that acts out its dreams. Similarly, persons with REM behavior disorder, an unusual sleep disorder in humans, become physically active during REM sleep.

Although the precise neuronal circuits generating the circadian and ultradian rhythms of sleep and arousal are not known, we do know some of the major cellular components. Many cholinergic neurons within the brain stem and basal forebrain fire in anticipation of either waking or REM sleep. These cholinergic neurons in turn project throughout the forebrain, including the thalamus, cerebral cortex, and hippocampus. The release of acetylcholine (ACh) depolarizes, and therefore activates, many of these target cells.

Noradrenergic and serotonergic neurons of the brain stem and histaminergic neurons of the hypothalamus also project widely throughout the nervous system and modulate neuronal excitability during different phases of the sleep-wake cycle. These cells fire in anticipation of the waking state and maintain a regular, almost pacemaker-like, discharge rate throughout waking. The discharge rate of the noradrenergic cells increases in response to novel stimuli, while that of the serotonergic cells increases in response to changes in blood pH. Finally, the ventral lateral preoptic nucleus of the anterior hypothalamus includes cells that inhibit ascending activating networks, thus promoting sleep.

Although the rate of firing of noradrenergic, serotonergic, and histaminergic neurons increases in anticipation of and during the waking state, it decreases ahead of REM sleep and may even become completely silent. These cells are therefore known as REM-OFF cells. Other neurons, some of which are cholinergic, discharge in anticipation of and during the period of REM sleep and are known as REM-ON cells (Figure 51–5).

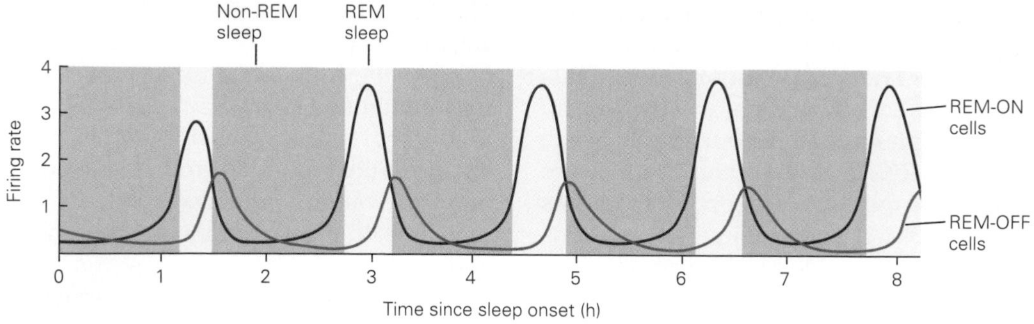

Figure 51–5 Firing rate of brain stem neurons involved in the onset and offset of REM sleep. Certain cholinergic neurons (**red line**) in the brain stem discharge strongly during periods of REM sleep but less so during non-REM sleep and thus are known as REM-ON cells. In contrast, certain noradrenergic and serotonergic cells (**blue line**) become almost completely silent near the onset of REM sleep and then reach their maximum activity at the offset of each REM period and therefore are known as REM-OFF cells. (Adapted, with permission, from McCarley and Massaquoi 1986.)

Presumably, the discharge of these REM-ON cells is responsible for the activation of the forebrain during REM sleep. Interestingly, the final step of Otto Loewi's experiment demonstrating that ACh is a chemical transmitter came to him in a dream. Thus ACh participated in its own discovery.

The cyclicity of REM and non-REM sleep can be modeled as an antagonistic interaction between REM-OFF (histaminergic, noradrenergic, and serotonergic) cells and REM-ON (cholinergic) cells.

During REM sleep phasic bursts of action potentials occur throughout the forebrain in association with rapid eye movements. These bursts of activity are strongest within the pontine and geniculate nuclei and the occipital (visual) cortex and therefore are known as ponto-geniculate-occipital (PGO) waves. These waves appear to be initiated by the phasic discharge of brain stem cholinergic neurons; the activation of nicotinic ACh receptors on cells in the forebrain results in a rapid depolarization of the postsynaptic cells. During waking PGO waves may result from activation of brain stem mechanisms mediating shifts in attention associated with eye movements.

Sleep-Related Activity in the EEG Is Generated Through Local and Long-Range Circuits

Sleep is associated with characteristic patterns of activity in the EEG. Non-REM sleep is dominated by sleep spindles, appearing as 1–2 second periods of 7–14 Hz waxing and waning oscillations, and delta (0.5–4 Hz) or slower (< 1 Hz) oscillations. How and where are these EEG rhythms generated?

Slices of forebrain isolated from the rest of the brain can generate activity similar to that which occurs during sleep. For example, thin slices of either the thalamus or the cerebral cortex generate spontaneous activity that resembles the EEG rhythms of non-REM sleep (Figure 51–6). Thus at least some of the spontaneous firing patterns of the forebrain during non-REM sleep result from local neuronal networks alone, without requiring external modulatory input. These firing patterns reflect the basal, or resting, state of the forebrain when it is relieved of the barrage of neurotransmitters from other structures in the waking state and REM sleep.

In fact the progression from waking to stage 1 to stage 4 sleep is the consequence of a gradual withdrawal of modulatory neurotransmitters, allowing forebrain neurons to gradually hyperpolarize and shift into the basal state and the generation of the slow EEG-rhythms of non-REM sleep. Once the activity of these neurons becomes slow and synchronized, cognitive function is reduced or abolished. The observation that waking and REM sleep are active states that must be maintained by ongoing activity in modulatory pathways fits well with our intuitive notion of sleep. We isolate ourselves from stimuli and relax into a hopefully blissful repose.

The purpose, if any, of rhythmic brain activity during sleep is not yet known. It may merely be the expression of the system properties of neural circuits that are idle during sleep. Or rhythmic activity may serve to keep cells active without the brain being sensitive to external stimuli. This activity could tune or recalibrate the brain during sleep—allowing useless information to be forgotten and important facts to be retained.

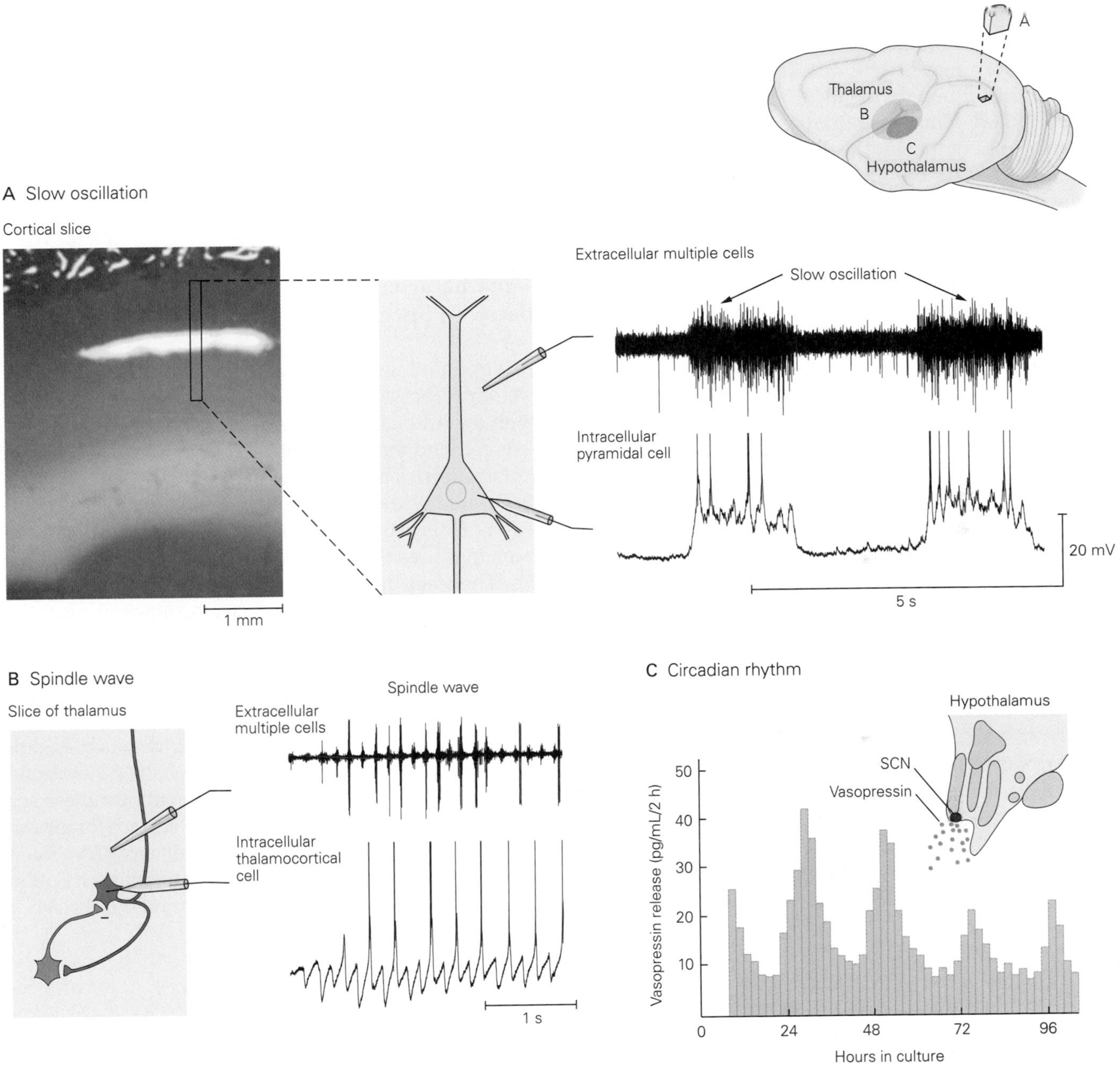

Figure 51–6 Cellular mechanisms of electroencephalogram rhythm generation during sleep.

A. The slow oscillation that underlies the slow waves of the EEG in vivo typically occurs during slow-wave sleep and is generated by the massively recurrent excitatory and inhibitory networks of the cerebral cortex. The slow oscillation is evident in vitro in extracellular recordings from a number of cortical cells made simultaneously with an intracellular recording of a single pyramidal cell. The picture of a cortical slice shows the sites of cell recordings. (Reproduced, with permission, from Sanchez-Vives and McCormick 2000.)

B. A spindle wave is evident in vitro in extracellular recordings from a number of cells made simultaneously with the intracellular recording of a single thalamocortical cell in a slice of the thalamus. This pattern of activity typically originates in the thalamus during slow-wave sleep and is transmitted to the cerebral cortex, where it appears in the EEG (see Figure 51–1A). Spindle waves are generated exclusively by the interaction of thalamic excitatory and inhibitory circuits. (Reproduced, with permission, from von Krosigk et al. 1993.)

C. A circadian rhythm is maintained in vitro as evidenced by rhythmic release of vasopressin from neurons in the isolated suprachiasmatic nucleus (**SCN**), demonstrating that these neurons have endogenous mechanisms for timing the 24-hour cycle. (Reproduced, with permission, from Earnest and Sladek 1987.)

Sleep Changes with Age

Sleep shows striking and characteristic changes with age. As every new parent quickly learns, the sleep of a newborn, although plentiful (16–18 hours a day), is distributed almost randomly throughout the day. What the parent may not realize, however, is that more than 50% (8–9 hours) of that sleep is spent in a REM-like state (Figure 51–7).

Sleep recordings from a premature infant exhibit an even higher percentage of REM sleep, indicating that in utero the fetus spends a large fraction of the day in a brain-activated but movement-inhibited state. As neuronal activity influences the development of functional circuits in the brain, it is reasonable to think that the spontaneous activity of the immature brain during sleep facilitates the development of circuits.

By approximately 4 months of age the average baby begins to show diurnal rhythms that are synchronized with day and night, much to the relief of weary parents. The total duration of sleep gradually declines, however, so that by 3 to 5 years of age the child may sleep 10 to 12 hours a day. At these early ages sleep is deep; stages 3 and 4 are prominent, with an abundance of delta waves in the EEG. As a result, children are not easily wakened by environmental stimuli.

Even though children ages 3 to 5 years may spend a large percent of their sleep in REM sleep, only approximately 33% of awakenings result in recall of dreams. These dream reports are brief, and contain virtually no story, self-representation, or interaction between the characters in the dream. However, by the age of 7 to 9 years the dream reports take on more of the qualities of those of adults, including the ability to analyze, abstract, manipulate, and construct visuospatial images or ideas. The content of dreams parallels the development of cognitive skills in the dreamer.

With age, sleep becomes less deep and more fragmented. The percent of time spent in stages 3 and 4 of non-REM sleep may drop dramatically, especially in old age. This results in a significant decrease in the perceived quality of sleep and an increase in daytime sleepiness. Disorders of sleep, such as insomnia and sleep apnea, also become more prevalent with age.

The Characteristics of Sleep Vary Greatly Between Species

Although all animals have circadian rest periods, the similarity between these and human sleep decreases with evolutionary distance. Nevertheless, some scientists contend that all animals, from fruit flies to man, do in fact sleep. The duration of sleep and the behaviors associated with it vary widely between species. Sleep seems essential to life, but its precise features have been modified to fit the requirements of each species.

The sleep habits of more than 90 mammals have been studied. Some sleep in well-protected burrows (eg, moles and rabbits), whereas others sleep in the open in herds. Giraffes sleep only approximately two hours a day, cats sleep approximately 13 hours, and the brown bat sleeps almost 20 hours. Some mammals (eg, cattle) sleep with their eyes open. Some, such as dolphins and porpoises, sleep with only half of their brain at a time. Presumably this adaptation allows these sea mammals to continually swim to the surface for air. All mammals have clearly recognizable non-REM sleep and nearly all have REM sleep. One notable exception is the spiny anteater, which has only non-REM sleep.

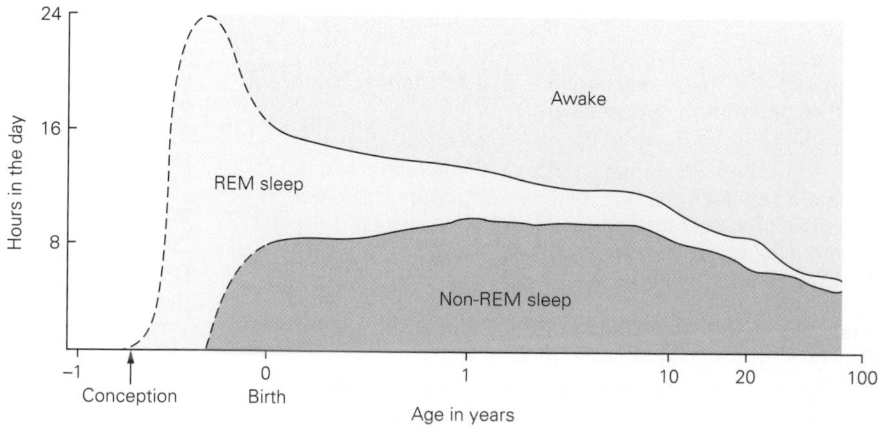

Figure 51–7 The amount of time spent each day in waking, REM sleep, and non-REM sleep changes over life. The proportion of the day spent in sleep decreases with age, with a particularly dramatic decrease in REM sleep during the first few years of life. The time spent in different sleep periods before birth is not well known, although data from premature infants suggest that babies in utero spend a large percentage of their time in a REM-like state. (Adapted, with permission, from Hobson 1989.)

Birds also have REM and non-REM sleep, although during REM sleep they do not lose muscle tone completely, allowing them to remain perched. A state resembling non-REM sleep is recognizable in reptiles, amphibians, and fish, although REM sleep is not evident.

Nocturnal animals are active at night, exploiting an ecological niche, and sleep during the daylight. Other species, such as humans, make use of the abundant sunlight during the day and are diurnal.

Sleep Disorders Have Behavioral, Psychological, and Neurological Causes

More than half of the population experiences significant difficulties with sleep at least on occasion, and as many as one in five persons suffers from chronic sleep problems. Disruption of sleep and waking is the most prevalent health disorder in the United States. Falling asleep while driving, for example, is thought to be responsible for at least 100,000 traffic accidents every year. Lack of sleep was a contributing factor in the disasters at the Three Mile Island and Chernobyl nuclear power plants.

Millions of people struggle through daily life sleepy, and many are irritable or unmotivated owing to disruptions in sleep. As a result, sleep disorders are common in general medical practice. Most sleep problems have mundane causes and may simply require a change in habit. Others involve complicating factors such as shift work, depression, or substance abuse. Some sleep disorders now provide new insights into brain function.

As sleep is organized into several cyclical, roughly 90-minute periods of REM and non-REM sleep, each component can be disrupted. The most common disorders are related to a breakdown in the transition between sleep and waking, such as difficulty falling asleep or early morning wakening. More than half of adults experience insomnia at some point each year. Their sleep is either too short, difficult to obtain, or not refreshing. The lack of adequate or fulfilling sleep often leads to another common complaint: daytime sleepiness.

Other sleep disorders may represent a breakdown in specific neural circuits. For example, sudden activation of the inhibitory descending motor pathways during the waking state can lead to bouts of cataplexy (loss of muscle tone), which is often associated with narcolepsy (described below). The opposite can also happen. In REM behavior disorder the descending inhibitory motor pathways do not function during REM sleep, such that the affected individual may jump up and move about during vivid dreams.

In other sleep disorders circadian rhythmicity may fail, resulting in a phase advance or phase delay in the sleep-wake cycle. Finally, sleep may be associated with inappropriate or unwanted behaviors such as night terrors, sleep walking, tooth grinding, bed wetting, and so on. These unusual behaviors disrupt sleep and are collectively known as *parasomnias*.

Insomnia Is the Most Common Form of Sleep Disruption

Insomnia, the most common form of sleep disruption, can be prolonged and severe or temporary and mild, as in response to short-term stress. The incidence of insomnia increases with age and is more common in women. Insomnia can manifest as difficulty falling asleep, difficulty staying asleep through the night, or early morning awakening before sufficient sleep is obtained. Insomnia may result from physical or emotional complications or simply from poor sleep habits (eg, consumption of excessive caffeine, alcohol, or food, or exercising vigorously before sleep). Insomnia is often associated with depression where early morning awakening is common.

Benzodiazepines, commonly used as anxiolytics (mild tranquilizers), are also commonly used for short-term treatment of insomnia. Benzodiazepines facilitate the opening of $GABA_A$ (γ-aminobutyric acid type A) receptor-channels through a binding site separate from that for GABA. Although these drugs facilitate sleep, they also suppress stage 4 sleep. Chronic use may be habit-forming and lead to a lightening and fragmentation of sleep. A related compound, zolpidem (sold under the trade name Ambien), binds selectively to a subset of benzodiazepine receptors, does not suppress deep sleep, and is considered relatively selective for facilitating sleep. It is therefore safer than general benzodiazepines for treatment of insomnia.

Over-the-counter sleep aids are often antihistamines (H_1 histamine receptor antagonists). Antihistamines are sedative in some individuals because they antagonize the activation of H_1 receptors, which normally excite thalamic and other central neurons. Muscarinic ACh receptor antagonists also have sedative effects, although these vary between individuals. Anticholinergic actions are common to many psychoactive drugs, such as tricyclic antidepressants, and therefore these drugs are used for insomnia. As discussed earlier, activation of muscarinic ACh receptors in the brain has a general arousal effect by exciting the principal neurons and, in some parts of the brain, by inhibiting GABAergic inhibitory interneurons.

Excessive Daytime Sleepiness Is Indicative of Disrupted Sleep

Sleepiness during the day is the primary complaint of individuals seeking help at hospital sleep centers. The invention of electric lights has allowed people to stay active well into the night. The increasing demands of work, family, and social life along with ever increasing opportunities for entertainment have led to a dramatic shortening in the time spent asleep, from an average of 10 to approximately 7 hours.

This trend has led to a chronic sleep deficit in the average adult that affects not only mood and general feelings of well being, but also work or school performance. Sleep deficit can be dangerous, as when driving or operating machinery. Telltale signs of insufficient sleep include unusually short sleep-onset latencies (less than 15 minutes), the need to sleep in on weekends, overuse of stimulants such as caffeine, and dependence on an alarm clock to wake up in the morning.

Excessive daytime sleepiness is a symptom of several underlying sleep disorders including sleep apnea, narcolepsy, and restless leg syndrome. Sleep apnea and restless leg syndrome are two of the most prevalent disorders that lead to daytime sleepiness, largely through a reduction in the quantity and quality of sleep. Narcolepsy is present in only a small fraction of the population but is devastating in its negative effects.

The Disruption of Breathing During Sleep Apnea Results in Fragmentation of Sleep

Reduction of muscle tone can result in either an annoying disturbance of sleep, as in snoring, or in greatly disturbed sleep, as in sleep apnea (cessation of breathing). Approximately 4% of middle-aged men (2% of middle-aged women) have sleep apnea. At older than age 65 years these percentages increase to more than 28% of men and 24% of women.

Sleep apnea is a serious condition, for it not only disrupts sleep but also can cause excessive sleepiness during the day, early morning headaches, depression, irritability, sexual dysfunction, and learning and memory difficulties. In severe cases sleep apnea can lead to cardiac dysfunction and be life-threatening.

The most common form of sleep apnea, *obstructive sleep apnea*, results from a physical obstruction of the pharynx. Breathing ceases for 10 or more seconds. A pathological condition involves at least 5 to 10 of these interruptions per hour. In *central sleep apnea* the disruption of breathing has a neurological origin. In either type of sleep apnea the decrease in blood oxygen tension and increase in CO_2 leads to an arousal response (but not complete awakening). The period of apnea ends with a deep breath, and the sufferer then falls back into a deeper sleep, only to repeat the cycle once again (Figure 51–8).

These frequent disruptions cause fragmentation of sleep, a general decrease in quality of sleep, and therefore daytime sleepiness. Because the affected individual usually does not become fully awake with each apneic period, he may be completely unaware of the problem except for the resultant daytime sleepiness or the concern of a friend or spouse who observes an apneic spell. This pattern is usually easy to diagnose in a sleep laboratory.

REM sleep is especially conducive to sleep apnea owing to the characteristic reduction in muscle tone, which facilitates collapse of the airway. During REM sleep responses to hypoxia are reduced, and the response to increases in carbon dioxide levels (hypercapnia) is completely lost. In addition, the brain stem mechanisms responsible for regulation of blood O_2 and CO_2 levels are weakened, allowing these levels to drop well below those that would be tolerated in the waking state. Obesity can be a precipitating factor for obstructive sleep apnea because airflow through the pharynx is typically reduced.

Obstructive sleep apnea is treated by keeping the pharynx open with positive pressure through a face mask. This treatment can lead to an almost immediate reversal of the symptoms, a more restful sleep, and a reduction in daytime sleepiness. However, most patients eventually reject use of the mask because they find it too uncomfortable or claustrophobic to use consistently.

Narcolepsy Is Characterized by Abnormal Activation of Sleep Mechanisms

Narcolepsy occurs in approximately 0.04% of the population or approximately 120,000 people in the United States. It is characterized by a breakdown in the transition between waking and sleep. Sleep and sleep mechanisms invade daytime periods, often at inappropriate times, and sleep at night is fragmented and disrupted by multiple awakenings. Narcolepsy is characteristically manifested in five symptoms, some or all of which may be seen in any one individual.

The most prevalent symptom is excessive daytime sleepiness and irresistible "sleep attacks" during the waking hours. These sleep attacks (usually less than 20 minutes) can come at any moment and sometimes are a source of embarrassment. For example, falling asleep during conversation or at work may lead to

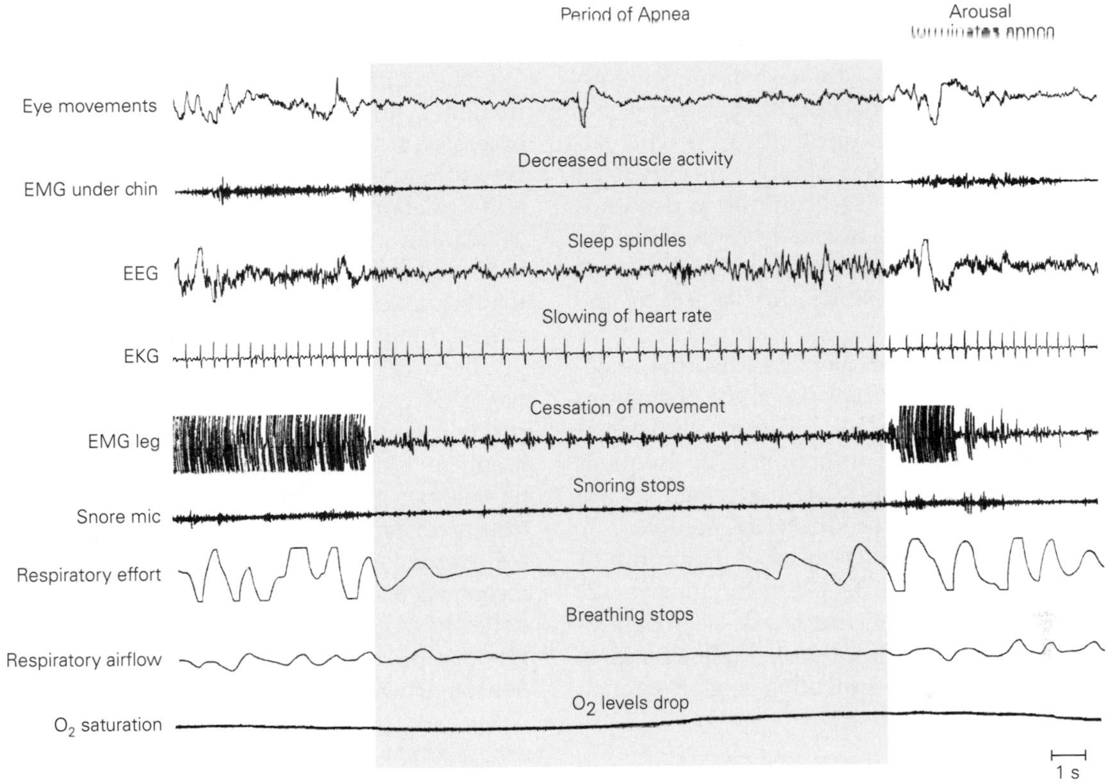

Figure 51–8 An episode of sleep apnea is captured in this polysomnogram, a simultaneous record of various bodily functions. Sleep apnea disrupts normal sleep patterns. The episode shown here includes cessation of breathing. Decreases in respiratory effort and airflow result in the cessation of snoring and a decrease in oxygen saturation. The slowing of the heart rate and appearance of sleep spindles during the apnea episode indicate that the individual is asleep. The period of apnea is preceded and terminated by arousal and leg movements. (**EEG**, electroencephalogram; **EKG**, electrocardiogram; **EMG**, electromyogram.)

the incorrect assumption that the narcoleptic is uninterested in the conversation or in doing a full day's work. Sleep attacks are precipitated by any behavior that is relatively passive and boring such as watching television, driving a car, or studying for finals. Unfortunately, sleeping does not completely alleviate the tendency to have sleep attacks.

A second symptom, cataplexy, occurs in approximately 70% of narcoleptic patients. Cataplexy is a sudden bilateral loss of muscle tone, typically in the knees and face and neck, leading to a sagging of the jaw and falling to the floor. Consciousness is preserved, however, and the sufferer is typically awake but feels either unable or barely able to move. The onset of a cataplexic episode occurs over a couple of seconds; the episode itself lasts for seconds but in rare instances can last minutes. Emotion, most typically laughter, can provoke an attack, perhaps owing to the fact that during laughter there is a general decrease in muscle tone. Cataplexy is thought to result from abnormal activation of the motor inhibition that normally occurs during periods of REM sleep.

Third, vivid dreamlike experiences may occur during the transition between sleep and waking. These events are known as either hypnagogic (sleep onset) or hypnopompic (sleep offset) hallucinations. What differentiates them from dreams is that the narcoleptic person is not fully asleep and is aware that he is not dreaming—the images seem real. The dreamlike experiences are typically bizarre, frightening, and unpleasant; they are predominantly visual, although auditory and tactile experiences are also frequent. As with dreams, sensations of smell or taste are rare. Hallucinations of this type may also occur in normal people at transitions between sleep and waking.

A fourth symptom, sleep paralysis, also typically occurs in the transition between sleep and waking (either going to sleep at night or waking in the morning). Unlike cataplexy it is not triggered by emotion and episodes last longer, sometimes up to 10 minutes. As sufferers are unable to make even the smallest of movements, such as opening their eyelids or lifting a finger, the experience is frightening and unpleasant. As with cataplexy it is assumed that sleep paralysis results from inappropriate activation of the inhibitory descending motor pathways that are normally responsible for inhibiting movement during REM sleep. Sleep paralysis also occurs in non-narcoleptics (up to 30% of the general population).

The final symptom of narcolepsy is disturbed nocturnal sleep. Although narcoleptics may fall asleep quickly and often immediately fall into REM sleep (Figure 51–9), their sleep is interrupted by frequent arousals. For most narcoleptics these awakenings are brief, but some may stay awake for hours at night.

A diagnosis of narcolepsy requires a minimum of either (1) daytime lapses into sleep and cataplexy or (2) a pattern of excessive daytime sleepiness, sleep paralysis, or hypnagogic or hypnopompic hallucinations, and a polysomnogram demonstrating a short latency to sleep and a period of REM sleep either at the beginning of sleep or shortly thereafter.

The different components of narcolepsy are treated with different pharmacological agents. The excessive sleepiness and sleep spells of narcolepsy are typically treated with central nervous stimulants such as amphetamines. These agents enhance the release of catecholamines and inhibit their reuptake. Cataplexy is treated with tricyclic antidepressants, which inhibit the reuptake of norepinephrine and serotonin and are potent inhibitors of REM sleep.

Both genetic and environmental factors contribute to narcolepsy. In only 1% of cases does narcolepsy run in a family and only approximately one-fourth of identical twins are concordant for narcolepsy. Thus narcolepsy genes appear to confer merely a susceptibility to narcolepsy, whereas environmental factors contribute strongly. By studying narcoleptic dogs, Emmanuel Mignot found that these animals have a defect in the gene coding for the hypocretin-2 receptor. Hypocretin-1 and -2 (also called orexin A and B) are neuropeptides produced in a small cluster of neurons

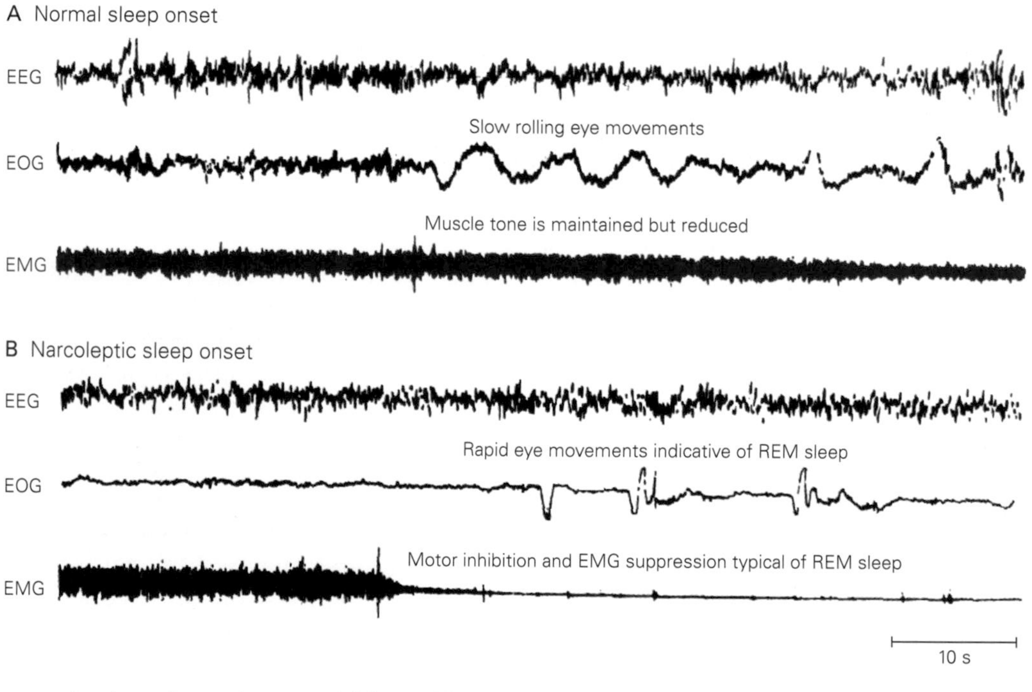

Figure 51–9 In narcoleptic patients sleep can initiate with REM sleep.

A. Sleep onset in a normal person is associated with slow rolling eye movements and a slow decrease in muscle tone.

B. Sleep onset in a narcoleptic is associated with a sudden decrease in muscle tone and the appearance of rapid eye movements typical of REM sleep. The REM sleep that occurs at the beginning of sleep usually lasts 10 to 20 minutes, after which sleep progresses through stages 1 through 4 of non-REM sleep. (**EEG**, electroencephalogram; **EMG**, electromyogram; **EOG**, electro-oculogram.)

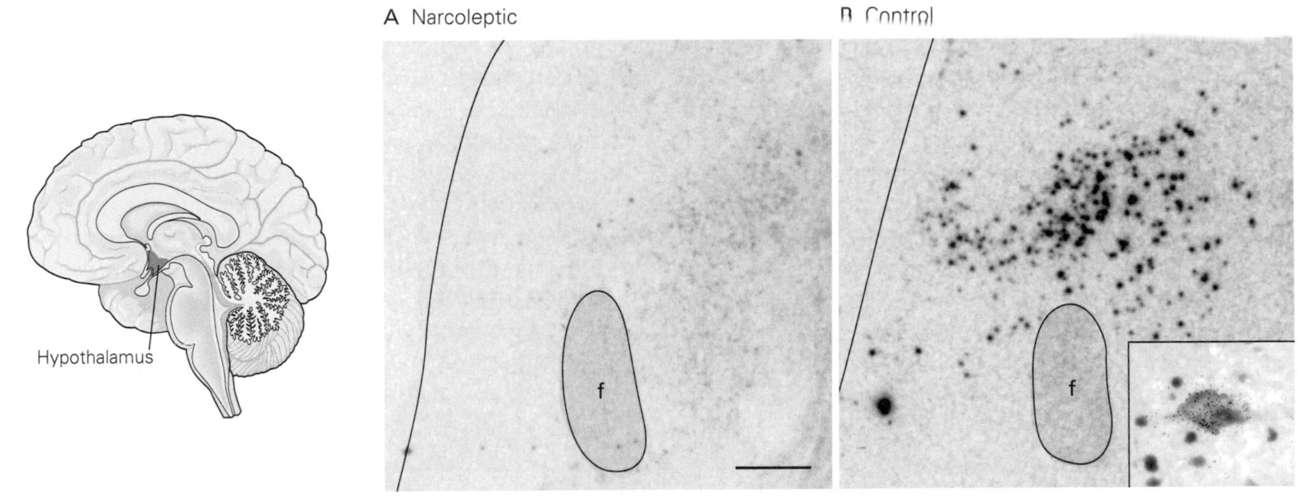

Figure 51–10 Narcolepsy is associated with a loss of hypothalamic neurons that produce the peptide hypocretin. A dramatic loss of neurons is evident in the brain of a narcoleptic compared to a normal brain. The inset illustrates the positive identification of a hypocretinergic cell from a normal person. (f, fornix.) (Reproduced, with permission, from Peyron et al. 2000.)

within the hypothalamus that project widely throughout the brain, including the brain stem nuclei responsible for REM sleep (eg, locus ceruleus). Activation of hypocretin receptors in locus ceruleus and other neurons has a slow excitatory effect. Through an unknown mechanism, a loss of this or other modulatory actions of hypocretin results in the abnormal differentiation of sleep and waking typical of narcolepsy.

To study the role of the hypocretin system in feeding behavior, Masashi Yanagisawa and collaborators knocked out the genes for both hypocretin-1 and -2 in mice and found that these mice displayed symptoms typical of narcolepsy. In narcoleptic humans the cerebral spinal fluid levels of hypocretin are remarkably reduced even though the hypocretin genes are not mutated. Immunocytochemical examination of the brains of deceased narcoleptics has revealed a striking loss of hypocretinergic neurons (Figure 51–10).

Restless Leg Syndrome and Periodic Leg Movements Disrupt Sleep

Restless leg syndrome occurs in approximately 8% of the population and is characterized by an irresistible urge to move the legs. This symptom occurs during the day but is usually worse at night while resting in bed. The patient may feel relief only by moving the legs either in bed or by walking about.

Approximately 80% of people suffering from restless leg syndrome also experience periodic leg movements in sleep, when the legs move for a few seconds every 10 to 20 seconds. These leg movements result in a lightening of sleep and therefore an increase in daytime sleepiness. The prevalence of restless leg syndrome and periodic leg movements increases greatly with age, becoming more common in the elderly.

Parasomnias Include Sleep Walking, Sleep Talking, and Night Terrors

Parasomnias are repeated disruptions of sleep that are relatively common and usually mild. They include sleep walking, sleep talking, confusional arousals, bed wetting, night terrors, and REM behavior disorder. Although not normally considered a sleep disorder, sudden infant death syndrome (SIDS) is an example of fatal respiratory failure that occurs during sleep (see Chapter 46).

Sleep walking, sleep talking, and confusional arousals are relatively common in children and typically occur during stages 3 and 4 sleep. These events may be precipitated by disturbing or arousing the child from deep sleep. For short events the EEG is a continued pattern of slow waves; for longer events the pattern changes to an "activated" pattern—low-voltage, desynchronized high-frequency activity—characteristic of waking. Usually sleepwalkers or talkers are unaware of an event and have no memory of it. Speech is largely incoherent during an event; remarkably sleep walkers are often able to avoid colliding with objects.

Night terrors also occur in stages 3 and 4 sleep and are common in children (approximately 2–3%). The child cries as if in great fear, perhaps with eyes wide open and heart rate greatly elevated, for several minutes or longer. Even though they may appear awake, they are actually asleep. During the episode they are inconsolable, and attempts to calm or wake the child may only cause the screams and fearful behavior to worsen. The child usually does not remember the night terror, in contrast to remembering nightmares. Thus night terrors are typically much more difficult for the parent than for the child.

During REM sleep descending inhibition of motor neurons in the spinal cord normally prevents people from acting out their vivid dreams. This descending pathway may be damaged in people suffering from REM behavior disorder (usually men and elderly people). During REM sleep the body may become rigid or extremely tense and may exhibit prominent muscle twitching in association with the phasic eye movements of REM sleep. If the dream has intense physical activity, the patient may even get out of bed and injure himself or his bed partner with his vigorous activity. The mechanisms underlying REM behavior disorder are not yet known.

Circadian Rhythm Sleep Disorders Are Characterized by an Activity Cycle That Is Out of Phase with the World

The most frequent circadian rhythm disorder involves problems with entrainment to the day-night cycle. A patient may find it impossible to fall asleep until very late at night, for example 3 a.m. (delayed sleep phase disorder or DSPD) or impossible to stay awake past the early evening hours, for example 7 p.m. (advanced sleep phase disorder or ASPD).

The most prevalent disruption of normal circadian rhythms occurs in those who work either part-time or full-time during the night. In some individuals forcing a lifestyle that is out of phase with the natural day-night cycle can lead to several medical problems, including unstable mood, vigilance impairments, colds, high blood pressure, stomach problems, and weight gain. In general, shift workers also experience a higher incidence of workplace and automobile accidents because of increased sleepiness.

In rare cases patients may lack an endogenous circadian rhythm or may not be able to synchronize their rhythm with that of the environment. As one can imagine, these disorders cause great difficulties for those afflicted.

An Overall View

For a behavior that involves up to 25 years of our lifetime, it is surprising how much we do not yet fully understand about the functions of sleep. Sleep is essential for life, at least for rats. A rat deprived of all sleep dies after approximately 3 to 4 weeks owing to a breakdown in metabolic processes. In fact, sleep deprivation can cause death even more quickly than food deprivation.

In practice we sleep because we are sleepy, just as we eat or drink because we are hungry or thirsty. But the function of sleep is not to relieve sleepiness. Intuitively we think of sleep as restorative, but exactly what is restored is unknown. In addition to a restorative function, other functions have been proposed, including energy conservation, memory consolidation and sorting, recalibration of neuronal networks, and behavioral suppression during periods of the day for which the animal is not well adapted.

One explanation for this diversity of function is that bodily functions have, over evolution, become segregated into different portions of the day/night cycle so as to make efficient use of resources. Indeed, studies of gene expression reveal that a massive reorganization of the molecular and cellular biology of neurons occurs in the transition from alertness to sleep, suggesting that a similar marked reorganization occurs during sleep. Sleep is therefore likely to have many functions, just as waking does.

In fact, it may be useful to turn the question "Why do we sleep?" on its head and ask instead, "Why do we wake up?" In general, periods of waking are generated to accomplish a goal, for example, the procurement of food and housing, having a family, building a society; otherwise rest is warranted. By keeping the animal inactive during periods in which it is not well-suited for wandering about, sleep may ensure adequate rest and the reservation of energy stores. Waking up and becoming active can cost at least an additional 10% of energy. Given scarce food resources, ceasing activity for a significant fraction of each day can lead to a small but significant increase in survival. Thus sleep may be a light and short version of hibernation, an easily generated and reversible period of rest and energy conservation.

Another idea is called the protection hypothesis. Most animals are adapted for activity during the day or night. Being active at the wrong period brings with it considerable risks both from other animals (eg, predators) or environmental conditions (eg, cold during the night or heat during the day, or unseen objects because of low light levels).

Sleep involves the entire organism and in fact involves the family and society as a whole. Even so, many neuroscientists believe that sleep is of and for the brain. One neural function that is often proposed for sleep is memory consolidation. Disruption of sleep has detrimental effects on some types of learning, particularly procedural memory, although the stressful effects of lost sleep are always a confounding factor.

One idea holds that the spontaneous activity occurring in the sleeping brain is a type of neuronal exercise machine—keeping the brain "in tune" for the requirements of daily activities. By passing spontaneous patterned activity throughout neuronal circuits during the night, the brain can recalibrate the strength of synaptic connections as well as the electrophysiological properties of single neurons, resulting perhaps in the retaining of important information and the forgetting of irrelevant information. The presence of spontaneous patterns of neuronal activity in all animals during sleep, which is energetically more costly than neuronal silence, suggests that this activity plays an important functional role in sleep. Indeed, the spontaneous patterns of activity occurring in the brain during REM sleep are the neural basis of dreams.

The importance of REM sleep is a particularly thorny issue. Patients on some forms of antidepressant may go years with a near complete suppression of REM sleep without any marked deficits in the ability to form new memories or otherwise function normally. REM sleep may allow for a more immediate response to the environment during sleep (which has obvious survival value in the wild) because animals awakened from REM sleep are more responsive and show better sensory and motor function than those awakened from non-REM sleep. In a group of sleeping animals at least one or more of them may be in this state of readiness at any given moment and therefore able to alert the pack of an intruder.

Both REM and non-REM sleep are highly regulated processes that the brain and body appear to crave. Deprivation of REM sleep results in "REM rebound" in which the loss is made up by excessive REM sleep in the following night's sleep. This regulation suggests that REM sleep, and sleep in general, plays one or more critical functions. It remains for us, or rather our brains, to discover the nature of these functions so that we may more fully understand the more ethereal third of our lives.

David A. McCormick
Gary L. Westbrook

Selected Readings

Borbely A. 1988. *Secrets of Sleep*. New York: Basic Books.

Hobson JA. 1988. *The Dreaming Brain*. New York: Basic Books.

Kryger MH, Roth T, Dement WC. 2010. *Principles and Practice of Sleep Medicine*. Philadelphia: Elsevier Saunders.

Lavie P. 1998. *The Enchanted World of Sleep*. A Barris (transl). New Haven: Yale Univ. Press.

References

Achermann P, Borbely AA. 2003. Mathematical models of sleep regulation. Front Biosci 8:683–693.

Andersen P, Andersson S. 1968. *Physiological Basis of the Alpha Rhythm*. New York: Appleton-Century Crofts.

Aschoff J. 1965. Circadian rhythms in man. Science 148: 1427–1432.

Aserinsky E, Kleitman N. 1953. Regularly occurring periods of eye motility and concomitant phenomena during sleep. Science 118:273–274.

Chemelli RM, Willie JT, Sinton CM, Elmquist JK, Scammell T, Lee C, Richardson JA, et al. 1999. Narcolepsy in orexin knockout mice: molecular genetics of sleep regulation. Cell 98:437–451.

Daan S, Beersma DG, Borbely AA. 1984. Timing of human sleep: recovery process gated by a circadian pacemaker. Am J Physiol 246:R161–183.

Dement W, Kleitman N. 1957. Cyclic variations in EEG during sleep and their relation to eye movements, body motility, and dreaming. Electroencephalogr Clin Neurophysiol Suppl 9:673–690.

Earnest DJ, Sladek CD. 1987. Circadian vasopressin release from perifused rat suprachiasmatic explants in vitro: effects of acute stimulation. Brain Res 422:398–402.

Emery P, Reppert SM. 2004. A rhythmic Ror. Neuron 43: 443–446.

Hardin PE. 2005. The circadian timekeeping system of *Drosophila*. Curr Biol 15:R714–722.

Hobson JA. 1989. *Sleep*. New York: Scientific American Library.

Hobson JA, Pace-Schott EF. 2002. The cognitive neuroscience of sleep: neuronal systems, consciousness and learning. Nat Rev Neurosci 3:679–693.

Lin L, Faraco J, Li R, Kadotani H, Rogers W, Lin X, Qiu X, et al. 1999. The sleep disorder canine narcolepsy is caused by a mutation in the hypocretin (orexin) receptor 2 gene. Cell 98:365–376.

Mahowald MW, Schenck CH. 2005. Insights from studying human sleep disorders. Nature 437:1279–1285.

McCarley RW, Massaquoi SG. 1986. A limit cycle mathematical model of the REM sleep oscillator system. Am J Physiol 251:R1011–1029.

McCormick DA, Bal T. 1997. Sleep and arousal: thalamocortical mechanisms. Annu Rev Neurosci 20:185–215.

Moruzzi G, Magoun HW. 1949. Brain stem reticular formation and activation of the EEG. Electroencephalogr Clin Neurophysiol Suppl 1:455–473.

Peyron C, Faraco J, Rogers W, Ripley B, Overeem S, Charnay Y, Nevsimalova S, et al. 2000. A mutation in a case of early onset narcolepsy and a generalized absence of hypocretin peptides in human narcoleptic brains. Nat Med 6:991–997.

Purves D, Augustine GA, Fitzpatrick D, Katz LC, LaMantia A-S, McNamara JO. 1997. *Neuroscience*. Sunderland, MA: Sinauer.

Purves D, Augustine GA, Fitzpatrick D, Hall W, LaMantia A-S, McNamara JO, Williams SM. 2004. *Neuroscience*, 3rd ed. Sunderland, MA: Sinauer.

Reppert SM, Weaver DR. 2002. Coordination of circadian timing in mammals. Nature 418:935–941.

Sanchez-Vives MV, McCormick DA. 2000. Cellular and network mechanisms of rhythmic recurrent activity in neocortex. Nat Neurosci 3:1027–1034.

Saper CB, Lu J, Chou TC, Gooley J. 2005. The hypothalamic integrator for circadian rhythms. Trends Neurosci 28: 152–157.

Saper CB, Scammell TE, Lu J. 2005. Hypothalamic regulation of sleep and circadian rhythms. Nature 437:1257–1263.

Siegel JM. 2000. In: MH Kryger, T Roth, WC Dement (eds). *Principles and Practice of Sleep Medicine*. Philadelphia: Elsevier Saunders.

Siegel JM. 2005. Clues to the functions of mammalian sleep. Nature 437:1264–1271.

Steriade MM, McCarley RW. 2005. *Brain Control of Wakefulness and Sleep*. New York: Plenum.

Steriade MM, McCormick DA, Sejnowski TJ. 1993. Thalamocortical oscillations in the sleeping and aroused brain. Science 262:679–685.

Steriade MM, Timofeev I, Grenier F. 2001. Natural waking and sleep states: a view from inside neocortical neurons. J Neurophysiol 85:1969–1985.

Stickgold R. 2005. Sleep-dependent memory consolidation. Nature 437:1272–1278.

von Krosigk M, Bal T, McCormick DA. 1993. Cellular mechanisms of a synchronized oscillation in the thalamus. Science 261:361–364.

Part VIII

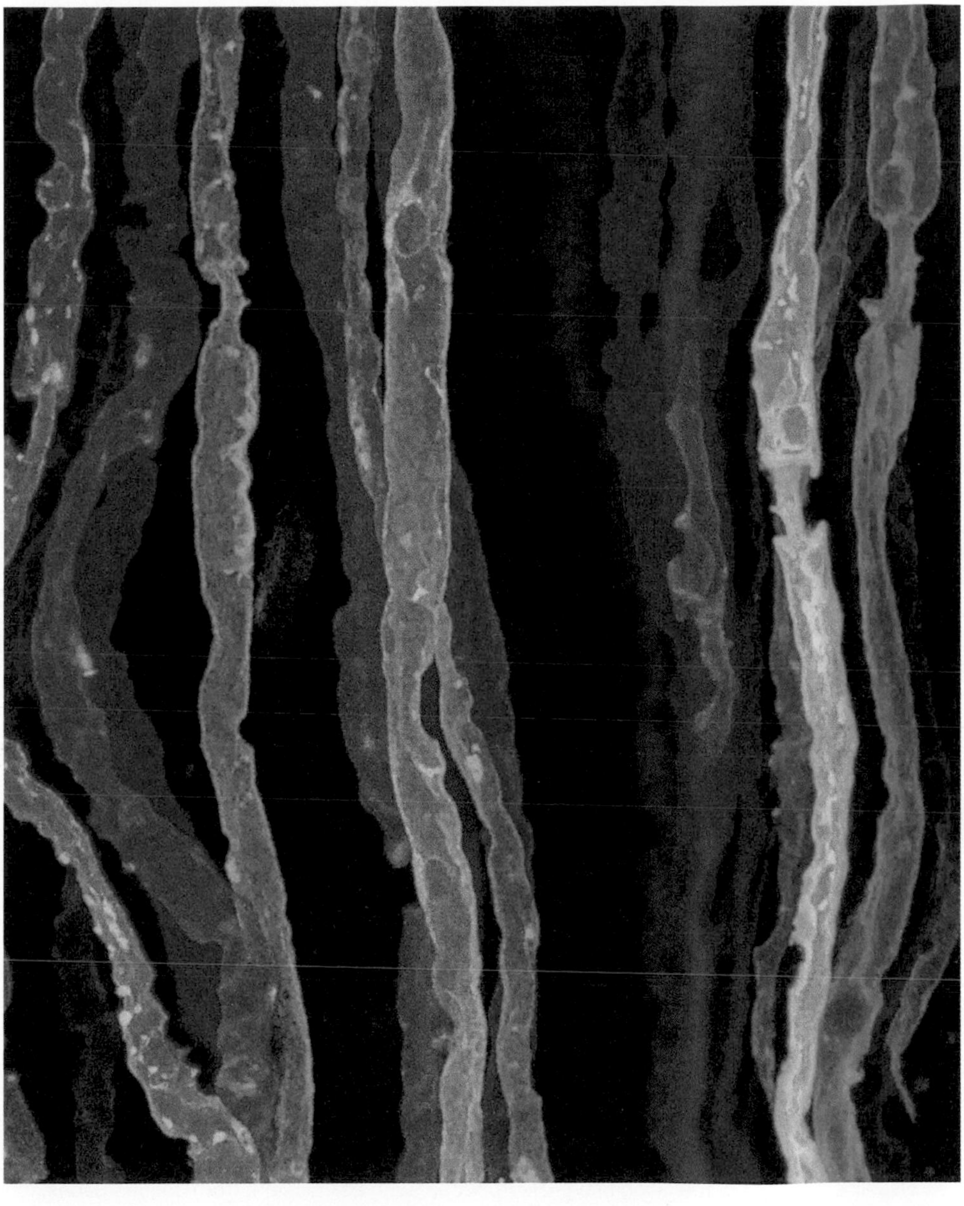

Preceding Page

Motor axons travel in parallel through a cranial nerve in a mouse. The *Brainbow* neuroimaging technique used to create this image permits labeling of individual neurons with distinct colors. The method has advanced dramatically our ability to map and visualize neurons in the living brain. (Reproduced, with permission, from Joshua Sanes. Image appeared in Livet J, Weissman TA, Kang H, Draft RW, Lu J, Bennis RA, Sanes JR, Lichtman JW. Nature 2007; 540:56-61)

VIII Development and the Emergence of Behavior

All of the innumerable behaviors controlled by the mature nervous system—from the perception of sensory input and the control of motor output to cognitive functions such as learning and memory—depend on precise interconnections formed by many millions of neurons during embryonic and postnatal development.

More than a century ago, Santiago Ramón y Cajal undertook a comprehensive series of anatomical studies on the structure and organization of the nervous system, and then set out to probe its development. Modern developmental neuroscientists follow in Ramón y Cajal's footsteps, trying to uncover the processes underlying the formation of neural circuits. In the intervening years technical advances have made it possible to extend this inquiry to the molecular and genetic levels. During the past few decades there have been many striking advances in understanding the molecular basis of neural development. These advances include the identification of proteins that determine how nerve cells acquire their identities, how they extend axons to target cells, form synaptic connections, and have also provided insight into how synaptic connections are modified by experience.

Development of the nervous system depends on the expression of particular genes at particular times and places. This spatial and temporal pattern of gene expression is regulated by both hardwired molecular programs and epigenetic processes. The factors that control neuronal differentiation originate both from cellular sources within the embryo and from the external environment. Internal influences include cell surface and secreted molecules that control the fate of neighboring cells, as well as transcription factors that act at the level of DNA to control gene expression. External factors include nutrients, sensory stimuli, and social experience, the effects of which are mediated through patterned changes in the activity of nerve cells. The interaction of these intrinsic and environmental factors is critical for the proper differentiation of each nerve cell.

The recent progress in defining the mechanisms that control the development of the nervous system is due largely to molecular biological studies of neural function. To take but one example, the molecular cloning of genes encoding extrinsic factors (eg, secreted proteins) and intrinsic determinants (eg, transcription factors) has provided unanticipated insight into the differentiation of the nervous system. Moreover, the function of specific genes can now be tested directly in transgenic animals or in animals in which individual genes have been inactivated by mutation.

Other important advances have emerged from the analysis of simple and genetically accessible organisms such as the fruit fly *Drosophila* and the nematode worm *Caenorhabditis elegans*. Most of the key molecules that control the formation of the nervous system are found to be conserved in organisms separated by millions of years of evolution. Thus, despite the great diversity of animal forms, the developmental programs that govern body plan and neural connectivity are conserved throughout phylogeny. It is now clear that mutations in these genes are responsible for some degenerative and even behavioral disorders. Thus, studies of neural development are beginning to provide practical insight into neurological diseases and to suggest rational strategies for restoring neural connections and function after disease or traumatic injury.

There is, however, one major way in which humans—and to a lesser extent other mammals—differ from invertebrates and lower vertebrates. Although humans are quite helpless at birth, their capacities to learn, reason, decide and abstract are prodigious. A newly-hatched bird or fly is not remarkably different in its behavioral repertoire from its adult self, but no one could say that about a person. This is largely because the nervous system of a newborn human is something of a rough draft. The hard-wired circuits that lay out its basic plan are then modified over a prolonged postnatal period by experience, acting via neural activity. In this way, the experience of each individual can leave indelible imprints on his or her nervous system and the cognitive abilities of the brain can be enhanced by learning. These processes act in all mammals, and neuroscientists now use mice to probe the mechanisms that underlie them—but they are especially prominent and prolonged in humans. It may be that the prolonged period during which experience can sculpt the human nervous system is the most important single factor in making its capabilities unique among all species.

In human infants the experience-dependent acquisition of cognitive abilities is a social feature illustrated by the fact that infants learn better from other people than from television programs. The social interactions help language development, and as language development progresses, it helps social interactions. Until recently, analysis of this late, experience-dependent remodeling of the nervous system was primarily the province of psychology. Over the past several decades, however, neuroanatomists and neurophysiologists have made strides in understanding cellular changes that underlie it. Perhaps most exciting, continued progress in genetic and molecular technologies are now being applied to the topic. The issues have been more complex and harder to define than those encountered at the early stages in neural development mentioned above, so the molecular revolution has been slower in coming to them—but the pace is now increasing rapidly. The implications of this new knowledge are great. For example, understanding how cognitive abilities are acquired during the preschool years helps us enhance the ability to educate all children. Moreover, there is increasing reason to believe that some behavioral disorders, such as autism or schizophrenia, may result in part from defects in the experience-dependent tuning of neural circuits during early postnatal life.

In Part VIII, we examine vertebrate neural development in a sequential manner. Beginning with the early stages of neural development, we concentrate on the factors that control the diversity and survival of nerve cells, guide axons, and regulate the formation of synapses. We then explain how interaction with the environment, both social and physical, modifies or consolidates the neural connections formed during early development. Depriving individuals of their normal environment during the early critical period of development can have profound consequences for the later maturation of the brain and thus for behavior. Finally, we examine factors, such as steroid hormones, that continue to influence the structure of the brain during early postnatal development and the biochemical changes that occur as the brain ages.

Part VIII

52

Patterning the Nervous System

A VAST ARRAY OF NEURONS AND GLIAL CELLS is produced during development of the vertebrate nervous system. Different neurons develop in discrete anatomical positions, acquire varied morphological forms, and establish connections with specific populations of target cells. The diversity of neurons is far greater than that of cells in any other organ of the body. The retina, for example, has dozens of classes of amacrine interneurons, and the spinal cord more than a hundred motor neuron classes. Nevertheless, the true number of neuronal classes in the mammalian central nervous system remains unclear—perhaps more than a thousand.

The diversity of neuronal cell types underlies the impressive computational properties of the mammalian nervous system. Yet, as we describe in this chapter and those that follow, the developmental principles that drive the differentiation of the nervous system are begged and borrowed from those used to direct the development in other tissues. In one sense the development of the nervous system merely represents an elaborate example of the basic challenge that pervades all of developmental biology: How to convert a single cell, the fertilized egg, into the highly differentiated cell types that characterize the mature organism.

Indeed, the convergence of developmental biology and neural science has led us to appreciate that superficial differences in the structure of the nervous systems of diverse species belie the expression of commonly shared principles and mechanisms of neural development that have been conserved throughout evolution. Much of what we know about the cellular and molecular bases of neural development in vertebrates comes from genetic studies of so-called simple organisms, most notably the fruit fly *Drosophila melanogaster* and the worm *Caenorhabditis elegans.*

Nevertheless, because the eventual goal of studies of neural development is surely to explain how the assembly of the nervous system directs and constrains human behavior, in this chapter and those that follow our description of the rules and principles of nervous system development focus primarily on vertebrate organisms.

The Neural Tube Becomes Regionalized Early in Embryogenesis

The nervous system begins to develop at a relatively late stage in the entire program of embryonic development. Well before it forms, however, the primitive embryo has generated three main cell, or germ, layers—the endoderm, mesoderm, and ectoderm.

The *endoderm* is the innermost germ layer that later gives rise to the gut tube, as well as to the lungs, pancreas, and liver. The *mesoderm* is the middle germ layer that gives rise to muscle, connective tissues, and much of the vascular system. The *ectoderm* is the outermost layer that gives rise to the skin as well as to the columnar epithelium of the neural plate, the precursor of the central and peripheral nervous systems.

Soon after the neural plate forms it begins to fold into a tubular structure, the *neural tube,* through a process called neurulation (Figure 52–1). The caudal region of the neural tube gives rise to the spinal cord, whereas the rostral region becomes the brain.

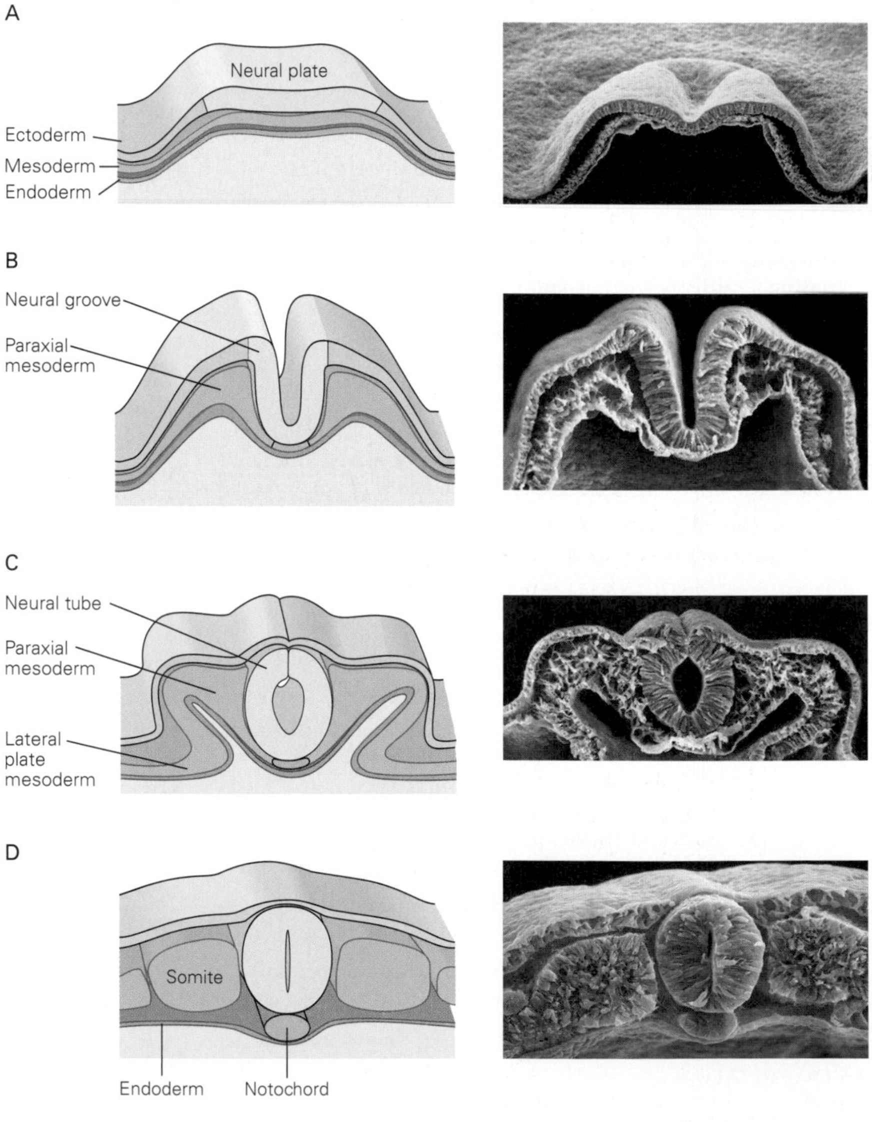

Figure 52–1 The neural plate folds to form the neural tube. (Electron micrographs of chick neural tube reproduced, with permission, from G. Schoenwolf.)

A. Early in embryogenesis three germ cell layers—the ectoderm, mesoderm, and endoderm—lie close together. The ectoderm gives rise to the neural plate, the precursor of the central and peripheral nervous systems.

B. The neural plate buckles at its midline to form the neural groove.

C. Closure of the dorsal neural folds forms the neural tube.

D. The neural tube lies over the notochord and is flanked by somites, an ovoid group of mesodermal cells that give rise to muscle and cartilage.

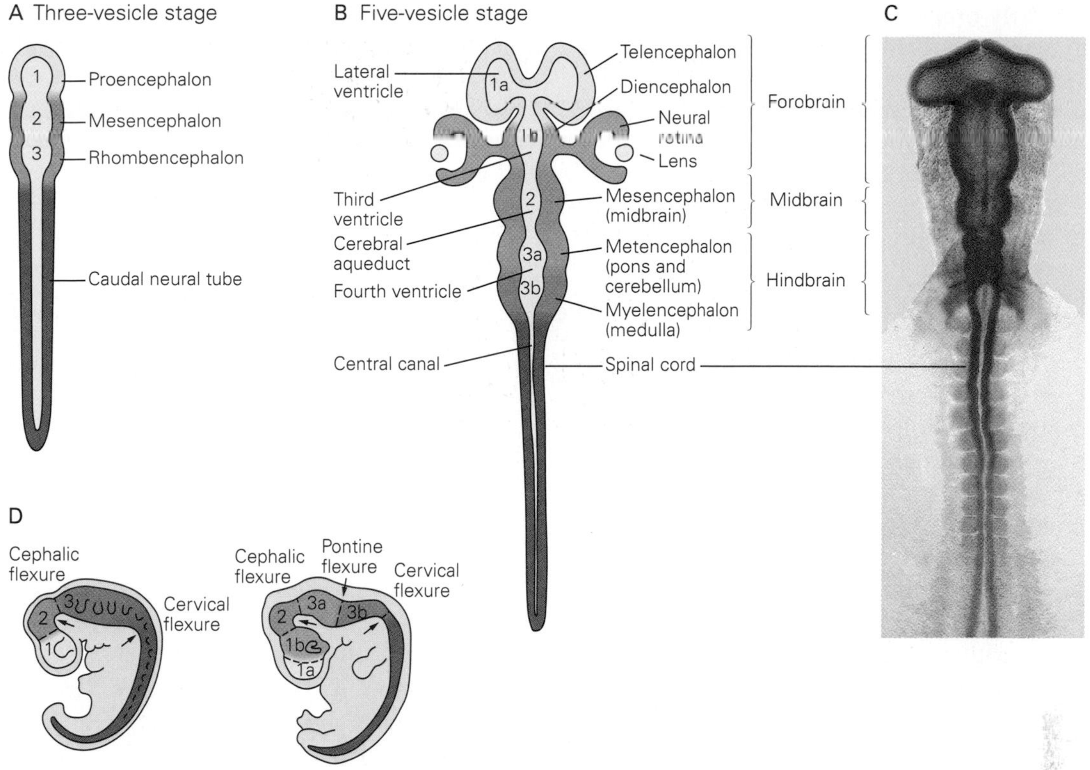

Figure 52–2 Sequential stages of neural tube development.

A. At early stages of neural tube development there are three brain vesicles.

B. Shortly after, two additional vesicles form, one in the forebrain (giving rise to regions 1a and 1b) and the other in the hindbrain (giving rise to regions 3a and 3b).

C. Top-down view of the neural tube of a chick embryo at the five-vesicle stage. (Reproduced, with permission, from G. Schoenwolf.)

D. The neural tube bends at the cephalic, pontine, and cervical flexures.

During these early stages of neural development cells divide rapidly, although cell proliferation is not uniform. Individual regions of the neural epithelium expand at different rates and begin to form the various specialized regions of the mature central nervous system. Differences in the rate of proliferation of cells in rostral regions of the neural tube result in the formation of three brain vesicles: the forebrain (or prosencephalic) vesicle, the midbrain (or mesencephalic) vesicle, and the hindbrain (or rhombencephalic) vesicle (Figure 52–2A).

At this early three-vesicle stage the neural tube flexes twice: once at the *cervical flexure,* at the junction of the spinal cord and hindbrain, and once at the *cephalic flexure,* at the junction of the hindbrain and midbrain. A third flexure, the *pontine flexure,* forms later, and later still the cervical flexure straightens out and becomes indistinct (Figure 52D). The cephalic flexure remains prominent throughout development, and its persistence is the reason why the orientation of the longitudinal axis of the forebrain deviates from that of the brain stem and spinal cord.

As the neural tube develops, two of the primary embryonic vesicles divide further, thus forming the five-vesicle stage (Figure 52–2B, C). The forebrain vesicle divides to form the telencephalon and diencephalon, and the hindbrain vesicle divides to form the metencephalon and myelencephalon. Together with the spinal cord these subdivisions make up the major functional regions of the mature central nervous system (see Chapter 15). These functional domains are the products of progressive patterning and subdivision of the neural tube, developmental events that are regulated by a variety of secreted signals.

Secreted Signals Promote Neural Cell Fate

As with other organs, the emergence of the neural plate is the culmination of a complex molecular program that involves the tightly orchestrated expression of specific genes within ectodermal cells. The entire nervous system derives from a restricted region of the ectoderm.

Early in development ectodermal cells are faced with the choice of whether to become neural or epidermal cells. This decision is arguably the most fundamental step of neural development, and one that has been the subject of intense study for nearly 100 years. Much of this interest has focused on a search for signals that control the fate of ectodermal cells.

We now know that two major classes of proteins work together to promote the differentiation of an ectodermal cell into a neural cell. The first are *inductive factors,* signaling molecules that are secreted by nearby cells. Some of these factors are freely diffusible and exert their actions at a distance, but others are tethered to the cell surface and act locally. The second are surface receptors that enable cells to respond to inductive factors. Activation of these receptors triggers the expression of genes that encode intracellular proteins—transcription factors, enzymes, and cytoskeletal proteins—which push ectodermal cells along the pathway to becoming neural cells.

The ability of a cell to respond to inductive signals, termed its *competence,* depends on the exact repertory of receptors, transduction molecules, and transcription factors expressed by the recipient cell. Thus a cell's fate is determined not only by the signals to which it is exposed—a consequence of when and where it finds itself in the embryo—but also by the profile of genes it expresses as a consequence of its prior developmental history. We will see in subsequent chapters that the interaction of localized inductive signals and intrinsic cell responses is evident at virtually every step throughout neural development.

Development of the Neural Plate Is Induced by Signals from the Organizer Region

The discovery that specific signals are responsible for triggering the formation of the neural plate was the first major advance in understanding the mechanisms that pattern the nervous system. In 1924 Hans Spemann and Hilde Mangold made the remarkable observation that the differentiation of the neural plate from uncommitted ectoderm depends on signals secreted by a specialized group of cells they called the *organizer region.*

Working with amphibian embryos they showed that organizer activity is restricted to a region of the embryo called the dorsal lip of the blastopore, which is destined to form the dorsal mesoderm. Spemann and Mangold demonstrated the crucial role of the organizer in forming the nervous system by transplanting small pieces of dorsal blastopore lip tissue underneath the ventral ectoderm of a host embryo, a region that normally gives rise to ventral epidermal tissue (Figure 52–3). By grafting organizer cells from a pigmented embryo into

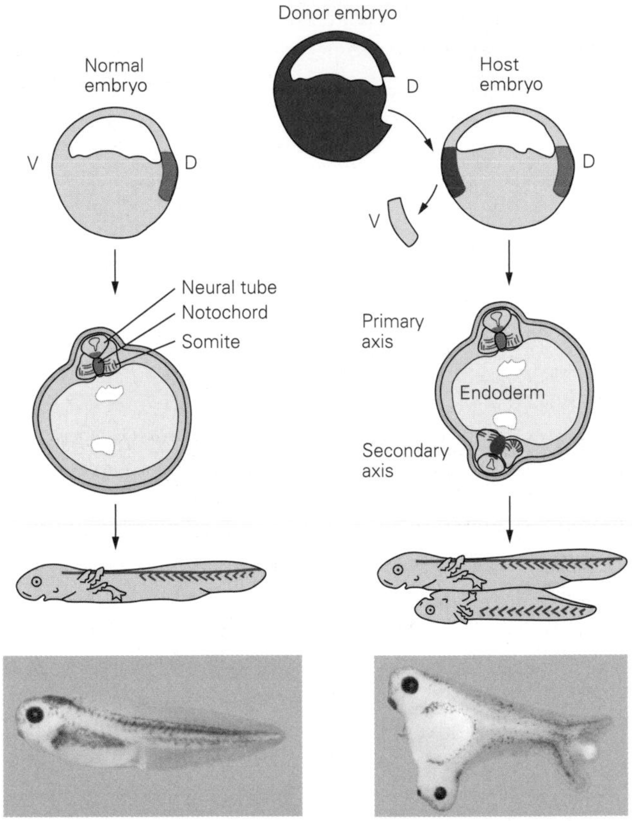

Figure 52–3 Signals from the organizer region induce a second neural tube. (Micrographs reproduced, with permission, from Eduardo de Robertis.)

Left: In the normal frog embryo cells from the organizer region (the dorsal blastopore lip) populate the notochord, floor plate, and somites. **Right:** Spemann and Mangold grafted the dorsal blastopore lip from an early gastrula stage embryo into a region of a host embryo that normally gives rise to the ventral epidermis. Signals from grafted cells induce a second embryonic axis, which includes a virtually complete neural tube. The donor tissue was from a pigmented embryo, whereas the host tissue was unpigmented, permitting the fate of grafted cells to be monitored by their characteristic pigmentation. Grafted cells themselves contribute only to the notochord, floor plate, and somites of the host embryo. As the embryo matures the secondary neural tube develops into a complete nervous system. In the *Xenopus* embryo shown in the micrograph, the second neural axis was induced by injection of an antagonist of bone morphogenetic protein (BMP), in effect substituting for the organizer signal (Figure 52–4). The primary neural axis is also apparent. (**V**, ventral; **D**, dorsal.)

an unpigmented host, they were able to distinguish the position and fate of donor and host cells.

Spemann and Mangold found that transplanted organizer cells followed their normal developmental program, generating midline mesoderm tissue such as the somites and notochord. But the transplanted cells also caused a striking change in the fate of the neighboring ventral ectodermal cells of the host embryo. Host ectodermal cells were induced to form a virtually complete copy of the nervous system (Figure 52–3). Spemann and Mangold went on to show that organizer cells were the only tissue that possessed this inductive effect.

These pioneering studies revealed that the nervous system is induced by signals from a highly restricted organizing center. As we will discuss, many aspects of neural tube patterning are now known to depend on signals secreted by other local organizing centers through actions similar in principle to that of the classical organizer region.

Neural Induction Is Mediated by Peptide Growth Factors and Their Inhibitors

For decades after Spemann and Mangold's pioneering studies, identification of the neural inducer constituted a Holy Grail of developmental biology. The search was marked by little success until the 1980s, when the advent of molecular biology and the availability of better markers of early neural tissue led to a breakthrough in our understanding of neural induction and its chemical mediators.

The first advance came from a simple finding: when the early ectoderm is dissociated into single isolated cells, effectively preventing cell-to-cell signaling, the cells readily acquire neural properties in the absence of added factors. The surprising implication of this finding was that the "default" fate of ectodermal cells is neural differentiation and that this fate is prevented by signals from neighboring ectodermal cells. In other words, the long sought-after "inducer" is actually a "de-repressor" of neural fate.

These ideas immediately raised two further questions. What ectodermal signal represses neural differentiation and what does organizer tissue provide to overcome the effects of the repressor? Studies of neural induction in frogs and chicks have now provided partial answers to these questions.

In the absence of signals from the organizer, ectodermal cells synthesize and secrete *bone morphogenetic proteins* (BMP), members of a large family of transforming growth factor β (TGFβ) related proteins. The BMPs, acting through serine/threonine kinase class receptors on ectodermal cells, suppress the potential for neural differentiation and promote epidermal differentiation. Key evidence for the role of BMPs as neural repressors came from experiments in which a truncated version of a BMP receptor, which blocks BMP signaling, was found to trigger the differentiation of neural tissue in the *Xenopus* frog embryo. Conversely, exposure of ectodermal cells to BMP signaling promoted differentiation as epidermal cells (Figure 52–4).

The identification of BMPs as suppressors of neuronal differentiation in turn raised the possibility that the ability of organizer tissue to induce neural differentiation in ectodermal cells might be mediated by factors that antagonize BMP signaling. Direct support for this idea came from the finding that cells of the organizer region express many secreted proteins that act as BMP antagonists. These proteins include noggin, chordin, follistatin, and even some variant BMP proteins. Each of these proteins has the ability to induce ectodermal cells to differentiate into neural tissue. Thus there is no single neural inducer. In fact, multiple classes of proteins are required for induction, as shown by the later finding that the exposure of ectodermal cells to fibroblast growth factors (FGFs) is also a necessary step in neural differentiation.

Together these studies have provided a molecular explanation of the cellular phenomena first described by Spemann and Mangold. Nevertheless, many details of the pathway of neural induction remain to be clarified. We know that transcription factors of the SoxB family, expressed in prospective neural plate cells, function as intermediaries in the acquisition of neural character. But other components of the pathway remain to be uncovered.

Rostrocaudal Patterning of the Neural Tube Involves Signaling Gradients and Secondary Organizing Centers

As soon as cells of the neural plate have been induced they begin to acquire regional characteristics that mark the first steps in the differentiation of the forebrain, midbrain, hindbrain, and spinal cord. Cells in each of these four major regions acquire diverse neuronal fates and identities.

The subdivision of the neural plate into its major functional domains is directed by a series of secreted inductive factors and follows the same basic principles of neural induction. These inductive factors are initially secreted from mesodermal and endodermal cells that flank the neural plate. Later, after neural tube closure, they are also secreted from secondary organizing

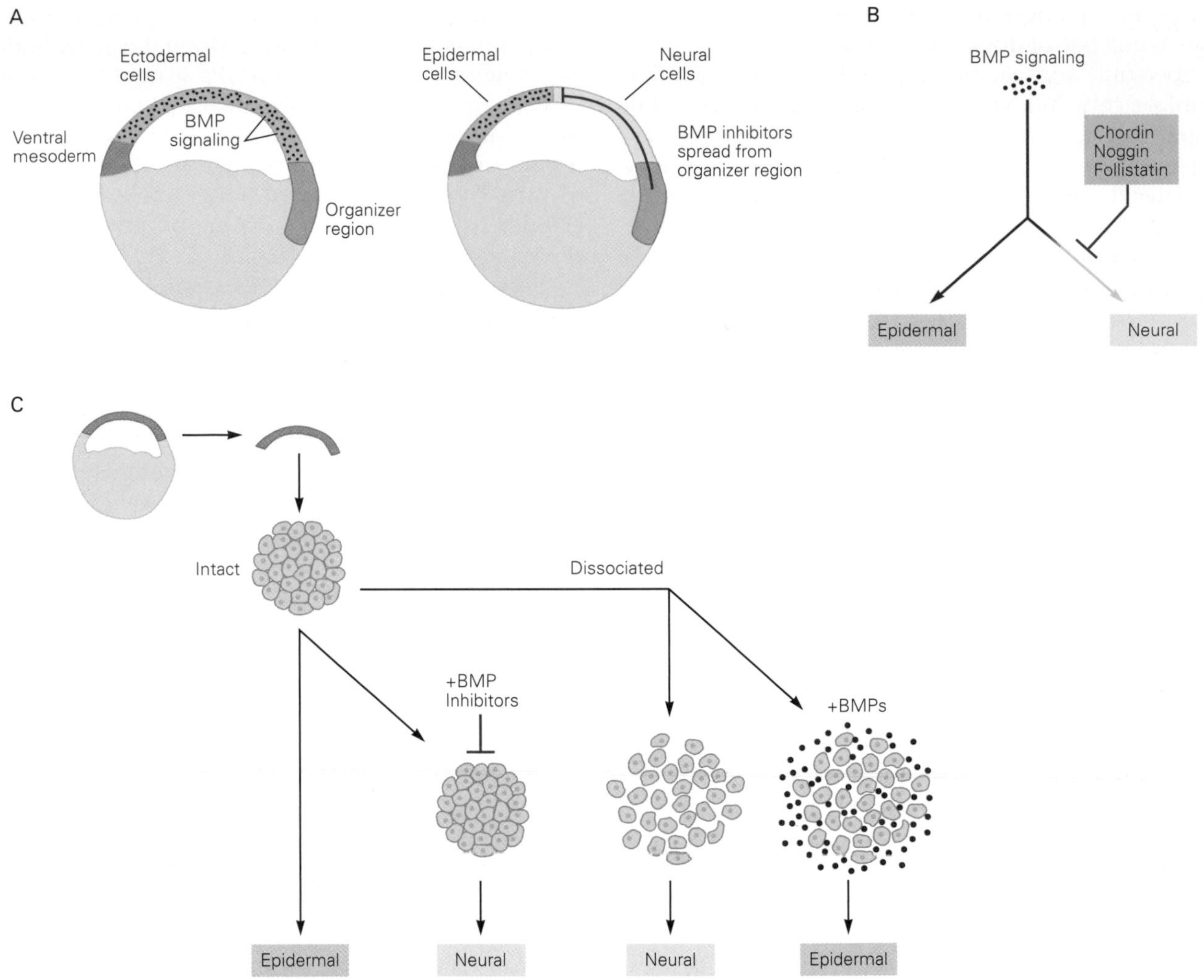

Figure 52–4 Inhibition of bone morphogenetic protein (BMP) signaling initiates neural induction.

A. In *Xenopus* frog embryos signals from the organizer region (**red line**) spread through the ectoderm to induce neural tissue. Ectodermal tissue that is beyond the range of organizer signals gives rise to epidermis.

B. BMP inhibitors secreted from the organizer region (including noggin, follistatin, and chordin) bind to BMPs and block the ability of ectodermal cells to acquire an epidermal fate, thus promoting neural character.

C. Ectodermal cells acquire neural or epidermal character depending on the presence or absence of BMP signaling. When ectodermal cell aggregates are exposed to BMP signaling they differentiate into epidermal tissue. When BMP signaling is blocked, either by dissociating ectodermal tissue into single cells or by addition of BMP inhibitors to ectodermal cell aggregates, the cells differentiate into neural tissue.

centers embedded within the neural tube. Some of these factors generate a broad rostrocaudal signaling gradient that can span the entire neural plate whereas others act more locally.

Neural plate cells in different regions of the neural tube respond to these inductive signals by expressing distinct transcription factors that gradually constrain the developmental potential of cells in each local domain. In this way neurons at different rostrocaudal levels acquire distinct identities and functions and the neural tube becomes subdivided along its rostrocaudal axis into functionally specific domains.

Signals from the Mesoderm and Endoderm Define the Rostrocaudal Pattern of the Neural Plate

The rostrocaudal patterning of the neural plate is initiated by factors secreted by mesodermal and endodermal tissues that flank the neural plate. One important class of factors is the Wnt proteins (an acronym based on their founding family members, the *Drosophila* Wingless protein and the mammalian *Int*1 proto-oncogene protein).

The net level of Wnt signaling activity is low at rostral levels of the neural plate and increases progressively in the caudal direction. This activity gradient arises because the mesoderm that flanks caudal regions of the neural plate expresses high levels of Wnt, whereas the endoderm that underlies the rostral region of the neural plate is a source of secreted proteins that inhibit Wnt signaling, much as BMP inhibitors attenuate BMP signaling at an earlier stage. Cells at progressively more caudal positions along the neural plate are exposed to increasing levels of Wnt activity and thus acquire a more caudal regional character, spanning the entire range from forebrain, to midbrain, to hindbrain and finally to spinal cord (Figure 52–5).

After the neural tube has acquired its initial rostrocaudal character, the mesoderm and endoderm secrete additional signals that further refine this pattern. At the very rostral margin of the neural tube a specialized group of cells, called the anterior neural ridge, secretes FGF that patterns the telencephalon, as we discuss later in the chapter. At more caudal levels of the neuraxis the secretion of retinoic acid and FGF from the mesoderm establishes distinct subdomains of the hindbrain and spinal cord.

Signals from Organizing Centers within the Neural Tube Pattern the Forebrain, Midbrain, and Hindbrain

The early influence of mesodermal and endodermal tissues on rostrocaudal neural pattern is further refined by signals from two specialized cell groups in the neural tube itself. One of these cell groups is called the *zona limitans intrathalamica* and appears as a pair of horn-like spurs within the diencephalon (Figure 52–6). Zona limitans intrathalamica cells secrete the protein sonic hedgehog (Shh), which patterns nearby cells that give rise to the nuclei of the thalamus. (The actions of sonic hedgehog are described in detail below in the context of its prominent role in spinal cord patterning.)

A second cell group, called the *isthmic organizer*, forms at the boundary of the hindbrain and midbrain. The isthmic organizer serves a key role in patterning these two domains of the neural tube as well as in specifying the neuronal subtypes within them. Dopaminergic neurons of the substantia nigra and ventral tegmental area are generated in the midbrain, just rostral to the isthmic organizer, whereas serotonergic neurons of the raphe nuclei are generated just caudal to the isthmic organizer, within the hindbrain. As an illustration of how these secondary neural signaling centers impose neural pattern, we describe the origin and signaling activities of the isthmic organizer.

The rostrocaudal positional character of the neural plate stems from the expression of homeodomain transcription factors. Cells in forebrain and midbrain domains of the neural plate express Otx2, whereas cells in the hindbrain domain express Gbx2. The point of transition of Otx2 and Gbx2 expression is located at the midbrain-hindbrain boundary (Figure 52–5) and marks the position at which the isthmic organizer will emerge after neural tube closure. At this boundary other transcription factors are expressed, notably En1 (an Engrailed class transcription factor).

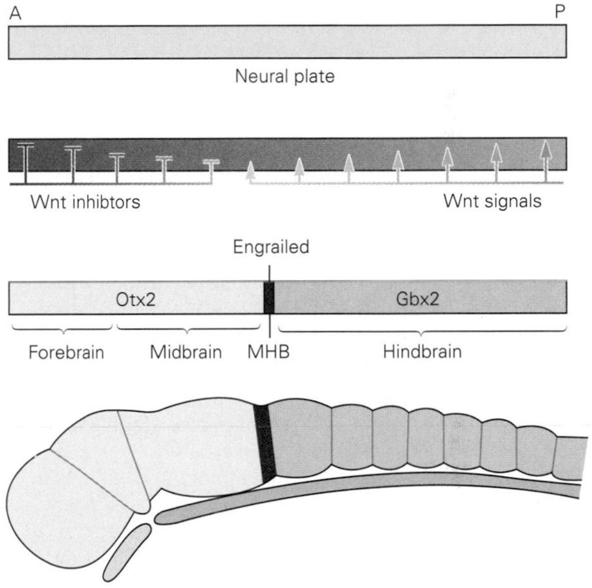

Figure 52–5 Early anteroposterior patterning signals establish distinct transcription factor domains and define the position of the midbrain-hindbrain boundary region. The anteroposterior pattern of the neural plate is established by exposure of neural cells to a gradient of Wnt signals. Anterior (**A**) regions of the neural plate are exposed to Wnt inhibitors secreted from the endoderm and thus perceive only low levels of Wnt activity. Progressively more posterior (**P**) regions of the neural plate are exposed to high levels of Wnt signaling from the paraxial mesoderm and to lower levels of Wnt inhibitors. In response to this Wnt signaling gradient and other signals, cells in anterior and posterior regions of the neural plate begin to express different transcription factors: Otx2 at anterior levels and Gbx2 at more posterior levels. The intersection of these two transcription factor domains marks the region of the midbrain-hindbrain boundary (**MHB**), where Engrailed transcription factors are expressed. (Adapted, with permission, from Wurst and Bally-Cuif 2001.)

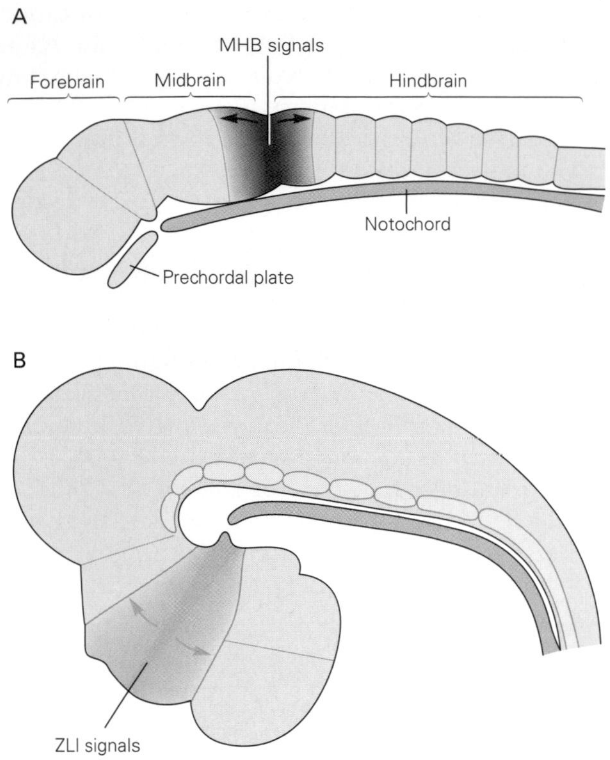

Figure 52–6 Local signaling centers in the developing neural tube. (Adapted, with permission, from Kiecker and Lumsden 2005.)

A. This side view of the early neural tube shows the location of the midbrain-hindbrain boundary (**MHB**), the source of secreted signals that pattern cell types in the midbrain and hindbrain. The prechordal plate and notochord are two nonneural signaling centers that influence the dorsoventral patterning of the neural tube.

B. This side view of the neural tube at a later stage shows the position of the zona limitans intrathalamica (**ZLI**) at the boundary within the caudal forebrain (diencephalon). The ZLI is a source of sonic hedgehog signals.

These transcription factors in turn control the expression of two signaling factors, Wnt1 and FGF8, by cells of the isthmic organizer. Wnt1 is involved in the proliferation of cells in the midbrain-hindbrain domain and in the maintenance of FGF8 expression. The spread of FGF8 from the isthmic organizer into the midbrain domain marked by Otx2 expression induces differentiation of dopaminergic neurons, whereas its spread into the hindbrain domain marked by Gbx2 expression triggers the differentiation of serotonergic neurons (Figure 52–7A).

The differential action of FGF8 illustrates an important economy in early neural patterning. The early actions of inductive signals impose discrete domains of transcription factor expression, and these transcriptional domains then allow cells to interpret the actions of the same secreted factor in different ways, producing different neuronal subtypes. In this way a relatively small number of secreted factors—FGFs, BMPs, hedgehog proteins, Wnt proteins, and retinoic acid—are used in different regions and at different times to program the vast diversity of neuronal cell types generated within the central and peripheral nervous systems.

Dorsoventral Patterning of the Neural Tube Involves Similar Mechanisms at Different Rostrocaudal Levels

As soon as the neural epithelium acquires its rostrocaudal character, cells located at different positions along its dorsoventral axis start to differentiate into various neuronal and glial cell types.

In contrast to the diversity of signals and organizing centers responsible for rostrocaudal patterning of developing neurons, there is a striking consistency in the strategies and principles that establish dorsoventral pattern. We focus initially on the mechanisms of dorsoventral patterning at caudal levels of the neural tube that give rise to the spinal cord, and then describe how similar strategies are used to pattern the forebrain.

Neurons in the spinal cord serve two major functions. They relay cutaneous sensory input to higher centers in the brain and they transform sensory input into motor output. The neuronal circuits that mediate these functions are segregated anatomically. Circuits involved in the processing of cutaneous sensory information are located in the dorsal half of the spinal cord, whereas those involved in the control of motor output are mainly located in the ventral half of the spinal cord. The neurons that form these circuits are generated at different positions along the dorsoventral axis of the spinal cord in a patterning process that begins with the establishment of distinct progenitor cell types.

In the ventral half of the neural tube motor neurons are generated close to the ventral midline, and most of the interneuron classes that control motor output are generated just dorsal to the position at which motor neurons appear (Figure 52–8). The dorsal half of the neural tube generates projection neurons and local circuit interneurons that process incoming sensory information. In addition, the dorsal neural tube gives rise to neural crest cells, a population of stem cells that migrate out of the neural tube into the periphery, where they serve as precursors to the entire peripheral nervous system.

How are the position and identity of spinal neurons established? The dorsoventral patterning of the neural tube is initiated by signals from mesodermal and ectodermal cells that lie close to the ventral and dorsal poles of the neural tube, and is perpetuated by signals from two midline neural organizing centers. Ventral patterning signals are initially provided by the notochord, a mesodermal cell group that lies immediately under the ventral neural tube, and this signaling activity is transferred to the floor plate, a specialized glial cell group that sits at the ventral midline of the neural tube itself. Dorsal signals are provided initially by cells of the epidermal ectoderm that span the dorsal midline of the neural tube, and subsequently by the roof plate, a glial cell group embedded at the dorsal midline of the neural tube (Figure 52–8D).

Thus neural patterning is initiated through a process of *homogenetic* induction, in which like begets like: Notochord signals induce the floor plate, which induces ventral neurons, and signals from ectoderm induce the roof plate, which induces dorsal neurons. This strategy ensures that inductive signals are positioned appropriately to control neural cell fate and pattern over a prolonged period of development, as tissues grow and cells move.

The Ventral Neural Tube Is Patterned by Sonic Hedgehog Protein Secreted from the Notochord and Floor Plate

Within the ventral half of the neural tube the identity and position of developing motor neurons and local interneurons depends on the inductive activity of the sonic hedgehog (Shh) protein, which is secreted by the notochord and subsequently by the floor plate (Figure 52–7A). Shh is a member of a family of secreted proteins related to the *Drosophila* hedgehog protein, which controls many aspects of embryonic development.

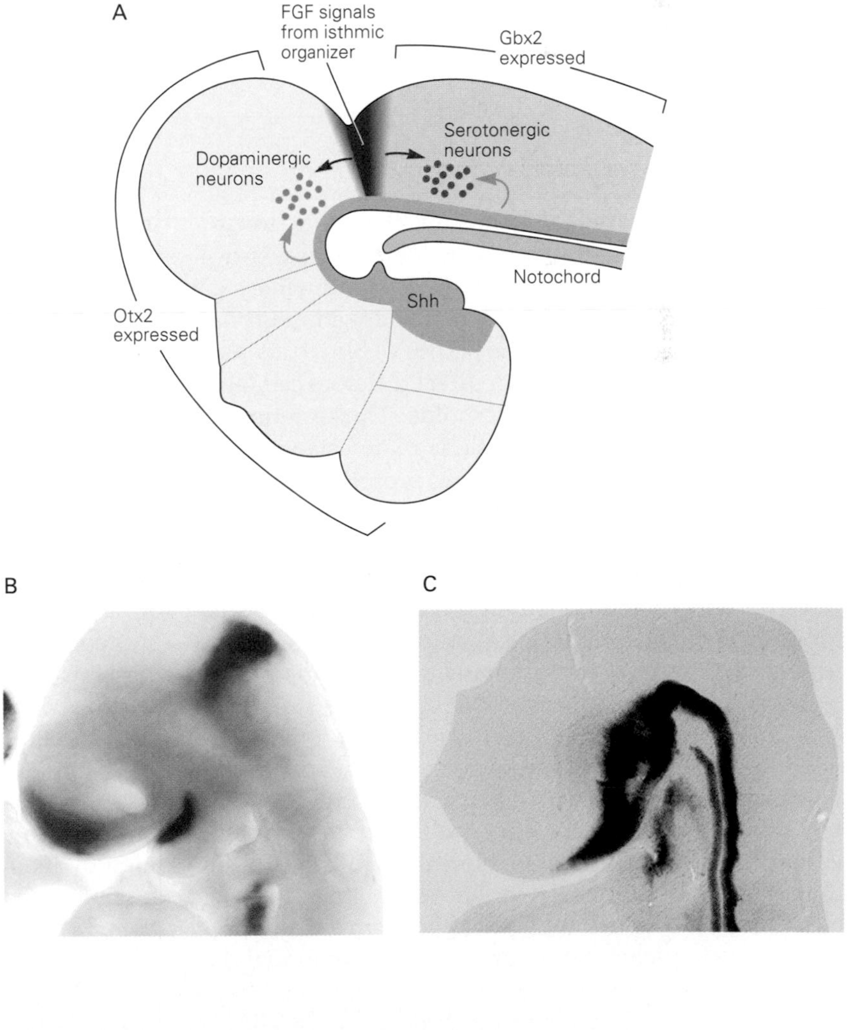

Figure 52–7 Signals from the midbrain-hindbrain boundary pattern neurons in the midbrain and hindbrain.

A. Fibroblast growth factor (**FGF**) signals from the isthmic organizer act in concert with sonic hedgehog (**Shh**) signals from the ventral midline to specify the identity and position of dopaminergic and serotonergic neurons. The distinct fates of these two classes of neurons result from the different transcriptional profiles of cells in the midbrain (Otx2) and hindbrain (Gbx2). (Adapted, with permission, from Wurst and Bally-Cuif 2001.)

B. Expression of the gene encoding FGF4 by cells at the midbrain-hindbrain boundary. (Image reproduced, with permission, from Gail Martin.)

C. Expression of the gene encoding Shh by cells at the ventral midline of the neural tube and by the notochord. (Image reproduced, with permission, from T. Lints and J. Dodd.)

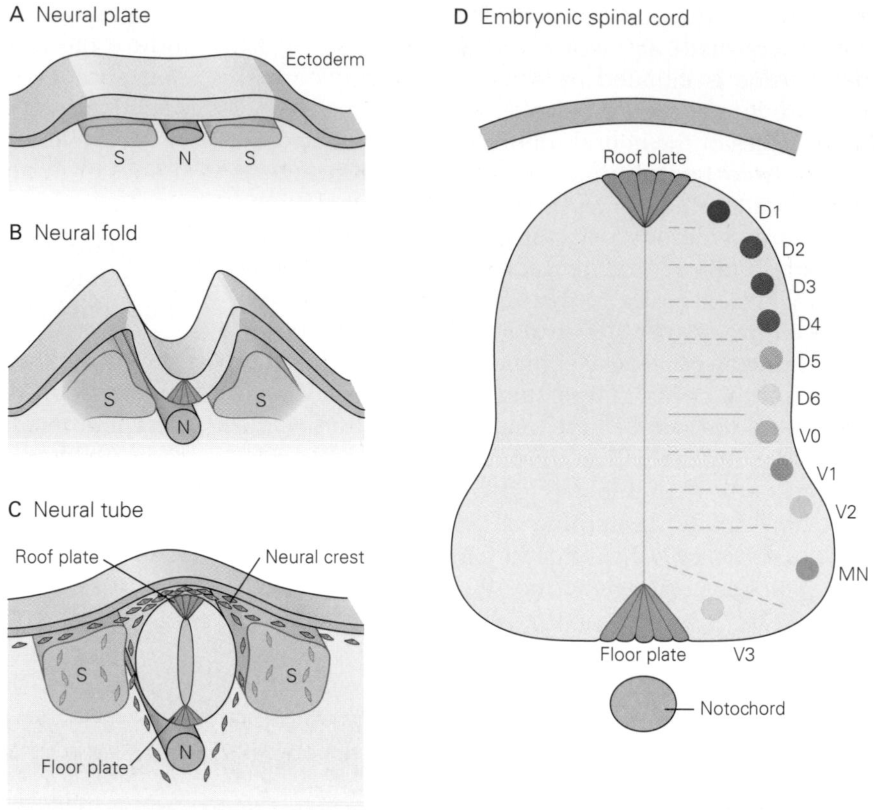

Figure 52–8 Stages in the early development of the spinal cord.

A. The neural plate is generated from ectodermal cells that overlie the notochord (**N**) and the future somites (**S**). It is flanked by the epidermal ectoderm.

B. The neural plate folds dorsally at its midline to form the neural fold. Floor plate cells (**blue**) differentiate at the ventral midline of the neural tube.

C. The neural tube forms by fusion of the dorsal tips of the neural folds. Roof plate cells form at the dorsal midline of the neural tube. Neural crest cells migrate from the neural tube into and past the somites before populating the sensory and sympathetic ganglia.

D. Distinct classes of neurons are generated at different dorsoventral positions in the embryonic spinal cord. Ventral interneurons (**V0–V3**) and motor neurons (**MN**) differentiate from progenitor domains in the ventral spinal cord. Six classes of early dorsal interneurons (**D1** to **D6**) develop in the dorsal half of the spinal cord. (Adapted, with permission, from Goulding et al. 2002.)

Shh signaling is necessary for the induction of each of the neuronal classes generated in the ventral half of the spinal cord. How can a single inductive signal specify the fate of at least half a dozen neuronal classes? The answer lies in the ability of Shh to act as a morphogen—a signal that can direct different cell fates at different concentration thresholds. The secretion of Shh from the notochord and floor plate establishes a ventral-to-dorsal gradient of Shh protein activity in the ventral neural tube, such that progenitor cells that occupy different dorsoventral positions within the neural epithelium are exposed to small (two- to threefold) differences in ambient Shh signaling activity. Different levels of Shh signaling activity direct progenitor cells in different ventral domains to differentiation as motor neurons and interneurons (Figure 52–9).

These findings raise two additional questions. How is the spread of Shh protein within the ventral neural epithelium controlled in such a precise manner? And how are small differences in Shh signaling activity converted into all-or-none decisions about the identity of progenitor cells in the ventral neural tube?

Active Shh protein is synthesized from a larger precursor protein, cleaved through an unusual autocatalytic process that involves a serine protease-like activity resident within the carboxy terminus of the precursor protein. Cleavage generates an amino terminal protein fragment that possesses all of the signaling activity of Shh. During cleavage the active amino terminal fragment is modified covalently by the addition of a cholesterol molecule. The addition of this lipophilic anchor tethers most of the Shh protein to the surface of notochord and floor plate cells. Nevertheless, a small fraction of the anchored protein is released from the cell surface and transferred from cell to cell within the ventral neural epithelium. In reality the molecular machinery that ensures the formation of a long-distance gradient of extracellular Shh protein is more complex, involving specialized transmembrane proteins that promote the release of Shh from the floor plate, as well as proteins that regulate Shh protein transfer between cells.

How does the gradient of Shh protein within the ventral neural tube direct progenitor cells along different pathways of differentiation? Shh signaling is initiated by its interaction with a transmembrane receptor complex that consists of a ligand-binding subunit called *patched* and a signal-transducing subunit called *smoothened* (named for the corresponding fly genes).

The binding of Shh to patched relieves its inhibition of smoothened and so activates an intracellular signaling pathway that involves several protein kinase enzymes, transport proteins, and most important the Gli proteins, a class of zinc finger transcription factors.

In the absence of Shh the Gli proteins are proteolytically processed into transcriptional repressors that prevent the activation of Shh target genes. Activation of the Shh signaling pathway inhibits this proteolytic processing, with the result that transcriptional activator forms of Gli predominate, thus directing the expression of Shh target genes. In this way an extracellular gradient of Shh protein is converted into a nuclear gradient of Gli activator proteins. The ratio of Gli repressor and activator proteins at different dorsoventral positions determines which target genes are activated.

What genes are activated by Shh-Gli signaling and how do they participate in the specification of ventral neuronal subtypes? The major Gli targets are genes encoding yet more transcription factors. One major class of Gli targets encodes homeodomain proteins, transcription factors that contain a conserved DNA-binding motif termed a *homeobox*. A second major class of target genes encodes proteins with a basic helix-loop-helix DNA-binding motif. Some homeodomain and basic helix-loop-helix proteins are repressed and others activated by Shh signaling, each at a particular concentration threshold. In this way cells in the ventral neural tube are allocated to one of five cardinal progenitor domains, each marked by its own transcription factor profile (Figure 52–9).

The transcription factors that define adjacent progenitor domains repress each other's expression. Thus,

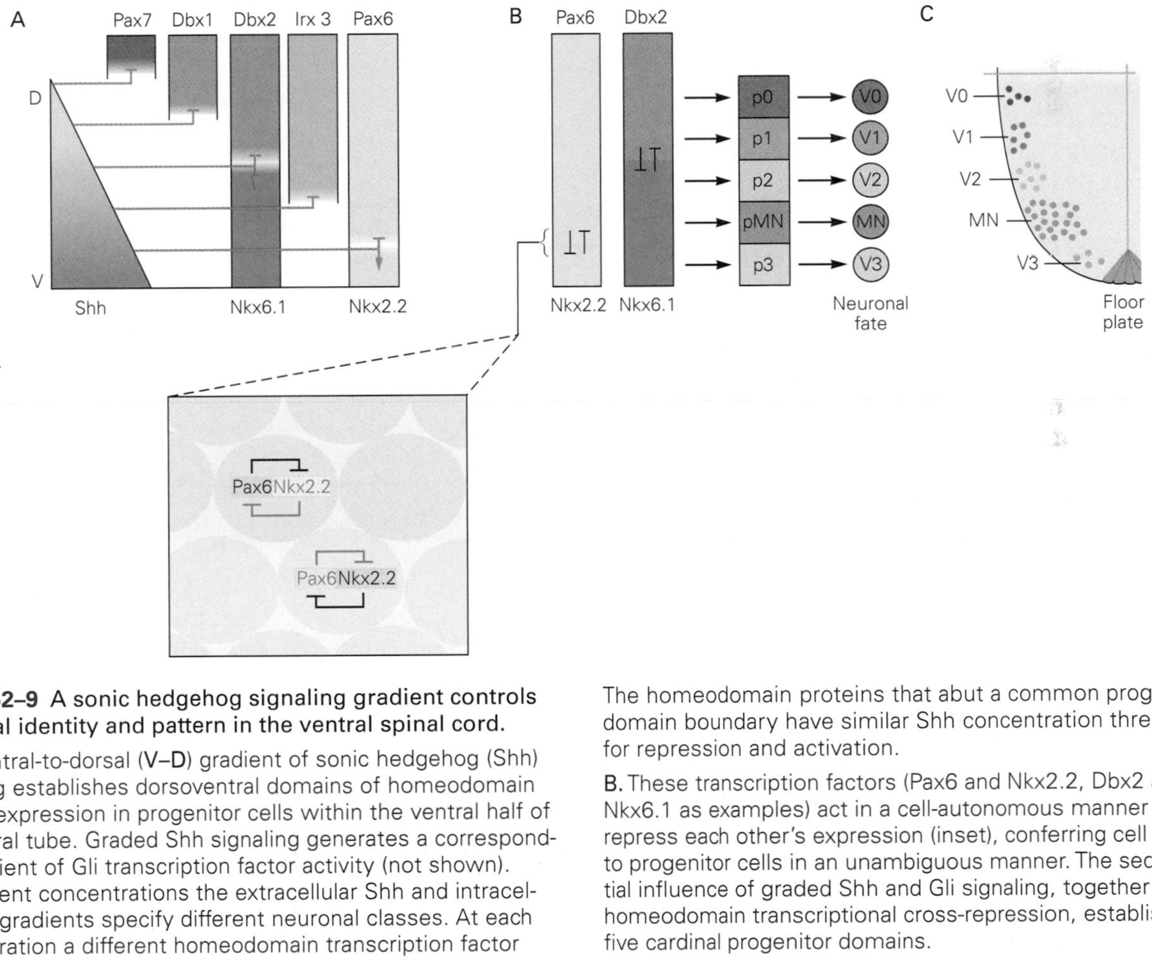

Figure 52–9 A sonic hedgehog signaling gradient controls neuronal identity and pattern in the ventral spinal cord.

A. A ventral-to-dorsal (**V–D**) gradient of sonic hedgehog (Shh) signaling establishes dorsoventral domains of homeodomain protein expression in progenitor cells within the ventral half of the neural tube. Graded Shh signaling generates a corresponding gradient of Gli transcription factor activity (not shown). At different concentrations the extracellular Shh and intracellular Gli gradients specify different neuronal classes. At each concentration a different homeodomain transcription factor (Pax7, Dbx1, Dbx2, Irx3, or Pax6) is repressed, with Pax7 the most sensitive and Pax6 the least sensitive to repression. Other homeodomain transcription factors (Nkx6.1 and Nkx2.2) are induced at different Shh and Gli signaling levels. The homeodomain proteins that abut a common progenitor domain boundary have similar Shh concentration thresholds for repression and activation.

B. These transcription factors (Pax6 and Nkx2.2, Dbx2 and Nkx6.1 as examples) act in a cell-autonomous manner to repress each other's expression (inset), conferring cell identity to progenitor cells in an unambiguous manner. The sequential influence of graded Shh and Gli signaling, together with homeodomain transcriptional cross-repression, establishes five cardinal progenitor domains.

C. The postmitotic neurons that emerge from these domains give rise to the five major classes of ventral neurons: the interneurons **V0–V3** and motor neurons (**MN**).

although a cell may initially express several transcription factors that could direct the cell along different pathways of differentiation, a minor imbalance in the starting concentration of the two factors is rapidly amplified through repression, and only one of these proteins is stably expressed. This winner-take-all strategy of transcriptional repression sharpens the boundaries of progenitor domains and ensures that an initial gradient of Shh and Gli activity will resolve itself into clear distinctions in transcription factor profile. The transcription factors that specify a ventral progenitor domain then direct the expression of downstream genes that commit progenitor cells to a particular postmitotic neuronal identity.

Studies of the logic of ventral neuronal patterning have thus shown that the fate of a neuron is determined in part by the actions of transcriptional repressors rather than activators. This principle operates in many other tissues and organisms, emphasizing that principles of neuronal patterning have been cobbled together from strategies that have proved useful in directing other aspects of embryonic development. Disruption of components of the Shh signaling pathway results in a wide variety of human diseases. Mutations in human Shh pathway genes result in defects in the development of ventral forebrain structures (holoprosencephaly), as well as neurological defects such as spina bifida, limb deformities, and certain cancers.

The Dorsal Neural Tube Is Patterned by Bone Morphogenetic Proteins

A signaling strategy based on graded morphogen levels activating sets of transcriptional programs has also been found to determine the patterning of cell types in the dorsal spinal cord. The differentiation of roof plate cells at the dorsal midline of the neural tube is triggered by BMP signals from epidermal cells that initially border the neural plate and later flank the dorsal neural tube.

After the neural tube has closed, roof plate cells themselves begin to express BMP as well as Wnt proteins. Wnt proteins promote the proliferation of progenitor cells in the dorsal neural tube. BMP proteins induce the differentiation of neural crest cells and later the generation of diverse populations of sensory relay neurons that settle in the dorsal spinal cord.

Dorsoventral Patterning Mechanisms Are Conserved Along the Rostrocaudal Extent of the Neural Tube

The strategies used to establish dorsoventral pattern in the spinal cord also control cell identity and pattern along the dorsoventral axis of the hindbrain and midbrain, as well as throughout much of the forebrain.

In the mesencephalic region of the neural tube Shh signals from the floor plate act in concert with the rostrocaudal patterning signals discussed earlier to specify dopaminergic neurons of the substantia nigra and ventral tegmental area as well as serotonergic neurons of the raphe nuclei (see Figure 52–7). In the forebrain Shh signals from the ventral midline and BMP signals from the dorsal midline act in combination to establish different regional domains. Shh signaling from the ventral midline sets up early progenitor domains that later produce neurons of the basal ganglia and some cortical interneurons, whereas BMP signaling from the dorsal midline is involved in establishing early neocortical character.

Local Signals Determine Functional Subclasses of Neurons

To this point we have seen how a uniform group of neural precursor cells, the neural plate, is progressively partitioned into discrete rostrocaudal and dorsoventral domains within the neural tube, and how cells in these domains are subject to specialized programs of neural differentiation. But how are cells within these domains able to generate the extraordinary diversity of neuronal classes that typifies the vertebrate central nervous system? We answer that question by focusing on development of the motor neuron.

Motor neurons can be distinguished from all other classes of neurons in the central nervous system by the simple fact that they have axons that extend out of the spinal cord into the periphery. Viewed in this light, motor neurons represent a coherent and distinct subtype. But motor neuron subtypes can be distinguished by their position within the central nervous system as well as by the target cells they innervate. The primary job of most motor neurons is to innervate skeletal muscles, of which there are approximately 600 in a typical mammal. From this it follows that there must be an equal number of motor neuron classes.

In this section we discuss the developmental mechanisms that direct the differentiation of these different functional subclasses. The details of motor neuron development are also important for understanding the basis of neurological disorders that affect these neurons, including spinal muscular atrophy and amyotrophic lateral sclerosis (Lou Gehrig disease). Similar principles drive the diversification of other neuronal classes.

Rostrocaudal Position Is a Major Determinant of Motor Neuron Subtype

Motor neurons are generated along much of the rostrocaudal axis of the neural tube, from the midbrain to the spinal cord. Distinct motor neuron subclasses develop at each rostrocaudal level (Figure 52–10), suggesting that one goal of the patterning signals that establish rostrocaudal positional identity within the neural tube is to make motor neurons different.

One major class of genes involved in specifying motor neuron subtypes is the *Hox* gene family. These homeobox genes encode a family of transcription factors that contain a homeodomain. Homeodomain proteins represent a major class of transcription factors that regulate developmental processes in organisms as diverse as yeast, plants, and mammals. The mammalian genome contains 39 *Hox* genes, organized in four chromosomal clusters. These genes derive from an ancestral *Hox* complex that also gave rise to the *HOM-C* gene complex in *Drosophila* (Figure 52–11).

Members of the vertebrate *Hox* gene family are expressed in overlapping domains along the rostrocaudal

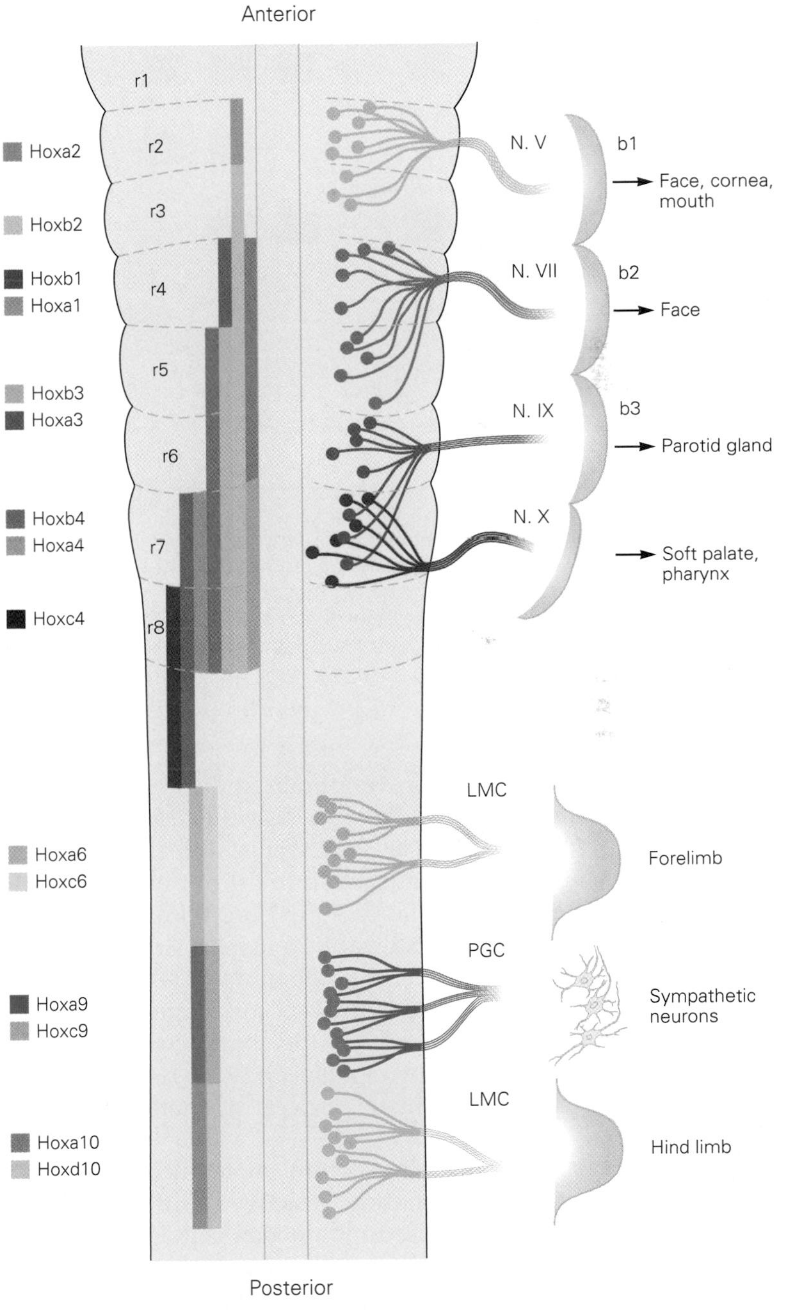

Figure 52–10 The anteroposterior profile of *Hox* gene expression determines the subtype of motor neurons in the hindbrain and spinal cord. Different Hox proteins are expressed in discrete but partially overlapping rostrocaudal domains of the hindbrain and spinal cord. The position of *Hox* genes on the four mammalian chromosomal clusters roughly corresponds to their domain of expression along the anteroposterior axis of the neural tube.

At hindbrain levels motor neurons sending axons into cranial nerves V (trigeminal), VII (facial), IX (glossopharyngeal), and X (vagus) are depicted. These cranial motor nerves project to peripheral targets in the branchial arches **b1–b3**. The hindbrain rhombomeres (**r1–r8**) and Hox profiles are shown on the left.

At spinal levels, motor neurons that send axons to the forelimb and hind limb are contained within the lateral motor columns (**LMC**), located at brachial and lumbar levels of the spinal cord, respectively. Preganglionic autonomic motor neurons (**PGC**) destined to innervate sympathetic ganglion targets are generated at thoracic levels. (Adapted, with permission, from Kiecker and Lumsden 2005.)

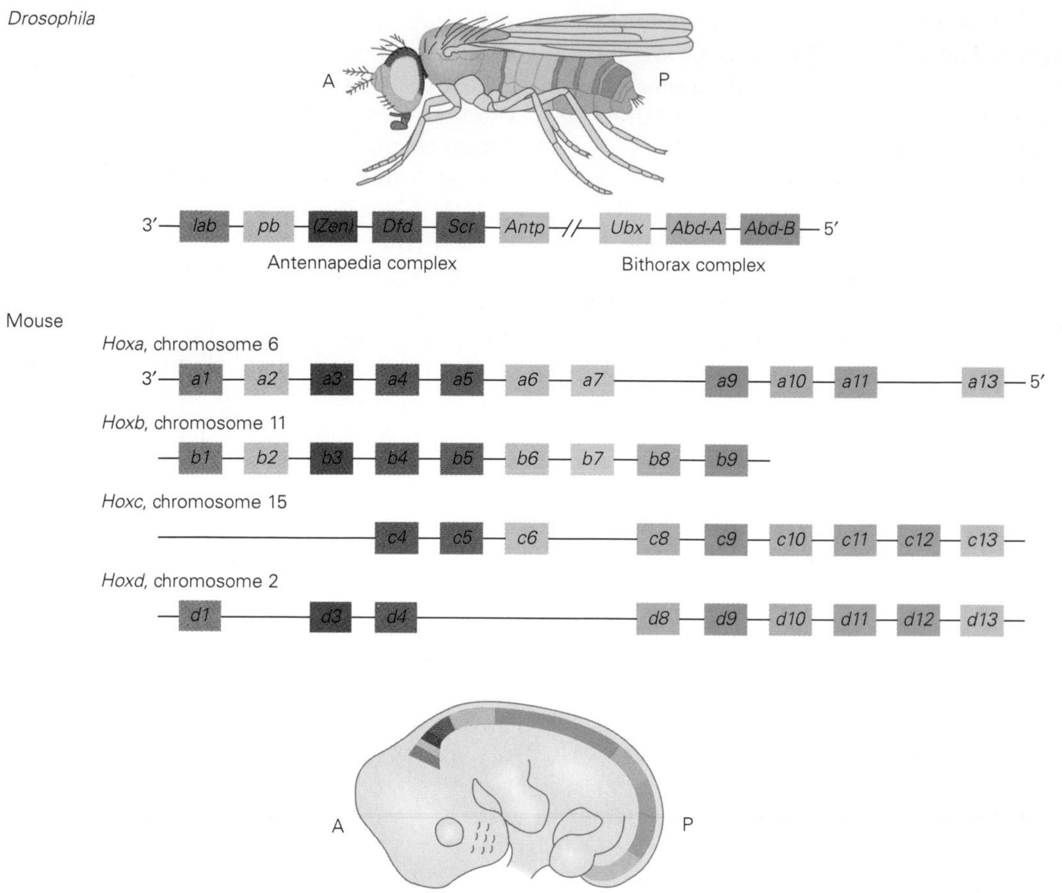

Figure 52–11 The clustered organization of *Hox* genes is conserved from flies to vertebrates. The diagram shows the chromosomal arrangement of *Hox* genes in the mouse and *HOM-C* genes in *Drosophila.* Insects have one ancestral *Hox* gene cluster, whereas higher vertebrates such as birds and mammals have four duplicate *Hox* gene clusters. The position of a given *Hox* or *HOM-C* gene on the chromosomal cluster is typically related to the position on the anteroposterior body axis where the gene is expressed. (Adapted, with permission, from Wolpert et al. 1988.)

axis of the developing midbrain, hindbrain, and spinal cord. As in *Drosophila,* the position of an individual *Hox* gene within its cluster predicts its rostrocaudal domain of expression within the neural tube. In most but not all cases, *Hox* genes located at more 3′ positions within the chromosomal cluster are expressed in more rostral domains, within the midbrain and hindbrain, whereas genes at more 5′ positions are expressed in progressively more caudal positions within the spinal cord (Figures 52–10 and 52–11). This spatial array of *Hox* gene expression determines many aspects of motor neuron subtype.

We illustrate how *Hox* genes control motor neuron identity by focusing on neurons generated in the hindbrain and spinal cord. The fundamental cellular building blocks of the hindbrain are termed *rhombomeres,* compartmental units that are arrayed along the rostrocaudal axis of the hindbrain (Figure 52–10). Genetic studies in the mouse have shown that specific *Hox* genes control the identity of neurons in individual rhombomeres. For example, *Hoxb1* is expressed at high levels in rhombomere 4, the domain that gives rise to facial motor neurons, but is absent from rhombomere 2, the domain that gives rise to trigeminal motor neurons (Figure 52–10).

In the mouse, mutations that eliminate the activity of *Hoxb1* change the fate of cells in rhombomere 4; there is a switch in the identity and connectivity of the motor neurons that emerge from this domain. In the absence of *Hoxb1* function cells in rhombomere 4 generate motor neurons that innervate trigeminal rather than facial targets, that is, the motor neuron subtype normally generated within rhombomere 2 (Figure 52–12).

Other studies of *Hox* gene function within the hindbrain have confirmed the general principle that motor neuron identity is controlled by the spatial distribution of *Hox* gene expression.

The challenge of connecting individual spinal motor neurons with particular muscles in the limbs and body wall demands an even more complex program of cellular and molecular differentiation. Spinal motor neurons are clustered within longitudinal columns that occupy discrete segmental positions, in register with their peripheral targets. Motor neurons that innervate forelimb and hindlimb muscles are found in the lateral motor columns at cervical and lumbar levels of the spinal cord, respectively. In contrast, motor neurons that innervate sympathetic neuronal targets are found within the preganglionic motor column at thoracic levels of the spinal cord. Within the lateral motor columns, motor neurons that innervate a single limb muscle are clustered together into discrete groups, termed *motor pools*. Because each limb in higher vertebrates contains more than 50 different muscle groups, a corresponding number of motor pools are required.

The identity of motor neurons in the spinal cord is controlled by the coordinate activity of *Hox* genes found at more 5′ positions within the chromosomal *Hox* clusters. For example, the spatial domains of expression and activity of Hox6 and Hox9 proteins establish the identities of motor neurons in the brachial lateral motor column and the preganglionic motor column. Hox6 proteins specify brachial lateral motor column identity, whereas Hox9 proteins specify preganglionic motor column identity. Motor neurons at the boundary of the forelimb and thoracic regions acquire an unambiguous columnar identity because the Hox6 and Hox9 proteins are mutually repressive (Figure 52–13), similar to the transcriptional cross-repression that occurs in the dorsoventral patterning of the spinal cord.

Local Signals and Transcriptional Circuits Further Diversify Motor Neuron Subtypes

How do motor neurons within the lateral motor columns develop more refined identities, directing their axons to specific limb muscles? Once again, *Hox* genes control this stage of motor neuron diversification. We illustrate this function of Hox proteins by considering the pathway that generates the distinct divisional and pool identities of neurons within the brachial lateral motor column that innervate the muscles of the forelimb (Figure 52–13A).

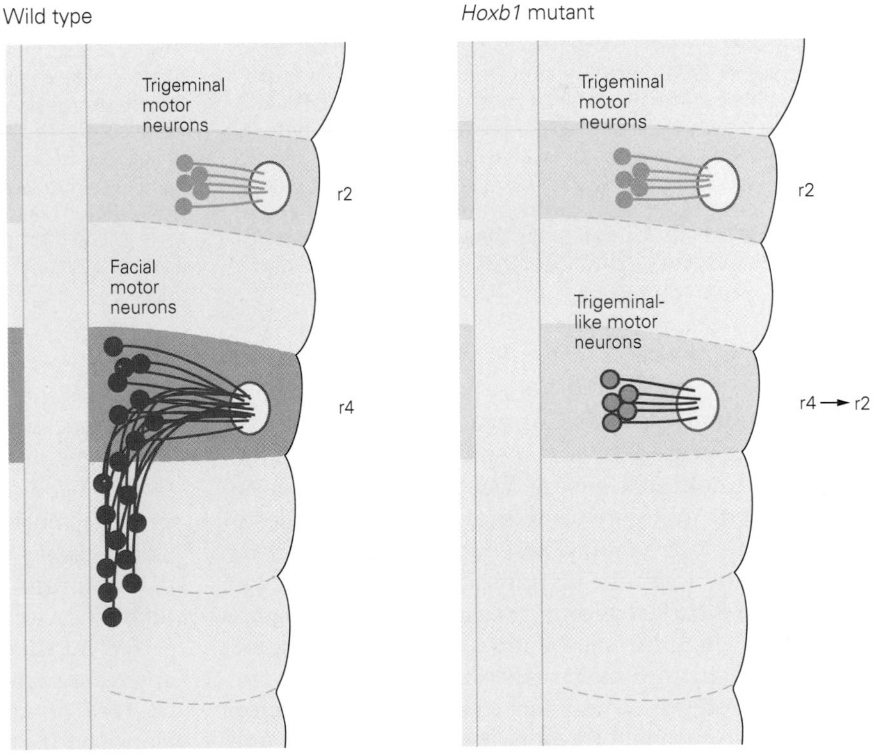

Figure 52–12 The mouse *Hoxb1* gene controls the identity and projection of hindbrain motor neurons. *Hoxb1* is normally expressed at highest levels by cells in rhombomere r4. In wild type mice trigeminal motor neurons are generated in rhombomere r2, and their cell bodies migrate laterally before projecting their axons out of the hindbrain at the r2 level. In contrast, the cell bodies of facial motor neurons generated in rhombomere r4 migrate caudally yet project their axons out of the hindbrain at the r4 level. In mouse *Hoxb1* mutants motor neurons generated in rhombomere r4 migrate laterally instead of caudally, acquiring the features of r2 level trigeminal motor neurons. Ellipses indicate axonal exit points. (Adapted, with permission, from Struder et al. 1996.)

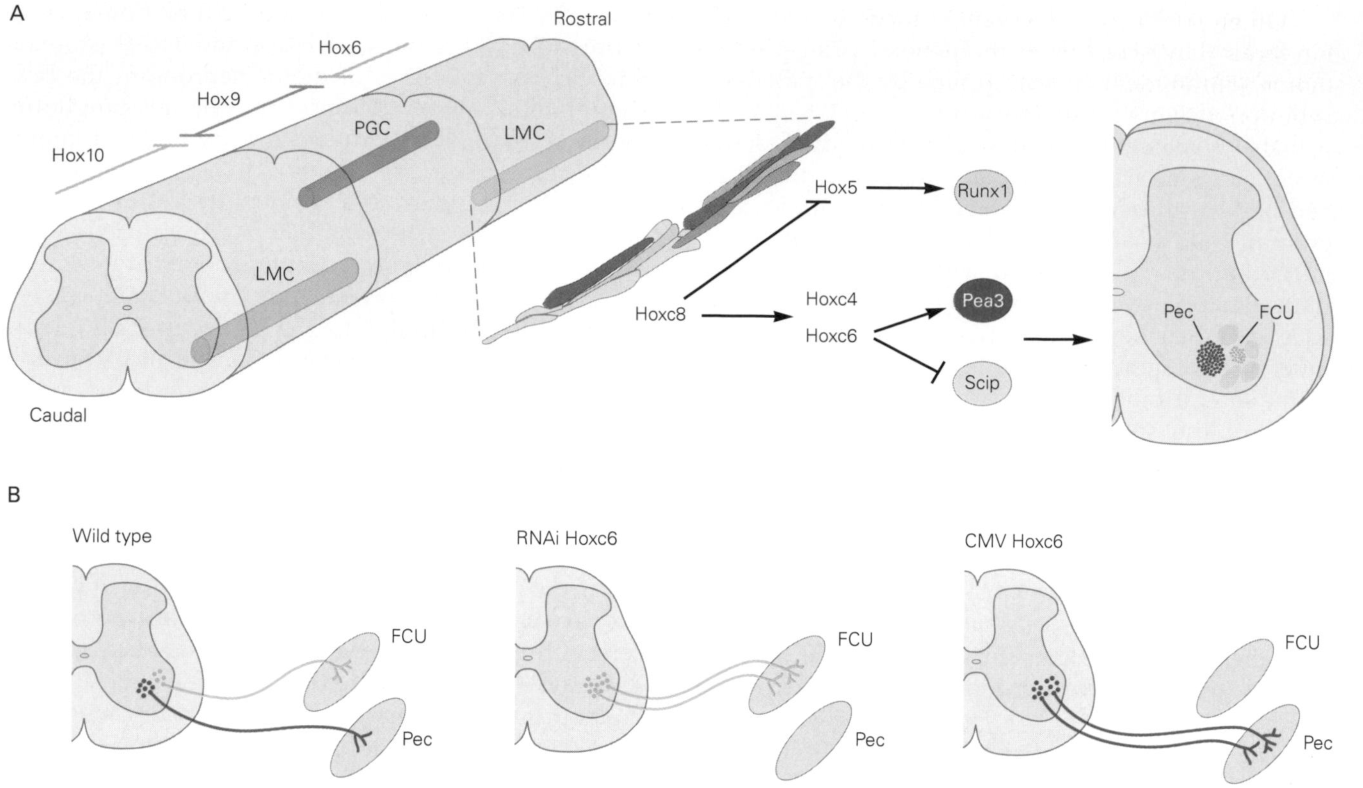

Figure 52–13 **Hox proteins control the identity of neurons in motor columns and pools.** (Adapted, with permission, from Daser et al. 2005.)

A. Hox6, Hox9, and Hox10 proteins are expressed in motor neurons at distinct rostrocaudal levels of the spinal cord and direct motor neuron identity and peripheral target connectivity. Hox6 activities control the identity of cells in the brachial lateral motor column (**LMC**), Hox9 controls the identity of cells in the preganglionic column (**PGC**), and Hox10 the identity of cells in the lumbar column (**LMC**). Cross-repressive interactions between Hox6, Hox9, and Hox10 proteins refine Hox profiles, and Hox activator functions define LMC and PGC identities. A more complex Hox transcriptional network controls motor pool identity and connectivity. Hox genes determine the rostrocaudal position of motor pools within the LMC. Hoxc8 is required in caudal LMC neurons to generate the motor pools for the pectoralis (**Pec**) and flexor carpi ulnaris (**FCU**) muscles; these neurons express the transcription factors Pea3 and Scip, respectively. The patterns of Hox expression in the Pec and FCU pools are established through a transcriptional network that appears to be driven largely by Hox cross-repressive interactions.

B. Changing the Hox code within motor pools changes the pattern of muscle connectivity. Alterations in the profile of Hox6 expression determine the expression of Pea3 and Scip and control the projection of motor axons to the Pec or FCU muscles. RNAi knock-down of Hox6 suppresses innervation of the Pec muscle so that motor axons innervate the FCU muscle only. Ectopic expression of Hoxc6 driven by a cytomegalovirus (CMV) promoter represses connectivity with FCU, so that motor axons innervate only the Pec muscle.

Additional repressive interactions between Hox proteins expressed by the neurons in different lateral motor columns ensure that neurons that populate different motor pools express distinct profiles of Hox protein expression. These Hox profiles direct the expression of downstream transcription factors as well as the axonal surface receptors that enable motor axons to respond to local cues within the limb that guide them to specific muscle targets (Figure 52–13A).

Hox proteins control the expression of receptors for guidance cues that direct motor axons into the limb. The expression of Hox6 proteins activates a retinoic acid signaling pathway that directs the expression of two homeodomain transcription factors, Is11 and Lhx1. These factors in turn assign motor neurons into two divisional classes and determine the pattern of expression of the ephrin receptors that guide motor axons in the limb. The axons of motor neurons in these two divisions project into the ventral and dorsal halves of the limb mesenchyme under the control of ephrin signaling (Figure 52–14). The mechanism by which ephrins direct axons along specific trajectories will be described in Chapter 54.

Not all motor neuron columns are determined by Hox protein activity, however. The median motor column is generated at all segmental levels of the spinal cord in register with axial muscles. Development of median motor column cells is controlled by Wnt4/5 signals secreted from the ventral midline of the spinal cord, and by the expression of the homeodomain proteins Lhx3 and Lhx4, which render neurons in this column immune to the segmental patterning actions of Hox proteins.

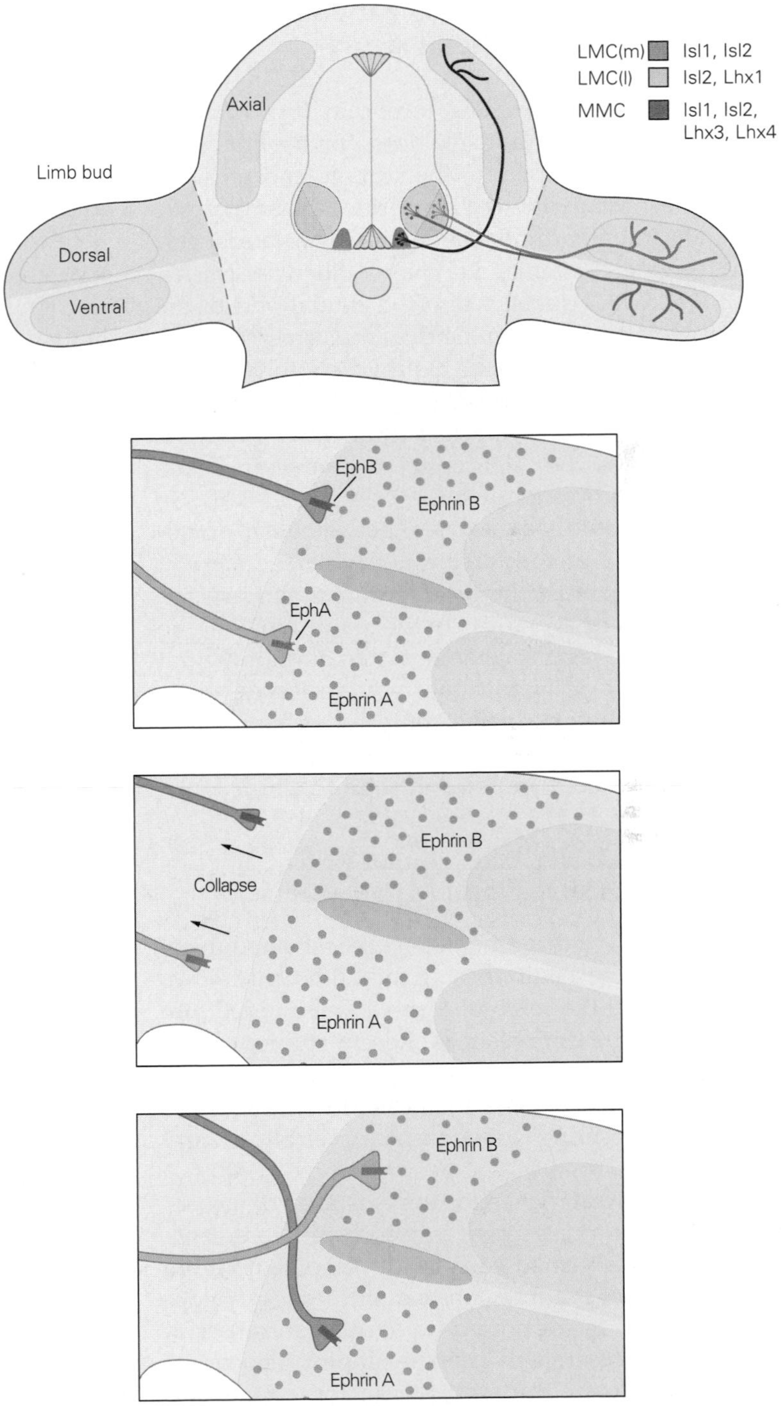

Figure 52–14 The axons of lateral motor column neurons are guided into the limb by ephrin class tyrosine kinase receptors. Motor neurons in the medial and lateral divisions of the lateral motor column (**LMC**) project axons into the ventral and dorsal halves of the limb mesenchyme, respectively. The profile of expression of LIM class homeodomain proteins regulates this dorsoventral projection. The LIM homeodomain protein Isl1 expressed by medial LMC neurons directs a high level of expression of EphB receptors, such that as the axons of these cells enter the limb they are prevented from projecting dorsally by the high level of repellant ephrin B ligands expressed by cells of the dorsal limb mesenchyme. These axons therefore project into the ventral limb mesenchyme. Conversely, the LIM homeodomain protein Lhx1 expressed by lateral LMC neurons directs a high level of expression of EphA receptors, such that as the axons of these cells enter the limb they are prevented from projecting ventrally by the high level of repellant ephrin A ligands expressed by cells of the ventral limb mesenchyme. These axons therefore project into the dorsal limb mesenchyme. (**MMC**, medial motor column.)

Thus in both the hindbrain and spinal cord the point-to-point connectivity of motor neurons with specific muscles emerges through tightly orchestrated programs of homeodomain protein expression and activity. In vertebrates these genes have evolved to direct neuron subtype and connectivity as well the basic body plan.

The Developing Forebrain Is Patterned by Intrinsic and Extrinsic Influences

Neurons in the mammalian forebrain form circuits that mediate emotional behaviors, perception, and cognition and participate in the storage and retrieval of memories. Much like the hindbrain, the embryonic forebrain is initially divided along its rostrocaudal axis into transversely organized domains called *prosomeres.* Prosomeres 1 to 3 develop into the caudal part of the diencephalon, from which the thalamus emerges. Prosomeres 4 to 6 give rise to the rostral diencephalon and telencephalon. The ventral region of the rostral diencephalon gives rise to the hypothalamus and basal ganglia, whereas the telencephalon gives rise to the neocortex and hippocampus.

We have described how signals establish dorsoventral domains of the forebrain that later give rise to the hypothalamus, the basal ganglia, and the telencephalon. Here we turn to the patterning of the neocortex itself, asking whether the developmental mechanisms and principles that govern the development of other regions of the central nervous system also control the emergence of cortical areas specialized for particular sensory, motor, and cognitive functions.

Inductive Signals and Transcription Factor Gradients Establish Regional Differentiation

From the time of Brodmann's classical anatomical description at the beginning of the 20th century we have known that the cerebral cortex is subdivided into many different functional areas. Recent studies of cortical development have begun to provide insight into the signaling mechanisms that establish these basic subdivisions, forming somatosensory, auditory, and visual areas.

There is now evidence for the existence of a cortical "protomap," a basic plan in which different cortical areas are established early in development before inputs from other brain regions can influence development. This view is supported by studies of transcription factor expression in the developing neocortex. Two homeodomain transcription factors, Pax6 and Emx2, are expressed in complementary anteroposterior gradients in the ventricular zone of the developing neocortex—high levels of Pax6 at anterior levels and high levels of Emx2 at posterior levels. These early patterns are established in part by a local rostral source of FGF signals, which promote Pax6 and repress Emx2 expression (Figure 52–15A).

The distinct spatial domains of expression of Pax6 and Emx2 also depend on cross-repressive interactions between the two transcription factors. The spatial distribution of Pax6 and Emx2 helps to establish the initial regional pattern of the neocortex. In mice lacking Emx2 activity there is an expansion of rostral neocortex—the motor and somatosensory areas—at the expense of the more caudal auditory and visual areas. Conversely, in mice lacking Pax6 activity visual and auditory areas are expanded at the expense of motor and somatosensory areas (Figure 52–15B).

Thus, as in the spinal cord, hindbrain, and midbrain, early neocortical patterns are established through the interplay between local inductive signals and gradients of transcription factor expression. How these gradients specify discrete functional areas in the neocortex remains unclear. Transcription factors that precisely mark individual neocortical areas early in development have not yet been identified, although surface adhesion proteins, such as the cadherins, are known to segregate to specific sensory and motor areas.

Afferent Inputs Also Contribute to Regionalization

In the adult neocortex different functional areas can be distinguished by differences in the layering pattern of neurons—the cytoarchitecture of the areas—and by their neuronal connections. One striking instance of regional distinctiveness in cell pattern is a grid-like array of neurons and glial cells termed "barrels" in the primary somatosensory cortex of rodents. Each cortical barrel receives somatosensory information from a single whisker on the snout of the animal, and the regular array of cortical barrels reflects the somatotopic organization of afferent information from the body surface, culminating in the projection of thalamic afferents to specific cortical barrels (Figure 52–16A).

Cortical barrels are evident soon after birth, and their development depends on a critical period of afferent input from the periphery; their formation is disrupted if the whisker field in the skin is eliminated during this critical period. Strikingly, if prospective visual cortical tissue is transplanted into the somatosensory cortex around the time of birth, barrels form in the transplanted tissue with a pattern that closely

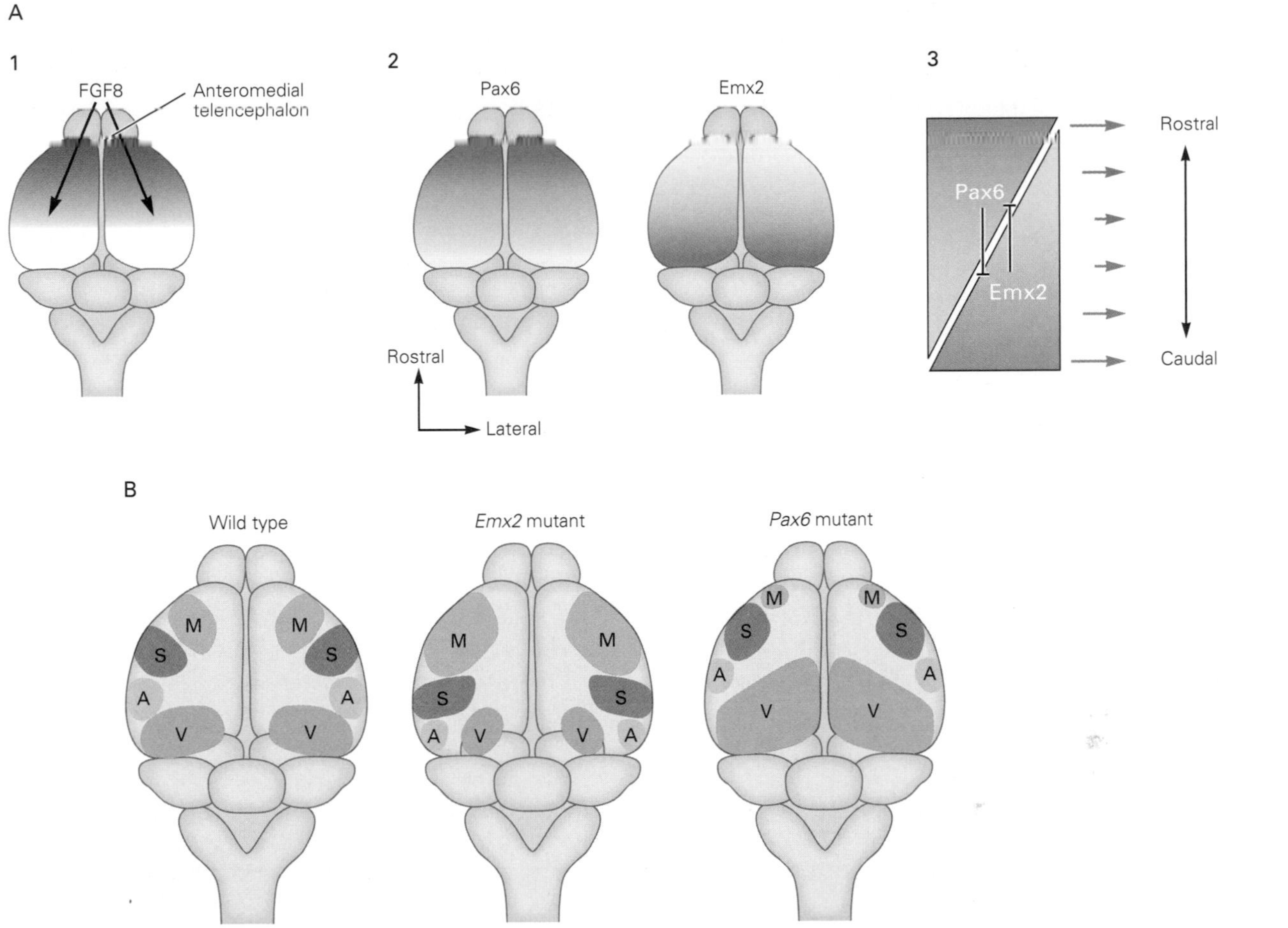

Figure 52–15 Anteroposterior gradients of expression of transcription factors establish discrete functional areas along the anteroposterior axis of the developing forebrain. (Adapted, with permission, from Hamasaki et al. 2004.)

A. (**1**) FGF8 signals from the anteromedial telencephalon establish the rostrocaudal pattern of the cerebral cortex. (**2**) A top-down view of the developing cerebral cortex in the mouse shows inverse rostrocaudal gradients of the transcription factors Pax6 and Emx2. (**3**) These two transcription factors mutually repress each other's expression.

B. Different functional areas develop at different rostrocaudal positions. Motor areas develop in the anterior region (**M**) and visual areas in more posterior regions (**V**). Genetic elimination of Emx2 function results in expansion of the motor areas and contraction in auditory (**A**) and visual areas. Conversely, elimination of Pax6 function results in an expansion of the visual areas and a contraction of motor and auditory areas. (**S**, somatosensory areas.)

resembles that of the normal somatosensory barrel field (Figure 52–16B). Together these findings demonstrate that afferent input superimposes aspects of neocortical patterning on the basic features of the protomap.

The nature of the input to different cortical areas influences neural function as well as cytoarchitecture. This can be shown by monitoring physiological and behavioral responses after rerouting afferent pathways of one sensory modality to a region of neocortex that normally processes a different modality. In animals in which retinal inputs are rerouted into the auditory pathway, the primary auditory cortex contains a systematic representation of visual space rather than of sound frequency (Figure 52–17). When these animals are trained to discriminate a visual from an auditory cue, they perceive a cue as visual when the rewired auditory cortex is activated by vision.

Thus brain pathways and neocortical regions are established through genetic programs during early development but later depend on afferent inputs for their specialized anatomical, physiological, and behavioral functions.

Figure 52–16 Sensory input regulates the organization of "barrels" in the developing somatosensory cortex in rodents. (Adapted, with permission, from Schlagger and O'Leary 1991.)

A. The barrel area of the rodent somatosensory cortex forms a somatotopic representation of the rows of whiskers on the animal's snout. Similar representations of the whisker field are present upstream—in the brain stem and in the thalamic nuclei that relay somatosensory inputs from the face to the cortex.

B. A barrel-like cellular organization is induced in developing visual cortex tissue that was grafted at an early postnatal stage into the somatosensory cortex.

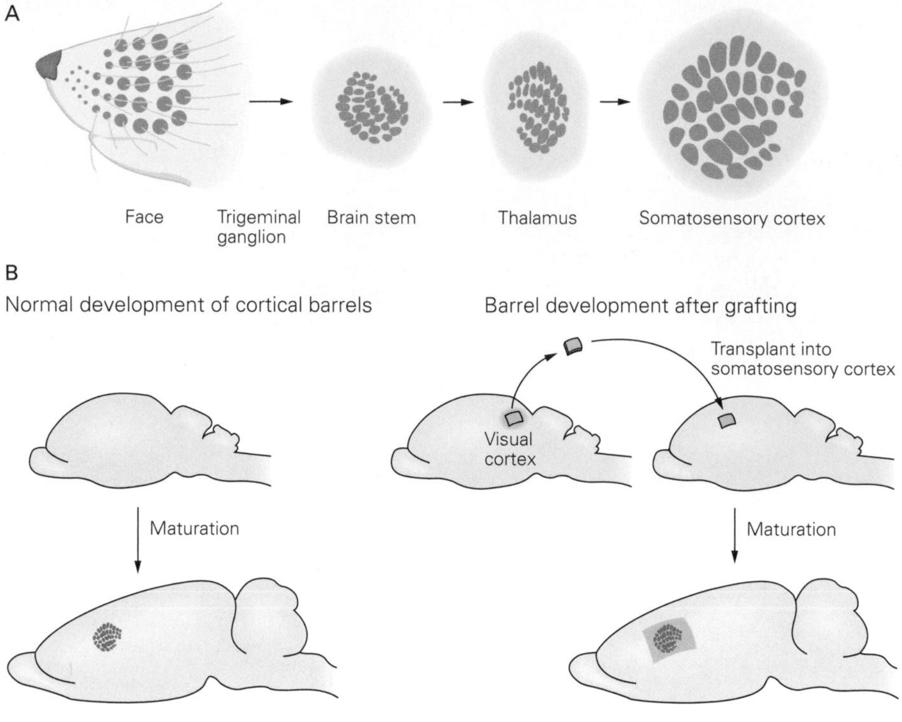

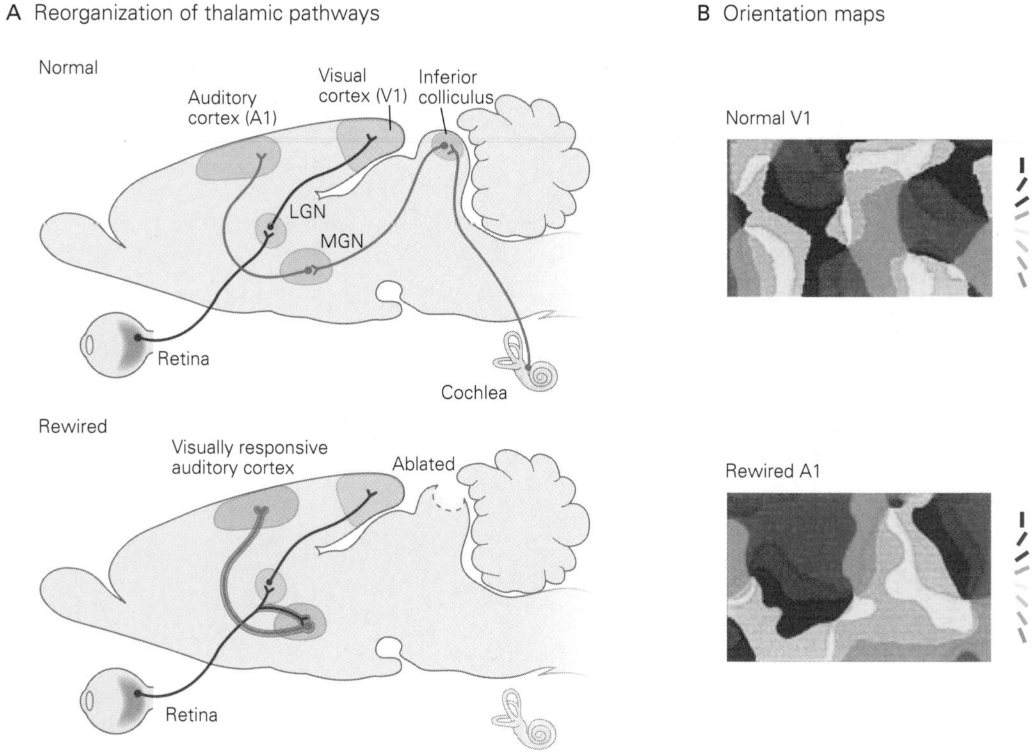

Figure 52–17 Rerouting thalamocortical input can recruit cortical areas for new sensory functions. (Adapted from Sharma, Angelucci, and Sur 2000.)

A. The visual pathway consists of afferent fibers from the retina that innervate the lateral geniculate nucleus (**LGN**) and superior colliculus. Axons from the LGN project to the primary visual cortex (**V1**). The auditory pathway projects from the cochlear nucleus (not shown) to the inferior colliculus, and then to the medial geniculate nucleus (**MGN**) and on to the primary auditory cortex (**A1**). Ablating the inferior colliculus in neonatal ferrets causes retinal afferents to innervate the MGN. As a consequence, the auditory cortex is reprogrammed to process visual information.

B. Visual orientation maps similar to those seen in normal V1 cortex are observed in rewired A1 auditory cortex of ferrets using optical imaging of intrinsic signals. The different colors represent different receptor field orientations (see bars at right). The pattern of activity in rewired A1 resembles that of normal V1.

An Overall View

The diverse functions of the mature vertebrate nervous system arise from regionally distinct subdivisions of the neural tube. Establishment of these subdivisions proceeds in four major developmental steps: (1) the generation of progenitor cells in the neural plate and neural tube, (2) the generation of regional differences within the neural tube that correspond to the major subdivisions of the mature nervous system, (3) the specification of distinct neuronal subtypes, and (4) the influence of neuronal inputs.

The early pattern of cell differentiation in the neural tube can be viewed as a series of inductive interactions in which signals provided by one cell group direct the fate of neighboring cells. The extensive diversification of cell types is orchestrated by a surprisingly small number of inducing factors that control programs of transcription factor expression in target cells. The developmental history of the cell, as well as the profile of transcription factors it expresses at a given time in development, determines its responsiveness to these inducing factors.

Despite differences in the organization of the nervous systems of invertebrates and vertebrates, the signaling molecules responsible for the differentiation and patterning of developing neurons have been conserved throughout animal evolution to a surprisingly high degree, reflecting an economical use of genetic information. Not only are the same signaling molecules used in many different organisms, but the receptors for these signals and the developmental programs they activate are also conserved. In addition, the same signals are used at many different developmental stages within one organism. Thus, the analysis of the development of the vertebrate nervous system has benefited greatly from genetic studies of flies and worms.

Thomas M. Jessell
Joshua R. Sanes

Selected Readings

Dessaud E, McMahon AP, Briscoe J. 2008. Pattern formation in the vertebrate neural tube: a sonic hedgehog morphogen-regulated transcriptional network. Development 135:2489–2503.

Goulding M. 2009. Circuits controlling vertebrate locomotion: moving in a new direction. Nat Rev Neurosci 10: 507–518.

Hamburger V. 1988. *The Heritage of Experimental Embryology. Hans Spemann and the Organizer.* New York: Oxford Univ. Press.

Jessell TM. 2000. Neuronal specification in the spinal cord: inductive signals and transcriptional codes. Nat Rev Genet 1:20–29.

Kiecker C, Lumsden A. 2005. Compartments and their boundaries in vertebrate brain development. Nat Rev Neurosci 6:553–564.

Lumsden A, Krumlauf R. 1996. Patterning the vertebrate neuraxis. Science 274:1109–1115.

Rakic P. 2002. Evolving concepts of cortical radial and areal specification. Prog Brain Res 136:265–280.

Stern CD. 2005. Neural induction: old problem, new findings, yet more questions. Development 132:2007–2021.

Sur M, Rubenstein JL. 2005. Patterning and plasticity of the cerebral cortex. Science 310:805–810.

Wurst W, Bally-Cuif L. 2001. Neural plate patterning: upstream and downstream of the isthmic organizer. Nat Rev Neurosci 2:99–108.

References

Bell E, Wingate RJ, Lumsden A. 1999. Homeotic transformation of rhombomere identity after localized Hoxb1 misexpression. Science 284:2168–2171.

Cholfin JA, Rubenstein JL. 2007. Patterning of frontal cortex subdivisions by Fgf17. Proc Natl Acad Sci USA 104:7652–7657.

Dasen JS, Tice BC, Brenner-Morton S, Jessell TM. 2005. A Hox regulatory network establishes motor neuron pool identity and target-muscle connectivity. Cell 123:477–491.

Goulding M, Lanuza G, Sapir T, Narayan S. 2002. The formation of sensorimotor circuits. Curr Opin Neurobiol 12:505–515.

Hamasaki T, Leingartner A, Ringstedt T, O'Leary DD. 2004. EMX2 regulates sizes and positioning of the primary sensory and motor areas in neocortex by direct specification of cortical progenitors. Neuron 43:359–372.

Horng S, Sur M. 2006. Visual activity and cortical rewiring: activity-dependent plasticity of cortical networks. Prog Brain Res 157:3–11

Ille F, Atanasoski S, Falkm S, Ittner LM, Marki D, Buchmann-Moller S, Wurdak H, Suter U, Taketo MM, Sommer L. 2007. Wnt/BMP signal integration regulates the balance between proliferation and differentiation of neuroepithelial cells in the dorsal spinal cord. Dev Biol 304:394–408.

Kiecker C, Lumsden A. 2005. Compartments and their boundaries in vertebrate brain development. Nat Rev Neurosci 6:553–564.

Levine AJ, Brivanlou, AH. 2007. Proposal of a model of mammalian neural induction. Dev Biol 308:247–256.

Lim Y, Golden JA. 2007. Patterning the developing diencephalon. Brain Res Rev 53:17–26.

Liu A, Niswander LA. 2005. Bone morphogenetic protein signalling and vertebrate nervous system development. Nat Rev Neurosci 6:945–954.

Lupo G, Harris WA, Lewis KE. 2006. Mechanisms of ventral patterning in the vertebrate nervous system. Nat Rev Neurosci 7:103–114.

Maden M. 2006. Retinoids and spinal cord development. J Neurobiol 66:726–738.

Mallamaci A, Stoykova A. 2006. Gene networks controlling early cerebral cortex arealization. Eur J Neurosci 23: 847–856.

Nordstrom U, Maier E, Jessell TM, Edlund T. 2006. An early role for WNT signaling in specifying neural patterns of Cdx and Hox gene expression and motor neuron subtype identity. PLoS Biol 4:1438–1452.

Rash BG, Grove EA. 2006. Area and layer patterning in the developing cerebral cortex. Curr Opin Neurobiol 16: 25–34.

Schlaggar BL, O'Leary DDM. 1991. Potential of visual cortex to develop an array of functional units unique to somatosensory cortex. Science 252:1556–1560.

Sharma K, Leonard AE, Lettieri K, Pfaff SL. 2000. Genetic and epigenetic mechanisms contribute to motor neuron pathfinding. Nature 406:515–519.

Sharma J, Angelucci A, Sur M. 2000. Induction of visual orientation modules in auditory cortex. Nature 404:841–847.

Song MR, Pfaff SL. 2005. Hox genes: the instructors working at motor pools. Cell 123:363–365.

Stamataki D, Ulloa F, Tsoni SV, Mynett A, Briscoe J. 2005. A gradient of Gli activity mediates graded Sonic Hedgehog signaling in the neural tube. Genes Dev 19:626–641.

Struder M, Lumsden A, Ariza-McNaughton L, Bradley A, Krumlauf R. 1996. Altered segmental identity and abnormal migration of motor neurons in mice lacking *Hoxb-1*. Nature 384:630–634.

von Melchner L, Pallas SL, Sur M. 2000. Visual behaviour mediated by retinal projections directed to the auditory pathway. Nature 404:871–876.

Wilson SI, Edlund T. 2001. Neural induction: toward a unifying mechanism. Nat Neurosci 24:1161–1168 Suppl.

Wolpert L, Beddinton R, Brockes J, Jessell TM, Lawrence PA, Meyerowitz E. 1998. *Principles of Development*. New York: Oxford Univ Press.

Wolpert L, Smith J, Jessell T, Lawrence P, Robertson E, Meyerowitz E. 2006. *Principles of Development*, 3rd ed. New York: Oxford Univ Press.

Wurst W, Bally-Cuif L. 2001. Neural plate patterning: upstream and downstream of the isthmic organizer. Nat Rev Neurosci 2:99–108.

53

Differentiation and Survival of Nerve Cells

In the preceding chapter we described how local inductive signals pattern the neural tube and establish the early regional subdivisions of the nervous system—the spinal cord, hindbrain, midbrain, and forebrain. Here we turn to the issue of how progenitor cells within these regions differentiate into neurons and glial cells, the two major cell types that populate the nervous system.

We discuss some of the molecules that specify neuronal and glial cell fates and how they are regulated. The basic mechanisms of neurogenesis endow cells with common neuronal properties, features that are largely independent of the region of the nervous system in which they are generated or the specific functions they perform. We also discuss the mechanisms by which developing neurons express neurotransmitters and synaptic receptors.

After the identity and functional properties of the neuron have begun to emerge, additional developmental processes determine whether the neuron will live or die. Remarkably, approximately half of the neurons generated in the mammalian nervous system are lost through programmed cell death. We examine the factors that regulate the survival of neurons and the possible benefits of widespread neuronal loss. Finally, we describe the existence of a core biochemical pathway that programs the death of nerve cells.

The Proliferation of Neural Progenitor Cells Involves Symmetric and Asymmetric Modes of Cell Division

The mature brain comprises billions of nerve cells and even more glial cells. Yet its precursor, the neural plate, initially comprises only a few hundred cells. From this simple comparison we infer that regulation of the proliferation of neural cells is a major driving force in shaping brain development. Histologists in the late 19th century showed that neural epithelial cells close to the ventricular lumen of the embryonic brain exhibit features of mitosis, and we now know that the proliferative zones surrounding the ventricles are the major regions involved in the production of neural cells in the cerebral cortex as well as other regions of the central nervous system.

At early stages of embryonic development most progenitor cells in the ventricular zone of the neural tube proliferate rapidly. Many of these early neural progenitors have the properties of stem cells: They can generate additional copies of themselves, a process called *self-renewal,* and also give rise to differentiated neurons and glial cells (Figure 53–1B). As with other types of stem cells, neural progenitor cells undergo stereotyped programs of cell division.

One mode of cell division is asymmetric: The progenitor produces one differentiated daughter and another daughter that retains its stem cell-like properties. This mode does not permit amplification of the stem cell population. In a second mode neural stem cells divide symmetrically to produce two stem cells, and in this way expand the population of proliferative progenitor cells. Both symmetric and asymmetric modes have been found in the embryonic cerebral cortex in vivo and in cortical cells grown in tissue culture (Figure 53–1C).

The incidence of symmetric and asymmetric cell division is influenced by signals in the local environment of the dividing cell, making it possible to control the probability of self-renewal or differentiation. Environmental factors can influence the outcome of progenitor cell divisions in two fundamental ways. They can act in an "instructive" manner, biasing the outcome of the division process and causing the stem cell to adopt one fate at the expense of others. Or they can act in a "selective" manner, permitting the survival and maturation of only certain cell progeny.

Radial Glial Cells Serve As Neural Progenitors and Structural Scaffolds

Radial glial cells are the earliest morphologically distinguishable cell type to appear within the primitive neural epithelium. Their cell bodies are located in the ventricular zone and their long process extends to the pial surface. As the brain thickens, the processes of radial glial cells remain attached to the ventricular and pial surfaces. After the generation of neurons is complete, many radial glial cells differentiate into astrocytes, a prominent class of glial cell in the mature brain. The elongated shape of the radial glial cell places it in a favorable position to serve as a scaffold for the migration of neurons that emerge from the ventricular zone (Figure 53–2).

The ventricular zone was once thought to contain two major cell types: radial glial cells and a set of neuroepithelial progenitors, which served as the primary source of neurons. This classical view has changed dramatically in the last few years. Radial glial cells are in fact progenitor cells that generate both neurons and astrocytes in addition to their role in neuronal migration (Figure 53–2). When radial glial cells are selectively labeled with fluorescent dyes or viruses, tracing of their clonal progeny reveals cell clusters that contain both neuronal and radial glial cells. These findings indicate that radial glial cells are able to undergo both asymmetric and self-renewing cell division, and serve as a major source of post-mitotic neurons as well as astrocytes. Radial glial cells may also serve as progenitors of neurons in the adult central nervous system.

The Generation of Neurons or Glial Cells Is Regulated by Delta-Notch Signaling and Basic Helix-Loop-Helix Transcription Factors

How do radial glial cells make the decision to self-renew, generate neurons, or give rise to mature astrocytes? The answer to this question involves an evolutionarily conserved signaling system.

In flies and vertebrates neural fate is regulated by a cell-surface signaling system, comprised of the transmembrane ligand delta and its receptor notch, which regulates a cascade of transcription factors of the basic helix-loop-helix (bHLH) family. This signaling system was revealed in genetic studies in *Drosophila.* Neurons emerge from within a larger cluster of ectodermal cells, each of which has the potential to generate neurons. This *proneural region* is defined by expression of proneural genes, which encode transcription factors of the bHLH class. Yet within the proneural region only certain cells form neurons; the others become epidermal support cells.

Initially the ligand delta and its receptor notch are expressed at similar levels by all proneural cells (Figure 53–3A). With time, however, notch activity is enhanced in one cell and suppressed in its neighbor. The cell in which notch activity is highest loses the potential to form a neuron and acquires an alternative fate.

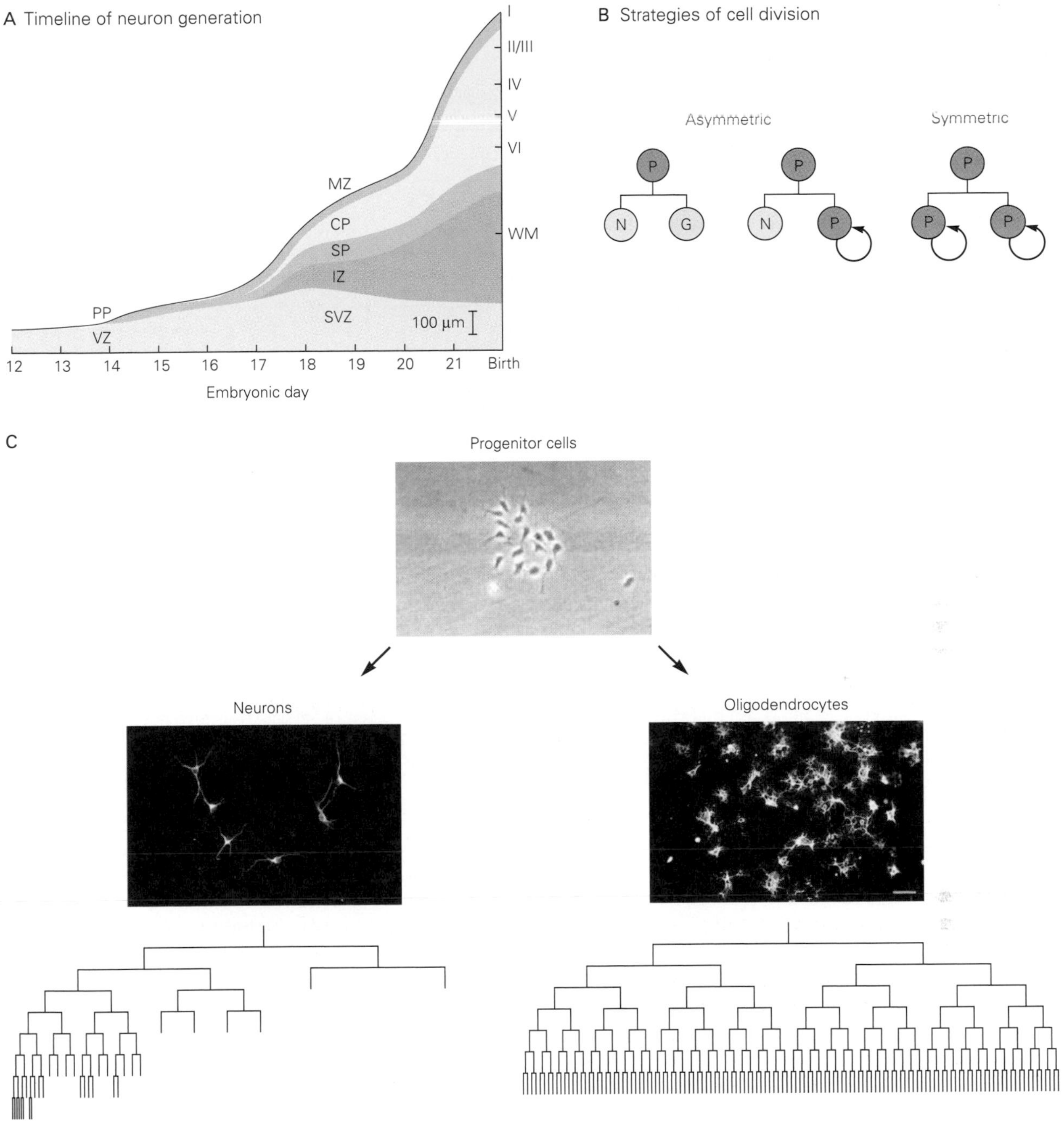

Figure 53–1 Neural progenitor cells have different modes of division.

A. Temporal sequence of neurogenesis in the mouse cerebral cortex. Neurons begin to accumulate in the cortical plate (**CP**) during the last 5 days of embryonic development. Within the cortical plate neurons populate the deep layers before settling in the superficial layers. (**MZ**, marginal zone; **PP**, preplate; **SP**, subplate; **IZ**, intermediate zone; **SVZ**, subventricular zone; **VZ**, ventricular zone; **WM**, white matter.)

B. Asymmetric and symmetric modes of cell division. A progenitor cell (**P**) undergoes asymmetric division to generate a neuron (**N**) and a glial cell (**G**) (left). A progenitor cell undergoes asymmetric division, giving rise to another progenitor cell and a neuron. This mode of division contributes to the generation of neurons at early stages of development, and of glial cells at later stages, typical of many regions of the central nervous system (middle). A progenitor cell undergoes symmetric division to generate two additional progenitor cells (right).

C. Time-lapse cinematography captures the divisions and differentiation of isolated cortical progenitor cells in the rodent. Lineage diagrams illustrate cells that undergo predominantly asymmetric division, giving rise to neurons (left), or symmetric division that gives rise to oligodendrocytes (right). (Modified, with permission, from Qian et al. 1998.)

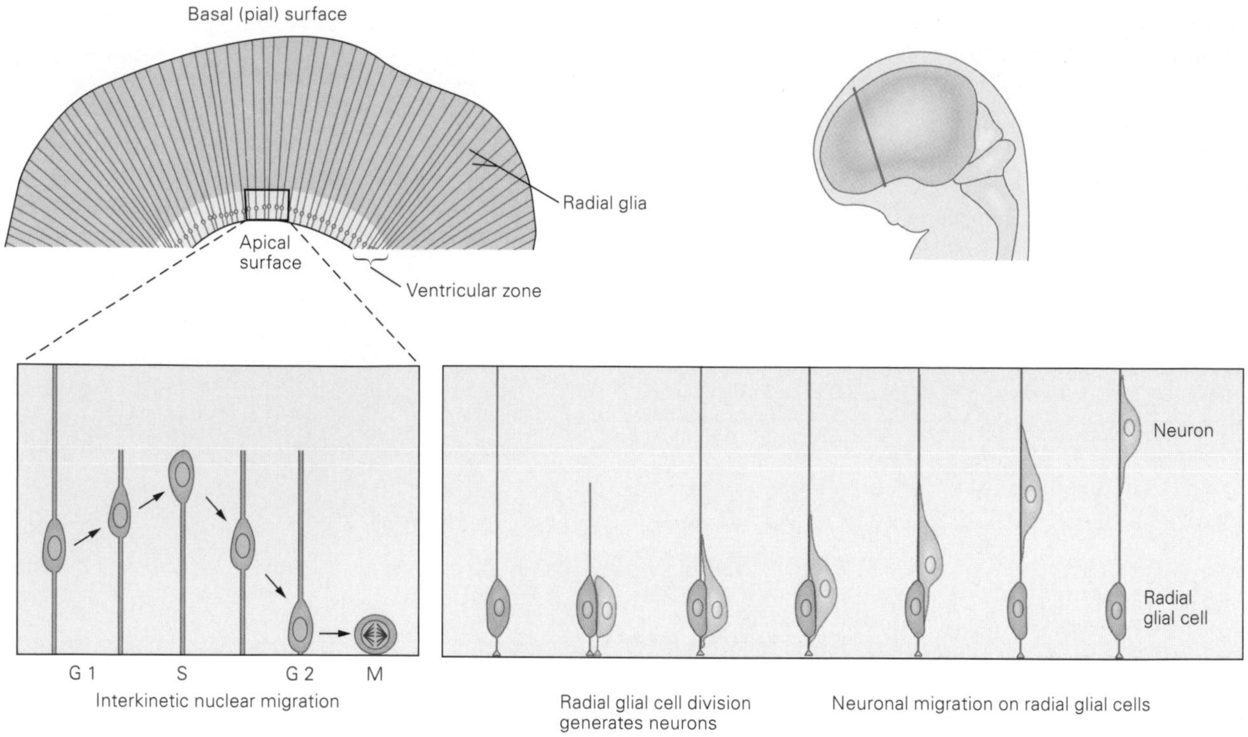

Figure 53–2 Radial glial cells serve as precursors to neurons in the central nervous system and also provide a scaffold for radial neuronal migration. Progenitor cells in the ventricular zone of the developing cerebral cortex have nuclei that migrate along the apical-basal axis as they progress through the cell cycle. **Left**: During the G1 phase nuclei rise from the inner (apical) surface of the ventricular zone. During the S phase they reside in the outer (basal) third of the ventricular zone. During the G2 phase they migrate apically, and mitosis occurs when the nuclei reach the ventricular surface. **Right**: During cell division radial glial cells give rise to postmitotic neurons that migrate away from the ventricular zone using radial glial cells as a guide.

The binding of Delta to Notch results in proteolytic cleavage of the Notch cytoplasmic domain, which then enters the nucleus. There it functions as a transcription factor, regulating the activity of bHLH transcription factors that suppress the ability of the cell to become a neuron and reduce the level of expression of the ligand Delta (Figure 53–3B). Through this feedback pathway a minor difference in the initial level of Notch signaling is rapidly amplified to generate an all-or-none difference in the status of Notch activation, and consequently the fates of the two cells. This basic logic of Delta-Notch and bHLH signaling has been conserved in vertebrate and invertebrate neural tissues.

How does Notch signaling regulate neuronal and glial production in mammals? At early stages in the development of the mammalian cortex Notch signaling promotes the generation of radial glial cells by activating members of the Hes family of bHLH transcriptional repressors. Two of these proteins, Hes1 and Hes5, appear to maintain radial glial cell character by activating the expression of an ErbB class tyrosine kinase receptor for neuregulin, a secreted signal that promotes radial glial cell identity. The Notch ligand Delta1 as well as neuregulin are expressed by newly generated cortical neurons; thus the radial glial cells depend on feedback signals from their neuronal progeny for continued production.

At later stages of cortical development Notch signaling continues to activate Hes proteins, but a change in the intracellular response pathway results in astrocyte differentiation. At this stage the Hes proteins work by activating a transcription factor, STAT3, which recruits the serine-threonine kinase JAK2, a potent inducer of astrocyte differentiation. STAT3 also activates expression of astrocyte-specific genes such as the glial-fibrillary acidic protein (GFAP).

The generation of oligodendrocytes, the second major class of glial cells in the central nervous system, follows many of the principles that control neuron and astrocyte production. Notch signaling regulates the expression of two bHLH transcription factors, Olig1 and Olig2, which have essential roles in the production of embryonic and postnatal oligodendrocytes.

The generation of cortical neurons requires that cells avoid exposure to notch signals (Figure 53–4). This task is achieved in part through the expression of numb, a cytoplasmic protein that antagonizes notch signaling. The key role of numb in neurogenesis was first shown in *Drosophila,* where it determines the neuronal fate of daughter cells of asymmetrically dividing progenitors. In the mammalian cortex numb, as with Notch,

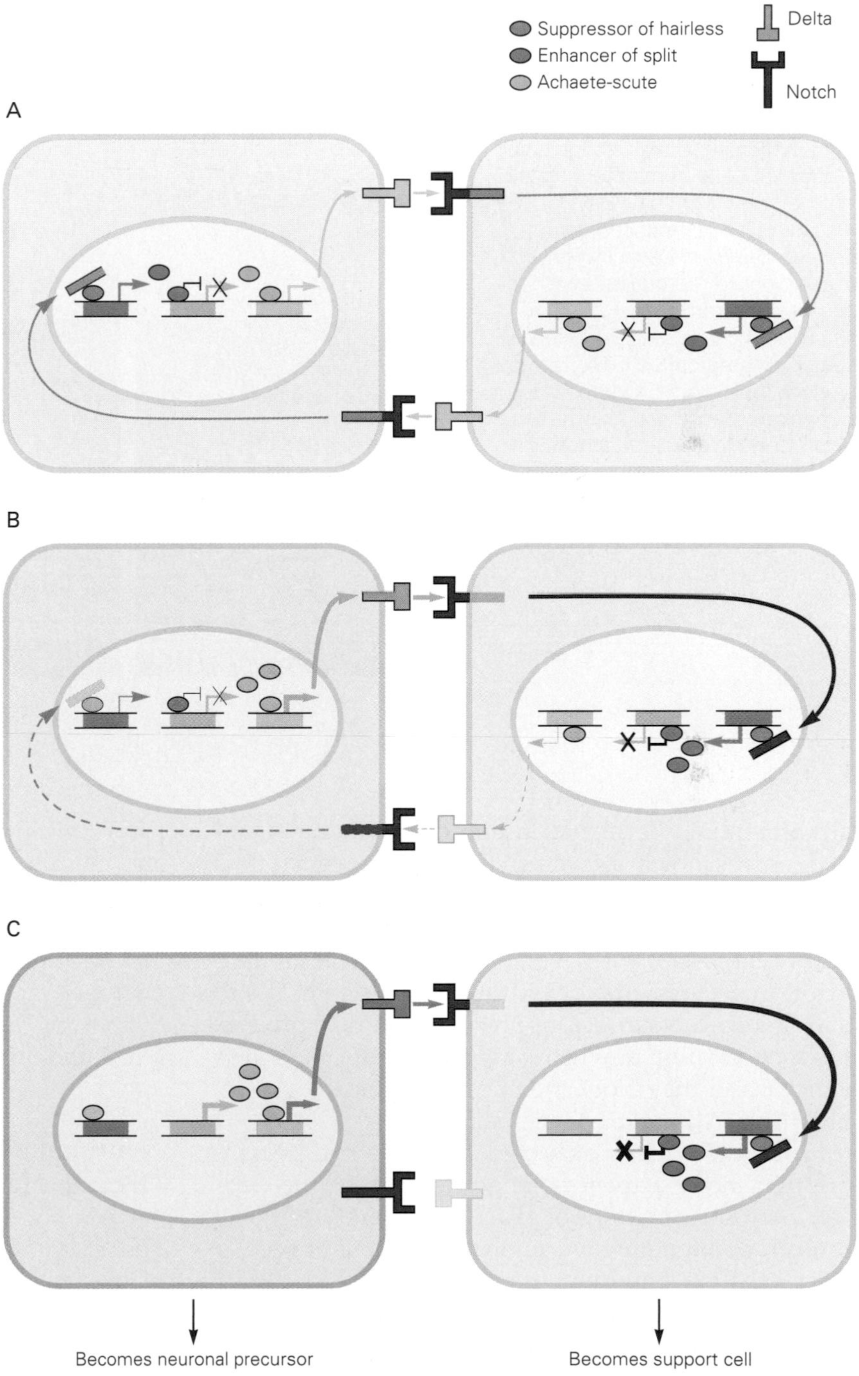

Figure 53–3 Delta acts as a ligand for Notch and determines neuronal fate.

A. At the onset of the interaction between two cells, the ligand Delta engages the receptor Notch. Delta and Notch are expressed at similar levels on each cell, and thus their initial signaling strength is equal.

B. A small imbalance in the strength of Delta-Notch signaling breaks the symmetry of the interaction. In this example the left cell provides a slightly greater Delta signal, thus activating Notch signaling in the right cell to a greater extent. On binding by Delta, the cytoplasmic domain of Notch is cleaved to form a proteolytic fragment called Notch-Intra, which enters the nucleus of the cell and initiates a basic helix-loop-helix (bHLH) transcriptional cascade that regulates the level of delta expression. Notch-Intra forms a transcriptional complex with a bHLH protein, suppressor of hairless, which binds to and activates the gene encoding a second bHLH protein, enhancer of split. Once activated, enhancer of split binds to and represses expression of the gene encoding a third bHLH protein, achaete-scute. Achaete-scute activity promotes expression of delta. Thus, by repressing achaete-scute, enhancer of split decreases transcriptional activation of the Delta gene and production of Delta protein. This diminishes the ability of the cell on the right to activate Notch signaling in the left cell.

C. Once the level of Notch signaling in the left cell has been reduced, suppressor of hairless no longer activates enhancer of split, and the level of expression of achaete-scute increases, resulting in enhanced expression of Delta and further activation of Notch signaling in the right cell. In this way a small initial imbalance in Delta-Notch signaling is rapidly amplified into a marked asymmetry in the level of Notch activation in the two cells. In the mammalian central nervous system cells with high levels of Notch activation are diverted from neuronal fates, whereas cells with low levels of Notch activation become neurons.

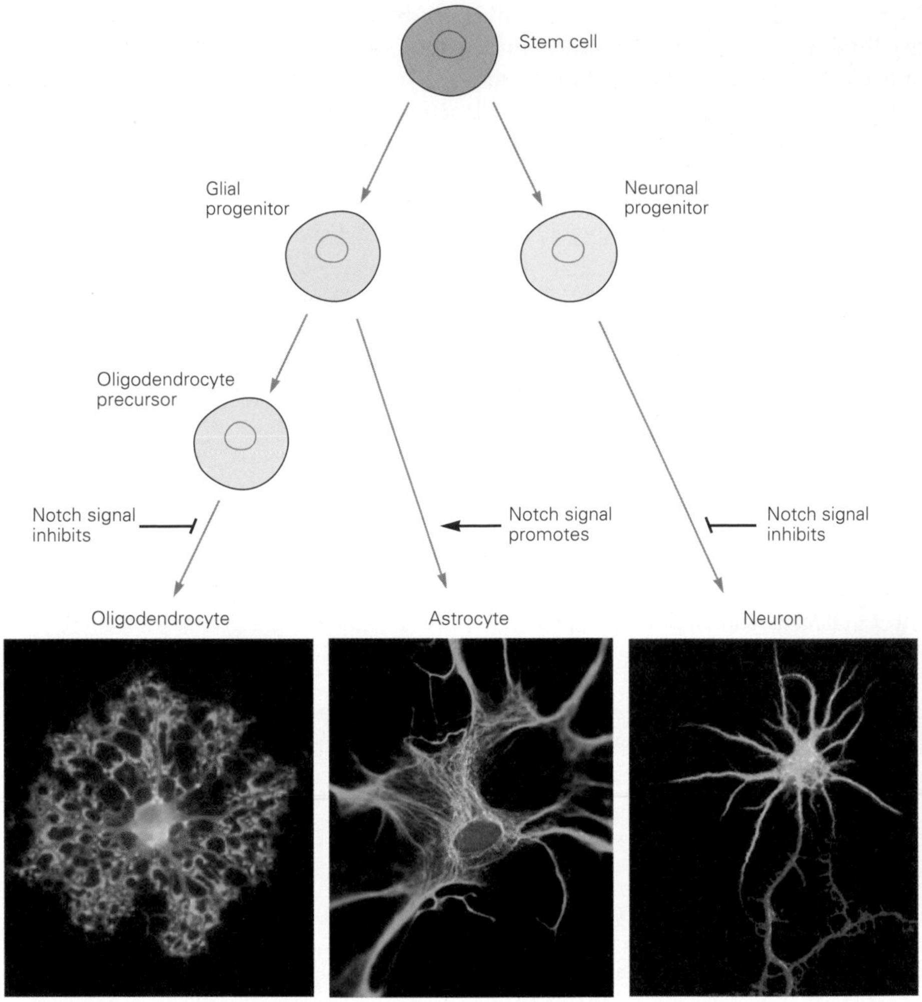

Figure 53–4 Notch signaling regulates the fate of cells in the developing cerebral cortex. Notch signaling has several roles in cell differentiation in the developing cerebral cortex. The activation of Notch signaling in glial progenitor cells results in the differentiation as astrocytes and inhibits differentiation as oligodendrocytes (left pathway). Notch signaling also inhibits progenitor cells from differentiating into neurons (right pathway). (Photo on left reproduced, with permission, from David H. Rowitch; middle photo reproduced, with permission, from Edward Nyatia and Dirk Michael Lang/SA Science Lens Competition(SAASTA); photo on right reproduced, with permission, from Masatoshi Takeichi, Riken Center for Developmental Biology.

is preferentially localized in neuronal daughters and antagonizes notch signaling. As a consequence, loss of numb activity causes progenitor cells to proliferate extensively. The inhibition of notch signaling results in the expression of several proneural bHLH transcription factors, notably Mash1, neurogenin-1, and neurogenin-2. Neurogenins promote neuronal production by activating downstream bHLH proteins such as neuroD, and they block the formation of astrocytes by inhibiting JAK and STAT signaling.

Although delta-notch signaling and bHLH transcription factor activators lie at the heart of the decision to produce neurons or glial cells, several additional transcriptional pathways augment this core molecular program. One important transcription factor, REST/NRSF, is expressed in neural progenitors and glial cells, where it represses the expression of neuronal genes. REST/NRSF rapidly degrades as neurons differentiate, permitting the expression of neurogenic bHLH factors and other neuronal genes. Homeodomain transcription factors of the SoxB class also play an important role in maintaining neural progenitors by blocking neurogenic bHLH protein activity. The differentiation of neurons therefore requires the avoidance of REST/NRSF and SoxB protein activity.

Neuronal Migration Establishes the Layered Organization of the Cerebral Cortex

The mammalian cerebral cortex develops in three main stages: a preplate, a cortical plate, and finally the mature pattern of layers. Neural precursors in the ventricular zone of the preplate differentiate into neurons that migrate along radial glial fibers before settling in the cortical plate. These migratory cells divide the preplate into a subplate and a marginal zone (Figure 53–5).

Once within the cortical plate, neurons become organized into well-defined layers. The laminar settling position of a neuron is correlated precisely with its *birthday*, a term that refers to the time at which a dividing precursor cell undergoes its final round of cell division and gives rise to a postmitotic neuron. Cells that migrate from the ventricular zone and leave the cell cycle at early stages give rise to neurons that settle in the deepest layers of the cortex. Cells that exit the cell cycle at progressively later stages migrate over longer distances and pass earlier-born neurons, before settling in more superficial layers of the cortex. Thus the layering of neurons in the cerebral cortex follows an inside-first, outside-last rule (Figure 53–6A).

Disruption in the migratory and settling programs of cortical neurons underlies much human cortical pathology (Figure 53–6C, D). In *lissencephaly* (Greek, smooth brain, referring to the characteristic smoothing of the cortical surface in patients with the disorder) neurons leave the ventricular zone but fail to complete their migration into the cortical plate. As a result, the mature cortex is typically reduced from six to four neuronal layers, and the arrangement of neurons in each remaining layer is disordered. Occasionally, lissencephaly is accompanied by the presence of an additional group of neurons in the subcortical white matter. Patients with lissencephalies from mutations in the *Lis1* and *doublecortin* genes often suffer severe mental retardation and intractable epilepsy. The Lis1 and doublecortin proteins have been localized to microtubules, suggesting they are involved in microtubule-dependent nuclear movement, although their precise functions in neuronal migration remain unclear.

Mutations that disrupt the reelin signaling pathway disrupt the final stage of neuronal migration through the cortical subplate. Reelin is an extracellular matrix protein that is secreted from the Cajal-Retzius cells, a class of neurons found in the preplate and marginal

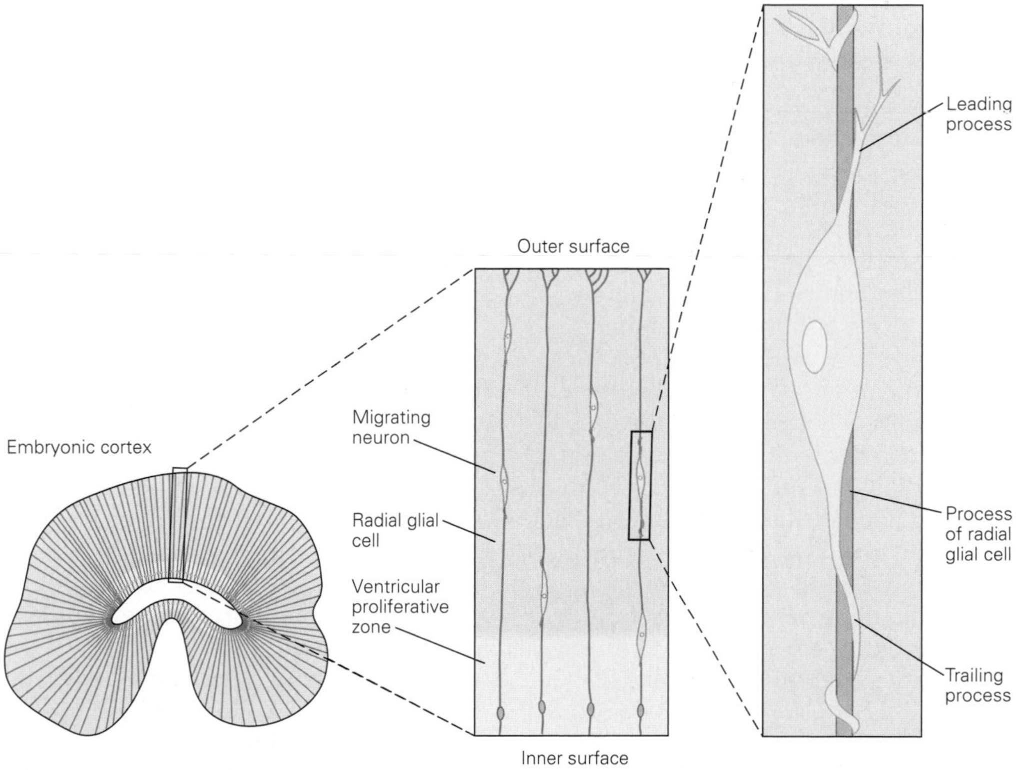

Figure 53–5 Neurons migrate along radial glial cells. After their generation from radial glial cells, newly generated neurons in the embryonic cerebral cortex extend a leading process that wraps around the shaft of the radial glial cell, thus using the radial glial cells as scaffolds during their migration from the ventricular zone to the pial surface of cortex.

zone. Signals from these cells are crucial for the migration of cortical neurons. In mice lacking functional reelin, neurons fail to detach from their radial glial scaffolds and pile up underneath the cortical plate, disobeying the inside-out migratory rule. As a consequence, the normal layering of cell types is inverted and the marginal zone is lost. Reelin acts through cell-surface receptors that include the ApoE receptor 2 and the very low-density lipoprotein receptor. The binding of reelin to these receptors activates an intracellular protein, Dab1, which transduces reelin signals. Cadherin-like adhesion proteins may also be involved in transducing reelin signals. Not surprisingly, the loss of proteins that transduce reelin signals produce similar migratory phenotypes.

Central Neurons Migrate Along Glial Cells and Axons to Reach Their Final Settling Position

The migration of neurons follows one of three major programs, termed *radial*, *tangential*, and *free* migration. With radial migration central neurons move along the long unbranched processes of radial glial cells. With tangential migration central neurons use axonal tracts as their guides. Free migration occurs in the peripheral nervous system without radial glia or axonal tracts.

Glial Cells Serve As a Scaffold in Radial Migration

Classical anatomical studies of cortical development in the primate brain in the 1970s provided evidence that neurons generated in the ventricular zone migrate to their settling position along a pathway of radial glial fibers. Radial glial cells serve as the primary scaffold for radial neuronal migration. Their cell bodies are located close to the ventricular surface and give rise to elongated fibers that span the width of the developing cerebral wall. Each radial glial cell has one basal end-foot in the ventricular zone at the apical surface and processes that terminate in multiple end-feet at the pial surface of the brain (Figure 53–5). Radial glial scaffolds are especially important in the development of the primate cortex, where neurons are required to migrate over long distances as the cerebral wall expands.

Most radial glial cells are transient structures; as we have seen, they give rise to neurons and eventually differentiate into astrocytes. A single radial glial cell scaffold can support the migration of up to 30 generations of cortical neurons.

What forces and molecules power neuronal migration on radial glial cells? After a neuron leaves the cell cycle its leading process wraps around the shaft of the radial glial cell and its nucleus translocates within the cytoplasm of the leading process. Although the leading process of the migrating neuron extends slowly and steadily, the nucleus moves in an intermittent, stepwise manner because of complex rearrangements of the cytoskeleton. A microtubular lattice forms a cage around the nucleus, and movement of the nucleus depends on a centrosome-like structure, termed a *basal body*, which projects a system of microtubules into the leading process, providing the conduit for nuclear movement (Figure 53–7A). Defects in neuronal migration that result from loss of *Lis1* or *doublecortin* (Figure 53–6) reflect the critical role of these genes in microtubular assembly and function.

Neuronal migration along radial glia also involves adhesive interactions between cells. Adhesive receptors such as integrins promote neuronal extension on radial glial cells. The migration of neurons along glial fibers is nevertheless different from the extension of axons driven by growth cones (see Chapter 54). In neuronal migration the leading process is devoid of the structured actin filaments that typify growth cones and more closely resembles an extending dendrite, an inference made first by Santiago Ramon y Cajal.

Axon Tracts Serve As a Scaffold for Tangential Migration

The second prominent mechanism of neuronal translocation in the developing brain is tangential migration. This form of migration is used to populate distinct regions of the nervous system and may have evolved as a mechanism for increasing the complexity of neuronal circuits. Its major cellular substrate appears to be preexisting axonal tracts that connect regions of neuronal generation with the final settling position of the neurons. In the developing cortex the axons of cortical projection neurons reach the internal capsule just as migratory neurons begin to enter the neocortex; at this intersection immigrating neurons are tightly associated with the bundles of axons that leave the cortex.

Neurons that use tangential migration follow precise routes of navigation and settling. This can best be seen in the ventral telencephalon, which contains two major sites of neuronal production, the medial and lateral ganglionic eminences. Some of the neurons generated in this region are destined to populate the basal

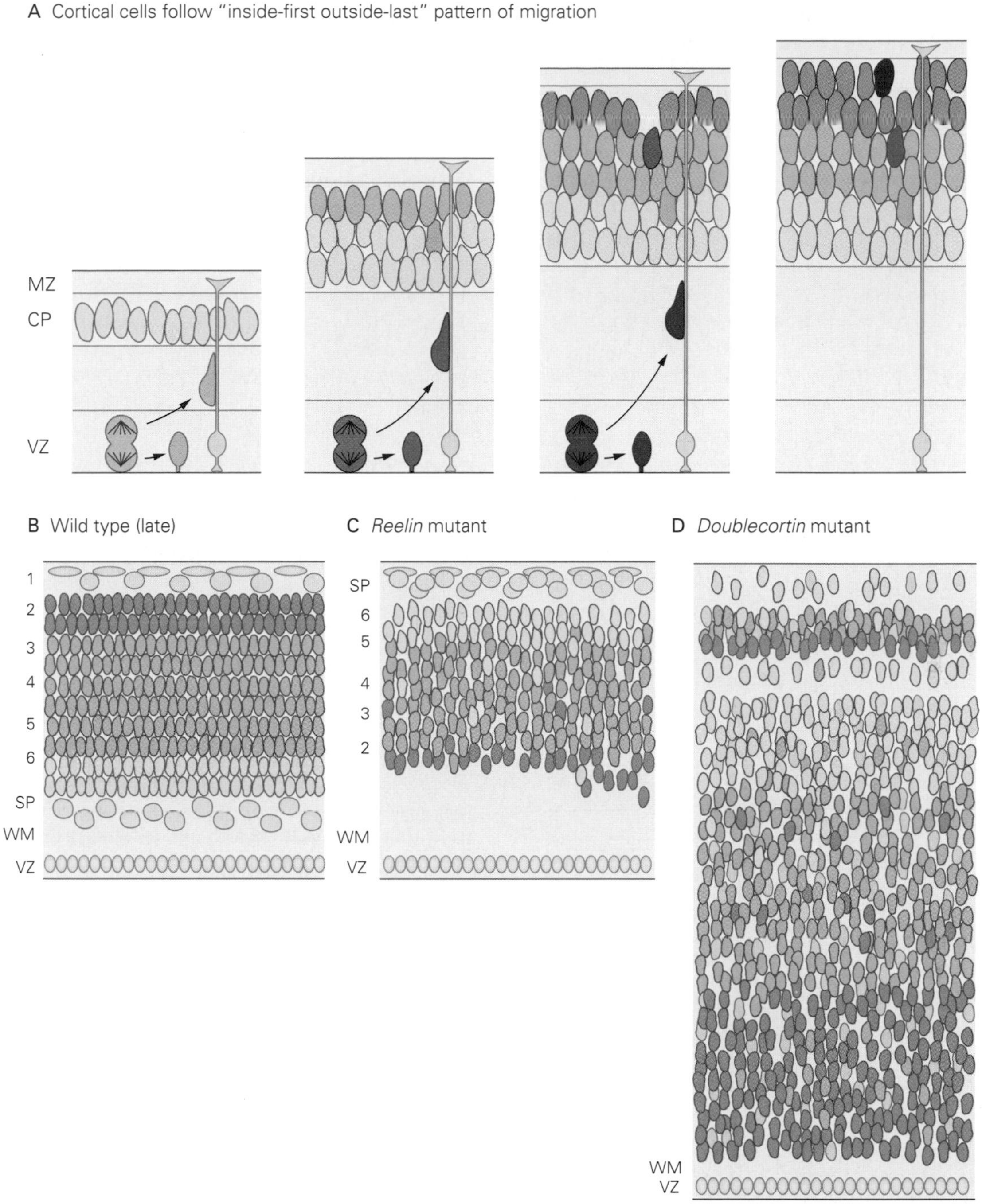

Figure 53–6 The migration of neurons in the cerebral cortex is responsible for the layered organization of the cortex. (Modified, with permission, from Olsen and Walsh 2002.)

A. During normal cortical development neurons use radial glial cells as migratory scaffolds as they enter the cortical plate. As they approach the pial surface, neurons stop migrating and detach from radial glial cells. (**CP**, cortical plate; **MZ**, marginal zone; **VZ**, ventricular zone.)

B. An orderly inside-out pattern of neuronal migration results in the formation of six neuronal layers in the mature cerebral cortex, arranged between the white matter (**WM**) and subplate (**SP**).

C. In the mouse mutant *reeler,* which lacks functional reelin protein, the layering of neurons in the cortical plate is severely disrupted and partially inverted. In addition, the entire cortical plate develops beneath the subplate.

D. In *doublecortin* (*dcx*) mutants the cortex is thickened, neurons lose their characteristic layered identity, and some layers contain fewer neurons. A similar disruption is observed in *Lis1* mutants, which underlies certain forms of human lissencephaly.

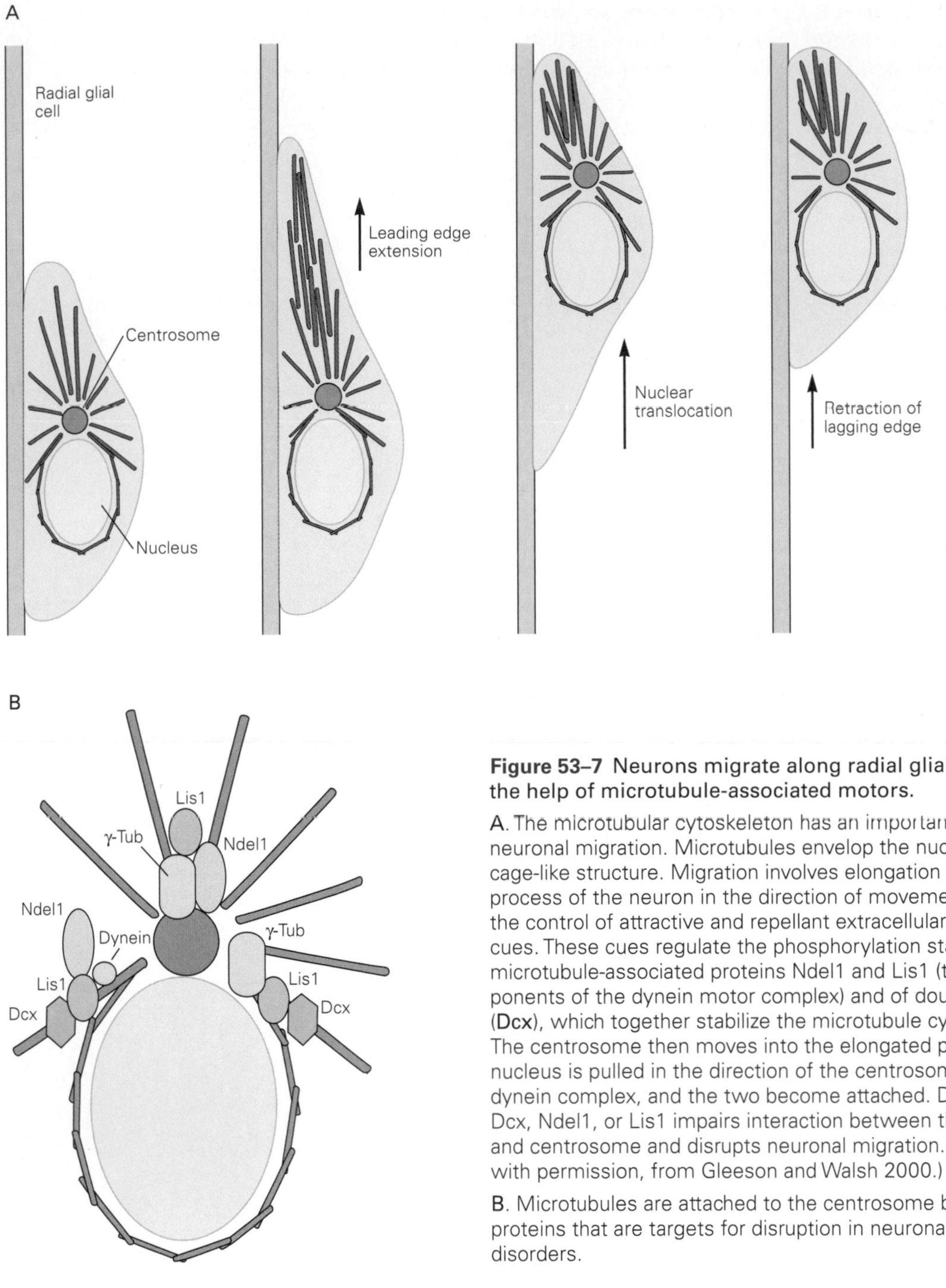

Figure 53–7 Neurons migrate along radial glial cells with the help of microtubule-associated motors.

A. The microtubular cytoskeleton has an important role in neuronal migration. Microtubules envelop the nucleus in a cage-like structure. Migration involves elongation of the leading process of the neuron in the direction of movement, under the control of attractive and repellant extracellular guidance cues. These cues regulate the phosphorylation status of the microtubule-associated proteins Ndel1 and Lis1 (two components of the dynein motor complex) and of doublecortin (**Dcx**), which together stabilize the microtubule cytoskeleton. The centrosome then moves into the elongated process, the nucleus is pulled in the direction of the centrosome by the dynein complex, and the two become attached. Disruption of Dcx, Ndel1, or Lis1 impairs interaction between the nucleus and centrosome and disrupts neuronal migration. (Modified, with permission, from Gleeson and Walsh 2000.)

B. Microtubules are attached to the centrosome by a series of proteins that are targets for disruption in neuronal migration disorders.

ganglia. Tangential migration of neurons from these ventral structures also provides the cerebral cortex, hippocampus, and olfactory bulb with interneurons.

Neurons generated in the medial ganglionic eminence migrate tangentially and settle in the neocortex where they give rise to many interneuron populations, including Cajal-Retzius neurons. Thus cortical neurons originate from two sources: Excitatory neurons from the cortical ventricular zone and interneurons from the medial ganglionic eminence. In contrast, neurons generated in the lateral ganglionic eminence migrate rostrally and contribute the periglomerular and granule interneurons of the olfactory bulb (Figure 53–8). In this rostral migratory stream neurons use neighboring neurons as substrates for migration (chain migration). In the adult brain neurons that follow the rostral migratory stream originate instead in the subventricular zone of the striatum.

Transcription factors control the character of ganglion eminence neurons and ensure their tangential migration. The homeodomain proteins Dlx1 and Dlx2 are expressed by cells in the ganglionic eminences. In mice lacking Dlx1 and Dlx2 activity the perturbation of neuronal migration leads to a profound reduction in the number of GABAergic interneurons in the cortex. Similarly, in mice lacking the gene encoding the homeodomain transcription factor Gsh2 the rostral migratory stream is disrupted and the arrival of interneurons in the olfactory bulb is delayed.

Neural Crest Cell Migration in the Peripheral Nervous System Does Not Rely on Scaffolding

The peripheral nervous system derives from neural crest stem cells, a small group of neuroepithelial cells at the boundary of the neural tube and epidermal ectoderm. Soon after their induction neural crest cells are transformed from epithelial to mesenchymal cells and begin to delaminate from the neural tube. They then migrate to many sites throughout the body. Neural crest cell migration does not rely on scaffolding (ie, radial glial cells or preexisting axon tracts) and thus is called free migration. This form of neuronal migration requires significant cytoarchitectural and cell adhesive changes and differs from most of the migratory events in the central nervous system.

Bone morphogenetic protein (BMP) signaling is critical for neural crest induction (see Chapter 52), as well as neural crest migration. Exposure of neural epithelial cells to BMPs triggers molecular changes that convert epithelial cells to a mesenchymal state, causing them to delaminate from the neural tube and migrate into the periphery. BMPs trigger changes in neural crest cells by inducing expression of transcription factors, notably the zinc finger proteins snail, slug, and twist, which have a conserved role in promoting epithelial-to-mesenchymal transitions. These transcription factors direct expression of proteins that regulate the properties of the cytoskeleton as well as enzymes that degrade extracellular matrix proteins. These enzymes give neural crest cells the ability to break down the basement membrane surrounding the epithelium of the neural tube, permitting them to embark on their migratory journey into the periphery.

As neural crest cells begin to delaminate, their expression of cell adhesion molecules changes. Alterations in expression of adhesive proteins, notably cadherins, permit neural crest cells to loosen their adhesive contacts with neural tube cells and begin the delamination process. Neural crest cells also begin to express integrins, receptors for extracellular matrix proteins such as laminins and collagens that are found along peripheral migratory paths.

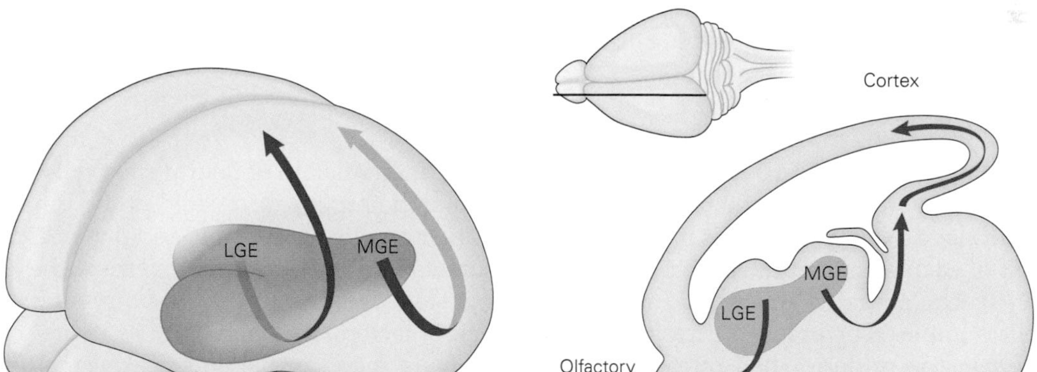

Figure 53–8 Interneurons generated in the ventral telencephalon migrate tangentially to the cerebral cortex. Neurons generated in the medial ganglionic eminences (**MGE**) migrate tangentially and settle in the neocortex. On arrival they give rise to interneurons, including Cajal-Retzius neurons. Neurons generated in the lateral ganglionic eminence (**LGE**) migrate rostrally and contribute the periglomerular and granule interneurons of the olfactory bulb. Neurons migrating to the olfactory bulb use neighboring migrating cells as substrates for migration (a process called chain migration). (Adapted from Rallu, Corbin and Fishell 2002.)

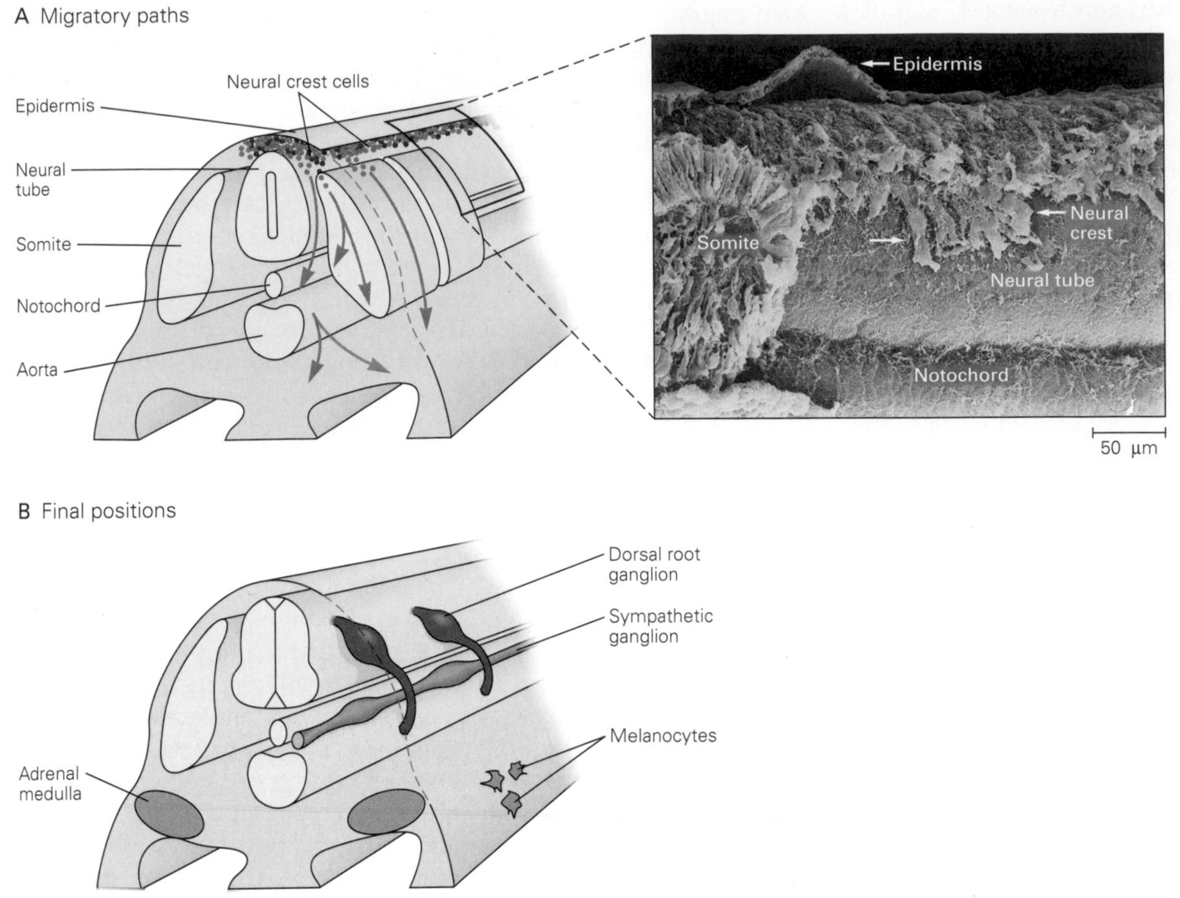

Figure 53–9 Neural crest cell migration in the peripheral nervous system.

A. A cross section through the middle part of the trunk of a chick embryo shows the main pathways of neural crest cells. Some migratory cells migrate along a superficial pathway, just beneath the ectoderm, and differentiate into pigment cells of the skin. Others migrate along a deeper pathway that takes them through the somites, where they coalesce to form dorsal root sensory ganglia. Still others migrate between the neural tube and somites, past the dorsal aorta. These cells differentiate into sympathetic ganglia and adrenal medulla. The scanning electron micrograph shows neural crest cells migrating away from the dorsal surface of the neural tube of a chick embryo. (Micrograph, used with permission, courtesy of K. Tosney.)

B. The final settling positions of neural crest cells, after they have completed their migration and undergone differentiation.

The first structures encountered by migrating neural crest cells are somites, epithelial cells that later give rise to muscle and cartilage. Neural crest cells pass through the anterior half of each somite but avoid the posterior half (Figure 53–9). The rostral channeling of migratory neural crest cells is imposed by ephrin B proteins, which are concentrated in the posterior half of each somite. Ephrins provide a repellant signal that interacts with EphB class tyrosine kinase receptors on neural crest cells to prevent their invasion. Neural crest cells that remain within the anterior sclerotome of the somite differentiate into sensory neurons of the dorsal root ganglia; those that migrate around the dorsal region of the somite approach the skin and give rise to melanocytes.

Differentiation of neural crest cells into dorsal root ganglion neurons is initiated at the time the cells emigrate from the neural tube, and depends on early exposure to Wnt signals secreted from the dorsal neural tube and somites as well as expression of neurogenin bHLH factors. In contrast, those neural crest cells that follow a more medial and ventral migratory path are exposed to BMPs secreted from the dorsal aorta and develop as sympathetic neurons that acquire a noradrenergic phenotype. BMPs promote noradrenergic neuronal differentiation by inducing the expression of a variety of transcription factors that include the bHLH protein Mash1, the homeodomain protein Phox2, and the zinc finger protein Gata2 (Figure 53–10).

The Neurotransmitter Phenotype of a Neuron Is Plastic

Neurons continue to develop after they have migrated to their final position, and no aspect of their later differentiation is more important than the choice of chemical neurotransmitter. The migratory pathway that a neural crest cell pursues to reach its final location exposes the cell to environmental signals that have a critical role in determining its transmitter phenotype.

The Transmitter Phenotype of a Peripheral Neuron Is Influenced by Signals from the Neuronal Target

The transmitter phenotype of autonomic neurons is plastic, and the final transmitter phenotype is determined in part by the end organs they innervate. Most sympathetic neurons use norepinephrine as their primary transmitter. However, those that innervate the exocrine sweat glands in the foot pads use acetylcholine, and even these neurons express norepinephrine at the time they first innervate the sweat glands of the skin. Only after their axons have contacted the sweat glands do they stop synthesizing norepinephrine and start producing acetylcholine.

When the sweat glands from the foot pad of a newborn rat are transplanted into a region that is normally innervated by noradrenergic sympathetic neurons, the synaptic neurons acquire cholinergic transmitter properties, indicating that cells of the sweat gland secrete factors that induce cholinergic properties in sympathetic neurons.

Several secreted factors trigger the switch from a noradrenergic to cholinergic phenotype in sympathetic neurons. The sweat gland secretes a cocktail of interleukin 6-like cytokines, notably cardiotrophin-1, leukemia inhibitory factor, and ciliary neurotrophic factor. Several aspects of neuronal metabolism that are linked to transmitter synthesis and release are controlled by these factors. The neurons stop producing the large dense-core granules characteristic of noradrenergic neurons and start making the small electron-translucent vesicles typical of cholinergic neurons (Figure 53–11).

The Transmitter Phenotype of a Central Neuron Is Controlled by Transcription Factors

Neurons that populate the central nervous system use two major neurotransmitters. The amino acid L-glutamate is the major excitatory transmitter and GABA is the major inhibitory transmitter. Distinct molecular programs are used to establish neurotransmitter phenotype in different brain regions and neuronal classes. We shall illustrate the general strategy for assignment of amino acid neurotransmitter phenotypes by focusing on neurons in the cerebral cortex and cerebellum.

The cerebral cortex contains glutamatergic pyramidal neurons that are generated within the cortical plate and rely on the bHLH factors neurogenin-1 and neurogenin-2 for their differentiation. In contrast, as

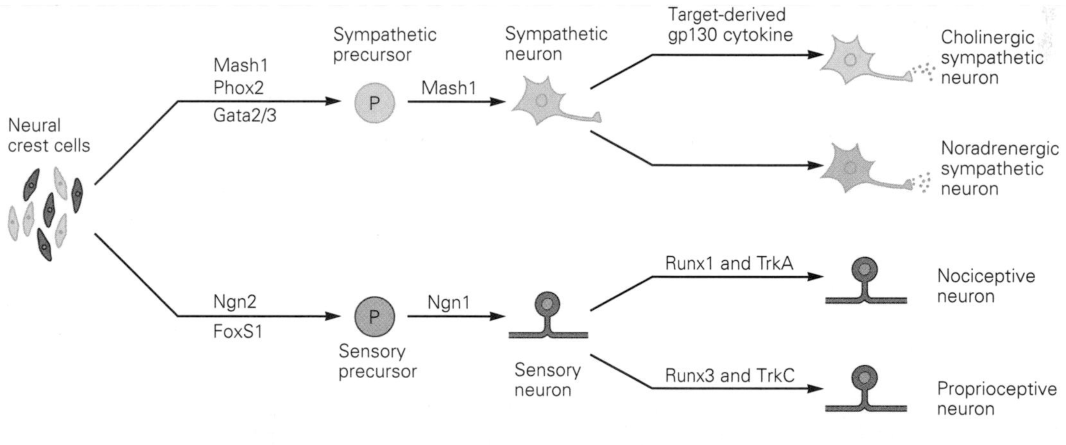

Figure 53–10 Neural crest cells differentiate into sympathetic and sensory neurons. The neuronal fates of trunk neural crest cells are controlled by transcription factor expression. Expression of the bHLH protein Mash1 directs neural crest cells along a sympathetic neuronal pathway. Sympathetic neurons can acquire noradrenergic or cholinergic transmitter phenotypes depending on the target cells they innervate and the level of gp130 cytokine signaling (see Figure 53–11). Two bHLH proteins, neurogenin-1 and -2, direct neural crest cells along a sensory neuronal pathway. Sensory neurons that express the transcription factor Runx1 and the tyrosine kinase receptor TrkA become nociceptors, whereas those that express Runx3 and TrkC become proprioceptors.

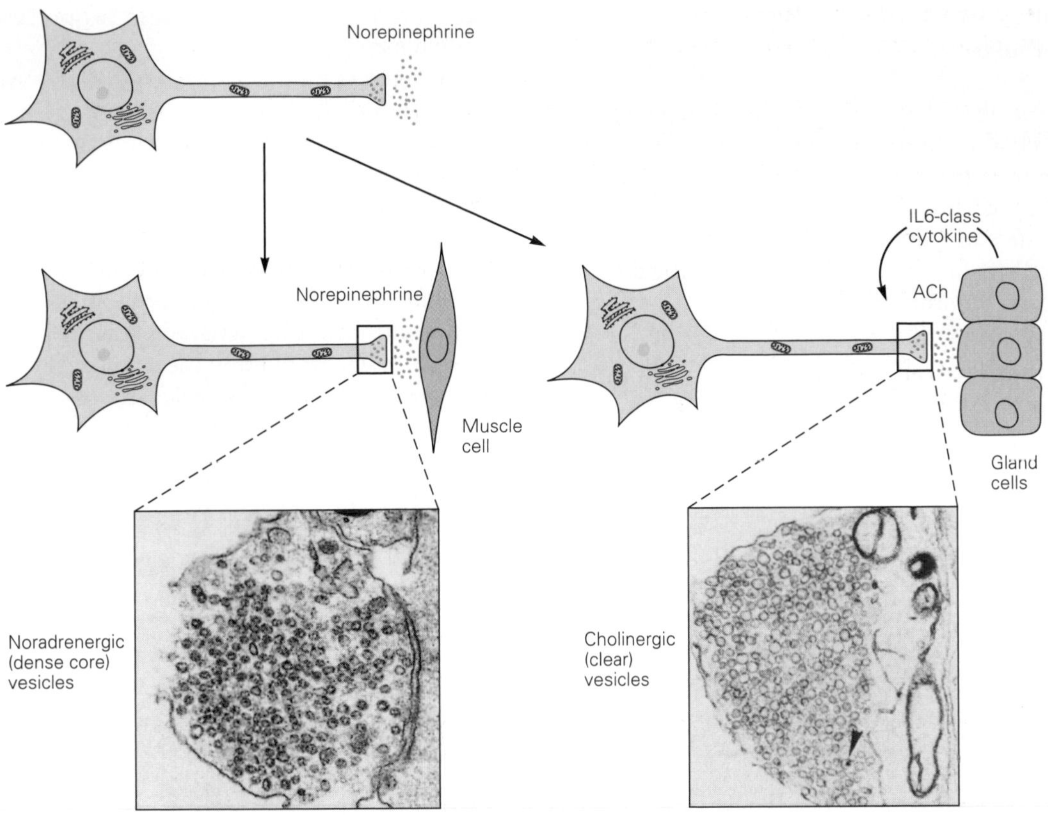

Figure 53–11 The target of sympathetic neurons determines neurotransmitter phenotype. Sympathetic neurons are initially specified with a noradrenergic transmitter phenotype. Most sympathetic neurons, including those that innervate cardiac muscle cells, retain this transmitter phenotype, and their terminals are packed with the dense-core vesicles in which norepinephrine is stored. But the sympathetic neurons that innervate sweat gland targets are induced to switch to a cholinergic transmitter phenotype; their terminals become filled with the small clear vesicles in which acetylcholine (**ACh**) is stored. Sweat gland cells direct the switch in transmitter phenotype by secreting members of the interleukin cytokine family. Several members of this family, including leukemia inhibitory factor (**LIF**) and ciliary neurotrophic factor (**CNTF**), are potent inducers of cholinergic phenotype in sympathetic neurons grown in cell culture. (Micrographs reproduced, with permission, courtesy of S. Landis.)

we discussed earlier in the chapter (see "Axons Tracts Serve As a Scaffold for Tangential Migration"), most GABAergic inhibitory interneurons migrate into the cortex from the ganglionic eminences, and their inhibitory transmitter character is specified by the bHLH protein Mash1 (Figures 53–12A) as well as by the Dlx1 and Dlx2 proteins.

Similarly, the cerebellum contains several different classes of inhibitory neurons (Purkinje, Golgi, basket, and stellate neurons) and two major classes of excitatory neurons (granule neurons and large cerebellar nuclear neurons). These inhibitory and excitatory neurons have different origins; GABAergic neurons derive from the ventricular zone, whereas glutamatergic neurons migrate into the cerebellum from the rhombic lip. The generation of GABAergic and glutamatergic neurons is controlled by two different bHLH transcription factors, Ptf1a for inhibitory and Math-1 for excitatory neurons (Figure 53–12B). These bHLH factors are expressed by neuroepithelial cells but not by mature neurons, implying that differentiation into glutamatergic and GABAergic neurons is initiated prior to neuronal generation.

The Survival of a Neuron Is Regulated by Neurotrophic Signals from the Neuron's Target

Not all neurons are destined to survive, and decisions about life and death are therefore aspects of a neuron's fate. The surprising and counterintuitive fact is that cell death is preprogrammed in most animal cells, including neurons.

The Neurotrophic Factor Hypothesis Was Confirmed by the Discovery of Nerve Growth Factor

The target of a neuron is a key source of factors essential for the neuron's survival. The critical role of target cells in neuronal survival was discovered in studies of the dorsal root ganglia.

In the 1930s Samuel Detwiler and Viktor Hamburger discovered that the number of sensory neurons in embryos is increased by transplantation of an additional limb bud into the target field and decreased if the limb target is removed. At the time these findings were thought to reflect an influence of the limb on the proliferation and subsequent differentiation of sensory neuron precursors. In the 1940s, however, Rita Levi-Montalcini made the startling observation that the death of neurons is not simply a consequence of pathology or experimental manipulation, but rather occurs during the normal program of embryonic development. Levi-Montalcini and Hamburger went on to show that removal of a limb leads to the excessive death of sensory neurons rather than a decrease in their production.

These early discoveries on the life and death of sensory neurons were quickly extended to neurons in the central nervous system. Hamburger found that

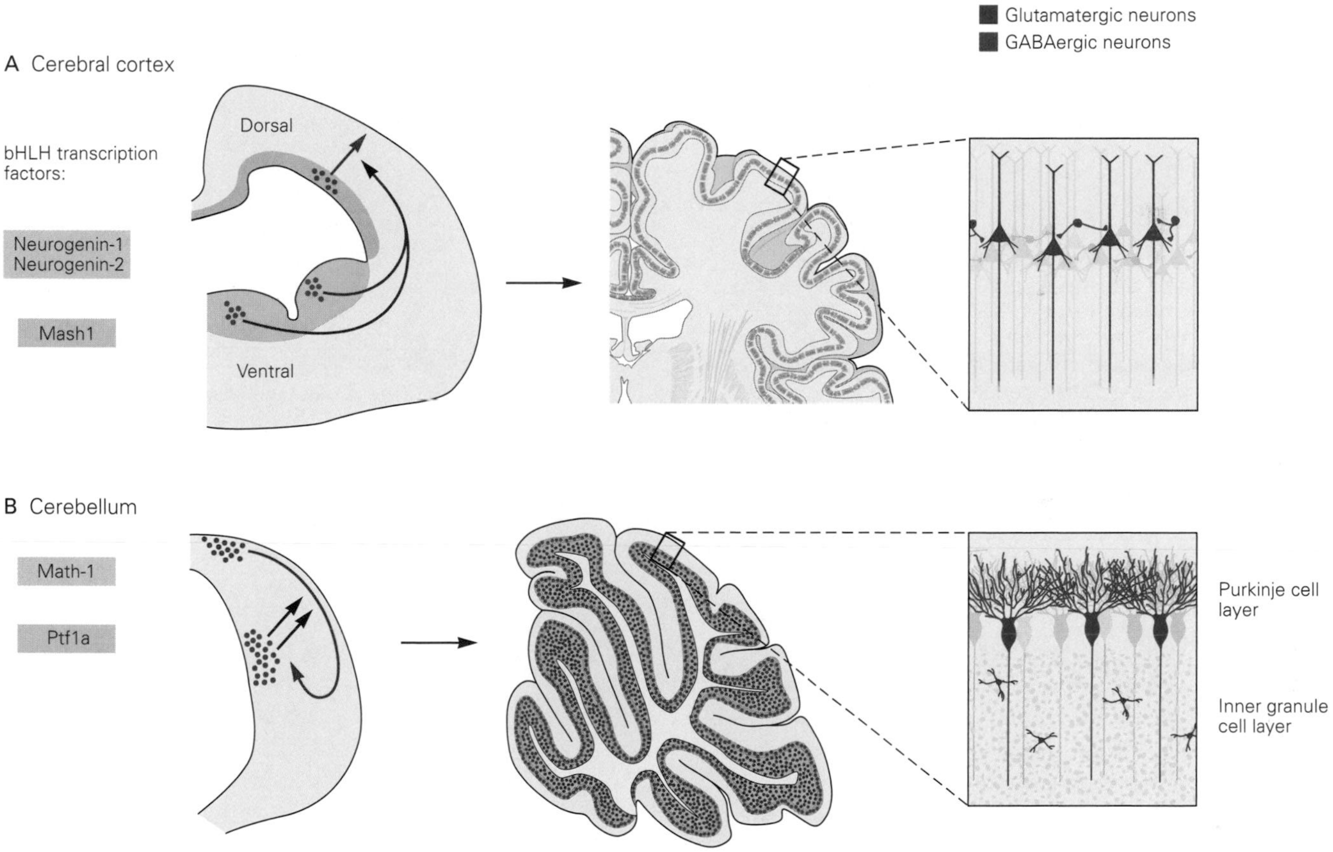

Figure 53–12 The neurotransmitter phenotype of central neurons is controlled by basic helix-loop-helix transcription factors.

A. In the cerebral cortex GABAergic and glutamatergic neurons derive from different proliferative zones and are specified by different basic helix-loop-helix (**bHLH**) transcription factors. Glutamatergic pyramidal neurons derive from the cortical ventricular zone, and their differentiation depends on the activities of neurogenin-1 and -2. The differentiation of GABAergic interneurons in the ganglionic eminences of the ventral telencephalon depends on the bHLH protein Mash1. These neurons migrate dorsally to supply the cerebral cortex with most of its inhibitory interneurons (see Figure 53–8).

B. In the developing cerebellum GABAergic and glutamatergic neurons also derive from different proliferative zones and are specified by bHLH transcription factors. Glutamatergic granule cells migrate into the cerebellum from the rhombic lip, settle in the inner granular layer (**IGL**), and are specified by the bHLH protein Math-1. GABAergic Purkinje neurons migrate from the deep cerebellar proliferative zone, settle in the Purkinje cell layer (**PCL**), and are specified by the bHLH protein Ptf1a.

approximately half of all motor neurons generated in the spinal cord die during embryonic development. Moreover, in experiments similar to those performed on sensory ganglia, Hamburger discovered that motor neuron death could be increased by removing a limb and reduced by adding an additional limb (Figure 53–13). These findings indicate that signals from target cells are critical for the survival of neurons within the central as well as peripheral nervous system. We now know that the phenomenon of neuronal overproduction, followed by a phase of neuronal death, occurs in most regions of the vertebrate nervous system. Blocking neuromuscular activity with drugs such as curare also reduces the extent of motor neuron death (Figure 53–13).

The early discoveries of Levi-Montalcini and Hamburger laid the foundations for the *neurotrophic factor hypothesis*. The core of this hypothesis is that cells at or near the target of a neuron secrete small amounts of an essential nutrient or trophic factor, and that the uptake of this factor by nerve terminals is needed for the survival of the neuron (Figure 53–14). This hypothesis was dramatically confirmed in the 1970s when Levi-Montalcini and Stanley Cohen purified the protein we now know as nerve growth factor (NGF) in the early 1970s and showed that this protein is made by target cells and supports the survival of sensory and sympathetic neurons in vitro. Moreover, neutralizing antibodies directed against NGF were found to cause a profound loss of sympathetic and sensory neurons in vivo.

Neurotrophins Are the Best Studied Neurotrophic Factors

The discovery of NGF prompted a search for additional neurotrophic factors. Today we know of over a dozen secreted factors that promote neuronal survival.

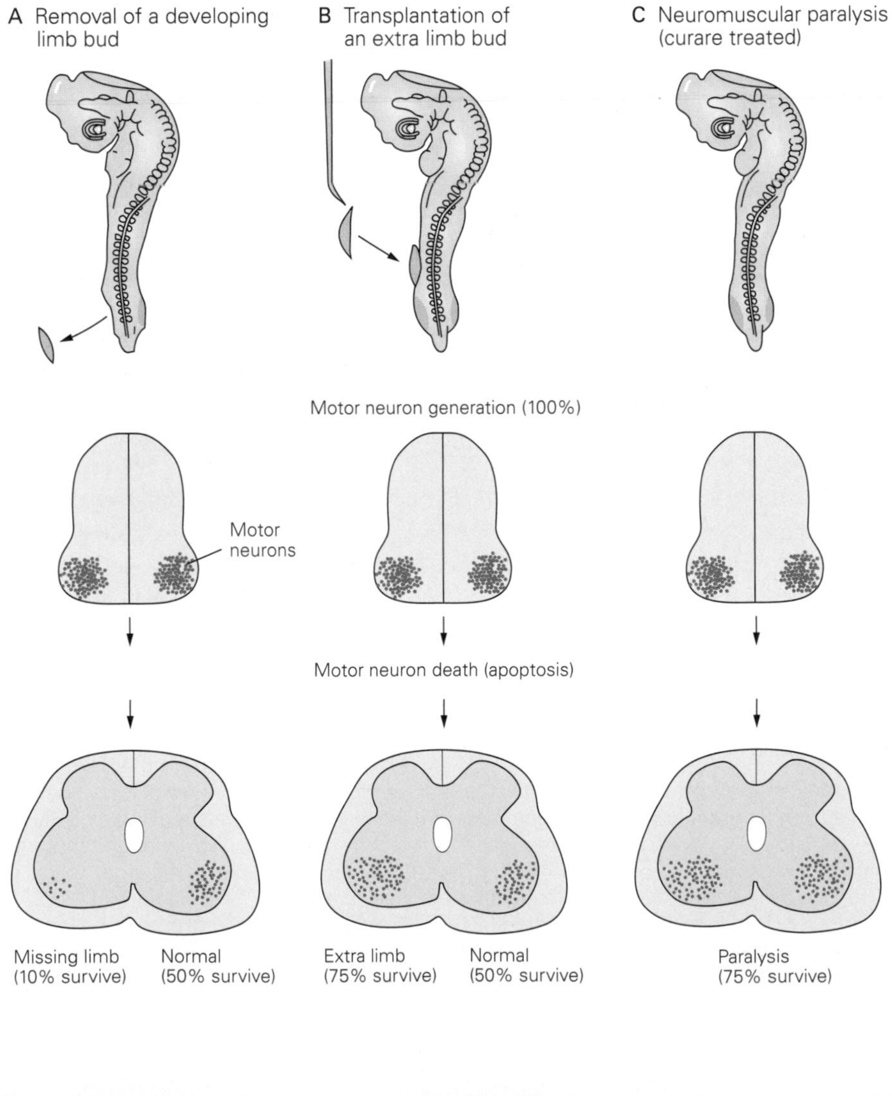

Figure 53–13 The survival of motor neurons depends on signals provided by their muscle targets. The role of the muscle target in motor neuron survival was demonstrated by Viktor Hamburger in a classic series of experiments performed in the chick embryo. (Adapted, with permission, from Purves and Lichtman 1985.)

A. A limb bud was removed from a 2.5-day-old chick embryo soon after the arrival of motor nerves. A section of the lumbar spinal cord 1 week later reveals few surviving motor neurons on the deprived side of the spinal cord. The number of motor neurons on the contralateral side with an intact limb is normal.

B. An extra limb bud was grafted adjacent to a host limb prior to the normal period of motor neuron death. A section of the lumbar spinal cord 2 weeks later shows an increased number of limb motor neurons on the side with the extra limb.

C. Blockade of nerve-muscle activity with the toxin curare, which blocks acetylcholine receptors, rescues many motor neurons that would otherwise die. Curare may act by enhancing the release of trophic factors from inactive muscle.

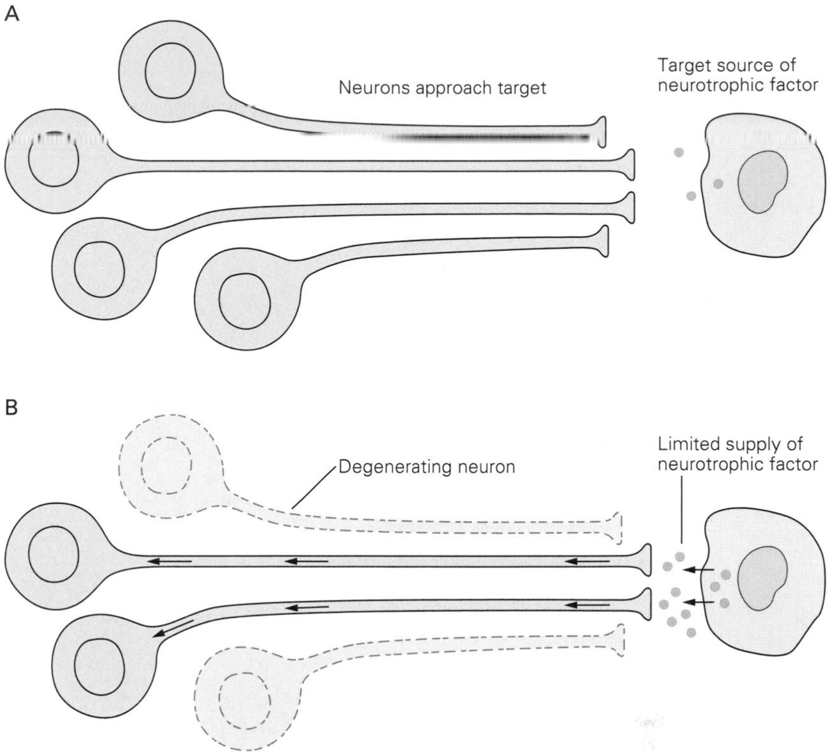

Figure 53–14 The neurotrophic factor hypothesis. (Adapted, with permission, from Reichardt and Farinas 1997.)

A. Neurons extend their axons to target cells, which secrete low levels of neurotrophic factors. (For simplicity only one target cell is shown.) The neurotrophic factor binds to specific receptors and is internalized and transported to the cell body, where it promotes neuronal survival.

B. Neurons that fail to receive adequate amounts of neurotrophic factor die through a program of cell death termed apoptosis.

The best studied of the neurotrophic factors are related to NGF and are called the neurotrophin family.

There are three main neurotrophins: NGF itself, brain derived neurotrophic factor (BDNF), and neurotrophin-3 (NT-3). Other classes of proteins that promote neuronal survival include members of the transforming growth factor β family, the interleukin 6-related cytokines, fibroblast growth factors, and even certain inductive signals we encountered earlier (BMPs and hedgehogs). Other neurotrophic factors, notably members of the glial cell line-derived neurotrophic factor (GDNF) family, are responsible for the survival of different types of sensory and sympathetic neurons (Figure 53–15).

Neurotrophins interact with two major classes of receptors, the Trk receptors and p75. Neurotrophins promote cell survival and promote cell death through activation of Trk receptors, whereas signaling through the p75 receptor promotes cell death. The Trk family comprises three membrane-spanning tyrosine kinases named TrkA, TrkB, and TrkC, each of which exists as a dimer (Figure 53–16).

As with other tyrosine kinase receptors, the binding of neurotrophins to Trk receptors leads to phosphorylation of an intracellular domain of the receptor, resulting in the dimerization of Trk proteins and phosphorylation of specific tyrosine residues in the activation loop of the kinase domain. Phosphorylation of these residues leads to a conformational change in the receptor and to phosphorylation of tyrosine residues that serve as docking sites for adaptor proteins. Activation of Trk receptors promotes the survival of neurons and also triggers their differentiation. These divergent biological responses involve different intracellular signaling pathways: neuronal differentiation largely by the mitogen-activated kinase (MAPK) enzymatic pathways and survival largely by the phosphatidylinositol-3 kinase pathway (Figure 53–17).

In contrast to the specificity of Trk receptor interactions, all neurotrophins bind the receptor p75 (Figure 53–16). The activation of p75 promotes neuronal survival through a pathway that involves activation of the NF-B enzyme. In the absence of exposure to neurotrophins, p75 receptor activation promotes neuronal death. Receptor p75 is a member of the tumor necrosis factor (TNF) receptor family and promotes cell death by activating proteases of the caspase family, which we discuss below.

Neurotrophin signaling is relayed from the axon terminal to the cell body of the neuron through a process that involves internalization of a complex of neurotrophin bound to Trk receptors. The retrograde

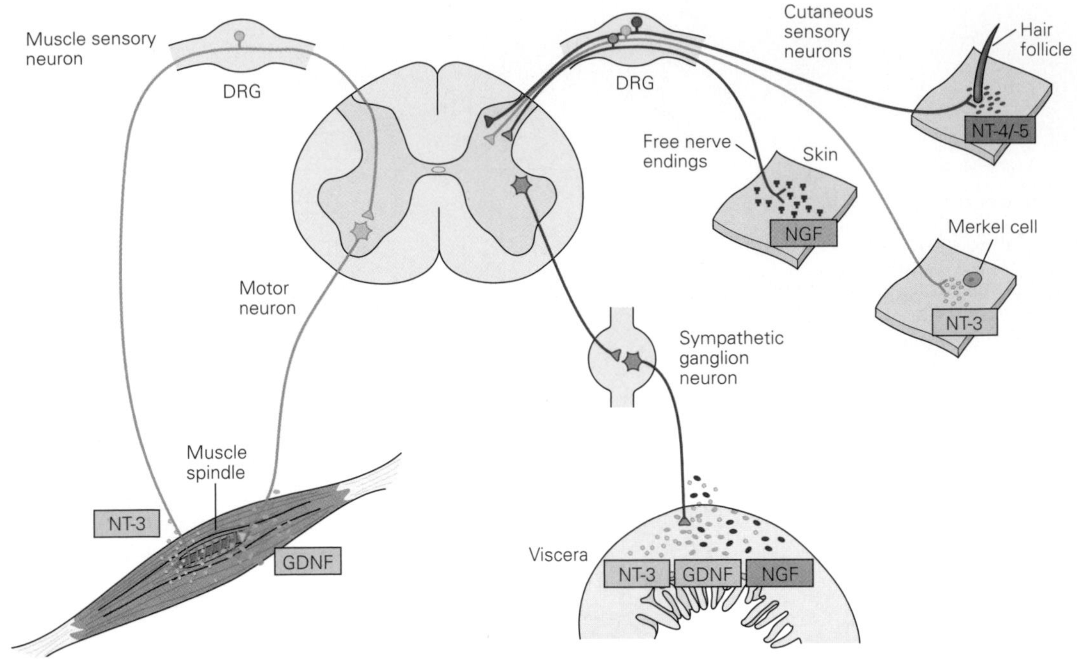

Figure 53–15 Different neurotrophic factors promote the survival of distinct populations of dorsal root ganglion neurons. Proprioceptive sensory neurons that innervate muscle spindles depend on neurotrophin-3 (**NT-3**); nociceptive neurons that innervate skin depend on nerve growth factor (**NGF**); mechanoreceptive neurons that innervate Merkel cells depend on neurotrophin-3; and those that innervate hair follicles depend on neurotrophin-4 and -5 (**NT-4/-5**). Motor neurons depend on glial cell line-derived neurotrophic factor (**GDNF**) and other factors. Sympathetic neurons depend on NGF, NT-3, and GDNF. (Adapted, with permission, from Reichardt and Farinas 1997.)

transport of this complex occurs in a class of endocytotic vesicles called signaling endosomes. The transport of these vesicles brings activated Trk receptors into cellular compartments able to activate signaling pathways and transcriptional programs essential for neuronal survival.

The picture is more complex for neurons in the central nervous system. The survival of motor neurons, for example, is not dependent on a single neurotrophic factor; different classes of motor neurons require neurotrophins, glial cell line-derived neurotrophic factor (GDNF), and interleukin-6-like proteins expressed by

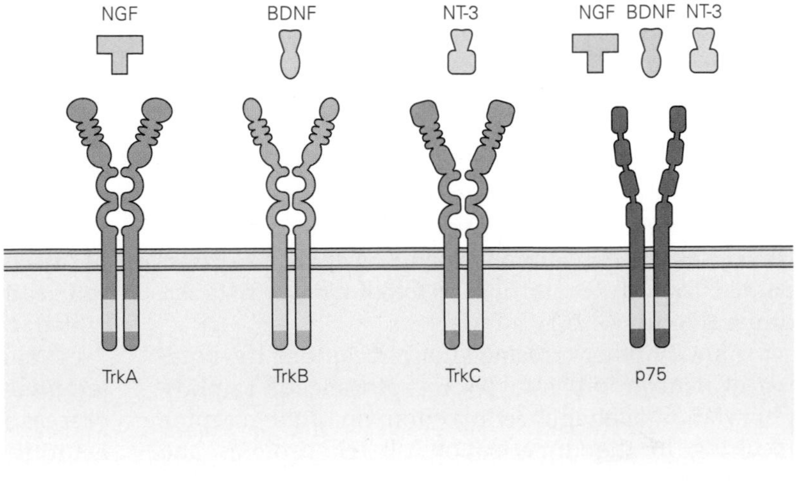

Figure 53–16 Neurotrophins and their receptors. Each of the three main neurotrophins interacts with a different transmembrane tyrosine kinase receptor (**Trk**). In addition, all three neurotrophins can bind to the low-affinity neurotrophin receptor p75. (**BDNF**, brain-derived neurotrophic factor; **NGF**, nerve growth factor; **NT-3**, neurotrophin-3.) (Adapted, with permission, from Reichardt and Farinas 1997.)

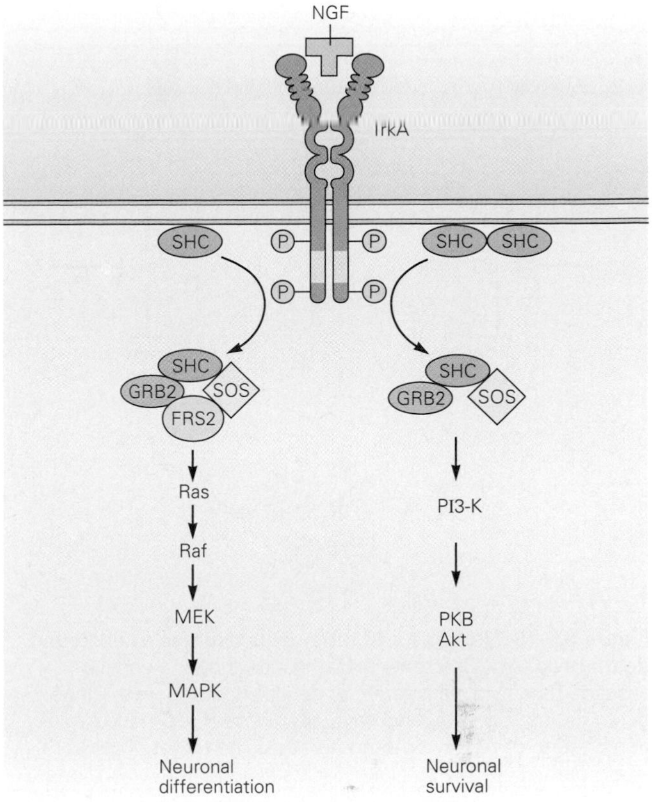

Figure 53–17 Binding of nerve growth factor to the TrkA receptor activates alternative intracellular signaling pathways. The binding of nerve growth factor (NGF) induces dimerization of the TrkA receptor, which triggers its phosphorylation at many different residues. Phosphorylation of TrkA results in the recruitment of the adaptor proteins SHC, GRB2, and SOS. The additional recruitment of FRS2 to this complex (left) activates a Ras kinase signaling pathway that promotes neuronal differentiation. In the absence of FRS2 (right) the complex activates a phosphatidylinositol-3 kinase (**PI3-K**) pathway that promotes neuronal survival. (**Akt/PKB**, protein kinase B; **MAPK**, microtubule-associated protein kinase; **MEK**, mitogen-activated/ERK kinase.) (Adapted, with permission, from Reichardt and Farinas 1997.)

muscles or peripheral glial cells. The survival of these neuronal classes depends on the exposure of axons to local neurotrophic factors.

Neurotrophic Factors Suppress a Latent Death Program in Cells

Neurotrophic factors were once believed to promote the survival of neural cells by stimulating their metabolism in beneficial ways, hence their name. It is now evident, however, that neurotrophic factors suppress a latent death program present in all cells of the body, including neurons.

This biochemical pathway can be considered a suicide program. Once it is activated, cells die by *apoptosis* (Greek, falling away): They round up, form blebs, condense their chromatin, and fragment their nuclei. Apoptotic cell deaths are distinguishable from *necrosis*, which typically results from acute traumatic injury and involves rapid lysis of cellular membranes without activation of the cell death program.

The first clue that deprivation of neurotrophic factors kills neurons by unleashing an active biochemical program emerged from studies that assessed neuronal survival after inhibition of RNA and protein synthesis. Exposure of sympathetic neurons to protein synthesis inhibitors was found to prevent the death of sympathetic neurons triggered by removal of NGF. These results sparked the idea that neurons are always capable of synthesizing proteins that are lethal and that NGF prevents their synthesis: Neurotrophins suppress an endogenous death program.

Key insights into the biochemical nature of the endogenous cell death program emerged from genetic studies of the nematode *Caenorhabditis elegans.* During the development of *C. elegans* a precise number of cells is generated and a fixed number of these cells die—the same number from embryo to embryo. The findings prompted a screen for genes that block or enhance cell death, which led to the identification of the cell death (*ced*) genes. Two of these genes, *ced-3* and *ced-4,* are needed for the death of neurons; in their absence every one of the cells destined to die instead survives. A third gene, *ced-9,* is needed for survival, and works by antagonizing the activities of *ced-3* and *ced-4* (Figure 53–18). Thus, in the absence of *ced-9* many additional cells die,

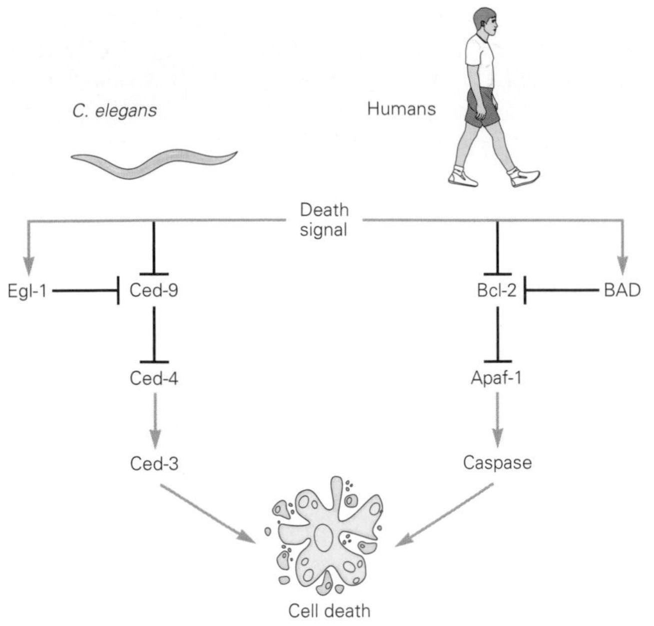

Figure 53–18 Neurons and other cells express a conserved death program. Different cellular insults trigger a genetic cascade that involves a series of death effector genes. These death genes and pathways have been conserved in the evolution of species from worms to humans. The target of the core death pathway is the activation of a set of proteolytic enzymes, the caspases. Caspases cleave many downstream and essential protein substrates (see Figure 53–19), resulting in the death of cells by a process termed *apoptosis*. Genetic analysis of the worm *Caenorhabditis elegans* indicates that the Ced-9 protein acts upstream and inhibits the activity of Ced-4 and Ced-3, two proteins that promote cell death. Many vertebrate homologs of Ced-9, the Bcl-2 family of proteins, have been identified. Some of these proteins, such as Bcl-2 itself, inhibit cell death, but others promote cell death by antagonizing the actions of the Bcl-2. The Bcl-2 class proteins act upstream of Apaf-1 (a vertebrate homolog of Ced-4) and the caspases (vertebrate homologs of Ced-3).

even though these deaths still depend on *ced-3* and *ced-4* activity.

The cell death pathway in *C. elegans* has been conserved in mammals. Similar proteins and pathways control the apoptotic death of central and peripheral neurons, indeed of all developing cells. The worm *ced-9* gene encodes a protein that is related to members of the mammalian Bcl-2 family, which protect lymphocytes and other cells from apoptotic death. The worm *ced-3* gene encodes a protein closely related to a class of mammalian cysteine proteases called caspases. The worm *ced-4* gene encodes a protein that is functionally related to a mammalian protein called apoptosis activating factor-1 or Apaf-1.

The mammalian apoptotic cell death pathway works in a way that resembles the worm pathway. The morphological and histochemical changes that accompany the apoptosis of mammalian cells result from the activation of caspases, which cleave specific aspartic acid residues within cellular proteins. Two classes of caspases regulate apoptotic death: the initiator and effector caspases. Initiator caspases (caspase-8, -9 and -10) cleave and activate effector caspases. Effector caspases (caspase-3 and -7) cleave other protein substrates, so triggering the apoptotic process. Perhaps 1% of all proteins in the cell serve as substrates for effector caspases. Their cleavage contributes to neuronal apoptosis through many pathways: by activation of proteolytic cascades, inactivation of repair, DNA cleavage, mitochondrial permeabilization, and initiation of phagocytosis.

The survival of mammalian neurons is determined by the balance between anti-apoptotic and pro-apoptotic members of the Bcl-2 family of proteins. Some Bcl-2-proteins such as BAX and BAK permeabilize mitochondrial outer membranes, causing the release of pro-apoptotic proteins such as cytochrome *c* into the cytosol. The release of cytochrome *c* induces Apaf-1 to bind and activate caspase-9, leading to the cleavage and activation of effector caspases. The binding of neurotrophic factors to their tyrosine kinase receptors is thought to lead to the phosphorylation of protein substrates that promote Bcl-2-like activities (Figure 53–19B). Thus withdrawal of neurotrophic factors from neurons changes the balance from anti-apoptotic to pro-apoptotic members of the Bcl-2 family, which triggers the neuron's demise.

The caspase cell death program can also be activated by many cellular insults, including DNA damage and anoxia (Figure 53–19A). The activation of cell-surface death receptors such as Fas by extracellular ligands results in the activation of caspase-8 or -10 as well as the recruitment of death effector proteins such as FADD. Recruitment of an initiator caspase to the Fas-FADD complex then leads to activation of effector caspases. Because many neurodegenerative disorders result in apoptotic death, pharmacological strategies to inhibit caspases are under investigation.

An Overall View

The nervous system generates an overabundance of neurons and superfluous cells. From beginning to end, intercellular signals provide crucial direction to the developing nervous system. After many years of descriptive embryology we now have the first molecular insights into two fundamental issues in neurogenesis: the mechanisms by which cells acquire neuronal and glial identities and those by which certain young neurons and glial cells survive at the expense of others.

Major insights into these aspects of neurogenesis have emerged from genetic studies of two invertebrate organisms: the fruit fly *Drosophila melanogaster* and the nematode worm *Caenorhabditis elegans*. This research has shown, once again, the striking phylogenetic conservation of the molecular machinery responsible for animal development. Yet insight into the trophic factors that promote the development and survival of nerve cells came first from studies of vertebrates. Moreover, research on neurotrophic factor signaling and the

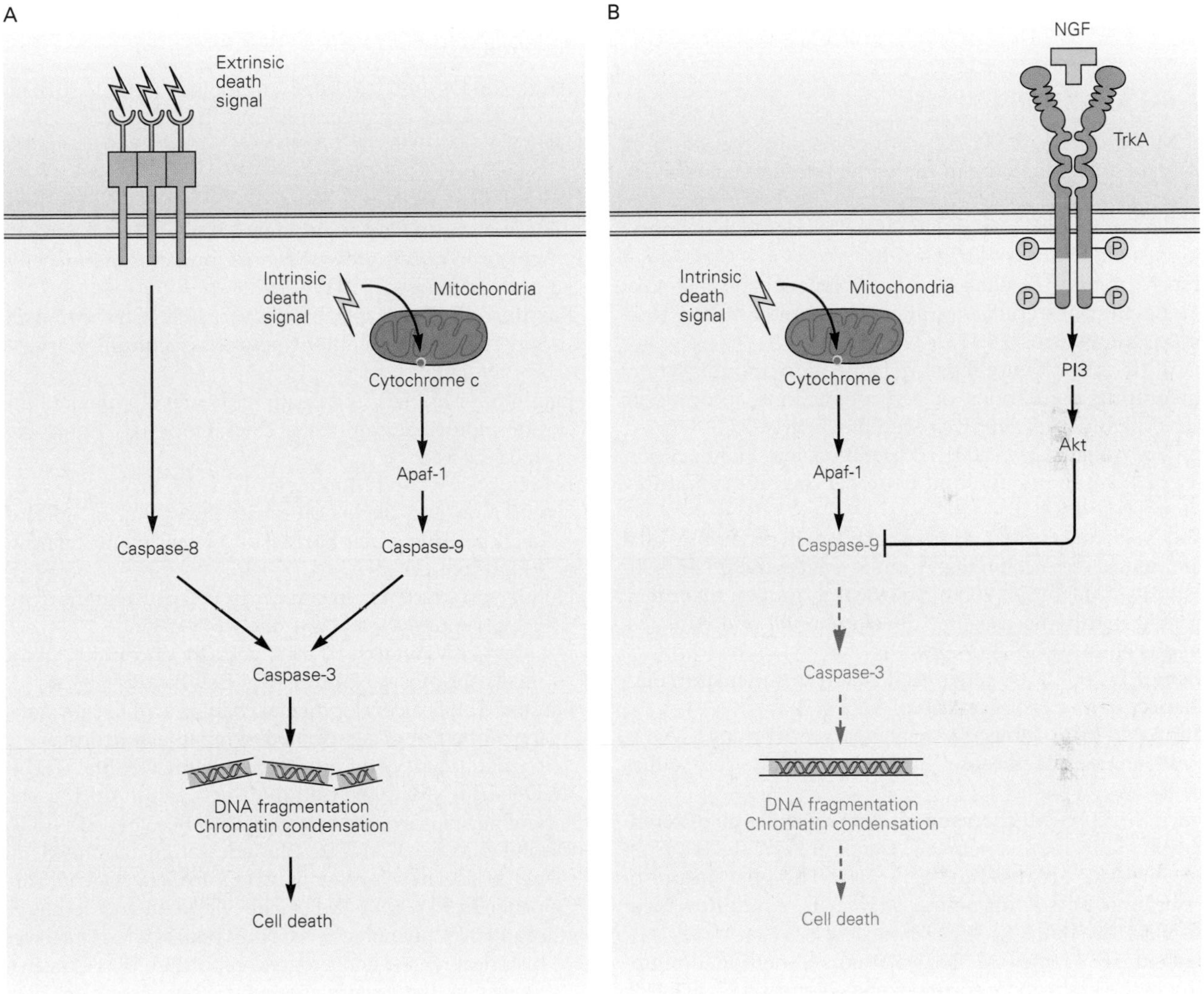

Figure 53–19 Neurotrophic factors suppress caspase activation and cell death. (Adapted, with permission, from Jesenberger and Jentsch 2002.)

A. Two types of pathways trigger cell death: extrinsic activation of surface membrane death receptors and intrinsic activation of a mitochondrial pathway. Both pathways result in activation of caspases such as caspase-8 and caspase-9, which initiate a proteolytic cleavage cascade that converges at the level of caspase-3 activation. Cleavage of the caspase precursor removes the caspase prodomain and produces a proteolytically active enzyme conformation.

The extrinsic pathway involves activation of death receptors by ligands such as tumor-necrosis factor (TNF) receptor 1 or Fas/CD95. The intrinsic pathway involves stress-induced signals such as DNA damage that initiate the release of cytochrome *c* from the mitochondrial intermembrane space. Cytochrome *c* binds to Apaf-1 and recruits and activates caspase-9.

B. Binding of neurotrophins to Trk receptors recruits the PI3 kinase pathway and Akt, suppressing the cell death pathway by inhibiting caspase-9. (**Akt**, protein kinase B [**PKB**].) This pathway is inhibited in developing neurons by neurotrophic factors explaining why their withdrawal leads to apoptosis.

biochemistry of cell death mechanisms is beginning to be applied to the search for treatment of neurodegenerative disorders.

Thomas M. Jessell
Joshua R. Sanes

Selected Readings

Bibel M, Barde YA. 2000. Neurotrophins: key regulators of cell fate and cell shape in the vertebrate nervous system. Genes Dev 14:2919–2937.

Bredesen DE, Rao RV, Mehlen P. 2006. Cell death in the nervous system. Nature 443:796–802.

Corbin JG, Nery S, Fishell G. 2001. Telencephalic cells take a tangent: non-radial migration in the mammalian forebrain. Nat Neurosci 4:1177–1182 Suppl.

Duband JL. 2006. Neural crest delamination and migration: integrating regulations of cell interactions, locomotion, survival and fate. Adv Exp Med Biol 589:45–77.

Feng Y, Walsh CA. 2001. Protein-protein interactions, cytoskeletal regulation and neuronal migration. Nat Rev Neurosci 2:408–416.

Gaiano N, Fishell G. 2002. The role of notch in promoting glial and neural stem cell fates. Annu Rev Neurosci 25:471–90.

Gleeson JG, Walsh CA. 2000. Neuronal migration disorders: from genetic diseases to developmental mechanisms. Trends Neurosci 23:352–359.

Guillemot F. 2007. Cell fate specification in the mammalian telencephalon. Prog Neurobiol 83:37–52.

Hoshino M. 2006. Molecular machinery governing GABAergic neuron specification in the cerebellum. Cerebellum 5:193–198.

Howard MJ. 2005. Mechanisms and perspectives on differentiation of autonomic neurons. Dev Biol 277:271–286.

Kriegstein AR, Alvarez-Buylla A. 2009 The glial nature of embryonic and adult neural stem cells. Annu Rev Neurosci 32:149–184.

Kriegstein AR, Noctor SC. 2004. Patterns of neuronal migration in the embryonic cortex. Trends Neurosci 27:392–399.

Kriegstein AR, Parnavelas JG. 2006. Progress in corticogenesis. Cereb Cortex 16:1–2 Suppl.

Marin O, Rubenstein JL. 2003. Cell migration in the forebrain. Annu Rev Neurosci 26:441–483.

Monuki ES, Walsh CA. 2002. Mechanisms of cerebral cortical patterning in mice and humans. Nat Neurosci 4:1199–1206 Suppl.

Nery S, Fishell G, Corbin, JG. 2002. The caudal ganglionic eminence is a source of distinct cortical and subcortical cell populations. Nat Neurosci 5:1279–1287.

Rallu M, Corbin JG, Fishell G. 2002. Parsing the prosencephalon. Nat Rev Neurosci 3:943–951.

Reichardt LF. 2006. Neurotrophin-regulated signaling pathways. Philos Trans R Soc Lond B Biol Sci 361:1545–1564.

Sun Y, Nadal-Vicens M, Misono S, Lin MZ, Zubiaga A, Hua X, Fan G, Greenberg ME. 2001. Neurogenin promotes neurogenesis and inhibits glial differentiation by independent mechanisms. Cell 104:365–376.

Wonders CP, Anderson SA. 2006. The origin and specification of cortical interneurons. Nat Rev Neurosci 7:687–696.

Yuan J, Yankner BA. 2000. Apoptosis in the nervous system. Nature 407:802–809.

References

Anderson DJ. 1997. Cellular and molecular biology of neural crest cell lineage determination. Trends Genet 13:276–280.

Detwiler SR. 1936. *Neuroembryology: An Experimental Study.* New York: Macmillan.

Doupe AJ, Landis SC, Patterson PH. 1985. Environmental influences in the development of neural crest derivatives: glucocorticoids, growth factors, and chromaffin cell plasticity. J Neurosci 5:2119–2142.

Furshpan EJ, Potter DD, Landis SC. 1982. On the transmitter repertoire of sympathetic neurons in culture. Harvey Lect 76:149–191

Hamburger V. 1975. Cell death in the development of the lateral motor column of the chick embryo. J Comp Neurol 160:535–546.

Hamburger V, Levi-Montalcini R. 1949. Proliferation differentiation and degeneration in the spinal ganglia of the chick embryo under normal and experimental conditions. J Exp Zool 111:457–501.

Henderson CE. 1996. Programmed cell death in the developing nervous system. Neuron 17:579–585.

Jesenberger V, Jentsch S. 2002. Deadly encounter: ubiquitin meets apoptosis. Nat Rev Mol Cell Biol 3:112–121.

Landis SC. 1980. Developmental changes in the neurotransmitter properties of dissociated sympathetic neurons: a cytochemical study of the effects of medium. Dev Biol 77:349–361.

Le Douarin NM. 1998. Cell line segregation during peripheral nervous system ontogeny. Science 231:1515–1522.

Olson EC, Walsh CA. 2002. Smooth, rough and upside-down neocortical development. Curr Opin Genet Dev 12:320–327.

Oppenheim RW. 1981. Neuronal cell death and some related regressive phenomena during neurogenesis: a selective historical review and progress report. In: WM Cowan (ed.), *Studies in Developmental Neurobiology: Essays in Honor of Viktor Hamburger,* pp. 74–133. New York: Oxford Univ. Press.

Qian X, Goderie SK, Shen Q, Stern JH, Temple S. 1998. Intrinsic programs of patterned cell lineages in isolated vertebrate CNS ventricular zone cells. Development 125:3143–3152.

Purves D, Lichtman JW. 1985. *Principles of Neural Developement,* p. 433. Sunderland, MA: Sinauer.
Reichardt LF. 2006. Neurotrophin-regulated signaling pathways. Philos Trans R Soc Lond B Biol Sci 361:1545–1564.
Shah NM, Groves AK, Anderson DJ. 1996. Alternative neural crest cell fates are instructively promoted by TGF beta superfamily members. Cell 85:331–343.

54

The Growth and Guidance of Axons

In the two preceding chapters we saw how neurons are generated in appropriate numbers, at correct times, and in the right places. These early developmental steps set the stage for later events that direct neurons to form functional connections with target cells. To form connections neurons have to extend long processes—axons and dendrites—which permit connectivity with postsynaptic cells and synaptic input from other neurons.

The growing axon may have to travel a long distance—up to several meters in a giraffe—and ignore many inappropriate neuronal partners before terminating in just the right region and recognizing its correct synaptic targets. In this chapter we examine how neurons elaborate axons and dendrites, and how axons are guided to their targets. In subsequent chapters we consider how neurons form synapses and how patterns of connections are shaped by activity.

We begin this chapter by discussing how certain neuronal processes become axons and others dendrites. We then consider the challenges that face an axon as it projects along tortuous pathways to its target. Finally, we illustrate general features of axonal guidance by describing the development of two well-studied axonal pathways: one that conveys visual information from the retina to the brain and another that conveys cutaneous sensory information from the spinal cord to the brain.

Differences in the Molecular Properties of Axons and Dendrites Emerge Early in Development

The processes of neurons vary enormously in their length, thickness, branching pattern, and molecular architecture. Nonetheless, most neuronal processes fit two functional categories: axons and dendrites. More than a century ago Santiago Ramón y Cajal hypothesized that this distinction underlies the ability of neurons to transmit information in a particular direction, an idea he formalized as the law of dynamic polarization.

Cajal wrote that "the transmission of the nerve impulse is always from the dendritic branches and the cell body to the axon." In the decades before electrophysiological methods were up to the task, this law provided a means of analyzing neural circuits histologically. Although exceptions have been found, Ramón y Cajal's law remains a basic principle that relates structure and function in the nervous system and highlights the importance of knowing how neurons acquire their polarized form.

Neuronal Polarity Is Established Through Rearrangements of the Cytoskeleton

Much of our knowledge about neuronal polarization comes from studies of neurons taken from the rodent brain and grown in tissue culture. Hippocampal neurons grown in isolation develop processes reminiscent of those seen in vivo: a single, long, cylindrical axon and several shorter, tapered dendrites (Figure 54–1A). Axons and dendrites soon acquire molecular distinctions, as cytoskeletal and synaptic proteins are targeted to these components. For example, a particular form of the Tau protein is localized in axons and the MAP2 protein in dendrites (Figure 54–1B)

Cultured neurons are especially useful for developmental studies because they initially show no obvious sign of polarization and acquire their specialized features gradually in a stereotyped sequence of cellular steps. This sequence begins with extension of several short processes, each equivalent to the others. Soon thereafter, one process is established as an axon and the remaining processes acquire dendritic features (Figure 54–1A).

How does this occur? Cytoskeletal proteins that maintain elongated processes and drive growth are central to this process. If the actin filaments in an early neurite are destabilized, the ensuing cytoskeletal rearrangements commit the neurite to becoming the axon, while the remaining neurites become dendrites. If the nascent axon is removed, one of the remaining neurites quickly assumes an axonal character. This sequence suggests that axonal specification is a key event in neuronal polarization and that signals from newly formed axons both suppress the generation of additional axons and promote dendrite formation.

The nature of the axonally derived signal that represses other axons is not known. But some insight into signals that control cytoskeletal arrangements has come from the study of a group of proteins encoded by the *Par* complex genes. As first shown in the nematode worm *Caenorhabditis elegans*, Par proteins are involved in diverse aspects of cytoskeletal reorganization, including the polarization of neuronal processes. Mammalian forebrain neurons lacking *Par3, Par4, Par6*, or relatives of *Par1* grow multiple processes that are intermediate in length between axons and dendrites and bear markers of both processes (Figure 54–1B).

Although neurons grown in culture are similar to those in the brain, they are deprived of key extrinsic cues and signals. Cultured neurons become randomly arranged with respect to each other, whereas in many regions of the developing brain neurons line up in rows, with their dendrites pointing in the same direction (Figure 54–2A). This difference in vivo and in vitro implies that extrinsic signals regulate the polarization machinery. In the developing brain the local release of semaphorins, and other axonal guidance factors that we discuss later in the chapter, may help to orient dendrites (Figure 54–2C). The job of the Par protein complex is to link these extracellular signals to the cellular machinery that rearranges the cytoskeleton, a process achieved in part through the regulation of proteins that modify actin or tubulin function. In fact both the Tau protein in axons and the MAP2 protein in dendrites associate with and affect microtubules.

If local signals are needed to polarize neurons in the brain, how is polarity established in the uniform environment of a tissue culture? One possible explanation is that minor variations in the intensity of signaling within a neuron, or in signals from its immediate environment, will activate Par proteins in one small domain of the neuron, triggering the nearest process to become an axon. If, by happenstance, one process grows slightly faster than its neighbors, its chances of becoming an axon increase markedly (Figure 54–2B). Presumably, this proto-axonal process emits signals that decrease the chance of other processes following suit, forcing them to become dendrites.

Dendrites Are Patterned by Intrinsic and Extrinsic Factors

Although processes destined to become axons and dendrites initially are indistinguishable, they soon acquire distinct features. Nascent dendrites grow at acute angles and their branches are generally more numerous and closer to the cell body than those of axons. In addition, small protrusions called spines extend from the distal branches of dendrites. Finally, some dendritic branches are retracted or "pruned" to give the arbor its final and definitive shape (Figure 54–3).

Although the core features of dendrite formation are common to many neurons, there is a striking variation in dendrite number, shape, and branching pattern among neuronal types. Indeed, the shape and form of its dendritic arbor is one of the main ways in which

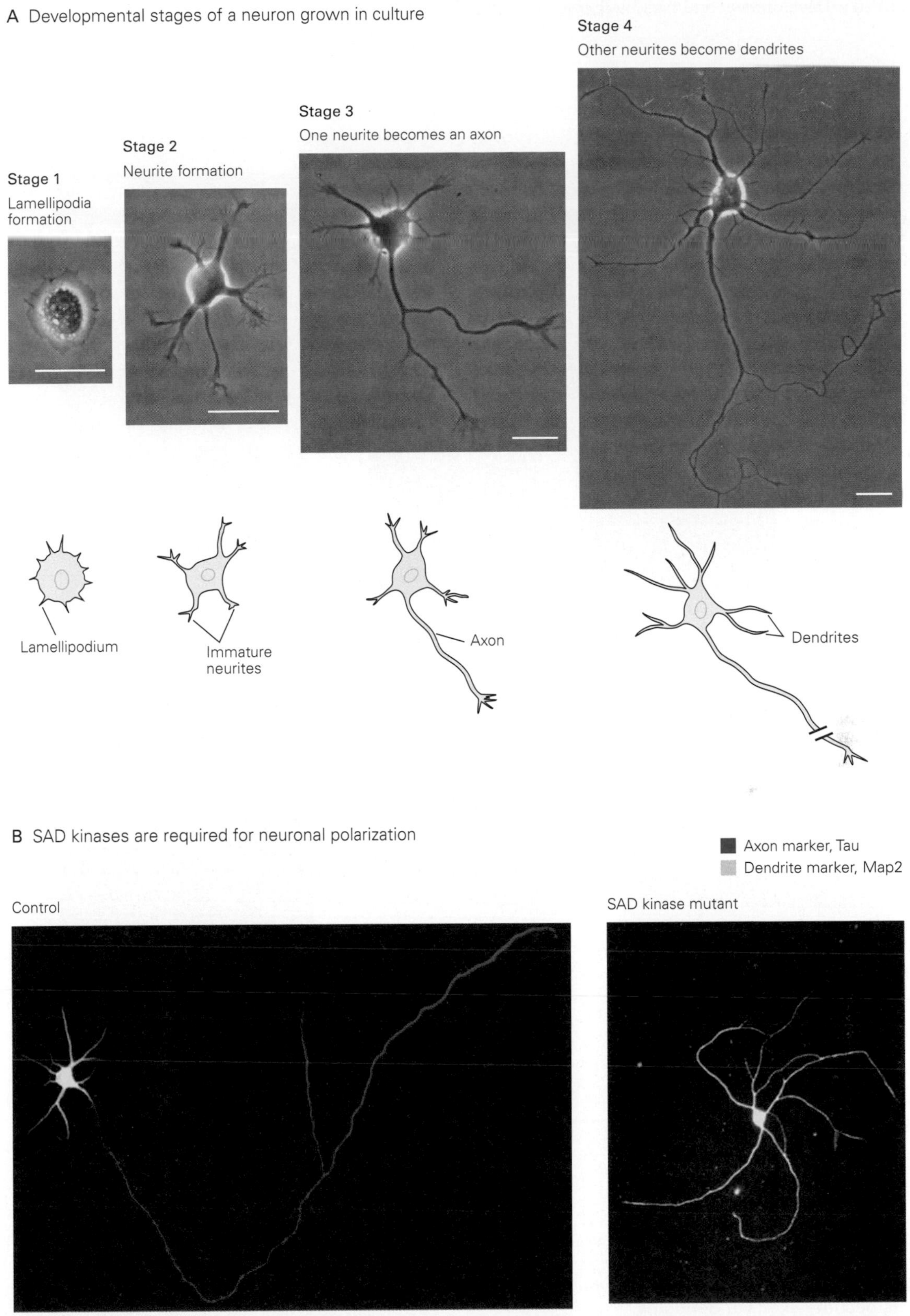

Figure 54–1 The differentiation of axons and dendrites marks the emergence of neuronal polarity.

A. Four stages in the polarization of a hippocampal neuron grown in tissue culture. (Adapted, with permission, from Kaech and Banker 2006.)

B. Hippocampal neurons grown in culture possess multiple short, thick dendrites that are enriched in the microtubule-associated protein MAP2. They also possess a single long axon that is marked by a dephosphorylated form of the microtubule-associated protein tau (left). A cultured neuron isolated from a mutant mouse lacks expression of a *Par* family gene (SAD kinase). The neuron generates neurites that co-express Tau and MAP2, markers of axons and dendrites respectively. The length and diameter of these neurites are intermediate in size between those of axons and dendrites (right). (Reproduced, with permission, from Kishi et al. 2005.)

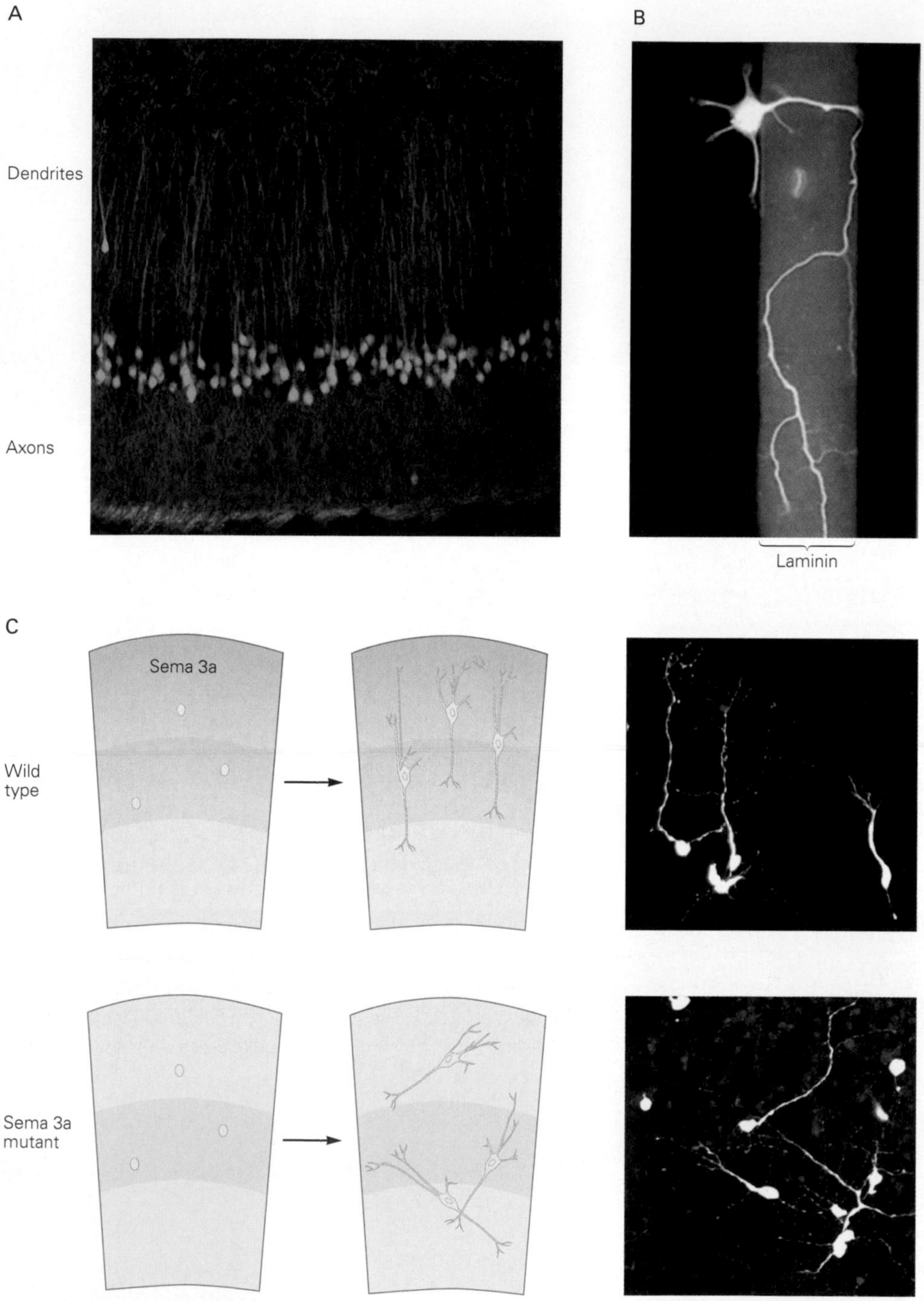

Figure 54–2 Extracellular factors determine whether neuronal processes become axons or dendrites.

A. Cortical pyramidal neurons in vivo display a common axonal and dendritic orientation. (Image reproduced, with permission, from Josh Sanes.)

B. Neurons growing on laminin acquire polarity. When a cortical neuron extends a process from a less attractive substrate onto laminin, the process grows faster and usually becomes an axon. (Image reproduced, with permission, from Paul Letourneau.)

C. In the developing neocortex semaphorin-3A (Sema 3A) is secreted by cells near the pial surface. Semaphorin-3A is an attractant for growing dendrites, helping to establish neuronal polarity and orientation. The parallel orientation of cortical pyramidal neurons is disrupted in mutant mice lacking functional semaphorin-3A. (Reproduced, with permission, from Polleux, Morrow, and Ghosh 2000.)

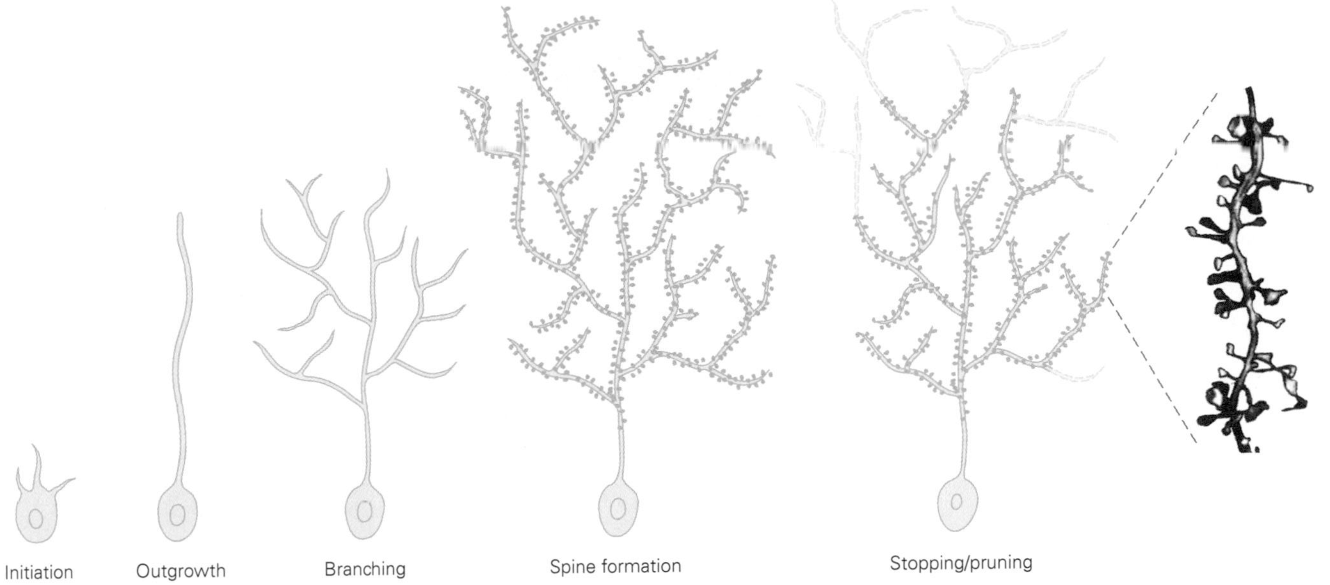

Figure 54–3 Dendritic branching develops in a series of steps. The outgrowth of dendrites involves the formation of elaborate branches from which spines develop. Certain branches and spines are later pruned to achieve the mature pattern of dendrite arborization. (Image of spines at right reproduced, with permission, from Stefan W. Hell.)

neurons can be classified. Cerebellar Purkinje cells can be distinguished from granule cells, spinal motor neurons, and hippocampal pyramidal neurons simply by looking at the pattern of their dendrites.

How is dendritic pattern established? Neurons must have intrinsic information about their shape because the patterns in tissue culture are strikingly reminiscent of those in vivo (Figure 54–4). The transcriptional programs that specify neuronal subtype (see Chapter 52) presumably also encode information about neuronal shape. A second mechanism for establishing the pattern of dendritic arbors is the recognition of one dendrite by others of the same cell. In the *Drosophila* nervous system repellent signaling between dendrites of the same neuron, mediated by the different isoforms of a recognition protein known as DS-CAM, helps to ensure that dendrites expand over a broad territory rather than bunching together.

The dendrites of neighboring neurons also provide cues. In many cases the dendrites of a particular class of neuron cover a surface with minimal overlap, a spacing pattern called *tiling*. The tiling of dendrites appears to result from specific inhibitory interactions among the dendrites of a particular class of neuron. Tiling allows each class of neuron to receive information from the entire surface or area it innervates. Tiling of a region by the dendrites of one class of neuron also avoids the confusion that could arise if the dendrites of many different neurons occupied the same area.

Thus interactions between dendrites establish an overall arborization pattern through a mixture of intrinsic and extracellular mechanisms. Once a cell process is committed to an axonal or dendritic character, it becomes sensitive to a variety of intrinsic and extrinsic signals that determine its trajectory. For dendrites these patterning signals determine neuronal morphology. For axons, which we consider next, the signals guide the axons to their targets.

The Growth Cone Is a Sensory Transducer and a Motor Structure

Once an axon forms it begins to grow toward its synaptic target. The key neuronal element responsible for axonal growth is a specialized structure at the tip of the axon called the *growth cone.* Both axons and dendrites use growth cones for elongation, but those linked to axons have been studied more intensively.

Ramón y Cajal discovered the growth cone and had the key insight that it was responsible for axonal pathfinding. With static images alone for inspiration (Figure 54–5A), he envisioned the growth cone to be "endowed with exquisite chemical sensitivity, rapid

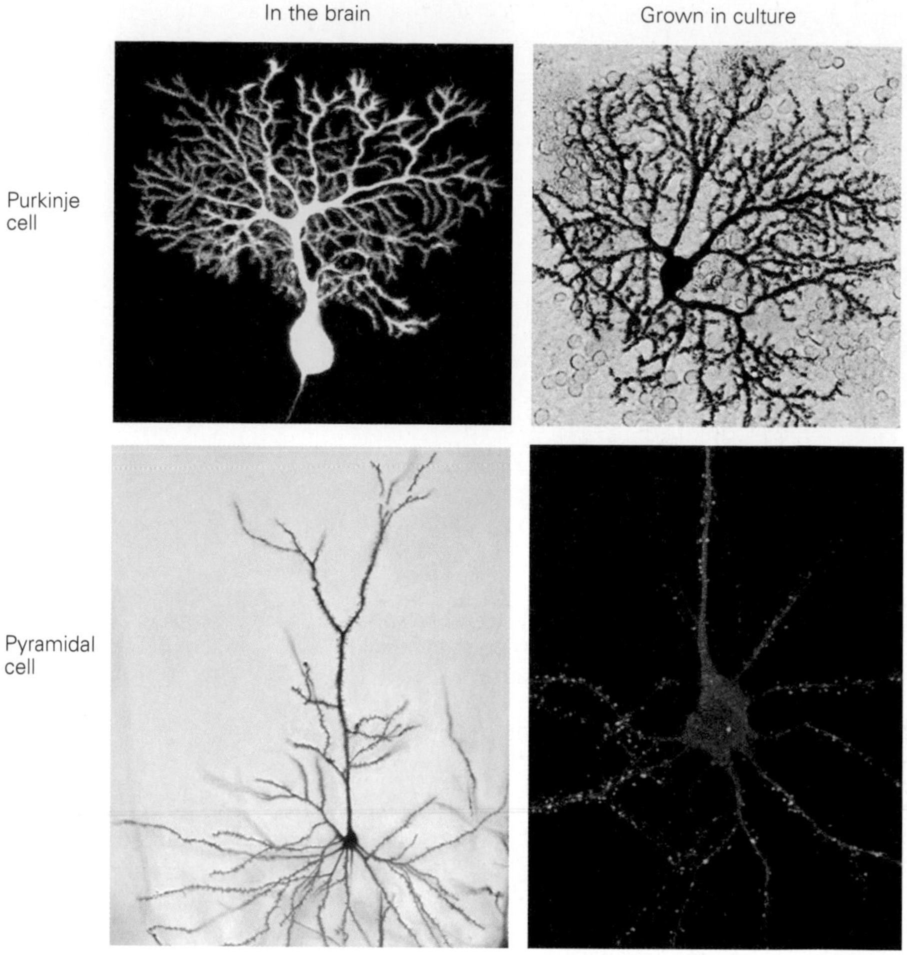

Figure 54–4 The morphologies of neurons are preserved in dissociated cell culture. Cerebellar Purkinje neurons and hippocampal pyramidal neurons have distinctive patterns of dendritic branching. These basic patterns are recapitulated when these two classes of neurons are isolated and grown in dissociated cell culture. (The image on the upper left is from David L. Becker; upper right from Yoshio Hirabayashi; lower left by Grazyna Gorney, reproduced, with permission, from Terry E. Robinson; the image in the lower right from Kelsey Martin. All images reproduced with permission.)

ameboid movements and a certain motive force, thanks to which it is able to proceed forward and overcome obstacles met in its way … until it reaches its destination."

Many studies over the past century have confirmed Ramón y Cajal's intuition. We now know that the growth cone is both a sensory structure that receives directional cues from the environment and a motor structure whose activity drives axon elongation. Ramón y Cajal also pondered "what mysterious forces precede the appearance of these processes … promote their growth and ramification … and finally establish those protoplasmic kisses … which seem to constitute the final ecstasy of an epic love story." In more modern and prosaic terms we now know that the growth cone guides the axon by transducing positive and negative cues into signals that regulate the cytoskeleton, thereby determining the course and rate of axonal outgrowth.

Growth cones have three main compartments. Their *central core* is rich in microtubules, mitochondria, and other organelles. Long slender extensions called *filopodia* project from the body of the growth cone. Between the filopodia lie *lamellipodia,* which are also motile and give the growth cone its characteristic ruffled appearance (Figure 54–5C).

Growth cones sense environmental signals through their filopodia: rod-like, actin-rich, membrane-limited structures that are highly motile. Their surface membranes bear receptors for the molecules that serve as directional cues for the axon. Their length—tens of micrometers in some cases—permits the filopodia to sample environments far in advance of the central core of the growth core. Their rapid movements permit them to compile a detailed inventory of the environment, and their flexibility permits them to navigate around cells and other obstacles.

When filopodia encounter signals in the environment, the growth cone is stimulated to advance, retract, or turn. Several motors power these orienting behaviors. One source of power is the movement of actin along myosin, an interaction similar to the one that powers the contraction of skeletal muscle fibers, although the actin and myosin of neurons are different from those in muscle. The assembly of actin monomers into polymeric filaments also contributes a propulsive force for filopodial extension. Acting in parallel, actin filaments constantly depolymerize at the base of filopodia. Depolymerization slows during periods of growth cone advance, leading to greater net forward motion. The movement of membranes along the substrate provides yet another source of forward motion.

The contribution of each type of molecular motor to the advance of the growth cone is likely to vary from one situation to another. With all of these motors the final step involves the flow of microtubules from the

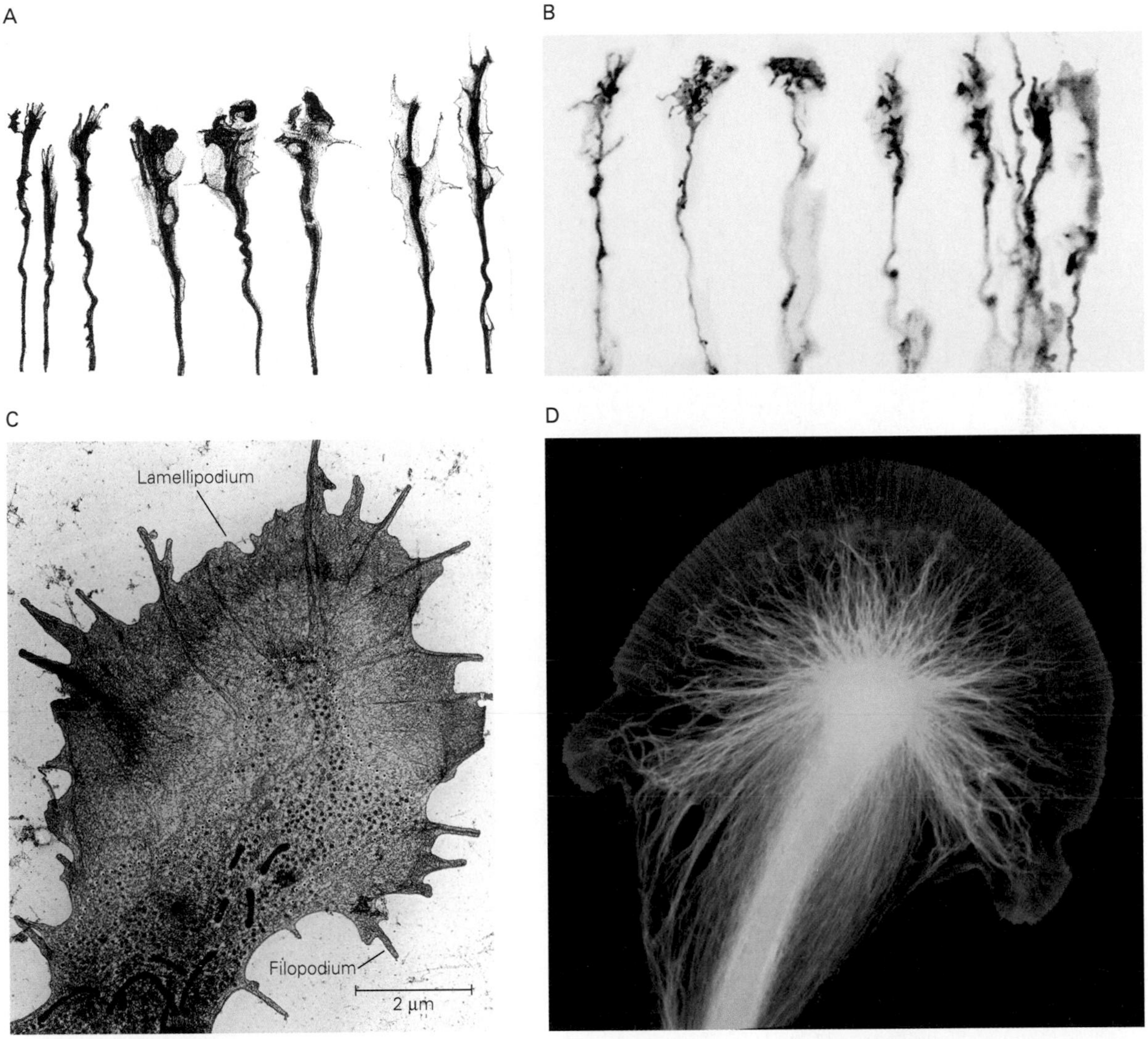

Figure 54–5 Neuronal growth cones.

A. Drawings of growth cones by Santiago Ramón y Cajal, who discovered these cellular structures and inferred their function.

B. The diverse morphologies of growth cones are visualized in dye-labeled retinal ganglion neurons in the mouse. Note the similarities with Cajal's drawings. (Reproduced, with permission, from Carol Mason and Pierre Godemont.)

C. The three main domains of the growth cone—filopodia, lamellipodia, and a central core—shown by whole-mount electron microscopy. (Reproduced, with permission, from Bridgman and Dailey 1989.)

D. The growth cone of a neuron from *Aplysia* in which actin and tubulin have been visualized. Actin (**purple**) is concentrated in lamellipodia and filopodia, whereas tubulin and microtubules (**aquamarine**) are concentrated in the central core. (Image reproduced, with permission, from Paul Forscher and Dylan Burnette.)

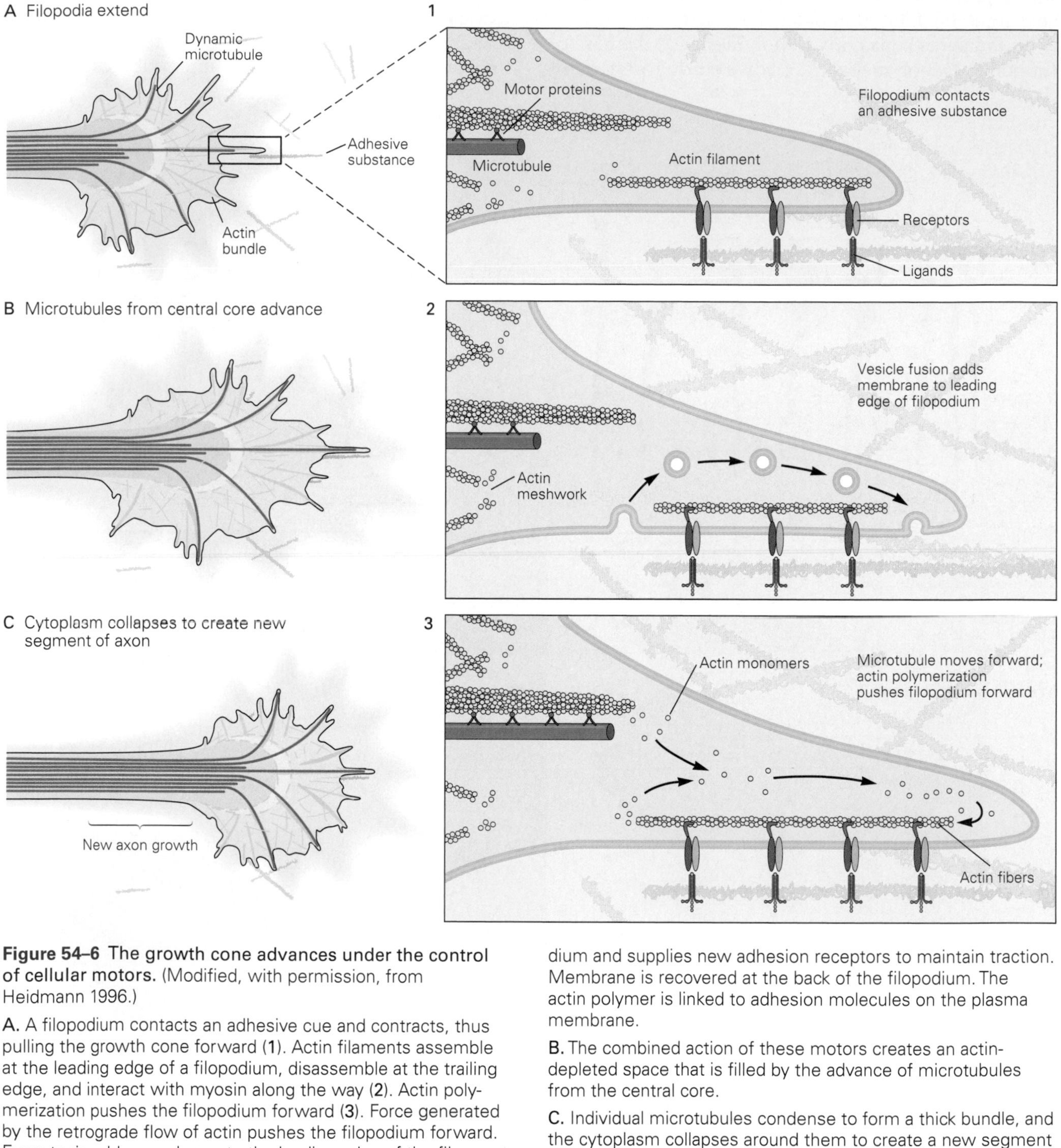

Figure 54–6 The growth cone advances under the control of cellular motors. (Modified, with permission, from Heidmann 1996.)

A. A filopodium contacts an adhesive cue and contracts, thus pulling the growth cone forward (**1**). Actin filaments assemble at the leading edge of a filopodium, disassemble at the trailing edge, and interact with myosin along the way (**2**). Actin polymerization pushes the filopodium forward (**3**). Force generated by the retrograde flow of actin pushes the filopodium forward. Exocytosis adds membrane to the leading edge of the filopodium and supplies new adhesion receptors to maintain traction. Membrane is recovered at the back of the filopodium. The actin polymer is linked to adhesion molecules on the plasma membrane.

B. The combined action of these motors creates an actin-depleted space that is filled by the advance of microtubules from the central core.

C. Individual microtubules condense to form a thick bundle, and the cytoplasm collapses around them to create a new segment of axonal shaft.

central core of the growth cone into the newly extended tip, thus moving the growth cone ahead and leaving in its wake a new segment of axon. New lamellipodia and filopodia form in the advancing growth cone and the cycle repeats (Figure 54–6).

Accurate pathfinding can occur only if the growth cone's motor action is linked to its sensory function. It is crucial therefore that the recognition proteins on the filopodia are signal-inducing receptors and not merely binding moieties that mediate adhesion. The binding of a ligand to its receptor affects growth in diverse ways. It stimulates the formation, accumulation, and even the breakdown of soluble intracellular molecules that function as second messengers. These second messengers affect the organization of the cytoskeleton, and in this way regulate the direction and rate of movement of the growth cone.

One important second messenger is calcium. The calcium concentration in growth cones is regulated by the activation of receptors on filopodia and this affects the organization of the cytoskeleton, which in turn modulates motility. Growth cone motility is optimal within a narrow range of calcium concentrations, called a *set point*. Activation of filopodia on one side of the growth cone leads to a concentration gradient of calcium across the growth cone, providing a possible basis for changes in the direction of growth.

Other second messengers that link receptors and motor molecules include cyclic nucleotides. These nucleotide second messengers modulate the activity of enzymes such as protein kinases, protein phosphatases, and rho-family guanosine triphosphatases (GTPases). In turn these messengers and enzymes regulate the activity of proteins that regulate the polymerization and depolymerization of actin filaments, thereby promoting or inhibiting axonal extension.

The critical role of intracellular signals in growth cone motility and orientation can be demonstrated using embryonic neurons grown in culture. Application of growth factors to one side of a growth cone activates receptors locally and leads to extension and turning of the growth cone toward the source of the signal. In essence, the factor attracts the growth cone. Yet when cyclic adenosine monophosphate (cAMP), levels in the neuron are decreased, the same stimulus acts as a repellent and the growth cone turns away from the signal (Figure 54–7). Other repulsive factors can become attractive when levels of the second messenger cyclic guanosine 3′-5′-monophosphate (cGMP) are raised.

Another strategy for coupling the sensory and motor functions of the growth cone is to engage the cytoskeleton directly, through the intracellular domain of receptors. Integrin receptors couple to actin in growth cones when they bind molecules associated with the surface of adjoining cells or the extracellular matrix, thereby influencing motility. Recently, it has been found that growth cones contain messenger RNAs as well as the machinery for protein synthesis. The activation of receptors can lead to local synthesis of new motor proteins precisely when and where they are needed. Thus the growth cone has many strategies

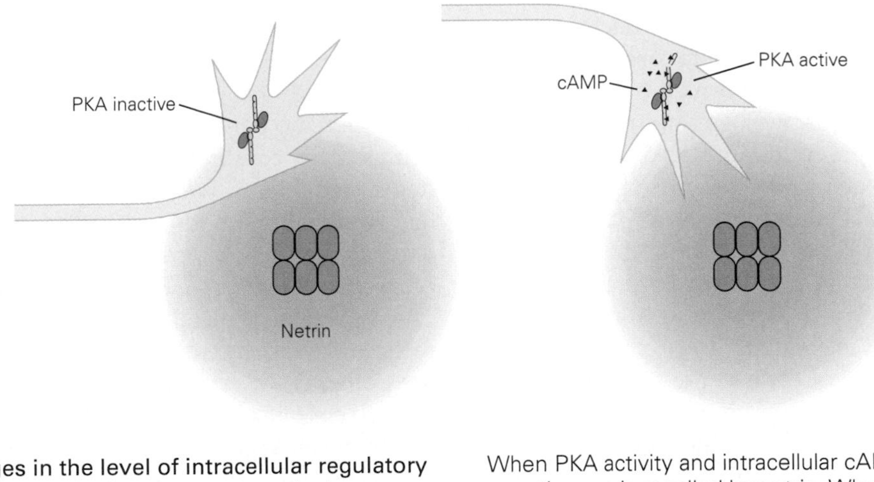

Figure 54–7 Changes in the level of intracellular regulatory proteins can determine whether the same extrinsic cue attracts or repels the growth cone. The state of protein kinase A (**PKA**) activity can alter the growth cone's response to an extracellular orienting factor, in this instance the protein netrin. When PKA activity and intracellular cAMP levels are low, the growth cone is repelled by netrin. When PKA activity is high, the resulting elevation in intracellular cAMP causes the growth cone to be attracted to a local source of netrin. (Adapted, with permission, from Ming et al. 1997.)

and mechanisms for integrating molecular signals to direct the axon in specific directions.

Molecular Cues Guide Axons to Their Targets

For much of the 20th century a debate raged between advocates of two very different views of how growth cones navigate embryonic terrains to reach their targets. A molecular view of axonal guidance was first articulated at the turn of the 20th century by the physiologist J. N. Langley. But by the 1930s many eminent biologists, including Paul Weiss, believed that axonal outgrowth was essentially random and that appropriate connections persisted largely because of productive, matching patterns of electrical activity in the axon and its target cell.

In our molecular age Weiss's ideas may seem simplistic but they were not unreasonable at the time. In tissue culture axons grow preferentially along mechanical discontinuities (scratches and bumps on a cover slip), and embryonic nerve trunks often align themselves with solid supports (blood vessels or cartilage). It seemed logical to Weiss that mechanical guidance, called *stereotropism,* could account for axonal patterning. We are quite comfortable today with the idea that electrical signals can be used to change the way current flows in a computer without the need to resolder connections. Likewise, patterns of activity and experience can strengthen or weaken neural connections without requiring the formation of new axonal pathways. Then why not consider that congruent activity, called *resonance* by Weiss, is involved in establishing appropriate connections?

Today few scientists believe that stereotaxis or resonance are crucial forces in neuronal connectivity. The tipping point that shifted opinion in favor of the molecular view was an experiment performed with frogs and other amphibia in the 1940s by Roger Sperry (ironically, a student of Weiss). Sperry manipulated the information carried from the eye to the brain by the axons of retinal ganglion cells. These axons terminate in their target areas—the lateral geniculate body in the thalamus and the superior colliculus (or optic tectum) in the midbrain—in such a way that an orderly retinotropic map of the visual field is created.

Because of the optics of the eye, the visual image on the retina is an inversion of the visual field. The retinal ganglion cells reinvert the image by the manner in which their axons terminate in the optic tectum, the main visual center in the brain of frogs (Figure 54–8A). If the optic nerve is cut the animal is blinded. In lower vertebrates cut retinal axons can reestablish projections to the tectum, whereupon vision is restored. This is not the case in mammals, as we will discuss in Chapter 57.

Sperry performed a simple yet profound experiment that demonstrated the organization of the retinotectal projection. He severed the optic nerve in a frog and then rotated the eye in its socket by 180 degrees before regeneration of the nerve. Remarkably, the frog exhibited orderly responses to visual input, but the behavior was wrong. When the frog was presented with a fly on the ground it jumped up, and when offered a fly above its head it struck downward (Figure 54–8B). Importantly, the animal never learned to correct its mistakes. Sperry suggested—and later verified with anatomical and physiological methods—that the retinal axons had reinnervated their original tectal targets, even though these connections provided the brain with erroneous spatial information that led to aberrant behavior. The inference of these experiments was that recognition between axons and their targets relied on molecular matching rather than functional validation and refinement of random connections.

But Weiss's ideas are by no means obsolete. Indeed, we now recognize that the activity of neural circuits can play a crucial role in shaping connectivity. The current view is that molecular matching predominates during embryonic development, and that activity and experience modify circuits after they have formed. In this chapter and the next we describe the molecular cues that guide the formation of neural connections, and then in Chapter 56 we examine the role of activity and experience in the fine-tuning of synaptic connections.

Sperry's conjecture, often called the *chemospecificity hypothesis,* prompted developmental neurobiologists to search for axonal and synaptic "recognition molecules." Success was limited for the first few decades, in part because these molecules are present in small amounts and on discrete subsets of neurons and there were no effective methods for isolating rare molecules from complex tissues. As with the search for neural inducers, advances in biochemical and molecular biological methods gradually made this task more feasible, and many proteins involved in the guidance of axons to their targets have now been discovered. These proteins typically consist of pairs of ligands and receptors: The ligands are presented by cells along the pathway an axon follows and the receptors by the growth cone itself.

In the most general terms, guidance cues can be presented on cell surfaces, in the extracellular matrix, or in soluble form. They act by either promoting or inhibiting outgrowth of the axon. Most receptors are embedded in

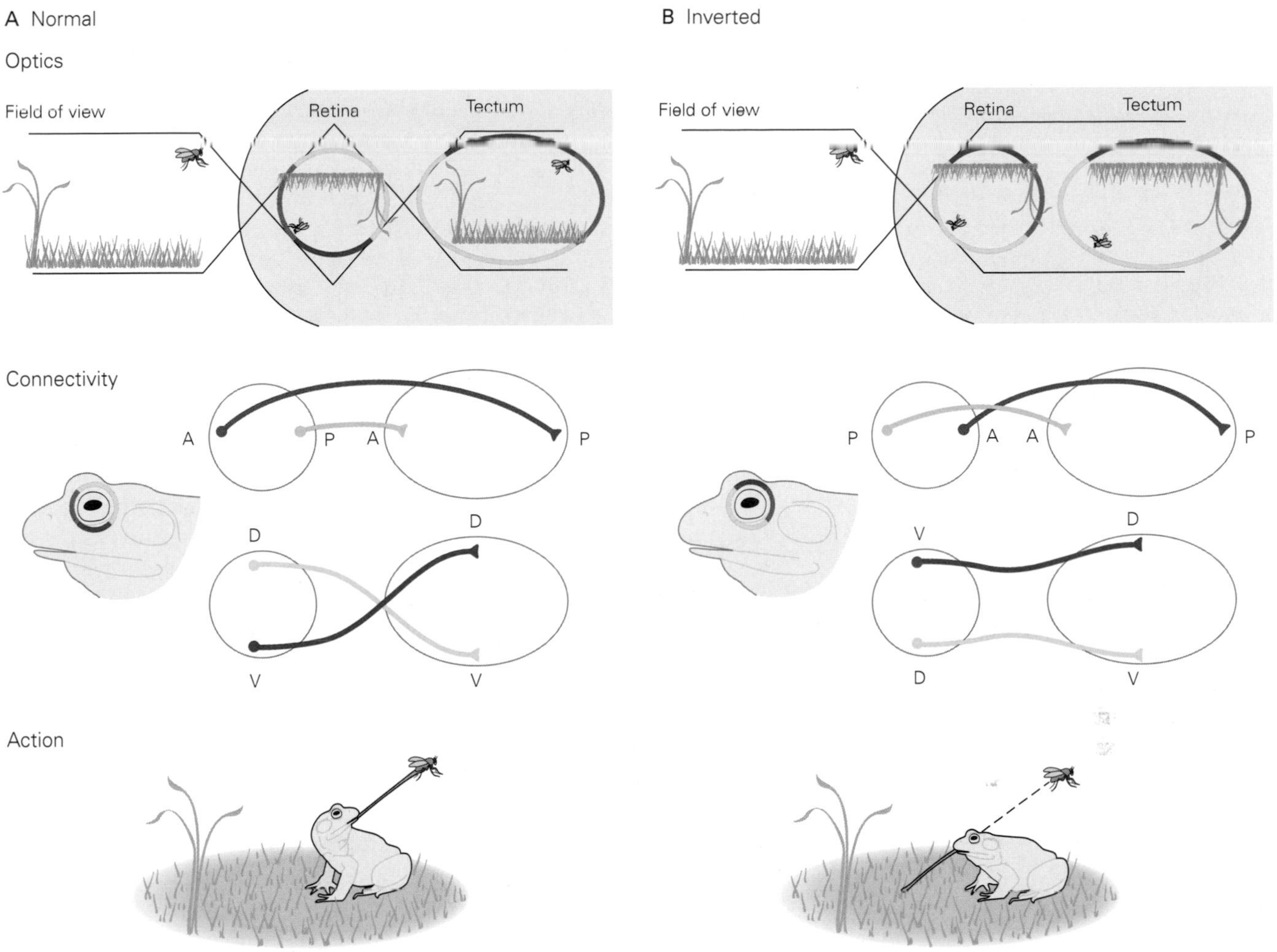

Figure 54–8 Roger Sperry's classical experiments on regeneration in the visual system provided evidence for chemoaffinity in the wiring of connections.

A. In the visual system of the frog the lens projects an inverted visual image onto the retina and the optic nerve then transfers the image, with an additional inversion, to the optic tectum. The orderly arrangement of inputs to the tectum is responsible for this transfer. Neurons in the anterior retina project axons to the posterior tectum, while neurons in the posterior retina project to the anterior tectum. Similarly, neurons in the dorsal retina project to the ventral tectum and neurons in the ventral retina project to the dorsal tectum. As a result, visually guided behaviors (here catching a fly) are accurate. (**A**, anterior; **D**, dorsal; **P**, posterior; **V**, ventral.)

B. If the optic nerve is cut, and the eye is surgically rotated in its socket before the nerve regenerates, visually guided behavior is aberrant. When a fly is presented overhead, the frog perceives it as below, and vice versa. The inversion of behavioral reflexes results from the connection of regenerating retinal axons to their original targets, even though these connections now transfer an inverted, inappropriate map of the world into the brain.

the growth cone membrane; they have an extracellular domain that selectively binds the cognate ligand and an intracellular domain that couples to the cytoskeleton, either directly or through intermediates such as second messengers. Activation of these receptors can promote or inhibit neurite outgrowth. A ligand presented to one side of the growth cone can result in turning. In this way the local distribution of environmental cues can steer the growth cone.

As a result of these recent discoveries, axon guidance—a process that appeared mysterious years ago—can now be viewed as the orderly consequence of protein-protein interactions that instruct the growth cone to grow, turn, and stop (Figures 54–9 and 54–10).

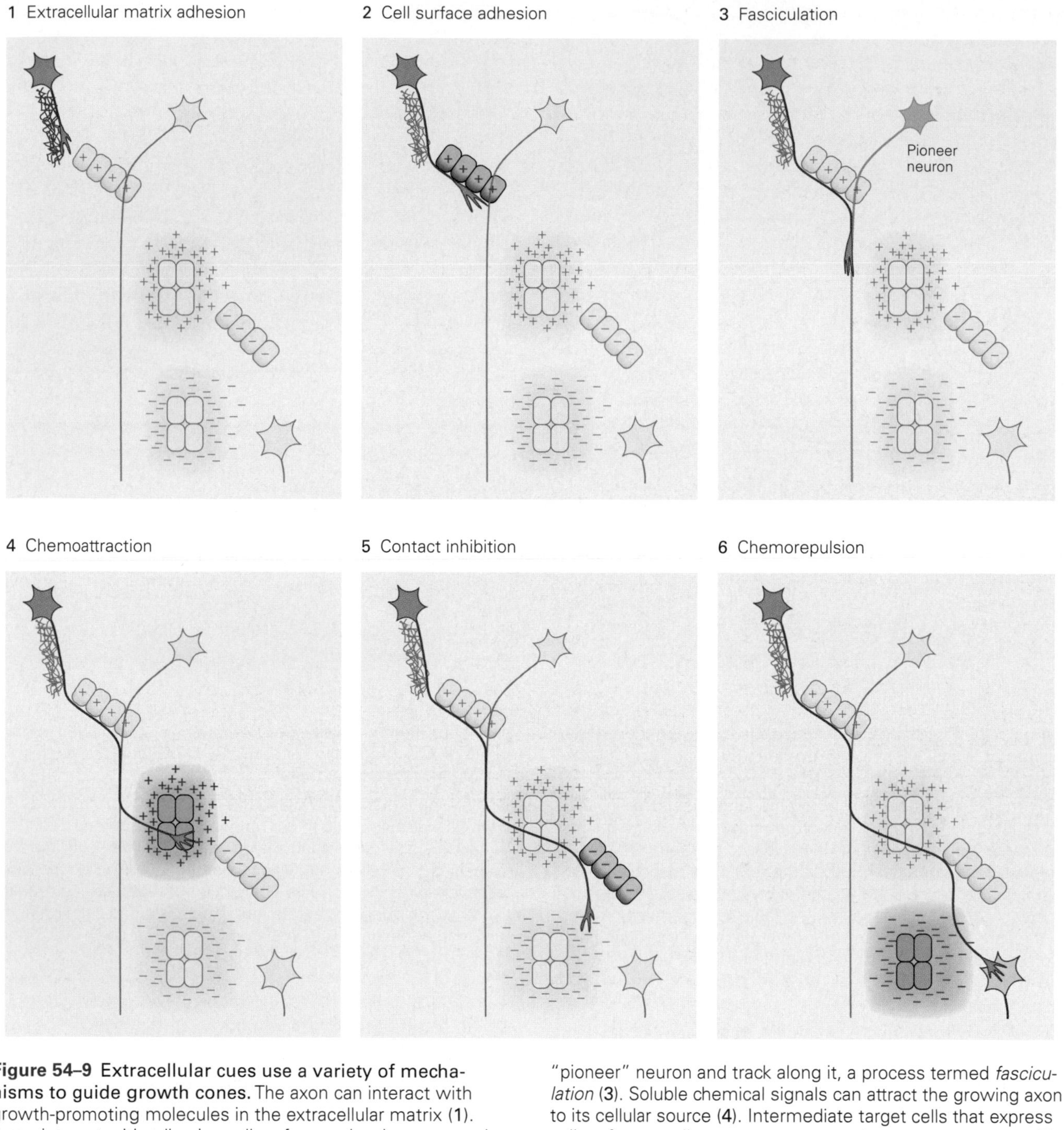

Figure 54–9 Extracellular cues use a variety of mechanisms to guide growth cones. The axon can interact with growth-promoting molecules in the extracellular matrix (**1**). It can interact with adhesive cell-surface molecules on neural cells (**2**). The growing axon can encounter another axon from a "pioneer" neuron and track along it, a process termed *fasciculation* (**3**). Soluble chemical signals can attract the growing axon to its cellular source (**4**). Intermediate target cells that express cell-surface repellent cues can cause the axon to turn away (**5**). Soluble chemical signals can repel the growing axon (**6**).

This limited set of instructions is sufficient, when presented with spatial precision, to choreograph growth cone behaviors with exquisite subtlety. Axonal guidance can therefore be explained by describing how and where ligands are presented and how the growth cone integrates this information to generate an orderly response. In the rest of the chapter we illustrate lessons learned by describing the journeys of two types of axons: the axons of retinal ganglion neurons and those of a particular class of sensory relay neurons in the spinal cord.

The Growth of Retinal Ganglion Axons Is Oriented in a Series of Discrete Steps

Sperry's experiment implied the existence of axon guidance cues but did not reveal where they were or how they worked. For a time, one prominent view was that recognition occurred mostly at or near the target and that mechanical forces or long-range chemotactic factors sufficed to get axons to the vicinity of the target.

We now know that axons reach distant targets in a series of discrete steps, making frequent decisions at closely spaced intervals along their route. To illustrate this point we shall trace in greater detail the path that Sperry was trying to understand, that of a retinal axon growing to the optic tectum.

Growth Cones Diverge at the Optic Chiasm

The first task of the axon of a retinal ganglion cell is to leave the retina. As it enters the optic fiber layer it extends along the basal lamina and glial end-feet positioned at the retina's edge. The growth of the axon is oriented from the outset, indicating that it can read directional cues in the environment. As it approaches the center of the retina it comes under the influence of attractants emanating from the optic nerve head (the junction of the optic nerve with the retina proper), which guide it into the optic stalk. It then follows the optic nerve toward the brain (Figure 54–11).

The first axons to travel this route follow the cells of the optic stalk, the rudiment of the neural tube that connects the retina to the diencephalon from which it arose. These "pioneer" axons then serve as scaffolds for later-arriving axons, which are able to extend accurately simply by following their predecessors (see strategy 3 in Figure 54–9). Once they reach the optic chiasm, however, the retinal axons must make a choice. Axons that arise from neurons in the nasal hemiretina of each eye cross the chiasm and proceed to the opposite side of the brain, whereas those from the temporal half are deflected as they reach the chiasm and so stay on the same side of the brain (Figure 54–12A).

This divergence in trajectory reflects the differential responses of axons from the nasal and temporal hemiretinas to guidance cues presented by midline chiasm cells. Some retinal axons contact and traverse chiasm cells, whereas others are inhibited by these cells and deflected away, thus remaining in the ipsilateral side. One of the key molecules presented by chiasm cells is a membrane-bound repellent of the ephrin-B family (Figure 54–12B), which also figures in later steps of retinal ganglion cell axon guidance.

The fraction of temporal retinal axons that project ipsilaterally varies among species: a few in lower vertebrates, some in rodents, and many in humans. These differences reflect placement of the eyes. In many animals the eyes point to the sides and monitor different parts of the visual world, so that information from the two eyes need not be combined. In humans both eyes look forward and sample largely overlapping regions of the visual world, so coordination of visual input is essential.

After crossing the optic chiasm, retinal axons assemble in the optic tract along the ventral surface of the diencephalon. Axons then leave the tract at different points. In most vertebrate species the tectum of the midbrain (called the superior colliculus in mammals) is the major target of retinal axons, but a small number of axons project to the lateral geniculate nucleus of the thalamus. In humans, however, most axons project to the lateral geniculate, a sizable number reach the colliculus, and small numbers project to the pulvinar, superchiasmatic nucleus, and pretectal nuclei. Within these targets different retinal axons project to different regions. As Sperry showed, the retinal axons form a precise retinotopic map on the tectal surface. Similar maps form in other areas innervated by retinal axons.

Having reached an appropriate position within the tectum, retinal axons need to find an appropriate synaptic partner. To achieve this last leg of their journey, retinal axons turn and dive into the tectal neuropil (Figure 54–11), descending along the surface of radial glial cells, which provide a scaffold for radial axonal growth. Although radial glial cells span the entire extent of the neuroepithelium, each retinal axon confines its synaptic terminals to a single layer. The dendrites of many postsynaptic cells extend through multiple layers and form synapses along their whole length, but retinal inputs are restricted to a small fraction of the target neuron's dendritic tree. These organizational features imply that layer-specific cues arrest axonal elongation and trigger arborization.

Axons therefore solve the problem of long-distance navigation by dividing their journey into short segments, and by recognizing and responding to

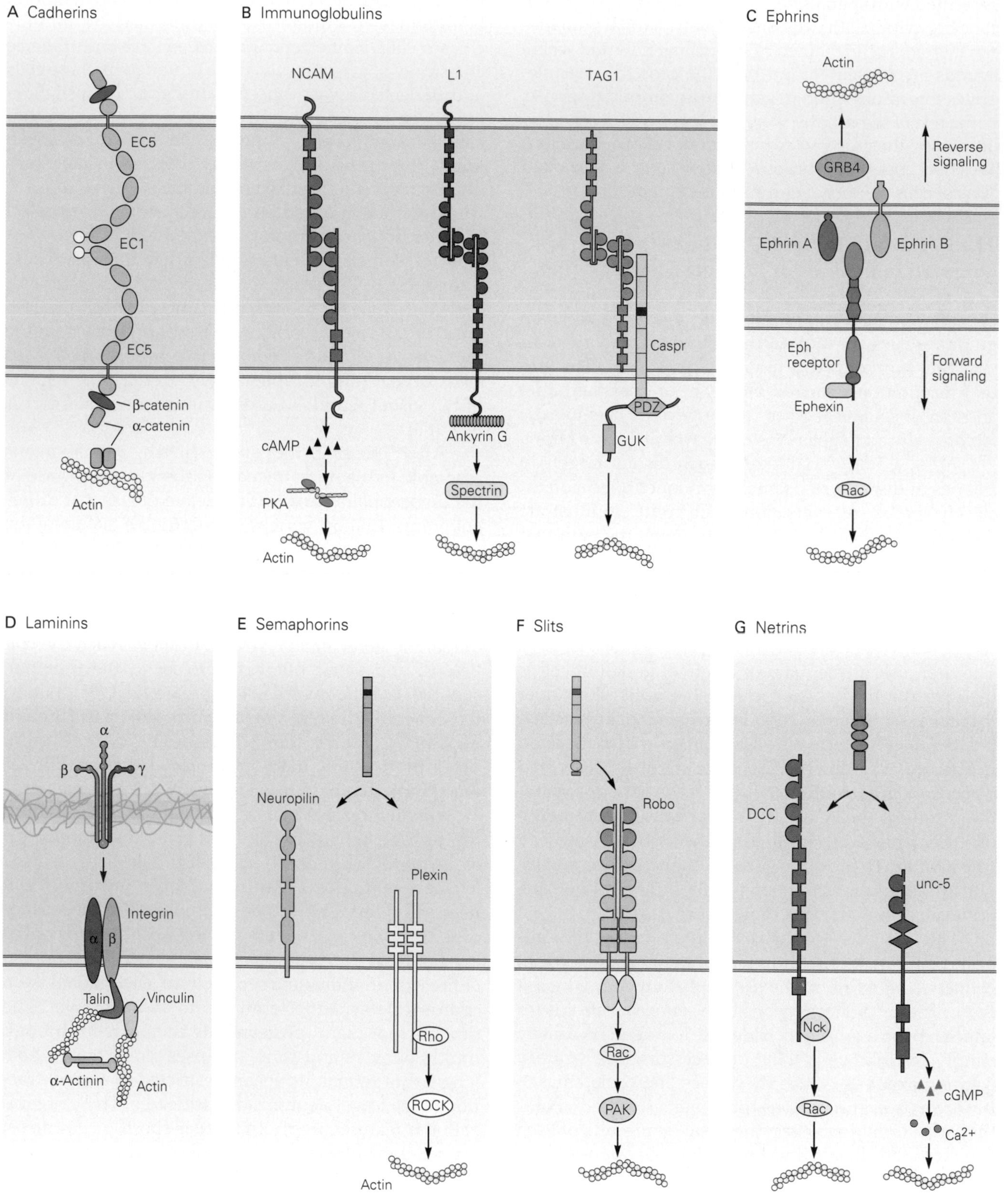
A Cadherins
EC5
EC1
EC5
β-catenin
α-catenin
Actin
B Immunoglobulins
NCAM
L1
TAG1
Caspr
PDZ
GUK
cAMP
PKA
Actin
Ankyrin G
Spectrin
C Ephrins
Actin
GRB4
Reverse signaling
Ephrin A
Ephrin B
Eph receptor
Forward signaling
Ephexin
Rac
D Laminins
α
β
γ
Integrin
α
β
Talin
Vinculin
α-Actinin
Actin
E Semaphorins
Neuropilin
Plexin
Rho
ROCK
Actin
F Slits
Robo
Rac
PAK
G Netrins
DCC
unc-5
Nck
Rac
cGMP
Ca2+

Figure 54–10 (Opposite) **Diverse molecular families control the growth and guidance of developing axons.**

A. A large family of classical cadherins promote cell and axonal adhesion, primarily through homophilic interactions between cadherin molecules on adjacent neurons. Adhesive interactions are mediated through interactions of the extracellular EC1 domains. Cadherins transduce adhesive interactions though their cytoplasmic interactions with catenins, which link cadherins to the actin cytoskeleton.

B. A diverse array of immunoglobulin superfamily proteins are expressed in the nervous system and mediate adhesive interactions. The three examples shown here, NCAM, L1, and TAG1, can bind both homophilically and heterophilically to promote axon outgrowth and adhesion. These proteins contain both immunoglobulin domains (**circles**) and fibronectin type III domains (**squares**). Homophilic interactions typically involve amino terminal immunoglobulin domains. Different Ig adhesion molecules interact with the cytoskeleton via diverse cytoplasmic mediators, only a few of which are shown here.

C. Different ephrin proteins bind to Eph class tyrosine kinase receptors. Class A ephrins are linked to the surface membrane through a glycosyl phosphatidylinositol tether, whereas class B ephrins are transmembrane proteins. Class A ephrins typically bind class A Eph kinases, and class B ephrins typically bind class B Eph kinases. Forward Eph signaling usually elicits repellant or inhibitory responses in receptive cells, whereas reverse ephrin signaling can elicit adhesive or inhibitory responses. Ephrin and Eph signaling involves many different cytoplasmic mediators.

D. Laminin proteins are bound to the extracellular matrix and promote cell adhesion and axon extension through interactions with integrin receptors. Integrins mediate adhesion and axon growth through interactions with the cytoskeleton via many intermediary proteins.

E. Semaphorin proteins can promote or inhibit axonal growth through interaction with a diverse array of plexin and neuropilin receptors, which transduce signals via rho class GTPases and downstream kinases.

F. Slit proteins typically mediate repellant responses through interaction with Robo class receptors, which influence axonal growth via intermediary GTPases such as Rac.

G. The secreted- or extracellular-matrix-associated netrin proteins mediate both chemoattractant and chemorepellent responses. Attractant responses are mediated through interaction with DCC (deleted in colorectal cancer) receptors, whereas repellent responses involve interactions with DCC and unc-5 co-receptors. Netrin receptors signal via GTPases and cGMP cascades.

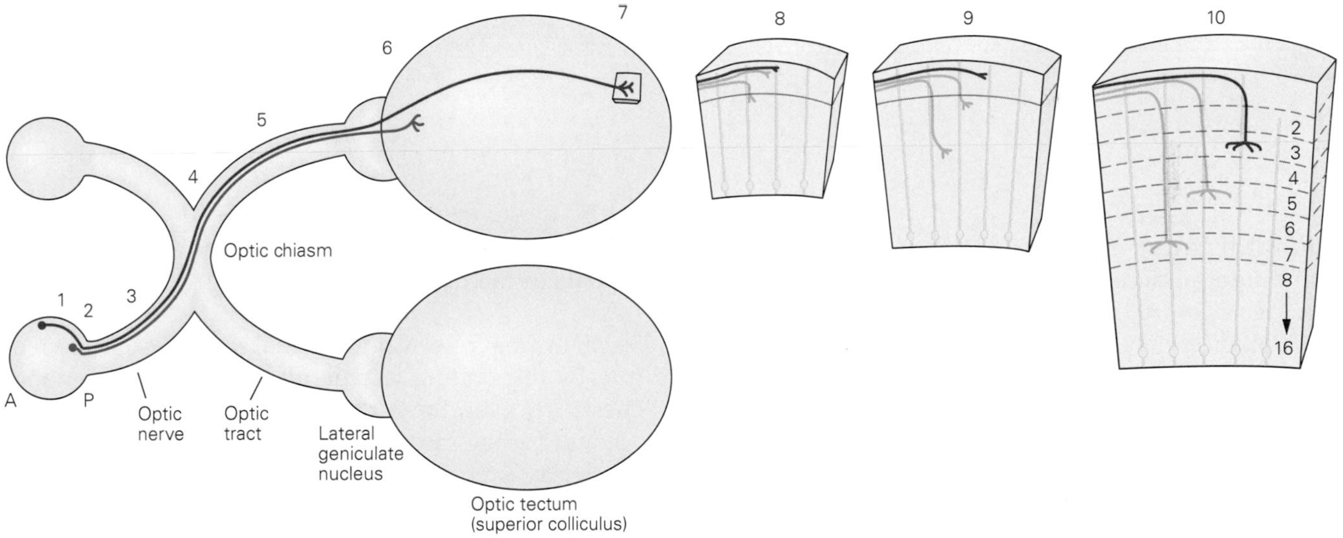

Figure 54–11 The axons of retinal ganglion cells grow to the optic tectum in discrete steps. Two neurons that carry information from the nasal half of the retina are shown. The axon of one crosses the optic chiasm to reach the contralateral optic tectum. The axon of the other also crosses the optic chiasm but projects to the lateral geniculate nucleus. The numbers indicate important landmarks on the axon's journey. The growing axon is directed toward the optic nerve head with the retina (**1**), enters into the optic nerve (**2**), extends through the optic nerve (**3**), swerves to remain ipsilateral (not shown) or cross to the contralateral side at the optic chiasm (**4**), extends through the optic tract (**5**), enters into the optic tectum or lateral geniculate nucleus (**6**), navigates to an appropriate rostrocaudal and dorsoventral position on the tectum (**7**), descends from the tectal surface (**8**), stops at an appropriate layer where a rudimentary terminal arbor is formed (**9**), and finally is refined (**10**).

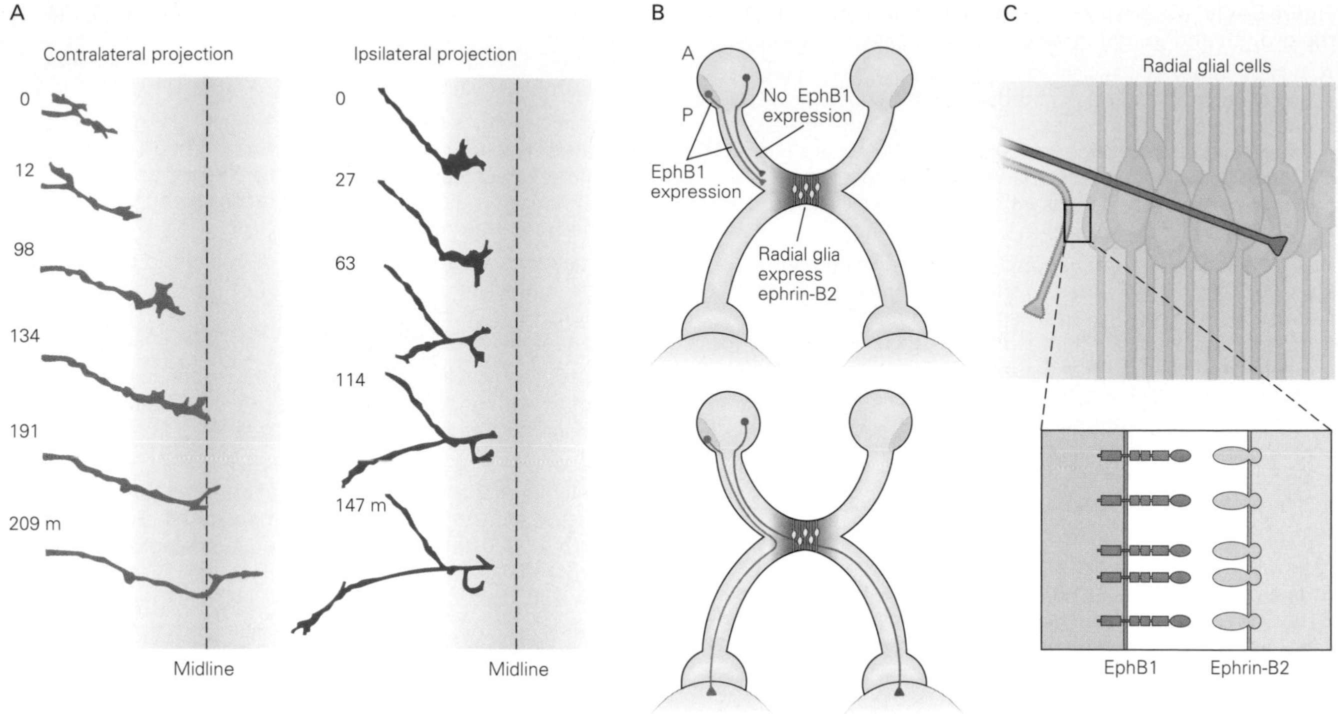

Figure 54–12 Axons of retinal ganglion neurons diverge as they reach the optic chiasm.

A. A time lapse series shows axons approaching the midline. Axons that arise from the nasal hemiretina cross the optic chiasm and project to the contralateral tectum (left). In contrast axons from the temporal hemiretina reach the chiasm but fail to cross and thus project toward the ipsilateral tectum (right). (Reproduced, with permission, from Godemont, Wong, and Mason 1994.)

B. The axons of temporal hemiretina neurons, which express the tyrosine kinase receptor EphB1, encounter ephrin-B2 expressed by midline radial glial cells at the optic chiasm and so are prevented from crossing the midline. The axons of nasal hemiretina neurons, which lack EphB1 receptors, are unaffected by the presence of ephrin-B2 and cross to the contralateral side. (**A**, anterior; **P**, posterior.)

C. Higher-power view illustrating the trajectories of retinal ganglion cell axons at the chiasm.

intermediate targets along the path to their final targets. Some intermediate targets, such as the optic chiasm, are "decision" regions where axons need to diverge.

Reliance on intermediate targets is an effective solution to the problem of long-distance axonal navigation but is not the only one. In some cases the first axons reach their targets when the embryo is small and the distance to be covered is short. These "pioneer" axons respond to molecular cues embedded in cells or the extracellular matrix along their way. The first axons to exit the retina fall within this class. Axons that appear later, when distances are longer and obstacles more numerous, can reach their targets by following the pioneers. Yet another guidance mechanism is a molecular gradient. Indeed, as we will see, gradients of cell-surface molecules in the tectum inform axons about their proper termination zone.

Ephrins Provide Gradients of Inhibitory Signals in the Brain

So far we have seen how retinal axons reach the tectum by responding to a series of discrete directional cues. However, these choices during growth do not account for the smoothly graded connections implied by Sperry's analysis of the retinotopic map in the tectum. The quest for the hypothetical "graded map molecules" became a major focus for developmental neurobiologists, and so we describe it in some detail.

A key breakthrough in the quest for these molecules came with the development of bioassays in which explants from defined portions of the retina were laid on substrates of tectal membrane fragments. The membrane fragments were taken from defined anteroposterior portions of the tectum and arranged in alternating stripes. Axons from the temporal (posterior) hemiretina were found to grow preferentially on membranes from anterior tectum, a preference similar to that exhibited in vivo (Figure 54–13). This preference was found to result from the presence of inhibitory factors in posterior membranes rather than from attractive or adhesive substances in anterior membranes. This observation was one of the first to emphasize the role of inhibitory or repellent substances in axon guidance.

This stripe assay permitted the characterization of an inhibitory cue, present in membranes from the posterior but not the anterior tectum. Independently, molecular biologists identified a family of receptor tyrosine kinases, the Eph kinases, and a large family of membrane-associated ligands, the ephrins. Both receptors and ligands are divided into A and B subfamilies. The ephrin-A proteins bind and activate EphA kinases; conversely, ephrin-B proteins bind and activate EphB kinases (Figure 54–14).

The two lines of research converged when the tectal inhibitory cue was identified as ephrin-A5. We now know that the Eph kinases and ephrins serve many functions in neural and nonneural tissues and that each class of proteins can serve as ligands or receptors, depending on cellular context. In the developing nervous system these proteins comprise a major group of repellent signals.

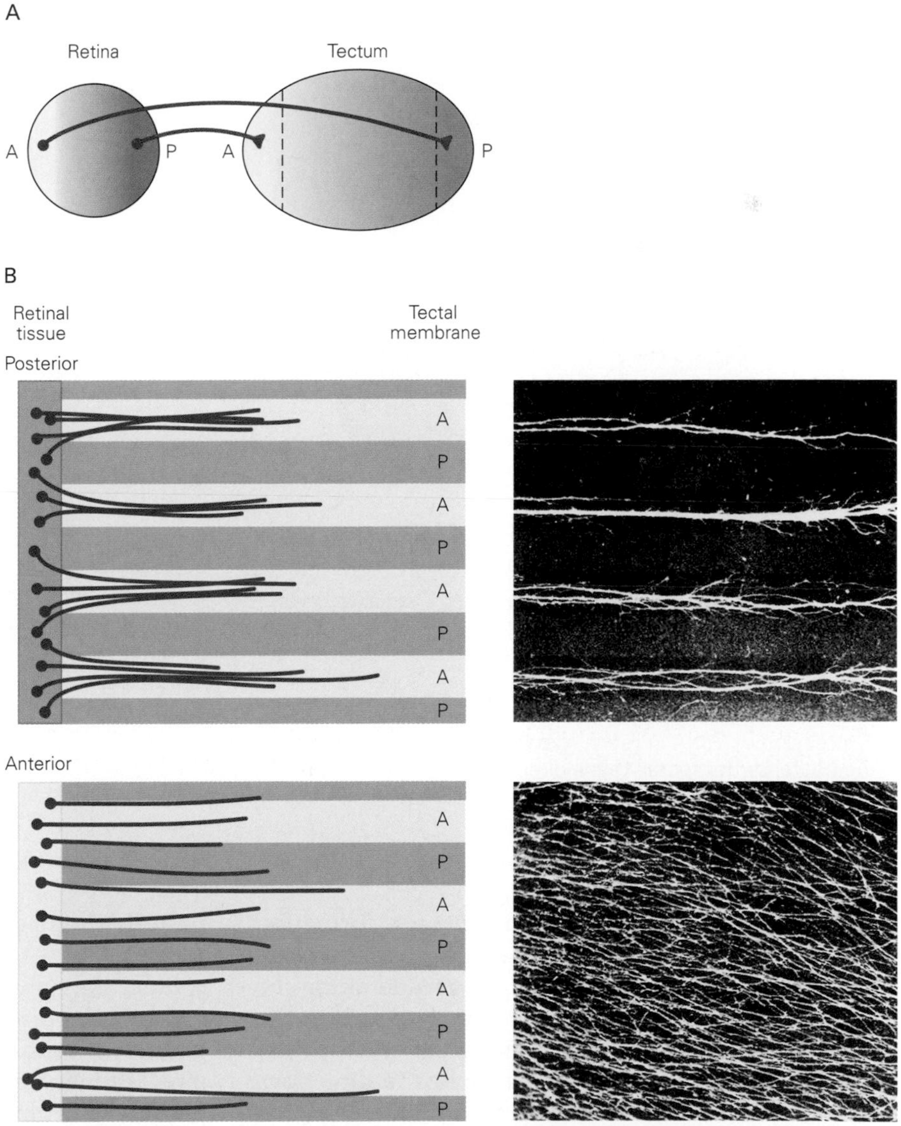

Figure 54–13 Repellant signals guide developing retinal axons in vitro.

A. Retinal ganglion axons from the posterior (temporal) hemiretina project into the anterior developing tectum. Conversely, axons from the anterior (nasal) hemiretina project into the posterior tectum.

B. Fragments of membrane were taken from specified anteroposterior portions of the tectum and arranged in alternating strips. Axons from explants of posterior retina grow selectively on the fragments from anterior tectum. The preferential growth of axons on anterior membrane results from an inhibitory cue in the posterior membrane. In contrast, axons from anterior retina grow on both anterior and posterior tectal membrane fragments. (**A**, anterior; **P**, posterior.) (Modified, with permission, from Walter, Henke-Fahle, and Bonhoeffer 1987.)

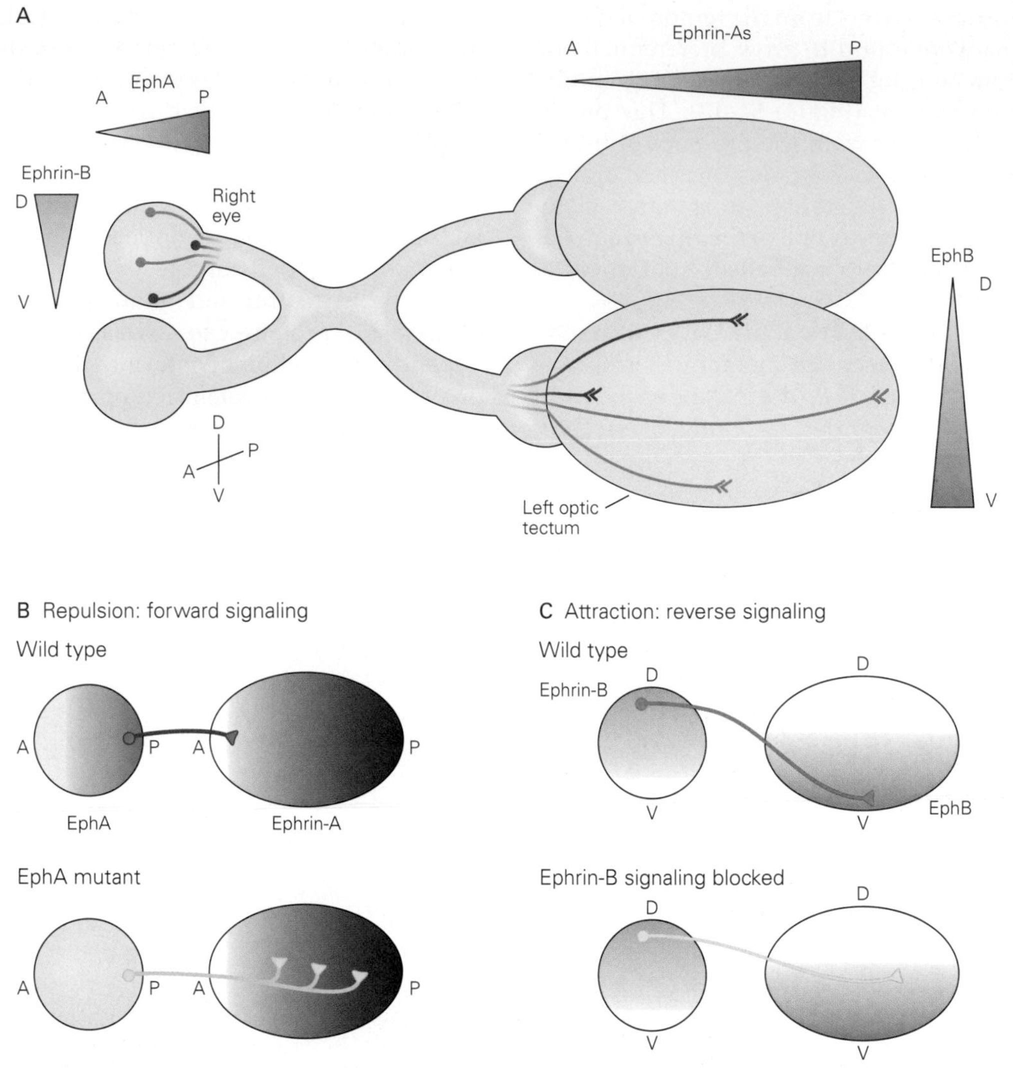

Figure 54–14 The formation of retinotopic maps in vivo depends on ephrin-Eph kinase signaling.

A. In the retina EphA receptors are expressed in an anteroposterior (A-P) gradient, and ephrin-B is expressed in a dorsoventral (D-V) gradient. In the tectum ephrin-A receptors are distributed in an anteroposterior gradient and EphB in a dorsoventral gradient.

B. Expression of EphA in retinal axons that derive from neurons in the posterior (temporal) retina directs axon growth to the anterior tectum through avoidance of ephrin-A proteins. In EphA mutant mice posterior retinal axons are able to project to a more posterior domain within the tectum.

C. EphB signaling directs the projection of dorsal retinal axons to the ventral tectum. Blocking ephrin-B signaling with soluble EphB protein causes dorsal axons to project to an abnormally dorsal domain within the tectum.

Ephrin-Eph interactions account for formation of the retinotopic map in the tectum. In the tectum ephrin-A2 and ephrin-A5 levels are graded along the anteroposterior axis, and in the retina the levels of the Eph receptors are also graded along the anteroposterior axis. These gradients run in opposite directions in the tectum: ephrin-A grades from anterior-low to posterior-high and in the retina Eph-A kinase from posterior-high to anterior-low (Figure 54–14A). Such counter-gradients account, at least in part, for topographic mapping. Axons from posterior retinal ganglion cells with high levels of receptors are repelled most strongly by the high level of ephrin-A in the posterior tectum and thus are confined to the anterior tectum. The less sensitive axons from the anterior retina are able to penetrate further into the posterior domain of the tectum. Ephrin-A2 and -A5 are therefore strong candidates for chemospecificity factors of the type postulated by Sperry.

The crucial role of ephrins and Eph kinases in the formation of retinotopic maps has been confirmed in vivo. Overexpression of ephrin-A2 in the developing optic tectum of chick embryos generates small patches of cells in the rostral tectum that are abnormally rich in ephrin-A2. Temporal retinal axons, which normally avoid the ephrin-rich caudal tectum, also avoid these patches in the rostral tectum, and they terminate in abnormal positions. In contrast, nasal retinal axons, which normally grow toward the caudal tectum, are not perturbed by encounters with excess ephrin.

Conversely, in mice with targeted mutations in the *ephrin-A2* and *ephrin-A5* genes some posterior retinal axons terminate in inappropriately posterior tectal regions (Figure 54–14B). Anterior retinal axons, which naturally express low levels of EphA proteins, project normally in these mutants. In mice lacking both ephrin-A proteins these deficits are more severe than with either single mutant. Thus the interaction of ephrin-A with EphA receptors is crucial for the targeting of retinal axons in the tectum. These ephrin/EphA pairs possess the properties of the recognition molecules that Sperry predicted were necessary to direct topographic mapping along the anteroposterior axis of the tectum.

But the retinal map is two-dimensional, so what establishes order along the dorsoventral axis? The ephrin/EphB pairs are involved in establishing this axis. Just as ephrin-A and EphA are graded along the anteroposterior axis, ephrin-B and EphB are graded along the dorsoventral axis, and genetic manipulation of ephrin-B and EphB levels affects dorsoventral mapping (Figure 54–14C). Thus the retinotopic map is arranged along rectangular coordinates with ephrin/EphA and ephrin/EphB labeling the anteroposterior and dorsoventral axes, respectively.

This simple view is satisfying, but the reality is more complex. First, Eph kinases are expressed in the tectum as well as in the retina, and ephrins are expressed in the retina as well as in the tectum. Thus, so-called "cis" interactions (Eph and ephrin on the same cell) as well as "trans" interactions (Eph on growth cone, ephrin on target cell) may be involved. Second, both ligands and receptors are present at multiple points along the optic pathway and play multiple roles. As we have seen, ephrin/EphB interactions affect not only dorsoventral mapping but also the decision of an axon to cross to the contralateral side at the optic chiasm. Finally, in visual circuits precise axonal mapping is regulated by patterns of neural activity, as discussed in the next two chapters. Nonetheless, we now have the initial outline of a molecular strategy for the formation of specific topographic projections from the eye to the brain.

Axons from Some Spinal Neurons Cross the Midline

One of the fundamental features of the central nervous system is the need to coordinate activity on both sides of the body. To accomplish this task certain axons need to project to the opposite side.

We have seen one example of axonal crossing in the optic chiasm. Another example that has been studied in detail is the axonal crossing of *commissural neurons* that convey sensory information from the spinal cord to the brain at the ventral midline of the spinal cord across the floor plate. After crossing, axons turn abruptly and grow up toward the brain. This simple trajectory raises several questions. How do these axons reach the ventral midline? On arrival how do they cross the midline? After crossing how do they *ignore* cues that axons on the other side are using to get to the midline? In other words, why do they turn toward the brain instead of crossing back?

Netrins Direct Developing Commissural Axons Across the Midline

Many of the neurons that send axons across the ventral midline are generated in the dorsal half of the spinal cord. The first task for these axons is to reach the ventral midline. Ramón y Cajal considered the possibility that chemotactic factors emitted by targets could attract axons, but this idea lay dormant for nearly a century. We now know that such chemotropic factors do exist and one of them, the protein netrin-1, mediates the chemoattractant activity of the floor plate. When presented in culture, netrin attracts commissural axons; when mice are deprived of netrin-1 function, axons fail to reach the floor plate (Figure 54–15).

The netrin protein is structurally related to the protein product of *unc-6,* a gene shown to regulate axon guidance in the nematode *C. elegans.* Two other *C. elegans* genes, *unc-5* and *unc-40,* encode receptors for the unc-6 protein. Vertebrate netrin receptors are related to the unc-5 and unc-40 receptors: The unc-5H proteins are homologs of unc-5, and DCC (deleted in colorectal cancer) and neurogenin are related to unc-40 (see Figure 54–10G). These receptors are members of the immunoglobulin superfamily, and their functions have

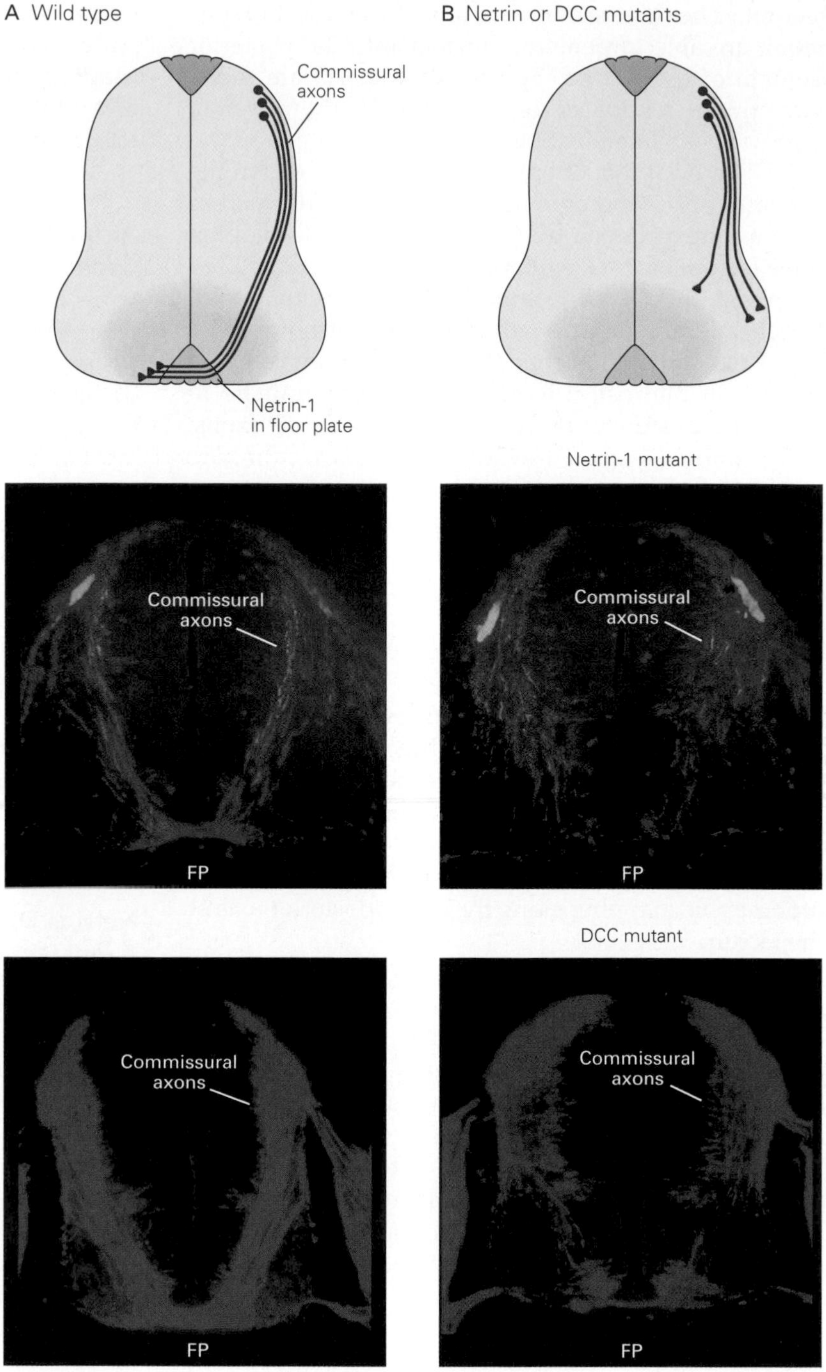

Figure 54–15 Netrin signaling attracts the axons of spinal commissural neurons to the floor plate. (Micrographs reproduced, with permission, from Marc Tessier-Lavigne.)

A. Netrin-1 is secreted by floor plate cells and attracts the axons of commissural neurons to the floor plate (**FP**) at the ventral midline of the spinal cord.

B. Most commissural axons fail to reach and cross the floor plate when netrin or DCC proteins are eliminated.

been remarkably conserved throughout animal evolution (Figure 54–16). This conservation supports the use of simple and genetically accessible invertebrates to unravel developmental complexities. In no area has this approach been more fruitful than in the analysis of axon guidance. Dozens of genes that affect this process were first identified and cloned in *Drosophila* and *C. elegans* and then shown to play important and related roles in mammals.

Other signaling systems work with netrins to guide commissural axons on this initial phase of their journey to the brain. For example, bone morphogenetic proteins secreted by the roof plate act as repellants and begin to direct commissural axons ventrally.

Chemoattractant and Chemorepellent Factors Pattern the Midline

Once commissural axons reach the midline, they find themselves exposed to the highest available level of netrin-1. Yet this netrin-rich environment does not keep the axons at the midline indefinitely. Instead they cross to the other side of the spinal cord, while at the same time their contralateral counterparts are navigating up the netrin chemoattractant gradient.

This puzzling behavior is explained by the fact that growth cones change their responsiveness to attractive and repellent signals as a consequence of exposure to floor plate signals. This switch illustrates an important property of intermediate targets involved in axon guidance. Factors presented by intermediate targets not only influence the growth of axons but also change the sensitivity of the growth cone, preparing it for the next leg of its journey.

Once axons arrive at the floor plate, they become sensitive to the chemorepellent signal slit, which is secreted by floor plate cells (Figure 54–17). Before commissural axons reach the floor plate the robo proteins that serve as slit receptors are kept inactive by expression of a related protein, rig-1. As axons reach the floor plate rig-1 is lost, unleashing robo activity and causing axons to respond to the repellant actions of slit. This repellant action propels growth cones *down* the slit gradient into the contralateral side of the spinal cord. In addition, activated robo forms a complex with DCC, which renders these netrin receptors incapable of responding to their ligand. The decreased sensitivity of growth cones to the attractive properties of the floor plate helps to account for the transient nature of the floor plate's influence on axons.

Finally, once axons have left the floor plate they turn rostrally toward their eventual synaptic targets in the brain. A rostrocaudal gradient of Wnt proteins expressed by floor plate cells appears to direct axon growth rostrally at the ventral midline (Figure 54–17D). Thus different cues guide commissural axons during distinct phases of their overall trajectory. This same process is presumably played out for hundreds and even thousands of classes of neurons to establish the mature pattern of brain wiring.

An Overall View

Many developmental processes shape precise patterns of connections in the nervous system, but none is more important than the guidance of axons from their origin to appropriate targets. The specificity required to achieve the correct wiring is extraordinary. Axons need to grow long distances, bypassing numerous targets along the way, before reaching and forming connections with appropriate synaptic partners.

The nervous system has devised elaborate mechanisms to achieve its basic wiring plan. At the cellular level one basic strategy is to break the long journey into manageable legs. Thus axons do not set off like explorers of old, crossing completely uncharted territory in search of distant goals. Instead, they receive guidance

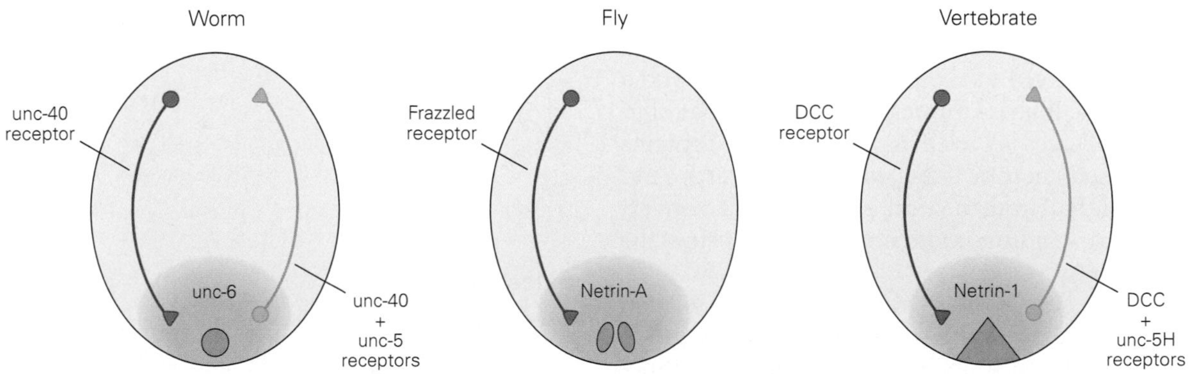

Figure 54–16 The expression and activity of netrins have been conserved throughout evolution. Netrins are secreted by ventral midline cells in worms, flies, and vertebrates and interact with receptors on cells or axons that migrate or extend along the dorsoventral axis. The netrin receptors unc-40 (worm), frazzled (fly), and deleted in colorectal cancer (DCC) (vertebrate) mediate netrin's attractant activity, whereas unc-5 class receptors mediate its repellent activity.

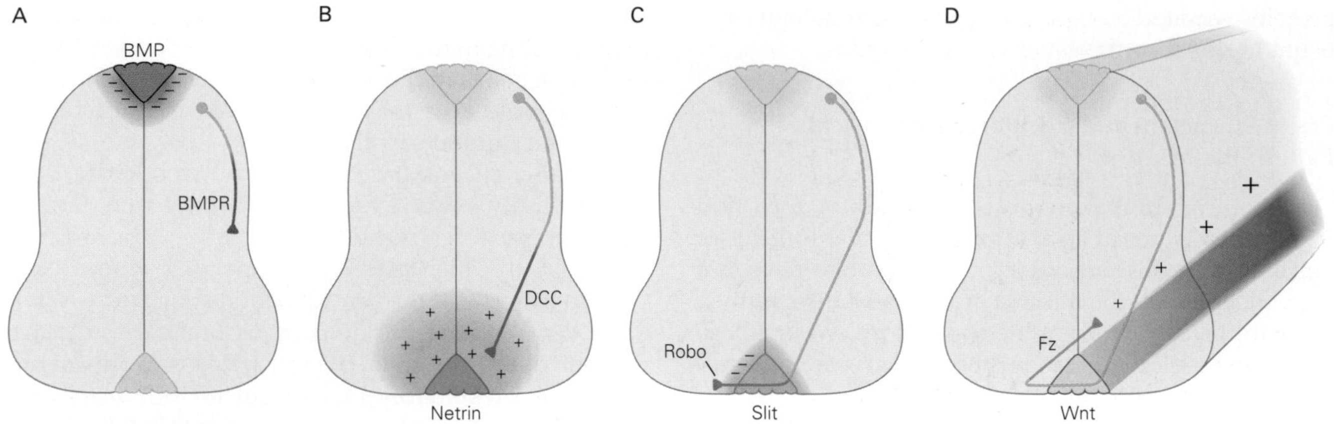
A
BMP
BMPR
BMP signaling directs axons ventrally, away from the roof plate.
B
DCC
Netrin
Netrin-DCC signaling attracts axons to the floor plate.
C
Robo
Slit
Slit interacts with Robo receptors on axons to prevent midline recrossing.
D
Fz
Wnt
Axons turn and travel rostrally, guided by Wnts.

Figure 54–17 Guidance cues expressed by roof plate and floor plate cells guide commissural axons in the developing spinal cord.

A. Bone morphogenetic proteins (**BMP**) secreted by roof plate cells interact with BMP receptors on commissural axons to direct the axons away from the roof plate.

B. Netrin expressed by floor plate cells attracts commissural axons to the ventral midline of the spinal cord. Sonic hedgehog has also been implicated in the ventral guidance of commissural axons.

C. Slit proteins secreted by floor plate cells interact with robo receptors on commissural axons to prevent these axons from recrossing the midline. Prior to crossing, but not after, commissural axons express robo3 (rig-1) in addition to robo1 and robo2. The rig-1 protein inactivates the robo receptors, preventing the axons from responding to the repellant effects of slits as they approach the ventral midline.

D. Wnt proteins secreted from floor plate cells and distributed in a rostrocaudal gradient interact with frizzled (**Fz**) proteins on commissural axons after midline crossing, guiding them toward the brain.

at intervals along the way. Some axons that grow early in the embryo, when distances are short, serve as scaffolds for later-growing axons. Other axons grow along epithelial surfaces or extracellular matrices. Often so-called guidepost cells or intermediate targets mark sites at which axons need to make divergent choices.

The axon receives and responds to these guidance clues with a specialized terminal apparatus, the growth cone. The growth cone is both a sensory and a motor structure. It bears numerous receptors that bind environmental cues as well as cytoskeletal proteins and actin-based motors that propel it forward. And it contains signal transduction systems that convert ligand-receptor binding into instructions that steer the growth cone.

In the past several years rapid progress has been made in the identification of molecules that guide axons. Guidance cues include soluble, membrane-bound, and extracellular matrix molecules. Many of the soluble molecules are members of gene families, such as the ephrins, netrins, slits, semaphorins, and laminins. Families of membrane-bound receptors on the growth cones include adhesion molecules, Eph kinases, neuropilins, plexins, robos, and integrins. Mutations in genes that encode these ligands and receptors can result in developmental neurological disorders.

Joshua R. Sanes
Thomas M. Jessell

Selected Readings

Barnes AP, Polleux F. 2009. Establishment of axon-dendrite polarity in developing neurons. Annu Rev Neurosci 32:347–381.

Black DL, Zipursky SL. 2008. To cross or not to cross: alternatively spliced forms of the Rob03 receptor regulate discrete steps in axonal midline crossing. Neuron 58: 297–298.

Dent EW, Gertler FB. 2003. Cytoskeletal dynamics and transport in growth cone motility and axon guidance. Neuron 40:209–227.

Egea J, Klein R. 2007. Bidirectional Eph-ephrin signaling during axon guidance. Trends Cell Biol 17:230–238.

Evans TA, Bashaw GJ. 2010. Axon guidance at the midline: of mice and flies. Curr Opin Neurobiol 20:79–85.

Lin AC, Holt CE. 2007. Local translation and directional steering in axons. EMBO J 26:3729–3736.

Lowery LA, Van Vactor D. 2009. The trip of the tip: understanding the growth cone machinery. Nat Rev Mol Cell Biol 10:332–343.

O'Donnell M, Chance RK, Bashaw GJ. 2009. Axon growth and guidance: receptor regulation and signal transduction. Annu Rev Neurosci 32:383–412.

Pak CW, Flynn KC, Bamburg JR. 2008. Actin-binding proteins take the reins in growth cones. Nat Rev Neurosci 9:136–147.

Petros TJ, Rebsam A, Mason CA. 2008. Retinal axon growth at the optic chiasm: to cross or not to cross. Annu Rev Neurosci 31:295–315.

Round J, Stein E. 2007. Netrin signaling leading to directed growth cone steering. Curr Opin Neurobiol 17:15–21.

Sánchez-Camacho C, Bovolenta P. 2009. Emerging mechanisms in morphogen-mediated axon guidance. Bioessays 31:1013–1025.

Schmid RS, Maness PF. 2008. L1 and NCAM adhesion molecules as signaling coreceptors in neuronal migration and process outgrowth. Curr Opin Neurobiol 18:245–250.

Tojima T, Hines JH, Henley JR, Kamiguchi H. 2011. Second messengers and membrane trafficking direct and organize growth cone steering. Nat Rev Neurosci 12: 191–203.

Zheng JQ, Poo MM. 2007. Calcium signaling in neuronal motility. Annu Rev Cell Dev Biol 23:375–404.

References

Barnes AP, Lilley BN, Pan YA, Plummer LJ, Powell AW, Raines AN, Sanes JR, Polleux F. 2007. LKB1 and SAD kinases define a pathway required for the polarization of cortical neurons. Cell 129:549–563.

Barnes AP, Polleux F. 2009. Establishment of axon-dendrite polarity in developing neurons. Annu Rev Neurosci 32:347–381.

Bridgman PC, Dailey ME. 1989. The organization of myosin and actin in rapid frozen nerve growth cones. J Cell Biol 108:95–109.

Dickson BJ, Gilestro GF. 2006. Regulation of commissural axon pathfinding by slit and its robo receptors. Annu Rev Cell Dev Biol 22:651–675.

Erskine L, Herrera E. 2007. The retinal ganglion cell axon's journey: insights into molecular mechanisms of axon guidance. Dev Biol 308:1–14.

Fazeli A, Dickinson SL, Hermiston ML, Tighe RV, Steen RG, Small CG, Stoeckli ET, et al. 1997. Phenotype of mice lacking functional Deleted in colorectal cancer (Dcc) gene. Nature 386:796–804.

Forscher P, Smith SJ. 1988. Actions of cytochalasins on the organization of actin filaments and microtubules in a neuronal growth cone. J Cell Biol 107:1505–1516.

Frisen J, Yates PA, McLaughlin T, Friedman GC, O'Leary DD, Barbacid M. 1998. Ephrin-A5 (AL-1/RAGS) is essential for proper retinal axon guidance and topographic mapping in the mammalian visual system. Neuron 20: 235–243.

Godement P, Wang LC, Mason CA. 1994. Retinal axon divergence in the optic chiasm: dynamics of growth cone behavior at the midline. J Neurosci 14:7024–7039.

Grueber WB, Jan LY, Jan YN. 2003. Different levels of the homeodomain protein cut regulate distinct dendrite branching patterns of Drosophila multidendritic neurons. Cell 112:805–818.

Harada T, Harada C, Parada LF. 2007. Molecular regulation of visual system development: more than meets the eye. Gene Dev 21:367–378.

Harrison RG. 1959. The outgrowth of the nerve fiber as a mode of protoplasmic movement. J Exp Zool 142:5–73.

Hattori D, Millard SS, Wojtowicz WM, Zipursky SL. 2008. Dscam-mediated cell recognition regulates neural circuit formation. Annu Rev Cell Dev Biol 24:597–620.

Heidemann SR. 1996. Cytoplasmic mechanisms of axonal and dendritic growth in neurons. Int Rev Cytol 165: 235–296.

Henley J, Poo MM. 2004. Guiding neuronal growth cones using Ca^{2+} signals. Trends Cell Biol 14:320–330.

Jan YN, Jan LY. 2010. Branching out: mechanisms of dendritic arborization. Nat Rev Neurosci 11:316–28.

Kaech S, Banker G. 2006. Culturing hippocampal neurons. Nat Protoc 1:2406–2415.

Kapfhammer JP, Grunewald BE, Raper JA. 1986. The selective inhibition of growth cone extension by specific neurites in culture. J Neurosci 6:2527–2534.

Keino-Masu K, Hinck L, Leonardo ED, Chan SS, Culotti JG, Tessier-Lavigne M. 1996. Deleted in colorectal cancer (DCC) encodes a netrin receptor. Cell 87:75–85.

Kidd T, Brose K, Mitchell KJ, Fetter RD, Tessier-Lavigne M, Goodman CS, Tear G. 1998. Roundabout controls axon crossing of the CNS midline and defines a novel subfamily of evolutionarily conserved guidance receptors. Cell 92:205–215.

Kishi M, Pan YA, Crump JG, Sanes JR. 2005. Mammalian SAD kinases are required for neuronal polarization. Science 307:929–932.

Kolodkin AL, Levengood DV, Rowe EG, Tai YT, Giger RJ, Ginty DD. 1997. Neuropilin is a semaphorin III receptor. Cell 90:753–762.

Letourneau PC. 1979. Cell-substratum adhesion of neurite growth cones, and its role in neurite elongation. Exp Cell Res 124:127–138.

Letourneau PC. 1996 The cytoskeleton in nerve growth cone motility and axonal pathfinding. Perspect Dev Neurobiol 4:111–123.

Loschinger J, Weth F, Bonhoeffer F. 2000. Reading of concentration gradients by axonal growth cones. Philos Trans R Soc Lond B Biol Sci 355:971–982.

Lumsden AG, Davies AM. 1983. Earliest sensory nerve fibres are guided to peripheral targets by attractants other than nerve growth factor. Nature 306:786–788.

Luo L, Flanagan JG. 2007. Development of continuous and discrete neural maps. Neuron 56:284–300.

McLaughlin T, O'Leary DD. 2005. Molecular gradients and development of retinotopic maps. Annu Rev Neurosci 28:327–355.

Ming GL, Song HJ, Berninger B, Holt CE, Tessier-Lavigne M, Poo MM. 1997. cAMP-dependent growth cone guidance by netrin-1. Neuron 19:1225–1235.

Polleux F, Morrow T, Ghosh A. 2000. Semaphorin 3A is a chemoattractant for cortical apical dendrites. Nature 404: 567–573.

Schmitt AM, Shi J, Wolf AM, Lu CC, King LA, Zou Y. 2006. Wnt-Ryk signalling mediates medial-lateral retinotectal topographic mapping. Nature 439:31–37.

Serafini T, Colamarino SA, Leonardo ED, Wang H, Beddington R, Skarnes WC, Tessier-Lavigne M. 1996. Netrin-1 is required for commissural axon guidance in the developing vertebrate nervous system. Cell 87:1001–1014.

Serafini T, Kennedy TE, Galko MJ, Mirzayan C, Jessell TM, Tessier-Lavigne M. 1994. The netrins define a family of axon outgrowth-promoting proteins homologous to C. elegans UNC-6. Cell 78:409–424.

Shelly M, Cancedda L, Heilshorn S, Sumbre G, Poo MM. 2007. LKB1/STRAD promotes axon initiation during neuronal polarization. Cell 129:565–577.

Sperry RW. 1943. Visuomotor coordination in the newt (*Triturus viridescens*) after regeneration of the optic nerve. J Compar Neurol 79:33–55.

Sperry RW. 1945. Restoration of vision after crossing of optic nerves and after contralateral transplantation of eye. J Neurophysiol 8:17–28.

Tada T, Sheng M. 2006. Molecular mechanisms of dendritic spine morphogenesis. Curr Opin Neurobiol 16:5–101.

Tessier-Lavigne M. 2002. Wiring the brain: the logic and molecular mechanisms of axon guidance and regeneration. Harvey Lect 98:103–143.

Walter J, Henke-Fahle S, Bonhoeffer F. 1987. Avoidance of posterior tectal membranes by temporal retinal axons. Development 101:909–913.

Weiss P. 1941. Nerve patterns: the mechanics of nerve growth. Growth 5:163–203. Suppl.

Zou Y, Lyuksyutova AI. 2007. Morphogens as conserved axon guidance cues. Curr Opin Neurobiol 17:22–28.

55

Formation and Elimination of Synapses

So far we have examined three stages in the development of the mammalian nervous system: the formation and patterning of the neural tube, the birth and differentiation of neurons and glial cells, and the growth and guidance of axons. One additional step must occur before the brain becomes functional: the formation of synapses. Only when synapses are formed and functional can the brain go about the business of processing information.

Three key processes drive synapse formation. First, axons make choices among many potential postsynaptic partners. By forming synaptic connections only on particular target cells, neurons assemble functional circuits that can process information. Usually synapses must be formed at specific sites on the postsynaptic cell; some axons form synapses on dendrites, others on cell bodies, and yet others on axons or nerve terminals. Cellular and subcellular specificity are evident throughout the brain, but we will illustrate the general features of synapse formation with a few well-studied classes of neurons.

Second, after cell-cell contacts have formed, the portion of the axon that contacts the target cell differentiates into a presynaptic nerve terminal, and the domain of the target cell contacted by the axon differentiates into a specialized postsynaptic apparatus. Precise coordination of pre- and postsynaptic differentiation depends on interactions between the axon and its target cell. Much of what we know about these interactions comes from studies of the neuromuscular junction, the synapse between motor neurons and skeletal muscle fibers. The simplicity of this synapse made it a favorable system to probe the structural and electrophysiological principles of chemical synapses, and this simplicity has also helped in the analysis of developing synapses. In this chapter we use the neuromuscular synapse to illustrate key features of synaptic development, and we also apply insights from this peripheral synapse to examine the synapses that form in the central nervous system.

Finally, once formed, synapses continue to mature, often undergoing major rearrangements. One striking aspect of later development is the wholesale elimination of a large fraction of synapses, a process that is usually accompanied by the growth and strengthening of surviving synapses. Like neuronal cell death (see Chapter 53), synapse elimination is a puzzling and seemingly wasteful step in neural development. It is increasingly clear, however, that it plays a key role in refining initial patterns of connectivity. We will discuss the main features of synapse elimination at the neuromuscular junction, where it has been studied intensively, as well as at synapses between neurons, where it also is prominent.

Throughout this chapter we emphasize the interplay of molecular programs and neural activity in shaping synaptic patterns. Synapse formation stands at an interesting crossroads in the sequence of events that assemble the nervous system. The initial steps in this process appear to be "hardwired" by molecular programs. However, as soon as synapses form, the nervous system begins to function, and the activity of neural circuits plays a critical role in subsequent development. Indeed, the information-processing capacity of the nervous system is refined through its use, most dramatically in early postnatal life but also into adulthood. In this sense the nervous system continues to develop throughout life. This discussion will be a useful prelude to Chapter 56, where we discuss how genes and the environment—nature and nurture—interact to customize nervous systems early in postnatal life.

Recognition of Synaptic Targets Is Specific

Once axons reach their designated target areas they must choose appropriate synaptic partners from the many potential targets within easy reach. Although synapse formation is thought to be a selective process at both cellular and subcellular levels, few of the molecules that confer synaptic specificity have been identified.

Recognition Molecules Promote Selective Synapse Formation

The specificity of synaptic connections is particularly evident when intertwined axons select subsets of target cells. In these cases axon guidance and selective synapse formation can be distinguished. The first report of such specificity came more than 100 years ago when J. N. Langley, studying the autonomic nervous system, proposed the first version of a chemospecificity hypothesis (see Chapter 54).

Langley observed that autonomic preganglionic neurons are generated at distinct rostrocaudal levels of the spinal cord. Their axons enter sympathetic ganglia together but form synapses with different postsynaptic neurons that innervate distinct targets. Using behavioral assays as a guide, Langley inferred that the axons of preganglionic neurons located in the rostral spinal cord form synapses on ganglion neurons that project their axons to relatively rostral targets such as the eye, whereas neurons that derive from more caudal regions of the spinal cord synapse on ganglion neurons that project to caudal targets such as the ear (Figure 55–1A). He then showed that similar patterns were reestablished after the preganglionic axons were severed and allowed to regenerate, leading him to postulate that some sort of molecular recognition was responsible (Figure 55–1B, C).

Electrophysiological studies later confirmed Langley's intuition about the specificity of synaptic connections in these ganglia. Moreover, this selectivity is apparent from early stages of innervation, even though specific types of postsynaptic neurons are interspersed within the ganglion. The reestablishment of selectivity in adults after nerve damage shows that specificity does not emerge through peculiarities of embryonic timing or neuronal positioning.

To illustrate the idea of target specificity in more detail we will consider the axons of developing retinal ganglion cells. These neurons differ in their response properties—some ganglion neurons respond to increases in light level (ON cells), others to decreases (OFF cells), others to moving objects, and still others to light of a particular color. The axons of all ganglion cells run through the optic nerve, forming parallel axonal pathways from the retina to the brain.

The response properties of each class of ganglion neurons depend on the synaptic inputs they receive from amacrine and bipolar interneurons, which in turn receive synapses from light-sensitive photoreceptors. All of the synapses from bipolar and amacrine cells onto ganglion cell dendrites occur in a narrow zone of the retina called the inner plexiform layer (see Chapter 26). Axons and dendrites therefore have the daunting task of recognizing their correct partners within a large crowd of inappropriate bystanders.

In the inner plexiform layer the processes of different amacrine and bipolar cell types, as well as the dendrites of functionally distinct ganglion cell types, branch and synapse in different sublayers. The dendrites of ON and OFF cells are restricted to inner and outer portions of the plexiform layer, respectively, and therefore receive synapses from different interneurons (Figure 55–2). There are a dozen sublayers within the

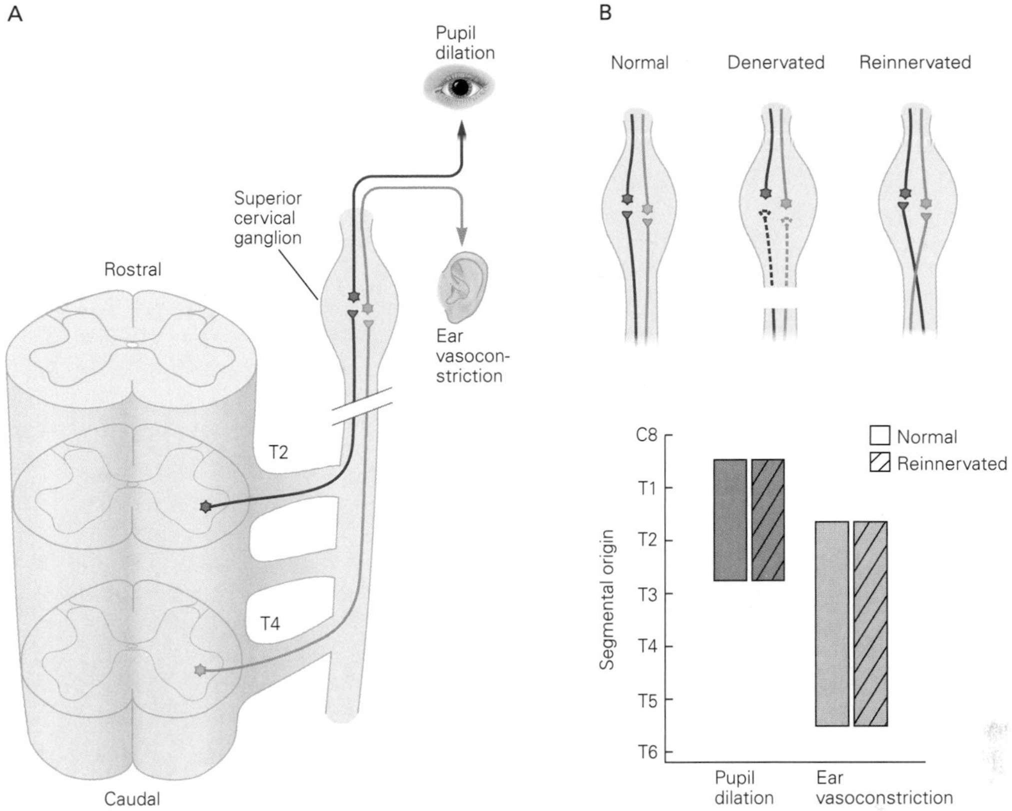

Figure 55–1 Preganglionic motor neurons regenerate selective connections with their sympathetic neuronal targets.

A. Preganglionic motor neurons arise from different levels of the thoracic spinal cord. Axons that arise from rostrally located thoracic neurons innervate superior cervical ganglion neurons that project to rostral targets, including the eye muscles. Axons that arise from neurons at caudal levels of the thoracic spinal cord innervate ganglion neurons that project to more caudal targets, such as the blood vessels of the ear. These two classes of ganglion neurons are intermingled in the ganglion, which suggested to J. N. Langley that preganglionic axons from different thoracic levels selectively form synapses with neurons that terminate in specific peripheral targets.

B. After nerve damage in adults, similar segment-specific patterns of connectivity are established through reinnervation, supporting the notion that synapse formation is selective. (Reproduced, with permission, from Nja and Purves 1977.)

inner plexiform layer, each with its own cohort of synapses. Similar lamina-specific connections are found in many other regions of the brain and spinal cord. For example, in the cerebral cortex distinct populations of axons confine their dendritic arbors and synapses to just one or two of the six main layers.

One clue to the establishment of lamina-specific synapses in the retina comes from the finding that subsets of ganglion neurons in the chick embryo express different classes of immunoglobulin-like adhesion molecules (see Chapter 54). These proteins promote homophilic interactions, that is, they bind to the same protein on other cell surfaces. Moreover, the amacrine and bipolar cells that contact a particular ganglion cell type in a specific sublamina often express the same adhesion molecules as their target cell (Figure 55–2B). When the characteristic adhesion molecule of a chick retinal ganglion neuron is removed, the cell's dendrites are no longer confined to a specific lamina. Conversely, the dendrites shift to a new lamina when they are forced to express a new immunoglobulin adhesion molecule. Thus a "like-binds-like" recognition system appears to contribute to this instance of synaptic specificity.

A different type of specificity is evident in the olfactory system. In the olfactory epithelium each neuron expresses just one of approximately 1,000 types of receptors. Neurons expressing one receptor are randomly distributed across a large sector of the epithelium, yet all of their axons converge on the dendrites of just a few target neurons in the olfactory bulb,

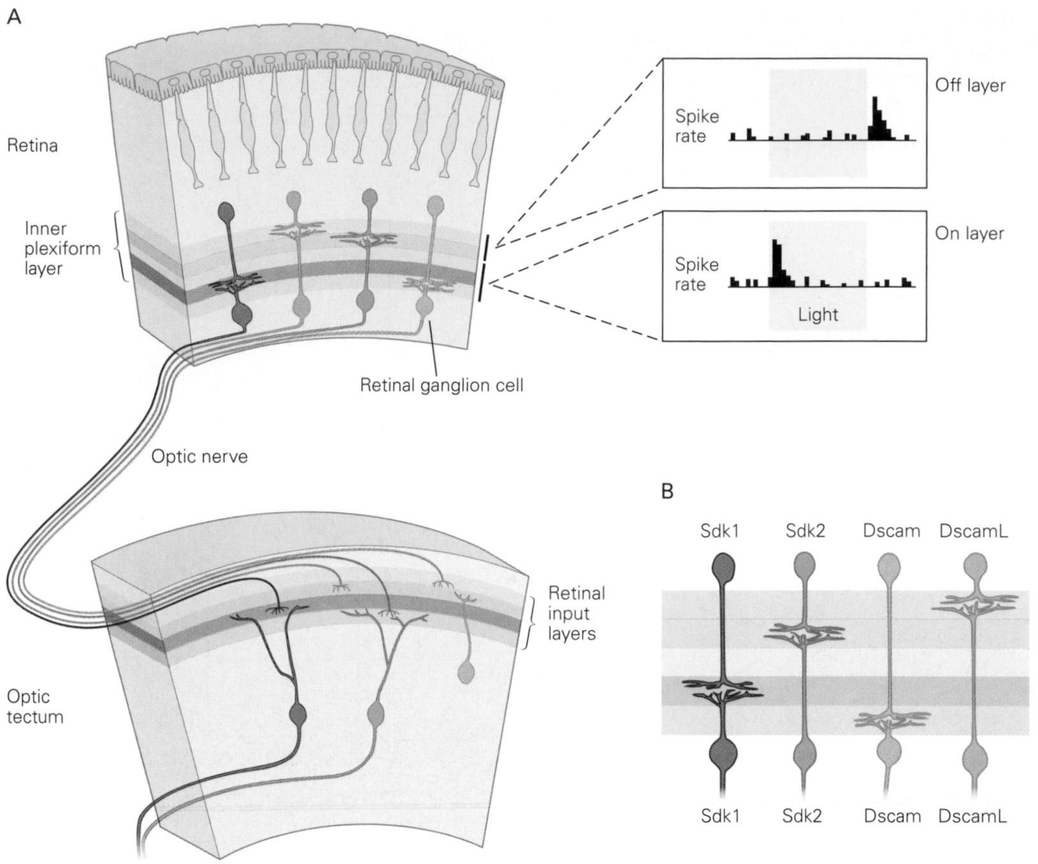

Figure 55–2 Retinal ganglion neurons form layer-specific synapses. (Reproduced, with permission, from Sanes and Yamagata 2009.)

A. The dendrites of retinal ganglion neurons receive input from the processes of retinal interneurons (amacrine and bipolar cells) in the inner plexiform layer, which is subdivided into at least 10 sublaminae. Specific subsets of interneurons and ganglion cells often arborize and synapse in just one layer. These lamina-specific connections determine which aspects of visual stimuli (their onset or offset) activate each type of retinal ganglion cell. The responses of OFF and ON retinal ganglion cells are shown on the right.

B. Immunoglobulin superfamily adhesion molecules (Sdk1, Sdk2, Dscam, and DscamL) are expressed by different subsets of amacrine and retinal ganglion neurons in the developing chick embryo. Amacrine neurons that express one of these four proteins form synapses with retinal ganglion cells that express the same protein. Manipulating Sdk or Dscam expression alters these patterns of lamina-specific arborization.

forming synapse-rich glomeruli (Figure 55–3A). When an individual olfactory receptor is deleted, the axons that normally express the receptor reach the olfactory bulb but fail to converge into specific glomeruli or to terminate on the appropriate postsynaptic cells (Figure 55–3B). Conversely, when neurons are forced to express a different odorant receptor, their axons form glomeruli at a different position within the olfactory bulb (Figure 55–3C).

Together these experiments suggest that olfactory receptors not only determine a neuron's responsiveness to specific odorants but also help the axon to form appropriate synapses on target neurons. Specific olfactory receptors may serve as recognition molecules, but it seems more likely that they influence the expression and activity of other receptor systems that contribute to the guidance of olfactory axons. In support of this view, recognition molecules have been found to regulate the interactions of olfactory axons with each other and with their targets.

Different Synaptic Inputs Are Directed to Discrete Domains of the Postsynaptic Cell

Nerve terminals not only discriminate among candidate targets, they also terminate on a specific portion of the target neuron. In many areas of the brain axons arriving in layered structures often confine their terminals to one layer, even if the dendritic tree of the postsynaptic cell traverses numerous layers. In the cerebellum the axons of different types of neurons terminate on distinct domains of the Purkinje neurons. Granule cell axons contact distal dendritic spines, climbing fiber axons contact proximal dendritic shafts, and basket cell axons contact the axon hillock and initial segment (Figure 55–4).

Such specificity presumably relies on molecular cues on the postsynaptic cell surface. For Purkinje neurons of the cerebellum one such cue is neurofascin, an adhesion molecule of the immunoglobulin superfamily. Neurofascin is present at high levels on the axonal initial segment and directs basket cells to form axons selectively on this axonal domain. Adhesion molecules can therefore also serve as recognition molecules for particular domains of a neuron. Since individual neurons can form synapses with several classes of pre- and postsynaptic cells, it follows that each neuronal subtype must express a variety of synaptic recognition molecules.

Neural Activity Sharpens Synaptic Specificity

So far we have emphasized the role of recognition molecules in the formation of synapses. Once synapses form, neural activity within the circuit plays a critical role in refining synaptic patterns. In the retinotectal system interactions between ephrins and Eph kinases result in formation of a crude retinotopic map in the tectum (see Chapter 54).

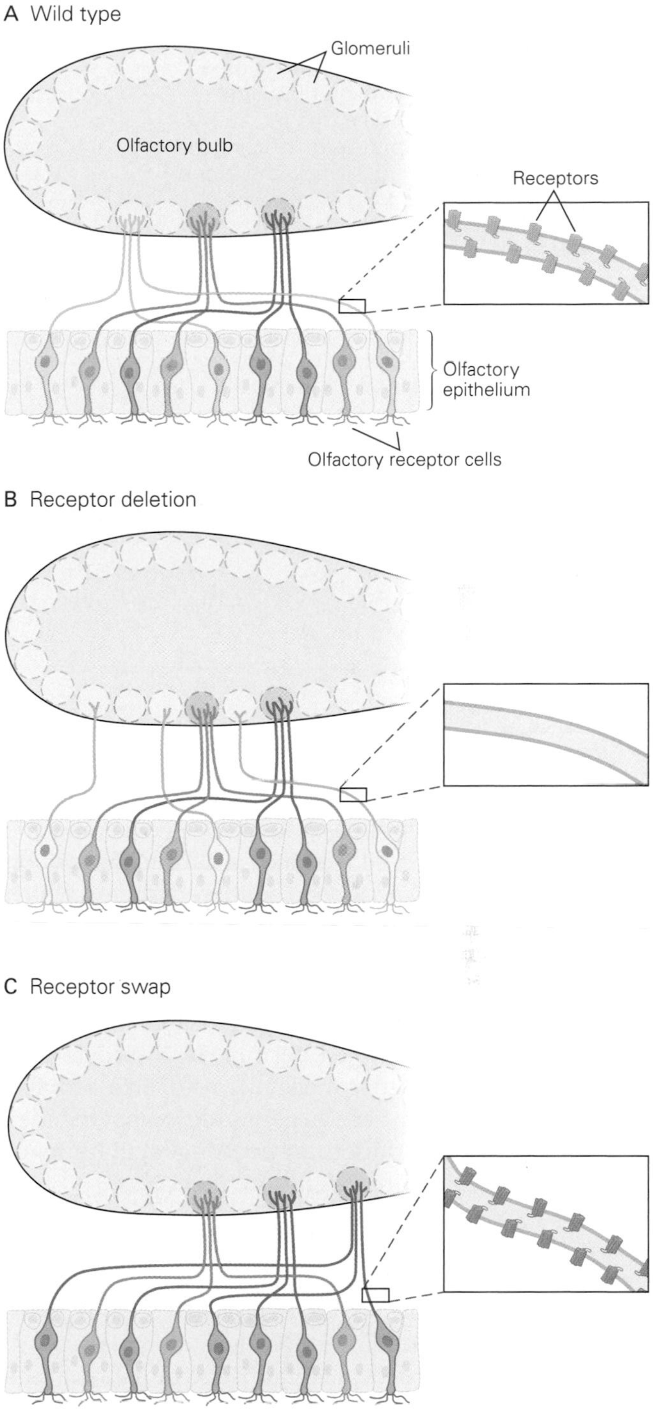

Figure 55–3 Olfactory receptors influence the targeting of sensory axons to discrete glomeruli in the olfactory bulb. (Adapted, with permission, from Sanes and Yamagata 2009.)

A. Each olfactory receptor neuron expresses one of approximately 1,000 possible odorant receptors. Neurons expressing the same receptor are distributed sparsely throughout the olfactory epithelium of the nose. The axons of these neurons form synapses with target neurons in a single glomerulus in the olfactory bulb.

B. In mouse mutants in which an odorant receptor gene has been deleted, the olfactory neurons that would have expressed the gene send their axons to other glomeruli, in part because these neurons now express other receptors.

C. When one odorant receptor gene replaces another in a set of olfactory sensory neurons, their axons project to a new glomerulus. Odorant receptor expression may set the overall activity level of the neuron, thus influencing the nature and level of expression of axonal guidance and recognition molecules.)

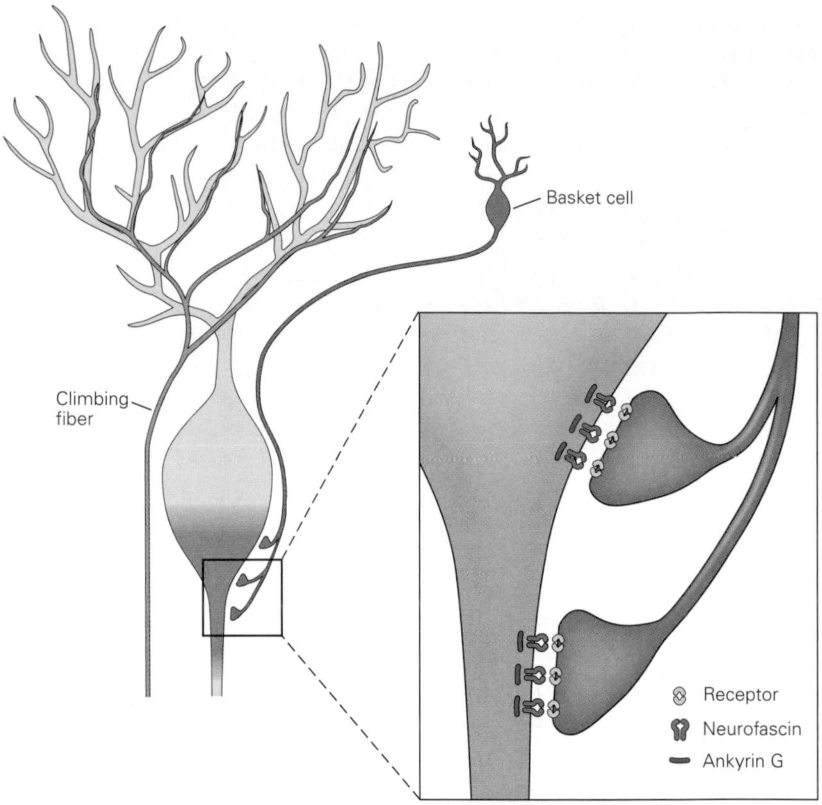

Figure 55–4 The axons of inhibitory interneurons in the cerebellum terminate on a distinct region of the cerebellar Purkinje cell. Many neurons form synapses on cerebellar Purkinje neurons, each selecting a distinct domain on the Purkinje cell. The axons of inhibitory basket cells form most of their synapses on the axon hillock and initial segment. Basket cells select these domains by recognizing neurofascin, a cell surface immunoglobulin superfamily adhesion molecule that is anchored to the initial segment of the axon by ankyrin G. When the localization of neurofascin is perturbed, basket cell axons fail to restrict synapse formation to the initial segment. (Adapted, with permission, from Huang 2006.)

But activity-dependent processes refine the axonal arbors of retinal ganglion cells, thus sharpening the tectal map (Figure 55–5). The axons of retinal ganglion neurons initially form broad diffuse arbors, which gradually become denser but more focused. This refinement is inhibited when the activity of synapses is blocked. Likewise, dendritic arbors of some retinal ganglion cells initially span multiple sublaminae in the inner plexiform layer, then become restricted to narrow ones. The molecular mechanisms of this activity-dependent refinement are largely unknown. One idea is that the level and pattern of neuronal activity regulates the expression of recognition molecules.

These examples illustrate a widespread phenomenon: Molecular cues control initial specificity but, once the circuit begins to function, specificity is sharpened through neural activity. In the two cases mentioned here, sharpening involves loss of synapses. We will return to the process of synapse elimination at the end of this chapter, and consider its consequences for behavior in the next chapter.

In a few cases neural activity can turn an inappropriate target into an appropriate one. This mechanism has been most clearly demonstrated in skeletal muscle, where mammalian muscle fibers can be divided into several categories according to their contractile characteristics. Muscle fibers of particular types express genes for distinctive isoforms of the main contractile proteins, such as myosins and troponins.

Few muscles are composed exclusively of a single type of fiber; most have fibers of all types. Yet the branches of an individual motor axon innervate muscle fibers of a single type, even in "mixed" muscles in which fibers of different types are intermingled (Figure 55–6A). This pattern, sometimes termed *motor unit homogeneity*, implies a remarkable degree of synaptic specificity. However, matching does not come about solely through recognition in the motor axon of the appropriate type of muscle fiber. The motor axon can also convert the target muscle fiber to an appropriate type. When a muscle is deinnervated at birth, before the properties of its fibers are fixed, a nerve that normally innervates a slow muscle can be redirected to reinnervate a muscle destined to become fast, and vice versa. Under these conditions the contractile properties of the muscle are partially transformed in a direction imposed by the firing properties of the motor nerve (Figure 55–6B, C).

Different patterns of neural activity are responsible for the switch in muscle properties. Most strikingly, direct electrical stimulation of a muscle with patterns normally evoked by slow or fast nerves leads to changes that are nearly as dramatic as those produced by cross-innervation (Figure 55–6D). Although activity-based conversion of the type used at the neuromuscular junction is unlikely to be a major contributor to synaptic specificity in the central nervous system, it raises the possibility that central axons can modify the properties of their synaptic targets, contributing to the diversification of neuronal subtypes and refining connectivity imposed by recognition molecules.

Principles of Synaptic Differentiation Are Revealed at the Neuromuscular Junction

The neuromuscular junction comprises three types of cells: a motor neuron, a muscle fiber, and Schwann cells. All three types are highly differentiated in the region of the synapse.

The process of synapse formation is initiated when a motor axon, guided by the multiple factors described in Chapter 54, reaches a developing skeletal muscle and approaches an immature muscle fiber. Contact is made and the process of synaptic differentiation begins. As the growth cone begins its transformation into a nerve terminal, the portion of the muscle surface opposite the nerve terminal begins to acquire its own specializations. As development proceeds, synaptic components are added and structural signs of synaptic differentiation become apparent in the pre- and postsynaptic cells and in the synaptic cleft. Eventually the neuromuscular junction acquires its mature and complex form (Figure 55–7A, B).

Three general features of neuromuscular junction development have provided clues about the molecular mechanisms that underlie synapse formation. First, nerve and muscle organize each other's differentiation. In principle, the precise apposition of pre- and postsynaptic specializations might be explained by independent programming of nerve and muscle properties. However, in muscle cells cultured alone

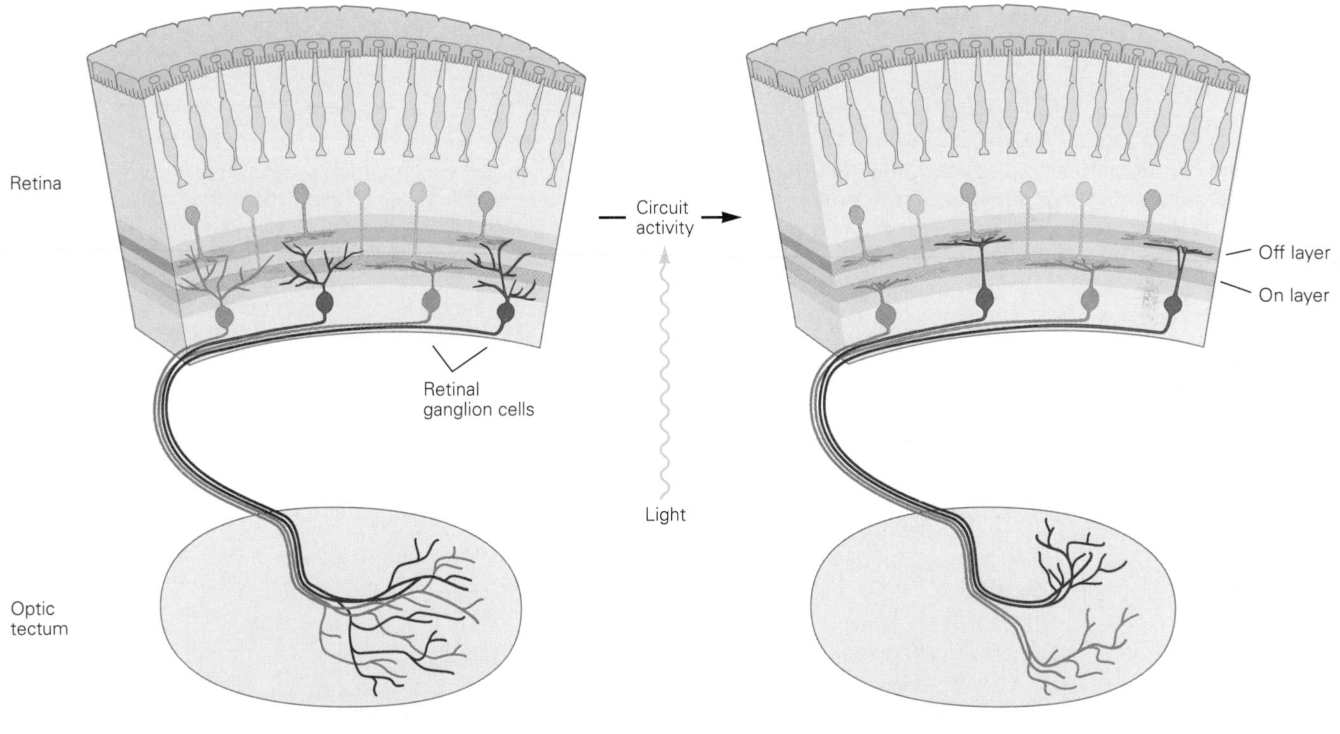

Figure 55–5 Electrical activity refines the specificity of synaptic connections in the retina. Some retinal ganglion cells initially form dendritic arbors that are limited to specific sublaminae in the inner plexiform layer of the retina, whereas others initially form diffuse arbors that are later pruned to form large specific patterns. Similarly, the axonal arbors of retinal ganglion cells initially innervate a large region of their target fields in the lateral geniculate nucleus and optic tectum. This expansive axonal arbor is then refined so as to concentrate many branches in a small region. Abolishing electrical activity in retinal ganglion cells decreases the remodeling of dendritic and axonal arbors.

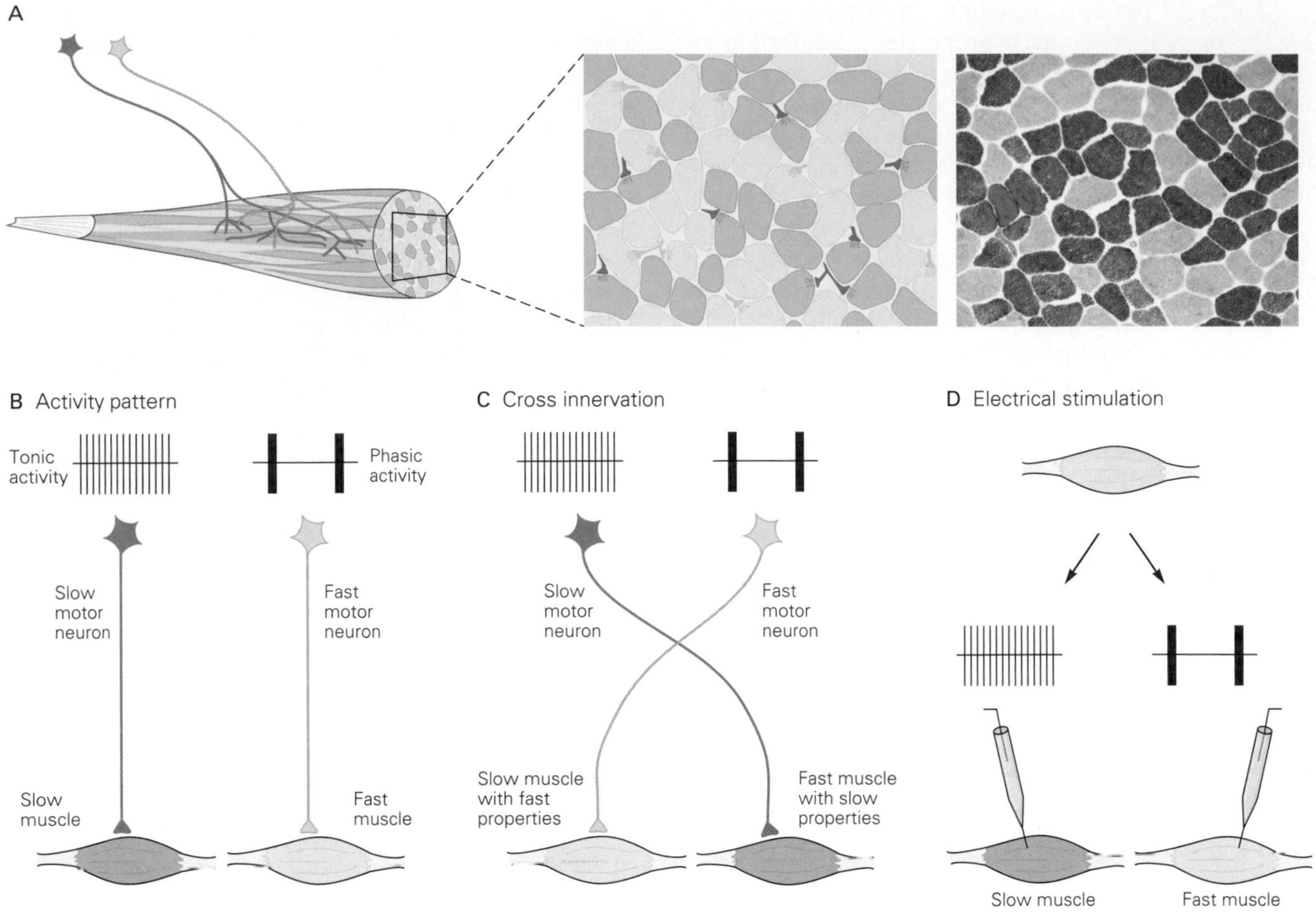

Figure 55–6 The pattern of motor neuron activity can change the biochemical and functional properties of skeletal muscle cells.

A. Muscle fibers have characteristic metabolic, molecular, and electrical properties that identify them as "slow" (tonic) or "fast" (phasic) types. The micrograph on the right shows a section of muscle tissue with histochemical staining for myosin ATPase. The middle sketch shows a section through the muscle, in which motor neurons (**green** and **brown**) form synapses on a single type of muscle fiber. (Photo reproduced, with permission, from Arthur P. Hays.)

B. Motor neurons that connect with fast and slow muscle fibers (fast and slow motor neurons) exhibit distinct patterns of electrical activity: steady low frequency (tonic) for slow and intermittent high-frequency bursts (phasic) for fast.

C. Cross-innervation experiments showed that some property of the motor neuron helps to determine whether muscle fibers are fast or slow. Cross-innervation was achieved by surgically rerouting fast axons to slow muscle and vice versa. Although the properties of the motor neurons are little changed, the properties of the muscle change profoundly. For example, fast motor neurons induce fast properties in the slow muscle. (Adapted, with permission, from Salmons and Sreter 1976.)

D. The effects of innervation by fast and slow nerves on muscle are mediated in part by their distinct patterns of activity. When a fast muscle is stimulated in a slow tonic pattern, the muscle acquires slow electrical and molecular properties. Conversely, fast phasic stimulation of a once slow muscle can convert it to a faster type.

acetylcholine (ACh) receptors are generally distributed uniformly on the surface, although some are clustered as in mature postsynaptic membranes. Yet when motor neurons are added to the cultures they extend neurites that contact the muscle cells more or less randomly, instead of seeking out the ACh receptor clusters. New receptor clusters appear precisely at the points of contact with the presynaptic neurites while preexisting uninnervated clusters eventually disperse (Figure 55–8). Thus factors on or released by motor axons exert a profound influence on the synaptic organization of the muscle cell. Likewise, muscles signal

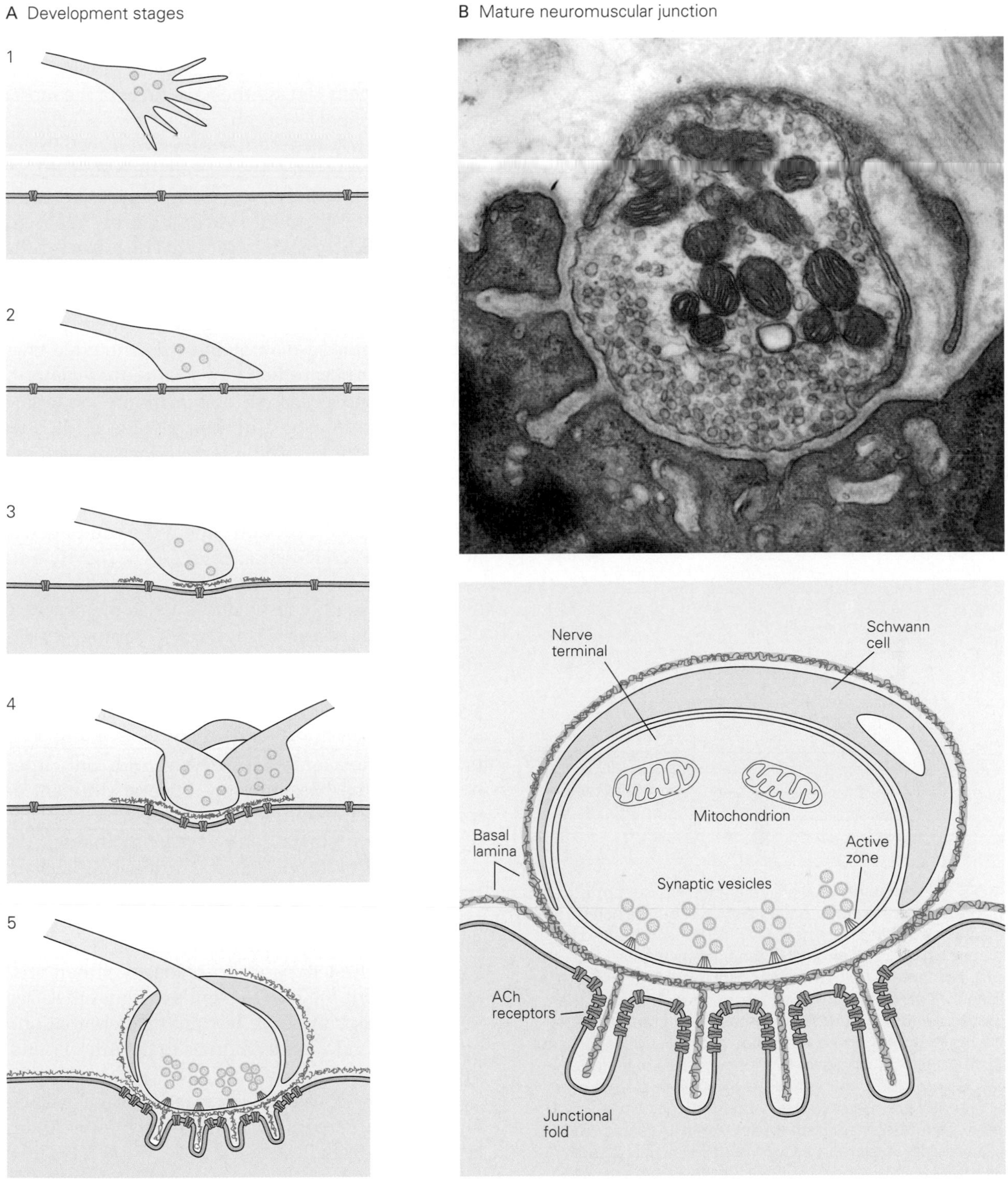

Figure 55–7 The neuromuscular junction develops in sequential stages.

A. A growth cone approaches a newly fused myotube (**1**) and forms a morphologically unspecialized but functional contact (**2**). The nerve terminal accumulates synaptic vesicles and a basal lamina forms in the synaptic cleft (**3**). As the muscle matures, multiple axons converge on a single site (**4**). Finally, all axons but one are eliminated and the surviving terminal matures (**5**). (Adapted, with permission, from Hall and Sanes 1993.)

B. At the mature neuromuscular junction, pre- and postsynaptic membranes are separated by a synaptic cleft that contains basal lamina and extracellular matrix proteins. Vesicles are clustered at presynaptic release sites, transmitter receptors are clustered in the postsynaptic membrane, and nerve terminals are coated by Schwann cell processes. (Image reproduced, with permission, courtesy of T. Gillingwater.)

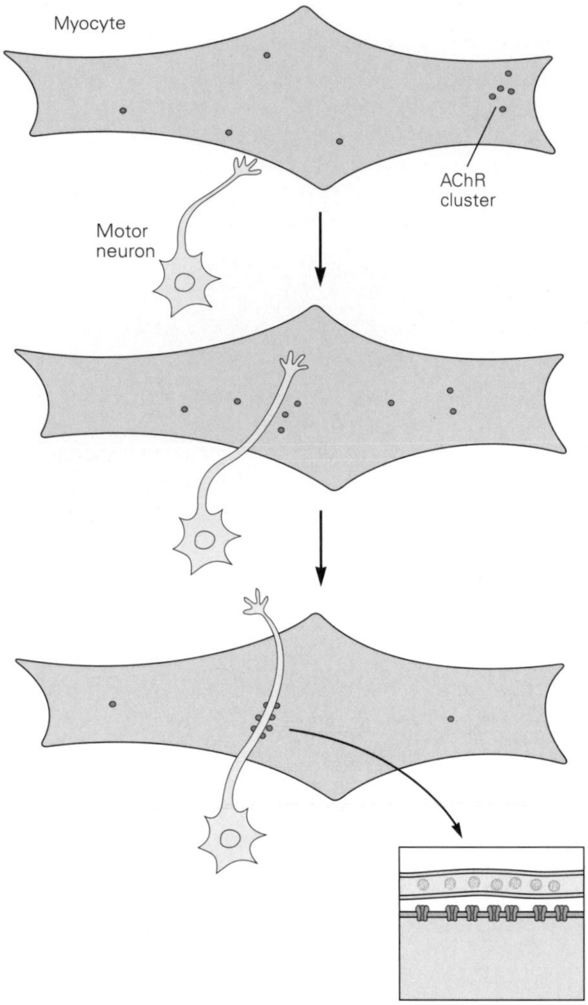

Figure 55–8 Nerve and muscle cells express synaptic components, but synaptic organization requires cell interactions. Acetylcholine receptors **(AChR)** are synthesized by muscle cells cultured without neurons. Many receptors are diffusely distributed, but some form high-density aggregates similar to those found in the postsynaptic membrane of the neuromuscular junction. When neurons first contact muscle they do not restrict themselves to the receptor-rich aggregates. Instead, new receptor aggregates form at sites of neurite-muscle contact, and many of the preexisting clusters disperse. Similarly, motor axons contain synaptic vesicles that cluster at sites of neurite contact with muscle cells. (Adapted, with permission, from Anderson and Cohen 1977; Lupa, Gordon, and Hall 1990.)

retrogradely to motor nerve terminals. When motor neurons in culture extend neurites, they assemble and transport synaptic vesicles, some of which form aggregates similar to those found in nerve terminals. When the neurites contact muscle cells, new vesicle clusters form opposite the muscle membrane, and most of the preexisting clusters disperse.

Second, as these studies showed, motor neurons and muscle cells can synthesize and arrange most synaptic components without each other's help. Uninnervated myotubes can synthesize functional ACh receptors and gather them into high-density aggregates. Likewise, motor axons can form synaptic vesicles and cluster them into varicosities in the absence of muscle. In fact, vesicles in growth cones can synthesize and release ACh in response to electrical stimulation, before the growth cone has reached its target cells. Thus the developmental signals that pass between nerve and muscle do not induce wholesale changes in cell properties; rather they assure that components of the pre- and postsynaptic machinery are organized at the correct time and in the right places. It is useful therefore to think of the intercellular signals that control synaptogenesis as organizers rather than inducers.

A third key feature of neuromuscular junction development is that new synaptic components are added in several distinct steps. The newly formed synapse is not simply a prototype of a fully developed synapse. Although nerve and muscle membrane form close contacts at early stages of synaptogenesis, only later does the synaptic cleft widen and the basal lamina appear. Similarly, ACh receptors accumulate in the postsynaptic membrane before acetylcholinesterase accumulates in the synaptic cleft, and the postsynaptic membrane acquires junctional folds only after the nerve terminal has matured. Several different axons innervate each myotube around the time of birth, but during early postnatal life all but one axon withdraws.

This elaborate sequence is unlikely to be orchestrated by the simple act of contact between nerve and muscle. More probably, multiple signals pass between the cells—the nerve sends a signal to the muscle that triggers the first steps in postsynaptic differentiation, at which point the muscle sends a signal that triggers the initial steps of nerve terminal differentiation. The nerve then sends further signals to the muscle, and this interaction continues.

We now consider retrograde (from muscle to nerve) and anterograde (from nerve to muscle) organizers in more detail.

Differentiation of Motor Nerve Terminals Is Organized by Muscle Fibers

Soon after the growth cone of a motor axon contacts a developing myotube, a rudimentary form of neurotransmission begins. The axon releases ACh in vesicular packets, the transmitter binds to receptors, and the muscle responds with depolarization and weak contraction.

The onset of transmission at the new synapse reflects the intrinsic capabilities of each synaptic partner. Nevertheless, these intrinsic capabilities cannot readily explain the marked increase in the rate of transmitter release that occurs after nerve-muscle contact is made, nor can they explain the accumulation of synaptic vesicles and the assembly of active zones in the small portion of the motor axon that contacts the muscle surface. These developmental steps require signals from muscle to nerve.

A clue to the source of these signals came from studies on the reinnervation of adult muscle. Although axotomy leaves muscle fibers denervated and leads to insertion of ACh receptors in nonsynaptic regions, the postsynaptic apparatus remains largely intact. It is still recognizable by its synaptic nuclei, junctional folds, and the ACh receptors, which remain far more densely packed in synaptic areas than in extrasynaptic areas of the cell. Damaged peripheral axons regenerate readily (unlike those in the central nervous system) and form new neuromuscular junctions that look and perform much like the original ones.

A century ago, Fernando Tello y Muñóz, a student of Santiago Ramón y Cajal, noted that the new junctions form at preexisting synaptic sites on the denervated muscle fibers even though the postsynaptic specializations occupy only 0.1% of the muscle fiber surface (Figure 55–9A). Later, electron microscopy showed that specialization in the axon occurs only in the terminals that contact the muscle. For example, active zones form directly opposite the mouths of the postsynaptic junctional folds. These findings imply that motor axons recognize signals associated with the postsynaptic apparatus.

When regenerating axons reach a muscle fiber they encounter the basal lamina of the synaptic cleft. To explore the significance of this association, muscles were damaged in vivo in a way that killed the muscle fibers but left their basal lamina intact. The necrotic fibers were phagocytized, leaving behind basal lamina sheaths on which synaptic sites were readily recognizable. At the same time that the muscle was damaged the nerve was cut and allowed to regenerate. Under these conditions motor axons reinnervated the empty basal lamina sheaths, contacting synaptic sites as precisely as they would have if muscle fibers were present. Moreover, nerve terminals developed at these sites and active zones even formed opposite struts of basal lamina that once lined junctional folds. These observations implied that components of the basal lamina organize presynaptic specialization (Figure 55–9B).

Several such molecular organizers have now been identified. Among the best studied are isoforms of the protein laminin. Laminins are major components of all basal laminae and promote axon outgrowth in many neuronal types (see Chapter 54). They are heterotrimers of α, β, and γ chains, comprising a family of at least five α, four β, and three γ chains. Muscle fibers synthesize multiple laminin isoforms and incorporate them into the basal lamina. Laminin-211, a heterotrimer containing the $\alpha 2$, $\beta 1$, and $\gamma 1$ chains, is the major laminin in the basal lamina, and its absence leads to severe muscular dystrophy. In the synaptic cleft, however, isoforms bearing the $\beta 2$ chain predominate (Figure 55–10A).

In vitro motor axons that encounter a deposit of $\beta 2$-containing laminin stop growing, accumulate synaptic vesicles, and acquire the ability to release neurotransmitter. Conversely, the development of nerve terminals and Schwann cells is perturbed in mutant mice that lack the $\beta 2$ laminin (Figure 55–10B). These laminins appear to act by binding to voltage-sensitive calcium channels that reside in the axon terminal membrane, where they couple activity to transmitter release. Laminins act on the extracellular domain of the channels whereas the intracellular segment recruits or stabilizes other components of the release apparatus.

Because presynaptic specialization proceeds to some extent in the absence of laminins, additional retrograde organizers of axonal specialization must exist. Among these are members of the fibroblast growth factor and collagen IV families, both produced by muscle cells. Thus target-derived proteins from multiple families collaborate to organize the presynaptic nerve terminal.

Differentiation of the Postsynaptic Muscle Membrane Is Organized by the Motor Nerve

Soon after myoblasts fuse to form myotubes, the genes that encode ACh receptor subunits are activated. Receptor subunits are synthesized, assembled into pentamers in the endoplasmic reticulum, and inserted into the plasma membrane. As noted above, some receptors spontaneously form aggregates, but the majority are distributed throughout the membrane at a low density, approximately 1,000 per μm^2.

Once synapse formation is complete, however, the distribution of the receptors changes drastically. The receptors become concentrated at the synaptic sites of the membrane (to a density up to 10,000 per μm^2) and depleted in the nonsynaptic membrane (reduced to 10 per μm^2 or less). This thousand-fold difference in ACh receptor density occurs a few tens of micrometers from the edge of the nerve terminal.

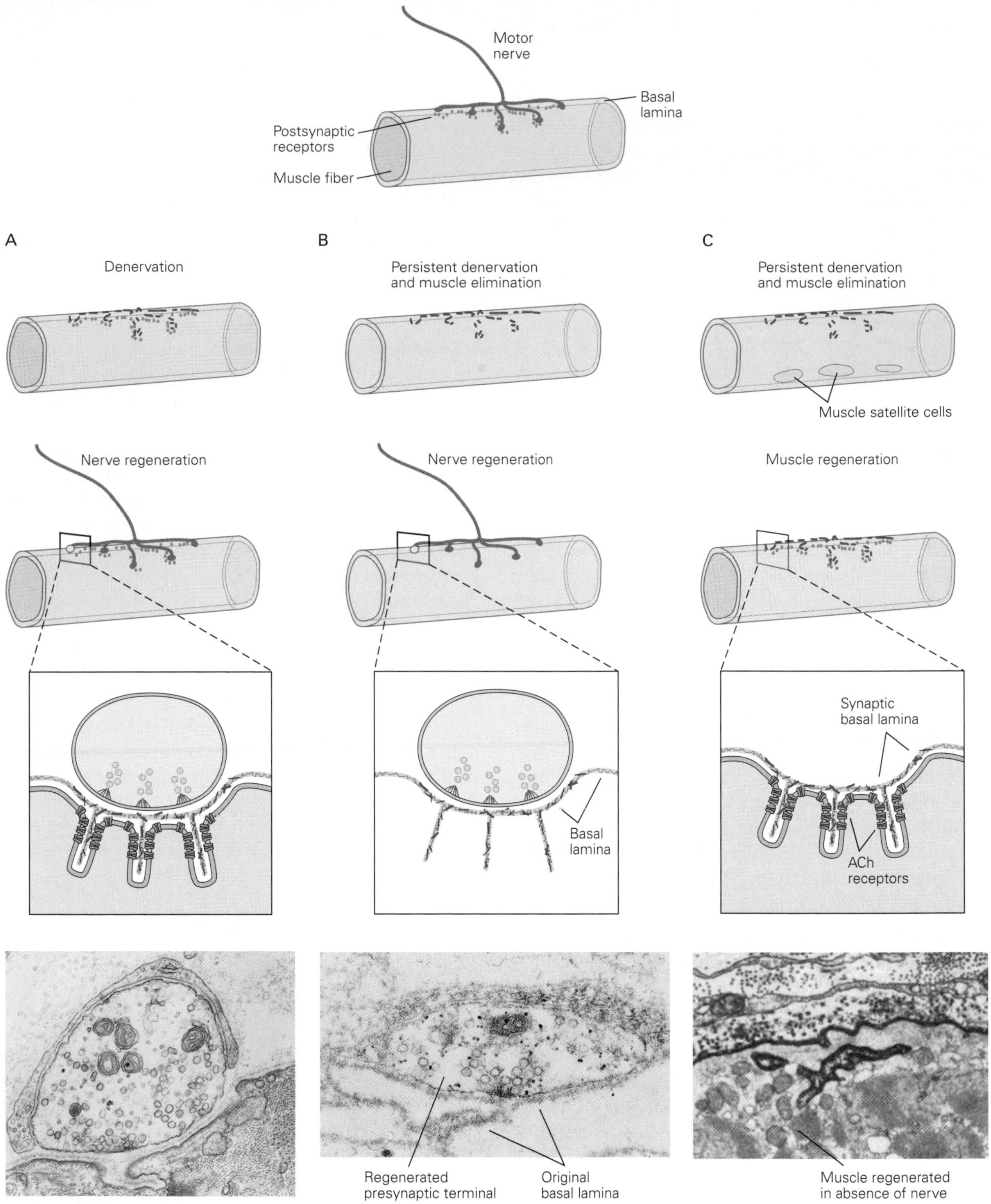

Figure 55–9 Synaptic portions of basal lamina contain proteins that organize developing nerve terminals.

A. After nerve damage motor axons regenerate and form new neuromuscular junctions. Nearly all of the new synapses form at the original synaptic sites. (Micrograph reproduced, with permission, from Glicksman and Sanes 1983.)

B. A strong preference for innervation at original synaptic sites persists even after the muscle fibers have been removed, leaving behind basal lamina "ghosts." Regenerated axons develop synaptic specialization on contact with the original synaptic sites on the basal lamina. (Micrograph reproduced, with permission, from Glicksman and Sanes 1983.)

C. Following denervation of a skeletal muscle fiber and elimination of mature muscle fibers, muscle satellite cells proliferate and differentiate to form new myofibers. The expression of ACh receptors on the regenerated myofiber surface is concentrated in the synaptic areas of basal lamina, even when reinnervation is prevented. (Micrograph reproduced, with permission, from Burden, Sargent, and McMahan 1979.)

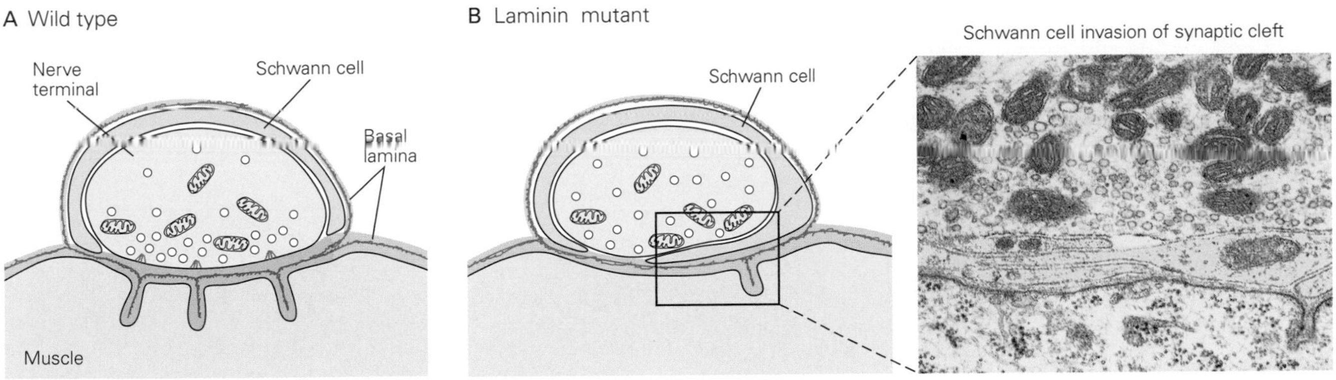

Figure 55–10 Different laminin isoforms are localized at synaptic and extrasynaptic areas of the basal lamina.

A. Different laminin isoforms are found in synaptic (**brown**) and extrasynaptic (**green**) areas of basal lamina. Isoforms, containing the β2 chain, are concentrated in the synaptic areas.

B. Maturation of neuromuscular junctions is impaired in mice lacking β2 laminins. These mutants have few active zones, and the synaptic cleft is invaded by Schwann cell processes (**blue**). (Micrograph reproduced, with permission, from Noakes et al. 1995.)

Appreciation of the critical role of the nerve in the redistribution of ACh receptors inspired a search for factors that might promote their clustering. This quest led to the discovery of a proteoglycan, agrin. Agrin is synthesized by motor neurons, transported down the axon, released from nerve terminals, and incorporated into the synaptic cleft (Figure 55–11A, B). Some agrin isoforms are also made by muscle cells, but the neuronal isoforms are about a thousand-fold more active in aggregating ACh receptors.

The phenotype of mutant mice lacking agrin shows that agrin has a central role in the organization of ACh receptors. Agrin mutants have grossly perturbed neuromuscular junctions and die at birth. The number, size, and density of ACh receptor aggregates are severely reduced in these mice (Figure 55–11C). Other components of the postsynaptic apparatus—including cytoskeletal, membrane, and basal lamina proteins—are also reduced. Interestingly, the differentiation of presynaptic elements is also perturbed. However, the defects in the presynaptic element do not result directly from lack of agrin in the motor neuron, but rather indirectly from the failure of the disorganized postsynaptic apparatus to generate signals for presynaptic specialization.

How does agrin work? Agrin's major receptor is a complex of a muscle-specific tyrosine kinase called MuSK (muscle-specific trk-related receptor with a kringle domain) and a coreceptor subunit called LRP4 (Figure 55–11A). MuSK is normally concentrated at synaptic sites in the muscle membrane, and muscles of mutant mice lacking MuSK do not have ACh receptor clusters (Figure 55–11C). Myotubes generated in vitro from these mutants express normal levels of ACh receptors, but these receptors cannot be clustered by agrin. MuSK therefore appears to be a critical component of the receptor for agrin. LRP4 functions together with MuSK, an adaptor protein Dok-7, and a cytoplasmic protein rapsyn. LRP4 forms a complex with MuSK and binds agrin efficiently. Dok-7 binds MuSK and signals to rapsyn, which is also necessary for ACh receptor clustering. Rapsyn is co-localized with ACh receptors in vivo, is present at ACh receptor clusters soon after they form, and can induce the aggregation of ACh receptors in vitro. In mice lacking rapsyn muscles form normally and ACh receptors accumulate in normal numbers but fail to aggregate at the synaptic sites on the membrane.

Thus an extracellular protein (agrin), transmembrane proteins (MuSK and LRP4), an adaptor protein (Dok-7), and a cytoskeletal protein (rapsyn) form a chain that links commands from the motor axon to ACh receptor clustering in the muscle membrane.

Nevertheless, postsynaptic differentiation can occur in the absence of this transduction pathway. This capacity was apparent in early studies on cultured muscle (see Figure 55–8) and is also seen in vivo: ACh receptor clusters form initially but then disperse in agrin mutants (Figure 55–11C). Clustering also occurs in muscles that lack innervation entirely. Conversely, no clustering occurs in mutant animals lacking MuSK, LRP4, Dok-7, or rapsyn. Thus the signaling pathway that initiates postsynaptic differentiation can be activated without agrin, but agrin is required to maintain clustering of ACh receptors.

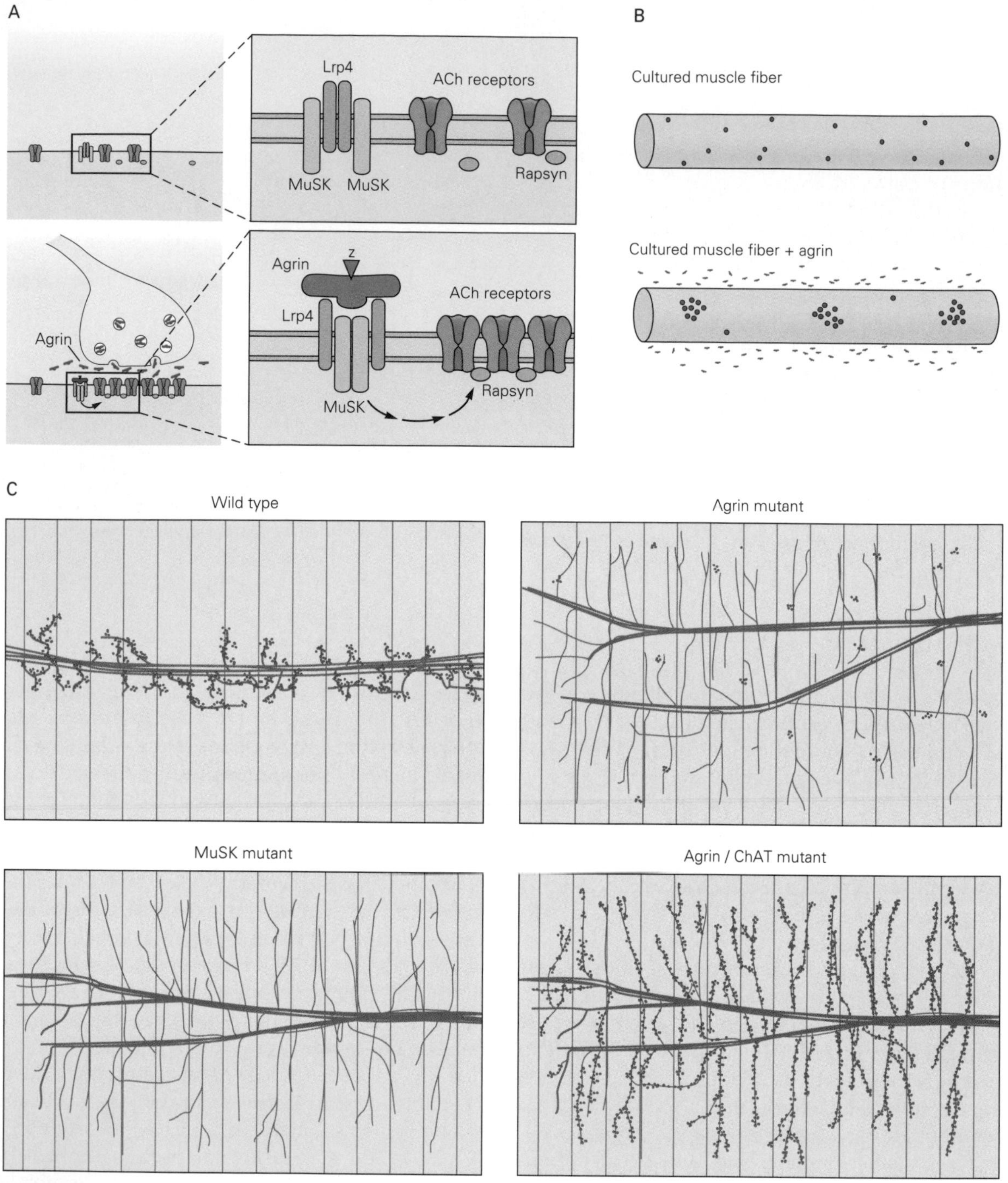

Figure 55–11 Agrin induces aggregation of ACh receptors at synaptic sites.

A. Agrin is a large (~400 kDa) extracellular matrix proteoglycan. Alternative splicing includes a "z" exon that confers the ability to cluster ACh receptors. When released by a nerve terminal, agrin binds Lrp4 on the muscle membrane, activating the membrane-associated receptor tyrosine kinase MuSK and triggering an intracellular cascade that results in ACh receptor clustering. Clustering is mediated by rapsyn, a cytoplasmic ACh receptor-associated protein. (Adapted, with permission, from DeChiara et al. 1996.)

B. Few ACh receptor clusters form on myofibers grown in culture under control conditions, but addition of agrin induces ACh receptor clustering. (Adapted, with permission, from Misgeld et al. 2005.)

C. Muscles from wild type neonatal mice and from three mutant types. Muscles were labeled for ACh receptors (**green**) and motor axons (**brown**). In wild type mice ACh receptor clusters have formed under each nerve terminal by birth, whereas in agrin mutants most clusters have dispersed. ACh receptors are also absent in MuSK mutant mice. When the genes for agrin and ChAT (choline acetyltransferase) are mutated, clusters of ACh receptors remain, indicating that agrin works by counteracting receptor dispersion mediated by ACh. All three mutant conditions also show axonal abnormalities, reflecting the inability of the muscle to supply retrograde factors. (**ACh**, acetylcholine; **MuSK**, muscle-specific trk-related receptor with a kringle domain.) (Adapted, with permission, from Gautam et al. 1996.)

The role of agrin is perhaps best understood in terms of the requirement that pre- and postsynaptic specializations be perfectly aligned. Acetycholine receptor aggregates persist in uninnervated muscles but disappear in agrin mutant muscles, suggesting that axons sculpt the postsynaptic membrane through the combined action of agrin and a dispersal factor. One major dispersal factor is ACh itself; clustering persists in mutants that lack both agrin and ACh (Figure 55–11C). Thus agrin may render ACh receptors immune to the declustering effects of ACh. Through a combination of positive and negative factors, the motor neuron ensures that the patches of postsynaptic membrane contacted by axon branches are rich in ACh receptors.

The Nerve Regulates Transcription of Acetylcholine Receptor Genes

Along with redistribution of ACh receptor in the plane of the membrane, the motor nerve orchestrates the transcriptional program responsible for expression of ACh receptor genes in muscle. To understand this aspect of transcriptional control, it is important to appreciate the geometry of the muscle.

Individual muscle fibers are often more than a centimeter long and contain hundreds of nuclei along their length. Most nuclei are far from the synapse, but a few are clustered beneath the synaptic membrane, so that their transcribed and translated products do not have far to go to reach the synapse. In newly formed myotubes most nuclei express genes encoding the ACh receptor α-, β-, δ-, and γ-subunits. In adult muscles, however, only synaptic nuclei express ACh receptor genes; nonsynaptic nuclei do not. This change in pattern occurs in three steps.

During early stages of synapse formation the ACh receptor subunit genes are expressed at higher levels in synaptic nuclei than in their nonsynaptic neighbors (Figure 55–12). Signals acting through MuSK are needed for this specialization. Around the time of birth, ACh receptor gene expression shuts down in nonsynaptic nuclei. This change reflects a repressive effect of the nerve, as originally shown by studies of denervated muscle. When muscle fibers are denervated, as happens when the motor nerve is damaged, the density of ACh receptors in the postsynaptic membrane increases markedly, a phenomenon termed *denervation supersensitivity.*

This repressive effect of the nerve is mediated by electrical activation of the muscle. Under normal conditions the nerve keeps the muscle electrically active, and active muscle synthesizes fewer ACh receptors than inactive muscle. Indeed, direct stimulation of denervated muscle through implanted electrodes decreases ACh receptor expression, preventing or reversing the effect of denervation (Figure 55–12B). Conversely, when nerve activity is blocked by application of a local anesthetic, the number of ACh receptors throughout the muscle fiber increases, even though the synapse is intact.

In essence, then, the nerve uses ACh to repress expression of ACh receptor genes extrasynaptically. Current that passes through the channel of the receptor leads to an action potential that propagates along the entire muscle fiber. This depolarization opens voltage-dependent Ca^{2+} channels, leading to an influx of Ca^{2+}, which activates a signal transduction cascade that reaches nonsynaptic nuclei and regulates transcription of ACh receptor genes. Thus the same voltage changes that produce muscle contraction over a period of milliseconds also regulate transcription of ACh receptor genes over a period of days.

The increase in transcription of ACh receptor genes in nuclei beneath the synapse, along with the decrease in nuclei distant from synapses, leads to localization of ACh receptor mRNA and thus preferential synthesis and insertion of ACh receptors near synaptic sites. This local synthesis is reminiscent of that seen at postsynaptic sites on dendritic spines in the brain. Local synthesis in muscle is advantageous since ACh receptors synthesized near the ends of fibers would never reach the synapse without degradation.

We have used the ACh receptor as an example of postsynaptic differentiation, but many components of the postsynaptic apparatus are regulated in similar ways—their aggregation depends on agrin and MuSK, and their transcription is enhanced in synaptic nuclei and repressed in extrasynaptic nuclei by electrical activity. Thus synaptic components have tailor-made regulatory mechanisms, but many of these components are regulated in parallel.

The Neuromuscular Junction Matures in a Series of Steps

The adult neuromuscular junction is dramatically different in its molecular architecture, shape, size, and functional properties from the simple nerve-muscle contact that initiates neurotransmission in the embryo. Maturation of the nerve terminal, the postsynaptic membrane, and the intervening synaptic cleft occurs in a complex series of steps. We illustrate this step-wise synaptic construction with a continued focus on the development of ACh receptors.

As we have seen, ACh receptors aggregate in the plane of the membrane as the neuromuscular

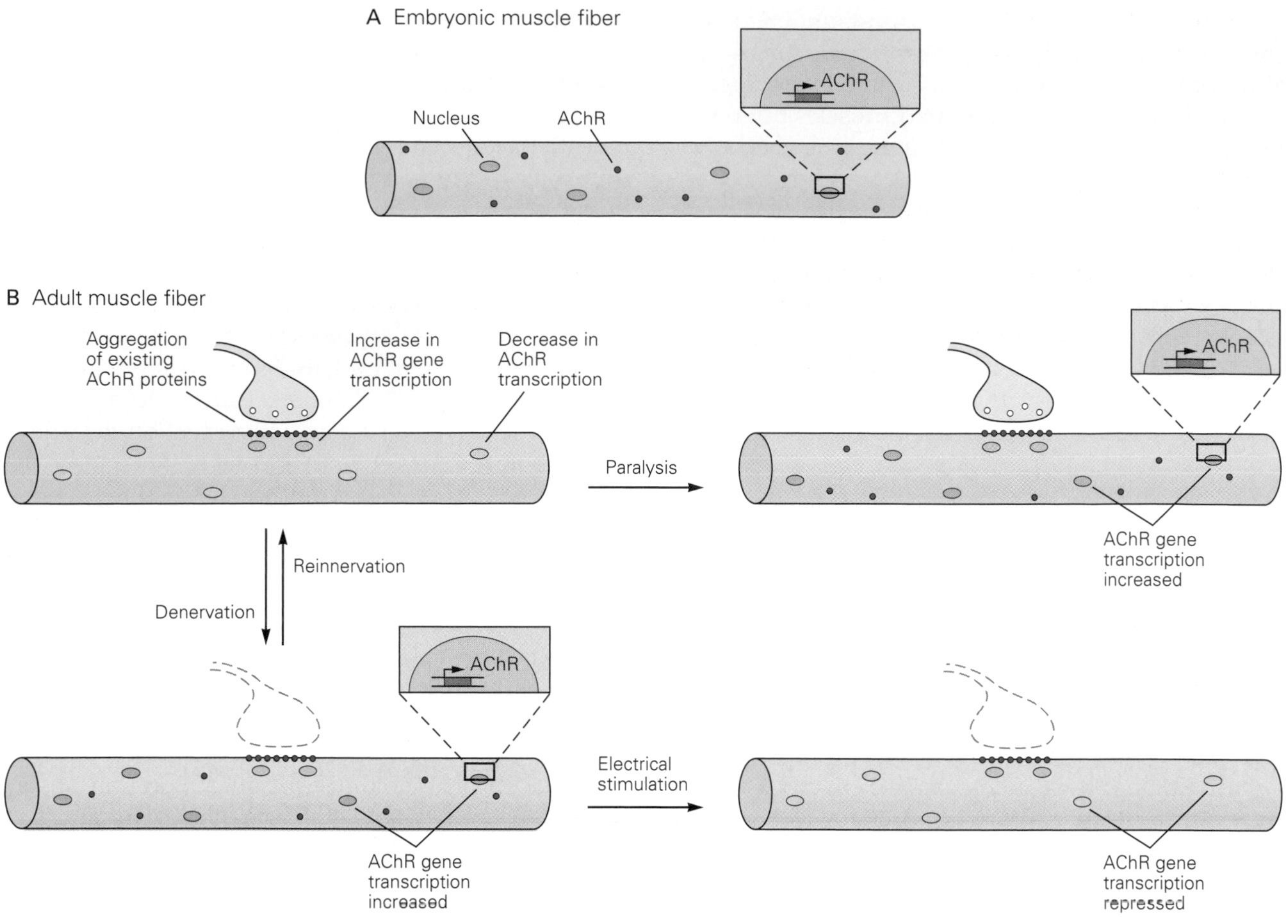

Figure 55–12 Clustering of ACh receptors at the neuromuscular junction results from transcriptional regulation and local protein trafficking.

A. Acetylcholine receptors (AChR) are distributed diffusely on the surface of embryonic myotubes.

B. After the muscle is innervated by a motor axon the number of receptors in extrasynaptic regions decreases, whereas receptor density at the synapse increases. This reflects the aggregation of preexisting receptors and enhanced expression of ACh receptor genes in nuclei that lie directly beneath the nerve terminal. In addition, the transcription of receptor genes is repressed in nuclei in extrasynaptic regions. Electrical activity in muscle represses ACh gene expression in nonsynaptic nuclei, leading to a lower density of ACh receptors in these regions. The nuclei at synaptic sites are immune to this repressive effect. Following denervation, ACh receptor gene expression is upregulated in extrasynaptic nuclei, although not to the high level attained by synaptic nuclei. Paralysis mimics the effect of denervation, whereas electrical stimulation of denervated muscle mimics the influence of the nerve and decreases the density of ACh receptors in the extrasynaptic membrane.

junction begins to form, and receptor gene transcription is enhanced in synaptic nuclei. A few days later activity begins to decrease the level of extrasynaptic receptors and the stability of receptors changes. In embryonic muscle ACh receptors are turned over rapidly (with a half-life of approximately 1 day) throughout the membrane, whereas in adult muscle they are relatively stable (with a half-life of approximately 2 weeks). The metabolic stabilization of ACh receptors helps concentrate them at synaptic sites and stabilize the postsynaptic apparatus.

During the first few postnatal days the composure of the ACh receptor changes, shuts off the δ gene and activates the ε gene. As a result, new ACh receptors inserted in the membrane are composed of α-, β-, δ-, and ε-subunits rather than α-, β-, δ-, and γ-subunits. This altered subunit composition tunes the receptor in a way that is suited to its mature function. However, although it occurs at the same time as the metabolic stabilization, the two changes are not causally linked.

These molecular changes in the postsynaptic membrane are accompanied by changes in its shape

(Figure 55–13). Soon after birth junctional folds begin to form in the postsynaptic membrane and ACh receptors become concentrated at the crests of the folds, along with rapsyn, whereas other membrane and cytoskeletal proteins are localized in the depths of the folds. The initial aggregate of ACh receptors appears to have a plaque-like appearance. Perforations that undergo fusion and fission eventually transform the dense plaque into a pretzel-shape that follows the branches of the nerve ending. Finally, the postsynaptic membrane enlarges and eventually contains many more ACh receptors than were present in the initial cluster. Each of these changes occurs while the synapse is functional, implying that ongoing activity plays an important role in synaptic maturation.

Central Synapses Develop in Ways Similar to Neuromuscular Junctions

Synapses in the central nervous system are structurally similar to neuromuscular junctions, and they function in a similar way. Their formation also adheres to the principles of development of the neuromuscular

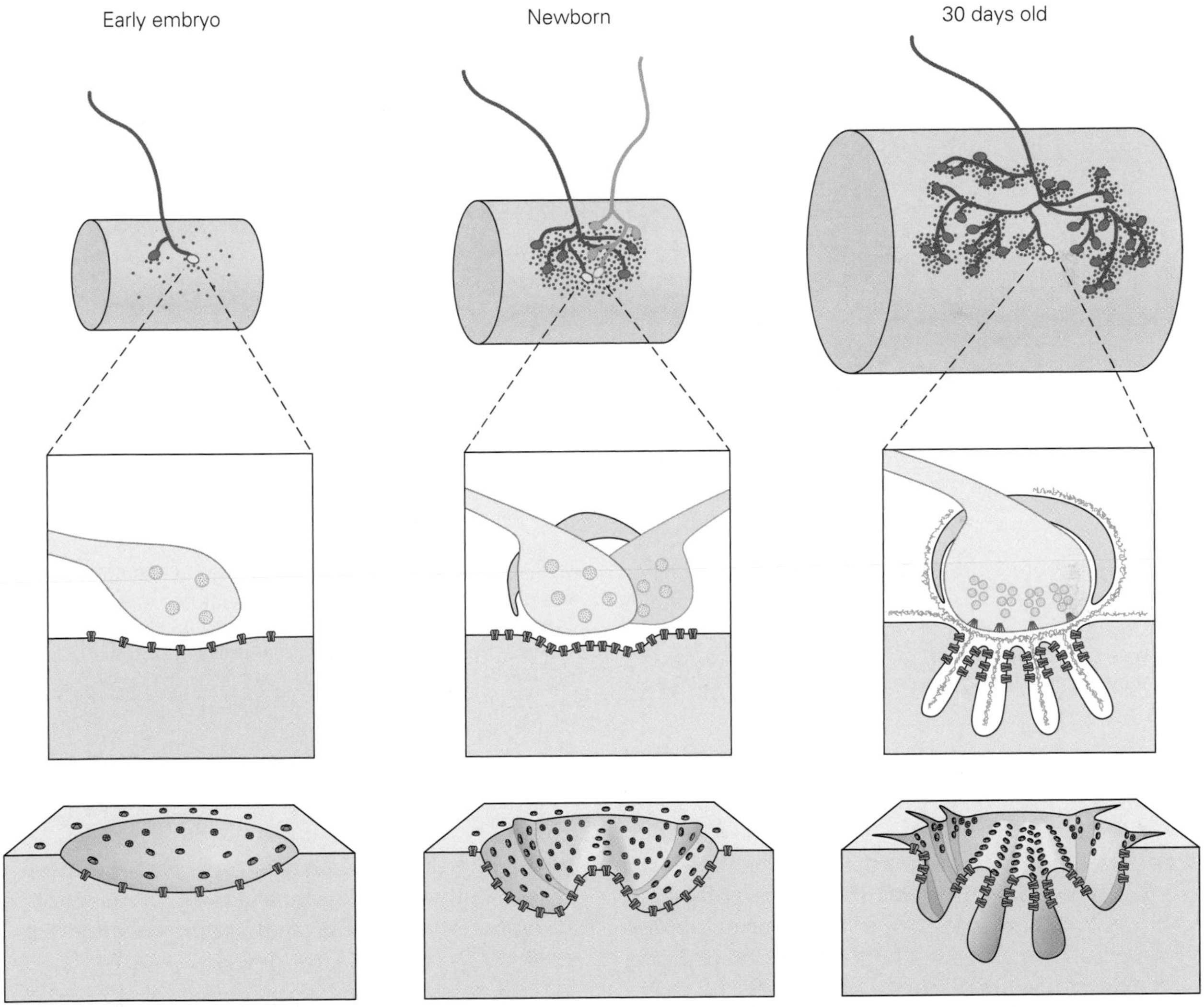

Figure 55–13 The postsynaptic membrane at the neuromuscular junction matures in stages. During early embryogenesis ACh receptors exist as loose aggregates. Later these aggregates condense into a plaque-like structure. After birth the dense cluster opens up as the nerve develops multiple terminals. These axon branches expand in an intercalary fashion as the muscle grows, and the plaque indents to form a gutter, which then invaginates to form folds. Receptors are concentrated at the crests of the folds. (Adapted, with permission, from Sanes and Lichtman 2001.)

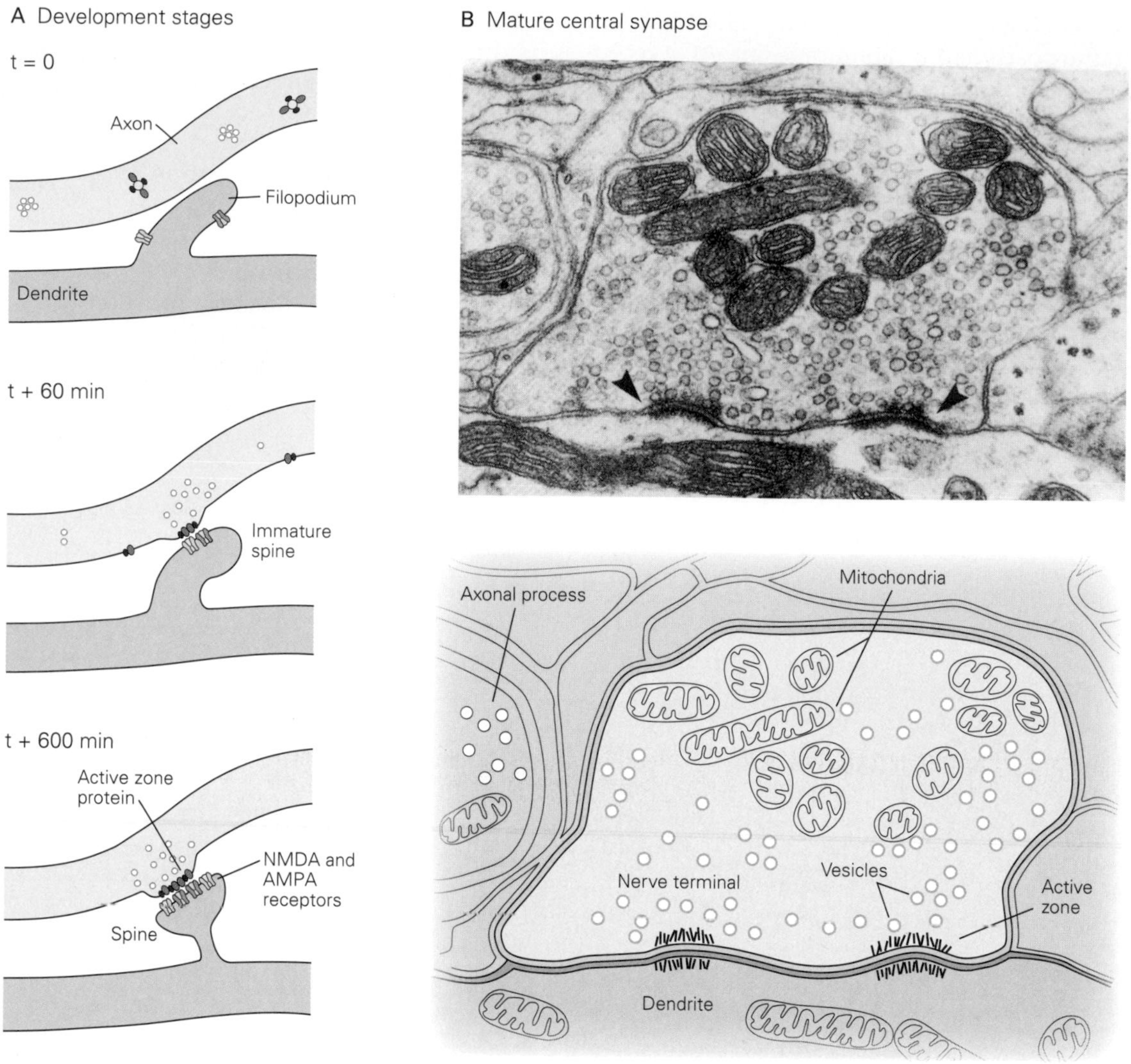

Figure 55–14 Ultrastructure of a synapse in the mammalian central nervous system.

A. Initial contact between an axon and a filopodium on a developing dendrite leads to a stable dendritic spine and an axo-dendritic synapse. This entire process can take as little as 60 minutes.

B. In a mature interneuron synapse in the cerebellum, synaptic vesicles in the nerve terminal are clustered at active zones (**arrows**) directly opposite receptor-rich patches of postsynaptic membrane. (Reproduced, with permission, from J.E. Heuser and T.S. Reese.)

junction: Pre- and postsynaptic elements regulate each other's differentiation by organizing presynthesized synaptic components rather than by inducing expression of specific genes, and synapses develop in a progressive series of steps (Figure 53–14).

Resolving whether this cellular parallel extends to the molecular level has proven difficult, because of the small size and relative inaccessibility of central synapses. But studies of cultured neurons suggest that the cellular logic of synapse formation is indeed conserved between neuromuscular junctions and central synapses, although different organizers are involved.

Neurotransmitter Receptors Become Localized at Central Synapses

The concentration of neurotransmitter receptors in the postsynaptic membrane is a feature shared by many synapses. In the brain, receptors for glutamate, glycine, GABA (γ-aminobutyric acid), and other neurotransmitters are concentrated in patches of membrane aligned with nerve terminals that contain the corresponding transmitter.

The processes by which these receptors become localized may be similar to those at the neuromuscular junction. In cultures of dissociated hippocampal neurons, for example, both glutamatergic and GABA-ergic nerve terminals appear to stimulate clustering of appropriate receptors in the postsynaptic membrane (Figure 55–15). The mediators of these effects are unknown. Moreover, nerves can induce expression of genes encoding glutamate receptors in central

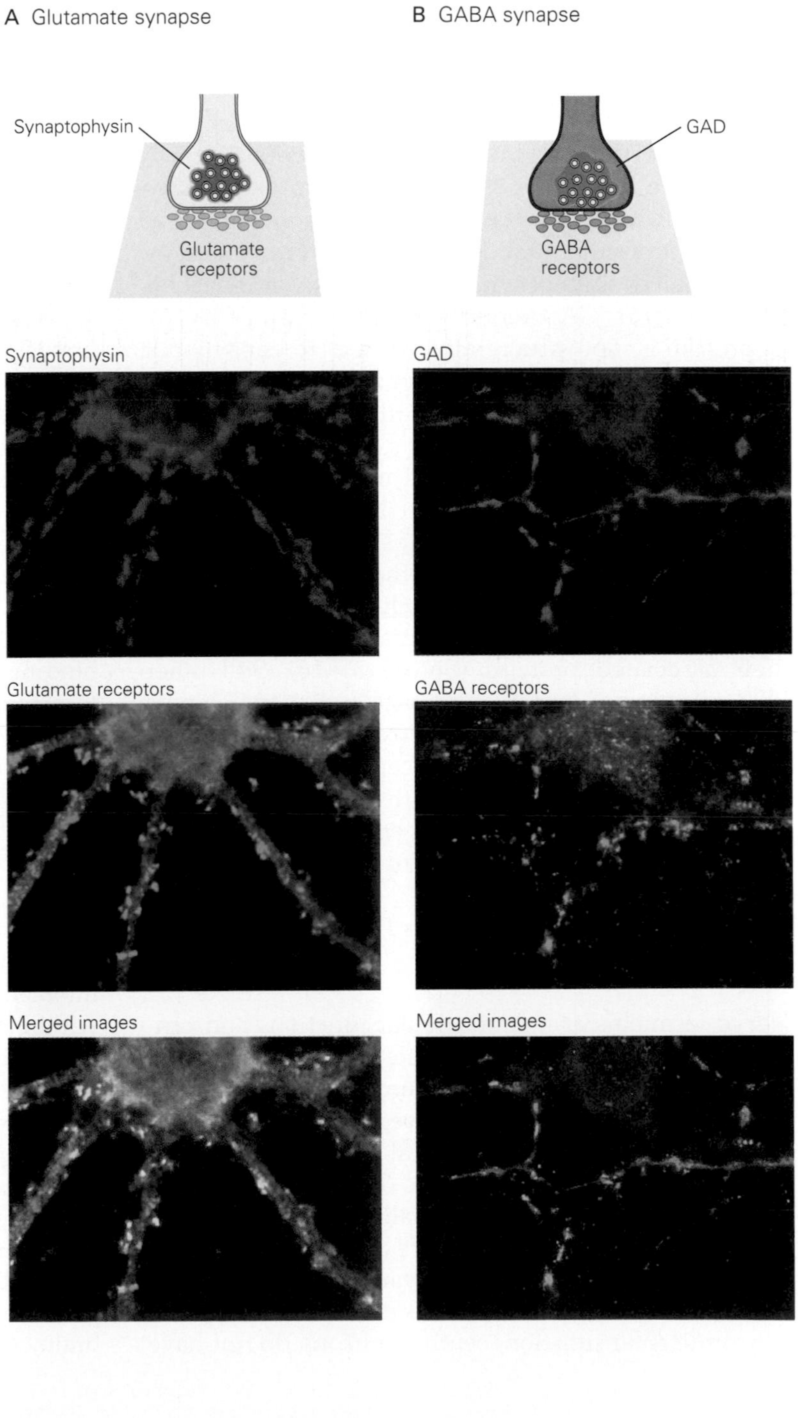

Figure 55–15 **Localization of neurotransmitter receptors in central neurons.** Glutamate and GABA receptors are localized at excitatory and inhibitory synapses in culture. Glutamate receptors are clustered underneath synaptophysin-labeled excitatory nerve terminals, but not all clusters of glutamate receptors are associated with nerve terminals. GABA receptors are clustered under inhibitory terminal boutons that express GAD67. (**GABA**, γ-aminobutyric acid; **GAD**, glutamic acid decarboxylase.) (Images reproduced, with permission, from A. M. Craig.)

neurons, much as occurs for ACh receptors in muscle. Finally, electrical activity also regulates expression of neurotransmitter receptors in neurons.

In forming receptor clusters, central neurons face an obvious challenge that myotubes do not: They are contacted by axon terminals from distinct classes of neurons that use different neurotransmitters. Thus the nerve terminal probably has an instructive role in the clustering of receptors. In cultures of hippocampal neurons, glutamatergic and GABAergic axons terminate on adjacent regions of the same dendrite. Initially glutamate and GABA receptors are dispersed, but soon each type becomes selectively clustered beneath terminals that release that neurotransmitter. This observation implies the existence of multiple clustering signals with parallel pathways of signal transduction.

In central neurons several distinct proteins have been found to play a role similar to that of rapsyn at the neuromuscular junction. One, gephyrin, is highly concentrated in the synaptic densities at glycinergic and some GABAergic synapses (Figure 55–16). Gephyrin is not structurally related to rapsyn but appears to have similar functions: it links the receptors to the underlying cytoskeleton. Its overexpression in nonneural cells leads to clustering of glycine receptors. Moreover, in gephyrin-deficient mutant mice glycine receptor clusters fail to form at inhibitory synapses. Similarly, a class of proteins that share conserved segments called PDZ domains—the prototypes being PSD-95 or SAP-90—facilitates clustering of NMDA-type (*N*-methyl-D-aspartate) glutamate receptors and their associated proteins (Figure 55–16). Still other PDZ-containing proteins interact with AMPA-type (α-amino-3-hydroxy-5-methylisoxazole-4-propionate) and metabotropic glutamate receptors. Different presynaptic signals may activate pathways that lead to the expression and localization of gephyrin, PSD-95, and other functionally related proteins.

Synaptic Organizing Molecules Pattern Central Nerve Terminals

Nerve terminals at neuromuscular junctions and central synapses are quite similar, reflecting the fact that the motor axon is part of a central neuron. Most of the major protein components of synaptic vesicles have now been isolated and appear to be identical at both types of synapses. Likewise, the mechanisms of transmitter release differ only quantitatively, not qualitatively.

However, the synaptic cleft differs dramatically. Whereas muscle fibers are ensheathed by a basal lamina that has a distinctive molecular structure at the neuromuscular junction, central neurons do not have a prominent basal lamina. Central synaptic clefts contain no detectable laminin or collagen. Instead, intercellular adhesion at central synapses may involve the interaction of matched adhesion molecules on pre- and postsynaptic membranes, with no intermediate matrix.

Several adhesion molecules link the pre- and postsynaptic membrane and also pattern presynaptic differentiation as synapses form. Among them is a class of proteins in postsynaptic membranes, the neuroligins. Their receptors on axonal membranes are the neurexins. The ability of neuroligins to promote presynaptic differentiation was first revealed by culturing neurons with nonneural cells engineered to express neuroligins. In culture synaptic vesicles form clusters at sites of contact with the neuroligin-expressing cells and they are capable of releasing neurotransmitter when stimulated (Figure 55–17). Conversely, neurotransmitter receptors in dendrites aggregate at sites that contact nonneural cells engineered to express neurexins. Thus neurexin-neuroligin interactions facilitate precise apposition of pre- and postsynaptic specializations. Differences among neurexin and neuroligin protein isoforms may also contribute to the matching of excitatory and inhibitory nerve terminals with excitatory and inhibitory neurotransmitter receptors.

How do neurexins and neuroligins work? Part of the answer is that their carboxy terminal tails bind to PDZ domains in proteins such as PSD-95 (Figure 55–16). Indeed, a remarkable number of proteins in both pre- and postsynaptic membranes have PDZ domain-binding motifs, notably adhesion molecules, neurotransmitter receptors, and ion channels. Moreover, many cytoplasmic proteins that possess PDZ domains are present in nerve terminals and beneath the postsynaptic membrane. Thus PDZ-containing proteins can serve as scaffolding molecules that link key components on both sides of the synapse. Interactions of proteins such as neurexins and neuroligins may provide a means of coupling the intercellular interactions required for synaptic recognition to the intracellular interactions required to cluster synaptic components within the cell membrane.

An indication of their critical role is that mutations of neurexin and neuroligin genes have been found in a small subset of patients with autism. However, even though neurexin-neuroligin interactions can organize synapses in culture, it remains unclear whether this is their primary role in vivo. Genetic deletion of neurexins or neuroligins has little effect on synapse size or number. Thus other transsynaptic ligand-receptor pairs may organize synaptic differentiation in the brain, with neuroligins and neurexins consolidating

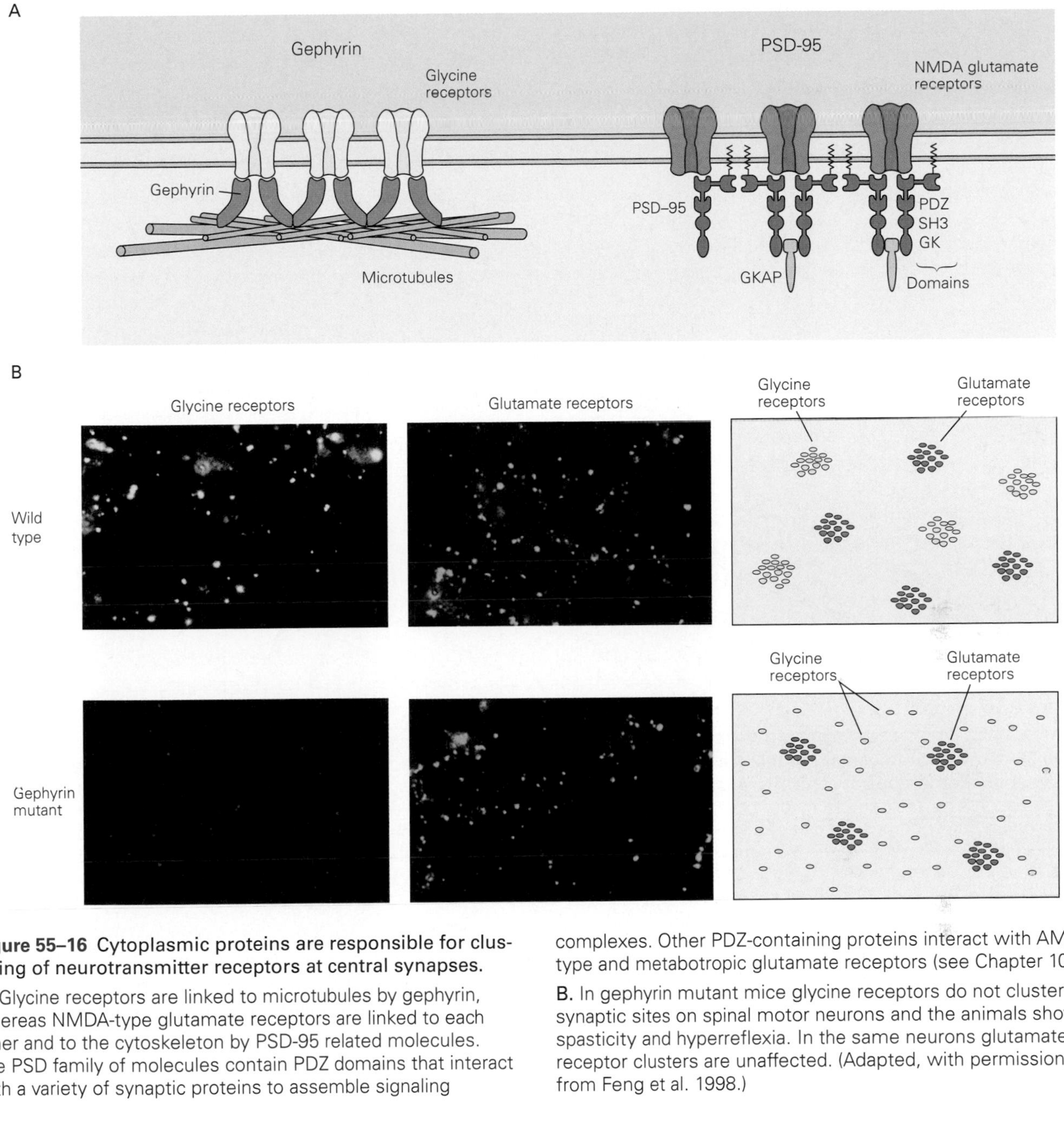

Figure 55–16 Cytoplasmic proteins are responsible for clustering of neurotransmitter receptors at central synapses.

A. Glycine receptors are linked to microtubules by gephyrin, whereas NMDA-type glutamate receptors are linked to each other and to the cytoskeleton by PSD-95 related molecules. The PSD family of molecules contain PDZ domains that interact with a variety of synaptic proteins to assemble signaling complexes. Other PDZ-containing proteins interact with AMPA-type and metabotropic glutamate receptors (see Chapter 10).

B. In gephyrin mutant mice glycine receptors do not cluster at synaptic sites on spinal motor neurons and the animals show spasticity and hyperreflexia. In the same neurons glutamate receptor clusters are unaffected. (Adapted, with permission, from Feng et al. 1998.)

these synapses at a later time and specifying their particular properties. Candidate synaptic organizers include adhesion molecules of the cadherin and immunoglobulin superfamilies, as well as ephrins and Eph kinases, and soluble members of the fibroblast growth factor and Wnt families of morphogens. Which of the many proteins capable of influencing synaptic differentiation in culture are actually crucial for synapse formation in vivo remains to be determined.

Glial Cells Promote Synapse Formation

We have focused on the pre- and postsynaptic partners at synapses, but the organization of synapses involves a third cellular element: glial cells. Schwann cells are the glia at neuromuscular junctions, and astrocytes are the glia at central synapses. Neurons form few synapses when cultured in isolation but many when glia are present (Figure 55–18A).

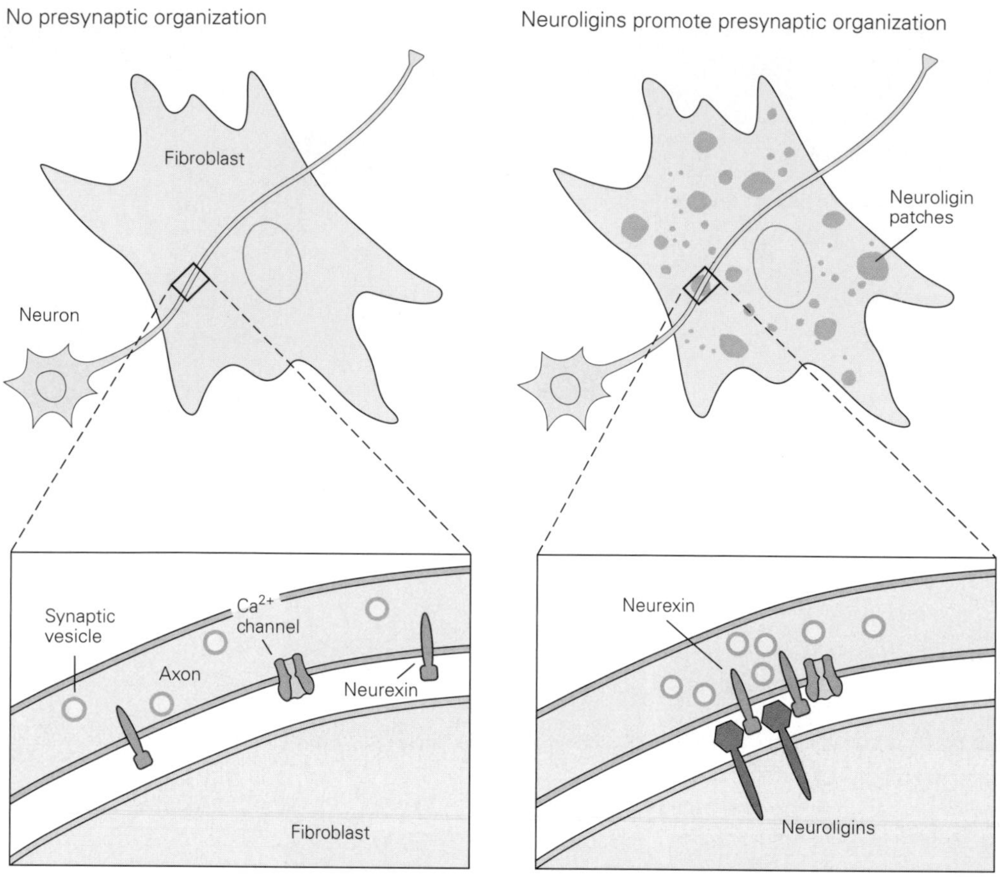

Figure 55–17 Macromolecular complexes link pre- and postsynaptic membranes at central synapses. Interactions between neurexins and neuroligins promote synaptic differentiation. When brain neurons are cultured with cells that express neuroligin, those segments of the axon that contact these cells form presynaptic specializations, marked by clustered neurexin, Ca^{2+} channels, and synaptic vesicles. Neurons grown with control cells lacking neuroligins lack such presynaptic specializations. (Adapted, with permission, from Scheiffele et al. 2000 and Graf et al. 2004.)

Glial cell surface and secreted molecules are both required for optimal synapse formation. Several glial-derived molecules that enhance synapse function have been isolated. One in particular is a large matrix protein, thrombospondin, and another a lipid, cholesterol. Others presumably remain to be discovered.

Some Synapses Are Eliminated After Birth

In adult mammals each muscle fiber bears only a single synapse. However, this is not the case in the embryo. At intermediate stages of development several axons converge on each myotube and form synapses at a common site. Soon after birth all inputs but one are eliminated.

The process of synapse elimination is not a consequence of neuronal death. It occurs long after the period of naturally occurring cell death (see Chapter 53). Each motor axon withdraws branches from some muscle fibers but strengthens its connections with others, thus focusing its increasing capacity for transmitter release on a decreasing number of targets. Moreover, axonal elimination is not targeted to defective synapses; all inputs to a neonatal myotube are morphologically and electrically similar, and each can activate the postsynaptic cell (Figure 55–19).

What is the purpose of the transient stage of polyneuronal innervation? One possibility is that it ensures that each muscle fiber is innervated. A second is that it allows all axons to capture an appropriate set of target cells. A third, intriguing idea is that synapse elimination provides a means by which activity can change the strength of specific synaptic connections. We begin to explore this idea in Chapter 56.

Like synapse formation, synapse elimination results from intercellular interactions. Every muscle

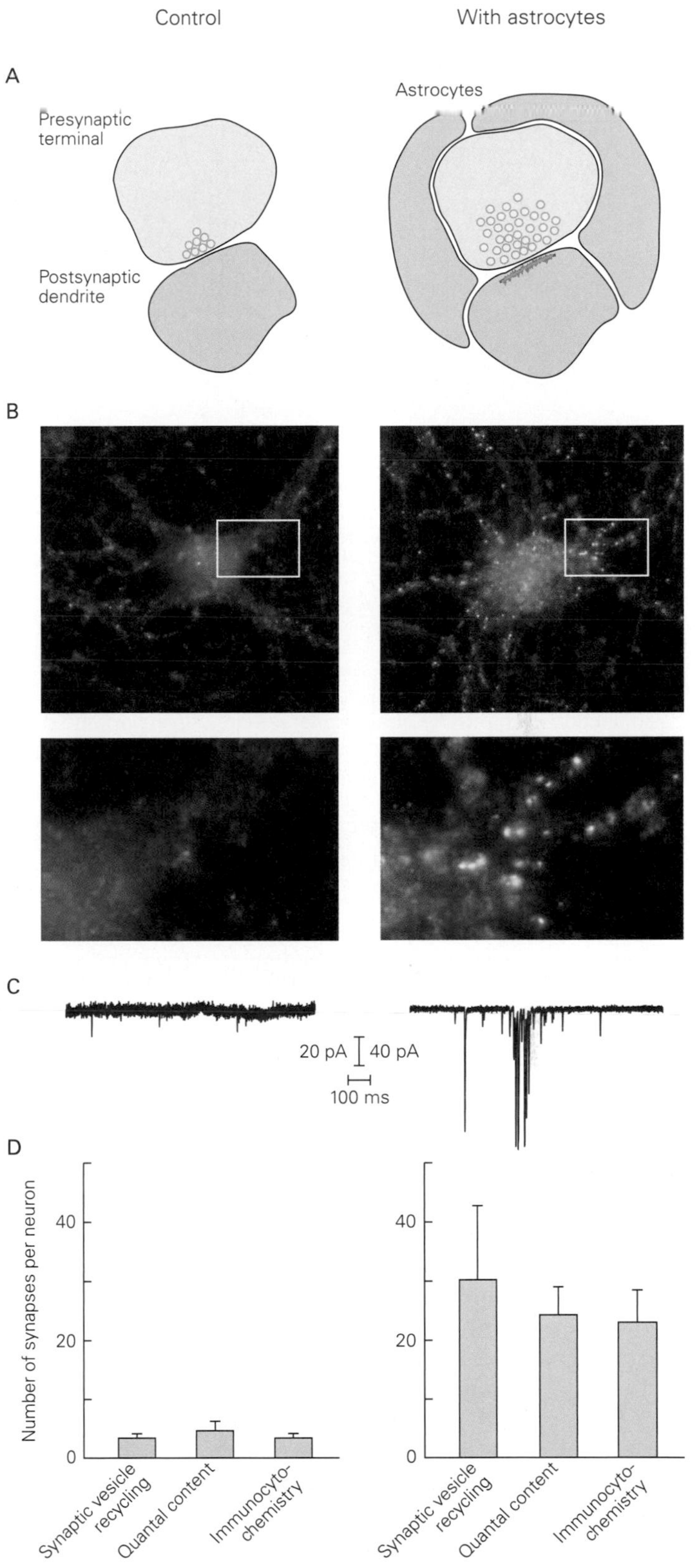

Figure 55–18 Signals from glial cells promote synapse formation.

A. Astrocytes promote the maturation of both pre- and postsynaptic elements of the synapse.

B. Neurons cultured with astrocytes form more synapses, as assessed by expression of synaptic proteins (**yellow dots**). (Reproduced, with permission, from Ben A. Barres.)

C. Retinal neurons cultured with astrocytes form a greater number of synapses, as shown by increased transmitter release.

D. Synapse formation is enhanced in the presence of astrocytes by three measures.

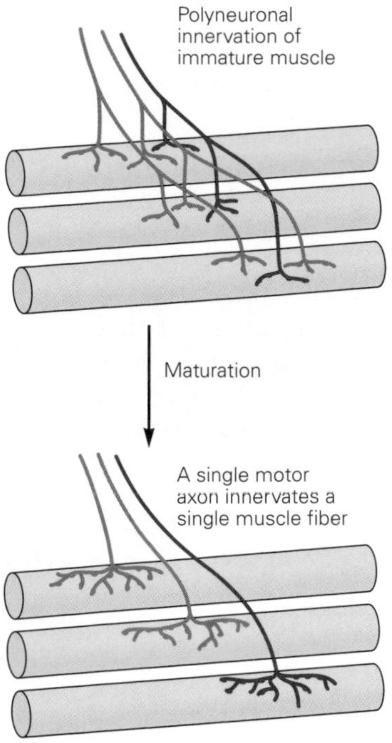

Figure 55–19 Some neuromuscular synapses are eliminated after birth. Early in the development of the neuromuscular junction each muscle fiber is innervated by several motor axons. After birth all motor axons but one withdraw from each fiber and the surviving axon becomes more elaborate. Synapse elimination occurs without any overall loss of axons—axons that "lose" at some muscle fibers "win" at others.

fiber ends up with exactly one input: None have zero, and very few have more than one. It is difficult to imagine how this could occur without feedback from the muscle cell. Moreover, the axons that remain after partial denervation at birth have a larger number of synapses than they did initially. Thus synapse elimination appears to be a competitive process.

What drives the competition and what is the reward? There is good evidence that neural activity plays a role: Paralysis of muscle reduces competition, whereas direct stimulation enhances it. These findings show that activity is involved, but they do not show that activity determines the outcome of the process, as all axons are affected similarly. Because the essence of the competitive process is that some synapses gain territory at the expense of others, differential activity among axons may be a determinant of axon winners and losers. Changing the activity of only a subset of axons in a living animal has been a technical challenge, but genetic approaches have made this possible in mice. In fact, when the activity of one of the inputs to a muscle fiber is decreased, that axon is highly likely to withdraw.

If the more active axon wins the competition, there is a new problem. Because all synapses made by an axon have the same activity pattern, one might predict that the least active axon in the muscle would eventually lose all of its synapses and the most active would retain all of its synapses. Yet this does not happen. Instead, all axons win at some sites and lose at others, so that every axon ends up innervating a substantial number of muscle fibers.

One possible resolution to this paradox is that the outcome of competition may not be determined by the number of synaptic potentials from the winning axon at a synapse but rather by the total amount of synaptic input that the axon provides to the muscle—a product of the number of impulses and the amount of transmitter released per impulse. In this case an axon that loses at several synapses might redistribute its resources (for example, synaptic vesicles) so that the remaining terminals would be strengthened and more likely to win at their synapses. Conversely, an axon that wins many competitions might find itself with insufficient vesicles to generate large synaptic potentials, and would eventually lose to competitors at some synapses. In this way the number of muscle fibers innervated by individual axons would vary little among axons, as observed.

If activity drives the competition, what is the object of the competition? One idea is that the mechanisms are similar to those that determine whether neurons live or die. The muscle might produce limited amounts of a trophic substance for which the axons compete. As the winner grows it either deprives the loser of its sustenance or gains enough strength to mount an attack on its competitor. Alternatively, the muscle might release a toxic or punitive factor. In these scenarios, although the muscle does contribute a factor in the competition, the outcome is entirely dependent on differences between axons. These differences could be related to activity. The more active axon might be better able to take up trophic factor or resist a toxin. Such positive and negative competitive interactions have been demonstrated at nerve-muscle synapses in culture although not in vivo.

The muscle, however, could play a selective role in synapse elimination rather than just providing a broadly distributed signal. This idea is based on studies in which individual neuromuscular junctions were observed at close intervals during the process of synapse elimination. Acetylcholine receptors and components of the postsynaptic cytoskeleton begin to disappear from parts of the maturing neuromuscular junction before nerve terminals withdraw. This suggests that differences in activity among competing axons may elicit different responses in postsynaptic ACh receptors. For example, the more active axon might trigger a signal from the muscle fiber that strengthens its adhesive interactions with the synaptic cleft, whereas the less active axon might elicit a signal that weakens those interactions.

The complexity of the brain makes direct demonstration of synapse elimination problematic, but electrophysiological evidence from many parts of the central nervous system indicates that synapse elimination is widespread. In autonomic ganglia synapse elimination has been documented directly and their rules seem similar to that found at neuromuscular junctions. Individual axons withdraw from some postsynaptic cells while simultaneously increasing the size of the synapses they form with other neurons.

An Overall View

The formation of synapses completes the hardwiring of the nervous system. To form a functional network, synaptic connections must be exquisitely specific: nerve terminals must recognize the proper target cell from numerous potential partners and often even a specific portion of the target cell's surface. Specificity starts with molecular recognition between partners and is enhanced by patterns of electrical activity.

The requirements for the synapse are stringent. The postsynaptic membrane must be responsive to the neurotransmitter that the nerve terminal releases. The apposition of pre- and postsynaptic elements must be precise at a molecular level, so that responses can occur on a time scale of milliseconds. And synaptic structure must be sufficiently stable to last a lifetime, yet sufficiently plastic to change with experience.

To meet these demands, synaptogenesis needs to be a highly interactive process. Although the pre- and postsynaptic cells can each synthesize synaptic components on their own, they exchange numerous signals to coordinate their activities spatially and temporally. In this chapter we have illustrated these interactions primarily with a focus on the neuromuscular junction. Motor nerve terminals use a combination of electrical and chemical signals to sculpt the postsynaptic apparatus of the muscle fiber. One key signal is agrin, which acts with the neurotransmitter ACh to sculpt the postsynaptic membrane. In turn, the muscle fiber provides signals that organize synaptic specialization in the nerve terminal, signals that include both soluble trophic factors and matrix-associated proteins such as the laminins.

Although central synapses are less accessible, it is becoming clear that they develop by the same general rules as neuromuscular junctions. Some developmentally important molecules found at the neuromuscular junction also regulate differentiation of central synapses, but the latter also use different signals such as the neurexins and neuroligins.

Finally, some of the synapses formed by a particular axon are eliminated, while others prosper. Axons begin by making small synapses on many targets, and end up with large synapses on relatively few targets. This rearrangement is often triggered by activity providing a means through which experience, translated into neural impulses, can modify neural circuits during early life.

Joshua R. Sanes
Thomas M. Jessell

Selected Readings

Barres BA. 2008. The mystery and magic of glia: a perspective on their roles in health and disease. Neuron 60:430–440.

Baudouin S, Scheiffele P. 2010. Neuroligin-neurexin complexes. Cell 141:908.

Craig AM, Graf ER, Linhoff MW. 2006. How to build a central synapse: clues from cell culture. Trends Neurosci 29:8–20.

Huang ZJ, Scheiffele P. 2008. GABA and neuroligin signaling: linking synaptic activity and adhesion in inhibitory synapse development. Curr Opin Neurobiol 18:77–83.

Huberman AD, Feller MB, Chapman B. 2008. Mechanisms underlying development of visual maps and receptive fields. Annu Rev Neurosci 31:479–509.

Sanes JR, Lichtman JW. 2001. Induction, assembly, maturation and maintenance of a postsynaptic apparatus. Nat Rev Neurosci 2:791–805.

Sanes JR, Yamagata M. 2009. Many paths to synaptic specificity. Annu Rev Cell Dev Biol 25:161–195.

References

Anderson, MJ, Cohen MW. 1977. Nerve-induced and spontaneous redistribution of acetylcholine receptors on cultured muscle cells. J Physiol 268:757–773.

Ango F, di Cristo G, Higashiyama H, Bennett V, Wu P, Huang ZJ. 2004. Ankyrin-based subcellular gradient of neurofascin, an immunoglobulin family protein, directs GABAergic innervation at Purkinje axon initial segment. Cell 119:257–272.

Balice-Gordon RJ, Lichtman JW. 1994. Long-term synapse loss induced by focal blockade of postsynaptic receptors. Nature 372:519–524.

Buffelli M, Busetto G, Bidoia C, Favero M, Cangiano A. 2004. Activity-dependent synaptic competition at mammalian neuromuscular junctions. News Physiol Sci 19:85–91.

Buller AJ, Eccles JC, Eccles RM. 1960. Interactions between motoneurons and muscles in respect of the characteristic speeds of their responses. J Physiol 150:417–439.

Burden SJ, Sargent PB, McMahan, UJ. 1979. Acetylcholine receptors in regenerating muscle accumulate at original synaptic sites in the absence of the nerve. J Cell Biol 82:412–425.

Christopherson KS, Ullian EM, Stokes CC, Mullowney CE, Hell JW, Agah A, Lawler J, Mosher DF, Bornstein P, Barres BA. 2005. Thrombospondins are astrocyte-secreted proteins that promote CNS synaptogenesis. Cell 120:421–433.

DeChiara TM, Bowen DC, Valenzuela DM, Simmons MV, Poueymirou WT, Thomas S, Kinetz E, et al. 1996. The receptor tyrosine kinase MuSK is required for neuromuscular junction formation in vivo. Cell 85:501–512.

Feng G, Tintrup H, Kirsch J, Nichol MC, Kuhse J, Betz H, Sanes JR. 1998. Dual requirement for gephyrin in glycine receptor clustering and molybdoenzyme activity. Science 282:1321–1324.

Fox MA, Sanes JR, Borza DB, Eswarakumar VP, Fassler R, Hudson BG, John SW, et al. 2007. Distinct target-derived signals organize formation, maturation, and maintenance of motor nerve terminals. Cell 129:179–193.

Fox MA, Umemori H. 2006. Seeking long-term relationship: axon and target communicate to organize synaptic differentiation. J Neurochem 97:1215–1231.

Garner CC, Waites CL, Ziv NE. 2006. Synapse development: still looking for the forest, still lost in the trees. Cell Tissue Res 326:249–262.

Gautam M, Noakes PG, Moscoso L, Rupp F, Scheller RH, Merlie JP, Sanes JR. 1996. Defective neuromuscular synaptogenesis in agrin-deficient mutant mice. Cell 85:525–535.

Glicksman MA, Sanes JR. 1983. Differentiation of motor nerve terminals formed in the absence of muscle fibres. J Neurocytol 12:661–671.

Graf ER, Zhang X, Jin SX, Linhoff MW, Craig AM. 2004. Neurexins induce differentiation of GABA and glutamate postsynaptic specializations via neuroligins. Cell 119:1013–1026.

Hall ZW, Sanes JR. 1993. Synaptic structure and development: the neuromuscular junction. Cell 72:99–121. Suppl.

Huang ZJ. 2006. Subcellular organization of GABAergic synapses: role of ankyrins and L1 cell adhesion molecules. Nat Neurosci 9:163–166.

Imai T, Suzuki M, Sakano H. 2006. Odorant receptor-derived cAMP signals direct axonal targeting. Science 314:657–661.

Kim E, Sheng M. 2004. PDZ domain proteins of synapses. Nat Rev Neurosci 5:771–781.

Lichtman JW, Colman H. 2000. Synapse elimination and indelible memory. Neuron 25:269–278.

Lupa MT, Gordon H, Hall ZW. 1990. A specific effect of muscle cells on the distribution of presynaptic proteins in neurites and its absence in a C2 muscle cell variant. Dev Biol 142:31–43.

McAllister AK. 2007. Dynamic aspects of CNS synapse formation. Annu Rev Neurosci 30:425–450.

McMahan UJ. 1990. The agrin hypothesis. Cold Spring Harb Sym Quant Biol 55:407–418.

Misgeld T, Kummer TT, Lichtman JW, Sanes JR. 2005. Agrin promotes synaptic differentiation by counteracting an inhibitory effect of neurotransmitter. Proc Natl Acad Sci U S A 102:11088–11093.

Mori K, Sakano H. 2011. How is the olfactory map formed and interpreted in the mammalian brain? Annu Rev Neurosci 34:467–499.

Nishimune H, Sanes JR, Carlson SS. 2004. A synaptic laminin-calcium channel interaction organizes active zones in motor nerve terminals. Nature 432:580–587.

Nja A, Purves D. 1977. Re-innervation of guinea-pig superior cervical ganglion cells by preganglionic fibres arising from different levels of the spinal cord. J Physiol 272:633–651.

Noakes PG, Gautam M, Mudd J, Sanes JR, Merlie JP. 1995. Aberrant differentiation of neuromuscular junctions in mice lacking s-laminin/laminin beta 2. Nature 374:258–262.

Okada K, Inoue A, Okada M, Murata Y, Kakuta S, Jigami T, Kubo S, et al. 2006. The muscle protein Dok-7 is essential for neuromuscular synaptogenesis. Science 312: 1802–1805.

Salmons S, Sreter FA. 1976. Significance of impulse activity in the transformation of skeletal muscle type. Nature 263:30–34.

Sanes JR, Lichtman JW. 1999. Development of the vertebrate neuromuscular junction. Annu Rev Neurosci 22:389–442.

Sanes JR, Lichtman JW. 2001. Induction, assembly, maturation and maintenance of a postsynaptic apparatus. Nat Rev Neurosci 2:791–805.

Sanes JR, Yamagata M. 2009. Many paths to synaptic specificity. Annu Rev Cell Dev Biol 25:161–195.

Scheiffele P, Fan J, Choih J, Fetter R, Serafini T. 2000. Neuroligin expressed in nonneuronal cells triggers presynaptic development in contacting axons. Cell 101:657–669.

Serizawa S, Miyamichi K, Takeuchi H, Yamagishi Y, Suzuki M, Sakano H. 2006. A neuronal identity code for the odorant receptor-specific and activity-dependent axon sorting. Cell 127:1057–1069.

Shen K, Fetter RD, Bargmann CI. 2004. Synaptic specificity is generated by the synaptic guidepost protein SYG-2 and its receptor, SYG-1. Cell 116:869–881.

Takeichi M. 2007. The cadherin superfamily in neuronal connections and interactions. Nat Rev Neurosci 8:11–20.

Torborg CL, Feller MB. 2005. Spontaneous patterned retinal activity and the refinement of retinal projections. Prog Neurobiol 76:213–235.

Vaughn JE. 1989. Fine structure of synaptogenesis in the vertebrate central nervous system. Synapse 3:255–285.

Walsh MK, Lichtman JW. 2003. In vivo time-lapse imaging of synaptic takeover associated with naturally occurring synapse elimination. Neuron 37:67–73.

Wu H, Xiong WC, Mei L. 2010. To build a synapse: signaling pathways in neuromuscular junction assembly. Development 137:1017–1033.

Yamagata M, Sanes JR. 2008. Dscams and Sidekicks direct lamina-specific synaptic connections in vertebrate retina. Nature 451:465–469.

56

Experience and the Refinement of Synaptic Connections

THE HUMAN NERVOUS SYSTEM IS FUNCTIONAL at birth: Newborn babies can see, hear, breathe, and suckle. However, the capabilities of human infants are quite rudimentary compared to those of other species. Wildebeest calves can stand and run within minutes of birth, and many birds can fly shortly after they hatch from their eggs. In contrast, a human baby cannot lift its head until it is 2 months old, cannot bring food to its mouth until it is 6 months old, and cannot survive without parental care for a decade.

What accounts for the delayed maturation of our motor, perceptual, and cognitive abilities? One main factor is that the embryonic connectivity of the nervous system, discussed in Chapters 52 through 55, is only a "rough draft" of the neural circuits that exist in our adult selves. After birth, embryonic circuits are refined by sensory stimulation—our experiences. This two-part sequence—genetically determined connectivity followed by experience-dependent reorganization—is a common feature of mammalian neural development, but in humans the second phase is especially prolonged.

At first glance this delay in human neural development might seem dysfunctional. Although it does exact a toll, it also provides an advantage. Because our mental abilities are shaped largely by experience, we gain the ability to custom fit our nervous systems to our individual bodies and unique environments. It could be argued that it is not the large size of the human brain but rather its experience-dependent maturation that makes our mental capabilities superior to those of other species.

The plasticity of the nervous system in response to experience endures throughout life. Nevertheless, periods of heightened susceptibility to modification, known as *sensitive periods*, occur at particular times in development. In some cases the adverse effects of deprivation or atypical experience early in life cannot easily be reversed by providing appropriate experience at a later age. Such necessary periods of development are referred to as *critical periods*. As we shall see, new discoveries are blurring the distinction between sensitive and critical periods, so we will use the term critical periods to refer to both.

Critical periods can most easily be appreciated from the perspective of behavior—the capacity to perceive the world around us, to learn a language, or to form strong social relationships. A 5-year-old child can quickly and effortlessly learn a second language, whereas a 15-year-old adolescent may become fluent but is likely to speak with an accent, even if he lives to be 90 years old. Likewise, when a cataract that deprives a child of vision is removed in early childhood, there are no lasting effects of the cataract, but when the surgery occurs at the age of 10 years, she is unlikely ever to have normal visual acuity. In each of these cases relevant experience must occur within a critical period if behavior is to develop normally.

The process of learning is also influenced by critical periods. One of the most striking illustrations of a lifelong behavior established during a critical period is imprinting, a form of learning in birds. Just after hatching, birds become indelibly attached, or imprinted, to a prominent moving object in their environment, typically their mother. The process of imprinting is important for the protection of the hatchling. Although the attachment is acquired rapidly and persists, imprinting can only occur during a critical period soon after hatching—in some species only a few hours. Thus postnatal development of the nervous system can be viewed as a series of critical periods.

We begin this chapter by examining the evidence that early experience shapes a range of human mental capacities, from our ability to make sense of what we see to our ability to engage in appropriate social interactions. To illustrate the neural basis of these experiential effects we describe the role of experience in the development of the visual system in experimental animals. Studies of the development of the visual system have provided our most detailed understanding of how experience shapes neural circuitry throughout the brain. We will see that experience is needed to refine patterns of synaptic connections and to stabilize these patterns once they have formed. Finally, we will consider recent evidence that critical periods may be less restrictive than once thought; in some cases they can be extended or "reopened".

Understanding experience-dependent plasticity and the extent to which critical periods can be reopened in adulthood has important practical consequences. First, much educational policy is based on the idea that early experience is crucial, so it is important to know exactly when a particular form of enrichment will be optimally beneficial. Second, medical treatment of many childhood conditions, such as congenital cataracts, is now predicated on the idea that early intervention is imperative if long-lasting deficits are to be avoided. Third, there is increasing concern that some behavioral disorders, such as autism, may be caused by impaired reorganization of neural circuits during critical periods. Finally, the possibility of reopening critical periods in adulthood is leading to new therapeutic approaches to neural insults such as stroke that previously were thought to have irreversible consequences.

Development of Human Mental Function Is Influenced by Early Experience

Early Experience Has Lifelong Effects on Social Behaviors

The conclusion that certain social or perceptual experiences are important for human development was first arrived at through studies of children who had been deprived of these experiences early in life. In rare cases children abandoned in the wild and later returned to human society have been studied. As might be expected, these children were socially maladjusted. Surprisingly, however, the defects proved to be generally irreversible.

In the 1940s the psychoanalyst René Spitz provided more systematic evidence that early interactions with other humans are essential for normal social development. Spitz compared the development of infants raised in a foundling home with the development of infants raised in a nursing home attached to a women's prison. Both institutions were clean and both provided adequate food and medical care. The babies in the prison nursing home were all cared for by their mothers, who, although in prison and away from their families, tended to shower affection on their infants in the limited time allotted to them each day. In contrast, infants in the foundling home were cared for by nurses, each of whom was responsible for several babies. As a result, children in the foundling home had far less contact with other humans than did those in the prison's nursing home.

The two institutions also differed in another respect. In the prison nursing home the cribs were open, so that the infants could readily watch other activities in the ward; they could see other babies play and observe the staff go about their business. In the foundling home the bars of the cribs were covered by sheets that prevented the infants from seeing outside. In reality, the babies in the foundling home were living under conditions of severe sensory and social deprivation.

Groups of newborn infants at the two institutions were followed through their early years. At the end of the first 4 months the infants in the foundling home fared better on several developmental tests than those in the prison nursing home, suggesting that intrinsic factors did not favor the infants in the prison nursing home. But by the end of the first year the motor and intellectual performance of the children in the foundling home had fallen far below that of children in the prison nursing home. Many of the children in the foundling home had developed a syndrome that Spitz called *hospitalism* and is now often called *anaclitic depression*. These children were withdrawn and displayed little curiosity or gaiety. Moreover, their defects extended beyond the emotional and cognitive. They were especially prone to infection, implying that the brain exerts complex controls over the immune system as well as behavior. By their second and third years, children in the prison nursing home were similar to children raised in normal families at home—they were agile, had a vocabulary of hundreds of words, and spoke in sentences. In contrast, the development of children in the foundling home was still further delayed—many were unable to walk or to speak more than a few words.

More recent studies of other similarly deprived children have confirmed these conclusions and shown that the defects are long-lasting. Longitudinal studies of orphans who were raised for several years in large impersonal institutions with little or no personal care, then adopted by caring families, have been especially revealing. Despite every effort of the adoptive parents, many of the children were never able to develop appropriate, caring relationships with family members or peers (Figure 56–1A). More recent imaging studies have revealed defects in brain structure correlated with, and presumably due to, this deprivation (Figure 56–1B).

As compelling as these studies on humans are, it is difficult to derive definitive conclusions. An influential set of studies that extended the analysis of social behavior to monkeys was carried out in the 1960s by two psychologists, Harry and Margaret Harlow. The Harlows reared newborn monkeys in isolation for 6 to 12 months, depriving them of contact with their mothers, other monkeys, or people. At the end of this period the monkeys were physically healthy but behaviorally devastated. They crouched in a corner of their cage and rocked back and forth like autistic children (Figure 56–1C). They did not interact with other monkeys, nor did they fight, play, or show any sexual interest. Thus a 6-month period of social isolation during the first 18 months of life produced persistent and serious disturbances in behavior. By comparison, isolation of an older animal for a comparable period was found to be without such drastic consequences. These results confirmed, under controlled conditions, the critical influence of early experience on later behavior. For ethical reasons, these studies would not be possible today.

Development of Visual Perception Requires Visual Experience

The dramatic dependence of the brain on experience and the ability of that experience to shape perception is evident in people born with cataracts. Cataracts are opacities of the lens that interfere with the optics of the eye but not directly with the nervous system; they are easily removed surgically. In the 1930s it became apparent that patients who had congenital binocular cataracts removed after the age of 10 years had permanent deficits in visual acuity and had difficulties perceiving shape and form, a condition called *amblyopia*. In contrast, when cataracts that develop in adults are removed decades after they form, normal vision returns immediately.

Likewise, children with *strabismus* (crossed eyes) do not have normal depth perception (*stereopsis*), an ability that requires the two eyes to focus on the same location at the same time. They can acquire this ability if their eyes are aligned surgically during the first few years of life, but not if surgery occurs later in adolescence. As a result of these observations, congenital cataracts are now usually removed, and strabismus is corrected surgically, in early childhood. Over the past few decades researchers have elucidated structural and physiological underpinnings of these critical periods.

Development of Binocular Circuits in the Visual Cortex Depends on Postnatal Activity

Because sensory experience of the world is transformed into patterns of electrical activity in the brain, one might imagine that electrical signals in neural circuits affect the brain's circuitry. But is this true? And if it is true, what changes occur and how does activity trigger them?

Our most detailed understanding of these links comes from studies of the neural circuits that mediate

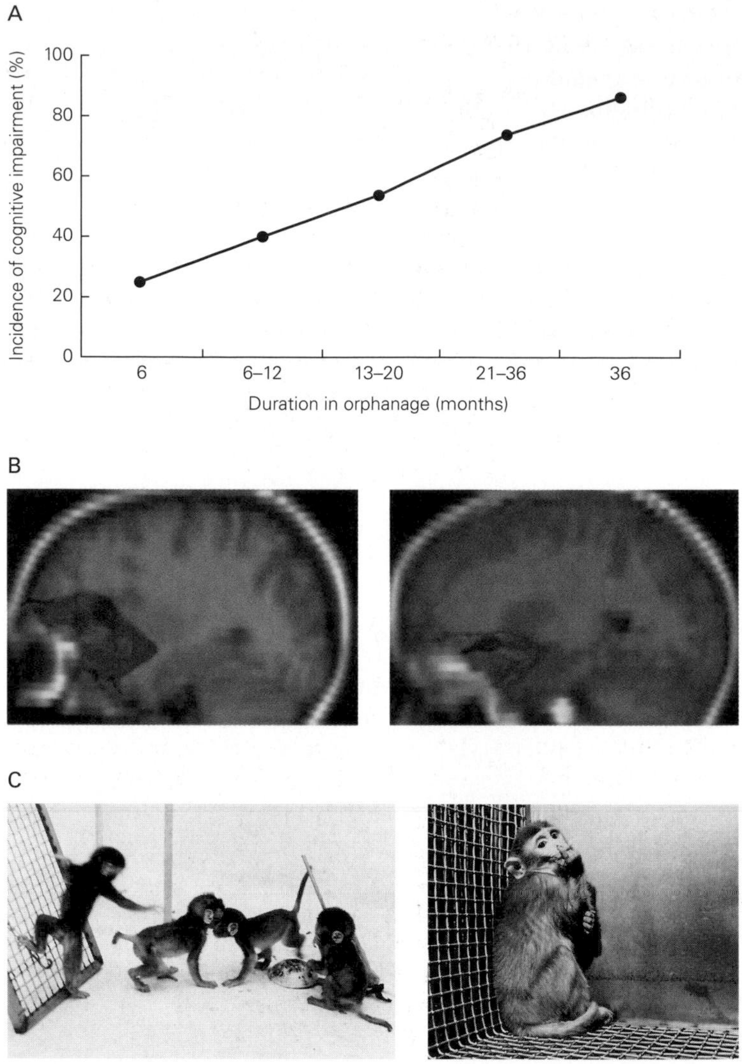

Figure 56–1 Early social deprivation has a profound impact on later brain structure and behavior.

A. Neurocognitive dysfunction is evident in children raised under conditions of social deprivation in orphanages. The incidence of cognitive impairment increases with the duration of stay in the orphanage. (Reproduced, with permission, from Behen et al. 2008.)

B. Diffusion tensor magnetic resonance imaging (MRI) scans show a well-developed and robust uncinate fasciculus (**red region**) in a normal child (left), whereas in a socially deprived child (right) it is thin and poorly organized. (Reproduced, with permission, from Eluvathingal et al. 2006.)

C. Early social interactions impact later social behavior patterns. Monkeys reared in the presence of their siblings acquire social skills that permit effective interactions in later life (left). A monkey reared in isolation never acquires the capacity to interact with others, and remains secluded and isolated in later life (right). (Adapted, with permission, from Harry F. Harlow, University of Wisconsin.)

binocular vision. The key figures in the early phases of this work were David Hubel and Torsten Wiesel, who undertook a set of studies on cats and monkeys to investigate how experience affects the structural and functional organization they had delineated (Figure 56–2).

Visual Experience Affects the Structure and Function of the Visual Cortex

In one influential study Hubel and Wiesel raised a monkey from birth to 6 months of age with one eyelid sutured shut, thus depriving the animal of vision in that eye. When the sutures were removed it became clear that the animal was blind in the deprived eye. They then performed electrophysiological recordings from cells along the visual pathway to determine where the defect arose. They found that retinal ganglion cells in the deprived eye, as well as neurons in the lateral geniculate nucleus that receive input from the deprived eye, responded well to visual stimuli and had essentially normal receptive fields.

In contrast, cells in the visual cortex were fundamentally altered. In the cortex of normal animals most neurons are binocularly responsive. In animals that had been monocularly deprived for the first 6 months, most cortical neurons did not respond to signals from the deprived eye (Figure 56–3). The few cortical cells that were responsive were not sufficient for visual perception. Not only had the deprived eye lost its ability to drive most cortical neurons, but this loss was permanent and irreversible.

Hubel and Wiesel went on to test the effects of visual deprivation imposed for shorter periods and at different ages. They obtained three types of results, depending on the timing and duration of the deprivation. First, monocular deprivation for a few weeks during the first 2 postnatal months led to loss of cortical responses from the deprived eye that was reversible after the eye had been opened, especially if the opposite eye was then closed to encourage use of the initially deprived eye. Second, monocular deprivation for a few weeks during the next months also resulted in a substantial loss of cortical responsiveness to signals from of the deprived eye, but in this case the effects were irreversible. Finally, deprivation in adults, even for periods of many months, had no effect on the responses of cortical cells to signals from the deprived eye or on visual perception. These results demonstrated that the cortical connections that control visual perception are established within a critical period of early development.

Are there structural correlates of these functional defects? To address this question we need to recall three basic facts about the anatomy of the visual cortex. First, inputs from the two eyes remain segregated in the lateral geniculate nucleus. Second, the geniculate inputs carrying information from the two eyes to the cortex terminate in alternating columns, termed *ocular dominance columns*. Third, lateral geniculate axons terminate on neurons in layer IVC of the primary visual cortex; convergence of input from the two eyes on a common target cell occurs at the next stage of the pathway, in cells above and below layer IVC (Figure 56–2).

To examine whether the architecture of ocular dominance columns depends on visual experience early in postnatal life, Hubel and Wiesel deprived newborn animals of vision in one eye and then injected a labeled amino acid into the normal eye. The injected label was incorporated into proteins in retinal ganglion cell bodies, transported along the retinal axons to the lateral geniculate nucleus, transferred to geniculate neurons, and then transported to the synaptic terminals of these axons in the primary visual cortex. After closure of one eye the columnar array of synaptic terminals relaying input from the deprived eye was reduced, whereas the columnar array of terminals relaying input from the normal eye was expanded (Figure 56–4). Thus sensory deprivation early in life alters the structure of the cerebral cortex.

How are these striking anatomical changes brought about? Does sensory deprivation alter ocular dominance columns after they have been established, or does it interfere with their formation? It is now clear that the mature pattern of ocular dominance columns in monkeys is not achieved until 6 weeks after birth (Figure 56–5). Only at this time do the terminals of fibers from the lateral geniculate nucleus become completely segregated in the cortex (Figure 56–6). Because the inputs are not well segregated at the time that

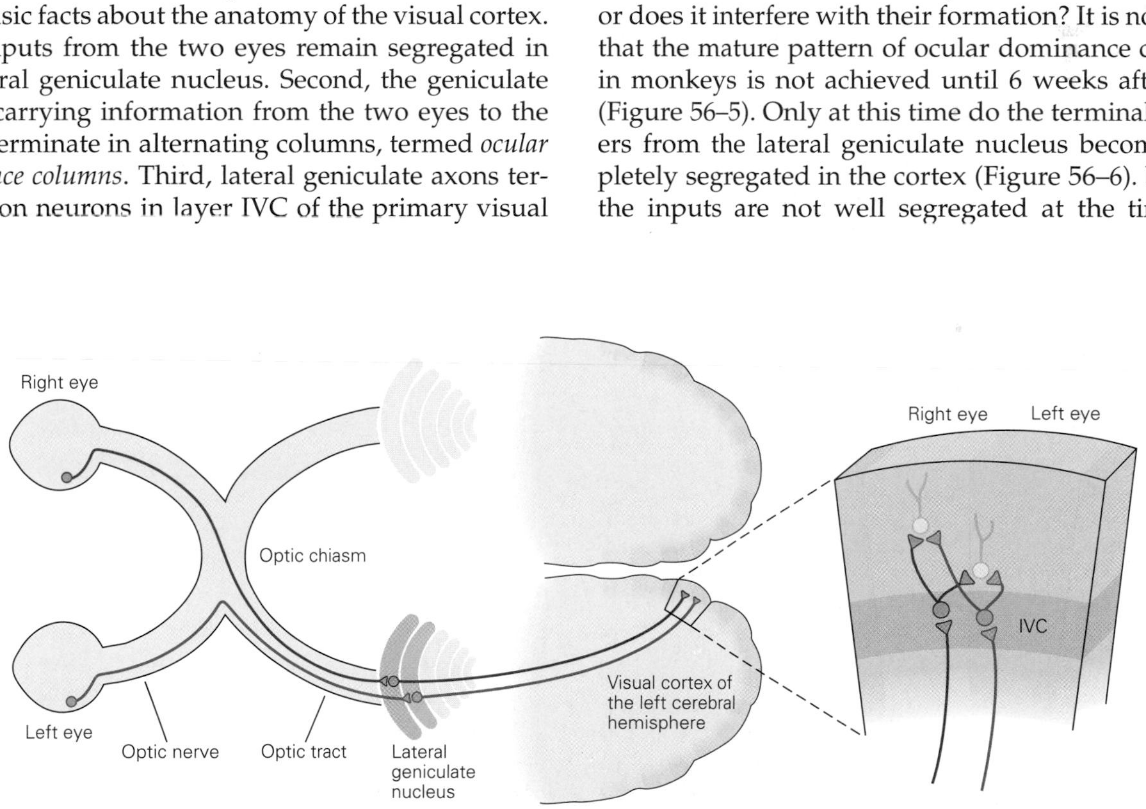

Figure 56–2 Afferent pathways from the two eyes project to discrete columns of neurons in the visual cortex. Retinal ganglion neurons from each eye send axons to separate layers of the lateral geniculate nucleus. The axons of neurons in the lateral geniculate nucleus project to neurons in layer IVC of the primary visual cortex. Neurons in layer IVC are organized in alternating sets of ocular dominance columns; each column receives input from only one eye. The axons of the neurons in layer IVC project to neurons in adjacent columns as well as to neurons in the upper and lower layers of the same column. As a result, most neurons in the upper and lower layers of the cortex receive information from both eyes.

visual deprivation exerts its effects, we can conclude that the deprivation perturbs the segregation of the inputs. We will see later that the remodeling of thalamic axonal arbors contributes to the perturbation of cortical columns.

Patterns of Electrical Activity Organize Binocular Circuits in the Visual Cortex

What determines the extent of ocular dominance columns? The crucial factor may be the existence of minor differences in the proportion of inputs from each eye that converge on common target cells at birth. If by chance the fibers conveying input from one eye are initially more numerous in one local region of cortex, those axons may have an advantage.

How might this occur? An attractive idea, based on a theory first proposed in the 1940s by Donald Hebb, is that connections are strengthened when pre- and postsynaptic elements at a synapse are active together. In the case of binocular interactions, neighboring axons from the same eye tend to fire in synchrony because they are activated by the same visual stimulus at any instant. The synchronization of their firing means that

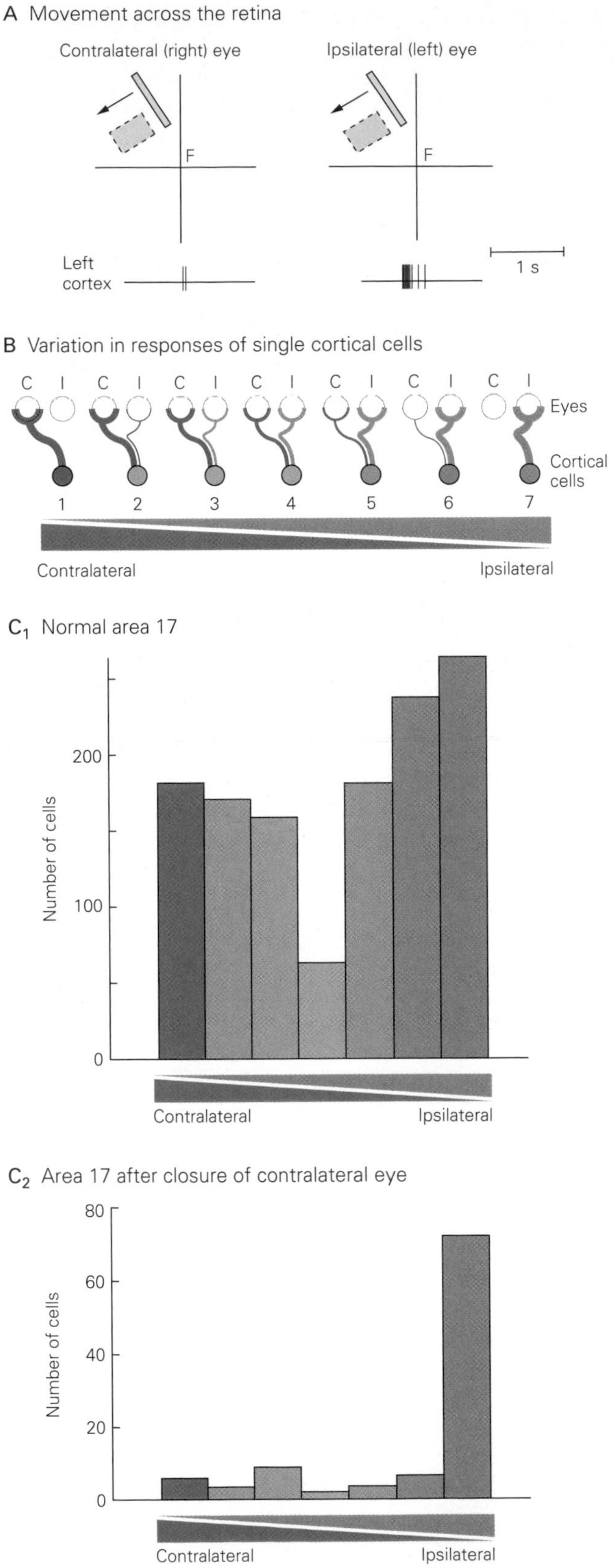

Figure 56–3 Responses of neurons in the primary visual cortex of a monkey to visual stimuli. (Adapted, with permission, from Hubel and Wiesel 1977.)

A. A diagonal bar of light is moved leftward across the visual field, traversing the receptive fields of a binocularly responsive cell in area 17 of visual cortex. Receptive fields measured through the right and left eye are drawn separately. The receptive fields of the two cells are similar in orientation, position, shape, and size, and respond to the same form of stimulus. Recordings (below) show that the cortical neuron responds more effectively to input from the ipsilateral eye. (**F**, fixation point.)

B. The responses of single cortical neurons in area 17 can be classified into seven groups. Neurons receiving input only from the contralateral eye (**C**) fall into group 1, whereas neurons that receive input only from the ipsilateral eye (**I**) fall into group 7. Other neurons receive inputs from both eyes, but the input from one eye may influence the neuron much more than the other (groups 2 and 6), or the differences may be slight (groups 3 and 5). Some neurons respond equally to input from both eyes (group 4). According to these criteria, the cortical neuron shown in part A falls into group 6.

C. Responsiveness of neurons in area 17 to stimulation of one or the other eye. The upper plot shows the responses of more than 1,000 neurons in area 17 in the left hemisphere of normal adult and juvenile monkeys. Neurons in layer IV that normally receive only monocular input have been excluded. The lower plot shows the responses of neurons in the left hemisphere of a monkey in which the contralateral (right) eye was closed from the age of 2 weeks to 18 months and then reopened. Most neurons respond only to stimulation of the ipsilateral eye.

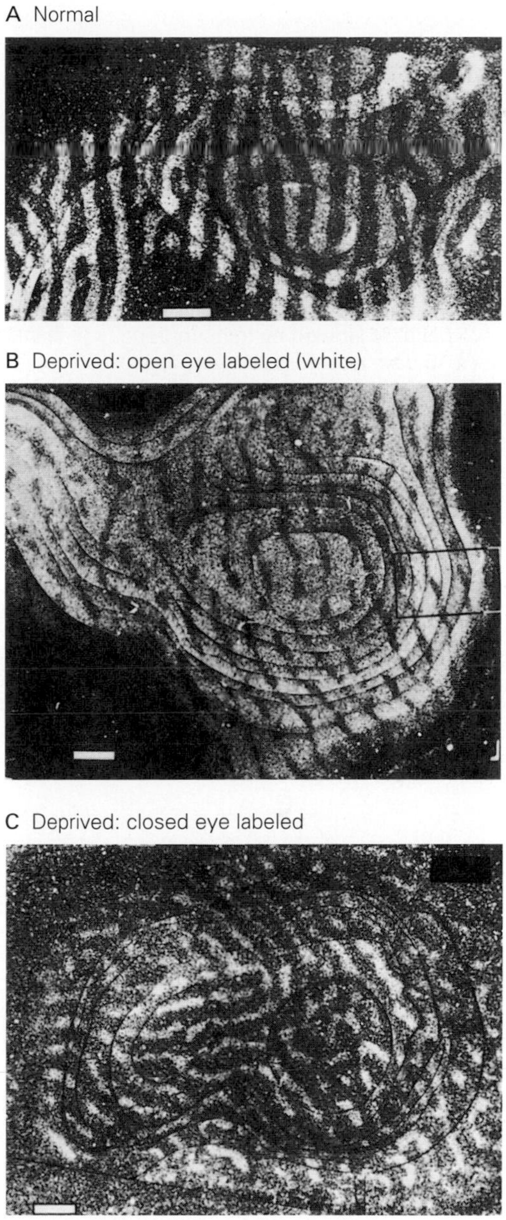

Figure 56–4 Visual deprivation of one eye during a critical period of development reduces the width of the ocular dominance columns for that eye. (Scale bars = 1 mm.) (Adapted, with permission, from Hubel et al. 1977.)

A. A tangential section through area 17 of the right hemisphere of a normal adult monkey, 10 days after the right eye was injected with a radiolabeled amino acid. Radioactivity is localized in stripes (**white areas**) in layer IVC of the visual cortex, indicating areas of termination of the axons from the lateral geniculate nucleus that carry input from the injected eye. The alternating unlabeled (dark) stripes correspond to regions of termination of the axons carrying signals from the uninjected eye. Labeled and unlabeled stripes are of equal width.

B. A comparable section through the visual cortex of an 18-month-old monkey whose right eye had been surgically closed at 2 weeks of age. Label was injected into the left eye. The wider white stripes are the labeled terminals of afferent axons carrying signals from the open (left) eye; the narrow dark stripes are terminals of axons with input from the closed (right) eye.

C. A section comparable to that in part B from an 18-month-old animal whose right eye had been shut at 2 weeks. Label was injected into the right eye, giving rise to narrow white stripes of labeled axon terminals and wide dark stripes of unlabeled terminals.

they cooperate in the depolarization and excitation of a target cell. This cooperative action maintains the viability of those synaptic contacts at the expense of the noncooperating synapses.

Cooperative activity promotes branching of axons and thus creates the opportunity for the formation of additional synaptic connections with cells in the target region. At the same time, the strengthening of synaptic contacts made by the axons of one eye will impede the growth of synaptic inputs from the opposite eye. In this sense fibers from the two eyes may be said to compete for a target cell. Together, cooperation and competition between axons ensure that two populations of afferent fibers will eventually innervate distinct regions of the primary visual cortex with little local overlap.

Competition and cooperation are not simply the outcome of neural activity per se, or of differences in absolute levels of activity among axons. Instead, they appear to depend on precise temporal patterns of activity in the competing (or cooperating) axons. The principle was dramatically illustrated by Hubel and Wiesel in a set of studies that examined stereoscopic

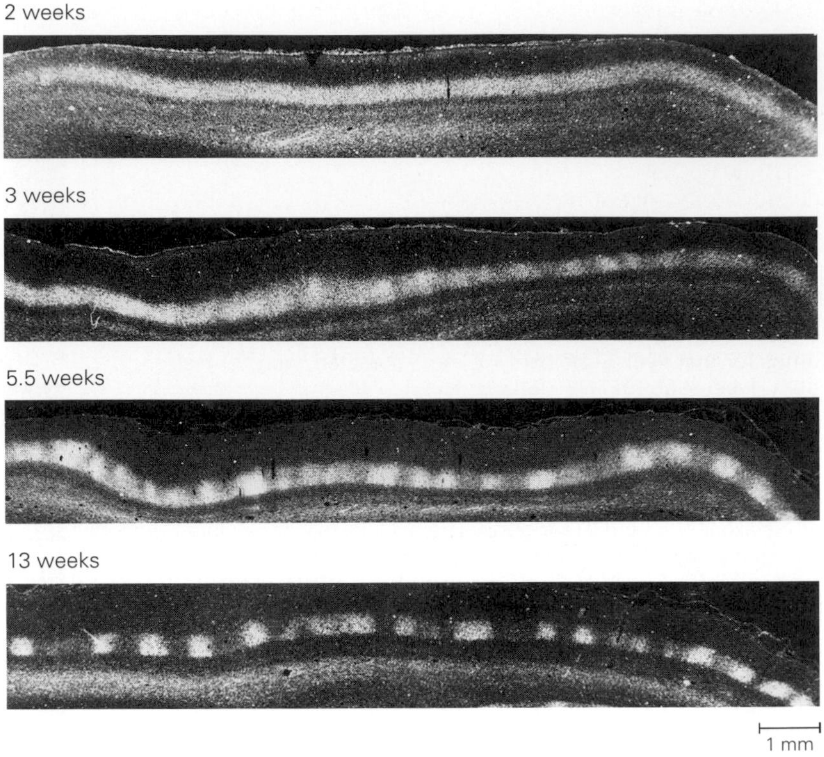

Figure 56–5 The development of ocular dominance columns. Autoradiographs of four stages in the postnatal development of ocular dominance columns in the visual cortex in a cat. The images show horizontal sections through columns in the cortex ipsilateral to an eye that was injected with a radiolabeled amino acid. The cells in the lateral geniculate nucleus that receive input from the injected eye become labeled by transneuronal transport. At 15 days after birth the terminals of labeled fibers are spread in a relatively uniform manner along layer IV and are intermingled with those of unlabeled fibers that convey signals from the contralateral eye. At 3 and 5.5 weeks some segregation of the terminals is visible, but only as modest differences in labeling density. At 13 weeks the borders of the labeled bands become more sharply defined as the fibers conveying inputs from each eye segregate. (Adapted, with permission, from LeVay, Stryker, and Shatz 1978.)

vision—the perception of depth. The brain normally computes depth perception by comparing the disparity in retinal images between the two eyes. When the eyes are improperly aligned, this comparison cannot be made and stereoscopy is impossible. Such misalignments occur in children who are "cross-eyed," or strabismic. As noted, this condition can be surgically repaired, but unless the surgery occurs during the first few years of life, the children forever remain incapable of stereoscopy.

Hubel and Wiesel examined the impact of strabismus on the organization of the visual system in cats. To render cats strabismic, the tendon of an extraocular muscle was severed in kittens. Both eyes remained fully functional but misaligned. Inputs from the two eyes that converged on a binocular cell in the visual cortex now carried information about different stimuli in slightly different parts of the visual field. As a result, cortical cells became monocular, driven by input from one eye or the other but not both (Figure 56–7). This finding suggested to Hubel and Wiesel that disruption of the synchrony of inputs led to competition rather than cooperation, so that cortical cells came to be dominated by one eye, presumably the one that had dominated it very slightly at the outset.

These physiological studies led investigators to test whether pharmacological blockade of electrical activity in retinal ganglion cells could affect neural connectivity in the visual system. Activity was blocked by injecting each eye with tetrodotoxin, a toxin that selectively blocks voltage-sensitive Na^+ channels. Signals from the two eyes were generated separately by direct electric stimulation of the bilateral optic nerves. In kittens ocular dominance columns are not established if activity in retinal ganglion neurons is blocked before the critical period of development. When the two optic nerves are stimulated synchronously, ocular dominance columns still fail to form. Only when the optic nerves are stimulated asynchronously are ocular dominance columns established.

If the development of ocular dominance columns indeed depends on competition between afferent fibers, might it be possible to induce the formation of columns where they normally are not present, simply by establishing competition between two sets of axons? This radical possibility was tested in frogs, where retinal ganglion neurons from each eye project only to the contralateral side of the brain. In normal frogs afferent fibers from the two eyes do not compete for the same cortical cells, so there is no columnar segregation of afferent inputs. To generate competition a third eye was transplanted early in larval development into a region of the frog's head near one of the normal eyes. The retinal ganglion neurons of the extra eye extended axons to the contralateral optic tectum. Remarkably, axon terminals from the transplanted and normal eyes segregated, generating a pattern of regular alternating columns (Figure 56–8).

This finding suggested that competition between two sets of afferent axons for the same population of cortical neurons drives their segregation into distinct target territories. The columnar segregation of retinal inputs in the frog brain is dependent on synaptic activity, presumably at the synapses between retinal axons and tectal neurons. Thus neural activity has powerful roles in fine-tuning visual circuits.

Reorganization of Visual Circuits During a Critical Period Involves Alterations in Synaptic Connections

The pioneering work of Hubel, Wiesel, and their colleagues showed that early experience is a critical

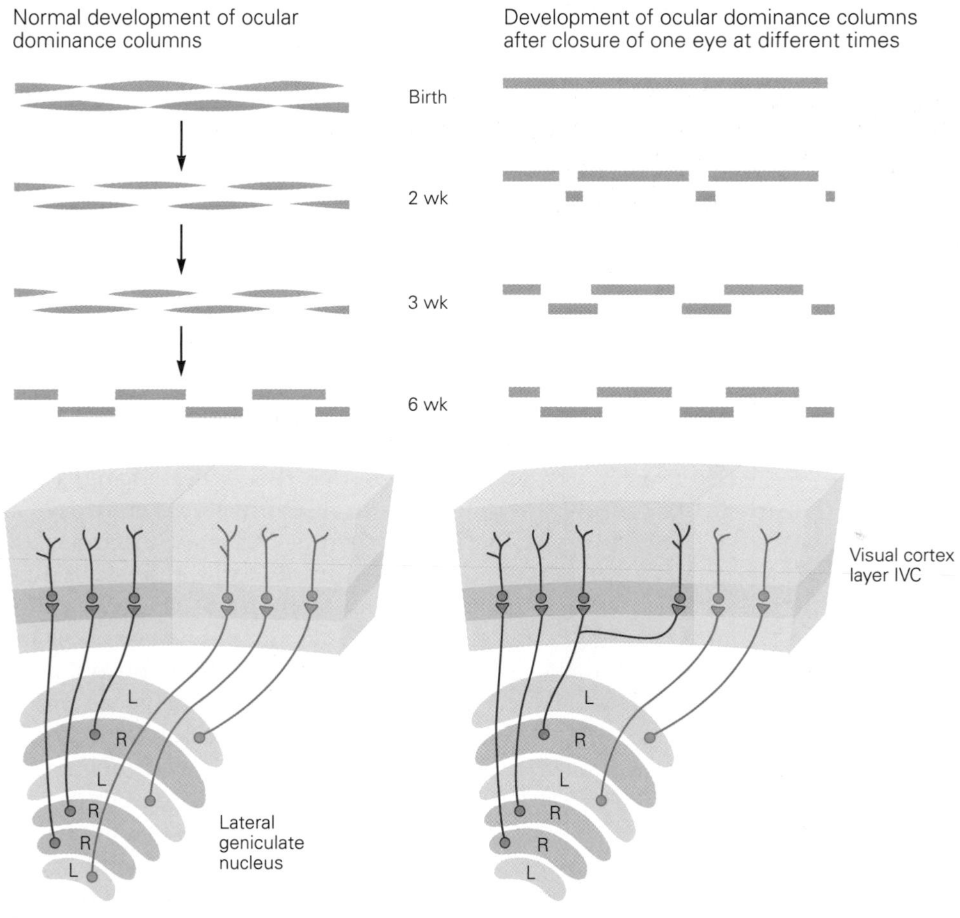

Figure 56–6 The effects of eye closure on the formation of ocular dominance columns. The top diagrams show the gradual segregation of the terminals of lateral geniculate afferents in layer IVC of the visual cortex under normal conditions (left) and when one eye is deprived of stimulation (right). The blue domains represent the areas of termination of inputs from one eye, the red domains are those of the other eye. The lengths of the domains represent the density of the terminals at each point along layer IVC. For clarity the columns are shown here as one above the other, whereas in reality they are side by side in the cortex. During normal development layer IVC is gradually divided into alternating sites of input from each eye. The consequences of depriving sight in one eye depend on the timing of eye closure. Closure at birth leads to dominance by the open eye (**red**) because at this point little segregation has occurred. Closure at 2, 3, and 6 weeks has a progressively weaker effect on the formation of ocular dominance columns because the columns become more segregated with time. (Adapted, with permission, from Hubel, Wiesel, and LeVay 1977.)

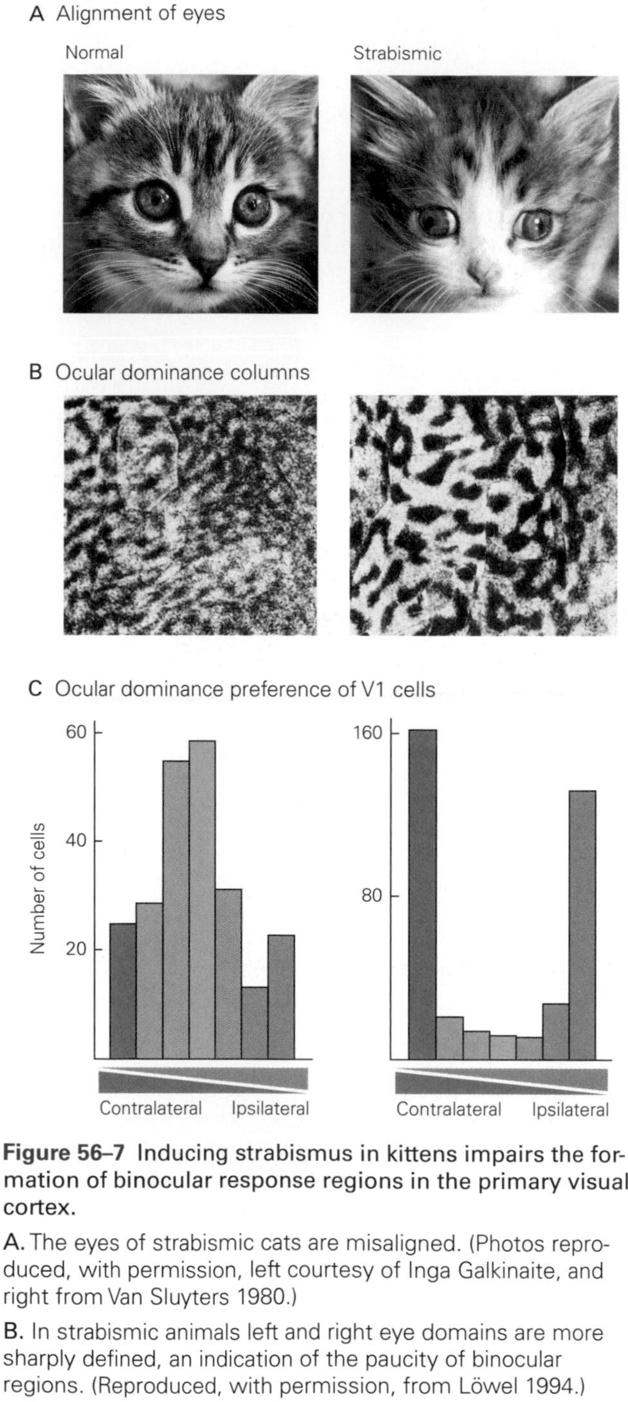

Figure 56–7 Inducing strabismus in kittens impairs the formation of binocular response regions in the primary visual cortex.

A. The eyes of strabismic cats are misaligned. (Photos reproduced, with permission, left courtesy of Inga Galkinaite, and right from Van Sluyters 1980.)

B. In strabismic animals left and right eye domains are more sharply defined, an indication of the paucity of binocular regions. (Reproduced, with permission, from Löwel 1994.)

C. Strabismic animals have fewer binocularly tuned neurons in the visual cortex. (Reproduced, with permission, from Hubel and Wiesel 1965.)

prerequisite for the emergence of normal structure and function in the visual cortex. However, despite four decades of research, many questions about the cellular and molecular mechanisms that underlie the critical period have remained unanswered. Hubel, Wiesel, and their disciples studied cats and monkeys, in which manipulations of cells and molecules are difficult. Recently, many investigators have begun to address these issues in mice because they are more amenable to mechanistic analysis.

Reorganization Depends on a Change in the Balance of Excitatory and Inhibitory Inputs

When one eye is closed or patched, the cortex no longer receives input from that eye. If the loss of input is prolonged for a few days before the eye is reopened, the cortex cannot be activated by input from the formerly deprived eye. Nor can the cells of the cortex be activated by direct stimulation of the corresponding optic nerve.

What converts this early loss of functional input into a permanent alteration of functional capability? One idea is that thalamic axons carrying information from the deprived eye lose their ability to activate cortical neurons. A decrease in efficacy of the thalamocortical synapse may contribute to this effect, but this is not the whole story. In cats and monkeys each thalamic axon carries input from only one eye (Figure 56–2). Because loss of responsiveness to the deprived eye occurs only if the other eye remains active, one might imagine that the earliest changes would occur where inputs from the two eyes converge on binocular cells. Local circuits connect the targets of the monocular thalamic inputs in layer IV to the binocular neurons in layers II/III and V. The first physiological changes following closure of one eye occur in layers II/III and V, not in layer IV. This implies that the loss of cortical responsiveness to the deprived eye results from a circuit alteration rather than from a simple loss of input.

What changes in cell function account for these changes in circuitry? At least three have been proposed. First, excitatory synapses within the primary visual cortex may decrease in strength, perhaps by undergoing long-term depression (LTD) (see Chapter 66). In fact, direct recording from cortical neurons shows that LTD does occur soon after eye closure. Second, inhibitory synapses may become stronger, leading to a net decrease in the level of excitation of cortical neurons by inputs from the closed eye. Third, an increase in inhibition within the cortex may alter network properties in a more subtle way, such as tuning the circuit to favor LTD.

The involvement of inhibition has been demonstrated by studies in the binocular region of mouse

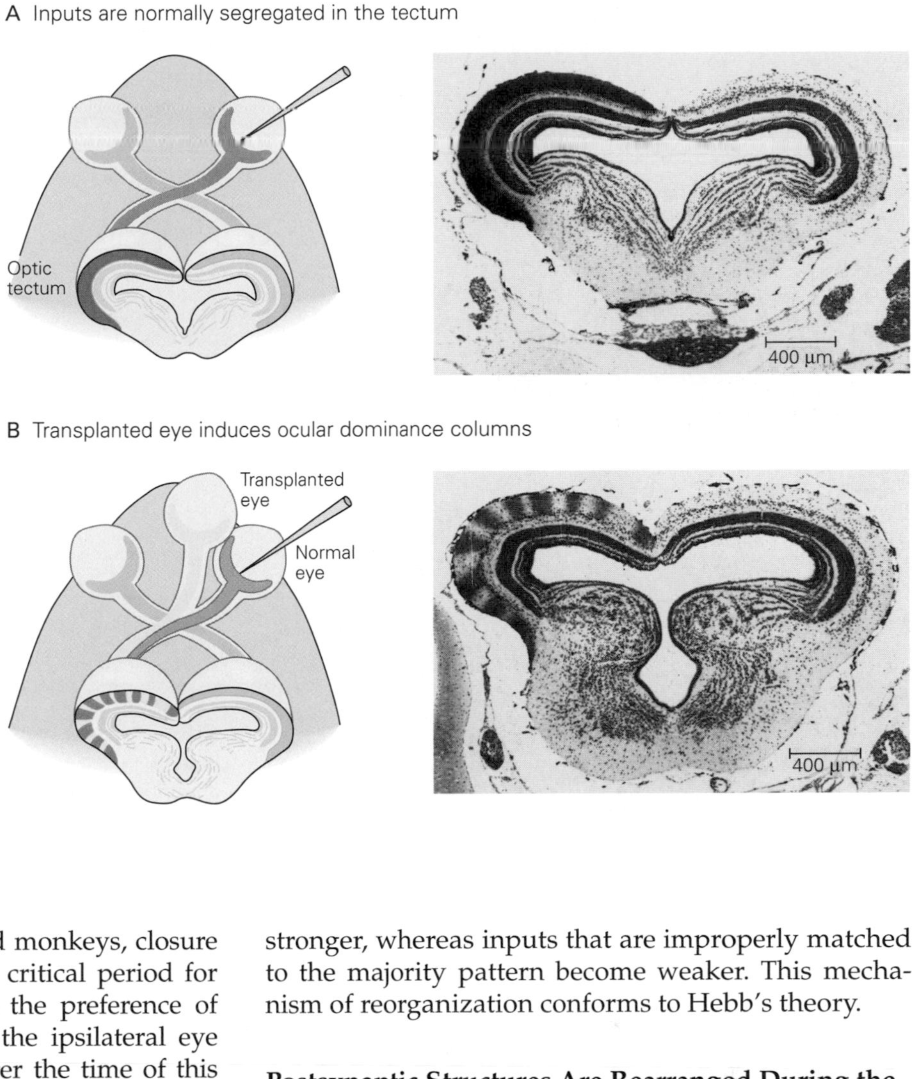

Figure 56–8 Ocular dominance columns can be experimentally induced in a frog by transplantation of a third eye. (Adapted, with permission, from Constantine-Paton and Law 1978.)

A. Three days before the transplant the right eye was injected with a radiolabeled amino acid. The autoradiograph in a coronal section of the hindbrain shows the entire superficial neuropil of the left optic lobe filled with silver grains, indicating the region occupied by synaptic terminals from the labeled (contralateral) eye.

B. Some time after a third eye was transplanted near the normal right eye the right eye was injected with a radiolabeled amino acid. The autoradiograph shows that the left optic lobe receives inputs from both the labeled eye and the transplanted eye. The normally continuous synaptic zone of the contralateral eye has become divided into alternating dark and light zones that indicate the sites of inputs from each eye.

visual cortex. In mice, as in cats and monkeys, closure of the contralateral eye during the critical period for ocular dominance markedly shifts the preference of binocular neurons to inputs from the ipsilateral eye (Figure 56–9). Closure before or after the time of this normal critical period, however, fails to alter the preference of the neurons. Physiological studies have shown that monocular deprivation potentiates inhibitory feedback onto the neurons that the deprived eye normally excites. Moreover, the critical period in which monocular deprivation elicits changes in preference can be advanced using a genetic method to enhance gamma-aminobutyric acid (GABA) signaling (Figure 56–10). Conversely, the period in which monocular deprivation enhances the preference for ipsilateral eye input can be delayed by delaying GABA signaling (Figure 56–10). Thus a balance of intracortical excitation and inhibition is required for reorganization during this critical period.

What explains the change in responsiveness? After one eye is closed responsiveness to the open eye increases. This increase involves enhanced efficacy of synaptic transmission, a process resembling long-term potentiation (see Chapters 66 and 67). Inputs firing together with the majority of their neighbors become stronger, whereas inputs that are improperly matched to the majority pattern become weaker. This mechanism of reorganization conforms to Hebb's theory.

Postsynaptic Structures Are Rearranged During the Critical Period

What are the structural correlates of the physiological changes that result in altered responsiveness of the visual cortex to input from the closed and open eyes? Particular attention has been paid to dendritic spines as potential sites of plasticity.

Spines are small protrusions from the dendrites of many cortical neurons on which excitatory synapses form. They are dynamic structures, and their appearance and loss are thought to reflect the formation and elimination of synapses. Spine motility is especially marked during early postnatal development, and increases in spine dynamics and number have been associated with changes in behavior.

Striking alterations in the motility and number of dendritic spines on neurons in the mouse visual cortex are observed following closure of one eye. Two days after eye closure in young mice the motility and

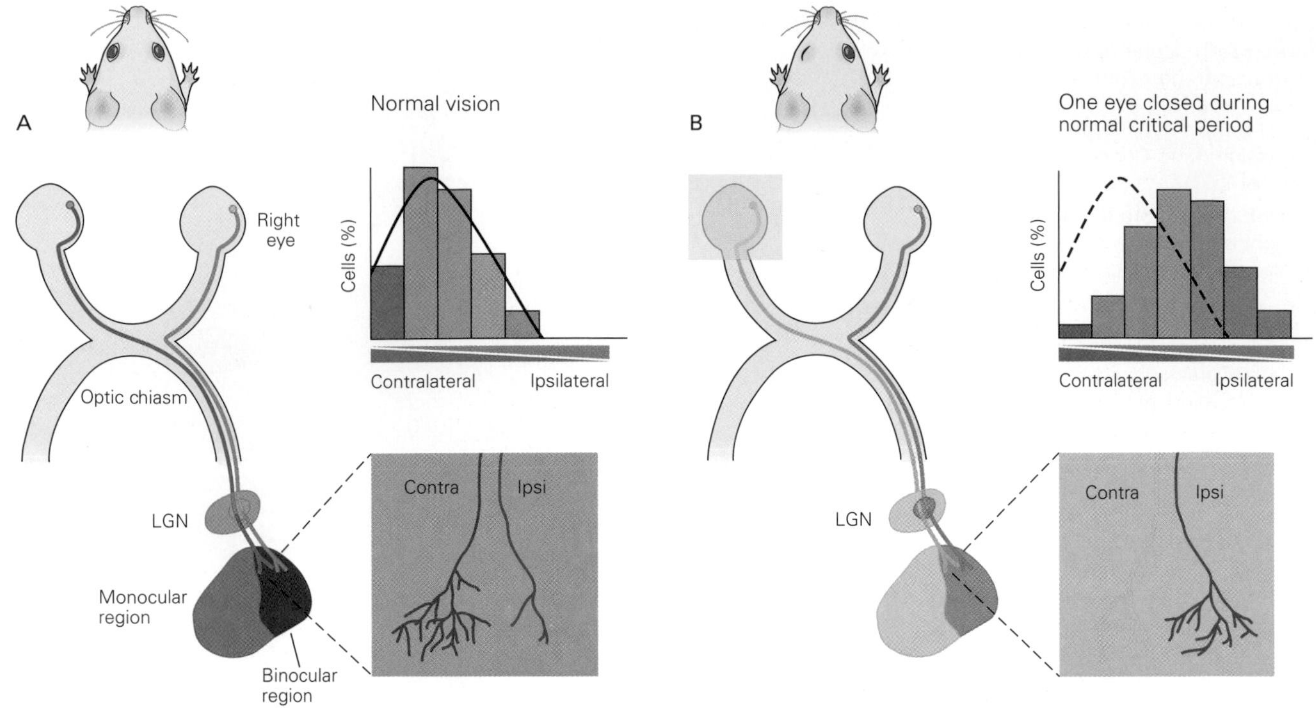

Figure 56–9 A critical period for ocular dominance plasticity is evident in mice. (Adapted, with permission, from Hensch et al. 2005.)

A. The visual cortex in mice contains a small region that receives thalamic (**LGN**) inputs from both eyes. In this binocular region most neurons are responsive to contralateral eye input, fewer respond to binocular inputs, and very few respond to ipsilateral eye input only.

B. When the contralateral eye has been closed during the normal critical period and then reopened, inputs from that eye are underrepresented and many more neurons respond to binocular or ipsilateral eye input. Eye closure before or after the time of the normal critical period does not elicit the same shift in responsiveness.

turnover of dendritic spines on neurons in the visual cortex increases, suggesting that synaptic connections are beginning to rearrange (Figure 56–11). A few days later the number of spines begins to change—the number of spines on the apical dendrites of pyramidal neurons initially decreases but after longer periods of deprivation increases again.

These alterations in spine motility and number can be correlated with three known features of the critical period. First, rather than occurring in layer IV, the changes occur primarily in superficial and deep layers of the cortex, where binocular cells lie. Second, they occur only in the portion of the visual cortex that normally receives binocular input. Third, they fail to occur following eye closure in adult mice (Figure 56–11).

Together these results support a model that links spine dynamics with critical period plasticity. According to this model, spine motility increases before physiological changes in responsiveness can be recorded. This condition may result from the imbalance of inputs to binocular neurons from the open and closed eyes, and it may reflect the first stages in synaptic rearrangement. In turn, the loss of spines, and presumably of synapses, corresponds in time and space to the loss of input from the closed eye and may provide a structural basis for the permanence of this loss. The later growth of new spines occurs as or after responsiveness to the open eye increases, and may underlie the adaptive rearrangement that permits the cortex to make the best use of the input available to it.

Thalamic Inputs Are Also Remodeled

How are local changes in spines related to the large-scale structural changes in ocular dominance columns shown in Figure 56–4? When developing axons from the lateral geniculate nucleus first reach the cortex, the terminal endings of several neurons overlap extensively. Each fiber extends a few branches over an area of the visual cortex that spans several future ocular dominance columns. As the cortex matures, axons retract some branches, expand others, and even form new branches (Figure 56–12A).

With time each geniculate neuron becomes connected almost exclusively to a group of neighboring cortical neurons within a single column. The arbors become segregated into columns through the pruning or retraction of certain axons and the sprouting of others. This dual process of axon retraction and sprouting occurs widely throughout the nervous system during development.

What happens after one eye is closed? Axons from a closed eye are at a disadvantage and a greater than normal proportion retract. At the same time, axons from the open eye sprout new terminals at sites vacated by fibers that would otherwise convey input from the closed eye (Figure 56-12B). If an animal is deprived of the use of one eye early during the critical period of axonal segregation, the normal processes of axon retraction and outgrowth are perturbed. In contrast, if an animal is deprived of the use of one eye only after the ocular dominance columns are almost fully segregated, axons conveying input from the open eye actually sprout collaterals in regions of the cortex that they had vacated earlier (see Figure 56–6).

Initially it was believed that rearrangements of thalamocortical axons in monocularly deprived animals caused the changes in cortical responsiveness to the open and closed eyes. We now know, through electrophysiological recording and assays of spine dynamics described above, that physiological changes and synaptic alterations precede these large-scale axonal rearrangements. So rather than causing the physiological changes, axonal remodeling may contribute to making these changes enduring and irreversible. The question then becomes: How do alterations in synaptic structure and function within the cortex lead to alterations in the input?

One idea is that activity regulates the secretion of neurotrophic factors by cortical neurons. Such factors may then regulate survival of some neurons at the expense of others (see Chapter 53) or promote the expansion of some axonal arbors at the expense of others. One such factor, brain-derived neurotrophic factor (BDNF), is indeed synthesized and secreted by cortical neurons. Administering excess BDNF, or interfering with its receptor trkB, modifies the formation of ocular dominance columns. Nevertheless, interpreting the actions of these trophic factors is not straightforward. BDNF and trkB signaling affect the cortex in many ways, including enhancing the growth of thalamocortical axons. BDNF can also speed the maturation of inhibitory circuits, which, as noted above, can

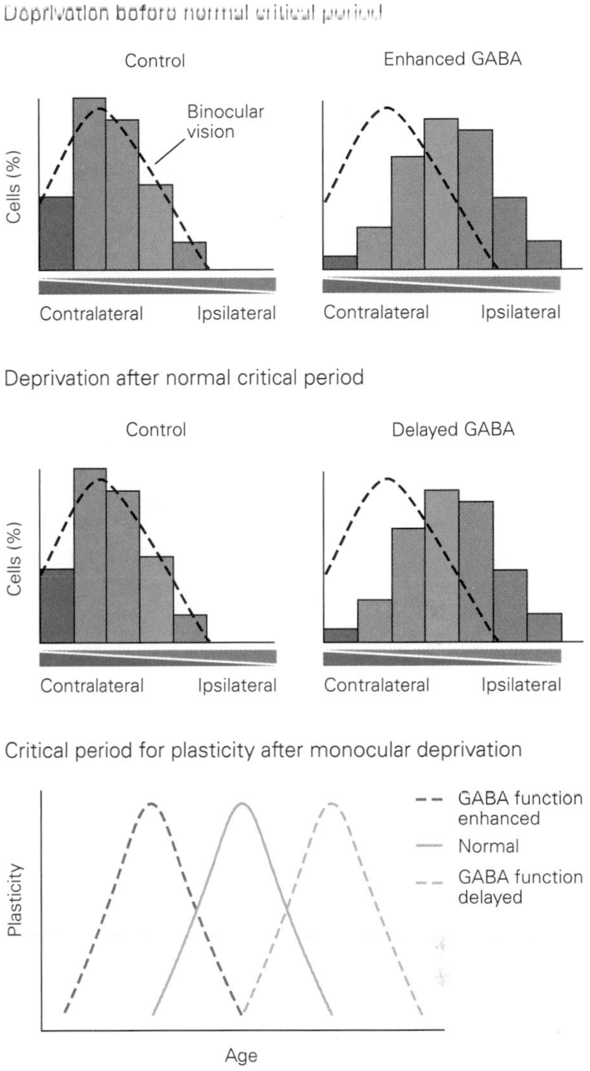

Figure 56–10 The timing of the critical period for ocular dominance plasticity in mice is sensitive to the level of GABAergic neurotransmission. Altering the status of GABA (γ-aminobutyric acid) synthesis and signaling shifts the period in which monocular deprivation can change the response properties of neurons in the visual cortex. Enhancing GABA signaling, through administration of benzodiazepines, shifts the critical period for monocular deprivation to an earlier developmental time. In contrast, delaying GABA signaling, by reducing GABA synthesis genetically and then administering benzodiazepines at a later time, shifts the critical period for monocular deprivation to a later developmental time. (Adapted, with permission, from Hensch et al. 1998.)

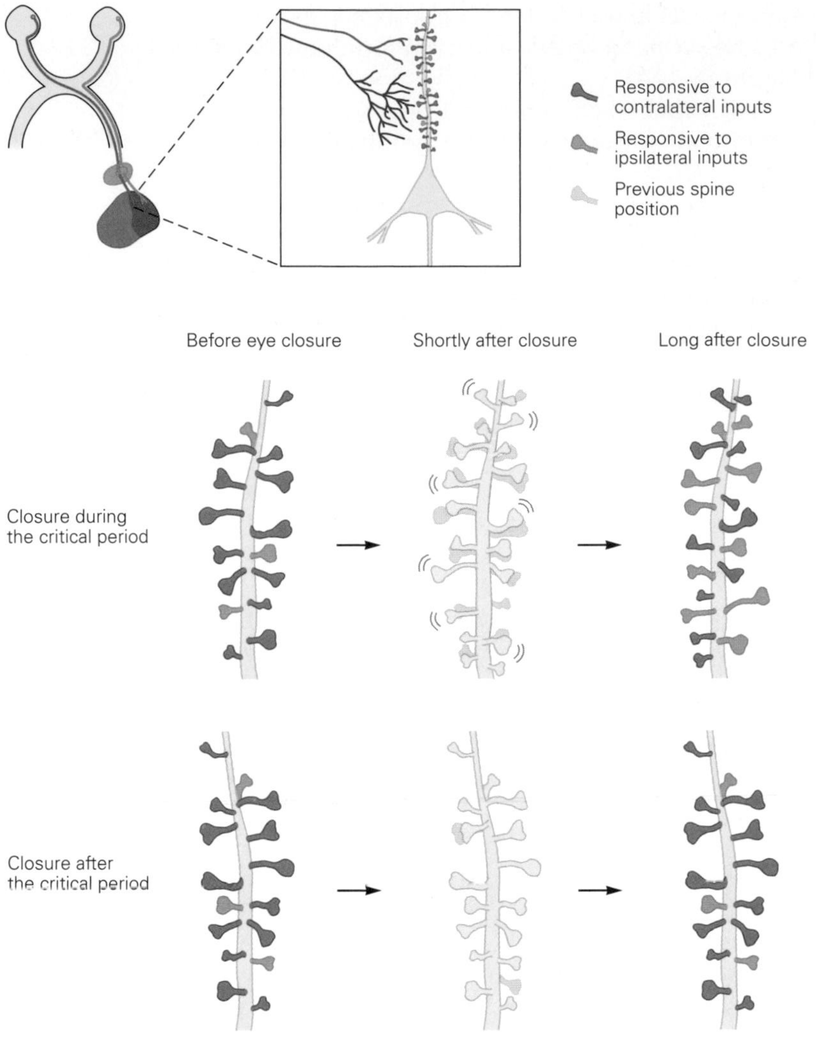

Figure 56–11 The motility of dendritic spines in the mouse visual cortex changes after one eye is closed. The dendrites of pyramidal neurons in the visual cortex have many spines, the density of which remains comparatively constant under normal conditions. Closure of one eye (contralateral in this example) during the critical period for binocular development enhances the motility of dendritic spines and over time results in an increase in the proportion of spines that receive synaptic input from the open eye. Similar changes in spine motility are not observed if the eye is closed after the critical period. (Reproduced, with permission, from Oray et al. 2004.)

influence plasticity. It remains unclear whether BDNF is a specific catalyst of the competition that preferentially promotes expansion of some arbors.

Synaptic Stabilization Contributes to Closing the Critical Period

A hallmark of critical periods is that the time interval in which experience affects the development of neural circuits is limited. What determines the timing of this remarkable biological response? To answer this question we must ask what opens the critical period and what closes it.

Opening of critical periods could result from maturation of systems required for plasticity. As we have mentioned, genetic studies indicate that maturation of inhibitory circuits in the visual cortex is required for initiation of the critical period for binocular development. Likewise, synapses that are modified by competitive interactions between the eyes, or by synchronous activity, may not undergo long-term potentiation or depression until they reach a sufficient level of maturity.

The factors that terminate the critical period have been studied in more detail. Since synapses and circuits are labile during critical periods, an obvious idea is that stabilizing factors bring this period of heightened plasticity to a close. The cellular and molecular landscape of the cortex changes in many ways as the brain matures, and several of these alterations may play roles. One parameter is the state of myelination of axons, which occurs around the time the critical period closes. Formation of myelin creates physical barriers to sprouting and axonal growth. Moreover, as discussed in detail in Chapter 57, myelin contains factors such as Nogo and myelin-associated glycoprotein that actively inhibit growth of axons. In mutant mice lacking Nogo or one of its receptors, NogoR, the critical period remains open into adulthood, suggesting that the appearance of these receptors normally contributes to closing the critical period (Figure 56–13).

Another possible agent of closure is the perineuronal net, a web of glycosaminoglycans that wraps certain classes of inhibitory neurons. These nets form around the time that the critical period closes. Infusion of the enzyme chondroitinase, which digests perineuronal nets, maintains plasticity. Thus critical periods may close once molecular barriers to synaptic growth and rearrangement come into play.

Why should there be an end to critical periods? Would it not be advantageous for the brain to maintain its ability to remodel into adulthood? Perhaps not—the ability of our brain to adapt to variations in sensory input, to gradual physical growth (eg, increases in the distance between the eyes affecting binocular correspondence), and to various congenital disorders is a valuable asset. At an extreme, if one eye is lost it is advantageous to devote all available cortical real estate to the remaining eye. Conversely, one would not want wholesale reorganization, possibly accompanied by loss of skills and memories, if vision through one eye were lost temporarily in adulthood due to disease or injury. So enhancing plasticity during a critical period may represent an adaptive compromise between flexibility and stability.

Segregation of Retinal Inputs in the Lateral Geniculate Nucleus Is Driven by Spontaneous Neural Activity In Utero

Some of the principles of development of the visual cortex we have discussed also govern the development of the lateral geniculate nucleus. The arbors of retinal ganglion cells from the two eyes are segregated into alternating layers in this nucleus, much as the projections from this nucleus are segregated in alternating ocular dominance columns in the visual cortex (Figure 56–14).

In both structures individual axons at first form terminals in multiple domains (layers in the geniculate nucleus, columns in the cortex). Later the terminals become segregated by a process of refinement. As in the cortex, the segregation of the inputs from each eye can be disrupted by applying tetrodotoxin to the optic nerves, indicating that activity is essential for segregation. In the lateral geniculate nucleus, however, the segregation of inputs is complete before birth.

Since segregation of retinal inputs in the lateral geniculate nucleus occurs before birth, vision cannot drive the neural activity essential for segregation. It turns out that the axons of retinal neurons are spontaneously active in utero, well before the eyes open. Neighboring ganglion cells fire in synchronous bursts that last a few seconds, followed by silent periods that may last for minutes. Sampling the activity of retinal ganglion neurons across the entire retina revealed that

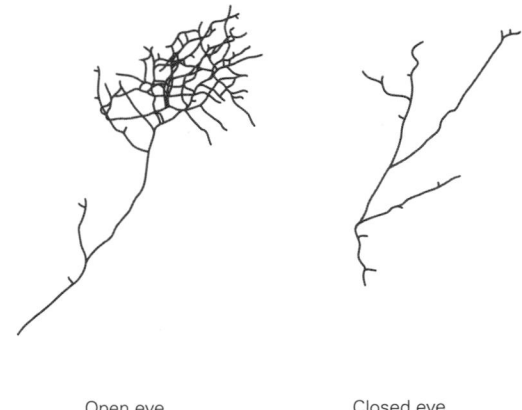

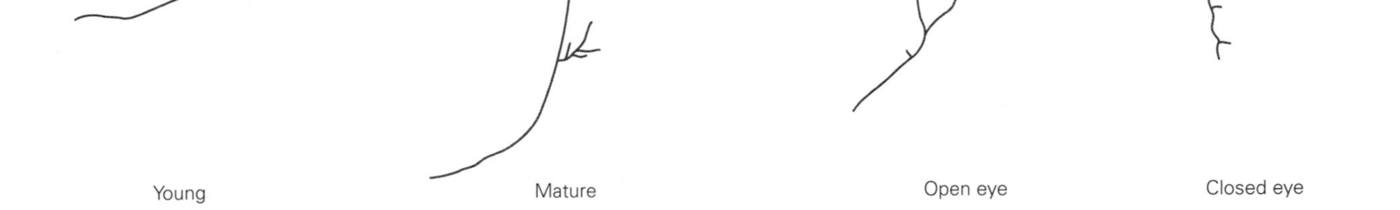

Figure 56–12 The branching of thalamocortical fibers in the visual cortex of kittens changes after the closure of an eye. (Adapted, with permission, from Antonini and Stryker 1993.)

A. During normal postnatal development the axons of lateral geniculate nucleus cells branch widely in the visual cortex. The branching eventually becomes confined to a small region.

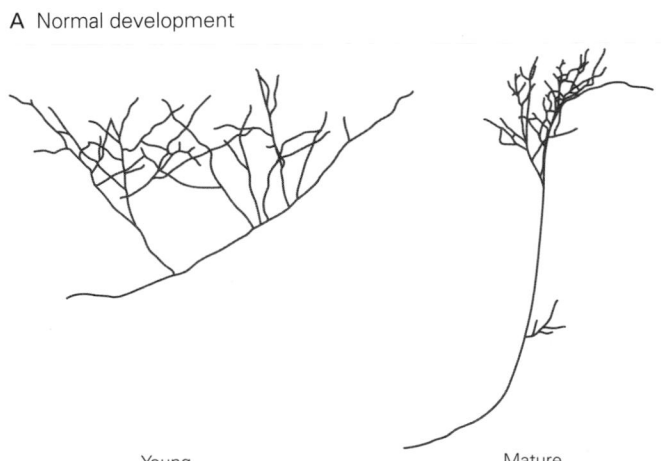

B. After one eye is closed the terminal arbors of neurons in the pathway from that eye are dramatically smaller compared to those of the open eye.

these bursts propagate across much of the retina in a wave-like manner (Figure 56–15). This pattern of ganglion cell activity appears to be coordinated by excitatory inputs from amacrine cells in the overlying layer of the retina (see Figure 26–3).

The spontaneous, synchronous firing of a select group of ganglion neurons excites a local group of neurons in the lateral geniculate nucleus. Such synchronized activity appears to strengthen these synapses at the expense of other nearby synapses. The fact that retinal ganglion neurons are spontaneously active in utero is an important clue to the development of many pathways in the brain that are refined before they have the chance to respond to environmental stimulation.

Activity-Dependent Refinement of Connections Is a General Feature of Circuits in the Central Nervous System

We have seen that neural activity is critical for segregating axons from the two retinas into distinct layers in the lateral geniculate nucleus and then into distinct columns in the visual cortex. Is this a special case, or does activity also affect maturation elsewhere in the visual system, and even in other parts of the brain? Studies of many systems show that activity-dependent control of refinement is a general property of neural circuits in the mammalian brain.

Many Aspects of Visual System Development Are Activity-Dependent

One well-studied example of activity-dependent development in the visual system is the sharpening of the topographic distribution of retinal ganglion cell axons onto their central targets, a topic we introduced in Chapter 54. Molecular cues such as ephrins guide

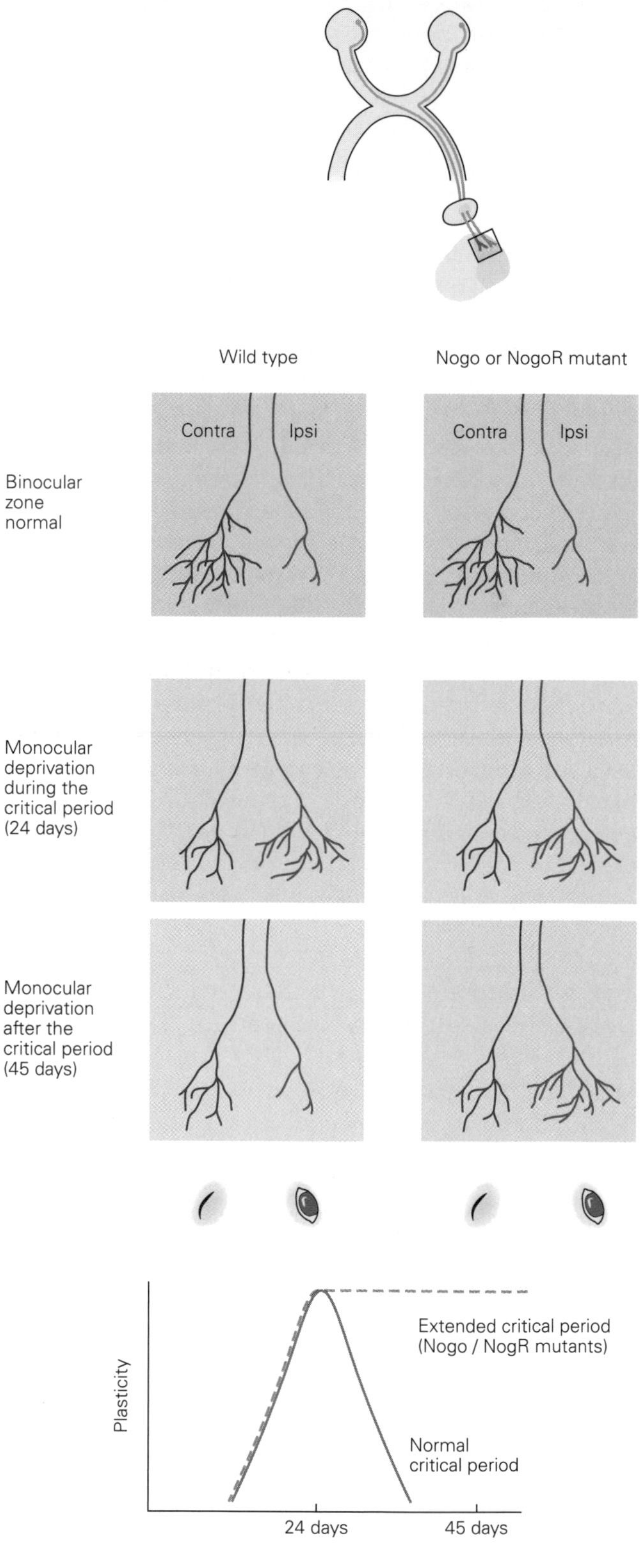

Figure 56–13 The critical period for monocular deprivation is extended in mice lacking Nogo signaling. The drawings show arborization patterns of thalamocortical axons carrying signals from contralateral and ipsilateral eyes to the binocular zone in visual cortex. Monocular deprivation during the critical period elicits a shift in ocular preference in neurons in the binocular zone in both wild type mice and mice mutant for Nogo or the Nogo receptor. After the normal critical period (at 45 days) monocular deprivation continues to elicit a marked shift in axonal input and ocular preference in mice mutant for Nogo-A or the Nogo receptor but not in wild type mice. The plot shows that elimination of Nogo signaling prevents closure of the critical period. (Adapted, with permission, from McGee et al. 2005.)

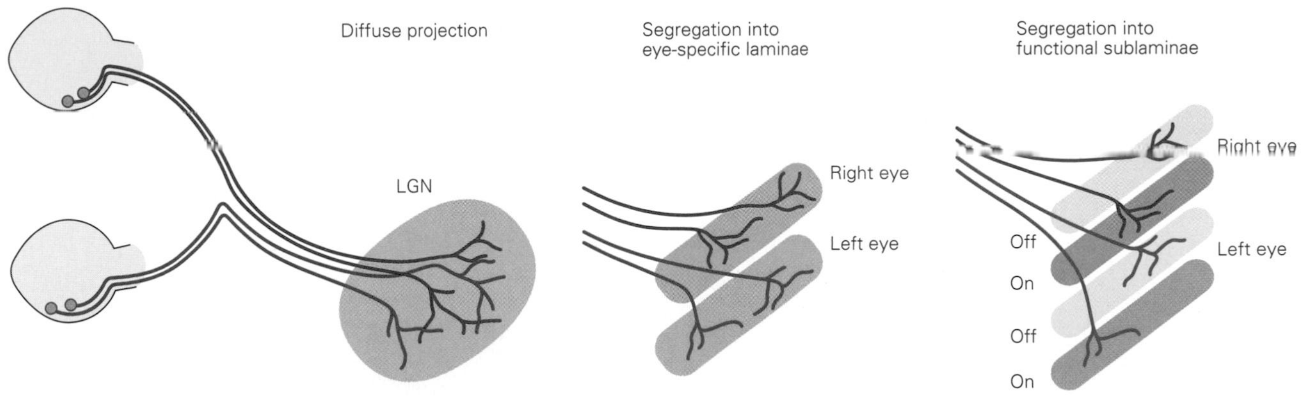

Figure 56–14 The terminals of retinal ganglion cells in the lateral geniculate nucleus become segregated during normal development. At early stages the terminals of axons from each eye intermingle. At later stages the inputs from the left and right eyes segregate into separate layers of the nucleus. In some species axons from one eye even segregate into functionally specialized sublayers (on and off layers in ferrets). (Adapted, with permission, from Sanes and Yamagata 1999.)

axons to appropriate sites in the tectum, but they are not sufficient to form the refined visual map.

Histological and physiological studies have found that the map formed initially in the superior colliculus (the equivalent of the optic tectum of lower vertebrates) is coarse, and that individual retinal ganglion cell axons have large, overlapping arbors. These axonal arbors are later pruned to their mature size, resulting in a more restricted and precise field of termination. If retinal activity is inhibited, only the initial coarse map forms.

Is it the pattern of activity or activity itself that is important in visual map formation? Put another way, is activity simply "permissive" for refinement, or is it "instructive," determining exactly which axons win or lose the competition? Many experiments show that the latter idea is closer to the truth.

In one study the accuracy of the retinotectal map was assessed in fish raised in a tank illuminated only by brief flashes from a strobe light. A control group was raised in a normal laboratory environment. The total light intensity presented to the fish was similar under both conditions, but the resulting pattern was very different. In control fish the images fell haphazardly on various parts of the retina as the fish swam around their tanks. This input produces local synchronous activity of the sort generated by the waves of spontaneous activity described above—neighboring ganglion cells tend to fire together, but there is little correlation with the firing patterns of distant ganglion cells. In these fish the map becomes precise. In contrast, stroboscopic illumination synchronously activates nearly all of the ganglion cells, and as a consequence the retinotectal map remains coarse.

Presumably, the tectum determines which retinal axons are near neighbors by judging which ones fire in synchrony, much as activity patterns in the lateral geniculate nucleus or visual cortex determine which axons carry signals from the same eye. This information is then used to refine the topographic map, through mechanisms similar to those in the cortex. When all of the axons fire in synchrony, the tectum cannot determine which axons are neighbors; refinement fails, and the map remains coarse.

Auditory Maps Are Refined During a Critical Period

Activity-dependent refinement is not unique to the visual system. Activity is essential for shaping patterns of connectivity in most regions of the central nervous system. In the auditory system, for example, inputs form orderly tonotopic maps in the cochlear nucleus, the inferior colliculus, and the auditory cortex, such that neurons responding best to low frequencies lie at one edge of each structure, while neurons tuned to high frequencies are at the other. These maps underlie our sense of pitch. In addition, neurons vary in their sensitivity to sounds sensed by the contralateral and ipsilateral ears, and this discrepancy helps us determine the point in horizontal space from which a sound arises (see Chapter 31).

These auditory patterns are analogous to the retinotopic maps of the visual system. And, like their visual analogs, these auditory connections can be refined or modified by experience. Thus, although tonotopic maps can form in silence, exposure of an animal to "white noise" impairs refinement of the tuning curves

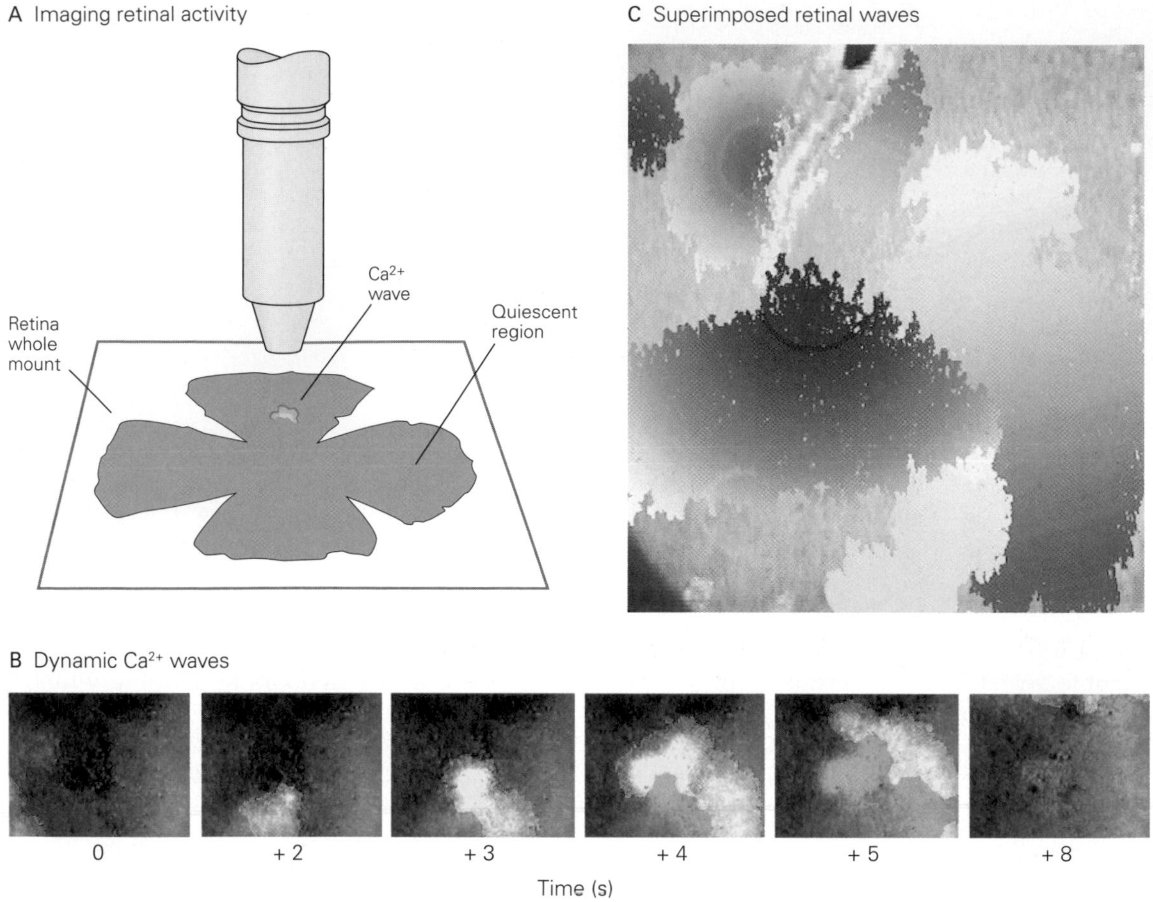

Figure 56–15 Correlated waves of neural activity in the developing retina.

A. Microscopic visualization of the activity of retinal ganglion neurons in a flat-mounted preparation of mammalian retina. Spontaneous waves of neural activity are visualized by monitoring Ca^{2+} transients (**yellow domain**) after loading of cells with dyes that change their fluorescent emission spectrum with changes in intracellular Ca^{2+} concentration.

B. These still images from a movie sequence show the propagation of one Ca^{2+} activity focus (**yellow domain**) across the retina. Images were taken 1 second apart. Many cells within the activity focus are activated synchronously (Reproduced, with permission, from Blankenship et al. 2009).

C. Retinal activity waves recorded over time are superimposed in this image. Discrete waves are indicated in different colors; the origin of a wave is indicated by a darker hue. These waves originate in different retinal foci and spread in distinct, unpredictable directions. (Reproduced, with permission, from Meister et al. 1991.)

of neurons in the inferior colliculus, while exposure to specific frequencies enhances representation of those frequencies in the map.

Neural circuit reorganization not only optimizes processing of information in one sensory modality but also brings information of multiple sensory modalities into register. Studies on barn owls have provided insight into how auditory and visual maps are coordinated during a critical period. During the day owls use vision to localize their prey—mice or other small rodents—but at night they rely on auditory cues, and at dusk both sensory channels are used. The localization of sound must be precise if owls are to succeed in finding prey, and it is intuitively obvious that the visual and auditory cues for the same location need to be consistent.

Auditory localization in owls, as in people, results in large part from computation of the temporal difference between a sound arriving at the two ears. This difference is only a few tens of microseconds, as expected from calculations based upon the speed of sound and the width of the head. Remarkably, the auditory system is sensitive to these extremely short interaural time differences (ITDs) and can calculate prey position from them (Figure 56–16). Moreover, many neurons in the optic tectum with receptive fields centered on a particular location are also tuned to ITDs that correspond to sounds emitted from that same point in space. The registration is imprecise at early stages but becomes progressively more precise during early adolescence as a consequence of the animal's experience.

Crucial insight into how this registration occurs came from experiments in which prisms were mounted over the eyes of owls of different ages. The prisms shifted the retinal image horizontally so that the visual map in the tectum reflected a world systematically displaced from its "actual" orientation. This change abruptly disrupted the correspondence between visual and auditory receptive fields. Over the next several weeks, however, the ITD to which tectal neurons responded optimally, ie, their auditory receptive fields changed until the visual and auditory maps came back into register (Figure 56–17). Thus the visual map instructs the auditory map.

Further experiments showed that this reorganization resulted from rewiring of connections between two deeper auditory nuclei (Figure 56–18). When prism goggles were placed on young owls, changes in ITD tuning were fully adaptive, in that the animals compensated completely for the effects of the prisms. In contrast, goggles placed on mature owls (older than 7 months of age) had little effect. Thus reorganization of this auditory projection occurs optimally during a critical juvenile period.

Distinct Regions of the Brain Have Different Critical Periods of Development

Not all brain circuits are stabilized at the same time. Even within the visual cortex the critical periods for organization of inputs differ among layers. As an example, the neural connections in layer IVC of the visual cortex of the monkey are not affected by monocular deprivation by the time the animal is two months old. In contrast, connections in the upper and lower layers continue to be influenced by sensory experience (or lack of it) for almost the entire first year after birth. Critical periods for other features of the visual system, such as orientation tuning, occur at different developmental stages (Figure 56–19A).

The timing of critical periods also varies between brain regions (Figure 56–19B). The adverse consequences of sensory deprivation for the primary sensory regions of the brain are generally fully realized early in postnatal development. In contrast, social experience can affect the intracortical connections over a much longer period. These differences may explain why certain types of learning are optimal at particular stages of development. For example, certain cognitive capacities—language, music, and mathematics—usually must be acquired well before puberty if they are to develop at all. In addition, insults to the brain at specific early stages of postnatal life may selectively affect the development of certain perceptual abilities and behavior.

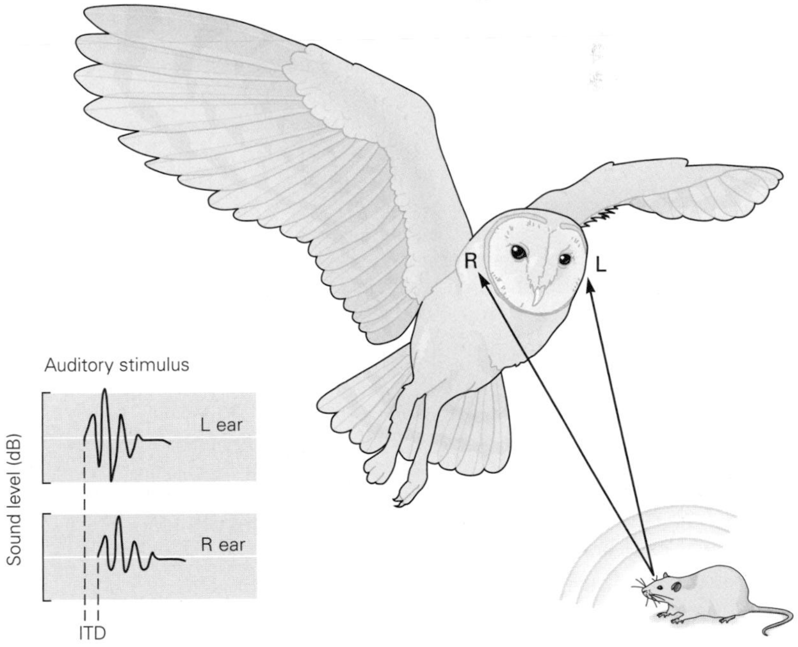

Figure 56–16 The barn owl uses interaural time differences to localize its prey. Sound waves generated by movements of a mouse are received by the owl's left and right ears. As the prey emits noise, the difference in the time of arrival of auditory stimuli at the two ears—the interaural time difference (ITD)—is used to calculate the precise position of the prey target. (Reproduced, with permission, from Knudsen 2002.)

Critical Periods Can Be Reopened in Adulthood

By definition critical periods are limited in time. However, it is now clear that they are less sharply defined than previously thought. Extending or reopening critical periods in adulthood could increase brain plasticity and make it possible to facilitate recovery from strokes and other insults that inactivate discrete regions of the nervous system.

Some of the best evidence for the view that critical periods can be extended comes from studies on matching of auditory and visual maps in owls. In initial experiments the realignment of auditory and visual maps following displacement of the visual field with prism goggles was largely restricted to an early sensitive period. However, three strategies dramatically enhance binaural tuning plasticity in adult owls.

First, when adult owls that had worn goggles as adolescents are refitted with the goggles, the auditory map again shifts to align with the new visual map (Figure 56–20A). In contrast, in adult owls that had not worn the goggles as adolescents, the use of goggles has little effect on the organization of the auditory map. Thus the events of map rearrangement during the normal critical period must leave a neural trace that permits rearrangement later in life. In fact, in the owls that wore prisms in early life, axonal projections to auditory nuclei that were normally pruned were maintained, providing a structural basis for the reorganization in adulthood.

A second method for inducing late plasticity is to displace the retinal image in small steps by having the owl wear a series of prism spectacles of progressively increasing strength. Under these conditions adjustment

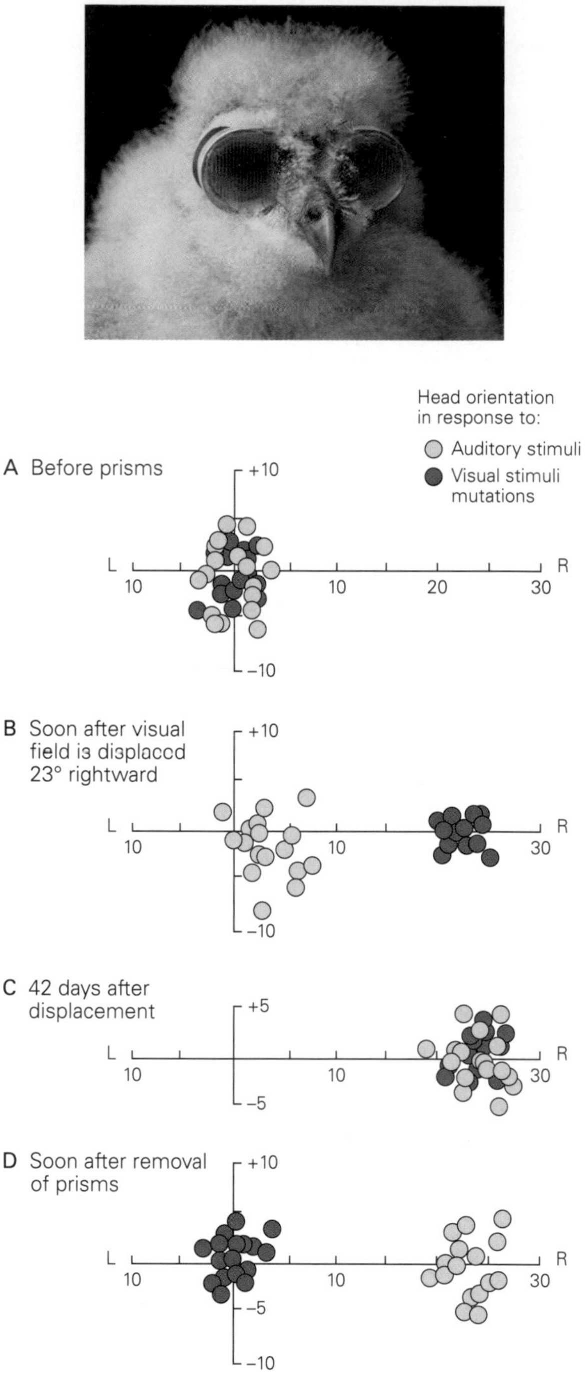

Figure 56–17 Reorganization of sensory maps in the optic tectum of owls after systematic displacement of the retinal image. The retinal image in adolescent owls can be displaced by prism goggles, which shift images from 5 to 30 degrees. (Modified, with permission, from Knudsen 2002.)

A. Before application of the prisms the visual and auditory neural maps coincide.

B. The prism goggles displace the retinal image by 23 degrees. Consequently, the neural and auditory maps are out of alignment.

C. The two brain maps are once again congruent 42 days after prism application because the auditory map has shifted to realign with the visual map.

D. Soon after the prisms are removed, the visual map reverts to its original position, but the auditory map remains in its shifted position.

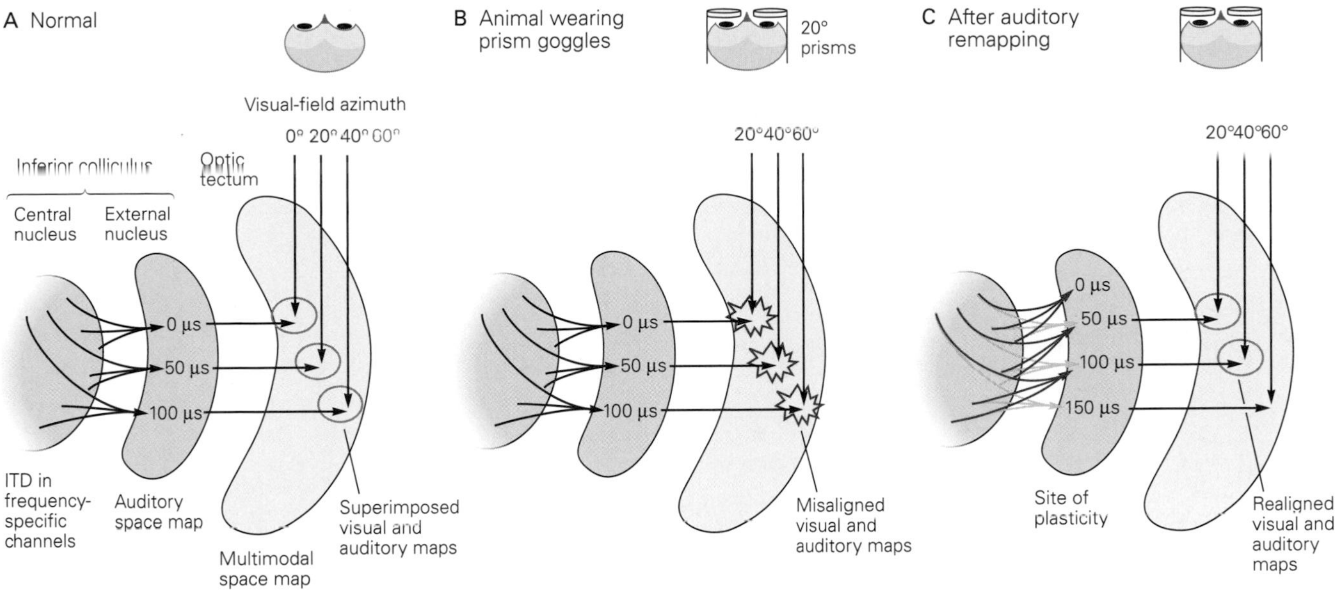

Figure 56–18 The effect of prism experience on information flow in the midbrain auditory localization pathway in the barn owl. (Modified, with permission, from Knudsen 2002.)

A. The auditory pathway in a normal owl. The interaural time difference (**ITD**) is measured and mapped in frequency-specific channels in the brain stem. This information ascends to the inferior colliculus, where a neural map of auditory space is created. The map is conveyed to the optic tectum where it merges with a map of visual space.

B. After an owl is fitted with prism goggles the visual and auditory space maps in the optic tectum become misaligned.

C. After reorganization of auditory maps, the visual and auditory maps are once again in alignment.

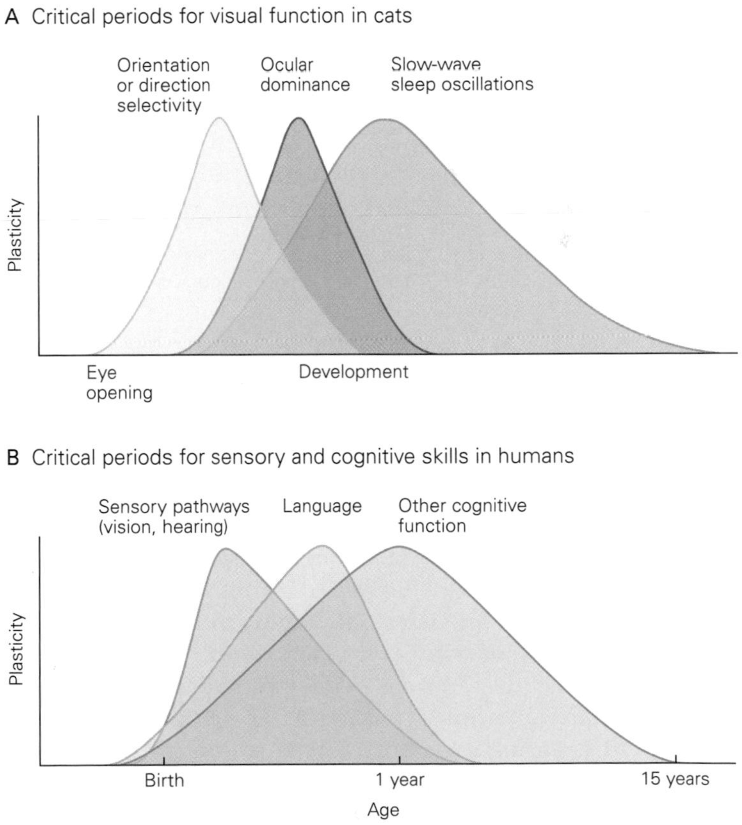

Figure 56–19 The timing of critical periods varies with brain function. (Reproduced, with permission, from Hensch 2005.)

A. In cats the critical periods for development of orientation or direction selectivity in visual neurons occur earlier than those for establishment of ocular dominance and slow-wave sleep oscillation.

B. In humans the timing of periods for development of sensory processing, language, and cognitive functions varies.

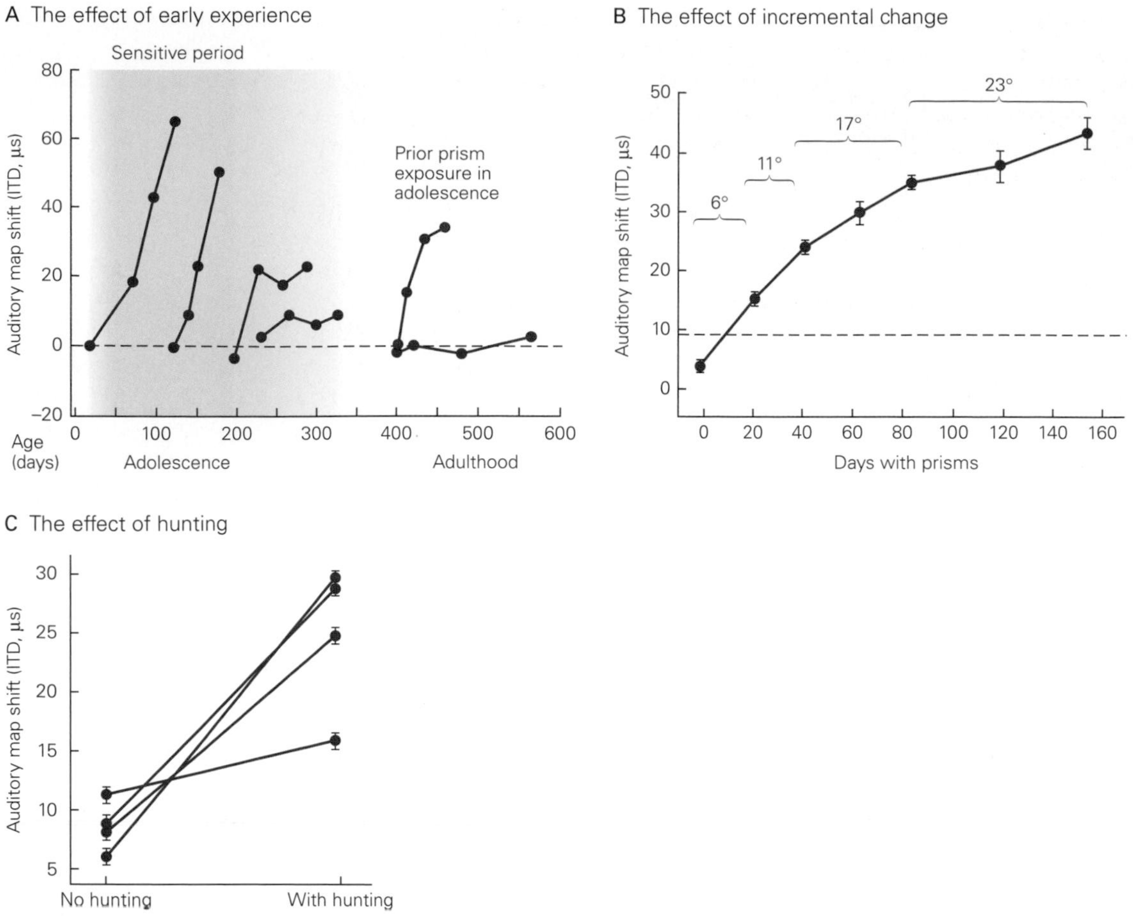

Figure 56–20 Specific behavioral regimes have different effects on the realignment of visual and auditory neural maps in the mature barn owl.

A. The remodeling of the auditory maps that results from wearing prism goggles for a brief period during adolescence leaves a neural trace that can be reactivated in the adult. When these birds are fitted with the goggles as adults, the auditory map is still able to realign with the visual map. (Reproduced, with permission, from Knudsen 2002.)

B. When an animal is fitted with a series of prisms, each of which produces a small displacement in the visual image, the auditory map is successfully brought into alignment. The dotted line shows the extent of realignment if the animal is fitted with a 23 degree prism on day 0. (Reproduced, with permission, from Linkenhoker and Knudsen 2002.)

C. If an adult owl has the opportunity to hunt live prey while wearing prism goggles, auditory remapping occurs, perhaps because of enhanced motivation to sharpen perception. (Reproduced, with permission, from Bergan et al. 2005.)

of the auditory map is typically two- to threefold greater than the response to a single large displacement of the retinal image (Figure 56–20B).

The third technique is to allow owls to hunt live prey. In earlier experiments on plasticity in the optic tectum of owls, the animals were housed and fed under standard laboratory conditions. However, when adult prism-wearing owls are allowed to capture live mice under low light conditions for 10 weeks, they exhibit far greater plasticity than owls fed dead mice (Figure 56–20C), albeit less than that exhibited by juvenile owls that did not hunt. So hunting increases the plasticity of binaural tuning in adult owls. This finding provides a dramatic demonstration that behavioral context affects the ability of the nervous system to reorganize. Whether this effect results from increased sensory information, attention, arousal, motivation, or reward needs to be resolved.

Recent data suggest that critical periods can also be extended or reopened in mammals. There have even been reports that the best-studied critical period, the period for formation of ocular dominance columns, can be modified. Human amblyopia can be ameliorated in adulthood by training. In addition, new insights into the molecular mechanisms underlying critical periods in mice have suggested pharmacological strategies to extend or reopen critical periods. Encouraging results have already been obtained with drugs that alter inhibitory circuitry, destabilize perineuronal nets, or neutralize the growth inhibiting properties of myelin.

How can we reconcile the strong evidence for critical periods with the newer evidence for reorganization of circuitry in adults? The plasticity of critical periods can be distinguished from plasticity in adulthood by its magnitude and by the ease with which it is triggered. These differences result from two factors. First, from early postnatal life into adolescence the molecular environment in the brain is conducive to axonal growth, and cellular mechanisms are optimal for promoting the formation, strengthening, weakening, and elimination of synapses. Under these conditions circuits can undergo fundamental changes in their architecture and biochemistry in response to the animal's experience. Conversely, in mature circuits molecular and structural elements promote stability and impede plasticity.

Second, in a developing circuit no particular pattern of connectivity is firmly entrenched, so there is less to overcome. The connections specified by genetic determinants are less precise and the connections themselves are relatively weak. The patterns of neural activity that are stimulated by experience sharpen and even realign these patterns of connectivity. Once a pattern of connectivity becomes established, strong activation of the established circuit impedes the development of alternative wiring. This difference may help explain the special circumstances needed to trigger plasticity in adulthood. Circuits can be altered by passive exposure of animals to unusual environments during the critical period, whereas adult plasticity may require that the animal pay attention to the stimulus. In sum, experience during critical periods has a potent effect on circuits because the cellular and molecular conditions are optimal for plasticity and because the instructed pattern of connectivity does not have to compete with a long-existing pattern.

An Overall View

Connections among neurons in the mammalian brain arise from two fundamentally different developmental programs: molecular guidance cues and patterned neural activity. Molecular cues guide axons to target regions and initiate the formation of synaptic connections. Once synaptic contact is established, however, continued development depends on the coordination of neural activity between pre- and postsynaptic neurons.

In many instances activity is stimulated by sensory experience, allowing a circuit to refine itself to suit a particular environment. This remarkable ability allows the nervous system to be, in essence, individualized so that it performs optimally. Conversely, it would be maladaptive to allow experience to trigger large-scale reorganization of the nervous system in adults, once behaviors have been established and skills learned. Perhaps for this reason, refinement of neural circuits in response to environmental conditions is largely restricted to critical periods in early development.

Activity-dependent reorganization has been studied in greatest detail in the visual system, particularly in the development of a coordinated binocular view of the world. If afferent fibers carrying input from the same region of the retina of one eye converge on a common cortical neuron, they have an advantage. Their synchronous firing strengthens the synapses of all cooperating fibers, while the synapses of the noncooperating fibers from the other eye decline.

These functional changes lead to local structural changes, for example in dendritic spines, and eventually to large-scale structural changes, with some axon terminals sprouting new synaptic contacts and others withdrawing entirely. As a consequence, overlap of inputs from the two eyes is eliminated and the inputs from the two eyes become segregated into alternating columns in the cortex. If vision is lost in one eye, the cortex reorganizes to devote most of its space to the open eye: Responsiveness to the deprived eye decreases and columns of cells receiving input from the deprived eye shrink, while responsiveness to the open eye increases and its columns expand. One can think of this reorganization as adaptive in that it ensures that as much of the cortex as possible ends up being used.

Studies of monocular deprivation have also provided insight into mechanisms that restrict plasticity in particular circuits to critical periods. A proper balance of excitation and inhibition may be necessary to initiate the critical period. During this period the segregation of afferent fibers and establishment of ocular dominance columns is affected dramatically by changing the balance of activity in the fibers from the two eyes. After the critical period existing connections stabilize and are much less susceptible to such modification. Myelination of axons and formation of matrix-rich nets around interneurons contribute to the stabilization. Studies of the development of ocular dominance columns suggest how other, more complex sensory experiences early in development might change the circuitry and structure of the growing brain.

Because of the enduring nature of neural changes early in life, critical periods are times of both great opportunity and great vulnerability. If the environment to which an animal is exposed during a critical period is representative of the environment it will experience as an adult, plasticity shapes the connectivity of a circuit to make optimal use of cortical real estate and process information optimally. However, maladaptive stimulation during this period can lead to lifelong defects. Social deprivation in early childhood, for example, has lasting effects on social behavior. Some behavioral disorders such as autism may also result in part from aberrant or defective circuit maturation during critical periods.

It has long been clear that reopening of critical periods could, if properly controlled, have numerous benefits. Therapies could be designed to reorganize and retrain the brain to compensate for losses incurred by injuries and disease. Maladaptive reorganization in childhood could be remedied. It might even be possible for adults to learn new skills with some of the effortless efficiency that children exhibit during their critical periods. These possibilities remain science fiction, but it is heartening that recent studies have begun to reveal ways of extending or reopening critical periods in animals, by training regimens or in a few cases pharmacological intervention.

Joshua R. Sanes
Thomas M. Jessell

Selected Readings

Harlow HF. 1958. The nature of love. Am Psychol 13:673–685.

Hensch TK. 2005. Critical period plasticity in local cortical circuits. Nat Rev Neurosci 6:877–888.

Huberman AD, Feller MB, Chapman B. 2008. Mechanisms underlying development of visual maps and receptive fields. Annu Rev Neurosci 31:479–509.

Katz LC, Schatz CJ. 1996. Synaptic activity and the construction of cortical circuits. Science 274:133–1138.

Knudsen EI. 2002. Instructed learning in the auditory localization pathway of the barn owl. Nature 417:322–328.

Wiesel TN. 1982. Postnatal development of the visual cortex and the influence of environment. Nature 299:583–591.

References

Antonini A, Stryker MP. 1993. Rapid remodeling of axonal arbors in the visual cortex. Science 260:1819–1812.

Barkat TR, Polley DB, Hensch TK. 2011. A critical period for auditory thalamocortical connectivity. Nat Neurosci 14:1189–1194.

Behen ME, Helder E, Rothermel R, Solomon K, Chugani HT. 2008. Incidence of specific absolute neurocognitive impairment in globally intact children with histories of early severe deprivation. Child Neuropsychol 14: 453–469.

Bergan JF, Ro P, Ro D, Knudsen EI. 2005. Hunting increases adaptive auditory map plasticity in adult barn owls. J Neurosci 25:9816–9820.

Blankenship A, Ford K, Johnson J, Seal R, Edwards R, Copenhagen D, Feller M. 2009. Synaptic and extrasynaptic factors governing glutamatergic retinal waves. Neuron 62:230–241.

Brainard MS, Knudsen EI. 1998. Sensitive periods for visual calibration of the auditory space map in the barn owl optic tectum. J Neurosci 18: 3929–3942.

Constantine-Paton M, Law MI. 1978. Eye-specific termination bands in tecta of three-eyed frogs. Science 202: 639–641.

Eluvathingal TJ, Chugani HT, Behen ME, Juhász C, Muzik O, Maqbool M, Chugani DC, Makki M. 2006. Abnormal brain connectivity in children after early severe socioemotional deprivation: a diffusion tensor imaging study. Pediatrics 117:2093–2100.

Feller MB, Wellis DP, Stellwagen D, Werblin S, Shatz, CJ. 1996. Requirement for cholinergic synaptic transmission in the propagation of spontaneous retinal waves. Science 272:1182–1187.

Frenkel MY, Bear MF. 2004. How monocular deprivation shifts ocular dominance in visual cortex of young mice. Neuron 44:917–923.

Galli L, Maffei L. 1988. Spontaneous impulse activity of rat retinal ganglion cells in prenatal life. Science 242: 90–91.

Hata Y, Stryker MP. 1994. Control of thalamocortical afferent rearrangement by postsynaptic activity in the developing visual cortex. Science. 265:1732–1735.

Hebb DO. 1949. *Organization of Behavior: A Neuropsychological Theory*. New York: Wiley.

Hensch TK, Fagiolini M, Mataga N, Stryker MP, Baekkeskov S, Kash SF. 1998. Local GABA circuit control of experience-dependent plasticity in developing visual cortex. Science 282:1504–1508.

Hofer S, Mrsic-Flogel T, Bonhoeffer T, Hubener M. 2006. Lifelong learning: ocular dominance plasticity in mouse visual cortex. Curr Opin Neurobio 16:451–459.

Hofer S, Mrsic-Flogel T, Bonhoeffer T, Hubener M. 2009. Experience leaves a lasting structural trace in cortical circuits. Nature 457:313–317.

Holtmaat A, Svoboda K. 2009. Experience-dependent structural synaptic plasticity in the mammalian brain. Nat Rev Neurosci 10:647–658.

Hubel DH, Wiesel TN. 1965. Binocular interaction in striate cortex of kittens reared with artificial squint. J Neurophysiol 28:1041–1059.

Hubel DH, Wiesel TN. 1977. Ferrier lecture: functional architecture of macaque monkey visual cortex. Proc R Soc Lond B Biol Sci 198:1–59.

Hubel DH, Wiesel TN, LeVay S. 1977. Plasticity of ocular dominance columns in monkey striate cortex. Philos Trans R Soc Lond B Biol Sci 278:377–409.

Kaneko M, Hanover JL, England PM, Stryker MP. 2008. TrkB kinase is required for recovery, but not loss, of cortical responses following monocular deprivation. Nat Neurosci 11:497–504.

Khibnik LA, Cho KK, Bear MF. 2010. Relative contribution of feed forward excitatory connections to expression of ocular dominance plasticity in layer 4 of visual cortex. Neuron 66:493–500.

Knudsen EI. 2002. Instructed learning in the auditory localization pathway of the barn owl. Nature 417:322–328.

Kuhl PK. 2004. Early language acquisition: cracking the speech code. Nat Rev Neurosci 5:831–843.

Levay S, Stryker MP, Shatz CJ. 1978. Ocular dominance columns and their development in layer IV of the cat's visual cortex. J Comp Neurol 179:223–244.

Linkenhoker BA, Knudsen EI. 2002 Incremental training increases the plasticity of the auditory space map in adult barn owls. Nature 419:293–296.

Löwel S. 1994. Ocular dominance column development: strabismus changes the spacing of adjacent columns in cat visual cortex. J Neurosci 14:7451–7468.

Maffei A, Nataraj K, Nelson SB, Turrigiano GG. 2006. Potentiation of cortical inhibition by visual deprivation. Nature 443:81–84.

Mataga N, Mizuguchi Y, Hensch TK. 2004. Experience-dependent pruning of dendritic spines in visual cortex by tissue plasminogen activator. Neuron 44:1031–1041.

McGee AW, Yang Y, Fischer QS, Daw NW, Strittmatter SM. 2005. Experience-driven plasticity of visual cortex limited by myelin and Nogo receptor. Science 309:2222–2226.

Meister M, Wong ROL, Baylor DA, Shatz CJ. 1991. Synchronous bursts of action potentials in ganglion cells of the developing mammalian retina. Science 252:939–943.

Moreau E. 1913. Histoire de la guerison d'un aveugle-ne. Ann Ocul (Paris) 149:81–118.

Nelson CA 3rd, Zeanah CH, Fox NA, Marshall PJ, Smyke AT, Guthrie D. 2007. Cognitive recovery in socially deprived young children: the Bucharest Early Intervention Project. Science 318:1937–1940.

Oray S, Majewska A, Sur M. 2004. Dendritic spine dynamics are regulated by monocular deprivation and extracellular matrix degradation. Neuron 44:1021–1030.

Pizzorusso T, Medini P, Berardi N, Chierzi S, Fawcett JW, Maffei L. 2002. Reactivation of ocular dominance plasticity in the adult visual cortex. Science 298:1248–1251.

Rakic P. 1981. Development of visual centers in the primate brain depends on binocular competition before birth. Science 214:928–931.

Sanes JR, Yamagata M. 1999. Formation of lamina-specific synaptic connections. Curr Opin Neurobiol 9:79–87.

Shatz CJ, Stryker MP. 1988. Prenatal tetrodotoxin infusion blocks segregation of retino-geniculate afferents. Science 242:87–89.

Spitz RA. 1945. Hospitalism: an inquiry into the genesis of psychiatric conditions in early childhood. Psychoanal Study Child 1:53–74.

Van Sluyters, RC and Levitt FB. 1980. Experimental strabismus in the kitten. J Neurophysio 43:686–699.

57

Repairing the Damaged Brain

For much of its history neurology has been a discipline of outstanding diagnostic rigor but little therapeutic efficacy. Simply put, neurologists have been renowned for their ability to localize lesions with great precision but until recently have had little to offer in terms of treatment. During the past decade this situation has begun to change.

Advances in our understanding of the structure, function, and chemistry of the brain's neurons, glial cells, and synapses have led to new ideas for treatment. Many of these are now in clinical trials and some are already available to patients. Developmental neuroscience is emerging as a major contributor to this sea change for three main reasons. First, efforts to preserve or replace neurons lost to damage or disease rely on recent advances in our understanding of the mechanisms that control the generation and death of nerve cells (see Chapters 52 and 53). Second, efforts to improve the regeneration of neural pathways following injury draw heavily on what we have learned about the growth of axons and the formation of synapses (see Chapters 54 and 55). Third, there is increasing evidence that some devastating brain disorders, such as autism and schizophrenia, are the result of disturbances in the formation of neural circuits in embryonic or early postnatal life. Accordingly, studies of normal development may provide an essential foundation for discovering precisely what has gone wrong in disease.

In this chapter we focus on the first two of these issues: How neuroscientists hope to augment the limited ability of neurons to recover normal function. We shall begin by describing how axons degenerate following the separation of the axon and its terminals from the cell body. The regeneration of severed axons is robust in the peripheral nervous system of mammals and in the central nervous system of lower vertebrates, but very poor in the central nervous system of mammals. Many investigators have sought the reasons for these differences in the hope that understanding them will lead to methods for augmenting recovery of the human brain and spinal cord following injury. Indeed, we shall see that several differences in regenerative capacity of mammalian neurons have been discovered, each of which has opened promising new approaches to therapy.

Next we shall consider an even more dire consequence of neural injury: the death of neurons. The inability of the adult brain to form new neurons has been a central dogma of neuroscience since the pioneering neuroanatomist Santiago Ramón y Cajal asserted that in the injured central nervous system, "Everything may die, nothing may be regenerated." This pessimistic view dominated neurology for most of the last century despite the fact that Ramón y Cajal added, "It is for the science of the future to change, if possible, this harsh decree." Remarkably, in the past few decades evidence has accumulated that neurogenesis does occur in certain regions of the adult mammalian brain. This discovery has helped accelerate the pace of research on ways to stimulate neurogenesis and to replace neurons following injury. Although this work is preliminary, and in some respects controversial, it now seems possible that in the future neuroscientists will be able to reverse Cajal's "harsh decree."

Damage to Axons Affects Neurons and Neighboring Cells

Because neurons have very long axons and cell bodies of modest size, most injuries to the central or peripheral nervous system involve damage to axons. Transection of the axon, either by cutting or by crushing, is called *axotomy*, and its consequences are numerous.

Axon Degeneration Is an Active Process

Axotomy divides the axon in two: a proximal segment that remains attached to the cell body and a distal segment that has lost this crucial attachment. Axotomy dooms the distal segment of the axon. Synaptic transmission soon fails at severed nerve terminals. After a delay, physical degeneration of the axon occurs and once it begins its progression is relatively rapid and inevitably proceeds to completion (Figure 57–1). Within the distal segment the neuronal membrane breaks down, the cytoskeleton is disassembled, and

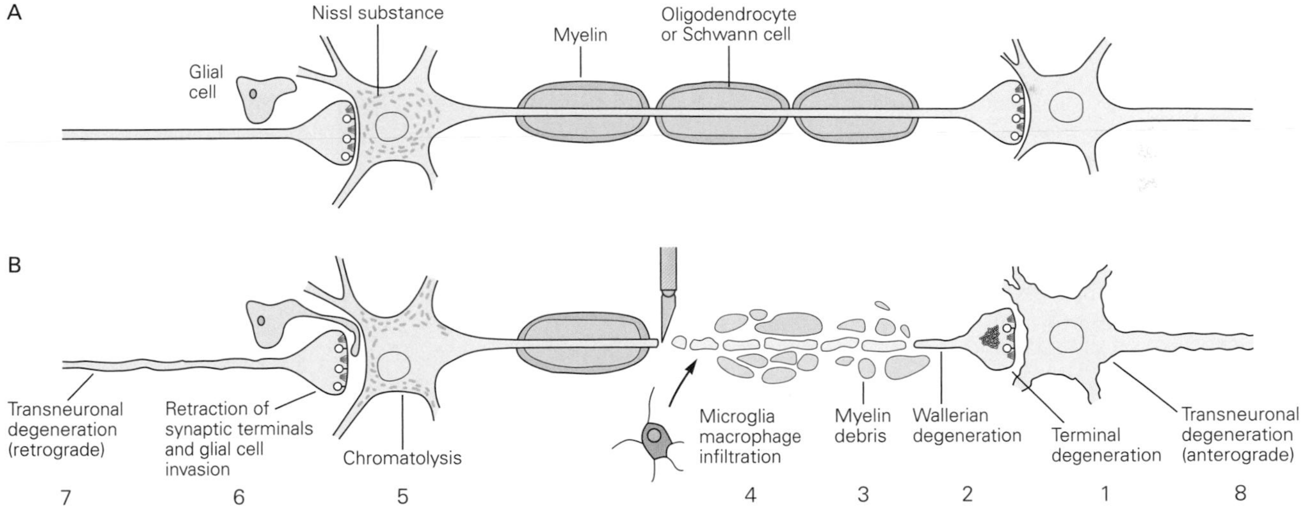

Figure 57–1 Axotomy affects the injured neuron and its synaptic partners.

A. A normal neuron with an intact functional axon wrapped by myelinating cells contacts a postsynaptic neuron. The neuron's cell body is itself a postsynaptic target.

B. After axotomy the nerve terminals of the injured neuron begin to degenerate (**1**). The distal axonal stump separates from the parental cell body, becomes irregular, and undergoes Wallerian degeneration (**2**). Myelin begins to fragment (**3**) and the lesion site is invaded by phagocytic cells (**4**). The cell body of the damaged neuron undergoes chromatolysis: The cell body swells and the nucleus moves to an eccentric position (**5**). Synaptic terminals that contact the damaged neuron withdraw and the synaptic site is invaded by glial cell processes (**6**). The injured neuron's inputs (**7**) and targets (**8**) can atrophy and degenerate.

cytoskeletal components are degraded. This degenerative response is the first step in an elaborate constellation of changes that were initially described in 1850 by Augustus Waller, changes that are now called *Wallerian degeneration*.

The degeneration of transected axons was long thought to be a passive process, the consequence of separation from the neuronal cell body, within which most of the cell's proteins are synthesized. Lacking a source of new protein, the distal stump would, in essence, wither away. But the discovery and analysis in mice of a spontaneously occurring mutant called *Wlds* (Wallerian degeneration slow) challenged this view (Figure 57–2). In the *Wlds* mutant the distal stumps of peripheral nerves persist for several weeks after transection, about 10-fold longer than in normal mice. The *Wlds* mutation results in the fusion of two normal proteins into a novel protein. One of the contributing proteins is normally involved in biosynthesis of a metabolic cofactor, nicotinamide adenine dinucleotide (NADH), and the other is normally involved in ubiquitination, the process that covalently modifies proteins for degradation.

It remains unclear how the presence of the *Wlds* fusion protein slows degeneration so dramatically, but its discovery has been important in several ways. First, the very fact that degeneration *can* be slowed proves that it is not a passive consequence of separation from the cell body, but is rather an actively regulated response. Second, the nature of the *Wlds* protein has already given us clues about the nature of the active process that drives Wallerian degeneration.

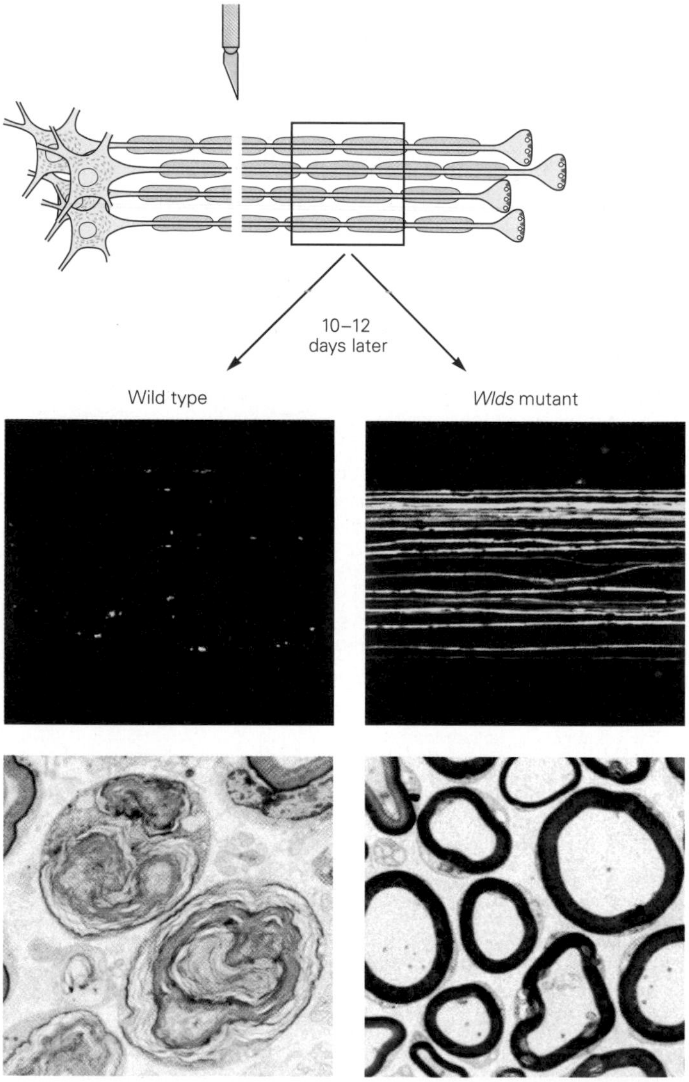

Figure 57–2 Axonal degeneration is delayed in *Wlds* mutant mice. After sectioning of a peripheral nerve in wild type animals, axons in the distal stump degenerate rapidly, as shown by disrupted axonal fragments (**yellow**) and the lack of myelinated axonal profiles at the electron micrographic level. In *Wlds* mutant mice the distal portion of severed axons persists for a long time. (Top two confocal micrographs reproduced, with permission, from Beirowski et al. 2004. Bottom two electron micrographs reproduced, with permission, from Michael Coleman.)

Third, and perhaps most importantly, insight into how the *Wlds* fusion protein acts may be useful in devising treatments for neurological disorders in which axonal degeneration is prominent. A fatal disease of motor neurons, amyotrophic lateral sclerosis, falls into this category. Other possibilities include some forms of spinal muscular atrophy, Parkinson disease, and even Alzheimer disease. Axon degeneration that occurs in these diseases, as well as after metabolic, toxic, or inflammatory insults, resembles the degeneration that follows acute trauma and may be regulated in similar ways. Expression of the *Wlds* fusion protein significantly delays axonal loss and can even extend the life span of certain mouse models of motor neuron disease. Thus, while methods for saving transected distal axons are unlikely to be useful clinically for treating patients who have suffered traumatic injury, the same techniques could be useful in treating neurodegenerative diseases.

We return now to the injured axon itself. Even though the proximal portion of the axon remains attached to the cell body, it too suffers. And in some cases the neuron itself dies by apoptosis, probably because axotomy isolates the neuronal cell body from its supply of target-derived trophic factors. Even when this does not occur, the cell body often undergoes a series of cellular and biochemical changes called the *chromatolytic reaction:* The cell body swells, the nucleus moves to an eccentric position, and the rough endoplasmic reticulum becomes fragmented (Figure 57–1B). Chromatolysis is accompanied by other metabolic changes, including an increase in protein and RNA synthesis as well as a change in the pattern of genes that the neuron expresses. These changes are reversible if regeneration is successful.

Axotomy Leads to Reactive Responses in Nearby Cells

Axotomy sets in motion a cascade of responses in numerous types of neighboring cells. Among the most important responses are those of the glial cells that ensheath the distal nerve segment. The myelin sheath becomes fragmented and eventually removed.

This process is rapid in the peripheral nervous system, where the myelin-producing Schwann cells break the myelin into small fragments and engulf it. Schwann cells, which then divide, secrete factors that recruit macrophages from the blood stream. The macrophages in turn assist in the disposal of debris. Schwann cells also produce growth factors that promote axon regeneration, a point to which we will return later.

In contrast, in the central nervous system the myelin-forming oligodendrocytes have little or no ability to dispose of myelin, and the blood-brain barrier prevents the entry of macrophages, so removal of debris depends on a limited quantity of resident macrophages called *microglia*. These differences in cellular properties explain the observation that Wallerian degeneration proceeds to completion much more slowly in the central nervous system.

Axotomy also affects postsynaptic neurons. When axotomy disrupts the major inputs to a cell—as happens in denervated muscle, or to neurons in the lateral geniculate when the optic nerve is cut—the consequences are severe. Usually the target atrophies and sometimes dies. When targets are only partially denervated, their responses are more limited. In addition, axotomy affects presynaptic neurons. In many instances synaptic terminals withdraw from the cell body or dendrites of chromatolytic neurons and are replaced by the processes of glial cells—Schwann cells in the periphery and microglia or astrocytes in the central nervous system. This process, called *synaptic stripping,* depresses synaptic activity and can impair functional recovery.

Although the mechanism of synaptic stripping remains unclear, two possibilities have been suggested. One is that postsynaptic injury causes axon terminals to lose their adhesiveness to synaptic sites so that they are subsequently wrapped by glia. The other is that glia initiate the process of synaptic stripping in response to factors released from the injured neuron or to changes in its cell surface. Whatever the trigger, the activation of microglia and astrocytes by axotomy clearly contributes to the stripping process. In addition, biochemically altered astrocytes, called reactive astrocytes, contribute to formation of a *glial scar* near sites of injury.

As a result of these transsynaptic effects, neuronal degeneration can propagate through a circuit in both anterograde and retrograde directions. For example, a denervated neuron that becomes severely atrophic can fail to activate its target, which in turn becomes atrophic. Likewise, when synaptic stripping prevents an afferent neuron from obtaining sufficient sustenance from its target cell, the afferent neuron's inputs are placed at risk. Such chain reactions help to explain how injury to one site in the central nervous system eventually affects regions far from the source of the injury.

Central Axons Regenerate Poorly After Injury

Central and peripheral nerves differ substantially in their ability to regenerate after injury. Peripheral nerves can often be repaired following injury. Although the

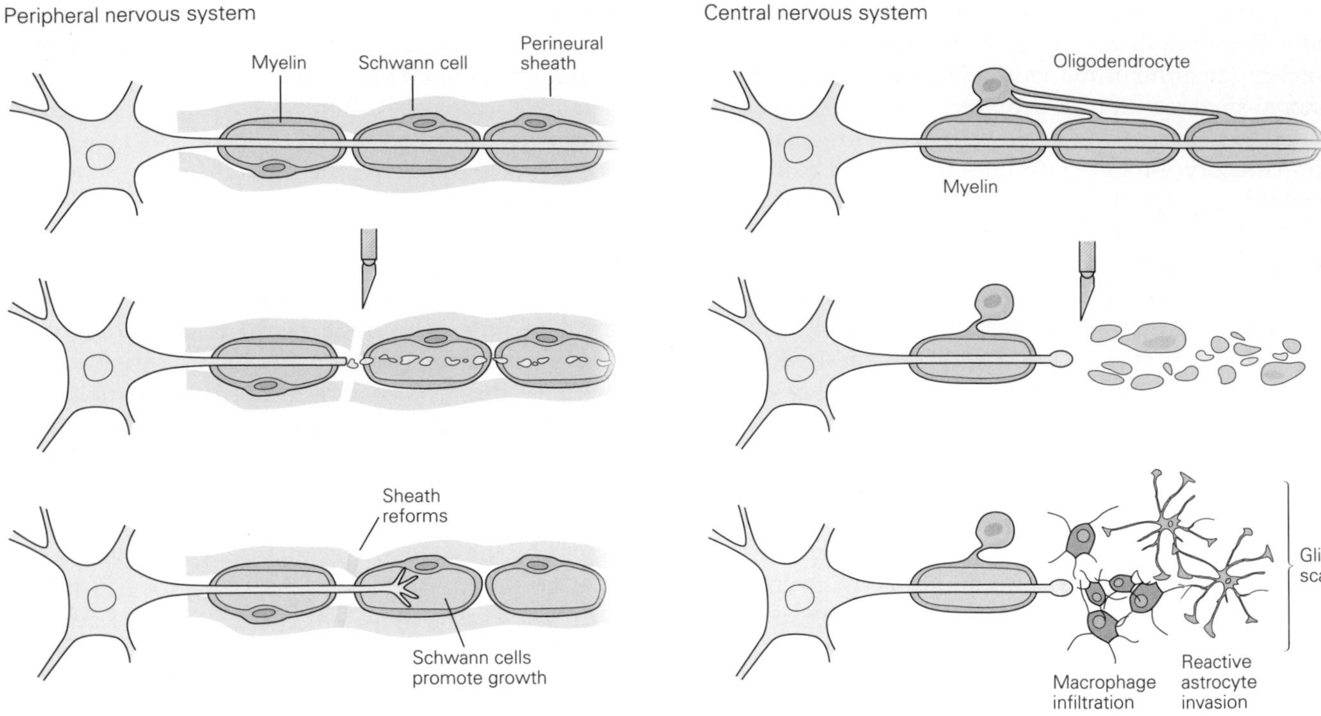

Figure 57–3 Axons in the periphery regenerate better than those in the central nervous system. After sectioning of a peripheral nerve, the perineural sheath reforms rapidly and Schwann cells in the distal stump promote axonal growth by producing trophic and attractant factors and expressing high levels of adhesive proteins. After sectioning of axonal tracts in the central nervous system, the distal segment disintegrates and myelin fragments. In addition, reactive astrocytes and macrophages are attracted to the lesion site. This complex cellular milieu, termed a *glial scar*, inhibits axonal regeneration.

distal segments of axons degenerate, connective tissue elements surrounding the distal stump generally survive. Axonal sprouts grow from the proximal stump, enter the distal stump, and grow along the nerve toward its targets (Figure 57–3). The mechanisms that drive this process are related to those that guide embryonic axons. Chemotropic factors secreted by Schwann cells attract axons to the distal stump, adhesive molecules within the distal stump promote axon growth along cell membranes and extracellular matrices, and inhibitory molecules in the perineural sheath prevent regenerating axons from going astray.

Once regenerated peripheral axons reach their targets they are able to form new functional nerve endings. Motor axons form new neuromuscular junctions; autonomic axons successfully reinnervate glands, blood vessels, and viscera; and sensory axons reinnervate muscle spindles. Finally, those axons that lost their myelin sheaths are remyelinated, and chromatolytic cell bodies regain their original appearance. Thus in all three divisions of the peripheral nervous system—motor, sensory, and autonomic—the effects of axotomy are reversible. This is not to imply that peripheral regeneration is perfect. In the motor system recovery of strength may be substantial, but recovery of fine movements is usually impaired. Some motor axons form synapses on inappropriate muscle fibers, some peripheral axons never find their targets, and some neurons die. Nevertheless, the regenerative capacities in the peripheral nervous system are impressive.

In contrast, in the central nervous system regeneration after injury is poor (Figure 57–3). The proximal stumps of damaged axons can form short sprouts, but these soon stall and form swollen endings called "retraction bulbs" that fail to progress. Long-distance regeneration is rare. The longstanding failure of central regeneration has led to the pessimistic view that injuries to the brain and spinal cord are largely irreversible, and that therapy must be restricted to rehabilitative measures.

For some time neurobiologists have been seeking the reasons why regenerative capacity in the central and peripheral nervous systems differs so dramatically. The goal of this work is to identify the crucial barriers to regeneration so that they can be overcome. These studies have begun to bear fruit, and there is now cautious optimism that the injured human brain and spinal cord have a regenerative capacity that can eventually be exploited.

Before discussing these new developments it is helpful to consider the problem of neural regeneration in a broader biological context. Is it the ability of peripheral axons to regenerate that is unusual, or the inability of central axons to do so? It is in fact the latter. Obviously, central axons grow well during development. More surprisingly, axons in immature mammals can also regenerate following transection in the brain or spinal cord. Moreover, regeneration is robust in the central nervous systems of lower vertebrates such as fish and frogs, as exemplified by the studies of Roger Sperry on restoration of vision following damage to the optic nerve (see Chapter 54).

So why have mature mammals lost this seemingly important capacity for repair? The answer may lie in what the mammalian brain *can* do peerlessly, which is to remodel its basic wiring diagram in accordance with experience during critical periods in early postnatal life, so that each individual's brain is optimized to deal with the changes and challenges of internal and external worlds (see Chapter 56). But once remodeling has occurred, it must be stabilized. It is obviously useful to reassign cortical space to one eye if the other is blinded in childhood, but we would not want our cortical connections similarly rearranged in response to a brief period of unusual illumination or darkness. Maintaining constancy in the face of small perturbations in connectivity may therefore have the unavoidable consequence of limiting the ability of central connections to regenerate in response to injury. In this view our limited regenerative capacity is the Faustian biological bargain we have made for the possession of many precisely wired circuits that underlie our superior intellectual powers.

Therapeutic Interventions May Promote Regeneration of Injured Central Neurons

In seeking reasons for the poor regeneration of central axons, one critical question is whether the poor recovery reflects an inability of neurons themselves to grow or an inability of the environment to support axonal growth. This issue was addressed by Albert Aguayo and his colleagues in the early 1980s. They inserted segments of a central nerve trunk into a peripheral nerve graft, and segments of a peripheral nerve into the brain or spinal cord, to find out how the translocated axons would respond.

Aguayo found that the axons in the translocated segments promptly degenerated, leaving "distal stumps" containing glia, support cells, and extracellular matrix. The results were striking. Spinal axons that regenerated poorly following spinal cord injury grew several centimeters when inserted into a peripheral nerve (Figure 57–4). Conversely, peripheral axons regenerated well through their own distal nerve trunk, but fared poorly when paired with a severed optic nerve (Figure 57–5).

Aguayo extended these studies to show that axons from multiple regions, including the retinal ganglion, olfactory bulb, brain stem, and mesencephalon, could each regenerate long distances if provided with a suitable environment. As we will see later, it turns out that regrowth of central axons is intrinsically limited. Nevertheless, these pioneering experiments focused attention on components of the central environment that inhibit regenerative ability and motivated an intensive search for the molecular culprits.

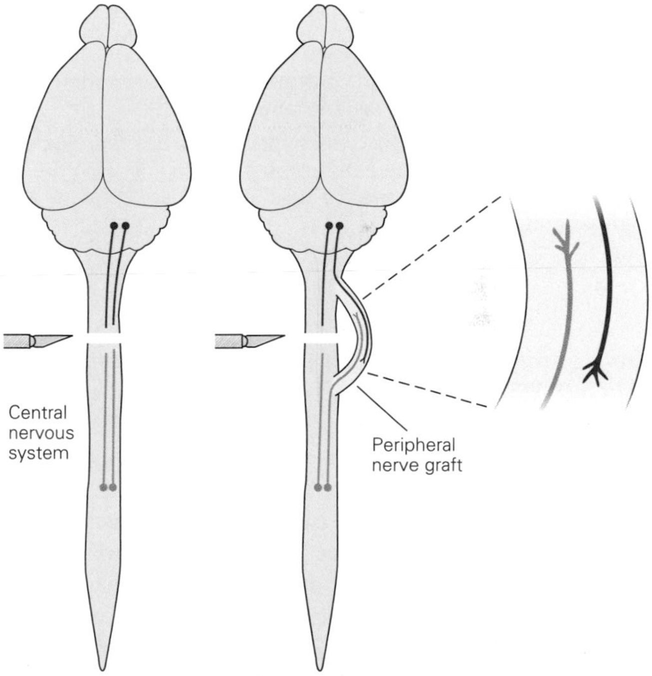

Figure 57–4 A transplanted peripheral nerve provides a favorable environment for the regeneration of central axons. *Left*: After sectioning of the spinal cord, ascending and descending axons fail to cross the lesion site. *Right*: Insertion of a bridging peripheral nerve graft that bypasses the lesion site promotes regeneration of both ascending and descending axons. (Adapted, with permission, from Aguayo 1981.)

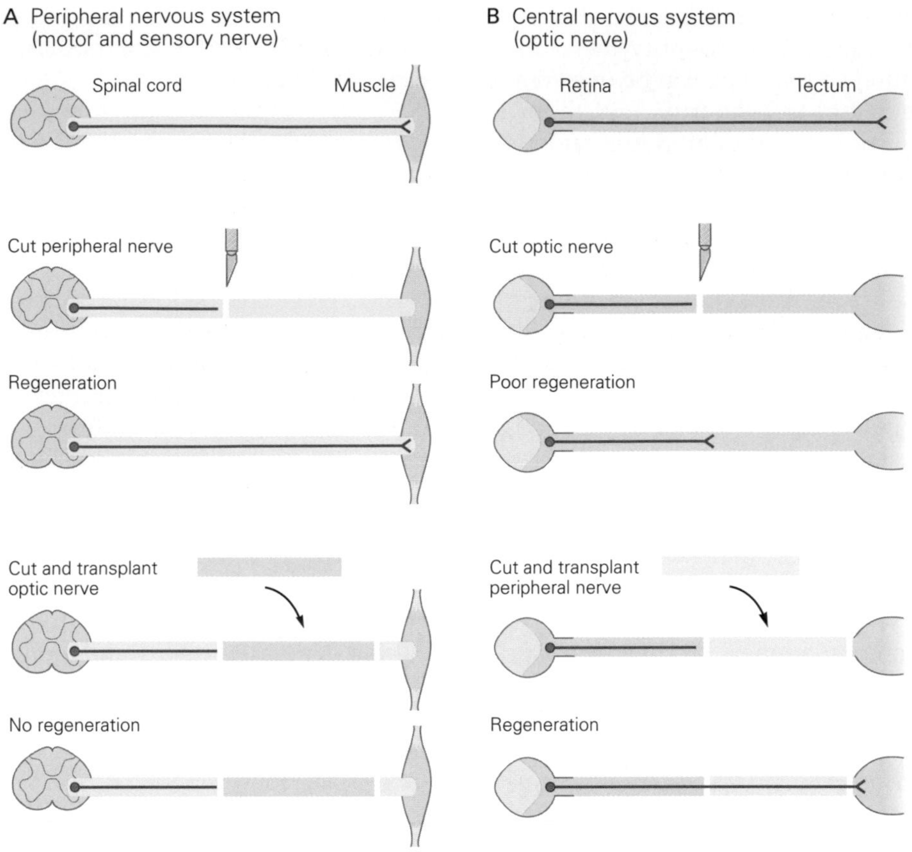

Figure 57–5 Peripheral and central nerves differ in their ability to support axonal regeneration.

A. In the peripheral nervous system severed axons regrow past the site of injury. Insertion of a segment of optic nerve into a peripheral nerve suppresses the ability of the peripheral nerve to regenerate.

B. In the central nervous system severed axons typically fail to regrow past the site of injury. Insertion of a section of peripheral nerve into a central nerve tract promotes regeneration.

Environmental Factors Support the Regeneration of Injured Axons

In probing the differences between peripheral and central growth environments, initial searches were influenced by the results of experiments performed by Ramón y Cajal's student Jorge Tello-Muñoz nearly a century before Aguayo's studies. Tello transplanted segments of peripheral nerves into the brains of experimental animals and found that injured central axons grew toward the implants, whereas they barely grew when implants were not available.

This result implied that peripheral cells provide growth-promoting factors to the injured areas; factors normally absent from the brain. Ramón y Cajal reasoned that central nerve pathways lacked "substances able to sustain and invigorate the indolent and scanty growth" similar to those provided by peripheral pathways. Numerous studies over the succeeding century identified constituents of peripheral nerves that are potent promoters of neurite outgrowth. These include components of Schwann cell basal laminae such as laminin, and cell adhesion molecules of the immunoglobulin superfamily. In addition, cells in denervated distal nerve stumps begin to produce neurotrophins and other trophic molecules. Together these molecules nourish neurons and guide growing axons in the embryonic nervous system, so it makes sense that they also promote the regrowth of axons. By contrast, central neuronal tissue is a poor source of these molecules, containing little laminin and low levels of trophic molecules. Thus in the embryo both central and peripheral nervous systems provide environments that promote axon outgrowth. But only the peripheral environment retains this capacity in adulthood, or is able to regain it effectively following injury.

The practical implications of this view are that supplementing the central environment with growth-promoting molecules might improve regeneration. To this end investigators have infused neurotrophins into areas of injury or inserted conduits rich in extracellular matrix molecules such as laminin. In some attempts Schwann cells themselves, or cells engineered to secrete trophic factors, have been grafted into sites of injury. In many of these cases injured axons grow slightly more extensively than they do under control conditions. Yet regeneration remains limited, with axons generally failing to extend long distances. More important, functional recovery is minimal.

What accounts for such disappointingly limited regeneration? One limitation appears to be the existence of inhibitory signaling pathways that block the growth-promoting activity of cytokine factors. In the optic nerve, for example, the poor regeneration of the axons of retinal ganglion neurons is accounted for in part by the state of activation of a cytokine signaling pathway. The axonal growth-promoting effects of cytokines such as ciliary neurotrophic factors (CNTFs) involve activation of a receptor GP130, and GP130 signaling is counteracted by the activity of a suppressor of cytokine signaling called SOCS3. Thus deletion of the SOCS3 gene in mice augments the ability of CNTF to promote regeneration of retinal ganglion cell axons in the optic nerve (Figure 57–6).

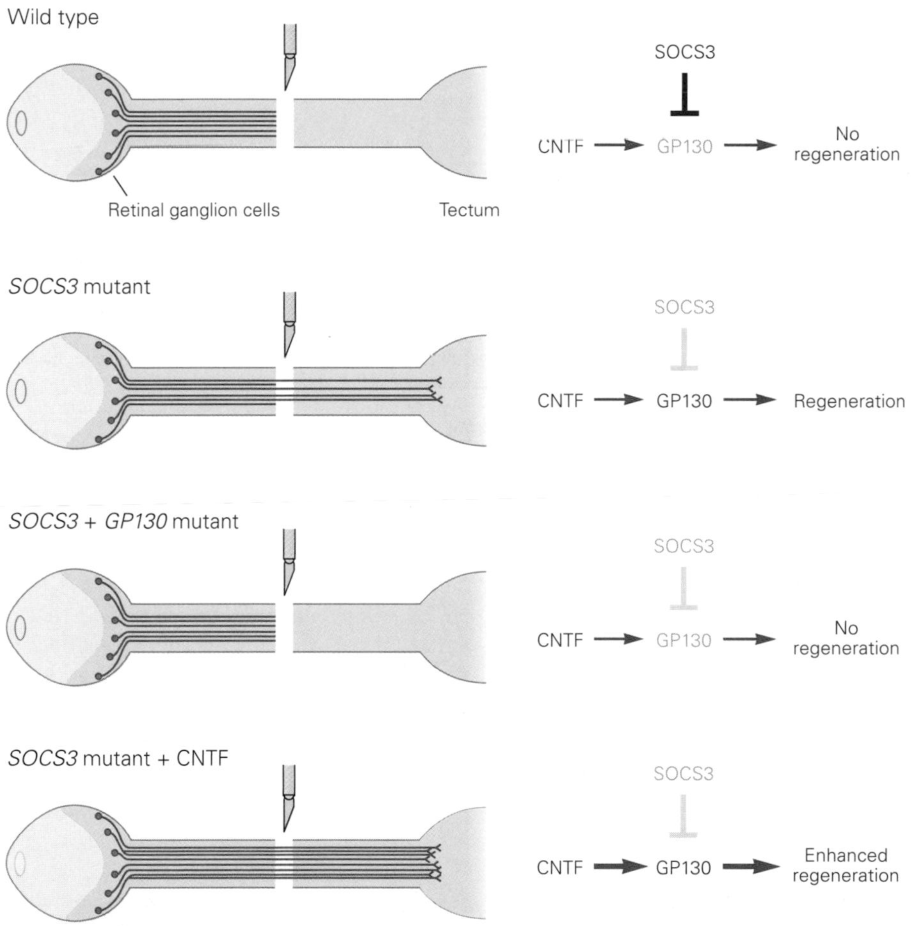

Figure 57–6 Signaling pathways that regulate axon regeneration in the optic nerve. The regeneration of retinal ganglion cell axons in the optic nerve is normally constrained by neuronal expression of the gene for SOCS3, which blocks the ability of ciliary neurotrophic factor (**CNTF**) to bind its receptor GP130 and thus blocks CNTF from promoting regeneration. In *SOCS3* mutant mice, ambient levels of CNTF are sufficient to improve optic nerve regeneration. Elimination of GP130 as well as SOCS3 blocks the capacity for regeneration. Addition of extra CNTF enhances the capacity for regeneration in *SOCS3* mutant mice. (Adapted, with permission, from Smith et al. 2009.)

Components of Myelin Inhibit Neurite Outgrowth

Fragments of central myelin are potent inhibitors of neurite outgrowth. Sprouting of spinal axon collaterals following injury is enhanced in rats treated to prevent myelin formation in the spinal cord (Figure 57–7). These findings implied that although both central and peripheral environments might contain a supply of growth-promoting elements, central nerves also contain inhibitory components. That myelin inhibits neurite growth may seem peculiar, but in fact myelination normally occurs postnatally, after axon extension is largely complete.

Searches for the inhibitory components of central myelin turned up an embarrassment of riches. Several classes of molecules found at higher levels in central myelin compared to peripheral myelin are able to inhibit neurite outgrowth when presented to cultured neurons. The first to be discovered was identified when an antibody generated against myelin proteins proved to be capable of partially neutralizing myelin's ability to inhibit neurite outgrowth. Use of this antibody to isolate the corresponding antigen yielded the protein now called Nogo. Two other proteins, myelin-associated glycoprotein (MAG) and oligodendrocyte-myelin glycoprotein (OMgp), initially isolated as major components of myelin, have been found to inhibit the growth of some neuronal types.

Intriguingly, Nogo, MAG, and OMgp each bind to common membrane receptors, NogoR and PirB (Figure 57–8). In mutant mice lacking PirB, regeneration of severed corticospinal axons is enhanced; the extent of axonal regeneration in mice lacking NogoR or its three ligands is uncertain. Identifying physiologically relevant constraints on regeneration may be complicated by the presence of still undiscovered inhibitors. But if many inhibitory components trigger the same intracellular signaling pathway, then interference with that pathway might neutralize the impact of many inhibitors in one fell swoop.

Injury-Induced Scarring Hinders Axonal Regeneration

Myelin debris is not the only source of growth-inhibiting material in the injured brain or spinal cord. As noted earlier, astrocytes become activated and proliferate following injury, acquiring features of reactive astrocytes that generate scar tissue at sites of injury. Scarring is an adaptive response that helps to limit the size of the injury, to reestablish the blood-brain barrier, and to reduce inflammation.

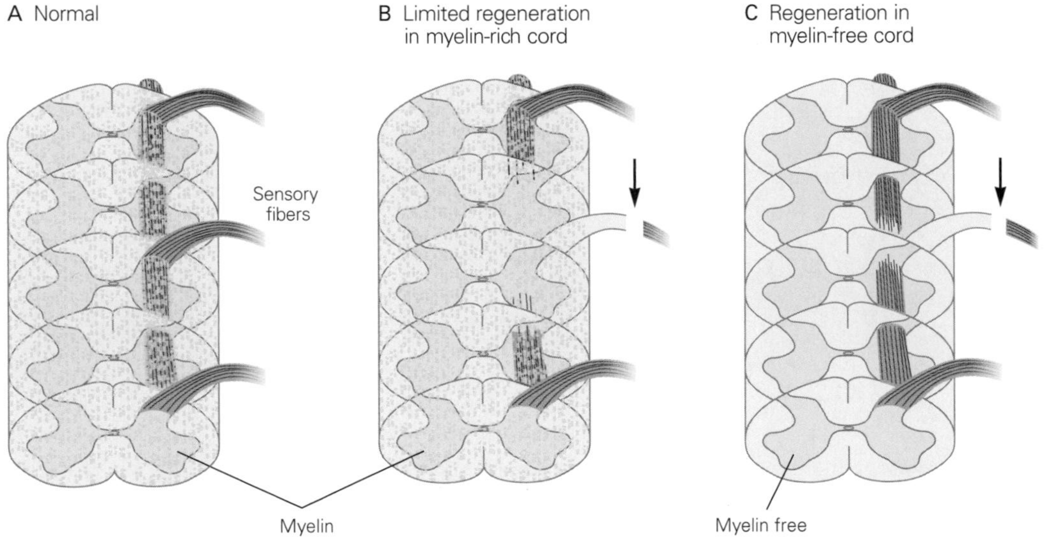

Figure 57–7 Myelin inhibits regeneration of central axons. (Adapted, with permission, from Schwegler, Schwab, and Kapfhammer 1995.)

A. Sensory fibers normally extend rostrally in a myelin-rich spinal cord.

B. Right dorsal root fibers were sectioned in 2-week-old normal rats. Regeneration of the fibers was assessed histochemically 20 days later. The central branches of the sectioned axons degenerated, leaving a portion of the spinal cord denervated. Little regeneration occurred in the myelin-rich cord.

C. Some littermates received local x-irradiation to block myelination. In these animals sensory fibers that entered the cord through neighboring uninjured roots sprouted new collaterals following denervation.

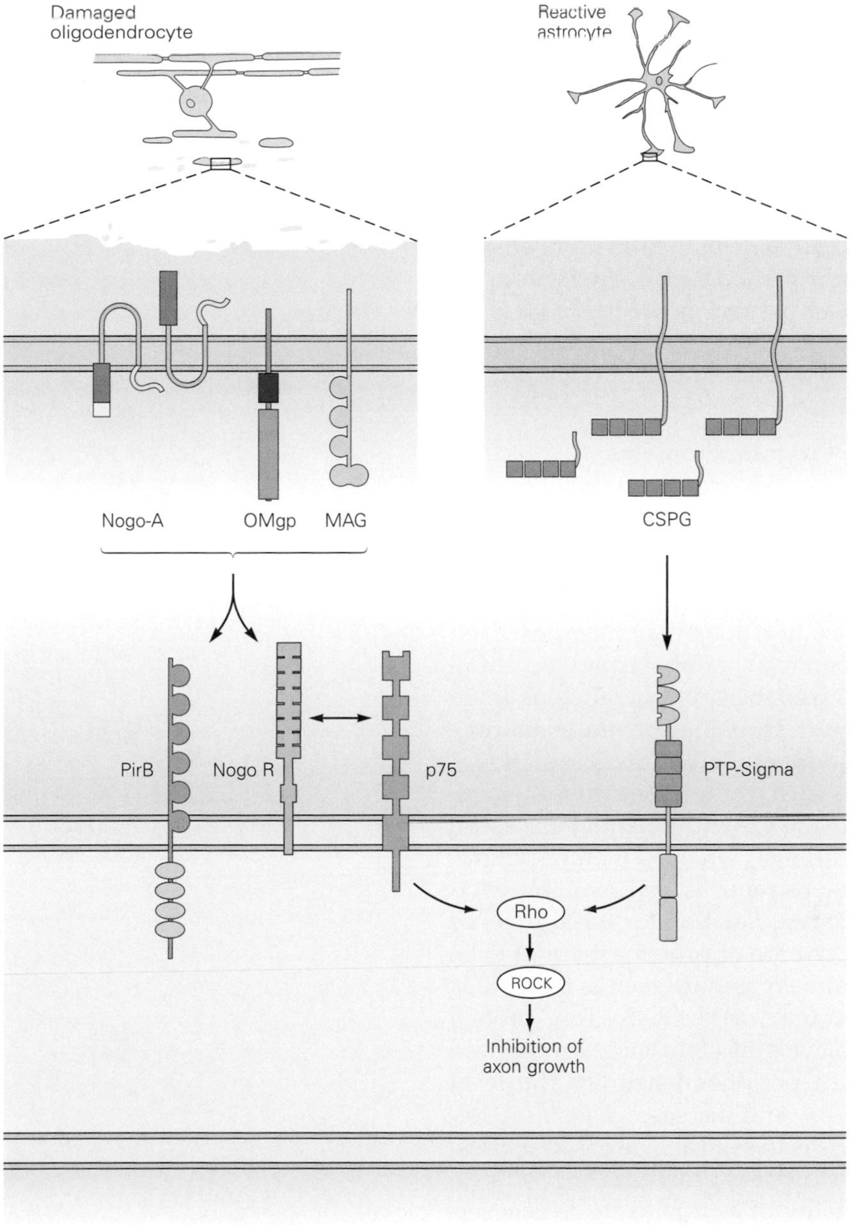

Figure 57–8 Myelin and glial scar components that inhibit regeneration of central axons. *Left*: Myelin contains the proteins Nogo-A, oligodendrocyte-myelin glycoprotein (**OMgp**), and myelin-associated glycoprotein (**MAG**). All three proteins are exposed when myelin breaks down. They can bind a receptor protein Nogo R, which can associate with the neurotrophin receptor p75, as well as an immunoglobulin-like receptor protein PirB. Inactivation of PirB results in a modest enhancement of corticospinal axon regeneration. *Right*: Chondroitin sulphate proteoglycans (**CSPG**) are major components of the glial scar and are thought to suppress axon regeneration through interaction with the receptor tyrosine phosphatase PTP-sigma, which activates intracellular mediators such as Rho and ROCK. (Adapted, with permission, from Yiu et al. 2006.)

But the scar itself hinders regeneration in two ways: through mechanical interference with axon growth and through growth-inhibiting effects of proteins produced by cells within the scar. Chief among these inhibitors are a class of chondroitin sulfate proteoglycans (CSPG) that are produced in abundance by reactive astrocytes and directly inhibit axon extension by interaction with tyrosine phosphatase receptors on axons (Figure 57–8). Attention has therefore focused on ways of dissolving the glial scar by infusion of an enzyme called *chondroitinase*, which breaks down the sugar chains on CSPG. This treatment promotes axon regeneration and functional recovery in animals. Drugs that reduce inflammation and decrease scarring, notably prednisolone, are also beneficial if administered shortly after injury, before the scar forms.

An Intrinsic Growth Program Promotes Regeneration

So far we have emphasized differences between the local environments of peripheral and central axons. However, environmental differences cannot completely account for the poor regeneration of central axons. Even though they can regenerate in peripheral nerves, central axons grow much less well than peripheral axons when navigating the same path. Thus adult central axons may be less capable than peripheral axons of regeneration.

In support of this idea, experiments in tissue culture have shown that the growth potential of central neurons decreases with age, whereas mature peripheral neurons extend axons robustly in a favorable environment. One potential explanation for this difference is variation in the expression of proteins thought to be critical for optimal axon elongation, such as the 43 kDa growth-associated protein or GAP-43. This protein is expressed at high levels in embryonic central and peripheral neurons. In peripheral neurons the level remains high in maturity and increases even more following axotomy, whereas in central neurons its expression decreases as development proceeds.

Is this reduced ability of central axons to regenerate irreversible? Hope for reversibility is provided by studies involving "conditioning lesions." Recall that primary sensory neurons in dorsal root ganglia have a bifurcated axon, with a peripheral branch that extends to skin, muscle, or other targets, and a central branch that enters the spinal cord. The peripheral branch regenerates well following injury, whereas the central branch regenerates poorly. However, the central branch will regenerate successfully if the peripheral branch is damaged several days before the central branch is damaged (Figure 57–9). Somehow prior injury or conditioning lesion activates an axonal growth program.

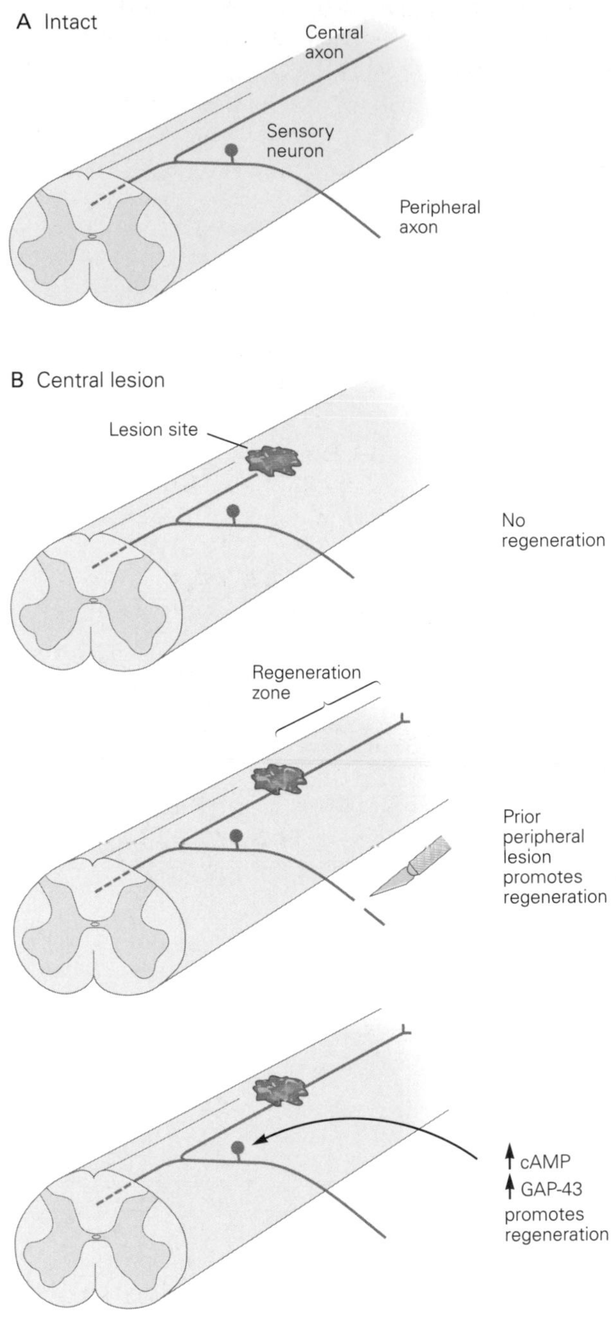

Figure 57–9 A conditioning lesion promotes regeneration of the central branch of a primary sensory neuron axon. After lesions of the spinal cord there is little regeneration of the central branch beyond the injury site. However, if the peripheral branch of the axon is sectioned before the central branch is damaged, the latter will grow beyond the lesion site. The impact of such a "conditioning lesion" can be mimicked by elevating levels of cyclic adenosine monophosphate (**cAMP**) or of the growth-associated protein GAP-43 in the peripheral branch.

One component of the growth program responsible for regeneration of the central branch appears to be cyclic adenosine monophosphate (cAMP). This second-messenger molecule activates enzymes that in turn promote neurite outgrowth. Levels of cAMP are high when neurons initially form circuits; they decline postnatally in central but not peripheral neurons. In some instances increased supplies of cAMP or proteins normally activated by cAMP can promote regeneration of central axons following injury. Accordingly, drugs that increase cAMP levels, or that activate targets of cAMP, are being actively considered as therapeutic agents to be administered following spinal cord injury. In addition, expression of GAP-43 can promote the regeneration of sensory axons past the site of a spinal cord lesion.

Formation of New Connections by Intact Axons Can Lead to Functional Recovery

So far we have discussed interventions designed to enhance the limited regenerative capacity of injured central axons. An alternative strategy focuses on the significant, although incomplete, functional recovery that can occur following injury even without appreciable regeneration of cut axons. If the basis for this limited recovery of function can be understood, it may be possible to enhance regeneration and function.

A rearrangement of existing connections in response to injury may contribute to recovery of function. We have learned that axotomy leads to changes in both the inputs to and the targets of the injured neuron. Although many of these changes are detrimental to function, some are beneficial. In particular, the central nervous system can, following injury, spontaneously undergo adaptive reorganization that helps it regain function. For example, after transection of the descending corticospinal pathway, which occurs with many traumatic injuries of the spinal cord, the cortex can no longer transmit commands to motor neurons below the site of the lesion. Over several weeks, however, intact corticospinal axons rostral to the lesion begin to sprout new terminal branches and form synapses on spinal interneurons whose axons extend around the lesion, thereby forming an intraspinal detour that contributes to limited recovery of function (Figure 57–10).

Similar instances of functional reorganization have been demonstrated in the motor cortex and brain stem. These compensatory responses attest to the latent plasticity of the nervous system. The ability of the nervous system to rewire itself is most vigorous during the critical periods of early postnatal life (see Chapter 56) but can also be reawakened by traumatic events in adulthood.

How can the nervous system's rewiring ability be improved? It is possible that some of the beneficial effects of grafts in experimental animals reflect reorganization of intact axons rather than regeneration of transected axons. As the nervous system's plasticity becomes better understood, therapeutic strategies that promote specific changes in circuitry may become possible. Perhaps most promising is an approach in which cellular or molecular interventions that promote growth are combined with behavioral therapies that result in circuit rewiring.

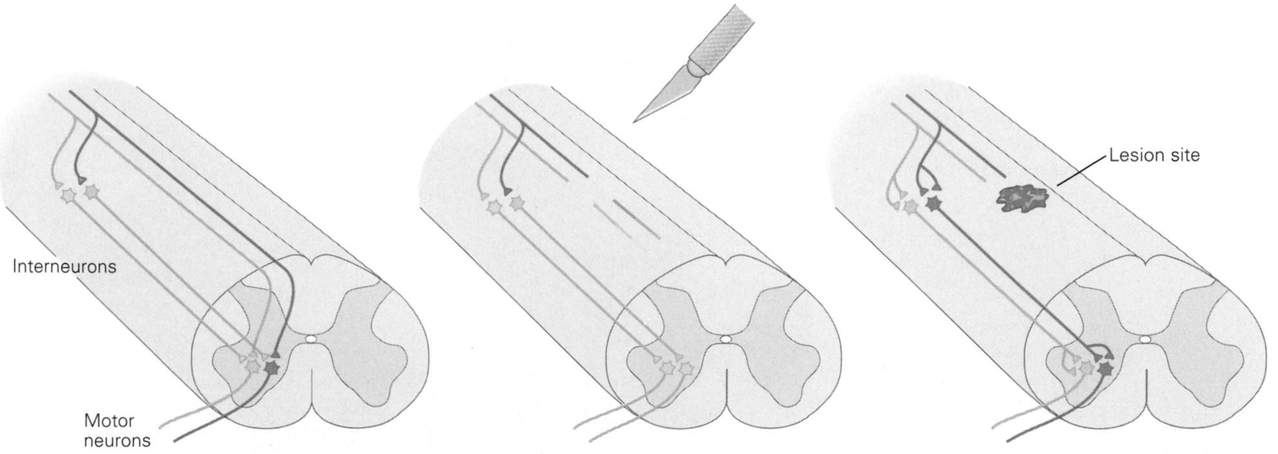

Figure 57–10 Function can be recovered after spinal cord injury through reorganization of spinal circuits. Severed corticospinal axons can reestablish connections with motor neurons by sprouting axon collaterals that innervate propriospinal interneurons whose axons bypass the lesion and contact motor neurons located caudal to the lesion site. (Adapted, with permission, from Bareyre et al. 2004.)

Neurons in the Injured Brain Die but New Ones Can Be Born

The failure to grow a new axon is by no means the worst fate that can befall an injured neuron. For many neurons axotomy leads to the death of the cell. Efforts to improve recovery following injury therefore need to consider neuronal survival as well as axonal regrowth. Since neuronal death is a frequent consequence of severe neural insults, such as stroke and neurodegenerative disease, improved ways of retaining or replacing neurons would have broad utility.

The loss of cells following injury is not unique to the nervous system, although in other tissues new cells are often effective at repairing damage. This regenerative capacity is most dramatic in the hematopoietic system, where a few stem cells can repopulate the entire adaptive immune system. In contrast, it has long been believed that the generation of neurons is complete by birth. Because of this, approaches to regeneration have often focused on finding ways to spare neurons that would otherwise die.

This traditional view is changing, prompted by Joseph Altman's discovery in the 1960s that neurogenesis continues into adulthood in some parts of the mammalian brain (Figure 57–11). This finding challenged fundamental tenets of existing dogma, and the idea that new neurons could form in the hippocampus and olfactory bulb of postnatal rodents was met with skepticism for three decades.

More recently, however, the application of better cell labeling technologies has amply confirmed Altman's results and extended them to nonhuman primates and, even in a limited way, to humans via material obtained at autopsy. In the dentate gyrus of the hippocampus, for example, precursor cells divide throughout life. Some die soon after they are born and others become glial cells, but a substantial minority differentiate into granule cells that are indistinguishable from those born at embryonic stages (Figure 57–12).

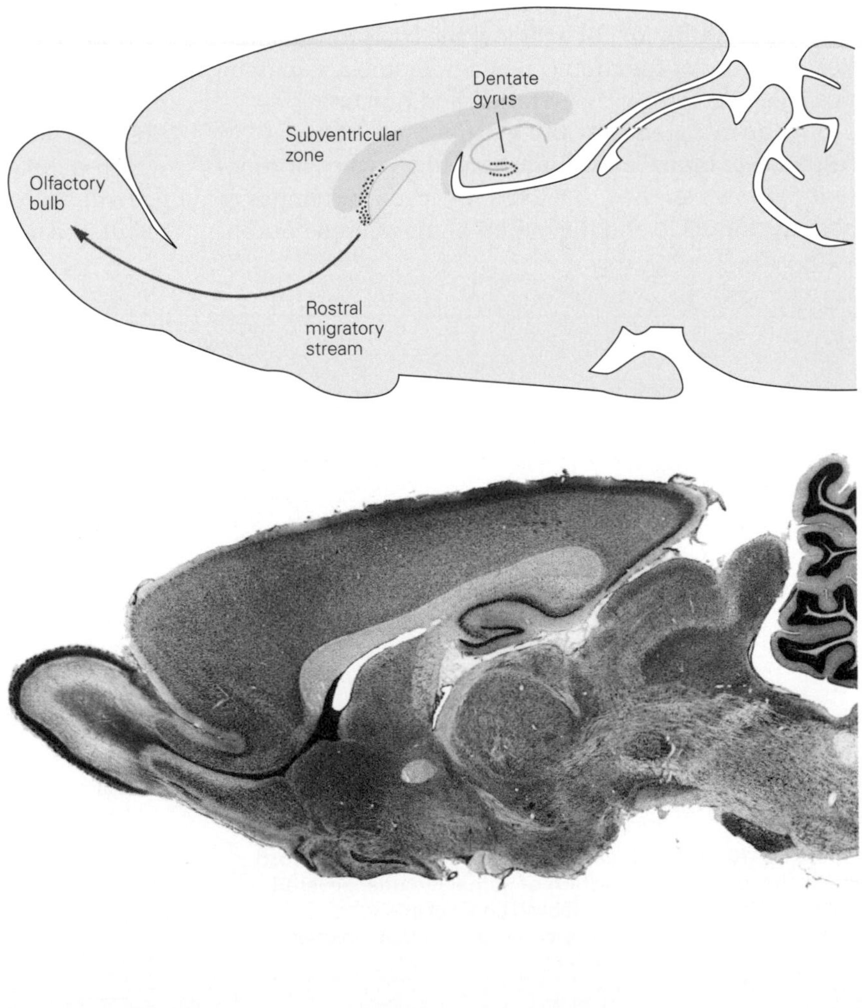

Figure 57–11 Neurons are born in the adult rodent brain at two sites. Neurons born in the subventricular zone migrate rostrally to populate the olfactory bulb. Neurons born in the hippocampus populate the dentate gyrus. (Bottom micrograph reproduced, with permission from Elsaesser and Paysan, 2007, and BrainMaps.org)

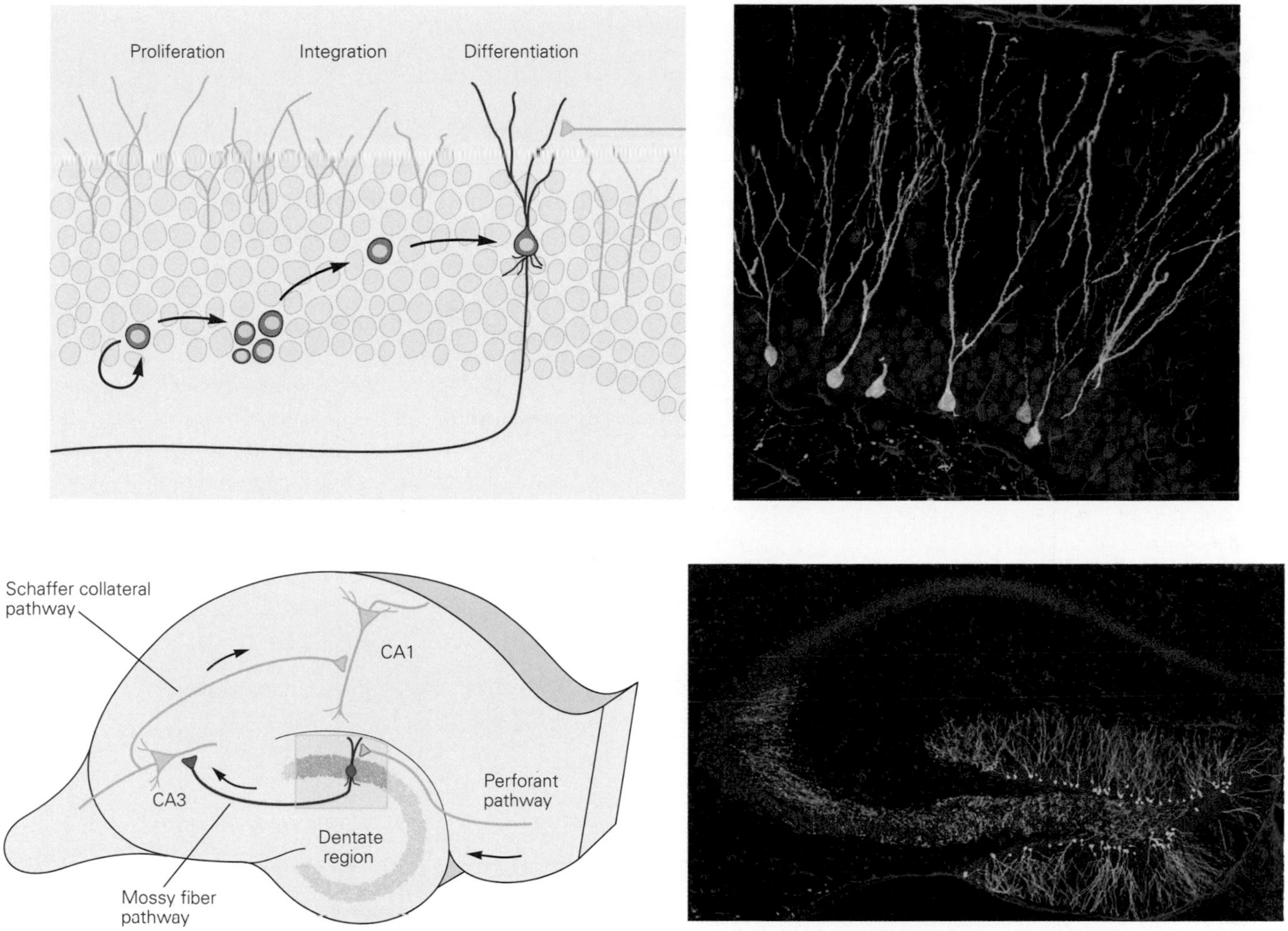

Figure 57–12 Neurons born in the germinal zone of the dentate gyrus in adult rodents are integrated into hippocampal circuits. The diagrams on the left show the pathways of neuronal differentiation and integration into dentate gyrus circuits. In the images on the right newly generated neurons and their dendritic arbors are labeled with a virus expressing green fluorescence protein. (Micrographs courtesy of F. Gage, reproduced with permission.)

New neurons are also added to the adult olfactory bulb. They are generated in a subventricular zone far from the bulb itself, then migrate to their destination (Figure 57–13). In both cases the new neurons extend axons and dendrites, form synapses, and become integrated into functional circuits. Thus neurons born at embryonic stages are gradually replaced by later-born neurons, so that the total number of neurons in these regions of the brain is maintained.

The function of neurons born in mature animals is not completely understood, but the cells appear able to recapitulate many of the properties of neurons that arise in the embryo. When the generation of new neurons in the adult is prevented, certain behaviors mediated by the olfactory bulb and hippocampus are degraded. Conversely, some behavioral alterations are accompanied by alterations in the tempo of adult neurogenesis. Adult neurogenesis can be decreased in animal models of depression and chronic stress, whereas enrichment of the habitat of an animal or an increase in the physical activity of otherwise sedentary rodents can increase the generation of new neurons.

Where do neurons generated in the adult brain come from? The principle that embryonic neurons and glia arise from multipotential progenitors also applies to neurons born in adults. Stem cells are the source of neurons in the adult as well as the embryo. The discovery and characterization of neurogenesis from adult stem cells has influenced research on recovery from injury in two important ways.

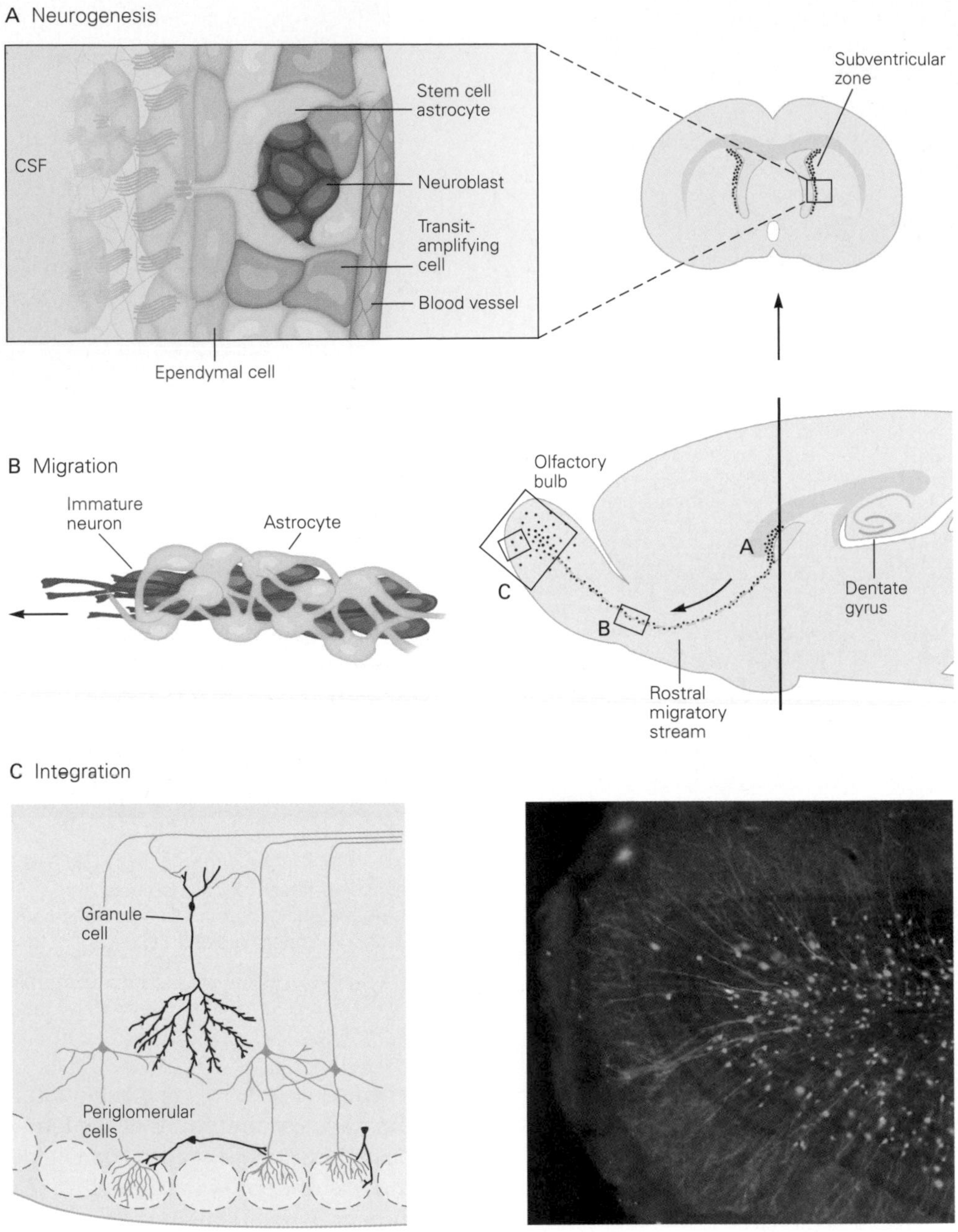

Figure 57–13 The origin and fate of neurons born in the adult ventricular zone. (Adapted, with permission, from Tavazoie et al. 2008.)

A. Neuroblasts develop in an orderly progression from astrocytic stem cells via a population of so-called transit-amplifying cells within a local niche close to blood vessels in the subventricular zone. (**CSF**, cerebrospinal fluid.)

B. Neuroblasts differentiate into immature neurons that migrate to the olfactory bulb using astrocytes as guides. They crawl along each other in a process called chain migration.

C. On arrival in the olfactory bulb, immature neurons differentiate into granule cells and periglomerular cells, two classes of olfactory bulb interneurons. (Image reproduced, with permission, from A. Mizrahi.)

First, the findings that endogenously generated neurons can differentiate and extend processes through the thicket of adult neuropil and can be integrated into functional circuits led researchers to speculate that the same could be true for transplanted neurons or precursors. In the past decade the idea of replacing lost neurons has progressed from science fiction to a tantalizingly testable hypothesis. Second, since neural precursors can be induced to divide and differentiate, strategies designed to augment this innate ability are now being considered, with the goal of producing neurons in large enough numbers to replace those lost to injury or neurodegenerative disease. At present such strategies are not part of clinical practice, but the intensity of the research devoted to these goals is reason for optimism.

Therapeutic Interventions May Retain or Replace Injured Central Neurons

Transplantation of Neurons or Their Progenitors Can Replace Lost Neurons

For many years neurologists have transplanted developing neurons into experimental animals to see if the new neurons could reverse the effects of injury or disease. These attempts have had promising results, most notably in the treatment of loss of dopaminergic cells in Parkinson disease, but their application to human patients has been fraught with difficulty.

One problem is the difficulty obtaining and growing developing neurons in sufficient numbers. Modifying neurons by introducing new genes so as to improve their chances of functioning in a new environment has also been challenging. In many cases the grafted neurons are already too mature to differentiate properly or to integrate effectively into functional circuits.

With the discovery that neural precursors transplanted into the adult brain differentiate into neurons, these obstacles may soon be overcome. Several classes of precursors have been transplanted successfully, including neural stem cells and committed precursors. In many cases these cells differentiate into neurons that are more characteristic of the transplant site than of their site of origin. This result supports the idea that the local environment plays a major role in determining neuronal cell type, and suggests that precursors need not be derived separately for each neuronal type. Conversely, the plasticity of such precursors is not unlimited, so differentiation along specific pathways needs to be established in culture before engrafting the cells.

To date this has been achieved most successfully with embryonic stem cells (ES cells). These cells are derived from early blastocyst stage embryos and can give rise to all cells of the body. In principle, the ability to direct the differentiation of ES cells along specific pathways in culture permits the generation of large numbers of cells for transplantation. Furthermore, methods for generating specific classes of neural precursors and neurons from ES cells have been devised. For example, it is possible to generate neurons that possess many or all of the properties of the spinal motor neurons that are lost in amyotrophic lateral sclerosis or to generate the dopaminergic neurons lost from the striatum in Parkinson disease, and so to engraft such neurons into the spinal cord or brain (Figure 57–14).

This technology has been enhanced recently by the molecular reprogramming of skin fibroblast cells to create induced pluripotent stem (iPS) cells (Figure 57–15). These iPS cells have a distinct advantage over ES cells; their production does not require use of embryos, effectively bypassing a minefield of practical, political, and ethical concerns that have hindered research using human ES cells. Another advantage of iPS cells is that they can be generated from an individual patient's own skin cells, neatly avoiding issues of immunological incompatibility. Many hurdles need to be overcome before iPS cells can be used clinically in regenerative medicine. Nevertheless, these cells are already being used in chemical screens to identify compounds that counteract the cellular defects that underlie human neurodegenerative disease.

Stimulation of Neurogenesis in Regions of Injury May Contribute to Restoring Function

What if, following injury in adults, one could stimulate endogenous neuronal precursors to produce neurons capable of replacing those that have been lost? Two recent findings suggest that this idea is not so far-fetched.

First, neural precursors capable of forming neurons in culture have been isolated from many parts of the adult nervous system, including the cerebral cortex and spinal cord, even though neurogenesis in adults is ordinarily confined to the olfactory bulb and hippocampus. This diversion of cell fate leads to the idea that in the adult, neurogenesis occurs in specialized niches that contain local permissive factors.

Second, the generation of new neurons can be stimulated by traumatic or ischemic injury (akin to stroke), even in areas such as the cerebral cortex or

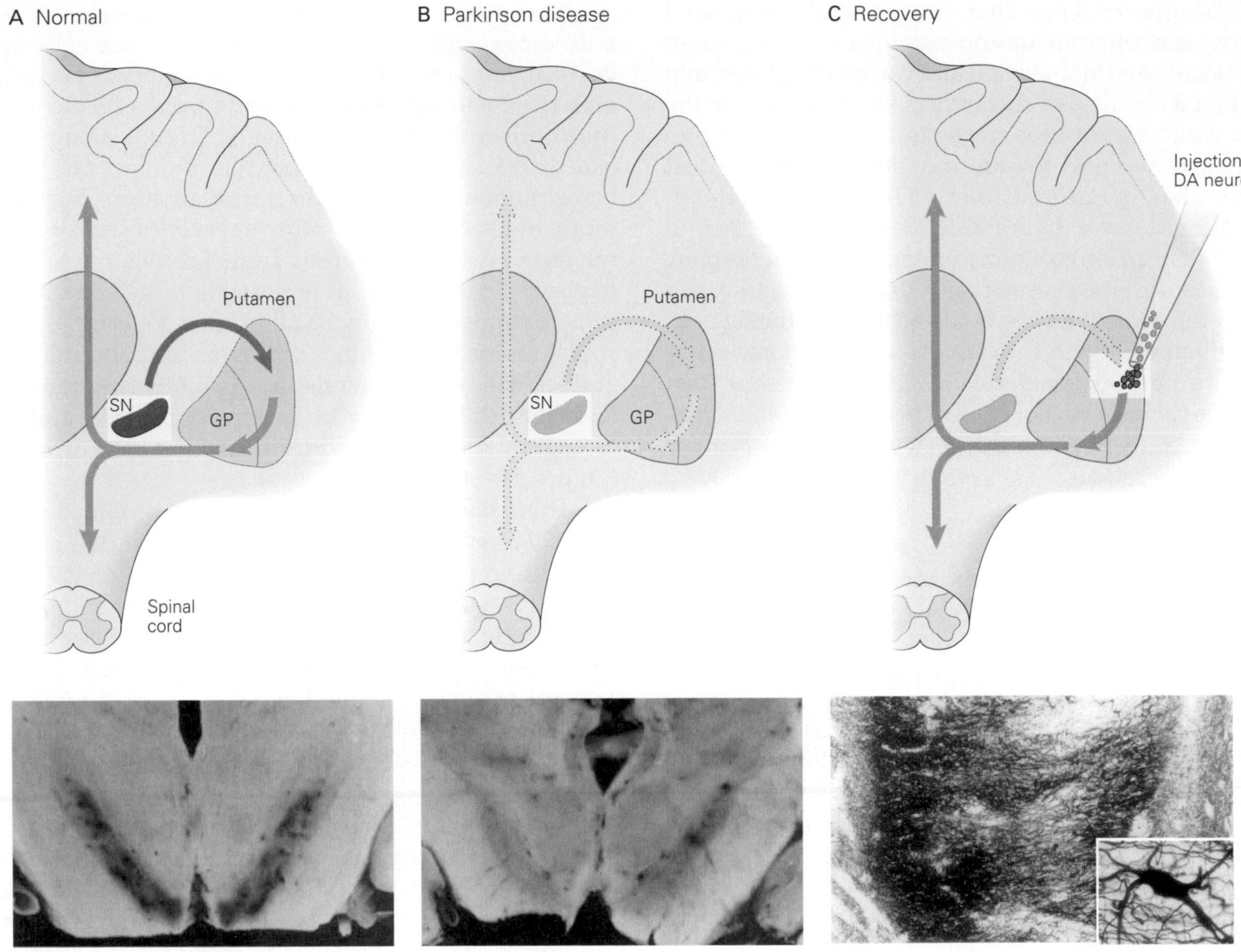

Figure 57–14 Loss of dopaminergic neurons in Parkinson disease can be treated by grafting embryonic cells into the putamen.

A. In the healthy brain dopaminergic projections from the substantia nigra (**SN**) innervate the putamen, which in turn activates neurons in the globus pallidus (**GP**). Pallidal outputs to the brain and spinal cord facilitate movement. The image below shows melanin-rich dopaminergic neurons in human substantia nigra.

B. In Parkinson disease the loss of dopaminergic neurons in the substantia nigra deprives the putamen-globus pallidus pathways of their drive. The image below shows the virtual absence of melanin-rich dopaminergic neurons in the substantia nigra of an individual with Parkinson disease.

C. Direct injection of embryonic dopaminergic neurons into the putamen reactivates the globus pallidus output pathways. The image below shows tyrosine hydroxylase expression in the cell bodies and axons of embryonic mesencephalic dopaminergic neurons grafted into the putamen of a human patient. (Image reproduced, with permission, from Kordower et al. 2000.)

spinal cord in which neurogenesis normally fails to occur. However, the fact that recovery after stroke and injury is poor demonstrates that spontaneous compensatory neurogenesis is insufficient for tissue repair. Injury-induced neurogenesis has been enhanced in experimental animals by administration of growth factors that promote neuronal production from progenitors grown in culture. If such interventions could be adapted to humans, the range of neurons subject to replacement would be greatly increased.

Transplantation of Nonneuronal Cells or Their Progenitors Can Improve Neuronal Function

Cells other than neurons are lost after brain injury. Among the most profound losses are those of oligodendrocytes, the cells that form the myelin sheath around central axons. The stripping of myelin continues long after traumatic injury and contributes to progressive loss of function of axons that may not have been injured directly.

Although the adult brain and spinal cord are capable of generating new oligodendrocytes and replacing lost myelin, this cellular production line is insufficient to restore function in many cases. Since several common neurological diseases, most notably multiple sclerosis, are accompanied by a profound state of demyelination, there is strong interest in providing the nervous system with additional oligodendrocyte precursors in order to augment remyelination.

Neural stem cells, multipotential progenitors, ES cells, and iPS cells can give rise not only to neurons but also to nonneural cells, including oligodendrocytes and their direct precursors. Indeed, at present human ES cells are being channeled into oligodendrocyte progenitor cells and implanted into injured spinal cords of experimental animals. Transplanted cells that differentiate into oligodendrocytes enhance remyelination and substantially improve the locomotor ability of experimental animals (Figure 57–16).

Restoration of Function Is the Aim of Regenerative Therapies

We need to bear in mind that efforts to replace central neurons or to enhance the regeneration of their axons would be of little use if these axons were unable to form functional synapses with their target cells.

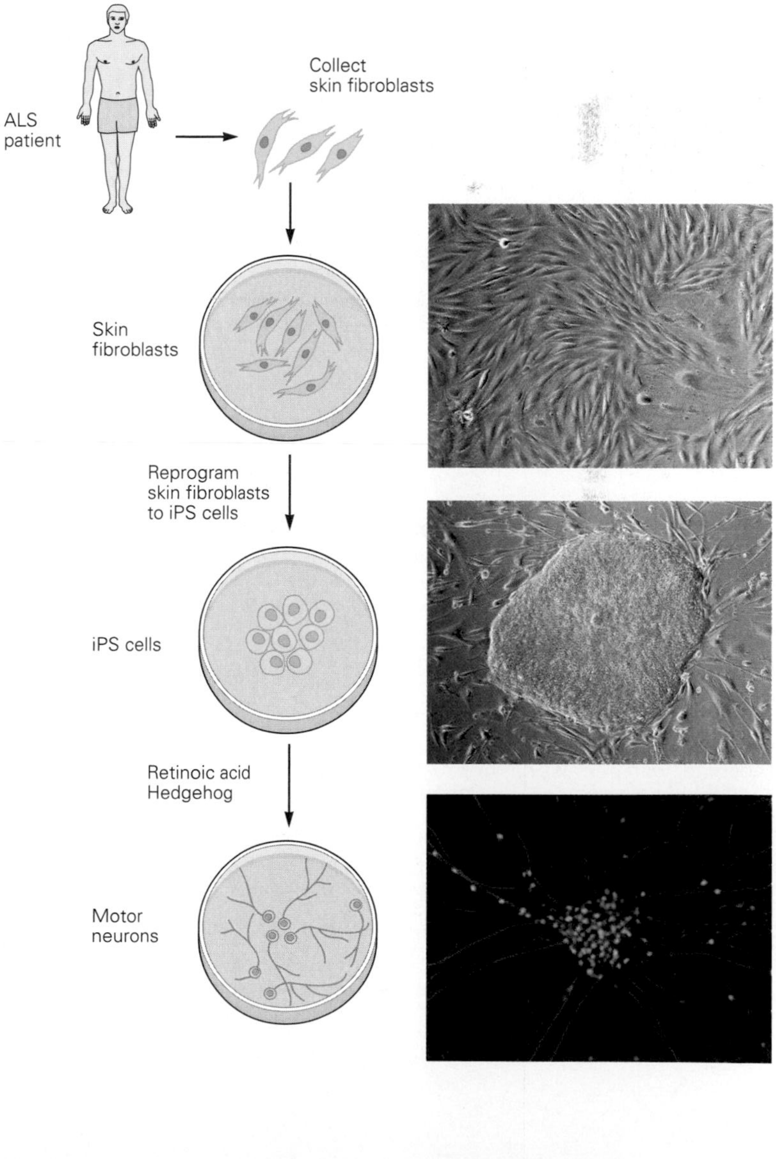

Figure 57–15 Fibroblasts from an individual with amyotrophic lateral sclerosis can be reprogrammed to generate spinal motor neurons. Human skin fibroblasts are used to generate induced pluripotent stem cells (**iPS**) that can then be directed to a motor neuron fate by exposure to retinoic acid and hedgehog signals. The images at right show (from top to bottom) cultured fibroblasts, an iPS cell clump, and differentiated motor neurons expressing characteristic nuclear transcription factors (**green**) and axonal proteins (**red**). (Cell images reproduced, with permission, from C. Henderson, H. Wichterle, G. Croft, and M. Weygandt.)

The same fundamental questions asked about axon regeneration in adults therefore apply to synaptogenesis: Can it happen, and if not, why not?

It has been difficult to address these questions because axonal regeneration following experimentally induced injury is usually so poor that the axons never reach appropriate target fields. However, several of the studies discussed earlier in this chapter offer hope that synapse formation is possible within the dense adult neuropil. In fact, axon branches that regenerate following injury can form synapses on nearby targets. For example, Aguayo and his colleagues found that retinal axons were able to regrow into the superior colliculus when they were channeled through a peripheral nerve that had been grafted into the optic nerve (Figure 57–17A). Remarkably, some collicular neurons fired action potentials when the eye was illuminated, showing that functional synaptic connections had been reestablished (Figure 57–17B).

Likewise, neurons that arise endogenously or are implanted by investigators can form and receive synapses, raising the possibility that behaviors can be restored. Thus there is reason to believe that if injured axons can be induced to regenerate, or new neurons supplied to replace lost ones, they will wire up in ways that help restore lost functions and behaviors.

An Overall View

Axons can regenerate and form new synapses following injury, but regeneration is far more widespread and effective in peripheral axons than in central axons. Recent studies have identified several key factors that limit regeneration of central axons. These include insufficient supplies of growth-promoting factors, pathways laden with growth-inhibitory factors, impenetrable scars, and an intrinsic reluctance of adult central axons to grow.

This is a discouraging array of obstacles, but by understanding them we can hope to manipulate them. If this can be done, it should be possible to enhance regeneration following injury and thus provide restoration of function to many patients for whom there is currently little hope.

Given the complexity of the problem, it is perhaps overly optimistic to expect that any single intervention will suffice. Instead, combined approaches may be

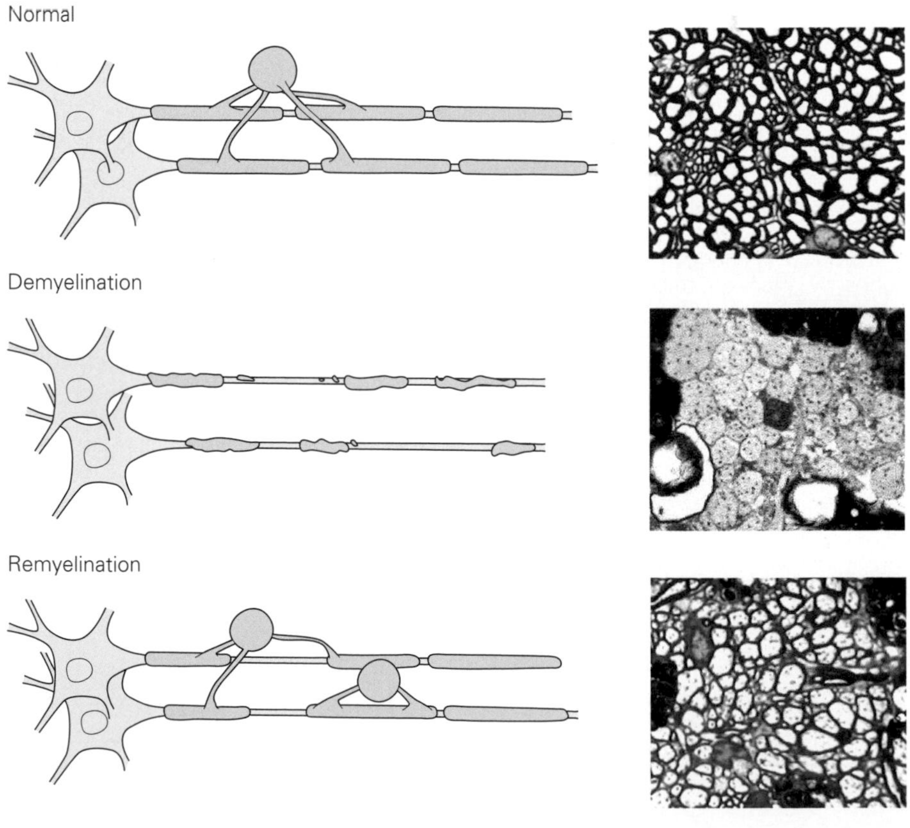

Figure 57–16 Restoration of myelination in the central nervous system by transplanted oligodendrocyte stem cells. In experiments on rodents with demyelinated axons, grafts of oligodendrocyte precursor cells can restore myelination to near normal. Sections through central nerve tracts are shown in the images at right. (Adapted, with permission, from Franklin and ffrench-Constant 2008.)

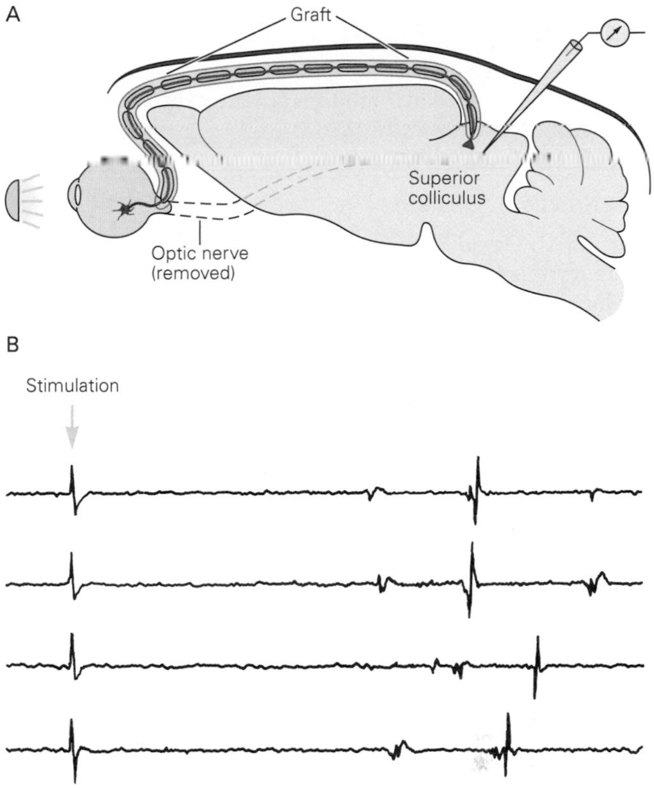

Figure 57–17 Regenerated retinal ganglion axons in the optic nerve can form functional synapses. (Reproduced, with permission, from Keirstead et al. 1989.)

A. A segment of optic nerve in an adult rat was removed and a segment of sciatic nerve was grafted in its place. The other end of the sciatic nerve was attached to the superior colliculus. Some retinal ganglion cell axons regenerated through the sciatic nerve and entered the superior colliculus.

B. Once the axons of the retinal ganglion neurons had regenerated, recordings were made from the superior colliculus. Flashes of light delivered to the eye elicited action potentials in collicular neurons, demonstrating that at least some regenerated axons had formed functional synapses.

needed. For example, the enzyme treatment that breaks down chondroitin proteoglycans in the glial scar is far more effective when combined with administration of neurotrophic factors. Likewise, implantation of cellular bridges that promote regeneration may need to be combined with administration of drugs to neutralize inhibitory factors that would otherwise halt growth as axons leave the bridge and enter the neuropil to form synapses.

Another consequence of axonal injury, and of many neurodegenerative diseases, is the death of neurons. This is particularly serious because in most parts of the brain and spinal cord the neurons we are born with are the only ones we will ever have. Here two new developments provide hope where there had been little: the discovery that new neurons are formed and integrated into functional circuits in a few parts of the brain, and the suite of technological advances that has allowed large numbers of neural precursors to be generated for implantation.

Finally, we should not avoid the relationship between the failure of regeneration following injury and the stabilization of connections that occurs at the end of critical periods. Myelination, which occurs largely at the end of a critical period, may have the secondary effect of preventing further, large-scale rearrangement of synaptic connections. Likewise, astrocytes may not only nurture synapses but also contribute proteoglycans that limit the ability of axons to reach out to new targets. Thus, caution will be needed to ensure that treatments aimed at fostering recovery following injury do not end up promoting formation of maladaptive circuits.

Joshua R. Sanes
Thomas M. Jessell

Selected Readings

Chen ZL, Yu WM, Strickland S. 2007. Peripheral regeneration. Annu Rev Neurosci 30:209–233.

Coleman M. 2005. Axon degeneration mechanisms: commonality amid diversity. Nat Rev Neurosci 6:889–898.

Takahashi K, Yamanaka S. 2006. Induction of pluripotent stem cells from mouse embryonic and adult fibroblast cultures by defined factors. Cell 126:663–676.

Winkler C, Kirik D, Bjorklund A. 2005. Cell transplantation in Parkinson's disease: how can we make it work? Trends Neurosci 28:86–92.

Yiu G, He Z. 2006. Glial inhibition of CNS axon regeneration. Nat Rev Neurosci 7:617–627.

References

Aguayo AJ, David S, Bray GM. 1981. Influences of the glial environment on the elongation of axons after injury: transplantation studies in adult rodents. J Exp Biol 95:231–240.

Alilain WJ, Horn KP, Hu H, Dick TE, Silver J. 2011. Functional regeneration of respiratory pathways after spinal cord injury. Nature 475:196–200.

Altman J. 1969. Autoradiographic and histological studies of postnatal neurogenesis. IV. Cell proliferation and migration in the anterior forebrain, with special reference to persisting neurogenesis in the olfactory bulb. J Comp Neurol 137:433–457.

Altman J, Das GD. 1965. Autoradiographic and histological evidence of postnatal hippocampal neurogenesis in rats. J Comp Neurol 124:319–335.

Atwal JK, Pinkston-Gosse J, Syken J, Stawicki S, Wu Y, Shatz C, Tessier-Lavigne M. 2008. PirB is a functional receptor for myelin inhibitors of axonal regeneration. Science 322:967–970.

Bareyre FM. 2008. Neuronal repair and replacement in spinal cord injury. J Neurol Sci 265:63–72.

Bareyre FM, Kerschensteiner M, Raineteau O, Mettenleiter TC, Weinmann O, Schwab ME. 2004. The injured spinal cord spontaneously forms a new intraspinal circuit in adult rats. Nat Neurosci 7:269–277.

Bierowski B, Berek L, Adalbert R, Wagner D, Grumme DS, Addicks K, Ribchester RR, Coleman MP. 2004. Quantitative and qualitative analysis of Wallerian degeneration using restricted axonal labelling in YFP-H mice. J Neurosci Methods 134:23–35.

Bradbury EJ, McMahon SB. 2006. Spinal cord repair strategies: why do they work? Nat Rev Neurosci 7:644–653.

Bradbury EJ, Moon LD, Popat RJ, King VR, Bennett GS, Patel PN, Fawcett JW, McMahon SB. 2002. Chondroitinase ABC promotes functional recovery after spinal cord injury. Nature 416:636–640.

Busch SA, Silver J. 2007. The role of extracellular matrix in CNS regeneration. Curr Opin Neurobiol 17:120–127.

Caroni P, Schwab ME. 1988. Antibody against myelin-associated inhibitor of neurite growth neutralizes nonpermissive substrate properties of CNS white matter. Neuron 1:85–96.

Carulli D, Laabs T, Geller HM, Fawcett JW. 2005. Chondroitin sulfate proteoglycans in neural development and regeneration. Curr Opin Neurobiol 15:116–120.

Dimos JT, Rodolfa KT, Niakan KK, Weisenthal LM, Mitsumoto H, Chung W, Croft GF, et al. 2008. Induced pluripotent stem cells generated from patients with ALS can be differentiated into motor neurons. Science 321:1218–1221.

Dunnett SB, Bjorklund A, Lindvall O. 2001. Cell therapy in Parkinson's disease—stop or go? Nat Rev Neurosci 2:365–369.

Elsaesser R, Paysan J. 2007. The sense of smell, its signaling pathways, and the dichotomy of cilia and microvilli in olfactory sensory cells. BMC Neurosci (Suppl 3):S1.

Ferretti P, Zhang F, O'Neill P. 2003. Changes in spinal cord regenerative ability through phylogenesis and development: lessons to be learnt. Dev Dyn 226:245–256.

Ferri A, Sanes JR, Coleman MP, Cunningham JM Kato AC. 2003. Inhibiting axon degeneration and synapse loss attenuates apoptosis and disease progression in a mouse model of motoneuron disease. Curr Biol 13:669–673.

Franklin RJ, French-Constant C. 2008. Remyelination in the CNS: from biology to therapy. Nat Rev Neurosci 9:839–855.

Galtrey CM, Fawcett JW. 2007. The role of chondroitin sulfate proteoglycans in regeneration and plasticity in the central nervous system. Brain Res Rev 54:1–18.

Imayoshi I, Sakamoto M, Ohtsuka T, Takao K, Miyakawa T, Yamaguchi M, Mori K, Ikeda T, Itohara S, Kageyama R. 2008. Roles of continuous neurogenesis in the structural and functional integrity of the adult forebrain. Nat Neurosci 10:1153–1161.

Keirstead HS, Nistor G, Bernal G, Totoiu M, Cloutier F, Sharp K, Steward O. 2005. Human embryonic stem cell-derived oligodendrocyte progenitor cell transplants remyelinate and restore locomotion after spinal cord injury. J Neurosci 25:4694–4705.

Keirstead SA, Rasminsky M, Fukuda Y, Carter DA, Aguayo AJ, Vidal-Sanz M. 1989. Electrophysiologic responses in hamster superior colliculus evoked by regenerating retinal axons. Science 246:255–257.

Kordower J, Sortwell C. 2000. Neuropathology of fetal nigra transplants for Parkinson's disease. Prog Brain Res 127:333–344.

Lee JK, Chan AF, Luu SM, Zhu Y, Ho C, Tessier-Lavigne M, Zheng B. 2009. Reassessment of corticospinal tract regeneration in Nogo-deficient mice. J Neurosci 29:8649–8654.

Liu BP, Cafferty WB, Budel SO, Strittmatter SM. 2006. Extracellular regulators of axonal growth in the adult central nervous system. Philos Trans R Soc Lond B Biol Sci 361:1593–1610.

Liu K, Tedeshi A, Park KK, He Z. 2011. Neuronal intrinsic mechanisms of axon regeneration. Annu Rev Neurosci 34:131–152.

Lois C, Alvarez-Buylla A. 1994. Long-distance neuronal migration in the adult mammalian brain. Science 264: 1145–1148.

Magavi SS, Leavitt BR, Macklis JD. 2000. Induction of neurogenesis in the neocortex of adult mice. Nature 405: 951–955.

Maier IC, Schwab ME. 2006. Sprouting, regeneration and circuit formation in the injured spinal cord: factors and activity. Philos Trans R Soc Lond B Biol Sci 361:1611–1634.

Schwab ME, Thoenen H. 1985. Dissociated neurons regenerate into sciatic but not optic nerve explants in culture irrespective of neurotrophic factors. J Neurosci 5:2415–2423.

Schwegler G, Schwab ME, Kapfhammer JP. 1995. Increased collateral sprouting of primary afferents in the myelin-free spinal cord. J Neurosci 15:2756–2767.

Smith PD, Sun F, Park KK, Cai B, Wang C, Kuwako K, Martinez-Carrasco I, Connolly L, He Z. 2009. SOCS3 deletion promotes optic nerve regeneration in vivo. Neuron 64:617–623.

Sohur US, Emsley JG, Mitchell BD, Macklis JD. 2006. Adult neurogenesis and cellular brain repair with neural progenitors, precursors and stem cells. Philos Trans R Soc Lond B Biol Sci 361:1477–1497.

Takahashi K, Tanabe K, Ohnuki M, Narita M, Ichisaka T, Tomoda K, Yamanaka S. 2007. Induction of pluripotent stem cells from adult human fibroblasts by defined factors. Cell 131:861–872.

Takahashi K, Yamanaka S. 2006. Induction of pluripotent stem cells from mouse embryonic and adult fibroblast cultures by defined factors. Cell 126:663–676.

Tavazoie M, Van der Verken L, Silva-Vargas V, Louissaint M, Colonna L, Zaidi B, Garcia-Verdugo JM, Doetsch F. 2008. A specialized vascular niche for adult neural stem cells. Cell Stem Cell 3:279–288.

Thuret S, Moon LD, Gage FH. 2006. Therapeutic interventions after spinal cord injury. Nat Rev Neurosci 7:628–643.

Wernig M, Zhao JP, Pruszak J, Hedlund E, Fu D, Soldner F, Broccoli V, Constantine-Paton M, Isacson O, Jaenisch R. 2008. Neurons derived from reprogrammed fibroblasts functionally integrate into the fetal brain and improve symptoms of rats with Parkinson's disease. Proc Natl Acad Sci U S A 105:5856–5861.

Yiu G, He Z. 2006. Glial inhibitors and intracellular signaling mechanisms. Nat Rev Neurosci 7:617–627.

Zhao C, Deng W, Gage FH. 2008. Mechanisms and functional implications of adult neurogenesis. Cell 132:645–660.

Zhou FQ, Snider WD. 2006. Intracellular control of developmental and regenerative axon growth. Philos Trans R Soc Lond B Biol Sci 361:1575–1592.

58

Sexual Differentiation of the Nervous System

FEW WORDS ARE MORE LOADED WITH meaning than the word "sex." Sexual activity is a biological imperative and a major human preoccupation. The physical differences between men and women that underlie partner recognition and reproduction are obvious to all of us, and their developmental origins are well understood. In contrast, our understanding of behavioral differences between the sexes is primitive. In many cases their very existence remains controversial, and the origins of those that have been clearly demonstrated remain unclear.

In this chapter we first briefly summarize the embryological basis of sexual differentiation. We then discuss at greater length the behavioral differences between the two sexes, focusing on those differences or dimorphisms for which some neurobiological basis has been found. These dimorphisms include physiological responses (erection, lactation), drives (maternal behavior), and even more complex behaviors (gender identity). In analyzing these dimorphisms we will discuss three issues.

First, what are the genetic origins of sexual differences? Human males and females have a complement of 23 chromosomal pairs, and only one differs between the sexes. Females have a pair of X chromosomes (and are therefore "XX"), whereas males have one copy of the X chromosome paired with a Y chromosome (XY). The other 22 chromosome pairs, called *autosomes,* are shared between males and females. We will see that some genetic determinants arise from the presence of a Y chromosome, while others arise from sex-specific patterns of autosomal gene expression that exert their impact during development.

Second, how are differences in genes and gene expression translated into differences between the brains of men and women? We will see that key intermediates are the sex hormones, a set of steroids that includes testosterone and estrogens. These hormones act during embryogenesis as well as postnatally, first organizing the physical development of both genitalia and brain regions, and later activating particular physiological and behavioral responses. Hormonal regulation is especially complex because the nervous system, which is profoundly influenced by sex steroids, also controls their synthesis. This feedback loop may help to explain how the external environment, including social and cultural factors, can ultimately shape sexual dimorphism at a neural level.

Third, what are the crucial neural differences that underlie sexually dimorphic behaviors? Clear physical and molecular differences between the brains of men and women have been found. These differences imply that neural circuitry differs between the sexes, and in a few cases these distinctions in connectivity are directly related to behavioral differences. In other cases, however, sexually dimorphic behaviors appear to result from differential usage of the same basic circuits.

Before proceeding we must define the usage of two words that are commonly confused with each other: *sex* and *gender*. As a descriptor of biological differences between men and women, the word *sex* is used in three ways. First, *anatomical sex* refers to overt differences including the differences in the external genitalia as well as other sexual characteristics such as the distribution of body hair. *Gonadal sex* refers to the presence of male or female gonads, the testes or ovaries. Finally, *chromosomal sex* refers to the distribution of the sex chromosomes between females (XX) and males (XY).

Whereas *sex* is a biological term, *gender* encompasses the collection of social behaviors and mental states that typically differ between males and females. *Gender role* is the set of behaviors and social mannerisms that is typically distributed in a sexually dimorphic fashion within the population. Toy preferences in children as well as distinctive attire are some examples of gender roles that can distinguish males from females. *Gender identity* is the feeling of belonging to the category of the male or female sex. Importantly, gender identity is distinct from *sexual orientation*, the erotic responsiveness displayed toward members of one or the other sex.

Are gender and sexual orientation genetically determined? Or are they social constructs molded by cultural expectations and personal experience? As the examples in this chapter will illustrate, we are still far from untangling the contributions of genes and environment to such complex phenomena. However, our recognition that genes and experience interact to shape neural circuits gives us a more realistic framework with which to answer this question compared to our predecessors, who were constrained by the simplistic view that genes and experience acted in mutually exclusive ways.

Genes and Hormones Determine Physical Differences Between Males and Females

Chromosomal Sex Directs the Gonadal Differentiation of the Embryo

Sex determination is the embryonic process whereby chromosomal sex directs the differentiation of the gonadal sex of the animal. Surprisingly, this process differs in fundamental ways within the animal kingdom and even among vertebrates. In most mammals, including humans, however, an XY genotype drives differentiation of the embryonic gonad into testes, whereas an XX genotype leads to ovarian differentiation. Hormones produced by the testes and ovaries subsequently direct sexual differentiation of the nervous system and the rest of the body.

It is the presence of the Y chromosome rather than the lack of a second X chromosome that is the crucial determinant of male differentiation. This was first evident in rare individuals born with two or even three X chromosomes in addition to a Y chromosome (XXY or XXXY). These individuals are men who exhibit male-typical traits. In fact, female cells do not have two active X chromosomes. Early in embryogenesis one of the two X chromosomes in each female cell is chosen at random for inactivation and the genes on it are rendered transcriptionally silent. Thus both male and female cells have a single active X chromosome and male cells also have a Y chromosome.

The sex-determining activity of the Y chromosome is encoded by the gene *SRY* (sex-determining region on Y) whose activity is required for masculinization of the embryonic gonads (Figure 58–1). Inactivation or deletion of *SRY* leads to complete sex reversal: Individuals are chromosomally male (XY) but externally indistinguishable from females. Conversely, in rare instances *SRY* translocates to another chromosome (to the X chromosome or an autosome) during spermatogenesis. Such sperm can fertilize eggs to produce individuals who are chromosomally female (XX) but externally male. However, such XX sex-reversed men are infertile, as many of the genes required for sperm function are located on the Y chromosome.

How does *SRY* instruct the undifferentiated gonads to develop into testes? The female differentiation program appears to be the default mode; patterning genes prime the body and gonads to develop along female-specific pathways. The *SRY* gene encodes a transcription factor that induces expression of genes, some of which prevent execution of the default program and initiate the process of male gonadal differentiation. One of the best-studied targets of the SRY transcription

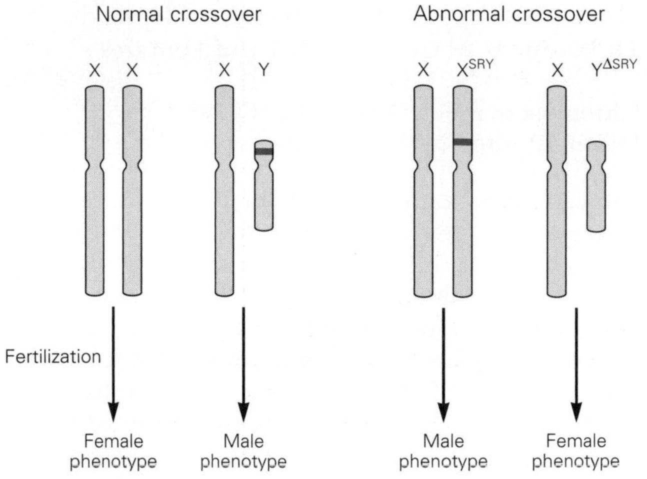

Figure 58–1 The role of the *SRY* gene in sex determination in humans. *SRY*, the sex-determining locus (**blue domain**), resides on the nonhomologous region of the short arm of the Y chromosome. The presence of *SRY* is determinative for male differentiation in many mammals, including primates and most rodents. Normally X- or Y-bearing sperm fertilize an oocyte to generate XX females or XY males, and the resulting phenotypic sex is concordant for the chromosomal sex. Rarely *SRY* translocates to the X chromosome or an autosome (not shown). In such cases XX^{SRY} offspring are phenotypically male while $XY^{\Delta SRY}$ offspring (the Δ indicating a gene deletion) are phenotypically female. (Modified, with permission, from Wilhelm, Palmer, and Koopman 2007.)

factor is another transcription factor, SOX9, which is required for differentiation of the testes. SOX9 in turn activates a variety of genes required for formation of testicular Sertoli cells. Thus SRY initiates a cascade of inductive interactions that ultimately lead to male-specific gonad development.

Gonads Synthesize Hormones That Promote Sexual Differentiation

The chromosomal complement of the embryo directs sexual differentiation of the gonads and in turn the gonads determine the sex-specific features of the nervous system and the rest of the body. They do this by secreting hormones. Gonadal hormones have two major roles. Their developmental role is traditionally referred to as *organizational* because the early effects of hormones on the brain and the rest of the body lead to major, generally irreversible, aspects of cell and tissue differentiation. Later some of the same hormones trigger physiological or behavioral responses. These influences, generally termed *activational*, are reversible.

One example of an organizational role of gonadal hormones is seen in the differentiation of structures that connect the gonads to the external genitalia. In males the Wolffian duct gives rise to the vas deferens, the seminal vesicles, and the epididymis. In females the Müllerian duct differentiates into the oviduct, the uterus, and the vagina (Figure 58–2). Initially both female (XX) and male (XY) embryos possess Wolffian and Müllerian ducts. In males the developing testes secrete a protein hormone, the Müllerian inhibiting substance (MIS), and a steroid hormone, testosterone. MIS leads to a regression of the Müllerian duct and testosterone induces the Wolffian duct to differentiate into its mature derivatives. In females the absence of MIS permits the Müllerian duct to differentiate into its adult derivatives, and the absence of circulating testosterone causes the Wolffian duct to resorb. Thus the Y chromosome overrides a female default program to generate male gonads, which in turn secrete hormones that override a female default program of genital differentiation.

The action of MIS is largely confined to embryos, but steroid hormones exert effects throughout life—that is, they have activational as well as organizational roles. All of the steroid hormones derive from cholesterol (Figure 58–3). The sex steroids can be divided into androgens, which generally promote male characteristics, and the estrogens plus progesterone that promote female characteristics. The testes produce mostly the androgen testosterone, while the ovaries produce mostly progesterone and an estrogen, 17-β-estradiol. The menstrual cycle is a good example of the activational function of estrogen and progesterone.

A glance at the metabolic relationships among steroid hormones (Figure 58–3) reveals a surprise. The female hormone progesterone is the precursor of the male hormone testosterone, and testosterone is the direct precursor of the female hormone 17-β-estradiol. Thus the enzymes that convert one hormone to the other control not only the level of the hormone but also the "sign" (male or female) of the hormonal effect. Aromatase, the enzyme that converts testosterone to estradiol, is present at high levels in the ovaries but not in the testes. Differential expression of aromatase is the reason for sexual dimorphism in circulating testosterone and estrogen. Aromatase is also expressed in various regions of the brain (Figure 58–4A), and many of the effects of testosterone on neurons are thought to occur after its conversion to estrogen. Testosterone is also converted by the enzyme 5α-reductase into another androgenic steroid, 5α-dihydrotestosterone (DHT), in various target tissues, including the external genitalia. In these tissues DHT is responsible for induction of secondary male characteristics such as facial and body hair and growth of the prostate. Later in life DHT is the culprit in male pattern baldness.

As one can imagine, mutations in genes encoding enzymes involved in steroid hormone biosynthesis have far-reaching consequences. The phenotypes dramatically illustrate both the organizational and activational effects of steroid hormones, as well as the difficulty of neatly distinguishing the two. Here we describe three disorders (Table 58–1).

The first, congenital adrenal hyperplasia or CAH, is a genetic deficiency in the synthesis of corticosteroids by the adrenal glands that results in overproduction of testosterone and related androgens. This condition is autosomal recessive and occurs once in 10,000–15,000 live births. In girls born with CAH, excess androgens lead to some masculinization of the external genitalia, a process called *virilization*. Virilization clearly reflects the organizational roles of steroids. This condition can be diagnosed at birth and resolved by surgical intervention. Treatment with corticosteroids reduces testosterone levels, permitting these females to undergo puberty and to be fertile.

A second genetic disorder, 5α-reductase II deficiency, can also affect sexual differentiation (Table 58–1). In male fetuses 5α-reductase II is expressed at high levels in the precursor of the external genitalia, where it converts circulating testosterone into DHT. The high local concentrations of DHT virilize the external genitalia. Clinical 5α-reductase II deficiency is inherited in an autosomal recessive manner, and males present at birth with ambiguous (under-virilized) or overtly feminized external genitalia. In many instances, therefore, chromosomally male patients (XY) with this condition are mistakenly raised as females until puberty, at which time the large increase in circulating testosterone virilizes the body hair, musculature, and, most dramatically, the external genitalia.

Steroid Hormones Act by Binding to Specific Receptors

The critical role of steroid receptors in controlling sexual differentiation is well illustrated by patients with a third disorder, complete androgen insensitivity syndrome or CAIS (Table 58–1). Testosterone, estrogen,

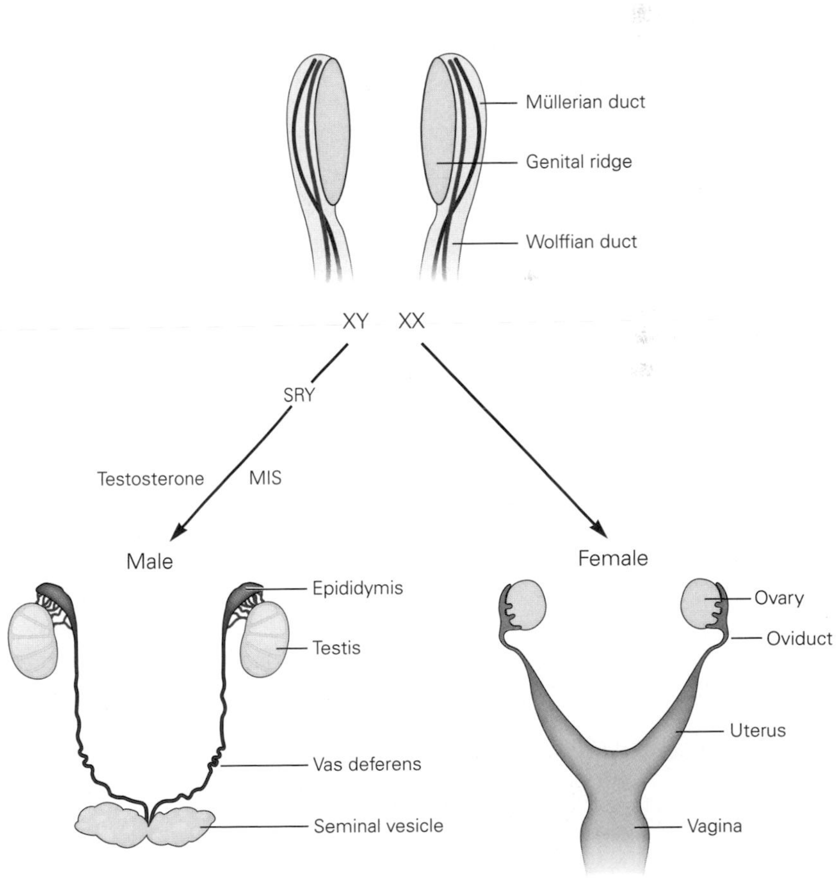

Figure 58–2 Sexual differentiation of the internal genitalia. Embryos of both sexes develop bilateral genital ridges (the gonadal anlagen) that can differentiate into either testes or ovaries; Müllerian ducts, which can differentiate into oviducts, the uterus, and the upper vagina; and Wolffian ducts, which can differentiate into the epididymis, the vas deferens, and the seminal vesicles. In XY embryos the expression of the *SRY* gene in the genital ridge induces differentiation of this tissue into testes and of the Wolffian ducts into the rest of the male internal genitalia, while the Müllerian ducts are resorbed. In XX embryos the *absence* of *SRY* permits the genital ridges to develop into ovaries and the Müllerian ducts to differentiate into the rest of the female internal genitalia; in the absence of circulating testosterone the Wolffian ducts degenerate. (**MIS**, Müllerian inhibiting substance.) (Modified, with permission, from Wilhelm, Palmer, and Koopman 2007.)

and progesterone are hydrophobic molecules that are able to diffuse across cell membranes, enter the bloodstream, enter cells in many organs, and bind to intracellular ligand-specific receptors. The receptors for these hormones are encoded by distinct but homologous genes.

A single gene encodes a receptor that binds the androgens testosterone and DHT. The androgen receptor binds DHT approximately threefold more tightly than testosterone, accounting for the greater potency of DHT. There is also a single receptor for progesterone (progesterone receptor), whereas two genes encode receptors that bind estrogens (estrogen receptors α and β). The estrogen receptors are present in many tissues of the body, including the brain (Figure 58–4B).

These receptor proteins are transcription factors that bind specific sites in the genome and modulate transcription of target genes. They contain several signature motifs, including a hormone-binding domain, a DNA-binding domain, and a domain that modulates the transcriptional activity of target genes (Figure 58–5A). Hormones activate the transcriptional activity by binding to the receptor. In the absence of ligand the receptors bind to protein complexes that sequester them in the cytoplasm. Upon binding of ligand the receptors dissociate from the complex and enter the nucleus, where they dimerize and bind to specific sequence elements in the promoter and enhancer regions of target genes, modulating their transcription (Figure 58–5B).

Patients with CAIS are chromosomally XY but carry a loss-of-function allele of the X-linked androgen receptor that abolishes cellular responses to testosterone and DHT. Because the pathway of sex determination via *SRY* remains functional, these patients have testes. However, because of androgen signaling, the Wolffian ducts do not develop, the testes fail to descend, and the external genitalia are feminized. In adulthood most of these patients opt for surgical removal of the testes and hormonal supplementation appropriate for females.

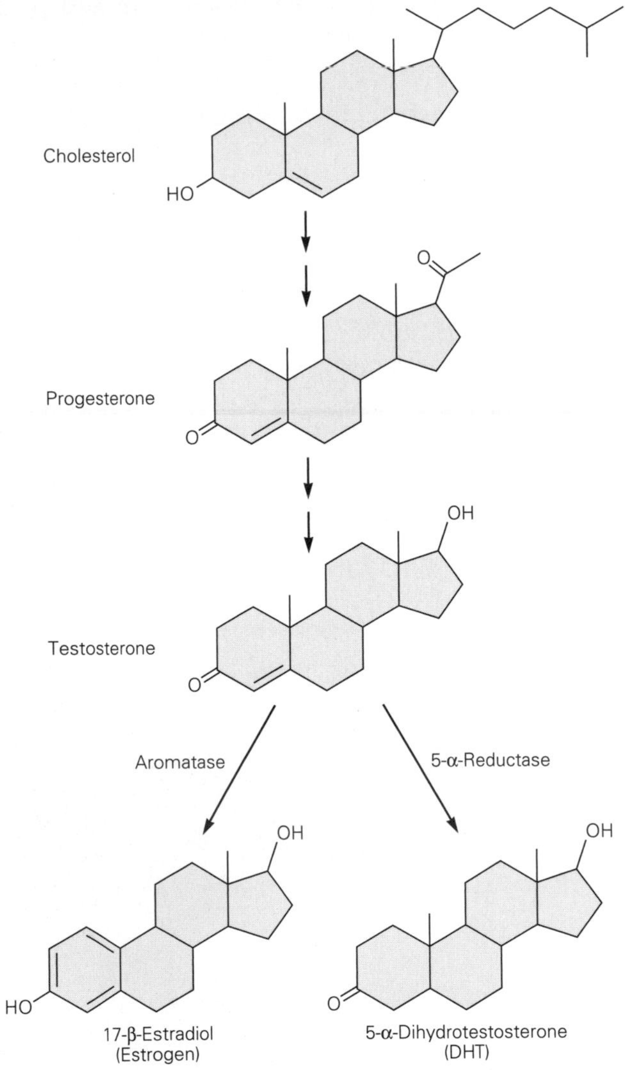

Figure 58–3 Steroid hormone biosynthesis. Cholesterol is the precursor of all steroid hormones and is converted via a series of enzymatic reactions into progesterone and testosterone. Testosterone or related androgens are obligate precursors of all estrogens in the body, a conversion that is catalyzed by aromatase. The expression of 5-α-reductase in target tissues converts testosterone into dihydrotestosterone, an androgen.

Sexual Differentiation of the Nervous System Generates Sexually Dimorphic Behaviors

Sex-specific behaviors occur because the nervous system differs between males and females. These differences arise from a combination of genetic factors, such as components of the sex determination pathways, as well as environmental factors, such as social experience. In many cases both genetic and environmental inputs act through the steroid hormone system to sculpt the nervous system. Many anatomical instances of sexual dimorphism have been documented, including differences in the numbers and size of neurons in particular structures as well as differences in the pattern and number of synapses.

It is challenging to trace the chain of causality from environmental or genetic factors to the development of neural dimorphisms and to link these differences to sex-specific behaviors. In this section we examine a few cases in which studies in experimental animals have provided insights. In later sections we ask

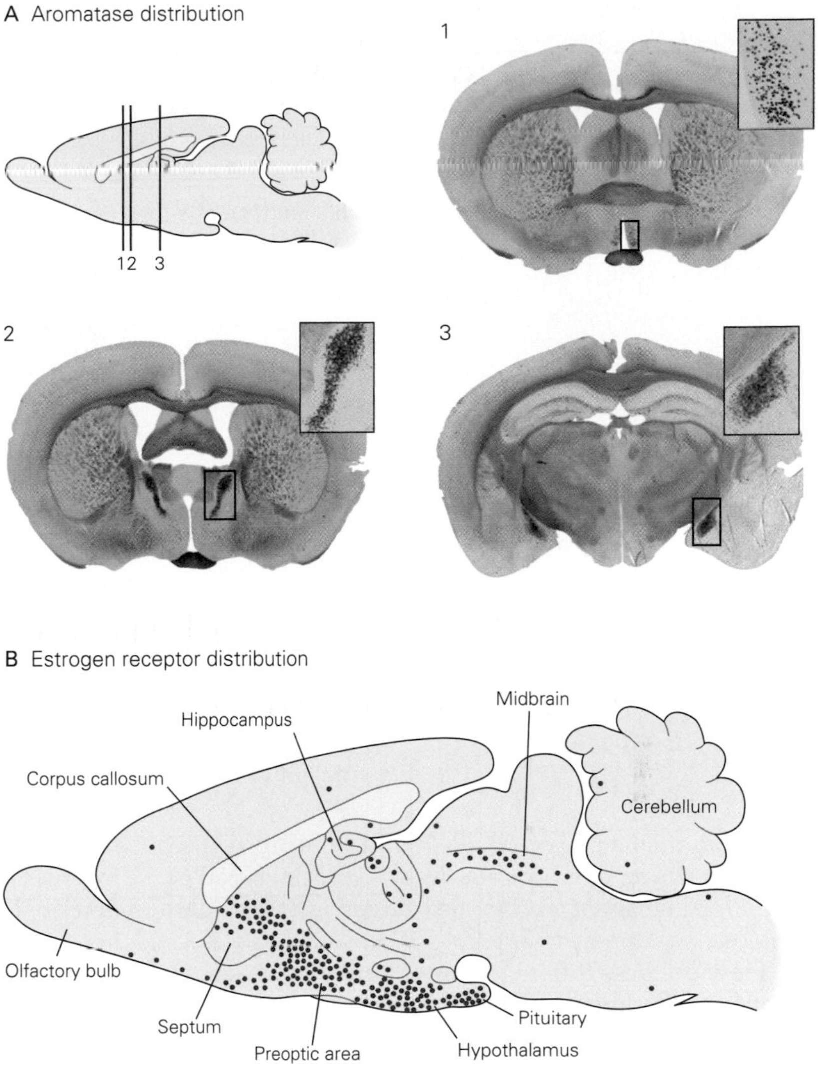

Figure 58–4 **Aromatase and estrogen receptors are expressed in specific regions of the brain.**

A. The enzyme aromatase, which catalyzes the conversion of testosterone into estrogen (see Figure 58–3), is expressed in discrete neuronal populations in the brain. Aromatase labeled with a reporter protein (**blue**) in transgenic mice is shown here in three coronal planes of the brain: in neurons in the preoptic hypothalamus (**1**), in the bed nucleus of the stria terminalis or BNST (**2**), and in the medial amygdala (**3**). These areas contain sexually dimorphic neurons that regulate sexual behavior, aggression, and maternal behaviors. (Modified, with permission, from Wu et al. 2009.)

B. This midsagittal section of an adult rat brain shows binding of estrogen to cells in various hypothalamic regions, including the preoptic area, which is sexually dimorphic. Additional estrogen binding is seen in the septum, hippocampus, pituitary, and midbrain. Other, more lateral areas such as the amygdala (not shown) also contain estrogen receptors.

whether similar mechanisms underlie sexually dimorphic behaviors in humans.

However, before proceeding we note that the ways in which chromosomal mechanisms of sex determination are linked to the cellular processes of sexual differentiation in the central nervous system vary widely among species. In insects sex differences in behavior are independent of hormonal secretion from the gonads, and instead rely exclusively on a sex determination pathway within individual neurons. This mode of sexual differentiation of the brain and behavior is particularly well understood in the fruit fly, where it has been demonstrated that the sex determination cascade initiates expression of a single transcription factor, fruitless, that specifies the entire repertory of male sexual behaviors (Box 58–1).

A Sexually Dimorphic Neural Circuit Controls Erectile Function

The lumbar spinal cord of many mammals, including humans, contains a sexually dimorphic motor center, the spinal nucleus of the bulbocavernosus (SNB). Motor neurons in the SNB innervate the bulbocavernosus muscle, which plays an important part in penile reflexes in males and vaginal movements in females.

In adult rats the male SNB contains many more motor neurons than the female SNB. In addition, male SNB motor neurons are larger in size and have larger dendritic arbors, with a corresponding increase in the number of synapses they receive. Like the SNB motor neurons, the bulbocavernosus muscle is larger in males than females; it is completely absent in the females of

Table 58–1 Three Clinical Syndromes That Highlight the Role of Androgens in Masculinization in Humans

	Complete androgen insensitivity syndrome (CAIS)	5-α-reductase II deficiency	Congenital adrenal hyperplasia (CAH)
Chromosomal sex	XY	XY	XX
Molecular basis	Nonfunctional androgen receptor, leading to inability to respond to circulating androgens.	Nonfunctional 5-α-reductase II, leading to deficit in conversion of testosterone to 5α-dihydrotestosterone (DHT) in target tissues.	Defect in corticosteroid synthesis, leading to increase in circulating androgens from the adrenals.
Gonad	Testis	Testis	Ovary
Wolffian derivatives	Vestigial	Present	Absent
Müllerian derivatives	Absent	Absent	Present
External genitalia:			
At birth	Feminized	Variably feminized	Variably virilized
After puberty	Feminized	Masculinized	Feminized
Gender identity	Female	Female or male	Female or male
Sexual partner preference	Male	Female or male	Female or male

some mammalian species. SNB motor neurons also innervate the levator ani muscle, which is involved in copulatory behavior and is also larger in males than females.

How do these differences arise? Initially the circuit is not sexually dimorphic. At birth male and female rats have similar numbers of neurons in the SNB and similar numbers of fibers in the bulbocavernosus and levator ani muscles. In females, however, many motor neurons in the SNB and many fibers in the bulbocavernosus and levator ani muscles die in early postnatal life. Thus this sexual dimorphism arises not by male-specific generation of cells but rather by female-specific cell death.

Perinatal injections of testosterone or DHT can rescue a significant number of the dying neurons and muscle fibers in the female rat. Conversely, treatment of male pups with an androgen receptor antagonist increases the number of dying neurons and muscle fibers. So at a deeper level we see that the dimorphism results from male-specific preservation of motor neurons and muscle fibers that would die in the absence of hormone.

Where does testosterone act to establish this structural dimorphism? Is it primarily a survival factor for the motor neurons, with muscle fibers dying secondarily because they lose their innervation? Or does testosterone act on muscles, which then provide a trophic factor to support the survival of SNB motor neurons? This issue has been examined in rats carrying a mutation of the androgen receptor (*tfm* allele) that reduces binding of ligand to 10% of normal. The receptor resides on the X chromosome, so all males that carry a mutant gene on their one and only X chromosome are feminized and sterile. For female heterozygotes, the situation is more complicated. As described earlier, one of the X chromosomes is randomly inactivated in each XX female.

Female heterozygotes are therefore mosaics: some cells express a functional androgen receptor allele, others the mutated allele. Each muscle fiber has many nuclei, so most bulbocavernosus muscle fibers in the heterozygous female express functional androgen receptors. Motor neurons have a single nucleus, however, so each neuron is either normal or receptor-deficient. If androgen receptors were required in the neuron, one would expect only receptor-expressing SNB motor neurons to survive, whereas if receptors were required only in muscles, one would expect surviving motor neurons to be a mixture of wild type and mutant.

In fact, the latter situation occurs, indicating that survival of SNB motor neurons does not depend on a neuron-autonomous function of the androgen receptor.

Rather, these neurons receive a trophic cue from the androgen-dependent bulbocavernosus and the levator ani muscles (Figure 58–7A). These cues may include the ciliary neurotrophic factor (CNTF) or a related molecule, because mutant male mice lacking a CNTF receptor exhibit a decreased number of SNB motor neurons, typical of females.

Male and female SNB motor neurons also differ in size. Androgens determine the differences in number and size of these neurons in different ways. Studies of *tfm* mutants showed that androgens exert an organizational effect during early postnatal life through a direct effect on muscle. Low levels of androgens during this critical period lead to an irreversible reduction in the number of SNB motor neurons. Later, androgens act directly on SNB motor neurons to increase the extent of their dendritic arbors. A loss of circulating testosterone, such as that occurring after castration, leads to a dramatic pruning of dendritic arbors; injection of supplemental testosterone to a castrated male rat can restore this dendritic branching pattern (Figure 58–7B). This effect persists in adulthood and is reversible, so it can be viewed as an activational influence. Thus androgens can exert diverse effects, even on a single neuronal type.

A Sexually Dimorphic Neural Circuit Controls Song Production in Birds

Several species of songbirds learn species-specific vocalizations that are used for courtship rituals and territorial marking (see Chapter 60). A set of interconnected brain nuclei controls the learning and production of birdsong (Figure 58–8A). In some songbird species both sexes sing and the structure of the song circuit is similar in males and females. In other species, such as zebra finches and canaries, males alone sing. In these species several song-related nuclei are significantly larger in the male than in the female.

The development of sexual dimorphism in song circuitry has been studied in detail in the zebra finch. In the adult male zebra finch the robust nucleus of the archistriatum (RA) contains fivefold more neurons than does the same nucleus in females. In addition,

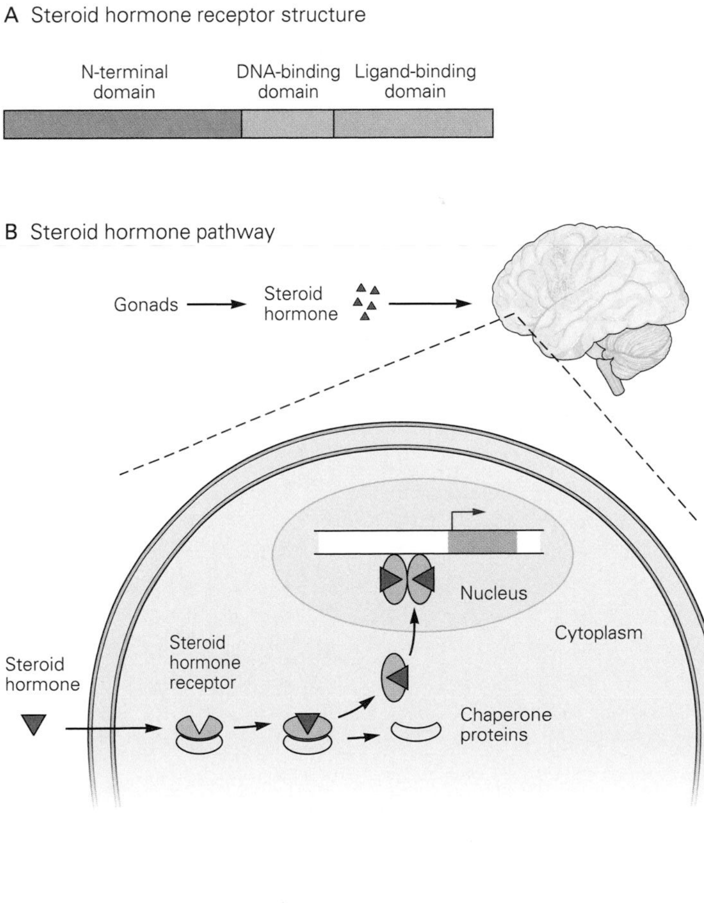

Figure 58–5 Steroid hormone receptors and their mechanism of action.

A. The canonical receptors for steroid hormones are ligand-activated transcription factors. These receptors have an N-terminal domain, which contains a transcriptional transactivator domain; a central DNA-binding domain; and a C-terminal ligand-binding domain, which may contain an additional transcriptional transactivator domain.

B. Sex steroid hormones are hydrophobic and enter the circulation by diffusing across the plasma membrane of steroidogenic cells in the gonads. They enter target cells in distant tissues such as the brain by passing through the plasma membrane and bind their cognate receptors. The steroid hormone receptor typically exists in a multiprotein complex with chaperone proteins in the cytoplasm of hormone-responsive cells. Ligand-binding promotes dissociation of the receptor from the chaperone complex and translocation into the nucleus. In the nucleus the receptor is thought to bind to hormone response elements as a homodimer to modulate transcription of target genes. (Modified, with permission, from Wierman 2007.)

Box 58–1 Genetic and Neural Control of Mating Behavior in the Fruit Fly

In the presence of a female fruitfly the adult male fly engages in a series of essentially stereotyped routines that usually culminate in copulation (Figure 58–6A). This elaborate male courtship ritual is encoded by a cascade of gene transcription within the brain and peripheral sensory organs that masculinizes the underlying neural circuitry.

Sex determination in the fly does not depend on gonadal hormones, as it does in vertebrates. Instead, it occurs cell autonomously throughout the body. In other words, sexual differentiation of the brain and the rest of the body is independent of gonadal sex. The male-specific Y chromosome of fruit flies does not bear a sex-determining locus. Instead, sex is determined by the ratio of X chromosome number to autosome number (X:A). A ratio of 1 is determinative for female differentiation, whereas a ratio of 0.5 drives male differentiation.

The X:A ratio sets into motion a cascade of gene transcription and alternative splicing programs that leads to the expression of sex-specific splice forms of two genes, *doublesex* (*dsx*) and *fruitless* (*fru*). The *dsx* gene encodes a transcription factor that is essential for sexual differentiation of the nervous system and the rest of the body, with the sex-specific splice variants responsible for male- and female-typical development.

The *fru* gene encodes a set of putative transcription factors that is generated by multiple promoters and alternative splicing. In males one particular mRNA (fru^M) is translated into functional proteins. In female flies alternative splicing results in the absence of such proteins.

Males carrying a genetically modified *fru* allele that can only be spliced in the female-specific manner (fru^F) have essentially normal, *dsx*-dependent sexual differentiation. These fru^F males therefore resemble wild type males externally. However, the loss of Fru^M in these animals abolishes male courtship behavior directed toward females. These data indicate that Fru^M is required for male courtship and copulation.

Conversely, transgenic female flies carrying a fru^M allele exhibit male mating behavior toward wild type females, indicating that fru^M is sufficient to inhibit female sexual responses and promote male mating.

Intriguingly, fru^F males do not court females and, like wild type females, do not reject mating attempts by wild type males or fru^M females. Similarly, fru^M females attempt to mate with both fru^M and wild type females. These data suggest that fru^M may also specify sexual partner preference, which in the case of wild type males would be directed to females.

In wild type females without fru^M the neural pathways are wired such that these flies exhibit sexually receptive behaviors toward males. When groups of fru^F males (or fru^M females) are housed together, they court each other vigorously, often forming long chains of flies attempting copulation.

To build the circuitry underlying male courtship rituals, fru^M appears to initiate cell-autonomous male-typical differentiation of the neurons in which it is expressed. This leads to overt neuroanatomic dimorphism in cell number or projections of several specific classes of neurons (Figure 58–6B). Many neurons that express fru^M are not distributed in dimorphic patterns. In these neurons fru^M may regulate the expression of particular classes of genes whose products drive a male-specific program of physiology and function.

Are neurons that express fru^M required for male courtship behavior? When synaptic transmission is genetically blocked in these neurons in adult males all components of courtship behavior are abolished. Importantly, these males continue to exhibit normal movement, flight, and other behaviors in response to visual and olfactory stimuli. These findings demonstrate that fru^M appears to be expressed in a neural circuit that is essential for and dedicated to male fly courtship.

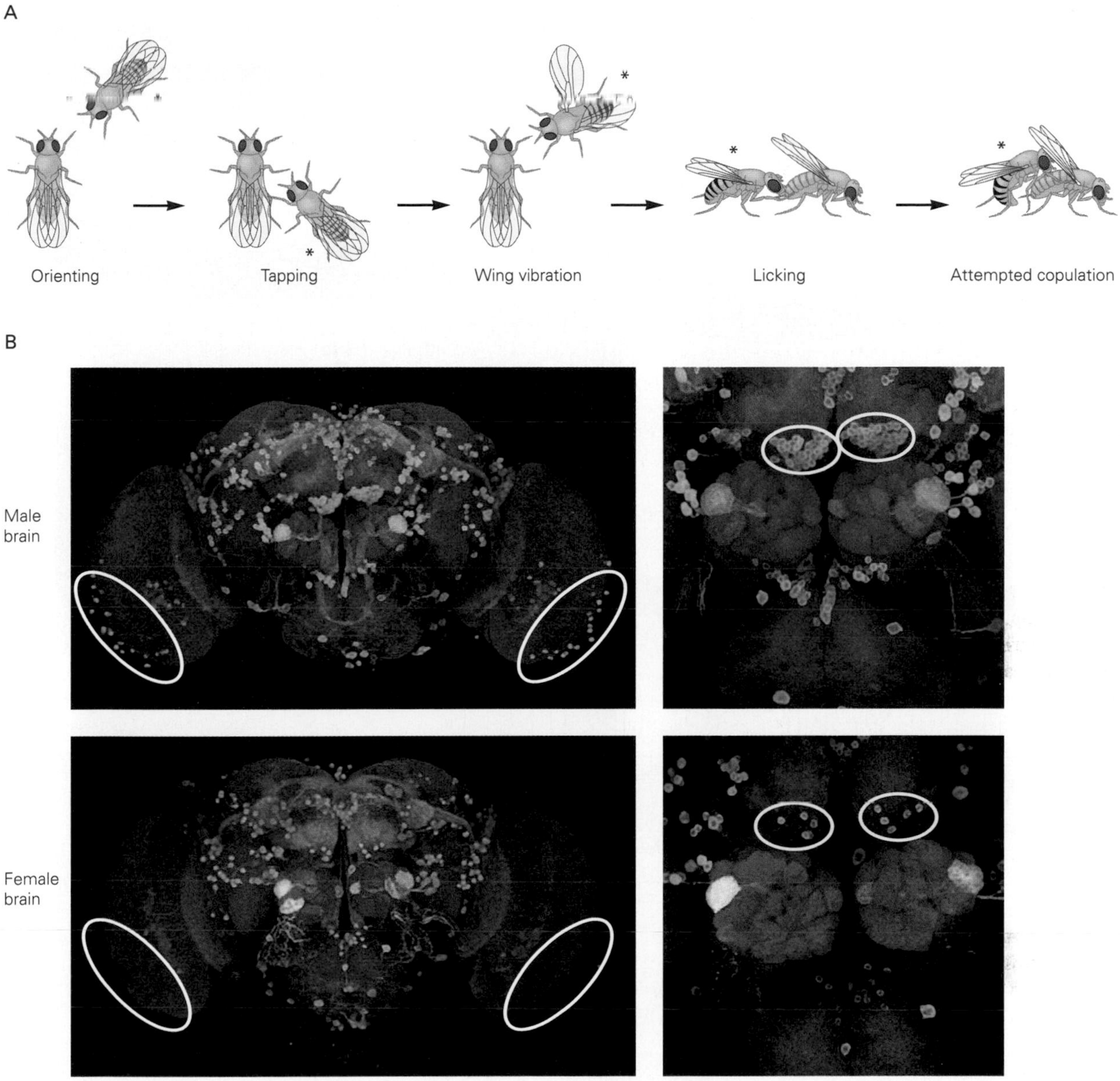

Figure 58–6 Control of male courtship in the fruit fly.

A. Male *Drosophila melanogaster* (labeled with **asterisk**) engage in a stereotyped sequence of behavioral routines that culminate in attempted copulation. The male fly orients toward the female and then taps her with his forelegs. This is followed by wing extension in the male and a species-specific pattern of wing vibrations that is commonly referred to as the fly courtship song. If the female fly is sexually receptive, she slows down and permits the male to lick her genitalia. The female then opens her vaginal plates in order to allow the male to initiate copulation. All steps in the male mating ritual require the expression of a sex-specific splice variant of the *fruitless* (*fru*) gene. (Modified, with permission, from Greenspan and Ferveur 2000.)

B. The *fru* gene encodes a male-specific splice variant that is necessary and sufficient to drive most steps in the male fly courtship ritual. *Fru* expression is visualized using a fluorescent reporter protein (**green**) in transgenic flies. *Fru*-expressing neuronal clusters are present in comparable numbers in the central nervous system of both male and female flies. However, there are sex differences in *Fru* expression as well. A cluster of *Fru*-expressing neurons is present in the male optic lobes (in the area within the **white ellipses**) but absent in the corresponding regions in the female brain. The two male antennal lobe regions (areas within **yellow ellipses**) contain about 30 neurons each, whereas each female region has only 4–5 neurons. (Modified, with permission, from Kimura et al. 2005.)

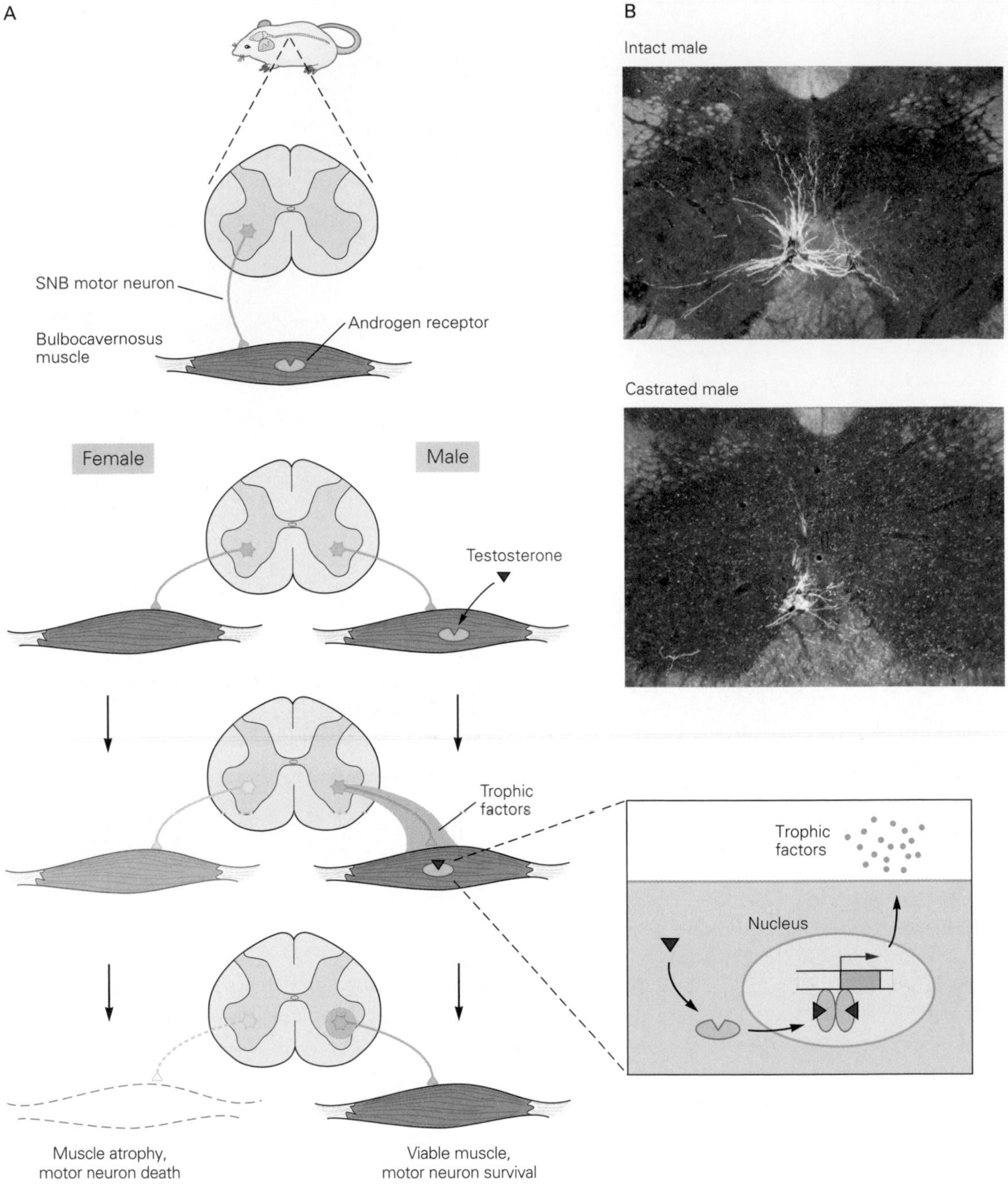

Figure 58–7 Sexual dimorphism in the spinal nucleus of the bulbocavernosus muscle.

A. The spinal nucleus of the bulbocavernosus (**SNB**) is found in the male lumbar spinal cord but is greatly reduced in the female. The motor neurons of the nucleus are present in both sexes at birth but the lack of circulating testosterone in females leads to death of the SNB neurons and their target muscles. It is thought that testosterone in the male circulation promotes the survival of the target muscles, which express the androgen receptor. In response to testosterone the muscles provide trophic support to the innervating SNB neurons. This muscle-derived survival factor is likely to be ciliary neurotrophic factor or a related member of the cytokine family. Thus testosterone acts on muscle cells to control the sexual differentiation of SNB neurons. (Reproduced, with permission, from Morris, Jordan, and Breedlove 2004.)

B. Dendritic branching of SNB neurons is regulated by circulating testosterone in adult male rats. In males the dendrites arborize extensively within the spinal cord (upper photo). The fact that the arbors are pruned in adult castrated male rats (lower photo) is evidence that this dendritic branching depends on androgens. The spinal cord is shown in transverse section and the SNB neurons and their dendrites are labeled by a retrograde tracer injected into target muscles. (Reproduced, with permission, from Cooke and Woolley 2005.)

the afferent projections to RA exhibit a striking sexual dimorphism—only in males does the RA receive input from high vocal centers (HVCs) (Figure 58–8B). These sex differences in cell number and connectivity of RA are not evident until after hatching, when in females a large number of RA neurons die and in males the axons of HVC neurons enter the RA nucleus.

These sexually dimorphic anatomical features are regulated by steroid hormones. When females are supplied with estrogen (or an aromatizable androgen such as testosterone) after hatching, the number of neurons in the RA and the termination pattern in the nucleus are similar to that of the male. However, early hormone administration to young females is not sufficient to masculinize the song nuclei to a size comparable to that of adult males, nor is it sufficient to induce singing in females. To achieve these functions, female birds that receive testosterone or estradiol after hatching must also receive testosterone or dihydrotestosterone (but not estrogen) as adults. Thus steroids play both organizational and activational roles in this system.

A Sexually Dimorphic Neural Circuit in the Hypothalamus Controls Mating Behavior

In many mammalian species the preoptic region of the hypothalamus and a reciprocally connected region, the bed nucleus of the stria terminalis (BNST), play important roles in sexually dimorphic mating behaviors. In male rodents and monkeys these areas are activated during mating behavior; surgical lesions that ablate the preoptic region or the BNST result in deficits in male sexual behavior in male rodents, and also disinhibit female-type sexual receptivity. Thus this region contains neurons that activate and inhibit female sexual behavior. Surgical lesioning of the preoptic hypothalamic region activates male mating routines and inhibits female sexual receptivity in rodents.

Both the preoptic hypothalamus and the BNST are sexually dimorphic, containing more neurons in males compared to females. The sexually dimorphic nucleus of the preoptic area (SDN-POA) also contains significantly more neurons in the male. A male-specific perinatal surge of testosterone promotes survival of neurons in the SDN-POA, whereas in females these same cells gradually die off in the early postnatal period. This development is similar to that in the sexually dimorphic nuclei of the rodent spinal cord and the songbird brain, suggesting that androgen control is a common mechanism for production of sex differences in the size of neuronal populations.

Curiously, the ability of brain testosterone to promote the survival of neurons is likely to be exerted via aromatization into estrogen and subsequent activation of the estrogen receptors (see Figure 58–5). How, then, is the neonatal female brain shielded from the effects of circulating estrogen? In newborn females there is very little estrogen in the circulation, and the small amount present is sequestered by binding to α-fetoprotein, a serum protein. This explains why female mice lacking α-fetoprotein exhibit male-specific behaviors and reduced female-typical sexual receptivity. In this case, then, structural sexual dimorphism does not result from differential effects of androgens and estrogens, but rather from sex differences in the level of hormone available to the target tissue.

Environmental Cues Control Some Sexually Dimorphic Behaviors

Sex-specific behaviors are usually initiated in response to sensory cues in the environment. There are many such cues, and distinct sensory modalities are used in a species-specific manner to elicit a similar response. Courtship rituals can be triggered by species-specific vocalizations, visual signals, odors, and even, in the case of weakly electric fish, by electric discharges. Recent genetic and molecular studies have led to significant insight into how sensory experience controls some of these behaviors in rodents. Here we discuss two examples: the regulation of partner choice by pheromones and the regulation of maternal behavior by experience during infancy.

Pheromones Control Partner Choice in Mice

Many animals rely on their sense of smell to move about, obtain food, and avoid predators. They also rely on pheromones—chemicals that are produced by an animal to affect the behavior of another member of the species. In rodents pheromones can trigger many sexually dimorphic behaviors, including mate choice and aggression (the propensity of males to fight over territory or mates and the tendency of nursing females to attack nest intruders).

Pheromones are detected by neurons in two distinct sensory tissues in the vertebrate nose: the main olfactory epithelium (MOE) and the vomeronasal organ (VNO) (Figure 58–9A). It is thought that sensory neurons in the MOE detect volatile odors whereas those in the VNO detect nonvolatile chemosensory cues. Removal of the olfactory bulb, the only synaptic target of neurons in the MOE and the VNO, abolishes mating as well as aggression in mice and other rodents. These and other studies indicate an essential role for olfactory stimulation in initiating mating and fighting.

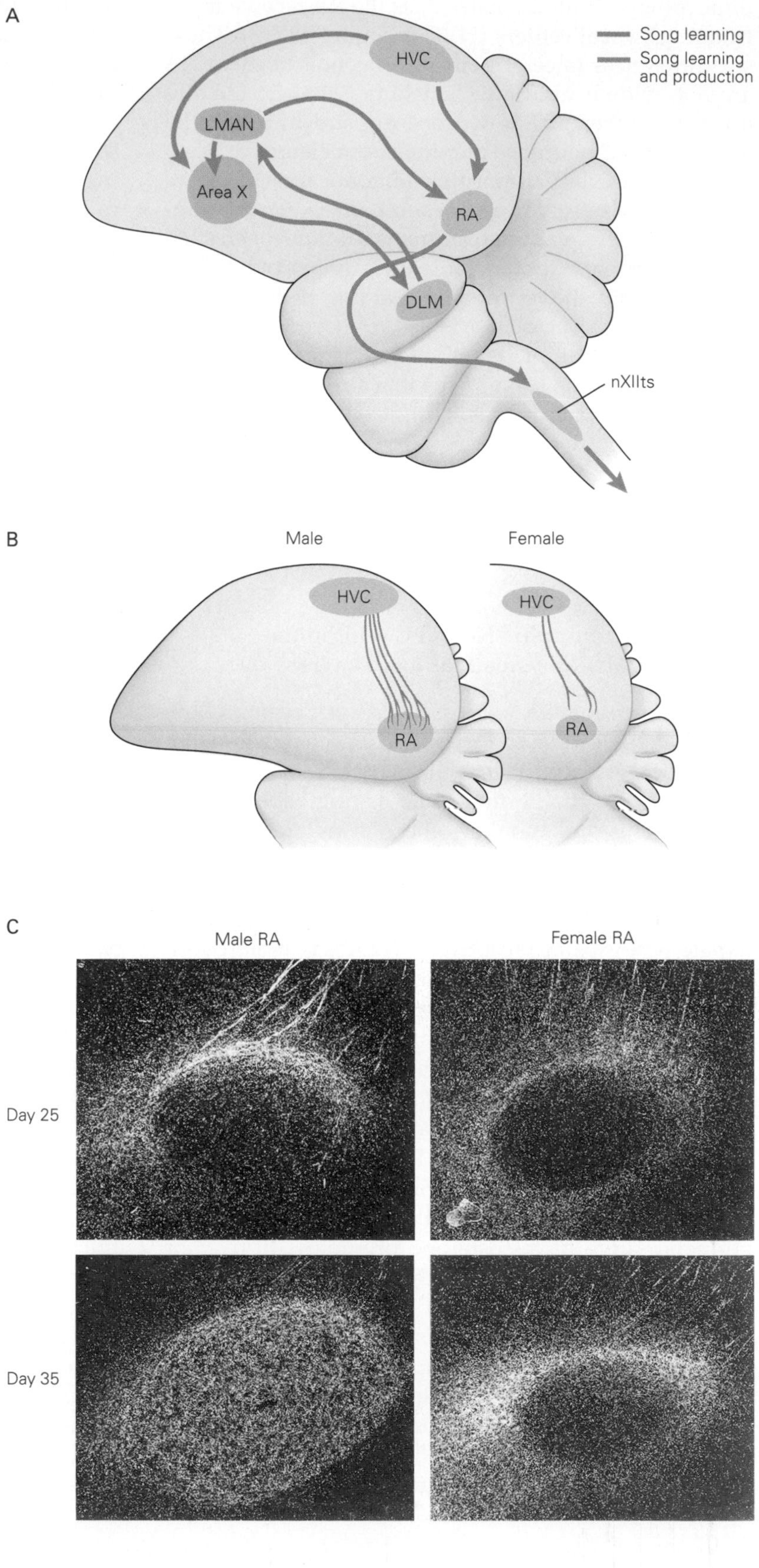

Figure 58–8 Sexual dimorphism in the avian song circuit.

A. Songbirds have a dedicated neural circuit for song production and learning, with distinct components contributing to learning or production. Many of these components are sexually dimorphic in songbirds in which only one sex sings. For example, in zebra finches the male sings, and the male high vocal center (**HVC**), robust nucleus of the archistriatum (**RA**), lateral magnocellular nucleus of the anterior neostriatum (**LMAN**), and area X are larger in volume and contain more neurons than the comparable regions in the female. (**DLM**, medial nucleus of the dorsolateral thalamus; **nXIIts**, hypoglossal nucleus.) (Reproduced, with permission, from Brainard and Doupe 2002.)

B. In the male the axons of HVC neurons terminate on neurons in the RA nucleus, whereas in females the axons terminate in a zone surrounding the nucleus. The sexual dimorphism in cell number and connectivity of these regions is regulated by estrogen. (Reproduced, with permission, from Morris, Jordan, and Breedlove 2004.)

C. The pattern of termination of the axons of HVC neurons in the RA nucleus varies in males and females at different ages after hatching. (Reproduced, with permission, from Konishi and Akutagawa 1985.)

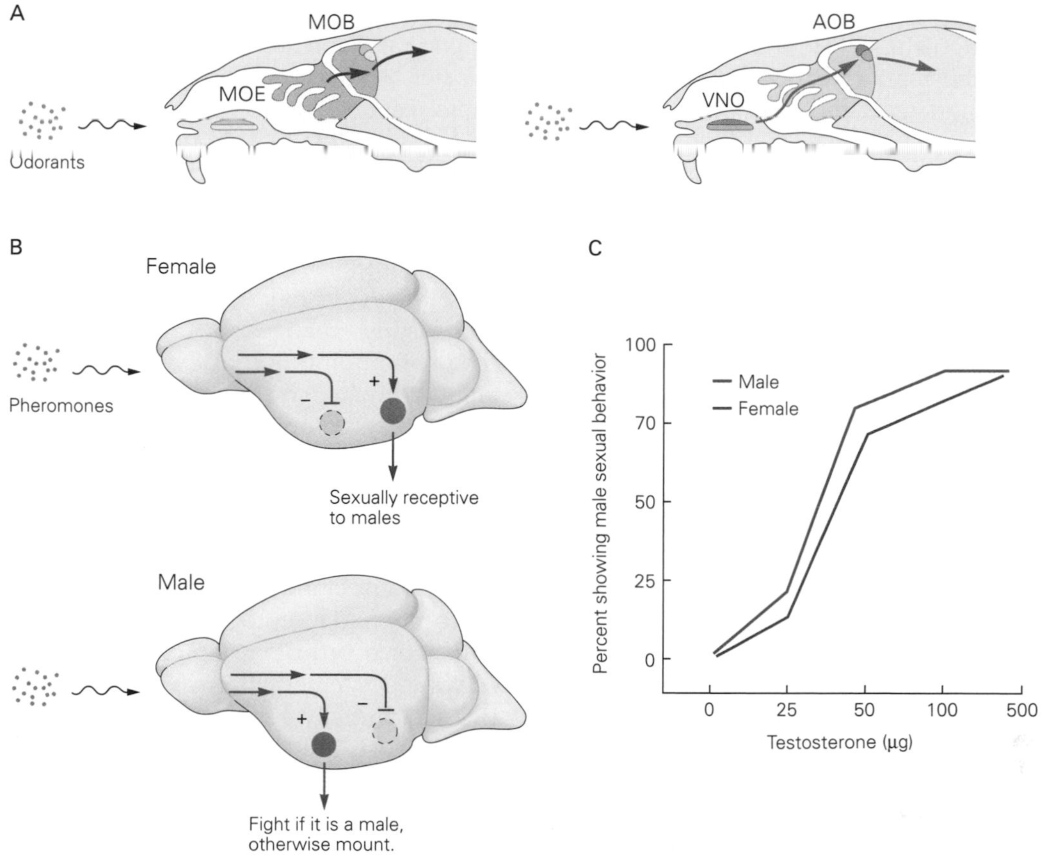

Figure 58–9 Pheromonal and hormonal control of male and female sexual behavior.

A. Odorants are detected by sensory neurons in the main olfactory epithelium (**MOE**), which projects to the main olfactory bulb (**MOB**), and by neurons in the vomeronasal organ (**VNO**), which projects to the accessory olfactory bulb (**AOB**). Many of the central connections of the MOE and VNO pathway are anatomically segregated. (Modified, with permission, from Dulac and Wagner 2006.)

B. Female mice possess the neural circuitry that can activate either male (**blue**) or female (**red**) mating behaviors. In wild type females pheromones activate female mating behavior and inhibit male-type mating. By contrast, in males pheromones activate a circuitry that will initiate fights with males and mating with females. (Modified, with permission, from Kimchi, Xu, and Dulac 2007.)

C. Testosterone activates male sexual behavior in male and female mice. The data are from a study in which the gonads of male and female mice were surgically removed in adulthood. None of the animals exhibited male sexual behavior with wild type females following surgery. After administration of testosterone, mating behavior was restored in castrated males, and females displayed male sexual behavior. This effect was dose-dependent; at the highest dose male and female mice exhibited comparable levels of male-type mating behavior toward wild type females. (Modified, with permission, from Edwards and Burge 1971.)

Genetically engineered disruption of pheromone responsiveness in the MOE or VNO reveals that these sensory tissues have a surprisingly complex role in the mating behavior of mice. A functional MOE is essential to trigger male sexual behavior, and an intact VNO is required for sex discrimination and directing the male to mate with females.

Key to these experiments is the fact that olfactory neurons in the MOE and the VNO use different signal transduction cascades to convert olfactory input into electrical responses. The cation channel Trpc2 appears essential for pheromone-evoked signaling in VNO neurons; it is not expressed in MOE neurons, which use a different signal transduction apparatus. Thus mice lacking the gene *trpc2* have a nonfunctional VNO and an intact MOE. Mating behavior directed to animals of the opposite sex appears unaltered in *trpc2* mutant males as well as females. However, both males and female mutants often exhibit male sexual behavior with members of either sex. For example, *trpc2* mutant females mate with females in a manner seemingly indistinguishable from wild type males, except of course the females cannot ejaculate. These and other findings suggest that the VNO is used to discriminate among sexual partners. When the VNO is inactivated animals can no longer distinguish between males and females, and mutants therefore exhibit male sexual behavior toward members of both sexes. Similarly, adult wild type females treated with testosterone also exhibit male sexual behavior toward females (Figure 58–9C).

One implication of these studies is that female mice possess the neural circuitry for male sexual behavior (Figure 58–9B). Activation of this neural circuit is inhibited in wild type females by sensory input from the VNO and by the lack of testosterone. Removal of the VNO or administration of testosterone activates male sexual behavior in females. Male mating behavior has been observed in females of many species, indicating that the findings in mice are likely to be of general relevance. Thus neural pathways for male and female mating behavior appear to be present in both sexes. The female-typical behavior of male rats following hypothalamic lesions is another example. In such cases it is the differential regulation of these circuits that underlies the sexually dimorphic expression of male and female sexual behaviors.

Early Experience Modifies Later Maternal Behavior

The preoptic area of the hypothalamus and the BNST are also important for another set of sexually dimorphic behaviors in females. Nursing rodents are good mothers, building a nest for their litter, crouching over the pups to keep them warm, and returning the pups to the nest when they happen to crawl away. Surgical lesioning of either the preoptic region or the BNST abolishes these maternal behaviors.

Studies of these behaviors have shed light on variations among individual females and how these differences exert lifelong effects on behavior of the offspring. Female lab rats exhibit distinct, stable forms of maternal care: Some lick and groom (LG) their pups frequently (high-LG mothers), whereas others lick and groom less frequently (low-LG mothers). Female offspring of high-LG mothers display high-LG activity when they themselves become mothers compared to female offspring of low-LG mothers (Figure 58–10). Moreover, pups of high-LG mothers show less anxiety-like behaviors in stressful conditions than do the pups of low-LG mothers.

These results suggested that levels of licking and grooming behavior and stress responses are genetically determined. However, studies by Michael Meaney and his colleagues provide an alternative explanation. When female rat pups are transferred from their mother to a foster mother at birth, their maternal behavior and stress responses as adults resemble those of their foster mother rather than those of their biological mother. Thus experience in infancy can lead to lifelong behavioral patterns. Because these patterns impact maternal behavior, their influence can endure over many generations.

How does brief and early experience lead to such long-lasting changes? One mechanism involves a covalent modification of the genome. Stress responses are coordinated by glucocorticoids acting on glucocorticoid receptors in the hippocampus. Throughout life tactile stimulation, including grooming, leads to transcriptional activation of the glucocorticoid receptor gene, which ultimately leads to reduced release of hypothalamic hormones that trigger stress responses. Tactile stimulation during early life also regulates the glucocorticoid receptor gene in a second way. A key site in the glucocorticoid receptor gene is methylated by the enzyme DNA methyltransferase, leading to gene inactivation. Initially gene methylation occurs in all pups, but pups reared by high-LG mothers are selectively demethylated. Thus in animals reared by high-LG mothers the effects of adult experience are potentiated. This is an example of epigenetic modification by which genes can be turned on or off more or less permanently. These animals exhibit blunted behavioral responses to stressful stimuli later in life.

What are the biological links between early experience and behavioral variation? A peptide hormone, oxytocin, plays a major role. Classical work showed that oxytocin regulates provision of milk by the mother, which occurs via reflex ejection in response to suckling (milk let-down). Oxytocin is synthesized by neurons in the hypothalamus and released into the general circulation through their projections in the posterior pituitary. It elicits smooth muscle contraction in the mammary gland, resulting in milk ejection. Oxytocin release from the pituitary is controlled by suckling, which provides a sensory stimulus that is conveyed to the hypothalamus by spinal afferent nerves.

Oxytocin and a related polypeptide hormone vasopressin also play important roles in regulating maternal bonding and other social behaviors (see Chapter 3). In these cases experience appears to modulate behaviors by affecting both release of oxytocin and levels of the oxytocin receptor in specific brain areas. In both rats and voles individual differences in the care females provide their offspring correlate with variations in oxytocin receptor level in specific brain areas. Especially noteworthy is that oxytocin receptor levels in

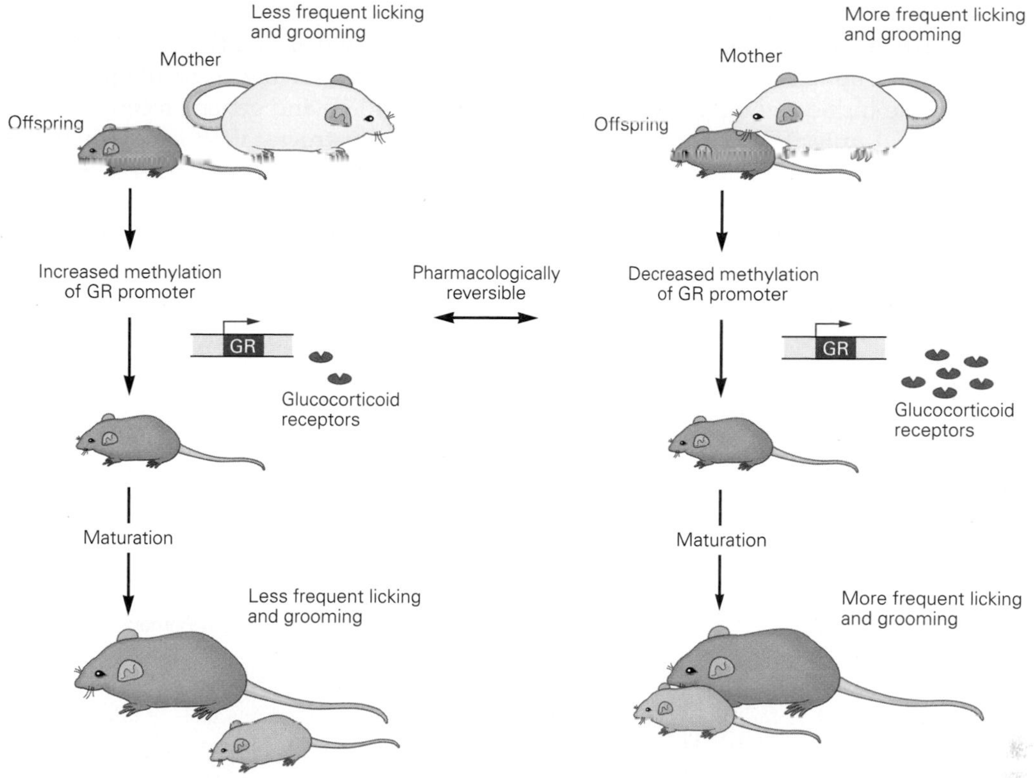

Figure 58–10 The regulation of maternal behavior by past social experience. In a common lab rat strain mothers lick and groom their pups at low or high frequencies, resulting in distinct epigenetic modifications at the glucocorticoid receptor (**GR**) promoter. Mothers that lick and groom at high frequency raise progeny with low levels of DNA methylation at the GR promoter, resulting in higher levels of GR expression in the hippocampus. Females raised by these mothers exhibit higher frequencies of licking and grooming behavior with their own pups. Mothers that lick and groom at low frequency raise progeny with high DNA methylation levels at the GR promoter and lower levels of hippocampal GR expression. Females nursed by these mothers subsequently exhibit similar low levels of licking and grooming of their pups. Pharmacological reversal of the epigenetic modifications at the GR promoter results in a corresponding change in both GR expression and maternal behavior. (Modified, with permission, from Sapolsky 2004.)

several regions are higher in female offspring reared by high-LG mothers than in female progeny of low LG-mothers. Thus sensory stimulation may affect activity of the oxytocin and vasopressin systems, which in turn regulate maternal and other social behaviors.

These experiments suggest powerful mechanisms by which early experience can influence later behavior. Are they applicable to humans? Two recent observations suggest they are. First, as discussed in Chapter 56, children raised for lengthy periods in orphanages with little individual care have long-lasting defects in a variety of social behaviors. Even years after placement in foster homes these children have, on average, lower levels of oxytocin and vasopressin in their serum than children raised with biological parents. Second, people who have suffered abuse as children often grow up to be poor parents. Postmortem studies have shown that adults who had been abused as children exhibited greater promoter methylation of their glucocorticoid receptor genes than adults in control populations. Although these studies are new and require replication, they provide tantalizing hints at the biological mechanisms that underlie the lifelong effects of early parental care.

Sexual Dimorphism in the Human Brain May Correlate with Gender Identity and Sexual Orientation

Are structural differences between the brains of male and female mammals also present in humans and, if so, might they be functionally important? Early studies revealed that a few structures are markedly larger in men: Onuf's nucleus in the spinal cord, the homolog of the spinal nucleus of the bulbocavernosus in rodents (Figure 58–7); the BNST, implicated in rodent mating behavior; and the interstitial nucleus of the anterior hypothalamus 3 (INAH3), related to the rodent SDN-POA discussed earlier (Figure 58–11).

Advances in high-resolution magnetic resonance imaging (MRI) and genetic technology have uncovered more subtle structural and molecular dimorphisms in the central nervous system. For example, structures

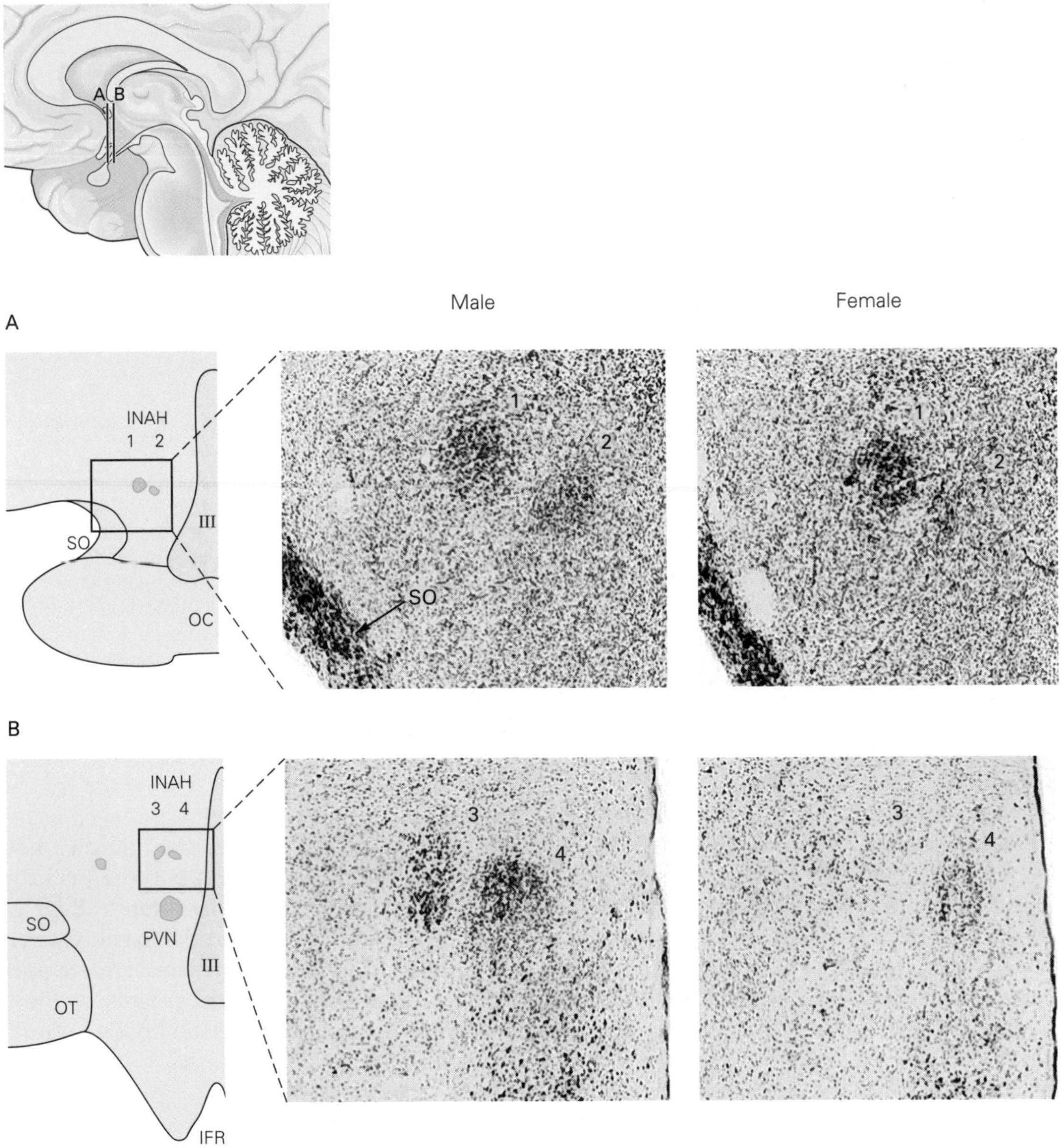

Figure 58–11 Sexual dimorphism in the interstitial nucleus of the anterior hypothalamus (INAH) 3 in the human brain. The human hypothalamus contains four small, discrete neuronal clusters, INAH1 through INAH4. While INAH1, INAH2, and INAH4 appear similar in men and women, INAH3 is significantly larger in men. The section in part A is 0.8 mm anterior to the section in part B. The photomicrographs show these nuclei in adult male and female brains. (**IFR**, infundibular recess; **III**, third ventricle; **OC**, optic chiasm; **OT**, optic tract; **PVN**, paraventricular nucleus; **SO**, supraoptic nucleus.) (Reproduced, with permission, from Gorski 1988.)

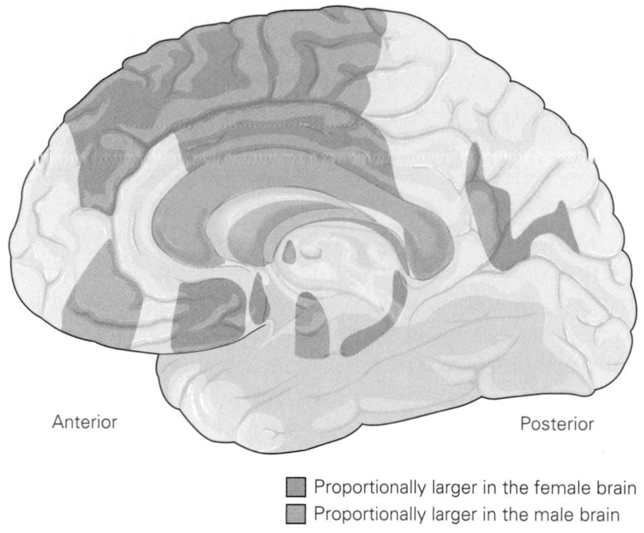

Figure 58–12 Sexual dimorphism is widespread in the adult human brain. A magnetic resonance imaging (MRI) study measured the volume of many brain regions in adult men and women. The volume of each region was normalized to the size of the cerebrum for both sexes. Sex differences were significant in many regions, including several cortical areas that likely mediate cognitive functions. (Modified, with permission, from Cahill 2006.)

such as the fronto-orbital cortex and several gyri—including the precentral, superior frontal, and lingual gyri—occupy a significantly larger volume in adult women compared to a cohort of adult men (Figure 58–12). Moreover, the frontomedial cortex, amygdala, and angular gyrus volumes are larger in men compared to women. Thus there are likely to be many sexual dimorphisms in the human brain.

What remains unclear is how these dimorphisms arise and how they relate to behavior. They might arise early from the organizational effects of hormones, or later as a result of experience. Structural differences arising before or soon after birth could underlie behavioral differences, whereas structural differences that arise later in life might be results of dimorphic behaviors.

Answers to these questions are fairly clear in a few cases. For example, studies of the development of neural circuits responsible for penile erection and lactation in rodents translate readily to humans. In contrast, differences in cognitive function, sexual partner preference, and gender identity are poorly understood. Little progress has been made in relating sex differences in cognitive functions to structural differences in the brain, in part because the very existence of cognitive differences remains a matter of controversy; if they exist at all, they are small and represent differences in means between highly variable male and female populations. On the other hand several lines of evidence have connected clear differences in gender identity and sexual orientation to dimorphisms in the brain.

Early insight into this issue came from observation of people with single-gene mutations that dissociate anatomical sex from gonadal and chromosomal sex, such as CAIS, CAH, and 5α-reductase deficiency (see Table 58–1). For example, girls with CAH experience an excess of testosterone during fetal life; the disorder is generally diagnosed at birth and corrected. Nevertheless, the early exposure to androgens is correlated with subsequent changes in gender-related behaviors. On average, girls with CAH tend to exhibit toy preferences and play typical of boys of equivalent age. There is also a small but significant increase in the incidence of homosexual and bisexual orientation in females treated for CAH as children, and a significant proportion of these females also express the desire to live as men, consistent with a change in gender identity. These findings suggest that early organizational effects of steroids affect gender-specific behaviors independent of chromosomal and anatomical sex.

In 5α-reductase II deficiency and CAIS many of the afflicted males show feminized external genitalia and are mistakenly raised as females until puberty. Thereafter their histories diverge. In 5α-reductase II deficiency the symptoms arise from a defect in testosterone processing largely confined to the developing external genitalia. At puberty a large increase in circulating testosterone virilizes the body hair, musculature, and most dramatically, the external genitalia. At this stage many but not all patients choose to adopt a male gender. In CAIS, in contrast, defects arise from a body-wide defect in the androgen receptor. These patients commonly seek medical advice after they fail to menstruate at puberty. Concordant with their feminized external phenotype, most CAIS patients have a female gender identity and a sexual preference for men. They opt for surgical removal of the testes and hormonal supplementation appropriate for females.

What accounts for the different outcomes? Among many possibilities, one is that the dramatic change in behavior in 5α-reductase II patients at puberty results from the effects of testosterone acting on the brain. In CAIS patients these effects do not occur because androgen receptors are absent from the brain. Clearly, however, this explanation does not rule out social and cultural upbringing as important factors in determining gender identity and sexual orientation.

A second set of studies probing the biology of sexual orientation assessed responses to pheromones. Pheromone perception in humans is quite different from that of mice, and is likely a less important sense. Humans do not have a functional VNO, and most of the genes implicated in pheromone reception in mice, such as *trpc2* and those encoding VNO receptors, are absent (or nonfunctional pseudogenes) in the human genome. To the extent that humans do sense pheromones they appear to use the main olfactory epithelium and bulb. Chemicals that appear to be human pheromones include androstadienone (AND), an odorous androgenic metabolite, and estratetraenol (EST), an odorous estrogenic metabolite. AND is present at 10-fold higher concentrations in male sweat compared to female sweat, whereas EST is present in the urine of pregnant women. Both compounds can produce sexual arousal, AND in heterosexual women and EST in heterosexual men, even at concentrations so low that there is no conscious olfactory perception.

Brain areas activated by AND and EST have been identified by positron emission tomography (PET) imaging. When AND is presented, certain hypothalamic nuclei are activated in heterosexual women but not heterosexual men, whereas when EST is presented, adjacent regions containing clusters of nuclei are activated in men but not women (Figure 58–13A).

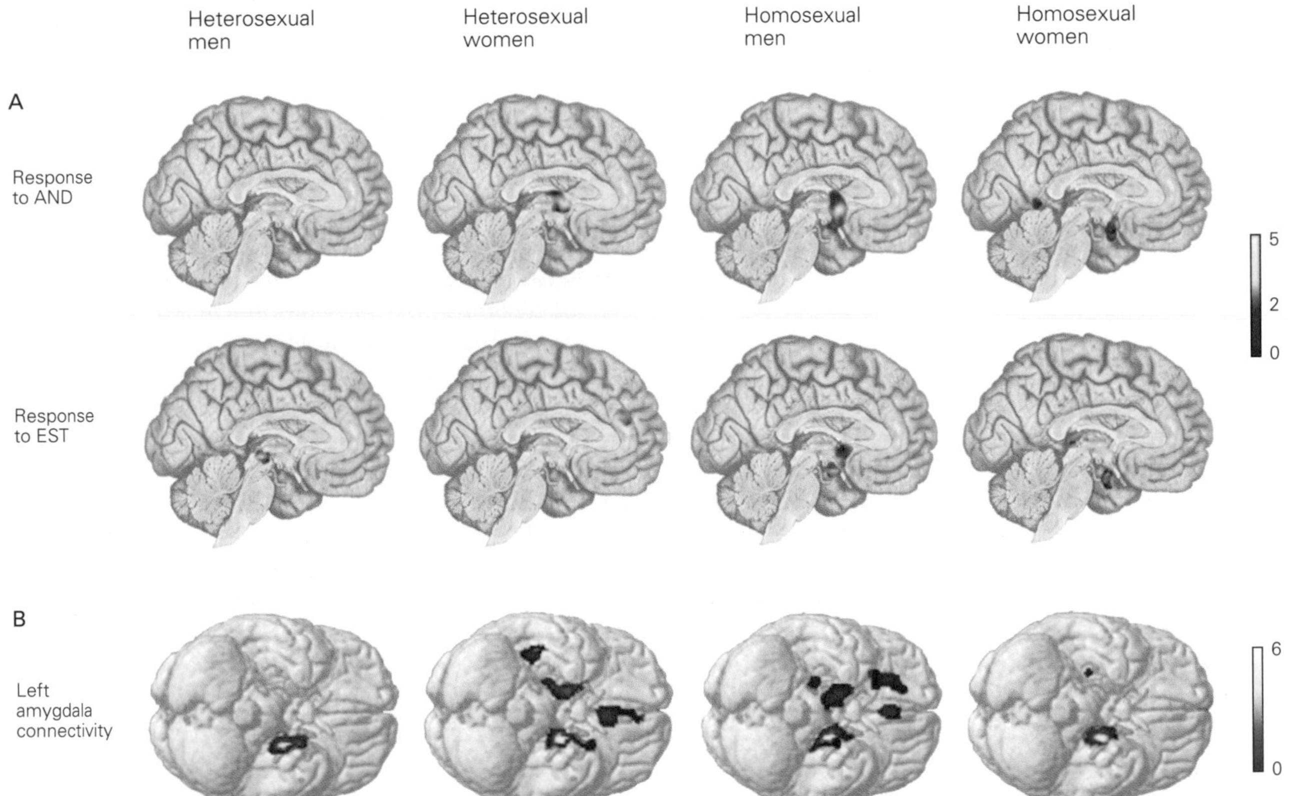

Figure 58–13 Some sexually dimorphic patterns of olfactory activation in the brain correlate with sexual orientation.

A. Positron emission tomography (PET) imaging was used to identify brain regions that were activated when subjects sniffed androstadienone (**AND**) or estratetraenol (**EST**) compared to nonodorous air. AND activated several hypothalamic centers in the brains of heterosexual women but not men, whereas EST activated several hypothalamic centers in heterosexual males but not females. Patterns of activation in the hypothalamus of homosexual men were similar to that of heterosexual women in response to AND, while similar patterns of activation were found in heterosexual men and homosexual women in response to EST. The color calibration on the right shows the level of putative neural activity. Because the same brain regions were selected to compare the figure does not illustrate maximal activation for each condition. (Modified, with permission, from Berglund, Lindstrom, and Savic 2006; Savic, Berglund, and Lindstrom 2005.)

B. Heterosexual and homosexual subjects were scanned while breathing unscented air, and a measure of covariance was used to estimate connectivity among regions. In heterosexual women and homosexual men the left amygdala was strongly connected to the right amygdala, whereas connectivity remained local in heterosexual men and homosexual women. Because the same brain regions were selected to compare, the figure does not illustrate maximal activation for each condition. (Modified, with permission, from Savic and Lindstrom 2008.)

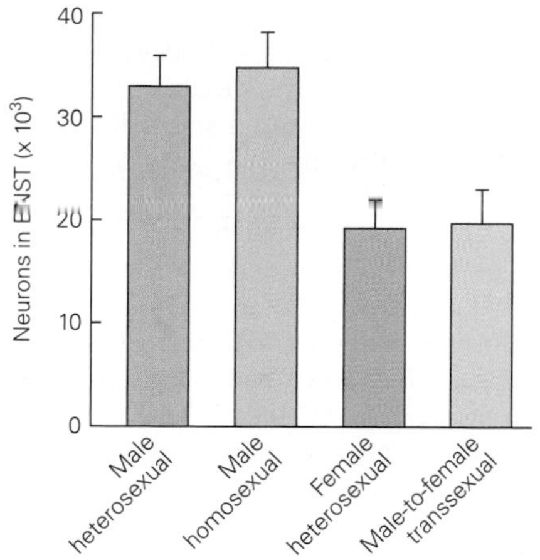

Figure 58–14 Sexual dimorphism in the human bed nucleus of the stria terminalis. The nucleus (BNST) has significantly more neurons in men compared to women regardless of male sexual orientation. Similar to women, male-to-female transsexuals have fewer neurons than men. In the one female-to-male transsexual brain available for postmortem analysis (not shown in the bar graph), the number of neurons is well within the normal range for men. (Modified, with permission, from Kruijver et al. 2000.)

In homosexual men and women there is a reversal of hypothalamic activation: AND but not EST activates hypothalamic centers in homosexual men, and conversely EST but not AND activates those areas in lesbian women. Heterosexual and homosexual brains therefore appear to process olfactory sensory information in different ways.

Do sexually dimorphic structures in homosexual brains correlate with anatomical sex or sexual orientation? Imaging studies have provided support for the view that the brains of homosexual men resemble those of heterosexual woman, and that the brains of homosexual women resemble those of heterosexual men (Figure 58–13B). Moreover, the volume of the sexually dimorphic BNST is small in male-to-female transsexuals compared to men, whereas female-to-male transsexuals appear to have a larger BNST compared to women (Figure 58–14). In these transgender individuals it remains possible that the structural dimorphism is a consequence rather than a cause of gender identity or sexual orientation. But they do raise the possibility that homosexual men and women are exposed prenatally to hormonal or other stimuli similar to those experienced by the other sex.

If prenatal influences do lead to dissociation of sex from gender, are those influences genetic? Other than the rare syndromes described earlier, attempts to find genetic bases for sexual orientation or gender identity have not been productive. Claimed genetic contributions are small and claims of associations with specific genomic loci have not been replicated. Thus, while the current weight of evidence favors some contribution of early, even prenatal, factors in these processes, their cause and relative weight remain unknown.

An Overall View

In most mammals, including humans, the sex determination pathway directs the differentiation of the testes in males and ovaries in females. The *SRY* gene on the Y chromosome is a master regulator that overrides a default female pathway to initiate formation of male gonads. The gonads then produce hormones that organize further differentiation of the body.

Of particular importance for generation of differences in the brain are the steroid hormones, including testosterone, estrogens, and progesterone. Again, the female pathway is often the default mode of differentiation, and at least during early life it is the absence of steroid hormones that permits feminization of brain and behavior to proceed. In many cases the underlying cellular phenomena resemble those that occur widely during normal development, such as apoptosis, neurite extension, synapse formation, and branch retraction. In sexually dimorphic structures these universal processes are brought under the control of sex steroids, so they occur to different extents in males and females. The effects of sex steroids are not confined to these irreversible organizational events during development; they also act in adult life to shape the behavioral repertoire of both sexes.

The link between sex differences in neuronal populations and behavior has been well established for behavioral responses such as erectile function and song production. Recent studies also provide insight into how individual variations in early experience are translated into adult variations in maternal behaviors. By contrast, we are only beginning to delineate the neural pathways underlying more complicated sexually dimorphic behaviors.

We do not yet understand how the nervous system generates various gender-related behaviors such as sexual orientation and gender identity. Here the relative contributions of genetic determinants and social experience remain to be determined. With advances in imaging and genetics, however, we are now poised to start linking specific neural pathways with sexually dimorphic complex social behaviors. These studies have the potential to yield insight into fundamental aspects of human nature such as our sexuality and the basis of many of our social interactions.

Nirao M. Shah
Thomas M. Jessell
Joshua R. Sanes

Selected Readings

Arnold AP. 2004. Sex chromosomes and brain gender. Nat Rev Neurosci 5:701–708.

Byne W. 2006. Developmental endocrine influences on gender identity: implications for management of disorders of sex development. Mt Sinai J Med 73:950–959.

Cahill L. 2006. Why sex matters for neuroscience. Nat Rev Neurosci 7:477–484.

Curley JP, Jensen CL, Mashoodh R, Champagne FA. 2010. Social influences on neurobiology and behavior: epigenetic effects during development. Psychoneuroendocrinology 36:352–371.

Dulac C, Wagner S. 2006. Genetic analysis of brain circuits underlying pheromone signaling. Annu Rev Genet 40:449–467.

Hines M. 2006. Prenatal testosterone and gender-related behavior. Eur J Endocrinol 155:S115–S121.

Morris JA, Jordan CL, Breedlove SM. 2004. Sexual differentiation of the vertebrate nervous system. Nat Neurosci 7:1034–1039.

Swaab DF. 2004. Sexual differentiation of the human brain: relevance for gender identity, transsexualism and sexual orientation. Gynecol Endocrinol 19:301–312.

Wilhelm D, Palmer S, Koopman P. 2007. Sex determination and gonadal development in mammals. Physiol Rev 87:1–28.

Wu MV, Shah NM. 2010. Control of musculinization of the brain and behavior. Curr Opin Neurobiol 21:116–123.

References

Bakker J, De Mees C, Douhard Q, Balthazart J, Gabant P, Szpirer J, Szpirer C. 2006. Alpha-fetoprotein protects the developing female mouse brain from masculinization and defeminization by estrogens. Nat Neurosci 9:220–226.

Berglund H, Lindstrom P, Savic I. 2006. Brain response to putative pheromones in lesbian women. Proc Natl Acad Sci U S A 103:8269–8274.

Brainard MS, Doupe AJ. 2002. What songbirds teach us about learning. Nature 417:351–358.

Byne W, Lasco MS, Kemether E, Shinwari A, Edgar MA, Morgello S, Jones LB, Tobet S. 2000. The interstitial nuclei of the human anterior hypothalamus: an investigation of sexual variation in volume and cell size, number and density. Brain Res 856:254–258.

Cohen-Kettenis PT. 2005. Gender change in 46, XY persons with 5α-reductase-2 deficiency and 17β-hydroxysteroid dehydrogenase-3 deficiency. Arch Sex Behav 34:399–410.

Cooke BM, Woolley CS. 2005. Gonadal hormone modulation of dendrites in the mammalian CNS. J Neurobiol 64:34–46.

Demir E, Dickson BJ. 2005. *Fruitless* splicing specifies male courtship behavior in *Drosophila*. Cell 121:785–794.

Edwards DA, Burge KG. 1971. Early androgen treatment and male and female sexual behavior in mice. Horm Behav 2:49–58.

Forger NG, de Vries GJ. 2010. Cell death and sexual differentiation of behavior: worms, flies, and mammals. Curr Opin Neurobiol 20:776–783.

Goldstein LA, Kurz EM, Sengelaub DR. 1990. Androgen regulation of dendritic growth and retraction in the development of a sexually dimorphic spinal nucleus. J Neurosci 10:935–946.

Gorski RA, Harlan RE, Jacobsen CD, Shryne JE, Southam AM. 1980. Evidence for the existence of a sexually dimorphic nucleus in the preoptic area of the rat. J Comp Neurol 193:529–539.

Greenspan RJ, Ferveur JF. 2000. Courtship in *Drosophila*. Annu Rev Genet 34:205–232.

Gregg C, Zhang J, Butler JE, Haif D, Dulac C. 2010. Sex-specific parent-of-origin allelic expression in the mouse brain. Science 329:682–685.

Kimchi T, Xu J, Dulac C. 2007. A functional circuit underlying male sexual behavior in the female mouse brain. Nature 448:1009–1014.

Kimura K, Ote M, Tazawa T, Yamamoto D. 2005. *Fruitless* specifies sexually dimorphic neural circuitry in the *Drosophila* brain. Nature 438:229–233.

Konishi M, Akutagawa E. 1985. Neuronal growth, atrophy and death in a sexually dimorphic song nucleus in the zebra finch brain. Nature 315:145–147.

Koopman P, Gubbay J, Vivian N, Goodfellow P, Lovell-Badge R. 1991. Male development of chromosomally female mice transgenic for *Sry*. Nature 351:117–121.

Kruijver FP, Zhou JN, Pool CW, Hofman MA, Gooren LJ, Swaab DF. 2000. Male-to-female transsexuals have female neuron numbers in a limbic nucleus. J Clin Endocrinol Metab 85:2034–2041.

Långström N, Rahman Q, Carlström E, Lichtenstein P. 2010. Genetic and environmental effects on same-sex sexual behavior: a population study of twins in Sweden. Arch Sex Behav 39:75–80.

LeVay S. 1991. A difference in hypothalamic structure between heterosexual and homosexual men. Science 253:1034–1037.

Leypold BG, Yu CR, Leinders-Zufall T, Kim MM, Zufall F, Axel R. 2002. Altered sexual and social behaviors in *trp2* mutant mice. Proc Natl Acad Sci U S A 99:6376–6381.

Liu YC, Salamone JD, Sachs BD. 1997. Lesions in medial preoptic area and bed nucleus of stria terminalis: differential effects on copulatory behavior and noncontact erection in male rats. J Neurosci 17:5245–5253.

Mandiyan VS, Coats JK, Shah NM. 2005. Deficits in sexual and aggressive behaviors in *Cnga2* mutant mice. Nat Neurosci 8:1660–1662.

Manoli DS, Foss M, Villella A, Taylor BJ, Hall JC, Baker BS. 2005. Male-specific *fruitless* specifies the neural substrates of *Drosophila* courtship behaviour. Nature 436:395–400.

McCarthy MM, Arnold AP. 2011. Reframing sexual differentiation of the brain. Nat Neurosci 14:677–683.

McGowan PO, Sasaki A, D'Alessio AC, Dymov S, Labonté B, Szyf M, Turecki G, Meaney MJ. 2009. Epigenetic regulation of the glucocorticoid receptor in human brain associates with childhood abuse. Nat Neurosci 12:342–348.

Nottebohm F, Arnold AP. 1976. Sexual dimorphism in vocal control areas of the songbird brain. Science 194:211–213.

Ohno S, Geller LN, Lai EV. 1974. TFM mutation and masculinization versus feminization of the mouse central nervous system. Cell 3:235–242.

Sapolsky RM. 2004. Mothering style and methylation. Nat Neurosci 7:791–792.

Savic I, Berglund H, Gulyas B, Roland P. 2001. Smelling of odorous sex hormone-like compounds causes sex-differentiated hypothalamic activations in humans. Neuron 31: 661–668.

Savic I, Berglund H, Lindstrom P. 2005. Brain response to putative pheromones in homosexual men. Proc Natl Acad Sci U S A 102:7356–7361.

Savic I, Lindstrom P. 2008. PET and MRI show differences in cerebral asymmetry and functional connectivity between homo- and heterosexual subjects. Proc Natl Acad Sci U S A 105:9403–9408.

Sekido R, Lovell-Badge R. 2009. Sex determination and *SRY*: down to a wink and a nudge? Trends Genet 25:19–29.

Shah NM, Pisapia DJ, Maniatis S, Mendelsohn MM, Nemes A, Axel R. 2004. Visualizing sexual dimorphism in the brain. Neuron 43:313–319.

Stockinger P, Kvitsiani D, Rotkopf S, Tirian L, Dickson BJ. 2005. Neural circuitry that governs Drosophila male courtship behavior. Cell 121:795–807.

Stowers L, Holy TE, Meister M, Dulac C, Koentges G. 2002. Loss of sex discrimination and male-male aggression in mice deficient for TRP2. Science 295:1493–1500.

Weaver IC, Cervoni N, Champagne FA, D'Alessio AC, Sharma S, Seckl JR, Dymov S, Szyf M, Meaney MJ. 2004. Epigenetic programming by maternal behavior. Nat Neurosci 7:847–854.

Wierman ME. 2007. Sex steroid effects at target tissues: mechanisms of action. Adv Physiol Educ 31:26–33.

Wu MV, Manoli DS, Fraser EJ, Coats JK, Tollkuhn J, Honda S, Harada N, Shah NM. 2009. Estrogen masculinizes neural pathways and sex-specific behaviors. Cell 139:61–72.

Zhang TY, Meaney MJ. 2010. Epigenetics and the environmental regulation of the genome and its function. Annu Rev Psychol 61:439–466, C1-3.

Zhang J, Webb DM. 2003. Evolutionary deterioration of the vomeronasal pheromone transduction pathway in catarrhine primates. Proc Natl Acad Sci U S A 100:8337–8341.

59

The Aging Brain

The average life span in the United States in 1900 was about 50 years. Today it is approximately 76 years for men and 81 for women (Figure 59–1), and is higher still in 30 other countries. These increases result largely from a reduction in infant mortality, the development of vaccines and antibiotics, better nutrition, improved public health measures, and advances in the treatment and prevention of heart disease and stroke. Because of increased life expectancy, along with the large cohort of "baby boomers" born after World War II, the elderly are the most rapidly growing segment of the U.S. population.

Increased longevity is a double-edged sword: Age-related cognitive alterations are increasingly prevalent. Their extent varies widely among individuals. For many, the alterations are mild and have relatively little impact on the quality of life—the momentary lapses we jokingly call "senior moments." Other cognitive impairments, although not debilitating, are troubling enough to hinder the ability of the elderly to manage their lives independently. At the far extreme are the severe dementias, which rob the elderly of memory and reasoning. Of these, Alzheimer disease is the most prevalent.

As the population ages, research on age-related changes in the brain has become a more prominent area of focus for neuroscientists, neurologists, and psychologists. The main aim of research on aging has been to find treatments for Alzheimer disease and other dementias, but it is also important to understand the normal process of cognitive decline with age. After all, age is the greatest susceptibility factor for a wide variety of neurodegenerative disorders. Understanding what happens to our brains as we age may not only improve the quality of life for the general population but may also provide clues that will eventually help us vanquish seemingly unrelated pathological changes.

With this in mind, we begin this chapter with a consideration of how the normal brain ages. We then proceed to consider the broad range of pathological changes in cognition, and finally focus on Alzheimer disease, the most common cause of severe memory loss and intellectual deterioration in the elderly.

The Structure and Function of the Brain Change with Age

As we grow old our bodies change—our hair thins, our skin wrinkles, and our joints creak. It is no surprise

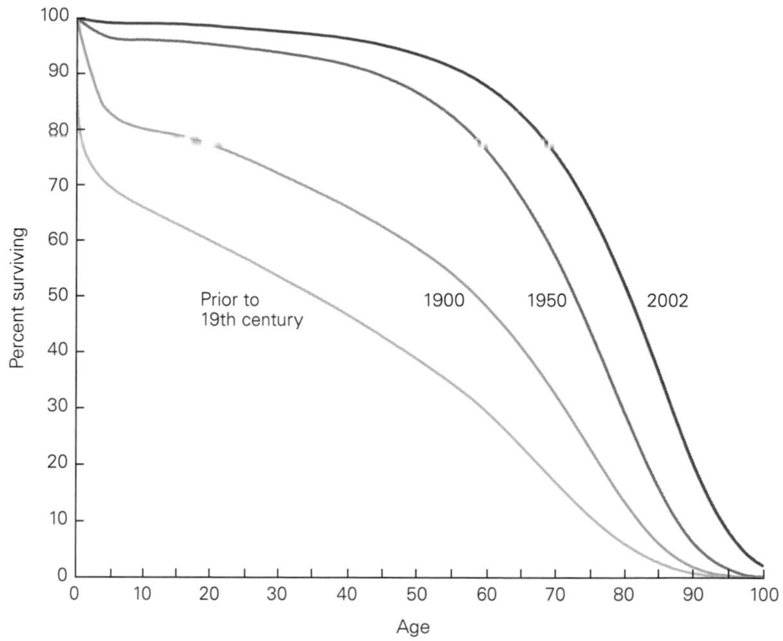

Figure 59–1 Human life span is increasing. Changes in human longevity illustrate the rapid extension in life span that has occurred in the United States over the past 100 years. (Modified, with permission, from Strehler 1975; Arias 2004.)

then that our brain also changes. Indeed, many of the behavioral alterations that occur with age affect almost everyone, providing evidence of underlying alterations in the nervous system.

For example, motor skills decline in the elderly. The posture of an old person is less erect than that of a young adult. Gait is slower and stride length is shorter. Postural reflexes are often sluggish, making individuals more susceptible to loss of balance. Although muscles weaken and bones become more brittle, these motor abnormalities result in large part from subtle processes that involve the peripheral and central nervous systems. Sleep patterns also change with age: Older people sleep less and wake more frequently. Mental functions ascribed to the forebrain, such as memory and problem-solving abilities, also decline.

Age-related declines in mental abilities are highly variable. First, there are considerable differences in the rate and severity of cognitive decline among individuals (Figure 59–2A). Although most people experience a gradual decline in mental agility, for some the decline is rapid, whereas others retain their cognitive powers throughout life. Giuseppe Verdi, Eleanor Roosevelt, and Pablo Picasso are well-known members of this latter, unusual category. Titian continued to paint masterpieces in his late 80s, and Sophocles is said to have written *Oedipus at Colonus* in his 92nd year. The rarity of completely preserved function suggests that its retention may reflect special properties in the life experiences or genes of these people. Accordingly, there has been great interest in studying rare individuals who retain nearly intact cognition into their tenth or even eleventh decade. These so-called "centenarians" may provide insight into environmental or genetic factors that protect against normal age-related cognitive decline or that protect against the more devastating pathological descent into dementia. For the moment, however, no such factors have been found.

Second, when data from many individuals are averaged, it is clear that some cognitive capacities decline significantly with age while others are largely spared (Figure 59–2B). For example, working and long-term memories, visuospatial abilities (measured by arranging blocks into a design or drawing a three-dimensional figure), and verbal fluency (as measured by rapid naming of objects or naming as many words as possible that start with a specific letter of the alphabet) usually decline with old age. On the other hand, measures of vocabulary, information, and comprehension often show minimal decline in normal individuals well into the 80s.

Age-related alterations in memory, motor activity, mood, sleep pattern, appetite, and neuroendocrine function result from alterations in the structure and function of the brain. Even the healthiest 80-year-old brain does not look like its 20-year-old self. Elderly people exhibit mild shrinkage in the volume of the brain and a loss in brain weight, as well as enlargement of the ventricles (Figure 59–3A). The decreases

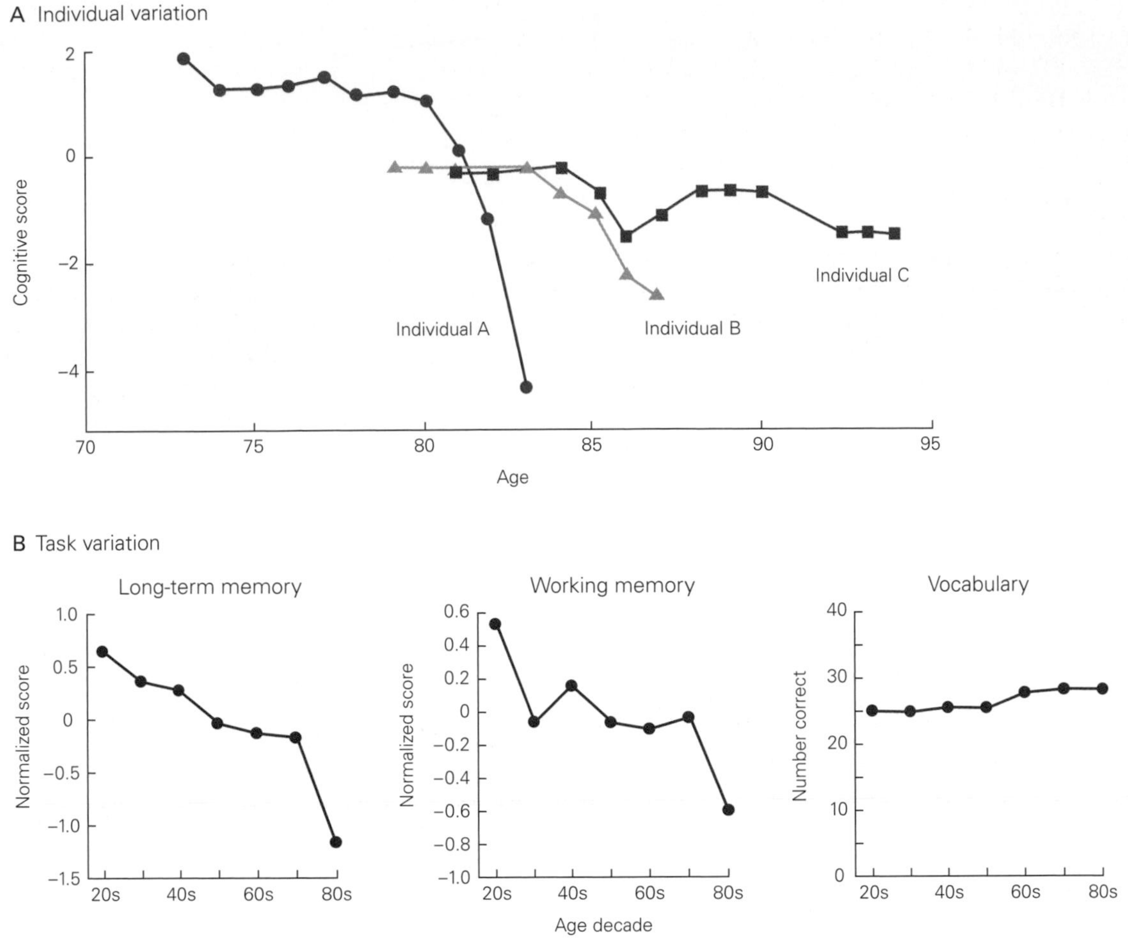

Figure 59–2 Variation in age-related cognitive decline.
A. Cognitive scores of three people who were given a battery of cognitive tests annually for decades. Person A declined rapidly. Persons B and C showed similar cognitive performances into their 80s but then diverged. (Adapted, with permission, from Rubin et al. 1998.)

B. Average scores on several cognitive tests administered to a large number of people. Long-term declarative memory and working memory decline throughout life, and more so in advanced age. In contrast, knowledge of vocabulary is maintained. (Reproduced, with permission, from Park et al. 1996.)

in brain weight average 0.2% per year from college age onward, and about 0.5% per year in the 70s. One might imagine that these changes result from death of neurons, and indeed some neurons are lost with age. For example, 25% or more of the motor neurons that innervate skeletal muscles die in generally healthy elderly individuals. This loss contributes to sarcopenia, the muscle weakness and atrophy that can be a serious clinical problem in the elderly.

In general, however, there is minimal neuronal loss in most parts of the brain, so brain shrinkage must arise from other factors. Indeed, analysis of the brain of humans and experimental animals reveals structural alterations in both neurons and glia. Myelin is fragmented and lost, leading to a decline in the integrity of white matter. At the same time, the density of the dendritic arbors of cortical and other neurons decreases, resulting in shrinkage of neuropil. In addition, levels of enzymes that synthesize some neurotransmitters, such as dopamine, norepinephrine, and acetylcholine, decrease with age, presumably resulting in functional defects in synapses that use these transmitters. Moreover, synapse structure is clearly aberrant, at least at the neuromuscular junction (Figure 59–4), raising the possibility that structural changes may also lead to functional deficits at central synapses. Finally, the number of synapses in the neocortex and many other regions of the brain declines (Figure 59–5).

These cellular changes lead to alterations in the integrity of the neural circuits that mediate our mental activities. Loss of synapses along with impairment in function of remaining synapses are thought to be important contributors to age-related cognitive decline. Changes in white matter are widespread but are especially notable in the prefrontal and temporal cortex. They may underlie alterations in executive functions and the ability to focus attention and to encode and store memory, functions that are localized in frontal-striatal systems and the temporal lobes. The loss of white matter may also help explain the recent finding that the elderly brain is less able to support synchronization of activity in widely separated areas that normally work together to carry out complex mental activities. Disruption of these large-scale networks could be an important cause of cognitive decline.

It was long thought that aging resulted from progressive deterioration of cells and tissues due to accumulated genetic damage or toxic waste products. In support of this idea, mitotic cells removed from animals and placed in a tissue culture dish divide only for a limited number of times before they age and die. This view of "preordained" aging has changed radically over the past decade, primarily as a result of studies in model organisms in which mutations that significantly extend life span have been found (Figure 59–6).

These dramatic discoveries establish that the aging process is under active genetic control. One such regulatory pathway that has been characterized includes

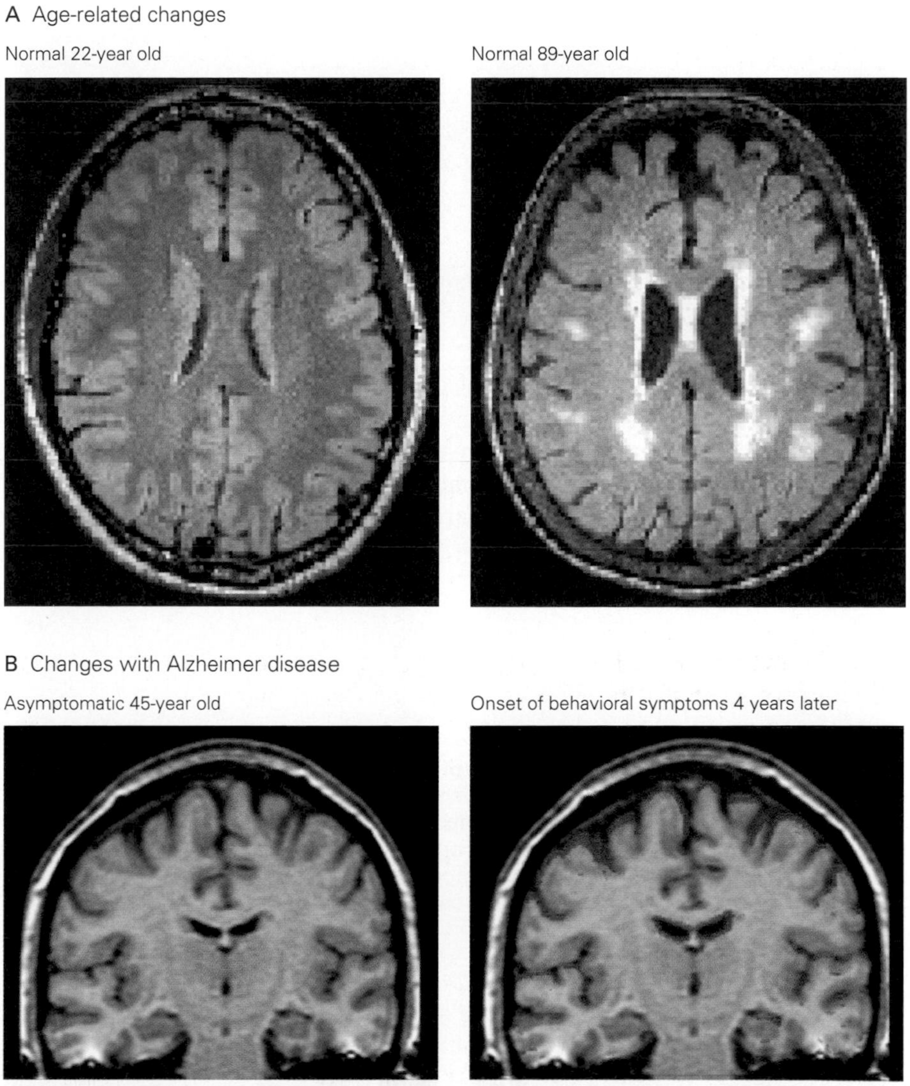

Figure 59–3 Magnetic resonance imaging reveals changes in brain structure during aging and at the onset of Alzheimer disease.

A. Images of normal 22- and 89-year-old brains reveal changes in the structure of the living brain. (Reproduced, with permission, from R. Buckner.)

B. Images of the same individual over a 4-year period illustrate the progressive shrinking of cortical structures and the beginnings of ventricular enlargement (**red**). Note that these structural changes are evident prior to the onset of behavioral symptoms. (Reproduced, with permission, from N. Fox.)

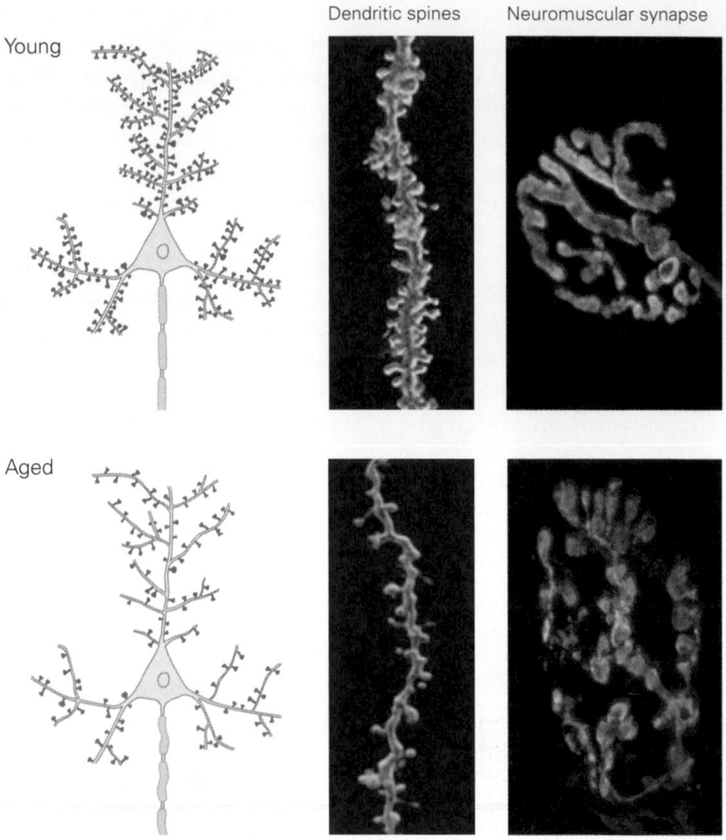

Figure 59–4 Age-related changes in dendritic and synaptic structure. Reconstructions of cortical pyramidal neurons in aging rodents show the loss of dendritic spines with age. Neuromuscular synapses in rodents also exhibit age-related changes in structure. (Spine images reproduced, with permission, from J. Luebke; synapse images reproduced, with permission, from G. Valdez.)

insulin and insulin-like growth factors, their receptors, and the signaling programs they activate. Disruption of these genes leads to increased resistance of cells to lethal oxidative damage. Presumably, the normal forms of these genes benefit the organism during the reproductive period and have therefore been selected by evolution. Their deleterious effects on longevity, once the animals are past reproductive age, may be an unfortunate side effect about which evolution cares little.

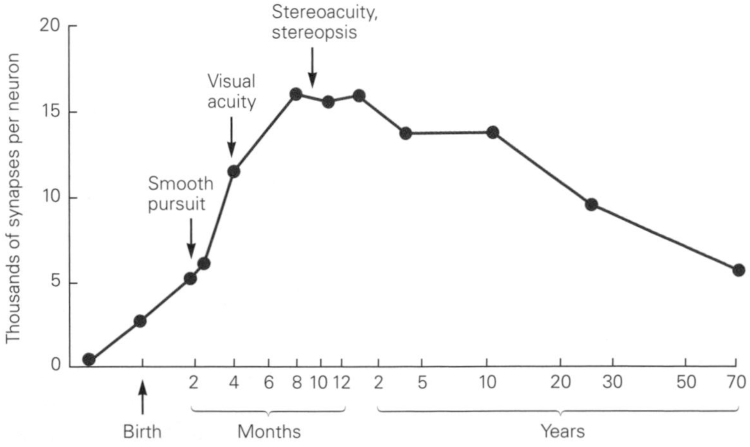

Figure 59–5 Age-related changes in synaptic density. Cognitive capacity during early development is accompanied by a marked increase in synapse density in different regions of the cerebral cortex. Developmental landmarks through age 10 months are indicated. The density of cortical synapses declines with age. (Adapted, with permission, from P. Huttenlocher.)

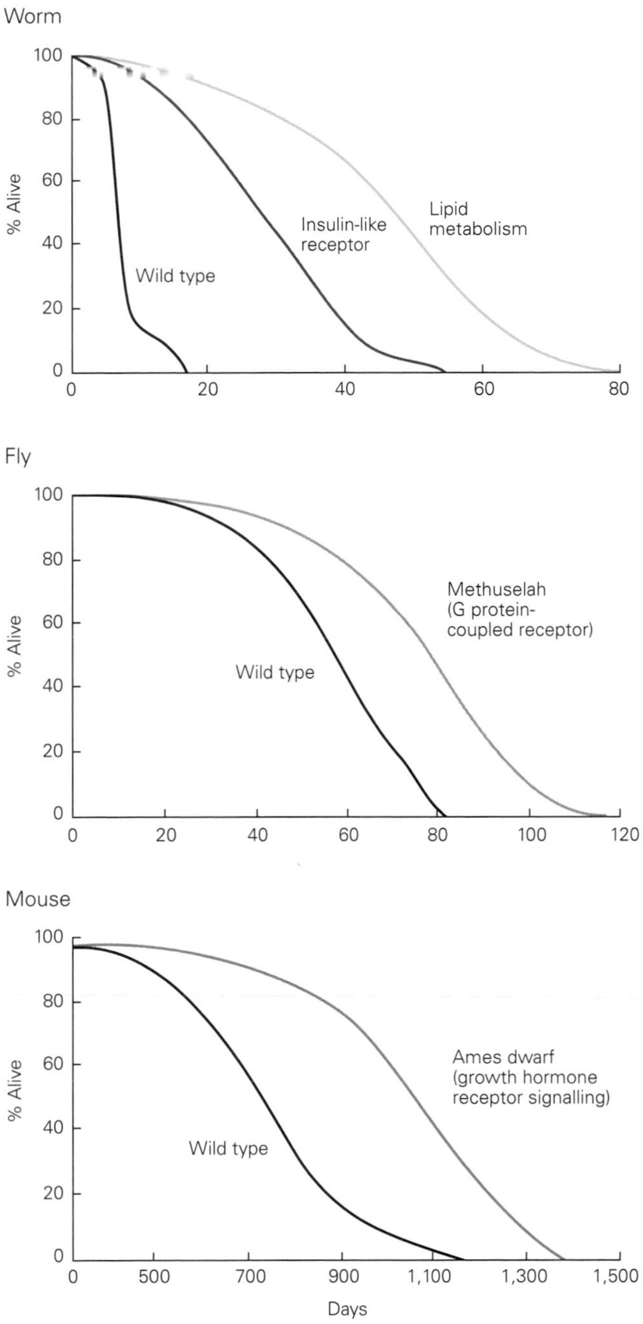

Figure 59–6 Life span can be increased through genetic mutation. Genetic mutations in specific receptors and signaling proteins markedly enhance life span in mutant strains of the worm, fly, and mouse, indicating that genetic regulatory mechanisms affect aging and life span. (Top reproduced, with permission, from Hekimi 2003; middle reproduced, with permission, from Yi 1998; bottom reproduced with permission, from Brown-Borg 1996.)

These findings have two major implications for understanding how aging affects the nervous system. First, the biochemical mechanisms that lead to, or protect from, the ravages of age are likely to underlie the changes in neurons that lead to cognitive decline. Research to explore this link between cellular change and cognitive functioning is now underway in model organisms. Second, and perhaps more excitingly, research on model organisms is leading to strategies for extending life span or health span (the period during which one remains generally healthy) by pharmacological intervention in the pathways uncovered by genetic studies.

For example, the best-validated environmental intervention for extending life span in organisms ranging from yeast to worms to primates is caloric restriction, a strategy unlikely to be broadly acceptable to people. However, it appears that caloric restriction acts through genes in the insulin pathway mentioned above, and may involve a set of enzymes called *sirtuins*. The sirtuins are activated by a compound called *resveratrol*, originally isolated from red wine, a longevity-promoting beverage. Resveratrol, in turn, retards some aspects of aging, including cognitive measures, when administered to mice. While it is unlikely that resveratrol will serve as a fountain of youth in humans, it nevertheless exemplifies the new chemistries that are currently under consideration. These chemical strategies use model organisms to explore not only the positive factors that lead to aging but also the inhibitory constraints that prevent model organisms and presumably humans from achieving their full life span in a reasonably healthy state.

Cognitive Decline Is Dramatic in a Small Percentage of the Elderly

In most people age-related cognitive changes do not seriously compromise the quality of life. In a subset of elderly people, however, cognitive decline reaches a level that can be viewed as pathological. At the lesser end of the pathological range is a constellation of changes known as mild cognitive impairment, or MCI. This syndrome is characterized by memory impairments that may be alarming to the individual but are not serious enough to affect daily life; general cognition remains intact.

Owing to its subtlety, MCI is difficult to diagnose, but longitudinal studies have convinced neurologists that it is a real condition. Approximately 15% of individuals diagnosed with MCI progress to Alzheimer disease within a few years of diagnosis, and an additional 50% of them will eventually succumb to Alzheimer disease.

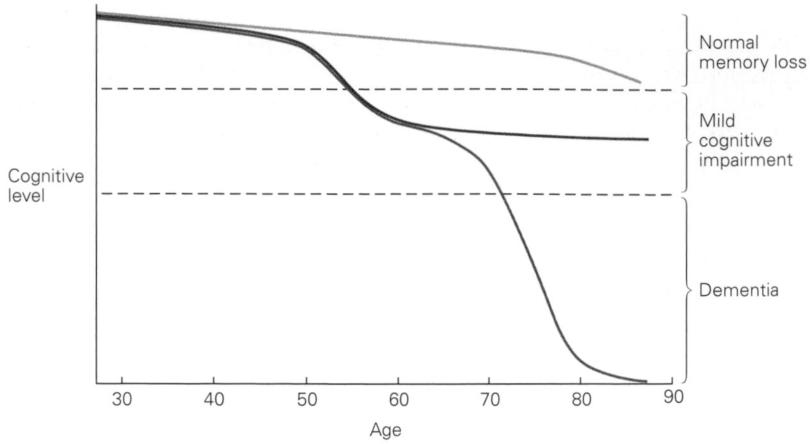

Figure 59–7 Cognitive performance can vary widely with age. Normal age-related memory loss does not impair cognitive abilities. Mild cognitive impairment is accompanied by a gradual and modest loss of cognitive abilities. Dementia is accompanied by a severe and accelerating loss of cognitive performance. The distinction between mild cognitive impairment and dementia becomes apparent only after the initial decline in cognitive performance. (From the National Institute on Aging: http://www.nia.nih.gov/alzheimers/publication/part-2-what-happens-brain-ad/changing-brain-ad)

Conversely, some elderly people with MCI remain at a stable plateau for decades (Figure 59–7). There is currently intense interest in learning how to distinguish individuals who will progress to more severe difficulties from those who will age relatively normally.

More troubling are the age-related or senile dementias. Senile dementia is a clinical syndrome in the elderly that involves progressive impairment of memory as well as cognitive faculties such as language, problem solving, judgment, calculation, or attention. Dementia syndromes are associated with a variety of diseases. The most common, Alzheimer disease, is discussed in detail below. The second most common cause of dementia in the elderly is cerebrovascular disease, particularly strokes that lead to focal ischemia and consequent infarction in the brain.

Large lesions in the cortex are often associated with language disturbances (aphasia), hemipareses, or neglect syndromes, depending on which portions of the brain are compromised. Small infarctions in white matter or deeper structures of the brain, termed *lacunes*, also occur as a consequence of hypertension. In small numbers they may be asymptomatic, or they may contribute to the normal cognitive decline of aging or underlie certain cases of mild cognitive impairment that do not progress to Alzheimer disease. As vascular lesions increase in number and size, however, their impact becomes heightened; eventually they can lead to dementia.

Numerous other conditions that can lead to dementia include Parkinson disease, alcoholism, drug intoxications, infections such as AIDS and syphilis, brain tumors, vitamin deficiencies (notably lack of vitamin B_{12}), thyroid disease, and a variety of other metabolic disorders. In some patients schizophrenia or depression may mimic a dementia syndrome. Emil Kraepelin chose the term "dementia praecox" to highlight the cognitive deficit in a disease that affects young people, a disease we now call schizophrenia. Although the clinical features of these dementias may resemble those of Alzheimer disease or cerebrovascular disease in some respects, the symptoms and tempo of dementia may vary, depending on the nature and site of the neurological abnormality. Because some dementias can be treated, it is important for the physician to probe the differential diagnoses of dementia with clinical history, examinations, and laboratory studies.

Alzheimer Disease Is the Most Common Senile Dementia

In 1901 Alois Alzheimer examined a middle-aged woman who had developed memory deficits and progressive loss of cognitive abilities. One of the first noticeable symptoms of this woman's illness was unprovoked suspicion of her husband's behavior. Her memory became increasingly impaired. She could no longer orient herself, even in her own home, and she hid objects in her apartment. At times she believed that people intended to murder her.

She was institutionalized in a psychiatric hospital and died less than five years after the onset of illness. Alzheimer performed an autopsy that disclosed specific alterations in the cerebral cortex, described below. The constellation of behavioral symptoms and physical alterations was subsequently given the name Alzheimer disease (AD).

The first case of the disease caught Alzheimer's attention because it occurred in middle age, but in general the disease afflicts the elderly. Most patients with AD exhibit the first clinical signs during their seventh decade. Early onset cases are often familial, and mutations have been discovered in many of these patients, as we shall discuss below. Late-onset cases are sporadic, and their cause remains unknown.

In both the sporadic and familial forms of AD there is a remarkably selective defect in declarative memory. At first, language, strength, reflexes, and sensory abilities and motor skills are nearly normal. Gradually, however, memory is lost along with cognitive abilities such as problem solving, language, calculation, and visuospatial perception. Unsurprisingly, these cognitive losses lead to other behavioral alterations, and some patients develop psychotic symptoms, such as hallucinations and delusions. In all patients mental functions and activities of daily living progressively become impaired; in the late stages these individuals are mute, incontinent, and bedridden.

Alzheimer disease affects approximately one-eighth of people older than 65 years. Five million people in the United States now suffer from dementia. Because the number of elderly is increasing rapidly, the population at risk for AD is the fastest growing segment of our society (Figure 59–8). During the next 25 years the number of people with AD in the United States will triple, as will the cost of caring for patients no longer able to care for themselves. Thus, AD is one of society's major public health problems.

The Brain in Alzheimer Disease Is Altered by Atrophy, Amyloid Plaques, and Neurofibrillary Tangles

Alzheimer disease is characterized by three dramatic abnormalities of the brain, all of which Alzheimer described. First, the brain is atrophied, with narrowed gyri, widened sulci, reduced brain weight, and enlarged ventricles (Figure 59–9). These changes, seen in mild form in cognitively intact elderly people who die from other causes, are severe in advanced AD. Moreover, neuron death is widespread in AD, whereas in normal aged brains it is minimal. Thus AD is a neurodegenerative disease.

Second, sections of brains of AD patients obtained at autopsy reveal extracellular plaques of dense material called *amyloid,* large aggregates of fibrillar peptides arranged as sheets (Figure 59–10). Amyloid can be detected when stained with dyes such as Congo red, and is refractive when viewed in polarized light or when stained with thioflavin and viewed with fluorescence optics. The extracellular deposits of amyloid are surrounded by swollen axons and dendrites. These neuronal processes in turn are associated with processes of astrocytes and microglia (inflammatory cells). Amyloid plaques also occur in the walls of cerebral blood vessels in the Alzheimer brain.

Third, neurons that are affected but still alive have cytoskeletal abnormalities, the most dramatic of which is the accumulation of neurofibrillary tangles (Figure 59–10). These tangles are filamentous inclusions in the cell bodies and proximal dendrites that contain paired helical filaments and 15 nm straight filaments. Other cytoskeletal abnormalities occur in axons and terminals (dystrophic neurites) and dendrites (neuropil threads). Both types of lesions include intracellular paired helical filaments, suggesting that these fibrillar inclusions result from common mechanisms.

In AD these alterations do not occur uniformly throughout the brain, but rather affect specific regions. The entorhinal area, the hippocampus, the neocortex, and the nucleus basalis are especially vulnerable

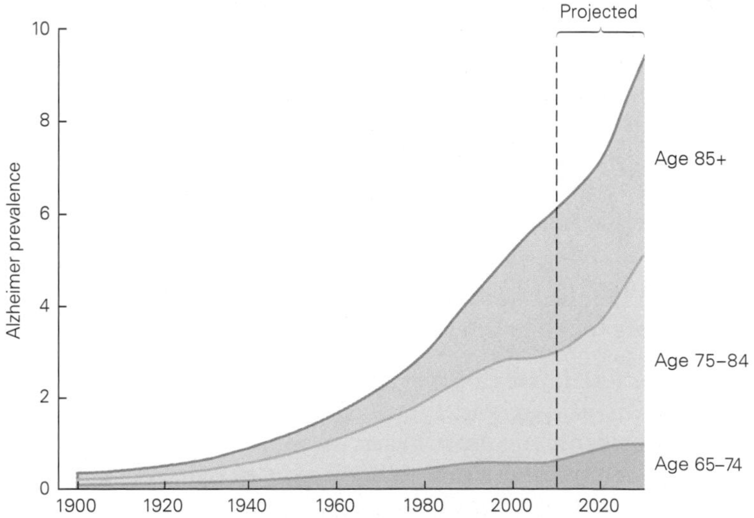

Figure 59–8 Alzheimer disease is a growing public health problem. As the population ages, Alzheimer disease is expected to become increasingly prevalent (prevalence is measured in millions). (Adapted, with permission, from Brumback and Leech 1994, Herbert et al. 2003.)

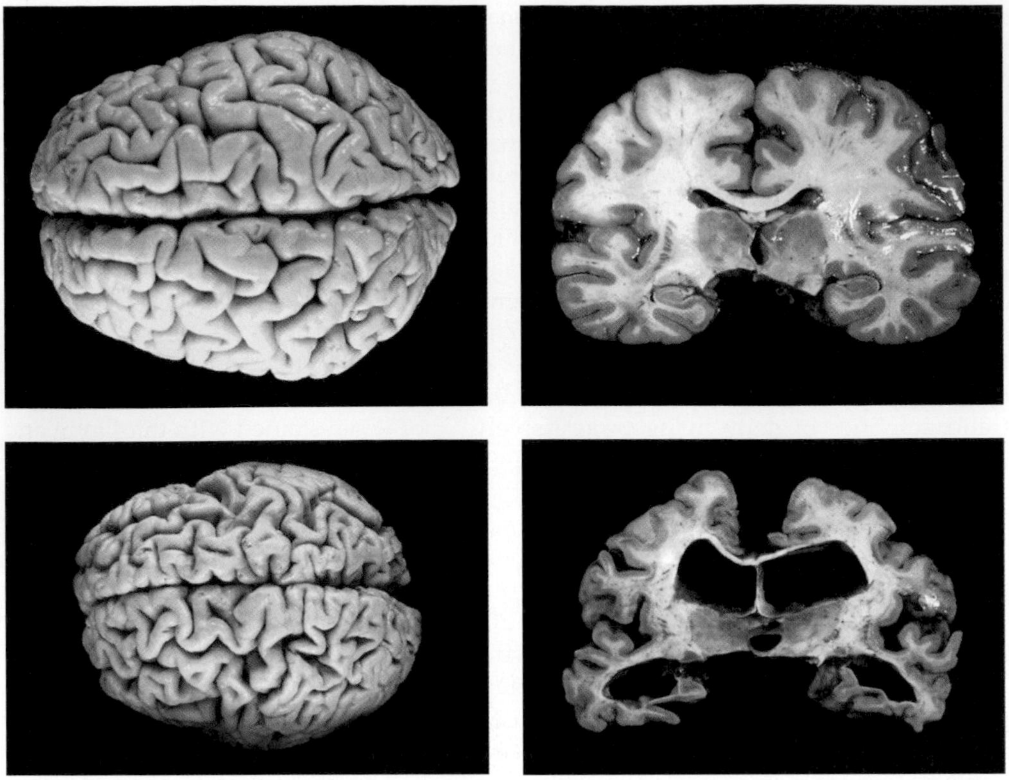

Figure 59–9 Overt pathological changes in the brain of individuals with Alzheimer disease. When compared to age-matched normal brains, the brain of an Alzheimer patient displays marked shrinkage and ventricular enlargement. (Whole brain photos from P. Anderson, University of Alabama at Birmingham, Department of Pathology; brain slice photos from A. C. McKee; all reproduced with permission.)

(Figure 59–11). Alterations in the entorhinal cortex and hippocampus are likely the structural underpinnings of problems with declarative memory that are the first symptoms of AD. These alterations contrast with those in frontostriatal circuits that correlate with age-related cognitive decline in normal subjects. Abnormalities in the basal forebrain cholinergic systems may contribute to cognitive difficulties and attention deficits that appear later in the progression of the disease. These anatomical differences, along with widespread neuronal death, argue against the idea, once prevalent, that AD is an extreme form of the normal aging processes.

Amyloid Plaques Contain Toxic Peptides That Contribute to Alzheimer Pathology

To characterize amyloid plaques, George Glenner, Konrad Beyreuther, and their colleagues isolated the plaques by centrifugation, based on their low solubility, and determined some of their components. The principal constituent turned out to be a group of small peptides that together were named Aβ.

Two main forms of the peptide were found. The predominant peptide is 40 amino acids in length and the minor one 42 amino acids (the original 40 residues plus two additional amino acids at the carboxy terminal end). Biochemical studies showed that the Aβ42 peptide nucleates more rapidly than Aβ40 into amyloid fibrils. In individuals with AD, amyloid deposition begins with Aβ42, while Aβ40 accumulates later. Moreover, when applied to neurons in culture, the Aβ42 peptide is more toxic than Aβ40. These results implicate Aβ42 as a key component of amyloid plaques.

In general, short peptides are formed by cleavage from a precursor protein, so researchers set out to isolate the protein from which Aβ was derived. The precursor was soon found and molecularly cloned, and named *amyloid precursor protein* or APP (Figure 59–12). APP is a large transmembrane glycoprotein that is present in the dendrites, cell bodies, and axons of many types of neurons as well as a variety of nonneuronal cells.

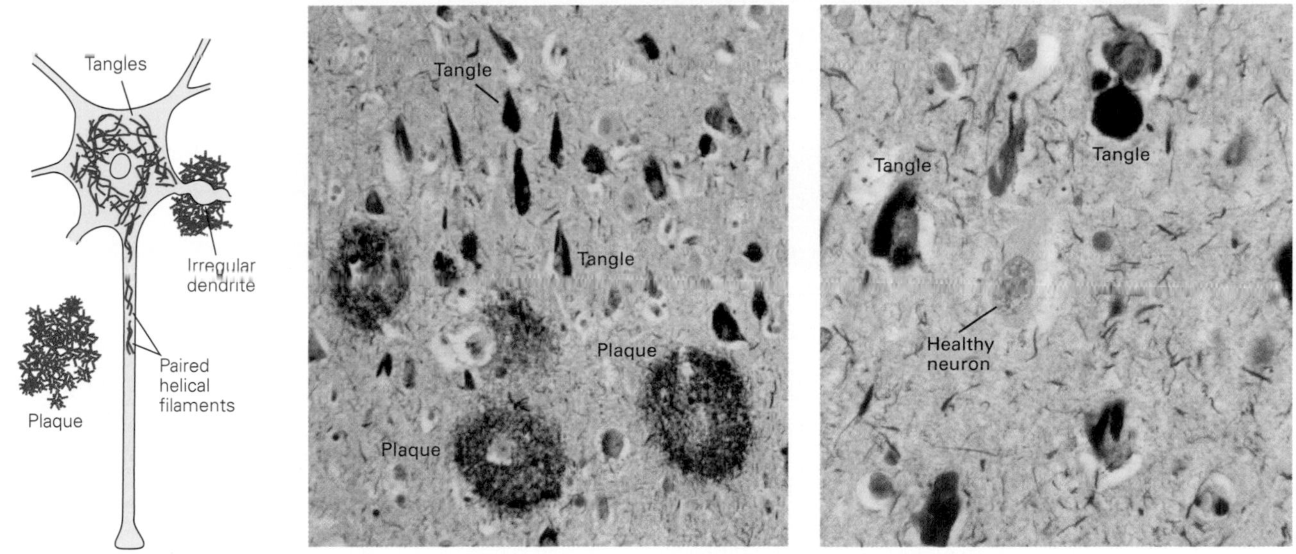

Figure 59–10 Plaques and tangles in the Alzheimer brain. A section of cerebral cortex from the brain of an individual with severe Alzheimer disease shows typical plaques and neurofibrillary tangles. (Images from James Goldman, reproduced with permission.)

Left: The diagram shows a neuron containing neurofibrillary tangles, composed of bundles of paired-helical filaments in the cell body and more paired helical filaments in the axon. Amyloid plaques are shown in the neuropil, one of them surrounding a dendrite, which displays an altered, swollen shape. Tangles are composed of abnormal polymers of hyperphosphorylated tau protein, and amyloid plaques are extracellular deposits of polymers of the amyloid beta (A4) peptide.

Middle: A section of neocortex from a patient with Alzheimer disease has been treated with a silver stain. The tissue shows neuronal cell bodies containing neurofibrillary tangles and neuropil containing amyloid plaques.

Right: A higher magnification of the cortex shows neurofibrillary tangles in neuronal cell bodies and, in contrast, a healthy neuron without a tangle. Note the many thin silver-positive cell processes in the neuropil; these are neuronal processes that contain paired helical filaments.

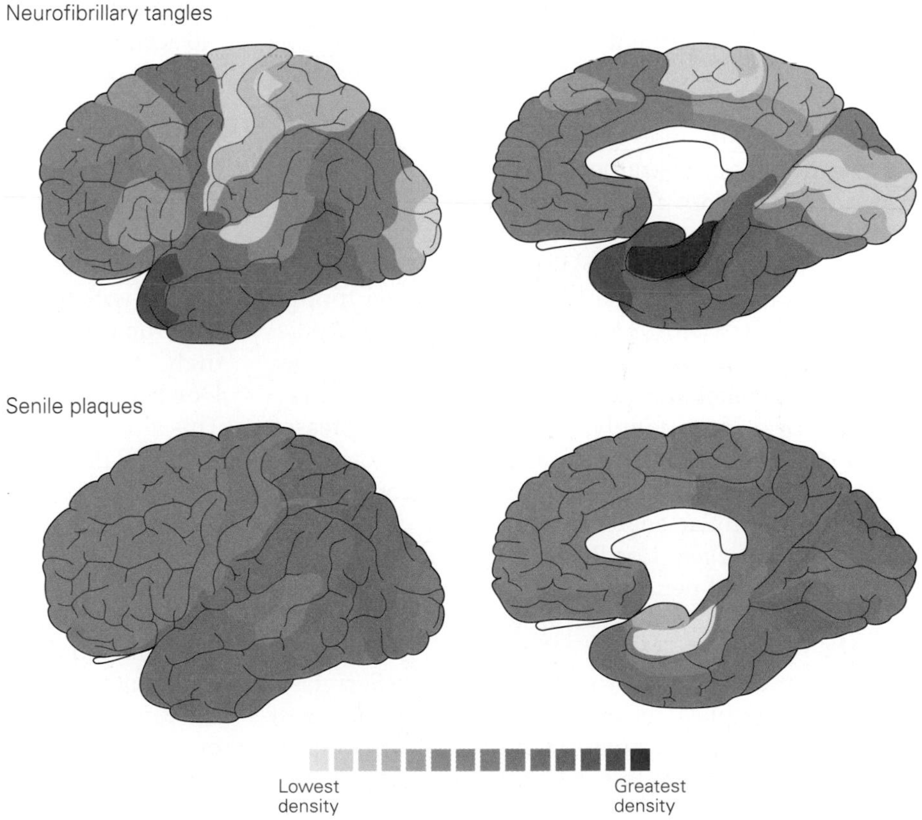

Figure 59–11 Neurofibrillary tangles and senile plaques are concentrated in different regions of the Alzheimer brain. Lateral and medial views of the cerebral hemispheres. (Adapted, with permission, from Arnold et al. 1991.)

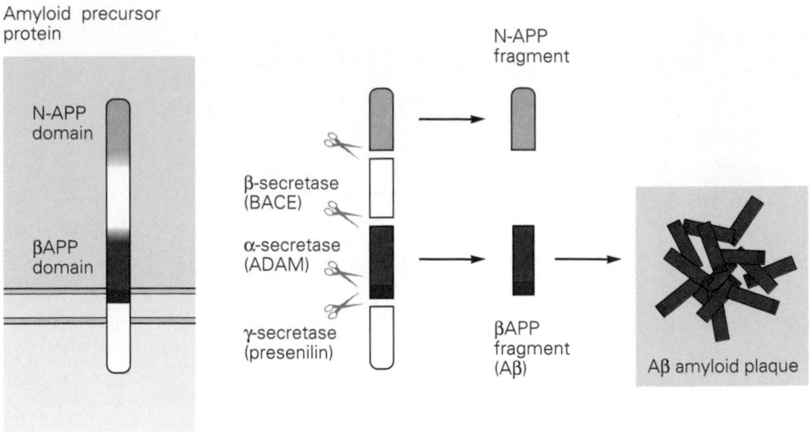

Figure 59–12 Processing of the amyloid precursor protein. The amyloid precursor protein (APP) is a transmembrane protein of uncertain function. Through proteolytic cleavage it generates many distinct proteolytic fragments. Proteolytic cleavage by γ- and β-secretases generate an intracellular fragment, an Aβ peptide, which can be 40 or 42 residues in length, and an amino-terminal fragment (N-APP) that may have distinct effects.

Despite intensive study, the normal functions of APP in the brain remain poorly understood.

Once APP was isolated it became possible to ask how it is processed to form Aβ peptides. The answer has turned out to be complex. Three proteolytic activities—α-, β-, and γ-secretases—cut APP into pieces. The β- and γ-secretases cleave APP to generate a soluble extracellular fragment that is released into the interstitial fluid, the Aβ peptides that include part of the transmembrane segment, and a cytosolic or intracellular fragment (Figure 59–12). The cleavage by γ-secretase is unusual in that it occurs in a membrane-spanning portion of APP, a region long thought to be immune from hydrolysis because it is surrounded by lipids rather than water. In nonneuronal cells α-secretase cleaves APP in the middle of the Aβ sequence. This cleavage prevents the formation of Aβ peptides and helps explain why Aβ peptides are largely confined to the nervous system even though APP is present in neuronal and nonneuronal cells alike.

The enzymes that account for α-, β-, and γ-secretases have been isolated and characterized. α-Secretase is a member of a large family of extracellular proteases called *ADAM* (A Disintegrin and Metalloproteinase) that are responsible for degrading many components of the extracellular matrix. β-secretase, called *β-site APP cleaving enzyme 1* or BACE1, is a transmembrane protein in central neurons and concentrated in synaptic areas. Brain cells derived from mutant mice lacking BACE1 do not produce Aβ peptides, proving that BACE1 is indeed the neuronal β-secretase. γ-Secretase, the most complicated of the three, and the most recently isolated, is actually a multiprotein complex that cleaves several different transmembrane proteins. As expected, given its peculiar ability to act within the membrane, γ-secretase itself includes membrane proteins. Two are called presenilin-1 and presenilin-2, reflecting their association with AD. Other components of the complex are nicastrin, Aph-1, and Pen-2, also transmembrane proteins.

Although the biochemical properties of Aβ and APP appeared interesting, the critical question remained: Are they causally related to the debilitating symptoms of AD? One might imagine that the disease is caused by Aβ accumulation, but Aβ might also form as a result of another pathological process or even be an innocuous correlate. Genetic evidence in humans and experimental animals has been critical in demonstrating that APP plays a central role in AD.

The first clue came from the observation that the APP gene lies on chromosome 21. Chromosome 21 is present in three copies (rather than the normal two) in people with Down syndrome. For this reason Down syndrome is also referred to as trisomy 21. Interestingly, it had long been known that most people with Down syndrome who live to the age of 40 develop AD. This association is consistent with the idea that excessive APP predisposes to AD.

More direct genetic evidence came from the analysis of patients with familial AD. Only a small number of cases of AD are familial, usually those in which onset occurs early, younger than age 60 years, and most of these are inherited as simple dominant mutations. As new methods of molecular cloning became available in the late 1980s, several groups began using them to identify the genes mutated in familial AD. Remarkably, the first three genes identified were those encoding APP, presenilin-1, and presenilin-2 (Figure 59–13). By now many different mutations have been found in all three genes, and the majority of them influence cleavage of APP, increasing the production of Aβ peptides or the proportion of the more toxic Aβ42 species.

Some APP mutations are amino acid substitutions flanking or within the Aβ region. Cells that express these mutant sequences secrete several-fold more Aβ peptide than cells expressing wild-type APP. Another APP mutation influences γ-secretase to selectively generate Aβ42 rather than Aβ40. Likewise, in most presenilin mutants the mutant γ-secretase has higher than normal activity or generates peptides with an increased ratio of Aβ42 to Aβ40. Thus mutants in the APP or presenilin genes do not lead to loss of the proteins but rather to increased production of Aβ42.

These human studies offer compelling evidence that cleavage of APP plays a key causative role in at least some cases of familial, early-onset AD, and point to a role for Aβ42. Because Aβ42-rich amyloid plaques are a cardinal feature of the far larger group of patients with sporadic, late-onset AD, it is likely that APP cleavage is also involved in generating symptoms in this larger group.

Finally, genetic studies of mice have strengthened the case that APP cleavage contributes to AD. Transgenic mice that express relatively high levels of wild-type or mutant APP exhibit structural, physiological, and behavioral abnormalities associated with AD. Transgenic expression of mutant APP forms identical to those found in familial AD leads to appearance of amyloid plaques in the hippocampus and cortex, swollen neurites in proximity to Aβ deposits, decreased density of synaptic terminals in the forebrain, decrements in synaptic transmission, and degeneration of neurons. Moreover, these transgenic mice are deficient in tasks assessing spatial and episodic-like memory. Alterations are more severe in transgenic mice that express altered forms of both APP and presenilin-1. These lines of mice are invaluable tools for addressing mechanistic issues about the pathogenesis of AD and for testing potential therapies. Moreover, AD-like alterations in transgenic mice appear in a year or less rather than over decades, as in humans.

Given the strong evidence that APP cleavage is involved in the pathogenesis of AD, the next question is how the accumulation of cleavage products

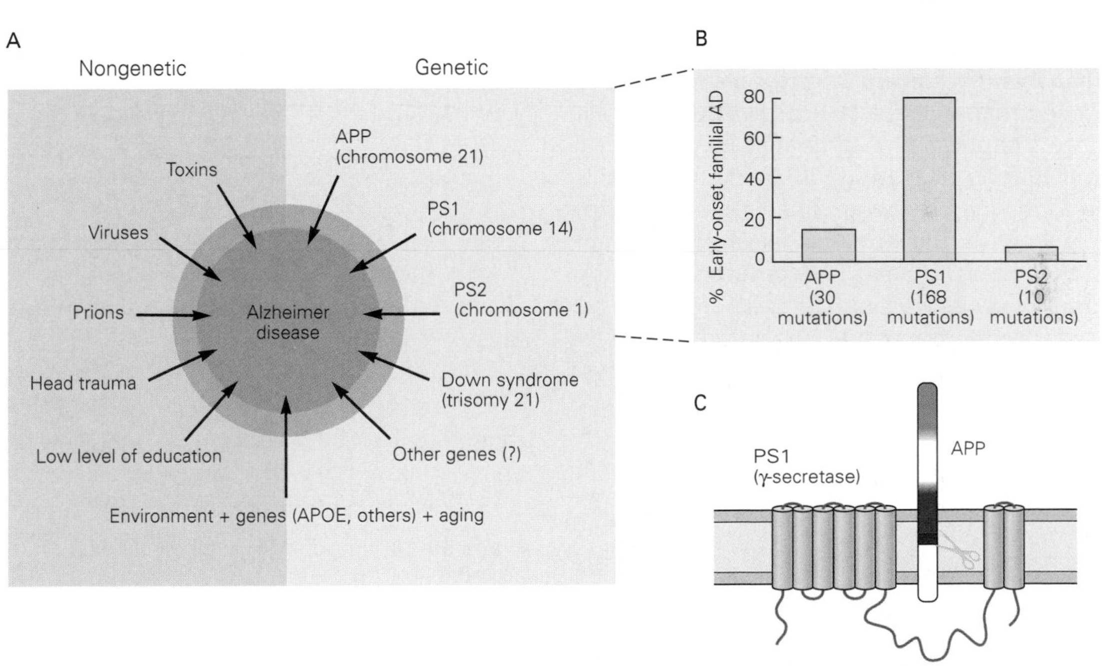

Figure 59–13 Environmental and genetic factors in Alzheimer disease.

A. Environmental and genetic factors. (**ApoE**, apolipoprotein E; **APP**, amyloid precursor protein; **PS1**, presenilin-1; **PS2**, presenilin-2.)

B. Specific genes involved in early-onset Alzheimer disease (AD).

C. Presenilin-1 is associated with APP proteins within the plasma membrane.

contributes to the symptoms. There are three sets of cleavage products: the secreted extracellular region (ectodomain), the Aβ peptide, and the cytoplasmic fragment. Greatest attention has been paid to the Aβ peptides, which were the first to be discovered. One view holds that Aβ in plaques, especially Aβ42, poisons neurons in the vicinity, leading to synaptic dysfunction, degeneration of axon terminals, and eventually death of neurons.

An alternative explanation is that aggregation of soluble forms of Aβ into plaques is the body's incompletely successful attempt to sequester toxic protein fragments. The Aβ peptides can bind to synaptic proteins and affect trafficking of postsynaptic neurotransmitter receptors, including glutamate receptors. Regulated trafficking of these receptors may be essential for forms of synaptic plasticity such as long-term depression and potentiation. As a result, memory defects in AD could involve interference by Aβ in plasticity. In turn, interference in synaptic function could lead to withdrawal and loss of synapses.

Involvement of Aβ peptides in AD does not mean that the other two cleavage products of APP, the cytoplasmic and extracellular fragments (Figure 59–12), have no role in AD. The cytoplasmic fragment can form a complex with other proteins, including Fe65, translocate to the nucleus, and influence transcription in ways that could be deleterious. Although there is little evidence that this mechanism contributes to AD, it is well established that Notch, a critical regulator of neurogenesis (see Chapter 53), is activated by γ-secretase cleavage and that its cleaved cytoplasmic fragment is transported to the nucleus, where it acts as a transcription factor. Likewise, the secreted extracellular fragment of APP appears to have toxic effects on nearby neurons. Thus it is possible that APP is a potent instigator of AD because the fragments generated from it by proteolytic cleavage damage neurons in different ways.

Neurofibrillary Tangles Contain Microtubule-Associated Proteins

Most research on the molecular and cellular basis of AD has focused on amyloid plaques but the neurofibrillary tangles have also been implicated in disease progression (Figure 59–10). Molecular analysis revealed that these abnormal inclusions in cell bodies and proximal dendrites contain aggregates of hyperphosphorylated isoforms of tau, a microtubule-binding protein that is normally soluble (Figure 59–14). Tau plays a key role in intracellular transport, particularly in axons, by binding to and stabilizing microtubules.

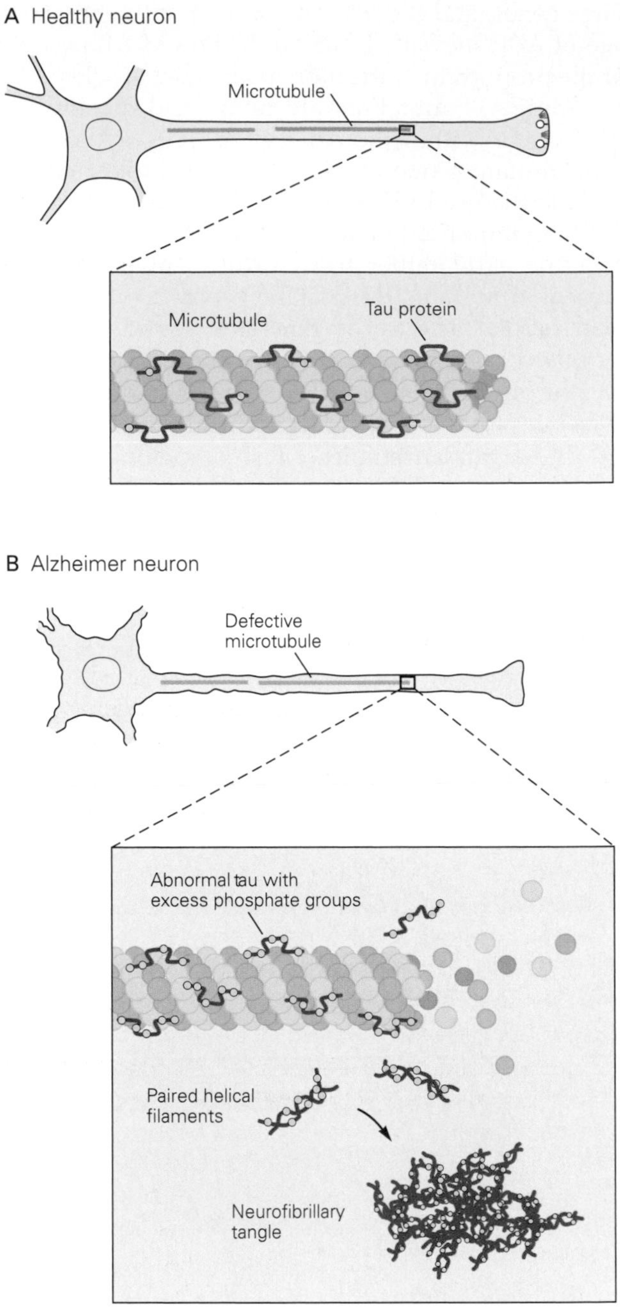

Figure 59–14 Neurofibrillary tangles contain mutant tau proteins.

A. In healthy neurons tau protein associates with normal microtubules but not paired helical filaments, and contributes to the structural integrity of the neuron.

B. In a diseased neuron the tau protein becomes hyperphosphorylated. As a consequence, phosphorylated tau loses its association with normal microtubules, which begin to disassemble, and instead associates with paired helical filaments, which become sequestered in neurofibrillary tangles (NFT).

Impairments in axonal transport compromise synaptic stability, trophic support, and other interactions. Eventually, affected nerve cells die and the neurofibrillary tangles remain in the extracellular space as tombstones of the cells destroyed by disease.

Although tangles are a defining feature of AD, it remains unclear what role they, and the hyperphosphorylated tau of which they are made, play in the pathogenesis of the disease. Whereas mutations of APP and presenilin genes can lead to AD, no mutations of the tau gene have been found in familial AD. This difference leads some to view tangles as a consequence or correlate, but not a cause, of AD symptoms.

Other observations suggest a more causal relationship. First, filamentous deposits of hyperphosphorylated tau are seen in a variety of neurodegenerative disorders. Second, mutations in the tau gene have been found to underlie another form of inherited dementia, frontotemporal dementia with Parkinson disease type 17 (FTPD17), which shares some features with AD but lacks plaques. Third, symptoms of AD correlate better with the number and distribution of tangles than that of plaques seen in autopsy material. For example, tangles are usually first evident in neurons of the entorhinal cortex, the likely site of early memory disturbance, before plaques appear in this area.

For many years controversy has raged between those who believe that Aβ is the main causal agent of AD and those who believe that tau-rich tangles play a major role. These advocates have been called "Baptists" and "Taoists," respectively. It now seems most likely that both Aβ and tau are involved, and that pathology results from their combined effects. For example, transgenic mice that express both mutant APP and mutant tau develop more severe AD-like behavioral deficits than mice overexpressing either alone. Moreover, there appears to be interplay between plaques and tangles. Thus injection of Aβ42 into specific brain regions of transgenic mice that express a mutant tau protein increases the number of tangles in nearby neurons, and a manipulation that reduces the number and size of plaques leads to a decrease in levels of hyperphosphorylated tau. Thus, even if tangles are not sufficient to "cause" AD, they are likely to play a role in symptoms and disease progression.

Risk Factors for Alzheimer Disease Have Been Identified

A few individuals develop AD because they bear mutant alleles of the APP or presenilin genes, but in most cases no genetic or environmental causes are obvious. Can we, then, predict who will get AD?

The major risk factor is age. The disease is present in a vanishingly small fraction of people younger than age 60 (these being mostly familial cases), 1–3% of those between ages 60 and 70, 3–12% of those between ages 70 and 80, and 25–35% of those older than age 85. Thus one safe prediction is that elderly people are prime candidates for AD. However, this statistical association is of little therapeutic use because modern medicine can do nothing to slow the passage of time. There has therefore been intense interest in other factors that affect the incidence of AD.

The most significant genetic risk factor discovered to date in sporadic late-onset AD is an allele of the gene *ApoE*. The ApoE protein is the major carrier of cholesterol and other lipids in the blood. The gene is expressed as three alleles, *ApoE2*, *ApoE3*, and *ApoE4*, which differ from each other at only a few amino acids (Figure 59–15). People with the *ApoE4* allele are at risk for AD. This allele is present in only a few percent of the general population but in 40–50% of those with AD. Put another way, carrying one *ApoE4* allele increases by about fourfold one's chance of developing AD, compared to people who carry only *ApoE2* or *ApoE3* alleles. The mechanism by which *ApoE4* predisposes one to AD is not known. Moreover, *ApoE4* is a risk factor for several neurological diseases, including Parkinson disease and multiple sclerosis, so it may act in ways that do not involve APP or Aβ directly.

Alzheimer Disease Can Be Diagnosed Well but Available Treatments Are Poor

Diagnosing AD at its early stages is challenging as its initial symptoms are similar to the changes that are part of normal age-related cognitive decline. Until recently, even diagnosis of more advanced AD was difficult. In the 1970s diagnostic error rates were approximately 30%, as judged by the best objective measure: the detection of plaques and tangles at autopsy. Indeed, until biological and genetic research provided a deeper understanding of the pathology, it remained somewhat controversial whether AD was best viewed as a discrete disease or as one end of a continuum that passed from normal aging through mild cognitive impairment to dementia.

During the past few decades the situation has improved, largely because of three factors. First, protocols for physical, neurological, and neuropsychological examination have become more sophisticated and standardized. Second, increased knowledge of the structural changes revealed by magnetic resonance imaging (MRI) have helped in diagnosing AD at early

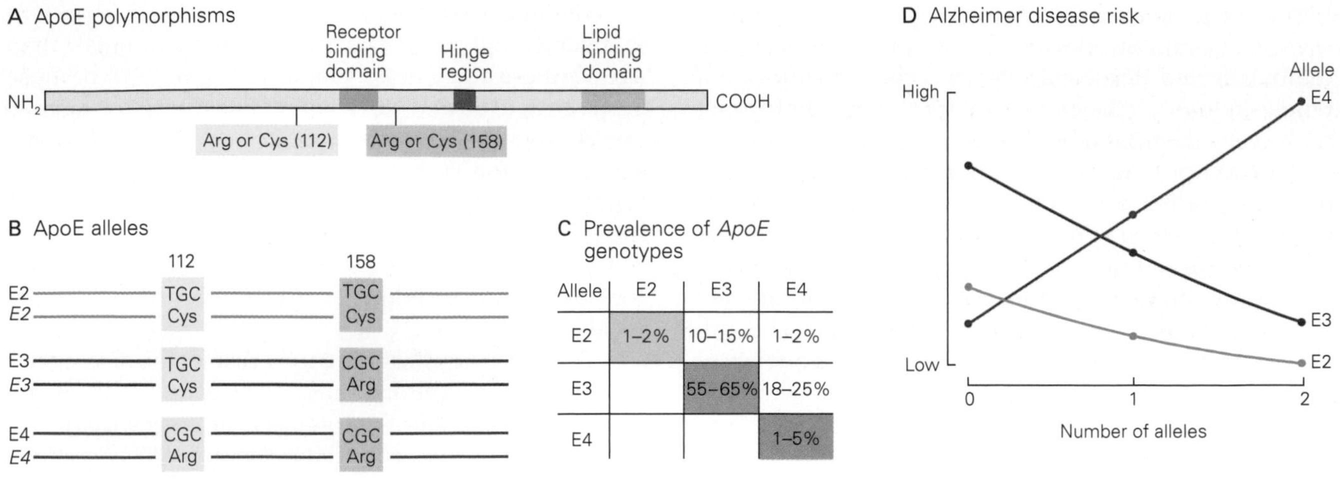

Figure 59–15 Polymorphisms in the *ApoE* gene are a prominent risk factor for Alzheimer disease.

A. Polymorphisms in the *ApoE* gene involve changes in amino acid sequence at two critical residues (112 and 158).

B. Changes in amino acid sequence in the three *ApoE* alleles.

C. Prevalence of *ApoE* genotypes in the general population.

D. *ApoE* alleles are risk factors for Alzheimer disease. Inheritance of one *ApoE4* allele increases by about fourfold the probability of progressing to Alzheimer disease. Inheritance of the *ApoE2* allele reduces the risk.

stages. For example, it is now possible to predict, with approximately 80% accuracy, which patients with mild cognitive impairment will proceed to AD based on the cortical thinning and ventricular enlargement visible by MRI. These imaging and diagnostic methods also assist in distinguishing dementia syndromes from each other and relating structural to functional defects. For example, early in a disease called *semantic dementia,* patients have difficulty naming objects, and MRI reveals atrophy of the temporal poles. In contrast, in AD initial difficulties center on memory, and MRI reveals initial alterations in the medial temporal cortex and hippocampus.

Third, and perhaps most promising, amyloid plaques can now be visualized by positron emission tomography (PET) using new compounds that avidly bind amyloid. The first of these, called *Pittsburgh compound B* (PIB), binds with high affinity to Aβ, and its radioactive form, labeled with short-lived isotopes of carbon or fluorine, is readily detected by PET (Figure 59–16). The availability of safe molecular markers of AD permits early stages of the disease to be studied, before clinical symptoms are present. Of equal importance, the ability to distinguish older adults with and without amyloid plaques permits, for the first time, detailed analyses of normal aging uncomplicated by confounding early-stage AD.

Improved diagnosis of AD is, of course, most useful if treatments are available that can halt or slow its progression at an early stage. Here the news is not so good. At present there is no cure for Alzheimer disease. Present-day therapies focus on treating associated symptoms, such as depression, agitation, sleep disorders, hallucinations, and delusions. One of the principal targets is the cholinergic system in the basal forebrain, a region of the brain that is severely damaged in Alzheimer disease. Several strategies have been developed to influence this cholinergic system. Acetylcholinesterase inhibitors increase levels of acetylcholine by inhibiting its breakdown, and represent one of the few drugs approved by the FDA for treatment of AD. Unfortunately, these drugs exert, at best, a modest effect on cognitive functions and the activities of daily living. Likewise, addition of precursors of acetylcholine (choline, lecithin, etc) or cholinergic agonists have not proven effective.

On the other hand, recent increases in our understanding of the biological basis of AD have highlighted several promising new therapeutic targets, all of which are being explored intensively. One approach is to develop drugs that reduce the activity of the β- and γ-secretases that cleave APP to generate Aβ peptides and the associated soluble extracellular and intracellular fragments. In fact, decreasing either β- or γ-secretase levels in transgenic mice that overexpress mutant APP decreases both Aβ deposition and age-associated memory abnormalities in these models. Accordingly, pharmaceutical companies are trying to develop drugs that will decrease levels of β- and γ-secretases in humans. An obstacle to this approach is that the secretases have other substrates in addition to APP, so decreasing their levels can have deleterious side effects. For example, one promising inhibitor of γ-secretase also decreased production of T and B cells of the immune system. As an alternative, it may be possible to find cleavage-inhibiting drugs that bind to critical sites on APP rather than to the secretases.

Other researchers are targeting the different proteins that have been implicated in AD: α-secretase, ApoE4, and tau. Because α-secretase cleaves in the middle of Aβ, it prevents Aβ accumulation. Researchers are exploring ways to increase α-secretase levels or activity. Conversely, ApoE4 predisposes to AD, whereas ApoE3 is innocuous or protective. Researchers are therefore seeking ways to convert the properties of ApoE4 into those of ApoE3, or to target the receptors through which it acts. Likewise, interventions that prevent hyperphosphorylation of tau could slow generation of neurofibrillary tangles, which appear to worsen neuronal health in a variety of neurodegenerative diseases.

Another approach is to decrease levels of Aβ through immunological means. Immunization with Aβ, which leads to generation of antibodies of Aβ, and passive transfer of antibodies to Aβ have been tested in transgenic mice models of Alzheimer disease. Both treatments reduce levels of Aβ and plaques. The mechanisms of enhanced Aβ clearance are not certain. Serum antibodies likely serve as a "sink" to extract low molecular weight Aβ peptides from the brain into the circulation, thus changing the equilibrium of Aβ in different compartments and promoting removal of Aβ from the brain. Alternatively, a small amount of Aβ antibody could reach the brain, bind Aβ, and recruit microglia to enter the affected regions and remove Aβ. Whatever the mechanism, Aβ immunotherapy in mice appears to reduce Aβ levels (Figure 59–17) and thus attenuate the otherwise severe impact of amyloid plaque on learning and cognition. These findings suggest that immunotherapeutic strategies may be successful in AD patients.

An Overall View

Aging affects the brain in many ways. Some changes are subtle, and the neurobiological basis of accompanying behavioral disturbances is unclear. Other problems are moderate, as in mild cognitive impairment (MCI). Some deficits are progressive and disabling as occurs in the various dementia syndromes. The most common dementia in the elderly is Alzheimer disease (AD), one of the most complex diseases in clinical medicine.

Alheimer disease is a common cause of morbidity and mortality in the elderly. In recent years there have been major advances in understanding this disease. Investigators have more accurately documented the relationship of MCI to early AD, identified genetic causes and risk factors, developed a variety of new diagnostic approaches that allow detection of amyloid plaques in living people, and clarified

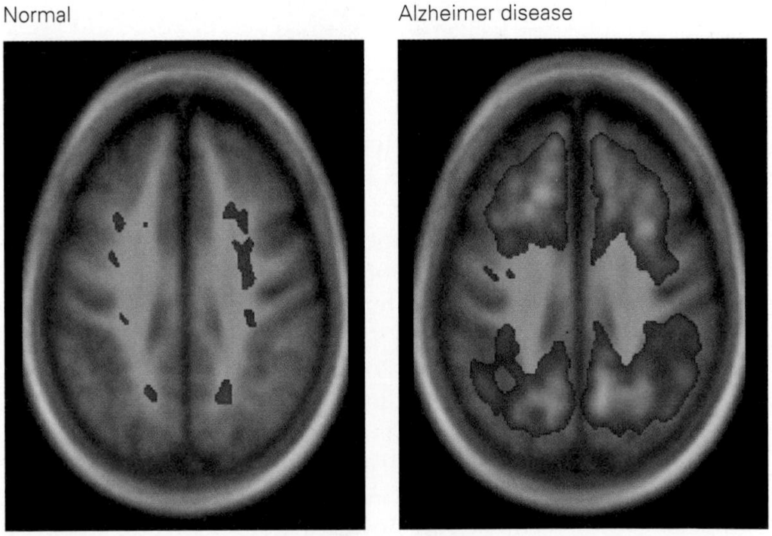

Figure 59–16 Visualizing Alzheimer disease in the living brain. The density of β-amyloid plaques is indicated by the **red** regions in these images made after administration of Pittsburgh compound B, a fluorescent analog of thioflavin T. (Reproduced, with permission, from R. Buckner.)

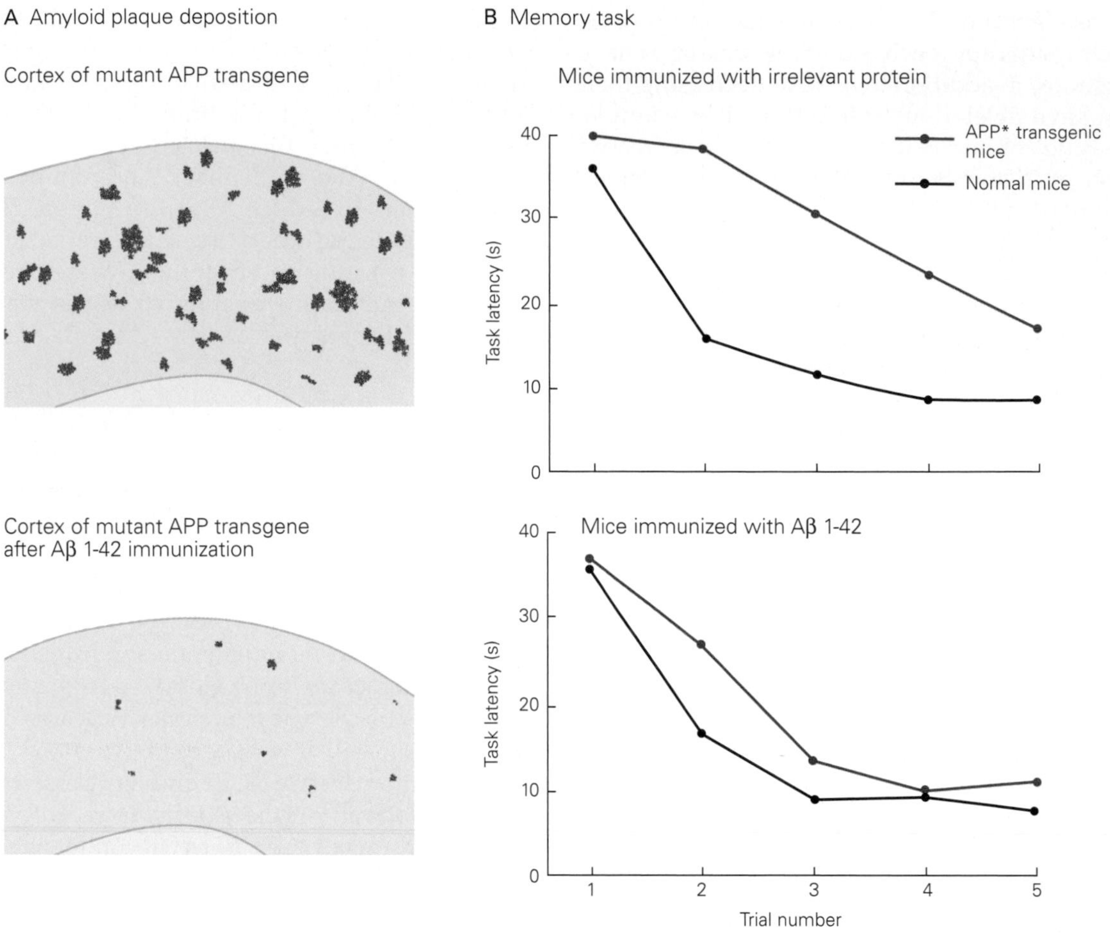

Figure 59–17 Immunization with antibodies to Aβ peptide clears Aβ plaque and preserves cognitive performance in transgenic mice expressing the peptide. (Adapted, with permission, from Brody 2008.)

A. Amyloid plaque deposition in the cerebral cortex of mice carrying a mutant APP transgene and in mice treated by Aβ vaccination. Note the reduction in Aβ plaque deposition.

B. Cognitive performance (a memory test) in APP transgenic mice immunized with an irrelevant protein or with Aβ vaccination. Mice vaccinated with Aβ perform at levels close to non-transgenic animals, whereas mice immunized with an irrelevant protein show severe impairment in memory.

the ways in which the character, distributions, and stages of pathology are related to clinical signs. The mechanisms that lead to formation of plaques and tangles have begun to be delineated and studies of in vitro and in vivo models systems have led investigators to identification of potential new targets for treatment.

We are now on the threshold of implementing novel therapies based on an understanding of the neurobiology, neuropathology, biochemistry, and genetics of this illness. Moreover, a variety of tools, including biomarkers, brain imaging, and measures of Aβ flux between brain and plasma compartments, are now being developed to assess efficacies of treatments. Over the next few years it seems possible that these discoveries will lead to the rational design of new therapies that can be tested in animal models. With perseverance and luck, some of these approaches may be introduced into the clinic to benefit AD patients, for whom medicine has so far had very little to offer.

Joshua R. Sanes
Thomas M. Jessell

Selected Readings

Brody DL, Holtzman DM. 2008. Active and passive immunotherapy for neurodegenerative disorders. Annu Rev Neurosci 31:175–193.

Buckner RL. 2004. Memory and executive function in aging and AD: multiple factors that cause decline and reserve factors that compensate. Neuron 44:195–208.

Corder EH, Saunders AM, Strittmatter WJ, Schmechel DE, Gaskell PC, Small GW, Roses AD, Haines JL, Pericak-Vance MA. 1993. Gene dose of apolipoprotein E type 4 allele and the risk of Alzheimer disease in late onset families. Science 261:921–923.

Goedert M, Spillantini MG. 2006. A century of Alzheimer's disease. Science 314:777–781.

Haass C, Selkoe DJ. 2007. Soluble protein oligomers in neurodegeneration: lessons from the Alzheimer's amyloid beta-peptide. Nat Rev Mol Cell Biol 8:101–112.

Kenyon C. 2005. The plasticity of aging: insights from long-lived mutants. Cell 120:449–460.

Perrin RJ, Fagan AM, Holtzman DM. 2009. Multimodal techniques for diagnosis and prognosis of Alzheimer's disease. Nature 461:916–22.

Tanzi RE, Bertram L. 2005. Twenty years of the Alzheimer's disease amyloid hypothesis: a genetic perspective. Cell 120:545–555.

References

Andrews-Hanna JR, Snyder AZ, Vincent JL, Lustig C, Head D, Raichle ME, Buckner RL. 2007. Disruption of large-scale brain systems in advanced aging. Neuron 56:924–935.

Arias E. 2004. United States Life Tables, 2001. *National Vital Statistics Reports,* Vol. 52, No. 14. National Center for Health Statistics, Hyattsville, MD.

Arnold SE, Hyman BT, Flory J, Damasio AR, Van Hoesen GW. 1991. The topographical and neuroanatomical distribution of neurofibrillary tangles and neuritic plaques in the cerebral cortex of patients with Alzheimer's disease. Cereb Cortex 1:103–116.

Bard F, Cannon C, Barbour R, Burke RL, Games D, Grajeda H, Guido T, et al. 2000. Peripherally administered antibodies against amyloid beta-peptide enter the central nervous system and reduce pathology in a mouse model of Alzheimer disease. Nat Med 6:916–919.

Bishop NA, Lu T, Yankner BA. 2010. Neural mechanisms of ageing and cognitive decline. Nature 464:529–35.

Brown-Borg H, Borg K, Meliska C, Bartke A. 1996. Dwarf mice and the ageing process. Nature 384:33.

Brumback RA and Leech RW. 1994. Alzheimer's disease: pathophysiology and hope for therapy. J Oklahoma Med Assoc 87:103–111

Bu G. 2009. Apolipoprotein E and its receptors in Alzheimer's disease: pathways, pathogenesis and therapy. Nat Rev Neurosci 10:333–344.

Cai H, Wang Y, McCarthy D, Wen H, Borchelt DR, Price DL, Wong PC. 2001. BACE1 is the major beta-secretase for generation of A–beta peptides by neurons. Nat Neurosci 4:233–234.

Cao X, Sudhof TC. 2001. A transcriptionally active complex of APP with Fe65 and histone acetyltransferase Tip60. Science 293:115–120.

Cleary JP, Walsh DM, Hofmeister JJ, Shankar GM, Kuskowski MA, Selkoe DJ, Ashe KH. 2005. Natural oligomers of the amyloid beta protein specifically disrupt cognitive function. Nat Neurosci 8:79–84.

Cohen E, Dillin A. 2008. The insulin paradox: aging, proteotoxicity and neurodegeneration. Nat Rev Neurosci 9:759–767.

Cohen E, Paulsson JF, Blinder P, Burstyn-Cohen T, Du D, Estepa G, Adame A, et al. 2009. Reduced IGF-1 signaling delays age-associated proteotoxicity in mice. Cell 139:1157–1169.

De Strooper B. 2010. Proteases and proteolysis in Alzheimer disease: a multifactorial view on the disease process. Physiol Rev 90:465–494.

De Strooper B, Saftig P, Craessaerts K, Vanderstichele H, Guhde G, Annaert W, Von Figura K, Van Leuven F. 1998. Deficiency of presenilin-1 inhibits the normal cleavage of amyloid precursor protein. Nature 391:387–390.

Dickstein DL, Kabaso D, Rocher AB, Luebke JI, Wearne SL, Hof PR. 2007. Changes in the structural complexity of the aged brain. Aging Cell 6:275–284.

Glenner GG, Wong CW. 1984. Alzheimer's disease: initial report of the purification and characterization of a novel cerebrovascular amyloid protein. Biochem Biophys Res Commun 120:885–890.

Goate A, Chartier-Harlin MC, Mullan M, Brown J, Crawford F, Fidani L, Giuffra L, et al. 1991. Segregation of a missense mutation in the amyloid precursor protein gene with familial Alzheimer's disease. Nature 349:704–706.

Hebert LE, Scherr PA, Bienias JL, Bennett DA, Evans DA. 2003. Alzheimer Disease in the US population: prevalence estimates using the 2000 census. Arch Neurobiol 60: 1119–1122.

Hekimi S, Guarente L. 2003. Genetics and the specificity of the aging process. Science 299:1351–1354.

Hsiao K, Chapman P, Nilsen S, Eckman C, Harigaya Y, Younkin S, Yang F, Cole G. 1996. Correlative memory deficits, Abeta elevation, and amyloid plaques in transgenic mice. Science 274:99–102.

Huttenlocher PR. 2002. *Neural Plasticity: The Effects of Environment on the Development of the Cerebral Cortex.* Cambridge, MA: Harvard University Press.

Kang J, Lemaire HG, Unterbeck A, Salbaum JM, Masters CL, Grzeschik KH, Multhaup G, Beyreuther K, Muller-Hill B. 1987. The precursor of Alzheimer's disease amyloid A4 protein resembles a cell-surface receptor. Nature 325: 733–736.

Kim J, Castellano JM, Jiang H, Basak JM, Parsadanian M, Pham V, Mason SM, Paul SM, Holtzman DM. 2009. Overexpression of low-density lipoprotein receptor in the brain markedly inhibits amyloid deposition and increases extracellular A beta clearance. Neuron 64:632–644.

Klunk WE, Engler H, Nordberg A, Wang Y, Blomqvist G, Holt DP, Bergstrom M, et al. 2004. Imaging brain amyloid in Alzheimer's disease with Pittsburgh Compound-B. Ann Neurol 55:306–319.

Lesne S, Koh MT, Kotilinek L, Kayed R, Glabe CG, Yang A, Gallagher M, Ashe KH. 2006. A specific amyloid-beta protein assembly in the brain impairs memory. Nature 440:352–357.

Levy-Lahad E, Wasco W, Poorkaj P, Romano DM, Oshima J, Pettingell WH, Yu CE, et al. 1995. Candidate gene for the chromosome 1 familial Alzheimer's disease locus. Science 269:973–977.

Markesbery WR, Schmitt FA, Kryscio RJ, Davis DG, Smith CD, Wekstein DR. 2006. Neuropathologic substrate of mild cognitive impairment. Arch Neurol 63:38–46.

Mattson MP, Akbari Y, LaFerla FM. 2003. Triple-transgenic model of Alzheimer's disease with plaques and tangles: intracellular A beta and synaptic dysfunction. Neuron 39:409–421.

Morgan D, Diamond DM, Gottschall PE, Ugen KE, Dickey C, Hardy J, Duff K, et al. 2000. A beta peptide vaccination prevents memory loss in an animal model of Alzheimer's disease. Nature 408:982–985.

Morris JC, McKeel DW Jr, Storandt M, Rubin EH, Price JL, Grant EA, Ball MJ, Berg L. 1991. Very mild Alzheimer's disease: informant-based clinical, psychometric, and pathologic distinction from normal aging. Neurology 41:469–478.

Nikolaev A, McLaughlin T, O'Leary DD, Tessier-Lavigne M. 2009. APP binds DR6 to trigger axon pruning and neuron death via distinct caspases. Nature 457:981–989.

Oddo S, Caccamo A, Shepherd JD, Murphy MP, Golde TE, Kayed R, Metherate R, Park DC, Smith AD, Lautenschlager G, Earles JL, Frieske D, Zwahr M, Gaines CL. 1996. Mediators of long-term memory performance across the life span. Psychol Aging 11:621–637.

Price JL, Davis PB, Morris JC, White DL. 1991. The distribution of tangles, plaques and related immunohistochemical markers in healthy aging and Alzheimer's disease. Neurobiol Aging 12:295–312.

Rubin EH, Storandt M, Miller JP, Kinscherf DA, Grant EA, Morris JC, Berg L. 1998. A prospective study of cognitive function and onset of dementia in cognitively healthy elders. Arch Neurol 55:395–401.

Strehler BL. 1975. Implications of Aging Research for Society. Proceedings of the 58th Annual Meeting of the Federation of American Societies for Experimental Biology, 1974. 34:5–8.

Valdez G, Tapia JC, Kang H, Clemenson GD, Gage FH, Lichtman JW, Sanes JR. 2010. Attenuation of age-related changes in mouse neuromuscular synapses by caloric restriction and exercise. Proc Natl Acad Sci U S A 107: 14863–14868.

Van Broeckhoven C, Haan J, Bakker E, Hardy JA, Van Hul W, Wehnert A, Vegter-Van der Vlis M, Roos RA. 1990. Amyloid beta protein precursor gene and hereditary cerebral hemorrhage with amyloidosis (Dutch). Science 248: 1120–1122.

Vincent B, Cisse MA, Sunyach C, Guillot-Sestier MV, Checler F. 2008. Regulation of betaAPP and PrPc cleavage by alpha-secretase: mechanistic and therapeutic perspectives. Curr Alzheimer Res 5:202–211.

Wilcock DM, Gharkholonarehe N, Van Nostrand WE, Davis J, Vitek MP, Colton CA. 2009. Amyloid reduction by amyloid-beta vaccination also reduces mouse tau pathology and protects from neuron loss in two mouse models of Alzheimer's disease. J Neurosci 29:7957–7965.

Yi, L, Seroude L, Benzer, S. 1998. Extended life-span and stress resistance in the *Drosophila* mutant Methuselah. Science 282:943–946.

Part IX

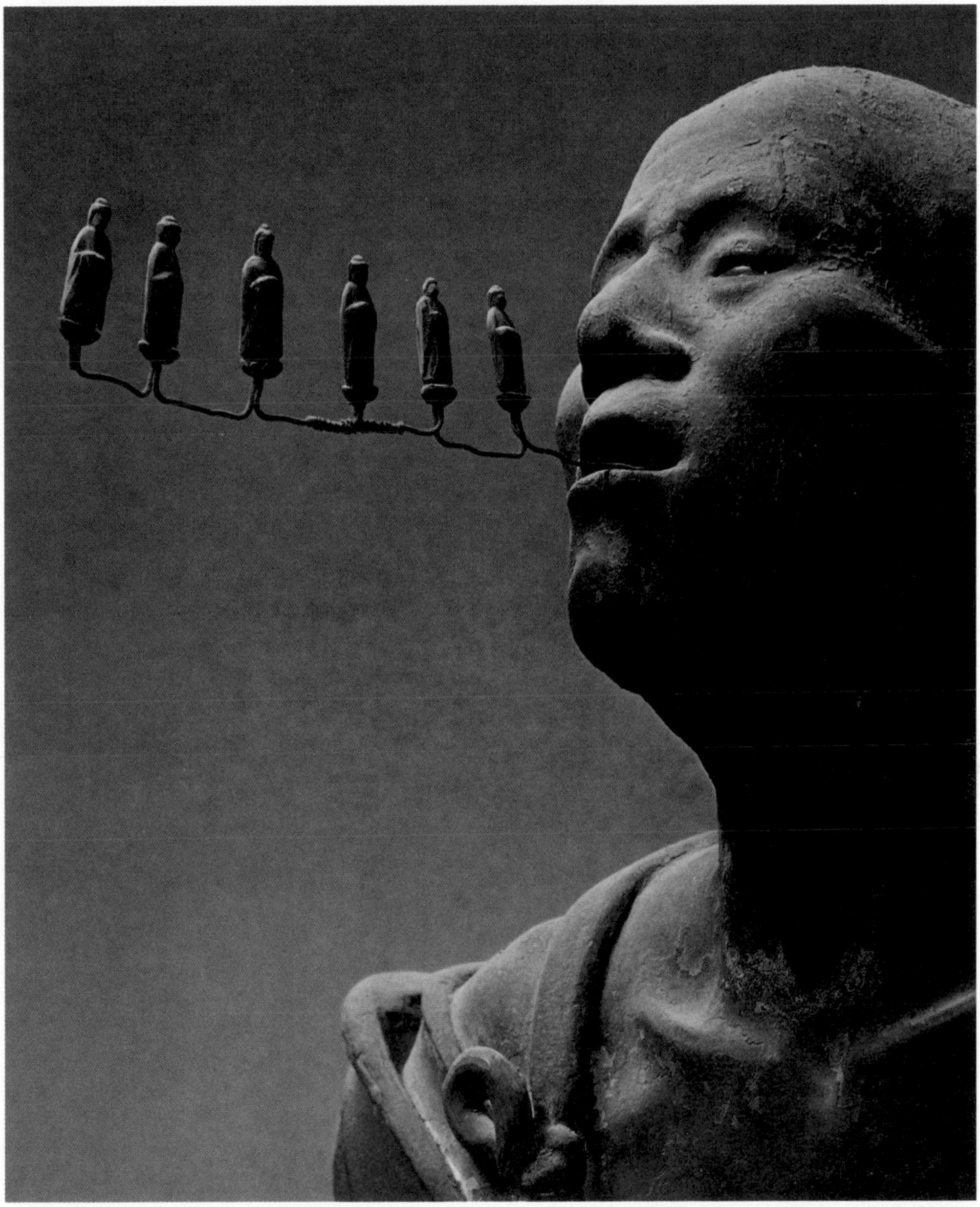

Preceding Page

Wooden sculpture of the itinerant Buddhist monk Kūya. This portrait by the 13th century sculptor Kōshō shows the monk reciting the *nembutsu*, or praise of the Buddha, which in Japan takes the form of six characters. Kuya taught that focused recitation of the nembutsu would lead to rebirth in the Pure Land, a state of spiritual illumination. The six small Buddhas issuing from his mouth represent the six syllables of the spoken prayer. This portrayal shows remarkable complexity of representation, with pieces of wood carved in the shape of figurines, symbolizing discrete components of speech, which together represent language, its underlying concept, and in this case a means to spiritual enlightenment. (Reproduced, with permission from Rokuharamitsuji-temple, Kyoto, Japan.)

IX Language, Thought, Affect, and Learning

Motor and sensory functions take up less than one-half of the cerebral cortex in humans. The rest of the cortex is occupied by the association areas, which coordinate events arising in the motor and sensory centers. Three association areas—the prefrontal, parietal-temporal-occipital, and limbic—are involved in cognitive behavior: speaking, thinking, feeling, perceiving, planning, learning, memory, and skilled movements.

Most of the early evidence relating cognitive functions to the association areas came from clinical studies of brain-damaged patients. Thus, the study of language in patients with aphasia yielded important information about how human mental processes are distributed in the two hemispheres of the brain and how they develop.

Genetic manipulation in experimental animals can now be used to evaluate the relative contribution of genes and learning to specific types of behavior. Even the highest cognitive abilities have a genetic component. Composing music is an excellent example. Music conforms to complex, unusually abstract rules that must be learned, yet clearly it has genetic components intertwined with its learned aspects. The great composer Johann Sebastian Bach had many children, five of whom were distinguished musicians and composers. His only grandson also was a composer and harpsichordist to the court of Prussia. In 1730, Bach proudly wrote that he was able to "put on a vocal and instrumental concert with my own family."

Much of today's neural science concerns cognitive neural science, a merger of neurophysiology, anatomy, developmental biology, cell and molecular biology, and cognitive psychology—a merger that has given rise to a new science of mind. Until two decades ago the study of higher mental function was approached in two complementary ways: through psychological observation and through invasive experimental physiology. In the first part of the 20th century, to avoid untestable concepts and hypotheses, psychology became rigidly concerned with behaviors defined strictly in terms of observable stimuli and responses. Orthodox behaviorists thought it unproductive to deal with consciousness, feeling, attention, or even motivation.

By concentrating only on observable actions, behaviorists asked: What can an organism do, and how does it do it? Indeed, careful quantitative analysis of stimuli and responses has contributed greatly to our understanding of the acquisition and use of "implicit" knowledge of perceptual and motor skills. However, humans and other higher animals also have "explicit" knowledge of facts and events. Thus we also need to ask: What does the animal know about the world, and how does it come to know it? How is that knowledge represented in the brain? And does explicit knowledge differ from implicit knowledge? Much perhaps most, knowledge is unconscious a great deal of the time. We need to know the nature of the unconscious processes, the systems that mediate them, and their influence on the nature of conscious mental activity. Finally, we need to know about the highest realms of conscious knowledge, the knowledge of oneself as an individual, a thinking and feeling human being.

The modern effort to understand the neural mechanisms of higher mental functions began at the end of the 18th century when Franz Joseph Gall, a German neuroanatomist, proposed that particular mental functions are discretely localized in the brain. By the mid-19th century, clinical neurologists, who regarded their patients as "natural experiments" in brain function, studied brain lesions at autopsy to discover where particular brain functions were located. In 1861, Pierre Paul Broca, using evidence from the damaged brains of aphasic patients, convinced the scientific establishment that speech is controlled by a specific area of the left frontal lobe. Soon afterward the control of voluntary movement was localized, and the various primary sensory cortices for vision, audition, somatic sensation, and taste were delineated.

Neural science is only beginning to analyze the nature of the internal representations that cognitive psychologists have insisted intervenes between stimulus and response, and the very real dynamic unconscious mental processes studied by psychoanalysts—only now beginning to address the subjective sense of individuality, will, and purpose that is common to us all. In the past, ascribing a particular behavioral feature to a mental process that could not be directly observed meant that the process must be excluded from study because no reliable technique was available to examine brain function in the context of behavior. In Part IX, we show that because the nervous system and even its unconscious mental processes have become more accessible to behavioral experiments, internal representations of experience can be explored in a controlled manner.

A key concern of cognitive psychology and psychoanalysis is the relative importance of genetic and learned factors in forming a mental representation of the world. These disciplines can be strengthened by the insights into behavior that neuroscience now offers. The task for the years ahead is to produce a psychology still concerned with problems of mental representation, cognitive dynamics, and subjective states of mind but grounded firmly in empirical neural science.

Part IX

60

Language

LANGUAGE IS UNIQUELY HUMAN and arguably our greatest skill and our highest achievement. Despite its complexity, all typically developing children master it by the age of three. What causes this universal developmental phenomenon, and why are children so much better at acquiring a new language than adults? Once language is mastered, what brain systems are involved in language processing, and how does brain damage produce the various disorders of language known as the aphasias?

For centuries these questions about language and the brain have prompted vigorous debate among theorists. In the last decade, however, an explosion of information regarding language has taken us beyond the nature–nurture debates and beyond the standard view of specialized brain areas responsible for language. Two factors are largely responsible for this change.

First, functional brain imaging techniques such as positron emission tomography (PET), functional magnetic resonance imaging (fMRI), electroencephalography, and magnetoencephalography have allowed us to examine activation patterns in the brain while the subject carries out language tasks—naming objects or actions, listening to sounds or words, or detecting grammatical anomalies. The results of these studies reveal a far more complex picture than the one first conceived of by Carl Wernicke in 1874, a picture in which multiple and relatively segregated brain systems cooperate functionally in language processing.

Second, behavioral and brain studies of language acquisition show that infants learn language in ways that had not been envisioned. Well before children produce their first words, they learn the sound patterns underlying the phonetic units, words, and phrase structure of the language they hear. Listening to language alters the infant brain early in development, and early language learning affects the brain for life. These new findings have led to a new view of language that encompasses its development, mature state, and dissolution in aphasia.

Humans are not the only species to communicate. Passerine birds attract mates with songs, bees code the distance and direction to honey by dancing, and monkeys signal a desire for sexual contact or fear at the approach of an enemy with coos and grunts. With language we accomplish all of the above and more. We use language to provide information and express our emotions, to comment on the past and future, and create fiction and poetry. Using sounds that have only an arbitrary association with the meanings they convey, we talk about anything and everything. No animal has a communication system that parallels human language either in form or in function. Language is the defining characteristic of humans, and living without it creates a totally different world, as patients with aphasia following a stroke experience so heartbreakingly.

Language Has Many Functional Levels: Phonemes, Morphemes, Words, and Sentences

What distinguishes language from other forms of communication? The key feature is a finite set of sounds that can be combined with infinite possibilities. This set of sounds or phonemes is used to create semantic units called morphemes. Each language has a distinctive set of phonemes and rules for combining them into morphemes and words. Words can be combined according to the rules of syntax into an infinite number of sentences.

Understanding language presents an interesting set of puzzles, one that even supercomputers have thus far not mastered. Computers even have difficulty with phonetic discrimination. For example, in English the sounds /r/ and /l/ differentiate the words *rock* and *lock*. In Japanese, however, this sound change does not alter the meaning of a word as the /r/ and /l/ sounds are used interchangeably. Similarly, Spanish speakers distinguish between the words *pano* and *bano*, whereas English speakers treat the /p/ and /b/ sounds at the beginning of these words as the same sounds. Given that many languages use identical sounds, but group them differently, children must discover how sounds are grouped to make meaningful differences in their language.

Phonetic units are sub-phonemic. As we have illustrated above with /r/ and /l/, they are both phonetic units but their phonemic status differs in English and Japanese. In English, the two are phonemically distinct, meaning that they change the meaning of a word. However, in Japanese /r/ and /l/ belong to the same phonemic category and are not distinct. Phonetic units are distinguished by subtle variations in vibrations of the vocal tract called *formant frequencies* (Figure 60–1). The patterns and timing of formant frequencies distinguish words that differ in only one phonetic unit, such as the words *pat* and *bat*. In normal speech, formant changes occur very rapidly, on the order of milliseconds. The auditory system has to track these rapid changes to distinguish semantically different sounds and understand speech. Identifying words in written language is easy because there are spaces between words. However, in speech there are no acoustic breaks between words. Thus speech requires a process that can detect words on the basis of something other than sounds bracketed by silence. Computers have a great deal of trouble recognizing words in the normal flow of speech.

Phonotactic rules specify how phonemes can be combined to form words. Both English and Polish use the phonemes /z/ and /b/, for example, but the combination *zb* is not allowed in English, whereas in Polish it is common (as in the name Zbigniew).

Morphemes are the smallest meaningful units of a language, best illustrated by prefixes and suffixes. In English, for example, the prefix *un* (meaning *not*) can be added to many adjectives to convey the opposite meaning (eg, *unimportant*). Suffixes often signal the tense or number of a word. For example, to pluralize in English we add *s* or *es* (*pot* becomes *pots*, *bug* becomes *bugs*, or *box* becomes *boxes*). To change the tense of a regular verb we add an ending to the word (eg, *play* can become *plays*, *playing*, and *played*). Irregular verbs do not follow the rule (eg, *go* becomes *went* rather than *goed*, and *break* becomes *broke* rather than *breaked*). Every language has a different set of rules for altering the tense and number of a word.

Finally, to create language, words have to be strung together. *Syntax* specifies word and phrase order for

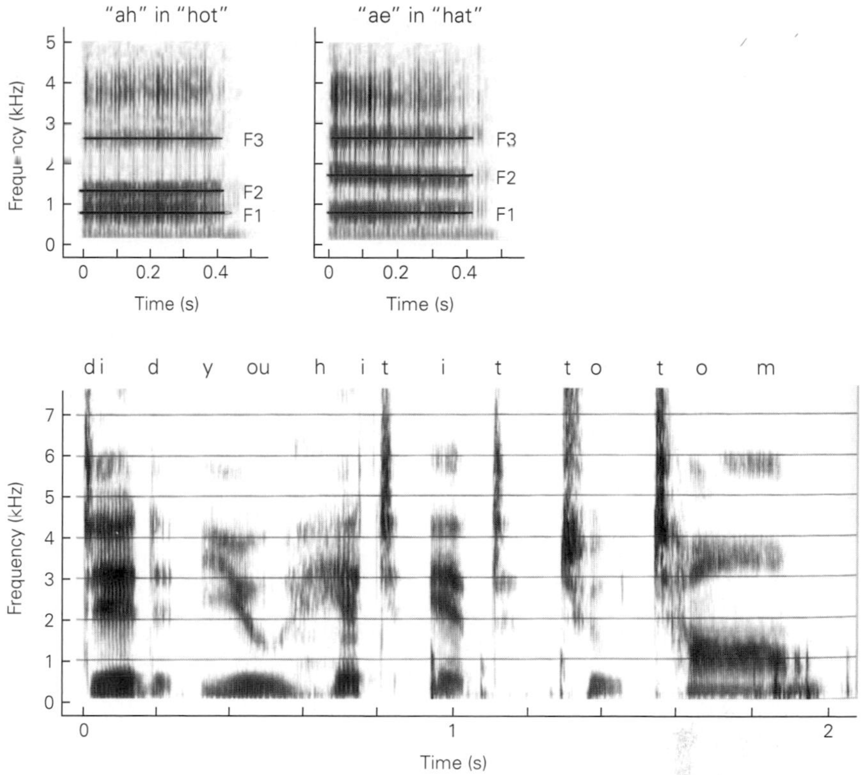

Figure 60–1 Formant frequencies. Formants, shown here as a function of time in a spectrographic analysis of speech, are systematic variations in the concentration of energy at various frequencies, and represent resonances of the vocal tract. The formant patterns for two simple vowels ("ah" and "ae") spoken in isolation are distinguished by differences in formant 2 (F2). Formant patterns for the sentence "Did you hit it to Tom?" spoken slowly and clearly illustrate the rapid changes that underlie normal speech. (Adapted, with permission, from Kuhl 2000.)

a given language. In English, for example, sentences typically conform to a subject–verb–object order (eg, *He eats cake*), whereas in Japanese, it is typically subject–object–verb (eg, *Kare wa keeki o tabemasu*, literally, *He cake eats*). Languages have systematic differences in the order of larger constituents (noun phrases and verb phrases) of a sentence, and in the order of words within constituents, as illustrated by the difference between English and French noun phrases. In English adjectives precede the noun (eg, *a very intelligent man*), whereas in French most follow the noun (eg, *un homme très intelligent*).

Language Acquisition in Children Follows a Universal Pattern

Regardless of culture, all children initially exhibit universal patterns of speech perception and production that do not depend on the specific language children hear (Figure 60–2). By the end of the first year infants have learned through exposure to a specific language which phonetic units convey meaning in that language and recognize likely words, even though they do not yet understand those words. By 12 months of age infants understand approximately 50 words and have begun to produce speech that resembles the native language. By the age of 3 years children know approximately 1,000 words (by adulthood 70,000), create long adult-like sentences, and can carry on a conversation.

In the last half of the 20th century debate on the nature and acquisition of language was ignited by a highly publicized exchange between a strong learning theorist and a strong nativist. In 1957 the behavioral psychologist B. F. Skinner proposed that language was acquired through learning. In his book *Verbal Behavior* Skinner argued that language, like all animal behavior, was a learned behavior that developed in children as a function of external reinforcement and careful parental shaping. By Skinner's account infants learn language as a rat learns to press a bar—through monitoring and management of reward contingencies. The nativist Noam Chomsky, writing a review of *Verbal Behavior*, took a very different position. Chomsky argued that traditional reinforcement learning has little to do with humans' abilities to acquire language. Instead, every individual has an innate "language faculty" that includes a universal grammar and a universal phonetics; exposure to a specific language triggers a "selection" process for one language.

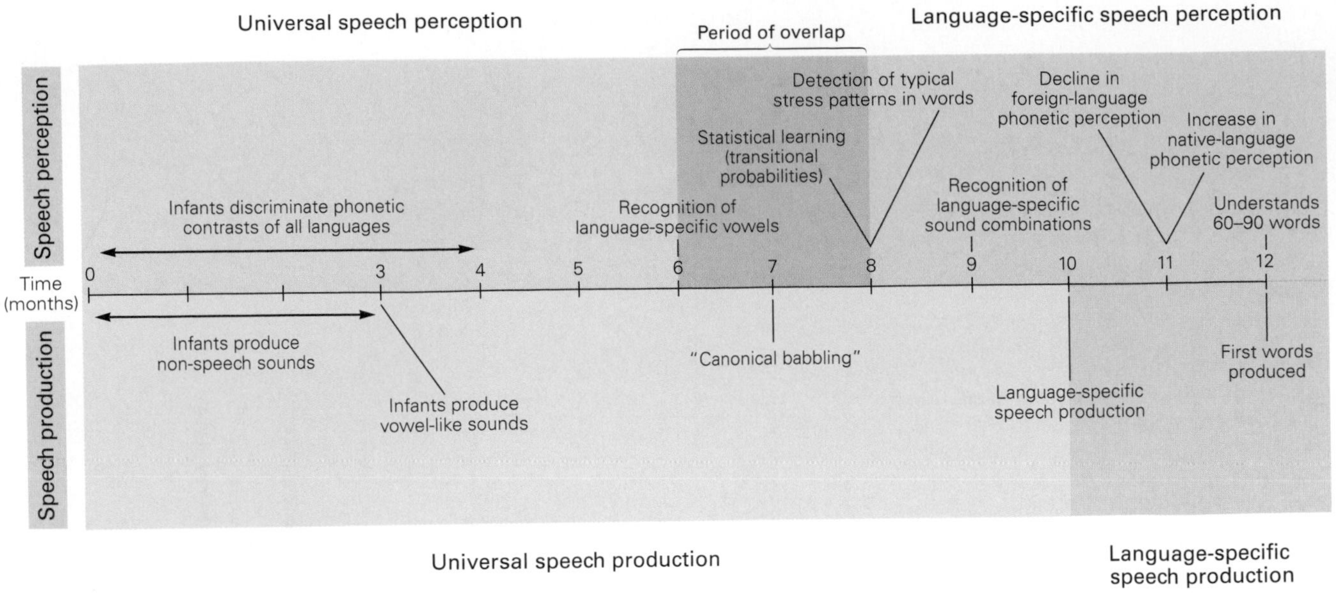

Figure 60–2 Language development progresses through a standard sequence in all children. Speech perception and production in children in various cultures initially follow a language-universal pattern. By the end of the first year of life, language-specific patterns emerge. Speech perception becomes language-specific before speech production. (Adapted, with permission, from Doupe and Kuhl 1999.)

More recent studies of language acquisition in infants and children have clearly demonstrated that the kind of learning going on in infancy does not resemble that described by Skinner with its reliance on external shaping and reinforcement. However, a nativist account such as Chomsky's, in which the language the infant hears triggers a choice among innate options, also does not capture the process.

The "Universalist" Infant Becomes Linguistically Specialized by Age 1 Year

In the early 1970s psychologist Peter Eimas showed that infants were especially good at hearing the acoustic changes that distinguish phonetic units in the world's languages. He showed that infants could discern slight acoustic changes at the boundaries between phonetic categories, and that they could do this for phonetic units in languages they had never experienced. The phenomenon is called *categorical perception*; adults have this ability only for phonetic units in languages in which they are fluent. Japanese people, for example, find it very difficult to hear the distinction between the American English /r/ and /l/ sounds. Both are perceived as Japanese /r/, and, as we have seen, Japanese speakers use the two sounds interchangeably when producing words.

Categorical perception was originally thought to occur only in humans, but in 1975 cognitive neuroscientist Patricia Kuhl showed that it exists in nonhuman mammals such as chinchillas and monkeys. Since then many studies have confirmed this result (as well as species differences). The studies suggest that the evolution of phonetic units was strongly influenced by preexisting auditory structures and capacities. Infants' ability to hear all possible differences in speech prepares them to learn any language; at birth they are linguistic "universalists."

Right before the onset of first words, infants' ability to discriminate nonnative phonetic units rapidly declines. By the end of the first year, infants fail to discriminate phonetic changes that they successfully recognized 6 months earlier. At the same time, infants become significantly more adept at hearing native-language phonetic distinctions. For example, when American and Japanese infants were tested between 6 and 12 months of age on the discrimination of the American English /r/ and /l/, American infants improved significantly between 8 and 10 months, whereas Japanese infants declined, suggesting that this is a sensitive period for phonetic learning.

Speech production develops simultaneously with speech perception (Figure 60–2). All infants, regardless of culture, produce sounds that are universal. Infants

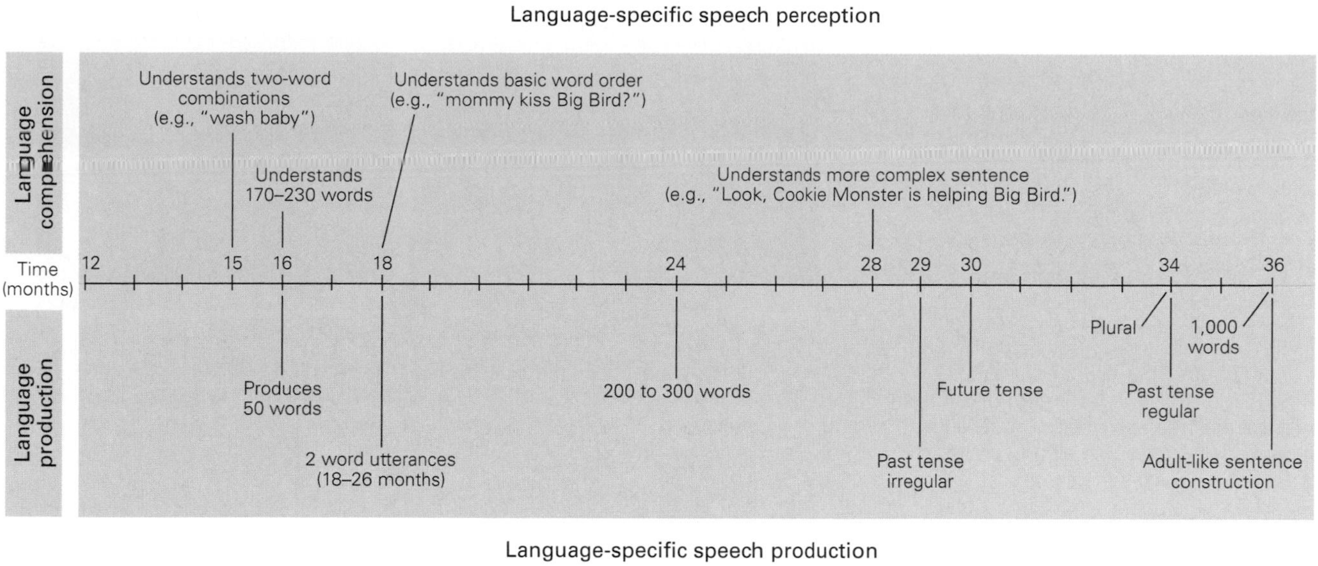

"coo" with vowel-like sounds at 3 months of age, and "babble" using consonant-vowel combinations at about 7 months of age. Toward the end of the first year language-specific patterns of speech production begin to emerge in infants' spontaneous utterances. As children approach the age of 2 years, they begin to mimic the sound patterns of their native language. Chinese toddlers' utterances reflect the pitch, rhythm, and phonetic structure of Mandarin, and the utterances of British toddlers sound distinctly British. Infants develop an ability to imitate the sounds they hear others produce as early as 20 weeks of age. Very early in development infants begin to master the subtle motor patterns required to produce their "mother tongue." Speech-motor patterns acquired in the earliest stages of language learning persist throughout life and influence the sounds, tempo, and rhythm of a second language learned later.

The second half of the first year appears to be a sensitive period for speech learning. If infants are exposed to a new language at this time, do they learn? Kuhl exposed American infants to Mandarin Chinese in the laboratory between 9 and 10 months of age and found that the infants learned if exposure occurred through interaction with a human being; infants exposed to the exact same material through television or audiotape with no live human interaction do not learn (Figure 60–3). When tested, the performance of the live-exposure group was statistically indistinguishable from that of infants raised in Taiwan who had listened to Mandarin for 10 months (Figure 60–3). These results established that at 9 months of age the right kind of exposure to a foreign language permits phonetic learning, supporting the view that this is a sensitive period for phonetic learning. The study also demonstrated, however, that social interaction appears to play an essential role in learning.

What causes the change in infants' perception between 6 and 12 months of age? Studies of infants suggest that early exposure to speech induces an implicit learning process that reduces the infant's initial ability to hear distinctions between foreign-language sounds. At 6 months of age infants begin to organize speech sounds into categories based on *phonetic prototypes*, ie, the most frequently occurring phonetic units in their language. Six-month-old infants in the United States and Sweden were tested with prototypical English and Swedish vowels to examine whether infants discriminated acoustic variations in the vowels, like those that occur when different talkers produce them. By 6 months of age the American and Swedish infants ignored acoustic variations around native-language prototypes. This "category perception" did not occur with nonnative prototypes. This explains why 11-month-old Japanese infants fail to discriminate English /r/ and /l/ after experience with Japanese. Brain imaging and behavioral tests on infants confirm this change between 7 and 11 months of age.

Language Uses the Visual System

Language is typically communicated through an auditory–vocal channel. However, deaf speakers communicate through a visual–manual channel. Natural

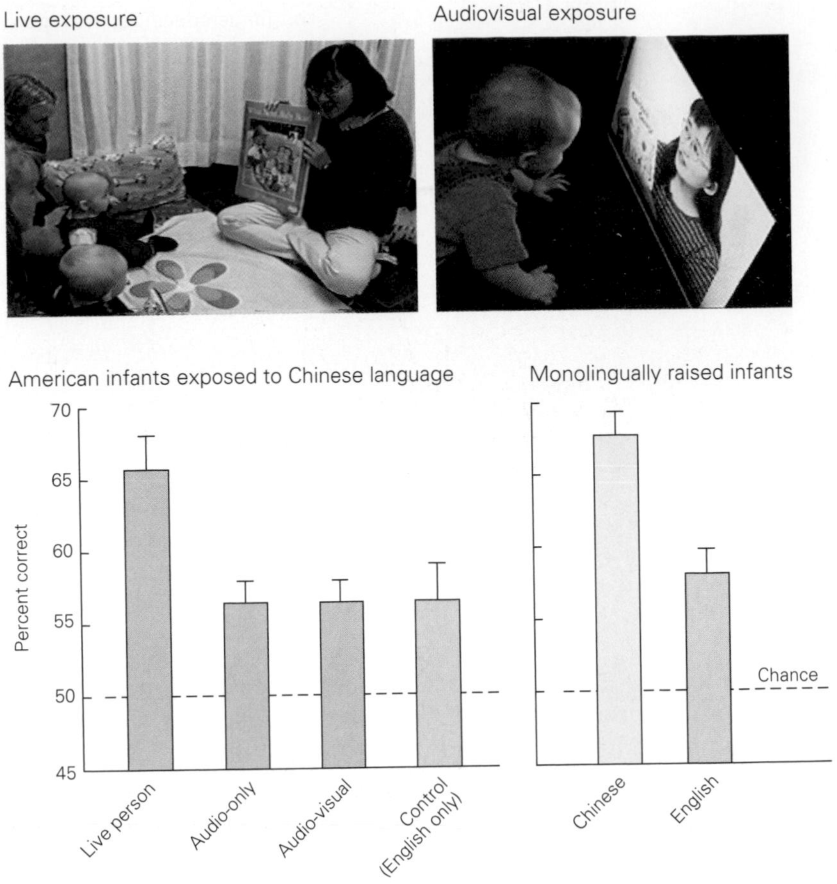

Figure 60–3 Infants can learn the phonemes of a nonnative language at 9 months of age. Three groups of American infants were exposed for the first time to a new language (Mandarin Chinese) in 12 25-minute sessions between the ages of 9 and 10.5 months. One group interacted with live native speakers of Mandarin; a second group was exposed to the identical material through television; and a third group heard tape recordings only. A control group had similar language sessions but heard only English. Performance on discrimination of Mandarin phonemes was tested in all groups after exposure (11 months). Only infants exposed to live Mandarin speakers discriminated the Mandarin phonemes. Infants exposed through TV or tapes showed no learning, and were indistinguishable from the controls (who heard only English). The performance of American infants exposed to live Mandarin speakers was equivalent to monolingual Taiwanese infants of the same age who had experienced Mandarin from birth. (Reproduced, with permission, from Kuhl, Tsao, and Liu 2003.)

signed languages, such as American Sign Language (Ameslan or ASL), are those invented by the deaf and vary across countries. Deaf infants "babble" with their hands at approximately the same time in development as hearing infants babble orally. Other developmental milestones, such as first words and two-word combinations, also occur on the developmental timetable of hearing infants.

Additional studies indicate that visual information of another kind, the face of the talker, is not only very helpful for communication but also affects the everyday perception of speech. We all experience the benefits of "lip-reading" at noisy parties—watching speakers' mouth movements helps us understand speech in a noisy environment. The most compelling laboratory demonstration that vision plays a role in everyday speech perception is the illusion that results when discrepant speech information is sent to the visual and auditory modalities. When subjects hear the sound /ba/ while watching a person pronounce "ga," they report hearing an intermediate articulation /da/. Such demonstrations support the idea that speech categories are defined both auditorily and visually, and that perception is governed by both sight and sound.

Prosodic Cues Assist Learning of Words and Sentences

Long before infants recognize that things and events in the world have names, they memorize the global sound patterns typical in their language. Infants use the *prosodic* cues in speech—the pitch, duration, and loudness changes—that occur in words to learn these patterns. In English, for example, a strong/weak pattern of stress is typical—as in the words "BAby," "MOMmy," "TAble," and "BASEball"—whereas in other languages a weak/strong pattern predominates. Six and 9-month-old infants given a listening choice between words in English or Dutch show a listening preference for native-language words at the age of 9 months (but not at six months).

Prosodic cues convey both linguistic information (differences in intonation and tone in languages such as Chinese) and paralinguistic information, such as the emotional state of the speaker. Even in utero infants learn by listening to the prosody of speech produced by their mothers. Certain sounds are transmitted through bone conduction to the womb; these are typically intense (above 80 dB), low-frequency sounds (particularly below 300 Hz, but as high as 1,000 Hz with some attenuation). Thus the prosodic patterns of speech, including voice pitch and the stress and intonation patterns characteristic of a particular language and speaker, are transmitted to the fetus, while the sound patterns that convey phonetic units and words are greatly attenuated. At birth infants demonstrate learning that depends on this prosodic information by showing listening preferences for (a) the language spoken by their mothers during pregnancy, (b) their mother's voice over that of another female, and (c) stories with a distinct tempo and rhythm read by the mother during the last 10 weeks of pregnancy.

Infants Use Transitional Probabilities to Identify Words in Continuous Speech

Seven- to 8-month-old infants recognize words using the probability that one syllable will follow another. The transitional probabilities between syllables in a word are high because the sequential order remains constant. In the word *potato,* for example, the syllable "ta" always follows the syllable "po" (probability of 1.0). Transitional probabilities between words, as between "hot" and "po" in the string "hot potato," are much lower.

Jenny Saffran showed that infants treat phonetic units and syllables with high transitional probabilities as word-like units. In one experiment infants heard 2-minute strings of pseudo-words, such as *tibudo, pabiku, golatu,* and *daropi,* without any acoustic breaks between them. They were then tested for recognition of these pseudo-words as well as new ones formed by combining the last syllable of one word with the two initial syllables of another word (such as *tudaro* formed from gola*tu* and *daro*pi). Infants recognized the original pseudo-words, indicating that they use the transitional probabilities to identify words.

These forms of learning clearly do not involve Skinnerian reinforcement. Caretakers do not manage the contingencies and gradually, through reinforcement strategies, shape the statistical analyses performed by infants. Conversely, language learning by infants also does not appear to reflect a process in which innately provided options are chosen based on language experience. Rather, infants learn language through detailed and sophisticated analysis of the language they hear, an analysis that reveals to them patterns of variation in natural language. The learning of these patterns in turn alters perception to favor the native language. What infants learn is constrained by the architecture of the brain, and language evolved to capitalize on infant learning. This mirrors the argument that the development of phonetic units was significantly influenced by the features of mammalian hearing, ensuring that infants would find it easy to discriminate phonemes, the fundamental units of meaning in language.

There Is a Critical Period for Language Learning

Children learn language more naturally and efficiently than adults, a paradox given that the cognitive skills of adults are superior. Why should this be the case?

Many consider language acquisition to be an example of a skill that is learned best during a *critical period* in development. Eric Lenneburg proposed that maturational factors at puberty caused a change in the neural mechanisms that control language acquisition. Evidence supporting this view comes from classic studies of Chinese and Korean immigrants to the United States who were immersed in English at ages ranging from 3 to 39 years. When asked to identify errors in sentences containing grammatical mistakes, an easy task for native speakers, second-language learners' performance declined with the age of arrival in the United States. A similar trend emerges when one compares individuals exposed to ASL from birth to those exposed between 5 and 12 years of age. Those exposed from birth were best at identifying errors in ASL, those exposed at age 5 were slightly poorer, and those exposed after the age of 12 years were substantially poorer.

What restricts our ability to learn a new language after puberty? Developmental studies suggest that prior learning plays a role. Learning a native language produces a *neural commitment* to detection of the acoustic patterns of that language, and this commitment interferes with later learning of a second language. Early exposure to language results in neural circuitry that is "tuned" to detect the phonetic units and prosodic patterns of that language. Neural commitment to native language enhances the ability to detect patterns based on those already learned (eg, phonetic learning supports word learning), but reduces the ability to detect patterns that do not conform. Learning the motor patterns required to speak a language also results in neural commitment. The motor patterns learned for one language are often incompatible with those required for pronunciation of the second language and thus can interfere with efforts to pronounce the second language without an accent.

Early in life two or more languages can be easily learned because interference effects are minimal until neural patterns are well established. We know little about how the brain handles the representation of two distinct languages when presented with both initially. The currently favored position is that experience, as well as maturation, are the major factors leading to the developmental critical period for language. Maturation can set the time when the window for learning "opens," but experience can be primarily responsible for determining when the window "closes." Both factors—a maturational development that enables learning and the neural commitment that results from learning—likely operate together to constrain learning a new language later in life.

We do not completely lose the ability later in life to learn a new language. Regardless of the age at which learning begins, second-language learning is improved by a training regime that mimics critical components of early learning—long periods of listening in a social context (immersion), the use of both auditory and visual information, and exposure to simplified and exaggerated speech resembling "motherese."

"Motherese" Enhances Language Learning

Everyone agrees that when adults talk to their children they sound unusual. Discovered by linguists and anthropologists in the early 1960s as they listened to languages spoken around the world, "motherese" (or "parentese," as fathers produce it as well) is a special speaking style used when addressing infants and young children. Motherese has a higher pitch, slower tempo, and exaggerated intonation contours, and is easily recognized.

Compared to adult-directed speech, the pitch of the voice is increased on average by an octave both in males and in females. Phonetic units are spoken more clearly and are acoustically exaggerated, thus increasing the acoustic separation of phonetic units. Adults speaking to infants exaggerate just those features of speech that are critical to their native language. Chinese mothers, for example, exaggerate the four tones in Mandarin that are critical to word meaning in Chinese. Evidence suggests that motherese does in fact assist infants' discrimination of phonetic units.

Infants prefer listening to infant-directed rather than adult-directed speech when given a choice. When infants are allowed to activate recordings of infant-directed or adult-directed speech, by turning left or right, they will turn in whatever direction is required to turn on infant-directed speech.

Several Cortical Regions Are Involved in Language Processing

Language Circuits in the Brain Were First Identified in Studies of Aphasia

Details of the neural basis of language first became apparent in the study of acquired language disorders known as aphasias. Focal brain lesions brought about by cerebrovascular diseases (stroke), head injury, and degenerative diseases such as Alzheimer and Pick disease cause the aphasias. Because language is unique to humans, animal models of language cannot be developed, and the study of aphasia remains an important source of information for elucidating the neural underpinnings of language.

The neural basis of language processing was first outlined in studies of the aphasias in the second half of the 19th century in France by Pierre Paul Broca and in Germany by Karl Wernicke. Based on their work and that of others, Wernicke formulated a model of neural processing of language (see Chapter 1). Most elements of this early model have stood the test of time. Prominent among these is the notion that in most individuals language processing depends more on structures in the left hemisphere than on those of the right. The left cerebral hemisphere is dominant for language in a majority of right-handed individuals and in a smaller but significant majority of left-handed individuals. Regardless of handedness, in more than 95% of individuals the grammar, lexicon, phonemic assembly, and phonetic production of language depend on the left hemisphere. Languages that rely on visual-motor signs rather than on auditory speech—signed languages such as ASL—also depend on the left hemisphere.

The early study of aphasia also revealed that damage to two brain areas, known as Broca's area in the left lateral frontal region and Wernicke's area in the left posterior superior temporal lobe, was associated with distinct profiles of language disorder, respectively Broca aphasia and Wernicke aphasia.

The Left Hemisphere Is Specialized for Phonetic, Word, and Sentence Processing

Although the conclusion that "we speak with the left hemisphere" is incontrovertible, the origin of that functional separation of the hemispheres during development is unclear. Whether left hemisphere specialization for language derives from a general tendency for the left hemisphere to engage in analytic processing or is a specific linguistic specialization is not known. Studies by neuroscientist Helen Neville have shown that the left hemisphere is activated not only by auditory stimuli but also by visual stimuli that have linguistic significance. Deaf individuals process visual information in the speech-processing regions of the left hemisphere. Such studies suggest that the speech-related regions of the left hemisphere are well suited to processing expression independent of the modality.

When in development does the left hemisphere become dominant in language processing? Evidence from a variety of sources suggests that left hemisphere specialization for language develops rapidly in infancy. We do not know if left hemisphere dominance for language is present at birth or whether experience with language is required to produce differentiation of the hemispheres; neuroimaging studies on this issue are in progress.

Prosody Engages Both Right and Left Hemispheres Depending on the Information Conveyed

Prosodic information can be linguistic, conveying semantic meaning as tones do in Mandarin Chinese or Thai, and also paralinguistic, expressing our attitudes and emotions. The pitch of the voice carries both kinds of information, and the brain's processing of each kind of information differs. Emotional changes in pitch engage the right hemisphere, primarily in right frontal and temporal regions. A different pattern of brain activity occurs when pitch is used to convey semantic information.

A number of neuroimaging studies have investigated the neural processing of semantic tone. In Thai speakers, for example, the left frontal lobe is consistently activated in response to changes in tone (Figure 60–4). In speakers of a non-tonal language, such as native speakers of American English, or speakers who use tone differently than do Thai speakers, such as Mandarin Chinese speakers, the Thai words do not activate these left hemisphere regions (Figure 60–4).

The fact that the left hemisphere plays the dominant role in phonemic and grammatical processing does not mean that the right hemisphere plays no role in language. Right hemisphere processing of emotional information helps convey a speaker's mood and intentions, and this helps interpret sentence meaning. Patients with right hemisphere lesions often produce speech with inappropriate stress, timing, and intonation, and their speech sounds emotionally flat; they also frequently fail to interpret the emotional cues in others' speech.

The right hemisphere also plays a role in discourse. Patients with damage in the right hemisphere have difficulty ordering sentences into a coherent narrative. They also have difficulty comprehending meaning when the full meaning depends on the relationships among sentences rather than on each sentence taken in isolation. For this reason these patients often fail to understand jokes, and this has an impact in their social lives.

Language Processing in Bilinguals Depends on Age of Acquisition and Language Use

How are multiple languages represented in the human brain? Modern neuroimaging techniques allow bilingual processing to be studied more directly and in greater detail than in earlier studies. They show that both the age at which a second language is acquired and the degree of proficiency in the second language affect how the brain processes multiple languages. In "late" bilinguals (those who learned a second language in adulthood) the second language and native language are processed in spatially separated areas in the language-sensitive left frontal region. In "early" bilinguals (those who acquired both languages as children) the two languages are processed in the same area.

The Model for the Neural Basis of Language Is Changing

On the basis of new observations and the contribution of Norman Geschwind in the 1960s, neurologists further developed Wernicke's model for the neural basis of language. In this revised model, which came to be known as the Wernicke-Geschwind model, Wernicke's area was presumed to analyze the acoustic signals making up words, while Broca's area organized the articulation of speech. The arcuate fasciculus was assumed to be a unidirectional pathway that helped speech production by bringing information from Wernicke's area to Broca's.

In the model both Wernicke's and Broca's areas interact with association areas. Acoustic cues contained in a spoken word are processed by the auditory pathways and reach Wernicke's area, where the meaning of a word is elaborated and then conveyed to higher brain structures, for example in sectors of the inferior parietal cortex. Eventually such patterns are converted into acoustic patterns and transferred by the arcuate fasciculus into Broca's area and turned into vocalizations.

In this model the ability to read and write also depends on Wernicke's and Broca's areas. In the case of reading, Wernicke's area receives signals from areas of visual cortex on the left and activates the corresponding auditory patterns. In the case of writing, auditory activity that represents these patterns is converted into motor outputs in the premotor region (Exner's area) just above Broca's area.

For several years the Wernicke-Gerschwind model provided a useful framework for the investigation of the neural basis of language processes. It also formed the basis for a practical classification of the aphasias that clinical neurologists still use today (Table 60–1). However, details of the model were called into question by the advent of structural magnetic resonance imaging, and the development of psycholinguistics.

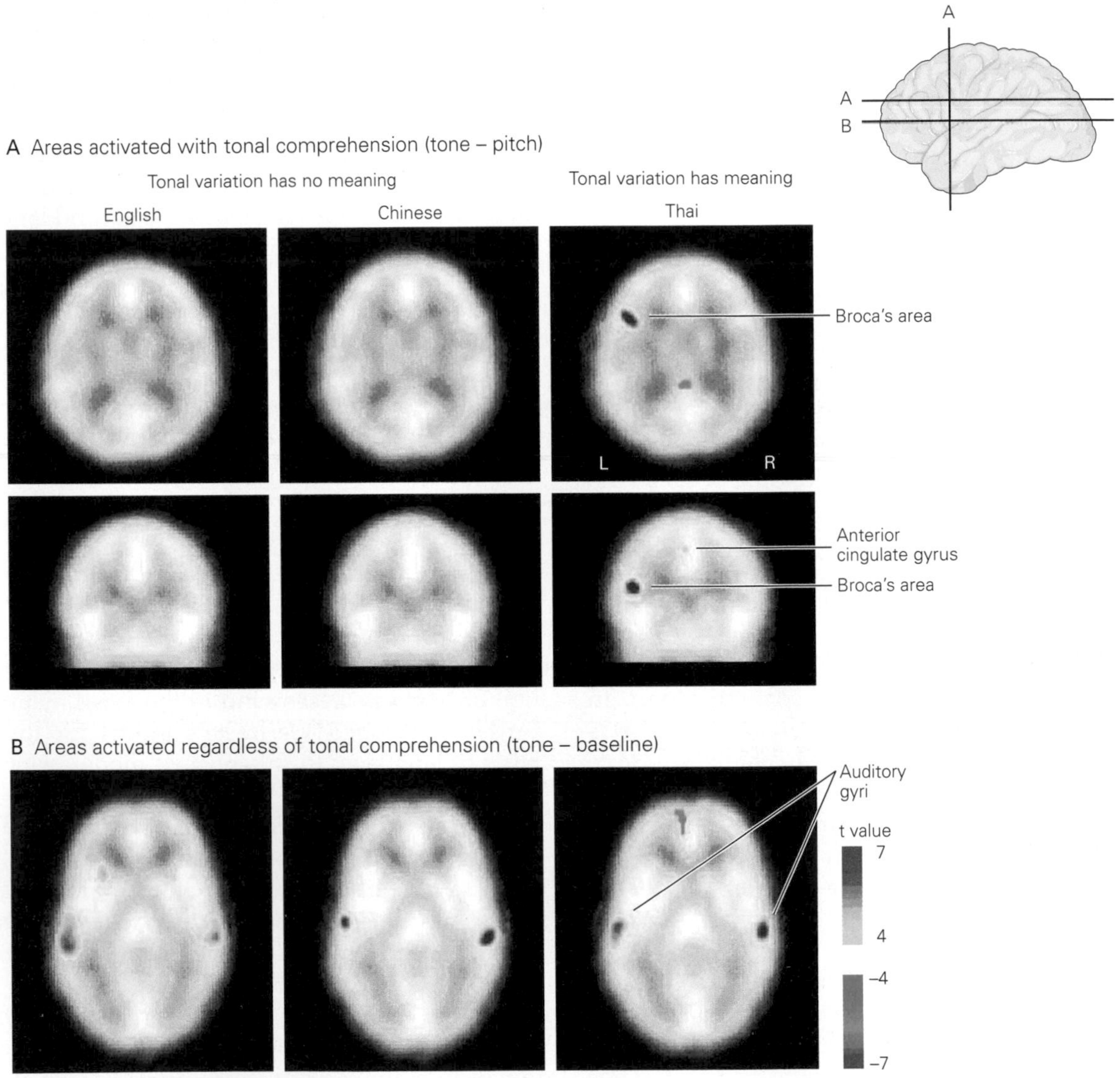

Figure 60–4 Brain activity patterns differ in speakers of tonal and nontonal languages. Positron emission tomography (PET) images show that cerebral blood flow (CBF) differs in Thai, Mandarin Chinese, and American English subjects listening to Thai variations in tone. (Reproduced, with permission, from Gandour et al. 2000.)

A. Only Thai listeners have CBF increases in the left Broca's area and also in the anterior cingulate gyrus. "Tone – pitch" means that the tone task and the pitch task are being compared using the standard subtraction technique (tone activation minus pitch activation). There is relatively more activation in the tone task compared to the pitch task (the pitch task was used as the reference baseline).

B. The "tone – baseline" condition compares the tone task with a "resting" condition, which is also standard procedure in these studies. All three groups show similar CFB increases in the auditory gyri.

Table 60–1 Differential Diagnosis of the Main Types of Aphasia

Type of aphasia	Speech	Comprehension	Capacity for repetition	Other signs	Region affected
Broca	Nonfluent, effortful	Largely preserved for single words and grammatically simple sentences	Impaired	Right hemiparesis (arm > leg); patient aware of defect and can be depressed	Left posterior frontal cortex and underlying structures
Wernicke	Fluent, abundant, well articulated, melodic	Impaired	Impaired	No motor signs; patient can be anxious, agitated, euphoric, or paranoid	Left posterior superior and middle temporal cortex
Conduction	Fluent with some articulatory defects	Intact or largely preserved	Impaired	Often none; patient can have cortical sensory loss or weakness in right arm	Left superior temporal and supramarginal gyri
Global	Scant, nonfluent	Impaired	Impaired	Right hemiplegia	Massive left perisylvian lesion
Transcortical motor	Nonfluent, explosive	Intact or largely preserved	Intact or largely preserved	Sometimes right-sided weakness	Anterior or superior to Broca's area
Transcortical sensory	Fluent, scant	Impaired	Intact or largely preserved	No motor signs	Posterior or inferior to Wernicke's area

Functional imaging techniques and the direct recording of electrical potentials from the exposed cerebral cortex of patients undergoing surgery for epilepsy opened the possibility for conducting studies in normal individuals engaged in language tasks, and the results of such studies led to revisions of the model.

Together the new approaches have contributed to a better definition of the neural systems responsible for language. The roles of Wernicke's and Broca's areas have expanded, and the arcuate fasciculus is now known to be a bidirectional tract that interconnects larger areas of sensory cortex with prefrontal and premotor areas. Just as importantly, additional areas of the left hemisphere have been found to be involved in language processing. These new areas are located in association areas of the left frontal, temporal, and parietal regions, which appear to provide connections between the processing of concepts and words. Other areas in prefrontal and cingulate areas are thought to exert executive control and mediate working-memory and attentional processes. An additional locus of speech production has been identified in the left insular region. In brief, in the revised version of the model the processing of language requires a far larger network of brain areas than was contemplated earlier.

As suggested by Hanna and Antonio Damasio, the new evidence indicates that three large systems interact to connect language reception and production with conceptual knowledge. Broca's and Wernicke's areas, selected sectors of insular cortex, and the basal ganglia form one system, a language *implementation system*. This system analyzes incoming auditory signals so as to activate conceptual knowledge and also supports phonemic and grammatical construction and controls speech production. It is anatomically surrounded by a second system, a *mediational system*, made up of numerous separate regions in the temporal, parietal, and frontal association areas. These regions act as brokers between the implementation system and a third system, a *conceptual system*, a collection of regions distributed throughout the association areas. In sum, a picture is emerging of a more complex neural network specialized in language processing (Figure 60–5).

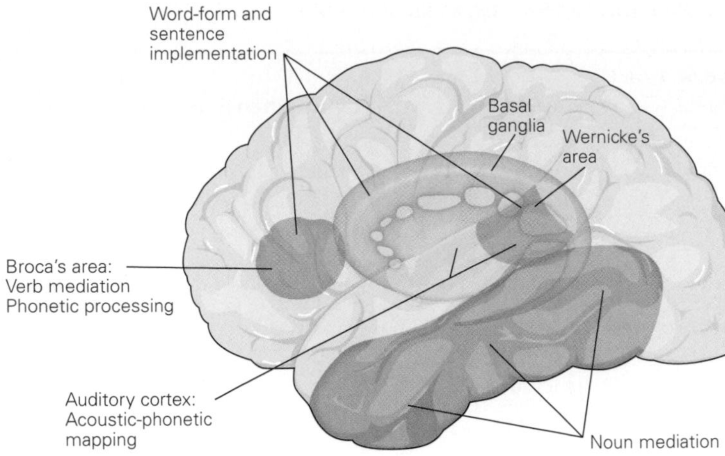

Figure 60–5 Language processing involves distributed neural networks. Imaging studies show that language processing involves a more complex and distributed network than previously thought. Particular brain areas are specialized for processing at the phonetic, word, or sentence level.

Brain Injuries Responsible for the Aphasias Provide Important Insights into Language Processing

Broca Aphasia Results from a Large Lesion in the Left Frontal Lobe

Broca aphasia is a disorder of speech production that includes impairments of grammatical processing. Patients have labored and slow speech, articulation is impaired, and the melodic intonation of normal speech is lacking (Table 60–2). Yet patients sometimes have considerable success at verbal communication even when they are difficult to understand because their selection of certain types of words, especially nouns, is often correct. By contrast, verbs as well as grammatical words such as prepositions and conjunctions are poorly selected or can be missing altogether. Another major sign of Broca aphasia is a defect in the ability to repeat complex sentences spoken by the examiner. In general, patients with Broca aphasia give the impression that they comprehend the words and sentences they hear, but suitable tests reveal that comprehension is incomplete.

Because most patients with Broca aphasia give the impression of understanding conversational speech, the condition was initially thought to be a deficit of production only. But Broca aphasics only comprehend sentences whose meaning can be derived from the meaning of the words used. They have difficulty comprehending sentences with meanings that depend mostly on grammar. Broca aphasics can understand *The apple that the girl ate was green* but have trouble understanding *The girl that the boy is chasing is tall*. This is because the patients can understand the first sentence without recourse to grammatical rules—girls eat apples, but apples do not eat girls; apples can be green, but girls cannot. The patients have difficulty with the second sentence, however, because both girls and boys can be tall, and either can chase the other. To understand the second sentence it is necessary to analyze its grammatical structure, something that Broca aphasics have difficulty doing.

Broca aphasia results from damage to Broca's area (the inferior left frontal gyrus, which contains Brodmann's areas 44 and 45); surrounding frontal fields (the external aspect of Brodmann's area 6, and areas 8, 9, 10, and 46); the underlying white matter, insula, and basal ganglia (Figure 60–6); and a small portion of the anterior superior temporal gyrus. A small sector of the insula, an island of cortex buried deep inside the cerebral hemisphere, can also be included in the correlates of Broca's aphasia. This is because patients who have lesions in a small part of the left insula have difficulty pronouncing phonemes in their proper order. They usually produce combinations of sounds that are very close to the target word, suggesting that they have trouble coordinating the articulatory movements necessary for speech. They have no difficulty perceiving speech sounds or recognizing their own errors and no trouble in finding words.

The structures damaged in Broca aphasia are part of a neural network involved in both the assembly of phonemes into words and the assembly of words into sentences. The network is presumably specialized for relational aspects of language, which include the grammatical structure of sentences and the proper use of grammatical vocabulary and verbs. The other

Table 60–2 Examples of Spontaneous Speech Production and Repetition for the Primary Types

Type of aphasia	Spontaneous speech	Repetition
	Stimulus (Western Aphasia Battery picnic picture): What do you see in this picture?	Stimulus: "The pastry cook was elated."
Broca	"O, yea. Det's a boy an' a girl . . . an' . . . a . . . car . . . house . . . light po' (pole). Dog an' a . . . boat. 'N det's a . . . mm . . . a coffee, an' reading. Det's a mm . . . a . . . det's a boy . . . fishin.'" (Elapsed time: 1 min 30 s)	"Elated."
Wernicke	"Ah, yes, it's, ah . . . several things. It's a girl . . . uncurl . . . on a boat. A dog . . .' S is another dog . . . Uh-oh . . . long's . . . on a boat. The lady, it's a young lady. An' a man a They were eatin.' 'S be place there. This . . . a tree! A boat. No, this is a . . . It's a house. Over in here . . . a cake. An' it's, it's a lot of water. Ah, all right. I think I mentioned about that boat. I noticed a boat being there. I did mention that before . . . Several things down, different things down . . . a bat . . . a cake . . . you have a . . ." (Elapsed time: 1 min 20 s)	"/I/ . . . no . . . In a fog."
Conduction	"Kay. I see a guy readin' a book. See a women /ka . . . he . . . /pourin' drink or something.' An' they're sittin' under a tree. An' there's a . . . car behind that an' then there's a house behind th' car. An' on the other side, the guy's flyn' a /fait . . . fait/(kite) See a dog there an' a guy down on the bank. See a flag blowin' in the wind. Bunch of /hi . . . a . . . /trees in behind. An a sailboat on th' river, river . . . lake. 'N guess that's about all . . . 'Basket there." (Elapsed time: 1 min 5 s)	"The baker was . . . What was that last word?" ("Let me repeat it: The pastry cook was elated.") "The baker-er was / vaskerin/ . . . uh . . ."
Global	(Grunt)	(No response)

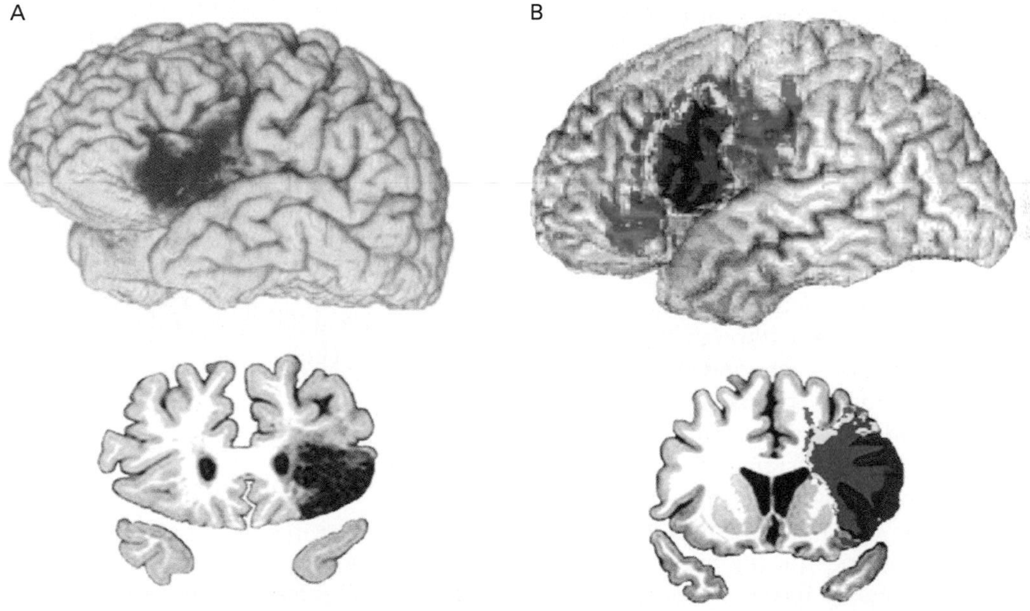

Figure 60–6 **Sites of lesions in Broca aphasia.** (Reproduced, with permission, from Hanna Damasio.)

A. **Top:** Three-dimensional MRI reconstruction of a lesion (an infarction) in the left frontal operculum (**dark gray**) in a patient with Broca aphasia. **Bottom:** Coronal MRI section of the same brain through the damaged area.

B. **Top:** Three-dimensional MRI overlap of lesions in 13 patients with Broca aphasia (**red** indicates that lesions in five or more patients share the same pixels). **Bottom:** Coronal MRI section of the same composite brain image through the damaged area.

cortical components of the network are located in lateral areas of the left frontal cortex (Brodmann's areas 47, 46, 9), the left parietal cortex (areas 40, 39), and sensorimotor areas above the Sylvian fissure between Broca's and Wernicke's regions (lower sector of areas 3, 1, 2, and 4). The critical subcortical component is in the left basal ganglia (head of the caudate nucleus and putamen). When damage is restricted to Broca's area alone or to its subjacent white matter, the result is the condition of Broca's area aphasia, a milder version of true Broca aphasia from which many patients are able to recover.

Wernicke Aphasia Results from Damage to Left Posterior Temporal Lobe Structures

The speech of patients with Wernicke aphasia is effortless, melodic, and produced at a normal rate, and is thus quite unlike that of patients with true Broca aphasia. The content of the speech, however, is often unintelligible because of frequent errors in the choice of words and phonemes, the order of which determines the word (Table 60–2).

Patients with Wernicke aphasia often shift the order of individual sounds and sound clusters, and add or subtract them to a word in a manner that distorts the intended phonemic plan. These errors are called *phonemic paraphasias* (paraphasia refers to any substitution of an erroneous phoneme or entire word for the intended, correct one). When phoneme shifts occur frequently and in close temporal proximity, words become unintelligible. Even when individual sounds are normally produced, Wernicke aphasics have great difficulty selecting words that accurately represent their intended meaning (known as a verbal or semantic paraphasia). For example, a patient might say *headman* when he means *president*.

Wernicke aphasics have difficulty comprehending the sentences uttered by others. Although this deficit is suggested by the Wernicke-Geschwind model, Wernicke's area is no longer seen as the center of auditory comprehension. The modern view is that Wernicke's area is part of a system that associates speech sounds with concepts. This system includes, in addition to Wernicke's area, the many parts of the brain that subserve grammar, attention, and the knowledge that is the source of the meanings of the words in the sentences.

Wernicke aphasia is usually caused by damage to the posterior section of the left auditory association cortex (Brodmann's area 22), although in severe and persisting cases there is involvement of the middle temporal gyrus and deep white matter (Figure 60–7).

Conduction Aphasia Results from Damage to a Specific Sector of Posterior Language Areas

Patients with conduction aphasia comprehend simple sentences and produce intelligible speech. However, like Broca and Wernicke aphasias, they cannot repeat sentences verbatim, they cannot assemble phonemes effectively (and thus produce many phonemic paraphasias) and cannot easily name pictures and objects. Speech production and auditory comprehension are less compromised than in the two other major aphasias (Table 60–2).

Persistent conduction aphasia is caused by damage to the left superior temporal gyrus and the inferior parietal lobe (Brodmann's areas 39 and 40). The damage can extend to the left primary auditory cortex (Brodmann's areas 41 and 42), the insula, and the underlying white matter.

A recent study by Buchsbaum and colleagues points to a specific subterritory, area Spt located at the boundary of areas 39 and 40, as the region of maximal lesion overlap in cases of conduction aphasia. Area Spt exhibits both auditory and motor responses. In brief, no evidence supports Wernicke's idea that conduction aphasia is caused by a simple interruption or disconnection of the arcuate fasciculus alone. The damage does compromise white matter, as Wernicke predicted, and destroys feed-forward and feedback projections that interconnect areas of temporal, parietal, insular, and frontal cortex. This connectional system seems to be part of the network required to assemble phonemes into words and to coordinate speech articulation.

In spite of the fact that the exact anatomical correlates of conduction aphasia are being revised and that the mechanism of the defect now appears more complex than that proposed in the Wernicke-Geschwind model, it is interesting to note that Wernicke correctly predicted both the main signs of the syndrome and the approximate location of the correlated lesion. The general model still holds.

Global Aphasia Results from Widespread Damage to Several Language Centers

Global aphasics are almost completely unable to comprehend language or formulate and repeat sentences, thus combining features of Broca, Wernicke, and conduction aphasias. Speech is reduced to a few words at best. The same word might be used repeatedly, appropriately or not, in a vain attempt to communicate an idea. Nondeliberate ("automatic") speech may be preserved, however. This includes stock expletives (which are used appropriately and with normal phonemic,

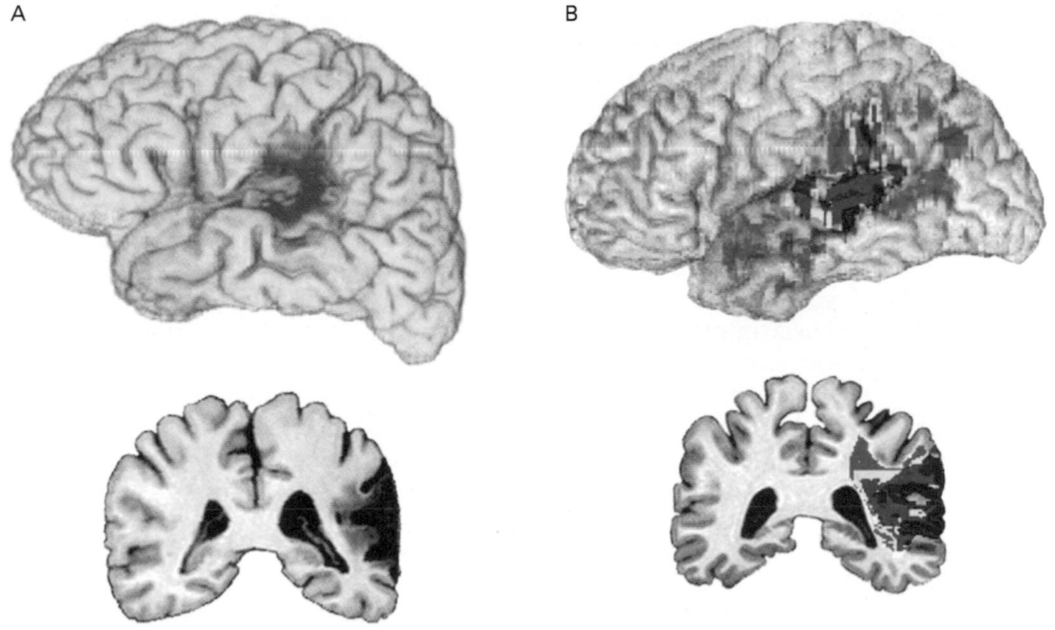

Figure 60–7 Sites of lesions in Wernicke aphasia.

A. **Top:** Three-dimensional MRI reconstruction of a lesion (an infarction) in the left posterior and superior temporal cortex (**dark gray**) in a patient with Wernicke aphasia. **Bottom:** Coronal MRI section of the same brain through the damaged area.

B. **Top:** Three-dimensional MRI overlap of lesions in 13 patients with Wernicke aphasia, obtained with the MAP-3 technique (**red** indicates that five or more lesions share the same pixels). **Bottom:** Coronal MRI section of the same composite brain image through the damaged area.

phonetic, and inflectional structures), routines such as counting or reciting the days of the week, and the ability to sing previously learned melodies and their lyrics. Auditory comprehension is limited to a small number of words and idiomatic expressions.

Classic global aphasia is accompanied by weakness in the right side of the face and paralysis of the right limbs. It involves damage in three regions: damage to the anterior language region and the basal ganglia and insula, leading to Broca aphasia; damage to the auditory areas of cortex, leading to conduction aphasia; and damage to the posterior language regions, producing Wernicke aphasia. Such widespread damage can only be caused by a stroke in the region supplied by the middle cerebral artery (Appendix C).

Transcortical Aphasias Result from Damage to Areas Near Broca's and Wernicke's Areas

The Wernicke-Geschwind model predicts that aphasias can be caused not only by damage to components of the language system but also to areas and pathways that connect those components to the rest of the brain. Patients with transcortical motor aphasia, such as Broca aphasics, speak nonfluently, but they can *repeat* sentences, even very long sentences.

Transcortical motor aphasia has been linked to damage to the left dorsolateral frontal area, a patch of association cortex anterior and superior to Broca's area, although there can be substantial damage to Broca's area itself. The left dorsolateral frontal cortex is involved in the allocation of attention and the maintenance of higher executive abilities, including the selection of words. For example, part of the left dorsolateral frontal cortex is activated in functional neuroimaging studies when subjects have to produce the names or actions associated with particular objects (eg, saying "kick" in response to "ball"), and damage to it leaves a patient unable to perform such a task, although they can produce words in ordinary conversation.

The aphasia can also be caused by damage to the left supplementary motor area, located high in the frontal lobe, directly in front of the primary motor cortex and buried mesially between the hemispheres. Electrical stimulation of the area in nonaphasic surgery patients causes the patients to make involuntary vocalizations or to be unable to speak, and functional neuroimaging studies have shown it to be activated in speech production. Thus the supplementary motor area appears to contribute to the initiation of speech, whereas the dorsolateral frontal regions contribute to ongoing control of speech, particularly when the task is difficult.

Transcortical sensory aphasics have fluent speech, impaired comprehension, and great trouble naming things. The aphasia differs from Wernicke aphasia in the same way that transcortical motor aphasia differs from Broca aphasia: Repetition is spared. In fact, patients with transcortical sensory aphasia might repeat and even make grammatical corrections in phrases and sentences they do not understand. The aphasia thus appears to be a deficit in semantic retrieval, without significant disruption of syntactic and phonological abilities.

Transcortical motor and sensory aphasias are believed to be caused by damage that spares the arcuate fasciculus. This would explain the sparing of repetition skills. Transcortical aphasias are thus the complement of conduction aphasia, behaviorally and anatomically. Transcortical sensory aphasia appears to be caused by damage to parts of the junction of the temporal, parietal, and occipital lobes, which connect the perisylvian language areas with the parts of the brain responsible for word meaning.

Finally, the growing attention given to degenerative brain conditions has permitted a characterization of the primary progressive aphasias (PPA). Their presentation tends to correspond to that of the classical aphasias. The main variants of PPA, as classified by Maria Luisa Gorno-Tempini and colleagues, are *nonfluent/agrammatic, semantic,* and *logopenic*.

The Classical Aphasias Have Not Implicated All Brain Areas Important for Language

The cortical sites damaged in the classical aphasias comprise only a portion of language-related areas in the brain. More recent research on aphasia has uncovered several other language-related regions in the cerebral cortex and in subcortical structures. For example, the anterior temporal and inferotemporal cortex have only recently become associated with language.

Damage to the *left* temporal cortex, in Brodmann's areas 21, 20, and 38, causes severe and pure naming defects—impairments of word retrieval without any accompanying grammatical, phonemic, or phonetic difficulty. When the damage is confined to the left temporal pole (Brodmann's area 38), the patient has difficulty recalling the names of unique places and persons but not names for common entities. When the lesions involve the mid temporal sector (areas 21 and 20), the patient has difficulty recalling both unique and common names. Finally, damage to the left posterior inferotemporal sector causes a deficit in recalling words for particular types of items—tools and utensils—but not words for natural things or unique entities. Recall of words for actions or spatial relationships is not compromised (Figure 60–8).

The left temporal cortex contains neural systems that hold the key to retrieving words denoting various categories of things ("tools," "eating utensils"), but not words denoting actions ("walking," "riding a bicycle"). These findings were obtained not only from studies of patients with brain lesions resulting from stroke, head injury, herpes encephalitis, and degenerative processes such as Alzheimer disease, but also from functional imaging studies of typical individuals and from electrical stimulation of these same temporal cortices during surgery.

Areas of frontal cortex in the mesial surface of the left hemisphere, which include the supplementary motor area and the anterior cingulate region (known as Brodmann's area 24), play an important role in the initiation and continuation of speech. Damage in these areas impairs the initiation of movement (akinesia) and causes mutism, a complete absence of speech. In aphasic patients the complete absence of speech is a rarity and is only seen during the very early stages of the condition. Patients with akinesia and mutism fail to communicate by words, gestures, or facial expression because the drive to communicate is impaired, not because the neural machinery of expression is damaged as in aphasia.

Damage to the left subcortical gray nuclei impairs grammatical processing in both speech and comprehension. The basal ganglia are closely interconnected with the frontal and parietal cortex and may have a role in assembling morphemes into words and words into sentences, just as they serve to assemble the components of complex movements into a smooth whole.

Certain brain lesions in adults can cause *alexia*, a disruption of the ability to read, or *agraphia*, a disruption of the ability to write (also known as word blindness). The two disorders may appear combined or separately, and they may or may not be associated with aphasia depending on the site of the causative lesion. Given the very recent emergence of writing (less than 5,000 years ago), and the even more recent emergence of near universal literacy (probably less than a century ago), it is unlikely that a special reading system evolved in the human brain in such a short period of evolutionary time. Therefore pure alexia without aphasia cannot be attributed to impairment of a

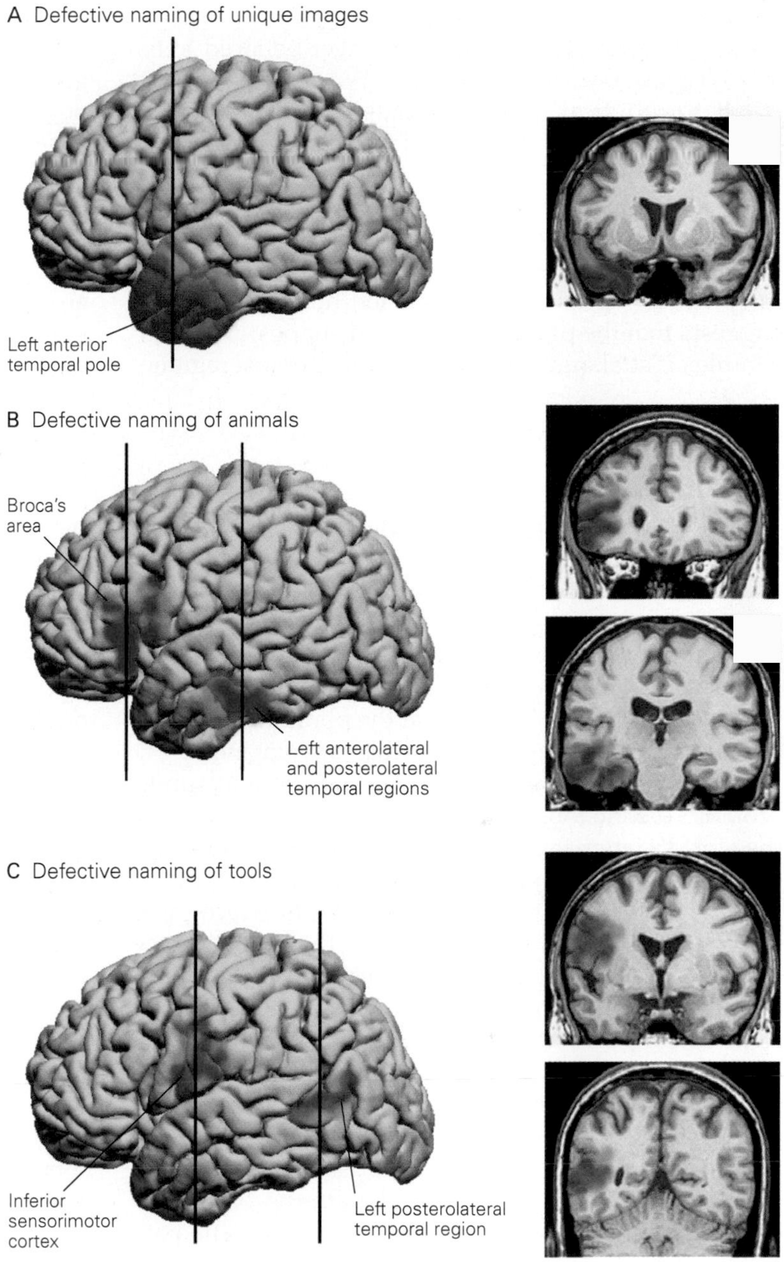

Figure 60–8 Regions of the brain other than Broca's and Wernicke's areas involved in language processing. The study used functional magnetic resonance imaging (fMRI) to study patients with selected brain lesions.

A. The left anterior temporal pole is the region of maximal overlap of lesions associated with impaired naming of unique images, such as the face of a person.

B. The left anterolateral and posterolateral temporal regions as well as Broca's region are the sites of maximal overlap of lesions associated with impaired naming of nonunique animals.

C. The left motor cortex and left posterolateral temporal cortex are the sites of maximal overlap of lesions associated with deficits in naming of tools.

special reading system in the brain, and is more likely to be caused by a disconnection between the visual and language systems.

Because vision is a bilateral brain process while language is lateralized, pure alexia requires a disruption in the transfer of visual information to the language areas of the left hemisphere. In 1892 the French neurologist Jules Dejerine studied an intelligent and highly articulate man who had recently lost the ability to read, even though he could spell, understand words spelled to him, copy written words, and recognize them after writing the individual letters. The patient could not see color in his right visual field, but his vision was otherwise intact in both visual fields.

Postmortem examination revealed damage in a region of the left occipital region that disrupted the transfer of visually related signals from *both* the left and right visual cortex to language areas in the left hemisphere. The postmortem also revealed some damage to the splenium, the posterior portion of the corpus callosum that interconnects left and right visual association cortices. This lesion is no longer believed to be involved in pure alexia, however. When the splenium is cut for surgical reasons without damaging visual cortices, patients can read words normally in the right visual field but not those in the left.

Functional imaging studies have shown that reading words and word-like shapes selectively activates extrastriate areas (secondary visual cortex) anterior to the primary visual cortex in the left hemisphere. This suggests that the processing of word shapes, like other complex visual qualities, requires that general region.

An Overall View

Advances in our understanding of language processing by the brain come from three sources: its acquisition in children, its study in typical individuals using noninvasive brain imaging techniques, and its dissolution in patients suffering brain injury. Studies on infants and children are demonstrating that children, even infants, master the details of language at the phonological, lexical, and syntactic levels very early in development.

Infants begin life capable of responding to subtle acoustic distinctions that cue phonetic differences in the world's languages, distinctions that likely capitalize on general auditory perceptual processes. Very rapidly, a powerful learning process causes infants to recognize statistical properties in the language they hear, allowing them to form phonetic categories, find words in the ongoing stream of discourse, and recognize the phrase structure of their native language, all before 10 months of age. Speech production takes a similar course, showing universal patterns early in life, which show differentiation by about 10 months of age. By the end of the first year, when the infant's first words appear, language learning evolves from universal patterns of speech perception and production to a language-specific pattern. Infant-directed speech ("motherese"), with its enhanced prosodic cues and its exaggerated phonetic units, may assist language learning in the young.

Early language learning being documented in experiments on infants and young children is unrelated to external reinforcement of the kind described by Skinner. Nor does it conform to the process described by Chomsky, by which innately provided options are chosen (or maintained) on the basis of experience. Infant language learning involves a more general sensory and cognitive ability that fine tunes the brain and alters both speech perception and production very early.

The processing of a native language differs from the processing of a foreign language. Taken together, studies show that highly diverse brain regions are involved in language processing and represent a progressive neural commitment to the features and properties of the native language. These findings, and studies of second language acquisition, suggest new models of the critical or sensitive period for language acquisition.

The difficulty in learning a second language later in life appears to be related to experience or expertise, in addition to age of acquisition. Language experience and use commit brain structure to patterns that reflect the primary language so that second language learning is difficult to the degree that it employs a totally different set of phonological and grammatical rules.

Behavioral and brain studies of infants and adults who have been systematically exposed to a foreign language are likely to elucidate the nature of the brain's plasticity for language over a lifetime. Studies of infants who are being raised in bilingual or trilingual homes are likely to answer questions about whether the human brain has limitless potential for language, or whether our ability to acquire multiple languages is constrained. These studies will not only advance our understanding of the neural basis of language but may elucidate general biological principles regarding human learning.

At the same time, studies on the nature of language dissolution in aphasia have made great progress since Broca's and Wernicke's seminal discoveries. They have given us a more complete understanding of linguistic processes and an appreciation of the complex ways in which they interconnect with systems for perception, motor control, conceptual knowledge, and intentions. The challenges to elucidating the neural basis of language remain formidable, although several developments offer the hope of continued progress in the near future.

Improvements in structural imaging will allow more precise and consistent delineation of lesions that affect specific features of language ability. Measurement of brain activity in typical subjects will become increasingly important in the future, as both the spatial and temporal resolution of these techniques improve and the experimental paradigms used to study language become more productive. Neurosurgical candidates whose brain functions must be mapped by stimulation during surgery or by recording from implanted electrode grids that remain in place during everyday activities will be an important source of fine-grained information.

Nevertheless, the data available from the past decade of research already suggest two important insights, as noted by Greg Hickok and David Poeppel: The recruitment of brain regions in language studies is highly dependent on the tasks used in the experiment, and language reception may be more bilaterally organized than previously appreciated.

A promising approach is to relate findings on the developmental time course of human language acquisition, plasticity for second language learning, and studies on language dissolution caused by brain trauma. Are the components of language that are learned earliest—those involving prosodic and phonetic learning in speech perception and production—most resistant to change when learning a second language, and also the least likely to suffer from the effects of trauma to the brain? Future research will address these issues.

Understanding the human capacity for language is important for the advancement of fundamental neuroscience and indispensable for the treatment of patients with aphasia, which is one of the most frequent impairments of higher function caused by stroke and head injury (the others are impairments of memory, emotion, and decision making). The astonishing feat of language is too complex to be understood with the tools of any single academic or medical specialty and, as several disciplines come together to study the underlying neural processes, we should expect further significant breakthroughs.

Patricia K. Kuhl
Antonio R. Damasio

Selected Readings

Damasio AR. 1992. Aphasia. N Engl J Med 326:531–539.

Damasio H, Grabowski TJ, Tranel D, Hichwa R, Damasio AR. 1996. A neural basis for lexical retrieval. Nature 380: 499–505.

Damasio H, Tranel D, Grabowski TJ, Adolphs R, Damasio AR. 2004. Neural systems behind word and concept retrieval. Cognition 92:179–229.

Doupe A, Kuhl PK. 1999. Birdsong and speech: common themes and mechanisms. Annu Rev Neurosci 22:567–631.

Gopnik A, Meltzoff AN, Kuhl PK. 2001. *The Scientist in the Crib: What Early Learning Tells Us About the Mind.* New York: Harper Collins.

Hauser M, Chomsky N, Fitch T. 2002. The faculty of language: what is it, who has it, and how did it evolve? Science 298:1569–1579.

Hickok G, Poeppel D. 2007. The cortical organization of speech processing. Nat Rev Neurosci 8:393–402.

Kuhl PK. 2004. Early language acquisition: cracking the speech code. Nat Rev Neurosci 5:831–843.

Kuhl PK, Rivera-Gaxiola M. 2008. Neural substrates of language acquisition. Annu Rev Neurosci 31:511–534.

Pinker S. 1994. *The Language Instinct.* New York: William Morrow.

References

Bates E, Wulfeck B, MacWhinney B. 1991. Cross-linguistic research in aphasia: an overview. Brain Lang 41:123–148.

Baynes K. 1990. Language and reading in the right hemisphere: highways or byways of the brain? J Cogn Neurosci 2:159–179.

Bishop DVM. 1983. Linguistic impairment after left hemidecortication for infantile hemiplegia. A reappraisal. Q J Exp Psychol 35A:199–207.

Broca P. 1861. Remarques sur le siegè de la faculté du langage articulé, suivies d'une observation d'aphemie (perte de la parole). Bull Société Anatomique de Paris 6:330–357.

Buchsbaum BR, Baldo J, Okada K, Berman KF, Dronkers N, D'Esposito M, Hickok G. 2011. Conduction aphasia, sensory-motor integreation, and phonological short-term memory—an aggregate analysis of lesion and fMRI data. Brain Lang 119:119–128.

Chomsky N. 1959. A review of B. F. Skinner's "Verbal Behavior." Language 35:26–58.

Cornell TL, Fromkin VA, Mauner G. 1993. A linguistic approach to language processing in Broca's aphasia: a paradox resolved. Curr Direct Psych Sci 2:47–52.

Damasio AR, Damasio H. 1992. Brain and language. Sci Am 267:89–95.

Damasio AR, Tranel D. 1993. Nouns and verbs are retrieved with differently distributed neural systems. Proc Natl Acad Sci U S A 90:4957–4960.

Dejerine J. 1892. Contribution a l'étude anatomopathologique et clinique des differentes varietés de cecité verbale. Memoires Soc Biol 4:61–90.

Dennis M, Whitaker HA. 1976. Language acquisition following hemidecortication: linguistic superiority of the left over the right hemisphere. Brain Lang 3:404–433.

Dronkers NF. 1996. A new brain region for coordinating speech articulation. Nature 384:159–161.

Eimas PD, Siqueland ER, Jusczyk P, Vigorito J. 1971. Speech perception in infants. Science 171:303–306.

Fernald A, Kuhl P. 1987. Acoustic determinants of infant preference for Motherese speech. Infant Behav Dev 10:279–293.

Flege JE. 1995. Second language speech learning: theory, findings, and problems. In: W. Strange (ed). *Speech Perception and Linguistic Experience*, pp. 233–277. Timonium, MD: York Press.

Flege JE, Yeni-Komshian GH, Liu S. 1999. Age constraints on second-language acquisition. J Mem Lang 41:78–104.

Fromkin V, Rodman R. 1997. *An Introduction to Language*, 6th ed. New York: Harcourt Brace Jovanovich.

Galaburda AM. 1994. Developmental dyslexia and animal studies: at the interface between cognition and neurology. Cognition 50:133–149.

Gandour J, Wong D, Hsieh L, Weinzapfel B, Van Lancker D, Hutchins GD. 2000. A crosslinguistic PET study of tone perception. J Cogn Neurosci 12:207–222.

Gardner H, Brownell H, Wapner W, Michelow D. 1983. Missing the point: the role of the right hemisphere in the processing of complex linguistic materials. In: E. Perecman (ed). *Cognitive Processes in the Right Hemisphere*, pp. 169–192. New York: Academic Press.

Geschwind N. 1970. The organization of language and the brain. Science 170:940–944.

Geschwind N. 1965. Disconnexion syndromes in animals and man. Brain 88:585–644.

Goodglass H. 1993. *Understanding Aphasia.* San Diego: Academic Press.

Gorno-Tempini ML, Hillis AE, Weintraub S, Kertesz A, Mendez M, Cappa SF, et al. 2011. Classification of primary progressive aphasia and its variants. Neurol 76: 1006–1014.

Imada T, Zhang Y, Cheour M, Tualal S, Ahonen A, Kuhl PK. 2006. Infant speech perception activates Broca's area: a developmental magnetoencephalography study. Neuroreport 17:957–962.

Iverson P, Kuhl PK, Akahane-Yamada R, Diesch E, Tohkura Y, Kettermann A, Siebert C. 2003. A perceptual interference account of acquisition difficulties for non-native phonemes. Cognition 87:B47–57.

Johnson J, Newport E. 1989. Critical period effects in sound language learning: the influence of maturation state on the acquisition of English as a second language. Cognit Psychol 21:60–99.

Jusczyk PW, Friederici AD, Wessels JMI, Svenkerud VY, Jusczyk AM. 1993. Infants' sensitivity to the sound patterns of native language words. J Mem Lang 32:402–420.

Knudsen EI. 2004. Sensitive periods in the development of the brain and behavior. J Cogn Neurosci 16:1412–1425.

Kuhl PK. 2000. A new view of language acquisition. Proc Natl Acad Sci U S A 97:11850–11857.

Kuhl PK, Andruski J, Christovich I, Chistovich L, Kozhevnikova E, Ryskina V, Stolyarova E, Sungberg U, Lacerda F. 1997. Cross-language analysis of phonetic units in language addressed to infants. Science 277:684–686.

Kuhl PK, Tsao F-M, Liu H-M. 2003. Foreign-language experience in infancy: effects of short-term exposure and social interaction on phonetic learning. Proc Natl Acad Sci U S A 100:9096–9101.

Kuhl PK, Williams KA, Lacerda F, Stevens KN, Lindblom B. 1992. Linguistic experience alters phonetic perception in infants by 6 months of age. Science 255:606–608.

Lenneberg E. 1967. *Biological Foundations of Language*. New York: Wiley.

Lesser RP, Arroyo S, Hart J, Gordon B. 1994. Use of subdural electrodes for the study of language functions. In: A. Kertesz (ed). *Localization and Neuro-Imaging in Neuropsychology*, pp. 57–72. San Diego: Academic Press.

Linebarger M, Schwartz M, Saffran E. 1983. Sensitivity to grammatical structure in so-called agrammatic aphasics. Cognition 13:361–392.

Liu H-M, Kuhl PK, Tsao F-M. 2003. An association between mothers' speech clarity and infants' speech discrimination skills. Dev Sci 6:F1-F10.

Mazoyer BM, Tzourio N, Frak V, Syrota A, Murayama N, Levrier O, Salamon G, Dehaene S, Cohen L, Mehier J. 1993. The cortical representation of speech. J Cogn Neurosci 5:467–479.

Miyawaki K, Strange W, Verbrugge R. Liberman AM, Jenkins JJ, Fujimura O. 1975. An effect of linguistic experience: the discrimination of [r] and [l] by native speakers of Japanese and English. Percept Psychophys 18:331–340.

Neville HJ, Coffey SA, Lawson D, Fischer A, Emmorey K, Bellugi U. 1997. Neural systems mediating American Sign Language: effects of sensory experience and age of acquisition. Brain Lang 57:285–308.

Newport EL, Aslin RN. 2004. Learning at a distance I. Statistical learning of non-adjacent dependencies. Cogn Psychol 48:127–162.

Ojemann G. 1994. Cortical stimulation and recording in language. In: A. Kertesz (ed). *Localization and Neuroimaging in Neuropsychology*, pp. 35–55, San Diego: Academic Press.

Penfield W, Roberts L. 1959. *Speech and Brain Mechanisms*. Princeton, NJ: Princeton University Press.

Peterson SE, Fox PT, Posner MI, Mintun M, Raichle ME. 1988. Positron emission tomographic studies of the cortical anatomy of single-word processing. Nature 331:585–589.

Pettito LA, Holowka S, Sergio LE, Levy B, Ostry DJ. 2004. Baby hands that move to the rhythm of language: hearing babies acquiring sign language babble silently on the hands. Cognition 93:43–73.

Saffran JR, Aslin RN, Newport EL. 1996. Statistical learning by 8-month old infants. Science 274:1926–1928.

Silva-Pereyra J, Rivera-Gaxiola M, Kuhl PK. 2005. An event-related brain potential study of sentence comprehension in preschoolers: semantic and morphosyntatic processing. Cogn Brain Res 23:247–258.

Skinner BF. 1957. *Verbal Behavior. Acton,* MA: Copely Publishing Group.

Stromswold K, Caplan D, Alpert N, Rauch S. 1996. Localization of syntactic comprehension using positron emission tomography. Brain Lang 52:452–473.

Tsao F-M, Liu H-M, Kuhl PK. 2004 Speech perception in infancy predicts language development in the second year of life: a longitudinal study. Child Dev 75: 1067–1084.

Wernicke C.1874. *Der Aphasische Symptomenkomplex*. Breslau: Kohn und Weigert.

Wertz RT, LaPointe LL, Rosenbek JC. 1984. *Apraxia of Speech in Adults: The Disorder and Its Management.* Orlando: Grune and Stratton.

Yeni-Komshian G, Flege JE, Liu S. 2000. Pronunciation proficiency in the first and second languages of Korean-English bilinguals. Biling Lang Cogn 3:131–149.

Zaidel E. 1990. Language functions in the two hemispheres following complete commissurotomy and hemispherectomy. In: F. Boiler, J. Grafman (eds). *Handbook of Neuropsychology*. New York: Elsevier.

Zurif EB, Caramazza A, Meyerson R. 1972. Grammatical judgments of agrammatic aphasics. Neuropsychology 10:405–417.

61

Disorders of Conscious and Unconscious Mental Processes

ALTHOUGH COGNITIVE NEUROSCIENCE emerged at the end of the 20th century as a major new discipline, a precise meaning of the term *cognition* can often appear elusive. The term is used in different ways in different contexts. At one extreme the "cognitive" in cognitive neuroscience has replaced the older term *information processing*. In this sense cognition is simply what the brain does. When cognitive neuroscientists speak of visual features or motor responses being represented by neural activity, they are using concepts of information processing. From this point of view the language of cognition provides a bridge between descriptions of neural activity and behavior because the same terms can be applied in both domains.

At the other extreme the term "cognition" refers to those higher level processes fundamental to the formation of conscious experience. This is what is meant in the term *cognitive therapy*, an approach to treatment pioneered by Aaron Beck and Albert Ellis and developed from *behavior therapy*. Rather than trying to change a patient's behavior directly, cognitive therapy has the aim of changing the patient's attitudes and beliefs (Box 61–1).

In common parlance the term "cognition" means thinking and reasoning, a usage closer to its Latin root *cognoscere* (getting to know or perceiving). Thus the *Oxford English Dictionary* defines it as "the action or faculty of knowing." Indeed, we know the world by applying thinking and reasoning to the raw data of our senses.

Used in this way there can be many kinds of disorders of cognition. After brain damage some patients can no longer understand the raw data supplied by their senses. This type of disorder was first delineated by Sigmund Freud and called an agnosia or loss of knowledge (see Chapter 17). Agnosias can take many different forms. A patient with visual agnosia can see perfectly well but is no longer able to recognize or make sense of what he sees. A patient with prosopagnosia has a specific problem recognizing faces. A patient with auditory agnosia might hear perfectly well but is unable to recognize spoken words.

Cognition is sometimes impaired from birth, so that a person has difficulty in acquiring knowledge. This might lead to general mental retardation or, if the problem is more localized, to specific learning difficulties such as dyslexia (difficulty learning about written language) or autism (difficulty in learning about other minds). Finally, cognition can become aberrant so that the knowledge acquired about the world is false. These disorders of thinking lead to false perceptions

Box 61–1 Cognitive Therapy

Dissatisfaction with psychological treatments based on Freud's theories of unconscious motivation intensified in the middle of the 20th century. Not only did these theories have no relevance to experimental psychology, but more importantly there was no empirical evidence that psychodynamic treatments actually worked.

The first form of alternative psychological therapy to emerge from laboratory studies is known as *behavior therapy*. The fundamental assumption of this approach is that maladaptive behavior is learned and can therefore be eliminated by applying the Pavlovian and Skinnerian principles of stimulus-response learning. So, for example, a child who has been attacked by a dog can become fearful of all dogs. This fearful response can be extinguished if the child learns that the conditioned stimulus (the sight of a dog) is not followed by the unconditioned stimulus (being bitten).

Behavior therapy was shown to be quick and effective for many disorders such as phobias. However, many mental disorders are better characterized in terms of maladaptive thinking rather than maladaptive behavior. In the 1960s Aaron Beck and Albert Ellis initiated a new kind of therapy in which the principles of learning are used to change thoughts rather than behavior. This is known as *cognitive therapy* or *cognitive behavior therapy*.

This form of therapy has been particularly successful in the treatment of depression. Depression is typically associated with negative thoughts (eg, remembering only the bad things that have happened to me) and negative attitudes (believing that I will never achieve my goals). Cognitive therapists teach their clients methods for reducing the frequency of these negative thoughts and changing their negative attitudes into positive ones.

(hallucinations) and false beliefs (delusions) associated with major mental illnesses such as schizophrenia.

Conscious and Unconscious Cognitive Processes Have Distinctive Neural Correlates

Cognition, deriving knowledge through thinking and reasoning, is one of the three components of consciousness. The other two are emotion and will. It used to be taken for granted that thinking and reasoning were under conscious voluntary control, and that cognition was not possible without consciousness. By the end of the 19th century, however, Freud developed a theory of unconscious mental processes and suggested that much human behavior was guided by motivations of which we are not aware.

Of more direct importance for neuroscience was the idea of *unconscious inferences*, originally proposed somewhat earlier by Helmholtz. Helmholtz was the first to carry out quantitative psychophysical experiments and to measure the speed with which signals are conducted in peripheral nerves. It had been thought that sensory signals arrived in the brain immediately (with the speed of light), but Helmholtz showed that nerve conduction was actually quite slow. He also noted that reaction times were even slower. These observations implied that a great deal of brain work intervened between sensory stimuli and conscious perception of an object. Helmholtz concluded that much of what goes on in the brain is not represented in consciousness and that what does enter consciousness (ie, what is perceived) depends on unconscious inferences. In other words, the brain uses evidence from the senses to decide on the most likely identity of the object that is causing these sensations but does this without our awareness.

This view was extremely unpopular with Helmholtz's contemporaries, and indeed still today. Most people believe that consciousness is necessary for making inferences and that moral responsibility can be assigned only to decisions that are based on conscious inferences. If inferences could be made without consciousness, there could be no ethical basis for praise or blame. Helmholtz's ideas about unconscious inferences were largely ignored.

Nevertheless, by the middle of the 20th century evidence began to accumulate in favor of the idea that most cognitive processing never enters consciousness. After the invention of electronic computers, the discipline of artificial intelligence (AI) was born and researchers began to study how and to what extent machines could perceive the world beyond themselves. It rapidly became clear that many apparently simple perceptual processes, when defined as a set of computations, are actually very complex.

Visual perception is the prime example. In the 1960s almost no one realized how difficult it would be to build machines that could recognize the shape and appearance of objects. We now know that it is very difficult. A fundamental question is how to work out which edges go with which object in a typical cluttered visual scene containing many overlapping objects. No one thought visual perception was difficult because it seemed so easy for us. I look out of the window and I see buildings, trees, flowers, and people. I am not aware of any mental processes behind this perception. Instead, my awareness of all these objects seems instantaneous and direct. The computational approach to vision revealed the underlying neural processes on which our seemingly effortless perception of the world depends. Similar processes underlie all sensory perception and especially the perception of sounds as speech. Most neural scientists now believe that only percepts, but not cognitive processing, are conscious phenomena.

The evidence for unconscious cognitive processes comes not only from artificial intelligence studies but also studies of cognition in people with brain damage. The effects of unconscious processes on behavior can be demonstrated most strikingly in certain neurological patients, such as those with "blind sight," a disorder first delineated in the 1970s by Lawrence Weiskrantz. These patients have lesions in the primary visual cortex and claim to see nothing in the part of the visual field served by the damaged area. However, when asked to guess, they are able to detect simple visual properties such as movement or color far better than is expected by chance. Despite having no sensory-based perception of objects in the blind parts of the visual field, these patients do have unconscious information about the objects and this information is available to guide their behavior.

Another example is unilateral neglect because of lesions in the right parietal lobe (see Chapter 17). Patients with this disorder have normal vision, but they ignore objects on the left side of the space in front of them. Some patients even ignore the left side of individual objects. In one experiment by John Marshal and Peter Halligan patients were shown two drawings of a house. The left side of one house was on fire (Figure 61–1). When asked if there were any differences between the houses, patients replied "no." But when asked which house they would prefer to live in, they chose the house that was not burning. This choice was thus made on the basis of information that was not represented in consciousness. These are just two examples of the abundant empirical evidence for the existence of unconscious cognitive processes in addition to the aspects of cognition familiar to us through introspection.

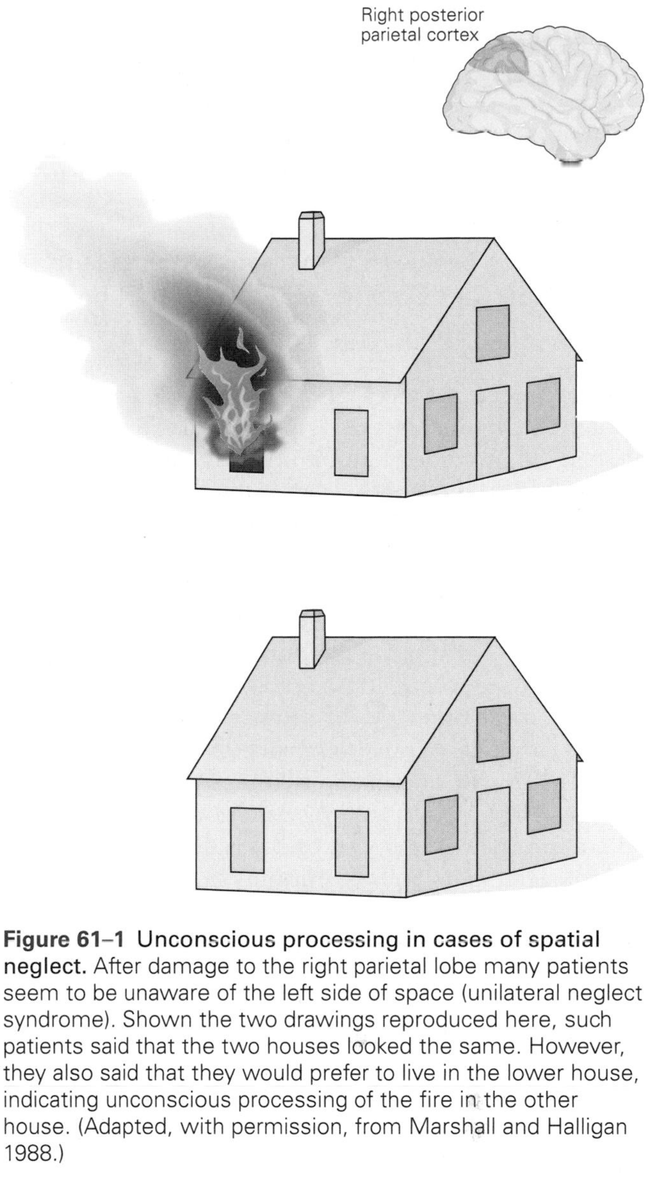

Figure 61–1 Unconscious processing in cases of spatial neglect. After damage to the right parietal lobe many patients seem to be unaware of the left side of space (unilateral neglect syndrome). Shown the two drawings reproduced here, such patients said that the two houses looked the same. However, they also said that they would prefer to live in the lower house, indicating unconscious processing of the fire in the other house. (Adapted, with permission, from Marshall and Halligan 1988.)

Currently one of the most exciting programs of research in neuroscience concerns the search for the *neural correlates of consciousness* (NCC) initiated by Francis Crick and Christopher Koch (see Chapter 17). The aim of this program is to demonstrate qualitative differences between the neural activity associated with conscious and unconscious cognitive processes. This research is important not only because it may give us answers to the difficult question of the function of consciousness but also because it is relevant to our understanding of many neurological and psychiatric disorders.

The weird experiences and delusional beliefs of patients with certain cognitive disorders were once dismissed as beyond understanding. Cognitive neuroscience provides us with a framework for understanding how these experiences and beliefs can arise from specific alterations in normal cognitive mechanisms.

Differences Between Conscious Processes in Perception Can Be Seen in Exaggerated Form after Brain Damage

In many circumstances perception can change without any change in sensory stimulation. This phenomenon is illustrated by ambiguous figures such as the Rubin figure and the Necker cube (Figure 61–2). In other circumstances a big change in sensory stimulation can occur without the observer being aware of this change—the perception remains constant. A compelling example of this is change blindness.

To demonstrate change blindness two versions of a complex scene are constructed. In one well-known example developed by Ron Rensink the picture consists of a military transport plane standing on an airport runway. In one of the two versions an engine is missing. If these two pictures are shown in alternation on a computer screen, but critically interspersed with a blank screen, it can take minutes to notice the difference even though it is obvious when pointed out. (See Figure 29–3 for another example.)

In light of these examples we can explore some simple questions about the relationship between neural activity and conscious and unconscious cognitive processes. We can identify the neural activity associated with changes in perception when there is no change in sensory stimulation. We can discover whether changes in sensory input are registered in the brain even if not represented in consciousness. We can ask whether there is some qualitative difference between the neural activity associated with conscious as opposed to unconscious processes.

Two important results have emerged from studies that seek to identify the neural activity associated with specific types of percepts. The first is that certain kinds of conscious percepts are related to neural activity in specific areas of the brain. When we perceive the faces in the Rubin figure, there is more activity in the area of the fusiform gyrus, which is specialized for the processing of faces. Those brain areas that are specialized for recognition of certain kinds of objects (faces, words, landscapes, etc.) or for certain visual features (color, motion, etc.) become more active when the object or the feature is consciously perceived (Figure 61–3).

This observation also applies to deviant perception (hallucinations). After degeneration of the peripheral visual system leading to blindness, some patients experience intermittent visual hallucinations (Charles Bonnet syndrome). These hallucinations vary from one patient to another. Some patients see colored patches, others see grid-like patterns, and some even see faces. Dominic ffytche has found that these hallucinations are associated with increased activity in the secondary visual cortex, and the content of the hallucination is related to the specific locus of activity (Figure 61–4).

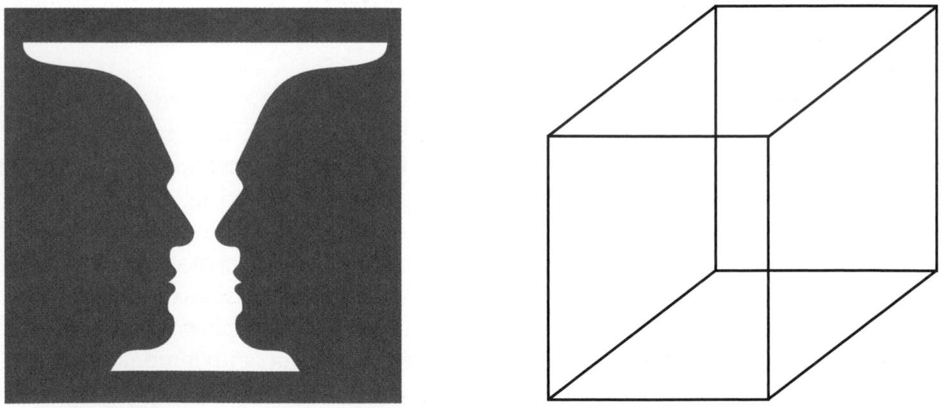

Figure 61–2 Ambiguous figures. If you stare at the figure on the left (the Rubin figure) you sometimes see a vase and sometimes two faces looking at each other. If you stare at the figure on the right (the Necker cube) you see a three-dimensional cube, but the front face of the cube is sometimes seen at the bottom left and sometimes at the top right. In each figure the brain finds two equally good, but mutually exclusive, interpretations of what is there. Our conscious perception spontaneously alternates between these two interpretations.

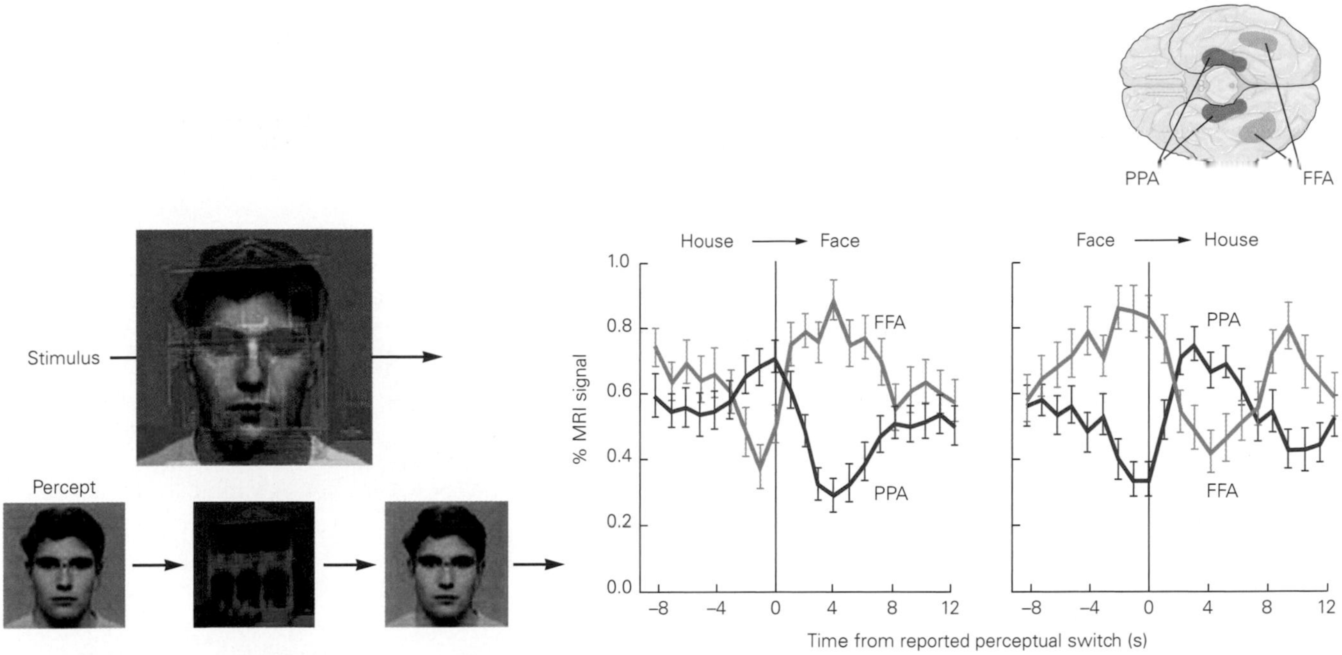

Figure 61–3 Neural activity associated with ambiguous visual information. An ambiguous stimulus was created by simultaneously presenting a face to one eye and a house to the other eye. Brain activity was measured while subjects observed these images. Subjects were instructed to press a button whenever a spontaneous switch in perception occurred (because of binocular rivalry). When the face is perceived (**left**), activity increases in the fusiform face area (**FFA**); when the house is perceived (**right**), activity increases in the parahippocampal place area (**PPA**). (Reproduced, with permission, from Tong et al. 1998.)

Schizophrenic patients frequently experience complex hallucinations, which usually have the form of voices talking to or about the patient. These hallucinations are associated with activity in the auditory cortex.

These observations suggest that conscious experience may result from activity in certain cortical regions. This idea is difficult to test experimentally. Nevertheless, in the 1950s the neurosurgeon Wilder Penfield showed that electrical stimulation of the cortex in patients undergoing neurosurgery can give rise to conscious experience. Transcranial magnetic stimulation of the cortex in the region of V5/MT can lead to seeing moving light flashes.

The second important conclusion drawn from studies that seek to correlate neural activity and specific percepts is that activity in a specialized area is necessary but not sufficient to yield conscious experience. For example, in the change blindness paradigm subjects are often unaware of large changes in the picture they are viewing. If the change involves a face, activity is elicited in the fusiform gyrus whether or not the subject is aware of the change. But when the sensory change is also perceived consciously there is, in addition, activity in parietal and frontal cortex (Figure 61–5).

These observations are relevant to our understanding of unilateral neglect. It may be that the damage in the right parietal cortex simply prevents the formation of conscious representations of objects on the left side of space, since objects on the left side still elicit neural activity in the visual cortex. That is, sensory activity may support an unconscious inference in patients that they would not want to live in the house that is burning on the left side.

In normal people stimuli that do not enter awareness can nevertheless elicit overt responses. A face with a fearful expression elicits a fear response in the autonomic nervous system, measured as an increase in skin conductance (galvanic response) because of sweating. This response occurs even if the face is immediately followed by another visual stimulus, such that the face is not consciously perceived. There may be an advantage to having a rapid but poor resolution system for avoiding dangerous things. We jump first and only later, on the basis of a slow, high-resolution system, become aware of the identity of the object that made us jump (see Chapter 48). Damage in one or the other of these two recognition systems can explain certain otherwise puzzling neurological and psychiatric disorders.

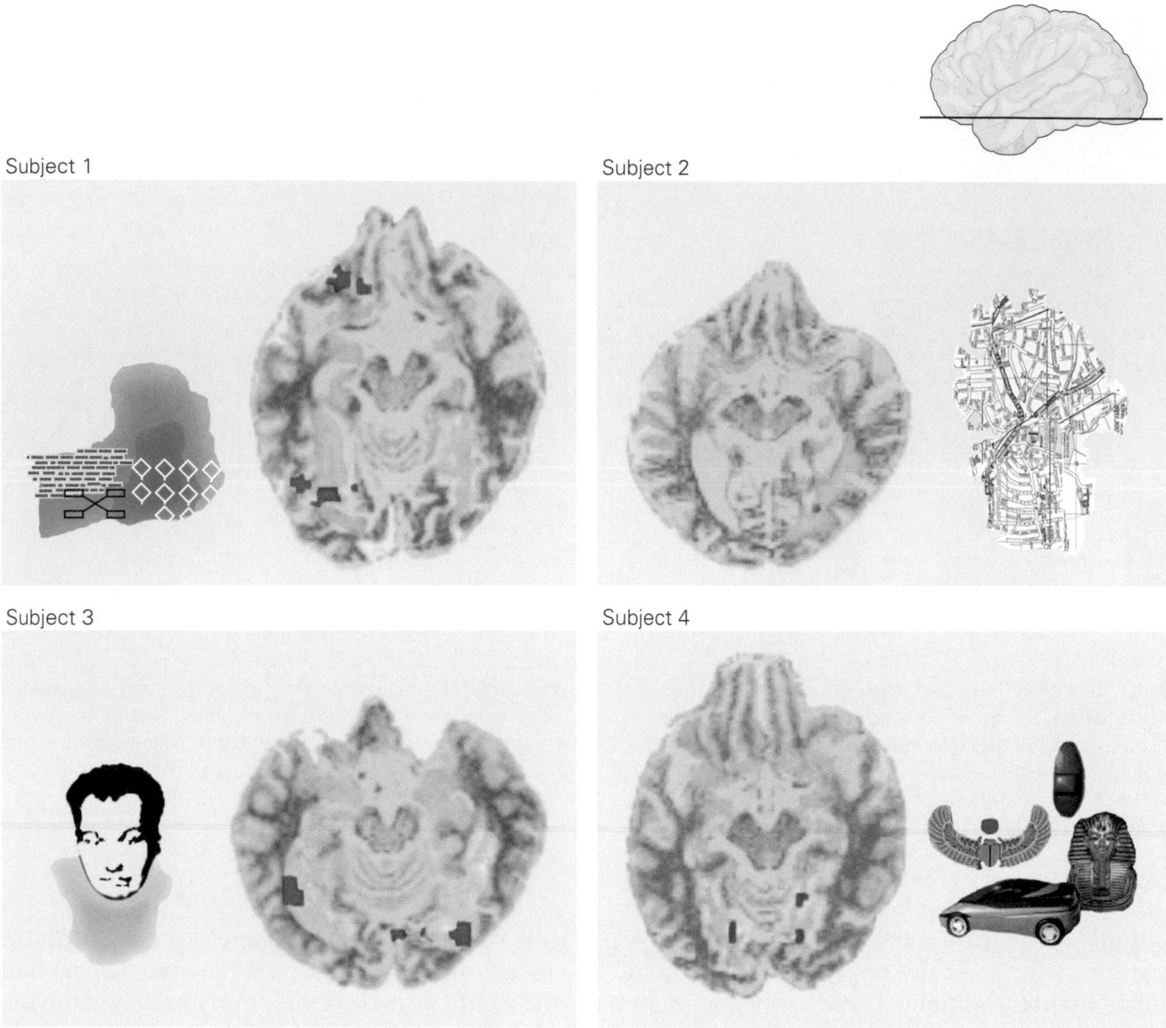

Figure 61–4 Neural activity associated with visual hallucinations. Some patients with damage to the retina experience visual hallucinations. The location of the neural activity and the content of the hallucination are related. The experience of colors, patterns, objects, or faces, is associated with heightened activity (**red**) in specific regions of inferior temporal cortex. The fusiform gyrus is shaded **blue** for reference. (Reproduced, with permission, from ffytche et al. 1998.)

Prosopagnosia is a perceptual disorder in which faces are no longer recognizable. The patient knows he is looking at a face but cannot recognize the face, even the face of his wife. The problem is specific to faces and the visual system. The patient may still be able to recognize his wife from her clothes, her gait, and her voice.

Actually, patients with prosopagnosia are able to identify faces but they do so unconsciously. They show autonomic responses to familiar faces and do better than chance when asked to guess whether or not faces shown to them belong to people who are familiar. In fact, they may use their awareness of the autonomic (emotional) responses elicited by a face to judge familiarity.

Capgras syndrome, a delusion that is occasionally observed in schizophrenic patients and in some neurological patients, shows the opposite pattern. These patients firmly believe that someone close to them, usually a husband or wife, has been replaced by an impostor. They claim that the person, although similar if not identical in appearance, is in fact someone else. Often this delusion is acted on with the demand that the impostor leave the house. In one extreme case a patient accused his stepfather of being a robot and subsequently decapitated him to look for batteries and microfilm in his head.

Haydn Ellis and Andy Young have suggested that this bizarre delusion is the mirror phenomenon of prosopagnosia. According to this view, the processing stream for face recognition is intact, but the stream that mediates the emotional response to the face is not functional. As a result, patients recognize the person in front of them but, because the emotional response is lacking, feel that there is something fundamentally wrong. This account has been partially confirmed by the observation that these patients do not have normal autonomic responses to familiar faces.

This explanation implies that Capgras delusions are not the consequence of disordered thinking but of disordered experience. A patient sees the face of his wife without having the normal emotional response. The conclusion that this is not his wife but an impostor is a cognitive response to this abnormal experience, the mind's attempt to explain experience.

The Control of Action Is Largely Unconscious

The sense that we are in control of our own actions is a major component of consciousness. But are we aware of all aspects of our own actions? David Milner and Mel Goodale studied intensively a patient known as D.F. who demonstrates a striking lack of awareness of certain aspects of her own action. As a result of damage to her inferior temporal lobe caused by carbon monoxide poisoning, D.F. suffers from *form agnosia*. She is unable to perceive the shapes of things. She cannot distinguish a square from an oblong card and cannot describe the orientation of a slot. Yet when she picks up the oblong card to place it through the slot she orients her hand and forms her grasp appropriately (Figure 61–6). D.F. is able to use sensory information about the shapes of objects to guide reaching and grasping movements, but this information is not conscious.

This unconscious guidance system is not unique to patients with brain damage. It is simply revealed more starkly in the case of D.F. by the damage to the system that normally brings visual information about shape into consciousness. Indeed, we can all make rapid and accurate grasping movements without being aware of the perceptual and motor information that

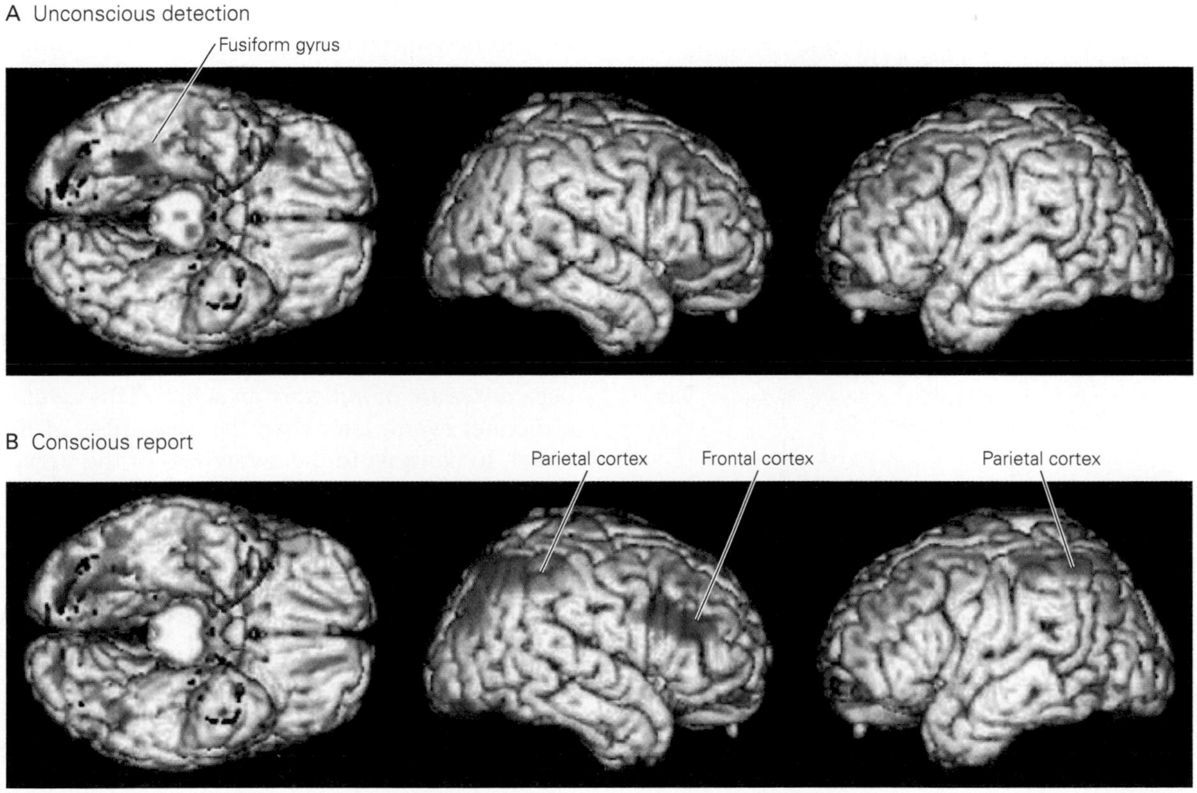

Figure 61–5 Brain activity with and without awareness. Activity in the fusiform face area increased when the face viewed by subjects changed, whether subjects were unaware of the change (**A**) or conscious of it (**B**). When subjects were aware of the change, activity in parietal and frontal cortex also increased. (Reproduced, with permission, from Beck et al. 2001.)

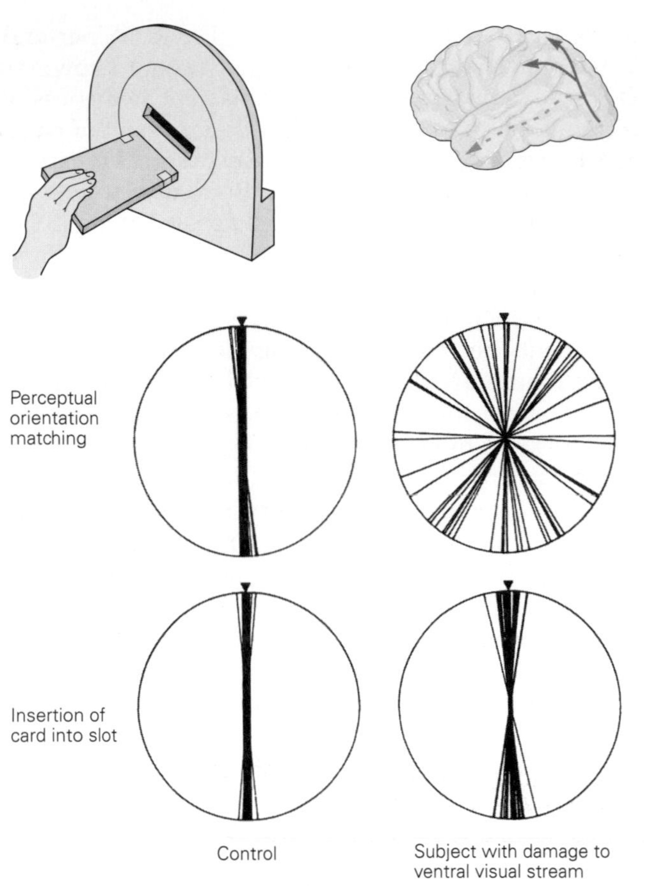

Figure 61–6 Action can be controlled by unconscious stimuli. As a result of damage to the inferior temporal cortex, the patient D.F. is unable to recognize objects based on their shape (form agnosia). She cannot align the tablet with the slot (perceptual matching) because she is not consciously aware of the orientation of either the tablet or the slot. When she is asked to put the tablet through the slot in a quick movement, she orients her hand rapidly and accurately, presumably because the brain mechanisms that drive the movement do not require the subject to identify intellectually the properties of the visual stimuli that guide the movement, but instead use visual mechanisms of which the subject is unaware. (Adapted, with permission, from Milner and Goodale 1995.)

is being used to control these movements. Sometimes we are not even aware of having made the movement. This largely unconscious system for visually guided reaching and grasping is analogous to, and probably overlaps with, the rapid but poor-resolution system associated with fear responses.

Although we may not be aware of the perceptual and motor controls of actions like reaching and grasping, we think we consciously control our actions because we decide on an action and then initiate it. But what aspects of an action are we actually aware of? In an influential experiment by Benjamin Libet subjects were asked to lift a finger "whenever they felt the urge to do so." During this experiment Libet used EEG to measure the "readiness potential," a change in brain activity that occurs up to one second before a subject makes any voluntary movement. The time at which subjects reported feeling the urge to lift a finger occurred hundreds of milliseconds *after* the beginning of this readiness potential.

Later studies by Patrick Haggard and Martin Eimer revealed that the time of awareness of the urge to act is correlated with the time at which the evoked potential in brain activity measured over the scalp ceases to be medially located and shifts toward the side of the brain that controls the movement, contralateral to the hand that will move. This observation suggests that we are not aware of intending to make a voluntary movement until the nature of that movement has been precisely specified in a motor plan.

The results of these experiments have generated much discussion among philosophers as well as neural scientists concerning the existence of free will. If brain activity can be used to predict when someone is going to act before they are aware of having the urge to perform that act, does this mean that these urges are predetermined and our experience of freely willing them is an illusion? The decision to act might still be made freely but made without awareness. The awareness of the choice comes later. This implies that the unconscious inferences proposed by Helmholtz occur in the motor domain as well as the sensory domain. However, even if we leave open the possibility that free will may operate unconsciously, we are left with the moral dilemma whether people can be held responsible for decisions that are made unconsciously.

Libet also measured the time at which his subjects became aware of *initiating* an action. This awareness is a distinct event, later than the awareness of the urge to act. In contrast to the awareness of the urge, which is later than the associated brain activity, awareness of initiating the act occurs before the act itself begins. The time at which we become aware of initiating a movement occurs some 80 ms before the movement actually starts (Figure 61–7), while any sensory feedback from the movement will occur 100 ms or so after the movement has actually started.

Thus the awareness of initiating a movement is much too early to be based on any sensory feedback. What we are aware of must be based on expected rather than actual sensory information. We are very surprised if the actual sensations do not match what we predicted, as when we pick up an object that is much lighter than anticipated (see Chapter 33). Furthermore, if the difference between predicted and actual sensations is small, the predicted sensation dominates our awareness.

Pierre Fourneret and Marc Jeannerod required subjects to draw a vertical line using a computer's mouse. The subjects could not see their hand and so could not see that the computer introduced a distortion in the line displayed on the screen. In one test subjects had to move their hand at an angle of 10 degrees to the left to produce a vertical line on the screen (Figure 61–8). In other tests different degrees and directions of distortion were applied. The striking result was that subjects were not aware that the direction of their movements did not match the direction of the line they saw on the screen. When subjects were asked to repeat a movement that had actually deviated 10 degrees to the left, but were not shown the line they were making on the screen, they actually performed the straightforward movement that they thought they had just made. It would seem that as long as the goal is realized (drawing a straightforward line), we are aware of the expected sensory feedback, not the actual sensory feedback.

The idea that we are normally aware of expectations about movements rather than the actual sensations helps us to understand otherwise bizarre experiences. For example, after the amputation of a limb, patients experience a phantom limb (see Chapter 17). Some patients believe they can move this phantom just as they could previously move the real limb. Amputees still experience the urge to move the missing limb, and they can select specific movements they want the missing limb to make. As a result, their unconscious sensorimotor systems predict the sensations they would feel if they were to make the movement. It is these predicted sensations that dominate our normal awareness of action and provide the basis for the sensation of a moving phantom limb.

The Conscious Recall of Memory Is a Creative Process

For most of us memory is the conscious reliving of a past experience in our imagination. From a behaviorist point of view, however, memory and learning are processes by which our past experience alters future behavior. Our behavior is often affected by past experience without our being aware of the memory or the influence it is having on us. Once again, such effects are seen in their most striking form in patients with damage to certain areas of the brain.

Some patients become densely amnesic after damage to the medial regions of the temporal lobe (see Chapter 67). These patients show no decline in intellect as measured by IQ tests but cannot remember anything for more than a few minutes. Although devastating, this memory impairment is actually rather circumscribed. The problem is largely manifested in *declarative memory*, and most severely in a type of declarative

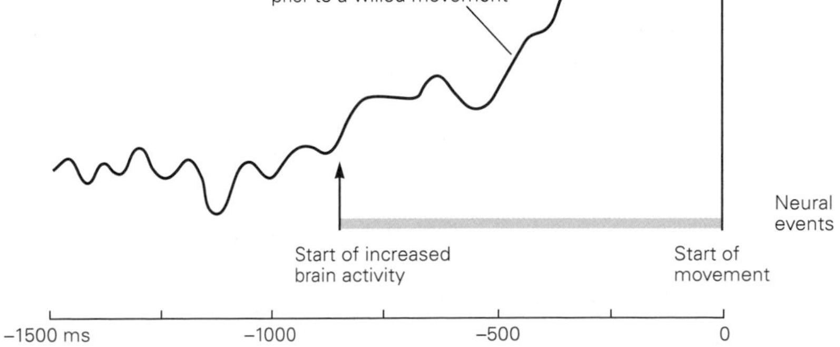

Figure 61–7 Mental time is not the same as neural time. When subjects are asked to lift a finger "whenever you feel the urge," a slow change in electrical activity in the brain is detected for up to a second before the finger movement begins (the readiness potential). However, subjects first become aware of the urge to lift their finger several hundred milliseconds *after* the first detectable change in brain activity. In contrast, their first awareness that the finger is moving is just *before* the actual movement begins. (Adapted, with permission, from Libet et al. 1983.)

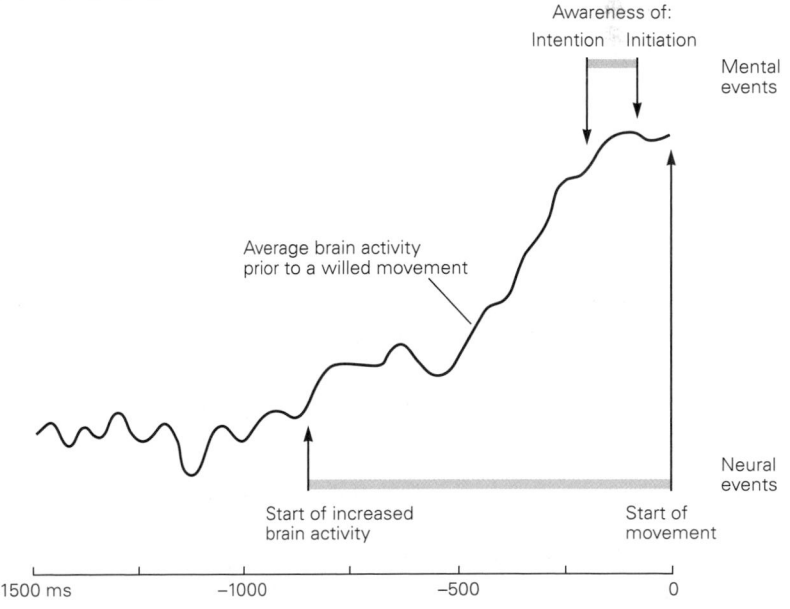

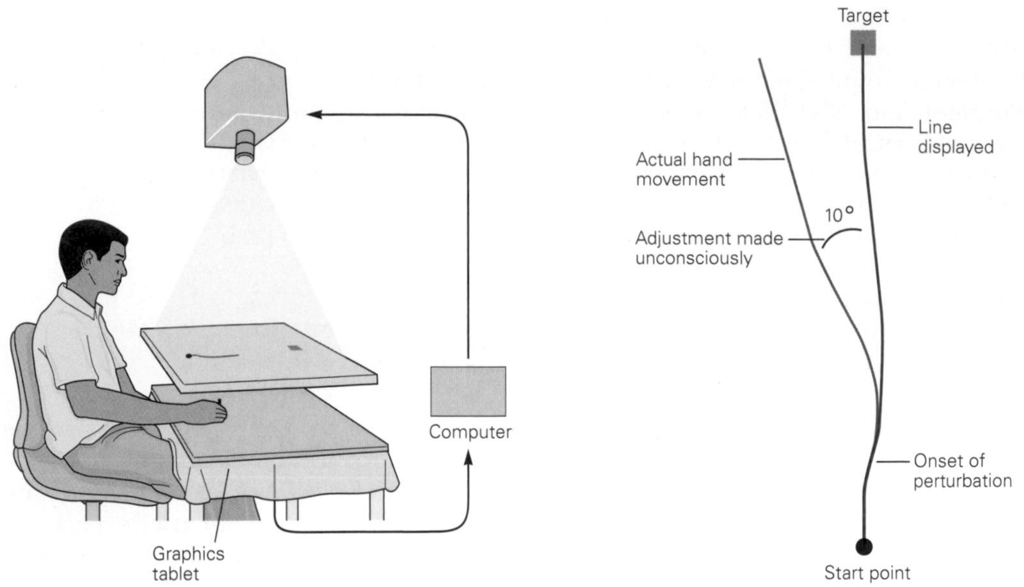

Figure 61–8 Actions can be modified unconsciously. Subjects are asked to draw a straight line with a computer mouse but cannot see their hand, only the line on the screen. The computer is programmed to systematically distort the line displayed on the screen. In the result shown here the subject had to move his hand 10 degrees to the left to produce a vertical line on the screen. Subjects are not aware of making such adjustments. (Adapted, with permission, from Fourneret and Jeannerod 1998.)

memory called *episodic memory*, the ability to recollect events in one's life (see Chapter 67). *Procedural memory*, in which consciousness has a minor role (see Chapter 66), remains intact. Thus patients still remember motor skills such as riding a bicycle and can often learn new motor skills at a normal rate. These different effects of brain damage on memory can lead to dramatic dissociations. A patient who has been learning some new skill everyday for a week will deny ever having performed the task before. He is then surprised to find how skillful he has become.

Normal people routinely learn skills unconsciously, although this is much more difficult to demonstrate convincingly. Several studies of procedural learning have used "choice reaction-time" paradigms. For example, subjects presented with four buttons that light up in sequence have to press as quickly as possible each button after it lights up. The subject is not told that the buttons light up in a particular sequence. Of course, knowledge of this sequence would enable the subject to predict which signal will come next and thus to respond more rapidly. In fact, responses do become faster once the sequence can be predicted, even when the subject is entirely unable to describe the sequence.

Another widely used protocol tests subjects' ability to recall lists of words they have memorized, a task that taps a form of declarative memory. In the recall phase a subject is presented with a list of the words that were on the study list plus new words. An amnesic patient has great difficulty with this type of task and may misclassify most of the previously seen words as new since she cannot recall seeing them before. Nevertheless, the brain activity elicited by reading old words is different from that elicited by the new words. Thus there is unconscious recognition of a difference, equivalent to that shown by patients with unilateral neglect or prosopagnosia. Normal subjects usually find this task easy, but they too will occasionally misclassify old words as new; as with amnesiacs, the evoked brain response registers the distinction lost to conscious retrieval (Figure 61–9).

Occasionally a subject misclassifies a new word as an old one. This misclassification amounts to a false memory. Such misclassifications are most likely to occur when the new word is semantically related to one or more of the old words. If the list of old words contained *big, great, huge,* then the new word *large* is likely to be identified as old. One explanation for this is that the perception of the new word *large* has been unconsciously primed by the previous presentation of the old words. Thus the new word *large* is processed easily and quickly. Because the subject is aware of this perceptual fluency, he concludes the word must be familiar and classifies it as old.

This observation emphasizes that memory is a creative process. Our conscious memories are constructed from both conscious recall and unconscious knowledge. To guard against false memories, as with false percepts, we use our knowledge about the world to determine what memories are plausible.

In some patients the process by which memories are screened seems to become dramatically disturbed. If asked what happened yesterday, most patients with amnesia will say that they cannot remember. However, a few will give elaborate accounts that do not correspond to reality. Such false memories are called confabulations. These memories can sometimes be extremely implausible. For example, one patient said that he had met Harold Wilson (a former British Prime Minister) and discussed a building job they were both working on.

In some cases these false memories are arbitrary constructions, as if the patient would rather make something up than admit that he does not know. In other cases the false memories are very specific and consistent. For example, one patient with brain damage caused by a fall, studied by Paul Burgess, became convinced that one of the nurses on the rehabilitation ward in England was the same nurse that had looked after him in the intensive care unit in the United States. He also believed that this nurse had stolen his watch and was having an affair with his wife. This patient was able to discuss all other subjects perfectly rationally but was entirely convinced of the truth of his memories about the nurse despite all evidence to the contrary.

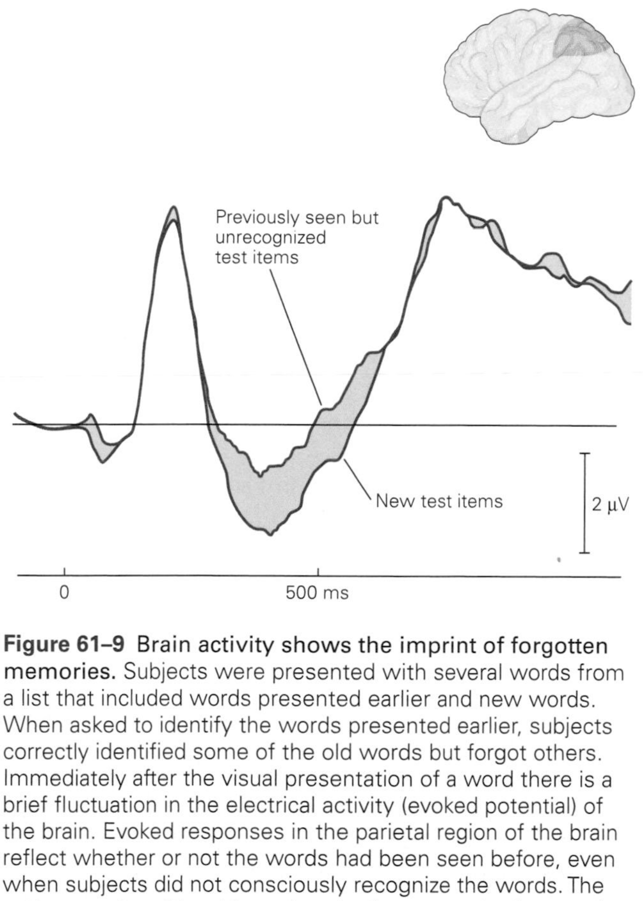

Figure 61–9 Brain activity shows the imprint of forgotten memories. Subjects were presented with several words from a list that included words presented earlier and new words. When asked to identify the words presented earlier, subjects correctly identified some of the old words but forgot others. Immediately after the visual presentation of a word there is a brief fluctuation in the electrical activity (evoked potential) of the brain. Evoked responses in the parietal region of the brain reflect whether or not the words had been seen before, even when subjects did not consciously recognize the words. The pattern produced by old words, whether recognized or not, is different from that produced by the new words. (Reproduced, with permission, from Rugg et al. 1998.)

False memories of this kind can be indistinguishable from the false beliefs expressed by patients with schizophrenia. Paranoid delusions similar to those described above are common, but some delusions can be even more obviously at odds with reality. One patient studied by Alan Baddeley believed he was a rock guitarist and a Russian chess grand master, even though he cannot play the guitar or chess and does not speak Russian. "But if you don't speak Russian, isn't that rather odd for a Russian chess player?" "Yes, well, I don't speak Russian, but I think it is possible that I've been hypnotized to forget things like the fact that I can speak Russian."

This patient's beliefs seem no longer to be constrained by his knowledge and experience of the world. Furthermore, the problem is self-sustaining as the patient's false beliefs become part of his knowledge of the world. Nevertheless, if our conscious perception and memory were too strongly constrained by our prior knowledge, we would never be able to see anything new or remember anything unusual. The neural mechanisms by which beliefs are acquired and fixed have as yet been only minimally investigated, but the various phenomena described above indicate how a research program might be initiated.

Behavioral Observation Needs to Be Supplemented with Subjective Reports

By the middle of the 20th century it had become clear that the classic behaviorist approach was inadequate for the exploration of many psychological processes. Language acquisition, selective attention, and working memory cannot be understood in terms of relations between stimuli and responses, however complex the relationships postulated.

The demonstration that some cognitive processes are unconscious requires that we move even further from behaviorism. If we want to explore the whole range of conscious and unconscious cognitive processes we will not be able to do so by focusing on overt behavior alone. We must not assume that a subject making purposeful, goal-directed actions is necessarily aware of the stimuli eliciting the action or even of the action itself. We must supplement behavioral observations with subjective reports. We have to ask the subject, "Did you see the stimulus? Did you move your hand?"

During the decades in which psychology was dominated by behaviorism, subjective reports were not considered an appropriate source of data. As a result, methods for recording subjective reports lag far behind methods for studying overt behavior. Regrettably, many studies of cognitive processes still make no systematic attempt to record subjective experience because of the long tradition of excluding subjective reports. One hundred years ago introspection was the major method for obtaining data in psychology. How else could one study consciousness? However, different schools of psychology obtained different results and, as John B. Watson emphasized, there seemed to be no objective way of deciding who was right. How can you independently confirm subjective experience? Thus the method fell into disrepute.

Subjective reports are usually verbal—our subject tells us in words what the experience was like for him or her. But they need not be verbal. In many experiments a human subject may indicate that he or she has seen the stimulus by pressing a button. Pressing a button is an observable behavior, but the behavior is an indicator of a conscious thought.

This kind of nonverbal report can also be used in experiments with monkeys. When presented with an ambiguous figure such as the Rubin vase, a monkey can be trained to press one button when it sees the face and another button when it sees the vase. The choice about which button to press must be based on introspection. Robert Hampton used this technique in a memory experiment. A monkey was asked to distinguish familiar and new objects. This task is typically presented in a forced-choice format. The monkey (or person) is presented with a familiar object and a new object and has to choose the familiar one. A correct choice might occur because the familiar object is consciously recognized. If no conscious recognition occurs then the monkey (or person) must guess. Some of these guesses may be right, because of cues arising from unconscious processes, but many will be wrong.

Incorrect guesses can be avoided if the response "Don't know" is permitted (indicated by not pressing either button). With this format the proportion of button presses that are wrong should be reduced because guesses have been eliminated. Here again the behavior of pressing the button is partially based on introspection: If I am aware that I do not know the answer, I will not press a button. Monkeys are able to improve their performance (and thus get more food rewards) when given the opportunity not to make a choice, suggesting that they know when they are guessing.

Brain Imaging Can Corroborate Subjective Reports

The problem of verifying subjective reports can be partially addressed with the use of brain imaging. Brain imaging studies have shown that neural activity occurs in localized areas of the brain during mental activity unaccompanied by any overt behavior. The content of such mental activity, such as imagining or daydreaming, can only be known from the subject's reports.

If we scan a subject while he says he is imagining moving his hand, activity will be detected in many parts of the motor system. In most motor regions this activity is less intense than the activity associated with an actual movement, but it is well above resting levels. Similarly, if a subject reports that she is imagining a face she has recently seen, activity can be detected in the "face recognition area" of the fusiform gyrus (Figure 61–10). In these examples the observed neural activity detected by the scanner provides independent confirmation of the experience reported by the subject. The content of consciousness can, in certain limited cases, be inferred from patterns of neural activity.

Malingering and Hysteria Can Lead to Unreliable Subjective Reports

When we record reports of subjective experience we are using the subject like a meter. Just as a meter can convert electrical resistance into the position of a pointer on a dial (reading 100 ohms) so a subject can convert the wavelength of a light source into the report of a color ("I see red.")

But there is a critical way in which the meter is not like a person. The meter does not experience red and cannot communicate meaning. And, while the meter might be faulty, it can never pretend to see red when it is really seeing blue. Most of the time we presume that subjective reports are true, that is, the subject is trying as far as possible to give an accurate description of his experience. But in some circumstances subjects might say "blue" even though what they saw was red. How could this arise and what is the status of the subjective report in such cases?

Consider a patient who has become amnesic as a result of extensive damage to the medial temporal cortex. Shown a photograph of someone whom he sees every day on the ward, the patient denies ever having

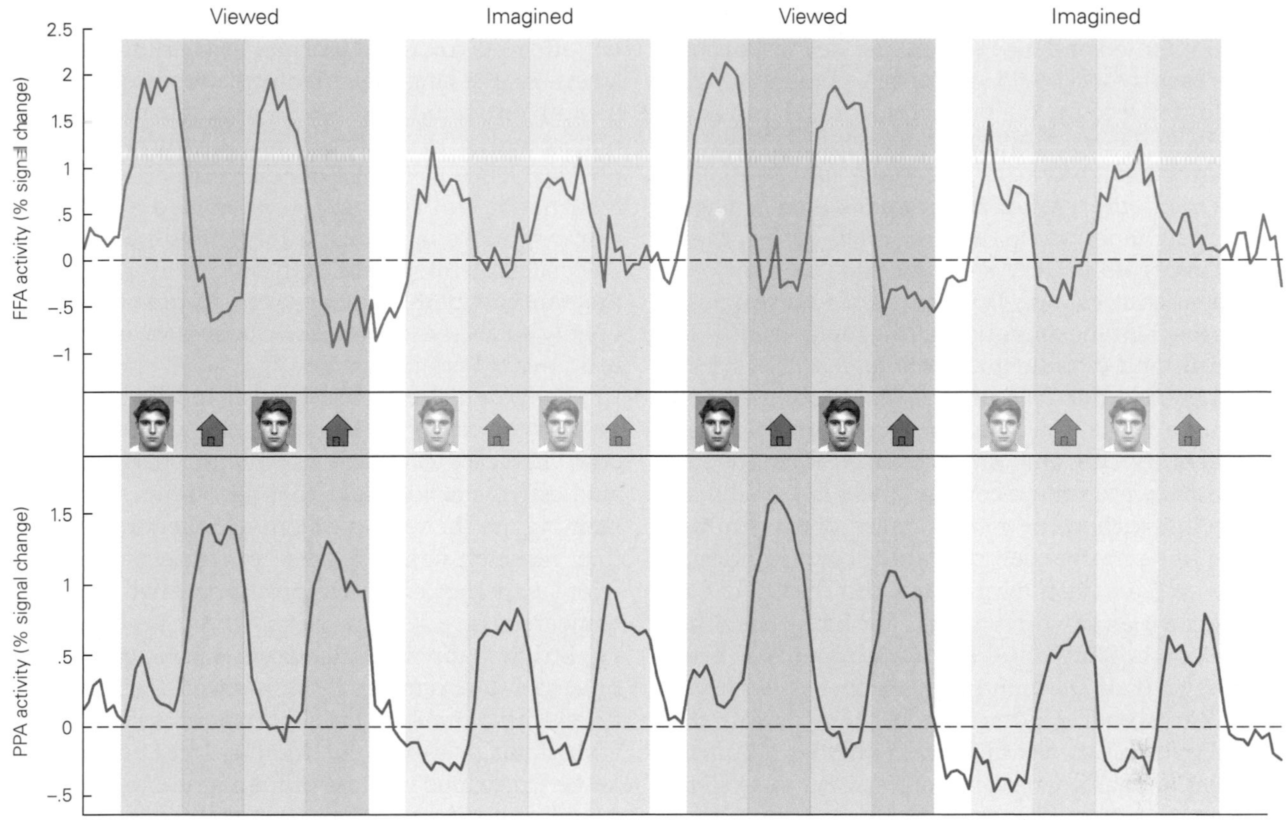

Figure 61–10 Imagining a face or a place correlates with activity in specific areas of the brain. Subjects were scanned while they viewed or imagined faces and houses. In the first block subjects alternately viewed a face or a house. When viewing a face, brain activity increases in the fusiform face area of the inferior temporal lobe (**FFA**). When viewing a house, brain activity increases in the parahippocampal place area of the inferior temporal cortex (**PPA**). In the next block subjects alternately *imagined* a face or a house. The same brain regions are active during both the imagining and direct viewing of faces and houses, although the activity is less pronounced during the imagined viewing. (Reproduced, with permission, from O'Craven and Kanwisher 2000.)

seen this person before. But physiological measurements (electroencephalogram or skin conductance) made at the same time show a response to the photo (but not to photos of people he has not seen before). We conclude that conscious memory processes have been damaged while unconscious processes remain intact. This patient's subjective report is an accurate account of his *conscious* experience, but there are things he "knows" that do not enter consciousness.

Another patient is brought in having been found wandering on the street. There is no evidence of brain damage, but he has lost his memory to the extent of no longer knowing anything about himself or his history. He, too, denies any knowledge of the familiar people he is shown in photographs, but when tested he shows physiological responses to these familiar people. In this case, because of the lack of detectable brain damage (and other features of the memory loss), we begin to wonder about the truthfulness of his statements. Perhaps the physiological responses indicate that he does consciously recognize people. Subsequently the patient is identified by the police, and we discover that he is wanted for a serious crime committed in the neighboring county. Our doubts about the reliability of his reports increase. Finally, our suspicions are confirmed when he foolishly tells a fellow patient, "It's so easy to fool those clinical psychologists."

In this case we have direct evidence that the patient was deliberately misleading us about his conscious experience. In many ways the ability to deceive is the pinnacle of all human attainments, for to deceive others we must not only be conscious of our own mental state but also of their state. Is there some way we could have discovered from our patient's behavior that he was deceiving us? One approach is to use a memory test of the kind discussed earlier. The patient studies a list of words. He then sees a new list consisting of the words he has just studied and new words, and he must decide whether each word is old or new. A genuine amnesic would not recognize any of the words. He would have to guess. Through unconscious priming effects he might perform slightly better than chance. The malingering patient can recognize the old words but will have a strong tendency to deny that he has seen them before. Unless he is very sophisticated, he may perform worse than chance. It seems we can distinguish between the genuine amnesic and the malingerer.

A third kind of patient also simulates amnesia (or some other disorder) but does so unconsciously and thus is not a malingerer. Such a case would be called hysterical or psychogenic amnesia. Like the malingerer his performance on the recognition test is worse than chance. Nonetheless, he is not aware of his simulation. The same mechanism probably occurs in normal people who have been hypnotized and then told that they have no memory for what has just happened. This phenomenon is sometimes referred to as a dissociated state; that part of the mind that records experiences and makes verbal reports has become dissociated from the part that is creating the simulation. Hysterical simulations can create sensory loss, such as hysterical blindness, and motor disorders, such as hysterical paralysis or hysterical dystonia, as well as hysterical memory loss.

We are still a long way from understanding the cognitive processes or underlying physiology of these disorders. A key problem is how to distinguish hysteria from malingering. From the standpoint of conscious experience the two disorders are quite different: The malingerer is aware that he is simulating whereas the hysterical patient is not. Yet the patients' subjective reports and overt behavior in the two cases are very similar. Is there no measure that can distinguish between these different disorders? This may be one situation where studies of neural activity are the only way to make the critical distinction between these different states of consciousness.

An Overall View

The study of mental disorders forces us to confront the conceptual gap between the mental and the physical. It is no longer possible to maintain that some mental disorders have mental causes and others physical causes. There is now abundant evidence that a physical cause (abnormal brain function) can create a mental disorder such as the false belief that "My wife has been replaced by an impostor" (Capgras syndrome).

Cognitive neuroscience has had a major impact on our attempts to bridge this gap because its descriptive language, the language of information processing, can be applied simultaneously to psychological and neural processes. In Cartesian terms information is not physical since it is not extended in space or time. Yet information can be stored in physical devices such as memory sticks or books. Information theory and the associated development of the computer provided the first hint that perhaps science can address the question of how subjective experience can emerge from activity in a physical brain.

The cognitive neuroscience approach has been applied to many different mental abnormalities in both neurological and psychiatric patients. These studies have made clear that perception, action, and memory are the result of many parallel processes, and that although some of these processes support conscious experience, the majority occur below the level of awareness.

Striking abnormalities occur when some of these processes are damaged while others remain intact. An example presented in this chapter is D.F., a patient with damage to inferior temporal cortex. She is no longer consciously aware of the shape of an object and hence cannot describe it or recognize what it is. She can nevertheless form her hand into the appropriate shape to pick up the object. From the perspective of cognitive neuroscience, her problem can be described in terms of two kinds of representations that are needed for performing the two kinds of tasks. For reaching and grasping an object, its shape needs to be represented in hand-centered coordinates relating to the position of the hand that will do the grasping. For recognizing an object, an object-centered representation is required that is independent of viewpoint. In D.F. the latter kind of representation has been damaged while the former remains intact.

Although the control of action is largely unconscious, we are very much aware of ourselves as inhabiting and owning our bodies and as agents of action that causes things to happen in the world. These experiences of the self can also be upset by brain abnormalities. Overactivity in the right hemisphere at the junction of the temporal and parietal cortex can create "out-of-the-body" experiences, the experience of looking at one's body from the outside. Damage to the right hemisphere can cause one to look on a limb as "not me." These abnormal experiences can be explained as the result of faulty neural representations of the body and its parts in space.

Even more striking is the disorder of the experience of the self described by patients with schizophrenia.

A patient with "delusions of control" experiences his actions as being under the control of an alien force: "My fingers pick up the pen, but I don't control them. What they do is nothing to do with me." This is not a problem of ownership. The patient knows it is his fingers that are moving. Instead, this is an abnormality in the experience of agency, the awareness of who or what is responsible for the fingers moving. Although we cannot yet describe the cause at the neural level, this symptom is associated with overactivity in parietal cortex, and there is increasing evidence that it is created by a failure to predict the sensory consequences of actions.

Many aspects of motor control occur without consciousness because the feedback sensations associated with movement are actively suppressed. This is because the sensory consequences of our own movements can be predicted on the basis of the information we use to generate the movements. This is why we cannot tickle ourselves. If I stroke the palm of my hand, the conscious sensation and the associated brain activity is greatly reduced in comparison to what occurs if someone else strokes my palm. I can predict what I am going to feel when I tickle myself. I cannot predict what I am going to feel if someone else tickles me. This is a rare example of cognitive neuroscience contributing to our understanding of conscious experience.

We now know why philosophers describe the experience of action as "thin and evasive." For patients with schizophrenia the experience of action is no longer thin and evasive, as the sensory consequences of their actions are not properly suppressed. When they make an active movement with their arm they experience all the sensations that normally occur only when their arm is moved passively by some external force. A cognitive model can thus explain the experience that leads patients with schizophrenia to believe that their actions are caused by alien forces. It remains to be seen whether this cognitive model can also help us understand the abnormality at the neural level.

Christopher D. Frith

Selected Readings

Frith CD. 2007. *Making Up the Mind: How the Brain Creates Our Mental World.* Oxford: Blackwell.

Gazzaniga MS (ed). 1995. *Cognitive Neuroscience: A Reader.* Oxford: Blackwell.

Koch C. 2004. *The Quest for Consciousness: A Neurobiological Approach.* Englewood, CO: Roberts.

Marr D. 1982. *Vision: A Computational Investigation into the Human Representation and Processing of Visual Information.* San Francisco: Freeman.

McCarthy R, Warrington EK. 1990. *Cognitive Neuropsychology: A Clinical Introduction.* London, San Diego: Academic Press.

Sacks O. 1970. *The Man Who Mistook His Wife for a Hat and Other Clinical Tales.* New York: Touchstone.

References

Antal A, Kincses TZ, Nitsche MA, Paulus W. 2003. Modulation of moving phosphene thresholds by transcranial direct current stimulation of V1 in human. Neuropsychology 41:1802–1807.

Baddeley AD, Thornton A, Chua SE, McKenna P. 1996. Schizophrenic delusions and the construction of autobiographical memory. In: DC Rubin (ed). *Remembering Our Past: Studies in Autobiographical Memory*, pp. 384–428. Cambridge, UK: Cambridge University Press.

Baddeley AD, Wilson BA. 1986. Amnesia, autobiographical memory and confabulation. In: DC Rubin (ed). *Autobiographical Memory*, pp. 225–252. Cambridge, UK: Cambridge University Press.

Bauer RM. 1994. Autonomic recognition of names and faces in prosopagnosia: a neuropsychological application of the Guilty Knowledge test. Neuropsychology 22:457–469.

Beck DM, Rees G, Frith CD, Lavie N. 2001. Neural correlates of change and change blindness. Nat Neurosci 4:645–650.

Beck JS. 1995. *Cognitive Therapy: Basics and Beyond.* New York: Guilford Press.

Blount G. 1986. Dangerousness of patients with Capgras syndrome. Nebr Med J 71:207.

Burgess PW, Baxter D, Rose M, Alderman N. 1986. Delusional paramnesic syndrome. In: PW Halligan, JC Marshall (eds). *Method in Madness: Case Studies in Cognitive Neuropsychiatry*, pp. 51–78. Hove, UK: Psychology Press.

Destrebecqz A, Cleeremans A. 2001. Can sequence learning be implicit? New evidence with the process dissociation procedure. Psychon B Rev 8:343–350.

Dierks T, Linden DE, Jandl M, Formisano E, Goebel R, Lanfermann H, Singer W. 1999. Activation of Heschle's gyrus during auditory hallucinations. Neuron 22:615–621.

Ellis HD, Young AW. 1990. Accounting for delusional misidentification. Br J Psychiat 157:239–248.

ffytche DH, Howard RJ, Brammer MJ, David A, Woordruff P, Williams S. 1998. The anatomy of conscious vision: an fMRI study of visual hallucinations. Nat Neurosci 1:738–742.

Fourneret P, Jeannerod M. 1998. Limited conscious monitoring of motor performance in normal subjects. Neuropsychology 36:1133–1140.

Frith C. 2005. The self in action: lessons from delusions of control. Conscious Cogn 14:752–770.

Glisky EL, Schacter DL. 1988. Long-term retention of computer learning in patients with memory disorders. Neuropsychology 26:173–178.

Haggard P, Eimer M. 1999. On the relation between brain potentials and awareness of voluntary movements. Exp Brain Res 126:128–133.

Hampton RR. 2001. Rhesus monkeys know when they remember. Proc Natl Acad Sci U S A 98:5359–5362.

Jacoby LL, Whitehouse K. 1989. An illusion of memory: false recognition influenced by unconscious perception. J Exp Psychol Gen 118:126–135.

Jeannerod M. 1994. The representing brain: neural correlates of motor intention and imagery. Behav Brain Sci 17: 187–202.

Kopelman MD. 1995. The assessment of psychogenic amnesia. In: AD Baddeley, BA Wilson, FN Watts (eds). *Handbook of Memory Disorders*. New York: Wiley.

Leopold DA, Logothetis NK. 1999. Multistable phenomena: changing views in perception. Trends Cogn Sci 3:254–264.

Libet B, Gleason CA, Wright EW, Pearl DK. 1983. Time of conscious intention to act in relation to onset of cerebral activity (readiness potential). The unconscious initiation of a freely voluntary act. Brain 106:623–642.

Marshall JC, Halligan PW. 1988. Blindsight and insight in visuo-spatial neglect. Nature 336:766–767.

Merskey H. 1995. *The Analysis of Hysteria: Understanding Conversion and Dissociation*, 2nd ed. London: Gaskell.

Milner AD, Goodale MA. 1995. *The Visual Brain in Action*. Oxford, UK: Oxford University Press.

O'Craven KM, Kanwisher N. 2000. Mental imagery of faces and places activates corresponding stimulus-specific brain regions. J Cogn Neurosci 12:1013–1023.

Öhman A, Soares JJ. 1994. "Unconscious anxiety": phobic responses to masked stimuli. J Abnorm Psychol 103: 231–240.

Penfield W, Perot P. 1963. The brain's record of auditory and visual experience: a final summary and discussion. Brain 86:595–696.

Rensink RA, O'Regan JK, Clark JJ. 1997. To see or not to see: the need for attention to perceive changes in scenes. Psychol Sci 8:368–373.

Rugg MD, Mark RE, Walla P, Schloerscheidt AM, Birch CS, Allan K. 1998. Dissociation of the neural correlates of implicit and explicit memory. Nature 392:595–598.

Schenk T. 2006. An allocentric rather than perceptual deficit in patient DF. Nat Neurosci 9:1369–1370.

Shergill SS, Samson G, Bays PM, Frith CD, Wolpert DM. 2005. Evidence for sensory prediction deficits in schizophrenia. Am J Psychiatry 162:2384–2386.

Tong F, Nakayama K, Vaughn JT, Kanwisher N. 1998. Binocular rivalry and visual awareness in human extrastriate cortex. Neuron 21:753–759.

Watson JB. 1930. *Behaviorism*. Chicago: University of Chicago Press.

Weiskrantz L. 1986. *Blindsight: A Case Study and Its Implications*. Oxford, UK: Oxford University Press.

62

Disorders of Thought and Volition: Schizophrenia

The success of neurobiology in providing insights into perception, cognition, and more recently emotion has inspired increasingly sophisticated biological investigations into disorders of thought and mood. In this chapter and the next we examine the four most serious disorders of thinking and mood: schizophrenia, depression, mania, and the anxiety states. These disorders involve disturbances in thought, self-awareness, perception, affect, volition, and social interaction.

In addition to being scientifically challenging, mental illness such as schizophrenia is of great social importance. Tragically this illness results in lifelong disability. The World Health Organization counts schizophrenia as one of the most significant contributors to disease burden (defined as healthy years of life lost to illness) worldwide. Fully 5% of people with schizophrenia commit suicide. Many more are homeless. The vast majority are unable to function successfully in school or in the workplace. Before the advent of psychopharmacologic therapies, schizophrenia and the mood disorders accounted for more than half of all hospital admissions in the United States. Even now schizophrenia accounts for approximately 30% of all hospitalizations.

The pattern of symptoms of schizophrenia are remarkably similar in all countries and cultures. The average prevalence worldwide ranges between 0.5 and 1%; the male-female ratio is 1.4:1. Diagnosis is usually made during late adolescence or early adulthood with the emergence of full symptoms, but in retrospect the illness begins far earlier with prodromal symptoms.

Diagnosis of Schizophrenia Is Based on Standardized Clinical Criteria

In medicine the understanding of a disease, and therefore its diagnosis, is ultimately based on identification of (1) etiological factors (such as microbes, toxins, or genetic risks) and (2) pathogenesis (mechanisms by which etiologic agents produce disease). Unfortunately, the etiology and pathogenesis of most mental disorders have not been determined. As a result, psychiatric diagnoses still rely on the patient's description of symptoms, the examiner's observations, a detailed natural history (the course of the illness over time), and the response to treatment.

This approach to psychiatric diagnosis began at the turn of the 20th century with the work of Emil Kraepelin in Germany. Influenced by Rudolf Virchow, the German pioneer of cellular pathology, and by Thomas Sydenham, the English clinician who focused attention on the natural history of medical diseases, Kraepelin studied mental disorders as specific disease processes. Even without knowledge about the etiology and pathogenesis, of diseases affecting thought, emotion, and behavior, he argued, such diseases could still be distinguished on the basis of signs, symptoms, and natural history.

Of course, the presentation of a single sign or symptom is not in itself evidence for disease because it may occur in healthy people. But when certain signs and symptoms occur together they form a syndrome, a condition that can be distinguished from normal behavior or from other clusters of signs and symptoms. The natural history of a disease is studied by tracing the onset of signs and symptoms in patients' lives and how they change with time. Thus a syndrome can emerge at a characteristic age or it can follow a characteristic clinical course. For example, Kraepelin recognized that most patients with schizophrenia (which he called dementia praecox) do not recover the level of functioning they had prior to the onset of the disease, whereas most patients with mood disorders experience cycles of relapse and at least partial recovery.

Since the 1980s the diagnosis of psychiatric disorders has been based on standardized criteria that have made diagnosis more reliable. Two different clinicians applying standardized criteria for schizophrenia are very likely to arrive at the same diagnosis. Nevertheless, without etiological or pathophysiological data and lacking objective tests, current diagnostic systems such as the *Diagnostic and Statistical Manual of Mental Disorders, 4th edition* (*DSM-IV*) of the American Psychiatric Association cannot define disease states in scientifically verifiable terms. With progress in such areas as genetics and neuroimaging, it eventually should be possible to arrive at objectively verifiable and thus valid diagnostic criteria for mental disorders.

The Symptoms of Schizophrenia Can Be Grouped into Positive, Negative, and Cognitive

It is useful to subdivide the symptoms of schizophrenia into three clusters because each may reflect different aspects of the pathophysiology and because each responds differently to the medications presently used. Positive or psychotic symptoms include mental phenomena that do not occur in healthy people, such as hallucinations and delusions. Negative (or "deficit") symptoms result from impairment of normal functions and can include blunted emotional responses, withdrawal from social interactions, impoverished content of thought and speech (Box 62–1), and a lack of motivation.

A third symptom cluster includes cognitive abnormalities—sometimes described as "disorganization symptoms." These symptoms impair working memory and executive functions—the ability to organize one's life. These cognitive symptoms typically persist even during otherwise successful treatment with medication and are thought to be significant contributors to long-term disability. Interestingly, cognitive symptoms can be found to some degree in persons at very high risk of developing schizophrenia but who have not yet experienced hallucinations or delusions, and in otherwise healthy relatives of patients with schizophrenia, suggesting that cognitive symptoms reflect genetic predispositions to schizophrenia.

The medications used to treat schizophrenia are called antipsychotic drugs and are most effective at diminishing the positive symptoms as well as psychotic symptoms that occur in mood disorders. None of the medications reliably benefits the cognitive symptoms.

Schizophrenia Is Characterized by Psychotic Episodes

The most dramatic manifestations of schizophrenia are psychotic symptoms, including hallucinations and delusions. Hallucinations are percepts that occur in the absence of appropriate sensory stimuli and can occur in any sensory modality. In schizophrenia the most common hallucinations are auditory. Typically, a patient hears voices, but noises or music are also common. Sometimes the voices will carry on a dialog and frequently are experienced as bullying and derogatory. Occasionally, voices will issue commands to the patient that can create a high risk of harm, including suicide. Neuroimaging studies of subjects experiencing auditory hallucinations suggest that areas normally involved in the processing of language are recruited during hallucinations. These include Broca's area in the frontal lobe and Wernicke's area in the superior temporal lobe of the cerebral cortex (see Chapter 60).

Delusions are firm beliefs that are not realistic and not explained by the patient's culture. They can be so powerful that sufferers cannot (or refuse to) compare their beliefs to what is actually happening in the world. Delusions can be quite varied in form. For some patients reality is distorted: The world is full of hidden signs meant only for them (delusions of reference), or they are being closely watched or persecuted (paranoid

Box 62–1 Schizophrenic Speech

Language disturbance is a central feature of schizophrenia and one of the primary behaviors by which it is diagnosed. Grammar is reasonably intact, but content can wander or be incoherent, a symptom that is commonly referred to as "loosening of associations." More bizarre but less common patterns of speech include neologisms (idiosyncratically invented words), blocking (sudden spontaneous interruptions), or clanging (associations based on the sounds rather than the meanings of words, such as "If you can make sense out of nonsense, well, have fun. I'm trying to make cents out of sense. I'm not making cents anymore. I have to make dollars.")

Examples of loosening of associations are:

"I'm supposed to be making a film, but I don't know what is going to be the end of it. Jesus Christ is writing a book about me."

"I don't think they care for me because two million camels . . . 10 million taxis . . . Father Christmas on the rebound."

Question: "How does your head feel?" Answer: "My head, well that's the hardest part of the job. My memory is just as good as the next working man's. I tell you what my trouble is, I can't read. You can't learn anything if you can't read or write properly. You can't pick up a nice book, I don't just mean a sex book, a book about literature or about history or something like that. You can't pick up and read it and find things out for yourself."

Several different types of loosening of associations have been proposed (such as derailment, incoherence, tangentiality, or loss of goal). However, it remains unclear whether these reflect disturbances in fundamentally different mechanisms or different manifestations of a common underlying disturbance, such as the inability to represent a "speech plan" to guide coherent speech. A disturbance of such a mechanism would be consistent with, and may parallel, impairment of control of other cognitive functions in schizophrenia, such as deficits in working memory.

delusions). Others experience bizarre delusions, for example that some entity is inserting or extracting thoughts from their brain or that their dental fillings are radio transmitters broadcasting what they say to nefarious groups. Psychotic symptoms can also occur in mood disorders and drug-induced delirium, but the other symptoms and clinical course of those states are not consistent with schizophrenia.

The full emergence of schizophrenia is often preceded by a period of early symptoms. In this prodromal period the patient can behave eccentrically, become socially isolated, exhibit blunted affect, poverty of speech, a poor attention span, and lack of motivation. Once the disease is fully manifest, periods of florid psychosis typically occur, accompanied by markedly disordered thinking and abnormalities in the regulation of emotion. These periods of overt psychosis are interspersed with periods of residual symptoms. After the first few episodes the patient rarely returns to full normal functioning.

Both Genetic and Nongenetic Risk Factors Contribute to Schizophrenia

Schizophrenia, like many other mental illnesses, runs in families. As early as 1930 Franz Kalman in Germany studied familial patterns of transmission and concluded that genes contribute significantly to schizophrenia. Three major strategies have been used to quantify the contribution of heredity to the risk of schizophrenia and to understand how genetic risk is transmitted.

In one strategy the rate of concordance for schizophrenia in monozygotic twin pairs, whose DNA sequences are 100% identical, is compared with that in dizygotic twin pairs, whose DNA sequences are on average 50% identical. Assuming that the familial environment is roughly identical for both types of twin pairs, then if genes play a significant role the concordance rates should be higher among monozygotic pairs than among dizygotic pairs. In fact, monozygotic twins have a concordance rate of nearly 50% for schizophrenia, whereas dizygotic twins have a concordance rate of approximately 15% (slightly higher than that for ordinary siblings, which also have on average 50% genetic identity).

Although these rates suggest an important role for genes in schizophrenia, they also demonstrate that genes are not completely determinative. If they were, the concordance rate for monozygotic twins would be 100% as it is in Huntington disease for example. Thus factors other than inherited DNA sequence, such as new mutations, epigenetic modification of DNA, environmental factors, and stochastic factors occurring during brain development, play a role in converting inherited genetic vulnerability into the disease.

To separate genetic factors and environmental influences more clearly, Seymour Kety, David Rosenthal, and Paul Wender examined children who were adopted at or shortly after birth in Denmark, a country where very accurate family and health records are kept. They found that the rate of schizophrenia in the biological family of an adoptee was much more strongly predictive of schizophrenia than the rate in the adoptive family. Kety and his colleagues also observed that some of the blood relatives of schizophrenic adoptees exhibited some symptoms of schizophrenia, such as social isolation, suspiciousness, eccentric beliefs, and magical thinking, even though they did not have full-blown schizophrenia. These symptoms are part of what is now called schizotypal personality disorder. Kety and his colleagues did not possess modern understandings of working memory, but it would have been interesting to know whether their sample also exhibited the cognitive abnormalities now documented in some relatives of people with schizophrenia. Overall the schizotypal symptoms are thought to be a mild, nonpsychotic form of the disease.

More recently, unaffected monozygotic twins and even siblings of patients with schizophrenia have been found to exhibit some neuroanatomic abnormalities similar to those with the disease. In one magnetic resonance imaging (MRI) study monozygotic twins discordant for schizophrenia had similar deficits in the dorsolateral prefrontal cortex and superior temporal gyrus.

Studies by Irving Gottesman of extended pedigrees of Danish patients with schizophrenia also support the importance of genes. Gottesman noted the correlations between the risk of schizophrenia in relatives and the percentage of the total genetic material each relative shared with the patient. He found a greater lifetime risk of schizophrenia among first-degree relatives (parents, siblings, and children, who share 50% of the relatives' DNA sequences) than among second-degree relatives (aunts, uncles, nieces, nephews, and grandchildren), who share 25% of their DNA sequences with the patient. Even third-degree relatives (who share only 12.5% of the patient's DNA sequences) were at higher risk for schizophrenia than the 1% of the population at risk for this disease (Figure 62–1).

With the advent of modern genomic technologies during the last decade, progress has been made in identifying variations in DNA sequence that contribute to the risk of schizophrenia. As with many common disorders, risk for schizophrenia has proven to be genetically heterogeneous, with no single gene proving necessary or sufficient. Two forms of genetic variation have been associated with schizophrenia: Variations in single nucleotide bases, and larger chromosomal deletions, duplications, or translocations. In most cases schizophrenia appears to result from the action of a large number of genes together with environmental risk

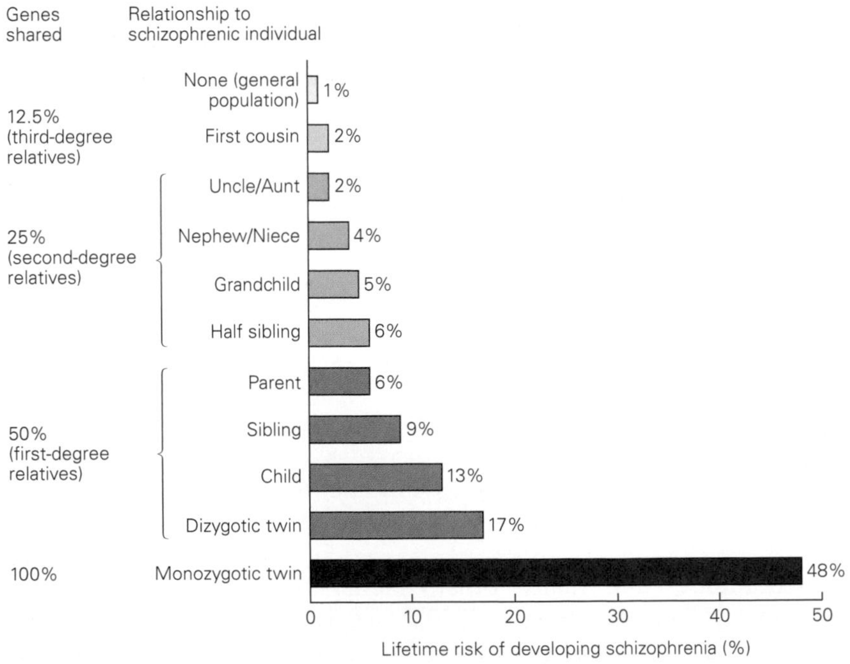

Figure 62–1 Lifetime risk of schizophrenia as a function of genetic relatedness to a person with schizophrenia. Note that risk increases with increased genetic relatedness but varies within categories of relatedness, reflecting epigenetic effects or new mutations. (Reproduced, with permission, from Gottesman 1991.)

factors. In a minority of cases schizophrenia risk is markedly elevated by chromosomal abnormalities such as a microdeletion on chromosome 22q11.2.

As with any genetically influenced disease, understanding how certain sequences at particular loci in the genome confer risk should provide important clues to pathophysiology, and thus treatment development. Because schizophrenia may result from abnormal developmental processes in the brain, knowing the time during development and adulthood when the genes that predispose to schizophrenia are expressed in the brain would be valuable, as it would suggest different avenues for investigation and might also suggest optimal times for therapeutic intervention.

The complexity of schizophrenia genetics is illustrated by a well-studied chromosomal translocation that was discovered in a large Scottish family. This translocation between chromosomes 1 and 11 inactivates a gene that came to be called Disrupted in Schizophrenia-1 (*Disc*-1) that appears to have significant roles in brain development. Within this multigenerational family, individuals who inherited the translocation exhibit serious mental illness but not necessarily schizophrenia. Some have bipolar disorder and others have major depression. Thus truncations in *Disc*-1 must interact with other genes and nongenetic factors to determine the ultimate phenotype.

Attempts to identify objectively measurable components of schizophrenia and other psychiatric disorders have focused on what have been called intermediate phenotypes or endophenotypes. Intermediate phenotypes may represent measurable structural brain abnormalities—cognitive abnormalities (such as deficits in working memory) measured by their neural correlates on functional neuroimaging—or they may represent measurable neurochemical abnormalities. If intermediate phenotypes can successfully be identified, they may simplify the search for risk genes because they may help identify more homogeneous populations for study than those identified by clinical symptoms and interviewing alone.

The search for modifiable environmental risk factors has also proved daunting because some environmental factors that correlate with the disease may be a result rather than a cause of schizophrenia and others may be proxies for the actual, but as yet undiscovered risks. For example, a consistent relationship has been found between schizophrenia and low socioeconomic status. However, the evidence suggests that schizophrenia itself impairs occupational and social success, leading to downward socioeconomic drift, rather than the alternative notion that stressors associated with poverty contribute to the disease. Other environmental risk factors, including season of birth, urban birth, maternal exposure to viral illness, paternal age, and perinatal complications, have been identified in population studies. Understanding the aspects of urban birth that might contribute to the risk of schizophrenia poses a significant challenge.

Neuroanatomic Abnormalities May Be a Causative Factor in Schizophrenia

Schizophrenia is characterized by certain abnormalities in brain anatomy that can be seen with structural and functional magnetic resonance imaging (fMRI). Thinning of specific areas of the prefrontal, temporal, and parietal cerebral cortex has been observed in many studies (Figure 62–2). The thinning of the prefrontal cortex is most pronounced in the dorsolateral prefrontal cortex, the brain region most critical for working memory.

Thinning in the temporal lobe has been traced to a loss of gray matter in the superior temporal gyrus, the temporal pole, the amygdala (amygdala reductions may be limited to males), and the hippocampus. These regions are normally involved in integrating cognition and emotion. The loss of gray matter is counterbalanced by an increase in the volume of the cerebral ventricles (Figure 62–3).

Structural abnormalities in the brain, such as loss of cortical gray matter, have been correlated with functional abnormalities both in cognitive performance tests and studies with positron emission therapy (PET) or fMRI. Impairment of functions that are dependent on the prefrontal cortex have been particularly well documented. For example, patients with schizophrenia have deficits in working memory and cognitive control, which are correlated in functional neuroimaging studies with lack of activity in the dorsolateral prefrontal cortex.

Loss of Gray Matter in the Cerebral Cortex Appears to Result from Loss of Synaptic Contacts Rather Than Loss of Cells

The observed loss of volume in the frontal and temporal cortical regions is not the result of cell death (loss of cell bodies) but rather a reduction in dendritic, axonal, and synaptic processes (neuropil). As a consequence, the density of cells in the cerebral cortex increases. More cells per unit volume and less total gray matter contribute to enlargement of the ventricular spaces.

Like the prefrontal and temporal cortex, the thalamus also appears smaller in patients with schizophrenia compared to nonaffected individuals. But cell counts in postmortem tissue suggest that, unlike the cerebral cortex, there may be loss of cell bodies in the mediodorsal nucleus of the thalamus. Because cells of

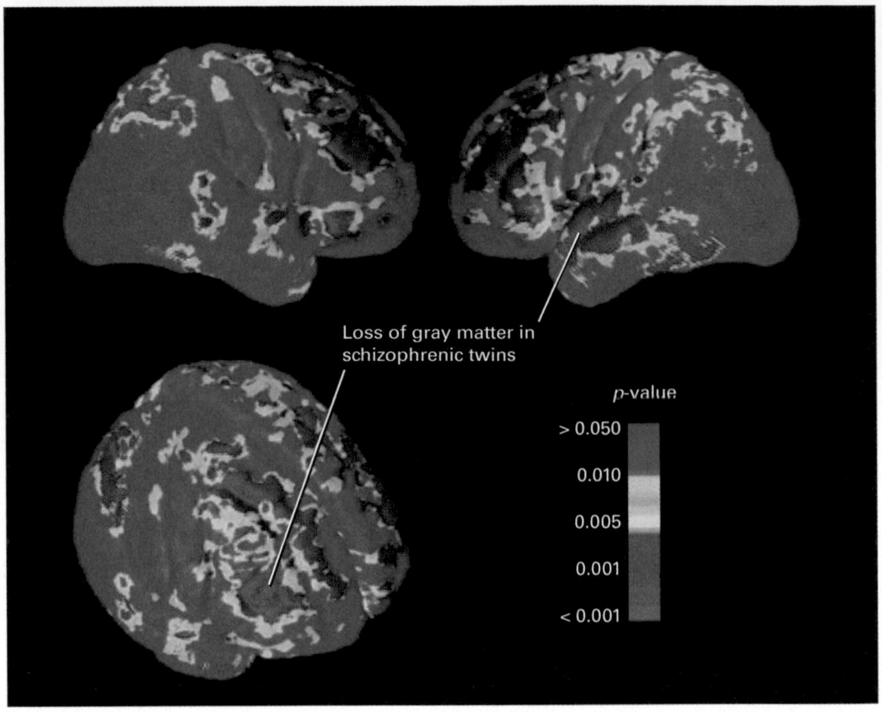

Figure 62–2 Gray matter loss in schizophrenia. Gray matter loss is well documented in schizophrenia; unaffected first-degree relatives also show some loss of cortical gray matter. A study of monozygotic and dizygotic twin pairs discordant for schizophrenia and healthy matched control twins showed that there are significant gray matter deficits in those at genetic risk for schizophrenia. However, among the affected members of twin pairs there are additional, disease-specific deficits in dorsolateral prefrontal, superior temporal, and superior parietal association areas. These reflect the influence of nongenetic factors (eg, developmental or environmental factors). The disease-specific gray matter loss correlates with symptom severity and degree of cognitive dysfunction rather than with duration of illness or drug treatment. The images here show regional deficits in gray matter in schizophrenic monozygotic twins relative to their healthy co-twins (n = 10 pairs) viewed from the right, left, and right-oblique perspectives. Differences in twins are illustrated by the pseudocolor scale superimposed on cortical surface maps, with pink and red indicating the greatest statistical significance. (Reproduced, with permission, from Cannon et al. 2002.)

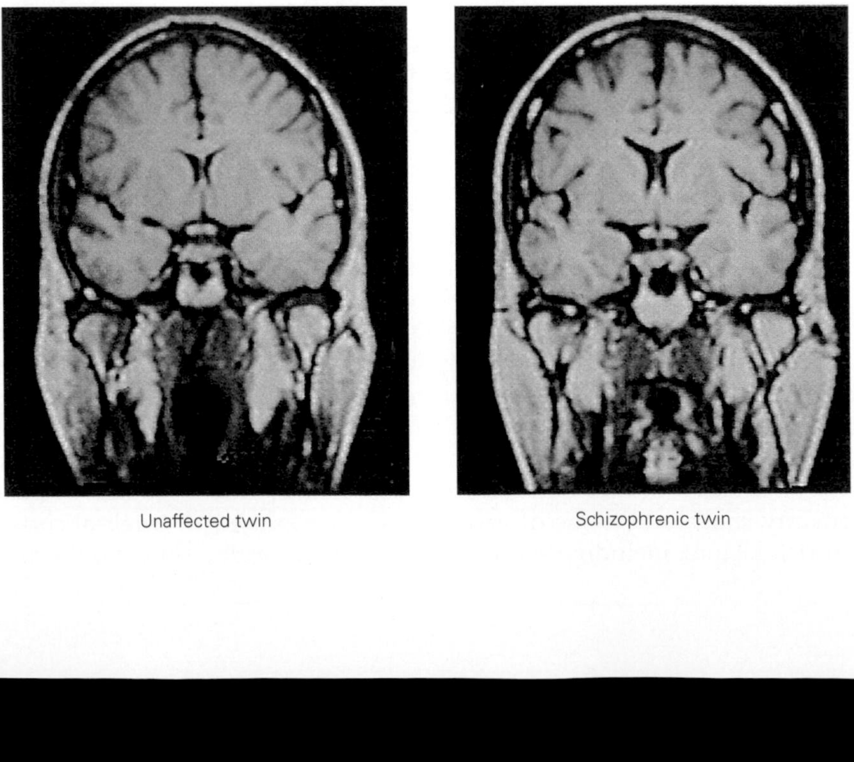

Figure 62–3 Enlargement of lateral ventricles in schizophrenia. This MRI compares monozygotic co-twins discordant for schizophrenia. The affected member of the twin pair has the characteristically enlarged ventricles of schizophrenia. Because there is a wide range of normal ventricular volumes in the population, an unaffected monozygotic twin serves as a particularly appropriate control subject. As with Figure 62–2, this comparison also illustrates the role of nongenetic factors in schizophrenia because monozygotic twins have identical genomes.

the mediodorsal nucleus send their axons to the dorsolateral prefrontal cortex, loss of these axonal terminals could in turn contribute to the reduction of cortical dendrites and the dendritic spines that usually receive these thalamocortical connections.

Pyramidal neurons, the most common type of excitatory neuron in the neocortex, receive excitatory input from the thalamus on dendritic spines. Thus the reduction in dendrites and dendritic spines (Figure 62–4) would likely signify a loss of synaptic contacts in the dorsolateral prefrontal cortex in schizophrenia. The loss of synaptic connections in this region could possibly explain the impairment of working memory and executive function that characterizes schizophrenia (Figure 62–5).

Abnormalities in Brain Development During Adolescence May Contribute to Schizophrenia

Because schizophrenia first occurs typically in late teenage years or in the early twenties, symptoms may be triggered by abnormalities in late stages of brain development. Early adulthood is an important period of brain development, as the brain matures in response to a variety of influences. These range from gonadal steroids in adolescence to stressful life experiences such as separating from parents and siblings for college or military service, or becoming independent by taking on adult responsibilities such as employment and sexual relationships.

During this period critical life events are accompanied by synaptic pruning that is part of the selective maintenance of those synaptic connections that are used effectively during normal brain development. Synaptic pruning may be particularly important in the prefrontal cortex. Moreover, the pruning coincides with major changes in dopaminergic neurotransmission in this brain area during late adolescence. The timing of these processes is consistent with the implication of both prefrontal cortex and the dopaminergic system in the pathogenesis of schizophrenia (Figure 62–5).

Although slow continued loss of gray matter in prefrontal and temporal cortex has been observed after diagnosis, cortical abnormalities and ventricular enlargement are generally observed at the time of first diagnosis, suggesting that the pathogenic processes underlying schizophrenia have been active long before psychotic symptoms emerge.

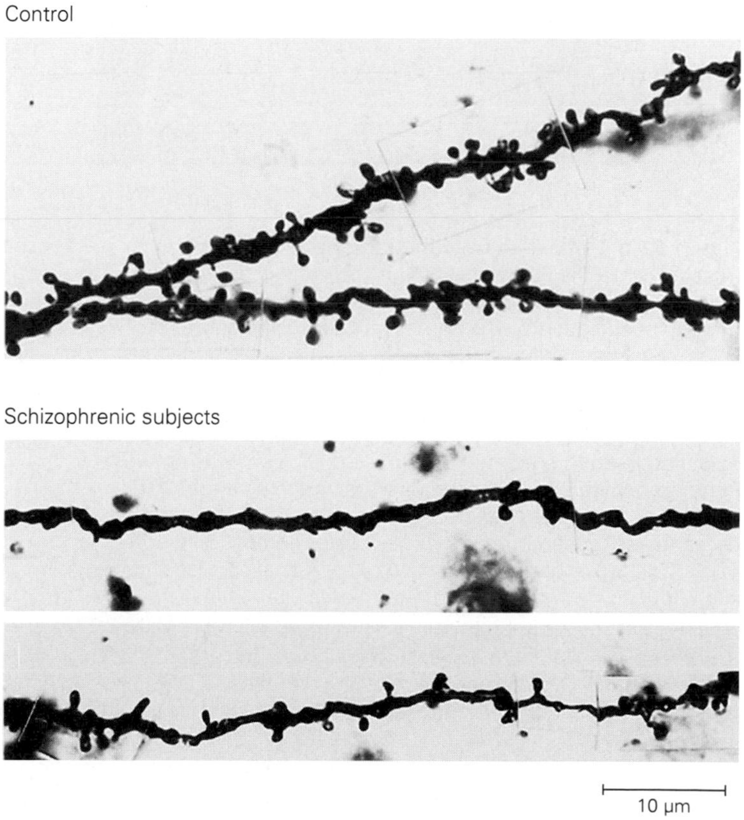

Figure 62–4 Decreased dendritic spine density in schizophrenia. Brightfield photomicrographs illustrate Golgi-impregnated basilar dendrites and spines of pyramidal neurons in layer III in the dorsolateral prefrontal cortex in a normal control subject and two subjects with schizophrenia. Note the loss of dendritic spines in the schizophrenic subjects. (Reproduced, with permission, from Glantz and Lewis 2000.)

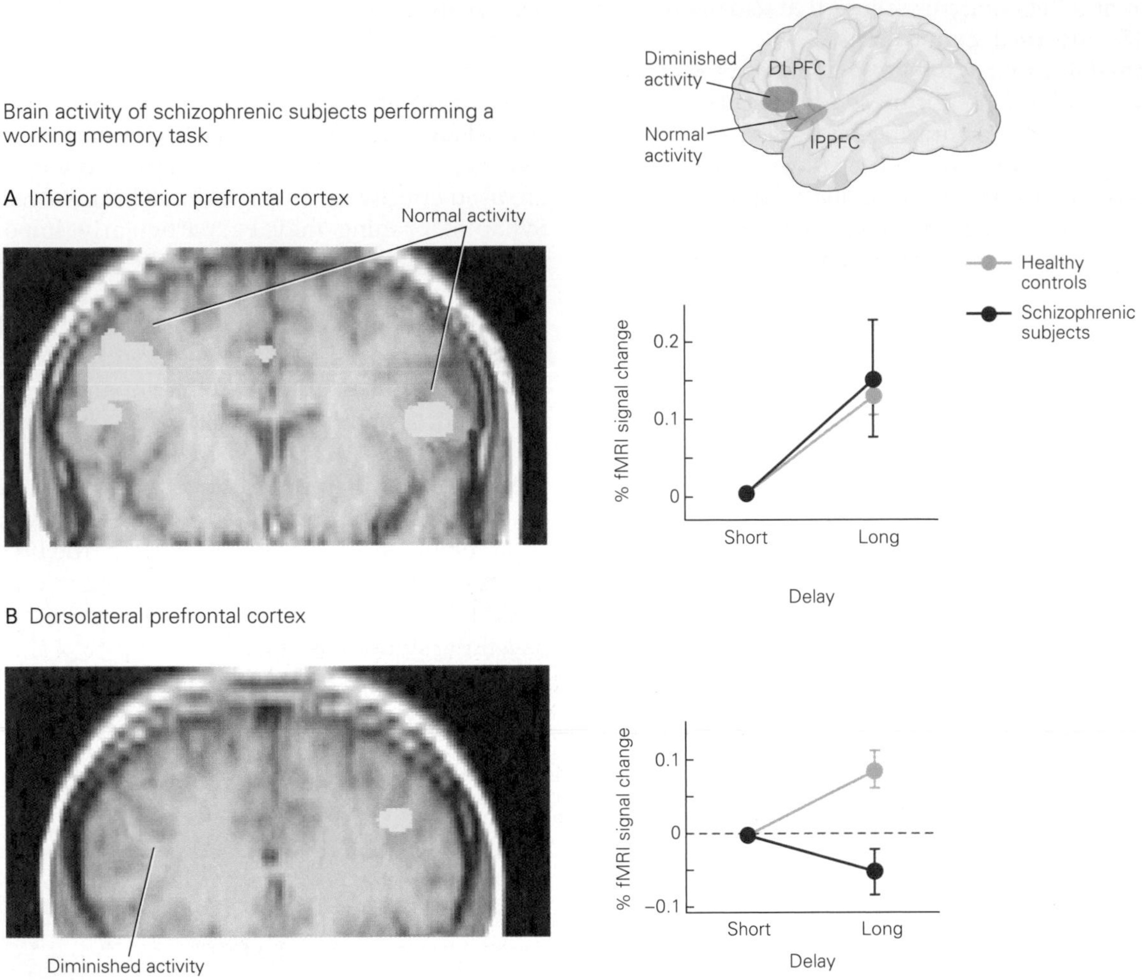

Figure 62–5 Deficits in the function of prefrontal cortex in schizophrenia. Functional MRI (fMRI) was used to examine activity in prefrontal cortex in patients with schizophrenia (first-episode patients who had never been given antipsychotic drugs) as well as healthy controls during performance of a working memory task. Subjects were presented with a sequence of letters and instructed to respond to a particular letter (the "probe" letter) only if it immediately followed another specified letter (the "contextual cue" letter). Demands on working memory were increased by increasing the delay between the cue and the probe letters. A longer delay places greater demands on working memory. The greater demand is hypothesized to require greater activation of prefrontal cortical circuits. (Reproduced, with permission, from Barch et al. 2001.)

A. In both schizophrenic patients and controls activation within Brodmann's area 44/46 increases normally with increases in demand on working memory, suggesting that these inferior posterior regions of prefrontal cortex (IPPFC) have intact function in schizophrenia. The plot shows the signal change that occurs in the "long-delay" and "short-delay" conditions in healthy controls and patients with schizophrenia based on the activity in the right side of the prefrontal cortex shown in the fMRI scan. Similar effects were observed for activity in the left-side.

B. There is less activity in Brodmann's area 46/49, a region of dorsolateral prefrontal cortex (DLPFC), in patients with schizophrenia relative to healthy controls. Unlike the areas of prefrontal cortex shown in part A, Brodmann's area 46/49 is not activated normally in subjects with schizophrenia. The plot shows that, unlike IPPFC, DLPFC in schizophrenic subjects fails to activate in the long-delay relative to the short-delay condition, consistent with the deficit in working memory function shown by patients with schizophrenia. Selective impairment of one region of prefrontal cortex alongside other regions that appear to have normal function suggests that the impairment is caused by a regionally specific process rather than a diffuse and nonspecific pathophysiological process.

Comparisons of middle-aged and older monozygotic twins that are discordant for schizophrenia (and in which the unaffected twin serves as a control) have shown that the severity of gray matter deficits in the prefrontal cortex correlate with severity of symptoms, not with the duration of illness. Of course, such studies cannot tell us whether the deficits were fully present at the onset of symptoms. To address this issue Judith Rapoport conducted a longitudinal study of those rare individuals with onset of schizophrenia in childhood and documented a correlation between progression of gray matter deficits and ventricular enlargement with time and duration of illness. In these subjects the normal loss of gray matter during adolescence, presumably related to normal processes of synaptic pruning, was exaggerated (Figure 62–6).

Antipsychotic Drugs Act on Dopaminergic Systems in the Brain

The antipsychotic drugs used to treat schizophrenia all act on the dopaminergic pathways of the forebrain. The first effective antipsychotic drug, chlorpromazine,

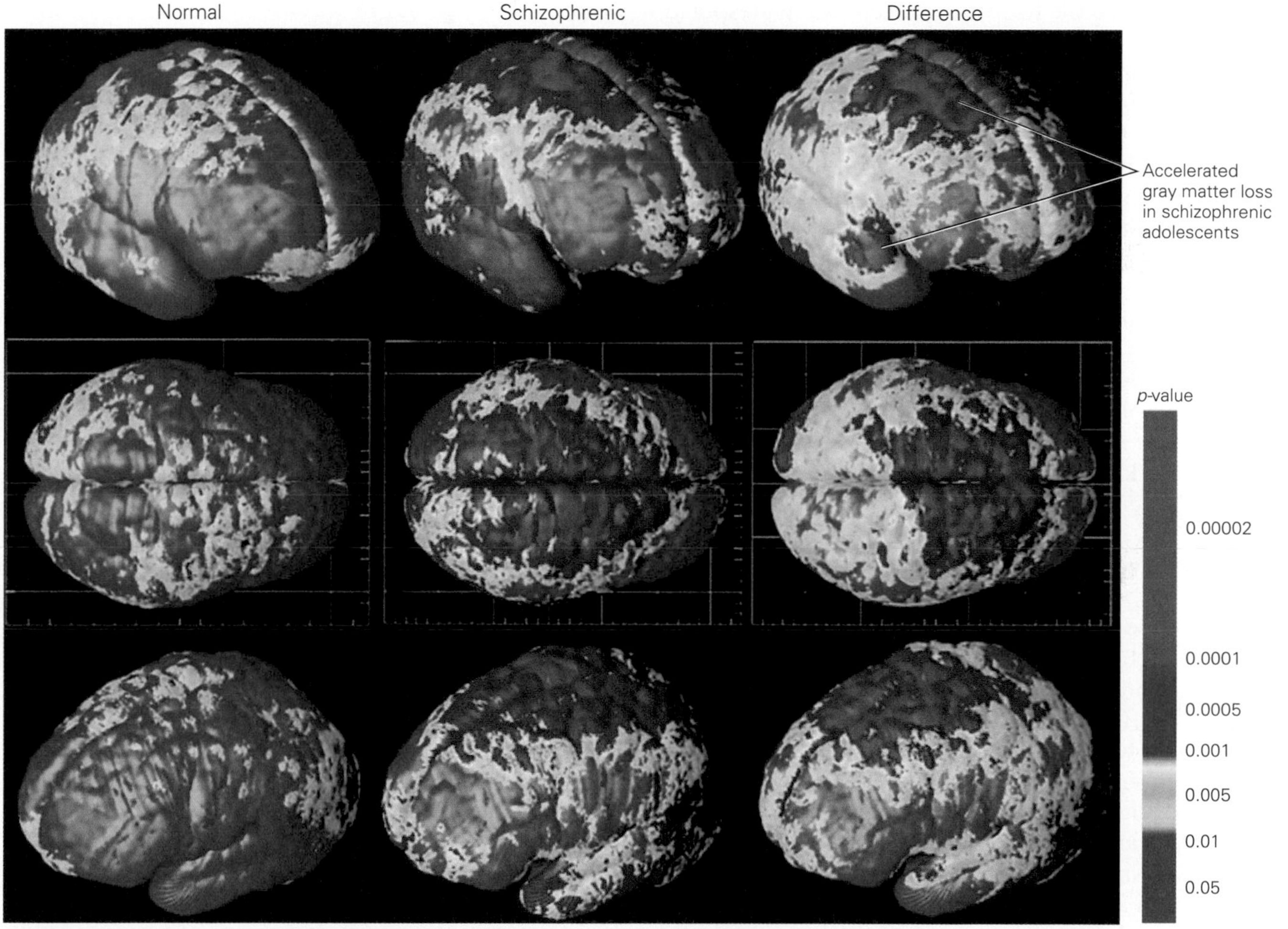

Figure 62–6 Normal loss of gray matter in adolescence is accelerated in adolescents with schizophrenia. The volume of gray matter in parietal, motor, supplementary motor, and superior frontal areas of cerebral cortex is progressively reduced during adolescence because of normal processes of synaptic pruning. In schizophrenic adolescents the loss of gray matter is more pronounced in broad regions of temporal cortex, including the superior temporal gyrus. The loss of gray matter attributable to schizophrenia (right column) can be determined by comparing the average rates of gray matter loss in normal and schizophrenic adolescents. Significant differences are shown in the pseudocolor scale superimposed on the cortical maps. (Reproduced, with permission, from Thompson et al. 2001.)

was developed for its antihistaminic and sedating effects and not for its psychiatric effects. Chlorpromazine was later found to be effective in treating the agitation of patients with schizophrenia and manic depressive illness. Based on these acute calming effects, chlorpromazine and many related drugs were initially described as major tranquilizers. By the mid 1960s, however, it became clear that these drugs were not simply acting as tranquilizers but were specifically reducing the positive symptoms of schizophrenia, such as hallucinations and delusions. They were also effective in treating the psychotic symptoms that can occur in mood disorders, such as mania or severe depression.

The antipsychotic drugs had less impact on the negative symptoms of schizophrenia and little or no impact on cognitive deficits. Patients did improve enough to leave the hospital. Indeed, the widespread use of antipsychotic drugs paved the way for the large-scale release of patients with schizophrenia from psychiatric institutions. Unfortunately, these patients did not return to their premorbid level of functioning. The recognition that the sedating properties of early antipsychotic drugs were undesirable side effects led to the development of newer less sedating antipsychotic compounds. In addition, all of the first-generation antipsychotic drugs, with the exception of clozapine, produced Parkinson-like side effects in the extrapyramidal tract such as stiffness, tremor, and difficulty initiating movements.

Because Parkinson disease is caused by the loss of dopaminergic neurons in the midbrain, the occurrence of Parkinson-like symptoms with antipsychotic drug treatment suggested to Arvid Carlsson that these drugs decreased dopaminergic transmission. Following up on this idea, Carlsson established that the antipsychotic drugs block dopamine receptors. Two families of dopamine receptors are known. The D_1 family, which in humans includes D_1 and D_5, are coupled to stimulatory G proteins that activate adenylyl cyclase. The D_2 family, which includes D_2, D_3, and D_4, are coupled to the inhibitory G protein (G_i) that inhibits the cyclase. The D_2 family of receptors has also been shown to signal through an independent pathway involving β arrestin$_2$ (β-arr$_2$) and Akt, a protein kinase previously known as protein kinase B. The family of D_1 receptors are expressed in the striatum and are the major type of dopamine receptor in the cerebral cortex and hippocampus, while the D_2 family of receptors is expressed most densely in the striatum, but also in the cerebral cortex, amygdala, and hippocampus. Correlations between receptor binding studies and clinical efficacy in reducing positive psychotic symptoms indicate that the D_2 family is the main target of the therapeutic actions of antipsychotic drugs on positive symptoms (Figure 62–7).

Antipsychotic drugs not only treat acute relapses of schizophrenia and other psychotic disorders, but continuous treatment with these drugs reduces hospitalization because it markedly increases the time between relapses. Unfortunately, the side effects that occur with administration limit their long-term use. A second generation of antipsychotic medications has been developed based on the observation that clozapine has less likelihood of causing Parkinsonian side effects than the other drugs and can also produce

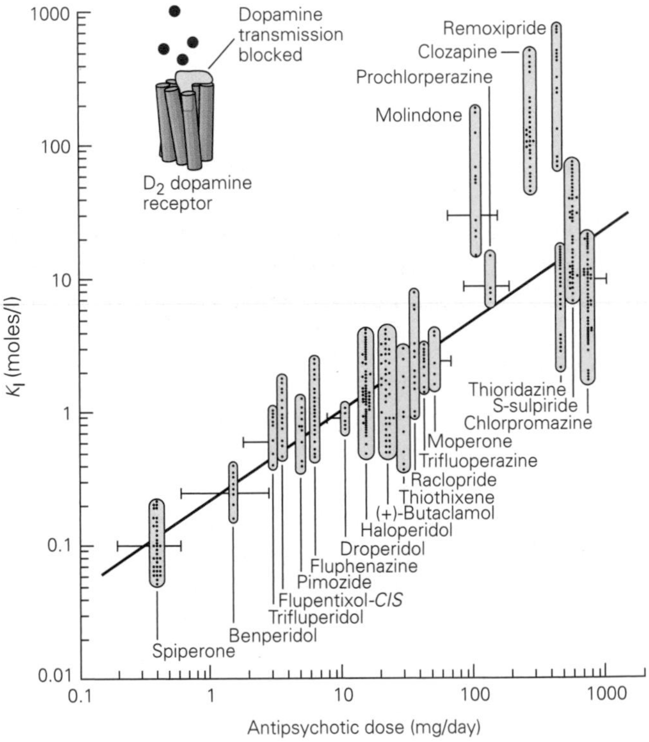

Figure 62–7 The potency of first-generation antipsychotic drugs in treating positive symptoms is strongly correlated with their affinity for D_2 dopamine receptors. On the horizontal axis is the average daily dose required to achieve similar levels of clinical efficacy. On the vertical axis is K_I, concentration of drug required to bind 50% of D_2 receptors in vitro. The higher the drug concentration required, the lower the affinity of the drug for the receptor. The measurements on the two axes are not entirely independent of each other as the ability of a drug to block dopamine D_2 receptors in vitro is often used to help determine doses to be tested in clinical trials. Clozapine, which does not fall on the line, has significantly greater efficacy than the others, although its mechanism of action is not well understood. (Adapted, with permission, from Seeman et al. 1976.)

therapeutic responses in some patients with schizophrenia for whom other drugs have not worked. (Unfortunately clozapine has other serious side effects that limit its use.)

Based on the properties of clozapine, some of the second-generation drugs were designed to have somewhat lower affinity for D_2 receptors than the first-generation drugs, and some also block the serotonin 5-HT_{2A} receptors, an action that was thought to protect against motor side effects. Recent large-scale clinical trials of the newer drugs have been disappointing, however, showing little incremental benefit over the older antipsychotic drugs. None of the newer drugs is equal to clozapine in efficacy.

Because drugs that reduce positive symptoms do so by blocking D_2 receptors, investigators have asked: What is the role of dopamine in the symptoms of schizophrenia? Although some drugs that block D_2 receptors reduce psychotic symptoms, other drugs that increase dopamine at synapses (such as amphetamine and cocaine) can produce psychotic symptoms, especially paranoid symptoms. Thus Carlsson suggested that dopaminergic systems are hyperactive in schizophrenia.

The most direct evidence for this idea comes from studies in the mid-1990s that found that amphetamine-produced increases in dopamine release were greater in schizophrenic patients than in healthy subjects. These studies suggest that abnormalities in amphetamine-sensitive processes—such as dopamine storage, vesicular transport, dopamine release, or dopamine reuptake by presynaptic neurons—might lead to hyperactivity in the subcortical dopaminergic systems and could contribute to the positive symptoms of schizophrenia, the symptoms that respond to antipsychotic drugs.

Although dopamine activity might increase in subcortical regions of the brain in schizophrenia, there is also some evidence that it might decrease in cortical regions and that this might contribute to the cognitive symptoms. In particular, the number of D_1 dopamine receptors in the prefrontal cortex is thought to be reduced in schizophrenia, an interesting idea because D_1 receptors have been shown to play a role in working memory and executive functions reliant on prefrontal cortex.

Glutamate, the major excitatory neurotransmitter in the brain, also has been implicated in schizophrenia, albeit indirectly. Phencyclidine and ketamine, which block the NMDA-type glutamate receptor and which were originally developed as anesthetic agents, produce psychotic symptoms. In healthy subjects ketamine also produces cognitive dysfunction that mimics, at least to a degree, the cognitive abnormalities seen in schizophrenia. This has led several investigators to explore the idea that decreased function of NMDA-type glutamate receptors might play a role in producing some of the positive and cognitive symptoms of schizophrenia. These studies indicate that positive and cognitive symptoms are probably the result of abnormalities in several transmitter systems that act either in parallel or in combination with dopamine.

An Overall View

Schizophrenia is a chronic, profoundly disabling disorder characterized by dramatic psychotic symptoms, as well as deficits in emotion, motivation, and cognition. The cognitive deficits impair the ability of people with schizophrenia to regulate their behavior in accordance with reasonable, stable goals. The result is that people with schizophrenia are frequently unable to hold down simple jobs, even at those times when antipsychotic drugs effectively control their hallucinations and delusions.

Once considered a purely psychological reaction to the family environment, it is now clear that schizophrenia is highly influenced by genetic risk factors; indeed, with modern genetic technologies the first convincing risk genes are being identified.

Postmortem studies and neuroimaging are documenting loss of gray matter in the prefrontal and temporal cerebral cortex. Functional neuroimaging is revealing the basis of the disabling cognitive symptoms. Despite this progress, the drugs that we have to treat schizophrenia, as useful as they are, still leave patients seriously symptomatic awaiting new discoveries from neural science.

Steven E. Hyman
Jonathan D. Cohen

Selected Readings

Cohen JD, Servan-Schreiber D. 1992. Context, cortex, and dopamine: a connectionist approach to behavior and biology in schizophrenia. Psychol Rev 99:45–77.

Harrison PJ. 1999. The neuropathology of schizophrenia. A critical review of the data and their interpretation. Brain 122:593–624.

Kerns JG, Berenbaum H. 2002. Cognitive impairments associated with formal thought disorder in people with schizophrenia. J Abnorm Psychol 111:211–224.
Lewis DA, Levitt P. 2002. Schizophrenia as a disorder of neurodevelopment. Annu Rev Neurosci 25:409–432.
Nestler EJ, Hyman SE, Malenka RJ. 2001. *Molecular Neuropharmacology. A Foundation for Clinical Neuroscience*. New York: McGraw-Hill.

References

Arnold SE, Trojanowski JQ, Gur RE, Blackwell P, Han LY, Choi C. 1998. Absence of neurodegeneration and neural injury in the cerebral cortex in a sample of elderly patients with schizophrenia. Arch Gen Psychiatry 55:225–232.
Barch DM, Carter CS, Braver TS, Sabb FW, MacDonald AW, Noll DC, Cohen JD. 2001. Selective deficits in prefrontal cortex function in medication-naïve patients with schizophrenia. Arch Gen Psychiatry 58:280–288.
Barch DM, Berenbaum H. 1996. Language production and thought disorder in schizophrenia. J Abnormal Psychiatry 105:81–88.
Beaulieu JM, Gainetdinov RR, Caron MG. 2009. Akt/GSK3 signaling in the action of psychotropic drugs. Annu Rev Pharmacol Toxicol 49:327–47.
Cannon TD, Thompson PM, van Erp TG, Toga AW. 2002. Cortex mapping reveals regionally specific patterns of genetic and disease-specific gray-matter deficits in twins discordant for schizophrenia. Proc Natl Acad Sci U S A 99:3228–3233.
Carter CS, Mintun M, Nichols T, Cohen JD. 1997. Anterior cingulate gyrus dysfunction and selective attentional dysfunction in schizophrenia: an 150-H20 PET study during Stroop task performance. Am J Psychiatry 154:1670–1675.
Chapman LJ, Chapman JP, Miller GA. 1964. A theory of verbal behavior in schizophrenia. In: BA Maher (ed). *Progress in Experimental Personality Research*. New York: Academic Press.
Geyer MA, Swerdlow NR, Mansbach RS, Braff DL. 1990. Startle response models of sensorimotor gating and habituation deficits in schizophrenia. Brain Res Bull 25: 485–498.
Glahn DC, Therman S, Manninen M, Huttunen M, Kaprio J, Lonnqvist J, Cannon TD. 2003. Spatial working memory as an endophenotype of schizophrenia. Biol Psychiatry 53:624–626.
Glantz LA, Lewis DA. 2000. Decreased dendritic spine density on prefrontal cortical pyramidal neurons in schizophrenia. Arch Gen Psychiatry 57:65–73.
Gottesman II. 1991. *Schizophrenia Genesis: The Origins of Madness*. New York: Freeman.
Green MF. 1996. What are the functional consequences of neurocognitive deficits in schizophrenia? Am J Psychiatry 153:321–330.
Heaton RK, Gladsjo JA, Palmer BW, Kuck, J, Marcotte, TD, Jeste DV. 2001. Stability and course of neuropsychological deficits in schizophrenia. Arch Gen Psychiatry 58:24–32.
Kane J, Honigfeld G, Singer J, Meltzer H. 1988. Clozapine for the treatment-resistant schizophrenic. A double-blind comparison with chlorpromazine. Arch Gen Psychiatry 45:789–796.
Kety SS, Rosenthal D, Wender PH, Schulsinger F. 1968. The types and prevalence of mental illness in the biological and adoptive families of adopted schizophrenics. J Psychiatry Res 6:345–362.
Laruelle M, Abi-Dargham A, van Dyck CH, Gil R, D'Souza CD, Erdos J, McCance E. 1996. Single photon emission computerized tomography imaging of amphetamine-induced dopamine release in drug-free schizophrenic subjects. Proc Natl Acad Sci U S A 93:9235–9240.
Lieberman JA, Stroup TS, McEvoy JP, Swartz MS, Rosenheck PA, Perkins DO, Keefe RS, Davis SM, Davis CE, Lebowitz BD, Severe J, Hsaio JK. 2005. Effectiveness of antipsychotic drugs in patients with chronic schizophrenia. N Engl J Med 353:1209–1223.
McGrath J, Saha S, Chant D, Welham J. 2008. Schizophrenia: a concise overview of incidence, prevalence, and mortality. Epidemiol Rev 30:67–76.
Millar JK, Wilson-Annan JC, Anderson S, Christie S, Taylor MS, Semple CA, Devon RS, et al. 2000. Disruption of two novel genes by a translocation co-segregating with schizophrenia. Hum Mol Genet 22:1415–1423.
Mortensen PB, Pedersen CB, Westergaard T, Wohlfahrt J, Ewald H, Mors O, Andersen PK, Melbye M. 1999. Effects of family history and place and season of birth on the risk of schizophrenia. N Engl J Med 340:603–608.
Owen MJ, Craddock N, O'Donovan MC. 2010. Suggestion of roles for both common and rare risk variants in genome-wide studies of schizophrenia. Arch Gen Psychiatry 67:667–673.
Popken GJ, Bunney WE Jr, Potkin SG, Jones EG. 2000. Subnucleus-specific loss of neurons in medial thalamus of schizophrenics. Proc Natl Acad Sci U S A 97:9276–9280.
Rajkowska G, Selemon LD, Goldman-Rakic PS. 1998. Neuronal and glial somal size in the prefrontal cortex: a postmortem morphometric study of schizophrenia and Huntington disease. Arch Gen Psychiatry 55:215–224.
Rapoport JL, Giedd JN, Blumenthal J, Hamburger S, Jeffries N, Fernandez T, Nicolxon R, Bedwell J, Lenane M, Zijdenbos A 1999. Progressive cortical change during adolescence in childhood-onset schizophrenia. A longitudinal magnetic resonance imaging study. Arch Gen Psychiatry 56:649–654.
Ripke S, Sanders AR, Kendler KS, Levinson DF, Sklar P, Holmans PA, Lin D-Y. 2011. Genome-wide association study identifies five new schizophrenia loci. Nat Genet 43: 969–976.
Seeman P, Lee T, Chau-Wong M, Wong K. 1976. Antipsychotic drug doses and neuroleptic/dopamine receptors. Nature 261:717–719.
Silver H, Feldman P, Biolker W, Gur RC. 2003. Working memory deficit as a core neuropsychological dysfunction in schizophrenia. Am J Psychiatry 160:1809–1816.
Suddath RL, Christison GW, Torrey EF, Casanova MF, Weinberger DR. 1990. Anatomical abnormalities in the

brains of monozygotic twins discordant for schizophrenia. N Engl J Med 322:789–794.

Thompson PM, Vidal C, Giedd JN, Gochman P, Blumenthal J, Nicolson R, Toga, AW, Rapoport J. 2001. Mapping adolescent brain change reveals dynamic wave of accelerated gray matter loss in very early-onset schizophrenia. Proc Natl Acad Sci U S A 98:11650–11655.

van Haren NE, Schnack HG, Cahn W, van den Heuvel MP, Lepage C, Collins L, Evans AC, Hulshoff Pol HE, Kahn RS. 2011 Changes in cortical thickness during the course of illness in schizophrenia. Arch Gen Psychiatry 68: 871–880.

Walsh T, McClellan JM, McCarthy SE, Addington AM, Pierce SB, Cooper GM, Nord AS, et al. 2008. Rare structural variants disrupt multiple genes in neurodevelopmental pathways in schizophrenia. Science 320:539–543.

63

Disorders of Mood and Anxiety

Emotions are transient responses to specific stimuli in the environment (eg, the presence of danger), the body (eg, pain), or, for humans, the mind (eg, a train of thought). When an emotional state is prolonged, it can become one's dominant emotional state over time, or mood. Mood thus may be independent of immediate personal and environmental circumstances.

Mood and anxiety disorders are the most common serious disorders of the brain. Mood disorders generally involve either depression or elation. Anxiety disorders involve abnormal regulation of a powerful emotion, fear. In both mood and anxiety disorders the core symptoms have a major emotional component and are accompanied by physiological, cognitive, and behavioral abnormalities.

We discuss disorders of mood and anxiety together because both involve negative emotional states and because they appear to involve overlapping neural circuits that include the amygdala and the anterior cingulate cortex. There also is evidence for overlapping risk factors between major depressive disorder and some anxiety disorders. Commonalities of circuitry and genetic risks, as well as the negative effects of long-term anxiety on a person's mood, may explain the observation that nearly 60% of patients with major depressive disorder also suffer from an anxiety disorder. Anxiety disorder most commonly precedes the onset of depression.

Because emotions are transient responses to stimuli that can be reproduced in the laboratory, they have proven more amenable than moods to neuroscientific study. Objective measurement of moods is difficult, compared with the more stereotypic physiological or behavioral components of emotional responses (see Chapter 48), and experimental approaches to regulating mood have had limited success. Good animal models exist for certain emotions, such as fear and pleasure, and because many features of these states appear to be conserved in evolution, the animal models are relevant to humans (see Chapter 48).

Animal models have allowed detailed investigation of the neural circuitry, physiology, and biochemistry underlying these states. For example, studies of rodent models of instinctive (unlearned) fear and learned fear (in which an animal learns to associate a previously neutral cue with a threat) have elucidated the "fear circuits" centered in the amygdala and the hypothalamus. These circuits activate the sympathetic nervous system to alter heart rate and blood pressure, stimulate secretion of stress hormones, and elicit species-specific defensive behaviors such as motionlessness ("freezing") in rodents and escape behaviors in other species. Such basic investigations are providing testable hypotheses for studies of fear and anxiety and their disorders in humans.

In contrast, neurobiological investigations of moods are less advanced. Although much evidence suggests that animals do have moods, developing empirical methods of ascertaining what those moods are and how they match human experience has been challenging. Most animal models of depression were not developed to investigate the pathophysiology of the human disease, but as empirical screens for antidepressant drugs. Many of these models are based on chronic stress; although chronic stress and depressed mood have many features in common, they are not identical.

The lack of well-validated animal models of moods and mood disorders has made it difficult to identify the neural circuitry responsible for the regulation and maintenance of moods. Much investigation of mood circuitry has perforce been carried out in humans using noninvasive technologies such as neuro-imaging.

The Most Common Disorders of Mood Are Unipolar Depression and Bipolar Disorder

In the 5th century BC moods were thought to depend on the balance of four humors—blood, phlegm, yellow bile, and black bile. An excess of black bile was believed to cause depression. In fact, the ancient Greek term for depression, *melancholia,* means black bile. Although this explanation of depression seems fanciful today, the underlying view that psychological disorders reflect physical processes is correct.

Only in the past three decades have relatively precise criteria for mood disorders been developed in parallel with those for thought and cognitive disorders (see Chapter 61). Disorders of mood are now classified based on symptoms, natural history (including age of onset, course, and outcome), patterns of familial transmission, and response to treatment. Based on these factors, one can distinguish between two major classes of disorders in people who suffer from depression. Unipolar depression is diagnosed in people who suffer only from depressive episodes; bipolar disorder is diagnosed in individuals in whom depression alternates with episodes of mania (Table 63–1).

Another important distinction is that between primary and secondary mood disorders. Mood disorders caused by drugs (eg, drugs used to treat hypertension) or pathophysiological processes that affect the brain (eg, hypothyroidism) are considered secondary to another condition. The onset of depression late in life also may be secondary to pathophysiological processes such as Parkinson disease or diffuse vascular disease affecting cerebral vessels. Although such cases are important, our discussion here focuses on mood disorders, unipolar and bipolar illnesses, arising as independent pathophysiological processes.

Unipolar Depression Often Begins Early in Life

The key clinical features of unipolar depression can be summarized in Hamlet's words, "How weary, stale, flat, and unprofitable seem to me all the uses of this world!" Untreated, an episode of depression typically lasts 4 to 12 months. The central feature of depression is an unpleasant (dysphoric) mood present most of the day, day in and day out, often accompanied by intense mental anguish, the inability to experience pleasure (anhedonia), and a generalized loss of interest in the world. Sadness is most typical, but anger, irritability, and loss of interest in usual pursuits can predominate in some patients.

Major depression is distinguished from normal sadness or grief by its severity, pervasiveness, duration, and associated symptoms, including physiological, behavioral, and cognitive symptoms (Table 63–1). Physiological symptoms include sleep disturbance, most often insomnia with early morning awakening, but occasionally excessive sleeping; loss of appetite and weight loss, but occasionally excessive eating; and decreased energy. Behaviorally, some depressed patients exhibit slowed motor movements, described

Table 63–1 Symptoms of Mood Disorders

Major Depression

A. Either depressed mood (1) or loss of interest or pleasure (2):
1. Depressed mood most of the day, nearly every day, as indicated by either subjective report (eg, "I feel sad or empty") or observation made by others (eg, "He appears tearful")
2. Markedly diminished interest or pleasure in all, or almost all, activities most of the day, nearly every day (as indicated by either subjective account or observation made by others)

B. At least four of the following symptoms are present nearly every day for at least 2 weeks:
1. Significant weight loss when not dieting, or weight gain (eg, a change of more than 5% of body weight in a month), or decrease or increase in appetite nearly every day
2. Insomnia or hypersomnia nearly every day
3. Psychomotor agitation or retardation nearly every day (observable by others, not merely subjective feelings of restlessness or being slowed down)
4. Fatigue or loss of energy nearly every day
5. Feelings of worthlessness or excessive or inappropriate guilt (which may be delusional) nearly every day (not merely self-reproach or guilt about being sick)
6. Diminished ability to think or concentrate, or indecisiveness, nearly every day (either by subjective account or as observed by others)
7. Recurrent thoughts of death (not just fear of dying), recurrent suicidal ideation without a specific plan, or a suicide attempt or a specific plan for committing suicide

Manic Episode

A. A distinct period of abnormally and persistently elevated, expansive, or irritable mood, lasting at least 1 week (or any duration if hospitalization is necessary).

B. During the period of mood disturbance three (or more) of the following symptoms have persisted (four if the mood is only irritable) and have been present to a significant degree:
1. Inflated self-esteem or grandiosity
2. Decreased need for sleep (eg, feels rested after only 3 hours of sleep)
3. More talkative than usual or pressure to keep talking
4. Flight of ideas or subjective experience that thoughts are racing
5. Distractibility (ie, attention too easily drawn to unimportant or irrelevant external stimuli)
6. Increase in goal-directed activity (either socially, at work or school, or sexually) or psychomotor agitation
7. Excessive involvement in pleasurable activities that have a high potential for painful consequences (eg, engaging in unrestrained buying sprees, sexual indiscretions, or foolish business investments)

Adapted from the *Diagnostic and Statistical Manual of Mental Disorders*, 4th ed.

as psychomotor retardation, whereas others can be extremely agitated. Cognitive symptoms are evident in both the content of thoughts (hopelessness, thoughts of worthlessness and of guilt, suicidal thoughts and urges) and in cognitive processes (difficulty concentrating, slow thinking, and poor memory).

In the most severe forms of depression psychotic symptoms can occur, including delusions (unshakable false beliefs that cannot be explained by a person's culture) and hallucinations. The psychotic symptoms of depression generally reflect the person's feelings that he or she is worthless or bad. A severely depressed person might, for example, believe that he or she is emitting a potent odor because he or she is rotting from the inside.

The most serious negative outcome from depression is suicide. Suicide is the eighth leading cause of death in the United States, and the third leading cause of death among young people 15 to 24 years of age. More than 90% of suicides are associated with mental illness, with depression being the leading cause.

In the standard classification of psychiatric disorders in the United States—the *Diagnostic and Statistical Manual of Mental Disorders, Fourth Edition* (*DSM-IV*) of the American Psychiatric Association—episodic, primary, unipolar depression that lasts for at least two weeks is classified as major depression. Major depression often begins early in life; approximately one-half of cases occur in those younger than 25 years of age, but first episodes are observed across the life span. Those who have had a first episode in childhood or adolescence have a particularly high likelihood of recurrence. Once a second episode has occurred, a pattern of repeated relapse and remission generally sets in. Some people do not recover completely from their first acute episode and have chronic, albeit milder, unremitting depression that can be punctuated by acute exacerbations. Chronic, somewhat milder depressions lasting more than 2 years are called *dysthymia*. Although the symptoms of dysthymia are less severe than those of a major depressive episode, the long duration of the symptoms makes this a very disabling illness.

Bipolar Disorder Includes Episodes of Mania

Bipolar disorder is named for its chief symptom, swings of mood between mania and depression. Mania is characterized by euphoria or irritability, a marked increase in energy and a decreased need for sleep, impulsiveness, and excessive engagement in goal-directed behaviors, often with poor judgment characterized by extreme optimism. For example, a person might go on spending sprees well beyond his or her means. During manic episodes self-esteem is inflated, often reaching delusional proportions; individuals might consider themselves to be royalty, prophets, or even deities.

Mania also affects cognition. During a manic episode a person often cannot stick to a topic and might jump quickly from idea to idea, making comprehension difficult. Speech is typically rapid and difficult to interrupt. Psychotic symptoms commonly occur during manic episodes and are generally consistent with the person's elevated mood. For example, people with mania can have delusions that they possess special powers. The symptoms that characterize the depressive episodes in bipolar disorder are indistinguishable from those in unipolar depressions.

Patients who have had at least one manic episode are considered to have bipolar disorder, even if they have not yet experienced a depressive episode. The onset of manic episodes tends to be relatively rapid, occurring over a period of a few days to a few weeks. Bipolar disorder generally begins in young adulthood, uncommonly in childhood. Most episodes lack a clear precipitant, but sleep deprivation can initiate a manic episode, suggesting a relationship between neural systems that regulate circadian rhythms and those that regulate moods. People with bipolar disorder have recurrent episodes of the illness, both manias and depression. However, the rate of cycling between mania, depression, and normal mood (euthymia) varies widely. Between periods of mania or depression some people with bipolar disorder are relatively free of symptoms, but a large fraction have residual symptoms. A few patients have severe, chronic symptoms despite treatment.

Mood Disorders Are Common and Disabling

The lifetime risk of major depressive disorder in the United States is 16.2%. Within any 1 year 6.6% of the population suffers major depression. The prevalence of depression differs in different countries and cultures, but the nature of the symptoms is remarkably similar around the world.

In childhood major depression occurs equally in males and females. After puberty, however, depression occurs more commonly in females independent of culture. In the United States the ratio of females to males with major depression is 1.7:1. Depression is the leading cause of disability worldwide.

In contrast to the high frequency of unipolar depression, bipolar disorder is less common, with a prevalence of 1% that exhibits relatively little variability from country to country. As with major depression, the symptoms are the same across countries and cultures. The risk of bipolar disorder is equivalent in males and females worldwide.

Both Genetic and Nongenetic Risk Factors Play an Important Role in Mood Disorders

As with schizophrenia, both bipolar disorder and major depression run in families with patterns of transmission that are inconsistent with simple Mendelian (single gene) dominant, recessive, or sex chromosome-linked modes of inheritance. One way to estimate the influence of genes on a disease phenotype is to measure the increased risk that results from relatedness to a person who has the disease. This increase in risk can be expressed as a *recurrence risk ratio*. The recurrence risk ratio provides a rough measure of the aggregate influence of genes on a trait but does not provide insight into how many genes might be involved.

Recurrence risk ratios demonstrate that genes contribute to the risk of unipolar depression but exert a much stronger influence on the risk of bipolar disorder (Table 63–2). As in schizophrenia (see Chapter 62), the concordance rates among monozygotic twin pairs (who are genetically identical) are less than 100%. Thus genes alone do not cause mood disorders but must interact with developmental or environmental factors to produce illness.

Overall the genetic risk for mood disorders, like that for schizophrenia, is genetically complex. Genetic linkage and association studies suggest there are multiple pathways of genetic risk for mood disorders, and thus no single gene will likely prove to be either necessary or sufficient.

Table 63–2 Recurrence Risk Ratios (λ) for Mood Disorders and Schizophrenia

Disorder	Siblings	Identical twins
Schizophrenia	9	48
Bipolar disorder	7	60
Major depression	2–3	16

λ measures the lifetime risk for a disorder as a multiple of the general population risk that results from the degree of relatedness to a person with the disorder. Thus for schizophrenia the base rate in the population is 1%. Given a sibling with schizophrenia there is a ninefold increase in risk (which in this case equals a 9% risk). Given an identical twin with the disorder, the relative risk is 48 times higher than in the general population. Schizophrenia and bipolar disorder are highly genetically influenced, major depression more moderately so.

From the point of view of prevention it is important to sort out the relative roles of genes and environmental risk factors because the latter can be modified. Much evidence suggests that stressful and adverse life events increase the risk of major depression; even here, however, genes may play a role in two ways because they shape a person's temperament. First, temperament plays a role in the kinds of situations into which people place themselves; second, genetic factors can influence the response that people have to adverse life experiences when they do occur. Such interactions between genetic and environmental factors complicate the task of isolating risk factors.

Specific Brain Regions and Circuits Are Involved in Mood Disorders

Because animal models of mood and mood regulation are not fully convincing, investigation of the circuitry involved in mood disorders has relied to a great extent on structural and functional imaging of humans, and to a lesser degree on postmortem analyses of human brains. Neuro-imaging studies of major depression and bipolar disorder have identified abnormalities in brain regions thought to be involved in emotion and cognition (Figure 63–1). Despite progress to date, imaging has not yet identified specific abnormalities in a neural system that can be used reliably to diagnose major depressive or bipolar disorder.

One brain region that has consistently been implicated in both major depressive and bipolar disorders is the gyrus of the anterior cingulate cortex. This structure runs parallel to the corpus callosum, along the medial surface of each cerebral hemisphere (Figure 63–1). It has two functional subdivisions. A rostral and ventral subdivision is thought to be involved in emotional processes and autonomic function; it has extensive connections to the hippocampus, the amygdala, orbital prefrontal cortex, anterior insula, and nucleus accumbens. A caudal subdivision is thought to be involved in cognitive processes and the control of behavior; it connects with the dorsal regions of prefrontal cortex, secondary motor cortex, and posterior cingulate cortex.

Abnormal function in both subdivisions of the anterior cingulate cortex has been documented in people with mood disorders (Figure 63–2). However, abnormal functioning during major depressive episodes and the depression phase of bipolar disorder has been most consistently found in the rostral subdivision, which is concerned with emotion, and especially in the subgenual region (the region ventral to the genu of the corpus callosum). Indeed, a decrease in activity of the subgenual anterior cingulate gyrus following antidepressant treatment correlates with the success of the treatment (Figure 63–3).

Neuro-imaging also implicates the amygdala and hippocampus in mood disorders. The involvement of the amygdala is not surprising given the wealth of evidence that this structure is involved in the processing of negative emotions, including fear (see Chapter 48). Enlargement of the amygdala has been found in depression, and increases in the basal level of activity in the amygdala have been observed in depression, bipolar disorder, and anxiety disorders. As in many disorders, the volume of the hippocampus may be reduced in depression. This change correlates with the duration of prior episodes of depression and not with the age of the person, consistent with the idea that protracted major depression might produce hippocampal atrophy. Nonetheless, until longitudinal studies are conducted we cannot be certain whether a small hippocampus is a risk factor for depression or a result of it.

Despite the findings that we have described, the use of neuro-imaging to study depression is still in its early stages. Most studies to date have been restricted to anatomical measurement of brain structures or to basal (unstimulated) brain activity in depressed subjects compared with healthy control subjects. Investigators are now beginning to use *activation paradigms*, in which brain activity is measured in response to specific cognitive or emotional stimuli.

Activation paradigms can be a powerful means of identifying brain circuits associated with specific normal and disordered function. For example, in healthy subjects the anterior cingulate cortex is activated by pain, cognitive conflict, and errors in task performance. Thus the anterior cingulate cortex may ascertain whether behavior is successfully proceeding toward desired goals, and perceived discrepancies between goals and outcomes could contribute to depression.

Depression and Stress Are Interrelated

In some cases depression follows a stressful experience; conversely, the experience of depression is itself stressful. Indeed, depression shares several features with chronic stress, including changes in appetite, sleep, and energy. Major depression and chronic stress may also share biochemical changes, such as persistent activation of the hypothalamic-pituitary-adrenal (HPA) axis (Figure 63–4).

In depressed individuals daily production of the glucocorticoid stress hormone cortisol and secretion of corticotrophin-releasing hormone (CRH) and adrenocorticotropic hormone (ACTH) can all be elevated. A *transient* increase in cortisol secretion, as occurs with acute stress, suppresses the immune system (saving energy and delaying inflammatory processes that might inhibit the fight-or-flight response), shifts the body to a catabolic state (making energy available to confront the cause of the stress), increases energy levels, sharpens cognition, and may increase confidence. However, a *chronic* increase may contribute to symptoms of depression. For example, people with Cushing disease (in which pituitary tumors secrete excess ACTH leading to excess cortisol) often experience depression and insomnia.

Feedback mechanisms within the HPA axis normally permit cortisol (or exogenously administered glucocorticoids) to inhibit CRH and ACTH secretion and therefore to suppress additional cortisol synthesis and secretion. In approximately one-half of people with major depression this feedback system

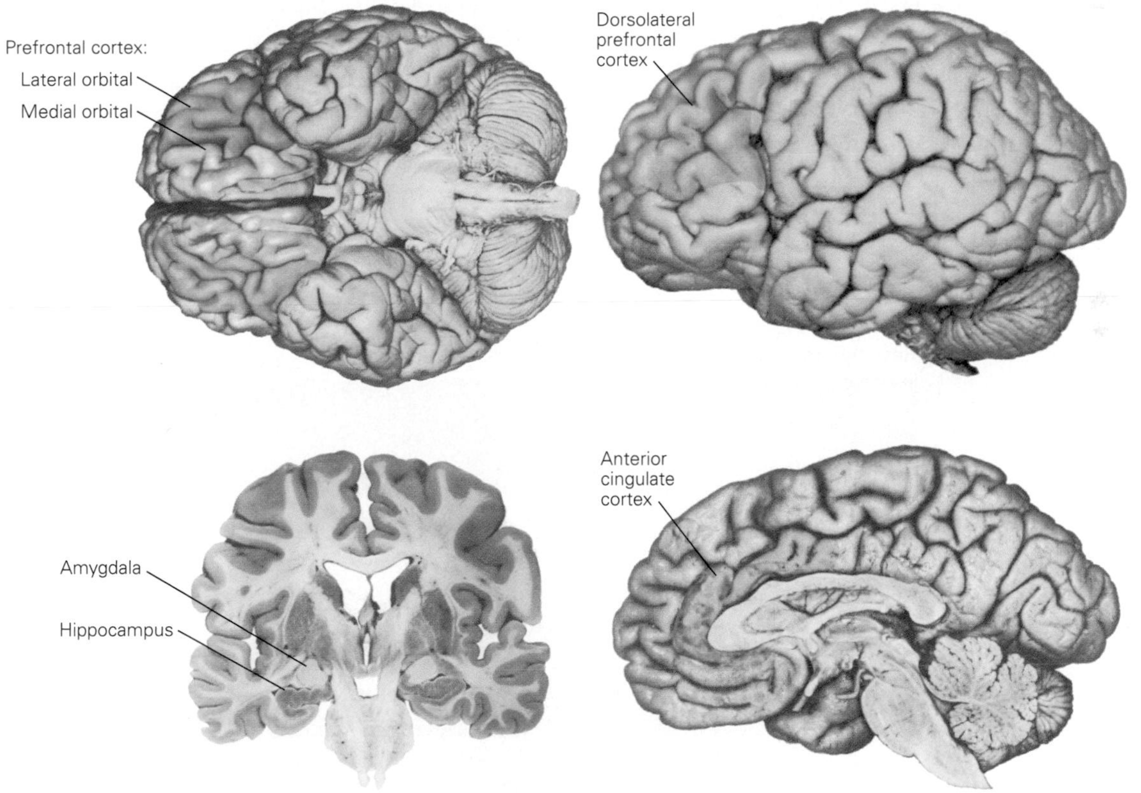

Figure 63–1 Brain centers of emotional dysfunction in patients with depression. Each of these interconnected structures plays a role in regulating emotion and physiological and behavioral responses to emotional stimuli. Abnormalities in one or more of these regions or in the interconnections among them are associated with failures of emotion regulation. (Reproduced, with permission, from Davidson, Putnam, and Larson 2000.)

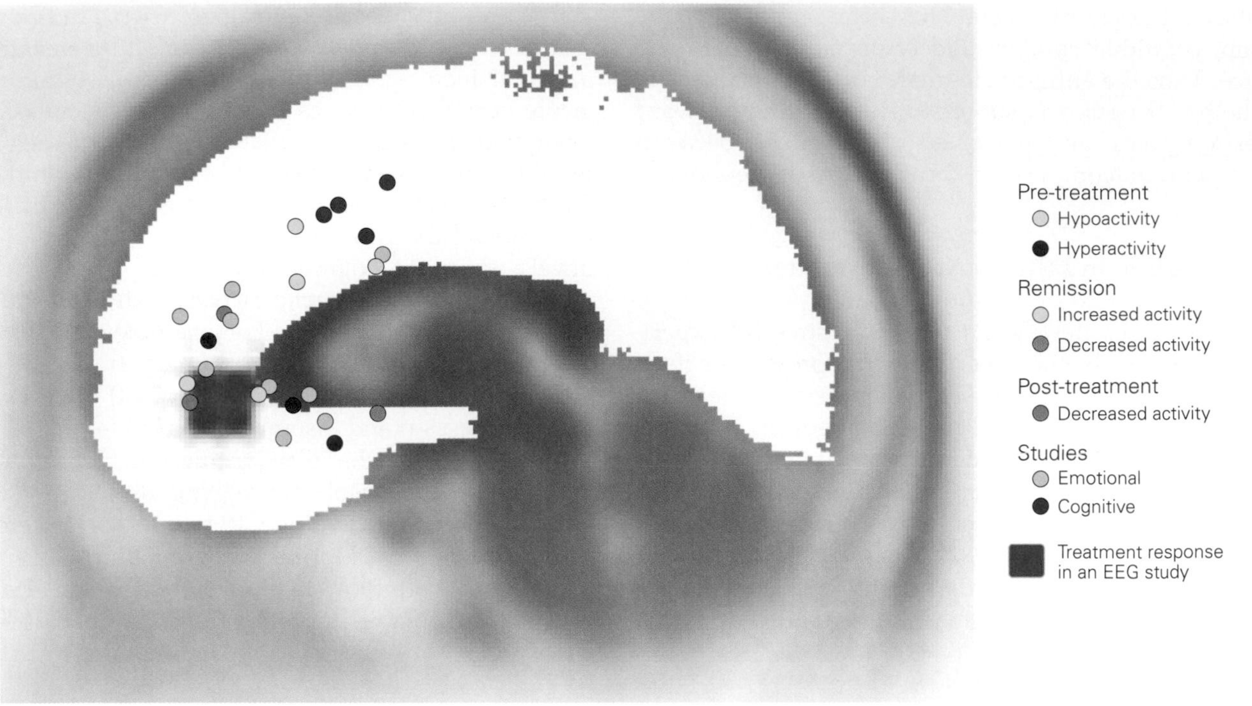

Figure 63–2 Involvement of the anterior cingulate cortex in depression. The figure summarizes the findings of several studies using brain imaging. Colored circles show sites of activation or deactivation before or after treatment of patients with depression. **Black circles** indicate pretreatment hyperactivity among patients who responded to treatment; **green circles** indicate posttreatment decreased activity in responders; **pink circles** indicate hypoactivity in depressed subjects; **yellow circles** indicate increased activity with remission of depression; and the sole **brown circle** indicates decreased activity with remission of depression. Studies involving emotional tasks (**blue circles**) and cognitive tasks (**purple circles**) in nonpsychiatric subjects are also shown. The large **red area** shows the location of treatment response observed in an electroencephalogram (EEG) study of depression. (Adapted, with permission, from Pizzagalli et al. 2001.)

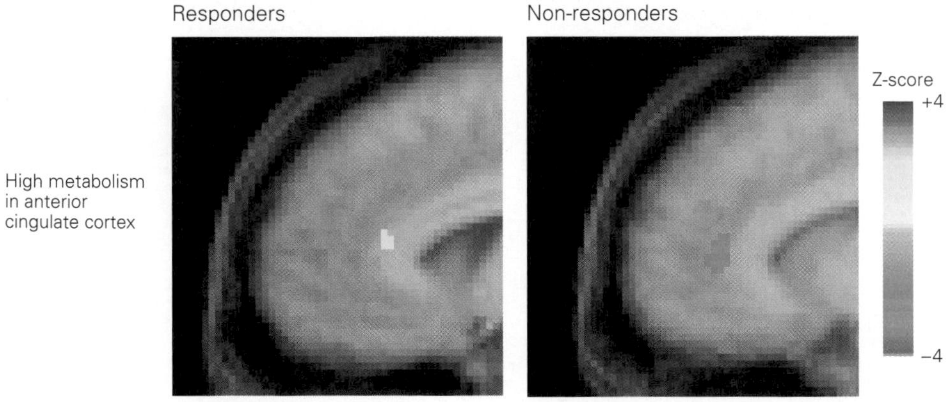

Figure 63–3 Increased activity in the anterior cingulate cortex predicts responsiveness to treatment with antidepressant drugs. Regional cerebral glucose metabolism was measured by positron emission tomography (PET) as a proxy for brain activity. Depressed patients with elevated metabolism in the rostral anterior cingulate cortex had better responses to antidepressant treatment than those who did not. Cingulate hypermetabolism may represent an adaptive response to depression that predicts antidepressant response. (Reproduced, with permission, from Mayberg et al. 1997).

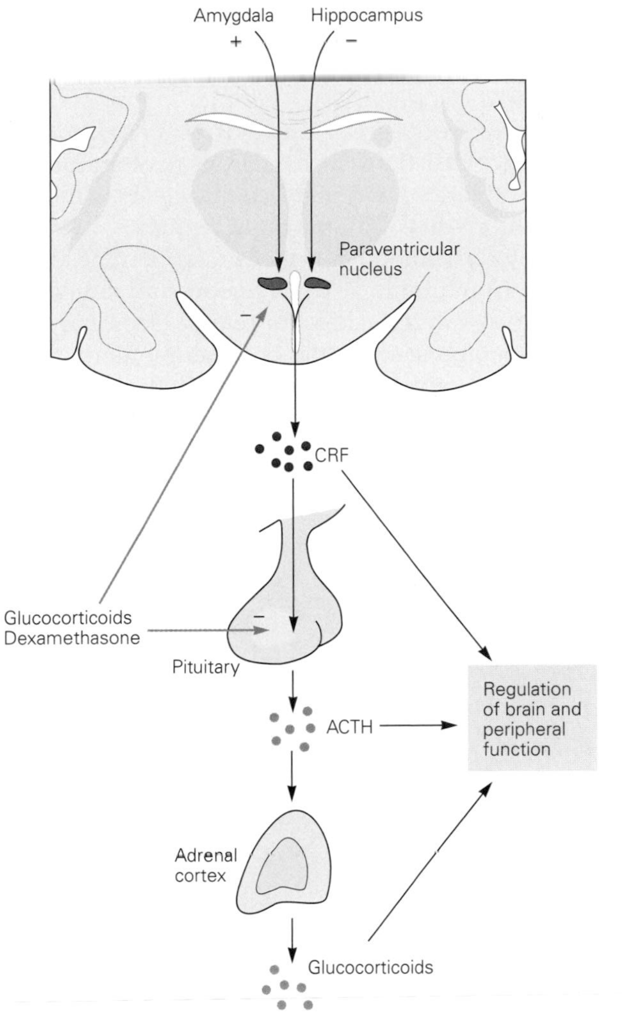

Figure 63–4 The hypothalamic-pituitary-adrenal axis. Neurons in the paraventricular nucleus of the hypothalamus synthesize and release corticotropin-releasing factor (**CRF**), the key regulatory hormone in this cascade. Secretion of CRF follows a circadian pattern, and the effects of stress are superimposed on this circadian pattern. Excitatory fibers from the amygdala convey information about stress and activate CRF secretion and biosynthesis; inhibitory fibers descend from the hippocampus. CRF enters the hypophyseal portal system and stimulates the corticotrophic cells of the anterior pituitary. These cells synthesize and release adrenocorticotropic hormone (**ACTH**), which enters the systemic circulation and ultimately stimulates the adrenal cortex to release glucocorticoids. In humans the major glucocorticoid is cortisol; in rodents it is corticosterone. Both cortisol and synthetic glucocorticoids such as dexamethasone act at the level of the pituitary and hypothalamus to inhibit further release of ACTH and CRF respectively. (Adapted, with permission, from Nestler, Hyman, and Malenka 2009.)

is impaired; their HPA axis becomes resistant to suppression even by potent synthetic glucocorticoids such as dexamethasone. Although readily measurable disturbances of the HPA axis are not sensitive or specific enough to be used as a diagnostic test for depression, the observed abnormalities suggest strongly that altered stress responses are an important component of depression in a large proportion of people with the illness.

If recurrent depression causes the decrease in hippocampal volumes described above, it may be that excessive cortisol secretion is the cause. Two theories have been offered to explain how depression might lead to hippocampal atrophy. One is that persistently elevated levels of glucocorticoids can damage mature neurons, perhaps making them more susceptible to glutamate excitotoxicity (see Chapter 43). The other is that elevated cortisol levels or some other aspect of chronic stress suppresses normal neurogenesis (the formation of new neurons), resulting in fewer cells being produced and thus a smaller hippocampus.

In many animals, as well as humans, new granule cells within the dentate gyrus of the hippocampus are produced during adult life. In rodents these new neurons are incorporated into neural circuits. Stressful or aversive experiences as well as glucocorticoids inhibit the proliferation of granule cell precursors and thus suppress normal rates of neurogenesis in the hippocampus. In contrast, antidepressants, including the selective serotonin reuptake inhibitors, increase the rate of neurogenesis. Thus depression might cause hippocampal atrophy by inhibiting neurogenesis and antidepressants might reverse this effect by treating the depression (therefore decreasing stress) and possibly by directly stimulating neurogenesis (by mechanisms that are not yet understood).

These hypothalamic and hippocampal abnormalities may contribute to the symptoms of depression and influence its course. Hypothalamic CRH secretion is under the stimulatory control of pathways from the amygdala and inhibitory pathways from the hippocampus. Damage to the hippocampus could lead to a vicious cycle in which loss of inhibitory control of CRH secretion would lead to greater cortisol release, producing additional hippocampal atrophy. In fact, depression can be accompanied by memory impairments that could be explained by hippocampal dysfunction, either by itself or in conjunction with disturbances in executive function involving the prefrontal cortex, such as failure of attentional mechanisms at the time of memory encoding.

Major Depression Can Be Treated Effectively

Three types of treatment are effective for major depressive disorder: antidepressant drugs, cognitive-behavioral psychotherapy, and electroconvulsive therapy.

Antidepressant Drugs Target Monoaminergic Neural Systems

The most widely used treatment for depression is antidepressant drugs that act initially on the monoaminergic systems in the nervous system. The monoamines—serotonin, norepinephrine, and dopamine—are synthesized in small nuclei within the brain stem (see Figure 46–2). Serotonergic and noradrenergic nuclei are concentrated in the caudal brain stem (Figures 63–5 and 63–6). Most dopamine in the brain is synthesized in more rostral nuclei, the substantia nigra and ventral tegmental area of the midbrain (see Figure 46–2E). Each of the monoaminergic nuclei projects widely throughout the brain; the serotonergic and noradrenergic axons descend into the spinal cord as well. This widespread connectivity permits monoaminergic neurons to produce coordinated responses and thus to influence functions such as arousal, attention, vigilance, motivation, and other cognitive and emotional states that involve multiple brain regions.

Serotonin, norepinephrine, and dopamine are synthesized from amino acid precursors and either packaged into synaptic vesicles for release (see Chapter 12) or else metabolized by the enzyme monoamine oxidase (MAO), which is associated with the outer leaflet of mitochondrial membranes. After release these neurotransmitters bind synaptic receptors or are cleared

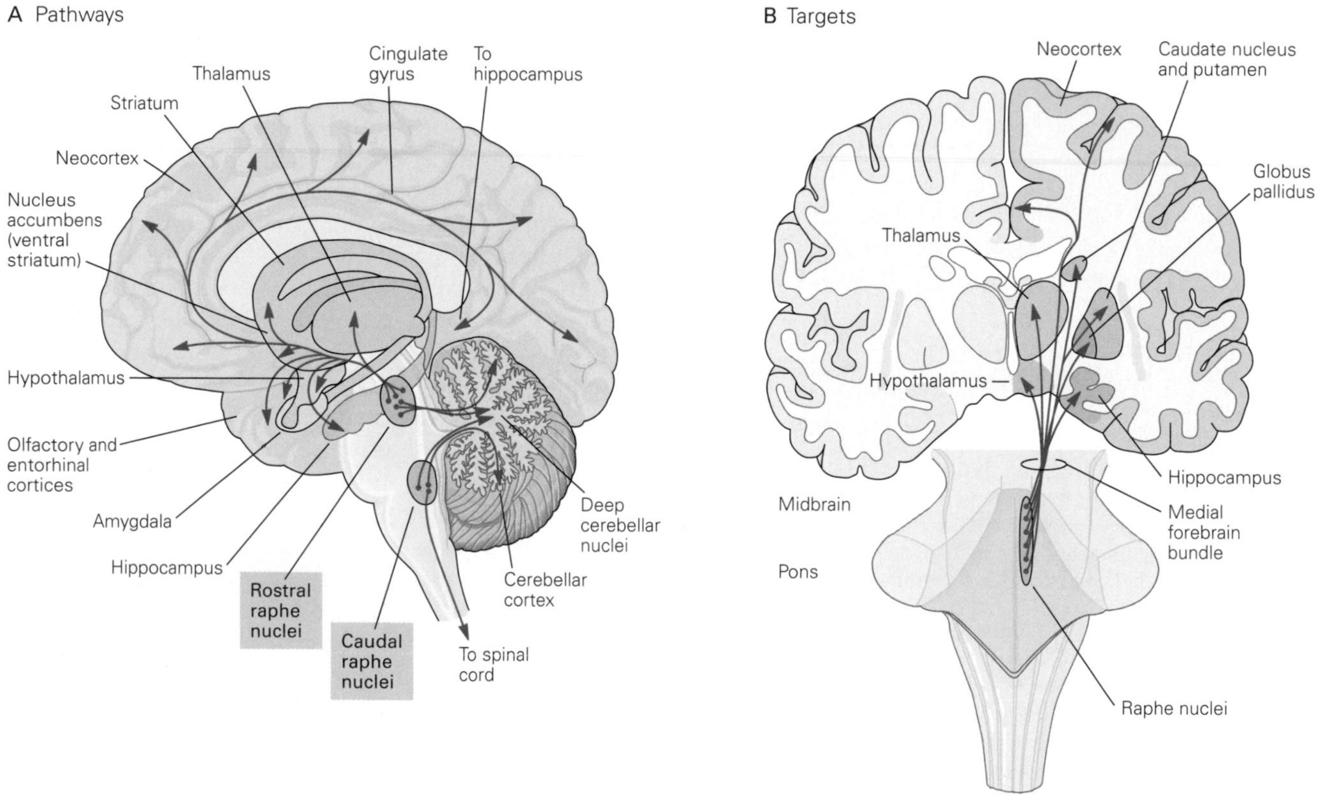

Figure 63–5 The major serotonergic systems in the brain arise in the raphe nuclei of the brain stem. Serotonin is synthesized in a group of brain stem nuclei called the raphe nuclei. These neurons project throughout the neuraxis, ranging from the forebrain to the spinal cord. The serotonergic projections are the most massive and diffuse of the monoaminergic systems, with single serotonergic neurons innervating hundreds of target neurons. (Adapted, with permission, from Heimer 1995.)

A. A sagittal view of the brain illustrates the raphe nuclei. In the brain these nuclei form a fairly continuous collection of cell groups close to the midline of the brain stem and extending along its length. In the drawing here they are shown in more distinct rostral and caudal groups. The rostral raphe nuclei project to a large number of forebrain structures.

B. This coronal view of the brain illustrates some of the major structures innervated by serotonergic neurons of the raphe nuclei.

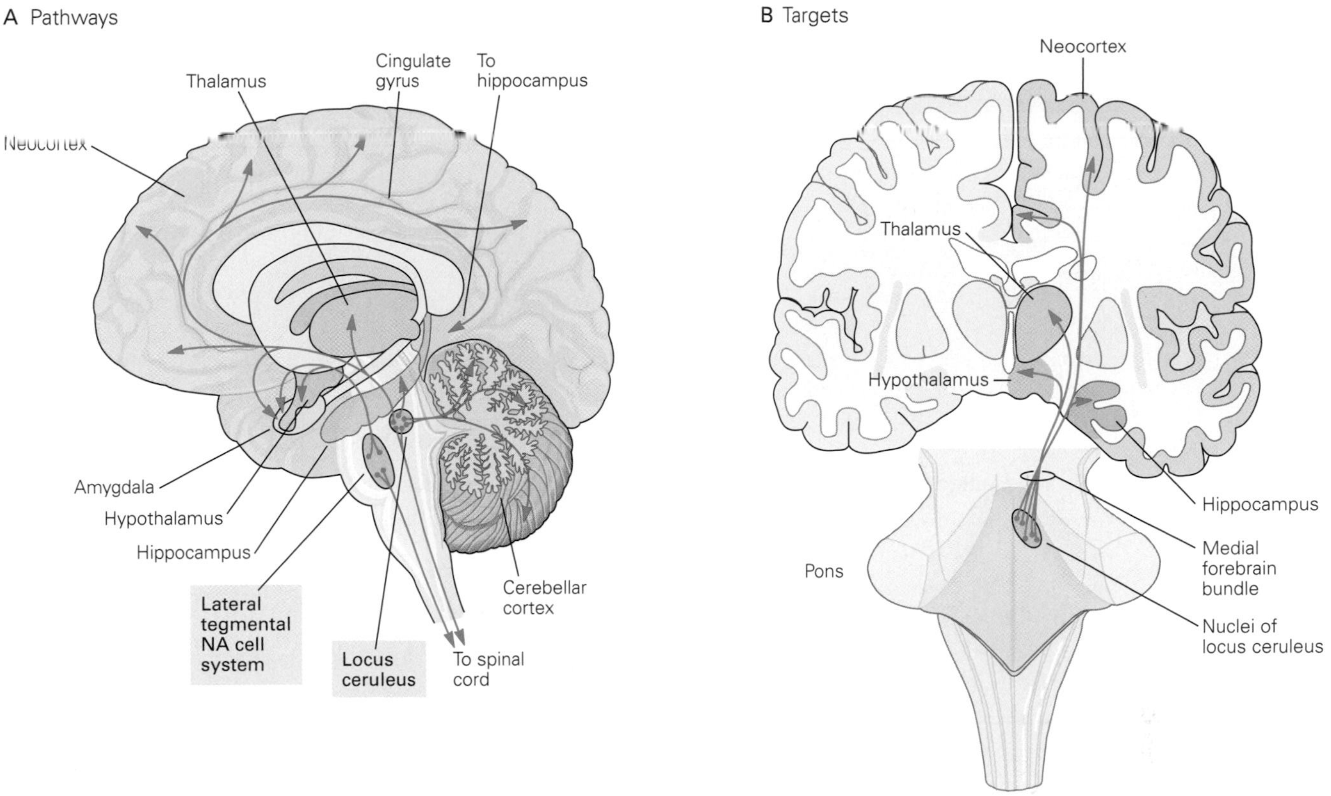

Figure 63–6 The major noradrenergic projection of the forebrain arises in the locus ceruleus. (Adapted, with permission, from Heimer 1995.)

A. Norepinephrine is synthesized in several brain stem nuclei, the largest of which is the nucleus locus ceruleus, a pigmented nucleus located just beneath the floor of the fourth ventricle in the rostrolateral pons. A lateral midsagittal view demonstrates the course of the major noradrenergic pathways from the locus ceruleus and lateral brain stem tegmentum. Axons from the locus ceruleus project rostrally into the forebrain and also into the cerebellum and spinal cord; axons from noradrenergic nuclei in the lateral brain stem tegmentum project to the spinal cord, hypothalamus, amygdala, and ventral forebrain.

B. A coronal section shows the major targets of neurons from the locus ceruleus.

from the synapse by specific transporters located on the presynaptic cell membrane.

Serotonin and norepinephrine each have a variety of receptors on the presynaptic terminals as well as postsynaptic target cells. There are at least 14 distinct serotonin receptors in humans, divided into seven major classes denoted 5-HT_1 through 5-HT_7 (Table 63–3). Norepinephrine receptors can be divided into two major classes, the α and β adrenergic receptors, with multiple subtypes (Table 63–4). With the exception of the 5-HT_3 receptor, serotonin, norepinephrine, and dopamine act on G protein-coupled receptors that initiate signaling cascades that produce long-term changes in the response properties of the postsynaptic neuron. It is thought that antidepressant drugs are able to alter the responsiveness of the brain to diverse cognitive and emotional stimuli by directly or indirectly influencing G protein-coupled receptors expressed in large numbers of neurons.

The most widely used antidepressant drugs fall into several major groupings, each of which affects the monoaminergic systems in different ways (Figure 63–7). The *monoamine oxidase inhibitors,* such as phenelzine and tranylcypromine, were the first effective antidepressants. They are highly effective against both depression and anxiety disorders but are rarely used today because of their side effects. MAO inhibitors may exert their effects on depression by blocking the capacity of MAO to break down norepinephrine, serotonin, or dopamine in presynaptic terminals, thus making extra neurotransmitter available for packaging into vesicles and for release.

Two forms of MAO, types A and B, are found in the brain. Type A is also found in the gut and liver,

Table 63–3 Serotonin Receptors

Receptor	G-Protein linkage	Locations in the brain
5-HT_{1A}	$G_{i/o}$	Cerebral cortex, hippocampus, septum, amygdala, dorsal raphe
5-HT_{1B}	$G_{i/o}$	Substantia nigra, basal ganglia
5-HT_{1D}	$G_{i/o}$	Substantia nigra, striatum, nucleus accumbens, hippocampus
5-HT_{1E}	$G_{i/o}$	Cerebral cortex, dorsal raphe, hippocampus
5-HT_{1F}	$G_{i/o}$	Cerebral cortex, dorsal raphe, hippocampus
5-HT_{2A}	$G_{q/11}$	Cerebral cortex, basal ganglia
5-HT_{2B}	$G_{q/11}$	No brain expression
5-HT_{2C}	$G_{q/11}$	Basal ganglia, substantia nigra, hippocampus
5-HT_{3}	Ligand-gated channel	Cerebral cortex, hippocampus, brain stem, spinal cord
5-HT_{4}	G_s	Striatum, nucleus accumbens, hippocampus
5-HT_{5A}	G_s	Cerebral cortex, hippocampus, cerebellum
5-HT_{5B}	Unknown	Cerebral cortex, hippocampus, cerebellum
5-HT_{6}	G_s	Cerebral cortex, striatum, olfactory tubercle, hippocampus
5-HT_{7}	G_s	Cerebral cortex, hypothalamus, thalamus

where it catabolizes bioactive amines that are present in foods. Inhibition of MAO-A permits bioactive amines such as tyramine to enter the bloodstream from foods that contain it in high concentrations, such as aged cheeses. These amines are taken up by sympathetic neurons through transporters, thus displacing endogenous monoamines. This process may result in massive release of norepinephrine and epinephrine, resulting in severe elevations of blood pressure. The MAO inhibitors that have been most widely used as antidepressants inhibit MAO-A and MAO-B nonselectively or MAO-A alone, and thus require that patients

Table 63–4 Norepinephrine Receptors

Receptor	G-Protein linkage	Locations in the brain
α_{1A}	$G_{q/11}$	Cerebral cortex, hippocampus
α_{1B}	$G_{q/11}$	Cerebral cortex, brain stem
α_{1D}	$G_{q/11}$	No brain expression
α_{2A}	$G_{i/o}$	Cerebral cortex, midbrain, caudal brain stem, spinal cord
α_{2B}	$G_{i/o}$	Diencephalon
α_{2C}	$G_{i/o}$	Cerebral cortex, basal ganglia, cerebellum, hippocampus
β_1	G_s	Cerebral cortex, cerebellar nuclei, brain stem, spinal cord
β_2	G_s	Hippocampus, piriform cortex, cerebellar cortex
β_3	$G_s/G_{i/o}$	No brain expression

avoid foods with a high monoamine content. A selective MAO-B inhibitor, selegiline, which has been used to treat Parkinson disease, has recently proved effective in treating depression. But at antidepressant doses, which are higher than for Parkinson disease treatment, it loses its selectivity.

The *tricyclic antidepressants,* such as imipramine, amitriptyline, and desipramine, inhibit either norepinephrine or serotonin transporters or both. These drugs are effective against depression and many anxiety disorders. But they also block many other neurotransmitter receptors, including the muscarinic acetylcholine, histamine H-1, and α_1 noradrenergic receptors, producing side effects such as dry mouth, drowsiness, urinary retention, and postural hypotension, thus limiting their use. Some newer drugs, such as venlafaxine and duloxetine, block both norepinephrine and serotonin but lack the tricyclic structure and the unwanted receptor interactions of the older drugs.

The *selective serotonin reuptake inhibitors,* such as fluoxetine, sertraline, and paroxetine, are widely used. As their name implies, they inhibit the uptake of serotonin selectively. They are effective for major depressive disorder, many anxiety disorders, and, in high doses, for obsessive-compulsive disorder.

In addition to their role in the pharmacologic treatment of mood disorders, the monoamine neurotransmitters may also play a role in pathogenesis. However, much of the evidence for such a link has come from the actions of antidepressant drugs themselves. Because effective treatments may exert their beneficial effects indirectly, the role of monoamines in pathogenesis remains quite uncertain.

Interest in the monoamines began in the 1950s when it was observed that reserpine, an alkaloid derived from the rauwolfia plant, then used to treat hypertension, precipitated depression in approximately 15% of people who received the drug. Reserpine depletes the brain of norepinephrine, serotonin, and dopamine by blocking the ability of presynaptic neurons to take up these neurotransmitters into synaptic vesicles. As a result, the neurotransmitters remain in the cytoplasm where they are degraded by monoamine oxidase. In a serendipitous discovery, iproniazid, a drug that was initially developed to treat tuberculosis, was found to have antidepressant properties. Because of its side effects, iproniazid itself is no longer in use, but it proved to be the prototype MAO inhibitor.

Because depression could be induced by reserpine, which depletes monoamines, and could be ameliorated by MAO inhibitors, which protects monoamines from degradation, the idea emerged that depression involved a decrease in the availability of monoamines. Further support for this idea came from the discovery of tricyclic antidepressants, which block the uptake of synaptically released norepinephrine and serotonin, thereby prolonging the action of these neurotransmitters within the synapse. These observations led to the hypothesis that depression results from a deficiency of monoaminergic synaptic transmission and that clinically effective antidepressants work by increasing the availability of monoamines at synapses.

A major weakness with this simple hypothesis comes from the observation that the inhibitory actions of antidepressants on monoamine uptake or on MAO are rapid and occur even with the first dose of medication, whereas several weeks of treatment are required to observe a lifting of the depression clinically. Attempts to explain this delay have led to several ideas. Enhancement of serotonergic or noradrenergic synaptic transmission stimulates a large number of pre- and postsynaptic receptors and activates downstream signaling pathways, some of which activate gene expression and ultimately protein synthesis. One general hypothesis is that, over weeks, newly synthesized proteins alter the responsiveness of neurons or cause the remodeling of synaptic connections in a manner that treats the depression. However, this hypothesis is not supported by any evidence of the genes and proteins that might be responsible or the cells and circuits in which they might exert their effects. One recently discovered mechanism by which antidepressants can regulate gene expression is by causing covalent modification of histone proteins and thus the conformation of chromatin. This type of mechanism might also contribute to the ability of antidepressant responses to persist even after treatment has been completed.

An additional hypothesis is based on the observation, described above, that antidepressant drugs enhance the rate of neurogenesis in the dentate gyrus of the hippocampus. According to this hypothesis the therapeutic delay in antidepressant response would result from the slow time course of development of new neurons and their incorporation into circuits. Some experiments suggest that inhibition of neurogenesis blocks the action of antidepressants in some rodent models of stress, but other experiments suggest that even if hippocampal neurogenesis plays a role in antidepressant action, it is not absolutely necessary.

The slow onset of existing antidepressant drugs is not only a scientific puzzle but also a serious clinical problem. While waiting for their symptoms to improve patients may become demoralized and a minority may be at increased risk of suicidal thoughts and acts. The search for rapidly acting antidepressants

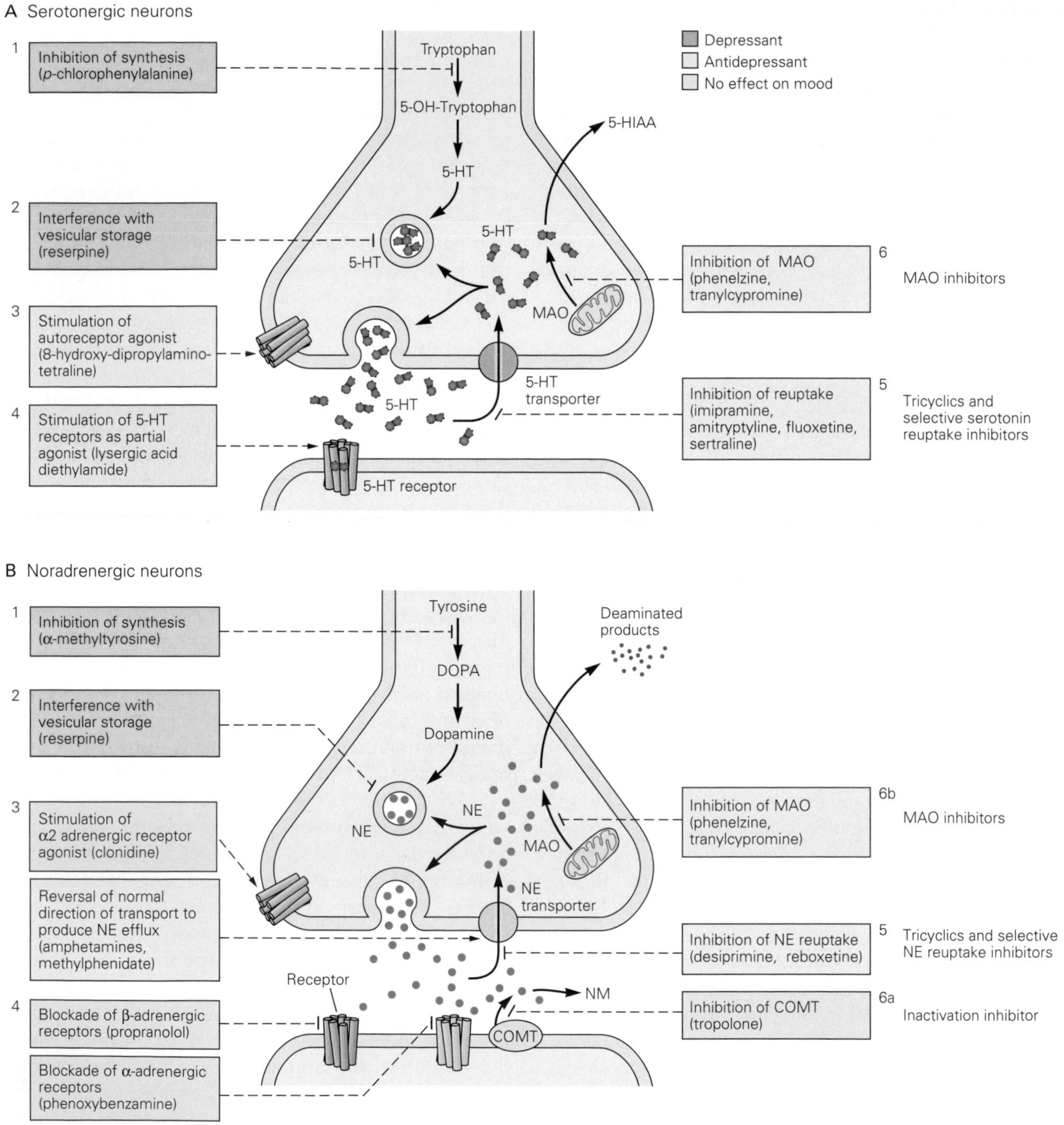
A Serotonergic neurons
Depressant
Antidepressant
No effect on mood
1
Inhibition of synthesis (p-chlorophenylalanine)
Tryptophan
5-OH-Tryptophan
5-HT
5-HIAA
2
Interference with vesicular storage (reserpine)
5-HT
5-HT
6
Inhibition of MAO (phenelzine, tranylcypromine)
MAO inhibitors
MAO
3
Stimulation of autoreceptor agonist (8-hydroxy-dipropylamino-tetraline)
5-HT transporter
5
Inhibition of reuptake (imipramine, amitryptyline, fluoxetine, sertraline)
Tricyclics and selective serotonin reuptake inhibitors
5-HT
4
Stimulation of 5-HT receptors as partial agonist (lysergic acid diethylamide)
5-HT receptor
B Noradrenergic neurons
1
Inhibition of synthesis (α-methyltyrosine)
Tyrosine
Deaminated products
DOPA
2
Interference with vesicular storage (reserpine)
Dopamine
3
Stimulation of α2 adrenergic receptor agonist (clonidine)
NE
NE
MAO
6b
Inhibition of MAO (phenelzine, tranylcypromine)
MAO inhibitors
Reversal of normal direction of transport to produce NE efflux (amphetamines, methylphenidate)
NE transporter
5
Inhibition of NE reuptake (desiprimine, reboxetine)
Tricyclics and selective NE reuptake inhibitors
Receptor
NM
6a
Inhibition of COMT (tropolone)
Inactivation inhibitor
COMT
4
Blockade of β-adrenergic receptors (propranolol)
Blockade of α-adrenergic receptors (phenoxybenzamine)

Figure 63–7 (Opposite) **Actions of antidepressant drugs at serotonergic and noradrenergic synapses.** The figure shows the pre- and postsynaptic sides of serotonergic and noradrenergic synapses. Serotonin and norepinephrine are synthesized from amino acid precursors by enzymatic cascades. The neurotransmitters are packaged in synaptic vesicles; free neurotransmitter within the cytoplasm is metabolized by monoamine oxidase, an enzyme that is associated with the abundant mitochondria found in presynaptic terminals. On release, serotonin and norepinephrine interact with several types of pre- and postsynaptic receptors (see Tables 63–3 and 63–4). Each neurotransmitter is cleared from the synapse by a specific transporter. The serotonin and norepinephrine transporters and monoamine oxidase are targets of antidepressant drugs.

A. Important sites of drug action at serotonergic synapses. Not all actions described are shown in the figure.

1. *Enzymatic Synthesis. p*-Chlorophenylalanine can inhibit the rate-limiting enzyme tryptophan hydroxylase, which initiates the cascade that converts tryptophan to 5-OH-tryptophan, the precursor of 5-hydroxytryptophan (**5-HT**, serotonin).

2. *Storage.* Reserpine and tetrabenazine interfere with the transport of serotonin and catecholamines into synaptic vesicles by blocking the vesicular monoamine transporter, $VMAT_2$. The cytoplasmic serotonin is degraded (see A. 6. below) and thus the neuron is depleted of neurotransmitter. Reserpine was used as an antihypertensive drug, but commonly caused depression as a side effect.

3. *Presynaptic Receptors.* Agonists at presynaptic receptors produce negative feedback on neurotransmitter synthesis or release. The agonist 8-hydroxy-diprolamino-tetraline (8-OH-DPAT) acts on $5\text{-}HT_{1A}$ receptors. The antimigraine triptan drugs (eg, sumatriptan) are agonists at $5\text{-}HT_{1D}$ receptors.

4. *Postsynaptic Receptors.* The hallucinogen lysergic acid diethylamide (LSD) is a partial agonist at $5\text{-}HT_{2A}$ receptors on the postsynaptic serotonergic neurons. Second-generation antipsychotic drugs, such as risperidone and olanzapine, are antagonists at $5\text{-}HT2_A$ receptors in addition to their ability to block D_2 dopamine receptors. The antiemetic compound ondansetron is an antagonist at $5\text{-}HT_3$ receptors, the only ligand-gated channel among the monoamine receptors. Its key site of action is in the medulla.

5. *Uptake.* The selective serotonin reuptake inhibitors, such as fluoxetine and sertraline, are selective blockers of the serotonin transporter. The tricyclic drugs have mixed actions; some, such as clomipramine, are relatively selective for the serotonin transporter. Uptake blockers increase synaptic concentrations of serotonin. Amphetamines enter monoamine neurons through the uptake transporter and interact with the vesicular transporter on synaptic vesicles to release neurotransmitter into the cytoplasm. The neurotransmitter is then pumped out of the neuron into the synapse through the uptake transporter acting in reverse.

6. *Degradation.* Phenelzine and tranylcypromine, both of which are effective for depression and panic disorder, block monoamine oxidase A and B (MAO_A and MAO_B). Moclobemide, effective against depression, is selective for MAO_A; selegiline, which has been used to treat Parkinson disease, is selective for MAO_B in low doses (5-HIAA, 5-hydroxyindoleacetic acid).

B. Important sites of drug action at noradrenergic synapses.

1. *Enzymatic synthesis.* The competitive inhibitor α-methyltyrosine blocks the reaction catalyzed by tyrosine hydroxylase that converts tyrosine to DOPA. A dithiocarbamate derivative, FLA 63 (not shown), blocks the reaction that converts DOPA to dopamine.

2. *Storage.* Reserpine and tetrabenazine interfere with the transport of norepinephrine, dopamine, and serotonin into synaptic vesicles by blocking the vesicular monoamine transporter $VMAT_2$. The cytoplasmic neurotransmitter is degraded (see A. 6. below) and thus the neuron is depleted of neurotransmitter.

3. *Presynaptic Receptors.* Agonists at presynaptic receptors produce negative feedback on neurotransmitter synthesis or release. Clonidine is an agonist at α_2 adrenergic receptors, inhibiting norepinephrine (**NE**) release. It has anxiolytic and sedative effects and is also used to treat attention deficit hyperactivity disorder. Yohimbine is an antagonist at α_2 adrenergic receptors; it induces anxiety.

4. *Postsynaptic Receptors.* Propranolol is an antagonist at β_2-adrenergic receptors that blocks many effects of the sympathetic nervous system. It is used to treat some forms of cardiovascular disease but is commonly used to block anxiety during performance situations. Phenoxybenzamine is an agonist at α-adrenergic receptors.

5. *Uptake.* Certain tricyclic antidepressants, such as desipramine, and newer norepinephrine selective reuptake inhibitors (**NRI**) such as reboxetine, selectively block the norepinephrine transporter, thus increasing synaptic norepinephrine. Amphetamines enter monoaminergic neurons through the uptake transporter and interact with the vesicular transporter on synaptic vesicles to release neurotransmitter into the cytoplasm. The neurotransmitter is then pumped out of the neuron into the synapse through the uptake transporter acting in reverse.

6. *Degradation.* At the postsynaptic neuron tropolone inhibits the enzyme catechol-*O*-methyltransferase (**COMT**), which inactivates norepinephrine (**6a**). Normetanephrine (**NM**) is formed by the action of COMT on norepinephrine. At the presynaptic neuron degradation by monoamine oxidase (**MAO**) is blocked by the monoamine oxidase inhibitors phenelzine and tranylcypromine (**6b**), as described in Figure 63–5.

has recently revealed that a single intravenous dose of ketamine, which blocks NMDA-type glutamate receptors, produces antidepressant effects within hours and that these effects persist for a week. Ketamine was developed as a dissociative anesthetic, a drug that distances a person from the experience of his body and produces other cognitive disturbances. However, in adults it may also produce psychotic-like symptoms and euphoria, and so is an abused street drug. A drug with such a profile of action is not likely to prove useful as an antidepressant, but it has led to promising new avenues of research focused on signaling initiated by NMDA receptors.

Overall, evidence for direct involvement of monoamines in pathogenesis remains scant. A large number of genetic studies attempting to link polymorphisms in genes that influence serotonergic function have remained inconclusive.

Psychotherapy Is Effective in the Treatment of Major Depression

Nonpharmacologic treatments are also effective in the treatment of major depression. Short-term symptom-focused psychotherapies have been developed for depression and tested in clinical trials. The best-studied psychotherapy used against depression is cognitive-behavioral therapy, which is effective in the treatment of mild and moderately severe major depression and in dysthymic disorder. Cognitive-behavioral therapy focuses on identifying and correcting distorted negative interpretations of events and automatic negative thinking that may initiate or perpetuate the depressed mood (see Box 61–1).

An important challenge is to understand what happens in the brain in response to such specialized forms of learning as cognitive-behavioral therapy. For example, such therapies may alter the activity of brain structures thought to mediate negative emotion, such as the amygdala and anterior cingulate cortex. The use of brain imaging techniques to demonstrate such changes may eventually help identify those patients who are particularly amenable to cognitive therapy and track their therapeutic progress, and my even be useful in training and therapy as a form of biofeedback.

Electroconvulsive Therapy Is Highly Effective Against Depression

Although it still conjures up negative images in the popular imagination, electroconvulsive therapy (ECT) administered with modern anesthesia is medically safe and remains the single most effective intervention for the acute treatment of serious major depression. It is also effective in both the depressed and manic phases of bipolar disorder. Electroconvulsive therapy is used when patients with major depression fail to respond to medication or when the patient is too debilitated to take medication.

Generally, six to eight treatments are given, most commonly on an outpatient basis, with unilateral lead placement. Bilateral placement can be used if unilateral is unsuccessful. Patients are anesthetized, and electrical stimulation is administered just to the degree that will produce electroencephalographic evidence of a generalized seizure. The major side effect is temporary memory impairment, with some retrograde amnesia. Amnesia is minimized by using unilateral lead placement and the lowest level of electrical stimulation needed. It is thought that electroconvulsive therapy increases the availability of biogenic amines in the brain, but its mechanism of action remains uncertain.

Motivated by the desire to improve on the therapeutic effects of ECT while diminishing its side effects, methods based on more focused forms of brain electrical stimulation are being explored. These include deep brain stimulation (DBS) using implanted electrodes and transcranial magnetic stimulation (TMS).

Bipolar Disorder Can Be Treated with Lithium and Several Drugs Initially Developed as Anticonvulsants

The discovery by John Cade in 1949 that lithium is effective in the treatment of mania initiated the modern era of psychopharmacology. In bipolar patients lithium not only treats acute episodes of mania but can also prevent recurrences of both mania and depression. It was thus the first "mood stabilizing" drug. Several drugs initially developed to treat epilepsy, such as valproic acid, were later shown to be effective in treating mania and in preventing recurrences of mania and depression.

The mechanism by which lithium stabilizes mood is not known. The two most promising ideas are based on lithium's ability to block enzymes involved in intracellular signaling pathways. Many neurotransmitter receptors indirectly activate phospholipase C through the G protein G_Q (eg, the α_1-norepinephrine, 5-HT_2 serotonin, and several muscarinic acetylcholine receptors). Phospholipase C hydrolyzes phosphatidylinositol 4,5-bisphosphate (PIP_2) to liberate two second messengers (Figure 63–8). PIP_2 is normally synthesized from free inositol. Central neurons cannot obtain free inositol from plasma because of the blood-brain barrier. They therefore must either recycle inositol, which requires the generation of inositol phosphates

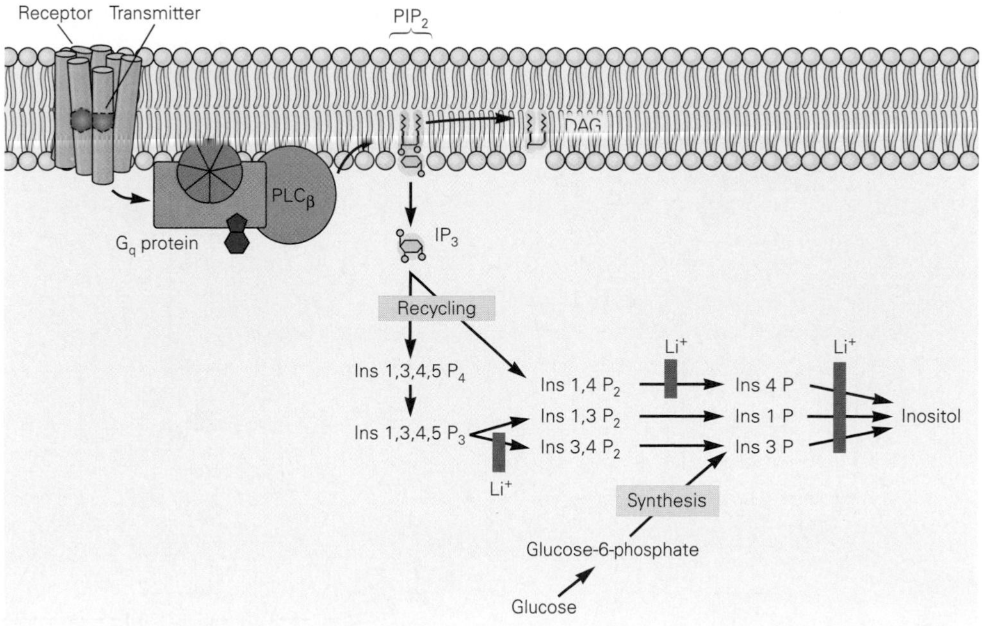

Figure 63–8 Lithium action on phosphatidylinositol pathways. A variety of neurotransmitter receptors are linked by the protein G_q (see Tables 63–3 and 63–4) to phospholipase $C_β$, which hydrolyzes phosphatidylinositol-4,5-biphosphate (**PIP_2**) to generate two second messengers, diacylglycerol (**DAG**) and inositol 1,4,5-triphosphate (**IP_3**). IP_3 releases Ca^{2+} from intracellular stores and subsequently is metabolized to forms that may not participate in neural signal transduction, including inositol 1,3,4,5-tetraphosphate (**Ins 1,3,4,5 P_4**). These are all metabolized to produce several inositol monophosphates, of which all are in turn metabolized by inositol monophosphate phosphatase, an enzyme that is inhibited by therapeutic concentrations of lithium (Li^+). De novo synthesis of inositol from glucose-6-phosphate also must pass through an inositol monophosphate intermediate. Thus in the presence of lithium the monophosphates derived from recycling of second messengers or from new synthesis cannot be dephosphorylated to yield free inositol. This should inhibit the ability of cells to regenerate PIP_2 and thus disrupt the second-messenger cascade. (Reproduced, with permission, from Nestler, Hyman, and Malenka 2009.)

by hydrolysis of phosphatidylinositols, or synthesize it from glucose-6-phosphate, a product of glycolysis.

Lithium inhibits several inositol phosphatases, including inositol-monophosphate-phosphatase, which is critical for the synthesis of the second messengers diacylglycerol (DAG) and inositol 1,4,5-triphosphate (IP_3) (Figure 63–8). As a result, lithium would appear to limit the ability of neurons to synthesize precursors of second messengers and therefore dampen the ability of neurons to fire at abnormally high rates. Alternatively, inositol depletion might alter gene expression that in turn would alter the response properties of critical neurons.

The second idea about how lithium stabilizes mood comes from the observation that lithium inhibits glycogen synthase kinase type 3 (GSK3), a critical enzyme in the Wnt signaling pathway (Figure 63–9). The Wnt signaling pathway plays important roles in brain development (see Chapter 53). How inhibition of this pathway might treat mania remains unknown.

Valproic acid is an anticonvulsant that also stabilizes mood. It appears to facilitate the actions of GABA (γ-aminobutyric acid), the key inhibitory neurotransmitter in the brain, possibly by increasing GABA release. The mechanisms by which anticonvulsants might treat bipolar disorder and the question of whether the mechanisms are shared with lithium remain important but unanswered.

Whatever the molecular mechanisms of lithium or the anticonvulsants, it seems likely that mood stabilizers dampen the dynamics of mood regulatory systems. Mood is regulated by the external environment as well as internal inputs, including the internal hormonal milieu, immune modulators, and circadian controls (eg, both the serotonergic and noradrenergic

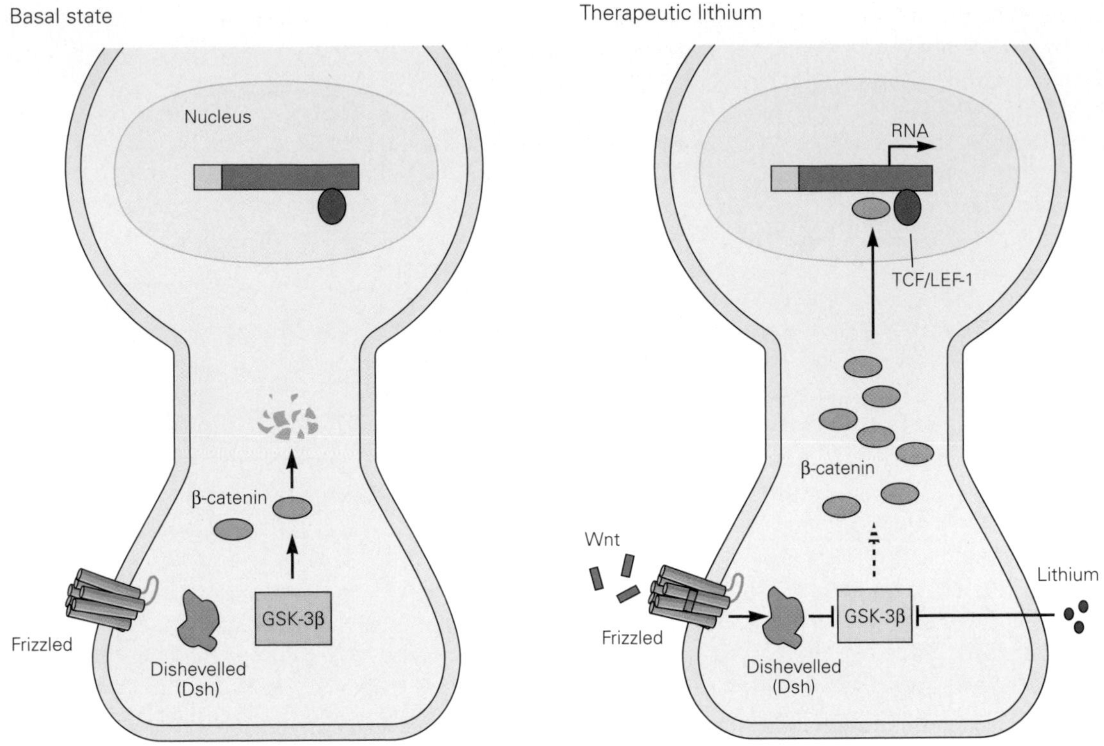

Figure 63–9 Lithium affects the Wnt signaling pathway. Wnt secretory proteins are involved in cell proliferation and differentiation. The Wnt protein was initially discovered as a critical molecule in *Drosophila* wing development but has been identified in the mammalian brain as well. Wnt binds receptors of the Frizzled family, initiating a signaling cascade to the nucleus that involves a cytosolic protein Dishevelled (**Dsh**) and glycogen synthase kinase 3β (**GSK-3β**). Phosphorylation by GSK-3β causes the degradation of another protein, β-catenin (left panel). GSK-3β is inhibited when Wnt binds Frizzled or when lithium is present in therapeutic concentrations, thus stabilizing β-catenin (right panel). When the level of β-catenin builds up, the protein translocates to the nucleus of the cell where it activates gene expression through a transcription complex TCF/LEF-1. Which genes might be induced by this pathway to stabilize mood is unknown. Interestingly, a Dsh knockout mouse exhibits abnormal social behavior and grooming. (Reproduced, with permission, from Nestler, Hyman, and Malenka 2009.)

systems show diurnal variations closely coupled with the sleep-wake cycle). The coupling of these systems is complex, involving dynamic interactions that are still poorly understood. Understanding these interactions is likely to give insight into the pathological cycle of bipolar disorder.

Anxiety Disorders Stem from Abnormal Regulation of Fear

Fear is a complex physiological, behavioral, cognitive, and, in humans, subjective response to a threatening stimulus. It evolved as an adaptive response to real threats and is usually transient. Anxiety is a longer-lasting response to danger signals that can arise either from immediate circumstances that signal well-defined danger or from vague indications of ill-defined events that are thought to have adverse consequences.

Anxiety can be highly adaptive; arousal, vigilance, and physical preparedness increase the likelihood of survival in dangerous situations. However, because many situations lack clear signs of safety, anxiety can persist. When anxiety persists beyond genuine risk, or when it produces a response out of proportion to the possible threat, the result can be distressing and disabling. Anxiety is the core symptom in several common psychiatric disorders. In the United States 28.5% of the population suffer from one or more anxiety disorders over the course of their lifetimes.

Anxiety disorders are distinguished from each other by the nature, intensity, and time course of symptoms, patterns of familial transmission, precipitating factors, the role of external cues in triggering episodes, and the constellation of associated symptoms. In some situations anxiety is not produced by a single eliciting stimulus but by an accumulation of cues. The currently recognized anxiety disorders are panic disorder, post-traumatic stress disorder, generalized anxiety disorder, social anxiety disorder (also called social phobia), simple phobias, and obsessive-compulsive disorder.

Panic disorder. The cardinal symptom of panic disorder is the unexpected panic attack consisting of a discrete period of intense fear accompanied by somatic symptoms such as palpitations, shortness of breath, sweating, paresthesias, and dizziness, and by a powerful fear of losing control or of dying (Table 63–5). Panic disorder is diagnosed when panic attacks recur and give rise to anticipatory anxiety about future attacks. People with panic disorder might restrict their lives progressively to avoid situations or places in which attacks occur or from which they might not be able escape should they experience an attack. It is common for patients to avoid crowds, bridges, and elevators; some individuals eventually stop leaving home altogether. A generalized phobic avoidance is called *agoraphobia*.

Post-traumatic stress disorder. Post-traumatic stress disorder (PTSD) follows an experience of severe danger or injury. First recognized in soldiers during World War I after combat trauma, it also occurs after civilian traumas such as violent assaults or serious accidents. It is characterized by emotional numbness to ordinary stimuli, punctuated by painful reliving of the traumatic episode, often initiated by sounds, images, or odors that trigger highly charged memories of the circumstances in which the trauma occurred. For example, a Vietnam War veteran with PTSD might experience intense symptoms after hearing a traffic helicopter pass overhead (recalling the heavy use of assault helicopters in that war). It is also characterized by disturbed sleep that can include nightmares, and by hyperarousal, such as an exaggerated startle response.

Generalized anxiety disorder. This disorder is characterized by chronic (months-long) worry and vigilance that is not warranted by circumstances. This worry is accompanied by physiological disturbances such as heightened sympathetic nervous system arousal (evidenced by an increase in heart rate) and by motor tension.

Social anxiety disorder. This disorder is characterized by a persistent fear of social situations or performance situations that expose a person to the scrutiny of others. The patient has an intense fear of acting in a way that will prove humiliating. Stage fright is a form of social anxiety that is limited to special circumstances, such as public speaking. Generalized social anxiety, as its name implies, involves adverse responses to most social situations and can therefore prove quite disabling.

Simple phobias consist of intense, excessive fear of specific stimuli, such as snakes, spiders, or height.

Obsessive-compulsive disorder. Obsessive-compulsive disorder (OCD) is characterized by obsessions (intrusive, unwanted thoughts) and compulsions (performance of highly ritualized behaviors intended to neutralize the negative thoughts and emotions resulting from the obsessions). The person experiences the obsessions as foreign and unwanted. Attempts to resist the urge to perform the compulsive acts result in high levels of anxiety. Typical symptom patterns are repetitive hand washing to neutralize fears of contamination (sometimes hours a day to the point of skin damage), or repeatedly checking the front door to see that it is locked.

Although current classifications of psychiatric disorders, including *DSM-IV*, place OCD among the anxiety disorders, family studies and imaging studies suggest that the disorder may share risk factors and dysfunction of striatal circuits with Tourette disorder, which is characterized by motor tics (involuntary, rapid movements) as well as vocal tics—grunts, noises, obscenities—and is often accompanied by obsessive-compulsive symptoms. Additional evidence for primary problems in striatal circuits, rather than the amygdala circuits implicated in other anxiety disorders, comes from the study of Sydenham chorea,

Table 63–5 Symptoms of a Panic Attack

A discrete period of intense fear or discomfort in which four (or more) of the following symptoms develop abruptly and reach a peak within 10 minutes:
Palpitations, pounding heart, or accelerated heart rate
Sweating
Trembling or shaking
Sensations of shortness of breath or smothering
Feeling of choking
Chest pain or discomfort
Nausea or abdominal distress
Feeling dizzy, unsteady, lightheaded, or faint
Derealization (feelings or unreality) or depersonalization (being detached from oneself)
Fear of losing control or going crazy
Fear of dying
Paresthesias (numbness or tingling sensations)
Chills or hot flushes

a movement disorder that can result from acute rheumatic fever. Interestingly, many patients with Sydenham chorea experience transient OCD-like symptoms. Sydenham chorea results from antibodies developed in response to a streptococcal infection, and the antibodies have been shown to bind to neurons in the striatum. OCD can be treated with high doses of selective serotonin reuptake inhibitor and by psychotherapy aimed at stopping intrusive thoughts and compulsive rituals.

Anxiety Disorders Have a Genetic Component

Panic disorder, generalized anxiety disorder, phobias, and OCD all run in families. First-degree relatives of individuals with panic disorder have a significantly greater risk of panic disorder than the general population or the first-degree relatives of unaffected control subjects.

Twin studies have concluded that panic disorder, generalized anxiety disorder, and probably phobias are explained to a large extent by genes. Twin studies also suggest overlapping genetic risk factors for depression and generalized anxiety disorder, which helps explain the observation that these two disorders often occur together.

In post-traumatic stress disorder genes appear to act in two important ways. They influence (1) the risk of developing the disorder after exposure to traumatic events and (2) the likelihood of individuals exposing themselves to dangerous situations.

Animal Models of Fear May Shed Light on Human Anxiety Disorders

Because many responses to fearful stimuli are conserved across mammalian species, animal models are potentially relevant to human disorders. In addition, because stimuli that elicit fear and anxiety can be readily produced in the laboratory, animal models are amenable to study. Studies using animal models have focused on two general classes of fear: innate fear and learned fear.

Studies of innate or instinctual fear exploit the natural tendencies of rats and mice to avoid open spaces or other situations that expose them to predators (Figure 63–10). Studies of learned or conditioned fear exploit the ability of rodents and other animals to form powerful associations between previously neutral cues and temporally linked danger. As described in Chapter 48, studies using these animal models have led to the outline of an amygdala-based fear circuitry that mediates defensive behaviors and appropriate physiologic responses to danger. They have been useful in designing noninvasive studies of human subjects with anxiety disorders, and as screens for anxiety-reducing drugs and genetic mutations that influence fear.

Our growing understanding of fear circuitry has generated testable hypotheses about the pathophysiology of

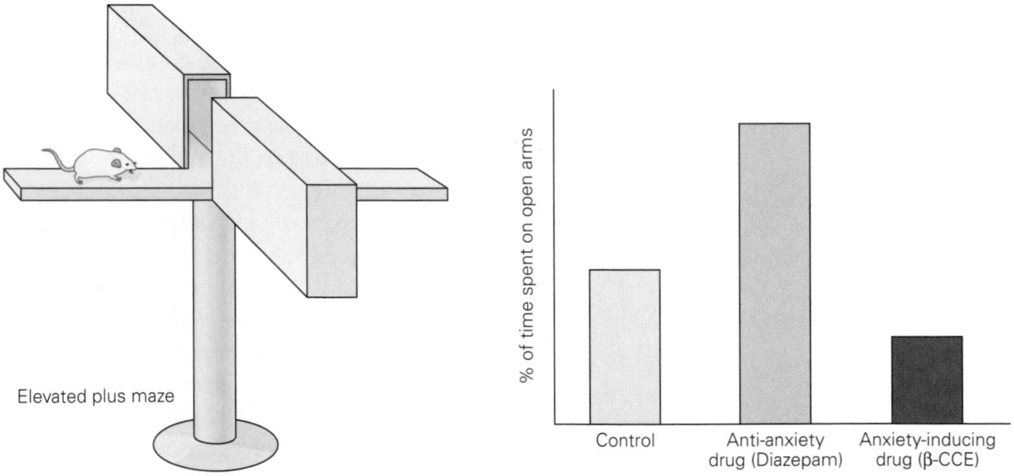

Figure 63–10 The effects of anxiety-reducing drugs can be tested on rodents in the elevated plus maze. The apparatus has two intersecting arms, one enclosed and the other open. A rat or mouse is placed at the intersection and the time spent on the open or enclosed arms is measured. Rodents normally prefer the closed arm. Rodents given benzodiazepine drugs, such as diazepam, which reduce anxiety in humans, spend more time in the open arm. Rodents given the benzodiazepine inverse agonist β-carboline (β-CCE), which strongly induces anxiety in humans, spend less time in the open arm. (Reproduced, with permission, from Nestler, Hyman, and Malenka 2009.)

human anxiety disorders such as post-traumatic stress disorder. For example, fear conditioning occurs normally in humans and is usually adaptive. By learning cues that signify danger and developing efficient responses, an individual minimizes future risk of harm. The central abnormality in post-traumatic stress disorder appears to be fear conditioning that is excessive, such that later minor cues are able to elicit fear responses. This dysregulated fear response alters other cognitive, emotional, and physiological responses. By mechanisms that are not yet well understood, it may alter basal levels of arousal, leading to exaggerated startle responses and disordered sleep. Other aspects of post-traumatic stress disorder, such as emotional numbing, are more difficult to model in experimental animals.

The unexpected panic attack—the hallmark of panic disorder—may represent a "false alarm" in which the fear circuitry is activated in the absence of a threat. Whether such abnormal activation originates from the fear circuitry itself or elsewhere in the nervous system is not known. Panic attacks can be produced in susceptible people by increasing partial pressure of carbon dioxide (PCO_2) in their blood or administering caffeine or drugs, which increase sympathetic outflow. Although these observations suggest a low threshold for activating the fear circuitry in persons with panic disorder, we do not yet understand the neurophysiologic mechanisms that trigger spontaneous panic attacks.

Panic attacks can be a source of fear conditioning. Initially, panic attacks are usually spontaneous, with no obvious relationship to the immediate context or environmental stimuli. However, environmental cues experienced in conjunction with a panic attack can become fear-associated stimuli. Later, these cues can trigger severe anticipatory anxiety or even a full panic attack.

With simple phobias and social anxiety the fear circuitry may be activated by cues that ordinarily signal very limited, if any, danger, such as risk of embarrassment. The experience can lead to avoidance of the cues. A person with a phobia of air travel might limit travel to surface transportation, and a person with stage fright might alter career plans to avoid public speaking.

Neuro-imaging Implicates Amygdala-Based Circuits in Human Fear and Anxiety

The understanding of the neural circuitry underlying fear and anxiety in animal models has guided neuroimaging studies of humans. In healthy subjects the amygdala is activated in response to stimuli that reliably induce fear, such as faces portraying fear, as well as during fear conditioning.

In a functional magnetic resonance imaging (fMRI) study of normal volunteers the presentation of a face portraying fear activated the dorsal subregion of the amygdala; this region contains what is thought to be the amygdala's main output nucleus, the central nucleus. When the same faces were shown only briefly to these subjects, followed by a neutral face (referred to as backward masking), the subjects did not report awareness of having seen the fearful face. Yet they exhibited physiological signs of fear (activation of the sympathetic nervous system). This test paradigm activates the basolateral subregion of the amygdala (which contains inputs from the thalamus and cerebral cortex) in healthy subjects similar to that of subjects with anxiety disorders (Figure 63–11).

Functional neuroimaging has also revealed heightened activity in the amygdala in specific anxiety disorders, including social anxiety disorder and post-traumatic stress disorder. In individuals with social anxiety disorder the increase in activity is induced by images of fearful faces; in individuals with post-traumatic stress disorder it is induced by narratives that are reminiscent of their trauma.

Structural imaging has also been used to study anxiety disorders. The most often replicated structural finding is diminished hippocampal volume in individuals with depression or post-traumatic stress disorder. Until longitudinal studies are performed, it is not clear whether a small hippocampus is a risk factor for post-traumatic stress disorder or a result of the disorder.

Anxiety Disorders Can Be Treated Effectively with Medications and Psychotherapy

Cognitive-behavioral therapies designed for specific anxiety disorders have proved as effective as medication in the treatment of anxiety disorders. For example, a person with cue-elicited anxiety, whether a simple phobia, phobic avoidance resulting from panic disorder, or social anxiety disorder, is coached to confront the phobic stimulus with adequate support and a new cognitive schema for coping with the fear. For many patients a combination of medication and cognitive-behavioral therapy may prove necessary.

Among the medications used for various anxiety disorders, drugs that were initially developed as antidepressants have proven highly efficacious and are the drugs of choice. The selective serotonin reuptake inhibitors are most widely used because they are easily tolerated. Simple phobias are best treated with cognitive-behavioral therapy rather than medication. The response of obsessive-compulsive disorder to treatment differs from those anxiety disorders in which amygdala-based

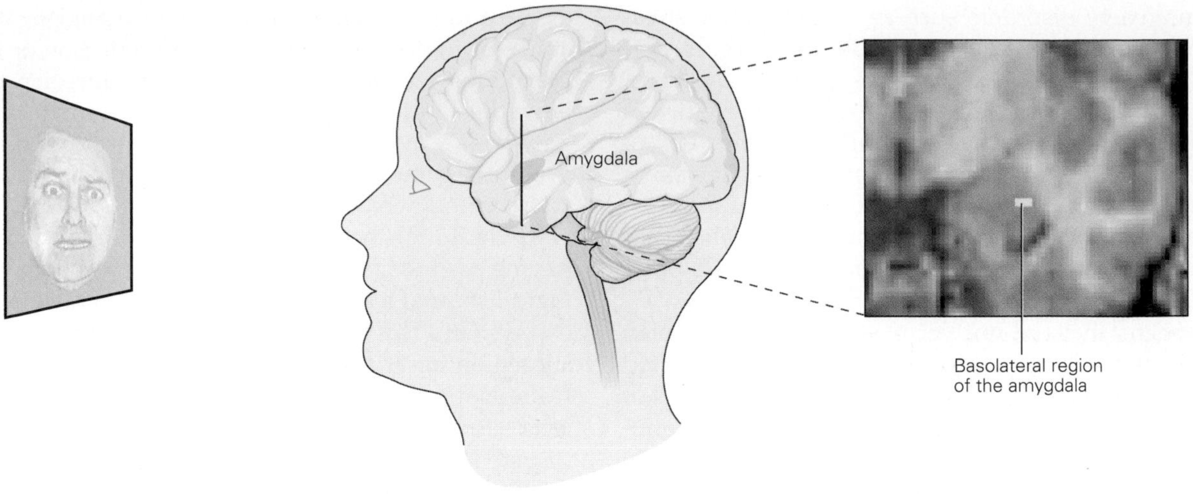

Figure 63–11 Amygdala activation in response to a masked presentation of a fearful stimulus. A human subject observes projected images while being scanned by magnetic resonance imaging. When a fearful face is presented for a very brief time followed by presentation of a neutral face (a protocol called *backward masking*), the subject is not consciously aware of the fearful face. Under these conditions the basolateral region of the amygdala predicts individual differences in trait anxiety in healthy subjects similar to those found in patients with anxiety disorders. (Reproduced, with permission, from Etkin et al. 2004.)

fear circuitry is thought to be the primary abnormality. Obsessive-compulsive disorder responds only to serotonin selective drugs at higher doses. Medications are generally combined with cognitive-behavioral therapy specially designed to inhibit compulsive behaviors.

Another class of drugs, the benzodiazepines, are occasionally used for generalized anxiety disorder, whereas higher doses are used for panic disorder. However, existing benzodiazepines can cause sedation; indeed, they are also used as hypnotics, and can degrade cognitive function. Moreover, benzodiazepines can cause dependence (as evidenced by worsened, so-called rebound anxiety) and insomnia when drugs are discontinued. In some individuals they can produce addiction (see Chapter 49). An advantage of the benzodiazepines is they react rapidly following a single dose, in contrast to the antidepressants, which can take weeks to become effective. Overall, they are second-line treatments to the selective serotonin reuptake inhibitors and other antidepressants, often used temporarily until the response to antidepressants takes effect.

The benzodiazepines produce their therapeutic effect by enhancing the inhibitory action of GABA at $GABA_A$ receptors. This receptor is ionotropic and selective for Cl^-. It is a pentamer, organized like barrel staves around an aqueous pore (Figure 63–12). Allosteric binding of benzodiazepine modifies the receptor complex, increasing the affinity of the GABA binding site for GABA. As a result, GABA-activated Cl^- channels open more frequently, enhancing the hyperpolarizing effect of GABA on the neuron. The sedative barbiturate drugs also bind the $GABA_A$ receptor complex, but at a site near the Cl^- channel. Barbiturates increase not only the affinity of the receptor for GABA but also channel open time, creating a greater risk of excessive central nervous system depression than is seen with benzodiazepines.

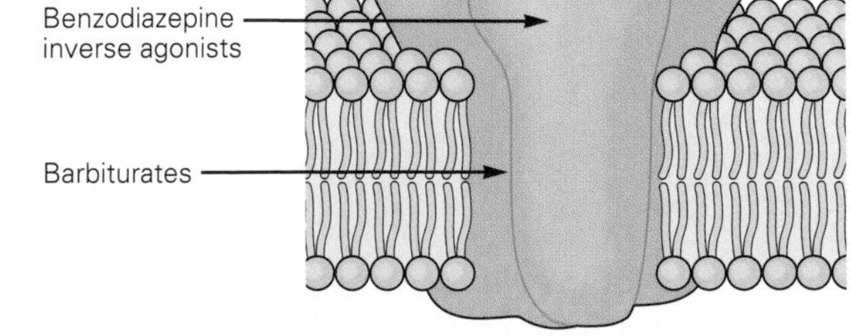

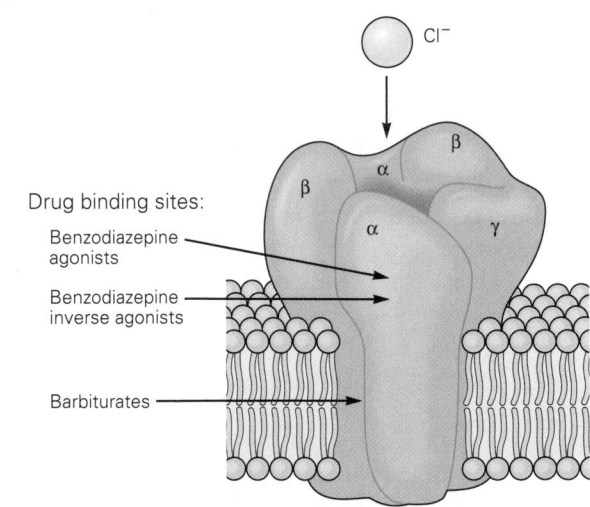

Figure 63–12 The $GABA_A$ receptor complex. The $GABA_A$ (γ-aminobutyric acid A) receptor is a pentamer arranged to form a Cl^- channel. In addition to the neurotransmitter GABA, the receptor binds several important drugs, including benzodiazepines and barbiturates, at physically separate sites.

An Overall View

Mood and anxiety disorders have long been misunderstood, even to the point that affected individuals can become objects of stigma. Because mood and anxiety disorders have a far greater impact on disability than on mortality (despite the risk of suicide), these disorders have too often been given low priority by health-care systems.

These unfortunate circumstances are beginning to change. Modern epidemiological and economic research has documented the enormous burden created by these disorders, which tend to begin early in life and to interfere with learning in young people and the ability to work in adults. Increased scientific understanding has also made a difference.

Although there is still a long way to go before we understand fully the neural basis of these disorders or the genetic, developmental, and environmental risk factors that give rise to them, there is little doubt that mood and anxiety disorders are real disorders of the brain. For example, compelling hypotheses concerning the neural circuits underlying anxiety disorders have been put forth and are being tested, and neuroimaging has provided important leads in the study of mood disorders.

The existing treatments for chronic mood and anxiety disorders are generally not curative. However, existing medications and cognitive-behavioral therapies can markedly improve symptoms, even to the point of remission for many individuals. The study of mood and anxiety disorders is a challenging frontier for neural science, but a challenge with very significant rewards for human health.

Steven E. Hyman
Jonathan D. Cohen

Selected Readings

American Psychiatric Association. 1994. *Diagnostic and Statistical Manual of Mental Disorders,* 4th ed. Washington, DC: American Psychiatric Association.

Davidson RJ, Pizzagalli D, Nitschke JB, Putnam K. 2002. Depression: perspectives from affective neuroscience. Annu Rev Psychol 53:545–574.

Delgado MR, Nearling KI, LeDoux JE, Phelps EA. 2008. Neural circuitry underlying the regulation of conditioned fear and its relation to extinction. Neuron 59:829–838.

Gordon JA, Hen R. 2004. Genetic approaches to the study of anxiety. Annu Rev Neurosci 27:193–222.

Yehuda R. 2002. Post-traumatic stress disorder. N Engl J Med 346:108–114.

References

Barlow DH, Gorman JM, Shear MK, Woods SW. 2000. Cognitive-behavioral therapy, imipramine, or their combination for panic disorder: a randomized controlled trial. JAMA 283:2529–2536.

Beaulieu JM, Gainetdinov RR, Caron MG. 2009. Akt/GSK3 signaling in the action of psychotropic drugs. Annu Rev Pharmacol Toxicol 49:327–347.

Berndt ER, Koran LM, Finkelstein SN, Gelenberg AJ, Kornstein SG, Miller IM, Thase ME, Trapp GA, Keller MB. 2000. Lost human capital from early-onset chronic depression. Am J Psych 157:940–947.

Bouton ME, Mineka S, Barlow DH. 2001. A modern learning theory perspective on the etiology of panic disorder. Psychol Rev 108:4–32.

David DJ, Samuels BA, Rainer Q, Wang JW, Marsteller D, Mendez I, Drew M, et al. 2009. Neurogenesis-dependent and -independent effects of fluoxetine in an animal model of anxiety/depression. Neuron 62:479–493.

Davidson RJ, Putnam KM, Larson CL. 2000. Dysfunction in the neural circuitry of emotion regulation–a possible prelude to violence. Science 289:591–594.

Dohrenwend BR, Turner JB, Turse NA, Adams BG, Koenen KC, Marshall R. 2006. The psychological risks of Vietnam for U.S. veterans: a revisit with new data and methods. Science 313:979–982.

Etkin A, Klemenhagen KC, Dudman JT, Rogan MT, Hen R, Kandel ER, Hirsch J. 2004. Individual differences in trait anxiety predict the response of the basolateral amygdala to unconsciously processed fearful faces. Neuron 44:1043–1055.

Frank E, Thase ME. 1999. Natural history and preventative treatment of recurrent mood disorders. Annu Rev Med 50:453–468.

Frodl TS, Koutsouleris N, Bottlender R, Forn C, Jager M, Scupin I, Reiser M, Holler HJ, Meisenzahl EM. 2008. Depression-related variation in brain morphology over 3 years. Effects of stress? Arch Gen Psychiatry 65:1156–1165.

Gross C, Hen R. 2004. The developmental origins of anxiety. Nat Rev Neurosci 5:545–552.

Heimer L. 1995. *The Human Brain and Spinal Cord,* 2nd ed. New York, Berlin: Springer-Verlag.

Hu H, Real E, Takamiya K, Kang MG, LeDoux J, Huganir RL, Malinow R. 2007. Emotion enhances learning via norepinephrine regulation of AMPA-receptor trafficking. Cell 131:160–173.

Hyman SE, Nestler EJ. 1996. Initiation and adaptation: a paradigm for understanding psychotropic drug action. Am J Psychiatry 153:151–162.

International Schizophrenia Consortium: Purcell SM, Wray NR, Stone JL, Visscher PM, O'Donovan MC, Sullivan PF, Sklar P, et al. 2009. Common polygenic variation contributes to risk of schizophrenia and bipolar disorder. Nature 460:748–762.

Kendler KS, Aggen SH, Knudsen GP, Røysamb E, Neale MC, Reichborn-Kjennerud T. 2011. The structure of genetic and environmental risk factors for syndromal and subsyndromal common DSM-IV axis I and all axis II disorders. Am J Psychiatry168:29–39.

Kessler RC, Berglund P, Demler O, Jin R, Koretz D, Merikangas KR, Rush AJ, Wlters EE, Wang PS. 2003. The epidemiology of major depressive disorder: results from the National Comorbidity Survey replication (NCS-R). JAMA 289:3095–3105.

Krishnan V, Nestler EJ. 2008.The molecular neurobiology of depression. Nature 455:894–902.

Li N, Lee B, Liu RJ, Banasr M, Dwyer JM, Iwata M, Li XY, Aghajanian G, Duman RS. 2010. mTOR-dependent synapse formation underlies the rapid antidepressant effects of NMDA antagonists. Science 329:959–964.

Low K, Crestani F, Keist R, Benke D, Brunig I, Benson JA, Fritschy JM, et al. 2000. Molecular and neuronal substrate for the selective attenuation of anxiety. Science 6:131–134.

Mayberg HS, Lozano AM, Voon V, McNeely HE, Seminowicz D, Hamani C, Schwalb JM, Kennedy SH. 2005. Deep brain stimulation for treatment-resistant depression. Neuron 45:651–660.

Mayberg HS, Brannan SK, Mahurin RK, Jerabek PA, Brickman JS, Tekell JL, Silva JA, McGinnis S, Glass TG, Martin CC, Fox PT. 1997. Cingulate function in depression: a potential predictor of treatment response. Neuroreport 8:1057–1061.

Mineka S, Watson D, Clark LA. 1998. Comorbidity of anxiety and unipolar mood disorders. Annu Rev Psych 49: 377–412.

Nestler EJ, Hyman SE, Malenka RJ. 2009. *Molecular Neuropharmacology. A Foundation for Clinical Neuroscience*, 2nd ed. New York: McGraw-Hill.

Nock MK. 2010. Self-injury. Annu Rev Clin Psychol 6:339–363.

Pizzagalli D, Pascual-Marqui RD, Nitschke JB, Oakes TR, Larson CL, Abercrombie HC, Schaefer SM, Koger JV, Benca RM, Davidson RJ. 2001. Anterior cingulate activity as a predictor of degree of treatment response in major depression: evidence from brain electrical tomography analysis. Am J Psychiatry 158:405–415.

Sheline YI, Sanghavi M, Mintun MA, Gado MH. 1999. Depression duration but not age predicts hippocampal volume loss in medically healthy women with recurrent major depression. J Neurosci 19:5034–5043.

Shin LM, Wright CI, Cannistraro PA, Weddig MM, McMullin K, Martis, B, Macklin ML, et al. 2005. A functional magnetic resonance imaging study of amygdala and medial prefrontal cortex responses to overtly presented fearful faces in posttraumatic stress disorder. Arch Gen Psychiatry 62:273–281.

Wray NR, Pergadia ML, Blackwood DH, Penninx BW, Gordon SD, Nyholt DR, Ripke S, et al. 2010. Genomewide association study of major depressive disorder: new results, meta-analysis, and lessons learned. Mol Psychiatry 2 November 2010; doi: 10.1038/mp.2010.109.

Zarate CA Jr, Singh JB, Carlson PJ, Brutsche NE, Ameli R, Luckenbaugh DA, Charney DS, Manji HK. 2006. A randomized trial of an N-methyl-D-aspartate antagonist in treatment-resistant major depression. Arch Gen Psychiatry 63:856–864.

64

Autism and Other Neurodevelopmental Disorders Affecting Cognition

DURING THE PAST CENTURY "MENTAL RETARDATION" was broadly used to label a variety of cognitive impairments that were linked to prenatal or early postnatal brain abnormalities. Some subgroups with easily identifiable physical features, such as Down syndrome, were recognized early on. In recent years syndromes that result from genetic anomalies but do not express obvious physical features, such as fragile X syndrome, have also been delineated.

Common to all of these disorders are mental impairments that persist throughout life, hampering development and learning, hence the terms "neurodevelopmental disorder" and "learning disability." Generally speaking, even if all mental functions seem to be affected, some tend to be more affected than others. This differential vulnerability gives interesting clues about the different origins and developmental time course of specific mental functions in normal development.

In this chapter we focus on autism and briefly consider Down syndrome, fragile X, and other neurodevelopmental disorders with a known genetic basis. Autism is especially interesting because it impairs brain functions that are highly sophisticated in human beings: social awareness and communication. Autism is also an exemplar of many psychiatric disorders: there is a striking range in severity of symptoms, an impressive heterogeneity of comorbid conditions, and no clear cut neuropathology. It is likely that autism will ultimately be viewed as a class of disorders each with different etiologies that include genetic and environmental factors and their interaction.

Autism Has Characteristic Behavioral Features

Autism has probably always been with us, but it was identified and labeled only in 1943 by Leo Kanner and by Hans Asperger in 1944. Where were the autistic people in the past? Rare historical documents suggest that some may have been valued as eccentrics or holy fools, but the majority were probably considered to suffer constitutional mental deficiency.

Today clinicians and researchers think of autism as a spectrum of disorders with three common diagnostic features, each showing a great deal of variability among individuals: impaired social interaction, impaired verbal and nonverbal communication, and restricted or circumscribed interests with stereotyped behaviors. The label "Asperger syndrome" is often used for individuals who exhibit the typical features of autism but have high verbal ability and no delay in language acquisition.

Autism and related disorders affect approximately 1% of the population, a far higher frequency than was previously recognized. Whether this reflects a better understanding and recognition of the range of disorders that actually belongs in this category or an actual increase in incidence is not entirely clear. The possibility that this increase is due to immunization or any simple environmental factor has been largely eliminated. Some studies indicate that the sperm of older fathers increases the incidence of autism as it does for schizophrenia. Risk also goes up with the age of the mother. As we shall see below, up to 10% of children with autism carry a genetic defect that results from a copy number variation, a mutation that arises in the germline.

Classification today is based on the three diagnostic criteria described above, which are more inclusive than those used in the earliest descriptions of the disease. Boys outnumber girls by 4 to 1, and by approximately 8 to 1 in cases of autism without intellectual disability. Although autism can occur in people with a high IQ, more than half the individuals with autism suffer from intellectual disability (defined as an IQ below 70). By definition, autism should be detectable before the child is 3 years old. Autism occurs in all countries and cultures and in every socioeconomic group.

Although autism is clearly a disorder that affects the brain, there are as yet no diagnostic biological markers and therefore diagnosis is based on behavioral criteria. Because behavior is highly changeable during development and depends on a number of factors, such as age, environment, social context, and availability and duration of remedial help, no single behavior could ever be diagnostic.

Some parents of an autistic child are aware that something is not quite right with their child from an early age. Other parents report that their babies first developed typically and then regressed in their development during the second year of life. A prospective study of siblings at genetic risk for autism showed that at age 6 months infants at genetic risk and later diagnosed autistic did not differ from those who were typically developing on measures of social interaction, such as gaze to faces, social smile, and vocalizations to others. However, differences from typically developing children increasingly emerged and were significant by 1 year of age. One of the earliest signs, near the end of the first year, is that the baby does not turn when called by name. Other early signs include the lack of preference for people over objects, and repetitive use of objects, such as spinning, and unusual visual exploration.

Beginning at approximately 18 months of age several other signs become clear. Most children with autism do not automatically direct their attention to the person or object that is the focus of other people's attention. Children with autism often fail to use pointing or other gestures to direct the attention of other people. They also fail to engage in ordinary make-believe play. Later, signs of delayed and abnormal language development are evident, with echoing of other people's speech (echolalia) and the use of idiosyncratic expressions. By the age of 3, typical cases of autism can be diagnosed reliably on the basis of this constellation of social and communication impairments, and rigid and repetitive behavior and interests. In cases where there is neither intellectual disability nor language delay (Asperger syndrome), diagnosis is typically not made until school age.

Like other neurodevelopmental disorders, autism is a lifelong disorder. Autism is not progressive, however. On the contrary, special educational programs and professional support often lead to marked improvements in behavior with age. The understanding and use of language by people with autism is quite variable. Even in individuals of high ability, language remains literal and conversational skills are lacking, as evident in poor turn-taking and poor understanding of irony. Most people with autism continue to find social situations difficult and are hampered in their ability to make friends or sustain lasting relationships.

A preference for routines and restricted behavior patterns remains throughout life, although the nature of obsessions and interests often undergo marked changes. In early childhood an individual may be drawn to shiny pieces of metal, in later childhood collect light bulbs, and in adulthood obsessively construct a novel dictionary. Hypersensitivity to touch, taste, sound, or vision is frequently mentioned in personal accounts and appears to play a role in restricting behavior by creating strong avoidances or preferences. Unfortunately, no neurobiological insight into these alterations in sensory function has yet emerged. People with autism are commonly susceptible to a variety of co-morbid psychiatric problems, particularly anxiety and depression. Nevertheless, reasonably good adaptation is possible when the environment is stable and highly structured.

There Is a Strong Genetic Component in Autism

Convincing data that autism has a strong genetic component come from studies of monozygotic twin pairs, who have identical genes. These studies show anywhere from 60% to 91% concordance of autism. The range is broad in part because some studies consider only the most serious forms of autism, whereas others consider the full spectrum of autism-like disorders. Dizygotic twins, in contrast, have been estimated to have 10–30% concordance when the full autism spectrum is considered. If a woman has one child with autism, the risk that a second child will have autism increases approximately 20-fold. Approximately 20% of siblings of a child with autism may also have autism. The risk increases if the second child is a male or if two prior children have disorders on the autism spectrum.

These family studies indicate that autism is not generally the result of mutations in a single gene but rather variation in many genes, giving rise to a complex pattern of inheritance. As in other polygenic disorders, it is likely that the genes responsible are not the same genes in all individuals but that different combinations are drawn from a larger pool of predisposing genes. This heterogeneity has made the identification of specific genes difficult.

Despite the difficulties, genomic regions have been implicated on several chromosomes. Of particular interest are mutations in two genes on the X chromosome in two sibling pairs with either autism or Asperger syndrome. These genes encode neuroligins, postsynaptic cell adhesion proteins important in synapse formation. These observations are intriguing because they are X-linked genes and may explain the male preponderance. The neuroligin discovery has recently been supported by a study of mice harboring mutations similar to the human mutations. These mice show impaired social interactions and, as a neural correlate, increased inhibitory synaptic transmission.

In addition to conventional mutations in specific genes, copy number variation has emerged as a potentially important genetic mechanism in autism. Copy number variation describes genomic deletions and duplications of pieces of a chromosome involving up to 100 consecutive genes on a chromosome. These deletions and duplications have recently been appreciated as a significant source of genetic variation in humans. Although copy number variants are almost always inherited, recent studies suggest that 10% of autistic patients carry a de novo gene copy number that neither parent carries. These are caused not by more common conventional mutations of discrete genes but by sporadic mutations of genomic structure in the germline in the cells that give rise to sperm and ova. Thus copy number variations may play an important role in autism (and other disorders) and perhaps explain the difficulties encountered in identifying autism-susceptibility genes.

Even though heritability, or the proportion of the phenotypic variance due to genetic factors, is very high for autism, environmental factors likely also play an important role, although no specific environmental factors have been conclusively identified. Infections by viruses (such as rubella, measles, influenza, herpes simplex, and cytomegalovirus) may contribute to the etiology of autism and perhaps represent environmental cues. The possibility that a genetic defect alters features of brain development by affecting the immune system is receiving greater attention. There is substantial evidence that mediators of immune functions such as cytokines and chemokines also play a role in brain development including synaptogenesis. Given the complexity of autism and its various forms, it is likely that a variety of etiologies will ultimately be discovered, some purely genetic, others that depend on genetic risk factors coupled with environmental factors, and some purely environmental causes.

Autism Has Characteristic Neurological Abnormalities

If autism is a developmental disorder of the brain, what parts of the nervous system are most severely affected? Research in this area is still in its infancy and no comprehensive picture of the neuropathology of autism is yet available. In fact, for a disorder with such a profound impact on the life of an individual, the brain, at least at a superficial level, looks relatively normal. However, more detailed quantitative analyses have begun to demonstrate consistent alterations in the size and time course of development of particular brain regions.

The first magnetic resonance imaging (MRI) studies of autism in the mid-1980s focused on the cerebellum and suggested that hypoplasia of the cerebellar vermis was characteristic of autism. These findings, however, have generally not been replicated. Other brain regions that have been found to be abnormal in autism include the cerebral cortex (although the salient portion of the cerebral cortex varies from study to study), medial temporal lobe structures such as the amygdala and hippocampus, and the corpus callosum (Figure 64–1).

The notion that cortical development may be altered in autism arose from clinical observations that before age 2 the head circumference of children with autism is often larger than typically developing controls. Approximately 20% of individuals with autism have unusually large heads (macrocephaly). These data would suggest that a large head and thus increased brain size might be a common, although by no means universal, feature of autism. There is, however, increasing evidence that an abnormal time course in development, not the outcome of brain development, is diagnostic of autism.

Several research groups have gathered provocative evidence for precocious growth of the brain, and particularly of the frontal lobe, during the first few

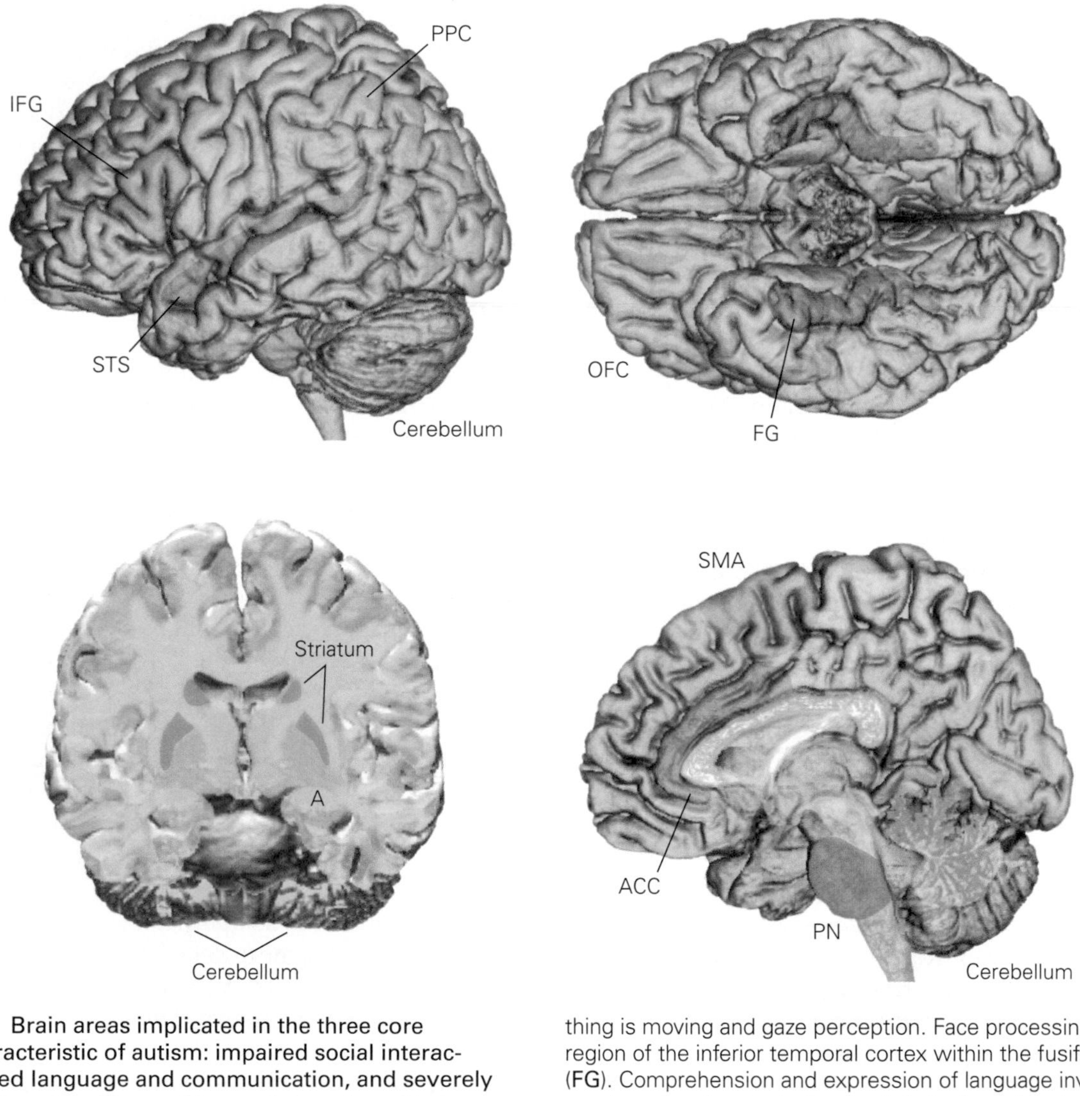

Figure 64–1 Brain areas implicated in the three core deficits characteristic of autism: impaired social interaction, impaired language and communication, and severely restricted interests with repetitive and stereotyped behaviors. Areas implicated in social deficits include the orbitofrontal cortex (**OFC**), the anterior cingulate cortex (**ACC**), and the amygdala (**A**). Cortex bordering the superior temporal sulcus (**STS**) has been implicated in mediating the perception that a living thing is moving and gaze perception. Face processing involves a region of the inferior temporal cortex within the fusiform gyrus (**FG**). Comprehension and expression of language involve a number of regions including the inferior frontal region, the striatum, and subcortical areas such as the pontine nuclei (**PN**). The striatum has also been implicated in the mediation of repetitive behaviors. A number of imaging and postmortem studies have indicated that the cerebellum may also be pathological in autism.

years of life of autistic children. Most studies show that at birth the brains of children with autism are either of normal size or perhaps slightly smaller than typically developing children and this is true again in adulthood. Clearly, the development of the brain is a precisely orchestrated process; if one or more brain regions develop out of sequence, patterns of brain connectivity and thus brain function could be seriously disturbed.

Beyond the cerebral cortex, other brain regions also show abnormal development. Perhaps most striking is the amygdala, a region of the temporal lobe that is involved in the detection of dangers in the environment and in modulating some forms of social interaction (see Chapter 48). Interestingly, in typically developing boys the amygdala develops over an unusually long period, increasing in size by nearly 40% between the ages of 8 and 18 years. The rest of the brain actually decreases in size during this same time period by approximately 10% because of refinement of connectivity and function. For boys with autism the amygdala reaches adult size by eight years of age. Thus whatever refinement of connectivity takes place in typically developing preadolescent and adolescent children may not occur in boys with autism.

Many studies have gone beyond simply evaluating the volume of the brain or brain regions and have analytically broken down a region of the brain into compartments representing grey matter and white matter. Alterations in white matter volume may actually be a more sensitive indicator of pathology in autism than grey matter differences. In fact, some researchers have proposed that the enlarged brain volume that has been reported in young children with autism can be accounted for, in large part, by disproportionate increases in white matter volume. Thus some studies have found a larger volume of white matter in boys with autism aged 2 to 3 years compared to controls. Interestingly, this difference was not found in adolescence, further evidence of an abnormality of early development.

As these studies illustrate, autism is not a disorder that affects a single brain region. The amount and kind of brain pathology in a particular individual may depend on whether the etiology is more genetic or environmental. Finally, the pathology of autism may not be apparent in the mature size and shape of the brain but in the time course of development of both the structure and connections of the brain.

The picture of the neuropathology of autism at a microscopic level is also not clear. This is in part because of the paucity of brains available for analysis. To date fewer than 200 brains have been subjected to microscopic analysis, and only a small fraction of these have undergone quantitative analysis. Another problem is the co-morbid occurrence of epilepsy. Approximately 30% of individuals with autism also have seizure disorders, and seizures damage the amygdala and many of the other brain regions that have been implicated in autism.

One reasonably consistent finding in autism has been the lower number of Purkinje cells in the cerebellum. Gaps in the orderly arrays of Purkinje cells are noticeable when using neural stains that mark cell bodies. Whether this reduction in cell number is because of autism, epilepsy, or the co-occurrence of both disorders is not clear. It is also not clear whether reduced numbers of Purkinje cells are characteristic of autism or a more general finding in neurodevelopmental disorders. Cerebellar alterations have been found in cases of idiopathic intellectual disability, Williams syndrome, and many other childhood disorders. A few cases of alterations of brain stem nuclei that are connected to the cerebellum, such as the olivary complex, have also been reported.

Microscopic abnormalities have also been observed in the autistic cerebral cortex, including defects in the migration of cells into the cortex, such as ectopias, nests of cells in white matter that failed to enter the cortex. It has also been proposed that the columnar organization of the autistic cortex is abnormal. These provocative findings are awaiting confirmation in larger studies using quantitative strategies. Finally, one study found fewer neurons in the mature amygdala of people with autism. Because this study was carried out with individuals that did not have co-morbid epilepsy, the change in the amygdala looks to be a real component of autistic neuropathology. It raises the possibility that autism may have a neurodegenerative component to its pathology.

There Are Distinctive Cognitive Abnormalities in Autism

Social Communication Is Impaired: The Mind Blindness Hypothesis

One cognitive theory of social communication, termed *theory of mind*, postulates that humans have a particularly well-developed ability to attribute mental states to others in an intuitive and fully automatic fashion. Watching a young man surreptitiously trying to open a car door without a key, you instantly understand that he believes he can break in while being unobserved, and expect him to run away as soon as he realizes someone is watching. Thus you explain and predict his behavior by inferring his mental states (desires, intentions, beliefs, knowledge). This so-called mentalizing ability is thought to have an identifiable biological basis and to depend on a dedicated brain mechanism. Further, it is postulated that this mentalizing mechanism is faulty in autism, with profound effects on social development.

It is now generally agreed that certain social insights typical of humans depend on the capacity to mentalize spontaneously. Spontaneous mentalizing allows us to appreciate that different people have different thoughts and that thoughts represent internal functions of the mind that are different from external reality. From an evolutionary point of view, the capacity to mentalize is extremely advantageous. It enables us to predict what other people are going to do next by "reading" their minds. It helps us to deceive and outsmart others, but also to teach and persuade, thus facilitating social and cultural learning.

The inability to mentalize, or "mind blindness," was first tested in autism with a simple puppet game, the Sally-Anne test. Young children with autism, unlike those with Down syndrome and unlike typically developing four-year-olds, cannot predict where a puppet will first look for an object that was moved while the puppet was out of the room. They are not able to imagine that the puppet will "think" that the object will be where the puppet had left it (Figure 64–2). Many autistic children eventually do learn to pass this task, but on average with a 5-year delay. Mentalizing acquired so slowly remains effortful and error-prone even in adulthood.

At the same time, young children with autism show excellent appreciation of physical causes and events. For instance, the child who is incapable of deceiving a character (by falsely telling him that a box is locked), is quite capable of locking the same box to prevent the thief from stealing its contents.

Variations of the Sally-Anne test and other mentalizing tasks have been used with children and adults with autism and Asperger syndrome since the mid 1980s (Figure 64–3). Compared to people with low-functioning autism, people with Asperger syndrome do much better when tested on mentalizing tasks, but they still show subtle difficulties. Whereas they solve many of these tests through effortful mentalizing, they show a lack of automatic mentalizing. This can be assessed by eye gaze anticipation. In contrast, there is some evidence that typically developing infants as young as 7 months show spontaneous mentalizing, and there is wide agreement that this automatic ability is well established from the second year of life.

Functional neuroimaging studies have scanned the brains of healthy subjects while they are engaged in tasks that necessitate thinking about mental states. A wide range of tasks using visual and verbal stimuli has been used in these studies. The results indicate that mentalizing is associated with the activation of a network of specific brain regions.

In one positron emission tomography (PET) study healthy adults viewed silent animations of geometric shapes. In some of the animations the triangles move in scripted scenarios designed to evoke mentalizing (for example, triangles tricking each other). In other animations the triangles move randomly and do not evoke mentalizing. Comparison of the scans made while subjects viewed the two types of animations reveals a specific network of four brain centers involved in mentalizing (Figure 64–4). Confirming the earlier PET study, more recent fMRI studies using the same animations also showed that in autism this network has reduced activation and weaker connectivity between its components.

One component of this network, the medial prefrontal cortex, is a region thought to be involved in monitoring one's own thoughts. A second component, in the temporoparietal region of the superior temporal lobe, is known to be activated by eye gaze and biological motion. Patients with lesions in this area in the left hemisphere are unable to pass the Sally-Anne test. The third region involves the amygdala, which is involved in the evaluation of social and nonsocial information for indications of danger in the environment. The fourth region involves the inferior temporal region, which is known to be involved in the perception of faces. All these components have been implicated in brain abnormalities in autistic individuals.

Other Social Mechanisms Contribute to Autism

The mind blindness hypothesis attributes all impairments in social communication to an inability to imagine the mental states of others. It has thus been influential as an example of how a specific cognitive deficit that explains a range of behavioral symptoms can arise from a neurophysiological or anatomical abnormality in specific networks of the brain.

The absence of preferential attention to social stimuli and mutual attention are widely acknowledged as early signs of autism. However, these may be distinct problems independent of mentalizing, given that mutual attention normally appears toward the end of the first year when signs of mentalizing are still sparse. Researchers have been considering the possibility

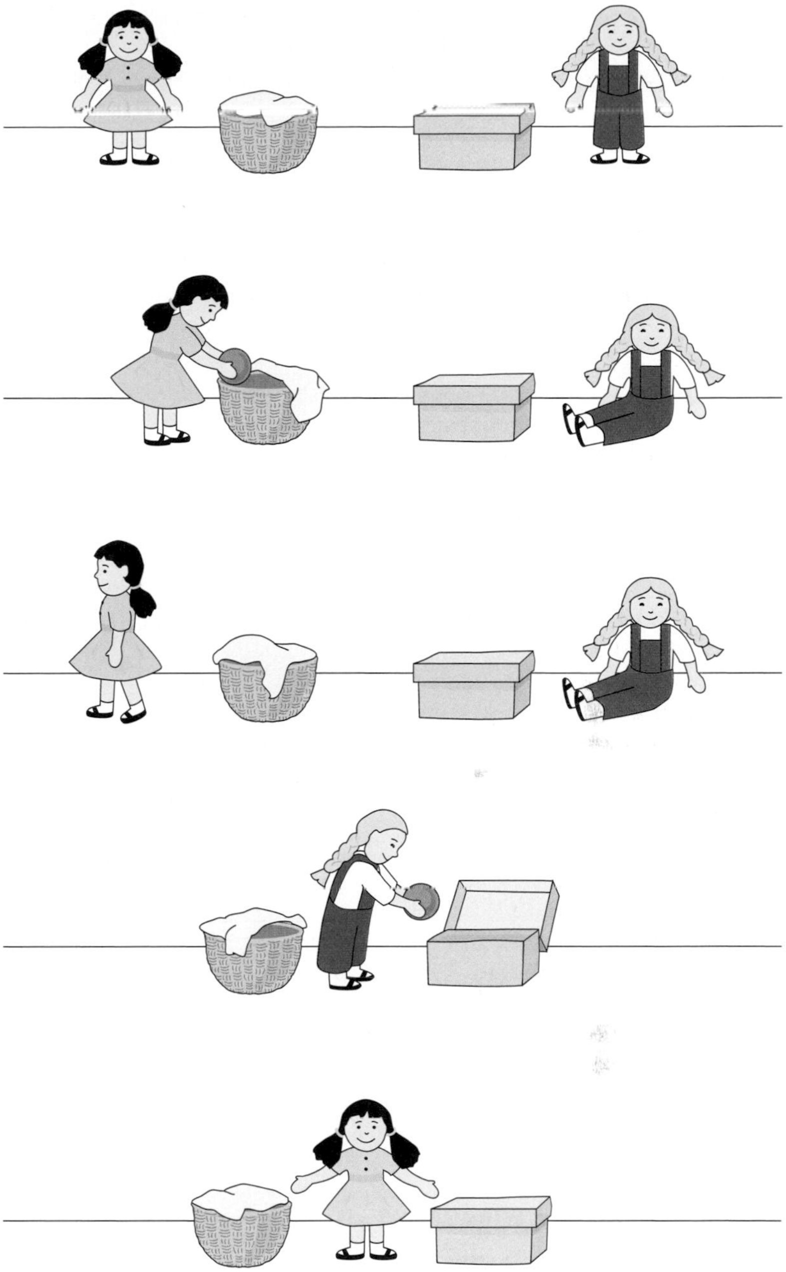

Figure 64–2 The Sally-Anne test. This first test of the "theory of mind" begins with a scripted performance using two dolls. Sally has a basket; Anne has a box. Sally puts a ball into her basket. She goes for a walk and leaves the room. While Sally is outside, naughty Anne takes the ball out of the basket and puts it into her box. Now Sally comes back from her walk and wants to play with her ball. Where will she look for the ball, the basket or the box? The answer, the basket, is obvious to most typically developing 4-year-olds but not to autistic children of the same or even higher mental age. (Adapted with permission, from Axel Scheffler.)

that a specific neural mechanism underlies attention to social stimuli, such as faces, voices, and biological motion. From birth normal infants prefer to attend to agents rather than other stimuli. An absence of this preference could lead to an inability to understand and interact with others. In favor of this hypothesis, researchers found that the gaze of individuals with autism is markedly abnormal when watching social scenes. One study found that autistic individuals fixate on people's mouths instead of the normal preference for eyes (Figure 64–5).

Imaging experiments have compared brain activity in autistic and normal subjects while they watch agents, their movements, their faces or voices. In these studies evidence has been accumulating in support of the idea that autistic individuals show atypical perception of eye movements, facial expressions, body gestures, and actions. This evidence implicates

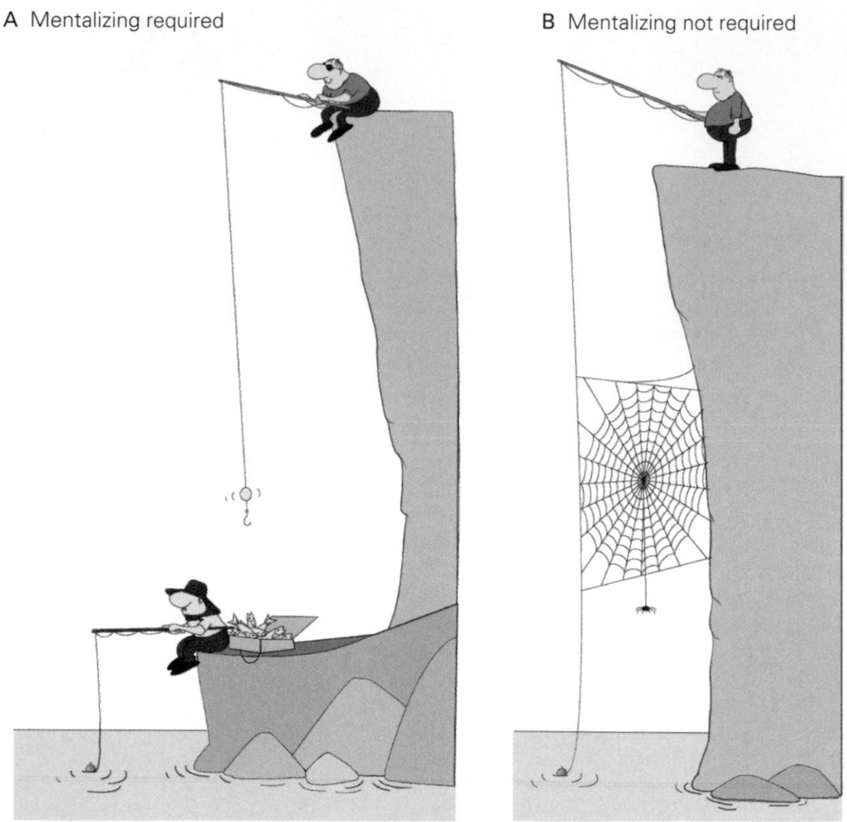

Figure 64–3 Examples of cartoons used in imaging studies of "mentalizing." Participants were asked to consider the meaning of each picture (silently) and then to explain them. In a functional magnetic resonance imaging (fMRI) study normal adults passively viewed cartoons that require mentalizing versus those that do not. A characteristic network of brain regions is activated in each subject (see Figure 64–4). (Reproduced, with permission, from Gallagher et al. 2000.)

the superior temporal sulcus region, a region of the brain that is known to have a role in the perception of intention of actions. In addition, frontal and parietal attentional brain systems that facilitate orientation to social stimuli appear to exert less top-down control in autism.

People with Autism Show a Lack of Behavioral Flexibility

Repetitive and inflexible behavior in autism may reflect abnormalities in the executive functions of the frontal lobe, a wide array of higher cognitive processes that includes the ability to disengage from a given task, to inhibit inappropriate responses, to plan and manage sequences of deliberate actions by staying on task, keeping multiple task demands in working memory, monitoring performance, and shifting attention from one task to another.

Even autistic individuals with normal or superior IQ have problems in planning, organizing, and flexibly switching between behaviors. Both low- and high-functioning individuals are stumped when asked to suggest different uses of one object such as a handkerchief (used to block a sneeze, to wrap loose objects, etc.). Flexible thinking is also poor in patients with acquired damage to the frontal lobe. In autism lack of flexible thinking appears to relate to a lack of behavioral flexibility in everyday life.

Difficulties in executive functioning are characteristic of other neurodevelopmental disorders: attention-deficit/hyperactive disorder, phenylketonuria, Tourette syndrome, dyslexia, and dyspraxia. For example, attention deficit hyperactive disorder is characterized by poor inhibitory control, whereas autism is characterized by poor flexibility, generativity, and planning. How the neural mechanisms underlying each of these difficulties differ is as yet unclear.

Some People with Autism Have Special Talents

One of the most fascinating features of autism is the existence of so-called "islets of ability", in at least 10% of the cases, in music, art, calculation, or memory.

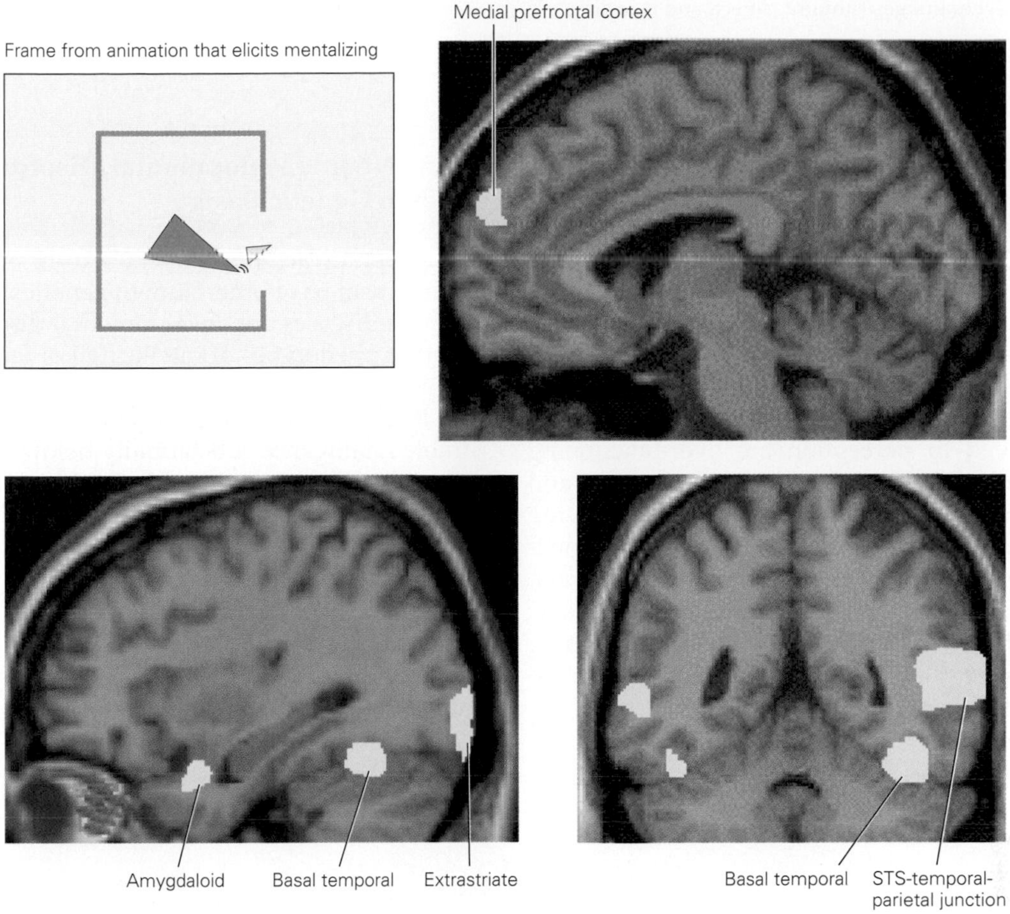

Figure 64–4 The mentalizing system of the brain. Healthy volunteers were presented with animated triangles that moved in such a way that viewers would attribute mental states to them. In the sample frame shown, the larger triangle was seen as encouraging the smaller triangle to leave the enclosure. They were also presented with animated triangles that moved in a more or less random fashion and thus would not elicit mentalizing. The highlighted areas show differences in the positron emission tomography (PET) scans of brain activation when these two viewing conditions were compared. (Reproduced, with permission, from Castelli et al. 2002.)

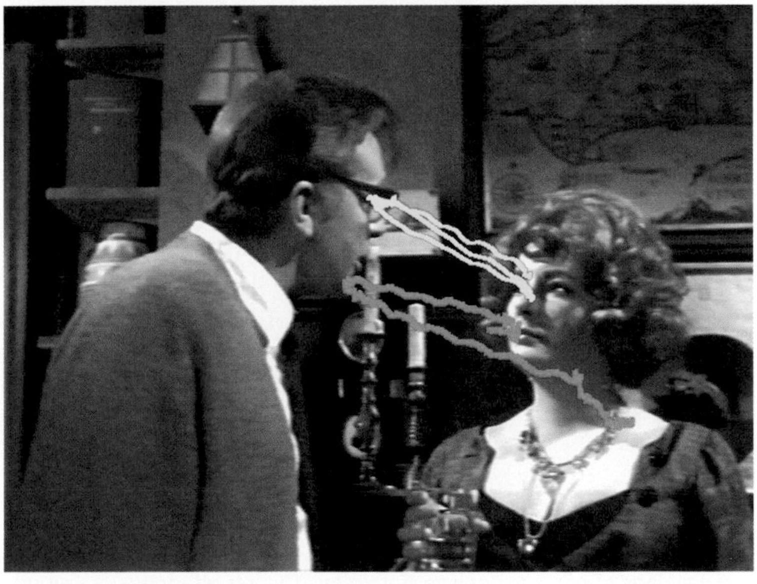

Figure 64–5 Individuals with autistic disorder often do not look into the eyes of others. Patterns of eye movements in individuals with autism were studied while the subjects watched clips from the film "Who's Afraid of Virginia Wolf?" When looking at human faces the subjects tended to look at the mouth rather than the eyes, and in scenes of intense interaction between people they tended to look at irrelevant places rather than at the faces of the actors. (Reproduced, with permission, from Klin et al. 2002.)

The frequency of superior rote memory for facts related to special interests is higher still. Approximately one-third of individuals with autism have perfect pitch, even when not musically trained. It is unknown what networks in the brain give rise to these phenomena.

One explanation for islets of ability is that information processing is preferentially geared to tiny details at the cost of seeing the bigger picture (the "weak central coherence" account). A similar idea is that brain regions involved in perception are over-functioning (the "enhanced perceptual functioning" account), and another idea is that there is a preference for processing details that suit "systemizing" such as calendar knowledge. Neuropsychological data support both explanations, but decisive experiments still remain to be done. The drawing by the gifted artist with high-functioning autism in Figure 64–6 shows beautifully detailed cityscapes, as well as detailed numerical patterns and dates.

Some Neurodevelopmental Disorders Have a Known Genetic Basis

It is generally accepted that 10% to 15% of individuals with autism have other known genetic diseases. Many of these diseases are developmental disorders leading to other phenotypes of intellectual or learning disability, which may overlap with autism.

Intellectual disability is generally defined as measurable intelligence substantially below the population mean that is associated with significant limitations in adaptive functioning before the age of 18 years. Adaptive functioning is defined as how well one copes, at a given age, with common demands of life and includes such things as communication, social and interpersonal skills, and self-care.

Intelligence is usually defined by the intelligence quotient (or IQ), as determined by a variety of

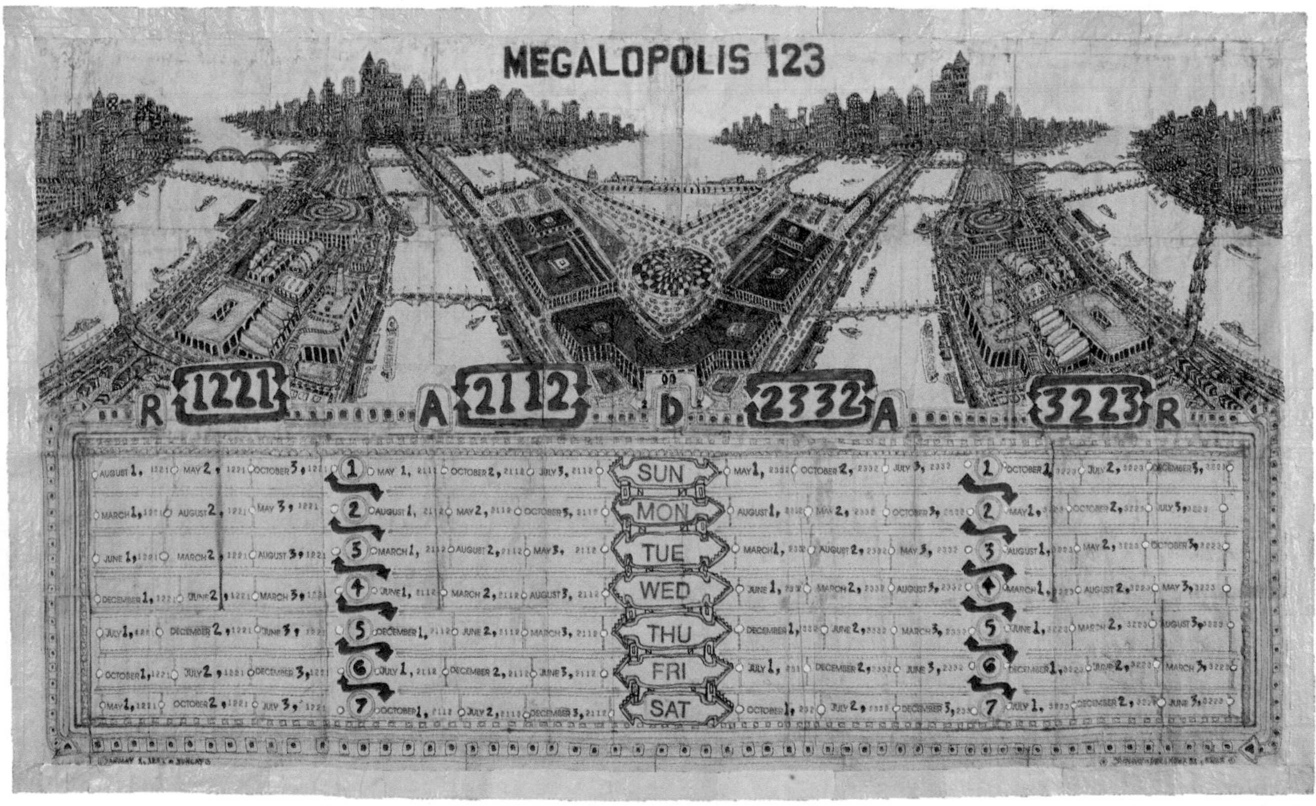

Figure 64–6 Strikingly beautiful art work by George Widener. He is a highly accomplished and much admired outsider artist. In the attention to detail this drawing resembles the drawings of other autistic savant artists. The intricate topographical detail of a symmetrically arranged city, with rivers, bridges and tall buildings, is combined with minutely executed and seemingly abstruse calendar sequences. Mastery of the calendar, and the ability to name the day of the week for any given date has often been described for autistic savants. The viewer of this drawing can partake in an otherwise very private world of space and time, numbers, and patterns. (Reproduced, with permission, from the Henry Boxer Gallery, London. www.outsiderart.co.uk.)

standardized tests, such as the Stanford-Binet or Wechsler Scales. These tests, in the general population, produce a range of scores that define a bell curve with the mean at 100 points. By definition an IQ below 2 standard deviations (below 70 points) is considered in the range of intellectual disability. Besides an IQ below 70, a person with intellectual disability also shows deficits in adaptive functioning. Like IQ, adaptive functioning is measured by standardized tests.

Fragile X Syndrome

Fragile X syndrome is a common form of chromosome X-linked intellectual disability. Patients show many similarities to autism, such as poor eye contact, a dislike of being touched, and repetitive behaviors. Its prevalence is approximately one in 4,000 boys and one in 8,000 girls. Estimates of the concurrence of autism and fragile X syndrome vary widely. In some early studies up to 25% of boys with autism were incorrectly diagnosed as having the fragile X syndrome. With the discovery of the gene for fragile X, diagnostic tests based on the genetic abnormality became available, lowering the percentage to approximately 3%. However, among children with fragile X syndrome, nearly 30% meet standard diagnostic criteria for autism.

The fragile X mutation is quite remarkable. The *FMR1* gene on the X chromosome includes the nucleotide triplet CGG. In normal individuals this triplet is repeated in approximately 30 copies. In fragile X syndrome patients the number of repeats is more than 200, with approximately 800 repeats being most common. As we have seen in Chapters 3 and 43, this expansion of trinucleotide repeats has since been recognized in other genes leading to neurological diseases, such as Huntington disease. When the number of CGG repeats exceeds 200, the *FMR1* gene becomes heavily methylated, and gene expression is shut off. Consequently, the fragile X mental retardation protein (FMRP) is lacking.

Lack of functional FMRP is considered responsible for fragile X syndrome. FMRP is a selective RNA-binding protein that renders messenger RNA dormant by blocking translation until protein synthesis is required. It is found at the base of dendritic spines together with ribosomes, where it regulates local dendritic protein synthesis that is needed both for synaptogenesis and for certain forms of long-lasting synaptic changes associated with learning and memory (see Chapters 66 and 67). Interestingly, a form of long-lasting synaptic change that requires local protein synthesis, the long-term depression of excitatory synaptic transmission, is actually enhanced in a mouse model of fragile X syndrome in which the gene encoding FMRP has been deleted. Loss of FMRP may enhance long-term depression by allowing excess translation of messenger RNAs (mRNAs) important for synaptic plasticity.

Indeed, mice lacking FMRP do not require new protein synthesis for the induction of long-term synaptic depression. An exciting implication of these data is that chemical antagonists of the type 5 metabotropic glutamate receptor, mGluR5, activation of which is required for this form of long-term depression, may lessen the excess protein translation and thus perhaps have a therapeutic benefit.

Rett Syndrome

Another single-gene disorder sometimes confused with autism is Rett syndrome, a devastating disorder that affects girls primarily. Affected children appear normal from birth until 6 to 18 months of age, when they regress, losing speech and hand skills that they had acquired. Rett syndrome is progressive, and initial symptoms are followed by repetitive hand movements, a loss of motor control, and intellectual retardation. Girls with Rett syndrome can live into adulthood but never regain speech or the ability to use their hands. Its prevalence is approximately one in 15,000 girls.

Rett syndrome is an X-linked inherited disease caused by mutations in the *MeCP2* gene, which normally encodes a transcription factor that binds to methylated cytosine bases in DNA, thus regulating gene expression and chromatin remodeling. Although loss of *MeCP2* alters expression of a wide range of genes, an important contributing factor to the Rett syndrome phenotype may be the result of the reduced expression of the gene that codes for brain-derived neurotropic factor (BDNF). In mice reduced expression of this secreted neurotrophic factor leads to a phenotype much like the mouse model of Rett syndrome; overexpression of BDNF can substantially improve the phenotype in *MeCP2* mutant mice.

One might think that such a global abnormality in gene expression would lead to an even more severe phenotype than that of Rett syndrome. It turns out that one copy of *MeCP2* is essential for survival. Boys who have a single X chromosome and thus a single copy of *MeCP2* die prenatally or soon after birth of encephalopathy if they carry a mutant form of *MeCP2*. Although girls carry two X chromosomes, only one is active in any given cell. Because the choice of which X chromosome is active is random, girls with a *MeCP2* mutation on one X chromosome are mosaics: Some of their cells express the normal protein whereas others express the abnormal form. The cells with the normal protein compensate and thus the phenotype develops into the Rett syndrome rather than the early lethal disease.

Down Syndrome

Down syndrome is the most common cause of birth defects in the United States and a major cause of intellectual disability. Each year approximately 100,000 infants worldwide are born with Down syndrome—approximately one in 1,000 births. Approximately 7% of children with Down syndrome also have autism.

Besides manifesting a characteristic set of facial and physical features, hypotonia, and congenital heart defects, Down syndrome is associated with cognitive defects and with early-onset Alzheimer disease. Among the cognitive deficits are poor spatial memory and difficulties in converting short-term to long-term memory. These memory defects are consistent with the fact that in individuals with Down syndrome the hippocampus is smaller than in typical development. The deficits are also the opposite of the exceptional short-term and long-term memory of many individuals with autism.

What are the specific genes that contribute to the cognitive symptoms of Down syndrome? Down syndrome results from the presence of an extra copy of chromosome 21 (trisomy of chromosome 21). Approximately 88% of these extra chromosomes are maternal in origin, 9% are paternal, and 3% occur at mitosis after fertilization. Studies of rare cases of partial trisomy of chromosome 21 suggest that the entire extra copy of the chromosome does not need to be expressed to have the full-blown syndrome.

A considerable part of the Down syndrome phenotype results from duplication of a 2-Mb region at segment 21q22.2 that contains 50 to 70 genes called *the critical Down region*. Examination of 27 transcripts that cover 80% of this region reveals several genes of potential interest for the cognitive deficit. These include a gene for two inwardly rectifying K^+ channels (*KCNJ6*, Homo sapiens potassium inwardly rectifying channel, subfamily J, member 6, also know as Kir3.2 or GIRK2) that are expressed in the developing and adult central nervous system, the gene for a kainate-type glutamate receptor mGluR5 (*GRM5*) which regulates a form of plasticity implicated in fragile X syndrome, the single-minded gene 2 (*SIM2*), and the gene for a dual-functioning protein kinase called *minibrain kinase* (*Mnbk*).

Prader-Willi and Angelman Syndrome and Other Disorders

Few errors that involve an entire chromosome are compatible with life. Among the autosomes, in addition to Down syndrome, only trisomy 18 and trisomy 13, each leading to severe intellectual disability, occur in an appreciable frequency, with a prevalence of one in 3,000 and one in 20,000 live births, respectively. Various numerical errors of the sex chromosomes occur but usually do not cause a significant degree of delay in cognitive development.

The only exception is Turner syndrome, which occurs in females missing an X chromosome. Girls who carry only the maternal X chromosome display a much higher prevalence of social-interaction difficulties similar to autism than do girls who carry the paternal X chromosome. This suggests genetic imprinting, where maternal and paternal copies of a gene are differentially expressed.

With imprinted genes, which represent only a small fraction (< 1%) of the genome, only one copy of the gene is expressed. In contrast, both the paternal and maternal alleles of nonimprinted genes are expressed. With paternally imprinted genes only the maternal allele is expressed. With maternally imprinted genes the opposite is true; only the paternally inherited allele is active. For example, with a maternally imprinted gene, either of the father's two alleles can be expressed in his children whereas the mother's alleles are silent. However, imprinting is reversible and is erased in the germ cells. Thus the same maternal alleles that are silenced in a mother's offspring can be active when they are transmitted by her son to his children.

Prader-Willi syndrome and Angelman syndrome, two related disorders with intellectual disability and possible connections with autism, are classic examples of imprinting. These two syndromes are usually caused by a specific deletion of the same region of chromosome 15 (Figure 64–7). However, individuals with Prader-Willi syndrome inherit the defective chromosome 15 from their father, whereas individuals with Angelman syndrome inherit the defective gene from their mother (see Chapter 3). Despite involving the same genetic mutation, the two syndromes have different symptoms. Prader-Willi syndrome is associated with mild intellectual disability, hypogonadism, and a hypothalamic abnormality that results in the inability to feel satiated from hunger, leading to morbid obesity. In contrast, Angelman syndrome is characterized by profound intellectual disability and an inappropriately happy demeanor with frequent laughing and smiling.

How can the same genetic deletion produce such different behavioral and physical changes? The answer lies in the differential patterns of imprinting of the paternal and maternal alleles of certain genes in this region of chromosome 15. If the paternal chromosome contains the deletion, as occurs in Prader-Willi syndrome, only the maternal alleles are present. Thus any maternal alleles that are normally turned off because of imprinting will not be expressed in the offspring. Similarly, if the maternal chromosome contains the deletion, as occurs in Angelman syndrome, those genes that are normally turned off because of paternal imprinting will not be expressed in the offspring. Because different sets of genes are imprinted in males and females, individuals with Prader-Willi syndrome and Angelman syndrome have defects in expression of distinct sets of genes. Therefore, despite having similar deletions of chromosome 15, individuals with Prader-Willi and Angelman syndromes have completely different phenotypes.

Although Prader-Willi syndrome likely involves the loss of more than one imprinted gene on chromosome 15, the cause of Angelman syndrome has been narrowed to a single gene encoding the E3 ubiquitin ligase enzyme. Imprinted genes on chromosome 15 may also predispose for autism, as linkage studies have shown some positive signal from the proximal long arm of chromosome 15. Indeed, a significant number of individuals with autism, perhaps as many as 1%, have maternal duplications of a portion of proximal chromosome 15 immediately adjacent to the Prader-Willi/Angelman syndrome region.

Other chromosome deletions that produce cognitive changes do not involve imprinted genes. Such deletions simply reduce the normal level of that gene's protein product by approximately 50%, because of the loss of one of the two alleles. Half the normal amount of some proteins is insufficient to support normal cellular function (known as *haploinsufficiency*), resulting in a particular behavioral phenotype. Most often these deletions involve varying degrees of intellectual disability and sometimes produce striking neuropsychiatric phenotypes.

One such example is Smith-Magenis syndrome, which results from the deletion of a single band on the short arm of chromosome 17. The syndrome is characterized by mild to moderate intellectual disability and

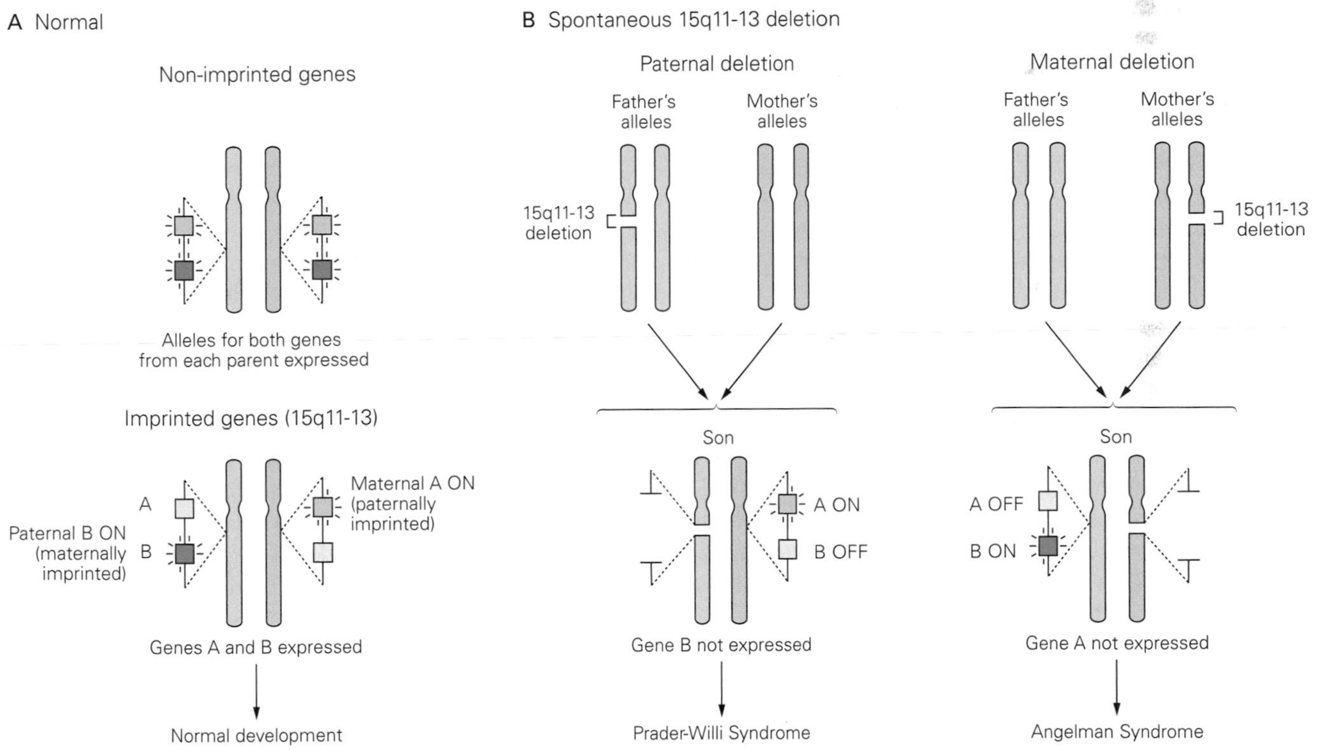

Figure 64–7 Imprinting in Prader-Willi and Angelman syndrome. Approximately 70% of Prader-Willi and Angelman syndrome patients inherit chromosome 15 from one parent with spontaneous (noninherited) deletions of the q11–13 interval. This interval contains imprinted genes with alleles that are either expressed or not depending on whether the chromosome was inherited from the father or mother. If the chromosome with the deletion is from the father, Prader-Willi syndrome occurs because maternally imprinted genes on the corresponding interval of the intact maternal chromosome (gene B, for example) are not expressed. If the chromosome with the deletion is from the mother, the gene for ubiquitin ligase (*UBE3A*) will not be expressed in offspring because of its normal inactivation on the paternal chromosome caused by imprinting; loss of expression of this gene leads to Angelman syndrome.

marked hypersomnolence. Smith-Magenis syndrome patients engage in a variety of unusual self-mutilations that they seem unable to resist, such as onychotillomania (self-mutilation of the finger and toe nails) and polyembolokoilomania (insertion of foreign objects into body orifices). They also repeat two stereotypic behaviors, spasmodically squeezing their upper body ("self hug") and hand licking and page flipping ("lick and flip"). What is most remarkable is that although most patients with Smith-Magenis syndrome have a 4-Mb deletion, four patients have been identified recently with a mutation in only one of the genes in this interval, *RAI1,* which is expressed in neurons. Once the function of *RAI1* becomes understood, it will be fascinating to consider how haploinsufficiency leads to the bizarre behaviors of Smith-Magenis syndrome.

Williams syndrome is also a segmental deletion but on the long arm of chromosome 7. Although no specific gene of the 25 to 30 genes within the deletion is singly responsible, the phenotype is nevertheless intriguing. Williams syndrome patients show specific dissociations of cognitive function, such as severe deficits in construction of visuospatial relations, yet have good language capabilities and do well in face recognition tests. However, the cognitive processes underlying these achievements differ from those used by typically developing children. Interestingly, Williams syndrome patients, regardless of family background and ethnicity, share somewhat similar personality traits marked by empathy and overfriendliness, making this syndrome in many ways the opposite of the stereotype of autism.

Probably hundreds of genes can lead to intellectual disability when mutated. Many of them encode proteins whose roles are central to brain development and function. For example, a form of lissencephaly ("smooth brain"), the loss of convolutions and gyri in the cerebral cortex, results from the mutation or deletion of the gene *LIS1,* which encodes a protein that normally participates in the regulation of cytoplasmic dynein heavy chains, which are essential for axonal transport (see Chapters 4 and 53). Intellectual disability also results from mutations of at least three genes with products that interact with Rho GTPases, leading to disruptions in signaling from the cell surface to the actin cytoskeleton that presumably alter neurite outgrowth. Mutations in Rab GTPases, which participate in vesicle fusion, also can lead to severe intellectual disability.

Other gene defects have much more subtle impacts on the nervous system and behavior. For example, Tony Monaco and co-workers studied an extended family, KE, in which a severe speech and language disorder is transmitted as an autosomal dominant condition because of a mutation in the gene *FOXP2,* which codes for a transcription factor. The *FOXP2* mutation causes faulty selection and sequencing of fine orofacial movements necessary for articulation, resulting in deficiencies in language processing and grammatical skills. *FOXP2* mutations have also been found in unrelated individuals with similar language deficits. Interestingly, nucleotide substitution rates in the *FOXP2* gene between species, a measure of evolutionary change, are accelerated in primates, suggesting that this gene had been a target of natural selection, possibly playing a significant role in the evolution of language in humans.

An Overall View

The study of neurodevelopmental disorders via cognitive neuroscience clearly illustrates the power of the synthesis of cognitive psychology and neuroscience and in fact moves this convergence into new directions. In the study of autism, for example, the mind blindness hypothesis has shown how cognitive theory can direct the search for the neural basis of a developmental disorder and how biological studies can open up a new window: the biology of social interactions.

A full understanding of the neurobiological basis of the many neurodevelopmental disorders that lead to intellectual disability will require the convergence of neuroscience, other medical disciplines, and functional genomics. A bottom-up approach—progressing from the identification of genes responsible for cognitive or behavioral disorders to an understanding of their effects on brain development—will clearly be crucial. At the same time, a top-down approach is needed, identifying the specific cognitive profile of each disorder and defining the critical neural circuits involved, using tools such as functional and structural brain imaging.

Autism is an example of a genetically complex disorder with a wide spectrum of manifestations, and the large differences between individual cases are often commented upon. Nevertheless, cognitive neuroscience has made advances in the difficult task of phenotyping patients and has helped pinpoint relevant brain regions and abnormal connections between them. This knowledge should be helpful in identifying the genetic and environmental risk factors that predispose to autism. Other developmental disorders that involve learning disabilities, especially those with much clearer patterns of inheritance than autism, are better suited to a bottom-up approach that begins with gene identification. Regardless of the approach, the underlying mechanisms that lead to cognitive and behavioral impairment in humans are most likely to be uncovered by research that combines cognitive psychology, neuroscience, and molecular genetics.

Uta Frith
Francesca G. Happé
David G. Amaral
Stephen T. Warren

Selected Readings

Amaral D, Geschwind D, Dawson G (eds). 2011. *Autism Spectrum Disorders.* Oxford: Oxford University Press.

Baron-Cohen S, Tager-Flusberg H, Cohen DJ. 2000. *Understanding Other Minds: Perspectives from Autism,* 2nd ed. Oxford: Oxford University Press.

Frith U. 2008. *Autism: A Very Short Introduction.* Oxford: Oxford University Press

Happé F, Frith U (eds). 2010. *Autism and Talent.* Oxford: Oxford University Press. (First published as a special issue of Philosophical Transactions of the Royal Society, Series B, Vol. 364, 2009).

References

Amaral DG, Schumann CM, Nordahl CW. 2008. Neuroanatomy of autism. Trends Neurosci 31:137–145.

Baron-Cohen S, Cox A, Baird G, Swettenham J, Nightingale N, Morgan K, Drew A, Charman T. 1996. Psychological markers in the detection of autism in infancy in a large population. Br J Psychiatry 168:158–163.

Baron-Cohen S, Leslie AM, Frith U. 1985. Does the autistic child have a 'theory of mind'? Cognition 21:37–46.

Bauman ML. 1999. Autism: clinical features and neurobiological observations. In: H Tager-Flusberg (ed). *Neurodevelopmental Disorders. (Developmental Cognitive Neuroscience),* pp. 383–399. Cambridge, MA: MIT Press.

Bear MF, Huber KM, Warren ST. 2004. The mGluR theory of fragile X syndrome. Trends Neurosci 27:370–377.

Cassidy SB, Morris CA. 2002. Behavioral phenotypes in genetic syndromes: genetic clues to human behavior. In: LA Barness (ed). *Advances in Pediatrics,* Vol. 49, pp. 59–86. Philadelphia, PA: Mosby.

Castelli F, Happé F, Frith CD, Frith U. 2002. Autism, Asperger syndrome and brain mechanisms for the attribution of mental states to animated shapes. Brain 125: 1839–1849.

Chelly J, Mandel J-L. 2001. Monogenic causes of X-linked mental retardation. Nat Rev Genet 2:669–680.

Courchesne E, Pierce K, Schumann CM, Redcay E, Buckwalter JA, Kennedy DP, Morgan J. 2007. Mapping early brain development in autism. Neuron 56:399–413.

Dawson G, Toth K, Abbott R, Osterling J, Munson J, Estes A, Liaw J. 2004. Early social attention impairments in autism: social orienting, joint attention, and attention to distress. Dev Psychol 40:271–283.

Folstein SE, Rosen-Sheidley B. 2001. Genetics of autism: complex etiology for a heterogeneous disorder. Nat Rev Genet 2:943–955.

Fombonne E. 2009. Epidemiology of pervasive developmental disorders. Pediatr Res 65:591–598.

Gallagher HL, Happé F, Brunswick N, Fletcher PC, Frith U, Frith, CD. 2000. Reading the mind in cartoons and stories: an fMRI study of 'theory of mind' in verbal and nonverbal tasks. Neuropsychologia 38:11–21.

Geschwind DH. 2011. Genetics of autism spectrum disorders. Trends Cogn Sci 15:409–416.

Happe F, Ehlers S, Fletcher P, Frith U, Johansson M, Gillberg C, Dolan R, Frackowiak R, Frith C. 1996. "Theory of mind" in the brain. Evidence from a PET scan study of Asperger syndrome. Neuroreport 8:197–201.

Hazlett HC, Poe M, Gerig G, Smith RG, Provenzale J, Ross A, Gilmore J, Piven J. 2005. Magnetic resonance imaging and head circumference study of brain size in autism: birth through age 2 years. Arch Gen Psychiatry 62:1366–1376.

Hill E. 2004. Executive dysfunction in autism. Trends Cogn Sci 8:26–32.

Jamain S, Quach H, Betancur C, Råstam M, Colineaux C, Gillberg IC, Soderstrom H, et al. 2003. Mutations of the X-linked genes encoding neuroligins NLGN3 and NLGN4 are associated with autism. Nat Genet 34:27–29.

Jin P, Alisch RS, Warren ST. 2004. RNA and microRNA in fragile X syndrome. Nat Cell Biol 6:1048–1053.

Kana RK, Keller TA, Cherkassky VL, Minshew NJ, Just MA. 2009. Atypical frontal-posterior synchronization of Theory of Mind regions in autism during mental state attribution. Soc Neurosci 4:135–52.

Klin A, Jones W, Schultz R, Volkmar F, Cohen, D. 2002. Defining and quantifying the social phenotype in autism. Am J Psychiatry 159:895–908.

Kovács ÁM, Téglás E, Endress AD. 2010. The social sense: susceptibility to others' beliefs in human infants and adults. Science 330:1830–1834.

Lai CS, Fisher SE, Hurst JA, Vargha-Khadem F, Monaco AP. 2001. A forkhead-domain gene is mutated in a severe speech and language disorder. Nature 413:519–523.

Malaspina D, Harlap S, Fennig S, Heiman D, Nahon D, Feldman D, Susser ES. 2001. Advancing paternal age and the risk of schizophrenia. Arch Gen Psychiatry 58: 361–367.

Malaspina D, Reichenberg A, Weiser M, Fennig S, Davidson M, Harlap S, Wolitzky R, et al. 2005. Paternal age and intelligence: implications for age-related genomic changes in male germ cells. Psychiatr Genet 15:117–125.

Nakamoto M, Nalavadi V, Epstein MP, Narayanan U, Bassell GJ, Warren ST. 2007. Fragile X mental retardation protein deficiency leads to excessive mGluR5-dependent internalization of AMPA receptors. Proc Natl Acad Sci U S A 104:15537–15542.

Nickl-Jockschat T, Habel U, Maria Michel T, Manning J, Laird AR, Fox PT, Schneider F, Eickhoff SB. 2011. Brain structure anomalies in autism spectrum disorder-a meta-analysis of VBM studies using anatomic likelihood estimation. Hum Brain Mapp Jun 20. DOI: 10.1002/hbm.21299

Ozonoff S, Iosif AM, Baguio F, Cook IC, Hill MM, Hutman T, Rogers SJ, Rozga A, Sangha S, Sigman M, Steinfeld MB, Young GS. 2010. A prospective study of the emergence of early behavioral signs of autism. J Am Acad Child Adolesc Psychiat 49:256–266.

Ozonoff S, Macari S, Young GS, Goldring S, Thompson M, Rogers SJ. 2008. Atypical object exploration at 12 months of age is associated with autism in a prospective sample. Autism 12:457–472.

Pelphrey KA, Shultz S, Hudac CM, Vander Wyk BC. 2011. Research review: constraining heterogeneity: the social brain and its development in autism spectrum disorder. J Child Psychol Psychiatry 52:631–644.

Redcay E, Courchesne E. 2005. When is the brain enlarged in autism? A meta-analysis of all brain size reports. Biol Psychiatry 58:1–9.

Ronald A, Hoekstra RA. 2011. Autism spectrum disorders and autistic traits: a decade of new twin studies. Am J Med Genet B Neuropsychiatr Genet 156B:255–274.

Samson D, Apperly IA, Chiavarino C, Humphreys GW. 2004. Left temporoparietal junction is necessary for representing someone else's belief. Nat Neurosci 7:499–500.

Schultz RT, Grelotti DJ, Klin A, Kleinman J, Van der Gaag C, Marois R, Skudlarski P. 2003. The role of the fusiform face area in social cognition: implications for the pathobiology of autism. Philos Trans R Soc Lond B Biol Sci 358:415–427.

Schumann CM, Hamstra J, Goodlin-Jones BL, et al. 2004. The amygdala is enlarged in children but not adolescents with autism; the hippocampus is enlarged at all ages. J Neurosci 24:6392–6401.

Sebat J, Lakshmi B, Malhotra D, Troge J, Lese-Martin C, Walsh T, Yamrom B, et al. 2007. Strong association of de novo copy number variation with autism. Science 316:445–449.

Senju A, Southgate V, White S, Frith U. 2009. Mindblind eyes: an absence of spontaneous theory of mind in Asperger syndrome. Science 325:883–885.

Slager RE, Newton TL, Vlangos CN, Finucane B, Elsea SH. 2003. Mutations in RAI1 associated with Smith-Magenis syndrome. Nat Genet 33:1–3.

Tabuchi K, Blundell J, Etherton MR, Hammer RE, Liu X, Powell CM, Südhof TC. 2007. A neuroligin-3 mutation implicated in autism increases inhibitory synaptic transmission in mice. Science 318:71–76.

65

Learning and Memory

IN HIS MASTERFUL NOVEL *One Hundred Years of Solitude* Gabriel Garcia Marquez describes a strange plague that invades a tiny village and robs people of their memories. The villagers first lose personal recollections, then the names and functions of common objects. To combat the plague, one man places written labels on every object in his home. But he soon realizes the futility of this strategy, because the plague eventually destroys even his knowledge of words and letters.

This fictional incident reminds us of how important learning and memory are in everyday life. Learning refers to a change in behavior that results from acquiring knowledge about the world, and memory is the process by which that knowledge is encoded, stored, and later retrieved. Marquez's story challenges us to imagine life without the ability to learn and remember. We would forget people and places we once knew, and no longer be able to use and understand language or execute motor skills we had once learned; we would not recall the happiest or saddest moments of our lives, and would even lose our sense of personal identity. Learning and memory are essential to the full functioning and independent survival of people and animals.

In 1861 Pierre Paul Broca discovered that damage to the posterior portion of the left frontal lobe (Broca's area) produces a specific deficit in language. Soon thereafter it became clear that other mental functions, such as perception and voluntary movement, are also mediated by discrete parts of the brain (see Chapter 1). This naturally led to the question: Are there discrete neural systems concerned with memory? If so, is there a "memory center" or is memory processing widely distributed throughout the brain?

Contrary to the prevalent view that cognitive functions are localized in the brain, many students of learning doubted that memory is localized. In fact, until the middle of the 20th century many psychologists doubted that memory is a discrete function, independent of perception, language, or movement. One reason for the persistent doubt is that memory storage involves many different parts of the brain. We now appreciate, however, that these regions are not all equally important. There are several fundamentally different types of memory, and certain regions of the brain are much more important for some types of storage than for others.

During the past several decades researchers have made significant progress in the analysis and understanding of learning and memory. In this chapter we focus on three insights. First, there are several forms of learning and memory, each with its distinctive cognitive properties and mediated by specific brain systems. Second, memory can be deconstructed into discrete encoding, storage consolidation, and retrieval processes. Finally, imperfections and errors in remembering can provide clues about the nature and function of learning and memory.

Memory can be classified along two dimensions: (1) the time course of storage and (2) the nature of the information stored. We shall first consider the time course.

Short-Term and Long-Term Memory Involve Different Neural Systems

Short-Term Memory Maintains Transient Representations of Information Relevant to Immediate Goals

When we reflect on the nature of memory we usually think of the long-term memory that William James referred to as "memory proper" or "secondary memory." That is, we think of memory as "the knowledge of a former state of mind after it has already once dropped from consciousness." This knowledge depends on the formation of a memory trace that is durable, in which the representation persists even when its content has been out of conscious awareness for a long period.

Not all forms of memory, however, constitute "former states of mind." In fact, the ability to store information depends on short-term memory, called working memory, which maintains current, albeit transient, representations of goal-relevant knowledge. In humans working memory consists of at least two subsystems—one for verbal information and another for visuospatial information. The functioning of these two subsystems is coordinated by a third system called the *executive control processes*. Executive control processes are thought to allocate attentional resources to the verbal and visuospatial subsystems, and to monitor, manipulate, and update stored representations.

We use the verbal subsystem when we attempt to keep speech-based (phonological) information in conscious awareness, as when we mentally rehearse a phone number just obtained from an operator. The verbal subsystem consists of two interactive components: a store that represents phonological knowledge and a rehearsal mechanism that keeps these representations active while we need them. Neuropsychological and neuroimaging data indicate that phonological storage depends on posterior parietal cortices, and rehearsal partially depends on articulatory processes in Broca's area.

The visuospatial subsystem of working memory retains mental images of visual objects and of the location of objects in space. The rehearsal of spatial and object information is thought to involve modulation of such representations in the parietal, inferior temporal, and extrastriate occipital cortices by the frontal and premotor cortices. Current research is concerned with whether visuospatial working memory might best be viewed as two subsystems, one for object knowledge and one for spatial knowledge.

Single-cell recordings in nonhuman primates indicate that some prefrontal neurons maintain spatial representations, others maintain object representations, and still others represent the integration of spatial and object knowledge. Although neurons concerned with working memory of objects tend to fall in the ventrolateral prefrontal cortex and those concerned with spatial knowledge tend to fall in the dorsolateral prefrontal cortex, all three classes of neurons are present in both prefrontal subregions (Figure 65–1).

Short-Term Memory Is Selectively Transferred to Long-Term Memory

In the mid-1950s startling new evidence about the neural basis of long-term memory emerged from the study of patients who had undergone bilateral removal of the hippocampus and neighboring regions in the medial temporal lobe as treatment for epilepsy. The first and best-studied case was a patient called H.M. studied by the psychologist Brenda Milner and the surgeon William Scoville. After H.M. died on December 2, 2008, his full name, Henry Molaison, was revealed to the world.

H.M., a 27-year-old man, had suffered for more than 10 years from untreatable temporal lobe epilepsy caused by brain damage sustained at age 7 years in a bicycle accident. As an adult his seizures rendered him unable to work or lead a normal life. At surgery Scoville removed the hippocampal formation, the

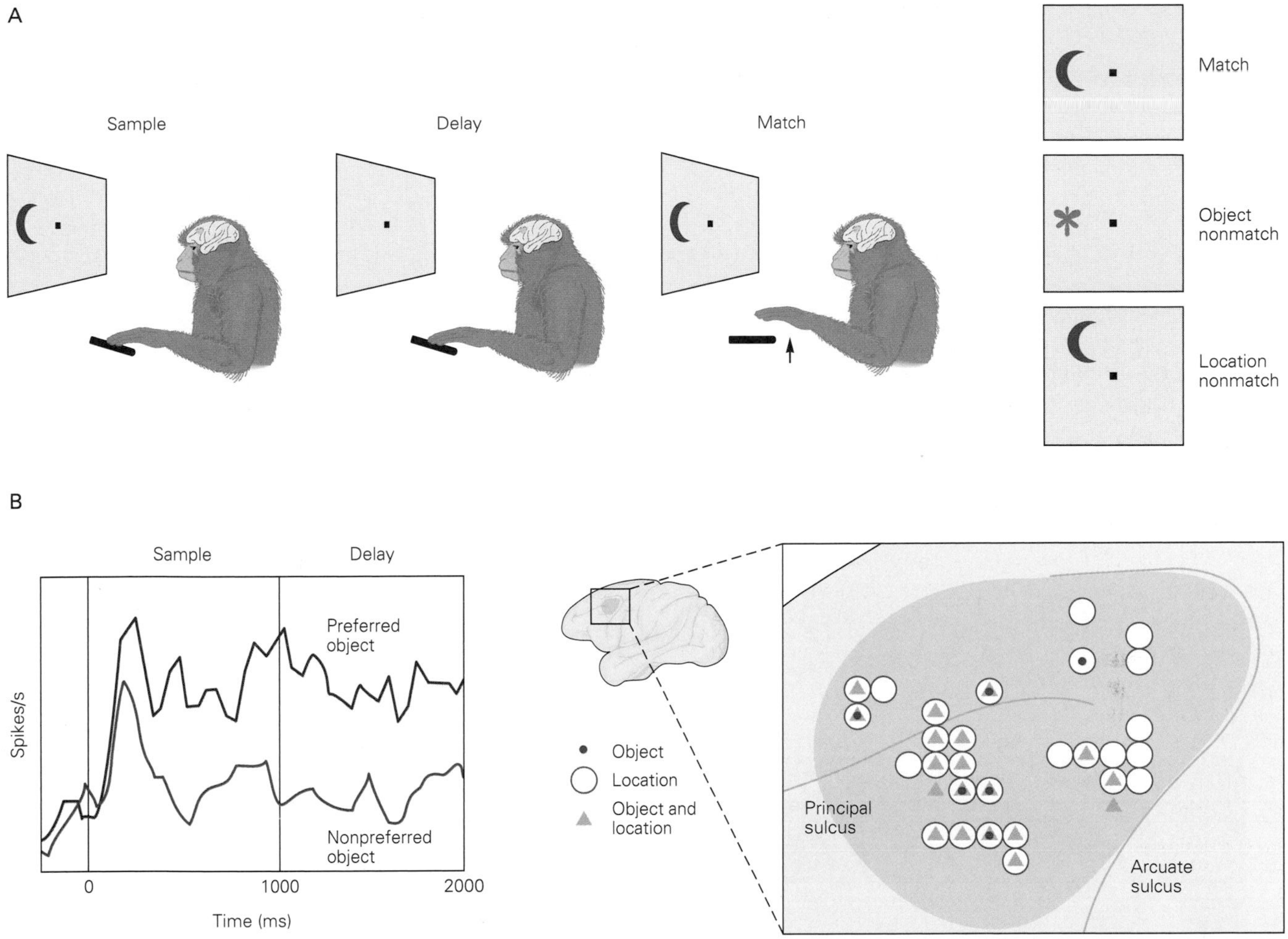

Figure 65–1 The prefrontal cortex maintains a working memory. (Adapted, with permission, from Rainer, Asaad, and Miller 1998.)

A. The role of prefrontal cortex in maintaining information in working memory is often assessed in monkeys using electrophysiological methods in conjunction with the delayed-match-to-sample (DMS) task. In this type of task each trial begins when the monkey grabs a response lever and fixates a small target at the center of a computer screen. An initial stimulus (the "sample") is briefly presented and must be held in working memory until the next stimulus (the "match") appears. In the task illustrated here the monkey was required to remember the sample ("what") and its location ("where") and release the lever only in response to stimuli that "matched" on both dimensions.

B. Neural firing rates in the primate lateral prefrontal cortex during the delay period in the task are often above baseline and represent responses to the type of stimulus (what), the location (where), and the integration of the two (what and where). At left is the activity of a prefrontal neuron to preferred objects (to which the neuron responds robustly) and to nonpreferred objects (to which the neuron responds minimally) during the task. Activity is robust when the monkey encounters the preferred object (sample) and during the delay. In the sketch at right the symbols represent recording sites where neurons that maintained each type of information (what, where, and what and where) were found. Typically, several types of neurons were found at one site; hence many symbols overlap and some symbols indicate more than one neuron.

amygdala, and parts of the multimodal association area of the temporal cortex bilaterally (Figure 65–2). After the surgery H.M.'s seizures were better controlled, but he was left with a devastating memory deficit (or amnesia). What was so remarkable about H.M.'s deficit was its specificity.

He still had normal working memory, for seconds or minutes, indicating that the medial temporal lobe is not necessary for transient memory. He also had long–term memory for events that had occurred before the operation. He remembered his name, the job he had held, and childhood events, although his memory of

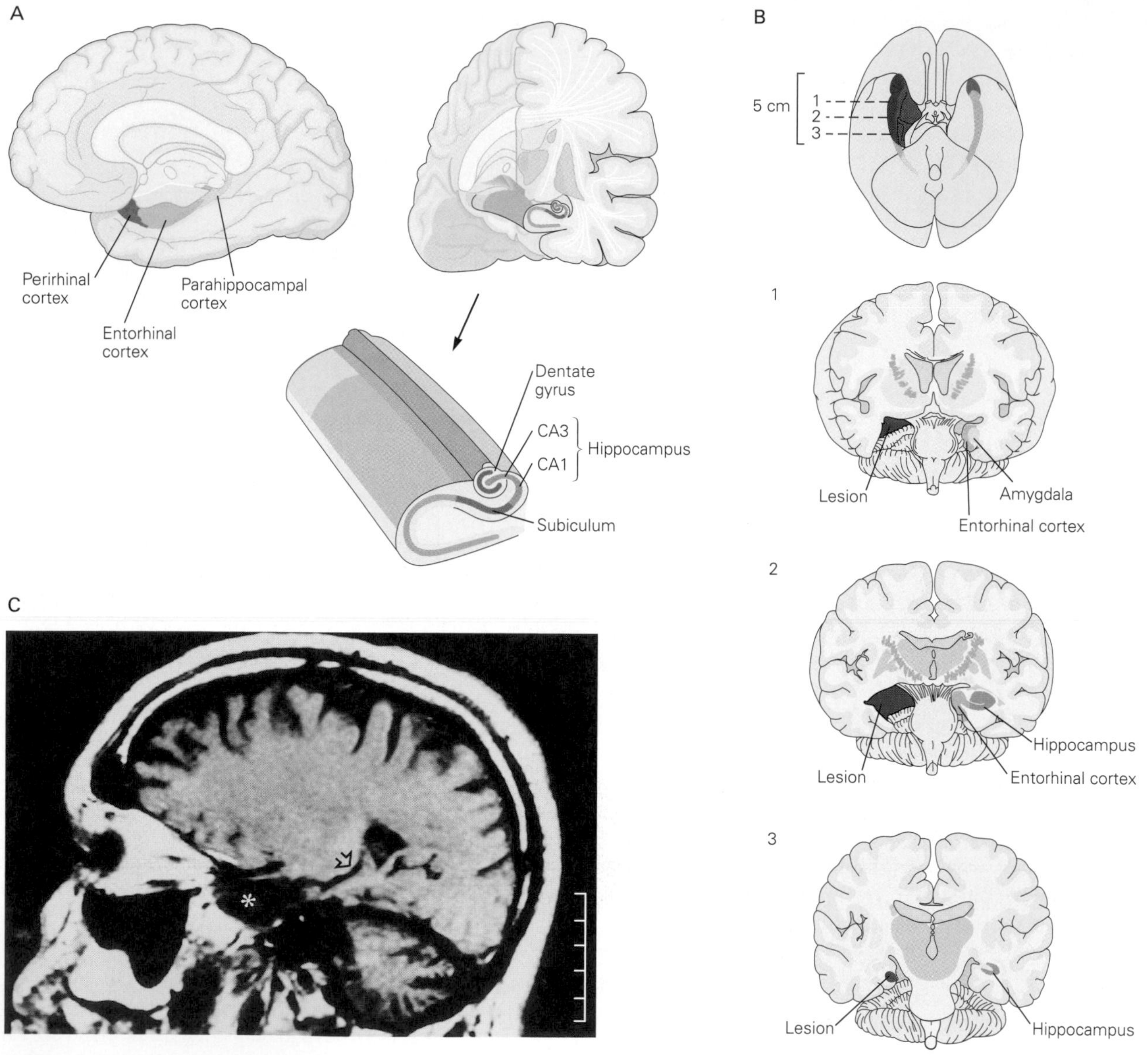

Figure 65–2 The medial temporal lobe and memory storage.

A. The key components of the medial temporal lobe important for memory storage.

B. The areas of temporal lobe resected (**gray shading**) in the patient known as H.M., viewed from the ventral surface of the brain (left hemisphere is on the right side of the image). Surgery was a bilateral, single-stage procedure, but to illustrate the structures that were removed the right side of the image is shown here intact. The longitudinal extent of the lesion is shown in a ventral view of the brain (**top**). Cross sections 1 through 3 show the estimated extent of areas of the brain removed from H.M. (Adapted, with permission, from Corkin et al. 1997.)

C. Magnetic resonance image (MRI) scan of a parasagittal section from the left side of H.M.'s brain. The calibration bar at the right of the panel has 1-cm increments. The **asterisk** indicates the resected portion of the anterior temporal lobes. The **arrowhead** points to the remaining portion of the intraventricular portion of the hippocampal formation. Approximately 2 cm of preserved hippocampal formation is visible bilaterally. Note also the substantial degeneration in the enlarged folial spaces of the cerebellum. (Adapted, with permission, from Corkin et al. 1997.)

information acquired in the years just before surgery was not robust. In addition, he retained a command of language, including his vocabulary, indicating that semantic memory was preserved. His IQ remained unchanged in the range of bright–normal.

What H.M. now lacked, and lacked dramatically, was the ability to transfer new information from working memory into long-term memory. He was unable to retain for lengthy periods information about people, places, or objects that he had just encountered. Asked to remember a new telephone number, H.M. could repeat it immediately for seconds to minutes because of his intact working memory. But when distracted, even briefly, he forgot the number. H.M. could not recognize people he met after surgery, even when he met them again and again. For several years he saw Milner every month, yet each time she entered the room he reacted as though he had never seen her before. H.M. is not unique. All patients with extensive bilateral lesions of the limbic association areas of the medial temporal lobe from either surgery or disease show similar long-term memory deficits.

H.M. is a historic case because his deficit provided the first clear link between memory and the medial temporal lobe, including the hippocampus. Given the large size of the hippocampus proper, the question next arose: How extensive does a bilateral lesion have to be to produce a memory deficit? Clinical evidence from several patients as well as data from experimental animals suggests that a lesion restricted to any of the major components of the system can have a significant effect on long-term memory. For example Larry Squire, David Amaral, and their colleagues found that the patient R.B. had only one detectable lesion after a cardiac arrest—destruction of the pyramidal cells in the CA1 region of the hippocampus. Nevertheless, R.B.'s memory deficits were qualitatively similar to those of H.M., although quantitatively much milder.

The different subregions of the medial temporal lobe, which together comprise the medial temporal lobe memory system, may not have equivalent roles, however. For example, some areas in the medial temporal lobe circuit may be particularly important for object recognition. Damage to the perirhinal cortex that spares the underlying hippocampus produces a greater deficit in object recognition than do selective lesions of the hippocampus that spare the overlying cortex.

In contrast, some theorists have argued that the hippocampus may be relatively more important for spatial representation than for object recognition. In mice and rats lesions of the hippocampus interfere with memory for space and context, and single neurons in the hippocampus encode specific spatial information (see Chapter 67). Functional imaging of the brain in healthy humans shows that activity increases in the right hippocampus when spatial information is recalled, and in the left hippocampus when words, objects, or people are recalled. These physiological findings are consistent with the clinical observation that lesions of the right hippocampus give rise to problems with spatial orientation whereas lesions of the left hippocampus cause defects in verbal memory.

Long-Term Memory Can Be Classified As Explicit or Implicit

Another crucial finding about H.M. was that not all types of long-term memory were impaired. Even though H.M. and other patients with damage to the medial temporal lobe had profound memory deficits, they were able to form and retain certain types of durable memories as well as healthy subjects.

For example, H.M. learned to draw the outlines of a star while looking at the star and his hand in a mirror (Figure 65–3). Like healthy subjects learning to remap hand-eye coordination, H.M. initially made many mistakes, but after several days of training his performance was error-free and comparable to that of healthy subjects. Nevertheless, he did not consciously remember having performed the task.

Later work by Squire and others made it clear that the long-term memory capabilities of H.M. and other amnesic patients are not limited to motor skills. These patients retain simple reflexive learning, including habituation, sensitization, classical conditioning, and operant conditioning (to be discussed later in this chapter). Furthermore, they are able to improve their performance on certain perceptual and conceptual tasks. For example, they do well with a form of memory called priming, in which perception of a word or object is improved by prior exposure. Thus, when shown only the first few letters of previously studied words, a subject with amnesia is able to generate the same number of words as normal subjects, even though the amnesic patient has no conscious memory of having recently studied the words (Figure 65–4).

Is this distinction between forms of long-term memory in amnesic patients a fundamental difference in normal memory function? To address this question the cognitive psychologists Peter Graf and Daniel Schacter examined healthy subjects and found two types of long-term memory that differed in whether conscious awareness was required for the recall.

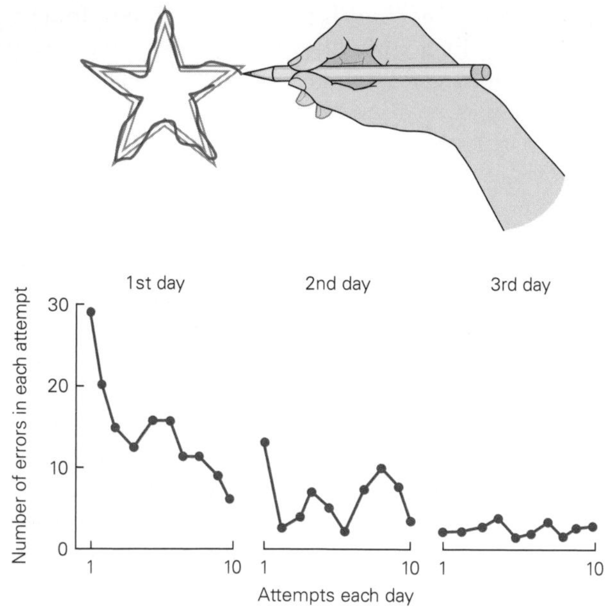

Figure 65–3 The amnesic patient H.M. could learn skilled movements. He was taught to trace between two outlines of a star while viewing his hand in a mirror. The graph plots the number of times, during each attempt, that he strayed outside the outlines as he drew the star. As with healthy subjects, H.M. improved considerably with repeated attempts despite the fact that he had no recollection of having performed the task before. (Reproduced, with permission, from Blakemore 1977.)

One type is an unconscious form of memory that is evident in the performance of a task and is known as *implicit memory* (also referred to as nondeclarative or procedural memory). Implicit memory is typically manifested in an automatic manner, with little conscious processing on the part of the subject. Different forms give rise to priming, skill learning, habit memory, and conditioning (Figure 65–5).

The other type is the deliberate or conscious retrieval of previous experiences as well as conscious recall of factual knowledge about people, places, and things. This type is known as *explicit memory* (or declarative memory). Explicit memory is highly flexible; multiple pieces of information can be associated under different circumstances. Implicit memory, however, is tightly connected to the original conditions under which the learning occurred.

Explicit Memory Has Episodic and Semantic Forms

The Canadian psychologist Endel Tulving first developed the idea that explicit memory can be further classified into episodic memory (the memory of personal experiences or autobiographical memory) and semantic memory (memory for facts). *Episodic memory* is used to recall that we saw the first flowers of spring yesterday or that we heard Beethoven's "Moonlight Sonata" several months ago. *Semantic memory* is used to learn the meanings of new words or concepts. The medial temporal lobe plays a critical role in both episodic and semantic memory, as is evident in patients like H.M., who have difficulties in forming and retaining new conscious memories of their personal experiences or the meanings of new concepts.

We have learned two additional important things about explicit memory. First, the brain does not have a single long-term store of explicit memories. Instead the storage of any item of knowledge is widely distributed among many brain regions and can be accessed independently (by visual, verbal, or other sensory clues).

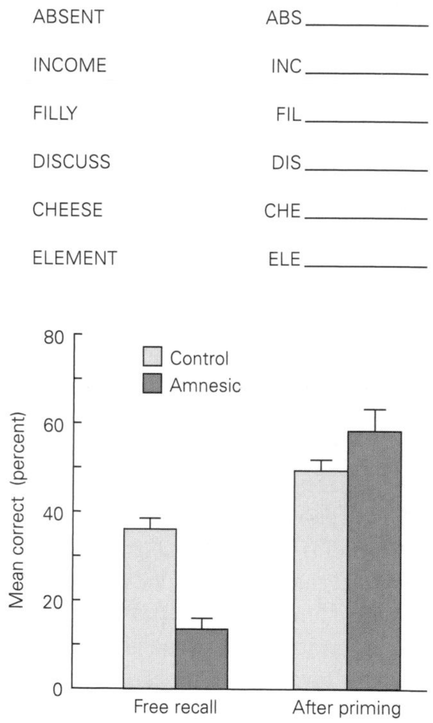

Figure 65–4 Amnesic and normal control subjects were tested on recall of words under two conditions. First they were presented with common words and then asked to recall the words (free recall). Amnesic patients did not do well on this test. However, when subjects were given the first three letters of a word and instructed simply to form the first word that came to mind (completion), the amnesic subjects performed as well as normal subjects. The baseline guessing rate in the word completion condition was 9%. (Reproduced, with permission, from Squire 1987.)

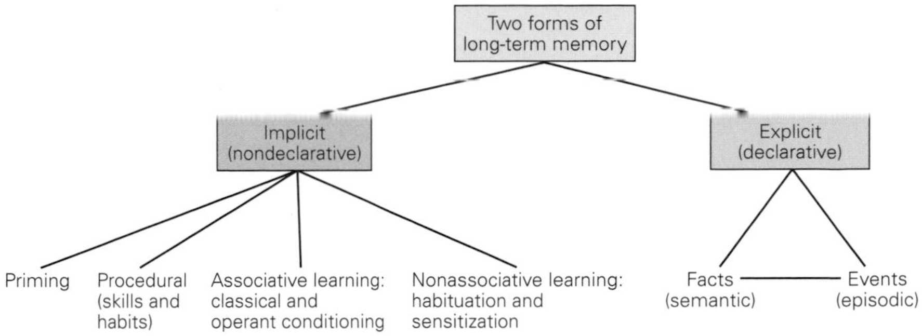

Figure 65–5 Long-term memory is either explicit (conscious) or implicit (subconscious).

Second, explicit memory is mediated by at least four related but distinct types of processing: encoding, storage, consolidation, and retrieval.

Explicit Memory Processing Involves at Least Four Distinct Operations

Encoding is the process by which new information is attended and linked to existing information in memory. The extent of this process is critically important for determining how well the learned material will be remembered. For a memory to persist and be well remembered, the incoming information must be encoded thoroughly, what the psychologists Fergus Craik and Robert Lockhart called "deep" encoding. This is accomplished by attending to the information and associating it with knowledge that is already well established in memory. Memory encoding also is stronger when one is well motivated to remember.

Storage refers to the neural mechanisms and sites by which memory is retained over time. One of the remarkable features about long-term storage is that it seems to have an almost unlimited capacity; there is no known limit to the amount of information in long-term storage. In contrast, working memory storage is very limited; psychologists believe that human working memory can hold only a few pieces of information at any one time.

Consolidation is the process that makes the temporarily stored and still labile information more stable. As we shall learn in the next two chapters, consolidation involves expression of genes and protein synthesis that give rise to structural changes at synapses.

Finally, *retrieval* is the process by which stored information is recalled. It involves bringing back to mind different kinds of information that are stored in different sites. Retrieval of memory is much like perception; it is a constructive process and therefore subject to distortion much as perception is subject to illusions (Box 65–1).

Retrieval of information is most effective when a retrieval cue reminds individuals of how they initially encoded an experience. For example, in a classic behavioral experiment Craig Barclay and colleagues asked some subjects to encode sentences such as "The man lifted the piano." On a later test, "something heavy" was a more effective cue for recalling piano than "something with a nice sound." Other subjects, however, encoded the sentence "The man tuned the piano." For them, "something with a nice sound" was a more effective retrieval cue for piano than "something heavy." Retrieval, particularly of explicit memories, also is partially dependent on working memory.

Episodic Knowledge Depends on Interaction Between the Medial Temporal Lobe and Association Cortices

Although studies of amnesic patients during the past few decades have refined our understanding of various types of memory, medial temporal lobe damage affects all four operations of memory—encoding, storage, consolidation, and retrieval—and thus it is often difficult to discern how the medial temporal lobe contributes to each. Positron emission tomography (PET) and functional magnetic resonance imaging (fMRI) allow us to scan the healthy brain in the process of building new memories or retrieving existing memories, and thus to identify specific regions that are active during different processes.

Functional MRI scans show that activity in the medial temporal lobe is greater when subjects engage in deep encoding (eg, attending to the meaning of information by judging whether a word is concrete or abstract) than when they engage in shallow encoding (eg, judging whether a word is presented in upper or lower case letters). Activity in parts of the left prefrontal cortex is also enhanced during deep encoding,

Box 65–1 The Transformation of Explicit Memories

How accurate is explicit memory? This question was explored by the psychologist Frederic Bartlett in a series of studies in the 1930s in which the subjects were asked to read stories and then retell them. The recalled stories were shorter and more coherent than the original stories, reflecting reconstruction and condensation of the original.

The subjects were unaware that they were editing the original stories and often felt more certain about the edited parts than about the unedited parts of the retold stories. They were not confabulating; they were merely interpreting the original material so that it made sense on recall.

Observations such as these lead us to believe that explicit memory, at least episodic (autobiographical) memory, is a constructive process like sensory perception. In fact, explicit memory is a product of the perceptual process. Sensory perception is not a passive recording of the external world but a process in which sensory signals produce information that is shaped by the way in which afferent pathways process those signals.

It is also constructive in the sense that individuals perceive the environment from the standpoint of a specific point in space as well as a specific point in their own history. As described in Chapter 27, optical illusions nicely illustrate the active role of perceptual processes in arriving at our personal knowledge of our surroundings.

Likewise, once information is stored, recall is not an exact copy of the information stored. Past experiences are used in the present as cues that help the brain reconstruct a past event. During recall we use a variety of cognitive strategies, including comparison, inference, shrewd guessing, and supposition, to generate a memory that not only seems coherent to us but is also consistent with other memories and with our "memory of the memory."

suggesting that frontal lobe and medial temporal lobe processing contribute to encoding episodic memory.

Anthony Wagner and his colleagues tested the relation between frontal and medial temporal lobe activity during encoding of an experience and the later remembering of the experience. Subjects were scanned using event-related fMRI while they learned a long series of words (event-related fMRI allows researchers to examine brain activity based on participants' responses to specific items or events). Their memory of the words was then tested outside the scanner to compare their recall with the activity recorded while learning the series of words. At the time of encoding, activity in several regions of the left prefrontal cortex was enhanced when subjects were studying words that they were later able to recall (Figure 65–6). Using similar methods to examine the encoding of memories of pictures, James Brewer and John Gabrieli and their colleagues found greater activity in the right prefrontal cortex during encoding of pictures that were later recalled compared to pictures that could not be recalled.

Both studies also revealed greater activity in the medial temporal lobe during encoding of stimuli that were subsequently remembered compared to those that were forgotten. This is further evidence that episodic learning depends on interaction between cognitive control processes in the prefrontal cortex and associative binding mechanisms in the medial temporal lobe.

Interaction between the medial temporal lobe and distributed cortical regions is also central in current thinking about memory consolidation. Recall that patient H.M., whose medial temporal lobe was surgically removed, could still recall childhood memories. In fact, early observations suggested that H.M. could recall many of the experiences of his life up until several years before his operation. These observations of H.M. and other amnesic patients with damage to the medial temporal lobe suggest that old memories are not stored in the medial temporal lobe itself; if they were, H.M. would not be able to recall his early experiences. Rather, they are stored in various other cortical regions.

According to Larry Squire and others, the medial temporal region may play a temporary role in the consolidation of memories, but after a sufficiently long period is no longer needed as memories can be retrieved directly from cortical regions. This finding is consistent with the fact that amnesic patients are better able to recall remote memories than memories from the period just before they became amnesic.

As with studies of encoding, studies of retrieval of episodic knowledge have implicated the prefrontal cortex and medial temporal lobe. In one study, monkeys were trained to associate a specific visual object with a preceding visual cue. During training the monkeys learn that they will receive a reward if they press a lever when a specific object is shown, but only when that object is preceded by the learned visual cue. Electrophysiological recordings reveal that, after training, the visual cue activates neurons in the monkey's inferior temporal cortex during the recall of the stored visual memory.

Importantly, even after the monkey has undergone brain surgery to prevent the afferent flow of visual information from primary visual cortex to inferior temporal cortex, the visual cue is able to elicit the correct behavioral response and to elicit firing in the inferior temporal cortex neurons. This implies that information about the visual cue must reach neurons in the inferior temporal cortex through a "top-down" pathway in which signals from the primary visual cortex activate neurons in prefrontal cortex that in turn activate neurons in the inferior temporal cortex. When this "top-down" pathway is also surgically interrupted, the monkeys fail to respond to the visual cue, which can no longer trigger activity in the inferior temporal cortex neurons (Figure 65–7). PET and fMRI scans of human subjects asked to recall or recognize previously studied words or pictures show activity in the anterior and lateral prefrontal cortex.

The retrieval of contextual or event details associated with episodic memory also involves activity in the medial temporal lobe, particularly in the hippocampus. Medial temporal lobe activity is thought to facilitate the activation of neocortical representations that were present during encoding. Consistent with this perspective, Yasushi Miyashita and colleagues have demonstrated that signals from the medial temporal lobe precede the recruitment of episodic knowledge in the neocortex. Mark Wheeler and colleagues and Lars Nyberg and colleagues observed similar patterns of activation in visual and auditory association areas during both the encoding and retrieval of pictures and sounds. As with encoding of episodic memory, retrieval involves a complex interaction between the medial temporal lobe and distributed cortical regions, including the prefrontal cortex and other high-level association areas.

Semantic Knowledge Is Stored in Distinct Association Cortices and Retrieval Depends on the Prefrontal Cortex

Semantic knowledge is our general knowledge about the world, encompassing facts, concepts, and information

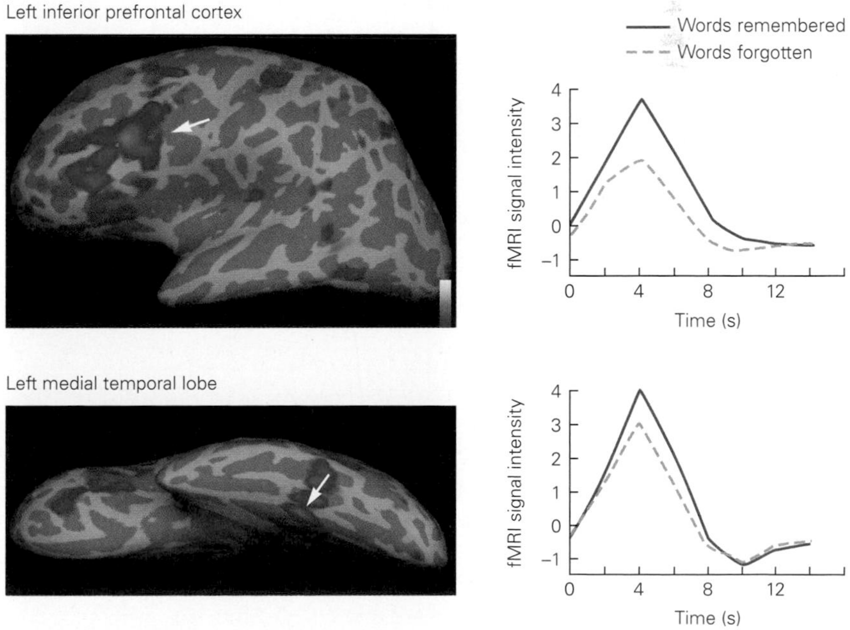

Figure 65–6 Activity in the prefrontal cortex and medial temporal lobe during an experience is essential to remembering the experience.

Neural activity during encoding of visual events (presentation of words) was measured using functional magnetic resonance imaging (fMRI). Subsequently, recall of the studied words was tested and each word was classified as either remembered or forgotten. The scans taken during encoding were then sorted into two groups: those made during encoding of words that were later remembered and those made during encoding of words that were later forgotten. This subsequent memory analysis reveals greater activation in regions of the left prefrontal cortex and medial temporal lobe during the encoding of words later remembered than those later forgotten (locations denoted by **white arrows**). At right are the observed fMRI responses in these regions for words later remembered (**red line**) and those later forgotten (**dashed line**). (Adapted from, with permission, from Wagner et al. 1998.)

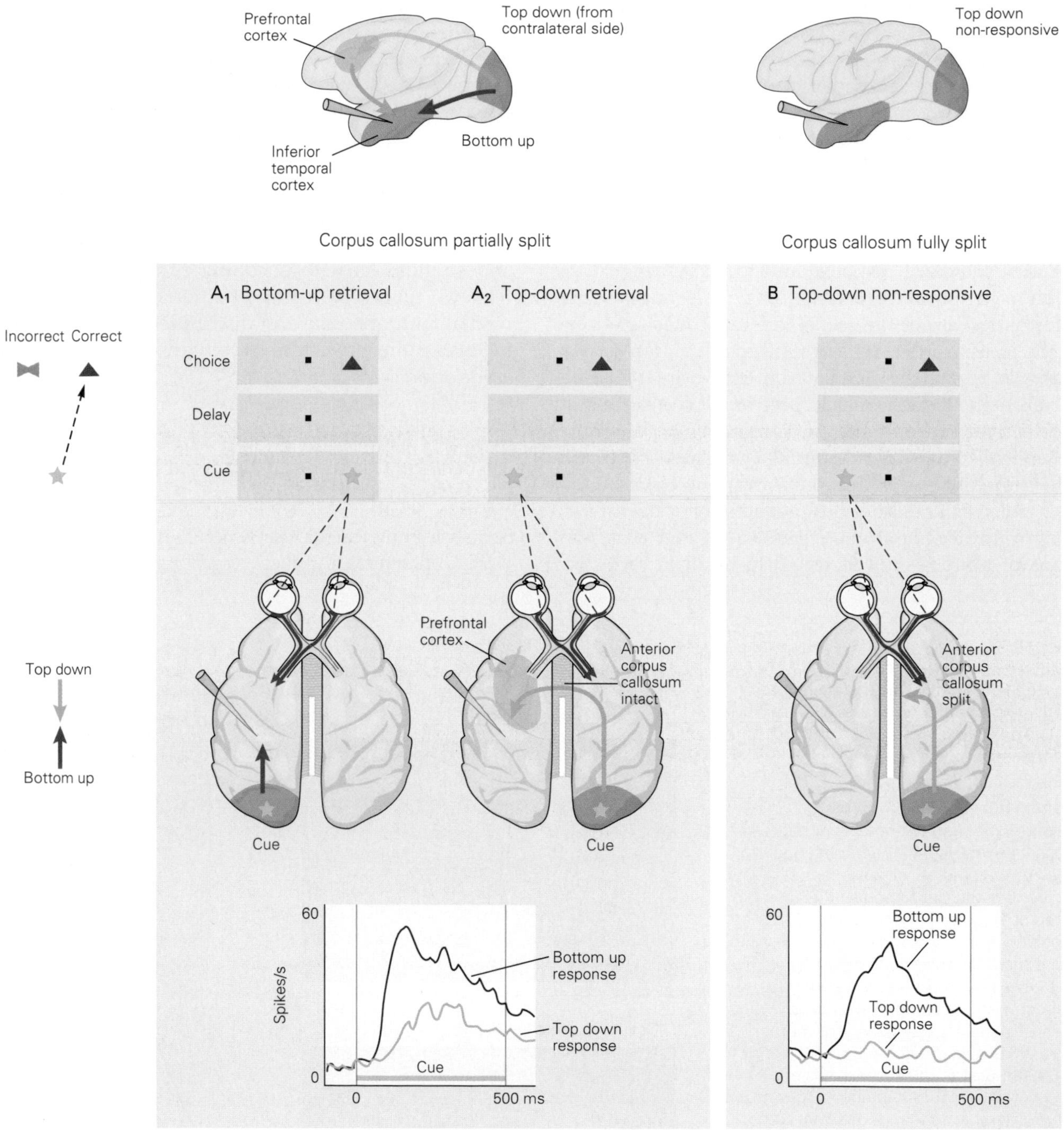
Prefrontal cortex
Top down (from contralateral side)
Bottom up
Inferior temporal cortex
Top down non-responsive
Corpus callosum partially split
Corpus callosum fully split
A1 Bottom-up retrieval
A2 Top-down retrieval
B Top-down non-responsive
Incorrect Correct
Choice
Delay
Cue
Top down
Bottom up
Prefrontal cortex
Anterior corpus callosum intact
Anterior corpus callosum split
Cue
60
Spikes/s
Bottom up response
Top down response
Cue
0
0
500 ms

about objects, as well as words and their meanings. Semantic knowledge is distinguished from episodic knowledge in that it is typically not associated with the context in which the information was acquired. It is stored in a distributed manner in the neocortex, including the lateral and ventral temporal lobes.

The organization and flexibility of semantic knowledge is remarkable. Consider the concept "elephant." When first learned through a picture it appears to be quite simple. With further learning, however, many images of elephants become associated with a name, at first spoken and then written. Later other pieces of information are associated: elephants are living things, they live in a particular environment and have unique patterns of behavior, they emit distinctive sounds and are often gray in color, and they perform in circuses. Given this associative structure—which would collectively correspond to the concept "elephant"—any one feature, such as the word *elephant*, can serve as a cue that leads to recovery of other associated features.

There is no single storage site for all of the semantic knowledge that we have acquired over our lifetime. Rather, the semantic components of a concept are distributed among many brain regions. Specific brain regions are dedicated to representing specific features (eg, form, color, or motion), such that a lesion in one region can impair a specific type of knowledge associated with a particular concept while sparing others.

Rosaleen McCarthy and Elizabeth Warrington described patients whose knowledge about living things was impaired while their knowledge about inanimate objects was intact. For example, one patient correctly defined towel as "material used to dry people," but incorrectly defined wasp as a "bird that flies." Other patients demonstrate the reverse deficit. The brain appears to organize semantic knowledge according to conceptual primitives, eg, form and function. Because some categories are particularly dependent on information about form (eg, living things) whereas others depend on knowledge of function (eg, inanimate things), focal brain damage can result in the loss of memory for particular semantic categories while sparing knowledge of others.

Neuroimaging studies using PET and fMRI provide more evidence about how different categories of knowledge are represented in the intact human brain. When people name pictures of animals there is greater activity in left inferior temporal regions, which represent information about the form of objects, than when they name pictures of tools. In contrast, tool naming is associated with activity in left premotor regions, which represent information about the patterns of motor

Figure 65–7 (Opposite) The prefrontal cortex contributes to recall of associated knowledge. (Reproduced, with permission, from Tomita et al. 1999.)

A. The experimental design includes "bottom-up" and "top-down" retrieval conditions. A monkey was trained to associate a specific object with a prior visual cue. During testing the monkey was shown a visual cue on a screen. After a delay the monkey was then shown one of several objects (choice). The monkey had to choose whether the object is the one that is associated with the visual cue (by releasing a lever). The posterior corpus callosum of the monkeys in the study was partially split so that the bottom-up sensory signal from visual cortex could not directly reach visual areas in the opposite hemisphere. **1**. In the bottom-up retrieval condition the retrieval cue and choice object are presented in the right visual hemifield contralateral to the recording site (electrode) in the left inferior temporal cortex. Because the left hemisphere processes the right visual field, visual information enters the primary visual cortex in the same hemisphere as the recording electrode. The monkey was able to choose the correct object associated with the cue (data not shown) indicating that bottom-up sensory signals are sufficient for retrieval. The bottom-up signal in response to the visual cue also elicits a large increase in neural firing rate in the inferior temporal cortex neurons. **2**. In the top-down retrieval condition the cue is presented in the left visual hemifield ipsilateral to the recording site, whereas the choice object is presented contralaterally in the right visual hemifield. Thus visual information about the cue enters the hemisphere opposite to the recording site. Because the posterior corpus callosum is cut, there is no direct bottom-up pathway from right visual cortex to left inferior temporal cortex. Nonetheless the visual cue is able to elicit a strong electrophysiological response in inferior temporal cortex neurons in the left hemisphere and the monkey is able to choose the correct object associated with the cue. In this condition visual information from the right hemisphere crosses over to the left hemisphere through the intact anterior portion of the corpus callosum. Top-down signals from prefrontal cortex, which carry information about the retrieval cue, elicit neuronal firing and retrieval of associated representations through feedback connections to the inferior temporal cortex.

B. When the corpus callosum is fully split, visual information from the contralateral hemisphere can no longer reach the ipsilateral prefrontal cortex. This prevents top-down retrieval signals from being transmitted to inferior temporal neurons. As a result, neurons in the left inferior temporal cortex are no longer activated by the presentation of the visual cue to the left hemifield. In addition, the monkeys no longer choose the correct object when the cue is presented to the contralateral visual hemifield. In contrast, left inferior temporal cortex neurons show a strong response when the cue is presented to the right visual hemifield because the bottom-up pathway from left visual cortex to left inferior temporal cortex is intact.

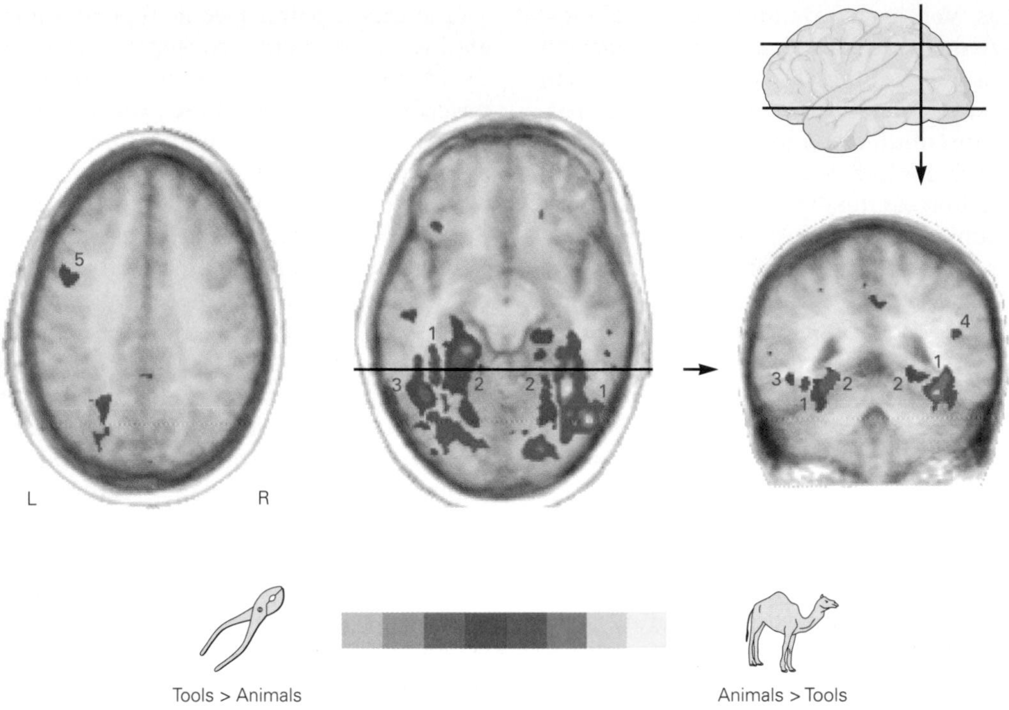

Figure 65–8 Neural correlates of category-specific knowledge. Functional magnetic resonance imaging (fMRI) data show neural activity associated with silent naming of animals and tools shown in pictures. Regions with greater activity when animals were named (shown in **yellow** and **red**) include the lateral fusiform gyrus (**1**) and right superior temporal sulcus (**4**). Regions with greater activity when tools were named (**blue**) include the medial fusiform gyrus (**2**), left middle temporal gyrus/inferior temporal sulcus (**3**), and left ventral premotor cortex (**5**). (Reproduced, with permission, from Martin and Chao 2001.)

movements associated with the use of an object, and in left middle temporal regions, which represent information about how objects move in space (Figure 65–8).

Implicit Memory Supports Perceptual Priming

Implicit memory stores forms of knowledge that are typically acquired without conscious effort and which guide behavior unconsciously. Priming is a type of implicit memory that operates in amnesic patients as well as healthy subjects, suggesting that it does not depend on medial temporal lobe structures.

Two types of priming have been proposed. *Conceptual priming* provides easier access to task-relevant semantic knowledge because that knowledge has been used before. It is correlated with decreased activity in left prefrontal regions that subserve initial retrieval of semantic knowledge. In contrast, *perceptual priming* occurs within a specific sensory modality, and according to Tulving and Schacter it depends on cortical modules that operate on sensory information about the form and structure of words and objects.

Damage to unimodal sensory regions of cortex impairs modality-specific perceptual priming. For example, one patient with an extensive lesion of the right occipital lobe failed to demonstrate visual priming for words but had normal explicit memory (Figure 65–9). This condition is the reverse of that found in amnesic patients such as H.M., and provides further evidence that the neural mechanisms of priming are distinct from those for explicit memory.

Visual priming is almost always correlated with decreased activity in higher-order visual (extrastriate) areas of cortex. Randy Buckner and his colleagues using fMRI found that activity in extrastriate cortex was greater during the initial exposure to an object than when the object was presented again later. These findings parallel the finding that activity in the left prefrontal cortex is reduced during conceptual priming. Most tasks include both perceptual and conceptual priming, and there probably are no sharp distinctions between the two.

Other forms of nondeclarative memory subserve the learning of habits, the learning of motor, perceptual, and cognitive skills, and the formation and expression of conditioned responses. In general, these forms of implicit memory are characterized by incremental learning, which proceeds gradually with repetition. The neural circuits that initiate habit, motor skill, and conditioned learning are independent of the medial temporal lobe system responsible for explicit memory.

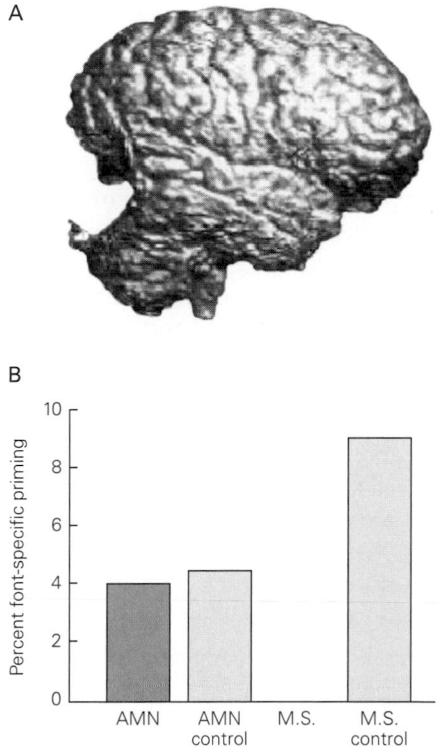

Figure 65–9 The right occipital cortex is required for visual priming for words. (Adapted with permission, from Vaidya et al. 1998.)

A. Structural magnetic resonance imaging (MRI) depicts the near complete removal of the right occipital cortex in a patient, M.S., who suffered pharmacologically intractable epilepsy with a right occipital cortical focus.

B. Font-specific priming is intact in amnesic patients (**AMN**) and their controls as well as in the controls for patient M.S., but not in M.S. himself. Font-specific priming is a form of visual priming in which the individual is better able to identify a briefly flashed word when the type font is identical to an earlier presentation, compared to identification when the font is different (priming equals performance when the font is the same minus performance when the font is different). The patient M.S. has normal explicit memory, even for visual cues (data not shown), but lacks implicit memory for specific properties of visually presented words.

For example, H.M. is able to acquire new visuomotor skills, like the mirror-tracing task (see Figure 65–3).

New perceptual, motor, or cognitive abilities are also learned through repetition. With practice, performance becomes more accurate and faster, and these improvements generalize to learning novel information. Skill learning moves from a cognitive stage, where knowledge is represented explicitly and the learner must pay a great deal of attention to performance, to an autonomous stage, where the skill can be executed without much conscious attention. As an example, driving a car initially requires that one pay attention to each component of the skill, but after practice one no longer attends to the individual components.

The learning of sensorimotor skills depends in part on the basal ganglia, cerebellum, and neocortex. Dysfunction of the basal ganglia in patients with Parkinson and Huntington disease impairs learning of motor skills. Patients with cerebellar lesions also have difficulties acquiring some motor skills, and functional imaging of healthy individuals during sensorimotor learning shows changes in the activity of the basal ganglia and cerebellum. Finally, skilled behavior can depend on structural changes in motor neocortex, as seen by the expansion of the cortical representation of the fingers in musicians (see Chapter 67).

Perceptual learning improves the ability to make sense of novel sensory inputs, as in learning to read mirror-reversed text or recognizing novel objects by reference to familiar categories. Amnesic patients with damage to the medial temporal lobe can learn to read mirror-reversed text but this learning is mildly impaired in Huntington disease and variably impaired in Parkinson disease. Patients with cerebellar lesions have no difficulty with perceptual learning, even though the learning of motor skills is impaired.

A neuroimaging study by Russell Poldrack and his colleagues suggests that extensive practice with mirror reading produces a shift in the parts of the brain involved in the task. In this study performance of the mirror-reading task before practice was correlated with activity in ventral visual processing regions as well as extensive activity in the parietal cortex. After practice, activity decreased in the parietal cortex but increased in the left inferior temporal cortex, a region associated with representing visual form (Figure 65–10). These results reflect a transition from having to mentally rotate the mirror-reversed words to the ability to read directly the reversed letters. Different neural processes are involved once skilled performance moves from the cognitive to the autonomous stage. Similar neural changes have been observed in imaging studies of motor and visual-motor skill learning.

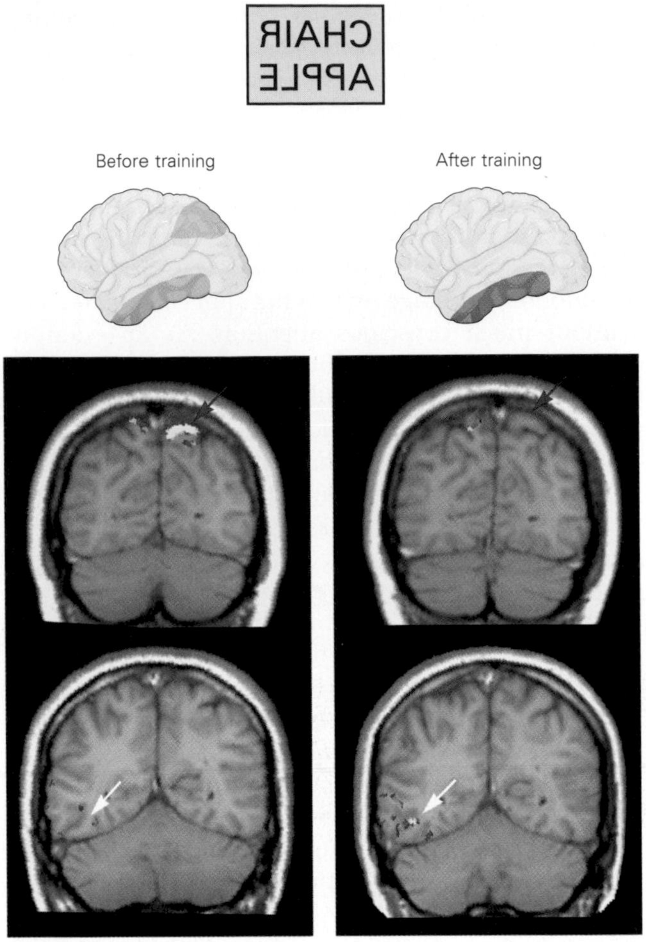

Figure 65–10 Perceptual learning involves a shift from cognitive to autonomous stages that use different neural pathways. Subjects are asked to read mirror-reversed text, something most people rarely encounter. Prior to training individuals rely on the parietal cortex (**red arrow**) and to a lesser extent the inferior temporal cortex (**white arrow**). After extensive training the processing pathways involved in the task appear to be different. Individuals rely less on the parietal cortex and more on the inferior temporal cortex. (Reproduced, with permission, from Poldrack et al. 1998.)

Implicit memory also underlies habit learning or Pavlovian associative conditioning, the gradual learning about the predictive relationship between a stimulus and a response (discussed later). Habit learning in humans has been studied using the probabilistic classification task, where subjects attempt to predict accurately one of two possible outcomes based on the presentation of a set of cues, with each cue having a probabilistic relation to each outcome. For example, subjects may be asked to predict the weather (rain or sunshine) based on a set of cue cards (Figure 65–11).

Because the associations between the cues and outcomes are probabilistic, thus requiring numerous trials to learn, explicit (conscious) memory of specific trials is not as useful for successful performance as the gradual accumulation of knowledge about the stimulus-outcome associations. Barbara Knowlton and colleagues have shown that, in contrast to patients with medial temporal lobe lesions, patients with basal ganglia disorders are severely impaired in this task.

Implicit Memory Can Be Associative or Nonassociative

Our consideration of implicit memory has so far focused on humans. But some forms of implicit memory can also be studied in nonhuman animals, and animal studies have distinguished two types of implicit memory: nonassociative and associative. With nonassociative learning an animal learns about the properties of a single stimulus. With associative learning the animal learns about the relationship between two stimuli or between a stimulus and a behavior.

Nonassociative learning results when a subject is exposed once or repeatedly to a single type of stimulus. Two forms of nonassociative learning are common in everyday life: habituation and sensitization. Habituation, a decrease in a response, occurs when a benign stimulus is presented repeatedly. For example, most people in the United States are startled when they first hear the sound of a firecracker on Independence Day, but as the day progresses they become accustomed to the noise and do not respond. Sensitization (or pseudo-conditioning) is an enhanced response to a wide variety of stimuli after the presentation of an intense or noxious stimulus. For example, an animal will respond more vigorously to a mild tactile stimulus after receiving a painful pinch. Moreover, a sensitizing stimulus can override the effects of habituation, a process called dishabituation. For example, after the startle response to a noise has been reduced by habituation, one can restore the intensity of response to the noise by delivering a strong pinch.

With sensitization and dishabituation the timing of stimuli is not important because no association between stimuli must be learned. In contrast, with two forms of associative learning the timing of the stimuli to be associated is critical. Classical conditioning involves learning a relationship between two stimuli, whereas operant conditioning involves learning a relationship between the organism's behavior and the consequences of that behavior.

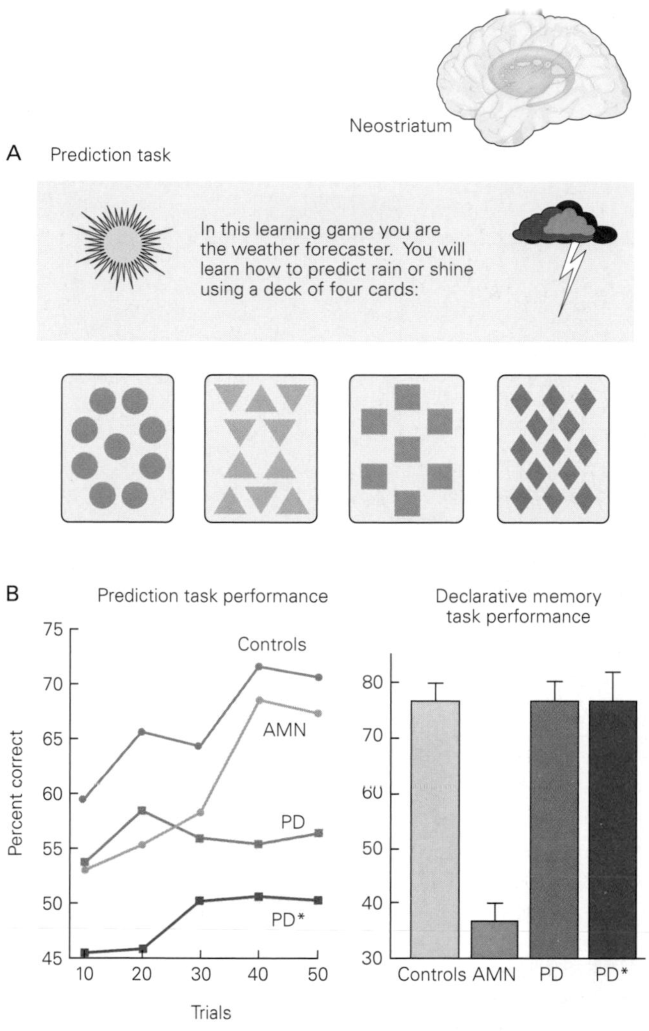

Figure 65–11 Learning predictive relationships involves the neostriatum.

A. Subjects are instructed to predict whether the weather will be rain or sunshine based on a set of cue cards. Each cue card has a probabilistic relation to each weather outcome (eg, predicting sunshine either 75, 57, 43, or 25% of the time). Subjects attempt to learn these relations during training and they are told after each trial whether their prediction is correct or incorrect.

B. Performance on the prediction task across the first 50 training trials is plotted on the left; performance results on a declarative memory test are shown on the right. Amnesic patients (**AMN**) initially learn the prediction task at the same rate as healthy control subjects, although their performance on the declarative memory task is impaired. By contrast, patients with Parkinson disease (**PD**), who suffer impairments in basal ganglia function, perform poorly on the prediction task but perform as well as controls on the declarative memory task. **PD*** identifies a subgroup of the Parkinsonian patients with the most severe symptoms. (Reproduced, with permission, from Knowlton, Mangels, and Squire 1996.)

Classical Conditioning Involves Associating Two Stimuli

Classical conditioning was first described at the turn of the century by the Russian physiologist Ivan Pavlov. The essence of classical conditioning is the pairing of two stimuli. The conditioned stimulus (CS), such as a light, a tone, or a touch, is chosen because it produces either no overt response or a weak response usually unrelated to the response that eventually will be learned. The reinforcement, or unconditioned stimulus (US), such as food or a shock, is chosen because it normally produces a strong and consistent response (the unconditioned response), such as salivation or withdrawal of the leg. Unconditioned responses are innate; they are produced without learning. Repeated presentation of a CS followed by a US gradually elicits a new or different response called the conditioned response.

One way of explaining conditioning is that repeated pairing of the CS and US causes the CS to become an anticipatory signal for the US. With sufficient experience an animal will respond to the CS as if it were anticipating the US. For example, if a light is followed repeatedly by the presentation of meat, eventually the sight of the light itself will make the animal salivate. Thus classical conditioning is the way an animal learns to predict events.

The probability of occurrence of a conditioned response decreases if the CS is repeatedly presented without the US. This process is known as extinction. If a light that has been paired with food is later repeatedly presented in the absence of food, it will gradually cease to evoke salivation. Extinction is an important adaptive mechanism; it would be maladaptive for an animal to continue to respond to cues that are no longer meaningful to it. The available evidence indicates that extinction is not the same as forgetting, but that something new is learned—the CS now signals that the US will not occur.

For many years psychologists thought that classical conditioning resulted as long as the CS preceded the US by a critical time interval. According to this view, each time a CS is followed by a US (reinforcing stimulus) a connection is strengthened between the internal representations of the stimulus and response or between the representations of one stimulus and another. The strength of the connection was thought to depend on the number of pairings of CS and US.

A substantial body of evidence now indicates that classical conditioning cannot be adequately explained simply by the fact that two events or stimuli occur one after the other (Figure 65–12). Indeed, it would not be

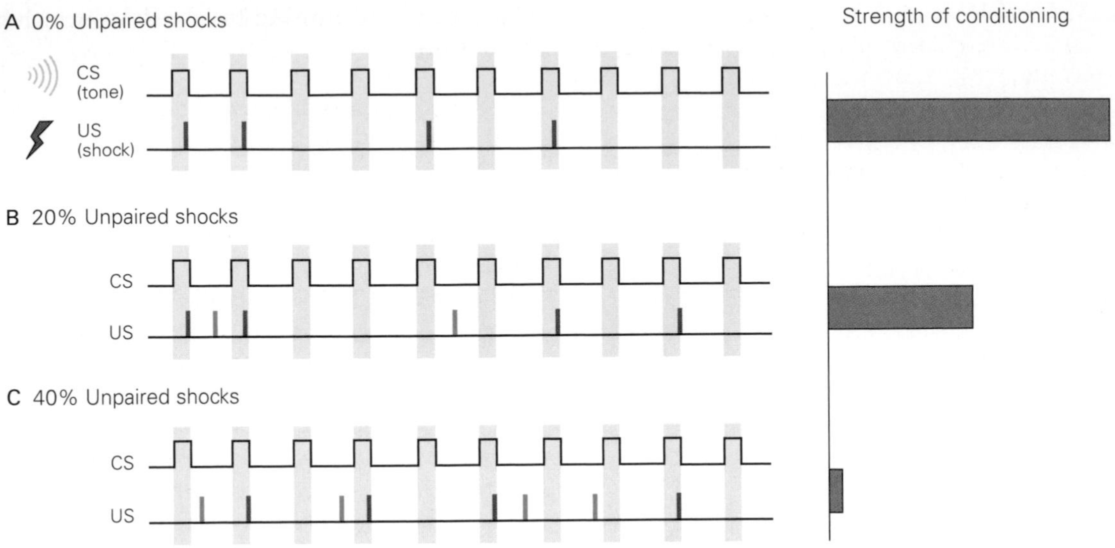

Figure 65–12 Classical conditioning depends on the degree to which two stimuli are correlated. In this experiment on rats a tone (the conditioned stimulus or CS) was paired with an electric shock (the unconditioned stimulus or US) in four out of 10 of the trials (**red ticks**). In some trial blocks the shock was presented without the tone (**green ticks**). The degree of conditioning was evaluated by determining how effective the tone alone was in suppressing lever-pressing to obtain food. Suppression of lever-pressing is a sign of a conditioned defensive response, freezing. (Adapted, with permission, from Rescorla 1968.)

A. Maximal conditioning occurred when the US was presented only with the CS.

B–C. Little or no conditioning was evident when the shock occurred without the tone as often as with it (40%). Some conditioning occurred when the shock occurred 20% of the time without the tone.

adaptive to depend solely on sequence. Rather, all animals capable of associative conditioning, from snails to humans, remember actual relationships rather than simply sequential events. Thus classical conditioning, and perhaps all forms of associative learning, enables animals to distinguish events that reliably occur together from those that are only randomly associated.

Lesions in several regions of the brain affect classical conditioning. A well-studied example is conditioning of the protective eyeblink reflex in rabbits, a form of motor learning. A puff of air to the eye naturally causes an eyeblink. A conditioned eyeblink can be established by pairing the puff with a tone that precedes the puff. The conditioned response (an eyeblink in response to a tone) is abolished by a lesion at either of two sites. Damage to the vermis of the cerebellum abolishes the conditioned response but does not affect the unconditioned response (eyeblink in response to a puff of air). Interestingly, neurons in the same area of the cerebellum show learning-dependent increases in activity that closely parallel the development of the conditioned behavior. A lesion in the interpositus nucleus, a deep cerebellar nucleus, also abolishes the conditioned eyeblink. Thus both the vermis and the deep nuclei of the cerebellum play an important role in conditioning the eyeblink and perhaps other simple forms of classical conditioning involving skeletal muscle movement.

Operant Conditioning Involves Associating a Specific Behavior with a Reinforcing Event

A second major paradigm of associative learning, discovered by Edgar Thorndike and systematically studied by B. F. Skinner and others, is operant conditioning (also called trial-and-error learning). In a typical laboratory example of operant conditioning a hungry rat or pigeon is placed in a test chamber in which the animal is rewarded for a specific action. For example, the chamber may have a lever protruding from one wall.

Because of previous learning, or through play and random activity, the animal will occasionally press the lever. If the animal promptly receives a positive reinforcer (eg, food) after pressing the lever, it will begin to press the lever more often than the spontaneous rate. The animal can be described as having learned that among its many behaviors (for example, grooming, rearing, and walking) one behavior is followed by food. With this information the animal is likely to press whenever it is hungry.

If we think of classical conditioning as the formation of a predictive relationship between two stimuli (the CS and the US), operant conditioning can be considered as the formation of a predictive relationship between an action and an outcome. Unlike classical conditioning, which tests the responsiveness of a reflex to a stimulus, operant conditioning tests behavior that occurs either spontaneously or without an identifiable stimulus. Operant behaviors are said to be emitted rather than elicited. In general, actions that are rewarded tend to be repeated, whereas actions followed by aversive, although not necessarily painful, consequences tend not to be repeated. Many experimental psychologists feel that this simple idea, called the law of effect, governs much voluntary behavior.

Because operant and classical conditioning involve different kinds of association—an association between an action and a reward or between two stimuli, respectively—one might suppose the two forms of learning are mediated by different neural mechanisms. However, because the laws of operant and classical conditioning are quite similar, the two forms of learning may use the same neural mechanisms. For example, timing is critical in both. In operant conditioning the reinforcer usually must closely follow the operant action. If the reinforcer is delayed too long, only weak conditioning occurs. Similarly, classical conditioning is generally poor if the interval between the conditioned and unconditioned stimuli is too long or if the unconditioned stimulus precedes the conditioned stimulus.

Associative Learning Is Constrained by the Biology of the Organism

Animals generally learn to associate stimuli that are relevant to their survival. For example, animals readily learn to avoid certain foods that have been followed by a negative reinforcement (eg, nausea produced by a poison), a phenomenon termed *taste aversion*.

Unlike most other forms of conditioning, taste aversion develops even when the unconditioned response (poison-induced nausea) occurs after a long delay, up to hours after the CS (specific taste). This makes biological sense, because the ill effects of infected foods and naturally occurring toxins usually follow ingestion only after some delay. For most species, including humans, taste-aversion conditioning occurs only when certain tastes are associated with illness. Taste aversion develops poorly if a taste is followed by a painful stimulus that does not produce nausea. Animals do not develop an aversion to a visual or auditory stimulus that has been paired with nausea.

Errors and Imperfections in Memory Shed Light on Normal Memory Processes

Memory allows us to revisit our personal past, provides access to a vast network of facts, associations, and concepts, and supports learning. But memory is not perfect. We often forget events rapidly or gradually, sometimes distort the past, and occasionally remember events that we would prefer to forget. In the 1930s the British psychologist Frederic Bartlett reported experiments in which people read and tried to remember complex stories. He showed that people often misremember many features of the stories, often distorting information based on their expectations about what should have happened (Box 65–1). Forgetting and distortion can provide important insights into the workings of memory.

Daniel Schacter classified memory's imperfections into seven basic categories, called "the seven sins of memory": transience, absent-mindedness, blocking, misattribution, suggestibility, bias, and persistence. Here we focus on six of these.

Absent-mindedness results from the lack of attention to immediate experience. Absent-mindedness during encoding is a likely source of common memory failures such as forgetting where one recently placed an object. Absent-mindedness also occurs when we forget to carry out a particular task such as picking up groceries on the way home from the office, even though we initially encoded the relevant information. Little is known about the neural bases of absent-mindedness.

Blocking refers to temporary inaccessibility of information stored in memory. People often have partial awareness of a sought-after word or image but are nonetheless unable to recall it accurately or completely. People sometimes feel that a blocked word is on "the tip of the tongue"—we are aware of the initial letter of the word, the number of syllables in it, or a like-sounding word. Determining which information is correct and which is incorrect requires a great deal of conscious effort.

In an fMRI study Anat Maril and her colleagues scanned people while they tried to recall the names of people or places in response to cues. When they entered a tip-of-the-tongue state, brain regions that have been implicated in cognitive tasks—the anterior cingulate and the right dorsolateral prefrontal cortex—showed intense activity. This activity likely reflects a subject's attempts to sort out correct from incorrect information and to resolve the memory block.

Absent-mindedness and blocking are sins of omission: At a moment when we need to remember information, it is inaccessible. However, memory is also characterized by sins of commission, situations in which some form of memory is present but wrong.

Misattribution refers to the association of a memory with an incorrect time, place, or person. False recognition, a type of misattribution, occurs when individuals report that they "remember" items or events that never happened. Such false memories have been documented in controlled experiments where people claim to have seen or heard words or objects that had not been presented previously but are similar in meaning or appearance to what was actually presented. Studies using PET and fMRI have shown that the hippocampus has similar levels of activity during both true and false recognition, which may be one reason why false memories sometimes feel like real ones.

Suggestibility refers to the tendency to incorporate external information into memory, usually as a result of leading questions or suggestions. Research using hypnotic suggestion indicates that various kinds of false memories can be implanted in highly suggestible individuals, such as remembering hearing loud noises at night. Studies with young adults have also shown that repeated suggestions to imagine a childhood experience can produce memories of episodes that never occurred. These findings are important theoretically because they highlight that memory is not simply a "playback" of past experiences. Despite these important theoretical and practical implications, next to nothing is known about the neural bases of suggestibility.

Bias refers to distortions and unconscious influences on memory that reflect one's general knowledge and beliefs. People often misremember the past to make it consistent with what they presently believe, know, or feel. As with suggestibility, however, almost nothing is known about the brain mechanisms of bias.

Persistence refers to obsessive memory, constant remembering of information or events that we might want to forget. Neuroimaging studies have illuminated some neurobiological factors that contribute to persistent emotional memories. For example, Larry Cahill and collaborators performed PET scans of subjects viewing a sequence of slides depicting an emotional story. The key results concerned activity in the amygdala, the almond-shaped structure located near the hippocampus and long known to be involved in emotional processing (see Chapter 48). The level of recall of the emotional components of the story was highly correlated with the level of activity in the amygdala during presentation of the story. This and related studies implicate the amygdala in the encoding and retrieval of emotionally charged experiences that can repeatedly intrude into consciousness.

Although persistence can be disabling, it also has adaptive value. The persistence of memories of disturbing experiences increases the likelihood that we will recall information about arousing or traumatic events at times when it may be crucial for survival.

Indeed, many memory imperfections may have adaptive value. For example, although the various forms of forgetting (transience, absent-mindedness, and blocking) can be annoying, a memory system that automatically retains every detail of every experience could result in an overwhelming clutter of useless trivia. This is exactly what happened in the fascinating case of Shereshevski, a mnemonist studied by the Russian neuropsychologist Alexander Luria. Shereshevski was filled with highly detailed memories of his past experiences and was unable to generalize or to think at an abstract level. A healthy memory system does not encode, store, and retrieve the details of every experience. Thus transience, absent-mindedness, or blocking allows us to avoid the unfortunate fate of Shereshevski.

An Overall View

We began this chapter by noting three key principles: (1) several different forms of learning and memory can be distinguished behaviorally, (2) memory can be analyzed in terms of discrete operations (encoding, storage, consolidation, and retrieval), and (3) imperfections and errors in remembering can provide telltale clues about learning and memory.

Considerable evidence supports the first principle, that there are different forms of memory, and we are learning that each involves different regions or combinations of regions in the brain. Thus working memory, which maintains goal-relevant information for short periods, has several neural components. Explicit memory involves the encoding and retrieval of two classes of knowledge: episodic memory, which represents personal experiences, and semantic memory, which represents general knowledge and facts. Explicit memory is typically retrieved deliberately and with some awareness that one is engaged in an act of remembering.

Implicit memory includes forms of perceptual and conceptual priming, as well as the learning of motor and perceptual skills and habits. It tends to be inflexible and expressed in the performance of tasks without conscious awareness. Implicit memory flows automatically in the course of perceiving, thinking, and acting.

Considerable progress also has been made concerning our second principle, that memory involves discrete encoding, storage, consolidation, and retrieval processes. Encoding of new memories depends critically on contributions from specific regions within the cortex and medial temporal lobe as shown most clearly in recent studies using fMRI.

The initiation of long-term storage of explicit memory requires the temporal lobe system, as highlighted by studies of amnesic patients such as H.M. Consolidation processes stabilize stored representations, rendering explicit memories no longer dependent on the medial temporal lobe. Retrieval of episodic memory involves the medial temporal lobe, as well as frontal and parietal cortices. Implicit memory, in contrast, involves a wide variety of brain regions, most often cortical areas that support the specific perceptual, conceptual, or motor systems recruited to process a stimulus or perform a task.

The third principle, that the past can be forgotten or distorted, is based on studies demonstrating that memory is not a faithful record of all details of every experience. Retrieved memories are the result of a complex interplay among various brain regions, and can be reshaped over time by multiple influences. Various forms of forgetting and distortion tell us much about the flexibility of memory that allows the brain to adapt to the physical and social environment.

Daniel L. Schacter
Anthony D. Wagner

Selected Readings

Baddeley AD. 1986. *Working Memory*. Oxford: Oxford Univ. Press.

Buckner RL, Wheeler ME. 2001. The cognitive neuroscience of remembering. Nat Rev Neurosci 2:624–634.

Eichenbaum H, Cohen NJ. 2001. *From Conditioning to Conscious Recollection: Memory Systems of the Brain*. Oxford: Oxford Univ. Press.

Goldman-Rakic S. 1995. Architecture of the prefrontal cortex and the central executive. Ann N Y Acad Sci 769:71–83.

Goldman-Rakic S. 1995. Functional organization of the human frontal cortex for mnemonic processing evidence from neuroimaging studies. In: J Grafman, F Boller, KJ Holyoak (eds). *Structure and Functions of the Human Prefrontal Cortex*, pp. 71–83. New York: New York Academy of Sciences.

Hardt O, Einarsson, EO, Nader K. 2010. A bridge over troubled water: reconsolidation as a link between cognitive and neuroscientific memory research traditions. Ann Rev Psychol 61:141–167.

Jonides J, Lewis RL, Nee DE, Lustig C, Berman MG, Moore KS. 2008. The mind and brain of short-term memory. Ann Rev Psychol 59:193–224.

Kamin LJ. 1969. Predictability, surprise, attention, and conditioning. In: BA Campbell, RM Church (eds). *Punishment and Aversive Behavior*, pp. 279–296. New York: Appleton–Century–Crofts.

McClelland JL, McNaughton BL, O'Reilly RC. 1995. Why there are complementary learning systems in the hippocampus and neocortex: insights from the successes and failures of connectionist models of learning and memory. Psychol Rev 102:419–457.

Miller EK, Cohen JD. 2001. An integrative theory of prefrontal cortex function. Annu Rev Neurosci 24:167–202.

Milner B, Squire LR, Kandel ER. 1998. Cognitive neuroscience and the study of memory. Neuron 20:445–468.

Muller R. 1996. A quarter of a century of place cells. Neuron 17:813–822.

Schwartz B, Robbins SJ. 1994. *Psychology of Learning and Behavior*, 4th ed. New York: Norton.

Schacter DL. 1996. *Searching for Memory: The Brain, the Mind and the Past*. New York: Harper Collins/Basic Books.

Schacter DL. 2001. *The Seven Sins of Memory: How the Mind Forgets and Remembers*. Boston: Houghton Mifflin.

Schacter DL, Addis, DR. 2007. The cognitive neuroscience of constructive memory: remembering the past and imagining the future. Philos Trans Roy Soc (B) 362:773–786.

Squire LR, Kandel ER. 1999. *Memory: From Mind to Molecules*. New York: WH Freeman.

Steinmetz JE, Lavond DG, Ivkovich D, Logan CG, Thompson RF. 1992. Disruption of classical eyelid conditioning after cerebellar lesions: damage to a memory trace system or a simple performance deficit? J Neurosci 12:4403–4426.

Tulving E. 1983. *Elements of Episodic Memory*. Oxford: Oxford Univ. Press.

Wixted JT, Squire LR. 2011. The medial temporal lobe and the attributes of memory. Trends Cog Sci 15:210–217.

References

Badre D, Wagner AD. 2007. Left ventrolateral prefrontal cortex and the cognitive control of memory. Neuropsychologia 45:2883–2901.

Barclay CR, Bransford JD, Franks JJ, et al. 1974. Comprehension and semantic flexibility. J Verb Learn Verb Behav 13: 471–481.

Bartlett FC. 1932. *Remembering: A Study in Experimental and Social Psychology*. Cambridge: Cambridge Univ. Press.

Blakemore C. 1977. *Mechanics of the Mind*. Cambridge, MA: Cambridge Univ. Press.

Brewer JB, Zhao Z, Desmond JE, et al. 1998. Making memories: brain activity that predicts how well visual experience will be remembered. Science 281:1185–1187.

Cahill L, Haier RJ, Fallon J, et al. 1996. Amygdala activity at encoding correlated with long-term, free recall of emotional information. Proc Natl Acad Sci U S A 93:8016–8021.

Corkin S. 2002. What's new with the amnesic patient H.M.? Nat Rev Neurosci 3:153–160.

Corkin S, Amaral DG, González RG, et al. 1997. H.M.'s medial temporal lobe lesion: findings from magnetic resonance imaging. J Neurosci 17:3964–3979.

Craik FIM, Lockhart RS. 1972. Levels of processing: a framework for memory research. J Verb Learn Verb Behav 11:671–684.

Domjan M, Burkhard B. 1986. *The Principles of Learning and Behavior*, 2nd ed. Monterey, CA: Brooks/Cole.

du Lac S, Raymond JL, Sejnowski TJ, Lisberger SG. 1995. Learning and memory in the vestibulo-ocular reflex. Annu Rev Neurosci 18:409–441.

Eldridge LL, Knowlton BJ, Furmanski CS, et al. 2000. Remembering episodes: a selective role for the hippocampus during retrieval. Nat Neurosci 3:1149–1152.

Hebb DO. 1966. *A Textbook of Psychology*. Philadelphia: Saunders.

Knowlton BJ, Mangels JA, Squire LR. 1996. A neostriatal habit learning system in humans. Science 273:1399–1402.

Luria AR. 1968. *The Mind of a Mnemonist*. New York: Basic Books.

Maril A, Wagner AD, Schacter DL. 2001. On the tip of the tongue: an event-related fMRI study of semantic retrieval failure and cognitive conflict. Neuron 31:653–660.

Martin A, Chao LL. 2001. Semantic memory and the brain: structure and processes. Curr Opin Neurobiol 11:194–201.

McCarthy RA, Warrington EK. 1990. *Cognitive Neuropsychology: A Clinical Introduction*. San Diego: Academic Press.

McGaugh JL. 1990. Significance and remembrance: the role of neuromodulatory systems. Psychol Sci 1:15–25.

Naya Y, Yoshida M, Miyashita Y. 2001. Backward spreading of memory-related signal in the primate temporal cortex. Science 291:661–664.

Nyberg L, Habib R, McIntosh AR, Tulving E. 2000. Reactivation of encoding-related brain activity during memory retrieval. Proc Natl Acad Sci U S A 97:11120–11124.

Pavlov IP. 1927. *Conditioned Reflexes: Investigation of the Physiological Activity of the Cerebral Cortex*. GV Anrep (transl). London: Oxford Univ. Press.

Penfield W. 1958. Functional localization in temporal and deep sylvian areas. Res Publ Assoc Res Nerv Ment Dis 36:210–226.

Petrides M. 1994. Frontal lobes and behavior. Curr Opin Neurobiol 4:207–211.

Phelps EA. 2006. Emotion and cognition: insights from studies of the human amygdala. Ann Rev Psychol 57:27–53.

Poldrack RA, Clark J, Pare-Blagoev EJ, et al. 2001. Interactive memory systems in the human brain. Nature 414:546–550.

Poldrack RA, Desmond JE, Glover GH, Gabrieli JDE. 1998. The neural basis of visual skill learning: an fMRI study of mirror-reading. Cereb Cortex 8:1–10.

Rainer G, Asaad WF, Miller EK. 1998. Memory fields of neurons in the primate prefrontal cortex. Proc Natl Acad Sci U S A 95:15008–15013.

Rescorla RA. 1968. Probability of shock in the presence and absence of CS in fear conditioning. J Comp Physiol Psychol 66:1–5.

Rescorla RA. 1988. Behavioral studies of Pavlovian conditioning. Annu Rev Neurosci 11:329–352.

Roediger HL III, McDermott KB. 1995. Creating false memories: remembering words not presented in lists. J Exp Psychol Learn Mem Cogn 21:803–814.

Schacter DL. 1987. Implicit memory: history and current status. J Exp Psychol Learn Mem Cogn 13:501–518.

Schacter DL, Guerin SA, St. Jacques PL. 2011. Memory distortion: an adaptive perspective. Trends Cog Sci 15:467–474.

Schacter DL, Wig GS, Stevens WD. 2007. Reductions in cortical activity during priming. Curr Opinion Neurobiol 17:171–176.

Skinner BF. 1938. *The Behavior of Organisms: An Experimental Analysis*. New York: Appleton–Century–Crofts.

Squire LR. 1987. *Memory and Brain*. New York: Oxford Univ. Press.

Thompson-Schill SL, Swick D, Farah MJ, et al. 1998. Verb generation in patients with focal frontal lesions: a neuropsychological test of neuroimaging findings. Proc Natl Acad Sci U S A 95:15855–15860.

Thorndike EL. 1911. *Animal Intelligence: Experimental Studies*. New York: Macmillan.

Tomita H, Ohbayashi M, Nakahara K, et al. 1999. Top-down signal from prefrontal cortex in executive control of memory retrieval. Nature 401:699–703.

Tulving E, Schacter DL. 1990. Priming and human memory systems. Science 247:301–306.

Vaidya CJ, Gabrieli JD, Verfaellie M, et al. 1998. Font-specific priming following global amnesia and occipital lobe damage. Neuropsychology 12:183–192.

Wagner AD. 2002. Cognitive control and episodic memory: contributions from prefrontal cortex. In: LR Squire, DL Schacter (eds). *Neuropsychology of Memory*, 3rd ed., pp. 174–192. New York: Guilford Press.

Wagner AD, Koutstaal W, Maril A, et al. 2000. Task-specific repetition priming in left inferior prefrontal cortex. Cereb Cortex 10:1176–1184.

Wagner AD, Paré-Blagoev EJ, Clark J, Poldrack RA. 2001. Recovering meaning: left prefrontal cortex guides controlled semantic retrieval. Neuron 31:329–338.

Wagner AD, Schacter DL, Rotte M, Koutstaal W, Maril A, Dale AM, Rosen BR, Buckner RL. 1998. Building memories: remembering and forgetting of verbal experiences as predicted by brain activity. Science 281:1188–1191.

Warrington EK, Weiskrantz L. 1982. Amnesia: a disconnection syndrome? Neuropsychologia 20:233–248.

Wheeler ME, Petersen SE, Buckner RL. 2000. Memory's echo: vivid remembering reactivates sensory-specific cortex. Proc Natl Acad Sci U S A 97:11125–11129.

White NM, McDonald RJ. 2002. Multiple parallel memory systems in the brain of the rat. Neurobiol Learn Mem 77:125–184.

66

Cellular Mechanisms of Implicit Memory Storage and the Biological Basis of Individuality

THROUGHOUT THIS BOOK WE HAVE EMPHASIZED that all behavior is a function of the brain and that malfunctions of the brain produce characteristic disturbances of behavior. Behavior is also shaped by experience. How does experience act on the neural circuits of the brain to change behavior? How is new information acquired by the brain and, once acquired, how is it remembered?

In the previous chapter we saw that memory is not a single process but has at least two major forms. Implicit memory operates unconsciously and automatically, as in the memory for habits and perceptual and motor skills, whereas explicit memory operates consciously, as in the memory for people, places, and objects. Long-term storage of explicit memory begins in the hippocampus and the medial temporal lobe of the neocortex, whereas long-term storage of implicit memory requires a family of structures: the neocortex for priming, the striatum for skills and habits, the amygdala for learned fear, the cerebellum for learned motor skills, and certain reflex pathways for nonassociative learning such as habituation and sensitization (Figure 66–1).

Over time, explicit memories are transferred to different regions of the neocortex. In addition, many cognitive, motor, and perceptual skills that we initially store in explicit memory ultimately become so ingrained with practice that they become stored as implicit memory.

The transference from explicit to implicit memory and the difference between them is dramatically demonstrated in the case of the English musician and conductor Clive Waring, who in 1985 sustained a viral infection of his brain (herpes encephalitis) that affected the hippocampus and temporal cortex. Waring was left with a devastating loss of memory for events or people he had encountered even a minute or two earlier.

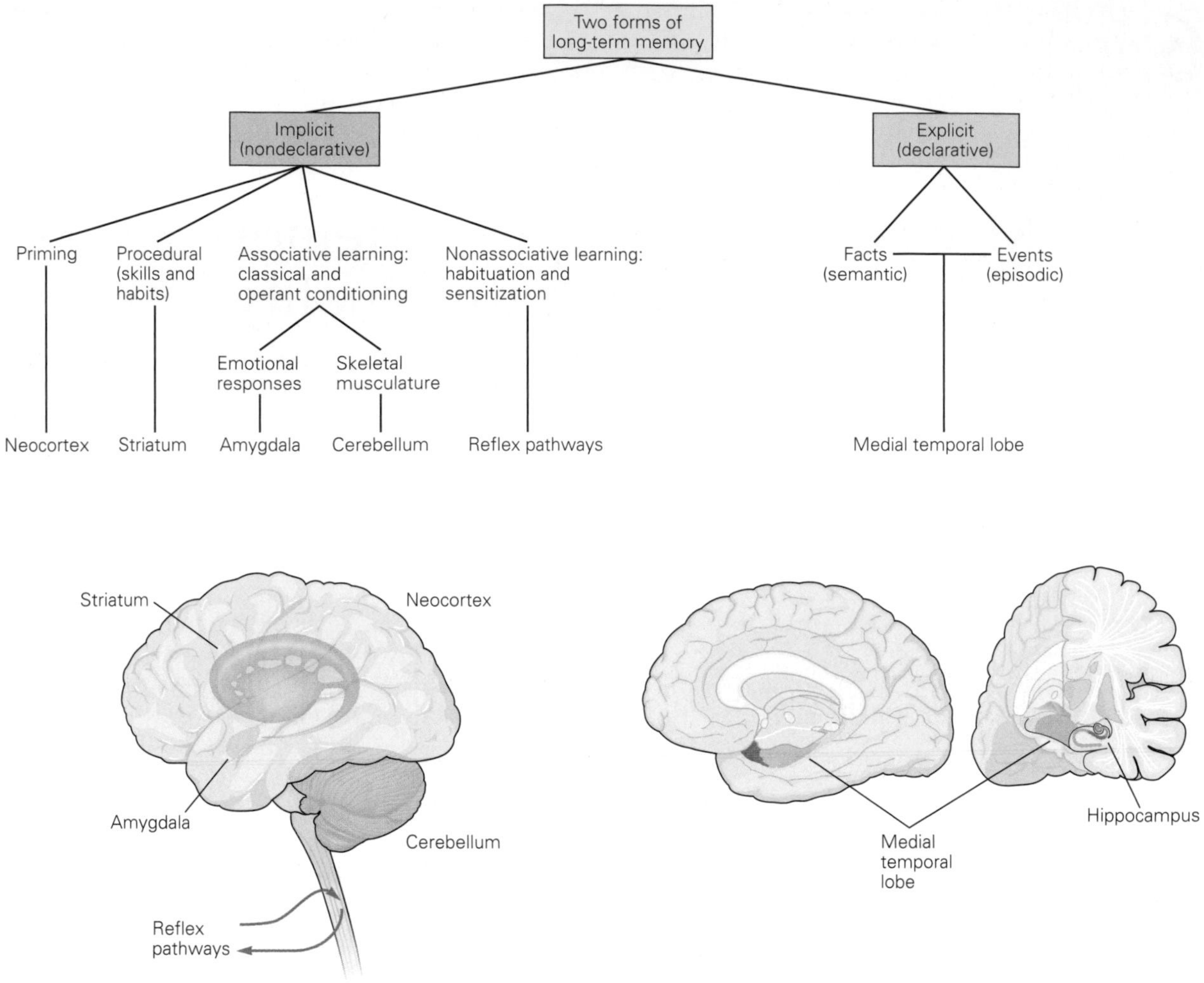

Figure 66–1 Two forms of long-term memory involve different brain systems. Implicit memory involves the neocortex, striatum, amygdala, cerebellum, and in the simplest cases the reflex pathways themselves. Explicit memory requires the medial temporal lobe and the hippocampus, as well as certain areas of neocortex (not shown).

Yet he could still read music, perform on the piano, and conduct a chorale. Under these circumstances it was clear that many aspects of his basic personality—the biological basis of his individuality—were still intact. Once a performance was completed, however, he could not remember a thing about it.

Similarly, William deKooning, the abstract expressionist painter, developed Alzheimer disease and severe disturbances of explicit memory. As the disease progressed and his memory for people, places, and objects deteriorated, he nevertheless continued to produce important and interesting paintings. This aspect of his creative personality was relatively untouched.

In this chapter we examine the cellular and molecular mechanisms that underlie implicit memory in invertebrate and vertebrate animals. In the next chapter we examine the biology of explicit memory storage in mammals.

Storage of Implicit Memory Involves Changes in the Effectiveness of Synaptic Transmission

Studies of elementary forms of implicit learning—habituation, sensitization, and classical conditioning—provided the groundwork for understanding the neural mechanisms of memory storage. Such learning has been analyzed in simple invertebrates and in a variety of vertebrate reflexes, such as the flexion reflexes, fear responses, and the eye blink. These simple forms of implicit learning involve changes in the effectiveness of the synaptic pathways that mediate the behavior.

Habituation Results from an Activity-Dependent Presynaptic Depression of Synaptic Transmission

Habituation is the simplest form of implicit learning. It occurs, for example, when an animal learns to ignore a novel stimulus. An animal reacts to a new stimulus with a series of orienting responses. If the stimulus is neither beneficial nor harmful, the animal learns to ignore it after repeated exposure.

The physiological basis of habituation was first investigated by Charles Sherrington while studying posture and locomotion in the cat. Sherrington observed a decrease in the intensity of certain reflexes in response to repeated electrical stimulation of the motor pathways. He suggested that this decrease, which he called *habituation*, is caused by diminished synaptic effectiveness in the stimulated pathways. Habituation was later investigated at the cellular level by Alden Spencer and Richard Thompson. They found close cellular and behavioral parallels between habituation of a spinal flexion reflex in cats (the withdrawal of a limb from a noxious stimulus) and habituation of more complex human behaviors. They showed that during habituation the strength of the input from local excitatory interneurons onto motor neurons in the spinal cord decreased. Connections to interneurons from sensory neurons innervating the skin were unaffected.

Because the organization of interneurons in the vertebrate spinal cord is quite complex, it was difficult to analyze further the cellular mechanisms of habituation in the flexion reflex. Progress required a simpler system. The marine mollusk *Aplysia californica*, which has a simple nervous system of about 20,000 central neurons, proved to be an excellent system for studying implicit forms of memory.

Aplysia has a repertory of defensive reflexes for withdrawing its respiratory gill and siphon, a small fleshy spout above the gill used to expel seawater and waste (Figure 66–2A). These reflexes are similar to the withdrawal reflex of the leg studied by Spencer and Thompson. Mild touching of the siphon elicits reflex withdrawal of both the siphon and gill. With repeated stimulation these reflexes habituate. As we shall see, these responses can also be dishabituated, sensitized, and classically conditioned.

The neural circuit mediating the gill-withdrawal reflex in *Aplysia* has been studied in detail. Touching the siphon excites a population of mechanoreceptor sensory neurons that innervate the siphon. The release of glutamate from sensory neuron terminals generates fast excitatory postsynaptic potentials (EPSPs) in interneurons and motor cells. The EPSPs from the sensory cells and interneurons summate on motor cells both temporally and spatially, causing them to discharge strongly, thereby producing vigorous withdrawal of the gill. If the stimulus is repeated, the monosynaptic EPSPs produced by sensory neurons in both interneurons and motor cells progressively decrease, paralleling the habituation of gill withdrawal. In addition, repeated stimulation also leads to a decrease in the strength of synaptic transmission from the excitatory interneurons to the motor neurons; the net result is that the reflex response diminishes (Figure 66–2B,C).

What reduces the effectiveness of synaptic transmission between the sensory neurons and their postsynaptic cells during repeated stimulation? Quantal analysis revealed that the amount of glutamate released from presynaptic terminals of sensory neurons decreases. That is, fewer synaptic vesicles are released with each action potential in the sensory neuron; the sensitivity of the postsynaptic glutamate receptors does not change. Because the reduction in transmission occurs in the activated pathway itself and does not require another modulatory cell, the reduction is referred to as *homosynaptic depression*. This depression lasts many minutes.

An enduring change in the functional strength of synaptic connections thus constitutes the cellular mechanism mediating short-term habituation. As change of this type occurs at several sites in the gill-withdrawal reflex circuit, memory is distributed and stored throughout the circuit. Depression of synaptic transmission by sensory neurons, interneurons, or both is a common mechanism underlying habituation of escape responses of crayfish and cockroaches as well as startle reflexes in vertebrates.

How much can the effectiveness of a synapse change and how long can the change last? In *Aplysia* a single session of 10 stimuli leads to short-term habituation of the withdrawal reflex lasting minutes. Four sessions separated by periods ranging from several hours to 1 day produce long-term habituation, lasting as long as 3 weeks (Figure 66–3).

Anatomical studies indicate that long-term habituation is caused by a decrease in the number of synaptic contacts between sensory and motor neurons. In naïve animals 90% of the sensory neurons make physiologically detectable connections with identified motor neurons. In contrast, in animals trained for long-term habituation the incidence of connections is reduced to 30%; the reduction in number of synapses persists for a week and does not fully recover even 3 weeks later.

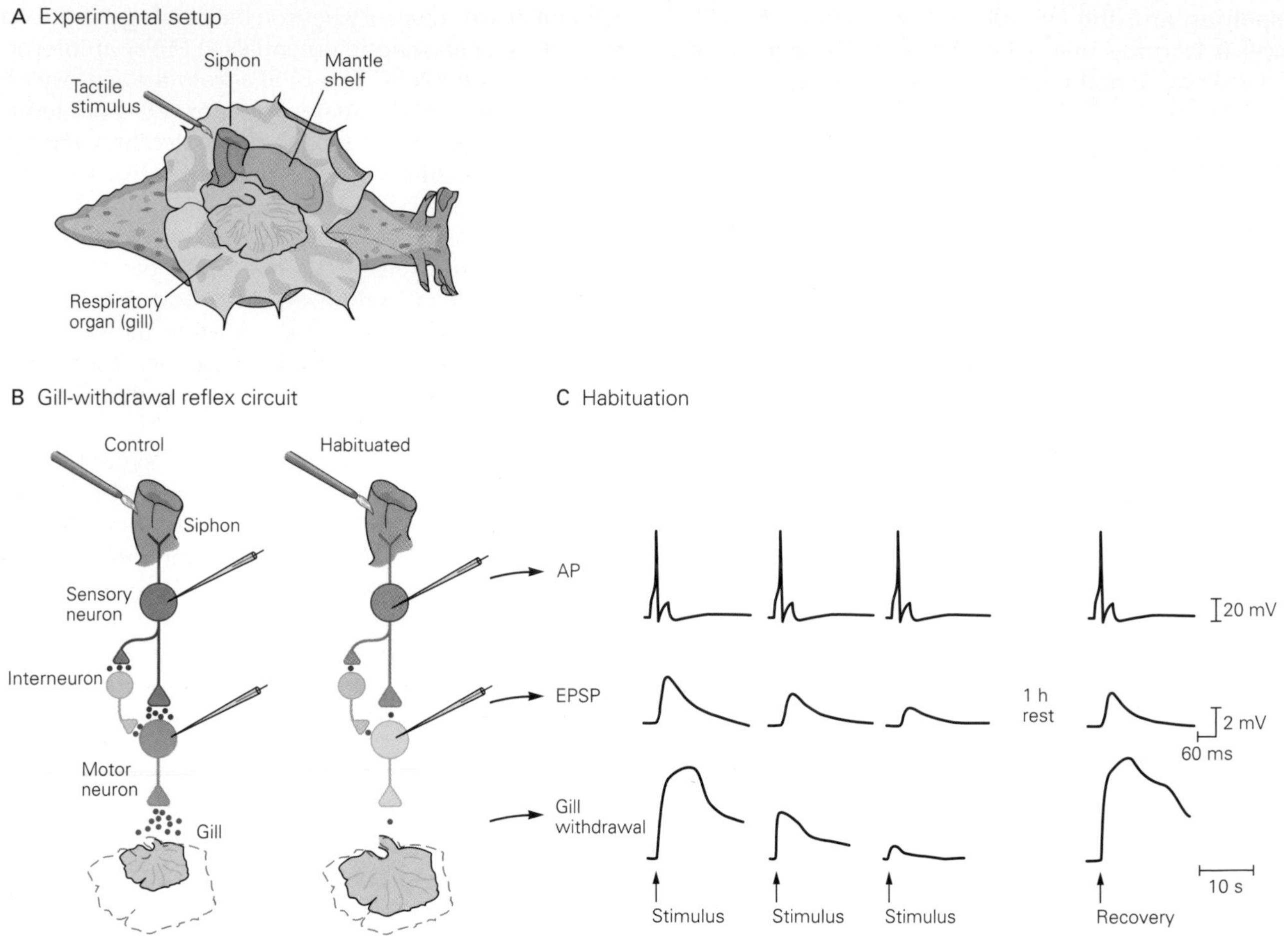

Figure 66–2 Short-term habituation of the gill-withdrawal reflex of the marine snail *Aplysia*.

A. A dorsal view of *Aplysia* illustrates the respiratory organ (gill) and the mantle shelf, which ends in the siphon, a fleshy spout used to expel seawater and waste. Touching the siphon elicits the gill-withdrawal reflex. Repeated stimulation leads to habituation.

B. This simplified circuit shows key elements of the gill-withdrawal reflex as well as sites involved in habituation. Approximately 24 mechanoreceptor neurons in the abdominal ganglion innervate the siphon skin. These sensory cells make excitatory synapses onto a cluster of six motor neurons that innervate the gill as well as on interneurons that modulate the firing of the motor neurons. (For simplicity only one of each type of neuron is illustrated here.) Touching the siphon leads to withdrawal of the gill (**dashed outline** shows original gill size; **solid outline** shows maximal withdrawal).

C. Repeated stimulation of the siphon sensory neuron (**top traces**) leads to a progressive depression of synaptic transmission between the sensory and motor neurons, seen as a decrease in size of the motor neuron EPSP with no change in the action potential (**AP**) in the presynaptic sensory neuron. In a separate experiment repeated stimulation of the siphon results in a decrease in gill withdrawal (habituation). One hour after repetitive stimulation both the EPSP and gill withdrawal have recovered. Habituation is now known to involve a decrease in transmitter release at many synaptic sites throughout the reflex circuit (part B). (Adapted, with permission, from Pinsker et al. 1970; Castellucci and Kandel 1974.)

As we shall see later, long-term sensitization of synaptic transmission is associated with an increase in the number of synapses between sensory and motor neurons.

Not all synapses are equally modifiable. In *Aplysia* the strength of some synapses rarely changes, even with repeated activation. In synapses specifically involved in learning (such as the connections between sensory and motor neurons in the withdrawal reflex circuit) a relatively small amount of training can produce large and enduring changes in synaptic strength.

Sensitization Involves Presynaptic Facilitation of Synaptic Transmission

When an animal repeatedly encounters a harmless stimulus, its responsiveness to the stimulus habituates.

In contrast, with a *harmful* stimulus the animal typically learns fear; it responds vigorously not only to the harmful stimulus but also to other concurrent stimuli, even harmless ones. As a result, defensive reflexes for withdrawal and escape become heightened. This enhancement of reflex responses is called *sensitization.*

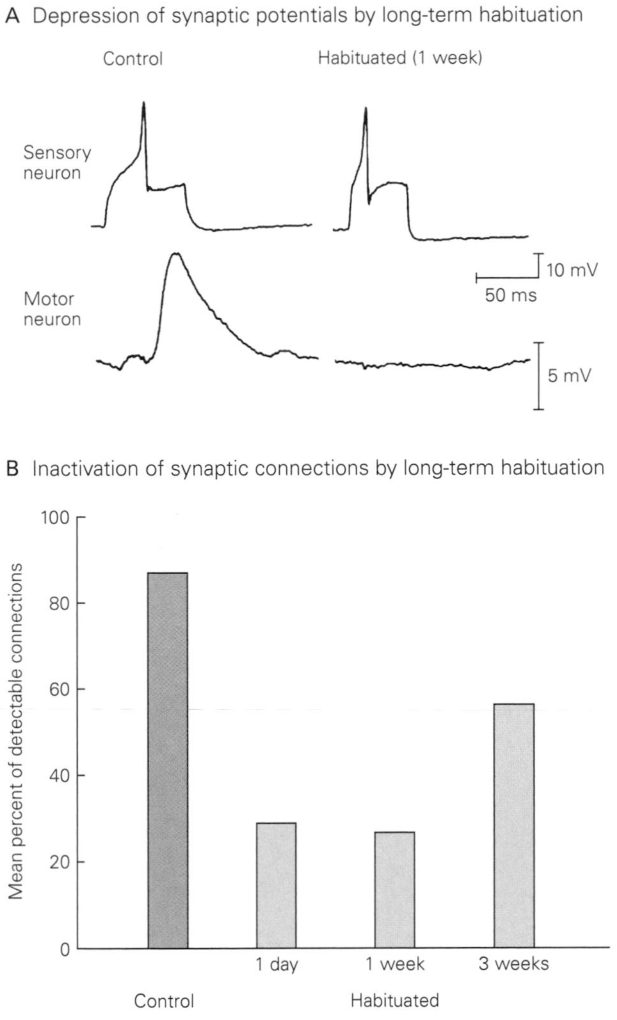

Figure 66–3 Long-term habituation of the gill-withdrawal reflex in *Aplysia*. (Adapted, with permission, from Castellucci, Carew, and Kandel 1978.)

A. Comparison of the action potentials and synaptic potentials in sensory and motor neurons, respectively, in an untrained animal (control) and one that has been subjected to long-term habituation. In the habituated animal 1 week after training no synaptic potential occurs in the motor neuron in response to the sensory neuron action potential.

B. The mean percentage of sensory neurons making physiologically detectable connections with motor neurons in habituated animals is decreased at three points in time after long-term habituation training.

Like habituation, sensitization can be transient or long lasting. A single shock to the tail of an *Aplysia* produces short-term sensitization of the gill-withdrawal reflex that lasts minutes; five or more shocks to the tail produce sensitization lasting days to weeks. Tail shock is also sufficient to overcome the effects of habituation and enhance a habituated gill-withdrawal reflex, a process termed *dishabituation*.

Sensitization and dishabituation result from an enhancement in synaptic transmission at several connections in the neural circuit of the gill-withdrawal reflex, including the connections made by sensory neurons with motor neurons and interneurons—the same synapses depressed by habituation (Figure 66–4A). Typically, modifiable synapses can be regulated bidirectionally, participate in more than one type of learning, and store more than one type of memory. The bidirectional synaptic changes that underlie habituation and sensitization are the result of different cellular mechanisms. In *Aplysia* the same synapses that are weakened by habituation through a homosynaptic process can be strengthened by sensitization through a *heterosynaptic* process that depends on modulatory interneurons activated by the harmful stimulus to the tail.

At least three groups of modulatory interneurons are involved in sensitization. The best studied use serotonin as a transmitter. The serotonergic interneurons form synapses on many regions of the sensory neurons, including axo-axonic synapses on the presynaptic terminals of the sensory cells. The serotonin released from the interneurons after a single tail shock binds to a type of receptor in the sensory neurons that is coupled to a stimulatory G protein that increases the activity of adenylyl cyclase. This action produces the second messenger cyclic adenosine monophosphate (cAMP), which in turn activates the cAMP-dependent protein kinase (PKA) (see Chapter 11). Serotonin also activates a second type of G protein-coupled receptor that leads to the hydrolysis of phospholipids and the activation of protein kinase C (PKC).

The protein phosphorylation mediated by PKA and PKC enhances the release of transmitter from sensory neurons through at least two mechanisms (Figure 66–4B). In one action PKA phosphorylates a K^+ channel, causing it to close. This broadens the action potential and thus enhances Ca^{2+} influx through voltage-gated Ca^{2+} channels, which in turn enhances transmitter release. In a second action protein phosphorylation through PKC enhances the functioning of the release machinery directly. Presynaptic facilitation in response to release of serotonin by a tail shock lasts for a period of many minutes. Repeated noxious stimuli can strengthen synaptic activity for days.

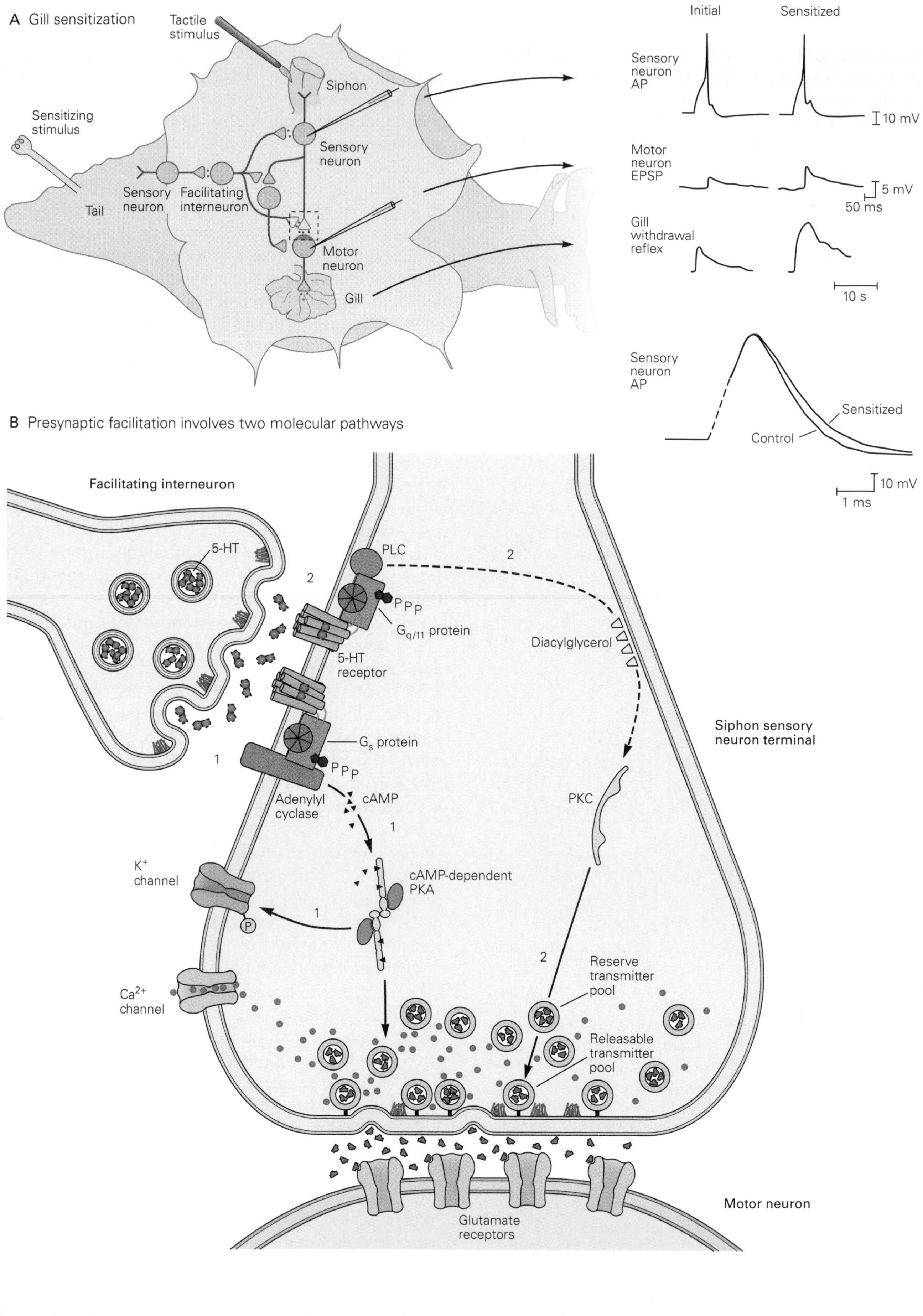
A Gill sensitization
Tactile stimulus
Siphon
Sensitizing stimulus
Sensory neuron
Tail
Sensory neuron
Facilitating interneuron
Motor neuron
Gill
Initial
Sensitized
Sensory neuron AP
10 mV
Motor neuron EPSP
5 mV
50 ms
Gill withdrawal reflex
10 s
Sensory neuron AP
Sensitized
Control
10 mV
1 ms
B Presynaptic facilitation involves two molecular pathways
Facilitating interneuron
5-HT
2
PLC
2
PPP
$G_{q/11}$ protein
Diacylglycerol
5-HT receptor
G_s protein
1
PPP
Adenylyl cyclase
cAMP
1
Siphon sensory neuron terminal
PKC
K^+ channel
cAMP-dependent PKA
P
1
2
Reserve transmitter pool
Ca^{2+} channel
Releasable transmitter pool
Motor neuron
Glutamate receptors

Classical Conditioning of Fear Involves Coordinated Pre- and Postsynaptic Facilitation of Synaptic Transmission

Classical conditioning is a more complex form of learning. Rather than learning about the properties of one stimulus, as in habituation and sensitization, the animal learns to associate one type of stimulus with another. As described in Chapter 65, an initial weak conditioned stimulus (such as the ringing of a bell) becomes highly effective in producing a response when paired with a strong unconditioned stimulus (such as presentation of food). In reflexes that can be enhanced by both classical conditioning and sensitization, like the defensive withdrawal reflexes of *Aplysia,* classical conditioning results in greater and longer-lasting enhancement.

For classical conditioning of the *Aplysia* gill-withdrawal reflex, a weak touch to the siphon serves as the conditioned stimulus while a strong shock to the tail serves as the unconditioned stimulus. When the gill withdrawal reflex is classically conditioned, gill withdrawal in response to siphon stimulation alone is greatly enhanced. This enhancement is even more dramatic than the enhancement produced in an unpaired pathway by tail shock alone (sensitization). In classical conditioning the timing of the conditioned and unconditioned stimuli is critical. To be effective, the conditioned stimulus (siphon touch) must *precede* (and predict) the unconditioned stimulus (tail shock), often within an interval of about 0.5 seconds (Figure 66–5).

The convergence in individual sensory neurons of the signals initiated by the conditioned and unconditioned stimuli is critical. A strong shock to the tail excites serotonergic interneurons that form synapses on presynaptic terminals of the siphon sensory neurons, resulting in presynaptic facilitation associated with sensitization (Figure 66–5A). However, when the tail shock (unconditioned stimulus) immediately follows a slight tap on the siphon (conditioned stimulus), the serotonin from the interneurons produces even greater presynaptic facilitation, a process termed *activity-dependent facilitation* (Figure 66–5B).

How does this work? During conditioning the modulatory interneurons activated by tail shock release serotonin shortly *after* siphon touch has triggered an action potential in the sensory neurons. The action potential triggers an influx of Ca^{2+} into the sensory neuron's presynaptic terminals, the Ca^{2+} binds to calmodulin, and the complex in turn binds to adenylyl cyclase. This primes the adenylyl cyclase so that it responds more vigorously to the serotonin released following the unconditioned stimulus at the tail. As a result, the production of cAMP is enhanced, which increases the amount of presynaptic facilitation. If the order of stimuli is reversed so that serotonin release precedes Ca^{2+} influx in the presynaptic terminals, there is no potentiation and no classical conditioning.

Thus the cellular mechanism of classical conditioning in the monosynaptic pathway of the withdrawal reflex is largely an elaboration of the mechanism of sensitization, with the added feature that the adenylyl cyclase serves as a *coincidence detector* in the presynaptic sensory neuron, recognizing the temporal order of

Figure 66–4 (Opposite) Short-term sensitization of the gill-withdrawal reflex in *Aplysia.*

A. Sensitization of the gill-withdrawal reflex is produced by applying a noxious stimulus to another part of the body, such as the tail. A shock to the tail activates tail sensory neurons that excite facilitating (modulatory) interneurons, which form synapses on the cell body and terminals of the mechanoreceptor sensory neurons that innervate the siphon. Through these axo-axonic synapses the modulatory interneurons enhance transmitter release from the siphon sensory neurons onto their postsynaptic gill motor neurons (presynaptic facilitation), thus enhancing gill withdrawal. Presynaptic facilitation results, in part, from a prolongation of the sensory neuron action potential (**bottom traces**). (Adapted, with permission, from Pinsker et al. 1970; Klein and Kandel 1980.)

B. Presynaptic facilitation in the sensory neuron is thought to occur by means of two biochemical pathways. The diagram shows details of the synaptic complex in the **dashed box** in part A.

Pathway 1: A facilitating interneuron releases serotonin (**5-HT**), which binds to metabotropic receptors in the sensory neuron terminal. This action engages a G protein (**G_s**), which in turn increases the activity of adenylyl cyclase. The adenylyl cyclase converts ATP to cAMP, which binds to the regulatory subunit of PKA, thus activating its catalytic subunit. The catalytic subunit phosphorylates certain K^+ channels, thereby closing the channels and decreasing the outward K^+ current. This prolongs the action potential, thus increasing the influx of Ca^{2+} through voltage-gated Ca^{2+} channels and thereby augmenting transmitter release.

Pathway 2: Serotonin binds to a second class of metabotropic receptor that activates the $G_{q/11}$ class of G protein that enhances the activity of phospholipase C (**PLC**). The PLC activity leads to production of diacylglycerol, which activates protein kinase C (**PKC**). Phosphorylation of presynaptic proteins by PKC results in the mobilization of vesicles containing glutamate from a reserve pool to a releasable pool at the active zone, increasing the efficiency of transmitter release.

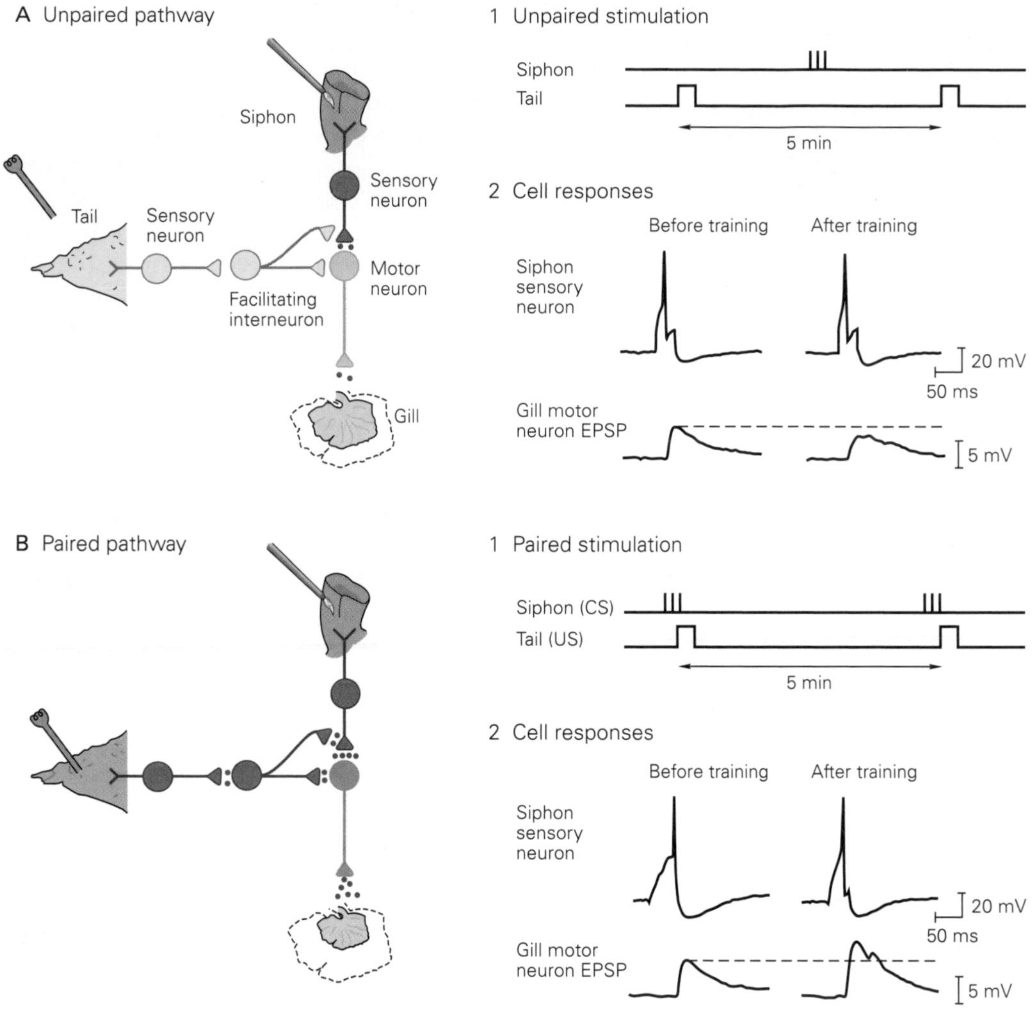

Figure 66–5 Classical conditioning of the gill-withdrawal reflex in *Aplysia*. (Adapted, with permission, from Hawkins et al. 1983.)

A. The siphon is stimulated by a light touch and the tail is shocked, but the two stimuli are not paired in time. The tail shock excites facilitatory interneurons that form synapses on the presynaptic terminals of sensory neurons innervating the mantle shelf and siphon. This is the mechanism of sensitization. **1.** The pattern of unpaired stimulation during training. **2.** Under these conditions the size of the motor neuron EPSP is only weakly facilitated by the tail shock. In this example the EPSP actually decreases slightly despite the tail shock because repeated unpaired stimulation of the siphon leads to synaptic depression.

B. The tail shock is paired with stimulation of the siphon. **1.** The siphon is touched (conditioned stimulus or CS) immediately prior to shocking the tail (unconditioned stimulus or US). As a result, the siphon sensory neurons are primed to be more responsive to input from the facilitatory interneurons in the unconditioned pathway. This is the mechanism of classical conditioning; it both amplifies the response of the conditioned pathway and restricts the amplification to that pathway. **2.** Recordings of EPSPs in an identified motor neuron produced by the siphon sensory neurons before training and one hour after training. After training the EPSP in the motor neuron produced by paired sensory input is considerably greater than either the EPSP before training or the EPSP following unpaired tail shock (shown in part A2). This produces a more vigorous gill withdrawal.

the physiological representations of both the unconditioned stimulus (tail shock) and conditioned stimulus (siphon touch).

In addition to the presynaptic component of activity-dependent facilitation, a postsynaptic component is triggered by Ca^{+} influx into the motor neuron when it is highly excited by the siphon sensory neurons. The properties of this postsynaptic mechanism are similar to those of long-term potentiation of synaptic transmission in the mammalian brain (discussed later in this chapter and in Chapter 67).

Long-Term Storage of Implicit Memory Involves Changes in Chromatin Structure and Gene Expression Mediated by the cAMP-PKA-CREB Pathway

Cyclic AMP Signaling Has a Role in Long-Term Sensitization

In all forms of learning practice makes perfect. Repeated experience converts short-term memory into a long-term form. In *Aplysia* the form of long-term memory that has been most intensively studied is long-term sensitization. Like the short-term form, long-term sensitization of the gill-withdrawal reflex involves changes in the strength of connections at several synapses, including those between sensory and motor neurons. However, it also involves the growth of new synaptic connections.

Five spaced training sessions (or repeated applications of serotonin) over approximately 1 hour produce long-term sensitization and long-term synaptic facilitation lasting 1 or more days; continued spaced training over several days produces sensitization that persists for 1 or more weeks. Long-term sensitization, like the short-term form, requires protein phosphorylation that is dependent on increased levels of cAMP (Figure 66–6).

The conversion of short-term memory into long-term memory, called *consolidation,* requires synthesis of messenger RNAs and proteins in the neurons in the circuit. Thus specific gene expression is required for long-term memory. The transition from short-term to long-term memory depends on the prolonged rise in cAMP that follows repeated applications of serotonin. This leads to prolonged activation of PKA, allowing the catalytic subunit of the kinase to translocate into the nucleus of the sensory neurons. It also leads indirectly to activation of a second protein kinase, the mitogen-activated protein kinase (MAPK), a kinase commonly associated with cellular growth (see Chapter 11). Within the nucleus the catalytic subunit of PKA phosphorylates and thereby activates the transcription factor CREB-1 (*c*AMP *r*esponse *e*lement *b*inding protein 1), which binds a promoter element called CRE (*c*AMP *r*ecognition *e*lement) (Figures 66–6 and 66–7).

To turn on gene transcription, phosphorylated CREB-1 recruits a transcriptional coactivator, CREB-binding protein (CBP), to the promoter region. CBP has two important properties that facilitate transcriptional activation: it recruits RNA polymerase II to the promoter, and it functions as an acetyltransferase, adding acetyl groups to certain lysine residues on its substrate proteins. One of the most important substrates of CBP are the histone proteins, which are components of nucleosomes, the fundamental building blocks of chromatin. The histones contain a series of positively charged basic residues that strongly interact with the negatively charged phosphates of DNA. This interaction causes DNA to become tightly wrapped around the nucleosomes, much like string is wrapped around a spool, thereby preventing necessary transcription factors from accessing their gene targets.

The binding of CBP to CREB-1 leads to histone acetylation, which causes a number of important structural and functional changes at the nucleosome level. For example, acetylation neutralizes the positive charge of lysine residues in the histone tail domains, decreasing the affinity of histones for DNA. Also, specific classes of transcriptional activators can bind to acetylated histones and facilitate the repositioning of nucleosomes at the promoter region. Together these and other types of chromatin modifications serve to regulate the accessibility of chromatin to the transcriptional machinery, and thus enhance the ability of a gene to be transcribed. As we will see in Chapter 67, a mutation in the gene encoding CBP underlies Rubinstein-Taybi syndrome, a disorder associated with mental retardation.

The turning on of transcription by PKA also depends on its ability to indirectly activate the MAPK pathway (see Chapter 11). MAPK phosphorylation of the transcription factor CREB-2 relieves an inhibitory action of CREB-2 on transcription (Figure 66–6B). The combined effects of CREB-1 activation and relief of CREB-2 repression induces a cascade of new gene expression important for learning and memory (Figure 66–7).

The presence of both a repressor (CREB-2) and an activator (CREB-1) of transcription at the first step in long-term facilitation suggests that the threshold for long-term memory storage can be regulated. Indeed, we see in everyday life that the ease with which short-term memory is transferred into long-term memory varies greatly with attention, mood, and social context.

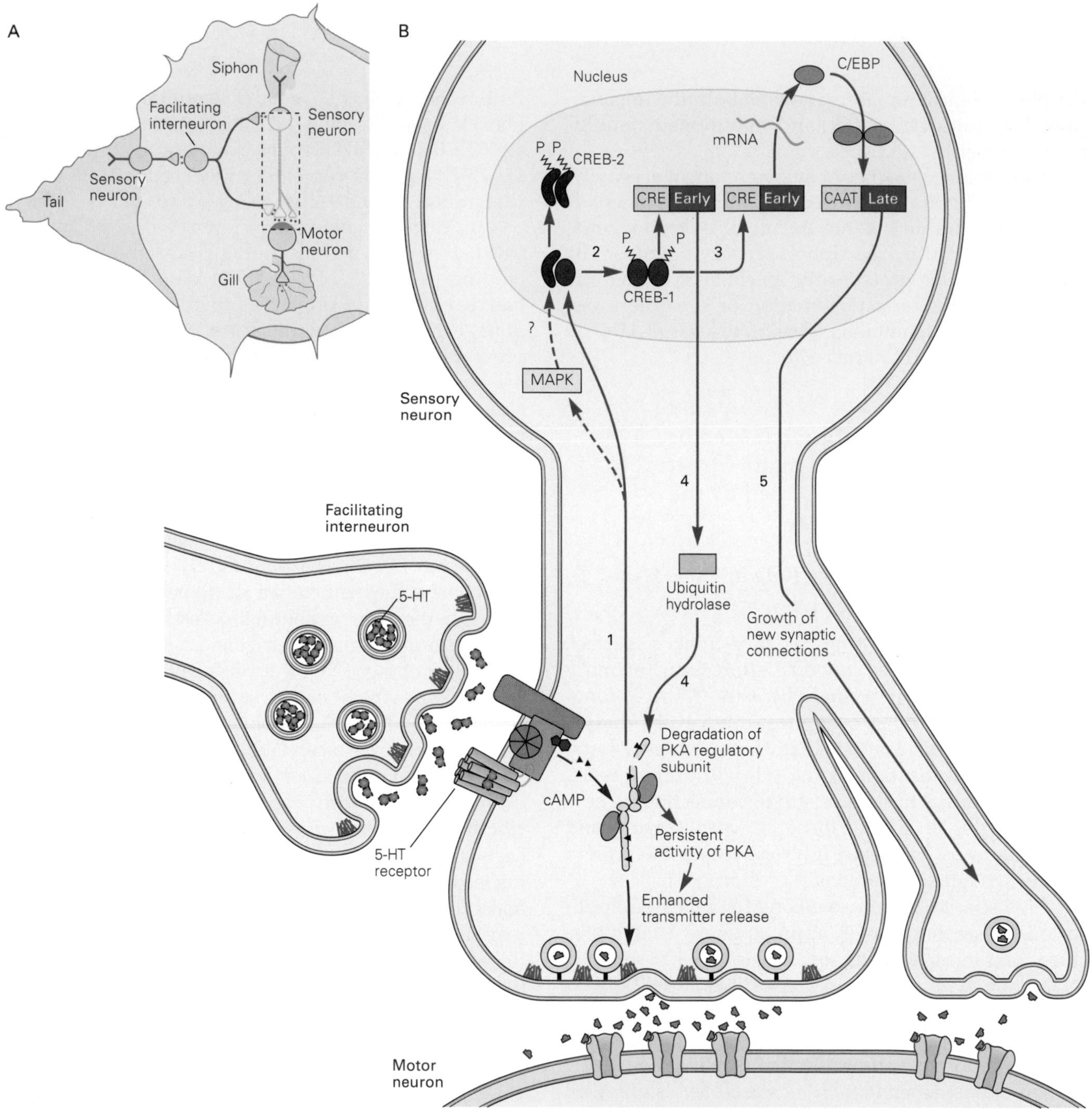

Figure 66–6 Long-term sensitization involves synaptic facilitation and the growth of new synaptic connections.

A. Long-term sensitization of the gill-withdrawal reflex of *Aplysia* following repeated tail shocks involves long-lasting facilitation of transmitter release at the synapses between sensory and motor neurons.

B. Long-term sensitization of the gill-withdrawal reflex leads to persistent activity of PKA, resulting in the growth of new synaptic connections. Repeated tail shock leads to more pronounced elevation of cAMP, producing long-term facilitation (lasting 1 or more days) that outlasts the increase in cAMP and recruits the synthesis of new proteins. This inductive mechanism is initiated by translocation of PKA to the nucleus (**pathway 1**), where PKA phosphorylates the transcriptional activator CREB-1 (cAMP response element binding protein 1) (**pathway 2**). CREB-1 binds cAMP regulatory elements (CRE) located in the upstream region of several cAMP-inducible genes, activating gene transcription (**pathway 3**). PKA also activates the mitogen-activated protein kinase (**MAPK**), which phosphorylates the transcriptional repressor CREB-2 (cAMP response element binding protein 2), thus removing its repressive action. One gene activated by CREB-1 encodes a ubiquitin hydrolase, a component of a specific ubiquitin proteasome that leads to the proteolytic cleavage of the regulatory subunit of PKA, resulting in persistent activity of PKA, even after cAMP has returned to its resting level (**pathway 4**). CREB-1 also activates the expression of the transcription factor C/EBP, which leads to expression of a set of unidentified proteins important for the growth of new synaptic connections (**pathway 5**).

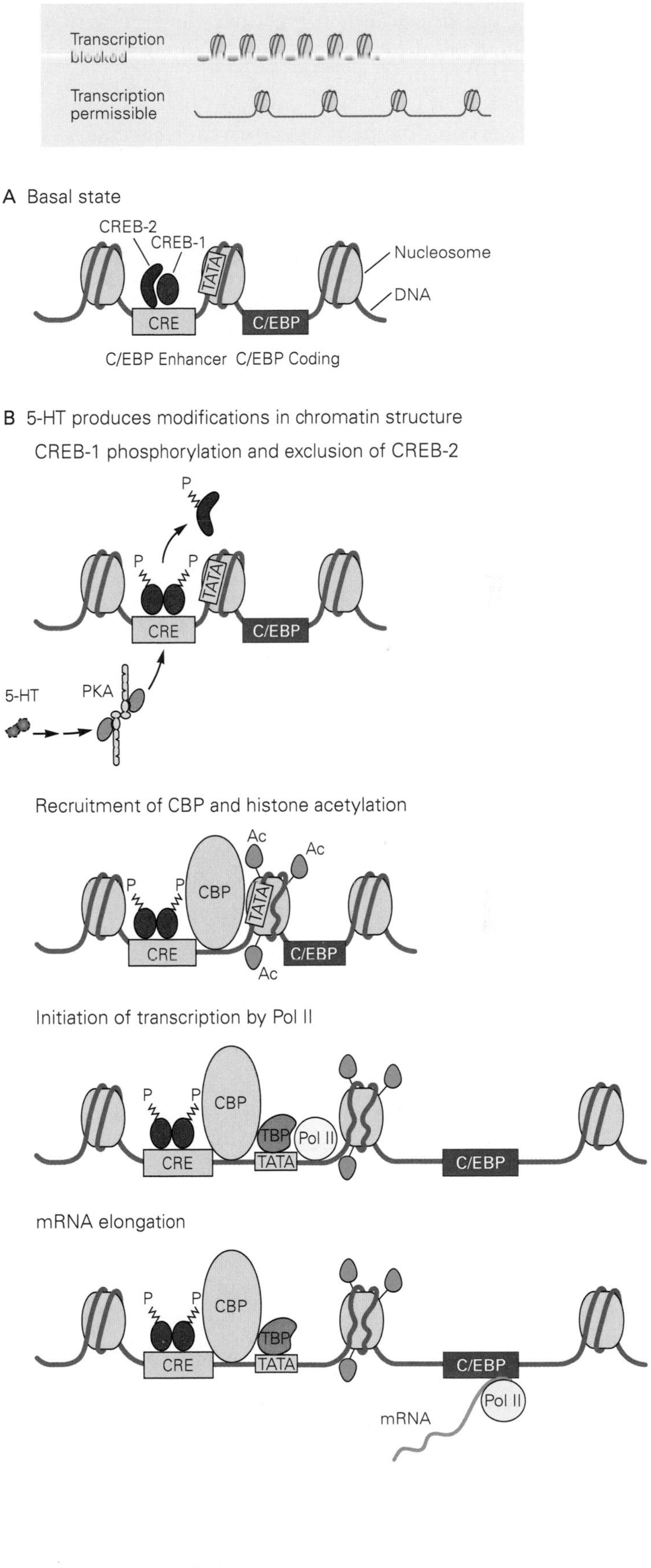

Figure 66–7 Regulation of histone acetylation by serotonin, CREB-1, and CBP.

A. Under basal conditions the activator CREB-1 (here in complex with CREB-2) occupies the binding site for CRE (cAMP recognition element) within the promoter region of its target genes. In the example shown here, CREB-1 binds to the CRE within the C/EBP promoter. In the basal state CREB-1 binding is not able to activate transcription because the TATA box, the core promoter region responsible for recruiting RNA polymerase II (**Pol II**) during transcription initiation, is inaccessible because the DNA is tightly bound to histone proteins in the nucleosome.

B. Serotonin (**5-HT**) activates PKA, which phosphorylates CREB-1 and indirectly enhances CREB-2 phosphorylation by MAPK, causing the repressor to dissociate from the promoter. This allows CREB-1 to form a complex at the promoter with CREB binding protein (**CBP**). Activated CBP acetylates specific lysine residues of the histones, causing them to bind less tightly to DNA. Along with other changes in chromatin structure, acetylation facilitates the repositioning of the nucleosome that previously blocked access of the Pol II complex to the TATA box. This repositioning allows Pol II to be recruited to initiate transcription of the C/EBP gene. (**TBP**, TATA binding protein).

Two of the genes expressed in the wake of CREB-1 activation and the consequential alteration in chromatin structure are important in the early development of long-term facilitation. One is a gene for ubiquitin carboxyterminal hydrolase. The other is a gene for a transcription factor, CAAT box enhancer binding protein (C/EBP), a component of a gene cascade necessary for synthesizing proteins needed for the growth of new synaptic connections (Figure 66–6, 66–7).

The hydrolase, which facilitates ubiquitin-mediated protein degradation (see Chapter 3), helps enhance activation of PKA. Protein kinase A is made up of four subunits; two regulatory subunits inhibit two catalytic subunits (see Chapter 11). With long-term training and the induction of the hydrolase, approximately 25% of the regulatory subunits are degraded in the sensory neurons. As a result, free catalytic subunits can continue to phosphorylate proteins important for the enhancement of transmitter release and the strengthening of synaptic connections, including CREB-1, long after cAMP has returned to its basal level (Figure 66–6B). Formation of a constitutively active enzyme is therefore the simplest molecular mechanism for long-term memory. With repeated training a second-messenger kinase critical for short-term facilitation can remain persistently active for up to 24 hours without requiring a continuous activating signal.

The second and more enduring consequence of CREB-1 activation is the activation of the transcription factor C/EBP. This transcription factor forms both a homodimer with itself and a heterodimer with another transcription factor called *activating factor*. Together these factors act on downstream genes that trigger the growth of new synaptic connections that support long-term memory.

With long-term sensitization the number of presynaptic terminals in the sensory neurons in the gill-withdrawal circuit doubles (Figure 66–8). The dendrites of the motor neurons also grow to accommodate the additional synaptic input. Thus long-term structural changes in both post- and presynaptic cells increase the number of synapses.

Long-term habituation, in contrast, leads to *pruning* of synaptic connections. The long-term inactivation of the functional connections between sensory and motor neurons reduces the number of terminals of each sensory neuron by one-third (Figure 66–8A).

Long-Term Synaptic Facilitation Is Synapse Specific

A typical neuron in the mammalian brain makes 10,000 synapses with a wide range of target cells. It is therefore generally thought that long-term memory storage should be synapse specific—that is, only those synapses that actively participate in learning should be enhanced. However, the finding that long-term facilitation involves gene expression—which occurs in the nucleus, an organelle that is far removed from a neuron's synapses—raises some fundamental questions regarding information storage.

Is long-term memory storage indeed synapse specific, or do the gene products recruited during long-term memory storage alter the strength of every presynaptic terminal in a neuron? And if long-term memory is synapse specific, what are the cellular mechanisms that enable the products of gene transcription to selectively strengthen just some synapses and not others?

Kelsey Martin and her colleagues addressed these questions regarding long-term facilitation by using a cell culture system consisting of an isolated *Aplysia* sensory neuron with a bifurcated axon that makes separate synaptic contacts with two motor neurons. The sensory neuron terminals on one of the two motor neurons were activated by focal pulses of serotonin, thus mimicking the neural effects of a shock to the tail. When only one pulse of serotonin was applied, those synapses showed short-term facilitation. The synapses on the second motor neuron, which did not receive serotonin, showed no change in synaptic transmission (Figure 66–9).

When five pulses of serotonin were applied to the same synapses, those synapses displayed both short-term and long-term facilitation, and new synaptic connections were formed with the motor neuron. Again the synapses that did not receive serotonin showed no enhancement of synaptic transmission (Figure 66–9B). Thus both short-term and long-term synaptic facilitation are synapse specific and manifested only by those synapses that receive the modulatory serotonin signal.

But how are the nuclear products able to enhance transmission at certain synapses only? Are the newly synthesized proteins somehow targeted to only those synapses that receive serotonin? Or are they shipped out to all synapses but used productively for the growth of new synaptic connections only at those synapses that have been activated—or marked—perhaps by only a single pulse of serotonin?

To test this question Martin and her colleagues again selectively applied five pulses of serotonin to the synapses made by the sensory neuron onto one of the motor neurons. This time, however, the synapses with the second motor neuron were simultaneously activated by a single pulse of serotonin (which by itself produces only short-term synaptic facilitation lasting

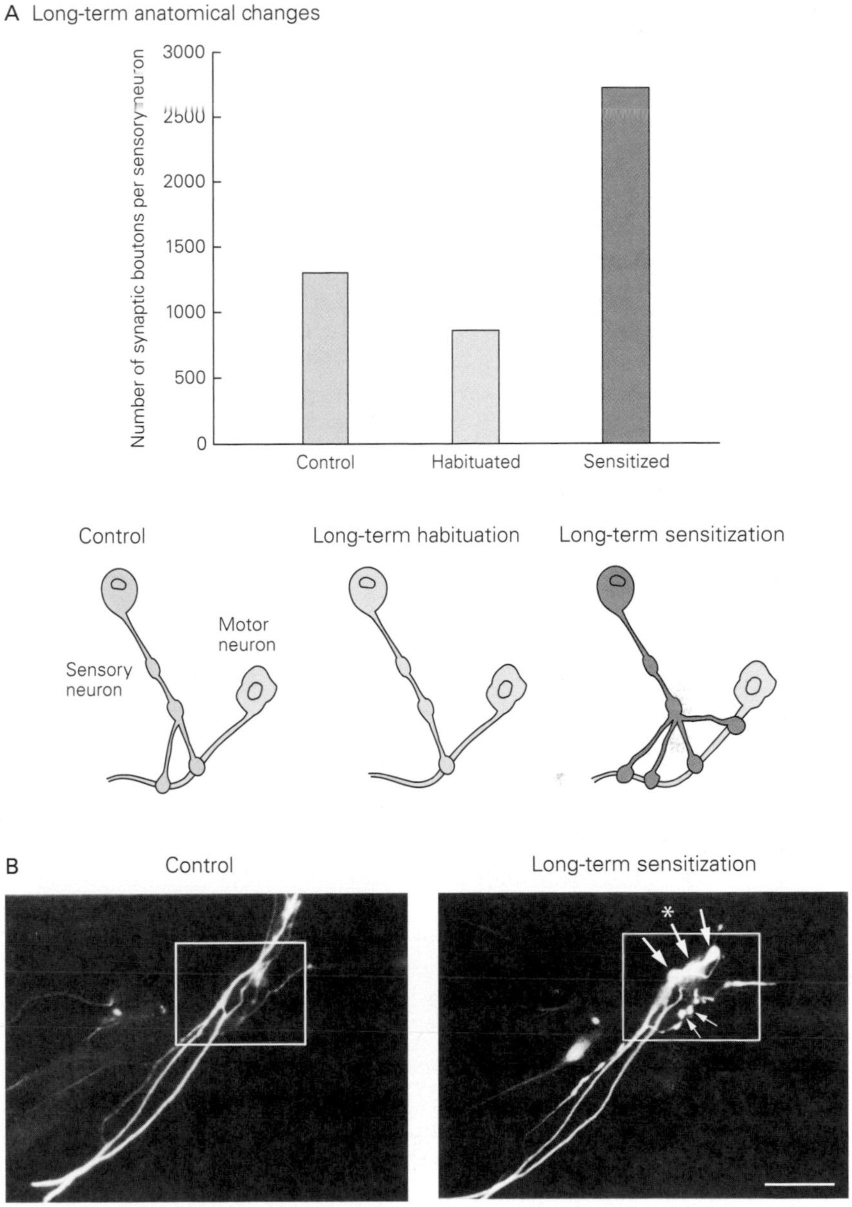

Figure 66–8 Long-term habituation and sensitization involve structural changes in the presynaptic terminals of sensory neurons.

A. Long-term habituation leads to a loss of synapses, and long-term sensitization leads to an increase in number of synapses. When measured either 1 day (shown here) or 1 week after training, the number of presynaptic terminals (or boutons) relative to control levels is increased in sensitized animals and reduced in habituated animals. The drawings below the graph illustrate changes in the number of synaptic contacts. Swellings or varicosities on sensory neuron processes are presynaptic terminals. (Adapted, with permission, from Bailey and Chen 1983.)

B. Fluorescence images of the axon of a sensory neuron contacting a motor neuron in culture before (**left**) and 1 day after (**right**) five brief exposures to serotonin. The resulting increase in varicosities simulates the synaptic changes associated with long-term sensitization. Prior to serotonin application no presynaptic varicosities are visible in the outlined area (control). After serotonin the growth of several new varicosities is apparent (**arrows**), indicative of formation of new synapses. Boutons can be seen at the arrows in the right, some of which contain a fully developed zone, identified by the asterisk, or have small, immature active zones. Scale bar = 50 μm. (Reproduced, with permission, from Glanzman, Kandel, and Schacher 1990.)

minutes). Under these conditions the single pulse of serotonin was sufficient to induce long-term facilitation and growth of new synaptic connections at the contacts between the sensory neuron and the second motor neuron. Thus application of the single pulse of serotonin onto the synapses at the second branch enabled those synapses to use the nuclear products produced in response to the five pulses of serotonin onto the synapses of the first branch, a process called *capture*.

These results suggest that newly synthesized gene products, both mRNAs and proteins, are delivered by a fast axonal transport mechanism to all the synapses of a neuron but are functionally incorporated only at synapses that have been tagged or marked by previous synaptic activity.

For a synapse to use the new proteins and mRNAs for long-term facilitation, it must first be marked by serotonin. Although one pulse of serotonin at a synapse is insufficient to turn on new gene expression in the cell body, it is sufficient to allow that synapse to make productive use of new proteins generated in the soma in response to the five pulses of serotonin at another synapse. This idea, developed by Martin and

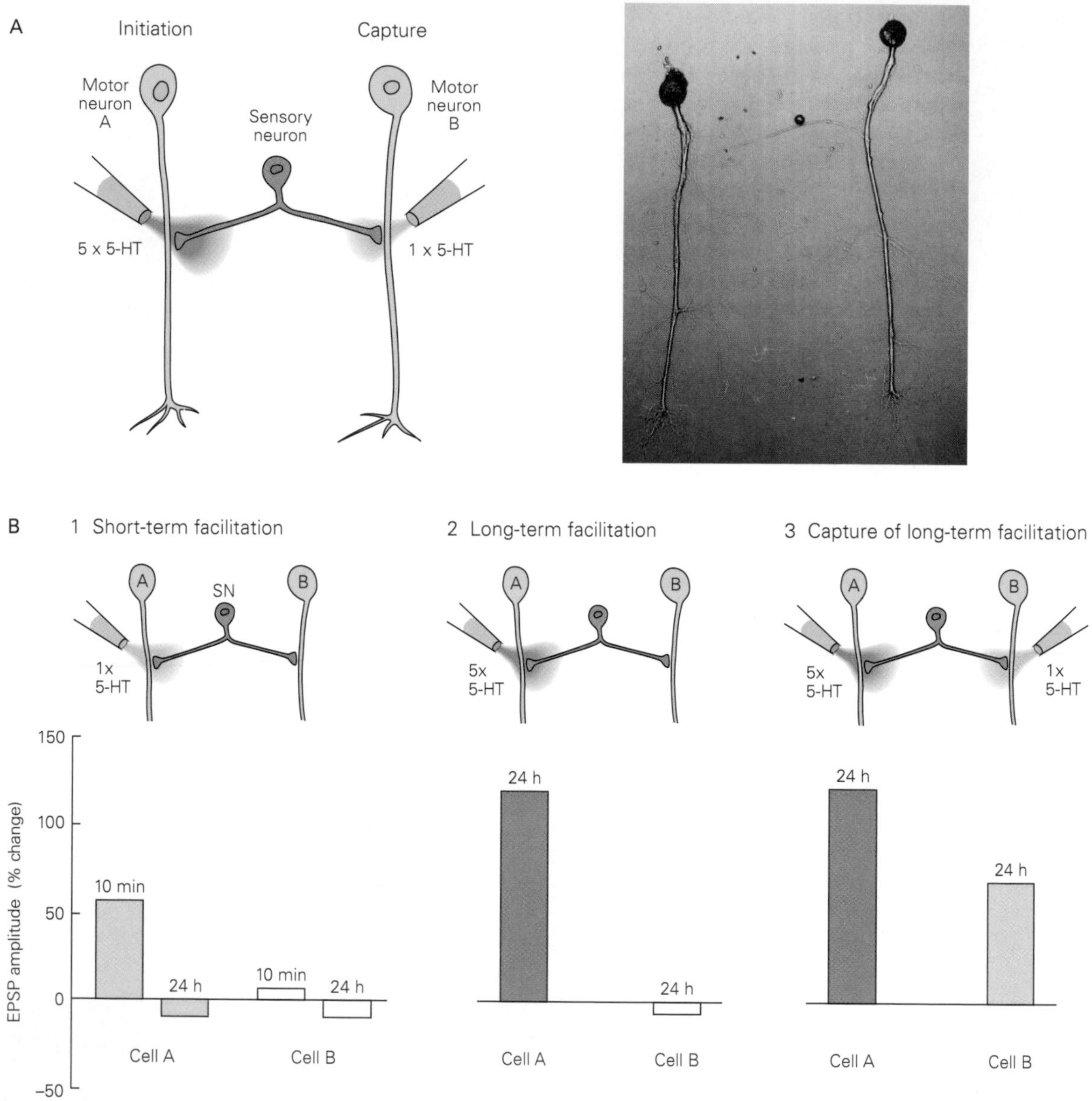

Figure 66–9 Long-term facilitation of synaptic transmission is synapse-specific. (Adapted, with permission, from Martin et al. 1997.)

A. The experiment uses a single presynaptic sensory neuron that contacts two postsynaptic motor neurons (**A** and **B**). The pipette on the left is used to apply five pulses of serotonin (**5-HT**) to a sensory neuron synapse with motor neuron A, initiating long-term facilitation at these synapses. The pipette on the right is used to apply one pulse of 5-HT to a sensory neuron synapse with motor neuron B, allowing this synapse to make use of (capture) new proteins produced in the cell body in response to the five pulses of 5-HT at the synapses with motor neuron A. The image at the right shows the actual appearance of the cells in culture.

B. 1. One pulse of 5-HT applied to the synapses with motor neuron A produces only short-term (10 min) facilitation of the excitatory postsynaptic potential (EPSP) in the neuron. By 24 hours the EPSP has returned to its normal size. There is no significant change in EPSP size in cell B. **2**. Application of five pulses of 5-HT to the synapses with cell A produces long-term (24 hour) facilitation of the EPSP in that cell but no change in the size of the EPSP in cell B. **3**. However, when five pulses of 5-HT onto the synapses with cell A are paired with a single pulse of 5-HT onto the synapses with cell B, cell B displays long-term facilitation and an increase in EPSP size after 24 hours.

her colleagues for *Aplysia* and independently by Frey and Morris for the hippocampus in rodents, is called *synaptic capture* or *synaptic tagging*.

These findings raise the question, what is the nature of the synaptic mark that allows the capture of the gene products for long-term facilitation? When an inhibitor of PKA was applied locally to the synapses receiving the single pulse of serotonin, those synapses could no longer capture the gene products produced in response to the five pulses of serotonin (Figure 66–10). This indicates that phosphorylation mediated by PKA is required for capturing the long-term process.

In the early 1980s Oswald Steward discovered that ribosomes, the machinery for protein synthesis, are situated locally at the synapse in addition to being present in the cell body. Martin examined the importance of local protein synthesis in long-term synaptic facilitation by applying a single pulse of serotonin together with an inhibitor of local protein synthesis onto one set of synapses while simultaneously applying five pulses of serotonin to the other set of synapses. Normally long-term facilitation and synaptic growth would persist for up to 72 hours in response to synaptic capture. In the presence of the protein synthesis inhibitor, synaptic capture could still generate long-term synaptic facilitation at the synapses exposed to only one pulse of serotonin for at least 24 hours (Figure 66–10B), but synaptic growth and facilitation at these synapses collapsed after 24 hours, indicating that the maintenance of learning-induced

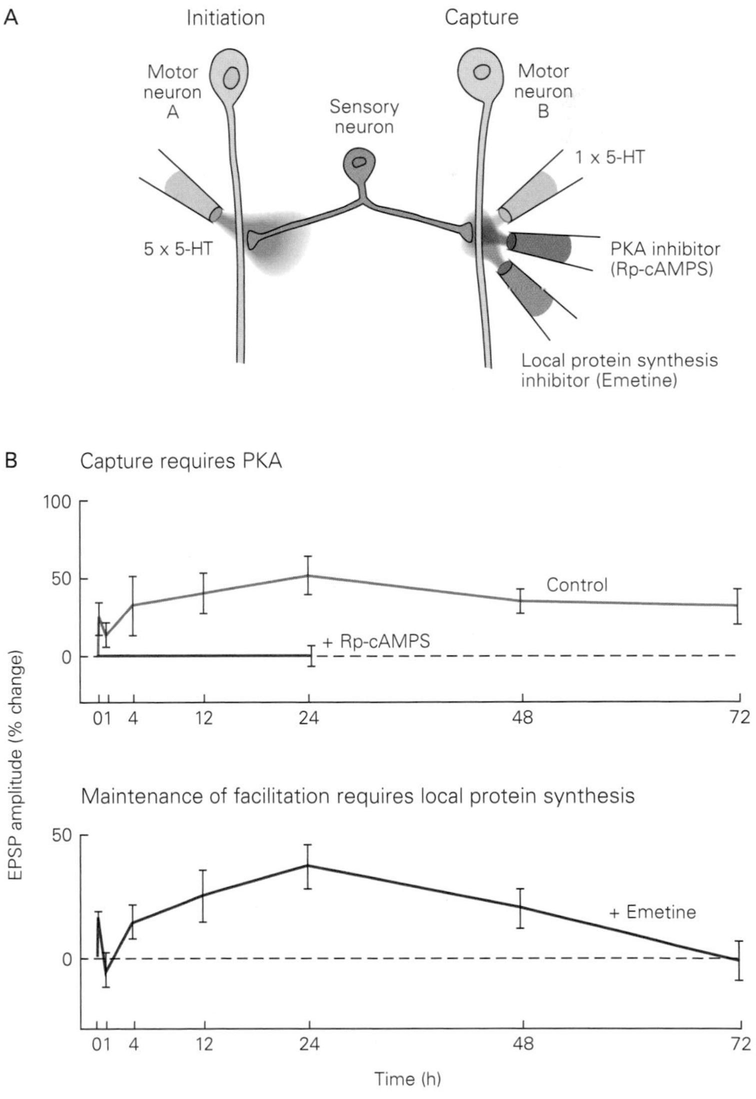

Figure 66–10 Long-term facilitation requires both cAMP-dependent phosphorylation and local protein synthesis. (Adapted, with permission, from Casadio et al., 1999.)

A. Five pulses of serotonin (**5-HT**) are applied to the synapses on motor neuron A and a single pulse is applied to those of cell B. Inhibitors of protein kinase A (**Rp-cAMPS**) or local protein synthesis (**emetine**) are applied to synapses on cell B.

B. Rp-cAMPS blocks the capture of long-term facilitation completely at the synapses on neuron B. Emetine has no effect on the capture of facilitation or the growth of new synaptic connections measured 24 hours after 5-HT application, but by 72 hours it fully blocks synaptic enhancement. The outgrowth of new synaptic connections is retracted and long-term facilitation decays after 1 day if capture is not maintained by local protein synthesis. (**Rp-cAMPS**, Rp-diastereomer of adenosine cyclic 3′,5′-phosphorothioate.)

synaptic growth requires new local protein synthesis at the synapse.

Martin and her colleagues thus found that regulation of protein synthesis at the synapse plays a major role in controlling synaptic strength at the sensory-to-motor neuron connection in *Aplysia.* As we shall see in Chapter 67, local protein synthesis is also important for the later phases of long-term potentiation of synaptic strength in the hippocampus.

These findings indicate there are two distinct components of synaptic marking in *Aplysia.* The first component, lasting about 24 hours, initiates long-term synaptic plasticity and synaptic growth, requires transcription and translation in the nucleus, and recruits local PKA activity, but does not require local protein synthesis. The second component, which stabilizes the long-term synaptic change after 72 hours, requires local protein synthesis at the synapse. How might this local protein synthesis be regulated?

Long-Term Facilitation Requires a Prion-Like Protein Regulator of Local Protein Synthesis for Maintenance

The fact that mRNAs are translated at the synapse in response to marking of that synapse by one pulse of serotonin suggests that these mRNAs may initially be dormant and under the control of a regulator of translation recruited by serotonin. Joel Richter found that in *Xenopus* (frog) oocytes the maternal mRNAs have a short tail of adenine nucleotides, poly(A), at their 3′ end and are silent until activated by the cytoplasmic polyadenylation element binding protein (CPEB), which binds to a site on mRNAs and recruits poly(A) polymerase, leading to the elongation of the poly(A) tail. Kausik Si and his colleagues found that serotonin increases the local synthesis of a novel, neuron-specific isoform of CPEB in *Aplysia* sensory neuron processes (Figure 66–11). The induction of CPEB is independent of transcription but requires new protein synthesis. Blocking CPEB locally at an activated synapse blocks the long-term maintenance of synaptic facilitation at the synapse but not its initiation and maintenance for 24 hours.

How might CPEB stabilize the late phase of long-term facilitation? Most biological molecules have a relatively short half-life (hours to days) compared to the duration of memory (days, weeks, even years). How then can the learning-induced alterations in the molecular composition of a synapse be maintained for such a long time? Most hypotheses rely on some type of self-sustained mechanism that can somehow modulate synaptic strength and synaptic structure.

Si and his colleagues found that the neuronal isoform of *Aplysia* CPEB indeed appears to have self-sustaining properties that resemble those of prion proteins. Prions were discovered by Stanley Prusiner, who demonstrated that these proteins were the causative agents of Jacob-Creutzfeldt disease, a terrible neurodegenerative human disease, and of mad cow disease. Prion proteins can exist in a soluble form and an aggregated form that is capable of self-perpetuation. *Aplysia* CPEB also has two conformational states, a soluble form that is inactive and an aggregated form that is active. This switch involves an N-terminal domain of CPEB that is rich in glutamine, similar to prion domains in other proteins.

In a naïve synapse CPEB exists in the soluble, inactive state, and its basal level of expression is low. However, in response to serotonin the local synthesis of CPEB increases until a threshold concentration is reached that switches CPEB to the aggregated, active state, which is then capable of activating the translation of dormant mRNAs. Once the active state is established, it becomes self-perpetuating by recruiting soluble CPEB to aggregates. Dormant mRNAs, made in the cell body and distributed cell-wide, are translated only at synapses with active CPEB.

Because the activated CPEB is self-perpetuating, it could promote a self-sustaining, synapse-specific long-term molecular change and provide a mechanism for the stabilization of learning-related synaptic growth and the persistence of memory storage (Figure 66–11). This proposed mechanism, albeit self-perpetuating, is different from conventional prion mechanisms, which are pathogenic (the aggregated state of most prion proteins causes cell death). By contrast, CPEB is a new form of a prion-like protein. It is a functional prion; the active self-perpetuating form of the protein does not kill cells but rather has an important physiological function.

Classical Fear Conditioning in Flies Uses the cAMP-PKA-CREB Pathway

Do the mechanisms for implicit memory found in *Aplysia* have parallels in other animals? Studies on fear learning in both the fruit fly *Drosophila* and mouse indicate that the molecular mechanisms of implicit memory are conserved throughout evolution.

The fruit fly is particularly convenient for the study of implicit memory storage because its genome is easily manipulated and, as first demonstrated by Seymour Benzer and his colleagues, the fly can be classically conditioned.

In a typical classical conditioning paradigm an odor is paired with repeated electrical foot shocks. The extent of learning is then examined by allowing

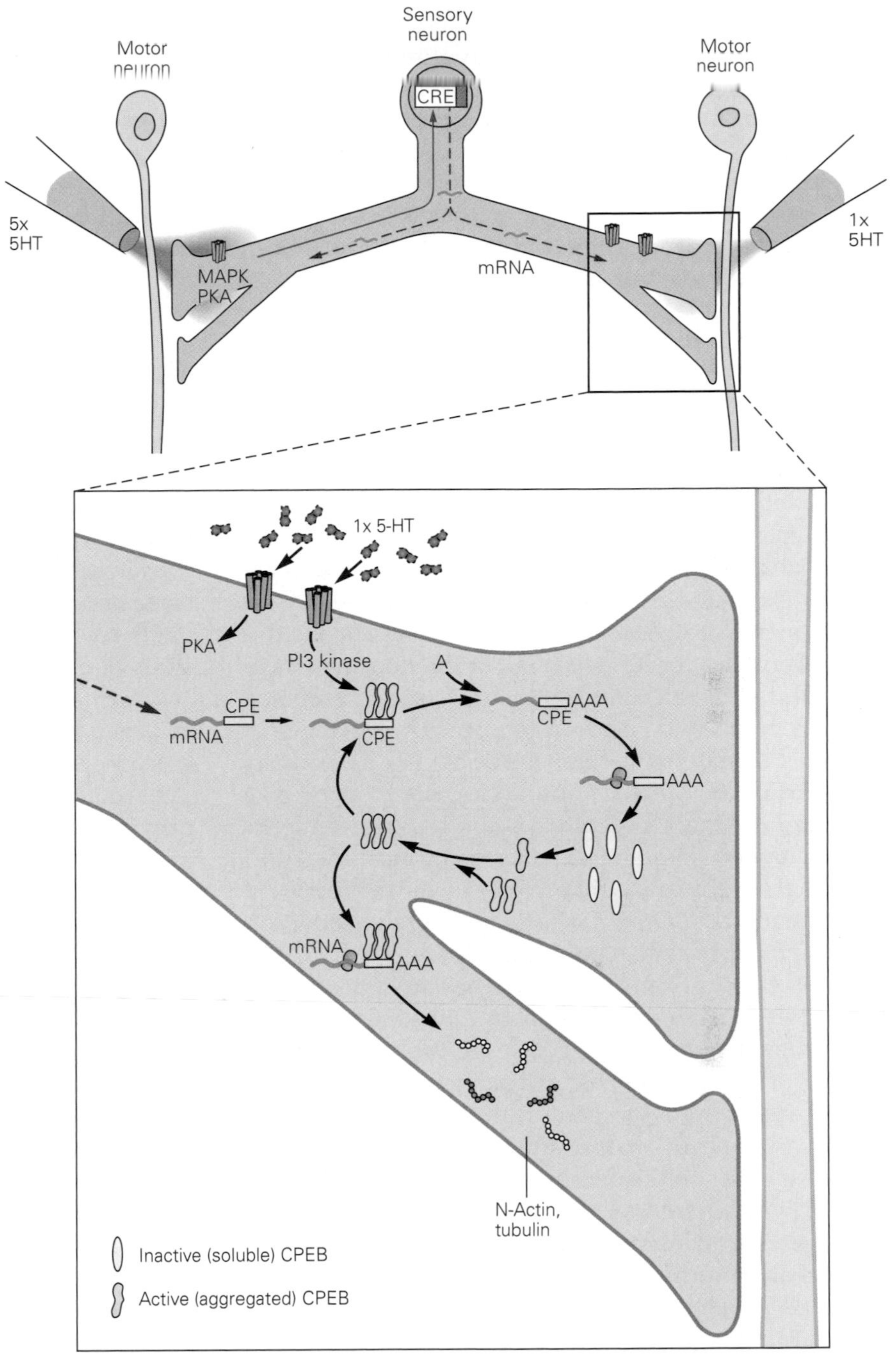

Figure 66–11 CPEB may be a self-perpetuating switch of protein synthesis at axon terminals and synapse-specific growth. According to this model (based on Bailey, Kandel, and Si, 2004) five pulses of serotonin (**5-HT**) set up a signal that goes back to the nucleus to activate synthesis of mRNA. Newly transcribed mRNAs and newly synthesized proteins made in the cell body are then sent to all terminals by fast axonal transport. However, only those terminals that have been marked by exposure to at least one pulse of serotonin can use the proteins productively to grow new synapses and produce long-term facilitation. The marking of a terminal involves two components: (**1**) protein kinase A (**PKA**), which is necessary for the immediate synaptic growth initiated by the proteins transported to the terminals, and (**2**) phosphoinositide 3 kinase (**PI3 kinase**), which initiates the local translation of mRNAs required to maintain synaptic growth and long-term facilitation past 24 hours. Some of the mRNAs at the terminals encode CPEB, a regulator of local protein synthesis. In the basal state CPEB is thought to exist in a largely inactive conformation as a soluble monomer that cannot bind to mRNAs. Through some as yet unspecified mechanism activated by serotonin and PI3 kinase, some copies of CPEB convert to an active conformation that forms aggregates. The aggregates function like prions in that they are able to recruit monomers to join the aggregate, thereby activating the monomers. The CPEB aggregates bind the cytoplasmic polyadenylation element (**CPE**) site of mRNAs. This binding recruits the poly(A) polymerase machinery and allows poly(A) tails of adenine nucleotides (A) to be added to dormant mRNAs. The polyadenylated mRNAs can now be recognized by ribosomes, allowing the translation of these mRNAs to several proteins. For example, in addition to CPEB, this leads to the local synthesis of N-actin and tubulin, which stabilize newly grown synaptic structures.

the flies to choose between two arms of a maze, where one arm contains the conditioned odor and the other arm contains an unpaired odor. Following training, a large fraction of wild-type flies avoids the arm with the conditioned odor. Several fly mutants have been identified that do not learn to avoid the conditioned odor. These learning-defective mutants have been given imaginatively descriptive names such as *dumb*, *dunce*, *rutabaga*, *amnesiac*, and *PKA-R1*. Of great interest, all of these mutants have defects in the cAMP cascade.

Olfactory fear conditioning depends on a region of the fly brain called the mushroom bodies. Neurons of the mushroom bodies, called Kenyon cells, receive olfactory input from the antennal lobes, structures similar to the olfactory lobes of the mammalian brain. The Kenyon cells also receive input from neurons that release dopamine in response to aversive stimuli, such as a foot shock. The dopamine binds to a metabotropic receptor (encoded by the *dumb* gene) that activates a stimulatory G protein and a specific type of Ca^{2+}/calmodulin-dependent adenylyl cyclase (encoded by the *rutabaga* gene), similar to the cyclase involved in classical conditioning in *Aplysia*. The convergent action of dopamine released by the unconditioned stimulus (foot shock) and a rise in intracellular Ca^{2+} triggered by olfactory input leads to the synergistic activation of adenylyl cyclase, producing a large increase in cAMP.

Recent experiments have demonstrated that flies can be classically conditioned when an odorant is paired with direct stimulation of the dopaminergic neurons, bypassing the foot shock. In these experiments the mammalian P2X receptor (an ATP-gated cation channel), is expressed as a transgene (see Box 3–3) in the dopaminergic neurons. The flies are then injected with a caged derivative of ATP. As a result the dopamine neurons can be excited to fire action potentials by shining light on the flies to release ATP from its cage and activate the P2X receptors. When the dopamine neurons are activated in the presence of an odor, the flies undergo fear conditioning; they learn to avoid the odor. Thus the unconditioned stimulus activates a modulatory signal mediated by dopamine that conveys aversive reinforcement, much as serotonin acts as an aversive reinforcement signal for learned fear in *Aplysia.*

A reverse genetic approach has also been used to explore memory formation in *Drosophila.* In these experiments various transgenes are placed under the control of a promoter that is heat-sensitive. The heat sensitivity permits the gene to be turned on at will. This was done in mature animals to minimize any potential effect on the development of the brain. When the catalytic subunit of PKA was blocked by transient expression of an inhibitory transgene, flies were unable to form short-term memory, indicating the importance of the cAMP signal transduction pathway for associative learning and short-term memory in *Drosophila.*

Long-term memory in *Drosophila* requires new protein synthesis just as in *Aplysia* and other animals. Like *Aplysia, Drosophila* expresses a CREB activator gene. Knockout of this gene selectively blocks long-term memory without interfering with short-term memory. Conversely, when the gene is overexpressed a training procedure that ordinarily produces only short-term memory produces long-term memory.

As in *Aplysia,* certain forms of long-term memory in *Drosophila* also involve CPEB and may depend on prion-like activity in this protein. Male flies learn to suppress their courtship behavior as a result of exposure to unreceptive females. When the N-terminal domain of CPEB is deleted genetically, there is a loss of long-term courtship memory. This N-terminal domain is rich in glutamine residues and corresponds to the glutamine rich prion-like domain of CPEB in *Aplysia.* Thus several molecular mechanisms involved in implicit memory are conserved from *Aplysia* to flies, and, as we will see next, this conservation extends to mammals.

Memory for Learned Fear in Mammals Involves the Amygdala

Innate fear, the ability to recognize and respond to danger, is necessary for survival. Not only snails and flies but all animals as well as humans need to distinguish predators from prey and hostile environments from safe ones. Because innate fear has been conserved throughout the evolution of species, one can readily discern and study fear in a variety of experimental animals.

At the beginning of the 20th century both Pavlov and Freud independently discovered that fear can also be learned. A previously neutral stimulus, such as a tone, can become associated with a fearful stimulus, such as a painful shock, so that the tone leads to conditioned fear, a form of what Freud called "signal anxiety." Both Freud and Pavlov also appreciated that learned fear—anticipatory defensive responses to danger signals—is biologically adaptive and therefore also conserved in evolution. Learned fear prepares the individual for fight or flight if there is even the suggestion of external danger.

From the work of Joseph LeDoux, Michael Davis, and Michael Fanselow we now have a good understanding of the neural circuits for both instinctive and learned fear in mammals. In particular, we know that both are centered on the amygdala, which participates in the detection and evaluation of a broad range of significant and potentially dangerous environmental stimuli (see Chapter 48). The amygdala receives information about unconscious fear responses (emotional state) directly and information about the cognitive processing of fear (feelings) indirectly by means of connections from the cingulate cortex.

In addition to its innate ability to respond to routine, natural threats, the amygdala-based defense system is also able to learn quickly about new dangers. It can associate a new neutral (conditioned) stimulus with a known threatening (unconditioned) stimulus on a single paired exposure and this learned fear can be remembered throughout life. The input nucleus of the amygdala, the lateral nucleus, is the site of convergence for the signals from the unconditioned stimulus (such as a shock) and the conditioned stimulus (such as a tone). Both signals are carried by a rapid direct pathway that goes directly from the thalamus to the amygdala and a slower indirect pathway that goes from the thalamus to the cortex and from there to the amygdala. These parallel pathways are important for conditioning of fear (Figure 66–12).

Long-term memory for learned fear in mammals requires CREB, as it does in *Aplysia* and *Drosophila*. In fact, in studies of the amygdala, Alcino Silva and his colleagues have found that neurons in the amygdala are recruited for long-term memory based on their basal levels of CREB expression. Neurons with large amounts of the CREB switch, required for long-term memory, are selectively recruited in fear learning. Indeed, the relative activity of CREB at the time of learning determines whether a neuron is recruited. Conversely, if those neurons with a large amount of CREB are selectively ablated after learning, the memory of fear is blocked.

Pavlovian classical conditioning modifies the strength of synaptic transmission in the amygdala. In response to a tone, an extracellular electrophysiological signal proportional to the excitatory synaptic response is recorded in the lateral nucleus. Following pairing of the tone with a shock, the electrophysiological response is enhanced because of an increase in synaptic transmission (Figure 66–13).

What causes the enhanced synaptic response of learned fear? This question has been addressed by examining synaptic transmission in isolated brain slices containing the input pathways and nuclei of the amygdala. High-frequency tetanic stimulation of either the direct or indirect pathways induces a long-lasting increase in the synaptic response to these inputs (Figure 66–14). This change is a form of homosynaptic plasticity called *long-term potentiation* (LTP), which we examine in detail in Chapter 67 in connection with explicit memory and the hippocampus, where this mechanism was first identified.

Long-term potentiation in the lateral nucleus of the amygdala is triggered by Ca^{2+} influx into the postsynaptic neurons in response to strong synaptic activity. The Ca^{2+} entry is mediated by the opening of both NMDA-type glutamate receptors and L-type voltage-gated Ca^{2+} channels in the postsynaptic cell. Calcium influx triggers a biochemical cascade that enhances synaptic transmission through both the insertion of additional AMPA-type glutamate receptors in the postsynaptic membrane and an increase in transmitter release from the presynaptic terminals. The persistence of the memory for learned fear and the synaptic changes also require both cAMP-dependent protein kinase and MAPK, which activate the transcription factor CREB to initiate gene expression, much like learned fear in *Aplysia* and *Drosophila*.

Are these experimentally induced activity-dependent synaptic changes important for the induction of learned fear or are they only corollary or parallel phenomena? Two types of genetic experiments support the idea that LTP provides a cellular mechanism for memory storage of learned fear. In one experiment genetic disruption of the GluN2B (NR2B) subunit of the NMDA receptor was found to interfere both with fear conditioning and

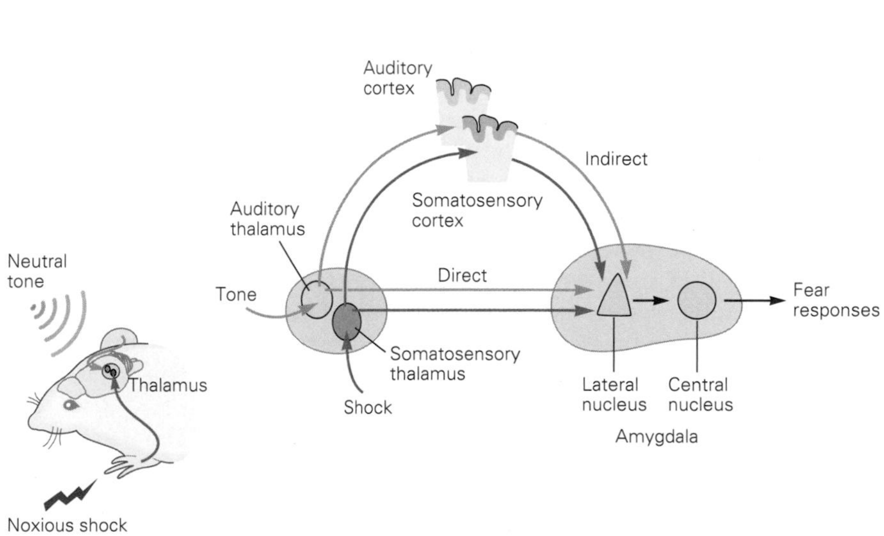

Figure 66–12 The neural pathways recruited during learned fear. The signal for the conditioned stimulus, here a neutral tone, is carried directly from the auditory thalamus to the lateral nucleus of the amygdala and by an indirect pathway via the auditory cortex. Similarly the signal for the unconditioned stimulus, here a shock, is conveyed through nociceptive pathways directly from the somatosensory part of the thalamus to the lateral nucleus and by an indirect pathway via the somatosensory cortex. The lateral nucleus in turn projects to the central nucleus, the output nucleus of the amygdala, which activates neural circuits that increase heart rate, produce other autonomic changes, and elicit defensive behaviors that constitute the fear state. (Reproduced, with permission, from Kandel 2006.)

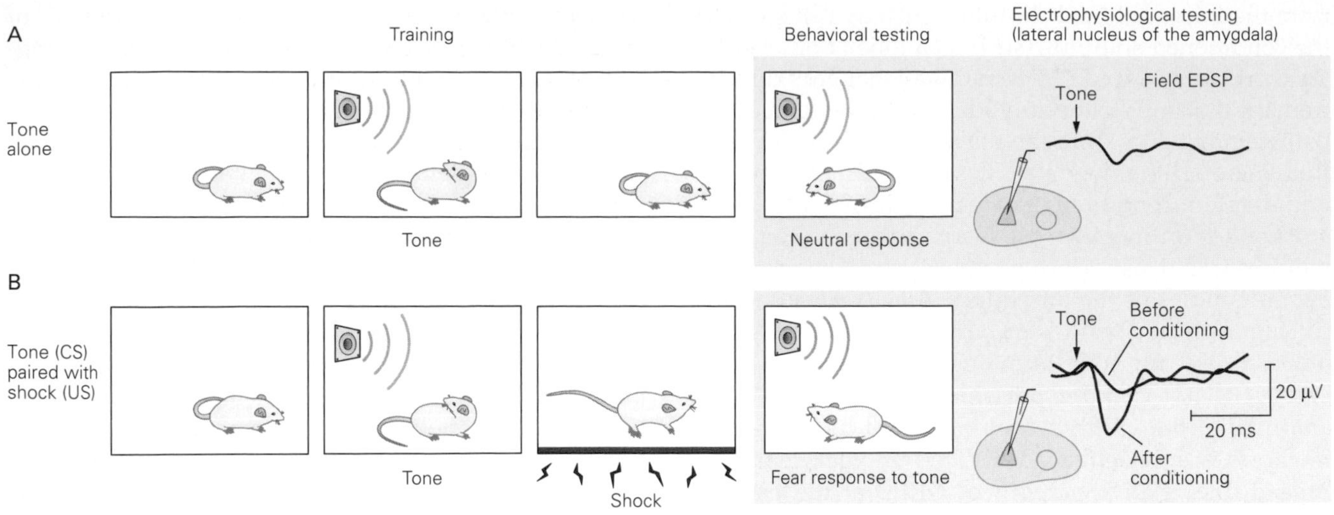

Figure 66–13 Learned fear produces parallel and correlated behavioral and electrophysiological changes.

A. An animal ordinarily ignores a neutral tone. The tone produces a small synaptic response in the amygdala recorded by an extracellular field electrode. This field EPSP is generated by the small voltage drop between the recording electrode in the amygdala and a second electrode on the exterior of the brain as excitatory synaptic current enters the dendrites of a large population of amygdala neurons.

B. When the tone is presented immediately before a foot shock (US), the animal learns to associate the tone (CS) with the shock. Now the tone alone will elicit what the shock previously elicited. Thus the tone causes the mouse to freeze, an instinctive fear response. After fear conditioning the electrophysiological response in the lateral nucleus of the amygdala to the tone is greater than the response prior to conditioning. (Reproduced, with permission, from Rogan et al. 2005.)

the induction of LTP in pathways that transmit the conditioned stimulus (tone) signal to the lateral amygdala. Moreover, this mutation affected only learned fear; it did not affect instinctive fear responses or routine synaptic transmission. Conversely, overexpression of the GluN2B subunit facilitated fear learning. Similarly, disruption of CREB signaling, a step downstream from Ca^{2+} influx, interfered with fear conditioning whereas enhancement of CREB activity facilitated learning.

Convincing evidence that LTP is important for learned fear comes from the finding that the size of the LTP elicited by electrical stimulation in slices of the amygdala isolated from animals previously trained for fear is reduced compared to the size of LTP in slices from animals that did not undergo prior fear training. This result is taken as evidence that fear learning recruits LTP: Because there is an upper limit to the amount by which synapses can be potentiated, the LTP induced by fear conditioning precludes further LTP in response to electrical stimulation. These results also suggest that artificially induced LTP and fear-induced LTP are related and are mutually exclusive.

A second line of experiments suggests that memory for a single emotional event requires the induction of LTP, and that a significant fraction of the total population of pyramidal cells in the lateral nucleus must express LTP to generate fear memory. In these experiments pyramidal neurons in the lateral nucleus were infected with a genetically engineered virus that did not damage the neurons but caused them to express AMPA receptors tagged with a fluorescent label. Fear conditioning led to an increase in insertion of the tagged AMPA receptors into the cell membrane, similar to what is seen during experimentally induced LTP in brain slices. When a different virus was used to express a C-terminal portion of the AMPA receptor that competes with and prevents the insertion of endogenous AMPA receptors, memory for learned fear was substantially reduced, even though the virus infected only 10% to 20% of the neurons in the lateral nucleus.

Habit Learning and Memory Require the Striatum

Habits are routines that are acquired gradually by repetition and are the result of a distinct form of implicit learning. A habit is a stimulus-response association, a behavior that is triggered simply by particular stimuli rather than by desire for (or fear of) some outcome.

In his classic book *The Principles of Psychology*, the great American psychologist William James characterized habit as the driving force of our daily operations—we are creatures of habit. As with all forms of implicit learning, habits are expressed in action alone, without conscious control, and not in verbal reports.

Many habits are learned early and retained throughout life. We learn to navigate through the world without conscious thought. Learned motor skills allow us to avoid objects in our path or to avoid bumping into people in a crowd. We learn through imitation, trial and error, practice and experience to dry ourselves and comb our hair after a shower, put on our clothes and even drive to work, all in a sequence that requires minimal attention. Much as proposed by Pavlov and the American psychologist Edward Thorndike, we can

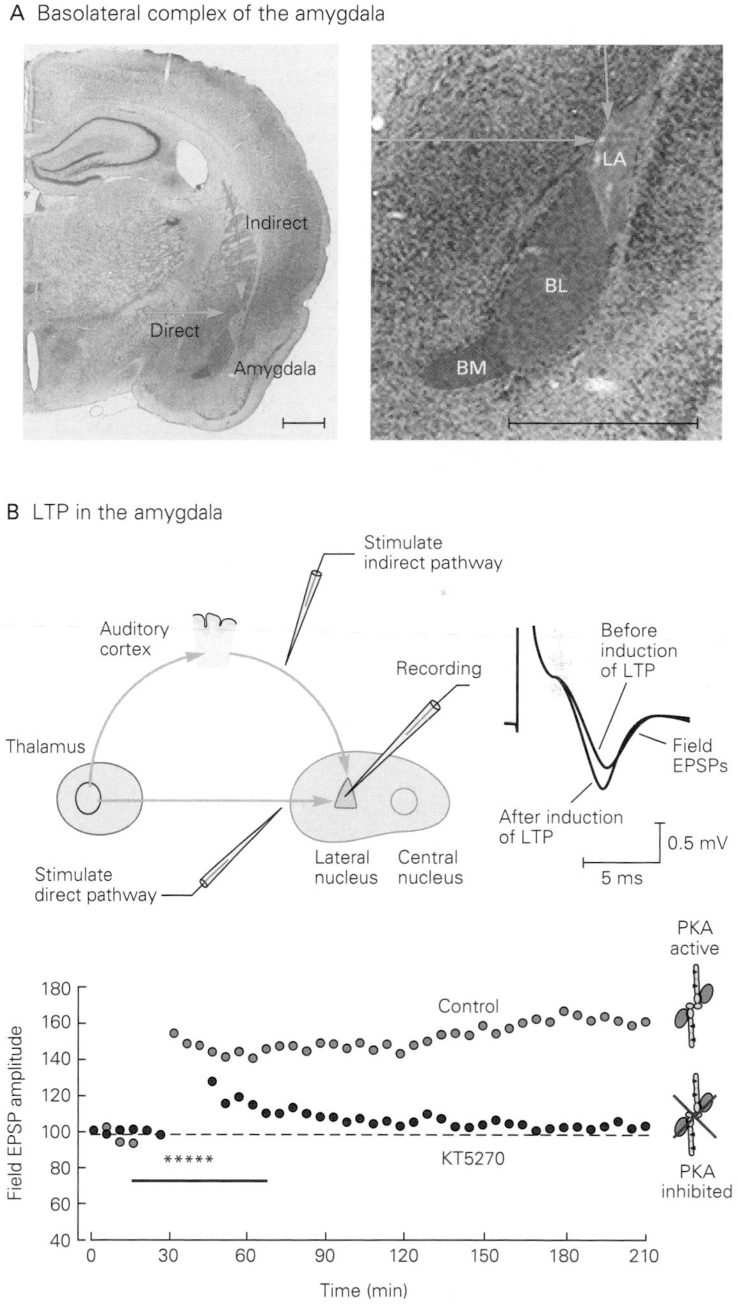

Figure 66–14 Long-term synaptic change in the amygdala may mediate fear conditioning.

A. A coronal brain slice from a mouse shows the position of the amygdala. The enlargement shows three key input nuclei of the amygdala—the lateral (**LA**), basolateral (**BL**), and basomedial (**BM**) nuclei—which together form the basolateral complex. These nuclei project to the central nucleus, which projects to the hypothalamus and brain stem. (Adapted, with permission, from Maren 1999.)

B. High-frequency tetanic stimulation of the direct or indirect pathway to the lateral nucleus initiates long-term potentiation (**LTP**). The drawing shows the position of the extracellular voltage recording electrode in the lateral nucleus, and the positions of two stimulating electrodes used to activate either the direct pathway (from the thalamus) or the indirect pathway (via the auditory cortex). The plot shows the amplitude of the extracellular field EPSP in response to stimulation of the indirect cortical pathway during the time course of the experiment. When a pathway is stimulated at a low frequency (once every 30 seconds), the field EPSP is stable. However, when five trains of high-frequency tetanic stimulation are applied (**asterisks**) the response is enhanced for a period of hours. The facilitation depends on PKA and is compromised when the PKA inhibitor KT5720 is applied (the **bar** shows period of drug application). Field EPSPs before and after induction of LTP are also shown. (Adapted, with permission, from Huang and Kandel 1998; Huang, Martin, and Kandel 2000.)

build up complex behaviors by combining simpler behaviors learned through repeated stimulus-response conditioning.

Many forms of habit learning depend on the four nuclei of the basal ganglia: the striatum, globus pallidus, substantia nigra, and subthalamic nucleus (see Chapter 43). The striatum, the input nucleus, has three subdivisions (at least in humans and other primates): the caudate nucleus, the putamen, and the ventral striatum. The caudate nucleus is involved in certain forms of procedural learning, including stimulus-response associations and some forms of skill learning. It and the ventral striatum malfunction in a variety of diseases in which habit learning is disordered, including obsessive-compulsive disorder and addiction.

Striatum-based implicit memory differs from hippocampus-based explicit memory in interesting ways. Mark Packard and his colleagues demonstrated fundamental differences in the neural structure underlying the two types of memory. They tested both types of memory using the same eight-arm maze (Figure 66–15). Explicit memory was tested with a "win-shift" foraging task. A rat was placed in the maze daily and removed after it had collected food from every arm, and this was repeated over several consecutive days. The rat's task was to minimize wasted effort by remembering where it had already found food (a win); to avoid revisiting those arms the rat had to shift its focus to the unvisited arms. In performing this task the animal has to acquire and use information about single events. It must remember the specific locations it has visited on a given day. This type of learning requires the hippocampus and is impaired by its lesion. Damage to the caudate nucleus has no effect on this behavior.

The same maze was then used to teach the rat a "win-stay" strategy, an example of implicit learning. With this task the animal needs to learn to visit four of the eight arms of the maze that are identified by a light at the entrance. Only these four arms contained a food reward. Over two weeks of training the animals learned to revisit only the arms that were lit. The win-stay task, in contrast to the win-shift task, is disrupted by damage to the caudate nucleus but not by damage to the hippocampus. The two tasks are superficially similar, but the win-stay task requires the animal to learn about regularities that are constant from day to day (lit arms always contain food) rather than to remember specific events on a given day (which unmarked arms it has already visited).

Examination of such striatum-dependent learning in mice has begun to shed light on the molecular mechanisms underlying habit learning. As is the case with many forms of implicit memory, striatum-based habit memory also requires CREB. Animals with selective impairment of CREB function in the striatum show impaired striatum-dependent learning.

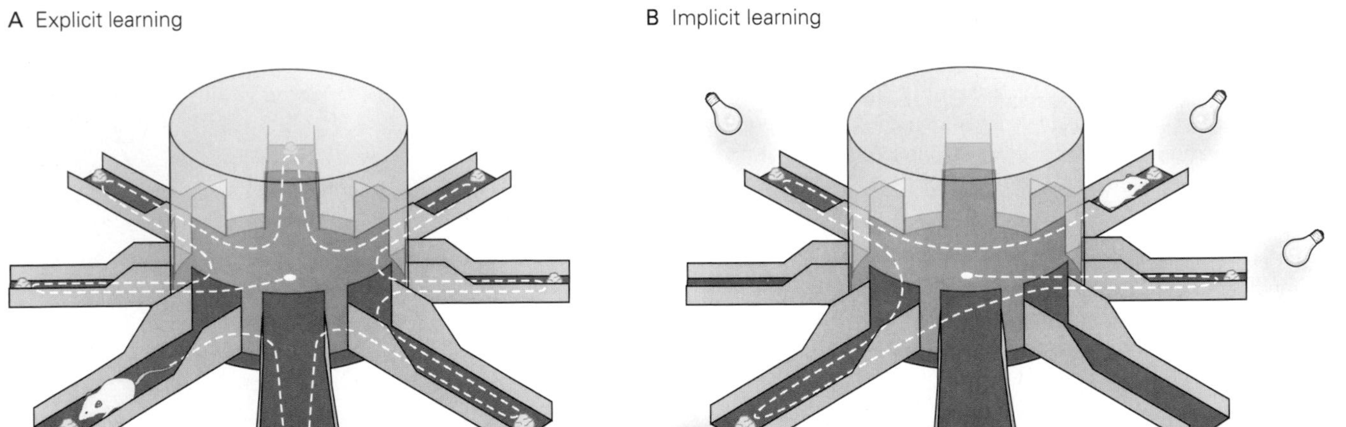

Figure 66–15 An eight-arm maze is used to demonstrate the difference between explicit and implicit learning. (Adapted, with permission, from Packard, Hirsh, and White 1989; Squire and Kandel 2008.)

A. In an explicit learning task a rat finds that food is available at the end of each arm. Initially a rat enters arms at random; with practice the animal will learn to find all of the eight morsels by entering each arm only once (by following a path similar to the one shown by the **dashed line**).

B. In an implicit learning task food is available only in four arms that are illuminated. The animal learns to visit each of these arms by associating the light with the food.

In the striatal learning system one likely locus of synaptic plasticity is the excitatory projection from the cortex to the striatum. This pathway undergoes a form of LTP that is mediated by NMDA receptors, much like that at the synaptic sites in the amygdala involved in learned fear. Like LTP in the amygdala, the persistence of LTP at corticostriatal synapses also requires CREB and is impaired in mice when CREB function in the striatum is selectively inhibited. The parallel impairment of synaptic plasticity and learning in the striatum is similar to what has been seen in *Drosophila* and *Aplysia* as well as in the mammalian amygdala, and supports the view that transcriptional-dependent alterations in synaptic strength provide a general mechanism of implicit memory.

Learning-Induced Changes in the Structure of the Brain Contribute to the Biological Basis of Individuality

To what extent do the anatomical alterations in synapses required for long-term memory storage alter the large-scale functional architecture of the mature brain? The answer is well illustrated by the fact that the maps of the body surface in the primary somatic sensory cortex differ among individuals in a manner that reflects the use of specific sensory pathways. This remarkable finding results from the expansion or retraction of the connections of sensory pathways in the cortex according to the specific experience of the individual (see Chapter 17).

The reorganization of afferent inputs as a result of behavior is also evident at lower levels in the brain, specifically at the level of the dorsal column nuclei, which contain the first synapses of the somatic sensory system. Therefore organizational changes probably occur throughout the somatic afferent pathway.

The process by which experience alters the somatosensory maps in the cortex is illustrated in an experiment in which adult monkeys were trained to use their middle three fingers at the expense of other fingers to obtain food. After several thousand trials of this behavior, the area of cortex devoted to the middle fingers expanded greatly (see Figure 66–16A). Thus practice may expand synaptic connections by strengthening the effectiveness of existing connections.

The normal development of the afferent input to cortical neurons in the somatosensory system may depend on different levels of activity in neighboring afferent axons. When the skin surfaces of two adjacent fingers in monkeys were surgically connected so that the connected fingers were always used together, thus ensuring that their afferent somatosensory axons were normally coactivated, the normally sharp discontinuity between the zones in the somatosensory cortex that receive inputs from these digits was abolished. Thus normal development of the boundaries of representation of adjacent fingers in the cortex may be guided not only genetically but also through experience. Fine tuning of cortical connections may depend on associative mechanisms such as LTP, similar to the role of cooperative activity in shaping the development of ocular dominance columns in the visual system (see Chapter 56).

This plasticity is evident in humans as well. Thomas Elbert explored the hand representation in the motor cortex of string instrument players. These musicians use their left hand for fingering the strings, manipulating the fingers in a highly individuated way. By contrast, the right hand, used for bowing, is used almost like a fist. The representation of the right hand in the cortex of string instrument players is the same as that of nonmusicians. But the representation of the left hand is greater than in nonmusicians and substantially more prominent in players who started to play their instrument prior to age 13 years (Figure 66–16B).

Because each of us is brought up in a somewhat different environment, experiencing different combinations of stimuli and developing motor skills in different ways, each individual's brain is uniquely modified. This distinctive modification of brain architecture, along with a unique genetic makeup, constitutes a biological basis for individuality.

An Overall View

A striking feature of implicit or procedural memory storage is that the recall of this memory is accomplished without recourse to conscious thought. Many aspects of personality, much of what we do in our daily life, is guided by implicit memory. These principles are consistent with a central tenet of psychoanalytic theory, the idea that we are unaware of much of our mental life. A great deal of what we experience—what we perceive, think, fantasize—cannot be directly accessed by conscious thought. Nor can we explain what often motivates our actions. The idea of unconscious mental processes not only is important in its own right but it is critical in the approach to neuroscientific studies of implicit memory storage and the resulting consequences for our individuality.

As we learned in Chapter 65, Brenda Milner made the remarkable discovery in 1954 that the medial temporal lobe, especially the hippocampus, mediates storage of what we now call explicit memory, the memory

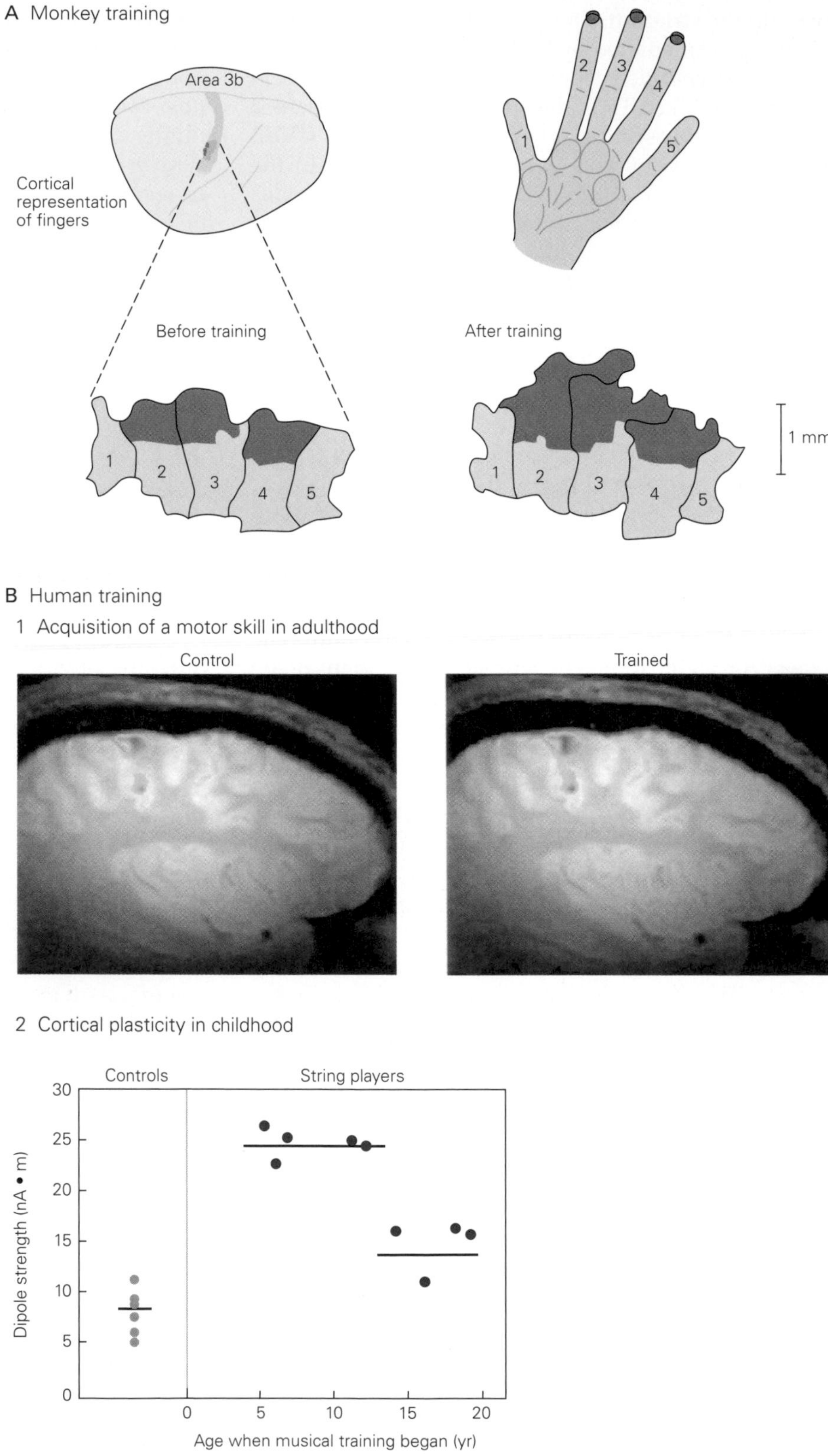

Figure 66–16 Training expands existing representation in the cortex of inputs from the fingers.

A. A monkey was trained for 1 hour per day to perform a task that required repeated use of the tips of fingers 2, 3, and occasionally 4. After training the portion of area 3b of the somatosensory cortex representing the tips of the stimulated fingers (**dark color**) is substantially greater than normal (measured 3 months prior to training). (Adapted, with permission, from Jenkins et al. 1990.)

B. 1. A human subject trained to do a rapid sequence of finger movements will improve in accuracy and speed after 3 weeks of daily training (10–20 min each day). Functional magnetic resonance imaging scans of the primary motor cortex (based on local blood oxygenation level-dependent signals) show that after 3 weeks of training the region activated in trained subjects (**orange region**) is larger than the region activated in control subjects who performed unlearned finger movements in the same hand. The change in cortical representation in trained subjects persisted for several months. (Reproduced, with permission, from Karni et al. 1998.)

2. The size of the cortical representation of the fifth finger of the left hand is greater in string players than in nonmusicians. The graph plots the dipole strength obtained from magnetoencephalography, a measure of neural activity. The increase is most pronounced in musicians that began musical training before age 13. (Reproduced, with permission, from Elbert et al. 1995.)

for people, objects, and places that is consciously recalled. In 1962 she made the further discovery that even though the patient H.M. had no conscious recall of new experiences with people, places, and objects, he was nonetheless fully capable of learning new perceptual and motor skills. This learning is stored in what we now call implicit memory, which is "recalled" only in performance and not typically reached through conscious recall.

Using the two memory systems together is the rule rather than the exception. The two systems overlap and are commonly used together in many learning experiences. Indeed, constant repetition often can transform explicit learning into implicit learning. For example, learning to drive an automobile at first involves conscious recollection; many aspects of driving eventually become an automatic and nonconscious motor activity.

Implicit memory itself comprises several processes that involve different brain systems. Acquisition of emotional states involves the amygdala; formation of new motor (and perhaps cognitive) habits requires the neostriatum; learning new motor behavior depends on the cerebellum; and simple reflex learning occurs directly in sensory and motor pathways. In different situations and learning experiences implicit memory formation depends on different combinations of these components of the nervous system. These implicit memory systems also work in parallel with the explicit memory system of the hippocampus so that with extensive experience explicit memory can essentially be carried forward by implicit memory systems.

In implicit memory, then, we have a biological manifestation of one component of unconscious mental life. How does this biologically delineated unconscious process relate to Freud's concept of the unconscious? In his later writings Freud used the term "unconscious" in different ways. Sometimes he used it in a strict way to refer to the *repressed* or *dynamic unconscious.* In this dynamic unconscious information about conflict and drive is prevented from reaching consciousness by powerful defensive mechanisms such as repression. This dynamic unconscious is what the classical psychoanalytic literature refers to simply as the unconscious.

At the same time, Freud proposed another component of unconscious activity, one concerned with habits and with perceptual and motor skills. This component fits our current understanding of implicit memory. According to Freud, an individual is not aware of most of the mental processes underlying our habits and as a result underlying these aspects of our personality. This idea is consistent with current neurological thinking that much of mental life is unconscious.

As these arguments make clear, the empirical study of unconscious psychic processes was severely limited for many years by the lack of suitable experimental methods. Today, however, biology has a wide range of empirical methods that are providing cellular and molecular insights that are expanding our understanding of a very wide range of mental activity.

Eric R. Kandel
Steven A. Siegelbaum

Selected Readings

Alberini CM. 2009. Transcription factors in long-term memory and synaptic plasticity. Physiol Rev 89:121–45.

Bailey CH, Kandel ER. 2008. Synaptic remodeling, synaptic growth and the storage of long-term memory in *Aplysia.* Prog Brain Res 169:179–198.

Busto GU, Cervantes-Sandoval I, Davis RL. 2010. Olfactory learning in *Drosophila*. Physiology (Bethesda) 25: 338–346.

Dudai Y. 2002. *Memory from A to Z.* Oxford: Oxford Univ. Press.

Hawkins RD, Kandel ER, Bailey CH. 2006. Molecular mechanisms of memory storage in *Aplysia.* Biol Bull 210:174–191.

Merzenich MM, Recanzone EG, Jenkins WM, Allard TT, Nudo RJ. 1988. Cortical representational plasticity. In: P Rakic, W Singer (eds). *Neurobiology of Neocortex,* pp. 41–67. New York: Wiley.

Sigurdsson T, Doyère V, Cain CK, LeDoux JE. 2007. Long-term potentiation in the amygdala: a cellular mechanism of fear learning and memory. Neuropharmacology 52:215–227.

Tubon CT Jr, Yin JCP. 2008. CREB responsive transcription and memory formation. In: Dudek SM (ed). *Transcriptional Regulation by Neuronal Activity , Part III,* pp. 377–397. New York: Springer.

References

Bailey CH, Chen MC. 1983. Morphological basis of long-term habituation and sensitization in *Aplysia.* Science 220: 91–93.

Bear MF, Connors BW, Paradiso MA. 2001. *Neuroscience: Exploring the Brain,* 2nd ed. Chicago, IL: Lippincott, Williams & Wilkins.

Casadio A, Martin KC, Giustetto M, Zhu H, Chen M, Bartsch D, Bailey CH, Kandel ER. 1999. A transcient, neuron-wide form of CREB-mediated long-term facilitation can be stabilized at specfic synapses by local protein synthesis. Cell 99:221–237.

Castellucci VF, Carew TJ, Kandel ER. 1978. Cellular analysis of long-term habituation of the gill-withdrawal reflex in *Aplysia californica*. Science 202:1306–1308.

Castellucci VF, Kandel ER. 1974. A quantal analysis of the synaptic depression underlying habituation of the gill-withdrawal reflex in *Aplysia*. Proc Natl Acad Sci U S A 71:5004–5008.

Claridge-Chang A, Roorda RD, Vrontou E, Sjulson L, Li H, Hirsh J, Miesenböck G. 2009. Writing memories with light-addressable reinforcement circuitry. Cell 139:405–415.

Eichenbaum H, Cohen NJ. 2001. *From Conditioning to Conscious Recollection: Memory Systems of the Brain*. Oxford: Oxford Univ. Press.

Elbert T, Pantev C, Wienbruch C, Rockstroh B, Taub E. 1995. Increased cortical representation of the fingers of the left hand in string players. Science 270:305–307.

Glanzman DL, Kandel ER, Schacher S. 1990. Target-dependent structural changes accompanying long-term synaptic facilitation in *Aplysia* neurons. Science 249:799–802.

Guan Z, Giustetto M, Lomvardas S, Kim J-H, Miniaci MC, Schwartz JH, Thanos D, Kandel ER. 2002. Integration of long-term–memory-related synaptic plasticity involves bidirectional regulation of gene expression and chromatin structure. Cell 111:483–493.

Hawkins RD, Abrams TW, Carew TJ, Kandel ER. 1983. A cellular mechanism of classical conditioning in *Aplysia:* Activity-dependent amplification of presynaptic facilitation. Science 219:400–405.

Hegde AN, Inokuchi K, Pei W, Casadio A, Ghirardi M, Chain DG, Martin KC, Kandel ER, Schwartz JH. 1997. Ubiquitin C-terminal hydrolase is an immediate-early gene essential for long-term facilitation in *Aplysia*. Cell 89:115–126.

Huang YY, Kandel ER. 1998. Postsynaptic induction and PKA-dependent expression of LTP in the lateral amygdala. Neuron 21:169–178.

Huang YY, Martin KC, Kandel ER. 2000. Both protein kinase A and mitogen-activated protein kinase are required in the amygdala for the macromolecular synthesis-dependent late phase of long-term potentiation. J Neurosci 20:6317–6325.

Jenkins WM, Merzenich MM, Ochs MT, Allard T, Guic-Robles E. 1990. Functional reorganization of primary somatosensory cortex in adult owl monkeys after behaviorally controlled tactile stimulation. J Neurophysiol 63:82–104.

Kandel ER. 2001. The molecular biology of memory storage: a dialogue between genes and synapses. Science 294:1030–1038.

Kandel ER. 2006. *In Search of Memory: The Emergence of a New Science of Mind*. New York: WW Norton.

Karni A, Meyer G, Rey-Hipolito C, Jezzard P, Adams MM, Turner R, Ungerleider LG. 1998. The acquisition of skilled motor performance: fast and slow experience-driven changes in primary motor cortex. Proc Natl Acad Sci U S A 95:861–868.

Keleman K, Krüttner S, Alenius M, Dickson BJ. 2007. Function of the *Drosophila* CPEB protein Orb2 in long-term courtship memory. Nat Neurosci 10:1587– 1593.

Klein M, Kandel ER. 1980. Mechanism of calcium current modulation underlying presynaptic facilitation and behavioral sensitization in *Aplysia*. Proc Natl Acad Sci U S A 77:6912–6.

Maren S. 1999. Long-term potentiation in the amygdala: a mechanism for emotional learning and memory. Trends Neurosci 22:561–567.

Martin KC, Casadio A, Zhu H, Yaping E, Rose JC, Chen M, Bailey CH, Kandel ER. 1997. Synapse-specific, long-term facilitation of *Aplysia* sensory to motor synapses: a function for local protein synthesis in memory storage. Cell 91:927–938.

McDonald RJ, White NM. 1993. A triple dissociation of memory systems: hippocampus, amygdala, and dorsal striatum. Behav Neurosci 107:3–22.

Packard MG, Hirsh R, White NM. 1989. Differential effects of fornix and caudate nucleus lesions on two radial maze tasks: evidence for multiple memory systems. J Neurosci 9:1465–1472.

Pavlov IP. 1927. *Conditioned Reflexes: An Investigation of the Physiological Activity of the Cerebral Cortex*. GV Anrep (transl). Oxford: Oxford Univ. Press.

Pinsker H, Kupferman I, Castelucci V, Kandel ER. 1970. Habituation and dishabituation of the gill-withdrawal reflex in *Aplysia*. Science 167:1740–1742.

Pittenger C, Fasano S, Mazzocchi-Jones D, Dunnett SB, Kandel ER, Brambilla R. 2006. Impaired bidirectional synaptic plasticity and procedural memory formation in striatum-specific cAMP response element-binding protein-deficient mice. J Neurosci 261:2808–2813.

Rogan MT, Leon KS, Perez DL, Kandel ER. 2005. Distinct neural signatures for safety and danger in the amygdala and striatum of the mouse. Neuron 46:309–20.

Si K, Giustetto M, Etkin A, Hsu R, Janisiewicz AM, Miniaci MC, Kim JH, Zhu H, Kandel ER. 2003. A neuronal isoform of CPEB regulates local protein synthesis and stabilizes synapse-specific long-term facilitation in *Aplysia*. Cell 115:893–904.

Si K, Lindquist S, Kandel ER. 2003. A neuronal isoform of the *Aplysia* CPEB has prion-like properties. Cell 115:879–891.

Spencer AW, Thompson RF, Nielson DR Jr. 1966. Response decrement of the flexion reflex in the acute spinal cat and transient restoration by strong stimuli. J Neurophysiol 29:240–252.

Squire LR, Kandel ER. 2008. *Memory: From Mind to Molecules*, 2nd ed. Greenwood Village: Roberts & Co.

Yin JCP, Wallach JS, Del Vecchio M, Wilder EL, Zhuo H, Quinn WG, Tully T. 1994. Induction of a dominant negative CREB transgene specifically blocks long-term memory in *Drosophila*. Cell 79:49–58.

67

Prefrontal Cortex, Hippocampus, and the Biology of Explicit Memory Storage

EXPLICIT MEMORY—THE CONSCIOUS recall of information about people, places, and objects—is what people commonly think of as memory. Sometimes called *declarative memory*, it binds our mental life together by allowing us to recall at will what we ate for breakfast, where we ate it, and with whom. It allows us to join what we did today with what we did yesterday or the week or month before that.

The two structures in the mammalian brain that are critical for encoding and storing explicit memories are the prefrontal cortex and the hippocampus. The prefrontal cortex mediates working memory (see Chapter 65). Information stored in working memory can be actively maintained for very short periods and then rapidly forgotten, such as a telephone number that is remembered only until it is dialed, or it can be stored elsewhere in the brain as long-term memory. The hippocampus stores declarative information in a more stable form for periods ranging from days to weeks to years, up to a lifetime. The ultimate storage site for all declarative memories is thought to be in the cerebral cortex. In this chapter we focus on the cellular and molecular mechanisms underlying working memory and long-term storage of explicit memories.

Working Memory Depends on Persistent Neural Activity in the Prefrontal Cortex

In vivo electrophysiological recordings from neurons in the prefrontal cortex of nonhuman primates have provided insights into the neural basis of working memory. Neuronal activity is measured while the animal is engaged in a delayed match-to-sample working memory task.

In such tasks the animal is initially shown an image (the sample) and must retain the image in working memory for seconds to minutes after the initial image is extinguished (the delay period). The monkeys are then shown a test image and must press a lever to indicate whether the test image matches the sample image.

Neurons in the prefrontal cortex fire persistently during the delay period, presumably contributing to the neural representation of the image in working memory. Two major mechanisms may contribute to this persistent neural activity: the intrinsic properties of neuronal membranes and recurrent synaptic connectivity.

Intrinsic Membrane Properties Can Generate Persistent Activity

In some cortical neurons a brief electrical stimulation can lead to persistent firing that lasts for seconds or even minutes after the end of the stimulus (Figure 67–1A). Moreover, the rate of firing can be a graded function of the intensity of the stimulation. This persistent firing is not affected by blockers of fast excitatory and inhibitory synaptic transmission, indicating that it depends on the intrinsic membrane properties of the neuron.

The intrinsic mechanism underlying persistent firing has been best characterized in neurons in the deep layers of the entorhinal cortex. Normally a brief depolarizing current pulse elicits a transient burst of action potentials in these neurons. However, when the entorhinal neurons are exposed to acetylcholine, which activates G-protein coupled muscarinic receptors, a brief depolarizing current elicits a prolonged train of action potentials that persists for tens of seconds, far longer than the current stimulus.

This maintained firing depends on the opening of a type of channel termed the *Ca^{2+}-activated nonselective* (CAN) cation channel. The opening of these channels requires two simultaneous events. First, the muscarinic receptor signaling cascade must be stimulated by extracellular acetylcholine; second, there must be an increase in intracellular Ca^{2+}, normally generated by the opening of voltage-gated Ca^{2+} channels during the firing of a brief burst of action potentials. Ca^{2+} then opens the CAN channel by binding to a site on the channel's cytoplasmic surface. As the cytoplasmic Ca^{2+} level remains elevated for some time after the burst of action potentials, the inward current through the CAN channels leads to a prolonged afterdepolarization following the burst of action potentials.

If the initial stimulation period is sufficiently intense, the Ca^{2+} influx will activate sufficient current through the CAN channels so that the afterdepolarization will trigger a second round of spikes. This in turn leads to more Ca^{2+} influx, which activates more CAN channels, leading to a larger afterdepolarization that can maintain firing that far outlasts the initial stimulus. Thus these CAN channels contribute to persistent firing by participating in a positive feedback loop with voltage-gated Ca^{2+} channels. Recent studies suggest that this mechanism of persistent firing also is observed in prefrontal cortex neurons.

Network Connections Can Sustain Activity

The second type of mechanism for sustained firing depends on recurrent synaptic connections within neural circuits. In the simplest case activity is maintained by recurrent excitatory connections within the active population of neurons. A network can comprise either long-range connections between distinct regions of the brain or local circuits (Figure 67–1B). The firing maintained through such chains is referred to as *reverberatory* activity.

Another circuit that can sustain activity depends on reciprocal inhibitory synapses between two populations of neurons (Figure 67–1B). Neurons in both populations fire spontaneously at a basal level that is normally held in check by the reciprocal inhibitory synapses. However, a brief excitatory input to one population of neurons will transiently enhance their firing rate, which leads to an increase in their inhibitory output onto the second population. As a result, the firing rate of the second population decreases. This decreases the inhibitory input onto the first population of neurons, further enhancing their rate of firing.

This mechanism of positive feedback, termed *disinhibition,* can lead to firing of the first population of neurons that outlasts the initial stimulus. A network of reciprocal inhibitory connections between distinct populations of neurons contributes to the sustained firing of oculomotor neurons such as those of the goldfish, which are responsible for remembering eye position. It is likely that persistent activity during working memory involves a combination of network and intrinsic mechanisms.

Working Memory Depends on the Modulatory Transmitter Dopamine

Although the relative importance of intrinsic activity versus network activity in working memory remains uncertain, it is clear that the efficiency of working memory and persistent activity in prefrontal cortex neurons depends on the state of activation of the D_1 type of dopamine receptors. These receptors are coupled to

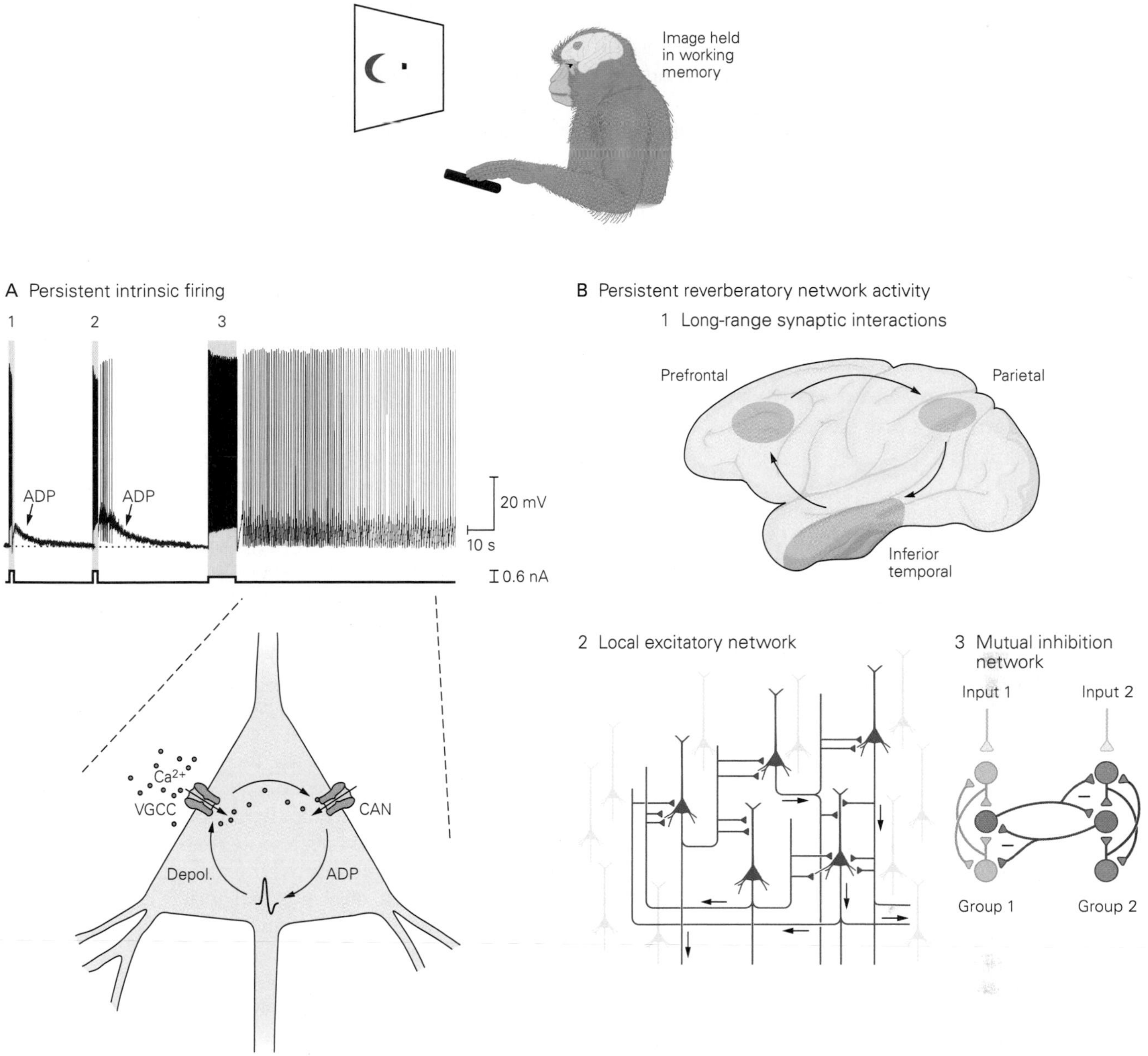

Figure 67–1 Mechanisms of persistent neuronal activity that may contribute to working memory. When a monkey performs a working memory task neurons in prefrontal cortex fire persistently during the delay period of the task.

A. Intrinsic mechanisms of graded persistent activity. A brief depolarizing stimulus to a pyramidal neuron in the entorhinal cortex elicits a short burst of action potentials followed by an afterdepolarization (**ADP**) (**1**). A slightly longer stimulus elicits a longer burst of spikes followed by a larger afterdepolarization (**2**). When the stimulus is further lengthened, the afterdepolarization is sufficient to trigger additional action potentials, leading to persistent firing for tens of seconds (**3**). The diagram illustrates a potential mechanism for the persistent firing. The influx of Ca^{2+} through voltage-gated Ca^{2+} channels (**VGCC**) during an action potential opens Ca^{2+}-activated nonselective cation (**CAN**) channels. The resulting inward current through the CAN channels produces an afterdepolarization that can lead to action potentials. The action potentials further activate VGCCs, perpetuating the cycle. The recordings were obtained in the presence of carbachol, which activates muscarinic acetylcholine (ACh) receptors and a downstream signaling cascade that enables the opening of CAN channels when intracellular Ca^{2+} is also elevated. (Reproduced, with permission, from Egorov et al. 2002.)

B. Recurrent networks of synaptically coupled neurons can lead to persistent reverberatory activity. **1**. Some network interactions occur between two widely separated populations of excitatory neurons in distinct brain regions. **2**. Other excitatory networks are local, illustrated here by reciprocally connected neighboring pyramidal neurons in neocortex. **3**. Persistent activity can be generated through mutual inhibition. This example consists of two populations of neurons, groups 1 and 2. Within each population the neurons are reciprocally connected by excitatory synapses. However, each population mutually inhibits the other. In this manner an excitatory input to group 1 leads to the silencing of group 2. The loss of inhibitory input from group 2 (a process termed *disinhibition*) in turn enhances the firing of group 1 (B1 and B2 reproduced, with permission, from Wang 2001; B3 reproduced, with permission, from Aksay et al. 2007.)

the G protein G_s and the production of cyclic adenosine monophosphate (cAMP).

Patricia Goldman-Rakic and colleagues have found that there is an inverted U-shaped relation between the extent of D_1 receptor activation and working memory: Working memory is most efficacious at intermediate levels of D_1 receptor activation. Defects in the dopaminergic regulation of working memory in prefrontal cortex are thought to contribute to the cognitive deficits associated with schizophrenia.

Explicit Memory in Mammals Involves Different Forms of Long-Term Potentiation in the Hippocampus

What neural mechanisms are responsible for long-term explicit memory mediated by the hippocampus and its associated structures in the medial temporal lobe of the mammalian brain? Unlike working memory, long-term storage of information by the hippocampus is not thought to depend on persistent neural firing but rather to involve long-lasting changes in the strength of synaptic connections.

The hippocampus receives multimodal sensory and spatial information from the nearby entorhinal cortex. The major output of the hippocampus is through the pyramidal neurons in the CA1 region, which project back to the entorhinal cortex and to the subiculum, another medial temporal lobe structure. The critical importance of CA1 neurons in learning and memory is seen in the profound memory loss exhibited by patients with lesions in this region, which has been complemented by numerous studies in animal models. Information from the entorhinal cortex reaches CA1 neurons along two excitatory pathways, one direct pathway and one indirect. Together these inputs are termed the *perforant pathways.*

The *direct pathway* has its origins in neurons of layer III of the entorhinal cortex. The axons of these neurons form synapses on the very distal apical dendrites of CA1 neurons (such perforant projections are also called the temporoammonic pathway). In the *indirect pathway* information from neurons of layer II of the entorhinal cortex reaches CA1 neurons through the *trisynaptic pathway.* In the initial leg of this pathway the axons of layer II neurons project through the *perforant pathway* to the granule cells of the dentate gyrus (an area considered part of the hippocampus). The granule cell axons project in the *mossy fiber pathway* to excite the pyramidal cells in the CA3 region of the hippocampus. Finally, the CA3 axons project through the *Schaffer collateral pathway* to make excitatory synapses on more proximal regions of CA1 pyramidal cell dendrites (Figure 67–2).

The fact that CA1 pyramidal neurons receive cortical information through two pathways has led to the view that CA1 neurons compare information in the indirect circuit with sensory input from the direct pathway. Lesion studies indicate that both direct and indirect inputs to CA1 may be necessary for normal learning and memory. Lesions of the indirect Schaffer collateral pathway limit the ability of mice to perform a complex spatial learning and memory task, although some form of spatial learning remains intact. Lesions of the direct pathway to CA1 do not appear to alter initial formation of memory, but inhibit the ability of an animal to store those initial memories as long-term memory, a process termed *consolidation*. Genetic inactivation of the direct path also interferes with episodic memory, in which an animal must learn about the temporal relation between two or more events.

In 1973 Timothy Bliss and Terje Lomø discovered that the initial stage of the trisynaptic pathway—the perforant pathway from layer II of the entorhinal cortex to the dentate granule neurons—is remarkably sensitive to previous activity. A brief high-frequency train of stimuli (a tetanus) gives rise to *long-term potentiation* (LTP), a long-lasting increase in the amplitude of the excitatory postsynaptic potentials (EPSPs) in the dentate granule neurons. (In Chapter 66 we saw how a similar form of synaptic potentiation at synapses in the amygdala contributes to fear conditioning.) Subsequent studies showed that brief high-frequency trains of stimulation can induce forms of LTP at all three synapses of the trisynaptic pathway as well as at the direct perforant path synapses with CA1 neurons (Figure 67–3). Long-term potentiation can last for days or even weeks when induced in the intact animal using implanted electrodes. LTP can also be examined in slices of hippocampus and in cell culture, where it can last several hours.

Studies in these different pathways have shown that LTP is not a single form of synaptic plasticity. Rather it comprises a family of processes that strengthen synaptic transmission at different hippocampal synapses through distinct cellular and molecular mechanisms. Indeed, even at a single synapse different forms of LTP can be induced by different patterns of synaptic activity. However, these distinct processes also share many important similarities.

All forms of LTP are induced by synaptic activity in the pathway that is being potentiated—that is, LTP is homosynaptic. However, the various forms of LTP differ in the relative importance of different receptors and ion channels. In addition, different forms of

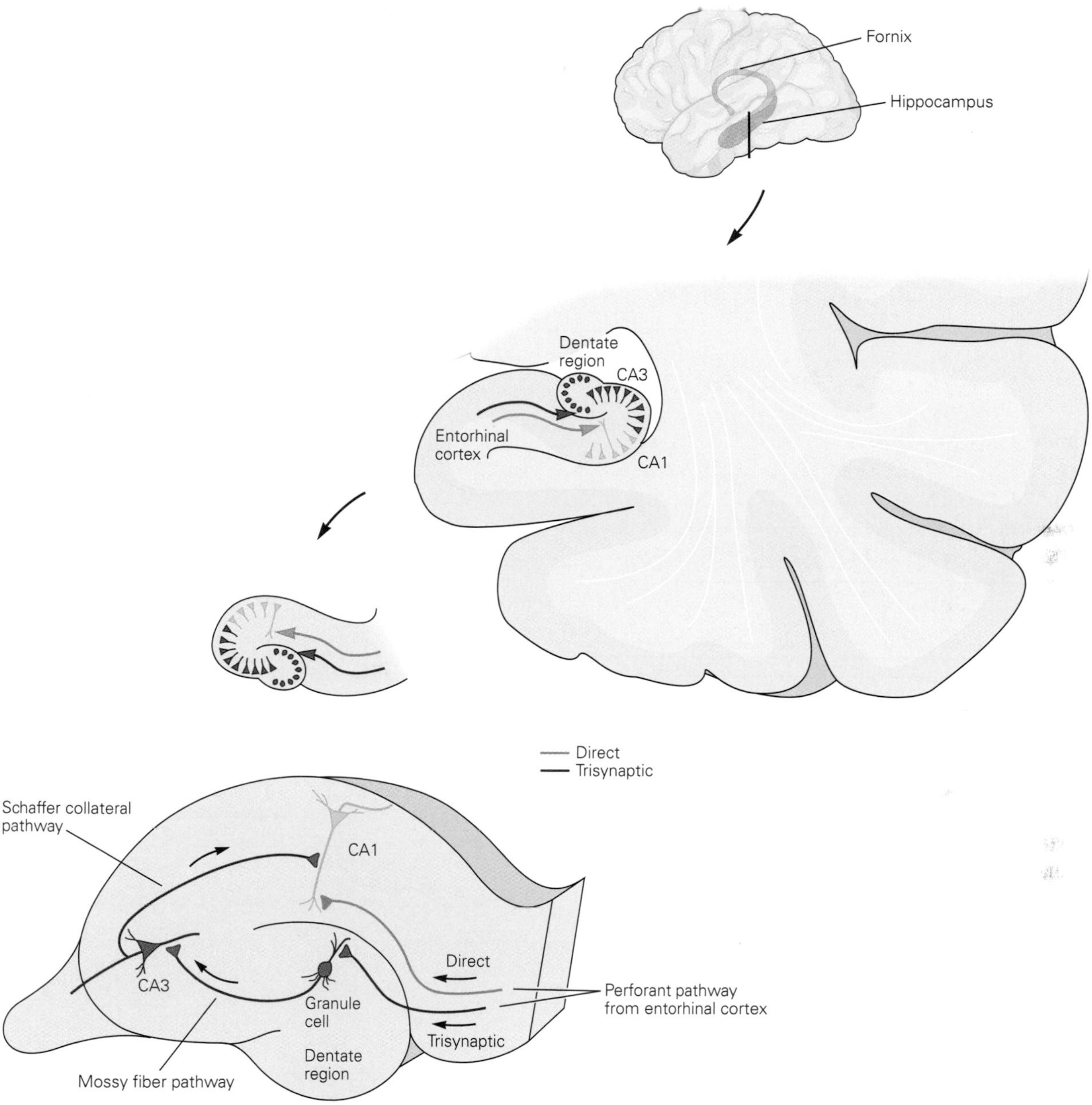

Figure 67–2 The hippocampal synaptic circuit is important for declarative memory. Information arrives in the hippocampus from entorhinal cortex through the *perforant pathways*, which provide both direct and indirect input to CA1 pyramidal neurons, the major output neurons of the hippocampus. (**Arrows** denote the direction of impulse flow.) In the indirect *trisynaptic pathway* neurons in layer II of entorhinal cortex send their axons through the perforant path to make excitatory synapses onto the granule cells of the dentate gyrus. The granule cells project through the mossy fiber pathway and make excitatory synapses with the pyramidal cells in area CA3 of the hippocampus. The CA3 cells excite the pyramidal cells in CA1 by means of the Schaffer collateral pathway. In the *direct pathway* neurons in layer III of entorhinal cortex project through the perforant path to make excitatory synapses on the distal dendrites of CA1 pyramidal neurons without intervening synapses.

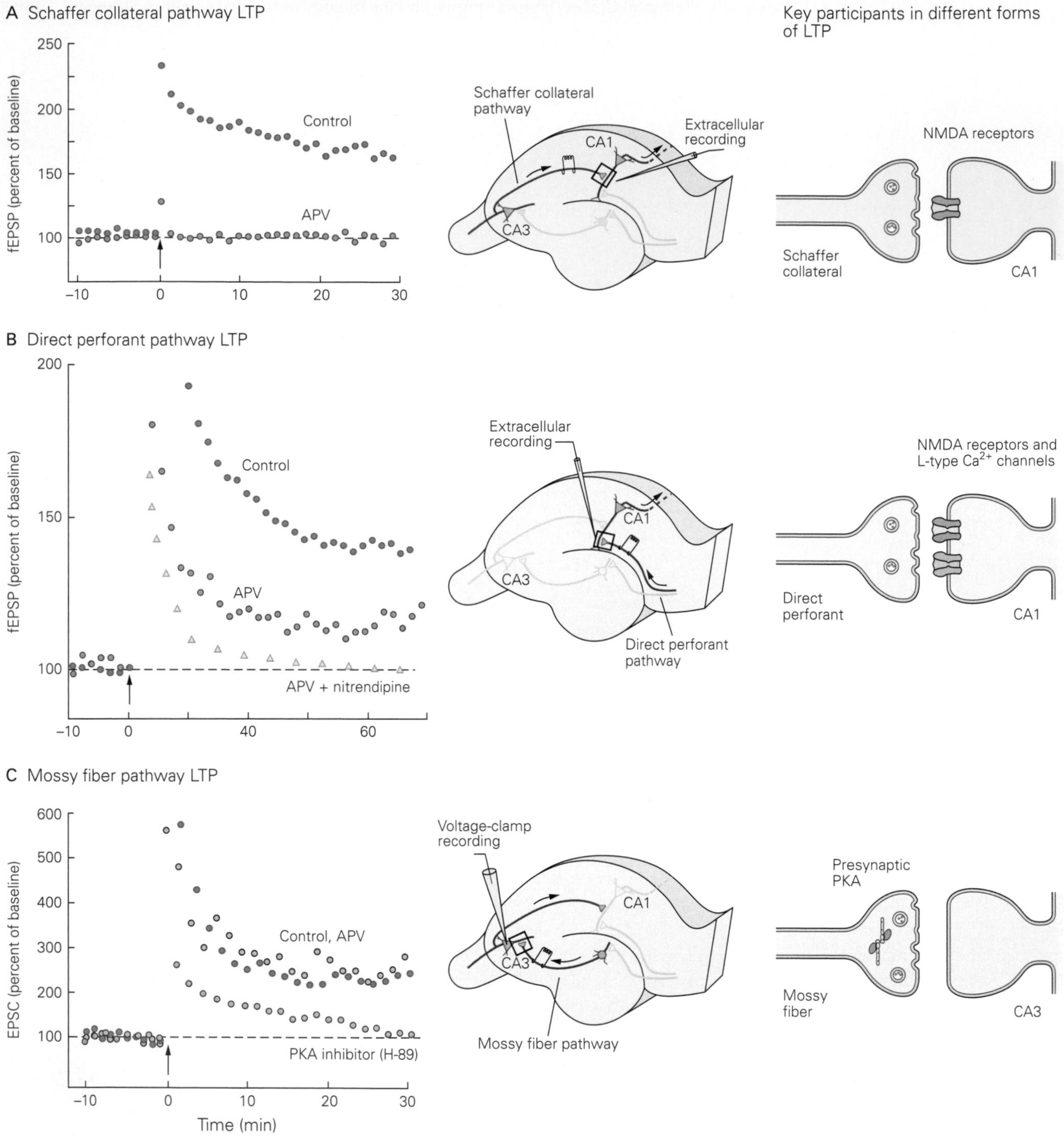

Figure 67–3 Different neural mechanisms underlie long-term potentiation at each of the three synapses in the trisynaptic pathway in the hippocampus. Long-term potentiation (LTP) is present at synapses throughout the hippocampus but depends to differing degrees on activation of NMDA-type glutamate receptors.

A. Tetanic stimulation of the Schaffer collateral pathway (at arrow) induces LTP at the synapses between presynaptic terminals of CA3 pyramidal neurons and their postsynaptic CA1 pyramidal neurons. The graph plots the size of the extracellular field EPSP (**fEPSP**) expressed as a percent of the initial baseline fEPSP prior to induction of LTP. At these synapses LTP requires activation of the NMDA receptors in the CA1 neurons as it is completely blocked when the tetanus is delivered in the presence of the NMDA receptor antagonist APV. (Reproduced, with permission, from Morgan and Teyler 2001.)

B. Tetanic stimulation of the direct pathway from entorhinal cortex to CA1 neurons generates LTP of the fEPSP that depends partially on activation of the NMDA receptors and partially on activation of L-type voltage-gated Ca^{2+} channels. It is therefore only partially blocked by APV. Addition of APV and nitrendipine, a dihydropyridine that blocks L-type channels, is needed to fully inhibit LTP. (Reproduced, with permission, from Remondes and Schuman 2003.)

C. Tetanic stimulation of the mossy fiber pathway induces LTP at the synapses with the pyramidal cells in the CA3 region. In this experiment the excitatory postsynaptic current was measured under voltage-clamp conditions. This LTP does not require activation of the NMDA receptors and so is not blocked by APV. It does require activation of protein kinase A and so is blocked by the kinase inhibitor H-89. (Reproduced, with permission, from Zalutsky and Nicoll 1990.)

LTP may recruit different second-messenger signaling pathways either in the presynaptic cell, altering transmitter release, or in the postsynaptic cell, altering its sensitivity to the neurotransmitter glutamate.

The similarities and differences in the mechanisms of LTP at the Schaffer collateral, mossy fiber, and entorhinal inputs to CA1 can be seen by examining the role of the postsynaptic NMDA type of glutamate receptor in the induction of LTP in the three pathways. In all three pathways synaptic transmission is persistently enhanced in response to a brief tetanic stimulation. However, the contribution of the NMDA receptor to the induction of LTP differs in the three pathways.

At the Schaffer collateral synapses with CA1 pyramidal neurons, the induction of LTP in response to a brief 100 Hz stimulation is completely blocked when the tetanus is applied in the presence of the NMDA receptor antagonist 2-amino-5-phosphonovaleric acid, (AP5 or APV). However, APV only partially inhibits the induction of LTP at the direct entorhinal synapses with CA1 neurons and has no effect on LTP at the mossy fiber synapses with CA3 pyramidal neurons (Figure 67–3). In the next two sections we consider the mechanisms of LTP in more detail, first in the mossy fiber pathway and then in the Schaffer collateral pathway.

Long-Term Potentiation in the Mossy Fiber Pathway Is Nonassociative

Glutamate released at the mossy fiber synapses binds to both the NMDA and AMPA type of glutamate receptors in the postsynaptic membrane of the CA3 neurons. However, under most conditions the NMDA receptors have only a minor role in synaptic transmission in this pathway. Moreover, as noted above, blocking these receptors has no effect on LTP (Figure 67–3C). Rather, LTP in the mossy fiber pathway is triggered by the large Ca^{2+} influx into the presynaptic terminals during a tetanus. In the presynaptic cell the Ca^{2+} influx activates a calcium/calmodulin–dependent adenylyl cyclase complex, thereby increasing the production of cAMP and activating protein kinase A. This leads to an increase in the release of glutamate from the mossy fiber terminals, resulting in LTP. Activity in the postsynaptic cell is not required for this form of LTP. Thus, mossy fiber LTP is nonassociative.

The increase in transmitter release is thought to depend on the ability of protein kinase A to phosphorylate RIM1α, a synaptic vesicle protein that interacts with several other presynaptic proteins important for exocytosis (see Chapter 12). Thus mossy fiber LTP is abolished in mice in which the gene for RIM1α has been deleted through genetic engineering. The importance of presynaptic protein kinase A in mossy fiber LTP resembles aspects of the synaptic changes responsible for associative learning in the gill-withdrawal reflex of *Aplysia* and amygdala-based learned fear in rodents (see Chapter 66). Another similarity with the synaptic changes in *Aplysia* is that induction of mossy fiber LTP is under the control of a system of modulatory inputs. Just as the activation of adenylyl cyclase by serotonin is important for long-term facilitation in *Aplysia,* mossy fiber LTP is facilitated by the binding of norepinephrine to β-adrenergic receptors, enhancing the activation of adenylyl cyclase.

Long-Term Potentiation in the Schaffer Collateral Pathway Is Associative

Like the mossy fiber terminals in the CA3 region, glutamate released from the Schaffer collateral terminals activates both AMPA and NMDA receptors in the postsynaptic membrane of CA1 pyramidal neurons. However, unlike the mossy fiber system, LTP in the Schaffer collateral pathway requires activation of the NMDA receptors in the postsynaptic cell, which triggers a complex postsynaptic signaling cascade.

The opening of the NMDA receptors, unlike the AMPA receptors, requires that two events occur simultaneously. First, like any ionotropic receptor, glutamate must bind to the NMDA receptor to open the channel. However, when the membrane is at the resting potential or only modestly depolarized by a weak synaptic input, glutamate binding by itself is not sufficient for the NMDA receptors to conduct ions because the pore of the receptor-channel is blocked by extracellular Mg^{2+} (Figure 67–4A; see Chapter 10). For the receptor to function efficiently, the postsynaptic membrane must undergo a significant depolarization to expel the bound Mg^{2+} by electrostatic repulsion. In this manner the receptor acts as a coincidence detector: It is functional only when action potentials in the presynaptic neuron release glutamate that binds to the receptor *and* the membrane potential of the postsynaptic cell is sufficiently depolarized.

Because of the Mg^{2+} blockade of the NMDA receptors, at negative voltages near the resting potential EPSPs are largely generated by the opening of AMPA receptors. The burst of strong synaptic activity during induction of LTP opens a large number of AMPA receptors, generating an EPSP that is sufficient to trigger a postsynaptic action potential. The action potential generates a large depolarization that is able to expel Mg^{2+} from the pore of the NMDA receptor, permitting the receptor to conduct cations and contribute to the postsynaptic depolarization.

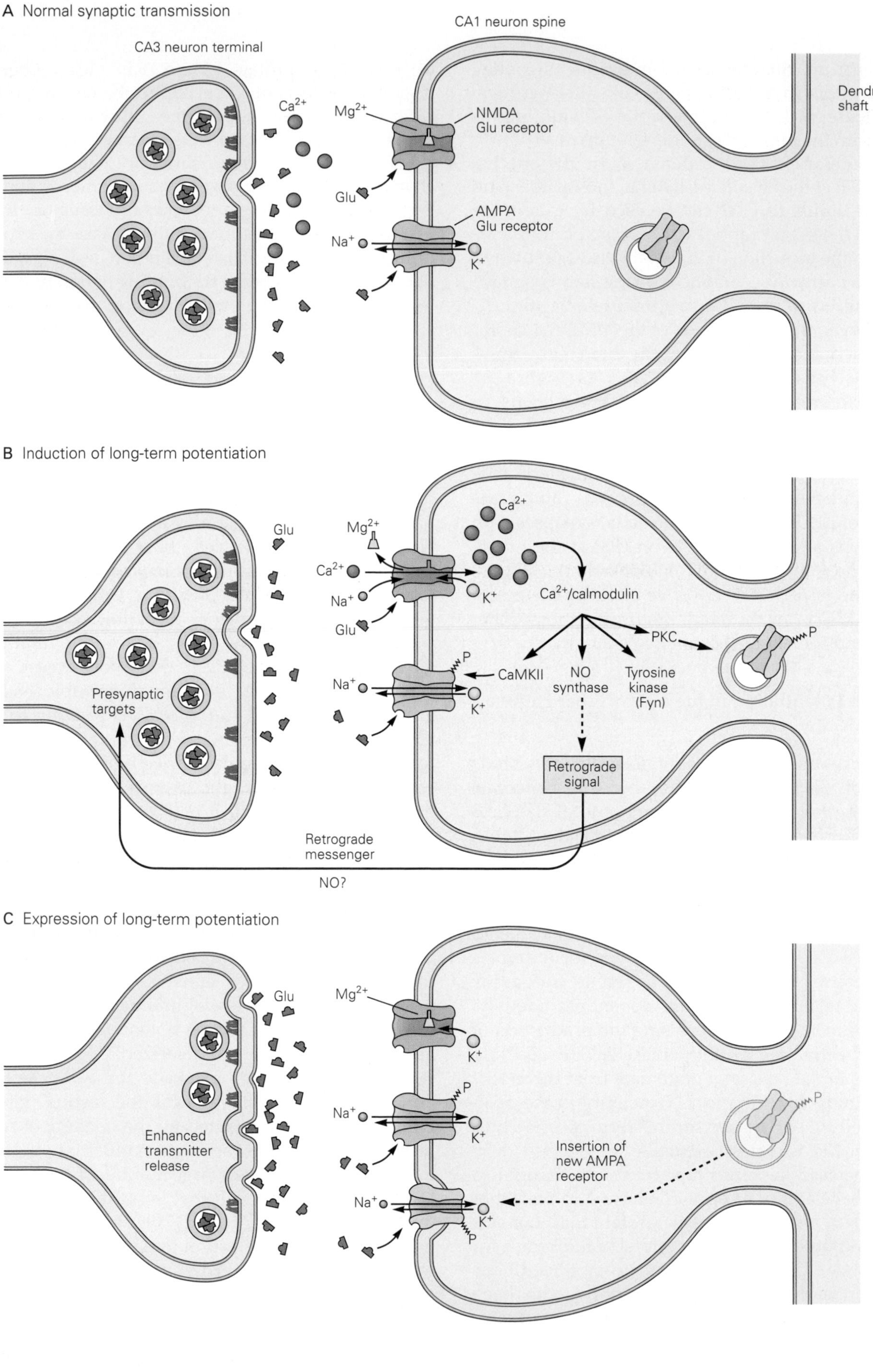

A Normal synaptic transmission
CA3 neuron terminal
CA1 neuron spine
Dendritic shaft
Ca^{2+}
Mg^{2+}
NMDA Glu receptor
Glu
AMPA Glu receptor
Na^+
K^+
B Induction of long-term potentiation
Glu
Mg^{2+}
Ca^{2+}
Na^+
K^+
Glu
Ca^{2+}/calmodulin
PKC
P
CaMKII
NO synthase
Tyrosine kinase (Fyn)
Presynaptic targets
Retrograde signal
Retrograde messenger
NO?
C Expression of long-term potentiation
Glu
Mg^{2+}
K^+
Na^+
P
Enhanced transmitter release
Insertion of new AMPA receptor

Why are the NMDA receptors required to induce LTP if the AMPA receptors are sufficient to produce a large postsynaptic depolarization? The answer lies in the fact that in addition to conducting monovalent Na^+ and K^+ ions, similar to the conductance properties of the AMPA receptors, the NMDA receptors also have a high permeability to Ca^{2+}. Thus activation of these receptors leads to a significant increase in the intracellular Ca^{2+} concentration in the postsynaptic cell. The Ca^{2+} elevation is vital to the induction of LTP; injection of a chemical chelator of Ca^{2+} into the postsynaptic CA1 cell blocks the induction of LTP. The increase in Ca^{2+} activates several downstream signaling pathways, including calcium/calmodulin–dependent protein kinase II (CaMKII), protein kinase C (PKC), and tyrosine kinases. These signaling pathways lead to changes that both enhance the response of the postsynaptic cell to glutamate and increase the amount of glutamate released from the presynaptic Schaffer collateral terminals (Figure 67–4B).

Neuroscientists often find it useful to distinguish between the mechanisms underlying the *induction* of LTP (the biochemical reactions activated by the tetanic stimulation) and those responsible for the *expression* of LTP (the long-term changes that take place at the synapse responsible for enhanced synaptic transmission). The mechanisms for the induction of LTP at the CA3-CA1 synapse are postsynaptic. What are the mechanisms involved in the expression of LTP at this synapse? Is the enhancement caused by an increase in transmitter release, an increased postsynaptic response to a fixed amount of transmitter, or some combination of the two?

Recent studies suggest that the cellular mechanisms underlying the expression of LTP vary depending on the precise pattern of activity that induces LTP. In many cases LTP that is induced solely by Ca^{2+} influx through NMDA receptors appears to be largely caused by an increase in the response of the postsynaptic membrane of the CA1 neuron to glutamate. But other patterns of stimulation elicit other forms of LTP at the same synapse and these also have presynaptic effects that enhance transmitter release.

One of the key pieces of evidence for a postsynaptic contribution to the expression of LTP at Schaffer collateral synapses comes from an examination of so-called "silent synapses" (Figure 67–5). In some recordings from pairs of hippocampal pyramidal neurons, stimulation of an action potential in one neuron fails to elicit a synaptic response in a second (postsynaptic) neuron when that neuron is at its resting potential (approximately –70 mV).

This result is not surprising as any given hippocampal presynaptic neuron is connected to only a small fraction of other neurons. However, what is surprising is that, in some neuronal pairs, when the second neuron is depolarized under voltage clamp to +30 mV, which removes the Mg^{2+} block from the NMDA receptors, stimulation of the presynaptic neuron elicits a large excitatory postsynaptic current (EPSC) in the postsynaptic neuron, mediated by the NMDA receptors. This result indicates that the two neurons were synaptically connected all along but the postsynaptic neuron contained only NMDA receptors at its synaptic contact with the presynaptic neuron. These connections are called silent synapses because they do not generate an EPSP at the normal resting potential of the cell as a result of the Mg^{2+} block of the NMDA receptors. Synapses from other presynaptic neurons on the same postsynaptic cell may have AMPA receptors in addition to NMDA receptors (nonsilent synapses).

The key finding from these experiments is seen following the induction of LTP. Pairs of neurons initially connected solely by silent synapses now often exhibit

Figure 67–4 (Opposite) A model for the induction of long-term potentiation at Schaffer collateral synapses.

A. During normal, low-frequency synaptic transmission glutamate released from the terminals of CA3 Schaffer collateral axons acts on both NMDA and AMPA receptors in the postsynaptic membrane of dendritic spines (the site of excitatory input) of CA1 neurons. Sodium and K^+ flow through the AMPA receptors but not through the NMDA receptors because their pore is blocked by Mg^{2+} at negative membrane potentials.

B. During a high-frequency tetanus the large depolarization of the postsynaptic membrane (caused by strong activation of the AMPA receptors) relieves the Mg^{2+} blockade of the NMDA receptors, allowing Ca^{2+}, Na^+, and K^+ to flow through these channels. The resulting increase of Ca^{2+} in the dendritic spine triggers calcium-dependent kinases—calcium/calmodulin–dependent kinase (**CaMKII**) and protein kinase C (**PKC**)—as well as the tyrosine kinase Fyn, leading to induction of LTP.

C. Second-messenger cascades activated during induction of LTP have two main effects on synaptic transmission. Phosphorylation through activation of protein kinases, including PKC, enhances current through the AMPA receptors, in part by causing insertion of new receptors into the spine synapses. In addition, the postsynaptic cell releases (in ways that are still not understood) retrograde messengers that activate protein kinases in the presynaptic terminal to enhance subsequent transmitter release. One such retrograde messenger may be nitric oxide (NO), produced by the enzyme NO synthase (shown in part B).

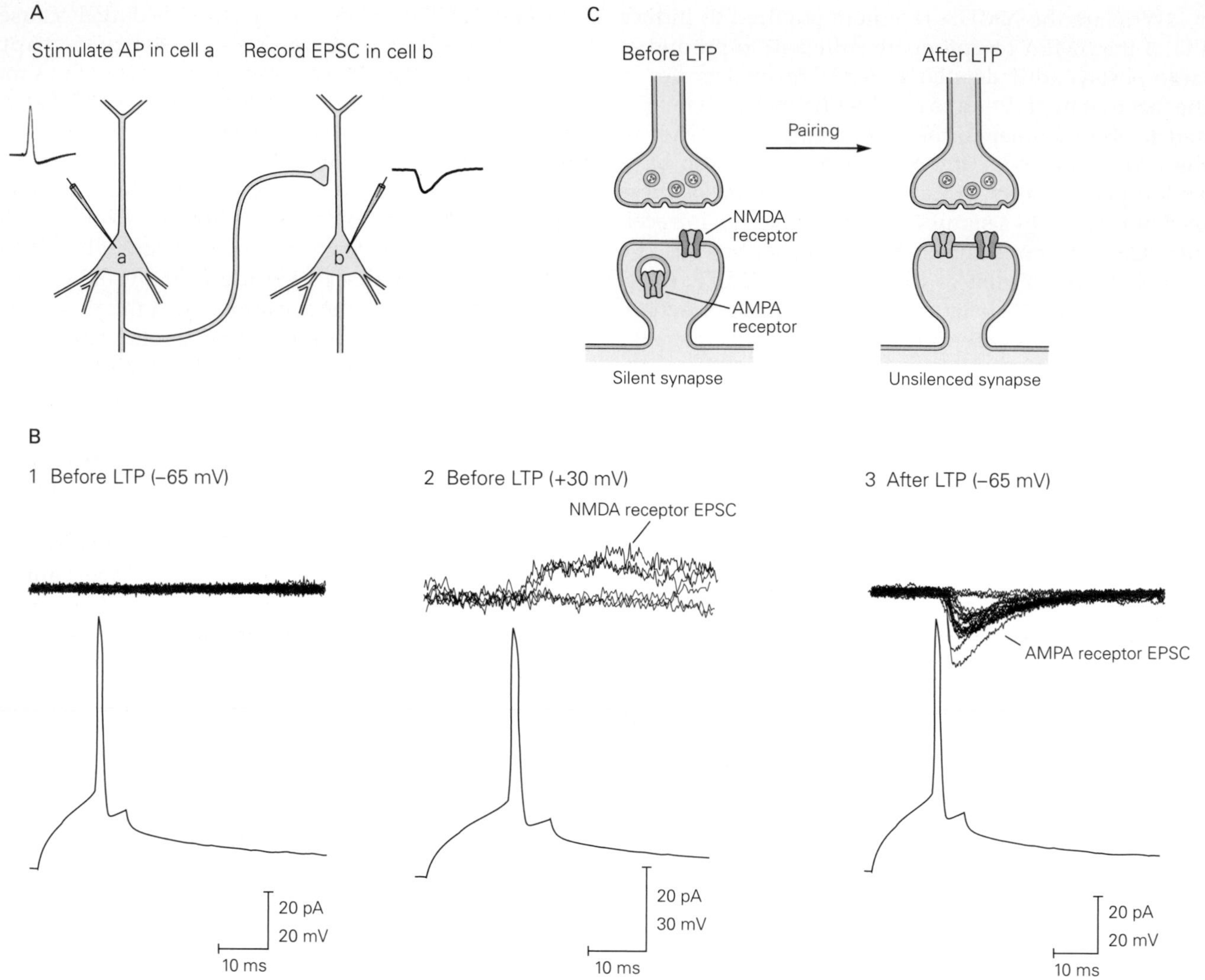

Figure 67–5 Unsilencing of silent synapses during long-term potentiation.

A. Intracellular recordings are obtained from a pair of hippocampal pyramidal neurons. An action potential is triggered in neuron *a* by a depolarizing current pulse and the resultant excitatory postsynaptic current (**EPSC**) produced in neuron *b* is recorded under voltage clamp conditions.

B. Effect of induction of LTP on silent synapses. Before induction of LTP there is no EPSC in cell *b* in response to an action potential in cell *a* when the membrane potential of neuron *b* is at its resting value of –65 mV (**1**). However, slow NMDA receptor-mediated EPSCs are observed when neuron *b* is depolarized by the voltage clamp to +30 mV (**2**). LTP is then induced by pairing action potentials in neuron *a* with postsynaptic depolarization in neuron *b* to relieve Mg^{2+} block of the NMDA receptors. After this pairing fast AMPA receptor-mediated EPSCs are seen at –65 mV (**3**).

C. Mechanism of the unsilencing of silent synapses. Prior to LTP the dendritic spine contacted by a presynaptic CA3 neuron contains only NMDA receptors. Following induction of LTP intracellular vesicles containing AMPA receptors fuse with the plasma membrane at the synapse, adding new receptors on the spine.

large EPSPs at the resting potential mediated by AMPA receptors. These results indicate that LTP must involve an increase in the response of AMPA receptors to glutamate at the previously silent synapses, a process Roberto Malinow refers to as "AMPAfication."

How does the induction of LTP increase the response of AMPA receptors at previously silent synapses? The strong synaptic stimulation used to induce LTP will trigger glutamate release at both silent and nonsilent synapses on the same postsynaptic neuron.

This leads to the opening of a large number of AMPA receptors at the nonsilent synapses, which in turn produces a large postsynaptic depolarization. The depolarization will propagate throughout the neuron to relieve Mg^{2+} block of the NMDA receptors at both the nonsilent and silent synapses. At the silent synapses the Ca^{2+} influx through the NMDA receptors activates a biochemical cascade that ultimately leads to the insertion of clusters of AMPA receptors in the postsynaptic membrane from a pool of intracellular receptors stored in recycling endosomal vesicles. The fusion of these vesicles with the plasma membrane is triggered by the phosphorylation by protein kinase C of the cytoplasmic tail of the endosomal AMPA receptors (Figure 67–4B,C).

As discussed earlier, LTP is not a unitary process even at a single synapse. At Schaffer collateral synapses LTP generated by a brief 100 Hz tetanus depends solely on Ca^{2+} influx through NMDA receptors, whereas LTP induced by a 200 Hz tetanus depends on Ca^{2+} influx through both NMDA receptors and L-type voltage-gated Ca^{2+} channels. (A similar mechanism contributes to LTP in the direct entorhinal pathway to CA1 neurons.) This high-frequency form of LTP is expressed both through presynaptic mechanisms that enhance glutamate release and through postsynaptic mechanisms that increase the membrane response to glutamate. Thus both the induction and expression of LTP depend on a family of presynaptic and postsynaptic processes.

Because induction of LTP requires Ca^{2+} influx into the postsynaptic cell, the increase in transmitter release during LTP implies that the presynaptic cell must receive information from the postsynaptic cell that LTP has been induced. There is now evidence that Ca^{2+}-activated second messengers in the postsynaptic cell, or perhaps Ca^{2+} itself, cause the postsynaptic cell to release one or more chemical messengers that diffuse to the presynaptic terminals to enhance release (see Figure 67–4B,C and Chapter 11). Importantly, these diffusible retrograde signals appear to affect only those presynaptic terminals that have been activated by the tetanic stimulation, thereby preserving synapse specificity.

Long-Term Potentiation in the Schaffer Collateral Pathway Follows Hebbian Learning Rules

The NMDA receptors endow LTP in the Schaffer collateral pathway with several interesting properties that have direct relevance to learning and memory. First, LTP in this pathway requires the near simultaneous activation of a large number of afferent axons, a feature called *cooperativity* (Figure 67–6). This requirement stems from the fact that relief of Mg^{2+} block of the NMDA receptor requires a large depolarization.

The second important property of LTP in the Schaffer collateral pathway is that it is *associative*.

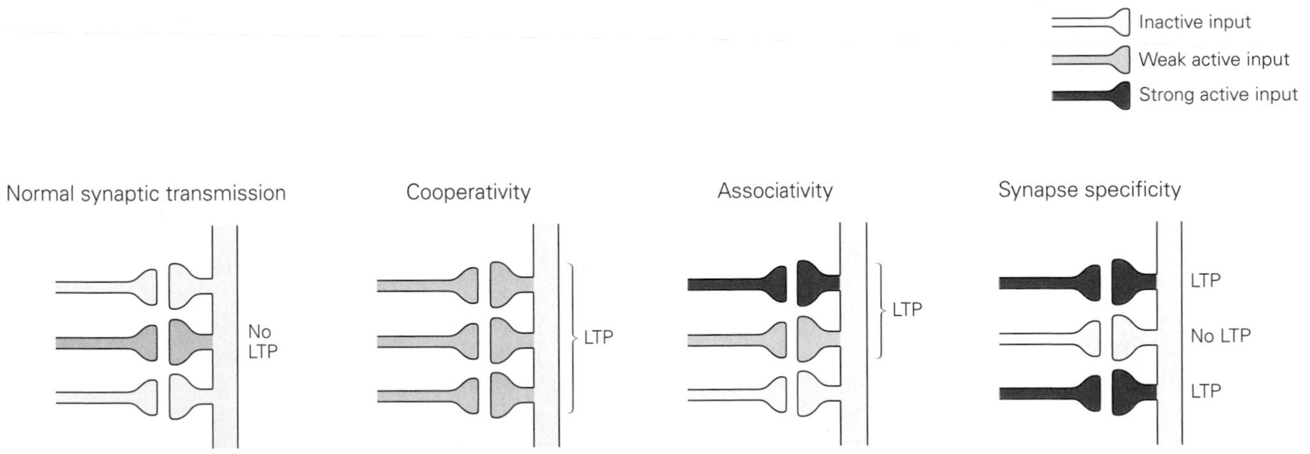

Figure 67–6 Long-term potentiation in CA1 pyramidal neurons of the hippocampus shows cooperativity, associativity, and synapse specificity. With normal synaptic transmission a single action potential in one or a few axons (weak input) leads to a small EPSP that is insufficient to expel Mg^{2+} from the NMDA glutamate receptor-channels and thus cannot induce LTP. This ensures that irrelevant stimuli are not remembered. The near-simultaneous activation of several weak inputs during strong activation (cooperativity) produces a suprathreshold EPSP that triggers action potential firing and results in LTP in all pathways. Stimulation of strong and weak inputs together (associativity) causes LTP in both pathways. In this way a weak input becomes significant when paired with a powerful one. An unstimulated synapse does not undergo LTP in spite of the strong stimulation of neighboring synapses. This ensures that memories are selectively formed at active synapses (synapse specificity).

A weak synaptic input normally does not produce enough postsynaptic depolarization to induce LTP. However, if that weak input is coactivated or paired with a strong synaptic input that does produce suprathreshold depolarization, then the large depolarization will be able to propagate to the synapse with weak input, leading to relief of the Mg^{2+} blockade of the NMDA receptors in the postsynaptic membrane at that site and the induction of LTP.

The third key property of LTP is that it is *synapse specific*. If a particular synapse is not activated during a period of strong synaptic stimulation, the NMDA receptors at that site will not be able to bind glutamate and thus will not be activated despite the strong postsynaptic depolarization. As a result, that synapse will not undergo LTP.

Each of these three properties of cooperativity, associativity, and synapse specificity underlies key components of memory storage. Cooperativity ensures that only events of a high degree of significance, those that activate sufficient inputs, will result in memory storage. Associativity, like associative Pavlovian conditioning, allows an event (or conditioned stimulus) that has little significance in and of itself to be endowed with a higher degree of meaning if that event occurs just before or simultaneously with another more significant event (an unconditioned stimulus). Finally, synapse specificity ensures that inputs that convey information not related to a particular event will not be strengthened to participate in a given memory.

The finding that the induction of LTP in the Schaffer collateral pathway requires that presynaptic activity be strong enough to elicit firing in the postsynaptic neuron provides evidence for *Hebb's rule*, proposed in 1949 by the psychologist Donald Hebb as a theoretical mechanism for how neuronal circuits are modified by experience: "When an axon of cell A . . . excites cell B and repeatedly or persistently takes part in firing it, some growth process or metabolic change takes place in one or both cells so that A's efficiency as one of the cells firing B is increased." A similar principle is involved in fine-tuning synaptic connections during the late stages of development (see Chapter 56).

The Hebbian nature of LTP is best illustrated by the phenomenon of spike timing-dependent plasticity. Under most circumstances hippocampal neurons do not produce the high-frequency trains of action potentials typically used to induce LTP. However, a form of LTP can be induced by pairing a single presynaptic stimulus with the firing of a single action potential in the postsynaptic cell. In fact, this coincidence detection is very strict. In agreement with Hebb's postulate, the pairing protocol produces LTP only if the postsynaptic cell fires a few milliseconds *after* the EPSP. That is, the presynaptic cell must fire before the postsynaptic cell. If the postsynaptic cell fires just before the EPSP, a long-lasting decrease in the size of the EPSP occurs (this long-term depression is described more fully below.) If the action potential occurs more than a hundred milliseconds before or after the EPSP, the synaptic strength will not change.

The pairing rules of spike timing-dependent plasticity result in large part from the cooperative properties of the NMDA receptor. If the postsynaptic spike occurs during the EPSP, the spike is able to relieve the Mg^{2+} blockade of the receptor at a time when the NMDA receptor-channel has been activated by the binding of glutamate. This leads to a large influx of Ca^{2+} through the receptor and the induction of LTP. However, if the postsynaptic action potential occurs prior to glutamate release, any relief from the Mg^{2+} block will occur when the gate of the receptor-channel is closed, because of the absence of glutamate. As a result there will be little influx of Ca^{2+} through the receptor to induce LTP.

These studies of the Schaffer collateral pathway indicate that two sequential associative mechanisms ensure that the induction of LTP is restricted to those synapses at which there is both presynaptic and postsynaptic activity, in accord with Hebb's learning rule. The first mechanism is the associative property of the NMDA glutamate receptor. The second is the selective action of retrograde messengers released from the postsynaptic cell at only those presynaptic sites that are active. As we saw in Chapter 66, these two associative mechanisms in series also contribute to associative classical conditioning in *Aplysia* and in the amygdala. Thus mechanisms of synaptic plasticity important for learning and memory have been conserved throughout evolution of the species at broad classes of synapses and for distinct forms of learning.

Long-Term Potentiation Has Early and Late Phases

Long-term potentiation has two phases. One train of action potentials produces a phase of LTP lasting 1 to 3 hours called *early LTP*. This component, which is the phase we have been considering up to now, does not require new protein synthesis, cAMP, or PKA activation. However, four or more trains of synaptic stimulation induce a late LTP that lasts up to 24 hours; this late LTP does require cAMP and PKA, as well as changes in gene transcription and the synthesis of new proteins (Figure 67–7).

Although the mechanisms for early LTP in the Schaffer collateral and mossy fiber pathways are quite different, the mechanisms for late LTP in the two pathways appear similar. In both pathways late LTP recruits the cAMP and PKA signaling pathway, which recruits the cAMP response element binding protein (CREB) transcription factor, leading to the synthesis of new mRNAs and proteins.

How do the synaptic mechanisms for the expression of early and late LTP differ? Quantal analysis (see Chapter 12) was used to examine synaptic transmission between a single presynaptic CA3 neuron and a single postsynaptic CA1 cell (Figure 67–8).

Prior to LTP a CA3 neuron typically forms only one functional synapse with a CA1 neuron. At this synapse a presynaptic action potential releases with low probability a single vesicle of transmitter. This weak connection between a single CA3 and single CA1 neuron means that a large number of CA3 neurons must be co-activated to trigger a spike in the postsynaptic CA1 cell. Following induction of early LTP, the probability that a presynaptic action potential will release a vesicle is increased (Figure 67–8C).

Induction of the late phase of LTP by direct application of a chemical analog of cAMP dramatically changes the response to synaptic stimulation. Under these conditions a presynaptic action potential elicits a very large EPSP through the release of multiple quanta of transmitter (Figure 67–8D). Because each release site (active zone) in the presynaptic terminal is thought to release at most one vesicle in an all-or-none fashion, the increase in the number of quanta indicates that late LTP recruits new presynaptic release sites apposed to new clusters of AMPA receptors in the postsynaptic membrane. Moreover, the formation of new synapses requires new protein synthesis, consistent with the idea that late LTP involves a growth process. Light microscopic imaging studies of live neurons in hippocampal slices provide direct evidence that LTP induces the formation of new dendritic spines, the sites of new excitatory synaptic input.

Like sensitization of the gill-withdrawal reflex in *Aplysia*, late LTP in the Schaffer collateral pathway is synapse specific. When two independent sets of synapses in the same postsynaptic CA1 neuron are stimulated

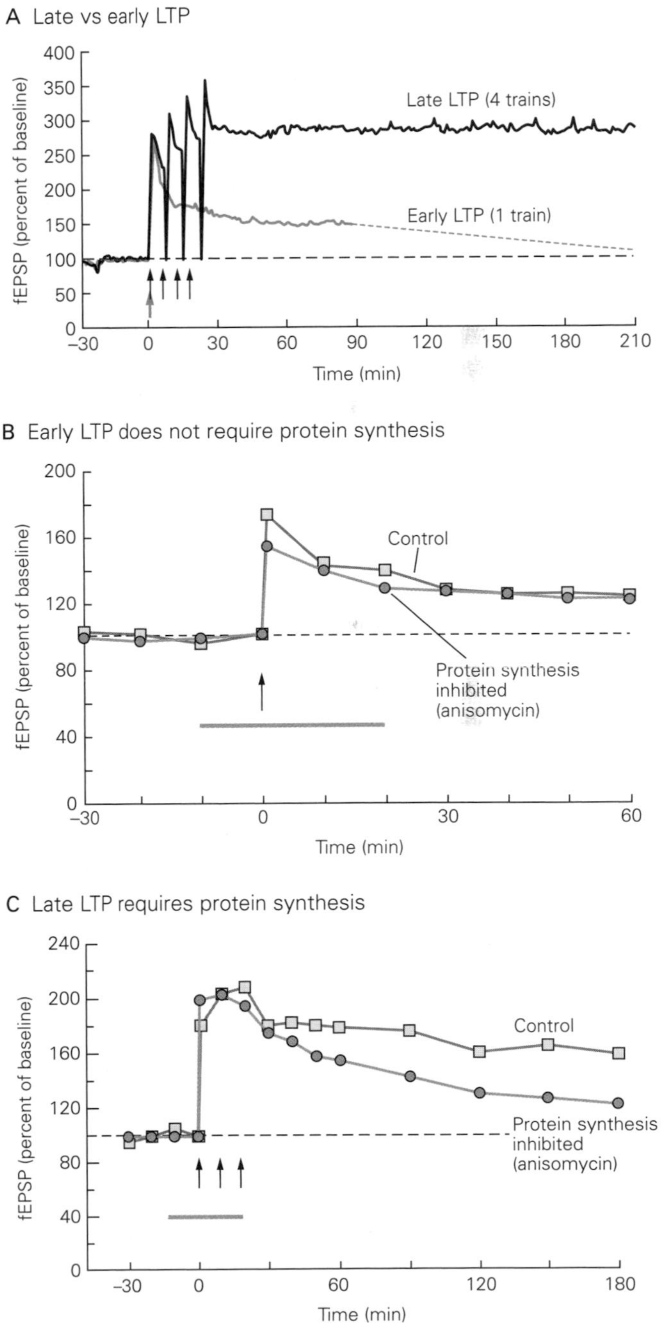

Figure 67–7 Early and late phases of long-term potentiation in the CA1 region of the hippocampus.

A. Early LTP is induced by a single tetanus lasting 1 second at 100 Hz. Late LTP is induced by four tetani given 10 minutes apart. Early LTP of the fEPSP lasts only 1 to 2 hours, whereas the late LTP lasts more than 8 hours (only the first 3.5 hours are shown). (Reproduced, with permission, from Kandel 2001.)

B. Early LTP induced by one tetanus is not blocked by anisomycin, an inhibitor of protein synthesis. Bar indicates application of anisomycin during the LTP induction protocol. (Reproduced, with permission, from Huang and Kandel 1994.)

C. Late LTP induced by three trains of stimulation is blocked by anisomycin. (Three or four trains can be used to induce late LTP.) (Reproduced, with permission, from Huang and Kandel 1994.)

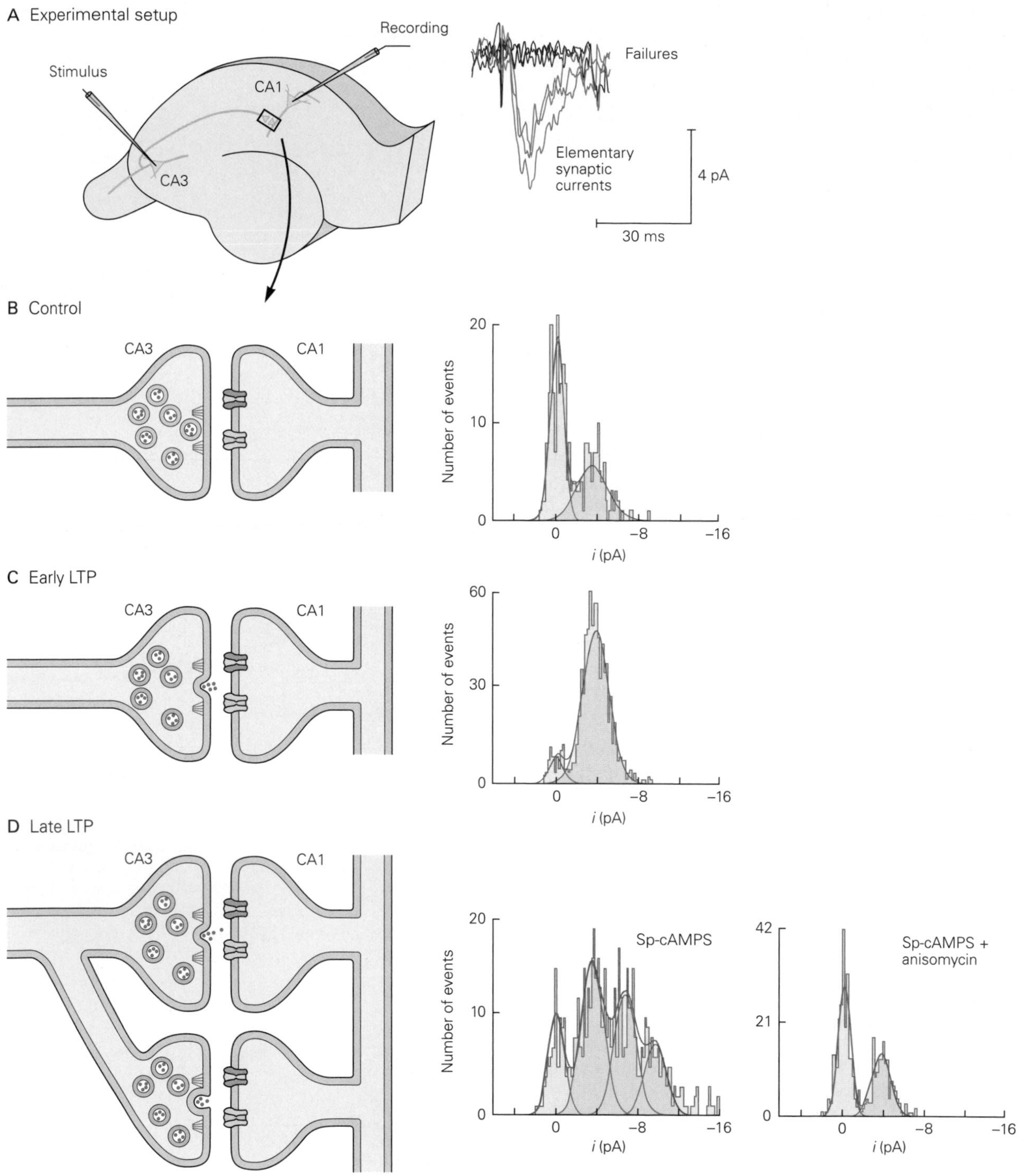
A Experimental setup
Recording
Stimulus
CA1
CA3
Failures
Elementary synaptic currents
4 pA
30 ms
B Control
CA3
CA1
Number of events
20
10
0
0
−8
−16
i (pA)
C Early LTP
CA3
CA1
Number of events
60
30
0
0
−8
−16
i (pA)
D Late LTP
CA3
CA1
Number of events
20
10
0
Sp-cAMPS
0
−8
−16
i (pA)
42
21
0
Sp-cAMPS + anisomycin
0
−8
−16
i (pA)

using two electrodes spaced some distance apart, the application of four trains of tetanic stimulation to one set of synapses induces late LTP only at the activated synapses; synaptic transmission at the second set of nonstimulated synapses is not altered. However, Uwe Frey and Richard Morris found that if a single tetanus is applied to the second set of synapses soon after the four tetani are applied to the first set, the single train is able to induce late LTP at the synapses it activates. This phenomenon is similar to the synapse-specific capture of long-term facilitation at the sensory-motor neuron synapses in *Aplysia* (see Chapter 66). At the Schaffer collateral synapses the single tetanus somehow marks the activated synapses allowing them to respond to, or capture, the new proteins synthesized in response to signals from the synapses that received the four tetani.

How can a few brief trains of synaptic stimulation produce such long-lasting increases in synaptic transmission? Studies from Todd Sacktor have shown that the maintenance of late LTP depends on a novel isoform of protein kinase C termed PKMζ (PKM zeta). Most isoforms of PKC contain both a regulatory domain and a catalytic domain (see Chapter 11). Binding of diacylglycerol, phospholipids, and Ca^{2+} to the regulatory domain of PKC relieves its inhibitory binding to the catalytic domain, which is then free to phosphorylate its protein substrates. In contrast, PKMζ lacks a regulatory domain and so is constitutively active.

Levels of PKMζ in the hippocampus are normally low. Tetanic stimulation that induces LTP leads to an increase in synthesis of PKMζ through enhanced translation of its mRNA. This mRNA is present in the CA1 neuron dendrites, enabling its local translation to rapidly alter synaptic strength. Blockade of PKMζ with a specific inhibitor does not block early LTP but does block late LTP. Moreover, application of the PKMζ blocker several hours after the LTP induction protocol can reverse late LTP after it has been established. This result indicates that the maintenance of late LTP requires the persistent and ongoing activity of PKMζ, which leads to the persistent increase in insertion of AMPA receptors in the postsynaptic membrane (Figure 67–9).

Spatial Memory Depends on Long-Term Potentiation in the Hippocampus

Long-term potentiation is an experimentally induced change in synaptic strength produced by strong direct stimulation of neural pathways. Does this form of synaptic change occur physiologically for explicit memory storage? If so, how does it affect the normal processing of information for memory storage in the hippocampus?

To date a large number of experimental approaches have shown that inhibiting LTP interferes with spatial memory. One spatial memory test uses a pool filled with an opaque fluid (the Morris water maze). To escape from the liquid a mouse must find a platform submerged below the surface of the fluid and completely

Figure 67–8 (Opposite) **Quantal analysis of early and late phases of long-term potentiation.** (Reproduced, with permission, from Bolshakov et al. 1997.)

A. When a single presynaptic CA3 cell is stimulated to fire an action potential, it produces a small excitatory postsynaptic current (EPSC) in a postsynaptic CA1 cell recorded under voltage clamp conditions. When the CA3 cell is stimulated successively at a frequency too low to induce LTP or LTD, the EPSC varies from stimulus to stimulus. The stimulus either evokes an EPSC (a success) or does not evoke any measurable response (a failure). The amplitude of the successes is equal to that of the miniature EPSC, the elementary or quantal response.

B. Before LTP, stimulation of the presynaptic cell results in many failures; the synapse has a low probability of releasing a vesicle. The distribution of the EPSC amplitudes can be approximated by two Gaussian curves, one centered on zero current (the failures) and the other centered on −4 pA (the successful responses). These histograms are consistent with the type of synapse illustrated here, in which a single CA3 cell makes a single synaptic connection with a CA1 cell. This connection has a single active zone from which a single vesicle is released in an all-or-none manner (failures or successes) in response to successive stimuli. The postsynaptic membrane contains both NMDA and AMPA receptors, the latter of which are responsible for the rapid EPSC at negative potentials.

C. Once early LTP has been induced, the probability of release increases significantly, leading to a decrease in the fraction of failures and an increase in the fraction of successes. The EPSC histogram is again fitted by two Gaussian curves, consistent with the view that there is still only a single release site that releases at most a single vesicle but now with a high probability of release. (This study examined LTP at non-silent synapses under conditions where insertion of new AMPA receptors was not observed.)

D. When late LTP is induced by prolonged application of a membrane-permeable analog of cAMP (Sp-cAMPS), the distribution of successful responses is no longer fitted by a single Gaussian curve. Instead, three or four Gaussian curves are fitted, suggesting that a single presynaptic action potential releases multiple quanta (synaptic vesicles) of transmitter. These effects are blocked by anisomycin, an inhibitor of protein synthesis. The increase in number of quanta is consistent with the growth of new sites of synaptic transmission between the presynaptic and postsynaptic neurons. (**Sp-cAMPS**, Sp-diastereomer of adenosine cyclic 3′,5′-phosphorothioate.)

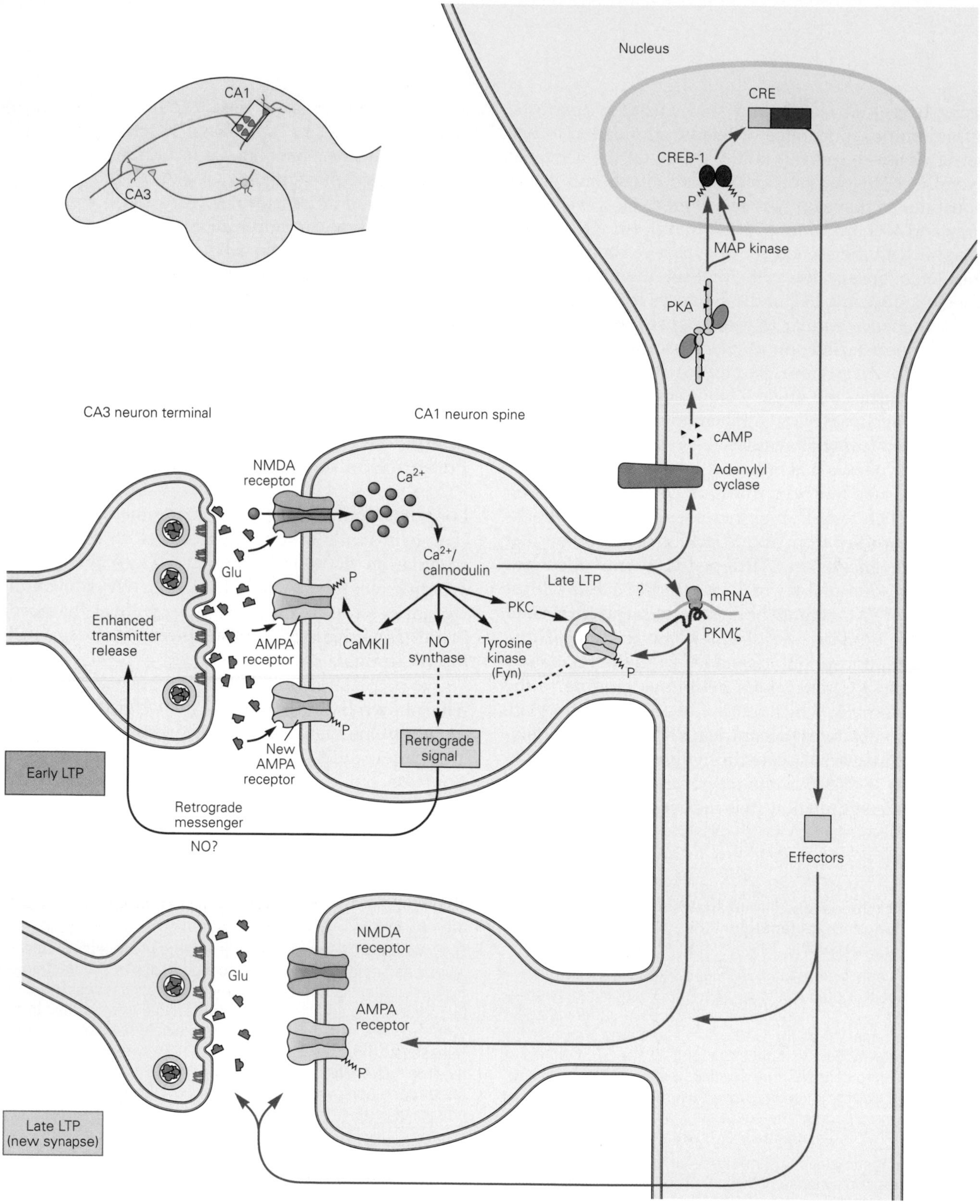

Figure 67–9 A model for the molecular mechanisms of early and late phases of long-term potentiation. A single tetanus induces early LTP by activating NMDA receptors, triggering Ca^{2+} influx into the postsynaptic cell and the activation of a set of second messengers. With repeated tetani the Ca^{2+} influx also recruits an adenylyl cyclase, which generates cAMP that activates PKA. This leads to the activation of MAP kinase, which translocates to the nucleus where it phosphorylates CREB-1. CREB-1 in turn activates transcription of targets (containing the CRE promoter) that are thought to lead to the growth of new synaptic connections. Repeated stimulation also activates translation in the dendrites of mRNA encoding PKMζ, a constitutively active isoform of PKC. This leads to a long-lasting increase in the number of AMPA receptors in the postsynaptic membrane. A retrograde signal, perhaps NO, is thought to diffuse from the postsynaptic cell to the presynaptic terminal to enhance transmitter release.

hidden from view. The animal is released at random locations around the pool and initially encounters the platform by chance. However, in subsequent trials the mouse quickly learns to locate the platform and then remembers its position based on spatial *contextual cues*—markings on the walls of the room in which the pool is located. This task requires the hippocampus. In a *noncontextual* version of this test the platform is raised above the water surface or marked with a flag so that it is visible, permitting the mouse to navigate directly to the platform using brain pathways that do not require an intact hippocampus.

When NMDA receptors are blocked by injection of a pharmacological antagonist into the hippocampus, the animal can find the visible platform in the noncontextual version of the task but cannot remember the location of the hidden platform in the contextual version. These experiments thus suggest that some mechanism involving NMDA receptors in the hippocampus, perhaps LTP, is involved in spatial learning. As we saw above, NMDA receptors are required for the induction but not for the persistence or maintenance of LTP. Similarly, injection of an NMDA receptor blocker into the hippocampus *after* an animal has learned a spatial memory task does not inhibit subsequent memory recall for that task.

As we also saw above, PKMζ is required for the maintenance of LTP but is not involved in its initial induction. Todd Sacktor and his colleagues have found a corresponding requirement for PKMζ in the persistence of memory. Thus injection of a pharmacological inhibitor of PKMζ into the hippocampus 1 day after an animal has been trained on a spatial task disrupts the memory for that task.

More direct evidence for the correlation of memory and LTP comes from experiments with mutant mice that have genetic lesions that interfere with LTP. One interesting mutation is produced by the genetic deletion of the NR1 subunit of the NMDA receptor. Neurons lacking this subunit fail to form functional NMDA receptors. Mice with a general deletion of the subunit die soon after birth, indicating the importance of these receptors for neural function. However, it is possible to generate lines of mutant mice in which the NR1 deletion is restricted to CA1 pyramidal neurons and occurs only 1 or 2 weeks after birth (Box 67–1). These mice survive into adulthood and show a loss of LTP in the Schaffer collateral pathway. This disruption is highly localized; nevertheless the mutant mice have a serious deficit in spatial memory (Figure 67–12).

Although it is perhaps not surprising that genetic manipulations can impair neuronal function, in some cases genetic changes can actually enhance both hippocampal LTP and spatial learning and memory. One of the first examples of such an enhancement comes from studies of a mouse mutant that overexpresses the NR2B subunit of the NMDA receptor. This subunit is normally present at early stages of development but is downregulated at adult hippocampal synapses. Receptors that incorporate this subunit allow more Ca^{2+} influx than those that do not. In mutant mice that overexpress the NR2B subunit LTP is enhanced, presumably because of an enhancement in Ca^{2+} influx. Importantly, learning and memory for several different tasks are also enhanced (Figure 67–13).

One concern with gene knockouts or transgene expression is that such mutations might lead to subtle developmental abnormalities. That is, changes in the size of LTP and spatial memory in the mutant animals could be the result of an early developmental alteration in the wiring of the hippocampal circuit rather than a change in the basic mechanisms of LTP. This possibility can be addressed by reversibly turning on and off a transgene that interferes with LTP (see Box 67–1).

Reversible gene expression has been used to explore the role of the enzyme CaMKII, whose function in LTP was discussed above. After a brief exposure to Ca^{2+}, CaMKII can be converted to a Ca^{2+} independent state through its autophosphorylation at threonine-286 (Thr286). This ability to become persistently active in response to a transient Ca^{2+} stimulus led to the suggestion that CaMKII may act as a simple molecular switch to maintain memory. Mutation of Thr286 to the negatively charged amino acid aspartate mimics the effect of autophosphorylation at Thr286 and converts the CaMKII to a Ca^{2+}-independent form.

Transgenic expression of this dominant mutation of CaMKII (CaMKII–Asp286) results in a systematic shift in the relation between stimulus frequency during a tetanus and the resultant change in synaptic strength during long-term plasticity. In the transgenic mice intermediate-frequency tetanic stimulation at 10 Hz, which normally induces a small amount of LTP, induces long-term depression of synaptic transmission in the Schaffer collateral pathway (Figure 67–14A). In contrast, Schaffer collateral LTP in response to a 100 Hz tetanus is not altered. The defect in synaptic plasticity with intermediate frequency stimulation is associated with an inability of the mutant mice to remember spatial tasks (Figure 67–14C). However, the defects in LTP and in spatial memory can be fully rescued when the mutant gene is switched off in the adult, thereby showing that the memory defect is not due to a developmental abnormality (Figure 67–14).

These several experiments using restricted knockout and overexpression of the NMDA receptor and

Box 67–1 Restricting Gene Knockout and Regulating Transgenic Expression

Biological analysis of learning requires the establishment of a causal relation between specific molecules and learning. In the past this relationship was difficult to demonstrate in mammals but now can be studied successfully in mice either by the use of transgenes or gene knockout.

With gene knockout, deletion of a specific gene is induced in embryonic stem cells through homologous recombination (see Figure 3–8). Experiments using transgenes and gene knockout have made it possible to examine the relationship of NMDA receptors and different second-messenger-dependent protein kinases to long-term potentiation in the hippocampus and to spatial learning.

Conventional gene knockout is unrestricted; animals inherit the genetic deletion in all of their cell types. Global genetic deletion may cause developmental defects that interfere with the later functioning of neural circuits important for memory storage. As a result, interpretation of the results from experiments using conventional gene knockout run into two types of problems.

First, it is often difficult to exclude the possibility that the abnormal phenotype observed in mature animals results directly or indirectly from a developmental defect rather than because that gene plays a specific, active role in learning and memory. Second, global gene knockout makes it difficult to attribute abnormal phenotypes to a particular type of cell or specific region within the brain.

Regional Control of Gene Expression

To improve the utility of gene knockout technology, methods have been developed that restrict deletions to cells in a specific tissue or at specific points in an animal's development. One method of regional restriction exploits the *Cre/loxP* system. The *Cre/loxP* system is a site-specific recombination system, derived from the P1 phage, in which the phage enzyme Cre recombinase catalyzes recombination between 34 bp *loxP* recognition sequences, which are normally not present in animal genomes.

The *loxP* sequences can be inserted into the genome of embryonic stem cells by homologous recombination such that they flank one or more exons of a gene of interest (called a *floxed* gene). When the stem cells are injected into an embryo, a mouse can be eventually bred in which the gene of interest is floxed and still functional in all cells of the animal.

A second line of transgenic mice can then be generated that expresses Cre recombinase under the control of a neural promoter sequence that is normally expressed in a restricted brain region. By crossing the Cre transgenic line of mice with the line of mice with the floxed gene of interest, the gene will only be deleted in those cells that express the Cre transgene (Figure 67–10).

In the example shown in Figure 67–10 the gene encoding the NR1 (or GluN1) subunit of the NMDA glutamate receptor has been flanked with *loxP* elements and then crossed with a mouse line expressing Cre recombinase under control of the *CaMKII* promoter, which normally is expressed in forebrain neurons. In this particular line expression was fortuitously limited to the CA1 region of the hippocampus, resulting in selective deletion of the NR1 subunit in this brain region. Because the *CaMKII* promoter only activates gene transcription postnatally, early developmental changes are minimized by this strategy.

Temporal Control of Gene Expression

In addition to regional restriction of gene expression, effective use of genetically modified mice requires control over the timing of gene expression. The ability to turn a transgene on and off gives the investigator an additional degree of flexibility and can exclude the possibility that any abnormality observed in the phenotype of the mature animal is the result of a developmental defect produced by the transgene. This can be done in mice by constructing a gene that can be turned on or off with a drug.

One starts by creating two lines of mice. Line 1 carries a particular transgene, for example *CaMKIIα-Asp286*, a mutated form of the gene *CaMKIIα* coding for a constitutively active kinase. Instead of being attached to its normal promoter, the transgene is attached to the promoter *tetO* that is ordinarily found only in bacteria (Figure 67–11).

This promoter cannot by itself turn on the gene; it needs to be activated by a specific transcriptional regulator. Thus the second line of mice expresses a second transgene that encodes a hybrid transcription factor, the tetracycline transactivator (tTA), which recognizes and binds to the *tetO* promoter. Expression of tTA is placed under the control of a region-specific promoter, such as the promoter for *CaMKIIα*.

When the two lines of mice are mated, some of the offspring will carry both transgenes. In these mice the tTA binds to the *tetO* promoter and activates the mutated *CaMKIIα* gene. This mutant causes abnormalities in long-term potentiation (see Figure 67–14).

But when the antibiotic doxycycline (similar to tetracycline) is administered, the drug binds to the transcription factor tTA, causing it to undergo a change in shape that makes it come off the promoter. In the presence of the antibiotic, cells stop expressing CaMKIIα-Asp286 and long-term potentiation returns to normal, demonstrating that the transgene exerts its effect by perturbing signaling in the adult brain rather than by interfering with neural development.

One can also generate mice that express a mutant form of tTA called reverse tTA (rtTA). This transactivator will not bind to *tetO* unless the animal is fed doxycycline. In this case the transgene is always turned off unless the drug is given.

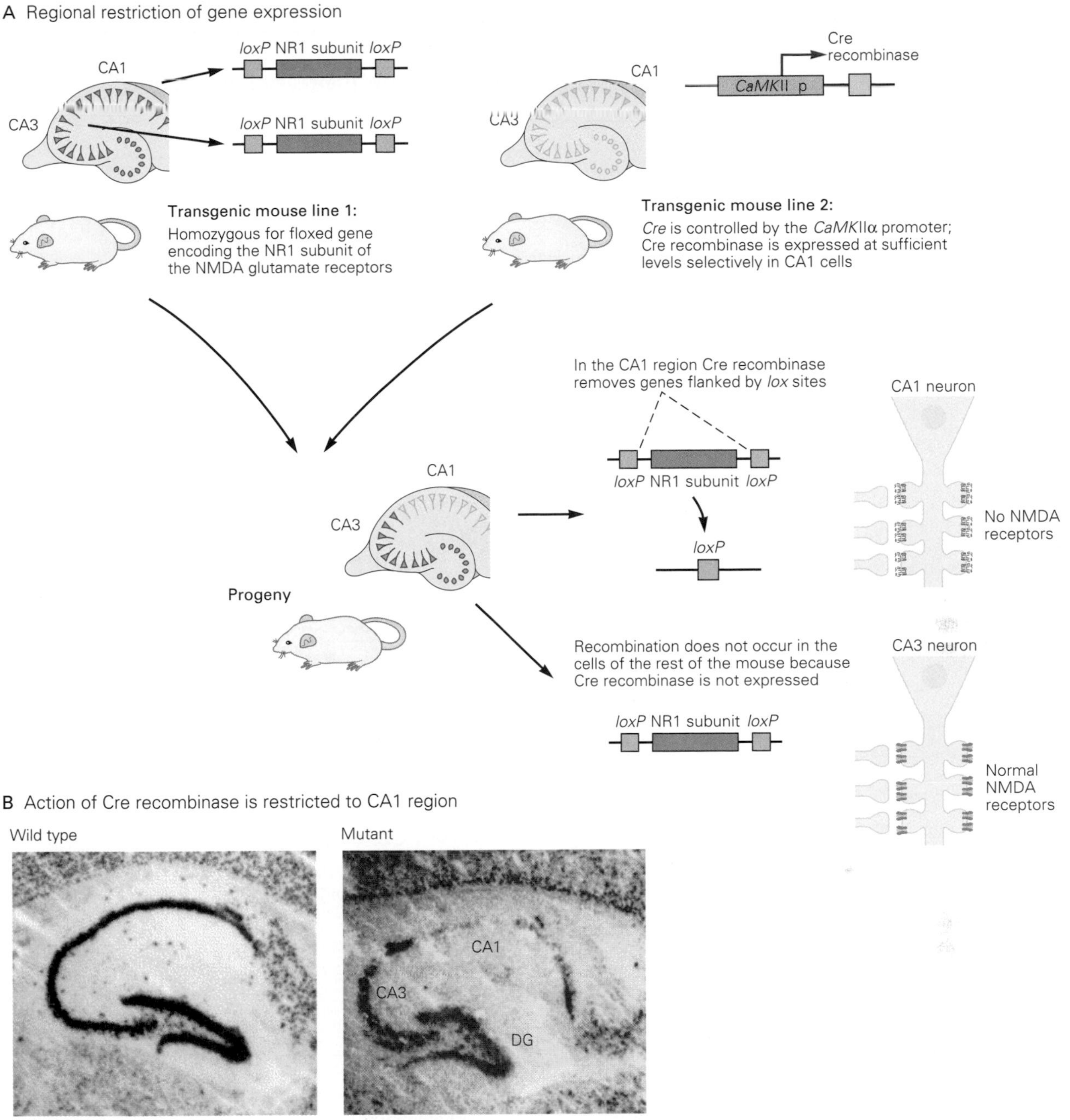

A Regional restriction of gene expression
loxP NR1 subunit loxP
CA1
CA3
loxP NR1 subunit loxP
Cre
recombinase
CA1
CaMKII p
Transgenic mouse line 1:
Homozygous for floxed gene encoding the NR1 subunit of the NMDA glutamate receptors
Transgenic mouse line 2:
Cre is controlled by the CaMKIIα promoter; Cre recombinase is expressed at sufficient levels selectively in CA1 cells
In the CA1 region Cre recombinase removes genes flanked by lox sites
CA1 neuron
CA1
CA3
loxP NR1 subunit loxP
loxP
No NMDA receptors
Progeny
Recombination does not occur in the cells of the rest of the mouse because Cre recombinase is not expressed
CA3 neuron
loxP NR1 subunit loxP
Normal NMDA receptors
B Action of Cre recombinase is restricted to CA1 region
Wild type
Mutant
CA1
CA3
DG

Figure 67–10 The *Cre/loxP* system for gene knockout.

A. A line of mice is bred in which the gene encoding the NR1 subunit of the NMDA receptor has been flanked by *loxP* genetic elements (transgenic mouse line 1). These so-called "floxed NR1" mice are then crossed with a second line of mice in which a transgene coding for Cre recombinase is placed under the control of a transcriptional promoter specific to a cell type or a tissue type (transgenic mouse line 2). In this example the promoter from the *CaMKIIα* gene is used to drive expression of the *Cre* gene. In progeny that are homozygous for the floxed gene and that carry the Cre recombinase transgene, the floxed gene will be deleted by *Cre*-mediated *loxP* recombination only in cell type(s) in which the promoter driving *Cre* expression is active.

B. In situ hybridization is used to detect mRNA for the NR1 subunit in hippocampal slices from wild-type and mutant mice that contain two floxed NR1 alleles and express Cre recombinase under the control of the *CaMKIIα* promoter. Note that NR1 mRNA expression (**dark staining**) is greatly reduced in the CA1 region of the hippocampus but remains normal in CA3 and the dentate gyrus (**DG**). (Reproduced, with permission, from Tsien, Huerta, and Tonegawa 1996.)

Box 67–1 Restricting Gene Knockout and Regulating Transgenic Expression (Continued)

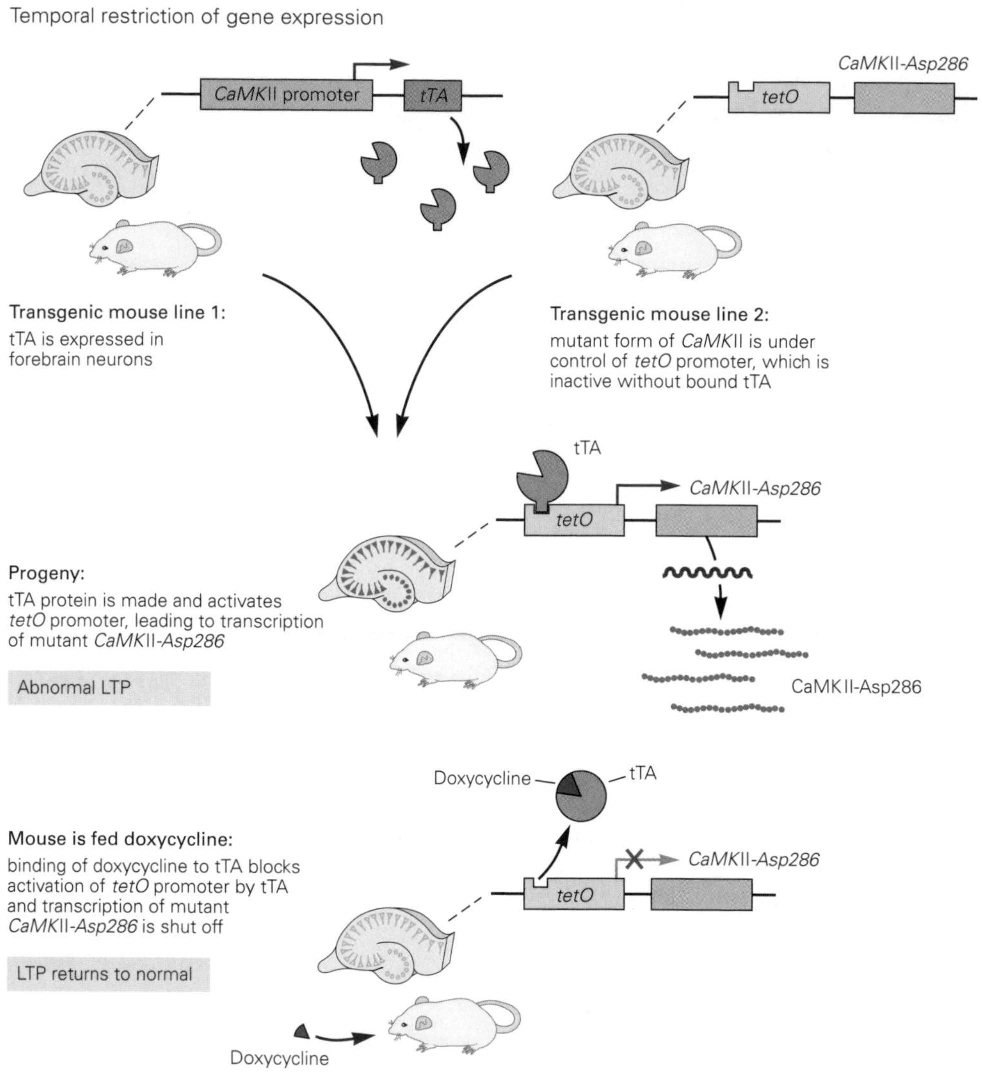
Temporal restriction of gene expression
CaMKII promoter
tTA
tetO
CaMKII-Asp286
Transgenic mouse line 1:
tTA is expressed in forebrain neurons
Transgenic mouse line 2:
mutant form of CaMKII is under control of tetO promoter, which is inactive without bound tTA
tTA
tetO
CaMKII-Asp286
Progeny:
tTA protein is made and activates tetO promoter, leading to transcription of mutant CaMKII-Asp286
Abnormal LTP
CaMKII-Asp286
Doxycycline
tTA
Mouse is fed doxycycline:
binding of doxycycline to tTA blocks activation of tetO promoter by tTA and transcription of mutant CaMKII-Asp286 is shut off
CaMKII-Asp286
tetO
LTP returns to normal
Doxycycline

Figure 67–11 The tetracycline system for temporal and spatial regulation of transgene expression. Two independent lines of transgenic mice are bred. One line expresses, under the control of the *CaMKIIα* promoter, the tetracycline transactivator (tTA), an engineered protein incorporating a bacterial transcription factor that recognizes the bacterial *tetO* operon. The second line contains a transgene of interest—here encoding a constitutively active form of CaMKII (*CaMKII–Asp286*) that makes the kinase persistently active in the absence of Ca^{2+}—whose expression is under control of *tetO*. When these two lines are mated the offspring express the tTA protein in a pattern restricted to the forebrain. When the tTA protein binds to *tetO* it will activate transcription of the downstream gene of interest. Tetracycline (or doxycycline) given to the offspring binds to the tTA protein and causes a conformational change that leads to the unbinding of the protein from *tetO*, blocking transgene expression. In this manner mice will express CaMKII–Asp286 in the forebrain, and this expression can be turned off by administering doxycycline to the mice. (Reproduced, with permission, from Mayford et al. 1996.)

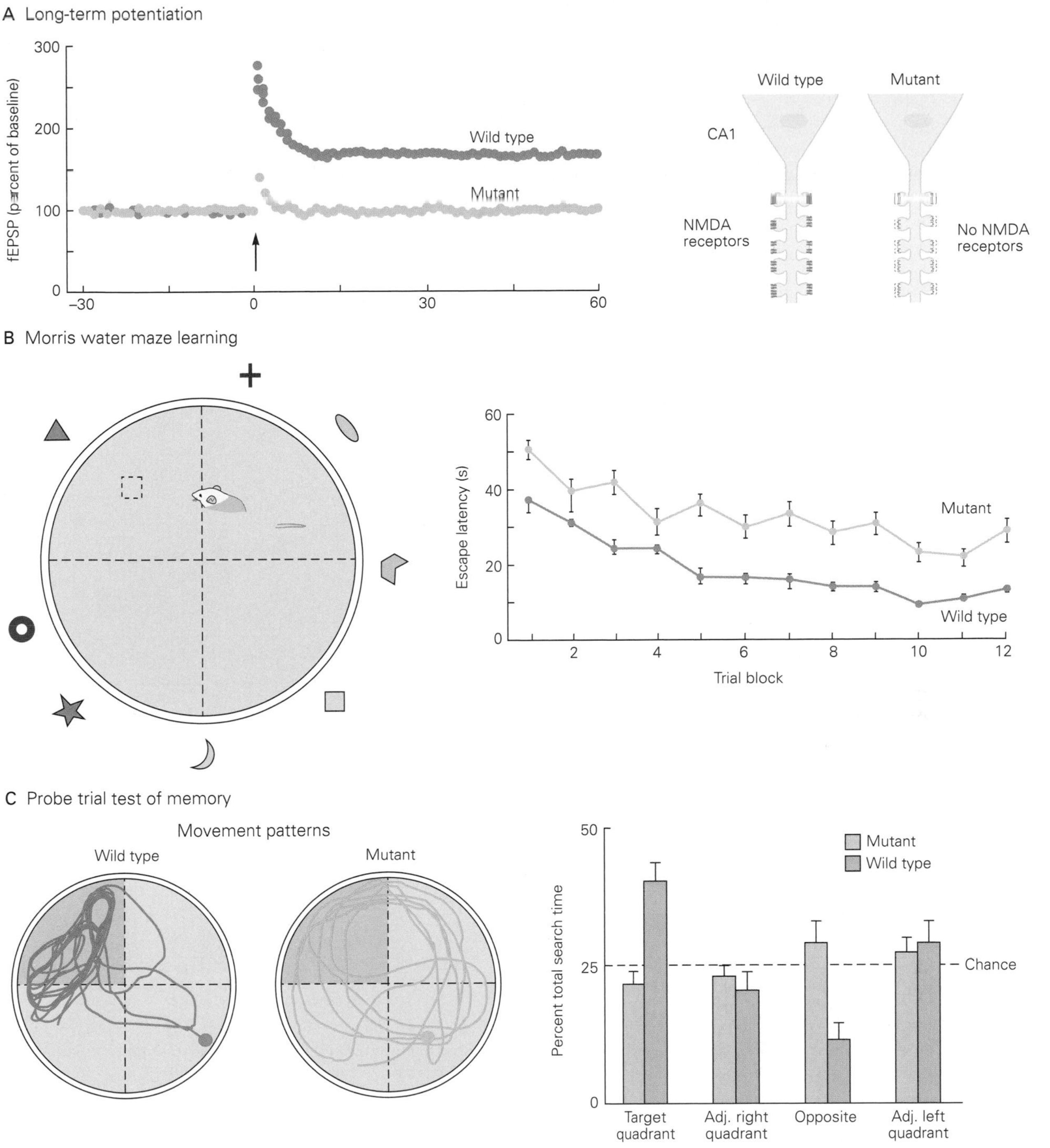

Figure 67–12 Long-term potentiation, and spatial learning and memory are impaired in mice that lack the NMDA receptor in the CA1 region of the hippocampus. (Reproduced, with permission, from Tsien, Huerta, and Tonegawa 1996.)

A. LTP is abolished in mice in which the NMDA receptor is selectively deleted in CA1 pyramidal neurons by knocking out the NR1 subunit gene. Field EPSPs were recorded in response to Schaffer collateral stimulation. Tetanic stimulation at 100 Hz for 1 s (**arrow**) caused a large potentiation in wild-type mice but failed to induce LTP in the NMDA receptor knockout (mutant) mice.

B. Mice that lack the NMDA receptor in CA1 pyramidal neurons have impaired spatial memory. A platform (**dashed square**) is submerged in an opaque fluid in a circular tank (the Morris water maze). To avoid remaining in the water the mice have to find the platform using spatial (contextual) cues on the walls surrounding the tank, and then climb onto the platform. The graph shows escape latency or the time required by mice to find the hidden platform in successive trials. The mutant mice display a longer escape latency in every block of trials (four trials per day) than do the wild-type mice. Also, mutant mice do not reach the optimal performance attained by the control mice after 12 training days, even though they show some improvement with training.

C. After the mice have been trained in the Morris maze the platform is taken away. In this probe trial the wild-type mice spend a disproportionate amount of time in the quadrant that formerly contained the platform (the target quadrant), indicating that they remember the location of the platform. Mutant mice spend an equal amount of time (25%) in all quadrants, ie, they perform at chance level, indicating deficient memory.

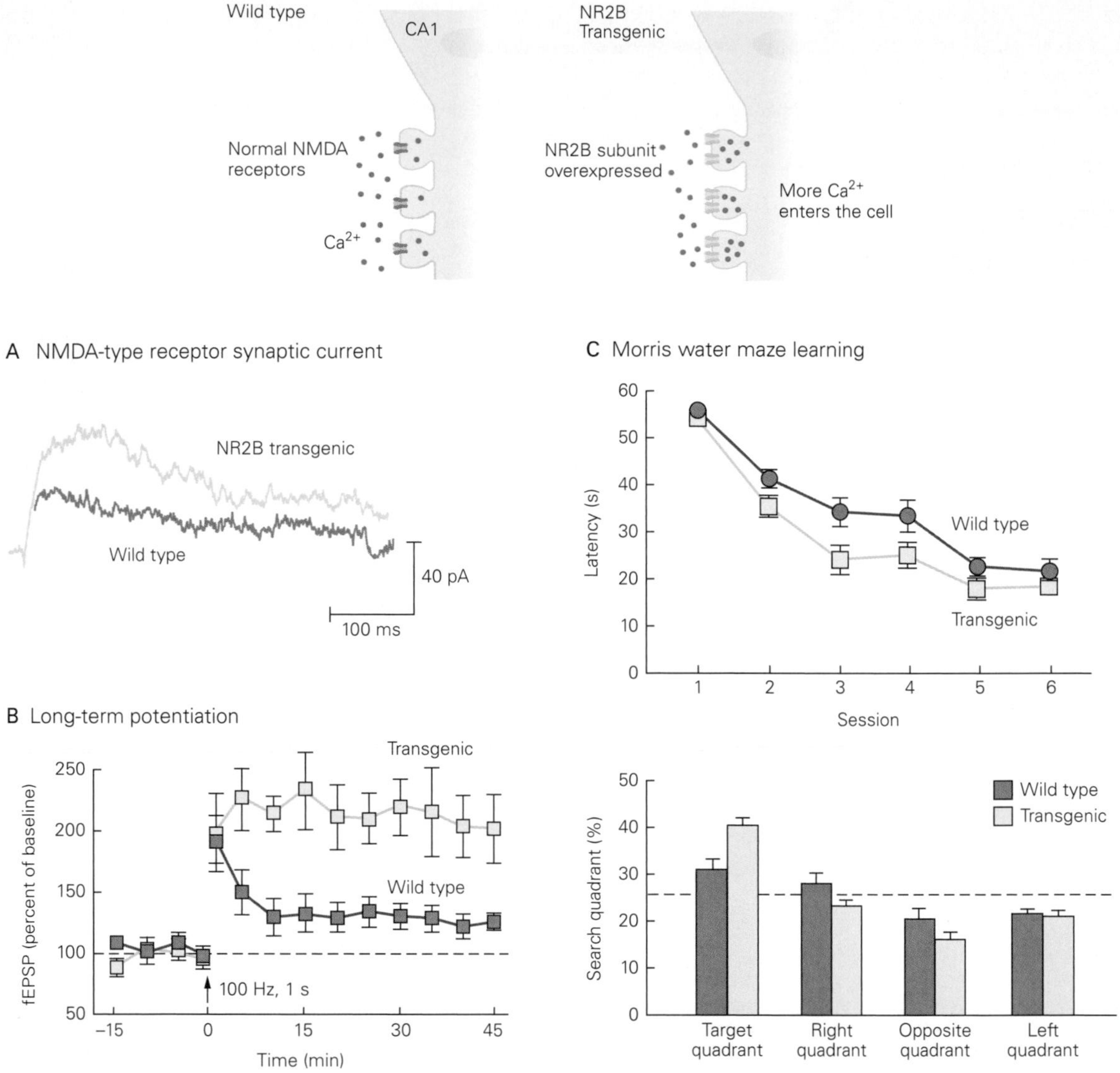

Figure 67–13 Learning and memory are enhanced in mice that overexpress the NR2B subunit of the NMDA glutamate receptor. (Reproduced, with permission, from Tang et al. 1999.)

A. The amplitude of the current generated by the NMDA receptors in response to a brief pulse of glutamate is enhanced and its time course prolonged in hippocampal neurons obtained from mice that contain a transgene that expresses higher levels of the NR2B subunit compared to wild-type mice.

B. Long-term potentiation produced by tetanic stimulation of the Schaffer collateral synapses is greater in the transgenic mice than in wild-type mice.

C. Spatial learning is enhanced in the transgenic mice as demonstrated in the **upper plot**. The rate of learning in a Morris water maze (the reduction in time to find the hidden platform, or escape latency) is faster in transgenic mice than in wild-type. Spatial memory is also enhanced in the transgenic mice as demonstrated in the probe trial (**lower plot**). Transgenic mice spend more time in the target quadrant, which previously contained the hidden platform, than do wild-type mice (see Figure 67–12C).

regulated overexpression of CaMKII-Asp286 make it clear that the molecular pathways important for LTP in the Schaffer collateral pathway are also required for spatial memory. However, in addition to receiving input through the Schaffer collaterals, CA1 neurons also receive excitatory input from the entorhinal cortex. Synaptic plasticity at the entorhinal inputs in CA1 may also contribute to spatial learning and memory. The HCN1 hyperpolarization-activated cation channel is strongly expressed in the very distal dendrites of CA1 neurons, the site of the entorhinal inputs. These channels are partially open at the resting potential, which decreases the membrane resistance (R_m) of the dendrite. This reduces the size of the EPSP in response to a given excitatory synaptic current ($\Delta V_{EPSP} = I_{EPSP} \times R_m$) and decreases the membrane time constant ($\tau_m = R_m \times C_m$). The net effect is a reduction in the spatial and temporal integration of EPSPs in the perforant path.

Mice lacking the HCN1 subunit show markedly enhanced temporal summation of EPSPs in the distal dendrites in response to a tetanus because of the

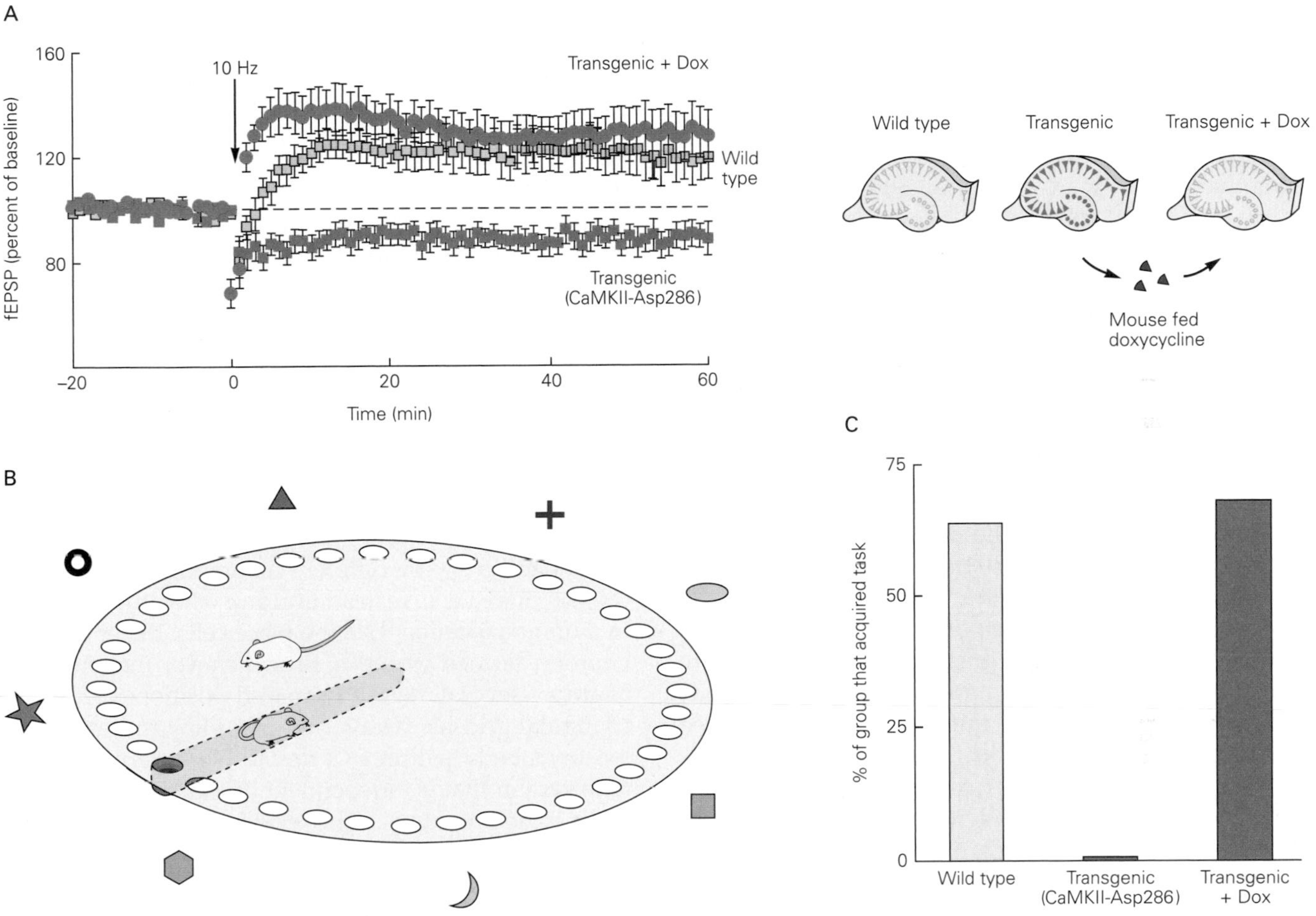

Figure 67–14 Deficits in long-term potentiation and spatial memory due to a transgene are reversible. (Reproduced, with permission, from Mayford et al. 1996.)

A. An LTP deficit is seen in hippocampal slices from transgenic mice that overexpress a constitutively active form of CaMKII, CaMKII-Asp286. Expression of this kinase is under control of *tetO* and the tTA transcription factor (see Box 67–1). Four groups of mice were tested: transgenic mice that are fed doxycycline (Dox), which blocks expression of the kinase; transgenic mice without doxycycline, in which the kinase is expressed; and wild-type mice with and without doxycycline. In wild-type mice a 10 Hz tetanus induces LTP; doxycycline has no effect (data are not shown). In the transgenic mice the tetanus fails to induce LTP but causes a small synaptic depression. In the transgenic mice that are fed doxycycline the deficit in LTP is reversed.

B. The effect of the kinase on spatial memory was tested in the Barnes maze. This consists of a platform with 40 holes, one of which leads to an escape tunnel that allows the mouse to exit the platform. The mouse is placed in the center of the platform. Mice do not like open, well-lit spaces and therefore try to escape from the platform by finding the hole that leads to the escape tunnel. The most efficient way of learning and remembering the location of the hole (and the only way of meeting the criteria set for the task by the experimenter) is by using distinctive markings on the four walls as cues for hippocampal-dependent spatial memory.

C. Transgenic mice that express the CaMKII-Asp286 kinase and receive doxycycline perform as well as wild-type mice in learning the Barnes maze task (approximately 65% of animals learn the task), whereas transgenic mice without the doxycycline (in which the kinase is highly expressed) do not learn the task.

increased membrane time constant. This contributes to a large increase in the magnitude of LTP at the perforant path synapses. In contrast, the same mice show relatively little change in EPSPs or LTP at the Schaffer collateral synapses, which are formed on more proximal regions of CA1 dendrites where expression of HCN1 is relatively modest. Importantly, the mutant mice get smarter, exhibiting a significantly faster rate at which they learn to find the hidden platform in the Morris maze relative to littermates that express normal levels of HCN1. Such experiments support the view that LTP at the most distal perforant path inputs to CA1 neurons also contributes to spatial learning and memory.

The preceding experiments demonstrate that a wide range of pharmacological and genetic manipulations that alter LTP are correlated with changes in spatial learning and memory. However, such results do not directly show that spatial learning and memory are actually associated with an enhancement in hippocampal synaptic transmission. Mark Bear and colleagues addressed this question by monitoring the strength of synaptic transmission at the Schaffer collateral CA1 synapses in vivo in rats using an array of extracellular recording electrodes.

Recordings were made of synaptic strength as rats were trained to avoid one side of a box through administration of a foot shock. These experiments show that after training there is a small but significant increase in the amplitude of synaptic transmission at a subset of the recording electrodes. Importantly, at electrode sites where the enhancement is greatest, LTP in response to tetanic stimulation through an independent electrode is diminished. This result implies that the enhanced synaptic transmission following spatial training is actually caused by the induction of LTP; because the amount of LTP at a given synapse is finite, the prior induction of LTP during learning occludes the subsequent induction of LTP by electrical stimulation. This effect is similar to the occlusion of LTP in the amygdala during fear learning, as discussed in Chapter 66.

A Spatial Map of the External World Is Formed in the Hippocampus

In 1971 John O'Keefe and John Dostrovsky made the remarkable discovery in rats that the hippocampus contains a cognitive map of an animal's spatial environment. An animal's familiarity with a particular environment is represented in the hippocampus by the firing pattern of populations of pyramidal cells, termed *place cells*, in the CA3 and CA1 regions. A place cell fires when an animal enters a certain location in a specific environment, the cell's *place field* (Figure 67–15). The population of place fields specify the environment. When the animal enters a new environment new place fields are formed within minutes and are stable for weeks to months. Thus, if one records the electrical activity of a number of place cells it is possible to predict where the animal is in its environment. In this manner the hippocampus is thought to constitute a cognitive map of the animal's surroundings.

O'Keefe's demonstration of place cells provided the first evidence for a neural representation of the environment that allows an animal to move deliberately around the world. The idea of a cognitive map was predicted earlier by the great cognitive psychologist Edward Tolman. He proposed that somewhere in the brain there must be a representation of the environment. This cognitive map is not topographic or egocentric in its organization, like the maps for touch or vision on the surface of the cerebral cortex. Rather the map is allocentric (or geocentric); it is fixed with respect to a point in the outside world.

How is the spatial map formed? What type of spatial information is carried by the afferent connections to the hippocampal place cells? In 2005 Edvard and May-Britt Moser and their colleagues in Norway discovered that neurons in the medial entorhinal cortex, whose axons form the perforant pathway to the hippocampus, map space in a very different manner from the hippocampal place cells. Instead of firing when the animal is in a unique location, like the place cells, the entorhinal neurons, termed *grid cells*, fire whenever the animal is at any of several, regularly spaced positions forming a triangular grid-like array. This grid allows the animal to locate its body within a Cartesian-like external coordinate system that is independent of context, landmarks, or specific markings. The gridded spatial information conveyed by the entorhinal inputs is transformed within the hippocampus into unique spatial locations represented by the firing of place cells.

Once the firing pattern of a population of hippocampal neurons is formed for a given environment, how is it maintained? Because the place cells are the same hippocampal pyramidal neurons that undergo experimental LTP, a natural question is whether LTP is important. This question was addressed in experiments in mice in which LTP was disrupted.

Surprisingly, in mice lacking the NR1 subunit of the NMDA receptor, hippocampal pyramidal neurons still fire in place fields despite the fact that LTP is blocked. Thus this form of LTP is not required for the transformation of spatial sensory information into place fields. However, place fields of hippocampal neurons in the mutant mice are larger and fuzzier in outline than

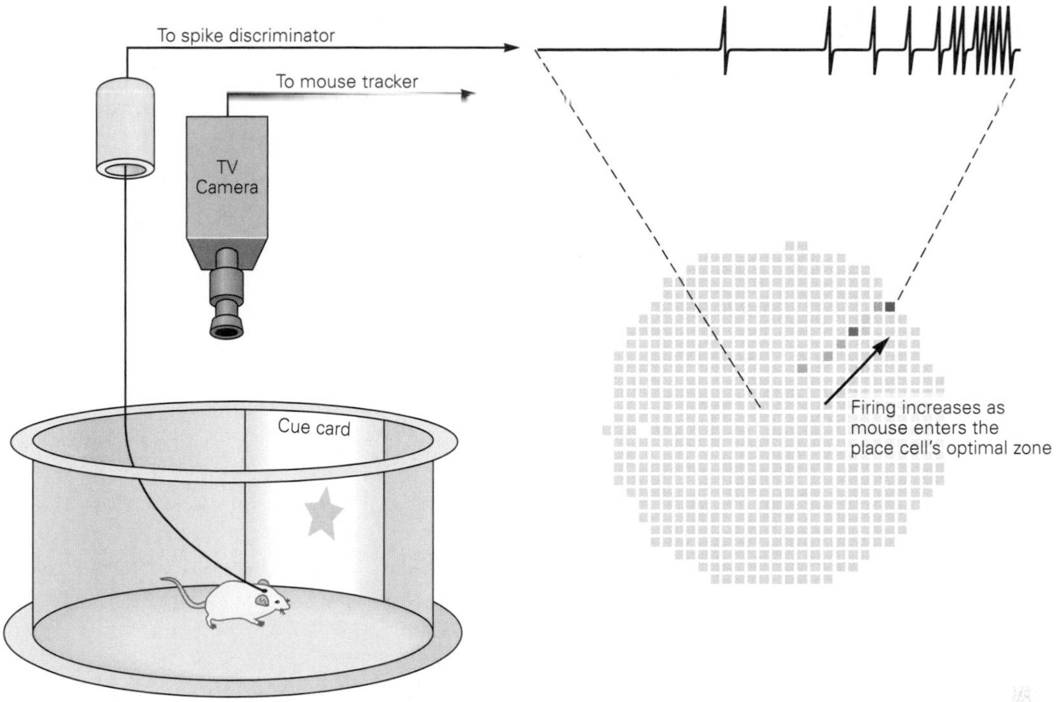

Figure 67–15 The firing patterns of pyramidal cells in the hippocampus create an internal representation of the animal's location in its surroundings. Electrodes implanted in the hippocampus of a mouse are attached to a recording cable, which is connected to an amplifier attached to a computer-based spike-discrimination program. The mouse is placed in a cylinder with an overhead TV camera that transmits to a device that detects the position of the mouse. The cylinder also contains a visual cue to orient the animal. Spikes in individual hippocampal pyramidal neurons (place cells) are detected by the spike discrimination program. The firing rate of each cell is then plotted as a function of the animal's location in the cylinder. This information is visualized as a two-dimensional map of color-coded firing rates for the cell, from which the cell's place field can be determined. Yellow, orange, red, green, blue, and purple pixels show regions with progressively increasing rates of firing. The place field is the location in space that elicits optimal firing in the cell. (Adapted, with permission, from Muller, Kubie, and Ranck 1987.)

those in normal animals. In a second experiment with mutant mice, late LTP and long-term spatial memory were selectively disrupted by expression of a transgene that encodes a protein inhibitor of protein kinase A. In these mice place fields also form but the firing patterns of individual cells are stable only for an hour or so (Figure 67–16). Thus late LTP is required not for the formation but for long-term stabilization of place fields.

These experiments raise a final question: To what degree do these maps of an animal's surroundings mediate explicit memory? In humans explicit memory is defined as the conscious recall of facts about people, places, and objects. Although consciousness cannot be studied empirically in the mouse, selective attention, which is required for conscious recall, can be examined.

When mice are presented with different behavioral tasks, the long-term stability of a neuron's place field correlates strongly with the degree of attention required to perform the task. When a mouse does not attend to the space it walks through, place fields form but are unstable after 3 to 6 hours. Animals with unstable place fields are unable to learn a spatial task. However, when a mouse is forced to attend to the space, for example as it forages for food, the place fields are stable for days.

How does this attentional mechanism work? Studies in primates have shown the importance of the prefrontal cortex and the modulatory dopaminergic system during attention. Indeed, the formation of stable place fields in mice requires the action of dopamine on the D_1/D_5 type of receptor, which stimulates adenylyl cyclase, leading to production of cAMP and activation of PKA. This demonstrates that, rather than being a form of implicit memory that is stored and recalled without conscious effort, long-term memory of a stably formed place field requires the animal to attend to its environment, as is the case for explicit memory in humans.

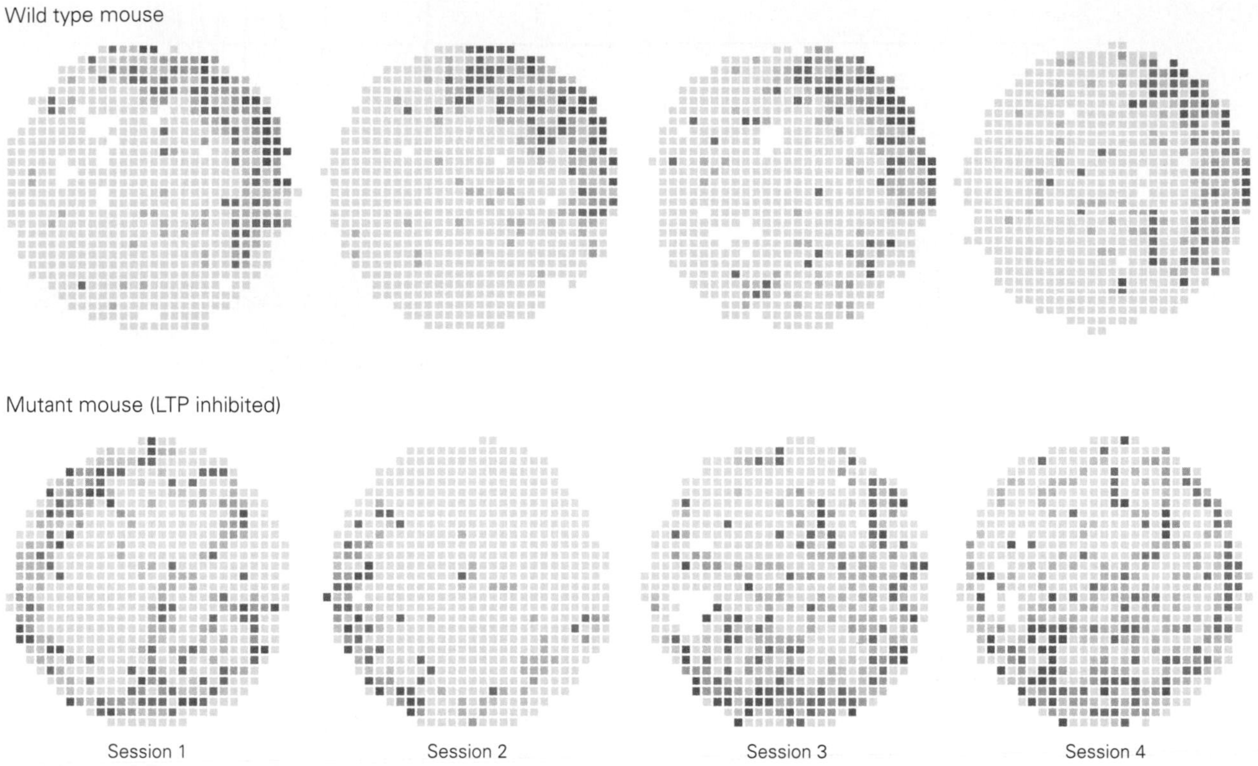

Figure 67–16 Disruption of long-term potentiation alters the stability of place field formation in hippocampal cells. Color-coded firing-rate maps (see Figure 67–15) show the place fields recorded in four successive sessions from a single hippocampal pyramidal neuron in a wild-type mouse and from a neuron in a mutant mouse that expresses the persistently active CaMKII (which inhibits the induction of LTP). Before each recording session the animal is taken out of the cylinder and sometime later reintroduced into it. In each of the four sessions the place field for the cell in the wild-type animal is stable. In this example the place cell fires whenever the animal is in the upper right region of the enclosure. By contrast, the place field of the cell in the mutant mouse is unstable across the different sessions. (Reproduced, with permission, from Rotenberg et al. 1996.)

Different Subregions of the Hippocampus Are Required for Pattern Separation and for Pattern Completion

Explicit memory is used to store facts (semantic memory) and episodes (episodic memory). Successful storage and recall of explicit memory requires the ability to distinguish between two closely related images, episodes, or spatial configurations—an ability called *pattern separation.* Explicit memory can also use partial cues to retrieve previously stored memories by filling in an incomplete pattern based on preexisting knowledge—an ability called *pattern completion.* Both capabilities are essential for optimal memory performance. We need to distinguish similar memories when the differences between them are important, and we need to recall memories when only partial clues for recall are available.

A variety of cell-physiological and computation studies, beginning with the theoretical work of David Marr in the 1970s, suggests that pattern completion depends on the recurrent connections between the CA3 pyramidal cells and that pattern separation depends on the direct projection from the entorhinal cortex to the dentate gyrus. The dentate's role in pattern separation was suggested because the number of granule cells in the dentate far exceeds the number of CA3 or CA1 pyramidal neurons. These ideas have now received support from genetic experiments by Susumu Tonegawa and his colleagues.

The importance of LTP between CA3 neurons is seen in studies performed on mice in which the NMDA glutamate receptor is selectively deleted in the CA3 neurons. These mice experience a selective loss of LTP at the recurrent synapses between CA3 neurons, with no change in LTP at the mossy fiber synapses onto the CA3 neurons or at the Schaffer collateral synapses between CA3 and CA1 neurons. Despite this deficit, the mice show normal learning and memory in the water maze. However, when the mice are asked to find a hidden platform with fewer than the normal number of spatial cues, their performance is impaired. This indicates that LTP at the recurrent synapses between CA3 neurons is important for pattern completion.

Similarly, the mechanism of pattern separation has been examined in mice in which a critical subunit of the NMDA receptor is selectively deleted from granule neurons in the dentate gyrus, or in which the neural activity of the granule neurons is blocked. Mutant mice lacking a functional NMDA receptor in the dentate gyrus have difficulty distinguishing between two similar contexts—that is, the mice cannot perform pattern separation.

One of the most unexpected findings in neuroscience has been the realization that neurogenesis is not limited to early stages of development. New neurons continue to be born throughout adulthood and become incorporated into neural circuits. However, adult neurogenesis is limited to two types of neurons in two brain regions: inhibitory granule cells in the olfactory bulb and the excitatory granule neurons of the dentate gyrus. When neurogenesis in the dentate is blocked, either by X-ray irradiation of specific brain regions or administration of a chemical that interferes with DNA synthesis, there is a variable effect on learning and memory; some forms of hippocampal-dependent memory are impaired whereas others appear intact. However, recent exciting results show that pattern separation specifically requires the participation of adult-born granule neurons. Moreover, procedures that stimulate neurogenesis enhance the ability of a mouse to perform pattern separation during a contextual memory task, which requires the animal to discriminate between closely related environments. Methods to enhance neurogenesis are now being explored as a means of treating different types of age-related memory loss.

Memory Also Depends on Long-Term Depression of Synaptic Transmission

If synaptic connections could only be enhanced and never attenuated, synaptic transmission might rapidly saturate—the strength of the synaptic connection might reach a point beyond which further enhancement is not possible. Yet individuals are able to learn and store new memories throughout a lifetime. This paradox led to the suggestion that neurons must have mechanisms to downregulate synaptic function to counteract LTP.

In fact such an inhibitory mechanism, termed *long-term depression* (LTD), was first discovered in the cerebellum, where it is important for motor learning. Since then, LTD has also been characterized at a number of synapses within the hippocampus. Whereas LTP is typically induced by a brief, high-frequency tetanus, the induction of LTD requires prolonged periods of low-frequency synaptic stimulation such as stimulation at 1 Hz for 15 minutes. LTD can also be induced by a pairing protocol, in which an EPSP is evoked after a postsynaptic cell fires an action potential. This suggests an anti-Hebbian learning rule: Synapses that do not contribute to the firing of a cell are weakened. Like LTP, a number of molecular and synaptic mechanisms are available to produce LTD.

Surprisingly many of the forms of LTD also require activation of the same receptors involved in LTP, namely the NMDA receptors (Figure 67–17A). Moreover, like LTP, LTD is thought to require Ca^{2+} influx through the NMDA receptors into the postsynaptic neuron. How can activation of a single type of receptor leading to elevated levels of a single second messenger, Ca^{2+}, produce both potentiation and depression?

A key difference lies in the protocols used to induce LTP or LTD. Compared to the high-frequency stimulation used to induce LTP, the low-frequency tetanus used to induce LTD produces a relatively modest postsynaptic depolarization and thus is much less effective at relieving the Mg^{2+} block of the NMDA receptors. As a result, the increase in the postsynaptic Ca^{2+} concentration is much smaller than observed during induction of LTP. This low concentration of Ca^{2+} is thought to be insufficient to activate CaMKII, the enzyme implicated in LTP. Rather, LTD is thought to result from the activation of the calcium-dependent phosphatase calcineurin, an enzyme complex that has a higher affinity for Ca^{2+} compared to that of CaMKII (see Chapter 11).

The activated calcineurin triggers a signaling cascade that activates still other phosphatases that dephosphorylate a number of proteins, including the GluA1 (also known as GluR1) subunit of the AMPA receptor. In addition to activating phosphatases, the LTD induction protocol also increases the phosphorylation of the GluA2 (or GluR2) subunit of the AMPA receptor by protein kinase C. The combined effects of dephosphorylation of GluA1 and phosphorylation of GluA2 trigger the endocytosis of the AMPA receptors, reducing the number of receptors in the postsynaptic membrane and thus reducing the size of the EPSP.

Distinct forms of LTD can be induced through the activation of metabotropic glutamate receptors. Such forms do not require activation of phosphatases but depend on activation of mitogen-activated protein (MAP)

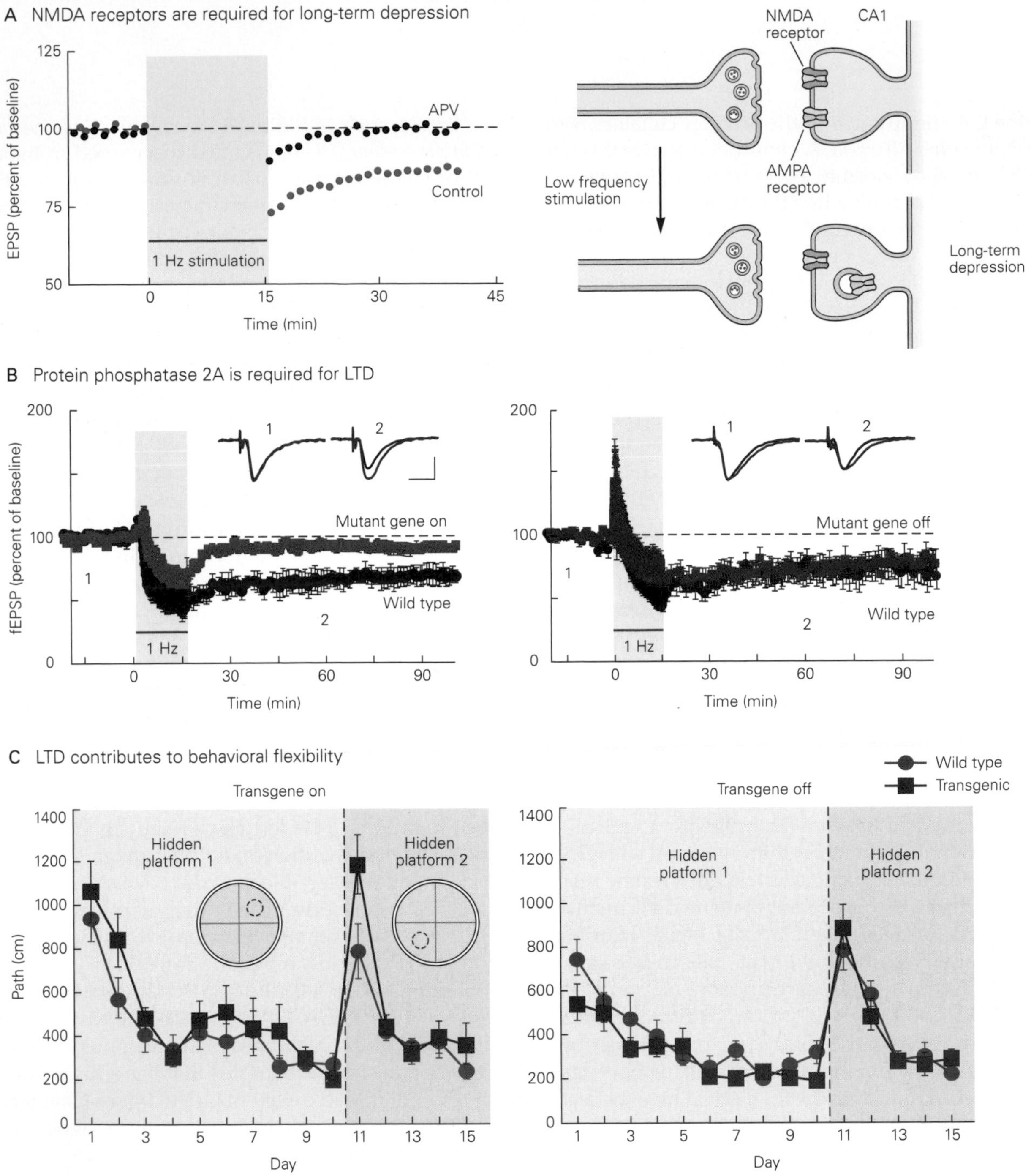

Figure 67–17 Long-term depression of synaptic transmission requires NMDA receptors and phosphatase activity.

A. Prolonged low-frequency stimulation (1 Hz for 15 minutes) of Schaffer collateral fibers produces a long-term decrease in the size of the field EPSP in the hippocampal CA1 region, a decrease that outlasts the period of stimulation (control). The diagram shows that long-term depression (**LTD**) results from removal of AMPA receptors from the postsynaptic membrane by endocytosis. This LTD is blocked when the 1 Hz stimulation is given in the presence of APV to block NMDA receptors. (Reproduced, with permission, from Dudek and Bear 1992.)

B. Long-term depression requires protein dephosphorylation. The plots compare LTD in the CA1 region of wild-type mice and transgenic mice that express a protein that inhibits phosphoprotein phosphatase 2A. Transgene expression is under control of the tTA system. In the absence of doxycycline, when the protein inhibitor is expressed, induction of LTD is inhibited (**left plot**). When inhibitor protein expression is turned off by administering doxycycline, a normal-sized LTD is induced (**right plot**).

C. Inhibition of phosphatase 2A alters behavioral flexibility. Transgenic mice expressing the phosphatase inhibitor learn the location of the submerged platform in the Morris maze at the same rate as wild-type mice (days 1 through 10). Learning is measured by the daily decrease in the path length the mice traverse as they search for the platform during training. At the end of day 10 the platform is moved to a new hidden location and the mice are retested (days 11–15). Now the transgenic mice require significantly longer path lengths to find the platform on the first day of retesting (day 11). When transgene expression is turned off with doxycycline, the transgenic mice display normal learning on all phases of the test. (Panels B and C reproduced, with permission, from Nicholls et al. 2008.)

kinase signaling pathways (see Chapter 11). These types of LTD lead to a reduction in synaptic transmission through a decrease in glutamate release from the Schaffer collateral terminals as well as through alterations in the trafficking of AMPA receptors in the postsynaptic cells.

Much less is known about the behavioral role of LTD compared to that of LTP, but some insight has come from recent studies using a transgenic mouse that expresses an inhibitor of protein phosphatase under regulated control. This mouse shows a deficit in NMDA receptor-dependent LTD when the transgene is expressed but shows normal LTD when transgene expression is suppressed (Figure 67–17B). In contrast, transgene expression does not affect LTP or forms of LTD that involve metabotropic glutamate receptors. The transgene-expressing mice also show normal learning the first time they are tested in the Morris maze. However, when the mutant mice are retested after the hidden platform has been moved to a new location, they show a decreased ability to learn the new location and tend to persevere in searching for the platform near the previously learned location (Figure 67–17C). This result suggests that LTD is needed for behavioral flexibility. Thus LTD may be necessary not only to prevent LTP saturation, but also as an active participant in memory storage.

Epigenetic Changes in Chromatin Structure Are Important for Long-Term Synaptic Plasticity and Learning and Memory

As is the case with long-term implicit memory, long-term explicit memory storage also requires covalent alterations in chromatin structure. Such changes are termed epigenetic. One form of epigenetic regulation involves acetylation of histone proteins, the protein component of the nucleosome repeat unit of chromatin. CREB binds to the cAMP-recognition element (CRE) promoter and recruits a transcriptional coregulator, the CREB-binding protein (CBP), which functions as a histone acetylase. Acetylation of the N-terminal tails of histones by CBP disrupts repressive chromatin structure and opens up the promoter region of target genes, allowing the binding of RNA polymerase II to initiate transcription (Figure 67–18A).

Mutations in CBP underlie Rubinstein-Taybi syndrome, a rare condition characterized by mental retardation and skeletal abnormalities. Rubinstein-Taybi syndrome can be modeled in mice by insertion of a truncated nonfunctional form of CBP into the mouse genome. These mice show a reduction in histone acetylation and impairment in the late phase of LTP that is associated with a deficit in certain forms of hippocampal-dependent long-term memory.

Whereas defects in histone acetylation result in memory impairment, enhancement of histone acetylation using inhibitors of histone deacetylase (HDAC) can enhance memory. Remarkably, in a mutant mouse line that undergoes significant hippocampal degeneration, memory capabilities that have been lost following neuronal death can be recovered by treatment of the mice with HDAC inhibitors, raising the possible clinical usefulness of these compounds, which were first developed as anticancer agents.

A second form of chromatin modulation that has been implicated in learning and memory involves DNA methylation (Figure 67–18B). Certain cytosine bases that precede guanine bases in DNA (CpG sites) can be methylated by DNA methyltransferases. DNA methylation recruits methyl-CpG-binding proteins that in turn bind transcriptional corepressor complexes that inhibit gene expression, in part because these complexes contain HDACs. DNA methylation is thought to be of particular importance during early development, when it helps initially to determine cell fate and maintain cell identity. Evidence that DNA methylation is important for proper development of the human nervous system is illustrated by the fact that mutations in the methyl-CpG-binding protein 2 underlie Rett syndrome, a pervasive neurodevelopmental disorder discussed in Chapter 64.

Recent experiments suggest that DNA methylation may also play an acute role in learning and memory in the adult. Thus contextual fear conditioning in mice causes an increase in methylation of the gene encoding the neurotrophin BDNF in the CA1 region of the hippocampus, which leads to changes in BDNF expression. Injection of pharmacological inhibitors of DNA methylation into the CA1 region both inhibits the change in BDNF expression and impairs fear memory 24 hours after conditioning. Consistent with findings for other forms of hippocampal-dependent learning and memory, the changes in DNA methylation require activation of the NMDA receptor. At present the mechanism linking NMDA receptor activation to changes in DNA methylation is unknown.

Are There Molecular Building Blocks for Learning?

Three key findings have emerged from cellular studies of implicit and explicit memory storage. First, the molecular mechanisms of some associative forms of

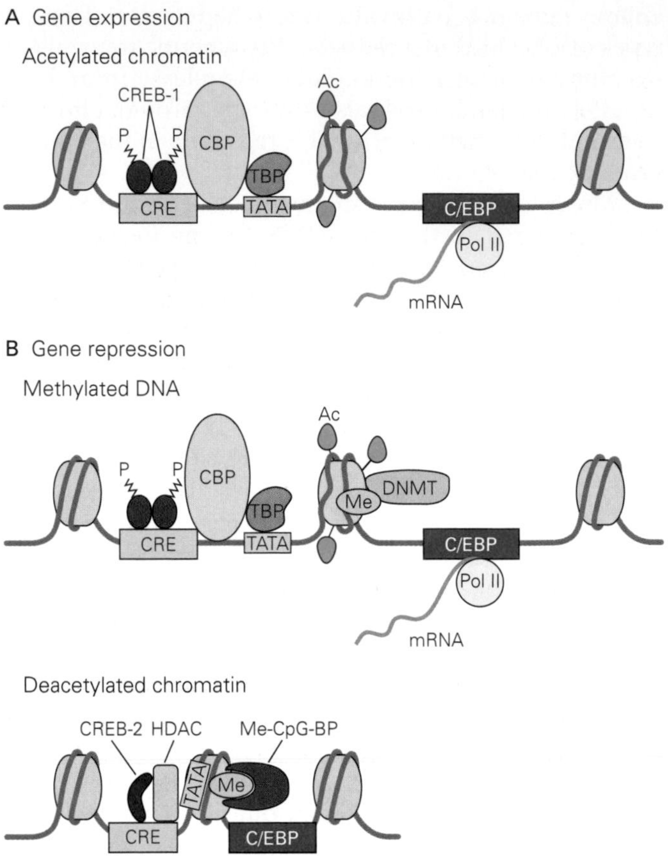

Figure 67–18 Long-term memory requires epigenetic alterations in chromatin structure.

A. Phosphorylation of CREB-1 following induction of the late phase of LTP in the hippocampus recruits the binding of CBP to the promoter region of target genes. In turn CBP acetylates certain positively charged lysine residues on the N-terminal tails of histone proteins, which form the nucleosome unit of chromatin. Acetylation loosens the binding of negatively charged DNA to the histones, allowing transcription to proceed and resulting in the late phase of LTP.

B. The induction of LTP also leads to changes in methylation of certain cytosine bases that precede guanine nucleotides (CpG sites) in DNA through the action of DNA methyltransferases (**DNMT**). This recruits methyl-CpG-binding proteins (**Me-CpG-BP**), which in turn recruit histone deacetylases (**HDAC**), leading to a decrease in histone acetylation, which, together with CREB-2, represses transcription.

synaptic plasticity are based on those of nonassociative forms in the same cell. This suggests that there may be molecular building blocks for synaptic plasticity. Simpler forms of plasticity might serve as components of more complex mechanisms, such as the joint recruitment of presynaptic and postsynaptic mechanisms of plasticity.

Second, the molecular mechanisms of elementary forms of associative learning, both implicit and explicit, are similar. The two synaptic mechanisms for memory storage we have considered—activity-dependent presynaptic facilitation for storing implicit memory and associative long-term potentiation for storing explicit memory—seem to derive from the associative properties of specific proteins (eg, the responsiveness of adenylyl cyclase or the NMDA receptor when two independent signals are simultaneously present).

Finally, despite their clear differences, implicit and explicit memory storage seem to rely on elements of a common multi-component genetic switch involving protein kinase A, CREB, and epigenetic changes in chromatin structure that convert labile short-term memory into long-term memory. Moreover, these mechanisms of synaptic plasticity do not operate in isolation. Rather, they are embedded in distributed neural circuits that have considerable computational power and thus can add substantial complexity to the actions of individual cells.

An Overall View

The demonstration that changes in the effectiveness of neural connections underlie memory, and thus learning, has revised our view of the relationship between social and biological processes in the shaping of an individual's behavior, both in health and disease. Until recently the majority view in medicine and psychiatry was that biological and social determinants of behavior act on separate components of the mind. For example, psychiatric illnesses were traditionally classified as either organic or functional. Organic mental illnesses included the dementias such as Alzheimer disease and the toxic psychoses such as those that follow the chronic use of alcohol. Functional mental illnesses included the various depressive syndromes, the schizophrenias, and the neuroses.

This distinction dates to the 19th century when neuropathologists examined the brains of patients coming to autopsy and found gross and readily demonstrable distortions in the architecture of the brain in some psychiatric diseases but not in others. Diseases that produce anatomical evidence of brain lesions were called *organic*; those lacking these features were called *functional*.

This distinction is no longer tenable, as the last two chapters of this book make clear. Everyday events—sensory stimulation, deprivation, and learning—can effectively weaken synaptic connections in some circumstances and strengthen them in others. We no longer think that only certain diseases ("organic diseases") affect mentation through biological changes in the brain whereas others ("functional diseases") do not. The basis of contemporary neural science is that all mental processes are biological and therefore any alteration in those processes is necessarily organic.

The question of the relative roles of nature and nurture in human behavior has shifted. We now ask, how do specific biological processes of the brain give rise to specific mental events and how in turn do social factors modulate the brain's biological structure? In the attempt to understand a particular mental illness it is more appropriate to ask, to what degree is this biological process determined by genetic and developmental factors? To what degree is it determined by a toxic or infectious agent, or by a developmental abnormality? To what degree is it socially determined? Even those mental disturbances that are considered most heavily determined by social factors must have a biological aspect, as it is the activity of the brain that is being modified by experience.

Insofar as social intervention works—whether through psychotherapy, counseling, or the support of family or friends—it must work by acting on the brain and quite likely on the strength of connections between nerve cells. Moreover, the absence of detectable structural changes does not rule out the possibility that important biological changes are nevertheless occurring. They may simply occur at a subcellular or even molecular level that is below the level of detection with the techniques available to us.

Demonstrating the biological nature of mental functioning requires more sophisticated anatomical methodologies than the light-microscopic histology of 19th-century pathologists. To clarify these issues it will be necessary to develop a neuropathology of mental illness that is based on anatomical structure *and* function. Imaging techniques—positron emission tomography and functional magnetic resonance imaging among others—have allowed the noninvasive exploration of the human brain on a cell-biological level, the level of resolution that is required to understand the physical mechanisms of mentation and therefore of mental disorders. This approach is being pursued in the study of schizophrenia and depression.

In studying the specific cellular changes that underlie memory storage, we should look for altered gene expression in abnormal as well as normal mental states. There is now substantial evidence that the susceptibility to major psychotic illnesses—schizophrenia and bipolar disorder—is heritable. Nevertheless, a sibling whose identical twin develops schizophrenia has only a 50% chance of also developing a psychosis. Thus environmental factors must also be important. The cell-biological data on learning and long-term memory reviewed in this chapter suggest that neurotic illnesses acquired by learning are likely to involve alterations in the *regulation* of gene expression (Figure 67–19).

Development, hormones, stress, and learning are all factors that alter gene expression by modifying the binding of transcriptional regulatory proteins to each other and to the regulatory regions of genes. It is likely that at least some neurotic illnesses (or components of them) result from effects of gene regulation that are reversible. It is intriguing to think, then, that insofar as psychotherapy is successful in changing behavior it does so by producing alterations in gene expression. If so, treatment of neurosis or character disorders by psychotherapeutic intervention would, if successful, also produce structural changes in the nervous system. Thus we face the attractive possibility, for which there is now preliminary evidence, that improved brain imaging techniques might ultimately be useful not only for diagnosing various psychiatric illnesses but also for monitoring the progress of psychotherapy.

When we consider together what we know about synapse formation and synaptic plasticity, it is clear there are two overlapping stages in the development and maintenance of synapses. The first stage, the initial steps of synapse formation, occurs primarily early in development and is under the control of genetic and developmental processes, commonly diffusible signals, cell matrix interactions, and cell-cell interactions. The second stage, the fine tuning of synapses by experience, occurs daily throughout later life. The activity-dependent mechanisms at work during critical periods of development are thought to be closely related to the activity-dependent cellular mechanisms involved in associative learning. Recent evidence indicates that age-related memory loss, including that which occurs

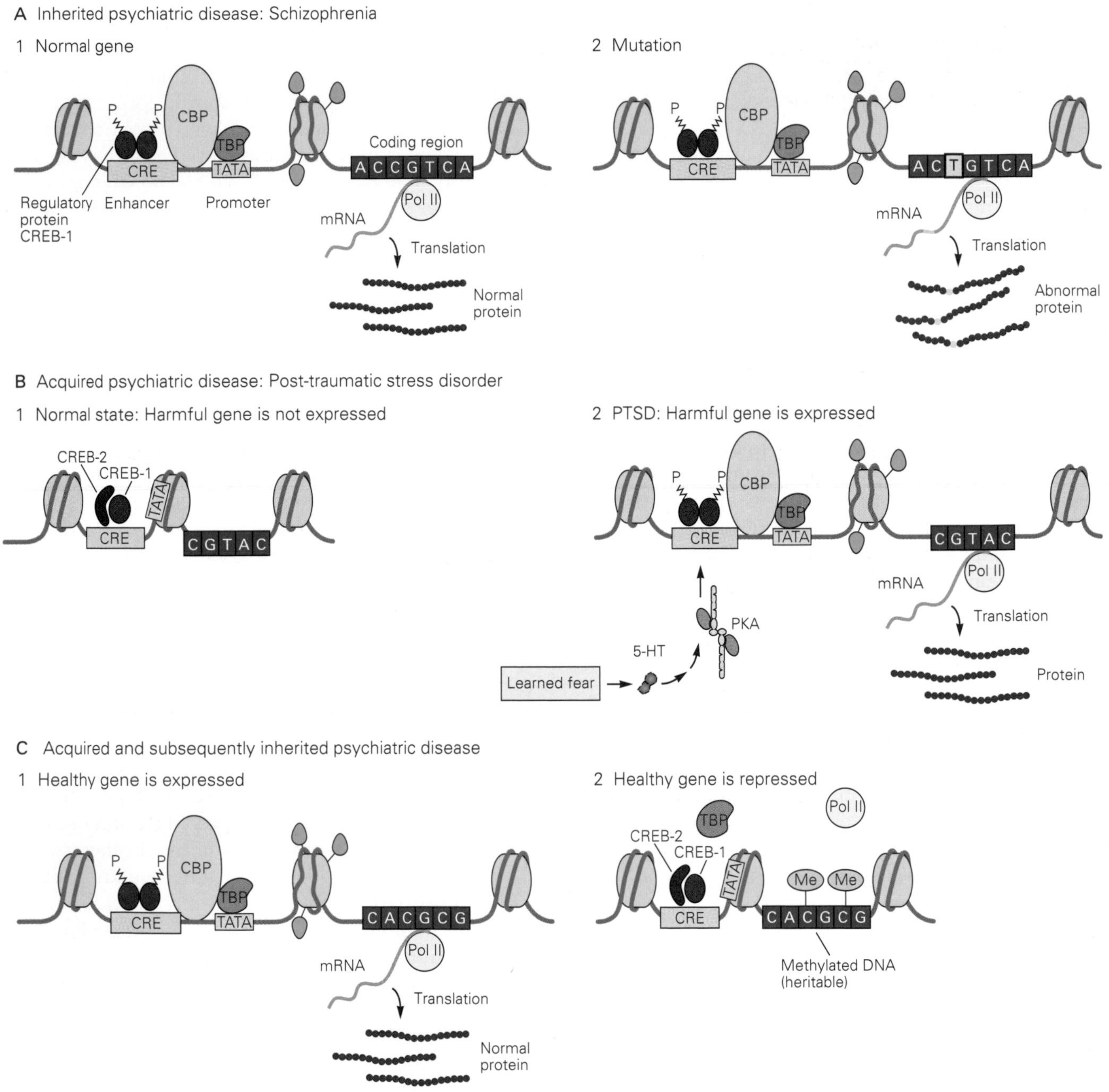
A Inherited psychiatric disease: Schizophrenia
1 Normal gene
P
P
CBP
TBP
CRE
TATA
Coding region
ACCGTCA
Regulatory protein CREB-1
Enhancer
Promoter
mRNA
Pol II
Translation
Normal protein
2 Mutation
P
P
CBP
TBP
CRE
TATA
ACTGTCA
mRNA
Pol II
Translation
Abnormal protein
B Acquired psychiatric disease: Post-traumatic stress disorder
1 Normal state: Harmful gene is not expressed
CREB-2
CREB-1
TATA
CRE
CGTAC
2 PTSD: Harmful gene is expressed
P
P
CBP
TBP
CRE
TATA
CGTAC
mRNA
Pol II
Translation
Protein
PKA
5-HT
Learned fear
C Acquired and subsequently inherited psychiatric disease
1 Healthy gene is expressed
P
P
CBP
TBP
CRE
TATA
CACGCG
mRNA
Pol II
Translation
Normal protein
2 Healthy gene is repressed
TBP
Pol II
CREB-2
CREB-1
TATA
Me
Me
CRE
CACGCG
Methylated DNA (heritable)

Figure 67–19 (Opposite) **Inherited and acquired illnesses both involve genetic changes.** Inherited illnesses result from the expression of altered genes, whereas acquired illnesses (neuroses) involve the modulation of normal gene expression by environmental stimuli. The gene illustrated here has two segments. A coding region is transcribed into mRNA by an RNA polymerase and the mRNA in turn is translated into a specific protein. A regulatory segment consists of enhancer and promoter regions (see Box 11–1). In this example the RNA polymerase can transcribe the gene when the regulatory proteins CREB-1 and CBP bind to the enhancer region. For binding to occur, CREB-1 must be phosphorylated (**P**).

A. Inherited psychiatric disease. **1.** Under normal conditions the phosphorylated CREB regulatory protein binds the enhancer segment, thereby activating transcription of the structural gene, leading to the production of the protein. **2.** A mutant form of the coding region of the structural gene, for example, in which a thymidine (**T**) has been substituted for cytosine (**C**), leads to transcription of an altered messenger RNA. This in turn produces an abnormal protein, giving rise to the disease state. This alteration in gene structure may become established in the germline and therefore heritable.

B. Acquired disease. **1.** If the regulatory protein for a normal structural gene is not phosphorylated, it cannot bind the promoter site and thus gene transcription cannot be initiated. **2.** A specific frightening experience can lead to the activation of a modulatory transmitter such as serotonin (**5-HT**), which leads to elevation of cAMP and activation of protein kinase A. The catalytic subunit phosphorylates the regulatory protein, which then can bind to the enhancer segment and thus initiate gene transcription. By this means an abnormal learning experience could lead to the altered expression of a protein that gives rise to symptoms of a psychiatric disorder such as post-traumatic stress disorder.

C. Heritable epigenetic changes. Certain experiences, for example extreme stress during early childhood, can lead to changes in DNA methylation, which alters gene expression. Such changes in methylation can be maintained even during DNA replication as a result of the activity of maintenance DNA methyltransferases. In some instances changes in DNA methylation can be passed from a mother to her offspring.

in the early stages of Alzheimer disease, may primarily result from a defect in synaptic plasticity. Drugs that enhance the ability to induce synaptic plasticity, and in particular LTP, offer a promising approach for the treatment of memory loss.

The finding that epigenetic changes play important roles in learning, memory and behavioral modifications adds a new dimension to our understanding of how environmental and social interactions can produce long-lasting changes in the nervous system. What is particularly striking is that these epigenetic changes allow environmental influences to be passed from a mother onto her offspring. Infant neglect and child abuse are extremely stressful for the developing child and are thought to contribute to cognitive and social deficits that lead to the later development of psychiatric illnesses such as anxiety states and depression.

We now know that early prenatal and postnatal environmental influences, including maternal behavior, can lead to persistent chromatin modifications in the form of direct methylation of the genes that encode hormones, growth factors, and receptors that are important for learning, memory, and emotional states. Moreover, females that experienced maltreatment during infancy later produce offspring that inherit this DNA methylation for at least one generation. Thus, not only our own experience, but that of our mothers, can have a direct and lasting influence on our genetic landscape.

The convergence of neurobiology, cognitive psychology, neurology, and psychiatry that we have emphasized throughout this book is filled with promise. Modern cognitive psychology has shown that the brain stores an internal representation of the world while neurobiology has shown that this representation can be understood in terms of the activity of individual nerve cells and their interconnections. This synthesis has given us a deeper understanding of perception, learning, and memory as well as profound new biological insight into the nature of mental illnesses.

Steven A. Siegelbaum
Eric R. Kandel

Selected Readings

Abel T, Nguyen PV, Barad M, Deuel TAS, Kandel ER, Bourtchouladze R. 1997. Genetic demonstration of a role for PKA in the late phase of LTP and in hippocampal based long-term memory. Cell 88:615–626.

Andersen P, Morris R, Amaral D, Bliss T, O'Keefe J. (eds). 2007. *The Hippocampus Book*. New York: Oxford Univ. Press.

Barco A, Bailey CH, Kandel ER. 2006. Common molecular mechanisms in explicit and implicit memory. J Neurochem 97:1520–1533.

Day JJ, Sweatt JD. 2011. Epigenetic mechanisms in cognition. Neuron 70:813–829.

Frey U, Morris RG. 1991. Synaptic tagging and long-term potentiation. Nature 385:533–536.

Hübener M, Bonhoeffer T. 2010. Searching for engrams. Neuron 67:363–371.

Kerchner GA, Nicoll RA. 2008. Silent synapses and the emergence of a postsynaptic mechanism for LTP. Nat Rev Neurosci 9:813–825.

Kessels HW, Malinow R. 2009. Synaptic AMPA receptor plasticity and behavior. Neuron 61:340–350.

Mansuy IM, Mayford M, Jacob B, Kandel ER, Bach ME. 1998. Restricted and regulated overexpression reveals calcineurin as a key component in the transition from short-term to long-term memory. Cell 92:39–49.

Morris RG. 2006. Elements of a neurobiological theory of hippocampal function: the role of synaptic plasticity, synaptic tagging and schemas. Eur J Neurosci 23:2829–2846.

Moser EI, Kropff E, Moser MB. 2008. Place cells, grid cells, and the brain's spatial representation system. Ann Rev Neurosci 31:69–89.

Nakazawa K, Quirk MC, Chitwood RA, Watanabe M, Yeckel MF, Sun LD, Kato A, et al. 2002. Requirement for hippocampal CA3 NMDA receptors in associative memory recall. Science 297:211–218.

Nakazawa K, Sun LD, Quirk MC, Rondi-Reig L, Wilson MA, Tonegawa S. 2003. Hippocampal CA3 NMDA receptors are crucial for memory acquisition of one-time experience. Neuron 38:306–315.

Sacktor TC. 2011. How does PKMζ maintain long-term memory? Nat Rev Neurosci 12:9–15.

Sahay A, Wilson DA, Hen R. 2011. Pattern separation: a common function for new neurons in hippocampus and olfactory bulb. Neuron 70:582–588.

Steward O, Schuman EM. 2001. Protein synthesis at synaptic sites on dendrites. Ann Rev Neurosci 24:299–325.

Winder DG, Mansuy IM, Osman M, Moallem TM, Kandel ER. 1998. Genetic and pharmacological evidence for a novel, intermediate phase of long-term potentiation suppressed by calcineurin. Cell 92:25–37.

References

Aksay E, Olasagasti I, Mensh BD, Baker R, Goldman MS, Tank DW. 2007. Functional dissection of circuitry in a neural integrator. Nat Neurosci 10:494–504.

Bliss TVP, Lomø T. 1973. Long-lasting potentiation of synaptic transmission in the dentate gyrus of the anesthetized rabbit following stimulation of the perforant path. J Physiol (Lond) 232:331–356.

Bolshakov VY, Golan H, Kandel ER, Siegelbaum SA. 1997. Recruitment of new sites of synaptic transmission during the cAMP-dependent late phase of LTP at CA3-CA1 synapses in the hippocampus. Neuron 19:635–651.

Bourtchouladze R, Frenguelli B, Blendy J, Cioffi D, Schutz G, Silva A. 1994. Deficient long-term memory in mice with a targeted mutation of the cAMP responsive element binding protein. Cell 79:59–68.

Dudek SM, Bear MF. 1992. Homosynaptic long-term depression in area CA1 of hippocampus and effects of *N*-methyl-D-aspartate receptor blockade. Proc Natl Acad Sci U S A 89:4363–4367.

Egorov AV, Hamam BN, Fransen E, Hasselmo ME, Alonso AA. 2002. Graded persistent activity in entorhinal cortex neurons. Nature 420:173–178.

Fischer A, Sananbenesi F, Wang X, Dobbin M, Tsai LH. 2007. Recovery of learning and memory is associated with chromatin remodelling. Nature 447:178–182.

Goldman-Rakic PS. 1995. Cellular basis of working memory. Neuron 14:477–485.

Grant SGN, O'Dell TJ, Karl KA, Stein PL, Soriano P, Kandel ER. 1992. Impaired long-term potentiation, spatial learning, and hippocampal development in *fyn* mutant mice. Science 258:1903–1910.

Gustafsson B, Wigström H, Abraham WC, Huang Y-Y. 1987. Long-term potentiation in the hippocampus using depolarizing current as the conditioning stimulus to single volley synaptic potential. J Neurosci 7:774–780.

Gustafsson B, Wigström H. 1988. Physiological mechanisms underlying long-term potentiation. Trends Neurosci 11:156–162.

Haftig T, Moser E. 2005. Microstructure of the spatial map in the entorhinal complex. Nature 436:801–808.

Hebb DO. 1949. *The Organization of Behavior: A Neuropsychological Theory.* New York: Wiley.

Huang Y-Y, Kandel ER. 1994. Recruitment of long-lasting and protein kinase A-dependent long-term potentiation in the CA1 region of hippocampus requires repeated tetanization. Learn Mem 1:74–82.

Huang Y-Y, Kandel ER, Varshavsky L, Brandon EP, Qi M, Idzerda RL, McKnight GS, Bourtchouladze R. 1995. A genetic test of the effects of mutations in PKA on mossy fiber LTP and its relation to spatial and contextual learning. Cell 83:1211–1222.

Huang Y-Y, Li X-C, Kandel ER. 1994. cAMP contributes to mossy fiber LTP by initiating both a covalently-mediated early phase and a macromolecular synthesis-dependent late phase. Cell 79:69–79.

Kandel ER. 2001. The molecular biology of memory storage: a dialog between genes and synapses. (Nobel Lecture) Bioscience Reports 21:565–611.

Malinow R. 2003. AMPA receptor trafficking and long-term potentiation. Philos Trans R Soc Lond B Biol Sci 358: 707–714.

Malinow R, Tsien RW. 1990. Presynaptic enhancement shown by whole cell recordings of LTP in hippocampal slices. Nature 357:134–139.

Mayford M, Bach ME, Huang Y-Y, Wang L, Hawkins RD, Kandel ER. 1996. Control of memory formation through regulated expression of a CaMKII transgene. Science 274:1678–1683.

McHugh TJ, Blum KI, Tsien JZ, Tonegawa S, Wilson MA. 1996. Impaired hippocampal representation of space in CA1-specific NMDAR1 knockout mice. Cell 87: 1339–1349.

McHugh TJ, Jones MW, Quinn JJ, Balthasar N, Coppari R, Elmquist JK, Lowell BB, Fanselow MS, Wilson MA, Tonegawa S. 2007. Dentate gyrus NMDA receptors mediate rapid pattern separation in the hippocampal network. Science 317:94–99.

Morgan SL, Teyler TJ. 2001. Electrical stimuli patterned after the theta-rhythm induce multiple forms of LTP. J Neurophysiol 86:1289–1296.

Muller RU, Kubie JL, Ranck JB Jr. 1987. Spatial firing patterns of hippocampal complex-spike cells in a fixed environment. J Neurosci 7:1935–1950.

Nakashiba T, Cushman JD, Pelkey KA, Renaudineau S, Buhl DL, McHugh TJ, Rodriguez Barrera V. 2012. Young dentate granule cells mediate pattern separation, whereas old granule cells facilitate pattern completion. Cell 149:188–201.

Nakashiba T, Young JZ, McHugh TJ, Buhl DL, Tonegawa S. 2008. Transgenic inhibition of synaptic transmission reveals role of CA3 output in hippocampal learning. Science 319:1260–1264.

Nicholls RE, Alarcon JM, Malleret G, Carroll RC, Grody M Vronskaya S, Kandel ER. 2008. Transgenic mice lacking NMDAR-dependent LTD exhibit deficits in behavioral flexibility. Neuron 58:104–117.

Nolan MF, Malleret G, Dudman JT, Buhl DL, Santoro B, Gibbs E, Vronskaya S, et al. 2004. A behavioral role for dendritic integration: HCN1 channels constrain spatial memory and plasticity at inputs to distal dendrites of CA1 pyramidal neurons. Cell 119:719–732.

O'Keefe J, Dostrovsky J. 1971. The hippocampus as a spatial map: preliminary evidence from unit activity in the freely-moving rat. Brain Res 34:171–175.

Remondes M, Schuman EM. 2003. Molecular mechanisms contributing to long-lasting synaptic plasticity at the temporoammonic-CA1 synapse. Learn Mem 10:247–252.

Rotenberg A, Mayford M, Hawkins RD, Kandel ER, Muller RU. 1996. Mice expressing activated CaMKII lack low frequency LTP and do not form stable place cells in the CA1 region of the hippocampus. Cell 87:1351–1361.

Rumpel S, LeDoux J, Zador A, Malinow R. 2005. Postsynaptic receptor trafficking underlying a form of associative learning. Science 308:83–88.

Schuman EM, Madison DV. 1991. A requirement for the intercellular messenger nitric oxide in long-term potentiation. Science 254:1503–1506.

Silva AJ, Paylor R, Wehner JM, Tonegawa S. 1992. Impaired spatial learning in α-calcium-calmodulin kinase II mutant mice. Science 257:206–211.

Silva AJ, Stevens CF, Tonegawa S, Wang Y. 1992. Deficient hippocampal long-term potentiation in α-calcium-calmodulin kinase II mutant mice. Science 257:201–206.

Tang YP, Shimizu E, Dube GR, Rampon C, Kerchner GA, Zhuo M, Liu G, Tsien JZ. 1999. Genetic enhancement of learning and memory in mice. Nature 401:63–69.

Tsien JZ, Chen DF, Gerber D, Tom C, Mercer EH, Anderson DJ, Mayford M, Kandel ER, Tonegawa S. 1996. Subregion and cell type-restricted gene knockout in mouse brain. Cell 87:1317–1326.

Tsien JZ, Huerta PT, Tonegawa S. 1996. The essential role of hippocampal CA1 NMDA receptor-dependent synaptic plasticity in spatial memory. Cell 87:1327–1338.

Tsien RW, Malinow R. 1990. Long-term potentiation: presynaptic enhancement following postsynaptic activation of Ca^{2+}-dependent protein kinases. Cold Spring Harbor Symp Quant Biol 55:147–159.

Wang XJ. 2001. Synaptic reverberation underlying mnemonic persistent activity. Trends Neurosci 24:455–463.

Weisskopf MG, Castillo PE, Zalutsky RA, Nicoll RA. 1994. Mediation of hippocampal long-term potentiation by cyclic AMP. Science 265:1878–1882.

Whitlock JR, Heynen AJ, Shuler MG, Bear MF. 2006. Learning induces long-term potentiation in the hippocampus. Science 313:1093–1097.

Zalutsky RA, Nicoll RA. 1990. Comparison of two forms of long-term potentiation in single hippocampal neurons. Science 248:1619–1624.

Appendices

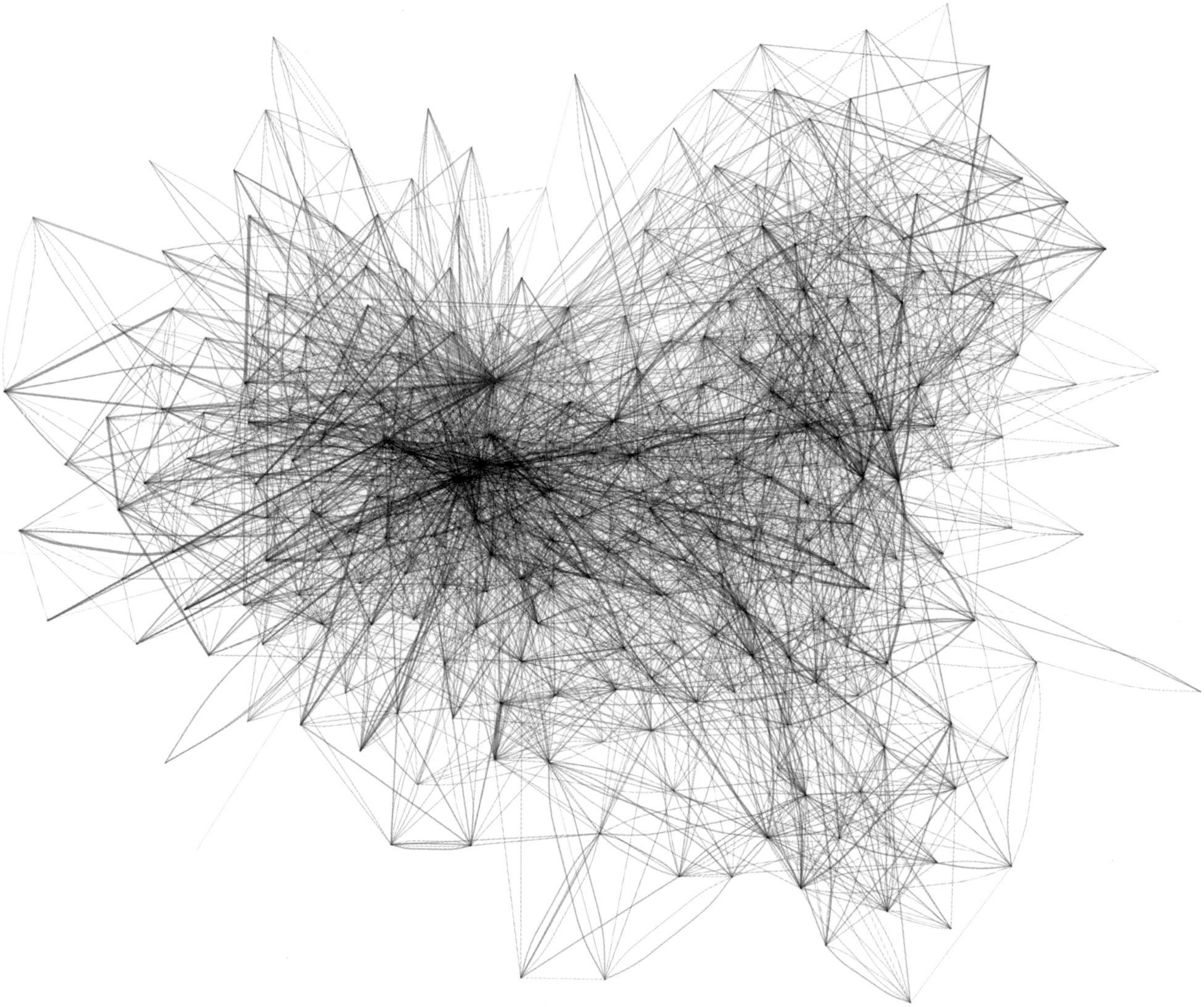

Preceding Page

Connectome of *Caenorhabditis elegans.* Behavior is determined by the connections between an organism's nerve cells. Networks of neurons, which in mammals reach an astounding degree of complexity, choreograph our simplest reflexes and our most profound insights. While exploration of neural networks in the mammalian brain is in its early stages, the complete set of neural connections—the connectome—has been almost entirely mapped for the nematode *C. elegans.* With only 302 neurons, 6393 chemical synapses, 890 gap junctions, and 1410 neuromuscular junctions, this simple animal provides a window into the operations carried out by a complete nervous system. In this image each point represents a neuron and the thickness of each line reflects the number of contacts between the neurons (from 1–37). Gap junctions are red, chemical synapses are blue, and neuromuscular junctions are magenta; all neuromuscular junctions are directed at one idealized point in the graph. For simplicity, directionality and neuron type are not shown. (Reproduced, with permission, from Eduardo Izquierdo, with data from White, JG, Southgate E, Thomson JN, Brenner S. 1986. The structure of the nervous system of the nematode *Caenorhabditis elegans*. Philosophical Transactions of the Royal Society B:Biological Sciences 314:1–340; and Varshney LR, Chen, BL, Paniaqua E, Hall DH, Chklovskii DB. 2011. Structural properties of the *C. elegans* neuronal network. PLoS Comput Biol 7:e1001066. doi:10.1371/journal.pcbi. 1001066)

Appendix A

Review of Basic Circuit Theory

FAMILIARITY WITH THE BASIC PRINCIPLES of electrical circuit theory is important for understanding the equivalent circuit model of the neuron developed in Chapters 6, 7, and 9. The appendix is divided into three parts:

1. The definition of basic electrical parameters.
2. A set of rules for elementary circuit analysis.
3. A description of current in circuits with capacitance.

Basic Electrical Parameters

Potential Difference (V or E)

Electrical charges exert an electrostatic force on other charges: like charges repel, opposite charges attract. The force decreases as the distance between two charges increases. *Work* is done when two charges that initially are separated are brought together. Negative work is done if their polarities are opposite and positive work if they are the same. The greater the values of the charges and the greater their initial separation, the greater the work done. (Work = $\int_{r1}^{0} f(r)\,dr$ where f is electrostatic force and r_1 is the initial distance between the two charges.)

Potential difference is a measure of this work: The *potential difference* between two points is the work that must be done to move a unit of positive charge (one coulomb) from one point to the other (ie, it is the potential energy of the charge). One volt (V) is the energy required to move one coulomb a distance of one meter against a force of one newton.

Current (I)

A potential difference exists within a system whenever positive and negative charges are separated. Charge separation may be generated by a chemical reaction (as in a battery) or by diffusion of two electrolyte solutions with different ion concentrations across a selectively permeable barrier, such as a cell membrane. If a charge separation exists within a conducting medium, charges move between the areas of potential difference: Positive charges are attracted to the region with a more negative potential, and negative charges to the region of positive potential.

Current is defined as the net movement of charge per unit time. According to convention, the direction of current is defined as the direction of flow of positive charge. In metallic conductors current is carried by negatively charged electrons, which move in the opposite direction of conventionally defined current. In nerve and muscle cells current is carried by both positive and negative ions in solution. One ampere (A) of current represents the movement of one coulomb (of charge) per second.

Conductance (g)

Any object through which electrical charges can flow is called a conductor. The unit of electrical conductance is the siemens (S). According to Ohm's law the current that flows through a conductor is directly proportional to the potential difference across it:[1]

$$I = V \times g$$

$$\text{Current } (A) = \text{Potential difference } (V) \times \text{Conductance } (S).$$

As charge carriers move through a conductor, some of their electrical potential energy is converted into thermal energy caused by their frictional interactions with the conducting medium.

Each type of material has an intrinsic property called *conductivity* (σ), which is determined by its molecular structure. Metallic conductors conduct electricity extremely well and thus have high conductivities. Aqueous solutions with high-ionized salt concentrations have somewhat lower conductivity, and lipids have very low conductivity—they are poor conductors of electricity and are therefore good insulators. The conductance of an object is proportional to σ times its cross-sectional area divided by its length:

$$g = (\sigma) \times \text{area}/\text{length}.$$

Length is defined as the direction along which one measures conductance. For example, the conductance measured along the cytoplasmic core of an axon is reduced if its length is increased or its diameter decreased (Figure A–1).

Electrical resistance (R) is the reciprocal of conductance and a measure of the resistance provided by an object to current. Resistance is measured in ohms (Ω):

$$1\ \Omega = 1/(1\ \text{S}).$$

[1]This formula for current flow is analogous to other formulas for describing flow (eg, bulk flow of a liquid caused by a hydrostatic pressure, flow of a solute in response to a concentration gradient, flow of heat in response to a temperature gradient, etc.). In each case flow is proportional to the product of a driving force times a conductance factor.

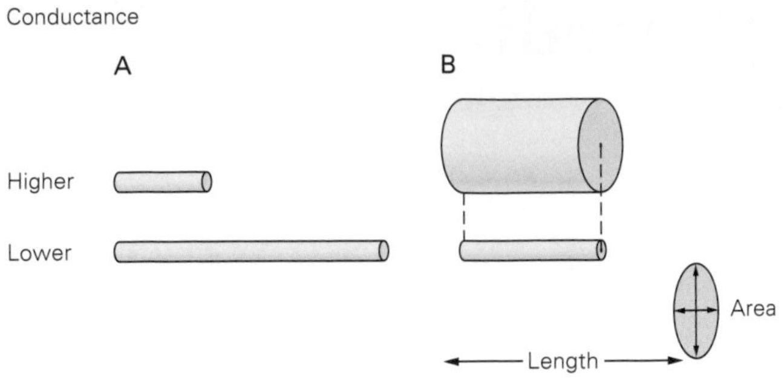

Figure A–1 The conductance of an object is determined by geometric factors, together with conductivity. Conductance is inversely proportional to the length of the conductor (**A**) and directly proportional to the cross-sectional area of the conductor (**B**).

Capacitance (C)

A capacitor consists of two conducting plates separated by an insulating layer. Its fundamental property is its ability to separate charges of opposite sign: Positive charges are stored on one plate, negative charges on the other. In the example in Figure A–2 a net excess of positive charges on plate x and an equal excess of negative charges on plate y results in a potential difference between the two plates.

This potential difference can be measured by determining how much work is required to move a positive test charge from y to x. Initially, the test charge is attracted by the negative charges on y and repelled by the more distant positive charges on x. The result of these electrostatic interactions is a force f that opposes the movement of the charge from y to x. However, as the test charge is moved toward x, the attraction by the negative charges on y diminishes and the repulsion by the positive charges on x increases, with the result that the net electrostatic force exerted on the test charge is constant everywhere between x and y. Work (W) is force times the distance (D) over which the force is exerted:

$$W = f \times D.$$

The work done in moving the test charge from one side of the capacitor to the other is equal to the difference in electrical potential energy, or potential difference, between x and y. In Figure A–2 it is shown as the shaded region in the plots.

Capacitance is measured in farads (F). The greater the density of charges on the capacitor plates, the greater the force acting on the test charge and the

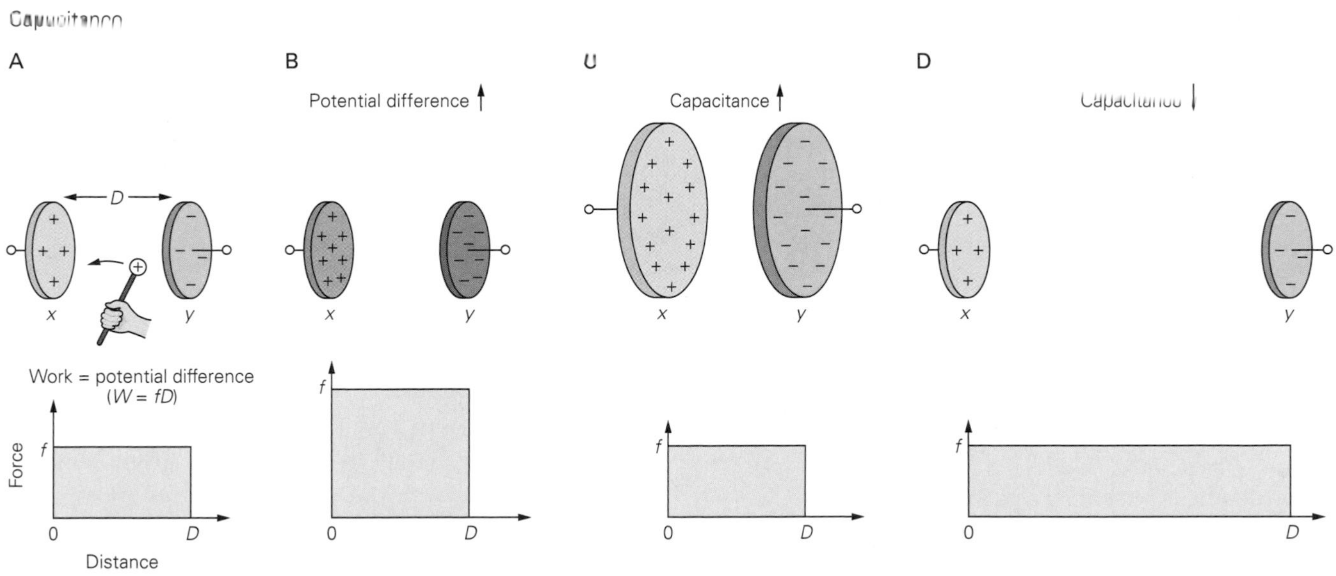

Figure A–2 The capacitance of a parallel-plate capacitor is determined by the area of the two plates and the distance between them.

A. A test charge moved between two charged plates must overcome a force. The work done against this force is the potential difference between the two plates.

B. Increasing the density of charge carriers increases the potential difference.

C. Increasing the area of the plates increases capacitance by increasing the number of charges required to produce a given potential difference.

D. Increasing the distance between the two plates decreases capacitance, decreasing the number of charges required to produce a given potential difference.

greater the resulting potential difference across the capacitor (see Figure A–2B). Thus, for a given capacitor there is a linear relationship between the amount of charge (Q) stored on its plates and the potential difference across it:

$$Q \text{ (coulombs)} = C \text{ (farads)} \times V \text{ (volts)} \qquad \textbf{(A–1)}$$

where C, the capacitance, is a constant.

The capacitance of a parallel-plate capacitor is determined by two features of its geometry: the area (A) of the two plates and the distance (D) between them. Increasing the area of the plates increases capacitance because a greater amount of charge must be deposited on each side to produce the same charge density, which is what determines the force f acting on the test charge (Figure A–2A and C). Increasing the distance between the plates does not change the force acting on the test charge, but it does increase the work that must be done to move it from one side of the capacitor to the other (Figure A–2A and D). Therefore, for a given charge separation between the two plates, the potential difference between them is proportional to the distance. Put another way, the greater the distance, the smaller the amount of charge that must be deposited on the plates to produce a given potential difference, and therefore the smaller the capacitance (Equation A–1).

These geometrical determinants of capacitance can be summarized by the equation

$$C \propto A/D.$$

As shown in Equation A–1, the separation of positive and negative charges on the two plates of a capacitor results in a potential difference between them. The converse of this statement is also true: The potential difference across a capacitor is determined by the net positive and negative charge on its plates. For the potential across a capacitor to change, the amount of electrical charges stored on the two conducting plates must change first.

Rules for Circuit Analysis

Familiarity with a few basic rules for electric circuit analysis will help in understanding the equivalent circuits used throughout the textbook.

Conductance

The symbol for a conductor is:

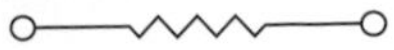

A variable conductor is represented as:

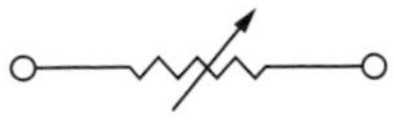

A pathway with infinite conductance (zero resistance) is called a *short circuit* and is represented by a line:

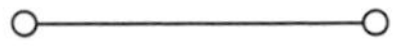

Conductances *in parallel* add:

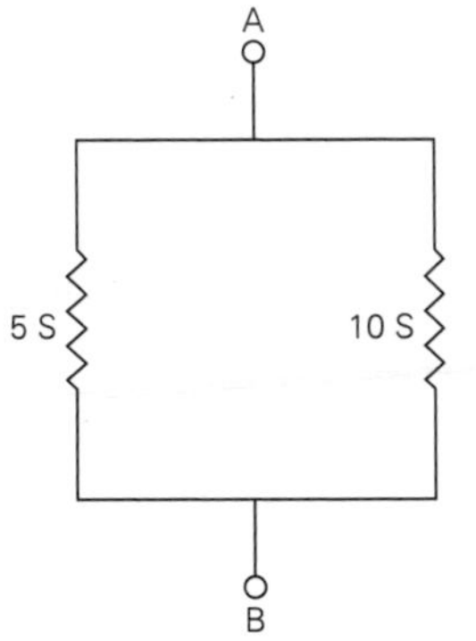

$g_{AB} = 15$ S

Conductances *in series* add reciprocally:

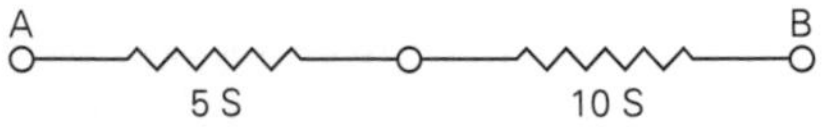

$$1/g_{AB} = 1/5 + 1/10 = 3/10$$
$$g_{AB} = 3.3 \text{ S}.$$

Resistances *in series* add, while resistances *in parallel* add reciprocally.

Current

An arrow denotes the direction of current (net movement of positive charge). Ohm's law is

$$I = V \times g = V/R.$$

When charge flows through a conductor, the end that the current enters is positive with respect to the end that it leaves:

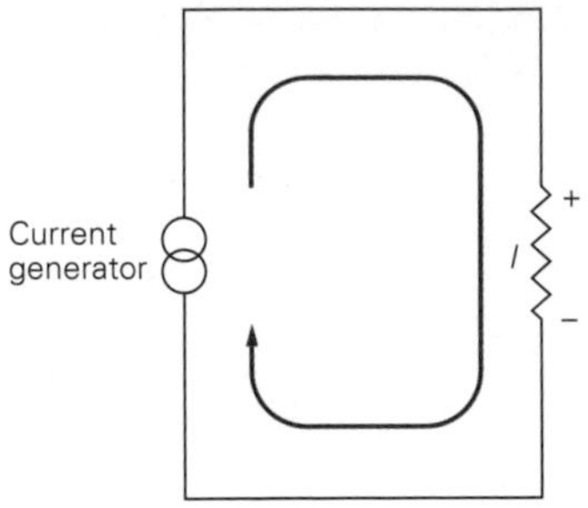

The algebraic sum of all currents entering or leaving a junction is zero. (We arbitrarily define current approaching a junction as positive, and current leaving a junction as negative.) In the following circuit for junction x

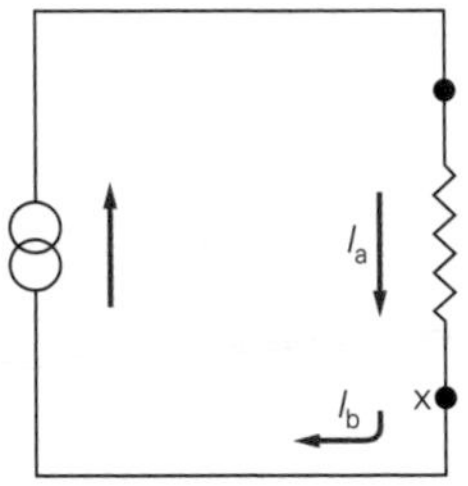

the currents are

$$I_a = +5 \text{ A}$$
$$I_b = -5 \text{ A}$$
$$I_a + I_b = 0.$$

In the following circuit for junction y

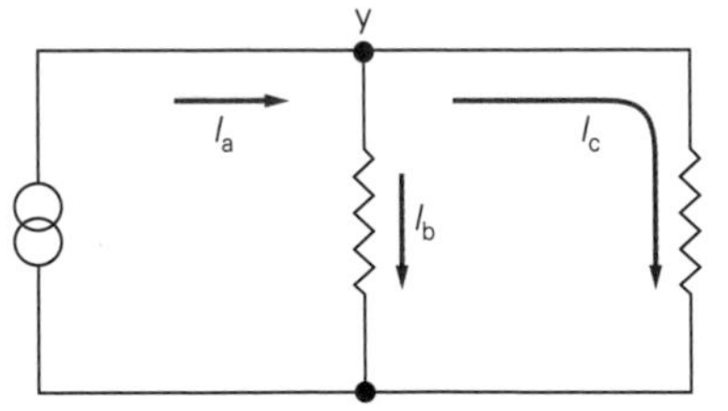

the currents are

$$I_a = +3 \text{ A}$$
$$I_b = -2 \text{ A}$$
$$I_c = -1 \text{ A}$$
$$I_a + I_b + I_c = 0.$$

Current follows the path of greatest conductance (least resistance). For conductance pathways in parallel, the current through each path is proportional to its conductance value divided by the total conductance of the parallel combination:

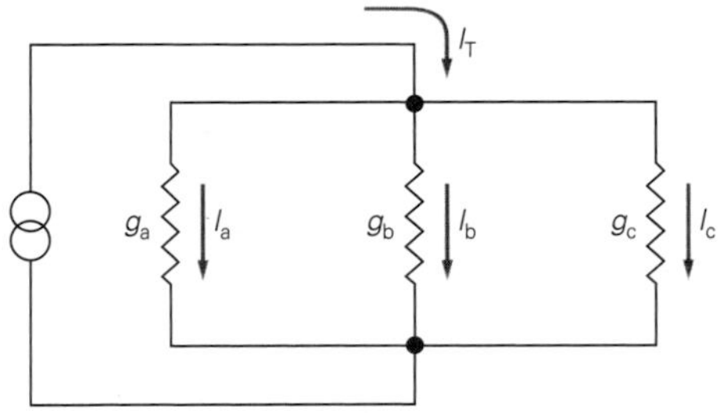

$$I_T = 10\text{ A}$$
$$g_a = 3\text{ S}$$
$$g_b = 2\text{ S}$$
$$g_c = 5\text{ S}$$

$$I_a = \frac{I_T \times g_a}{g_a + g_b + g_c} = 3\text{ A}$$

$$I_b = \frac{I_T \times g_b}{g_a + g_b + g_c} = 2\text{ A}$$

$$I_c = \frac{I_T \times g_c}{g_a + g_b + g_c} = 5\text{ A}.$$

Capacitance

The symbol for a capacitor is:

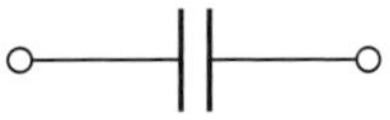

The potential difference across a capacitor is proportional to the charge stored on its plates:

$$V_C = Q/C.$$

Potential Difference

The symbol for a battery or electromotive force (E) is

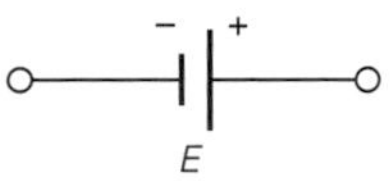

The positive pole is always represented by the longer bar.

Batteries in series add algebraically, but attention must be paid to their polarities. If their polarities are the same, their absolute values add:

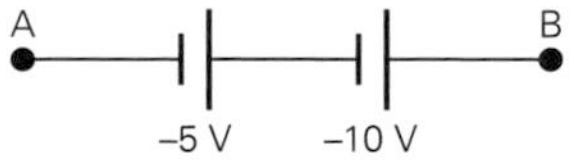

$$V_{AB} = -15\text{ V}.$$

If their polarities are opposite, they subtract:

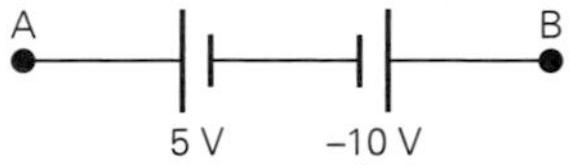

$$V_{AB} = -5\text{ V}.$$

(Here the convention used for potential difference is that $V_{AB} = V_A - V_B$.)

A battery drives a current around the circuit from its positive to its negative terminal:

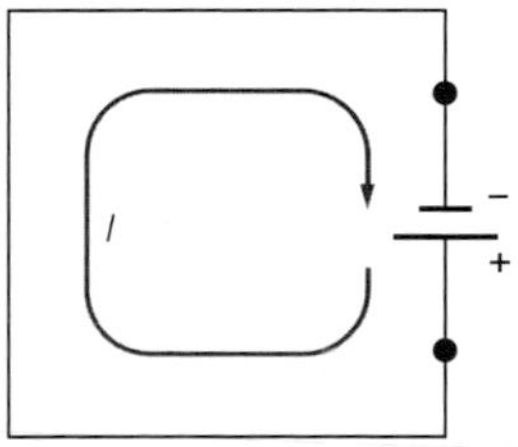

For purposes of calculating the total resistance of a circuit, the internal resistance of a battery is set at zero.

The potential differences across parallel branches of a circuit are equal:

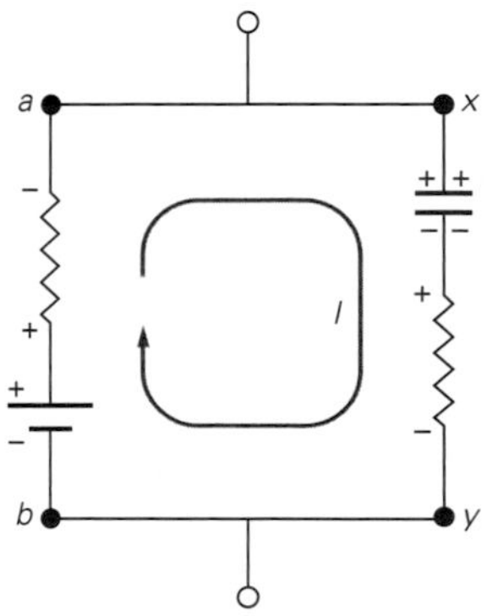

$$V_{ab} = V_{xy}.$$

As one goes around a closed loop in a circuit, the algebraic sum of all the potential differences is zero:

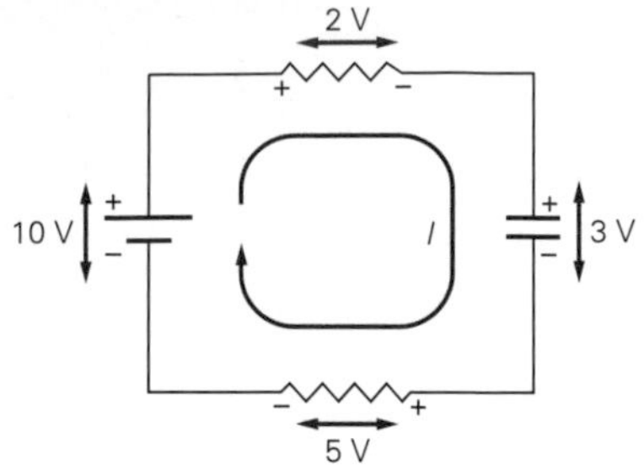

Thus,

$$2\text{ V} + 3\text{ V} + 5\text{ V} - 10\text{ V} = 0.$$

Current in Circuits with Capacitance

Circuits that have capacitive elements are much more complex than those which have only batteries and conductors because in capacitive circuits current varies with time. The time dependence of changes in current and voltage in capacitive circuits is illustrated qualitatively in the following three examples.

Circuit with Capacitor

Current does not cross the insulating gap in a capacitor; rather, it builds up positive and negative charges on the capacitor plates. However, we can measure a current into and out of the terminal of a capacitor. Consider the circuit shown in Figure A–3A. When switch S is closed, the battery E moves a net positive charge onto plate a, and an equal amount of net positive charge is withdrawn from plate b. The result is a counterclockwise current in the circuit (Figure A–3B).

Because this current flows into or out of the terminals of a capacitor, it is called a *capacitive current* (I_c). Because there is no resistance in this circuit, the battery E can generate a very large amplitude of current that will charge the capacitance to a value $Q = E \times C$ instantaneously (Figure A–3D).

Circuit with Resistor and Capacitor in Series

Now consider what happens if a resistor is added in series with the capacitor (Figure A–4A). The maximum current that can be generated when switch S is closed (Figure A–4B) is now limited by Ohm's law ($I = V/R$). Therefore the capacitor charges more slowly. When the potential across the capacitor has finally reached the value $V_c = Q/C = E$ (Figure A–4C), there is no longer a difference in potential around the loop (ie, the battery voltage E is equal and opposite to the voltage across the capacitor, V_c). The two thus cancel out, and no net potential difference is left to drive a current around the loop.

The potential difference is greatest, and current is at a maximum, immediately after the switch is closed. As the capacitor begins to charge, the net potential difference ($V_c + E$) available to drive a current becomes smaller and current decreases. This results in an exponential change in voltage as well as current across the resistor and the capacitor. Note that in this circuit resistive current must equal capacitative current at all times (see earlier section, Rules for Circuit Analysis).

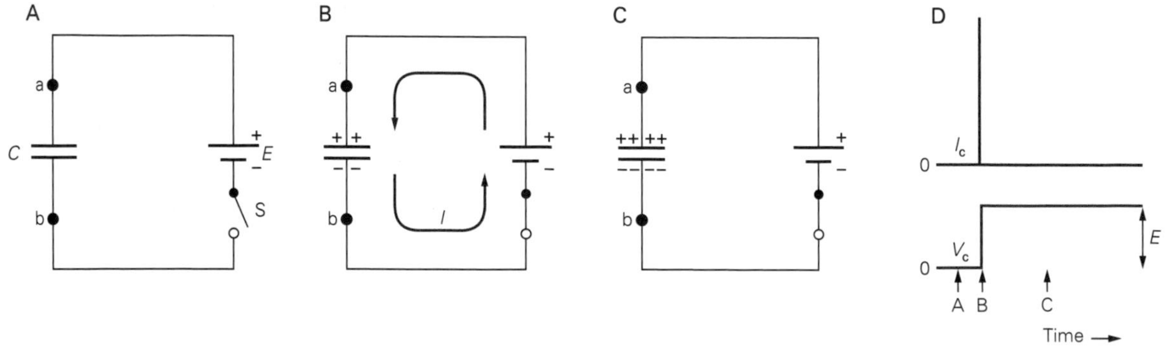

Figure A–3 Time course of charging a capacitor.

A. Circuit before the switch (**S**) is closed.

B. After the switch is closed.

C. After the capacitor has become fully charged.

D. Time course of changes in current (I_c) and potential difference across the capacitor (V_c) in response to closing of the switch.

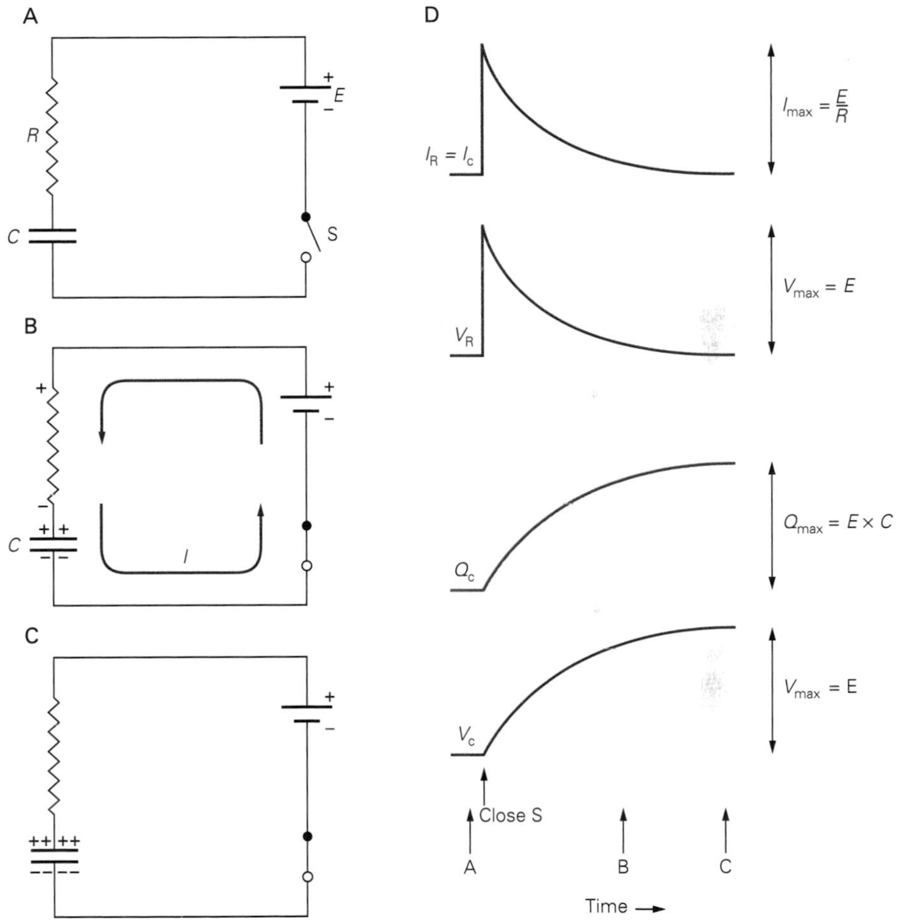

Figure A–4 Time course of charging a capacitor (*C*) in series with a resistor (*R*) from a constant voltage source (*E*).

A. Circuit before the switch (**S**) is closed.

B. Shortly after the switch is closed.

C. After the capacitor has settled at its final potential.

D. Time course of changes in current (*I*), charge deposited on the capacitor (Q_c), and potential differences across the resistor (V_R) and capacitor (V_c) after closing the switch.

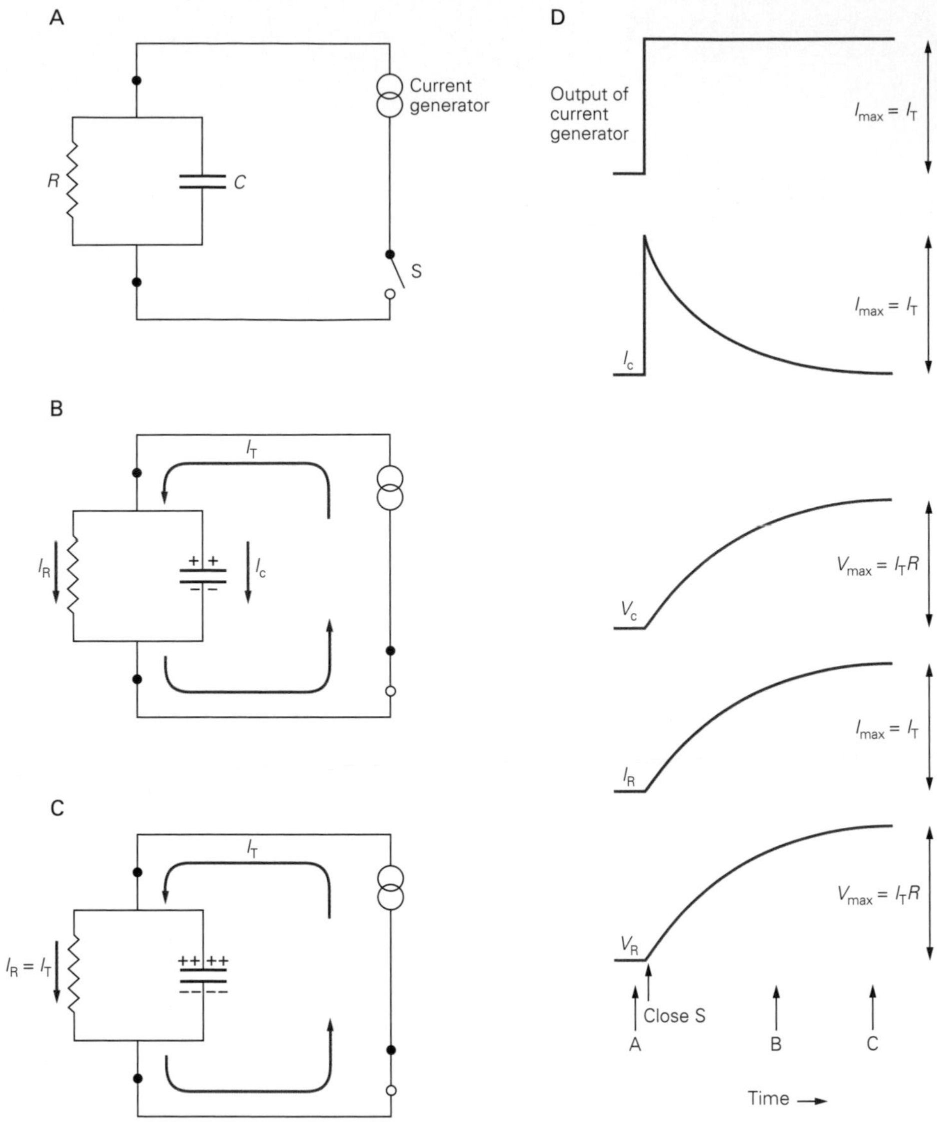

Figure A–5 Time course of charging a capacitor (C) in parallel with a resistor (R) from a constant current source.

A. Circuit before the switch (S) is closed.

B. After the switch is closed.

C. After the charge deposited on the capacitor has reached its final value.

D. Time course of changes in I_c, V_c, I_R, and V_R after closing of the switch.

Circuit with Resistor and Capacitor in Parallel

Consider now what happens if we place a parallel resistor and capacitor in series with a constant-current generator that generates a total current I_T (Figure A–5A). When the switch (S) is closed, charge starts to flow around the loop (Figure A–5B). In the first instant of time after the current begins to flow, all the charge flows into the capacitor (ie, $I_T = I_c$). However, as charge builds up on the plates of the capacitor, a potential difference V_c is generated.

Because the resistor and capacitor are in parallel, the potential across them must be equal; thus part of the total current begins to flow through the resistor, such that $I_R \times R = V_R = V_c$. As less and less charge flows into the capacitor, the rate of charging slows; this accounts for the exponential shape of the curve of voltage versus time. Eventually, the voltage reaches a plateau and no longer changes. When this occurs, all the charge flows through the resistor and $V_c = V_R = I_T \times R$ (Figure A–5C).

Steven A. Siegelbaum
John Koester

Appendix B

The Neurological Examination of the Patient

THE KEY TO THE ANALYSIS OF SIGNS and symptoms referable to the nervous system is a rigorous neurological examination of the patient. This examination begins with an assessment of the patient's mental functioning.

Mental Status

Alertness and Attentiveness

A patient's level of consciousness is defined in terms of responses to stimuli. Rather than simply using terms such as *lethargy*, *obtundation*, *stupor*, and *coma*, the examiner needs to note the minimal stimulus that elicits a response (eg, voice, shaking the patient, applying pain) and the response (eg, sustained alertness vs. fleeting eye opening with mumbling).

An impaired attention span is usually apparent during history taking. It can be tested more formally by having the patient repeat a series of numbers or count backward from 20. Sequential digit testing is sensitive, but the test is not specific; difficulty may connote impairment of immediate (working) memory.

Inattentiveness so severe that meaningful interaction with the environment is impossible is characteristic of *delirium*. Such patients are often agitated.

Behavior, Mood, and Thought

Neuropsychiatric abnormalities can be identified in this part of the mental status examination. Affect, the outward expression of mood, may be manifested in clothing, facial expression, amount and type of activity, and stream of conversation. If depression is suspected, the patient should be specifically queried; mood may be more disturbed than affect suggests.

Schizophrenic patients may demonstrate indifference, flattening of affect, or inappropriate mood. They may appear hostile and paranoid. Behavior sometimes suggests hallucinations even when they are denied. Schizophrenic speech may reveal loosening of associations, incoherence, blocking, stereotypy, or distractibility.

Slowing of speech and activity is a manifestation of medial frontal lobe damage (abulia). Lesions of the frontal lobe also produce social disinhibition, inappropriate jocularity, and difficulty sustaining goal-directed behavior.

Orientation and Memory

People aware of their own identity as well as of the basic facts of their surroundings (hospital, home address, city, state; time of day, day of week, month, year) are said to be "oriented to person, place, and time." Memory impairment secondary to brain injury or a dementing illness is usually greater for recent than remote events; such patients are disoriented to place and time but not to person. Disorientation is neither a sensitive nor a specific marker of amnesia, however.

Memory is clinically categorized as immediate (working), recent, and remote. A sensitive test for recent memory is to have the patient repeat three unrelated words (eg, Chicago, orange, thirty-three) and then repeat them after 5 minutes. If unable to recall the words, the patient is asked to select the words from a list. Amnestic disorders tend to affect recall more than recognition. Long-term memory can be tested by having the patient recall people or events from the past and then verifying the answers.

Conventional testing identifies disturbances of explicit memory (see Chapter 67). Amnestic or dementing illnesses are less likely to affect implicit memory systems such as procedural memory (remembering how to perform a skilled motor act).

Cognitive Abilities

Intellectual skills are assessed in standardized IQ tests, which are subject to educational and cultural bias. Tests include calculation, word similarities, word opposites, and proverb interpretation.

Language Disorders

Aphasia is a disturbance of language unexplained by an impairment of the neural machinery for hearing, vision, or vocalizing (see Chapter 60). Clinical subtypes of aphasia can be identified by assessing six basic components of language: spontaneous speech, speech comprehension, naming, repetition, writing, and reading (Figure B–1).

Spontaneous Speech

The patient's speech may be abnormal in a number of ways. *Fluency,* the amount of speech produced over time, may be reduced. *Prosody,* the musical qualities of speech (pitch, accent, rhythm), can also be impaired. In *paraphasias* incorrect words are substituted for correct ones. Patients with *literal* (or phonemic) paraphasia use words that phonetically resemble the intended word but contain one or more substituted syllables (eg, "hosicle" instead of "hospital"). Those with *verbal* (or semantic) paraphasia use real but unintended words (eg, "hotel" instead of "hospital"). In some patients paraphasic errors are simply occasional contaminants of speech; in others, they almost entirely replace it.

Even in the absence of paraphasias the content of aphasic speech may be difficult to grasp. Severely restricted vocabulary may be reflected by logorrheic but empty speech as well as by hesitation before certain words. *Paragrammatic* speech preserves some semblance of syntax despite such profoundly restricted semantic content. By contrast, *agrammatic* (or telegrammatic) speech omits relational words (such as prepositions or conjunctions).

Speech Comprehension

Casual conversation with the patient may not reveal abnormalities of speech comprehension, which can be mild, moderate, or severe. Specific testing is required. Assessment of speech comprehension should not depend on the patient's verbal responses to commands or questions. A wrong answer to a question could signify a paraphasic error rather than failure of comprehension. If a simple or complex command is followed, it can be presumed that the command was understood. However, failure to follow a command could have explanations other than impaired comprehension, for example, paralysis, apraxia, pain, or negativism.

A more reliable method of testing speech comprehension is to ask yes-or-no questions. Even patients with severely restricted speech output can usually indicate affirmative or negative. Both the patient and the examiner must of course know the correct answers. Still another way of testing speech comprehension is to ask the patient to point to objects or body parts.

As with abnormal speech output, semantic and syntactic (relational) comprehension can be dissociated. Syntactic comprehension can be assessed by asking the patient to handle objects. For example, after identifying a comb, a pen, and a key, ask the patient to put the key *on top* of the comb or the comb *between* the key and the pen.

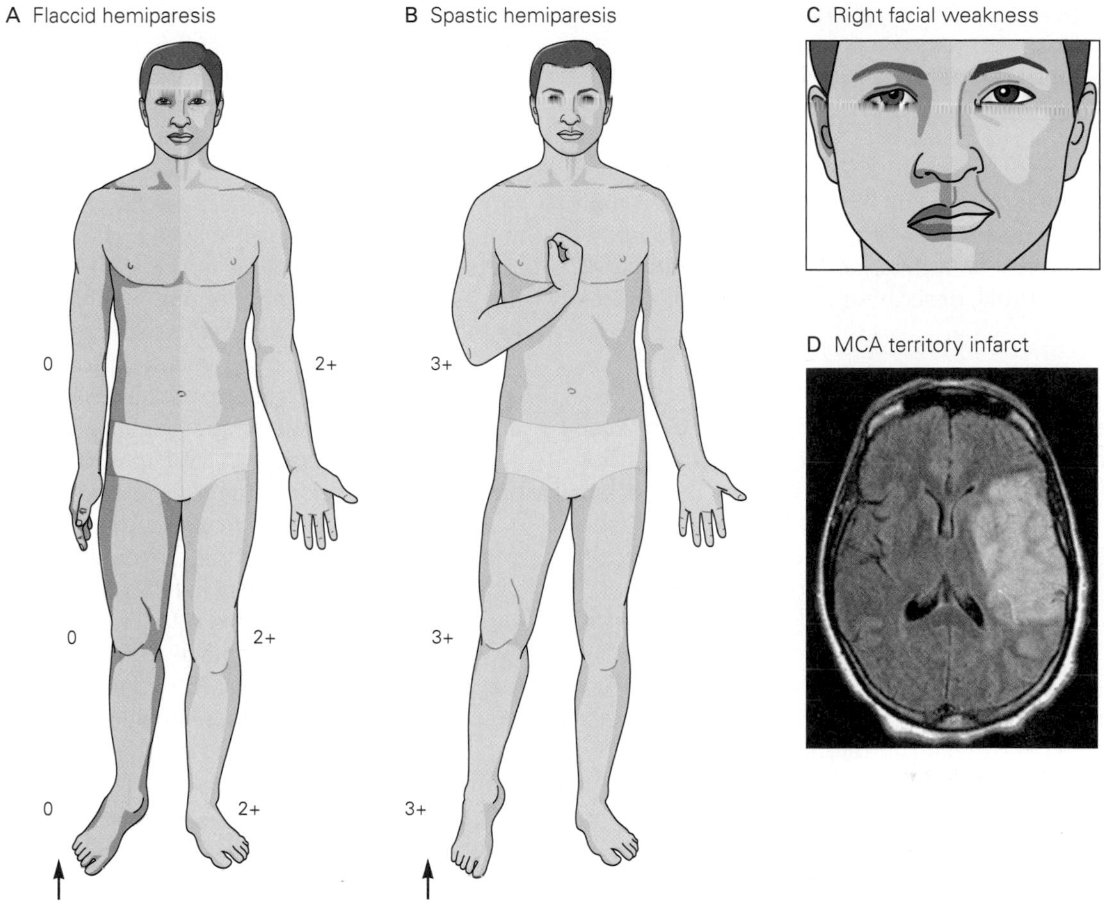

Figure B–1 A stroke in the left middle cerebral artery (MCA) territory producing contralateral hemiparesis and aphasia.

A. The patient develops sudden right-sided weakness involving face, arm, and leg. Examination reveals left gaze preference and weakness of extensor muscles of the right arm, more pronounced distally than proximally, and to a lesser degree weakness of flexors of the right leg. In the first few days tendon reflexes may be absent at the right triceps, knee, and ankle. A right Babinski reflex is present (arrow). Numbers indicate the strength of the reflex, where 2+ is normal. (See the section on Deep Tendon Reflexes.)

B. In weeks to months the patient may develop tonic flexure posture of the right arm and extensor posture of the right leg. Tendon reflexes on the right will become brisk with a positive Babinski reflex.

C. There is weakness of the right side of the face, characterized by widening of the palpebral fissure because of a lax lower lid, blunting of the right nasolabial fold, and drooping of the right corner of the mouth. There may also be acute weakness of the forehead with decreased furrowing of the brow, but this usually resolves quickly as the upper facial motor neurons receive bilateral supranuclear innervation. The patient has a nonfluent aphasia. Speech is effortful and telegraphic, and the prosody is abnormal. The patient cannot repeat words or phrases and becomes easily frustrated but can follow simple commands.

D. Site of stroke is on the left parieto-frontal region. Note that the left is shown on the right in diagnostic brain scans.

Naming

Patients with adequate vision can be shown objects, body parts, colors, or pictures of actions (confrontation naming). A variety of abnormal responses indicate anomia, the loss of the ability to recall or recognize the names of things. Some patients exhibit paraphasias. Some hesitate and grope for the correct word (tip-of-the-tongue phenomenon). Some patients describe rather than name an object. For example, instead of saying "necktie," the patient says, "It's what you wear around your neck."

Repetition

The patient is asked to repeat sentences such as "In the winter the President lives in Washington." Syntactically complex sentences may be particularly difficult (for example, "If he were to come, I would go out"). Errors most often consist of paraphasic substitutions.

Writing

Testing of writing begins by having patients sign their names. More specific tests of writing include dictated sentences, words, or letters, as well as spontaneous writing; for example, describing what is seen in a room.

Reading

Reading ability is tested by having the patient read aloud simple sentences, words, or letters. Reading comprehension can be tested by having the patient follow written commands that were previously successfully executed as oral commands or by having the patient answer written yes-or-no questions.

Praxis

Praxis refers to performance of a learned motor act. In its broadest sense *apraxia* refers to impaired motor activity not explained by weakness, incoordination, abnormal tone, bradykinesia, movement disorder, dementia, aphasia, or poor cooperation. Failure to perform an act is not evidence of apraxia. To be apractic the act must be performed incorrectly, or components of the act must be performed imprecisely. Parts of the act might be omitted, sequenced abnormally, or incorrectly oriented in space. There are three types of testing: (1) gesture ("Show me how you would throw a ball"); (2) imitation ("Watch how I point upward, then you do it"); and (3) use of an actual object ("Here is a spoon. Show me how you would use it").

Apraxias are traditionally classified as limb-kinetic, ideational, and ideomotor. With limb-kinetic apraxia the act is understood but motor execution is faulty. With ideational apraxia the idea of the act—the neural representation of the act, or *engram*—is disrupted. With ideomotor apraxia the idea of the act and the motor components of its execution are functionally disconnected. Such patients might be unable to imitate using a hammer but able to accurately describe its use and, if given a hammer, use it correctly.

Gnosia and Spatial Manipulation

Agnosia is a failure of recognition not explained by impaired primary sensation (tactile, visual, auditory) or cognitive impairment. It has been described as "perception stripped of its meaning." Agnosia differs from anomia in that the patient not only fails to name an object but also cannot select it from a group or match it to a picture. With tactile agnosia (astereognosis), touch threshold is normal yet patients cannot identify what they are touching.

Comparable agnosias exist in the visual and auditory spheres. However, because the responsible lesions are likely to be bilateral, visual and auditory agnosias are rare. *Simultanagnosia* is the inability to recognize the meaning of a whole scene or object, even though its individual components are correctly recognized.

The left hemisphere usually processes language and the right hemisphere processes spatial information. Right hemispheric (particularly parietal) lesions impair spatial perception and manipulation; patients have difficulty reading maps or finding their way about (*topographagnosia*), or difficulty copying simple pictures or shapes or drawing simple objects such as a flower or a clock face (*constructional apraxia* or *apractagnosia*).

Even more striking is spatial hemineglect syndrome. Patients with damage to the right hemisphere may ignore objects to the left of midline, including the left side of the body (personal neglect syndrome). They may fail to recognize severe hemiplegia (*anosognosia*) or even to acknowledge left body parts as their own (*asomatognosia*). Asked to bisect a line, such patients indicate a point to the right of midline. A copied picture might be missing the left half, and a drawn clock face might have all the numbers neatly arranged on the right.

A subtle manifestation of spatial neglect is *extinction*. Patients are able to recognize a stimulus (visual, auditory, or tactile) on either side when it is presented alone but unable to recognize the stimulus when it is presented on one side while the opposite side is also stimulated.

Cranial Nerve Function

Several of the cranial nerves are multifunctional; their motor, sensory, and autonomic functions must be assessed separately. The optic nerve is actually a central nervous system tract, and the accessory nerve is anatomically an aberrant spinal nerve (the motor neurons reside in the upper spinal cord).

Olfactory Nerve (Cranial N. I)

When patients complain that foods no longer taste right, the first step is to look into the nose for possible obstruction of airflow. Each nostril is then tested separately, using non-noxious odorants such as coffee or soap. (Pungent substances such as ammonia will stimulate trigeminal nociceptors.) Failure to smell anything is termed *anosmia*. Unpleasant distortion of an innocuous odorant is termed *parosmia*.

There are several cerebral representations for olfaction in the brain. As a result anosmia is most often secondary to local nasal disease, or to lesions affecting olfactory fibers as they pass through the cribriform plate (see Figure 32–1).

Optic Nerve (Cranial N. II)

Visual Acuity

Visual acuity is tested with Snellen's chart (at 20 feet) or a hand-held card (at 14 inches). The eyes are tested separately; if acuity is severely reduced, finger counting, detection of hand movement, or light perception should be assessed. Refractive errors are identified by having patients wear their glasses or look through a pinhole. Inspection of the eyes and funduscopic examination will often identify ocular lesions impairing acuity, such as corneal scarring, cataracts, glaucoma, diabetic retinopathy, or macular degeneration.

Visual Fields

The eyes are tested separately. The examiner faces the patient and holds an object equidistant between the patient's and the examiner's eyes to compare his or her own experience with that of the patient. A test object is moved slowly inward from the periphery, and the patient is asked to indicate when it is first seen; or the patient can be told to count fingers in different visual quadrants. Stimuli are presented simultaneously to the right and left fields to identify spatial neglect (extinction).

Visual field testing provides very accurate localization of structural lesions (see Figure 25–5). Monocular visual impairment, including either field defect or scotoma (an area of visual loss surrounded by preserved vision), localizes a lesion to the optic nerve, the retina, or other ocular structures. Bitemporal hemianopia, if caused by a single lesion, places that lesion at the optic chiasm. Homonymous hemianopia, quadrantanopia, or bilateral congruent scotomas indicate a lesion behind the chiasm in the contralateral optic tract, lateral geniculate nucleus of the thalamus, optic radiation, or primary visual cortex.

Funduscopy

Using an ophthalmoscope, the examiner focuses successively on the cornea, anterior chamber, lens, and vitreous body, and then surveys the optic disk, retinal vessels, and the retina itself. Optic atrophy refers to disk pallor; its many causes include glaucoma, optic nerve compression, infarction, and multiple sclerosis.

In papilledema (optic disk swelling) the disk margins become blurred and elevated. Papilledema can be the result of local pathology, for example the inflammatory demyelination of optic neuritis, in which case visual acuity is acutely impaired by swelling of the optic nerve head. When papilledema is the result of increased intracranial pressure, the normal blind spot becomes enlarged but visual acuity is not initially affected; over time, however, the visual fields become constricted and visual acuity is impaired. In addition, the ratio of the diameter of retinal veins to arteries (normally approximately 3:2) increases, and there may be retinal hemorrhages and whitish exudates.

Other abnormalities identified by funduscopy include arterial narrowing (hypertension), exudates (diabetes mellitus, blood dyscrasias), microaneurysms (diabetes mellitus), subhyaloid hemorrhages (located between the retina and the vitreous membrane and associated with subarachnoid hemorrhage), tubercles and other granulomas, phakomas (glial collections, associated with the hereditary diseases neurofibromatosis and tuberous sclerosis), pigmentary changes (retinitis pigmentosa), and emboli (seen within arteriolar branches of the central retinal artery).

Oculomotor, Trochlear, and Abducens Nerves (Cranial N. III, IV, VI)

Pupils

The pupillary light reflex is tested by directing a bright light into each eye and observing the bilateral response. Both pupils should constrict to bright light in either eye. The accommodation reflex and pupillary near response are tested by having the patient converge onto an object held close to the eyes; the pupils should constrict.

Anisocoria (unequal pupils) signifies either a parasympathetic lesion affecting the larger pupil or a sympathetic lesion affecting the smaller pupil. A parasympathetic lesion is indicated by marked pupillary dilatation, loss of the light reflex, or both, as well as involvement of extraocular muscles innervated by the oculomotor nerve. A sympathetic lesion is indicated by pupillary constriction, preservation of the light reflex, and signs of Horner syndrome (ptosis and, in some cases, loss of sweating over the ipsilateral face). A pupil with both parasympathetic and sympathetic denervation will be mid-position and unreactive to light.

A unilateral lesion involving the optic nerve or retina is indicated when neither pupil constricts in response to light directed into the affected eye, but both pupils constrict when light is directed into the unaffected eye (afferent pupillary defect). The pupils react equally because the pupillary light reflex is consensual (Figure B–2A; and see Figure 45–7).

The afferent end of the accommodation reflex pathway is in visual areas of the occipital lobe, which communicate with the parasympathetic component (the Edinger-Westphal nucleus) of the oculomotor nucleus by a route separate from the light reflex pathway. Lesions that selectively interrupt the light reflex pathway (for example, Argyll-Robertson pupils, seen most often with neurosyphilis) destroy the light reflex but do not impair the accommodation reflex.

Extraocular Eye Movement

The examiner looks for (1) paresis producing conjugate limitation of gaze in a particular direction (both eyes are equally affected so there is no diplopia); (2) paresis affecting one or more extraocular muscles (producing disconjugate eye movements with diplopia); and (3) spontaneous involuntary eye movements (eg, nystagmus).

The patient is asked to look to the right, to the left, and up and down in each horizontal direction. When the eyes follow a moving target they move more slowly (pursuit velocity) than when shifting from one static object to another (saccadic velocity). The two types of movement are controlled by separate anatomical and physiological mechanisms that can be selectively affected by lesions of the cerebrum, brain stem, or cerebellum (see Figures 39–2, 39–9, and 39–14).

Horizontal gaze palsy usually indicates a lesion of the frontal eye field (FEF) or the pontine paramedian reticular formation (PPRF) (see Figures 39–6, 39–9, and 39–10). If the FEF is affected the eyes will be deviated toward the side of the lesion. If the PPRF is affected the eyes will be deviated away from the side of the lesion.

Vertical gaze paresis—limitation of conjugate upward and downward gaze—indicates damage to the midbrain, either the rostral interstitial nucleus of the median longitudinal fasciculus or the posterior commissure.

Monocular limitation of adduction with preserved convergence (internuclear ophthalmoplegia) indicates damage to the ipsilateral median longitudinal fasciculus. There is often horizontal nystagmus in the contralateral abducting eye (see Figure B–2).

Disconjugate eye movements indicate impairment of particular cranial nerves or extraocular muscles (see Figures 39–4, 39–5, 39–6, and 39–7). If the eye cannot move outward there is a lesion involving either the abducens nerve (N. VI) or the lateral rectus muscle. If the eye cannot move downward when deviated inward there is a lesion of the trochlear nerve (N. IV) or the superior oblique muscle. Any other monocular limitations in movement are caused by a lesion of the oculomotor nerve (N. III) or one of its muscles of innervation (an exception is internuclear ophthalmoplegia).

The oculomotor nerve controls the levator palpebrae muscle, and ptosis is a common sign of lesions of this nerve. Unlike the mild Horner syndrome, oculomotor denervation can result in total eye closure.

The oblique muscles mediate intorsion and extorsion when the eye is either in mid-position or abducted. A compensatory head tilt (away from the side of the lesion) is therefore a feature of trochlear nerve palsy.

Nystagmus

Involuntary repetitive eye movements, or nystagmus, can be either unilateral or bilateral. Pendular nystagmus, with roughly equal velocity in either direction, is most often the result of severe visual impairment during early childhood. Rhythmical nystagmus, a slow drift in one direction followed by a rapid corrective movement in the other, can be present with the eyes at rest and the gaze fixed; it tends to be accentuated by ocular deviation, with the fast component in the direction of gaze.

Horizontal or rotatory nystagmus on primary gaze is most often associated with vestibular lesions, peripheral or central. Vertical nystagmus (the fast component directed upward or downward) suggests a brain stem lesion. Horizontally directed nystagmus on lateral gaze is often a benign side effect of certain drugs, particularly sedatives and anticonvulsants.

Trigeminal Nerve (Cranial N. V)

The three divisions of the trigeminal nerve carry sensation from the face, anterior scalp, eye, and much of the nasal and oral cavities. Fibers in the mandibular division innervate the muscles of mastication (see Figures 45–2 and 45–3).

The examiner initially checks sensations at the forehead, the malar region, and the chin, defining the outer borders of any deficit found. Decreased sensation confined to the entire trigeminal area indicates a peripheral lesion involving the nerve root or the trigeminal ganglion. Decreased sensation confined to

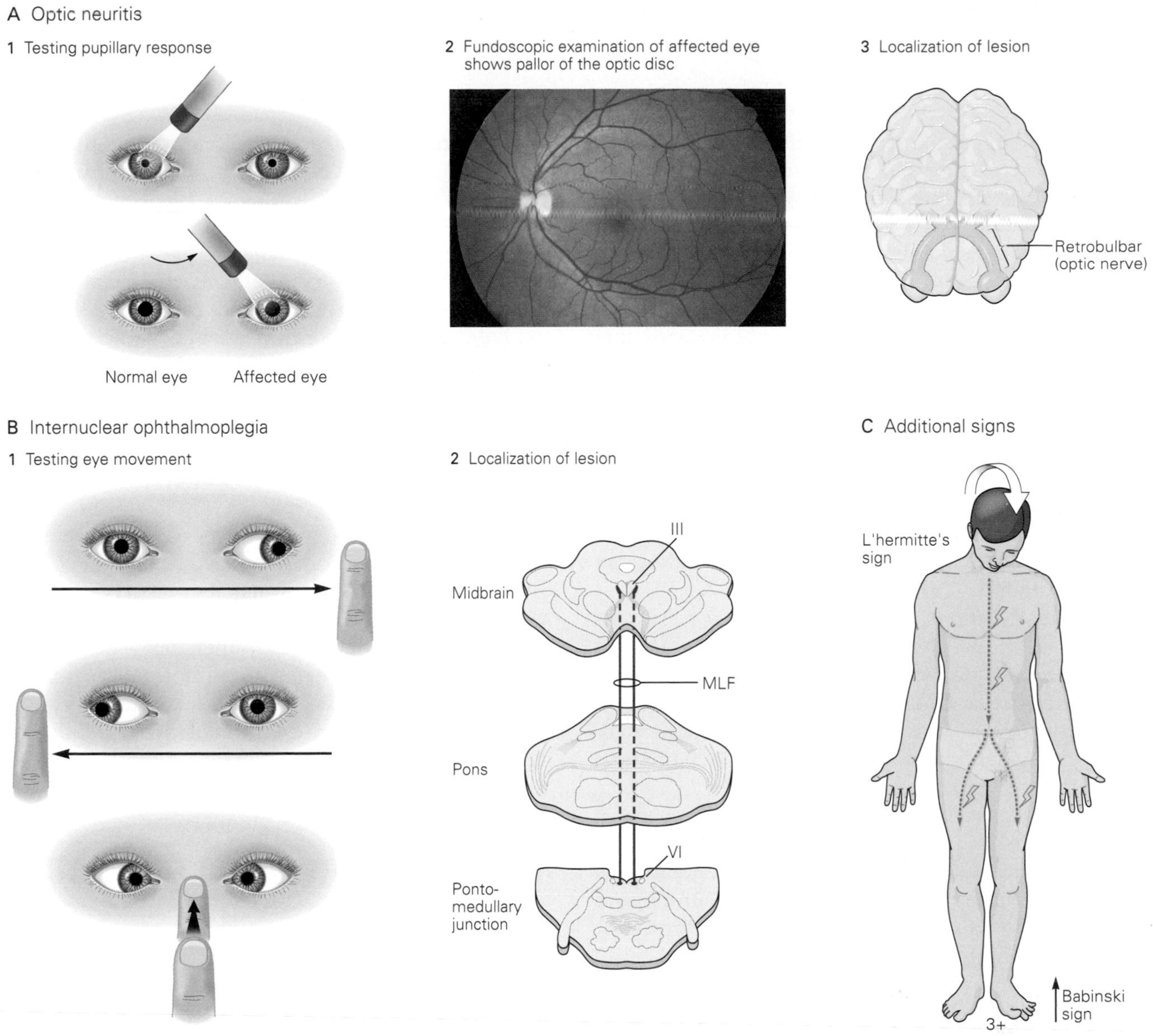

Figure B–2 Multiple sclerosis produces protean symptoms that wax and wane.

A. A common early symptom of multiple sclerosis (**MS**) is transient blurred vision in one eye as a result of optic neuritis, inflammation of the optic nerve that occurs during the acute phase of an MS lesion. **1.** Shining a light in the normal eye produces both direct and consensual pupillary constriction, but when the light is swung to the affected eye, both pupils dilate because the patient perceives a relative dimming of light intensity. This is referred to as a de-afferented pupil. At no time with a de-afferented pupil is there anisocoria. A positive "swinging flashlight test" indicates a de-afferented pupil. **2.** To determine the site of the lesion the examiner must use an ophthalmoscope to evaluate the possibility of a corneal or lenticular opacity, vitreous hemorrhage, retinal detachment, or ischemic retinopathy. **3.** If the funduscopic examination is normal, or reveals a slight elevation or blurring of the optic nerve head, the lesion is localized to the visual pathway behind the eye. Lack of a homonymous visual field defect involving the other eye localizes the lesion proximal to the optic chiasm, therefore placing the lesion in the retrobulbar segment of the optic nerve consistent with the diagnosis of optic neuritis.

B. The condition known as internuclear ophthalmoplegia (**INO**) is frequently the result of MS. The patient complains of double vision. **1.** The patient attempts to visually follow a finger moving from side to side. The abducting eye follows but the adducting eye fails to track past the midline. The abducting eye may demonstrate nystagmus. The possibility of a lesion involving the oculomotor nucleus (N. III) is tested by examining convergence. The patient looks at the target finger placed directly in front and follows as the finger is brought toward the patient's nose. Normal adduction during convergence rules out a lesion of the nerve or nucleus. Additionally, the pupils will be observed to constrict as a result of the near response. **2.** INO indicates a lesion of the medial longitudinal fasciculus (**MLF**), the white matter tract that links the third nerve (oculomotor) nucleus in the midbrain with the sixth nerve (abducens) nucleus in the pons to coordinate lateral gaze. Because these tracts are crossed and near the midline, most cases of INO are bilateral.

C. As the result of an MS plaque involving the posterior columns of the cervical cord, patients may experience an electric shock-like sensation traveling down the spine and possibly into the limbs when the examiner flexes the neck (L'hermitte sign). Because MS is a disease of central white matter, lesions may cause upper motor neuron signs, such as brisk reflexes or a Babinski sign.

one division suggests a more distal lesion. If pain and temperature are decreased, but touch is preserved, the lesion involves the spinal trigeminal tract and nucleus in the lower brain stem or upper cervical cord. If touch is also impaired, the lesion involves the principal trigeminal nucleus in the pons. If impaired sensation extends beyond the borders of the trigeminal area, the lesion is suprasegmental in the upper brain stem, thalamus, or parietal lobe.

Because the corneal reflex is consensual (the efferent end of the reflex pathway is in the facial nerve), a purely trigeminal lesion results in a decreased response in both eyes when the affected side is stimulated and a normal response in both eyes when the unaffected side is stimulated. Unilateral weakness of eye closure occurs in the affected eye when either cornea is stimulated.

Unilateral lesions of the trigeminal nerve or its third division cause the opened jaw to deviate toward the ipsilateral side because of ipsilateral pterygoid muscle weakness. Unilateral suprasegmental lesions are unlikely to cause jaw deviation because motor neurons of the trigeminal motor nucleus receive bilateral innervation from the primary motor cortex.

The jaw jerk is produced by tapping downward on the chin when the jaw is slightly open. Like other tendon reflexes it is decreased or absent with lesions of the nuclear or peripheral nerve (lower motor neurons) and brisk with lesions of the corticobulbar tract or motor cortex (upper motor neurons).

Facial Nerve (Cranial N. VII)

The facial nerve supplies facial muscles, including the frontalis ("wrinkle your forehead"), orbicularis oculi ("close your eyes tightly"), orbicularis oris ("close your lips tightly"), levator anguli oris ("show your teeth"), and platysma ("show your teeth and grimace"). With mild lesions there may not be frank weakness but rather a wider opening between the upper and lower eyelids and a flattening of the nasolabial fold ipsilaterally.

More proximal lesions can involve (1) a branch to the stapedius muscle of the middle ear (resulting in an increased sensitivity to loud sounds, or hyperacusis), (2) the chorda tympani branch to the sublingual and submandibular salivary glands and the tongue (resulting in decreased taste over the tongue's anterior two-thirds, usually tested with sugar or salt), or (3) the greater petrosal branch to the lacrimal gland and nasal mucosa (resulting in decreased lacrimation).

In most people motor neurons innervating the upper facial muscles, particularly the frontal muscle, receive projections from the motor cortex of both hemispheres, whereas those innervating the lower facial muscles receive only contralateral projections. Thus suprasegmental lesions tend to spare the frontal muscle and sometimes eye closure (upper-motor-neuron facial weakness), whereas lower brain stem or nerve damage tends to involve all the facial muscles (lower-motor-neuron facial weakness).

Following peripheral nerve injury such as Bell's palsy or trauma, aberrant reinnervation may produce synkinesis of the eye and mouth. Eye closure results in involuntary elevation of the angle of the mouth on the affected side, whereas baring the teeth results in involuntary closure of the ipsilateral eye.

Vestibulocochlear Nerve (Cranial N. VIII)

The auditory and vestibular nerves run together as the eighth cranial nerve. Both carry information from the labyrinths of the inner ear. The auditory (cochlear) nerve conveys sound information from the cochlea, whereas the vestibular nerve conveys equilibrium information from the utricle, saccule, and semicircular canals (see Figure 40–1).

Auditory Function

Neurons in the cochlear nucleus project both ipsilaterally and contralaterally. Thus unilateral deafness signifies a lesion of the cochlear nucleus, the auditory nerve, or the ear. Deafness from peripheral lesions is of two types. *Conduction deafness* is the result of obstruction or disease of the external auditory canal, the tympanic membrane, or the middle ear. *Sensorineural deafness* is the result of damage to the cochlea, the cochlear nerve, or the cochlear nuclei. Conduction deafness preferentially affects low tones; sensorineural deafness preferentially affects high tones. Patients with cochlear nerve or cochlear nucleus lesions may have only mildly impaired hearing for pure tones yet severe difficulty in discriminating speech because of its tonal complexity. Both peripheral and central lesions cause tinnitus.

The auditory examination begins with a simple screening test in which the ability of each ear to detect a watch ticking or two fingers rubbed together is compared. The Weber and Rinne tests help to distinguish conduction from sensorineural deafness. In the Weber test a 512 Hz tuning fork is placed midline on the forehead. With conduction deafness the sound will be heard best on the hearing-impaired side, whereas with sensorineural deafness the sound will be heard best on the normal side. In the Rinne test the tuning fork is placed over the mastoid; when the patient reports that the sound is no longer heard, it is held close to the external auditory meatus. In normal subjects and in those with nerve deafness air conduction will outlast bone conduction. With conduction deafness bone conduction will outlast air conduction. The Weber test is most useful when deafness is unilateral and the Rinne test when deafness is bilateral.

Vestibular Function

The vestibular nerve carries impulses from hair cells in the semicircular canals to the vestibular nuclei in the brain stem. Widespread projections from the vestibular nuclei communicate with the spinal cord, the cerebellum, eye movement control centers, and the forebrain.

Tests of vestibular function involve labyrinthine stimulation, either by head movement, head positioning, or temperature. In some patients vertigo, nystagmus, and sometimes nausea and vomiting are precipitated by any rapid movement of the head. In others, particularly those with benign positional vertigo, vertigo is triggered (after a latency of up to half a minute) by lying on the affected ear.

In the caloric test the ear is irrigated alternately with water several degrees centigrade above and below body temperature. With the head elevated 30 degrees the normal response consists of nystagmus (and vertigo), with the fast component directed away from the cold stimulus but toward the warm stimulus. There are two main patterns of abnormal response. Nystagmus may be absent or briefer in response to a cold or warm stimulus in the same ear; this *canal paresis* is associated with peripheral vestibular lesions. Conversely, a reduced response may occur when cold water is instilled into one ear or warm water is instilled into the other ear; this *directional preponderance* is associated with lesions of central vestibular pathways.

When pointing to objects, vertiginous patients whose eyes are closed tend to deviate toward the side of the lesion (*past-pointing*). Similarly, when walking in place with closed eyes, they tend to rotate toward the affected side.

Glossopharyngeal and Vagus Nerves (Cranial N. IX, X)

Assessment of the ninth and tenth cranial nerves is usually limited to examination of the palate and pharynx. Nasal speech suggests palatal weakness. Hoarseness or a reduced cough suggests laryngeal weakness.

Choking on saliva while talking suggests pharyngeal weakness. Difficulty swallowing (dysphagia) solid food suggests mechanical obstruction such as esophageal carcinoma; dysphagia for liquids as well as solids or for only liquids suggests neurological dysfunction. Dysphagia can be checked by asking the patient to swallow a small amount of water.

When the patient says, "ah" with the mouth open and the tongue relaxed, the palate should rise symmetrically, the uvula should remain in the midline, and the pharyngeal walls should contract symmetrically. With unilateral palatal or pharyngeal weakness, phonation causes the uvula to deviate toward the normal side. The gag reflex is tested by gently touching each side of the pharynx with a cotton-tipped applicator. As with the pupillary and corneal reflexes, the response is bilateral. The response of the palatal and pharyngeal muscles to phonation and tactile stimulation therefore reveals whether a lesion is unilateral or bilateral, and whether the damaged nerves are efferent, afferent, or both.

With unilateral laryngeal lesions the abnormal vocal cord may be positioned in adduction, in which case there may be no symptoms; if it is positioned in abduction there will be hoarseness or aphonia but normal breathing. With bilateral lesions the vocal cords may be positioned in abduction, in which case there will be hoarseness or aphonia but normal breathing; if they are positioned in adduction there will be inspiratory phonation (stridor) and life-threatening respiratory obstruction.

Spinal Accessory Nerve

The sternocleidomastoid is the only major striated muscle with ipsilateral cortical representation. Following destructive cerebral lesions weakness in the sternocleidomastoid is unusual but may occur ipsilaterally; contralateral trapezius weakness may also occur. The sternocleidomastoid is tested by having patients press their chin against resistance in the direction of the contralateral shoulder. Bilateral damage causes weakness of forward head flexion. Trapezius weakness is demonstrated by assessing shoulder elevation or shrugging or by observing winging of the upper scapula.

Hypoglossal Nerve (Cranial N. XII)

The hypoglossal nerve innervates the muscles of the tongue. It arises near the midline of the medulla oblongata and exits the posterior fossa through the hypoglossal foramen. Each hypoglossal nucleus receives bilateral projections from the motor cortex.

Inspection of the tongue may reveal atrophy or fasciculations, either of which indicates damage to lower motor neurons, either peripherally or in the medulla. Tongue atrophy, if unilateral, causes reduction in size on one side with excessive ridging and wrinkling of the affected side. Fasciculations in the tongue can be difficult to tell from normal tongue movements or tremor. These small local contractions are nonrhythmic and make the tongue resemble a *bag of worms*. They should be present when the tongue is completely at rest.

With unilateral weakness because of lesions of upper or lower motor neurons the tongue deviates toward the weak side. If there is no deviation, weakness is assessed by having the patient push the tongue into each cheek while the examiner pushes against the cheek. With unilateral lesions of upper motor neurons there may be no deviation and little evident weakness, yet patients may experience dysarthria (imperfect articulation), particularly with the lingual consonants (*tay* for anterior tongue, *kay* for the posterior tongue). Bilateral tongue weakness causes dysarthria, dysphagia, and sometimes even difficulty breathing.

Bilateral lesions of the lower brain stem can result in *bulbar palsy*. The tongue is paralyzed, atrophic, and fasciculating. There is no movement of the palate or pharynx with phonation, and the gag reflex is absent. With unilateral supranuclear lesions these muscles are often spared or only mildly impaired because of the bilateral cortical projections to lower brain stem motor neurons.

Bilateral lesions of the cerebrum or upper brain stem, however, can result in severe dysarthria and dysphagia because of effects on the corticobulbar pathway. The tongue is paralyzed but neither atrophic nor fasciculating. The palate and pharynx do not move with phonation, but the gag reflex is hyperactive. Such a patient is said to have *pseudobulbar palsy*. An interesting and unexplained feature of this syndrome is lability or hyperreflexia of emotional response. A remark that would normally produce a mild chuckle precipitates embarrassed peals of laughter, and asking a question such as "How are you feeling?" may result in explosive weeping.

Musculoskeletal System

Observations of spontaneous and commanded movements can reveal patterns of weakness that localize a lesion. Weakness of extensor muscle groups of the arm and flexors of the leg on the same side suggests a lesion of the corticospinal tract on the contralateral side. If the weakness is acute, the limbs may be flaccid; if chronic, there may be increased tone and brisk tendon reflexes (spasticity) (see Figure B–1).

Weakness of both legs (paraparesis) or of both legs and both arms (quadriparesis) may be the result of a lesion of the spinal cord or of widespread dysfunction of the peripheral nervous system or muscles. Lesions of the spinal cord may be associated with a sensory level (see section on Sensory Systems) or bladder dysfunction, and lesions above the spinal cord may be accompanied by signs of brain stem or cortical dysfunction. Peripheral neuropathies tend to produce a generally symmetrical pattern of limb weakness. As a rule, weakness that begins or is greater in the distal arms or legs suggests peripheral neuropathy, whereas weakness of the proximal limb muscles (shoulder and girdle) suggests myopathy (Figure B–3).

Weakness confined to a single limb may reflect plexopathy or mononeuropathy. Examining the strength of individual muscle groups innervated by specific nerves is key, and a chart of muscle innervation by nerve, trunk, and root can be a great aid in localization.

Observing Spontaneous Movement

The motor examination begins with observations of spontaneous movement, which may reveal patterns of weakness but may also reveal spontaneous uncontrolled movements such as tremor, athetosis, chorea, myoclonus, or dystonia. Fasciculations of individual muscle groups can sometimes be enhanced by directly tapping the muscle with a reflex hammer. If unilateral atrophy of limb musculature is suspected, the circumference of the limb should be measured and compared to the same region of the opposite limb.

Detecting a Lesion in the Corticospinal Tract

The patient's arms are held outstretched with palms upward and eyes closed. Mild corticospinal lesions may cause one arm to drift below the level of the other, with pronation of the upturned palm. A subtle sign of corticospinal pathology is clumsiness of fine finger movements, brought out by asking the patient to rapidly and steadily tap the forefinger against the thumb (finger-repetitive test), and then to tap each finger against the thumb in rapid succession (finger-successive test). One should compare the facility with which this is performed by each hand, bearing in mind that most people will be slightly more adept with their dominant side (see Figure B–1).

Testing Muscle Tone

With the patient relaxed, the arms are passively flexed and extended around the elbow and wrist joints. Muscle tone may be flaccid, which is usual following acute paralysis, lower motor neuron lesions, or myopathy; or it may be increased, often with a characteristic give-way relaxation after initial resistance (*clasp-knife* effect), reflecting spasticity and an upper motor neuron lesion.

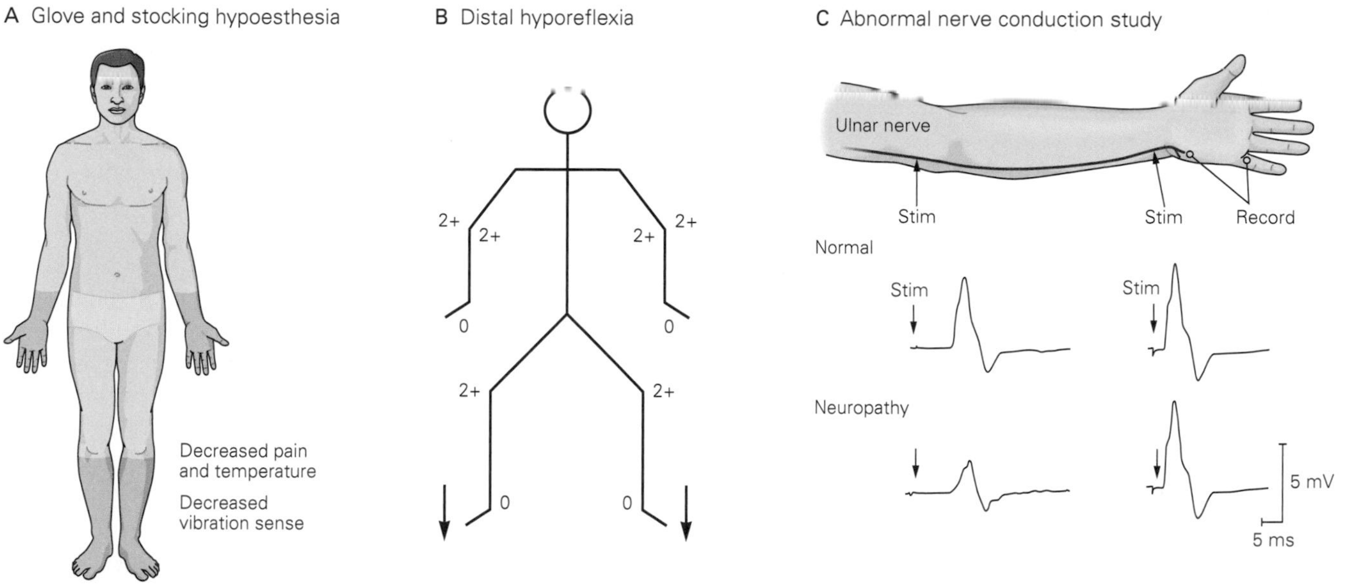

Figure B–3 Sensorimotor neuropathy associated with diabetes.

A. The patient initially complains of numbness in the distal legs, but with progression the hands also become involved. Diabetic neuropathy is an axonal neuropathy that affects both myelinated small fibers and unmyelinated C fibers. Because these sensory fibers subserve pain and temperature sensation, examination reveals decreased pain and temperature sensation. The findings are initially in the feet, but the signs and symptoms gradually ascend; by the time numbness extends to just below the knee, the hands are usually also involved in a "glove and stocking" distribution. Loss of sensation for vibration is also detectable.

B. Weakness of the limbs develops late and is greatest distally, especially in the intrinsic muscles of the feet and hands. The Achilles reflexes are diminished early, and finger flexor responses can be diminished by the time sensory changes are apparent in the hands.

C. Nerve conduction studies demonstrate changes characteristic of an axonal neuropathy. When the ulnar nerve is stimulated above the elbow or at the wrist, and the evoked hypothenar muscle response is measured in the hand, the evoked compound muscle action potential is reduced in amplitude but the latencies are normal.

Tone in the lower limbs may be tested in the supine patient by abruptly lifting the thigh. If the heel lifts briefly off the bed, tone is normal; if the leg rises rigidly off the bed, tone is increased; if the heel drags along the sheets, tone is decreased. Resistance to movement in all directions and throughout range of movement (*lead-pipe rigidity*) is characteristic of Parkinson disease; it may be accompanied by *cogwheeling*, a stepwise *ratcheting* that reflects the tremor of Parkinson disease superimposed on increased tone (Figure B–4).

Testing Muscle Strength

Muscle power is graded on a scale of 0 to 5 (0 = no contraction, 1 = contraction but no movement, 2 = contraction but not against gravity, 3 = movement against gravity but not against even minimal resistance, 4 = movement against minimal to moderate resistance, 5 = normal). Testing includes flexion and extension of the head; abduction, adduction, and rotation of the shoulders; flexion and extension of the elbows, wrists, and fingers; intrinsic hand muscle movements; and flexion and extension of the hip, knee, ankle, and toes. Comparison is made between right versus left, proximal versus distal, and arms versus legs.

Sensory Systems

Establishing Boundaries and Comparing Sides Are Crucial to the Sensory Examination

As in the motor examination, patterns and symmetry are key. Distal symmetrical sensory loss is characteristic of peripheral neuropathies. Brain stem lesions, for example of the lateral medulla, produce pain and temperature loss ipsilaterally on the face and contralaterally on the body. Bilateral loss of all sensation below a

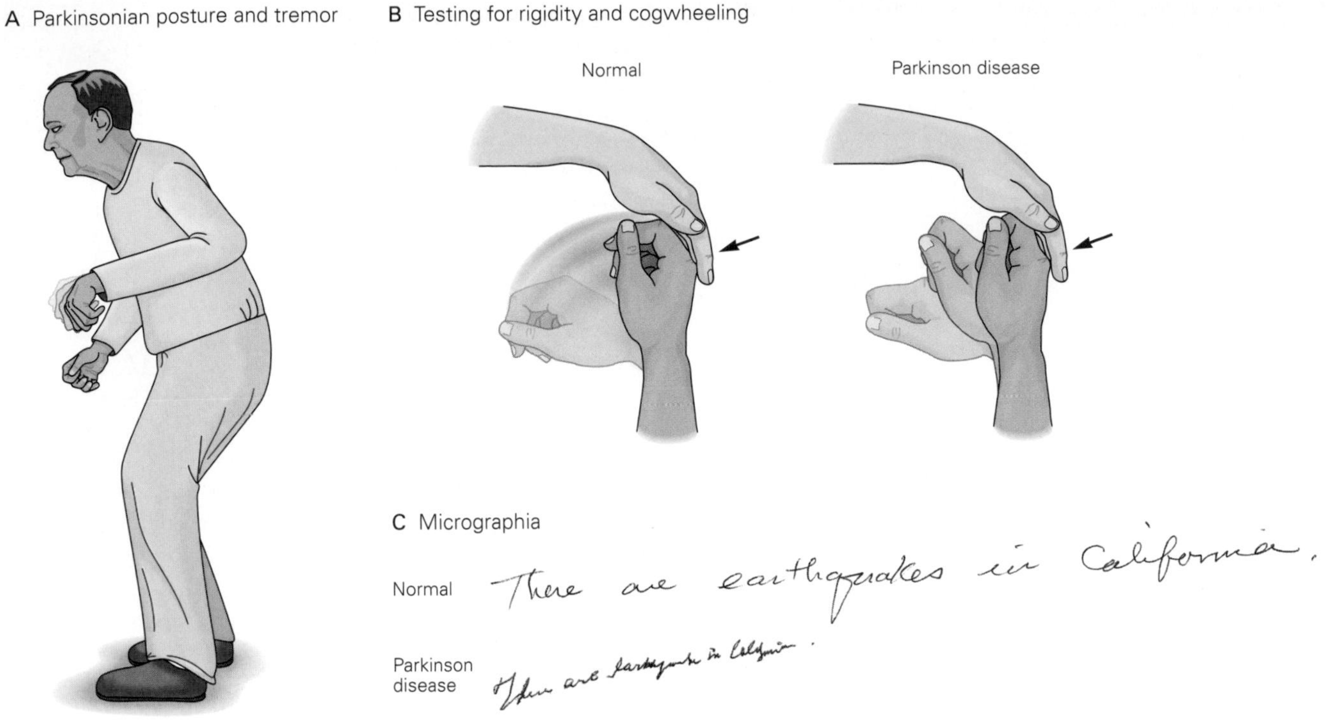

Figure B–4 Parkinson disease is manifested by akinesia, rigidity, and tremor.

A. Characteristic features of Parkinson disease include a stooped flexed posture, akinesia manifested as decreased arm swing when walking, and a resting tremor of four to five cycles per second (often involving the hands and typically with the forefinger rubbing against the thumb producing a *pill rolling* gesture).

B. Even at early stages, passively flexing and extending the patient's wrist while asking him to pretend to write using the other hand will produce a stiffness of muscle tone that feels to the examiner like bending a lead rod (*lead pipe rigidity*). If a tremor is present, the examiner will feel a *cogwheel* or ratcheting motion rather than a smooth excursion.

C. An early manifestation is micrographia, manifested as a change in handwriting and demonstrated by asking the patient to write a sentence.

trunk level is characteristic of spinal cord lesions; the *sensory level*, the upper border of the area of sensory loss, is usually one or two segments higher on the back than on the chest. Preservation of sensation in the sacrum (sacral sparing) indicates an intraparenchymal lesion while loss of sensation indicates an extraparenchymal compressive lesion. Sacral sensory loss (saddle anesthesia) suggests a lesion of the cauda equina or conus medullaris.

Ipsilateral hyperalgesia, an increased sensitivity to pain, may be a result of nerve root irritation at the level of the lesion. Sensory loss develops throughout the root distribution as the lesion expands, and pain and temperature loss occurs in the contralateral leg when a spinal cord lesion produces spinothalamic tract dysfunction. There may also be ipsilateral loss of proprioception because of dorsal column dysfunction. Spinal cord lesions arising within the cord, as in syringomyelia, can damage crossing spinothalamic fibers, causing segmental pain and temperature loss (for example, in a cape-like distribution throughout the shoulders and upper back if damage is in the upper cervical cord, or in the hands if damage is in the lower cervical cord) (Figure B–5).

Testing Pain Sensation

Pain is tested with a safety pin or the sharp end of a broken applicator stick, which should be disposed of after use. Pressing a pin against the bony part of a limb will be felt more sharply than a similar stimulus applied to a fleshy part. A single application of the pin should suffice; repetitive stimulation will increase the stimulus strength through temporal summation in receptor neurons.

Testing proceeds from head to toe in an orderly pattern, comparing locations on each side. Test spots should include proximal and distal upper and lower limbs, both front and back. Bearing in mind the sensory dermatomes (see Figure 22–9), a reasonable strategy is to test over the deltoid (C5), dorsal forearm (C6), thenar eminence (C6, but also median nerve), tip of the little finger (C8, ulnar nerve), medial forearm (T1), and axilla (T2). On the chest one should probe on either side of the midline and test along the back if a sensory level is detected on the chest or abdomen. Because C5 to T1 roots innervate the arms and hands, there is a C4/T2 boundary above the nipple line, and lower cervical cord lesions may produce a sensory level in this region. The lower limbs are tested over the thigh (L2), medial calf (L4), dorsum of the foot (L5), and lateral malleolus or sole of the foot (S1).

If areas of decreased sensation are detected, finer testing is necessary to map the borders and determine whether the lesion involves nerves, roots, or the central nervous system. In addition to anesthesia, patients may report either a dull sensation (hypalgesia), which may be as significant as anesthesia and just as useful in mapping patterns of deficit, or possibly hyperalgesia, which sometimes indicates the upper level of a spinal cord lesion.

Temperature Testing

Pain and temperature are both carried centrally in the spinothalamic tract, so areas lacking hot or cold sensation will most often lack pain sensation as well. If pinprick testing has uncovered a deficit, testing temperature sensation by applying a cold tuning fork to the

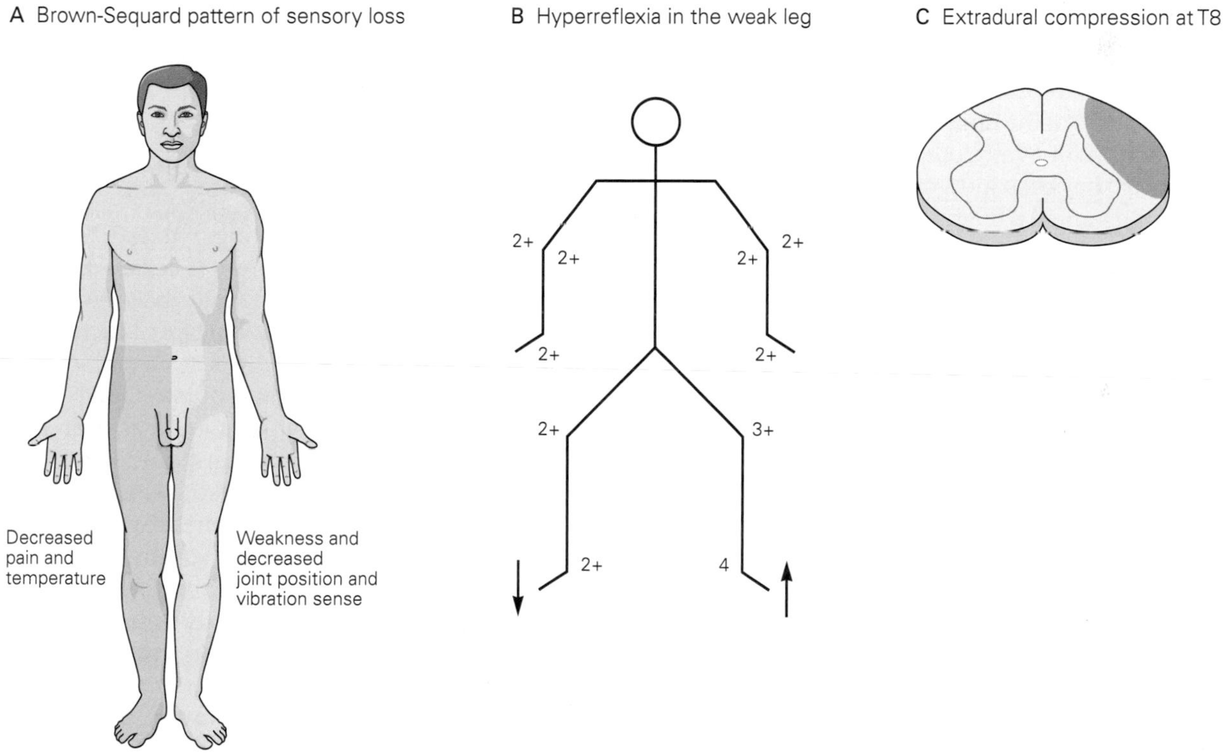

Figure B–5 Back pain with weakness and numbness in spinal cord compression.

A. Spinal cord compression by a tumor can produce a Brown-Séquard syndrome. The primary symptom is leg weakness, but there may be a radicular pattern of numbness on the side ipsilateral to the compression because of injury of the sensory root, and loss of pain and temperature sensation in the contralateral leg because of compression of the spinothalamic tract. Position and vibration sensation may be diminished in the ipsilateral leg because of compression of the dorsal columns.

B. The weak leg ipsilateral to the lesion has brisk tendon reflexes and a Babinski reflex as a result of involvement of the corticospinal tract.

C. The physical examination is suggestive of a lesion on the left side of the thoracic cord at the level of approximately T8. A magnetic resonance imaging scan confirms extradural cord compression by a tumor mass at T8.

skin for several seconds can be a very useful procedure to confirm involvement of spinothalamic modalities.

Touch Testing

Testing light touch sensation is not helpful in localizing central lesions because touch sensation is carried by several spinal tracts, but it is very helpful in localizing peripheral lesions of nerves or roots. Testing should follow the procedure for testing pain by stroking lightly with a finger or a cotton wisp. Deficits may include a simple decrease in sensation (hypesthesia), a distorted or abnormal sensation (dysesthesia), or even a painful sensation (allodynia).

Testing Proprioception

With eyes closed one can still sense the position of one's arms and legs because of proprioceptive nerve endings in the joints that convey sensory information by way of the dorsal columns of the spinal cord. To test position sense in the elbow and shoulder, ask the patient to extend the arms with eyes closed and to touch the forefinger to the tip of the nose.

Position sense in the fingers (or wrist) is tested by asking the patient with eyes closed to identify whether the finger (or wrist) has been moved up or down by the examiner. Grasp the patient's finger at the sides rather than the dorsal and palmar surfaces to ensure that the patient does not use pressure sense to judge direction of movement. Position sense is very sensitive; only 1 to 2 millimeters of displacement is required. In rare instances of loss of proprioception the arms may drift into odd dystonic postures (pseudoathetosis) when the eyes are closed.

To test the hip and knee joints, ask the supine patient with eyes closed to identify when the leg has been moved to a new position, or to point to the big toe as the leg is moved to a series of positions. Proprioception of the big toe is tested as for the fingers.

The Romberg test for balance is performed by asking the patient to stand unassisted with feet together and eyes closed. The test is considered positive if the patient loses balance. Although dorsal column lesions produce a positive test, so will a variety of other conditions, including inner ear dysfunction and cerebellar lesions. Sensory ataxia, a gait disorder resulting from uncertainty concerning limb position, indicates posterior column lesions.

Testing Vibration Sensation

Vibration is tested with a 128 Hz tuning fork held against the bony wrist and the lateral malleolus of the ankle. Place the stem firmly against the patient's wrist or ankle and instruct the patient to signal when the vibration has stopped. To ensure that sensation has not ceased because of habituation, promptly remove and replace the fork to test whether the patient can still feel vibration; when the patient declares the vibration has stopped, place the fork against your own wrist to confirm that it is no longer vibrating. Vibration sensation can also be tested at the toes, knees, and elbows. Decreased vibratory sensation at the toes and ankles is a sensitive measure of sensory peripheral neuropathy (see Figure B–3).

Complete spinal cord transection will produce bilateral hyperesthesia at the level of the lesion and loss of sensation in all modalities beginning several segments below. Hemisection of the spinal cord (Brown-Séquard syndrome) produces ipsilateral loss of vibration and position sense and contralateral loss of pain and temperature a few levels below the lesion (see Figure B–5). Central cord lesions, such as syringomyelia, injure the spinothalamic fibers as they cross just anterior to the spinal canal, producing bilateral loss of pain and temperature at the level of the lesion while sparing other modalities such as light touch and proprioception.

Testing Cortical Processing of Touch

Sensory information originating in the pathways tested above is processed in the cerebral cortex. But findings from tests of perception will only be significant once the elementary sensory pathways for touch have been found to be intact.

The patient, with arms outstretched and eyes closed, is asked to state which hand has been touched. The examiner lightly touches first one hand, then the other, and then both simultaneously. Patients suffering from spatial neglect may correctly identify single touches on both sides but consistently fail to report a touch on one side when both sides are touched simultaneously (double simultaneous stimulation). This deficit, termed sensory extinction, implicates a lesion of the contralateral parietal lobe.

Graphesthesia is tested by having the patient with eyes closed identify numbers from 1 to 10 traced on the palm of each hand using a pointed but blunt instrument. The traced numbers should be right side up with respect to the patient.

The patient's ability to identify objects by touch (stereognosis) is tested by asking the patient with eyes closed to identify a common object such as a key, comb, or coin that is placed in the palm. The patient is permitted to manipulate the object with his fingers. As always, performance on the right is compared to the left.

Two-point discrimination is tested by first applying a single stimulus, then two stimuli simultaneously and asking the patient with eyes averted to identify these correctly. The separation that can be discriminated will vary with the density of sensory innervation over different skin regions; thus the fingertips can detect the smallest separations. The same areas on both sides should be compared.

Motor Coordination

Testing coordination and involuntary movement assesses cerebellar and basal ganglia function. Involuntary movements include tremors (repetitive, oscillatory motions), myoclonus (sudden twitching of muscle groups), asterixis (periodic lapse of muscle tone), chorea (rapid, chaotic twitching), athetosis ("wormian" writhing motions), dystonia (athetotic-like movements with held postures), and ballism (proximal flinging movements of the arms).

These movements are best observed with the patient at rest with arms outstretched. Asterixis is brought out by having the patient hold hands dorsiflexed at the wrist in the position used by traffic policeman to command "stop." Periodic lapse of posture (the "wave good-bye" sign) is positive for asterixis. Tremors are classified as resting, postural, and action. Postural tremors can be assessed by having the patient hold the arms in the outstretched posture, whereas action tremors can be assessed by having the patient touch first the examiner's finger and then his own nose. Resting tremors are best assessed by observing the patient seated, lying down, or walking with arms hanging down.

The term *ataxia* (literally, disorder) refers to a variety of impairments of coordination as well as unsteady gait most often following a cerebellar lesion. Cerebellar lesions cause ipsilateral rebound, dysmetria, and dysdiadochokinesia. *Rebound* is tested by applying downward pressure against the patient's outstretched arms and releasing abruptly. If rebound is present, the arms will fly up rather than return to the neutral position. *Dysmetria* consists of overshooting or undershooting the target. In the arms dysmetria is detected with the same finger-to-finger and finger-to-nose test used to detect action tremor, which often coexists. In the legs dysmetria (and action tremor) can be detected by having the patient place a heel on the opposite knee and run it down the shin.

Dysdiadochokinesia, the inability to maintain a steady rhythmic movement, is identified by having the patient perform rapid successive movements (for example, tapping the thumb and index finger together, or one hand against the other, or tapping a foot on the floor) and rapid alternating movements (for example, alternately pronating and supinating the hands or alternately tapping the toe and heel of one foot on the floor).

Gait and Stance

The patient is asked to stand and walk normally 5 to 10 paces, then turn around and walk back. Observations should be made of posture, arm swing, foot position, step size, and dexterity of motion, especially during turning. During walking the insteps of both feet normally line up along an imaginary line; when there is an increase in the distance between the two feet, the gait is broad-based and suggestive of cerebellar disease or proprioceptive loss.

With *flaccid hemiparesis* the affected arm has diminished swing and the affected leg may drag (footdrop). When footdrop occurs in isolation, as for example with peroneal nerve injury, the patient may have a "steppage" gait, lifting the leg higher than normal to compensate for foot dragging. With *spastic hemiparesis* the affected side shows hemiparetic posture, with the arm flexed at the elbow and wrist and leg extended and inverted (see Figure B–1). Gait therefore has a circular form (circumduction) as the patient swings the affected leg off the ground by throwing his body to the opposite side. The foot describes a circular motion with each step. With *spastic paraparesis* or quadriparesis, as occurs with cerebral palsy, bilateral extensor tone may produce toe-walking or scissoring as a result of bilateral circumduction. Parkinsonian gait is characterized by a forward stoop, loss of arm swing, shuffling, and festination (acceleration, as if the patient were trying to catch up with his center of gravity) (see Figure B–4).

Myopathic gait is characterized by waddling, the result of bilateral hip abductor weakness. *Antalgic gait* refers to gait in which compensatory maneuvers (eg, favoring one leg) are adopted to minimize pain. Subtle signs of hemiparesis can be detected with the use of *stressed gaits,* such as walking on toes, heels, or the outside edges of the feet. Note the position of the arms during these gaits for evidence of synkinesia.

Synkinesia or *overflow movement* is said to occur when the ipsilateral arm and hand posture mimics the position of the foot. Such associated movements are normal in very young children and tend to be prominent in cases of cerebral palsy, but are not normal in adults. Unilateral hand-foot overflow movements can be seen in mild cases of hemiparesis.

Balance

Patients are asked to walk a straight line as though on a tight rope, one foot in front of the other. Any deviation from a straight path is noted. This test is sensitive for cerebellar ataxia of gait, as occurs with alcohol intoxication, and is thus the basis of the field sobriety test. However, patients with lesions of the cerebellum for any cause will demonstrate a *drunken gait*, as can patients with labyrinthine dysfunction, dizziness, weakness, balance trouble, or proprioceptive problems.

Patients with severe cerebellar ataxia or vertigo may not be able to stand with feet together. After examining and establishing the stability of the patient's stance, the patient is told to close his eyes. The Romberg test may identify more subtly impaired stance.

Deep Tendon Reflexes

Examining tendon reflexes can confirm whether weakness is due to damage of lower or upper motor neurons. Increased reflexes indicate damage in upper motor neurons; diminished reflexes indicate damage to lower motor neurons (see Figure B–1). Rating is on a scale of 0 to 5, where 0 = absent, 1 = reduced, 2 = normal, 3 = brisk without clonus, 4 = transient clonus, and 5 = sustained clonus. Reflexes of 4 or 5 are usually pathological, but hypoactive reflexes are often normal.

Both sides are compared and reproducible asymmetry is always significant. Tendon reflexes are elicited by tapping a stretched tendon to activate the muscle spindle. The muscle to be tested should be relaxed and not under active contraction. If a tendon response appears to be absent, the response may be enhanced by having the patient perform some task, for example interlocking the fingers of both hands and attempting to pull them apart as the examiner elicits the reflex.

Tendon Reflexes in the Arms

To elicit a biceps reflex the arm is flexed 90 degrees at the elbow; pressure is applied to the biceps tendon using an extended forefinger and then a phasic stretch is elicited by striking the forefinger with the reflex hammer. To elicit the triceps reflex the elbow is also held at 90 degrees and the tendon is struck directly with the hammer. The brachioradial muscle is tested by holding the patient's hand with the elbow flexed and striking the radius just above the wrist.

Finger flexors are tested by having the patient gently flex the fingers against the examiner's outstretched forefinger and then striking the forefinger with the hammer to apply a sudden extension. Brisk reflexes may be associated with reflex spread. For example, stretching the finger flexors may cause the thumb to flex as well, and flicking the nail of the patient's forefinger may similarly trigger finger and thumb flexion (Hoffmann reflex).

Tendon Reflexes in the Legs

The patellar reflex is best elicited with the patient either sitting with legs crossed or supine. The leg is lifted from behind the knee and the patellar tendon is struck below the knee. If the patella reflex is very brisk, clonus may be elicited by extending the leg and, while holding the patella between thumb and forefinger, applying a sharp downward stretch. Reflex spread may include a crossed adductor response, elicited in the supine patient by pressing on the medial knee to slightly spread (abduct) the leg and then striking the hand with the hammer. Adduction of both legs suggests pathological briskness.

The ankle reflex is best elicited with the leg triple-flexed (at the hip, knee, and ankle). The ankle is then dorsiflexed by applying pressure to the ball of the foot with the hand. Striking either this hand or the Achilles tendon with the reflex hammer will produce a sudden stretch of the gastrocnemius tendon and trigger the reflex. In this position it is easy to observe clonus, if present. Ankle clonus usually accompanies spasticity.

Asymmetrical Superficial Reflexes

The plantar response is conveniently tested following the ankle reflex. A blunt instrument (a key or wooden applicator stick) is used to stroke up along the lateral edge of the sole and across the plantar surface. The big toe should be observed for extension and the remaining toes for possible fanning, an *extensor plantar response* (Babinski reflex). A flexor motion or no toe motion at all can be normal, but a neutral response on one side may be significant in the presence of a clear flexor response on the other side. Babinski reflex indicates a corticospinal lesion (see Figure B–1).

Abdominal reflexes are elicited by drawing a blunt instrument across the abdomen several inches to one side of the umbilicus and then repeating the maneuver on the other side. A normal response is movement of the umbilicus toward the side of stimulation. Symmetrically absent responses are not significant, but an asymmetrically absent response can be associated with upper motor neuron lesions.

Frontal Lobe Reflexes

Several so-called frontal release signs or primitive reflexes have been described. These include the snout reflex, elicited by tapping the mouth gently with the reflex hammer and observing whether the lips purse; the palmomental reflex, elicited by scratching the palm and observing contraction of the mentalis muscle; and the grasp reflex, triggered by stroking the palm and triggering an involuntary grasp. These responses are often associated with frontal lobe lesions, but, with the exception of the grasp reflex, they are also present in many normal adults.

Arnold R. Kriegstein
John C.M. Brust

Appendix C

Circulation of the Brain

The brain is highly vulnerable to disturbance of its blood supply. Anoxia lasting only seconds causes neurological symptoms; when it lasts minutes it can cause irreversible neuronal damage. Blood flow to the central nervous system must efficiently deliver oxygen, glucose, and other nutrients and remove carbon dioxide, lactic acid, and other metabolites. The cerebral vasculature has special anatomical and physiological features that protect the brain. However, when these mechanisms fail, the result is a stroke. Broadly defined, the term *stroke,* or *cerebrovascular accident,* refers to the neurological symptoms or signs that result from diseases involving blood vessels. These are usually focal and acute.

The Blood Supply of the Brain Can Be Divided into Arterial Territories

Each cerebral hemisphere is supplied by an *internal carotid artery,* which arises from the common carotid artery beneath the angle of the jaw, enters the cranium through the carotid foramen, traverses the cavernous sinus (giving off the *ophthalmic artery*), penetrates the dura, and then divides into the anterior and middle cerebral arteries (Figure C–1).

The large surface branches of the *anterior cerebral artery* supply the cortex and white matter of the inferior frontal lobe, the medial surface of the frontal and parietal lobes, and the anterior corpus callosum (Figure C–2). Smaller penetrating branches—including the so-called *recurrent artery of Heubner*—supply the deeper cerebrum and diencephalon, including limbic structures, the head of the caudate, and the anterior limb of the internal capsule.

The large surface branches of the *middle cerebral artery* supply most of the cortex and white matter of the hemisphere's convexity, including the frontal, parietal, temporal, and occipital lobes, and the insula

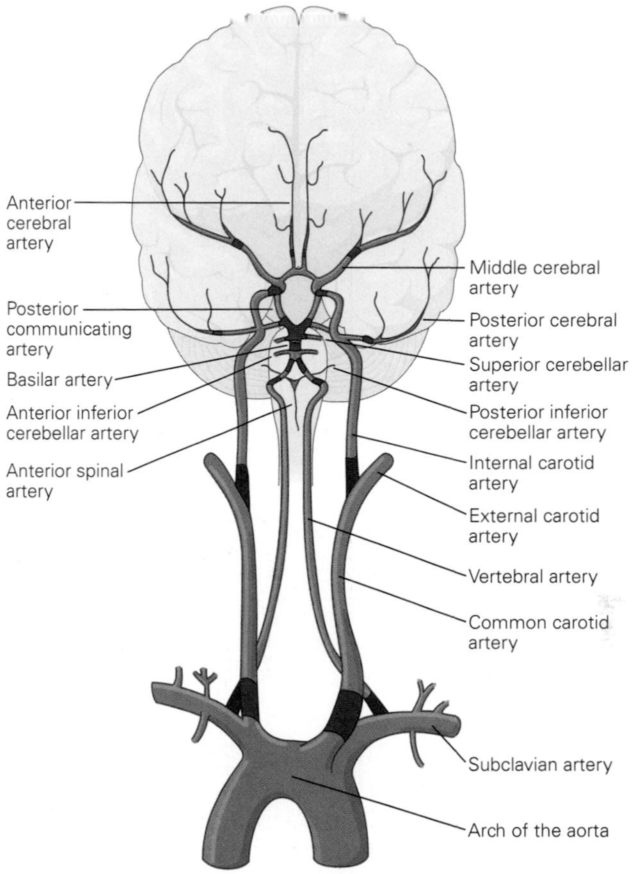

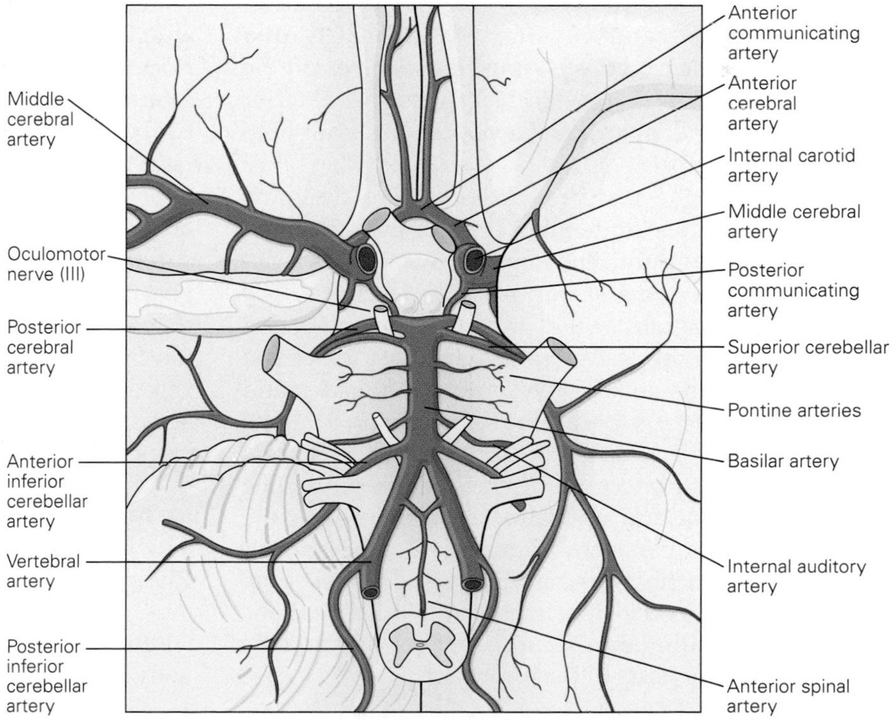

Figure C–1 The blood vessels of the brain. The circle of Willis is made up of the proximal posterior cerebral arteries, posterior communicating arteries, internal carotid arteries just before their bifurcations, proximal anterior cerebral arteries, and anterior communicating artery. **Black areas** are common sites of atherosclerosis and occlusion.

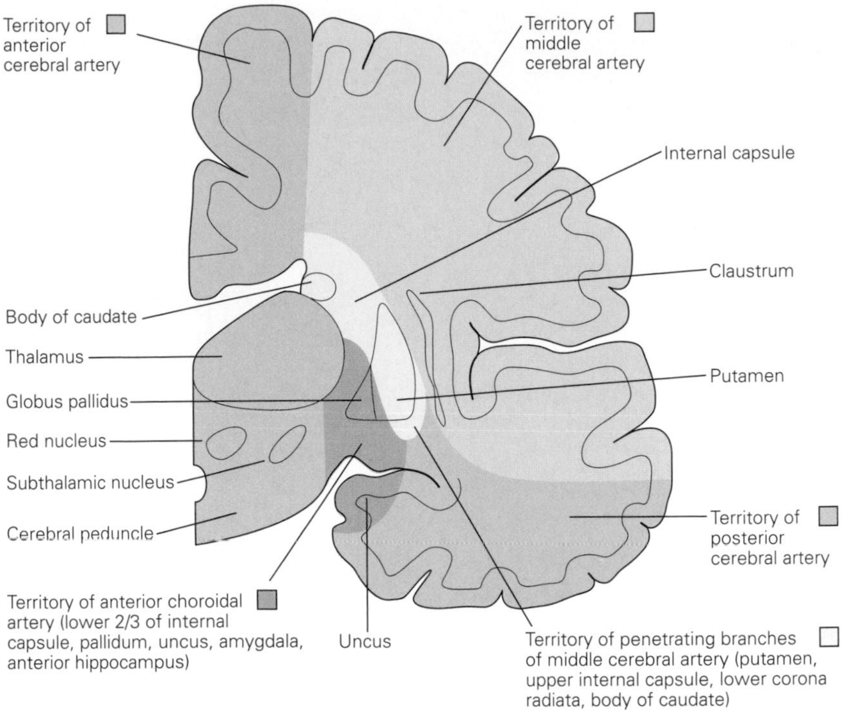

Figure C–2 Cerebral arterial areas.

(Figure C–2). Smaller penetrating branches (the *lenticulostriate arteries*) supply the deep white matter and diencephalic structures, such as the posterior limb of the internal capsule, putamen, outer globus pallidus, and body of the caudate. After the internal carotid emerges from the cavernous sinus, it also gives off the *anterior choroidal artery,* which supplies the anterior hippocampus and, at a caudal level, the posterior limb of the internal capsule.

Left and right vertebral arteries arise from the subclavian arteries and enter the cranium through the foramen magnum. Each gives off an *anterior spinal artery* and a *posterior inferior cerebellar artery.* The vertebral arteries join at the junction of the pons and medulla to form the *basilar artery,* which at the pontine level gives off the *anterior inferior cerebellar artery* and the *internal auditory artery* and at the midbrain level the *superior cerebellar artery.* The basilar artery then divides into the two *posterior cerebral arteries,* which supply the inferior temporal and medial occipital lobes and the posterior corpus callosum (Figure C–2). The smaller penetrating branches of these vessels (the *thalamoperforate* and *thalamogeniculate arteries*) supply diencephalic structures, including the thalamus and the subthalamic nuclei, as well as parts of the midbrain.

Interconnections between blood vessels (*anastomoses*) protect the brain when part of its vascular supply is blocked (Figure C–3). At the *circle of Willis,* which provides an overlapping blood supply, the two anterior cerebral arteries are connected by the anterior communicating artery, and the posterior cerebral arteries are connected to the internal carotid arteries by the posterior communicating arteries. Other important anastomoses include connections between the ophthalmic artery and branches of the external carotid artery through the orbit, and connections at the brain surface between branches of the middle, anterior, and posterior cerebral arteries (sharing *border zones* or *watersheds*). The small penetrating vessels arising from the circle of Willis and proximal major arteries tend to lack anastomoses. The deep brain regions they supply are therefore referred to as *end zones* (no source of overlapping blood supply).

The Cerebral Vessels Have Unique Physiological Responses

Although the human brain constitutes only 2% of total body weight, it receives approximately 15% of the cardiac output and consumes approximately 20% of the oxygen used by the entire body. These values reflect the high metabolic rate and oxygen requirements of the brain. The total blood flow to the brain is 750 to 1000 mL/min; approximately 350 mL of this amount flows through each carotid artery and approximately 100 to 200 mL flow through the vertebrobasilar arterial system. Flow per unit mass of gray matter (somata and dendrites) is approximately four times that of white matter (axons).

Cerebral vessels are capable of altering their own diameter and can respond to altered physiological conditions. Two main types of autoregulation exist. Brain arterioles constrict when the systemic blood pressure is raised and dilate when it is lowered. These adjustments help maintain optimal cerebral blood flow. The result is that normal people have a constant cerebral blood flow between mean arterial pressures of 60 to 150 mm Hg. Above or below these pressures cerebral blood flow rises or falls linearly.

The second type of autoregulation involves blood or tissue gases and pH. When arterial carbon dioxide (CO_2) is raised, brain arterioles dilate and cerebral blood flow increases; with hypocarbia, vasoconstriction results and cerebral blood flow decreases. The response is sensitive: Inhalation of 5% CO_2 increases blood flow by 50%; 7% CO_2 doubles it. Changing arterial O_2 causes an opposite and less pronounced response. Breathing pure O_2 lowers blood flow by approximately 13%; 10% O_2 raises it by 35%. The mechanism of these responses is uncertain. The vasodilatory action of arterial CO_2 is probably mediated by alterations in extracellular pH. Local concentrations of K^+ and adenosine, both of which cause vasodilation, may play a role.

Whatever the mechanism, these responses protect the brain by increasing the delivery of oxygen and the removal of acidic metabolites under conditions of hypoxia, ischemia, or tissue damage. They also allow nearly instantaneous adjustments of regional cerebral

A

B

C

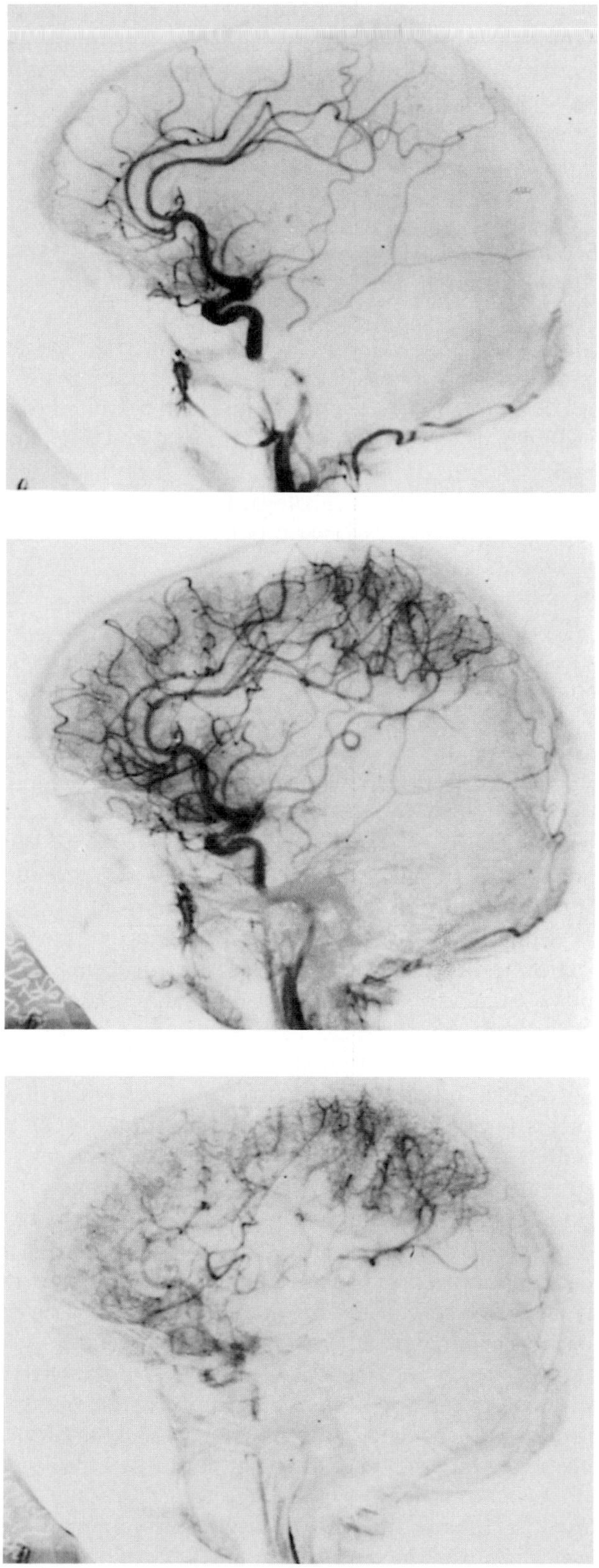

Figure C–3 Angiograms demonstrate the importance of anastomoses in allowing retrograde filling after occlusion of the middle cerebral artery. (Reproduced, with permission, from Margaret Whelan and Sadek K. Hilal.)

A. Occlusion of the middle cerebral artery results in no filling in the middle cerebral distribution.

B. Retrograde filling of the middle cerebral artery has begun via distal anastomotic branches of the anterior cerebral artery.

C. Retrograde filling of the middle cerebral artery continues at a time when little contrast material is seen in the anterior cerebral artery.

blood flow to meet the demands of rapidly changing oxygen and glucose metabolism that accompany normal brain activities. For example, viewing a complex scene increases oxygen and glucose consumption in the visual cortex of the occipital lobes. The resulting increased CO_2 concentration and lowered pH in the area rapidly increase local blood flow.

A Stroke Is the Result of Disease Involving Blood Vessels

Diseases of blood vessels are among the most frequent serious neurological disorders, ranking third as a cause of death in the adult population in the United States and probably first as a cause of chronic functional incapacity. Approximately two million Americans today are impaired by the neurological consequences of cerebrovascular disease, many between 25 and 64 years of age.

Strokes are either occlusive (closure of a blood vessel) or hemorrhagic (bleeding from a vessel). Insufficiency of blood supply is termed *ischemia*; if it is temporary, symptoms and signs may clear with little or no pathological evidence of tissue damage. Ischemia results in more than simply *anoxia,* because a reduced blood supply deprives tissue not only of oxygen but also of glucose. In addition, it prevents the removal of potentially toxic metabolites such as lactic acid. When ischemia is sufficiently severe and prolonged, neurons die; this condition is called *infarction.*

Hemorrhage may occur at the surface of the brain (extraparenchymal), for example from rupture of saccular aneurysms at the circle of Willis, causing subarachnoid hemorrhage. Alternatively, hemorrhage may be intraparenchymal, for example from rupture of vessels damaged by chronic hypertension—and may cause a blood clot or *hematoma* within the cerebral hemispheres, brain stem, or cerebellum. Hemorrhage may result in ischemia or infarction. Because of its mass, an intracerebral hematoma may limit the blood supply of adjacent brain tissue. By mechanisms that are not understood, subarachnoid hemorrhage may cause reactive vasospasm of cerebral surface vessels, leading to further ischemic brain damage.

Although most occlusive strokes are caused by atherosclerosis and thrombosis and most hemorrhagic strokes are associated with hypertension or aneurysms, strokes of either type may occur at any age from many other causes, including cardiac disease, trauma, infection, neoplasm, blood dyscrasia, vascular malformation, immunological disorder, and exogenous toxins.

Clinical Vascular Syndromes May Follow Vessel Occlusion, Hypoperfusion, or Hemorrhage

Infarction Can Occur in the Middle Cerebral Artery Territory

Infarction in the territory of the middle cerebral artery (Figure C–4) causes the most frequently encountered stroke syndrome, with contralateral weakness, sensory loss, and visual field impairment (homonymous hemianopia), and, depending on the hemisphere involved, either language disturbance (left) or impaired spatial perception (right). Weakness and sensory loss affect the face and arm more than the leg because of the somatotopy of the motor and sensory cortex (pre- and postcentral gyri). The face- and arm-control areas are on the convexity of the hemisphere, whereas the leg-control area is on the medial surface.

Motor and sensory loss are greatest in the hand because the more proximal limbs and the trunk tend to have greater representation in both hemispheres. Paraspinal muscles, for example, are rarely weakened in

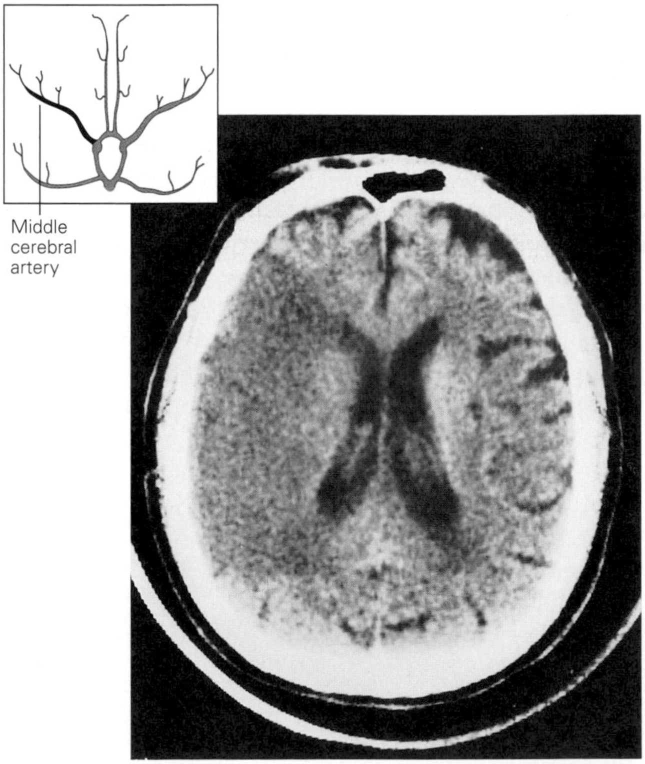

Figure C–4 Computed tomography scan showing infarction (dark area) in the territory of the middle cerebral artery. (Reproduced, with permission, from Allan J. Schwartz.)

unilateral cerebral lesions. Similarly, the facial muscles of the forehead and the muscles of the pharynx and jaw are represented in both hemispheres and therefore are usually spared. Tongue weakness is variable. If weakness is severe (plegia), muscle tone is usually decreased at first but gradually increases over days or weeks to spasticity with hyperactive tendon reflexes. A Babinski sign, reflecting upper motor neuron disturbance, is usually present. When weakness is mild, or during recovery, there may be clumsiness or slowness of movement out of proportion to loss of strength; such motor disability may resemble parkinsonian bradykinesia or even cerebellar ataxia.

Acute paresis of contralateral conjugate gaze often occurs as a result of damage to the convexity of the frontal cortex anterior to the motor cortex (the frontal eye field). For reasons that are unclear, this gaze palsy persists for only one or two days, even when other signs remain severe.

Sensory loss tends to involve discriminative and proprioceptive modalities more than affective modalities (pain and temperature sensation), which may be impaired or altered but are usually not lost completely. Joint position sense may be severely disturbed, causing limb ataxia, and there may be loss of two-point discrimination, astereognosis (inability to recognize an object by tactile sensation alone), or extinction (failure to appreciate a touch stimulus if a comparable stimulus is delivered simultaneously to the unaffected side of the body).

Homonymous hemianopia is the result of damage to the optic radiations, the deep fiber tracts connecting the thalamic lateral geniculate nucleus to the visual (*calcarine*) cortex. If the parietal radiation is primarily affected, the visual field loss may be an inferior quadrantanopia, whereas in temporal lobe lesions quadrantanopia may be superior.

In more than 95% of right-handed persons and most of those who are left handed, the left hemisphere is dominant for language. Destruction of left frontal, parietal, or temporal opercular (*perisylvian*) cortex in left-dominant people causes aphasia, which takes several forms depending on the degree and distribution of the damage. Frontal opercular lesions tend to produce particular difficulty with speech output and writing while preserving at least partially language comprehension (*Broca aphasia*). Infarction of the posterior superior temporal gyrus tends to cause severe difficulty in speech comprehension and reading (*Wernicke aphasia*). When damage to the opercular cortex is widespread, a severe disturbance of mixed type occurs (*global aphasia*). Left-hemisphere convexity damage, especially parietal, also causes motor apraxia, a disturbance of learned motor acts not explained by weakness or incoordination.

Right-hemisphere convexity infarction, especially parietal, causes disturbances of spatial perception. Patients may have difficulty in copying simple diagrams (*constructional apraxia*), interpreting maps or finding their way about (*topographagnosia*), or putting on their clothing properly (*dressing apraxia*). Awareness of space and the patient's own body on the side contralateral to the lesion may be particularly impaired (*hemi-inattention* or *hemineglect*). Patients also fail to acknowledge their hemiplegia (*anosognosia*), left arm (*asomatognosia*), or any external object to the left of their own midline.

Particular types of language or spatial dysfunction tend to result from occlusion of one of the several main pial branches of the middle cerebral artery, not the proximal stem. In these circumstances other signs (eg, weakness or visual field defect) may be absent. Similarly, occlusion of the rolandic branch of the middle cerebral artery causes motor and sensory loss affecting the face and arm without disturbing vision, language, or spatial perception.

Infarction Can Occur in the Anterior Cerebral Artery Territory

Infarction in the territory of the anterior cerebral artery (Figure C–5) causes weakness and sensory loss qualitatively similar to that of convexity lesions, but infarction in this territory affects mainly the distal contralateral leg. Urinary incontinence may be present, but it is uncertain whether this is because of a lesion of the paracentral lobule (medial hemispheric motor and sensory cortices) or a more anterior region necessary for the inhibition of bladder emptying. Damage to the supplementary motor cortex disturbs speech. Involvement of the anterior corpus callosum causes apraxia of the left arm (*sympathetic apraxia*), which is attributed to disconnection of the left (language-dominant) hemisphere from the right motor cortex.

Bilateral infarction in the territory of the anterior cerebral artery (occurring, for example, when both arteries arise anomalously from a single trunk) causes abulia, a severe behavioral disturbance consisting of profound apathy, motor inertia, and muteness, and attributable to destruction of the inferior frontal lobes (orbitofrontal cortex), deeper limbic structures, supplementary motor cortices, and cingulate gyri.

Infarction Can Occur in the Posterior Cerebral Artery Territory

Infarction in the territory of the posterior cerebral artery (Figure C–6) causes contralateral homonymous

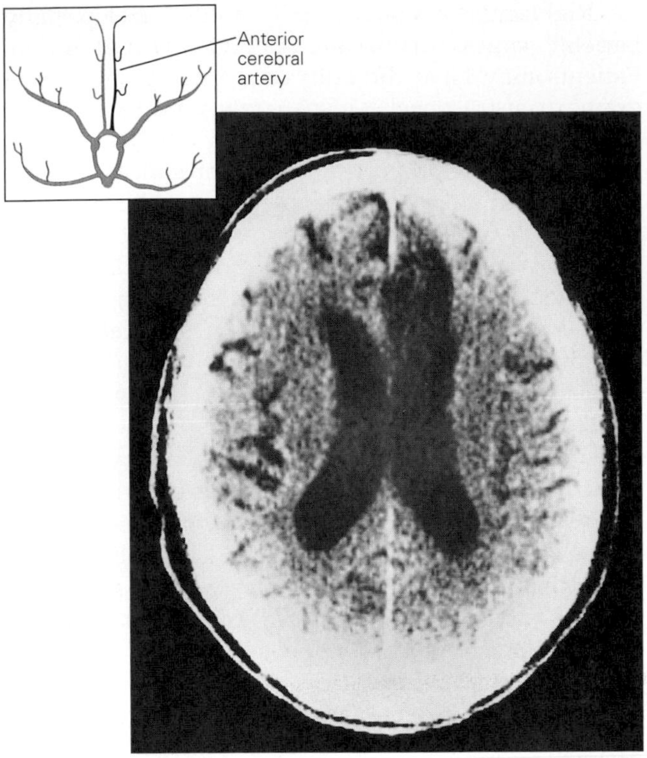

Figure C–5 Computed tomography scan showing infarction (dark area) in the territory of the anterior cerebral artery. (Reproduced, with permission, from Allan J. Schwartz.)

hemianopsia by destroying the medial occipital cortex. Macular (central) vision tends to be spared because the occipital pole, where macular vision is represented, receives anastomotic blood supply from the middle cerebral artery. If the lesion is on the left and the posterior corpus callosum is affected, alexia—the inability to read—may be present without aphasia or agraphia. A possible explanation for the alexia is the disconnection of the right occipital cortex (visual processing) from the language-dominant left hemisphere. If infarction is bilateral (eg, following thrombosis at the point where both posterior cerebral arteries arise from the basilar artery), there may be cortical blindness that is not recognized by the patient (Anton syndrome), or memory disturbance as a result of bilateral damage to the inferomedial temporal lobes.

If the posterior cerebral artery occlusion is proximal, the following structures may be damaged: the thalamus, causing contralateral hemisensory loss and sometimes dysesthesia (altered touch sensation) and spontaneous pain (thalamic pain syndrome); the subthalamic nucleus, causing contralateral severe proximal chorea (hemiballism); or even the midbrain, with ipsilateral oculomotor palsy and contralateral hemiparesis or ataxia from involvement of the corticospinal tract or the crossed superior cerebellar peduncle (dentatothalamic tract).

The Anterior Choroidal and Penetrating Arteries Can Become Occluded

Anterior choroidal artery occlusion can cause contralateral hemiplegia and sensory loss from involvement of the posterior limb of the internal capsule and homonymous hemianopia from involvement of the thalamic lateral geniculate nucleus.

The deeper cerebral white matter and diencephalon are supplied by small penetrating arteries, which arise from the circle of Willis or the proximal portions of the middle, anterior, and posterior cerebral arteries. Occlusion of these end-arteries causes small infarcts (less than 1.5 cm in diameter) called *lacunes* with characteristic syndromes. For example, lacunes in the pyramidal tract area of the internal capsule cause

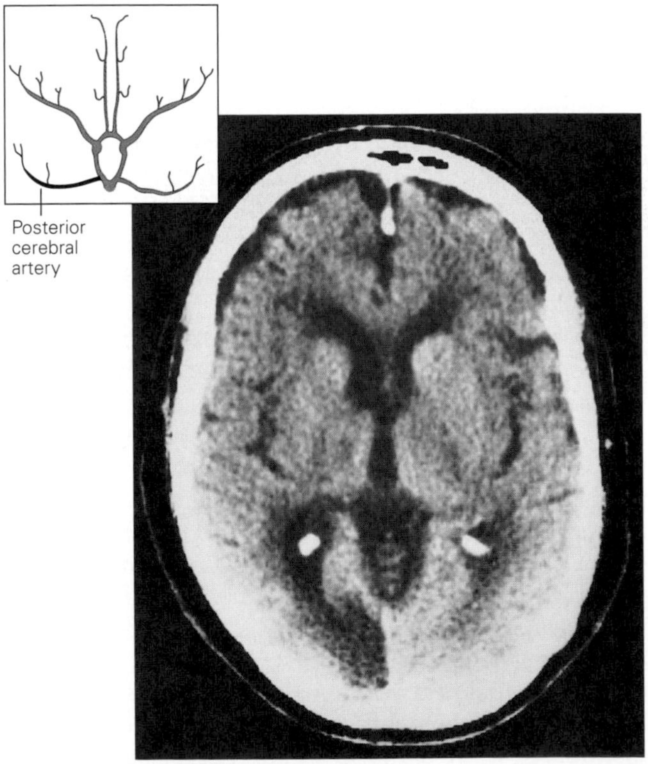

Figure C–6 Computed tomography scan showing infarction (dark area) in the territory of the posterior cerebral artery. (Reproduced, with permission, from Allan J. Schwartz.)

pure hemiparesis, with face, arm, and leg weakness of equal severity but little or no sensory loss, visual field disturbance, aphasia, or spatial disruption. Lacunes in the ventral posterior nucleus of the thalamus produce pure hemisensory loss, with involvement of pain, temperature, proprioceptive, and discriminative modalities and with little motor, visual, language, or spatial disturbance. Most lacunes occur in redundant areas (eg, nonpyramidal corona radiata) and so are not symptomatic. If bilateral and numerous, however, they may cause a characteristic syndrome (*état lacunaire*) of progressive dementia, shuffling gait, and pseudobulbar palsy (spastic dysarthria and dysphagia, with lingual and pharyngeal paralysis and hyperactive palate and gag reflexes, plus lability of emotional response, with abrupt crying or laughing out of proportion to mood).

Infarction restricted to structures supplied by the recurrent artery of Heubner or other deep penetrating branches of the anterior cerebral artery (the anterior caudate nucleus and, less predictably, the anterior putamen and anterior limb of the internal capsule) results in varying combinations of psychomotor slowing, dysarthria, agitation, contralateral neglect, and, when left hemispheric, language disturbance.

The Carotid Artery Can Become Occluded

Atherothrombotic vessel occlusion often occurs in the internal carotid artery rather than the intracranial vessels. Particularly in a patient with an incomplete circle of Willis, infarction may include the territories of both the middle and anterior cerebral arteries, with arm and leg weakness and sensory loss equally severe. Alternatively, infarction may be limited to the distal shared territory (border zones) of these vessels, destroying motor cortex at the upper cerebral convexity and producing weakness limited to the arm or the leg.

The Brain Stem and Cerebellum Are Supplied by Branches of the Vertebral and Basilar Arteries

Branches of the vertebral and basilar arteries consist of three groups: (1) paramedian branches, including the anterior spinal artery, supply midline structures; (2) short circumferential branches supply more lateral structures, including the inferior, middle, and superior cerebellar peduncles; and (3) long circumferential arteries—the posterior inferior, anterior inferior, and superior cerebellar arteries—also supply lateral brain stem structures and the cerebellar peduncles, as well as the cerebellum itself. Most of the midbrain is supplied by branches of the posterior cerebral artery. The interpeduncular branches, the most medial branches located between the basilar artery bifurcation and the posterior communicating arteries, supply paramedian midbrain structures. Lateral to this group are the thalamoperforate branches, which supply the inferior, medial, and anterior thalamus and the subthalamic nucleus. Further laterally are the thalamogeniculate branches, which supply lateral and dorsal structures in the midbrain and thalamus. In some people the midbrain also receives blood from the superior cerebellar, posterior communicating, and anterior choroidal arteries. After passing around the midbrain, the posterior cerebral artery enters the middle fossa to supply the occipital and inferior temporal lobes. It does not supply the cerebellum.

Damage to specific brain stem structures produces a variety of syndromes (Figure C–7). With the exception of the lateral medullary syndrome of Wallenberg, however, most original descriptions of these syndromes were based on patients with neoplasms. Brain stem infarction more often follows occlusion of the vertebral or basilar arteries themselves rather than their medial or lateral branches; resulting syndromes and signs tend to be less stereotyped than originally described.

Generally speaking, a lesion of the posterior fossa is suggested by (1) bilateral long tract (motor or sensory) signs, (2) crossed (eg, left face and right limb) motor or sensory signs, (3) cerebellar signs, (4) stupor or coma (from involvement of the ascending reticular activating system), (5) disconjugate eye movements or nystagmus, and (6) involvement of cranial nerves not usually affected by unilateral hemispheric infarcts (eg, unilateral deafness or pharyngeal weakness). Sometimes a lesion involving only a single tiny structure can be localized accurately by symptomatology. For example, internuclear ophthalmoplegia implicates a lesion of the median longitudinal fasciculus. Other lesions produce more ambiguous symptoms. For example, infarction limited to the upper pontine corticospinal tract can produce contralateral face, arm, and leg weakness indistinguishable from that caused by a small infarct in the internal capsule.

Infarcts Affecting Predominantly Medial or Lateral Brain Stem Structures Produce Characteristic Syndromes

Medullary and pontine syndromes are conveniently viewed as lateral or medial (Figure C–7). Infarction of the lateral medulla follows occlusion of the vertebral artery or less often the posterior inferior cerebellar artery. Symptoms and signs include (1) vertigo, nausea, vomiting, and nystagmus (from involvement of

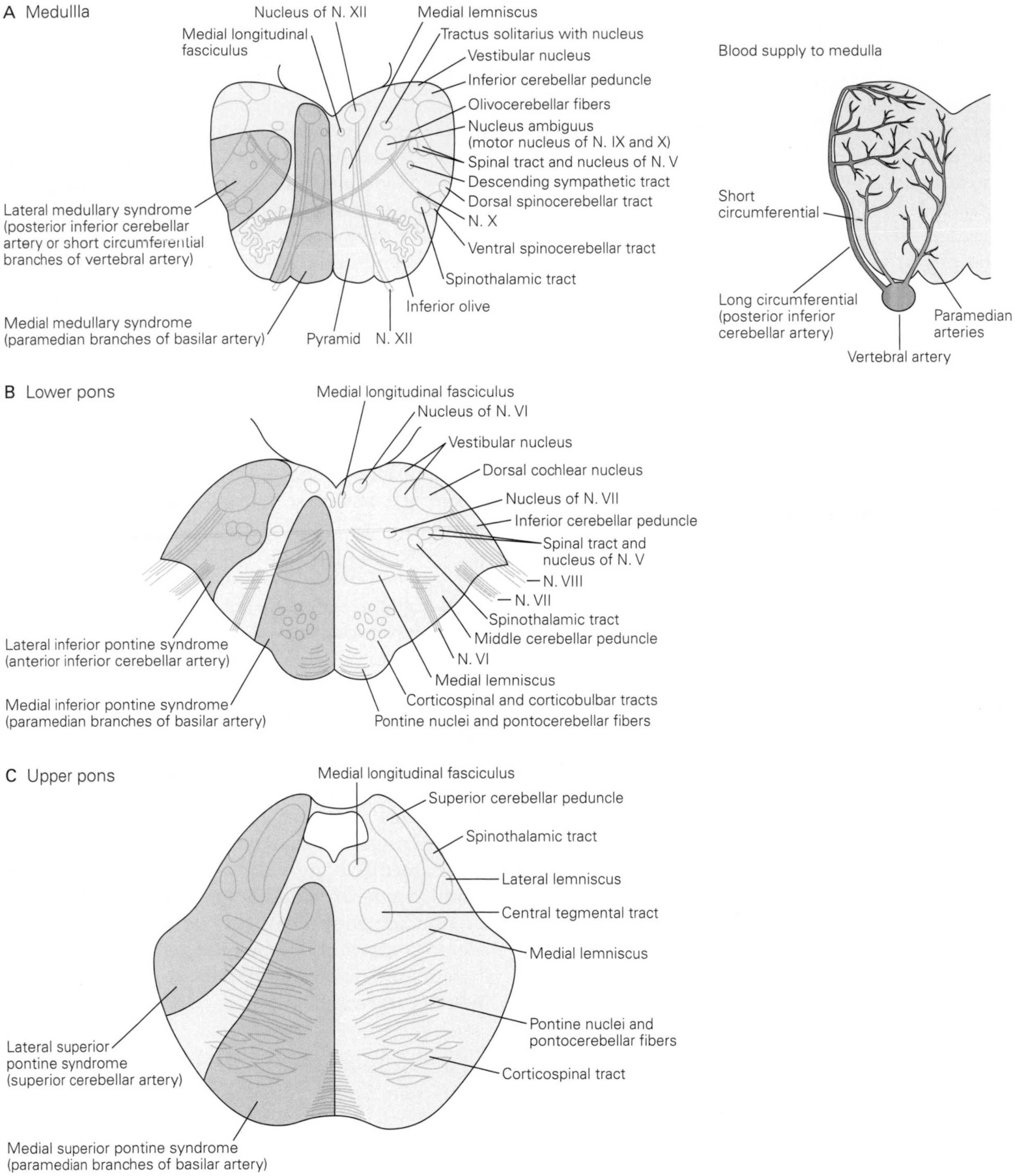
A Medullla
Nucleus of N. XII
Medial lemniscus
Medial longitudinal fasciculus
Tractus solitarius with nucleus
Vestibular nucleus
Inferior cerebellar peduncle
Olivocerebellar fibers
Nucleus ambiguus (motor nucleus of N. IX and X)
Spinal tract and nucleus of N. V
Descending sympathetic tract
Dorsal spinocerebellar tract
N. X
Ventral spinocerebellar tract
Spinothalamic tract
Inferior olive
Lateral medullary syndrome (posterior inferior cerebellar artery or short circumferential branches of vertebral artery)
Medial medullary syndrome (paramedian branches of basilar artery)
Pyramid
N. XII
Blood supply to medulla
Short circumferential
Long circumferential (posterior inferior cerebellar artery)
Paramedian arteries
Vertebral artery
B Lower pons
Medial longitudinal fasciculus
Nucleus of N. VI
Vestibular nucleus
Dorsal cochlear nucleus
Nucleus of N. VII
Inferior cerebellar peduncle
Spinal tract and nucleus of N. V
N. VIII
N. VII
Spinothalamic tract
Middle cerebellar peduncle
N. VI
Medial lemniscus
Corticospinal and corticobulbar tracts
Pontine nuclei and pontocerebellar fibers
Lateral inferior pontine syndrome (anterior inferior cerebellar artery)
Medial inferior pontine syndrome (paramedian branches of basilar artery)
C Upper pons
Medial longitudinal fasciculus
Superior cerebellar peduncle
Spinothalamic tract
Lateral lemniscus
Central tegmental tract
Medial lemniscus
Pontine nuclei and pontocerebellar fibers
Corticospinal tract
Lateral superior pontine syndrome (superior cerebellar artery)
Medial superior pontine syndrome (paramedian branches of basilar artery)

Figure C–7 Syndromes of brain stem vascular lesions (indicated on the left in each figure).

the vestibular nuclei); (2) ataxia of gait and ipsilateral limbs (inferior cerebellar peduncle or the cerebellum itself); (3) decreased pain and temperature (but not touch) sensation on the ipsilateral face (spinal tract and nucleus of the trigeminal nerve) and the contralateral body (spinothalamic tract); (4) dysphagia, hoarseness, ipsilateral weakness of the palate and vocal cords, and ipsilaterally decreased gag reflex (nucleus ambiguus, or glossopharyngeal and vagus outflow tracts); and (5) ipsilateral Horner syndrome (descending sympathetic fibers). Involvement of the nucleus solitarius can cause ipsilateral loss of taste, and hiccups are often present. The symptoms and signs for infarcts affecting different levels of the brain stem are listed in Table C–1.

Infarction of the medial medulla causes contralateral hemiparesis (from involvement of the corticospinal tract), ipsilateral tongue weakness with dysarthria and deviation toward the paretic side (hypoglossal nucleus or outflow tract), and contralateral impaired proprioception and discriminative sensation with preserved pain and temperature sensation (medial lemniscus).

Infarction of the lateral pons affects caudal structures when the anterior inferior cerebellar artery is occluded and rostral structures when the superior cerebellar artery is occluded (Figure C–8). Symptoms of caudal damage resemble those of lateral medullary infarction, with vertigo, nystagmus, gait and ipsilateral limb ataxia, crossed face-and-body pain and temperature loss, Horner syndrome, and ipsilateral loss of taste. There is also unilateral tinnitus and deafness (from involvement of the cochlear nuclei). Involvement of more medial structures can cause ipsilateral gaze paresis or facial weakness. Symptoms of rostral damage include gait and ipsilateral limb ataxia, Horner syndrome, and crossed sensory loss, which at this level includes touch as well as pain and temperature sensation on the ipsilateral face (from involvement of the primary sensory nucleus or entering sensory fibers of the trigeminal nerve). There may also be ipsilateral jaw weakness with deviation to the paretic side (trigeminal motor nucleus and outflow tract). Vertigo, deafness, and face weakness are not present.

Infarction of the medial pons, whether caudal or rostral, causes contralateral hemiparesis (from involvement of the corticospinal tract). Caudal lesions affecting the facial nucleus or outflow tract cause ipsilateral facial weakness. Rostral lesions result in contralateral facial weakness. There may also be ipsilateral gaze paresis (paramedian pontine reticular formation or abducens nucleus, together comprising the *pontine gaze center*) or abducens paresis (sixth nerve outflow tract); internuclear ophthalmoplegia and limb and gait ataxia are often present. Contralateral impairment of proprioception and discriminative touch is most prominent with caudal lesions. Rapid involuntary movements of the palate—so-called *palatal myoclonus*—has been attributed to involvement of the central tegmental tract; the involuntary movements may spread to include the pharynx, larynx, face, eyes, or respiratory muscles.

Midbrain syndromes are viewed as ventral (or peduncle), tegmental, and dorsal (including the collicular, pretectal, and tectal areas) (Figure C–9). Because the vertebral and basilar arteries themselves are usually the site of occlusion, pure forms of these stereotypic syndromes are infrequently encountered clinically. Unilateral ventral lesions cause *Weber syndrome,* characterized by ipsilateral paresis of adduction and vertical gaze and pupillary dilation (involvement of oculomotor nerve outflow tract) and contralateral face, arm, and leg paresis (corticospinal and corticobulbar tracts). Unilateral tegmental lesions cause *Claude syndrome,* characterized by oculomotor paresis (oculomotor nucleus) and contralateral ataxia and tremor (often referred to as *rubral tremor* but probably the result of damage to projections from the cerebellum to the thalamus). Lesions affecting both the peduncle and tegmentum produce combinations of oculomotor paresis, ataxia, and weakness (*Benedikt syndrome*). Dorsal midbrain lesions, which are infrequently vascular and rarely unilateral, cause *Parinaud syndrome,* characterized by impaired vertical gaze—especially upward (posterior commissure and the rostral interstitial nucleus of the median longitudinal fasciculus)—and loss of the pupillary light reflex (pretectal structures).

Because the vertebral and basilar arteries themselves are usually the site of occlusion, pure forms of these stereotypic syndromes are infrequently encountered clinically.

Bilateral brain stem lesions can be devastating. Paramedian infarction of the upper brain stem can destroy the reticular activating system and cause stupor or coma. Bilateral infarction of the rostral basis pontis destroys descending corticospinal and corticobulbar fibers, causing paralysis of all muscles except eye movements; if the tegmentum is spared such patients remain awake and communicate with their eyes (the locked-in state).

Infarction Can Be Restricted to the Cerebellum

Infarcts of the inferior cerebellum, which has extensive vestibular connections, can cause vertigo, nausea, and nystagmus without other symptoms, suggesting disease of the inner ear or vestibular nerve. More superior cerebellar infarcts produce gait and ipsilateral limb ataxia.

Table C–1 Syndromes of Brain Stem Infarction

	Symptoms	Structure involved
Medulla		
Lateral	Vertigo, nystagmus	Vestibular nuclei
	Ataxia of gait and ipsilateral limbs	Inferior cerebellar peduncle and cerebellum
	Decreased pain and temperature sensation on ipsilateral face	Spinal tract and nucleus of trigeminal nerve
	Decreased pain and temperature on contralateral body	Spinothalamic tract
	Dysphagia, hoarseness	Nucleus ambiguus
	Ipsilateral Horner syndrome	Descending sympathetic fibers
	Ipsilateral loss of taste	Nucleus solitarius
Medial	Contralateral hemiparesis	Corticospinal tract
	Ipsilateral tongue weakness	Hypoglossal nucleus and emerging fibers of N. XII
	Decreased proprioception and discriminative sensation on contralateral body	Medial lemniscus
Pons		
Lateral	Ataxia of gait and ipsilateral limbs	Middle cerebellar peduncle and cerebellum
	Decreased pain, temperature, and touch sensation on ipsilateral face	Primary sensory nucleus of trigeminal nerve
	Deafness, tinnitus	Cochlear nuclei
	Decreased pain and temperature sensation on contralateral body	Spinothalamic tract
	Ipsilateral jaw weakness	Trigeminal motor nucleus
	Ipsilateral Horner syndrome	Descending sympathetic fibers
Medial	Contralateral hemiparesis	Corticospinal tract
	Ipsilateral facial weakness	Facial nucleus and emerging fibers of N. VII
	Ipsilateral gaze paresis	Paramedian pontine reticular formation or abducens nucleus
	Ipsilateral abducens paresis	Abducens nucleus and emerging fibers of N. VI
	Internuclear ophthalmoplegia	Median longitudinal fasciculus
	Limb and gait ataxia	Nuclei and crossing cerebellar fibers of the basis pontis
	Decreased proprioception and discriminative sensation on contralateral body	Medial lemniscus
Midbrain[1]		
Ventral	Ipsilateral pupillary dilation and paresis of adduction and vertical gaze	Emerging fibers of oculomotor nerve
	Contralateral face weakness and hemiparesis	Corticobulbar and corticospinal tracts
Tegmental	Ipsilateral oculomotor paresis	Oculomotor nucleus
	Contralateral limb ataxia and tremor	Cerebellar projections to red nucleus and thalamus
Dorsal	Bilateral paresis of upward gaze and loss of pupillary light reflex (Parinaud syndrome)	Posterior commissure, rostral interstitial nucleus of the median longitudinal fasciculus, and pretectal structures

[1]See Figure C–9.

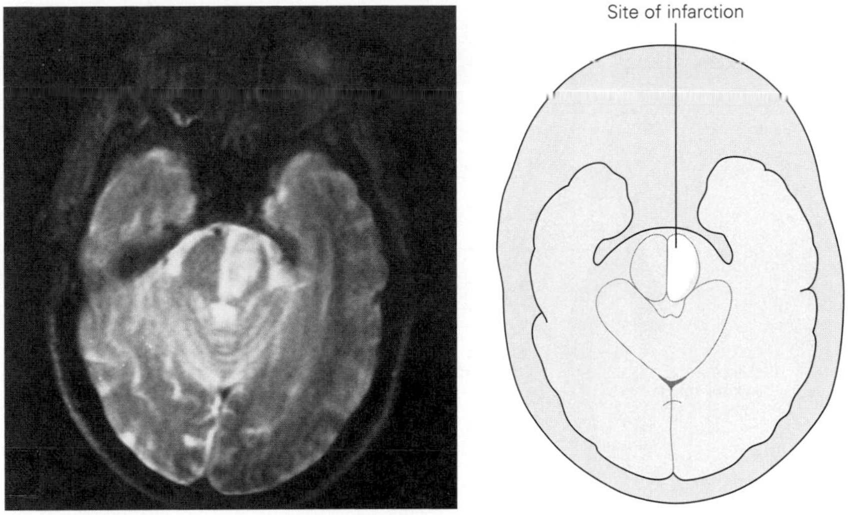

Figure C–8 **Magnetic resonance imaging shows a lesion (white highlight) in the ventral portion of one half of the pons.** The lesion stops abruptly at the midline, suggesting unilateral occlusion of one or more paramedian vessels.

Infarction Can Affect the Spinal Cord

Vascular anatomy explains the characteristic pattern of spinal cord infarction (Figure C–10). Vessel occlusion is usually in a proximal segmental artery. Because of the anastomotic continuity of the posterior spinal arteries, infarction tends to be limited to the anterior spinal artery territory. Thus paraparesis or quadriparesis (corticospinal tracts), loss of bladder and bowel control, and loss of pain and temperature sensation below the lesion (spinothalamic tracts) are common; but proprioception and discriminative touch (dorsal columns) are spared.

If the cervical or lumbar spinal cord is involved, atrophic weakness of upper or lower extremity muscles (anterior horns) can occur. Because the anterior spinal artery gives off sulcal arteries that alternately enter the left and right halves of the spinal cord, infarction can sometimes produce a Brown-Séquard syndrome, with ipsilateral weakness and contralateral loss of pain and temperature sensation.

Diffuse Hypoperfusion Can Cause Ischemia or Infarction

Brain ischemia or infarction may accompany diffuse hypoperfusion (shock). In such circumstances the most vulnerable regions are often the border zones between large arterial territories and the end zones of deep penetrating vessels. Whatever the cause of reduced cerebral perfusion, signs tend to be bilateral. Paralysis and sensory loss may be present in both arms (from bilateral infarction of the cortex at the junction of the middle and anterior arterial supply, affecting the arm control area of the motor and sensory cortex).

Disturbed vision or memory may result (from infarction of the occipital or inferior temporal lobes at the junction of the middle and posterior cerebral arterial supply). There may also be ataxia (from cerebellar border zone infarction) or abnormal movements such as chorea or myoclonus (presumably from involvement

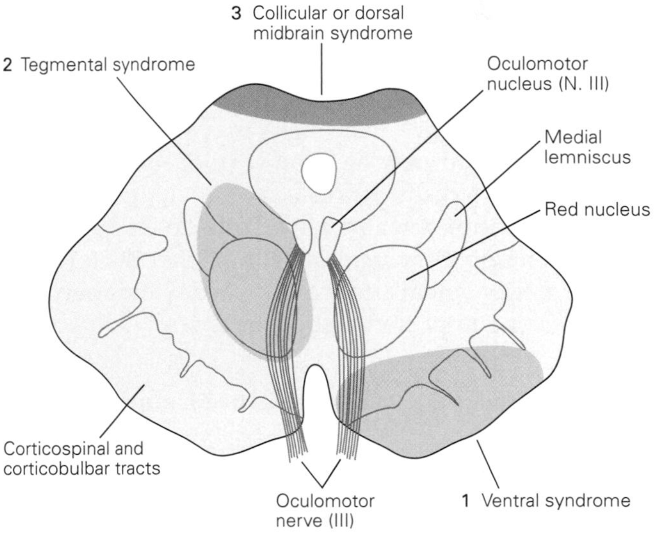

Figure C–9 **The three midbrain syndromes.** Syndromes of midbrain infarction are conveniently characterized as ventral (1), tegmental (2), or dorsal (3).

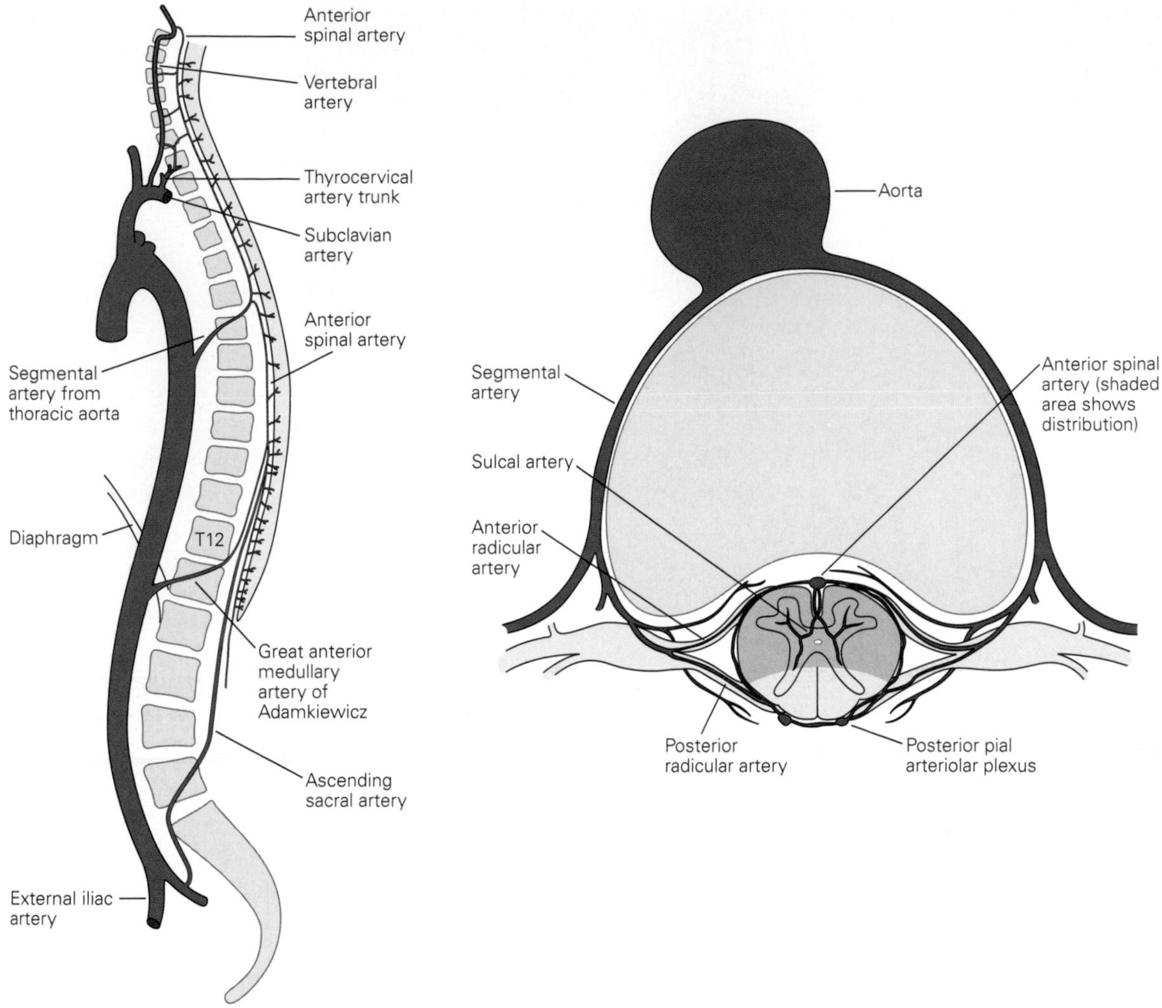

Figure C–10 Major sources of blood supply to the spinal cord. (Anterior spinal rami are not shown.)

of the basal ganglia). Such signs may exist alone or in combination and may be accompanied by aphasia or other cognitive disturbances.

Hypotension can also cause spinal cord infarction, most often upper thoracic, affecting either the territory of the anterior spinal artery or the border zone between the anterior and posterior spinal arteries.

Cerebrovascular Disease Can Cause Dementia

Cerebral infarction causes dementia by a number of mechanisms:

1. Infarcts may be critically located. For example, thalamic or inferomedial temporal damage (posterior cerebral artery, usually bilateral) can cause amnesia; hemispheric convexity damage (middle cerebral artery) can cause cognitive or behavioral impairment not explained by disruption of language or spatial discrimination; and bilateral inferomedial frontal lobe damage (anterior cerebral artery) can cause abulia and impaired memory.
2. Multiple scattered infarcts, none sufficient to cause significant cognitive loss, can produce additive effects culminating in dementia. In such patients at least 100 cc of brain volume has usually been destroyed.
3. Small vessel disease, affecting especially the deep cerebral white matter, can cause either scattered lacunes or more diffuse ischemic lesions. When such lesions are severe enough to cause dementia, there is often altered behavior, pseudobulbar palsy, pyramidal signs, disturbed gait, and urinary incontinence.

The Rupture of Microaneurysms Causes Intraparenchymal Stroke

The two most common causes of hemorrhagic stroke, hypertensive intraparenchymal hemorrhage and rupture of a saccular aneurysm, tend to occur at particular sites and to cause recognizable syndromes. Hypertensive intracerebral hemorrhage is the result of damage to the same small penetrating vessels that, when occluded, cause lacunes; in the case of hemorrhage the damaged vessels develop weakened walls (Charcot-Bouchard microaneurysms) that eventually rupture. The most common sites are the putamen, thalamus, pons, internal capsule and corona radiata, and cerebellum. Large diencephalic hemorrhages tend to cause stupor and hemiplegia and have a high mortality rate.

With putamenal hemorrhage (Figure C–11) the eyes are usually deviated ipsilaterally (because of disruption of capsular pathways descending from the frontal eye field), whereas with thalamic hemorrhage (Figure C–12) the eyes tend to be deviated downward and the pupils may not react to light (because of involvement of midbrain pretectal structures essential for upward gaze and pupillary light reactivity). Small hemorrhages may not impair alertness, and with small thalamic hemorrhages sensory loss may exceed weakness. Moreover, computerized tomography reveals that small thalamic hemorrhages can cause aphasia when on the left and hemineglect when on the right.

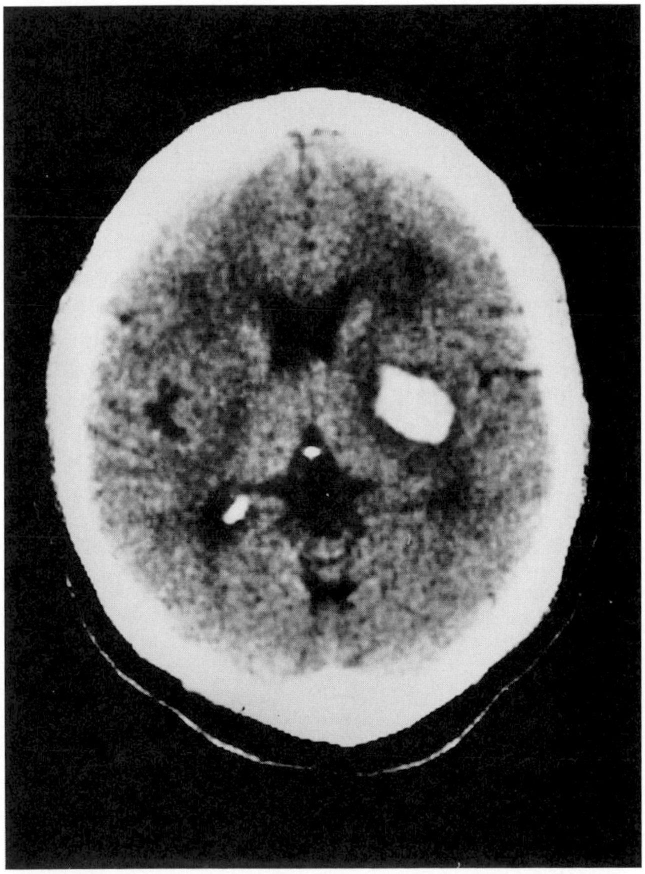

Figure C–11 Computed tomography scan showing hemorrhage (white area) in the putamen. (Reproduced, with permission, from Allan J. Schwartz.)

Pontine hemorrhage, unless quite small, usually causes coma (by disrupting the reticular activating system) and quadriparesis (by transecting the corticospinal tracts). Eye movements, spontaneous or reflex (eg, to ice water in either external auditory canal) are absent, and pupils are pinpoint in size, reflecting transection of descending sympathetic pathways. Pupillary light reactivity is usually preserved, however, for the pathway mediating this reflex, from retina to midbrain, is intact. Respirations may be irregular, presumably because the caudal reticular formation is involved. These strokes are nearly always fatal.

Cerebellar hemorrhage, which tends to occur in the region of the dentate nucleus, typically causes a sudden inability to stand or walk (astasia-abasia), with ipsilateral limb ataxia. There may be ipsilateral abducens palsy, or horizontal gaze palsy, or facial weakness, presumably from pontine compression. Long-tract motor and sensory signs are usually absent, however. As swelling increases, further brain stem damage may cause coma, ophthalmoplegia, miosis, and irregular respiration, with fatal outcome.

The Rupture of Saccular Aneurysms Causes Subarachnoid Hemorrhage

Saccular aneurysms (not to be confused with hypertensive Charcot-Bouchard microaneurysms) are most often found at the junction of the anterior communicating artery with an anterior cerebral artery, the junction of a posterior communicating artery with an internal carotid artery, and the first bifurcation of a middle cerebral artery in the sylvian fissure. Each aneurysm, upon rupture, tends to cause not only sudden severe headache but also a characteristic syndrome. By producing a hematoma directly over the oculomotor nerve as it traverses the base of the brain, a ruptured posterior communicating artery aneurysm often causes ipsilateral pupillary dilation with loss of light reactivity. A middle cerebral artery aneurysm may, by either hematoma or secondary infarction, cause a clinical picture resembling that of middle cerebral artery occlusion. After rupture of an anterior communicating

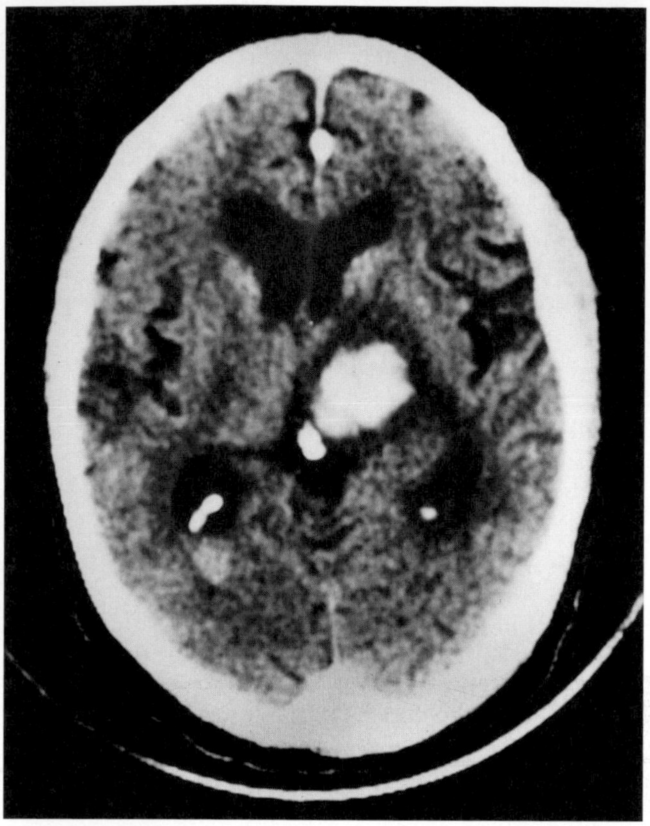

Figure C–12 Computed tomography scan showing thalamic hemorrhage (white area) surrounded by edema or infarction (dark zone). (Reproduced, with permission, from Allan J. Schwartz.)

artery aneurysm, there may be no focal signs but only decreased alertness or behavioral changes.

Posterior fossa aneurysms most often occur at the rostral bifurcation of the basilar artery or at the origin of the posterior inferior cerebellar artery. They cause a variety of cranial nerve and brain stem signs. Rupture of an aneurysm at any site may cause abrupt coma; the reason is uncertain but may be related to sudden increased intracranial pressure and functional disruption of vital pontomedullary structures.

Stroke Alters the Vascular Physiology of the Brain

After a stroke, cerebral blood flow and cerebrovascular responses to changes in blood pressure or arterial gases are altered. There may be vasomotor paralysis with loss of autoregulation in response to blood pressure changes and then blunted responses to alterations in arterial O_2 or CO_2. This kind of physiological abnormality is especially likely in brain areas that are ischemic but not yet infarcted; such an area often surrounds acutely infarcted brain tissue and is called the *ischemic penumbra*. Lowered blood pressure in this setting can, by critically reducing perfusion in the penumbra, convert ischemia to infarction. The use of cerebral vasodilators can also produce an unintended response, increasing cerebral blood flow in regions distant from the ischemic region without affecting vessels within the ischemic region. Blood may therefore be shunted from ischemic to normal brain.

Strategies for restoring cerebral perfusion in patients with acute ischemic stroke (for example, giving recombinant tissue-type plasminogen activator to degrade the clot causing the infarction) are based on the assumption that an ischemic penumbra represents salvageable tissue, even if infarction within it does not.

John C. M. Brust

Selected Readings

Brust JCM. 2010. Cerebral infarction. In: LP Rowland, TA Pedley (eds), *Merritt's Textbook of Neurology*, 12th ed., pp. 268–275, Philadelphia, PA: Lippincott Williams & Wilkins.

Zazulia AR, Markham J, Powers WJ. 2011. Cerebral blood flow and metabolism in human cerebrovascular disease. In: JP Mohr, PA Wolf, JC Grotta, MA Moskowitz, MR Mayberg, R von Kummer (eds), *Stroke: Pathophysiology, Diagnosis and Management*, 5th ed., pp. 44–67, Philadelphia, PA: Elsevier Saunders.

Zivin JA. 2004. Approach to cerebrovascular disease. In: L Goldman, D Ausiello (eds), *Cecil Textbook of Medicine*, 22nd ed., pp. 2280–2287, Philadelphia, PA: Saunders.

Appendix D

The Blood–Brain Barrier, Choroid Plexus, and Cerebrospinal Fluid

To function optimally, neurons of the central nervous system and their supporting glia require a highly specialized environment. The fluids that bathe the central nervous system's interstitial and cerebrospinal compartments are regulated by the blood–brain and blood–cerebrospinal fluid (CSF) barriers. Evidence for these barriers was first obtained in the 19th century when it was observed that acidic vital dyes stain the brain if the dye is injected into the cerebrospinal fluid but not if injected into the blood stream.

The interstitial fluid in the brain and the cerebrospinal fluid in the intraventricular and subarachnoid spaces are separately compartmentalized. Homeostasis of these fluid compartments and ultimately the intracellular compartment of brain cells is regulated to a great degree by the blood–brain and blood–CSF barriers (Figure D–1). Endothelial cells of the cerebral microvasculature form the blood–brain barrier that regulates the movement of molecules between the blood and interstitial fluid compartments. Epithelial cells of the choroid plexus produce the cerebrospinal fluid and regulate its composition.

These barriers exclude toxic substances and protect neurons from circulating neurotransmitters such as norepinephrine and glutamate, the blood levels of which can increase greatly after a meal or in response to stress. The selective exclusion by the blood–brain barrier results primarily from specialized anatomical properties of the endothelial cells that limit the passive diffusion of water-soluble substances from the blood into the interstitial and cerebrospinal fluid compartments. As a result, many metabolites required for brain growth and function must be transported selectively across the brain endothelial and choroid epithelial cell surfaces. Specific transporters deliver energy substrates, essential amino acids, and peptides to the brain and remove metabolites.

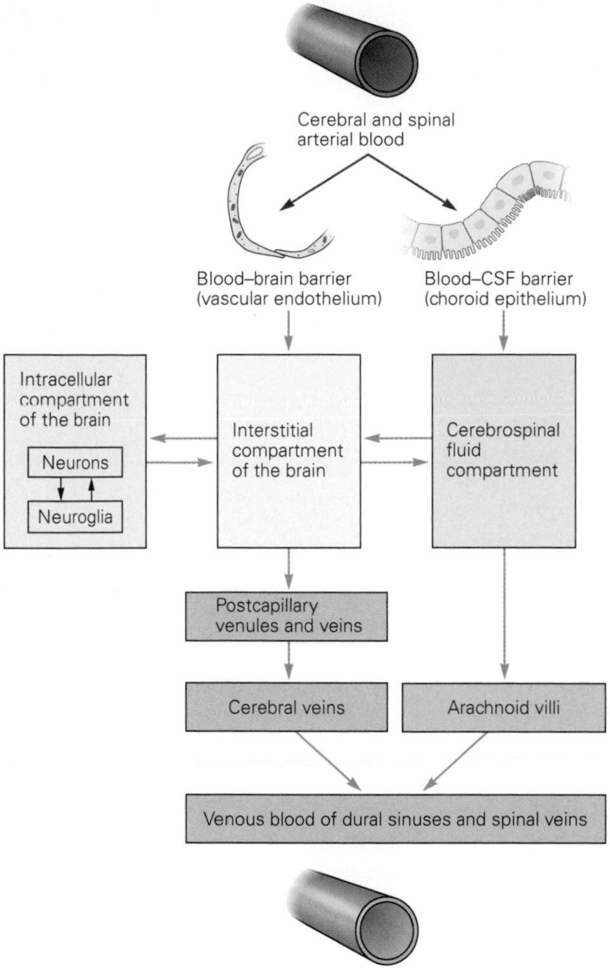

Figure D–1 Relationships between intracranial fluid compartments and the blood–brain and blood–cerebrospinal fluid (CSF) barriers. The tissue elements indicated in parentheses form the barriers. Arrows indicate the direction of fluid flow under normal conditions. (Adapted, with permission, from Carpenter 1978.)

The Blood–Brain Barrier Regulates the Interstitial Fluid in the Brain

Distinctive Properties of the Endothelial Cells of Brain Capillaries Account for the Blood–Brain Barrier

The small blood vessels of the brain are composed primarily of endothelial cells that continuously line the vessel luminal surface. On the abluminal side the endothelial cells are associated with pericytes, smooth muscle-like cells imbedded within the basement membrane of microvessels. Perivascular astrocytes extend processes that ensheathe most of the abluminal microvessel surface to form a microvessel-astroglial complex (Figure D–2). The endothelial cells and their extensive intercellular junctions are the principal component of the barrier (Figure D–3).

In capillaries of peripheral organs and in the relatively few brain capillaries that do not contribute to the barrier (eg, those of the circumventricular organs), blood-borne polar molecules diffuse across vessel walls by multiple mechanisms. This diffusion occurs through spaces between endothelial cells, through specialized cytoplasmic fenestrations, or by fluid-phase or receptor-mediated endocytosis.

Fluid-phase endocytosis is a relatively nonspecific process by which endothelial cells (and most other cells) engulf and then internalize molecules encountered in the extracellular space by vesicular endocytosis. *Receptor-mediated endocytosis* is a specific process in which a ligand binds to a membrane receptor on the external surface of a cell, is internalized by means of clathrin-coated vesicles, and is transported across the cell membrane. Once within the cell the vesicle may traverse the cell, fuse with the cell membrane on the opposite cell surface and release its contents to the extracellular space, or fuse with an intracellular endosome and release its contents.

Endothelial cells of blood–brain barrier vessels are relatively deficient in vesicular transport and they are also nonfenestrated. Instead they are interconnected by complex arrays of tight junctions (Figure D–3B), which block diffusion across vessel walls. All generic endothelial cells are interconnected by a modest number of tight junctional complexes and normally have low transendothelial resistance (5–10 ohm-cm^2). In the vessels of the blood–brain barrier, however, extensive arrays of tight junctions generate high transendothelial resistance (2,000 ohm-cm^2), excluding particles as small as K^+ ions (Figure D–4).

Tight Junctions Are a Major Feature of the Anatomical Blood–Brain Barrier Composition and Structure

Tight junctions of the blood–brain barrier are composed of three principal transmembranous proteins—claudins, occludins, and junctional adhesion molecules—as well as numerous cytoplasmic accessory proteins (Figure D–5).

Claudin (~22 kDa) has four transmembrane domains and forms the backbone of tight junctional complexes. Of the more than 20 members of the claudin gene family, isoforms 1 and 5 are expressed at the junctions of the blood–brain barrier. Occludin (~65 kDa) is a tight junctional protein, also has four transmembrane domains, and is recruited to junctional complexes by claudins. Claudins and occludins interact intimately at the junctional membrane to influence junctional complexity and tightness. Junctional adhesion molecules (JAMs) are located lateral to the claudins and occludins and mediate cell-cell adhesive interactions required for junctional assembly. JAMs also play an important role in the transmigration of inflammatory cells across barrier endothelial cells.

Numerous accessory proteins positioned on the cytoplasmic side of tight junctions mediate interactions between the transmembrane junctional and cytoskeletal proteins and modulate dynamic junctional properties. The zona occludin proteins link the occludins and claudins to the actin cytoskeleton (Figure D–5). They also form a scaffold for other regulatory proteins such as cingulin, a myosin-like protein, and AF-6, a target of the small G protein Ras. It is currently believed that changes in protein-protein interactions at the cytoplasmic junctional–cytoskeletal interface, resulting from gene transcription and protein phosphorylation events, modulate tight junction structure and function.

The Blood–Brain Barrier Is Permeable in Three Ways

Normal development and brain function require many substances that must cross brain microvessels. Entry into the brain is achieved primarily in three ways: (1) by diffusion of lipid soluble substances, (2) by facilitative and energy-dependent receptor-mediated transport of specific water-soluble substances, and (3) by ion channels.

Diffusion of Lipid-Soluble Substances

The brain is separated from the blood only by the large surface of endothelial cell membrane (approximately 180 cm^2/g in gray matter). This membrane permits the efficient exchange of lipid-soluble gases such as oxygen (O_2) and carbon dioxide (CO_2), an exchange limited only by the surface area of the blood vessels and by cerebral blood flow. Barrier vessels are impermeable to molecules with poor lipid-solubility such as mannitol. The permeability coefficient of the blood–brain barrier for many substances is directly proportional to the lipid-solubility of the substance as measured by the oil–water partition coefficient (Figure D–6).

An example of the relationship of permeability and lipid-solubility is the correlation between the relative abuse potential of psychoactive drugs such as nicotine and heroin and their lipid-solubility. Increasing the lipid-solubility of drugs enhances their delivery to the brain. Drugs with great lipid-solubility, however, are poorly soluble in blood and bind to serum albumin

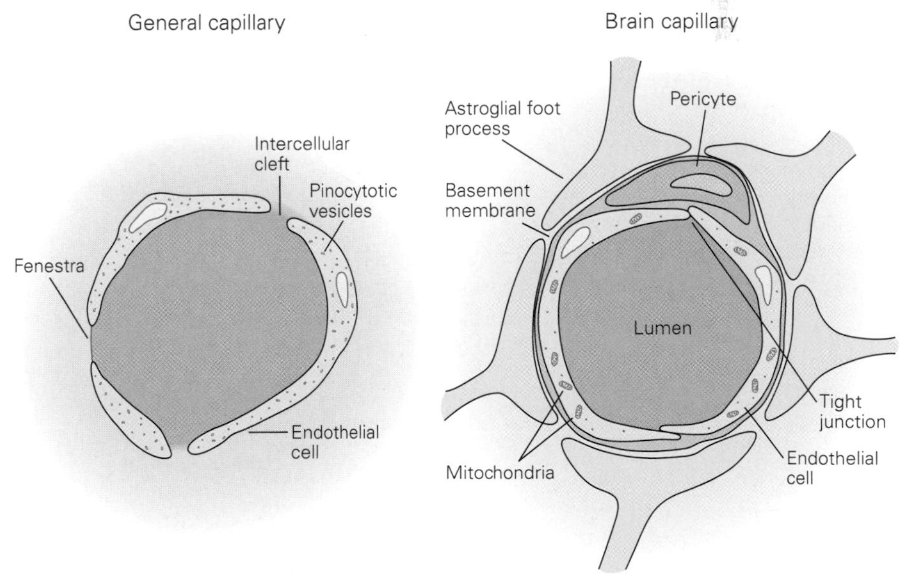

Figure D–2 **Ultrastructural features of endothelial cells of brain capillaries and general (systemic) capillaries.** The endothelial cells of brain barrier capillaries are relatively lacking in pinocytotic vesicles, contain an increased number of mitochondria to support energy-dependent transport properties, and are interconnected by very complex interendothelial tight junctions (see Figure D–5). These anatomical features in conjunction with specific transport systems (see Figure D–7) result in highly selective transport of water-soluble compounds across the barrier endothelium. Astroglial foot processes almost completely surround the brain capillaries and are thus believed to influence barrier-specific endothelial differentiation. In contrast, systemic capillaries have interendothelial clefts, fenestrae, and prominent pinocytotic vesicles. These features of systemic capillaries allow relatively nonselective diffusion across the capillary wall. (Reproduced, with permission, from Goldstein and Betz 1986.)

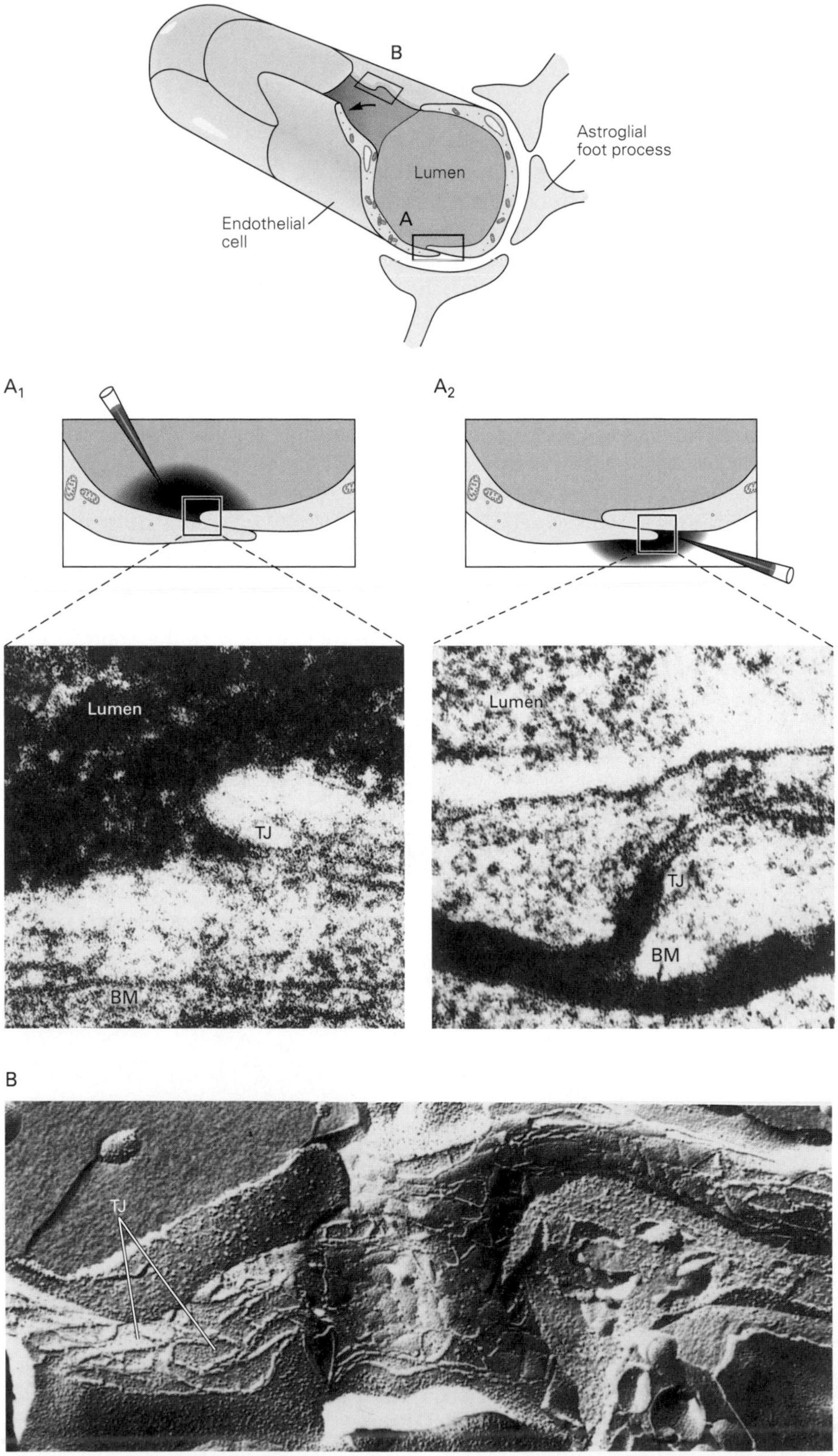

Figure D–3 Tight junctions between endothelial cells are the basis of the anatomical blood–brain barrier.

A. 1. When injected into arteries that supply the brain, the electron-dense tracer horseradish peroxidase is easily visualized within the brain vessel lumens (**dark staining at top**) but is excluded from entering the brain by interendothelial tight junctions (**TJ**). The luminal space appears at the top of the electron micrographs in both 1 and 2. (Reproduced, with permission, from Reese and Karnovsky 1967.) **2.** When injected into the subarachnoid space, horseradish peroxidase readily diffuses between the perivascular astroglial foot processes and across the abluminal basement membrane (**BM**) but fails to penetrate the interendothelial tight junction. (Reproduced, with permission, from Brightman and Reese 1969.)

B. This freeze-fracture photomicrograph of isolated brain microvessels shows complex arrays of interendothelial tight junctions (**TJ**). (Reproduced, with permission, from Shivers et al. 1984.)

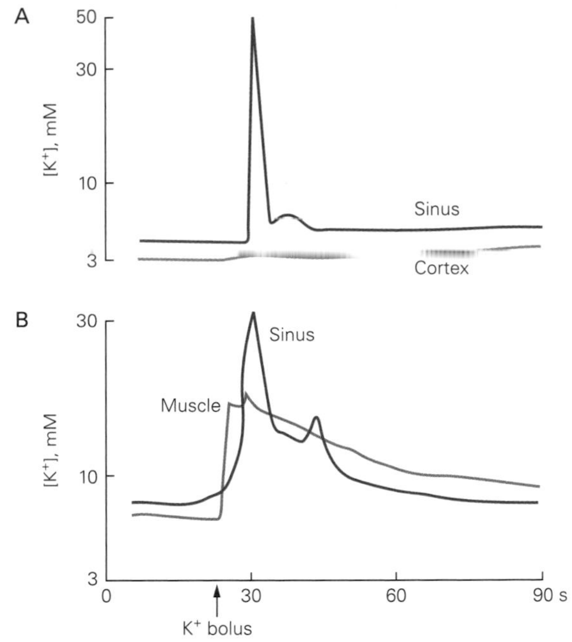

Figure D–4 **Time course of K^+ entry into tissue extracellular fluid following arterial injection.** The time course of K^+ entry into the cerebral cortex and neck muscle is compared to the cerebral venous outflow in the sagittal sinus following bolus injection of potassium chloride (**KCl**) in the aortic arch.

A. In the cerebral cortex the K^+ concentration remains essentially unchanged because of the blood–brain barrier to ions.

B. In the neck muscle K^+ diffuses rapidly across nonbarrier vessels into the extracellular space of the muscle. (Reproduced, with permission, from Hansen et al. 1977.)

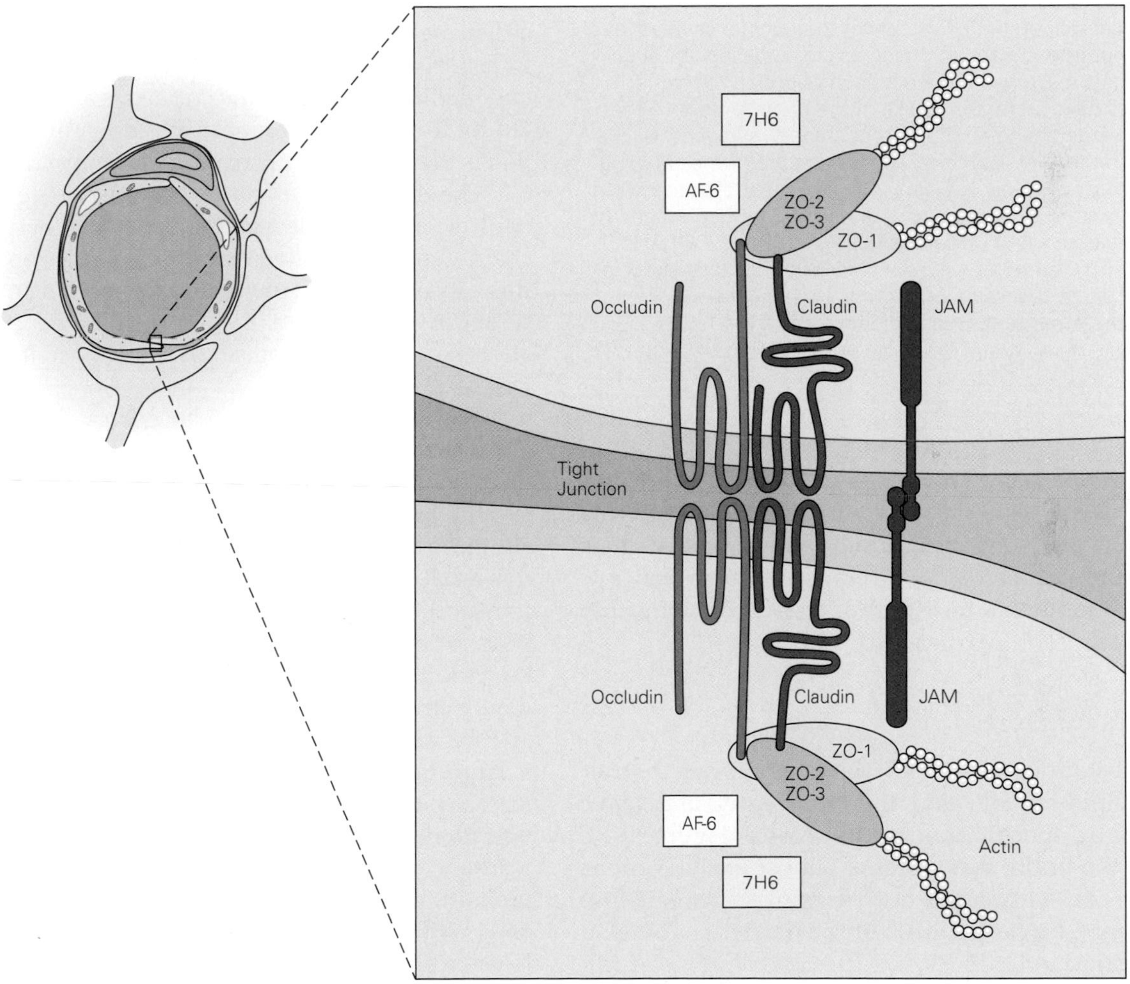

Figure D–5 **Protein interactions at the tight junctions between barrier endothelial cells.** Occludin, claudin, and junctional adhesion molecules (**JAM**) are membrane-spanning junctional proteins. Claudins on adjacent endothelial cells bind homotypically and mediate interendothelial adhesive interactions. Occludins interact with claudins to enhance and modulate interendothelial permeability. JAMs localize to the periphery of junctional complexes and mediate inflammatory cell transmigration across barrier endothelial cells. The cytoplasmic accessory proteins represented by zona occludins (**ZO-1**, **ZO-2**, and **ZO-3**), **AF-6**, and **7H6**, regulate the interaction of junctions with cytoskeletal components and modulate junction function via interactions with signal transduction proteins in the membrane and cytoplasm. (Adapted, with permission, from Huber et al. 2001.)

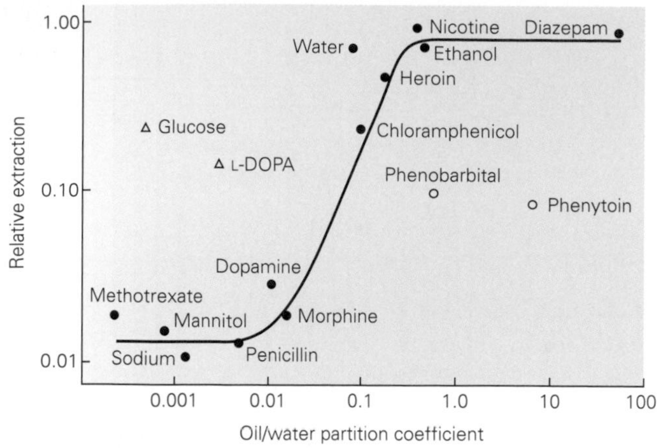

Figure D–6 The oil–water partition coefficient correlates with brain uptake of many compounds. The coefficient is an index of lipid solubility. Brain uptake of a substance is determined by comparing the extraction of the substance relative to a highly permeable tracer during a single passage through the cerebral circulation. In general, compounds with higher coefficients have a greater uptake in the brain. Uptake of the anticonvulsants phenobarbital and phenytoin is lower than predicted from their lipid-solubility partly because of their binding to plasma proteins. This explains why the onset of anticonvulsant activity from these agents is slower than that of diazepam. Uptake of glucose and L-dihydroxyphenylalanine (L-DOPA) is greater than indicated by their lipid solubility because specific carriers facilitate their transport into the brain capillary. (Reproduced, with permission, from Goldstein and Betz 1986.)

protein, properties that reduce delivery to the brain. Lipid-solubility is not an accurate indicator of the permeability of some hydrophilic substances, such as glucose and vinca alkaloids, because of the presence of selective endothelial transport or enzyme systems that increase or inhibit permeability.

Facilitative and Energy-Dependent Transport

Most substances that cross the blood–brain barrier are not lipid-soluble and therefore enter and leave the brain by specific transport systems (Figure D–7). Because the brain uses glucose almost exclusively as its source of energy, the hexose transporter (glucose transporter isotype-1, Glut1) of the barrier endothelial cells is abundant.

Like other transporters Glut1 consists of 12-transmembrane segments. It is a facilitative, saturable, and stereospecific transporter that functions at both the luminal and abluminal endothelial cell membranes. Because it is not energy-dependent, it cannot move glucose against a concentration gradient. In fact, the net flux of glucose is driven by the higher concentration of glucose in the plasma. More than 99% of the glucose that enters barrier endothelial cells is shuttled across for use by neurons and glia.

Monocarboxylic acids such as β-hydroxybutyrate serve as the brain's primary energy source during early development in suckling neonates and in response to starvation in mature animals. These acids are transported across the barrier endothelial cells by the monocarboxylic acid transporter-1 (MCT1).

Amino acids are transported across barrier endothelial cells primarily by three distinct carrier systems. These systems (L, A, and ASC) were initially characterized by their different patterns and mechanisms of transport, and by their preference for different amino acid analogs. The *L-system* preferentially transports large neutral amino acids with branched or ringed side chains such as leucine and valine. This Na^+-independent, facilitative transport system is located at luminal and abluminal endothelial cell membranes. It also transports L-DOPA L-dihydroxyphenylalanine), the dopamine precursor that is the mainstay for treating Parkinson disease.

The *A-system* preferentially transports glycine and neutral amino acids with short linear or polar side chains, such as alanine or serine. Unlike the L-system this carrier is Na^+-dependent, and pumps amino acids down a Na^+ gradient that is maintained by Na^+-K^+-adenosine triphosphatase (ATPase), an ionic pump that uses ATP.

The *ASC-system* is also an energy-dependent and Na^+-dependent transporter that preferentially recognizes alanine, serine, and cysteine. A-system and ASC-system expression and function are localized at the abluminal endothelial cell surface. As a consequence of this localization these carriers are the primary means of transport of small neutral amino acids out of brain up a concentration gradient.

Another transport system found to be most abundant in brain barrier microvessels belongs to a family of ATP-binding cassette transporters (ABC transporters), a large family of transmembrane proteins expressed in many cell types. The first member of this family was identified for the ability to impart multiple drug resistance (MDR) to tumor cells. The MDR transporter limits the entry into cells of a wide range of natural and synthetic hydrophobic toxins (eg, vinca alkaloids, actinomycin-D) and therapeutic compounds (eg, cyclosporin). The ability of MDR transporters to pump certain steroid hormones suggests a physiologic role. MDR transporters are expressed by barrier endothelial cells but not by endothelial cells of most other tissues. This explains why MDR substrates do not readily cross the blood–brain barrier. Mice genetically engineered to lack MDR1a gene expression are much more sensitive than wild-type controls to centrally acting toxic compounds, indicating that MDR gene expression at the blood–brain barrier protects the brain from circulating neurotoxins.

Ion Channels and Exchangers

Specific ion channels and ion transporters mediate electrolyte movement across the blood–brain barrier. A nonselective luminal ion channel that is inhibited by both amiloride and atrial natriuretic peptide has been revealed in both in vivo studies of transport across brain microvessels and patch-clamp studies of cultured brain endothelial cells. Na^+/H^+ and Cl^-/bicarbonate (HCO_3^-) exchangers also appear to function at the luminal membrane.

The abluminal membrane of brain endothelial cells has a relatively high concentration of Na^+-K^+-ATPase that pumps K^+ from the interstitial fluid into the endothelial cell and pumps Na^+ out of the cell. This ion exchange uses ATP energy. In conjunction with K^+ channels in astrocytes, this abluminal endothelial pump may play an important role in removing extracellular K^+ released during neuronal activity (see Chapter 6).

Endothelial Enzyme Systems Form a Metabolic Blood–Brain Barrier

Transport systems and carriers are not the only mechanisms for regulating the composition of the interstitial fluid. Certain enzyme systems specific to the blood–brain barrier are also important. The first recognized and best characterized is the barrier to L-DOPA.

Plasma L-DOPA enters brain endothelial cells by means of the L-system amino acid transporter. The relatively large amounts of DOPA decarboxylase and monoamine oxidase in barrier endothelial cells rapidly metabolize L-DOPA to 3,4-dihydroxyphenylacetic acid, thereby inhibiting the entry of L-DOPA to brain

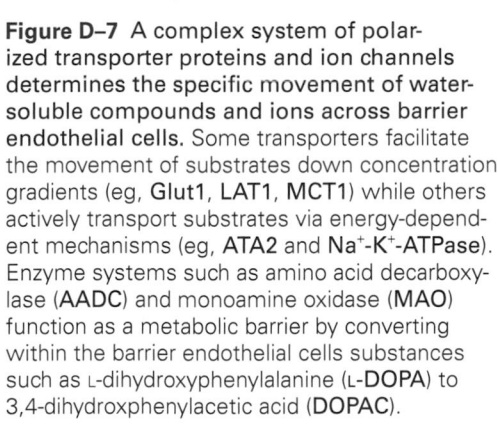

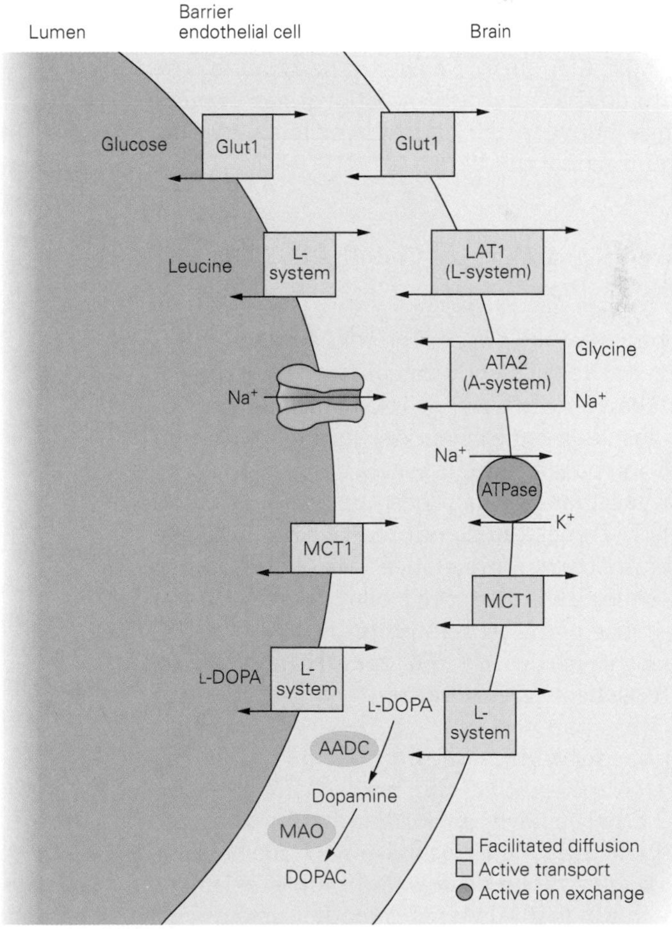

Figure D–7 A complex system of polarized transporter proteins and ion channels determines the specific movement of water-soluble compounds and ions across barrier endothelial cells. Some transporters facilitate the movement of substrates down concentration gradients (eg, **Glut1**, **LAT1**, **MCT1**) while others actively transport substrates via energy-dependent mechanisms (eg, **ATA2** and **Na^+-K^+-ATPase**). Enzyme systems such as amino acid decarboxylase (**AADC**) and monoamine oxidase (**MAO**) function as a metabolic barrier by converting within the barrier endothelial cells substances such as L-dihydroxyphenylalanine (**L-DOPA**) to 3,4-dihydroxphenylacetic acid (**DOPAC**).

(Figure D–7). This explains why effective therapy for Parkinson disease requires that L-DOPA be given together with an inhibitor of DOPA decarboxylase.

Other blood-borne amines, including catecholamines, are inactivated by monoamine oxidases of the barrier endothelium. Another barrier enzyme, γ-glutamyl transpeptidase, detoxifies glutathione-bound compounds and vasoactive leukotrienes.

Some Areas of the Brain Lack a Blood–Brain Barrier

Not all cerebral blood vessels are impermeable. Leaky structures include the posterior pituitary and the circumventricular organs: the area postrema, subfornical organ, laminar terminalis, subcommissural organ, and median eminence.

The absence of the blood–brain barrier in these regions is consistent with their physiologic functions. Neurosecretory products of the posterior pituitary have to pass efficiently across endothelial cells into the circulation. The subfornical organ is a chemoreceptor-rich area that monitors the blood level of angiotensin II to regulate water balance and other homeostatic functions.

These regions are isolated from the rest of the brain by specialized ependymal cells called *tanycytes* located along the ventricular surface close to the midline. The tanycytes are coupled by tight junctions and prevent free exchange between the circumventricular organs and the cerebrospinal fluid.

Brain-Derived Signals Induce Endothelial Cells to Express a Blood–Brain Barrier

The developing brain expresses the cellular and molecular signals that induce endothelial expression of the blood–brain barrier phenotype. The neural anlagen of the brain is vascularized early in development through the invasion of proliferating vessels derived from an extraneural vascular plexus. These perineural vessels are composed of fenestrated endothelial cells that have no blood–brain barrier properties. The fenestrations are lost soon after the endothelial cells penetrate neural tissue. The subsequent expression of different blood–brain barrier properties on the endothelium occurs gradually, consistent with a maturational cascade.

The brain parenchymal signals that induce endothelial barrier formation are not known. Of the principal cell types within the brain, astrocytes are thought to be particularly important for this function because of their intimate association with the abluminal surface of brain blood vessels and from experimental evidence in blood–brain barrier model systems.

Diseases Can Alter the Blood–Brain Barrier

A variety of pathological situations are associated with altered blood–brain barrier function. Many brain tumors, especially highly malignant ones, contain vessels with poorly developed blood–brain barriers. Such vessels are excessively leaky and lack the differentiated transport properties of normal blood–brain barrier vessels. The abnormal permeability accounts for the accumulation of interstitial fluid (ie, vasogenic edema) commonly associated with brain tumors. The abnormal properties of tumor endothelial cells are presumably due to either the absence of normal interactions between astrocytes and capillaries or by the secretion of growth factors and cytokines by tumor cells. Factors secreted by tumors that enhance vessel proliferation and permeability include vascular endothelial growth factor (VEGF), hepatocyte growth factor/scatter factor (HGF/SF), and matrix metalloproteinases.

The blood–brain barrier is also altered in bacterial meningitis. The barrier is normally impermeable to antibiotics such as penicillin. Bacterial meningitis, abscesses, and their associated inflammatory responses cause partial breakdown of the blood–brain barrier. This barrier response appears to be mediated in part by the accumulation of vasoactive eicosanoids; inflammatory cytokines such as tumor necrosis factor, interleukins, and macrophage chemoattractant protein-1; and matrix metalloproteinases that degrade capillary basement membranes. This barrier dysfunction accounts for many adverse neurological effects of meningitis but it also enhances the delivery of antibiotics that inefficiently penetrate across an intact barrier.

Because development and function of the normal brain are closely linked to specific anatomical, biochemical, and transport properties of the blood–brain barrier, specific defects in genes that code for barrier endothelial proteins might account for inherited brain disorders. The first disorder of blood–brain barrier transport to be recognized involves insufficient endothelial transport of glucose because of sporadic mutations in the *glut1* gene causing Glut1 haploinsufficiency. Patients with this syndrome are normal at birth but soon develop poorly controlled seizures, diminished brain growth, and mental retardation in association with a substantially diminished concentration of cerebrospinal fluid glucose.

Cerebrospinal Fluid Is Secreted by the Choroid Plexuses

Cerebrospinal fluid is secreted in the cerebral ventricles mainly by the choroid plexuses (Figure D–8A),

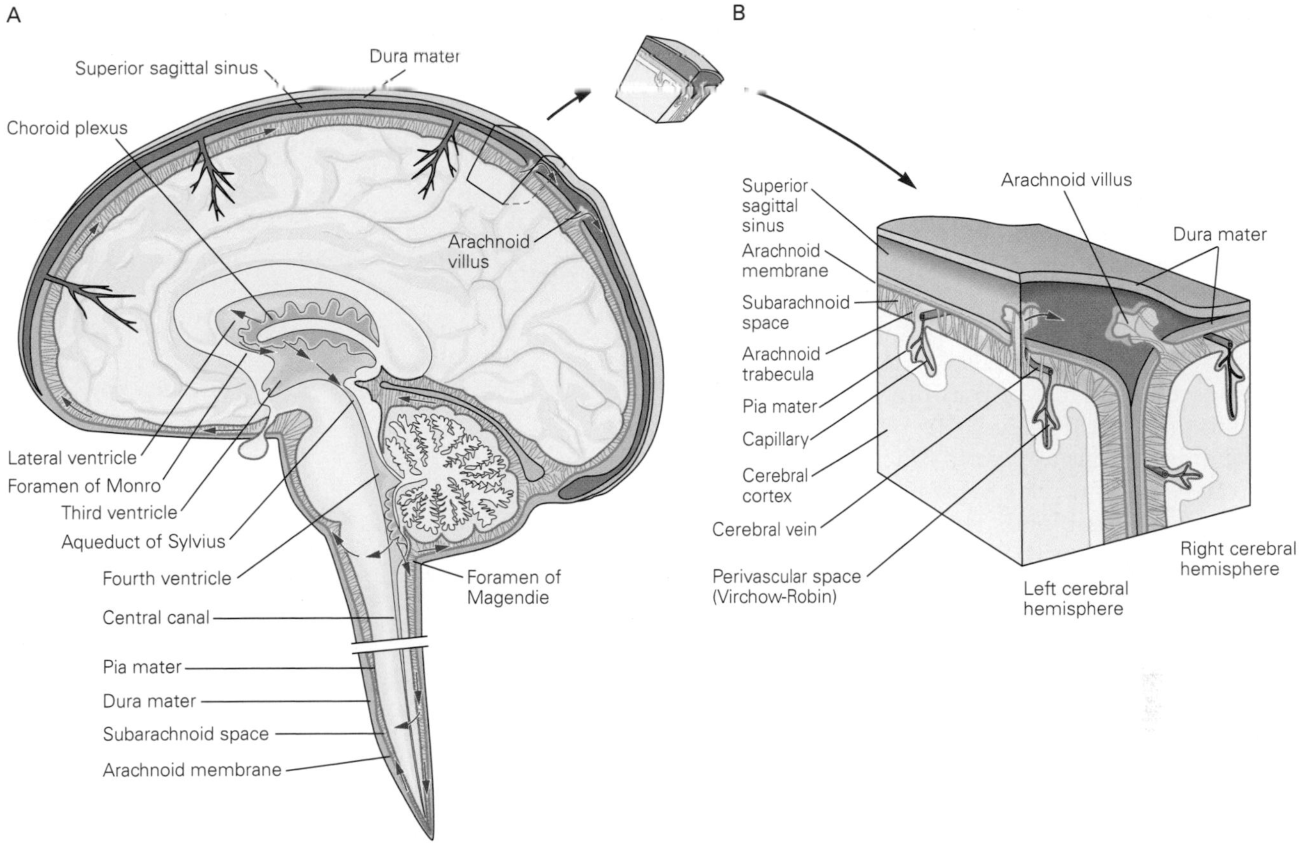

Figure D–8 Distribution of cerebrospinal fluid.

A. Sites of formation, circulation, and absorption of cerebrospinal fluid (CSF). All spaces containing CSF communicate with each other. Choroidal and extrachoroidal sources of the fluid exist within the ventricular system, which is lined by permeable ependymal cells. The CSF circulates to the subarachnoid space and is absorbed into the venous system via the arachnoid villi. Arachnoid villi adjacent to the spinal roots supplement the absorption into the intracranial venous sinuses. (Adapted, with permission, from Fishman 1992.)

B. The subarachnoid space is bounded externally by the arachnoid membrane and internally by the pia mater, which penetrates the surface of the brain along with blood vessels to form Virchow-Robin spaces. (Adapted, with permission, from Carpenter 1978.)

capillary networks that are surrounded by cuboidal or columnar epithelium. The CSF flows from the lateral ventricles through the interventricular foramina of Monro into the third ventricle. From there it flows into the fourth ventricle through the cerebral aqueduct of Sylvius and then through the foramina of Magendie and Luschka into the subarachnoid space. The subarachnoid space lies between the arachnoid and the pia mater, which, together with the dura mater, form the three meningeal layers that cover the brain (Figure D–8B). Within the subarachnoid space, fluid flows down the spinal canal and also upward back over the convexity of the brain (Figure D–8A).

The CSF flowing over the brain extends into the sulci and the depths of the cerebral cortex in extensions of the subarachnoid space along blood vessels called the Virchow-Robin spaces. Small solutes diffuse freely between the interstitial fluid and the CSF in these perivascular spaces and across the ependymal lining of the ventricular system, facilitating the movement of metabolites from deep within the hemispheres to cortical subarachnoid spaces and the ventricular system. This flow of interstitial fluid across the ependymal surface into the ventricular system (extrachoroidal cerebrospinal fluid production) is believed to account for at most a small percentage of total CSF production.

The total volume of CSF is estimated to be approximately 140 mL. Under normal conditions the lateral and third ventricles contain approximately 12 mL and the spinal subarachnoid space approximately 30 mL as measured by computed tomography. The remaining 100 mL is in the subarachnoid space and the major cisterns of the brain (eg, cisterna magna, mesencephalic cistern).

The CSF is absorbed through the arachnoid granulations and villi. Arachnoid granulations consist of clusters of villi that typically form visible herniations of the arachnoid membrane through the dura and into the lumen of the superior sagittal sinus and other venous structures (Figure D–8). The villi themselves are visible microscopically and positioned between the CSF and venous blood. Cells of the villus membrane contain vacuoles that transport fluid from one side of the cell to the other (Figure D–9).

The granulations appear to function as valves that allow one-way flow of CSF from the subarachnoid spaces into venous blood. This one-way flow of CSF is sometimes called bulk flow because all constituents of CSF leave with the fluid, including small molecules, proteins, microorganisms, and red blood cells. The rate of formation of CSF in adults is 0.35 mL per minute or approximately 500 mL per day, so that the entire volume of CSF is turned over three or four times a day.

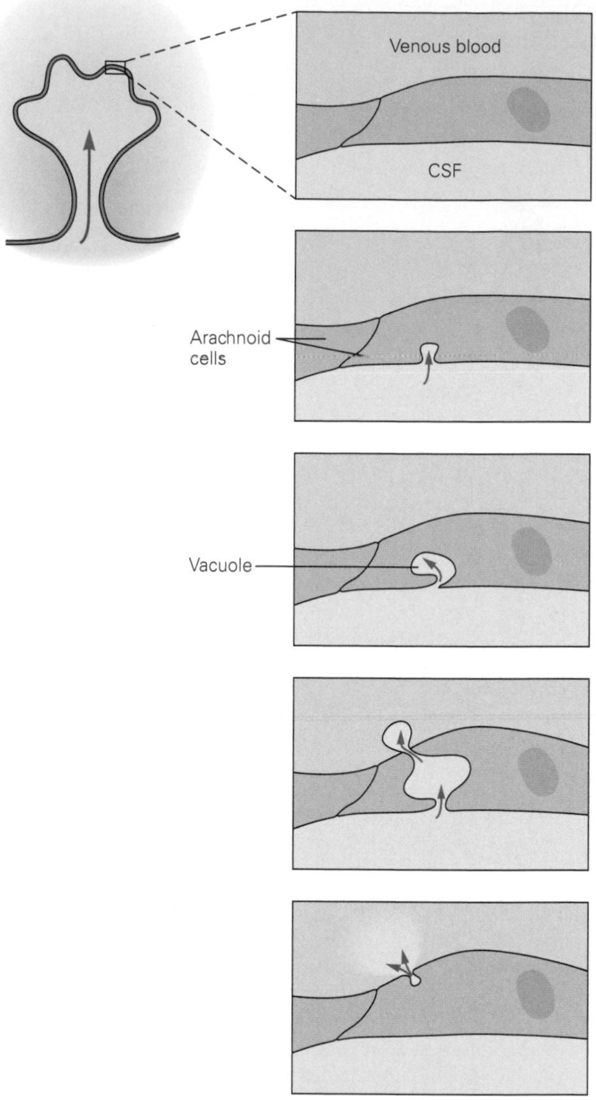

Figure D–9 Transport of cerebrospinal fluid within the arachnoid villi is achieved by giant vacuoles in the arachnoid cells. This mechanism could account for the one-way bulk flow of CSF from the subarachnoid space to the venous system. Some vacuoles are large enough to encompass red blood cells. (Adapted, with permission, from Fishman 1992.)

Cerebrospinal Fluid Has Several Functions

The CSF communicates with brain interstitial fluid and therefore helps maintain a constant extracellular environment for neurons and glia. The one-way flow of CSF from the ventricular system into the subarachnoid space and into the venous sinuses is a major route for removing potentially harmful brain metabolites.

The CSF also provides a mechanical cushion to protect the brain from impact with the bony calvarium when the head moves. By its buoyant action the CSF allows the brain (average weight 1400 g) to float, thereby reducing its effective weight in situ to less than 50 g.

The CSF may also serve as a lymphatic system for the brain and as a conduit for polypeptides that are secreted by hypothalamic neurons and act at remote sites in the brain. The pH of CSF affects both pulmonary ventilation and cerebral blood flow, another example of the homeostatic role of CSF.

Epithelial Cells of the Choroid Plexuses Account for the Blood–Cerebral Spinal Fluid Barrier

The choroid plexuses are structurally similar to the distal and collecting tubules of the kidney, using capillary filtration and epithelial secretory mechanisms to maintain the chemical stability of the CSF. The capillaries that traverse the choroid plexuses are freely permeable to plasma solutes. A barrier exists, however, at the choroid epithelial cells. The transport and exchange of substances by the choroid plexuses are bidirectional, accounting for both continuous production of CSF and active transport of metabolites out of the central nervous system into the blood (Figure D–10).

The cerebrospinal and extracellular fluids of the brain are in a steady state under normal physiological circumstances. The concentrations of K^+, Ca^{2+}, bicarbonate, and glucose in the CSF are lower than in blood plasma, and CSF is also more acidic (Table D–1). These differences are a result of regulation of the constituents of CSF by active transport at the choroid plexus epithelium. Under normal conditions blood plasma and CSF are in osmotic equilibrium, because water follows the osmotic gradient that is created by active transport of solutes.

Choroid Plexuses Nurture the Developing Brain

The choroid plexuses appear as epithelial invaginations soon after neural tube closure where the lateral, third, and fourth ventricles will eventually form. They become vascularized and begin producing CSF before the brain becomes well vascularized. The ultimate vascularity of the choroid plexuses is high. In the mature rat blood flow per gram of tissue is as much as fivefold higher in the choroid plexus than in cerebral cortex.

Production of CSF during early brain development is believed to have multiple functions. The hydrodynamic and pressure effects of CSF production may specifically influence the developing brain's three-dimensional shape and laminar organization. The CSF may be a source of nutrition for the developing prevascularized brain, as the choroid epithelial cells deliver substances from blood to the CSF for the developing brain. Initially this blood-to-CSF transfer occurs relatively nonspecifically through a transcellular tubular-cisternal endoplasmic reticular system. It becomes more selective as the choroid epithelial cells differentiate to create a mature blood–CSF barrier. The choroid epithelial cells also synthesize and secrete proteins that may have paracrine effects on the development of neighboring neuroepithelial cells.

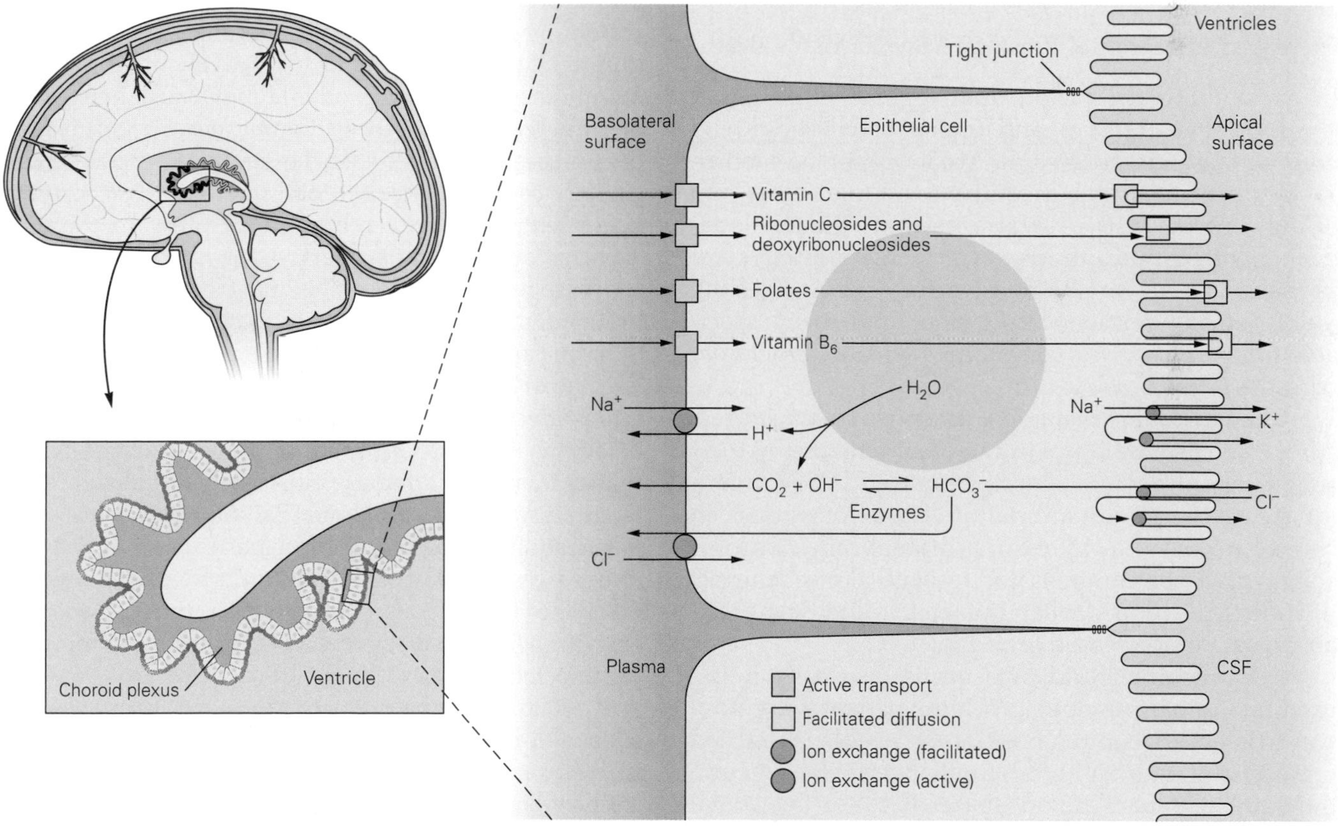

Figure D–10 The blood–cerebral spinal fluid barrier. The flow of molecules across the blood–CSF barrier is regulated by several mechanisms in the epithelial cells of the choroid plexus. Some micronutrients such as vitamin C are transported into epithelial cells by an energy-dependent active transporter located at the basolateral membrane and released into the CSF at the apical surface by facilitated diffusion, which requires no energy. Essential ions are also exchanged between CSF and blood plasma. Transport of an ion in one direction is linked to the transport of a different ion in the opposite direction, as in the exchange of Na^+ ions for K^+ ions. (Adapted, with permission, from Spector and Johanson 1989.)

Table D–1 Comparison of Serum and Cerebrospinal Fluid

	CSF*	Serum*
Water content (%)	99	93
Protein (mg/dL)	35	7000
Glucose (mg/dL)	60	90
Osmolarity (mOsm/L)	295	295
Na^+ (mEq/L)	138	138
K^+ (mEq/L)	2.8	4.5
Ca^{2+} (mEq/L)	2.1	4.8
Mg^{2+} (mEq/L)	0.3	1.7
Cl^- (mEq/L)	119	102
pH	7.33	7.41

*Average or representative values.
(Reproduced, with permission, from Fishman 1992.)

Increased Intracranial Pressure May Harm the Brain

In considering the factors that regulate intracranial pressure, the cranium and spinal canal should be regarded as a closed system. According to the Monro-Kellie doctrine, an increase in the volume of any one of the contents of the calvarium—brain tissue, blood, CSF, or other brain fluids—will increase intracranial pressure because the bony calvarium rigidly fixes the total cranial volume. Mass lesions and their associated interstitial edema commonly increase intracranial pressure.

Changes in arterial and intracranial venous pressures may also influence intracranial pressure by their actions on intracranial blood volume and CSF dynamics. Acute changes in arterial or venous pressures can change intracranial pressure dramatically. Chronic changes may be compensated by several mechanisms, including venous collateralization and increased absorption or decreased formation of CSF.

Cerebrospinal fluid pressure is ordinarily measured by lumbar puncture. With the patient lying sideways (lateral decubitus position), a needle is inserted between the fourth and fifth lumbar vertebrae and into the lumbar subarachnoid space. Because the spinal cord extends only to the first lumbar vertebra, there is no risk of injuring the spinal cord. When the CSF flows freely through the needle, the hub of the needle is attached to a manometer, and the fluid is allowed to rise. The normal pressure is 65 to 195 mm CSF (or water), or 5 to 15 mm Hg.

In using the lumbar CSF pressure as a guide to intracranial pressure, it is assumed that pressures are equal throughout the neuraxis. Normally this is reasonable; but in many diseases (eg, brain tumor or obstruction of CSF pathways) this may not be true. For this reason, and also because the lumbar needle cannot be left in place for prolonged periods, catheters are sometimes inserted into the lateral ventricles to measure pressure there (Figure D–11).

Equally effective are pressure-sensitive transducers that can be inserted under the skull in the epidural or subarachnoid space for continuous monitoring of intracranial pressure. Continuous monitoring has the advantage of identifying waves of transiently elevated intracranial pressure that can occur in certain disorders, such as normal pressure hydrocephalus.

Brain Edema Is an Increase in Brain Volume Because of Increased Water Content

Brain edema may be local (eg, from a surrounding contusion, infarct, or tumor) or generalized. The brain is divided into compartments by relatively noncompliant membranes. Local brain edema may cause herniation of brain tissue across these membranes. Specific examples include herniation of the cingulate gyrus across the falx cerebri, temporal lobe uncus across the cerebellar tentorium, or cerebral cortex outward through calvarial defects after surgery.

Vasogenic edema is the most common form of brain edema. It is attributed to increased permeability of brain capillary endothelial cells, which increases the volume of the extracellular fluid. White matter is generally affected more than gray because of the tendency of edema fluid to accumulate along tracts of white matter. Vasogenic edema is most easily visualized using magnetic resonance imaging. Pathological increases in permeability of the blood–brain barrier also can be visualized by computerized tomography and magnetic resonance imaging after intravenous administration of contrast agents that selectively enter the brain through the affected vessels

Cytotoxic edema refers to the intracellular swelling of injured neurons, glia, and endothelial cells. It occurs in hypoxia from asphyxia or global cerebral ischemia after cardiac arrest because failure of the ATP-dependent Na^+-K^+ pump allows Na^+, and therefore water, to accumulate within cells. Another cause of cytotoxic edema is water intoxication, a consequence of the acute systemic hypo-osmolarity caused by drinking excessive amounts of water or administration of hypotonic intravenous fluids. Acute hyponatremia, which can be induced for example by inappropriate secretion of antidiuretic hormone or renal salt-wasting from secretion of atrial natriuretic hormone, can cause cellular swelling and brain edema. Under these circumstances water moves from extracellular to intracellular sites. Cytotoxic edema may also accompany vasogenic edema in encephalitis, trauma, and stroke.

A family of water channels, the aquaporins, regulate fluid homeostasis in the brain and other organs by facilitating the movement of water through cellular membranes. The 11 known aquaporins (AQP0 to AQP10) consist of two tandem repeats of three transmembrane α-helixes and two connecting loops, each containing an asparagine-proline-alanine motif, that form a membrane pore of 3–6 Å diameter (Figure D–12).

Six family members (AQP1, AQP3, AQP4, AQP5, AQP8, AQP9) exist in the rodent brain. The AQP4 protein is produced by ependymal cells and astrocytes but not neurons. It appears in the endothelial cells and perivascular processes of astrocytes concurrent with the development of the blood–brain barrier; expression is altered in disorders producing blood–brain barrier dysfunction and cerebral edema. The AQP4 and AQP9 channels are found in astrocyte processes in periventricular regions and in the glia limitans bordering the subarachnoid space and thus may have a role in facilitating movement of water between CSF and brain parenchyma. The AQP1 channel appears to transport water at the choroid plexus during CSF formation.

Hydrocephalus Is an Increase in Volume of the Cerebral Ventricles

Hydrocephalus has three possible causes: oversecretion of cerebrospinal fluid, impaired absorption of CSF, or obstruction of CSF pathways. Oversecretion of CSF is rare but is thought to occur in some functioning tumors of the choroid plexus (papilloma) because removal of the tumor may relieve the hydrocephalus. These tumors are associated with subarachnoid hemorrhage and high CSF protein content, which could also impair the absorption of CSF.

Impaired absorption of CSF may result from any condition that raises intracranial pressure, such as thrombosis of cerebral veins or sinuses. Impaired CSF absorption at the arachnoid villi is a common cause of communicating hydrocephalus (enlargement of the entire ventricular system without obstruction of CSF flow) following subarachnoid hemorrhage, trauma, or bacterial meningitis.

Impaired CSF absorption is also believed to be the cause of normal-pressure hydrocephalus, which is characterized by dementia, urinary incontinence, and a disorder of gait called *apraxia*. Brain imaging reveals communicating hydrocephalus, and routine lumbar puncture typically shows normal intracranial pressure. However, continuous intracranial pressure monitoring reveals episodic elevations in intracranial pressure, suggesting that intermittent intracranial hypertension causes the condition. The clinical symptoms are

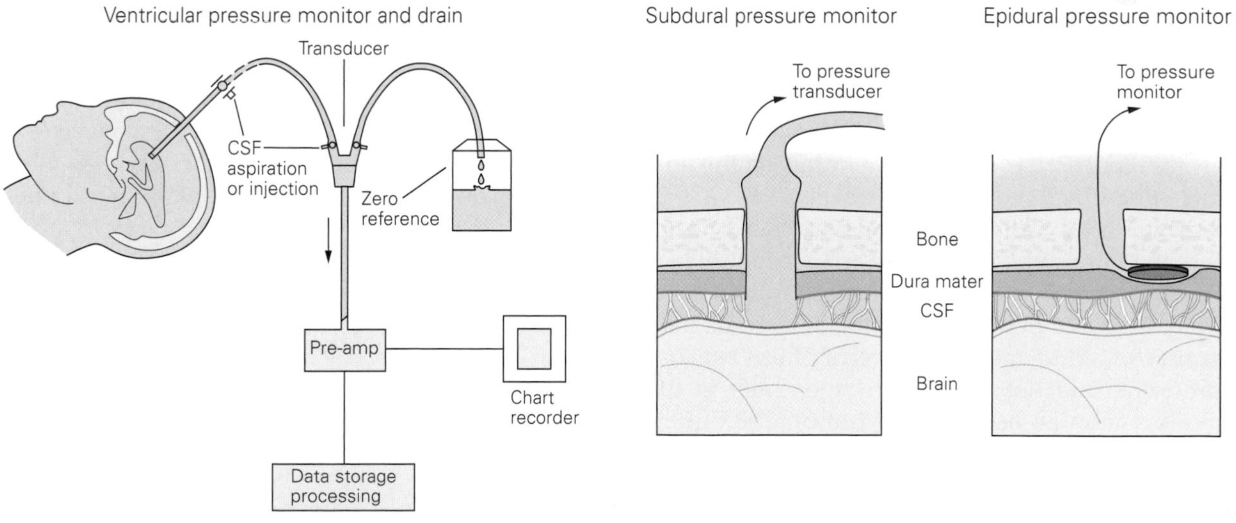

Figure D–11 Techniques for continuous measurement of intracranial pressure. (Adapted, with permission, from Jennett and Teasdale 1981.)

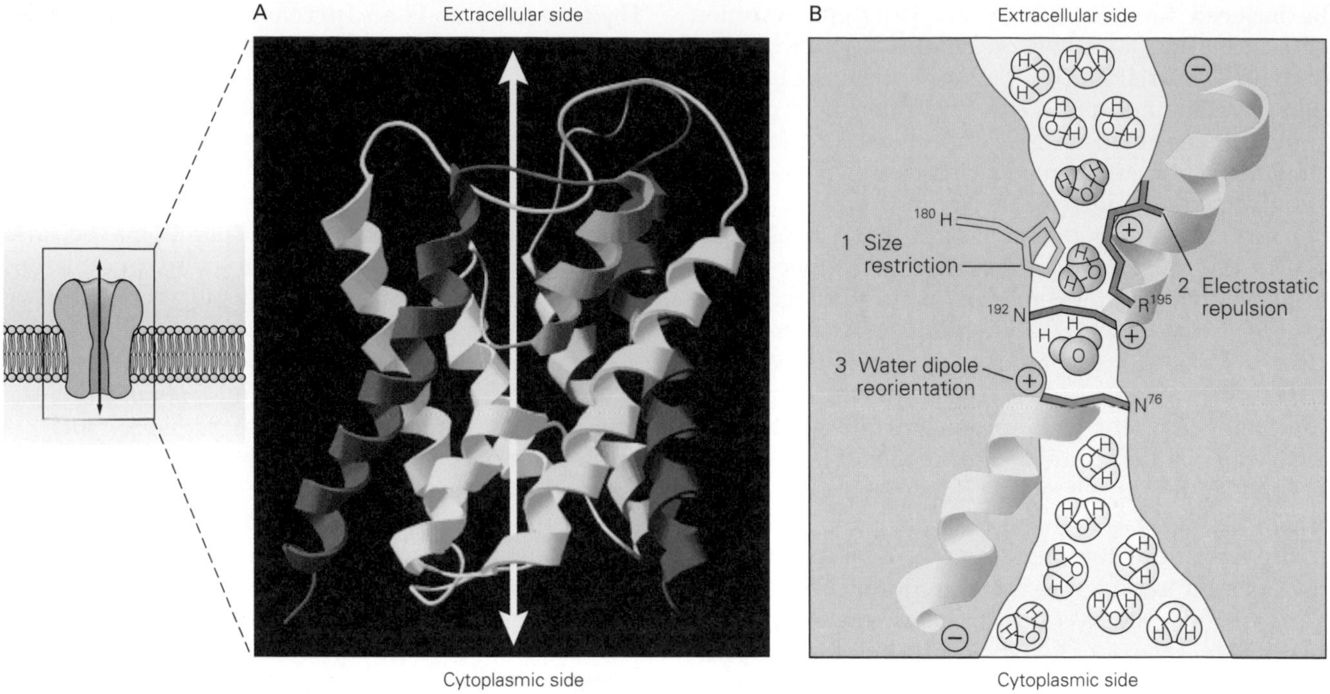

Figure D–12 Water transport across cell membranes in the brain is facilitated by membrane-spanning water channels called aquaporins (AQP).

A. Model of a transmembranous AQP1 subunit. The amino-terminus is **dark blue** and the carboxy terminus is **dark orange**. Six long membrane-spanning helixes surround two hemipores (loops with short helixes depicted in **light blue** and **light orange**) that meet in the center of the lipid membrane bilayer. The **arrow** indicates the aqueous channel through the protein.

B. Physicochemical features of the AQP1 water channel. Three water molecules (**purple**) represent transient interactions with the pore-lining at discrete sites. Bulk water molecules (**blue**) occur in the extracellular and intracellular spaces. Three features of the channel make it selective for water. **1.** The pore narrows 8 Å above the channel midpoint to a diameter of 2.8 Å. **2.** At the narrowest region of the pore conserved residue (Arg-195) forms a barrier to cations, including protonated water (H_3O^+). **3.** Two short helixes meet at the channel midpoint, providing positively charged dipoles that reorient traversing water molecules, disrupting hydrogen bonding in the single-file chain of traversing water molecules and preventing the formation of proton conductance. (Adapted, with permission, from Kozono et al. 2002.)

believed to result from the effects of the expanded lateral ventricles and abnormal absorption of CSF through the ventricular ependymal lining on the surrounding subcortical white matter tracts.

Obstruction of CSF pathways may result from tumors, congenital malformations, or scarring. A particularly vulnerable site for all three mechanisms is the narrow aqueduct of Sylvius. Aqueductal stenosis may result from congenital malformations or gliosis because of intrauterine infection or hemorrhage. Later in life the aqueduct may be occluded by tumor. The outlets of the fourth ventricle may be obstructed by congenital atresia of the foramina of Luschka and Magendie, which may lead to enlargement of all four ventricles (Dandy-Walker syndrome). Obstruction of flow at the basilar cisterns, resulting from conditions such as intraventricular hemorrhage or meningitis, can also cause enlargement of the entire ventricular system. In early life the cranial vault enlarges with the ventricles; after the sutures fuse, cranial volume is fixed and hydrocephalus develops at the expense of brain volume.

John J. Laterra
Gary W. Goldstein

Selected Readings

Bradbury MWB (ed). 1992. *Physiology and Pharmacology of the Blood-Brain Barrier*. New York: Springer Verlag.

Del-Bigio MR. 1993. Neuropathological changes caused by hydrocephalus. Acta Neuropathol Berl 85:573–585.

Doczi T. 1993. Volume regulation of the brain tissue: a survey. Acta Neurochir (Wien) 121:1–9.

Doyle DJ, Mark PW. 1992. Analysis of intracranial pressure. J Clin Monit 8:81–90.

Dziegielewska KM, Ek J, Habgood MD, Saunders NR. 2001. Development of the choroid plexus. Microsc Res Tech 52:5–20.

Fishman RA. 1992. *Cerebrospinal Fluid in Diseases of the Nervous System*. Philadelphia: Saunders.

Furuta Y, Piston DW, Hogan BLM. 1997. Bone morphogenic proteins (BMPs) as regulators of dorsal forebrain development. Development 124:2203–2212.

Katzman R, Pappius HM. 1973. *Brain Electrolytes and Fluid Metabolism*. Baltimore: Williams & Wilkins.

Keep RF, Xiang J, Betz AL. 1993. Potassium transport at the blood-brain and blood–CSF barriers. Adv Exp Med Biol 331:43–54.

Laterra J, Stewart PA, Goldstein GW. 1991. Development of the blood-brain barrier. In: RA Polin, WW Fox (eds). *Neonatal and Fetal Medicine—Physiology and Pathophysiology*, 2nd ed. Philadelphia: W.B. Saunders.

Lyons MK, Meyer FB. 1990. Cerebrospinal fluid physiology and the management of increased intracranial pressure. Mayo Clin Proc 65:684–707.

Mooradian AD, Morin AM, Cipp LJ, Haspel HC. 1991. Glucose transport is reduced in the blood-brain barrier of aged rats. Brain Res 551:145–149.

Nilsson C, Lindvall-Axelsson M, Owman C. 1992. Neuroendocrine regulatory mechanisms in the choroid plexus-cerebrospinal fluid system. Brain Res Rev 17: 109–138.

Rapoport SI. 1976. *Blood-Brain Barrier in Physiology and Medicine*. New York: Raven Press.

Ropper AH, Kennedy SF (eds). 1988. *Neurological and Neurosurgical Intensive Care*. Maryland: Aspen Publishers.

Segal MB. 1993. Extracellular and cerebrospinal fluids. J Inherit Metab Dis 16:617–638.

Vannucci SJ, Maher F, Simpson IA. 1997. Glucose transporter proteins in brain: delivery of glucose to neurons and glia. Glia 21:2–21.

References

Badaut J, Lasbennes F, Magistretti PJ, Regli L. 2002. Aquaporins in brain: distribution, physiology and pathophysiology. J Cereb Blood Flow Metab 22:367–378.

Betz AL, Goldstein GW. 1986. Specialized properties and solute transport in brain capillaries. Annu Rev Physiol 48:241–250.

Borgesen SE, Gjetrris F. 1982. The predictive value of conductance to outflow of CSF in normal pressure hydrocephalus. Brain 105:65–86.

Borgesen SE, Gjetrris F. 1987. Relationships between intracranial pressure, ventricular size, and resistance to CSF outflow. J Neurosurg 67:535–539.

Brightman MW, Reese TS. 1969. Junctions between intimately apposed cell membranes in the vertebrate brain. J Cell Biol 40:648.

Carpenter MB. 1970. *Human Neuroanatomy*, 7th ed. Baltimore, MD: William & Wilkins.

Cunningham LA, Wetzel M, Rosenberg G. 2005. Multiple roles for MMPs and TIMPs in cerebral ischemia. Glia 50:329–339.

DeVivo DC, Trifiletti R, Jacobson RI, Harik SI. 1990. Glucose transporter deficiency causing persistent hypoglycorrhachia: A unique cause of infantile seizures and acquired microcephaly. Ann Neurol 29:414–415.

Duelli R, Enerson BE, Gerhart DZ, Drewes LR. 2000. Expression of large amino acid transporter LAT1 in rat brain endothelium. J Cereb Blood Flow Metab 20:1557–1562.

Ehrlich P. 1885. *Das Sauerstoff-Bedurfnis des Organismus. Eine Farbenanalytische Studie*. Berlin: Hirschwold.

Fishman RA. 1975. Brain edema. N Engl J Med 293:706–711.

Friedemann U. 1942. Blood-brain barrier. Physiol Rev 22:125–145.

Gerhart DZ, Enerson BE, Zhdankina OY, Leino RL, Drewes LR. 1997. Expression of monocarboxylate transporter MCT1 by brain endothelium and glia in adult and suckling rats. Am J Physiol 273:E207-E213.

Goldman E. 1909. Die äussere und innere Sekretion des gesunden und kranken Organismus im Lichte der "vitalen Färbung." Beitr Klin Chirurg 64:192–265.

Goldstein GW, Betz AL. 1986. The blood-brain barrier. Sci Am 255:74–83.

Guerin C, Laterra J, Hruban R, Brem H, Drewes LR and Goldstein GW. 1990. The glucose transporter and blood-brain barrier of human brain tumors. Ann Neurol 28:758–765.

Guerin C, Laterra J, Drewes L, Brem H, Goldstein GW. 1992. Vascular expression of glucose transporter in experimental brain neoplasms. Am J Pathol 140:114–125.

Hansen AJ, Lund-Andersen H, Crone C. 1977. K^+-permeability of the blood-brain barrier, investigated by aid of a K^+-sensitive microelectrode. Acta Physiol Scand 101:438–435.

Huber JD, Egleton RD, Davis TP. 2001. Molecular physiology and pathophysiology of tight junctions in the blood-brain barrier. Trends Neurosci 24:719–725.

Jennett B, Teasdale G. 1981. *Management of Head Injuries*. Philadelphia, PA: FA Davis Company.

Klepper J, Willemsen M, Verrips A, et al. 2001. Autosomal dominant transmission of GLUT1 deficiency. Hum Mol Genet 10:63–68.

Kniesel U, Wolburg H. 2000. Tight junctions of the blood-brain barrier. Cell Mol Neurobiol 20:57–76.

Kozono D, Yasui M, King LS, Agre P. 2002. Aquaporin water channels: atomic structure and molecular dynamics meet clinical medicine. J Clin Invest 109:1395–1399.

Lal B, Indurti RR, Couraud P-O, Goldstein GW, Laterra J. 1994. Endothelial cell implantation and survival within experimental gliomas. Proc Natl Acad Sci U S A 21:9695–9699.

Lee SR, Wang X, Tsuji K, Lo EH. 2004. Extracellular proteolytic pathophysiology in the neurovascular unit after stroke. Neurol Res 26:854–861.

Nico B, Frigeri A, Nicchia GP, Quondamatteo F, Herken R, Errede M, Ribatti D, Svelto M, Roncali L. 2001. Role of aquaporin-4 water channel in the development and integrity of the blood-brain barrier. J Cell Sci 114:1297–1307.

Pellerin L, Pellegri G, Martin JL, Magistretti PJ. 1998. Expression of monocarboxylate transporter mRNAs in mouse brain: Support for a distinct role of lactate as an energy substrate for the neonatal vs. adult brain. Proc Natl Acad Sci U S A 95:3990–3995.

Reese TS, Karnovsky MJ. 1967. Fine structural localization of a blood-brain barrier to exogenous peroxidase. J Cell Biol 34:207.

Resnick L, Berger JR., Shapshak P, Tourtellotte WW. 1988. Early penetration of the blood-brain barrier by HIV. Neurology 38:9–14.

Rubin LL, Hall DE, Porter S, Barbu K, Cannon C, Horner HC, Janatpour M et al. 1991. A cell culture model of the blood-brain barrier. J Cell Biol 115:1725–1735.

Schinkel AH, Smit JJM, van Tellingen O, Beijnen JH, Wagenaar E, van Deemter L, Mol CA et al. 1994. Disruption of the mouse mdr1a P-glycoprotein gene leads to a deficiency in the blood-brain barrier and to increased sensitivity to drugs. Cell 77:491–502.

Shivers RR, Betz AL, Goldstein GW. 1984. Isolated rat brain capillaries posses intact, structurally complex interendothelia tight junction; freeze-fracture verification of tight junction integrity. Brain Res 324:313–322.

Spector R, Johanson CE. 1989. The mammalian choroid plexus. Sci Am 261:68–74.

Stanimirovic D, Satoh K. 2000. Inflammatory mediators of cerebral endothelium: a role in ischemic brain inflammation. Brain Pathol 10:113–126.

Stewart PA, Wiley MJ. 1981. Developing nervous tissue induces formation of blood-brain barrier characteristics in invading endothelial cells: a study using quail-chick transplantation chimeras. Dev Biol 84:183–192.

Svendgaard NA, Bjorklund A, Hardebo JE, Stenevi U. 1975. Axonal degeneration associated with a defective blood-brain barrier in cerebral implants. Nature 255:334–336.

Takanaga H, Tokuda N, Ohtsuki S, Hosoya K, Terasaki T. 2002. ATA2 is predominantly expressed as system A at the blood-brain barrier and acts as brain to blood efflux transport for L-proline. Mol Pharmacol 61:1289–1296.

Wagner CA, Lang F, Broer S. 2001. Function and structure of heterodimeric amino acid transporters. Am J Physiol Cell Physiol 281:C1077-C1093.

Wahl M, Unterberg A, Baerthmann A, Schilling L. 1988. Mediators of blood-brain barrier dysfunction and formation of vasogenic brain edema. J Cereb Blood Flow Metab 8:621–634.

Wolburg H, Neuhaus J, Kniesel U, Krauss B, Schmid EM, Ocalan M, Farrell C, Risau W. 1994. Modulation of tight junction structure in blood-brain barrier endothelial cells. J Cell Sci 107:1347–1357.

Appendix E

Neural Networks

BY ITSELF A SINGLE NEURON is not intelligent. But a vast network of neurons can think, feel, remember, perceive, and generate the many remarkable phenomena that are collectively known as "the mind." How does intelligence emerge from the interactions between neurons? This is the central question motivating the study of neural networks. In this appendix we provide a brief historical review of the field, introduce some key concepts, and discuss two influential models of neural networks, the perceptron and the cell assembly.

Starting from the 1940s researchers have proposed and studied many brain models in which sophisticated computations are performed by networks of simple neuron-like elements. Most models are based on two shared principles. First, our immediate experience is rooted in ongoing patterns of action potentials in brain cells. Second, our ability to learn from and remember past experiences is based at least partially on long-lasting modifications of synaptic connections. Although these principles are widely accepted by neuroscientists, they immediately suggest many difficult questions.

For example, to our conscious minds, perceiving an object or moving a limb is experienced as a single, unitary event. But in the brain either act is the result of a collection of a stupendous number of neural events—the discharge of action potentials or the release of neurotransmitter vesicles—indiscernible by the conscious mind. How are these events united into a coherent perception or movement?

Storage of our immediate experience in long-term memory is presumed to occur with changes in synaptic connections. But how exactly is a memory divided up and distributed across many synapses? If some synapses are used to store more than one memory, how then is interference between memories avoided? When past experiences are recalled from memory, how might synaptic connections evoke a pattern of firing that is similar to a pattern that occurred in the past? Finally, when we reason, daydream, or otherwise float in the stream of consciousness, our mental state is not directly tied to any immediate sensory stimulus or motor output. How do networks of neurons dynamically generate the patterns of activity related to such mental states?

These are profound questions. Many hypothetical answers have been proposed in the form of neural network models, a body of work that spans many decades and which we survey here. Although they are far from being tested conclusively, these hypotheses have influenced the research of a number of experimental neuroscientists and are being developed further today by theoretical neuroscientists.

Early Neural Network Modeling

Perhaps the first attempt to explain behavior in terms of synaptic connectivity was Sherrington's reflex arc. A reflex behavior is defined as a rapid, involuntary, and stereotyped response to a specific stimulus (see Chapter 35). For any reflex behavior one can generally identify a reflex arc, a chain of synapses starting from a sensory neuron and ending with a motor neuron. The sequential activation of neurons in this chain is a series of causes and effects that connect the stimulus to the response. The reflex arc can be regarded as an ancestor of neural network models.

In 1938 Rafael Lorente de Nó, a student of Santiago Ramón y Cajal, argued that synaptic loops ("internuncial chains") were the basic circuits of the central nervous system. A synaptic loop is a chain of synapses that starts and ends at the same neuron. It is a closed chain, in contrast to the open chain of a reflex arc. Lorente de Nó suggested that the purpose of these loops was to sustain "reverberating" activity patterns. In fact, Sherrington's student, Graham Brown, in his studies of spinal cord rhythmicity, proposed a related view of the brain, involving intrinsic generation of neural activity rather than stimulus-response relationships. These scientists emphasized that the brain has an intrinsic dynamic richer than that of reflex arcs, which are inactive until stimulated by the outside world.

In an influential book published in 1949, Donald Hebb proposed the idea of a "cell assembly" as a functional unit of the nervous system and discussed the form of synaptic plasticity that would become known as Hebb's rule. (The rule had previously been formulated by several other thinkers, of whom the earliest was perhaps the philosopher Alexander Bain in 1873.) Hebb argued that repeated synaptic communication between neurons could strengthen the connections between the neurons, creating synaptic loops that were capable of supporting the reverberating activity patterns of Lorente de Nó.

These ideas of Sherrington, Graham Brown, Lorente de Nó, and Hebb were later formalized in mathematical models of neural networks. Two famous classes of models are perceptrons and associative memory networks. *Perceptrons* have been popular as models of the visual system because they illustrate how recognition of an object can be decomposed into many feature detection events. A perceptron can be organized hierarchically, so that the decomposition process begins with simple features at the bottom of the hierarchy and proceeds to complex features at the top, as is thought to occur in the visual system (see Chapter 28).

Associative memory networks have been used to model how the brain stores and recalls long-term memories. Central to these models is Hebb's concept of the cell assembly, a group of excitatory neurons mutually coupled by strong synapses. Memory storage occurs with the creation of a cell assembly by Hebbian synaptic plasticity (see Chapter 66), and memory recall occurs when the neurons in a cell assembly are activated by a stimulus.

The perceptron and the cell assembly have very different synaptic connectivities. As in Sherrington's reflex arc, the polysynaptic pathways in a perceptron all travel in the same overall direction, from the input layer to the output layer. The perceptron generalizes the reflex arc, because it allows many synapses to diverge from a neuron and converge onto a neuron.

The perceptron is a special case of a *feed-forward network*, defined as one with no synaptic loops. As noted above, a synaptic loop is defined as a polysynaptic pathway that starts and ends at the same neuron. Networks with loops are called *recurrent* or *feedback networks*, to distinguish them from feed-forward networks. A cell assembly typically contains loops, and is therefore recurrent.

Lorente de Nó and Hebb postulated that neural activity can persist longer in the brain by circulating through synaptic loops. Thus a cell assembly can maintain a persistent activity pattern resembling patterns observed by neurophysiologists in studies of short-term and working memory. In other words, loops could be important for the generation of persistent mental states in the brain, which are required for behaviors in which stimulus and response are separated by a long time delay. In contrast, the direct pathways of the perceptron are suited for modeling behavioral responses that immediately follow a stimulus.

Only very simple neural networks are described in this appendix. The "neurons" in these models are much simpler than biological neurons, and the "synapses" do not do justice to the intricacies of biological synapses. When modeling a complex system, simplifying its elements helps one to focus on the properties that emerge from the interactions between them. This strategy has historically been used by neural networks researchers focusing on emergent properties of brain function. More realistic models of how neurons integrate synaptic inputs are described in Appendix F.

Neurons Are Computational Devices

Action potentials and synaptic potentials are dynamic events that involve a complex interplay between the membrane voltage of a neuron and the opening and closing of its ion channels. Computational neuroscientists often ignore these complexities in their thinking and instead rely on the following simplification: *A neuron fires an action potential when a sufficiently large number of excitatory synapses onto it are activated simultaneously.*

This statement is based on the fact that a single excitatory postsynaptic potential is typically much smaller in amplitude (less than 0.5 mV) than the gap of many millivolts that separate the resting potential from the threshold for an action potential. Therefore, many simultaneous excitatory postsynaptic potentials need to sum in the postsynaptic neuron to drive its voltage over the threshold for firing.

The above simplification of the conditions for neuronal firing has inspired a great deal of mathematical formalism. In 1943 Warren McCulloch and Walter Pitts proposed a model of the computation performed by a neuron and the excitatory synapses converging onto it. The McCulloch-Pitts neuron takes multiple inputs and produces a single output. All inputs and the output are binary variables, 0 or 1. The neuron is characterized by a single parameter θ, its threshold. If a subset of θ or more inputs is equal to 1, then the neuron's output is 1; otherwise the output is 0.

In the biological interpretation of the McCulloch-Pitts model each input variable represents the activation of an excitatory synapse at the neuron. The input is equal to 1 when the excitatory synapse is activated. The parameter θ is used to model the threshold of a biological neuron and is equal to the minimum number of excitatory synapses that must be simultaneously activated to produce an action potential. In this interpretation the McCulloch-Pitts model formalizes the above caricature of a biological neuron.

Two McCulloch-Pitts neurons can be connected so that the output of one neuron is the input of another. This corresponds to the biological fact that excitatory synapses converging onto a neuron are activated by the discharging of the presynaptic neurons. By making many such connections, it is possible to construct a model of a neural network.

In the McCulloch-Pitts model, neurons are either active ("1") or inactive ("0"). This is admittedly a crude way of describing neural activity, because it does not distinguish between active neurons with different firing rates. But this coarse description is used not only by theorists but also by experimental neurophysiologists, who often speak of active and inactive neurons in the exploratory phases of their experiments before they make precise measurements of firing rates. Although the graded nature of firing rates can be captured using more realistic model neurons (Box E–1), here we will limit ourselves to the McCulloch-Pitts model to minimize the use of mathematical equations.

This simplification also allows the application of ideas from Boolean logic, in which the binary values 0 and 1 correspond to "false" and "true." Boolean logic, named after the British mathematician George Boole, is a formalization of deductive reasoning that is based on manipulations of binary variables that represent truth values. Boolean logic is the mathematical foundation of digital electronic circuits. Using their model, McCulloch and Pitts argued that the activity of each neuron signifies the truth of some logical proposition. They concluded that neurons (and by extension networks of neurons) perform logical computations.

A Neuron Can Compute Conjunctions and Disjunctions

If we accept the idea that biological neurons can perform logical computations, then it is natural to ask what types of computations are possible. We will answer this question by studying the behavior of the McCulloch-Pitts model neuron. Of course, biological neurons are more complex and therefore likely to be more powerful computational devices. But by analyzing the McCulloch-Pitts neuron we can expect to establish lower bounds on the computational power of biological neurons. In other words, if a computation is possible for a McCulloch-Pitts neuron it should be possible for a biological neuron, although the converse is not necessarily true.

Box E–1 Mathematics of Neural Networks

The McCulloch-Pitts neuron is simple enough that its behavior can be described in words. More sophisticated models require the precision of mathematics for a clear formulation.

The linear-threshold (LT) model neuron corrects a shortcoming of the McCulloch-Pitts neuron that all excitatory inputs are equally effective in bringing the neuron to its firing threshold; the number of active inputs is important, but their identities are not. For a biological neuron in which some synapses are stronger than others, such a simplification is not realistic.

To model this aspect of synaptic function, the LT neuron takes the weighted sum of its inputs, where the weights of the sum represent synaptic strengths. If the sum exceeds a threshold, the LT neuron becomes active.

To model a network of LT neurons, assume that their activities at time t are given by the N variables, $x_1(t)$, $x_2(t)$ ..., $x_N(t)$ which take on the values 0 or 1, that is, a neuron is either active ("1") or silent ("0"). Then the activities at time $t + 1$ are given by

$$x_i(t+1) = H\left(\sum_{j=1}^{N} W_{ij} x_j(t) - \theta_j\right) \qquad \textbf{(E–1)}$$

where H is the Heaviside step function defined by $H(u) = 1$ for $u \geq 0$ and $H(u) = 0$ otherwise, W_{ij} is the strength or weight of the synapse between neuron i and the presynaptic neuron j, and θ_j is the threshold of neuron i. For a network of N neurons, the synaptic weights W_{ij} form an $N \times N$ matrix, and the thresholds θ_j an N-dimensional vector.

The LT and McCulloch-Pitts models are equivalent if the synaptic strengths of the LT model satisfy two conditions. First, the strengths of all excitatory synapses must equal one to yield the uniformity of strengths discussed above. Second, each inhibitory synapse must be so strong that activating it is enough to keep the LT neuron below threshold, no matter how many excitatory inputs are active. This second condition is in accord with the behavior of inhibition in the original McCulloch-Pitts neuron and could be regarded as a crude model of shunting inhibition (see Chapter 10).

The LT neuron of Equation E–1 can perform many different types of computation, depending on the choice of synaptic weights and thresholds. By arguments similar to those given in the main text, any Boolean function can be realized by combining LT neurons into a network. A perceptron network can be implemented by a synaptic weight matrix in which certain elements are constrained to be zero. (Such elements would give rise to "backwards" pathways in the perceptron model illustrated in Figure E–1.) An associative memory network can be constructed by choosing W_{ij} to be a correlation matrix (see Box E–3).

The LT neuron is either active or inactive, but the firing rates of biological neurons are continuously graded quantities. This can be modeled by replacing the Heaviside step function H in Equation E–1 by some other function F with graded output. Neural activity is described by continuously graded variables r_1 ... r_N rather than binary variables, which are interpreted as rates of action-potential firing. Furthermore, time can be treated continuously in the differential equation

$$\tau \frac{dr_i}{dt} + r_i = F\left(\sum_{j=1}^{N} W_{ij} r_j - \theta_j\right) \qquad \textbf{(E–2)}$$

rather than discretely as in Equation E–1. This type of model is discussed in more detail in Appendix F.

In Equation E–2 the soma of the neuron is regarded as a device that converts input current into the cell's rate of firing. This point of view is often taken by electrophysiologists, who characterize a neuron by its *f-I* curve, plotted by injecting current into a neuron and recording the resulting firing rate. The dendrite of the neuron is assumed to linearly combine the currents produced by its synapses, a good approximation in some biological neurons. Each synapse generates a current that is proportional to the firing rate of its presynaptic neuron.

Equation E–2 is still quite crude in its description of neural activity as an overall firing rate. More sophisticated models have differential equations governing voltages and conductances and generate individual action potentials. For example, the voltages in the numerical simulations of Figure E–5 were generated by leaky integrate-and-fire model neurons. More about this and other spiking model neurons can be found in works listed in the bibliography at the end of the appendix, as well as in Appendix F.

Suppose that the threshold parameter θ of a McCulloch-Pitts neuron is set at a high value, equal to the total number of inputs. Then the neuron is active if, and only if, all of its synaptic inputs are active. In other words, the output of the neuron is the *conjunction* of its input variables, which is also known as the logical AND operation. Alternatively, the threshold can be set at a low value, equal to one, such that activation of one or more synaptic inputs is enough to activate the neuron. In this case the output of the neuron is the *disjunction* of its input variables, which is also known as the logical OR operation.

Although a McCulloch-Pitts neuron can compute some logical functions, it cannot compute others. A famous example is the exclusive-or (XOR) operation. By definition the XOR operation on two inputs results in "1" if, and only if, exactly one of its inputs is "1." Thus if both inputs are "1," the XOR function outputs "0," while the OR function outputs "1." Proving that a single McCulloch-Pitts neuron cannot compute the XOR operation is left as an exercise to the reader. However, XOR can be computed by a network of McCulloch-Pitts neurons, as is explained below.

A Network of Neurons Can Compute Any Boolean Logical Function

What functions can be computed by a network of McCulloch-Pitts neurons? Conjunctions and disjunctions are basic building blocks of Boolean logic. The original definition of a McCulloch-Pitts neuron included both inhibitory and excitatory synapses. It turns out that synaptic inhibition can be used for the operation of negation (logical NOT).

Consider a neuron that is spontaneously active and receives a single strong inhibitory synapse. When the inhibitory synapse is inactive, the neuron is spontaneously active. But when the inhibitory synapse is active, the neuron is inactive, silenced by inhibition. In other words, the neuron responds with 1 when its input is 0 but with 0 when its input is 1. This is exactly the NOT operation.

It is well known that any function of Boolean logic can be synthesized by combining the AND, OR, and NOT operations. Because McCulloch-Pitts neurons can compute all of these operations, it follows that networks of McCulloch-Pitts neurons can compute any function of Boolean logic, including XOR.

Why is it important that these models compute Boolean functions? Boolean logic lies at the heart of modern digital computers. The computers on our desktops, and in fact all digital electronic circuits, are designed to implement Boolean logic. When a digital computer runs a software program, it simply executes sequences of logical operations. Thus networks of McCulloch-Pitts neurons can compute the same functions as digital computers.[1]

These facts about networks of McCulloch-Pitts neurons were discovered in the 1940s and 1950s when neural network models played a role in the formal theory of automata and computation. This line of research showed that neural network models have great computational power in principle. Nevertheless, a difficult question remains: How are computations actually performed by brains? This question cannot be answered by formal arguments alone. It is now being addressed both by theoretical and experimental neuroscientists who try to understand how the brain works, and by computer scientists and engineers who create artificial systems that emulate capabilities of the brain.

The notion that a neuron is a device for computing conjunctions and disjunctions is prominent in the ensuing discussion of neural network models of the visual system.

Perceptrons Model Sequential and Parallel Computation in the Visual System

The term *perceptron* was coined in the 1950s by Frank Rosenblatt to describe his neural network models of visual perception. In a perceptron neurons are organized in layers (Figure E–1).[2] The first layer is the input to the network and the last layer the output. Each layer sends synapses only to the next layer, so that information flows in the "forward" direction from the input to the output. Although perceptrons can be constructed from various kinds of model neurons, we will use the simple McCulloch-Pitts neurons.

The computations in a perceptron, as in the visual system, occur through both sequential and parallel processing of information. The layers of a perceptron can be regarded as a sequence of steps in a computation. The neurons within each layer perform similar operations that are executed in parallel during a single

[1]A formal model of a digital computer called a *Turing machine* is more powerful than a network of McCulloch-Pitts neurons because it has a memory with an infinite capacity. But any real digital computer has finite memory and is therefore less powerful than the idealized Turing machine.

[2]There is some variation in the use of the term "*perceptron*". Some people call the network in Figure E–1 a "multilayer perceptron," and use "perceptron" to refer only to a network with a single layer of synapses. Here we use perceptron as a generic term covering both multilayer and single-layer perceptrons.

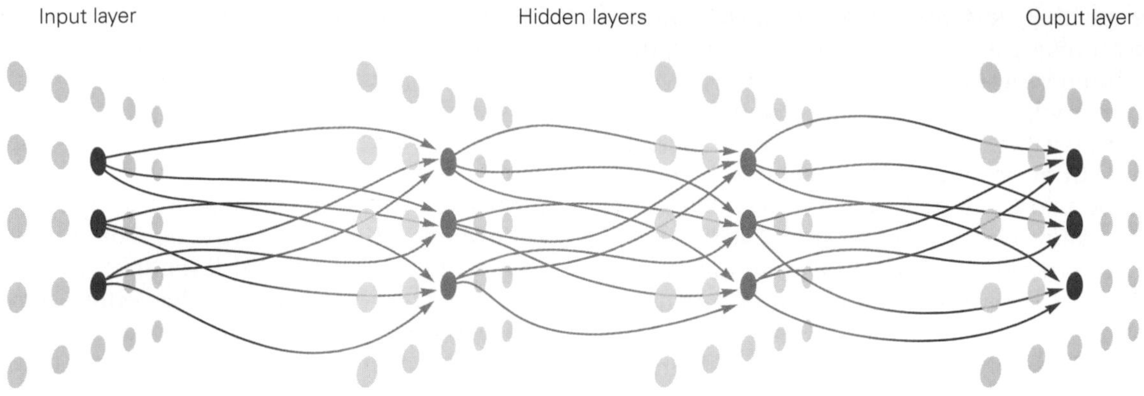

Figure E–1 The perceptron model. A perceptron is a network of idealized neurons arranged in layers with synaptic connections from each layer to the succeeding one. In general, any number of "hidden layers" may intervene between the input and output. Each disk represents a neuron. An arrow pointing from the presynaptic neuron to the postsynaptic neuron represents a synapse. There are no loops in the network.

step of the computation. Because vision is often quite fast compared to other cognitive tasks, it may require only a few sequential steps, but each step involves a large number of operations performed by many neurons working in parallel. It is natural to represent this kind of computation by a perceptron with a small number of layers, each with many neurons.

Simple and Complex Cells Could Compute Conjunctions and Disjunctions

We shall develop the analogy between perceptrons and the visual system by exploring its implications for primary visual cortex (V1). As discussed in Chapter 27, the "simple cells" of V1 respond selectively to stimuli in the visual field that have a certain spatial orientation. A simple cell responds to a bar of light close to a particular orientation but not to bars with other orientations.

In a classic 1962 paper David Hubel and Torsten Wiesel described this property of orientation selectivity in V1 and also proposed the first model of how it is achieved. They assumed that what they called a "simple" cortical cell receives synaptic inputs from cells in the lateral geniculate nucleus (LGN) and suggested that orientation selectivity of the simple cell in V1 depends on the spatial arrangement of the receptive fields of the LGN cells. Thus, if the center-surround receptive fields of the LGN cells were arranged along a straight line (see Figure 27–3), a bar of light with the same orientation as this line would activate all the LGN inputs of the simple cell simultaneously, driving the cortical simple cell that receives these inputs above the threshold for firing action potentials. Conversely, a bar of light at nonpreferred orientations would stimulate only some of the LGN inputs, leaving that simple cell below threshold for firing.

The preceding model of a simple cell can be interpreted as a McCulloch-Pitts neuron computing an AND operation (Figure E–2A) because a simple cell fires when *all* of its LGN inputs are activated. Recall that a McCulloch-Pitts neuron computes a conjunction if its threshold is set sufficiently high, and intuitively it makes sense that a high threshold goes along with high selectivity.

In addition to simple cells, V1 also contains "complex" cells, also first described by Hubel and Wiesel. Like simple cells, complex cells are orientation selective, but their responses are not sensitive to the location of the stimulus within the receptive field, whereas simple cells are quite sensitive to the precise alignment of the stimulus within the excitatory subregions of their receptive field.

Hubel and Wiesel proposed that a complex cell receives synaptic input from simple cells with similar orientation selectivity (Figure E–2C). The receptive fields of the simple cells add together to form the receptive field of the complex cell. If a visual stimulus with the preferred orientation activates any one of the simple cells, the complex cell is driven over the threshold for firing. This model is intended to explain why spatial location of the stimulus in the receptive field is not a factor in activating the complex cell.

This model of a complex cell can be interpreted as a McCulloch-Pitts neuron computing an OR operation (Figure E–2B) since a complex cell fires when *any* of its simple cell inputs is activated. A McCulloch-Pitts neuron computes a disjunction if its threshold is set sufficiently low, and it makes sense that a low threshold is appropriate for nonselective responses.

In effect, Hubel and Wiesel imagined simple and complex cells as McCulloch-Pitts neurons, although they did not use such language. For a McCulloch-Pitts neuron the threshold determines whether responses are selective or invariant. The simple cell's high threshold is responsible for the cell's orientation selectivity, while the complex cell's low threshold accounts for the invariance of its response to the location of the stimulus within its receptive field.

The Primary Visual Cortex Has Been Modeled As a Multilayer Perceptron

If the Hubel-Wiesel model is extended to many neurons, each with a receptive field that covers a different location in the visual field and tuned to a preferred orientation, then it amounts to a perceptron with three layers of neurons (Figure E–3).

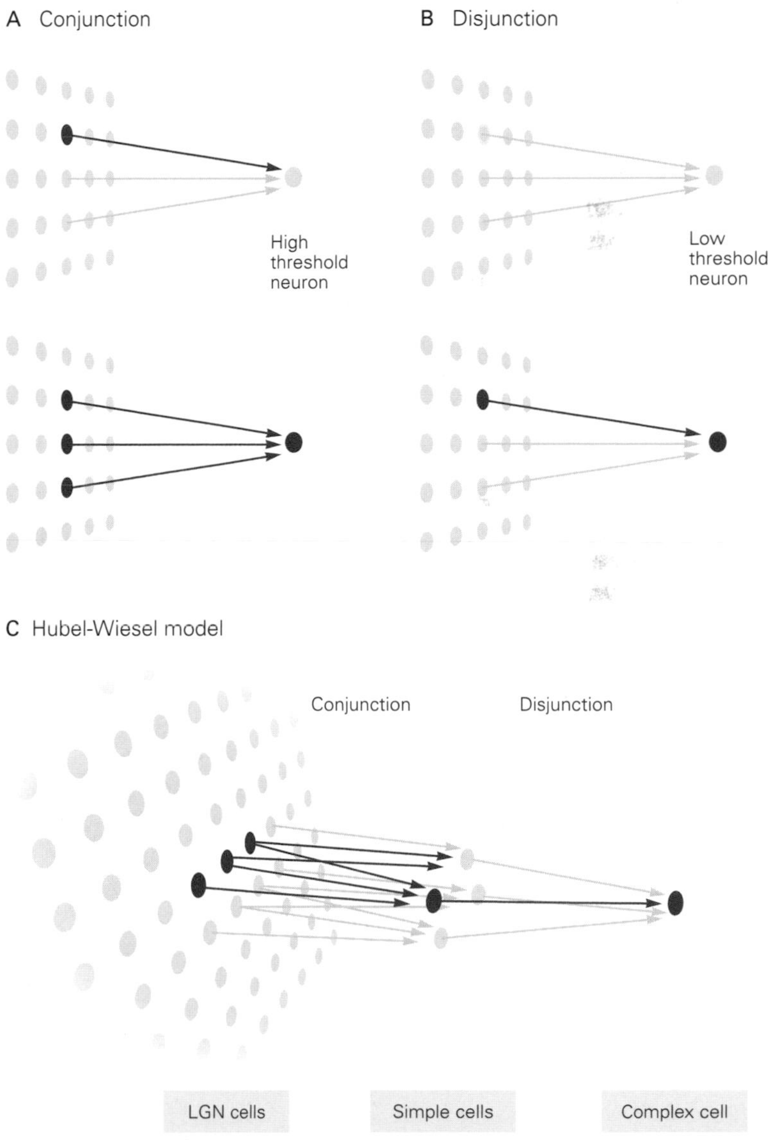

Figure E–2 A perceptron implementing conjunction (AND), disjunction (OR), and the Hubel-Wiesel neurobiological model of simple and complex cells in visual cortex. Neurons are represented by disks and synapses by arrows. Active neurons and synapses are colored red.

A. A neuron with a high threshold can compute the conjunction of three inputs. The neuron does not respond to only one input (**top**) or two inputs (not shown). It becomes active only when all three inputs are active (**bottom**).

B. A neuron with a low threshold can compute a disjunction of three inputs. The neuron remains inactive if all of its inputs are inactive (**top**). It becomes active if a single input neuron is active (**bottom**) or more than one input neuron is active (not shown).

C. In this realization of the Hubel-Wiesel model a disjunction neuron (**right**) receives inputs from a set of conjunction neurons (**middle**), which in turn receive inputs from a grid of neurons (**left**). The neurons in the grid represent lateral geniculate nucleus (LGN) cells, which are assumed to be either all ON-center or OFF-center cells and retinotopically organized so that the location of each cell in the grid corresponds to the location of its receptive field on the retina. A horizontally oriented visual stimulus activates three LGN cells in a row, which activate a "simple cell" (conjunction) that in turn activates a "complex cell" (disjunction). Like actual simple cells of primary visual cortex, each conjunction neuron responds selectively to stimuli with a particular orientation (horizontal in this case) and at a particular location. Likewise, like actual complex cells, the disjunction neuron responds selectively to stimuli with a particular orientation but is invariant to the exact location of the stimulus.

Indeed, like this perceptron, visual areas of the brain generally have a retinotopic organization: Neighboring cells have receptive fields that cover adjacent areas in the visual field. This means that a sheet of cortical tissue functions like a map of the visual field, and patterns of activity can actually resemble images. Similarly, each layer of the model in Figure E–3 is retinotopically organized so that at any moment a map of the overall activity pattern of its neurons depicts the stimulus image. Connections between the layers respect the spatial arrangements of receptive fields described above and shown in Figure E–2. The thresholds are set to yield conjunctions and disjunctions in simple cell and complex cell layers, respectively.

The structure of the model is idealized in a number of ways to facilitate understanding. All cells are arranged in uniformly spaced grids. Furthermore, the simple cell and complex cell layers each have a number of "feature maps." Each cell in a feature map detects exactly the same feature but in a different location of the visual field (Figure E–3). In the cortex the cells detecting different features would be intermingled, but in the model they are segregated for convenience.

A map of active neurons in the LGN layer of the model accurately represents the visual stimulus, whereas the simple and complex cell layers contain more abstract representations of the stimulus because of the orientation selectivity of neurons. In particular, the representation of the stimulus in the complex cell layer is robust and does not reflect small variations in the stimulus (see Figure E–3).

Selectivity and Invariance Must Be Explained by Any Model of Vision

The dichotomy between selectivity and invariance has been important in our discussion of the primary visual cortex and simple stimuli like bars. More generally, this dichotomy is relevant throughout the visual system and even for complex stimuli like entire objects. Let's step back and think about the computations that the entire visual system must accomplish.

Even though the act of seeing appears effortless for humans and animals, vision is a difficult computational problem. In spite of enormous progress in

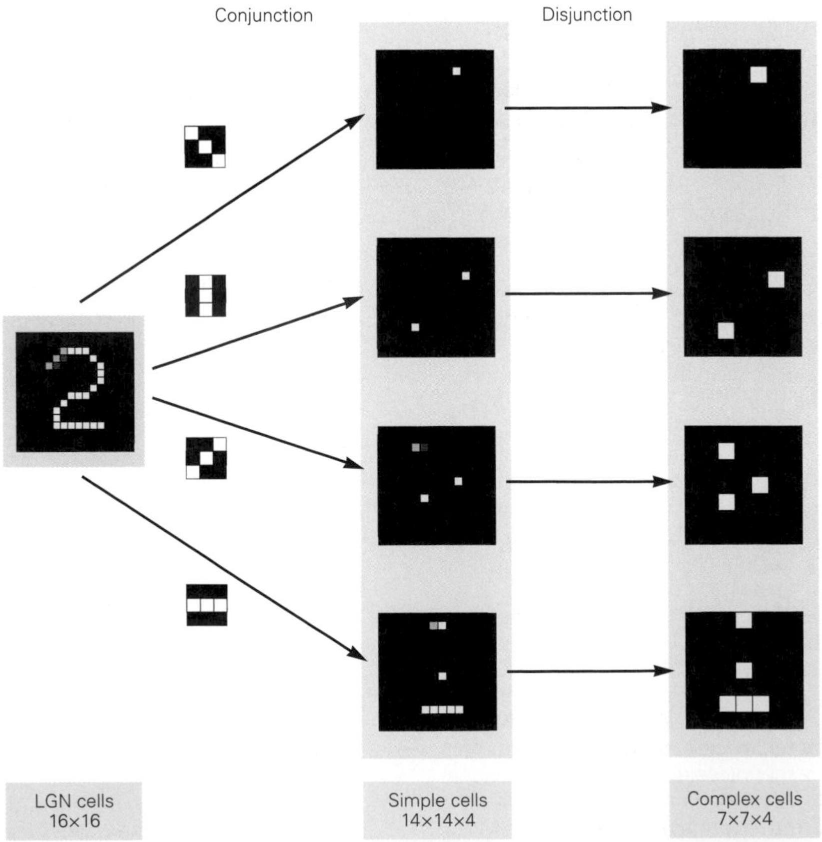

Figure E–3 A perceptron implementing the Hubel-Wiesel model of selectivity and invariance. The network in Figure E–2C can be extended to grids of many cells by specifying synaptic connectivity at all locations in the visual field. The resulting network can be repeated four times, one for each preferred orientation (horizontal, vertical, and two diagonals). This yields four retinotopically organized grids of simple cells, one for each preferred orientation, as well as four grids of complex cells. Each grid is called a *feature map*. Throughout the network the responses to two slightly different images of the numeral 2 are superimposed for comparison. A **yellow pixel** indicates a neuron that responds to both stimuli. A **red pixel** indicates a neuron that responds to one of the stimuli, and a **green pixel** indicates a neuron that responds to the other.

In the LGN layer the difference between the two stimuli is evident (see red and green pixels at the top of the numeral). In the simple cell layer the bottom two feature maps show different responses to the images (red and green pixels), but the top two are the same (all yellow pixels). Finally, the responses of the complex cells are the same for both images (all yellow pixels). Thus invariance and selectivity occur together in one network, although the invariance is limited (it does not hold for all distortions) and the selectivity is fairly simple.

algorithms, speed, and memory capacity, modern digital computers are still far from equaling the performance of biological vision systems. In particular, one of the main functions of vision is the recognition of objects. One reason this task is difficult for computers is that the images of a single object are highly variable. Factors such as lighting, location, and distance all cause changes in retinal images that the visual system must *ignore* in order to recognize an object—recognition requires some invariance in responding. However, the visual system cannot ignore all changes because it has to distinguish between different objects—it must therefore also be selective for certain aspects of images. Although the properties of invariance and selectivity may seem conflicting, they are somehow reconciled by the visual system.

How does the visual system accomplish object recognition? Neurophysiologists have investigated this question by recording from high-level visual areas, such as inferotemporal cortex. To give one example of their findings, certain inferotemporal neurons respond selectively to images of faces. These face-selective neurons have large receptive fields and the exact location of the face within the receptive field is not a factor in the cells' responses. Instead, the responses appear to be closely related to complex features or entire objects rather than simple features like bars or edges.

How are selectivity and invariance achieved by the face-selective neurons? According to one theory, all visual areas of cortex are arranged in a hierarchy (see Figure 28–2) and the Hubel-Wiesel model of simple and complex cells in the primary visual cortex (V1) can be generalized to the higher levels of the visual system. In this hierarchical model V1 is at the bottom and areas in the inferotemporal cortex are near the top. Neurons near the bottom of the hierarchy are selective for simple features, have small receptive fields, and are sensitive to small changes in stimulus location. Neurons near the top of the hierarchy are selective for complex features, have large receptive fields, and are invariant to large changes in stimulus location. Neuronal connections from each level to the next are organized so as to carry out computations analogous to the ones performed by simple and complex cells in V1. As we shall see, this hierarchical conception of visual recognition of objects has been formulated precisely in a number of neural network models.

Visual Object Recognition Could Be Accomplished by Iteration of Conjunctions and Disjunctions

Could perceptrons be used to model not just V1 but also the rest of the visual system? We introduced the idea that conjunctions create selectivity in V1 and disjunctions create invariance. Repeated alternation between conjunctions and disjunctions can be used to build up progressively greater selectivity and invariance, culminating in invariant recognition of entire objects.

Indeed, this idea was implemented in 1980 by Kunihiko Fukushima in the *Neocognitron,* a network model designed to recognize handwritten digits. Handwritten numbers may be less complex than images of natural stimuli such as faces or animals, but they are still quite challenging to recognize, as postal workers or anyone who has ever graded handwritten exams can attest. Indeed, digits produced by different writers often look very different, and even repetitions by a single writer can vary considerably.

The Neocognitron has a multilayer, feedforward architecture like that of a perceptron (although inhibition is treated somewhat differently).[3] The first layer functions like a retina in which neurons represent an image of a handwritten digit, and subsequent layers contain multiple feature maps (Figure E–4). Although the first layers are analogous to the layers of simple cells and complex cells of the network in Figure E–3, the subsequent layers are meant to model visual areas of cortex beyond V1. Using Boolean logic as an approximation of the operations performed by the elements in the Neocognitron, one can say that layers alternate between computing conjunctions and disjunctions.[4] In other words, the conjunction-disjunction scheme of the Hubel-Wiesel model is cascaded to form a hierarchical system. In the output layer retinotopic organization disappears completely. There are only 10 output neurons, each of which is selective for one of the digits "0" through "9." In a number of simulations the output neurons show an impressive degree of invariance to the location of the digit in the retina as well as to distortions of the digit.

A similar model was later developed by Yann LeCun and his colleagues. This model, called *LeNet,* adheres closely to the standard definition of a perceptron. The backpropagation algorithm was used to change the synaptic strengths of LeNet so as to reduce the error rate in recognizing images (Box E–2). LeNet achieved sufficient accuracy in recognizing handwritten characters to be used in some commercial applications.

[3]The strengths of the synapses in the Neocognitron were not specified by its designer. Instead, the Neocognitron learned from a sequence of visual stimuli through synaptic modifications based on a model of Hebbian plasticity (see Box E–2).

[4]Boolean logic is just an approximation, as the model neurons in the Neocognitron are actually analog rather than binary.

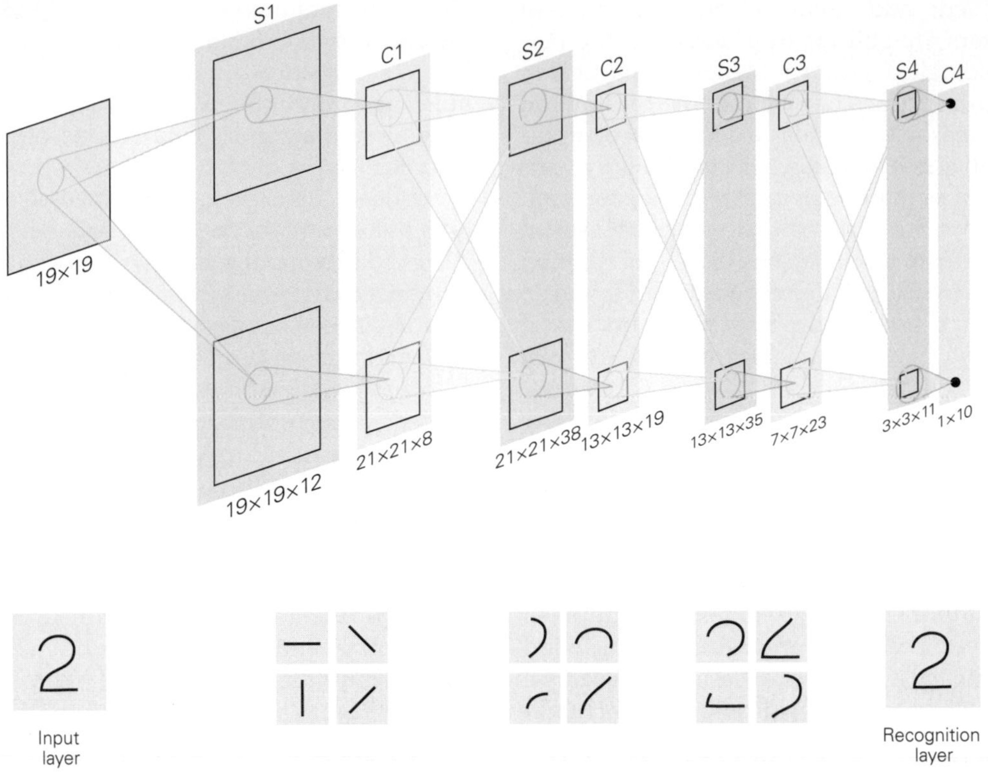

Figure E–4 **The Neocognitron model of digit recognition.** Each layer in the network is composed of a set of feature maps, and alternating layers contain "S-cells" or "C-cells." All feature maps are retinotopically organized because each cell receives input from neighboring cells of the previous layer. Each cell in a feature map detects the same feature but at different locations in the image.

An S-cell is analogous to a simple cell in the Hubel-Wiesel neurobiological model. It detects conjunction of features detected by C-cells in the previous layer. A C-cell is analogous to a complex cell in the Hubel-Wiesel model. It can be activated by any of the S-cells in the previous layer, which detect the same feature but at slightly different locations in the image. Receptive fields of cells become larger until the retinotopic organization vanishes completely in the final (recognition) layer.

The Neocognitron was constructed for the purpose of recognizing images of handwritten digits. Accordingly, the output neurons are detectors for the digits "0" through "9" and are highly invariant to small variations. Each S-cell layer generates more complex feature selectivity, and each C-cell layer yields more spatial invariance.

The images at the bottom are examples of preferred stimuli of cells in each layer. S1 and C1 cells respond selectively to oriented bars; S2 and C2 cells are selective for more complex features, such as the conjunction of bars; S3 and C3 cells are selective for still more complex features.

Its descendants are still being used today in the field of computer vision and are competitive with other state-of-the-art approaches.

In the Neocognitron and LeNet the Hubel-Wiesel neurobiological model of V1 is elaborated to the entire process of object recognition. In spite of several decades of intense scrutiny, there remain significant hurdles to testing neural network models of visual processing. To test a model two questions must be addressed. Are there synaptic connections in the brain like those of the model? Is the model a good approximation without other types of connections that are not included? Much experimental evidence concerning these questions is rather indirect and circumstantial. In particular, anatomical techniques for determining the connectivity of cortical circuits are still in their infancy. For example, there is no direct anatomical evidence for the hypothesis that simple cells in V1 are driven by LGN neurons with receptive fields lined up in a row, as originally proposed by Hubel and Wiesel, although there is some indirect physiological evidence.

As mentioned earlier, attempts have been made to arrange visual areas of cortex in a hierarchy that is consistent with the known anatomical connections between areas. When the visual system is modeled as a perceptron, only "bottom-up" connections are included. In

Box E–2 Learning in Neural Networks

The brain can perform many computational tasks that are beyond the capabilities of today's electronic computers, but it is also remarkable for another reason: It is a self-assembled system, wiring up its own synaptic connections, unlike an electronic computer that is actually built by external agents (humans or machines).

To emulate this process of self-assembly or self-organization, many neural models are equipped with dynamic processes that continually reorganize their synaptic connections. Some processes create or eliminate neurons or their connections, whereas others adjust the strengths of existing synaptic connections or change other properties of neurons.

To describe the process of self-organization, it is helpful to introduce some terminology for describing the synaptic organization of neural networks. The term *synaptic weight* is often used to refer to the strength of a particular synaptic connection, whereas the term *synaptic weight matrix* applies to the set of all synaptic weights in a network. The strength of the synapse onto neuron i from neuron j is written as W_{ij}. This is the element of the weight matrix located at the intersection of row i and column j (see Box E–1).

In many neural network models the weight matrix evolves in time according to a *synaptic plasticity rule*, a mathematical model governing the modifications of synaptic strengths. This is often called a *learning rule*, although strictly speaking, learning is a behavior of a network rather than a synapse.

The network typically starts out in a naïve state, that is, the weight matrix is initialized with random values. Then the network is exposed to a series of stimuli, each of which causes the weight matrix to be modified by the learning rule. Learning rules can take many forms. Much effort has been devoted to devising them and exploring their properties. The Hebbian rule is popular in neurobiological models; with this rule synapses are modified based on temporally contiguous activity of presynaptic and postsynaptic neurons.

It is common to apply the same learning rule to all synapses (or sometimes all excitatory synapses). In spite of this uniformity, the weight matrix becomes heterogeneous because the learning rule depends on activity, and activity patterns are typically nonuniform across a network. Therefore, very complex networks can be produced by a simple learning rule.

In some cases the life of the network is separated into training and operating phases. In the training phase synapses change, whereas in the operating phase the learning rules are turned off. This is analogous to natural development in which plasticity seems particularly strong in juvenile animals. In other cases the learning rules may be turned off gradually. In fully online learning the learning rules are never turned off, so that the network is always able to adapt to new situations.

It is commonly assumed that reorganization of neural networks in the brain is a decentralized process in which synapses are modified as a result of the interaction of the pre- and postsynaptic neurons rather than in response to signals from some central authority. The Hebbian rule is an example. A consequence of such localized self-organization is that one synapse on a neuron can be modified while another remains unchanged. Such specificity is generally observed in biological experiments on Hebbian plasticity, although some exceptions have been reported.

In addition to signaling in the pre- to postsynaptic direction, retrograde messengers such as nitric oxide may also play a role in synaptic plasticity (see Chapter 11), although their role has not been extensively explored in models. The diffuse neuromodulatory systems also have effects on synaptic plasticity (see Chapter 13), and some neural network models have attempted to include interaction between global signals from a central source and local signals as a factor in synaptic modification.

Learning rules are sometimes classified as unsupervised or supervised. *Supervised learning* involves an external "teacher" that evaluates the performance of the entire network and sends a reward or error signal that somehow reaches the synapses. The learning rule is devised so that it produces synaptic modifications that improve the performance of the network as evaluated by the teacher.

One of the most popular supervised learning methods is known as *backpropagation*. When implemented in a perceptron an error signal is propagated back through the network, starting with the output neurons and moving toward the input neurons. The synapses are then modified based on neural activity and the backpropagated error signal.

Backpropagation has been used by engineers for practical applications, such as a computer system for recognizing handwritten numbers based on LeNet. However, it is unclear whether backpropagation is a biologically plausible learning mechanism, even if it may be useful for engineers.

Using *Unsupervised learning* rules, such as the Hebbian rule, the network learns from sensory inputs without an explicit error signal. These learning rules can have a number of computational functions, such as associative learning, discovering useful stimulus features, or reducing the dimensionality of complex stimuli. They have been used to model the self-organization of feature maps in the primary visual cortex during the course of neural development (see Box E–3), as well as to train networks like the Neocognitron.

reality, however, there are also "top-down" connections. In some cases, such as the pathways between LGN and V1, the top-down connections far outnumber the bottom-up ones. It is thought that top-down connections are important for allowing cognitive factors such as expectation to influence perception.

Given these uncertainties and limitations, how useful are perceptrons as models of vision? Although, perceptrons are simplistic—they encompass only a subset of the connections in the visual system—they may capture some essence of the way that neural circuits perform visual computations. Indeed, perceptrons perform impressively on visual tasks such as recognizing handwritten digits, although they still fall short of human performance. Such engineering applications show how far one can push the simple ideas embodied in the perceptron.

Neural networks like the Neocognitron and LeNet model the visual system as a perceptron organized into a hierarchy of feature detectors. These models propose an answer to one of the questions posed at the beginning of this appendix: How is the psychological event of recognizing an object related to the huge number of neural events that underlie it? In a hierarchical perceptron the recognition of an object involves a relatively small number of sequential steps, each of which consists of a large number of operations executed in parallel. Each operation is very simple, carried out by a neuron that is activated when its synaptic inputs drive it above threshold. The sequential steps alternate between selectivity for more complex features and invariance to small distortions of these features. The neurons at the end of this sequence are selective for entire objects, ignoring variations in their appearance. Thus object recognition can be considered as an emergent property of the network, one that requires the coordinated activation of many neurons, located at many different steps.

Fifty years after Rosenblatt's pioneering work it is clear that perceptrons have been important in developing models of computations in the visual system. In the study of visual perception, as in other fields of science, formal models have proved to be valuable aids to experimentalists.

Associative Memory Networks Use Hebbian Plasticity to Store and Recall Neural Activity Patterns

The sight of a familiar face evokes a name. A simple odor triggers the vivid recollection of a past meal and the persons who were there. These everyday experiences illustrate that the facts and ideas stored in our memories are associated with each other. Philosophers and psychologists have argued that association is the basic principle of all mental activity. Neuroanatomists have studied the way that neurons are bound together in a web of synaptic connections. The two traditions converge in an intuitively appealing idea: Perhaps synaptic connections are the material substrate of mental associations.

This idea has been formalized in a number of neural network models of associative memory. A fundamental assumption in these models is that information is transferred back and forth between neural activity and synaptic connections. When novel information first enters the brain it is encoded in a pattern of neural activity. If this information is stored as memory, the neural activity leaves a trace in the brain in the form of modified synaptic connections. The stored information can be recalled when the modified connections again become active. This scheme assumes that synaptic connections remain stable for long periods of time, whereas neural activity is ephemeral and represents immediate experience only.

The transfer of information from neural activity to synapses is hypothesized to occur through Hebbian synaptic plasticity: A long-lasting increase in synaptic efficacy is induced if the presynaptic neuron repeatedly participates in the firing of its postsynaptic neuron (Box E–3). Some prominent forms of long-term potentiation involving the NMDA-type glutamate receptor are regarded as Hebbian (see Chapter 67). Conversely, the transfer of information from synapses to neural activity is thought to occur through a process of pattern completion in which activity spreads through an assembly of neurons coupled by synaptic loops. This idea is explained in more detail below.

Hebbian Plasticity May Store Activity Patterns by Creating Cell Assemblies

How might Hebbian plasticity transfer information from neural activity into the synapses of a neural network? One scenario is illustrated in Figure E–5, which depicts a population of excitatory neurons that could represent pyramidal neurons in the hippocampus or neocortex. It is common to assume that Hebbian plasticity modifies the synapses between pyramidal neurons but does not modify synapses involving inhibitory neurons. According to this theory, inhibitory neurons play only a supporting role in memory storage and recall by helping to prevent overexcitation of the network, or "confused" recall of multiple memories

Box E–3 Mathematical Models of Hebbian Plasticity

Associative memory networks were developed by a number of researchers.[1] In their modern form they have two essential features. First, the synaptic strengths are specified by a special type of matrix, called a correlation matrix. Second, the neurons are nonlinear, which enhances the ability of the models to perform the operation of pattern completion described in the main text.[2]

To store an activity pattern in long-term memory in a nonlinear network of the form written in Equation E–1 in Box E–1, synaptic strengths are changed by the *Hebbian rule*:

$$\Delta W_{ij} \propto x_i x_j \qquad \textbf{(E–3)}$$

This synaptic learning rule is Hebbian because it depends on the simultaneous activation of the postsynaptic neuron i and the presynaptic neuron j. (For binary neurons the change in Equation E–3 is only nonzero if x_i and x_j are both equal to 1.) If Equation E–3 is repeatedly applied with activity patterns drawn from an ensemble, then W_{ij} becomes proportional to the statistical *correlation* between the activities of neurons i and j (hence the term *correlation matrix*).

A popular modification of the basic Hebbian rule is to replace Equation E–3 by the *Covariance rule*:

$$\Delta W_{ij} \propto (x_i - \langle x_i \rangle)(x_j - \langle x_j \rangle) \qquad \textbf{(E–4)}$$

where $\langle x_i \rangle$ is the average activity of neuron i. When this is applied to an ensemble of activity patterns, W_{ij} becomes proportional to the statistical *covariance* between the activities of neurons i and j.

[1]See J.A. Anderson and E. Rosenfeld, *Neurocomputing: Foundations of Research*, 1988, IT Press.

[2]These two properties were first combined in associative memory networks by Shun-ichi Amari and Kaoru Nakano working independently in 1972.

The number of patterns that can be stored in synaptic connections is limited because the patterns eventually interfere with each other (see Figure E–6). The maximal number that can be stored is called the *capacity* of the network. In 1985 Daniel Amit, Hanoch Gutfreund, and Haim Sompolinsky introduced techniques from the statistical physics of disordered systems to calculate memory capacity. Later researchers used these techniques to find that the covariance rule of Equation E–4 is generally superior to the basic Hebbian rule of Equation E–3 because it reduces interference between patterns and therefore enhances storage capacity.

Physiologists have found that Hebbian plasticity can depend on the precise timing of presynaptic and postsynaptic spiking. One example of such a mechanism is spike timing-dependent plasticity (see Chapter 67). To incorporate this dependence, models more sophisticated than Equations E–3 and E–4 have been proposed (see the bibliography at the end of the appendix).

The main text of this appendix focuses on the use of the Hebbian rule in models of associative memory. However, the Hebbian rule has also been used to model the development of retinotopic maps in visual areas of cortex. Also, it is believed that Hebbian plasticity allows neuronal activity to influence the patterning and refinement of connections during neural development (see Chapter 56). In 1973 Christoph von der Malsburg advanced a neural network model of primary visual cortex in which Hebbian plasticity underlies the self-organization of orientation maps when the model network is exposed to visual stimuli.

In 1982 Teuvo Kohonen proposed a simplification of von der Malsburg's model, known as the self-organizing map (SOM). Kohonen showed how the SOM served as a general method of mapping the abstract high-dimensional space of stimuli onto a low-dimensional neural representation, as in a sheet of cortical tissue. Kohonen's learning rule causes neighboring neurons in the network to develop preferences for similar stimuli. This yields a low-dimensional map of the stimulus space based on similarities between sensory inputs.

at the same time. For simplicity, inhibitory neurons are not included in the model in Figure E–5.

The initial state of this network has no connections between neurons (Figure E–5A). This should not be taken literally. It depicts an initial situation in which synapses exist but are all very weak. Now suppose that three neurons are stimulated by synapses from sources outside the circuit (Figure E–5B). This situation corresponds roughly to activation of a distributed pattern of neural activity in the brain by a sensory stimulus, as is often observed in neurophysiological studies. Every synapse between a pair of active neurons is therefore exposed to coincident presynaptic and postsynaptic activity, thus strengthening the synapses.

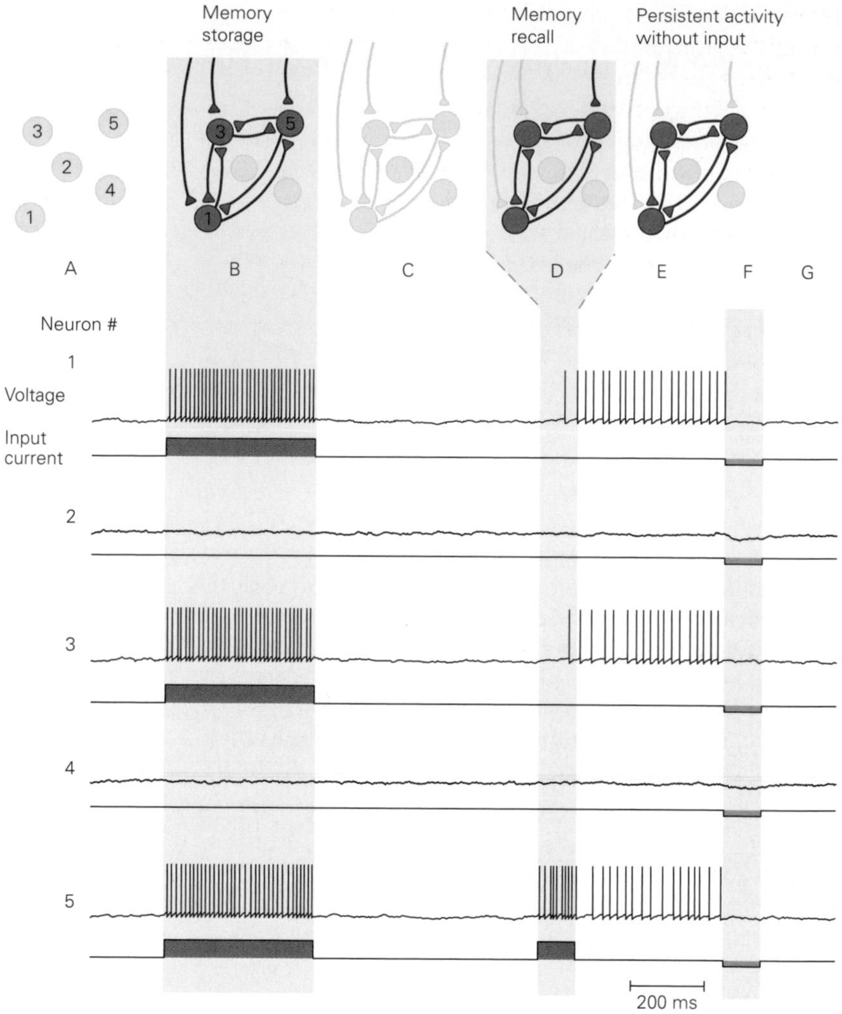

Figure E–5 Associative memory and persistent activity in a network of model neurons. Numerical simulations were done using the leaky integrate-and-fire model neuron described in Appendix F. This model neuron generates spike times but not the detailed shape of the action potential.

A. The synaptic connections between five neurons are initially very weak or nonexistent, and here are not drawn at all. Neurons 1, 3, and 5 are about to be activated by external input.

B. Input current activates the three neurons and Hebbian plasticity causes the synaptic connections between the neurons to strengthen, a form of associative memory storage.

C. When the input current ceases neuronal activity also ceases. The Hebbian strengthening of connections occurs during this interval after some time delay.

D. Input current stimulates just one of the original three neurons, but the excitatory connections complete the entire pattern. All three neurons of the pattern become activated.

E. Even after the input current has ended, the neurons remain persistently active.

F. A nonselective inhibitory input to all the neurons (circuit not depicted) quenches the persistent activity pattern.

G. The circuit returns to a quiescent state.

After this strengthening has occurred, a group of three neurons that are strongly coupled by excitatory synapses form a *cell assembly* (Figure E–5C). Neuroscientists generally use this term rather imprecisely. One must look to mathematical models of networks for more precise definitions, which generally have something to do with the presence of strong mutual excitatory interactions within a group of neurons. The word "assembly" emphasizes that the group did not initially exist but was constructed through the strengthening of the synapses of the neurons in the group, which in turn was caused by the simultaneous activation of the neurons.

In effect, the information in the original activity pattern is transferred to the pattern of strong synapses in the cell assembly. If the synaptic changes persist, the information is maintained even after the original activity pattern has ceased. It could be said that the network has learned an activity pattern by storing it into its synaptic strengths. Because of this, the cell assembly can replicate the original activity pattern, as will be explained below.

Cell Assemblies Can Complete Activity Patterns

If inputs are limited to one neuron in the three-cell assembly, the neuron starts to generate action potentials (Figure E–5D). Although the external inputs to the other two neurons do not change, they also become activated after a short latency because they are driven by synaptic input from the first neuron. This spreading of activation from one neuron to the other two is an example of *pattern completion*. Researchers have scaled up the same idea to very large networks.

Such a neural process is thought to be responsible for the psychological phenomenon of memory retrieval. Consider the example of seeing a friend and remembering his name and occupation. Partial information triggers recall of more information based on the completion of a neural activity pattern.

In the simulation in Figure E–5, stimulating any one out of the three neurons would result in completion of the entire pattern. This is a kind of symmetry and is analogous to the way in which memory retrieval can be symmetric; it is equally possible for a face to evoke recall of a name and vice versa. Symmetric pattern completion is possible for a cell assembly because of the lack of directionality in its connectivity. Activity can spread in any direction within a cell assembly except that activity in the last layer cannot spread backward to the rest of the network.

In the CA3 region of the hippocampus, a brain area that has been implicated in episodic memory (see Chapter 65), pyramidal neurons make synapses onto each other in a recurrent fashion, and Hebbian plasticity has been observed at these synapses. Therefore CA3 seems a prime candidate for a network containing cell assemblies, as many theorists have speculated in the past. The hypothesis that Hebbian synaptic plasticity stores memories as cell assemblies in CA3 has been investigated in studies of hippocampal place cells in rodents, the connections between which are thought to store spatial memories (see Chapter 67). Susumu Tonegawa and his colleagues created mutant mice in which a subunit of the NMDA-type glutamate receptor was deleted from CA3 pyramidal neurons. Long-term potentiation was impaired at these synapses, supporting the idea that the NMDA receptor is critical for Hebbian synaptic plasticity. Interestingly, mutant mice are still able to form spatial memories but have difficulty recalling them if some of the original visual landmarks are missing. Tonegawa and his colleagues interpreted this deficit in recall as impaired pattern completion, and ascribed it to impaired formation of cell assemblies in CA3.

Cell Assemblies Can Maintain Persistent Activity Patterns

Up to now our discussion of memory storage in synaptic connections has focused on long-term memory. Recall of a long-term memory occurs through the reactivation of a previous activity pattern, triggered by activation of a subset of the pattern. Once the activity pattern has been reactivated it can persist even after the extrinsic drive has ended because the neurons excite each other through their mutual excitatory connections.

Such persistent activity could also function as a short-term memory trace of the input that activated it. Short-term memory is generally regarded as distinct from long-term memory. For example, the famous patient H.M. lost the ability to store new long-term memories but had intact short-term memory, evidence that these are two distinct functions (see Chapter 65).

A classic example of short-term memory is the temporary memorization of a phone number for a few seconds after reading or hearing it. After dialing the phone number the information is rapidly lost from memory. If the phone number becomes too long, as when dialing internationally, it can be difficult to retain for even a few seconds. As this example illustrates, short-term memories last for only a very short time and contain limited information. In contrast, long-term memories can last a lifetime, and our brains seem to have virtually unlimited capacity for them.

As described in Chapter 67, similar short-term persistent activity has been observed in the primate brain during the performance of delayed-match-to-sample tasks that are designed to test short-term memory. For example, in each trial of an experiment a monkey views a sample image on a screen, then a blank screen during a delay period, and then another image. The monkey is trained to indicate whether the second image matches the first. In the primary visual cortex neural activity is observed only when the images are presented. However, in higher-level areas, such as inferotemporal and prefrontal cortex, persistent activity is also observed during the interval between images (see Figure 28–11). By sampling many neurons during this delay period, neurophysiologists have recorded distinct activity patterns corresponding to different sample images, suggesting that these activity patterns encode information about previously viewed images.

To summarize, the cell assembly concept has been used to explain both long-term and short-term memory. According to this concept a long-term memory is stored as strengthened connections between neurons in a cell assembly, while a short-term memory is maintained by persistent activity of the neurons in a cell assembly. Whether these ideas are correct remains uncertain, and some of their problematic aspects will be noted later. It should also be noted that not all associative memory networks depend on persistent activity. For example, in the network in Figure E–5 some numerical parameters could be changed so that pattern completion occurs during the stimulus presentation but not after the stimulus is gone.

Interference Between Memories Limits Capacity

Figure E–5 illustrates the storage and retrieval of a single activity pattern. In fact, however, a single network can store multiple patterns. If Hebbian synaptic modifications store multiple patterns, many cell assemblies are created. A stored pattern can be retrieved by stimulating some of the neurons in the corresponding cell assembly, leading to completion of the entire activity pattern.

However, the storage capacity of a network is not infinite. If the cell assemblies are completely nonoverlapping (share no neurons in common) they will not interfere with each other (Figure E–6A), and in these cases the number of patterns that can be stored is equal to the total number of neurons in the network divided by the size of a cell assembly.

Higher storage capacity can be achieved if the cell assemblies overlap (share neurons). However, overlap means there is the possibility of interference (Figure E–6B). Interference can lead to corruption of memories, so that the activity patterns expressed by the network deviate from the original patterns that were stored by Hebbian plasticity. If we attempt to store too many patterns in the network, interference eventually becomes catastrophic—the stored patterns disappear altogether. Therefore interference effects limit the storage capacity of the network, and mathematical theorists have studied these effects in detail.

Synaptic Loops Can Lead to Multiple Stable States

To describe how cell assembly can maintain different types of activity patterns, we use the concept of *multistability*, a term from dynamical systems theory.

In Figure E–5 the circuit is active during interval E but quiescent during interval G. During the quiescent and active states there is no external input, yet the circuit has two very different firing patterns. Thus the network possesses two possible stable states (active and inactive) for a single input, a phenomenon known as *bistability*. The transient currents at interval F in Figure E–5 switch the circuit from one stable state to the other.

A network with multiple cell assemblies is said to be *multistable* because activation of any one cell assembly produces a distinct stable state of the network. When a multistable system is at a steady state, this state depends on past as well as present input. This dependence on the past explains why the transient inputs of Figure E–5 can have a lasting effect on activity.

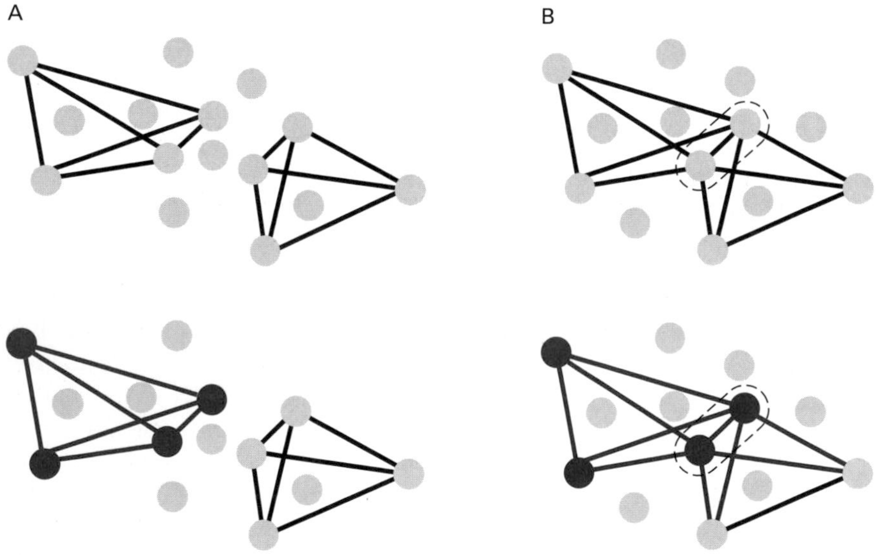

Figure E–6 The potential for interference between overlapping associative memory networks. Each link in the diagram represents a bidirectional pair of excitatory synapses.

A. Two nonoverlapping cell assemblies. Each assembly is a group of neurons that is fully coupled by strong excitatory synapses. Because the cell assemblies share neither neurons nor synapses in common, they are completely independent. One cell assembly alone can be activated (**red**) or both assemblies can be activated simultaneously (not shown).

B. Two overlapping cell assemblies. Because some neurons are involved in both cell assemblies (**dashed line**), there is potential for interference. Activation of one cell assembly could potentially spread to the other cell assembly (**lower drawing**). This can be prevented. If the threshold for neural activation is sufficiently high, the neurons belonging uniquely to the second cell assembly remain below threshold. Conversely, if the threshold is low, then it will be impossible to activate a single cell assembly without the other (not shown).

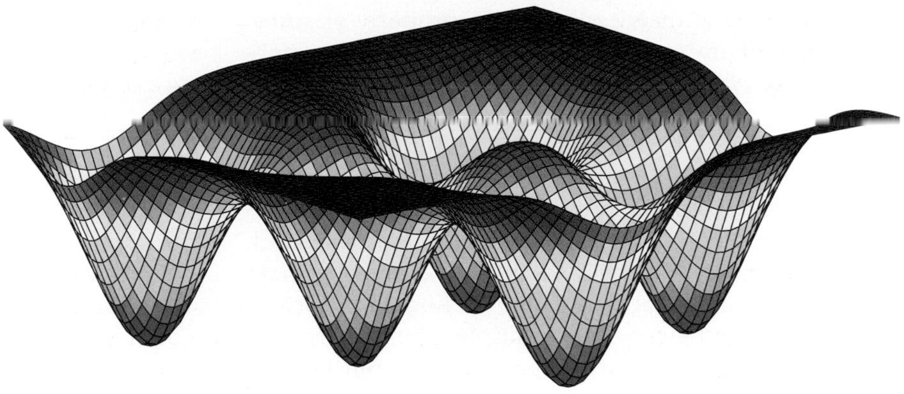

Figure E–7 Multiple stable states can be depicted as minima of an energy-like function. The dynamics of a multistable dynamical system can be visualized as descent on an energy landscape with multiple valleys. In a neural network model, this landscape would represent the space of all potential activity patterns and the valleys, or "attractors" (ie, the patterns that are stable and "attract" the activity). Such attractors could represent memories or, more generally, solutions to a computational problem.

Multistability is caused by the connectivity of the cell assemblies. More generally, networks that contain synaptic loops (a cell assembly is a special case of this) can have multiple stable states. In contrast, a perceptron is a type of network that has no loops and does not exhibit multistability. A network with multiple stable states is often called an *attractor neural network*, borrowing a term from dynamical systems theory.[5] A stable steady state is called an attractor of the dynamics because dynamical trajectories (the temporal evolution of the activity of the network) that start from similar initial conditions will converge (are attracted) to the stable state.

Symmetric Networks Minimize Energy-Like Functions

Further insight into multistability can be gained from a physical analogy. If the curved surface shown in Figure E–7 is slippery, a small object placed on the surface will slide downhill, ultimately coming to rest near the bottom of a valley, assuming that there is a little friction to damp the motion. The object could end up in any one of the valleys, depending on its starting point. Therefore the dynamics of the object is multistable.

The object's motion can be understood using the physical concept of energy. Because the gravitational potential energy of the object is a linear function of its height, the surface can be regarded as a graph of energy versus location in the horizontal plane. The object behaves as if its goal were to minimize its potential energy, in the sense that its downhill motion causes the potential energy to decrease until a minimum is reached. The multiple stable states correspond to the multiple minima of the energy.

In an influential paper published in 1982, John Hopfield constructed a mathematical function that assigns a numerical value to any activity pattern of a neural network model. He proved mathematically that this number is guaranteed to decrease as the activity of the network evolves in time until a stable state is reached. Because of this property, Hopfield's function represents the "energy of the network," and we will call it an *energy function*.[6] The energy of the network is analogous to the height of the sliding object in Figure E–7, and the activity of the network is analogous to the horizontal location of the sliding object. Of course, Figure E–7 is an impoverished depiction of a network energy function because the activity pattern of a network of n neurons is an n-dimensional vector, not a two-dimensional location in the horizontal plane.

As a special case, Hopfield applied the energy function to associative memory networks, showing that the process of memory recall by pattern completion (Figure E–5) is analogous to an object sliding down an energy landscape (Figure E–7).

Hopfield's construction of the energy function required that the interactions between neurons be symmetric: Any connection from one neuron to another is mirrored by another connection of equal strength in the opposite direction. This is the case, for example, in the cell assemblies of Figure E–5. Although perfect symmetry of interactions is not biologically plausible,

[5]Some apply the term *attractor network* rather loosely to any recurrent network, whereas others restrict application to recurrent networks with multistability.

[6]It should be stressed that this is an analogy, that the energy function is distinct from energy in the sense of physics. A minimum of the network energy function might actually correspond to an activity pattern in which neurons are firing at high rates and using large amounts of energy.

approximate symmetry might be a property of some biological neural networks, so that Hopfield's networks might be regarded as an idealization of them.

In 1986 Hopfield and David Tank pointed out that a neural network with an energy function can be used to perform a type of computation known as *optimization*. Many interesting problems in computer science can be formulated as the optimization of some kind of function. For example, in the traveling salesman problem, a salesman would like to find the shortest route by which he can visit multiple cities and return to his starting point. In this problem the function to be optimized is the length of the route. Hopfield and Tank showed how to construct a network that finds solutions to the traveling salesman problem. The energy of their network is equal to the distance of the route, which is encoded by the activity of the network. Because the network converges to a minimum of the energy, it effectively searches for an optimal solution to the traveling salesman problem.

This general approach was applied by many others to construct neural networks that solve a variety of optimization problems. The Hopfield-Tank approach could be viewed as an extension of the cell assembly to a general method of encoding a computational problem in the connections of a recurrent network, which solves the problem by converging to a steady state.

Hebbian Plasticity May Create Sequential Synaptic Pathways

In the simulations in Figure E–5 it is assumed that synapses between pairs of neurons are strengthened when the two neurons are active simultaneously. If signaling flows in both directions between the neurons, the synapses in both directions will be strengthened, preserving the symmetry of the interactions between the neurons.

However, Hebb actually argued that a synapse is strengthened when the presynaptic neuron is activated immediately before the postsynaptic neuron (activity in the presynaptic cell leads to an excitatory postsynaptic potential that contributes to firing the postsynaptic action potential). Hebbian plasticity that depends on temporal order has been observed in spike timing-dependent plasticity (see Chapter 67). The temporal asymmetry of this learning rule can lead to synaptic connectivities that are asymmetric, as opposed to those shown in Figure E–5.

Such asymmetry in the connectivity could be appropriate for the storage and recall of motor sequences, needed in skills such as playing a musical instrument, and which consist of temporally structured steps. Motor sequences are presumably created by sequential activation of groups of neurons. One can imagine storing a sequence in a network by giving it extrinsic inputs that activate neurons in some order. Hebbian plasticity would lead to a set of strengthened connections that are organized like the perceptron of Figure E–1. Later on the sequence could be recalled by activating the first group of neurons, which would activate the second group, and so on. The network would generate the sequence that had been stored by extrinsic input. This would be another example of pattern completion, one in which the pattern is a temporal sequence rather than a stable state as in Figure E–5.

In this hypothetical example the strong connections all point in the same direction, so that the interactions in the network are asymmetric. The network is unable to generate the same sequence in the opposite order because of the asymmetry. This is consistent with the fact that many well-practiced motor sequences are difficult to carry out in reverse order.

It seems plausible that symmetric and asymmetric connections could be important for storing different types of associations. The memory of a telephone number is sequential and asymmetric; remembering it forward is much easier than trying to remember it backward. But other types of associations are more symmetric: A face may evoke a name as easily as a name evokes a face.

In associative memory networks long-term memories are stored through modifications of synaptic strengths that last for long times. But such Hebbian style long-term potentiation is just one type of modification of biological synapses (see Chapter 67). The strengths of biological synapses can change more transiently. Diverse types of transient modification—short-term facilitation, short-term depression, augmentation, and so on—have been classified by their time scales and other properties. It is natural to speculate that these different forms of synaptic alteration could be used by the brain for a whole spectrum of memory processes with different time scales. In this view a firm distinction between short-term and long-term memory is too simplistic.

Previously we explained that a cell assembly supports both short-term and long-term memories. Does this mean that one can only maintain short-term memories of items that have already been stored as long-term memories? Everyday experience suggests that one can briefly maintain a short-term memory of a telephone number that has never been encountered before, for which no long-term memory exists. This issue could perhaps be solved if, as suggested above, the sharp distinction between short-term and long-term memory were replaced by a spectrum of memory processes with different time scales.

As noted in the introduction, the idea that persistent activity is maintained by cell assemblies, or more generally by synaptic loops, dates back to Hebb and Lorente de Nó. Many researchers have developed detailed and realistic simulations based on this idea, simulations that are more convincing than the simple one shown in Figure E–5. But demonstrating empirically that a specific example of persistent activity in the brain is caused by synaptic loops has been difficult. Persistent activity could also arise as an intrinsic property of the biophysics of single neurons, rather than an emergent property of networks. Hence the biological mechanisms of persistent activity are still controversial.

An Overall View

Perceptrons and associative memory networks are two historic types of neural network models still in use today. A perceptron is a layered network with no synaptic loops. Its layers represent sequential steps of a computation, where each layer can be regarded as many operations performed in parallel. The visual system has been modeled as a perceptron in which neurons are feature detectors and are hierarchically organized. According to this hierarchical perceptron model, visual recognition of an object is a sequential process in which each step consists of many feature detection events executed in parallel.

Because perceptrons lack synaptic loops, their dynamical behaviors are relatively simple. But the dynamics of the brain can evolve in ways that are dissociated from immediate sensory stimuli or motor actions. These rich intrinsic dynamics are likely to depend on loops in the synaptic connectivity of the brain. Hebbian plasticity is thought to create cell assemblies, which contain synaptic loops. These loops can endow a neural network with the property of multistability, and also lead to persistent activity patterns resembling those observed in neurophysiology experiments on short-term memory. Finally, symmetric neural networks, which contain synaptic loops, have been used to solve optimization problems and could therefore be viewed as a general class of computational devices.

Although decades have passed since perceptrons and associative memory networks were invented, it is still unclear how well these models explain visual perception and the storage and recall of memories. Given that these are some of the deepest and most complex issues in neuroscience, perhaps it is not surprising that testing the models experimentally is difficult. But given today's rapid progress in developing new experimental methods, one could imagine that neural network models will eventually come to play as central a role in systems neuroscience as the Hodgkin-Huxley model of the action potential plays in cellular neurophysiology.

Sebastian Seung
Rafael Yuste

Selected Readings

Anderson JA, Pellionisz A, Rosenfeld E. 1990. *Neurocomputing 2: Directions of Research.* Cambridge, MA: MIT Press.

Anderson JA, Rosenfeld E. 1988. *Neurocomputing: Foundations of Research.* Cambridge, MA: MIT Press.

Churchland PS, Sejnowski TJ. 1992. *The Computational Brain.* Cambridge, MA: MIT Press.

Dayan P, Abbott LF. 2001. *Theoretical Neuroscience.* Cambridge, MA: MIT Press.

Hebb DO. 1949. *The Organization of Behavior.* New York: Wiley.

Hopfield JJ, Tank DW. 1986. Computing with neural circuits: a model. Science 233:625–633.

McClelland JL, Rumelhart DE. 1986. *Parallel Distributed Processing, Vol. 2: Psychological and Biological Models.* Cambridge, MA: MIT Press.

Minsky ML. 1967. *Computation: Finite and Infinite Machines.* Englewood Cliffs, NJ: Prentice-Hall.

Rolls ET, Treves A. 1998. *Neural Networks and Brain Function.* New York: Oxford Univ. Press.

Rumelhart DE, McClelland JL. 1986. *Parallel Distributed Processing, Vol. 1: Explorations in the Microstructure of Cognition.* Cambridge, MA: MIT Press.

Trappenberg TP. 2002. *Fundamentals of Computational Neuroscience.* New York: Oxford Univ. Press.

References

Abbott LF, Nelson SB. 2000. Synaptic plasticity: taming the beast. Nat Neurosci 3:1178–1183.

Amari S-I. 1972. Learning patterns and pattern sequences by self-organizing nets of threshold elements. IEEE Trans Comput C-21:1197–1206.

Amit DJ, Gutfreund H, Sompolinsky H. 1985. Spin-glass models of neural networks. Phys Rev A32:1007–1018.

Bain A. 1873. *Mind and Body: The Theories of Their Relation.* New York: Appleton.

Ben-Yishai R, Bar-Or RL, Sompolinsky H. 1995. Theory of orientation tuning in visual cortex. Proc Natl Acad Sci U S A 92:3844–3848.

Bonhoeffer T, Staiger V, Aertsen A. 1989. Synaptic plasticity in rat hippocampal slice cultures: local "Hebbian" conjunction of pre- and postsynaptic stimulation leads to distributed synaptic enhancement. Proc Natl Acad Sci U S A 86:8113–8117.

Cohen MA, Grossberg S. 1983. Absolute stability of global pattern formation and parallel memory storage by competitive neural networks. IEEE Trans Syst Man Cybern SMC 13:815–826.

Felleman DJ, Van Essen DC. 1991. Distributed hierarchical processing in the primate cerebral cortex. Cerebr Cortex 1:1–47.

Ferster D, Miller KD. 2000. Neural mechanisms of orientation selectivity in the visual cortex. Annu Rev Neurosci 23:441–471.

Fukushima KM. 1980. Neocognitron: a self-organizing neural network model for a mechanism of pattern recognition unaffected by shift in position. Biol Cybern 36:193–202.

Griniasty M, Tsodyks MV, Amit DJ. 1993. Conversion of temporal correlations between stimuli to spatial correlations between attractors. Neural Comput 5:1–17.

Hopfield JJ. 1982. Neural networks and physical systems with emergent collective computational abilities. Proc Natl Acad Sci U S A 79:2554–2558.

Hubel DH, Wiesel TN. 1962. Receptive fields, binocular interaction and functional architecture in the cat's visual cortex. J Physiol 160:106–154.

Kohonen T. 1989. *Self-organization and Associative Memory*. Berlin: Springer-Verlag.

LeCun Y, Boser B, Denker JS, Henderson D, Howard RE, Hubbard W, Jackel LD. 1989. Backpropagation applied to handwritten zip code recognition. Neural Comput 1:541–551.

Leutgeb S, Leutgeb JK, Moser MB, Moser EI. 2005. Place cells, spatial maps and the population code for memory. Curr Opin Neurobiol 15:738–746.

Lorente de Nó R. 1938. Analysis of the activity of the chains of internuncial neurons. J Neurophysiol 1:207–244.

Major G, Tank DW. 2004. Persistent neural activity: prevalence and mechanisms. Curr Opin Neurobiol 14:675–684.

McNaughton BL. 1996. Deciphering the hippocampal polyglot: the hippocampus as a path integration system. J Exp Biol 199:173–185.

Nakazawa K, Quirk MC, Chitwood RA, Watanabe M, Yeckel MF, Sun LD, Kato A, et al. 2002. Requirement for hippocampal CA3 NMDA receptors in associative memory recall. Science 297:211–218.

Riesenhuber M, Poggio T. 1999. Hierarchical models of object recognition in cortex. Nat Neurosci 2:1019–1025.

Shapley R, Hawken M, Ringach DL. 2003. Dynamics of orientation selectivity in the primary visual cortex and the importance of cortical inhibition. Neuron 38:689–699.

Somers D, Nelson SB, Sur M. 1995. An emergent model of orientation selectivity in cat visual cortical simple cells. J Neurosci 15:5448–5465.

Tsodyks M, Feigelman M. 1988. Enhanced storage capacity in neural networks with low level of activity. Europhys Lett 6:101–105.

Appendix F

Theoretical Approaches to Neuroscience: Examples from Single Neurons to Networks

In one way or another all scientific researchers construct models. The role of theory is to develop, refine, and investigate these models to uncover new insights and to make new predictions. Theoretical (or computational) neuroscience explores the application of mathematical and computational methods to the study of neural systems.

Defining models of neural systems in mathematical terms assures that the models are self-consistent, with clearly revealed assumptions and limitations. Formulating models mathematically also allows the powerful techniques of mathematics and physics and the extraordinary capacity of modern computers to be used to understand model behavior. This power allows the implications of the models to be worked out fully, revealing features that are surprising and nonintuitive.

What makes a model good? Clearly it must be based on biological reality, but modeling necessarily involves an abstraction of that reality. It is important to appreciate that a more detailed model is not necessarily a better model. A simple model that allows us to think about a phenomenon more clearly is more powerful than a model with underlying assumptions and mechanisms that are obscured by complexity. The purpose of modeling is to illuminate, and the ultimate test of a model is not simply that it makes predictions that can be tested experimentally, but whether it leads to better understanding. No matter how detailed, no model can capture all aspects of the phenomenon being studied. As theoretical neuroscientist Idan Segev has said, borrowing from Picasso's description of art, modeling is the lie that reveals the truth.

Appendix E introduced two ideas that are central in theoretical neuroscience: the perceptron and the attractor. In this appendix we extend the discussion of theoretical neuroscience by considering the effect of synaptic input on neuron models that produce action potentials, by showing how inhibition and excitation can interact in network models to produce interesting and nonintuitive effects, and by presenting a model of decision-making. These examples convey a sense of how theoretical neuroscience research is done, and how it can shed light on the types of computations that neurons and networks of neurons can perform.

Single-Neuron Models Allow Study of the Integration of Synaptic Inputs and Intrinsic Conductances

Models of single neurons include some of the most detailed, accurate, and complex simulations performed in the field of theoretical neuroscience. Single-neuron modeling is used to reveal how the many different voltage- and ligand-dependent conductances expressed by a neuron interact to generate patterns of activity ranging from transient and sustained firing to the production of subthreshold oscillations and action-potential bursts. Because membrane conductances are nonlinear, interactions between them can be complex. Modeling studies allow these interactions to be mapped out and understood.

Another major focus of single-neuron modeling is to understand the functional consequences of the complex and beautiful morphology of neurons. One goal of this work is to understand how the specific location of a synapse or group of synapses on the dendritic arbor, in interaction with the voltage-dependent conductances in dendrites, affects the efficacy of synapses to drive a neuron to fire. Synaptic plasticity is also a major target of dynamically detailed modeling of neurons. In this regard backpropagating action potentials, which provide information to the synapses about the timing of somatic action potentials, are of particular interest. This work, and of course its experimental counterpart, has revealed the roles of nonlinear summation, subthreshold boosting, and dendritic spiking in the integration of inputs across the dendrite.

Single-neuron modeling studies are also valuable for understanding the effects of complex patterns of synaptic inputs on neuronal activity. In an experimental setting it is difficult to control large numbers of synaptic inputs precisely enough to perform analogous studies. Neurons are often studied in fairly inactive tissue slices or isolated in cell cultures. In vitro experiments can tell us how a particular neuron responds to the activation of one or a few synapses (from paired recordings, for example) or to synchronous activation of many synapses (through extracellular stimulation). Studying neurons with controlled synaptic input is ideal for exploring their basic electrophysiological characteristics, but not for understanding how they operate in vivo. We typically want to know how the neuron reacts to the complex input patterns that it receives from thousands of afferent fibers in a live animal. Theoretical studies allow us to bridge the gap between what we know from reduced experimental protocols and what we need to know to understand functioning neural circuits: the response properties of neurons in their natural environment.

Appendix E considered a neuron model in which synchronous presynaptic action potentials are counted and compared with a threshold to determine output. Here we examine how the large quantity of constant synaptic input in vivo modifies this picture, focusing on the effects of synchronization and timing of presynaptic inputs on the response of a neuron. Action potentials are also known as *spikes*, and we use the two terms interchangeably.

The role of spike synchronization in neural coding and signaling is actively debated. Synchronization of spikes has been proposed as a mechanism by which attention might enhance signals of particular interest, based on the observation that synchronous action potentials drive a neuron more strongly than the same number of action potentials spread over time. However, it is unlikely that all inputs to a neuron would ever be synchronized. Instead, we assume that the neuron receives a "background" of many asynchronous inputs, and that a small number of these inputs, which we call the signaling inputs, become synchronized by a particular signal or drive. Thus we need to study the effects of various degrees of synchronization in subsets of signaling inputs in a background of asynchronous input. Studying the effects of spike timing in more realistic conditions allows us to assess more accurately the role that timing may play in neural coding of information and in synaptic plasticity.

We will compare the sensitivity of neurons to the numbers and timing precision of synchronous signaling inputs in a quiet slice-like setting and in an active environment of asynchronous background inputs resembling that found in vivo. We will use a simple but useful model of the postsynaptic neuron known as the *integrate-and-fire model* in which inputs are integrated until a threshold voltage is reached, at which point a spike is emitted and the voltage is then reset to a lower value (Box F–1). By studying the responses of this model neuron we can compare the impacts of spike synchronization with and without asynchronous background input.

Neurons Show Sharp Threshold Sensitivity to the Number and Synchrony of Synaptic Inputs in Quiet Conditions Resembling In Vitro

We first explore the sensitivity of our integrate-and-fire model neuron to the number of synchronous signaling inputs it receives in the absence of any background asynchronous input. Under these conditions 43 synchronous presynaptic inputs are required to elicit an action potential (Figure F–1A).

Box F–1 The Integrate-and-Fire Model

The integrate-and-fire model is a model of real neurons that is simplified in three essential ways. It consists of a single compartment (typically only a cell body); its relationship between membrane current and membrane potential is linear; and it fires action potentials through a threshold-crossing rule.

Nevertheless, the model captures three essential features of the biophysics of neurons: membrane resistance, membrane capacitance, and action potential generation. In the model the membrane potential V for a neuron receiving a synaptic current I is governed by the equation

$$C_{\mathrm{m}} \frac{dV}{dt} = \frac{V_{\mathrm{rest}} - V}{R_{\mathrm{m}}} + I \qquad \textbf{(F–1)}$$

where C_{m} is the membrane capacitance, R_{m} the membrane resistance, V_{rest} the resting potential of the neuron, and I the current arising from synaptic inputs. This is the same equation used in Chapter 6 to describe passive changes in the membrane potential of a neuron.

Action potentials are generated by augmenting the equation with a rule: When the membrane potential reaches a threshold value, V_{th}, an action potential is generated and the membrane potential is reset to a value V_{reset}. After this the membrane potential is held at V_{reset} for a refractory period and then released to obey Equation F–1 once more.

To generate spontaneous background synaptic input in the single-neuron model, I is modeled to duplicate the effects of a large population of excitatory and inhibitory synapses being activated by constant-rate Poisson spike trains. For the network example, I for each neuron represents synaptic currents activated by other neurons in the network.

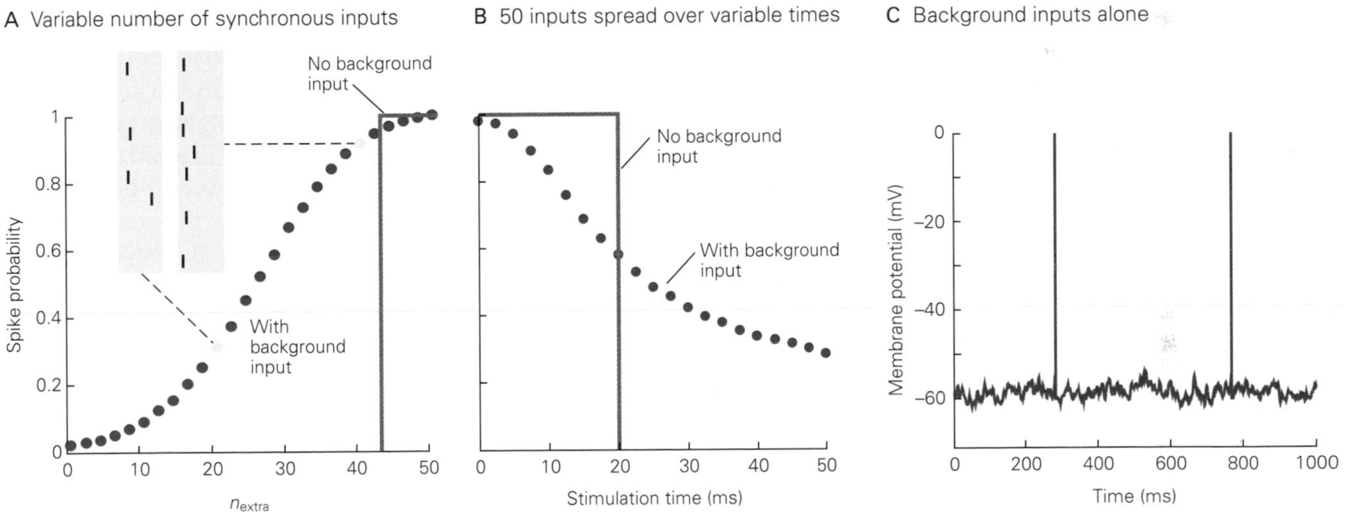

Figure F–1 Responses of an integrate-and-fire model neuron to synchronous input.

A. The plot shows the probability of a postsynaptic action potential or spike in response to synchronous input from n_{extra} excitatory synapses, both with and without any background (asynchronous) synaptic input. Without background input there is a sharp threshold: 42 synchronous inputs never give a spike, whereas 43 such inputs always do. With background input there is a much more gradual change in spike probability with the number of synchronous inputs and an increased sensitivity to small numbers of such inputs. The inset shows sample raster plots of postsynaptic spikes from 10 trials in the presence of background input plus either 20 synchronous excitatory synapses (**left**) or 40 (**right**). (Each row represents one trial; each vertical dash represents the time of occurrence of a postsynaptic action potential.)

B. The plot shows the probability of a postsynaptic action potential being generated by 50 signaling inputs with varying degrees of synchrony. Spreading the inputs uniformly over the stimulation time varies the degree of synchrony. With no background synaptic input there is a sharp threshold, so that if all inputs fire within 20 ms they always generate a spike; otherwise they never do. With an asynchronous background the transition is much more gradual, so that even with relatively little synchrony there is a significant probability of evoking a spike.

C. Asynchronous background input alone drives a low level of firing even in the absence of any signaling input, as seen by the two spikes that occur in the 1 second sample trace. The peaks of the action potentials have been clipped at 0 mV.

The number 43 depends on the particular model parameters we have chosen, but a more general property is also revealed. For the model in Appendix E the probability of producing a spike rises as a sharp step from 0 to 1, meaning that fewer than 43 synchronous presynaptic action potentials will never produce a response, whereas 43 or more will always produce a postsynaptic spike. Thus, when synchronous input appears alone without any asynchronous inputs, the neuron has a sharp threshold sensitivity to the number of synchronous action potentials it receives.

How sensitive is the neuron to timing of the signaling synaptic inputs? To address this question we look at what happens when the synchronous action potentials are spread over a finite period of time, thereby slightly desynchronizing them. When 50 input spikes are spread evenly over intervals ranging from zero to 50 ms, the model neuron responds only if the 50 input spikes are contained within an interval of 20 ms or less (Figure F–1B), indicating that it is quite sensitive to the interval over which the 50 input spikes are spread. Not surprisingly, the 20 ms interval matches the membrane time constant of the model neuron. Thus in the absence of asynchronous input this model neuron is highly sensitive to both the number and timing of its synchronous or nearly synchronous inputs.

Neurons Show Graded Sensitivity to the Number and Synchrony of Synaptic Inputs in Noisy Conditions Resembling In Vivo

What is the effect of background synaptic activity on the sensitivity of a neuron to synchronous signaling input? To address this question we again introduce either synchronous or slightly desynchronized signaling input, but this time we add it to ongoing asynchronous background input.

The nature and impact of ongoing background activity, which varies across brain areas, is a subject of intense experimental and theoretical investigation. Experiments that use different recording techniques do not always agree on the spontaneous firing rates even of neurons in the same area, and conflicting values are reported for the total synaptic conductance produced by spontaneous activity. Nevertheless, in studies of the cerebral cortex all researchers agree that background activity is large enough to cause significant fluctuations in the membrane potentials of recorded neurons, sometimes large enough to drive firing.

The background synaptic input we are discussing contains both excitatory and inhibitory components. In some cortical areas the background input appears as occasional bursts amidst relative quiet. In many other cortical areas the background input drives constant, ongoing voltage fluctuations. In these areas there is evidence that the excitatory and inhibitory components are individually quite large but roughly balance or cancel each other out. This cancellation is subject to fluctuations in which excitatory or inhibitory drive momentarily dominates. In the next section we illustrate how a network of deterministic model neurons can generate such fluctuations spontaneously. Here we obtain similar fluctuations by randomly generating presynaptic action potentials.

Ongoing background activity affects how a neuron integrates its signaling inputs. It also acts as a source of noise that usually limits, but in some cases enhances, the sensitivity and precision of responses to signaling inputs. For the single-neuron model we are using the asynchronous background synaptic input has three primary impacts. First, it alters the neuronal membrane potential, in our case raising it from a resting value of 20 mV below threshold to approximately 5 mV below threshold. This effect is caused by the fact that the cancellation or balance between excitation and inhibition is, even on average, only approximate. Because the model neuron is now closer to threshold, it becomes more sensitive to additional input.

Second, the continual activation of both excitatory and inhibitory synaptic conductances by ongoing input increases the overall conductance of the neuron. This lowers its effective time constant, allowing for quicker responses, and also reduces the sensitivity of the neuron to other synaptic input. However, for our model parameters the lowering of sensitivity is more than compensated by the fact that the baseline membrane potential is raised by 15 mV.

Third, background synaptic input introduces fluctuations in the membrane potential that generate a low rate of background firing and add a level of noise to responses to signaling inputs (Figure F–1C).

To study the effect of synchronous signaling input in the presence of this background, we add a number of extra presynaptic spikes at a particular point in time. The addition of 20 synchronous spikes produces a postsynaptic response on 4 out of 10 trials, whereas adding 40 synchronous inputs generates a spiking response on 7 of 10 trials (Figure F–1A). By accumulating results like these over many repeated trials, we can determine how often (on what fraction of trials or, equivalently, with what probability) a postsynaptic action potential is evoked within a short time interval (10 ms) following the synchronous presynaptic input.

Recall that in the absence of background input the model neuron showed sharp threshold sensitivity to the number of synchronized input spikes. This sharp threshold is lost when background input is added, but it is replaced by a higher sensitivity to small numbers of synchronized presynaptic action potentials (Figure F–1A). Rather than requiring at least 43 synchronous excitatory inputs to generate an output, the probability that the neuron will fire in the presence of background activity rises smoothly from zero. The neuron has a significant probability of responding to as few as 10 synchronous presynaptic action potentials.

Ongoing asynchronous background input also alters the probability of evoking a postsynaptic action potential when presynaptic action potentials are not perfectly synchronous but are spread uniformly over a finite stimulation time. Just as the neuron lost its step-like threshold for the number of presynaptic action potentials required to elicit a spike, it also loses its sharp sensitivity to the relative timing of these inputs (Figure F–1B). The neuron responds approximately 30% of the time to 50 additional action potentials even when they are spread over 50 ms. Thus the results in Figures F–1A and F–1B show that background input makes the neuron more sensitive to small numbers of presynaptic spikes but less sensitive to their synchrony (the degree to which they are tightly grouped in time).

Neuronal Messages Depend on Intrinsic Activity and Extrinsic Signals

The issue of whether to think of spike timing or firing rates as the dominant carrier of the "neural code" has been debated extensively, but it is often difficult to understand exactly what is being debated. Action potentials in a particular pathway carry information by virtue of their times of occurrence; they have no other attribute that can be varied systematically.

A steady signal can be adequately represented by neuronal firing rates because there is no temporal structure for spike times to encode. For rapidly fluctuating signals, however, spikes times can be important because they carry information about the timing and amplitude of such fluctuations. Either way we must remember that neurons respond in the context of the active environment in which they operate.

As we see from Figure F–1, inferences made from observations of neurons in a silent environment (without background synaptic input) may underestimate the responsiveness of a neuron to weak excitation. Similarly the ability of the neuron to sharply delineate different levels of input may be overestimated and the neuron's sensitivity to spike timing exaggerated.

Network Models Provide Insight into the Collective Dynamics of Neurons

Models of networks of neurons, or neural circuits, help us understand how large populations of neurons can work together to perform tasks. Using models, theorists have learned how networks can sustain particular patterns of *reverberating* activity or generate oscillatory or chaotic firing.

Network models address such issues as how neurons in primary sensory areas produce their responses, how cortical maps form and are modified by sensory experience, how populations of neurons represent information collectively and combine multisensory data, how objects are identified and classified, how memories stored in modified synaptic strengths can be read out, how motor responses are generated, and how evidence is integrated and used to make decisions.

Appendix E discusses basic ideas of how feed-forward circuitry (circuitry with no synaptic loops) may underlie the response properties of simple and complex cells in the primary visual cortex, and how recurrent circuitry (circuitry with synaptic loops) can create a *cell assembly* with strong mutual excitation among its neurons, allowing the assembly's activity to persist in the absence of a stimulus (thus forming an *attractor*). Here we continue these discussions with examples from network modeling.

We will examine how recurrent loops change both the gain and dynamics of responses to inputs, how a fully recurrent network can have hidden within it an effectively feed-forward structure that allows changes in gain to be separated from changes in dynamics, and how these ideas can give insight into aspects of visual cortex function. We also show how the basic idea of attractors can be extended to create a model of decision-making. Before we consider these examples, we show what can happen when model neurons like the one discussed previously are linked together into a network.

Balanced Networks of Active Neurons Can Generate the Ongoing Noisy Activity Seen In Vivo

When constructing and analyzing large networks it is typically not practical to model the constituent neurons with a high level of detail. Instead, the multitude of synaptic conductances and the complexity of dendritic morphology seen in real neurons are usually distilled down to a bare minimum.

In network models individual neurons are often modeled as integrate-and-fire neurons (see Box F–1) but may also be modeled as *firing-rate neurons*, meaning that only the rate at which a neuron fires is modeled, and not the timing of individual spikes (Box F–2). We employ both neuron models here. Simplifying the descriptions of individual neurons allows us to focus on effects that arise through network interactions.

What happens if we link together a large number of integrate-and-fire neurons through excitatory and inhibitory synapses? Such models typically involve thousands or even hundreds of thousands of neurons connected randomly and sparsely so that the probability of any two neurons being connected is less than 10%. Excitatory and inhibitory neurons are included in roughly the 4:1 proportion seen in cortical circuits.

The activity in such networks takes a number of different forms as shown by Carl van Vreeswijk and Haim Sompolinsky and by Nicolas Brunel. When the synaptic connections are weak, the bulk of the neurons are silent; but some fire in steady, regular sequences of action potentials that are not synchronized with the activity of other neurons of the network (Figure F–2A). As the strengths of the synapses, both excitatory and inhibitory, are increased, the network can transition into a state where the silent neurons start to fire, and the action potentials appear in irregular, asynchronous patterns (Figure F–2B). This form of activity provides a model of the background activity seen in real neural circuits.

The irregular, asynchronous activity depends on the sparseness of the synaptic connections in the network and on a balance between excitatory and inhibitory inputs received by a cell. These inputs arise from many other excitatory and inhibitory neurons that are themselves firing irregularly. Overall these inputs are balanced—on average, excitation and inhibition cancel—but constant fluctuations in input drive the cell to fire at irregular times. Thus the network self-consistently maintains irregular firing in all of its neurons. If the balance of

Box F–2 Firing-Rate Models

A network in which neurons and the interactions between them are described in terms of firing rates has two critical elements. The first is the relationship between the total synaptic current I that a neuron receives and its firing rate r. For current that is constant, this relationship is given in terms of a firing-rate function, $r = F(I)$.

When the current varies with time we assume that the firing rate lags behind but approaches this function exponentially, with a time constant τ, so that

$$\tau\frac{dr}{dt} = -r + F(I).$$

because this is a considerable simplification in the transformation from spiking to firing rate, the time constant τ does not have a straightforward biophysical interpretation and must represent the temporal response properties of the system as a whole, including (but not limited to) the effects of both membrane and synaptic time constants.

The second element needed to construct a network model is the relationship between I and the activity of other neurons in the network. The total current for each neuron is the sum of terms representing each of its inputs. The contribution of an individual presynaptic neuron to I is given by the product of its firing rate and a weight factor that characterizes the strength and type of the synapse through which it acts. The weights for excitatory synapses are positive whereas those for inhibitory synapses are negative.

If the network we are studying receives input from other areas outside the local network, this is included as an additional term in I that we denote by h.

As an example of a firing-rate model, consider a network of two populations of cells. A population of excitatory neurons all fire at a rate r_E and a population of inhibitory neurons fire at rate r_I. The external inputs to these two populations are denoted by h_E and h_I.

The strength of the synaptic connections between neurons of the excitatory population is denoted by w_{EE}, that between the inhibitory neurons by w_{II}, and the connections from the excitatory to the inhibitory and from the inhibitory to the excitatory populations have strengths given by w_{IE} and w_{EI}, respectively.

The resulting equations for the firing rates of the two populations are

$$\tau_E\frac{dr_E}{dt} = -r_E + F(w_{EE}r_E - w_{EI}r_I + h_E) \quad \textbf{(F–2)}$$

$$\tau_I\frac{dr_I}{dt} = -r_I + F(-w_{II}r_I + w_{IE}r_E + h_I). \quad \textbf{(F–3)}$$

Equations similar to these were used for Figures F–3, F–5 through F–7, and in Box F–3.

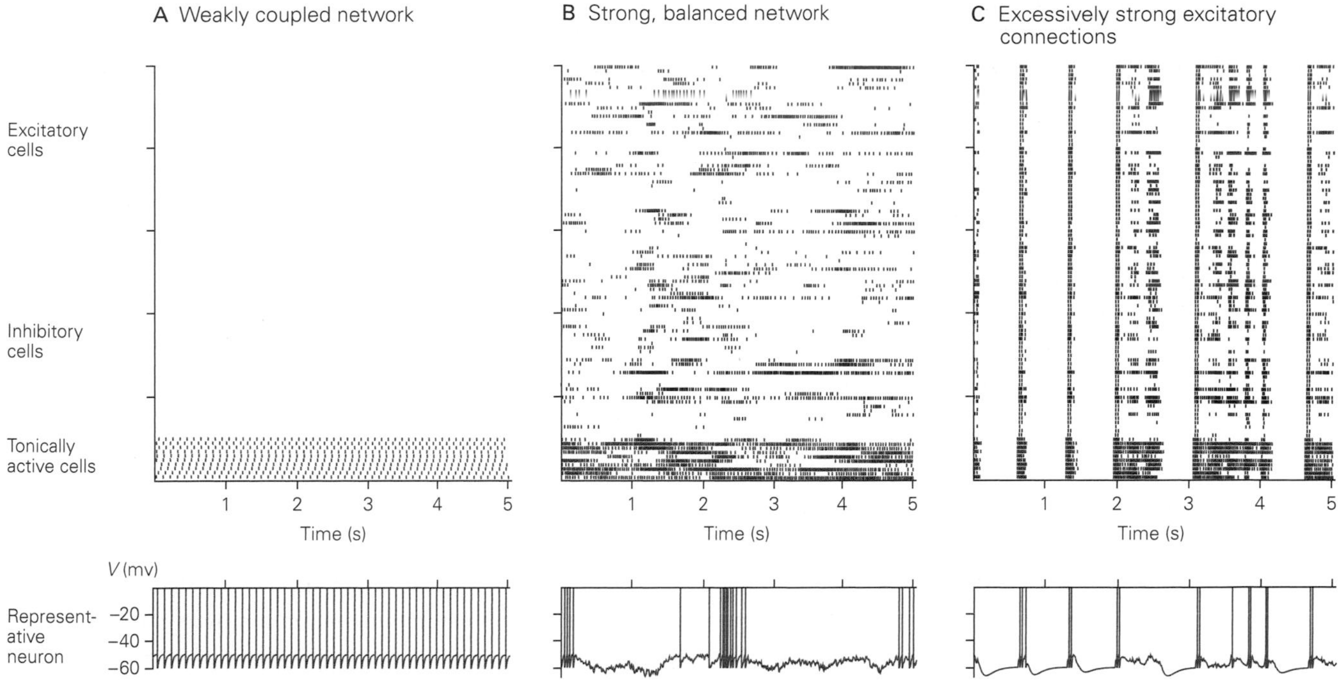

Figure F–2 Activity in networks of spiking neurons. The raster plots show a representative sample of neurons in a network of integrate-and-fire model neurons (only a fraction of network neurons are shown). Each row is a separate neuron, and each dot in a given row represents an action potential fired by that neuron. The voltage traces below the raster plots show a single representative neuron. The trace in part A denotes a tonically active excitatory neuron, while the traces in parts B and C are for nontonically active excitatory neurons. A tonically active neuron is one that receives a constant input current in addition to input from the network but is otherwise identical to the other excitatory neurons. The peaks of the action potentials are clipped at 0 mV.

Individual neurons may fire at regular intervals (regular firing) or at random times (irregular firing). In addition, neurons tend to fire independently rather than synchronizing their spike times (asynchronous firing).

A. In a weakly coupled network the tonically active neurons show regular asynchronous firing while all other neurons are silent.

B. A network with strong but balanced excitation and inhibition exhibits irregular, asynchronous spiking.

C. A network with excessively strong excitation shows seizure-like activity with the synchronous firing of a large fraction of the neurons.

excitation and inhibition is not maintained, a network-model form of epilepsy can arise (Figure F–2C). In this case the asynchronous activity is interrupted by gaps and periods of synchronous firing across the population. It is interesting that network models of ongoing spontaneous activity suffer quite easily from seizure-like activity, just like real neural circuits.

Irregular, asynchronous firing, much like the background firing seen in many cortical areas, can arise in network models with different patterns of synaptic connectivity, such as when the probability of connection between two neurons decreases with the distance between them or with the difference between their selectivities to stimulus properties. The major requirement is that inhibition must balance excitation, so that the mean input cannot drive the cell to fire and instead firing is induced by input fluctuations. In addition, connectivity should be sparse so that the firing of different cells does not become synchronized.

What can structured network circuitry achieve? In the following discussion we provide a few illustrative answers to this question. For this analysis we switch from a network of spiking model neurons to one in which the activities of network neurons are described by firing rates (Box F–2). Networks of spiking model neurons can display patterns of activity that cannot be reproduced by firing-rate models, but there is good agreement between the two types of models for the steady-state asynchronous activity we discuss here and in the following sections. Describing neuronal responses in terms of firing rates makes the mathematical analysis of neural networks much easier.

Feed-forward and Recurrent Networks Can Amplify or Integrate Inputs with Distinct Dynamics

The relative roles played by feed-forward and recurrent circuitry in shaping neuronal responses is a subject of debate in neuroscience. For example, neurons in layer IV of the primary visual cortex receive afferent inputs from the lateral geniculate nucleus of the thalamus, which relays visual information from the eyes, but they also receive abundant innervation from other cortical neurons. Are the tuning properties of these neurons—the dependence of their firing rates on stimulus parameters such as the orientation of a light or dark edge—determined mainly by feed-forward input from the lateral geniculate nucleus, or are they strongly shaped by recurrent cortical feedback?

The answer is not immediately obvious because feed-forward circuits and circuits in which tuning is strongly shaped by recurrence (recurrent networks) can produce the same types of response selectivity or tuning. Intracellular recording in vivo, in which voltage responses and their changes under experimental perturbations are studied, can more clearly distinguish the two types of circuits. However, given only firing rate responses, the differences between feed-forward and recurrent circuits are easiest to detect by examining response dynamics rather than static response properties. For this reason, here we discuss the dynamics of network responses in various forms of feed-forward and recurrent circuits.

A feed-forward circuit can modify input signals, creating a wide variety of response selectivities or amplifying a weak input without significantly altering response dynamics. For example, if one set of neurons forms strong excitatory synapses with another set, a weak input to the first set can yield a strong response in the second. This occurs with only a small dynamic change, namely the small delay required for the first set of neurons to integrate the input and produce spikes that propagate to drive the second set of neurons.

Similarly, recurrent circuits can modify input signals, but typically with larger dynamic changes. An example of this is a circuit that amplifies its inputs through recurrent excitatory loops. Consider a population of neurons that excites itself. The population's response to an external input can be significantly amplified because the recurrent excitation adds to the external drive. However, unlike feed forward amplification the recurrent excitation is accompanied by a general slowing of the population's response dynamics, which arises as follows.

A population responds to a pulse of input with a pulse of activity that then decays away. The recurrent excitation adds back some of the activity that would otherwise decay, slowing the decay of the population's activity. The population's response to a sustained input is similarly slowed; the ultimate response to input is amplified by a factor roughly equal to the degree of slowing (ie, a threefold slowing yields a threefold amplification) (Figure F–3A). This can be understood by thinking of the sustained input as a continuous sequence of pulse inputs. We imagine that the response to the sequence of pulses is just the sum of the responses to each individual pulse. (This is not quantitatively correct but provides a useful qualitative representation.) Because individual pulse responses decay more slowly, the overall level to which they sum is increased, but the rise of activity to this level occurs more slowly.

A network with recurrent excitation and inhibition can also have inhibitory loops through which a population of neurons inhibits itself. In this case responses are sped up rather than slowed down, and they are reduced in amplitude (Figure F–3B). The reduction in response amplitude occurs because the decay of the response to a pulse of input is accelerated: In addition to the decay that would otherwise occur, inhibition subtracts even more from the activity. Because the responses to individual pulses decay more quickly, the overall level to which they sum is decreased, but the rise of activity to this level occurs more quickly.

If recurrent excitation is increased to the point where activity set up by a transient input can sustain itself indefinitely, decay does not occur at all and the response is infinitely slowed. This requires fine-tuning of network parameters. The resulting circuit, known as an *integrator network*, has some interesting properties. The response of an integrator network to a transient pulse of input is a change in firing rate that lasts forever in the absence of further input but which becomes part of an ongoing integral if further input is applied (Figure F–3C). If the transient excitation in the network is not perfectly tuned but instead is slightly weaker, the input produces a change in firing rate that decays very slowly. Such approximate integrators are used to model neural circuits that remember signals.

What happens if the amount of excitation is increased beyond the point of perfect tuning that achieves an integrator? The examples shown in Figure F–3 all start and end in a resting state with zero activity. When excitation is overly strong, such a resting state, whether or not it is characterized by zero activity, becomes unstable. This means that after any small perturbation, induced for example by a transient input, the system will drive itself further away from this state rather than relaxing back to it.

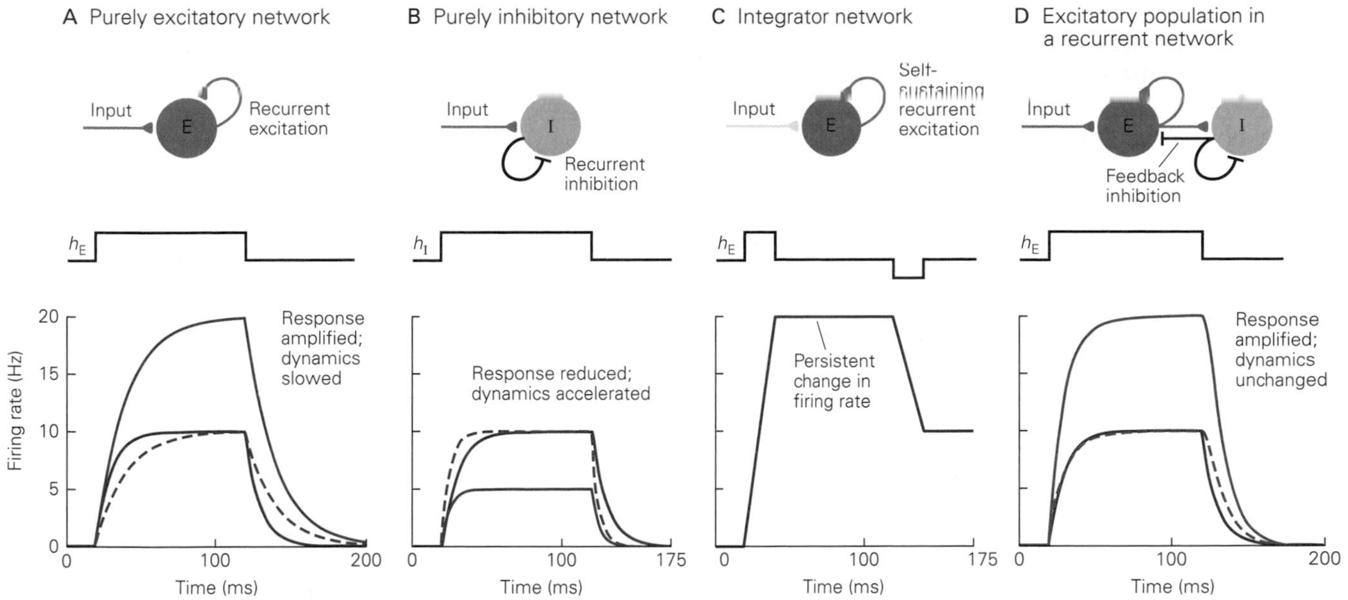

Figure F–3 Responses in excitatory and inhibitory networks of firing-rate neurons.

A. Response of a purely excitatory recurrent network to a square step of input (h_E). The **blue curve** is the response without excitatory feedback. Adding recurrent excitation increases the response but makes it rise and fall more slowly (**solid red curve**). The **dashed red curve** is a smaller copy of the solid red curve (scaled by a factor of 0.5) so that the time course of the solid red and blue curves can be compared more easily.

B. Response of a purely inhibitory recurrent network to a square step of input (h_I). The **blue curve** shows the response without recurrent inhibition. Adding recurrent inhibition decreases the response but makes it rise and fall more rapidly (**solid red curve**). The **dashed red** curve is a larger (2X) copy of the solid red curve.

C. Response of an integrator network to two input pulses (h_E). The response is the integral of the input and remains constant when the input is not present.

D. Response of the excitatory population in a mixed excitatory/inhibitory recurrent network to input to the excitatory neurons (h_E). The excitatory population excites both itself and the inhibitory population, whereas the inhibitory population inhibits both itself and the excitatory population, thus providing feedback inhibition to the excitatory population. The **blue curve** shows the response without recurrent connections (ie, without recurrent excitation or feedback inhibition). Adding the excitatory and inhibitory recurrent connections increases the response amplitude with little change in its time course (**solid red curve**). The **dashed red curve** is a scaled copy of the solid red curve as in part A.

Nonlinear processes ultimately stabilize a new pattern of activity, which is determined primarily by the network's own recurrent excitation rather than by the input and which can be self-sustaining in the absence of an input.

Fixed patterns of activity established and maintained by recurrent circuitry are attractors, as described in Appendix E. Attractors are often used as models for the persistent neural activity thought to hold items in working memory. If many different activity patterns are each strongly self-excitatory, a network can generate far more complex, chaotic dynamics. It has been argued that this can create a rich set of temporal patterns in areas of cortex such as primary motor cortex that can be harnessed by signals from motor planning areas to drive complex movement patterns.

Balanced Recurrent Networks Can Behave Like Feedforward Networks

Anatomical and electrophysiological studies of neurons in layer IV of the primary visual cortex (and in other sensory areas) have revealed many more recurrent than feed-forward connections in this layer. This discovery might seem to rule out feed-forward networks as relevant models of cortical circuits. However, function need not follow numbers.

A prominent hypothesis, supported by considerable evidence, is that the feed-forward inputs provide the driving input to layer IV neurons while the recurrent inputs amplify and modulate but do not drive responses. Feed-forward circuits are also relevant in another way: Under appropriate circumstances, strongly recurrent circuits can act effectively in a feed-forward manner.

To see how this works, we study a network consisting of two coupled populations, one excitatory and one inhibitory. To simplify the discussion we let the two projections from the excitatory population (to itself and to the inhibitory population) have the same strength, and likewise the two inhibitory projections. Thus we can speak of the strength of excitation (or inhibition)—meaning excitation (or inhibition) onto both excitatory and inhibitory neurons—without having to distinguish multiple projections of each type. Although this simplification dictates the specific results, it does not affect the overall conclusions as to how recurrent circuits can act in a feedforward manner and thus dissociate amplification from changes in dynamics.

We suppose the network is at a fixed point, meaning that there are steady excitatory and inhibitory firing rates in response to a steady feed-forward input, and that this fixed point is stable—after small transient perturbations the network will return to the fixed point. We suddenly increase the level of feed-forward input to the excitatory population (Figure F–3D). In this recurrent network the excitatory activity is amplified by the recurrent circuitry. Surprisingly, however, the time course of the increase is little different from that without recurrent circuitry. With different parameters the recurrently amplified response can exactly match the timing of, or even be faster than, the response without recurrent circuitry. Thus the recurrent circuit can amplify responses without any slowing of the temporal dynamics.

Apparently the mechanism of amplification is different from the recurrent amplification we considered previously. What is this mechanism? At the fixed point the difference between the excitation and inhibition received by a population is exactly that required to sustain the population's firing rates. Any change in the balance between excitation and inhibition drives a change in the firing rates until a new balance is restored. Increasing the feed forward input to the excitatory population shifts the balance toward excitation, thus driving up both excitatory and inhibitory firing rates. Similarly, an excess of inhibition drives down both excitatory and inhibitory firing rates.

Let us represent the firing rates as differences from the fixed-point firing rates. In this representation firing rates may be either positive or negative. We can then formally represent any pattern of excitatory and inhibitory firing rates as a weighted combination of two activity patterns. In the differential pattern excitatory and inhibitory cells have equal and opposite firing rates. In the common pattern excitatory and inhibitory cells have identical firing rates. Given some excitatory and inhibitory firing rates, if we weight the common pattern so that its common firing rate is the average of the excitatory and inhibitory rates, and weight the differential pattern so that it captures the difference between excitatory and inhibitory firing rates, then the sum of the two weighted patterns equals the given firing rates.

The advantage of expressing the activities in terms of these two patterns is that it allows a deeper insight into the dynamics. A shift in the network's balance toward excitation involves an increase in the size of the differential pattern, that is, the signed difference between excitatory and inhibitory firing rates increases. This imbalance in turn drives an increase in the size of the common pattern, that is, both excitatory and inhibitory firing rates increase. Similarly, a shift in the balance toward inhibition involves a decrease in the differential pattern, which decreases the common pattern. The network thus behaves precisely as it would if the differential activity pattern made a feed-forward synaptic connection to the common activity pattern, that is, imbalances drive balanced responses. Furthermore, there is no corresponding feedback from the common pattern onto the differential pattern. Balanced responses do not drive imbalances, nor does the differential pattern act on itself—imbalances do not drive further imbalance.

Thus the network of Figure F–3D, which appears to be fully recurrent when viewed in terms of the neurons, can be seen to have a hidden feed-forward structure when viewed in terms of differential and common activity patterns (it is hidden in the sense that it is not readily apparent in the synaptic connectivity of the network). This feed-forward pathway allows one activity pattern to excite the other without feedback (Figure F–4). The amplification driven by this "hidden" feedforward connection occurs with little dynamical slowing, whereas amplification as a result of a self-excitatory loop is achieved at the cost of slowing of the dynamics. This description is mathematically precise when the relationship of a neuron's firing rate to its input (see Box F–2) can be taken to be linear, and it provides a useful intuition for understanding this type of network behavior more generally.

The strength of the amplification depends on two factors. One is the strength of the feed-forward connection from the differential to the common pattern, which is given by the sum of the excitatory and inhibitory synaptic strengths. The other is the strength of any remaining feedback loops. If we assume that inhibition is stronger than excitation, this results in a loop by which the common pattern inhibits itself (Figure F–4),

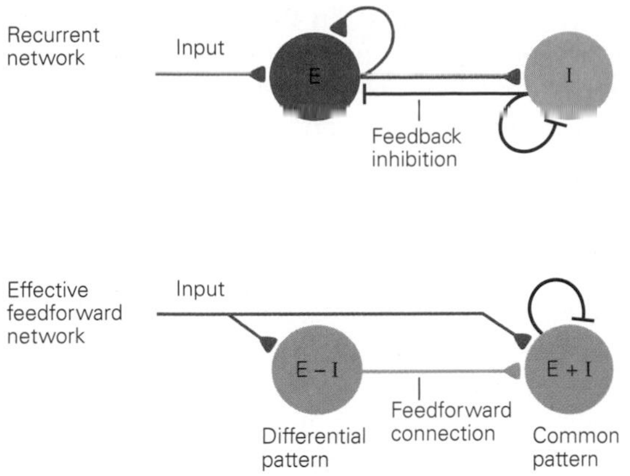

Figure F–4 An excitatory/inhibitory recurrent circuit is equivalent to a feed-forward circuit from a differential pattern (E − I) to a common pattern (E + I). The input to E in the recurrent circuit becomes equal input to both the E − I and E + I patterns. The inhibitory loop within the E + I pattern arises if the inhibitory projections are stronger than the excitatory.

because raising both excitatory and inhibitory rates produces a net inhibition of both the excitatory and inhibitory populations. This self-inhibition of the common pattern suppresses rather than amplifies responses; its strength is given by the difference between excitatory and inhibitory synaptic strengths. Thus the strongest amplification arises when both excitation and inhibition are strong but reasonably balanced.

This form of amplification can occur for each of many different spatial patterns of activity in a network of many neurons. In each spatial pattern an imbalance of excitatory and inhibitory activity can provide feed-forward drive to common excitatory and inhibitory activity, with different spatial patterns having different strengths of this drive and thus different degrees of amplification. This mechanism has been proposed to underlie observations of spontaneous activity in the primary visual cortex of anesthetized cats (that is, activity in the absence of a visual stimulus).

Despite the absence of a visual stimulus, spatial patterns of activity resembling responses to structured visual inputs make a larger contribution to the overall spontaneous activity than patterns unrelated to these visual responses. If we think of spontaneous activity as being driven by unstructured inputs to the visual cortex that equally drive many different patterns, then the patterns that resemble visually driven responses are being amplified by the visual cortical circuit more than other patterns. What is the mechanism underlying this amplification?

Preliminary analysis suggests that the dynamics of the amplified patterns are not significantly slowed. In a model network with balanced excitatory and inhibitory connections that preferentially target cells with similar orientation selectivity, the spatial patterns that resemble visually driven responses have the largest effective feed-forward weights and so are amplified relative to other spatial patterns, without dynamical slowing, by the mechanism shown in Figure F–3D. This provides a possible explanation for the amplification of activity patterns that resemble visual responses in the absence of a visual stimulus.

Paradoxical Effects in Balanced Recurrent Networks May Underlie Surround Suppression in the Visual Cortex

In this section we discuss another effect that can arise in networks in which excitation and inhibition are both strong but relatively balanced. We consider a network that satisfies two criteria.

First, the excitatory recurrence is strong enough to make the excitatory network unstable by itself. That is, if the network is at a stable fixed point, and if inhibitory firing rates were kept frozen at their fixed-point levels, then after small perturbations of excitatory firing rates the excitatory network would drive itself even further away from its fixed-point rates. Second, feedback inhibition (inhibition driven by the excitatory cells) stabilizes the network. A slight change in excitatory firing rates drives a sufficient change in inhibitory firing rates to push the excitatory rates back to their fixed-point levels, despite the tendency of the excitatory network to "run away" on its own.

We refer to a network meeting these two criteria as an *inhibition-stabilized network*. The strong recurrent excitation received by excitatory cortical neurons and the instability of cortical activity when inhibition is blocked suggest that cortical circuits may indeed be stabilized in this way.

Inhibition-stabilized networks provide a possible explanation for a paradoxical experimental observation. The region of visual space within which an appropriate visual stimulus can elicit a response in a neuron in the primary visual cortex (V1) is known as the center region of the cell's receptive field. For many V1 neurons, increasing the size of the stimulus so that it also covers the surrounding region (the *surround*) reduces the response, a phenomenon known as *surround suppression*. However, a stimulus covering only the surround and not the center yields no response.

It is believed that stimulation of the center of a neuron's receptive field drives external excitatory input relayed from the eyes to both excitatory and inhibitory neural populations in the local cortical circuit, whereas a surround stimulus excites neighboring regions of cortex that send excitation more strongly to the inhibitory population within the local circuit. We might therefore expect that a stimulus in the surround should increase firing in the local inhibitory population, which in turn would suppress responses in the excitatory population.

Instead, experiments by David Ferster and colleagues indicate that a surround stimulus reduces both the excitation *and* the inhibition that a V1 neuron receives. That is, surround suppression is actually mediated by a reduction in the excitation of a cell, which has a larger effect than a concurrent reduction in inhibition. The reduction in inhibition suggests that the firing rate of the inhibitory population, like that of the excitatory population, is reduced by the surround stimulus, and this has been directly confirmed by Xue-Mei Song and Chao-Yi Li. Thus we arrive at the paradoxical result: A surround stimulus that is believed to drive external excitation to an inhibitory population causes a net decrease in the inhibitory population's firing rate.

This paradox can be explained by the presence in the cortex of strong recurrent excitation that is stabilized by inhibition, as shown in a model constructed by Misha Tsodyks and colleagues in a different context. The inhibitory neurons receive such strong drive from the excitatory neurons that their activity is determined more by the excitatory neurons than by any external input.

To see this, consider an inhibition-stabilized network composed of two populations of neurons, one excitatory and the other inhibitory (as in Figure F–3D), each initially firing at steady rates in response to a constant center stimulus (Figure F–5A). Adding a surround stimulus provides additional excitation to the inhibitory neurons from external sources. This transiently increases inhibitory neurons firing (Figure F–5B), which in turn lowers the firing rates of the excitatory neurons in the network (Figure F–5C), causing a withdrawal of recurrent excitatory input to the inhibitory neurons. Precisely when the network is inhibition-stabilized, this withdrawal of recurrent excitatory input to the inhibitory neurons exceeds the increase in excitation from external sources that started the process, so that the ultimate result, paradoxically, is that inhibitory firing rates are also lowered (Figure F–5D).

It is natural to think that, with inhibitory firing rates lowered, excitatory firing rates should then rise back above their initial levels, but this does not occur. To understand this we must understand one more point about an unstable excitatory subnetwork. Recall that an increase in excitatory firing recruits so much extra recurrent excitation that, in the absence of changes in inhibitory firing, it would drive excitatory firing still higher. So too a decrease in excitatory firing withdraws so much recurrent excitation that excitatory firing rates would fall still lower in the absence of changes in inhibitory firing. The lowering of inhibitory firing rates decreases feedback inhibition, thus compensating for the deficiency of excitation and so stabilizing the lower firing rates of the excitatory population. The network thus arrives at a new stable fixed point in which both excitatory and inhibitory cells have lower firing rates than they did before additional external excitation was added to the inhibitory population.

This paradoxical result, in which adding excitatory input to the inhibitory cells results in a decrease in their steady state firing rate, is actually another instance of a hidden feed-forward connection by which a small differential or imbalance between excitation and inhibition can drive a large common response of both excitation and inhibition. In the present case the addition of excitatory input to the inhibitory cells drives a negative imbalance, which in turn drives a large negative common response, that is, a decrease in both excitatory and inhibitory rates. However, the increase in input also directly drives an increase in inhibitory firing rates. Thus there are two competing effects on inhibitory firing. The instability of the excitatory subnetwork turns out to be precisely equivalent to the condition in which the feed-forward effect is larger than the direct input effect, so that the net effect is a decrease in inhibitory firing rates.

The effect shown in Figure F–5 matches the observations we described earlier. When a stimulus in the receptive field surround results in additional excitatory input to inhibitory neurons, both the excitation and the inhibition in the recorded neurons is reduced. This finding and the theoretical analysis of it (only a portion of which is discussed here) provide strong evidence that the cortex operates in a regime in which recurrent excitation by itself is strong enough to be unstable but is stabilized by recurrent inhibition.

Recurrent Networks Can Model Decision-Making

As a final example of network modeling, we turn to circuits that select between different behaviors, that is, circuits that make decisions. Suppose the driver of an automobile needs to decide whether to turn right or left. Assume that there are two populations of excitatory neurons, one active when the decision is a right turn, the other when it is a left turn. Under some circumstances no decision needs to be made, so neither population should be highly active.

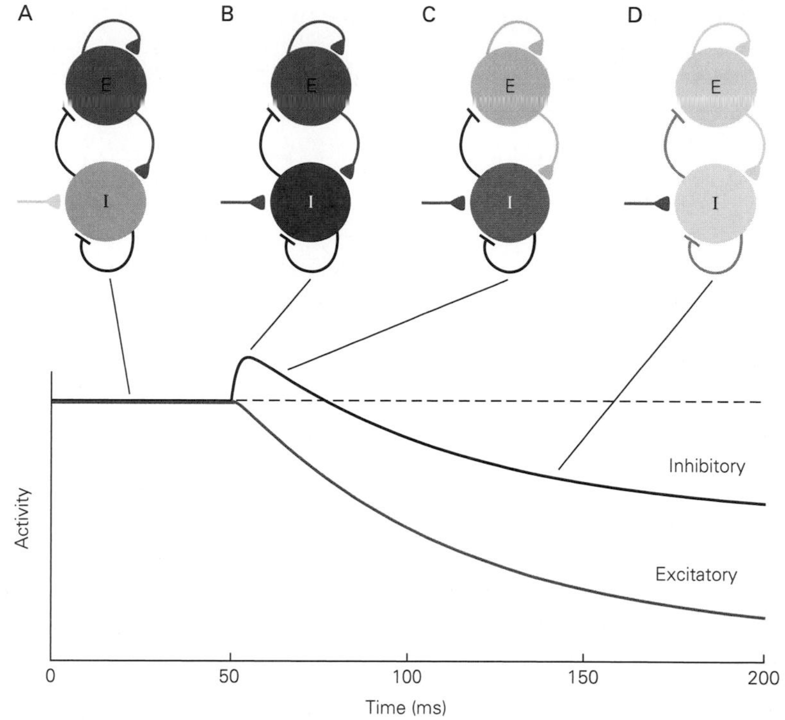

Figure F–5 Sequence of events following addition of a surround stimulus to a center stimulus in an inhibition-stabilized network model of primary visual cortex. The circuit consists of a population of excitatory neurons (E) that recurrently excite one another, and a population of inhibitory neurons (I) that recurrently inhibit one another (**red/pink synapses** are excitatory, **black/grey synapses** are inhibitory). The excitatory cells excite the inhibitory neurons, which in turn provide feedback inhibition to the excitatory cells. Stronger colors indicate higher levels of activity of a neuron or synapse. At all times the network receives a steady input driven by a steady center stimulus (not shown). The plot below is a continuous-time plot of excitatory and inhibitory firing rates. The points in time at which conditions A–D occur are indicated. (Adapted, with permission, from Ozeki et al. 2009.)

A. The circuit before the addition of the surround input. The populations are firing at steady rates in response to the center stimulus. The surround input is not yet activated.

B. After the surround input is activated at 50 ms, inhibitory firing rates initially increase.

C. This additional inhibitory input drives down excitatory firing rates, resulting in withdrawal of recurrent excitation from both excitatory and inhibitory neurons and a corresponding decrease in inhibitory firing rates.

D. When the network is inhibition-stabilized, this withdrawal of recurrent excitation to the inhibitory neurons is larger than the surround-induced increase of external excitation. Thus, in the end the inhibitory neurons receive less excitation than they did initially, and accordingly their firing rate is decreased.

A decision can be biased or unbiased by sensory input. If, for example, the sensory stimulus is a road sign that says "turn left," the sensory input should bias the decision toward a left turn. If the sensory stimulus is an obstacle in the middle of a three-lane highway, there is a need to turn but the direction may be arbitrary. In this case the sensory input should evoke a decision without biasing it. Between these extremes, inputs may provide a range of biasing effects.

To model decision-making in this context we follow the work of X. J. Wang, who has modeled decision-making circuits extensively. A network model of the kind of decision-making described above must have the following properties. First, in the absence of relevant sensory stimuli there should be a stable pattern of spontaneous activity corresponding to no decision. Second, a sensory stimulus requiring a decision should eliminate or destabilize the no-decision state and introduce two new stable firing patterns corresponding to the two possible actions. Third, sensory stimuli should be capable of biasing the outcome so that one of these decision states is more likely to occur than the other.

In our model different decision states are represented by two recurrently connected networks of excitatory neurons, both of which excite a single population of inhibitory neurons that return feed-back

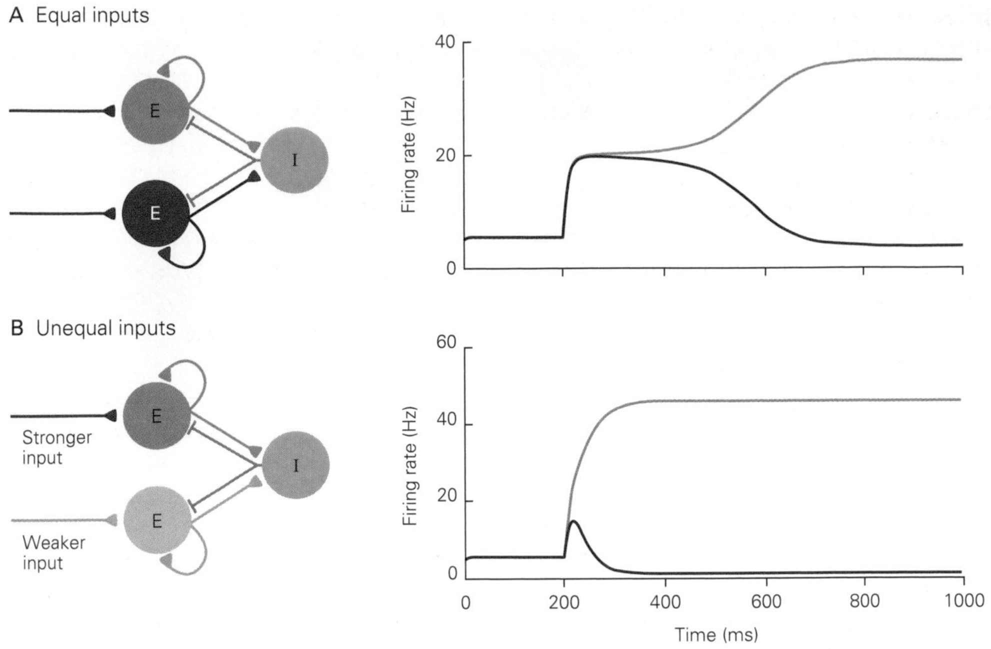

Figure F–6 A decision-making network. Two excitatory populations of neurons are active during two different decisions. An inhibitory population receives excitation from both excitatory populations and returns inhibition to both of them. A stimulus is presented at 200 ms. Before this time the network is in the no-decision state, in which excitatory populations have low firing rates.

A. In response to an unbiased stimulus the firing rates of both populations initially rise but then separate. The firing rate of the orange population ends up at a high value because small random fluctuations (too small to see) raise it slightly higher than the firing rate of the purple population. This small difference was then amplified by the network, leading to a large difference in the two rates. Ultimately, only the firing rate of the orange population remains high, corresponding to the decision.

B. A stimulus biased in favor of the orange population generates a larger input to one excitatory population than the other. Note that the decision state is reached more rapidly than in the case of equal inputs (part A).

inhibition to both of them (Figure F–6A). In the absence of sensory stimuli the network stays in a no-decision state in which the neurons have low activity. In this state we assume that the neurons have a low level of input, and their activity reflects an equilibrium involving this input, recurrent excitation, and feedback inhibition. A stimulus that induces a decision takes the form of excitatory drive to both excitatory populations of the network.

When there is no bias favoring one decision over the other, the inputs to the two excitatory populations are equal. Nevertheless, the model does make a decision—the firing rate of one population rises to and remains at a high level, while that of the other population falls back to a low firing rate after an initial rise (Figure F–6A). This occurs because the stimulus-generated inputs force both excitatory networks away from their no-decision firing rates. With the no-decision state eliminated, only two stable states remain available to the system, each corresponding to a different decision. One population ends up at a higher rate because small random fluctuations in the firing rates happen to favor that group (a small amount of noise was added to the model to generate these fluctuations). As a result of the fluctuations, each decision occurs 50% of the time.

When the stimulus is biased in favor of one population, the input to that population is higher than the input to the other. As a result, the firing rate of the favored population rises and remains high, while that of the other population falls after a brief and small rise (Figure F–6B). A strong-enough stimulus bias will produce the favored decision almost 100% of the time.

The latency from the time of the stimulus to the time a decision occurs can be determined by examining the divergence between the firing rates of the two neuronal populations. A decision is made more rapidly when the stimulus is biased than when it is unbiased

(Figure F–6). This situation is similar to what is observed in the experiments on perceptual decision-making. In these experiments a monkey is trained to report the perceived direction of dots that move in many different directions on a screen. The monkey's performance depends on the coherence of motion of the dots. On most trials the dots have an overall tendency to move in one of two possible directions, introducing a type of stimulus bias. In some trials the coherence is zero, but the monkey still has to choose a direction of motion from these two possibilities. This situation is analogous to that shown in Figure F–6A.

There is experimental evidence that neural populations representing the two choice possibilities may be located in the posterior parietal cortex, specifically the lateral intraparietal area. Neurons recorded in this area by Michael Shadlen and collaborators during perceptual decision experiments involving moving dots behave like the model neurons in Figure F–6. Neural activity is initially driven by the sensory stimulus but then increases for one decision and decreases for the other. The final decision is preceded by a ramping activity that is relatively slow in the case of zero coherence of motion of the dots. This may be an indication of the existence of a period during which fluctuations are accumulating until a decision is made.

How does the model shown in Figure F–6 work and how was it constructed? The model relies on two key elements: bistability and inhibition-mediated competition between the two populations of excitatory neurons. Bistability is the ability of a network to sustain activity corresponding to either of two different states, typically one with a low rate of firing and one with a high rate. Persistent firing at a high rate is made possible by strong recurrent excitation. Bistability requires the level of activity of a neuron to depend on its recurrent input in a nonlinear way. In the example of Figure F–6 the nonlinearity is assured by a sigmoidal neuronal response curve that makes the firing rate relatively insensitive to changes in input both at low firing rates (when mean voltage is well below threshold) and at high firing rates (when rates saturate) but highly sensitive at intermediate firing rates. At an intermediate level of firing the high sensitivity to changes in input renders the excitatory feedback unstable, forcing the network to high or low firing rates. At high or low firing rates the excitatory feedback becomes stable because of the weakened neuronal sensitivity, allowing a stable firing rate.

In a bistable network low and high firing rates are stable in the presence of small transient input pulses. Even if these transient inputs modify the firing rate of the network, the firing rate returns to its initial state after the input pulse terminates. However, larger input pulses can induce transitions from one firing rate to the other (Figure F–7).

The other crucial component in the model is inhibition. The decision model in Figure F–6 consists of two populations of excitatory neurons, each of which can be bistable, and an inhibitory population that is driven by both excitatory populations and reciprocally inhibits both of them. The purpose of the inhibitory population is to avoid the state in which both excitatory populations fire at high rates, which would correspond to making both decisions at once. This state is avoided by introducing sufficiently strong inhibition of the two excitatory populations. The resulting model is described mathematically in Box F–3. It and models

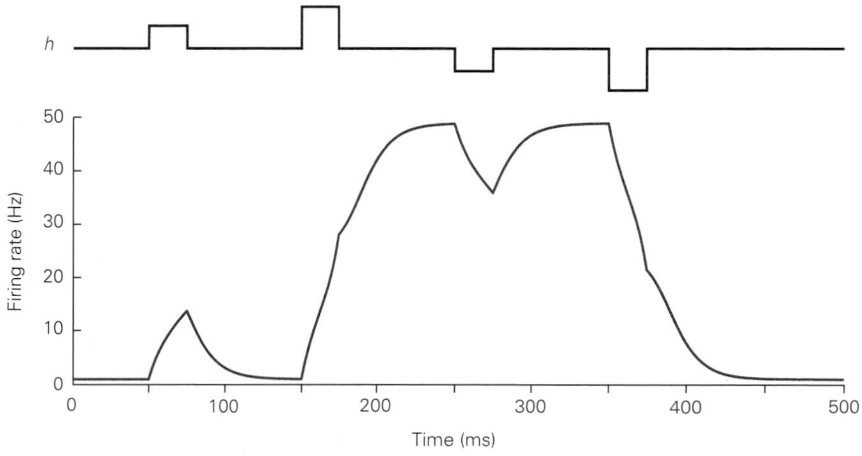

Figure F–7 A bistable network can alternate between two different states. The network starts in a low firing state. The first input pulse is too small to induce a transition from this state, but the larger second pulse flips the network into the high firing state. The third pulse is again too small to induce a transition, but the final pulse flips the network back to the low firing state.

Box F–3 The Decision Model

In the decision network r_a and r_b denote the firing rates of the excitatory populations a and b, each representing a unique decision, and r_I is the firing rate of an inhibitory population. As in Figure F–6A, we assume for simplicity that there is no excitatory coupling between the excitatory populations and that each receives identical input from the inhibitory population.

The equations of the model are:

$$\tau\frac{dr_a}{dt} = -r_a + \Gamma(w_{EE}r_a - w_{EI}r_I + h_a) \qquad \textbf{(F–4)}$$

$$\tau\frac{dr_b}{dt} = -r_b + F(w_{EE}r_b - w_{EI}r_I + h_b). \qquad \textbf{(F–5)}$$

A small amount of random (white) noise is added to the right side of these equations. To avoid having a third differential equation for inhibitory firing rates, we use the approximation that the inhibition responds instantaneously and assume that r_I is proportional to the sum of the excitatory rates r_a and r_b.

Without input ($h_a = h_b = 0$) the firing rates of the two excitatory populations are equal and low. As a result, neither action is preferred or taken. This is the same no-decision state seen during the initial 200 ms period of the simulations in Figure F–6.

To induce a decision we introduce excitatory inputs corresponding to a sensory stimulus. Sufficiently large but equal inputs ($h_a = h_b > 0$) result in two stable states that correspond to the two decision states, $r_a > r_b$ or $r_a < r_b$. The state corresponding to the previous no-decision outcome has now disappeared.

To introduce a bias into the decision, we make h_a and h_b different. For example, if h_a is significantly larger than h_b, only the stable state $r_a > r_b$ survives. For smaller biases there are regimes in which two stable states correspond to the two decisions, but the system is more likely to enter one stable state than the other.

like it provide an elegant way of simulating decision making, including such features as the time required to make a decision and the frequency of errors.

Laurence F. Abbott
Stefano Fusi
Kenneth D. Miller

Selected Reading

Dayan P, Abbott LF. 2001. *Theoretical Neuroscience: Computational and Mathematical Modeling of Neural Systems.* Cambridge, MA: MIT Press.

Destexhe A, Paré D. 1999. Impact of network activity on the integrative properties of neocortical pyramidal neurons in vivo. J Neurophysiol 81:1531–1547.

Fusi S, Asaad WF, Miller EK, Wang X-J. 2007. A neural circuit model of flexible sensori-motor mapping: learning and forgetting on multiple timescales. Neuron 54:319–333.

Goldman MS. 2009. Memory without feedback in a neural network. Neuron 61(4):621–634.

Holt GR, Softky WR, Koch C, Douglas RJ. 1996. Comparison of discharge variability in vitro and in vivo in cat visual cortex neurons. J Neurophysiol 75:1806–1814.

Mascaro M, Amit DJ. 1999. Effective neural response function for collective population states. Network 10: 351–373.

Rapp M, Yarom Y, Segev I. 1992. The impact of parallel fiber background activity on the cable properties of cerebellar Purkinje cells. Neural Comput 4:518–532.

Salinas E, Sejnowski TJ. 2002. Integrate-and-fire neurons driven by correlated stochastic input. Neural Comput 14:2111–2155.

Shadlen MN, Newsome WT. 1994. Noise, neural codes and cortical organization. Curr Opin Neurobiol 4:569–579.

Shriki O, Hansel D, Sompolinsky H. 2003. Rate models for conductance-based cortical neuronal networks. Neural Comput 15:1809–1841.

Softky WR, Koch C. 1993. The highly irregular firing of cortical cells is inconsistent with temporal integration of random EPSPs. J Neurosci 13:334–350.

Trefethen LN, Embree M. 2005. *Spectra and Pseudospectra: The Behavior of Nonnormal Matrices and Operators.* Princeton, NJ: Princeton Univ. Press.

Troyer TW, Miller KD. 1997. Physiological gain leads to high ISI variability in a simple model of a cortical regular spiking cell. Neural Comput 9:971–983.

Wang X-J. 2002. Probabilistic decision making by slow reverberation in cortical circuits. Neuron 36:955–968.

Wilson HR, Cowan JD. 1972. Excitatory and inhibitory interactions in localized populations of model neurons. Biophys J 12:1–24.

References

Brunel N. 2000. Dynamics of networks of randomly connected excitatory and inhibitory spiking neurons. J Physiol Paris 94:445–463.

Kenet T, Bibitchkov D, Tsodyks M, Grinvald A, Arieli A. 2003. Spontaneously emerging cortical representations of visual attributes. Nature 425:954–956.

Murphy B, Miller KD. 2009. Balanced amplification: a new mechanism of selective amplification of neural activity patterns. Neuron 61:635–648.

Ozeki H, Finn I, Schaffer ES, Miller KD, Ferster D. 2009. Surround suppression in cat visual cortex: evidence that V1 operates as an inhibition-stabilized network. Neuron 62:578–592.

Shadlen MN, Newsome WT. 2001. Neural basis of a perceptual decision in the parietal cortex (area LIP) of the rhesus monkey. J Neurophysiol 86:1916–1936.

Song XM, Li CY. 2008. Contrast-dependent and contrast-independent spatial summation of primary visual cortical neurons of the cat. Cerebr Cortex 18:331–336.

Tsodyks MV, Skaggs WE, Sejnowski TJ, McNaughton BL. 1997. Paradoxical effects of external modulation of inhibitory interneurons. J Neurosci 17:4382–4388.

van Vreeswijk C, Sompolinsky H. 1996. Chaos in neuronal networks with balanced excitatory and inhibitory activity. Science 274:1724–1726.

Wang X. 2008. Decision making in recurrent neuronal circuits. Neuron 60:215–234.

Index

The letters b, f, and t following a page number indicate box, figure, and table.

A

B

C

D

F

H

I

N

O

Q

R

S

T

U

V

W

X

Y

Z